P9-ART-585

RUBIN'S PATHOLOGY:

Clinicopathologic Foundations of Medicine

SIXTH EDITION

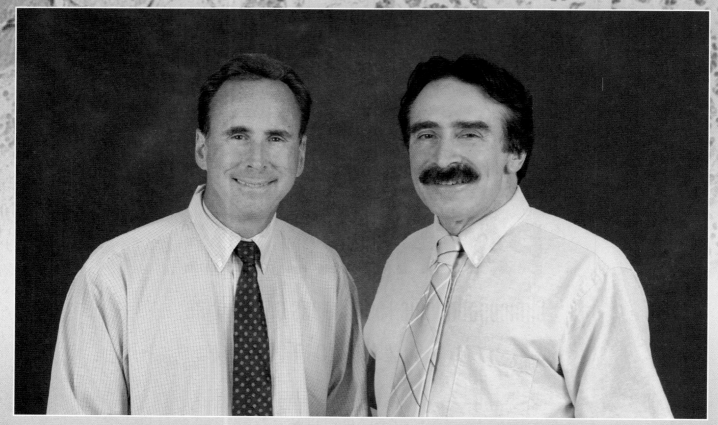

Editors Raphael Rubin, M.D., *left* and David S. Strayer, M.D., Ph.D., *right*.

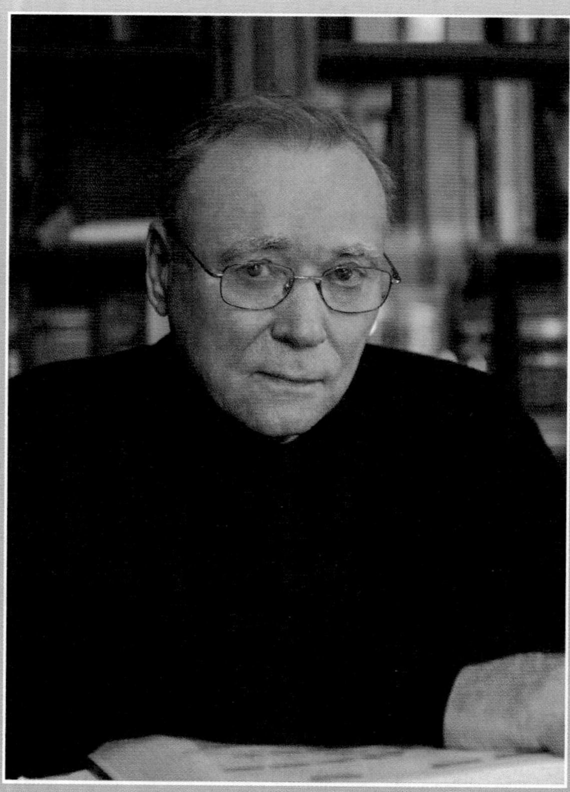

Founder and Consulting Editor Emanuel Rubin, M.D.

RUBIN'S

PATHOLOGY:

Clinicopathologic Foundations of Medicine

SIXTH EDITION

EDITORS:

Raphael Rubin, M.D.
Professor of Pathology

David S. Strayer, M.D., Ph.D.
Professor of Pathology

Department of Pathology and Cell Biology
Jefferson Medical College of Thomas Jefferson University
Philadelphia, Pennsylvania

FOUNDER AND CONSULTING EDITOR:

Emanuel Rubin, M.D.
Gonzalo Aponte Distinguished Professor of Pathology
Chairman Emeritus of the Department of Pathology and Cell Biology
Jefferson Medical College of Thomas Jefferson University
Philadelphia, Pennsylvania

Wolters Kluwer | Lippincott Williams & Wilkins
Health
Philadelphia • Baltimore • New York • London
Buenos Aires • Hong Kong • Sydney • Tokyo

Acquisitions Editor: Susan Rhyner
Product Manager: Sirkka Howes
Marketing Manager: Joy Fisher-Williams
Manufacturing Manager: Margie Orzech
Designer: Steve Druding
Compositor: Aptara, Inc.

Sixth Edition

351 West Camden Street
Baltimore, MD 21201

Two Commerce Square
2001 Market Street
Philadelphia, PA 19103

Printed in China

9 8 7 6 5 4 3 2 1

Library of Congress Cataloging-in-Publication Data

Rubin's pathology : clinicopathologic foundations of medicine / Editors, Raphael Rubin, M.D., David S. Strayer, M.D., Ph.D., Professor of Pathology Professor of Pathology, Department of Pathology and Cell Biology, Jefferson Medical College of Thomas Jefferson University Philadelphia, Pennsylvania, Founder and Consulting Editor, Emanuel Rubin, M.D., Gonzalo Aponte, Distinguished Professor of Pathology, Chairman Emeritus of the Department of Pathology and Cell Biology, Jefferson Medical College of Thomas Jefferson University, Philadelphia, Pennsylvania. — Sixth Edition.
p. ; cm.
Pathology : clinicopathologic foundations of medicine
Includes bibliographical references and index.
Summary: "The highly acclaimed foundation textbook Rubin's Pathology: Clinicopathologic Foundations of Medicine, now in its sixth edition, provides medical students with a lucid discussion of basic disease processes and their effects on cells, organs, and people. The streamlined coverage includes only what medical students need to know and provides clinical application of the chapter concepts. Icons signal discussions of pathogenesis, pathology, epidemiology, etiological factors, and clinical features. Rubin's Pathology is liberally illustrated with full-color graphic illustrations, gross pathology photos, and micrographs. The sixth edition is completely updated with expanded and revised context. A suite of exciting online tools for students includes a fully searchable e-text with all images, 140 interactive case studies, 1500 audio review questions, summary podcast lectures, and a selection of mobile flash cards for iPhone, iPod, and BlackBerry from the new Rubin's Pathology Mobile Flash Cards. Resources for faculty include a 600 question test generator and chapter outlines and objectives"—Provided by publisher.
ISBN 978-1-60547-968-2 (hardback : alk. paper) 1. Pathology. I. Rubin, Raphael, editor. II. Strayer, David S. (David Sheldon), 1949- editor. III. Rubin, Emanuel, 1928- editor. IV. Title: Pathology : clinicopathologic foundations of medicine.
[DNLM: 1. Pathologic Processes. QZ 4]
RB111.E856 2012
616.07—dc22

2010052493

DISCLAIMER

Care has been taken to confirm the accuracy of the information present and to describe generally accepted practices. However, the authors, editors, and publisher are not responsible for errors or omissions or for any consequences from application of the information in this book and make no warranty, expressed or implied, with respect to the currency, completeness, or accuracy of the contents of the publication. Application of this information in a particular situation remains the professional responsibility of the practitioner; the clinical treatments described and recommended may not be considered absolute and universal recommendations.

The authors, editors, and publisher have exerted every effort to ensure that drug selection and dosage set forth in this text are in accordance with the current recommendations and practice at the time of publication. However, in view of ongoing research, changes in government regulations, and the constant flow of information relating to drug therapy and drug reactions, the reader is urged to check the package insert for each drug for any change in indications and dosage and for added warnings and precautions. This is particularly important when the recommended agent is a new or infrequently employed drug.

Some drugs and medical devices presented in this publication have Food and Drug Administration (FDA) clearance for limited use in restricted research settings. It is the responsibility of the health care provider to ascertain the FDA status of each drug or device planned for use in their clinical practice.

To purchase additional copies of this book, call our customer service department at **(800) 638-3030** or fax orders to **(301) 223-2320**. International customers should call **(301) 223-2300**.

Visit Lippincott Williams & Wilkins on the Internet: http://www.lww.com. Lippincott Williams & Wilkins customer service representatives are available from 8:30 am to 6:00 pm, EST.

The publisher specially acknowledges the past work and contributions of Professor F. Stephen Vogel to the chapter on neuropathology. Dr. Vogel appreciates the publisher's previous recognition of its erroneous use of his work in the 4th and 5th editions, and wishes to publicly express his satisfaction with the authorship and content of the chapter as it appears in this 6th edition.

CCS0211

DEDICATION

We dedicate this book to our wives and families, whose tolerance, love and support sustained us throughout this endeavor; to our colleagues, from whom we have learned so much; to our chapter authors who have given so much of themselves to produce this new edition; and to students everywhere, upon whose curiosity and energy the future of medical science depends.

CONTRIBUTORS

Michael F. Allard, MD
Professor of Pathology and Laboratory Medicine
University of British Columbia
Cardiovascular Pathologist
Department of Pathology and Laboratory Medicine
The iCAPTURE Centre
St. Paul's Hospital
Vancouver, British Columbia, Canada

Mary Beth Beasley, MD
Associate Professor of Pathology
Mount Sinai Medical Center
New York, New York

Thomas W. Bouldin, MD
Professor of Pathology and Laboratory Medicine
Chair for Faculty and Trainee Development
University of North Carolina at Chapel Hill
Director of Neuropathology
McLendon Clinical Laboratories
University of North Carolina Hospitals
Chapel Hill, North Carolina

Diane L. Carlson, MD
Assistant Attending
Department of Pathology
Memorial Sloan-Kettering Cancer Center
New York, New York

Ivan Damjanov, MD, PhD
Professor of Pathology
The University of Kansas School of Medicine
Pathologist
Department of Pathology
University of Kansas Medical Center
Kansas City, Kansas

Jeffrey M. Davidson, PhD
Professor of Pathology
Vanderbilt University School of Medicine
Senior Research Career Scientist
Medical Research Service
Veterans Affairs Tennessee Valley Healthcare System
Nashville, Tennessee

David E. Elder, MD, ChB, FRCPA
Professor of Pathology and Laboratory Medicine
University of Pennsylvania School of Medicine
Director of Anatomic Pathology
Hospital of the University of Pennsylvania
Philadelphia, Pennsylvania

Alina Dulau Florea, MD
Assistant Professor of Pathology
Thomas Jefferson University
Philadelphia, Pennsylvania

Gregory N. Fuller, MD, PhD
Professor of Pathology
Chief of Neuropathology
The University of Texas M.D. Anderson Cancer Center
Houston, Texas

Roberto A. Garcia, MD
Assistant Professor of Pathology
The Mount Sinai School of Medicine
Chief of Orthopaedic and Soft Tissue Pathology
The Mount Sinai Hospital
New York, New York

J. Clay Goodman, MD
Professor of Pathology and Neurology
Walter Henrick Moursund Chair in Neuropathology
Associate Dean of Undergraduate Medical Education
Baylor College of Medicine
Houston, Texas

Avrum I. Gotlieb, MD, CM, FRCP
Professor of Laboratory Medicine and Pathology
University of Toronto
Staff Pathologist
Laboratory Medicine Program
University Health Network
Toronto, Ontario, Canada

Philip N. Hawkins, PhD, FRCP, FRCPath, FMedSci
Professor of Medicine
Centre for Amyloidosis and Acute Phase Proteins
University College London Medical School
Head, National Amyloidosis Centre
Royal Free Hospital
London, England, United Kingdom

Steven K. Herrine, MD
Professor of Medicine
Thomas Jefferson University
Philadelphia, Pennsylvania

J. Charles Jennette, MD
Brinkhous Distinguished Professor and Chair of Pathology and Laboratory Medicine
University of North Carolina, School of Medicine
Chief of Service
Department of Pathology and Laboratory Medicine
University of North Carolina Hospitals
Chapel Hills, North Carolina

Lawrence C. Kenyon, MD, PhD
Associate Professor of Pathology, Anatomy and Cell Biology
Thomas Jefferson University
Pathologist and Neuropathologist
Department of Pathology, Anatomy and Cell Biology
Thomas Jefferson University Hospital
Philadelphia, Pennsylvania

Robert Kisilevsky, MD, PhD, FRCPC, FRSC
Professor Emeritus
Department of Pathology and Molecular Medicine
Queen's University
Kingston, Ontario, Canada

Michael J. Klein, MD
Professor of Pathology and Laboratory Medicine
Weill Medical College of Cornell University
Pathologist-in-Chief and Director of Pathology and Laboratory Medicine
Hospital for Special Surgery
New York, New York

David S. Klimstra, MD
Chief of Surgical Pathology
Department of Pathology
Memorial Sloan-Kettering Cancer Center
New York, New York

Gordon K. Klintworth, MD, PhD
Professor of Pathology
Joseph A.C. Wadsworth Research Professor of Ophthalmology
Duke University
Durham, North Carolina

Amber Chang Liu, MSc
University of Toronto
Toronto, Ontario, Canada

Peter A. McCue, MD
Professor of Pathology
Thomas Jefferson University
Director of Anatomic Pathology
Thomas Jefferson University Hospital
Philadelphia, Pennsylvania

Bruce McManus, MD, PhD, FRSC
Professor of Pathology and Laboratory Medicine
University of British Columbia
Director, Providence Heart and Lung Institute
St. Paul's Hospital
Vancouver, British Columbia, Canada

Maria J. Merino, MD
Chief of Translational Pathology
Department of Pathology
National Cancer Institute
Bethesda, Maryland

Anna Marie Mulligan, MB, MSc, FRCPath
Assistant Professor of Laboratory Medicine and Pathobiology
University of Toronto
Anatomic Pathologist
Department of Laboratory Medicine
St. Michael's Hospital
Toronto, Ontario, Canada

Hedwig S. Murphy, MD, PhD
Associate Professor of Pathology
University of Michigan
Staff Pathologist
Department of Pathology and Laboratory Medicine
Veterans Affairs Ann Arbor Health System
Ann Arbor, Michigan

George L. Mutter, MD
Associate Professor of Pathology
Harvard Medical School
Pathologist
Department of Pathology
Brigham and Women's Hospital
Boston, Massachusetts

Victor J. Navarro, MD
Professor of Medicine, Pharmacology and Experimental Therapeutics
Medical Director, Liver Transplantation
Director, Transplant Hepatology Fellowship
Departments of Gastroenterology and Hepatology
Thomas Jefferson University
Philadelphia, Pennsylvania

Frances P. O'Malley, MB, FRCPC
Professor of Laboratory Medicine and Pathobiology
University of Toronto
Staff Pathologist
Department of Pathology and Laboratory Medicine
Mount Sinai Hospital
Toronto, Ontario, Canada

Stephen Peiper, MD
Peter A. Herbut Professor and Chairman of Pathology, Anatomy and Cell Biology
Thomas Jefferson University, Jefferson Medical College
Philadelphia, Pennsylvania

Jaime Prat, MD, PhD, FRCPath
Professor of Pathology
Director of Pathology
Autonomous University of Barcelona
Director of Pathology
Hospital de la Santa Creu i Sant Pau
Barcelona, Spain

Martha Quezado, MD
Staff Pathologist
Laboratory of Pathology
National Cancer Institute
National Institutes of Health
Bethesda, Maryland

Jeffrey E. Saffitz, MD, PhD
Mallinckrodt Professor of Medicine
Harvard Medical School
Chairman, Department of Pathology
Beth Israel Deaconess Medical Center
Boston, Massachusetts

Alan L. Schiller, MD
Professor of Pathology
Mount Sinai School of Medicine
Chairman, Department of Pathology
Mount Sinai Hospital
New York, New York

David A. Schwartz, MD, MSHyg, FCAP
Associate Clinical Professor of Pathology
Vanderbilt University School of Medicine
Nashville, Tennessee

Gregory C. Sephel, PhD
Associate Professor of Pathology
Vanderbilt University School of Medicine
Nashville, Tennessee

Elias S. Siraj, MD
Associate Professor of Medicine
Section of Endocrinology
Temple University School of Medicine
Program Director, Endocrinology Fellowship
Temple University Hospital
Philadelphia, Pennsylvania

Edward B. Stelow, MD
Associate Professor of Pathology
University of Virginia
Charlottesville, Virginia

Craig A. Storm, MD
Assistant Professor of Pathology
Dartmouth Medical School
Hanover, New Hampshire
Staff Dermatopathologist
Department of Pathology
Dartmouth-Hitchcock Medical Center
Lebanon, New Hampshire

William D. Travis, MD
Professor of Pathology
Weill Medical College of Cornell University
Attending Thoracic Pathologist
Memorial Sloan Kettering Cancer Center
New York, New York

Riccardo Valdez, MD
Assistant Professor of Pathology
Section Head, Hematopathology
Department of Laboratory Medicine and Pathology
Mayo Clinic
Scottsdale, Arizona

Jeffrey S. Warren, MD
Aldred S. Warthin Endowed Professor of Pathology
Director, Division of Clinical Pathology
University of Michigan Medical School
University of Michigan Hospitals
Ann Arbor, Michigan

Bruce M. Wenig, MD
Professor of Pathology
Albert Einstein College of Medicine
Bronx, New York
Chairman
Department of Pathology and Laboratory Medicine
Beth Israel Medical Center
St. Luke's and Roosevelt Hospitals
New York, New York

Kevin Jon Williams, MD
Professor of Medicine
Chief, Section of Endocrinology, Diabetes, and Metabolism
Temple University School of Medicine
Philadelphia, Pennsylvania

Robert Yanagawa, MD, PhD
Resident in Surgery
Division of Cardiac Surgery
University of Toronto, Faculty of Medicine
Toronto, Ontario, Canada

Mary M. Zutter, MD
Professor of Pathology and Cancer Biology
Vanderbilt University
Director of Hematopathology
Vanderbilt University Medical Center
Nashville, Tennessee

PREFACE

We prepare this sixth edition of *Rubin's Pathology: Clinicopathologic Foundations of Medicine* amid a whirlwind of major changes in medicine and medical education. These changes are taking place simultaneously with larger metamorphoses in ecologic, societal, information technology and scientific spheres. In aggregate, current developments are profoundly altering almost every aspect of the practice of medicine. Our goals as authors, scientists, educators and practicing clinicians are to help medical students to learn what they need in order to practice patient care in the near future, and to prepare them for even greater changes that we foresee on the horizon.

A critical challenge that has guided the preparation of this edition is our recognition of the fact that students in medical school are overwhelmed with subject matter, from organ-based physiology to molecular biology, from genetics to developmental therapeutics, from anatomy to immunology, from biochemistry to proteomics. Ever mindful of the need to avoid the burdensome detail that characterizes some other textbooks, we have sought to present to students what they must know, all the while eschewing abstruse discussions of medical minutiae, masses of experimental data and alluring but unproven hypotheses. We have tried to be instructive and formative of key precepts of pathology, and to stimulate thought and interest, without punishing students with superfluous information. This textbook provides a foundation for the understanding of pathology and pathogenesis of disease, in order to guide future medical practice. It is not intended to train bench scientists.

There is still a great deal to learn, and much of what needs to be learned reflects the changes that were mentioned above in the world around us. Environmental changes, i.e., alterations in climate, forestation, vertebrate and invertebrate animal populations and human contact with them, exposure to industrial and other chemicals, etc., all contribute to changing patterns of disease. This has been underscored by the rapid emergence of new infectious diseases, such as SARS (see Chapter 9); heightened appreciation for the effects of chemicals on human health, such as the dramatic effects on acute cardiovascular mortality of barring smoking in public places (see Chapter 8); and many others.

Societal changes, in particular evolving patterns of human travel and migration, have caused physicians in the industrialized world to encounter diseases that were once considered to be curiosities, confined geographically elsewhere. The genetic heterogeneity of the human race is an overlay on these population fluxes, and contributes to the increasing array of hitherto unknown diseases, disease susceptibilities and individual symptomatic presentations.

Scientific evolution, which now incorporates analyses of vast quantities of data generated by automated studies of gene expression, protein-protein interaction, DNA sequencing and much more, challenges students to understand its relevance to human health and disease. At the same time, an expanding cornucopia of targeted therapeutics, from antibodies to small molecules that hone in on specific molecular participants in disease processes, redefines treatment strategies. These therapies also generate new understanding of pathogenetic mechanisms, cause previously unknown complications of these treatments themselves and, perhaps vexingly, give us a greater appreciation of the plasticity of disease processes as they adapt to our best therapeutic agents.

The emergence of bioinformatics, with its endless quantities of data, will stimulate attempts to harness computational power to analyze biological and therapeutic problems. This field is still in its infancy, but will probably play an important role in medicine in the years to come.

Finally, information technology is impacting medical education as never before. Electronic learning aids abound. Medical instruction must identify new ways to reach and interact with technologically sophisticated students, and to improve the presentation of the instructional material itself. Accordingly, we have developed a host of resources that are designed to help students to learn and their instructors to teach. These include, for each chapter, electronic flash cards that can be displayed using smart phones, audio questions downloadable to MP3 players for self assessment, portable case histories to illustrate chapter materials, searchable online full text and more. An e-book suitable for personal and tablet computers will be available as well, simultaneously with the printed textbook.

In recognition of this exciting and challenging environment, this 6th edition of *Rubin's Pathology* has been greatly modified, and extensively revised, compared with its predecessor. Many chapters in areas in which extensive new information is available have been largely or completely rewritten and reorganized. The chapters on cell injury (Chapter 1), neoplasia (Chapter 5), breast (Chapter 19), hematopathology (Chapter 20), obesity and diabetes (Chapter 22), amyloidoses (Chapater 23) and neuropathology (Chapter 28) thus largely represent newly written, up-to-date presentations of their subjects. Countless new gross photographs, photomicrographs and drawings have been added, to present the material better and more intelligibly. Almost every chapter reflects major changes in authorship, including Chapters 3-6, 9, 10, 13-15, 17-23 and 25-28. We welcome the participation of all these new authors, who join those who helped prepare previous editions. These outstanding individuals represent among the best minds in Pathology and in medical education in North America and abroad. Their diligent and selfless efforts made this book.

Pathology in the 21st century is a dynamic and exciting discipline. Classical approaches to teaching, and understanding, pathology no longer suffice. Presentation of this material must now encompass the full range of instructional aids and must recognize that pathology and pathogenesis are inseparable. Together, they are an indispensable part of the foundation of all clinical medicine. Any textbook such as this is at best a snapshot of a moving object. We, the editors, together with all of the contributors, have provided an authoritative instructional and reference text that represents the state of the field in 2011. We emphasize what is understood, but do not shy away from describing the limits of current knowledge. As we view this field from the perspective of academic pathologists, the gaps in our understanding seem to expand exponentially, even as we continue to learn more and more. New knowledge generates ever more questions, and the inquisitive mind will find in this textbook a springboard to further exploration. We hope that our students and colleagues will share the excitement of discovery that we have been privileged to experience in our education and careers.

We acknowledge with gratitude the seminal and continuing contribution of Dr. Emanuel Rubin, the Founder and Consulting Editor of this volume that bears his name. Finally, it has been our honor and pleasure to work with the people at Lippincott, Williams & Wilkins, particularly Susan Rhyner, Sirkka Howes and Kelley Squazzo. Their energy, ingenuity and—most importantly—sense of humor, made this book possible.

David S. Strayer
Raphael Rubin
Philadelphia, 2011

ACKNOWLEDGMENTS

Many dedicated people, too numerous to list, provided insight that made this 6th Edition of *Rubin's Pathology* possible. The editors would like especially to thank the managing and editorial staff at Lippincott Williams & Wilkins and in particular Susan Rhyner, Sirkka Howes and also Kelley Squazzo, whose encouragement and support throughout all phases of this endeavor have not only touched us greatly personally but have been a key to the successful publication of this text and its ancillaries.

The editors also acknowledge contributions made by our colleagues who participated in writing previous editions and those who offered suggestions and ideas for the current edition.

Stuart A. Aaronson
Mohammad Alomari
Adam Bagg
Karoly Balogh
Sue Bartow
Douglas P. Bennett
Marluce Bibbo
Hugh Bonner
Patrick J. Buckley
Stephen W. Chensue
Daniel H. Connor
Jeffrey Cossman
John E. Craighead
Mary Cunnane
Giulia DeFalco
Hormuz Ehya
Joseph C. Fantone
John L. Farber
Kevin Furlong
Antonio Giordano
Barry J. Goldstein
Stanley R. Hamilton
Terrence J. Harrist
Arthur P. Hays
Serge Jabbour
Robert B. Jennings
Kent J. Johnson
Anthony A. Killeen
Michael J. Klein
William D. Kocher
Robert J. Kurman
Ernest A. Lack
Antonio Martinez-Hernandez
Steven McKenzie
Wolfgang J. Mergner
Frank A. Mitros
Adebeye O. Osunkoya
Juan Palazzo
Robert O. Peterson
Roger J. Pomerantz
Timothy R. Quinn
Stanley J. Robboy
Brian Schapiro
Roland Schwarting
Stephen M. Schwartz
Benjamin H. Spargo
Charles Steenbergen, Jr.
Steven L. Teitelbaum
Ann D. Thor
John Q. Trojanowski
Benjamin F. Trump
Jianzhou Wang
Beverly Y. Wang

CONTENTS

1 Cell Adaptation, Cell Injury and Cell Death

David S. Strayer • Emanuel Rubin

Pathology ***is the study of structural and functional abnormalities that are expressed as diseases of organs and systems.*** Classic theories attributed disease to imbalances or noxious effects of humors on specific organs. In the 19th century, Rudolf Virchow, often referred to as the father of modern pathology, proposed that injury to the smallest living unit of the body, the cell, is the basis of all disease. To this day, clinical and experimental pathology remain rooted in this concept.

Teleology—the study of design or purpose in nature—has long since been discredited as part of scientific investigation. Although facts can only be established by observation, to appreciate the mechanisms of injury to the cell, teleologic thinking can be useful in framing questions. As an analogy, it would be impossible to understand a chess-playing computer without an understanding of the goals of chess and prior knowledge that a particular computer is programmed to play it: it would be futile to search for the sources of defects in the specific program or overall operating system without an appreciation of the goals of the device. In this sense, it is helpful to understand the problems with which the cell is confronted and the strategies that have evolved to cope with them.

A living cell must maintain the ability to produce energy. Thus, the most pressing need for any free living cell, prokaryotic or eukaryotic, is to establish a structural and functional barrier between its internal milieu and a hostile environment. The **plasma membrane** serves this purpose in several ways:

- It maintains a constant internal ionic composition against very large chemical gradients between the interior and exterior compartments.
- It selectively admits some molecules while excluding or extruding others.
- It provides a structural envelope to contain the informational, synthetic and catabolic constituents of the cell.
- It provides an environment to house signal transduction molecules that mediate communication between the external and internal milieus.

At the same time, to survive, a cell must be able to adapt to adverse environmental conditions, such as changes in temperature, solute concentrations or oxygen supply; the presence of noxious agents; and so on. The evolution of multicellular organisms eased the hazardous lot of individual cells by establishing a controlled extracellular environment in which temperature, oxygenation, ionic content and nutrient supply are relatively constant. It also permitted the luxury of cell differentiation for such widely divergent functions as energy storage (liver cell glycogen and adipocytes), communication (neurons), contractile activity (heart muscle), synthesis of proteins or peptides for export (liver, pancreas and endocrine cells), absorption (intestine) and defense from foreign invaders (polymorphonuclear leukocytes, lymphocytes and macrophages).

Cells encounter many stresses as a result of changes in their internal and external environments. ***Patterns of response to such stresses comprise the cellular basis of disease.*** If an injury exceeds the adaptive capacity of the cell, the cell dies. A cell exposed to persistent sublethal injury has limited available responses, the expression of which we interpret as evidence of cell injury. In general, mammalian cells adapt to injury by conserving resources: decreasing or ceasing differentiated functions and focusing exclusively on their own survival. ***From this perspective, pathology is the study of cell injury and the expression of a cell's preexisting capacity to adapt to such injury.*** Such an orientation leaves little room for the concept of parallel—normal and pathologic—biologies.

Reactions to Persistent Stress and Cell Injury

Persistent stress often leads to chronic cell injury. In general, permanent organ injury is associated with the death of individual cells. By contrast, the cellular response to persistent sublethal injury, whether chemical or physical, reflects adaptation of the cell to a hostile environment. Again, these changes are, for the most part, reversible on discontinuation of the stress. In response to persistent stress, a cell dies or adapts. It is thus our view that at the *cellular level* it is more appropriate to speak of chronic adaptation than of chronic injury. The major adaptive responses are atrophy, hypertrophy, hyperplasia, metaplasia, dysplasia and intracellular storage. In addition, certain forms of neoplasia may follow adaptive responses.

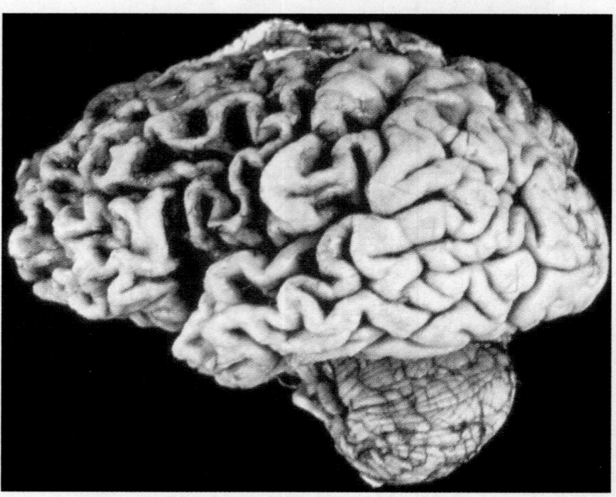

FIGURE 1-1. Atrophy of the brain. Marked atrophy of the frontal lobe is noted in this photograph of the brain. The gyri are thinned and the sulci conspicuously widened.

Atrophy Is an Active Response to an Altered Environment That Results in Reduced Function or Size of Cells or Organs

Clinically, atrophy is often noted as decreased size or function of an organ, which may occur under both pathologic and physiologic circumstances. Thus, for example, atrophy may result from disuse of skeletal muscle or from loss of hormonal signals following menopause. It may also be an adaptive response whereby a cell accommodates changes in its environment, all the while remaining viable. However, most commonly atrophy is a consequence of harmful processes such as those involved in some chronic diseases and biological aging (see later).

One must distinguish atrophy of an organ from cellular atrophy. Reduction in an organ's size may reflect reversible cell atrophy or irreversible loss of cells. For example, renewing physical activity to a disused limb may cause atrophic muscle cells to resume their usual size and function. By contrast, atrophy of the brain in Alzheimer* disease is secondary to extensive cell death; the size of the organ cannot be restored (Fig. 1-1). Atrophy occurs under a variety of conditions as outlined below (Table 1-1).

Reduced Functional Demand

A common form of atrophy follows reduced functional demand. For example, after immobilization of a limb in a cast as treatment for a bone fracture or after prolonged bed rest, the limb's muscle cells atrophy and muscular strength is reduced.

Inadequate Supply of Oxygen

***Interference with blood supply to tissues is called* ischemia.** Resulting oxygen deprivation may be insufficient to kill cells, in which case, cells may remain viable but functionally

*A note about eponymous diseases (i.e., diseases named after a person). Although in common usage the diseases that carry the names of Alzheimer, Parkinson, Cushing, etc., are cited as possessives (e.g., Alzheimer's disease, Parkinson's disease), medical convention requires that these diseases be so identified *without the possessive proper noun* ("Classification and nomenclature of morphological defects". *Lancet* 1975;1:513). In this text, we honor this convention.

Table 1-1

Conditions Associated With Atrophy

Disease or Condition	Examples of Conditions in Which Atrophy Occurs
Aging	Most organs that do not continuously turn over; most common setting for atrophy to occur
Chronic disease	Prototype for atrophy occurring in chronic disease is cancer; also seen in congestive heart failure, chronic obstructive pulmonary disease, cirrhosis of the liver and AIDS
Ischemia	Hypoxia, decreased nutrient availability, renal artery stenosis
Malnutrition	Generalized atrophy
Decreased functional demand	Limb immobilization, as in a fracture
Interruption of trophic signals	Denervation atrophy following nerve injury; menopause effect on the endometrium and other organs
Increased pressure	Decubitus ulcers, passive congestion of the liver

impaired. Under such circumstances, cell atrophy is common. It is frequently seen around the inadequately perfused margins of ischemic necrosis (infarcts) in the heart, brain and kidneys following vascular occlusion in these organs.

Insufficient Nutrients

Starvation or malnutrition leads to wasting of skeletal muscle and adipose tissue. At the microscopic level this is manifested as cell atrophy. It is striking that reduction in mass is particularly prominent in cells that are not vital to the survival of the organism. One cannot dismiss the possibility that a portion of the cell atrophy attributed to partial ischemia reflects a lack of nutrients.

Interruption of Trophic Signals

The functions of many cells depend on signals transmitted by chemical mediators. The endocrine system and neuromuscular transmission are the best examples. The actions of hormones or, for skeletal muscle, synaptic transmission, place functional demands on cells. These can be eliminated by removing the source of the signal (e.g., via ablation of an endocrine gland or denervation). If the anterior pituitary is surgically resected, loss of thyroid-stimulating hormone (TSH), adrenocorticotropic hormone (ACTH, also called corticotropin) and follicle-stimulating hormone (FSH) results in atrophy of the thyroid, adrenal cortex and ovaries, respectively. Atrophy secondary to endocrine insufficiency is not restricted to pathologic conditions; the endometrium atrophies when estrogen levels decrease after menopause (Fig. 1-2). Even cancer cells may undergo atrophy, to some extent, by hormonal deprivation. Androgen-dependent prostatic cancer partially regresses after administration of testosterone antagonists. Certain types of thyroid cancer may stop growing if one inhibits pituitary TSH secretion by administering thyroxine. If neurologic damage (e.g., from poliomyelitis or traumatic spinal cord injury) leads to denervation of muscle, the neuromuscular transmission necessary for muscle tone is lost and affected muscles atrophy.

Persistent Cell Injury

Persistent cell injury is most commonly caused by chronic inflammation associated with prolonged viral or bacterial infections. Chronic inflammation may be seen in a variety of other circumstances, including immunologic and granulomatous disorders. A good example is the atrophy of the gastric mucosa that occurs in association with chronic gastritis (see Chapter 13). Similarly, villous atrophy of the

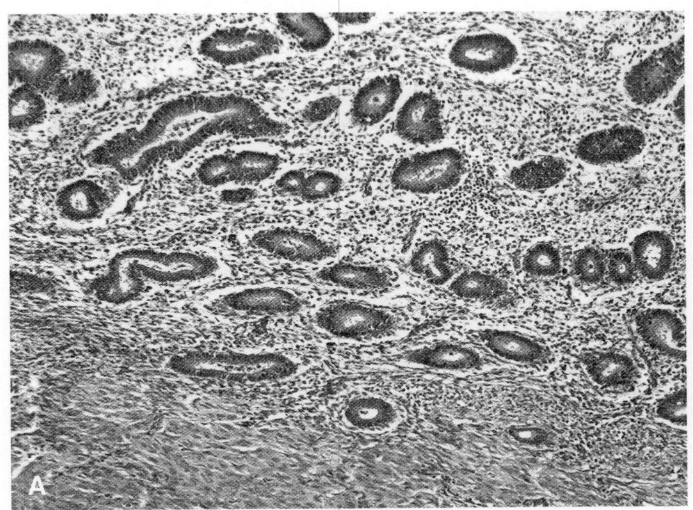

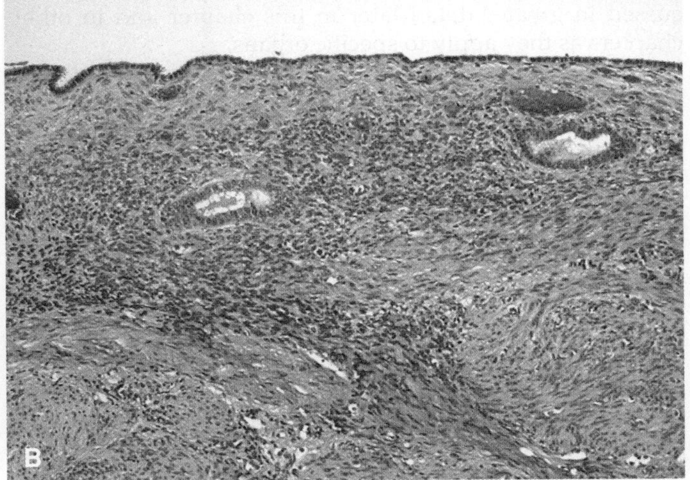

FIGURE 1-2. Atrophy of the endometrium. A. A section of the normal uterus from a woman of reproductive age reveals a thick endometrium composed of proliferative glands in an abundant stroma. **B.** The endometrium of a 75-year-old woman (shown at the same magnification) is thin and contains only a few atrophic and cystic glands.

small intestinal mucosa follows chronic inflammation of celiac disease.

Increased Pressure

Even physical injury, such as prolonged pressure in inappropriate locations, produces atrophy. Prolonged bed rest may lead to sustained pressure on the skin, causing atrophy of the skin and consequent decubitus ulcers (bed sores). Heart failure leads to increased pressure in sinusoids of the liver because the heart cannot pump the venous return from that organ efficiently. Accordingly, the cells in the center of the liver lobule, which are exposed to the greatest pressure, become atrophic.

Aging

In addition to conspicuous loss of skeletal muscle and adipose tissue, one of the hallmarks of aging (see below) is decreased size and number of nonreplicating cells, such as those of the brain and heart. The size of all parenchymal organs decreases with age. The size of the brain is invariably decreased, and in the very old the size of the heart may be so diminished that the term **senile atrophy** has been used.

Chronic Disease

Oftentimes, people afflicted with wasting chronic diseases such as cancer, congestive heart failure or acquired immunodeficiency syndrome (AIDS) demonstrate generalized atrophy of many tissues. Tissue loss exceeds what can be attributed to decreased caloric intake and reflects alterations in cytokines and other mediators.

Atrophy Is an Active Process

The size of cells and organs reflects an equilibrium between anabolic and catabolic processes and involves changes both in production and destruction of cellular constituents. In its most basic sense, atrophy is a cell's reversible restructuring of its activities to facilitate its own survival and adapt to conditions of diminished use. The molecular mechanisms are discussed in greater detail later in this chapter and in other chapters as they apply to specific organs.

Atrophy has been most extensively studied in adipose tissue and skeletal muscle, which respond rapidly to changes in demand for energy storage and contractile force, respectively. Striated muscle cells allow study of atrophy and hypertrophy (see below) without the confounding influence of cell proliferation. When a muscle is immobilized and the need for contraction decreases ("unloading"), myocytes institute selective adaptive mechanisms:

- **Protein synthesis:** Shortly after unloading, protein synthesis decreases, because of decreased protein elongation by ribosomes. This effect is specific; whereas synthesis of some proteins is decreased, production of other proteins that are important in mediating this adaptation may increase.
- **Protein degradation:** Particular ubiquitin-related specific protein degradation pathways (see below) are activated. These mediate the atrophic response in several ways. They lead to decreases in certain contractile proteins and in the specific transcription factors that drive expression of contractile protein genes. These increases in specific protein elimination are transient. If the atrophic state is maintained, cells reach a new equilibrium in which mass remains decreased and rates of protein synthesis and degradation realign.
- **Gene expression:** There are selective decreases in transcription of genes for, among other things, contractile activities. Transcription of some genes is actually upregulated, particularly those encoding proteins that mediate protein degradation.
- **Signaling:** The checks and balances that control the levels of upregulation and downregulation of intracellular signaling species change.
- **Energy utilization:** A selective decrease in the use of free fatty acids as an energy source for muscle has been noted during the response to unloading.

Atrophy is thus an active and specific adaptive response, and is not a passive shutdown of cellular processes. Moreover, it is reversible; restoring the environment that existed before atrophy developed allows cells to return to their normal size and function.

Hypertrophy Is an Increase in Cell Size and Functional Capacity

When trophic signals or functional demand increases, adaptive changes to satisfy these needs lead to increased cellular size (hypertrophy) and, in some cases, increased cellular number (hyperplasia; see below).

In some organs (e.g., heart, skeletal muscle), such adaptive responses are accomplished mainly by increased cell size (Fig. 1-3). In other organs (e.g., kidney, thyroid), cell numbers and cell size may both increase. This section deals with the mechanisms and consequences when cells enlarge to meet increased functional demands on them. Some mechanisms involved in the hypertrophic response are cell type specific, whereas others are more general. Also, cells that can divide use some of the same mechanisms to stimulate mitosis that nondividing cells use to increase their size.

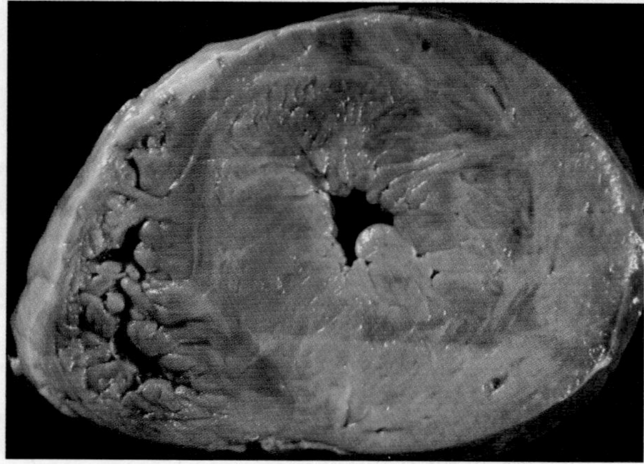

FIGURE 1-3. Myocardial hypertrophy. Cross-section of the heart of a patient with long-standing hypertension shows pronounced, concentric left ventricular hypertrophy.

Mechanisms of Cellular Hypertrophy

Whether the stimulus to enlarge is increased work load or increased endocrine or neuroendocrine mediators, there are certain processes that usually contribute to generating cellular hypertrophy.

Cellular Remodeling in Hypertrophy
When cells are stimulated to increase their mass, one of the first activities is enhanced proteasomal degradation of selected cellular proteins. Thus, proteins that do not contribute to the specific need for hypertrophy are degraded, even as production of proteins that promote hypertrophy tends to increase.

Signaling Mechanisms in Hypertrophy
Although signals that elicit hypertrophic responses vary, depending on the cell type and circumstances, the example of skeletal muscle hypertrophy illustrates some critical general principles. Thus, many types of signaling may lead to cell hypertrophy:

- **Growth factor stimulation:** Each tissue responds to different signals. In many cases certain growth factors appear to be key initiators of hypertrophy. For example, insulin-like growth factor-I (IGF-I) is increased in load-induced muscle hypertrophy, and in experimental settings may elicit hypertrophy even if load does not increase.
- **Neuroendocrine stimulation:** In some tissues, adrenergic signaling may be important in initiating or facilitating hypertrophy.
- **Ion channels:** Ion fluxes may activate adaptation to increased demand. Calcium channel activity, in particular, may stimulate a host of downstream enzymes (e.g., calcineurin) to produce hypertrophy.
- **Other chemical mediators:** Depending on the particular tissue, such factors as nitric oxide (NO•), angiotensin II, and bradykinin may support cell hypertrophic responses.
- **Oxygen supply:** Clearly increased functional demand on cells requires increased energy supply. Angiogenesis is stimulated when a tissue oxygen deficit is sensed and may be an indispensable component of adaptive hypertrophy.
- **Hypertrophy antagonists:** Just as some mechanisms foster cellular hypertrophy, others inhibit it. Atrial natriuretic factors, high concentrations of NO• and many other factors either brake or prevent cell adaptation by hypertrophy.

Effector Pathways

Whatever mechanisms initiate the signaling process to stimulate hypertrophy, there are a limited number of downstream pathways that mediate the effects of such signaling:

- **Increased protein degradation:** This was discussed above.
- **Increased protein translation:** Shortly after a prohypertrophic signal is received, production of certain proteins increases. This occurs very quickly and without changes in RNA levels, via increased translational efficiency. Activities of translational initiators and elongation factors are often stimulated in the early phases of hypertrophy to provide a rapid increase in the proteins needed to meet the increased functional demand.
- **Increased gene expression:** Concentrations of key proteins are also increased by upregulation of transcription of their corresponding genes. Many of the signaling pathways activated by cytokines, neurotransmitters and so forth activate an array of transcription factors. Thus, for example, the phosphatase calcineurin dephosphorylates transcription factor NFAT (*n*uclear *f*actor of *a*ctivated *T* cells), thereby facilitating its movement to the nucleus. As a result, transcription of target genes increases. Hypertrophy may also involve increased transcription of genes encoding growth-promoting transcription factors, such as Fos and Myc.
- **Survival:** Among the functions activated during hypertrophy is inhibition of cell death. Thus, stimulation of several receptors increases the activity of several kinases (Akt, PI3K and others; see below). These in turn promote cell survival, largely by inhibiting programmed cell death (apoptosis; see below).
- **Ancillary functions:** In some situations hypertrophy may involve changes in a cell's relation to its environment, such as remodeling extracellular matrix.
- **Recruitment of satellite cells:** Skeletal muscle hypertrophy includes recruiting perimuscular satellite cells to fuse with the muscle syncytia, providing additional nuclei, which are needed to support the expanded protein synthetic needs of the enlarging muscle.

Mechanisms of Hypertrophy Vary According to the Stimulus

Hypertrophy of skeletal muscle and heart may follow different pathways, depending on the requirements imposed by the increased functional demand. For instance, increased endurance of skeletal muscle entails increased aerobic activity (increased oxygen consumption). By contrast, the response to increased resistance (e.g., weightlifting) results in stimulation of signaling that does not necessitate increased oxygen supply (Fig. 1-4).

Similarly, cardiac hypertrophy may occur in response to exercise **(physiologic hypertrophy)** or increased vascular resistance **(pathologic hypertrophy).** Each stimulus involves different soluble mediators that in turn activate distinct cellular signaling pathways, with much different consequences (see Chapter 11).

In sum, the diverse stimuli that lead to cell hypertrophy stimulate adaptive cellular remodeling, increase protein production, facilitate cell function and promote cell survival.

Postmitotic Cells May Turn Over

Historically, neurons, cardiac myocytes and skeletal muscle cells were considered to be incapable of mitosis and, throughout their life span, remained in their original differentiated state. This view has generally been interpreted to imply that neurons and myocytes cannot be replaced, and therefore that the brain, heart and skeletal muscle cannot respond to cell loss or increased demand by adding cells.

The Concept of Postmitotic Cells and Terminal Differentiation

These paradigms are today considered only partially correct. Whereas neurons and cardiac myocytes may not undergo mitosis, recent studies have demonstrated the presence of committed progenitor cells, which proliferate and differentiate in response to cell death and injury or, in the case of striated muscle, increased functional demand.

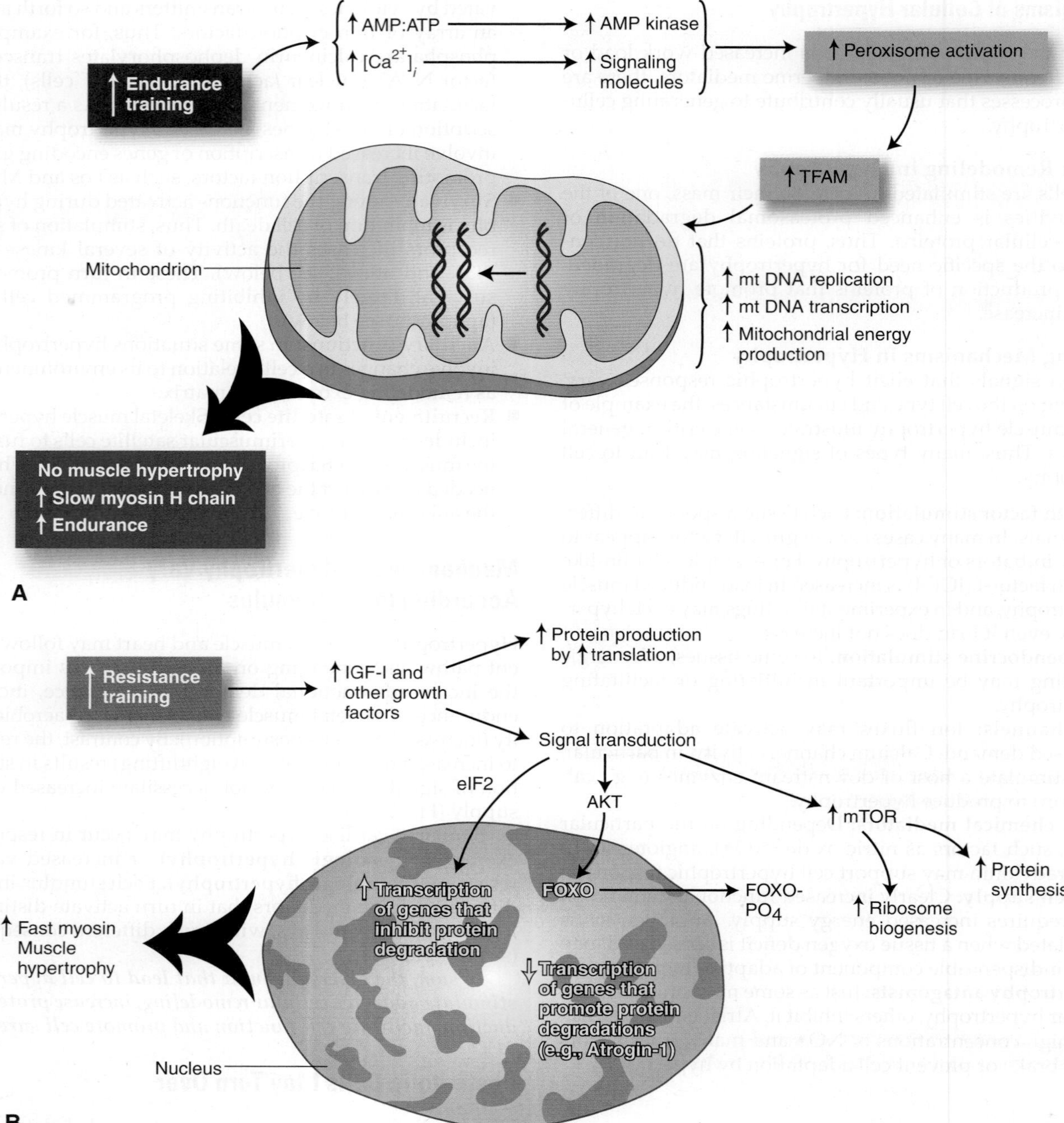

FIGURE 1-4. Mechanisms involved in muscle hypertrophy. A. Endurance training. Muscle strengthening for endurance entails repeated or prolonged exercise with small loads and leads to increases in the adenosine monophosphate–to–adenosine triphosphate (AMP:ATP) ratio, leading to increased AMP kinase activity. Such training also increases cytosol calcium concentration ($[Ca^{2+}i]$), which increases a number of cellular signaling intermediates. Consequent peroxisome activation increases the transcription factor–activating mitochondrial energy production (TFAM). Increased TFAM in turn activates both replication and transcription of mitochondrial DNA. The consequence is increase in muscle slow myosin H chain and improved endurance without muscle cell hypertrophy. **B. Resistance training.** Muscle strengthening by lifting weights, in which load, but not repetition, is increased, leads to muscle cell hypertrophy. This is mediated by increased insulin-like growth factor-I (IGF-I) and other growth factors (such as growth hormone), which act via a series of cellular intermediates such as transcription elongation factor eIF2, protein kinase B (AKT) and mammalian target of rapamycin (mTOR). Each of these mediates changes in gene expression and metabolism. AKT phosphorylates and inactivates the forkhead transcription factor FOXO, causing it to leave the nucleus and causing decreased transcription of genes involved in protein degradation (e.g., Atrogin-1). Simultaneously, increased eIF2 activity activates transcription of genes that inhibit protein degradation. The consequence is increased fast myosin H chain and increased myocyte size (hypertrophy).

These newer concepts also suggest a natural, albeit low, rate of cell loss and replacement in organs that had previously been considered "postmitotic," or "terminally differentiated." If this equilibrium is tilted to favor cell loss, organ atrophy may result, as seen in the heart, muscle and brain of the very aged. The equilibrium may also be shifted toward predominance of progenitor cell activity, as occurs in muscle hypertrophy.

Proteasomes Are Key Participants in Cell Homeostasis, Response to Stress and Adaptation to Altered Extracellular Environments

Cellular responses to alterations in their milieu were once studied exclusively by analyzing changes in gene expression and protein production. The issue of protein degradation was either ignored or relegated to the nonspecific proteolytic activities of lysosomes. However, it has become clear that cellular homeostasis requires mechanisms that allow the cell to destroy certain proteins selectively. Although there is evidence that more than one such pathway may exist, the best understood mechanism by which cells target specific proteins for elimination is the ubiquitin (Ub)–proteasomal apparatus.

Proteasomes

There are two different types of these cellular organelles, 20S and 26S. The degradative unit is the 20S core, to which two 19S "caps" are attached, to form the 26S proteasome. There are at least 32 different proteins in the proteasomal complex. They are arrayed, as shown in Fig. 1-5, with a 19S subunit at the entrance and another at the exit of the barrel-like structure, of which the 20S subunit forms the proteolytic center.

Proteins targeted for destruction are modified as described below, and recognized by one 19S subunit. They are then degraded in an adenosine triphosphate (ATP)-requiring process, with the adenosine triphosphatases (ATPases) in the first 19S unit and a unique proteolytic core located within the 20S subunit. The products of this process are peptides that are 3 to 25 amino acids in size, which are released through the lower 19S subunit. These peptides may be further degraded by cytosolic proteases.

The importance of proteasomes is underscored by the fact that they may comprise up to 1% to 2% of the total mass of the cell. These structures are evolutionarily highly conserved and are described in all eukaryotic cells. ***Mutations in key proteins that lead to interference with normal proteasomal function are lethal.***

The 20S proteasomes are important in degradation of **oxidized proteins** (see below). In 26S proteasomes, **ubiquitinated proteins** are degraded. A variant type of proteasome, the immunoproteasome, is formed in response to cellular production of interferon-γ (IFN-γ). Immunoproteasomes tend to gravitate to the endoplasmic reticulum and are important in processing proteins to 8- or 9-amino-acid peptides to be attached to major histocompatibility complex type I for presentation to the immune system as antigens (see Chapter 4).

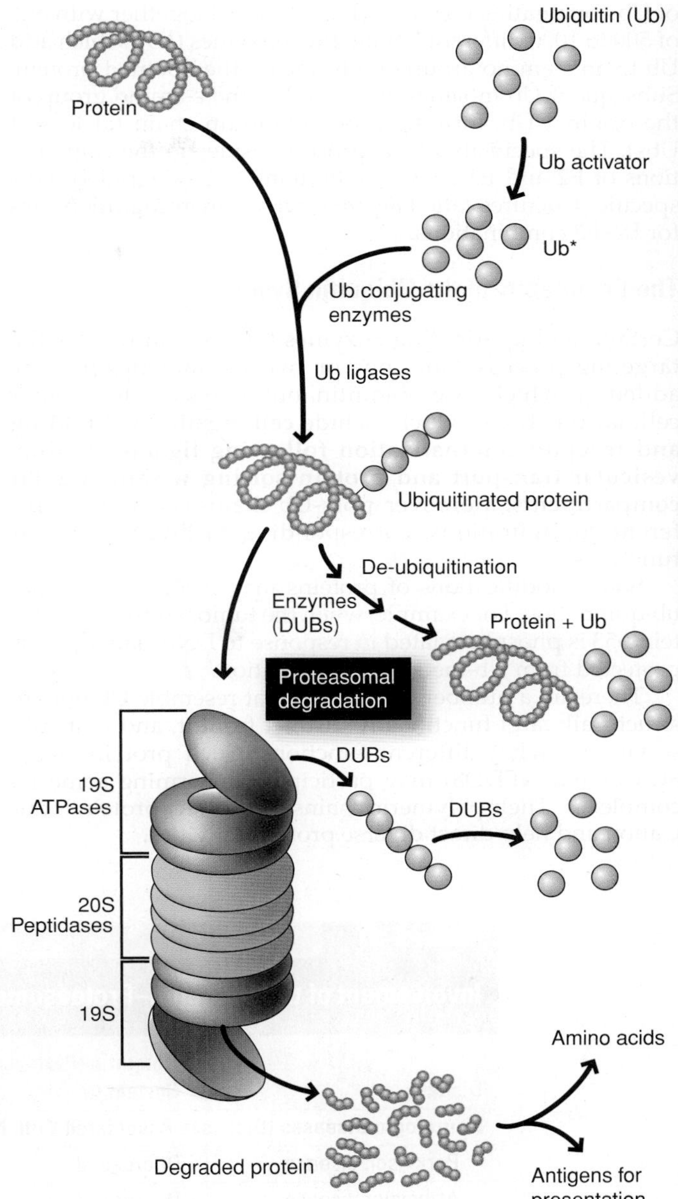

FIGURE 1-5. Ubiquitin–proteasome pathways. The mechanisms by which ubiquitin (Ub) targets proteins for specific elimination in proteasomes are shown here. Ub is activated (Ub*) by E1 ubiquitin activating enzyme, then transferred to an E2 (ubiquitin conjugating enzyme). The E2–Ub* complex interacts with an E3 (ubiquitin ligase) to bind a particular protein. The process may be repeated multiple times to append a chain of Ub moieties. These complexes may be deubiquitinated by deubiquitinating enzymes (DUBs). If degradation is to proceed, 26S proteasomes recognize the poly-Ub-conjugated protein via their 19S subunit and degrade it into oligopeptides. In the process, Ub moieties are returned to the cell pool of ubiquitin monomers.

Ubiquitin and Ubiquitination

Proteins to be degraded are flagged by attachment to small chains of ubiquitin molecules. Ub is a 76-amino acid protein that is the key to selective protein elimination; it is conjugated to proteins as a flag to identify those proteins to be destroyed. The process of attaching Ub to proteins is called ubiquitination (or, ubiquitylation).

A cascade of enzymes is involved (Fig. 1-5). Ub-activating enzyme, E1, binds Ub and then transfers it to one of dozens of Ub-conjugating enzymes (E2). These act together with one of 500 to 1000 different Ub-ligating enzymes (E3), which add Ub to an ε-amino group of a lysine on the doomed protein. Subsequent Ub moieties are added to the ε-amino group of the original Ub, forming a polyubiquitin chain (at least 4 Ubs). The specificity of the process resides in the combinations of E2 and E3 enzymes. Proteins to be degraded have specific structures called ***degrons***, which are recognition sites for E2–E3 combinations.

The Complexity of the Ubiquitin System

Certain deubiquitinating enzymes (DUBs) can reverse the targeting process. Only one or two Ub moieties may be added, in which case ubiquitination plays a role in other cellular functions, which include **cell membrane budding and receptor internalization following ligand binding, vesicular transport and protein sorting within cellular compartments.** Moreover, poly-Ub chains can assume different configurations, corresponding to diverse cellular functions.

Some modifications of proteins may protect them from ubiquitination. For example, when the tumor suppressor protein p53 is phosphorylated in response to DNA damage, it is protected from Ub-mediated degradation.

There are a number of proteins that resemble Ub but are structurally and functionally distinct from it, and that subserve somewhat different functions. Such proteins (e.g., SUMO and NEDD8) may participate in forming some E3 complexes. Their polymeric chains may direct protein localization and help direct diverse protein activities.

Why Ubiquitination Matters

Ubiquitination and specific protein elimination not only are important for normal cellular homeostasis but also are fundamental to cellular adaptation to stress and injury, as the following sections will show. In some cases, mutations in Ub pathway constituents are the primary causes of specific diseases, whereas in many instances altered ubiquitin– proteasome system activity plays an important role in the pathogenesis of diseases (Table 1-2). For example, defective ubiquitination is involved in several important neurodegenerative diseases. Mutations in parkin, a ubiquitin ligase, are implicated in the pathogenesis of Parkinson disease, in which undegraded parkin accumulates as Lewy bodies (see Chapter 28).

Regulation of ubiquitination may be important in tumor development. Thus, human papilloma virus strains that are associated with human cervical cancer (see Chapters 5 and 18) produce E6 protein, which inactivates the p53 tumor suppressor. This inactivation is implicated in the genesis of cervical cancer. E6 accomplishes this feat by binding an E3 (ubiquitin ligase) and facilitating its association with p53. As a result, increased ubiquitination of p53 accelerates its degradation. Finally, there is increasing evidence to suggest that impaired ubiquitination may be involved in some cellular degenerative changes that occur in aging and in a variety of storage diseases.

Ubiquitination also plays a role in gene expression. Nuclear factor-κB (NFκB) is an important transcriptional activator that is activated in two different ways by the ubiquitin–proteasome system. First, inactive precursor forms of the two NFκB subunits are ubiquitinated and cleaved to their active forms.

Table 1-2

Involvement of the Ubiquitin–Proteasome System in Disease

Disease	Ubiquitin–Proteasome System Activity	Anatomic Effect
Neurologic Diseases (Diseases Associated With Neuron Loss)		
Parkinson disease	Decreased	Lewy bodies
Alzheimer disease	Decreased	Amyloid plaques, neurofibrillary tangles
Amyotrophic lateral sclerosis	Decreased	Superoxide dismutase aggregates in motor neurons
Huntington disease	Decreased	Polyglutamine inclusions
Autoimmune Diseases		
Sjögren syndrome	Decreased	Chronic inflammation
Metabolic Diseases		
Type II diabetes mellitus	Increased	Insulin insensitivity
Cataract formation	Decreased	Aggregated oxidized proteins
Muscle Wasting		
Aging	Increased	Atrophy
Cancer and other chronic disease	Increased	Atrophy
Cardiovascular		
Ischemia/reperfusion	Decreased	Myocyte apoptosis
Pressure overload	Decreased	Myocyte apoptosis

This is an example of incomplete protein degradation by the ubiquitin–proteasome system. Also, the inhibitor of NFκB, called IκB, is degraded by ubiquitination. This step releases NFκB, which mediates expression of genes that promote cell survival. Proteasome inhibition permits persistence of the IκB–NFκB complex and therefore decreases NFκB-induced transcriptional activation. In the case of cancer cells, inhibiting proteasomal function would impair tumor cell survival and is consequently a target for pharmaceutical manipulation.

Autophagy Is a Multifaceted Cellular Autodigestive System That Is Important in Both Cellular Adaptation and Pathogenesis of Disease

Autophagy (from the Greek, "auto," *self*; "phagy," *eat*) comprises degradative pathways that operate through the transfer of cytoplasmic constituents to lysosomes for degradation. This process, which rids cells of materials such as misfolded proteins, microorganisms and damaged organelles, is one of the most evolutionarily conserved cellular operations. Material destined for self-cannibalization is sequestered in vesicles (autophagosomes) that fuse with a lysosome.

There are three recognized types of autophagy, which are illustrated in Fig. 1-6. Autophagy normally acts as a cellular housekeeper. It is upregulated when the cell is stressed (e.g., by starvation, hypoxia, growth factor deprivation, etc.). Under these conditions, it represents an alternative source of nutrients for energy production and structural reconstitution for cell survival. However, the autophagic pathway can also be called upon to kill cells, in which case it generates a caspase-independent form of cell death **(autophagic cell death).** In addition to its role in cellular adaptation to such adversity, autophagy also is important for the ability of cells to clear intracellular microorganisms, such as mycobacteria.

Autophagy in Disease

Oligomeric and aggregated proteins are poorly degraded by the proteasomal pathway. In this context, autophagy is important for the elimination of mutant or altered proteins that form aggregates. Such proteins are particularly involved in neurodegenerative diseases such as Huntington disease, Parkinson disease and Alzheimer disease. Thus, defects in autophagy are thought to play a key role in these disorders. Interference with autophagy is also thought to contribute to a variety of conditions, including degenerative and inflammatory diseases, cancer and aging (Table 1-3). Regulation of autophagy has been associated with a large family of genes, termed ATG genes, mutations of which are thought to contribute to many of these conditions.

Molecular Chaperones Are Important in Maintaining Cell Homeostasis

To ensure proper functional activity, proteins must achieve particular three-dimensional configurations by folding appropriately. This process is controlled by both the amino acid

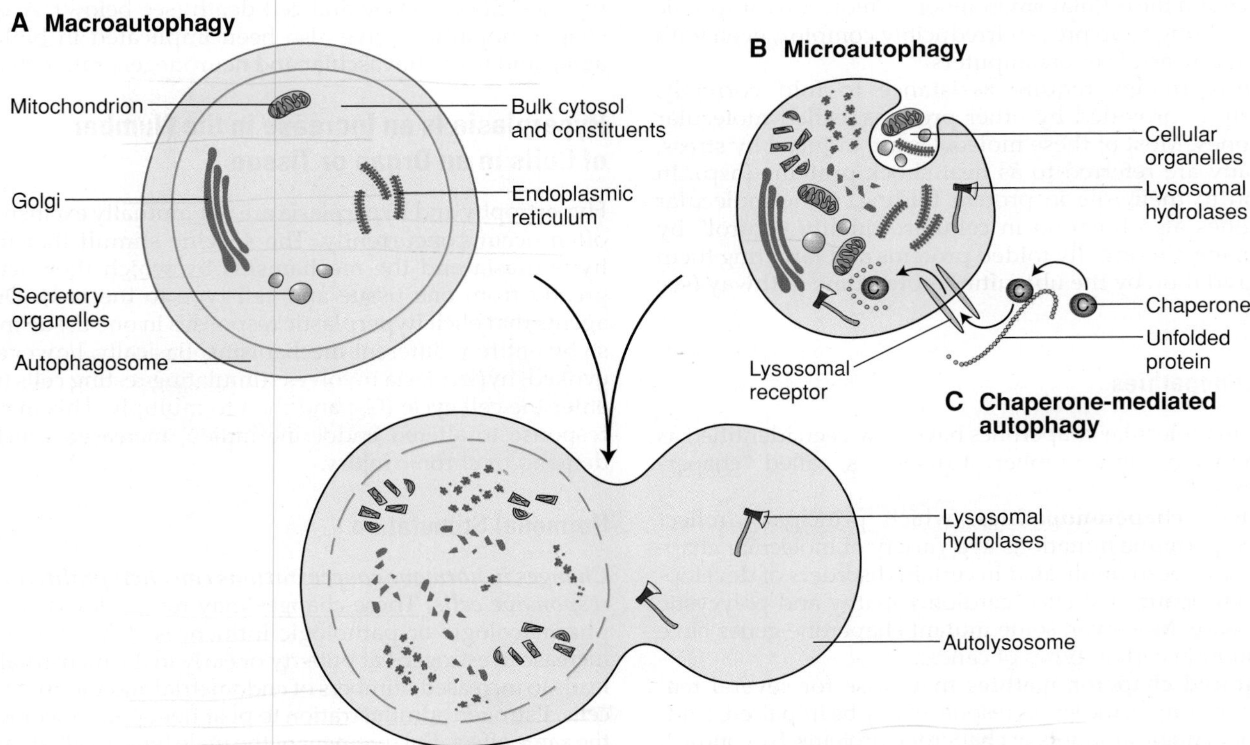

FIGURE 1-6. Types of autophagy. A. Macroautophagy, in which an autophagosome surrounds bulk cytosol and cytoplasmic organelles. **B. Microautophagy**, in which selected organelles or foreign materials (e.g., microbial pathogens) are engulfed by lysosomes. **C. Chaperone-mediated autophagy**, in which selected cellular macromolecules are conducted to lysosomes by chaperones (e.g., hsc70), which are recognized by lysosomal receptor proteins (e.g., LAMP-2A). The targeted material is destroyed by lysosomal degradation.

Table 1-3

Normal and Abnormal Autophagy in Human Disease

Disease	Normal Autophagy	Impaired Autophagy
Cancer	Removes damaged organelles and abnormal proteins	Some cancers are associated with mutant autophagy genes
	Helps maintain chromosome stability	Mutant p53 decreases autophagy
	May help cancer cells survive cytotoxicity of chemotherapy and generalized low nutrients	Acquired mutations that activate oncogenes like AKT, PI3K and Bcl-2 inhibit autophagy
Cardiac disease	Facilitates adaptation to ischemia and to increased peripheral vascular resistance	A form of familial cardiomyopathy may involve mutation in a gene controlling autophagosome–lysosome fusion
Neurodegenerative diseases	Maintains intracellular homeostasis and prevents protein accumulation	Accumulation of proteins or incompletely functional autophagosomes leads to toxic protein accumulation
		Several inherited diseases involve abnormal autophagosome motility or fusion
Liver disease	May allow elimination of abnormally folded proteins, in part by eliminating organelles in which they accumulate	Overly active autophagy may cause liver injury
Miscellaneous diseases		Inherited or acquired mutations in several genes involved in autophagy may be important in tuberous sclerosis, some forms of Crohn disease, Paget disease of bone and other inherited diseases

PI3K = phosphatidylinositol 3-kinase.

sequence and the cellular environment. Predictions of specific protein folding have proven irreducibly complex, even with the most powerful supercomputers.

Many proteins require assistance to fold correctly. This help is provided by other proteins, called molecular chaperones. Most of these molecules are induced by stress, and many are referred to as heat shock proteins (hsp). In addition to their role in protein folding, some molecular chaperones also function in cellular "quality control" by recognizing abnormally folded proteins and targeting them for degradation by the ubiquitin–proteasome pathway (see above).

Chaperonopathies

Defects in molecular chaperones have now been identified as etiologic factors in a number of disorders, called "chaperonopathies."

Genetic chaperonopathies, which principally reflect inherited germline mutations in a variety of molecular chaperones, have been implicated in certain disorders of development, neuropathies, dilated cardiomyopathy and polycystic liver disease. Moreover, some mutant chaperone genes have been found in certain types of cancer.

Acquired chaperonopathies may arise for several reasons. For example, the stress response may be impaired, leading to inadequate amounts of chaperone proteins. By contrast, levels of substrate (misfolded or degraded proteins) may exceed the capacity of the chaperone system. Chaperone molecules may also be sequestered in protein deposits, or inactivated by exogenous toxins (e.g., an enzyme from a virulent strain of *Escherichia coli* cleaves Hsp70). Chaperones may also contribute to tumorigenesis through effects on proteins that regulate the cell cycle and cell death (see below). Acquired chaperonopathies have also been implicated in biological aging and in cardiovascular and neurodegenerative diseases.

Hyperplasia Is an Increase in the Number of Cells in an Organ or Tissue

Hypertrophy and hyperplasia are not mutually exclusive and often occur concurrently. The specific stimuli that induce hyperplasia and the mechanisms by which they act vary greatly from one tissue and cell type to the next. Diverse agents that elicit hyperplastic responses in one tissue may do so by entirely different mechanisms. Basically, however it is evoked, hyperplasia involves stimulating resting cells (G_0) to enter the cell cycle (G_1) and then to multiply. This may be a response to altered endocrine milieu, increased functional demand or chronic injury.

Hormonal Stimulation

Changes in hormone concentrations can elicit proliferation of responsive cells. These changes may reflect developmental, pharmacologic or pathologic influences. Thus, the normal increase in estrogens at puberty or early in the menstrual cycle leads to increased numbers of endometrial and uterine stromal cells. Estrogen administration to postmenopausal women has the same effect. Enlargement of the male breast, called gynecomastia, may occur in liver failure, when the liver's inability to metabolize endogenous estrogens leads to their accumulation, or in men given estrogens as therapy for prostate cancer. Ectopic hormone production may be a tumor's first presenting symptom, e.g., erythropoietin secretion by renal tumors leads to hyperplasia of erythrocytes in the bone marrow.

Increased Functional Demand

Hyperplasia, like hypertrophy, may be a response to increased physiologic demand. At high altitudes low atmospheric oxygen content causes compensatory hyperplasia of erythrocyte precursors in the bone marrow and increased erythrocytes in the blood (secondary polycythemia) (Fig. 1-7). In this fashion, increased numbers of cells compensate for the decreased oxygen carried by each erythrocyte. The number of erythrocytes promptly falls to normal on return to sea level. Similarly, chronic blood loss, as in excessive menstrual bleeding, also causes hyperplasia of erythrocytic elements.

Immune responsiveness to many antigens may lead to lymphoid hyperplasia (e.g., the enlarged tonsils and swollen lymph nodes that occur with streptococcal pharyngitis). The hypocalcemia that occurs in chronic renal failure produces increased demand for parathyroid hormone in order to increase blood calcium. The result is hyperplasia of the parathyroid glands.

Chronic Injury

Persistent injury may result in hyperplasia. Long-standing inflammation or chronic physical or chemical injury is often accompanied by a hyperplastic response. For instance, pressure from ill-fitting shoes causes hyperplasia of the skin of the foot, so-called corns or calluses. If one considers that a key function of the skin is to protect underlying structures, such hyperplasia results in thickening of the skin and enhances the skin's functional capacity. Chronic inflammation of the bladder (chronic cystitis) often causes hyperplasia of the bladder epithelium, visible as white plaques on the bladder lining.

Inappropriate hyperplasia can itself be harmful—witness the unpleasant consequences of psoriasis, which is characterized by conspicuous hyperplasia of the skin (Fig. 1-7D). Excessive estrogen stimulation, whether from endogenous sources or from medication, may lead to endometrial hyperplasia.

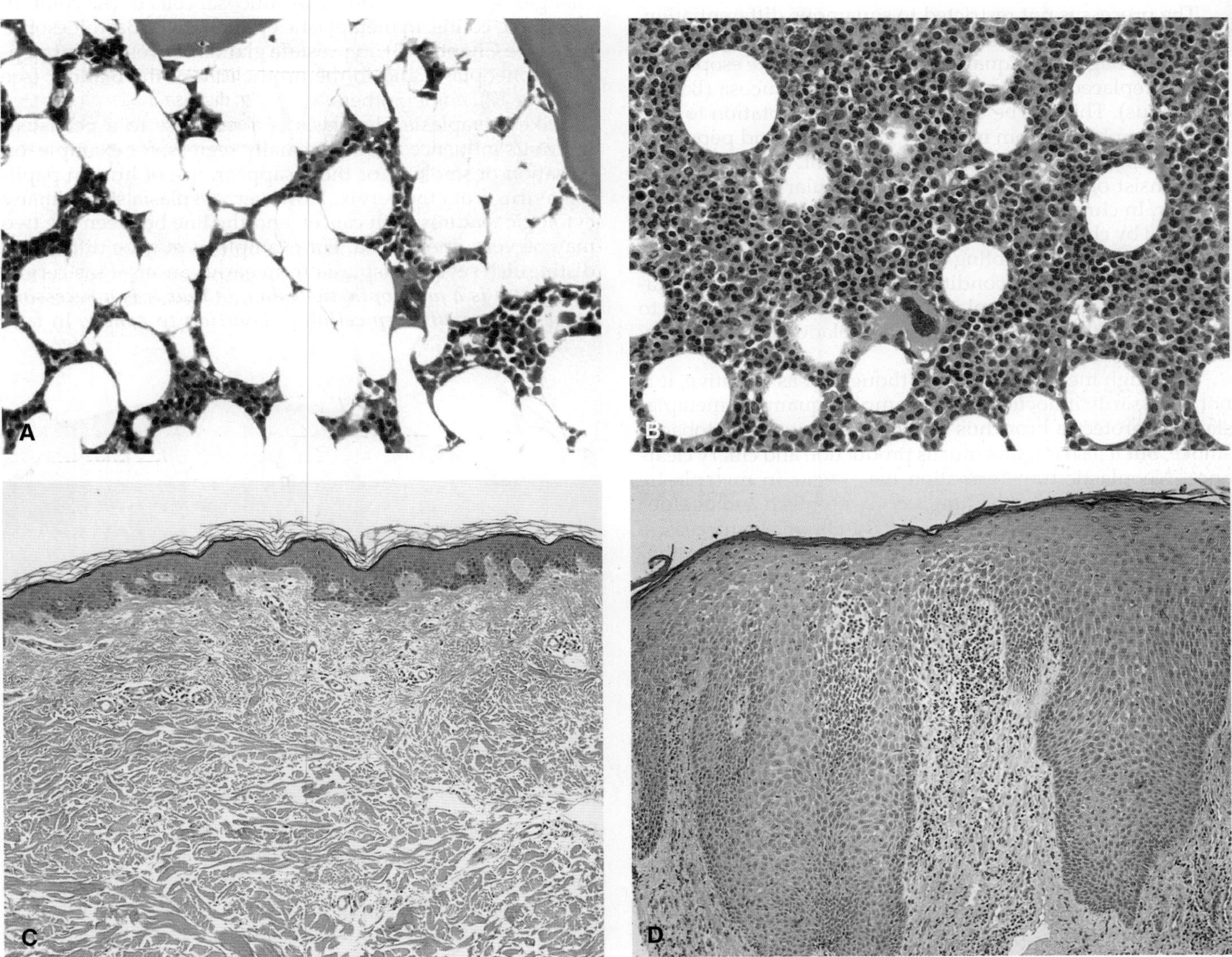

FIGURE 1-7. Hyperplasia. A. Normal adult bone marrow. B. Hyperplasia of the bone marrow. Cellularity is increased; fat is decreased. **C. Normal epidermis. D. Epidermal hyperplasia** in psoriasis, shown at the same magnification as in C. The epidermis is thickened, owing to an increase in the number of squamous cells.

The cellular and molecular mechanisms responsible for hyperplastic responses clearly relate to control of cell proliferation. These topics are discussed in Chapters 3 and 5, and under the heading of liver regeneration in Chapter 14.

Metaplasia Is Conversion of One Differentiated Cell Type to Another

Metaplasia is usually an adaptive response to chronic, persistent injury. That is, a tissue will assume the phenotype that provides it the best protection from the insult. Most commonly, glandular epithelium is replaced by squamous epithelium. Columnar or cuboidal lining cells may be committed to mucus production, but may not be adequately resistant to the effects of chronic irritation or a pernicious chemical. For example, prolonged exposure of the bronchial epithelium to tobacco smoke leads to squamous metaplasia. A similar response is associated with chronic infection in the endocervix (Fig. 1-8). In molecular terms, metaplasia involves replacing the expression of one set of differentiation genes with another.

The process is not restricted to squamous differentiation. When highly acidic gastric contents reflux chronically into the lower esophagus, the squamous epithelium of the esophagus may be replaced by stomach-like glandular mucosa (Barrett esophagus). This can be thought of as an adaptation to protect the esophagus from injury by gastric acid and pepsin, to which the normal gastric mucosa is resistant. Metaplasia may also consist of replacement of one glandular epithelium by another. In chronic gastritis, a disorder of the stomach characterized by chronic inflammation, atrophic gastric glands are replaced by cells resembling those of the small intestine. The adaptive value of this condition, known as intestinal metaplasia, is not clear. Metaplasia of transitional epithelium to glandular epithelium occurs when the bladder is chronically inflamed (cystitis glandularis).

Although metaplasia may be thought of as adaptive, it is not necessarily innocuous. For example, squamous metaplasia may protect a bronchus from injury caused by tobacco smoke, but it also impairs mucus production and ciliary clearance. Neoplastic transformation may occur in metaplastic epithelium; cancers of the lung, cervix, stomach and bladder often arise in such areas. However, if the chronic injury ceases, there is little stimulus for cells to proliferate, and the epithelium does not become cancerous.

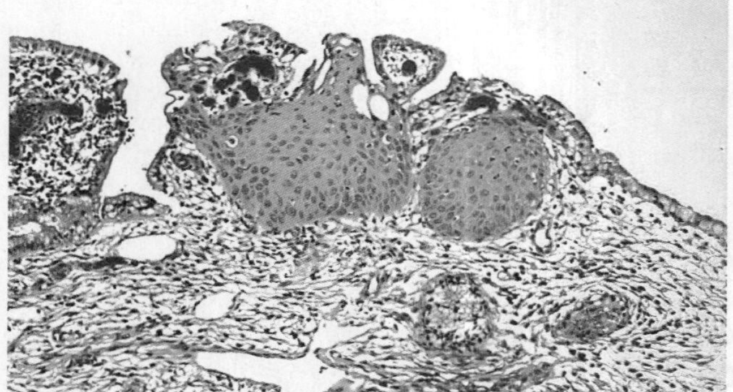

FIGURE 1-8. Squamous metaplasia. A section of endocervix shows the normal columnar epithelium at both margins and a focus of squamous metaplasia in the center.

Metaplasia is usually fully reversible. If the noxious stimulus is removed (e.g., when one stops smoking), the metaplastic epithelium eventually returns to normal.

Dysplasia Is Disordered Growth and Maturation of the Cellular Components of a Tissue

The cells that comprise an epithelium normally exhibit uniformity of size, shape and nucleus. Moreover, they are arranged in a regular fashion; for example, a squamous epithelium progresses from plump basal cells to flat superficial cells. In dysplasia, this monotonous appearance is disturbed by (1) variation in cell size and shape; (2) nuclear enlargement, irregularity and hyperchromatism; and (3) disarray in the arrangement of cells within the epithelium (Fig. 1-9). Dysplasia occurs most often in hyperplastic squamous epithelium, as seen in epidermal actinic keratosis (caused by sunlight) and in areas of squamous metaplasia, such as in the bronchus or the cervix. It is not, however, exclusive to squamous epithelium. For example, dysplastic changes occur in the columnar mucosal cells of the colon in ulcerative colitis, in metaplastic epithelium of Barrett esophagus (see Chapter 13), in prostate glands of prostatic intraepithelial neoplasia and in the urothelium of the bladder (see Chapter 17), among others.

Like metaplasia, dysplasia is a response to a persistent injurious influence and will usually regress, for example, on cessation of smoking or the disappearance of human papillomavirus from the cervix. However, dysplasia shares many cytologic features with cancer, and the line between the two may be very fine indeed. For example, it may be difficult to distinguish severe dysplasia from early cancer of the cervix. ***Dysplasia is a preneoplastic lesion, in that it is a necessary stage in the multistep cellular evolution to cancer.*** In fact,

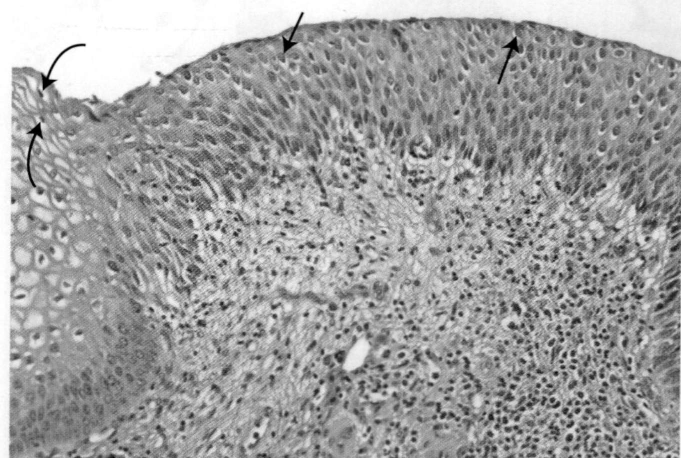

FIGURE 1-9. Dysplasia. Dysplastic epithelium of the uterine cervix lacks normal polarity, and individual cells show hyperchromatic nuclei and a greater than normal nucleus-to-cytoplasm ratio. Normal cervical epithelium is at left. Compare, for example, the size and hyperchromaticity of nuclei in the dysplastic cells (*straight arrows*) with the characteristics of normal counterparts (*curved arrows, left*) at comparable height in the adjacent normal cervix. In dysplasia, cellular arrangement is disorderly, largely lacking appropriate histologic maturation, from the basal layers to the surface.

dysplasia is included in the morphologic classifications of the stages of intraepithelial neoplasia in a variety of organs (e.g., cervix, prostate, bladder). Severe dysplasia is considered an indication for aggressive preventive therapy to cure the underlying cause, eliminate the noxious agent or surgically remove the offending tissue.

As in the development of cancer (see Chapter 5), dysplasia results from sequential mutations in a proliferating cell population. The fidelity of DNA replication is imperfect, and occasional mutations are inevitable. When a particular mutation confers a growth or survival advantage, progeny of the affected cell will tend to predominate. In turn, their continued proliferation provides greater opportunity for additional mutations. Accumulation of such mutations progressively distances the cell from normal regulatory constraints. ***Dysplasia is the morphologic expression of the disturbance in growth regulation.*** However, unlike cancer cells, dysplastic cells are not entirely autonomous, and with intervention, tissue appearance may still revert to normal.

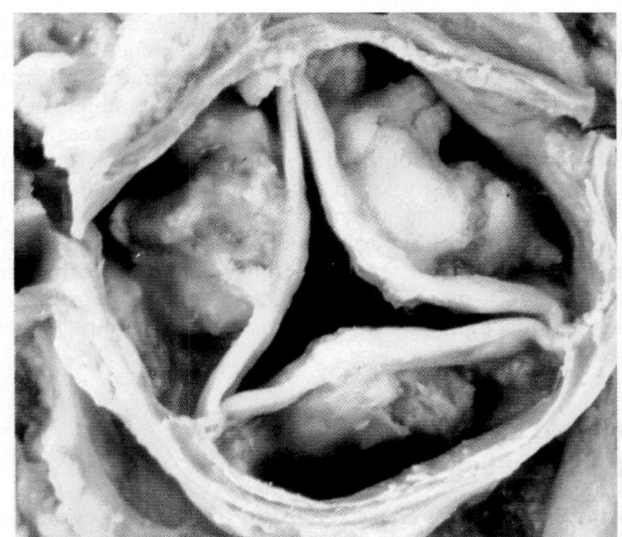

FIGURE 1-10. Calcific aortic stenosis. Large deposits of calcium salts are evident in the cusps and the free margins of the thickened aortic valve, as viewed from above.

Calcification May Occur as Part of Normal Development or as a Reflection of an Abnormal Process

The deposition of mineral salts of calcium is, of course, a normal process in the formation of bone from cartilage. As we have learned, calcium entry into dead or dying cells is usual because of the inability of such cells to maintain a steep calcium gradient. This cellular calcification is not ordinarily visible except as inclusions within mitochondria.

"Dystrophic" calcification refers to the macroscopic deposition of calcium salts in injured tissues. This type of calcification does not simply reflect an accumulation of calcium derived from the bodies of dead cells but rather represents an extracellular deposition of calcium from the circulation or interstitial fluid. Dystrophic calcification apparently requires the persistence of necrotic tissue; it is often visible to the naked eye and ranges from gritty, sandlike grains to firm, rock-hard material. In many locations, such as in cases of tuberculous caseous necrosis in the lung or lymph nodes, calcification has no functional consequences. However, dystrophic calcification may also occur in crucial locations, such as in the mitral or aortic valves (Fig. 1-10). In such instances, calcification leads to impeded blood flow because it produces inflexible valve leaflets and narrowed valve orifices (mitral and aortic stenosis). Dystrophic calcification in atherosclerotic coronary arteries contributes to narrowing of those vessels. Although molecules involved in physiologic calcium deposition in bone (e.g., osteopontin, osteonectin and osteocalcin) are reported in association with dystrophic calcification, the underlying mechanisms of this process remain obscure.

Dystrophic calcification also plays a role in diagnostic radiography. Mammography is based principally on the detection of calcifications in breast cancers; congenital toxoplasmosis, an infection involving the central nervous system, is suggested by the visualization of calcification in the infant brain.

"Metastatic" calcification reflects deranged calcium metabolism, in contrast to dystrophic calcification, which has its origin in cell injury. Metastatic calcification is associated with an increased serum calcium concentration **(hypercalcemia)**. In general, almost any disorder that increases the serum calcium level can lead to calcification in such inappropriate locations as the alveolar septa of the lung, renal tubules and blood vessels. Metastatic calcification is seen in various disorders, including chronic renal failure, vitamin D intoxication and hyperparathyroidism.

The formation of stones containing calcium carbonate in sites such as the gallbladder, renal pelvis, bladder and pancreatic duct is another form of pathologic calcification. Under certain circumstances, the mineral salts precipitate from solution and crystallize about foci of organic material. Those who have suffered the agony of gallbladder or renal colic will attest to the unpleasant consequences of this type of calcification.

Hyaline Refers to Any Material That Has a Reddish, Homogeneous Appearance When Stained With Hematoxylin and Eosin

The student will encounter the term **hyaline** in classic descriptions of diverse and unrelated lesions. Standard terminology includes hyaline arteriolosclerosis, alcoholic hyaline in the liver, hyaline membranes in the lung and hyaline droplets in various cells. The various lesions called hyaline actually have nothing in common. Alcoholic hyaline is composed of cytoskeletal filaments; the hyaline found in arterioles of the kidney is derived from basement membranes; and hyaline membranes consist of plasma proteins deposited in alveoli. The term is anachronistic and of questionable value, although it is still used as a morphologic descriptor.

Mechanisms and Morphology of Cell Injury

All cells have efficient mechanisms to deal with shifts in environmental conditions. Thus, ion channels open or close, harmful chemicals are detoxified, metabolic stores such as fat or glycogen may be mobilized and catabolic processes lead to the segregation of internal particulate materials. It is when environmental changes exceed the cell's capacity to maintain normal homeostasis that we recognize acute cell injury. If the stress is removed in time or if the cell can withstand the assault, cell injury is reversible, and complete structural and functional integrity is restored. For example, when circulation to the heart is interrupted for less than 30 minutes, all structural and functional alterations prove to be reversible. The cell can also be exposed to persistent sublethal stress, as in mechanical irritation of the skin or exposure of the bronchial mucosa to tobacco smoke. In such instances, the cell has time to adapt to reversible injury in a number of ways, each of which has its morphologic counterpart. On the other hand, if the stress is severe, irreversible injury leads to death of the cell. The precise moment at which reversible injury gives way to irreversible injury, the "point of no return," cannot be identified at present.

Hydropic Swelling Is a Reversible Increase in Cell Volume

Hydropic swelling is characterized by a large, pale cytoplasm and a normally located nucleus (Fig. 1-11). The greater volume reflects an increased water content. Hydropic swelling reflects acute, reversible cell injury and may result from such varied causes as chemical and biological toxins, viral or bacterial infections, ischemia, excessive heat or cold and so on.

By electron microscopy, the number of organelles is unchanged, although they appear dispersed in a larger volume. The excess fluid accumulates preferentially in the cisternae of the endoplasmic reticulum, which are conspicuously dilated, presumably because of ionic shifts into this compartment (Fig. 1-12). Hydropic swelling is entirely reversible when the cause is removed.

Hydropic swelling results from impairment of cellular volume regulation, a process that controls ionic concentrations in the cytoplasm. This regulation, particularly for sodium, involves three components: (1) the plasma membrane, (2) the plasma membrane sodium pump and (3) the supply of ATP. The plasma membrane imposes a barrier to the flow of sodium (Na^+) down a concentration gradient into the cell and prevents a similar efflux of potassium (K^+) from the cell. The barrier to sodium is imperfect and the relative leakiness to that ion permits the passive entry of sodium into the cell. To compensate for this intrusion, the energy-dependent plasma membrane sodium pump (Na^+/K^+-ATPase), which is fueled by ATP, extrudes sodium from the cell. Injurious agents may interfere with this membrane-regulated process by (1) increasing the permeability of the plasma membrane to sodium, thereby exceeding the capacity of the pump to extrude sodium; (2) damaging the pump directly; or (3) interfering with the synthesis of ATP, thereby depriving the pump of its fuel. In any event, the accumulation of sodium in the cell leads to an increase in water content to maintain isosmotic conditions, and the cell then swells.

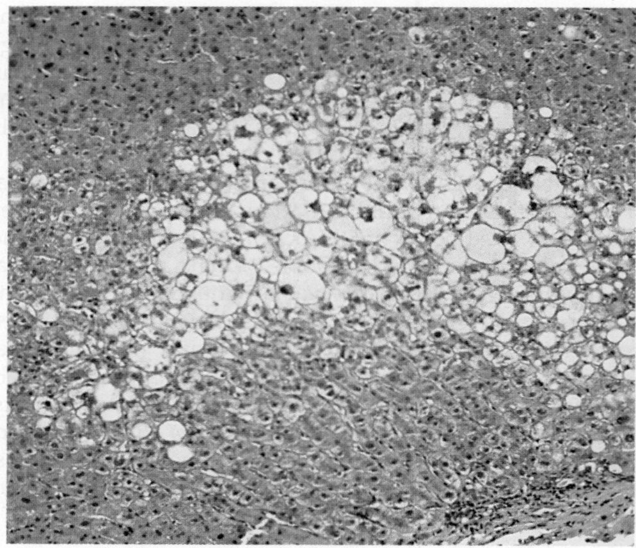

FIGURE 1-11. Hydropic swelling. A needle biopsy of the liver of a patient with toxic hepatic injury shows severe hydropic swelling in the centrilobular zone. The affected hepatocytes exhibit central nuclei and cytoplasm distended (ballooned) by excess fluid.

Subcellular Changes in Reversibly Injured Cells

- **Endoplasmic reticulum:** The cisternae of the endoplasmic reticulum are distended by fluid in hydropic swelling (Fig. 1-12). In other forms of acute, reversible cell injury, membrane-bound polysomes may undergo disaggregation

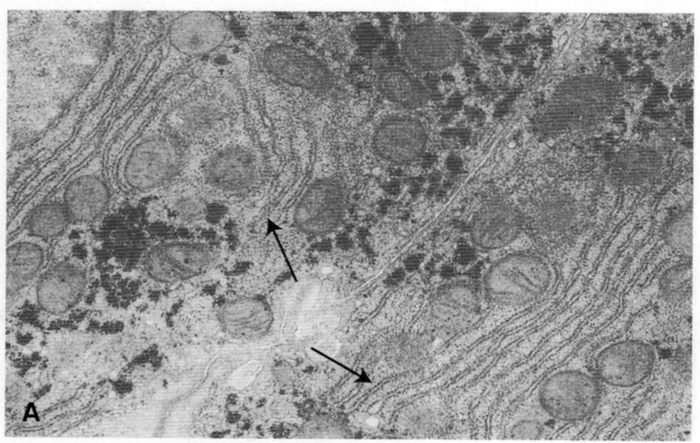

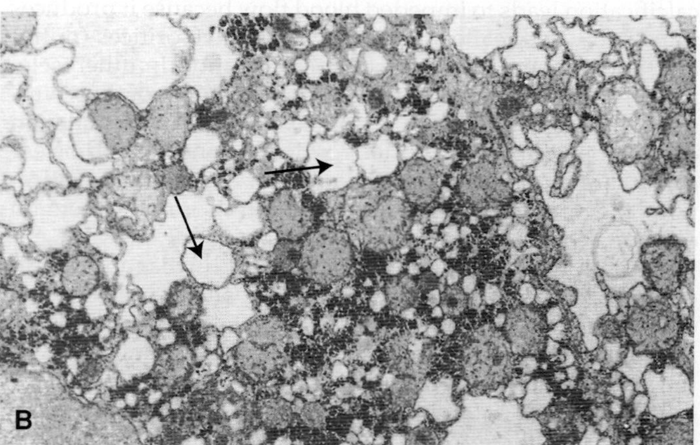

FIGURE 1-12. Ultrastructure of hydropic swelling of a liver cell. A. Two apposed normal hepatocytes with tightly organized, parallel arrays of rough endoplasmic reticulum (*arrows*). **B.** Swollen hepatocyte in which the cisternae of the endoplasmic reticulum are dilated by excess fluid (*arrows*).

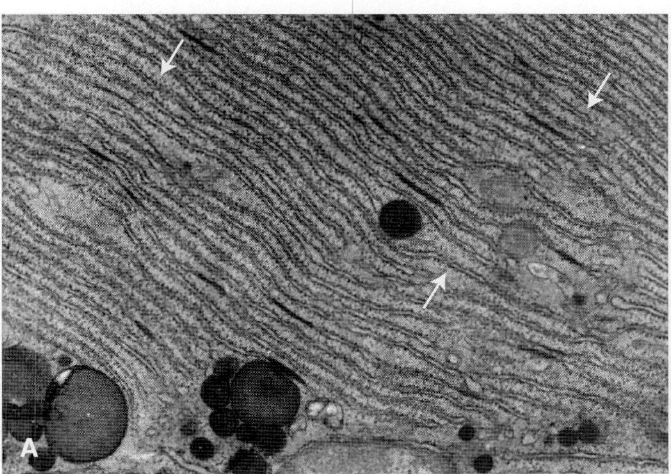

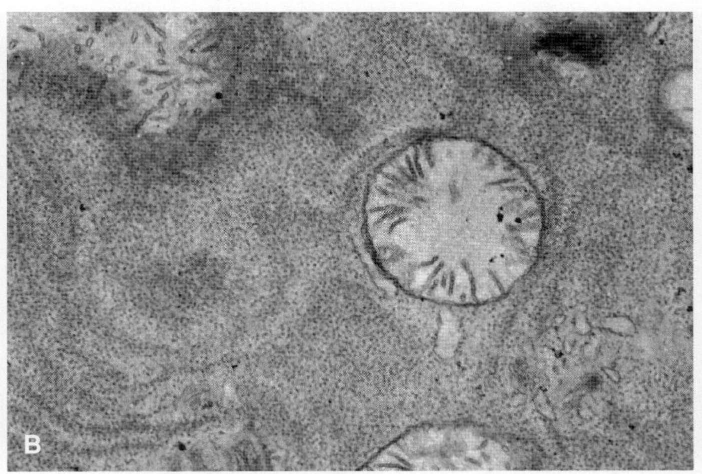

FIGURE 1-13. Disaggregation of membrane-bound polyribosomes in acute, reversible liver injury. A. Normal hepatocyte, in which the profiles of endoplasmic reticulum (*arrows*) are studded with ribosomes. **B.** An injured hepatocyte, showing detachment of ribosomes from the membranes of the endoplasmic reticulum and the accumulation of free ribosomes in the cytoplasm.

and detach from the surface of the rough endoplasmic reticulum (Fig. 1-13).

- **Mitochondria:** In some forms of acute injury, particularly ischemia, mitochondria swell (Fig. 1-14). This enlargement reflects the dissipation of the energy gradient and consequent impairment of mitochondrial volume control. Amorphous densities rich in phospholipid may appear in the mitochondria, but these effects are fully reversible on recovery.
- **Plasma membrane:** Blebs of the plasma membrane—that is, focal extrusions of the cytoplasm—are occasionally noted. These can detach from the membrane into the external environment without the loss of cell viability.
- **Nucleus:** In the nucleus, reversible injury is reflected principally in nucleolar change. The fibrillar and granular components of the nucleolus may segregate. Alternatively, the granular component may be diminished, leaving only a fibrillar core.

These changes in cell organelles (Fig. 1-15) are reflected in functional derangements (e.g., reduced protein synthesis and impaired energy production). ***After withdrawal of an acute stress that has led to reversible cell injury, by definition, the cell returns to its normal state.***

Ischemic Cell Injury Usually Results From Obstruction to the Flow of Blood

When tissues are deprived of oxygen, ATP cannot be produced by aerobic metabolism and is instead generated inefficiently by anaerobic metabolism. Ischemia initiates a series of chemical and pH imbalances, which are accompanied by

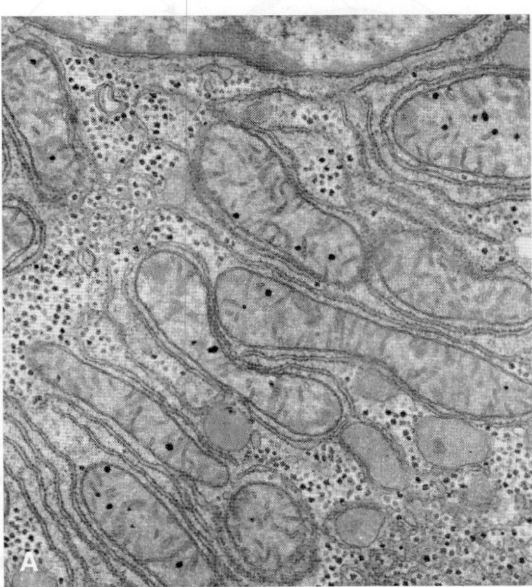

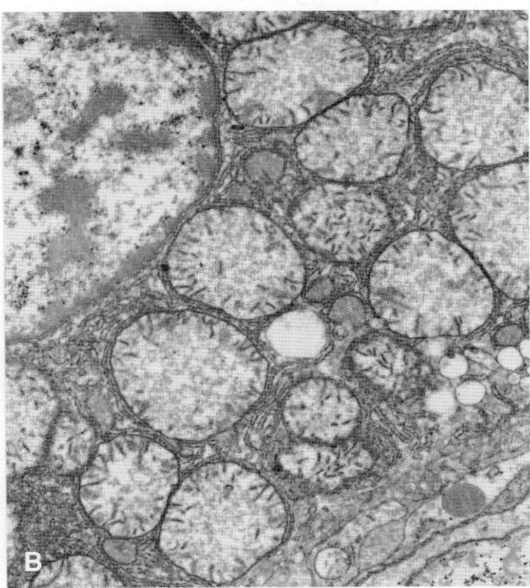

FIGURE 1-14. Mitochondrial swelling in acute ischemic cell injury. A. Normal mitochondria are elongated and display prominent cristae, which traverse the mitochondrial matrix. **B.** Mitochondria from an ischemic cell are swollen and round and exhibit a decreased matrix density. The cristae are less prominent than in the normal organelle.

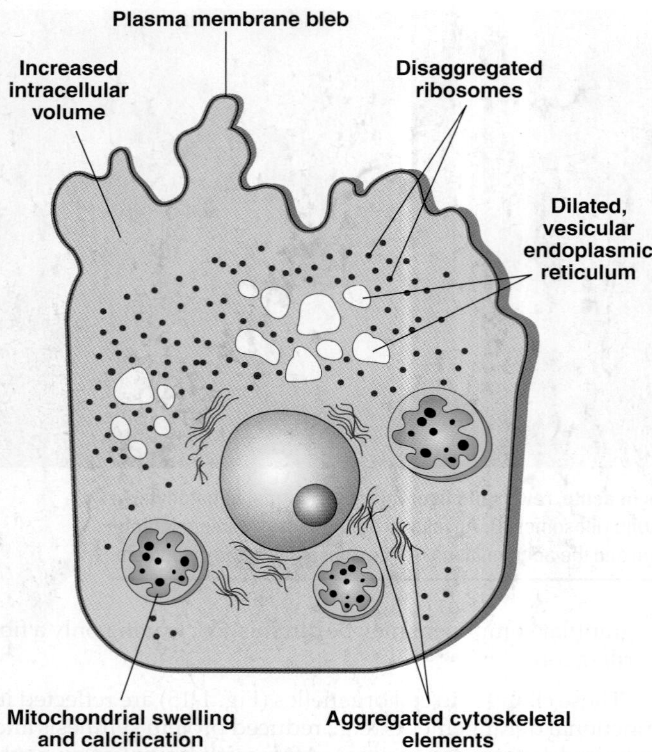

FIGURE 1-15. Ultrastructural features of reversible cell injury.

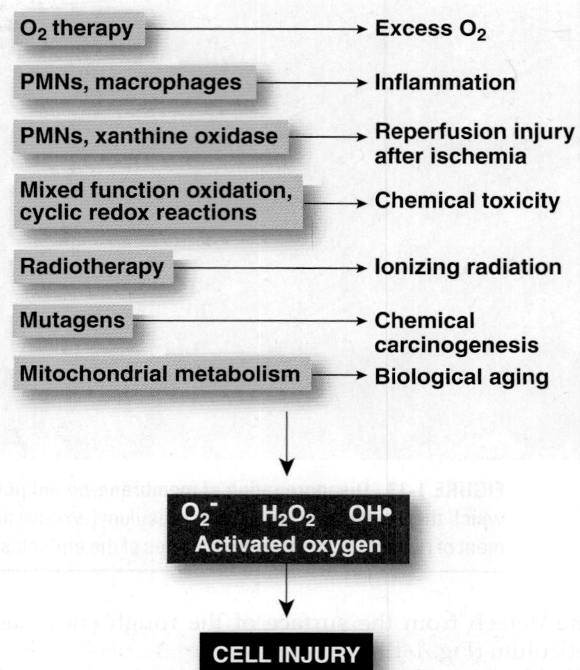

FIGURE 1-16. The role of activated oxygen species in human disease. *H_2O_2* = hydrogen peroxide; *O_2* = oxygen; *O_2^-* = superoxide; *OH•* = hydroxyl radical; *PMNs* = polymorphonuclear neutrophils.

enhanced generation of injurious free radical species. The damage produced by short periods of ischemia tends to be reversible if the circulation is restored. However, cells subjected to long episodes of ischemia become irreversibly injured and die. The mechanisms of cell damage are discussed below.

Oxidative Stress Is a Key Trigger for Cell Injury and Adaptive Responses

For human life, oxygen is both a blessing and a curse. Without it, life is impossible, but its metabolism can produce partially reduced oxygen species that react with virtually any molecule they reach.

Reactive Oxygen Species

Reactive oxygen species (ROS) have been identified as the likely cause of cell injury in many diseases (Fig. 1-16). The inflammatory process, whether acute or chronic, can cause considerable tissue destruction. In such circumstances partially reduced oxygen species produced by phagocytic cells are important mediators of cell injury. Damage to cells resulting from oxygen radicals formed by inflammatory cells has been implicated in diseases of the joints and of many organs, including the kidneys, lungs and heart. The toxicity of many chemicals may reflect the formation of toxic oxygen species. For example, the killing of cells by ionizing radiation is most likely the result of the direct formation of hydroxyl (OH•) radicals from the radiolysis of water (H_2O). There is also evidence of a role for reactive oxygen species in the formation of mutations during chemical carcinogenesis. Finally, oxidative damage has been implicated in biological aging (see below).

ROS have also been implicated in normal cell signaling, including modulation of gene regulation, activation of mitogen-activated protein (MAP) kinases, reversible protein

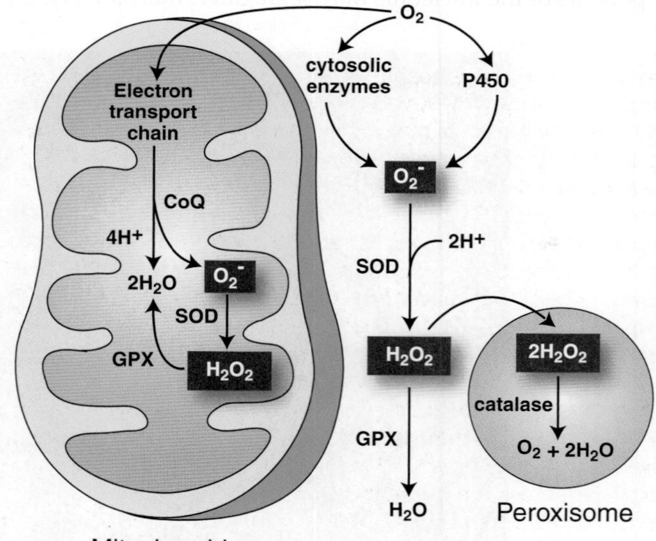

FIGURE 1-17. Mechanisms by which reactive oxygen radicals are generated from molecular oxygen and then detoxified by cellular enzymes. *CoQ* = coenzyme Q; *GPX* = glutathione peroxidase; *H^+* = hydrogen ion; *H_2O* = water; *H_2O_2* = hydrogen peroxide; *O_2* = oxygen; *O_2^-* = superoxide; *SOD* = superoxide dismutase.

Table 1-4

Reactive Oxygen Species (ROS)

Molecule	Attributes
Hydrogen peroxide (H_2O_2)	Forms free radicals via Fe^{2+}-catalyzed Fenton reaction Diffuses widely within the cell
Superoxide anion (O_2^-)	Generated by leaks in the electron transport chain and some cytosolic reactions Produces other ROS Does not readily diffuse far from its origin
Hydroxyl radical (OH•)	Generated from H_2O_2 by Fe^{2+}-catalyzed Fenton reaction The intracellular radical most responsible for attack on macromolecules
Peroxynitrite (ONOO•)	Formed from the reaction of nitric oxide (NO) with O_2^- Damages macromolecules
Lipid peroxide radicals (RCOO•)	Organic radicals produced during lipid peroxidation
Hypochlorous acid (HOCl)	Produced by macrophages and neutrophils during respiratory burst that accompanies phagocytosis Dissociates to yield hypochlorite radical (OCl^-)

Fe^{2+} = ferrous iron.

modifications (e.g., phosphorylation and dephosphorylation) and so forth. However, when present in excess under pathologic conditions, ROS may exert profound deleterious effects on signaling pathways. Among these pathways are those leading to cell death via apoptosis (see below).

Cells also may be injured when oxygen is present at concentrations greater than normal. In the past, this occurred largely under therapeutic circumstances in which oxygen was given to patients at concentrations greater than the normal 20% of inspired air. The lungs of adults and the eyes of premature newborns were the major targets of such oxygen toxicity.

Oxygen (O_2) has a major metabolic role as the terminal acceptor for mitochondrial electron transport. Cytochrome oxidase catalyzes the four-electron reduction of O_2 to H_2O. The resultant energy is harnessed as an electrochemical potential across the mitochondrial inner membrane.

Complete reduction of O_2 to H_2O involves the transfer of four electrons. There are three partially reduced species that are intermediate between O_2 and H_2O, representing transfers of varying numbers of electrons (Fig. 1-17). They are O_2^-, superoxide (one electron); H_2O_2, hydrogen peroxide (two electrons); and OH•, the hydroxyl radical (three electrons). For the most part these ROS are produced principally by leaks in mitochondrial electron transport, with an additional

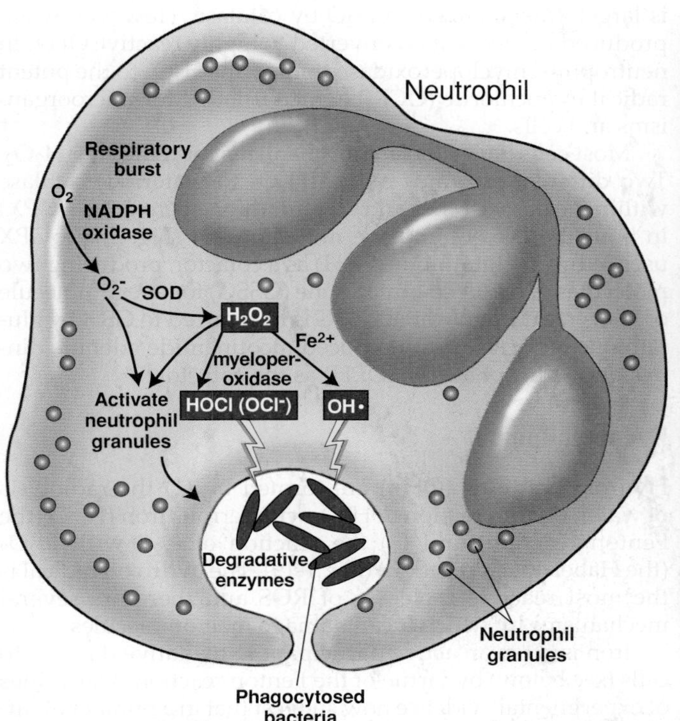

FIGURE 1-18. Generation of reactive oxygen species in neutrophils as a result of phagocytosis of bacteria. *Fe^{2+}* = ferrous iron; *H_2O_2* = hydrogen peroxide; *HOCl* = hypochlorous acid; *NADPH* = nicotinamide adenine dinucleotide phosphate; *OCl^-* = hypochlorite radical; *OH•* = hydroxyl radical; *SOD* = superoxide dismutase.

contribution from the mixed-function oxygenase (P450) system. The major forms of ROS are listed in Table 1-4.

Superoxide

The superoxide anion (O_2^-) is produced principally by leaks in mitochondrial electron transport or as part of the inflammatory response. In the first instance, the promiscuity of coenzyme Q (CoQ) and other imperfections in the electron transport chain allow the transfer of electrons to O_2 to yield O_2^-. In the case of phagocytic inflammatory cells, activation of a plasma membrane oxidase produces O_2^-, which is then converted to H_2O_2 and eventually to other ROS (Fig. 1-18). These ROS have generally been viewed as the principal effectors of cellular oxidative defenses that destroy pathogens, fragments of necrotic cells or other phagocytosed material (see Chapter 2). There is now evidence to suggest that their main role in cellular defenses may be as signaling intermediates, to elicit release of proteolytic and other degradative enzymes. It is these enzymes that are probably the most critical effectors of neutrophil-mediated destruction of bacteria and other foreign materials.

Hydrogen Peroxide

O_2^- anions are catabolized by superoxide dismutase (SOD) to produce H_2O_2. Hydrogen peroxide is also produced directly by a number of oxidases in cytoplasmic peroxisomes (Fig. 1-17). By itself, H_2O_2 is not particularly injurious, and it is largely metabolized to H_2O by catalase. However, when produced in excess, it is converted to highly reactive OH•. In neutrophils, myeloperoxidase transforms H_2O_2 to the potent radical hypochlorite (OCl^-), which is lethal for microorganisms and cells.

Most cells have efficient mechanisms for removing H_2O_2. Two different enzymes reduce H_2O_2 to water: (1) catalase within the peroxisomes and (2) glutathione peroxidase (GPX) in both the cytosol and the mitochondria (Fig. 1-17). GPX uses reduced glutathione (GSH) as a cofactor, producing two molecules of oxidized glutathione (GSSG) for every molecule of H_2O_2 reduced to water. GSSG is re-reduced to GSH by glutathione reductase, with reduced nicotinamide adenine dinucleotide phosphate (NADPH) as the cofactor.

Hydroxyl Radical

Hydroxyl radicals (OH•) are formed by (1) the radiolysis of water, (2) the reaction of H_2O_2 with ferrous iron (Fe^{2+}) (the Fenton reaction) and (3) the reaction of O_2^- with H_2O_2 (the Haber-Weiss reaction) (Fig. 1-19). The hydroxyl radical is the most reactive molecule of ROS and there are several mechanisms by which it can damage macromolecules.

Iron is often an active participant in oxidative damage to cells (see below) by virtue of the Fenton reaction. Many lines of experimental evidence now suggest that in a number of different cell types H_2O_2 stimulates iron uptake and so increases production of hydroxyl radicals.

- **Lipid peroxidation:** The hydroxyl radical removes a hydrogen atom from the unsaturated fatty acids of membrane phospholipids, a process that forms a free lipid radical (Fig. 1-20). The lipid radical, in turn, reacts with molecular oxygen and forms a lipid peroxide radical. This peroxide radical can, in turn, function as an initiator, removing another hydrogen atom from a second unsaturated fatty acid. A lipid peroxide and a new lipid radical result and a chain reaction is initiated. Lipid peroxides are unstable and break down into smaller molecules. The destruction of the unsaturated fatty acids of phospholipids results in a loss of membrane integrity.
- **Protein interactions:** Hydroxyl radicals may also attack proteins. The sulfur-containing amino acids cysteine and methionine, as well as arginine, histidine and proline, are especially vulnerable to attack by OH•. As a result of oxidative damage, proteins undergo fragmentation, cross-linking, aggregation and eventually degradation.
- **DNA damage:** DNA is an important target of the hydroxyl radical. A variety of structural alterations include strand breaks, modified bases and cross-links between strands. In most cases, the integrity of the genome can be reconstituted by the various DNA repair pathways. However, if oxidative damage to DNA is sufficiently extensive, the cell dies.

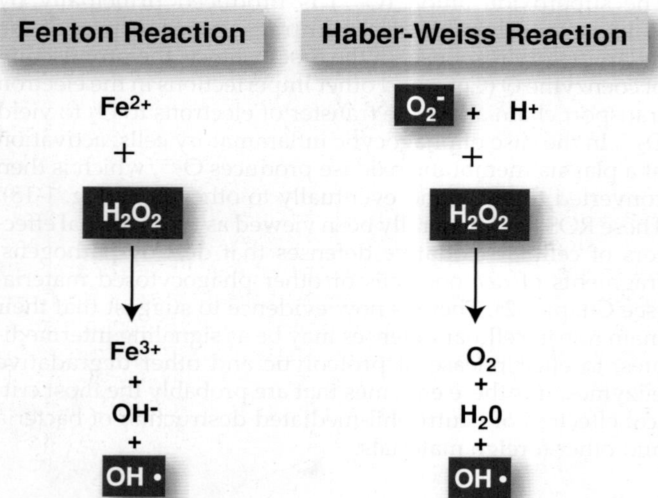

FIGURE 1-19. Fenton and Haber-Weiss reactions to generate the highly reactive hydroxyl radical. Reactive species are shown in red. Fe^{2+} = ferrous iron; Fe^{3+} = ferric iron; H^+ = hydrogen ion; H_2O_2 = hydrogen peroxide; OH^- = hydroxide; OH• = hydroxyl radical.

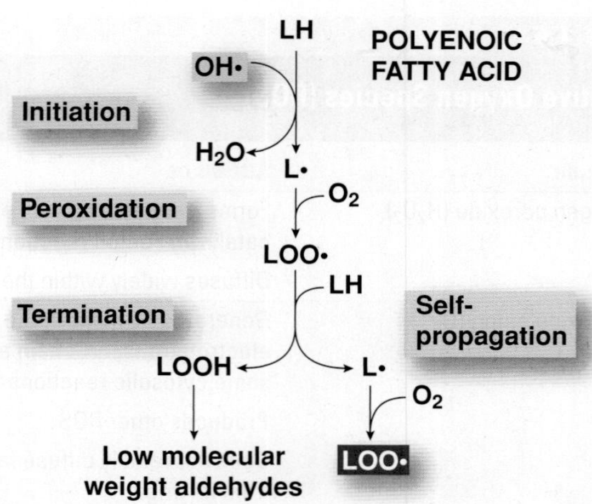

FIGURE 1-20. Lipid peroxidation initiated by the hydroxyl radical (OH•). H_2O = water; O_2 = oxygen; *L•* = lipid radical; *LOO•* = lipid peroxy radical; *LOOH* = lipid peroxide.

Fig. 1-21 summarizes the mechanisms of cell injury by activated oxygen species.

Peroxynitrite

Peroxynitrite ($ONOO^-$) is formed by the interaction of two free radicals, namely, superoxide (O_2^-) and nitric oxide (NO•): $NO\bullet + O_2^- \rightarrow ONOO^-$.

$ONOO^-$ attacks a wide range of biologically important molecules, including lipids, proteins and DNA. Nitric oxide, a molecule generated in many tissues, is a potent vasodilator and mediator of a number of important biological processes. Thus, the formation of peroxynitrite occupies an important place in free radical toxicology.

The Effectiveness of Cellular Defenses Against Oxygen Free Radicals May Determine the Outcome of Oxidative Injury

Cells manifest potent antioxidant defenses against ROS, including detoxifying enzymes and exogenous free radical scavengers (vitamins). The major enzymes that convert ROS to less reactive molecules are SOD, catalase and GPX.

Detoxifying Enzymes

- **SOD** is the first line of defense against O_2^-, converting it to H_2O_2 and O_2 (H^+ = hydrogen ion) ($2O_2^- + 2H^+ \rightarrow O_2 + H_2O_2$).

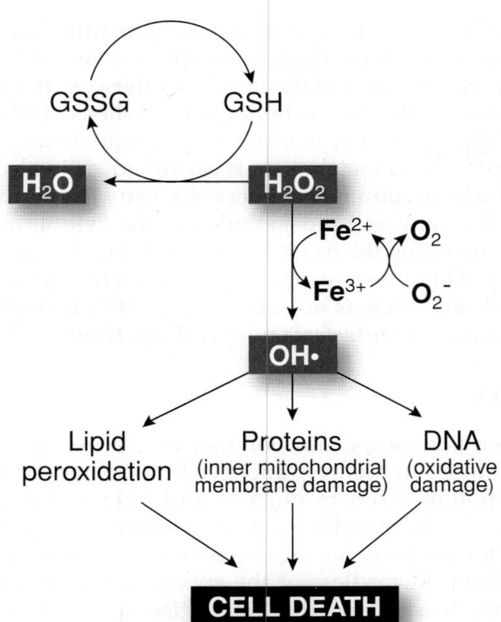

FIGURE 1-21. Mechanisms of cell injury by activated oxygen species. *Fe^{2+}* = ferrous iron; *Fe^{3+}* = ferric iron; *GSH* = glutathione; *GSSG* = glutathione; *H_2O_2* = hydrogen peroxide; *O_2* = oxygen; *O_2^-* = superoxide anion; *OH•* = hydroxyl radical.

- **Catalase**, principally located in peroxisomes, is one of two enzymes that complete the dissolution of O_2^- by eliminating H_2O_2 and, therefore, its potential conversion to OH• ($2H_2O_2 \rightarrow 2H_2O + O_2$).
- **GPX** catalyzes the reduction of H_2O_2 and lipid peroxides in mitochondria and the cytosol ($H_2O_2 + 2GSH \rightarrow 2H_2O +$ GSSG).

Scavengers of ROS

- **Vitamin E (α-tocopherol)** is a terminal electron acceptor and, therefore, blocks free radical chain reactions. Given that it is fat soluble, it exerts its activity in lipid membranes, protecting them against lipid peroxidation.
- **Vitamin C (ascorbate)** is water soluble and reacts directly with O_2, OH• and some products of lipid peroxidation. It also serves to regenerate the reduced form of vitamin E.
- **Retinoids,** the precursors of vitamin A, are lipid soluble and function as chain-breaking antioxidants.
- **NO•** is the product of constitutive or inducible nitric oxide synthases (NOSs). Although it may bind to superoxide to form highly reactive peroxynitrite, nitric oxide is also a major mechanism by which ROS are contained. NO• may accomplish this in several ways. Chelation of iron and scavenging of free radicals have been suggested, but recent studies suggest that the ability of NO• to increase proteasomal activity, and thus decrease cellular iron uptake by the transferrin receptor, may be involved.

Mutations May Impair Cell Function Without Causing Cell Death

There is evidence that mutations in genes that encode proteins responsible for certain cellular activities may lead to a wide array of clinical syndromes, but do not necessarily involve the death of affected cells. Increasingly, such mutations provide pathogenetic links among seemingly unrelated clinical diseases.

Chaperonopathies

As indicated above, molecular chaperones are important in maintaining correct protein folding, recognizing misfolded or improperly modified proteins and providing for their degradation. An array of diseases, called **chaperonopathies**, have been linked to mutations in the genes that encode these chaperones or other molecules that participate in these processes. The organ systems affected and the presenting symptom complexes of these diseases are diverse. A mutation in a chaperone cofactor is responsible for a form of X-linked retinitis pigmentosa. Hereditary spastic paraplegia is related to a mutation in heat shock protein (hsp60), a mitochondrial chaperone. In von Hippel-Lindau disease, a mutation in the gene for VHL protein leads to poor chaperone binding to VHL. Consequent VHL protein misfolding inactivates the tumor suppressor activity of the complex of which it is a part and leads to development of tumors of the adrenal, kidney and brain.

Channelopathies

Channelopathies are disorders of cell membrane ion channels and may be either inherited or acquired. Ion channels are transmembrane pore-forming proteins that allow ions, principally Na^+, K^+, calcium (Ca^{2+}) and chloride (Cl^-), to flow in or out of the cell. These functions are critical for numerous physiologic processes, such as control of the heartbeat, muscular contraction and relaxation and regulation of insulin secretion in pancreatic β cells. For example, activation and inactivation of sodium and potassium channels are responsible for the action potential in neurons, and calcium channels are important in contraction and relaxation of cardiac and skeletal muscle. Mutations in over 60 ion channel genes are known to cause a variety of diseases, including cardiac arrhythmias (e.g., short and long QT syndromes) and neuromuscular syndromes (e.g., myotonias, familial periodic paralysis). As an example, a number of inherited human disorders affecting skeletal muscle contraction, heart rhythm and functions of the nervous system are attributable to mutations in genes that encode voltage-gated sodium channels. Channelopathies have also been implicated in certain pediatric epilepsy syndromes. In addition, nonexcitable tissues may also be affected. In pancreatic β cells, ATP-sensitive potassium channels regulate insulin secretion, and mutations in these channel genes lead to certain forms of diabetes.

Manifestations of various channelopathies may reflect either gain of function (epilepsy, myotonia) or loss of function (weakness). Different mutations that affect the same ion channel may result in different disorders. For example, inherited mutations in a single sodium channel in skeletal muscle can result in either hyperkalemic or hypokalemic periodic paralysis. By contrast, in some instances, mutations in different genes may lead to the same phenotype. As an example, mutations in different skeletal muscle sodium channels may all result in hyperkalemic periodic paralysis.

Acquired channelopathies have also been identified in various other disorders, including some cancers and autoimmune neurologic conditions. Voltage-sensitive sodium, potassium and calcium channels have been shown to play a role in the onset, proliferation and malignant progression of a variety of cancers, including those of the prostate, colon and brain (Fig. 1-22).

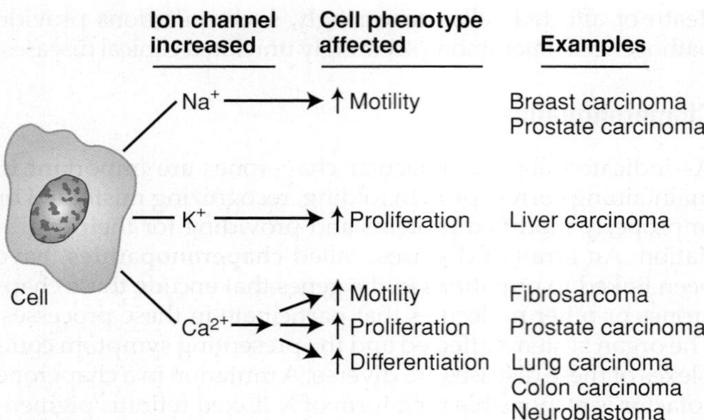

FIGURE 1-22. Association of defects in ion channel function (channelopathies) with malignant diseases. Acquired alterations in the functionality of particular ion channels (left) affect cellular motility, proliferation and differentiation (center). Specific channelopathies have been associated with certain types of malignancies (right).

Autoantibodies (see Chapter 4) have been demonstrated to be involved in disorders of both ligand-gated ion channels (receptors) and voltage-gated ones. Myasthenia gravis and autoimmune neuropathy have been related to autoantibodies against nicotinic acetylcholine receptors, which control ion channels. Autoantibodies directed against voltage-gated calcium and potassium channels are implicated in diverse neuromuscular disorders.

Intracellular Storage Is Retention of Materials Within the Cell

The substance that accumulates in the cell may be normal or abnormal, endogenous or exogenous, harmful or innocuous.

- **Nutrients,** such as fat, glycogen, vitamins and minerals, are stored for later use.
- **Degraded phospholipids,** which result from turnover of endogenous membranes, are stored in lysosomes and may be recycled.
- **Substances that cannot be metabolized** accumulate in cells. These include (1) endogenous substrates that are not further processed because a key enzyme is missing (hereditary storage diseases), (2) insoluble endogenous pigments (e.g., lipofuscin and melanin), (3) aggregates of normal or abnormal proteins and (4) exogenous particulates, such as inhaled silica and carbon or injected tattoo pigments.
- **Overload of normal body constituents,** including iron, copper and cholesterol, injures a variety of cells.
- **Abnormal proteins** may be toxic when they are retained within a cell. Examples are Lewy bodies in Parkinson disease and mutant α1-antitrypsin.

Fat

Bacteria and other unicellular organisms continuously ingest nutrients. By contrast, mammals do not need to eat continuously. They eat periodically and can survive a prolonged fast because they store nutrients in specialized cells for later use—fat in adipocytes and glycogen in the liver, heart and muscle.

Abnormal accumulation of fat is most conspicuous in the liver (see Chapter 14). Briefly, liver cells always contain some fat, because free fatty acids released from adipose tissue are taken up by the liver. There, they are oxidized or converted to triglycerides. Most of the newly synthesized triglycerides are secreted by the liver as lipoproteins. When delivery of free fatty acids to the liver is increased, as in diabetes, or when intrahepatic lipid metabolism is disturbed, as in alcoholism, triglycerides accumulate in liver cells. Fatty liver is identified morphologically as lipid globules in the cytoplasm. Other organs, including the heart, kidney and skeletal muscle, also store fat. ***One must recognize that fat storage is always reversible and there is no evidence that the excess fat in the cytoplasm per se interferes with cell function.***

Glycogen

Glycogen is a long-chain polymer of glucose, formed and largely stored in the liver and to a lesser extent in muscles. It is depolymerized to glucose and liberated as needed. Glycogen is degraded in steps by a series of enzymes, each of which may be deficient as a result of an inborn error of metabolism. Regardless of the specific enzyme deficiency, the result is a glycogen storage disease (see Chapter 6). These inherited disorders affect the liver, heart and skeletal muscle and range from mild and asymptomatic conditions to inexorably progressive and fatal diseases (see Chapters 11, 14 and 27).

The amount of glycogen stored in cells is normally regulated by the blood glucose concentration, and hyperglycemic states are associated with increased glycogen stores. Thus, in uncontrolled diabetes, hepatocytes and epithelial cells of the renal proximal tubules are enlarged by excess glycogen.

Inherited Lysosomal Storage Diseases

Like glycogen catabolism, breakdown of certain complex lipids and mucopolysaccharides (glycosaminoglycans) takes place by a sequence of enzymatic steps. Since these enzymes are located in the lysosomes, their absence results in lysosomal storage of incompletely degraded lipids, such as cerebrosides (e.g., Gaucher disease) and gangliosides (e.g., Tay-Sachs disease) or products of mucopolysaccharide catabolism (e.g., Hurler and Hunter syndromes). These disorders are all progressive but vary from asymptomatic organomegaly to rapidly fatal brain disease. See Chapter 6 for the metabolic bases of these disorders and Chapters 26 and 28 for specific organ pathology.

Cholesterol

The human body has a love–hate relationship with cholesterol. On the one hand, it is a critical component of all plasma membranes. On the other hand, when stored in excess, it is closely associated with atherosclerosis and cardiovascular disease, the leading cause of death in the Western world (see Chapter 10).

Briefly, the initial lesion of atherosclerosis (fatty streak) reflects accumulation of cholesterol and cholesterol esters in macrophages within the arterial intima. As the disease progresses, smooth muscle cells also store cholesterol. Advanced lesions of atherosclerosis are characterized by extracellular deposition of cholesterol (Fig. 1-23A).

In a number of disorders characterized by elevated blood levels of cholesterol (e.g., familial hypercholesterolemia or primary biliary cirrhosis), macrophages store cholesterol. When clusters of these cells in subcutaneous

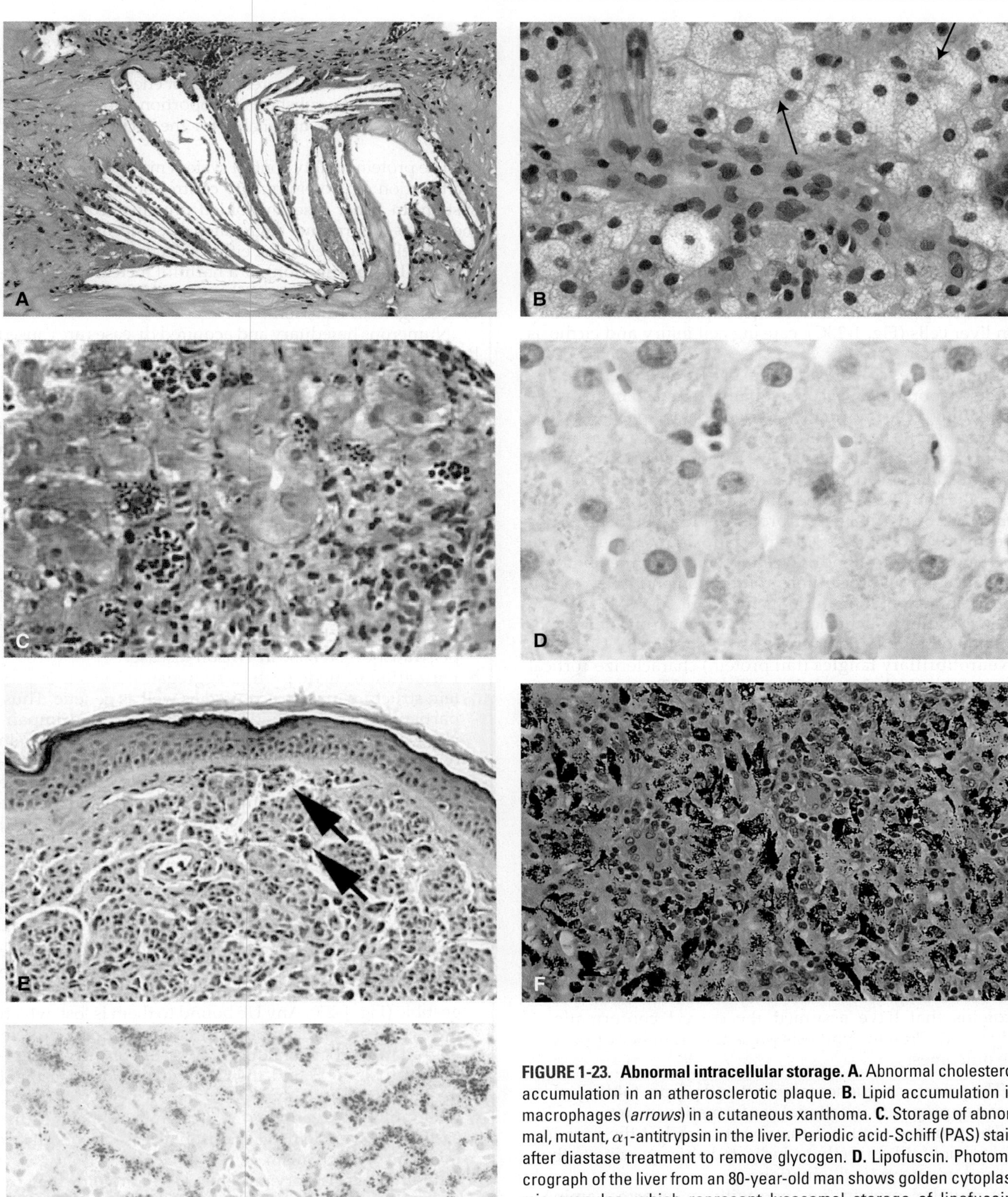

FIGURE 1-23. Abnormal intracellular storage. A. Abnormal cholesterol accumulation in an atherosclerotic plaque. **B.** Lipid accumulation in macrophages (*arrows*) in a cutaneous xanthoma. **C.** Storage of abnormal, mutant, α_1-antitrypsin in the liver. Periodic acid-Schiff (PAS) stain after diastase treatment to remove glycogen. **D.** Lipofuscin. Photomicrograph of the liver from an 80-year-old man shows golden cytoplasmic granules, which represent lysosomal storage of lipofuscin. **E.** Melanin storage (*arrows*) in an intradermal nevus. **F.** Carbon pigment storage. A mediastinal lymph node, which drains the lungs, exhibits numerous macrophages that contain black anthracotic (carbon) pigment. This material was inhaled and originally deposited in the lungs. **G.** Iron storage in hereditary hemochromatosis. Prussian blue stain of the liver reveals large deposits of iron within hepatocellular lysosomes.

tissues become grossly visible, they are termed **xanthomas** (Fig. 1-23B).

Abnormal Proteins

Numerous acquired and inherited diseases are characterized by the intracellular accumulation of abnormal proteins. The deviant tertiary structure of the protein may result from an inherited mutation that alters the normal primary amino acid sequence or may reflect an acquired defect in protein folding. The following are examples:

- **α_1-Antitrypsin deficiency** is a heritable disorder in which mutations in the coding gene for α_1-antitrypsin yield an insoluble protein that is not easily exported. It accumulates in liver cells (Fig. 1-23C), causing cell injury and cirrhosis (see Chapter 14).
- **Prion diseases** comprise a group of neurodegenerative disorders (spongiform encephalopathies) caused by the accumulation of abnormally folded prion proteins. The anomaly reflects the conversion of the normal α-helical structure to a β-pleated sheet. Abnormal prion proteins may result from an inherited mutation or from exposure to the aberrant form of the protein (see Chapter 28). The function of normal prion protein is not yet clear. It has been reported to have SOD-like antioxidant activity, a role in T-lymphocyte–dendritic cell interactions, the ability to enhance neural progenitor proliferation and a key role in development of long- term memory.
- **Lewy bodies** (α-synuclein) are seen in neurons of the substantia nigra in Parkinson disease (Chapter 28).
- **Neurofibrillary tangles** (tau protein) characterize cortical neurons in Alzheimer disease (Chapter 28).
- **Mallory bodies** (intermediate filaments) are hepatocellular inclusions in alcoholic liver injury (Chapter 14).

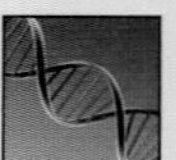

MOLECULAR PATHOGENESIS: Translation of mRNA by ribosomes produces a linear chain of amino acids that lacks a defined three-dimensional structure. In order to perform its specific function, each protein must be folded into its own native three-dimensional conformation. Curiously, it is energetically more favorable for the cell to produce many foldings and then edit the protein repertoire than to produce only a single functional conformation. Molecular chaperones associate with polypeptides in the endoplasmic reticulum and promote correct folding, after which they dissociate from those proteins that have assumed the correct conformation (Fig. 1-24). Protein synthesis presents a number of possible outcomes:

- The primary sequence is correct and proper folding into the appropriate functional conformation occurs.
- The primary sequence may be correct, but the protein does not fold correctly, as indicated above, owing to the random energetic fluctuations.
- A mutated protein (i.e., one with an incorrect amino acid sequence) does not fold correctly.
- A conformationally correct protein may become unfolded or misfolded due to an unfavorable environment (e.g., altered pH, high ionic strength, oxidation, etc.).

Protein misfolding is an intrinsic tendency of proteins and occurs continuously. The misfolded protein load is eliminated by protein quality control systems, including the ubiquitin–proteasome system and autophagic pathways. Evolutionary preference for energy conservation has dictated that a substantial proportion of newly formed proteins are rogues unsuitable for the society of civilized cells.

The protein quality control system may fail because of a malfunction of protein quality control or overload of this system. In either case, misfolded proteins accumulate in the cell as amorphous aggregates or as fibrils. They may lead to cell injury, reflecting either a decrease in a necessary activity **(loss of function)** or a harmful increase in a cellular enterprise that alters a delicate balance of forces within the cell **(gain of function).**

Numerous hereditary and acquired diseases are caused by evasion of the quality control system designed to promote correct folding and eliminate faulty proteins. Misfolded proteins can injure the cell in a number of ways:

- **Loss of function:** Certain mutations prevent correct folding of crucial proteins, which then do not function properly or cannot be incorporated into the correct site. For example, some mutations that lead to cystic fibrosis cause misfolding of an ion channel protein, which is then degraded. Failure of the protein to reach its destination at the cell membrane results in a defect in chloride transport that produces the disease cystic fibrosis. Other examples of loss of function include mutations of the low-density lipoprotein (LDL) receptor in certain types of hypercholesterolemia and mutations of a copper transport ATPase in Wilson disease.
- **Formation of toxic protein aggregates:** Defects in protein structure may be acquired as well as genetic. Thus, particularly in nondividing cells, age-related impairment of cellular antioxidant defenses leads to protein oxidation, which commonly alters protein tertiary structure, exposing interior hydrophobic amino acids that are normally hidden. In situations of mild to moderate oxidative stress, 20S proteasomes recognize the exposed hydrophobic moieties and degrade these proteins. However, if oxidative stress is severe, these proteins aggregate by virtue of a combination of hydrophobic and ionic bonds. Such aggregates are insoluble and tend to sequester Fe^{2+} ions, which in turn help generate additional ROS (see above), after which aggregate size increases. Whether or not the proteins contained in the aggregates are ubiquitinated, the aggregates are indigestible (Fig. 1-25). Any Ub bound to them is lost, which may cause a cellular deficit in Ub and impair protein degradation in general. Both by virtue of their generation of toxic ROS and their inhibition of proteasomal degradation, these aggregates may lead to cell death. Accumulation of amyloid β protein in Alzheimer disease and α-synuclein in Parkinson disease may occur by this type of mechanism.
- **Retention of secretory proteins:** Many proteins that are destined to be secreted from the cell require a correctly folded conformation to be transported through cellular compartments and released at the cell membrane. Mutations in genes that encode such proteins (e.g., α_1-antitrypsin) eventuate in cell injury because of massive accumulation of misfolded proteins within the liver cell. Failure to secrete this antiprotease into the circulation

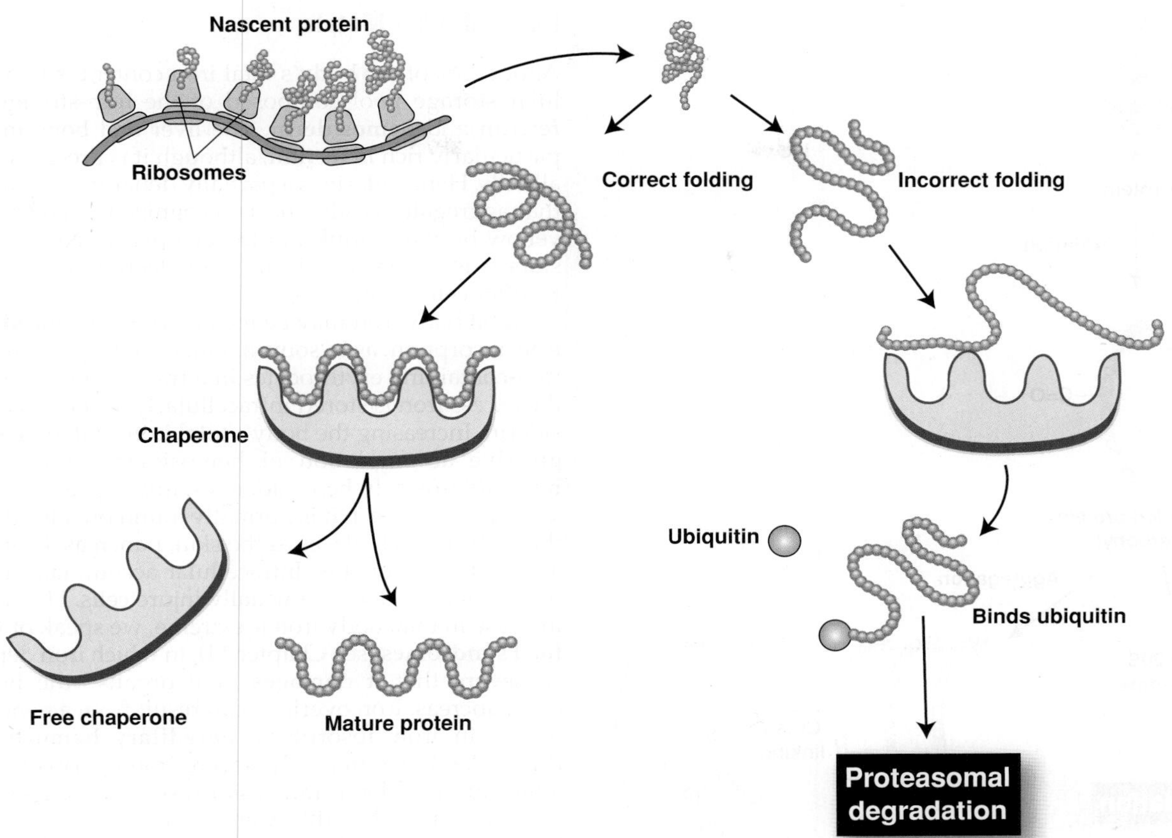

FIGURE 1-24. Differential handling of protein that is correctly folded (*left arrows*) and protein that is incorrectly folded (*right arrows*). Correctly folded proteins are chaperoned from the ribosomes that produce them to their ultimate cellular destination. Incorrectly folded proteins bind to ubiquitin, an association that directs the protein to proteasomes, where the misfolded protein is degraded.

also leads to unregulated proteolysis of connective tissue in the lung and loss of pulmonary parenchyma (emphysema).

- **Extracellular deposition of aggregated proteins:** Misfolded proteins tend to exhibit a β-pleated conformation in place of random coils or α-helices. These abnormal proteins often form insoluble aggregates, which may be visualized as extracellular deposits, the appearance depending on the specific disease. These accumulations often assume the forms of various types of amyloid and produce cell injury in systemic amyloidoses (see Chapter 23) and a variety of neurodegenerative diseases (see Chapter 28).

Lipofuscin

Lipofuscin is a mixture of lipids and proteins containing a golden-brown pigment called ceroid. It tends to accumulate by accretion of oxidized, cross-linked proteins and is indigestible. Lipofuscin occurs mainly in postmitotic cells (e.g., neurons, cardiac myocytes) or in cells that cycle infrequently (e.g., hepatocytes) (Fig. 1-23D). It is often more conspicuous in conditions associated with atrophy of an organ.

Although it was previously thought to be benign, there is increasing evidence that lipofuscin may be both a result and a cause of increasing oxidant stress in cells. It may impair both proteasomal function and lysosomal degradation of senescent or poorly functioning organelles. Consequently, inefficient or poorly functioning mitochondria may accumulate, generate more ROS and perpetuate the cycle.

Melanin

Melanin is an insoluble, brown-black pigment found principally in the epidermal cells of the skin, but also in the eye and other organs (Fig. 1-23E). It is located in intracellular organelles known as melanosomes and results from the polymerization of certain oxidation products of tyrosine. The amount of melanin is responsible for the differences in skin color among the various races, as well as the color of the eyes. It serves a protective function owing to its ability to absorb ultraviolet light. In white persons, exposure to sunlight increases melanin formation (tanning). The hereditary inability to produce melanin results in the disorder known as **albinism.** The presence of melanin is also a marker of the cancer that arises from melanocytes (melanoma). Melanin is discussed in detail in Chapter 24.

Exogenous Pigments

Anthracosis refers to the storage of carbon particles in the lung and regional lymph nodes (Fig. 1-23F). Virtually all urban dwellers inhale particulates of organic carbon generated by

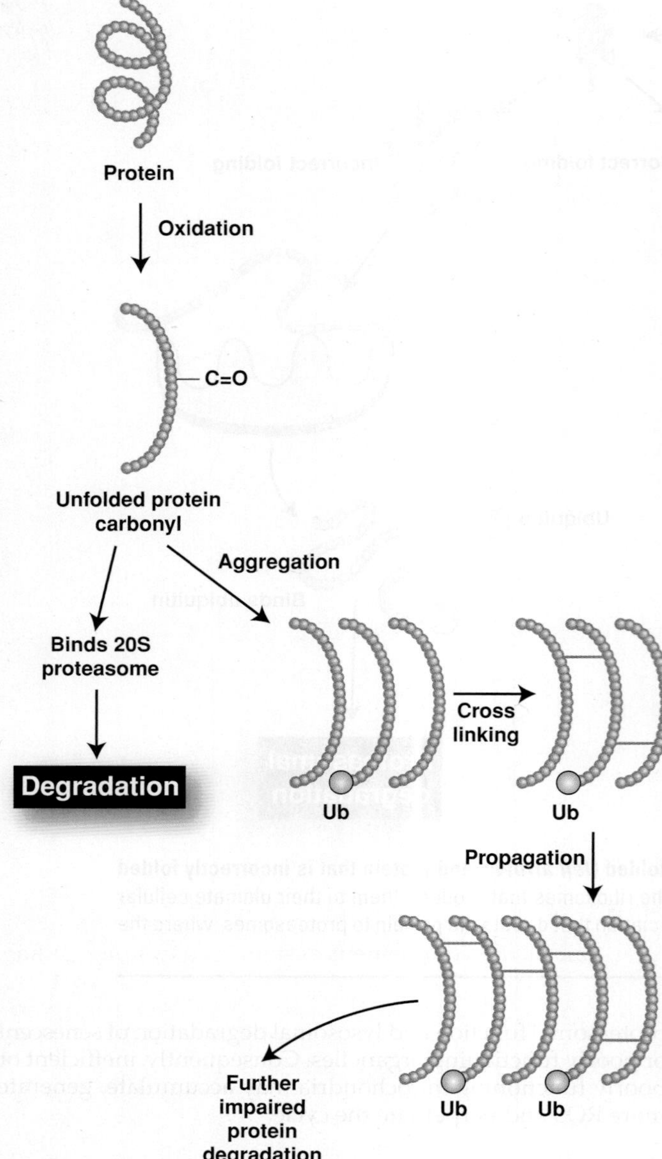

FIGURE 1-25. Mechanism of accumulation and elimination of oxidized proteins. On exposure to reactive oxygen species (ROS), proteins become oxidized to protein carbonyls. This forces a change in protein tertiary structure, exposing hydrophobic residues ordinarily on the protein interior. These protein carbonyls may be eliminated by 20S proteasomes without ubiquitination or, especially if the oxidant stress is heavy, they may aggregate on the basis of hydrophobic interactions. Some aggregated proteins may be ubiquitinated, but such aggregates cannot be degraded. With further accretion, aggregate substituents undergo cross-linking and continue to enlarge. *Ub* = ubiquitin.

the burning of fossil fuels. These particles accumulate in alveolar macrophages and are also transported to hilar and mediastinal lymph nodes, where the indigestible material is stored indefinitely within macrophages. Although the gross appearance of the lungs of persons with anthracosis may be alarming, the condition is innocuous.

Tattoos are the result of the introduction of insoluble metallic and vegetable pigments into the skin, where they are engulfed by dermal macrophages and persist for a lifetime.

Iron and Other Metals

About 25% of the body's total iron content is in an intracellular storage pool composed of the iron-storage proteins **ferritin** and **hemosiderin**. The liver and bone marrow are particularly rich in ferritin, although it is present in virtually all cells. Hemosiderin is a partially denatured form of ferritin that aggregates easily and is recognized microscopically as yellow-brown granules in the cytoplasm. Normally, hemosiderin is found mainly in the spleen, bone marrow and Kupffer cells of the liver.

Total body iron may be increased by enhanced intestinal iron absorption, as in some anemias, or by administration of iron-containing erythrocytes in a transfusion. In either case, the excess iron is stored intracellularly as ferritin and hemosiderin. Increasing the body's total iron content leads to progressive accumulation of hemosiderin, which is called **hemosiderosis.** In hemosiderosis, iron is present not only in the organs in which it is normally found but also throughout the body, in such places as the skin, pancreas, heart, kidneys and endocrine organs. Intracellular accumulation of iron in hemosiderosis does not usually injure cells. However, if the increase in total body iron is extreme, we speak of **iron overload syndromes** (see Chapter 14), in which iron deposition is so severe that it damages vital organs—the heart, liver and pancreas. Iron overload can result from a genetic abnormality in iron absorption, **hereditary hemochromatosis** (Fig. 1-23G). Alternatively, severe iron overload may occur after multiple blood transfusions, such as in treating hemophilia or certain hereditary anemias.

Excessive iron storage in some organs is also associated with increased risk of cancer. The pulmonary siderosis encountered among certain metal polishers is accompanied by a greater incidence of lung cancer. Hemochromatosis leads to a higher incidence of liver cancer.

Excess accumulation of lead, particularly in children, causes mental retardation and anemia. The storage of other metals also presents dangers. In Wilson disease, a hereditary disorder of copper metabolism, storage of excess copper in the liver and brain leads to severe chronic disease of those organs.

Ischemia/Reperfusion Injury Reflects Oxidative Stress

Ischemic Injury

Ischemia, defined as interruption of blood flow (e.g., myocardial infarct or stroke), results in cell injury or death by necrosis or apoptosis, or both. Loss of blood flow causes a decrease in cellular O_2 and an increase in cellular CO_2. Moreover, cells are deprived of key nutrients, such as glucose. A number of deleterious events occurs, including acidosis, generation of ROS, loss of glycogen stores, disruption of intracellular Ca^{2+} homeostasis and increased intracellular Ca^{2+}, mitochondrial injury and DNA damage. These changes can be tolerated by the cell for a short period of time, but after a critical threshold has been passed, cell death by necrosis or apoptosis, or both, becomes inevitable.

Although sudden and complete ischemia may result in cell death before adaptive mechanisms can come into play, repeated episodes of ischemia, exemplified by recurrent angina secondary to coronary artery disease, lead to adaptive responses. In the heart, these responses have been collectively termed ischemic preconditioning. Hypoxia-inducible factor (HIF) is the master regulator of transcriptional responses to hypoxia. This transcription factor, which is induced by lowered intracellular O_2 tension, activates a number of genes whose protein products limit production of ROS, Ca^{2+} accumulation and ATP depletion. As a result, HIF induction exerts a protective effect against mitochondrial injury, DNA damage and oxidative stress, thereby promoting the survival of the ischemic cell.

Reperfusion Injury

Reperfusion is the restoration of blood flow following a period of ischemia. Although reperfusion is beneficial in salvaging cells that have remained viable, the process itself results in pathologic consequences, to which the term "reperfusion injury" is applied.

Ischemia/reperfusion (I/R) injury reflects the interplay of transient ischemia, consequent tissue damage and exposure of damaged tissue to the oxygen that arrives when blood flow is reestablished (reperfusion). Initially, ischemic cellular damage leads to generation of free radical species. Reperfusion then provides abundant molecular O_2 to combine with free radicals to form ROS. Evolution of I/R injury also involves many other factors, including inflammatory mediators (tumor necrosis factor-α [TNF-α], interleukin-1 [IL-1]), platelet-activating factor (PAF), NOS and NO•, intercellular adhesion molecules, dysregulation of Ca^{2+} homeostasis and many more.

Xanthine Oxidase

Xanthine dehydrogenase may be converted by proteolysis during a period of ischemia into xanthine oxidase. On reperfusion, oxygen returns and the abundant purines derived from ATP catabolism during ischemia provide substrates for xanthine oxidase. This enzyme requires oxygen to catalyze the formation of uric acid; ROS are byproducts of this reaction. Inhibitors of xanthine oxidase (e.g., allopurinol) are in clinical trials to test their ability to limit tissue damage after reperfusion.

The Role of Neutrophils

An additional source of ROS during reperfusion is the neutrophil. Reperfusion prompts endothelial cells to move preformed P-selectin to the cell surface, allowing neutrophils to bind intercellular adhesion molecule-1 (ICAM-1) on the endothelial membrane and roll along endothelial cells (see Chapter 2). Neutrophils release large quantities of ROS and hydrolytic enzymes, both of which may injure the previously ischemic cells.

The Role of Nitric Oxide

There are two major forms of NOS: a constitutive form, which is common to endothelial cells and parenchymal cells (e.g., hepatocytes, neurons), and an inducible form (iNOS), mostly found in inflammatory cells. Nitric oxide dilates the microvasculature by relaxing smooth muscle, inhibits platelet aggregation and decreases adhesion between leukocytes and the endothelial surface. These activities are all mediated by the ability of NO• to decrease cytosolic Ca^{2+}, both by extrusion of calcium from the cell and by its sequestration within intracellular stores.

NO• also reacts with O_2^- to form the highly reactive species, $ONOO^-$. Normally, O_2^- is detoxified by SOD and little $ONOO^-$ is produced. However, I/R stimulates iNOS and the NO• produced inactivates SOD, thereby increasing the amount of NO• and favoring production of $ONOO^-$. The free radical gives rise to DNA strand breaks and lipid peroxidation in cell membranes.

NO• is a double-edged sword in I/R injury, however. Ischemia causes release of metal cations. Resulting Fe^{2+} ions play an important role in continuing to generate ROS during I/R injury. As noted above, NO• decreases transferrin-mediated iron uptake, and so may also partly protect cells from I/R injury.

Inflammatory Cytokines

I/R injury leads to release of cytokines, which both promote inflammation and modulate its severity. In this context proinflammatory cytokines such as TNF-α, IL-1 and IL-6 are thought to be important. These (1) promote vasoconstriction, (2) stimulate the adherence of neutrophils and platelets to endothelium and (3) have effects at sites distant from the ischemic insult itself.

Platelets

Platelets adhere to the microvasculature of injured tissue and release a number of factors that play a role in both tissue damage and cytoprotection. These include cytokines, TGF-β, serotonin and NO•.

Complement

Activation of the complement system (see Chapter 2) has been demonstrated during I/R. As a result, membrane attack complexes are deposited and chemotactic agents and proinflammatory cytokines are produced. The net result is recruitment and adhesion of neutrophils.

We can put reperfusion injury in perspective by emphasizing that there are three different degrees of cell injury, depending on the duration of the ischemia:

- With short periods of ischemia, reperfusion (and, therefore, the resupply of oxygen) completely restores the structural and functional integrity of the cell. Cell injury in this case is completely reversible.
- With longer periods of ischemia, reperfusion is not associated with restoration of cell structure and function but rather with deterioration and death of the cells. In this case, lethal cell injury occurs during the period of reperfusion.
- Lethal cell injury may develop during the period of ischemia itself, in which case reperfusion is not a factor. A longer period of ischemia is needed to produce this third type of cell injury. In this case, cell damage does not depend on the formation of ROS.

Proteasomes and Ischemia/Reperfusion Injury

Many of the cytokines that mediate tissue damage in I/R injury are expressed under the control of NFκB. In a number of experimental models, proteasomal activity is decreased after I/R. This effect stabilizes the NFκB–IκB complex (see above) and limits tissue damage.

Cell Death

Cell death is not simply an academic exercise; manipulation of cell viability by biochemical and pharmacologic intervention is currently a major area of research. For example, if we understand the biochemistry of ischemic death of cardiac myocytes, which is responsible for the leading cause of death in the Western world, we may be able to prolong myocyte survival after a coronary occlusion until circulation is restored.

Mechanisms that mediate the principal pathways of cell death may overlap. To appreciate the means by which cell death occurs and its potential therapeutic manipulation, it is important to understand how the process manifests morphologically.

Necrotic Cell Death Results From Exogenous Cell Injury and Is Reflected in Geographic Areas of Cell Death

At the cellular level, necrosis is characterized by cell and organelle swelling, ATP depletion, increased plasma membrane permeability, release of macromolecules from the cell and, eventually, cell death. The response to this process is usually acute inflammation, which itself may generate further cell injury (see Chapter 2). The stimuli that initiate the pathways leading to necrosis are highly variable and produce diverse recognizable histologic and cytologic patterns. However, as we shall see below, most instances of necrosis share certain mechanistic similarities.

Coagulative Necrosis

Coagulative necrosis is a morphologic term that refers to light microscopic alterations in dead or dying cells (Fig. 1-26). Shortly after a cell's death, its outline is maintained. When stained with the usual combination of hematoxylin and eosin, the cytoplasm of a necrotic cell is more deeply eosinophilic than usual. In the nucleus, chromatin is initially clumped and is then redistributed along the nuclear membrane. Three morphologic changes follow:

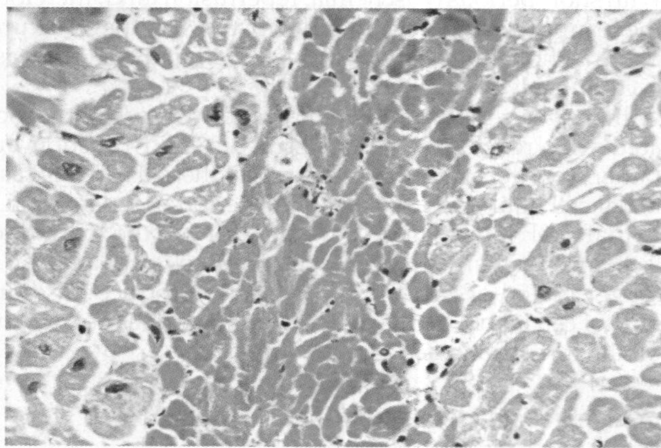

FIGURE 1-26. Coagulative necrosis. Photomicrograph of the heart in a patient with an acute myocardial infarction. In the center, the deeply eosinophilic necrotic cells have lost their nuclei. The necrotic focus is surrounded by paler-staining, viable cardiac myocytes.

- **Pyknosis:** The nucleus becomes smaller and stains deeply basophilic as chromatin clumping continues.
- **Karyorrhexis:** The pyknotic nucleus breaks up into many smaller fragments scattered about the cytoplasm.
- **Karyolysis:** The pyknotic nucleus may be extruded from the cell or it may manifest progressive loss of chromatin staining.

Early ultrastructural changes in a dying or dead cell reflect an extension of alterations associated with reversible cell injury (Figs. 1-13 and 1-14). In addition to the nuclear changes described above, the dead cell features dilated endoplasmic reticulum, disaggregated ribosomes, swollen and calcified mitochondria, aggregated cytoskeletal elements and plasma membrane blebs.

After a variable time, depending on the tissue and circumstances, the lytic activity of intracellular and extracellular enzymes causes the cell to disintegrate. This is particularly the case when necrotic cells have elicited an acute inflammatory response.

The appearance of necrotic tissue has traditionally been described as **coagulative necrosis** because of its similarity to coagulation of proteins that occurs upon heating. Although this term is based on obsolete concepts, it remains useful as a morphologic descriptor.

Whereas the morphology of individual cell death tends to be uniform across different cell types, the tissue responses are more variable. This diversity is described by a number of terms that reflect specific histologic patterns that depend on the organ and the circumstances.

Liquefactive Necrosis

When the rate of dissolution of necrotic cells is considerably faster than the rate of repair, the resulting morphologic appearance is termed **liquefactive necrosis.** Polymorphonuclear leukocytes of the acute inflammatory reaction contain potent hydrolases capable of digesting dead cells. A sharply localized collection of these acute inflammatory cells, generally in response to bacterial infection, produces rapid cell death and tissue dissolution. The result is often an **abscess** (Fig. 1-27), which is a cavity formed by liquefactive necrosis

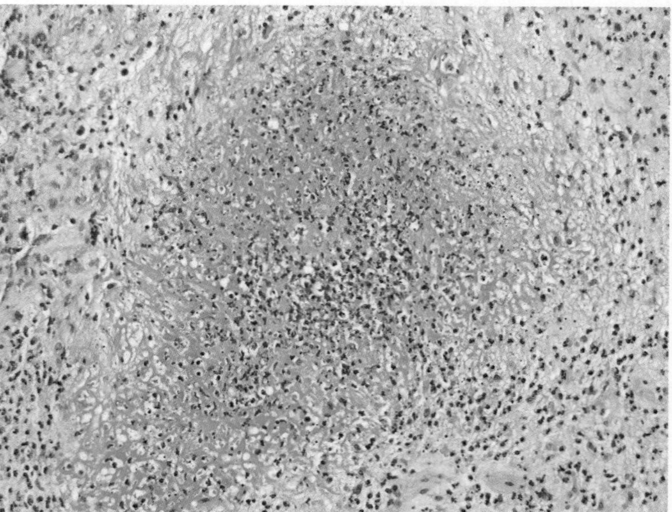

FIGURE 1-27. Liquefactive necrosis in an abscess of the skin. The abscess cavity is filled with polymorphonuclear leukocytes.

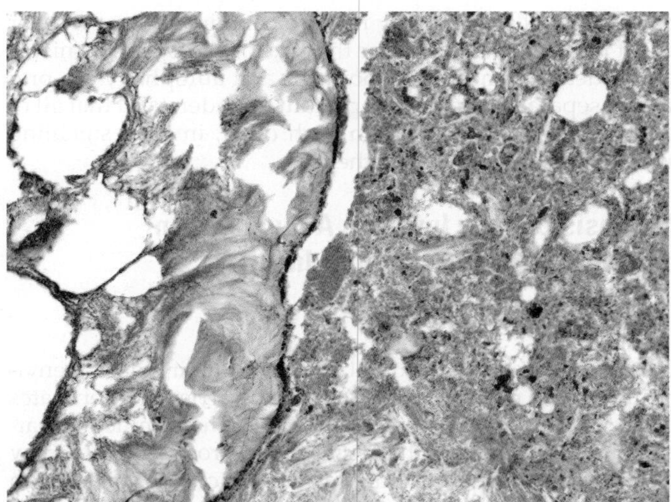

FIGURE 1-28. Fat necrosis. Photomicrograph of peripancreatic adipose tissue from a patient with acute pancreatitis shows an island of necrotic adipocytes adjacent to an acutely inflamed area. Fatty acids are precipitated as calcium soaps, which accumulate as amorphous, basophilic deposits at the periphery of the irregular island of necrotic adipocytes.

in a solid tissue. Eventually an abscess is walled off by a fibrous capsule that contains its contents.

Coagulative necrosis of the brain may occur after cerebral artery occlusion, and is often followed by rapid dissolution—liquefactive necrosis—of the dead tissue by a mechanism that cannot be attributed to the action of an acute inflammatory response. It is not clear why coagulative necrosis in the brain and not elsewhere is followed by disappearance of the necrotic cells, but the phenomenon may be related to the presence of more abundant lysosomal enzymes or different hydrolases specific to the cells of the central nervous system. Liquefactive necrosis of large areas of the central nervous system can lead to an actual cavity or cyst that will persist for the life of the person.

Fat Necrosis

Fat necrosis specifically affects adipose tissue and most commonly results from pancreatitis or trauma (Fig. 1-28). The unique feature determining this type of necrosis is the presence of triglycerides in adipose tissue. The process begins when digestive enzymes, normally found only in the pancreatic duct and small intestine, are released from injured pancreatic acinar cells and ducts into the extracellular spaces. On extracellular activation, these enzymes digest the pancreas itself as well as surrounding tissues, including adipose cells:

1. Phospholipases and proteases attack the plasma membrane of fat cells, releasing their stored triglycerides.
2. Pancreatic lipase hydrolyzes the triglycerides, which produces free fatty acids.
3. Free fatty acids bind calcium and are precipitated as calcium soaps. These appear as amorphous, basophilic deposits at the edges of irregular islands of necrotic adipocytes.

Grossly, fat necrosis appears as an irregular, chalky white area embedded in otherwise normal adipose tissue. In the case of traumatic fat necrosis, triglycerides and lipases are released from the injured adipocytes. In the breast, fat necrosis secondary to trauma is not uncommon and may mimic a tumor, particularly if some calcification has occurred.

Caseous Necrosis

Caseous necrosis is characteristic of tuberculosis (Fig. 1-29). The lesions of tuberculosis are tuberculous granulomas, or tubercles. In the center of such granulomas, the accumulated mononuclear cells that mediate the chronic inflammatory reaction to the offending mycobacteria are killed. In caseous necrosis, unlike coagulative necrosis, the necrotic cells fail to retain their cellular outlines. They do not, however, disappear by lysis, as in liquefactive necrosis. Rather, the dead cells persist indefinitely as amorphous, coarsely granular, eosinophilic debris. Grossly, this debris is grayish white, soft and friable.

Giant cells
Lymphocytes
Granuloma
Epithelioid cells
Caseous necrosis
A
LYMPH NODE

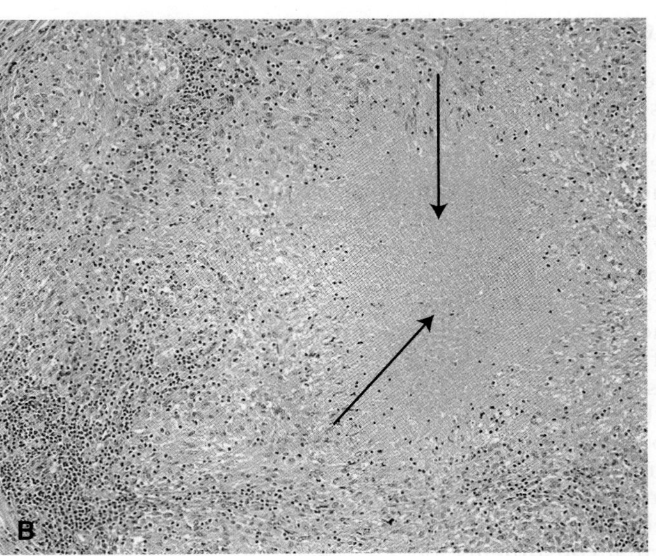

FIGURE 1-29. Caseous necrosis in a tuberculous lymph node. A. The typical amorphous, granular, eosinophilic, necrotic center is surrounded by granulomatous inflammation. **B.** Photomicrograph showing a tuberculous granuloma with central caseous necrosis (*arrows*).

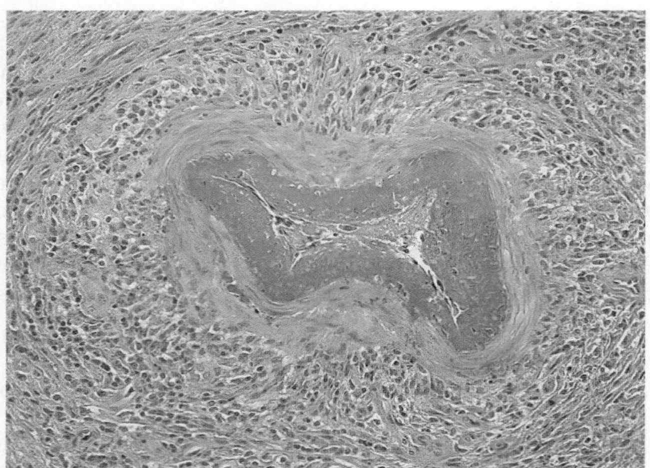

FIGURE 1-30. Fibrinoid necrosis. An inflamed muscular artery in a patient with systemic arteritis shows a sharply demarcated, homogeneous, deeply eosinophilic zone of necrosis.

It resembles clumpy cheese, hence the name **caseous necrosis.** This distinctive type of necrosis is generally attributed to the toxic effects of the mycobacterial cell wall, which contains complex waxes (peptidoglycolipids) that exert potent biological effects.

Fibrinoid Necrosis

Fibrinoid necrosis is an alteration of injured blood vessels, in which insudation and accumulation of plasma proteins cause the wall to stain intensely with eosin (Fig. 1-30). The term is something of a misnomer, however, because the eosinophilia of the accumulated plasma proteins obscures the underlying alterations in the blood vessel, making it difficult, if not impossible, to determine whether there truly is necrosis in the vascular wall.

Cells May Participate Actively in Their Own Death

Cell death is a field that has excited growing interest, both as an area of investigation and as an important target for therapeutic manipulation. Three main avenues leading to cell death have been delineated: necrosis, apoptosis and, most recently, autophagy. These processes had formerly been viewed as separate, nonintersecting roads. Necrosis was defined as accidental cell death caused by a hostile environment to which a cell could not adapt effectively. It was thus seen as a passive process in which the cell was more sinned against than sinning itself. Apoptosis is a form of cellular suicide in which the cell participates actively in its own demise. It has been appreciated as a mechanism by which individual cells utilize their own signaling systems to sacrifice themselves for the preservation of the organism. Autophagy (see above) is also an active signaling process that is elicited when a stressful environment requires autodigestion of a portion of the cell's macromolecular constituents.

There is increasing agreement that the various forms of cell death are not strictly separate, but rather share molecular effectors and signaling pathways. Cell processes incriminated in one may be co-conspirators with the others, and a particular cell's death may involve combinations of two, or all, of these mechanisms. For the sake of clarity, mechanisms of cell death by necrosis, apoptosis and autophagy are presented separately, but it is important to understand that all of these processes borrow from each other, involve signaling and collaborate with each other.

Necrosis Usually Involves Accumulation of a Number of Intracellular Insults

Ischemic Cell Death

Cells exist in a skewed equilibrium with their external environment. The plasma membrane is the barrier that separates the extracellular fluid from the internal cellular milieu. Whatever the nature of the lethal insult, cell necrosis is heralded by disruption of the permeability barrier function of the plasma membrane. Normally, extracellular concentrations of sodium and calcium are orders of magnitude greater than intracellular concentrations. The opposite holds for potassium. The selective ion permeability requires (1) considerable energy, (2) structural integrity of the lipid bilayer, (3) intact ion channel proteins and (4) normal association of the membrane with cytoskeletal constituents. When one or more of these elements is severely damaged, the resulting disturbance of the internal ionic balance is thought to represent the "point of no return" for the injured cell.

The role of calcium in the pathogenesis of cell death deserves special mention. Ca^{2+} concentration in extracellular fluids is in the millimolar range (10^{-3} M). By contrast, cytosolic Ca^{2+} concentration is 1/10,000 of that outside cells, i.e., about 10^{-7} M. Many crucial cell functions are exquisitely regulated by minute fluctuations in cytosolic free calcium concentration ($[Ca^{2+}]i$). Thus, massive influx of Ca^{2+} through a damaged plasma membrane ensures loss of cell viability.

The processes by which cells undergo death by necrosis vary according to the cause, organ and cell type. The best studied and most clinically important example is ischemic necrosis of cardiac myocytes. The mechanisms underlying the death of cardiac myocytes are in part unique, but the basic processes that are involved are comparable to those in other organs. Some of the unfolding events may occur simultaneously; others may be sequential (Fig. 1-31).

1. **Interruption of blood supply decreases delivery of O_2 and glucose.** Anoxia, whether it arises from ischemia (e.g., coronary artery atherosclerosis) or other causes (e.g., blood loss from trauma), decreases delivery of both oxygen and glucose to myocytes. For most cells, but especially for cardiac myocytes (which do not store much energy), this combined insult is formidable.
2. **Anaerobic glycolysis leads to overproduction of lactate and decreased intracellular pH.** The lack of O_2 during myocardial ischemia both blocks production of ATP and inhibits mitochondrial oxidation of pyruvate. Instead of entering the citric acid cycle, pyruvate is reduced to lactate in the cytosol by a process called anaerobic glycolysis. Lactate accumulation lowers intracellular pH. Consequent acidification of the cytosol initiates a downward spiral of events that propels the cell toward disaster.
3. **Distortion of the activities of pumps in the plasma membrane skews the ionic balance of the cell.** Na^+ accumulates because the lack of ATP renders the Na^+/K^+ ion exchanger inactive, an effect that leads to activation of the

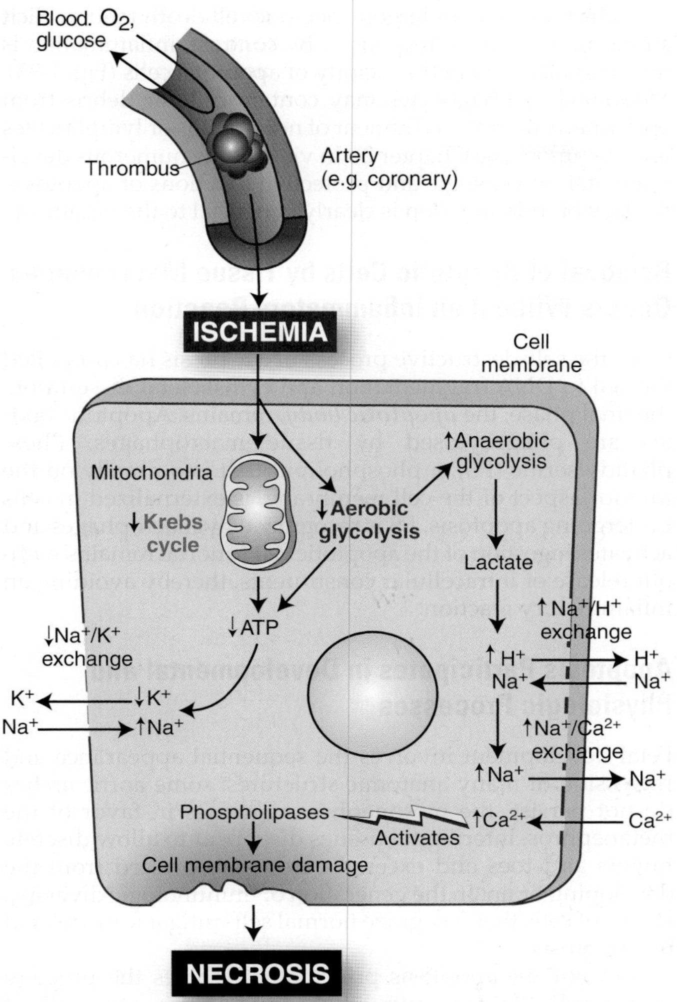

FIGURE 1-31. Mechanisms by which ischemia leads to cell death. *ATP* = adenosine triphosphate; *Ca^{2+}* = calcium ion; *H+* = hydrogen ion; *K^+* = potassium ion; *Na^+* = sodium ion; *O_2* = oxygen.

Na^+/H^+ ion exchanger. This pump is normally quiescent, but when intracellular acidosis threatens, it pumps H^+ out of the cell in exchange for Na^+ to maintain proper intracellular pH. The resulting increase in intracellular sodium activates the Na^+/Ca^{2+} ion exchanger, which increases calcium entry. Ordinarily, excess intracellular Ca^{2+} is extruded by an ATP-dependent calcium pump. However, with ATP in very short supply, Ca^{2+} accumulates in the cell.

4. **Activation of phospholipase A_2 (PLA_2) and proteases disrupts the plasma membrane and cytoskeleton.** High calcium concentrations in the cytosol of an ischemic cell activate PLA_2, leading to degradation of membrane phospholipids and consequent release of free fatty acids and lysophospholipids. The latter act as detergents that solubilize cell membranes. Both fatty acids and lysophospholipids are also potent mediators of inflammation (see Chapter 2), an effect that may further disrupt the integrity of the already compromised cell.

   Calcium also activates a series of proteases that attack the cytoskeleton and its attachments to the cell membrane. As the cohesion between cytoskeletal proteins and the plasma membrane is disrupted, membrane blebs form, and the shape of the cell is altered. The combination of electrolyte imbalance and increased cell membrane permeability causes the cell to swell, a frequent morphologic prelude to dissolution of the cell.
5. **Lack of O_2 impairs mitochondrial electron transport, thereby decreasing ATP synthesis and facilitating production of ROS.** Under normal circumstances, about 3% of the oxygen entering the mitochondrial electron transport chain is converted to ROS. During ischemia, generation of ROS increases because of (1) decreased availability of favored substrates for the electron transport chain, (2) damage to elements of the chain and (3) reduced activity of mitochondrial SOD. Among other effects, ROS cause peroxidation of cardiolipin, a membrane phospholipid that is unique to mitochondria and is sensitive to oxidative damage by virtue of its high content of unsaturated fatty acids. This attack inhibits the function of the electron transport chain and decreases its ability to produce ATP.
6. **Mitochondrial damage promotes the release of cytochrome c to the cytosol.** In normal cells the mitochondrial permeability transition pore (MPTP) opens and closes sporadically. Ischemic injury to mitochondria causes sustained opening of the MPTP, with resulting loss of cytochrome c from the electron transport chain. This process further diminishes ATP synthesis and may, under some circumstances, also trigger apoptotic cell death (see below).
7. **The cell dies.** When the cell can no longer maintain itself as a metabolic unit, necrotic cell death occurs. The line between reversible and irreversible cell injury (i.e., the "point of no return") is not precisely defined, but it is probably reached at about the time that the MPTP opens. Although this event by itself is not necessarily lethal, by the time it occurs, disruption of the electron transport chain has become irreparable and eventually necrotic cell death is inevitable.

Necrosis May Involve Active Signaling

Although in some instances necrotic cell death is instantaneous, or at least rapid, in other circumstances, necrosis is mediated via signaling cascades. For example, a family of pathogen recognition receptors has been identified that is responsible for recognizing a variety of bacterial and other components. This recognition triggers signaling pathways that can result in damage to mitochondria, lysosomes and cell membranes, and are independent of caspase-mediated apoptosis (see below). Crucial players in these signaling pathways include ROS, a serine-threonine kinase called RIP1 and extracellular ligands for cell membrane receptors (e.g., TNF-α and Fas ligand [FasL]). The latter has been implicated in apoptosis (see below), but when that process is inhibited by blocking caspase activity, these ligands may initiate necrosis signaling cascades.

Pharmacologic interference with a number of events involved in the pathogenesis of cell necrosis may eventually preserve cell viability after an ischemic insult and is the subject of intensive investigation.

Apoptosis, or Programmed Cell Death, Is a Signaling Mechanism by Which Cells Commit Suicide

Apoptosis is a pattern of cell death that is triggered by a variety of extracellular and intracellular stimuli and carried to its conclusion by organized cellular signaling

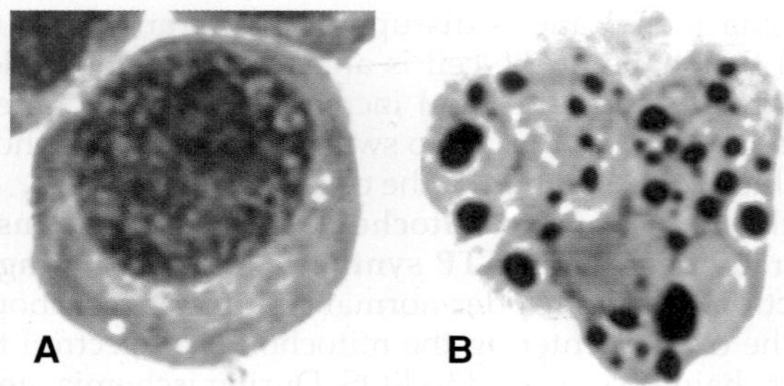

FIGURE 1-32. Apoptosis. A viable leukemic cell **(A)** contrasts with an apoptotic cell **(B)** in which the nucleus has undergone condensation and fragmentation.

cascades. It is part of the balance between the life and death of cells and determines that a cell dies when it is no longer useful or when it may be harmful to the larger organism. It is also a self-defense mechanism; cells that are infected with pathogens or in which genomic alterations have occurred are destroyed. In this context, many pathogens have evolved mechanisms to inactivate key components of the apoptotic signaling cascades. Apoptosis detects and destroys cells that harbor dangerous mutations, thereby maintaining genetic consistency and preventing the development of cancer. By contrast, as in the case of infectious agents that overcome antimicrobial resistance, successful clones of tumor cells often devise mechanisms to circumvent apoptosis.

Morphology of Apoptosis

Apoptotic cells are recognized by nuclear fragmentation and pyknosis, generally against a background of viable cells. Importantly, individual cells or small groups of cells undergo apoptosis, whereas necrosis characteristically involves larger geographic areas of cell death. Ultrastructural features of apoptotic cells include (1) nuclear condensation and fragmentation, (2) segregation of cytoplasmic organelles into distinct regions, (3) blebs of the plasma membrane and (4) membrane-bound cellular fragments, which often lack nuclei (Fig. 1-32).

Cells that have undergone necrotic cell death tend to elicit strong inflammatory responses. By contrast, inflammation is not generally seen in the vicinity of apoptotic cells (Fig. 1-33). Mononuclear phagocytes may contain cellular debris from apoptotic cells, but recruitment of neutrophils or lymphocytes is uncommon (see Chapter 2). In view of the numerous developmental, physiologic and protective functions of apoptosis, the lack of inflammation is clearly beneficial to the organism.

Removal of Apoptotic Cells by Tissue Macrophages Occurs Without an Inflammatory Reaction

Once the self-destructive process of apoptosis has propelled the cell to DNA fragmentation and cytoskeletal dissolution, the final phase, the ***apoptotic body***, remains. Apoptotic bodies are phagocytosed by tissue macrophages. Phosphatidylserine (PS), a phospholipid that is normally on the interior aspect of the cell membrane, is externalized in cells undergoing apoptosis. PS is recognized by macrophages and activates ingestion of the apoptotic cell's mortal remains without release of intracellular constituents, thereby avoiding an inflammatory reaction.

Apoptosis Participates in Developmental and Physiologic Processes

Fetal development involves the sequential appearance and regression of many anatomic structures: some aortic arches do not persist, the mesonephros regresses in favor of the metanephros, interdigital tissues disappear to allow discrete fingers and toes and excess neurons are pruned from the developing brain. In the generation of immunologic diversity, clones of cells that recognize normal self-antigens are deleted by apoptosis.

Physiologic apoptosis principally involves the progeny of stem cells that are continuously dividing (e.g., stem cells of the hematopoietic system, gastrointestinal mucosa and epidermis). Apoptosis of mature cells in these organs prevents overpopulation of the respective cell compartments by removing senescent cells and thus maintaining the normal architecture and size of the organ systems.

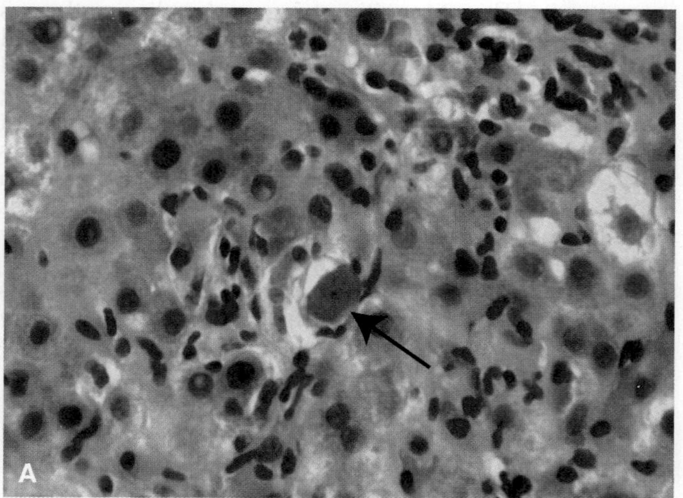

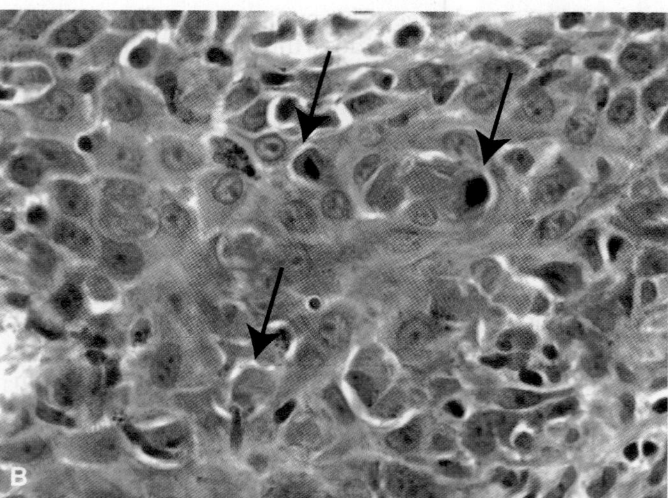

FIGURE 1-33. Histopathologic illustrations of apoptosis in the liver in viral hepatitis (A) and in the skin in erythema multiforme (B). Apoptotic cells are highlighted by *arrows*.

Apoptosis Eliminates Obsolescent Cells

A normal turnover of cells in many organs is essential to maintain the size and function of that cellular compartment. For example, as cells are continuously supplied to the circulating blood, older and less functional white blood cells must be eliminated to maintain the normal complement of the cells. Indeed, the pathologic accumulation of polymorphonuclear leukocytes in chronic myelogenous leukemia results from a mutation that inhibits apoptosis and therefore allows these cells to persist. In the mucosa of the small intestine, cells migrate from the depths of the crypts to the tips of the villi, where they undergo apoptosis and are sloughed into the lumen.

Apoptosis also maintains the balance of cellularity in organs that respond to trophic stimuli, such as hormones. An illustration of such an effect is the regression of lactational hyperplasia of the breast in women who have stopped nursing their infants. On the other side of the reproductive divide, postmenopausal women suffer atrophy of the endometrium after hormonal support has withered.

Apoptosis Deletes Mutant Cells

The integrity of an organism requires that it be able to recognize irreparable damage to DNA, after which the damaged cells must be eliminated by apoptosis. There is a finite error rate in DNA replication, owing to the infidelity of DNA polymerases. In addition, environmental stresses such as ultraviolet (UV) light, ionizing radiation and DNA-binding chemicals may also alter DNA structure. There are several means, the most important of which is probably p53, by which the cell recognizes genomic abnormalities and "assesses" whether they can be repaired. If the DNA damage is too severe to be repaired, a cascade of events leading to apoptosis is activated and the cell dies. This process protects an organism from the consequences of a nonfunctional cell or one that cannot control its own proliferation (e.g., a cancer cell).

Cancer cells must evade apoptosis many times during oncogenesis. Many tumors evolve mechanisms to circumvent or inhibit the apoptosis that might otherwise eliminate cells with the accumulated multiple mutations that are characteristic of cancer (see Chapter 5).

Apoptosis Is a Defense Against Dissemination of Infection

When a cell "detects" episomal (extrachromosomal) DNA replication, as in a viral infection, it tends to initiate apoptosis. This effect can be viewed as a means to eliminate infected cells before they can spread the virus. Many viruses have evolved protective mechanisms to manipulate cellular apoptosis. Viral gene products that inhibit apoptosis have been identified for many viruses, including human immunodeficiency virus (HIV), human papillomavirus, adenovirus and many others. In some cases these viral proteins bind and inactivate certain cellular proteins (e.g., p53) that are important in signaling apoptosis. In other instances, they may act at various points in the signaling pathways that activate apoptosis.

Apoptosis Comprises Several Signaling Pathways

Apoptosis reflects several different pathways that lead to similar endpoints. ***Extrinsic apoptosis*** reflects the activation of certain receptors by their ligands (e.g., Fas receptor [CD95] by FasL or TNF-α receptor by TNF-α). The ***intrinsic pathway***, by contrast, is triggered by diverse intracellular stresses and is characterized by a central role for mitochondria. Apoptosis may also be related to inflammatory processes or infectious agents. Both intracellular and extracellular ***infectious agents*** may elicit this type of apoptosis, and they may do so differently. A fourth type of apoptosis is the ***perforin/granzyme pathway***. This mechanism of apoptosis is caused by interactions of cytotoxic T cells with their cellular target and is activated by the transfer of granzyme B from the killer cell to its intended victim. These pathways are not rigid categories, but rather are paradigms that collectively encompass important features of diverse signaling mechanisms that lead to apoptosis. In fact, the different routes to apoptosis intersect and overlap.

Receptor–Ligand Interactions at the Cell Membrane May Trigger Apoptosis

Prominent examples of initiation of apoptosis at the cell membrane are the binding of TNF-α to its receptor (TNFR) and the recognition of FasL by its receptor, Fas. TNF-α is most often a soluble cytokine, whereas FasL is usually situated at the plasma membrane of certain cells, such as cytotoxic effector lymphocytes.

TNFR and Fas become activated upon binding their ligands. Specific amino acid sequences in the cytoplasmic tails of these transmembrane receptors, called death domains, act as docking sites for the corresponding death domains of other proteins that transmit proapoptotic intracellular signals that lead to apoptosis (Fig. 1-34A). After binding to the receptors, the latter proteins activate downstream signaling molecules, especially procaspase-8, which is converted to its activated form, caspase-8. In turn, caspase-8 activates downstream caspases in the apoptosis pathway.

The ultimate caspases activated in this process are the "effector" or "executioner" caspases, namely, caspases-3, -6 and -7. Caspase-3 is the most commonly activated effector caspase. In turn, it activates those enzymes that are responsible for nuclear fragmentation (e.g., caspase-activated DNase [CAD], which is responsible for degrading chromosomal DNA). Caspase-3 also destabilizes the cytoskeleton as the cell begins to fragment into apoptotic bodies.

Granzymes Released by Cytotoxic T Lymphocytes Cause Cell Killing by Activating Apoptosis

Activation of caspase signaling also occurs when killer lymphocytes, mainly cytotoxic T cells, recognize a cell as foreign. These lymphocytes release perforin and granzyme B. Perforin, as its name suggests, punches a hole in the plasma membrane of a target cell, through which proteins from the lymphocyte may enter the target cell. Granzyme B cleaves proteins at aspartate residues. In this capacity it directly activates procaspases, especially procaspase-10 (Fig. 1-34B), and also procaspase-3.

Granzyme B has also been shown to alter the balance of proapoptotic and antiapoptotic activities at the mitochondrial membrane. It activates Bid and, in so doing, increases mitochondrial cytochrome c release. Granzyme A, another constituent of cytotoxic T cells released into target cells, has been shown to trigger apoptosis by caspase-independent mechanisms. It activates a DNA nicking enzyme, called

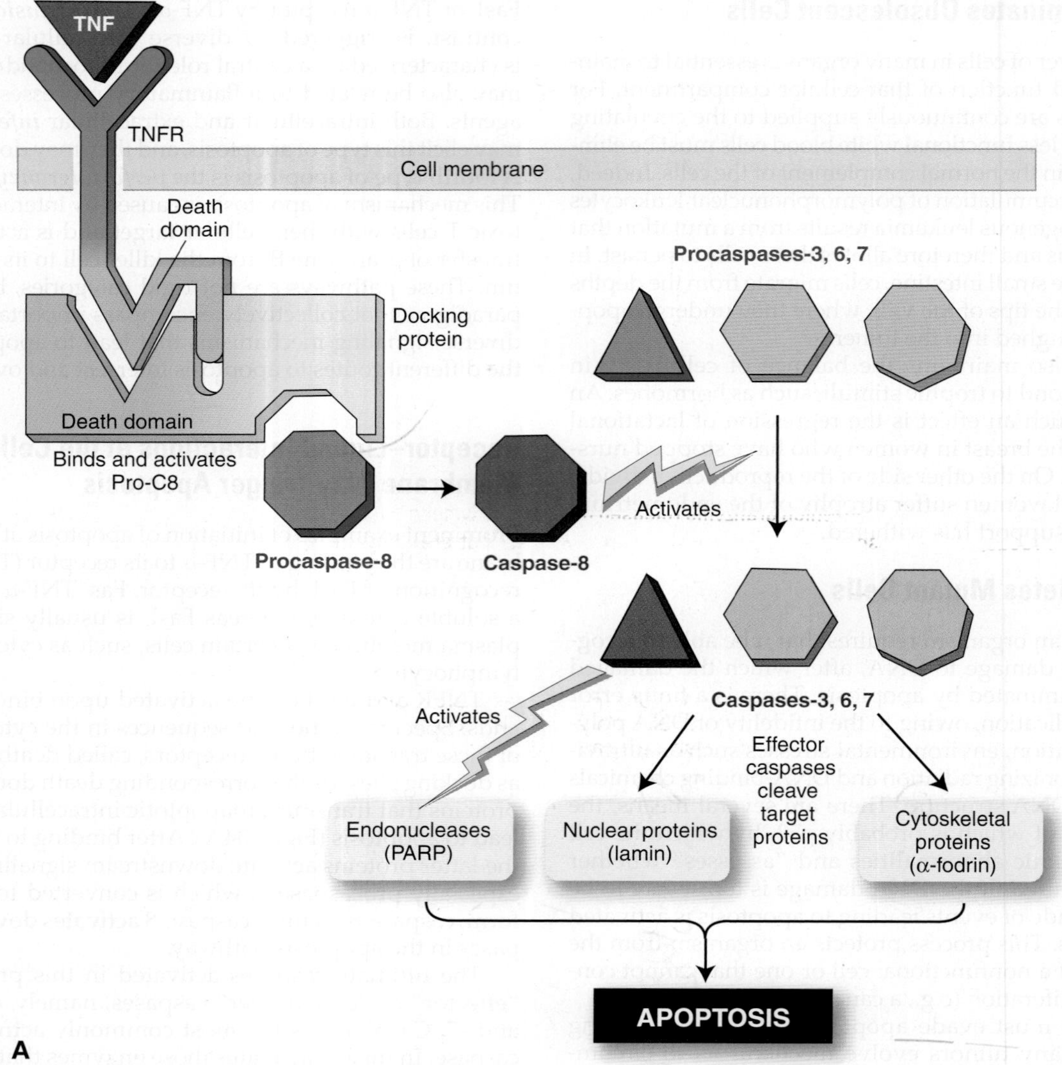

FIGURE 1-34. Mechanisms by which apoptosis may be initiated, signaled and executed. A. Ligand–receptor interactions that lead to caspase activation. *TNF* = tumor necrosis factor; *TNFR* = tumor necrosis factor receptor; *PARP* = poly-ADP-ribosylpolymerase. (*continued*)

NM23-H1, leading to apoptotic degradation of the cell's genomic DNA.

Cytochrome C Is a Key Player in Many Intracellular Pathways Signaling Apoptosis

Cytochrome (Cyt) c is normally bound by a phospholipid, **cardiolipin** (CL), to the inner mitochondrial membrane. Cyt c participates in many mitochondrial processes, including electron transport and membrane fluidity. ROS (e.g., superoxide) may elicit apoptosis by opening the MPTPs in the outer mitochondrial membrane. This process may involve oxidation of CL, resulting in Cyt c release through the permeability transition pore (see below).

The formation of nitric oxide radical (NO•) has similar consequences. ROS also activate neutral sphingomyelinase, a cytosolic enzyme that releases ceramide from sphingomyelin in the plasma membrane. In turn, ceramide stimulates cellular stress responses (stress-activated protein kinases), which then activate procaspase-8.

The Mitochondrial Membrane Helps Regulate the Intrinsic Pathway of Apoptosis

Mitochondrial proteins of the Bcl-2 family are the keys to this balance between cell life and death, and are divided into two groups based on the consequences of their overexpression or preponderance. The antiapoptotic members of this family include Bcl-2, Bcl-X_L and others (Table 1-5). Proapoptotic proteins of this family include Bad, Bak, Bax and others, and are in turn divided into two groups, based on their mechanisms of action. Some of these proapoptotic proteins may be thought of as activators (e.g., Bad, Bim, Bik, Puma, Noxa). They participate in apoptosis by turning on the others (especially Bak and Bax) (Table 1-5).

Antiapoptotic members of the Bcl-2 family exist as homodimers or as heterodimers in uneasy marriages with particular members of the proapoptotic side of the family (e.g., Bax, Bak). Such heterodimeric unions favor cell survival by sequestering the destructive activity of the proapoptotic proteins (Fig. 1-34C).

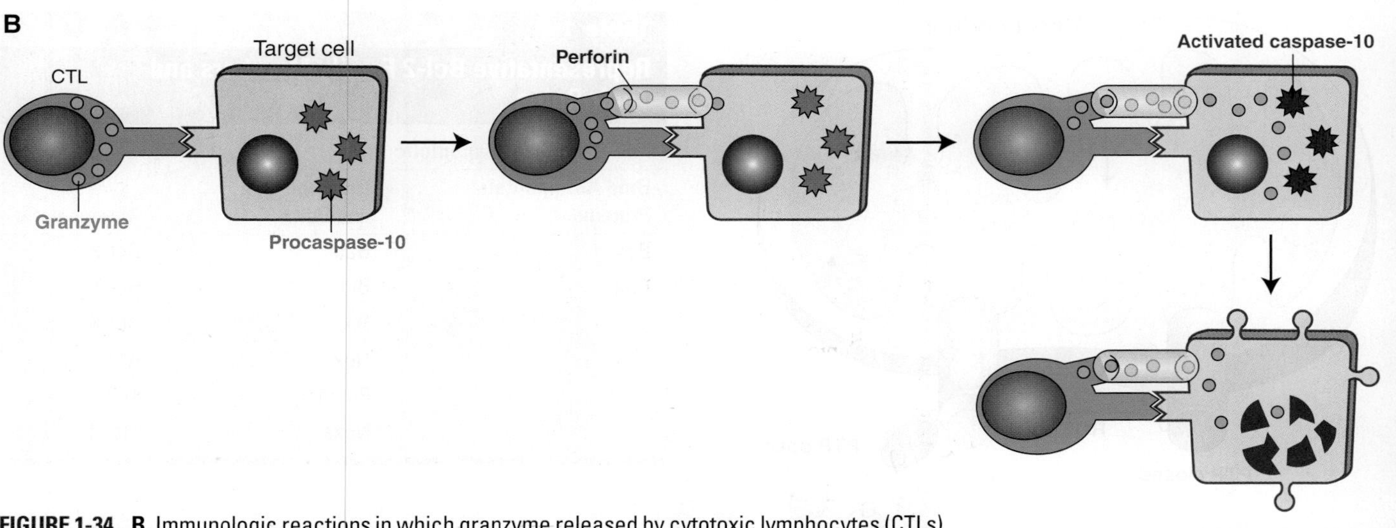

FIGURE 1-34. B. Immunologic reactions in which granzyme released by cytotoxic lymphocytes (CTLs) causes apoptosis. Procaspase-10 is shown as an example of procaspases that are activated by granzyme B.

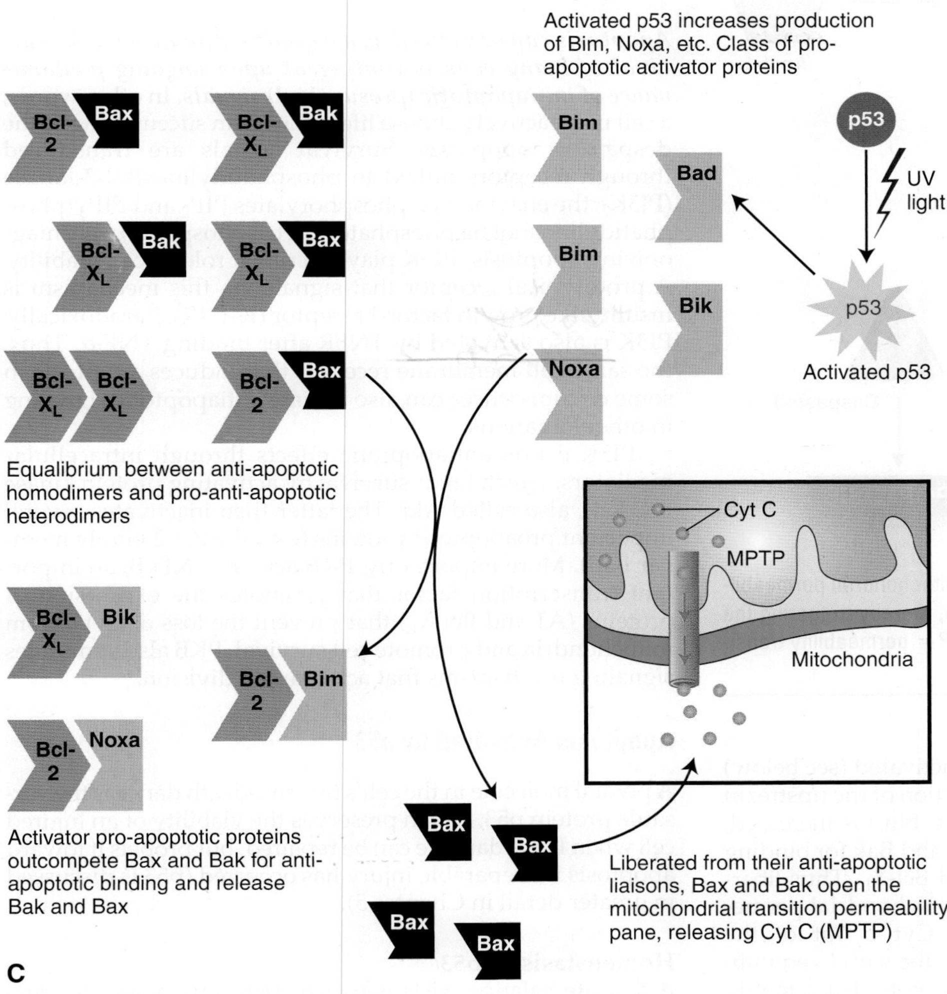

FIGURE 1-34. C. The equilibrium between proapoptotic and antiapoptotic members of the Bcl-2 family of proteins reflects binding of antiapoptotic members to themselves (homodimers) or to the proapoptotic proteins Bak and Bax. Activation of p53, for example, increases production of proapoptotic members of the Bcl-2 family (e.g., Bim, Puma; see Table 1-5), which outcompete Bax and Bak for binding to Bcl-2 and Bcl-X_L, freeing Bax and Bak to open the mitochondrial permeability pore (MPTP). (*continued*)

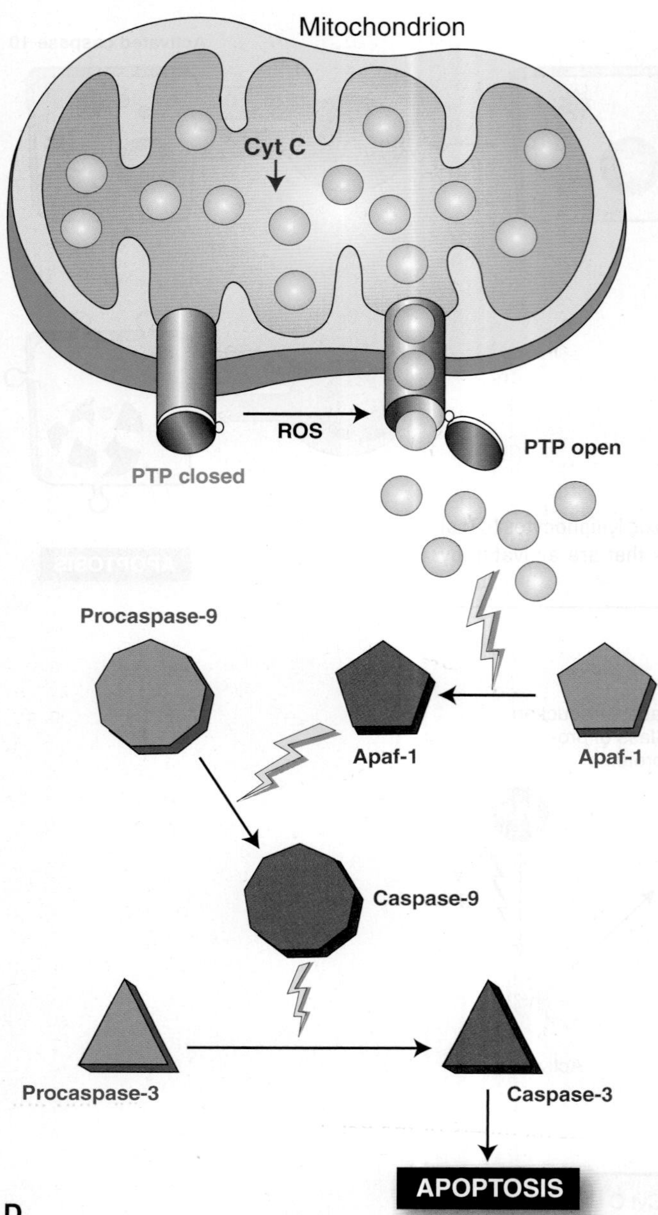

FIGURE 1-34. (*Continued*) **D.** Opening of the mitochondrial permeability transition pore, leading to Apaf-1 activation, thereby triggering the apoptotic cascade. *Cyt C* = cytochrome c; *PTP* = permeability transition pores; *ROS* = reactive oxygen species.

However, when, for example, p53 is activated (see below) by stimuli such as UV irradiation, production of the upstream proapoptotic proteins (e.g., Noma, Puma, Bim) is increased, and these femmes fatale outcompete Bax and Bak for binding to their antiapoptotic minders, Bcl-2 and Bcl-X_L. Thus liberated, Bax and Bak may then open the mitochondrial permeability transition pore, which allows Cyt c out of the mitochondria into the cytosol. In parallel, the shift in equilibrium between proapoptotic and antiapoptotic Bcl-2 family members to favor apoptosis releases Apaf-1 from a complex with Bcl-2, leading to activation of Apaf-1. Procaspase-9 is then activated. A complex of Cyt c, Apaf-1 and the now active caspase-9 is sometimes called the **apoptosome.** Its formation

Table 1-5

Representative Bcl-2 Family Members and Their Roles

Proapoptotic		
Bind Antiapoptotic Proteins	**Displace Bax and Bak**	**Antiapoptotic**
Bax	Bad	Bcl-2
Bak	Bid	Bcl-X_L
	Bik	Bcl-X
	Nox	A1
	Puma	Ku70
	Noxa	Mcl-1

activates procaspase-3 to caspase-3 (Fig. 1-34D), which in turn activates enzymes that degrade DNA (DNases; see above).

The Equilibrium Between Proapoptotic and Antiapoptotic Signals

Apoptosis can be viewed as a default pathway, and the survival of many cells is contingent upon ongoing predominance of antiapoptotic (prosurvival) signals. In other words, a cell must actively choose life rather than succumbing to the despair of apoptosis. Survival signals are transduced through receptors linked to phosphatidylinositol-3-kinase (PI3K), the enzyme that phosphorylates PIP_2 and PIP_3 (phosphatidylinositol bisphosphate and trisphosphate). By antagonizing apoptosis, PI3K plays a critical role in cell viability. A prototypical receptor that signals via this mechanism is insulin-like growth factor-I receptor (IGF-IR). Paradoxically, PI3K is also activated by TNFR after binding TNF-α. Thus, the same cell membrane receptor that induces apoptosis in some circumstances can also initiate antiapoptotic signaling in other situations.

PI3K exerts antiapoptotic effects through intracellular mediators, which favor survival by activating protein kinase B (PKB), also called Akt. The latter then inactivates several important proapoptotic proteins (e.g., the Bcl-2 family member Bad). More importantly, PKB activates NFκB, an important transcription factor that promotes the expression of proteins (A1 and Bcl-X_L) that prevent the loss of Cyt c from mitochondria and promote cell survival. PKB also stimulates signaling mechanisms that activate cell division.

Apoptosis Activated by p53

A pivotal molecule in the cell's life-and-death dance is the versatile protein p53, which preserves the viability of an injured cell when DNA damage can be repaired, but propels it toward apoptosis if irreparable injury has occurred (p53 is discussed in greater detail in Chapter 5).

Homeostasis of p53

A delicate balance exists between stabilization and destruction of p53. Thus, p53 binds to several proteins (e.g., Mdm2), which promote its degradation via ubiquitination. The ability of p53 to avoid this pernicious association depends on certain structural changes in the protein in response to stress,

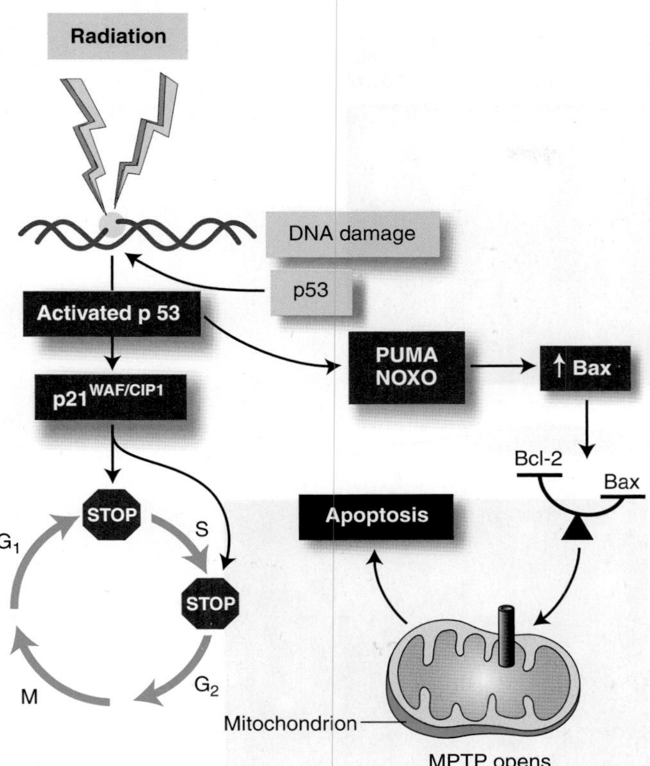

FIGURE 1-35. p53-mediated apoptosis. p53 is recruited to areas of DNA damage following, for example, external irradiation. Activated p53 activates p21WAF/CIP1, which halts cell cycle progression at the G_1/S and G_2/M transition points. If DNA damage is irreparable, p53 activates transcription of NOXA and PUMA, which alter the balance of proapoptotic and antiapoptotic Bcl-2 family proteins at the mitochondrial membrane in favor of apoptosis. The MPTP is opened (see Fig. 1-34C), leading to apoptosis.

DNA damage and so forth. These molecular modifications decrease its interaction with Mdm2, thereby enhancing survival of p53 and permitting its accumulation.

Function of p53

After it binds to areas of DNA damage, p53 activates proteins, particularly $p21^{WAF/CIP1}$, that arrest the cell in the G_1 stage of the cell cycle, allowing time for DNA repair to proceed. It also directs DNA repair enzymes to the site of injury. If the DNA damage cannot be repaired, p53 activates mechanisms that lead to apoptosis (Fig. 1-35).

One of the principal mechanisms by which p53 causes cell death is by altering the balance of Bcl-2 family members at the mitochondria. In its capacity as a transcription factor, it downregulates transcription of the antiapoptotic protein Bcl-2 and upregulates transcription of the proapoptotic genes *bax* and *bak*. It may also increase production of Noxa and Puma, which are necessary for p53-mediated opening of the MPTP. In addition, certain DNA helicases and other enzymes are activated by p53-mediated recognition of DNA damage, an effect that leads to translocation of a number of proapoptotic proteins (e.g., Fas) from the cell membrane to the cytosol.

p53 itself may also bind Bcl-2 and Bcl-X_L, thereby altering the balance of proapoptotic and antiapoptotic forces at the mitochondrial membrane. Thus, ionizing radiation causes translocation of p53 to the mitochondrial membrane. This function of p53 is mediated through its DNA-binding domain but is independent of transcriptional activation.

Stress also leads to accumulation of p53. Activation of certain oncogenes, such as *c-myc*, increases the amount of an Mdm2-binding protein ($p14^{ARF}$), thereby protecting p53 from Mdm2-induced destruction. Additional forms of stress that lead to p53 accumulation include hypoxia, depletion of ribonucleotides and loss of cell–cell adhesion during oncogenesis.

Inactivation of p53

Proteins of a number of oncogenic viruses inactivate p53 by binding to it. In fact, p53 was first identified as a cellular protein that coprecipitated with one such protein (SV40 large T antigen). Inactivating mutations of p53 are the most common DNA alterations in human cancer (see Chapter 5), which underscores its role as a switch that allows repair of DNA but triggers cellular suicide if that proves to be impossible.

Release of Ca^{2+} from the Endoplasmic Reticulum May Trigger Apoptosis

Cells maintain a large gradient of calcium concentration ($[Ca^{2+}]$) relative to the extracellular space. The extracellular space has about 4 orders of magnitude greater $[Ca^{2+}]$ than does the cytosol. Often, ligand-induced and other changes in cytosolic calcium concentration ($[Ca^{2+}]$i) are important secondary signals in cellular activation and mitosis. However, changes in $[Ca^{2+}]$i may also induce apoptosis. The endoplasmic reticulum (ER) stores considerable calcium, which may be released in response to various stimuli. Under certain circumstances, when ER Ca^{2+} release is activated, and particularly if Ca^{2+} release is prolonged, apoptosis ensues.

The proximity of the ER to mitochondria is key to this process. Ca^{2+} released by ER may be taken up by mitochondria. Resulting increases in mitochondrial $[Ca^{2+}]$ cause the MPTP to open, with release of Cyt c and activation of signaling, as described in the intrinsic cascade of apoptosis (see above). There is evidence that both proapoptotic and antiapoptotic members of the Bcl-2 family of proteins are important in regulating ER $[Ca^{2+}]$.

Furthermore, sustained release of Ca^{2+} from ER stores leads to release of caspase-12. This protein, which is bound to ER membrane, becomes activated upon its release. Activated caspase-12 in turn activates caspase-9 in the apoptosome (see above), in turn triggering the executioner caspases (mainly caspase-3).

Apoptosis Is Central to Many Disease Processes

When the regulation of apoptosis goes awry, there is the devil to pay. Apoptosis is central to the correct execution of embryologic development, elimination of self-reactive B- and T-lymphocyte clones and many other normal body functions. As a self-protective mechanism, apoptosis is an important guardian against uncontrolled cell proliferation (e.g., cancer) arising from accumulated DNA mutations (see Chapter 5).

Insufficient Apoptosis

If a major protein that mediates the defense of the organism, such as p53, is mutated, the protection afforded by apoptosis is compromised. Further mutations may accumulate without adequate impediment. Such pathways are commonly considered to be important in the development and progression

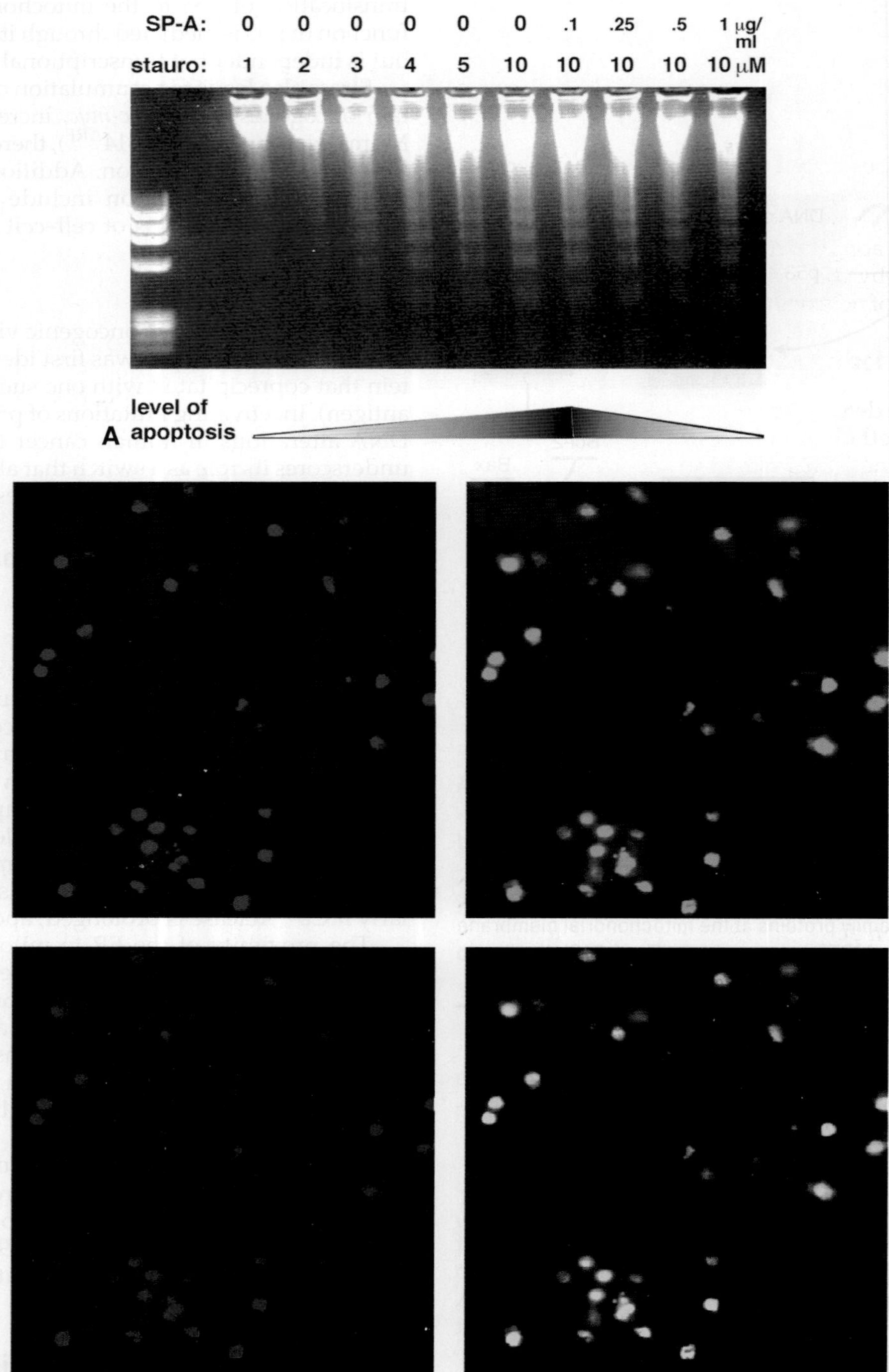

FIGURE 1-36. DNA fragmentation in apoptosis. A. Agarose gel electrophoresis of DNA isolated from lung epithelial cells treated with different amounts of staurosporine, which induces apoptosis, and with different amounts of surfactant protein-A (SP-A), which protects these cells from apoptosis. The schematic at the bottom illustrates the degree of apoptosis observed in these cells as a function of the concentrations of these two agents. At low concentrations of staurosporine or at high concentrations of SP-A, genomic DNA is largely unfragmented and thus remains at the top of the gel. By contrast, internucleosomal cleavage of DNA, such as occurs in apoptosis, is reflected in multiple, regularly spaced genomic DNA fragments, resembling a ladder. This phenomenon is called "laddering." **B. Fluorescence visualization of apoptotic cells.** Cultured human neurons were exposed to HIV-1 envelope glycoprotein (gp120), which elicits apoptosis in these cells. Panels illustrate (*upper left*) DAPI visualization of all nuclei in the culture; (*upper right*) Neuro-Trace (NT), a fluorescent Nissl stain, highlighting neurons; (*lower left*) fluorescent TUNEL assay, to visualize cells that contain breaks in their genomic DNA elicited by the gp120; and (*lower right*) overlay of NT and TUNEL, in which doubly positive cells (i.e., neurons undergoing apoptosis) are yellow.

of tumors (see Chapter 5). As another example, the ability of some viruses to block apoptosis allows those pathogens to replicate with less interference and so disseminate more widely than would otherwise be possible.

Excessive Apoptosis

In some cases, decreases in cell numbers due to "excessive" apoptosis may be fundamental to the development of certain diseases. For example, some neurodegenerative diseases are characterized by the accumulation of intracellular proteins within neurons, thereby triggering apoptosis and leading to diminished numbers of neurons and loss of specific functions.

Quantitative Assays for Apoptosis

Apoptotic cells can be detected by demonstrating fragmented DNA. A popular method involves the demonstration of nucleosomal "laddering." This virtually diagnostic pattern of DNA degradation, which is characteristic of apoptotic cell death, results from cleavage of chromosomal DNA at nucleosomes by activated endonucleases. Since nucleosomes are regularly spaced along the genome, a pattern of regular bands can be seen when fragments of cellular DNA are separated by electrophoresis (Fig. 1-36A).

Other assays are also used to detect and quantitate apoptosis. One is the TUNEL assay (terminal deoxyribonucleotidyl transferase [TdT]-mediated deoxyuridine triphosphate [dUTP]-digoxigenin nick end labeling), in which TdT transfers a fluorescent nucleotide to exposed breakpoints in DNA. Apoptotic cells that incorporate the labeled nucleotide are visualized by fluorescence microscopy (Fig. 1-36B) or flow cytometry. Apoptotic cells that have extruded some of the DNA have less than their normal diploid content. Automated measurement of DNA content in individual cells by flow cytometry thus produces a population distribution according to DNA content (cytofluorography). Other means of detecting apoptosis depend on quantitating the activated forms of enzymes that signal apoptosis, including the nuclear proteins PARP and lamin A.

Summary of Apoptosis

In summary, cells are continually poised between survival and apoptosis: their fate rests on the balance of powerful intracellular and extracellular forces, whose signals constantly act upon and counteract each other. Often, apoptosis functions as a self-protective programmed mechanism that leads to a cell's suicide when its survival may be detrimental to the organism. At other times, apoptosis is a pathologic process that contributes to many disorders, especially degenerative diseases. Thus, pharmacologic manipulation of apoptosis is an active frontier of drug development.

Autophagy Is an Additional Form of Programmed Cell Death

The phenomenon of autophagy has been described earlier as a mechanism by which the cell sequesters and recycles damaged organelles and macromolecules. There is a body of evidence that suggests that autophagic mechanisms can, in certain settings, be recruited to kill cells as a caspase-independent form of programmed cell death. Thus, autophagic cell death is now proposed as a legitimate alternative to apoptosis.

Autophagic cell death may involve excessive removal of cell organelles, thereby irrevocably interfering with vital cellular functions. Autophagy may also destroy selected proteins that sustain survival of the cell. In this context, experimental inhibition of autophagy and interference with the activity of genes involved with autophagic processes have prevented cell death induced by a variety of agents. Nevertheless, at this time, it remains controversial whether autophagy is responsible for a type of programmed cell death, and the extent to which such cell death occurs.

Ionizing Radiation Causes Oxidative Stress

The term "ionizing radiation" connotes an ability to cause radiolysis of water, thereby directly forming hydroxyl radicals. As noted above, hydroxyl radicals interact with DNA and inhibit DNA replication. For a nonproliferating cell, such as a hepatocyte or a neuron, the inability to divide is of little consequence. For a proliferating cell, however, the prevention of mitosis is a catastrophic loss of function. Once a proliferating cell can no longer divide, it dies by apoptosis, which rids the body of those cells that have lost their prime function. Direct mutagenic effects of ionizing radiation on DNA are also important. The cytotoxic effects of ionizing radiation are dose dependent. Whereas exposure to significant sources of radiation impairs the replicating capacity of cycling cells, massive doses of radiation may kill both proliferating and quiescent cells directly. Fig. 1-37 summarizes the mechanisms of cell killing by ionizing radiation.

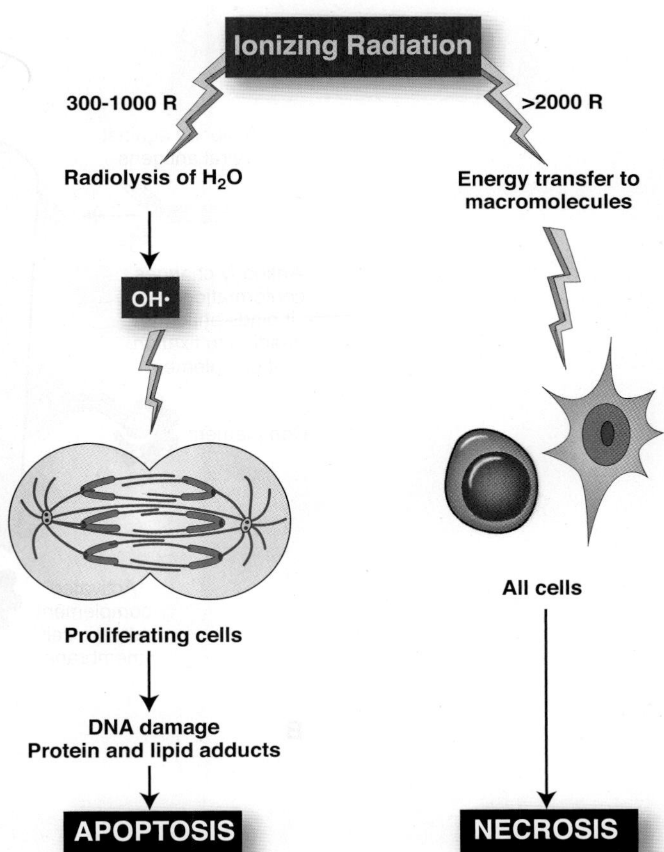

FIGURE 1-37. Mechanisms by which ionizing radiation at low and high doses causes cell death. *H_2O* = water, *OH•* = hydroxyl radical; *R* = rads.

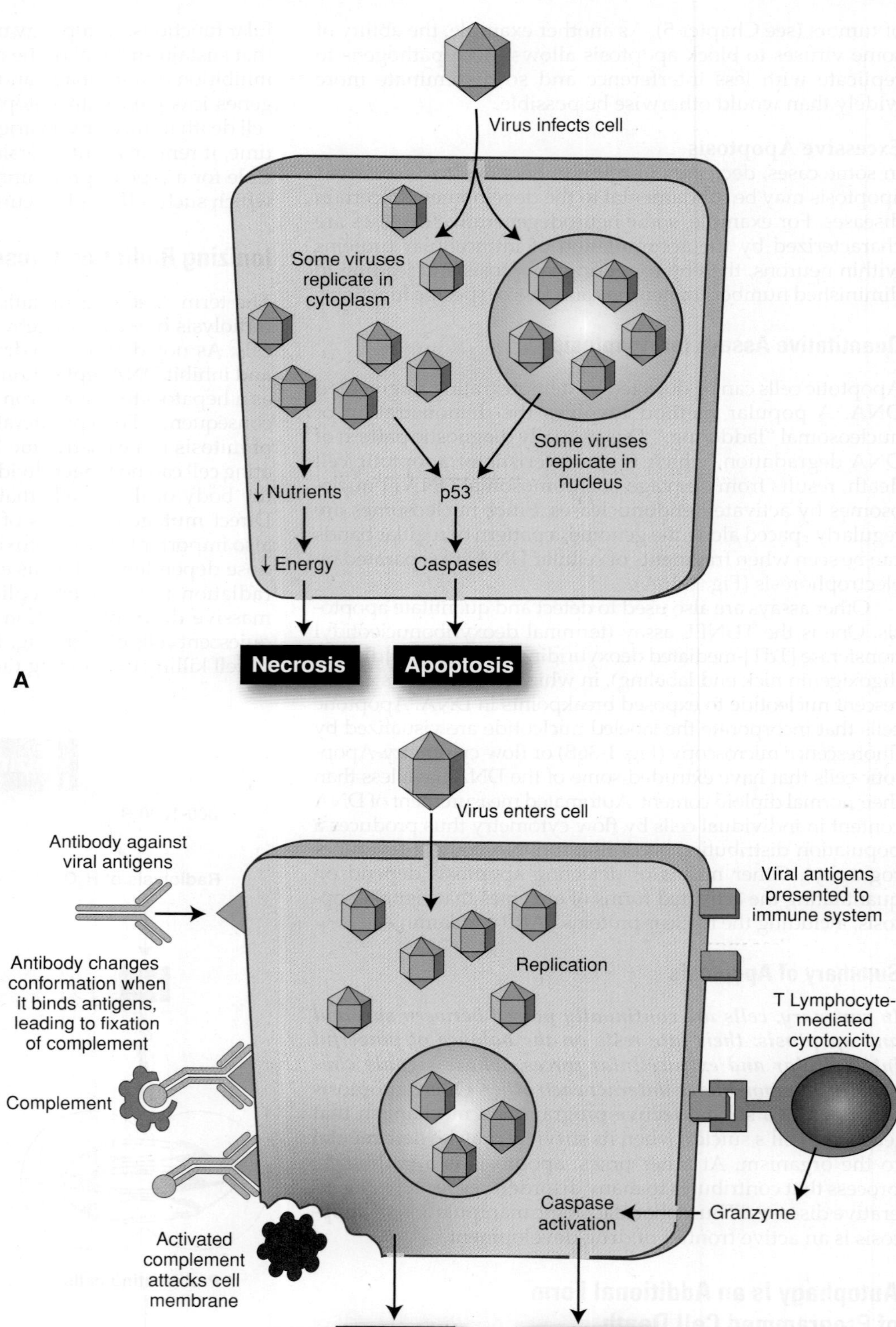

FIGURE 1-38. Cell injury caused by virus infection. A. Direct injury caused by virus infection, involving both depletion of cellular resources and activation of apoptotic signaling mechanisms. **B.** Mechanisms that lead to immunologically mediated destruction of virus-infected cells.

Viral Cytotoxicity May Be Direct or It May Be Immunologically Mediated

The means by which viruses cause cell injury and death are as diverse as viruses themselves. Unlike bacteria, a virus requires a cellular host to (1) house it; (2) provide enzymes, substrates and other resources for viral replication; and (3) serve as a source for dissemination when mature virions are ready to be spread to other cells. Viruses have evolved mechanisms by which they avoid biting the hand that feeds them (at least until they are ready for other hands). The ability of a virus to persist in an infected cell necessitates a parasitic, albeit temporary, relationship with the host cell. During this vulnerable phase, the virus plays a game of cat and mouse with the immune system as a device to evade elimination of the infected cell. This period is followed by a phase in which the virus disseminates, either by budding (which does not necessarily destroy the cell) or by lysis (which does). In some viral infections (e.g., herpes simplex, measles, zoster-varicella), infection of a host cell may last for many years or a lifetime, in which case the cell is not destroyed. There are patterns of cellular injury related to viral infections that deserve a brief mention:

- **Direct toxicity:** Viruses may injure cells directly by subverting cellular enzymes and depleting the cell's nutrients, thereby disrupting the normal homeostatic mechanisms. The mechanisms underlying virus-induced lysis of cells, however, are probably more complex (Fig. 1-38A).
- **Manipulation of apoptosis:** During their replicative cycle, and before virion assembly is complete, there are many viral activities that can elicit apoptosis. For example, apoptosis is activated when the cell detects episomal (extrachromosomal) DNA replication. Since viruses must avoid cell death before they have produced infectious progeny, they have evolved mechanisms to counteract this effect by upregulating antiapoptotic proteins and inhibiting proapoptotic ones. Some viruses also encode proteins that induce apoptosis once daughter virions are mature (Fig. 1-38A).
- **Immunologically mediated cytotoxicity:** Both humoral and cellular arms of the immune system protect against the harmful effects of viral infections by eliminating infected cells. Thus, presentation of viral proteins to the immune system in the context of a major histocompatibility complex (MHC) on cell surfaces leads to immune responses against the invader and elicits killer cells and antiviral antibodies. These arms of the immune system eliminate virus-infected cells by inducing apoptosis or by lysing the cell with complement (Fig. 1-38B) (see Chapter 4).

Chemicals May Injure Cells Directly and Indirectly

Innumerable chemicals can damage almost any cell in the body. The science of toxicology attempts to define the mechanisms that determine both target cell specificity and the mechanism of action of such chemicals. Toxic chemicals either (1) interact directly with cellular constituents without requiring metabolic activation or (2) are themselves not toxic but are metabolized to yield an ultimate toxin that interacts with the target cell. Whatever the mechanism, the result is usually necrotic cell death (see below).

Liver Necrosis Caused by the Metabolic Products of Chemicals

Studies of a few compounds that produce liver cell injury in rodents have enhanced our understanding of how chemicals injure cells. These studies have focused principally on those compounds that are converted to toxic metabolites. Carbon tetrachloride (CCl_4) and acetaminophen are well-studied hepatotoxins. Each is metabolized by the mixed-function oxidase system of the endoplasmic reticulum and each causes liver cell necrosis. These hepatotoxins are metabolized differently, and it is possible to relate the subsequent evolution of lethal cell injury to the specific features of this metabolism.

Carbon Tetrachloride

CCl_4 metabolism is a model system for toxicologic studies. CCl_4 is metabolized via the hepatic mixed-function oxygenase system (P450) to a chloride ion and a highly reactive trichloromethyl free radical ($CCl_3\bullet$).

$$CCl_4 + e^- \xrightarrow{P450} CCl_3\bullet + Cl^-$$

Like the hydroxyl radical, the trichloromethyl radical is a potent initiator of lipid peroxidation, although it may also interact with other macromolecules. However, in view of the rapidity with which CCl_4 kills cells (hours), peroxidative damage to the plasma membrane is the most likely culprit.

Acetaminophen

Acetaminophen, an important constituent of many analgesics, is innocuous in recommended doses, but when consumed to excess it is highly toxic to the liver. Overdose, both suicidal and accidental, is a common cause of acute liver failure. Most acetaminophen is enzymatically converted in the liver to nontoxic glucuronide or sulfate metabolites. Less than 5% of acetaminophen is ordinarily metabolized by isoforms of cytochrome P450 to NAPQI (*N*-acetyl-*p*-benzoquinone imine), a highly reactive quinone (Fig. 1-39). However, when large doses of acetaminophen overwhelm the glucuronidation pathway, toxic amounts of NAPQI are formed. NAPQI is responsible for acetaminophen-related toxicity by virtue of its conjugation with either GSH or sulfhydryl groups on liver proteins to form thiol esters. The latter cause extensive cellular dysfunction and lead to injury. At the same time, NAPQI depletes the antioxidant GSH, rendering the cell more susceptible to free radical–induced injury. Thus, conditions that deplete GSH (e.g., starvation) enhance the toxicity of acetaminophen. In addition, acetaminophen metabolism is accelerated by chronic alcohol consumption, an effect mediated by an ethanol-induced increase in the 3A4 isoform of P450. As a result, toxic amounts of NAPQI rapidly accumulate and may destroy the liver.

To summarize, metabolism of hepatotoxic chemicals by mixed-function oxidation leads to cell injury through covalent binding of reactive metabolites and peroxidation of membrane phospholipids. Lipid peroxidation is initiated by (1) a metabolite of the original compound (as with CCl_4) or (2) ROS formed during the metabolism of the toxin (as with acetaminophen), the latter augmented by weakened antioxidant defenses.

Chemicals That Are Not Metabolized

Directly cytotoxic chemicals interact with cellular constituents; prior metabolic conversion is not needed. The critical cellular targets are diverse and include, for example,

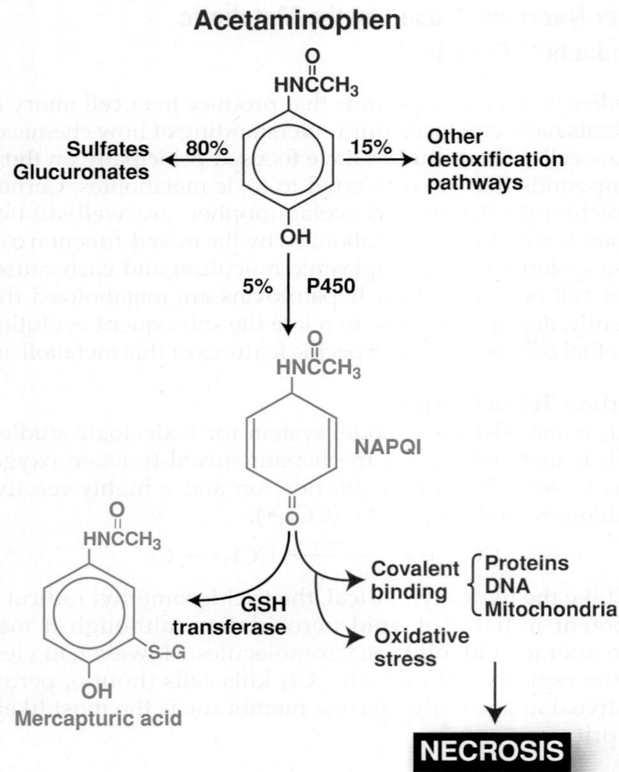

FIGURE 1-39. Chemical reactions involved in acetaminophen hepatotoxicity. *GSH* = glutathione; *NAPQI* = *N*-acetyl-*p*-benzoquinone imine.

mitochondria (heavy metals and cyanide), cytoskeleton (phalloidin, paclitaxel) and DNA (chemotherapeutic alkylating agents). Also, interaction of directly cytotoxic chemicals with glutathione (alkylating agents) weakens the cell's antioxidant defenses.

Biological Aging

The actress Bette Davis once remarked that old age is not for sissies. What she did not mention was that old age tends to be a consequence of living in modern society. It is rarely encountered in the wild among animals or in primitive human societies. From an evolutionary perspective, the aging process presents conceptual difficulties. Since animals in the wild usually do not attain their maximum life span, how did longevity come about? Biological longevity, which is generally interpreted as the extension of life well beyond the period of reproduction and childrearing, would not be expected to impart a selective advantage to a species and so should not significantly impact evolution. Nonetheless, it is clear that most humans survive well beyond their reproductive years. What determines lifespan? How do organisms change as a function of age?

Biological aging can be defined as a constellation of deleterious functional and structural changes that are inevitable consequences of longevity. Importantly, aging must be distinguished from disease. Although the aging process may increase vulnerability to many diseases, it is independent of the pathogenesis of any specific illness.

Maximal Life Span Has Remained Unchanged

Millennia ago the psalmist sang of a natural life span of 70 years, which with vigor may extend to 80. By contrast, it is estimated that the usual age at death of Neolithic humans was 20 to 25 years, and the average life span today in some underdeveloped regions is often barely 10 years more.

The difference between humans in primitive and in more developed environments is analogous to that observed between animals in their natural habitat and those in a zoo (Fig. 1-40). After an initial high mortality during maturation, animals in the wild experience a progressive linear decline in survival, ending at the maximum life span of the species. This steady decrease in the number of mature animals does not reflect aging but rather sporadic events, such as encounters with beasts of prey, accidental trauma, infection, starvation and so on. On the other hand, survival in the protected environment of a zoo is characterized by slow attrition until old age, at which time the steep decline in numbers is attributable to the aging process. ***Although such an environment offers protection from predation, it does not alter the maximum attainable life span significantly.*** An analogous situation is seen in studies of the human death rate. Less than a century ago, the steep linear slope of mortality in adults principally reflected random accidents and infections. With improved safety and sanitation, antibiotics and other drugs, and better diagnostic and therapeutic methods, the age-adjusted death rate in the United States has declined by 35% since 1970. In 2007, life expectancy at the time of birth was 80.4 years for women and 75.3 years for men.

Yet, the maximum human life span remains constant at about 105 years, although a very small proportion of the population may live longer than that. Even if diseases associated with old age, such as cardiovascular disease and cancer, were eliminated, only a modest increase in average life expectancy would be seen. A long period of good health and low mortality rate would be followed by a precipitously increased mortality owing to biological aging itself. Given the current life expectancy, the prevention or cure of the causes of premature death would have little impact on mean longevity.

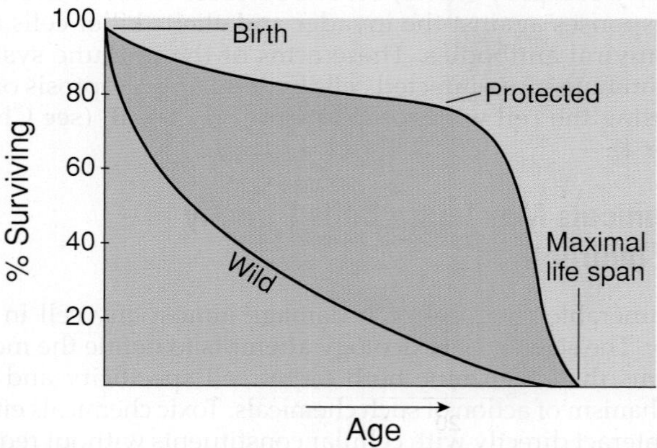

FIGURE 1-40. Life span of animals in their natural environment compared with that in a protected habitat. Note that both curves reach the same maximal life span.

Why do women live longer than men? Greater female longevity is almost universal in the animal kingdom. The male-to-female ratio at birth is 106:100, but from that time on, more women than men survive at every age, and at age 75 the male-to-female ratio is approximately 2:3. At the cellular level, somatic cells from females are no hardier than those from males. Factors involved in the difference in average human longevity include the greater male mortality from violent causes and greater susceptibility to cardiovascular disease, cancer, respiratory illness and cirrhosis in middle and old age. Historical differences between the sexes in cigarette smoking and alcoholism also contribute to the gender gap in longevity. Thus, men who escape these hazards can look forward to a longevity that is only slightly less than that in women.

Aging Is Characterized by Functional and Structural Deterioration

The insidious effects of aging can be detected in otherwise healthy persons. In many sports, an athlete in his or her 30s may be considered "old." Even in the absence of specific diseases or vascular abnormalities, beginning in the fourth decade of life there is a progressive decline in many physiologic functions (Fig. 1-41), including such easily measurable parameters as muscular strength, cardiac reserve, nerve conduction time, pulmonary vital capacity, glomerular filtration and vascular elasticity. These functional deteriorations are accompanied by structural changes. Lean body mass decreases and the proportion of fat rises. Constituents of the connective tissue matrix are progressively cross-linked. Lipofuscin ("wear and tear") pigment accumulates in organs such as the brain, heart and liver.

For some parameters the most noticeable impact of aging is on the effective response to increased functional demand. Thus, although resting pulse rate may be unchanged, maximal increases with exercise decline with age, and the time that is required for the heart rate to return to normal is prolonged. Similarly, elderly people may show impaired adaptation to an ingested carbohydrate load; fasting blood glucose levels are often similar to those seen in younger people, but they rise higher after a carbohydrate meal and return to normal more slowly.

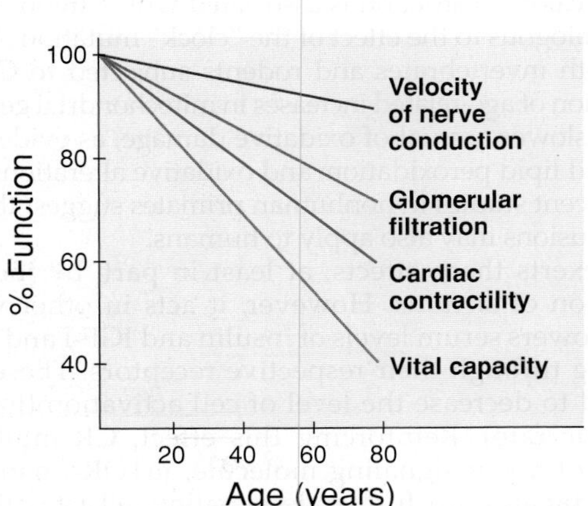

FIGURE 1-41. Decrease in human physiologic capacities as a function of age.

Diverse Experimental Systems Are Used to Elucidate Different Aspects of the Physiology of Aging

The study of biological aging focuses on the nature and causes of the processes that underlie the progressive loss of physiologic and structural robustness. There is no general agreement as to the mechanisms by which aging occurs. However, experimental observations in cultured cells, lower animals and humans have identified a number of factors that influence the progression of age-related changes.

Tissue Culture Studies

Cells in culture lend themselves to a variety of genetic and environmental manipulations that facilitate the isolation and identification of important influences on the ability of cells to replenish those that have been lost. In this context normal cultured human fibroblasts undergo about 50 population doublings, after which they stop dividing and are irreversibly arrested in the G_1 phase of the cell cycle. This process is called **replicative senescence**. Moreover, cells from persons afflicted with a syndrome of precocious aging, such as progeria (see below), display a conspicuously reduced number of population doublings in vitro. However, if normal cells in culture are exposed to an oncogenic virus or a chemical carcinogen, they continue to replicate indefinitely (i.e., they are **immortalized**).

Although immortalization does not in itself confer tumorigenic capacity, it is a step in that direction (see Chapter 5). Thus, an increase in a cell's replicative abilities may rescue it from senescence at the cost of leading it down the road toward tumor development. However, as we shall see below, some factors that facilitate carcinogenesis may also accelerate cell loss and impair cellular longevity.

Whole Animal Models

Most experiments on the aging of animals are performed in the roundworm (*Caenorhabditis elegans*), the fruit fly (*Drosophila*) and rodents, because of their short life spans and the ease of manipulation. Much less work has been done in higher mammals, but interesting correlations have been drawn from studies in humans and in nonhuman primates (see below).

Telomeres, Telomerase and Senescence

Telomeres are a series of short repetitive nucleotide sequences (TTAGGG in vertebrates) located at the 3′ ends of the DNA in chromosomes. Since DNA polymerase, which replicates DNA from the 5′ end to the 3′ end, cannot copy the linear chromosomes all the way to their tips, telomeres tend to shorten with each cell division. In this way, telomeres serve several important functions. They protect genes that are important for cell viability and replication that are near the termini of chromosomes from being lost with repeated cell divisions. It may be said that they act as a "replicative clock" (i.e., they keep track of and limit the number of divisions a cell may undergo).

To overcome these end replication limitations, many eukaryotic cells express a ribonucleoprotein enzyme, **telomerase,** which extends the length of telomeres at the ends of chromosomes and allows continued cell division. Because human cells have short telomeres, continued telomerase expression occurs in tissues that undergo frequent self-renewal (e.g., the gastrointestinal mucosa). In other cells the shortening of telomeres with each cycle of cell division functions as a tumor-suppressing mechanism, limiting cell proliferative capacity in vivo. Many human tumors thus display continued expression of telomerase (see Chapter 5).

Telomere shortening in blood mononuclear cells has been found to correlate as a marker with the presence of several age-related diseases, such as atherosclerosis and Alzheimer disease. The appearance of very short telomeres in hematopoietic progenitor cells, which normally proliferate rapidly, has been reported in aplastic anemia, a disorder characterized by replicative failure of those cells.

However, a simple explanation of the role of replicative senescence in either aging or tumor suppression is unlikely. First, many species (e.g., mice) have very long telomeres, and yet they age, obviously independently of telomere shortening. Because of these long telomeres, murine tumors do not require telomerase. By contrast, shortened telomeres are seen in a number of conditions associated with tumor development, such as Barrett esophagus, cirrhosis of the liver, some myeloproliferative syndromes and the preinvasive (in situ) stages of some forms of human cancers.

Although the potential connection between replicative senescence as a mechanism of aging and its role in tumor suppression is alluring, it remains conjectural. At this time, it may be useful to consider telomere shortening as an unindicted coconspirator in aging.

Genetic and Environmental Factors Influence Aging

In the roundworm, *C. elegans*, single-gene mutations (*Age* mutations) have been identified that extend life span up to fivefold, a greater increase than has been reported for any other model. In addition to prolonging the life span, *Age* mutations in *C. elegans* also confer a complex array of other phenotypes. For example, the so-called clock *(clk)* mutations slow most functions that relate to the overall metabolic rate (cell cycle progression, swimming, food pumping, etc.) (see below). *Age* mutations also confer resistance to both environmental (extrinsic) and intrinsic stresses, including ROS, heat shock and UV radiation. Thus, genes that prolong life in *C. elegans* apparently act to reduce the accumulation of cellular "injuries" that tend to shorten the worm's life span.

In experiments with *Drosophila,* strains of long-lived flies can be readily created by breeding the oldest flies with each other. In such studies, the better health of the aged flies is associated with a "trade-off" of decreased fitness in the young flies, as evidenced by decreased activity and fertility compared to wild-type flies. Thus, the original population seems to have a set of alleles that yields greater fitness at a young age and decreased fitness at an older one, a phenomenon termed **antagonistic pleiotropy**. This doctrine also applies to the protection against cancer by tumor suppressor mechanisms that may also compromise the ability of the organism to reach old age.

Sirtuins and Aging

Sirtuins are a family of proteins that have been highly conserved throughout evolution. Mammals have seven such proteins, the most studied of which is Sirt1. These proteins are NAD-dependent deacetylases that have a wide range of functions. Under most circumstances, Sirt1 promotes cell survival and stress resistance (see below), although in some settings,

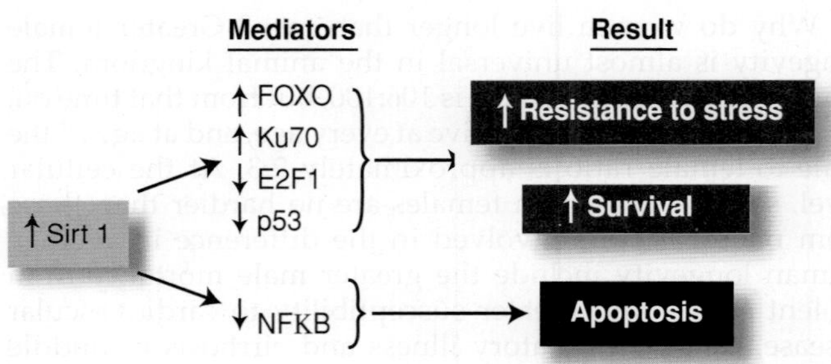

FIGURE 1-42. Sirtuin-1 and its activities. Sirtuins are NAD/NADH-dependent protein deacetylating enzymes. When activated, they increase the activities of the forkhead transcription factor FOXO and the antiapoptotic Bcl-2 homolog Ku70. The activities of E2F1 and p53 are decreased. As a result, cells display improved resistance to stress and survival. Activity of the transcription factor nuclear factor-κB (NFκB) may also be decreased. Lower levels of NFκB may favor apoptosis.

it may downregulate the prosurvival factor NFκB, thereby facilitating apoptosis (Fig. 1-42). In both *C. elegans* and *Drosophila*, overexpression of *sirt1* homologs increases life span about 50%. In mammals, manipulations that extend life span are associated with increased levels of Sirt1 (see below).

Sirt1 deacetylase activity promotes cell survival by inhibiting apoptosis in several ways. It activates a protein called Ku70, leading to increased Bax sequestration in the cytosol. As a consequence, Bax cannot activate the mitochondrial permeability transition pore. Sirt1 also activates a transcription factor, FOXO1, which directs increased transcription of DNA repair enzymes while repressing transcription of proapoptotic proteins. Among its many functions, Sirt1 also inactivates p53. Sirt1 thus is likely to act in many ways and may play an important role in fostering longevity.

Caloric Restriction, Sirtuins and Extended Life Span

Caloric restriction (CR) in rodents and lower species has long been known to increase longevity. Unfortunately, there is currently little evidence to support the extension of human life span by CR, although studies in nonhuman primates do show a lower incidence of age-related diseases in monkeys treated with CR. There is evidence to indicate that the extension of rodent life span by caloric restriction is associated with a hypometabolic state, analogous to the effect of the "clock" mutations in *C. elegans*. Both invertebrates and rodents subjected to CR show attenuation of age-related increases in mitochondrial generation of ROS; slower accrual of oxidative damage, as evidenced by decreased lipid peroxidation; and oxidative alterations of proteins. Recent studies in nonhuman primates suggest that similar conclusions may also apply to humans.

CR exerts these effects, at least in part, by increasing expression of sirtuins. However, it acts in other ways as well. It lowers serum levels of insulin and IGF-I and inhibits signaling through their respective receptors. These activities tend to decrease the level of cell activation (increased metabolic rate). Reinforcing this effect, CR inhibits the activity of a key signaling molecule, mTOR (mammalian target of rapamycin), further decelerating cell activation (Fig. 1-43). Interestingly, recent reports suggest that rapamycin (which also lowers mTOR activity) increases longevity in rodents.

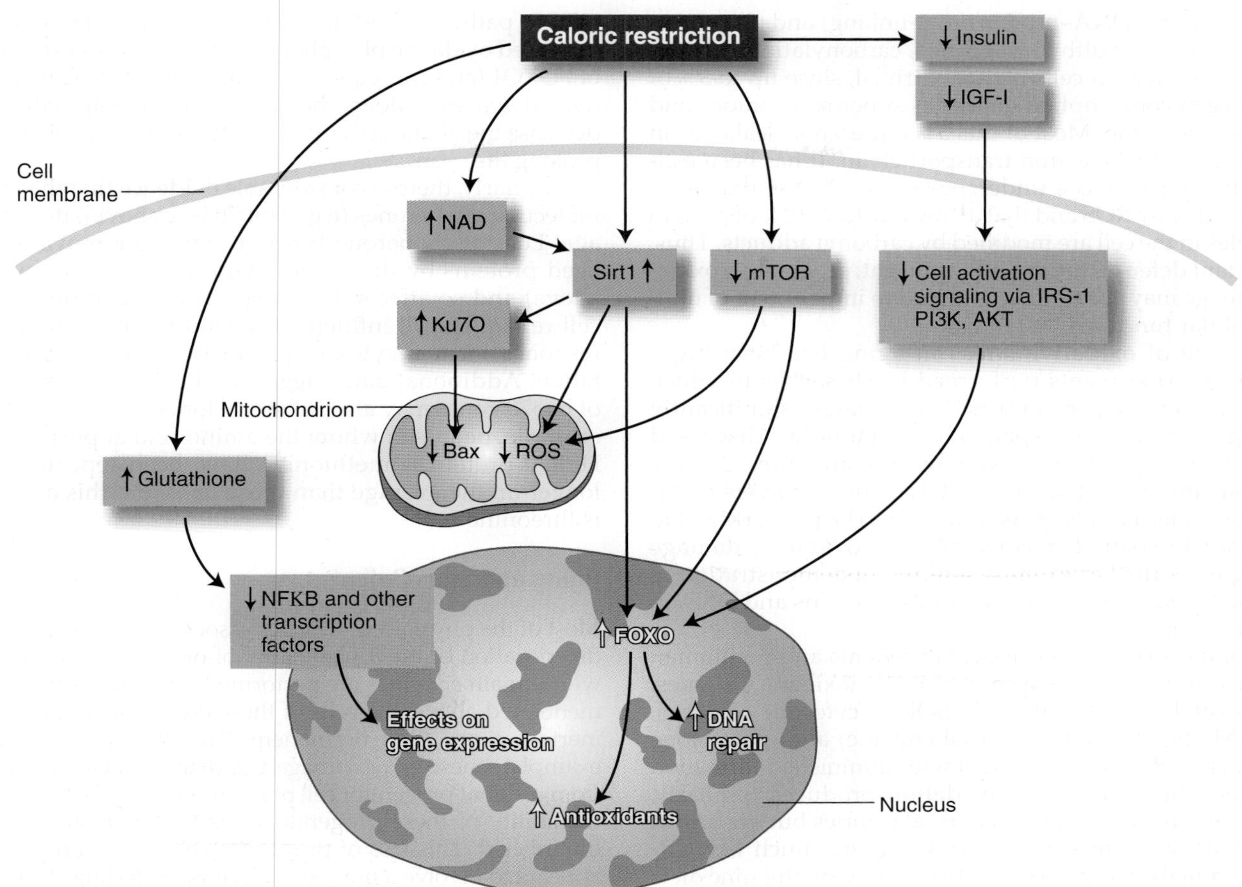

FIGURE 1-43. Consequences of caloric restriction on cell metabolism and survival pathways. Caloric restriction (CR) promotes cellular resistance to stress, inhibits apoptosis, promotes DNA repair and increases cellular production of antioxidants. CR lowers blood insulin-like growth factor-I (IGF-I) and insulin levels, in turn decreasing signaling by these factors through insulin response substrate-1 (IRS-1), phosphoinositol-3-kinase (PI3K) and AKT. It also decreases activity of the mammalian target of rapamycin (mTOR) and increases Sirt1. All these functions increase the activity of FOXO, leading to improved DNA repair and increased antioxidant production. As indicated in Fig. 1-42, increased Sirt1 activity also promotes survival by increasing Ku70 and thus inhibiting Bax. CR increases cellular stores of the antioxidant glutathione (GSH). This, in turn, may decrease nuclear factor-κB (NFκB) activity.

p53 and Aging

p53, a versatile molecule that is involved in apoptosis (see above), cell cycle control, tumor suppression (see Chapter 5) and transcriptional regulation, also plays a role in aging. It is normally present in the cytosol complexed with Mdm2, an E3 ubiquitin ligase that regulates p53 levels by directing its proteasomal degradation. In response to DNA damage, telomere shortening, oxidative stress, oncogene activation and other stimuli, Mdm2 may be degraded, thereby releasing p53. Acting via several intermediates that are tumor suppressor proteins, p53 directs both cell cycle arrest and apoptosis. While such activities are beneficial in preventing cells with severe DNA damage and oncogene activation from surviving, they also suggest that p53 activation may curtail longevity. In fact, shortened life expectancies, such as may be seen in mice lacking Ku70 or several tumor suppressor genes, can be rectified by knocking out p53. Conversely, mice with increased p53 expression or decreased Mdm2 have shortened life spans and are prone to accelerated development of degenerative changes, such as atrophy of organs, skin and bones and poor tolerance to stress (see below). Thus, the tumor suppressor activity of p53 may perversely be associated with decreased longevity.

Some epidemiologic observations in people support this possibility. In humans, there is a pleomorphism of p53 at codon 72. Some populations, generally near the equator, are homozygous for proline in that position, whereas people farther north tend to have arginine instead. Although the latter genotype of p53 provides more effective protection against cancer, after correcting for that, people homozygous for proline at codon 72 show 40% increased survival. Thus, a measure of protection from tumors may be purchased at the cost of decreased longevity.

The Impact of Stress on Aging

Oxidative stress is an invariable consequence of life in an atmosphere rich in oxygen. An important hypothesis holds that the loss of function that is characteristic of aging is caused by progressive and irreversible accrual of molecular oxidative damage. Such lesions may be manifested as (1) peroxidation of membrane lipids, (2) DNA modifications (strand breaks, base alterations, DNA–protein cross-linking) and (3) protein oxidation (loss of sulfhydryl groups, carbonylation). Oxidative stress in normal cells is hardly trivial, since up to 3% of total oxygen consumption generates superoxide anions and hydrogen peroxide. Most of this 3% represents "leakage" in the mitochondrial electron transport chain. It has been estimated that a single cell undergoes some 100,000 attacks on DNA per day by ROS and that at any one time 10% of protein molecules in the cell are modified by carbonyl adducts. Thus, antioxidant defenses are not fully efficient; progressive oxidative damage may accumulate and lead to impairment of multiple cellular functions.

The role of oxidative stress in aging has been highlighted by experiments performed in *Drosophila* in which overexpression of genes for SOD or catalase significantly prolongs the fly's life span. Furthermore, as discussed above, virtually all long-lived worms and flies display increased antioxidant defenses. SOD activity in livers of different primates has also been reported to be proportional to maximal life span. The correlation of oxidative damage with aging is further exemplified by the demonstration of increased oxidative damage to lipids, proteins and DNA in aged animals.

Caloric restriction (see above) in rodents and nonhuman primates increases the expression of antioxidant enzymes, such as catalase, SOD1 (Cu/Zn SOD, a cytosolic enzyme), SOD2 (Mn SOD, a mitochondrial enzyme) and glutathione peroxidase. CR is also associated with diminished formation of protein, lipid and DNA oxidation products. Similarly, rodents fed diets that contain normal calories but are low in methionine show increased longevity, very much like CR-treated animals. The protective effect of low-methionine diets has been attributed to reduced generation of ROS and diminished oxidative injury to cellular macromolecules. Interestingly, tissue amino acid levels were measured among eight mammalian species and compared to species longevity. Only methionine levels demonstrated a significant relationship with life span: species with lower tissue methionine levels lived longer.

Stress comes in many forms, and per se it is not an unmitigated villain in an organism's life-and-death struggle. Thus, episodic stress may prolong survival and lead to improved stress resistance. *C. elegans* worms selected for the highest levels of expression of heat shock proteins in response to stress survive longer. It was noted above that ischemic conditioning strengthens the heart and improves cardiac survival in the face of oxygen deprivation.

Lest one become too comfortable with the idea that aging basically represents accumulated oxidative or other injury, it should be emphasized that a number of studies have been done in many hundreds of thousands of people given antioxidant dietary supplements. These studies have failed to demonstrate any significant impact of antioxidants on human life span, disease development or health.

Accelerated Aging Is Associated With Accelerated Metabolism

Many of the factors that extend life in experimental systems are associated with decelerated metabolism, decreased mitochondrial activity and improved adaptation to stress. Conditions that lead to increased cellular metabolic activity are also associated with decreased longevity. Thus, increased IGF-I, insulin and growth hormone signaling and increased activation of the mTOR pathway lead to increased utilization of glucose, increased oxidative phosphorylation and decreased activation of FOXO1 (and consequently in impaired FOXO1-related oxidant defenses). Along the same lines, manipulations that decrease metabolic activity (e.g., CR or a low-methionine diet) prolong life span.

Similarly, there is considerable evidence that the levels of molecular chaperones (e.g., HSP70 [see above]) decline with age. Loss of chaperone function impairs removal of damaged proteins by the ubiquitin–proteasomal pathway (see above) and so affects many aspects of organ function and cell repair. Hsp70 influences several facets of the immune response, such as cytokine production and antigen presentation. Additional data suggest that allelic polymorphisms of hsp70 genes may also influence longevity in humans. For example, people in whom the amino acid at position 493 of HSP70 protein is methionine have been reported to live longer on the average than those in whom this amino acid is threonine.

Aging and Stem Cells

Most of the physiologic changes associated with aging involve deterioration of the functionality of organs (e.g., heart, brain) whose main activities are performed by nondividing cells. As mentioned above, the cells of these organs are not mitotically inert, nor are they permanent. Turnover does occur. For example, senescent or damaged cardiac myocytes are replaced from resident progenitor cell populations. However, with aging the ability of these progenitor cells to replenish lost cells is diminished. This loss of progenitor cell regenerative capacity appears to involve a number of factors, including (1) impaired DNA repair mechanisms and (2) accumulation of mitotic inhibitors, such as the tumor suppressors $p16^{INK4A}$, $p14^{ARF}$ and p53. In particular, the activities of $p16^{INK4A}$ and $p14^{ARF}$ are regulated by a group of proteins called polycomb (PcG). Engineered loss of PcG proteins leads to premature impairment of stem cell function and organ failure (Fig. 1-44). The balance between PcG and those cell cycle control proteins changes in response to stimuli such as DNA damage. Many human diseases of premature aging involve loss of proteins that are important in DNA repair processes (see below). Decreased function of the tumor suppressor $p14^{ARF}$ has been associated in mice with decreased frailty, and loss of this gene promotes continued robust hematopoietic and other stem cell activity with increasing age.

Diseases of Premature Aging

In humans, the modest correlation in longevity between related persons and the excellent concordance of life span among identical twins lend credence to the concept that aging is influenced by genetic factors. The existence of heritable diseases associated with accelerated aging buttresses this notion. The entire process of aging, including features such as male-pattern baldness, cataracts and coronary artery disease, is compressed into a span of less than 10 years in a genetic syndrome termed **Hutchinson-Guilford progeria** (Fig. 1-45). The cause of progeria is apparently a mutation in the *LMNA* gene, whose product is a protein termed **lamin A**. The mutant gene codes for a defective precursor of the lamin A protein, which has been termed **progerin.** This abnormal protein accumulates in the nucleus from one cell generation to the next, thereby interfering with its structural integrity, resulting in a

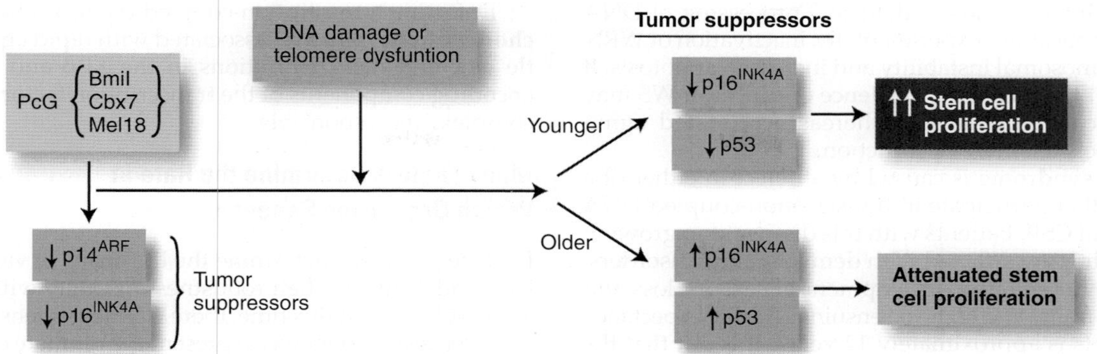

FIGURE 1-44. Polycomb group protein (PcG) effects on stem cell function in younger and older individuals. PcG, a complex of three proteins, generally inhibits the functioning of the cell cycle control proteins p14^{ARF} and p16^{INK4A}. The PcG complex may be activated by a number of cell injury–related stimuli. In younger individuals, it inhibits p14^{ARF}- and p16^{INK4A}-mediated cell cycle control, facilitating stem cell proliferation to repair or replace the injured tissue. In older individuals, poorer PcG activity leads to a different response to such injury: increased activity of p14^{ARF} and p16^{INK4A} leads to lower stem cell proliferative activity and less effective stem cell proliferation.

lobulated shape. The buildup of progerin also interferes with the organization of nuclear heterochromatin, a component that is thought to regulate the expression of numerous genes. Interestingly, the nuclear changes in cells from patients with progeria were corrected by treating the cells with inhibitors of farnesyltransferase, an enzyme that prevents progerin from becoming farnesylated. Experimental suppression of the production of progerin has also corrected the nuclear changes in cultured cells from patients with progeria.

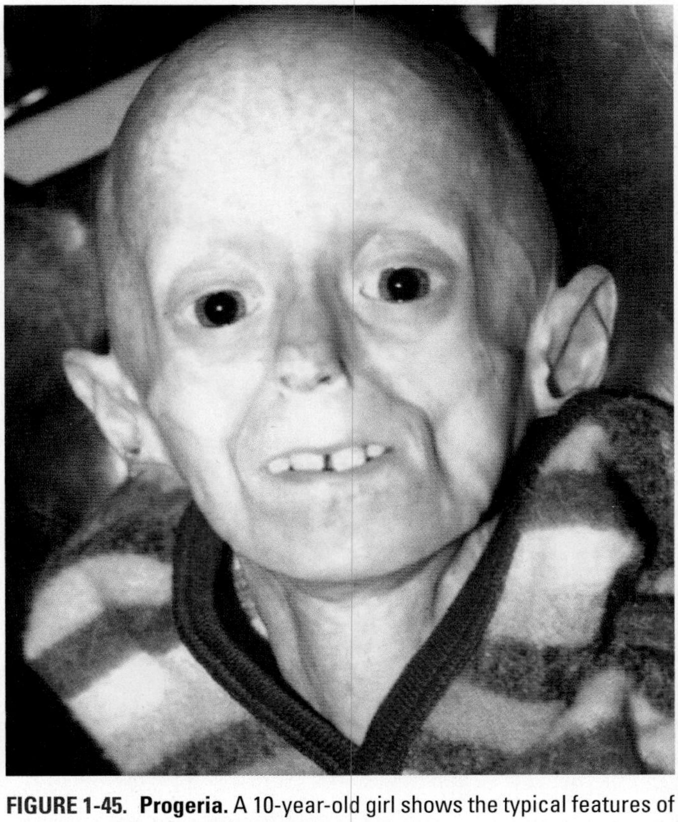

FIGURE 1-45. Progeria. A 10-year-old girl shows the typical features of premature aging associated with progeria.

Hutchinson-Guilford progeria is now recognized to be one of about 10 disorders associated with mutations in the *LMNA* gene, comprising a group termed "laminopathies." It is not known whether changes in lamin A contribute to the aging process, but cell nuclei from aged persons demonstrate defects similar to those seen in cells from patients with progeria.

Werner syndrome (WS) is a rare autosomal recessive disease characterized by early cataracts, hair loss, atrophy of the skin, osteoporosis and atherosclerosis. Affected persons are also at increased risk for the development of a variety of cancers. Patients typically die in the fifth decade from either cancer or cardiovascular disease. This phenotype of patients with WS gives the impression of premature aging. WS is caused by loss of function of the Werner (WRN) gene, which codes for a protein with multiple DNA-dependent enzymatic activities, including ATPase, helicase, exonuclease and strand annealing. There is experimental evidence that WRN plays a role in the resolution of replication blockage and in telomere

Table 1-6

Experimental Factors That Influence Biological Aging

Factors That Increase Longevity	Factors That Decrease Longevity
Mutations in p53, p14^{ARF}, p16^{INK4A}, etc.	Increased p53 activation
Decreased metabolic rate	Increased metabolic rate
Caloric restriction	Increased oxidative stress
Increased Sirt1	Increased mTOR activity
Age mutations	Increased cell cycle control proteins
Increased antioxidant defenses Episodic stress Genetic factors	Genetic factors

mTOR = mammalian target of rapamycin.

maintenance. Its loss leads to defective processing of DNA damage and replication. Experimentally, inactivation of WRN results in chromosomal instability and increased apoptosis. It is thought that the increased incidence of cancer in WS may reflect chromosomal changes, whereas accelerated aging probably reflects telomere dysfunction.

Cockayne syndrome is caused by a defect in either of a pair of genes that participate in transcription-coupled DNA repair, CSA and CSB. Patients with this disease stop growing early in life. They are afflicted with demyelinating disorders, leading to very premature development of sensory loss and cataracts, with frailty and cachexia ensuing. The life expectancy of such patients is approximately 12 years. It is felt that the enzyme defects responsible for this syndrome lead to cells accumulating DNA damage, causing defects in transcription and eventuating in cell death.

Defective transcription-coupled repair is also seen in **trichodystrophy**, which is associated with rapid aging and brittle hair and nails. Mutations in the XPB and XPD genes, encoding components of the transcription factor IIH helicase complex, are responsible.

Many Factors Determine the Rate at Which Organisms Senesce

Diverse processes determine the life spans of various organisms and influence their robustness or frailty with advancing age (Table 1-6). At this time, there is little consensus, save that senescence and longevity represent the ultimate expression of the interplay of many mechanisms that are involved in cell injury, repair and death. A unitary explanation for biological aging remains elusive.

2 Inflammation

Hedwig S. Murphy

Inflammation is a reaction, both systemic and local, of tissues and microcirculation to a pathogenic insult. It is characterized by elaboration of inflammatory mediators and movement of fluid and leukocytes from the blood into extravascular tissues. This response localizes and eliminates altered cells, foreign particles, microorganisms and antigens and paves the way for the return to normal structure and function.

The clinical signs of inflammation, termed *phlogosis* by the Greek physician Galen, and *inflammation* in Latin, were described in classical times. In the first century AD, the Roman encyclopedist Aulus Celsus described the four cardinal signs of inflammation, namely, **rubor** (redness), **calor** (heat), **tumor** (swelling) and **dolor** (pain). These features correspond to inflammatory events of vasodilation, edema and tissue damage. According to medieval concepts, inflammation represented an imbalance of various "humors," including blood, mucus and bile. Modern appreciation of the vascular basis of inflammation began in the 18th century with John Hunter, who noted dilation of blood vessels and appreciated that pus was accumulated material derived from the blood. Rudolf Virchow first described inflammation as a reaction to prior tissue injury. To the four cardinal signs he added a fifth: **functio laesa** (loss of function). Virchow's pupil Julius Cohnheim was the first to associate inflammation with emigration of leukocytes through the walls of the microvasculature. At the end of the 19th century, the role of phagocytosis in inflammation was emphasized by the eminent Russian zoologist Eli Metchnikoff. Finally, the importance of chemical mediators was described in 1927 by Thomas Lewis, who showed that histamine and other substances increased vascular permeability and caused migration of leukocytes into extravascular spaces. More recent studies have elucidated the molecular and genetic bases of acute and chronic inflammation.

Overview of Inflammation

The primary function of the inflammatory response is to eliminate a pathogenic insult and remove injured tissue components, thereby allowing tissue repair to take place. The body attempts to contain or eliminate offending agents, thereby protecting tissues, organs and, ultimately, the whole body from damage. Specific cells are imported to attack and

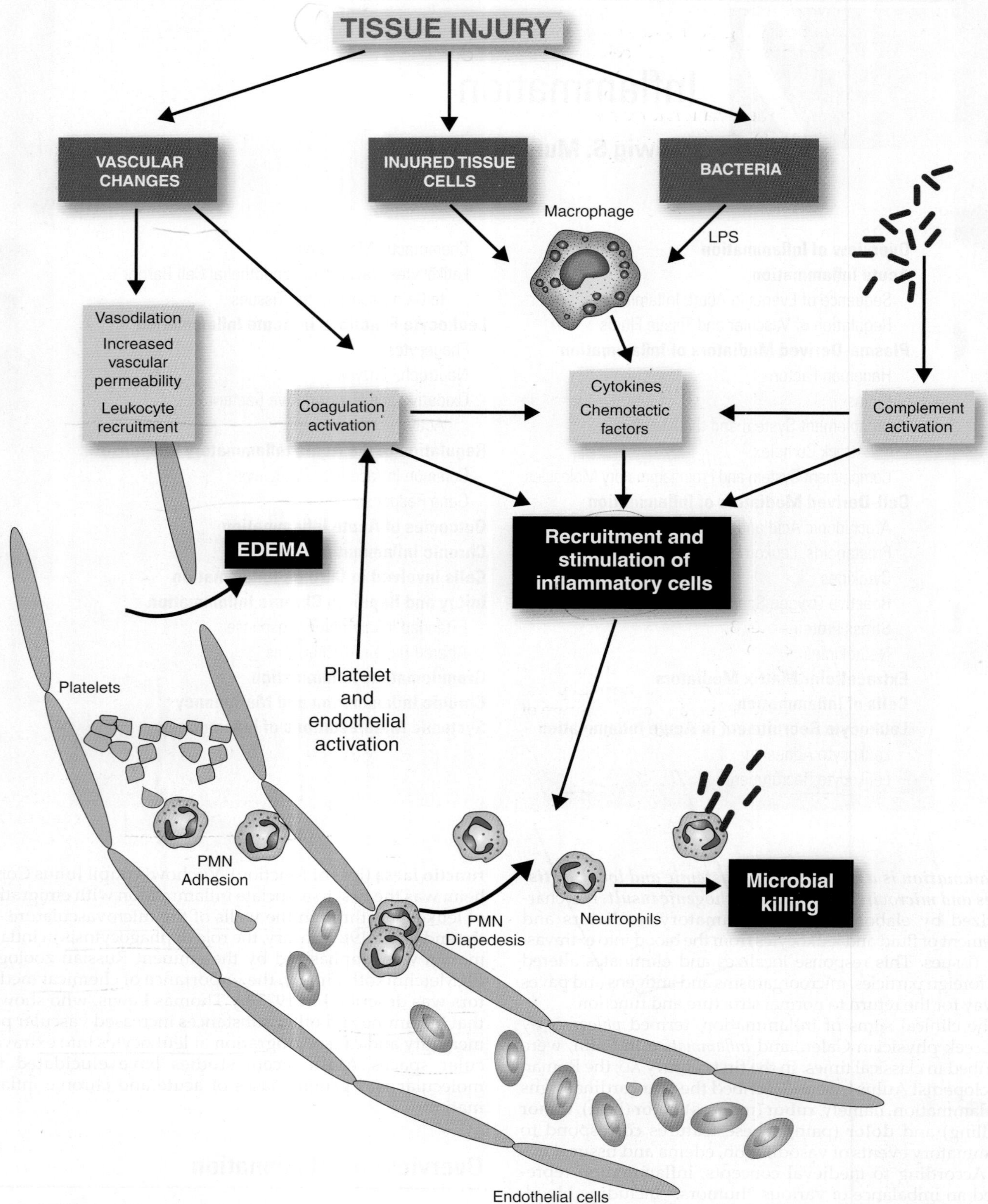

FIGURE 2-1. The inflammatory response to injury. Chemical mediators and cells are released from plasma following tissue injury. Vasodilation and vascular injury lead to leakage of fluid into tissues (edema). Platelets are activated to initiate clot formation and hemostasis and to increase vascular permeability via histamine release. Vascular endothelial cells contribute to clot formation, retract to allow increased vascular permeability and anchor circulating neutrophils via their adhesion molecules. Microbes (*red rods*) initiate activation of the complement cascade, which, along with soluble mediators from macrophages, recruit neutrophils to the site of tissue injury. Neutrophils eliminate microbes and remove damaged tissue so that repair can begin. *PMN* = polymorphonuclear neutrophil.

destroy injurious agents (e.g., infectious organisms, toxins or foreign material), enzymatically digest and remove them, or wall them off. During this process, damaged cells and tissues are digested and removed to allow repair to take place. The response to many damaging agents is immediate and stereotypic. The character of the inflammatory response is "modulated" depending on several factors, including the nature of the offending agent, duration of the insult, extent of tissue damage and microenvironment.

- **Initiation** of an inflammatory response results in activation of soluble mediators and recruitment of inflammatory cells to the area. Molecules are released from the offending agent, damaged cells and the extracellular matrix that alter the permeability of adjacent blood vessels to plasma, soluble molecules and circulating inflammatory cells. This stereotypic, immediate response leads to rapid flooding of injured tissues with fluid, coagulation factors, cytokines, chemokines, platelets and inflammatory cells, neutrophils in particular (Figs. 2-1 and 2-2). This overall process is termed **acute inflammation.**
- **Amplification** depends on the extent of injury and activation of mediators such as kinins and complement components. Additional leukocytes and macrophages are recruited to the area.
- **Destruction** of the damaging agent brings the process under control. Enzymatic digestion and phagocytosis reduce or eliminate foreign material or infectious organisms. At the same time, damaged tissue components are also removed and debris is cleared away, paving the way for repair to begin (see Chapter 3).
- **Termination** of the inflammatory response is mediated by intrinsic anti-inflammatory mechanisms that limit tissue damage and allow for repair and a return to normal physiologic function. Alternatively, depending on the nature of the injury and the specific inflammatory and repair response, a scar may develop in place of normal tissue. Importantly, intrinsic mechanisms are in place to terminate the inflammatory process; to prevent further influx of fluid, mediators and inflammatory cells; and to avoid digesting normal cells and tissue.

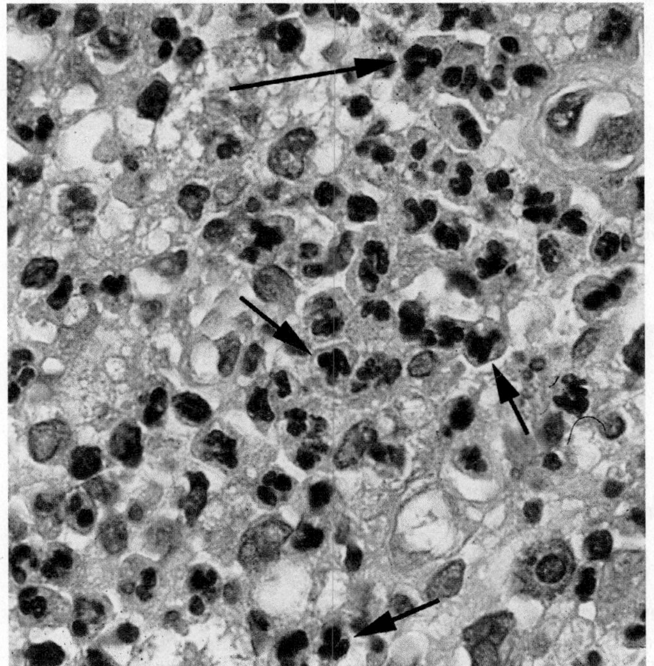

FIGURE 2-2. Acute inflammation with densely packed polymorphonuclear neutrophils (PMNs) with multilobed nuclei (*arrows*).

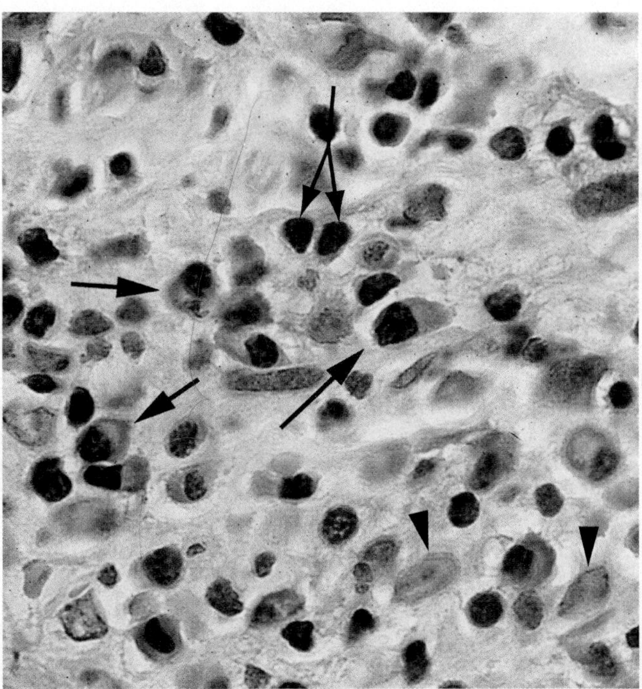

FIGURE 2-3. Chronic inflammation. Lymphocytes (*double-headed arrow*), plasma cells (*arrows*) and a few macrophages (*arrowheads*) are present.

Certain types of injury trigger a sustained immune and inflammatory response with the inability to clear injured tissue and foreign agents. Such a persistent response is termed **chronic inflammation.** Chronic inflammatory infiltrates are composed largely of lymphocytes, plasma cells and macrophages (Fig. 2-3). Acute and chronic inflammatory infiltrates often coexist.

Although inflammation usually works to defend the body, it may also be harmful. Acute inflammatory responses may be exaggerated or sustained, with or without clearance of the offending agent. Tissue damage may result: witness the ravages of bacterial pneumonia owing to acute inflammation or joint destruction in septic arthritis. Chronic inflammation may also damage tissue and lead to scarring and loss of function. Indeed, chronic inflammation is the basis for many degenerative diseases.

Impaired inflammatory responses may lead to uncontrolled infection, as in immunocompromised hosts. Several congenital diseases are characterized by deficient inflammatory responses due to defects in inflammatory cell function or immunity.

Acute Inflammation

The acute inflammatory response begins with direct injury or stimulation of cellular or structural components of a tissue, including:

- Parenchymal cells
- Microvasculature

- Tissue macrophages and mast cells
- Mesenchymal cells (e.g., fibroblasts)
- Extracellular matrix (ECM)

A Sequence of Events Follows Initiation of Acute Inflammation

- ***Immediately, in response to injury or insult, blood vessels rapidly and transiently constrict and then dilate.*** Under the influence of nitric oxide, histamine and other soluble agents, vasodilation occurs, allowing increased blood flow and expansion of the capillary bed.
- ***Increased vascular permeability leads to accumulation of fluid and plasma components in tissues affected by inflammation.*** Fluid exchange occurs normally between intravascular and extravascular spaces, with the endothelium forming a permeability barrier. Endothelial cells are connected to each other by tight junctions and separated from the tissue by a limiting basement membrane (Fig. 2-4). ***Disruption of this barrier function is a hallmark of acute inflammation.*** One of the earliest responses to tissue injury occurs at the level of capillaries and postcapillary venules. Specific inflammatory mediators are produced at the site of injury and act directly upon blood vessels to increase vascular permeability. Vascular leakage is caused by endothelial cell contraction, endothelial cell retraction and alterations in transcytosis. Endothelial cells are also damaged, either by direct injury to the cells or indirectly by leukocyte-mediated damage. There may be extensive loss of the permeability barrier, and fluid and cells may leak into the extravascular space, termed **edema** (Fig. 2-4).
- **Intravascular stimulation of platelets and inflammatory cells, and release of soluble mediators.** Specific inflammatory mediators produced at sites of injury stimulate platelets and intravascular inflammatory cells. Kinins, complement and components of the coagulation cascade are activated (Figs. 2-1, 2-5), further increasing vascular permeability and edema.

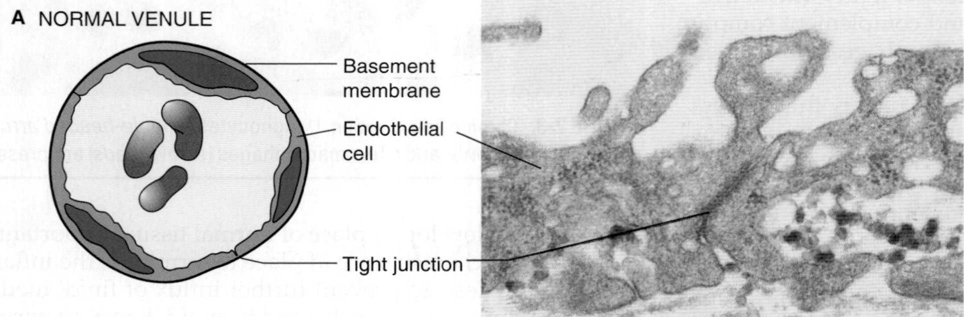

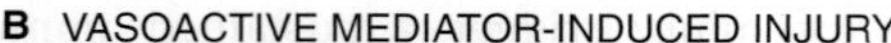

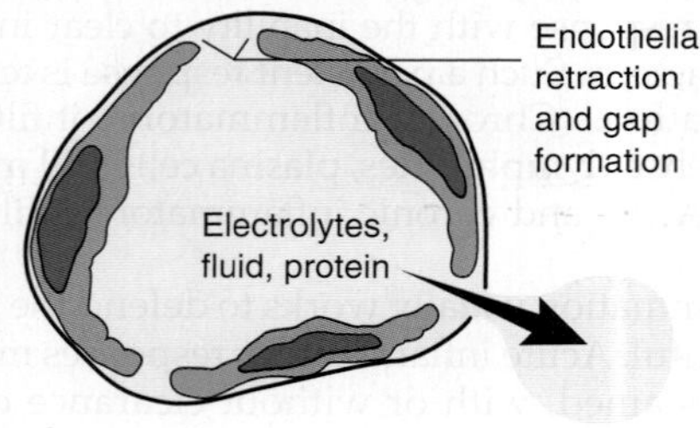

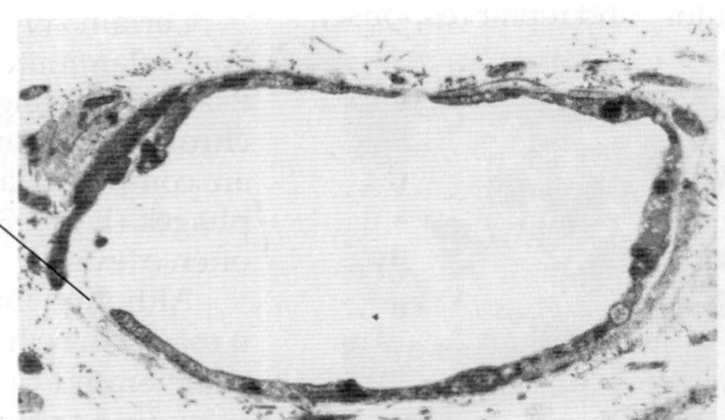

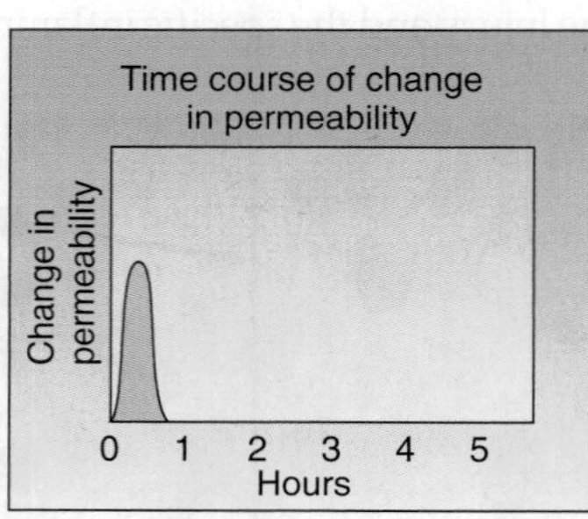

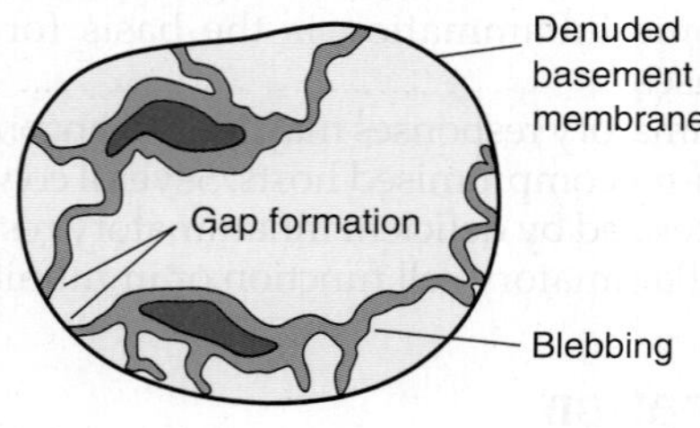

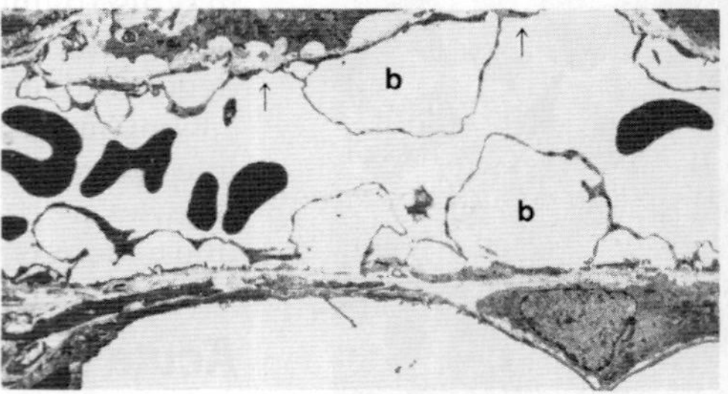

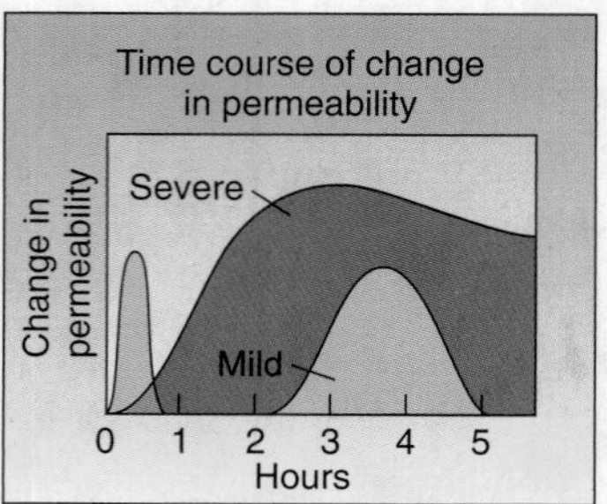

FIGURE 2-4. Responses of the microvasculature to injury. A. The wall of the normal venule is sealed by tight junctions between adjacent endothelial cells. **B.** During mild vasoactive mediator-induced injury, the endothelial cells separate and permit the passage of the fluid constituents of the blood. **C.** With severe direct injury, the endothelial cells form blebs (*b*) and separate from the underlying basement membrane. Areas of denuded basement membrane (*arrows*) allow a prolonged escape of fluid elements from the microvasculature.

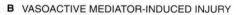

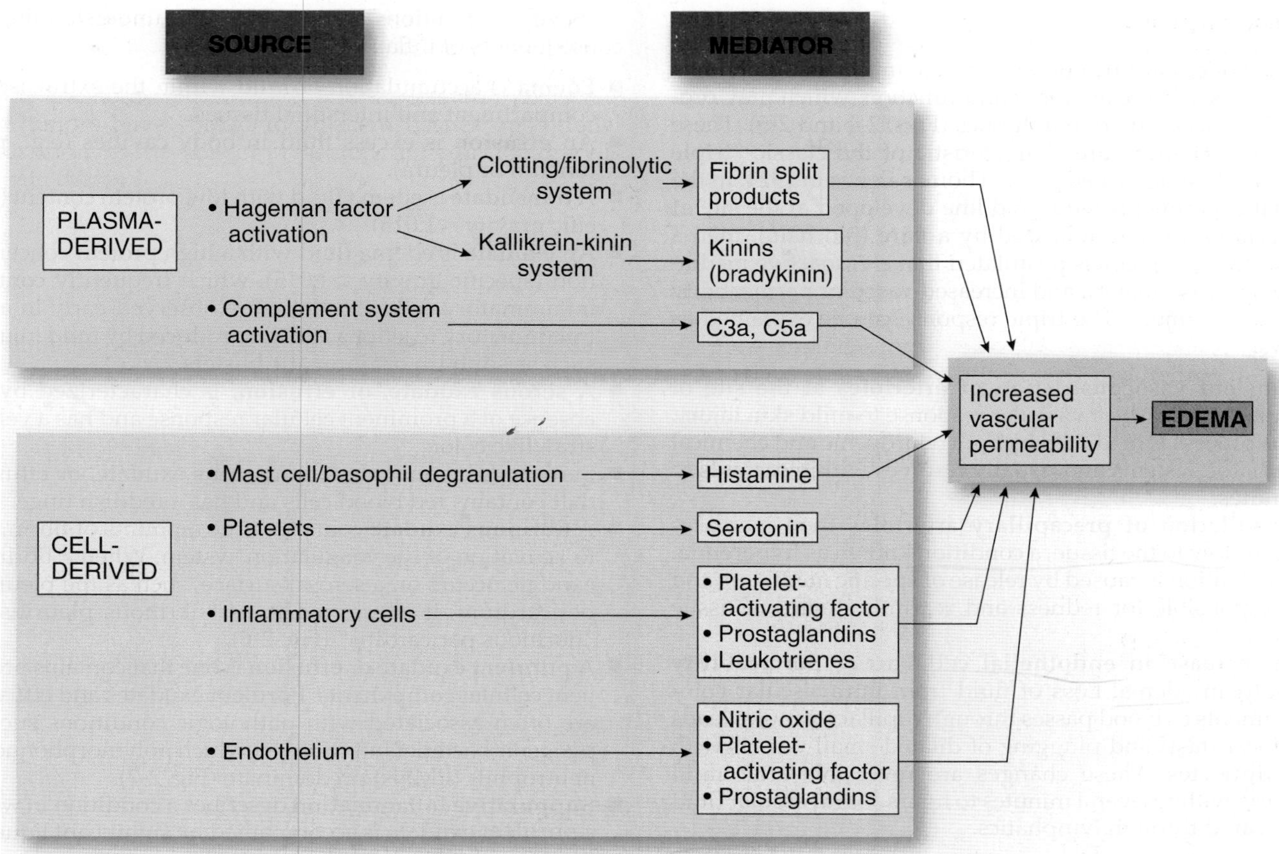

FIGURE 2-5. Inflammatory mediators of increased vascular permeability.

- **Recruitment of neutrophils to the injured site.** The vascular changes, vasodilation and edema increase the concentration of red blood cells and leukocytes within the capillary network. Chemotactic factors then recruit leukocytes, especially neutrophils, from the vascular compartment into the injured tissue (Figs. 2-1 and 2-2). Once present in tissues, recruited leukocytes initiate the process of eliminating offending agents so that damaged components can be removed and tissue repair can commence. These cells secrete additional mediators, which either enhance or inhibit the inflammatory response.

Intravascular and Tissue Fluid Levels Are Regulated by a Balance of Forces

Under normal circumstances, there is continual movement of fluid from the intravascular compartment to the extravascular space. Fluid that accumulates in the extravascular space is then cleared through lymphatics and returned to the circulation. Regulation of fluid transport across vascular walls is described in part by the **Starling principle**. According to this law, interchange of fluid between vascular and extravascular compartments results from a balance of forces that draw fluid into the vascular space or out into tissues (Chapter 7). These forces include:

- **Hydrostatic pressure** results from blood flow and plasma volume. Increased hydrostatic pressure forces fluid out of the vasculature.
- **Oncotic pressure** reflects the plasma protein concentration and draws fluid into vessels.
- **Osmotic pressure** is determined by relative amounts of sodium and water in vascular and tissue spaces.
- **Lymph flow**, the passage of fluid through the lymphatic system, continuously drains fluid out of tissues and into lymphatic spaces.

Noninflammatory Edema

When the balance of forces that regulate fluid transport is altered, flow into the extravascular compartment or clearance through lymphatics is disrupted. The net result is fluid accumulation in the interstitial spaces **(edema)**. This excess fluid expands the spaces between cells and ECM elements and leads to tissue swelling. A range of clinical conditions, either systemic or organ specific, are associated with edema. Obstruction of venous outflow **(thrombosis)** or decreased right ventricular function (congestive heart failure) cause back-pressure in the vasculature, thereby increasing hydrostatic pressure (Chapter 7). Loss of albumin (kidney disorders) or decreased synthesis of plasma proteins (liver disease, malnutrition) reduces plasma oncotic pressure. Any abnormality of sodium or water retention will alter osmotic pressure and the balance of fluid forces. Finally, obstruction of lymphatic flow may occur in various clinical settings but is most commonly due to surgical removal of lymph nodes or tumor obstruction. This fluid accumulation is referred to as **lymphedema.**

Inflammatory Edema

Among the earliest responses to tissue injury are alterations in microvasculature anatomy and function, which may promote fluid accumulation in tissues (Figs. 2-4 and 2-5). These pathologic changes are characteristic of the classic "triple response" first described by Sir Thomas Lewis in 1924. In the original experiments a dull red line developed at the site of mild trauma to skin, followed by a **flare** (red halo), then a **wheal** (swelling). Lewis postulated that a vasoactive mediator caused vasodilation and increased vascular permeability at the site of injury. The triple response can be explained as follows:

1. **Transient vasoconstriction of arterioles** at the site of injury is the earliest vascular response to mild skin injury. This process is mediated by both neurogenic and chemical mediator systems and usually resolves within seconds to minutes.
2. **Vasodilation of precapillary arterioles** then increases blood flow to the tissue, a condition known as **hyperemia**. Vasodilation is caused by release of specific mediators and is responsible for redness and warmth at sites of tissue injury.
3. **An increase in endothelial cell barrier permeability** results in edema. Loss of fluid from intravascular compartments as blood passes through capillary venules leads to local stasis and plugging of dilated small vessels with erythrocytes. These changes are reversible after mild injury: within several minutes to hours, extravascular fluid is cleared through lymphatics.

The vascular response to injury is a dynamic event that involves sequential physiologic and pathologic changes. **Vasoactive mediators,** originating from both plasma and cells, are generated at sites of tissue injury (Fig. 2-5). These mediators bind to specific receptors on vascular endothelial and smooth muscle cells, causing vasoconstriction or vasodilation. Vasodilation of arterioles increases blood flow and can exacerbate fluid leakage into the tissue. Vasoconstriction of postcapillary venules increases capillary bed hydrostatic pressure, potentiating edema formation. Vasodilation of venules decreases capillary hydrostatic pressure and inhibits movement of fluid into extravascular spaces.

After injury, vasoactive mediators bind specific receptors on endothelial cells, causing reversible endothelial cell contraction and gap formation (Fig. 2-4B). This break in the endothelial barrier leads to extravasation (leakage) of intravascular fluids into the extravascular space. Mild direct injury to the endothelium results in a biphasic response: an early change in permeability occurs within 30 minutes after injury, followed by a second increase in vascular permeability after 3 to 5 hours. When damage is severe, exudation of intravascular fluid into the extravascular compartment increases progressively, peaking 3 to 4 hours after injury.

Severe direct injury to the endothelium, such as is caused by burns or caustic chemicals, may result in irreversible damage. In such cases, the vascular endothelium separates from the basement membrane, resulting in cell blebbing (blisters or bubbles between the endothelium and the basement membrane). This leaves areas of basement membrane naked (Fig. 2-4C), disrupting the barrier between the intravascular and extravascular spaces.

Several definitions are important for understanding the consequences of inflammation:

- **Edema** is accumulation of fluid within the extravascular compartment and interstitial tissues.
- An **effusion** is excess fluid in body cavities (e.g., peritoneum or pleura).
- A **transudate** is edema fluid with low protein content (specific gravity <1.015).
- An **exudate** is edema fluid with a high protein concentration (specific gravity >1.015), which frequently contains inflammatory cells. Exudates are observed early in acute inflammatory reactions and are produced by mild injuries, such as sunburn or traumatic blisters.
- A **serous exudate,** or **effusion,** is characterized by the absence of a prominent cellular response and has a yellow, strawlike color.
- **Serosanguineous** refers to a serous exudate, or effusion, that contains red blood cells and has a reddish tinge.
- A **fibrinous exudate** contains large amounts of fibrin, due to activation of the coagulation system. When a fibrinous exudate occurs on a serosal surface, such as the pleura or pericardium, it is referred to as "fibrinous pleuritis" or "fibrinous pericarditis" (Fig. 2-6).
- **A purulent exudate or effusion** is one that contains prominent cellular components. Purulent exudates and effusions are often associated with pathologic conditions such as pyogenic bacterial infections, in which polymorphonuclear neutrophils (PMNs) predominate (Fig. 2-7).
- **Suppurative inflammation** describes a condition in which a purulent exudate is accompanied by significant liquefactive necrosis; it is the equivalent of pus.

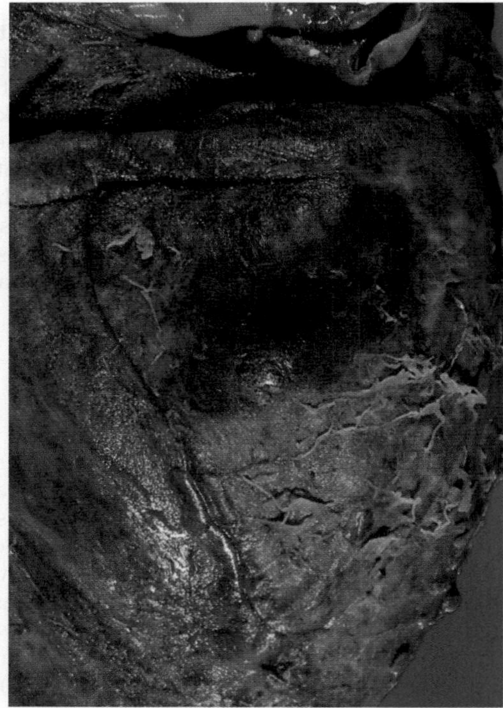

FIGURE 2-6. Fibrinous pericarditis. The heart from a patient who died in renal failure and uremia exhibits a shaggy, fibrinous exudate covering the entire visceral pericardium.

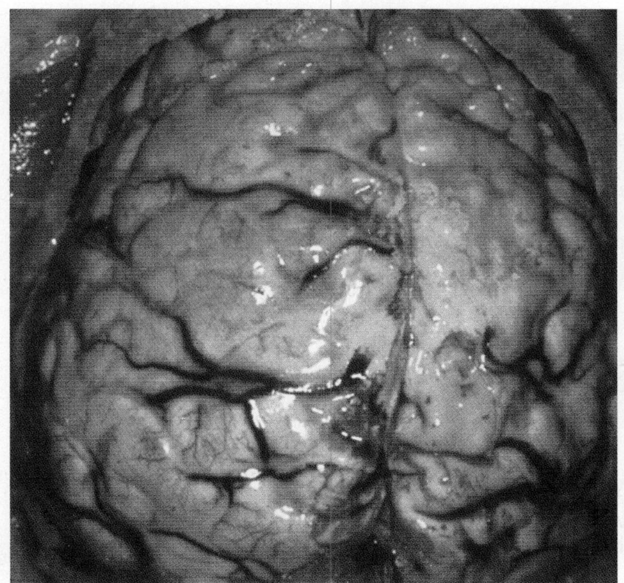

FIGURE 2-7. Purulent exudate. In this patient with bacterial meningitis, a viscid, cream-colored, acute inflammatory exudate is present within the subarachnoid space.

Plasma-Derived Mediators of Inflammation

Many chemical mediators are integral to initiation, amplification and termination of inflammatory processes (Fig. 2-8). Cell- and plasma-derived mediators work in concert to activate cells by binding specific receptors, activating cells, recruiting cells to sites of injury and stimulating release of additional soluble mediators. These mediators themselves are relatively short-lived, or are inhibited by intrinsic mechanisms, effectively turning off the response and allowing the process to resolve. Thus, these are important "on" and "off" control mechanisms of inflammation. Cell-derived mediators are considered below.

Plasma contains the elements of three major enzyme cascades, each composed of a series of proteases. Sequential activation of proteases results in release of important chemical mediators. These interrelated systems include (1) the **coagulation cascade**, (2) **kinin generation** and (3) the **complement system** (Fig. 2-9). The coagulation cascade is discussed in Chapters 10 and 20; the kinin and complement systems are presented here.

Hageman Factor Is a Key Initiator of Vasoactive Responses

Hageman factor (clotting factor XII), generated within the plasma, is activated by exposure to negatively charged surfaces such as basement membranes, proteolytic enzymes,

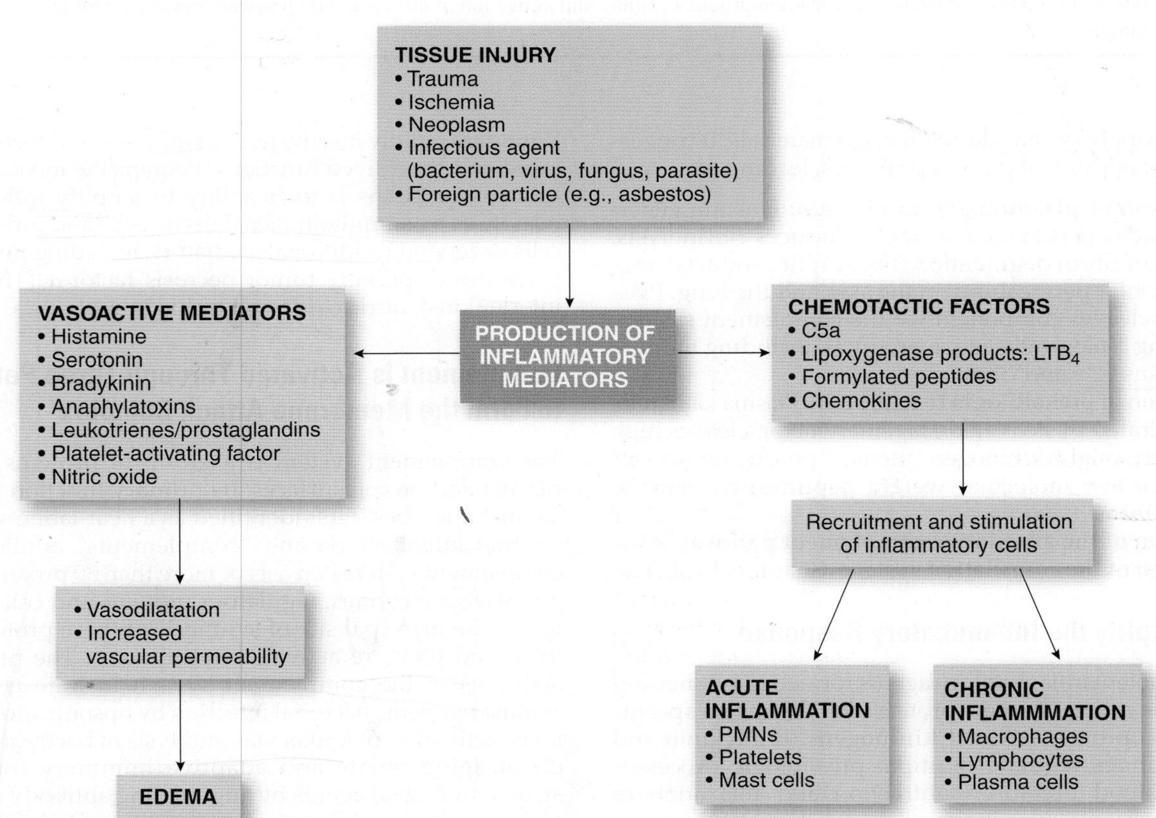

FIGURE 2-8. Mediators of the inflammatory response. Tissue injury stimulates the production of inflammatory mediators in plasma and released in the circulation. Additional factors are generated by tissue cells and inflammatory cells. These vasoactive and chemotactic mediators promote edema and recruit inflammatory cells to the site of injury. *PMNs* = polymorphonuclear neutrophils.

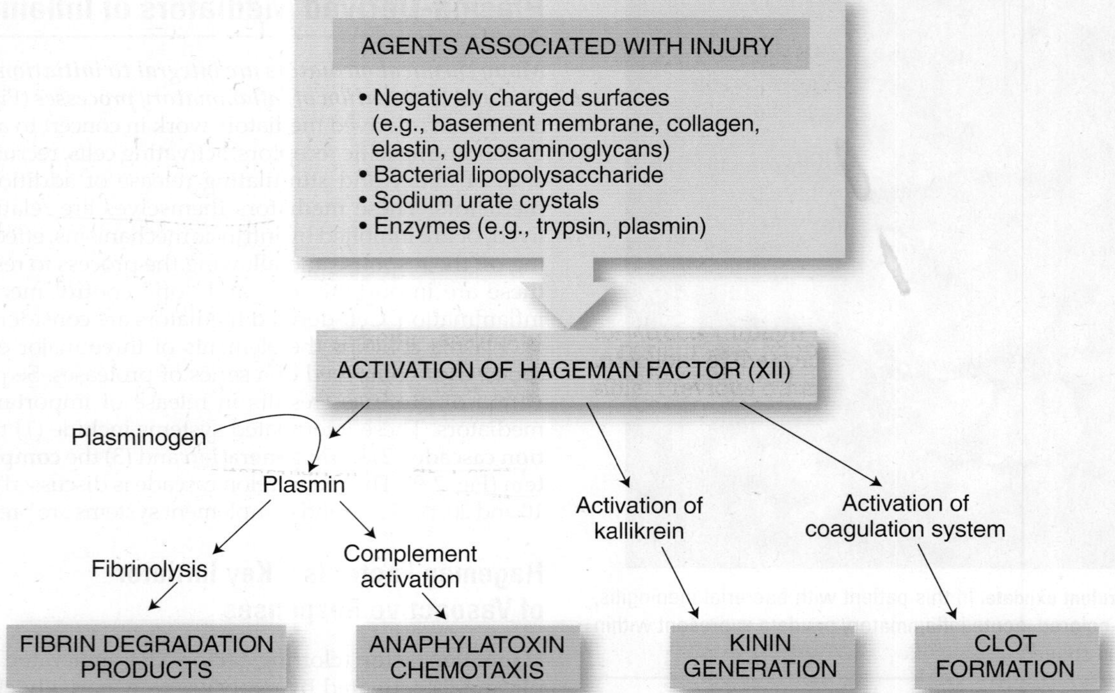

FIGURE 2-9. Hageman factor activation and inflammatory mediator production. Hageman factor activation is a key event leading to conversion of plasminogen to plasmin, resulting in generation of fibrin split products and active complement products. Activation of kallikrein produces kinins and activation of the coagulation system results in clot formation.

bacterial lipopolysaccharide and foreign materials. It triggers activation of additional plasma proteases, leading to:

- **Conversion of plasminogen to plasmin:** Plasmin generated by activated Hageman factor induces fibrinolysis. Products of fibrin degradation (fibrin split products) augment vascular permeability in the skin and the lung. Plasmin also cleaves components of the complement system, generating biologically active products, including the anaphylatoxins C3a and C5a.
- **Conversion of prekallikrein to kallikrein:** Plasma kallikrein, also generated by activated Hageman factor, cleaves high molecular weight kininogen, thereby producing several vasoactive low molecular weight peptides, collectively termed **kinins**.
- **Activation of the alternative complement pathway**
- **Activation of the coagulation system** (Chapters 10 and 20)

Kinins Amplify the Inflammatory Response

Kinins are potent inflammatory agents formed in plasma and tissue by the action of serine protease kallikreins on specific plasma glycoproteins termed **kininogens.** Bradykinin and related peptides regulate multiple physiologic processes including blood pressure, contraction and relaxation of smooth muscle, plasma extravasation, cell migration, inflammatory cell activation and inflammatory-mediated pain responses. The immediate effects of kinins are mediated by two receptors: B_1 receptors are induced by inflammatory mediators and are selectively activated by bradykinin metabolites; B_2 receptors are expressed constitutively and widely. Kinins are rapidly inactivated by kininases, and therefore have rapid and short-lived functions. Perhaps the most significant function of kinins is their ability to amplify inflammatory responses by stimulating local tissue cells and inflammatory cells to generate additional mediators, including prostanoids, cytokines (especially tumor necrosis factor-α [TNF-α] and interleukins), nitric oxide and tachykinins.

Complement Is Activated Through Three Pathways to Form the Membrane Attack Complex

The complement system is a group of proteins found in plasma and on cell surfaces. Its primary function is defense against microbes. First identified as a heat-labile serum factor that kills bacteria and "complements" antibodies, the complement system consists of more than 30 proteins including plasma enzymes, regulatory proteins and cell lysis proteins. The principal site of synthesis of these proteins is the liver, and they are activated in sequence. The physiologic activities of the complement system include (1) defense against pyogenic bacterial infection by opsonization, chemotaxis, activation of leukocytes and lysis of bacteria and cells; (2) bridging innate and adaptive immunity for defense against microbial agents by augmenting antibody responses and enhancing immunologic memory; and (3) disposal of immune products and products of inflammatory injury by clearance of immune complexes from tissues and removal of apoptotic cells. Certain complement components, **anaphylatoxins,** are vasoactive mediators. Other components fix opsonins on cell surfaces and still others induce cell lysis by generating the lytic complex C5b-9 **(membrane attack complex [MAC])**. The proteins involved in activating the complement system are themselves activated by three convergent pathways termed **classical, mannose-binding lectin (MBL)** and **alternative**.

The Classical Pathway

Activators of the classical pathway include antigen–antibody (Ag–Ab) complexes, products of bacteria and viruses, proteases, urate crystals, apoptotic cells and polyanions (polynucleotides). The proteins of this pathway are C1 through C9, the nomenclature following the historical order of discovery. Ag–Ab complexes activate C1, initiating a cascade that leads to formation of the MAC, which proceeds as follows (Fig. 2-10):

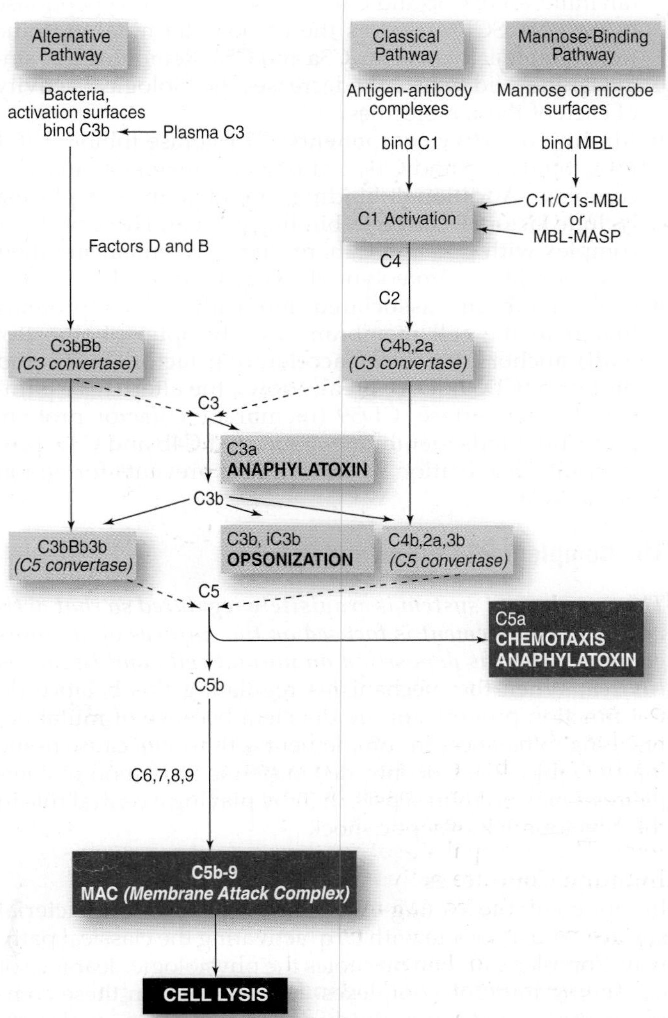

FIGURE 2-10. Complement activation. The alternative, classical and mannose-binding pathways lead to generation of the complement cascade of inflammatory mediators and cell lysis by the membrane attack complex (MAC). *MBL* = mannose-binding lectin; *MBL-MASP* = *M*BL-*a*ssociated *s*erine *p*rotease.

1. **Antibodies bound to antigens on bacterial cell surfaces bind the C1 complex.** The C1 complex consists of C1q, two molecules of C1r and two molecules of C1s. Antibodies in the immune complexes bind C1q, triggering activation of C1r and C1s.
2. **C1s first cleaves C4, which binds the bacterial surface and then cleaves C2.** The resulting cleaved molecules form the C4b2a enzyme complex, also called **C3 convertase,** which remains covalently bound to the bacterial surface. This anchors the complement system at specific tissue sites. If a covalent bond is not formed, the complex is inactivated, aborting the complement cascade in normal host cells or tissues.
3. **C3 convertase cleaves C3 into C3a and C3b.** This is a critical step in generating biologically active complement components. C3a is released as an **anaphylatoxin**. C3b reacts with cell proteins to localize, or "fix" on the cell surface. C3b and its degradation products, especially iC3b, on the surface of pathogens, enhance phagocytosis. This process of coating a pathogen with a molecule that enhances phagocytosis is **opsonization**, and the molecule that does this is referred to as an **opsonin**.
4. **The complex of C4b, C2a and C3b (termed C5 convertase) cleaves C5 into C5a and C5b.** C5a also is an anaphylatoxin, and C5b acts as the nidus for subsequent sequential binding of C6, C7 and C8 to form the MAC.
5. **The MAC assembles on target cells.** The MAC directly inserts into the plasma membrane by hydrophobic binding of C7 to the lipid bilayer. The resulting cylindrical transmembrane channel disrupts the barrier function of the plasma membrane and leads to cell lysis.

The Mannose-Binding Pathway

The mannose- or lectin-binding pathway has some components in common with the classical pathway. It is initiated by binding of microbes bearing terminal mannose groups to MBL, a member of the family of calcium-dependent lectins, called the **collectins**. This multifunctional acute phase protein has properties similar to those of immunoglobulin (Ig) M (IgM) antibody (it binds to a wide range of oligosaccharide structures), IgG (it interacts with phagocytic receptors) and C1q. This last property enables it to interact with either C1r-C1s or with a serine protease called MASP (*M*BL-*a*ssociated *s*erine *p*rotease) to activate complement as follows (Fig. 2-10):

1. **MBL interacts with C1r and C1s to generate C1 esterase activity.** Alternatively and preferentially, MBL forms a complex with a precursor of the serine protease, MASP. MBL and MASP bind to mannose groups on glycoproteins or carbohydrates on bacterial cell surfaces. After MBL binds a substrate, the MASP proenzyme is cleaved into two chains and expresses a C1-esterase activity.
2. **C1-esterase activity, either from C1r/C1s–MBL interaction or MBL–MASP, cleaves C4 and C2, leading to assembly of the classical pathway C3 convertase.** The complement cascade then continues as described for the classical pathway.

Alternative Pathway

The alternative pathway is initiated by derivative products of microorganisms such as endotoxin (from bacterial cell surfaces), zymosan (yeast cell walls), polysaccharides, cobra venom factor, viruses, tumor cells and foreign materials. Proteins of the alternative pathway are called "factors," followed by a letter. Activation of this pathway proceeds as follows (Fig. 2-10):

1. **A small amount of C3 in plasma cleaves to C3a and C3b.** This C3b is covalently bound to carbohydrates and proteins on microbial cell surfaces. It binds factor B and factor D to form the alternative pathway C3 convertase, C3bBb. This C3 convertase is stabilized by **properdin**.
2. **C3 convertase generates additional C3b and C3a.** Binding of a second C3b molecule to C3 convertase converts it to a C5 convertase, C3bBb3b.
3. **As in the classical pathway, cleavage of C5 by C5 convertase generates C5b and C5a and leads to assembly of the MAC.**

The Complement System Is Tightly Regulated to Generate Proinflammatory Molecules

Biological Activities of Complement Components

The end point of complement activation is formation of the MAC and cell lysis. Cleavage products generated at each step both catalyze the next step in the cascade and themselves have additional properties that render them important inflammatory molecules:

- **Anaphylatoxins** (C3a, C4a, C5a): These proinflammatory molecules mediate smooth muscle contraction and increase vascular permeability (Fig. 2-11).
- **Opsonins** (C3b, iC3b): Bacterial opsonization is the process by which a specific molecule (e.g., IgG or C3b) binds to the surface of the bacterium. The process enhances phagocytosis by enabling receptors on phagocytic cell membranes (e.g., Fc receptor or C3b receptor) to recognize and bind the opsonized bacterium. Viruses, parasites and transformed cells also activate complement by similar mechanisms, an effect that leads to their inactivation or death.
- **Proinflammatory molecules** (MAC, C5a): These chemotactic factors also activate leukocytes and tissue cells to generate oxidants and cytokines and induce degranulation of mast cells and basophils.
- **Lysis** (MAC): C5b binds C6 and C7, and subsequently C8 to the target cell; C9 polymerization is catalyzed to lyse the cell membrane.

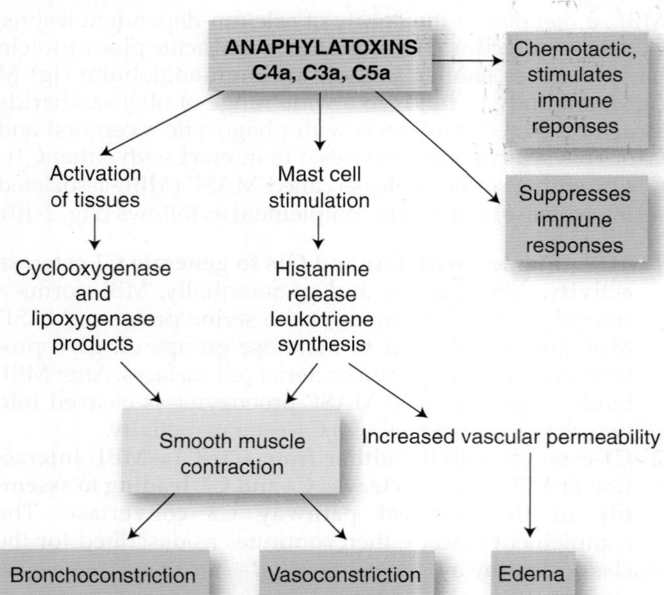

FIGURE 2-11. Biological activity of the anaphylatoxins. Complement activation products, generated during activation of the complement cascade, regulate vascular permeability, cell recruitment and smooth muscle contraction.

Regulation of the Complement System

Proteins in serum and on cell surfaces protect the host from indiscriminate injury by regulating complement activation. There are four major mechanisms for this:

- **Spontaneous decay:** C4b2a and C3bBb and their cleavage products, C3b and C4b, decrease by decay.
- **Proteolytic inactivation:** Plasma inhibitors include factor 1 (an inhibitor of C3b and C4b) and serum carboxypeptidase N (SCPN). SCPN cleaves the carboxy-terminal arginine from anaphylatoxins C4a, C3a and C5a. Removing this single amino acid markedly decreases the biological activity of each of these molecules.
- **Binding of active components:** C1 esterase inhibitor (C1 INA) binds C1r and C1s, forming an irreversibly inactive complex. Additional binding proteins in the plasma include factor H– and C4b-binding protein. These proteins complex with C3b and C4b, respectively, enhancing their susceptibility to proteolytic cleavage by factor I.
- **Cell membrane–associated molecules:** Two proteins linked to the cell membrane by glycophosphoinositol (GPI) anchors are decay-accelerating factor (DAF) and protectin (CD59). DAF breaks down the alternative pathway C3 convertase; CD59 (membrane cofactor protein, protectin) binds membrane-associated C4b and C3b, promotes its inactivation by factor I and prevents formation of the MAC.

The Complement System and Disease

The complement system is exquisitely regulated so that activation of complement is focused on the surfaces of microorganisms, whereas deposition on normal cells and tissues is limited. When the mechanisms regulating this balance do not function properly, or are deficient because of mutation, resulting imbalances in complement activity can cause tissue injury (Table 2-1). Uncontrolled systemic activation of complement may occur in sepsis, thereby playing a central role in the development of septic shock.

Immune Complexes

Immune complexes (Ag–Ab complexes) form on bacterial surfaces and associate with C1q, activating the classical pathway. Complement then promotes the physiologic clearance of circulating immune complexes. However, when these complexes are formed continuously and in excess (e.g., in chronic immune responses), the relentless activation of complement results in its consumption and, therefore, net depletion of complement. Complement inefficiency, whether due to complement depletion, deficient complement binding or defects in complement activation, results in immune deposition and inflammation, which in turn may trigger autoimmunity.

Table 2-1

Hereditary Complement Deficiencies

Complement Deficiency	Clinical Association
C3b, iC3b, C5, MBL	Pyogenic bacterial infections
	Membranoproliferative glomerulonephritis
C3, properdin, MAC proteins	Neisserial infection
C1 inhibitor	Hereditary angioedema
CD59	Hemolysis, thrombosis
C1q, C1r and C1s, C4, C2	Systemic lupus erythematosus
Factor H and factor I	Hemolytic-uremic syndrome
	Membranoproliferative glomerulonephritis

MAC = membrane attack complex; MBL = mannose-binding lectin.

Infectious Disease

Defense against infection is a key role of complement products. Defective functioning of the complement system leads to increased susceptibility to infection.

- Defects in antibody production, complement proteins or phagocyte function are associated with increased susceptibility to pyogenic infection by organisms such as *Haemophilus influenzae* and *Streptococcus pneumoniae*.
- Deficiencies in MAC formation are associated with increased infections, particularly with meningococci.
- Deficiency of complement MBL results in recurrent infections in young children.

Thick capsules may protect some bacteria from lysis by complement. Furthermore, bacterial enzymes can inhibit the effects of complement components, especially C5a, or increase catabolism of components, such as C3b, thereby reducing formation of C3 convertase. Viruses, on the other hand, may use cell-bound components and receptors to facilitate cell entry. *Mycobacterium tuberculosis,* Epstein-Barr virus, measles virus, picornaviruses, human immunodeficiency virus (HIV) and flaviviruses use complement components to target inflammatory or epithelial cells.

Inflammation and Necrosis

The complement system amplifies the inflammatory response. Anaphylatoxins C5a and C3a activate leukocytes, and C5a and MAC activate endothelial cells, inducing generation of oxidants and cytokines that are harmful to tissues when present in excess (Chapter 1). Nonviable or injured tissues cannot regulate complement normally.

Complement Deficiencies

The importance of an intact and appropriately regulated complement system is exemplified in people who have acquired or congenital deficiencies of specific complement components or regulatory proteins (Table 2-1). The most common congenital defect is a C2 deficiency, which is inherited as an autosomal codominant trait. Acquired deficiencies of early complement components occur in patients with some autoimmune diseases, especially those associated with circulating immune complexes. These include certain forms of membranous glomerulonephritis and systemic lupus erythematosus. Deficiencies in early components of complement (e.g., C1q, C1r, C1s and C4) are strongly associated with susceptibility to systemic lupus erythematosus; patients lacking the middle (C3, C5) components are prone to recurrent pyogenic infections, membranoproliferative glomerulonephritis and rashes; those who lack terminal complement components (C6, C7, or C8) are vulnerable to infections with *Neisseria* species. Such differences in susceptibility underscore the importance of individual complement components in host protection from bacterial infection. Congenital defects in proteins that regulate the complement system (e.g., C1 inhibitor and SCPN) result in chronic complement activation. C1 inhibitor deficiency is also associated with the syndrome of hereditary angioedema.

Cell-Derived Mediators of Inflammation

Circulating platelets, basophils, PMNs, endothelial cells monocyte/macrophages, tissue mast cells and the injured tissue itself are all potential cellular sources of vasoactive mediators. In general, these mediators are (1) derived from metabolism of phospholipids and arachidonic acid (e.g., prostaglandins, thromboxanes, leukotrienes, lipoxins, platelet-activating factor [PAF]), (2) preformed and stored in cytoplasmic granules (e.g., histamine, serotonin, lysosomal hydrolases) or (3) derived from altered production of normal regulators of vascular function (e.g., nitric oxide and neurokinins).

Arachidonic Acid and Platelet-Activating Factor Are Derived From Membrane Phospholipids

Phospholipids and fatty acid derivatives released from plasma membranes are metabolized into mediators and homeostatic regulators by inflammatory cells and injured tissues (Fig. 2-12). As part of a complex regulatory network, prostanoids, leukotrienes and lipoxins, which are derivatives of arachidonic acid, both promote and inhibit inflammation (Table 2-2). Net impact depends on several factors, including levels and profiles of prostanoid production, both of which change during an inflammatory response.

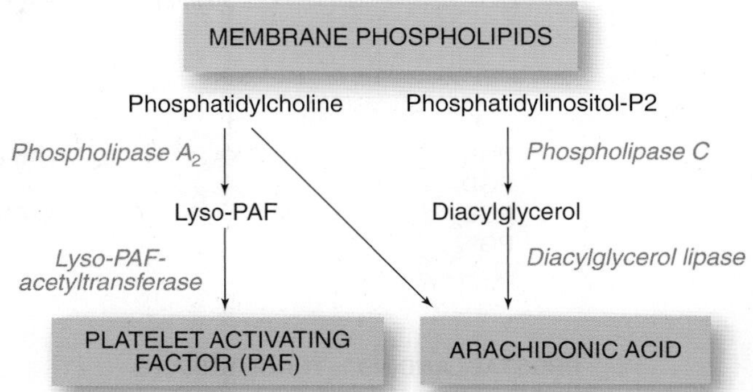

FIGURE 2-12. Cell membrane–derived mediators. Platelet-activating factor (PAF) is derived from choline-containing glycerophospholipids in the membrane. Arachidonic acid derives from phosphatidylinositol phosphates and from phosphatidyl choline.

Table 2-2

Biological Activities of Arachidonic Acid Metabolites

Metabolite	Biological Activity
PGE_2, PDG_2	Induce vasodilation, bronchodilation; inhibit inflammatory cell function
PGI_2	Induces vasodilation, bronchodilation; inhibits inflammatory cell function
$PGF_{2\alpha}$	Induces vasodilation, bronchoconstriction
TXA_2	Induces vasoconstriction, bronchoconstriction; enhances inflammatory cell functions (esp. platelets)
LTB_4	Chemotactic for phagocytic cells; stimulates phagocytic cell adherence; enhances microvascular permeability
LTC_4, LTD_4, LTE_4	Induce smooth muscle contraction; constrict pulmonary airways; increase microvascular permeability

P . . . = prostaglandin; LT . . . = leukotriene; TXA_2 = thromboxane A_2.

Arachidonic Acid

Depending on the specific inflammatory cell and the nature of the stimulus, activated cells generate arachidonic acid by one of two pathways (Fig. 2-12). One pathway involves liberation of arachidonic acid from the glycerol backbone of cell membrane phospholipids (in particular, phosphatidylcholine) by stimulus-induced activation of phospholipase A_2 (PLA_2). The other is metabolism of phosphatidylinositol phosphates to diacylglycerol and inositol phosphates by phospholipase C. Diacylglycerol lipase then cleaves arachidonic acid from diacylglycerol. Once generated, arachidonic acid is further metabolized through two pathways: (1) **cyclooxygenation**, with subsequent production of prostaglandins and thromboxanes; and (2) **lipoxygenation**, to form leukotrienes and lipoxins (Fig. 2-13).

Corticosteroids are widely used to suppress tissue destruction associated with many inflammatory diseases, including allergic responses, rheumatoid arthritis and systemic lupus erythematosus. They induce synthesis of an inhibitor of PLA_2 and block release of arachidonic acid in inflammatory cells. Although corticosteroids (e.g., prednisone) are widely used to suppress inflammatory responses, their prolonged administration can have significant harmful effects, including increased risk of infection, damage to connective tissue and adrenal gland atrophy.

Platelet-Activating Factor

Another potent inflammatory mediator derived from membrane phospholipids is PAF, synthesized by virtually all activated inflammatory cells, endothelial cells and injured tissue cells. During inflammatory and allergic responses, PAF is derived from choline-containing glycerophospholipids in the cell membrane, initially by the catalytic action of PLA_2, followed by acetylation by an acetyltransferase (Fig. 2-12). In plasma, PAF-acetylhydrolase regulates PAF activity.

PAF has diverse functions. It stimulates platelets, neutrophils, monocyte/macrophages, endothelial cells and vascular smooth muscle cells. PAF induces platelet aggregation and degranulation at sites of tissue injury and enhances release of serotonin, thereby altering vascular permeability. Because PAF primes leukocytes, it enhances functional responses (e.g., O_2 production, degranulation) to a second

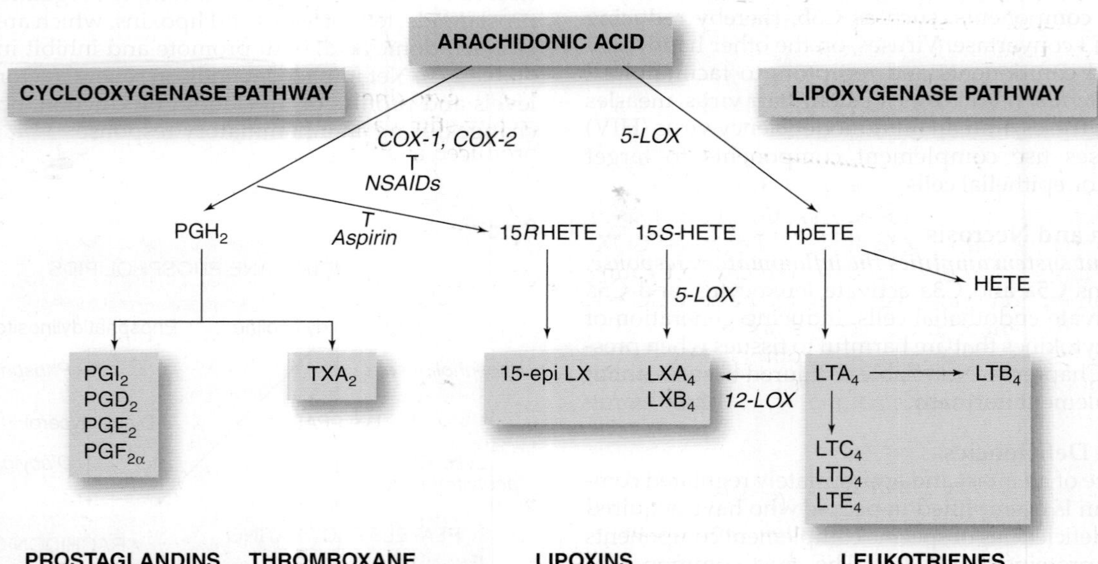

FIGURE 2-13. Biologically active arachidonic acid metabolites. The cyclooxygenase (COX) pathway of arachidonic acid metabolism generates prostaglandins (PG. . .) and thromboxane (TXA_2). The lipoxygenase (LOX) pathway forms lipoxins (LX. . .) and leukotrienes (LT. . .). Aspirin (acetylsalicylic acid) blocks the formation of 5-HETE (*HETE* = hydroxyicosatetraenoic acid). NSAIDs (nonsteroidal anti-inflammatory drugs) block COX-1 and COX-2. *HpETE* = 5-hydroperoxyeicosatetraenoic acid.

stimulus and induces adhesion molecule expression, specifically of integrins. PAF is also an extremely potent vasodilator, augmenting permeability of microvasculature at sites of tissue injury. PAF generated by endothelial cells cooperates with P-selectin. When P-selectin lightly tethers a leukocyte to an endothelial cell, PAF from the endothelial cell binds its receptor on the leukocyte and induces intracellular signaling.

Prostanoids, Leukotrienes and Lipoxins Are Biologically Active Metabolites of Arachidonic Acid

Prostanoids

Arachidonic acid is further metabolized by cyclooxygenases 1 and 2 (COX-1, COX-2) to generate prostanoids (Fig. 2-13). **COX-1** is constitutively expressed by most cells and increases upon cell activation. It is a key enzyme in the synthesis of prostaglandins, which in turn (1) protect the gastrointestinal mucosal lining, (2) regulate water/electrolyte balance, (3) stimulate platelet aggregation to maintain normal hemostasis and (4) maintain resistance to thrombosis on vascular endothelial cell surfaces. **COX-2** expression is generally low or undetectable, but increases substantially upon stimulation, generating metabolites important in inducing pain and inflammation.

The early inflammatory prostanoid response is COX-1 dependent; COX-2 takes over as the major source of prostanoids as inflammation progresses. Both COX isoforms generate prostaglandin H (PGH_2), which is then the substrate for production of prostacyclin (PGI_2), PGD_2, PGE_2, $PGF_{2\alpha}$ and TXA_2 (thromboxane). The profile of prostaglandin production (i.e., the quantity and variety produced during inflammation) depends in part on the cells present and their state of activation. Thus, mast cells produce predominantly PGD_2; macrophages generate PGE_2 and TXA_2; platelets are the major source of TXA_2; and endothelial cells produce PGI_2. Prostanoids affect immune cell function by binding G-protein–coupled cell surface receptors, leading to activation of a range of intracellular signaling pathways in immune cells and resident tissue cells. The repertoire of prostanoid receptors expressed by various immune cells differs, so the functional responses of these cells may be modified differently according to the prostanoids present.

Inhibition of COX is one mechanism by which nonsteroidal anti-inflammatory drugs (NSAIDs), including aspirin, indomethacin and ibuprofen, exert their potent analgesic and anti-inflammatory effects. NSAIDS block COX-2–induced formation of prostaglandins, thereby mitigating pain and inflammation. However, they also affect COX-1, lead to decreased homeostatic functions and so affect the stomach and kidneys adversely. This complication led to development of COX-2–specific inhibitors.

Leukotrienes

Slow-reacting substance of anaphylaxis (SRS-A) has long been recognized as a smooth muscle stimulant and mediator of hypersensitivity reactions. It is, in fact, a mixture of leukotrienes, the second major family of derivatives of arachidonic acid (Fig. 2-13). The enzyme 5-lipoxygenase (5-LOX) leads to synthesis of 5-hydroperoxyeicosatetraenoic acid (5-HpETE) and leukotriene A_4 (LTA_4) from arachidonic acid; the latter is a precursor for other leukotrienes. In neutrophils and certain macrophage populations, LTA_4 is metabolized to LTB_4, which has potent chemotactic activity for neutrophils, monocytes and macrophages. In other cell types, especially mast cells, basophils and macrophages, LTA_4 is converted to LTC_4 and thence to LTD_4 and LTE_4. These three cysteinyl-leukotrienes (1) stimulate smooth muscle contraction, (2) enhance vascular permeability and (3) are responsible for many of the clinical symptoms associated with allergic-type reactions. They thus play a pivotal role in the development of asthma. Leukotrienes exert their action through high-affinity specific receptors that may prove to be important targets of drug therapy.

Lipoxins

Lipoxins, the third class of products of arachidonic acid, are made within the vascular lumen by cell–cell interactions (Fig. 2-13). They are proinflammatory, trihydroxytetraene-containing eicosanoids that are generated during inflammation, atherosclerosis and thrombosis. Several cell types synthesize lipoxins from leukotrienes. LTA_4, released by activated leukocytes, is available for transcellular enzymatic conversion by neighboring cell types. When platelets adhere to neutrophils, LTA_4 from neutrophils is converted by platelet 12-lipoxygenase, forming lipoxin A_4 and B_4 (LXA_4 and LXB_4). Monocytes, eosinophils and airway epithelial cells generate 15*S*-hydroxyeicosatetraenoic acid (15*S*-HETE), which is taken up by neutrophils and converted to lipoxins via 5-LOX. Activation of this pathway can also inhibit leukotriene biosynthesis, thereby providing a regulatory pathway.

Aspirin initiates transcellular biosynthesis of a group of lipoxins termed "aspirin-triggered lipoxins," or 15-epimeric-lipoxins (15-epi-LXs). When aspirin is administered in the presence of inflammatory mediators, 15*R*-HETE is generated by COX-2. Activated neutrophils convert 15*R*-HETE to 15-epi-LXs, which are anti-inflammatory lipid mediators. Thus, this is another pathway where aspirin exerts a beneficial effect.

Cytokines Are Low Molecular Weight Proteins Secreted by Cells

Many cytokines, including interleukins, growth factors, colony-stimulating factors, interferons and chemokines, are produced at sites of inflammation (Fig. 2-14).

Cytokines

Cytokines produced at sites of tissue injury regulate inflammatory responses, ranging from initial changes in vascular permeability to resolution and restoration of tissue integrity. These molecules are inflammatory hormones that have **autocrine** (affecting themselves), **paracrine** (affecting nearby cells) and **endocrine** (affecting cells in other tissues) functions. While most cells produce cytokines, they differ in their cytokine repertoire. ***Through production of cytokines, macrophages are pivotal in orchestrating tissue inflammatory responses.***

Lipopolysaccharide (LPS), a molecule derived from the outer cell membrane of Gram-negative bacteria, is one of the most potent activators of macrophages. It also activates endothelial cells and leukocytes (Fig. 2-15). LPS binds specific cellular receptors, either directly or after binding a serum LPS-binding protein (LBP). It is a potent stimulus for production of TNF-α and interleukins (IL-1, IL-6, IL-8, IL-12 and

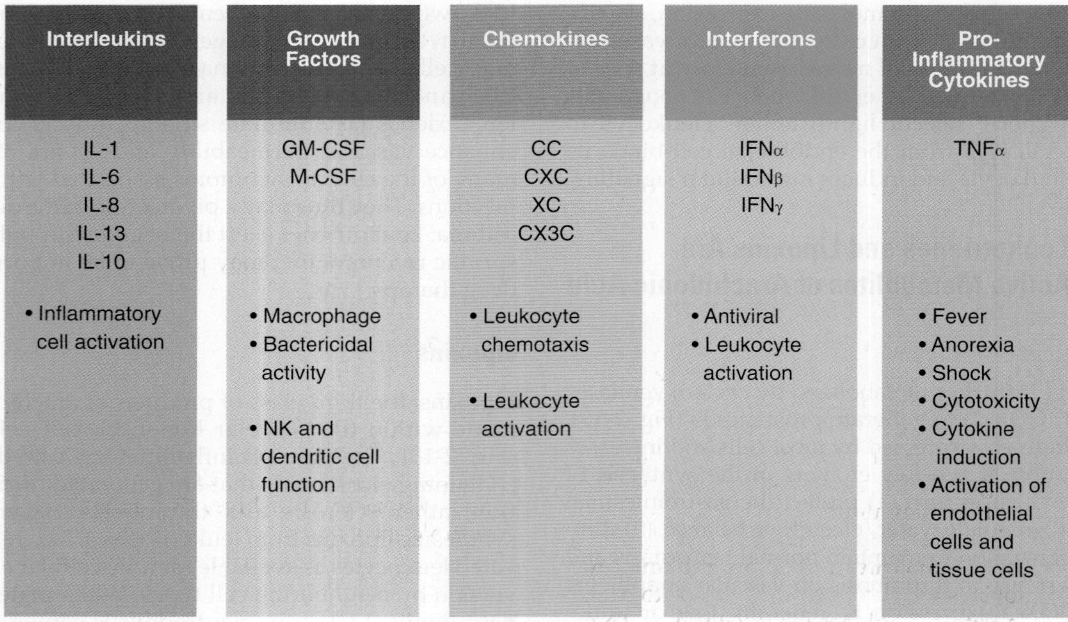

FIGURE 2-14. Cytokines important in inflammation. *GM-CSF* = granulocyte–macrophage colony-stimulating factor; *IL* = interleukin; *NK* = natural killer; *IFN* = interferon; *TNF* = tumor necrosis factor.

others). Macrophage-derived cytokines modulate endothelial cell–leukocyte adhesion (TNF-α), leukocyte recruitment (IL-8), the acute phase response (IL-6, IL-1) and immune functions (IL-1, IL-6, IL-12).

IL-1 and TNF-α, produced by macrophages as well as other cells, are central to development and amplification of inflammatory responses. These cytokines activate endothelial cells to express adhesion molecules and release cytokines, chemokines and reactive oxygen species (ROS; see below). TNF-α induces priming and aggregation of neutrophils. IL-1 and TNF-α are also among the mediators of fever, catabolism of muscle, shifts in protein synthesis and hemodynamic effects associated with inflammatory states (Fig. 2-15).

Interferon-γ (IFN-γ), another potent stimulus for macrophage activation and cytokine production, is produced by a subset of T lymphocytes as part of the immune response (Chapter 4). It is also synthesized by natural killer (NK) cells in the primary host response to intracellular pathogens (e.g., *Listeria monocytogenes*) and certain viral infections. NK cells migrate into tissues at sites of injury. When exposed to IL-12 and TNF-α, NK cells are activated to produce IFN-γ. Thus, an amplification pathway exists by which activated tissue macrophages produce TNF-α and IL-12, stimulating IFN-γ production by NK cells, with subsequent stimulation of additional macrophages.

Chemokines

Chemotactic cytokines, or chemokines, direct cell migration **(chemotaxis)**. Accumulation of inflammatory cells at sites of tissue injury requires their migration from vascular spaces into extravascular tissue. During this migration, the cell extends a pseudopod toward increasing chemokine concentration. At the leading front of the pseudopod, marked changes in levels of intracellular calcium are associated with assembly and contraction of cytoskeleton proteins. This

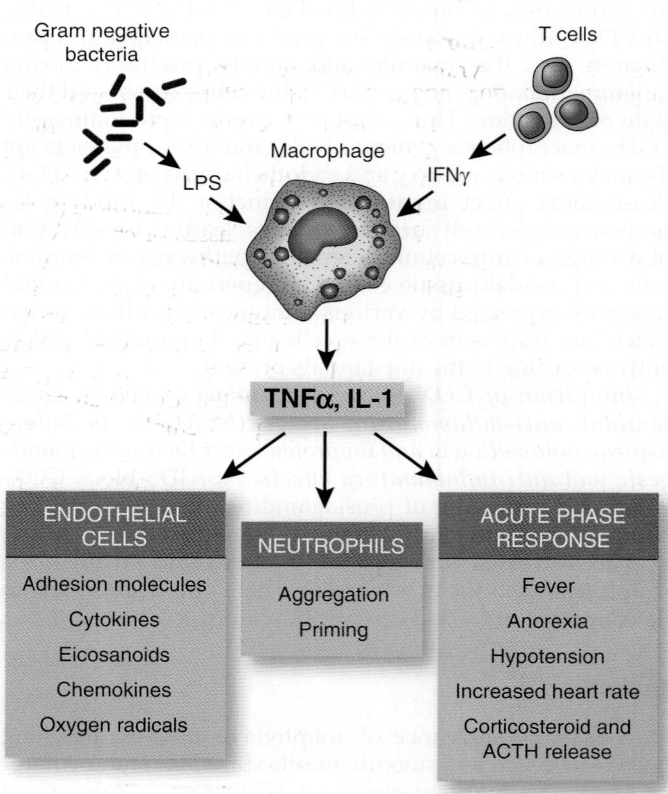

FIGURE 2-15. Central role of interleukin (IL)-1 and tumor necrosis factor (TNF)-α in inflammation. Lipopolysaccharide (LPS) and IFN-γ activate macrophages to release inflammatory cytokines, principally IL-1 and TNF-α, responsible for directing local and systemic inflammatory responses. *ACTH* = adrenocorticotrophic hormone.

process draws the remaining tail of the cell along the chemical gradient. The most important chemotactic factors for PMNs are:

- C5a, derived from complement
- Bacterial and mitochondrial products, particularly low–molecular-weight N-formylated peptides (such as *N*-formyl-methionyl-leucyl-phenylalanine [FMLP])
- Products of arachidonic acid metabolism, especially LTB_4
- Chemokines

Chemokines are a large class of cytokines (over 50 known members) that regulate leukocyte trafficking in inflammation and immunity. Unlike other cytokines, chemokines are small molecules that interact with G-protein–coupled receptors on target cells. These secreted proteins are produced by a variety of cell types, either constitutively or after induction, and differ widely in biological action. This diversity is based on specific cell types targeted, specific receptor activation and differences in intracellular signaling.

Two functional classes of chemokines have been distinguished: **inflammatory chemokines** and **homing chemokines**. Inflammatory chemokines are produced in response to bacterial toxins and inflammatory cytokines (especially IL-1, TNF-α and IFN-γ) by a variety of tissue cells as well as by leukocytes themselves. These molecules recruit leukocytes during host inflammatory responses. Homing chemokines are constitutively expressed and upregulated during disease states and direct trafficking and homing of lymphocytes and dendritic cells to lymphoid tissues during an immune response (Chapter 4).

Structure and Nomenclature

Chemokines are synthesized as secretory proteins consisting of approximately 70 to 130 amino acids, with four conserved cysteines linked by disulfide bonds. The two major subpopulations, termed CXC or CC chemokines (formerly called α and β chemokines), are distinguished by the position of the first two cysteines, which are either separated by one amino acid (CXC) or are adjacent (CC). Two additional classes of chemokines, each with a single member, have been identified. Lymphotactin has two instead of four conserved cysteines (XC), and fractaline (or neurotactin) has three amino acids between the first two cysteines (CX_3C). Chemokines are named according to their structure, followed by "L" and the number of their gene (CCL1, CXCL1, etc.). However, many of the traditional names for chemokines persist in current usage. Chemokine receptors are named according to their structure, "R," and a number (CCR1, CXCR1, etc.); most receptors recognize more than one chemokine and most chemokines bind more than one receptor. Receptor binding by chemokines may lead to agonistic or antagonistic activity. The same chemokine may act as an agonist at one receptor and an antagonist at another. Leukocyte recruitment or lymphocyte homing is modulated by combinations of these agonistic and antagonistic activities.

Anchoring and Activity

Chemokines function as immobilized or soluble molecules. They generate a chemotactic gradient by binding to proteoglycans of the ECM or to cell surfaces. As a result, high concentrations of chemokines persist at sites of tissue injury. Specific receptors on the surface of migrating leukocytes bind to matrix-bound chemokines and associated adhesion molecules, which tends to move cells along the chemotactic gradient to the injury site. This process of responding to a matrix-bound chemoattractant is **haptotaxis.** Chemokines are also displayed on cytokine-activated vascular endothelial cells. This process can augment very late antigen-4 (VLA-4) integrin-dependent adhesion of leukocytes, resulting in their firm arrest. As soluble molecules, chemokines control leukocyte motility and localization within extravascular tissues by establishing a chemotactic gradient. The multiplicity and combination of chemokine receptors on cells allows an extensive variety in biological function. Neutrophils, monocytes, eosinophils and basophils share some receptors but express other receptors exclusively. Thus, specific chemokine combinations can recruit selective cell populations.

Chemokines in Disease

Chemokines are implicated in a variety of acute and chronic diseases. These include disorders with a pronounced inflammatory component, in which case multiple chemokines are expressed in inflamed tissues. Examples are rheumatoid arthritis, ulcerative colitis, Crohn disease, pulmonary inflammation (chronic bronchitis, asthma), autoimmune diseases (multiple sclerosis, rheumatoid arthritis, systemic lupus erythematosus) and vascular diseases, including atherosclerosis.

Reactive Oxygen Species Are Signal-Transducing, Bactericidal and Cytotoxic Molecules

ROS are chemically reactive molecules derived from oxygen. Normally, they are rapidly inactivated, but when generated inappropriately, they can be toxic to cells (Chapter 1). ROS activate signal-transduction pathways and combine with proteins, lipids and DNA, which can lead to loss of cell function and cell death. Leukocyte-derived ROS, released within phagosomes, are bactericidal. ROS important in inflammation include superoxide ($O_2\bullet$, O_2^-), nitric oxide (NO•), hydrogen peroxide (H_2O_2) and hydroxyl radical (OH•) (Fig. 2-16).

Superoxide

Molecular oxygen is converted to superoxide anion (O_2^-) by several pathways: (1) within cells, O_2^- occurs spontaneously near the inner mitochondrial membrane; (2) in vascular endothelial cells, O_2^- is generated by flavoenzymes such as xanthine oxidase, as well as lipoxygenase and cyclooxygenase; and (3) in the setting of inflammation, leukocytes as well as endothelial cells use a reduced nicotinamide adenine dinucleotide phosphate (NADPH) oxidase to produce O_2^-.

Within endothelial cells, xanthine oxidase, a purine-metabolizing enzyme, converts xanthine and hypoxanthine to uric acid, thereby generating O_2^-. This pathway is a major intracellular source of O_2^- in neutrophil-mediated cell injury. Proinflammatory mediators, including leukocyte elastase and several cytokines, convert xanthine dehydrogenase to the active xanthine oxidase. Intracellular O_2^- interacts with nuclear factor-κB (NFκB), activating protein-1 (AP-1) and other molecules to activate signal transduction pathways. It is further metabolized to other free radicals, particularly OH•, which contribute to inflammation-related cell injury.

The NADPH oxidase of phagocytic cells, neutrophils and macrophages is a multicomponent enzyme complex that generates high concentrations of extracellular and intracellular O_2^-, mainly for bactericidal and cytotoxic functions. This oxidase uses NADH and NADPH as substrates for electron transfer to molecular oxygen. A similar enzyme complex is present in vascular endothelial cells, where it generates significant, albeit lower, concentrations of O_2^-.

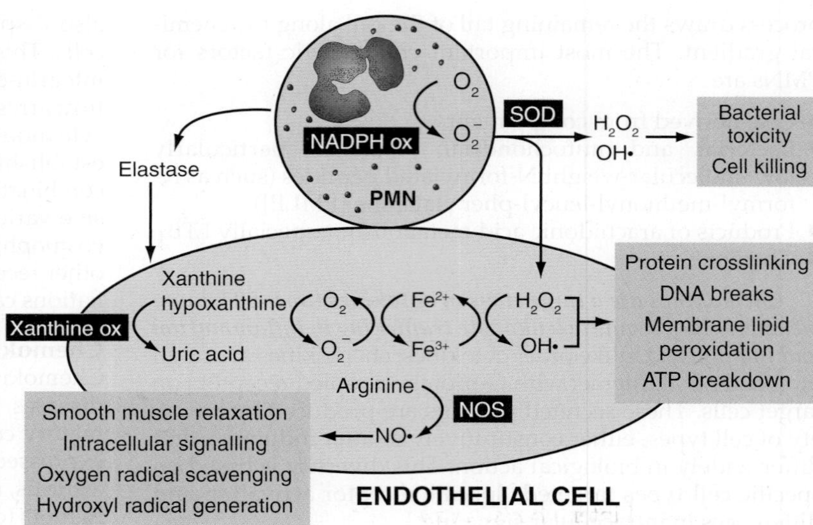

FIGURE 2-16. Biochemical events in neutrophil–endothelial cell interactions. When neutrophils are in firm contact with endothelial cells, oxygen radicals and other active molecules generated by both cells interact. Superoxide (O_2^-) generated by the neutrophil NADPH oxidase (NADPHox) is converted to toxic hydrogen peroxide (H_2O_2) and hydroxyl radical (OH•). Within the endothelial cell, xanthine oxidase (xanthine ox) converts xanthine to uric acid, ultimately generating O_2^- from molecular oxygen. Nitric oxide synthase (NOS) generates nitric oxide (NO•) from arginine. Reactive oxygen species contribute to numerous cellular events. *ATP* = adenosine triphosphate; *Fe^{2+}* = ferrous iron; *Fe^{3+}* = ferric iron; *PMN* = polymorphonuclear neutrophil.

Nitric Oxide

NO• is synthesized by nitric oxide synthase (NOS), which promotes oxidation of the guanidino nitrogen of L-arginine in the presence of O_2. There are three main NOS isoforms: **constitutively expressed neuronal** (nNOS) and **endothelial** (eNOS) forms and an **inducible** (iNOS) isoform. Inflammatory cytokines increase expression of iNOS, generating intracellular and extracellular NO•. NO• has diverse roles in the physiology and pathophysiology of the vascular system, including:

- NO• generated by eNOS acts as **endothelium-derived relaxing factor** (EDRF), mediating vascular smooth muscle relaxation.
- In physiologic concentrations, NO• alone and in balance with O_2^-, is an intracellular messenger.
- NO• prevents platelet adherence and aggregation at sites of vascular injury, reduces leukocyte recruitment and scavenges oxygen radicals.
- Excessive production of NO•, especially in parallel with O_2^-, generates the highly reactive and cytotoxic species, peroxynitrite (ONOO•).

Stress Proteins Protect Against Inflammatory Injury

When cells are subjected to stress conditions, many suffer irreversible injury and die. Others may be severely damaged. However, mild heat treatment prior to lethal injury provides tolerance to subsequent injury. This phenomenon reflects increased expression of the heat shock family of stress proteins (HSPs). Stress proteins belong to multigene families and are named according to molecular size, for example, Hsp27, Hsp70 and Hsp90. They are upregulated by diverse stresses, including oxidative/ischemic stress and inflammation, and are associated with protection during sepsis and metabolic stress. Protein damage and misfolded proteins are common denominators in injury and disease. Protection from many kinds of nonlethal stresses is mediated by HSPs, which act as molecular chaperones, increasing protein expression by enhancing folding of nascent proteins and preventing misfolding. Potential functions of stress proteins include suppression of proinflammatory cytokines and NADPH oxidase, increased nitric oxide–mediated cytoprotection and enhanced collagen synthesis.

Neurokinins Link the Endocrine, Nervous and Immune Systems

The neurokinin family of peptides includes substance P (SP) and neurokinins A (NKA) and B (NKB). These peptides are distributed throughout the central and peripheral nervous systems and represent a link between the endocrine, nervous and immune systems. A wide range of biological processes is associated with these peptides, including plasma protein extravasation and edema, vasodilation, smooth muscle contraction and relaxation, salivary secretion, airway contraction and transmission of nociceptive responses. As early as 1876, Stricker noted an association between sensory afferent nerves and inflammation. ***It is now recognized that injury to nerve terminals during inflammation evokes an increase in neurokinins, which in turn influence production of inflammatory mediators, including histamine, NO• and kinins.*** The actions of neurokinins are mediated by activation of at least three classes of receptors—NK1, NK2 and NK3—which are widely distributed throughout the body. The neurokinin system is linked to inflammation in the following settings:

- **Edema formation:** SP, NKA and NKB induce edema by promoting release of histamine and serotonin from mast cells.
- **Thermal injury:** SP and NKA are produced after thermal injury occurs and mediate early edema.
- **Arthritis:** SP is widely distributed in nerves in joints where it mediates vascular permeability. SP and NKA can modulate the activity of inflammatory and immune cells.
- **Airway inflammation:** SP and NKA have been implicated in bronchoconstriction, mucosal edema, leukocyte adhesion and activation and increased vascular permeability.

Extracellular Matrix Mediators

Interactions of cells and extracellular matrix regulate tissue responses to inflammation. The extracellular environment consists of a macromolecular matrix specific to each tissue. During injury, resident inflammatory cells interact with this matrix, using this scaffolding for migration along a chemokine gradient. Collagen, elastic fibers, basement membrane proteins, glycoproteins and proteoglycans are among the structural macromolecules of the ECM (Chapter 3). Matricellular proteins

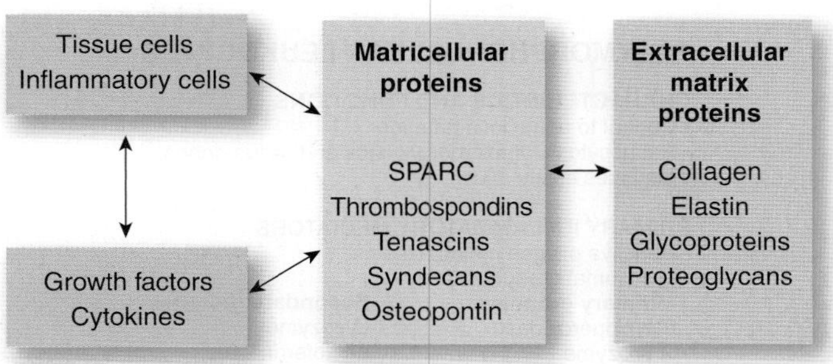

FIGURE 2-17. Dynamic relationship associates cells, soluble mediators and matricellular proteins with the extracellular matrix. *SPARC* = secreted protein acidic and rich in cysteine.

are secreted macromolecules that link cells to the ECM or that disrupt cell–ECM interactions. Cytokines and growth factors influence associations among cells, ECM and matricellular proteins (Fig. 2-17). Matricellular proteins include:

- **SPARC (secreted protein acidic and rich in cysteine)** is a multifunctional glycoprotein that organizes ECM components and modulates growth factor activity. It affects cell proliferation, migration and differentiation and is counteradhesive, especially for endothelial cells.
- **Thrombospondins** are secreted glycoproteins that modulate cell–matrix interactions, influence platelet aggregation and support neutrophil chemotaxis and adhesion.
- **Tenascins C, X and R** are counteradhesive proteins expressed during development, tissue injury and wound healing.
- **Syndecans** are heparan sulfate proteoglycans implicated in coagulation, growth factor signaling, cell adhesion to the ECM and tumorigenesis.
- **Osteopontin** is a phosphorylated glycoprotein important in bone mineralization. It also (1) mediates cell–matrix interactions, (2) activates cell signaling (particularly in T cells), (3) is chemotactic for and supports adhesion of leukocytes and (4) has anti-inflammatory effects via regulation of macrophage function.

Cells of Inflammation

Leukocytes are the major cellular components of the inflammatory response and include neutrophils, T and B lymphocytes, monocytes, macrophages, eosinophils, mast cells and basophils. Specific functions are associated with each of these cell types, but they overlap and vary as inflammation progresses. ***Inflammatory cells and resident tissue cells interact with one another in a continuous response during inflammation.***

Neutrophils

The polymorphonuclear neutrophil, or PMN, is the major cellular participant in acute inflammation. PMNs have granulated cytoplasm and a nucleus with two to four lobules, are stored in bone marrow, circulate in the blood and rapidly accumulate at sites of injury or infection (Fig. 2-18A). Neutrophil receptors recognize the Fc portion of IgG and IgM; complement components C5a, C3b and iC3b; arachidonic acid metabolites; chemotactic factors; and cytokines. In tissues, PMNs phagocytose invading microbes and dead tissue and then undergo apoptosis, an event that corresponds to the resolution phase of acute inflammation.

Endothelial Cells

Endothelial cells, a monolayer of cells lining blood vessels, help to separate intravascular and extravascular spaces. They produce antiplatelet and antithrombotic agents that maintain blood vessel patency and also vasodilators and vasoconstrictors that regulate vascular tone. Injury to a vessel wall interrupts the endothelial barrier and exposes local procoagulant signals (Fig. 2-18B).

Endothelial cells are gatekeepers in inflammatory cell recruitment: they may promote or inhibit tissue perfusion and inflammatory cell influx. Inflammatory agents such as bradykinin and histamine, endotoxin and cytokines induce endothelial cells to reveal adhesion molecules that anchor and activate leukocytes, present major histocompatibility complex (MHC) class I and II molecules and generate key vasoactive and inflammatory mediators. These mediators include:

- **Nitric oxide (NO•):** Originally identified as "endothelial-derived relaxation factor," NO• is a low–molecular-weight vasodilator that inhibits platelet aggregation, regulates vascular tone by stimulating smooth muscle relaxation and reacts with ROS to create highly reactive radical species (see above).
- **Endothelins:** Endothelins-1, -2 and -3 are low–molecular-weight peptides produced by endothelial cells. They are potent vasoconstrictor and pressor agents, which induce prolonged vasoconstriction of vascular smooth muscle.
- **Arachidonic acid–derived contraction factors:** Oxygen radicals generated by the hydroperoxidase activity of cyclooxygenase and prostanoids such as TXA_2 and PGH_2 induce smooth muscle contraction.
- **Arachidonic acid-derived relaxing factors:** The biological opponent of TXA_2, PGI_2 inhibits platelet aggregation and causes vasodilation.
- **Cytokines:** IL-1, IL-6, TNF-α and other inflammatory cytokines are generated by activated endothelial cells.
- **Anticoagulants:** Heparinlike molecules and thrombomodulin inactivate the coagulation cascade (Chapters 10 and 20).
- **Fibrinolytic factors:** Tissue-type plasminogen activator (t-PA) promotes fibrinolytic activity.
- **Prothrombotic agents:** von Willebrand factor facilitates adhesion of platelets, and tissue factor activates the extrinsic clotting cascade.

Monocyte/Macrophages

Circulating monocytes (Fig. 2-18C) are bone marrow–derived cells that have a single lobed or kidney-shaped nucleus. They may exit the circulation to migrate into tissue and become resident macrophages. In response to inflammatory mediators, they accumulate at sites of acute inflammation, where they take up and process microbes. Monocytes/macrophages produce potent vasoactive mediators, including prostaglandins and leukotrienes, PAF and inflammatory cytokines, and are especially important for maintaining chronic inflammation.

Dendritic Cells

Dendritic cells are derived from bone marrow progenitors, circulate in the blood as immature precursors and then are widely distributed in tissues where they differentiate. These highly efficient antigen-presenting cells stimulate naive T cells. Antigens bind to the **major histocompatibility complex**

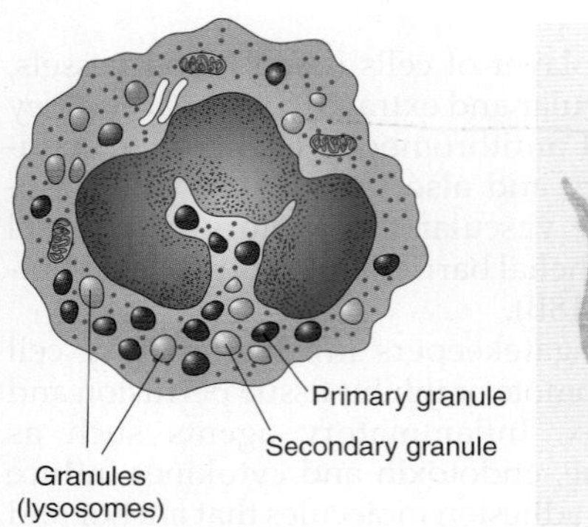

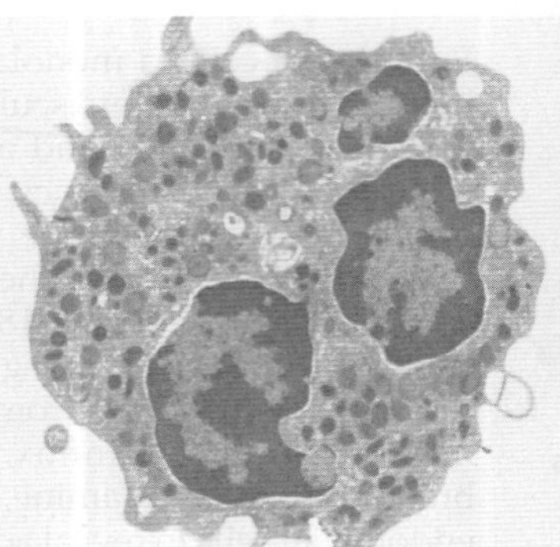

A

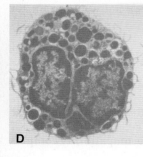

POLYMORPHONUCLEAR LEUKOCYTES

CHARACTERISTICS AND FUNCTIONS
- Central to acute inflammation
- Phagocytosis of microorganisms and tissue debris
- Mediates tissue injury

PRIMARY INFLAMMATORY MEDIATORS
- Reactive oxygen metabolites
- Lysosomal granule contents

Primary granules	Secondary granules
Myeloperoxidase	Lysozyme
Lysozyme	Lactoferrin
Defensins	Collagenase
Bactericidal/permeability increasing protein	Complement activator
Elastase	Phospholipase A_2
Cathepsins Protease 3	CD11b/CD18
Glucuronidase	CD11c/CD18
Mannosidase	Laminin
Phospholipase A_2	

Tertiary granules
Gelatinase
Plasminogen activator
Cathepsins
Glucuronidase
Mannosidase

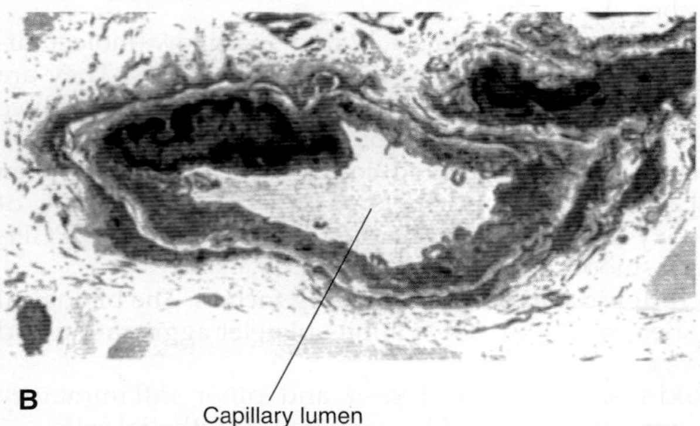

B

ENDOTHELIAL CELLS

CHARACTERISTICS AND FUNCTIONS
- Maintains vascular integrity
- Regulates platelet aggregation
- Regulates vascular contraction and relaxation
- Mediates leukocyte recruitment in inflammation

PRIMARY INFLAMMATORY MEDIATORS
- von Willebrand factor
- Nitric oxide
- Endothelins
- Prostanoids

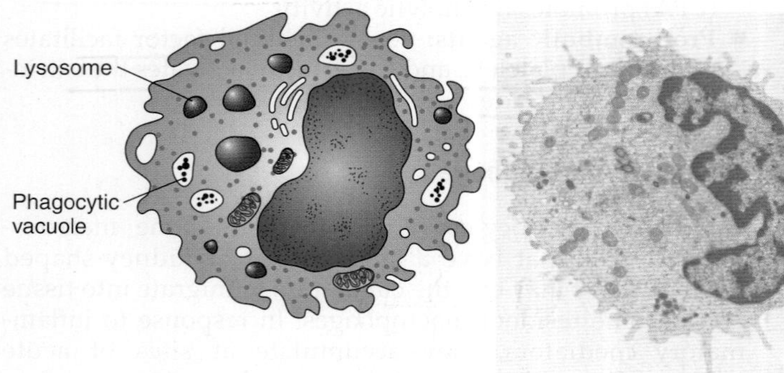

C

MONOCYTE/MACROPHAGE

CHARACTERISTICS AND FUNCTIONS
- Regulates inflammatory response
- Regulates coagulation/fibrinolytic pathway
- Regulates immune response (see Chapter 4)

PRIMARY INFLAMMATORY MEDIATORS
- Cytokines
  - -IL-1
  - -TNF-α
  - -IL-6
  - -Chemokines (e.g., IL-8, MCP-1)
- Lysosomal enzymes
  - -Acid hydrolases
  - -Serine proteases
  - -Metalloproteases (e.g., collagenase)
- Cationic proteins
- Prostaglandins/leukotrienes
- Plasminogen activator
- Procoagulant activity
- Oxygen metabolite formation

D

MAST CELL (BASOPHILS)

CHARACTERISTICS AND FUNCTIONS
- Binds IgE molecules
- Contains electron-dense granules

PRIMARY INFLAMMATORY MEDIATORS
- Histamine
- Leukotrienes (LTC, LTD, LTE)
- Platelet-activating factor
- Eosinophil chemotactic factors
- Cytokines (e.g., TNF-α IL-4)

FIGURE 2-18. Cells of inflammation: morphology and function. A. Neutrophil. **B.** Endothelial cell. **C.** Monocyte/macrophage. **D.** Mast cell. *IL* = interleukin; *MCP-1* = monocyte chemoattractant protein-1; *TNF-α* = tumor necrosis factor-α.

class II on dendritic cells and are presented to lymphocytes, which are subsequently activated.

Mast Cells and Basophils

Mast cell products play an important role in regulating vascular permeability and bronchial smooth muscle tone, especially in allergic hypersensitivity reactions (Chapter 4). Mast cells are found in connective tissues and are especially prevalent at lung and gastrointestinal mucosal surfaces, the dermis and the microvasculature. Basophils circulate in small numbers and can migrate into tissue.

Granulated mast cells and basophils (Fig. 2-18D) contain cell surface receptors for IgE. When IgE-sensitized mast cells or basophils are stimulated by antigen, physical agonists such as cold and trauma, or cationic proteins, inflammatory mediators in their dense cytoplasmic granules are secreted into extracellular tissues. These granules contain acid mucopolysaccharides (including heparin), serine proteases, chemotactic mediators for neutrophils, and eosinophils and histamine, a primary mediator of early increased vascular permeability. Histamine binds specific H_1 receptors in the vascular wall, inducing endothelial cell contraction, gap formation and edema, an effect that can be inhibited pharmacologically by H_1-receptor antagonists. Stimulation of mast cells and basophils also leads to release of products of arachidonic acid metabolism, including LTC_4, LTD_4 and LTE_4, and cytokines, such as TNF-α and IL-4.

Eosinophils

Eosinophils circulate in blood and are recruited to tissue similarly to PMNs. They are often seen in IgE-mediated reactions, such as hypersensitivity, allergic and asthmatic responses (Fig. 2-19A). Eosinophils contain leukotrienes and PAF, as well as acid phosphatase and peroxidase. They express IgA receptors and contain large granules with eosinophil major basic protein, both of which are involved in defense against parasites.

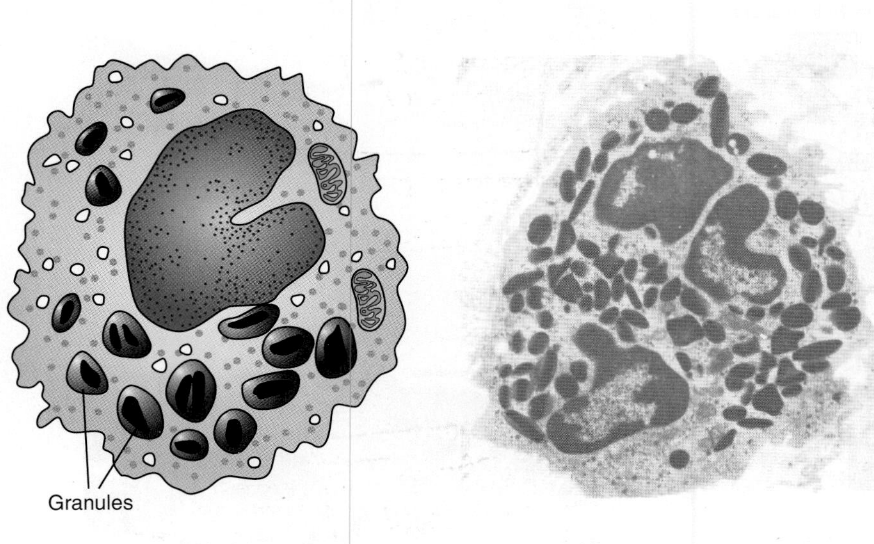

EOSINOPHILS

CHARACTERISTICS AND FUNCTIONS

- Associated with:
  - -Allergic reactions
  - -Parasite-associated inflammatory reactions
  - -Chronic inflammation
- Modulates mast cell-mediated reactions

PRIMARY INFLAMMATORY MEDIATORS

- Reactive oxygen metabolites
- Lysosomal granule enzymes (primary crystalloid granules)
  - -Major basic protein
  - -Eosinophil cationic protein
  - -Eosinophil peroxidase
  - -Acid phosphatase
  - -β-glucuronidase
  - -Arylsulfatase B
  - -Histaminase
- Phospholipase D
- Prostaglandins of E series
- Cytokines

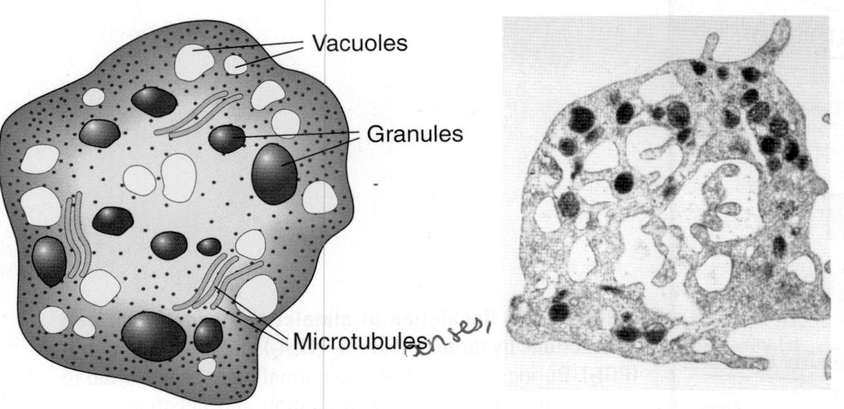

PLATELETS

CHARACTERISTICS AND FUNCTIONS

- Thrombosis; promotes clot formation
- Regulates permeability
- Regulates proliferative response of mesenchymal cells

PRIMARY INFLAMMATORY MEDIATORS

- Dense granules
  - -Serotonin
  - -Ca^{2+}
  - -ADP
- α-granules
  - -Cationic proteins
  - -Fibrinogen and coagulation proteins
  - -Platelet-derived growth factor (PDGF)
- Lysosomes
  - -Acid hydrolases
- Thromboxane A_2

FIGURE 2-19. More cells of inflammation: morphology and function. A. Eosinophil. **B.** Platelet. *ADP* = adenosine diphosphate.

Platelets

Platelets play a primary role in normal homeostasis and in initiating and regulating clot formation (Chapter 20). They are sources of inflammatory mediators, including potent vasoactive substances and growth factors that modulate mesenchymal cell proliferation (Fig. 2-19B). These cells are small (averaging about 2 mm in diameter), lack nuclei and contain three distinct kinds of inclusions: (1) **dense granules**, rich in serotonin, histamine, calcium and adenosine diphosphate (ADP); (2) **α-granules**, containing fibrinogen, coagulation proteins, platelet-derived growth factor (PDGF) and other peptides and proteins; and (3) **lysosomes**, which sequester acid hydrolases.

Platelets adhere, aggregate and degranulate when they contact fibrillar collagen (e.g., after vascular injury that exposes interstitial matrix proteins) or thrombin (after activation of the coagulation system) (Fig. 2-20). Degranulation is associated with release of serotonin (5-hydroxytryptamine), which, like histamine, directly increases vascular permeability. In addition, the arachidonic acid metabolite TXA_2, produced by platelets, plays a key role in the second wave of platelet aggregation and mediates smooth muscle constriction. On activation, platelets, as well as phagocytic cells, secrete cationic proteins that neutralize the negative charges on endothelium and promote increased permeability.

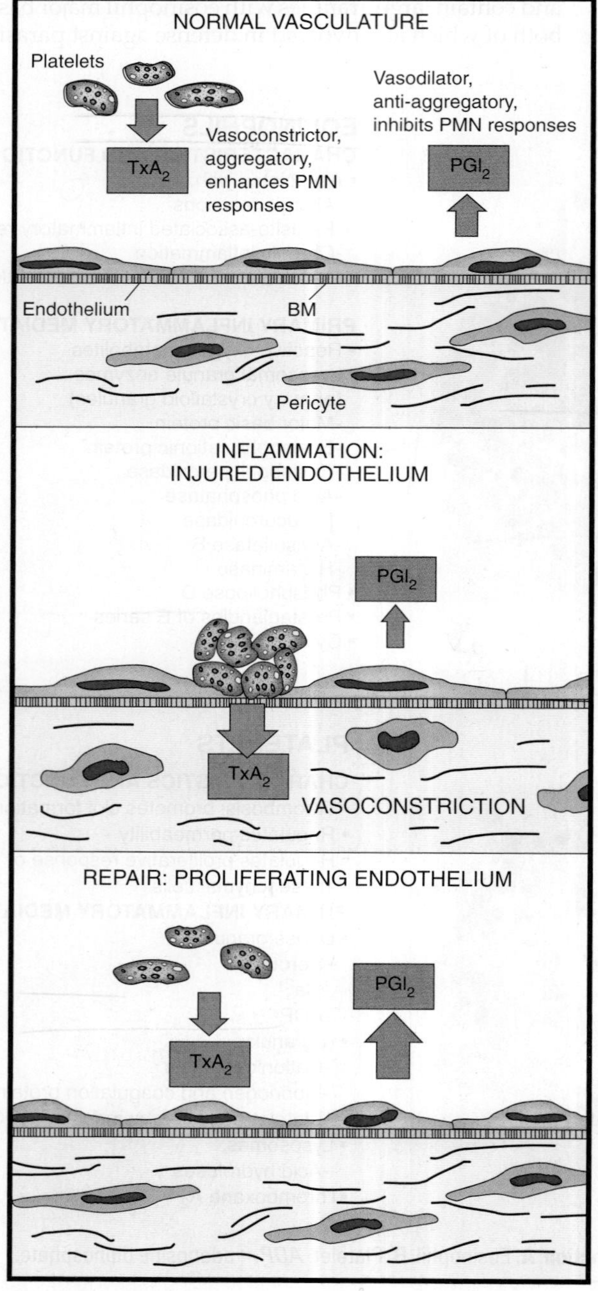

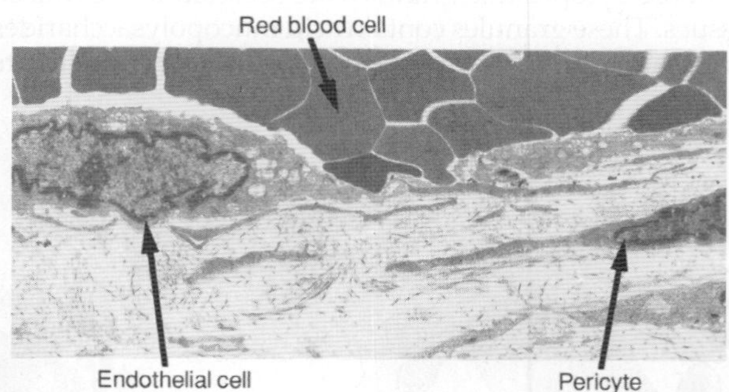

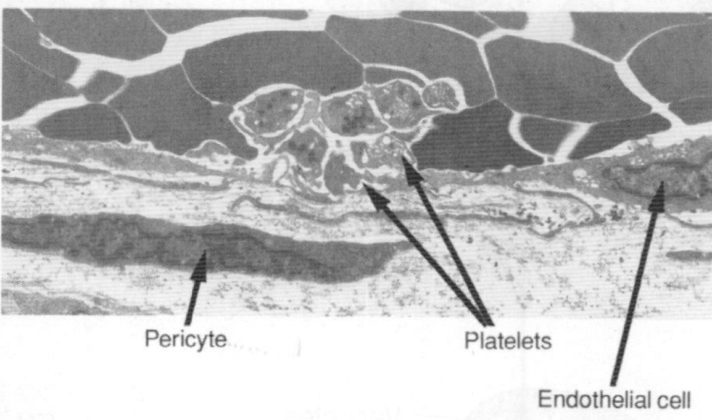

FIGURE 2-20. Regulation of platelet and endothelial cell interactions by thromboxane A_2 (TXA_2) and prostaglandin I_2 (PGI_2). During inflammation, the normal balance is shifted to vasoconstriction, platelet aggregation and polymorphonuclear neutrophil (PMN) responses. During repair, the prostaglandin effects predominate. *BM* = basement membrane.

Leukocyte Recruitment in Acute Inflammation

An essential feature of inflammation is accumulation of leukocytes, particularly PMNs, in affected tissues. Leukocytes adhere to vascular endothelium, becoming activated in the process. They then flatten and migrate from the vasculature, through the endothelial cell layer and into surrounding tissue. In the extravascular tissue, PMNs ingest foreign material, microbes and dead tissue (Fig. 2-21).

Leukocyte Adhesion to Endothelium Results From Interaction of Complementary Adhesion Molecules

Leukocyte recruitment to postcapillary venules begins with interaction of leukocytes with endothelial cell selectins, which are redistributed to endothelial cell surfaces during activation. This interaction, called **tethering**, slows leukocytes in the blood flow (Fig. 2-22). Leukocytes then move along the vascular endothelial cell surface with a saltatory movement, termed **rolling**. PMNs become activated by proximity to the endothelium and by inflammatory mediators, and adhere strongly to intercellular adhesion molecules (ICAMs) on the endothelium **(leukocyte arrest)**. As endothelial cells separate, leukocytes **transmigrate** through the vessel wall and, under the influence of chemotactic factors, leukocytes migrate to the site of injury.

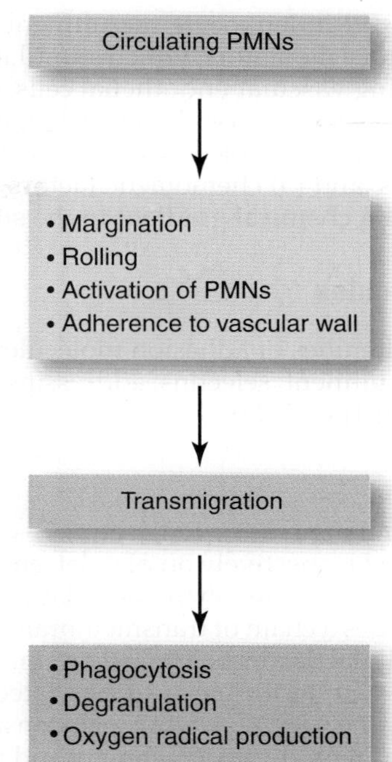

FIGURE 2-21. Leukocyte recruitment and activation. *PMNs* = polymorphonuclear neutrophils.

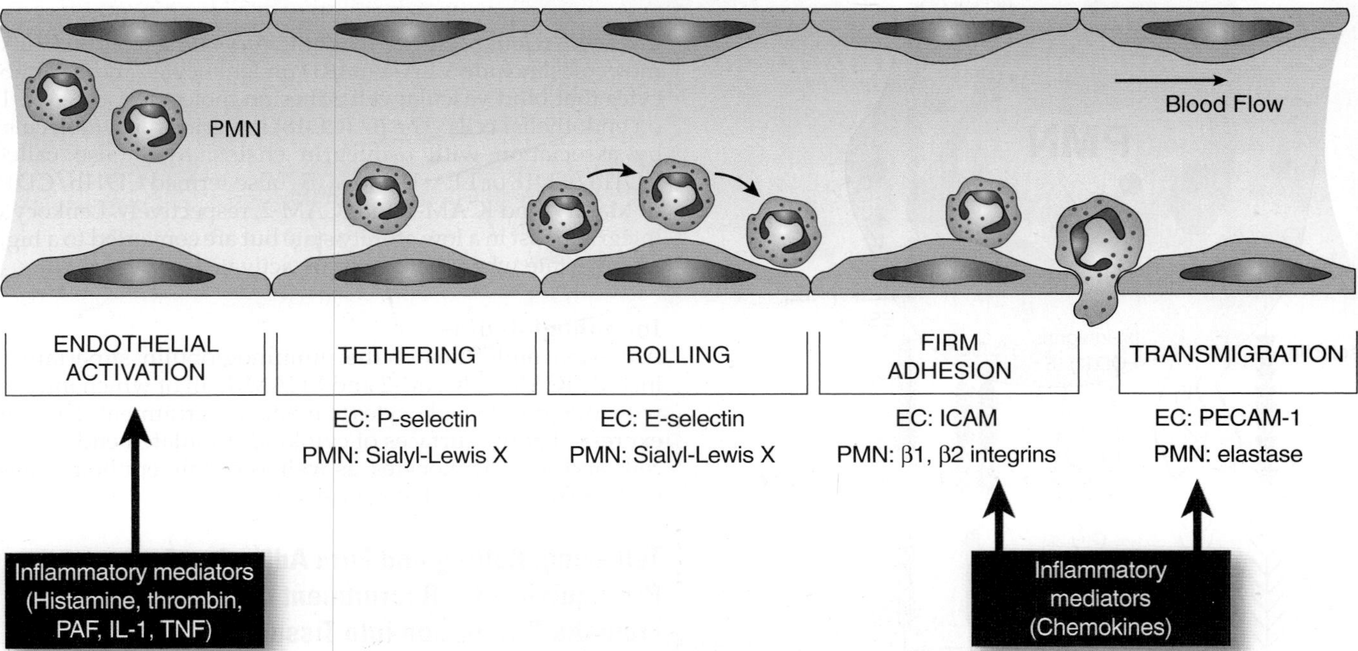

FIGURE 2-22. Neutrophil adhesion and extravasation. Inflammatory mediators activate endothelial cells to increase expression of adhesion molecules. Sialyl-Lewis X on neutrophil P-selectin glycoprotein-1 (PSGL-1) and E-selectin ligand (ESL-1) binds to P- and E-selectins to facilitate tethering and rolling of neutrophils. Increased integrins on activated neutrophils bind to intercellular adhesion molecule-1 (ICAM-1) on endothelial cells to form a firm attachment. Endothelial cell attachments to one another are released and neutrophils then pass between separated cells to enter the tissue. *EC* = endothelial cell; *IL* = interleukin; *PAF* = platelet-activating factor; *PMN* = polymorphonuclear neutrophil; *TNF* = tumor necrosis factor.

Events involved in leukocyte recruitment are regulated by (1) inflammatory mediators, which stimulate resident tissue cells, including vascular endothelial cells; (2) expression of adhesion molecules on vascular endothelial cell surfaces, which bind to reciprocal molecules on the surfaces of circulating leukocytes; and (3) chemotactic factors, which attract leukocytes along a chemical gradient to the site of injury.

Adhesion Molecules

Four molecular families of adhesion molecules are involved in leukocyte recruitment: selectins, addressins, integrins and immunoglobulins (Fig. 2-23).

Selectins

The selectin family includes P-selectin, E-selectin and L-selectin, expressed respectively on platelet, endothelium and leukocyte surfaces. Selectins share a similar molecular structure, which includes a chain of transmembrane glycoproteins with an extracellular lectin-binding domain. This calcium-dependent or C-type lectin binds to sialylated oligosaccharides, specifically the sialyl-Lewis X moiety on addressins, the binding of which allows rapid attachment and rolling of cells.

P-selectin (CD62P, GMP-140, PADGEM) is preformed and stored within Weibel-Palade bodies of endothelial cells and α-granules of platelets. On stimulation with histamine, thrombin or specific inflammatory cytokines, P-selectin is rapidly transported to the cell surface, where it binds to sialyl-Lewis X on leukocyte surfaces. Preformed P-selectin can be delivered quickly to the cell surface, allowing rapid adhesive interaction between endothelial cells and leukocytes.

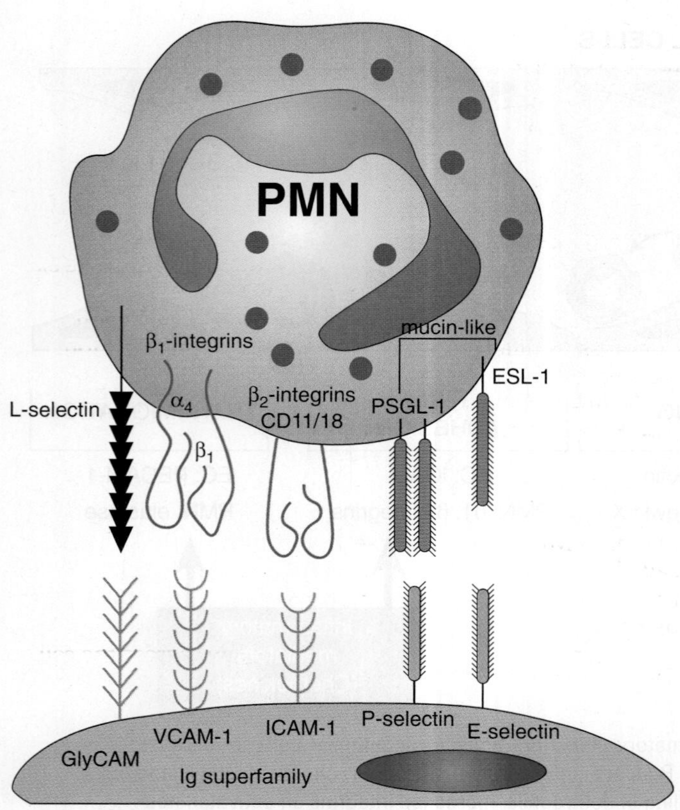

FIGURE 2-23. Leukocyte and endothelial cell adhesion molecules. *GlyCAM* = glycan-bearing cell adhesion molecule; *ICAM-1* = intercellular adhesion molecule-1; *VCAM* = vascular cell adhesion molecule.

E-selectin (CD62E, ELAM-1) is not normally expressed on endothelial cell surfaces but is induced by inflammatory mediators, such as cytokines or bacterial LPS. E-selectin mediates adhesion of neutrophils, monocytes and certain lymphocytes via binding to Lewis X or Lewis A.

L-selectin (CD62L, LAM-1, Leu-8) is expressed on many types of leukocytes. It was originally defined as the "homing receptor" for lymphocytes. It binds lymphocytes to high endothelial venules (HEVs) in lymphoid tissue, thereby regulating their trafficking through this tissue. L-selectin binds glycan-bearing cell adhesion molecule-1 (GlyCAM-1), mucosal addressin cell adhesion molecule-1 (MadCAM-1) and CD34.

Addressins

Vascular addressins are mucinlike glycoproteins including GlyCAM-1, P-selectin glycoprotein-1 (PSGL-1), E-selectin ligand (ESL-1) and CD34. They possess sialyl-Lewis X, which binds the lectin domain of selectins. Addressins are expressed at leukocyte and endothelium surfaces. They regulate localization of leukocyte subpopulations and are involved in lymphocyte activation.

Integrins

Chemokines, lipid mediators and proinflammatory molecules activate cells to express the integrin family of adhesion molecules (Chapter 3). Integrins have transmembrane α and β chains arranged as heterodimers. They participate in cell–cell interactions and cell–ECM binding. β_1, β_2, and β_7 integrins are involved in leukocyte recruitment. *V*ery *l*ate *a*ctivation (VLA) molecules include VLA-4 ($\alpha 4\beta 1$) on leukocytes and lymphocytes that bind vascular cell adhesion molecule-1 (VCAM-1) on endothelial cells. The $\beta 2$ (CD18) integrins form molecules by association with α-integrin chains: $\alpha_1\beta_2$ (also called CD11a/CD18 or LFA-1) and $\alpha_m\beta_2$ (also termed CD11b/CD18 or Mac-1) bind ICAM-1 and ICAM-2, respectively. Leukocyte integrins exist in a low affinity state but are converted to a high affinity state when these cells are activated.

Immunoglobulins

Adhesion molecules of the immunoglobulin superfamily include ICAM-1, ICAM-2 and VCAM-1, all of which interact with integrins on leukocytes to mediate recruitment. They are expressed at the surfaces of cytokine-stimulated endothelial cells and some leukocytes, as well as certain epithelial cells, such as pulmonary alveolar cells.

Tethering, Rolling and Firm Adhesion Are Prerequisites for Recruitment of Leukocytes From the Circulation into Tissues

For a rolling cell to adhere, there must first be a selectin-dependent reduction in rolling velocity. Early increases in rolling depend on P-selectin, whereas cytokine-induced E-selectin initiates early adhesion. Integrin family members function cooperatively with selectins to facilitate rolling and subsequent firm adhesion of leukocytes. Leukocyte integrin binding to the Ig superfamily of ligands expressed on vascular endothelium further retards leukocytes, increasing the length of exposure of each leukocyte to endothelium. At the same time, engagement of adhesion molecules activates intracellular signal transduction. As a result, leukocytes and vascular endothelial cells are further activated, with subsequent upregulation of L-selectin and integrin binding. The net result is firm adhesion.

Recruitment of specific subsets of leukocytes to areas of inflammation may result from unique patterns or relative densities of adhesion molecules on cell surfaces. For subsets of leukocytes, each cell type can express specific adhesion molecules. Cytokines or chemokines specific to the inflammatory process induce the display of adhesion molecules on vascular endothelium and changes in the affinity of these molecules for their ligands. For example, in allergic or asthmatic inflammation, cytokine induction of VCAM-1 on endothelial cells increases recruitment of VLA-4–bearing eosinophils in preference to neutrophils, which do not express VLA-4.

Leukocyte recruitment in some tissues may not follow this paradigm. In the liver, leukocytes may not need to roll in the narrow sinusoids before adhering to endothelium. Leukocyte adherence to arterioles and capillaries also has different requirements, reflecting the different hydrodynamic forces in these vessels.

Chemotactic Molecules Direct Neutrophils to Sites of Injury

Leukocytes must be accurately positioned at sites of inflammatory injury to carry out their biological functions. For specific subsets of leukocytes to arrive in a timely fashion, they must receive very specific directions. ***Leukocytes are guided through vascular and extravascular spaces by a complex interaction of attractants, repellants and adhesion molecules.*** **Chemotaxis** is a dynamic and energy-dependent process of directed cell migration. Blood leukocytes are recruited by chemoattractants released by endothelial cells. They then migrate from the endothelium toward the target tissue, down a gradient of one chemoattractant in response to a second more distal chemoattractant gradient.

Neutrophils must integrate the various signals to arrive at the correct site at the correct time to perform their assigned tasks. The most important chemotactic factors for PMNs are C5a, bacterial and mitochondrial products (particularly low–molecular-weight N-formylated peptides such as FMLP), products of arachidonic acid metabolism (especially LTB_4), products of ECM degradation and chemokines. The latter represent a key mechanism of leukocyte recruitment because they generate a chemotactic gradient by binding to ECM proteoglycans. As a result, high concentrations of chemokines persist at sites of tissue injury. In turn, specific receptors on migrating leukocytes bind matrix-bound chemokines, moving the cells along the chemotactic gradient to the site of injury.

Chemotactic factors for other cell types, including lymphocytes, basophils and eosinophils, are also produced at sites of tissue injury and may be secreted by activated endothelial cells, tissue parenchymal cells or other inflammatory cells. They include PAF, transforming growth factor-β (TGF-β), neutrophilic cationic proteins and lymphokines. ***The cocktail of chemokines presented within a tissue largely determines the type of leukocyte attracted to the site.*** Cells arriving at their destination must then be able to stop in the target tissue. Contact guidance, regulated adhesion or inhibitory signals may determine the final arrest of specific cells in specific tissue locations.

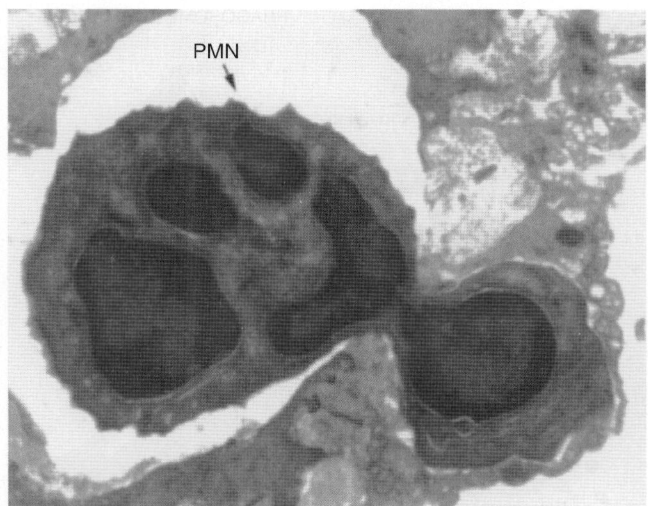

FIGURE 2-24. Transmission electron micrograph demonstrates neutrophil transmigration. A neutrophil exits the vascular space by diapedesis across the vascular endothelium. *PMN* = polymorphonuclear neutrophil.

Leukocytes Traverse the Endothelial Cell Barrier to Gain Access to Tissues

Leukocytes adherent to the vascular endothelium emigrate by **paracellular diapedesis** (i.e., passing between adjacent endothelial cells). Responding to chemokine gradients, neutrophils extend pseudopods and insinuate themselves between the endothelial cells and out of the intravascular space (Fig. 2-24). Vascular endothelial cells are connected by tight junctions and adherens junctions. CD31 (platelet endothelial cell adhesion molecule **[PECAM-1]**) on endothelial cell surfaces binds to itself to keep cells together. These junctions separate under the influence of inflammatory mediators, intracellular signals generated by adhesion molecule engagement and signals from the adherent neutrophils. Neutrophils mobilize elastase to their pseudopod membranes, inducing endothelial cells to retract and separate at the advancing edge of the neutrophil, a process facilitated by PMN-elicited increases in endothelial cell intracellular calcium.

Neutrophils also migrate through endothelial cells, by **transcellular diapedesis**. Instead of inducing endothelial cell retraction, PMNs may squeeze through small circular pores in endothelial cell cytoplasm. In tissues that contain fenestrated microvessels, such as gastrointestinal mucosa and secretory glands, PMNs may traverse thin regions of endothelium, called **fenestrae**, without damaging endothelial cells. In nonfenestrated microvessels, PMNs may cross the endothelium using endothelial cell caveolae or pinocytotic vesicles, which form small, membrane-bound passageways across the cell.

Leukocyte Functions in Acute Inflammation

Leukocytes Phagocytose Microorganisms and Tissue Debris

Many inflammatory cells—including monocytes, tissue macrophages, dendritic cells and neutrophils—recognize, internalize and digest foreign material, microorganisms or

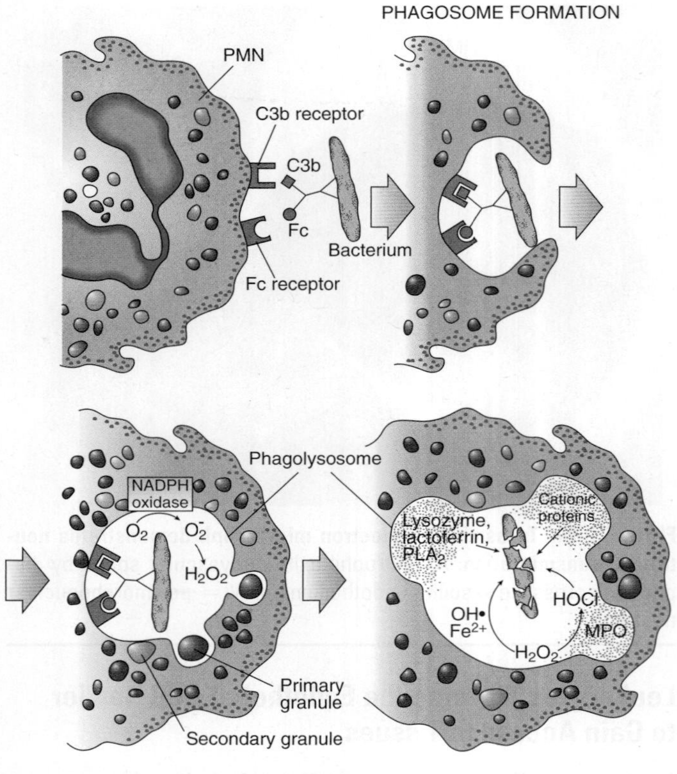

FIGURE 2-25. Mechanisms of neutrophil bacterial phagocytosis and cell killing. Opsonins such as C3b coat the surface of microbes, allowing recognition by the neutrophil C3b receptor. Receptor clustering triggers intracellular signaling and actin assembly within the neutrophil. Pseudopods form around the microbe to enclose it within a phagosome. Lysosomal granules fuse with the phagosome to form a phagolysosome into which the lysosomal enzymes and oxygen radicals are released to kill and degrade the microbe. *Fe^{2+}* = ferrous iron; *HOCl* = hypochlorous acid; *MPO* = myeloperoxidase; *PLA_2* = phospholipase A_2; *PMN* = polymorphonuclear neutrophil.

cellular debris by the process of **phagocytosis**. This term, first used over a century ago by Elie Metchnikoff, is now defined as ingestion by eukaryotic cells of large (usually >0.5 μm) insoluble particles and microorganisms. **Phagocytes** are the effector cells. The complex process involves a sequence of transmembrane and intracellular signaling events:

1. **Recognition:** Phagocytosis is initiated when specific receptors on the surface of phagocytic cells recognize their targets (Fig. 2-25). Phagocytosis of most biological agents is enhanced by, if not dependent on, their coating **(opsonization)** with plasma components **(opsonins)**, particularly immunoglobulins or C3b. Phagocytic cells possess specific opsonic receptors, including those for immunoglobulin Fcγ and complement components. Many pathogens have evolved mechanisms to evade phagocytosis by leukocytes. Polysaccharide capsules, protein A, protein M or peptidoglycans around bacteria can prevent complement deposition or antigen recognition and receptor binding.
2. **Signaling:** Clumping of opsonins at bacterial surfaces causes phagocyte plasma membrane Fcγ receptors to cluster. Subsequent phosphorylation of immunoreceptor tyrosine-based activation motifs (ITAMs), located in the cytosolic domain or γ subunit of the receptor, triggers intracellular signaling via tyrosine kinases that associate with the Fcγ receptor (Fig. 2-26).
3. **Internalization:** For Fcγ receptor or CR3, actin assembly occurs directly under the phagocytosed target. Polymerized actin filaments push the plasma membrane forward. The plasma membrane remodels to increase surface area and to form pseudopods surrounding the foreign material. The resulting phagocytic cup engulfs the foreign agent. The membrane then "zippers" around the opsonized particle to enclose it in a vacuole called a **phagosome** (Figs. 2-25 and 2-26).
4. **Digestion:** The phagosome with the foreign material fuses to cytoplasmic lysosomes to form a **phagolysosome**, into which lysosomal enzymes are released. The acid pH within the phagolysosome activates these hydrolytic enzymes, which then degrade the phagocytosed material. Some microorganisms have evolved mechanisms for evading killing by neutrophils by preventing lysosomal degranulation or inhibiting neutrophil enzymes.

Neutrophil Enzymes Are Required for Antimicrobial Defense and Débridement

Although PMNs are critical for degrading microbes and cell debris, they also contribute to tissue injury (Fig. 2-27). PMN release of their granule contents at sites of injury is a double-edged sword. On the one hand, débridement of damaged tissue by proteolytic breakdown is beneficial. On the other hand, degradative enzymes can damage endothelial and epithelial cells and degrade connective tissue.

Neutrophil Granules

The armamentarium of enzymes required for degradation of microbes and tissue is generated and contained within PMN cytoplasmic granules. Neutrophil primary, secondary and tertiary granules are differentiated morphologically and biochemically: each granule has a unique spectrum of enzymes (Fig. 2-18A).

- **Primary granules (azurophilic granules):** Antimicrobial and proteinase activity of these granules can directly activate other inflammatory cells. Potent acid hydrolases and neutral serine proteases digest a number of macromolecules. Lysozyme and PLA_2 degrade bacterial cell walls and biological membranes and are important in killing bacteria. Myeloperoxidase, a key enzyme in the metabolism of hydrogen peroxide, generates toxic oxygen radicals.
- **Secondary granules (specific granules):** These contain PLA_2, lysozyme and proteins that initiate killing of specific cells. In addition, their contents include the cationic protein, lactoferrin, a vitamin B_{12}-binding protein and a matrix metalloproteinase (collagenase) specific for type IV collagen.
- **Tertiary granules (small storage granules, C granules):** These granules are released at the leading front of neutrophils during chemotaxis. They are the source of enzymes that promote migration of cells through basement membranes and tissues including proteinases cathepsin, gelatinase and urokinase-type plasminogen activator (u-PA).

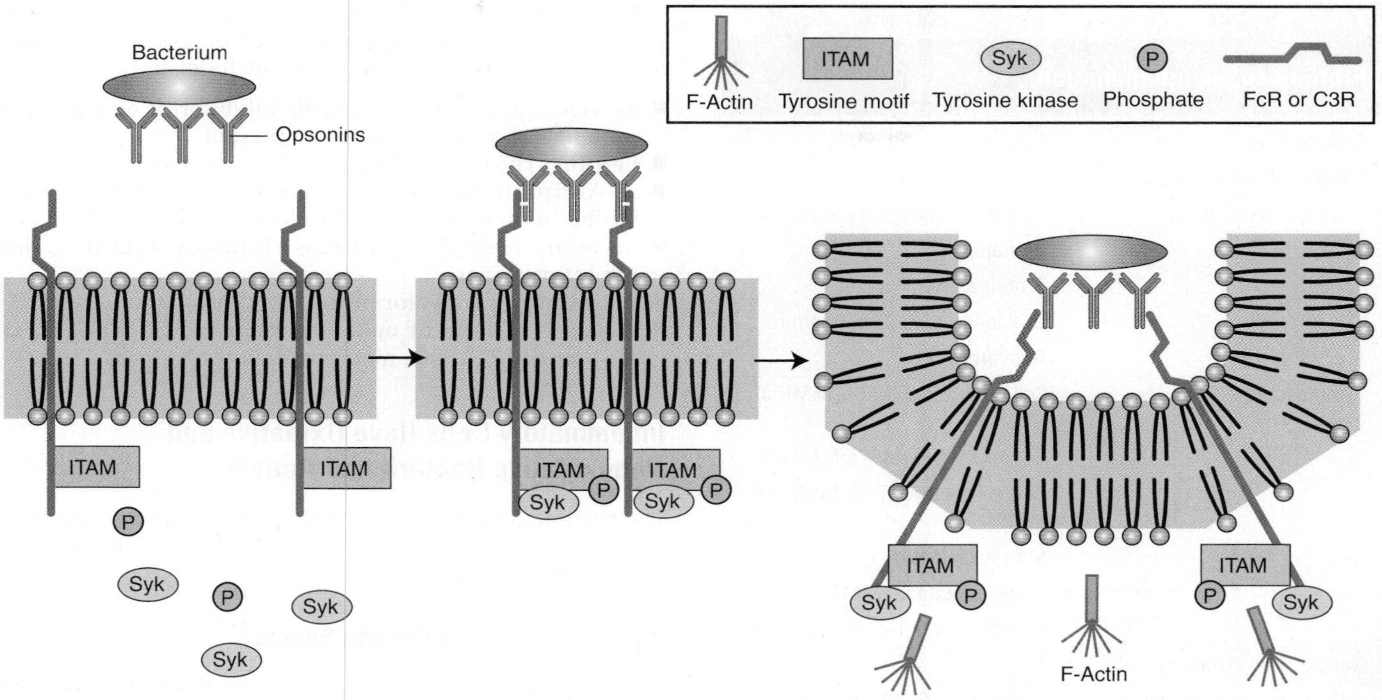

FIGURE 2-26. Intracellular signaling during leukocyte phagocytosis. Opsonins coating the surface of microbes or foreign material are recognized by the neutrophil C3b receptor. Receptor clustering triggers phosphorylation of immunoreceptor tyrosine-based activation motifs (ITAMs) on the receptor and tyrosine kinases initiate intracellular signaling. Polymerized actin filament aggregates beneath the plasma membrane to form a pseudopod to enclose the foreign agent.

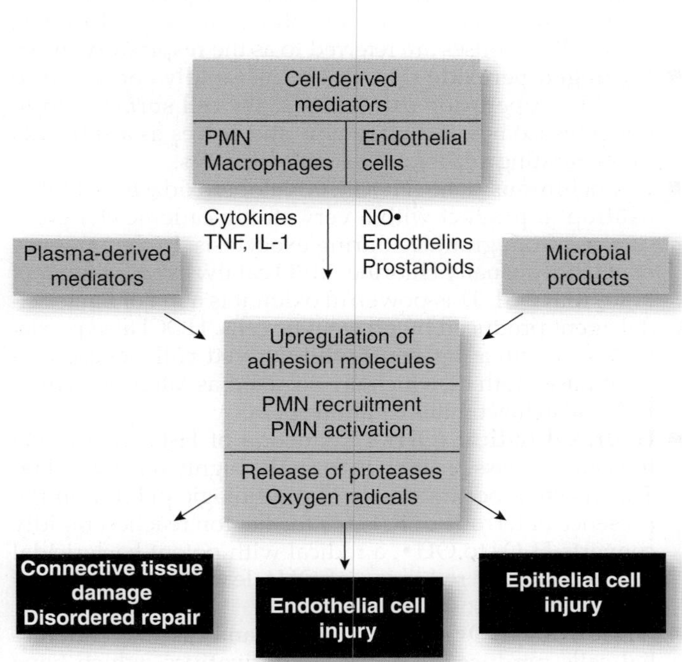

FIGURE 2-27. Leukocyte-mediated inflammatory injury. *IL* = interleukin; *LPS* = lipopolysaccharide; *NO•* = nitric oxide; *PMN* = polymorphonuclear neutrophil; *TNF* = tumor necrosis factor.

Proteinases

Proteolytic enzymes (proteinases) cleave peptide bonds in polypeptides; they are stored in cytoplasmic granules and secretory vesicles of neutrophils. As these cells leave the circulation, they release proteinases that enable them to penetrate the ECM and migrate to sites of injury, there to degrade matrix, cell debris and pathogens. Neutrophils, however, are not the only source of proteinases. These enzymes are also made by most inflammatory cells, including monocytes, eosinophils, basophils, mast cells and lymphocytes, and tissue cells, including vascular endothelium.

Proteinases are classified by their catalytic activity into four groups: serine proteinases and metalloproteinases are neutral enzymes that function in extracellular spaces; cysteine proteinases and aspartic proteinases are acidic and act in the acidic milieu of lysosomes (Table 2-3). These enzymes target a variety of intracellular and extracellular proteins, including (1) inflammatory products; (2) debris from damaged cells, microbial proteins and matrix proteins; (3) microorganisms; (4) plasma proteins, including complement components, clotting factors, immunoglobulins and cytokines; (5) matrix macromolecules (e.g., collagen, elastin, fibronectin and laminin); and (6) lymphocytes and platelets.

Serine Proteinases

Serine proteinases degrade extracellular proteins, cell debris and bacteria. Human leukocyte elastase (HLE) is primarily responsible for degrading fibronectin. Cathepsin G (CG) converts angiotensin I to angiotensin II, thereby mediating

Table 2-3

Proteinases in Inflammation

Enzyme Class	Examples
Neutral Proteinases	
Serine proteinases	Human leukocyte elastase
	Cathepsin G
	Proteinase 3
	Urokinase-type plasminogen Activator
Metalloproteinase	Collagenases (MMP-1, MMP-8, MMP-13)
	Gelatinases (MMP-7, MMP-9)
	Stromelysins (MMP-3, MMP-10, MMP-11)
	Matrilysin (MMP-7)
	Metalloelastase (MMP-12)
	ADAMs-7, -9, -15, -17
Acidic Proteinases	
Cysteine proteinases	Cathepsins, S, L, B, H
Aspartic proteinases	Cathepsin D

MMP = matrix metalloproteinase; ADAM = *A* protein with *d*isintegrin *a*nd *m*etalloproteinase domains.

smooth muscle contraction and vascular permeability. u-PA dissolves fibrin clots to generate plasmin at wound sites, degrades ECM proteins and activates procollagenases to create a path for leukocyte migration. Although serine proteinases are most important in digesting ECM molecules, they also modify cytokine activity: they solubilize membrane-bound cytokines and receptors by cleaving active cytokines from inactive precursors. They also detach cytokine receptors from cell surfaces, thus regulating cytokine bioactivity.

Metalloproteinases

There are at least 25 members identified (Chapter 3). Matrix metalloproteinases (**MMPs**, matrixins) degrade all ECM components, including basement membranes. They are subclassified according to substrate specificity into interstitial collagenases, gelatinases, stromelysins, metalloelastases and matrilysin. Proteins with disintegrin and metalloproteinase domains (ADAMs) regulate neutrophil infiltration by targeting the disintegrins. These molecules are polypeptides that disrupt integrin-mediated binding of cells to each other and to ECM.

Cysteine Proteinases and Aspartic Proteinases

These acid proteinases function primarily within lysosomes of leukocytes to degrade intracellular proteins.

Proteinase Inhibitors

The proteolytic environment is regulated by a battery of inhibitors. During wound healing these antiproteases protect against tissue damage by limiting protease activity. ECM remodeling occurs in the context of a balance between enzymes and inhibitors. In chronic wounds, continuous influx of neutrophils, with their proteases and ROS, may overwhelm and inactivate these inhibitors, allowing continuation of proteolysis (Chapter 3). Known proteinase inhibitors include:

- **α_2-Macroglobulin:** Nonspecific inhibitor of all classes of proteinases, primarily found in plasma
- **Serpins:** The major inhibitors of serine proteinases
- **α_1-Antiproteases** (α_1-antitrypsin, α_1-antichymotrypsin): Inhibit human leukocyte elastase and cathepsin G
- **Secretory leukocyte proteinase inhibitor (SLPI), Elafin:** Inhibit proteinase 3
- **Plasminogen activator inhibitors (PAIs):** Inhibit u-PA
- **Tissue inhibitors of metalloproteinases (TIMP-1, -2, -3, -4):** Specific for tissue matrix metalloproteinases

Inflammatory Cells Have Oxidative and Nonoxidative Bactericidal Activity

The bactericidal activity of PMNs and macrophages is mediated in part by production of ROS and in part by oxygen-independent mechanisms.

Bacterial Killing by Oxygen Species

Phagocytosis is accompanied by metabolic reactions in inflammatory cells that lead to production of several oxygen metabolites (Chapter 1). These products are more reactive than oxygen itself and contribute to the killing of ingested bacteria (Fig. 2-25).

- **Superoxide anion** (O_2^-): Phagocytosis activates a NADPH oxidase in PMN cell membranes. NADPH oxidase is a multicomponent electron transport complex that reduces molecular oxygen to O_2^-. Activation of this enzyme is enhanced by prior exposure of cells to a chemotactic stimulus or LPS. NADPH oxidase activation increases oxygen consumption and stimulates the hexose monophosphate shunt. Together, these cell responses are referred to as the **respiratory burst**.
- **Hydrogen peroxide** (H_2O_2): O_2^- is rapidly converted to H_2O_2 by superoxide dismutase at the cell surface and in phagolysosomes. H_2O_2 is stable and serves as a substrate for generating additional reactive oxidants.
- **Hypochlorous acid** (HOCl): Myeloperoxidase (MPO), a neutrophil product with a very strong cationic charge, is secreted from granules during exocytosis. In the presence of a halide, usually chlorine, MPO catalyzes conversion of H_2O_2 to HOCl. This powerful oxidant is a major bactericidal agent produced by phagocytic cells. HOCl also participates in activating neutrophil-derived collagenase and gelatinase, both of which are secreted as latent enzymes. HOCl also inactivates α_1-antitrypsin.
- **Hydroxyl radical** (OH•): Reduction of H_2O_2 occurs via the Haber-Weiss reaction to form the highly reactive OH•. This reaction occurs slowly at physiologic pH, but in the presence of ferrous iron (Fe^{2+}) the Fenton reaction rapidly converts H_2O_2 to OH•, a radical with potent bactericidal activity. Further reduction of OH• leads to formation of H_2O (Chapter 1).
- **Nitric oxide** (NO•): Phagocytic cells and vascular endothelial cells produce NO• and its derivatives, which have diverse effects, both physiologic and nonphysiologic. NO• and other oxygen radical species interact with one another to balance their cytotoxic and cytoprotective effects. NO• can react with oxygen radicals to form toxic molecules such

Table 2-4

Congenital Diseases of Defective Phagocytic Cell Function Characterized by Recurrent Bacterial Infections

Disease	Defect
Leukocyte adhesion deficiency (LAD)	LAD-1 (defective β_2-integrin expression or function [CD11/CD18]) LAD-2 (defective fucosylation, selectin binding)
Hyper-IgE-recurrent infection, (Job) syndrome	Poor chemotaxis
Chediak-Higashi syndrome	Defective lysosomal granules, poor chemotaxis
Neutrophil-specific granule deficiency	Absent neutrophil granules
Chronic granulomatous disease	Deficient NADPH oxidase, with absent H_2O_2 production
Myeloperoxidase deficiency	Deficient HOCl production

H_2O_2 = hydrogen peroxide; HOCl = hypochlorous acid; Ig = immunoglobulin.

as peroxynitrite and *S*-nitrosothiols, or it can scavenge O_2^-, thereby reducing the amount of toxic radicals.

Monocytes, macrophages and eosinophils also produce oxygen radicals, depending on their state of activation and the stimulus to which they are exposed. Production of ROS by these cells contributes to their bactericidal and fungicidal activity and their ability to kill certain parasites. The importance of oxygen-dependent mechanisms in bacterial killing is exemplified in **chronic granulomatous disease** of childhood. In this hereditary deficiency of NADPH oxidase, failure to produce O_2^- and H_2O_2 during phagocytosis makes these persons susceptible to recurrent infections, especially with Gram-positive cocci. Patients with a related genetic deficiency in MPO cannot produce HOCl and show increased susceptibility to fungal infections with *Candida* (Table 2-4).

Nonoxidative Bacterial Killing

Phagocytes, particularly PMNs and monocytes/macrophages, have substantial antimicrobial activity that is oxygen independent. This activity mainly involves preformed bactericidal proteins in cytoplasmic granules. These include lysosomal acid hydrolases and specialized noncatalytic proteins unique to inflammatory cells.

- **Lysosomal hydrolases:** Neutrophil primary and secondary granules and lysosomes of mononuclear phagocytes contain hydrolases, including sulfatases and phosphatases, and other enzymes capable of digesting polysaccharides and DNA.
- **Bactericidal/permeability-increasing protein (BPI):** This cationic protein in PMN primary granules can kill many Gram-negative bacteria but is not toxic to Gram-positive bacteria or to eukaryotic cells. BPI inserts into the outer membrane of bacterial envelopes and increases its permeability. Activation of certain phospholipases and enzymes then degrades bacterial peptidylglycans.
- **Defensins:** Primary granules of PMNs and lysosomes of some mononuclear phagocytes contain this family of cationic proteins, which kill an extensive variety of Gram-positive and Gram-negative bacteria, fungi and some enveloped viruses. Some of these polypeptides can also kill host cells. Defensins are chemotactic for phagocytic leukocytes, immature dendritic cells and lymphocytes, so they help to mobilize and amplify antimicrobial immunity.
- **Lactoferrin:** Lactoferrin is an iron-binding glycoprotein found in the secondary granules of neutrophils, and in most body secretory fluids. Its iron-chelating capacity allows it to compete with bacteria for iron. It may also facilitate oxidative killing of bacteria by enhancing OH• formation.
- **Lysozyme:** This bactericidal enzyme is found in many tissues and body fluids, in primary and secondary granules of neutrophils and in lysosomes of mononuclear phagocytes. Peptidoglycans of Gram-positive bacterial cell walls are exquisitely sensitive to degradation by lysozyme; Gram-negative bacteria are usually resistant to it.
- **Bactericidal proteins of eosinophils:** Eosinophils contain several granule-bound cationic proteins, the most important of which are major basic protein (MBP) and eosinophilic cationic protein. MBP accounts for about half of the total protein of the eosinophil granule. Both proteins are ineffective against bacteria but are potent cytotoxic agents for many parasites.

Defects in Leukocyte Function

The importance of acute inflammatory cells in protection from infection is underscored by the frequency and severity of infections in settings when PMNs are greatly decreased or defective. ***The most common such deficit is iatrogenic neutropenia resulting from cancer chemotherapy.*** Functional impairment of phagocytes may occur at any step in the sequence: adherence, emigration, chemotaxis or phagocytosis. These disorders may be acquired or congenital. Acquired diseases, such as leukemia, diabetes mellitus, malnutrition, viral infections and sepsis, are often accompanied by defects in inflammatory cell function. Table 2-4 shows representative examples of congenital diseases linked to defective phagocytic function.

Regulation of the Acute Inflammatory Response

Infection, foreign agents and injured tissue are the triggers for acute inflammatory responses. The specificity and intensity of inflammatory mediators, both humoral and cellular, affect tissue responses to the offending agents. Left unchecked, acute inflammation can cause serious tissue injury and death (witness the lethality of pneumococcal pneumonia). However, genetic and biochemical regulation mitigates "bystander" effects of acute inflammation, thereby allowing resolution and repair.

Soluble Mediators Activate Common Intracellular Pathways

Plasma- and cell-derived proinflammatory mediators amplify tissue responses and represent a positive feedback loop, with progressive amplification of the response and subsequent tissue injury. Complement factors, proinflammatory cytokines and, in some cases, immune complexes activate signal

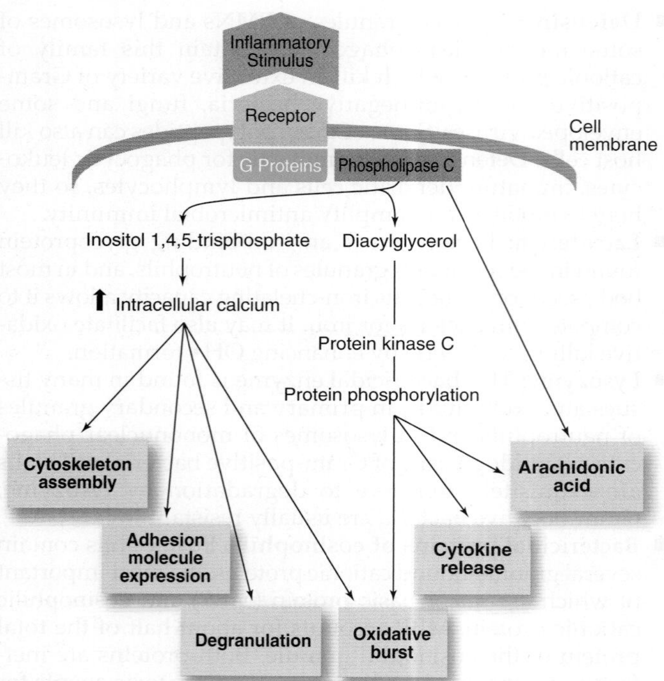

FIGURE 2-28. G-protein–mediated intracellular signal transduction pathway common to many inflammatory stimuli.

transduction pathways that control gene expression of proinflammatory mediators, including TNF-α, IL-1, chemokines and adhesion molecules. Secreted cytokines then propagate the response by activating other cell types using these and similar pathways. The process by which diverse stimuli lead to the functional responses of inflammatory cells is referred to as **stimulus–response coupling**. Stimuli can include microbial products and the many plasma- or cell-derived inflammatory mediators described in this chapter. Although intracellular signaling pathways are complex and vary with cell type and stimulus, some common intracellular pathways are associated with inflammatory cell activation by soluble mediators, including G-protein, TNF receptor (TNFR) and JAK-STAT pathways (Figs. 2-28, 2-29 and 2-30, respectively).

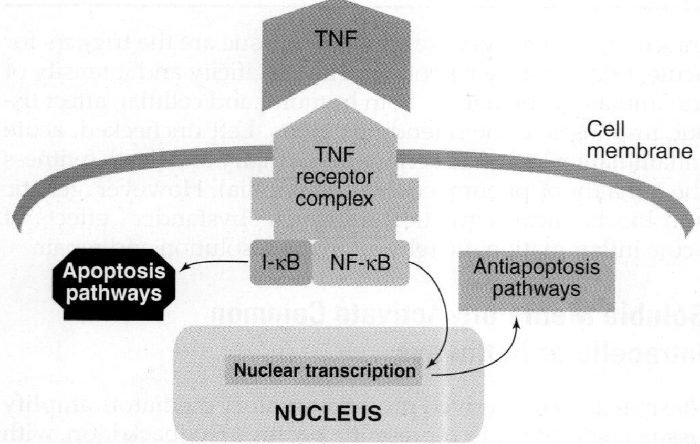

FIGURE 2-29. Tumor necrosis factor (TNF) receptor–mediated intracellular signal transduction pathway.

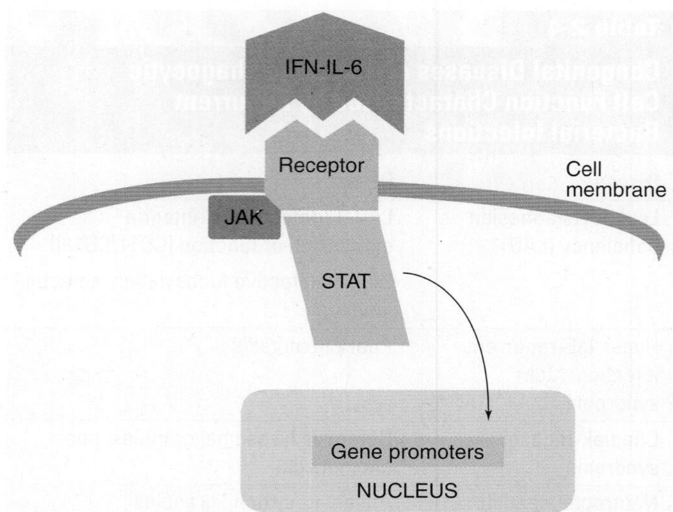

FIGURE 2-30. JAK-STAT–mediated intracellular transduction pathway. *IFN* = interferon; *IL* = interleukin.

G-Protein Pathways

Many chemokines, hormones, neurotransmitters and other inflammatory mediators signal via guanine nucleotide-binding (G) proteins (Fig. 2-28). G proteins vary in their intracellular connections but common activities include:

- **Ligand–receptor binding:** Binding of a stimulatory factor to a specific cell membrane receptor creates a ligand–receptor complex. Exchange of guanosine diphosphate (GDP) for guanosine triphosphate (GTP) activates the G protein, which dissociates into subunits that, in turn, activate phospholipase C and phosphatidylinositol-3-kinase (PI3K).
- **Phospholipid metabolism of cell membranes:** Phospholipase C hydrolyzes a plasma membrane phosphoinositide (phosphatidylinositol bisphosphate [PIP_2]) to generate diacylglycerol and inositol trisphosphate (IP_3).
- **Elevated cytosolic free calcium:** IP_3 induces release of stored intracellular calcium. In conjunction with influx of calcium ions from the extracellular environment, IP_3 increases cytosolic free calcium, a key event in inflammatory cell activation.
- **Protein phosphorylation and dephosphorylation:** Specific tyrosine kinases bind the ligand–receptor complex and initiate a series of protein phosphorylations.
- **Protein kinase C activation:** Protein kinase C and other protein kinases activate several intracellular signaling pathways, often leading to activation of gene transcription.

Tumor Necrosis Factor Receptor Pathways

TNF is central to the development of inflammation and its symptoms. It induces tumor cell apoptosis and regulates immune functions (Fig. 2-29). TNF and related proteins interact with two cell surface receptors to form a multiprotein-signaling complex at the cell membrane. This complex can trigger (1) apoptosis-related enzymes, **caspases** (Chapter 1); (2) inhibitors of apoptosis; or (3) activation of a nuclear transcription factor, **NFκB**. NFκB activation is regulated by association with and disassociation from IκB, the NF-κB inhibitor.

IκB binding to NFκB prevents the latter from translocating to the nucleus, where it can function as a transcriptional activator. This latter pathway is critical to regulation of TNF-mediated events during inflammation.

JAK-STAT Pathway

This pathway provides a direct signaling route from extracellular polypeptides (e.g., growth factors) or cytokines (e.g., interferons or interleukins) through cell receptors to gene promoters in the nucleus. Ligand–receptor interactions generate transcription complexes composed of JAK-STAT (Janus kinase–signal transducer and activator of transcription proteins). STAT proteins translocate to the nucleus, where they interact with gene promoters (Fig. 2-30).

Microbial Organisms and Damaged Cells Trigger the Gene Response

Four phases of gene expression in inflammation are shown in Fig. 2-31. These include:

1. **Initiation** of an inflammatory response, often by microbial products
2. **Gene activation** to induce proinflammatory mediators
3. **Reprogramming** to silence acute proinflammatory genes and to activate anti-inflammatory mediators
4. **Gene silencing** to promote resolution of the inflammatory response and allow recovery of tissue integrity

Initiation of Inflammation

An infectious agent or damaged cells provides the triggers to activate signaling pathways leading to the inflammatory response. Families of **pattern-recognition receptors** (PRRs) recognize **pathogen-associated microbial patterns** (PAMPs) and **danger-associated molecular patterns** (DAMPs) drive a coordinated immune response.

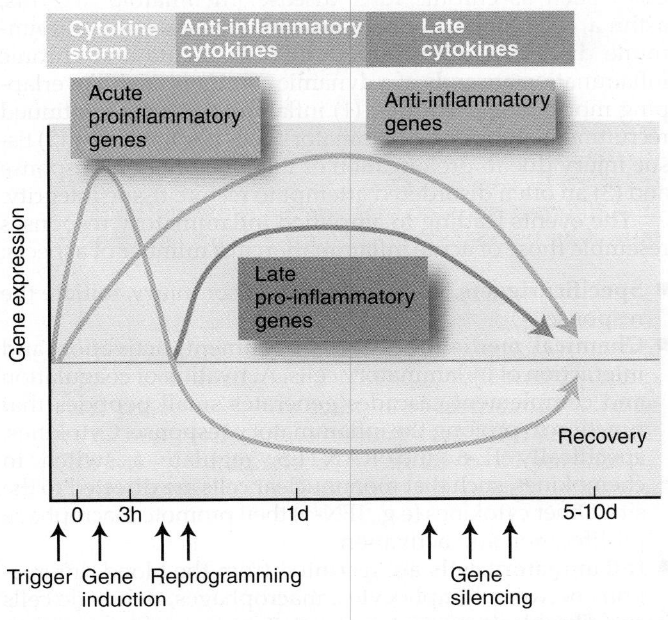

FIGURE 2-31. Time course of gene expression in the activation and regulation phases of the acute inflammatory response.

Toll-Like Receptors

Toll-like receptors (TLRs) are found on immune, inflammatory and tissue cells including mononuclear, endothelial and epithelial cells. TLRs on the cell surface (TLR1, -2, -4, -5 and -6) recognize bacterial cell wall components and viruses. Genetic polymorphisms of TLRs are related to specific cellular responses. For example, TLR4 is important for recognition and initiation of immune responses elicited by LPS of Gram-negative bacteria. TLR3, TLR7 and TLR9 are localized to endoplasmic reticulum and recognize viral RNA. Although TLR engagement activates intracellular pathways that defend against microbial organisms, this engagement may lead to excessive activation of cytokine cascades, notably contributing to the development of septic shock. Thus, IL-1 and TLR signaling have been implicated in a range of inflammatory and infectious diseases, and have prompted the development of TLR antagonists.

Nucleotide-Binding and Oligomerization Domain-Like Receptors

These intracellular soluble proteins also act as sensors for microbes (PAMPs) and cell injury (DAMPs). They form large molecular complexes termed **inflammasomes**, linked to the proteolytic activation of proinflammatory cytokines.

Retinoic Acid Inducible Gene-1–Like Receptors

Located in macrophages, dendritic cells and fibroblasts, these cytoplasmic RNA helicases survey for microbes and recognize viral RNA in the cytoplasm.

Gene Activation

The primary function of PRRs is to activate three major signaling pathways:

1. NFκB pathway
2. Mitogen-activated protein kinase/activator protein-1 (MAPKs/AP-1) pathway
3. Interferon regulatory factor (IRF) pathway

Activation of NFκB leads to induction of proinflammatory cytokines. MAPK activates AP-1, which induces proinflammatory cytokines. IRFs activate type 1 IFNs and proinflammatory mediators. Via these signal transduction pathways, microbial recognition leads to activation of transcription factors, which in turn bind specifically to sequences in gene promoters. TLRs engage microbes, activating immune cells by signaling from the plasma membrane via NFκB and AP-1. In a second pathway, TLRs signal from endosomes via activation of IRFs to induce type 1 interferons. Activation of retinoic acid inducible gene-1 (RIG-1) by cytoplasmic viral RNA binding activates NFκB and IRF3 to increase interferon transcription. The soluble cytoplasmic retinoic acid inducible gene-1-like receptors (RLRs) activate NFκB and induce signaling pathways, leading to interferon 1 transcription and inflammatory cytokine production.

Negative Regulators of Acute Inflammation

A process of natural resolution of acute inflammation occurs whereby the initial stimulus is removed and inflammatory cells undergo apoptosis. A combination of decreased production of proinflammatory mediators plus expression of anti-inflammatory mediators serves to brake the process. Removal of damaged tissue and cell debris allows proper healing to take place. The response to injury is variable, though, and genetics and the sex and age of a patient determine the response to injury, extent of healing and, in particular, progression to chronic inflammatory disease. Negative regulators of inflammation include:

- **Gene silencing and reprogramming:** Inflammation is associated with gene reprogramming, which silences acute proinflammatory gene expression, increases anti-inflammatory gene expression and allows the inflammatory process to progress toward resolution Notably, there are repressed transcription and sustained gene silencing of TNF-α, IL-1β and other proinflammatory genes and simultaneous increases in gene expression of anti-inflammatory factors such as IL-1 receptor antagonist (IL-1RA), TNF-α receptors, IL-6 and IL-10.
- **Cytokines:** IL-6, IL-10, IL-11, IL-12 and IL-13 limit inflammation by reducing production of the powerful proinflammatory cytokine, TNF-α. In some instances, this effect occurs by preventing degradation of IκB, thereby inhibiting cell activation and further release of inflammatory mediators.
- **Protease inhibitors:** Secretory leukocyte proteinase inhibitor (SLPI) and TIMP-2 are particularly important in reducing the responses of a variety of cell types, including macrophages and endothelial cells, and in decreasing connective tissue damage.
- **Lipoxins:** Lipoxins and aspirin-triggered lipoxins are anti-inflammatory lipid mediators that inhibit leukotriene biosynthesis.
- **Glucocorticoids:** Stimulation of the hypothalamic-pituitary-adrenal axis leads to release of immunosuppressive glucocorticoids. These have transcriptional and posttranscriptional suppressive effects on inflammatory response genes.
- **Kininases:** Kininases in plasma and blood degrade the potent proinflammatory mediator bradykinin.
- **Phosphatases:** One of the most common mechanisms used in signal transduction to regulate inflammatory cell signaling is rapid and reversible protein phosphorylation. Phosphatases and associated regulatory proteins provide a balancing, dephosphorylating system.
- **Transforming growth factor-β (TGF-β).** Apoptotic cells, particularly neutrophils, induce TGF-β expression. TGF-β suppresses proinflammatory cytokines and chemokines, induces a switch in arachidonic acid–derived mediators to production of lipoxin and resolvin (resolution phase interaction products; omega-3 polyunsaturated fatty acid), causes recognition and clearance of apoptotic cells and debris by macrophages and stimulates anti-inflammatory cytokines and fibrosis.

Outcomes of Acute Inflammation

As a result of regulatory components and the short life span of neutrophils, acute inflammatory reactions are usually self-limited, and they resolve. Ideally, the source of tissue injury is eliminated, inflammation recedes and normal tissue architecture and physiologic function are restored. The outcome of inflammation depends on the balance between cell recruitment, cell division, cell emigration and cell death. For tissue to return to normal, this process must be reversed: the stimulus to injury removed, proinflammatory signals turned off, acute inflammatory cell influx ended, tissue fluid balance restored, cell and tissue debris removed, normal vascular function restored, epithelial barriers repaired and the ECM regenerated. As signals for acute inflammation wane, PMN apoptosis limits the immune response and resolution begins.

However, inflammatory responses can lead to other outcomes:

- **Scar:** If a tissue is irreversibly injured, normal architecture is often replaced by a scar, despite elimination of the initial pathologic insult (Chapter 3).
- **Abscess:** If the area of acute inflammation is walled off by inflammatory cells and fibrosis, PMN products destroy the tissue, forming an abscess (Chapter 1).
- **Lymphadenitis:** Localized acute and chronic inflammation may cause secondary inflammation of lymphatic channels **(lymphangitis)** and lymph nodes **(lymphadenitis).** The inflamed lymphatic channels in the skin appear as red streaks, and the lymph nodes are enlarged and painful. Microscopically, affected lymph nodes show hyperplasia of lymphoid follicles and proliferation of mononuclear phagocytes in the sinuses (sinus histiocytosis).
- **Persistent inflammation:** Failure to eliminate a pathologic insult or inability to trigger resolution results in persistent inflammation. This may be evident as a prolonged acute response, with continued influx of neutrophils and tissue destruction, or more commonly as chronic inflammation.

Chronic Inflammation

When acute inflammation does not resolve or becomes disordered, chronic inflammation occurs. Inflammatory cells persist, stroma responds by becoming hyperplastic and tissue destruction and scarring lead to organ dysfunction. This process may be localized, but more commonly it progresses to disabling diseases such as chronic lung disease, rheumatoid arthritis, asthma, ulcerative colitis, granulomatous diseases, autoimmune diseases and chronic dermatitis. Acute and chronic inflammation are ends of a dynamic continuum with overlapping morphologic features: (1) inflammation with continued recruitment of chronic inflammatory cells is followed by (2) tissue injury due to prolongation of the inflammatory response and (3) an often disordered attempt to restore tissue integrity.

The events leading to amplified inflammatory responses resemble those of acute inflammation in a number of aspects:

- **Specific triggers,** microbial products or injury, initiate the response.
- **Chemical mediators** direct recruitment, activation and interaction of inflammatory cells. Activation of coagulation and complement cascades generates small peptides that function to prolong the inflammatory response. Cytokines, specifically IL-6 and RANTES, regulate a switch in chemokines, such that mononuclear cells are directed to the site. Other cytokines (e.g., IFN-γ) then promote macrophage proliferation and activation.
- **Inflammatory cells** are recruited from the blood. Interactions between lymphocytes, macrophages, dendritic cells and fibroblasts generate antigen-specific responses.
- **Stromal cell activation and extracellular matrix** remodeling occur, both of which affect the cellular immune response.

Varying degrees of fibrosis may result, depending on the extent of tissue injury and persistence of the pathologic stimulus and inflammatory response.

Chronic inflammation is not synonymous with chronic infection, but if the inflammatory response cannot eliminate an injurious agent, infection may persist. Chronic inflammation does not necessarily require infection: it may follow an acute inflammatory or immune response to a foreign antigen. Signals that result in an extended response include:

- **Bacteria, viruses and parasites:** These agents can provide signals to support persistence of inflammatory responses, which in this case may be directed toward isolating the invader from the host.
- **Apoptosis:** Since apoptotic neutrophils induce an anti-inflammatory response, defects in recognition or response to these cell remnants may lead to chronic inflammation.
- **Defective gene silencing:** Delayed and/or persistent expression of late proinflammatory genes contribute to prolongation of inflammatory responses. In this case, the gene silencing phase does not occur, the cytokine onslaught persists and pathologic inflammation develops.
- **Trauma:** Extensive tissue damage releases mediators capable of inducing an extended inflammatory response.
- **Cancer:** Chronic inflammatory cells, especially macrophages and T lymphocytes, may be the morphologic expression of an immune response to malignant cells. Chemotherapy may suppress normal inflammatory responses, increasing susceptibility to infection.
- **Immune factors:** Many autoimmune diseases, including rheumatoid arthritis, chronic thyroiditis and primary biliary cirrhosis, are characterized by chronic inflammatory responses in affected tissues. This may be associated with activation of antibody-dependent and cell-mediated immune mechanisms (Chapter 4). Such autoimmune responses may account for injury in affected organs.

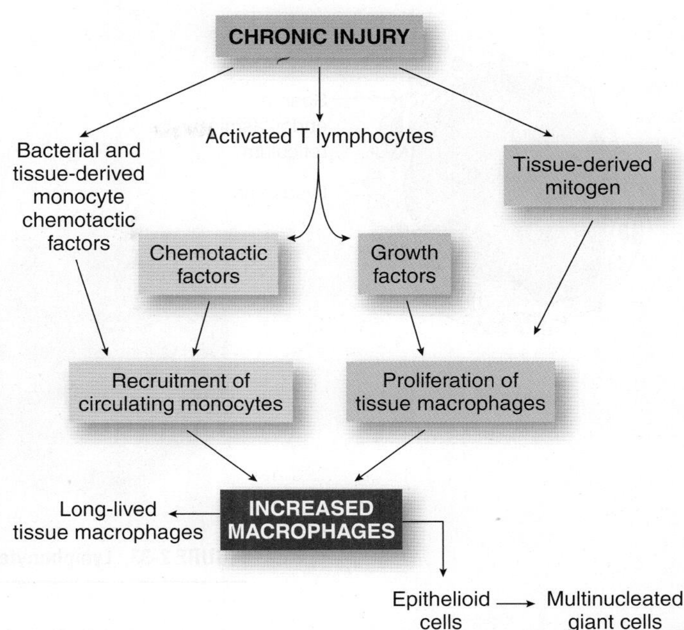

FIGURE 2-32. Accumulation of macrophages in chronic inflammation.

Cells Involved in Chronic Inflammation

The cellular components of chronic inflammatory responses are recruited from the circulation (macrophages, lymphocytes, plasma cells, dendritic cells and eosinophils) and affected tissues (fibroblasts, vascular endothelial cells).

Monocytes/Macrophages

Activated macrophages and their cytokines are central to initiating inflammation and prolonging responses that lead to chronic inflammation (Fig. 2-18C). Macrophages produce inflammatory and immunologic mediators and regulate reactions leading to chronic inflammation. They also regulate lymphocyte responses to antigens and secrete other mediators that modulate fibroblast and endothelial cell proliferation and activities.

The **mononuclear phagocyte system** includes promonocytes and their precursors in the bone marrow, blood monocytes and different types of histiocytes and macrophages, particularly Kupffer cells. Under the influence of chemotactic stimuli, IFN-γ and bacterial endotoxins, resident tissue macrophages are activated and proliferate, while circulating monocytes are recruited and differentiate into tissue macrophages (Fig. 2-32).

Within different tissues, resident macrophages differ in their armamentarium of enzymes and can respond to local inflammatory signals. Blood monocyte granules contain serine proteinases like those found in neutrophils. Circulating monocytes synthesize additional enzymes, particularly MMPs. When monocytes enter tissue and further differentiate into macrophages, they acquire the ability to generate additional MMPs and cysteine proteinases but lose the ability to produce serine proteinases. The activity of these enzymes is central to the tissue destruction that may occur in chronic inflammation. For example, in emphysema resident macrophages generate proteinases, particularly MMPs with elastolytic activity, which destroy alveolar walls and recruit blood monocytes into the lung. ***Other macrophage products include oxygen metabolites, chemotactic factors, cytokines and growth factors.***

Lymphocytes

Naive lymphocytes home to secondary lymphoid organs, where they encounter antigen-presenting cells and become antigen-specific lymphocytes. Plasma cells and T cells leaving secondary lymphoid organs circulate in the vascular system and are recruited into peripheral tissues.

T cells regulate macrophage activation and recruitment by secreting specific mediators (lymphokines), modulate antibody production and cell-mediated cytotoxicity and maintain immunologic memory (Fig. 2-33). NK cells, as well as other lymphocyte subtypes, help defend against viral and bacterial infections.

Plasma Cells

Plasma cells are rich in rough endoplasmic reticulum and are the primary source of antibodies (Fig. 2-34). Production of antibody to specific antigens at sites of chronic inflammation is important in antigen neutralization, clearance of foreign

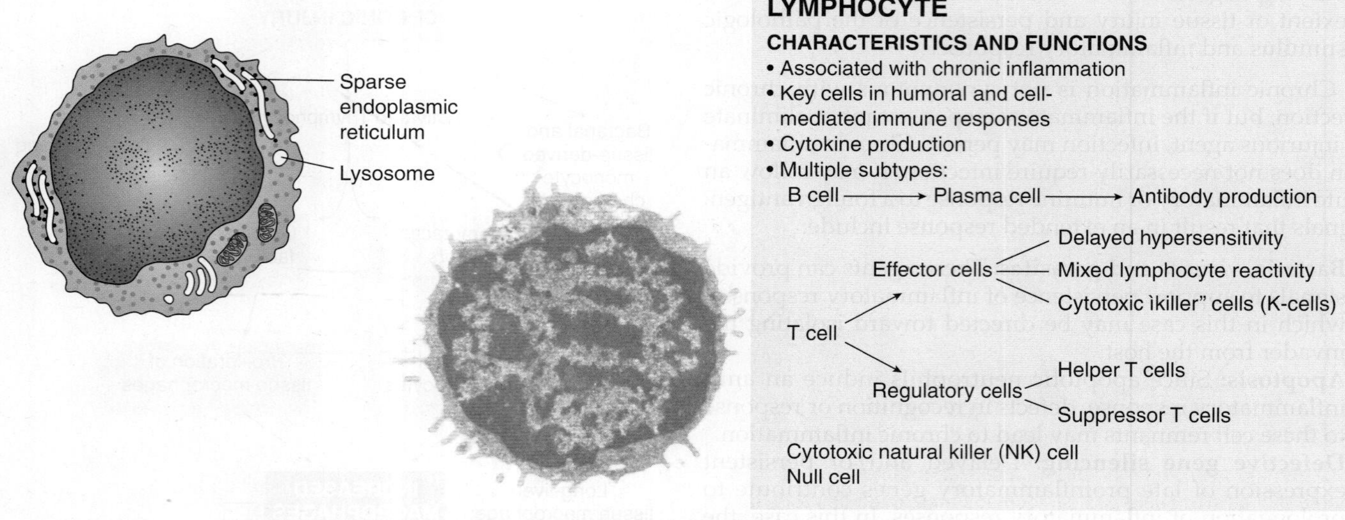

FIGURE 2-33. Lymphocyte: morphology and function.

antigens and particles and antibody-dependent cell-mediated cytotoxicity (Chapter 4).

Dendritic Cells

Dendritic cells are professional antigen-presenting cells that trigger immune responses to antigens (Chapter 4). They phagocytose antigens and migrate to lymph nodes, where they present those antigens. Recognition of antigen and other costimulatory molecules by T cells results in recruitment of specific cell subsets to the inflammatory process. During chronic inflammation, dendritic cells are present in inflamed tissues, where they help prolong responses.

Acute Inflammatory Cells

Neutrophils are characteristically involved in acute inflammation but may also be present during chronic inflammation if there is ongoing infection and tissue damage. Eosinophils are particularly prominent in allergic-type reactions and parasitic infestations.

Fibroblasts

Fibroblasts are long-lived, ubiquitous cells whose chief function is to produce components of the ECM (Fig. 2-35). They are derived from mesoderm or neural crest and can differentiate into other connective tissue cells, including chondrocytes, adipocytes, osteocytes and smooth muscle cells. Fibroblasts are the construction workers of the tissue, rebuilding the scaffolding of ECM upon which tissue is reestablished.

Fibroblasts not only respond to immune signals that induce their proliferation and activation but also are active players in the immune response. They interact with inflammatory cells, particularly lymphocytes, via surface molecules and receptors on both cells. For example, when CD40 on fibroblasts binds its ligand on lymphocytes, both cells are activated. Activated fibroblasts produce cytokines, chemokines and prostanoids, creating a tissue microenvironment that further regulates the behavior of inflammatory cells in the damaged tissue. (Fibroblast function in wound healing is discussed more fully in Chapter 3.)

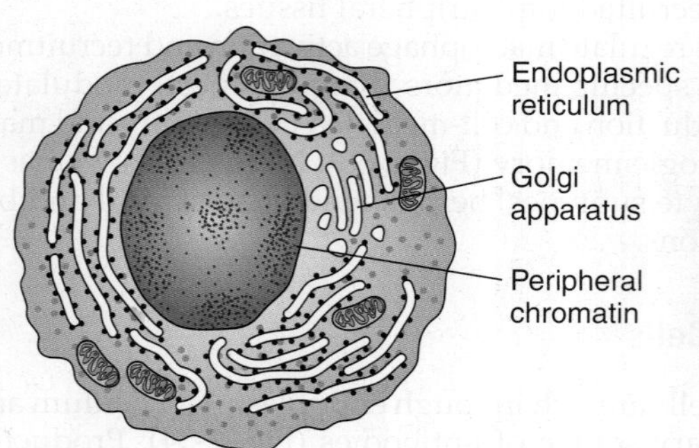

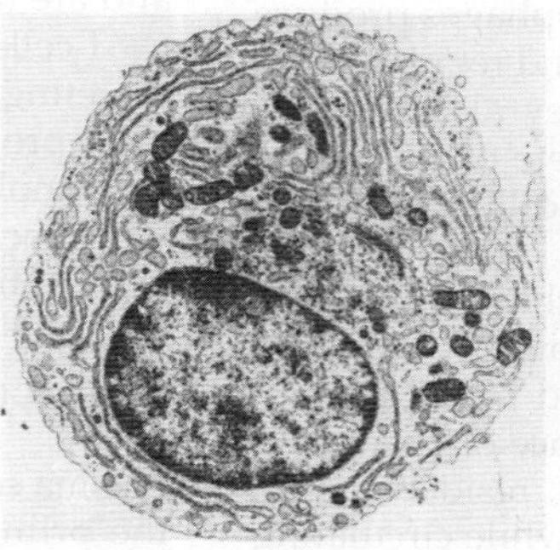

FIGURE 2-34. Plasma cell: morphology and function.

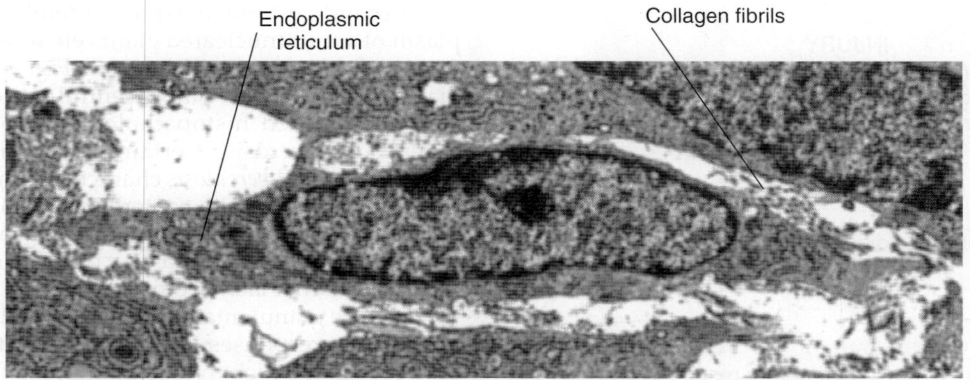

Endoplasmic reticulum
Collagen fibrils
FIBROBLAST
CHARACTERISTICS AND FUNCTIONS
• Produce extracellular matrix proteins
• Mediate chronic inflammation and wound healing
PRIMARY INFLAMMATORY MEDIATORS
• IL-6
• IL-8
• Cyclooxygenase-2
• Hyaluronan
• PGE2
• CD40 expression
• Matricellular proteins
• Extracellular proteins

FIGURE 2-35. Fibroblast: morphology and function. *IL* = interleukin.

Injury and Repair in Chronic Inflammation

Chronic inflammation is mediated by both immunologic and nonimmunologic mechanisms and is frequently observed in conjunction with reparative responses, namely, granulation tissue and fibrosis.

An Extended Inflammatory Response May Lead to Persistent Injury

The primary role of neutrophils in inflammation is host defense and débridement of damaged tissue. The neutrophil response, however, is a double-edged sword: neutrophil products protect the host by participating in antimicrobial defense and débridement of damaged tissue; however, if they are not appropriately regulated, these same products may prolong tissue damage and promote chronic inflammation. Neutrophil enzymes are beneficial when they are digesting phagocytosed organisms intracellularly, but these same enzymes can be destructive if they are released extracellularly. Thus, when neutrophils accumulate, connective tissue may be digested by their enzymes.

Persistent tissue injury produced by inflammatory cells is important in the pathogenesis of several diseases (e.g., pulmonary emphysema, rheumatoid arthritis, certain immune complex diseases, gout and acute respiratory distress syndrome). Phagocytic cell adherence, escape of reactive oxygen metabolites and release of lysosomal enzymes together enhance cytotoxicity and tissue degradation. Proteinase activity is significantly elevated in chronic wounds, creating a proteolytic environment that prevents healing.

Altered Repair Mechanisms Prevent Resolution

Repair processes initiated as part of inflammation can restore normal architecture and function. Early reparative efforts mimic wound healing. However, if inflammation is prolonged or exaggerated, repair may be incompletely effective and cause altered tissue architecture and tissue dysfunction. For example:

- Ongoing proliferation of epithelial cells can result in metaplasia. Goblet cell metaplasia, for example, characterizes the airways of smokers and asthmatics.
- Fibroblast proliferation and activation leads to increased ECM. Because ECM components such as collagen now occupy space normally devoted to tissue cells, organ function is altered (Chapter 3).
- The ECM may be abnormal. Matrix degradation and production change the normal mix of extracellular proteins. Thus, elastin degradation is important in development of emphysema.
- Altered ECM (e.g., fibronectin) can be a chemoattractant for inflammatory cells and present an altered scaffolding to cells.

Granulomatous Inflammation

Neutrophils ordinarily remove agents that incite acute inflammatory responses. However, there are circumstances in which reactive neutrophils cannot digest those substances. Such a situation is potentially dangerous, because it can lead to a vicious circle of (1) phagocytosis, (2) failure of digestion, (3) death of the neutrophil, (4) release of the undigested provoking agent and (5) rephagocytosis by a newly recruited neutrophil (Fig. 2-36). ***Granuloma formation is a protective response to chronic infection (e.g., fungal infections, tuberculosis, leprosy, schistosomiasis) or the presence of foreign material (e.g., suture or talc), isolating a persistent offending agent, preventing its dissemination and restricting inflammation, thereby protecting the host tissues.*** Some autoimmune diseases are also associated with granulomas, diseases such as rheumatoid arthritis and Crohn disease. In some cases such as sarcoidosis, no inciting agent has yet been identified.

The principal cells involved in granulomatous inflammation are macrophages and lymphocytes (Fig. 2-37). Macrophages are mobile cells that continuously migrate through extravascular connective tissues. After amassing substances that they cannot digest, macrophages lose their motility and accumulate at the site of injury to form nodular collections of pale, epithelioid cells: **granulomas**.

2 | Inflammation

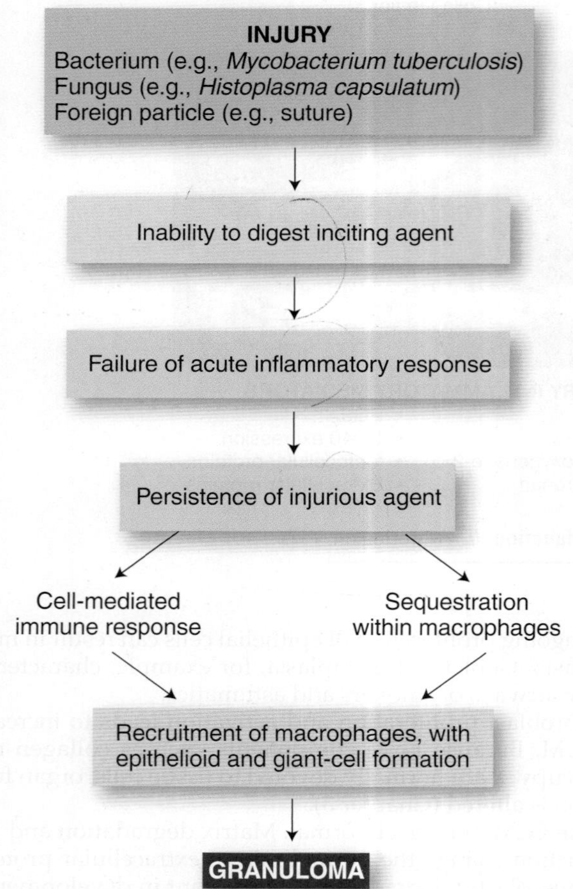

FIGURE 2-36. Mechanism of granuloma formation.

Multinucleate giant cells are formed by cytoplasmic fusion of macrophages. When the nuclei of such giant cells are arranged around the periphery of the cell in a horseshoe pattern, the cell is called a **Langhans giant cell** (Fig. 2-38). Frequently, a foreign agent (e.g., silica or a *Histoplasma* spore) or other indigestible material is identified within the cytoplasm of a multinucleated giant cell, in which case the term **foreign body giant cell** is used (Fig. 2-39). Foreign body giant cells tend to have more central nuclei. Granulomas are further classified histopathologically by the presence or absence of necrosis. Certain infectious agents such as *Mycobacterium tuberculosis* characteristically produce necrotizing granulomas, the centers of which are filled with an amorphous mixture of debris and dead microorganisms and cells. Other diseases such as sarcoidosis are characterized by granulomas that lack necrosis.

Immune granulomas, formed during delayed-type hypersensitivity responses, contain activated T cells and macrophages, which initiate granuloma formation. CD4+ T cells then recruit and organize cells at the site using CXCL chemokines to develop Th1-type granulomas and CCL chemokines to develop Th2-type granulomas. Several T cell cytokines stimulate macrophage function (e.g., IFN-γ), whereas others inhibit macrophage activation (e.g., IL-4, IL-10). Thus, lymphocytes are vital for regulating development and resolution of inflammatory responses.

The fate of a granulomatous reaction depends on the toxicity and immunogenicity of the inciting agent. Cell-mediated immune responses to an inciting agent may modify a granulomatous reaction by recruiting and activating more macrophages and lymphocytes. Finally, under the influence of T cell cytokines such as IL-13 and TGF-β, the granuloma burns out and becomes a fibrotic nodule.

Chronic Inflammation and Malignancy

Several chronic infectious diseases are associated with development of malignancies. For example, schistosomiasis of the urinary bladder leads to squamous cell carcinoma of that organ. Inflammation that is not specifically linked to infection may also be a risk factor for cancer. Patients with reflux esophagitis or ulcerative colitis are at higher risk for adenocarcinoma in those organs. The environment created by chronic inflammation promotes malignant transformation by a number of mechanisms (Chapter 5):

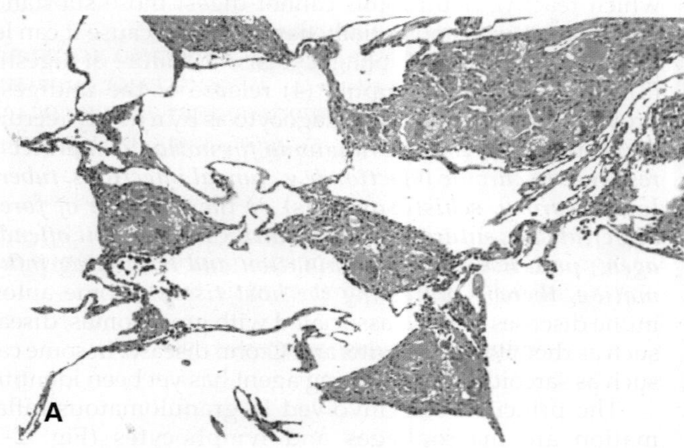

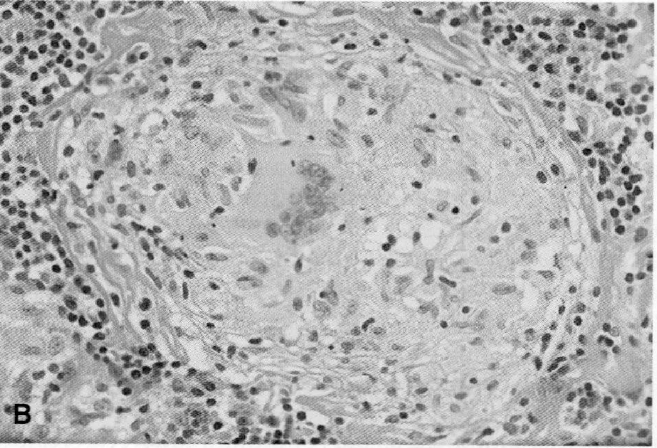

FIGURE 2-37. Granulomatous inflammation. A. Section of lung from a patient with sarcoidosis reveals numerous discrete granulomas. **B.** A higher-power photomicrograph of a single granuloma in a lymph node from the same patient depicts a multinucleated giant cell amid numerous pale epithelioid cells. A thin rim of fibrosis separates the granuloma from the lymphoid cells of the node.

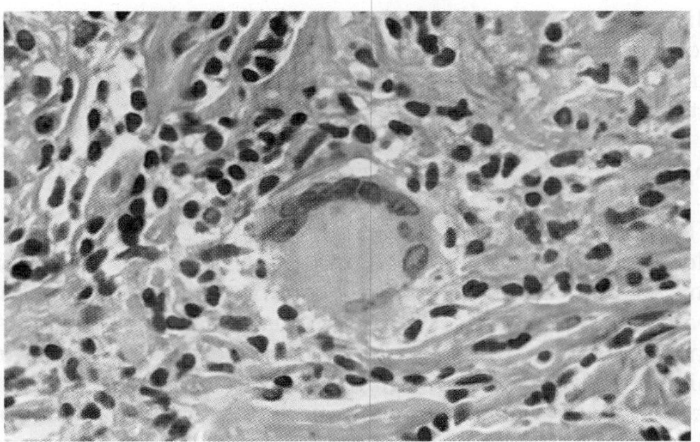

FIGURE 2-38. A Langhans giant cell shows nuclei arranged on the periphery of an abundant cytoplasm.

- **Increased cell proliferation:** Chronically stimulated cell division increases the likelihood of transforming mutations in the proliferating cells.
- **Oxygen and NO• metabolites:** Inflammatory metabolites, such as nitrosamines, may cause genomic damage.
- **Chronic immune activation:** Chronic antigen exposure alters the cytokine milieu by suppressing cell-mediated immune responses. This creates a more permissive environment for malignant growth.
- **Angiogenesis:** Growth of new vessels is associated with inflammation and wound healing and is required for maintenance of neoplastic lesions.
- **Inhibition of apoptosis:** Chronic inflammation suppresses apoptosis. Increased cell division and decreased apoptosis facilitate survival and expansion of mutated cell populations.

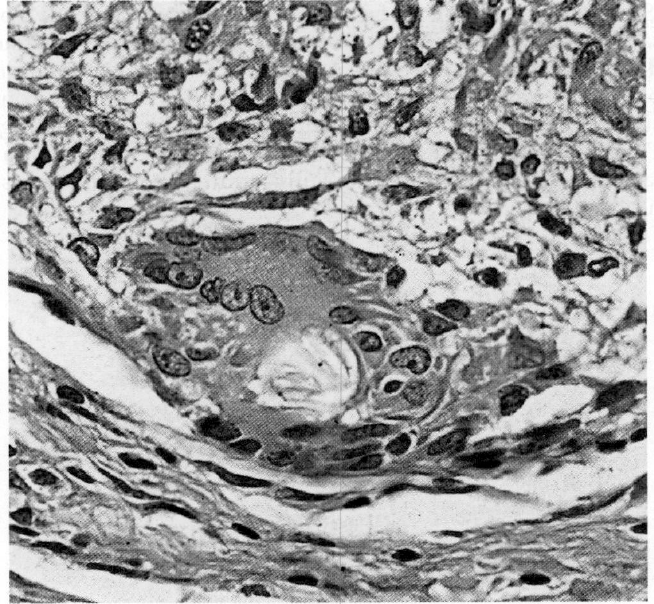

FIGURE 2-39. A foreign body giant cell has numerous nuclei randomly arranged in the cytoplasm.

Systemic Manifestations of Inflammation

An effective inflammatory response will (1) limit the area of injury, (2) clear the inciting pathologic agent and damaged tissue and (3) restore tissue function. However, under certain conditions, local injury may result in prominent systemic effects that can themselves be debilitating. These effects often result when a pathogen enters the bloodstream, a condition acting synergistically, are directly or indirectly responsible for both local and systemic effects of inflammation. The symptoms associated with inflammation, including fever, myalgia, arthralgia, anorexia and somnolence, are attributable to these cytokines. The most prominent systemic manifestations of inflammation, termed the **systemic inflammatory response syndrome (SIRS)**, are activation of the hypothalamic-pituitary-adrenal axis, leukocytosis, or the acute phase response, fever and shock.

Hypothalamic-Pituitary-Adrenal Axis

Many of the systemic effects of inflammation are mediated via the hypothalamic-pituitary-adrenal axis, a key component in the response to chronic inflammation and chronic immune disease. Inflammation results in release of anti-inflammatory glucocorticoids from the adrenal cortex. Loss of adrenal function can increase the severity of inflammation.

Leukocytosis

Leukocytosis, defined as an increase in circulating leukocytes, commonly accompanies acute inflammation. Immature PMNs ("band" forms) may also be seen in the peripheral blood (Chapter 20). Leukocytosis is most commonly associated with bacterial infections and tissue injury, and is caused by release of specific mediators from macrophages and perhaps other cells. These mediators accelerate release of PMNs, even immature PMNs, from the bone marrow. Subsequently, macrophages and T lymphocytes are stimulated to produce a group of proteins (called "colony-stimulating factors") that induce proliferation of bone marrow hematopoietic precursor cells. Occasionally, if circulating levels of PMNs and their precursors are very high, a **leukemoid (i.e., leukemia-like) reaction** may occur, which may be confused with leukemia.

In contrast to bacterial infections, viral infections (including infectious mononucleosis) are characterized by **lymphocytosis**, an absolute increase in the number of circulating lymphocytes. Parasitic infestations and certain allergic reactions cause eosinophilia (i.e., increased blood eosinophils).

Leukopenia

Leukopenia is an absolute decrease in circulating white cells. It is occasionally seen during chronic inflammation, especially in patients who are malnourished or who suffer from a chronic debilitating disease such as disseminated cancer. Leukopenia may also be caused by typhoid fever and certain viral and rickettsial infections.

Acute Phase Response

The acute phase response is a regulated physiologic reaction that occurs in inflammatory conditions. It is characterized clinically by fever, leukocytosis, decreased appetite and

Table 2-5

Acute Phase Proteins

Protein	Function
Mannose-binding protein	Opsonization/complement activation
C-reactive protein	Opsonization
α_1-Antitrypsin	Serine protease inhibitor
Haptoglobin	Binds hemoglobin
Ceruloplasmin	Antioxidant, binds copper
Fibrinogen	Coagulation
Serum amyloid A protein	Apolipoprotein
α_2-Macroglobulin	Antiprotease
Cysteine protease inhibitor	Antiprotease

altered sleep patterns, and chemically by changes in plasma levels of acute phase proteins. These proteins (Table 2-5) are synthesized primarily by the liver and released in large numbers into the circulation in response to an acute inflammatory challenge. Changes in plasma levels of acute phase proteins are mediated primarily by IL-1, IL-6 and TNF-α. Increased plasma levels of some acute phase proteins lead to an accelerated **erythrocyte sedimentation rate** (ESR), which is a qualitative index used clinically to monitor the activity of many inflammatory diseases.

Fever

Fever is a clinical hallmark of inflammation. Release of **pyrogens** (molecules that cause fever) by bacteria, viruses or injured cells may directly affect hypothalamic thermoregulation. More importantly, they stimulate production of endogenous pyrogens, namely, cytokines—including IL-1α, IL-1β, TNF-α and IL-6—and interferons, with local and systemic effects. IL-1 stimulates prostaglandin synthesis in hypothalamic thermoregulatory centers, thereby altering the "thermostat" that controls body temperature. Inhibitors of cyclooxygenase (e.g., aspirin) block the fever response by inhibiting IL-1–stimulated PGE_2 synthesis in the hypothalamus. TNF-α and IL-6 also increase body temperature by a direct action on the hypothalamus. Chills (the sensation of cold), rigor (profound chills with shivering and piloerection) and sweats (to allow heat dissipation) are symptoms associated with fever.

Pain

The process of pain is associated with (1) **nociception** (i.e., detection of noxious stimuli and transmission of this information to the brain), (2) pain perception and (3) suffering and pain behavior. Nociception is primarily a neural response initiated in injured tissues by specific nociceptors, which are high-threshold receptors for thermal, chemical and mechanical stimuli. Most chemical mediators of inflammation described in this chapter—including ions, kinins, histamine, NO•, prostanoids, cytokines and growth factors—activate peripheral nociceptors directly or indirectly. Kinins, especially bradykinin, are formed following tissue trauma and in inflammation; they activate primary sensory neurons via B_2 receptors to mediate pain transmission. Another kinin, des-arg bradykinin, activates B_1 receptors to produce pain only during inflammation. Cytokines, particularly TNF-α, IL-1, IL-6 and IL-8, produce pain hypersensitivity to mechanical and thermal stimuli. Prostaglandins and growth factors may directly activate nociceptors but appear to be most important in enhancing nociceptor sensitivity. Pain perception and subsequent behavior arise in response to this enhanced sensitivity to both noxious and normally innocuous stimuli.

Shock

Under conditions of massive tissue injury or infection that spreads to the blood (sepsis), significant quantities of cytokines, especially TNF-α, and other chemical mediators of inflammation may be generated in the circulation. Persistence of these mediators affects the heart and the peripheral vascular system by causing generalized vasodilation, increased vascular permeability, intravascular volume loss and myocardial depression with decreased cardiac output (SIRS) (Chapter 7). As a consequence, cardiac output may not satisfy the body's need for oxygen and nutrients **(cardiac decompensation)**. In severe cases, activation of coagulation pathways may cause microthrombi throughout the body, consuming clotting components and predisposing to bleeding. This condition is termed **disseminated intravascular coagulation** (Chapter 20). The net result is multisystem organ dysfunction and death.

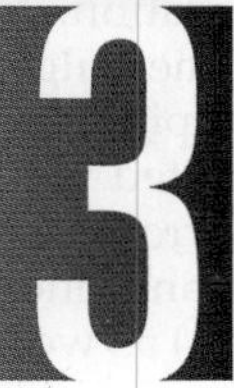

Repair, Regeneration and Fibrosis

Gregory C. Sephel • Jeffrey M. Davidson

Damaged tissue heals, whether by scarring or regeneration, in ways that ensure the immediate survival of the organism. Observations regarding the repair of wounds (i.e., wound healing) date to physicians in ancient Egypt and battle surgeons in classic Greece. The clotting of blood to prevent exsanguination was recognized as the first necessary event in wound healing. Later studies of wound infection led to the discovery that inflammatory cells are primary actors in the repair process. The importance of extracellular matrix, specifically collagen, in tissue integrity and wound healing was first recognized through study of scurvy, a disease that claimed the lives of millions (see Chapter 8). In May of 1747, Dr. James Lind, a surgeon in England's Royal Navy, conducted what is thought to be the first controlled clinical trial. Aboard the HMS Salisbury, he separated scurvy-ridden sailors into six treatment groups and observed that sailors given oranges and lemons derived the greatest benefit. In 1907 the role of vitamin C began to be clarified when Norwegians Axel Holst and Theodor Frolich discovered that guinea pigs, like humans, were unable to synthesize vitamin C (ascorbic acid). Ascorbate was eventually found necessary for prolyl hydroxylase, an enzyme required for proper folding and stabilization of the collagen triple helix, an important step in building a strong scar.

The topic of regeneration elicits thoughts of flatworms, starfish and amphibians. However, the human liver's ability to regenerate has long been known and was the basis of the Greek myth of Prometheus, whose liver regenerated daily. Modern concepts of regeneration and cell differentiation progressed in the later half of the 20th century. In the 1950s John Gurdon and others asked if all cells maintained the same genes during differentiation, or if genes were lost as cells differentiate. Gurdon eventually determined that even somatic cell nuclei transplanted into a Xenopus egg could form a normal adult organism. Current studies on epigenetic control of gene expression, stem and progenitor cell biology and directed control of differentiation patterns in cells are rapidly advancing the fields of regenerative healing and tissue engineering.

The study of wound healing now encompasses a variety of cells, matrix proteins, growth factors and cytokines, which regulate and modulate the repair process. Nearly every stage in the repair process is redundantly controlled, and there is no one rate-limiting step, except uncontrolled infection. Extracellular matrix will be presented here in some detail as it occupies a central role in both repair and regeneration. Matrix deposition is a key process in tissue repair, and matrix composition is an important functional factor in the niche environment that maintains stem and progenitor cells during regeneration and in the tissue microenvironments where stem or progenitor cells differentiate. ***Successful healing maintains tissue function and repairs tissue barriers, preventing blood loss and infection, but is usually accomplished through collagen deposition or scarring (fibrosis).*** Advances in our understanding of growth factors, extracellular matrix and stem cell biology are improving healing, and offer the possibility of restoring injured tissues to their normal architecture and of engineering replacement tissues.

Successful repair relies on a crucial balance between the *yin* of matrix deposition and the *yang* of matrix degradation. ***Regeneration is favored when matrix composition and architecture are unchanged.*** Thus, wounds that do not heal may reflect excess proteinase activity, decreased matrix accumulation or altered matrix assembly. Conversely, fibrosis and scarring may result from reduced proteinase activity or increased matrix accumulation. Whereas formation of new collagen during repair is required for increased strength of the healing site, chronic fibrosis is a major component of diseases that involve chronic injury.

The Basic Processes of Healing

Many of the basic cellular and molecular mechanisms required for wound healing are found in other processes involving dynamic tissue changes, such as development and tumor growth. Three key cellular mechanisms are necessary for wound healing:

- **Cellular migration**
- **Extracellular matrix organization and remodeling**
- **Cell proliferation**

Migration of Cells Initiates Repair

Cells That Migrate to the Wound

Migration of cells into a wound and activation of local cells are initiated by mediators that are released either de novo by resident cells or from reserves stored in granules of **platelets** and **basophils.** These granules contain cytokines, chemoattractants, proteases and mediators of inflammation, which together (1) control vascular supply, (2) degrade damaged tissue and (3) initiate the repair cascade. Platelets are activated when exposed to von Willebrand factor and collagen exposed at sites of endothelial damage, and their ensuing aggregation, in combination with fibrin cross-linking, limits blood loss. Activated platelets release platelet-derived growth factor (PDGF) and other molecules that facilitate adhesion, coagulation, vasoconstriction, repair and clot resorption. **Mast cells** are bone marrow–derived cells whose granules contain high concentrations of heparin. They reside in connective tissue near small blood vessels and respond to foreign antigens by releasing the contents of their granules, many of which are angiogenic. **Resident macrophages,** tissue-fixed mesenchymal cells and epithelial cells also release mediators that contribute to and perpetuate the early response. Their numbers are increased through proliferation and recruitment to the site of injury. ***The following are characteristic cell migrations of skin wounds* (Fig. 3-1):**

- **Leukocytes** arrive at the wound site early by adherence to activated endothelium and migrate rapidly into tissue by forming small focal adhesions (focal contacts). A family of small peptide chemoattractants **(chemokines)** is capable of restricted or broad recruitment of particular leukocytes (see Chapter 2).
- **Polymorphonuclear leukocytes** from the bone marrow invade the wound site within the first day. They degrade and destroy nonviable tissue by releasing their granular contents and generating reactive oxygen species.
- **Monocytes/macrophages** arrive shortly after neutrophils but persist for days or longer. They phagocytose debris and orchestrate the developing granulation tissue by release of cytokines and chemoattractants.
- **Fibroblasts, myofibroblasts, pericytes and smooth muscle cells** are recruited and propagated by growth factors and matrix degradation products, arriving in a skin wound by day 3 or 4. These cells mediate synthesis of connective tissue matrix (fibroplasia), tissue remodeling, vascular integrity, wound contraction and wound strength.
- **Endothelial cells** form nascent capillaries by responding to growth factors and are visible in a skin wound together with fibroblasts beyond day 3. Development of capillaries is needed for gas exchange, delivery of nutrients and influx of inflammatory cells.
- **Epidermal cells** move across the surface of a skin wound. Reepithelialization is delayed if the migrating epithelial cells must reconstitute a damaged basement membrane. In open wounds, keratinocytes migrate between provisional matrix (see below) and preexisting or newly formed stromal collagen, which is coated with plasma glycoproteins, fibrinogen and fibronectin. The phenotype of the epithelial layer is altered if basement membrane is lacking.
- **Stem cells** from bone marrow, and with respect to skin, stem cells or **progenitor cells** in the hair follicle and within the basal epidermal layer, provide renewable sources of epidermal and dermal cells capable of differentiation, proliferation and migration. Stem cells for epidermal regeneration reside in the bulge region of the hair follicle and the interfollicular epidermis (Fig. 3-1.5). Dermal progenitors are also associated with the lower hair shaft and the follicular bulb. Marrow-derived, multipotential progenitors of fibroblasts and endothelium are recruited to sites of injury (Fig. 3-1.1) as well, although they appear to play a temporary role in repair. These cells form new blood vessels and new epithelium and regenerate skin structures, such as hair follicles and sebaceous glands.

Mechanisms of Cell Migration

Cell migration uses the most important mechanism of wound healing (i.e., receptor-mediated responses to chemical signals **[cytokines]** and insoluble substrates of the extracellular matrix). Ameboid locomotion of the rapidly migrating leukocytes is powered by broad, wave-like, membrane extensions called **lamellipodia.** Slower-moving cells, such as fibroblasts, extend narrower, finger-like membrane protrusions labeled **filopodia.** Cell polarization and membrane extensions are initiated by growth factors or chemokines, which trigger a response by binding to their specific receptors on the cell surface. **Actin fibrils** polymerize and form a network at the membrane's leading edge, thereby propelling lamellipodia and filopodia forward, with traction by engaging the extracellular matrix substrate. Actin-related proteins modulate actin assembly, and numerous actin-binding proteins act like molecular tinker toys, rapidly constructing, stabilizing and destabilizing actin networks.

The leading edge of the cell membrane impinges upon adjacent extracellular matrix and adheres to it through transmembrane adhesion receptors termed **integrins** (see Chapter 2). These molecules show significant redundancy; many different integrin heterodimer combinations recognize the same matrix components (e.g., collagen, laminin, fibronectin). Focal contacts develop via adherence of the integrin extracellular domain to the connective tissue matrix. In vitro, focal adhesions form under the cell body, whereas smaller focal contacts form at the leading edge of migrating cells. The focal contact anchors actin stress fibers, against which myosins pull to extend or contract the cell body. As the cell moves forward, older adhesions at the rear are weakened or destabilized, allowing the trailing edge to retract.

Over 50 proteins have been associated with formation of adhesion plaques. The cytoplasmic domain of integrins is the trigger for a protein cascade that anchors actin stress fibers. The Rho family of guanosine triphosphatases (GTPases; Rho, Rac, Cdc42) are molecular switches that interact with surface receptors to regulate matrix assembly, generate focal adhesions and organize the actin cytoskeleton.

Integrins transmit intracellular signals that also regulate cellular survival, proliferation and differentiation. These functions are affected by other cell activators (e.g., cytokines), which alter the binding properties of the extracellular portion of integrins by signaling through their cytoplasmic portions. In this manner, cytokines can also influence organization and tension in matrix and tissue. Conversely, integrin binding is essential for many growth factor receptor signaling processes. Thus, growth factors and integrins share several common signaling pathways, but integrins are unique in their ability to organize and anchor cytoskeleton. Cytoskeletal connections are involved in cell–cell and cell–matrix connections

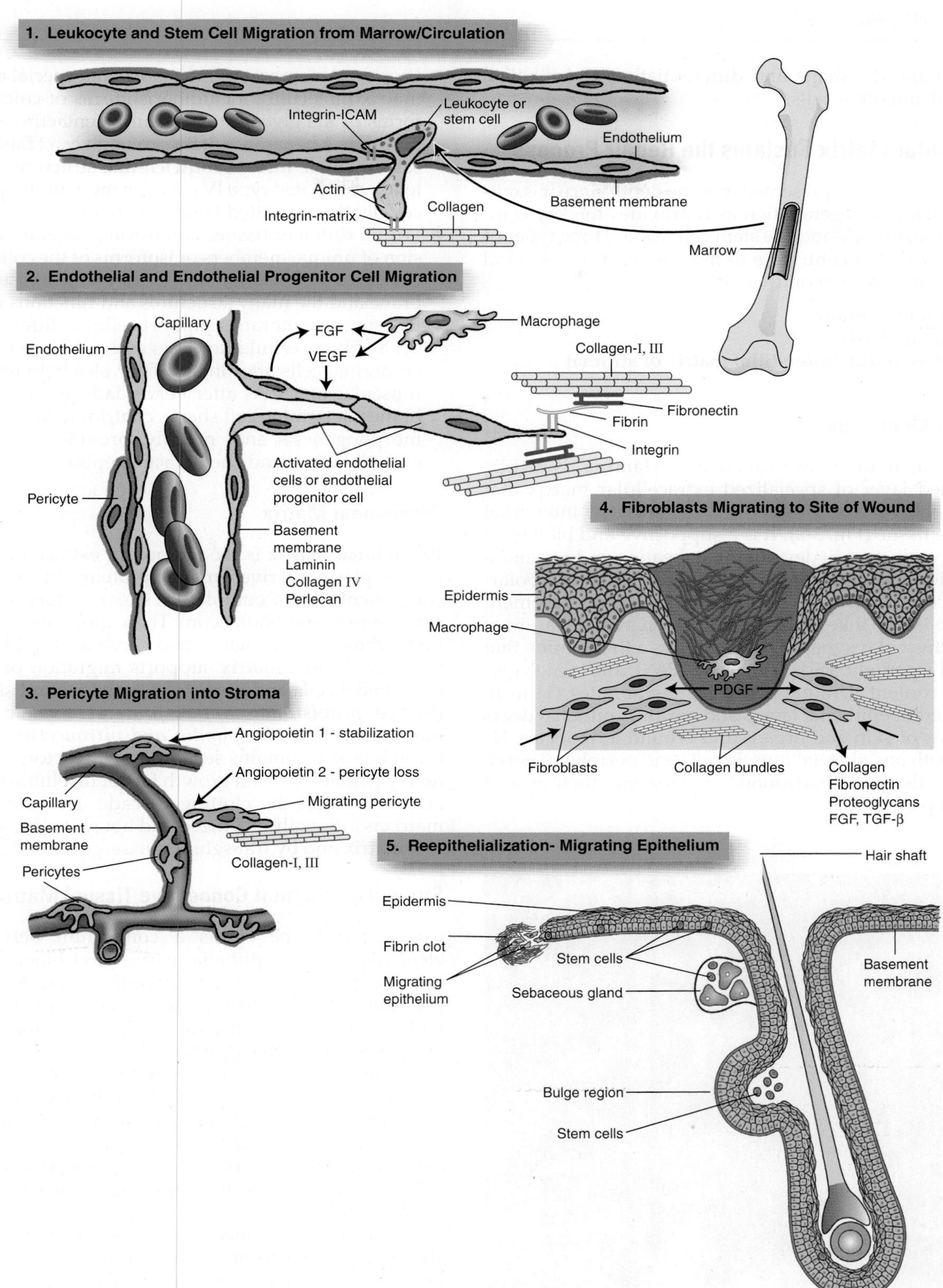

FIGURE 3-1. Resident and migrating cells initiate repair and regeneration. 1. After cytokine activation of capillary endothelium, leukocytes and bone marrow–derived circulating stem cells attach to, and migrate between, capillary endothelial cells; penetrate the basement membrane; and enter the interstitial matrix in response to chemotactic signals. **2.** Under the influence of angiogenic factors, capillary endothelial cells lose their connection with the basement membrane and migrate through the matrix to form new capillaries. Pericytes and basement membranes are required to stabilize new and existing capillary structures. **3.** Pericytes detach from capillary endothelial cells and their basement membranes to migrate into the matrix. **4.** Under the influence of growth factors such as platelet-derived growth factor (PDGF) and transforming growth factor-β (TGF-β), fibroblasts and smooth muscle actin-containing myofibroblasts become bipolar and migrate through the matrix to the site of injury. **5.** During reepithelialization, groups of basal keratinocytes extend beyond multilayered epidermis and basement membranes, and migrate between the fibrin eschar and the granulation tissue above the wound dermis. FGF = fibroblast growth factor; VEGF = vascular endothelial growth factor.

and determine the shape and differentiation of epithelial, endothelial and other cells.

Extracellular Matrix Sustains the Repair Process

Extracellular matrix is presented in some depth since it is critical for repair and regeneration as it provides the key components of scar tissue and the stem cell niche. Three types of extracellular matrix contribute to the organization, physical properties and function of tissue:

- **Basement membrane**
- **Provisional matrix**
- **Connective tissue (interstitial matrix or stroma)**

Basement Membranes

Basement membrane, also called **basal lamina**, is a thin, well-defined layer of specialized extracellular matrix that separates cells that synthesize it from adjacent interstitial connective tissue (Fig. 3-2). It is a supportive and biological boundary important in development, healing and regeneration, providing key signals for cell differentiation and polarity and contributing to tissue organization. Basement membrane is also a key structural and functional feature of the neuromuscular synapse. It appears as a thin lamina that stains by the periodic acid–Schiff stain (PAS), due to high glycoprotein content. Unique basement membranes (1) form under different epithelial layers and around epithelial ducts and tubules of skin and organs and around adipocytes, (2) cover smooth and skeletal muscle cells and peripheral nerve Schwann cells and (3) surround capillary endothelium and associated pericytes.

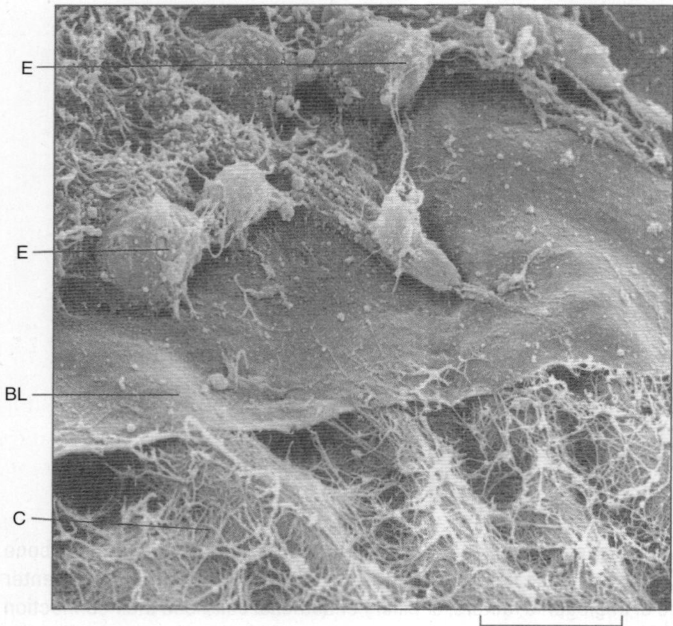

FIGURE 3-2. Scanning electron micrographs of basement membrane. Basement membrane (BL, basal lamina) separating chick embryo corneal epithelial cells (E) from underlying stromal connective tissue with collagen fibrils (C).

- Basement membranes are made from special extracellular matrix molecules, including isoforms of collagen IV, isoforms of the glycoprotein laminin, entactin/nidogen and perlecan, a heparan sulfate proteoglycan (Table 3-1). They self-assemble into a sandwich-like structure with a covalently associated type IV collagen mesh built upon the noncovalently associated laminin network.
- Within different tissues and during development, expression of unique members or isoforms of the collagen IV and laminin families imparts diversity to the basement membrane and the many structures and functions it supports.
- Basement membranes support cellular differentiation and act as filters, cellular anchors and a surface for migrating epidermal cells after injury. They also help reform neuromuscular junctions after nerve damage. Basement membranes determine cell shape, contribute to developmental morphogenesis and, notably, provide a repository for growth factors and chemotactic peptides.

Provisional Matrix

Provisional matrix is the temporary extracellular organization of plasma-derived matrix proteins and tissue-derived components that accumulate at sites of injury (e.g., hyaluronan, tenascin and fibronectin). These molecules associate with preexisting stromal matrix and serve to stop blood or fluid loss. Provisional matrix supports migration of leukocytes, endothelial cells and fibroblasts to the wound site. ***Plasma-derived provisional matrix proteins include fibrinogen, fibronectin, thrombospondin and vitronectin.*** The platelet thrombus also contains several growth factors, most prominently platelet-derived growth factor. Insoluble fibrin is generated through the clotting cascade, and the provisional matrix is internally stabilized and bound to the adjacent stromal matrix and by transglutaminase-generated cross-links.

Stromal (Interstitial Connective Tissue) Matrix

Connective tissue forms a continuum between tissue elements such as epithelia, nerves and blood vessels and provides physical protection by conferring resistance to compression or tension. Connective tissue stroma is also important for cell migration and as a medium for storage and exchange of bioactive proteins.

Connective tissue contains both extracellular matrix elements and individual cells that synthesize the matrix. The cells are primarily of mesenchymal origin and include fibroblasts, myofibroblasts, adipocytes, chondrocytes, osteocytes and endothelial cells. Bone marrow–derived cells (e.g., mast cells, macrophages, transient leukocytes) are also present.

The extracellular matrix of connective tissue, also called **stroma** or **interstitium**, is defined by fibers formed from a large family of collagen molecules (Table 3-2). Of the fibrillar collagens, type I collagen is the major constituent of bone. Type I and type III collagens are prominent in skin; type II collagen is predominant in cartilage. Elastic fibers, which impart elasticity to skin, large blood vessels and lungs, are decorated by microfibrillar proteins such as fibrillin. The so-called **ground substance** represents a number of molecules, including glycosaminoglycans (GAGs), proteoglycans, matricellular proteins and fibronectin, which are important in many biological functions of connective tissue and in the support and modulation of cell attachment.

Table 3-1

Basement Membrane Constituents and Organization

Basement Membrane Components	Chains	Molecular Structure	Molecular Associations	Basement Membrane Aggregate Form
Perlecan (heparan sulfate proteoglycan)	1 protein core 3 heparan sulfate GAG chains	GAG chains	Laminin, collagen IV, fibronectin, growth factors (VEGF, FGF), chemokines	Integrin receptors in plasma membrane
Laminin	16 isoforms Heterotrimers with α-, β-, γ-chains 5 α-chains, 3 β-chains, 3 γ-chains	α β γ	Integrin, dystroglycan and other receptors on variety of cells (epithelium, endothelium, muscle, Schwann cells, adipocytes) Forms self-associated noncovalent network that organizes basement membranes Laminin, nidogen/entactin, perlecan, agrin, fibulin	
Nidogen/ entactin	2-member family monomeric		Collagen IV, laminin, perlecan, fibulin Stabilizes basement membrane through association of laminin and collagen IV networks	
Collagen IV	≥3-member family Heterotrimers Chains selected from 2 or 3 of 6 unique α-chains	3 single chains form α-helical tail of collagenous regions and association of the 3 globular regions	Integrin receptors on many cells Forms covalent self-associated network Collagen IV, perlecan nidogen/entactin, SPARC	

FGF = fibroblast growth factor; GAG = glycosaminoglycan; SPARC = secreted protein acidic and rich and cysteine; VEGF = vascular endothelial growth factor.

Collagens

Collagen is the most abundant protein in the animal kingdom; it is essential for the structural integrity of tissues and organs. If its synthesis is reduced, delayed or abnormal, wounds fail to heal, as in scurvy or **nonhealing wounds.** Excess collagen deposition leads to **fibrosis.** Fibrosis is the basis of connective tissue diseases such as scleroderma and keloids, and of compromised tissue function seen in chronic damage to many organs, including kidney, lung, heart and liver.

The collagen superfamily of insoluble extracellular proteins are the major constituents of connective tissue in all organs, most notably cornea, arteries, dermis, cartilage, tendons, ligaments and bone. There are at least 27 distinct collagen molecules, each made from a triple helix of three collagen α-chains that form homo- or heterotrimers. All collagen chains have helical segments, largely composed of glycine, proline and hydroxyproline, in which every third amino acid is glycine (Gly-X-Y). The collagen domain that determines this glycine repeat and ascorbate-dependent, posttranslational formation of hydroxyproline are critical for this triple helical structure. The action of lysyl oxidase on lysine and hydroxylysine generates covalent collagen crosslinks.

Collagen synthesis exemplifies the complexity of posttranslational protein modification. Each molecule is made by self-association of three α-chains that wind around each other to form a triple helix. The triple helix includes members from an α-chain family that is unique for each collagen type.

Table 3-2

Collagen Molecular Composition and Structure

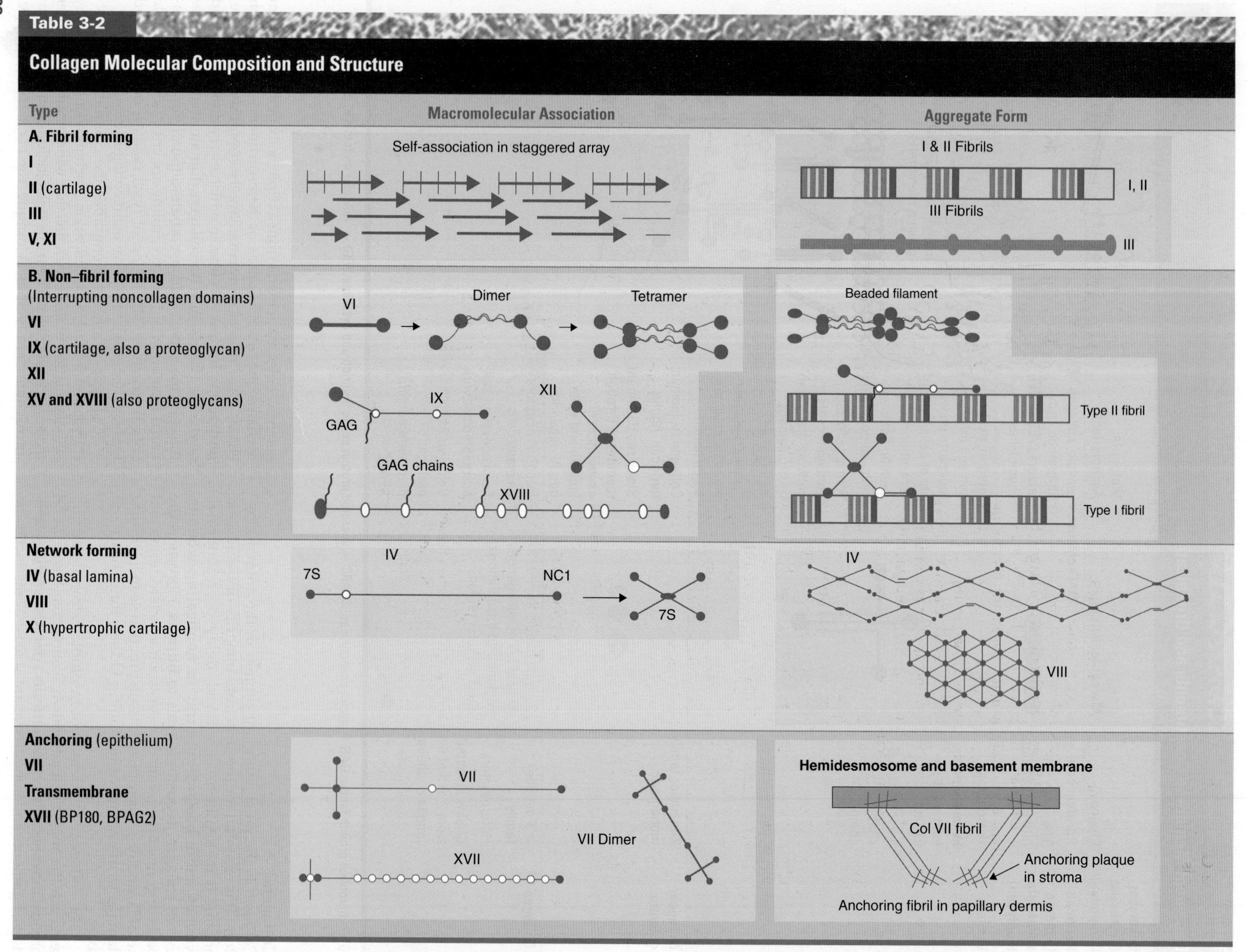

Type	Macromolecular Association	Aggregate Form
A. Fibril forming **I** **II** (cartilage) **III** **V, XI**		
B. Non–fibril forming (Interrupting noncollagen domains) **VI** **IX** (cartilage, also a proteoglycan) **XII** **XV and XVIII** (also proteoglycans)		
Network forming **IV** (basal lamina) **VIII** **X** (hypertrophic cartilage)		
Anchoring (epithelium) **VII** **Transmembrane** **XVII** (BP180, BPAG2)		

Collagen molecules lose stability when errors occur that change the Gly-X-Y sequence, in which case the unstable triple helix is more vulnerable to proteinase activity.

Successful collagen synthesis usually results from a series of posttranslational modifications: (1) alignment of the three chains; (2) ascorbate-dependent hydroxylation of proline and lysine; (3) triple helix formation; (4) cleavage of noncollagenous terminal peptides; (5) molecular alignment and microfibril association; and (6) covalent cross-linking, mediated by the copper-dependent enzyme lysyl oxidase. Mutations of fibrillar collagens cause diseases of bone (osteogenesis imperfecta), cartilage (chondroplasias), skin, joints and blood vessels (Ehlers-Danlos syndrome) (Chapters 6 and 26). Mutant basement membrane collagens lead to blistering (epidermolysis bullosa, Chapter 24) and kidney diseases (Alport syndrome, Chapter 16).

Fibrillar collagens include types I, II, III, V and XI. Types I, II and III are the most abundant, and appear as continuous fibrils. They are formed from a quarter-staggered packing of cross-linked collagen molecules, whose triple helix is uninterrupted (Table 3-2). These fibrillar collagens turn over slowly in most tissues, and are largely resistant to proteinase digestion, except by specific matrix metalloproteinases (MMPs). Type I fibril size and structure can be modified by incorporation of type V molecules, which nucleate formation of type I fibrils, or association with type III molecules, while type XI collagen nucleates type II fibrils. Mutant fibrillar collagens, lacking nonhelical interruptions, cause diseases from lethal to minor and involve skin, blood vessels, bone or cartilage. Type I is the most abundant collagen, and mutations in the genes for this molecule cause assembly defects in the triple helix that can lead to increased bone fractures, hyperextensible ligaments and dermis or easy bruising (Chapter 6).

Nonfibrillar collagens (Table 3-2) contain globular domains in addition to triple helical domains. These interruptions of the triple helical segments confer structural variability and flexibility not possessed by fibrillar collagens. Nonhelical domains enable small collagens (IX, XII) to associate with fibrillar collagens, modulating fiber packing of a linear collagen. Collagen VI forms beaded filament structures (VI) that encircle fibrillar collagens I and II, is found close to cells and associates with elastin in elastic fibers; mutations are associated with certain myopathies, as it helps bind muscle cells to basement membrane. Other nonfibrillar collagens act as **transmembrane** proteins (XVII) in hemidesmosomes that attach epidermal cells to basement membrane and are **fibrillar anchors** (VII) linking hemidesmosome and basement membrane to underlying stroma. **Network-forming collagens** facilitate formation of flexible, "chicken-wire" networks of basement membrane collagen (IV) or more ordered hexagonal networks (VIII, X) in other tissues. Mutations in collagen IV cause the abnormal glomerular basement membranes seen in Alport syndrome. Proteolytic fragments of collagen (matrikines) exhibit a different set of biological properties that are also important in tissue remodeling. For example, fragments of basement membrane collagens IV, XV and XVIII inhibit angiogenesis and tumor growth.

The collagens were once called **scleroproteins,** meaning both white and hard; yet in the cornea, layers of collagen can be transparent. The cornea consists of 10 to 20 orthogonally stacked layers of composites of type I and type V collagens (Fig. 3-3), the fibrils being uniform and smaller sized than the predominantly type I + type III composite collagen fibers in skin. Each layer has parallel, uniform-sized collagen fibers oriented at right angles to the underlying layer. In healing, injured corneas form disorganized white collagenous scars, which are opaque and interfere with vision. The structure of the cornea is remarkable to those who have seen only the loose, random, basket weave–like network of dermal collagen or the parallel arrays of collagen in tendons and ligaments. Yet structured orientation of collagen in human skin has long been known. Plastic surgeons use wrinkle (Langer) lines, which indicate the primary orientation of the underlying dermal collagen, to promote inconspicuous healing by reducing lateral tension on the wound site (gape). The tensile strength of skin that is broken parallel to creases and wrinkle lines exceeds that which is broken perpendicular to these lines, further suggesting a structured orientation of dermal collagen. Scars have an inappropriate arrangement of thicker, poorly woven collagen fibers.

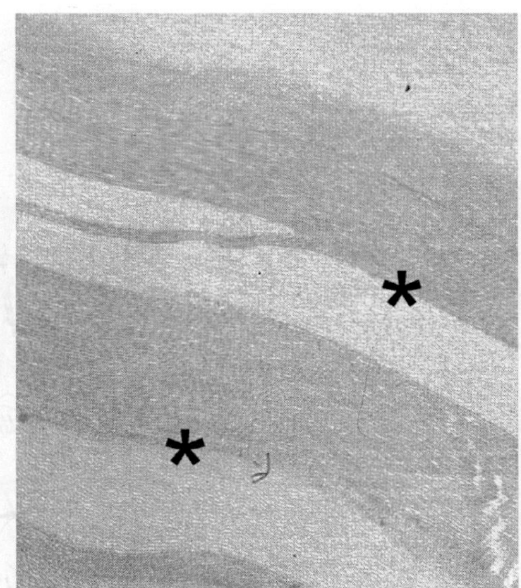

FIGURE 3-3. Human cornea, near center. Collagen fibers are highly organized in the cornea. Multiple plywood-like arrays of collagen fibers are of similar width and layers are sharply demarcated between asterisks (*). This precise organization is critical to the transparency and refractive index of the cornea.

Elastin and Elastic Fibers

Elastin is a secreted matrix protein that, unlike other stromal proteins, is not glycosylated (Table 3-3). Elastin allows deformable tissues such as skin, uterus, ligament, lung, elastic cartilage and aorta to stretch and bend with recoil. Its lack of carbohydrate, its extensive covalent cross-linking and its hydrophobic amino acid sequence make it the most insoluble of all vertebrate proteins. The elastic fiber is crucial for the function of several vital tissues, yet it is not efficiently replaced during repair of skin and lung. The absence, impaired assembly or slow accumulation of functional elastin following damage to skin or lung is offset by the fact that it is degraded with difficulty and turns over slowly. Nevertheless, elastic fibers are damaged by aging and sun exposure, conditions that lead to age-related loss of dermal suppleness and sagging.

Elastin stability results from its (1) hydrophobicity, (2) extensive covalent cross-linking (mediated by lysyl oxidase, the same enzyme that cross-links collagen) and (3) resistance to most proteolytic enzymes. Unlike skin and lung damage, the artery wall can rapidly form new concentric rings of elastic lamellae in response to hypertension and other injuries. Veins that are transplanted in coronary artery bypass surgery rapidly generate new elastic lamellae in the process of arterialization.

Table 3-3

Noncollagenous Matrix Constituents of Stroma

Stromal Connective Tissue Components	Chains	Molecular Structure	Molecular Associations	Tissue Structures
Fibronectin	Dimeric protein Chains chosen from ~20 splice variants of one gene	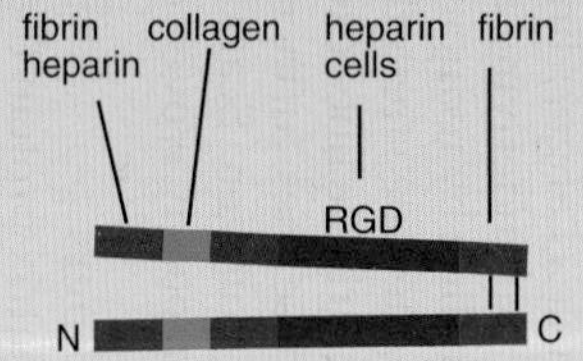 fibrin heparin; collagen; heparin cells; fibrin; RGD; N; C	Integrin receptors of many cells (RGD-binding site) Plasma fibronectin is soluble Cellular fibronectin can self-associate into fibrils at cell surface and also binds collagen, heparin, decorin, fibrin, certain bacteria (opsonin), LTBPs	Cell cytoplasm; 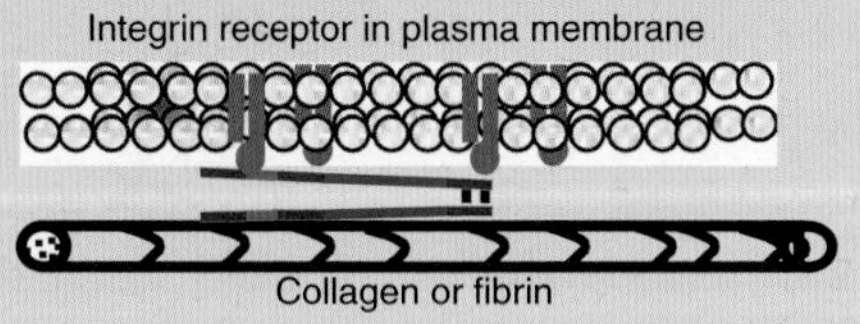 Integrin receptor in plasma membrane; Collagen or fibrin
Elastin	Monomer with several splice variants, 1 gene	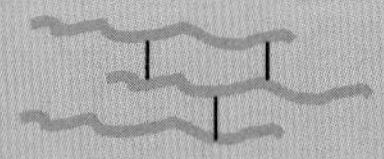 Elastin cross-links to form fiber	Self-association to form cross-linked amorphous fibers Formed on scaffold of microfibrillar polymers	Elastin fiber with microfibril polymers 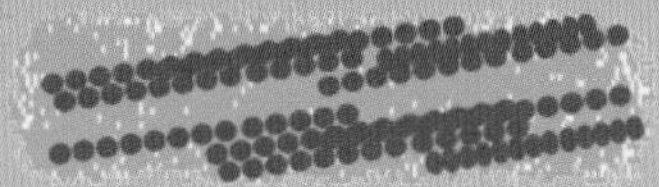
Fibrillins	Large glycoproteins—most common microfibrils needed for elastin fiber assembly	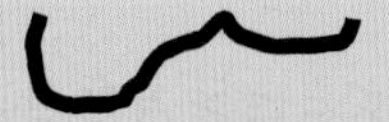	Forms beaded polymer Other microfibrillar proteins: LTBPs, fibulins, emilins, MAGP 1 and 2, lysyl oxidase	
Versican (hyaluronan-binding proteoglycans)	Family of 4 related genes Aggrecan found in cartilage Protein core decorated with 10–30 chondroitin sulfate and dermatan sulfate GAG chains	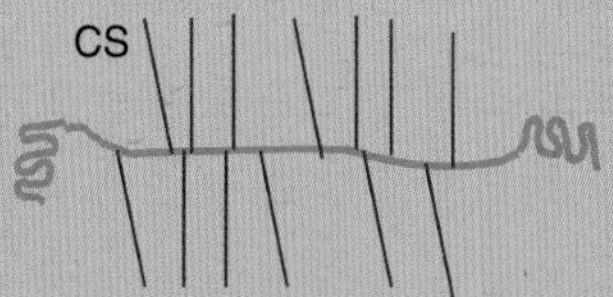 CS	Proteoglycans linked to hyaluronan via link protein to form very large composite structure	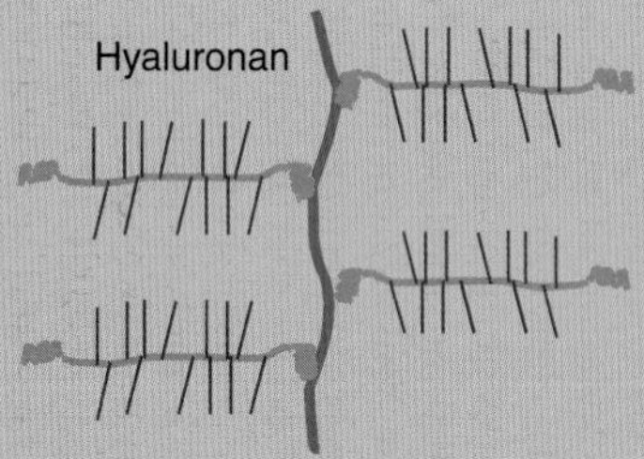 Hyaluronan
Decorin (small leucine-rich proteoglycans)	1 protein core, 1 gene One chondroitin sulfate or dermatan sulfate GAG chain Biglycan and fibromodulin structurally related, genetically distinct	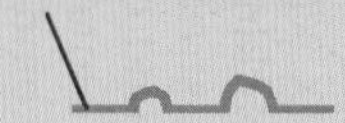	Collagen I and II, fibronectin, TGF-β, thrombospondin	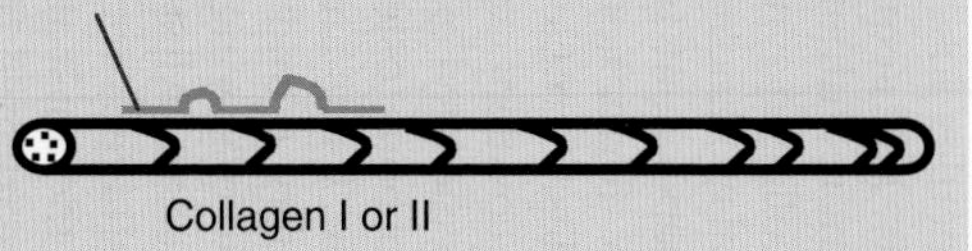 Collagen I or II

GAG = glycosaminoglycan; LTBPs = latent transforming growth factor-β–binding proteins; MAGP = microfibril-associated growth protein; RGD = Arg-Gly-Asp; TGF-β = transforming growth factor-β.

This observation illustrates the difference in the elastin synthetic capabilities of the vascular smooth muscle cell and those of dermal or lung fibroblasts.

Elastin is deposited as fibrils, which are complexed with several different glycoproteins (microfibrils) that decorate the perimeter of the elastic fiber. The best-characterized microfibrillar protein is **fibrillin** (Table 3-3). When mutated, abnormal fibrillin demonstrates decreased binding and reduced activation of transforming growth factor-β, leading to Marfan syndrome, with pleomorphic manifestations that include dissecting aortic aneurysm (Chapter 6).

Matrix Glycoproteins

Matrix glycoproteins contribute essential biological functions to basement membrane and stromal connective tissue. In general, these are large (150,000 to 1,000,000 kd) multimeric and multidomain proteins, with long arms that bind other matrix molecules and support or modulate cell attachment. Matrix glycoproteins help to (1) organize tissue topography, (2) support cell migration, (3) orient cells and (4) induce cell behavior. The principal matrix glycoprotein of basement membrane is **laminin,** and that of stromal connective tissue is **fibronectin.**

LAMININS: The laminins are a versatile family of basement membrane glycoproteins whose cross-like structure is formed by products of three related gene subfamilies to form α, β and γ heterotrimers (Table 3-1). There are 15 known laminin isoforms, which are formed from varying combinations of the five α-, three β- and three γ-chains. Expression of laminin isoforms in specific tissues contributes to the heterogeneity of tissue morphology and functions, in part, by supporting cell attachment via binding to membrane sulfated glycolipids or transmembrane integrin receptors. Laminin molecules self-polymerize into sheets initiating basement membrane formation by association with type IV collagen sheets and other basement membrane molecules.

The appropriate formation of epidermal laminin is key for normal epidermal function and reepithelialization of wounds. Epidermal integrity is imparted by hemidesmosomes, which develop from the binding of basement membrane laminin to epithelial integrin and collagen VII. The latter forms the anchoring fibril that connects the epidermal cell and basement membrane to the dermal connective tissue. Mutations in epidermal laminin, integrin, collagen VII or collagen XVII produce a potentially fatal skin blistering disease, termed **epidermolysis bullosa.**

FIBRONECTINS: Fibronectins are versatile, adhesive glycoproteins widely distributed in stromal connective tissue and deposited in wound provisional matrix (Table 3-3). Fibronectin chains form a V-shaped homo- or heterodimer linked at the C terminus by two disulfide bonds. Specific fibronectin domains bind bacteria, collagen, heparin, fibrin, fibrinogen and the cell matrix receptor integrin. Indeed, the integrin receptor family has been partly defined by studies showing its specific binding to fibronectin. The multifunctional dimer is designed to link matrix molecules to one another or to cells. Thrombi support cell migration on the high concentration of plasma-derived fibronectin that links fibrin strands, and the complex is stabilized by cross-linking of factor XIII (transglutaminase) to other provisional and dermal matrix components.

Two classes of fibronectin are formed by a single gene but from different sources: (1) the insoluble cellular form and (2) a hepatocyte-derived, soluble form in plasma. Though coded by one gene, as many as 24 fibronectin variants may be formed by alternative splicing. Clot-bound fibronectin supports platelet adhesion and may interact with collagen to promote keratinocyte attachment and migration during reepithelialization of corneal and cutaneous wounds by aiding collagen. Fibronectin synthesized by mesenchymal cells such as fibroblasts is assembled into insoluble fibrils with the aid of integrin receptors and collagen fibrils. Polymerized cellular fibronectin is found in granulation tissue and loose connective tissue. Excisional wound clotting and reepithelialization are unaffected by experimentally knocking out plasma fibronectin, suggesting that cellular fibronectin and other factors can compensate for its absence.

Glycosaminoglycans

Glycosaminoglycans (GAGs) are long, linear polymers of specific repeating disaccharides arranged in sequence that are also known as mucopolysaccharides. GAG chains are named by the disaccharide subunits in the polymer. GAG chains are negatively charged, due to the presence of carboxylate groups and, save for hyaluronan, the attachment of disaccharide modification with N- or O-linked sulfate groups. GAGs have the potential for exceptional diversity and biologic specificity owing to epimerization and variability in modifications (e.g., acetylation and sulfation). When sulfated GAG chains are O-linked to serine residues of protein cores, they are called **proteoglycans** (see below). GAG storage disorders result from autosomal recessive (or X-linked) deficiency of one of several lysosomal hydrolases that degrade GAGs, leading to intracellular accumulation within lysosomes. The 12 known mucopolysaccharidoses are slowly evolving disorders of connective tissue that significantly decrease life expectancy; affect ossification of cartilage, skeletal structure, stature and facies; and may cause psychomotor problems or even mild retardation.

Hyaluronan

Hyaluronan, the only GAG not covalently linked to a protein, is a linear polymer of 2000 to 25,000 disaccharides of glucosamine and glucuronic acid. Its uronic acid content makes hyaluronan very hydrophilic, and its high molecular mass creates a viscous solution. Hyaluronan can associate with protein cores of proteoglycans (defined below) that contain hyaluronan-binding regions and with hyaluronan-binding proteins at the cell surface. Certain proteoglycans bind ionically via a linking protein along the hyaluronan backbone to form large, hyaluronan/proteoglycan composites, such as **aggrecan** and **versican** (Table 3-3), molecules found in cartilage and stromal tissues. The hydrated viscosity of hyaluronan imparts resilience and lubrication to joints and connective tissue, and pericellular accumulation of these molecules facilitates cell migration through the extracellular matrix. Hyaluronan is highly prevalent in the stroma during embryonic development, and it is an early addition to the provisional matrix. The negatively charged carboxylate backbone of hyaluronan binds large amounts of water, creating a viscous gel that produces turgor in the matrix. As a biomaterial, hyaluronan can be chemically modified to act as a temporary dermal filler, joint lubricant or replacement for vitreous humor. Its synthesis occurs at the cell surface, and hyaluronan receptors send signals to the cell. Concentrations of hyaluronan are higher during dynamic tissue change associated with inflammation, wound repair, morphogenesis or cancer.

Proteoglycans

Proteoglycans are a diverse family of proteins with varying numbers, types and sizes of attached glycosaminoglycan chains linked by O-glycosidic bonds to serines or threonines.

They have a higher carbohydrate content than matrix glycoproteins, and though not branched, demonstrate substantial diversity through numerous carbohydrate modifications such as sulfation, unique linkages and varying sequences. Individual proteoglycans differ in size, core proteins, choice of GAG chains and tissue distribution.

Proteoglycans participate in matrix organization, structural integrity and cell attachment. Though their protein core often has biological activity, the properties of several proteoglycans are largely mediated by the GAG chains themselves. Heparan sulfate GAG chains of basement membrane (perlecan, collagen XVIII) and cell-associated proteoglycans (syndecan, glypican) modulate the availability and actions of heparin-binding growth factors, such as vascular endothelial growth factor (VEGF), fibroblast growth factor (FGF) and heparin-binding epidermal growth factor (HB-EGF). PDGF is also more weakly bound to these highly charged molecules. A group of small proteoglycans, which share a core protein domain of leucine-rich repeats, regulates transforming growth factor-β (TGF-β) activity and fibril formation in collagens I and II (Table 3-3). Sequestered growth factors are released when proteoglycans are degraded.

Tissue expression of extracellular matrix proteins and proteoglycans is shown in Table 3-4.

Table 3-4

Tissue Expression of Extracellular Matrix Molecules

Tissue or Body Fluid	Primary Mesodermal Cell	Prominent Collagen Types	Noncollagenous Matrix Proteins	Glycosaminoglycans Proteoglycans (PGs)
Plasma			Fibronectin, fibrinogen, vitronectin	Hyaluronan
Dermis	Fibroblast	I, III, V, VI, XII	Fibronectin, elastin, fibrillin	Hyaluronan, decorin, biglycan, versican
Reticular/papillary				
Epidermal junction		VII, XVII (BP 180), anchoring fibrils, hemidesmosome		
Muscle	Muscle cell	I, III, V, VI, VIII, XII	Fibronectin, elastin, fibrillin	Aggrecan, biglycan, decorin, fibromodulin
Peri-, epimysium	Fibroblast			
Aortic media/adventitia				
Tendon	Fibroblast	I, III, V, VI, XII	Fibronectin, tenascin (myotendon junction), elastin, fibrillin	Decorin, biglycan, fibromodulin, lumican, versican
Ligament	Fibroblast	I, III, V, VI	Fibronectin, elastin, fibrillin	Decorin, biglycan, versican
Cornea	Fibroblast	I, III, V, VI, XII		Lumican, keratocan, mimecan, biglycan, decorin
Cartilage	Chondrocyte hypertrophic cartilage	II, IX, VI, VIII, X, XI	Anchorin CII, fibronectin, tenascin	Hyaluronan, aggrecan, biglycan, decorin, fibromodulin, lumican, perlecan (minor)
Bone	Osteocyte	I, V	Osteocalcin, osteopontin, bone sialoprotein, SPARC (osteonectin)	Decorin, fibromodulin, biglycan
Basement membrane zones	Epithelial, endothelial adipocytes, Schwann cell, muscle cells (endomysium), pericytes	IV, XV, XVIII	Laminin, nidogen/entactin	Heparan sulfate proteoglycans, perlecan Collagen XVIII (vascular), agrin (neuromuscular junctions)

SPARC = secreted protein acidic and rich in cysteine.

Remodeling Is the Long-Lasting Phase of Repair

As repair proceeds, inflammatory cells become fewer in number and capillary formation is completed. In remodeling, equilibrium between collagen deposition and degradation is restored. Matrix metalloproteinases are the main remodeling enzymes, but neutrophil protease and serine proteases are also present.

A large family of 25 proteinases, MMPs, are central to wound healing, as they enable cells to migrate through stroma by degrading matrix proteins (see Table 2-3). They participate in cell–cell communication and activation or inactivation of bioactive molecules (e.g., immune system components, matrix fragments, growth factors) and influence cell growth and apoptosis. MMPs are synthesized as inactive proenzymes (zymogens) and require extracellular activation by already activated MMPs or serine proteinases. MMPs are named numerically (e.g., MMP-1, MMP-2) or by the matrix proteins they degrade, such as collagenase, stromelysin and gelatinase. MMPs cleave diverse extracellular substrates, many of which are degraded by more than one MMP. As with integrins, such redundancy emphasizes the importance of these molecules in regulatory control. ***The list of molecules needed for wound healing is indistinguishable from the list of MMP substrates.*** These include:

- Clotting factors
- Extracellular matrix proteins
- Latent growth factors and growth factor–binding proteins
- Receptors for matrix molecules and cell–cell adhesion molecules
- Immune system components
- Other MMPs, other proteinases, and proteinase inhibitors
- Chemotactic molecules

Most MMPs are closely regulated at the transcriptional level, except for MMP-2 (gelatinase A), which is often constitutively expressed. Transcription is regulated by (1) integrin signaling, (2) cytokine and growth factor signaling, (3) binding to certain matrix proteins or (4) tensional force on a cell. As the site of their substrates suggests, MMPs are secreted into and activated within the pericellular environment or the extracellular matrix or are membrane bound. Membrane-bound MMPs are transmembrane molecules or are linked to glycosylphosphatidylinositol (GPI). MMP-1 and -2 associate with integrins, thereby facilitating cell migration.

MMPs can also disrupt cell–cell adhesion and release, activate or inactivate bioactive molecules stored in the matrix. These include growth factors, chemokines, growth factor–binding proteins, angiogenic/antiangiogenic factors and bioactive cryptic fragments of matrix proteins released when their parent matrix molecules are degraded **(matrikines).**

Once secreted, MMP activity can be limited by diffusion, specific inhibitors, reduced activation and substrate specificity. There is a family of tissue inhibitors of metalloproteinases (TIMPs), in addition to the plasma-derived proteinase inhibitor, α_2-macroglobulin. A related family of membrane-bound proteases, ADAMs (a disintegrin and metalloproteinase) function to shed growth factors, chemokines and receptors on cell or neighboring cell surfaces.

Cell Proliferation Is Evoked by Cytokines and Matrix

Early in tissue injury, there is a transient increase in cellularity, which replaces damaged cells. Cell proliferation also initiates and perpetuates **granulation tissue,** a specialized vascular tissue formed transiently during repair (see below). Cells of granulation tissue derive from transient cell populations, including circulating leukocytes, and from resident capillary endothelial and mesenchymal cells (fibroblasts, myofibroblasts, pericytes and smooth muscle cells). Local and marrow-derived progenitor cells may also populate wounds, differentiating into endothelial and fibroblast populations. Terminally differentiated cells (e.g., cardiac myocytes, neurons) do not for the most part contribute to repair or regeneration (discussed below).

Growth factors and small chemotactic peptides (chemokines) provide soluble autocrine and paracrine signals for cell proliferation, differentiation and migration. Signals from soluble factors and extracellular matrix also work collectively to influence cell behavior.

Behaviors of cells in healing wounds—proliferation, migration and altered gene expression—are largely initiated by three receptor systems that share integrated signaling pathways:

- **Protein tyrosine kinase receptors** for peptide growth factors
- **G protein–coupled receptors** for chemokines and other factors
- **Integrin receptors** for extracellular matrix

Tyrosine kinase receptors, growth factor matrix integrin receptors and G protein–coupled receptors act in concert to direct cell behavior. These distinct receptor families bind unrelated ligands yet transmit signals within a network of cascading and intersecting intracellular signaling pathways that amplify the messages, often activating similar processes. Even different processes, such as proliferation, differentiation and migration, may share signals, such as those that initiate cytoskeletal changes. The myriad intracellular signaling mechanisms that regulate cell growth, survival and proliferation are beyond the scope of the current discussion. It is important to recognize that tissue responses are governed by the integration of signals from all these systems.

Repair

Outcomes of Injury Include Repair and Regeneration

Repair and regeneration follow inflammatory responses, inflammation itself being the primary response to tissue injury (see Chapter 2). To understand how inflammation influences repair, it is useful to review the various possible outcomes of acute inflammation. *Transient* acute inflammation may resolve completely, with locally injured parenchymal elements regenerating without significant scarring. Thus, after a moderate sunburn, occasional acute inflammatory cells may accompany transient vasodilation under solar-injured epidermis. By contrast, *progressive* acute inflammation, with eventual macrophage-predominant infiltrates, is central to the sequence of collagen elaboration and repair. Complete regeneration may occur with injury to liver or bone: normal hepatic structure is restored after self-limited hepatic insult due to a toxic drug.

Organization is a pathologic outcome of fibrinogen leakage from blood vessels during an inflammatory response. It occurs in serous cavities, like the peritoneum, when fibrin

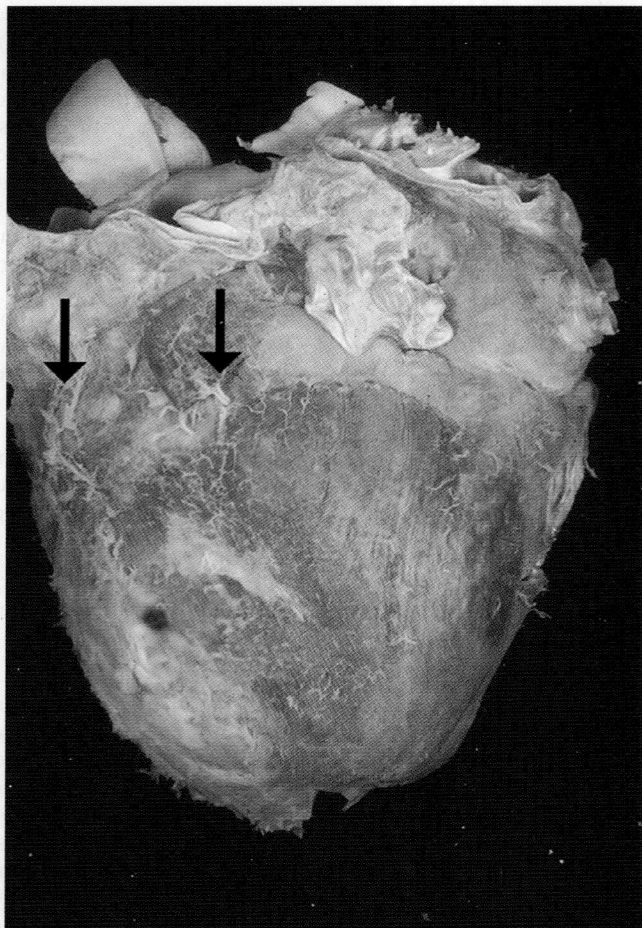

FIGURE 3-4. Organized strands of collagen in constrictive pericarditis (*arrows*). Excess collagen distorts the biomechanical properties of the heart.

strands are formed and not degraded. In pericarditis, fibroblasts invade fibrin matrix and secrete and organize collagen within fibrin strands, thus binding visceral and parietal pericardium together (Fig. 3-4). This constricts ventricular filling of the heart and may require surgical intervention. Fibrin strands may become organized in the peritoneal cavity after intra-abdominal surgery. Such "adhesions" (threads of collagen) can trap loops of bowel and cause intestinal obstruction.

Wound Healing Exhibits a Defined Sequence

Wound healing resulting in scar formation remains the predominant mode of repair. Given that wounds in the skin and extremities are easily accessible, they have been extensively studied as models. Healing within hollow viscera and body cavities, though less accessible for study, generally parallels the repair sequence in skin, as illustrated in Figs. 3-5 and 3-6 and Table 3-5.

Thrombosis

A thrombus (clot)—a **scab** or **eschar** after it dries—forms a barrier on wounded skin to invading microorganisms. This barrier also prevents loss of plasma and tissue fluid. Formed primarily from provisional matrix, including plasma fibrin, the thrombus is also rich in fibronectin. At the site of injury, fibrin is bound by fibronectin and they are soon cross-linked by factor XIII (FXIII), a transglutaminase. Binding provides local tensile strength and maintains closure. The thrombus contains contracting platelets, an initial source of growth factors. FXIII cross-links other matrix proteins, such as collagens and fibronectin, which aids in storage of latent growth factors and affects MMP degradation of matrix. Excess transglutaminase may cause undue scarring. FXIII deficiencies are associated with poor wound healing and bleeding. Much later, the thrombus is digested, after which it is undermined by regenerating epithelium. The scab then detaches.

Inflammation

Repair sites vary in the amount of local tissue destruction. For example, surgical excision of a skin lesion leaves little or no devitalized tissue. Demarcated, localized necrosis accompanies medium-sized myocardial infarcts. By contrast, widespread, irregularly defined necrosis is a feature of a large third-degree burn. Initially, an acute, neutrophil-dominated, inflammatory response liquefies the necrotic tissue. Acute inflammation persists as long as necessary, since necrotic material must be removed for repair to progress. Before granulation tissue appears, exudative, spent neutrophils may form pus or become trapped in the eschar. Plasma-derived fibronectin then binds collagen and cell membranes to facilitate phagocytosis. Fibronectin and cell debris are chemotactic for macrophages and fibroblasts (Figs. 3-5 and 3-7). ***The repair process begins when macrophages predominate at the site of injury.*** Macrophages ingest proteolytic products of neutrophils and secrete collagenase, thus facilitating liquefaction. Macrophages can assume proinflammatory (M1) or anti-inflammatory (M2) phenotypes. M2 cells make growth factors that stimulate fibroblast proliferation, collagen secretion and neovascularization.

Fibroblasts are also early responders to injury. These collagen-secreting cells are involved in inflammatory, proliferative and remodeling phases of wound repair. Fibroblasts are capable of further differentiation to contractile myofibroblasts (see below).

Granulation Tissue

Granulation tissue is the transient, specialized organ of repair, which replaces the provisional matrix. Like a placenta, it is only present where and when needed. It is deceptively simple, with a glistening and pebbled appearance (Fig. 3-8). Microscopically, a mixture of fibroblasts and red blood cells first appears, followed by development of provisional matrix and patent single cell-lined capillaries, which are surrounded by fibroblasts and inflammatory cells.

A key step in the process is recruitment of monocytes to the site of injury by chemokines and fragments of damaged matrix. Later, plasma cells are conspicuous, even predominating. Activated macrophages release growth factors and cytokines (Table 3-5, and see below) that direct angiogenesis, activate fibroblasts to form new stroma and continue the degradation and removal of the provisional matrix. However, macrophages may not be obligatory for wound repair: in mice lacking mature macrophages, functioning neutrophils repair skin wounds normally and without scarring.

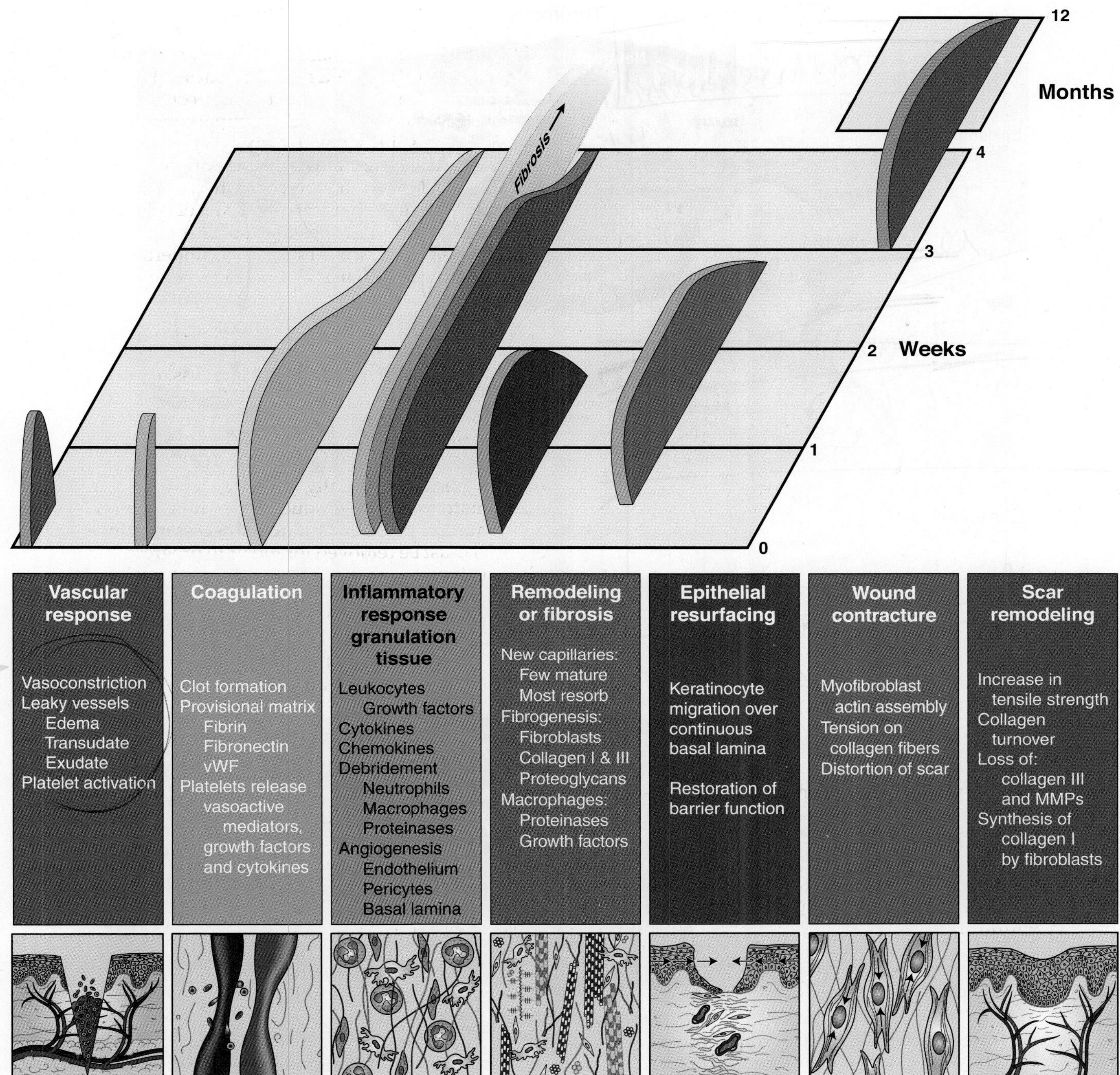

FIGURE 3-5. The sequential phases of the healing process.

Granulation tissue is fluid-rich, and its cellular constituents supply antibacterial peptides **(defensins)** and growth factors. It is highly resistant to bacterial infection, allowing the surgeon to create anastomoses at such nonsterile sites as the colon, in which fully one third of the fecal contents consist of bacteria.

Fibroblast Proliferation and Matrix Accumulation

Early granulation tissue matrix contains hyaluronan, proteoglycans, glycoproteins and type III collagen (Figs. 3-5, 3-6 and 3-7. Cytokines released by cells in the damaged area cause vascular leakage and attract inflammatory cells. About 2 to 3 days after injury, activated fibroblasts and capillary sprouts are seen. Fibroblasts in the wound change from oval to bipolar, as they begin to produce collagen (Figs. 3-7 and 3-9) and other matrix proteins, such as fibronectin. Secretion of type III collagen predominates initially but is rapidly overwhelmed by type I collagen incorporation into fibrils, which forms larger-diameter fibrils with greater tensile strength. Eventually, the matrix resumes it original composition of predominantly type I collagen and 15% to 20% type III collagen.

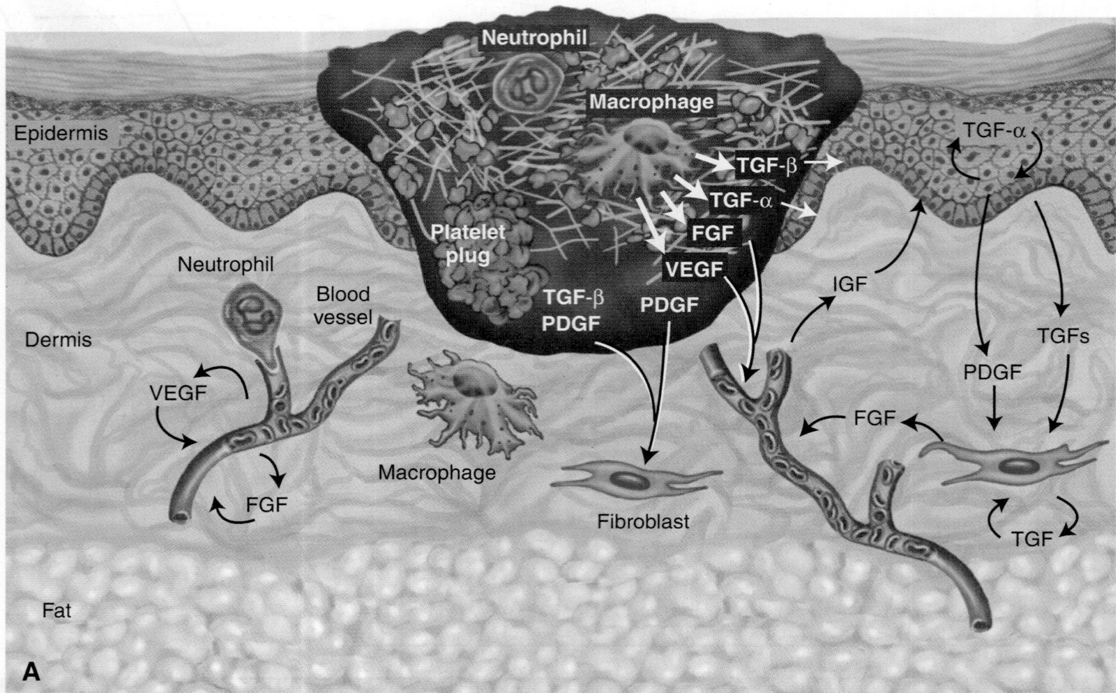

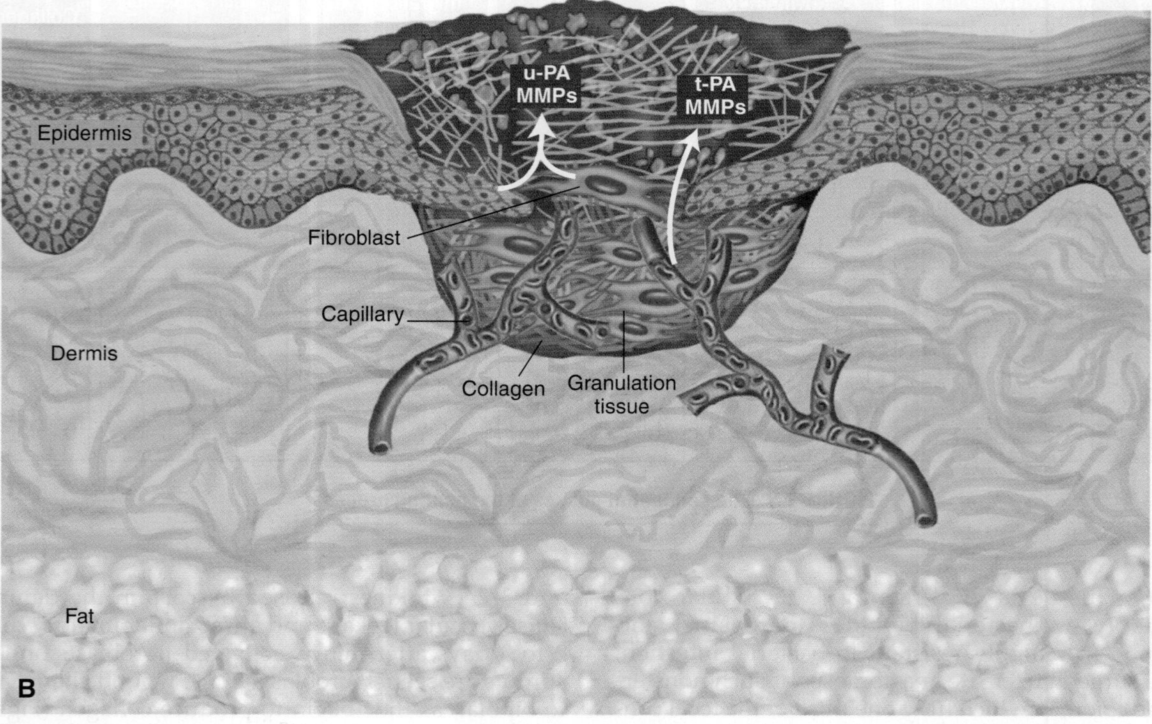

FIGURE 3-6. Cutaneous wound healing. A. 2 to 4 days. Growth factors controlling migration of cells are illustrated. Extensive redundancy is present, and no growth factor is rate limiting. Most factors have multiple effects, as listed in Table 3-6. Growth factor signals first arise from platelets, but activated macrophages, resident tissue cells and the matrix itself release a complex interplay of interacting signals. **B. 4 to 8 days.** Capillary blood vessels proliferate and the epidermal keratinocytes penetrate along the granulation tissue below the thrombus. The upper, acellular portion will become an eschar or scab. Fibroblasts deposit a collagen rich matrix. FGF = fibroblast growth factor; IGF = insulin-like growth factor; MMPs = matrix metalloproteinases; PDGF = platelet-derived growth factor; TGF-β = transforming growth factor-β; t-PA = tissue plasminogen activator; u-PA = urokinase-type plasminogen activator; VEGF = vascular endothelial growth factor.

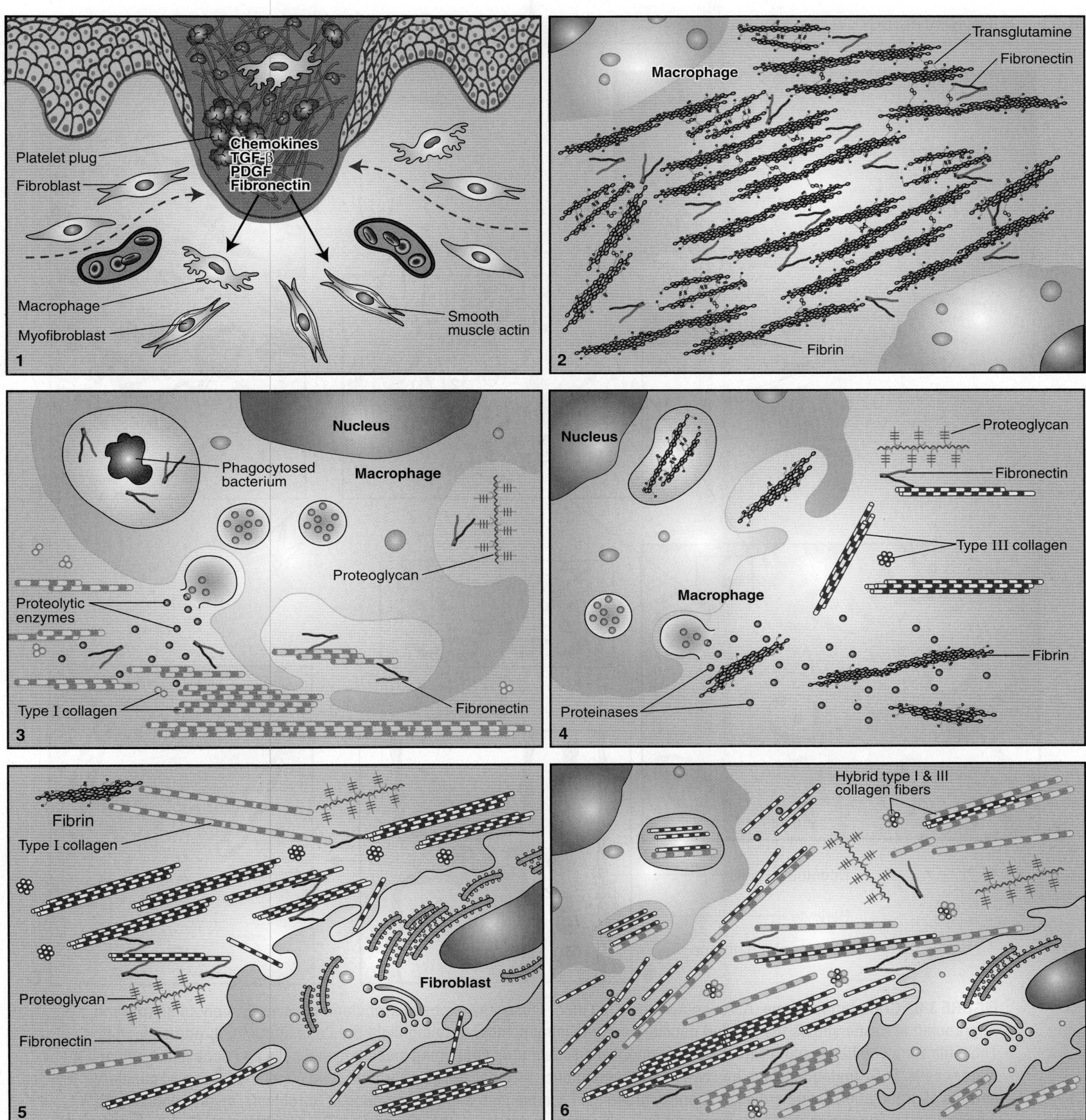

FIGURE 3-7. Summary of the healing process. 1. Inflammatory cell migration. A low-power view of the wound site depicts the migration of macrophages, fibroblasts and smooth muscle actin-containing myofibroblasts as they migrate to the wound from the surrounding tissue into the provisional matrix. Fibronectin, growth factors, chemokines, cell debris and bacterial products are chemoattractants for a variety of cells that are recruited to the wound site (2 to 4 days). The initial phase of the repair reaction typically begins with hemorrhage into the tissues. **2.** A **fibrin clot** forms from plasma and platelets, and it fills the gap created by the wound. Fibronectin in the extravasated plasma binds fibrin, collagen and other extracellular matrix components within fibrin strands that are cross-linked by the action of transglutaminase (factor XIII). This cross-linking provides a provisional mechanical stabilization of the wound (0 to 4 hours). Neutrophils rapidly infiltrate in the presence of bacteria or damaged tissue. **3. Macrophages** recruited to the wound area further process cell remnants and damaged extracellular matrix. The binding of fibronectin to cell membranes, collagens, proteoglycans, DNA and bacteria (opsonization) facilitates phagocytosis by these macrophages and contributes to the removal of debris (1 to 3 days). **4.** During the intermediate phase of the repair reaction, recruited **fibroblasts** deposit a new extracellular matrix of primarily smaller collagen type III fibers at the wound site, while the initial fibrin clot is lysed by a combination of extracellular proteolytic enzymes and phagocytosis (2 to 4 days). **5.** Concurrent with fibrin removal by macrophages, there is continued fibroblast production of a **temporary matrix** including proteoglycans, glycoproteins such as polymerized cellular fibronectin and fibers enriched in type III collagen (2 to 5 days). Integrin receptors act to form polymers of fibronectin, and integrins and fibronectin help form collagen fibrils. **6. Final phase of the repair reaction.** Gradually the fibroblasts convert to production of thicker collagen fibers rich in type I collagen and the temporary, thinner collagen III–enriched fibers are turned over, leading to the stronger definitive matrix (5 days to weeks).

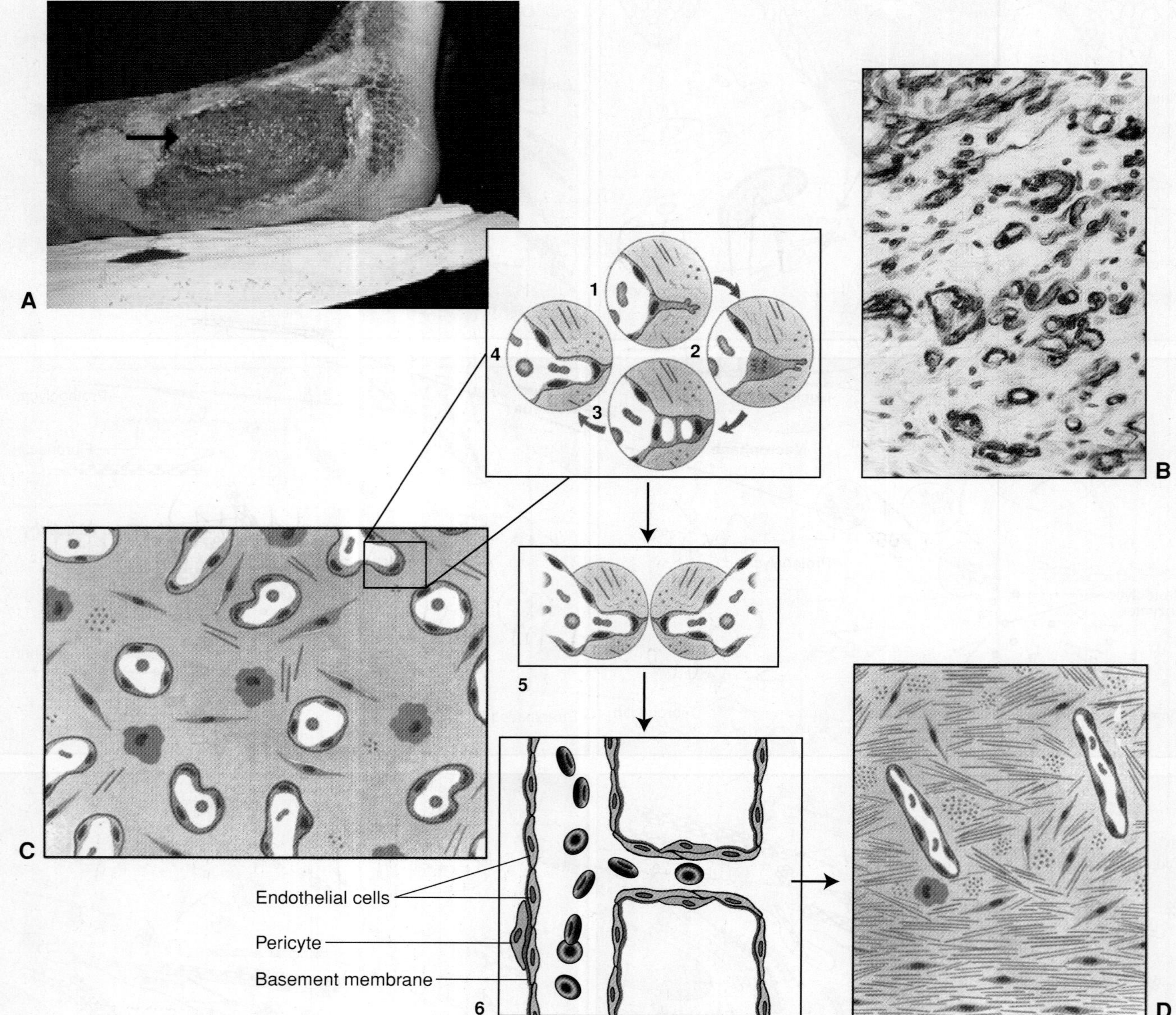

FIGURE 3-8. Granulation tissue. A. A venous stasis leg ulcer illustrates exposed granulation tissue. **B.** A photomicrograph of granulation tissue shows thin-walled capillary sprouts immunostained to highlight the basement membrane collagens. The infiltrating capillaries penetrate a loose connective tissue matrix containing mesenchymal cells and occasional inflammatory cells. **C.** Granulation tissue has two major components: stromal cells and proliferating capillaries. Initially, capillary sprouts of granulation tissue are a key feature, growing in a loose matrix in the presence of fibroblasts, myofibroblasts and macrophages. The macrophages are derived from monocyte migration to the wound site. The fibroblasts derive from adjacent tissue or from circulating fibrocytes; myofibroblasts derive from fibroblasts, mesenchymal stem cells or pericytes; and the capillaries arise primarily from adjacent vessels by division of the lining endothelial cells (steps 1 to 6), in a process termed ***angiogenesis.*** Endothelial cells put out cell extensions, called ***pseudopodia***, that grow toward the wound site. Cytoplasmic growth enlarges the pseudopodia, and eventually the cells divide. Vacuoles formed in the daughter cells eventually fuse to create a new lumen. The entire process continues until the sprout encounters another capillary sprout, with which it will connect. At its peak, granulation tissue is the most richly vascularized tissue in the body. **D.** Once repair has been achieved, most of the newly formed capillaries are reabsorbed, leaving a pale, avascular scar rich in collagen.

As matrix accumulation peaks at 5 to 7 days, production of TGF-β increases synthesis of collagen and fibronectin and decreases MMP transcription and matrix degradation. Extracellular cross-linking of newly synthesized collagen progressively increases wound strength. In the absence of macrophages, neutrophils may subserve these functions.

Growth Factors and Fibroplasia

The discovery of EGF and later identification of at least 20 other growth factors have explained many of the rapidly changing events in repair and regeneration. Redundancy and interaction among growth factors, other cytokines and MMPs

Table 3-5

Extracellular Signals in Wound Repair

Phase	Factor(s)	Source	Effects
Coagulation	XIIIa	Plasma	Cross-linking of fibrin thrombus
	TGF-α, TGF-β, PDGF, ECGF, FGF	Platelets	Chemoattraction and activation of subsequent cells
Inflammation	TGF-β, chemokines TNF-α, IL-1, SDF-1, PDGF	Neutrophil, macrophages, lymphocytes	Attract monocytes and fibroblasts; differentiate fibroblasts and stem cells
Granulation tissue formation	Basic FGF, TGF-β, PDGF	Monocytes then fibroblasts	Various factors are bound to proteoglycan matrix
Angiogenesis	VEGFs, FGFs, HGF	Monocytes, macrophages, fibroblasts	Development of blood vessels
	PDGF		Pericyte growth
Contraction	TGF-β1, β2	Macrophages, fibroblasts, keratinocytes	Myofibroblasts differentiate, bind to each other and to collagen and contract
Reepithelialization	KGF, HGF, EGF, HB-EGF, TGF-α	Macrophages, platelets, fibroblasts, keratinocytes	Epithelial proliferation, migration and differentiation
Maturation, fibroplasia, arrest of proliferation	TGF-β1, PDGF, CTGF	Macrophages, fibroblasts, keratinocytes	Accumulation of extracellular matrix, fibrosis, tensile strength
	Heparan sulfate proteoglycan (HSPG)	Endothelium Secretory fibroblasts	HSPG: Capture of TGF-β , VEGF and basic FGF in basement membrane
	Decorin proteoglycan		Decorin: Capture of TGF-β, stabilization of collagen structure, downregulation of migration, proliferation
	Interferon	Plasma monocytes	Suppresses proliferation of fibroblasts and accumulation of collagen
	Increased local oxygen	Repair process	Suppression of release of cytokines
Remodeling	FGF, KGF	Platelets, fibroblasts, keratinocytes, macrophages	Induction of MMPs
	MMPs, t-PAs, u-PAs	Sprouted capillaries, epithelial cells, fibroblasts	Remodeling by permitting ingrowth of vessels and restructuring of ECM
	Tissue inhibitors of MMPs	Local, not further defined	Balance the effects of MMPs in the evolving repair site

CTGF = connective tissue growth factor; ECGF = endothelial cell growth factor; ECM = extracellular matrix; EGF = epidermal growth factor; FGF = fibroblast growth factor; HB-EGF = heparin-binding EFG; HGF = hepatocyte growth factor; IL = interleukin; KGF = keratinocyte growth factor (FGF-7); MMPs = matrix metalloproteinases; PDGF = platelet-derived growth factor; SDF-1 = stromal cell–derived factor-1; TGF = transforming growth factor; TNF = tumor necrosis factor; t-PA = tissue plasminogen activator; u-PA = urokinase-type plasminogen activator; VEGF = vascular endothelial growth factor.

are illustrated in Tables 3-5, 3-6 and 3-7. Each has a predominant function in repair, so redundancy is limited. Specificity derives from (1) selective expression from members of large families (e.g., FGF and TGF-β), (2) temporal expression of different tyrosine kinase receptors and isotypes in unrelated cell populations, (3) variation in response pathways or intensity by distinct receptors and (4) latency or activation of growth factors (Table 3-5). Tables 3-6 and 3-7 show how growth factors control specific events in repair.

Several growth factor ligands are presented to their tyrosine kinase receptors while bound to extracellular matrix components such as heparan sulfate proteoglycans. There are some domains in matrix molecules in the laminin, collagen, tenascin and decorin families that bind weakly to growth factor receptors. Signals generated by these interactions are spatially restricted, persistent and concentrated, and may influence proliferation or migration differently from soluble ligands, though matrix molecules exert far greater effects by binding to integrins.

Growth factors expressed early in wound responses (VEGF, FGF, PDGF, EGF, keratinocyte growth factor [KGF]) support migration, recruitment and proliferation of cells involved in fibroplasia, reepithelialization and angiogenesis. Growth factors that peak later (TGF-β, insulin-like growth factor-I [IGF-I]) sustain the maturation phase and remodeling of granulation tissue. Tissue regeneration is also driven by signaling networks, which, in cooperation with matrix, support self-renewal, maintenance and differentiation of stem cells.

Wound outcomes vary after exogenous growth factors are added to wounds. PDGF is effective in accelerating healing in neuropathic diabetic foot ulcers; topical application of single growth factors in a bolus form generally does not prevent scars and does not consistently speed or improve healing,

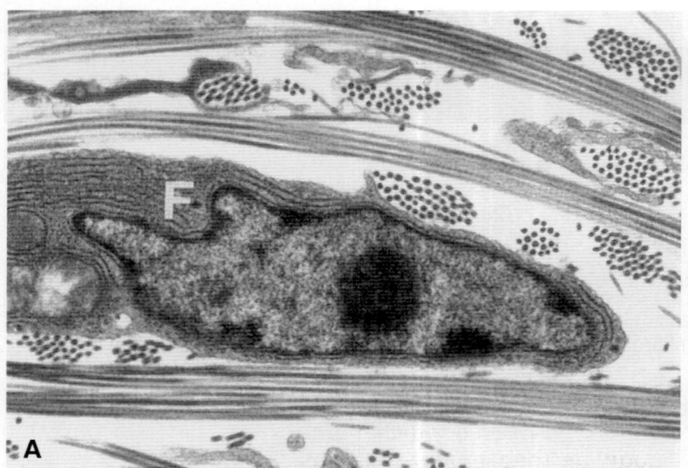

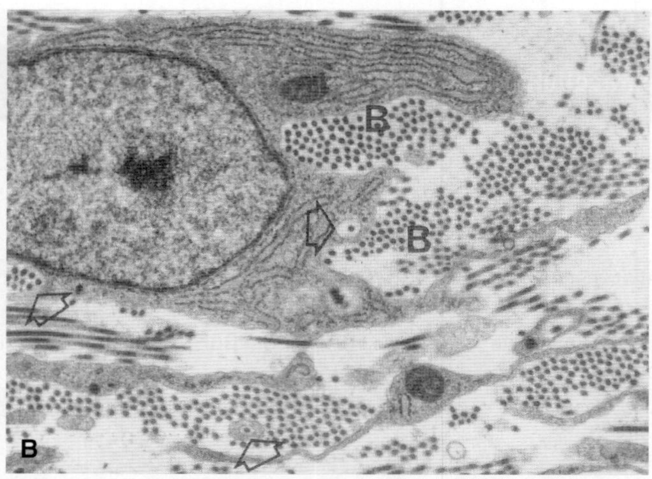

FIGURE 3-9. Fibroblasts and collagen fibers. Electron micrographs. A. Chick embryo fibroblast (F) lying between collagen fibers. The collagen fibers are seen as crosswise strands traversing the field and along the long axis, at a right angle, as dots. **B.** A chick embryo dermal fibroblast with abundant endoplasmic reticulum consistent with secretory activity and cell surface–associated collagen fibril bundles (B); some bundles are enveloped by fibroblast membrane and cytoplasm, indicating that collagen fibers can be assembled and extruded from long cellular processes (*arrows*). The fibrils are visualized on the long axis as dots.

compared to accepted methods of chronic wound management. Progress in cell culture, matrix and growth factor biology have sped the engineering of skin substitutes that express many growth factors and can improve clinical results for chronic wounds.

Growth factor participation in the early phases of repair is reasonably well understood, but the mechanisms for limiting and terminating repair are not well defined. Diminishing anoxia as repair progresses and reduced matrix turnover may trigger the denouement of the repair process. Recent evidence suggests that cytokines that bind to the CXCR3 receptor may

Table 3-6

Growth Factors Control Various Stages in Repair

Attraction of Monocytes/ Macrophages	**PDGFs, FGFs, TGF-β, MCP-1**
Attraction of fibroblasts	PDGFs, FGFs, TGF-β, CTGF, EGFs, SDF-1
Proliferation of fibroblasts	PDGFs, FGFs, EGFs, IGF, CTGF,
Angiogenesis	VEGFs, FGFs, HGF
Collagen synthesis	TGF-β, PDGFs, IGF, CTGF
Collagen secretion	PDGFs, FGFs, CTGF
Epithelial migration and proliferation	KGF, TGF-α, HGF, IGF of epithelium–epidermis
Resolution of repair	IP-9, IP-10

CTGF = connective tissue growth factor; EGF = epidermal growth factor; FGF = fibroblast growth factor; HGF = hepatocyte growth factor; IGF = insulin-like growth factor; IP-9/10 = interferon-γ–inducible protein 9/10; KGF = keratinocyte growth factor; MCP-1 = macrophage chemotactic protein-1; PDGF = platelet-derived growth factor; SDF-1 = stromal cell–derived factor-1; TGF = transforming growth factor; VEGF = vascular endothelial growth factor.

Table 3-7

Growth Factors, Enzymes and Other Factors Regulate Progression of Repair and Fibrosis

Secretion of collagenase	PDGF, EGF, IL-1, TNF, proteases
Movement of surface and stromal cells	t-PA (tissue plasminogen activator) u-PA (urokinase-type plasminogen activator) MMPs (matrix metalloproteinases) MMP-1 (collagenase 1) MMP-2 (gelatinase A) MMP-3 (stromelysin 1) MMP-8 (collagenase 2) MMP-13 (collagenase 3) MT1-MMP (MMP-14; membrane bound) MMP-19
Maturation or stabilization of blood vessels	Angiopoietins (Ang1, Ang2); PDGF
Inhibition of collagenase production Increase of TIMP production	TGF-β
Reduction in collagen production and turnover	Hypoxia
Collagen cross-linking and maturation	Lysyl oxidase, integrin receptors, fibronectin polymers, small proteoglycans

EGF = epidermal growth factor; IL = interleukin; PDGF = platelet-derived growth factor; TGF = transforming growth factor; TIMP = tissue inhibitor of metalloproteinases; TNF = tumor necrosis factor.

be important for regression of granulation tissue and limiting scarring. Finally, increased storage and decreased release of growth factors may stabilize the matrix, which may then transmit mechanical signals that reduce the effects of growth factors. Granulation tissue eventually becomes scar tissue, as the equilibrium between collagen synthesis and breakdown comes into balance within weeks of injury. Fibroblasts continue to alter scar appearance for several years.

Angiogenesis

The Growth of Capillaries

At its peak, granulation tissue has more capillaries per unit volume than any other tissue. New capillary growth is essential for delivery of oxygen and nutrients. New capillaries form by angiogenesis (i.e., sprouting of endothelial cells from preexisting capillary venules) (Fig. 3-8) and create the granular appearance for which granulation tissue is named. Less often, new blood vessels form de novo from angioblasts (endothelial progenitor cells [EPCs]). The latter process, known as **vasculogenesis,** is primarily associated with ontogeny.

Angiogenesis in wound repair is tightly regulated. Quiescent capillary endothelial cells are activated by loss of basement membrane and local release of cytokines and growth factors. The basement membranes surrounding endothelial cells and pericytes must be degraded before those cells can migrate into the provisional matrix. Endothelial passage through the matrix requires the cooperation of plasminogen activators, matrix MMPs and integrin receptors. The growth of new capillaries is supported by proliferation and fusion of endothelial cells (Fig. 3-8), and recent studies suggest that limited numbers of bone marrow–derived endothelial progenitor cells may also be recruited, at least transiently, to support growing vessels.

Migration of cells into a wound site is directed by soluble ligands (by **chemotaxis**) and proceeds along adhesive matrix substrates (by **haptotaxis**). Once capillary endothelial cells are immobilized, cell–cell contacts form, and an organized basement membrane develops on the exterior of the nascent capillary. Association with pericytes and signals from angiopoietin I, TGF-β and PDGF establish a mature vessel phenotype and help form nonleaky capillaries. New capillaries that have not matured are leaky and may undergo apoptosis.

Experimentally, stimulation of angiogenesis in cell culture requires extracellular matrix and growth factors, mainly VEGF. Loss of even one VEGF allele causes lethal defects in embryonic vasculature. In vivo, angiogenesis is initiated by hypoxia and a redundancy of cytokines, growth factors and various lipids, which stimulate or regulate VEGF. The transcription factor Hif-1α, whose stability is exquisitely regulated by tissue oxygen tension, is the main trigger for VEGF expression. Activated granulation tissue macrophages and endothelial cells produce basic FGF and VEGF, and wound epidermal cells release VEGF in response to KGF. Because the chief target of VEGF is endothelial cells, VEGF is critical for embryonic vascular development and angiogenesis, endothelial survival, differentiation and migration. Splice variants of VEGF concentrate along soluble and matrix-bound gradients to ensure appropriate vessel branching.

The binding of angiogenic growth factors to heparan sulfate–containing GAG chains is crucial to angiogenesis. Association with heparan sulfate chains affects the availability and action of growth factors and vessel pattern formation by (1) creating a storage reservoir of VEGF and basic FGF in capillary basement membranes and (2) using cell surface proteoglycan receptors to regulate VEGF and FGF receptor congregation, as well as signal delivery and intensity.

Angiogenesis and Receptor Cross-Talk

Surface integrin receptors sense changes in extracellular matrix and can react by modulating cellular responses to growth factors. This cross-talk is possible because integrin and growth factor signals converge to trigger many of the same signaling cascades that support cell survival, proliferation, differentiation and migration. Unlike growth factors, integrin receptors drive cell locomotion by organizing cytoskeletal changes at the membrane. When exposed to growth factors or the loss of an organized basement membrane, quiescent endothelial cells express new integrins that modulate their migration on provisional matrix proteins. Capillary sprouting relies principally on β_1-type integrins, although survival and spatial organization of the capillary network are regulated by other integrins, such as $\alpha v\beta 3$, responding to the composition and structure of their extracellular matrix ligands. Without appropriate matrix or sufficient growth factor signaling, endothelial cells are vulnerable to apoptotic cues.

Reepithelialization

The epidermis constantly renews itself by keratinocyte mitosis at the basal layer. The squamous cells then cornify or keratinize as they mature, move toward the surface and are shed a few days later. Maturation requires an intact layer of basal cells that are in direct contact with one another and the basement membrane. If cell–cell contact is disrupted, basal epithelial cells divide to reestablish contact with other basal cells. In denuded epidermis, hair follicles become the primary source of regenerating epithelium (Fig. 3-1). Once reestablished, the epithelial barrier demarcates the scab from the newly covered wound. When epithelial continuity is reestablished, the epidermis resumes its normal cycle of maturation and shedding.

Epithelialization protects against infection and fluid loss. Epithelial cells cover or close wounds either by migrating to cover the damaged surface or, less often, by a cinching process called **purse-string closure,** augmenting fibroblast/myofibroblast-mediated wound contraction. Skin provides the best-studied example of epithelial repair. The basal layer of skin epithelial cells, also called **epidermal cells** or **keratinocytes**, contributes important cytokines (interleukin [IL]-1, VEGF, TGF-α, PDGF, TGF-β) that initiate healing and local immune responses. To begin migration, keratinocytes must differentiate before forming a new covering over the wound. These cells normally bind laminin in the underlying basement membrane by hemidesmosome protein complexes containing $\alpha 6\beta 4$ integrin. Several members of the collagen family, namely, type XVII collagen (BP-180) and collagen type VII, also termed **anchoring fibril** (Table 3-2), are associated with the hemidesmosome complex. The anchoring fibril connects the hemidesmosome–basement membrane complex to the dermal connective tissue collagen fibers. Mutations in collagen XVII, epidermal basement membrane laminin, integrin $\alpha 6\beta 4$ or collagen VII produce a potentially fatal skin blistering disease, termed **epidermolysis bullosa,** while autoantibodies against the transmembrane collagen XVII (BP180, BPAG2) cause acquired blistering disorders like **bullous pemphigoid** (see Chapter 24).

Epithelial cells are connected at their lateral edges by **tight junctions** and **adherens junctions** composed of cadherin receptors. Cadherins are calcium-dependent, integral membrane proteins that form extracellular cell–cell connections and anchor intracellular cytoskeletal connections. In adherens junctions, they bind stable actin bundles to a cytoplasmic complex of α-, β- and γ-catenins. The layer of actin that encircles the epithelial cytoplasm creates lateral tension and strength and is called the **adhesion belt.** ***The shape and strength of epithelial sheets result from the tension of cytoskeletal connections to basement membrane and cell-to-cell connections.***

Cellular migration is the predominant means by which wound surfaces are reepithelialized. Groups of basal and suprabasilar keratinocytes originate at the margin of a wound and migrate along the provisional matrix, while progenitor cells in the adjacent basal layer or in hair follicles or sweat glands undergo mitosis, leading to epidermal thickening and hypertrophy. With basement membrane loss, cells come in contact with unfamiliar stromal or provisional matrix components, which stimulates cell locomotion and proteinase expression. As a result, β1 integrins that recognize stromal collagens shift from the lateral to the basal epithelial surface. Keratinocytes at the leading edge of the wound margin become migratory and secrete MMPs that facilitate their detachment from the basement membrane and remodeling of the granulation tissue surface. Cells are thought to migrate along a soluble chemical gradient **(chemotaxis),** due to matrix concentration or adhesion **(haptotaxis),** and matrix pliability or stiffness **(durotaxis).**

Epithelial motility is activated by assembly of actin fibers at focal adhesions organized by integrin receptors. Distinct sets of integrins bind to components of the wound, stromal or basement membrane matrices and direct the migrating cells along the margin of viable dermis. Movement through cross-linked fibrin apposed to the dermis also requires activation of plasmin from plasminogen to degrade fibrin. In addition to degrading fibrinogen and fibrin, plasmin activates specific MMPs. Proteolytic cleavage of stromal collagens I and III and laminin at focal adhesion contacts can release adhesion or enable keratinocyte migration. Migrating keratinocytes eventually resume their normal phenotype and become less hypertrophic after re-forming a confluent layer and attaching to their newly formed basement membrane.

Wound Contraction

As they heal, open wounds contract and deform. A central role in wound contraction is played by a specialized cell of granulation tissue, the **myofibroblast** (Fig. 3-10). This modified fibroblast is indistinguishable from collagen-secreting fibroblasts by conventional light microscopy. Unlike the latter, myofibroblasts express α-smooth muscle actin, desmin, vimentin and a particular fibronectin splice variant (ED-A) that forms polymerized cellular fibronectin. Myofibroblasts respond to agents that cause smooth muscle cells to contract or relax. In short, they look like fibroblasts but behave like smooth muscle cells. ***Myofibroblasts are responsible for normal wound contraction and its deforming pathologic cousin, wound contracture.*** Myofibroblasts usually appear about the third day of wound healing, in parallel with the sudden appearance of contractile forces, which then gradually diminish over the next several weeks. Myofibroblasts are increased in fibrosis and hypertrophic scars, particularly burn scars. Myofibroblasts and fibroblasts (and other mesenchymal cells) sense the stress exerted by the stiffness of the extracellular matrix on the integrin receptors to the actin stress fibers, triggering contraction via intracellular α-smooth muscle actin. Myofibroblasts further exert their contractile effects by formation of specific cell–cell contacts. By contrast, fibroblasts tend to be solitary cells. They lack α-smooth muscle actin, and are surrounded by collagen fibers but with less of the ED-A fibronectin variant. Myofibroblasts may originate as pericytes, vascular smooth muscle cells or fibrocytes/marrow progenitor cells.

Wound Strength

Skin incisions and surgical anastomoses in hollow viscera ultimately develop 75% of the strength of the unwounded site. Despite a rapid increase in tensile strength at 7 to 14 days, by the end of 2 weeks the wound still has a high proportion of type III collagen and has only about 20% of its ultimate strength. Most of the strength of the healed wound results from synthesis and intermolecular cross-linking of type I collagen during the remodeling phase. A 2-month-old incision, although healed, is still obvious. Incision lines and suture marks are distinct, vascular and red. By 1 year, the incision is white and avascular but usually still identifiable. As the scar fades further, it is often slowly deformed into an irregular line by stresses in the skin.

Regeneration

Regeneration is restoring an injured tissue or lost appendage to its original state. Regeneration and tissue maintenance require a population of self-renewing stem or precursor cells that can differentiate and replicate.

The adult human body is made up of several hundred types of well-differentiated cells, yet it maintains the remarkable potential to rebuild itself by replenishing dying cells and to heal itself by recruiting or activating cells that repair or regenerate injured tissue. Epithelial cells in the skin and gastrointestinal tract turn over rapidly, but—except for the cycling uterus—tissue remodeling is much slower in the adult. Some regeneration may be viewed as partially recapitulating embryonic morphogenesis from pluripotent stem cells. Unlike the newt, humans cannot replace lost limbs, but there are notable examples of regenerative processes. These are unfortunately limited to a number of adult tissues. Unique cells in bone marrow, epidermis, intestine and liver maintain sufficient developmental plasticity to orchestrate tissue-specific regeneration. There is a great medical need to develop regenerative capabilities in joint cartilage, brain neural tissue, heart myocardium and pancreatic beta cells. The power to replenish or regenerate tissue is derived from a small number of long-lived unspecialized cells, or **stem cells,** unique in their capacity for self-renewal and for producing clonal progeny that differentiate into more specialized cell types.

Embryonic and Adult Stem Cells Are Key to Regeneration

Embryonic stem (ES) cells, up to the stage of the preimplantation blastocyst, can differentiate into all cells of the adult

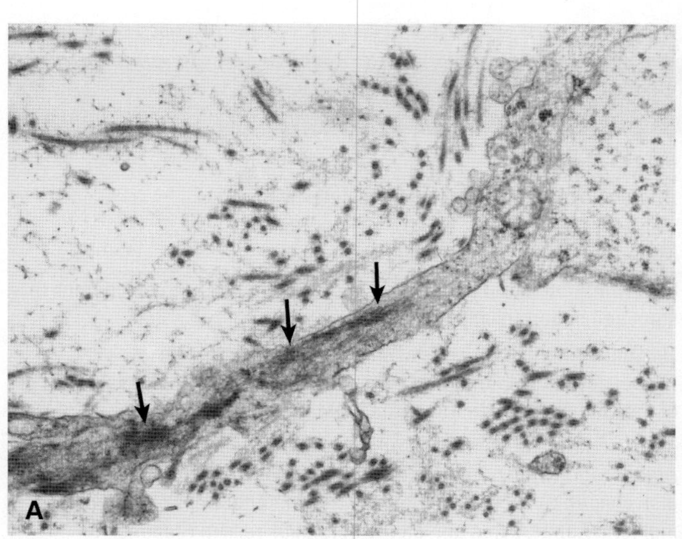

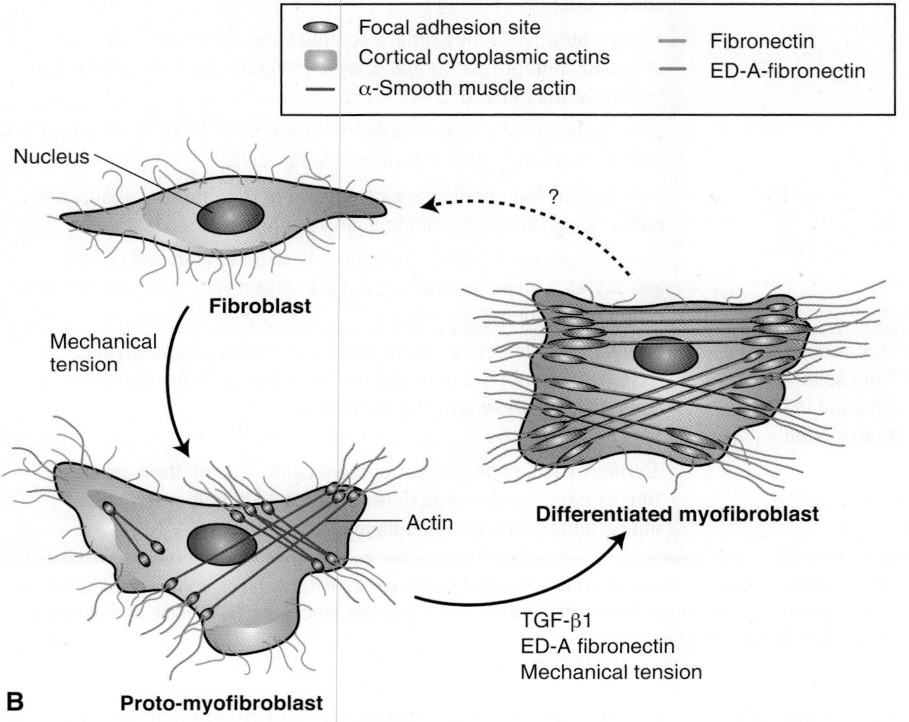

FIGURE 3-10. Myofibroblasts. Myofibroblasts have an important role in the repair reaction. These cells derive from pericytes or fibroblasts, with features intermediate between those of smooth muscle cells and fibroblasts, and they are characterized by the presence of discrete bundles of α-smooth muscle actin in the cytoplasm (*arrows*). Their clustered integrin receptors adhere tightly to and aid in formation of insoluble fibrils of cellular fibronectin, which align the cytoskeleton and bind collagen fibers, generating contractile forces important in wound contraction. **B. Development of myofibroblast from fibroblast.**

organism *and* preserve small populations of more restricted stem cells. Cells that are able to divide indefinitely, without terminally differentiating, inhabit many adult tissues and have been identified in tissues not known to regenerate. These **adult stem cells** may inhabit a specific tissue or be seeded there from circulating cells of bone marrow origin. Either way, the recently appreciated presence of stem cells in many tissues underscores the importance of a permissive and supportive environment for stem cell–driven regeneration (Table 3-8). Multipotential stem cells of adult tissues have a more restricted range of cell differentiation than ES cells and can be isolated from autologous tissue, reducing concerns of immunologic rejection after implantation. More recently, regulators of transcription patterns active in embryonic stem cells have been used to induce pluripotency in cells of adult tissues.

With the exception of the hematopoietic system, adult stem cells are difficult to identify and categorize. Imperfect choices must thus be made on the basis of characteristics such as morphology, developmental tissue of origin, the organ or tissue the cells were isolated from, genetic or immunologic markers or the capacity to differentiate into multiple or restricted lineages. Exceptions arise for several reasons: (1) any organ or tissue may contain more than one type of stem cell, (2) similar stem cells may be found in different organs and (3) a stem cell found in tissue may have originated in the bone marrow. Distinguishing between stem cell types using morphology and genetic or phenotypic markers for identification can be difficult and misleading because of the small number of stem cells present in a tissue, shared features between the cells, variance in marker expression through stages of development, the

Table 3-8

Adult Stem Cells Described in Mammals

	Cell Type	Role in Body
Bone marrow–derived stem cells	*Hematopoietic stem cells* (HSCs)	*Bone marrow* mesenchymal stem cells (MSCs)
	–Multipotent	MSC–Multipotent* endothelial progenitors
Adult tissue stem cells (some may be bone marrow derived)	*Constantly renewing (labile) cells*	*Epidermis*: unipotent basal keratinocyte stem cell and multipotent stem cell of hair follicle bulge
	–Epithelial-like cells (ectoderm or endoderm derived)	*Gut:* multipotent crypt cells of small and large intestine *Cornea:* corneal epithelial stem cells are located in the basal layer of the limbus between the cornea and the conjunctiva
	Persistent (stable) cells –Epithelial, parenchyma, neural (endoderm or ectoderm derived)	*Liver:* hepatocyte compensatory hyperplasia for maintenance, for regeneration and in response to surgical resection (other liver cells also divide); Oval cells (bipotent liver progenitor cells), canal of Hering, form hepatocytes and biliary epithelial cells in response to severe chemical damage
		Kidney: putative kidney renal interstitial and epithelial (Bowman capsule) stem/progenitor cells, which may be resident cells and/or bone marrow derived
		Lung: putative lung bronchioalveolar progenitor or stem cells that form bronchiolar Clara cells and alveolar cells
		Ear: mammalian cochlea are not known to regenerate sensory hair cells, though some nonmammalian vertebrates do
		Neural stem cells: multipotent, thought to be ependymal cells or astrocytes; subventricular zone of the lateral ventricle; subgranular zone of dentate gyrus
Tissue mesenchymal (mesoderm-derived) stem cells outside bone marrow	Progenitors of connective tissue cells; isolated from several tissues, although bone marrow origin cannot be excluded	*Skeletal:* satellite cells—between sarcolemma and overlying basement membrane of myofiber—also derived from pericytes or bone marrow mesenchymal stem cells
	Muscle cells	*Cardiac*: cardiac progenitor or stem cells—multipotent cardiomyocytes capable of limited differentiation and proliferation after injury; bone marrow mesenchymal stem cells

*These may be the same as multipotent adult progenitor cells (MAPCs), which represent bone marrow stromal cells whose differentiation is influenced by in vitro growth conditions. These cells are capable of seeding tissues outside the bone marrow by one or more of several possible processes: (1) specific progenitors or multipotent progenitors, (b) transdifferentiation, (c) cell fusion and (d) dedifferentiation.

possibility of cell fusion and the inherent phenotypic plasticity of stem cells.

Stem cells may be more generally defined by common properties that reflect their exquisite regulation, including:

- Ability to divide without limit, avoid senescence and maintain genomic integrity
- Capacity to undergo slow or intermittent division or remain quiescent
- Ability to propagate by self-renewal and differentiation
- Absence of lineage markers
- In some cases, specific anatomic localization
- Shared presence of growth and transcription markers common to uncommitted cells

Self-Renewal

Self-renewal is the defining property of adult stem cells and of early ES cells in vivo. Stem cell populations are small and the cells are difficult to purify. It has been difficult for investigators to agree on consensus definitions of specific (cell surface) markers for stem cell populations. Criteria such as increased nuclear:cytoplasmic ratio or (small) cell size can help to identify stem cells within tissues. The final definition depends on the ability of these cells to differentiate into multiple tissue types, in vitro or in vivo. Once stem cells are removed from their native microenvironments and placed in cell culture, they may modify their phenotype. The movement of bone marrow–derived stem cells to tissue is often studied using marked transplanted cells inserted into tissues of an irradiated host. Stem cells achieve self-renewal by asymmetric cell division, which produces a new stem cell and a daughter cell that is able to proliferate transiently and to differentiate. In contrast to stem cells, **progenitor** cells (transit amplifying cells) have little or no capability for self-renewal.

Cancer cells, like stem cells, undergo self-renewal, but unlike stem cells, cancer cells do so in an unregulated manner, as they fail to differentiate terminally or revert to quiescence. A cancer cell's capacity for self-renewal may be acquired early in tumorigenesis, or tumors may arise from resident stem cells, multipotent hematopoietic stems cells or even partially committed progenitor cells that somehow reacquire some characteristics of stem cells. Perpetuation of inflammatory processes could provide triggers that release stem or progenitor cells from their normal controls by modifying soluble and matrix-based signals of the microenvironment.

Stem Cell Differentiation Potential

The ability of ES cells to differentiate into all lineages diminishes as the embryo develops. Cells from the zygote and the first few divisions of the fertilized egg are **totipotent:** they can form any of approximately 200 different cell types in the adult body and the cells of the placenta. Nuclei of adult somatic cells can be totipotent, as dramatically proven by nuclear transplantation cloning experiments in amphibians and now several species of domesticated mammals, but this should not be confused with stem cell potency. ES cells from the inner cell mass of the blastocyst are **pluripotent**, meaning they may differentiate into nearly all cell lineages within any of the three germ layers. Totipotency is usually defined experimentally by showing that when a single ES cell is transplanted into an enucleated oocyte, it can give rise to a new organism through germline transmission. Postembryonically, implanted ES cells can also form teratomas. Pluripotent stem cells of the postfertilization zygote, such as neural crest cells, may differentiate into many cell types, but are not totipotent. Those adult cells that must self-renew throughout the lifetime of the organism are **multipotent**, or able to differentiate into several cell types within one lineage or one of the germ layers. Hematopoietic stem cells, for example, are lineage-restricted multipotent stem cells: they can form all the cells found in blood (Table 3-8). Marrow stromal cells (also known as mesenchymal stem cells) are multipotent stem cells that can be induced to differentiate into multiple cell types in vitro (endothelial progenitors, adipocytes, chondrocytes, osteoblasts, myoblasts) derived from a single cell lineage, the mesoderm germ layer.

Progenitor cells are **stable cells** that are distinguished from stem cells because they lack significant capacity for self-renewal; however, they maintain the potential for differentiation and rapid proliferation. They are sometimes referred to as **unipotent** stem cells, as exemplified by the basal keratinocyte of skin, but some may be multipotent or oligopotent.

In addition to normal differentiation pathways within a single tissue, cells of one tissue may **transdifferentiate** into cells of another tissue. Transdifferentiation, or **plasticity**, is controversial but may be induced experimentally by specific in vitro conditions or by seeding transplanted bone marrow stem cells into different tissue microenvironments, which are not stringent conditions. Somatic stem or progenitor cells, resident in several mesenchymal tissues but of uncertain origin, maintain the capacity to transdifferentiate. Epithelial-to-mesenchymal transformation occurs repeatedly during embryonic development as sheets of cells must be mobilized to form other tissues. In the adult, injured epithelium (renal tubules, pulmonary) can transform into fibroblasts under the influence of TGF-β, leading to scarring and fibrosis. An alternative but less popular hypothesis for tissue-specific differentiation by a circulating cell involves fusion of a circulating stem cell with a resident injured cell, as has been described in animal experiments. There is no consensus that either transdifferentiation or fusion contribute to either tissue homeostasis or regeneration.

Stem cell technology has advanced to the stage where it can be used to construct new tissues such as cartilage, skin, bone and blood vessels in vitro. Many current applications of stem cells rely on differentiation or action in situ of cells that undergo minimal differentiation. These approaches rely less upon the pluripotentiality and more upon the ability of progenitor cells to act as effector cells to alter the course of tissue repair. Progenitors recruited to wounds from the blood are present transiently during the repair process, but rarely undergo engraftment.

Bone marrow contains hematopoietic, mesenchymal and endothelial stem cells, providing a multifaceted regenerative capacity. Bone marrow stem cells, which are set aside during embryonic development, replenish the hematopoietic population. Endothelial stem cells from bone marrow have been implicated in tissue angiogenesis and may supplement endothelial hyperplasia during regeneration of blood vessels. Moreover, bone marrow–derived mesenchymal stem cells may populate repairing tissue in other parts of the body, though these may be difficult to discern from resident stem cells in the tissue (Table 3-8).

Skin epithelium and hair follicles regenerate from stem cells in basal epidermis and the bulge region of the hair follicle. Intestinal epithelium turns over rapidly and is replenished by intestinal stem cells that reside in the crypts of Lieberkühn. Liver reconstitution after partial hepatectomy is a hyperplastic response by mature differentiated hepatocytes of the remaining lobes and is not thought to involve stem cells. However, there is evidence for stem, or progenitor, cell–driven liver regeneration when hepatocytes are damaged by viral hepatitis or toxins. This regeneration is thought to arise from "oval cells" in the small bile ducts. These putative stem cells have characteristics of both hepatocytes (α-fetoprotein and albumin) and bile duct cells (γ-glutamyl transferase and duct cytokeratins) and may reside in terminal ductal cells in the canal of Hering.

Influence of Environment on Stem Cells

Stem cells exist in **microenvironments** or **niches** that provide sustaining signals from extracellular matrix and neighboring cells to limit their differentiation and to ensure their perpetuation. The mere presence of adult stem cells or progenitor cells is not solely sufficient for tissue regeneration when tissue is damaged. Many tissues contain resident progenitor cells, yet do not heal by regeneration. The method of repair is also influenced by the environment of the injury, that is, the growth factors, cytokines, proteinases and composition of the extracellular matrix. Whether a wound is repaired by regeneration or scarring and fibrosis is at least partly determined by the concentration, duration and composition of environmental signals present during inflammation. Skin healing during the first or second fetal trimester and maintenance regeneration of adult epidermis or intestinal epithelium generally occur without inflammation present and within an innate extracellular matrix. In such instances, normal structures and architecture are assembled in the absence of fibrosis or scarring. Wounds, however, produce physical damage, inflammatory growth factors and matrix changes that influence the response away from regeneration to scarring. Spinal cord injury, as an example, provides a particularly difficult challenge. Injury-induced cellular reactions lead to glial scar development, blocking axonal regeneration and complicating the possibility that an appropriately differentiated stem cell might drive regeneration and reestablish normal tissue function. Fibrosis, an urgent response to tissue damage, is a key impediment to regeneration.

Differentiated Cells Can Revert to Pluripotency

The amphibian studies of John Gurdon 50 years ago, later confirmed in many mammals, showed that cells do not lose DNA when they differentiate. Thus, ***is it possible to revert individual differentiated mammalian or human cells to pluripotency***? Cell differentiation involves controlled regulation of gene expression within an existing DNA sequence. This is accomplished through (1) **epigenetic modification** to DNA without changing or rearranging the sequence; (2) reduced expression of pluripotency associated genes, including the Polycomb group proteins; and (3) increased expression of lineage development genes. Epigenetic modifications include nucleic acid modifications within the DNA sequence, such as methylation, the presence of chromatin-associated proteins and modification of histone proteins.

Epigenetic modifiers establish transcriptional states necessary for cell differentiation and are heritable by progeny **(imprinting).** Interplay between epigenetic modifiers and lineage-determining transcription factors is necessary for the progressive differentiation states in a cell lineage. Differentiation is controlled at many levels. It may involve cell–cell contact and extracellular signals, but coactivation and coregulation of transcription factors associated with potency or lineage and epigenetic modifications are also key to the final state of a cell.

Investigators began to identify the reprogramming factors capable of reverting a somatic cell to an embryonic cell following successful somatic cell nuclear transfer into an oocyte, which progressed from the early amphibian studies to the more recent (1997) cloning of a sheep. Reversion to pluripotency from a fully differentiated cell (induced pluripotent stem [iPS] cell) has now been shown in mouse and human cells, by transcriptional overexpression of select combinations of four or fewer **pluripotency-associated genes** (OCT4, SOX2, Kruppel-like factor 4, MYC, estrogen-related receptor-β, NANOG or Lin28 homolog). OCT4 appears to be the most essential factor and MYC and KLF4 the least essential. These findings hold future promise for autologous cell therapies, but broad clinical application must await methods to safely generate such cells and accurately characterize their tumor-forming potential, pluripotency and extent of epigenetic reprogramming.

Cells Can Be Classified by Their Proliferative Potential

Different cells divide at different rates. Some mature cells do not divide at all, whereas others complete a cycle every 16 to 24 hours.

LABILE CELLS: Labile cells are found in tissues that are in a constant state of renewal. Tissues in which more than 1.5% of the cells are in mitosis at any one time are composed of labile cells. However, not all the cells in these tissues are continuously cycling. Stable cells are also constituents of labile tissues that are programmed to divide continuously. Labile tissues self-renew constantly, and typically form physical barriers between the body and the external environment. These include epithelia of the gut, skin, cornea, respiratory tract, reproductive tract and urinary tract. Hematopoietic cells of the bone marrow and lymphoid organs involved in immune defense are also labile. Polymorphonuclear nucleocytes and reticulocytes are terminally differentiated cells that are rapidly renewed. ***Under appropriate conditions, tissues composed of labile cells regenerate after injury, provided enough stem cells remain.***

STABLE CELLS: Stable cells populate tissues that normally are renewed very slowly but are populated with progenitor cells capable of more rapid renewal after tissue loss. Liver, bone and proximal renal tubules are examples of stable cell populations. Stable cells populate tissues in which fewer than 1.5% of cells are in mitosis. Stable tissues (e.g., endocrine glands, endothelium and liver) do not have conspicuous stem cells. Rather, their cells require an appropriate stimulus to divide. ***The potential to replicate, not the actual number of steady state mitoses, determines the ability of an organ to regenerate.*** For example, the liver, a stable tissue with less than one mitosis for every 15,000 cells, recovers through rapid hepatocyte hyperplasia after loss of up to 75% of its mass.

PERMANENT CELLS: are terminally differentiated, have lost all capacity for regeneration and do not enter the cell cycle. Traditionally, neurons, chondrocytes, cardiac myocytes and cells of the lens were considered permanent cells. Recent studies have confirmed that, if lost, cardiac myocytes and neurons may be replaced from progenitors, but not from division of existing cardiac myocytes or mature neurons. Permanent cells do not divide, but most of them do renew their organelles. The extreme example of permanent cells is the lens of the eye. Every lens cell generated during embryonic development and postnatal life is preserved in the adult without turnover of its constituents.

Conditions That Modify Repair

Local Factors May Influence Healing

Location of the Wound

In addition to its size and shape, the location of a wound also affects healing. In sites where scant tissue separates skin and bone (e.g., over the anterior tibia), a wound in the skin cannot contract. Skin lesions in such areas, particularly burns, often require skin grafts because their edges cannot be apposed. Complications or other treatments, like infection, obesity, diabetes, chemotherapy, glucocorticoids or ionizing radiation, also slow repair processes.

Blood Supply

Lower extremity wounds of diabetics often heal poorly or may even require amputation because advanced atherosclerosis in the legs (peripheral vascular disease) and defective angiogenesis compromise blood supply and impede repair. Varicose veins of the legs slow venous return and can also cause edema, formation of thick (fibrin) cuffs around microvessels, ulceration and nonhealing. Bed sores (decubitus ulcers) result from prolonged, localized, dependent pressure, which diminishes both arterial and venous blood flow and results in intermittent ischemia. Joint (articular) cartilage is largely avascular and has limited diffusion capacity. Often it cannot mount a vigorous inflammatory response, so that articular cartilage repairs poorly in the face of progressive, age-related wear and tear.

Systemic Factors

No specific effect of age alone on repair has been found, although there is evidence that stem cell reserves are reduced by aging. Scarring peaks during adolescence and diminishes with age. Healing also declines in postmenopausal women. Although reduced collagen and elastin may make the skin of a 90-year-old person fragile and so heal slowly, that person's colon resection or cataract extraction heals normally because the bowel and eye are practically unaffected by age.

Coagulation defects, thrombocytopenia and anemia impede repair. Local thrombosis decreases platelet activation, reducing the supply of growth factors and limiting the healing cascade. The decrease in tissue oxygen that accompanies severe anemia also interferes with repair. Exogenous corticosteroids retard wound repair by inhibiting collagen and protein synthesis and by exerting anti-inflammatory effects.

Fibrosis and Scarring Contrasted

Successful wound repair that leads to localized, transient scarring promotes rapid resolution of local injury. By contrast, in many chronic diseases inflammation persists and progresses to diffuse **fibrosis**, or excessive deposition of matrix proteins, particularly collagen. Inhaled smoke or inhaled silica particles induce chronic inflammation in the lung. Immunologically mediated inflammation of joints initiates rheumatoid arthritis. Inflammatory and noninflammatory factors lead to glomerulosclerosis in the kidney, including infection, hypertension and diabetes.

Ongoing insult or inflammation, mediated via the interplay of monocytes and lymphocytes, results in persistent high levels of cytokines, growth factors and locally destructive enzymes such as matrix metalloproteinases. Whatever the cause, fibrosis of parenchymal organs such as the lungs, kidney or liver disrupts normal architecture and impedes function. The functional unit (alveolus, hepatic lobule or renal glomerulus or tubule) is replaced by disordered collagen. Such fibrosis and resulting dysfunction are largely irreversible, and require removing the inciting stimulus or treatment, as in rheumatoid arthritis, to suppress inflammation and so minimize joint damage. Otherwise, tissue architecture and mechanics are so impaired that regenerative processes cannot reverse the injury. Fetal wound healing is regenerative because it is scarless.

Fibrosis is the pathologic consequence of persistent injury, and causes loss of function. Often it is the final common result of diverse diseases or injuries, the causes of which cannot be ascertained from the end result. As an example, scars of former glomeruli develop following bacterial or immunologic injury to the kidney, the specific cause being no longer identifiable. Scarring, however, is often beneficial: the scar resulting from a surgical incision in skin, though cosmetically unattractive, holds the skin together.

Prevention of fibrosis requires either blocking the stimulus of matrix production or increasing the level of matrix degradation. TGF-β and connective tissue growth factor (CTGF) are regulators of matrix production and have been associated with fibrotic connective tissue diseases. Approaches to controlling fibrotic progression to end-stage kidney disease have therefore targeted profibrotic factors such as TGF-β and plasminogen activator inhibitor (PAI-1). If PAI-1 is inhibited, it fails to block activation of plasminogen. As a result, plasmin degradation of extracellular matrix is increased, directly or through activating MMPs. Matrix deposition in the glomerulus is reduced, protecting the glomerulus from scarring and obliteration. Interestingly, inhibition of PAI could also reduce the incidence of **intra-abdominal adhesions**, a persistent problem of abdominal surgery and the main cause of intestinal obstruction. The adhesions are initiated by fibrin deposition when mesothelial lining is disrupted or heals ineffectively. If the fibrin matrix is not dissolved by plasmin within a few days, the fibrinous adhesion is invaded by fibroblasts and eventually transformed into a permanent fibrotic adhesion with collagen, capillaries and nerves.

There is accumulating evidence that resolution of the fibrotic process may not derive merely from reducing activating signals or developing an appropriate level of tensile strength and elasticity. Members of the CXCL3 family of cytokines that includes interferon-γ–inducible protein 9 (IP-9) and IP-10 are produced by fibroblasts and epithelial cells among other cell types. Increases in these proteins are associated with reduced fibrosis, while their absence can lead to exaggerated scarring.

Specific Sites Exhibit Different Repair Patterns

Skin

Healing in the skin involves both repair, primarily dermal scarring, and regeneration, principally of the epidermis and its appendages and vasculature. The salient features of primary and secondary healing are provided in Fig. 3-11.

Primary healing occurs when the surgeon closely approximates the edges of a wound. The actions of myofibroblasts are minimized due to the lack of mechanical strain, and regeneration of the epidermis is optimal, since epidermal cells need migrate only a minimal distance.

Secondary healing proceeds when a large area of hemorrhage and necrosis cannot be totally corrected surgically. In this situation, myofibroblasts contract the wound, and subsequent scarring repairs the defect.

The success and method of healing following a burn wound depends on the depth of the injury. If it is superficial or does not extend beyond the upper dermis, stem cells from sweat glands and hair follicles will regenerate the epidermis. If deep dermis is involved, the regenerative elements are destroyed and surgery with epidermal or keratinocyte grafts are necessary to cover or heal the wound site and reduce scarring and severe contractures. Cytokines produced by the grafted epidermis may contribute to the improved outcome.

Cornea

The cornea differs from skin in its stromal organization, vascularity and cellularity. Like skin, corneal stratified squamous epithelium is continually renewed by a stem cell population, at the periphery of the corneal limbus. Chemical injury to the cornea results in scarring, due to the distortion of the precisely arranged collagen fibers, effectively blinding the eye. Parenthetically, the cornea, because of its relative avascularity, was the first organ or anatomic structure to be successfully transplanted. Trachoma, an infectious human disease caused by an inflammatory response to *Chlamydia trachomatis*, is the world's

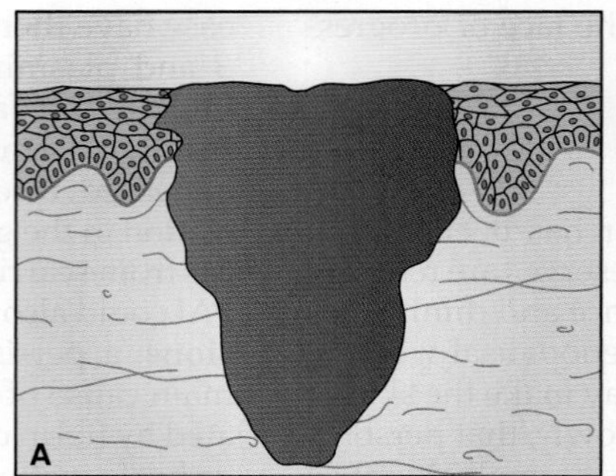

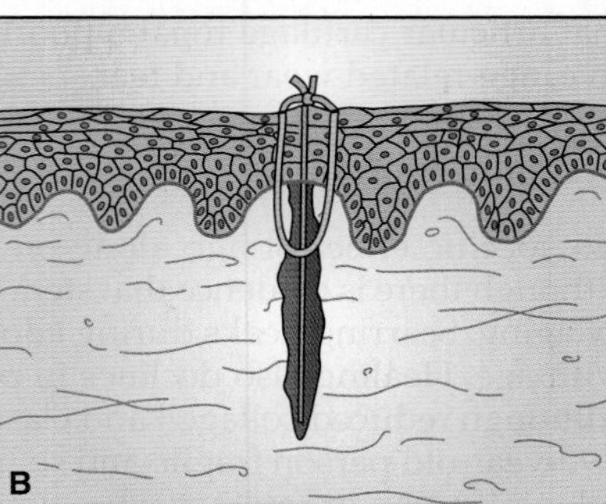

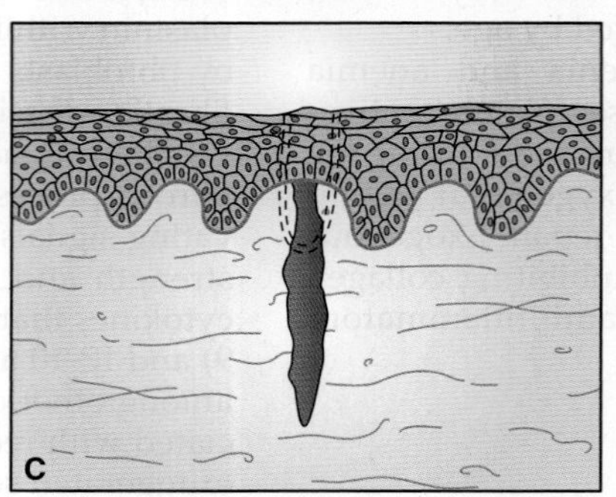

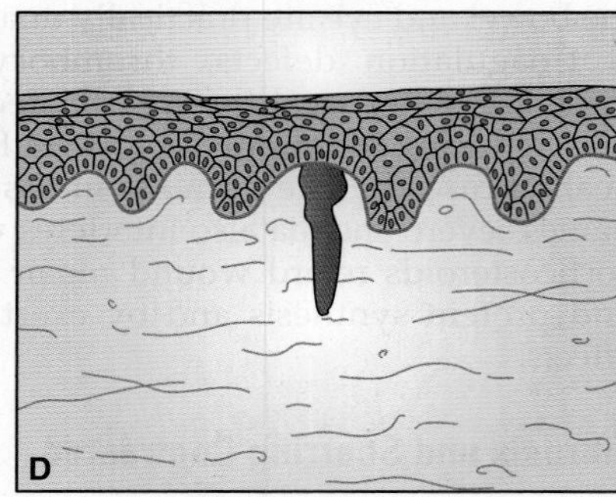

HEALING BY PRIMARY INTENTION (WOUNDS WITH APPOSED EDGES)

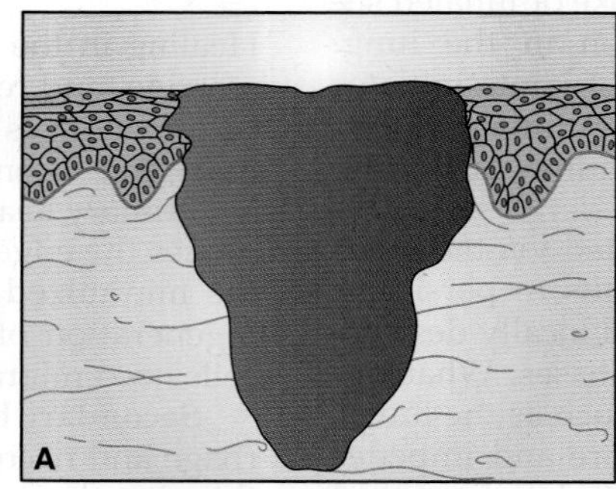

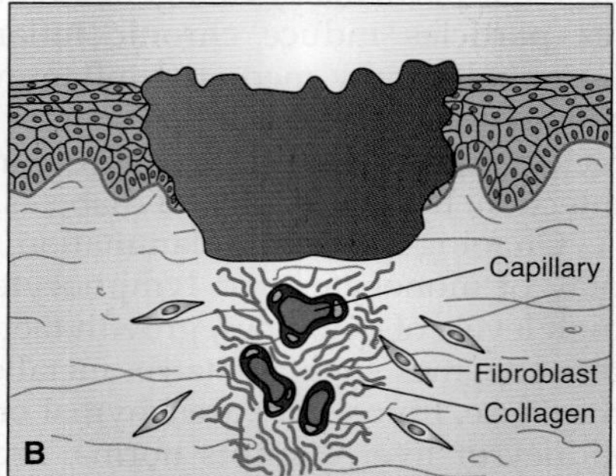

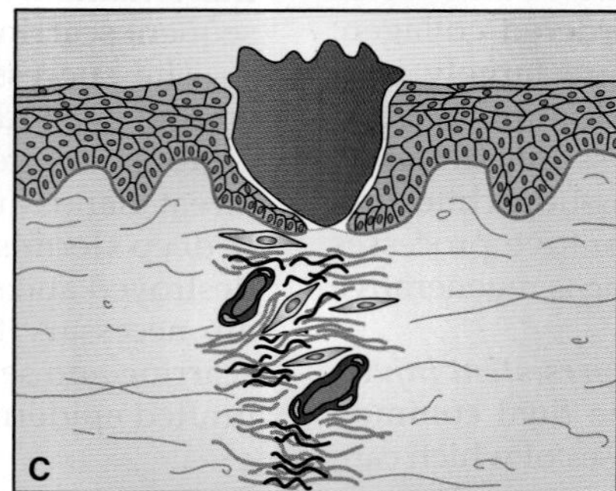

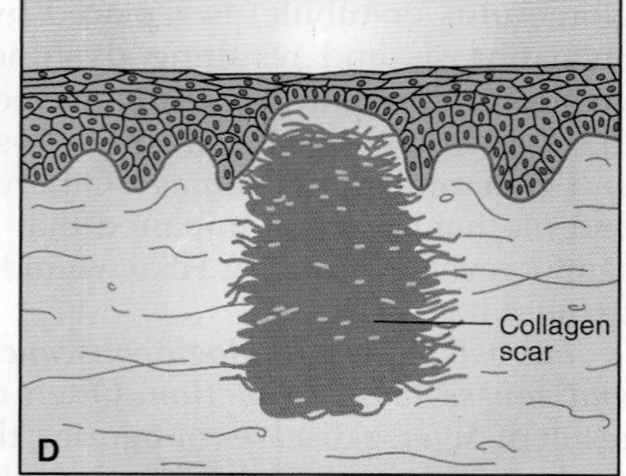

HEALING BY SECONDARY INTENTION (WOUNDS WITH SEPARATED EDGES)

FIGURE 3-11. Top. Healing by primary intention. A. An initial open, incised wound **(B)** with closely apposed wound edges held together with a suture and minimal tissue loss. **C.** There is decreased granulation tissue. Such a wound requires only minimal cell proliferation and neovascularization to heal. **D.** The result is a narrow, linear scar. **Bottom. Healing by secondary intention. A.** A gouged wound left to heal the open defect, in which the edges remain far apart and in which there is substantial tissue loss. **B.** The healing process requires wound contraction, extensive cell proliferation, matrix accumulation and neovascularization (granulation tissue) to heal. **C.** The wound is reepithelialized from the margins, and collagen fibers are deposited throughout the granulation tissue. **D.** Granulation tissue is eventually resorbed, leaving a large collagenous scar that is functionally and esthetically imperfect.

most common cause of blindness, resulting from scarring and opacity of the cornea (see Fig. 29-1).

Liver

The liver has tremendous regenerative capacity, even though the normal liver almost totally lacks mitoses and virtually all hepatocytes are in cell cycle phase G_0. After resection, liver regenerates by compensatory hyperplasia of hepatocytes. The necessary conditions for hepatic regeneration are complex (see Chapter 14). Suffice it to say here that regeneration ceases when the normal ratio of liver to total body weight is reestablished; the molecular switch that regulates this ratio is unknown. Transplant donation of the right hepatic lobe from a living donor is followed by complete regeneration of the normal liver in both the recipient and the donor.

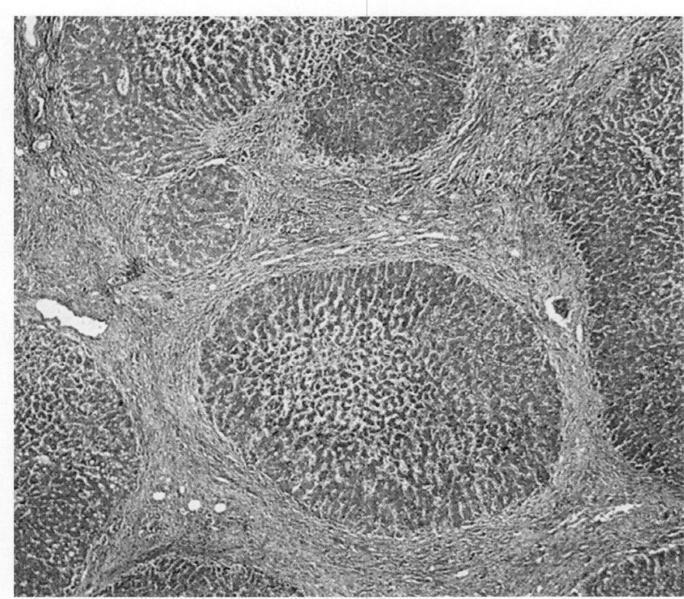

FIGURE 3-12. Cirrhosis of the liver. The consequence of chronic hepatic injury is the formation of regenerating nodules separated by fibrous bands. A microscopic section shows regenerating nodules (*red*) surrounded by bands of connective tissue (*blue*).

Acute chemical injury or fulminant viral hepatitis causes widespread necrosis of hepatocytes. However, if the connective tissue stroma, vasculature and bile ducts survive, liver parenchyma regenerates, and normal form and function are restored. Small cells at the canal of Hering, oval cells, are thought to be the stem cells responsible for such liver regeneration (Table 3-8). By contrast, in chronic injury in viral hepatitis or alcoholism, broad collagenous scars develop within the hepatic parenchyma, termed **cirrhosis** of the liver (Fig. 3-12). Hepatocytes form regenerative nodules that lack central veins and expand to obstruct blood vessels and bile flow. Despite adequate numbers of regenerated hepatocytes, architectural disarray impairs liver function and patients suffer variably severe symptoms of hepatic insufficiency.

Kidney

Although the kidney has limited regenerative capacity, removal of one kidney (nephrectomy) is followed by compensatory hypertrophy of the remaining kidney. If renal injury is not extensive and the extracellular matrix framework is not destroyed, tubular epithelium will regenerate. In most renal diseases, however, the matrix is disrupted, leading to incomplete regeneration with scar formation. The regenerative capacity of renal tissue is maximal in cortical tubules, less in medullary tubules and nonexistent in glomeruli. Recent data suggest that tubule repair occurs not from bone marrow–derived cells but as a result of proliferation of endogenous renal progenitor cells.

Cortical Renal Tubules

Tubular epithelium normally turns over and cells are shed into the urine. No reserve cell has been identified, and simple division accomplishes replacement. The outcome of injury hinges on the integrity of the tubular basement membrane. As long as the basement membrane is continuous, surviving tubular cells in the vicinity of a wound flatten, acquire a squamous-like appearance and migrate into the injured area along the basement membrane. Mitoses are frequent, and occasional clusters of epithelial cells project into the lumen. The flattened cells soon become more cuboidal, and differentiated cytoplasmic elements appear. Tubular morphology and function return to normal in 3 to 4 weeks.

Tubulorrhexis

Following tubulorrhexis, or rupture of the tubular basement membrane, events resemble those in tubular damage with an intact basement membrane, except that interstitial changes are more prominent. Fibroblasts proliferate, increased extracellular matrix is deposited and tubular lumens collapse. Some tubules will regenerate and others will become fibrotic with consequent focal losses of functional nephrons.

Medullary Renal Tubules

Medullary diseases of the kidney are often associated with extensive necrosis, which involves tubules, interstitium and blood vessels. The necrotic tissue sloughs into the urine. Healing by fibrosis produces urinary obstruction within the kidney. Although there is some epithelial proliferation, there is no significant regeneration. With injury to tubular epithelium, these cells can undergo epithelial–mesenchymal transformation, leading to interstitial fibrosis. TGF-β and CTGF have been implicated in this pathology.

Glomeruli

Unlike tubules, glomeruli do not regenerate. Necrosis of glomerular endothelial or epithelial cells, whether focal, segmental or diffuse, heals by scarring (Fig. 3-13). Mesangial cells are related to smooth muscle cells and seem to have some capacity for regeneration. Following unilateral nephrectomy, glomeruli in the remaining kidney enlarge by both hypertrophy and hyperplasia. Podocyte progenitor cells in the Bowman capsule may replace lost podocytes.

Lung

The epithelium lining the respiratory tract can regenerate to some degree, if the underlying extracellular matrix framework is not destroyed. Superficial injuries to tracheal and bronchial epithelia heal by regeneration from adjacent epithelium. The progenitor cell has not been clearly identified, although bronchioalveolar stem cells have been proposed. The outcome of alveolar injury ranges from complete regeneration of structure and function to incapacitating fibrosis. As with the liver, the degree of cell necrosis and the extent of the damage to the extracellular matrix framework determine the outcome (Fig. 3-14).

Alveolar Injury With Intact Basement Membranes

Alveolar injury following, for example, infections, shock and oxygen toxicity produces variable alveolar cell necrosis. Alveoli are flooded with an inflammatory exudate rich in plasma proteins. As long as the alveolar basement membrane is intact, healing is by regeneration. Neutrophils and macrophages clear the alveolar exudate, but if they fail to do so, it is organized by granulation tissue, and intra-alveolar fibrosis results. Alveolar type II pneumocytes (the alveolar reserve cells) migrate to denuded areas and divide to form cells with features intermediate between type I and type II pneumocytes.

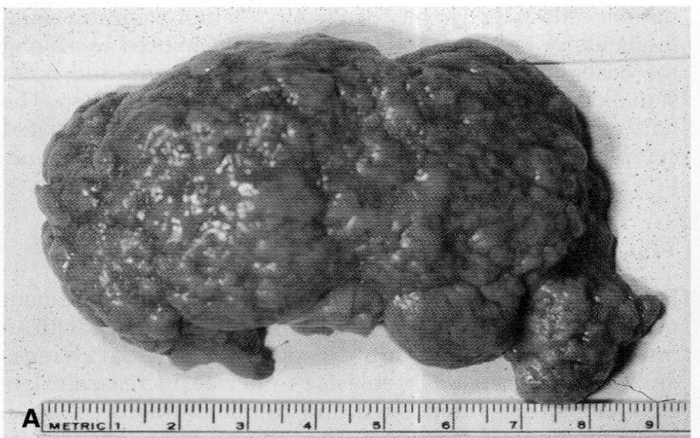

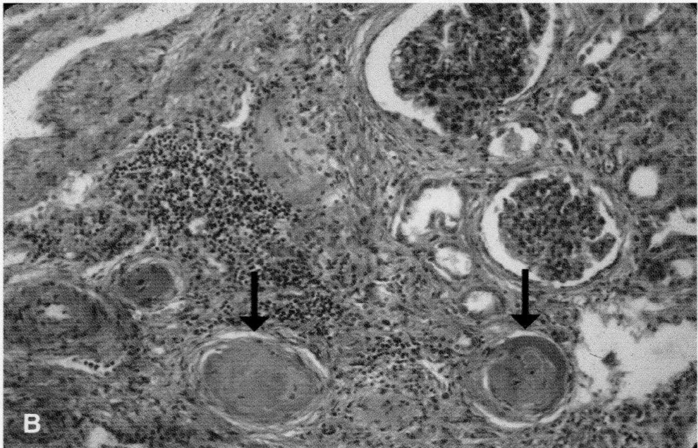

FIGURE 3-13. Scarred kidney. A. Repeated bacterial urinary tract infections have scarred the kidney. **B.** Many glomeruli have been destroyed and appear as circular scars (*arrows*).

These cells cover the alveolar surface and establish contact with other epithelial cells. Mitosis then stops and the cells differentiate into type I pneumocytes. Bone marrow–derived cells or putative lung bronchioalveolar progenitor or stem cells may participate by differentiating into bronchiolar Clara cells and alveolar cells (Table 3-8).

Alveolar Injury With Disrupted Basement Membranes
Extensive damage to alveolar basement membranes evokes scarring and fibrosis. Mesenchymal cells from alveolar septae proliferate and differentiate into fibroblasts and myofibroblasts. The role of macrophage products in inducing fibroblast proliferation in the lung is well documented. The myofibroblasts and fibroblasts migrate into the alveolar spaces, where they secrete extracellular matrix components, mainly type I collagen and proteoglycans, to produce pulmonary fibrosis. The most common chronic pulmonary disease is emphysema, which involves airspace enlargement and the destruction of alveolar walls. Ineffective replacement of elastin is associated with irreversible loss of tissue resiliency and function.

Heart

Cardiac myocytes had long been considered permanent, nondividing, terminally differentiated cells. There is recent evidence that cardiomyocytes, while not able to sufficiently repair damaged myocardium, are able to regenerate at a very low rate. The origin of these cells, whether they reside in the myocardium or migrate there following injury from sites unknown, is not resolved. For practical purposes, myocardial necrosis, from whatever cause, heals by the formation of granulation tissue and eventual scarring (Figs. 3-14 and 3-15). Not only does myocardial scarring result in the loss of contractile elements, but also the fibrotic tissue decreases the effectiveness of contraction in the surviving myocardium.

Nervous System

Mature neurons have been historically considered as permanent and postmitotic cells. Recent studies documented limited regenerative capacity in the brain, but have not altered well-established observations regarding the poor reparative capabilities of the nervous system. Following trauma, only regrowth and reorganization of the surviving neuronal cell processes can reestablish neural connections. Although the peripheral nervous system has the capacity for axonal regeneration, the central nervous system lacks this ability. The olfactory bulb and hippocampal dentate gyrus regions of adult mammalian brain are now known to regenerate via neural precursor or stem cells. Multipotent precursor cells have also been seen elsewhere in the brain, raising hope that repair of neural circuitry may eventually be possible (Table 3-8).

Central Nervous System
Damage to the brain or spinal cord is followed by growth of capillaries and gliosis (i.e., proliferation of astrocytes and microglia). Gliosis in the central nervous system is the equivalent of scar formation elsewhere; once established, it is permanent. In spinal cord injuries, axonal regeneration can be seen up to 2 weeks after injury. After 2 weeks, gliosis has taken place and attempts at axonal regeneration end. In the central nervous system, axonal regeneration occurs only in the hypothalamohypophysial region, where glial and capillary barriers do not interfere. Axonal regeneration seems to require contact with extracellular fluid containing plasma proteins.

Peripheral Nervous System
Neurons in the peripheral nervous system can regenerate axons, and under ideal circumstances, interruption in the continuity of a peripheral nerve may result in complete functional recovery. However, if cut ends are not in perfect alignment or are prevented from establishing continuity by inflammation or a scar, a traumatic neuroma results (Fig. 3-16). This bulbous lesion consists of disorganized axons and proliferating Schwann cells and fibroblasts. The regenerative capacity of the peripheral nervous system can be ascribed to (1) the fact that the blood-nerve barrier, which insulates peripheral axons from extracellular fluids, is not restored for 2 to 3 months, and (2) the presence of Schwann cells with basement membranes. Laminin, a basement membrane component, and nerve growth factor (NGF) guide and stimulate neurite growth.

Fetal Wound Repair

Surgery can now be performed in utero. Wounds produced in the first and second trimesters of pregnancy heal without

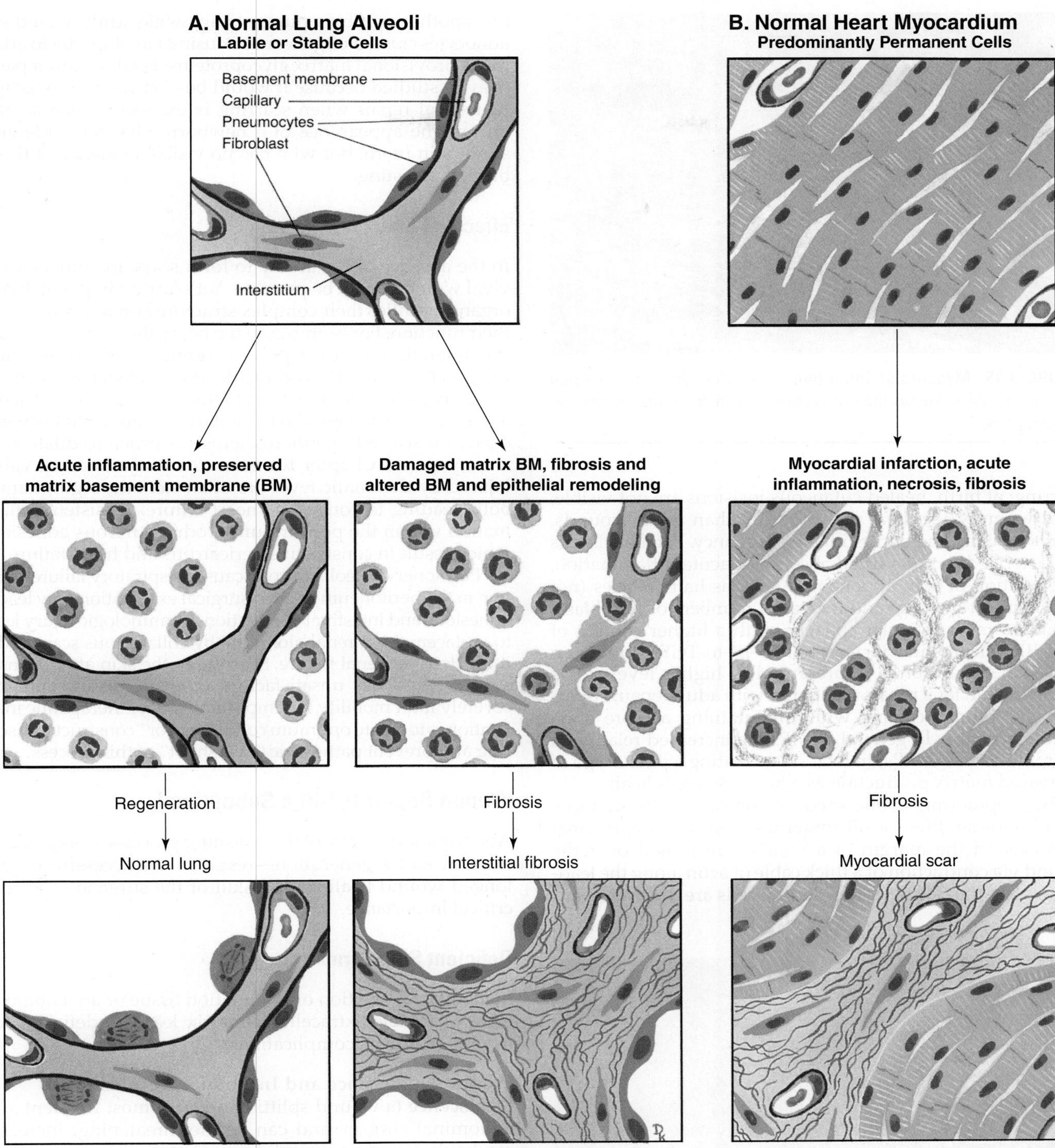

FIGURE 3-14. Examples of fibrotic and regenerative repair. A. The lung alveoli are lined with type I and type II epithelial cells (pneumocytes) that lie on a basement membrane. If the basement membrane remains intact following lung damage, there is rapid reepithelialization and return to normal lung architecture. If the basement membrane is damaged, type II epithelial cells proliferate on the underlying extracellular matrix, and fibroblasts and myofibroblasts are recruited and deposit a collagen-rich matrix leading to fibrosis. **B.** Though small numbers of cardiac stem cells have been described, regeneration of myocardium is rarely observed. By and large cardiomyocytes are terminally differentiated and not capable of renewal. Myocardial damage due to infarction and acute inflammation is repaired by fibrosis and scar formation, increasing chances of arrhythmia or heart failure.

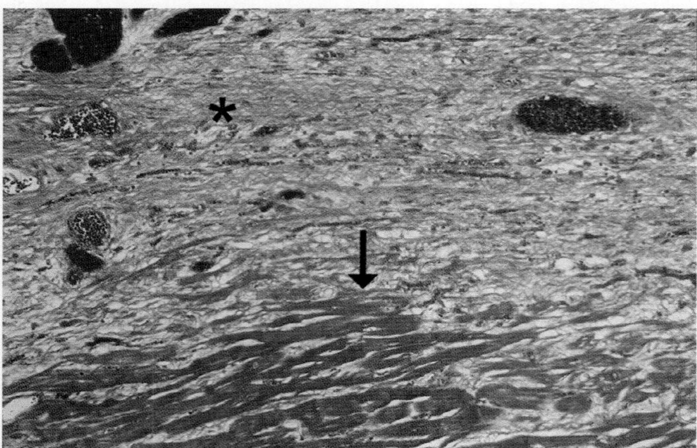

FIGURE 3-15. Myocardial infarction. A section through a healed myocardial infarct shows mature fibrosis (*) and disrupted myocardial fibers (*arrow*).

scarring; at birth, healed cutaneous incisions are not visible. Fetal wounds also heal more rapidly than adult wounds. Adult-type healing occurs in late pregnancy. Fetal healing is characterized by the virtual absence of acute inflammation, regeneration of skin appendages such as hair follicles (not seen in adult healing) and increased numbers of fibroblasts making a more reticular collagen with a higher content of type III collagen and increased TGF-β_3-to-TGF-β_1 ratios in fetal skin. Hyaluronan is preserved at higher levels for a longer time in fetal repair, compared with adult repair, apparently inhibiting scarring while maintaining a more open matrix structure. In general, MMPs are increased relative to their inhibitors (TIMPs) in fetal skin, creating a phenotype of decreased matrix production as a key to scarless healing.

Fetal epidermis is bilayered, in contrast to the multiple layers of the stratified adult epidermis. Embryonic epidermal cells around the margin of a wound are pulled over the wound via contraction of a thick cable of actin along the leading edge of the cells. Fetal epidermal cells are drawn toward one another as if by a purse-string, while adult wound keratinocytes crawl along the matrix using lamellipodia to attach to the provisional matrix glycoproteins. Fetal wound repair is heavily studied because it would be very helpful to recapitulate fetal repair when scarring is excessive, such as after burns. The appearance of a newborn who has undergone surgery in utero, but who has no visible evidence of this at birth, is arresting.

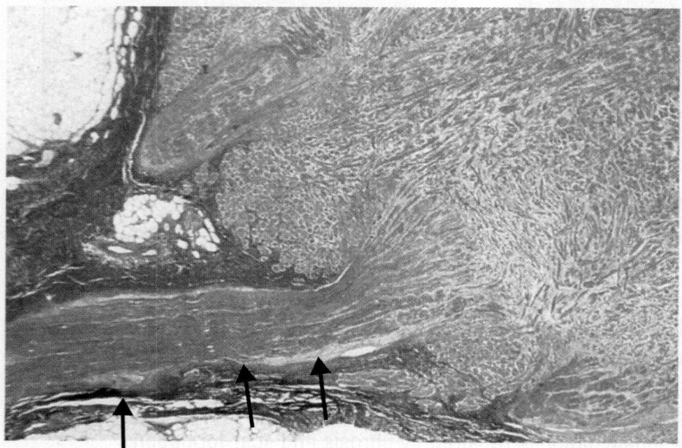

FIGURE 3-16. Traumatic neuroma. In this photomicrograph, the original nerve (*arrows*) enters the neuroma. The nerve is surrounded by dense collagenous tissue, which appears dark blue with this trichrome stain. Excessive repair obstructs axonal reconnection.

Effects of Scarring

In the absence of the ability to form scars, mammalian survival would hardly be possible. Yet scarring in parenchymal organs modifies their complex structure and never improves their function. For example, in the heart, the scar of a myocardial infarction serves to prevent rupture of the heart, but it reduces the amount of contractile tissue. If extensive enough, it may cause congestive heart failure or lead to a ventricular aneurysm (see Chapter 11). Similarly, an aorta that is weakened and scarred by atherosclerosis is prone to dilate as an aneurysm (see Chapter 10). Scarred mitral and aortic valves injured by rheumatic fever are often stenotic, regurgitant or both, leading to congestive heart failure. Persistent inflammation within the pericardium produces fibrous adhesions, which result in constrictive pericarditis and heart failure.

Pulmonary alveolar fibrosis causes respiratory failure. Infection in the peritoneum or even surgical exploration may lead to adhesions and intestinal obstruction. Immunologic injury leads to replacement of renal glomeruli by collagenous scars and, if it is extensive, renal failure. Scarring in the skin after burns or surgery produces unsatisfactory cosmetic results and may severely limit mobility. An important goal of therapeutic intervention is to create optimum conditions for "constructive" scarring and prevent pathologic "overshoot" of this process.

Wound Repair Is Often Suboptimal

Abnormalities in any of three healing processes—repair, contraction and regeneration—result in unsuccessful or prolonged wound healing. The skill of the surgeon is often of critical importance.

Deficient Scar Formation

Inadequate formation of granulation tissue or an inability to form a suitable extracellular matrix leads to deficient scar formation and its complications.

Wound Dehiscence and Incisional Hernias

Dehiscence (a wound splitting open) is most frequent after abdominal surgery and can be life-threatening. Increased mechanical stress on an abdominal wound from vomiting, coughing or bowel obstruction may cause dehiscence of that wound. Systemic factors predisposing to dehiscence include metabolic deficiency, hypoproteinemia and the general inanition that often accompanies metastatic cancer. **Incisional hernias** of the abdominal wall are defects caused by weak surgical scars due to insufficient deposition of extracellular matrix or inadequate cross-linking in the collagen matrix. Loops of intestine may be trapped within incisional hernias.

Ulceration

Wounds can ulcerate if an intrinsic blood supply is inadequate or if vascularization is insufficient during healing. For

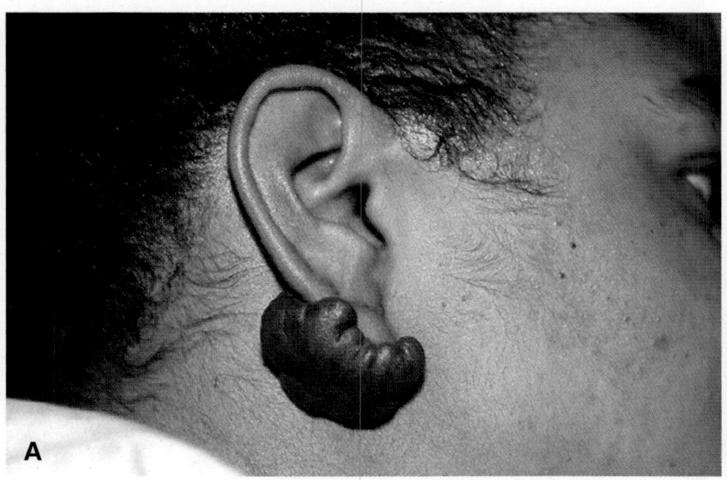

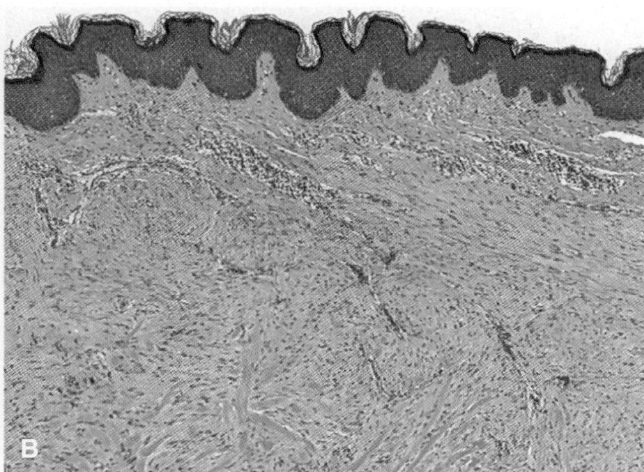

FIGURE 3-17. Keloid. A. A light-skinned black woman developed a keloid as a reaction to having her earlobe pierced. **B.** Microscopically, the dermis is markedly thickened by the presence of collagen bundles with random orientation and abundant cells.

example, leg wounds in people with varicose veins or severe atherosclerosis often ulcerate. Nonhealing wounds also develop in areas devoid of sensation because of persistent trauma. Such **trophic** or **neuropathic** ulcers are commonly seen in diabetic peripheral neuropathy. Occasionally they occur in patients with spinal involvement from tertiary syphilis or leprosy. Diabetes also reduces cellular responsiveness to growth factors, making it difficult to stimulate the healing process.

Excessive Scar Formation

Excessive deposition of extracellular matrix, mostly excessive collagen, at the wound site results in a hypertrophic scar. **Keloids** are exuberant scars that tend to progress beyond the site of initial injury and recur after excision (Fig. 3-17). Histologically, both of these types of scars exhibit broad and irregular collagen bundles, with more capillaries and fibroblasts than is normal for a scar of the same age. The rate of collagen synthesis and number of reducible cross-links remain high. This situation suggests a "maturation arrest," or block, in the healing process, a hypothesis that is supported by the overexpression of fibronectin in these lesions and the fact that, unlike normal scars, these scars do not reduce collagen synthesis if glucocorticoids are administered.

Keloids are unsightly, and attempts at surgical repair are always problematic, the outcome likely being a still larger keloid. Keloids are generally restricted to adolescence and early adulthood and to the upper trunk, neck and head, with the exception of the scalp. Dark-skinned persons are more frequently affected, suggesting a genetic basis for this condition. By contrast, **hypertrophic scars** are not associated with race or heredity, but the severity of scarring can decline with age.

Excessive Contraction

A decrease in the size of a wound depends on the presence of myofibroblasts, development of cell–cell contacts and sustained cell contraction. An exaggeration of these processes is termed **contracture** and results in severe deformity of a wound and surrounding tissues. Interestingly, regions that normally show minimal wound contraction (e.g., the palms, soles and anterior aspect of the thorax) are often prone to contractures. Contractures are particularly conspicuous when serious burns heal, and can be severe enough to compromise the movement of joints. In the alimentary tract, a contracture (stricture) can obstruct the passage of food in the esophagus or block the flow of intestinal contents.

Several diseases are characterized by contracture and irreversible fibrosis of the superficial fascia, including Dupuytren contracture (palmar contracture), Lederhosen disease (plantar contracture) and Peyronie disease (contracture of the cavernous tissues of the penis). In these diseases, there is no known precipitating injury, even though the basic process is similar to contracture in wound healing.

4 Immunopathology

Jeffrey S. Warren • David S. Strayer

The chief role of the immune system is to protect the host from invasion by foreign agents. Immune responses can be elicited by a wide range of agents including toxins, drugs, chemicals, viruses, bacteria, parasites and transplanted foreign tissues. Immune responses are characterized by their capacity to (1) distinguish self from nonself, (2) discriminate among potential invaders (specificity) and (3) generate immune memory and amplification responses (i.e., the ability to recall previous exposures and mount an intensified or anamnestic response).

Humans possess physical barriers such as (1) regionally adapted epithelia (e.g., thick skin, ciliated respiratory epithelium and a nearly impervious urothelium), (2) chemical–mechanical barriers (e.g., antibacterial lipids and mucus) and (3) indigenous microbial flora that compete with potential pathogens. Patterned hemodynamic responses, cell surface–associated and soluble mediator systems (e.g., complement and coagulation systems) and non–antigen-specific phagocytes (e.g., resident macrophages, neutrophils) are integral to **host defense** (see Chapter 2). Host defenses that are not antigen specific are components of the "**innate**" immune system. The antigen-specific or "**adaptive**" immune system encompasses lymphocytes, plasma cells, antigen-presenting cells (APCs), specific effector molecules (e.g., immunoglobulins) and a vast array of regulatory mediators.

As noted above, the defining features of adaptive immunity include specificity, memory and the capacity for amplification. Specificity and immunologic memory are direct results of activation by antigens of clonal lymphocytes that bear specific receptors. There are many linkages among the various layers of host defense. For example, an antibody can specifically bind to an epitope on a bacterium, leading to complement fixation and then generation of chemotactic peptides that attract non–antigen-specific phagocytic neutrophils.

It is important to consider the relationships of specific immune system components within the general rubrics of acute and chronic inflammation, cell injury and cell death. For example, immediate (type I) hypersensitivity reactions are immunoglobulin (Ig) E mediated, depend on generation of vasoactive compounds and feature inflammatory infiltrates rich in eosinophils. A type III hypersensitivity reaction, which is immune complex mediated, is characterized by an acute inflammatory infiltrate (mainly neutrophils). Type IV hypersensitivity reactions are triggered by antigen exposure and involve chronic inflammatory infiltrates (mononuclear phagocytes and T lymphocytes). Recognition of these mechanistic and morphologic relationships can be helpful diagnostically and therapeutically.

Biology of the Immune System

The Cells That Comprise the Immune System Derive From Hematopoietic Stem Cells

The cellular components of the immune and hematopoietic systems are derived from pluripotent **hematopoietic stem cells** (HSCs). Near the end of the first month of embryogenesis, HSCs appear in the extraembryonic erythropoietic islands adjacent to the yolk sac. At 6 weeks, the primary site of hematopoiesis shifts from extraembryonic blood islands to fetal liver and then to bone marrow. The latter process begins at 2 months and by 6 months has completely shifted to bone marrow. Although there are well-defined sequential changes in the primary site of hematopoiesis, there are periods of overlap. By 8 weeks of gestation, **lymphoid progenitors** derived from HSCs that are fated to become T cells circulate to the thymus where they differentiate into mature T lymphocytes. Lymphoid progenitors destined to become B cells differentiate first within fetal liver (8 weeks) and later within bone marrow (12 weeks). In the development of both thymus-derived T lymphocytes and bone marrow–derived B lymphocytes, the microenvironments (e.g., thymic epithelium, bone marrow stromal cells, growth factors) are critical. Mature lymphocytes exit the thymus and bone marrow and "home" to peripheral lymphoid tissues (e.g., lymph nodes, spleen, skin and mucosa). The population of peripheral lymphoid tissues by mature T and B lymphocytes and the rapid deployment and recirculation of mature lymphocytes to different, often remote, parts of the immune system are anatomically specific. **Lymphocyte homing and recirculation** are orchestrated by a series of leukocyte and endothelial surface molecules called **selectins** and **addressins**. The processes of lymphocyte development and homing/recirculation are important for understanding immune responses, genetic immunodeficiency states, regional host defense and the underpinnings of modern therapeutics (e.g., HSC transplantation).

The cells of the immune system express a vast array of surface molecules that are important in cellular differentiation and cell-to-cell communication. These surface molecules also serve as markers of cellular identity. The International Workshop on Human Leukocyte Differentiation Antigens is responsible for nomenclature of these markers and assigns them so-called cluster of differentiation or cluster designation (CD) numbers. Currently, some 300 different molecules have been assigned CD numbers.

Hematopoietic Stem Cells

Pluripotent HSCs account for between 0.01% and 0.1% of nucleated bone marrow cells. They exhibit characteristic light-scattering properties as assessed by flow cytometry, usually express **CD34** cell surface protein and lack cell surface molecules that characterize more mature lymphocyte subpopulations (e.g., CD2, CD3 and others). Hematopoietic stem cells differentially express more than 2000 different genes involved in a wide variety of cellular functions. Recently, a smaller population of $CD34^-$ HSCs was described. It is clear that stem cells cycle, replicate and give rise to progenitor cells. As these cells differentiate into lymphocytes, red blood cells, neutrophils and so forth, they lose proliferative capacity (Fig. 4-1). Two prevailing models of lymphopoiesis/hematopoiesis suggest that primitive stem cells give rise to committed progenitors (the **hierarchical model**) or that stem cells can develop into progenitor cells or back to stem cells (the **cell cycle or continuum model**). Circulating $CD34^+$ HSCs account for 0.01% to 0.1% of mononuclear peripheral blood cells. Bone marrow and blood HSCs are heterogeneous in terms of selected lymphocyte marker expression, myeloid markers, activation antigens and their capacity to engraft bone marrow. Infusion of sufficient numbers of peripheral blood HSCs into transplant recipients leads to faster marrow recovery than occurs in patients who have received marrow-derived HSCs. HSCs are quantified following harvest and before infusion into recipient patients. In clinical HSC transplantation, it is now common practice for donors to receive recombinant growth factors prior to HSC harvest. This practice leads to higher yields of harvested HSCs, decreased time to engraftment and improved success in engraftment. The proportion of bone marrow transplant recipients who receive harvested peripheral blood HSCs rather than marrow-derived HSCs has increased dramatically in recent years.

Lymphopoiesis and Hematopoiesis

As noted above, all mature lymphoid and hematopoietic cells are derived from a common population of pluripotential HSCs (Fig. 4-1). Each step in lymphopoiesis and hematopoiesis depends on a microenvironment that encompasses specific structural features and a complex array of growth factors. The primary branch point in differentiation is between lymphoid progenitors and myeloid progenitors. The former ultimately give rise to T lymphocytes, B lymphocytes, and natural killer (NK) cells, whereas the latter develop into granulocytic, erythroid, monocytic–dendritic and megakaryocytic colony-forming units (GEMM-CFUs). Downstream, CFUs become more lineage specific. Examples include CFU-GM (granulocyte-monocyte), CFU-Eo (eosinophil), CFU-E (erythrocyte) and so forth. "CFU" refers to a cell that ultimately gives rise to a specified population of "offspring," such as granulocytes, erythrocytes, monocytes, dendritic cells and megakaryocytes.

Lymphocytes

There are three major types of lymphocytes—T cells, B cells and NK cells—which account for 25% of peripheral blood leukocytes. Approximately 80% of blood lymphocytes are T cells, 10% B cells and 10% NK cells. The relative proportions of lymphocytes in the peripheral blood and central and peripheral lymphoid tissues vary. In contrast to the blood, only 30% to 40% of splenic and bone marrow lymphocytes are T cells.

T Lymphocytes

T lymphocytes can be subdivided into subpopulations by virtue of their specialized functions, surface CD molecules

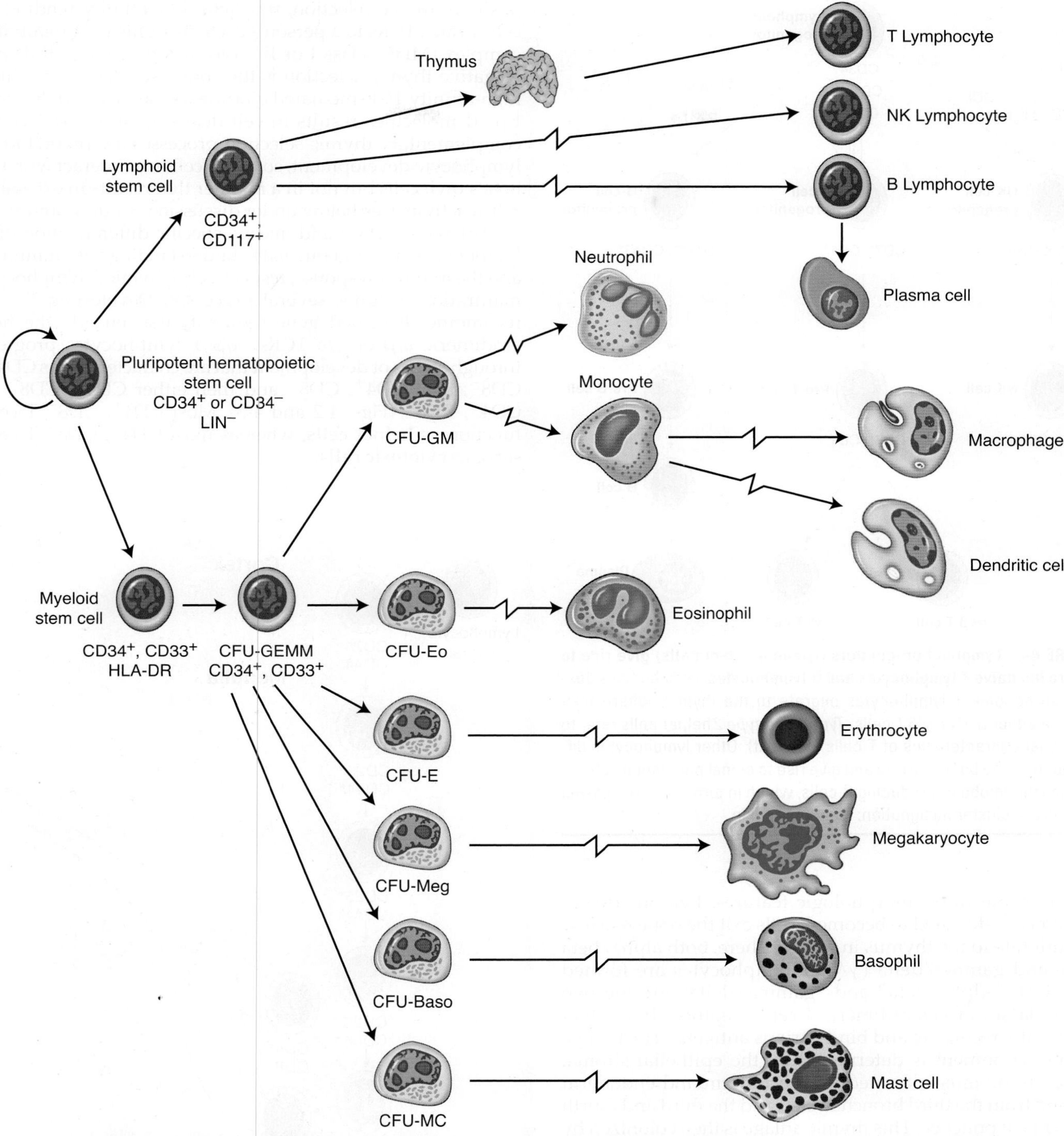

FIGURE 4-1. Pluripotent hematopoietic stem cells differentiate into either lymphoid or myeloid stem cells and, in the case of myeloid stem cells, into lineage-specific colony-forming units (CFUs). Under the influence of an appropriate microenvironment, CFUs give rise to definitive cell types. Lymphoid progenitors are precursors of natural killer (NK) cells, T lymphocytes, and B lymphocytes. B lymphocytes give rise to plasma cells. Lin- = lineage-negative; CD = cluster designation; CFU-GEMM = granulocytic, erythroid, monocytic–dendritic, and megakaryocytic colony-forming units; HLA = human leukocyte antigen.

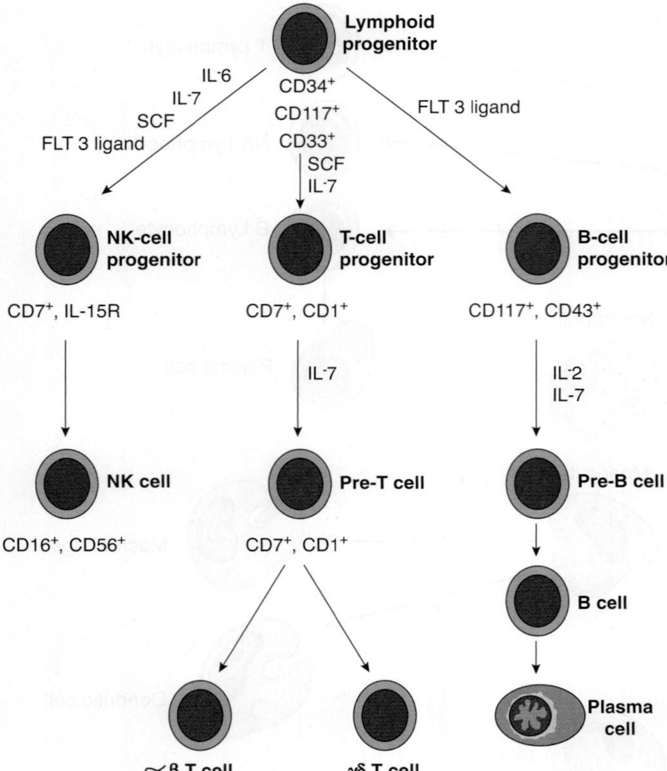

FIGURE 4-2. Lymphoid progenitors (lymphoid stem cells) give rise to mature but naïve T lymphocytes and B lymphocytes. Lymphocytes destined to become T lymphocytes migrate to the thymus where they become either α/β or γ/δ T cells. *Type 1* and *type 2* helper cells refer to functional characteristics of T cells (see text). Other lymphocytes differentiate in the bone marrow and give rise to clonal populations of surface immunoglobulin-producing B cells, which in turn can form plasma cells. CD = cluster designation; IL = interleukin.

and, in some cases, morphologic features. Lymphoid progenitor cells destined to become T cells exit the bone marrow and migrate to the thymus in waves. There, both alpha/beta (α/β) and gamma/delta (γ/δ) T lymphocytes are formed (Fig. 4-2). "Alpha/beta" and "gamma/delta" are the two major classes of heterodimeric T-cell receptors (TCRs) that specifically recognize and bind various antigens. The thymic microenvironment is determined by the epithelial stroma. The early thymus is formed from ectoderm and endoderm derived from the third bronchial cleft and the third and fourth pharyngeal pouches. This thymic anlage is then colonized by HSCs that give rise to T cells, macrophages and dendritic cells. The thymic cortex is composed of a meshwork of epithelial cell processes that surround groups of immature thymocytes that bear *both* CD4$^+$ and CD8$^+$ surface molecules (Fig. 4-3). As T lymphocytes mature, they percolate into thymic medulla where, in close proximity to nested groups of epithelial cells, they form more mature cells that are *either* CD4$^+$ or CD8$^+$.

The thymic corticomedullary junction contains many bone marrow HSC-derived macrophages and dendritic cells. Much of the **positive selection** of thymocytes occurs in the cortex; **negative selection** tends to occur through exposure of developing thymocytes to corticomedullary dendritic cells. In positive thymic selection, transient, low-affinity binding of cell surface TCRs to a person's own major histocompatibility complex (MHC) class I or II molecules prevents cell death. Negative thymic selection is the converse process in which high-affinity TCR-mediated binding to one's own MHC class I or II molecules results in cell death by apoptosis. These complementary thymic selection processes are pivotal to T-lymphocyte development, so that T cells can interact with the host's own cells but not in a manner that results in excessive self-reactivity (see below under discussion of autoimmunity).

Thymic selection and lineage-specific differentiation of T lymphocytes are fundamental to understanding autoimmunity and the immune response, respectively. Thymic T-lymphocyte maturation includes several processes. Developing T cells recombine dispersed gene segments that encode the heterodimeric α/β or γ/δ TCRs. α/β T lymphocytes progress through stages of development that are characterized as CD4$^-$, CD8$^-$, then CD4$^+$, CD8$^+$ and then either CD4$^+$, CD8$^-$ or CD4$^-$, CD8$^+$ (Figs. 4-2 and 4-3). Most CD4$^+$, CD8$^-$ T cells function as **helper cells**, whereas most CD4$^-$, CD8$^+$ T cells serve as **cytotoxic cells**.

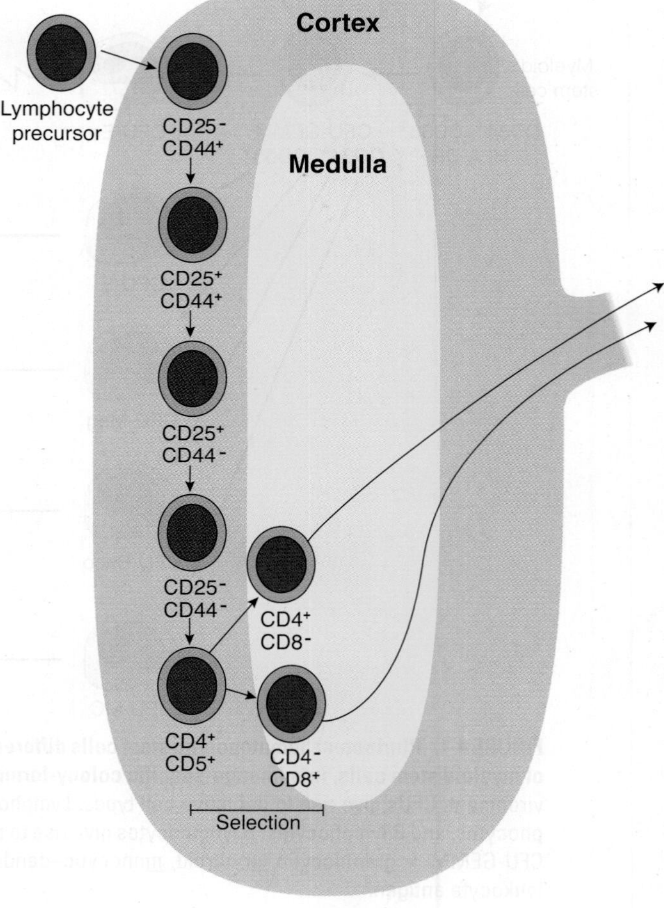

FIGURE 4-3. Lymphoid progenitors that are destined to become mature, but naïve, T cells differentiate as they percolate through the thymus. Peripheral CD4$^+$ and CD8$^+$ T cells are derived from thymic precursor cells that are simultaneously CD3$^+$, CD4$^+$ and CD8$^+$.

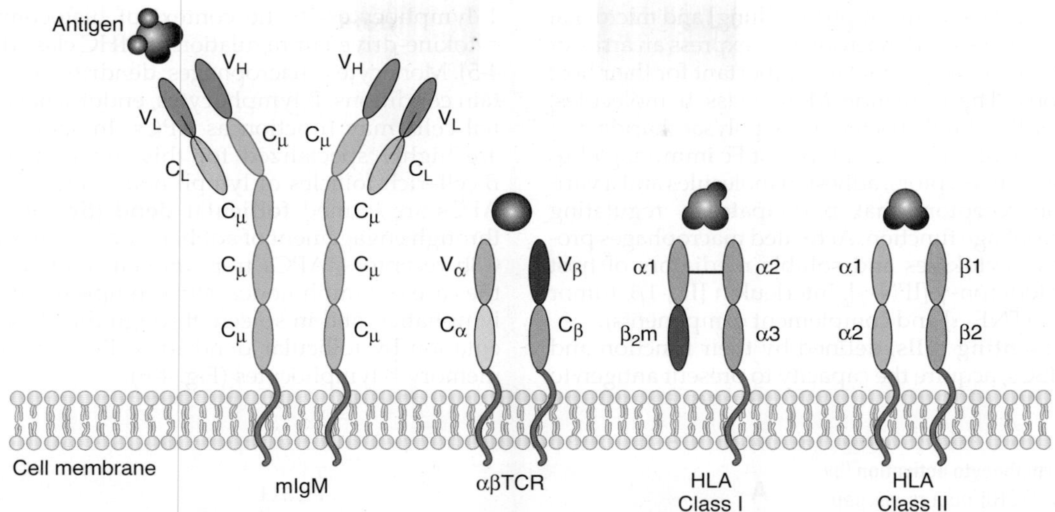

FIGURE 4-4. The antigen-binding sites of T-cell receptors (TCRs) and membrane immunoglobulin (mIg) are formed by the alignment of N-terminal variable domains of two peptide chains. Each variable (V) domain is derived from a transcript that is the product of a random VJ (TCR) or V(D)J (Ig) gene segment rearrangement. The antigen-binding grooves of major histocompatibility complex (MHC) molecules are formed by the alignment of the $\alpha1$ and $\alpha2$ domains of class I and the $\alpha1$ and $\beta1$ domains of class II molecules. C indicates a constant domain and β_2m represents β_2 microglobulin, which is a component of an intact human leukocyte antigen (HLA) class I molecule.

T lymphocytes exit the thymus and populate peripheral lymphoid tissues. In the thymus, antigen-specific TCRs are formed and expressed in conjunction with **CD3**, an essential accessory molecule that includes several subunits. Nearly 95% of circulating T lymphocytes express α/β TCRs. In turn, circulating α/β T cells also express either **CD4** or **CD8**. A smaller population (5%) of T cells expresses γ/δ TCRs and CD3 but neither CD4 nor CD8.

B Lymphocytes

B lymphocytes differentiate in the bone marrow into antibody-secreting plasma cells. Similar to T-lymphocyte development, the microenvironment of either the fetal liver or bone marrow is critical to B-lymphocyte development. In both sites only B lymphocytes that survive pass through the multiple steps necessary to produce surface immunoglobulin. Conversely, when surface immunoglobulin binds too avidly to self-antigens, developing B cells are negatively selected and eliminated.

Analogous to T cells, B lymphocytes express a surface antigen-binding receptor, **membrane immunoglobulin** (mIg), with the same antigen-binding specificity as the soluble immunoglobulin that will ultimately be secreted by the corresponding terminally differentiated plasma cells. Like T cells, B lymphocytes also exhibit a degree of heterogeneity (e.g., $CD5^+$ [B]) and $CD5^-$ [B2]).

T- and B-Cell Activation

TCRs, along with immunoglobulins and MHC class I and class II molecules (see below), confer specificity to the immune system by virtue of their capacity to bind specifically to foreign antigens (TCRs, Igs) or interact with self-cells (MHC). TCR, immunoglobulin and a portion of the MHC class I molecule are encoded by members of the immunoglobulin supergene family. The structural variability and, in turn, high specificity of TCRs and immunoglobulins are achieved through genetic recombination of segmented TCR and Ig genes. As noted above, an individual TCR is a heterodimer that forms an antigen-binding site (Fig. 4-4). The proteins that constitute TCRs and immunoglobulins each possess an amino-terminal antigen-binding variable (V) domain and a carboxy-terminal constant (C) domain. TCRs anchor the antigen to the cell surface, whereas immunoglobulins either anchor the receptor to the B-cell surface as mIg or, in the case of soluble immunoglobulin, mediate its biological function (Fig. 4-4).

NK Cells

NK cells recognize target cells mainly via antigen-independent mechanisms. They are believed to form in both the thymus and bone marrow. NK cells bear several types of class I MHC molecule receptors, which when engaged actually *inhibit* the NK cell's capacity to secrete cytolytic products. Certain tumor cells and virus-infected cells bear reduced numbers of MHC class I molecules and thus do not inhibit NK cells. In this scenario, NK cells engage virus-infected or tumor cells and secrete complement-like cytolytic proteins (perforin), granzymes A and B and other lytic molecules. NK cells also secrete granulysin, a cationic protein that induces target cell apoptosis.

In another example of linkage between different facets of the immune system, NK cells can also lyse target cells via antibody-dependent cellular cytotoxicity (ADCC). In ADCC, NK cells, through their Fc receptors, bind to the Fc domain of IgG that is specifically bound to antigen on surfaces of target cells. As with T and B cells, NK cells exhibit a degree of heterogeneity (e.g., $CD16^+$, $CD16^-$).

Mononuclear Phagocytes, Antigen-Presenting Cells and Dendritic Cells

Mononuclear phagocytes, chiefly **monocytes**, account for 10% of circulating white blood cells. Circulating monocytes give rise to resident tissue macrophages including, among others,

Kupffer cells (liver, alveolar macrophages [lung] and microglial cells [brain]). Monocytes and macrophages express an array of specific cell surface molecules that are important for their host defense functions. These include MHC class II molecules, CD14 (a receptor that binds bacterial lipopolysaccharide and can trigger cell activation), several types of Fc immunoglobulin receptors, toll-like receptors, adhesion molecules and a variety of cytokine receptors that participate in regulating monocyte/macrophage function. Activated macrophages produce a variety of cytokines and soluble mediators of host defense (e.g., interferon-γ [IFN-γ], interleukin [IL]-1β, tumor necrosis factor-α [TNF-α] and complement components).

Antigen-presenting cells, defined by their function and derived from HSCs, acquire the capacity to present antigen to T lymphocytes in the context of histocompatibility, after cytokine-driven upregulation of MHC class II molecules (Fig. 4-5). Monocytes, macrophages, dendritic cells and, under certain conditions, B lymphocytes, endothelial cells and epithelial cells may function as APCs. In some locations, APCs are highly specialized for this function. For instance, in B-cell–rich follicles of lymph nodes and spleen, specialized APCs are termed **follicular dendritic cells**. In these sites, through engagement of antibody and complement via Fc and C3b receptors, APCs trap antigen–antibody complexes. In the case of lymph nodes, such complexes arrive via afferent lymphatics, and in spleen, through the blood. Antigen presentation by follicular dendritic cells leads to generation of memory B lymphocytes (Fig. 4-6).

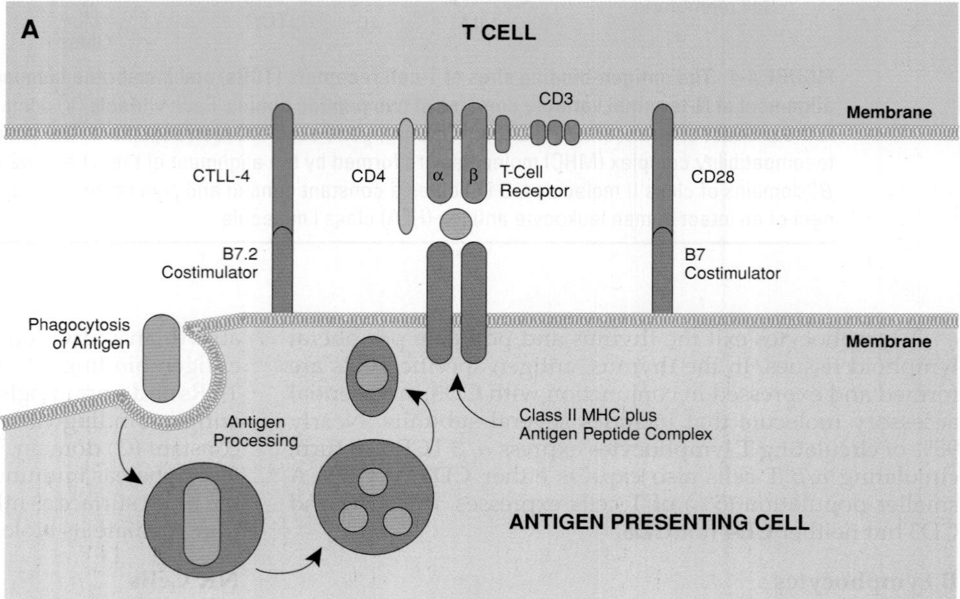

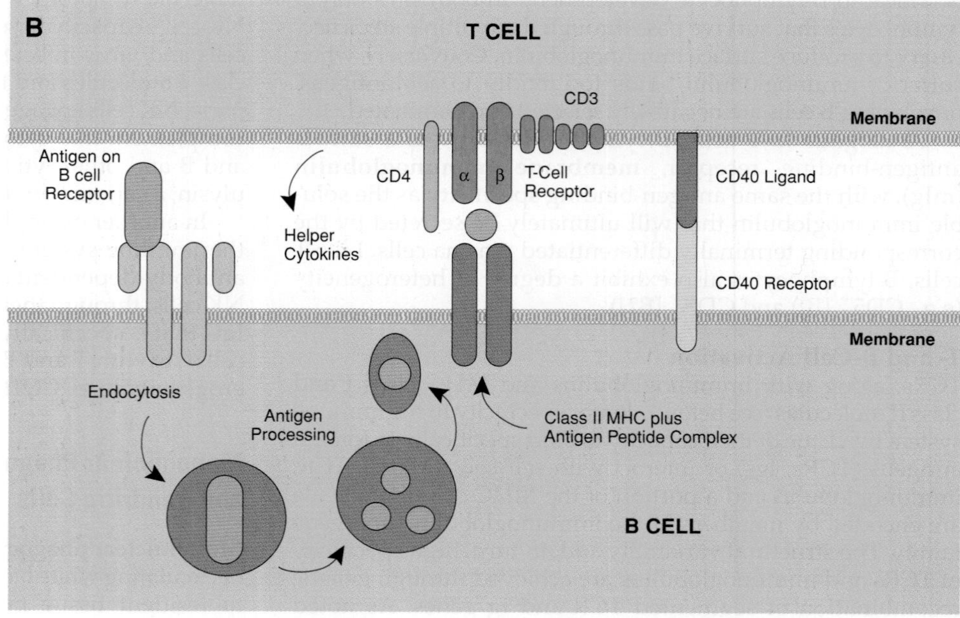

FIGURE 4-5. A. T-lymphocyte activation (by the T-cell receptor [TCR]) occurs via peptides cleaved from the phagocytized antigen (antigen processing) and presented to the TCR in the context of a histocompatible class II major histocompatibility complex (MHC) molecule. T-cell activation also requires accessory or costimulatory signals from cytotoxic lymphoid line (CTLL)-4 or CD28. **B.** A similar process applies to B-cell–T-cell interactions. The B-lymphocyte antigen receptor is membrane immunoglobulin.

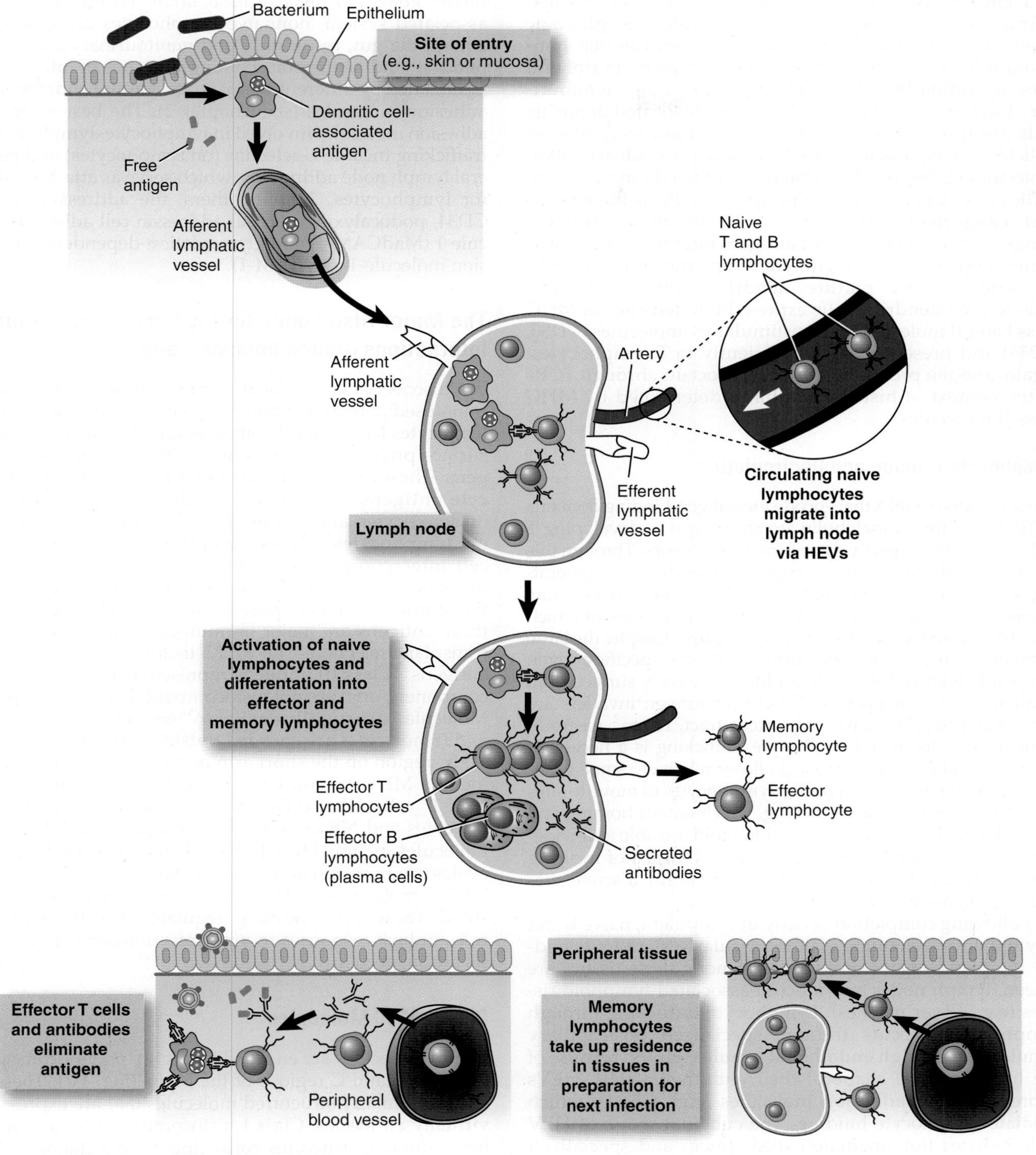

FIGURE 4-6. In an integrated immune response, antigen is processed and presented by a dendritic cell, which migrates via the afferent lymphatics to a regional lymph node. Within the regional lymph node antigen is presented to lymphocytes, which in turn are activated and may migrate (via homing mechanism) to specific peripheral sites. HEVs = high endothelial venules.

Dendritic cells are specialized APCs that are termed "dendritic" by virtue of their spider-like morphologic appearance. They are found in B-lymphocyte–rich lymphoid follicles, in thymic medulla and in many peripheral sites, including intestinal lamina propria, lung, genitourinary tract and skin (Fig. 4-6). Peripherally located dendritic cells are less mature than the APCs found in lymphoid follicles and express lower levels of accessory cell activation molecules (CD80 [B7-1], CD86 [B7-2]) than do mature dendritic cells. An example of a peripheral APC is the **epidermal Langerhans cell**. Upon exposure to an antigen, Langerhans cells engulf that antigen, migrate to a regional lymph node through an afferent lymphatic and differentiate into a more mature dendritic cell. Langerhans cell–derived dendritic cells express high densities of MHC class I and II molecules and costimulatory molecules (CD80, CD86) and present antigens efficiently to T lymphocytes. Again, antigen presentation to T cells occurs through TCRs in the context of histocompatibility determined by MHC class II molecules.

Lymphocyte Homing and Recirculation

The segments of DNA that encode the antigen-binding domains of TCRs and immunoglobulin are rearranged in developing T cells and B cells, respectively, to form "new" genes. Through this combinatorial process and a variety of other diversity-generating mechanisms, a large number of different antigen receptors is generated. Adults possess about 10^{12} lymphocytes, of which only 10% are in the circulation at a given time. Despite the large number of lymphocytes, the number with any specific antigen receptor is relatively small. In addition, the body surfaces that frequently serve as portals of entry for foreign invaders are very large (e.g., skin, 2 m^2; respiratory tract, 100 m^2; gastrointestinal tract, 400 m^2). Lymphocyte trafficking is a necessary aspect of host defense because it allows relatively small numbers of any set of antigen-specific lymphocytes to move to sites of "need." Lymphocyte trafficking, which entails homing and recirculation, has evolved to provide rapid, flexible and widespread distribution of lymphocytes and a means of focusing specific immunologic processes in anatomically discrete sites (e.g., lymph node cortex).

Following completion of early development, naïve B and T lymphocytes circulate via the vascular system to secondary lymphoid organs and tissues. Among these tissues are spleen, lymph nodes and mucosa-associated lymphoid tissues (e.g., Peyer patches). Lymphocyte trafficking through lymph nodes occurs through specialized postcapillary venules termed **high endothelial venules** (HEVs) because of the high cuboidal shape of their endothelial cells. HEVs express cellular adhesion molecules (e.g., CD31), which mediate lymphocyte binding. The cuboidal shape of HEV cells reduces flow-mediated shear forces and specialized intercellular connections facilitate egress of lymphocytes out of the vascular space. Lymphocytes that do not find their cognate antigen as they percolate through secondary lymphoid tissues reenter the circulation through efferent lymphatics and the thoracic duct.

By contrast, lymphocytes that have engaged an antigen leave the secondary lymphoid tissue, enter the circulation via lymphatics and the thoracic duct and then preferentially bind peripheral tissues (e.g., lymph nodes or mucosa-associated lymphoid tissue) from which the activating antigen was introduced. ***Hence, there are at least two major circuits, namely, lymph node and mucosa associated.*** Within the mucosa-associated system, nonnaïve lymphocytes can distinguish among the gut, respiratory and genitourinary tracts. Lymphocyte (and neutrophil) homing into sites of inflammation is mediated by different sets of leukocyte and endothelial cell adhesion molecules (see Chapter 2). The best-understood adhesion molecules involved in lymphocyte–lymphoid tissue trafficking include L-selectins (on lymphocytes) and peripheral lymph node addressins, which serve as attachment sites for lymphocytes. Among others, the addressins include CD34, podocalyxin, mucosal addressin cell adhesion molecule-1 (MadCAM-1) and glycosylation-dependent cell adhesion molecule-1 (GlyCAM-1).

The Major Histocompatibility Complex Coordinates Interactions Among Immune Cells

The discovery that sera of multiparous women and multiply-transfused patients contain antibodies against foreign blood leukocytes led to identification of an intricate system of cell surface proteins known as **major histocompatibility antigens.** These antigens are also referred to as **human leukocyte antigens** (HLAs) because they were first identified on leukocytes and are expressed in high concentrations on lymphocytes. HLAs orchestrate many of the cell–cell interactions fundamental to immune responses. As described above, productive interactions between cells of the immune system require histocompatibility. Conversely, these antigens are major immunogens and thus targets in transplant rejection. The MHC includes class I, II and III antigens. (Class III antigens represent certain complement components and are not histocompatibility antigens per se.) Molecules structurally similar to "traditional" MHC class I and II molecules are encoded outside of the more restricted MHC region on the short arm of chromosome 6. Examples include MHC-1b and CD1d, which can activate so-called "NK T" cells. NK T cells have characteristics of both T lymphocytes and NK cells. Other nontraditional MHC class I molecules include HLA-E, HLA-F and HLA-G. These molecules are more tissue restricted than HLA-A, HLA-B and HLA-C molecules, and their functions are not as well understood. These molecules may regulate NK-cell activity, and roles in host responses to viral infections and tumorigenesis are suspected.

Class I MHC Molecules

Class I molecules are encoded by highly polymorphic genes in the A, B and C regions of the MHC (Fig. 4-7). These loci encode similarly structured molecules that are expressed in virtually all tissues. Class I histocompatibility antigens are heterodimeric structures consisting of two chains, a 44-kd polymorphic transmembrane glycoprotein and a 12-kd nonpolymorphic molecule called β_2-microglobulin. The latter is a superficial surface protein lacking a membrane component and is noncovalently associated with the larger heavy chain. β_2-Microglobulin is encoded by a gene on chromosome 15. Structural polymorphism occurs primarily in the extracellular domains of the α-chain. MHC-I alleles are expressed codominantly, so tissues bear class I antigens inherited from each parent. These antigens are recognized by cytotoxic T cells during graft rejection or T-lymphocyte–mediated killing of virus-infected cells.

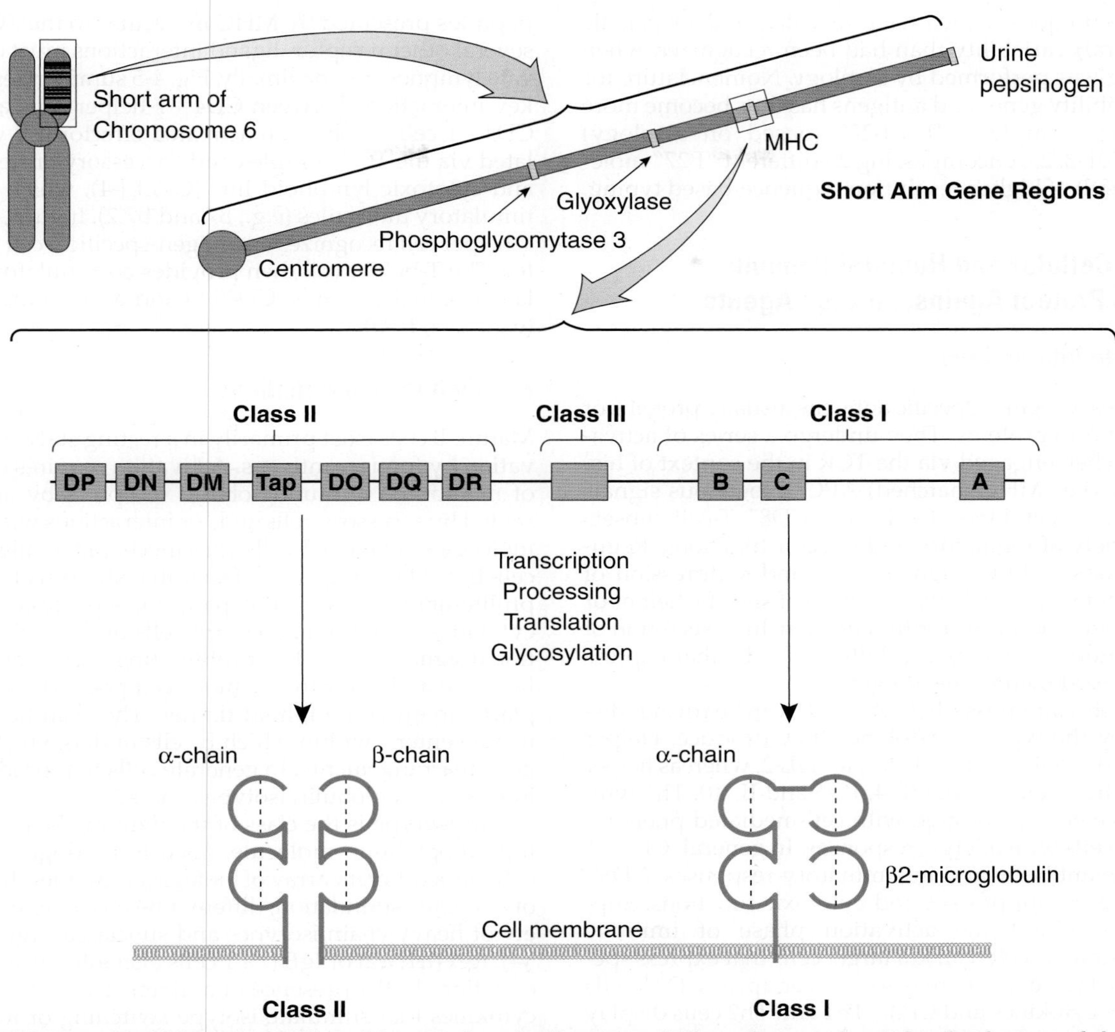

FIGURE 4-7. The highly polymorphic loci that encode major histocompatibility antigens are located on the short arm of chromosome 6. Class I and class II molecules exhibit different structures, but each participates in fundamentally important cell–cell interactions. Class III genes encode some complement components that are not formally histocompatibility antigens.

Class II MHC Molecules

Class II molecules are encoded by multiple loci in the D region: DP, DN, DM, DO, DQ and DR. The D region loci encode structurally similar molecules that are expressed primarily on accessory cells involved in antigen presentation. As noted above, the chief APCs include monocytes, macrophages, dendritic cells and B lymphocytes. Class II antigens have also been referred to as "Ia" (immunity-associated) antigens. Class II molecules are heterodimers that consist of two noncovalently linked glycoprotein chains. The 34-kd β-chain possesses a single disulfide bond; its extracellular domain is the major site of class II antigenic variability. The 29-kd α-chain has two disulfide bonds. Both chains are transmembrane proteins. As with class I antigens, D alleles are expressed codominantly and tissues bear antigens from each parent.

Clinical Tissue Typing

"Histocompatibility, HLA, or tissue typing" laboratories now use several approaches to identify the class I and class II antigens expressed by both potential donor tissues and recipient tissues prior to organ transplantation. Class I antigens have been defined serologically: antisera against various antigens are tested against donor (or recipient) lymphocytes. The system of nomenclature for class I antigens is based on the locus of origin (A1, A2, A3, B4, B6, C1, C2, etc.). Tissue typing reveals the two different antigens codominantly expressed at each locus, and one antigen (double dose) when there is homozygosity. Accordingly, a tissue might express A1, A2, B4, B6, DR3 and DR4 antigens. All loci are not universally typed in clinical laboratories. Tissue typing laboratories also quantify already formed antibodies to HLAs. These antibodies circulate in potential organ or tissue transplant recipients who have been immunized via previous blood transfusion, transplant or pregnancy. Increasingly, tissue-typing laboratories use molecular methods, including DNA sequencing, to identify class I and II antigens. Clinical outcomes for some types of grafts (e.g., HSC) have improved as a result of DNA sequence-level high-resolution typing.

Class II antigens were traditionally defined by serologic and functional assays, but these have largely been replaced by molecular techniques, which have revealed greater genetic (and structural) variability than had been recognized when tissue typing was performed by serology. Nomenclature for histocompatibility genes and antigens has thus become more complex; for example, "HLA-B27" (based on serology) became B*2701-2725, encompassing 25 different "B27" molecules, as a result of higher-resolution sequence-based typing.

Integrated Cellular and Humoral Immune Responses Protect Against Foreign Agents

T-Lymphocyte Interactions

T lymphocytes recognize specific antigens, usually proteins or haptens bound to proteins. They undergo a series of activation events when engaged via the TCR in the context of histocompatible (i.e., MHC-matched) APC. Exogenous signals are delivered by cytokines. $CD4^+$ and $CD8^+$ T-cell subsets exhibit a variety of regulatory and effector functions. Regulatory functions include augmentation and suppression of immune responses, usually via secretion of specific helper or suppressor cytokines. Effector functions include secretion of proinflammatory cytokines and killing of cells that express foreign or altered membrane antigens.

$CD4^+$ T cells, and possibly $CD8^+$ cells, can be further distinguished by the types of cytokines they produce. Helper type 1, or "Th1," cells produce IFN-γ and IL-2, whereas helper type 2, or "Th2," cells secrete IL-4, IL-5 and IL-10. Th1 lymphocytes have been associated with cell-mediated phenomena and Th2 cells with allergic responses. In general, $CD4^+$ T cells promote antibody and inflammatory responses. $CD8^+$ cells largely exert suppressor and cytotoxic functions. Suppressor cells inhibit the activation phase of immune responses; cytotoxic cells can kill target cells that express specific antigens. However, there is some overlap, as $CD8^+$ cells secrete helper cytokines and $CD4^+$ Th1 and Th2 cells display cross-regulatory suppression.

An important aspect of T-cell antigen recognition is the requirement for antigen to be presented on the surfaces of other cells in association with a histocompatible membrane protein (Figs. 4-5 and 4-6). As noted above, T cells bear membrane receptor complexes (α/β TCRs plus CD3 accessory molecules) on their surfaces. For maximal immune responses, the TCR–CD3 complex must interact with a foreign antigen in the context of cell-to-cell histocompatibility. Thus, antigens are presented to T cells by accessory cells (APCs) that bear appropriate histocompatibility molecules. Antigens may also be presented to T cells by cells that do not "present" antigens but rather express on their surface a foreign or altered self-protein in association with an appropriate histocompatibility molecule.

$CD8^+$ cells (cytotoxic T cells) recognize antigens in conjunction with HLA class I molecules, whereas $CD4^+$ cells (T-helper cells) recognize antigens together with class II molecules. The membrane CD4 and CD8 molecules of α/β T cells help to stabilize binding interactions. γ/δ T cells may also acquire CD8 outside the thymus and then use class I antigens for binding target cells. ***Foreign class I and class II molecules, which are not histocompatible with the host (e.g., transplanted histocompatibility antigens), are themselves potent immunogens and can be recognized by host T cells.*** This is why optimal tissue transplantation requires that donor and recipient be HLA matched. In addition to binding foreign peptides presented by MHC molecules to the TCR complex, several other receptor–ligand interactions must occur to activate lymphocytes maximally. Fig. 4-5 summarizes some of the key interactions between $CD4^+$ T-helper cells and APCs. A $CD4^+$ T cell becomes an activated effector cell when stimulated via the TCR complex and "accessory" receptors (CD28 and cytotoxic lymphoid line [CTLL]-4), which engage costimulatory molecules (e.g., B7 and B7.2). In turn, an activated T-helper cell recognizes an antigen-specific B cell via its receptor. The T-helper cell then provides costimulatory and regulatory signals, such as CD40 ligand and "helper" cytokines (e.g., IL-4, IL-5).

B-Lymphocyte Interactions

Mature B cells exist primarily in a resting state, awaiting activation by foreign antigens. Activation requires cross-linking of membrane immunoglobulin receptors by antigens presented by accessory cells and/or interactions with membrane molecules of helper T cells via a mechanism called cognate T-cell–B-cell help (Fig. 4-5). The initial stimulus leads to B-cell proliferation and clonal expansion, a process amplified by cytokines from both accessory cells and T cells. If no additional signal is provided, proliferating B cells return to a resting state and enter the memory cell pool. These events take place largely in lymphoid tissues. They can be seen as germinal centers, within which B cells undergo further somatic gene rearrangements, to generate cells that produce the various immunoglobulin isotypes and subclasses.

An **isotype** is the class of the defining heavy chain of an immunoglobulin molecule. Each immunoglobulin isotype exhibits a different array of biological activities. In the absence of antigenic stimulation, different B-cell clones express a variety of heavy-chain isotypes and subclasses: IgG ($\gamma1$, $\gamma2$, $\gamma3$, $\gamma4$), IgA ($\alpha1$, $\alpha2$) or IgE (ε). T cells also influence B-cell differentiation. In the presence of antigen, T cells produce helper cytokines that stimulate isotype switching or induce proliferation of previously committed isotype populations. For example, IL-4 induces switching to the IgE isotype.

The final stage of B-cell differentiation into antibody-synthesizing plasma cells requires exposure to additional products of T lymphocytes (e.g., IL-5, IL-6), especially in the case of protein antigens. However, some polyvalent agents induce B-cell proliferation and differentiation into plasma cells directly, bypassing the requirements for B-cell growth and differentiation factors. Such agents are called **polyclonal B-cell activators** because they do not interact with antigen-binding sites and hence are not specific antigens. Examples of polyclonal B-cell activators are bacterial products (lipopolysaccharide, staphylococcal protein A) and certain viruses (Epstein-Barr virus [EBV], cytomegalovirus [CMV]).

The predominant type of immunoglobulin produced during an immune response changes with age. Newborns tend to produce predominantly IgM. By contrast, older children and adults initially produce IgM following antigenic challenge but rapidly shift toward IgG synthesis.

Mononuclear Phagocyte Activities

Mononuclear phagocyte is a general term applied to phagocytic cell populations in virtually all organs and connective tissues. Among these cells are macrophages, monocytes, Kupffer cells of the liver and lung alveolar macrophages. The older term "histiocyte" is synonymous with **macrophage**, either a circulating or a fixed tissue macrophage. Subpopulations of macrophages exhibit different functions and phenotypes. Precursor cells (monoblasts and promonocytes) arise in bone marrow, enter the circulation as monocytes and then migrate into tissues, where they reside as tissue macrophages. In the lung, liver and spleen, numerous macrophages populate sinuses and pericapillary zones to form an effective filtering system that removes effete cells and foreign particulate material from blood. This system, formerly known as the "reticuloendothelial system," is now termed the **mononuclear phagocyte system**. In addition to their "housekeeping" functions, macrophages are critical in inducing immune responses and in maintenance and resolution of inflammatory reactions.

Macrophages are important accessory cells by virtue of their expression of class II histocompatibility antigens. They ingest and process antigens for presentation to T cells in conjunction with class II MHC molecules. The subsequent T-cell responses are further amplified by macrophage-derived cytokines. One of the best-characterized cytokines is IL-1, which, among a pleiotropic set of activities, promotes expression of IL-2 receptor on T cells, augmenting T-cell proliferation, which is driven by IL-2 (also known as T-cell growth factor). Among many effects of IL-1 on other tissues is preparation of the body to combat infection. For example, IL-1 induces fever and promotes catabolic metabolism.

Macrophages are major participants in subacute and chronic inflammatory reactions. During persistent inflammation, increased numbers of monocytes are recruited from the bone marrow. Under chemotactic influence, they migrate into sites of inflammation, where they mature into macrophages. Both recruited and resident tissue macrophages proliferate in these foci, where they secrete proteins, lipids, nucleotides and reactive oxygen and nitrogen metabolites. Functionally, these molecules are digestive, opsonic, cytotoxic, growth promoting and growth inhibiting.

The functional activities of macrophages and the spectrum of molecules that they produce are regulated by external factors, such as T-cell–derived cytokines. Macrophages exposed to such factors become "activated"; that is, they acquire a greater capacity to produce reactive oxygen metabolites, kill tumor cells and eliminate intracellular microorganisms.

If an agent that incites an inflammatory process is difficult to digest, a granulomatous reaction may ensue (see Chapter 2). Under such conditions, macrophages mature further, to become "epithelioid" cells and multinucleated giant cells. Macrophages can fuse to form multinucleate syncytia called **giant cells**. Different inciting agents elicit different types of giant cells. For example, granulomas caused by mycobacteria often contain Langhans-type giant cells, which have a semicircular arrangement of nuclei. Giant cells of foreign body granulomas exhibit a random distribution of nuclei. Both epithelioid cells and giant cells are poor phagocytes; they mainly sequester foreign material.

Clinical Evaluation of Immune Status

Suspicion of an immunodeficiency disorder should trigger a careful assessment of immune function. Immunodeficiency disorders are typically suggested by recurrent chronic or unusual infections. Alternatively, persons who consistently present with localized edema and itching following contact with an object in their environment may be suspected of having a **hypersensitivity response** to an antigen associated with that object.

Defects in the humoral immune system can result in a patient having difficulty clearing encapsulated bacteria from the bloodstream, resulting in life-threatening infections. Bacteria commonly seen in these immunocompromised patients include *Streptococcus pneumoniae*, *Haemophilus influenza* and *Neisseria meningitidis*. Defects in humoral immunity may be primary and present from soon after birth, or they may be acquired. They are quite diverse and include such diseases as selective IgA deficiency; common variable immune deficiency, in which immunoglobin levels are depressed; and the acquired immune deficiency state caused by human immunodeficiency virus (HIV)-1, in which immunoglobulin levels are elevated but disordered due to immune dysregulation and therefore ineffective. Patients with asplenia, whether secondary to a functional defect or frank absence of the spleen, are also at greatly increased risk of overwhelming bacteremia, especially with encapsulated bacteria.

The cellular immune system fights viral infections, participates in immune surveillance and may prevent or delay malignancy. The most dramatic example for the role of T lymphocytes is in advanced HIV-1 disease, acquired immunodeficiency syndrome (AIDS), in which $CD4^+$ T cells are severely depleted. Such patients develop opportunistic infections with fungi such as cryptococcus, viruses such as CMV and adenovirus and mycobacteria such as *Mycobacterium tuberculosis* and *Mycobacterium avium-intracellulare* complex.

Total Immunoglobulin Concentration Is Determined by Electrophoresis

Total aggregate concentration of IgG, IgA and IgM can be estimated by serum protein electrophoresis (SPEP). Serum proteins are separated by electrophoresis, stained with dyes that bind to proteins and quantitated by densitometry. Characteristic electrophoretic patterns of a normal person and a person with hypogammaglobulinemia are contrasted in Fig. 4-8. Immunoglobulins comprise the gammaglobulin fraction, which migrates toward the cathode and is reduced in patients with hypogammaglobulinemia.

Individual immunoglobulin (i.e., IgG, IgA, IgM) concentrations can be measured by quantitating individual isotypes using specific antibodies. Quantitation allows identification of selective immunoglobulin subclass deficiencies and, like SPEP, provides a measure of total serum immunoglobulin concentration. There are numerous conditions characterized by selective deficiencies of serum IgM, IgG, IgA or secretory IgA.

Antibody-Dependent Immunity Can Be Assessed by Testing for Antibodies Against Specific Antigens

Subtle humoral immune deficiencies are detected by quantitating circulating antibodies to specific antigens to which most people have been exposed via vaccination or common environmental contact (e.g., multivalent pneumococcal vaccine, tetanus toxoid, diphtheria toxoid, rubella virus). These serologic methods may be useful in highlighting deficiencies in specific facets of the humoral immune system, even if total serum immunoglobulin levels are normal. It may be useful to vaccinate a patient with a "killed" vaccine such as pneumococcal vaccine and then recheck levels of antibody to these specific antigens, usually 4 weeks postvaccination. Such an

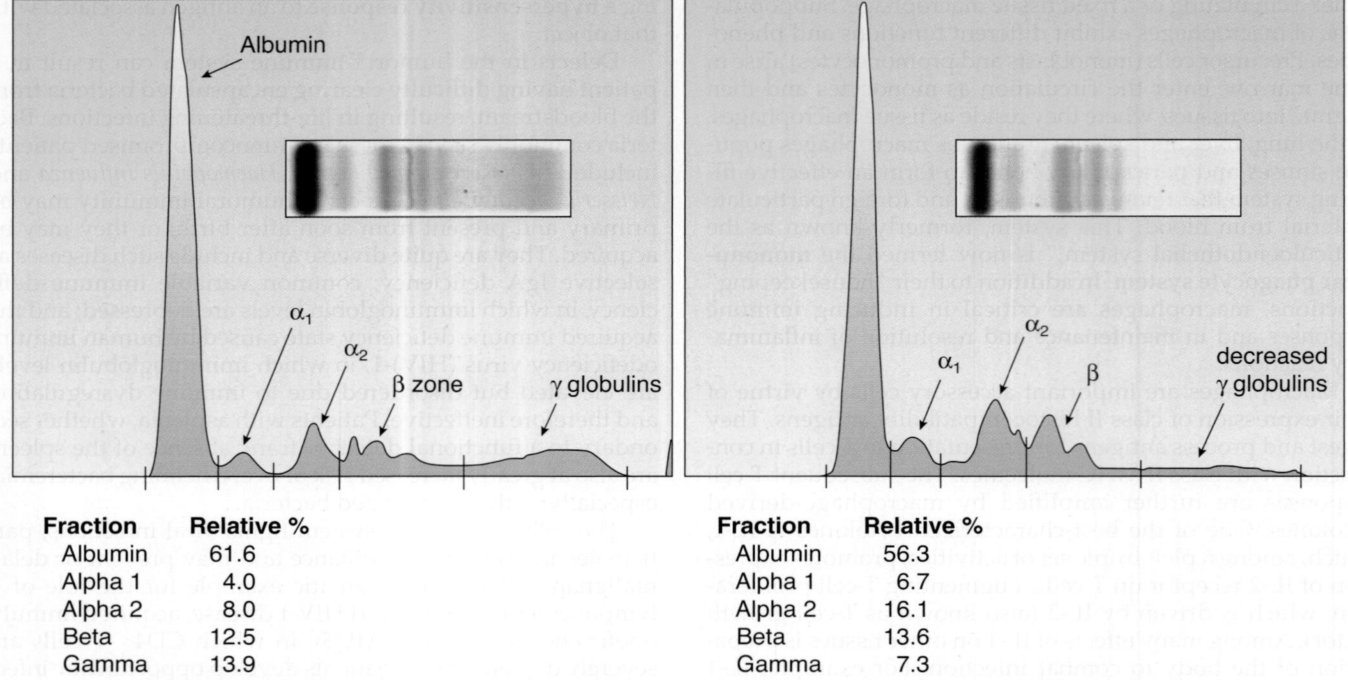

Fraction	Relative %
Albumin	61.6
Alpha 1	4.0
Alpha 2	8.0
Beta	12.5
Gamma	13.9

Fraction	Relative %
Albumin	56.3
Alpha 1	6.7
Alpha 2	16.1
Beta	13.6
Gamma	7.3

FIGURE 4-8. Normal (*left*) and hypogammaglobulinemic (*right*) serum protein electrophoresis (SPEP) patterns. SPEP provides a rapid means to evaluate several major protein components of serum.

immunologic challenge allows the clinician to assess this facet of the immune response.

Cell-Mediated Immunity Can Be Assessed Using Peripheral Blood T Cells or Skin Sensitivity Testing

Since the large majority (approximately 80%) of blood lymphocytes are T cells, the total lymphocyte count is a crude index of the ability of the body to generate adequate numbers of T cells. Screening of T-cell function can be done by skin testing for delayed-type hypersensitivity to antigens with which most people are assumed to have come into contact previously. After intradermal injection of small amounts of such antigens (e.g., *Candida albicans*), a normal response typically involves development of a specified area of redness and/or induration within a characteristic time frame.

More sophisticated analyses of T-cell function may involve in vitro studies using purified blood lymphocyte preparations. For example, T-cell proliferation in response to specific or nonspecific stimuli can provide an indication of T-lymphocyte function. Normal T (and B) cells proliferate in response to particular mitogenic stimuli. As cell proliferation entails new DNA synthesis, it can be measured by adding labeled nucleotides to the tissue culture medium. Thus, a strong proliferative response to plant lectin phytohemagglutinin (PHA) indicates that T-cell recognition is likely to be intact. Weak proliferation in response to PHA suggests qualitative or quantitative defects in T cells, or a problem in regulation of T-cell proliferation.

Lymphocyte Populations Are Quantitated by Flow Cytometry

Another approach to assessing T- and B-cell arms of the immune system is quantitating B and T lymphocytes in the blood, usually by flow cytometry. Blood lymphocytes are treated with antibodies against specific B- or T-cell membrane antigens, many of which belong to the system of "**cluster designation**," or CD, antigens. For example, CD20 is a B-cell antigen, whereas a commonly used marker of T cells is CD3. T cells are often further subcategorized by expression of CD4 (helper T cells) or CD8 (effector T cells). CD4 is not unique to T cells; it is also expressed by some mononuclear phagocytes. Lymphocyte subpopulation quantitation is commonly used to follow patients infected with HIV-1 by serial measurement of $CD4^+$ T cells.

Monoclonal antibodies against individual antigens are conjugated to fluorescent dyes such as fluorescein or rhodamine (fluorophores) and bind to the cells bearing those antigens. A flow cytometer dispenses cells in microdroplets that each have one cell. As each cell falls, it passes through narrow-band laser beams that excite a specific fluorophore. If the cell carries the antigen recognized by the fluorophore-labeled antibody, that fluorophore is excited to emit light of a particular wavelength, which is measured by a detector. The flow cytometer counts cells emitting light of that wavelength(s) and measures the intensity of those emissions. Current flow cytometers may have as many as 10 lasers, allowing simultaneous analysis of that number of cell membrane markers.

Such quantitation of T-lymphocyte populations is routinely used to follow the clinical status of patients infected with HIV-1 and to assess the effectiveness of highly active antiretroviral therapy (HAART, see later).

Molecular Evaluation of Immune Status Facilitates Diagnosis of Rare Immune System Defects

A large number of specific, often rare, immunodeficiency disorders have been defined on the basis of mutations within genes that encode various cell membrane–associated cell–cell communication molecules (e.g., β_2-integrins), cytosolic signal transduction molecules (e.g., Janus kinase 3), cytosolic enzymes (e.g., adenosine deaminase) and transcription factors involved in the regulation of host defense genes. More than 100 specific genetic defects that can result in impaired immune status have been identified (see below). Careful clinical evaluation of patients suspected of harboring a rare molecular defect is very important because most of these assays require expertise for correct interpretation and are exceedingly expensive.

Immunologically Mediated Tissue Injury

Immune responses not only protect against invasion by foreign organisms but may also cause tissue damage. Thus, many inflammatory diseases are examples of "friendly fire" in which the immune system attacks the body's own tissues. A variety of foreign substances (e.g., dust, pollen, viruses, bacteria) may act as antigens and provoke protective immune responses. In certain situations, the protective effects of an immune response give way to deleterious effects associated with a spectrum of lesions. Such lesions can produce manifestations that range from temporary discomfort to substantial injury. For example, in the process of phagocytizing and destroying bacteria, phagocytic cells (neutrophils and macrophages) often cause injury to surrounding tissue. An immune response that leads to tissue injury or disease is broadly called a **hypersensitivity** reaction. Many diseases are categorized as immune disorders or immunologically mediated conditions, in which an immune response to a foreign or self-antigen causes injury. Immune- or hypersensitivity-mediated diseases are common and include such entities as hives (urticaria), asthma, hay fever, hepatitis, glomerulonephritis and arthritis.

Hypersensitivity reactions are classified according to the type of immune mechanism (Table 4-1). Type I, II and III hypersensitivity reactions all require formation of a specific antibody to an exogenous (foreign) or an endogenous (self) antigen. An exception is a subset of type I reactions. The antibody isotype determines the mechanism by which tissue injury occurs.

- In most **type I**, or **immediate-type hypersensitivity, reactions,** IgE antibody is formed and binds to high-affinity receptors on mast cells and/or basophils via its Fc domain. Subsequent binding of antigen and cross-linking of IgE triggers rapid (immediate) release of products from these cells, leading to the characteristic manifestations of such diseases as urticaria, asthma and anaphylaxis.
- In **type II hypersensitivity reactions**, IgG or IgM antibody is formed against an antigen, usually a protein on a cell surface. Less commonly, the antigen is an intrinsic structural component of the extracellular matrix (e.g., part of the basement membrane). Such antigen–antibody coupling activates complement, which in turn lyses the cell (**cytotoxicity**) or damages the extracellular matrix. In some type II reactions, other antibody-mediated effects are operative.
- In **type III hypersensitivity reactions**, the antibody responsible for tissue injury is also usually IgM or IgG, but the mechanism of tissue injury differs. The antigen circulates in the vascular compartment until it is bound by antibody. The resulting immune complex is deposited in tissue. Complement activation at sites of antigen–antibody deposition leads to leukocyte recruitment, which is responsible for the subsequent tissue injury. In some type III reactions, antigen is bound by antibody in situ.
- **Type IV reactions**, or **cell-mediated** or **delayed-type, hypersensitivity reactions,** do not involve antibodies. Rather, antigen activation of T lymphocytes, usually with the help of macrophages, causes release of products by these cells, thereby leading to tissue injury.

Table 4-1

Modified Gell and Coombs Classification of Hypersensitivity Reactions

Type	Mechanism	Examples
Type I (anaphylactic type): immediate hypersensitivity	IgE antibody-mediated mast cell activation and degranulation	Hay fever, asthma, hives, anaphylaxis
	Non–IgE mediated	Physical urticarias
Type II (cytotoxic type): cytotoxic antibodies	Cytotoxic (IgG, IgM) antibodies formed against cell surface antigens; complement usually involved	Autoimmune hemolytic anemias, Goodpasture disease
	Noncytotoxic antibodies against cell surface receptors	Graves disease
Type III (immune complex type): immune complex disease	Antibodies (IgG, IgM, IgA) formed against exogenous or endogenous antigens; complement and leukocytes (neutrophils, macrophages) often involved	Autoimmune diseases (SLE, rheumatoid arthritis), many types of glomerulonephritis
Type IV (cell-mediated type): delayed-type hypersensitivity	Mononuclear cells (T lymphocytes, macrophages) with interleukin and lymphokine production	Granulomatous disease (tuberculosis)
		Delayed skin reactions (poison ivy)

Ig = immunoglobulin; SLE = systemic lupus erythematosus.

Many immunologic diseases are mediated by more than one type of hypersensitivity reaction. Thus, in hypersensitivity pneumonitis, lung injury results from hypersensitivity to inhaled fungal antigens and involves types I, III and IV hypersensitivity reactions.

Type I or Immediate Hypersensitivity Reactions Are Triggered by IgE Bound to Mast Cells

Immediate-type hypersensitivity is manifested by a localized or generalized reaction that occurs immediately (within minutes) after exposure to an antigen or "allergen" to which the person has previously been sensitized. The clinical manifestations of a reaction depend on the site of antigen exposure and extent of sensitization. For example, when a reaction involves the skin, the characteristic local reaction is a "wheal and flare," or **urticaria.** When the conjunctiva and upper respiratory tract are involved, sneezing and conjunctivitis result and we speak of **hay fever** (**allergic rhinitis**). In its generalized and most severe form, immediate hypersensitivity reactions are associated with bronchoconstriction, airway obstruction and circulatory collapse, as seen in anaphylactic shock. There is a high degree of genetically determined variability in susceptibility to type I hypersensitivity reactions. A variety of linkages and candidate genes have been identified. Particularly susceptible individuals are said to be "atopic."

Type I hypersensitivity reactions usually feature IgE antibodies that are formed by a $CD4^+$, Th2 T-cell–dependent mechanism and that bind avidly to Fc-epsilon ($Fc\varepsilon$) receptors on mast cells and basophils. The high avidity of IgE binding accounts for the term **cytophilic** antibody. Once exposed to a specific allergen that elicits IgE, a person is sensitized; subsequent exposures to that allergen or a cross-reacting epitope induce immediate hypersensitivity reactions. After IgE is elicited, repeat exposure to antigen typically induces additional IgE antibody, rather than antibodies of other classes, such as IgM or IgG.

IgE can persist for years bound to $Fc\epsilon$ receptors on mast cells and basophils, a feature unique to these cells. Upon subsequent reexposure, recognition of the soluble antigen or allergen by IgE coupled to its surface $Fc\epsilon$ receptor activates the mast cell or basophil. The potent inflammatory mediators that are released mediate the manifestations of type I hypersensitivity reactions. As shown in Fig. 4-9, the antigen (allergen) binds the Fab region of the IgE antibody. To activate the cell, the antigen must cross-link more than one IgE antibody molecule.

Most cells and basophils can also be activated by agents other than antibodies. For example, some individuals may develop urticaria after exposure to an ice cube (physical urticaria). The complement-derived anaphylatoxic peptides, C3a and C5a, can directly stimulate mast cells by a different receptor-mediated process (Fig. 4-9). These cell-activating events trigger release of stored granule constituents and rapid synthesis and release of other mediators. Some compounds, such as melittin (from bee venom), and some drugs (e.g., morphine) activate mast cells directly and induce release of granular constituents.

Regardless of how mast cell activation is initiated, cytosolic calcium influx is required. A rise in cytosolic free calcium is associated with increases in cyclic adenosine 3′,5′-monophosphate (cAMP), activation of several metabolic pathways within the mast cell and subsequent secretion of both preformed and newly synthesized products.

A number of potent mediators are released from granules within minutes. Because they are preformed and stored in granules, they exert immediate biological effects upon release. Of the granule constituents listed in Fig. 4-9, the biogenic amine **histamine** is particularly important. It induces constriction of vascular and nonvascular smooth muscle, causes microvascular dilation and increases venule permeability. These effects are largely mediated through H_1 histamine receptors. Histamine also increases gastric acid secretion through H_2 histamine receptors, and provokes the wheal-and-flare reaction in the skin. In the lungs, it causes the early manifestations of immediate hypersensitivity, including bronchospasm, vascular congestion and edema. Other preformed products released from mast cell granules include heparin, a series of neutral proteases (trypsin, chymotrypsin, carboxypeptidase and acid hydrolases) and at least two chemotactic factors: a neutrophil chemotactic factor and an eosinophil chemotactic factor. The latter is responsible for the accumulation of eosinophils, a characteristic finding in immediate hypersensitivity. The synthesis and secretion of cytokines by mast cells, by other recruited inflammatory cells and even by indigenous cells (e.g., epithelium) are important in the so-called "**late-phase**" reaction of immediate hypersensitivity. Late-phase responses typically last 2 to 24 hours, are marked by a mixed inflammatory infiltrate and are mediated by many cytokines including IL-1, IL-3, IL-4, IL-5, IL-6, TNF, granulocyte-macrophage colony-stimulating factor (GM-CSF) and the macrophage-inflammatory proteins (MIP)-1α and MIP-1β.

Activation of mast cells also increases synthesis of potent inflammatory mediators, particularly the various products of the arachidonic acid pathway that are formed after activation of phospholipase A_2. Products of cyclooxygenase (prostaglandins D_2, E_2 and F_2 and thromboxane) and lipoxygenase (leukotrienes B_4, C_4, D_4, E_4) are made. Arachidonic acid derivatives, which are also generated by a variety of other cell types, induce smooth muscle contraction, vasodilation and edema. Leukotrienes C_4, D_4 and E_4, previously known as "slow-reacting substances of anaphylaxis" (SRS-As), are important in the delayed bronchoconstriction phase of anaphylaxis. Leukotriene B_4, a potent chemotactic factor for neutrophils, macrophages and eosinophils, is formed during anaphylaxis and is involved in attracting inflammatory cells into tissues.

Another inflammatory mediator synthesized by mast cells is **platelet-activating factor** (PAF), a lipid derived from membrane phospholipids. As its name implies, PAF is a potent inducer of platelet aggregation and release of vasoactive amines from platelets. It is also a potent neutrophil chemotaxin. It has a broad range of activities and can activate all types of phagocytic cells.

As mentioned above, activated T cells, specifically Th2 T cells, produce cytokines that have important roles in allergic responses. Activated Th2 T-cell subsets produce IL-4, IL-5 and IL-13, leading to IgE production and increased numbers of mast cells and eosinophils. In allergy-prone people, a similar response occurs via T-cell clones that produce IL-4, IL-6 and IL-2, concentrations of which are also increased in allergic individuals. These persons also have reduced levels of IFN-γ, which suppresses development of Th2 clones and subsequent production of IgE.

In summary, type I (immediate) hypersensitivity reactions are characterized by a specific cytophilic antibody (IgE), which binds to high-affinity receptors on basophils and mast

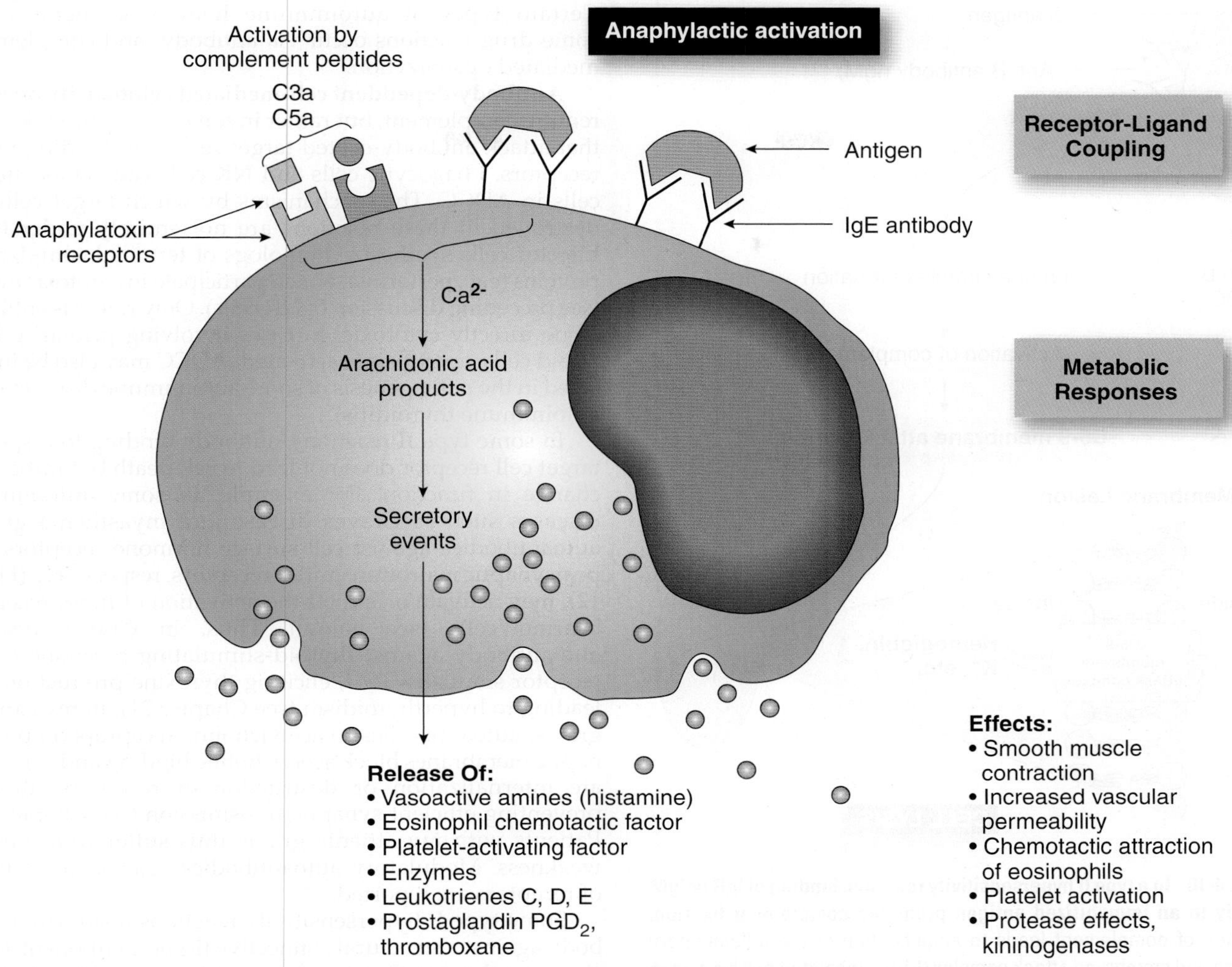

FIGURE 4-9. In a type I hypersensitivity reaction, allergen binds to cytophilic surface IgE antibody on a mast cell or basophil and triggers cell activation and the release of a cascade of proinflammatory mediators. These mediators are responsible for smooth muscle contraction, edema formation and the recruitment of eosinophils. Ca^{2+} = calcium ion; Ig = immunoglobulin; PGD_2 = prostaglandin D_2.

cells and reacts with a specific antigen (allergen). Activated mast cells and basophils release preformed (granule) products and synthesize mediators that cause the classic manifestations of immediate hypersensitivity and the late-phase reaction.

Type II Hypersensitivity Reactions Are Mediated by Antibodies Against Fixed Cellular or Extracellular Antigens

IgG and IgM typically mediate type II reactions. An important characteristic of these antibodies is their ability to activate complement through the immunoglobulin Fc domain. There are several antibody-dependent mechanisms of tissue injury.

The prototypic model of antibody-mediated erythrocyte cytotoxicity is illustrated in Fig. 4-10. IgM or IgG antibody binds an antigen at the erythrocyte membrane. At sufficient density, the bound immunoglobulin fixes complement via C1q and the classical pathway (see Chapter 2). Activated complement can destroy target cells by several mechanisms. Complement products can lyse target cells directly, via C5b-9 complement complexes (Fig. 4-10). This complex, called the **membrane attack complex,** inserts like the staves of a barrel into the plasma membrane and forms holes or ion channels, destroying the permeability barrier and inducing cell lysis. This type of complement-mediated cell lysis is exemplified by certain types of autoimmune hemolytic anemias resulting from antibodies against erythrocyte blood group antigens. In transfusion reactions that result from major blood group incompatibilities, hemolysis occurs through activation of complement.

Complement and antibody molecules can also destroy a target cell by **opsonization**. Target cells coated (opsonized) with immunoglobulin and/or C3b molecules are bound by phagocytes that express Fc or C3b receptors. Complement activation near a target cell surface leads to formation and covalent bonding of C3b (Fig. 4-11). Many phagocytic cells, including neutrophils and macrophages, have cell membrane

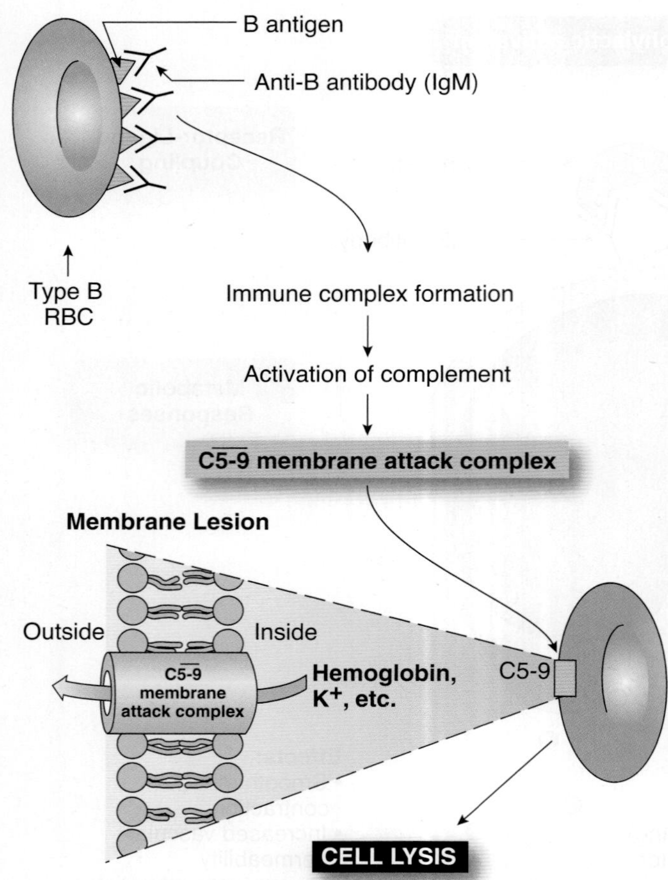

FIGURE 4-10. In a type II hypersensitivity reaction, binding of IgG or IgM antibody to an immobilized antigen promotes complement fixation. Activation of complement leads to amplification of the inflammatory response and membrane attack complex (MAC)-mediated cell lysis. Ig = immunoglobulin; K^+ = potassium ion; RBC = red blood cell.

Fc and C3b receptors. By binding to its receptor, immunoglobulin or C3b bridges the target and effector (phagocytic) cells, thereby enhancing phagocytosis and subsequent intracellular destruction of the antibody- or complement-coated cell. Certain types of autoimmune hemolytic anemias and some drug reactions occur via antibody- and complement-mediated opsonization.

Antibody-dependent cell-mediated cytotoxicity does not require complement, but rather involves cytolytic leukocytes that attack antibody-coated target cells after binding via Fc receptors. Phagocytic cells and NK cells can act as effector cells in ADCC. The mechanisms by which target cells are destroyed in these reactions are not entirely understood. Effector cells synthesize homologs of terminal complement proteins (e.g., perforins), which participate in cytotoxic events (see preceding discussion of NK cells). Only rarely is antibody alone directly cytotoxic. In cases involving primarily lymphoid cells, apoptosis is activated. ADCC may also be implicated in the pathogenesis of some autoimmune diseases (e.g., autoimmune thyroiditis).

In some type II reactions, antibody binding to a specific target cell receptor does not lead to cell death but rather to a change in function. For example, in some autoimmune diseases such as Graves disease and myasthenia gravis, autoantibodies against cell surface hormone receptors and postsynaptic neurotransmitter receptors, respectively (Fig. 4-12), may activate or inhibit the activation of those receptor-bearing cells (see below). Thus, in Graves disease, autoantibody against thyroid-stimulating hormone (TSH) receptor simulates TSH, eliciting thyroxine production and leading to hyperthyroidism (see Chapter 21). In myasthenia gravis, autoantibodies to acetylcholine receptors on postsynaptic membranes block acetylcholine binding and/or mediate internalization or destruction of receptors, thereby preventing efficient synaptic transmission (see Chapter 27). Patients with myasthenia gravis thus suffer from muscle weakness. Modulatory autoantibodies against many types of receptors are reported.

Some type II hypersensitivity reactions result from antibody against a structural connective tissue component. Classic examples are Goodpasture syndrome and the bullous skin diseases, pemphigus and pemphigoid (see Chapter 24). In these diseases, circulating antibody binds intrinsic connective tissue antigens and evokes a destructive local inflammatory response. In Goodpasture syndrome, antibody binds the noncollagenous domain of type IV collagen, which is a major structural component of pulmonary and glomerular basement membranes (Fig. 4-13). Local complement activation results in neutrophil chemotaxis, tissue injury and

FIGURE 4-11. In a type II hypersensitivity reaction, opsonization by antibody or complement leads to phagocytosis via either Fc or C3b receptors, respectively. Ig = immunoglobulin; PMN = polymorphonuclear neutrophil; RBC = red blood cell.

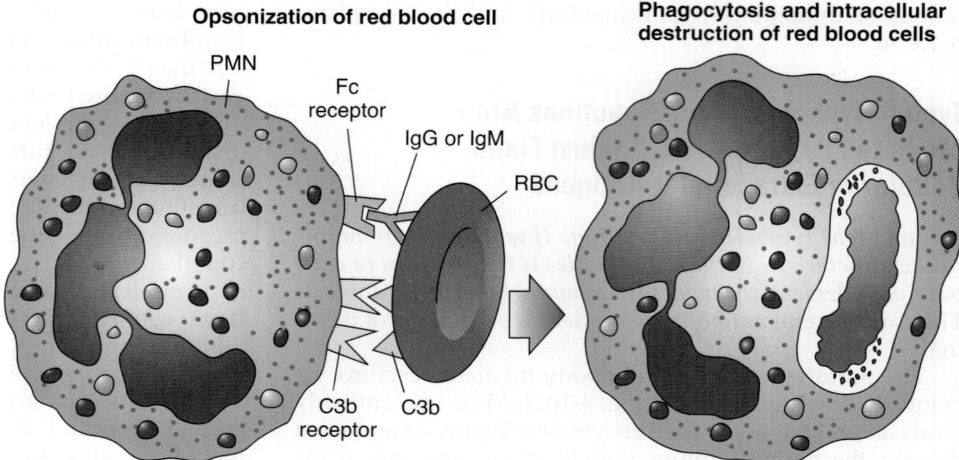

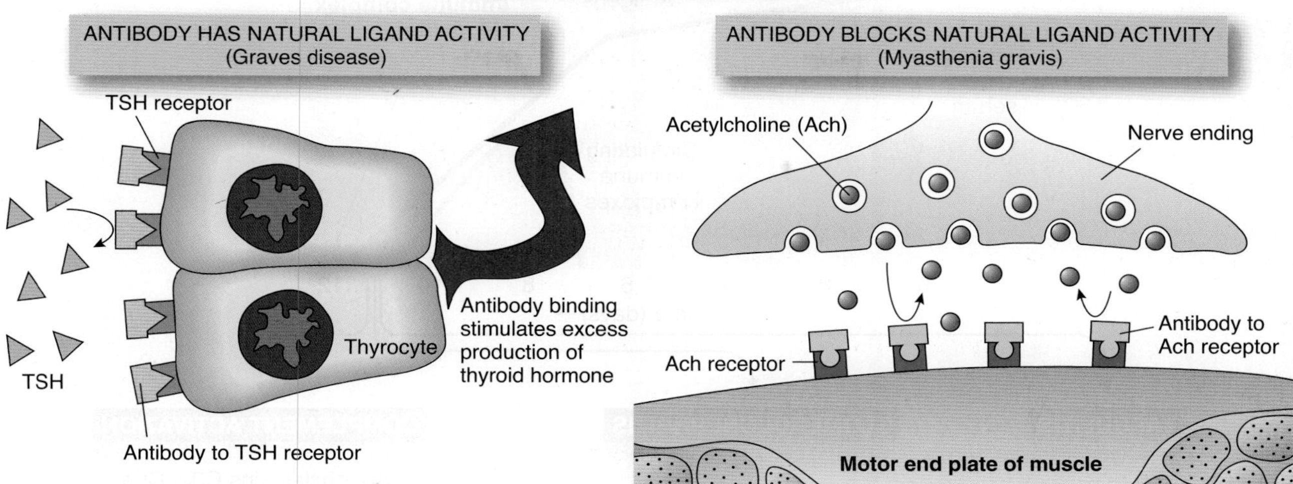

FIGURE 4-12. In a type II hypersensitivity reaction, antibodies bind to a cell surface receptor and induce activation (e.g., thyroid-stimulating hormone [TSH] receptors in Graves disease) or inhibition/destruction (e.g., acetylcholine receptors in myasthenia gravis).

pulmonary hemorrhage and glomerulonephritis. Direct complement-mediated damage to glomerular and alveolar basement membranes via membrane attack complexes may also be involved.

In summary, type II hypersensitivity reactions are directly or indirectly cytotoxic through action of antibodies against antigens on cell surfaces or in connective tissues. Complement participates in many of these cytotoxic events. Lysis is mediated directly by complement, indirectly by opsonization and phagocytosis or via chemotactic attraction of phagocytic cells, which produce a large variety of tissue-damaging products. Complement-independent reactions, such as ADCC, also play a role in type II hypersensitivity reactions.

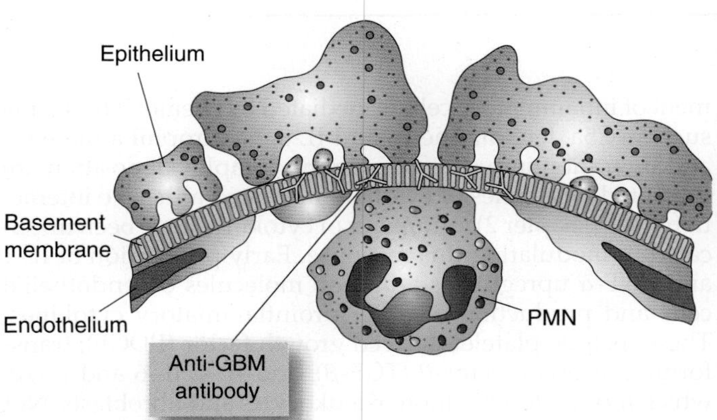

FIGURE 4-13. Goodpasture syndrome. In a type II hypersensitivity reaction, antibody binds to a surface antigen, activates the complement system and leads to the recruitment of tissue-damaging inflammatory cells. Several complement-derived peptides (e.g., C5a) are potent chemotactic factors. GBM = glomerular basement membrane; PMN = polymorphonuclear neutrophil.

In Type III Hypersensitivity Reactions Immune Complex Deposition or Formation in Situ Leads to Complement Fixation and Inflammation

IgG, IgM and occasionally IgA antibody against a circulating antigen or an antigen that is deposited or "planted" in a tissue can cause a type III response. Physicochemical characteristics of the immune complexes, such as size, charge and solubility, in addition to immunoglobulin isotype, determine whether an immune complex deposits in tissue and fixes complement. "Phlogistic" (inflammatory) immune complexes elicit inflammatory responses by activating complement, leading to recruitment of neutrophils and monocytes to the site. These activated phagocytes release tissue-damaging mediators, such as proteases and reactive oxygen intermediates.

Immune complexes have been implicated in many human diseases (Fig. 4-14). The most compelling cases are those in which demonstration of immune complexes in injured tissue correlates with development of injury. Examples include cryoglobulinemic vasculitis associated with hepatitis C infection, Henoch-Schönlein purpura (in which IgA deposits are found at sites of vasculitis) and systemic lupus erythematosus (SLE) (anti–double-stranded DNA in vasculitic lesions). In many diseases, immune complexes can be detected in plasma but there is no tissue injury. The physicochemical properties of circulating immune complexes frequently differ from those of complexes deposited in tissues. In some cases, vascular permeability may determine the localization of circulating immune complexes. Diseases that seem to be most clearly attributable to immune complex deposition are autoimmune diseases of connective tissue, such as SLE and rheumatoid arthritis, some types of vasculitis and many varieties of glomerulonephritis.

Serum sickness is an acute, self-limited disease that typically occurs 6 to 8 days after injection of a foreign protein.

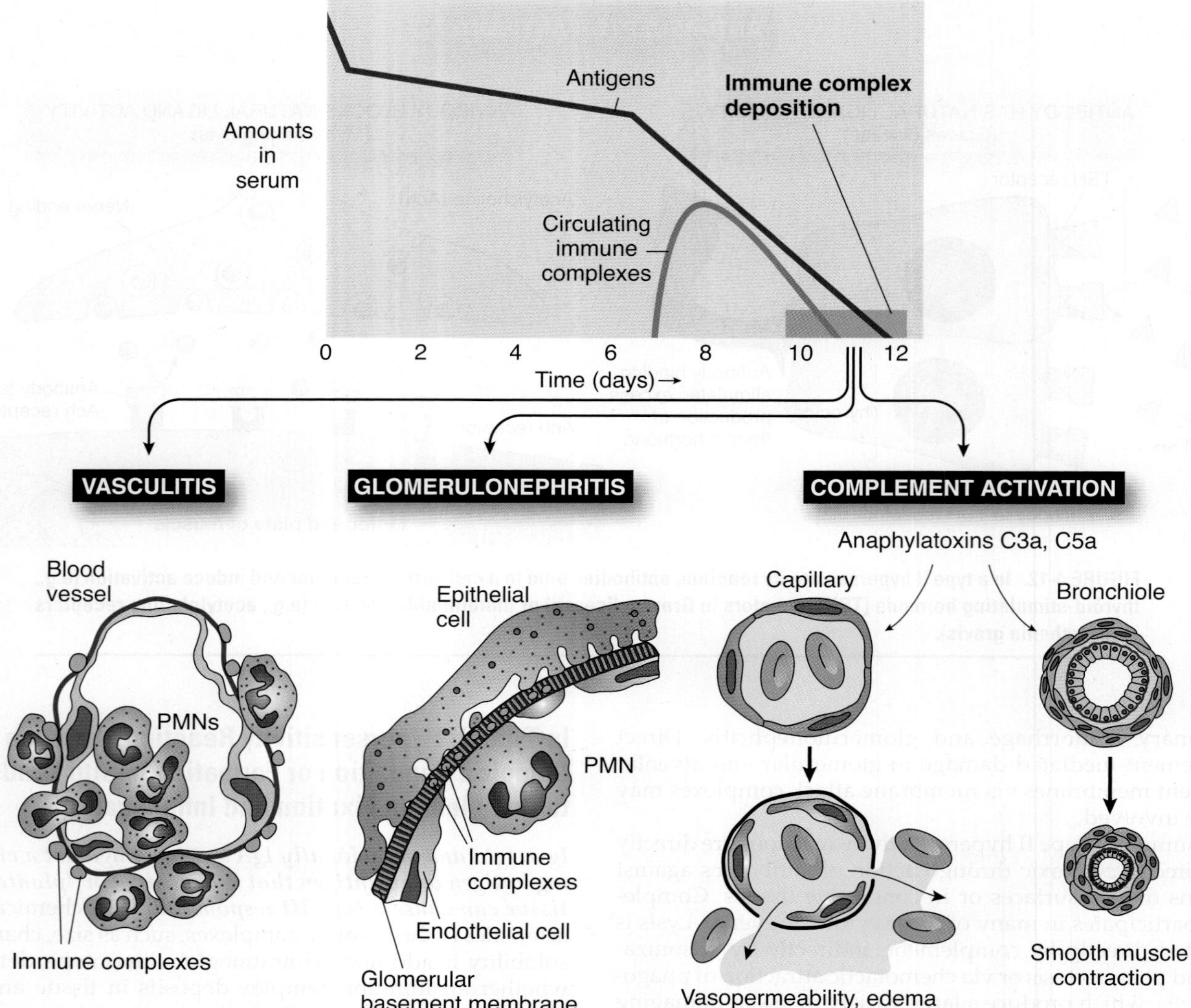

FIGURE 4-14. In type III hypersensitivity, immune complexes are deposited and can lead to complement activation and the recruitment of tissue-damaging inflammatory cells. The ability of immune complexes to mediate tissue injury depends on size, solubility, net charge and ability to fix complement. PMN = polymorphonuclear neutrophil.

Human serum sickness is uncommon, but sometimes occurs in patients who have received foreign proteins therapeutically (e.g., antilymphocyte globulin). It is characterized by fever, arthralgias, vasculitis and acute glomerulonephritis. In experimental acute serum sickness, levels of exogenously injected antigen in the circulation remain constant until about day 6, after which they fall rapidly (Fig. 4-14). At the same time, immune complexes (containing IgM or IgG bound to antigen) appear in the circulation. Some of these circulating complexes deposit in tissues such as renal glomeruli and blood vessel walls. They are rendered more soluble by their interaction with the complement system, which enhances tissue deposition. Interaction of immune complexes with complement also generates C3a and C5a, which increase vascular permeability.

Once phlogistic immune complexes are deposited in tissues, they trigger an inflammatory response. Local activation of complement by immune complexes results in formation of C5a, which is a potent neutrophil chemoattractant. Recruitment of inflammatory cells is mediated by chemotactic agents such as C5a, leukotriene B_4 and IL-8. Neutrophil adherence and migration into sites of immune complex deposition are mediated by a series of cytokine-mediated adhesive interactions (see Chapter 2). A number of cytokines have been implicated in modulating this response. Early production of IL-1 and TNF-α upregulates adhesion molecules on endothelial cells and production of other proinflammatory cytokines. These include platelet-derived growth factor (PDGF); transforming growth factor-β (TGF-β); and IL-4, IL-6 and IL-10, which modulate activation of leukocytes and fibroblasts. Not all cytokines are proinflammatory; IL-10, in particular, downregulates inflammatory responses.

Upon arrival, neutrophils are activated through contact with, and ingestion of, immune complexes. Activated leukocytes release many inflammatory mediators, including proteases, reactive oxygen intermediates and arachidonic acid products, which collectively produce tissue injury. The tissue injury associated with experimental serum sickness mimics

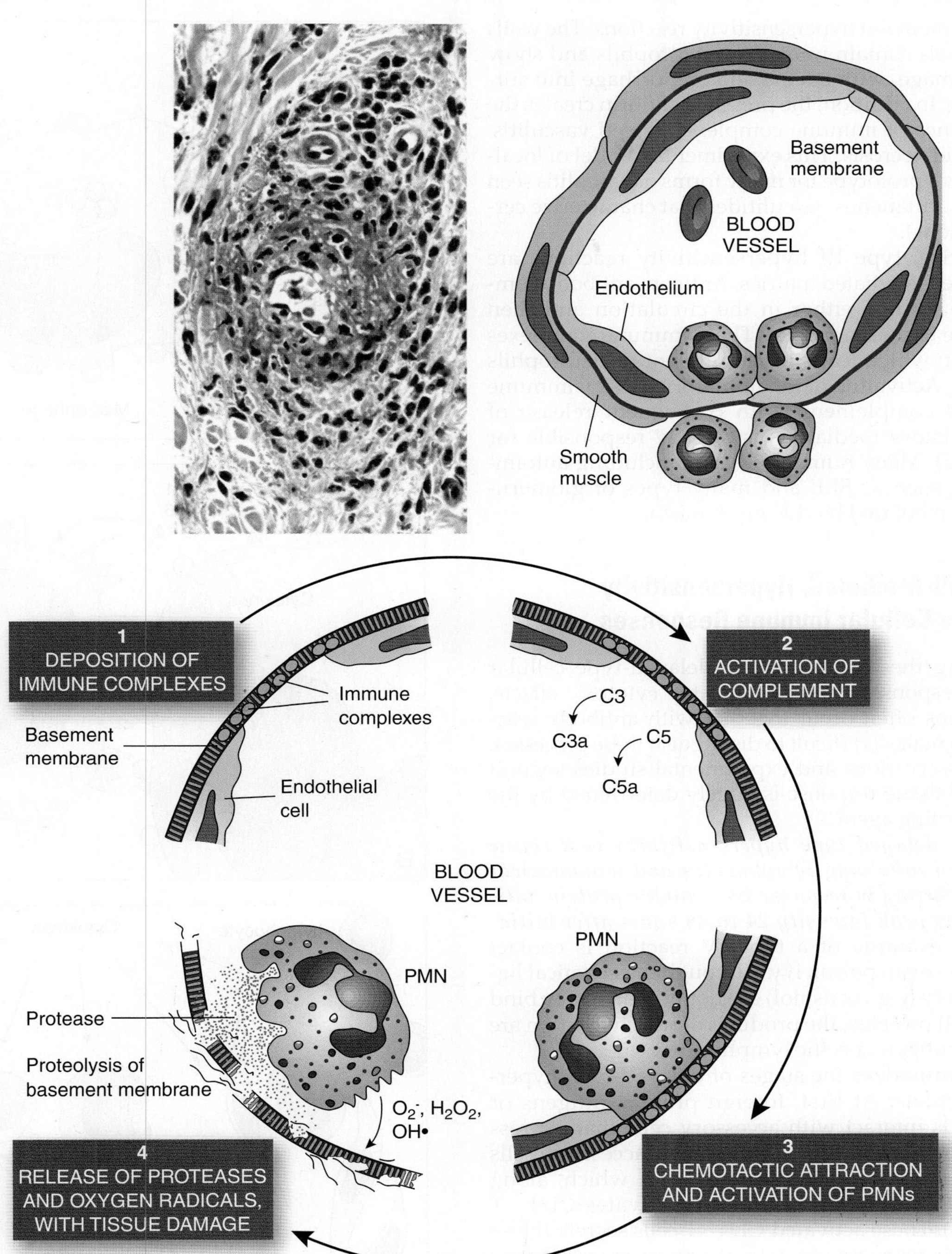

FIGURE 4-15. The Arthus reaction is a type III hypersensitivity reaction characterized by the deposition of immune complexes and the induction of an acute inflammatory response within blood vessel walls. Some vasculitic lesions exhibit fibrinoid necrosis. H_2O_2 = hydrogen peroxide; O_2^- = superoxide ion; OH• = hydroxyl radical; PMN = polymorphonuclear neutrophil.

that seen in many types of human vasculitis and glomerulonephritis.

The **Arthus reaction** has been characterized in an experimental model of vasculitis in which a localized injury is induced by immune complexes (Fig. 4-15). This reaction is classically seen in dermal blood vessels after local injection of an antigen to which an individual was previously sensitized. The circulating antibody and locally injected antigen diffuse down concentration gradients toward each other to form immune complex deposits in walls of small blood vessels. Resulting vascular injury is mediated by complement fixation, followed by recruitment and activation of neutrophils, which release their tissue-damaging mediators. Because injury in the Arthus reaction is caused by recruited neutrophils and their products, 2 to 10 hours are required for evidence of tissue injury. This is in marked contrast to more rapid type I (immediate) hypersensitivity reactions. The walls of affected vessels contain numerous neutrophils and show evidence of damage, with edema and hemorrhage into surrounding tissue. In addition, the presence of fibrin creates the classic appearance of immune complex–induced vasculitis, namely, fibrinoid necrosis. This experimental model of localized vasculitis is a prototype for many forms of vasculitis seen in humans (e.g., cutaneous vasculitides that characterize certain drug reactions).

To summarize, type III hypersensitivity reactions are immune complex–mediated injuries. Antigen–antibody complexes may be formed either in the circulation and then deposited in the tissues, or in situ. These immune complexes fix complement, which leads to recruitment of neutrophils and monocytes. Activation of inflammatory cells by immune complexes and complement, with consequent release of potent inflammatory mediators, is directly responsible for injury (Fig. 4-15). Many human diseases, including autoimmune diseases such as SLE and many types of glomerulonephritis, are mediated by this mechanism.

Type IV, or Cell-Mediated, Hypersensitivity Reactions Are Cellular Immune Responses

Included among these reactions are delayed-type cellular inflammatory responses and cell-mediated cytotoxic effects. Type IV reactions often occur together with antibody reactions, which can make it difficult to distinguish these processes. Both clinical observations and experimental studies suggest that the type of tissue response is largely determined by the nature of the inciting agent.

Classically, delayed-type hypersensitivity is a tissue reaction, mainly involving lymphocytes and mononuclear phagocytes, occurring in response to a soluble protein antigen and reaching peak intensity 24 to 48 hours after initiation. A classic example of a type IV reaction is contact sensitivity response to poison ivy. Although the chemical ligands in poison ivy (e.g., urushiol) are not proteins, they bind covalently to cell proteins, the products of which reaction are recognized by antigen-specific lymphocytes.

Fig. 4-16 summarizes the stages of delayed-type hypersensitivity reactions. At first, foreign protein antigens or chemical ligands interact with accessory cells that express class II HLA molecules (Fig. 4-16A). Such accessory cells (macrophages, dendritic cells) secrete IL-12, which, along with processed and presented antigen, activates CD4$^+$ T cells (Fig. 4-16B). These activated CD4$^+$ T cells secrete IFN-γ and IL-2, which respectively activate more macrophages and elicit T-lymphocyte proliferation (Fig. 4-16C). The protein antigens are actively processed into short peptides within phagolysosomes of macrophages and then presented on the cell surface in conjunction with class II HLA molecules. Processed and presented antigens are recognized by MHC-restricted, antigen-specific CD4$^+$ T cells, which become activated and synthesize an array of cytokines. Such activated CD4$^+$ cells are referred to as Th1 cells. In turn, the cytokines recruit and activate lymphocytes, monocytes, fibroblasts and other inflammatory cells. If the antigenic stimulus is eliminated, the reaction resolves spontaneously after about 48 hours. If the stimulus persists (e.g., poorly biodegradable mycobacterial cell wall components), an attempt to sequester the inciting agent may result in a granulomatous reaction.

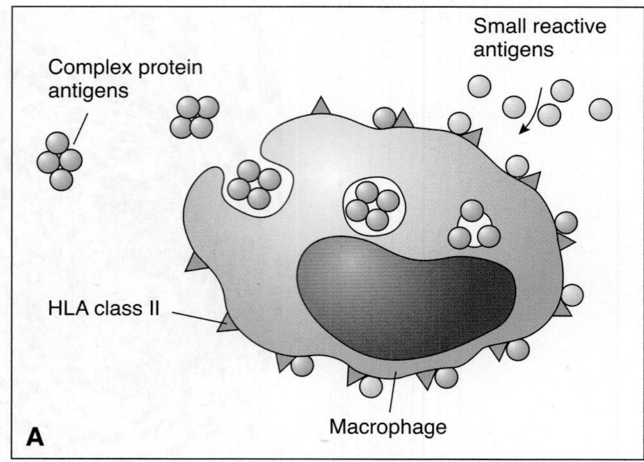

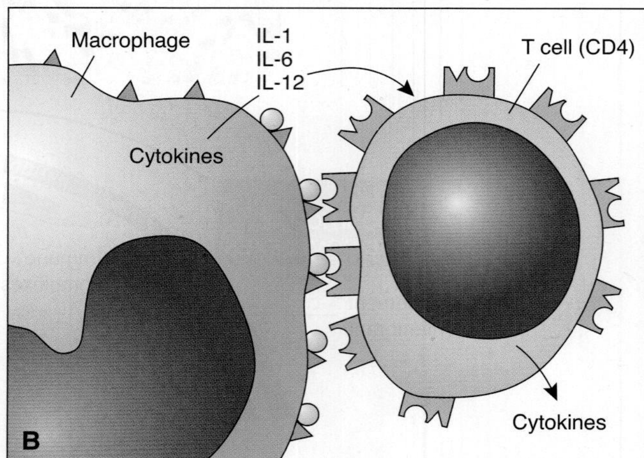

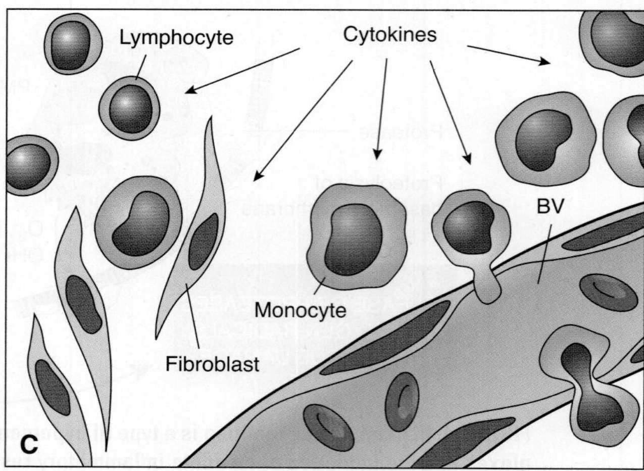

FIGURE 4-16. In a type IV (delayed-type) hypersensitivity reaction, complex antigens are phagocytized, processed and presented on macrophage cell membranes in conjunction with class II major histocompatibility complex (MHC) antigens. A. Antigen-specific, histocompatible, cytotoxic T lymphocytes bind the presented antigens and are activated. **B, C.** Activated cytotoxic T cells secrete cytokines that amplify the response. BV = blood vessel.

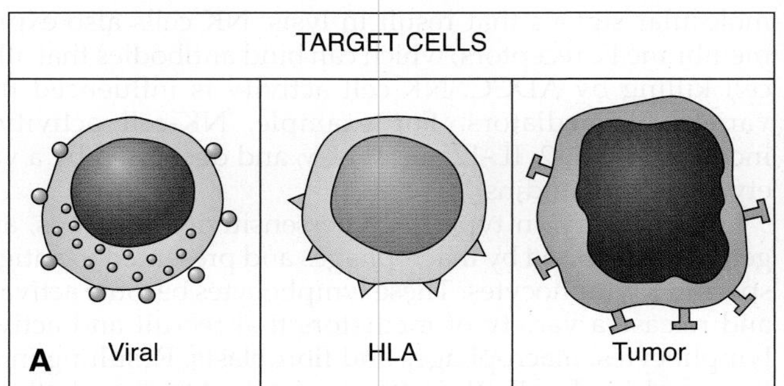

TARGET ANTIGENS
- Virally-coded membrane antigen
- Foreign or modified histocompatibility antigen
- Tumor-specific membrane antigens

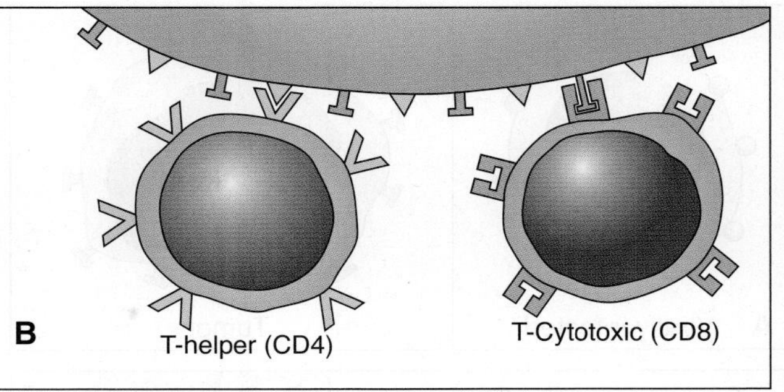

RECOGNITION OF ANTIGEN BY T CELLS
- T-helper cells recognize antigen plus class II molecules
- T-cytotoxic/killer cells recognize antigen plus class I molecules

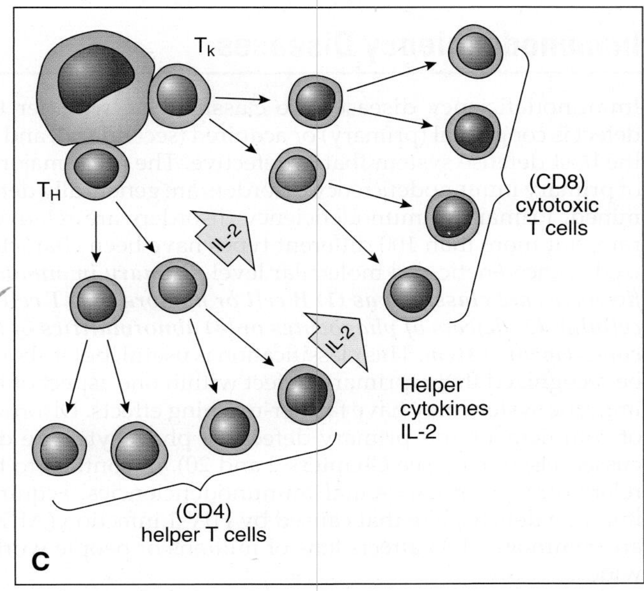

ACTIVATION AND AMPLIFICATION
- T-helper cells activate and proliferate, releasing helper molecules (e.g., IL-2)
- T-cytotoxic/killer cells proliferate in response to helper molecules

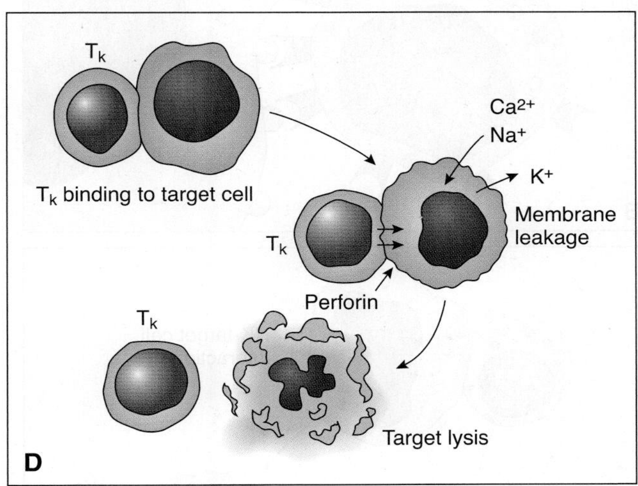

TARGET CELL KILLING
- T-cytotoxic/killer cells bind to target cell
- Killing signals perforin release and target cell loses membrane integrity
- Target cell undergoes lysis

FIGURE 4-17. In T-cell–mediated cytotoxicity, potential target cells include (A) virus-infected host cells, malignant host cells and foreign (histoincompatible transplanted) cells. **B.** Cytotoxic T lymphocytes recognize foreign antigens in the context of human leukocyte antigen (HLA) class I molecules. **C.** Activated T cells secrete lytic compounds (e.g., perforin and other mediators) and cytokines that amplify the response. **D.** Apoptosis (target cell killing) is mediated by perforin and involves influx of Ca^{2+} (calcium ion) and Na^+ (sodium ion), and efflux of K^+ (potassium ion); IL = interleukin.

Another mechanism by which T cells (especially CD8$^+$) *mediate tissue damage is direct cytolysis of target cells* (Fig. 4-17). This immune mechanism is important in destroying and eliminating cells infected by viruses, transplanted tissues and, possibly, tumor cells.

Fig. 4-17 summarizes the events in T-cell–mediated cytotoxicity. In contrast to delayed-type hypersensitivity reactions, cytotoxic CD8$^+$ T cells specifically recognize target antigens in the context of class I MHC molecules (Fig. 4-17). In the case of virus-infected cells and tumor cells, foreign antigens are actively presented together with self-MHC antigens. In graft rejection, foreign MHC antigens are themselves potent activators of CD8$^+$ T cells. Once activated by antigen, cytotoxic cell proliferation is aided by helper cells and mediated by soluble growth factors such as IL-2 (Fig. 4-17C). Expanded populations of antigen-specific cytotoxic cells are thus generated. Actual cell killing occurs via several mechanisms (Fig. 4-17D; see also Chapter 1). Cytolytic T cells (CTLs) secrete perforins that form pores in target cell membranes and introduce granzymes that activate intracellular caspases, leading to apoptosis. CTLs can also kill targets via engagement of Fas ligand (by the CTL) and Fas (on the target). Fas ligand–Fas interaction triggers apoptosis of the Fas-bearing cell.

The defining characteristics of NK cells have been described, but the extent to which such cells participate in tissue-damaging reactions is unclear. Some evidence indicates

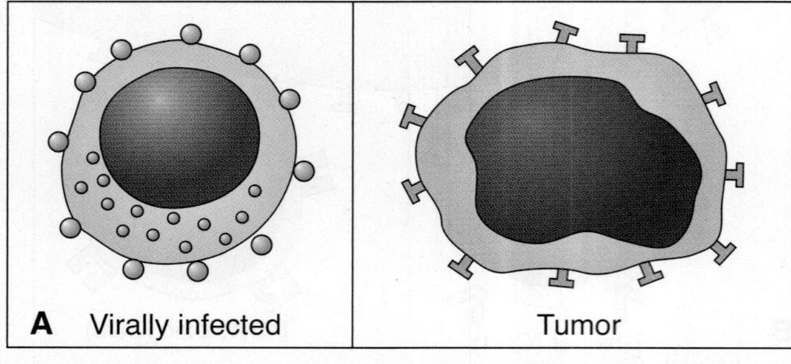

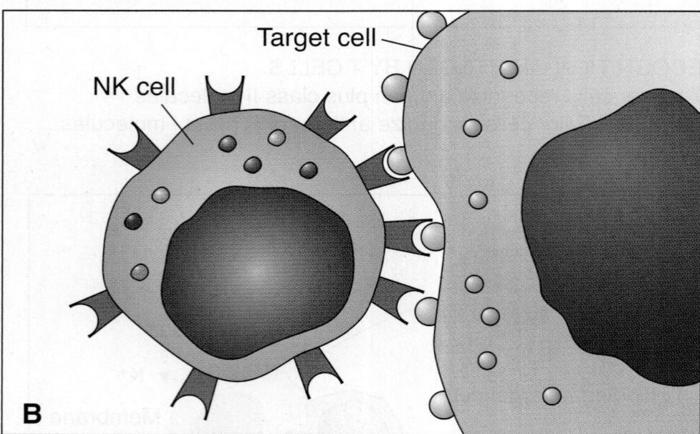

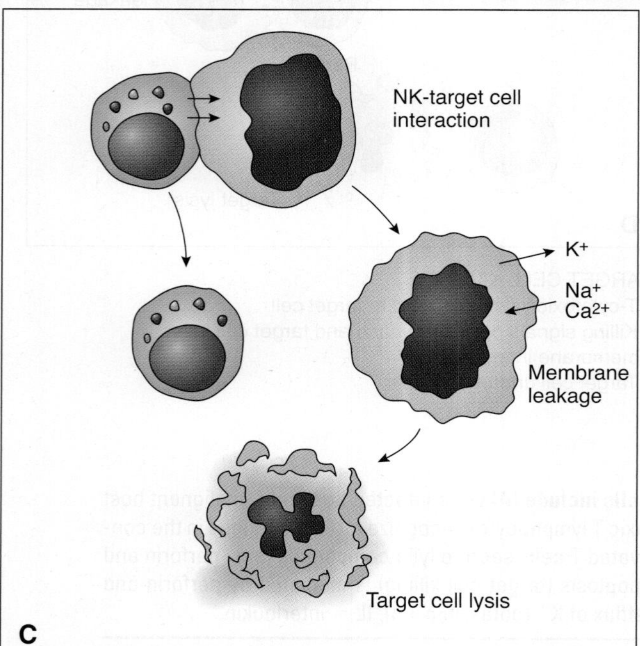

FIGURE 4-18. In natural killer (NK)-cell–mediated cytotoxicity, potential target cells include virus-infected and neoplastic cells (A). NK cells bind target cells **(B)**, are activated and secrete lytic compounds **(C)**. Ca^{2+} = calcium ion; K^{+} = potassium ion; Na^{+} = sodium ion.

that NK cells exert both effector and immunoregulatory functions. Fig. 4-18 summarizes target cell killing by NK cells. NK cells can recognize a variety of target cells. Target molecules include membrane glycoproteins expressed by certain virus-infected cells and tumor cells. In a series of events similar to those described for cytotoxic T cells, NK cells bind to target cells through their membrane receptors and then deliver molecular signals that result in lysis. NK cells also express membrane Fc receptors, which can bind antibodies that allow cell killing by ADCC. NK-cell activity is influenced by a variety of mediators. For example, NK-cell activity is increased by IL-2, IL-12 and IFN-γ, and decreased by a variety of prostaglandins.

In summary, in type IV hypersensitivity reactions, antigens are processed by macrophages and presented to antigen-specific T lymphocytes. These lymphocytes become activated and release a variety of mediators that recruit and activate lymphocytes, macrophages and fibroblasts. Resulting injury is caused by T cells themselves, macrophages or both. No antibodies are involved. The chronic inflammation in many autoimmune diseases—including type 1 diabetes, chronic thyroiditis, Sjögren syndrome and primary biliary cirrhosis—is largely the result of type IV hypersensitivity.

Immunodeficiency Diseases

Immunodeficiency diseases are classified by whether the defect is congenital (primary) or acquired (secondary), and by the host defense system that is defective. The great majority of primary immunodeficiency disorders are genetically determined. Primary immunodeficiency disorders are relatively rare, but more than 100 different types have been characterized at the genetic and molecular level. ***Primary immunodeficiencies are classified as (1) B cell or humoral, (2) T cell or cellular, (3) defects of phagocytes or (4) abnormalities of the complement system.*** This classification is useful, but it should be recognized that a primary defect within one aspect of the immune system may have farther-reaching effects. Disorders of complement and primary defects of phagocytes are discussed elsewhere (see Chapters 2 and 20). In contrast to the relative rarity of congenital immunodeficiencies, acquired immune deficits, like that caused by HIV-1 infection (AIDS), are common: AIDS affects tens of millions of people worldwide.

Functional defects in lymphocytes can be localized to particular stages in the ontogeny of the immune system, or to interruption of discrete immune activation events (Fig. 4-19). The explosive growth of knowledge regarding molecular mechanisms of immunodeficiency disorders has led to improved diagnosis, clinical management and therapeutic strategies. Identification of specific molecular defects and mechanistic understanding of the pathophysiology of various disorders have also provided great insight into the function of the immune system. A detailed classification scheme for primary immunodeficiency disorders is available via the World Health Organization (WHO). The most efficient diagnostic approach is a careful history with particular attention to age of onset, types of infection and judicious laboratory testing.

Primary Antibody Deficiency Diseases Are Characterized by Impaired Production of Antibodies

Patients with these diseases are subject to recurrent bacterial infections, a limited number of specific types of viral infections (e.g., echovirus infections of the central nervous

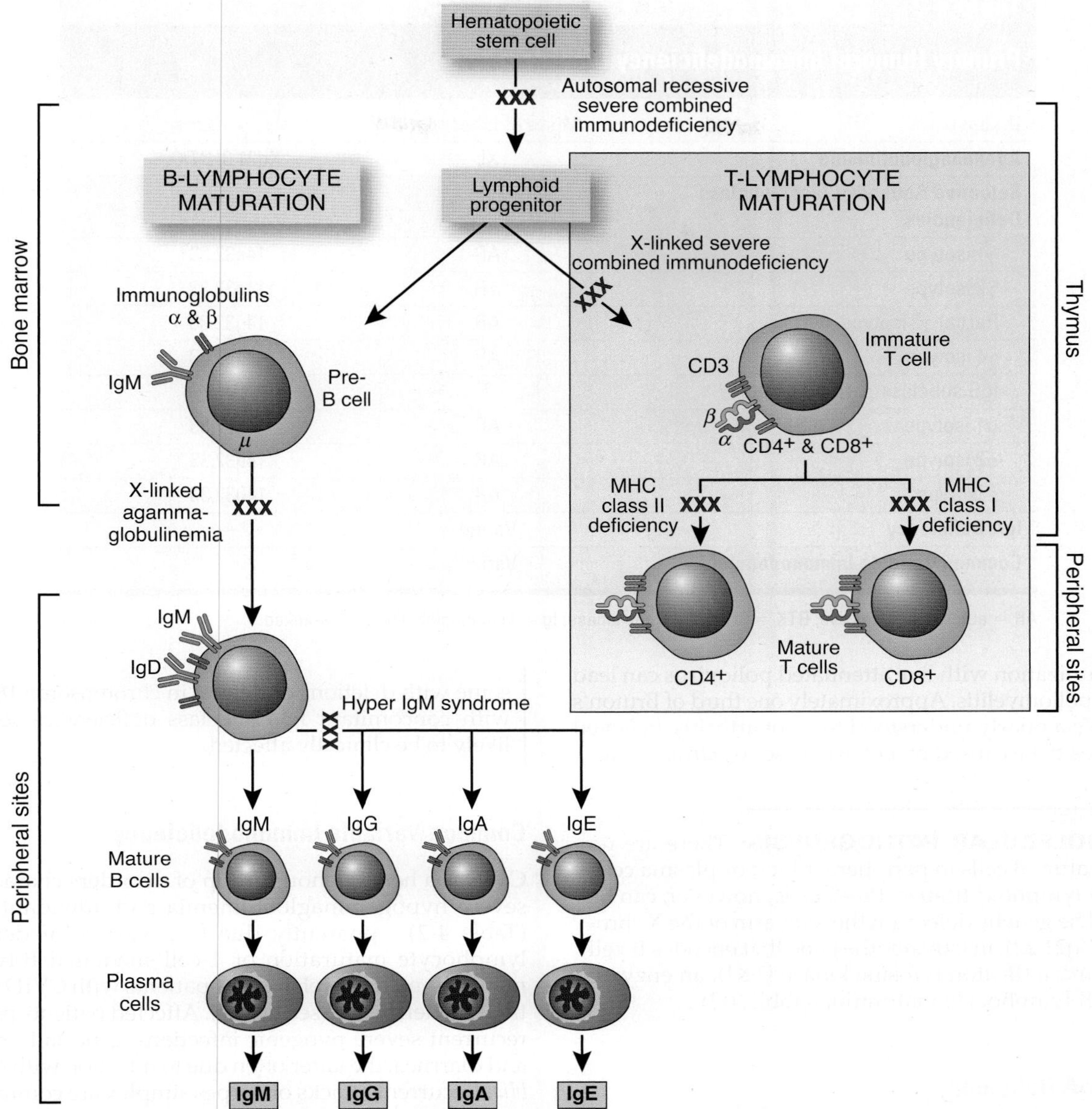

FIGURE 4-19. Hematopoietic stem cells give rise to lymphoid progenitor cells that, in a predetermined manner, populate either the bone marrow or thymus. Many primary immunodeficiency disorders have been characterized at both genetic and molecular mechanistic levels. In a number of immunodeficiency disorders, a discrete molecular defect results in a form of "maturational arrest" in the development of fully differentiated and functional lymphocytes.

system [CNS] in patients with Bruton agammaglobulinemia) and subnormal serum concentrations of either all or specific isotypes of immunoglobulin. There are a variety of immunoglobulin isotype and subclass deficiencies (Table 4-2). These include selective deletions of immunoglobulin heavy chains and selective loss of light-chain expression. In addition, some patients have normal levels of immunoglobulins but fail to make antibodies against specific antigens, usually polysaccharides. The clinical manifestations of these entities are highly variable; some patients suffer from life-threatening bacterial infections, varying from meningitis to mucosal infections, whereas other patients are asymptomatic.

Bruton X-Linked Agammaglobulinemia

Bruton X-linked agammaglobulinemia (XLA) typically presents in male infants at 7 to 9 months old, at which time maternal antibody levels have declined. As many as 10% of XLA patients do not present until they are teenagers and recent studies suggest that as many as 10% of adults classified as having "common variable immunodeficiency (CVID)" (see below) actually have XLA. These patients develop recurrent infections of mucosal tracts, pyoderma, meningitis and septicemia. Severe hypogammaglobulinemia involves all immunoglobulin isotypes. Occasional patients develop viral hepatitis or chronic enterovirus infections of the CNS or large

Table 4-2

Primary Humoral Immunodeficiency Disorders

Disease	Mode of Inheritance	Locus/Gene
Agammaglobulinemia	XL	Xq21.3/*BTK*
Selective Antibody Class/Subclass Deficiencies		
γ1 isotype	AR	14q32.33
γ2 isotype	AR	14q32.33
Partial γ3 isotype	AR	14q32.33
γ4 isotype	AR	14q32.33
IgG subclass ± IgA deficiency	?	—
α1 isotype	AR	14q32.33
α2 isotype	AR	14q32.33
ε isotype	AR	14q32.33
IgA Deficiency	Varied	—
Common Variable Immunodeficiency	Varied	—

AR = autosomal recessive; BTK = Bruton tyrosine kinase; Ig = immunoglobulin; XL = X-linked.

joints. Immunization with live attenuated poliovirus can lead to paralytic poliomyelitis. Approximately one third of Bruton's patients have a poorly understood form of arthritis, believed in some cases to be caused by enteroviruses or *Ureaplasma.*

MOLECULAR PATHOGENESIS: There are no mature B cells in peripheral blood or plasma cells in lymphoid tissues. Pre-B cells, however, can be detected. The genetic defect, on the long arm of the X chromosome (Xq21.22), inactivates the gene that encodes B-cell tyrosine kinase (Bruton tyrosine kinase [TK]), an enzyme critical to B-lymphocyte maturation (Table 4-2).

Selective IgA Deficiency

Selective IgA deficiency is the most common primary immunodeficiency syndrome. It is characterized by normal serum levels of IgG and IgM and low serum (<7 mg/dL) and secretory concentrations of IgA. Its incidence ranges from 1:18,000 in Japanese to 1:400 among Europeans. Patients are often asymptomatic but occasionally present with respiratory or gastrointestinal infections of varying severity. They also display a strong predilection for allergies, autoimmune diseases and collagen vascular disorders. Patients with selective IgA deficiency are at risk for allergic, occasionally anaphylactic, reactions to IgA-containing transfused blood products.

MOLECULAR PATHOGENESIS: Patients with IgA deficiency have peripheral blood B cells that coexpress IgA, IgM and IgD; their varied and poorly understood defects result in an inability to synthesize and secrete IgA (Table 4-2). There may be a common origin with CVID (see below). Some cases have been associated with drug exposures (e.g., phenytoin, D-penicillamine) and some with deletions or defects in chromosome 18. Patients with concomitant IgG subclass deficiencies seem more likely to be clinically affected.

Common Variable Immunodeficiency

CVID is a heterogenous group of disorders characterized by severe hypogammaglobulinemia and attendant infections (Table 4-2), apparently due to a variety of defects in B-lymphocyte maturation or T-cell–mediated B-lymphocyte maturation. Many relatives of patients with CVID have selective IgA deficiency (see below). Affected patients present with recurrent severe pyogenic infections, especially pneumonia and diarrhea, the latter often due to infection with *Giardia lamblia*. Recurrent attacks of herpes simplex are common; herpes zoster develops in one fifth of patients. The disease appears years to decades after birth, with a mean age at onset of 25 years. The incidence is estimated to be between 1:50,000 and 1:200,000. Inheritance patterns are variable. CVID features a variety of maturational and regulatory defects of the immune system. Cancers are increased in CVID, including a 50-fold greater incidence of gastric cancer. Interestingly, lymphoma is 300 times more frequent in women with this immunodeficiency than in affected men. Malabsorption due to lymphoid hyperplasia and inflammatory bowel diseases occurs more frequently than in the general population. CVID patients are also susceptible to other autoimmune disorders, including hemolytic anemia, neutropenia, thrombocytopenia and pernicious anemia.

Transient Hypogammaglobulinemia of Infancy

Prolonged hypogammaglobulinemia occurs in transient hypogammaglobulinemia of infancy after maternal antibodies in the infant have reached their nadir. Some affected infants develop recurrent infections and require therapy, but all eventually produce immunoglobulins. These infants possess mature B cells that are temporarily unable to produce antibodies. The defect is not well understood but is thought to represent delayed helper T-cell signal-generating capacity.

Hyper-IgM Syndrome

This syndrome is often classified as a humoral immunodeficiency because immunoglobulin production is disordered. Patients have subnormal IgG, IgA and IgE levels and elevated IgM concentrations. There is an X-linked form that results from defects in CD40 ligand (so-called type 1 hyper-IgM) and an autosomal recessive form due to defects in CD40 (so-called type 3 hyper-IgM). Infants with the X-linked form of this disease exhibit pyogenic and opportunistic infections, especially with *Pneumocystis jiroveci* (formerly *Pneumocystis carinii*). They also tend to develop autoimmune diseases involving the formed elements of blood, especially autoimmune hemolytic anemia, thrombocytopenic purpura and recurrent, severe neutropenia.

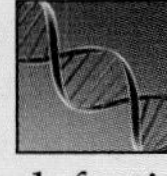

MOLECULAR PATHOGENESIS: Circulating B cells bear only IgM and IgD. The "switch" to other heavy-chain isotypes from IgD/IgM appears to be defective. Interaction of CD40 receptor on B-cell membranes with CD40 ligand is required for isotype switching (Fig. 4-19).

Primary T-Cell Immunodeficiency Diseases Typically Result in Recurrent or Protracted Viral and Fungal Infections

DiGeorge Syndrome

In its complete form, the DiGeorge syndrome is one of the most severe T-cell immunodeficiency disorders. It is typically recognized shortly after birth in infants with conotruncal congenital heart defects and severe hypocalcemia (due to **hypoparathyroidism**). Some patients exhibit characteristically abnormal facial features. Infants who survive the neonatal period are subject to recurrent and/or chronic viral, bacterial, fungal and protozoal infections.

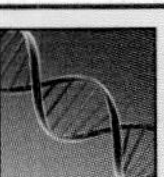

MOLECULAR PATHOGENESIS: The syndrome is caused by defective development of the third and fourth pharyngeal pouches, which give rise to the thymus and parathyroid glands and influence conotruncal cardiac development. Most patients have a point deletion in the long arm of chromosome 22. DiGeorge syndrome is considered to be a form of the "22q11 deletion syndrome." In the absence of a thymus, T-cell maturation is interrupted at the pre–T-cell stage. The immunologic defect has been corrected by transplanting thymic tissue. Most affected patients have a partial DiGeorge syndrome, in which a small remnant of thymus is present. With time, these individuals recover T-cell function without treatment. Some individuals with 22q11 mutations are not immunodeficient but suffer only from conotruncal cardiac defects.

Chronic Mucocutaneous Candidiasis

Chronic mucocutaneous candidiasis is the result of a congenital defect in T-cell function. It is characterized by susceptibility to candidal infections and is associated with an endocrinopathy (hypoparathyroidism, Addison disease, diabetes mellitus). Although most T-cell functions are intact, there is an impaired response to *Candida* antigens.

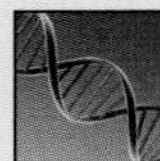

MOLECULAR PATHOGENESIS: The causes of the immunologic defect in chronic mucocutaneous candidiasis are a series of defects in T-cell development. Recent studies suggest that patients with this disorder react to *Candida* antigens differently from normal individuals. Unlike normal responses in which type 1 (IL-2/IFN-γ) T cells predominate and effectively control candidal infections, affected patients mount a type 2 (IL-4/IL-6) helper T-cell response, which is ineffective in resisting the organism.

Combined Immunodeficiency Diseases Exhibit Reduced Immunoglobulins and Defects in T-Lymphocyte Function

Severe combined immunodeficiencies are conspicuously heterogenous and represent life-threatening disorders (Table 4-3).

Table 4-3

Severe Combined Immunodeficiency: Molecular Lesions

Disease	Locus/Gene
T–/–B+/–NK+/–	
IL2RG *JAK3*	Cytokine receptor common γ-chain tyrosine kinase JAK3
T–/–B+/–NK+/–	
CD3D	CD3 complex, δ subunit
CD3E	CD3 complex, ε subunit
CD3G	CD3 complex, γ subunit
CIITA	MHC class II transactivator
RFXANK	MHC class II transactivator
FRX5	MHC class II transactivator
RXAP	MHC class II transactivator
ZAP70	TCR-associated protein of 70 kd
TAP1	Transporter-associated antigen processing 1
TAP2	Transporter-associated antigen processing 2
T–/–B–/–NK–/–	
ADA *PNP*	Adenosine deaminase Purine nucleotide phosphorylase
T–/–B–/–NK+/–	
RAG1 *RAG2*	Recombinase-activating gene 1 Recombinase-activating gene 2

MHC = major histocompatibility complex; TCR = T-cell receptor.

4 | Immunopathology

Severe Combined Immunodeficiency

Severe combined immunodeficiency (SCID) encompasses a large and heterogeneous group of disorders associated by deficiencies in T-cell and B-cell development and function. Affected patients present in the first few months of life with recurrent, often severe infections, diarrhea and failure to thrive. Some forms of SCID are also marked by nonimmunologic developmental defects. SCID is usually fatal within the first year of life unless the immune system can be reconstituted with a hematopoietic stem cell transplantation.

MOLECULAR PATHOGENESIS: SCID is consistently marked by defective T-cell development and/or function. In some types of SCID, B-cell development is also affected. Since B cells require T-cell–derived signals for optimal antibody production, most patients have defective cellular and humoral immunity. NK-cell development and function are variably affected. Current classifications for SCID include the following categories: T–/–B+/–NK–/–; T–/–B+/–NK+/–; T–/–B–/–NK–/–; and T–/–B–/–NK+/–.

The most common form of SCID in the United States (50% of cases) is due to mutations within *IL2RG; IL2RG* encodes the cytokine receptor common γ-chain, which is shared by receptors for IL-2, IL-4, IL-7, IL-9, IL-15 and IL-21. Defects in this gene result in complete absence of T cells and NK cells (90% of cases) but normal numbers of B cells. Immunoglobulin production is severely impaired because of the T-cell defect. Signaling downstream of the 1L receptors with the common γ-chain requires activation of JAK3 tyrosine kinase. Not surprisingly, T–/–B+/–NK– SCID patients with mutations in *JAK3* have been identified.

More than a dozen molecular lesions have been described in T–/–B+/–NK+ SCID patients. For instance, mutations in genes (*CD3D, CD3E, CD3G*) that encode each subunit (δ, ε, γ) of the TCR-associated CD3 complex have been described. These patients have all shown defects in T-lymphocyte function but the clinical features have varied. Another group of T–/–B+/–NK+ SCID patients are deficient of $CD4^+$ T cells in association with various defects in expression of MHC class II molecules. Yet another group of T–/–B+/–NK– SCID patients are deficient in $CD8^+$ T cells. Among this group of patients, mutations in *ZAP70, TAP1* and *TAP2* have been described. *ZAP70* (TCR-associated protein of 70 kd) is a tyrosine kinase involved in TCR signaling; *TAP1* and *TAP2* are required for shuttling of cytosolic peptide onto naïve HLA class I molecules for subsequent presentation to TCRs.

Mutations in the genes for adenosine deaminase (*ADA*) and purine nucleoside phosphorylase (*PNP*), enzymes in the purine nucleotide salvage pathway, result in T–/–B–/–NK– SCID. ADA deficiency accounts for 15% of all SCID patients in the United States. PNP deficiency is very rare.

Rare patients with T–/–B–/–NK+ SCID have a variety of mutations within genes that encode DNA-binding proteins involved in immunoglobulin and TCR gene rearrangement. Some of these patients suffer from radiation sensitivity in addition to immunodeficiency.

Molecular lesions are identified in approximately 95% of patients with SCID. This observation suggests that additional molecular lesions account for the remaining 5%.

Autoimmunity and Autoimmune Diseases

Autoimmune Disease Involves Immune Responses Against Self-Antigens

Autoimmunity implies that the immune system no longer effectively differentiates between self- and non–self-antigens. It was classically interpreted as an abnormal immune response that invariably caused disease, but it is now clear that autoimmune responses are common and are necessary in order to regulate the immune system. Anti-idiotype antibodies (antibodies against antigen-binding sites of immunoglobulins) are important in regulating the immune response; their presence is by definition an autoimmune response. When these "normal" regulatory mechanisms are in some way disrupted, uncontrolled production of autoantibodies or abnormal cell–cell recognition leads to tissue injury. Autoimmune disease results. ***Identification of specific autoantibodies may help to diagnose autoimmune diseases, but it is also necessary to show that the autoimmune reaction (whether cellular or humoral) is directly related to the disease process.*** Autoimmune diseases may be organ specific or generalized. At present, relatively few diseases (e.g., Hashimoto thyroiditis, type 1 diabetes, SLE) fit this rigorous criterion.

An abnormal autoimmune response to self-antigens implies a loss of **immune tolerance**. Immune tolerance describes a situation in which there is no measurable (or clinically evident) immune response to specific (usually self) antigens. The reasons for loss of tolerance in autoimmune diseases are not understood. Experimental studies suggest that tolerance to self-antigens is an active process and requires contact between self-antigens and immune cells. In the fetus, tolerance is readily established to antigens that cause vigorous immune responses in adults. There is extensive evidence that induction and maintenance of tolerance are active and ongoing processes, produced via several mechanisms. Thus, tolerance is an active state in which a potentially harmful immune response is blocked or prevented. Induction of tolerance to an antigen is partly related to the dose of antigen to which cells are exposed.

Putative mechanisms of tolerance are either central or peripheral. In **central tolerance** self-reactive T and B lymphocytes are "deleted" during their maturation in the thymus and bone marrow, respectively. Developing self-reactive T cells recognize self-peptides in the context of compatible MHC molecules and are induced to undergo apoptosis. These T cells are said to have been "negatively selected." In the bone marrow, a similar process occurs to B cells. **Peripheral tolerance** is important in regulating T cells that escape intrathymic negative selection. These T lymphocytes are held in check in the periphery through anergy, suppression and/or activation-induced cell death.

Theories of Autoimmunity

MOLECULAR PATHOGENESIS:

Inaccessible Self-Antigens

The simplest hypothesis to explain the loss of tolerance in autoimmune disease states that an immune reaction develops to a self-antigen not normally "accessible" to the immune system. Intracellular antigens are not exposed or released until some type of tissue injury "releases" or "exposes" them. At that time, an immune response develops (e.g., formation of antibodies against spermatozoa, lens tissue and myelin). Whether these autoantibodies induce injury directly is another matter. There is no evidence that antisperm antibodies induce generalized injury, aside from a localized orchitis. Thus, although autoantibodies may form against normally "sequestered" antigens, they appear to be pathogenic only infrequently.

Abnormal T-Cell Function

Autoimmune reactions have been suggested to develop as a result of abnormalities in the T-lymphocyte system. Most immune responses require T-cell participation to activate antigen-specific B cells. Alterations in the numbers or functional activities of helper or suppressor T cells would thus be expected to influence one's ability to mount an immune response. In fact, defects, particularly in suppressor T cells, are described in many autoimmune diseases. For example, there are reports of defective suppressor T-cell activity in human and experimental SLE. Lymphocytotropic antibodies have also been reported in patients with lupus. Abnormalities in suppressor T-cell function characterize other autoimmune diseases, including primary biliary cirrhosis, thyroiditis, multiple sclerosis, myasthenia gravis, rheumatoid arthritis and scleroderma. However, the critical question is whether these alterations in suppressor T-cell function cause these diseases or whether they are epiphenomena. Defects in suppressor T-cell function have also been found in persons with no evidence of autoimmune disease.

There has also been interest in abnormalities in helper T-cell function in autoimmune disease. Helper T cells are defined by their role in antigen-specific B-cell activation. It is believed that these cells maintain the helper T-cell tolerance induced by low doses of antigen. Recent evidence indicates that these cells become autoreactive in many autoimmune diseases. One key mechanism in autoimmunity is DNA hypomethylation caused by drugs and other agents. This effect leads to upregulation of leukocyte function antigen-1 (LFA-1) and B-cell activation independent of antigen. An example of this T-cell autoreactivity and loss of antigen specificity is drug-induced lupus. Experimentally, it is also possible to "break" this type of tolerance by altering an antigen so that the helper cell is activated and triggers the B cells. An example is when an antigen is modified by partial degradation or complexing with a carrier protein. Some rheumatic diseases are marked by autoantibodies to partially degraded connective tissue proteins, such as collagen or elastin. In some drug-induced hemolytic anemias, antibody against a drug causes hemolysis when the drug binds to erythrocyte membranes.

Molecular Mimicry

Another mechanism by which helper T-cell tolerance is overcome involves antibodies against foreign antigens that cross-react with self-antigens. Here helper T cells function "correctly" and do not induce autoantibody formation. Rather, the efferent limb of the immune response is abnormal. Thus, in rheumatic heart disease, antibodies against streptococcal bacterial antigens cross-react with antigens from cardiac muscle, a phenomenon known as **molecular mimicry.**

Polyclonal B-Cell Activation

Loss of tolerance may also involve polyclonal B-cell activation, in which B lymphocytes are directly activated by complex substances that contain many antigenic sites (e.g., bacterial cell walls and viruses). Development of rheumatoid factor in rheumatoid arthritis, anti-DNA antibodies in lupus erythematosus and other autoantibodies has been described after bacterial, viral and parasitic infections.

Tissue Injury in Autoimmune Diseases

Autoimmune diseases have traditionally been considered to be prototypical immune complex diseases, with immune complexes forming in the circulation or in tissues. Thus, type II (cytotoxic) and type III (immune complex) hypersensitivity reactions are implicated as the cause of tissue injury in many types of autoimmune diseases. Although it is probably true that these hypersensitivity reactions explain most autoimmune tissue injury, the story is more complicated. In some types of autoimmune diseases, T cells sensitized to self-antigens (such as thyroglobulin) may directly cause tissue injury (type IV reaction), but it is not clear to what extent.

Another mechanism of tissue injury is ADCC. Antibodies against an antigen expressed at the cell membrane lead to destruction of that cell. Thus, antibodies against parietal cell H^+/K^+-ATPase seem to be important in the pathogenesis of atrophic gastritis.

However, not all autoantibodies cause disease via cytotoxicity. In antireceptor antibody diseases, such as Graves disease and myasthenia gravis, antibody binds a receptor but the disease process reflects either activation or inactivation of the receptor, rather than cell loss. In Graves disease, autoantibody against the TSH receptor acts as an agonist to stimulate thyroid hormone production, whereas in myasthenia gravis the autoantibody either prevents acetylcholine binding to its receptor or leads to damage of the receptor, thereby impairing neuromuscular synaptic transmission. Anti-insulin receptor antibodies have also been described in acanthosis nigricans and ataxia telangiectasia, in which some patients develop a type of diabetes characterized by extreme insulin resistance.

Type III hypersensitivity reactions (immune complex disease) explain tissue injury in some types of autoimmune diseases. The prototypical disease in this category is SLE. In this disorder, DNA–anti-DNA complexes formed in the circulation (or at local sites) are deposited in tissues, where they induce inflammation and injury, such as occurs in vasculitis and glomerulonephritis. Other examples are rheumatoid arthritis, scleroderma, polymyositis/

dermatomyositis and Sjögren syndrome, all of which are characterized by immune phenomena and are classified as "collagen vascular diseases." Their clinical manifestations are systemic, and many organs and tissues are typically involved. By contrast, cytotoxic (type II–mediated) autoimmune reactions are, for the most part, organ specific.

Systemic Lupus Erythematosus Is a Prototypical Systemic Immune Complex Disease

SLE is a chronic, autoimmune, multisystem, inflammatory disease that may involve almost any organ but characteristically affects skin, joints, serous membranes and kidneys. Autoantibodies are formed against a variety of self-antigens, including plasma proteins (complement components, clotting factors) and protein–phospholipid complexes, cell surface antigens (lymphocytes, neutrophils, platelets, erythrocytes), intracellular cytoplasmic components (microfilaments, microtubules, lysosomes, ribosomes, RNA) and nuclear DNA, ribonucleoproteins and histones. The most important diagnostic autoantibodies are those against nuclear antigens—in particular, antibody to double-stranded DNA and to a soluble nuclear antigen complex, Sm (Smith) antigen, that is part of the spliceosome. High titers of these two **antinuclear antibodies** (ANAs) are nearly pathognomonic of SLE but are not directly cytotoxic. Antigen–antibody complexes deposit in tissues, leading to the characteristic vasculitis, synovitis and glomerulonephritis. For this reason, SLE is a prototype of type III hypersensitivity reactions. Occasionally, directly cytotoxic antibodies are present, particularly antibodies against cell surface antigens of leukocytes and erythrocytes. There is also evidence that cell-mediated immune responses are involved.

The prevalence of SLE varies worldwide. In North America and northern Europe, it is 40:100,000. In the United States, it appears to be more common and severe in blacks and Hispanics, although socioeconomic factors may in part be responsible. Over 80% of cases are in women of childbearing age, and SLE may affect as many as 1 in 700 women in this age group.

MOLECULAR PATHOGENESIS: The etiology of SLE is unknown. The presence of numerous autoantibodies, particularly ANAs, suggests a breakdown in immune surveillance mechanisms and loss of tolerance. Some manifestations of SLE result from tissue injury due to immune complex–mediated vasculitis. Other clinical manifestations (e.g., thrombocytopenia or the secondary antiphospholipid syndrome) are caused by autoantibodies to serum components or cell membrane molecules. However, the diagnostically helpful ANAs are not incriminated in the pathogenesis of SLE. Disordered cellular immunity also appears to play role in SLE. There appear to be many factors that predispose to development of SLE (Fig. 4-20).

Although there was at one time interest in C-type viral particles in experimental murine models of SLE, most evidence argues against a viral etiology for human SLE. The clear female preponderance in SLE is shared by many autoimmune diseases, and sex hormones may be involved. Immune responses in animals are strongly influenced by these hormones. In murine models of SLE, estrogens accelerate disease progression, while androgens have a moderating effect. Whether human SLE is influenced similarly is controversial. Experimentally, estrogens reportedly increase the likelihood of overcoming immunologic tolerance.

Genetic predisposition to lupus is suggested by a higher prevalence in some ethic groups, some families and monozygotic twins. The latter exhibit 20% to 30% concordance, suggesting that both genetic and environmental factors play a role. The incidence of SLE (and other autoimmune diseases) is higher among people who express certain MHC class II DR and DQ antigens. These gene products participate in two unlinked functions, namely, immune regulation and the effector limb of immune responses. Thus, the HLA-B8 haplotype is often associated with both autoimmune diseases and with those DR antigens in certain immunoregulatory abnormalities. These disorders include abnormal lymphocyte responses to antigens, decreased numbers of circulating suppressor cells and increased circulating B cells. Among the effector functions associated with these HLA haplotypes is a decrease in C3b receptors on cells that clear circulating immune

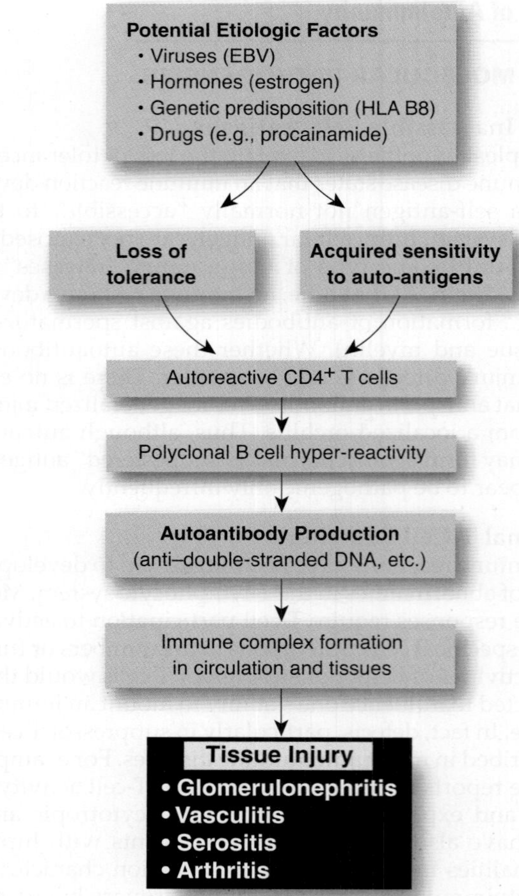

FIGURE 4-20. The pathogenesis of systemic lupus erythematosus is multifactorial. EBV = Epstein-Barr virus; HLA = human leukocyte antigen.

complexes. A critical role for the D/DR region in the pathogenesis of SLE is supported by the observation that inherited deficiencies of certain complement components, particularly C2, C4 and C1q, are associated with an increased incidence of SLE. The genes that encode these early complement components are within the HLA region, close to the D/DR locus.

Production of autoantibodies against many antigens is characteristic of SLE, but precise mechanisms underlying B-cell hyperreactivity are unknown. Two general hypotheses have been advanced. One attributes the disease to a nonspecific, polyclonal B-cell activation, although the nature of the stimulus is speculative. The second hypothesis holds that the antibodies formed in SLE represent a response to specific antigenic stimulation. Support for the latter theory comes from the observation that with time the antibodies of SLE demonstrate gene rearrangements and mutations that are typical of an antigen-driven response. Moreover, a patient with SLE often has antibodies to more than one epitope on a single antigen, further suggesting a primary role for an antigen-driven process. Although inciting antigens have not been identified, a number of factors render normal body constituents more immunogenic, including infection, ultraviolet light exposure and other environmental agents that damage cells. Foreign (e.g., viral) antigens might induce molecular mimicry, although direct evidence is lacking.

Whether or not autoimmunity in SLE is primarily driven by antigens, the variety of autoantibodies strongly suggests a general disturbance of immune tolerance. $CD4^+$ T cells become autoreactive following DNA hypomethylation. These autoreactive $CD4^+$ T cells overexpress the LFA-1 (CD11a) cell adhesion molecule, which stabilizes the interaction between T cells and APCs such as macrophages. These autoreactive $CD4^+$ T cells have been best described in mouse models; no consistent defect in this suppressor T-cell population has been found in humans. Among other immunologic abnormalities noted in SLE are increased circulating levels of IL-6, which in these patients is associated with B-cell differentiation.

There is good reason to believe that a significant portion of injury in lupus is due to deposition of circulating immune complexes against self-antigens, particularly against DNA: the occurrence of circulating immune complexes that contain nuclear antigen; the presence of those immune complexes in injured tissues, as identified by immunofluorescence; and the observation that immune complexes can be extracted from tissues that contain nuclear antigens. Additional evidence suggests that under certain conditions immune complex formation also occurs in situ—that is, in tissues rather than in the circulation. Examples include antibodies against connective tissue components and perhaps the membranous form of lupus glomerulonephritis. Type II hypersensitivity reactions are also implicated in lupus, since cytotoxic antibodies against leukocytes, erythrocytes and platelets have been described.

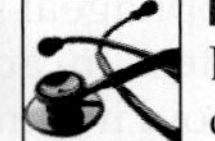

PATHOLOGY AND CLINICAL FEATURES: Because circulating immune complexes deposit in almost all tissues, virtually every organ in the body may be involved.

Joint disease is the most common manifestation of SLE; over 90% of patients have polyarthralgia. An inflammatory synovitis occurs, but unlike rheumatoid arthritis, joint destruction is unusual.

Skin involvement (see Chapter 24) is common. An erythematous rash in sun-exposed sites, a malar "butterfly" rash, is characteristic. Microscopically, a perivascular lymphoid infiltrate and liquefactive degeneration of the basal cells are seen. Immunofluorescence studies reveal immunoglobulin and complement deposition at the dermal–epidermal junction ("lupus band").

Renal disease, in particular glomerulonephritis, affects three fourths of patients with SLE. Immune complexes between DNA and IgG antibodies to double-stranded DNA deposit in glomeruli and lead to various forms of glomerulonephritis (see Chapter 16). Although glomerulonephritis is the most common renal manifestation of SLE, interstitial nephritis or (rarely) vasculitis can also be seen. In many of these cases, immunoglobulins and complement are detectable in the interstitium and in renal blood vessels.

Serous membranes are commonly involved in SLE. More than one third of patients have pleuritis and pleural effusion. Pericarditis and peritonitis occur, but less frequently.

Disorders of the respiratory system occur frequently, with clinical manifestations ranging from pleural disease to upper airway and pulmonary parenchymal disease. Pneumonitis is thought to be caused by deposition of immune complexes in alveolar septa and is associated with patchy acute inflammation. Progressive interstitial fibrosis develops in some patients. An increased incidence of pulmonary hypertension has also been reported.

Cardiac involvement (see Chapter 11) is often seen in SLE, although congestive heart failure is rare and is usually associated with myocarditis. All layers of the heart may be involved, with pericarditis being the most common finding. **Libman-Sacks endocarditis**, which is usually not clinically significant, is characterized by small nonbacterial vegetations on valve leaflets. These lesions should be differentiated from the larger, bulkier vegetations of bacterial endocarditis or the vegetations of rheumatic endocarditis, which are confined to the lines of valve closure.

CNS disease can be a life-threatening complication of lupus. Vasculitis leads to hemorrhage and infarction of the brain, which may sometimes be fatal.

Antiphospholipid antibodies are identified in one third of patients with SLE. This finding is associated with thromboembolic complications, including stroke, pulmonary embolism, deep venous thrombosis, portal vein thrombosis and spontaneous abortions.

Other organ involvement is less common and is often due to **vasculitis.** Lesions in the spleen are characterized by thickening and concentric fibrosis of the penicillary arteries, the so-called "onion-skin" pattern.

The clinical course of SLE is very variable, typically with exacerbations and remissions. Because of immunosuppressive therapies, better recognition of mild forms of the disease and improved antihypertensive medications, overall 10-year survival approaches 90%. Patients with severe renal or CNS disease or with systolic hypertension have the worst prognosis.

Drug-Induced Lupus Also Involves Immune Complex Deposition

A syndrome that resembles SLE may be precipitated in some people by the use of certain medications, most notably procainamide (for arrhythmias), hydralazine (for hypertension) and isoniazid (for tuberculosis). Drug-induced lupus ranges from asymptomatic laboratory abnormalities (positive ANA test) to a syndrome that is clinically similar to SLE. Unlike SLE, drug-induced lupus shows no sex predominance and most patients are over 50 years old. Factors that predispose to this syndrome include large daily doses of the offending drug, slow drug-acetylator status and (in hydralazine-induced lupus) HLA-DR4 genotype. As in SLE, deposition of immune complexes is a feature of drug-induced lupus. Patients with drug-induced lupus typically exhibit constitutional signs, polyarthritis, pleuritis and antinuclear antibodies. In addition, they may develop rheumatoid factor, false-positive tests for syphilis and a positive direct antiglobulin (Coombs) test. Renal and CNS involvement rarely occur in drug-induced lupus, and antibodies to double-stranded DNA and Sm antigen are uncommon. Autoantibodies to histones account for the positive ANA test result and are typical of drug-induced lupus. As in idiopathic SLE, autoreactive $CD4^+$ T cells have been implicated in polyclonal B-cell activation. The syndrome usually resolves when the offending drug is discontinued.

Chronic Discoid Lupus

The most common variety of localized lupus erythematosus is a skin disorder, although identical lesions can occur in some cases of SLE. Erythematous, depigmented and telangiectatic plaques occur most commonly on the face and scalp. Deposition of immunoglobulins and complement at the dermal–epidermal interface in chronic discoid lupus is similar to that in SLE. However, unlike SLE, uninvolved skin contains no immune deposits. Although ANAs develop in about one third of patients, antibodies to double-stranded DNA and Sm antigen are not seen. Most patients with discoid lupus are not otherwise ill, but up to 10% eventually show features of SLE.

Subacute Cutaneous Lupus

Subacute cutaneous lupus is characterized by papular and annular lesions, principally on the trunk. The disorder is aggravated by exposure to ultraviolet light (via sunlight), although lesions eventually resolve without scarring. Antibodies to a ribonucleoprotein complex (SS-A or Ro antigen) and an association with HLA-DR3 genotype are characteristic.

Sjögren Syndrome Targets the Salivary and Lacrimal Glands

Sjögren syndrome (SS) is an autoimmune disorder characterized by **keratoconjunctivitis sicca** (dry eyes) and **xerostomia** (dry mouth) without other connective tissue disease. This definition separates primary SS from secondary types that are occasionally associated with other disorders of connective tissue, such as SLE, rheumatoid arthritis, scleroderma and polymyositis. The primary type is also frequently associated with involvement of other organs, including the thyroid, lung and kidney.

Primary SS is the second most common connective tissue disorder after SLE and affects up to 3% of the population. Like most autoimmune diseases, it occurs mostly in women, 30 to 65 years old. There are strong associations between primary SS and certain MHC types, notably HLA-B8, Dw3, HLA-DR3, DRw-52 and HLA-Dw2, as well as MT2, a B-cell alloantigen. Familial clustering occurs, and affected families have a high incidence of other autoimmune diseases.

MOLECULAR PATHOGENESIS: The cause of SS is unknown. Autoantibodies, particularly ANAs against DNA or nonhistone proteins, are typical in patients with SS. Autoantibodies to soluble nuclear nonhistone proteins, especially antigens SS-A (Ro) and SS-B (La), are found in half of patients with primary SS and are associated with more-severe extraglandular and glandular manifestations. Autoantibodies to DNA or histones are rare; their presence suggests secondary SS associated with lupus. Organ-specific autoantibodies (e.g., against salivary gland antigens) are quite uncommon. As in SLE, it is controversial whether autoantibodies in SS mainly reflect polyclonal B-cell activation or are essentially antigen driven, although these processes are not mutually exclusive.

SS has become the focus for investigation of possible viral etiology for autoimmune disease. Particular attention has been paid to possible roles of EBV and human T-cell leukemia virus-1 (HTLV-1). Although it is still difficult to assign a role for EBV in the pathogenesis of SS, there is evidence that reactivation of this virus may be involved in perpetuating SS, polyclonal B-cell activation and development of lymphoma. In Japan, seropositivity for HTLV-1 among patients with SS is 23%, compared with 3.4% among unselected blood donors. Conversely, more than three quarters of HTLV-1 seropositive people had evidence of SS.

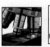

PATHOLOGY AND CLINICAL FEATURES: SS is characterized by intense lymphocytic infiltrates in the salivary and lacrimal glands (see Chapter 25, Fig. 5-29). Focal lymphocytic infiltrates in these glands are initially periductal. Most lobules are affected, especially the centers of the lobules. Well-defined germinal centers are rare. The lymphoid infiltrates destroy acini and ducts. The latter often become dilated and filled with cellular debris. Preservation of the glandular stroma helps to differentiate SS from lymphoma. The lymphocytic infiltrates in the glands are predominantly $CD4^+$ T cells, but a few B cells are also present. Late in the disease, the glands atrophy and may be replaced by hyalinized fibrotic tissue. Owing to the absence of tears, corneas become dry and fissured, and may ulcerate. Lack of saliva causes atrophy, inflammation and cracking of the oral mucosa. The pathology of the salivary and lacrimal glands is described in greater detail in Chapter 25.

Involvement of extraglandular sites is also common in SS. Pulmonary disease occurs in most patients, particularly bronchial gland atrophy in association with lymphoid infiltration. This causes thick tenacious secretions, focal atelectasis, recurrent infections and bronchiectasis. The gastrointestinal tract can also be affected, and many patients have difficulty swallowing (dysphagia). Esophageal submucosal glands are infiltrated by lymphocytes. In addition, atrophic gastritis occurs secondary to lymphoid infiltration of the gastric mucosa. Liver disease, especially primary biliary cirrhosis, is present in 5% to 10% of patients with SS and is associated with nodular lymphoid infiltrates and destruction of intrahepatic bile ducts (see Chapter 14). Interstitial nephritis and chronic thyroiditis occasionally accompany SS. SS is associated with a 40-fold increased risk of lymphoma, probably through B-cell clonal expansion.

Scleroderma (Progressive Systemic Sclerosis) Is Characterized by Vasculopathy and Excessive Collagen Deposition in the Skin and Internal Organs

Organs most affected are the lung, gastrointestinal tract, heart and kidneys. Scleroderma is four times as common in women, mostly 25 to 50 years of age, as in men. Familial clusters have been reported. There is an association between HLA-DQB1 and formation of the autoantibodies that are characteristic of this disease.

MOLECULAR PATHOGENESIS: Again, the cause of scleroderma is unknown. Patients with scleroderma exhibit abnormalities of humoral and cellular immune systems. Circulating B lymphocytes are normal in number, but hypergammaglobulinemia and cryoglobulinemia suggest that they may be hyperactive. ANAs are common but usually at lower titers than in SLE. Antibodies commonly found in scleroderma include nucleolar autoantibodies (primarily against RNA polymerase); antibodies to Scl-70, a nonhistone nuclear protein topoisomerase; and anticentromere antibodies, which are associated with the "CREST" variant of the disease (see below). The Scl-70 autoantibody is the most common and specific for the diffuse form of scleroderma, and is seen in 60% of these patients. However, there is no correlation between ANA titer and disease severity. Rheumatoid factor is commonly present in scleroderma and autoantibodies are occasionally directed against other issues, such as smooth muscle, thyroid gland and salivary glands. Antibodies against collagen types I and IV have also been described.

Cellular immune derangements are also seen in patients with progressive systemic sclerosis. Reduced circulating $CD8^+$ T-suppressor cells, evidence of T-cell activation, alterations in functions mediated by IL-1 and elevated IL-2, and soluble IL-2 receptor occur in active disease. Increased levels of IL-4 and IL-6 have also been described. Tissues exhibit active mononuclear inflammation, which precedes development of the vasculopathy and fibrosis characteristic of this disease. In these infiltrates, increased numbers of $CD4^+$ and $\gamma\delta+$ T cells (which adhere to fibroblasts) are present, as well as macrophages. Mast cells (degranulated) are also present in skin of scleroderma patients. The incidence of other autoimmune disorders, such as thyroiditis and primary biliary cirrhosis, is increased in patients with progressive systemic sclerosis. Circulating male fetal cells have been demonstrated in blood and blood vessel walls of many women with scleroderma who bore male children many years before the disease began. It has been suggested that scleroderma in these patients is similar to graft-versus-host disease (GVHD).

Progressive systemic sclerosis is characterized by widespread excessive collagen deposition. The cause remains unclear, but emerging evidence suggests that there is expansion and activation of fibrogenic clones of fibroblasts. These clones behave autonomously and display augmented procollagen synthesis, including increased circulating type III collagen aminopropeptide. Several factors may be responsible for this fibroblast activation. The $\gamma\delta+$ T cells adhere to fibroblasts and may activate them via cytokine generation. TGF-β is elevated in tissues of these patients, as are IL-1 and IL-4, all of which stimulate fibroblast proliferation and collagen biosynthesis. IL-6—which upregulates several matrix metalloproteinases and is important in modulation of collagen metabolism—is also elevated. Activated fibroblasts themselves produce cytokines and growth factors, such as IL-1, prostaglandin E (PGE), TGF-β and PDGF, which may in turn serve to activate other fibroblasts. Finally, activated fibroblasts also express the intercellular adhesion molecule-1 (ICAM-1), which may be important in T-cell and macrophage adherence and activation.

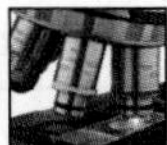

PATHOLOGY: The skin in scleroderma initially shows edema and then induration. The thickened skin exhibits a striking increase in collagen fibers in the reticular dermis; thinning of the epidermis with loss of rete pegs; atrophy of dermal appendages (Fig. 4-21A); hyalinization and obliteration of arterioles; and variable mononuclear infiltrates, primarily of T cells. The stage of induration may progress to atrophy or revert to normal. Increased collagen deposition can also occur in synovia, lungs, gastrointestinal tract, heart and kidneys.

Lesions in arteries, arterioles and capillaries are typical, and in some cases may be the first demonstrable pathology in this disease. Initial subintimal edema with fibrin deposition is followed by thickening and fibrosis of the vessel and reduplication or fraying of the internal elastic lamina. Involved vessels may become severely narrowed or occluded by thrombi.

The kidneys are involved in more than half of patients with scleroderma. They show marked vascular changes, often with focal hemorrhage and cortical infarcts (see Chapter 16). Among the most severely affected vessels are the interlobular arteries and afferent arterioles. Early fibromuscular thickening of the subintima causes luminal narrowing, which is followed by fibrosis (Fig. 4-21B). Fibrinoid necrosis is commonly seen in afferent arterioles. Glomerular alterations are nonspecific and focal changes range from necrosis extending from the afferent arterioles to fibrosis. There is diffuse deposition of immunoglobulin, complement and fibrin in affected vessels early in the disease, probably because of increased vascular permeability.

Diffuse interstitial fibrosis is the primary abnormality in lungs. The disease can progress to end-stage pulmonary fibrosis, so-called honeycomb lung (see Chapter 12).

Most patients with scleroderma have patchy myocardial fibrosis, and in about one fourth of cases, more than 10% of the myocardium is involved. These lesions result from focal myocardial necrosis, which may reflect focal ischemia secondary to a Raynaud-like reactivity of coronary microvasculature.

Progressive systemic sclerosis can involve any portion of the gastrointestinal tract. Esophageal dysfunction is the most common and troublesome gastrointestinal complication. Atrophy of smooth muscle and fibrous replacement are seen

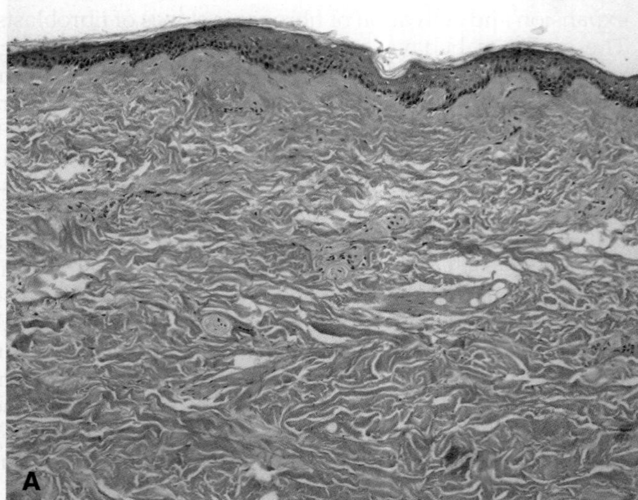

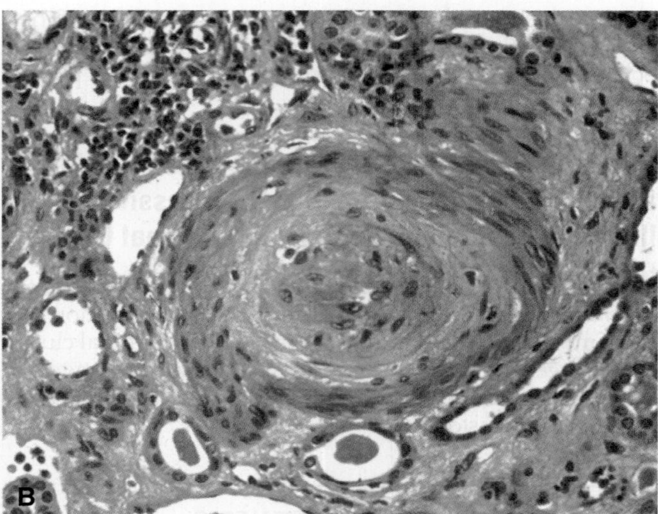

FIGURE 4-21. Sceroderma. A. Dermal fibrosis in scleroderma. Dense collagen accumulation beneath the epidermis. Note the absence of dermal appendages. **B. Scleroderma that affects the kidney is manifested by vascular involvement.** Here, the interlobular artery exhibits marked luminal narrowing due to pronounced intimal thickening.

in the lower esophagus. The small bowel is often involved, with patchy fibrosis, principally of the muscular layers.

CLINICAL FEATURES: Scleroderma presents as two distinct clinical categories, a **generalized (progressive systemic)** form and a **limited variant**. Progressive systemic sclerosis (diffuse scleroderma) is characterized by severe and progressive disease of skin and early onset of all or most of the associated abnormalities of visceral organs. Symptoms usually begin with Raynaud phenomenon, namely, intermittent episodes of ischemia of the fingers, marked by pallor, paresthesias and pain. These symptoms are accompanied, or followed, by edema of the fingers and hands, tightening and thickening of the skin, polyarthralgia and complaints referable to involvement of specific internal organs. The typical patient with generalized scleroderma exhibits "stone facies," owing to tightening of facial skin and restricted motion of the mouth. Progression of vascular lesions in the fingers leads to ischemic ulceration of the fingertips, with subsequent shortening and atrophy of the digits. Many patients suffer from painful tendinitis, and joint pain is common. Esophageal involvement causes hypomotility and dysphagia. Fibrosis in the small bowel interferes with intestinal mobility, with consequent bacterial overgrowth and secondary malabsorption. Pulmonary fibrosis causes dyspnea on exertion in more than half of patients, and may progress to dyspnea at rest and eventually to respiratory failure. Patients with long-standing disease are at risk for development of pulmonary hypertension and cor pulmonale. Although most patients with scleroderma have some myocardial fibrosis, congestive heart failure is uncommon. However, ventricular arrhythmias can cause sudden death.

The vascular involvement of the kidneys in generalized scleroderma is responsible for so-called scleroderma renal crisis: the sudden onset of malignant hypertension, progressive renal insufficiency and, frequently, microangiopathic hemolytic anemia. The syndrome reflects ischemic injury to the kidneys and usually occurs in the first few years of the disease. It is marked by conspicuously elevated levels of circulating renin.

The so-called limited form of scleroderma is a milder disease. Typically, such patients exhibit skin involvement, particularly the face and fingers. A variant within the spectrum of limited scleroderma is CREST syndrome, which is characterized by calcinosis, Raynaud phenomenon, esophageal dysmotility, sclerodactyly and telangiectasia. The limited variant usually does not entail severe systemic involvement early in disease but later can progress, primarily in the form of diffuse interstitial lung fibrosis. Patients with limited scleroderma often show circulating anticentromere antibodies.

Mixed Connective Tissue Disease Combines Features of SLE, Scleroderma and Dermatomyositis

The exact incidence of mixed connective tissue disease (MCTD) is unknown. Between 80% and 90% of patients are female, and most are adults (mean age, 37 years). Those symptoms that are characteristic of SLE include rash, Raynaud phenomenon, arthritis and arthralgias. The characteristics of scleroderma are swollen hands, esophageal hypomotility and pulmonary interstitial disease. Some patients also develop symptoms suggestive of rheumatoid arthritis. Patients with MCTD have been reported to respond well to corticosteroid therapy, although some studies have challenged this assertion.

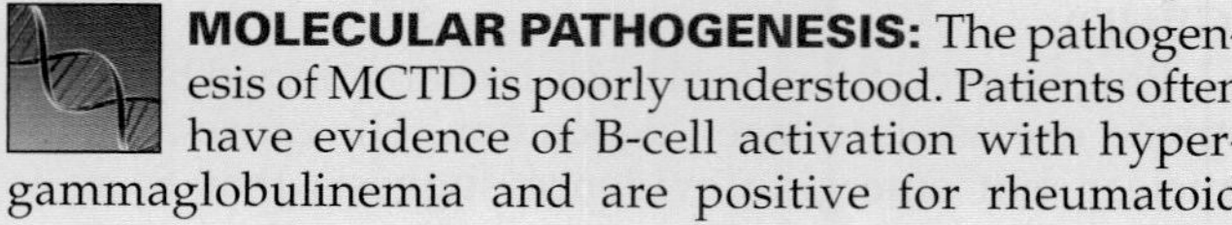

MOLECULAR PATHOGENESIS: The pathogenesis of MCTD is poorly understood. Patients often have evidence of B-cell activation with hypergammaglobulinemia and are positive for rheumatoid factor. ANAs are present but, differently from SLE, they do not usually bind double-stranded DNA. The most distinctive ANA is directed against an extractable nuclear antigen. Specifically, patients with MCTD have high titers of antibody to uridine-rich ribonucleoprotein (anti-U1-RNP) in the absence of other extractable nuclear antigens, including PM-1 and Jo-1. Anti-RNP antibodies may occasionally be detected in SLE, but usually in lower titer than in MCTD.

The cause of the formation and maintenance of the high titer of anti-RNP antibody is unclear. However, there is an association with HLA-DR4 and HLA-DR2 genotypes, suggesting a role for T cells in the autoantibody production. There is no direct evidence that these antibodies induce the characteristic involvement of the various organ systems.

There is also controversy over whether MCTD is a separate disease or a heterogeneous collection of patients with nonclassical presentations of SLE, scleroderma or polymyositis. For example, in some patients, MCTD seems to evolve into typical scleroderma. Other patients develop renal disease consistent with SLE. Still others differentiate into rheumatoid arthritis. Thus, MCTD may be an intermediate stage in the progression to a recognized autoimmune disease. Patients whose disease remains undifferentiated may make up a distinct subset. Thus, it remains unclear whether MCTD is a distinct entity or simply an overlap of symptoms in patients with other types of collagen vascular diseases.

Immune Reactions to Transplanted Tissues

Antigens encoded by the MHC on chromosome 6 are critical immunogenic molecules that can stimulate rejection of transplanted tissues. Thus, optimal graft survival occurs when recipient and donor are closely matched with regard to histocompatibility antigens. In practice, an exact HLA match is obtained infrequently, except in the case of transplantation between monozygotic twins. Vigilant monitoring of the functional status of the graft and immunosuppressive therapy is thus required after transplantation. In recent years, therapeutic advances have greatly improved transplant success rates, even when there is a degree of histoincompatibility. When graft-versus-host immune reactions (rejection) occur, any combination of immune responses may injure the graft. Renal allograft rejection is also discussed in Chapter 16.

MOLECULAR PATHOGENESIS: T-cell–mediated and antibody-mediated reactions are both important in the pathophysiology of transplant rejection. Antigen-presenting cells, specifically those bearing foreign MHC molecules in the graft, are recognized by host $CD8^+$ cytotoxic T lymphocytes, which mediate tissue injury; and host $CD4^+$ T-helper cells, which augment antibody production, induce IFN-γ production and activate macrophages. IFN-γ enhances MHC expression, amplifying tissue injury. Host APCs also process foreign donor antigens, leading to $CD4^+$-mediated delayed-type hypersensitivity and $CD4^+$-mediated antibody production.

Transplant rejection reactions are usually categorized as "hyperacute," "acute" and "chronic" rejection, based on the clinical tempo of the response and pathophysiologic mechanisms involved. However, in practice, the features of each overlap, creating ambiguity in diagnosis. Categorization of transplant rejection is also complicated by the toxicity of immunosuppressive drugs and by the potential for mechanical problems (e.g., vascular thrombosis) or recurrence of original disease (e.g., some types of glomerulonephritis). The next sections illustrate rejection in the context of renal transplantation. Similar responses occur in other transplanted tissues, although rejection as applied to each tissue type has its own unique features.

Hyperacute Rejection Occurs Within Minutes to Hours After Transplantation

Hyperacute rejection manifests clinically as a sudden cessation of urine output, with fever and pain at the graft site. This form of rejection is mediated by preformed anti-HLA antibodies and complement activation products, including chemotactic and other inflammatory mediators. This immediate rejection is catastrophic and necessitates prompt surgical removal of the kidney. The histologic features of hyperacute rejection in transplanted kidneys are vascular congestion, fibrin–platelet thrombi within capillaries, neutrophilic vasculitis with fibrinoid necrosis, prominent interstitial edema and neutrophil infiltrates (Fig. 4-22A). Fortunately, hyperacute rejection is not common when appropriate pretransplantation antibody screening is performed.

Acute Rejection Occurs Within the First Few Weeks or Months After Transplantation

Acute rejection is characterized by abrupt onset of azotemia and oliguria, which may be associated with fever and graft tenderness. Acute rejection most typically involves both cell-mediated and humoral mechanisms of tissue damage. If detected in its early stages, acute rejection can be reversed with immunosuppressive therapy. Needle biopsy is often needed to differentiate acute rejection from acute tubular necrosis or toxicity associated with immunosuppressive treatment. Findings vary depending on whether the rejection is primarily cellular or humoral. In acute cellular rejection, microscopy reveals interstitial infiltrates of lymphocytes and macrophages, edema, lymphocytic tubulitis and tubular necrosis (Fig. 4-22B). The acute humoral form, sometimes called rejection vasculitis, shows vascular damage consisting of arteritis, fibrinoid necrosis and thrombosis. Blood vessel involvement is an ominous sign because it usually means the rejection episode will be refractory to therapy.

Chronic Rejection Appears Months to Years After Transplantation

In chronic rejection, patients typically develop progressive azotemia, oliguria, hypertension and weight gain over a period of months. Chronic rejection may be the consequence of repeated episodes of cellular rejection, either asymptomatic or clinically apparent. The main histologic features are arterial and arteriolar intimal thickening causing vascular stenosis or obstruction, thickened glomerular capillary walls, tubular atrophy and interstitial fibrosis (Fig. 4-22C). There are

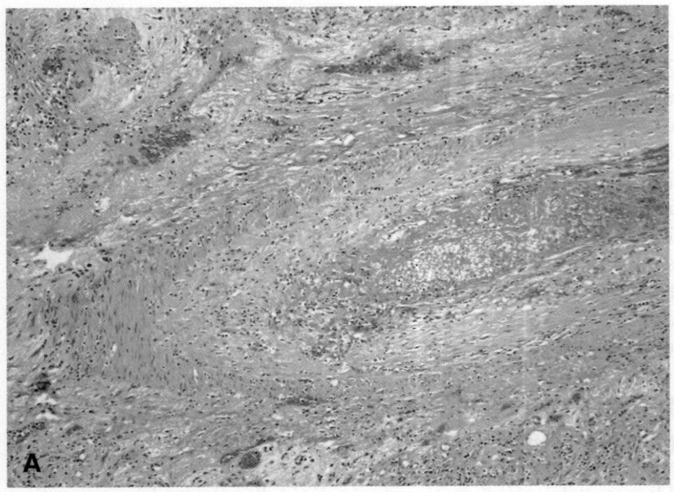

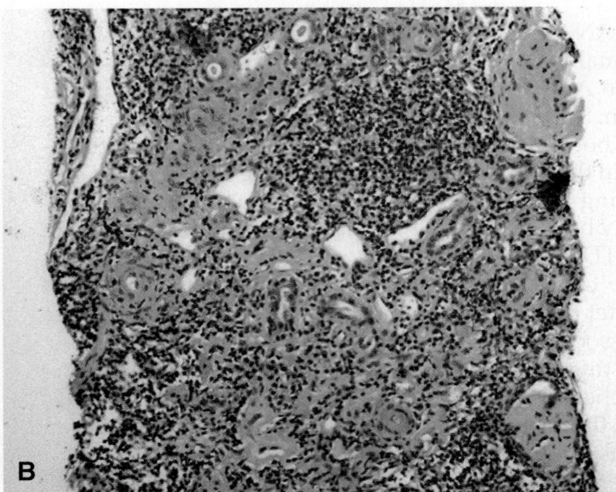

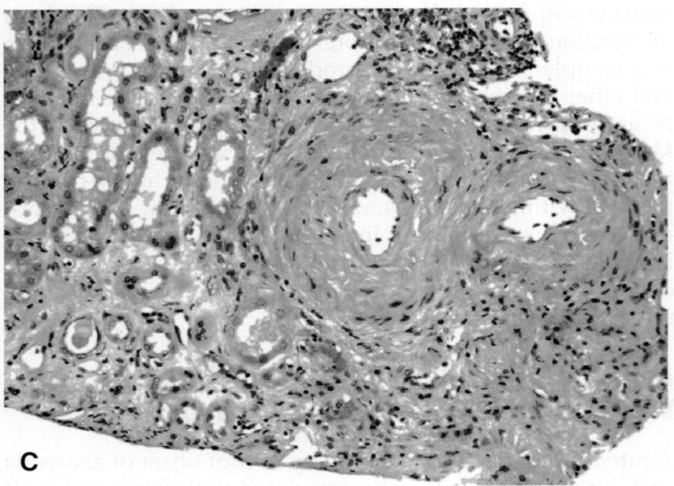

FIGURE 4-22. There are three major forms of renal transplant rejection. A. Hyperacute rejection occurs within minutes to hours after transplantation and is characterized, in part, by neutrophilic vasculitis, intravascular fibrin thrombi and neutrophilic infiltrates. **B. Acute cellular rejection** occurs within weeks to months after transplantation and is characterized by tubular damage and mononuclear leukocyte infiltration. **C. Chronic rejection** is observed months to years after transplantation and is characterized by tubular atrophy, patchy interstitial mononuclear cell infiltrates and fibrosis. In this example, arteries show fibrointimal thickening.

scattered interstitial mononuclear infiltrates, and tubules contain proteinaceous casts. Chronic rejection represents an advanced state of organ injury and does not respond to therapy. The histologies of acute and chronic rejection may overlap and vary in degree, and unambiguous pathologic distinction may not be possible on biopsy.

Graft-Versus-Host Disease Occurs When Donor Lymphocytes Recognize and React to the Recipient

The advent of transplantation of allogenic (donor) bone marrow or HSCs makes possible treatment of diseases that had previously been considered terminal or untreatable. In order for the transplanted bone marrow to engraft in the new the host, the recipient's bone marrow and immune system must be "conditioned" (usually ablated) by cytotoxic drugs, sometimes plus radiation. If the grafted cells include immunocompetent lymphocytes, these cells may react to—"reject"—host tissues, causing GVHD. GVHD can also occur if a profoundly immunodeficient patient is transfused with blood products containing HLA-incompatible lymphocytes.

The major organs affected in GVHD are skin, gastrointestinal tract and liver. The skin and intestine show mononuclear cell infiltrates and epithelial cell necrosis. The liver displays periportal inflammation, damaged bile ducts and liver cell injury. Clinically, acute GVHD manifests as rash, diarrhea, abdominal cramps, anemia and liver dysfunction. Chronic GVHD is characterized by dermal sclerosis, sicca syndrome (see above: dry eyes and mouth due to chronic inflammation of lacrimal and salivary glands) and immunodeficiency. Treatment of GVHD requires immunosuppression. Patients, especially those with chronic GVHD, may be at a higher risk for potentially life-threatening opportunistic infections (e.g., invasive aspergillosis).

Human Immunodeficiency Virus and Acquired Immunodeficiency Syndrome

AIDS is the most common immunodeficiency state worldwide. It is mainly caused by HIV-1, although a small minority of patients, primarily in western Africa, are infected with HIV-2. If untreated, people infected with HIV-1 are subject to a variety of immunologic defects, the most devastating of which is virtually complete eventual loss of cellular immunity, leading to catastrophic opportunistic infections. The relentless progression of HIV infection is now recognized as a continuum that extends from an initial asymptomatic state to the immune depletion that characterizes patients with overt AIDS, and the entire spectrum of the infection is often referred to as HIV/AIDS. The basic lesion is infection of $CD4^+$ (helper) T lymphocytes by HIV, which leads to depletion of this cell population and consequent impaired immune function and dysregulation. As a result, patients with AIDS usually die of opportunistic or other infections. There is also a high incidence of malignant tumors, mainly B-cell lymphomas and Kaposi sarcoma. Finally, infection of the CNS with HIV often leads to an array of syndromes ranging from minor cognitive or motor neuron disorders to frank dementia.

AIDS was first described in the United States in 1981, in a report of *P. carinii* (now termed *P. jiroveci*) pneumonia in homosexual men. The onset of this human epidemic is uncertain: although antibodies to HIV have been found in stored blood from the Congo Republic dating to 1959, sporadic cases of diseases that can retrospectively be attributed to HIV certainly occurred in Africa during the 1960s. By the late 1970s, clusters of strange infectious diseases in New York and Miami among homosexual men, intravenous drug users and Haitians are now recognized as having been caused by HIV. By 1982, these unusual infections were associated with Kaposi sarcoma and considered to reflect an underlying immune deficiency. Thus, the acronym "AIDS" was coined. At the same time, it became clear that AIDS was spread by contact with blood of persons suspected of bearing an infectious agent. In addition to homosexual men and intravenous drug users who shared needles, people at risk were identified among recipients of whole blood and blood products, especially hemophiliacs, heterosexual contacts and infants born to female drug users. In 1983, the responsible virus, now called HIV-1, was identified. Development of a first-generation serologic test to detect antibodies to HIV-1 in 1985 permitted accurate diagnosis and allowed donated blood products to be screened for HIV-1 antibodies and to be processed to inactivate HIV.

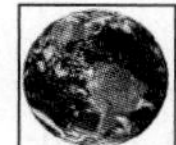

EPIDEMIOLOGY: Although AIDS most likely originated in sub-Saharan Africa, it is now a worldwide pandemic. The spread of HIV is attributable to the ease of international travel and enhanced population mobility, which in many societies coincided with a rapid increase in sexual promiscuity and sexually transmitted diseases. Presently, over 40 million people are infected with HIV. The World Health Organization estimated that, since its onset, the AIDS epidemic has killed over 25,000,000 people and continues to cause over 2,000,000 deaths yearly, worldwide.

Although the highest prevalence is in sub-Saharan Africa (Fig. 4-23), no country is free of HIV-1. An estimated 0.6% of the adult population in North America is HIV positive, and over 55,000 new infections and 23,000 deaths occur every year.

Although homosexual men once were by far the largest group of HIV-positive people in the United States, they now account for just over half of new cases. Most other cases are occurring in intravenous drug users and their sexual partners. The majority of AIDS patients in the United States are men, although the prevalence of HIV-1 infection in women continues to increase.

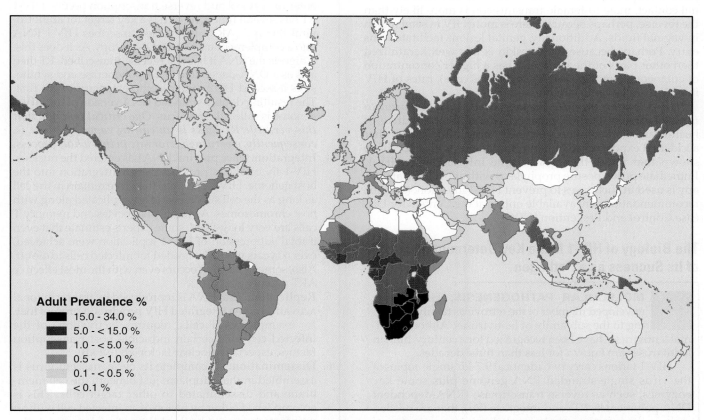

FIGURE 4-23. Prevalence of human immunodeficiency virus (HIV) infection among the adult population worldwide. World Health Organization (WHO) figures from 2006 demonstrate the extent of the HIV pandemic throughout the world.

Inhabitants of sub-Saharan Africa suffer more from the ravages of AIDS than in other regions. Although accurate statistics from this area are not as readily available as in industrialized countries, in parts of sub-Saharan Africa it is estimated that 25% of the population is HIV positive. The epidemiologic pattern differs from that in the United States in that African patients rarely report homosexuality or intravenous drug use and AIDS in Africa shows only a slight male predominance, indicating a predominant heterosexual spread of the infection.

Many cases of AIDS have been reported in western Europe and South America, largely in homosexual men, intravenous drug users and their sexual partners and prostitutes. AIDS is being reported increasingly in Asia, and some countries on that continent (Thailand, India and China) have witnessed huge proportionate increases in HIV infections.

HIV Is Transmitted by Contact With Blood and Certain Body Fluids, and Through Sexual Activity

Save for intravenous drug users and transfusion recipients, AIDS is mainly transmitted as a venereal disease, both homosexually and heterosexually. Transmission to newborns via breast milk is a concern in the developing world. Significant amounts of HIV have been isolated from blood, semen, vaginal secretions, breast milk and cerebrospinal fluid. Except for the latter, HIV in these fluids is present in both lymphocytes and free virus.

The virus is transmitted from semen through tears in the rectal mucosa, particularly in anal-receptive partners, and it can infect epithelial cells of the rectum directly. In heterosexual contact, male-to-female transmission is more likely than the reverse, perhaps because there is more HIV in semen than in vaginal fluids. Additionally, genital lesions facilitate virus entry. Perhaps because the foreskin is less well keratinized than other parts of the penis and has a higher concentration of cutaneous dendritic cells (Langerhans cells), rates of HIV infection are lower in circumcised men.

HIV-1 is not transmitted by nonsexual, casual exposure to infected persons. Further, prospective studies of hundreds of health care workers who sustained "needle sticks" or other accidental exposures to blood from patients with AIDS have shown that fewer than 1% became infected with HIV-1. Immediate postexposure prophylaxis with antiretroviral therapy is used in such cases to prevent HIV-1 infection. (Specific recommendations are available online at the Centers for Disease Control and Prevention [CDC].)

The Biology of HIV-1 Is the Key Determinant of Its Success as a Pathogen

MOLECULAR PATHOGENESIS: HIV-1 is an enveloped member of the retrovirus family, belonging to the subfamily of lentiviruses. Although animal lentiviruses have been recognized for a century, human lentiviruses are known for less than three decades.

HIV-1 virions carry two identical 9.7-kb single copies of the virus single-stranded RNA genome plus some key enzymes, such as reverse transcriptase (RNA-dependent DNA polymerase, RT) and integrase (IN), that are needed early in the infectious cycle (see below), in a core of viral proteins. The outermost layer, the envelope, is derived from the host cell membrane, in which are found virally encoded glycoproteins (gp120 and gp41). In addition to *gag*, *pol* and *env* genes present in all replication-competent RNA viruses, HIV-1 has six other genes that code for proteins that control viral replication and certain host cell functions. Mononuclear phagocytes and $CD4^+$ helper T lymphocytes are the main targets for HIV-1 infection, although the virus can enter other cells, such as B lymphocytes, astrocytes, endothelial cells and intestinal epithelium.

The replicative cycle of HIV-1 is depicted in Fig. 4-24.

1. **Binding:** Free HIV or an infected lymphocyte can transmit the virus to an uninfected cell. The HIV envelope glycoprotein gp120, either on the free virus or on the surface of an infected cell, binds the CD4 molecule on the surface of helper T lymphocytes and other cells, plus specific β-chemokine receptors. The most important of these chemokine receptors are CCR5 (on many phagocytic cells) and CXCR4 (on T lymphocytes). Virus binding to both CD4 and a chemokine receptor mediates HIV entry. However, HIV-1 can enter dendritic cells (DCs) via C-type lectin receptors (e.g., DC-SIGN). There is also evidence that CCR3 may be important in HIV-1 infection in the CNS (see below) and elsewhere.
2. **Internalization:** Upon binding to CD4, gp120 undergoes a conformational change, to uncover its CCR5 (or CXCR4) binding domain. Thereupon, viral gp41 forms a loop, fusing virus and cell membranes. The virus capsid, genome and those enzymes needed for the early phase of the infectious cycle enter the cell.
3. **DNA synthesis:** The virus genome, plus viral RT and IN, enter the cytosol and reverse transcription occurs. HIV-1 RT has several functions, and is a key target for antiretroviral therapy (ART). It reverse-transcribes HIV-1 RNA into a complementary DNA (cDNA) copy. As it does this, it digests the RNA it has just reverse-transcribed. RT then acts as a DNA-dependent DNA polymerase and synthesizes a second DNA strand complementary to the first. The resulting double-stranded DNA version of the HIV-1 genome is called the provirus. ***One critical function that this versatile RT lacks is an editing capacity. There is, consequently, a very high error rate in this whole process.***
4. **Integration:** Once proviral DNA has entered the nucleus, HIV-1 IN catalyzes provirus cDNA integration into the host genome. HIV-1 genomes therefore remain in the cell as long as the cell survives and are replicated along with host chromosomes. As tissue phagocytes and memory T cells are very long-lived, some experts estimate that even if total suppression of HIV-1 replication were achieved, over 60 years would be needed for infected cells to die off. Also, some replication occurs even with the most effective ART regiments.
5. **Replication:** Viral RNA is reproduced by transcriptional activation of the integrated HIV provirus, a process that, for example, for T cells, requires "activation" of the infected cell plus certain inducible host transcription factors, especially nuclear factor-κB (NFκB).
6. **Dissemination:** To complete its cycle, nascent virus is assembled in the cytoplasm just beneath the cell membrane and disseminated to other target cells. This is accomplished either by fusion of an infected cell with an uninfected one or by budding of virions from the plasma membrane of infected cells (Fig. 4-25).

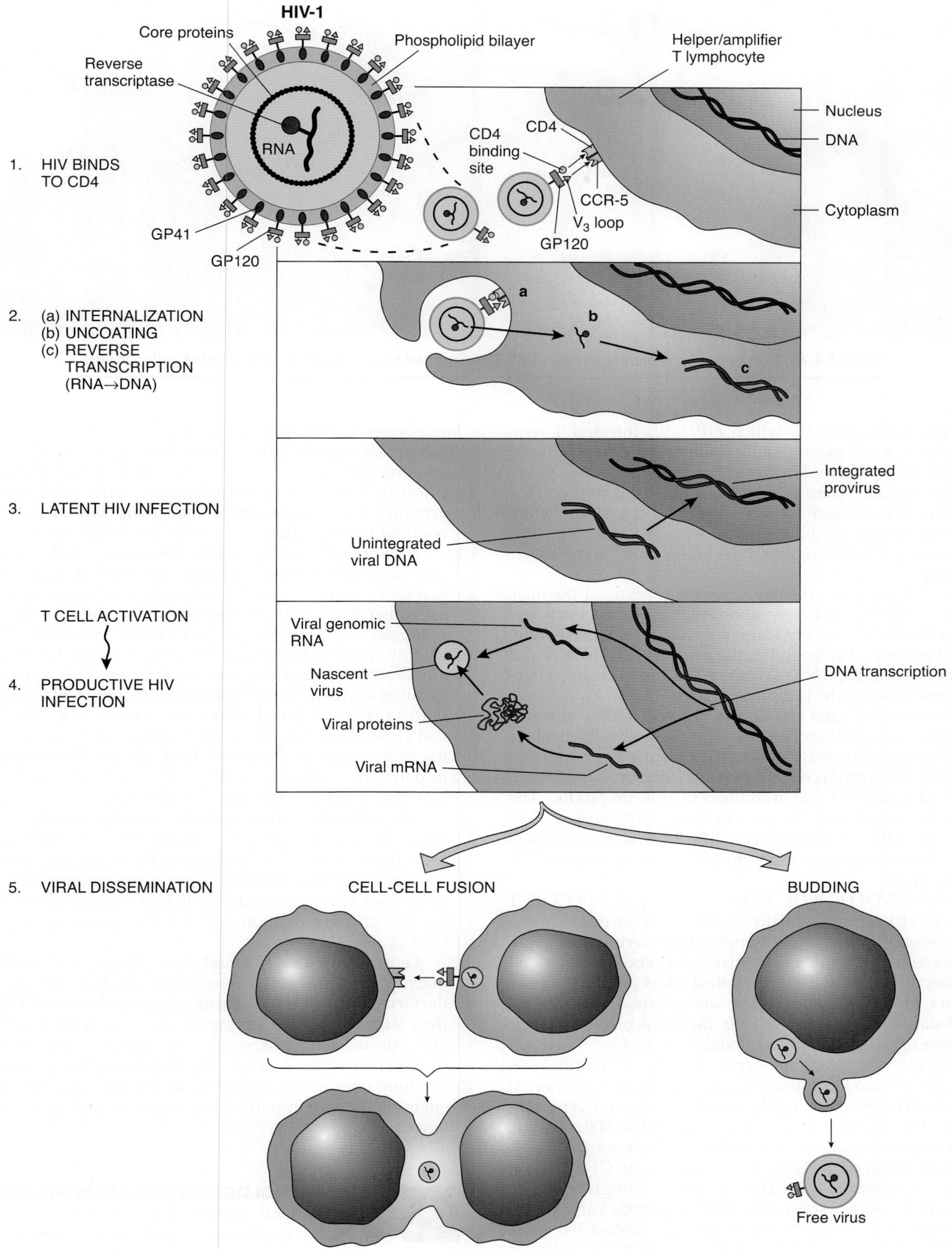

FIGURE 4-24. The life cycle of human immunodeficiency virus-1 (HIV-1) is a multistep process.

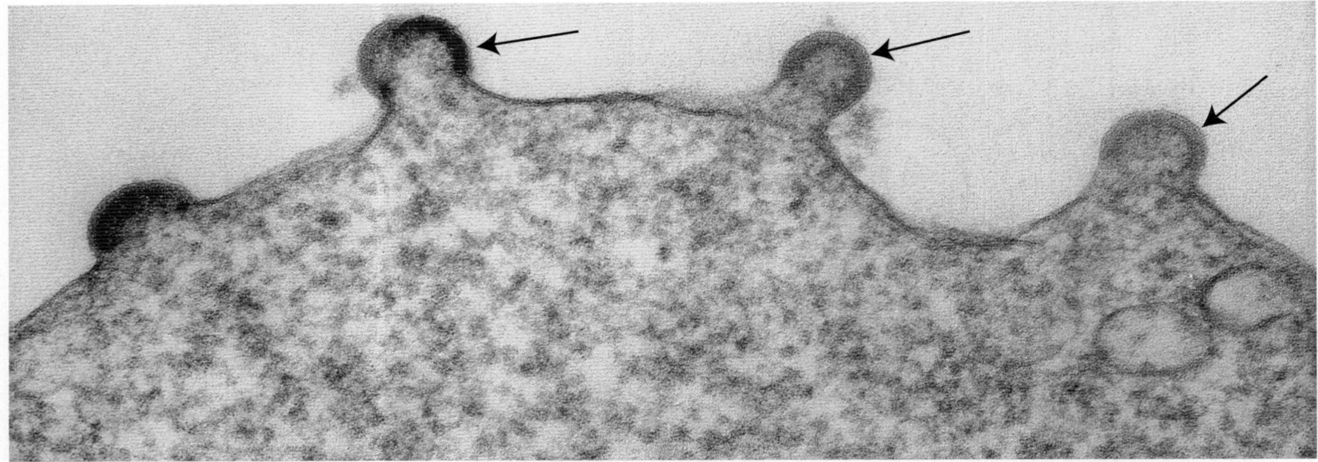

FIGURE 4-25. Human immunodeficiency virus-1 (HIV-1) virions can be seen budding from infected cells (*arrows*).

The mechanism by which HIV kills infected T lymphocytes is still incompletely understood. Virus-induced apoptosis and autophagy may be involved. Other possibilities include immune clearance of infected cells and the actions of secondary mediators such as cytokines. Whatever the mechanism(s), there is a clear association between increasing viral burden and declining $CD4^+$ lymphocyte counts.

HIV-1 persists, effectively, for the lifetime of the host. Even in the face of low or undetectable plasma virus levels, a latent or quiescent form of the virus remains in long-lived memory T cells and tissue phagocytes. There is also evidence that the CNS may serve as a reservoir for potential reseeding of the periphery.

Initiation of viral replication in latent HIV-1 infection depends on induction of host proteins during T-cell activation. Viral transcription may be activated by many T-cell mitogens and cytokines produced by monocyte/macrophages, including TNF-α and IL-1, and in addition, by proteins produced by other viruses that infect patients with AIDS, such as herpesvirus, EBV, adenovirus and CMV. Thus, immune system activation by a variety of infectious agents may promote HIV replication.

IMMUNOLOGY OF AIDS: The destruction of $CD4^+$ T cells by HIV-1 can essentially disable the entire immune system because this subset of lymphocytes exerts critical regulatory and effector functions that involve both cellular and humoral immunity. ***Thus, in typical AIDS patients, all elements of the immune system are eventually perturbed, including T cells, B cells, NK cells, the monocyte/macrophage lineage of cells and immunoglobulin production.***

Of the two functional types of $CD4^+$ T lymphocytes (i.e., helper and amplifier [or inducer] cells), those affected first in HIV infection are the amplifier subset. Eventually, total $CD4^+$ lymphocyte counts fall to less than 500 cells/μL, and helper-to-suppressor T-cell ratios decline from a normal of 2.0 to as little as 0.5. Numbers of $CD8^+$ (cytotoxic/suppressor) cells are variable, although in AIDS, most of these cells seem to be of the cytotoxic variety.

Defects in T-cell function are manifested by weak responses in skin testing with a variety of antigens (delayed hypersensitivity) and impaired proliferative responses to mitogens and antigens in vitro. Moreover, the deficiency of $CD4^+$ cells reduces levels of IL-2, the cytokine produced in response to antigens that stimulate cytotoxic T-cell killing. ***Thus, patients with AIDS cannot generate the antigen-specific cytotoxic T cells that are required to clear viruses and other infectious agents.***

Humoral immunity is also abnormal. Production of antibodies in response to specific antigenic stimulation is markedly decreased, often to less than 10% of normal. B cells also show poor proliferative responses in vitro to mitogens and antigens. Yet, sera of patients with AIDS usually show high levels of polyclonal immunoglobulins, autoantibodies and immune complexes. This apparent paradox is probably explained by the concurrent infection with polyclonal B-cell–activating viruses (e.g., EBV or CMV), which constantly stimulate B cells nonspecifically to produce immunoglobulins. Lack of $CD4^+$ lymphocytes impairs the cytotoxic T-cell proliferation that normally would eliminate B cells infected with EBV.

NK-cell activity is severely decreased in AIDS as well. Since these cells kill both virus-infected cells and tumor cells, this defect may contribute to the malignant tumors and viral infections that plague these patients. Suppression of NK-cell activity is related both to a decrease in NK-cell number and to reduction in IL-2 levels, owing to a loss of $CD4^+$ cells.

Lentiviruses tend to target macrophages, and infected macrophages may serve as reservoirs for dissemination of the virus. Interestingly, some macrophages express CD4 on their surfaces. Unlike T lymphocytes, which are killed by HIV, infected macrophages generally survive. Macrophages from patients with AIDS display impaired phagocytosis of immune complexes and opsonized particles, decreased chemotaxis and impaired responses to antigenic challenges.

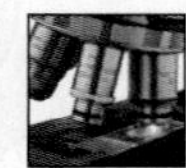 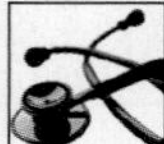

PATHOLOGY AND CLINICAL FEATURES: Patients recently infected with HIV-1 may have an acute, usually self-limited flu-like illness termed the **acute retroviral syndrome**. It clinically resembles infectious mononucleosis. This occurs 2 to 3 weeks after exposure to HIV, before appearance of antibodies against the virus. Less commonly, patients present with neurologic symptoms that suggest encephalitis, aseptic meningitis or a neuropathy. Fever, myalgia, lymphadenopathy, sore throat and a macular rash are common. Most of these symptoms resolve within 2 to 3 weeks, although lymphadenopathy, fever and myalgia may persist for a few months. Seroconversion occurs 1 to 10 weeks after the onset of this acute illness. Thus, the standard HIV-1 enzyme immunoassay (EIA) and Western blot testing, which depends on the presence of anti–HIV-1 *gag* antibodies, is negative during the initial stage of the infection. Most patients recover from this initial illness as their immune system mounts a cytotoxic T-cell counterattack, although a small percentage progress rapidly to frank AIDS within a few months. After the initial acute syndrome, most newly infected individuals enter a period of latency and slow immune system decline that averages approximately 10 years before they reach a state of serious immune compromise. If symptoms go unrecognized or untreated, the outcome will eventually be fulminant immunodeficiency and its fatal complications (Fig. 4-26).

Persistent generalized lymphadenopathy is palpable lymph node enlargement at two or more extrainguinal sites, persisting for more than 3 months in a person infected with HIV. The disorder develops either as part of the acute HIV syndrome or within a few months of seroconversion. The most common sites of involvement are the axillary, inguinal and posterior cervical nodes, although almost any group of lymph nodes can be affected. Many cells within the affected lymph nodes, especially follicular dendritic cells, harbor actively replicating virus. Biopsy reveals reactive changes with follicular hyperplasia, but are not diagnostic. Persistent generalized lymphadenopathy does not have any prognostic significance with respect to progression of HIV infection to AIDS.

Most patients infected with HIV express detectable viral antigens and antibodies within 6 months. Patients will generally experience an initial period of intense viremia with very high viral loads during the acute retroviral syndrome and a corresponding sharp drop in their absolute number of $CD4^+$ T cells (Fig. 4-27). As a patient's immune system begins to recognize the new infection, viral load drops and $CD4^+$ T-cell count begins to climb. This control of HIV-1 infection occurs via a vigorous cytotoxic T-cell response. Viral replication continues but is constrained by the immune response. The immune system and the HIV-1 load eventually enter into a sort of uneasy equilibrium, during which the HIV-1 viral RNA load stays fairly constant at the "viral set point." During this time infected persons are generally asymptomatic.

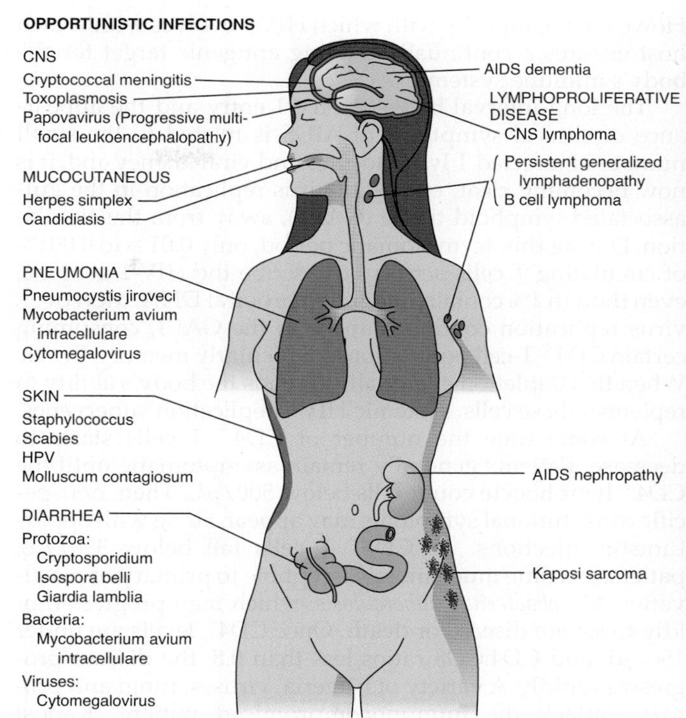

FIGURE 4-26. Human immunodeficiency virus-1 (HIV-1)–mediated destruction of the cellular immune system results in acquired immunodeficiency syndrome (AIDS). The infectious and neoplastic complications of AIDS can affect practically every organ system. CNS = central nervous system; HPV = human papilloma virus.

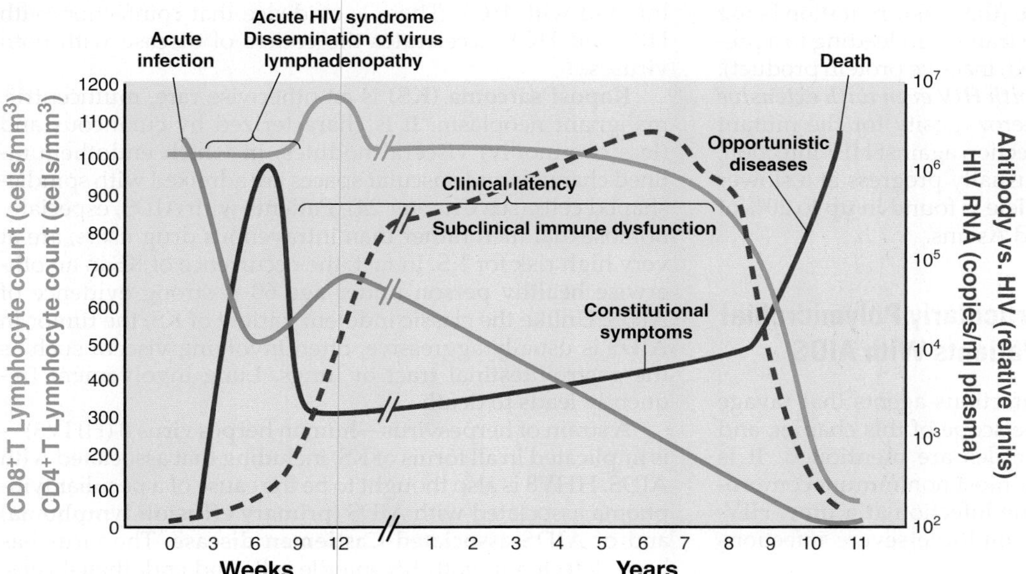

FIGURE 4-27. Generalized time course of human immunodeficiency virus-1 (HIV-1) infection. The time frame of the important events in the development of HIV-1 infection are shown, including the clinical syndrome, virus loads and $CD4^+$ and $CD8^+$ lymphocyte population dynamics over time.

However, the rapidity with which HIV-1 evolves within each host ensures a continually moving antigenic target for the body's immune system.

The long interval between HIV-1 entry and the appearance of clinical symptoms of AIDS is related to the small number of infected T lymphocytes and viral latency and, it is now becoming clear, extensive virus replication in the gut-associated lymphoid tissue (GALT), away from the circulation. During this asymptomatic period, only 0.01% to 0.001% of circulating T cells actively transcribe the HIV-1 genome, even though 1% contain integrated proviral DNA. Moreover, virus replication continues apace in the GALT, consuming certain $CD4^+$ T-cell populations, particularly memory T cells. When this depletion eventually exceeds the body's ability to replenish these cells, systemic HIV-1 replication supervenes.

At some time the number of $CD4^+$ T cells starts to decrease. Patients generally remain asymptomatic until the $CD4^+$ lymphocyte count falls below $500/\mu L$. Then, nonspecific constitutional symptoms may appear, along with opportunistic infections. As $CD4^+$ T cells fall below $350/\mu L$, patients become much more susceptible to primary or reactivation *Mycobacterium tuberculosis,* which may progress rapidly to severe disease or death. Once $CD4^+$ levels are under $150/\mu L$ and CD4:CD8 ratios less than 0.8, the disease progresses rapidly. A variety of bacteria, viruses, fungi and protozoa attack the immunocompromised patient. Kaposi sarcoma and lymphoproliferative disorders may appear, and neurologic disease is common.

Symptoms of CNS dysfunction occur in one third of AIDS patients and postmortem studies of patients who have died of AIDS reveal CNS pathology in more than three fourths of cases. HIV is thought to enter the brain via infected blood monocytes shortly after it enters the body. It then resides there in microglial cells and perivascular macrophages. HIV infection of neurons is not common, but HIV gene products produced by infected brain phagocytes are very toxic for neurons, and cause apoptosis via several mechanisms. ART drugs cross the blood-brain barrier poorly, so CNS HIV-1 infection may progress independently of HIV-1 infection outside the CNS, and despite good control of HIV-1 in the periphery. Longer survival among the HIV-positive population has led to greater numbers of patients with discernible neurologic deficits.

About 1% of whites are homozygous for asymptomatic major deletions in the CCR5 gene (the major mutation being a 32-base-pair deletion, causing a frameshift leading to a premature stop codon and a truncated, inactive protein product). ***These people remain uninfected with HIV even with extensive exposure to the agent.*** Even heterozygosity for the mutant CCR5 allele provides partial protection against HIV infection, and if infections do occur, they usually progress at a slower pace. Interestingly, the mutant allele is found in up to 20% of whites but is absent in blacks and Asians.

Opportunistic Infections, Particularly Polymicrobial Infections, Are Common in Patients With AIDS

Discussion of the diversity of infectious agents that ravage patients with AIDS is beyond the scope of this chapter, and only a few representative examples are mentioned. It is important to recognize that while most nonimmunocompromised patients will have only one infection at a time, HIV-1–infected patients can develop multiple severe infections simultaneously.

The majority of patients with HIV-1/AIDS suffer from opportunistic pulmonary infections, although this has been greatly reduced through the use of prophylactic antibiotics. *P. jiroveci* (formerly *P. carinii*) pneumonia may occur in patients with advanced HIV-1 disease. Lung infection with CMV and *M. avium-intracellulare* are less common. Patients with AIDS are also susceptible to *Legionella* infections.

Diarrhea occurs in over 75% of patients, often representing simultaneous infections with more than one organism. The most frequent pathogens are protozoans, including *Cryptosporidium, Isospora belli* and *Giardia lamblia. M. avium-intracellulare* and *Salmonella* species are the most common bacterial causes of diarrhea in AIDS patients. CMV infection of the gastrointestinal tract can manifest as a colitis associated with watery diarrhea in patients whose CD4 counts are under 50 cells/mm^3.

Cryptococcal meningitis is a devastating complication, and represents 5% to 8% of all opportunistic infections in patients with AIDS. CNS complications include cerebral toxoplasmosis; primary CNS lymphoma; encephalitis caused by herpes simplex, varicella or CMV; and progressive multifocal leukoencephalopathy, which is caused by the JC virus.

Virtually all patients with AIDS develop some form of skin disease, infections being the most prominent. *Staphylococcus aureus* is the most common, causing bullous impetigo, deeper purulent lesions (ecthyma) and folliculitis. Many of these *S. aureus* isolates carry virulence factors such as the Panton-Valentine leukocidin, which may increase the risk of bacterial invasion and severe disease. Chronic mucocutaneous herpes simplex infection is so characteristic of AIDS that it is considered an index infection in establishing the diagnosis. Skin lesions produced by *Molluscum contagiosum* and human papilloma virus (HPV) are also common, as are scabies and infections with *Candida* species. A varicella zoster eruption in someone under the age of 50 should raise the question of a possible occult HIV-1 infection.

Among the most common causes of death in patients with HIV/AIDS is hepatitis C virus (HCV) infection (see Chapter 14). In some studies, over one quarter of deaths among HIV-positive individuals are from hepatitis C. A very high percentage of HIV-positive intravenous drug abusers are also infected with HCV. There is evidence that coinfection with HIV and HCV accelerates the course of disease with both viruses.

Kaposi sarcoma (KS) is an otherwise rare, multicentric, malignant neoplasm. It is characterized by cutaneous and (less commonly) visceral nodules, in which endothelium-lined channels and vascular spaces are admixed with spindle-shaped cells (see Chapter 24). Patients with AIDS, especially homosexual men rather than intravenous drug users, are at very high risk for KS. In fact, the occurrence of KS in an otherwise healthy person under age 60 is strong evidence of AIDS. Unlike the classic indolent variety of KS, the tumor in AIDS is usually aggressive, often involving viscera such as the gastrointestinal tract or lungs. Lung involvement frequently leads to death.

A strain of herpesvirus—human herpes virus 8 (HHV8)—is implicated in all forms of KS, including that associated with AIDS. HHV8 is also thought to be the cause of a peculiar lymphoma associated with AIDS (**primary effusion lymphoma**) and of **AIDS-associated Castleman disease**. The virus has been detected in both KS spindle cells and endothelial cells.

The finding of HHV8 in the blood strongly predicts later development of KS. In fact, 75% of HIV-infected persons with HHV8 in the blood developed KS within 5 years. It is thought that HHV8 is sexually transmitted, as almost all homosexual HIV carriers are infected, but only a quarter of heterosexual drug users with HIV infection harbor HHV8.

B-cell lymphoproliferative diseases are common in patients with AIDS. Congenital and acquired immunodeficiency states are associated with B-cell hyperplasia, usually manifested as generalized lymphadenopathy. This lymphoproliferative syndrome may be followed by the appearance of high-grade B-cell lymphomas. In fact, patients who have been subjected to immunosuppressive therapy for renal transplants are at a 35-times-greater risk of developing lymphoma, and in one third of these cases the tumor is confined to the CNS. The lymphomas in chronically immunodeficient patients may manifest as an invasive polyclonal B-cell proliferation or as a monoclonal B-cell lymphoma. Many patients exhibit serologic evidence of infection with EBV and the EBV genome has been demonstrated in the lymphoma cells.

B-cell hyperplasia and generalized lymphadenopathy precede malignant lymphoproliferative disease. HIV-associated lymphomas are usually the large cell variety, as in other immunodeficiency conditions, although small cell lymphomas are sometimes seen. A conspicuous feature of lymphomas associated with AIDS is their predilection for extranodal sites, particularly primary lymphomas of the brain. In addition, lymphomas of the gastrointestinal tract, liver and bone marrow are frequent. The EBV genome has also been demonstrated in many AIDS-related lymphomas, especially in the CNS.

Efforts at Immunization to Limit Spread of HIV-1 Infection Have to Date Been Unsuccessful

Enormous energy and resources have been applied to vaccine development to prevent HIV-1 infection. To date, no approach to vaccination has provided more than a glimmer of hope. This failure reflects many factors, including the antigenic diversity of HIV-1 strains (Fig. 4-28). More mundane measures, such as careful screening of transfused blood products, condoms, male circumcision (see above) and prophylactic ART treatment of babies born to HIV-positive mothers, have helped to slow the spread of the virus.

The Introduction of Combination Antiretroviral Therapy Has Helped Many HIV-Positive People Live Longer and Healthier Lives

HIV infection represents a novel challenge in treatment. Human lentivirus infections have not been therapeutic targets in the past. Thus, new strategies have had to be developed to treat patients with HIV/AIDS. Therapy focuses on HIV proteins that are obligatory for HIV replication and sufficiently different from normal cellular proteins to offer clear targets for pharmacotherapy. Initial agents were designed to inhibit the function of HIV RT and protease (PR). Combining compounds that inhibit RT with drugs that inhibit PR has been the

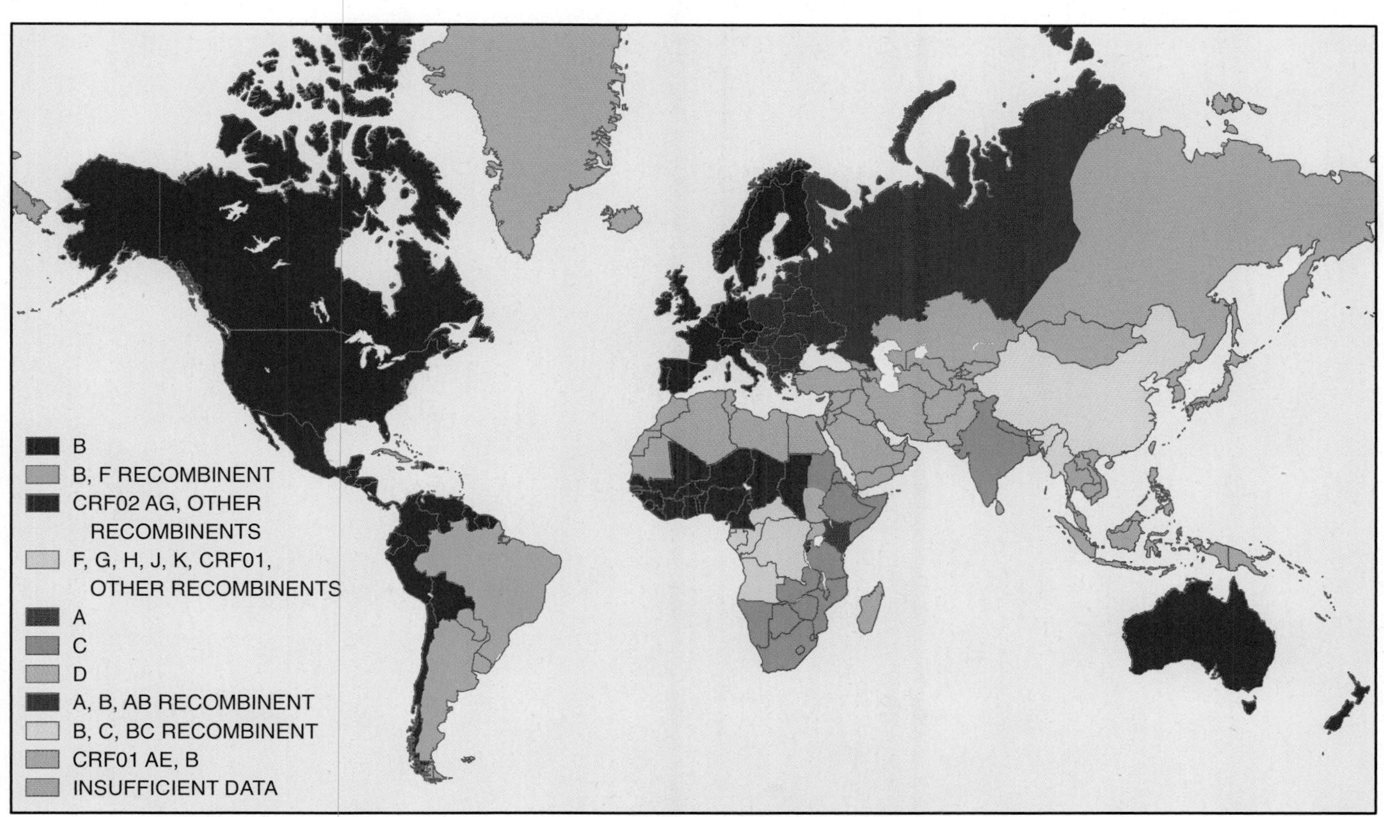

FIGURE 4-28. Diversity of human immunodeficiency virus-1 (HIV-1) antigens worldwide. The dominant HIV-1 serotypes (clades), by country; 2005 figures from the World Health Organization (WHO).

mainstay of ART. Use of ART revolutionized AIDS treatment, reducing AIDS-related mortality and increasing all indices of health in HIV-1–infected patients. Newer medications that target CCR5 and HIV-1 IN have recently been added to the antiretroviral therapeutic armamentarium.

As mentioned above, HIV-1 RT lacks an editing function, so that HIV mutates much more often than most other viruses. This high mutation rate facilitates avoidance of immune attack and enhances its ability to generate functional mutations that are resistant to ART. Although combining three or more drugs in most ART regimens depresses viral replication, HIV mutants resistant to multiple chemotherapeutic agents contribute now a high percentage of primary HIV isolates in the United States. Further, ART drugs do not cross the blood-brain barrier well, and the CNS may be a sanctuary for the virus. Thus, continuing development of antiretrovirals is needed to stay ahead of the virus's adaptability to the evolving therapeutic environment.

Quantitation of HIV-positive cells in the body has led to the conclusion that eradication of the virus from the body is not a realistic expectation with the types of chemotherapy currently available. Even ART patients with no detectable blood HIV-1 continue to deplete their memory $CD4^+$ T cells. Finally, although ART may eliminate HIV-positive cells from the blood, even temporary interruption of therapy invariably leads to viral rebound (i.e., reactivation of HIV from reservoirs outside the circulation to produce a high circulating viral load).

HIV-2 Causes a Clinical Syndrome Similar to That Caused by HIV-1

In 1985, otherwise healthy prostitutes in Senegal were discovered to harbor antibodies that cross-reacted with a monkey retrovirus, now termed **simian immunodeficiency virus** (SIV). A year later, a retrovirus similar to HIV-1 was isolated from West African patients with AIDS who were negative for antibodies against HIV-1. Antibodies to this new retrovirus, now termed HIV-2, also cross-reacted with SIV antigens. Frozen sera from West Africa dating to the 1960s have been shown to contain antibodies to HIV-2. In Guinea-Bissau, infection with HIV-2 has been shown in 8% of pregnant women, 10% of male blood donors and more than one third of prostitutes. The infection has now also been reported from other parts of Africa, Europe and the United States.

HIV-2 is morphologically similar to HIV-1, and the immunodeficiency state associated with HIV-2 infection is indistinguishable from AIDS caused by HIV-1. The risk factors for infection in both diseases seem to be similar. However, HIV-2 is felt to be derived from a different nonhuman primate virus from HIV-1, and is more difficult to transmit than HIV-1. People infected with HIV-2 tend to progress to AIDS more slowly than those infected with HIV-1.

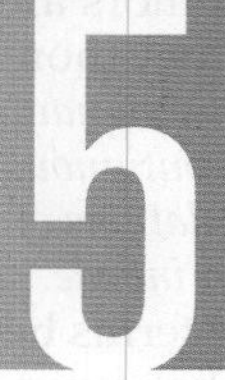

5 Neoplasia

David S. Strayer • Emanuel Rubin

THE PATHOLOGY OF NEOPLASIA

A **neoplasm** (Greek, *neo,* "new," + *plasma,* "thing formed") is the autonomous growth of tissues that have escaped normal restraints on cell proliferation and exhibit varying degrees of fidelity to their precursors. However, in some instances (e.g., follicular lymphoma; see Chapter 20), the accumulation of neoplastic cells reflects an escape from the mechanisms regulating cell survival and death. As well, some tumors (e.g., promyelocytic leukemia) involve impaired differentiation. The structural resemblance of the neoplastic cell to its cell of origin usually enables specific conclusions about its source and potential behavior. In view of their space-occupying properties, solid neoplasms are termed **tumors** (Gr., *swelling*). Tumors that remain localized are considered **benign,** whereas those that spread to distant sites are termed **malignant,** or **cancer.** The neoplastic process entails not only cell proliferation but also variable modification of the differentiation of the involved cell types. Thus, in a sense, cancer may be viewed as a burlesque of normal development.

Cancer is an ancient disease. Evidence of bone tumors has been found in prehistoric remains, and the disease is mentioned in early writings from India, Egypt, Babylonia and Greece. Hippocrates is reported to have distinguished benign from malignant growths. He also introduced the term *karkinos,* from which our term **carcinoma** is derived. In particular, Hippocrates described cancer of the breast, and in the 2nd century AD, Paul of Aegina commented on its frequency.

The incidence of neoplastic disease increases with age, and greater longevity in modern times, reflecting largely improved control of infectious and cardiovascular diseases, necessarily enlarges the population at risk. In previous centuries, on average, humans did not live long enough to develop many cancers that are particularly common in middle and old age, such as those of the prostate, colon, pancreas and kidney. If all cancer deaths caused by tobacco smoke are removed from the statistics, there has been no increase in the overall age-adjusted cancer death rate in men in the past half century, and there has been a continually decreasing rate in women. In part, this stability and decline in cancer death rates reflects improved early detection techniques (e.g., Pap smears). However, the age-adjusted incidence of specific cancers has fluctuated moderately over this time period.

In general, neoplasms are irreversible, and their growth is, for the most part, autonomous. Several observations are important:

- Neoplasms are derived from cells that normally maintain a proliferative capacity. Thus, mature neurons and cardiac myocytes do not give rise to tumors.
- A tumor may express varying degrees of differentiation, from relatively mature structures that mimic normal tissues to a collection of cells so primitive that the cell of origin cannot be identified.
- The stimuli responsible for the uncontrolled proliferation may not be identifiable.
- Neoplasia arises from mutations in genes that regulate cell growth, death or DNA repair.

Benign Versus Malignant Tumors

By definition, benign tumors do not penetrate (invade) adjacent tissue borders, nor do they spread (metastasize) to distant sites. They remain as localized overgrowths in the area in which they arise. As a rule, benign tumors are more differentiated than malignant ones—that is, they more closely resemble their tissue of origin. *By contrast, malignant tumors, or cancers, have the added property of invading contiguous tissues and metastasizing to distant sites, where subpopulations of malignant cells take up residence, grow anew and again invade.*

In common usage, the terms **benign** and **malignant** refer to the overall biological behavior of a tumor rather than to its morphologic characteristics. In most circumstances, malignant tumors have the capacity to kill, whereas benign ones spare the host. However, so-called benign tumors in critical locations can be deadly. For example, a benign intracranial tumor of the meninges (meningioma) can kill by exerting pressure on the brain. A minute benign tumor of the ependymal cells of the third ventricle (ependymoma) can block the circulation of cerebrospinal fluid, resulting in lethal hydrocephalus. A benign mesenchymal tumor of the left atrium (myxoma) may kill suddenly by blocking the mitral valve orifice. In certain locations, the erosion of a benign tumor of smooth muscle can lead to serious hemorrhage—witness the peptic ulceration of a stromal tumor in the gastric wall. On rare occasions, a functioning, benign endocrine adenoma can be life-threatening, as in the case of the sudden hypoglycemia associated with an insulinoma of the pancreas or the hypertensive crisis produced by a pheochromocytoma of the adrenal medulla. Conversely, certain types of malignant tumors are so indolent that they pose no threat to life. In this category are many cancers of the breast and prostate.

The biological behavior of some types of tumors may not necessarily reflect, or correlate with, their histologic appearance. In some cases, a tumor that displays histologic characteristics of malignancy may not metastasize or be capable of killing a patient. Basal cell carcinomas of the skin are examples of this type of tumor: they may invade subjacent structures locally but do not generally metastasize and are not life-threatening. Conversely, there are tumors that display the histologic characteristics of benignity but may be lethal. Aggressive meningiomas are nonmetastasizing, benign tumors. They may cause death by virtue of local invasiveness that may compromise vital structures. In the case of many endocrine tumors, the metastatic potential of a neoplasm is not predictable from its histology, and a tumor's benign or malignant nature can only be determined retrospectively, based on the presence or absence of metastases.

Classification of Neoplasms

In any language, the classification of objects and concepts is pragmatic and useful only insofar as its general acceptance permits effective prognostication. Similarly, the nosology of tumors reflects historical concepts, technical jargon, location, origin, descriptive modifiers and predictors of biological behavior. Although the language of tumor classification is neither rigidly logical nor consistent, it still serves as a reasonable mode of communication.

Benign Tumors Carry the Suffix "oma"

The primary descriptor of any tumor, benign or malignant, is its cell or tissue of origin. The classification of benign tumors is the basis for the names of their malignant variants. *The suffix "oma" for benign tumors is preceded by reference to the cell or tissue of origin.* For example, a benign tumor that resembles

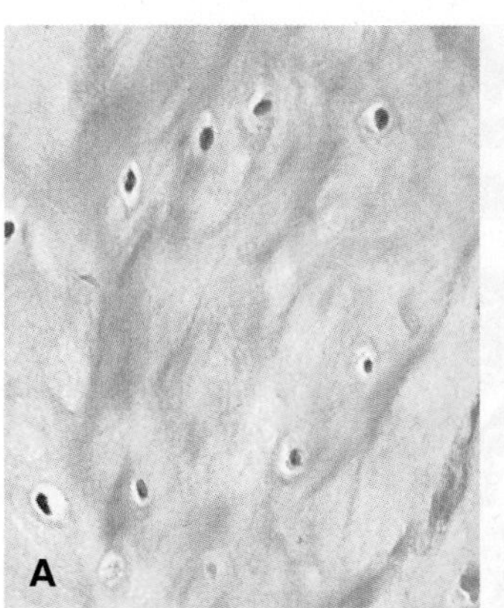

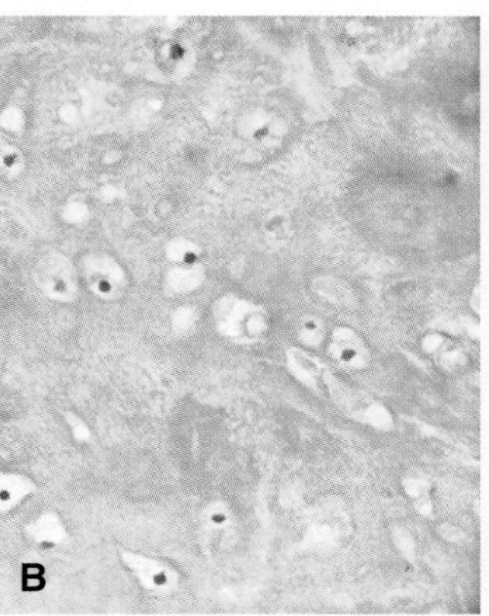

FIGURE 5-1. Benign chondroma. A. Normal cartilage. **B.** A benign chondroma closely resembles normal cartilage.

chondrocytes is called a **chondroma** (Fig. 5-1). If the tumor resembles the precursor of the chondrocyte, it is labeled **chondroblastoma.** When a chondroma is located entirely within the bone, it is designated **enchondroma.**

Tumors of epithelial origin are given a variety of names based on what is believed to be their outstanding characteristic. Thus, a benign tumor of the squamous epithelium may be called simply **epithelioma** or, when branched and exophytic, may be termed **papilloma.** Benign tumors arising from glandular epithelium, such as in the colon or the endocrine glands, are named **adenoma.** Accordingly, we refer to a **thyroid adenoma** (Fig. 5-2) or a **pancreatic islet cell adenoma.** In some instances, the predominating feature is the gross appearance, in which case we speak, for example, of an **adenomatous polyp** of the colon.

Benign tumors that arise from germ cells and contain derivatives of different germ layers are labeled **teratoma.** These tumors occur principally in the gonads and occasionally in the mediastinum and may contain a variety of structures, such as skin, neurons and glial cells, thyroid, intestinal

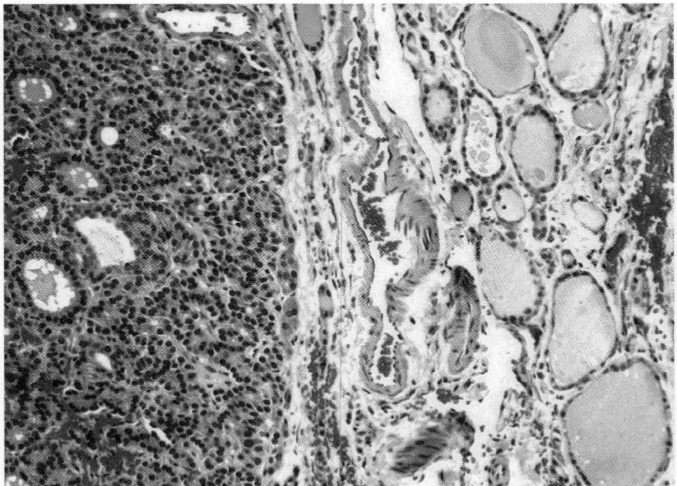

FIGURE 5-2. Benign thyroid adenoma. The follicles of a thyroid adenoma (*left*) contain colloid and resemble those of the normal thyroid tissue (*right*).

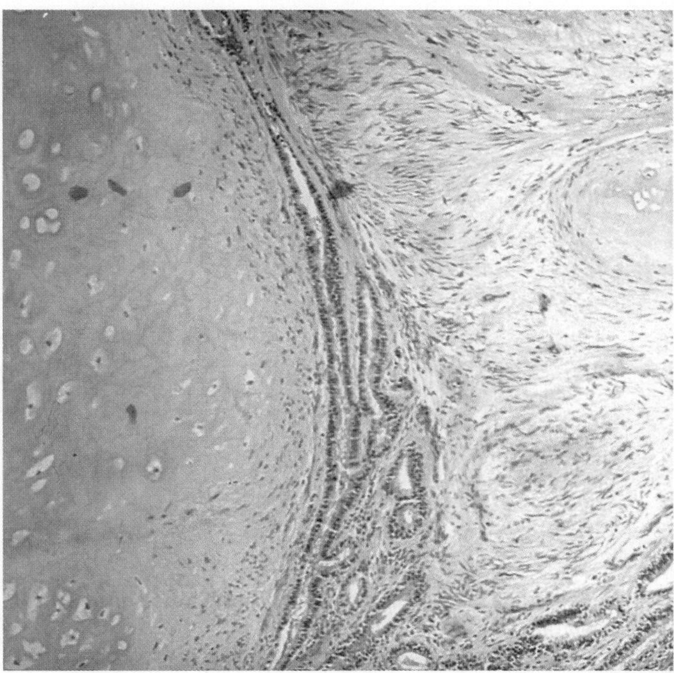

FIGURE 5-3. Hamartoma of the lung. The tumor contains islands of hyaline cartilage and clefts lined by cuboidal epithelium embedded in a fibromuscular stroma.

epithelium and cartilage. Localized, disordered differentiation during embryonic development results in a **hamartoma,** a disorganized caricature of normal tissue components (Fig. 5-3). Such tumors, which are not strictly neoplasms, contain varying combinations of cartilage, ducts or bronchi, connective tissue, blood vessels and lymphoid tissue. Ectopic islands of normal tissue, called **choristoma,** may also be mistaken for true neoplasms. These small lesions are represented by pancreatic tissue in the wall of the stomach or intestine, adrenal rests under the renal capsule and nodules of splenic tissue in the peritoneal cavity. Certain benign growths, recognized clinically as tumors, are not truly neoplastic but rather represent overgrowth of normal tissue elements. Examples are vocal cord polyps and skin tags.

Malignant Tumors Are Mostly Carcinomas or Sarcomas

In general, the malignant counterparts of benign tumors usually carry the same name, except that the suffix **"carcinoma"** *is applied to epithelial cancers and* **"sarcoma"** *to those of mesenchymal origin.* For instance, a malignant tumor of the stomach is a **gastric adenocarcinoma** or **adenocarcinoma of the stomach** (Fig. 5-4). **Squamous cell carcinoma** is an invasive tumor of the skin or other organs lined by a squamous epithelium (e.g., the esophagus). In addition, squamous cell carcinoma arises in the metaplastic squamous epithelium of the bronchus or endocervix. **Transitional cell carcinoma** is a malignant neoplasm of the bladder or ureters. By contrast, we speak of **chondrosarcoma** (Fig. 5-5) or **fibrosarcoma.** Sometimes the name of the tumor suggests the tissue type of origin, as in **osteogenic sarcoma.** Some tumors display neoplastic elements of different cell types but are not germ cell tumors. For

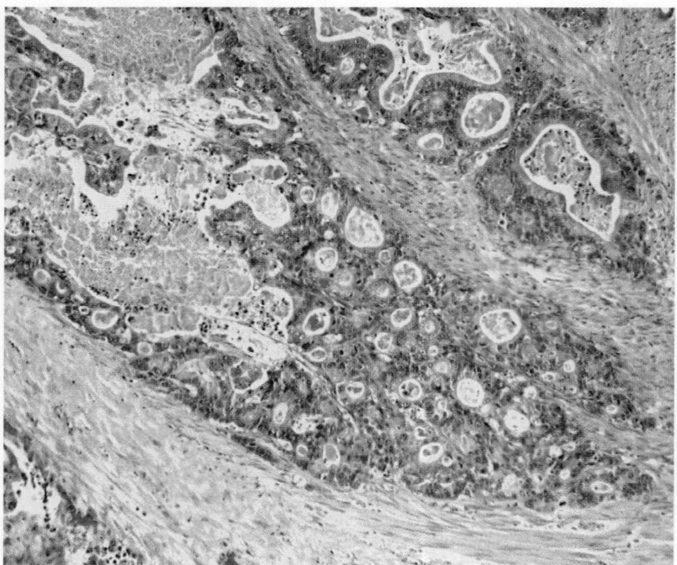

FIGURE 5-4. Adenocarcinoma of the stomach. Irregular neoplastic glands infiltrate the gastric wall.

example, **fibroadenoma** of the breast, composed of epithelial and stromal elements, is benign, whereas, as the name implies, **adenosquamous carcinoma** of the uterus or the lung is malignant. A rare malignant tumor that contains intermingled carcinomatous and sarcomatous elements is known as **carcinosarcoma.**

The persistence of certain historical terms adds a note of confusion. **Hepatoma** of the liver, **melanoma** of the skin, **seminoma** of the testis and the lymphoproliferative tumor, **lymphoma,** are all highly malignant. Tumors of the hematopoietic system are a special case in which the relationship to the blood is indicated by the suffix "emia." Thus, **leukemia** refers to a malignant proliferation of leukocytes.

Secondary descriptors (again, with some inconsistencies) refer to a tumor's morphologic and functional characteristics. For example, the term **papillary** describes a frond-like structure (Fig. 5-6). **Medullary** signifies a soft, cellular tumor with little connective tissue stroma, whereas **scirrhous** or **desmoplastic** implies a dense fibrous stroma (Fig. 5-7). **Colloid** carcinomas secrete abundant mucus, in which islands of tumor cells float. **Comedocarcinoma** is an intraductal neoplasm in which necrotic material can be expressed from the ducts. Certain visible secretions of the tumor cells lend their characteristics to the classification—for example, production of mucin or serous fluid. A further designation describes the gross appearance of a cystic mass. From all these considerations we derive such common terms as **papillary serous cystadenocarcinoma** of the ovary, **comedocarcinoma** of the breast, **adenoid cystic carcinoma** of the salivary glands, **polypoid adenocarcinoma** of the stomach and **medullary carcinoma** of the thyroid. Finally, tumors in which historically the histogenesis was poorly understood are often given an eponym—for example, Hodgkin disease, Ewing sarcoma of bone or Brenner tumor of the ovary.

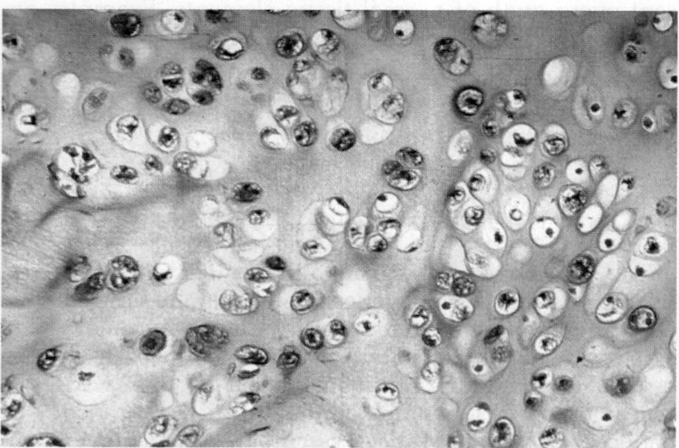

FIGURE 5-5. Chondrosarcoma of bone. The tumor is composed of malignant chondrocytes, which have bizarre shapes and irregular hyperchromatic nuclei, embedded in a cartilaginous matrix. Compare with Fig. 5-1.

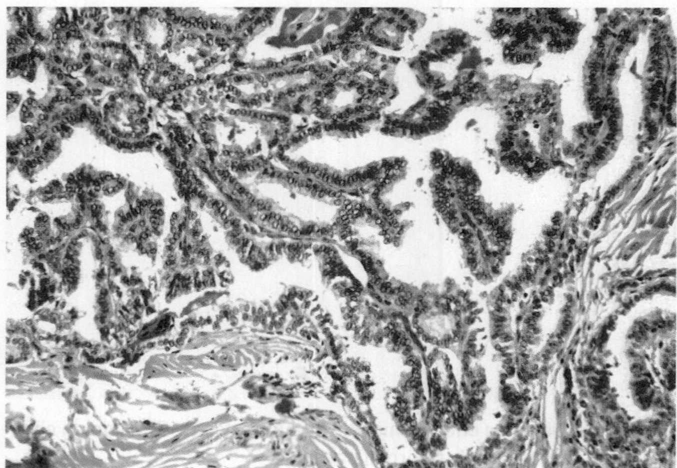

FIGURE 5-6. Papillary adenocarcinoma of the thyroid. The tumor exhibits numerous fronds lined by malignant epithelial cells.

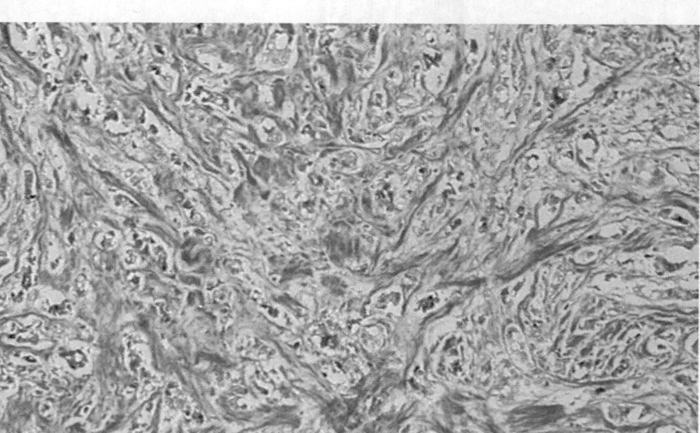

FIGURE 5-7. Scirrhous adenocarcinoma of the breast. A trichrome stain shows nests of cancer cells (*red*) embedded in a dense fibrous stroma (*blue* in this trichrome stain for collagen).

Histologic Diagnosis of Malignancy

There are no reliable molecular indicators of malignancy, and the "gold standard" for diagnosis of cancer remains routine microscopy. The distinction between benign and malignant tumors is, from a practical point of view, the most important diagnostic challenge faced by the pathologist. In most cases, the differentiation poses few problems; in a few, careful study is required before an accurate diagnosis is secure. However, there remain tumors that defy the diagnostic skills and experience of any pathologist; in these cases, the correct diagnosis must await the clinical outcome. In effect, the criteria used to assess the true biological nature of any tumor are based not on scientific principles but rather on a historical correlation of histologic and cytologic patterns with clinical outcomes. Although general criteria for malignancy are recognized, they must be used with caution in specific cases. For example, a reactive proliferation of connective cells termed **nodular fasciitis** (Fig. 5-8) has a more alarming histologic appearance than many fibrosarcomas, and misdiagnosis can lead to unnecessary surgery. Conversely, many well-differentiated endocrine adenocarcinomas are histologically indistinguishable from benign adenomas.

Benign Tumors Resemble Their Parent Tissue

Benign tumors tend to be histologically and cytologically similar to their tissues of origin. For example, **lipomas,** despite their often lobulated gross appearance, seem to be composed of normal adipocytes (Fig. 5-9). **Fibromas** are composed of mature fibroblasts and a collagenous stroma. **Chondromas** exhibit chondrocytes dispersed in a cartilaginous matrix. **Thyroid adenomas** form acini and produce thyroglobulin. The gross structure of a benign tumor may depart from the normal and assume papillary or polypoid configurations, as in papillomas of the bladder and skin and adenomatous polyps of the colon. *However, the lining epithelium of a benign tumor resembles that of the normal tissue.* Although many benign tumors are circumscribed by a connective tissue capsule, many equally benign neoplasms are not encapsulated. Unencapsulated benign tumors include papillomas and polyps of the visceral organs, hepatic adenomas, many endocrine adenomas and hemangiomas. *Remember that the definition of a benign tumor resides above all in its inability to invade adjacent tissue and to metastasize.*

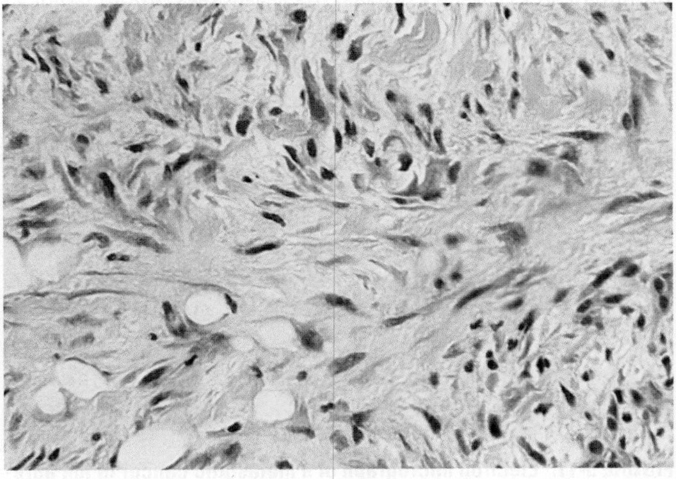

FIGURE 5-8. Nodular fasciitis. This cellular reactive lesion contains atypical and bizarre fibroblasts, which may be mistaken for a fibrosarcoma.

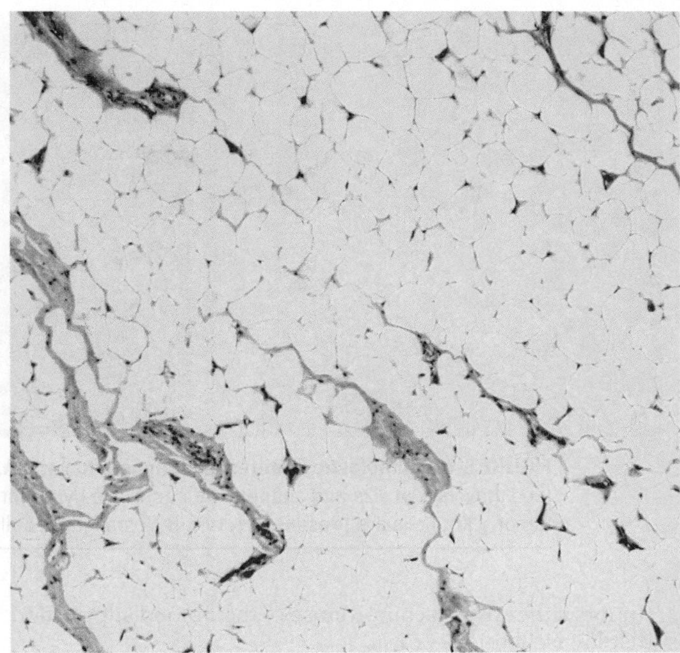

FIGURE 5-9. Lipoma. This subcutaneous, nodular tumor of adipocytes is microscopically indistinguishable from normal fat.

Malignant Tumors Depart From the Parent Tissue Morphologically and Functionally

Despite the histologic divergence of malignant tumors from their tissue of origin, an accurate identification of their source depends not only on the location but also on a morphologic resemblance to a normal tissue. Some of the histologic features that favor malignancy include the following:

- **Anaplasia or cellular atypia:** These terms refer to the lack of differentiated features in a cancer cell. In general, the degree of anaplasia correlates with the aggressiveness of the tumor. Cytologic evidence of anaplasia includes (1) variation in the size and shape of cells and cell nuclei **(pleomorphism);** (2) enlarged and hyperchromatic nuclei with coarsely clumped chromatin and prominent nucleoli; (3) atypical mitoses; and (4) bizarre cells, including tumor giant cells (Fig. 5-10). Many of these features are preceded by a preneoplastic dysplastic epithelium, which may lead to carcinoma in situ (see Chapter 1).
- **Mitotic activity:** Abundant mitoses are characteristic of many malignant tumors but are not a necessary criterion. However, in some cases (e.g., leiomyosarcomas), the diagnosis of malignancy is based on the finding of even a few mitoses.
- **Growth pattern:** In common with many benign tumors, malignant neoplasms often exhibit a disorganized and random growth pattern, which may be expressed as uniform sheets of cells, arrangements around blood vessels, papillary structures, whorls, rosettes and so forth. Malignant

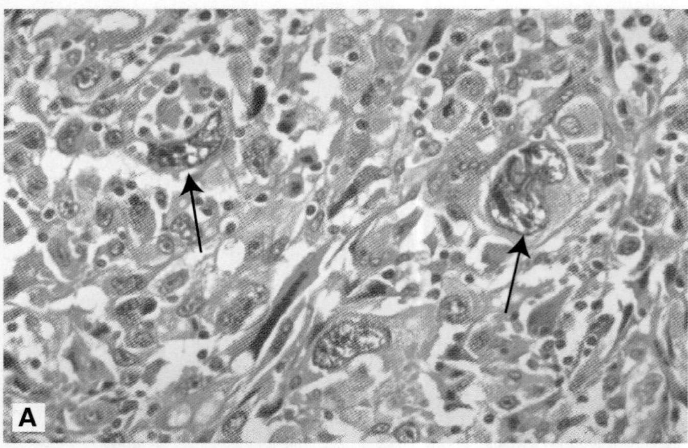

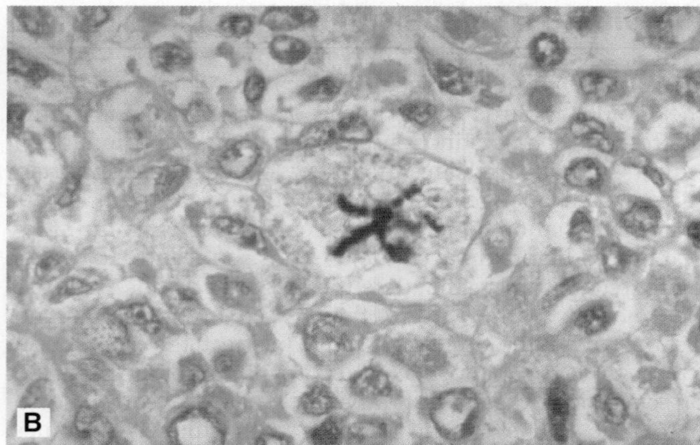

FIGURE 5-10. Anaplastic features of malignant tumors. A. The cells of this anaplastic carcinoma are highly pleomorphic (i.e., they vary in size and shape). The nuclei are hyperchromatic and are large relative to the cytoplasm. Multinucleated tumor giant cells are present (*arrows*). **B.** A malignant cell in metaphase exhibits an abnormal mitotic figure.

tumors suffer from a compromise of their blood supply and display ischemic necrosis.

- **Invasion:** Malignancy is proved by the demonstration of invasion, particularly of blood vessels and lymphatics. In some circumstances (e.g., squamous carcinoma of the cervix or carcinoma arising in an adenomatous polyp), the diagnosis of malignant transformation is made on the basis of local invasion.
- **Metastases:** The presence of metastases identifies a tumor as malignant. In metastatic disease that was not preceded by a clinically diagnosed primary tumor, the site of origin is often not readily apparent from the morphologic characteristics of the tumor. In such cases, electron microscopic examination and the demonstration of specific tumor markers may establish the correct origin.

Ultrastructural, Immunohistologic and Molecular Studies May Help to Identify the Origin of Tumors

Electron Microscopy

There are no specific determinants of malignancy or even of neoplasia itself that can be detected by electron microscopy. Although this technique may aid in identifying poorly differentiated cancers, whose classification is problematic by routine light microscopy, electron microscopy has largely been supplanted in tumor diagnosis by immunohistochemical staining. Nonetheless, carcinomas often exhibit desmosomes and specialized junctional complexes, structures that are not typical of sarcomas or lymphomas. The presence of melanosomes or premelanosomes signifies a melanoma, whereas small, membrane-bound granules with dense cores are features of endocrine neoplasms (Fig. 5-11). Another example of a diagnostically useful granule is the characteristic crystal-containing granule of an insulinoma derived from the pancreatic islets.

Tumor Markers

Tumor markers are products of malignant neoplasms that can be detected in the cells themselves or in body fluids. The ultimate tumor marker would be one that allows the unequivocal distinction between benign and malignant cells, but unfortunately no such marker exists. Nevertheless, some markers are often useful in identifying the cell of origin of a metastatic or poorly differentiated primary tumor. Metastatic tumors may be so undifferentiated microscopically as to preclude even the distinction between an epithelial and a mesenchymal origin. Tumor markers rely on the preservation of characteristics of the progenitor cell or the synthesis of specialized proteins by the neoplastic cell to make this distinction. Determination of cell lineage of undifferentiated tumors is more than an academic exercise, because therapeutic decisions may be based on their appropriate identification. For example, the treatment of carcinomas usually involves surgery, whereas malignant lymphomas are treated with radiation therapy and chemotherapy. Among these diagnostically useful markers are such diverse products as immunoglobulins, fetal proteins, enzymes, hormones and cytoskeletal and junctional proteins.

In addition to their use in identifying the lineages of malignancies, tumor-associated antigens are also used in other ways. Circulating prostate-specific antigen (PSA) is widely used to screen for prostatic carcinoma. Blood levels of

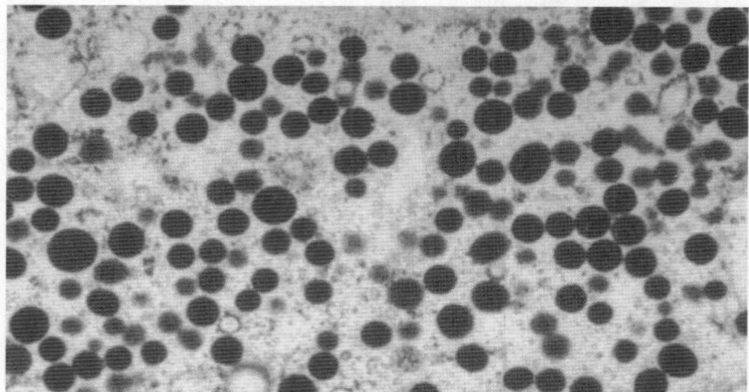

FIGURE 5-11. Electron micrograph of a metastatic cancer of the adrenal medulla (pheochromocytoma). The neuroendocrine origin of this poorly differentiated tumor was identified by the presence of characteristic cytoplasmic secretory granules.

tumor antigens are helpful in following the development of metastases and progression of the tumor after the primary neoplasm has been treated. Representative examples include carcinoembryonic antigen (CEA) for gastrointestinal tumors, cancer antigen (CA) 125 for ovarian carcinoma and prostate-specific antigen (PSA) for prostate cancer. Some tumor antigens may also be used to make important therapeutic decisions (e.g., estrogen/progesterone receptors and HER2/neu in breast cancer, epidermal growth factor receptor [EGFR] for lung cancer and c-kit for gastrointestinal stromal tumors). Tumor antigens may also be useful therapeutic targets, as illustrated by HER2/neu for breast cancer and CD20 for B-cell lymphoma.

The first demonstration of an antigen in tissue sections was reported in 1942, when Coons and coworkers used fluorescent antibodies to demonstrate a pneumococcal antigen. Some 25 years later, the visualization of tissue-bound antibody by light microscopy was facilitated by the development of horseradish peroxidase (HPO)-conjugated antibodies by Nakane and Pierce. HPO-linked antibodies were applied to tissue sections, followed by a colored substrate (usually diaminobenzidine [DAB]) for the enzyme. The product was detected as a color (in the case of DAB, brown). Counterstaining with hematoxylin facilitated localization within the specimen of the detected antigen. The specificity of the immunoperoxidase technique was greatly enhanced by the discovery in 1975 of an efficient technique for producing monoclonal antibodies by Köhler and Milstein. About the same time, the application of avidin–biotin high-affinity complexes to tissue immunostaining, combined with immunoperoxidase, increased the utility of the technique and is still used today.

Over the last 20 years, various fluorescence methodologies have been developed to detect alterations in chromosomal DNA. The method most used today is fluorescence in situ hybridization (FISH).

The following represent examples of the application of immunohistochemical methods in the diagnosis of tumors.

- **Carcinomas** uniformly express **cytokeratins (CKs),** which are intermediate filaments belonging to a multigene family of proteins. Lineage-associated markers are often useful in establishing the origin of a poorly differentiated carcinoma. For example, prostatic carcinomas consistently express the glycoprotein **PSA.** Most colon cancers produce **CEA** and CK20. Some thyroid carcinomas demonstrate **thyroglobulin,** and breast cancers frequently show nuclear receptors for **estrogen** and **progesterone.** Expression of the sialylated form of the **Lewis a antigen** (CA 19-9) has been associated with pancreatic and gastrointestinal cancers, whereas **CA 125** is a sensitive marker for ovarian cancers.
- **Neuroendocrine tumors** share positivity for cytokeratins with other carcinomas. However, they can be identified by their content of **chromogranins,** a family of proteins found in neurosecretory granules. Other markers for neuroendocrine differentiation are **synaptophysin** and Leu-7 (CD57). Specific antibodies exist for a number of peptide hormones, such as gastrin, bombesin, adrenocorticotropic hormone (ACTH), insulin, glucagon, somatostatin and serotonin.
- **Malignant melanomas** may be unpigmented and appear similar to other poorly differentiated carcinomas. They can often be distinguished by immunohistochemical studies (Fig. 5-12). Melanomas express HMB-45 and S-100 protein, but unlike most carcinomas, they are not positive for cytokeratins.
- **Soft tissue sarcomas** express the intermediate filament **vimentin.** Since this marker is also present in numerous nonmesenchymal tumors, its expression is meaningful only in concert with other markers and morphologic criteria. **Desmin,** another useful intermediate filament, is present in benign and malignant neoplasms originating from either smooth or striated muscle fibers. **Muscle-specific actin** is another marker for muscle tissue. **Neurofilament proteins** are excellent markers for tumors originating from neurons, including neuroblastomas and ganglioneuroma. **Glial fibrillary acidic protein** (GFAP), the first intermediate filament discovered, is strongly expressed on astrocytes and in most glial cell neoplasms.
- **Malignant lymphomas** are generally positive for **leukocyte common antigen** (LCA, CD45). Markers for lymphomas and leukemias were originally grouped by so-called cluster designations (CDs), at present numbering over 200, but are used today to identify a wide variety of both lymphoid and nonlymphoid cell types. Antibodies to

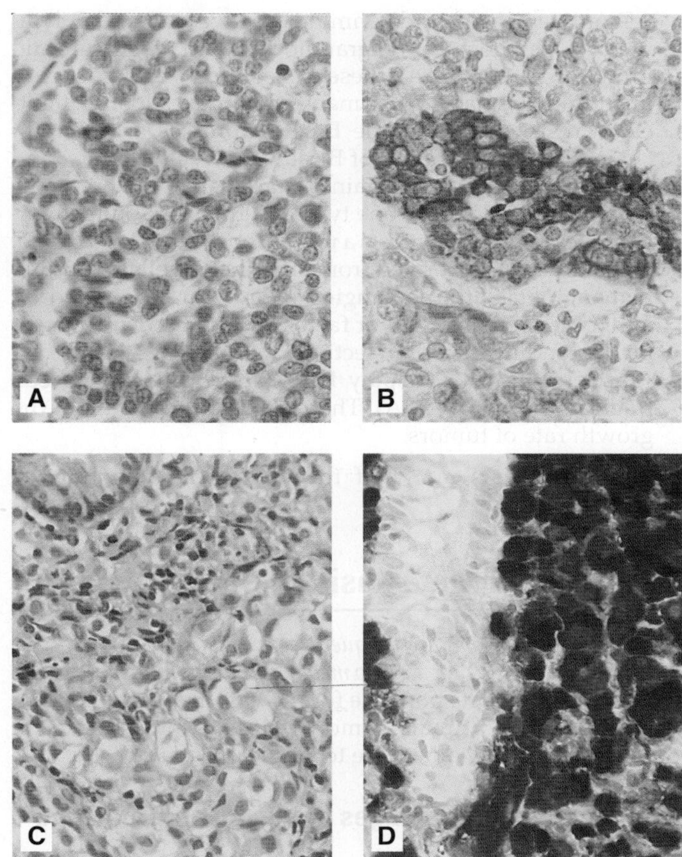

FIGURE 5-12. Tumor markers in the identification of undifferentiated neoplasms. A. A poorly differentiated metastatic bladder cancer is difficult to identify as a carcinoma with the hematoxylin and eosin stain. **B.** A section of the tumor depicted in *A* is positive for cytokeratin with an immunoperoxidase stain and is identified as carcinoma. **C.** A metastasis to the colon of an undifferentiated malignant melanoma is not pigmented, and its origin is unclear. **D.** An immunoperoxidase stain of the tumor shown in *C* reveals numerous cells positive for S-100 protein, a commonly used marker for cells of melanocytic origin.

CD antigens help to discriminate between T and B lymphocytes, monocytes and granulocytes and the mature and immature variants of these cells. B-cell malignancies, including plasmacytomas, manifest immunoglobulin light-chain restriction. A single B cell expresses κ or λ light chains. The proliferation of B cells positive for both κ and λ light chains argues against malignancy, whereas the demonstration of only one type of light chain on the lymphocytes strongly suggests a monoclonal B-cell lymphoma.

- **Vascular tumors** derived from endothelial cells, including hemangiomas and hemangiosarcomas, are identified by antibodies against CD31 or **factor VIII–related antigen,** or by the binding of certain lectins.
- **Proliferating cells** display **Ki-67** and **proliferating cell nuclear antigen** (PCNA). These are used to highlight the growth rate of tumors.

Table 5-1 lists many of the commonly used tumor markers.

Invasion and Metastasis

The two properties that are unique to cancer cells are the ability to invade locally and the capacity to metastasize to distant sites. These characteristics are responsible for the vast majority of deaths from cancer; the primary tumor itself (e.g., breast or colon cancer) is generally amenable to surgical resection.

Direct Extension Damages the Involved Organ and Adjacent Tissues

Most carcinomas begin as localized growths confined to the epithelium in which they arise. As long as these early cancers do not penetrate the basement membrane on which the epithelium rests, such tumors are termed ***carcinoma in situ*** (Fig. 5-13). In this stage, it is unfortunate that in situ tumors are asymptomatic, because they are invariably curable. When the in situ tumor acquires invasive potential and extends directly through the underlying basement membrane, it can compromise neighboring tissues and metastasize. In situations in which cancer arises from cells that are not confined by a basement membrane—such as connective tissue cells, lymphoid elements and hepatocytes—an in situ stage is not defined.

Malignant tumors characteristically grow within the tissue of origin, where they enlarge and infiltrate normal structures. They may also extend directly beyond the confines of that organ to involve adjacent tissues. The growth of the cancer is occasionally so extensive that replacement of the normal tissue results in functional insufficiency of the organ. Such a situation is not uncommon in primary liver cancer. Brain tumors, such as astrocytomas, infiltrate the brain until they compromise vital regions. The direct extension of malignant tumors within an organ may also be life-threatening because of their location. A common example is the intestinal obstruction produced by cancer of the colon (Fig. 5-14).

The invasive growth pattern of cancers often leads to their direct extension outside the tissue of origin, in which case the tumor may secondarily impair the function of an adjacent organ. Squamous carcinoma of the cervix frequently grows beyond the genital tract to obstruct the

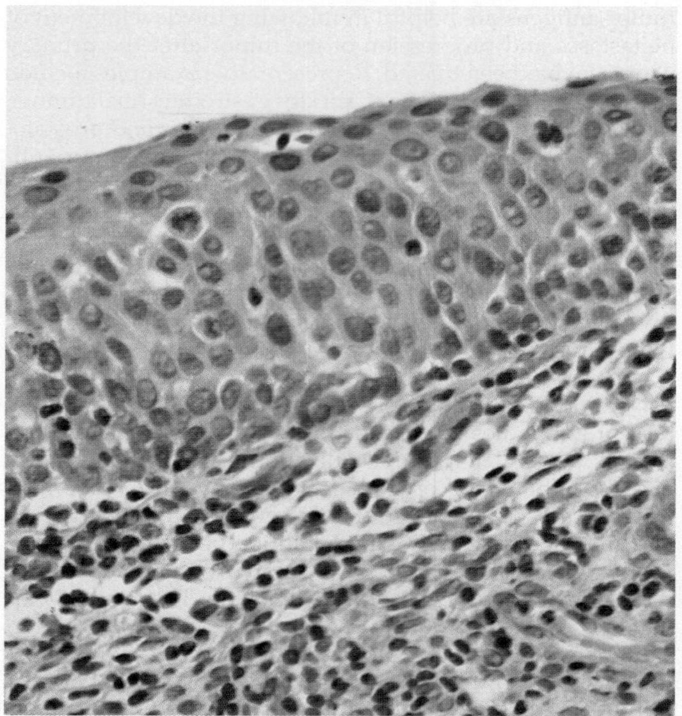

FIGURE 5-13. Carcinoma in situ. A section of the uterine cervix shows neoplastic squamous cells occupying the full thickness of the epithelium and confined to the mucosa by the underlying basement membrane.

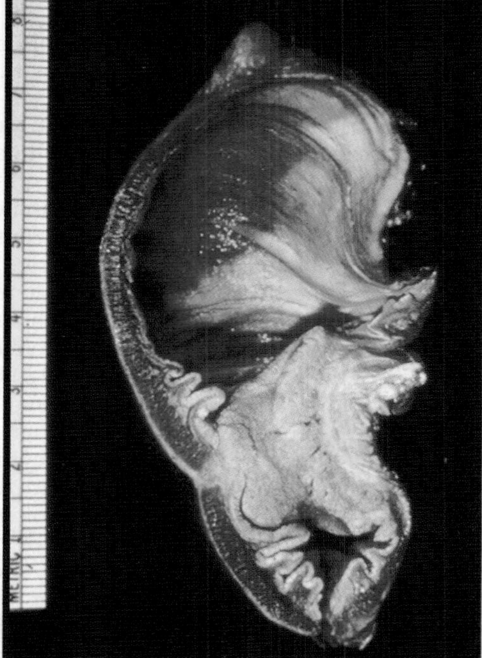

FIGURE 5-14. Adenocarcinoma of the colon with intestinal obstruction. The lumen of the colon at the site of the cancer is narrow. The colon above the obstruction is dilated.

Table 5-1

Frequently Used Markers to Identify Tumors

Marker	Target Cells
Epithelial Cells	
Cytokeratins (CKs)	Carcinomas, mesothelioma
CK7	Many non-GI adenocarcinomas
CK20	Gastrointestinal and ovarian carcinomas, urothelial carcinomas, Merkel cell tumor
Epithelial membrane antigen (EMA)	Carcinomas, mesothelioma, some large cell lymphomas
Ber-Ep4	Most carcinomas, but not in mesothelioma
B72.3 (tumor associated)	Many adenocarcinomas, but not in mesothelioma
Carcinoembryonic antigen (CEA)	Many adenocarcinomas of endodermal origin but not in others (e.g., renal, mesothelioma)
Mesothelial Cells	
Cytokeratins CK5/6	Mesothelioma
Vimentin	Mesothelioma
HBME	Mesothelioma, thyroid tumors
Calretinin	Mesothelioma
Melanocytes	
HMB-45	Malignant melanoma
S-100 protein	Malignant melanoma, glial cells
Mel A	Malignant melanoma
Neuroendocrine and Neural Cells	
Chromogranins, particularly chromogranin A	Neuroendocrine tumors
Synaptophysin	Neuroendocrine tumors
CD57	Neuroendocrine tumors, T and NK cells, Schwann cells
Glial Cells	
Glial fibrillary acidic protein (GFAP)	Astrocytoma and other glial tumors
Mesenchymal Cells	
Vimentin	Most sarcomas
Desmin	All types of muscle tumors
Muscle-specific actin	Muscle tumors, myofibroblast tumors
CD99	Ewing sarcoma, peripheral neuroectodermal tumors (PNETs), acute lymphoid and myeloid leukemias
Specific Organs	
Prostate-specific antigen (PSA)	Prostatic cancer
Prostate-specific alkaline phosphatase (PSAP)	Prostate cancer
Thyroglobulin	Thyroid cancer
α-Fetoprotein (AFP)	Hepatocellular carcinoma, yolk sac tumor
HepPar 1	Hepatocellular carcinoma
WT1	Wilms tumor, some mesotheliomas
Placental alkaline phosphatase (PLAP)	Seminoma, embryonal carcinoma
Human chorionic gonadotropin (hCG)	Trophoblastic tumors
CA19-9	Pancreatic and gastrointestinal carcinomas
CA125	Ovarian carcinoma, endometrial carcinoma, some other nongynecologic tumors (pancreas, mesothelioma)
Calcitonin	Medullary carcinoma of the thyroid
CD Markers	
CD1	Some T-cell leukemias, Langerhans cell proliferations
CD2	T cells, T-cell malignancies
CD3	T cells, T-cell malignancies
CD4	T cells, T-cell malignancies, monocytes, monocytic malignancies
CD5	T cells, some B-cell malignancies
CD8	Suppressor T cells, some T-cell malignancies
CD10 (common ALL antigen, CALLA)	Acute lymphoblastic leukemia, some B-cell lymphomas, renal cell carcinomas
CD15	Reed-Sternberg cells, some T cells, some myeloid leukemias, many adenocarcinomas, but not in mesothelioma
CD19	B cells, B-cell malignancies
CD20	B cells, B-cell malignancies
CD30	Hodgkin disease, anaplastic large cell lymphoma

(*continued*)

Table 5-1

Frequently Used Markers to Identify Tumors (*Continued*)

Marker	Target Cells
CD33	Myeloid leukemias
CD34	Acute myeloid or lymphoblastic leukemias, some spindle cell tumors
CD117 (c-Kit)	Chronic myeloid leukemia, gastrointestinal stromal tumors, seminomas, also tumors of lung, breast, endometrium, urinary bladder
Non-CD Leukemia/Lymphoma Markers	
κ Light chain	B-cell malignancies
λ Light chain	B-cell malignancies
TdT	Acute lymphoblastic leukemia
Bcl-1 and cyclin D1	Mantle cell lymphoma
Endothelial Markers	
von Willebrand factor (vWF)	Vascular neoplasms
CD31	Vascular neoplasms, endothelial cells
CD34	Bone marrow stem cells, vascular neoplasms (endothelial cells)
Lectins	Vascular neoplasms
CD43	Almost all leukocytes
CD56	NK cells

CA = cancer antigen; CD = cluster designation; GI = gastrointestinal; TdT = terminal deoxynucleotidyl transferase.

ureters or produce vesicovaginal fistulas. Neglected cases of breast cancer are often complicated by extensive skin ulceration. Even small tumors can produce severe consequences when they invade vital structures. A small lung cancer can cause a bronchopleural fistula when it penetrates the bronchus or exsanguinating hemorrhage when it erodes a blood vessel. The agonizing pain of pancreatic carcinoma results from direct extension of the tumor to the celiac nerve plexus. Tumor cells that reach serous cavities (e.g., those of the peritoneum or pleura) spread easily by direct extension or can be carried by the fluid to new locations on the serous membranes. The most common example is the seeding of the peritoneal cavity by certain types of ovarian cancer (Fig. 5-15).

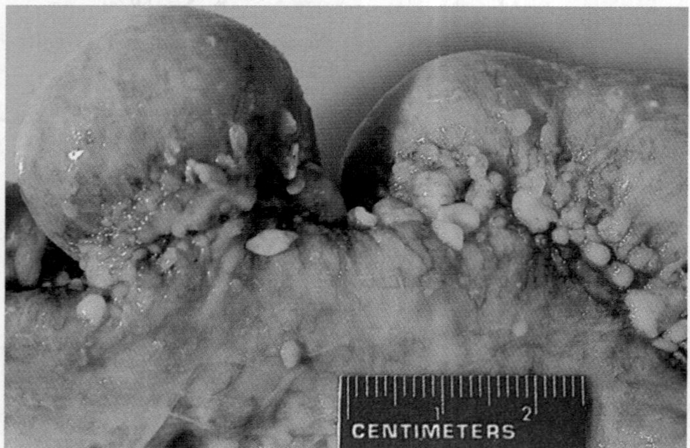

FIGURE 5-15. Peritoneal carcinomatosis. The mesentery attached to a loop of small bowel is studded with small nodules of metastatic ovarian carcinoma.

Metastatic Spread Is the Most Common Cause of Cancer Deaths

Metastasis (Greek, "displacement") is the migration of malignant cells from one site to another noncontiguous site. The invasive properties of malignant tumors bring them into contact with blood and lymphatic vessels. *In the same way that they can invade parenchymal tissue, neoplastic cells can also penetrate vascular and lymphatic channels, through which they disseminate to distant sites.* In general, metastases resemble the primary tumor histologically, although they are occasionally so anaplastic that their cell of origin is obscure.

Hematogenous Metastases

Cancer cells commonly invade capillaries and venules, whereas thicker-walled arterioles and arteries are relatively resistant. Before they can form viable metastases, circulating tumor cells must lodge in the vascular bed of the metastatic site (Fig. 5-16). Here they presumably attach to the walls of blood vessels, either to endothelial cells or to naked basement membranes. For many tumors this sequence of events explains why the liver and the lung are so frequently the sites of metastases. Because abdominal tumors seed the portal system, they lead to hepatic metastases; other tumors penetrate systemic veins that eventually drain into the vena cava and hence to the lungs. In this respect, some tumor cells released into the venous system survive passage through the microcirculation and are thus transported to more distant organs. For instance, tumor cells may traverse the liver and produce pulmonary metastases, and neoplastic cells may also survive passage through the pulmonary microcirculation to reach the brain, bones (Fig. 5-17) and other organs through arterial dissemination. Neoplastic cells arrested in the microcirculation penetrate the vessel walls at the site of metastasis.

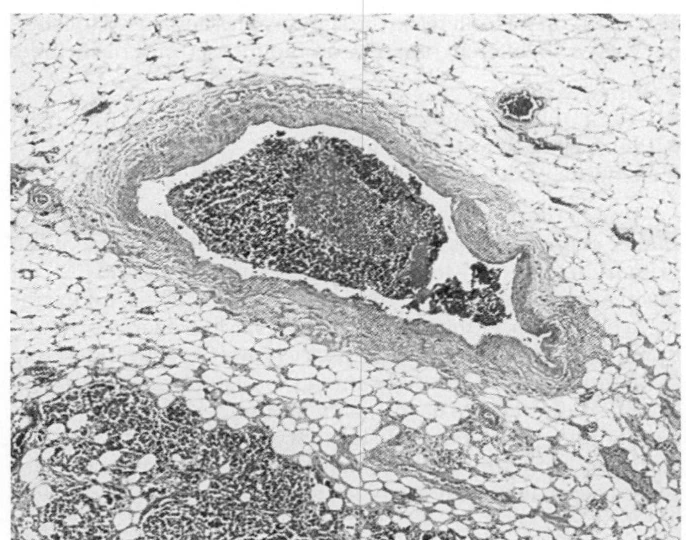

FIGURE 5-16. Hematogenous spread of cancer. A malignant tumor (*bottom*) has invaded adipose tissue and penetrated into a small vein.

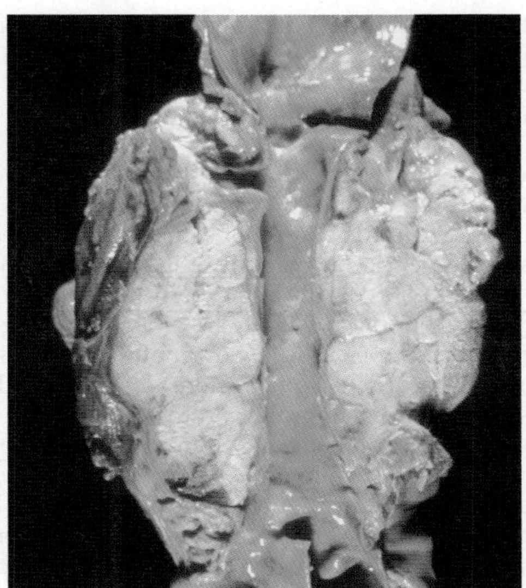

FIGURE 5-18. Metastatic carcinoma in periaortic lymph nodes. The aorta has been opened and the nodes bisected.

Lymphatic Metastases

A historical dogma of metastatic spread held that epithelial tumors (carcinomas) preferentially metastasize through lymphatic channels, whereas mesenchymal neoplasms (sarcomas) are distributed hematogenously. This distinction is no longer considered valid because of clinical observations of metastatic patterns and the demonstration of numerous connections between the lymphatic and vascular systems. Tumors arising in tissues that have a rich lymphatic network (e.g., the breast) often metastasize by this route, although the particular properties of specific neoplasms may play a role in the route of spread.

Basement membranes envelop only large lymphatic channels; they are lacking in lymphatic capillaries. Thus, invasive tumor cells may penetrate lymphatic channels more readily than blood vessels. Once in lymphatic vessels, the cells are carried to the regional draining lymph nodes, where they initially lodge in the marginal sinus and then extend throughout the node. Lymph nodes bearing metastatic deposits may be enlarged to many times their normal size, often exceeding the diameter of the primary lesion. The cut surface of the lymph node usually resembles that of the primary tumor in color and consistency and may also exhibit the necrosis and hemorrhage commonly seen in primary cancers (Fig. 5-18).

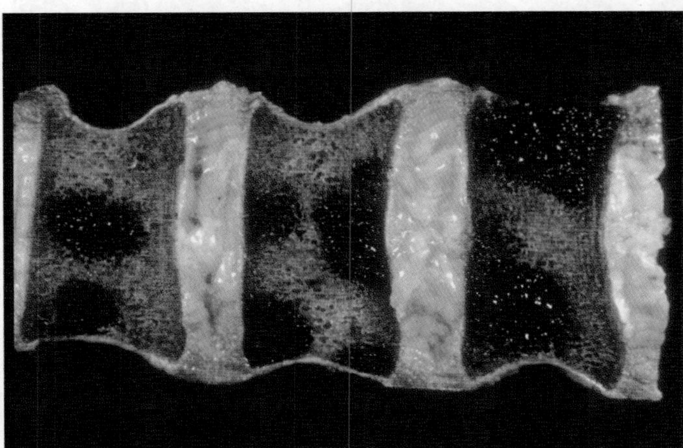

FIGURE 5-17. Multiple pigmented metastases in the vertebral bodies in a patient who died of malignant melanoma.

The regional lymphatic pattern of metastatic spread is most prominently exemplified by breast cancer. The initial metastases are almost always lymphatic, and these regional lymphatic metastases have considerable prognostic significance. Cancers that arise in the lateral aspect of the breast characteristically spread to axillary lymph nodes; those arising in the medial portion drain to the internal mammary thoracic lymph nodes.

Lymphatic metastases are occasionally found in lymph nodes distant from the site of the primary tumor. For example, occasional abdominal cancers may initially be signaled by the appearance of an enlarged supraclavicular node. A graphic example of the relationship of lymphatic anatomy to the spread of malignant tumors is afforded by cancers of the testis. Rather than metastasizing to inguinal nodes, as do other tumors of the male external genitalia, testicular cancers typically involve the draining abdominal periaortic nodes. The explanation lies in the descent of the testis from an intra-abdominal site to the scrotum, during which it is accompanied by its own lymphatic supply.

Seeding of Body Cavities

Malignant tumors that arise in organs adjacent to body cavities (e.g., ovaries, gastrointestinal tract and lung) may shed malignant cells into these spaces. Such body cavities principally include the peritoneal and pleural cavities, although occasional seeding of the pericardial cavity, joint space and subarachnoid space is observed. Similar to tissue culture, tumors in these sites grow in masses and often produce fluid (e.g., ascites, pleural fluid), sometimes in very large quantities.

Mucinous adenocarcinoma may also secrete copious amounts of mucin in these locations.

Target Organs in Metastatic Disease

It was recognized more than a century ago that the distribution of metastases in breast cancer is not random. In 1889, Paget proposed that the spread of tumor cells to specific secondary sites depends on compatibility between the tumor cells (the seed) and favorable microenvironment factors in the secondary site (the soil). By contrast, others have argued that metastatic spread depends solely on anatomic factors and the blood flow to an organ. Today, there is evidence that both mechanisms operate, depending on the tumor. For example, cancers of the breast, prostate and thyroid metastasize to bone, a tropism that suggests a favored "soil." Conversely, despite their size and abundant blood flow, neither the spleen nor skeletal muscle is a common site of metastases. There is evidence that tumor-associated stromal cells in fact "plow the road" for tumor spread to particular sites that are suitable to the metastatic survival of implants from that tumor (see below). Yet for many cancers, the vascular anatomy unquestionably influences the pattern of metastatic spread. Malignant tumors of the gastrointestinal tract commonly metastasize to the first vascular bed they encounter, namely, the liver. Similarly, lung cancers often spread to the brain. Additional factors that influence homing of cancer metastases are discussed later.

The Staging and Grading of Cancers

In an attempt to predict the clinical behavior of a malignant tumor and to establish criteria for therapy, many cancers are classified according to cytologic and histologic grading schemes or by staging protocols that describe the extent of spread.

Cancer Staging Refers to the Extent of Spread

The choice of a surgical approach or the selection of treatment modalities is principally influenced by the stage of a cancer. Moreover, most statistical data related to cancer survival are also based on this criterion. The significant criteria used for staging vary with different organs. Commonly used criteria include:

- Tumor size
- Extent of local growth, whether within or out of the organ
- Presence of lymph node metastases
- Presence of distant metastases

These criteria have been codified in the international **TNM cancer staging system,** in which "T" refers to the size of the primary tumor, "N" to regional node metastases and "M" to the presence and extent of distant metastases. Thus, for example, a breast cancer that is staged at T3N2M0 is a large primary tumor (T3) that has involved axillary lymph nodes moderately (N2), but has not detectably spread to distant sites (M0). The specific definitions of each T, N or M number vary among different tumors. As well, some tumor types, like central nervous system (CNS) tumors and hematologic malignancies, are staged according to different systems.

Cancer Grading Reflects the Organization and Cytology of Tumors

Well-differentiated tumors are referred to as low grade, whereas poorly differentiated neoplasms are regarded as high grade. Cytologic and histologic grading, which are necessarily subjective and at best semiquantitative, are based on the degree of anaplasia and on the number of proliferating cells. The degree of anaplasia is determined from the shape and regularity of the cells and from the presence of distinct differentiated features, such as functioning gland-like structures in adenocarcinomas or epithelial pearls in squamous carcinomas. The presence of such characteristics identifies a tumor as well differentiated. By contrast, the cells of "poorly differentiated" malignancies bear little resemblance to their normal counterparts. Evidence of rapid or abnormal growth is provided by (1) large numbers of mitoses, (2) atypical mitoses, (3) nuclear pleomorphism and (4) tumor giant cells. Most grading schemes classify tumors into three or four grades of increasing malignancy (Fig. 5-19). The general correlation

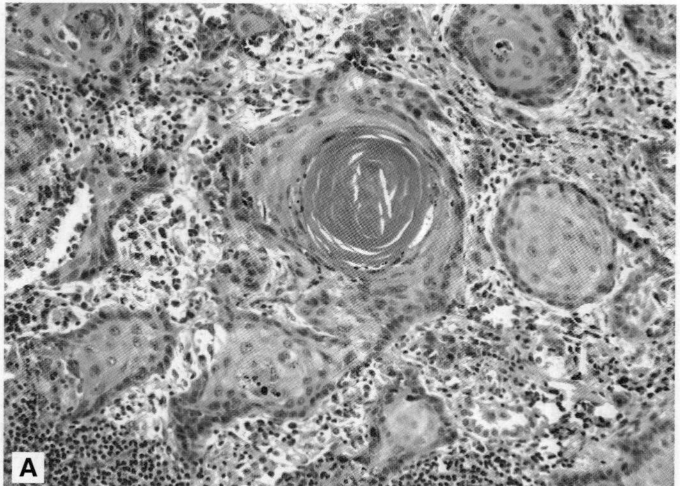

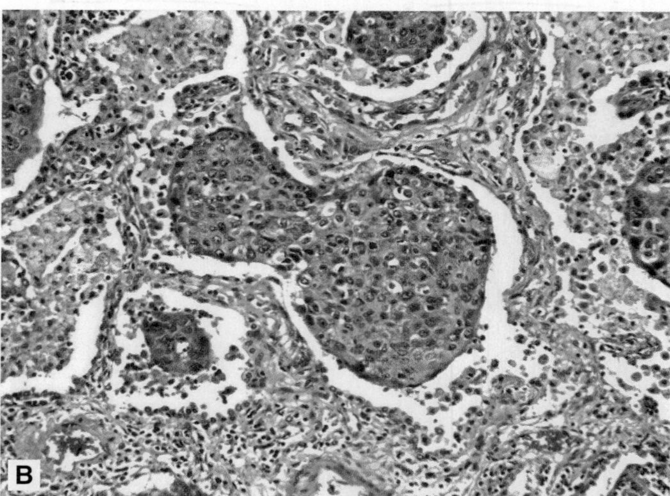

FIGURE 5-19. Cytologic grading of squamous cell carcinoma of the lung. A. Well-differentiated (grade 1) squamous cell carcinoma. The tumor cells bear a strong resemblance to normal squamous cells and synthesize keratin, as evidenced by epithelial pearls. **B.** Poorly differentiated (grade 3) squamous cell carcinoma. The malignant cells are difficult to identify as being of squamous origin.

between the cytologic grade and the biological behavior of a neoplasm is not invariable: there are many examples of tumors of low cytologic grades that exhibit substantial malignant properties.

THE BIOLOGY AND MOLECULAR PATHOGENESIS OF CANCER

Normal cells, even those that divide the most rapidly (e.g., myelocytes, intestinal mucosal cells), are exquisitely controlled in the rate and location of their proliferation and accumulation. Cancer arises with accumulated DNA mutations within a single cell. When enough mutations have occurred, the cell escapes growth control and eventually acquires additional mutations that permit local invasion and subsequent spread through vascular and lymphatic channels.

For most of recorded history, the genesis of cancer was considered to be simply due to a mysterious act of God. That is, the causation of cancer was not inherently comprehensible. However, in the late 18th century, specific causes of cancer were first identified. John Hill of London proposed that exposure to tobacco caused cancer. Shortly thereafter, Sir Percival Pott described scrotal cancer caused by soot among chimney sweeps in London. More than a century later, bladder cancer was reported in aniline dye workers in Germany.

In modern times, the major milestones in our understanding of tumor development include:

- 1911: F. Peyton Rous first described an avian cancer as being caused by a filterable agent (virus).
- 1920s: Human exposure to x-rays via fluoroscopy led to cancer.
- 1941: Berenblum first proposed the two-step (initiation/promotion) theory of chemical carcinogenesis.
- 1953: Watson and Crick identified DNA as the genetic material of cells and elucidated the structure of DNA.
- 1971: A. G. Knudson reported the involvement of two mutated alleles of the retinoblastoma (Rb) gene in the development of retinoblastomas and termed these genes tumor suppressors.
- 1974: The gene responsible for defective DNA repair in the skin disease xeroderma pigmentosum was linked to visceral cancers.
- 1976: Bishop and Varmus demonstrated mammalian genetic homologs, called proto-oncogenes, of viral transforming genes (oncogenes). When mutated, these cellular genes may be changed into growth-promoting genes (*c-onc*) that can lead to cancer.

In recent years, numerous other processes that impact on carcinogenesis have been identified. These include epigenetic changes, microRNAs, DNA methylation, covalent modification of histones and the role of apoptosis. Thus, the final answers to the pathogenesis of cancers remain elusive, and substantial research remains to be conducted.

Diverse Experimental Approaches Are Used to Study Tumorigenesis

Modern research into the molecular pathogenesis of cancer depends largely upon certain types of experimental models. The student of medicine is well advised to be aware of the means by which we come to our understanding of oncogenesis and the limitations of those experimental systems.

- **Cell culture:** In vitro studies may involve normal cells, cancer cells or a mixture of both. Like a freeze-frame vignette of a motion picture, cell culture studies permit careful analysis of individual influences, but their weakness is their inability to assess such influences in the context of an affected organ or animal.
- **Tumor transplants:** Transplantation of tumors into experimental animals permits study of various therapies (e.g., chemotherapy or immune manipulation). Tumor cells may also be transplanted to study certain facets of tumor growth, invasion and metastasis. The host can be manipulated to evaluate its interaction with the tumor as well.
- **Oncogenesis in animals:** The early phases of tumor pathogenesis may be studied by treating experimental animals with cancer-causing agents, such as chemicals, viruses, radiation, etc. This allows for study of early molecular events in oncogenesis in the context of a whole animal.
- **Genetically engineered organisms:** The DNA of experimental animals can be engineered to express, or lack, selected genes. Among these are genes thought to be involved in the pathogenesis of cancer. Because these experiments rely upon germline transmission of the genetic alterations, they illuminate the connections between embryonic development and later occurrence of cancer. Genetically modified yeast and *Candida elegans* (a roundworm) have been used extensively to elucidate signaling mechanisms related to tumorigenesis.
- **Molecular analyses:** The study of human tumors encompasses studies of DNA structure, gene expression, epigenetic factors, signaling pathways, metabolism, cell–matrix interactions and other possible influences on tumor biology. Given the current availability of high-throughput analyses, these types of studies often generate gargantuan amounts of data. Understanding how such data relate to specific aspects of tumor biology requires extensive and intensive computational resources.

Normal Processes That Regulate Cells and Inhibit Oncogenesis

What is a gene? Even before the discovery of the structure of DNA, the gene was defined as the unit of heredity. With the discovery that DNA was the genetic material and that DNA was transcribed into messenger RNA (mRNA), which was then translated into proteins, the terminology changed to define a gene as a segment of DNA that encoded a protein. However, the idea of a gene is now being reexamined because regions of the genome previously thought to be "noncoding" are now known to produce new classes of RNAs that influence gene expression. Moreover, regulatory DNA sequences may be located adjacent to, at a large distance from and even within the protein-coding sequences. Epigenetic phenomena elsewhere in the cell may also exert significant regulatory influences on gene expression. The contemporary notion of a gene and its regulation entails interdependent structures and layers and webs of control involving DNA sequences, RNA species, regulatory proteins and a complex signaling apparatus. Thus, the precise definition of a gene remains unsettled.

Mutations and Polymorphism: DNA replication is not perfect, and with each cell division about 1 nucleotide in 10^9 differs from the original. Thus, although the vast majority (99.6%) of base pairs in somatic cells are identical within the human race, two humans differ on the average by about 2.4×10^7 base pairs out of a total of 6×10^9 base pairs. In this way, the genetic determinants of "humanness" comprise almost all of the human genome and only the remainder can change without compromising an individual's (or progeny's) viability.

Variations in DNA sequences may result from germline changes or acquired alterations in somatic DNA as a result of single nucleotide substitutions or insertion or deletion of one or more nucleotides. **Polymorphisms** are defined as variations in DNA sequence that occur with a frequency of over 1% of the population and are not associated with known diseases. **Mutations** are comparable genetic changes that contribute to disease. (Mechanisms and types of DNA sequence variations are described in Chapter 6.)

Normal Cell Cycle Regulation Is an Important Defense Against Tumorigenesis

Since most cancers are characterized by uncontrolled cellular proliferation, an understanding of the functioning of normal cell cycle machinery is important. Cell replication follows a tightly orchestrated program. Myriad intracellular signal transduction pathways connect extracellular signals (growth factors, cytokines, etc.) with genes that regulate the cell cycle.

Cells may be cycling or quiescent. Those that replicate continuously (e.g., intestinal mucosa, hematopoietic progenitor cells) always transition from mitosis (M phase) to G_1, which is the antechamber to further cell division. By contrast, cells that replicate infrequently (e.g., hepatocytes) are in a quiescent phase, G_0. Upon stimulation by cytokines or events such as cell injury, cells in G_0 may enter G_1, after which they progress to cell division (Fig. 5-20).

DNA replication occurs in S phase, which is followed by G_2 and ultimately M. Cells progress directly from M phase into G_1 when they are in an actively dividing mode. Transit from one phase to another of the cell cycle is regulated at **checkpoints,** namely, times at which progression in the cell cycle can be prevented by specific proteins. Thus, during G_1, the commitment to enter S phase occurs at a **restriction point (R),** wherein the cell monitors its internal and external environment and "decides" whether to proceed with replication. The R point is regulated by **cyclins,** so named for their cyclic expression and degradation during the cell cycle. Cyclins activate a family of related protein kinases, **cyclin-dependent kinases (CDKs).** CDKs 2, 4 and 6 phosphorylate a family of **retinoblastoma proteins** (pRb). pRb phosphorylation unleashes transcription factors of the **E2F** family. E2F then drives the cell past the R point. Other cyclins and CDKs regulate S to G_2 and G_2 to M transitions.

CDKs are also regulated by **cyclin-dependent kinase inhibitors (CKIs).** Expression of CKIs can be induced by senescence, contact inhibition, extracellular antimitogenic factors (e.g., transforming growth factor-β [TGF-β]) and the tumor suppressor protein p53 (see below). The latter senses DNA damage at two checkpoints and suspends cell cycle transit until the damage is repaired. Should DNA repair fail, p53 activates apoptosis.

Recent data emphasize that phase transitions in the cell cycle are heavily influenced by ubiquitin conjugation and

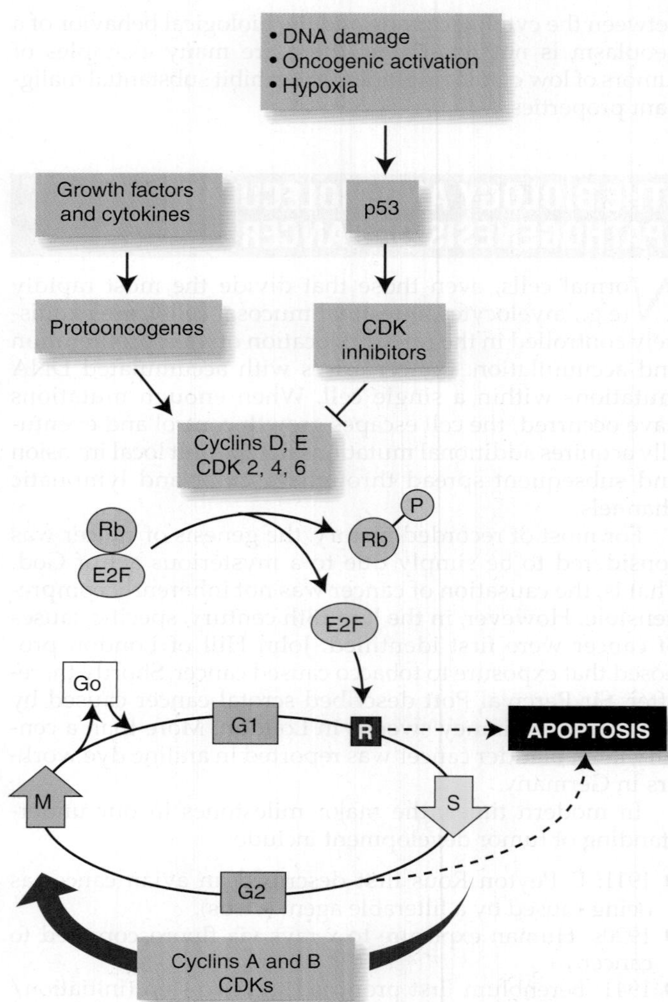

FIGURE 5-20. Regulation of the cell cycle. Cells are stimulated to enter G_1 from G_0 by growth factors and cytokines via proto-oncogene activation. A critical juncture in the transition of cells from G_1 to S phase is the restriction point (R). A major regulatory event in this process is the phosphorylation of retinoblastoma (Rb) by cyclin-dependent kinases (CDKs), which causes the release of the transcriptional activator E2F. CDKs are suppressed by CDK inhibitors (CKIs) that are regulated by p53. Tumor suppressor proteins block cell cycle progression largely within G_1. Interruption of cell cycle progression during G_1 and G_2 may lead to apoptosis as a default pathway. S, G_2 and M phases are also regulated by cyclins, CDKs and CKIs.

subsequent proteolysis via proteasomes. Under normal circumstances, the ubiquitin/proteasome system degrades phosphorylated CDKs, thereby preventing potentially harmful accumulation of these enzymes. Thus, inactivating mutations of this system lead to increased CDK activity and impair control of the cell cycle.

Loss of R point control deregulates progression through the cell cycle. Cancer cells often display loss of R point control through mechanisms such as (1) amplification/overexpression of cyclins/CDKs, (2) loss of CKIs and (3) mutational inactivation of p53 or pRb proteins.

Cells commonly suffer DNA damage from a variety of insults (e.g., reactive oxygen species [ROS], ionizing radiation) or harmful mutations. Survival of the organism necessitates the removal or repair of damaged DNA before mitosis. Cells have evolved mechanisms that recognize such injured DNA and that direct the cell into DNA repair or, as a default pathway, death. Progression of the cell cycle is impeded at three checkpoints: (1) during G_1, before entry into S phase, (2) as DNA is being replicated in S phase and (3) in G_2, before commencing mitosis. Of note, most cancer cells lack R points (see above), which suggests that they have evaded this aspect of cell cycle control.

Retinoblastoma Protein

One of the most important pathways in the cell's commitment to division involves pRb, which principally acts at the G_1/S boundary. It inhibits progression of the cell cycle by binding to the E2F transcription factor. The E2F family is composed of transcription factors that mediate cell entry into, and transit through, S phase. Under normal circumstances, pRb binds to E2F, thereby blocking its activity. Phosphorylation alters the conformation of pRb, so that E2F is released and the cell cycle can progress. The Rb system thus integrates many growth signals that promote cell cycle progression.

Cyclin-Dependent Kinases

Inhibitors of CDKs and specific phosphatases also inhibit cell cycle transit. These include $p14^{ARF}$, $p16^{INK4a}$ and $p21^{WAF}$. The expression of CKIs and inhibition of specific phosphatase activities activate cell cycle transit signals at appropriate checkpoints (Fig. 5-20).

p53

As mentioned in Chapter 1, p53 has been characterized as "the guardian of the genome." It coordinates cellular responses to DNA damage, mediates activation of G_1/S and G_2/M checkpoints and initiates the default program of apoptosis. The mechanisms underlying the actions of p53 include:

1. Normally, low levels of p53 are maintained by a ubiquitin (Ub) ligase, MDM2 (murine double minute), which binds p53 to Ub and leads to subsequent proteasomal degradation (see Chapter 1).
2. The protein kinases ATM (ataxia telangiectasia mutated) and ATR (ATM and Rad3 related) recognize DNA damage and phosphorylate p53. Activation of p53 through these kinases or via telomere dysfunction (see Chapter 1) contributes to cell cycle arrest.
3. Activation of a cell cycle checkpoint requires a period of arrest to permit DNA repair. When p53 is phosphorylated, it dissociates from MDM2 and translocates to the nucleus.
4. In this location, p53 further promotes cell cycle arrest by stimulating production of the CKI $p21^{WAF}$.
5. If DNA repair cannot be achieved, p53 promotes apoptosis (Fig. 5-21).

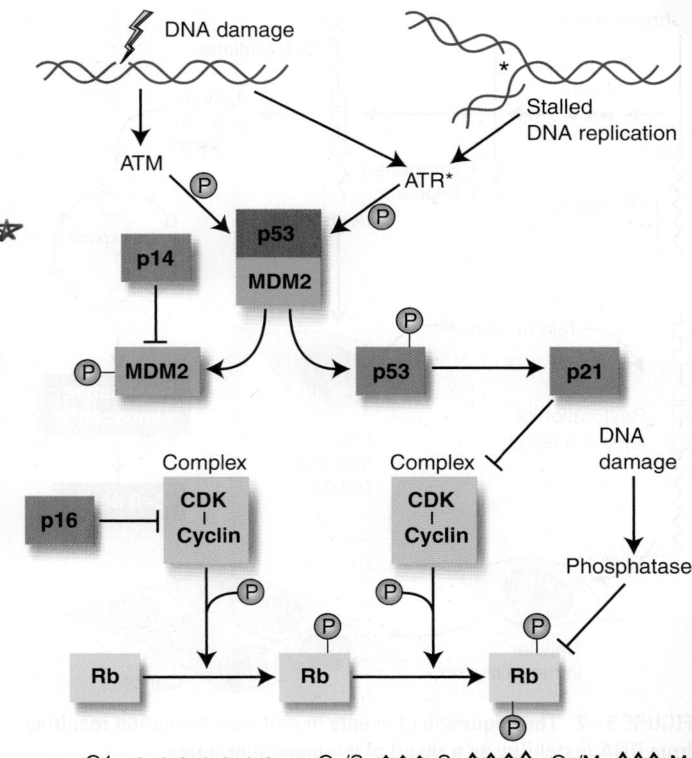

FIGURE 5-21. Linkage of DNA damage and replication stress to cell cycle arrest, via p53. Both DNA damage and other interference with DNA replication activate the kinases ATM (ataxia telangiectasia mutated) and ATR (ATM and Rad3 related). These kinases phosphorylate p53, releasing it from binding to its inhibitor, MDM2. Activated p53 stimulates p21 (also called $p21^{WAF1}$), thereby inhibiting the activity of a cyclin–CDK complex that phosphorylates pRb molecules that have already been phosphorylated by a different CDK–cyclin complex. p21 thus prevents hyperphosphorylation of pRb. Oncogene activity or genotoxic stresses can activate p14 and p16 (also called $p14^{ARF}$ and $p16^{INK4a}$), which block MDM2 or the first of the cyclin–CDK complexes mentioned above. The activities of p14 and p16 lead to decreased phosphorylation of pRb. DNA damage also activates protein phosphatases that dephosphorylate pRb. Phosphorylation of pRb is permissive for cell cycle progression through G_1/S and G_2/M checkpoints.

DNA Repair Prevents Mutations From Being Transmitted From One Cell Generation to the Next

The DNA of approximately one hundred trillion cells that constitute the human body is under relentless assault by both internal and exogenous stresses, including environmental chemicals and radiation, reactive oxygen species and infidelity of DNA polymerase. To preserve and protect their integrity, cells have evolved mechanisms that continuously repair this damage. Such mechanisms involve a variety of enzyme families that detect and repair different types of DNA injury so that damage does not threaten the viability and functionality of the cells. These enzymes also communicate with cell cycle checkpoint regulators to ensure that resulting mutations are not transmitted to daughter cells. Among the enzyme families are those that attend to such DNA modifications as single nucleotide substitutions, single- and double-strand breaks and DNA mismatches.

Telomeres Are Key Regulatory Structures That Trigger Senescence

Telomeres are repetitive DNA sequences at the 3′ ends of chromosomes, which tend to shorten with each successive mitosis (see Chapter 1). This process leads to cellular senescence,

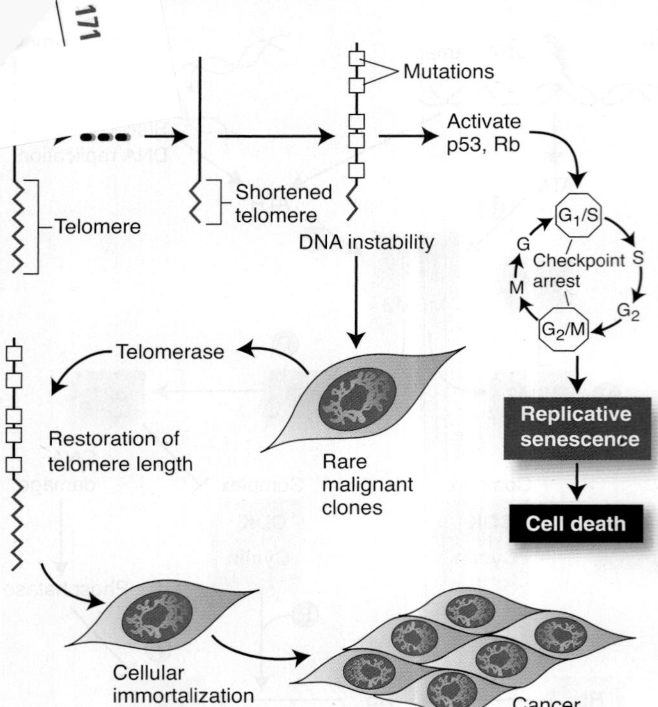

FIGURE 5-22. The sequence of events in cell transformation resulting from DNA instability as a result of telomere shortening.

corresponding to exhaustion of proliferative capacity in cultured cells. Such telomere attrition leads to nonspecific DNA instability, as telomere shortening eventually leads to cell death. Pathways mediated by checkpoint arrest via p53 and pRb also mediate replicative senescence. The majority of DNA changes that result from telomere exhaustion are lethal for the cell. However, rare malignant clones can emerge in which telomerase is activated, thereby maintaining telomere length and avoiding senescence. The result is cell immortalization, which experimentally may lead to malignant transformation (Fig. 5-22).

Microsatellites Are DNA Sequences That Are Excessively Prone to Mutation

Microsatellites are short sequences of up to 6 base pairs, which can be repeated up to 100 times. They are common in the human genome and are particularly useful in determining the degree of relationship between alleles. Microsatellites are inordinately prone to mutations, including changes in the numbers of repeats, especially during meiotic replication in germ cells. In most instances, these mutations are rectified by DNA mismatch repair enzymes. On occasion, however, mutations escape the repair process in the germline or in somatic cells, in which case they may be linked to the development of cancer (see below).

The Mechanisms Used to Repair Genetic Damage Depend Upon the Type of DNA Injury

There are several pathways by which damaged DNA is repaired. The principal ones are:

- **Mismatch repair:** This pathway is mainly involved in the repair of errors in DNA replication. These may include single base mismatches or errors in larger segments that may be caused by slippage during DNA replication. Incorrect bases are recognized and rectified by a family of enzymes (e.g., MSH2, MLH1) that stop DNA replication, correct the mistake and then allow replication to continue.
- **Nucleotide base excision repair:** These pathways mostly operate on DNA lesions caused by endogenous agents (e.g., ROS) or exogenous factors (e.g., ultraviolet [UV] light, chemicals). DNA repair through these means corrects bulky lesions in DNA that disturb the helical architecture of double-stranded DNA. The damaged area is excised and replaced, using the opposite strand as a template.
- **Double-strand break repair:** One of the most important dangers to the integrity of the genome is a DNA double-strand break (DSB). DSBs may occur as a result of several kinds of DNA damage, or during DNA replication. The impact of such major damage lies in its ability to produce conspicuous cytogenetic abnormalities, including deletions, amplifications and translocations of chromosomes. The mechanisms by which DSBs are repaired involve a complex cascade of proteins, which participate in homologous recombination, or end-joining from a different region of DNA on a different chromosome.

The Role of Disturbances in Cellular Control Mechanisms in Tumor Development and Progression

Genomic Instability Is an Important Contributor to Cancer Development

The pathogenesis of cancer involves multiple genetic events, and genomic instability is essential to the generation of mutations. In many neoplasms, three mechanisms of genetic instability are appreciated, namely, (1) chromosomal instability; (2) microsatellite instability, often the result of abnormal DNA mismatch repair; and (3) aberrant DNA methylation (see below).

The most important of these, although not universal, is probably chromosomal instability (CI). CI is characterized by an increased rate of additions or deletions of entire chromosomes, or portions thereof, that produce variability in cellular karyotypes. CI may result in **aneuploidy** (an imbalance in chromosome number), **gene amplification** (increased number of gene copies) and **loss of heterozygosity** (LOH, loss of one allele out of a pair).

LOH may result from loss of an entire chromosome, deletion of a segment of DNA bearing the gene in question or inactivation of that gene. As a result, the phenotype corresponding to the remaining allele is the only one for that locus. If that remaining allele is abnormal, the lack of a second allele to counterbalance it means that its abnormal phenotype is unopposed. Moreover, the phenotype of the remaining allele may promote the development of cancer. Typically, about one fourth of alleles are lost in malignancies.

Although the precise mechanisms responsible for CI are unclear in many cases, defects in chromosome segregation during mitosis commonly play an important role.

Role of Defects in DNA Repair Systems

An understanding of how defects in DNA repair contribute to oncogenesis was derived in part from observations made in familial cancer syndromes. For example, a type of colon cancer syndrome, hereditary nonpolyposis colon cancer (HNPCC, Lynch syndrome), entails a 75% lifetime risk for colon cancer. The large majority of HNPCC patients have mutations in MLH1 or MSH2 DNA mismatch repair enzymes (see above).

Xeroderma pigmentosum (XP), a hereditary syndrome characterized by enhanced sensitivity to UV light and development of skin cancer, reflects defects in nucleotide excision repair (NER) enzymes. In some common types of spontaneous lung cancer, a majority of cases exhibit mutant proteins involved in NER.

Double-Strand Break Repair and Cancer

As mentioned above, detection of DSBs and initiation of repair processes involves the ATM protein. Mutations in ATM and other enzymes involved in DSB repair are associated with a high frequency of malignant tumors. The specific mechanisms whereby mutations in the proteins that constitute the DSB apparatus lead to tumors remain subjects of investigation.

Oncogenes Are Counterparts of Normal Genes

Origin of Oncogenes

The concept of oncogenes was originally derived from studies of animal tumor viruses. Early research on transforming retroviruses showed that a limited number of viral genes could impart a neoplastic phenotype to virally infected cells. It was subsequently demonstrated that the transfer of specific genes from human tumor cells **(oncogenes)** into rodent cells in vitro could impart to those recipient cells a transformed phenotype. The transforming genes were discovered to be mutant versions of normal human genes involved in cellular growth regulation, proliferation, gene expression, etc., and were termed **proto-oncogenes.** Transforming retroviral oncogenes were designated with a *v-* (e.g., v-*onc*), and their cellular counterparts were denoted with a *c-* (e.g., c-*myc*, c-*jun*, c-*src*).

Mechanisms of Activation of Cellular Oncogenes

There are three general mechanisms by which proto-oncogenes become activated:

- A mutation in a proto-oncogene leads to **constitutive production of an abnormal protein.**
- Increased expression of a proto-oncogene causes **overproduction of a normal gene product.**
- Activation or expression of proto-oncogenes is regulated by numerous auto-inhibitory mechanisms that safeguard against inappropriate activity. Many mutations in proto-oncogenes render them **insensitive to normal auto-inhibitory and regulatory constraints** and lead to constitutive activation.

Activation by Mutation

Mutations by which proto-oncogenes are converted to oncogenes may involve (1) point mutations, (2) deletions or (3) chromosomal translocations. The first oncogene identified in a human tumor was activated c-*ras* from a bladder cancer. This gene was found to have a remarkably subtle alteration, namely, a point mutation in codon 12, a change that results in the substitution of valine for glycine in the ras protein. Subsequent studies of other cancers have revealed point mutations involving other codons of the *ras* gene, suggesting that these positions are critical for the normal function of the ras protein. Since the discovery of mutations in c-*ras*, alterations in other growth-regulatory genes have been described.

Activating, or gain-of-function, mutations in proto-oncogenes are usually somatic rather than germline alterations. Germline mutations in proto-oncogenes, which are known to be important regulators of growth during development, are ordinarily lethal in utero. There are several exceptions to this rule. For example, c-*ret* is incriminated in the pathogenesis of certain heritable endocrine cancers, and c-*met*, which encodes the receptor for hepatocyte growth factor, is associated with a hereditary form of renal cancer.

Activation by Chromosomal Translocation

Chromosomal translocations (i.e., the transfer of a portion of one chromosome to another) have been implicated in the pathogenesis of several human leukemias and lymphomas. The first and still the best-known example of an acquired chromosomal translocation in a human cancer is the **Philadelphia chromosome,** which is found in 95% of patients with chronic myelogenous leukemia (Fig. 5-23). The c-*abl* proto-oncogene on chromosome 9 is translocated to chromosome 22, where it is placed in juxtaposition to a site known as the breakpoint cluster region (*bcr*). The c-*abl* gene and *bcr* region unite to produce a hybrid oncogene that codes for an aberrant protein with very high tyrosine kinase activity, which generates mitogenic and antiapoptotic signals. The chromosomal translocation that produces the Philadelphia chromosome is an example of oncogene activation by formation of a chimeric (fusion) protein.

In 75% of patients with Burkitt lymphoma (a type of B-cell lymphoma; see Chapter 20), there is a translocation of c-*myc*, a proto-oncogene involved in cell cycle progression, from its site on chromosome 8 to a position on chromosome 14 (Fig. 5-23C). This translocation places c-*myc* adjacent to genes that control transcription of the immunoglobulin heavy chains. As a result, the c-*myc* proto-oncogene is activated by the promoter/enhancer sequences of these immunoglobulin genes and is consequently expressed constitutively rather than in a regulated manner. In 25% of patients with Burkitt lymphoma, the c-*myc* proto-oncogene remains on chromosome 8 but is activated by translocation of immunoglobulin light-chain genes from chromosome 2 or 22 to the 3′ end of the c-*myc* gene. In either case, a chromosomal translocation does not create a novel chimeric protein but stimulates the overproduction of a normal gene product. In Burkitt lymphoma the excessive amount of the normal c-*myc* product, probably in association with other genetic alterations, leads to the emergence of a dominant clone of B cells, driven relentlessly to proliferate as a monoclonal neoplasm. Many other hematopoietic malignancies, lymphomas and solid tumors reflect activation of oncogenes by chromosomal translocation. Although some malignant conditions are **initiated** by chromosomal translocations, during the **progression** of many cancers, myriad chromosomal abnormalities take place (translocations, breaks, aneuploidy, etc.).

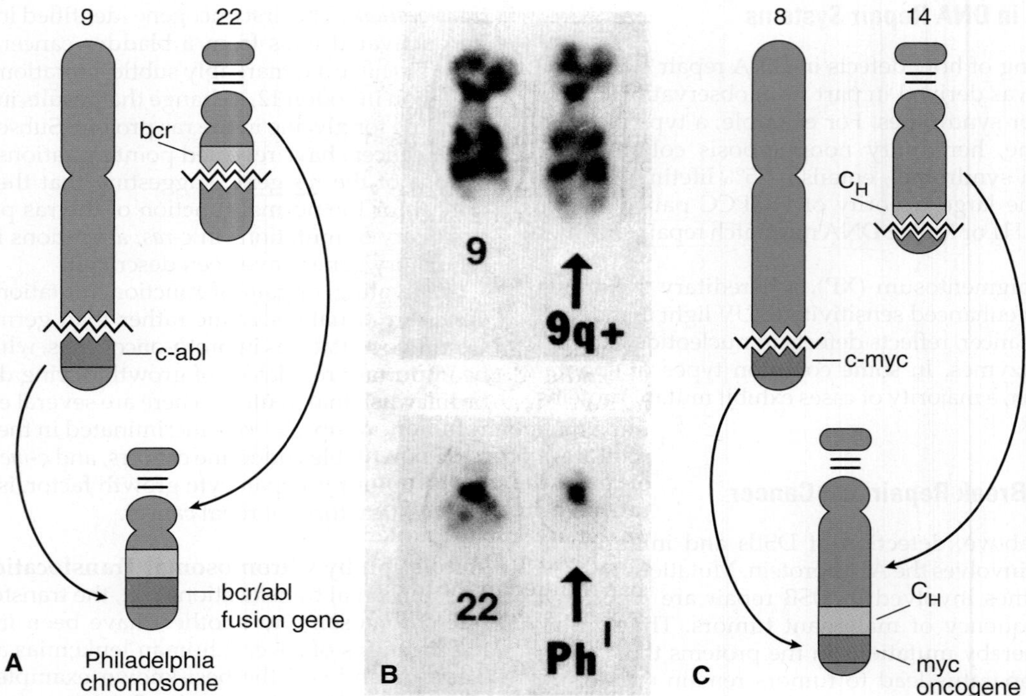

FIGURE 5-23. Oncogene activation by chromosomal translocation. A. Chronic myelogenous leukemia. Breaks at the ends of the long arms of chromosomes 9 and 22 allow reciprocal translocations to occur. The c-*abl* proto-oncogene on chromosome 9 is translocated to the breakpoint region (*bcr*) of chromosome 22. The result is the Philadelphia chromosome, (Ph^1), which contains a new fusion gene coding for a hybrid oncogenic protein (bcr-abl), presumably involved in the pathogenesis of chronic myelogenous leukemia. **B.** Karyotypes of a patient with chronic myelogenous leukemia showing the results of reciprocal translocations between chromosomes 9 and 22. The Philadelphia chromosome is recognized by a smaller-than-normal chromosome 22 (22q−). One chromosome 9 (9q+) is larger than its normal counterpart. **C.** Burkitt lymphoma. In this disorder, chromosomal breaks involve the long arms of chromosomes 8 and 14. The c-*myc* gene on chromosome 8 is translocated to a region on chromosome 14 adjacent to the gene coding for the constant region of an immunoglobulin heavy chain (C_H). The expression of c-*myc* is enhanced by its association with the promoter/enhancer regions of the actively transcribed immunoglobulin genes.

Activation by Gene Amplification

Chromosomal alterations that result in an increased number of gene copies (i.e., gene amplification) have been found primarily in human solid tumors. Such aberrations are recognized as (1) **homogeneous staining regions (HSRs)** (Fig. 5-24A); (2) **abnormal banding regions** on chromosomes; or (3) **double minutes,** which are visualized as multiple, small, paired, cytoplasmic bodies (Fig. 5-24B). In some cases, gene amplification involves proto-oncogenes. For example, HSRs derived from the N-*myc* proto-oncogene may be seen in neuroblastomas. The presence of N-*myc* HSRs is associated with up to a 700-fold amplification of this gene and is a marker of advanced disease with a poor prognosis. Activation of *myc*-family proto-oncogenes by means of gene amplification has also been demonstrated in small cell carcinoma of the lung, Wilms tumor and hepatoblastoma.

The *erb B* proto-oncogene is amplified in up to a third of breast and ovarian cancers. The *erb B2* gene (also designated *HER2/neu*) encodes a receptor-type tyrosine kinase that shows close structural similarity to the EGF receptor. Amplification of *erb B2* in breast and ovarian cancer may be associated with poor overall survival and decreased time to relapse. In this context an antibody targeted against HER2/neu (trastuzumab) is now used as adjunctive therapy for breast cancers that overexpress this protein.

Mechanisms of Oncogene Action

Oncogenes can be classified according to the roles of their normal counterparts (proto-oncogenes) in the biochemical pathways that regulate growth and differentiation. These include the following (Figs. 5-25 and 5-26):

- Growth factors
- Cell surface receptors
- Intracellular signal transduction pathways
- DNA-binding nuclear proteins (transcription factors)
- Cell cycle proteins (cyclins and cyclin-dependent protein kinases)
- Inhibitors of apoptosis (bcl-2)

In general, mutations that result in increased activity of a mutant gene are called **gain-of-function mutations.**

Oncogenes and Growth Factors

The binding of soluble extracellular growth factors to their specific surface receptors initiates signaling cascades that eventuate in entry of the cell into the mitotic cycle. A few proto-oncogenes encode growth factors that stimulate tumor cell growth. In some instances a growth factor acts upon the same cell that produces it **(autocrine stimulation).** Other growth factors act upon the receptors of neighboring cells

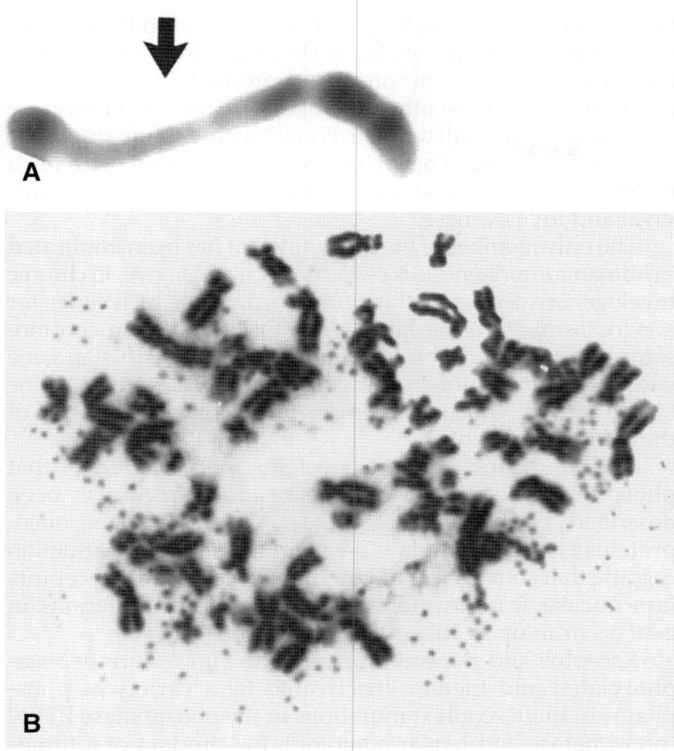

FIGURE 5-24. Chromosomal alterations in human solid tumors. **A.** Homogeneously staining region (HSR; *arrow*) in a chromosome from an ovarian carcinoma. **B.** Double minutes in a karyotype of a soft tissue sarcoma appear as multiple small bodies.

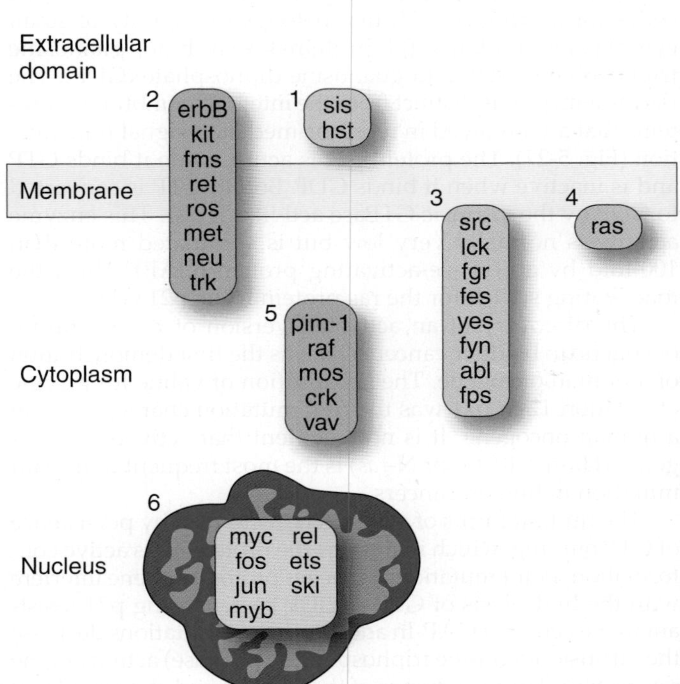

FIGURE 5-26. Cellular compartments in which oncogene or proto-oncogene products reside. (*1*) Growth factors, (*2*) transmembrane growth factor receptors (tyrosine kinase), (*3*) membrane-associated kinases, (*4*) *ras* GTPase family, (*5*) cytoplasmic kinases, (*6*) nuclear transcriptional regulators. GTP = guanosine triphosphate.

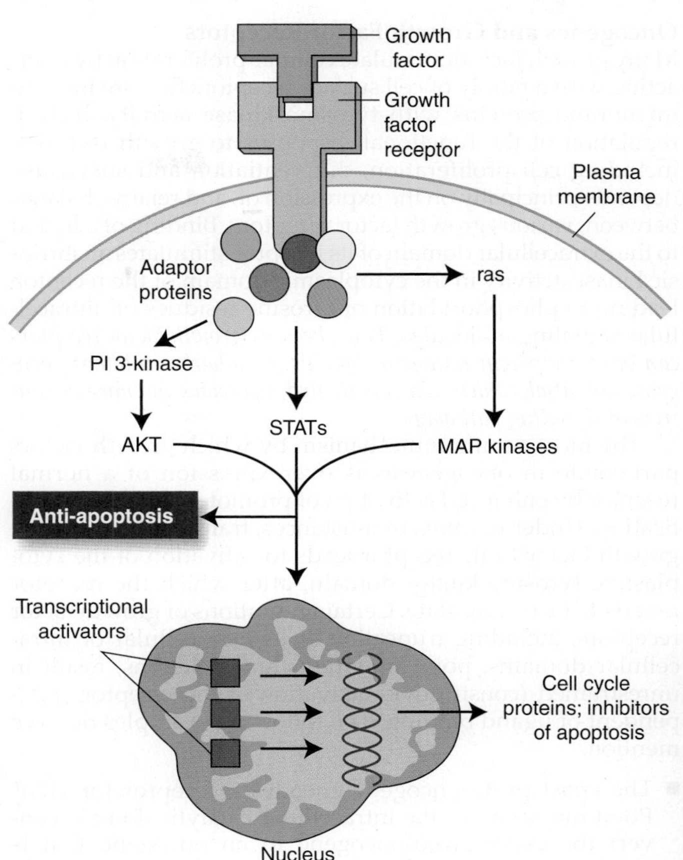

FIGURE 5-25. Signaling pathways controlling proliferation and apoptosis. The activation of growth factor receptors by their ligands causes the binding of adaptor proteins and the activation of a series of intracellular signaling molecules leading to transcriptional activation, the induction of cell cycle proteins and inhibition of apoptosis. Key targets include *ras,* mitogen-activated protein (MAP) kinases, signal transducer and activator transcription factors (STATs), phosphatidylinositol 3-kinase (PI3-kinase) and the serine/threonine kinase AKT.

(paracrine stimulation). Examples of growth factors involved in neoplastic transformation include platelet-derived growth factor (PDGF) and fibroblast growth factor (FGF).

PDGF is the protein product of the c-*sis* proto-oncogene and is a potent mitogen for fibroblasts, smooth muscle cells and glial cells. Cells derived from human sarcomas and glioblastomas (malignant glial cell tumors) produce PDGF-like polypeptides; their normal counterparts do not. Thus, a normal human gene (c-*sis*) that encodes a growth factor (PDGF) acquires transforming capacity when it is constitutively expressed in a cell that responds to this signal.

An oncogene (*HST*) that codes for a protein with homology to FGF has been identified in human stomach cancer and Kaposi sarcoma. In rodent models, neoplastic cells often express TGF-α.

Mutational activation of growth factor genes is not well characterized in human cancers. Nevertheless, whether caused by genetic or epigenetic mechanisms, cancer cells generally produce a mixture of growth factors with autocrine or paracrine activity, including insulin-like growth factor-I (IGF-I), PDGF, TGF-α, FGF, colony-stimulating factor-1 (CSF-1) and hepatocyte growth factor (HGF).

Oncogenes and Growth Factor Receptors

Many growth factors stimulate cellular proliferation by interacting with a family of cell surface receptors that are integral membrane proteins with tyrosine kinase activity. In fact, regulation of the functional responses to growth factors—including cell proliferation, differentiation and survival—depends principally on the expression of, and relative balance between, various growth factor receptors. Binding of a ligand to the extracellular domain of its receptor stimulates an intrinsic kinase activity in the cytoplasmic domain of the receptor, leading to phosphorylation of tyrosine residues on intracellular signaling molecules. *Thus, because growth factor receptors can generate potent mitogenic signals, they harbor a latent oncogenic potential, which, when activated, overrides the normal controls of signaling pathways.*

The most common mechanism by which growth factors participate in oncogenesis is overexpression of a normal receptor by enhanced activation of promoters or gene amplification. Under normal circumstances, transient binding of a growth factor to its receptor leads to activation of the cytoplasmic tyrosine kinase domain, after which the receptor reverts to its resting state. Certain mutations of growth factor receptors, including truncation of its extracellular or intracellular domains, point mutations and deletions, result in unrestrained (constitutive) activation of the receptor, independent of ligand binding. The following examples deserve mention.

- The c-*met* proto-oncogene encodes a receptor for HGF. Point mutations in the intracellular catalytic domain convert the c-*met* proto-oncogene to an oncogene that is involved in papillary renal cancers.
- Germline point mutations in c-*ret* lead to constitutive activation of the receptor and are associated with the multiple endocrine neoplasia (MEN) syndromes and familial medullary thyroid carcinoma (see Chapter 21).
- Patients with germline mutations in the catalytic domain of the c-*kit* tyrosine kinase tend to develop gastrointestinal stromal tumors (GISTs).
- Another abnormality of a growth factor receptor can result from chromosomal translocations that produce hybrid proteins with constitutive tyrosine kinase activity. In the case of the PDGF receptor, a chromosomal translocation [t(5;12)] generates a fusion protein between the cytoplasmic domain of the PDGF receptor and a motif encoded by c-*tel*. The abnormal receptor has been found in patients with myelomonocytic leukemia.

Epigenetic changes that result in increased synthesis of growth factors and their receptors are equally important as mutations and overexpression of growth factor receptors in the pathogenesis of human cancers. In some human malignancies (e.g., breast, ovarian and stomach cancers), amplification of *HER2/neu* results in autocrine activation that is mediated by overexpression of this growth factor receptor. Of greater importance in human cancers are epigenetic changes that cause increased synthesis of growth factors and receptors.

Oncogenes and Nonreceptor Protein Kinases

A number of proteins with tyrosine kinase activity are loosely associated with the inner aspect of the plasma membrane. Although they possess tyrosine kinase activity, they are neither integral membrane proteins nor growth factor receptors. The prototype of a viral oncogene that codes for mutant forms of these protein kinases is v-*src* (Fig. 5-26). A number of other oncogenes (*abl, lck, yes, fgr, fps, fes*) belong to the *src* family. The homologous c-*src* proto-oncogene product is expressed in most cells, whereas other members of the *src* family are expressed in specialized cell types, such as hematopoietic cells and epithelia. The *src* enzymes are activated by most receptor tyrosine kinases and influence cell proliferation, survival and invasiveness.

The only member of the *src* family that has been implicated in human tumorigenesis is c-*abl*. As discussed above, in chronic myelogenous leukemia this proto-oncogene, which codes for a cytoplasmic tyrosine kinase, is translocated from chromosome 9 to the *bcr* of chromosome 22. The *bcr-abl* fusion gene encodes a mutant protein with conspicuously elevated tyrosine kinase activity, which is necessary for the oncogenic action of the chimeric protein.

Soluble cytoplasmic oncoproteins (*raf, mos, pim*-1) that phosphorylate serine/threonine residues have also been described. The best studied of the soluble cytoplasmic oncoproteins is *raf*, which plays a role in the signal transduction cascade that converts ligand binding by cell surface receptors into nuclear transcriptional activation. Point mutations in c-*raf* occur in up to 10% of human cancers.

Receptor and nonreceptor tyrosine kinases are dephosphorylated and thereby inactivated by a variety of phosphatases. In this context mutations in the phosphatase PTEN (phosphatase and tensin homolog), the product of a tumor suppressor gene (see below), have been linked to a variety of human malignancies.

Ras Oncogenes

Ras is an effector molecule in the signal transduction cascade that couples the activation of growth factor receptors to changes in nuclear gene transcription. The *ras* proto-oncogene codes for a product, p21, that belongs to a family of small cytoplasmic proteins (G proteins) that bind guanosine triphosphate (GTP) and guanosine diphosphate (GDP). The ras protein, p21, is distinct from the integral membrane G proteins that are involved in receptor-mediated signal transduction (Fig. 5-27). The protein p21 is active when it binds GTP and is inactive when it binds GDP. Bound GTP is converted to GDP by the intrinsic GTPase activity of p21. This enzyme activity is normally very low but is stimulated more than 100-fold by a GTPase-activating protein (GAP). Thus, the inactivating switch for the ras protein is the p21 GTPase.

The discovery of an activated version of the *ras* proto-oncogene in bladder cancer cells was the first demonstration of a human oncogene. The substitution of valine for glycine at position 12 in p21 was the first mutation characterized in a human oncogene. It is now evident that activation of *ras* genes (Ha-*ras*, Ki-*ras* or N-*ras*) is the most frequent dominant mutation in human cancers.

The mutant forms of p21 are characterized by persistence of GTP binding, which maintains the protein in its active conformation. Point mutations in the *ras* proto-oncogene interfere with the hydrolysis of GTP to GDP by rendering p21 resistant to the action of GAP. In addition, some mutations decrease the intrinsic adenosine triphosphatase (ATPase) activity of the ras protein. The persistence of the GTP-bound state results in uncontrolled stimulation of *ras*-related functions, because p21 is locked in the "on" position.

This phenomenon, in which cancer cells require continued expression of an activated oncogene, has been called "oncogene addiction." By contrast, it has recently been

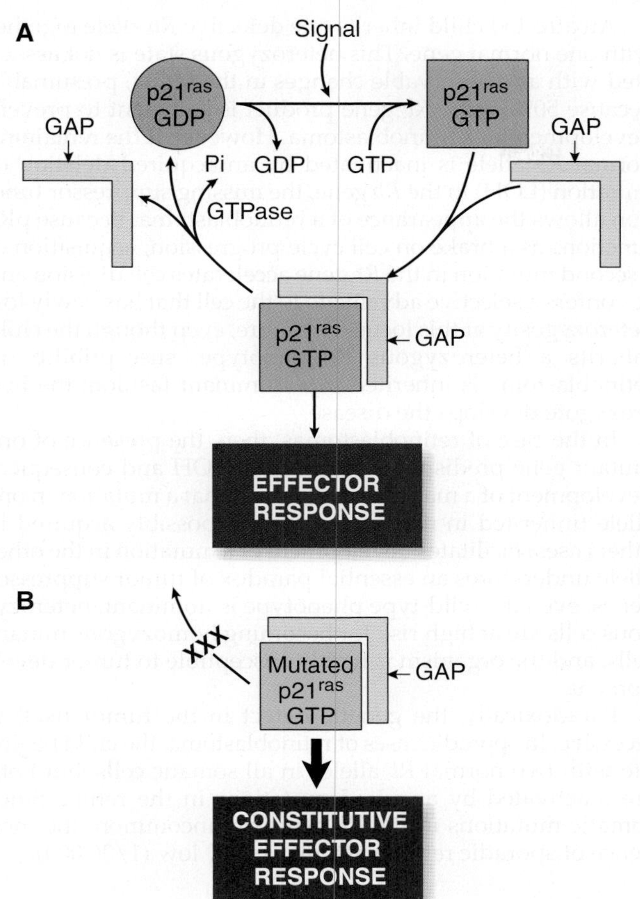

FIGURE 5-27. Mechanism of action of ras oncogene. A. Normal. The ras protein p21 exists in two conformational states, determined by the binding of either guanosine diphosphate (GDP) or guanosine triphosphate (GTP). Normally, most of the p21 is in the inactive GDP-bound state. An external stimulus, or signal, triggers the exchange of GTP for GDP, an event that converts p21 to the active state. Activated p21, which is associated with the plasma membrane, binds GTPase-activating protein (GAP) from the cytosol. The binding of GAP has two consequences. In association with other plasma membrane constituents, it initiates the effector response. At the same time, the binding of GAP to p21 GTP stimulates by about 100-fold the intrinsic GTPase activity of p21, thereby promoting the hydrolysis of GTP to GDP and the return of p21 to its inactive state. **B.** Mutated ras protein is locked into the active GTP-bound state because of an insensitivity of its intrinsic GTPase to GAP or because of a lack of the GTPase activity itself. As a result the effector response is exaggerated, and the cell is transformed.

shown that mutated *ras* (in this case, *Kras*) depends upon a normal protein (in this case, STK33) to maintain a neoplastic phenotype. This requirement for a normal (i.e., nononcogene) protein may be called "nononcogene addiction." Yet things are not so simple. In the case of *Kras*, nononcogene addiction also involves a complex set of dependencies, including pathways related to mitotic functions and proteasomal activity.

Oncogenes and Nuclear Regulatory Proteins

A number of nuclear proteins encoded by proto-oncogenes are intimately involved in the sequential expression of genes that regulate cellular proliferation and d
of these proteins can bind to DNA, wh
expression of other genes. The transitc
eral proto-oncogenes is necessary f
through specific points in the cell cy
binding of PDGF to cultured fibrobl
leave G_0 and enter the G_1 phase of the cell cycle.
thereafter, several genes, including c-*myc*, c-*fos* and c-*jun*, are expressed. Proto-oncogenes that are expressed early in the cell cycle, such as *myc* and *fos*, render the cells competent to receive the final signals for mitosis and are, therefore, termed **competence genes.** In general, competence genes play a role in (1) progression from G_1 to S phase in the cell cycle, (2) stability of the genome, (3) apoptosis and (4) positive or negative effects on cellular maturation. However, the cells are not yet fully programmed to divide after the expression of these genes and will enter S phase and mitosis only after further stimulation by other factors, such as EGF or IGF-I **(progression factors).**

The proteins encoded by c-*fos* and c-*jun* are components of AP-1, a transcription factor that activates the expression of a variety of genes. Mutations of the *jun* protein eliminate a negative regulatory domain, thereby prolonging its half-life and stimulating progression through G_1. Few mutations of c-*jun* have been identified in human tumors, but overexpression of the protein has been described in lung and colorectal cancers.

Although nuclear proteins encoded by proto-oncogenes can promote cellular proliferation, in some circumstances they stimulate differentiation. A rapid increase in c-*fos* expression follows the induction of differentiation in a variety of cells in vitro, including several hematopoietic cell lines and teratocarcinomas.

c-*Myc* is a nuclear protein that binds to a variety of other proteins and DNA to regulate gene transcription. Among other proteins, such targets include p53 and ornithine decarboxylase. As discussed above, the translocation characteristic of Burkitt lymphoma (t8:14) constitutively activates c-*myc* expression. c-*Myc* is also overexpressed in many human malignant tumors (e.g., adenocarcinoma of lung and breast).

Tumor Suppressor Genes Negatively Regulate Cell Growth

The concept of oncogenes, addressed above, postulates genetic alterations that accelerate cell proliferation. An additional mechanism by which genetic alteration contributes to carcinogenesis is a mutation that creates a deficiency of a normal gene product **(tumor suppressor)** that exerts a negative regulatory control of cell growth and thereby suppresses tumor formation **("loss-of-function mutations").** Such genes encode negative transcriptional regulators of virtually every process in multistep carcinogenesis, from cell division through invasion and metastasis.

Since both alleles of tumor suppressor genes must be inactivated to produce the deficit that allows the development of a tumor, it is inferred that the normal suppressor gene is dominant. In this circumstance, the heterozygous state is sufficient to protect against cancer. The loss of heterozygosity (see above) in a tumor suppressor gene by deletion or somatic mutation of the remaining normal allele predisposes to tumor development.

e of Tumor Suppressor Genes in Carcinogenesis

nor suppressor genes are incriminated in the pathogene-s of both hereditary and spontaneous cancers in humans. Two such genes serve as good examples. The Rb and p53 gene products serve to restrain cell division in many tissues, and their absence or inactivation is linked to the development of malignant tumors. *Thus, the mechanisms underlying the development of some tumors associated with germline and somatic mutations involve the same cellular gene products.*

Retinoblastoma Gene

Retinoblastoma, a rare childhood cancer, is the prototype of a human tumor whose origin is attributed to the inactivation of a specific tumor suppressor gene. About 40% of cases are associated with a germline mutation; the remainder are not hereditary. In patients with hereditary retinoblastoma, all somatic cells carry one missing or mutated allele of a gene (the *Rb* gene) located on the long arm of chromosome 13. By contrast, both alleles of the *Rb* gene are inactive in all the retinoblastoma cells. Thus, the *Rb* gene exerts a tumor suppressor function, and the development of hereditary retinoblastoma has been attributed to two genetic events (Knudson's "two-hit" hypothesis) (Fig. 5-28). As mentioned above, the nuclear protein p105Rb is phosphorylated by the activated cyclin/CDK complex, thereby inducing the release of E2F transcription factor, which allows G_1–S phase transition. Additionally, certain products of human DNA viruses (e.g., human papillomavirus [HPV]) inactivate p105Rb by binding to it. *The function of* Rb *genes is a critical checkpoint in the cell cycle, and inactivating mutations in* Rb *permit unregulated cell proliferation.*

An affected child inherits one defective *Rb* allele together with one normal gene. This heterozygous state is not associated with any observable changes in the retina, presumably because 50% of the *Rb* gene product is sufficient to prevent development of a retinoblastoma. However, if the remaining normal *Rb* allele is inactivated by an acquired deletion or mutation (LOH) in the *Rb* gene, the missing suppressor function allows the appearance of a retinoblastoma. Because pRb functions as a brake on cell cycle progression, acquisition of a second mutation in the *Rb* gene accelerates cell division and so confers a selective advantage to the cell that has newly lost heterozygosity at this locus. Therefore, even though the child inherits a heterozygous Rb genotype, susceptibility to retinoblastoma is inherited in a dominant fashion: the heterozygote develops the disease.

In the case of retinoblastomas, then, the presence of one mutant gene predisposes to eventual LOH and consequent development of a malignancy. The fact that a mutation in one allele (inherited in the case of *Rb*, but possibly acquired in other cases) facilitates development of a mutation in the other allele underscores an essential paradox of tumor suppressor genes: even if a wild-type phenotype is dominant, heterozygous cells are at high risk for becoming homozygous mutant cells, and the organism is highly susceptible to tumor development.

Paradoxically, the genetic defect in the tumor itself is recessive. In sporadic cases of retinoblastoma, the child begins life with two normal *Rb* alleles in all somatic cells, but both are inactivated by acquired mutations in the retina. Since somatic mutations in the *Rb* gene are uncommon, the incidence of sporadic retinoblastoma is very low (1/30,000).

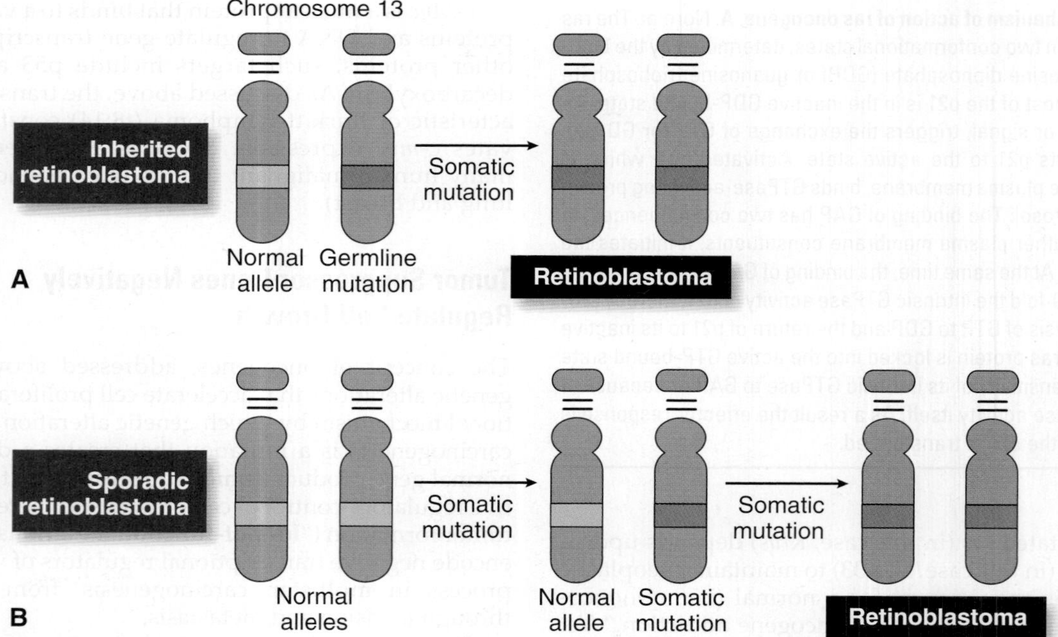

FIGURE 5-28. The "two-hit" origin of retinoblastoma. A. A child with the inherited form of retinoblastoma is born with a germline mutation in one allele of the retinoblastoma gene located on the long arm of chromosome 13. A second somatic mutation in the retina leads to the inactivation of the functioning *Rb* allele and the subsequent development of a retinoblastoma. **B.** In sporadic cases of retinoblastoma, the child is born with two normal *Rb* alleles. It requires two independent somatic mutations to inactivate *Rb* gene function and allow the appearance of a neoplastic clone.

Children who inherit a mutant *Rb* gene also have a 200-fold increased risk of developing mesenchymal tumors in early adult life, and more than 20 different cancers have been described. Chromosomal analysis has demonstrated abnormalities of the *Rb* locus in 70% of cases of osteosarcoma and in many instances of small cell lung cancer; carcinomas of the breast, bladder and pancreas; and other human tumors. Many types of *Rb* mutations have been described, including point mutations, insertions, deletions and translocations. In addition, epigenetic events, such as promoter hypermethylation (see below), may inactivate *Rb*.

The tumor suppressor activity of pRb is actually more complex than a simple description allows. pRb actually belongs to a family of three proteins, which have separate functions. These proteins can bind to numerous transcription factors and either antagonize or augment their functions. Rb proteins also modify chromatin structure, and the complexity of this gene is illustrated by the fact that pRb binds to many other signaling molecules.

The p53 Gene Family

The *p53* tumor suppressor gene is a principal mediator of growth arrest, senescence and apoptosis (Fig. 5-29). In response to DNA damage, oncogenic activation of other proteins and other stresses (e.g., hypoxia), p53 levels rise and prevent cells from entering the S phase of the cell cycle, thereby allowing time for DNA repair to take place. In this manner p53 acts as a "guardian of the genome" by restricting uncontrolled cellular proliferation under circumstances in which cells with abnormal DNA might propagate.

The p53 protein is a transcriptional factor that promotes the expression of a number of other genes involved in the control of cell cycle progression and apoptosis. DNA damage and other stresses (e.g., hypoxia) upregulate the expression of *p53*, which in turn enhances the synthesis of CKIs. The latter inactivates cyclin/CDK complexes, thereby leading to cell arrest at the G_1/S checkpoint. Cells arrested at this checkpoint may either repair the DNA damage and then reenter the cycle, or undergo apoptosis. The stimulation of gene transcription by p53 results in the synthesis of proteins (CIP1, GADD45) (Fig. 5-29) that enhance DNA repair by binding to proliferating cell nuclear antigen (PCNA, see above). Thus, *upregulation of p53 as a tumor suppressor has two important and related consequences: arrest of cell cycle progression and promotion of DNA repair*.

The *p53* gene is located on the short arm of chromosome 17, and its protein product is present in virtually all normal tissues. This gene is deleted or mutated in 75% of cases of colorectal cancer and frequently in breast cancer, small cell carcinoma of the lung, hepatocellular carcinoma, astrocytoma and numerous other tumors. *In fact, mutations of p53 seem to be the most common genetic change in human cancer.* Inactivating mutations of *p53*, which are largely missense mutations that impair the ability of p53 to bind to DNA, allow cells with damaged DNA to progress through the cell cycle. Many human cancers exhibit inactivation of both *p53* alleles. By contrast, in some cancers, the malignant cells express one normal *p53* allele and one mutant version. In these cases, the mutant p53 protein forms complexes with the normal p53 protein and thereby inactivates the function of the normal suppressor. When a mutant allele inactivates the normal one,

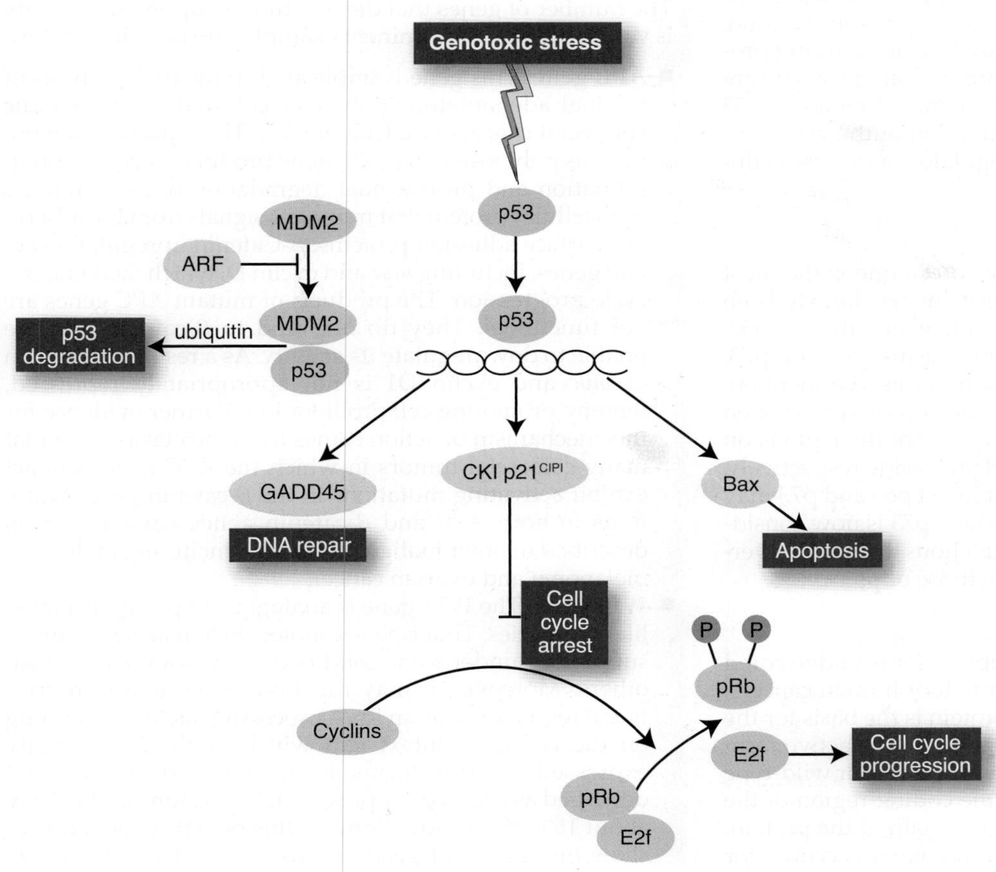

FIGURE 5-29. p53 regulation of genomic integrity. In response to genotoxic stress (e.g., ionizing radiation, carcinogens, mutagens), p53 binds to DNA and upregulates transcription of several genes. Cyclin-dependent kinase inhibitor (CKI) $p21^{CIP1}$ induces cell cycle arrest by preventing the release of E2F from retinoblastoma protein (pRB). GADD45 promotes DNA repair. Bax induces apoptosis, particularly if DNA repair fails. Importantly, cells with loss or mutation of *p53* do not undergo cell cycle arrest and DNA repair, but rather proliferate, generate additional mutations and increase the risk for the development of malignant tumors. MDM2 (murine double minute) binds to p53 and targets it for ubiquitin-mediated degradation. ARF inhibits MDM2/p53 binding. Reduction in p53 levels in some malignant neoplasms is associated with overexpression of MDM2 or absence of ARF.

the mutant allele is said be a **dominant negative** gene. Theoretically, a cell containing one mutant *p53* allele (i.e., a heterozygote) might have a growth advantage over the normal cells, a situation that would increase the number of cells at risk for a second mutation (loss of heterozygosity) and the development of cancer.

Negative regulation of p53 is principally accomplished by its binding to the MDM2 protein. The formation of the MDM2–p53 complex not only inhibits the function of p53 but also targets it for degradation via the ubiquitin pathway. In turn, MDM2 is inhibited by binding to ARF (p14), a tumor suppressor protein that is upregulated by any oncogenic stimulus (e.g., *myc, ras*) that induces *Rb* phosphorylation (which enhances E2F activity). Some cancers in which both *p53* alleles are structurally normal overexpress MDM2, thereby increasing p53 degradation. Other tumors in which p53 is intact do not express functional $p14^{ARF}$, thereby allowing unopposed MDM2-mediated proteolysis of p53. As in the case of *Rb*, certain DNA viral products in tumors (e.g., HPV E6) bind to p53 and promote its degradation. *Thus, most human cancers display either inactivating mutations of p53 or abnormalities in the proteins that regulate p53 activity.*

Although p53 tumor suppressor activity leads to cell cycle arrest, apoptosis and cellular senescence, these activities are only a part of a more complex tapestry of p53 functions, which are only now beginning to be appreciated. Among these additional activities are response to metabolic stress (lack of nutrients); regulation of autophagy and the redox state; production of ROS; and both promotion limitation of longevity.

Since p53 is so important in the life and death of cells, it is understandable that both its activity and protein levels are tightly regulated. In addition to numerous feedback loops, there are posttranslational modifications (phosphorylation, acetylation, etc.), natural antisense transcripts, binding proteins and small regulatory RNAs. Thus, mutations in p53 are only the tip of the iceberg as determinants of levels of p53 activity. In addition to being the "guardian of the genome," p53 may be considered a "master regulator of diverse cellular processes."

The p53 Family

Like a gathering of relations among whom one is the most boisterous, the family of p53-like proteins has largely been dominated by its most conspicuous member—that is, p53. However, there are several important cousins, p63 and p73, as well as some derivative proteins that deserve mention. Just as the region on chromosome 17 that encodes p53 is often mutated or deleted in human cancers, so are the regions on chromosomes 1 and 3 where p73 and p63 reside respectively. Some experimental data suggest that intact p63 and p73 may partly compensate for loss of p53. In fact, p73 is now considered to be a tumor suppressor with functions that partly overlap, and that are partly distinct from, those of p53.

Mutant p53s and Their Significance

The importance of p53 as a tumor suppressor is underscored by the fact that it is mutated in over half of human cancers. The structure of the wild-type p53 protein is the basis for the impact of mutations in p53 on oncogenesis. The active form of p53 is a homotetramer (i.e., an association of four wild-type p53 molecules). The largest part of the coding region of the p53 gene codes for the DNA-binding domain of the protein. Missense mutations in this DNA-binding region account for the vast majority of p53 mutations. Mutated p53 molecules are incorporated as equal partners in the p53 tetramers. In so doing, the mutant p53 moieties inactivate the tumor suppressor activity of the entire tetramer.

Interestingly, the treachery of mutant p53 molecules extends far beyond simple inactivation of tumor suppressor function. The aberrant protein also functions as an oncogene, modulating gene transcription. In addition, it protects cells from apoptosis. Mutant p53 also activates proinflammatory cytokines and extracellular matrix modulators. It blocks ATM-mediated (see above) protection against double-stranded DNA breaks. A common denominator underlying the effects of mutant p53 is its widespread stimulation of genes involved with cell proliferation. Moreover, mutant p53 activates cellular mechanisms that are responsible for resistance to chemotherapeutic drugs. In many cases, including tumors of the hematopoietic system, breast, urinary bladder and head and neck, a majority of studies report that mutations of p53 are associated with a poorer prognosis. Along these lines, it should be noted that some splice variants of p53 and p73, particularly those lacking the N-terminal domains, appear to inhibit aspects of their tumor suppressor activities and to act in part as oncogenes.

Li-Fraumeni syndrome *is an inherited predisposition to develop cancers in many organs owing to germline mutations of* p53. People with this condition carry germline mutations in one *p53* allele, but their tumors display mutations at both alleles. This situation is similar to that determining inherited retinoblastoma and is another example of the two-hit hypothesis (Fig. 5-28) and LOH (see above).

Other Tumor Suppressor Genes

The number of genes that display tumor suppressor activity is very large. A few prominent examples are described below.

- ***APC* gene:** This gene is implicated in the pathogenesis of familial adenomatous polyposis coli and most sporadic colorectal cancers (see Chapter 13). The wild-type adenomatous polyposis coli (*APC*) gene product causes the ubiquitination and proteasomal degradation of β-catenin, an intracellular protein that transmits signals from E-cadherin cell surface adhesion proteins. β-Catenin upregulates several genes, including *myc* and cyclin D, which facilitate cell cycle progression. The products of mutant *APC* genes are not functional. They do not bind to β-catenin and are unable to downregulate its activity. As a result, expression of *myc* and cyclin D1 is not appropriately repressed, thereby promoting cell proliferation. Further evidence for this mechanism of action comes from the observation that many colorectal tumors in which the *APC* gene is intact exhibit activating mutations in the β-catenin gene. Mutations in both *APC* and β-catenin genes have also been described in other malignant tumors, including malignant melanoma and ovarian cancer.
- ***WT1* gene:** The *WT1* gene is analogous to p53 in its Janus-like properties. That is, it is a molecule that acts as a tumor suppressor under some conditions and as an oncogene in others. Moreover, it may function either as a transcriptional regulator or as an RNA processing factor, depending on the cellular context and which of the 24 normally expressed WT1 isoforms is involved. WT1 was first described as a tumor suppressor in Wilms tumors, but only about 15% of sporadic forms of this pediatric renal cancer show mutated *WT1* genes. However, most Wilms tumors

produce, and often overproduce, normal WT1 protein. The contrary behavior of WT1 is best described in the context of acute myelogenous leukemia (AML). In normal primitive hematopoietic cells, WT1 overexpression leads to growth arrest and decreased hematopoiesis, consistent with tumor suppressor activity. Such tumor suppressor activity has also been demonstrated in some cases of AML. By contrast, normal WT1 is highly expressed in a variety of acute and chronic leukemias (see Chapter 20). Overexpression of WT1 in AML patients heralds poorer survival and a higher incidence of relapse after treatment. It is important that tumors of many types display increased expression of nonmutated WT1 (Table 5-2). WT1 exerts at least part of its oncogenic activity via its antiapoptotic properties. The function of WT1 depends to a great extent on its association with many other proteins involved with cell survival and growth. Thus, the apparently contradictory consequences of overproduction of this protein clearly depend on the context.

- ***BRCA1* and *BRCA2*:** *BRCA1* (breast cancer-1) and *BRCA2* are two tumor suppressor genes encoding proteins that are important in repair of DNA DSBs by homologous recombination, cell cycle checkpoint control and regulation of certain mitotic phases. Germline mutations in these genes create genomic instability in cells of both the breast and ovary. By age 70, women who inherit mutations in *BRCA1* suffer an 80% cumulative risk of breast cancer and a 35% cumulative risk of ovarian cancer. In women who have germline *BRCA2* mutations, the lifetime cumulative risk of breast cancer is 50% and of ovarian cancer is 10% to 15%. Fortunately, only about 5% of breast cancers in the United States reflect mutations in *BRCA1* or *BRCA2* (see Chapter 19). The large majority of women with germline mutations in *BRCA1* or *BRCA2* are heterozygous in their germline, and the breast and ovarian cancers that develop exhibit somatic mutations in the remaining normal allele (LOH, see above). The incidence of mutations in these genes in sporadic breast cancer is unclear, but it has been suggested that about 4% of sporadic ovarian cancers show mutated *BRCA* genes.

Table 5-2

Tumor Types Associated With Production of WT1

Cancer Type	Approximate Percentage Overexpressing WT1
Colorectal	70
Breast	85
Lung	90
Pancreas	75
Kidney	80
Thyroid	95
Ovary, serous	100
Ovary, endometrioid	25
Leukemia	75
Mesothelioma	80
Esophagus, squamous	90
Astrocytoma	90

- ***PTEN*.** Phosphatase and tensin homolog detected on chromosome 10 (or *PTEN*) is a potent tumor suppressor gene. It is the second most frequently mutated gene in human cancer, after p53. Normal PTEN is essential for maintenance of chromosomal stability, and its loss causes conspicuous changes in chromosomes. Although the mechanisms by which PTEN fosters the stability of the genome are completely different from those of p53, PTEN is now regarded as a "new guardian of the genome."

  Germline loss of PTEN leads to several tumor syndromes, the best known of which is Cowden syndrome. All are characterized by multiple benign hamartomas and greater than normal risk of cancer. However, the importance of PTEN is in its suppression of sporadic (i.e., nonhereditary) tumor development. Monoallelic loss or mutation in *PTEN* is commonly seen in a variety of tumors, including astrocytomas, and cancers of the breast, colon, lung and prostate. Homozygous mutations of *PTEN* are also frequent in many tumors, especially endometrial carcinomas and glioblastomas.

  PTEN protein appears to have myriad functions, including effects on response to DNA damage, apoptosis, cell cycle progression, aging, chemotaxis and angiogenesis. PTEN's profound effects on cell signaling are seen in most cancers. Importantly, the PTEN network does not function in isolation, but interfaces with other pathways of tumor suppression and oncogenic signaling. In this context, PTEN and p53 physically interact and regulate each other. A further connection to tumor development is the fact that mutated *ras* inhibits PTEN expression.

  PTEN is a phosphatase that dephosphorylates both proteins and lipids. Its normal network embraces the panoply of signals that connect growth factor–triggered signals from receptors at the cell surface to nuclear transcription factors that mediate many cellular functions. Normally PTEN dephosphorylates phosphoinositol trisphosphate (PIP3), a lipid signaling intermediate that activates numerous targets (Fig. 5-30). Levels of PTEN protein are normally maintained at a steady, high point. Thus, anything that changes PTEN protein levels, whether inactivation of one or both alleles, altered promoter activity or other epigenetic change, may lower the concentration of the protein to a point where it is unable to modulate levels of PIP3 effectively. Decreased PTEN activity permits PIP3 to accumulate and thereby constitutively activate a variety of signaling pathways involved in cell proliferation and survival, which are key in cancer development.
- ***NF-1*.** Neurofibromatosis (NF) type 1 is related to germline mutations of the *NF-1* gene, which encodes *neurofibromin,* a negative regulator of *ras*. Inactivation of *NF-1* permits unopposed *ras* function and thereby promotes cell growth. Patients with neurofibromatosis-1 are at a substantial risk for the development of neurogenic sarcomas.
- ***VHL*.** Germline inactivation of the von Hippel-Lindau (*VHL*) gene is associated with a syndrome of the same name, involving a constellation of tumors that include renal cell carcinomas, glioblastomas, pheochromocytomas, islet cell tumors of the pancreas and others. Inactivation of both alleles of the *VHL* gene, by mutation or promoter hypermethylation, may also occur in sporadic renal cell carcinomas.

  VHL protein is part of a ubiquitin ligase that targets transcription factors, called hypoxia-inducible factors (HIFs; see Chapter 1), for degradation. The defect in Ub

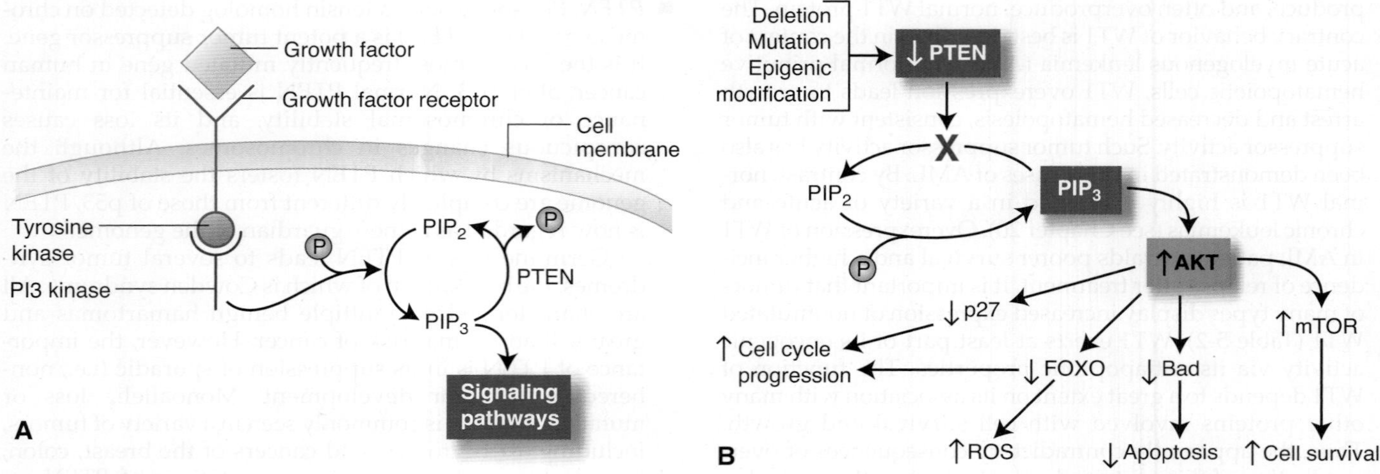

FIGURE 5-30. Signaling function of PTEN. A. Normal. Binding of a growth factor to its receptor leads to phosphorylation of phosphatidylinositol-bisphosphate (PIP2) to produce the important signaling molecule phosphatidylinositol-trisphosphate (PIP3). The level of PIP3 is regulated by its dephosphorylation by PTEN. **B. Decrease in PTEN.** If activity of PTEN is decreased by mutation or by epigenetic means, PIP3 accumulates, thereby activating Akt, a central signaling intermediate. As a result, p27, Bad and FOXO are not activated, thereby promoting cell cycle progression and decreasing apoptosis. At the same time, activation of mTOR stimulates cell survival. Loss of PTEN activity thus facilitates the development of uncontrolled cell proliferation and cancer.

conjugation leads to increased HIF, which activates transcription of genes important in cellular responses to low oxygen environments. These include those that (1) increase cellular intake of glucose for anaerobic glycolysis, (2) stimulate angiogenesis (vascular endothelial growth factor [VEGF]; see Chapter 10) and (3) activate several critical growth factors.

The carcinogenicity associated with the inactivation of VHL is caused in large part by the action of HIF in promoting tumor growth. Interestingly, similar activation of HIF occurs in the often oxygen-starved cores of many tumors, in the absence of *VHL* mutation. In those settings, HIF degradation is impaired by decreased activity of a cofactor for the ubiquitination reaction.

The normal VHL protein has additional tumor suppressor activities independent of HIF. These include (1) promoting apoptosis, (2) increasing cellular immobilization by adherence to matrix proteins and (3) repressing certain cell activation responses.

- ***FHIT.*** The fragile histidine triad (FHIT) tumor suppressor protein cleaves certain nucleotides into adenosine monophosphate (AMP) and adenosine diphosphate (ADP), but it is not clear how much its tumor suppressor activity relates to this enzymatic function. Loss of FHIT is associated with cancers of the gastrointestinal (GI) tract, lung, head and neck, breast, kidney and cervix. Certain acute leukemias are particularly related to aberrant FHIT expression. Most mutations in the *FHIT* gene are acquired deletions; its locus is the most fragile site in the human genome for chromosome breakage.

  Unlike most tumor suppressors except for APC, the FHIT protein does not bind DNA. Rather, it (like APC) enhances microtubule assembly. It is also felt to promote apoptosis via caspase-8 activation (see Chapter 1).

The aforementioned descriptions of tumor suppressor genes are only representative examples of a very large number of genes and networks that normally exert negative control of the processes that lead to tumor development, especially cell proliferation. It is beyond the scope of this discussion to address the full range of tumor suppressor activities, such as cell cycle control genes (e.g., p14, p16), cell spindle assembly, etc.

Organ Specificity of Abnormalities in Tumor Suppressor Genes and Oncogenes

Many of the inherited germline mutations cited above (e.g., *BRCA1* or *VHL* genes) lead to specific tumor syndromes. Other acquired abnormalities, such as amplification of *ErbB2* or mutations in *ras*, are associated with particular tumor types and not others. Although we have achieved a basic understanding of how such changes may lead to tumors, it remains unclear why alterations in certain genes tend to affect some organs but not others. Thus, the importance of BRCA1 in repair of DNA double-strand breaks is well established, but it is obscure why germline *BRCA1* mutations lead only to breast and ovarian cancers, and why only women are affected but not men. Additional studies may provide insights that could be therapeutically applicable to preventing or treating tumors that arise in these contexts.

Disturbances in Telomeres Contribute to Cancer

When chromosomal DNA is replicated, the DNA polymerase that is responsible for producing an identical copy of the original template begins at the 5′ end of the DNA strand to be copied and replicates the DNA toward the 3′ end, but often fails to reach that 3′ end. Thus, each time a cell divides, its DNA strands are shortened (see Chapter 1). If this process remains unchecked, further shortening of DNA strands would lead to the loss of critical coding sequences. Moreover, the unpaired chromosome ends would be subject to the action of the cell's DNA repair apparatus, an effect that could lead to aneuploidy via end-to-end recombination. These fates are prevented because the terminal portions of chromosomes are capped by nucleoprotein complexes, which are called **telomeres.** These structures contain strings of repetitive TTAGGG sequences. In normal cells some of these repeats are lost with each cell division, causing chromosomes to become shortened by a progressive decrease in telomere length.

As described in Chapter 1, ongoing telomere shortening in normal cells eventually reaches a critical length, thereby leading to senescence. If such critical shortening and uncapping of telomeres occurs in the context of acquired impairment of cell cycle checkpoint regulation (e.g., loss of $p16^{INK4a}$ or p53), chromosomes are susceptible to instability resulting from the types of rearrangements mentioned above (breakpoint–fusion–bridge cycles). Resulting chromosomal instability promotes carcinogenesis by facilitating chromosomal rearrangements, which in turn can eventuate in aneuploidy, translocations, amplifications and deletions. Thus, telomere attrition leads to sufficient genomic instability to set the stage for the development of mutations in sufficient numbers for cells to cross the borderline from benign to malignant.

The solution to the problem of cellular senescence and chromosomal instability resides in an enzyme with reverse transcriptase activity, referred to as **telomerase.** In normal human cells, the levels of this enzyme are insufficient to maintain telomere length, and each cell division therefore leads to progressive telomere attrition. However, in normal cells that divide frequently, telomerase makes a DNA copy of an RNA telomere template and affixes it to the 3′ end of the replicating DNA strand. In this way, telomerase preserves telomere length and chromosomal integrity in the face of continuing cell division. Not surprisingly, then, normal cells that express telomerase include those that need to continue to divide for the lifetime of the individual (e.g., hematopoietic progenitor cells, gastrointestinal epithelium and germ cells).

The cancer cell, presumably as a protective adaptation to genomic instability, reactivates telomerase, and 80% of human tumors display increased telomerase activity. A high level of this activity actually protects the cancer cell by suppressing the development of further, potentially lethal, chromosomal instability. *Thus, telomerase activation permits—but does not directly cause—the emergence of cancer* (Fig. 5-31).

Epigenetic Mechanisms May Both Impede and Foster Tumor Development

Mendelian genetics, as powerful as it is in explaining inheritance, cannot account for the enormous variability of phenotypes within any population. One explanation for this diversity is encompassed by the term **epigenetics,** *which is defined as changes in gene expression that are independent of DNA base sequence.* In addition to defining structural changes in the coding sequences of genes that contribute to cancer development, recent years have witnessed an increased appreciation of the major contribution of epigenetic influences to carcinogenesis. This may be understood as the twilight of somatic genetics and the dawn of a new era of cancer research. Several of these epigenetic factors are discussed below.

- **DNA methylation:** The most widely recognized epigenetic factor is DNA methylation. This process was first discovered as a global decrease in methylated DNA in human cancers, after which increased methylation of tumor suppressor genes was described. Thus, it was appreciated that DNA methylation could suppress gene expression.

  Development of an organism and differentiation of its cells to serve specific functions depends on selective expression and silencing of genes. During adult life, it is necessary for gene expression to vary according to tissue, cell type and other circumstances. This genetic regulation is largely achieved by DNA methylation.

  DNA methylation is concentrated on cytosines that precede guanines, an arrangement called CpGs. (The "p" corresponds to interbase phosphodiester bonds.) Regions rich in CpGs, called CpG islands, are particularly common (about 60%) in human gene promoter regions. Cytosine methylation in these islands is especially important in development, X chromosome inactivation in females and genomic imprinting (see Chapter 6). Increasing evidence indicates that the level of methylation—as both hypomethylation and hypermethylation—is an important actor in the drama of carcinogenesis.

  Hypermethylation: Many cancers are distinguished by hypermethylation of CpG islands in the promoter regions of tumor suppressor genes, such as *Rb, VHL* and *BRCA1.* Promoter hypermethylation has also been identified in genes that influence carcinogenesis by virtue of their roles in cell cycle transit, apoptosis, DNA repair and angiogenesis (see above). Patterns of hypermethylation vary according to tumor type, and suppression of certain genes by hypermethylation may represent a second hit, resulting in a functional loss of heterozygosity.

  Hypermethylation also illustrates the yin and yang of cancer pathogenesis. Noncoding regions of the human genome contain numerous repetitive sequences that are CpG rich and are heavily methylated under normal conditions. This effect protects chromosomal stability by silencing noncoding DNA (see later) and transposable DNA elements.

  Hypomethylation: As mentioned above, most cancers exhibit global hypomethylation, when compared to their normal tissue counterparts. This occurs in repetitive DNA sequences, as well as in exons and introns of protein-encoding genes. The extent of DNA hypomethylation increases as the malignant process advances from a benign proliferation to a malignant tumor. Undermethylation of DNA destabilizes DNA structure and favors recombination during mitosis, leading to increased deletions, translocations, chromosomal rearrangements and aneuploidy, all of which contribute to malignant transformation. Hypomethylation of genes associated with cell proliferation may increase the transcription of such genes. It has also been demonstrated that progressive hypomethylation of sequences in latent human tumor viruses (e.g., HPV, Epstein-Barr virus) has been linked to tumor development.
- **Histone modifications.** Chromatin is a complex of DNA and proteins that constitutes chromosomes. It packages DNA into a structure that permits mitosis and meiosis and regulates gene expression. Among the most important DNA-associated proteins are histones, a family of proteins that associate with DNA to form nucleosomes, which stabilize the three-dimensional structure of DNA. Covalent changes in the structure of histones via methylation, acetylation and other modifications influence numerous gene activities, including transcription, DNA repair and DNA replication. Methylation of histones leads to variable consequences, depending on the amino acid involved, but

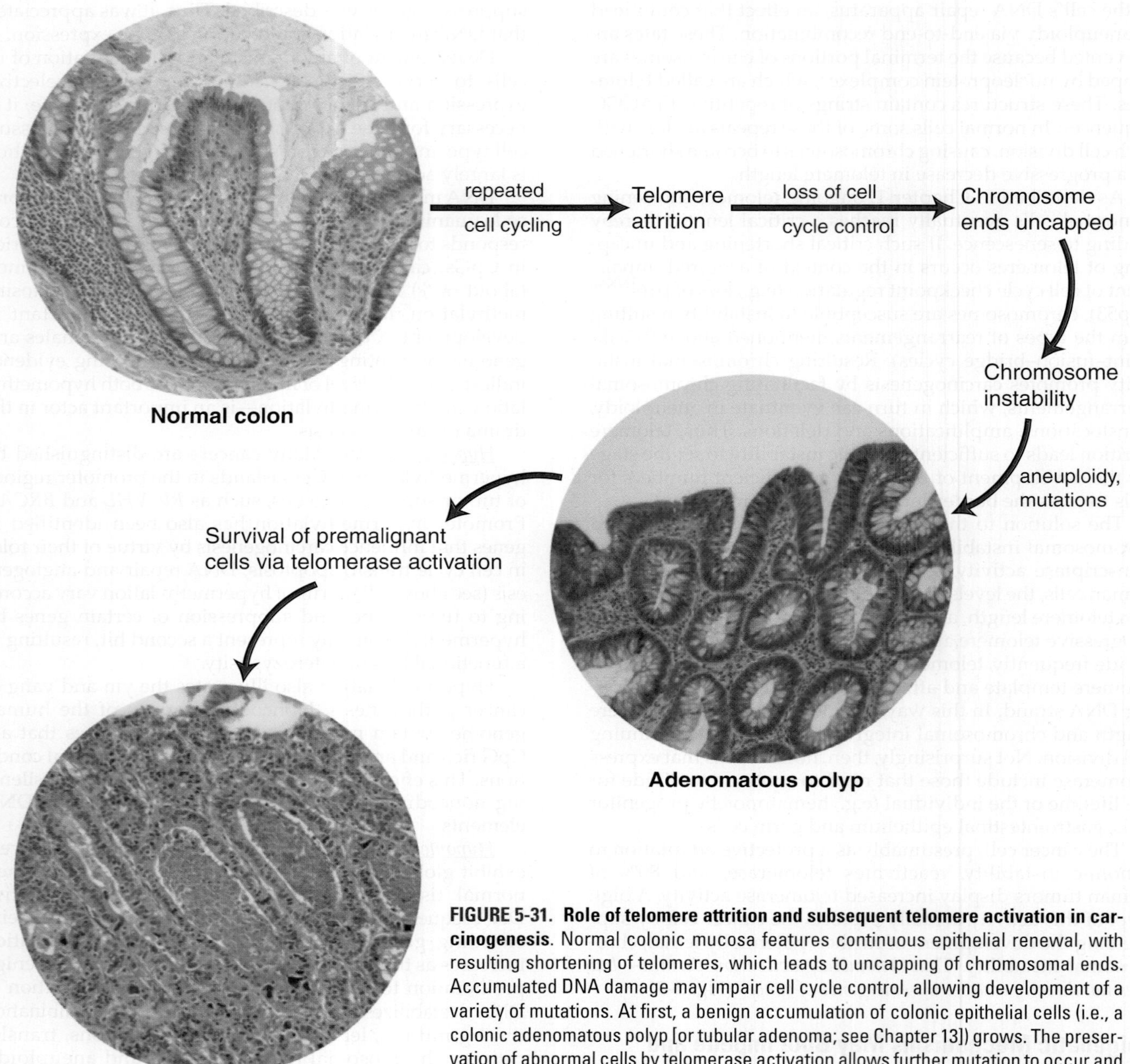

FIGURE 5-31. Role of telomere attrition and subsequent telomere activation in carcinogenesis. Normal colonic mucosa features continuous epithelial renewal, with resulting shortening of telomeres, which leads to uncapping of chromosomal ends. Accumulated DNA damage may impair cell cycle control, allowing development of a variety of mutations. At first, a benign accumulation of colonic epithelial cells (i.e., a colonic adenomatous polyp [or tubular adenoma; see Chapter 13]) grows. The preservation of abnormal cells by telomerase activation allows further mutation to occur and eventuates in malignant transformation.

histone acetylation is generally associated with transcriptional activation. As a corollary, histone deacetylation is associated with transcriptional silencing. Therefore, the combination of histone modification and DNA methylation comprises an intricate regulatory network whose disruption plays an important role in oncogenesis.

- **MicroRNA (miRNA) and cancer:** Not too long ago, the theory of the genetic basis of cancer envisioned an equilibrium between genes encoding proteins that either pushed a cell toward malignancy or protected it from that push. Life is not so simple. The discovery that most noncoding DNA (previously considered "junk DNA") is actually transcribed into untranslated RNA species and that these RNAs exert a regulatory function in gene expression has added fuel to the fire that threatens to consume "traditional" concepts of cancer genetics. Among the mass of untranslated RNA molecules produced are miRNAs, which are double-stranded, 22-base-pair-long RNA species, of which more than 1000 are currently described. These are made by RNA polymerase II from DNA sequences that may occur anywhere in the genome, including introns, exons and noncoding regions.

  miRNAs bind to mRNAs, to which they are complementary. Such binding may result in cleavage or degradation of the targeted transcript. The relationship between miRNAs and mRNAs is promiscuous in that any individual miRNA may regulate multiple mRNAs, and each mRNA can bind a number of miRNAs. Interestingly, about half of DNA sequences coding for miRNAs reside at fragile genomic sites and regions prone to amplification and loss of heterozygosity.

miRNAs have been shown to play an important role in the regulation of cell differentiation and proliferation, and it should then be obvious that altered miRNA levels may be linked to the development of cancer. It has been demonstrated that miRNAs are important for the growth and development of a number of human tumors, including those of the lung, colon, breast, pancreas and hematopoietic system. Like other epigenetic factors, miRNAs can function either as oncogenes or tumor suppressors, depending on the gene they target. The full panoply of miRNA activities remains to be elucidated, but their importance in cancer biology is unquestionable.

Cancer Cells Display Altered Metabolism

Almost a century ago, Otto Warburg recognized that cancer cells preferentially generate energy via cytoplasmic aerobic glycolysis, as opposed to mitochondrial oxidative phosphorylation. Given an adequate supply of glucose, such glycolysis can produce ATP faster than can mitochondrial mechanisms. Thus, many cancer cells take up much more glucose than do their normal counterparts. This observation is exploited by positron emission tomography (PET), which uses radiolabeled glucose analogs to visualize tumors.

Cancer cell growth requires higher levels of lipid and macromolecule biosynthesis (proteins, DNA) than are characteristic of these cells' more indolent normal relatives. In this context, glycolysis generates metabolic intermediates that supply the building blocks needed for those enhanced biosynthetic requirements. This is achieved by shunting mitochondrial function, at least in part, from energy generation to biosynthesis. Instead of being used to generate ATP, pyruvate produced by glycolysis is used to synthesize molecules for other anabolic pathways.

Importantly, networks composed of oncogenes and tumor suppressor genes influence the metabolic shift in cancer. The downstream effectors, phosphoinositide 3-kinase (PI3K), Akt and mTOR (see above), manage activities that support biosynthesis, a process that is normally regulated by the tumor suppressor PTEN (see above). Many cancers contain activating mutations in PI3K and are characterized by the loss of PTEN. Resulting activation of Akt and mTOR signaling pathways leads to enhanced metabolic activity, including increased cell receptors for glucose and amino acids, to enhance their availability for the tumor cell's biosynthetic needs. Diverse oncogenes (e.g., c-*myc*, *HRAS*, c-*src*) also strongly influence multiple metabolic pathways essential for cancer cell growth.

Several other tumor suppressors, including TSC1 and p53, and a number of kinases are implicated in metabolic control. For instance, PI3K has tumor-promoting activity, whereas AMPK may function as a tumor suppressor (see Fig. 5-32 for a more detailed summary of metabolic pathways in cancer cells).

Disturbances in Programmed Cell Death Play Key Roles in Oncogenesis

The total number of cells in any organ reflects a balance between cell division and cell death, and interference with this intricate equilibrium can result in the development of cancer. There are two principal mechanisms of programmed cell death, namely, apoptosis and autophagy (see Chapter 1), the dysregulation of which has been implicated in tumor development.

Apoptosis

Normally, apoptosis eliminates damaged or abnormal cells. Cancer cells therefore often evolve mechanisms to disable apoptosis. There are many known pro- and antiapoptotic proteins that have been found to interact in a head-spinning number of ways. To make this topic understandable, we will restrict ourselves to illustrative examples. These include both loss-of-function mutations in p53 and gain-of-function mutations in the Bcl-2 family of oncogenes that inhibit apoptosis. Stimulation of apoptosis by a number of oncogenes may occur if DNA damage control systems are operational. Moreover, a number of anticancer drugs operate by facilitating the process of apoptosis.

The prototypical example of the role of apoptosis in human cancer is follicular lymphoma (see Chapter 20), in which an inhibitor of apoptosis, Bcl-2, is constitutively activated by translocation to the promoter region of the immunoglobulin heavy chain [t(14:8)]. As a result, the normal equilibrium between the life and death of B lymphocytes is altered in favor of the former, thereby allowing accumulation of excess neoplastic B cells.

Increased expression of Bcl-2 has also been described in some other tumor types, including lung cancer and non-Hodgkin lymphoma. Chromosomal translocation is not the only mechanism by which Bcl-2 expression can be altered. Methylation and suppression of miRNAs that regulate Bcl-2 expression have been reported. Similarly, any impairment of p53 function, whether by mutation or epigenetic mechanisms, can decrease expression of proapoptotic Bcl-2 binding partners (see Chapter 1) and, in so doing, promote tumor formation.

The issue of apoptosis and cancer is further complicated by the phenomenon of **oncogene-mediated apoptosis.** Although the transcription factor Myc is generally considered to be an oncogene product, it also induces a default apoptosis pathway. Thus, promotion of cell proliferation by deregulated production of Myc is usually balanced by increased apoptosis. Induction of apoptosis by Myc acts as a "molecular safety valve" that blocks cancer development. For Myc-stimulated tumor development to occur, some cells producing Myc at high levels must also survive by overexpressing Bcl-2 or other antiapoptotic proteins.

This example illustrates the complexity inherent in the control of the on/off switch of apoptosis in cancer development.

Autophagy

Autophagy (see Chapter 1) was first considered to be a process characterized by bulk, nonselective degradation of cell constituents. However, it is now clear that it plays a role in many processes, including cancer. Autophagy operates in two ways: it may be nonselective or selective. Nonselective autophagy sequesters and catabolizes cytoplasmic components randomly, whereas selective autophagy detects and digests specific cell constituents. In this way, autophagy not only is a response to nutrient deprivation but also participates in many other processes, including tumor suppression. It is also a double-edged sword, as its activation facilitates tumor cell survival in a nutrient-poor environment. Expression of certain oncogenes, such as *ras*, may stimulate autophagy, leading to cellular senescence or death. *Autophagy thus*

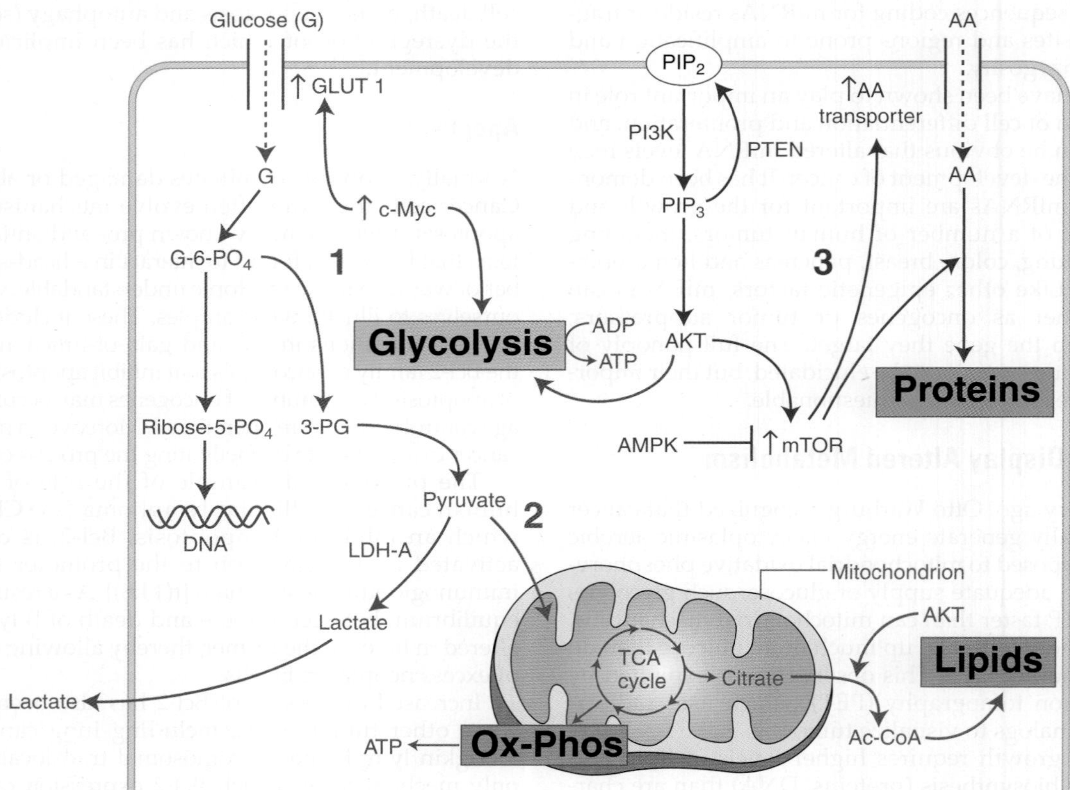

FIGURE 5-32. Cancer cell metabolism. *1.* Entry of glucose (G) into the cancer cell is facilitated by c-*myc*–mediated increases in the glucose transporter, GLUT1. Most glucose is metabolized by glycolysis, which leads to production of pyruvate, which is in turn converted to lactate. As part of this process, glucose-6-phosphate (G-6-PO4) and 3-phosphoglycerate (3-PG) are generated, both of which are precursors for ribose-5-phosphate (Ribose-5-PO4), an important building block in nucleic acid synthesis. *2.* Some of the pyruvate generated from glucose metabolism enters mitochondria, to be part of the tricarboxylic acid (TCA) cycle, which drives oxidative phosphorylation to produce adenosine triphosphate (ATP). Citrate from this cycle is exported to the cytosol, where it is incorporated into lipids; this process is stimulated by activated Akt. *3.* Activation of phosphoinositide 3-kinase (PI3K) leads to phosphoinositol trisphosphate (PIP3) production (which is decreased by PTEN), which in turn activates Akt, leading to increased glycolysis and activation of mTOR. The latter is inhibited by the tumor suppressors AMPK and TSC1/2. mTOR stimulates amino acid (AA) uptake through specific cell membrane transporters and eventuates in increased protein synthesis.

represents an alternative pathway of programmed cell death in preventing cancer.

Numerous tumor suppressor proteins, such as PTEN and the tuberous sclerosis proteins (TSC1, TSC2), constitutively facilitate autophagy. A number of oncogenes (Akt, Bcl-2, mTOR) impair autophagy, underscoring its importance as an antioncogenic process. Important genes involved in autophagy, such as beclin-1, are commonly mutated in many human cancers. Interestingly, several antineoplastic medications strongly promote autophagy. Although the connection between autophagy and cancer is not fully understood, impairment of the tumor suppressor function of autophagy may result in accumulation of materials within the cell that cause chromosomal instability, which ultimately may lead to cancer development.

Cellular Senescence Helps to Prevent Cancer

Cellular senescence is the loss of a cell's ability to complete the mitotic cycle, with irreversible arrest of cell cycle progression. However, the ability of senescent cells to remain viable for extended periods of time sets them apart from cells undergoing rapid apoptotic demise (see Chapter 1). The Rb and p53 tumor suppressors are the critical arbiters of cellular senescence.

Oncogene-Induced Cellular Senescence

Some impediments to tumor development that are not related to oncogenes have been discussed above. These include cell death by apoptosis and autophagy, and telomere-induced senescence. However, in recent years, oncogene-induced senescence (OIS) has been shown to constrain tumor formation in many types of cancer. Consistent with this role for OIS, senescent cells stimulate the tumor suppressor functions of both p53 and Rb.

To put OIS into the context of cancer, one should appreciate that the vast majority of cells sustaining an oncogenic mutation never become cancers. A simple calculation of mutation rates indicates that, in the human body, such mutations occur several times per minute, which contrasts with the relative infrequency of cancer in a human lifespan. A major barrier to the development of cancer appears to be cellular senescence.

Earlier studies showed that after activated Ras enhanced proliferation of affected cells, an irreversible growth arrest (i.e., cellular senescence) occurred. This senescence could be avoided by crippling p53 and Rb pathways, suggesting that such OIS actually evolved as a means to prevent tumors. Subsequently, activating alterations in other oncogenes were found to induce OIS in vivo. Benign tumors demonstrate such senescence, whereas advanced malignant tumors do not. Thus, lacking further mutations, OIS prevents benign cell proliferations from progressing to malignancy.

Despite extensive ongoing research, there is no single paradigm that explains all the data related to OIS. Although a variety of signals have been demonstrated via Rb and p53, it appears that senescence actually occurs by an exceedingly complex signaling network (Fig. 5-33).

If a cell manages to avoid the senescence program following oncogene activation, by whatever sequence of events,

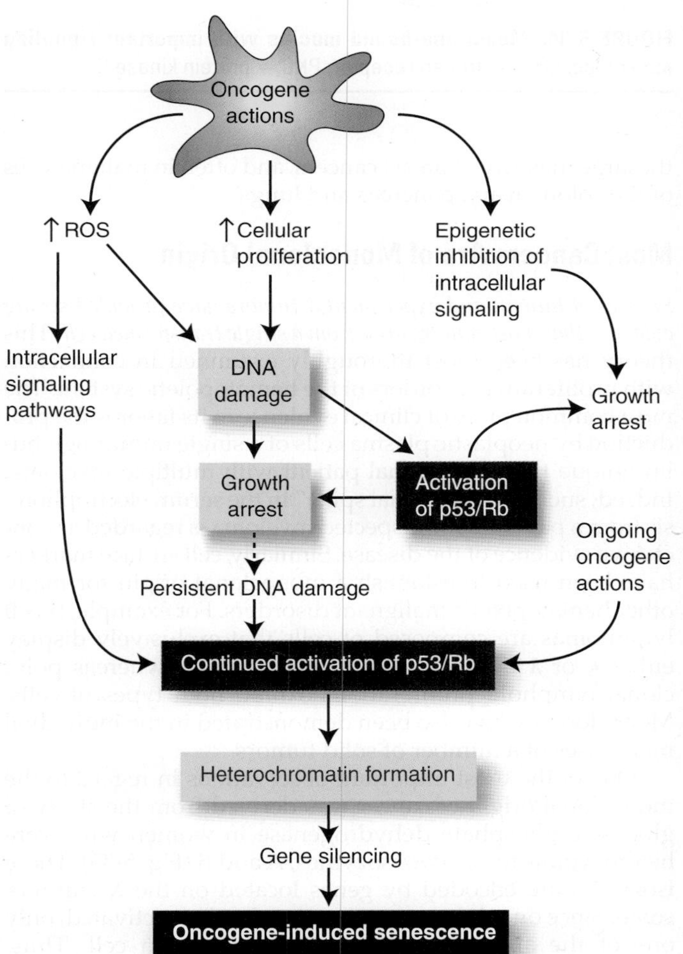

FIGURE 5-33. A hypothetical paradigm for oncogene-induced senescence (OIS). Oncogenic stress can elicit cellular responses that eventuate in cellular senescence. The factors that participate in this process activate p53 and pRb, and multiple pathways are needed to sustain this activation. Chromatin remodeling may then silence important genes and solidify the growth arrest.

that cell continues to proliferate and may be said to have been immortalized (see Chapter 1). If an immortalized cell accumulates further mutations in vivo, the proliferation that results may progress through dysplasia, in situ carcinoma and eventual invasion and metastasis. Thus, **multistep carcinogenesis** is a notion that reflects the necessity for tumor cells to acquire and accumulate mutations that both stimulate proliferation and inactivate cell senescence mechanisms.

Signal Transduction Translates Intra- and Extracellular Stimuli Into Cellular Activities

In recent years, many signaling pathways have been shown to participate in the development and spread of cancers. Several such pathways have been discussed in the section on oncogenes (see above), including receptor tyrosine kinases, nonreceptor G proteins and protein kinases. Here, we present several examples of how signal transduction relates to cancer biology.

Steroid Hormones

Some three centuries ago, the Italian physician Ramazzini observed that nuns had a particularly high incidence of breast cancer. This curiosity is now recognized to reflect the unopposed estrogen stimulation of breast epithelium, uninterrupted by pregnancy and lactation. Both estrogens and progesterone bind to specific cytoplasmic receptors. The resulting hormone–receptor complexes are then translocated to the nucleus, where they act as transcription factors that foster proliferation of responsive cells. Antiestrogen therapy for estrogen receptor–positive, progesterone receptor–positive tumors reduces the risk of recurrence after surgery. Other nuclear receptors have been identified in breast cancer, including those that bind androgens, corticosteroids, vitamins A and D, fatty acids and some dietary lipids. The interactions of these signaling pathways with each other and with other signaling pathways are highly complicated and not well understood.

The influence of androgens is most conspicuous in the case of prostate cancer, in which they stimulate growth by binding to the androgen receptor. This receptor pathway engages in cross-talk with other important pathways that affect the cell cycle, apoptosis and differentiation. Such interactions involve EGF, IGF-1, FGF, VEGF, TGF-β and other important signaling species. Removing androgen stimulation, whether by surgical or pharmacologic means, inhibits the growth of prostate cancer, although in most cases the tumors eventually become androgen insensitive.

Transforming Growth Factor-β

TGF-β, an extracellular cytokine in the microenvironment of cancer cells that triggers important regulatory pathways, is an example of cell communication mediators that strongly influence the pathogenesis of tumors. Its role in the genesis of cancer appears to be important, although cell and tissue responses to this cytokine are highly contextual. Normally, TGF-β tends mainly to suppress tumor development by modulating cell proliferation, survival, adhesion and differentiation. It also inhibits mitogenesis induced by constituents of the extracellular matrix. However, frankly malignant cells often acquire the capacity to evade or even to manipulate

Table 5-3

Transforming Growth Factor-β (TGF-β) and Cancer

Promotes	Inhibits
Normal Tumor-Suppressive Effects	
Apoptosis	Inflammation
Differentiation	Mitogenesis induced by extracellular matrix
Maintenance of cell number	
Failure of Tumor Suppression	
Autocrine mitogens	Immune surveillance
Motility	
Invasion and Metastasis	
Recruitment of myofibroblasts	
Malignant cell extravasation	
Modification of microenvironment	
Mobilization of osteoclasts	

Normally, TGF-β compels homeostasis and exerts tumor-suppressive activity through effects on the target cells themselves or the extracellular matrix. Failure of this activity by TGF-β permits production of growth factors, evasion of immune surveillance and establishment of factors that facilitate tumor cell invasion and metastasis.

TGF-β pathways for their own nefarious ends. Abnormal signaling in the TGF-β pathway can actually stimulate proliferation of tumor cells, facilitate their evasion of host defense mechanisms (see below) and foster invasion and metastasis.

Cancer cells may develop the ability to circumvent TGF-β–related suppressive activity via mutations in genes for TGF-β receptors or by interfering with downstream signaling by mutation or by promoter methylation of key proteins. Under these circumstances, cancer cells can hijack the regulatory activities of TGF-β to further their needs, such as tumor growth, invasion and metastasis. The loss of the tumor suppressor function of TGF-β through inactivating mutations of genes in its core pathway has been described in cancers of the colon, prostate, stomach, breast, pancreas and ovary and many others. A summary of the effects of TGF-β in cancer is presented in Table 5-3.

Other cytokines (e.g., granulocyte/monocyte colony-stimulating factor [GM-CSF] and interleukin-3 [IL-3] may contribute to tumor development simply by overexpression, especially for hematopoietic malignancies.

Membrane-Bound Mucins

Traditionally, mucins have been thought to be exclusively extracellular molecules charged with establishing an interface between many epithelial surfaces and the exterior. However, it is now recognized that membrane-bound mucins comprise a large family of glycoproteins that are frequently overproduced in a variety of cancers. The extracellular domains of these membrane-bound mucins (MUCs) lubricate and protect the cell surface. The cytoplasmic domains of these transmembrane glycoproteins function as scaffolds for interaction with signaling molecules that influence cell proliferation and survival (Fig. 5-34). In this context, MUC1 is overexpressed in

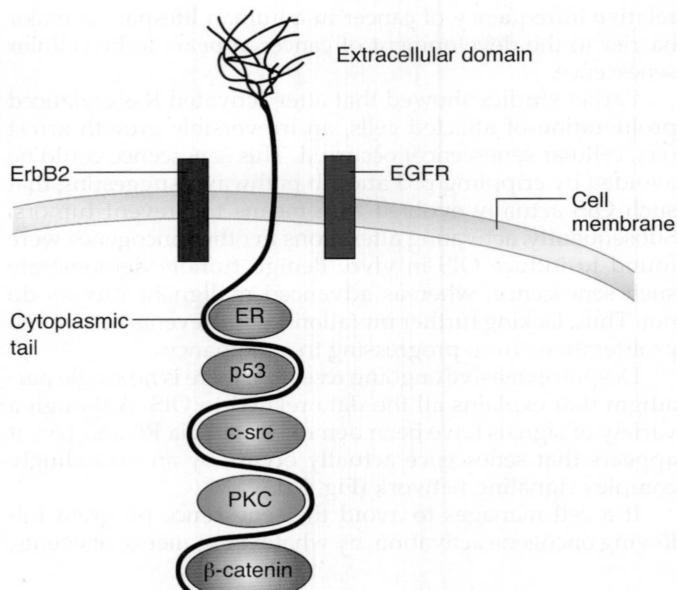

FIGURE 5-34. Membrane-bound mucins with important signaling molecules. ER = estrogen receptor; PKC = protein kinase C.

the large majority of breast cancers, and often in malignancies of the colon, ovary, pancreas and lungs.

Most Cancers Are of Monoclonal Origin

Studies of human and experimental tumors have provided strong evidence that most cancers arise from a single transformed cell. This theory has been most thoroughly examined in connection with proliferative disorders of the hematopoietic system. The most common piece of clinical evidence in its favor is the production by neoplastic plasma cells of a single immunoglobulin unique to an individual patient with multiple myeloma. Indeed, such a "monoclonal spike" in the serum electrophoresis from a patient with suspected myeloma is regarded as conclusive evidence of the disease. Similarly, cell surface markers have been used to establish a monoclonal origin for many other hematopoietic malignant disorders. For example, B-cell lymphomas are composed of cells that exclusively display either κ or λ light chains on their surfaces, whereas polyclonal lymphoid proliferations exhibit both types of cells. Monoclonality has also been demonstrated in the individual metastases of a number of solid tumors.

One of the most important observations in regard to the monoclonal origin of cancer was derived from the study of glucose-6-phosphate dehydrogenase in women who were heterozygous for its two isozymes, A and B (Fig. 5-35). These isozymes are encoded by genes located on the X chromosome. Since one X chromosome is randomly inactivated, only one of the alleles is expressed in any given cell. Thus, although the genotypes of all cells are the same, their phenotypes vary with regard to the expression of isozyme A or B. An examination of benign uterine smooth muscle tumors (leiomyomas, or "fibroids") revealed that all the cells in an individual tumor expressed either A or B but not both, indicating that each tumor was derived from a single progenitor cell. Although oligoclonal tumors have been described, they are distinctly uncommon.

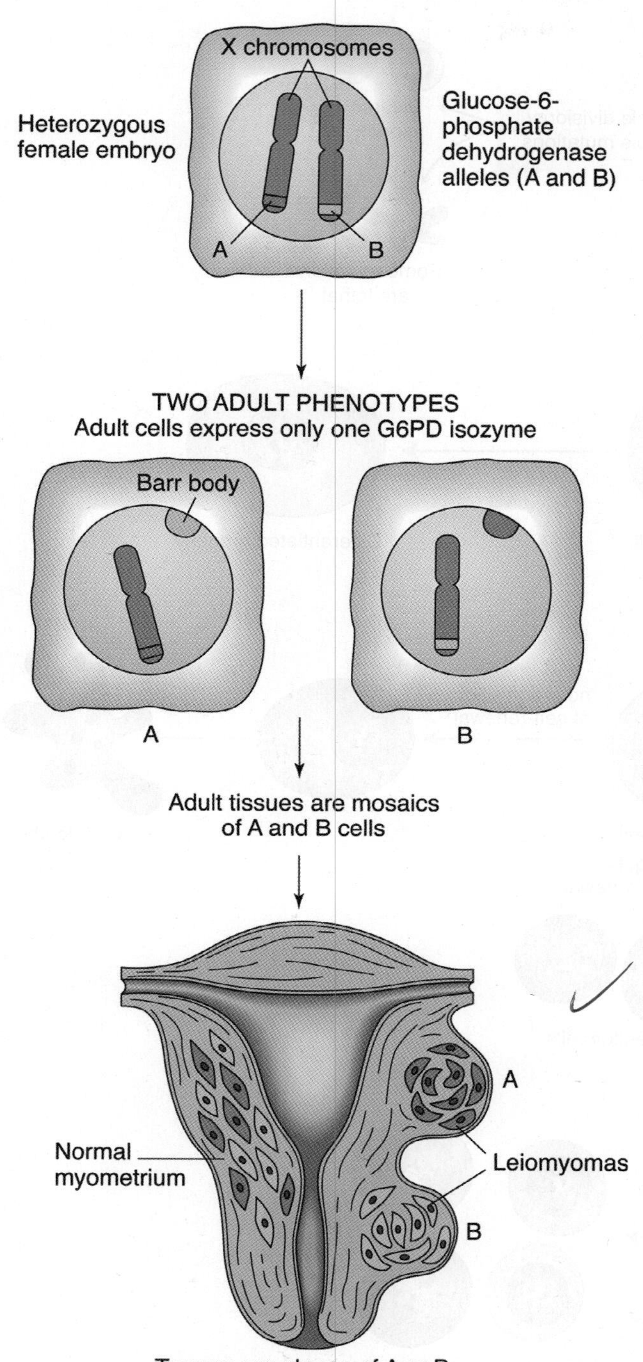

FIGURE 5-35. Monoclonal origin of human tumors. Some females are heterozygous for the two alleles of glucose-6-phosphate dehydrogenase (G6PD) on the long arm of the X chromosome. Early in embryogenesis, one of the X chromosomes is randomly inactivated in every somatic cell and appears cytologically as a Barr body attached to the nuclear membrane. As a result, the tissues are a mosaic of cells that express either the A or the B isozyme of G6PD. Leiomyomas of the uterus have been shown to contain one or the other isozyme (A or B) but not both, a finding that demonstrates the monoclonal origin of the tumors.

Most Tumors Are Heterogeneous in Their Appearance and Cellular Composition

Although almost all tumors begin as single clones of neoplastic cells, as they grow their cells show considerable genetic and phenotypic variation. This phenomenon is called **tumor heterogeneity.** Diversity of cells among a tumor population has broad implications for tumor progression and dissemination, as well as for responses to chemotherapy and the development of resistance to these agents. Several theories, which are not necessarily mutually exclusive, have been proposed to account for the diversity of cells in tumors.

Clonal Evolution

The original concept used to explain tumor heterogeneity holds that tumor cells progressively accumulate new mutations as they proliferate. A tumor in which many cells are dividing can thus, over time, generate a diverse population of genetically different cells. Some of these cells may be destined for the ignominy of cell death, whereas others may flourish as genetically distinct subclones of the original malignant cells (Fig. 5-36A). Darwinian-style selection governs which subclones will succeed and which will die, which will metastasize and which will remain localized.

Cancer Stem Cells

Only a minute proportion of the cells in a malignant tumor can produce a new tumor when they are transplanted into an immunologically deficient animal. Like somatic stem cells, which are capable of both self-renewal and differentiation, malignant cells with such capabilities are called **cancer stem cells.** The existence of cancer stem cells (CSCs) has been most convincingly demonstrated in acute myeloblastic leukemia (AML), although there is also strong evidence for their existence in a few solid tumors. In AML, far less than 1% of the leukemic cells express hematopoietic stem cell markers ($CD34^+$, $CD38^-$). Importantly, these are the only cells among the entire leukemic population that are capable of reestablishing a leukemia in an appropriate transplant recipient host. Comparable, but not identical, data have been obtained from studies of cancers of the breast, colon and brain.

Although the issue remains controversial, it appears that—at least in hematopoietic malignancies—CSCs may arise by transformation of normal hematopoietic stem cells or of lineage-committed progenitor cells. In the latter case, the transformed cells recapitulate at least parts of the normal stem cell program (Fig. 5-36B).

The significance of the fact of CSCs lies in their inherently low mitotic rate, which allows them to evade destruction by cytotoxic chemotherapeutic agents that preferentially kill rapidly dividing cells. Thus, although chemotherapy may destroy the bulk of a malignant tumor, residual CSCs may survive to regenerate the cancer.

Epigenetic Cancer Cell Plasticity

As important as CSCs are in some tumors, the evil machinations of malignancy have improvised even more devious approaches to maintaining and growing tumors. Thus, for some tumors (e.g., malignant melanomas), heterogeneity of tumor cell populations and the ability to regenerate a malignancy may entail

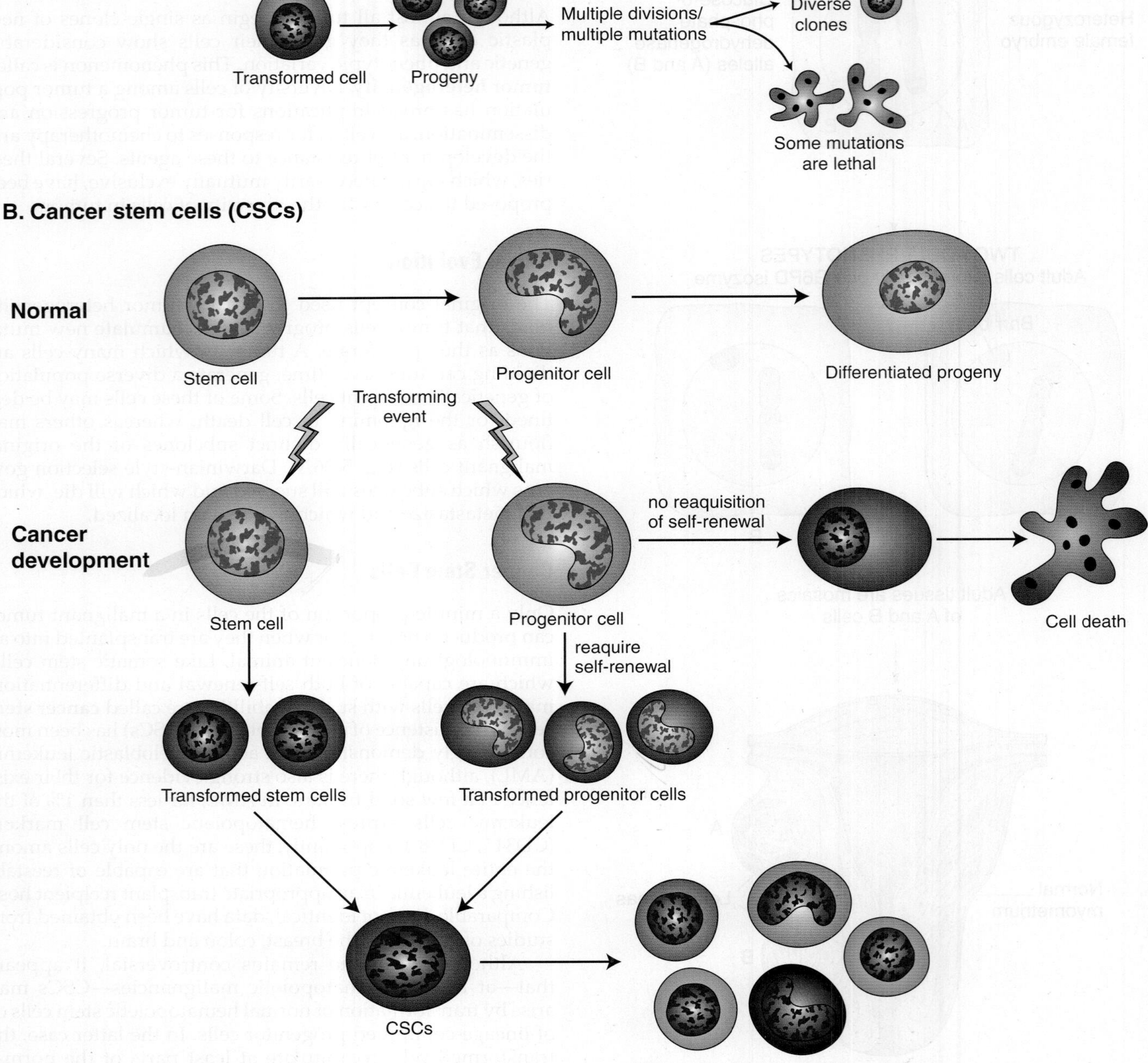

FIGURE 5-36. Paradigms of tumor heterogeneity. A. Clonal evolution. Proliferating tumor cells eventually develop a variety of mutations, with different individual cells acquiring different mutations, leading to heterogeneity in the tumor cell population. Some such mutations are inconsistent with cell survival, while others facilitate cancer progression. **B. Cancer stem cells.** Normally (*above*) stem cells give rise to committed progenitor cells. These then produce terminally differentiated cells. An oncogenic stimulus (*below*) to a stem cell may lead to an expanded pool of transformed stem cells. These become cancer stem cells (CSCs). Alternatively, the oncogenic stimulus may affect a committed progenitor cell. If the latter recapitulates a program of self-renewal, the resulting transformed progenitor may become a CSC. If it does not activate the self-renewal program, resulting differentiated progeny will be produced and eventually die. CSCs generated either via transformation of stem cells or transformation of committed progenitors may then be the antecedents of a heterogeneous malignant cell population.

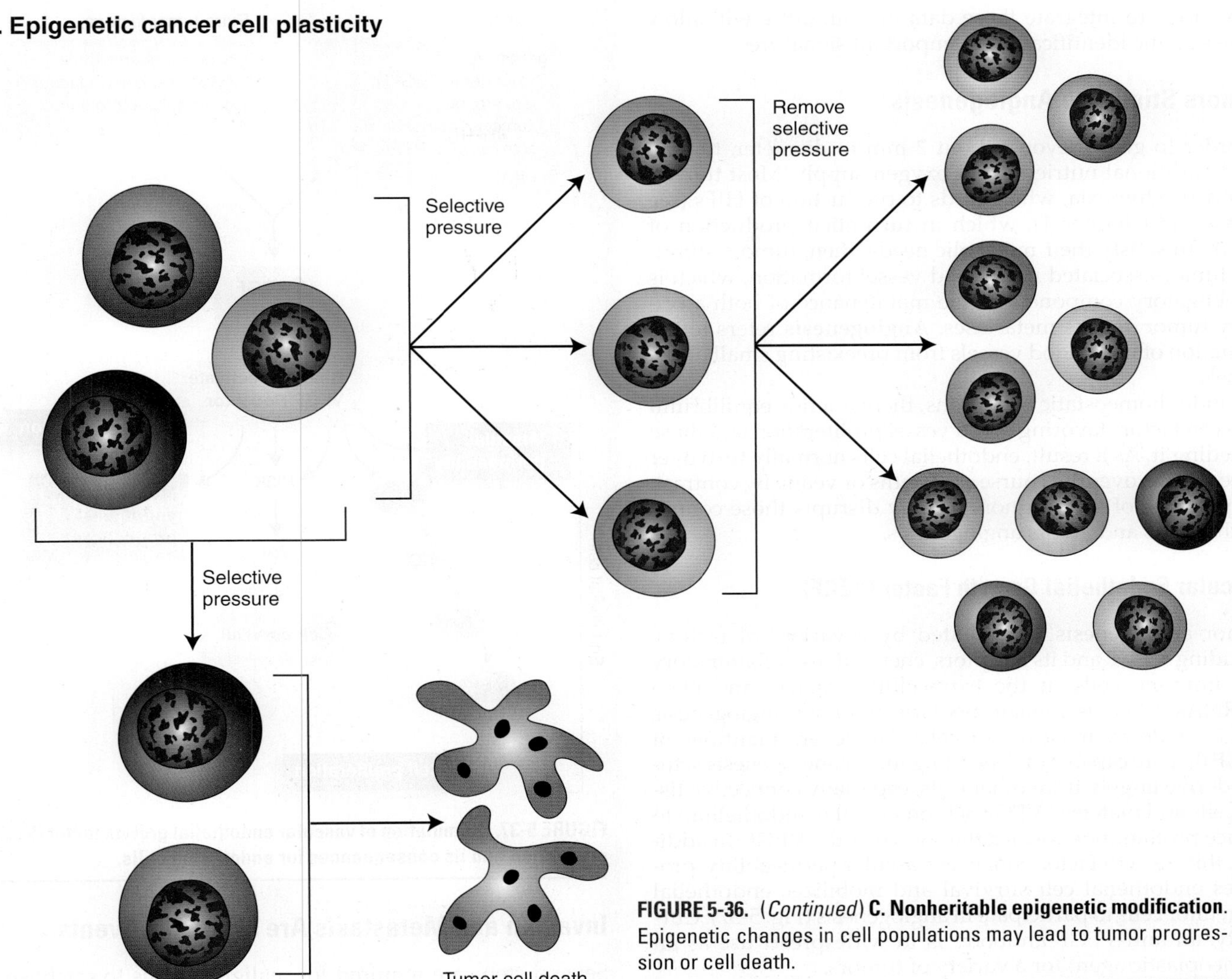

FIGURE 5-36. (*Continued*) **C. Nonheritable epigenetic modification.** Epigenetic changes in cell populations may lead to tumor progression or cell death.

epigenetic changes (e.g., the expression of proteins that covalently modify histones), which cells may switch on and off. Thus, a slowly proliferating population of tumor cells may alternate between different epigenetic states and so fluctuate between the ability to reconstitute a tumor and the lack of such ability. This type of deviousness allows for diverse populations of tumor cells to alternate between slowly dividing, tumor-reconstituting cells and rapidly dividing, nonreconstituting cells. Furthermore, tumor cells may achieve such metamorphoses without needing to incur further mutations.

The implications of this phenomenon are substantial. Some malignant tumors may represent constantly shifting therapeutic targets, with incredible plasticity in adapting to a changing chemotherapeutic milieu via the ability to shift phenotypes rapidly to evade antineoplastic drugs, and then to shift back to reemerge from a defensive posture and reassert an aggressive nature.

Gene Expression Signatures May Help Characterize the Biology of Tumors

The holy grail of cancer therapeutics is the identification of specific vulnerabilities of individual tumors to defined treatments, based on the tumor's distinctive individuality. The advent of high-throughput sequencing technologies opens the possibility of a new overview of the genetic landscape of tumors. It is thus becoming feasible to interrogate the unbelievable diversity of various tumors, looking for specific changes in genes that influence tumorigenesis. To allow interpretation of some 25,000 possible mutations in protein-encoding genes and up to 1000 mutations in noncoding regions, categorization of the affected genes by pathway analysis may be applied. Such an approach may paint a more detailed picture of the characteristics that are common among most malignant cells (e.g., autocrine mitogenic signaling, avoiding programmed cell death, independence of exogenous signals that limit growth and acquisition of the abilities to stimulate blood vessel growth and to invade and metastasize). The categories of alterations that are profiled as tumor signatures include variations in gene copy numbers, single nucleotide polymorphisms (SNPs), whole genome sequencing, description of mutations, methylation status of DNA and status of histones.

To date, many attempts at describing the gene signatures of specific tumors have been made, with the intention of predicting prognosis or identifying susceptibility to chemotherapy. However, the clinical applicability of such signatures remains doubtful. It is anticipated that the further development of technology to integrate these data meaningfully will allow more specific identification of important signatures.

Tumors Stimulate Angiogenesis

In order to grow beyond about 2 mm in diameter, tumors need additional nutrients and oxygen supply. Most tumors experience hypoxia, which leads to production of HIFs (see above and Chapter 1), which in turn elicit production of VEGF. To satisfy their metabolic needs, then, tumors stimulate tumor-associated new blood vessel formation, which is an obligatory component in the maintenance of both a primary tumor and its metastases. **Angiogenesis** refers to the formation of new blood vessels from preexisting small blood vessels.

Under homeostatic conditions, there is a fine equilibrium between factors favoring blood vessel proliferation and those impeding it. As a result, endothelial cells normally turn over quite slowly, over the course of months or years. By contrast, the presence of solid tumors usually disrupts those control mechanisms and favors angiogenesis.

Vascular Endothelial Growth Factor (VEGF)

Tumor angiogenesis is mediated by a variety of factors, including **VEGF** and its receptors, chemokines, inflammatory and immune cells in the extracellular matrix and even mi-RNAs. VEGF is a major mediator of tumor angiogenesis and is made by most tumor cells. However, quantities of VEGF that are capable of generating tumor angiogenesis actually derive largely from other cells, especially connective tissue cells and platelets. VEGF acts on vascular endothelium to induce proliferation toward the source of the VEGF. In addition, this growth factor enhances vascular permeability, promotes endothelial cell survival and mobilizes endothelial progenitor cells to participate in angiogenesis (Fig. 5-37). Currently, an anti-VEGF antibody is in widespread use as an antineoplastic agent for a variety of tumors.

Inflammatory Cytokines and Chemokines

Bone marrow–derived immune and inflammatory cells, including macrophages, neutrophils, natural killer cells, dendritic cells and myeloid precursor cells, all produce numerous soluble angiogenic factors. Equally important are tumor-associated stromal fibroblasts. However, the contribution of these cells to the growth of tumor blood vessels reflects the context of the tumor. In some settings, these cells assume a Dr. Jekyll–like antineoplastic phenotype and produce antitumor and antiangiogenic activities. In other settings, they become Mr. Hyde and generate proangiogenic and protumor microenvironments. As if this were not sufficiently complex, cells such as dendritic cells and myeloid-derived suppressor cells are capable of trans-differentiating into endothelial cells.

Notch signaling, an important developmental pathway, and specific angiogenesis-related miRNAs have also been shown to impact angiogenesis. In addition, angiostatic molecules) e.g., interferons, thrombospondin and certain chemokines) have been demonstrated to be active in the tumor microenvironment. The ability of tumors to grow and ocure adequate nutrients and oxygen by recruiting new ssels reflects a skewing of the delicate equilibrium ly exists between angiogenic and antiangiogenic

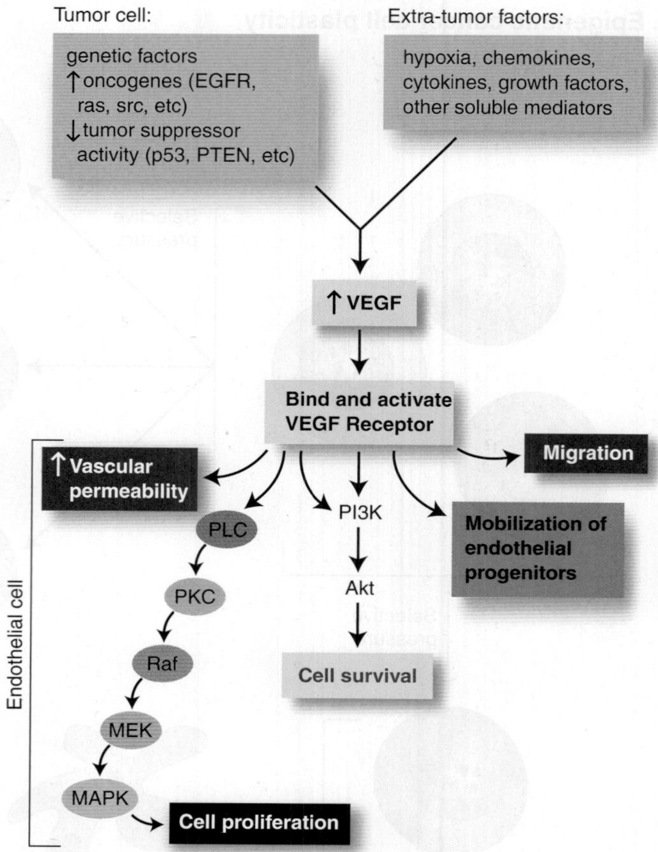

FIGURE 5-37. Stimulation of vascular endothelial growth factor (VEGF) production and its consequences for endothelial cells.

Invasion and Metastasis Are Multistep Events

Several steps are required for malignant cells to establish a metastasis (Fig. 5-38):

1. Invasion of the basement membrane underlying the tumor
2. Movement through extracellular matrix
3. Penetration of vascular or lymphatic channels
4. Survival and arrest within circulating blood or lymph
5. Exit from the circulation into a new tissue site
6. Survival and growth as a metastasis

Cancer cells evolve into subclones via genetic and epigenetic mechanisms, after which they interact with tumor-associated inflammatory cells. The latter may either be present in the extracellular matrix or be of bone marrow origin. In turn, these interactions become tumor ecosystems that stimulate signaling pathways for invasion and far-flung metastases. These microenvironments serve as communication points among cancer and mesenchymal cells, ligands and receptors, and signaling networks in a variety of different cells. The complexity of the processes of invasion and metastasis is evidenced by the heterogeneity of tumor cells, the consequences of oncogenes and tumor suppressors, the manifold functions of their products and the overlapping nature of the signaling pathways.

Invasion

Inherent in the definition of a malignant cell is its capacity to invade surrounding tissue. In epithelial tumors, invasion requires disruption of, and penetration through, the underlying basement membrane and passage through the extracellular matrix. Similarly, circulating cells destined to establish metastases must reproduce these same events to exit from the vascular or lymphatic compartment and establish residence at a distant site.

Movement through the extracellular matrix (ECM) requires proteases secreted by cancer cells and nonmalignant tumor-associated cells (see below). Under the influence of the extracellular signals noted above, the cancer cells develop protrusions that contain an actin core and integrins. These projections, called **invadopodia,** express matrix metalloproteinases (MMPs) and other proteolytic enzymes. Integrins in the ECM may not only function as mechanical anchors but also promote the development of invadopodia. The invadopodia clearly play a role in degrading the ECM and they offer a guide to the perplexed cell in navigating its microenvironment, through exploration of cell–cell and cell-matrix adhesions and by sensing chemoattractive molecules.

Tumor-Associated Host Cells

Host cells associated with tumors constitute about half of all cells within tumor masses. Such components include macrophages, leukocytes, fibroblasts, vascular endothelial cells, neural cells and fat cells (Fig. 5-39). Many of these cells are originally resident in the ECM, whereas others are of bone marrow origin. Importantly, all of these nontumor cells can influence the behavior of the cancer, both at its site of origin and at locations of metastases.

The ecosystems represented by the heterogeneity of tumor-associated cells have important prognostic implications and may eventually influence the development of therapies. However, the situation is complicated by the fact that many of the products of these cells have mutually opposite effects on tumor cell invasiveness, and a single paradigm or explanation is presently beyond reach.

Macrophages and Leukocytes

Human cancers usually contain abundant tumor-associated macrophages, which appear to promote tumor cell invasion and metastasis through inflammation and angiogenesis. In addition, these macrophages produce proinvasive enzymes that digest the basement membrane, including MMPs, urokinase plasminogen activator (u-PA) and cathepsins. Penetration of cancer cells through basement membranes and ECM is facilitated by expression of adhesion molecules that link cancer cells to diverse nonmalignant tumor-associated cells.

Adipocytes

The stroma in which many tumors arise contains adipocytes. Cross-talk between these cells and tumor cells frequently facilitates early stromal invasion by the malignant cells. Fat cells near tumors often express a particular MMP that assists the cancer cell in traversing the surrounding connective tissue.

Carcinoma in situ

Basement membrane

A cancer cell becomes capable of invasion (expresses surface adhesion molecules)

Tumor cell adhesion molecules bind to underlying extracellular matrix

Tumor cells disrupt and invade extracellular matrix

Release of proteolytic enzymes

Repeated binding to and dissolution of extracellular matrix

Tumor cells metastasize by way of blood vessels or lymphatics

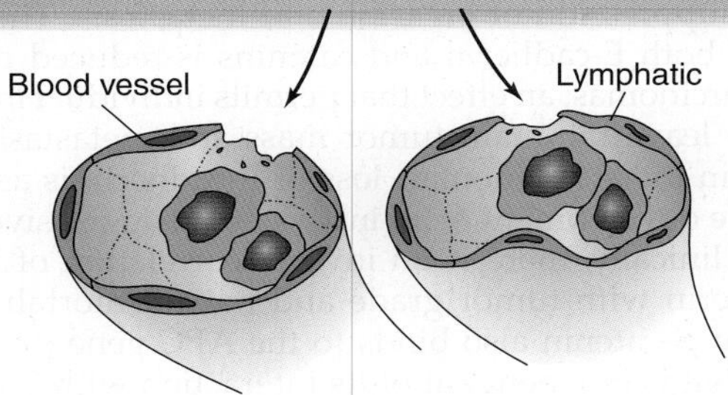

FIGURE 5-38. Mechanisms of tumor invasion and metastasis. The mechanism by which a malignant tumor initially penetrates a confining basement membrane and then invades the surrounding extracellular environment involves several steps. The tumor first acquires the ability to bind components of the extracellular matrix. These interactions are mediated by the expression of a number of adhesion molecules. Proteolytic enzymes are then released from the tumor cells, and the extracellular matrix is degraded. After moving through the extracellular environment, the invading cancer penetrates blood vessels and lymphatics by the same mechanisms.

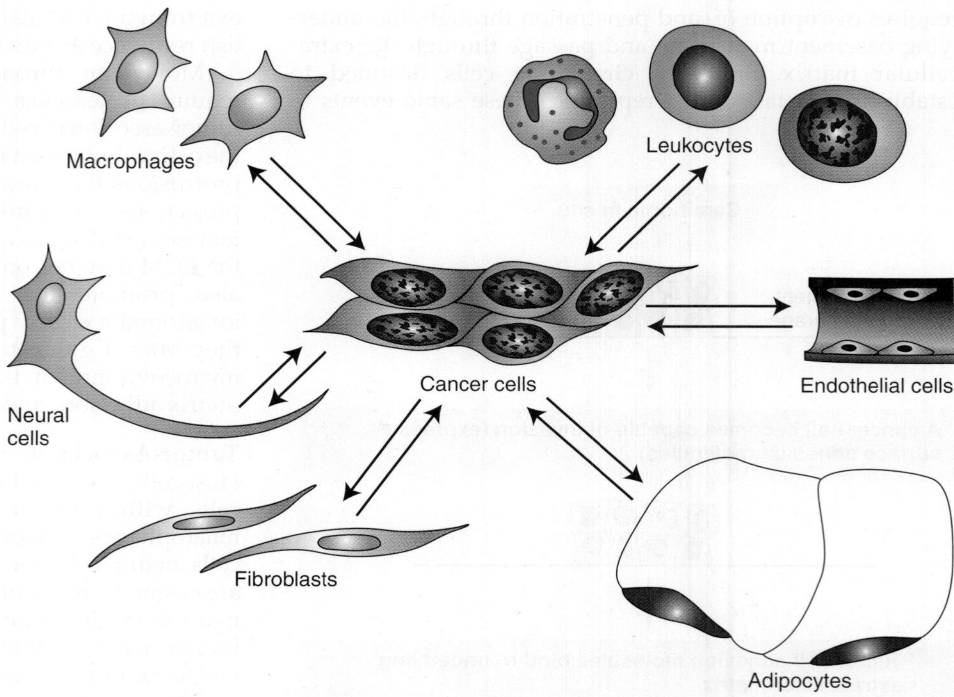

FIGURE 5-39. The cancer cell ecosystem. The developing tumor cells interact with the nonmalignant cells in their environment, via production of soluble and other mediators.

Leptin produced by adipocytes (see Chapter 23) also stimulates macrophages to secrete proinflammatory cytokines, which, in turn, promote invasion and metastasis.

Adhesion Molecules

The entire metastatic sequence, from the initial binding of the tumor cell to the underlying extracellular matrix to the growth in a distant location, depends on the expression of numerous adhesion molecules by the malignant cells. The display of such surface molecules varies with (1) the type of tumor, (2) the individual clone (tumor heterogeneity), (3) the stage of the malignant progression and (4) the specific step in the metastatic process. The main families of cell adhesion molecules are listed in Table 5-4.

INTEGRINS: Integrins are transmembrane receptors (see Chapter 3) that mediate cell–matrix and cell–cell attachment. The binding of integrins to their ligands also stimulates intracellular signaling and gene expression, which play a role in cell migration, proliferation, differentiation and survival. In addition, integrins affect the expression, localization and activation of collagenases (MMPs; see below) and can guide these enzymes to their targets in the extracellular matrix, where they degrade connective tissue and pave the way for the spread of tumor cells. Integrins can confer specificity to tumor cell homing to metastatic sites, and so influence the locations of metastases.

Table 5-4

Families of Adhesion Molecules That Regulate Tumor Cell Invasiveness and Metastasis

Type of Adhesion Molecule	Functions
Integrins	Interactions between cells and between cells and extracellular matrix
Selectins	Binding between tumor cells and nonmalignant tumor-associated cells
Cadherins	Interaction among tumor cells
Immunoglobulin cell adhesion molecule (IgCAM) superfamily	Binding both among tumor cells and between tumor cells and tumor-associated cells

IMMUNOGLOBULIN SUPERGENE FAMILY: A number of intercellular adhesion molecules belong to this superfamily, including intercellular adhesion molecule-1 (ICAM-1), MUC18, vascular cell adhesion molecule-1 (VCAM-1) and neural cell adhesion molecule (NCAM). The expression of ICAM-1 correlates positively with the aggressiveness of a variety of tumor cell types. Variation in expression of ICAM-1, VCAM-1 and NCAM has been shown to correlate with metastatic potential and prognosis.

CADHERINS AND CATENINS: Cadherins are a family of cell–cell adhesion molecules, which are calcium (Ca^{2+})-dependent transmembrane glycoproteins. The best-characterized of the cadherins, E-cadherin, is expressed on the surface of all epithelia and mediates cell–cell adhesion by mutual **zipper** interactions. Catenins (α, β and γ) are proteins that interact with the intracellular domain of E-cadherin and create a mechanical linkage between that molecule and the cytoskeleton, which is essential for effective epithelial cell interactions. Overall, cadherins and catenins are paramount in the suppression of invasion and metastasis. The expression of both E-cadherin and catenins is reduced or lost in most carcinomas, an effect that permits individual malignant cells to leave the main tumor mass and metastasize. As a result, in most carcinomas, loss of E-cadherin is associated with the development of an invasive and aggressive phenotype. Clinically, there is an inverse correlation of levels of E-cadherin with tumor grade and patient mortality. Interestingly, β-catenin also binds to the APC gene product, an effect that is independent of its interaction with E-cadherin and α-catenin. Mutations in either the APC or β-catenin gene are implicated in the development of colon cancer (see later and Chapter 13).

Proteolytic Enzymes

A breach of the basement membrane that separates an epithelium from the underlying mesenchymal compartment is the first event in tumor cell invasion. The basement membrane is composed of a number of extracellular matrix components, including type IV collagen, laminin and proteoglycans (see Chapter 3). Stromal and inflammatory cells associated with cancers elaborate a variety of proteases that degrade one or more of the basement membrane components. Such enzymes include u-PA and MMPs, including collagenases.

u-PA converts serum plasminogen to plasmin, a serine protease that degrades laminin and activates type IV procollagenase. u-PA activity is balanced by plasminogen activator inhibitor (PAI); changes in the expression of u-PA, the u-PA receptor and PAI have been reported in different cancers.

The MMPs comprise a family of zinc-dependent endopeptidases that are susceptible to tissue inhibitors of MMPs (TIMPs). MMPs include interstitial collagenases, stromelysins, gelatinases and membrane-type MMPs. These enzymes are synthesized and secreted by normal cells under conditions associated with physiologic tissue remodeling, such as wound healing and placental implantation. Under these circumstances, a balance between MMPs and TIMPs is strictly regulated. By contrast, the invasive and metastatic phenotypes of cancer cells are characterized by dysregulation of this balance.

A direct correlation between increased expression of MMPs and augmented invasive capacity or metastatic potential of tumor cells has been observed in many cancers. In addition, many of these same tumors exhibit decreased TIMP expression. MMPs are present in either tumor cells or surrounding stromal cells or both, depending on the particular neoplasm. In some instances, MMPs secreted by stromal cells are bound to integrins on the surface of the tumor cells, thereby providing a particularly high local concentration of protease activity at the site of tumor invasion. Deregulated MMP activity permits entry of cancer cells into, and their passage through, the extracellular matrix.

Epithelial-Mesenchymal Transition

As described above, invasion and metastasis by most epithelial tumor cells necessitate escape from the confines of the mucosa in which they originate. Tumor cells must then follow a trail through surrounding connective tissue that has been blazed by a variety of proteases. To accomplish these tasks, the epithelial cancer cells assume a phenotype that permits enhanced motility. They then resume their original identity in a new location. This chameleon-like change is both reversible and temporary, and is called the **epithelial-mesenchymal transition (EMT)**. During this process, the malignant epithelial cells, which are nonmotile and are encased in cell collectives via cell–cell tight junctions, disrupt these bonds and adopt a new guise as single, nonpolarized, mobile mesenchymal cells.

This transformation is orchestrated by a molecular team that includes loss of E-cadherin and by intrinsic signals, such as new gene mutations, and extrinsic signals, including growth factors (TGF-β, hepatocyte growth factor [HGF], EGF, IGF-1 and fibroblast growth factor). With such a diversity of triggers, it is not surprising that the complexity of effector pathways exceeds our current analytic skills. What is clear is that cancer cells undergoing EMT hijack cellular mechanisms that recapitulate processes that occur during ontogeny. Despite the importance of EMT, some cancer cells seem to invade without it and may assume ameboid forms or invade as a collection of cells.

Cell Collections and Solitary Cells in Metastasis

Cancer cells destined for a metastatic fate migrate either in packs or as single explorers. Solitary cells that have already undergone EMT represent only a small component of the entire primary tumor. As lone travelers, however, these cells move more rapidly than do cell clusters and intravasate (penetrate) into blood vessels, which provide a route for migration to faraway body sites. By contrast, compact cell collections preferentially transfer to the lymph nodes, where they generally remain in place. Collective cell migration to lymph nodes appears to be independent of spread through blood vessels, and each may be the preferred mode of dissemination for specific tumors. For example, head and neck tumors and breast cancers mostly spread initially to regional lymph nodes, whereas sarcomas prefer blood-borne metastasis. However, metastases may in turn metastasize and single cells may exfiltrate and disseminate widely via the bloodstream. This phenomenon is the basis of currently used assays to quantitate single tumor cells in the peripheral blood, the results of which are used both as prognostic indicators and to guide choice of chemotherapy.

Metastasis Is a Series of Complex Processes by Which Tumors Disseminate

Following their invasion of surrounding tissue, malignant cells may spread to distant sites by a process that includes a number of steps:

1. **Invasion of the circulation:** After invading interstitial tissue, malignant cells penetrate lymphatic or vascular channels. In lymph nodes, communications between lymphatics and venous tributaries allow the cells access to the systemic circulation. Most tumor cells do not survive their journey in the bloodstream, and fewer than 0.1% remain to establish a new colony.
2. **Escape from the circulation:** Circulating tumor cells may arrest mechanically in capillaries and venules, where they attach to endothelial cells. This adherence causes retraction of the endothelium, thereby exposing the underlying basement membrane to which tumor cells now bind. Clumps of tumor cells may also arrest in arterioles, where they grow within vascular lumens. In both situations, tumor cells eventually extravasate by mechanisms similar to those responsible for local invasion.
3. **Local growth:** In a hospitable site, the extravasated cancer cells grow in response to autocrine, angiogenic and possibly local growth factors produced by the host tissue. The newly established metastatic colony must also escape detection and destruction by host defenses (see below). The metastasis can metastasize again, either within the same organ or to distant sites.

Tumor Cell Arrest in the Circulation

While circulating, tumor cells associate with diverse formed constituents in the blood, including polymorphonuclear leukocytes, immune cells and platelets. These blood cells protect tumor cells from shear, immune and other stresses in the circulation. Such associations are mediated by adhesion molecules such as integrins, selectins (see Chapter 2) and a glycoprotein called CD44 at the surface of tumor cells. Tumor cells produce a factor that activates platelets via production of thrombin, and including fibrin and von Willebrand factor as bridging

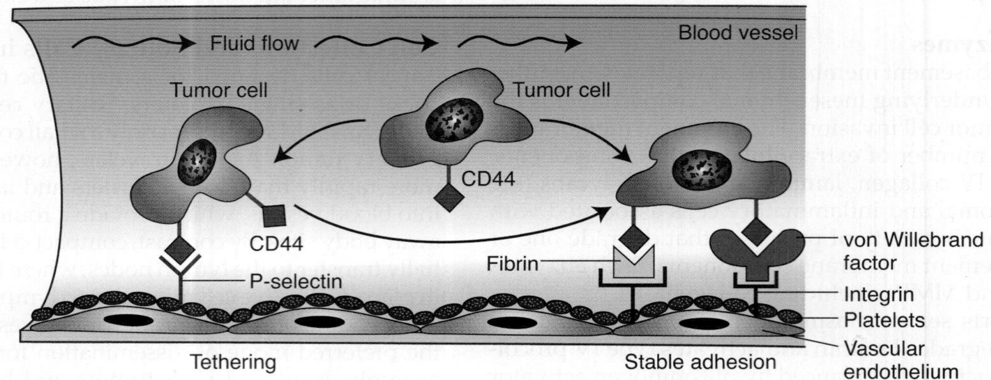

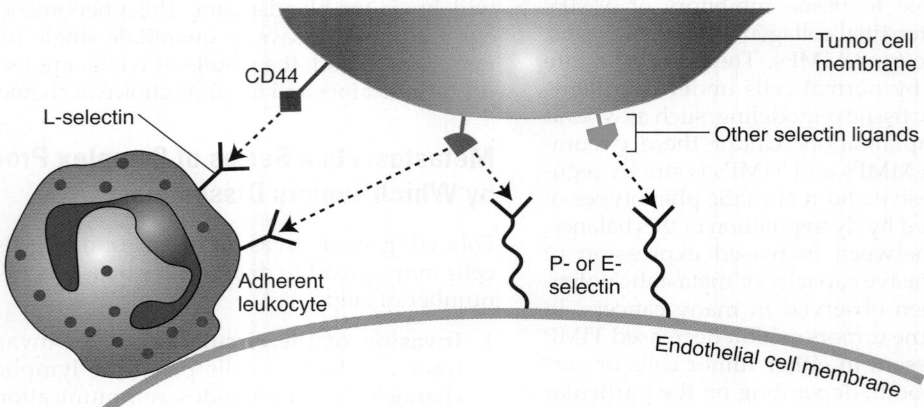

FIGURE 5-40. Mechanisms of tumor cell arrest in the circulation. A. Tumor cell adhesion to surface-anchored platelets. B. Adhesion of tumor cells to activated endothelial cells and endothelium-adherent leukocytes.

proteins. The binding of tumor cells to platelets requires P-selectin and platelet integrins, which recognize tumor cell CD44 via von Willebrand factor and fibrin. Similar interactions mediate tumor cell recognition and tethering to endothelial cells and to endothelial-bound leukocytes (Fig. 5-40).

Tumor Dormancy

It is well known that metastases may become clinically apparent many years, even decades, after a primary tumor mass is removed. This is particularly the case in breast cancers and malignant melanomas. It is also clear that some primary tumors may exist for many years before they are detected clinically. The presence of cancers, whether primary or metastatic, that do not enlarge to the point of being clinically detectable is termed **tumor dormancy.** Whatever the mechanism, the tumor cells have been hypnotized into a somnolent state, in which they inhabit the G_0 phase of the cell cycle.

The growth of cancer is not necessarily exponential and is often interrupted by quiescent intervals. This situation applies both to the primary tumor and to metastases. In both settings, the time course of the expansion of the tumor into a clinically detectable mass is highly variable, likely reflecting fluctuations in stimulating or permissive signals on the one hand, the actions of inhibitory factors on the other or both.

Although tumor dormancy is a well-established observation, the mechanisms underlying this phenomenon are poorly understood. One theory holds that growth arrest, possibly a result of extracellular and intracellular signaling, is responsible for the lack of tumor expansion. A different view postulates a static equilibrium between cell death and cell proliferation in dormant tumors. According to the latter theory, awakening of the transformed cells reflects the incursion of a disruptive stimulus that alters the equilibrium to favor cell proliferation.

Factors that have been implicated in tumor dormancy and in escape from tumor dormancy include angiogenesis, immune surveillance, apoptosis after oncogene inactivation (in cells that are oncogene addicted; see above), local processes such as inflammation, activation of cancer stem cells and adhesion molecules such as integrins. Importantly, more than 20 **metastasis suppressor genes** are known. These have the ability to prevent the various segments of the metastatic pathway. Thus, tumor dormancy has many faces, as reflected by the panoply of pathways by which tumor cells may be blocked from propagating and may be subsequently awakened (Fig. 5-41).

Currently, resection of many tumors in patients without evidence of distant metastases is often followed by adjuvant therapies that are directed against undetected micrometastases. Such treatments are usually of short duration and may not affect dormant tumor foci. Future cancer therapies may

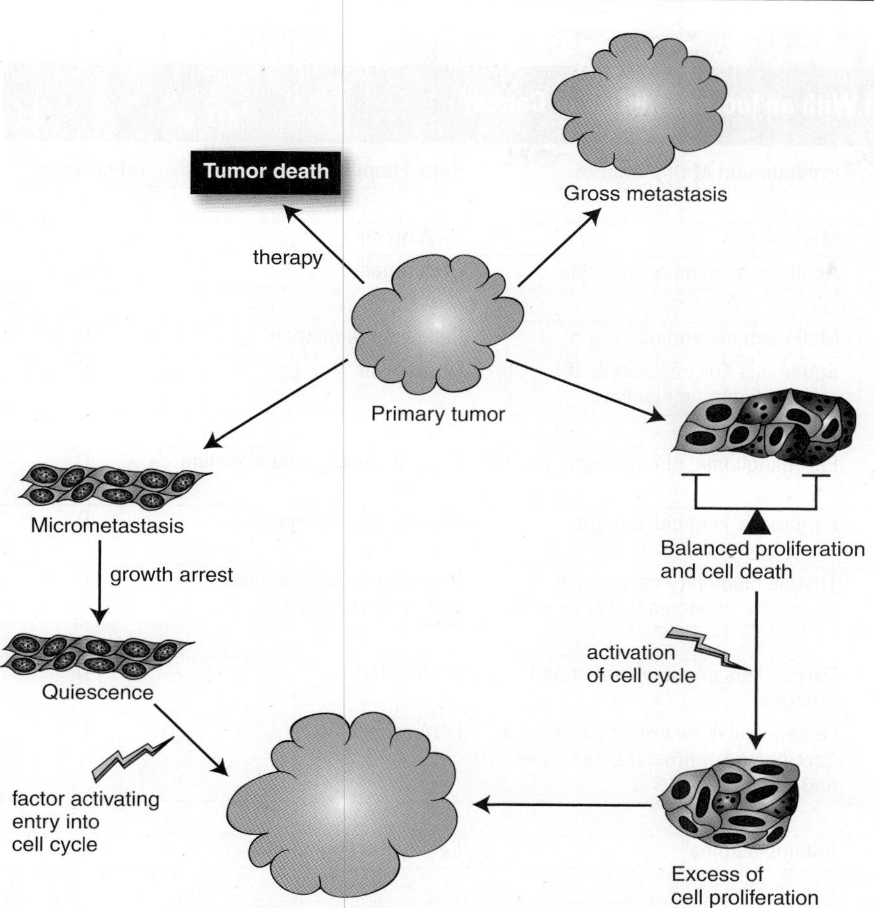

FIGURE 5-41. The fate of foci of cancer micrometastases. A primary cancer may be killed by therapies, such as radiation or chemotherapy, or it may be surgically removed. The tumor may produce a grossly evident metastasis. A number of factors may cause minute, clinically inapparent, metastatic foci of tumor cells to enter G_0 (*green*), but may be reactivated to enter the cell cycle (*blue*) and form a clinically detectable metastasis. Micrometastasis may also entail a balance between cell proliferation (*blue*) and cell death (*red*). If this equilibrium is disturbed in favor of tumor cell proliferation, the result may be a grossly evident mass of metastatic tumor.

actually exploit the characteristics of tumor dormancy. Approaches along these lines may focus on maintaining the dormant state in micrometastases, eradicating dormant cells by altering the equilibrium that sustains dormancy in favor of cell death or by forcing dormant foci into more active cycling to facilitate their targeting by conventional chemotherapy.

Interaction Between Malignant Cells and Surrounding Stroma May Drive Cancer Progression

The interactions between cancer cells and stroma in the processes of invasion and metastasis are discussed above. However, such interactions are even more complex and lead to feedback between stroma and cancers that can be lethal for tumor-associated fibroblasts. It has been proposed that transformed cells induce oxidative stress in nearby fibroblasts, which in turn are subject to mitochondrial dysfunction, autophagy of these poorly functioning mitochondria and then increased aerobic glycolysis by these cells. Consequently, the damaged fibroblasts provide nutrients such as lactate to enhance mitochondrial biogenesis and oxidative metabolism in the cancer cells themselves ("reverse Warburg effect"). Reactive oxygen species and nitric oxide from the injured fibroblasts, when transmitted to cancer cells, also may induce genomic instability in the latter, further promoting their malignant behavior. Thus, tumor cells may employ oxidative stress by stromal fibroblasts to enhance their own survival by using nutrients produced by the fibroblasts to drive proliferation and to propel their mutagenic evolution to a more aggressive phenotype.

Inherited Cancer Syndromes Encompass a Wide Variety of Tumors

Heritable cancer syndromes attributed to germline mutations make up only 1% of all cancers. These mutations principally involve tumor suppressor genes and DNA repair genes. As previously discussed for *Rb*, transmission of a single mutated allele of a tumor suppressor gene results in a heterozygous offspring. Since such persons are at a high risk for LOH (i.e., inactivation of the normal allele), they suffer a conspicuous susceptibility to various types of cancer. Thus, inheritance of cancer susceptibility in such cases is said to be dominant. However, in the tumor cells, both tumor suppressor alleles are inactivated. By contrast, a number of inherited cancer syndromes, mostly involving DNA repair genes, display classical recessive inheritance.

The hereditary tumors can be arbitrarily divided into three categories:

1. Inherited malignant tumors (e.g., Rb, WT, and many endocrine tumors)
2. Inherited tumors that remain benign or have a malignant potential (e.g., APC)
3. Inherited syndromes associated with a high risk of malignant tumors (e.g., Bloom syndrome, ataxia telangiectasia)

Most of these conditions are discussed in detail in the chapters dealing with specific organs, and selected examples are given in Table 5-5. In many cases, the underlying genetic defect responsible for the tumor development has been

Table 5-5

Selected Hereditary Conditions Associated With an Increased Risk of Cancer

Syndrome	Gene	Predominant Malignancies	Gene Function	Inheritance*
Chromosomal Instability Syndromes				
Bloom syndrome	*BLM*	Many sites	DNA repair	R
Fanconi anemia	?	Acute myelogenous leukemia	DNA repair	R
Hereditary Skin Cancer				
Familial melanoma	*CDKN2 (p16)*	Malignant melanoma	Cell cycle regulation	D
Xeroderma pigmentosum	*XP group*	Squamous cell carcinoma of skin; malignant melanoma	DNA repair	R
Endocrine System				
Hereditary paraganglioma and pheochromocytoma	*SDHD*	Paraganglioma; pheochromocytoma	Oxygen sensing and signaling	D
Multiple endocrine neoplasia (MEN) type 1	*MEN1*	Pancreatic islet cell tumors	Transcriptional regulation	D
MEN type 2	*RET*	Thyroid medullary carcinoma; pheochromocytoma (MEN type 2A)	Receptor tyrosine kinase; cell cycle regulation	D
Breast Cancer				
Breast/ovary cancer syndrome	*BRCA1*	Carcinomas of ovary, breast and prostate	DNA repair	D
Site-specific breast cancer	*BRCA2*	Female and male breast carcinoma; carcinomas of prostate, pancreas and ovary	DNA repair	D
Nervous System				
Retinoblastoma	*Rb*	Retinoblastoma	Cell cycle regulation	D
Phacomatoses				
Neurofibromatosis type 1	*NF1*	Neurofibrosarcomas; astrocytomas; malignant melanomas	Regulator of ras-mediated signaling	D
Neurofibromatosis type 2	*NF2*	Meningiomas; schwannomas	Regulator of cytoskeleton	D
Tuberous sclerosis	*TSC1*	Renal cell carcinoma; astrocytoma	Regulator of cytoskeleton	D
Gastrointestinal System				
Familial adenomatous polyposis	*APC*	Colorectal carcinoma	Cell cycle regulation; migration and adhesion	D
Hereditary nonpolyposis colorectal carcinoma (HNPCC; Lynch syndrome)	*hMSH2, hMSH6, hMLH1, hPMS1, hPMS2*	Carcinomas of colon, endometrium, ovary and bladder; malignant melanoma	DNA repair	D
Juvenile polyposis coli	*DPC4/SMAD4*	Colorectal carcinoma; endometrial carcinoma	TGF-β signaling	D
Peutz-Jeghers syndrome	*LKB1/STK11*	Stomach, small bowel and colon carcinomas	Serine threonine kinase	D
Kidney				
Hereditary papillary renal cell carcinoma	*MET*	Papillary renal cell carcinoma	Receptor tyrosine kinase; cell cycle regulation	D
Wilms tumor	*WT*	Wilms tumor	Transcriptional regulation	D
Von Hippel-Lindau	*VHL*	Renal cell carcinoma	Regulator of adhesion	D
Multiple Sites				
Carney complex	*PRKARIA*	Testicular neoplasms; thyroid carcinoma	cAMP signaling	D
Cowden syndrome	*PTEN*	Colorectal, breast and thyroid carcinomas	Protein tyrosine phosphatase	D
Li-Fraumeni syndrome	*TP53*	Breast carcinoma; soft tissue sarcomas; brain tumors; leukemia	Transcriptional regulation	D
Werner syndrome	*WRN*	Soft tissue sarcomas	DNA repair	R
Ataxia-telangiectasia	*ATM*	Lymphoma; leukemia	Cell signaling and DNA repair	R

* D, autosomal dominant; R, autosomal recessive.

ATM = mutated AT (gene); cAMP = cyclic adenosine 3′,5′-monophosphate; PTEN = phosphatase and tensin homolog; TGF-β = transforming growth factor-β.

identified. Some disorders that are difficult to classify, called **phacomatoses** (e.g., tuberous sclerosis, neurofibromatosis), have both developmental and neoplastic features. The tumors associated with these syndromes mostly involve the nervous system.

Although only a small proportion of all cancers show a Mendelian pattern of inheritance, certain cancers exhibit an undeniable tendency to run in families. It is estimated that in the case of many tumors, other members of the family of an affected person have a twofold to threefold increase in the risk of developing the same cancer. This predisposition is particularly marked for cancers of the breast and colon. The interplay of heredity and environment is exemplified by the case of lung cancer. Smokers who are closely related to a person with lung cancer have a higher risk of developing lung cancer themselves than smokers without this familial background.

Viruses and Human Cancer

Despite the existence of viral oncogenes, the number of human cancers definitely associated with viral infections is limited. Nevertheless, it is estimated that viral infections are responsible for 15% of all human cancers. The strongest associations between the presence of viruses and the development of cancer in humans are as follows:

- Human T-cell leukemia virus type I (HTLV-I) **(RNA retrovirus)** and T-cell leukemia/lymphoma
- HPV **(DNA)** and carcinoma of the cervix
- Hepatitis B virus (HBV, **DNA**) and hepatitis C virus (HCV, **RNA**) and primary hepatocellular carcinoma
- Epstein-Barr virus (EBV, DNA) and certain forms of lymphoma and nasopharyngeal carcinoma
- Human herpes virus 8 (HHV 8, **DNA**) and Kaposi sarcoma

Worldwide, infections with hepatitis B and C viruses and HPVs alone account for 80% of all virus-associated cancers.

Human T-Cell Leukemia Virus-I Is a Lymphotropic Agent

The one human cancer that has been firmly linked to infection with an RNA retrovirus is the rare adult T-cell leukemia, which is endemic in southern Japan and the Caribbean basin and occurs sporadically in other parts of the world. The etiologic agent, HTLV-I, is tropic for $CD4^+$ T lymphocytes and has also been incriminated in the pathogenesis of a number of neurologic disorders. It is estimated that leukemia develops in fewer than 5% of persons infected with HTLV-I and exhibits a latency period on the order of 40 years for its development. A closely related virus, HTLV-II, has been associated with only a few cases of lymphoproliferative disorders.

The HTLV-I genome contains no known oncogene and does not integrate at specific sites within the host genome. Oncogenic stimulation by HTLV-I is mediated principally by the viral transcriptional activation protein tax. Tax protein not only increases the transcription from its own viral genome but also promotes the activity of other genes involved in cell proliferation. These include genes that code for IL-2 and its receptor, GM-CSF, and the proto-oncogenes c-*fos* and c-*sis*. Tax also downregulates p53 and some cell cycle control proteins. Lymphocyte transformation in vitro by HTLV-I is initially polyclonal and only later monoclonal. Tax therefore probably initiates transformation, but additional genetic events are required for the appearance of the complete malignant phenotype.

DNA Viruses Encode Proteins That Bind Regulatory Proteins

Four DNA viruses (HPV, EBV, HBV and HHV 8) are incriminated in the development of human cancers. The transforming genes of oncogenic DNA viruses exhibit virtually no homology with cellular genes, whereas those of animal RNA retroviruses (oncogenes) are derived from, and are homologous with, their cellular counterparts (proto-oncogenes). As discussed above, oncogenic DNA viruses have genes that encode protein products that bind to, and inactivate, the products of tumor suppressor genes (e.g., *Rb, p53*).

Human Papilloma Virus

HPVs induce lesions in humans that progress to squamous cell carcinoma. They manifest a pronounced tropism for epithelial tissues, and their full productive life cycle occurs only in squamous cells. More than 140 distinct HPVs have been identified, and most are associated with benign lesions of squamous epithelium, including warts, laryngeal papillomas and condylomata acuminata (genital warts) of the vulva, penis and perianal region. Occasionally, condylomata acuminata and laryngeal papillomas undergo malignant transformation to squamous cell carcinoma. Although warts of the skin invariably remain benign, in a rare hereditary disease termed **epidermodysplasia verruciformis,** HPV produces benign flat warts that commonly progress to squamous carcinoma. At least 20 HPV types are associated with cancer of the uterine cervix, especially HPVs 16 and 18 (see Chapter 18). This association holds for both ectocervical squamous carcinoma and endocervical adenocarcinoma. A newly available vaccine protects against infection with most oncogenic HPV types and is expected to reduce the incidence of cervical cancer.

In recent years, HPV, especially HPV 16, has been identified in about 25% of head and neck squamous cell carcinomas. These include tumors of the tonsils and oropharynx, as well as the larynx. A similar colocalization has been reported for non-small cell lung carcinomas. Since all of these tumors are also associated with cigarette smoking, the role of HPV in carcinogenesis at these sites is mysterious. However, there are data that demonstrate a high incidence of HPV in adenocarcinomas of the lung that arise in nonsmokers. It has been suggested that in at least some of such cases, congenital HPV infection of the respiratory tract may be acquired at the time of delivery, by passage through the birth canal of an HPV-infected woman.

The major oncoproteins encoded by HPV are E5, E6 and E7. E6 binds to p53 and targets it for degradation. E7 binds to Rb, thereby releasing its inhibitory effect on cell cycle progression. E5 has been shown to activate the epidermal growth factor receptor. During the last half century, a cell line derived from cervical cancer, termed *HeLa cells,* has maintained worldwide popularity in the study of cancer. Interestingly, these cells have been found to express HPV-18 E6 and E7, and inactivation of these oncoproteins results in growth arrest. Thus, after many years growing in vitro in innumerable laboratories these cancer cells remain dependent on the expression of HPV proteins.

Epstein-Barr Virus

EBV is a human herpesvirus that is so widely disseminated that 95% of adults in the world have antibodies to it. EBV infects B lymphocytes, transforming them into lymphoblasts. In a small proportion of primary infections with EBV, this lymphoblastoid transformation is manifested as infectious mononucleosis (see Chapter 9), a short-lived benign lymphoproliferative disease. However, EBV is also intimately associated with the development of certain human cancers. A number of EBV genes are implicated in lymphocyte immortalization, including Epstein-Barr nuclear antigens (EBNAs) and latent infection–associated membrane proteins (LMPs). The EBNAs maintain the EBV genome in its episomal state and activate the transcription of viral and cellular genes. LMP1 interacts with cellular proteins that normally transduce signals from the tumor necrosis factor (TNF) receptor, a critical pathway in lymphocyte activation and proliferation. *Both EBNAs and LMPs can be demonstrated in most EBV-associated cancers.*

BURKITT LYMPHOMA: EBV was the first virus to be unequivocally linked to the development of a human tumor. In 1958 Burkitt described a form of childhood lymphoma in a geographical belt across equatorial Africa, which he suggested might have a viral etiology. A few years later, Epstein and Barr discovered viral particles in cell lines cultured from patients with Burkitt lymphoma (BL).

African BL is a B-cell tumor, in which the neoplastic lymphocytes invariably contain EBV and manifest EBV-related antigens (see Chapter 20). The tumor has also been recognized in non-African populations, but in those cases, only about 20% contain the EBV genome. The localization of BL to equatorial Africa is not understood, but it has been suggested that prolonged stimulation of the immune system by endemic malaria may be important. Under normal circumstances, the EBV-stimulated B-lymphocyte proliferation is controlled by suppressor T cells. The lack of an adequate T-cell response often reported in chronic malarial infections might result in uncontrolled B-cell proliferation, thereby providing the background for further genetic events that lead to the development of lymphoma. As discussed above, one of these is known to be a chromosomal translocation, in which the c-*myc* proto-oncogene is deregulated by being brought into proximity with an immunoglobulin promoter region. In addition, EBV proteins have been shown to inhibit apoptosis and activate signaling pathways involved in cell proliferation. A postulated sequence in the multistep pathogenesis of African BL is as follows:

1. Infection and polyclonal lymphoblastoid transformation of B lymphocytes by EBV
2. Proliferation of B cells and inhibition of suppressor T cells induced by malaria
3. Deregulation of the c-*myc* proto-oncogene by chromosomal translocation in a single transformed B lymphocyte and effects on other signaling pathways
4. Uncontrolled proliferation of a malignant clone of B lymphocytes

NASOPHARYNGEAL CARCINOMA: Nasopharyngeal carcinoma is a variant of squamous cell carcinoma that is particularly common in certain parts of Asia. EBV DNA and EBNA are present in virtually all of these cancers. It is thought that epithelial cells are exposed to EBV by lysis of infected lymphocytes traveling through lymphoid-rich epithelium. The pathogenesis of nasopharyngeal carcinoma may be related to infection with EBV in early childhood, with reactivation at 40 to 50 years of age and the appearance of tumors 1 to 2 years thereafter. One of the EBV proteins in this tumor has been shown to activate the EGF receptor signaling. Fortunately, 70% of patients with this disease are cured by radiation therapy alone.

OTHER EBSTEIN BARR VIRUS–ASSOCIATED TUMORS: EBV markers have been identified in about half of cases of classical Hodgkin lymphoma, in which the virus infects Reed-Sternberg cells. A number of T-cell lymphomas have also been found to harbor EBV. Interestingly, 5% of gastric carcinomas also show evidence of the presence of EBV.

POLYCLONAL LYMPHOPROLIFERATION IN IMMUNODEFICIENT STATES: Congenital or acquired immunodeficiency states can be complicated by the development of EBV-induced B-cell proliferative disorders. These lesions may be clinically and pathologically indistinguishable from true malignant lymphomas, but they differ in that most of them are polyclonal. The incidence of lymphoid neoplasia in immunosuppressed renal transplant recipients is 30 to 50 times that of the general population. In virtually all cases of lymphoproliferations associated with organ transplantation, EBNA or EBV genomic material is present in the neoplastic tissue. Similar B-cell lymphoproliferative disorders are seen in a number of other acquired immunodeficiencies, notably, acquired immunodeficiency syndrome (AIDS). Occasionally, a true monoclonal lymphoma may develop in the background of an EBV-induced lymphoproliferative disorder. As in the case of Burkitt lymphoma, the deficiency of T cells directed against EBV-infected B cells permits the survival of the latter.

Congenital immunodeficiency states, including X-linked lymphoproliferative syndrome (XLP), Wiskott-Aldrich syndrome and ataxia telangiectasia, are associated with EBV infections and aggressive lymphoproliferations. In the familial disorder XLP, clinical immunodeficiency is commonly inapparent until the onset of a particularly severe, and often fatal, form of infectious mononucleosis. In many of these patients who survive infectious mononucleosis, lymphoproliferative disorders and lymphomas ensue. Patients with XLP lack EBV-specific immune responses, including the formation of cytotoxic T cells that normally eliminate EBV-infected B cells.

Hepatitis B Virus and Hepatitis C Virus

Epidemiologic studies have established a strong association between chronic infection with HBV, a DNA virus, and HCV, an RNA virus, and the development of primary hepatocellular carcinoma (see Chapter 14). Two mechanisms have been invoked to explain the mechanism of carcinogenesis in virus-related liver cancer. One theory holds that the continued hepatocyte proliferation that accompanies chronic liver injury eventually leads to malignant transformation. However, a small subset of patients with HBV infection develop hepatocellular carcinoma in noncirrhotic livers. A second theory implicates a virally encoded protein in the pathogenesis of HBV-induced liver cancer. Transgenic mice expressing HBx, a small viral regulatory protein, also develop liver cancer, but without evident preexisting liver cell injury and inflammation.

The *HBx* gene product has been shown in vitro to upregulate a number of cellular genes. In addition, like other DNA viral oncoproteins, HBx binds to and inactivates p53. The underlying mechanisms in HBV-induced carcinogenesis are still controversial and require further investigation.

It has not been shown that HCV is directly oncogenic. However, some data suggest that expression of HCV core protein may contribute to the pathogenesis of hepatocellular carcinoma.

Human Herpesvirus 8

Kaposi sarcoma (KS) is a vascular tumor that was originally described in elderly eastern European men and later observed in sub-Saharan Africa (see Chapter 10). Kaposi sarcoma is today the most common neoplasm associated with AIDS. The neoplastic cells contain sequences of a novel herpesvirus, HHV 8, also known as KS-associated herpesvirus (KSHV). Interestingly, HHV 8 is present in virtually all specimens of Kaposi sarcoma, whether from HIV-positive or HIV-negative patients. In the United States, about 6% of the population carries HHV 8, but in the absence of a concomitant HIV-1 infection, does not exhibit any risk of KS. Importantly, 60% to 80% of the black population in sub-Saharan Africa is seropositive for HHV 8, but only a small proportion develop KS. In view of these discrepancies, and of the failure of KS tumors to grow in immunodeficient mice or tissue culture, many do not consider KS to be a true neoplasm. Rather, it may represent a proliferative disease induced by this virus. In addition to infecting the spindle cells of Kaposi sarcoma, HHV 8 is lymphotropic and has been implicated in two uncommon B-cell lymphoid malignancies, namely, **primary effusion lymphoma** and **multicentric Castleman disease.**

Like other DNA viruses, the HHV 8 viral genome encodes proteins that interfere with the p53 and Rb tumor suppressor pathways. Viral proteins have also been found to demonstrate antiapoptotic properties and to accelerate cell cycle transit. Moreover, antiviral drugs that inhibit HHV 8 lytic infection provide strong protection from the development of KS.

Chemical Carcinogenesis

The field of chemical carcinogenesis originated some two centuries ago in descriptions of an occupational disease (this was not the first recognition of an occupation-related cancer, since a specific predisposition of nuns to breast cancer was appreciated even earlier). The English physician Sir Percival Pott gets credit for relating cancer of the scrotum in chimney sweeps to a specific chemical exposure, namely, soot. Today we realize that other products of the combustion of organic materials are responsible for a man-made epidemic of cancer, namely, lung cancer in cigarette smokers.

The experimental production of cancer by chemicals dates to 1915, when Japanese investigators produced skin cancers in rabbits with coal tar. Since that time, the list of organic and inorganic carcinogens has grown exponentially. Yet a curious paradox existed for many years. Many compounds known to be potent carcinogens are relatively inert in terms of chemical reactivity. *The solution to this riddle became apparent in the early 1960s, when it was shown that most, although not all, chemical carcinogens require metabolic activation before they can react with cell constituents.* On the basis of those observations and the close correlation between mutagenicity and carcinogenicity, an in vitro assay using *Salmonella* organisms for screening potential chemical carcinogens—the Ames test—was developed a decade later. Subsequently, a variety of genotoxicity assays have been developed and are still used to screen chemicals and new drugs for potential carcinogenicity.

Chemical Carcinogens Are Mostly Mutagens

Associations between exposure to a specific chemical and human cancers have historically been established on the basis of epidemiologic investigations. These studies have numerous inherent disadvantages, including uncertainties in estimated doses, variability of the population, long and variable latency and dependence on clinical and public health records of questionable accuracy. As an alternative to epidemiologic studies, investigators turned to the use of studies involving animals. Indeed, such studies are legally required before the introduction of a new drug. Yet the logarithmic increase in the number of chemicals synthesized every year makes even this method prohibitively cumbersome and expensive. The search for rapid, reproducible and reliable screening assays for potential carcinogenic activity has centered on the relationship between carcinogenicity and mutagenicity.

*A **mutagen** is an agent that can permanently alter the genetic constitution of a cell.* The Ames test uses the appearance of frameshift mutations and base-pair substitutions in a culture of bacteria of a *Salmonella* sp. Mutations, unscheduled DNA synthesis and DNA strand breaks are also detected in rat hepatocytes, mouse lymphoma cells and Chinese hamster ovary cells. Cultured human cells are now used increasingly for assays of mutagenicity. About 90% of known carcinogens are mutagenic in these systems. Moreover, most, but not all, mutagens are carcinogenic. This close correlation between carcinogenicity and mutagenicity presumably occurs because both reflect damage to DNA. Although not infallible, in vitro mutagenicity assays have proved to be valuable tools in screening for the carcinogenic potential of chemicals.

Chemical Carcinogenesis Is a Multistep Process

Studies of chemical carcinogenesis in experimental animals have shed light on the distinct stages in the progression of normal cells to cancer. Long before the genetic basis of cancer was appreciated, it was demonstrated that a single application of a carcinogen to the skin of a mouse was not, by itself, sufficient to produce cancer. However, when a proliferative stimulus was then applied locally, in the form of a second, noncarcinogenic, irritating chemical (e.g., a phorbol ester), tumors appeared. The first effect was termed **initiation.** The action of the second, noncarcinogenic chemical was called **promotion.** Subsequently, further experiments in rodent models of a variety of organ-specific cancers (liver, skin, lung, pancreas, colon, etc.) expanded the concept of a two-stage mechanism to our present understanding of *carcinogenesis as a multistep process that involves numerous mutations.*

From these studies, one can abstract four stages of chemical carcinogenesis:

1. **Initiation** likely represents a mutation in a single cell.
2. **Promotion** reflects the clonal expansion of the initiated cell, in which the mutation has conferred a growth advantage. During promotion the altered cells remain dependent on the continued presence of the promoting stimulus. This stimulus may be an exogenous chemical or physical

agent or may reflect an endogenous mechanism (e.g., hormonal stimulation [breast, prostate] or the effect of bile salts [colon]).

3. **Progression** is the stage in which growth becomes autonomous (i.e., independent of the carcinogen or the promoter). By this time, sufficient mutations have accumulated to immortalize cells.
4. **Cancer,** the end result of the entire sequence, is established when the cells acquire the capacity to invade and metastasize.

The morphologic changes that reflect multistep carcinogenesis in humans are best exemplified in epithelia, such as those of the skin, cervix and colon. Although initiation has no morphologic counterpart, *promotion and progression are represented by the sequence of hyperplasia, dysplasia and carcinoma in situ.*

Chemical Carcinogens Usually Undergo Metabolic Activation

The International Agency for Research in Cancer (IARC) has listed about 75 chemicals as human carcinogens. Chemicals cause cancer either directly or, more often, after metabolic activation. The direct-acting carcinogens are inherently reactive enough to bind covalently to cellular macromolecules. A number of organic compounds, such as nitrogen mustard, *bis*(chloromethyl)ether and benzyl chloride, as well as certain metals are included in this category. Most organic carcinogens, however, require conversion to an ultimate, more reactive compound. This conversion is enzymatic and, for the most part, is effected by the cellular systems involved in drug metabolism and detoxification. Many cells in the body, particularly liver cells, possess enzyme systems that can convert procarcinogens to their active forms. Yet each carcinogen has its own spectrum of target tissues, often limited to a single organ. The basis for organ specificity in chemical carcinogenesis is not well understood.

POLYCYCLIC AROMATIC HYDROCARBONS: The polycyclic aromatic hydrocarbons, originally derived from coal tar, are among the most extensively studied carcinogens. In this class are such model compounds as benzo(a)pyrene, 3-methylcholanthrene and dibenzanthracene. These compounds have a broad range of target organs and generally produce cancers at the site of application. The specific type of cancer produced varies with the route of administration and includes tumors of the skin, soft tissues and breast. Polycyclic hydrocarbons have been identified in cigarette smoke, and so it has been suggested, but not proved, that they are involved in the production of lung cancer.

Polycyclic hydrocarbons are metabolized by cytochrome P450–dependent mixed function oxidases to electrophilic epoxides, which in turn react with proteins and nucleic acids. The formation of the epoxide depends on the presence of an unsaturated carbon–carbon bond. For example, vinyl chloride, the simple two-carbon molecule from which the widely used plastic polyvinyl chloride is synthesized, is metabolized to an epoxide, which is responsible for its carcinogenic properties. Workers exposed to the vinyl chloride monomer in the ambient atmosphere later developed hepatic angiosarcomas.

ALKYLATING AGENTS: Many chemotherapeutic drugs (e.g., cyclophosphamide, cisplatin, busulfan) are alkylating agents that transfer alkyl groups (methyl, ethyl, etc.) to macromolecules, including guanines within DNA. Although such drugs destroy cancer cells by damaging DNA, they also injure normal cells. Thus, alkylating chemotherapy carries a significant risk of solid and hematologic malignancies at a later time.

AFLATOXIN: In contrast to the polycyclic hydrocarbons, which are for the most part formed either by the combustion of organic material or synthetically, a heterocyclic hydrocarbon, aflatoxin B_1, is a natural product of the fungus *Aspergillus flavus*. Like the polycyclic aromatic hydrocarbons, aflatoxin B_1 is metabolized to an epoxide, which can bind covalently to DNA. Aflatoxin B_1 is among the most potent liver carcinogens recognized, producing tumors in fish, birds, rodents and primates. Since *Aspergillus* spp. are ubiquitous, contamination of vegetable foods exposed to the warm moist conditions, particularly peanuts and grains, may result in the formation of significant amounts of aflatoxin B_1. It has been suggested that in addition to hepatitis B and C, aflatoxin-rich foods may contribute to the high incidence of cancer of the liver in parts of Africa and Asia. In rodents exposed to aflatoxin B_1, the resulting liver tumors exhibit a specific inactivating mutation in the *p53* gene (G:C → T:A transversion at codon 249). Interestingly, human liver cancers in areas of high dietary concentrations of aflatoxin carry the same *p53* mutation.

AROMATIC AMINES AND AZO DYES: Aromatic amines and azo dyes, in contrast to the polycyclic aromatic hydrocarbons, are not ordinarily carcinogenic at the point of application. However, they commonly produce bladder and liver tumors, respectively, when fed to experimental animals. Both aromatic amines and azo dyes are primarily metabolized in the liver. The activation reaction undergone by aromatic amines is N-hydroxylation to form the hydroxylamino derivatives, which are then detoxified by conjugation with glucuronic acid. In the bladder, hydrolysis of the glucuronide releases the reactive hydroxylamine. Occupational exposure to aromatic amines in the form of aniline dyes has resulted in bladder cancer.

NITROSAMINES: Carcinogenic nitrosamines are a subject of considerable study because it is suspected that they may play a role in human gastrointestinal neoplasms and possibly other cancers. The simplest nitrosamine, dimethylnitrosamine, produces kidney and liver tumors in rodents. Nitrosamines are also potent carcinogens in primates, although unambiguous evidence of cancer induction in humans is lacking. However, the extremely high incidence of esophageal carcinoma in the Hunan province of China (100 times higher than in other areas) has been correlated with the high nitrosamine content of the diet. There is concern that nitrosamines may also be implicated in other gastrointestinal cancers because nitrites, commonly added to preserve processed meats and other foods, may react with other dietary components to form nitrosamines. In addition, tobacco-specific nitrosamines have been identified, although a contribution to carcinogenesis has not been proved. Nitrosamines are activated by hydroxylation, followed by formation of a reactive alkyl carbonium ion.

METALS: A number of metals or metal compounds can induce cancer, but the carcinogenic mechanisms are unknown. Divalent metal cations, such as nickel (Ni^{2+}), lead (Pb^{2+}), cadmium (Cd^{2+}), cobalt (Co^{2+}) and beryllium (Be^{2+}), are electrophilic and can, therefore, react with macromolecules. In addition, metal ions react with guanine and phosphate groups of DNA. A metal ion such as Ni^{2+} can depolymerize polynucleotides. Some metals can bind to purine and pyrimidine bases through covalent bonds or pi electrons of the bases. These reactions all occur in vitro, and the extent to which they occur in vivo is not known. Most metal-induced cancers occur in an occupational setting (see Chapter 8).

Endogenous and Environmental Factors Influence Chemical Carcinogenesis

Chemical carcinogenesis in experimental animals involves consideration of genetic aspects (species and strain, age and sex of the animal), hormonal status, diet and the presence or absence of inducers of drug-metabolizing systems and tumor promoters. A similar role for such factors in humans has been postulated on the basis of epidemiologic studies.

METABOLISM OF CARCINOGENS: **Mixed-function oxidases** are enzymes whose activities are genetically determined, and a correlation has been observed between the levels of these enzymes in various strains of mice and their sensitivity to chemical carcinogens. Since most chemical carcinogens require metabolic activation, agents that enhance the activation of procarcinogens to ultimate carcinogens should lead to greater carcinogenicity, whereas those that augment the detoxification pathways should reduce the incidence of cancer. In general, this is the case experimentally. Since humans are exposed to many chemicals in the diet and environment, such interactions are potentially significant.

SEX AND HORMONAL STATUS: These factors are important determinants of susceptibility to chemical carcinogens but are highly variable and in many instances not readily predictable. In experimental animals, there is sex-linked susceptibility to the carcinogenicity of certain chemicals. However, the effects of sex and hormonal status on chemical carcinogenesis in humans are not clear.

DIET: The composition of the diet can affect the level of drug-metabolizing enzymes. Experimentally, a low-protein diet, which reduces the hepatic activity of mixed-function oxidases, is associated with decreased sensitivity to hepatocarcinogens. In the case of dimethylnitrosamine, the decreased incidence of liver tumors is accompanied by an increased incidence of kidney tumors, an observation that emphasizes the fact that the metabolism of carcinogens may be regulated differently in different tissues.

Physical Carcinogenesis

The physical agents of carcinogenesis discussed here are UV light, asbestos and foreign bodies. Radiation carcinogenesis is discussed in Chapter 8.

Ultraviolet Radiation Causes Skin Cancers

Among fair-skinned persons, a glowing tan is commonly considered the mark of a successful holiday. However, this overt manifestation of the alleged healthful effects of the sun conceals underlying tissue damage. The harmful effects of solar radiation were recognized by ladies of a bygone era, who shielded themselves from the sun with parasols to maintain a "roses-and-milk" complexion and to prevent wrinkles. The more recent fad for a tanned complexion has been accompanied not only by cosmetic deterioration of facial skin but also by an increased incidence of the major skin cancers.

Cancers attributed to sun exposure, namely, basal cell carcinoma, squamous carcinoma and melanoma, occur predominantly in persons of the white race. The skin of persons of the darker races is protected by the increased concentration of melanin pigment, which absorbs UV radiation. In fair-skinned people, the areas exposed to the sun are most prone to develop skin cancer. Moreover, there is a direct correlation between total exposure to sunlight and the incidence of skin cancer.

UV radiation is the short-wavelength portion of the electromagnetic spectrum adjacent to the violet region of visible light. It appears that only certain portions of the UV spectrum are associated with tissue damage, and a carcinogenic effect occurs at wavelengths between 290 and 320 nm. *The effects of UV radiation on cells include enzyme inactivation, inhibition of cell division, mutagenesis, cell death and cancer.*

The most important biochemical effect of UV radiation is the formation of **pyrimidine dimers** in DNA, a type of DNA damage that is not seen with any other carcinogen. Pyrimidine dimers may form between thymine and thymine, between thymine and cytosine or between cytosine pairs alone. Dimer formation leads to a cyclobutane ring, which distorts the phosphodiester backbone of the double helix in the region of each dimer. Unless efficiently eliminated by the nucleotide excision repair pathway, genomic injury produced by UV radiation is mutagenic and carcinogenic.

Xeroderma pigmentosum, an autosomal recessive disease, exemplifies the importance of DNA repair in protecting against the harmful effects of UV radiation. In this rare disorder, sensitivity to sunlight is accompanied by a high incidence of skin cancers, including basal cell carcinoma, squamous cell carcinoma and melanoma. Both the neoplastic and nonneoplastic disorders of the skin in xeroderma pigmentosum are attributed to an impairment in the excision of UV-damaged DNA.

Asbestos Causes Mesothelioma

Pulmonary asbestosis and asbestosis-associated neoplasms are discussed in Chapter 12. Here we review possible mechanisms of carcinogenesis attributed to asbestos. In this context, it is not conclusively established whether the cancers related to asbestos exposure should be considered examples of chemical carcinogenesis or of physically induced tumors, or both.

Asbestos, a material widely used in construction, insulation and manufacturing, is a family of related fibrous silicates, which are classed as "serpentines" or "amphiboles." Serpentines, of which chrysotile is the only example of commercial importance, occur as flexible fibers; the amphiboles, represented principally by crocidolite and amosite, are firm narrow rods.

*The characteristic tumor associated with asbestos exposure is **malignant mesothelioma** of the pleural and peritoneal cavities.* This cancer, which is exceedingly rare in the general population, has been reported to occur in 2% to 3% (in some studies even more) of heavily exposed workers. The latent period (i.e., the interval between exposure and the appearance of a tumor) is usually about 20 years but may be twice that figure. It is reasonable to surmise that mesotheliomas of both pleura and peritoneum reflect the close contact of these membranes with asbestos fibers transported to them by lymphatic channels.

The pathogenesis of asbestos-associated mesotheliomas is obscure. Thin crocidolite fibers are associated with a considerably greater risk of mesothelioma than shorter and thicker amosite fibers or flexible chrysotile fibers. However, the distinction between these fibers in the causation of human disease should not be taken as absolute, particularly since mixtures of these fibers are characteristically found in human lungs.

An association between cancer of the lung and asbestos exposure is clearly established in smokers. A slight increase in the prevalence of lung cancer has been reported in nonsmokers exposed to asbestos, but the small number of cases renders an association questionable. Claims that exposure to asbestos increases the risk of gastrointestinal cancer have not withstood statistical analysis of the collected data. In any case, the widespread adoption of strict safety standards will undoubtedly relegate the hazards of asbestos to historical interest.

Foreign Bodies Produce Experimental Cancer

The implantation of inert materials induces sarcomas in certain experimental animals. However, *humans are resistant to foreign body carcinogenesis, as evidenced by the lack of cancers following the implantation of prostheses constructed of plastics and metals.* A few reports of cancer developing in the vicinity of foreign bodies in humans probably reflect scar formation, which in some organs seems to be associated with an increased incidence of cancers. Despite numerous contrary claims in lawsuits, there is no evidence that a single traumatic injury can lead to any form of cancer.

The general mechanisms underlying the development of neoplasia are summarized in Fig. 5-42.

Dietary Influences on Cancer Development Are Highly Controversial

About a quarter of a century ago, respected epidemiologists suggested that approximately one third of cancers in the United States could be prevented by changes in diet. Numerous epidemiologic studies have attempted to identify possible relationships between dietary factors and the occurrence of a variety of cancers. Such investigations have particularly emphasized the roles of dietary fats, red meat and fiber. The results of studies comparing different ethnic groups or societies across international borders have often not been accepted as accurate and in fact have sometimes yielded misleading conclusions. Prospective, cohort studies comparing like populations are usually more reliable.

Some such cohort studies have indicated correlations between consumption of animal (but not vegetable) fat and increased risk of breast cancer. This relationship was limited to premenopausal women, and there is a suggestion that nonlipid components of food containing animal fats may be involved.

In the case of colon cancer, consumption of red meat has been associated with increased risk; total fat and animal fat intake are not correlated independently of red meat intake. At one time, it was thought that intake of dietary fiber protected from colorectal cancer and other malignancies, but these conclusions have not withstood the test of time.

An association between the risk of aggressive (but not indolent) prostate cancer and the consumption of red meat has been claimed. However, further studies of this matter are needed.

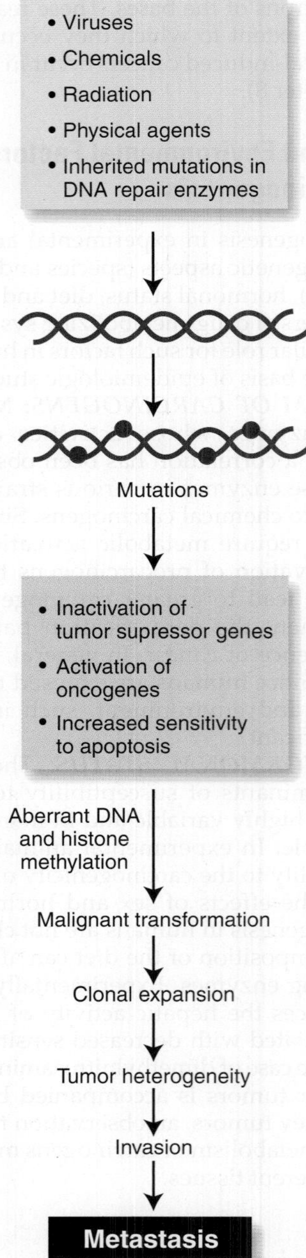

FIGURE 5-42. Summary of the general mechanisms of cancer.

Despite claims that eating fruits and vegetables helps to prevent cancer, there is little evidence that these dietary constituents protect from tumor development. Although there is a popular notion that high intake and blood concentrations of vitamin D may be associated with a lower incidence of some cancers, a recent review indicates that this is not the case. Several epidemiologic studies have provided preliminary data suggesting that a folate-rich diet decreases the risk of colorectal cancer.

In conclusion, the beneficial effects of dietary constituents on cancer risk are at best limited and are often controversial. The consequences of a specific type of diet on longevity are largely limited to reduced cardiovascular disease.

Physical activity and obesity are closely correlated with diet, and the dissection of independent effects of these influences by epidemiologic techniques has proven to be exceedingly difficult. The best evidence that physical activity decreases the risk of developing cancer exists for breast and colon malignancies. The same is true for obesity, which adds risk for endometrial, esophageal and kidney cancer. However, it is generally agreed that the evidence for these associations is not sufficient to allow for specific recommendations for changes in lifestyle in order to decrease cancer risk.

Tumor Immunology

The immune system represents a means of distinguishing self from nonself molecules, and has proven to be very effective in combating infectious agents. The concept of tumors as nonself structures, with unique tumor-specific antigens that can elicit protective immunologic responses, has been extensively demonstrated in experimental animals. Yet the relevance of such studies to human cancer remains unproven.

Most human cancers reflect somatic mutations that are capable of producing mutant proteins, which may potentially be targets of the immune system. In addition, normal proteins may be overexpressed, and posttranslational modifications of normal proteins may produce altered antigens. Tumor antigens not associated with oncogenic viruses may be categorized as follows:

- **Tumor-specific antigens (TSAs):** These represent somatic mutations or alterations in protein (and other) processing, unique to tumors.
- **Tumor-associated antigens (TAAs):** These reflect the production of normal proteins, either in excess or in a setting different from their normal expression.

Tumor-Specific Antigens

Most TSAs reside in mutated intracellular proteins. Theoretically, these proteins, or antigenic fragments thereof, can be presented to the immune system as a result of protein processing and degradation, and so could offer immunologic targets. Such proteins may be obligatory to establish and/or maintain a malignant phenotype, and so are likely to be produced despite evolving tumor heterogeneity (see above). However, most TSAs tend to be specific for individual patients' tumors, and not for tumor types, making immunologic targeting for therapy complicated and highly personalized. Nevertheless, since TSAs are expressed only by the cancer cells and not in normal tissues, there should be no preexisting immune tolerance to them and they are theoretically excellent candidates for tumor immunotherapy. These conclusions hold true for normal proteins that undergo aberrant posttranslational modifications, such as altered glycosylation, lipid association, etc.

Tumor-Associated Antigens

TAAs are molecules that are shared between cancer cells and normal cells. These include the following:

- **Oncospermatogonial antigens:** These molecules are normally only seen in testicular germ cells but may be produced by malignant cells. Since the testis is an immunologically privileged site, such molecules are not normally exposed to the immune system. However, immune reactivity of both cell- and antibody-mediated limbs to these antigens tends to be weak.
- **Differentiation antigens:** These molecules are seen on normal cells of the same derivation as the cancer cells. As an example, CD20, which is a normal B-cell differentiation antigen, is expressed by some lymphomas, and anti-CD20 antibody (rituximab) is effective treatment for such tumors.
- **Oncofetal antigens:** These antigens are produced by normal embryonic and fetal structures and by a variety of cancers (e.g., carcinoembryonic antigen, α-fetoprotein).
- **Overexpressed antigens:** These are normal proteins that are overproduced in certain malignant cells (e.g., prostate-specific antigen, HER2/neu).

Since TAAs represent a class of antigens that is principally recognized as "self" by the immune system, and so have elicited tolerance, they do not lead to effective immunologic responses.

To date, the evidence for natural control of neoplasia by immunologically mediated mechanisms (immune surveillance) in humans is scanty. Most interest in this area is directed toward possible therapeutic applications.

The potential development of effective cancer immunotherapy is complicated by tumor mechanisms to evade immunologically mediated destruction (Table 5-6). Among tumors' escape routes from immune attack are production of immunosuppressive cytokines, resistance to lysis by cytotoxic lymphocytes, inhibition of apoptotic signaling and changes in antigenic profiles. Interestingly, there is substantial evidence implicating mutant p53 as protecting cancer cells from granzyme-mediated apoptosis (see Chapter 1) caused by cytotoxic T lymphocytes (CTLs).

Another effect of cancer immunotherapy that must be overcome is related to tumor heterogeneity. Antibodies or CTLs directed against tumor antigens may lead to selective

Table 5-6

Potential Pathways for Tumor Cell Avoidance of Immunologically Mediated Destruction

Related to CTLs
Development of immune tolerance
Failure of helper T cells
Low numbers of sensitized CTLs
Lack of specificity for malignant cells
Barriers to entry of CTLs into tumor environment
Impairment of signal transduction in T cells
Deficiencies in CTL cytolytic activity
Regulatory T cells block antitumor activity
Related to Tumor Cells
Failure of tumor cells to stimulate latent lymphocyte reactivity
Low levels of tumor antigen production
Weak immunogenicity of tumor antigens
Decreased MHC antigens on tumor cell membranes
Elaboration of immunosuppressive molecules by tumors
Resistance of cancer cells to apoptosis and other cell death mechanisms
Tumor cells cause CTLs to undergo apoptosis

CTL = cytotoxic T lymphocyte; MHC = major histocompatibility complex.

emergence of malignant clones that have lost these antigens. Nevertheless, major efforts to develop new immune therapies for cancer continue.

Systemic Effects of Cancer on the Host

The symptoms of cancer are, for the most part, referable to the local effects of either the primary tumor or its metastases. However, in a minority of patients, cancer produces remote effects that are not attributable to tumor invasion or to metastasis, and are collectively termed **paraneoplastic syndromes.** Although such effects are rarely lethal, in some cases they dominate the clinical course. It is important to recognize these syndromes for several reasons. First, the signs and symptoms of the paraneoplastic syndrome may be the first clinical manifestation of a malignant tumor. Second, the syndromes may be mistaken for those produced by advanced metastatic disease and may, therefore, lead to inappropriate therapy. Third, when the paraneoplastic syndrome itself is disabling, treatment directed toward alleviating those symptoms may have important palliative effects. Finally, certain tumor products that result in paraneoplastic syndromes provide a means of monitoring recurrence of the cancer in patients who have had surgical resections or are undergoing chemotherapy or radiation therapy.

Fever

It is not uncommon for cancer patients to present initially with fever of unknown origin that cannot be explained by an infectious disease. Fever attributed to cancer correlates with tumor growth, disappears after treatment and reappears on recurrence. The cancers in which this most commonly occurs are Hodgkin disease, renal cell carcinoma and osteogenic sarcoma, although many other tumors are occasionally complicated by fever. Tumor cells may themselves release pyrogens or the inflammatory cells in the tumor stroma can produce IL-1.

Anorexia and Weight Loss

A paraneoplastic syndrome of anorexia, weight loss and cachexia is very common in patients with cancer, often appearing before its malignant cause becomes apparent. For example, a small asymptomatic pancreatic cancer may be suspected only on the basis of progressive and unexplained weight loss. Although cancer patients often decrease their caloric intake because of anorexia and abnormalities of taste, restricted food intake does not explain the profound wasting so common among them. The mechanisms responsible for this phenomenon are poorly understood. It is known, however, that unlike starvation, which is associated with a lowered metabolic rate, cancer is often accompanied by an elevated metabolic rate. It has been demonstrated that TNF-α and other cytokines (interferons, IL-6) can produce a wasting syndrome in experimental animals.

Endocrine Syndromes

Malignant tumors may produce a number of peptide hormones whose secretion is not under normal regulatory control. Most of these hormones are normally present in the brain, gastrointestinal tract or endocrine organs. Their inappropriate secretion can cause a variety of effects.

CUSHING SYNDROME: Ectopic secretion of ACTH by a tumor leads to features of Cushing syndrome, including hypokalemia, hyperglycemia, hypertension and muscle weakness (see Chapter 21). ACTH production is most commonly seen with cancers of the lung, particularly small cell carcinoma. It also complicates carcinoid tumors and other neuroendocrine tumors, such as pheochromocytoma, neuroblastoma and medullary thyroid carcinoma.

INAPPROPRIATE ANTIDIURESIS: The production of arginine vasopressin (antidiuretic hormone [ADH]) by a tumor may cause sodium and water retention to such an extent that it is manifested as water intoxication, resulting in altered mental status, seizures, coma and sometimes death. The tumor that most often produces this syndrome is small cell lung carcinoma. It is also reported with carcinomas of the prostate, gastrointestinal tract and pancreas and with thymomas, lymphomas and Hodgkin disease.

HYPERCALCEMIA: A paraneoplastic complication that afflicts 10% of all cancer patients, hypercalcemia, is usually caused by metastatic disease of bone. However, in about one tenth of cases it occurs in the absence of bony metastases. The most common cause of paraneoplastic hypercalcemia is the secretion of a parathormone-like peptide by an epithelial tumor, usually squamous cell lung carcinoma or breast adenocarcinoma. In multiple myeloma and lymphomas, hypercalcemia is attributed to the secretion of osteoclast activating factor. Other mechanisms of hypercalcemia involve the production of prostaglandins, active metabolites of vitamin D, TGF-α and TGF-β.

HYPOCALCEMIA: Cancer-induced hypocalcemia is actually more common than hypercalcemia and complicates osteoblastic metastases from cancers of the lung, breast and prostate. The cause of hypocalcemia is not known. Low calcium levels have been reported in association with calcitonin-secreting medullary carcinoma of the thyroid.

GONADOTROPIC SYNDROMES: Gonadotropins may be secreted by germ cell tumors, gestational trophoblastic tumors (choriocarcinoma, hydatidiform mole) and pituitary tumors. Less commonly, gonadotropin secretion is observed with hepatoblastomas in children and cancers of the lung, colon, breast and pancreas in adults. High gonadotropin levels lead to precocious puberty in children, gynecomastia in men and oligomenorrhea in premenopausal women.

HYPOGLYCEMIA: The best-understood cause of hypoglycemia associated with tumors is excessive insulin production by pancreatic islet cell tumors. Other tumors, especially large mesotheliomas, fibrosarcomas and primary hepatocellular carcinoma, are associated with hypoglycemia. The cause of hypoglycemia in nonendocrine tumors is not established, but the most likely candidate is production of somatomedins (IGFs), a family of peptides normally produced by the liver under regulation by growth hormone.

Neurologic and Neuromuscular Syndromes

Neurologic disorders are common in cancer patients, usually resulting from metastases or from endocrine or electrolyte disturbances. Vascular, hemorrhagic and infectious conditions affecting the nervous system are also common. However, additional neurologic complications of malignancies are known and may appear before the underlying tumor is detected. Many of these are mediated by autoimmune mechanisms.

Sensory Neuropathy and Encephalomyeloneuritis
Patients afflicted with this paraneoplastic syndrome complain of numbness and paresthesias and, conversely, variably acute aching and pain. These may be focal, but often affect all extremities over time, and are often complicated by disorders of gait, confusion and weakness. This syndrome may occur in patients with small cell lung cancer (SCLC; see Chapter 12) and is caused by circulating antibodies against Hu, an RNA-binding protein. High titers of anti-Hu antibodies are almost exclusively detected in people with SCLC. Lymphocytic infiltration of dorsal root ganglia is seen. Symptoms tend to be treatable when the primary tumor is treated.

Limbic Encephalitis
This condition may mimic herpes encephalitis, with seizures, memory deficits and a predilection for temporal lobe involvement. Anti-Hu antibodies in SCLC are often the culprits, although other autoantibodies causing this syndrome may be associated with other tumors (e.g., testicular) cancer. There are some forms in which antibodies to voltage-gated potassium channels are involved, in which immune suppression, in addition to antineoplastic chemotherapy, may ameliorate the CNS symptoms.

Paraneoplastic Autonomic Neuropathies
These are rare, but affect a quarter of patients with anti-Hu antibodies, and may be the initial presentation of the tumor. Systems affected, sometimes severely, include vascular tone, bowel and bladder. Antibodies against the nicotinic acetylcholine receptor are sometimes responsible.

Progressive Cerebellar Degeneration
This paraneoplastic syndrome may be the presenting symptom of an underlying malignancy and can be devastating. It occurs most often in association with breast cancer and, less often, Hodgkin lymphoma. Progressive cerebellar degeneration (PCD) often is caused by an antibody against a leucine zipper protein, Yo, although a number of other autoantibodies have been implicated. People afflicted with paraneoplastic PCD vary greatly in their responses to therapeutics, in part as a function of the particular autoantibody involved.

Vision Loss
Loss of sight may occur as an unusual paraneoplastic syndrome, most often caused by loss of retinal photoreceptors. SCLC is the tumor most often responsible, by virtue of eliciting an antibody against a photoreceptor antigen, recoverin.

Opsoclonus-Myoclonus
Nonvoluntary spasms of ocular and other muscles characterize this syndrome. Among children, about half of cases of this disorder are associated with neuroblastoma. About 10% of adults with opsoclonus-myoclonus will have a malignancy, most often Hodgkin lymphoma.

Diseases of Upper and Lower Motor Neurons
These syndromes may be paraneoplastic in origin. Diverse tumor associations have been reported, the most frequent being lymphoproliferative diseases and anti-Hu antibodies. Weakness is the most common presenting symptom. As many as 10% of patients presenting with amyotrophic lateral sclerosis have internal malignancies.

Subacute Motor Neuropathy
This is a disorder of the spinal cord, characterized by slowly developing lower motor neuron weakness without sensory changes. It is so strongly associated with cancer that an intensive search for an occult neoplasm, often a lymphoma, should be made in patients who present with these symptoms.

Peripheral Neuropathies
An array of peripheral neuropathies may be paraneoplastic in origin. Sensorimotor neuropathy, most likely attendant to lung cancer, is not associated with detectable antibodies. Some types of lymphoproliferative disorders associated with paraproteins, especially the sclerosing variant of plasma cell myeloma, may develop peripheral neuropathies.

Neuromuscular Junction Disorders
The most common association is with thymomas. About 15% of patients with myasthenia gravis have thymomas, and about half of patients with thymomas suffer from myasthenia gravis. Autoantibodies against the nicotinic acetylcholine receptor are the principal cause of this syndrome.

Eaton-Lambert Syndrome
This is an uncommon myasthenic disorder that is strongly associated with SCLC. Although the symptoms superficially resemble those of true myasthenia gravis, muscle strength improves with exercise, and there is a poor response to anticholinesterase therapy. Thymoma has a well-recognized association with **myasthenia gravis,** but a wide variety of other tumors have on occasion been linked to this disorder of the neuromuscular junction.

Hematologic Syndromes

The most common hematologic complications of neoplastic diseases result either from direct infiltration of the marrow or from treatment. However, hematologic paraneoplastic syndromes, which antedate the modern era of chemotherapy and radiation therapy, are well described.

Erythrocytosis
Cancer-associated erythrocytosis (polycythemia) is a complication of some tumors, particularly renal cell carcinoma, hepatocellular carcinoma and cerebellar hemangioblastoma. Interestingly, benign kidney disease, such as cystic disease or hydronephrosis, and uterine myomas can lead to erythrocytosis. Elevated erythropoietin levels are found in the tumor and in the serum in about half of patients with erythrocytosis.

Anemia
One of the most common findings in patients with cancer is anemia, but the mechanism underlying this disorder is not clear. The anemia is usually normocytic and normochromic, although iron-deficiency anemia is common in cancers that bleed into the gastrointestinal tract, such as colorectal cancers. Pure red cell aplasia, often associated with thymomas, and megaloblastic anemia are sometimes encountered.

Autoimmune hemolytic anemia may be associated with B-cell neoplasms and with solid tumors, particularly in the elderly. In fact, autoimmune hemolytic anemia in an older person suggests the possibility of an underlying neoplasm. **Microangiopathic hemolytic anemia** is occasionally seen, often in association with disseminated intravascular coagulation and thrombotic thrombocytopenic purpura.

Leukocytes and Platelets

Paraneoplastic granulocytosis, characterized by a peripheral granulocyte count over 20,000/μL, is a finding that may lead to an erroneous diagnosis of leukemia. This condition is usually caused by the secretion of a colony-stimulating factor by the tumor.

Eosinophilia and basophilia are sometimes occasionally noted in association with cancer. Hodgkin disease, in particular, may show eosinophilia in one fifth of cases. Basophilia may be seen in chronic myelogenous leukemia and other myeloproliferative diseases.

Thrombocytosis, with platelet counts above 400,000/μL, occurs in one third of cancer patients. Tumor production of thrombopoietin or IL-6 may be responsible. Platelet counts usually return to normal with successful treatment of the malignant disease.

The Hypercoagulable State

The association between cancer and venous thrombosis was noted almost 150 years ago by Trousseau. Since then, other abnormalities resulting from a hypercoagulable state (e.g., disseminated intravascular coagulation and nonbacterial thrombotic endocarditis) have been recognized. The cause of this hypercoagulable state is still debated.

VENOUS THROMBOSIS: This condition is most distinctly associated with carcinoma of the pancreas, in which there is a 50-fold increased incidence of this complication. Tumors of the breast, ovary, prostate, gastrointestinal tract and other organs, especially mucinous adenocarcinomas, are occasionally complicated by venous thrombosis, especially in the deep veins of the legs. Thromboembolism is not infrequent in this context, and is a leading cause of death in cancer patients.

DISSEMINATED INTRAVASCULAR COAGULATION: The widespread appearance of thrombi in small vessels in association with cancer may come to attention because of the chronic occurrence of thrombotic phenomena or an acute hemorrhagic diathesis. This complication is most commonly found with acute promyelocytic leukemia and adenocarcinomas.

NONBACTERIAL THROMBOTIC ENDOCARDITIS: The presence of noninfected verrucous deposits of fibrin and platelets on the left-sided heart valves occurs in cancer patients, particularly in debilitated persons (see Chapter 11). Although the effects on the heart are usually not of clinical importance, emboli to the brain and rarely the coronary arteries present a great danger. Paraneoplastic endocarditis may develop early in the course of a cancer and signal its presence long before the tumor would otherwise become symptomatic. This cardiac complication is most common with solid tumors but may occasionally be noted with leukemias and lymphomas.

Gastrointestinal Syndromes

Malabsorption of a variety of dietary components is an occasional paraneoplastic symptom, and half of cancer patients develop some histologic abnormalities of the small intestine, even though the tumor may not directly involve the bowel.

Hypoalbuminemia may result from a paraneoplastic depression of albumin synthesis by the liver or, in rare cases, a protein-losing enteropathy.

Nephrotic Syndrome

Nephrotic syndrome, as a consequence of renal vein thrombosis or amyloidosis, is a well-known complication of cancer. The nephrotic syndrome, in the form of minimal-change disease, may also complicate cancer, especially Hodgkin lymphoma. Membranous glomerulonephritis can occur, especially in adenocarcinomas of the gastrointestinal tract and lung.

Cutaneous Syndromes

Diverse dermatologic manifestations may complicate internal malignancies, often preceding detection of the tumor itself. Pigmented lesions and keratoses are well-recognized paraneoplastic effects.

- **Acanthosis nigricans** is marked by hyperkeratosis and pigmentation of the axilla, neck, flexures and anogenital region. *It is of particular interest because more than half of patients with acanthosis nigricans have cancer.* The development of the disease may precede, accompany or follow the detection of the cancer. Over 90% of cases occur in association with gastrointestinal carcinomas, and more than half accompany cancers of the stomach.
- **Dermatomyositis or polymyositis** has a five- to sevenfold greater incidence in cancer patients than in the general population. The association is most conspicuous in affected men older than 50 years, among whom more than 70% have cancer. In most cases, the muscle disorder and cancer present within a year of each other. In men, lung and GI cancers are most often associated with dermatomyositis, whereas in women, the most common association is with breast cancer.
- **Sweet syndrome** is a combination of elevated neutrophil count, acute fever and painful red plaques in the anus, neck and face. About one fifth of cases occur with malignancies, particularly those of the hematopoietic system.

There are numerous additional dermatologic syndromes that accompany internal malignancies. Some of these are listed in Table 5-7.

Amyloidosis

About 15% of cases of amyloidosis occur in association with cancers, particularly with multiple myeloma and renal cell carcinoma but also with other solid tumors and lymphomas (see Chapter 23). The presence of amyloidosis implies a poor prognosis; in patients with myeloma, amyloidosis is associated with a median survival of 14 months or less.

Table 5-7

Examples of Dermatologic Manifestations of Internal Malignancies

Cutaneous Disease	Commonly Associated Tumors
Acquired ichthyosis	Hodgkin and other lymphomas, myeloma
Palmar hyperkeratosis	Carcinomas of esophagus, breast, ovary
Acanthosis paraneoplastica	Cancer of head and neck, lungs, esophagus
Xanthomas	Hematologic malignancies, especially myeloma
Pyoderma gangrenosum	Hematologic malignancies, stomach cancer
Pemphigus, often involving internal organs	B-cell tumors, including Castleman disease
Hypertrichosis lanuginosa acquisita	Lung cancer
Erythema gyratum repens	Lung, colon, bladder, breast cancers

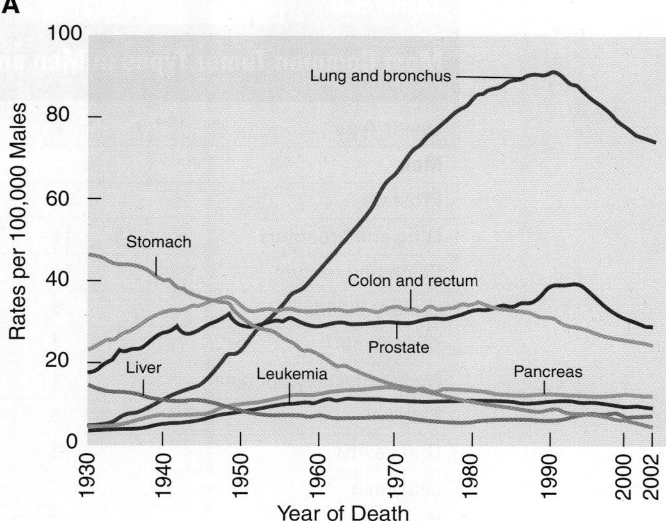

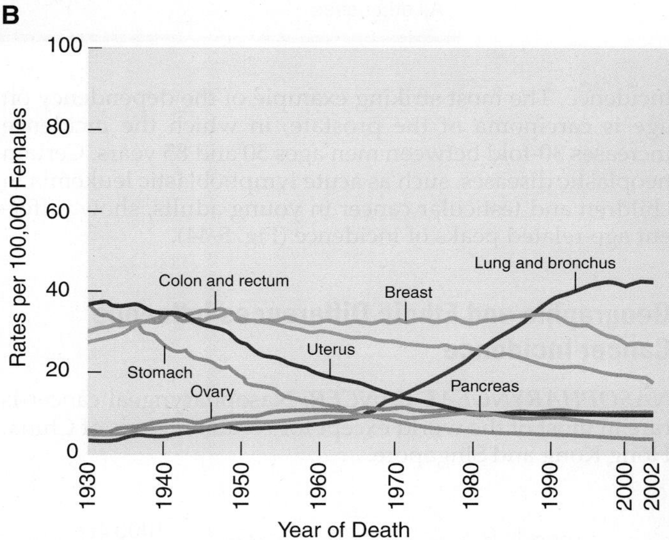

FIGURE 5-43. Cancer death rates in the United States, 1930 to 2002, among men (**A**) and women (**B**).

Epidemiology of Cancer

The mere compilation of raw epidemiologic data is of little use unless they are subjected to careful analysis. In evaluating the relevance of epidemiologic observations to cancer causation, the Hill criteria are germane:

- Strength of the association
- Consistency under different circumstances
- Specificity
- Temporality (i.e., the cause must precede the effect)
- Biological gradient (i.e., there is a dose-response relationship)
- Plausibility
- Coherence (i.e., a cause-and-effect relationship does not violate basic biological principles)
- Analogy to other known associations

It is not mandatory that a valid epidemiologic study satisfy all these criteria, nor does adherence to them guarantee that the hypothesis derived from the data is necessarily true. However, as a guideline they remain useful.

Cancer accounts for one fifth of the total mortality in the United States and is the second leading cause of death after cardiovascular diseases and stroke. For most cancers, death rates in the United States have largely remained flat for more than half a century, with some notable exceptions (Fig. 5-43). The death rate from cancer of the lung among men has risen dramatically from 1930, when it was an uncommon tumor, to the present, when it is by far the most common cause of death from cancer in men. As discussed in Chapter 8, the entire epidemic of lung cancer deaths is attributable to smoking. Among women, smoking did not become fashionable until World War II. Considering the time lag needed between starting to smoke and the development of cancer of the lung, it is not surprising that the increased death rate from lung cancer in women did not become significant until after 1965. In the United States, the death rate from lung cancer in women now exceeds that for breast cancer, and it is now, as in men, the most common fatal cancer. By contrast, for reasons difficult to fathom, cancer of the stomach, which in 1930 was by far the most common cancer in men and was more common than breast cancer in women, has shown a remarkable and sustained decline in frequency. Similarly, there has been a conspicuous decline in the death rate from cancer of the uterus corpus and cervix, possibly explained by better screening, diagnostic techniques and therapeutic methods. Overall, after decades of steady increases, the age-adjusted mortality as a result of all cancers has now reached a plateau. The ranking of the incidence of tumors in men and women in the United States is shown in Table 5-8.

Individual cancers have their own age-related profiles, but for most, increased age is associated with an increased

Table 5-8

Most Common Tumor Types in Men and Women

Tumor Type	%	Tumor Type	%
Men		**Women**	
Prostate	33	Breast	32
Lung and bronchus	14	Lung and bronchus	12
Colon and rectum	11	Colon and rectum	11
Urinary bladder	6	Uterine corpus	6
Melanoma	4	Ovary	4
Non-Hodgkin lymphoma	4	Non-Hodgkin lymphoma	4
Kidney	3	Melanoma	3
Oral cavity	3	Thyroid	3
Leukemia	3	Pancreas	2
Pancreas	2	Urinary bladder	2
All other sites	17	All other sites	20

incidence. The most striking example of the dependency on age is carcinoma of the prostate, in which the incidence increases 30-fold between men ages 50 and 85 years. Certain neoplastic diseases, such as acute lymphoblastic leukemia in children and testicular cancer in young adults, show different age-related peaks of incidence (Fig. 5-44).

Geographic and Ethnic Differences Influence Cancer Incidence

NASOPHARYNGEAL CANCER: Nasopharyngeal cancer is rare in most of the world except for certain regions of China, Hong Kong and Singapore.

ESOPHAGEAL CARCINOMA: The range in incidence of esophageal carcinoma varies from extremely low in Mormon women in Utah to a value some 300 times higher in the female population of northern Iran. Particularly high rates of esophageal cancer are noted in a so-called Asian esophageal cancer belt, which includes the great land mass stretching from Turkey to eastern China. Interestingly, throughout this region, as the incidence rises, the proportional excess in males decreases; in some of the areas of highest incidence there is even a female excess. The disease is also more common in certain regions of sub-Saharan Africa and among blacks in the United States. The causes of esophageal cancer are obscure, but it is known that it disproportionately affects the poor in many areas of the world,

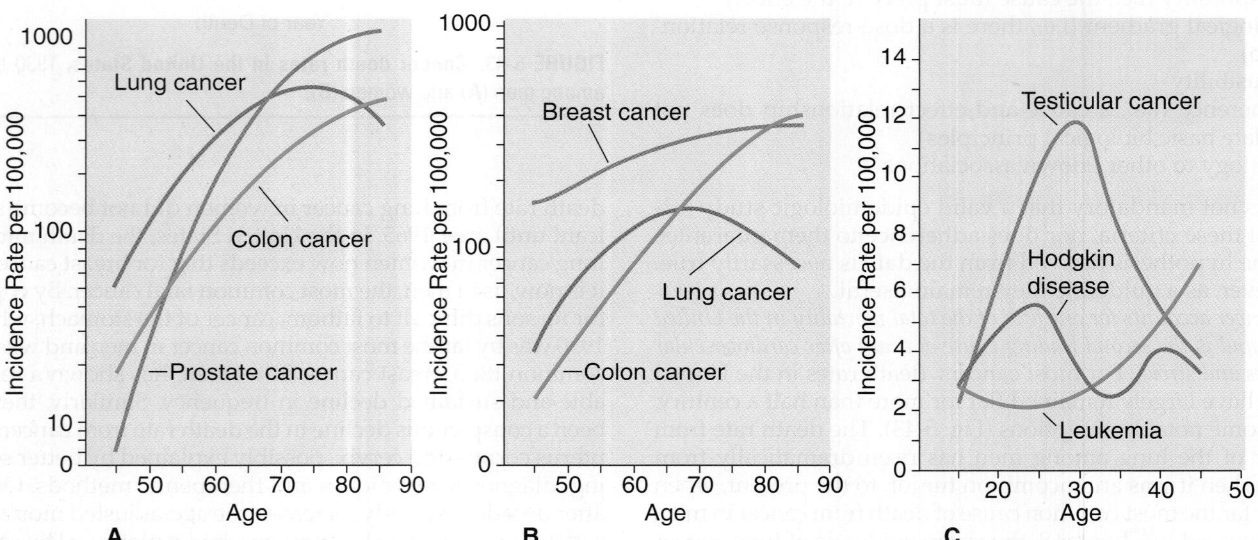

FIGURE 5-44. Incidence of specific cancers as a function of age. A. Men. **B.** Women. **C.** Testicular cancer in men and Hodgkin disease and leukemia in both sexes. The incidence of these cancers in *C* peaks at younger ages than do those in *A* and *B*.

and the combination of alcohol abuse and smoking is associated with a particularly high risk.

STOMACH CANCER: The highest incidence of stomach cancer occurs in Japan, where the disease is almost 10 times as frequent as it is among American whites. A high incidence has also been observed in Latin American countries, particularly Chile. Stomach cancer is also common in Iceland and eastern Europe.

COLORECTAL CANCER: The highest incidence of colorectal cancer is found in the United States, where it is three or four times more common than in Japan, India, Africa and Latin America. It had been theorized that the high fiber content of the diet in low-risk areas and the high fat content in the United States are related to this difference, but this concept has been seriously questioned.

LIVER CANCER: There is a strong correlation between the incidence of primary hepatocellular carcinoma and the prevalence of hepatitis B and C. Endemic regions for both diseases include large parts of sub-Saharan Africa and most of Asia, Indonesia and the Philippines. It must be remembered that levels of aflatoxin B_1 are high in the staple diets of many of the high-risk areas.

SKIN CANCER: As noted above, the rates for skin cancers vary with skin color and exposure to the sun. Thus, particularly high rates have been reported in northern Australia, where the population is principally of English origin and sun exposure is intense. Increased rates of skin cancer have also been noted among the white population of the American Southwest. The lowest rates are found among persons with pigmented skin (e.g., Japanese, Chinese and Indians). The rates for African blacks, despite their heavily pigmented skin, are occasionally higher than those for Asians because of the higher incidence of melanomas of the soles and palms in former population.

BREAST CANCER: Adenocarcinoma of the breast, the most common female cancer in many parts of Europe and North America, shows considerable geographic variation. The rates in African and Asian populations are only one fifth to one sixth of those prevailing in Europe and the United States. Epidemiologic studies have contributed little to our understanding of the etiology of breast cancer.

CERVICAL CARCINOMA: Striking differences in the incidence of squamous carcinoma of the cervix exist between ethnic groups and different socioeconomic levels. For instance, the very low rate in Ashkenazi Jews of Israel contrasts with a 25 times greater rate in the Hispanic population of Texas. In general, groups of low socioeconomic status have a higher incidence of cervical cancer than the more prosperous and better educated. This cancer is also directly correlated with early sexual activity and multiparity, and is rare among women who are not sexually active, such as nuns. It is also uncommon among women whose husbands are circumcised. A strong association with infection by HPVs has been demonstrated, and cervical cancer should be classed as a venereal disease.

CHORIOCARCINOMA: Choriocarcinoma, an uncommon cancer of trophoblastic differentiation, is found principally in women, following a pregnancy, although it can occur in men as a testicular tumor. The rates of this disease are particularly high in the Pacific rim of Asia (Singapore, Hong Kong, Japan and the Philippines).

PROSTATIC CANCER: Very low incidences of prostatic cancer are reported for Asian populations, particularly Japanese, whereas the highest rates described are in American blacks, in whom the disease occurs some 25 times more often. The incidence in American and European whites is intermediate.

TESTICULAR CANCER: An unusual aspect of testicular cancer is its universal rarity among black populations. Interestingly, although the rate in American blacks is only about one-fourth that in whites, it is still considerably higher than the rate among African blacks.

CANCER OF THE PENIS: This squamous carcinoma is virtually nonexistent among circumcised men of any race but is common in many parts of Africa and Asia. It is usually associated with HPV infection.

CANCER OF THE URINARY BLADDER: The rates for transitional cell carcinoma of the bladder are fairly uniform. Squamous carcinoma of the bladder, however, is a special case. Ordinarily far less common than transitional cell carcinoma, it has a high incidence in areas where schistosomal infestation of the bladder (bilharziasis) is endemic.

BURKITT LYMPHOMA: Burkitt lymphoma, a disease of children, was first described in Uganda, where it accounts for half of all childhood tumors. Since then, a high frequency has been observed in other African countries, particularly in hot, humid lowlands. It has been noted that these are areas where malaria is also endemic. High rates have been recorded in other tropical areas, such as Malaysia and New Guinea, but European and American cases are encountered only sporadically.

MULTIPLE MYELOMA: This malignant tumor of plasma cells is uncommon among American whites but displays a three to four times higher incidence in American and South African blacks.

CHRONIC LYMPHOCYTIC LEUKEMIA: Chronic lymphocytic leukemia is common among elderly persons in Europe and North America but is considerably less common in Japan.

Studies of Migrant Populations Give Clues to Cancer Development

Although planned experiments on the etiology of human cancer are hardly feasible, certain populations have unwittingly performed such experiments by migrating from one environment to another. Initially at least, the genetic characteristics of such persons remained the same, but the new environment differed in climate, diet, infectious agents, occupations and so on. *Consequently, epidemiologic studies of migrant populations have provided many intriguing clues to the factors that may influence the pathogenesis of cancer.* The United States, which has been the destination of one of the greatest population movements of all time, is the source of most of the important data in this field.

COLORECTAL, BREAST, ENDOMETRIAL, OVARIAN AND PROSTATIC CANCERS: Emigrants from low-risk areas in Europe and Japan to the United States exhibit an increased risk of colorectal cancer in the United States. Moreover, their offspring continue at higher risk and reach the incidence levels of the general American population. This rule for colorectal cancer also prevails for cancers of the breast, endometrium, ovary and prostate.

CANCER OF THE LIVER: As noted above, primary hepatocellular carcinoma is common in Asia and Africa, where it has been associated with hepatitis B and C. In

American blacks and Asians, however, the neoplasm is no more common than in American whites, a situation that presumably reflects the relatively low prevalence of chronic viral hepatitis in the United States.

HODGKIN DISEASE: In general, in poorly developed countries the childhood form of Hodgkin disease is the one reported most often. In developed Western countries, by contrast, the disease is most common among young adults, except in Japan. Such a pattern is characteristic of certain viral infections. Further evidence for an environmental influence is the higher incidence of Hodgkin disease in Americans of Japanese descent than that in Japan.

6 Developmental and Genetic Diseases

Stephen Peiper • David S. Strayer

Glossary

The following terms are used in the text or figures of this chapter:

Allele—One of multiple forms of a physical genetic locus

Alternative splicing—A regulatory mechanism by which variations in the incorporation of a gene's exons, or coding regions, into messenger RNA (mRNA) lead to the production of more than one related protein, or isoform

Autosomes—All of the nuclear chromosomes except for the sex chromosomes

Base pair (bp)—The association of nucleotide bases of opposite strands of DNA within a chromosome. An attached number (e.g., 12 bp) denotes the size of a sequence of DNA.

Centromere—The constricted region near the center of a chromosome, which has a critical role in cell division

Codon—A three-base sequence of DNA or RNA that specifies a single amino acid

Conservative mutation—A change in a DNA or RNA sequence that leads to the replacement of one amino acid with a biochemically similar one

Epigenetic—Changes in phenotype or gene expression due to mechanisms other than changes in DNA nucleotide sequence, such as methylation of regulatory sequences and histone modification

Exon—A region of a gene that codes for (i.e., encodes) a protein

Frame-shift mutation—Addition or deletion of a number of DNA bases not a multiple of 3 that disrupts boundaries of nucleotides in codons, thus shifting the reading frame of the gene. Codons downstream from the mutation are changed. The resulting protein is abnormal. Introduction of a premature stop codon or removal of a normal translational termination may alter protein size.

Gain-of-function mutation—A mutation that produces a protein that takes on a new or enhanced function

Genomics—The study of the functions and interactions of all the genes in the genome, including their interactions with environmental factors

Genotype—An individual's complete genetic constitution, including the combination of alleles

Haplotype—A group of physically linked genes on one chromosome that are inherited together

Hemizygous—Having a gene on one chromosome for which there is no counterpart on the opposite chromosome

Heterozygous—Having two different alleles at a specific autosomal (or X chromosomal in a female) gene locus

Homozygous—Having two identical alleles at a specific autosomal (or X chromosomal in a female) gene locus

Intron—A region of a gene that is in the intervening sequences between exons, and that does not contribute to the open reading frame that encodes a protein

Linkage disequilibrium—The nonrandom association in a population of alleles at nearby loci

Loss-of-function mutation—A mutation that decreases a protein's production and/or function

Missense mutation—A change in one DNA base that alters the amino acid encoded by a codon

Monogenic—Caused by a mutation in a single gene

Motif—A DNA-sequence pattern within a gene that, because of its similarity to sequences in other known genes, suggests a possible function of the gene, its protein product, or both

Multifactorial—Caused by the interaction of multiple genetic and environmental factors

Nonconservative mutation—A change in the DNA or RNA sequence that leads to the replacement of one amino acid with a very dissimilar one

Nonsense mutation—A 1 base change to a stop codon, leading to a truncated protein

Penetrance—The likelihood of an altered phenotype in a person with a certain mutant gene

Phenotype—The clinical consequence of a specific gene(s), environmental factors, or both

Point mutation—The substitution of a single DNA base in the normal DNA sequence

Regulatory mutation—A mutation in a region of the genome in multiple identical or closely related copies

Repeated sequence—A stretch of bases that occurs in the genome in multiple identical or closely related copies

Silent mutation—Substitution of a single DNA base, typically in the third position of a codon, that produces no change in the amino acid sequence of the encoded protein

Single-nucleotide polymorphism (SNP)—A variation (substitution, deletion or insertion) in DNA sequence in which a single nucleotide alteration occurs at a site in the genome that is different among members of a species. The majority of SNPs have only two alleles.

Stop codon—A codon that leads to the termination of a protein rather than the addition of an amino acid. The three stop codons are TGA, TAA and TAG.

It has been known since biblical times that certain disorders are inherited or related to disturbances in intrauterine development. The earliest sanitary codices contain guidelines on how to choose a healthy spouse, how to conceive healthy children and what to do or not do during pregnancy. Nevertheless, most of our scientific understanding of developmental and genetic disorders comes from only the past three decades, and the growth of molecular genetics has provided tools for unraveling etiologies and pathogeneses of these disorders.

Insight into the genetic basis of inherited disorders has been revolutionized in the postgenome era. The Human Genome Project provided a draft of the 3-billion-nucleotide human genome in 2003. Among its many findings, the project found that (1) the human genome contains about 24,000 genes, (2) only 1.1% to 1.4% of the genome encodes proteins, (3) the human genome contains more duplicated segments than are found in other mammals and (4) fewer than 7% of protein families could be identified as restricted to vertebrates. These data have facilitated the characterization of genetic bases of human diseases, including identifying therapeutic targets and disease susceptibility (and prevention) and essentially creating the field of pharmacogenomics. Thus, the identification of genes related to human disease has increased from fewer than 200 discoveries per year in the early 1990s when the genome project began to almost 2000 yearly in 2005. Among the many goals will be to understand the role of human variation in disease.

Diseases that present during the perinatal period may be caused solely by factors in the fetal environment, solely by genomic abnormalities or by interactions between genetic defects and environmental influences. For example, in phenylketonuria a genetic deficiency of phenylalanine hydroxylase causes mental retardation only if an infant is exposed to dietary phenylalanine.

Developmental and genetic disorders are classified as follows:

- **Errors of morphogenesis**
- **Chromosomal abnormalities**
- **Single-gene defects**
- **Polygenic inherited diseases**

A fetus may also be injured by **adverse transplacental influences** or deformities and injuries caused by intrauterine trauma or during parturition. After birth, acquired diseases of infancy and childhood are also important causes of morbidity and mortality.

Magnitude of the Problem

Each year, about one quarter of a million babies in the United States are born with a birth defect. Worldwide, at least 1 in 50 newborns has a major congenital anomaly, 1 in 100 has a single-gene abnormality and 1 in 200 has a major chromosomal abnormality.

In more than two thirds of all birth defects, the cause is not apparent (Fig. 6-1). No more than 6% of total birth defects can be attributed to uterine factors; maternal disorders such as metabolic imbalances or infections during pregnancy; and other environmental exposures (e.g., to drugs, chemicals and radiation). Most of the rest reflect by genomic defects, either hereditary traits or spontaneous mutations, and a smaller number by chromosomal abnormalities. While approximately 70% of birth defects are the result of unknown causes, application of newer technologies will continue to elucidate the mechanism of complex genetic diseases.

Chromosomal abnormalities account for only a small fraction of birth defects in newborns, but up to 50% of fetuses spontaneously aborted early in pregnancy have chromosomal abnormalities. ***The incidence of specific numerical chromosomal abnormalities in abortuses is several times higher than in term infants, indicating that most such chromosomal defects are lethal.*** Thus, only a small number of children with cytogenetic abnormalities are born alive.

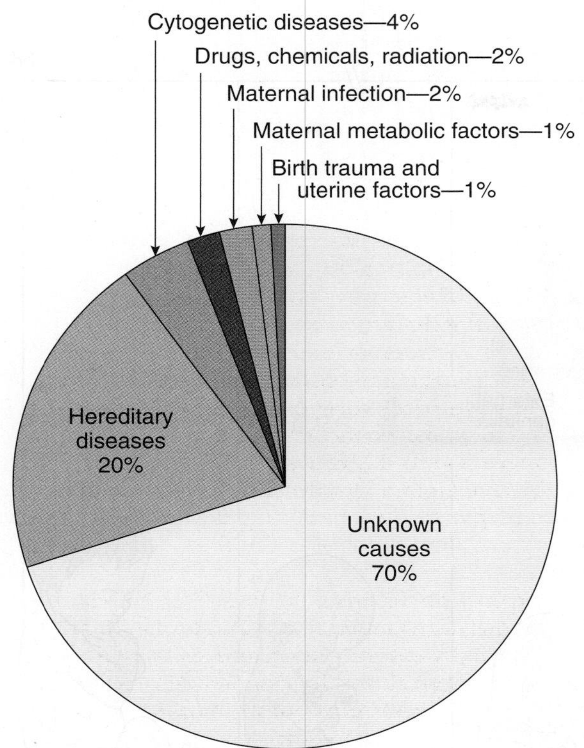

FIGURE 6-1. Causes of birth defects in humans. Most birth defects have unknown causes.

In Western countries, developmental and genetic birth defects account for half of deaths in infancy and childhood. In less developed countries, 95% of infant mortality is due to environmental causes such as infectious diseases and malnutrition. Further reductions in birth anomalies in industrialized societies will require genetic counseling, early prenatal diagnosis, identification of high-risk pregnancies and avoidance of potential teratogens. Prenatal dietary folic acid supplements have reduced the incidence of congenital neural tube defects.

Principles of Teratology

Teratology is the study of developmental anomalies (Greek *teraton,* "monster"). **Teratogens** are chemical, physical and biological agents that cause developmental anomalies. There are few proven teratogens in humans. However, many drugs and chemicals are teratogenic in animals and should thus be treated as potentially dangerous for humans.

Malformations are morphologic defects or abnormalities of an organ, part of an organ or anatomic region due to perturbed morphogenesis. Exposure to a teratogen may result in a malformation, but this is not invariably the case. Such observations have led to the formulation of general principles of teratology:

- **Susceptibility to teratogens is variable.** The key determinants of this variability are the genotypes of the fetus and the mother. Experimental data for this concept come from the fact that certain strains of inbred mice are susceptible to some teratogens while others are not. An example of human variability in the vulnerability to teratogens is the fetal alcohol syndrome, which affects some children of alcoholic mothers but not others.
- **Susceptibility to teratogens is specific for each embryologic stage.** Most agents are teratogenic only at particular times in development (Fig. 6-2). For example, maternal rubella infection only causes fetal abnormalities if it occurs during the first trimester of pregnancy.
- **The mechanism of teratogenesis is specific for each agent.** Teratogenic drugs may inhibit crucial enzymes or receptors, interfere with formation of mitotic spindles or block energy production, thereby inhibiting metabolic steps critical for normal morphogenesis. Many drugs and viruses affect specific tissues (e.g., neurotropism, cardiotropism) and so damage some developing organs more than others.
- **Teratogenesis is dose dependent.** Because multiple sites of action may determine the outcome of exposure, all established teratogens should be avoided during pregnancy; an absolutely safe dose cannot be predicted for every woman.
- **Teratogens produce death, growth retardation, malformation or functional impairment.** The outcome depends on the interaction between the teratogenic influences, the maternal organism and the fetal–placental unit.

Identifying human teratogens entails (1) population surveys, (2) prospective and retrospective studies of single malformations and (3) investigation of reported adverse effects of drugs or other chemicals. The list of proven teratogens is long and includes most cytotoxic drugs, alcohol, some antiepileptic drugs, heavy metals and thalidomide. Many drugs and chemicals have been declared safe for use during pregnancy because they were not teratogenic in laboratory animals. However, the fact that a drug is not teratogenic for mice or rabbits does not necessarily mean that it is innocuous for humans: thalidomide was found not to be teratogenic in mice and rats but it caused complex human malformations when many pregnant women ingested it during their first trimester of pregnancy. Interestingly, long after thalidomide was known to be teratogenic in humans, its teratogenicity in rabbits and monkeys was also demonstrated.

Errors of Morphogenesis

Normal intrauterine and postnatal development depends on sequential activation and repression of genes. A fertilized ovum (zygote) has all the genes of an adult organism, but most of them are inactive. As zygotes enter cleavage stages of development, individual genes or sets of genes are specifically activated at the stages of embryogenesis at which they are needed. Thus, ***abnormal gene activation or structure in early embryonic cells can cause early death.***

The cells that form two-cell and four-cell embryos (blastomeres) are equipotent: each can give rise to an adult organism. If embryonic cells separate at this stage, identical twins or quadruplets result. Since blastomeres are equipotent and interchangeable, loss of a single blastomere at this stage does not have serious sequelae. On the other hand, if one blastomere carries lethal genes, the others probably do as well. Activation of such genes is invariably fatal. Furthermore, a noxious exogenous agent affects all blastomeres and also causes death. We conclude that adverse environmental influences on preimplantation-stage embryos exert an all-or-nothing effect: either a conceptus dies or development proceeds uninterrupted, since the interchangeable blastomeres replace the loss. ***As a rule,***

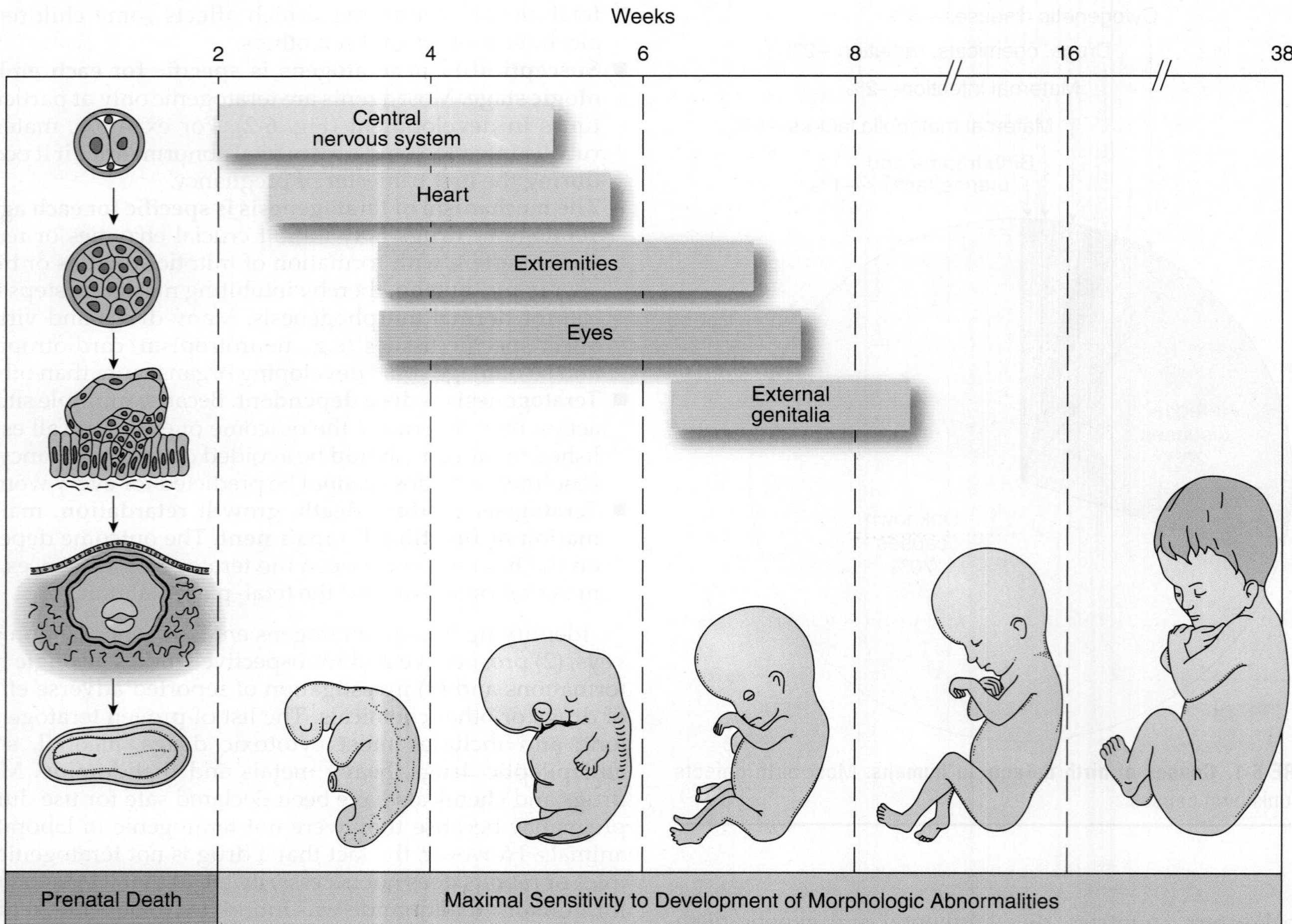

FIGURE 6-2. Sensitivity of specific organs to teratogenic agents at critical stages of human embryogenesis. Exposure to adverse influences in preimplantation and early postimplantation stages of development (*far left*) leads to prenatal death. Periods of maximal sensitivity to teratogens (*horizontal bars*) vary for different organ systems but overall are limited to the first 8 weeks of pregnancy.

exogenous toxins acting on preimplantation-stage embryos do not produce errors of morphogenesis and do not cause malformations* (Fig. 6-2). *The most common consequence of toxic exposure at the preimplantation stage is death of the embryo, which often passes unnoticed or is perceived as heavy, albeit delayed, menstrual bleeding.

Injury during the first 8 to 10 days after fertilization may cause incomplete separation of blastomeres, to yield conjoined twins ("Siamese twins") linked, for example, at the head (craniopagus), thorax (thoracopagus) or rump (ischiopagus). If conjoined twins are asymmetric, one is well developed and one rudimentary or hypoplastic. The latter is always abnormal and is externally attached to, or internally within, the body of the better-developed sibling (fetus in fetu). Some congenital teratomas, especially in the sacrococcygeal area, are actually asymmetric monsters.

Most complex developmental abnormalities affecting several organ systems are due to injuries that occur between implantation of the blastocyst and early organogenesis. This period is characterized by rapid cell division, cell differentiation and formation of so-called **developmental fields,** in which cells interact and determine each other's developmental fate. This process leads to irreversible differentiation of groups of cells. Complex morphologic movements form organ primordia (anlage), and organs are then interconnected in functionally active systems. ***The stage of embryonic development most susceptible to teratogenesis is formation of primordial organ systems, and many major developmental abnormalities are probably due to faulty gene activity or the effects of exogenous toxins*** (Fig. 6-2). Disorganized or disrupted morphogenesis may have minor or major consequences at the level of (1) cells and tissues, (2) organs or organ systems and (3) anatomic regions.

- **Agenesis** is the complete absence of an organ primordium. It may manifest as (1) total lack of an organ (e.g., unilateral or bilateral renal agenesis); (2) absence of part of an organ, as in agenesis of the corpus callosum of the brain; or (3) lack of tissue or cells in an organ, as in the absence of testicular germ cells in congenital infertility ("Sertoli cell only" syndrome).
- **Aplasia** is the persistence of an organ anlage or rudiment, without the mature organ. Thus, in aplasia of the lung the main bronchus ends blindly in nondescript tissue composed of rudimentary ducts and connective tissue.
- **Hypoplasia** means reduced size due to incomplete development of all or part of an organ. Micrognathia (small jaw) and microcephaly (small brain and head) are common examples.
- **Dysraphic anomalies** are defects caused by failure of apposed structures to fuse. In spina bifida, the spinal canal

does not close completely, and overlying bone and skin do not fuse, leaving a midline defect.

- **Involution failures** denote persistence of embryonic or fetal structures that should have involuted during development. A persistent thyroglossal duct is the result of incomplete involution of the tract that connects the base of the tongue with the developing thyroid.
- **Division failures** are caused by incomplete cleavage of embryonic tissues, when that process depends on programmed cell death. Fingers and toes are formed at the distal end of the limb bud by the loss of cells between the cartilage-containing primordia. If these cells do not undergo apoptosis, the fingers will be conjoined or incompletely separated (syndactyly).
- **Atresia** reflects incomplete formation of a lumen. Many hollow organs originate as cell strands and cords whose centers are programmed to die, to yield a central cavity or lumen. Esophageal atresia is characterized by partial occlusion of the lumen, which was not fully established in embryogenesis.
- **Dysplasia** is caused by abnormal organization of cells in tissues, which causes abnormal histogenesis. (This is different from the "dysplasia" of precancerous epithelial lesions [see Chapters 1 and 5].) Tuberous sclerosis is characterized by abnormal development of the brain, in which aggregates of normally developed cells are arranged into grossly visible "tubers."
- **Ectopia, or heterotopia,** denotes a normally formed organ that is outside its normal anatomic location. Thus, an ectopic heart is not in the thorax. Heterotopic parathyroid glands can be within the thymus in the anterior mediastinum.
- **Dystopia** refers to inadequate migration of an organ that remains where it was during development, rather than migrating to its proper site. Thus, the kidneys originate in the pelvis, then move cephalad out of the pelvis. Dystopic kidneys remain in the pelvis. Dystopic testes remain in the inguinal canal and do not descend into the scrotum (cryptorchidism).

Developmental anomalies caused by interference with morphogenesis are often multiple:

- A **polytopic effect** occurs when a noxious stimulus affects several organs that are simultaneously in critical stages of development.
- A **monotopic effect** refers to a single localized anomaly that results in a cascade of pathogenetic events.
- A **developmental sequence anomaly** (anomalad or complex anomaly) is a pattern of defects related to a single anomaly or pathogenetic mechanism: different factors lead to the same consequences through a common pathway. In the Potter complex (Fig. 6-3), pulmonary hypoplasia, external signs of intrauterine fetal compression and morphologic changes of the amnion are all related to oligohydramnios (a

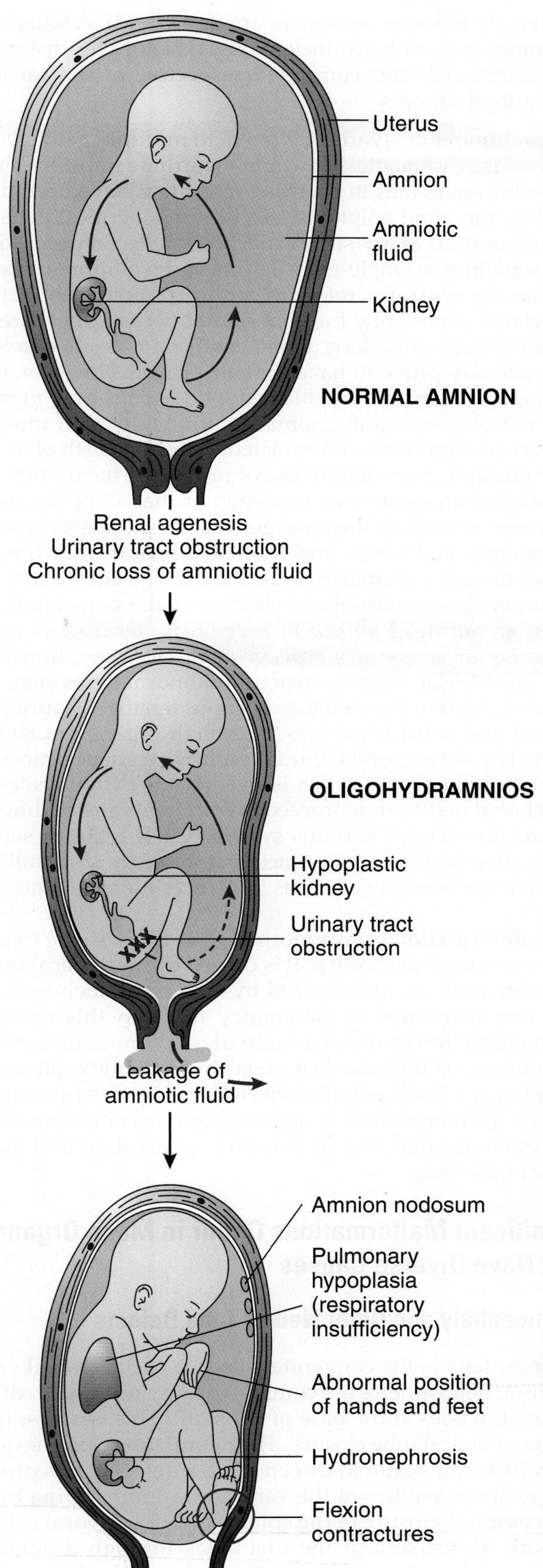

FIGURE 6-3. Potter complex. The fetus normally swallows amniotic fluid and, in turn, excretes urine, thereby maintaining its normal volume of amniotic fluid. In the face of urinary tract disease (e.g., renal agenesis or urinary tract obstruction) or leakage of amniotic fluid, the volume of amniotic fluid decreases, a situation termed **oligohydramnios.** Oligohydramnios results in a number of congenital abnormalities termed **Potter complex,** which includes pulmonary hypoplasia and contractures of the limbs. The amnion has a nodular appearance. In cases of urinary tract obstruction, congenital hydronephrosis is also seen, although this abnormality is not considered part of Potter complex.

severely reduced amount of amniotic fluid). A fetus in an amniotic sac with insufficient fluid develops the distinctive features of Potter complex irrespective of the cause of oligohydramnios.

A **developmental syndrome** refers to multiple pathogenetically related anomalies. The term **syndrome** implies a single cause for anomalies in diverse organs that have been damaged by the same polytopic effect during a critical developmental period. Many such syndromes reflect chromosomal abnormalities or single-gene defects. A **developmental association,** or **syntropy,** refers to multiple anomalies that are associated statistically but that do not necessarily share the same pathogenesis. Many anomalies that now seem unrelated may one day prove to have the same cause. However, until such associations are established, one should bear in mind that not all congenital anomalies in a child with multiple defects are necessarily interrelated. Thus, the birth of a child with multiple anomalies does not prove that the mother was exposed to an exogenous teratogen or that all of the anomalies were caused by the same genetic defect. The recognition of specific syndromes, and their distinction from random associations, is essential to assess the risk of recurrence of similar anomalies in subsequent children of the same family.

After the third month of pregnancy, teratogens rarely cause major errors of morphogenesis. However, functional and, to a lesser degree, structural abnormalities may still occur in children exposed to exogenous teratogens during the second and third trimesters. Although organs are already formed by the end of the third month of pregnancy, most still restructure and mature, as is needed for extrauterine life. Functional maturation proceeds at different rates in different organs: the central nervous system (CNS) requires several years after birth to attain functional maturity so is still susceptible to adverse exogenous influences for some time after birth.

A **deformation** is an abnormality of form, shape or position of a part of the body that is caused by mechanical forces. Most anatomic defects caused by adverse influences in the last two trimesters of pregnancy fall into this category. Responsible forces may be external (e.g., amniotic bands in the uterus) or intrinsic (e.g., fetal hypomobility caused by CNS injury). Thus, equinovarus foot can be due to compression by the uterine wall in oligohydramnios or to spinal cord abnormalities that lead to defective innervation and movement of the foot.

Significant Malformations Occur in Many Organs and Have Diverse Causes

Anencephaly and Other Neural Tube Defects

Anencephaly is the congenital absence of the cranial vault. Cerebral hemispheres are completely missing or are reduced to small masses at the base of the skull. This is a dysraphic defect of neural tube closure. The neural tube closes sequentially in a craniocaudad direction, so a defect in this process causes abnormalities of the vertebral column. **Spina bifida** is incomplete closure of the spinal cord or vertebral column or both. Protrusion of the meninges through a defect in the vertebral column is termed **meningocele.** In a **myelomeningocele** a meningocele is complicated by herniation of the spinal cord itself. Neural tube defects are discussed in Chapter 28.

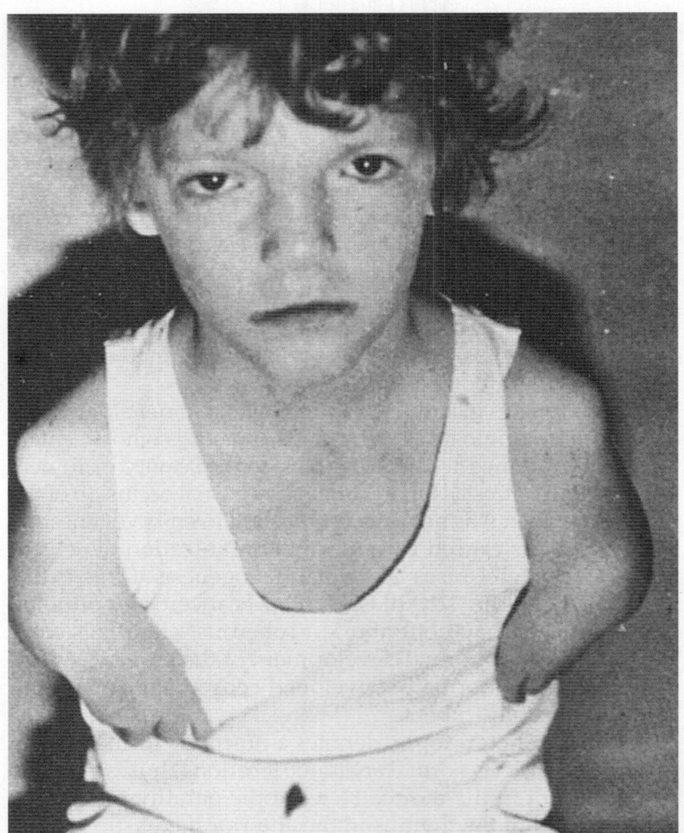

FIGURE 6-4. Thalidomide-induced deformity of the arms.

Thalidomide-Induced Malformations

Limb-reduction deformities, involving any number of extremities, are rare congenital defects of mostly obscure origin that affect 1 in 5000 liveborn infants. They have been known for ages: a Goya depiction of a typical example is in the Louvre Museum in Paris. In the 1960s, a sudden increase in the incidence of limb-reduction deformities in Germany and England was linked to maternal ingestion of a sedative, thalidomide, early in pregnancy. This derivative of glutamic acid is teratogenic between the 28th and 50th days of pregnancy. Many children born to mothers exposed to thalidomide had skeletal deformities and pleomorphic defects in other organs, mostly the ears **(microtia** and **anotia)** and heart. Typically, their arms were short and malformed (Fig. 6-4) and resembled the flippers of a seal **(phocomelia).** Sometimes limbs were completely missing **(amelia).** The CNS was unaffected, and these children had normal intelligence. Once the link between phocomelia and thalidomide was established, the drug was banned (1962), but not before an estimated 3000 malformed children were born. Thalidomide hinders limb growth by hindering angiogenesis and, perhaps, inducing caspase-8–dependent apoptosis. The same properties make the drug potentially useful for treating malignancies.

Fetal Hydantoin Syndrome

Of children born to mothers taking antiepileptic drugs, such as hydantoin, during pregnancy, 10% show characteristic facial features, hypoplasia of nails and digits and various congenital heart defects. Since this syndrome occurs only two to three times more often in treated epileptics than in untreated ones, it is uncertain whether all the defects reflect adverse effects of the drug. Nevertheless, that fetal susceptibility to this disorder appears to correlate with fetal levels of the microsomal detoxifying enzyme epoxide hydrolase. Presumably, accumulation of poorly detoxified reactive intermediates of hydantoin metabolism promotes teratogenesis.

Fetal Alcohol Syndrome

Fetal alcohol syndrome is caused by maternal consumption of alcoholic beverages during pregnancy. It is a complex of abnormalities including (1) growth retardation, (2) CNS abnormalities and (3) characteristic facial dysmorphology. As not all children harmed by maternal alcohol abuse show all these abnormalities, the term **fetal alcohol effect** is also used.

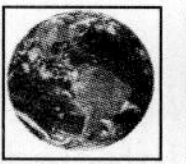
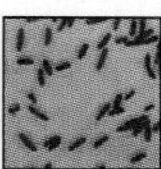

EPIDEMIOLOGY AND ETIOLOGIC FACTORS: An injurious effect of intrauterine exposure to alcohol was noted in biblical times and was reported during the historic London gin epidemic (1720 to 1750). However, a specific syndrome was only identified in 1968. The prevalence of fetal alcohol syndrome in the United States and Europe is 1 to 3 per 1000 live births. However, in populations with very high rates of alcoholism, such as some tribes of Native Americans, incidence may be 20 to 150 per 1000. ***It is thought that abnormalities related to fetal alcohol effect, particularly mild mental deficiency and emotional disorders, are far more common than the full-blown fetal alcohol syndrome.*** The minimum amount of alcohol needed to cause fetal injury is not well established, but children with the entire spectrum of fetal alcohol syndrome are usually born to mothers who are chronic alcoholics. Heavy alcohol consumption during the first trimester of pregnancy is particularly dangerous. The mechanism by which alcohol damages the developing fetus remains unknown.

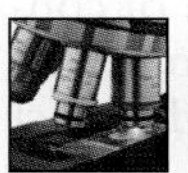
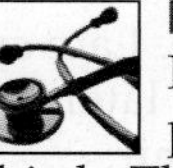

PATHOLOGY AND CLINICAL FEATURES: Infants born to alcoholic mothers often show prenatal growth retardation, which continues after birth. They may also have microcephaly, epicanthal folds, short palpebral fissures, maxillary hypoplasia, thin upper lip, micrognathia and a poorly developed philtrum. One third may have cardiac septal defects, although these often close spontaneously. Minor abnormalities of joints and limbs may occur.

Fetal alcohol syndrome is the most common cause of acquired mental retardation. One fifth of children with fetal alcohol syndrome have intelligence quotients (IQs) below 70, and 40% are between 70 and 85. Even if their IQ is normal, these children tend to have short memory spans and exhibit impulsive behavior and emotional instability (see Chapter 8).

TORCH Complex

The acronym TORCH refers to a complex of similar signs and symptoms produced by fetal or neonatal infection with* Toxoplasma *(T), rubella (R), cytomegalovirus (C) and Herpes simplex virus (H). The letter "O" in TORCH represents "others." The term was coined to alert pediatricians to the fact that these fetal and newborn infections may be indistinguishable from each other and that testing for all TORCH agents, and for some possible others as well, should be done (Fig. 6-5). "Other" agents include syphilis, tuberculosis, listeriosis, leptospirosis, varicella-zoster virus and Epstein-Barr virus. Human immunodeficiency virus (HIV) and human parvovirus (B19) have been suggested as additions to the list.

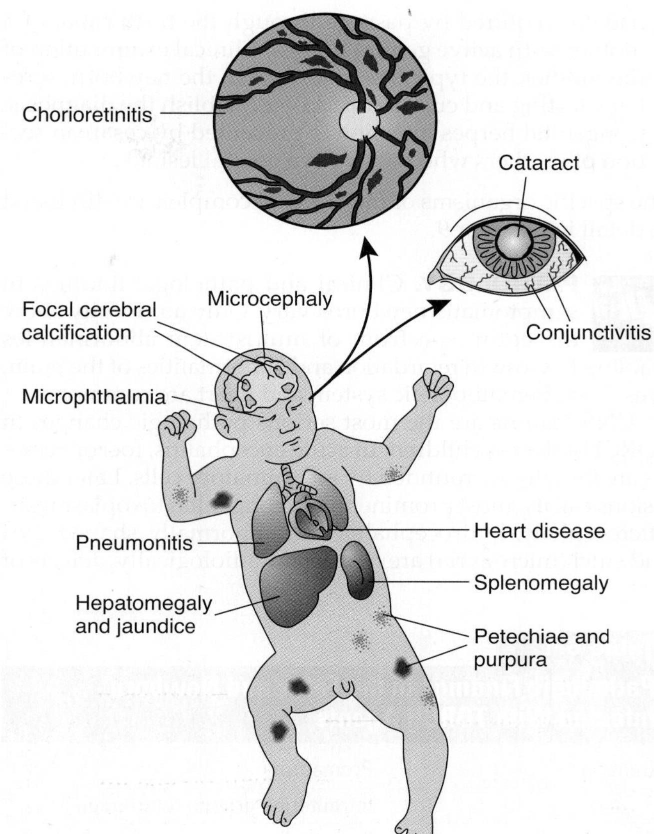

FIGURE 6-5. TORCH complex. Children infected in utero with *Toxoplasma*, rubella virus, cytomegalovirus, or herpes simplex virus show remarkably similar effects.

Infections with TORCH agents are common and occur in 1% to 5% of all liveborn infants in the United States. They are major causes of neonatal morbidity and mortality. The severe damage inflicted by these organisms is largely irreparable, and prevention (if possible) is the best approach. Unfortunately, titers of serum antibodies against TORCH agents in infants or mothers are usually not diagnostic, and a precise etiology cannot always be identified.

- **Toxoplasmosis:** Asymptomatic toxoplasmosis is common, and 25% of women in their reproductive years have antibodies to this organism. However, intrapartum *Toxoplasma* infection occurs in only 0.1% of all pregnancies.
- **Rubella:** Vaccination against rubella in the United States has virtually eliminated congenital rubella. Fewer than 10 cases are reported each year.
- **Cytomegalovirus (CMV):** In the United States, two thirds of women of childbearing age have antibodies to CMV, and up to 2% of newborns are infected congenitally. As most normal infants have maternally derived antibodies, CMV is diagnosed by urine culture.
- **Herpesvirus:** Intrauterine infection with herpes simplex virus type 2 (HSV-2) is uncommon. Neonatal infection is

usually acquired by passage through the birth canal of a mother with active genital lesions. Clinical examination of the mother, the typical skin lesions in the newborn, serologic testing and culture for HSV-2 establish the diagnosis. Congenital herpes infection is prevented by cesarean section of mothers who have active genital lesions.

The specific organisms of the TORCH complex are discussed in detail in Chapter 9.

PATHOLOGY: Clinical and pathologic findings in symptomatic newborns vary. Only a minority show the entire spectrum of multisystem abnormalities (Table 6-1). Growth retardation and abnormalities of the brain, eyes, liver, hematopoietic system and heart are common.

CNS lesions are the most serious pathologic changes in TORCH-infected children. In acute encephalitis, foci of necrosis are initially surrounded by inflammatory cells. Later these lesions calcify, most prominently in congenital toxoplasmosis. Microcephaly, hydrocephalus and abnormally shaped gyri and sulci (microgyria) are frequent. Radiologically, defects of cerebral matter (porencephaly), missing olfactory bulbs and other major brain defects may be identified. Psychomotor retardation, neurologic defects and seizures occur with severe CNS injury.

Ocular defects are also prominent in TORCH infections, particularly with rubella, in which over two thirds of patients have cataracts and microphthalmia. Glaucoma and retinal malformations (coloboma) may occur. Choroidoretinitis is common with rubella, *Toxoplasma* and CMV; is usually bilateral; and on funduscopy appears as pale, mottled areas surrounded by a pigmented rim. Keratoconjunctivitis is the most common eye lesion in neonatal herpes infection.

Cardiac anomalies occur in many children with the TORCH complex, mostly in congenital rubella. Patent ductus arteriosus and various septal defects are the most common cardiac abnormalities. Pulmonary artery stenosis and complex cardiac anomalies are occasionally seen.

Table 6-1

Pathologic Findings in the Fetus and Newborn Infected With TORCH Agents

General	Prematurity
	Intrauterine growth retardation
Central nervous system	Encephalitis
	Microcephaly
	Hydrocephaly
	Intracranial calcifications
	Psychomotor retardation
Ear	Inner ear damage with hearing loss
Eye	Microphthalmia (R)
	Chorioretinitis (TCH)
	Pigmented retina (R)
	Keratoconjunctivitis (H)
	Cataracts (RH)
	Glaucoma (R)
	Visual impairment (TRCH)
Liver	Hepatomegaly
	Liver calcifications (R)
	Jaundice
Hematopoietic system	Hemolytic and other anemias
	Thrombocytopenia
	Splenomegaly
Skin and mucosae	Vesicular or ulcerative lesions (H)
	Petechiae and ecchymoses
Cardiopulmonary system	Pneumonitis
	Myocarditis
	Congenital heart disease
Skeleton	Various bone lesions

T = *Toxoplasma*; R = rubella virus; C = cytomegalovirus; H = herpesvirus.

Congenital Syphilis

The organism that causes syphilis, *Treponema pallidum*, is transmitted to the fetus by a mother who has been infected during pregnancy or, possibly, in the 2 years before the pregnancy, although the actual risk is not known. About 1 in 2000 liveborn infants in the United States have congenital syphilis. In pregnant syphilitic women, stillbirth occurs in one third, and two thirds of infants carried to term manifest congenital syphilis.

T. pallidum may invade a fetus any time in pregnancy. Early infections mostly cause abortion, and grossly visible signs of congenital syphilis appear only in fetuses infected after the 16th week of pregnancy. As spirochetes grow in all fetal tissues, clinical presentations vary.

Children with congenital syphilis are normal at first, or show changes like those of the TORCH complex. Early lesions in various organs teem with spirochetes. They show perivascular infiltrates of lymphocytes and plasma cells, and granuloma-like lesions termed **gummas.** Many infants are asymptomatic, only to develop the typical stigmata of congenital syphilis in the first few years of life. Late symptoms of congenital syphilis appear many years later and reflect slowly evolving tissue destruction and repair:

- **Rhinitis:** A conspicuous mucopurulent nasal discharge, "snuffles," is almost always present as an early sign of congenital syphilis. The nasal mucosa is edematous and tends to ulcerate, leading to nosebleeds. Destruction of the nasal bridge eventually results in flattening of the nose, so-called **saddle nose.**
- **Skin:** A maculopapular rash is common early in congenital syphilis. Palms and soles are usually affected (as in secondary syphilis of adults), although it may involve the entire body or any part. Cracks and fissures **(rhagades)** occur around the mouth, anus and vulva. Flat raised plaques **(condylomata lata)** around the anus and female genitalia may develop early or after a few years.
- **Visceral organs:** A distinctive pneumonitis, characterized by pale hypocrepitant lungs **(pneumonia alba),** may develop in the neonatal period. Hepatosplenomegaly, anemia and lymphadenopathy may also be observed in early congenital syphilis.
- **Teeth:** The buds of incisors and sixth-year molars develop early in postnatal life, the time when congenital syphilis is particularly aggressive. Thus, the permanent incisors may

be notched **(Hutchinson teeth)** and molars malformed **(mulberry molars).**

- **Bones:** Periosteal inflammation with new bone formation **(periostitis)** is common, especially in the anterior tibia. This causes a distinctive outward curving **(saber shins).**
- **Eye:** Progressive corneal vascularization **(interstitial keratitis)** is an especially vexing complication of congenital syphilis, occurring as early as 4 years of age and as late as 20 years. The cornea eventually scars and becomes opaque.
- **Nervous system:** The nervous system is commonly involved, with symptoms starting in infancy or after 1 year. **Meningitis** predominates in early congenital syphilis, causing convulsions, mild hydrocephalus and mental retardation. **Meningovascular syphilis** is common later and may lead to deafness, mental retardation, paresis and other complications. **Hutchinson triad** is a combination of deafness, interstitial keratitis and notched incisor teeth.

The diagnosis of congenital syphilis is suggested by clinical findings plus a history of maternal infection. Serologic confirmation of active infection in newborns may be difficult because of transplacental transfer of maternal immunoglobulin (Ig) G. Penicillin is the drug of choice for intrauterine and postnatal syphilis. Given during intrauterine life or the first 2 years of postnatal life, it gives an excellent prognosis, and most symptoms of congenital syphilis are prevented.

Chromosomal Abnormalities

Cytogenetics is the study of chromosomes and their abnormalities. The current system of classification is the International System for Human Cytogenetic Nomenclature (ISCN).

The Normal Chromosomal Complement Is 44 Autosomes and 2 Sex Chromosomes

Cytogenetic analysis can be done on any dividing cell but most studies use circulating lymphocytes, which are easily stimulated to undergo mitosis. The dividing cells are treated with colchicine to arrest them in metaphase, then spread on glass slides to disperse the chromosomes. Staining facilitates identification of chromosomes and their distinctive bands.

Chromosome Structure

Chromosomes are classified by their length and the positions of their constrictions, or **centromeres,** seen on Giemsa stain. The centromere is the point at which the two identical strands of chromosomal DNA, the **sister chromatids,** attach to each other during mitosis. The location of the centromere is used to classify chromosomes as **metacentric, submetacentric** or **acrocentric.** The centromere in **metacentric chromosomes** (1, 3, 19 and 20) is exactly in the middle. In **submetacentric chromosomes** (2, 4 through 12, 16 through 18 and X), it divides chromosomes into short (p, from French, *petit*) and long arms (q, the next letter in the alphabet). **Acrocentric chromosomes** (13, 14, 15, 21, 22 and Y) have very short arms or stalks and satellites attached to an eccentrically located centromere (Fig. 6-6).

Stains are used to classify chromosomes into seven groups, A to G. Group A contains two large metacentric and a large submetacentric chromosome, group B has two large submetacentric chromosomes, group C includes six submetacentric chromosomes, etc.

In Fluorescence in Situ Hybridization DNA Probes Identify DNA Sequences

Fluorophore-labeled DNA probes used vary in size from individual genes or small regions of chromosomes (Figs. 6-6 and 6-7). Fluorescence in situ hybridization (FISH) is also employed to see if genetic material is lost or gained. Using probes with different fluorophores, one can identify chromosomal translocations. In **multicolor FISH,** or **spectral karyotyping,** such probes hybridize to whole chromosomes,

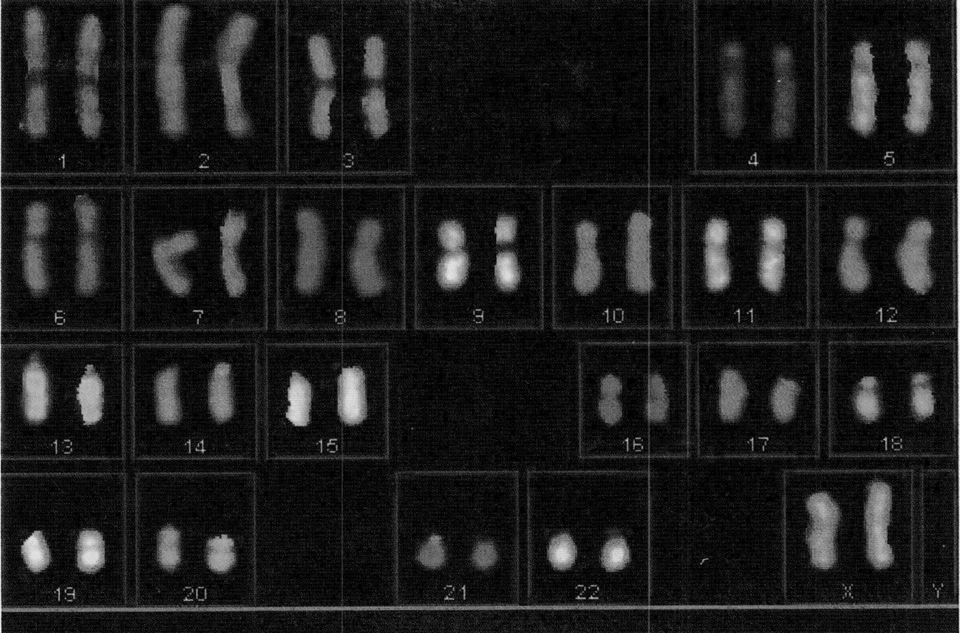

FIGURE 6-6. Spectral karyotype of human chromosomes.

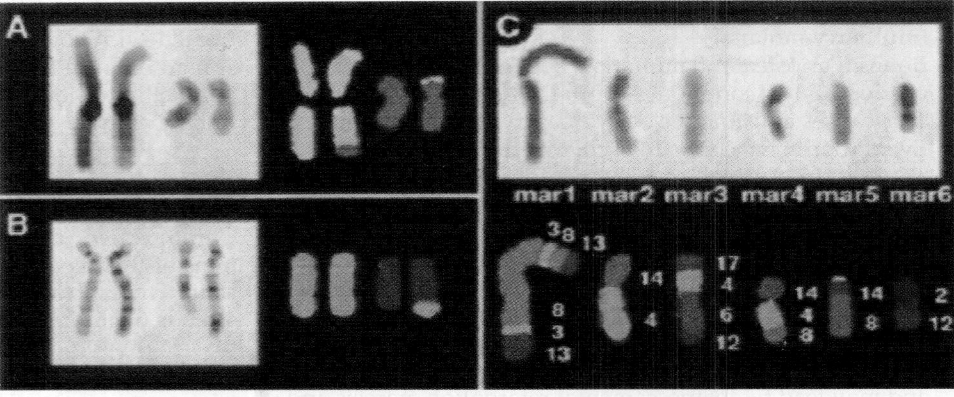

FIGURE 6-7. Translocations in human chromosomes demonstrated by spectral karyotyping. A. Balanced translocation: t(1; 11). **B.** Unbalanced karyotype: derivative chromosome 12 with chromosome 4 material attached (partial trisomy for 49 and partial monosomy for 12q). **C.** Characterization of marker chromosomes from an aneuploid breast cancer showing multiple translocations.

which facilitates detection of gross chromosomal abnormalities (Figs. 6-6 and 6-7).

Chromosomal Banding

To identify each chromosome individually, special stains delineate specific bands of different staining intensity on each chromosome. ***The pattern of bands is unique to each chromosome and makes it possible to (1) pair two homologous chromosomes, (2) recognize each chromosome and (3) identify defects on each segment of a chromosome.***

Chromosome bands are labeled as follows:

- **G bands** are highlighted using Giemsa stain (hence "G").
- **Q bands** stain with Giemsa and fluoresce when treated with quinacrine (thus, "Q").
- **R bands,** on appropriate staining, present as reverse (hence "R") images of G and Q bands; that is, dark G bands are light R bands and vice versa.
- **C banding** stains centromeres (hence "C") and other portions of chromosomes with constitutive heterochromatin. By contrast, facultative heterochromatin forms the inactive X chromosome (Barr body).
- **Nucleolar organizing region (NOR) staining** demonstrates secondary constrictions (stalks) of chromosomes with satellites.
- **T banding** stains the terminal (hence "T") ends of chromosomes.

Structural Chromosomal Abnormalities May Arise During Somatic Cell Division (Mitosis) or During Gametogenesis (Meiosis)

Changes in chromosome structure that occur in somatic cells during mitosis may (1) not affect a cell's basic functions and thus be silent, (2) interfere with one or more key cellular activities and lead to cell death or (3) change a key cell function (e.g., increase mitotic activity) so as to lead to dysfunction without cell death (see Chapter 5).

Structural chromosomal abnormalities that arise during gametogenesis are also important because they are transmitted to all somatic cells of an individual's offspring and may result in heritable diseases. During normal meiosis, homologous chromosomes (e.g., two chromosomes 1) form pairs, termed **bivalents.** By a normal process known as crossing over, parts of these chromosomes are exchanged, thus rearranging genetic constituents of each chromosome.

The International System for Human Cytogenetic Nomenclature designates chromosomal translocations. A translocation between chromosome "W" and "Z" is t(W;Z). The location on Giemsa-banded chromosomes "W" and "Z" (i.e., short arm p and long arm q) is also included in the nomenclature: t(W;Z) (band/"subband" on p or q of W; band/"subband" on p or q of Z).

Translocation is an abnormal process in which nonhomologous chromosomes (e.g., chromosomes 3 and 21) cross over and exchange genetic material. Two major types of chromosomal translocations are recognized: reciprocal and robertsonian.

Reciprocal Translocations

Reciprocal translocation is an exchange of acentric chromosomal segments between different (nonhomologous) chromosomes (Fig. 6-8). Reciprocal translocations are **balanced** if there is no net loss of genetic material: each chromosomal segment is translocated in its entirety. If this is present in gametes (sperm or ova), all somatic cells in progeny keep the abnormal chromosomal structure. ***Balanced translocations are not usually associated with loss of genes or disruption of vital gene loci, so most carriers of balanced translocations are phenotypically normal.*** Balanced reciprocal translocations can be inherited for many generations. Reciprocal translocations are particularly well demonstrated by current banding techniques.

Offspring of carriers of balanced translocations, however, are at risk because they will have unbalanced karyotypes and may show severe phenotypic abnormalities (Fig. 6-9). The abnormal positions of the exchanged chromosomal segments may disturb meiosis and lead to abnormal segregation of chromosomes. In a translocation carrier, formation of bivalents may be disturbed. For translocated segments to pair completely, a cross-like structure (quadriradial) is formed between the two chromosomes with the translocations and their two normal homologs. Unlike a normal bivalent, which typically resolves as each chromosome migrates to the opposite pole, a quadriradial can divide along several different planes. Some resulting gametes carry unbalanced chromosomes and, on fertilization, yield zygotes with combinations of partial trisomy and monosomy for segments of the translocated chromosomes.

Reciprocal translocations are detected in about 1 in 625 newborns. While most patients with balanced translocations are asymptomatic, 6% have an associated disorder, such as

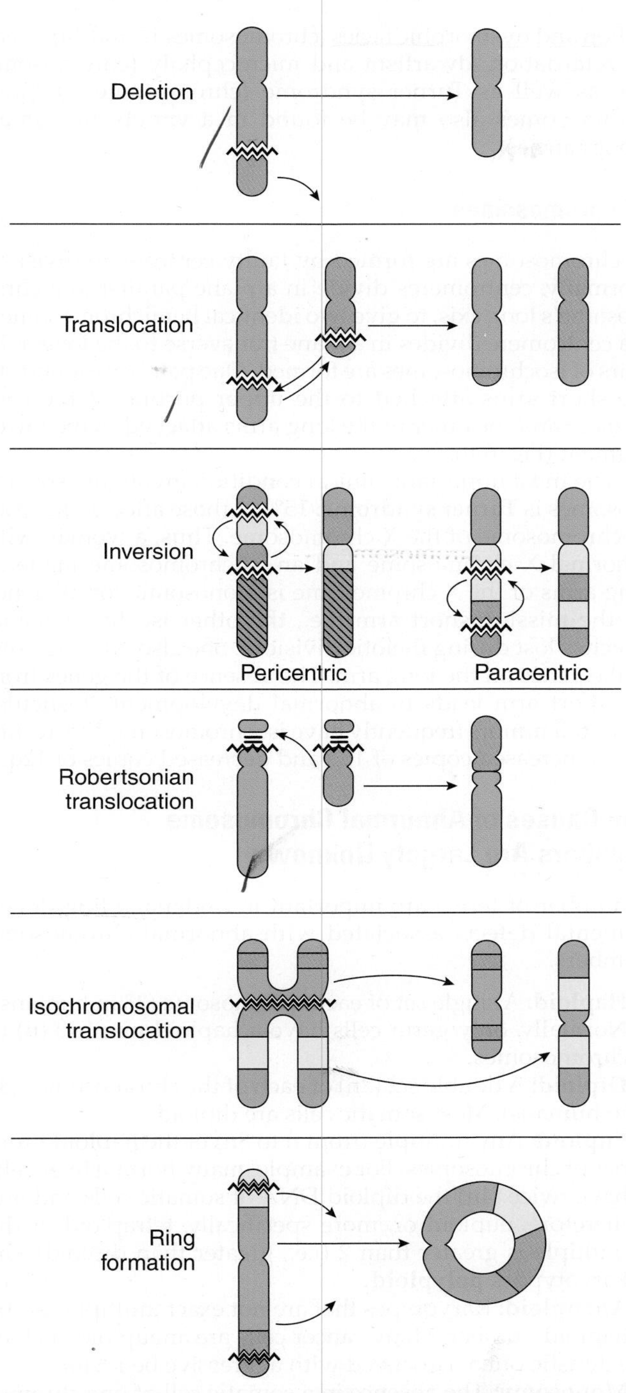

FIGURE 6-8. Structural abnormalities of human chromosomes. The deletion of a portion of a chromosome leads to the loss of genetic material and a shortened chromosome. A reciprocal translocation involves breaks on two nonhomologous chromosomes, with exchange of the acentric segments. An inversion requires two breaks in a single chromosome. If the breaks are on opposite sides of the centromere, the inversion is **pericentric;** it is **paracentric** if the breaks are on the same arm. A robertsonian translocation occurs when two nonhomologous acrocentric chromosomes break near their centromeres, after which the long arms fuse to form one large metacentric chromosome. Isochromosomes arise from faulty centromere division, which leads to duplication of the long arm (iso q) and deletion of the short arm, or the reverse (iso p). Ring chromosomes involve breaks of both telomeric portions of a chromosome, deletion of the acentric fragments and fusion of the remaining centric portion.

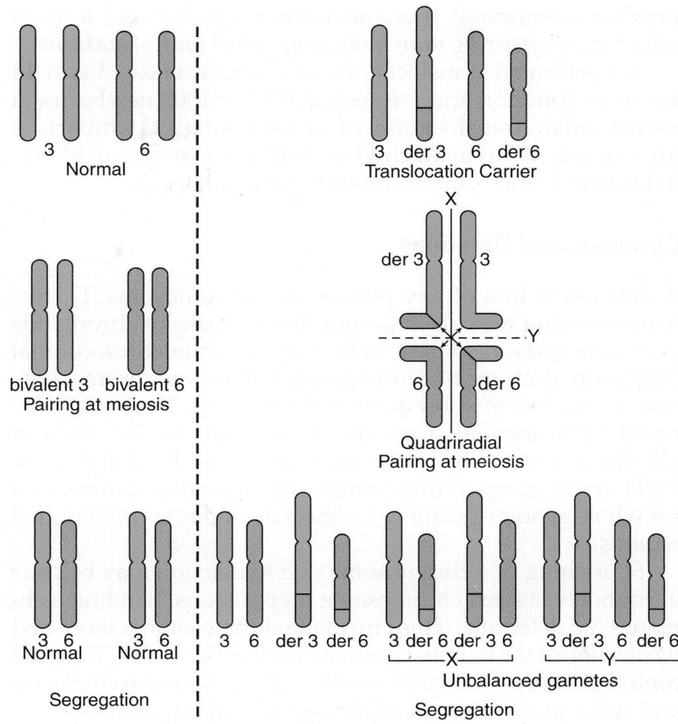

FIGURE 6-9. Meiotic segregation in a reciprocal balanced translocation involving chromosomes 3 and 6. The pairing of homologous chromosomes 3 and 6 in normal meiosis forms bivalents, which then segregate uniformly to create two gametes, each of which bears a single chromosome 3 and chromosome 6. Here the translocation carrier carries a balanced exchange of portions of the long arms of chromosomes 3 and 6. The chromosomes that carry the translocated genetic material are termed **derivative chromosomes** (der 3 and der 6). Diploid germ cells contain pairs of homologous chromosomes 3 and 6, each of which consists of one normal chromosome and one that carries a translocation. During meiosis, instead of the normal pairing into two bivalents, a quadriradial structure, containing all four chromosomes, is formed. In this circumstance, the chromosomes can segregate along several different planes of cleavage, shown as *X* and *Y*. In addition, the chromosomes can segregate diagonally (*arrows*). As a result, six different gametes can be produced, four of which are unbalanced and can result in congenital abnormalities.

autism, decreased intellectual ability and congenital abnormalities. In such instances, it is likely that the abnormalities are the result of disruption of a gene located at the breakpoint of the translocation.

Robertsonian Translocations

Robertsonian translocation (centric fusion) involves the centromere of acrocentric chromosomes. When two nonhomologous chromosomes are broken near the centromere, they may exchange two arms to form one large metacentric chromosome and a small chromosomal fragment. The latter lacks a centromere and is usually lost in subsequent divisions. As in reciprocal translocation, robertsonian translocation is balanced if there is no significant loss of genetic material. The carrier is also usually phenotypically normal, but may be infertile. *If a carrier is fertile, however, his or her gametes may*

produce unbalanced translocations (Figs. 6-7 and 6-8), in which case offspring may have congenital malformations.

Robertsonian translocations of chromosomes 13 and 14 are most common and are seen in 0.97 of 1000 newborns. A robertsonian translocation of chromosome 21 imparts a greater risk of having a child with Down syndrome. Maternal transmission is more common than paternal.

Chromosomal Deletions

A deletion is loss of any portion of a chromosome. Disturbances during meiosis in germ cells or breaks of chromatids during mitosis in somatic cells may generate chromosomal fragments that are not incorporated into any chromosome and so are lost in subsequent cell divisions. They may also result from unequal crossover during meiosis. Deletions of specific genes or chromosomal regions can be detected by FISH. Array comparative genomic hybridization can be used for whole genome profiling to detect deletions in unidentified regions.

Shortening of a chromosome due to deletion may be clear in routinely stained chromosome preparations. Banding techniques can determine if the arm of the chromosome is shortened by deletion of the terminal portion or a double break in the more central portions. The latter event leads to intercalary deletion and subsequent fusion of adjoining residual fragments.

Embryogenesis may be normal or abnormal. For example, in **cri du chat syndrome,** the short arm of chromosome 5 is deleted. Deletions may be related to several human cancers, including some hereditary forms of cancer. Thus, some familial **retinoblastomas** are associated with deletions in the long arm of chromosome 13 (see Chapter 5). **Wilms tumor aniridia syndrome** is associated with deletions in the short arm of chromosome 11. Other diseases associated with deletions include male infertility associated with chromosome Y deletions, approximately two thirds of cases with Duchenne muscular dystrophy (chromosome Xp) and the Prader-Willi syndrome.

Chromosomal Inversions

In chromosomal inversions, a chromosome breaks at two points and a segment inverts and then reattaches. **Pericentric inversions** result from breaks on opposite sides of the centromere; **paracentric inversions** involve breaks on the same arm of the chromosome (Fig. 6-8). During meiosis, homologous chromosomes that carry inversions do not exchange segments of chromatids by crossing over as readily as normal chromosomes, because of interference with pairing. Although this is of little consequence for the phenotype of the offspring, it may be important in evolutionary terms, since it may lead to clustering of certain hereditary features.

Ring Chromosomes

Ring chromosomes are formed by a break involving both telomeric ends of a chromosome, deletion of the acentric fragments and end-to-end fusion of the remaining centric portion of the chromosome (Fig. 6-8). The consequences depend primarily on the amount of genetic material lost because of the break. The abnormally shaped chromosome may impede normal meiotic division, but in most instances, this chromosomal abnormality is of no consequence. Ring chromosomes have been associated with epilepsy (chromosome 20), mental retardation and dysmorphic facies (chromosomes 13 and 14), mental retardation, dwarfism and microcephaly (chromosome 15), as well as Turner syndrome (chromosome X). Ring chromosomes also may be found in a variety of human malignancies.

Isochromosomes

Isochromosomes are formed by faulty centromere division. Normally, centromeres divide in a plane parallel to a chromosome's long axis, to give two identical hemichromosomes. If a centromere divides in a plane transverse to the long axis, pairs of isochromosomes are formed. One pair corresponds to the short arms attached to the upper portion of the centromere and the other to the long arms attached to the lower segment (Fig. 6-8).

The most important clinical condition involving isochromosomes is **Turner syndrome:** 15% of those affected have an isochromosome of the X chromosome. Thus, a woman with a normal X chromosome and an isochromosome made of long arms of the X chromosome is monosomic for all genes on the missing short arm (i.e., the other isochromosome, which is lost during meiotic division). She also has three sets of the genes on the long arm. The absence of the genes from the short arm leads to abnormal development. Testicular germ cell tumors frequently have isochromosome 12p, resulting in increased copies of 12p and decreased copies of 12q.

The Causes of Abnormal Chromosome Numbers Are Largely Unknown

A number of terms are important in understanding developmental defects associated with abnormal chromosome numbers.

- **Haploid:** A single set of each chromosome (23 in humans). Normally, only germ cells have a haploid number (n) of chromosomes.
- **Diploid:** A double set (2n) of each of the chromosomes (46 in humans). Most somatic cells are diploid.
- **Euploid:** Any multiple (from n to 8n) of the haploid number of chromosomes. For example, many normal liver cells have twice (4n) the diploid DNA of somatic cells and are, therefore, euploid or, more specifically, tetraploid. If the multiple is greater than 2 (i.e., greater than diploid), the karyotype is **polyploid.**
- **Aneuploid:** Karyotypes that are not exact multiples of the haploid number. Many cancer cells are aneuploid, a characteristic often associated with aggressive behavior.
- **Monosomy:** The absence in a somatic cell of one chromosome of a homologous pair. For example, in Turner syndrome there is a single X chromosome.
- **Trisomy:** The presence of an extra copy of a normally paired chromosome. For example, Down syndrome is caused by the presence of three chromosomes 21.

Nondisjunction

Nondisjunction is a failure of paired chromosomes or chromatids to separate and move to opposite poles of the spindle at anaphase, during mitosis or meiosis. *Numerical chromosomal abnormalities arise primarily from nondisjunction.* Nondisjunction leads to aneuploidy if only one pair of chromosomes fails to separate. It results in polyploidy if the entire set does not divide and all the chromosomes are segregated into a single daughter cell. In somatic cells, aneuploidy secondary to nondisjunction leads to one daughter cell with trisomy (2n + 1) and the other with monosomy (2n − 1) for the affected chromosome pair. Aneuploid germ cells have two copies of the same chromosome (n + 1) or lack the affected chromosome entirely (n − 1).

Anaphase lag is a special form of nondisjunction in which a single chromosome or chromatid fails to pair with its homolog during anaphase. It lags behind the others on the spindle and so is not incorporated into the daughter cell nucleus. In anaphase lag causing loss of one chromosome, one daughter cell is monosomic for the missing chromosome; the other is euploid.

Pathogenesis of Numerical Aberrations

The causes of chromosomal aberrations are obscure. Exogenous factors, such as radiation, viruses and chemicals, affect mitotic spindles or DNA synthesis and disturb mitosis and meiosis in experimental animals. However, how or whether these factors cause human chromosomal abnormalities is unknown. Autoantibodies and chromosomal anomalies may occur in families with autoimmune thyroid disorders. Such familial meiotic failure and chromosomal anomalies suggest genetic predispositions to faulty cell division. However, these hypotheses are unproved, and only two phenomena are known to contribute to numerical aberrations.

- **Nondisjunction during meiosis is more common in people with structurally abnormal chromosomes.** This is probably related to the fact that such chromosomes do not pair or segregate during gametogenesis as readily as do normal ones.
- **Maternal age is a key factor in some nondisjunction syndromes, particularly trisomy 21.**

Chromosomal Aberrations at Various Stages of Pregnancy

Chromosomal abnormalities identified at birth differ from those in early spontaneous abortions. At birth, the common chromosomal abnormalities are trisomies 21 (most frequent), 18, 13 and X or Y (47,XXX; 47,XXY; and 47,XYY). About 0.3% of all liveborn infants have a chromosomal abnormality. The most common chromosomal abnormalities in spontaneous abortions are 45,X (most frequent), then trisomies 16, 21 and 22. However, trisomy of almost any chromosome can be seen in spontaneous abortions. ***Up to 35% of spontaneous abortions have a chromosomal abnormality.*** The reason for these differences is presumably related to survival in utero. Very few fetuses with 45,X survive to term, and trisomy 16 is nearly always lethal in utero; a fetus with trisomy 21 has a better chance of surviving to birth.

Effects of Chromosomal Aberrations

Most major chromosomal abnormalities are incompatible with life. They are usually lethal to a developing conceptus and cause early death and spontaneous abortion. Embryos with significant loss of genetic material (e.g., autosomal monosomies) rarely survive pregnancy. Monosomy of the X chromosome (45,X) may be compatible with life, but over 95% of such embryos are lost during pregnancy. Absence of any X chromosome (i.e., 45,Y) invariably leads to early abortion.

Autosomal trisomies lead to several developmental abnormalities. Affected fetuses usually die during pregnancy or shortly after birth. Trisomy 21, which defines Down syndrome, is an exception, and people with Down syndrome may survive for years. Trisomy of the X chromosome may result in abnormal development but is not lethal.

Mitotic nondisjunction in embryonic cells early in development results in **mosaicism,** in which chromosomal aberrations are transmitted in some cell lineages but not others. ***The body thus has two or more karyotypically different cell lines.*** Mosaicism may involve autosomes or sex chromosomes, and the phenotype depends on the chromosome involved and the extent of mosaicism. Autosomal mosaicism is rare, probably because it is usually lethal. On the other hand, mosaicism involving sex chromosomes is common and is found in patients with gonadal dysgenesis who present with Turner or Klinefelter syndrome.

Nomenclature of Chromosomal Aberrations

Structural and numerical chromosomal abnormalities are classified by:

1. Total number of chromosomes
2. Designation (number) of affected chromosomes
3. Nature and location of the defect on the chromosome (Table 6-2)

Table 6-2

Chromosomal Nomenclature

Numerical designation of autosomes	1–22
Sex chromosomes	X, Y
Addition of a whole or part of a chromosome	+
Loss of a whole or part of a chromosome	−
Numerical mosaicism (e.g., 46/47)	/
Short arm of chromosome (petite)	p
Long arm of chromosome	q
Isochromosome	I
Ring chromosome	R
Deletion	del
Insertion	ins
Translocation	t
Derivative chromosome (carrying translocation)	der
Terminal	ter
Representative Karyotypes	
Male with trisomy 21 (Down syndrome)	47,XY, +21
Female carrier of fusion-type translocation between chromosomes 14 and 21	45,XX, −14, −21, +t(14q21q)
Cri du chat syndrome (male) with deletion of a portion of the short arm of chromosome 5	46,XY, del(5p)
Male with ring chromosome 19	46,XY, r(19)
Turner syndrome with monosomy X	45,X
Mosaic Klinefelter syndrome	46,XY/47,XXY

Table 6-3

Clinical Features of the Autosomal Chromosomal Syndromes*

Syndromes	Features
Trisomic Syndromes	
Chromosome 21 (Down syndrome 47,XX or XY, +21: 1/800)	Epicanthic folds, speckled irides, flat nasal bridge, congenital heart disease, simian crease of palms, Hirschsprung disease, increased risk of leukemia
Chromosome 18 (47,XX or XY, +18: 1/8000)	Female preponderance, micrognathia, congenital heart disease, horseshoe kidney, deformed fingers
Chromosome 13 (47,XX or XY, +13: 1/20,000)	Persistent fetal hemoglobin, microcephaly, congenital heart disease, polycystic kidneys, polydactyly, simian crease
Deletion Syndromes	
5p– syndrome (cri du chat 46,XX or XY, 5p−)	Cat-like cry, low birth weight, microcephaly, epicanthic folds, congenital heart disease, short hands and feet, simian crease
11p– syndrome (46,XX or XY, 11p–)	Aniridia, Wilms tumor, gonadoblastoma, male genital ambiguity
13q– syndrome (46,XX or XY, 13q–)	Low birth weight, microcephaly, retinoblastoma, congenital heart disease

*All of these syndromes are associated with mental retardation.

Karyotypes are described sequentially by:

1. Total number of chromosomes
2. Sex chromosome complement
3. Any abnormality

The short arm of a chromosome is designated **p,** and the long arm, **q.** Addition of chromosomal material, be it an entire chromosome or a part of one, is indicated by a plus sign (+) before the number of the affected chromosome. A minus sign (−) denotes loss of part or all of a chromosome. Or loss (deletion) of part of a chromosome may be designated by **del,** followed by the location of the deleted material on the affected chromosome. A translocation is written as a **t,** followed by brackets containing the involved chromosomes. Chromosomal aberrations in structure or number occur in 5 to 7 of 1000 liveborn infants; most are balanced translocations and are asymptomatic.

Numerical Autosomal Aberrations in Liveborn Infants Are Virtually All Trisomies

Structural aberrations that may result in clinical disorders include translocations, deletions and chromosomal breakage (Table 6-3).

Trisomy 21 (Down Syndrome)

Trisomy 21 is the most common cause of mental retardation. Liveborn infants are only a fraction of all conceptuses with this defect. Two thirds abort spontaneously or die in utero. Life expectancy is also reduced. Advances in treating infections, congenital heart defects and leukemia—the leading causes of death with Down syndrome—have increased life expectancy.

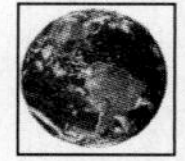

EPIDEMIOLOGY: ***Incidence of trisomy 21 rises dramatically with increasing maternal age: children of older mothers are at much greater risk for Down syndrome*** (Fig. 6-10). Up to their mid-30s, women have a constant risk of giving birth to a trisomic child of about 1 per 800 to 1000 liveborn infants. The incidence then increases sharply, to 1 in 30 at age 45 years. The risk of a mother having a second child with Down syndrome is 1%, regardless of maternal age, unless the syndrome is associated with translocation of chromosome 21. Still, most (80%) children with Down syndrome are born to mothers younger than 35 years of age, perhaps because this population has an overall higher incidence of pregnancy.

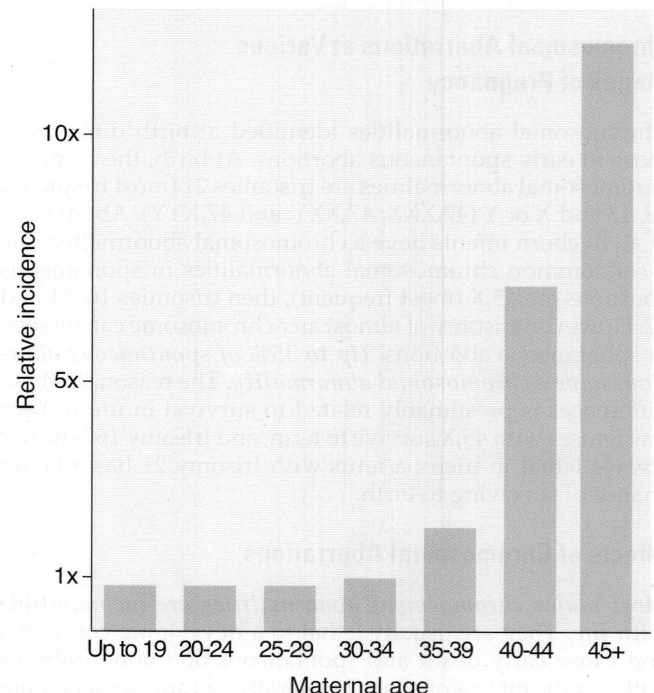

FIGURE 6-10. Incidence of Down syndrome in relation to maternal age. A conspicuous increase in the frequency of this disorder is seen over the age of 35 years.

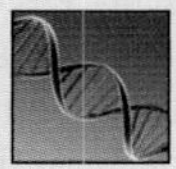

MOLECULAR PATHOGENESIS: Chromosome 21 is the smallest human autosome, with less than 2% of all human DNA. It has an acrocentric structure, and all genes of known function (except for ribosomal RNA) are on the long arm (21q). Based on studies of inherited translocations, in which only a part of chromosome 21 is duplicated, the region on chromosome 21 responsible for the full Down syndrome phenotype is in band 21q22.2, a 4-Mb region of DNA termed the **Down syndrome critical region** (DSCR). Genes in the DSCR that might be involved in Down syndrome have recently been identified. They encode transcription factors of the nuclear factor of activated T cells (NFAT, see Chapter 1) family, which are known to influence somatic development.

There are three mechanisms by which three copies of the genes on chromosome 21 that cause Down syndrome may be present in somatic cells:

- **Nondisjunction** in the first meiotic division of gametogenesis accounts for 92% to 95% of patients with trisomy 21. The extra chromosome 21 is maternal in about 95% of such children. Virtually all maternal nondisjunction seems to result from events in the first meiotic division (meiosis I).
- **Translocation** of an extra long arm of chromosome 21 to another acrocentric chromosome causes about 5% of cases of Down syndrome.
- **Mosaicism** for trisomy 21 is caused by nondisjunction during mitosis of a somatic cell early in embryogenesis and accounts for 2% of children born with Down syndrome.

How increasing maternal age increases the risk of bearing a child with trisomy 21 is poorly understood. It is known that the maternal age effect is related to maternal nondisjunction events, which implies that the defect lies in oocyte meiosis. Down syndrome associated with translocation or mosaicism is not related to maternal age.

Down syndrome caused by translocation of an extra portion of chromosome 21 occurs in two situations. Either parent may be a phenotypically normal carrier of a balanced translocation, or a translocation may arise de novo during gametogenesis. These translocations are typically robertsonian, tending to involve only acrocentric chromosomes, with short arms consisting of a satellite and stalk (chromosomes 13, 14, 15, 21 and 22). Translocations between these chromosomes are particularly common since they cluster during meiosis and so are subject to breakage and recombination more than other chromosomes. The most common translocation in Down syndrome (50%) is fusion of the long arms of chromosomes 21 and 14, t(14q;21q), followed in frequency (40%) by similar fusion involving two chromosomes 21, t(21q;21q).

If the translocation is inherited from a parent, a balanced translocation has been converted to an unbalanced one (Fig. 6-7B). Then, one would expect a one-third chance of Down syndrome among offspring of a carrier of a balanced robertsonian translocation. However, early loss of most embryos with trisomy 21 means that the actual incidence is only 10% to 15% with a maternal translocation and less than 5% if the father is the carrier.

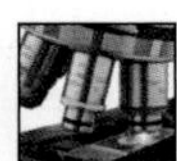 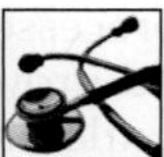

PATHOLOGY AND CLINICAL FEATURES: Diagnosis of Down syndrome is ordinarily made at birth by the infant's flaccid state and characteristic appearance. Diagnoses are confirmed by cytogenetic analysis. Over time, a typical constellation of abnormalities appears (Fig. 6-11).

- **Mental status:** Children with Down syndrome are invariably mentally retarded. Their IQs decline relentlessly and progressively with age. Mean IQs are 70 below the age of 1 year, and decline during the first decade of life to a mean of 30. The major defect seems to be an inability to develop

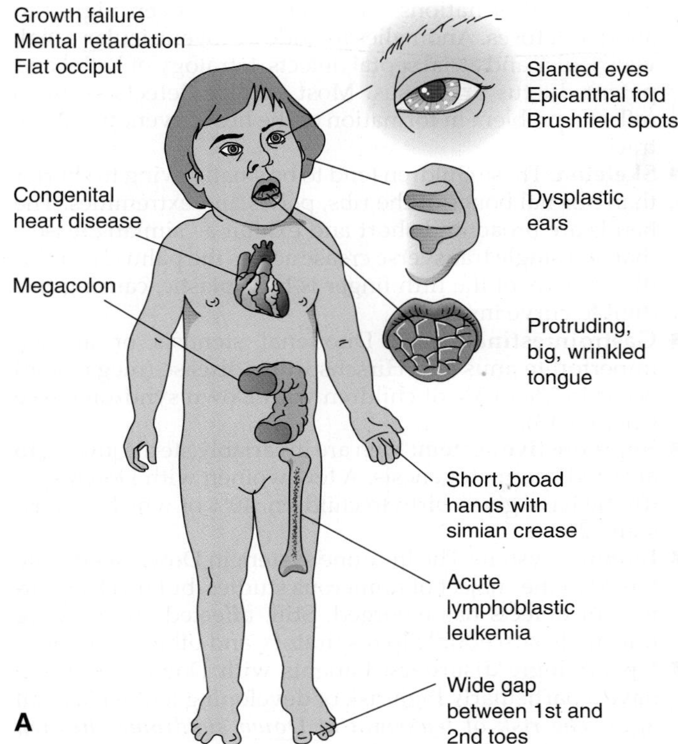

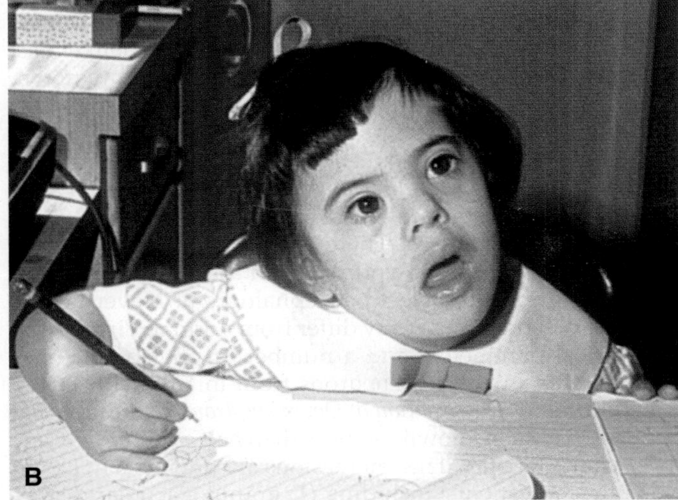

FIGURE 6-11. **A.** Clinical features of Down syndrome. **B.** A young girl with the facial features of Down syndrome.

more-advanced cognitive strategies and processes, problems that become more apparent as a child grows older. These children were once described as gentle and affectionate, but these personality stereotypes are now thought to be doubtful.

- **Craniofacial features:** Face and occiput tend to be flat, with a low-bridged nose, reduced interpupillary distance and oblique palpebral fissures. Epicanthal folds of the eyes impart an Asian appearance, which accounts for the obsolete term **mongolism.** Irides are speckled with **Brushfield spots.** Ears are enlarged and malformed. A prominent tongue, which typically lacks a central fissure, protrudes through an open mouth.
- **Heart:** One third of children with Down syndrome have cardiac malformations. The incidence is even higher in aborted fetuses. Anomalies include atrioventricular canal, ventricular and atrial septal defects, tetralogy of Fallot and patent ductus arteriosus. Most cardiac defects seem to reflect a problem in formation of the heart's venous inflow tract.
- **Skeleton:** These children tend to be small, owing to shorter than normal bones of the ribs, pelvis and extremities. The hands are broad and short and exhibit a "simian crease," that is, a single transverse crease across the palm. The middle phalanx of the fifth finger is hypoplastic, causing this digit to curve inward.
- **Gastrointestinal tract:** Duodenal stenosis or atresia, imperforate anus and Hirschsprung disease (megacolon) occur in 2% to 3% of children with Down syndrome (see Chapter 13).
- **Reproductive system:** Men are invariably sterile, owing to arrested spermatogenesis. A few women with Down syndrome have given birth to children, 40% of which had trisomy 21.
- **Immune system:** The immune system in Down syndrome has been the subject of numerous studies, but no clear pattern of defects has emerged. Still, affected children are unusually susceptible to respiratory and other infections.
- **Hematologic disorders:** Patients with Down syndrome have a particularly high risk of developing leukemia at all ages. ***The risk of leukemia in Down syndrome children younger than the age of 15 years is about 15-fold greater than normal.*** In children younger than 3 years, acute nonlymphocytic leukemia predominates. Most leukemias occur later and are usually acute lymphoblastic leukemias. The basis for the high incidence of leukemia is unknown, but leukemoid reactions (transient pronounced neutrophilia) are frequent in the newborn with Down syndrome. Interestingly, leukemias that develop in patients who are mosaic for Down syndrome are invariably trisomic for chromosome 21.
- **Neurologic disorders:** There is no clear pattern of neuropathology in Down syndrome, nor are there characteristic changes on the electroencephalogram. Nevertheless, neurons in trisomy 21 may differ from normal. Virtually all electrical parameters and a number of physiologic ones are altered in cultured neurons from infants with Down syndrome. *The association of Down syndrome with Alzheimer disease* has been known for more than half a century. By age 35, characteristic Alzheimer lesions are universal in Down syndrome patients, including (1) granulovacuolar degeneration, (2) neurofibrillary tangles, (3) senile plaques and (4) loss of neurons (see Chapter 28). The senile plaques and cerebral blood vessels of both Alzheimer disease and Down syndrome always contain the same fibrillar amyloid protein (β-amyloid protein). The similarity between the neuropathologies of Down syndrome and Alzheimer disease is also reflected in the appearance of dementia in one fourth to one half of older patients with Down syndrome and progressive loss of many intellectual functions that cannot be attributed to mental retardation alone.
- **Life expectancy:** During the first decade of life, the presence or absence of congenital heart disease largely determines survival in Down syndrome. Only about 5% of those whose hearts are normal die before age 10, but about 25% with heart disease die by then. If patients reach age 10, the age at death is about 55, which is 20 years or more lower than that of the general population. Only 10% reach age 70.

Trisomies of Chromosomes 18, 13 and 22

Trisomy 18, at 1 in 8000 live births, is the second most common autosomal syndrome. It results in mental retardation and affects females four times as often as males. Virtually all infants with trisomy 18 have congenital heart disease and die in the first 3 months of life.

Trisomies 13 and 22 are rare and both are associated with mental retardation, congenital heart disease and other abnormalities. Syndromes associated with trisomies of chromosomes 8 and 9 have also been described.

Translocation Syndromes

The prototypical translocation that causes partial trisomy is Down syndrome. Many other partial trisomies are reported, the best documented being 9p trisomy. In this disorder, the short arm of chromosome 9 may be translocated to one of several autosomes. Many kindreds with this syndrome are described. Carriers of a balanced chromosome 9 translocation are asymptomatic but may pass an unbalanced translocation on to their offspring. The disorder is characterized by mental retardation, microcephaly and other craniofacial abnormalities. A reciprocal translocation between the long arms of chromosomes 22 and 11 is also well known. Offspring of carriers may have an extra chromosome with parts of both 11 and 22, in which case they have partial trisomy of both chromosomes, leading to microcephaly and other anomalies.

Chromosomal Deletion Syndromes

Deletion of an entire autosomal chromosome (i.e., monosomy) is usually not compatible with life. However, several syndromes arise from deletions of parts of several chromosomes (Table 6-3). In most cases, the congenital syndromes are sporadic, but in a few instances, reciprocal translocations have been shown in the parents. Virtually all of these deletion syndromes are characterized by low birth weight, mental retardation, microcephaly and craniofacial and skeletal abnormalities. Cardiac and urogenital malformations are common.

- **5p– syndrome (cri du chat):** This is the best-known deletion syndrome, because the high-pitched cry of the infant is like that of a kitten and calls attention to the disorder. Most cases are sporadic, but reciprocal translocations have been reported in some parents.
- **11p– syndrome:** Deletion of the short arm of chromosome 11, specifically band 11p13, leads to absence of the iris (aniridia) and is often accompanied by Wilms tumor.

- **13q− syndrome:** Loss of the long arm of chromosome 13 is associated with retinoblastoma owing to the loss of the *Rb* tumor suppressor gene (see Chapter 5).
- **Other deletion syndromes:** Deletions of both short and long arms of chromosome 18 are documented, producing varying patterns of mental retardation and craniofacial anomalies. Loss of material from chromosomes 19, 20, 21 and 22 is usually associated with ring chromosomes. Syndromes associated with 21q− and 22q− are the most common and often resemble Down syndrome.
- **Deletions and rearrangements of subtelomeric sequences:** Telomeres are a repetitive sequence $(TTAGGG)_n$ at the ends of chromosomes. Subtelomeric regions of chromosomes are rich in genes. Deletions and rearrangements of these regions can only be demonstrated by FISH, are major causes of mild to severe mental retardation and dysmorphic features and are found in about 5% of such patients.

Chromosomal Breakage Syndromes

Several recessive syndromes show frequent chromosomal breakage and rearrangements and entail significant risk of leukemia and other cancers. These include xeroderma pigmentosum, Bloom syndrome (congenital telangiectatic erythema with dwarfism), ataxia telangiectasia and Fanconi anemia (constitutional aplastic pancytopenia). Acquired chromosome breaks and translocations occur with leukemias and lymphomas, the best documented of which are chronic myelogenous leukemia, t(9;22), and Burkitt lymphoma, mostly t(8;14) (see Chapters 5 and 20).

Numerical Aberrations of Sex Chromosomes Are Much More Common Than Those of Autosomes, Save for Trisomy 21

The reasons are not entirely clear, but additional sex chromosomes (Fig. 6-12) cause less severe clinical manifestations than do extra autosomes and are less likely to disturb critical stages of development. Additional X chromosomes probably cause less severe phenotypes because of **lyonization,** a normal process in which each cell only has one active X chromosome.

The contrast between the X and Y chromosomes is striking: the X chromosome is one of the larger chromosomes, with 6% of all DNA, but the Y chromosome is very small. More than 1300 genes have been identified on the X chromosome; the Y chromosome has fewer than 400 genes, one of which is the testis-determining gene (*SRY,* also known as *TDF*).

The Y Chromosome

In humans, unlike some lower organisms, it appears that genes on the Y chromosome are the key determinants of gender phenotype. Thus, the phenotype of people who are XXY (Klinefelter syndrome; see below) is male, and those who are XO (Turner syndrome) are female. The testis-determining gene (*SRY,* sex-determining region Y) is an intronless gene near the end of the short arm of the Y chromosome. The *SRY* gene encodes a small nuclear protein with a DNA-binding domain. This protein complexes with another protein (SIP-1) to form a transcriptional activator of autosomal genes that directs development of a male phenotype. Mutations in *SRY* lead to XY females, while translocations that add *SRY* to an X chromosome produce XX males.

A small proportion of infertile men with azoospermia or severe oligospermia have small deletions in regions of the Y chromosome. However, the size and location of these deletions are variable and do not correlate with the severity of spermatogenic failure.

The X Chromosome

Males carry only one X chromosome but the same amounts of X chromosome gene products as do females. This seeming discrepancy is explained by the **Lyon effect:**

- In females, one X chromosome is irreversibly inactivated early in embryogenesis and is detectable in interphase nuclei as a heterochromatic clump of chromatin attached to

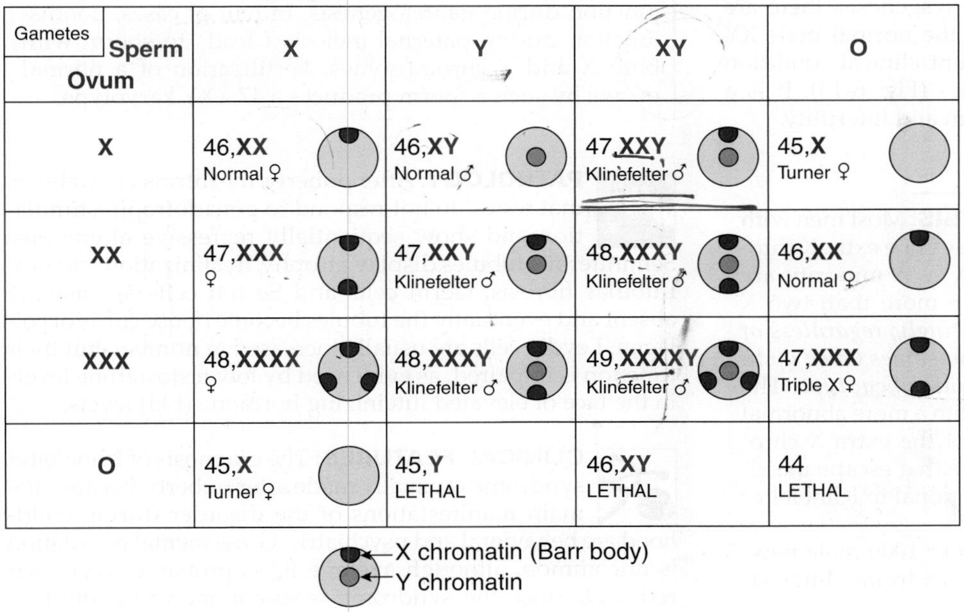

Gametes: Ovum \ Sperm	X	Y	XY	O
X	46,XX Normal ♀	46,XY Normal ♂	47,XXY Klinefelter ♂	45,X Turner ♀
XX	47,XXX ♀	47,XXY Klinefelter ♂	48,XXXY Klinefelter ♂	46,XX Normal ♀
XXX	48,XXXX ♀	48,XXXY Klinefelter ♂	49,XXXXY Klinefelter ♂	47,XXX Triple X ♀
O	45,X Turner ♀	45,Y LETHAL	46,XY LETHAL	44 LETHAL

X chromatin (Barr body)
Y chromatin

FIGURE 6-12. Numerical aberrations of sex chromosomes. Nondisjunction in either the male or female gamete is the principal cause of these abnormalities.

…ear membrane, termed the **Barr body.** The …romosome is extensively methylated at gene …ons and transcriptionally repressed. Nevertheless, …ant minority of X-linked genes escape inactivation …ntinue to be expressed by both X chromosomes. The pr…bility that an X chromosome is inactive seems to correlate with expression levels of *XIST*, an X-linked gene expressed only by the inactive partner.

- Either the paternal or maternal X chromosome is inactivated randomly.
- Inactivation of the X chromosome is virtually complete.
- X chromosome inactivation is permanent and transmitted to progeny cells, so paternally or maternally derived X chromosomes are propagated clonally. ***All females are thus mosaic for paternal and maternal X chromosomes.*** Mosaicism in females for glucose-6-phosphate dehydrogenase was key to demonstrating the monoclonal origin of neoplasms (see Chapter 5).

The issue is not quite so simple, however. If one X chromosome is entirely nonfunctional, persons with XXY (Klinefelter) or XO (Turner) karyotypes should be phenotypically normal. They are not, and the fact that they show phenotypic abnormalities indicates that inactivated X chromosomes still function, at least in part. Indeed, a part of the short arm of the X chromosome is known to escape X inactivation. This **pseudoautosomal region** can pair with a homologous region on the short arm of the Y chromosome and undergo meiotic recombination between the two. Genes in this location are present in two functional copies in both males and females. Thus, patients with Turner syndrome (45,X) are haploinsufficient for these genes, and those with more than two X chromosomes (e.g., Klinefelter patients) have more than two functional copies. A gene in this region, *SHOX*, is associated with height, and its haploinsufficiency in Turner syndrome may explain the short stature of Turner patients. Several other genes outside the pseudoautosomal region also escape X inactivation. ***Mental retardation in phenotypic boys and girls with extra X chromosomes correlates roughly with the number of X chromosomes.***

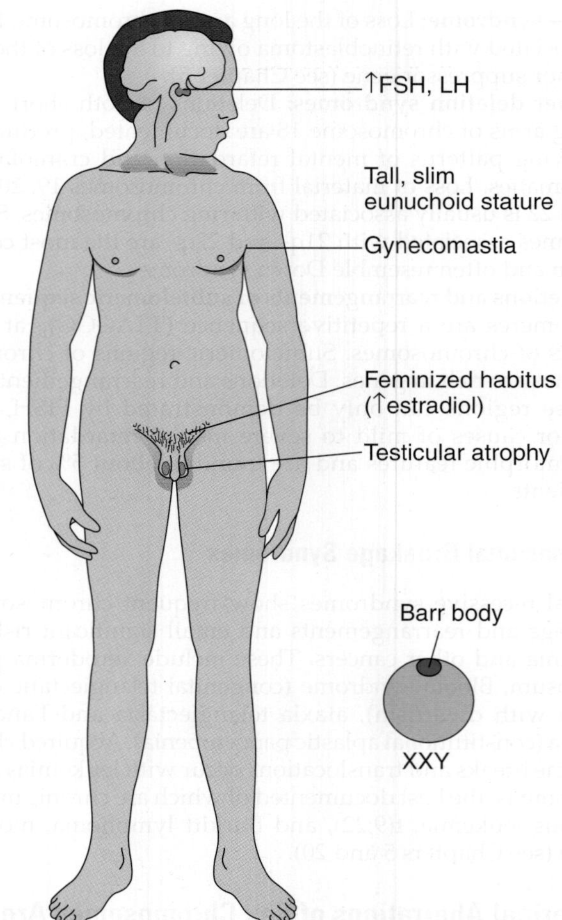

FIGURE 6-13. Clinical features of Klinefelter syndrome. FSH = follicle-stimulating hormone; LH = leuteinizing hormone.

Klinefelter Syndrome (47,XXY)

In Klinefelter syndrome, or testicular dysgenesis, there are one or more X chromosomes beyond the normal male XY complement. This is the most important clinical condition involving trisomy of sex chromosomes (Fig. 6-13). It is a prominent cause of male hypogonadism and infertility.

MOLECULAR PATHOGENESIS: Most men with Klinefelter syndrome (80%) have one extra X chromosome (i.e., they are 47,XXY). A minority are mosaics (e.g., 46,XY/47,XXY) or have more than two X chromosomes (e.g., 48,XXXY). ***Interestingly, regardless of the number of supernumerary X chromosomes (even up to four), the Y chromosome ensures a male phenotype.*** The additional X chromosomes correlate with a more abnormal phenotype, despite the inactivation of the extra X chromosomes. Presumably, the same genes that escape inactivation in normal females are still functional in Klinefelter syndrome.

Klinefelter syndrome occurs in 1 per 1000 male newborns, about the incidence of Down syndrome. Interestingly, half of all 47,XXY conceptuses are miscarried. The additional X chromosome(s) is a result of meiotic nondisjunction during gametogenesis. In half of cases, nondisjunction during paternal meiosis I leads to sperm with both X and Y chromosomes. Fertilization of a normal oocyte by such a sperm produces a 47,XXY karyotype.

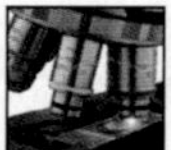

PATHOLOGY: After puberty, the intrinsically abnormal testes do not respond to gonadotropin stimulation and show sequentially regressive alterations. Seminiferous tubules display atrophy, hyalinization and peritubular fibrosis. Germ cells and Sertoli cells are usually absent and eventually the tubules become dense cords of collagen. Leydig cells are usually increased in number, but their function is impaired, as evidenced by low testosterone levels in the face of elevated luteinizing hormone (LH) levels.

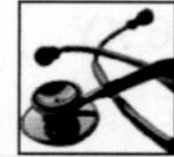

CLINICAL FEATURES: The diagnosis of Klinefelter syndrome is usually made after puberty, because the main manifestations of the disorder during childhood are behavioral and psychiatric. Gross mental retardation is uncommon, although average IQ is probably somewhat reduced. Since the syndrome is so common, it should be suspected in all boys with some mental deficiency or severe behavioral problems.

Children with Klinefelter syndrome tend to be tall and thin, with relatively long legs (eunuchoid body habitus). Normal testicular growth and masculinization do not occur at puberty, and testes and penis remain small. Feminine characteristics include a high-pitched voice, gynecomastia and a female pattern of pubic hair (female escutcheon). Azoospermia results in infertility. All of these changes are due to hypogonadism and a resulting lack of androgens. Serum testosterone is low to normal, but LH and follicle-stimulating hormone are remarkably high, indicating normal pituitary function. High circulating estradiol levels increase the estradiol-to-testosterone ratio, which determines the degree of feminization. Treatment with testosterone will virilize these patients but does not restore fertility.

The XYY Male

Interest in the XYY phenotype (1 per 1000 male newborns) comes from studies in penal institutions suggesting that this karyotype was significantly more prevalent there than in the general population. However, the idea that XYY "supermales" show antisocial behavior because of an extra Y chromosome has not been substantiated in other studies and the topic remains controversial. The only features of the XYY phenotype that are agreed on are tall stature, a tendency toward cystic acne and some problems in motor and language development. Aneuploidy of the Y chromosome is a consequence of meiotic nondisjunction in the father.

Turner Syndrome

Turner syndrome is the spectrum of abnormalities that results from **complete or partial X chromosome monosomy in a phenotypic female.** It occurs in about 1 in 5000 liveborn females. In three-quarters of cases, the single X chromosome of Turner syndrome is of maternal origin, suggesting that the meiotic error tends to be paternal. The incidence of the syndrome does not correlate with maternal age, and the risk of producing a second affected female infant is not increased.

The 45,X karyotype is one of the most common aneuploids in human conceptuses, but almost all are aborted spontaneously: up to 2% of abortuses show this aberration. As Turner patients survive normally after birth, why is the missing X chromosome lethal during fetal development? Perhaps the inactivated X chromosome in normal females (or the Y chromosome in males) protects against early demise of the embryo. It is believed that homologs of Y genes in the pseudoautosomal region of the X chromosome escape inactivation and are critical to the survival of a female conceptus.

About half of Turner patients lack an entire X chromosome (monosomy X). The remainder are mosaics or have structural X chromosome aberrations, such as isochromosome of the long arm, translocations and deletions. Mosaics with a 45,X/46,XX karyotype (15%) tend to have milder phenotypic manifestations of Turner syndrome and may even be fertile. In about 5% of patients, the mosaic karyotype is 45,X/46,XY, in which case an original male zygote was subsequently modified by a mitotic nondisjunction. Such persons are at a 20% risk of developing a germ cell cancer and should have prophylactic removal of the abnormal gonads.

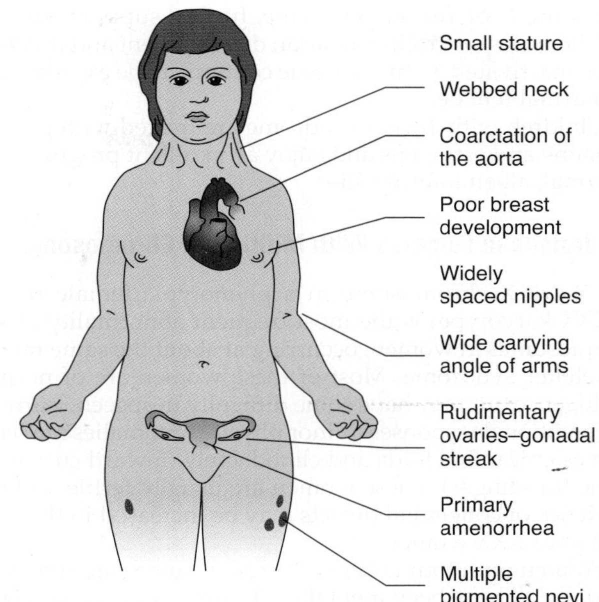

FIGURE 6-14. Clinical features of Turner syndrome.

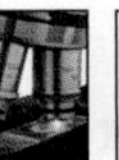 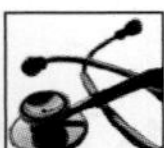

PATHOLOGY AND CLINICAL FEATURES: The clinical hallmarks of Turner syndrome are sexual infantilism with primary amenorrhea and sterility (Fig. 6-14). The disorder is usually discovered when absence of menarche brings the child to medical attention. Virtually all of these women are under 5 ft (152 cm) tall. Other clinical features include a short, webbed neck (pterygium coli); low posterior hairline; wide carrying angle of the arms (cubitus valgus); broad chest with widely spaced nipples; and hyperconvex fingernails. Half of patients have anomalies on urograms, the most common being horseshoe kidney and malrotation. Many have facial abnormalities, including a small mandible, prominent ears and epicanthal folds. Defective hearing and vision are common, and up to 20% may be mentally defective. Pigmented nevi become prominent as the patient ages. For unknown reasons, women with Turner syndrome are at a greater risk for chronic autoimmune thyroiditis and goiter.

Cardiovascular anomalies occur in almost half of Turner patients: coarctation of the aorta in 15% and a bicuspid aortic valve in up to one third. Essential hypertension occurs in some patients, and dissecting aneurysm of the aorta is occasionally a cause of death.

Ovaries of women with Turner syndrome show a curious acceleration of normal aging. Normal female fetal ovaries initially contain 7 million oocytes each, less than half of which survive until birth. Relentless loss of oocytes continues, so that at menarche only about 5% (400,000) remain. At menopause a mere 0.1% survive. Ovaries of fetuses with Turner syndrome contain oocytes at first, but they lose them rapidly. None remain by 2 years of age. The ovaries become fibrous streaks, whereas the uterus, fallopian tubes and vagina develop normally. Thus, menopause in children with Turner syndrome may be considered to occur long before menarche.

Interestingly, families are known in which several women have premature menopause and show deletions of portions of the long arm of one X chromosome. These data, with observations of Turner syndrome, further support the idea that the genes controlling ovarian development and function in the inactivated X chromosome continue to be expressed in the normal female.

Children with Turner syndrome are treated with growth hormone and estrogens and enjoy an excellent prognosis for a normal, albeit infertile, life.

Syndromes in Females With Multiple X Chromosomes

One extra X chromosome in a phenotypic female (i.e., a 47,XXX karyotype) is the most frequent abnormality of sex chromosomes in women, occurring at about the same rate as Klinefelter syndrome. Most of these women are of normal intelligence but may have some difficulty in speech, learning and emotional responses. Minor physical anomalies are seen, such as epicanthal folds and clinodactyly (inward curvature of the fifth finger). These women are usually fertile, but the incidence of congenital defects may be increased in the children of 47,XXX women.

Women with four and five X chromosomes are reported. Virtually all have been mentally retarded. They superficially resemble women with Down syndrome and do not mature sexually. Women with supernumerary X chromosomes have additional Barr bodies, indicating inactivation of all but one X chromosome. Clearly, some genes on inactivated X chromosomes are still expressed.

Single-Gene Abnormalities Confer Traits That Segregate Sharply Within Families

The classic laws of mendelian inheritance, named in honor of Gregor Mendel, are:

- **A mendelian trait** is determined by two copies of the same gene, called alleles, located at the same locus on two homologous chromosomes. In the case of the X and Y chromosomes in males, a trait is determined by just one allele.
- **Autosomal genes** are those located on one of the 22 autosomes.
- **Sex-linked traits** are encoded by loci on the X chromosome.
- **A dominant phenotypic trait** requires the presence of only one allele of a homologous gene pair and is seen whether the allelic genes are homozygous or heterozygous.
- **A recessive phenotypic trait** demands that both alleles be identical, that is, homozygous.
- In **codominance** both alleles in a heterozygous gene pair are fully expressed and contribute to the phenotype (e.g., the AB blood group genes).

Mendelian traits are classified as:

1. **Autosomal dominant**
2. **Autosomal recessive**
3. **Sex-linked dominant**
4. **Sex-linked recessive**

Diseases due to sex-linked dominant genes are rare and of little practical significance.

Mutations

To make proteins, DNA is transcribed into RNA, which is processed into mRNA, which in turn is translated by ribosomes. A change in DNA can lead to a corresponding change in the amino acid sequence of a specific protein or interference with its synthesis.

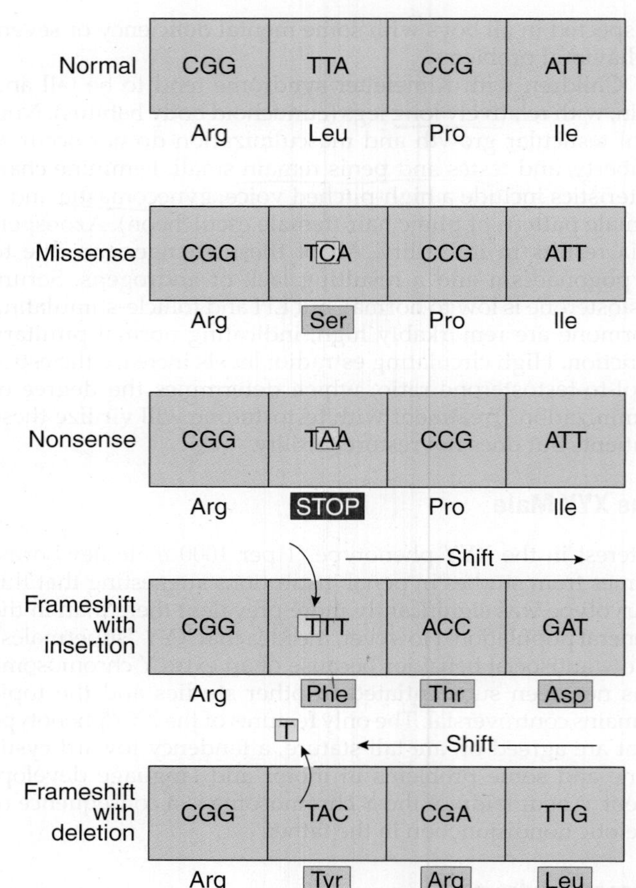

FIGURE 6-15. Point mutations that alter the reading frame of DNA. A variety of mutations in the second codon of a normal sequence of four amino acids is depicted. With a missense mutation, a change from T to C substitutes serine (Ser) for leucine (Leu). With a nonsense mutation, a change from T to A converts the leucine codon to a stop codon. A shift in the reading frame to the right results from insertion of a T, thus changing the sequence of all subsequent amino acids. Conversely, deletion of a T shifts the reading frame one base to the left and also changes the sequence of subsequent amino acids. Arg = arginine; Asp = aspartate; Ile = isoleucine; Phe = phenylalanine; Pro = proline; Thr = threonine; Tyr = tyrosine.

A mutation is a stable heritable change in DNA. The consequences of mutations are highly variable. Some have no functional consequences, but others are lethal and so are not transmitted to the next generation. Between these extremes is a broad range of DNA changes that account for the genetic diversity of any species. ***About 1 in 1000 base pairs is polymorphic in the human genome,*** and evolution is based on the accumulation over time of such nonlethal mutations that alter the ability of a species to adapt to its environment. The genetics of human disease focuses on mutations that impair protein function detectably. The major types of mutations (Fig. 6-15) are:

- **Point mutations:** If one base replaces another, a **point mutation** occurs. If it is in the coding region (the part of the gene that is translated into a protein), a point mutation has three possible consequences:

1. In a **synonymous mutation** the altered codon still encodes the same amino acid. For example, CGA and CGC both code for arginine.
2. A **missense mutation** (three fourths of base changes in the coding region) occurs when the new codon codes for a different amino acid. In sickle cell anemia, an adenine-to-thymine change in the β-globin gene replaces glutamic acid (GAG) with valine (GUG).
3. A **nonsense mutation** (4%) stops translation; that is, a codon for an amino acid is changed to a termination codon, yielding a truncated protein. For example, TAT codes for tyrosine, but TAA is a stop codon.

- **Frameshift mutations:** Amino acids are encoded by trinucleotide sequences. If the number of nucleotides in a gene is changed by an insertion or deletion, and if the number of bases added or deleted is not a multiple of 3, ***the reading frame of the message is changed.*** Then, even though the downstream sequence is the same, it will code for a different amino acid sequence and an unscheduled termination signal. Frameshift mutations can also alter transcription, splicing or processing of mRNA.
- **Large deletions:** When a large segment of DNA is deleted, the coding region of a gene may be entirely removed, in which case the protein product is absent. A large deletion may also appose coding regions of nearby genes, giving rise to a fused gene that codes for a hybrid protein in which part or all of one protein is followed by part or all of another.
- **Expansion of unstable trinucleotide repeat sequences:** The human genome contains frequent tandem trinucleotide repeat sequences, some of which are associated with disease. The number of copies of certain repetitive trinucleotide sequences varies among individuals, representing allelic polymorphism of the genes in which they are found. As a rule, the number of repeats below a particular threshold does not change during mitosis or meiosis; but above this threshold, the number of repeats can contract or, more commonly, expand. A number of distinct trinucleotide expansions have been identified in human disease (Table 6-4).

Identification of a family of genetic diseases resulting from expansion of trinucleotide repeats has generated a new molecular category of disease. The number of trinucleotide repeats increases with each successive generation, as does the severity of the disease and a younger age at onset. This mechanism is known as **genetic anticipation.** The majority of known trinucleotide repeat diseases result from expansions of a CAG codon, which encodes glutamine, in the open reading frame of the gene, resulting in a polyglutamine tract in the protein product. ***All of these disorders are associated with degeneration of neuronal cells.***

Fragile X Syndrome

The prototypic trinucleotide repeat disease is fragile X syndrome, in which the number of CCG repeats is increased. It is transmitted as an X-linked dominant trait with variable penetrance and is ***the most common cause of inherited mental retardation*** (see below). Numbers of CGG repeats are increased in a noncoding region adjacent to the *FMR1* gene on the X chromosome, which is required for neural development. The incidence is 1 per 4000 males and 1 per 4000 to 6000 females, as phenotype penetrance is variable. The expanded CGG repeat silences the *FMR1* gene by methylation of the FMR1 promoter through an unknown mechanism. The abnormal repeat is also associated with an inducible "fragile site" on the X chromosome, which appears in cytogenetic studies as a nonstaining gap or an apparent chromosomal break. The phenotype includes slow intellectual development and physical abnormalities, such as an elongated face and prominent ears.

Huntington Disease

Huntington disease (HD) is the most common genetic cause of chorea. It is also associated with abnormalities of muscle coordination and psychomotor and cognitive functions. The disease is transmitted as an autosomal dominant trait. HD is caused by expansion of a CAG repeat within the coding sequence of the *IT15* gene, which codes for the protein **huntingtin.** In normal people, 10 to 30 repeats is the rule, while those affected by the disease have 40 or more. CAG codes for glutamine, and abnormal expansion of the polyglutamine tract in HD confers a toxic gain of function to huntingtin. Although the precise mechanism by which mutant huntingtin causes selective neuronal loss is not understood, there is evidence to suggest that altered protein–protein interactions are responsible. In addition to HD, expanded CAG repeats are involved in a number of other neurodegenerative disorders (Table 6-4).

Myotonic Dystrophy

Myotonic dystrophy (MD), the most common form of autosomal muscular dystrophy (see Chapter 27), is caused by expansion of a CTG repeat in the 3′-untranslated region of the

Table 6-4

Representative Diseases Associated With Trinucleotide Repeats

Disease	Location	Sequence	Normal Length	Premutation	Full Mutation
Huntington disease	4p16.3	CAG	10–30	—	40–100
Kennedy disease	Xq21	CAG	15–25	—	40–55
Spinocerebellar ataxia	6p23	CAG	20–35	—	45–80
Fragile X syndrome	Xq27.3	CGG	5–55	50–200	200–1000
Myotonic dystrophy	19q13	CTG	5–35	37–50	50–2000
Friedreich ataxia	9q13	GAA	7–30	—	120–1700

MD gene on chromosome 19q. It is inherited as an autosomal dominant. Having up to 35 CTG repeats is normal, but MD patients may have up to 2000. The structure of the protein product of the gene, a serine/threonine protein kinase genetically related to kinases for classes of small G proteins, is unchanged. The abnormality is likely to reflect altered processing of mRNAs due to cis-acting sequences in the 3′-untranslated region, which is increasingly understood as a critical posttranscriptional regulator of protein production.

Friedreich Ataxia

Friedreich ataxia (FA) is an autosomal recessive degenerative disease affecting the CNS and the heart that is associated with expansion of a GAA repeat in the *frataxin* gene (see Chapter 28), which encodes a mitochondrial protein. Affected people have 120 to 1700 repeats in the first intron (noncoding) of the frataxin gene.

Functional Consequences of Mutations

A biochemical pathway represents the sequential actions of a series of enzymes, which are coded for by specific genes. A typical pathway can be represented by the conversion of a substrate (A) through intermediate metabolites (B and C) to the final product (D).

A	→	B → C	→	D
initial substrate		intermediary metabolites		end-products

A single gene defect can have several consequences:

- **Failure to complete a metabolic pathway:** The end-product (D) is not formed because an enzyme that is required for the completion of a metabolic sequence is missing:

  $$A \rightarrow B \rightarrow C - // \rightarrow (D)\ (\downarrow)$$

  An example of the failure to complete a metabolic pathway is **albinism,** a pigment disorder caused by a deficiency of tyrosinase. This enzyme catalyzes the conversion of tyrosine to melanin (via intermediate formation of dihydroxyphenylalanine [DOPA]). Without tyrosinase, the end-product, melanin, is not formed, and an affected person (an "albino") has no pigment in all organs that normally contain it, primarily the eyes and skin.
- **Accumulation of unmetabolized substrate:** The enzyme that converts the initial substrate into the first intermediary metabolite may be missing, in which case the initial substrate accumulates in excess.

  $$A\ (\rightarrow)^{\sim} // \rightarrow B\ (\downarrow)\ C\ (\downarrow)\ (D)\ (\downarrow)$$

  Thus, in **phenylketonuria,** an inborn deficiency of phenylalanine hydroxylase causes dietary phenylalanine to accumulate and reach toxic concentrations that interfere with postnatal brain development and cause severe mental retardation.
- **Storage of an intermediary metabolite:** An intermediary metabolite, which is normally quickly processed into the final product and so is usually present only in minute amounts, accumulates in large quantities if the enzyme for its metabolism is lacking.

  $$A \rightarrow B\ (\rightarrow)^{\sim} \rightarrow // \rightarrow C\ (\downarrow)\ D\ (\downarrow)$$

  This type of genetic disorder is exemplified by von Gierke disease, a glycogen storage disease that results from deficiency of glucose-6-phosphatase. The inability to convert glucose-6-phosphate into glucose leads to its alternative conversion to glycogen.
- **Formation of an abnormal end-product:** A mutant gene codes for an abnormal protein. In sickle cell anemia, valine replaces glutamate in the β-globin part of hemoglobin.

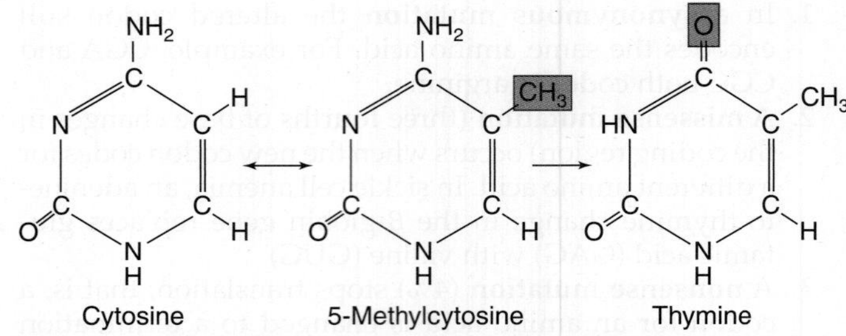

FIGURE 6-16. 5-Methylcytosine is formed from cytosine. Spontaneous deamination of 5-methylcytosine produces thymine.

Mutation Hotspots

Certain regions of the genome mutate at a much higher rate than average. The best-characterized hotspot is the dinucleotide pair CG, which is prone to undergo mutation to form TG. Methylation of cytosine in CG dinucleotides is a common means of regulating gene expression: the methylation product, 5-methylcytosine, represses gene transcription. Such 5-methylcytosine can undergo spontaneous deamination to thymine (Fig. 6-16). If this occurs in a gamete, it can become a fixed, heritable trait in the offspring.

Autosomal Dominant Disorders Are Expressed in Heterozygotes

If only one mutated allele is sufficient to cause disease when its paired allele on the homologous autosome is normal, the mutant trait is considered to be dominant. The features of autosomal dominant traits are (Fig. 6-17):

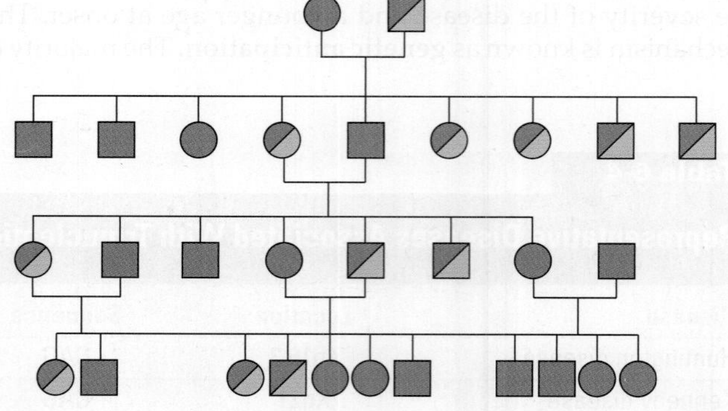

FIGURE 6-17. Autosomal dominant inheritance. Only symptomatic persons transmit the trait to the next generation, and heterozygotes are symptomatic. Both males and females are affected.

- Males and females are affected equally, as the mutant gene is on an autosomal chromosome. Thus, father-to-son transmission (which is absent in X-linked dominant disorders) may occur.
- The trait encoded by the mutant gene can be transmitted to successive generations (unless reproductive capacity is compromised).
- Unaffected members of a family do not transmit the trait to their offspring. Unless the disease represents a new mutation, everyone with the disease has an affected parent.
- Proportions of normal and diseased offspring of patients with the disorder are on average equal, because most affected persons are heterozygous, whereas their normal mates do not harbor the defective gene.

New Mutations Versus Inherited Mutations

As noted above, autosomal dominant diseases may result from a new mutation rather than transmission from an affected parent. Nevertheless, offspring of patients with a new dominant mutation have a 50% risk for the disease. ***With dominant autosomal disorders the ratio of new mutations to transmitted ones varies with the effect of the disease on fertility.*** The more a disease impairs reproduction, the greater the proportion of affected people who will represent new mutations. A dominant mutation causing 100% infertility would have to be a new mutation. If reproductive capacity is only partly impaired, the proportion of new mutations is lower. Thus, **tuberous sclerosis** is an autosomal dominant condition in which mental retardation limits reproductive potential, and new mutations account for 80% of cases. If a dominant disease has little effect on fertility (e.g., familial hypercholesterolemia), virtually all affected persons will have pedigrees showing classic vertical transmission of the disorder.

Biochemical Basis of Autosomal Dominant Disorders

There are several major mechanisms by which the presence of one mutant allele may cause disease even when the other allele is normal.

- If the gene product is rate limiting in a complex metabolic network (e.g., a receptor or an enzyme), having half of the normal amount of gene product may not be enough to maintain a normal phenotype. This is known as **haploinsufficiency.** For example, familial hypercholesterolemia is caused by insufficient low-density lipoprotein (LDL) uptake receptors on hepatocytes.
- In some diseases, the presence of an extra copy of an allele gives rise to a phenotype. An example of this is Charcot-Marie-Tooth disease type IA, which is caused by duplication of the peripheral myelin protein-22 gene.
- A mutant protein may be constitutively activated. For example, mutations in the *RET* proto-oncogene in families with multiple endocrine neoplasia type 2 increase activity of a tyrosine kinase that stimulates cell proliferation.
- Mutations in genes for structural proteins (e.g., collagens, cytoskeletal constituents) result in abnormal molecular interactions and disrupt normal morphologic patterns. Such a situation is exemplified by osteogenesis imperfecta and hereditary spherocytosis.

More than 1000 human diseases are inherited as autosomal dominant traits, although most are rare. Examples of human autosomal dominant diseases are given in Table 6-5.

Table 6-5

Representative Autosomal Dominant Disorders

Disease	Frequency	Chromosome
Familial hypercholesterolemia	1/500	19p
von Willebrand disease	1/8000	12p
Hereditary spherocytosis (major forms)	1/5000	14, 8
Hereditary elliptocytosis (all forms)	1/2500	1, 1p, 2q, 14
Osteogenesis imperfecta (types I–IV)	1/10,000	17q, 7q
Ehlers-Danlos syndrome type III	1/5000	2q
Marfan syndrome	1/10,000	15q
Neurofibromatosis type 1	1/3500	17q
Huntington chorea	1/15,000	4p
Retinoblastoma	1/14,000	13q
Wilms tumor	1/10,000	11p
Familial adenomatous polyposis	1/10,000	5q
Acute intermittent porphyria	1/15,000	11q
Hereditary amyloidosis	1/100,000	18q
Adult polycystic kidney disease	1/1000	16p

Inherited Connective Tissue Diseases Are Often Autosomal Dominant Traits

This discussion is limited to three of the most common and best-studied entities that affect connective tissue: Marfan syndrome, Ehlers-Danlos syndrome and osteogenesis imperfecta. Even in these well-delineated disorders, clinical symptomatology often overlaps. For instance, some patients exhibit the joint dislocations typical of Ehlers-Danlos syndrome, but other members of the same family suffer from multiple fractures characteristic of osteogenesis imperfecta. Yet others in the family, with the same genetic defect, may have no symptoms. Thus, current classifications based on clinical criteria will eventually be replaced by references to specific gene defects, as with the hemoglobinopathies.

Marfan Syndrome

Marfan syndrome is an autosomal dominant, inherited disorder of connective tissue with a variety of abnormalities in many organs, including the heart, aorta, skeleton, eyes and skin. One third of cases represent sporadic mutations. The incidence in the United States is 1 per 10,000.

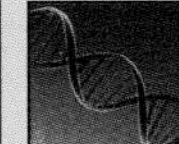

MOLECULAR PATHOGENESIS: The cause of Marfan syndrome is a missense mutation in the gene for *fibrillin-1 (FBN1)*, on the long arm of chromosome 15 (15q21.1). Fibrillin is a family of collagen-like connective tissue proteins. There are now about a dozen genetically distinct fibrillins, and over 100 mutations are known. It is widely distributed in many tissues in the form of a fiber system termed **microfibrils,** which are thread-like filaments that form larger fibers and are organized into rods, sheets and interlaced networks. **Microfibrillar fibers** are scaffolds for elastin deposition during embryonic development, after which they are part of elastic tissues (e.g., elastin is deposited on lamellae of microfibrillar fibers in the concentric rings of elastin in the aortic wall). By immunofluorescent microscopy, abnormal microfibrillar fibers are visualized in all tissues affected in Marfan syndrome.

Fibrillin-1 is a large, cysteine-rich glycoprotein that forms 10-nm microfibrils in the extracellular matrix of many tissues. Interestingly, the ciliary zonules that suspend the lens of the eye are devoid of elastin but consist almost exclusively of microfibrillar fibers (fibrillin). Dislocation of the lens is a characteristic feature of Marfan syndrome.

Deficiencies in the amount and distribution of microfibrillar fibers have been shown in the skin and fibroblast cultures of patients with Marfan syndrome, which renders the elastic fibers incompetent to resist normal stress. A transgenic mouse hemizygous for fibrillin-1 has been shown to be a phenocopy of Marfan syndrome in humans. Fibrillin also binds to transforming growth factor-β (TGF-β), a multifunctional protein that regulates cellular proliferation and is upregulated in a variety of inflammatory diseases. Increased levels of TGF-β are seen in the aorta, cardiac valves and lungs of patients with Marfan syndrome and may be the result of decreased fibrillin-1, which normally sequesters this cytokine. Treating the fibrillin-1–deficient mice with a TGF-β antagonist decreases the severity of their "Marfan phenotype," suggesting a potential therapeutic approach in this disease that does not directly focus on the target of the genetic mutation.

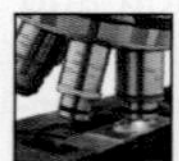 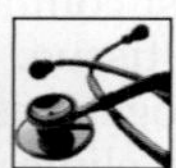

PATHOLOGY AND CLINICAL FEATURES: People with Marfan syndrome are usually (but not always) tall, and lower body length (pubis to sole) is more than upper body length. A slender habitus, which reflects a paucity of subcutaneous fat, is complemented by long, thin extremities and fingers, leading to the term **arachnodactyly** (spider fingers) (Fig. 6-18). Overall, affected patients resemble figures in paintings by El Greco.

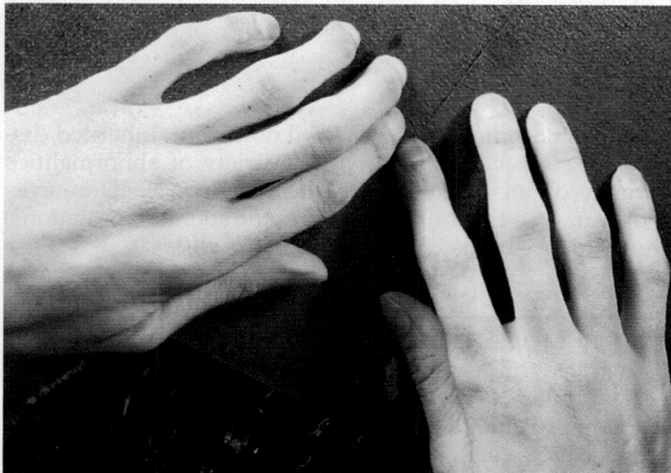

FIGURE 6-18. Long, slender fingers (arachnodactyly) in a patient with Marfan syndrome.

- **Skeletal system:** Skulls in Marfan syndrome are usually long (dolichocephalic), with prominent frontal eminences. Disorders of the ribs are conspicuous, causing pectus excavatum (concave sternum) and pectus carinatum (pigeon breast). Tendons, ligaments and joint capsules are weak, leading to hyperextensibility of the joints (double-jointedness), dislocations, hernias and kyphoscoliosis; the last is often severe.
- **Cardiovascular system:** ***The most important vascular defect is in the aorta, where the tunica media is weak.*** Weakness of the media leads to variable dilation of the ascending aorta and a high incidence of dissecting aneurysms, usually of the ascending aorta. These may rupture into the pericardial cavity or extend down the aorta and rupture into the retroperitoneal space. Dilation of the aortic ring results in aortic regurgitation, which may be severe enough to produce angina pectoris and congestive heart failure. The mitral valve may have redundant leaflets and chordae tendineae—leading to mitral valve prolapse syndrome (see Chapter 10). Cardiovascular disorders are the most common causes of death in Marfan syndrome.

  The aorta shows conspicuous fragmentation and loss of elastic fibers, with increased metachromatic mucopolysaccharide. Focally, the elastic tissue defect results in discrete pools of amorphous metachromatic material, reminiscent of that seen in Erdheim (idiopathic) cystic medial necrosis of the aorta. Smooth muscle cells are enlarged and lose their orderly circumferential arrangement.
- **Eyes:** Ocular changes are common in Marfan syndrome. These include dislocation of the lens (ectopia lentis), severe myopia due to elongation of the eye and retinal detachment.

Untreated men with Marfan syndrome usually die in their 30s, and untreated women often die in their 40s. However, antihypertensive therapy and replacement of the aorta with prosthetic grafts have increased life expectancy to almost normal longevity.

Ehlers-Danlos Syndromes

Ehlers-Danlos syndromes (EDSs) are rare inherited disorders of connective tissue that feature remarkable hyperelasticity and fragility of the skin, joint hypermobility and often a bleeding diathesis. Paganini is rumored to have had Ehlers-Danlos syndrome owing to his renowned flexibility on the violin fingerboard. The disorder is clinically and genetically heterogeneous. Different forms may be inherited as an autosomal dominant or recessive (autosomal or X-linked) trait depending on the specific mutation.

MOLECULAR PATHOGENESIS: Ten types of EDS have been established. ***They all share a generalized defect in collagen, including abnormalities in its structure, synthesis, secretion and degradation.*** In EDS types I to IV, VI and X, collagen fibrils are increased in size, with unusually small bundles, features that are consistent with the presence of abnormal collagen. Such changes involve type III collagen in EDS IV and type I collagen in EDS VII. EDS VII arises from mutations that alter the amino-terminal cleavage sites of either the 1 or 2 procollagen chain of type I collagen.

Deficiencies of specific collagen-processing enzymes, including lysyl hydroxylase and lysyl oxidase, cause EDS VI and IX, respectively. Deficiency of the *ADAMTS2* gene, which encodes a metallopeptidase that is critical for processing procollagen, is a rare cause of EDS. Deficiency of tenascin X, which is normally expressed in connective tissues, may also cause EDS. ***Whatever the underlying biochemical defect, the result is deficient or defective collagen.*** Depending on the type of EDS, these molecular lesions are associated with conspicuous weakness of supporting structures of the skin, joints, arteries and viscera.

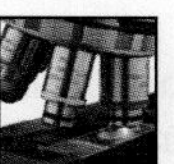
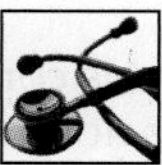

PATHOLOGY AND CLINICAL FEATURES: All types of EDS are characterized by soft, fragile, hyperextensible skin. Patients typically can stretch their skin many centimeters and trivial injuries can lead to serious wounds. Sutures do not hold well, so surgical incisions often dehisce. Hypermobility of the joints allows unusual extension and flexion (e.g., as in the "human pretzel" and other contortionists). EDS IV is the most dangerous variety, owing to a tendency of the large arteries, bowel and gravid uterus to spontaneously rupture. Death from such complications is common in the third and fourth decades of life.

Ehlers-Danlos syndrome VI causes severe kyphoscoliosis, blindness from retinal hemorrhage or rupture of the globe and death from aortic rupture. Severe periodontal disease, with loss of teeth by the third decade, characterizes EDS VIII. EDS IX features development of bladder diverticula during childhood, with a danger of bladder rupture and skeletal deformities.

Many people with clinical abnormalities suggesting EDS do not match any of the documented types of this disorder. Further genetic and biochemical characterization of such cases is likely to expand the classification of EDS.

Osteogenesis Imperfecta

Osteogenesis imperfecta (OI), or brittle bone disease, is a group of inherited disorders in which a generalized abnormality of connective tissue is expressed principally as fragility of bone. OI is inherited as an autosomal dominant trait, although rare cases are transmitted as autosomal recessive traits.

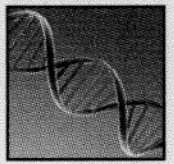

MOLECULAR PATHOGENESIS: ***Genetic defects in the eight types of OI are heterogeneous, but all affect type I collagen synthesis, helical structure or, rarely, other structural proteins in bone.*** The genes most commonly involved are *COL1A1* and *COL1A2*, which are required to form mature type I collagen. Point mutations may disrupt formation of the α-helical structure of type I collagen by converting glycines that occur at every third amino acid position to bulkier amino acids. Or, alterations in the C-terminus and certain deletions can disrupt formation of mature type I collagen fibrils. Some patients have no family history and represent founders resulting from a sporadic mutation.

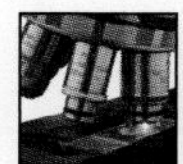
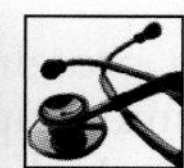

PATHOLOGY

- **Type I** OI appearanc bones occur during infanc to walk. Such patients h "fragile as a china doll." have blue sclerae as th imparts translucence to visible. A high incidence of fractures and fusion of the bones of the m their mobility.
- **Type II** OI is usually fatal in utero or shortly after birth. Affected infants have a characteristic facies and skeletal abnormalities. Those who are born alive usually die of respiratory failure within their first month.
- **Type III** OI causes progressive deformities. It is ordinarily detected at birth by the baby's short stature and misshapenness caused by fractures in utero. Dental defects and hearing loss are common. Unlike other OI types, type III is often an autosomal recessive trait.
- **Type IV** OI is like type I, but sclerae are normal and the phenotype is more variable.
- **Types V and VI** OI have clinical manifestations that are similar to those of type IV but have histologic features that are distinguishing: a "fish bone" appearance to the bone.
- **Types VII and VIII** OI have an autosomal recessive pattern of inheritance and are associated with abnormalities in the *CRTAP* gene and the *LEPRE1* gene, respectively.

Osteogenesis imperfecta is discussed in further detail in Chapter 26.

Neurofibromatosis

The neurofibromatoses include two distinct autosomal dominant disorders characterized by the development of multiple neurofibromas, which are benign Schwann cell tumors of peripheral nerves (see Chapter 28). These disorders involve all cells derived from the neural crest, including melanocytes in addition to Schwann cells and endoneurial fibroblasts. Thus, criteria for diagnosing neurofibromatosis type 1 include disorders of pigmentation as well as neural tumors.

Neurofibromatosis Type I (von Recklinghausen Disease)

Neurofibromatosis type I (NF1) is characterized by (1) disfiguring neurofibromas, (2) areas of dark pigmentation of the skin (café au lait spots), (3) pigmented lesions of the iris (Lisch nodules), (4) freckles in the groin or axilla, (5) gliomas of the optic nerve and (6) skeletal abnormalities, including thinning of the cortices of long bones. It is one of the more common autosomal dominant disorders, affecting 1 in 3500 persons of all races. The NF1 gene has a very high rate of mutation and half of cases are sporadic rather than familial. NF1 was first described in 1882 by von Recklinghausen, but references to it can be found as early as the 13th century.

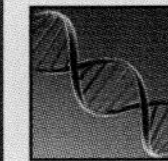

MOLECULAR PATHOGENESIS: Germline mutations in the NF1 gene, on the long arm of chromosome 17 (17q11.2), include deletions, missense mutations and nonsense mutations. The gene product, *neurofibromin*, belongs to a family of GTPase-activating

...APs), which inactivate the ras protein (see ...). In this sense, NF1 is a classic tumor suppres-... ***loss of GAP activity permits uncontrolled ras ...tion, which presumably predisposes to formation of ...ofibromas.***

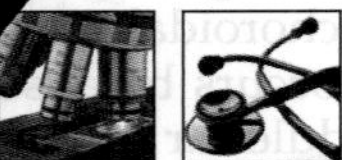

PATHOLOGY AND CLINICAL FEATURES: Clinical manifestations of NF1 are highly variable and difficult to explain entirely on the basis of a single gene defect. They include:

- **Neurofibromas:** More than 90% of patients with NF1 have cutaneous and subcutaneous neurofibromas by late childhood or adolescence. These tumors may total more than 500 and appear as soft, pedunculated masses, usually about 1 cm in diameter (Fig. 6-19). However, on occasion they may reach alarming proportions (up to 25 cm) and dominate the physical appearance of a patient. Subcutaneous neurofibromas are soft nodules along the course of peripheral nerves. **Plexiform neurofibromas** only occur in the context of NF1. These tumors usually involve larger peripheral nerves but on occasion arise from cranial or intraspinal nerves. Plexiform neurofibromas are often large, infiltrative tumors that cause severe disfigurement of the face or an extremity. The pathology of neurofibromas is discussed in Chapter 28. ***In 3% to 5% of NF1 patients, a neurofibrosarcoma will develop in a neurofibroma, usually a larger one of the plexiform type.*** Other neurogenic tumors, such as meningioma, optic glioma and pheochromocytoma, occur more often in NF1.

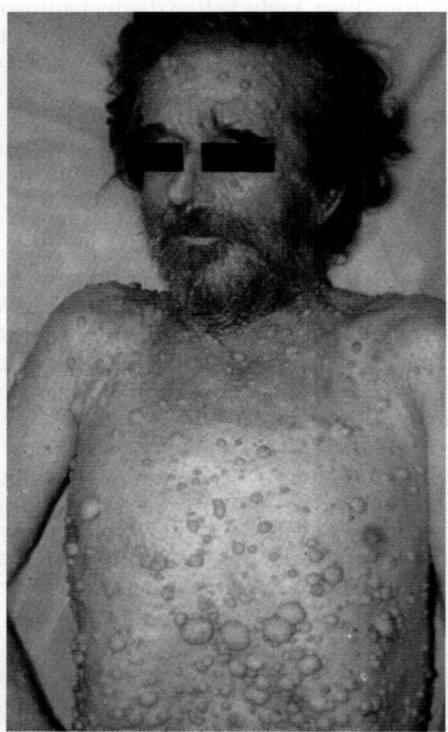

FIGURE 6-19. Neurofibromatosis type I. Multiple cutaneous neurofibromas are noted on the face and trunk.

- **Café au lait spots:** Although normal people may have occasional light brown patches on the skin, more than 95% of persons with NF1 display six or more such lesions. These are over 5 mm before puberty and more than 1.5 cm thereafter. Café au lait spots tend to be ovoid, with the longer axis oriented parallel to a cutaneous nerve. Numerous freckles, particularly in the axilla, are also common.
- **Lisch nodules:** Over 90% of patients with NF1 have pigmented nodules of the iris, which are masses of melanocytes. These lesions are thought to be hamartomas.
- **Skeletal lesions:** A number of bone lesions occur frequently in NF1. These include malformations of the sphenoid bone and thinning of the cortices of the long bones, with bowing and pseudarthrosis of the tibia, bone cysts and scoliosis.
- **Mental status:** Mild intellectual impairment is common in patients with NF1, but severe retardation is not part of the syndrome.
- **Leukemia:** The risk of malignant myeloid disorders in children with NF1 is 200 to 500 times normal. In some patients, both alleles of the NF1 gene are inactivated in leukemic cells.

Neurofibromatosis Type II (Central Neurofibromatosis)

Neurofibromatosis type II (NF2) is a syndrome defined by bilateral tumors of the eighth cranial nerve (acoustic neuromas) and, commonly, by meningiomas and gliomas. NF2 is much less common than NF1, occurring in 1 in 50,000 people. Most patients have bilateral acoustic neuromas, but the condition can be diagnosed in the presence of a unilateral eighth nerve tumor if two of the following are present: neurofibroma, meningioma, glioma, schwannoma or juvenile posterior lenticular opacity.

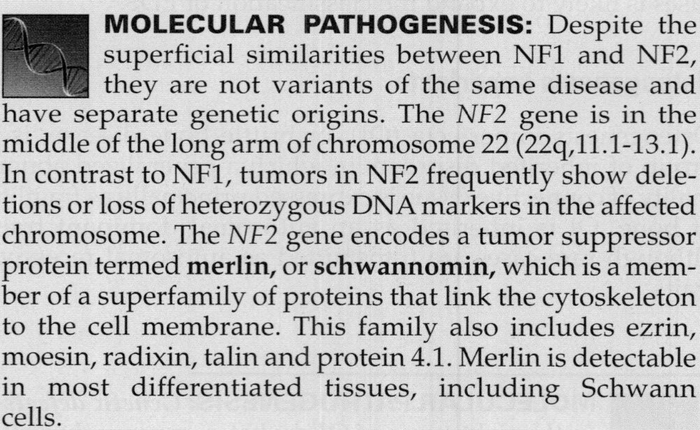

MOLECULAR PATHOGENESIS: Despite the superficial similarities between NF1 and NF2, they are not variants of the same disease and have separate genetic origins. The *NF2* gene is in the middle of the long arm of chromosome 22 (22q,11.1-13.1). In contrast to NF1, tumors in NF2 frequently show deletions or loss of heterozygous DNA markers in the affected chromosome. The *NF2* gene encodes a tumor suppressor protein termed **merlin, or schwannomin,** which is a member of a superfamily of proteins that link the cytoskeleton to the cell membrane. This family also includes ezrin, moesin, radixin, talin and protein 4.1. Merlin is detectable in most differentiated tissues, including Schwann cells.

Achondroplastic Dwarfism

Achondroplastic dwarfism is an autosomal dominant, hereditary disease of epiphyseal chondroblastic development that leads to inadequate enchondral bone formation. This distinctive form of dwarfism is characterized by short limbs with a normal head and trunk. The affected person has a small face, a bulging forehead and a deeply indented bridge of the nose. Achondroplastic dwarfism is not rare, occurring in 1 per 3000 live births.

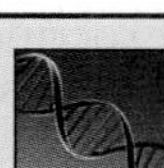

MOLECULAR PATHOGENESIS: Achondroplasia is associated with mutations in the basic fibroblast growth factor receptor 3 gene (*FGFR3*). This inactivating mutation removes the negative regulatory activity of this receptor on bone growth, resulting in an abnormality of cartilage formation and increased osteogenesis. New founder mutations in *FGFR3* are more frequent with advanced paternal age, are derived from the father and are developed during spermatogenesis. Achondroplasia is discussed in Chapter 26.

Familial Hypercholesterolemia

Familial hypercholesterolemia is an autosomal dominant disorder characterized by high levels of LDLs in the blood and deposition of cholesterol in arteries, tendons and skin. It is one of the most common autosomal dominant disorders, affecting 1 in 500 adults in the United States in its heterozygous form. Only 1 person in 1 million is homozygous for the disease. ***In this disease there is a striking acceleration of atherosclerosis and its complications*** (see Chapter 10).

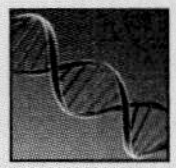

MOLECULAR PATHOGENESIS: In familial hypercholesterolemia the gene on the short arm of chromosome 19 that codes for the cell surface receptor that removes LDL from the blood is mutated. Over 150 different mutations in the LDL receptor gene are known. The LDL receptor is (1) synthesized in the endoplasmic reticulum (ER), (2) transferred to the Golgi, (3) transported to the cell surface and (4) internalized in coated pits by receptor-mediated endocytosis after it binds LDL. Genetic defects in each of these steps are known:

- **Class 1:** This is the most common defect. It leads to failure of synthesis of nascent LDL receptor protein in the ER, mostly due to large deletions in the gene (null alleles).
- **Class 2:** These mutations prevent transfer of the nascent receptor from the ER to the Golgi (transport-defective alleles), preventing it from appearing at the cell surface.
- **Class 3:** LDL receptors of class 3 mutations are expressed on the cell surface but are defective in the ligand-binding domain (binding-defective alleles).
- **Class 4:** These are rare mutations. LDL binding to the receptor is normal, but the receptor does not cluster in coated pits. Thus, receptor internalization by endocytosis is blocked (internalization-defective alleles).
- **Class 5:** Internalized LDL–receptor complexes remain within the endosome, and the receptor does not recycle to the plasma membrane (recycling-defective alleles).

Hepatocytes are the main cell type expressing LDL receptor. After LDLs bind the receptor, they are internalized and degraded in lysosomes, freeing cholesterol for further metabolism. If LDL receptor function is impaired, high levels of LDLs circulate, are taken up by tissue macrophages and accumulate to form occlusive arterial plaques (atheromas) and papules or nodules of lipid-laden macrophages (xanthomas) (see Chapter 10).

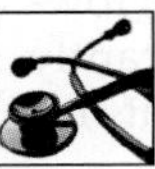

CLINICAL FEATURES: Heterozygous and homozygous familial hypercholesterolemia are distinct clinical syndromes, reflecting a clear gene-dosage effect.

Autosomal Recessive

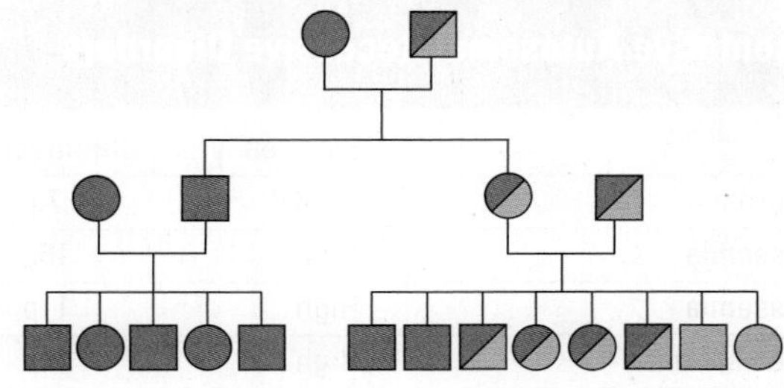

■● Homozygote with disease

◩◓ Heterozygote without disease (silent carrier)

FIGURE 6-20. Autosomal recessive inheritance. Symptoms of the disease appear only in homozygotes, male or female. Heterozygotes are asymptomatic carriers. Symptomatic homozygotes result from the mating of asymptomatic heterozygotes.

In heterozygotes, blood cholesterol (mean, 350 mg/dL; normal, <200 mg/dL) is elevated at birth. Tendon xanthomas develop in half the patients before age 30, and symptoms of coronary heart disease often occur before age 40. In homozygotes, blood cholesterol content is extremely high (600 to 1200 mg/dL) and virtually all patients have tendon xanthomas and generalized atherosclerosis in childhood. Untreated homozygotes typically die of myocardial infarction before 30 years of age.

Autosomal Recessive Disorders Cause Symptoms in People Who Have Defective Alleles on Both Homologous Chromosomes

Most genetic metabolic diseases show autosomal recessive inheritance (Fig. 6-20; Table 6-6). The fact that recessive genes are uncommon and the need for two mutant alleles to cause clinical disease determine the key characteristics of autosomal recessive inheritance. Some of the salient features of such disorders are:

- The more infrequent the mutant gene in the general population, the lower the chance that unrelated parents carry the trait. ***Rare autosomal recessive disorders often derive from consanguineous parents.***
- Both parents are usually heterozygous for the trait and are clinically normal.
- Symptoms appear in about 25% of their children. Half of all offspring are heterozygous for the trait and are asymptomatic. Thus, two thirds of unaffected offspring are heterozygous carriers.
- As in autosomal dominant disorders, autosomal recessive traits are transmitted equally to males and females.
- Symptoms of autosomal recessive disorders are ordinarily less variable than in autosomal dominant diseases. Recessive traits therefore present more commonly in childhood, while dominant disorders may initially appear in adults.
- The variability in clinical expression of many autosomal recessive diseases may reflect residual functionality of the affected enzyme. This variability is manifested in (1) different degrees of clinical severity, (2) age at onset or (3) the existence of acute and chronic forms of the specific disease.

Table 6-6

Representative Autosomal Recessive Disorders

Disease	Frequency	Chromosome
Cystic fibrosis	1/2500	7q
α-Thalassemia	High	16p
β-Thalassemia	High	11p
Sickle cell anemia	High	11p
Myeloperoxidase deficiency	1/2000	17q
Phenylketonuria	1/10,000	12q
Gaucher disease	1/1000	1q
Tay-Sachs disease	1/4000	15q
Hurler syndrome	1/100,000	22p
Glycogen storage disease Ia (von Gierke disease)	1/100,000	17
Wilson disease	1/50,000	13q
Hereditary hemochromatosis	1/1000	6p
α_1-Antitrypsin deficiency	1/7000	14q
Oculocutaneous albinism	1/20,000	11q
Alkaptonuria	<1/100,000	3q
Metachromatic leukodystrophy	1/100,000	22q

Most mutant genes responsible for autosomal recessive disorders are rare in the general population, since those homozygous for the trait often die before reproductive age. However, a few lethal autosomal recessive diseases, such as sickle cell anemia and cystic fibrosis (CF), are common. Heterozygosity for the sickle cell trait may increase resistance to malaria. There is no known survival advantage to possession of a mutant CF gene.

New mutations for recessive diseases are difficult to identify clinically because heterozygotes are asymptomatic. Nonconsanguineous mating of two such heterozygotes would occur by chance, and many generations later, if at all.

Biochemical Basis of Autosomal Recessive Disorders

Autosomal recessive diseases are usually due to deficiencies in enzymes rather than in structural proteins. A mutation that inactivates an enzyme rarely causes an abnormal phenotype in heterozygotes: most cellular enzymes operate at substrate concentrations well below saturation, so an enzyme deficiency is easily corrected simply by increasing the amount of substrate. In autosomal recessive diseases caused by impaired catabolism of dietary substances (e.g., phenylketonuria, galactosemia) or cellular constituents (e.g., Tay-Sachs, Hurler), increased substrate concentrations in heterozygotes overcome partial lack of the enzyme. By contrast, loss of both alleles in a homozygote results in complete loss of enzyme activity, which cannot be corrected by such mechanisms.

Cystic Fibrosis

Cystic fibrosis (CF) is the most common lethal autosomal recessive disorder in the white population. CF is characterized by (1) chronic pulmonary disease; (2) deficient exocrine pancreatic function; and (3) other complications of inspissated mucus in several organs, including the small intestine, liver and reproductive tract. The disease results from a defective chloride channel, the cystic fibrosis transmembrane conductance regulator (CFTR).

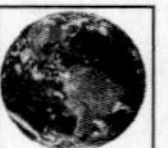

EPIDEMIOLOGY: More than 95% of cases occur in whites; the disease is rarely found in blacks and almost never in Asians. About 1 in 25 whites is a heterozygous carrier, and the incidence of the disease is 1 in 2500. Among the white population, incidence of CF varies with geography. It is highest in northern European Celtic populations such as Ireland and Scotland, and much lower among southern Europeans. Ashkenazi Jews have a high incidence of CF.

MOLECULAR PATHOGENESIS: The CFTR gene is on the long arm of chromosome 7 (7q31.2) (Table 6-6). It encodes a protein of 1480 amino acids that is a member of the adenosine triphosphate (ATP)-binding cassette transporter (ABC transporter) superfamily of membrane transporters, which is phylogenetically one of the oldest gene families. Designated the CFTR, it functions as a halide ion transporter in most epithelial cells. It has two ATP-hydrolyzing domains that drive the transporter function. It also has two domains, containing six hydrophobic helices in each, that anchor the transporter as a transmembrane spanning protein. There are two R domains, which have phosphorylation sites for cyclic adenosine 3′,5′-monophosphate (cAMP)-dependent protein kinase A and regulate chloride channel activity by increasing ATP binding.

CFTR activity is regulated by the balance between kinase and phosphatase activities (i.e., phosphorylation and dephosphorylation). Phosphorylation of the R domain, mostly by cAMP-dependent protein kinase A, stimulates chloride channel activity by enhancing ATP binding. Secretion of chloride anions by mucus-secreting epithelial cells controls the parallel secretion of fluid and, consequently, the viscosity of the mucus. In normal mucus-secreting epithelia, cAMP activates protein kinase A, which phosphorylates the regulatory domain of CFTR and permits channel opening. The most common mutation in the white population is a deletion of 3 base pairs, which deletes a phenylalanine residue (ΔF_{508}), producing an abnormally folded protein that is degraded. ΔF_{508} accounts for 70% of CFTR mutations in the white population. Mutations in the *CFTR* gene that disturb chloride channel function fall into several functional groupings (Fig. 6-21):

- **Failure of CFTR synthesis:** Mutations that result in premature termination signals interfere with synthesis of the full-length CFTR protein. As a result, there is no CFTR-mediated chloride secretion in involved epithelia.
- **Failure of CFTR transport to the plasma membrane:** Some mutations prevent proper folding of the nascent protein, so it is then targeted for proteasomal degradation rather than for transport to the plasma membrane (see Chapter 1). The ΔF_{508} mutation is of this class. However, the role of this mutation in CF varies significantly by geography and ethnicity. In Denmark, it accounts for

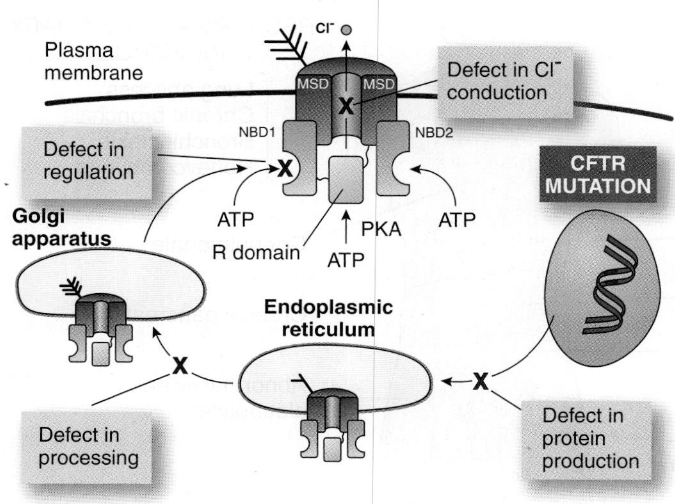

FIGURE 6-21. Cellular sites of the disruptions in the synthesis and function of cystic fibrosis transmembrane conductance regulator (CFTR) in cystic fibrosis (CF). ATP = adenosine triphosphate; Cl^- = chloride ion; MSD = membrane-spanning domain; NBD = nucleotide-binding domain; PKA = protein kinase A.

almost 90% of CF cases, but only 30% among Ashkenazi Jews. Analysis of haplotypes suggests that F_{508} originated 50,000 years ago in the Middle East, from where it progressively spread throughout Europe.

- **Defective ATP binding to CFTR:** Certain mutations allow CFTR proteins to reach the plasma membrane but affect ATP-binding domains, thus interfering with regulation of the channel and decreasing, but not abolishing, chloride secretion.
- **Defective chloride secretion by mutant CFTR:** Mutations in the channel pore inhibit chloride secretion.

The relationship between these genotypes (more than 1000 mutations are known) and the clinical severity of CF is complicated and not always consistent. The best correlation relates to pancreatic insufficiency. Severe symptoms are generally found in those with pancreatic insufficiency (85% of all cases of CF), whereas in milder cases pancreatic function is preserved. Class I and class II mutations are generally found among severely affected patients. By contrast, milder forms of CF feature class III and class IV mutations.

All pathologic consequences of CF reflect the abnormally thick mucus, which obstructs airway lumina, pancreatic and biliary ducts and the fetal intestine. CF was once called **mucoviscidosis.** Normal CFTR corrects the defect in chloride secretion in cultured cells from CF patients.

PATHOLOGY: CF affects many organs that produce exocrine secretions.

RESPIRATORY TRACT: ***Lung disease is responsible for most morbidity and mortality associated with CF.*** The earliest lesion is obstruction of bronchioles by mucus, with secondary infection and inflammation of bronchiolar walls. Recurrent cycles of obstruction and infection result in **chronic bronchiolitis** and **bronchitis,** which increase in severity as the disease progresses. Bronchial mucous glands undergo hypertrophy and hyperplasia, and airways are distended by thick and tenacious secretions. Widespread **bronchiectasis** is apparent by age 10 and often earlier. Late in the disease, large bronchiectatic cysts and lung abscesses are common. Secondary pulmonary hypertension may complicate the chronic bronchitis.

PANCREAS: Most patients (85%) with CF have a form of **chronic pancreatitis,** and in long-standing cases, little or no functional exocrine pancreas remains. Inspissated secretions in central pancreatic ducts produce secondary dilation and cystic change of the distal ducts (Fig. 6-22). Recurrent pancreatitis leads to loss of acinar cells and extensive fibrosis. At autopsy, the pancreas is often simply cystic fibroadipose tissue containing islets of Langerhans. The finding of pancreatic cysts and fibrosis led to the original name of cystic fibrosis.

LIVER: Inspissated mucous secretions in the intrahepatic biliary system obstruct the flow of bile in the drainage areas of the affected ducts and lead to focal **secondary biliary cirrhosis,** which is seen in one fourth of patients at autopsy. Inspissated concretions are seen in bile ducts and ductules, as are chronic portal inflammation and septal fibrosis. Sometimes (<5%), hepatic lesions are sufficiently widespread to lead to the clinical manifestations of biliary cirrhosis.

GASTROINTESTINAL TRACT: Shortly after birth, a normal newborn passes the intestinal contents that have accumulated in utero (meconium). The most important lesion of the gut in CF is small bowel obstruction in the newborn, **meconium ileus,** which is caused by failure to pass meconium in the immediate postpartum period. This occurs in 5% to 10% of newborns with CF and has been attributed to the failure of pancreatic secretions to digest meconium, possibly augmented by the greater viscosity of small bowel secretions.

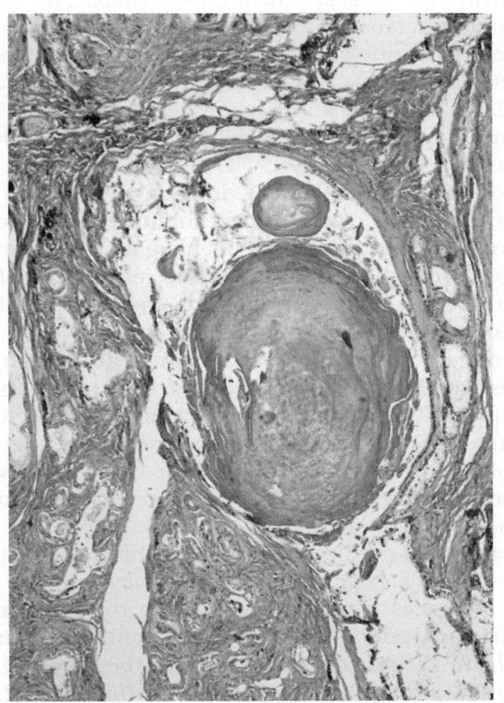

FIGURE 6-22. Intraductal concretion and atrophy of the acini in the pancreas of a patient with cystic fibrosis.

FIGURE 6-23. Clinical features of cystic fibrosis.

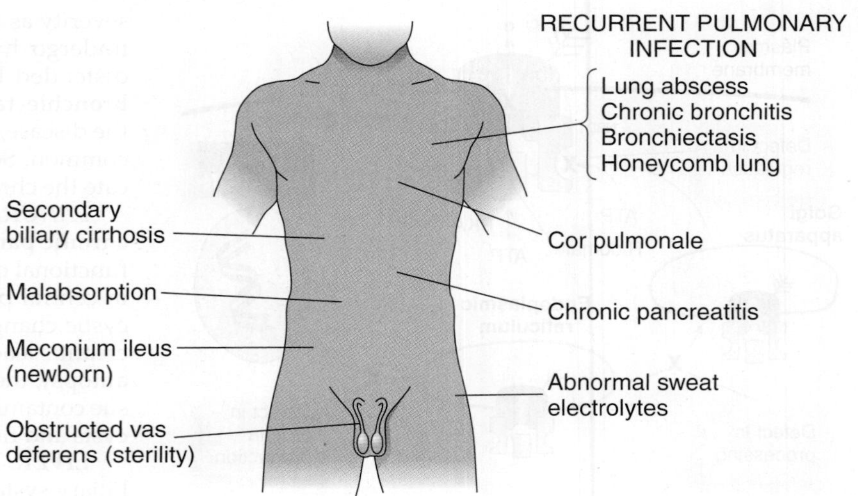

REPRODUCTIVE TRACT: Almost all boys with CF have atrophy or fibrosis of the reproductive duct system, including the vas deferens, epididymis and seminal vesicles. These lesions are due to luminal obstruction by inspissated secretions early in life and even in utero. Thus, only 2% to 3% of males are fertile, with spermatozoa absent from the semen in the rest.

A minority of women with CF are fertile, and many of them suffer from anovulatory cycles as a result of poor nutrition and chronic infections. Moreover, the cervical mucous plug is abnormally thick and tenacious.

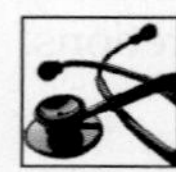

CLINICAL FEATURES: ***The diagnosis of CF is most reliably made by detecting increased concentrations of electrolytes in the sweat and by genetic studies that demonstrate the disease-causing mutations.*** The decreased chloride conductance characteristic of CF results in failure of chloride reabsorption by the cells of the sweat gland ducts and hence to accumulation of sodium chloride in the sweat (Fig. 6-23). Children with CF have been described as "tasting salty" and may even display salt crystals on their skin after vigorous sweating.

The clinical course of CF is highly variable. At one extreme, death may result from meconium ileus in the neonatal period, whereas some patients have reportedly survived to age 50. Improved medical care and recognition of milder cases of CF have helped to prolong the average life span, which is now about 30 years of age.

Pulmonary symptoms of CF begin with cough, which becomes productive of large amounts of tenacious and purulent sputum. Repeated infectious bronchitis and bronchopneumonia become progressively more frequent, and eventually shortness of breath develops. Respiratory failure and cardiac complications of pulmonary hypertension (cor pulmonale) are late sequelae.

The most common organisms that infect the respiratory tract in CF are *Staphylococcus* and *Pseudomonas* spp. As the disease advances, *Pseudomonas* may be the only organism cultured from the lung. ***In fact, recovery of*** **Pseudomonas sp.,** ***particularly the mucoid variety, from the lungs of a child with chronic pulmonary disease is virtually diagnostic of CF.*** Infection with *Burkholderia cepacia* is associated with **cepacia syndrome,** a very severe pulmonary infection that is highly resistant to antibiotics and is commonly fatal.

Failure of pancreatic exocrine secretion leads to fat and protein malabsorption, causing bulky, foul-smelling stools (steatorrhea), nutritional deficiencies and growth retardation.

Postural drainage of airways, antibiotic therapy and pancreatic enzyme supplementation are the mainstays of treatment. Molecular prenatal diagnosis of CF is now accurate in 95% of cases.

In Lysosomal Storage Diseases Unmetabolized Normal Substrates Accumulate in Lysosomes Because of Deficiencies of Specific Acid Hydrolases

Lysosomes are membrane-bound collections of hydrolytic enzymes that are used for controlled intracellular digestion of macromolecules. Lysosomal digestive enzymes are called "acid hydrolases" since their optimal activities are at acidic pHs (pH 3.5 to 5.5). This environment is maintained by an ATP-dependent proton pump in the lysosomal membrane. These enzymes degrade virtually all types of biological macromolecules. Extracellular macromolecules that are incorporated by endocytosis or phagocytosis and intracellular constituents that are subjected to autophagy are digested in lysosomes to their basic components (see Chapter 1). End-products may be transported across lysosomal membranes into the cytosol, where they are reused in the synthesis of new macromolecules.

Virtually all lysosomal storage diseases result from mutations in genes for lysosomal hydrolases. A deficiency in one of the more than 40 acid hydrolases can result in an inability to catabolize the normal macromolecular substrate of that enzyme. As a result, undigested substrates accumulate in, and engorge, lysosomes, expanding the lysosomal compartment of the cell. Resulting lysosomal distention occurs at the expense of other critical cellular components, particularly in the brain and heart, and can lead to a failure of cell function.

Lysosomal storage diseases are classified according to the material retained in the lysosomes. Thus, when accumulated substrates are sphingolipids, they are **sphingolipidoses.** Storage of mucopolysaccharides (glycosaminoglycans) leads to the **mucopolysaccharidoses.** More than 30 lysosomal storage diseases are known, but we limit our discussion to the more important ones.

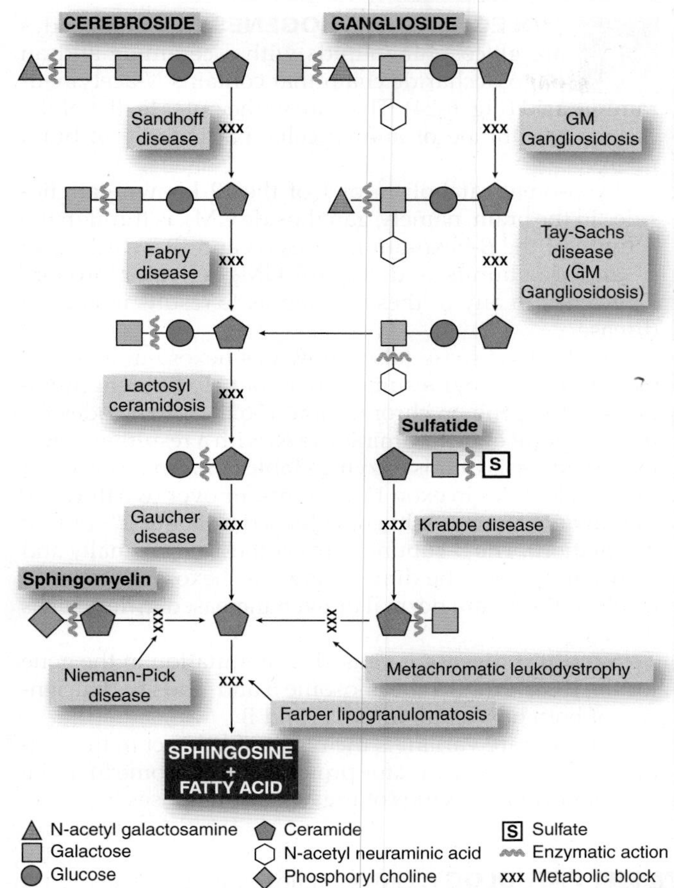

FIGURE 6-24. Disturbances of lipid metabolism in various sphingolipidoses.

Sphingolipidoses are lysosomal storage diseases in which lipids derived from the turnover of obsolete cell membranes accumulate. Cerebrosides, gangliosides, sphingomyelin and sulfatides are sphingolipid components of the membranes of a variety of cells. These substances are degraded within lysosomes by complex pathways to sphingosine and fatty acids (Fig. 6-24). Deficiencies of many of the acid hydrolases that mediate specific steps in these pathways lead to accumulation of undigested intermediate substrates in the lysosomes.

Gaucher Disease

Gaucher disease is characterized by accumulation of glucosylceramide, mainly in macrophage lysosomes. The disorder was first described in 1882 in a doctoral thesis by Gaucher, but its familial occurrence was not recognized for some 20 years.

MOLECULAR PATHOGENESIS: The abnormal enzyme is glucocerebrosidase, a lysosomal acid β-glucosidase. The enzyme deficiency can be traced to a variety of single base mutations in the β-glucosidase gene, on the long arm of chromosome 1 (1q21) (Table 6-6). Each of the three clinical types of the disease (see below) exhibits heterogeneous mutations in the β-glucosidase gene, although the molecular basis for the phenotypic differences remains to be firmly established.

The glucosylceramide that accumulates in Gaucher cells of the spleen, liver, bone marrow and lymph nodes derives principally from catabolism of membranes of senescent leukocytes, which are rich in cerebrosides. When membrane degradation is blocked by a lack of glucocerebrosidase, glucosylceramide, the intermediate metabolite, accumulates. The glucosylceramide of Gaucher cells in the brain is believed to originate from turnover of plasma membrane gangliosides of cells in the CNS.

PATHOLOGY: The hallmark of this disorder is the **Gaucher cells,** lipid-laden macrophages characteristically seen in the red pulp of the spleen, liver sinusoids, lymph nodes, lungs and bone marrow, although they may appear in virtually any organ. These cells are derived from resident macrophages in the respective organs, for example, Kupffer cells in the liver and alveolar macrophages in the lung. In the uncommon variants of Gaucher disease with involvement of the CNS, Gaucher cells originate from periadventitial cells in Virchow-Robin spaces.

Gaucher cells are large (20 to 100 μm) with eccentric nuclei and clear cytoplasm (Fig. 6-25) that has a characteristic fibrillar appearance, which has been likened to "wrinkled tissue paper" and is intensely positive with periodic acid–Schiff (PAS) stain. The material is stored within enlarged lysosomes and appears as parallel layers of tubular structures.

Splenic enlargement is virtually universal in Gaucher disease. In the adult form of the disorder, splenomegaly may be massive, weighing up to 10 kg. The cut surface of the enlarged spleen is firm and pale and often contains sharply demarcated infarcts. The red pulp shows nodular and diffuse infiltrates of Gaucher cells and moderate fibrosis.

The liver is usually enlarged by Gaucher cells within sinusoids, but hepatocytes are not affected. In severe cases, hepatic fibrosis and even cirrhosis may ensue. Bone marrow involvement is variable but leads to radiologic abnormalities in 50% to 75% of cases (see Chapter 26).

Gaucher cells may also be found in many other organs, including lymph nodes, lungs, endocrine glands, skin,

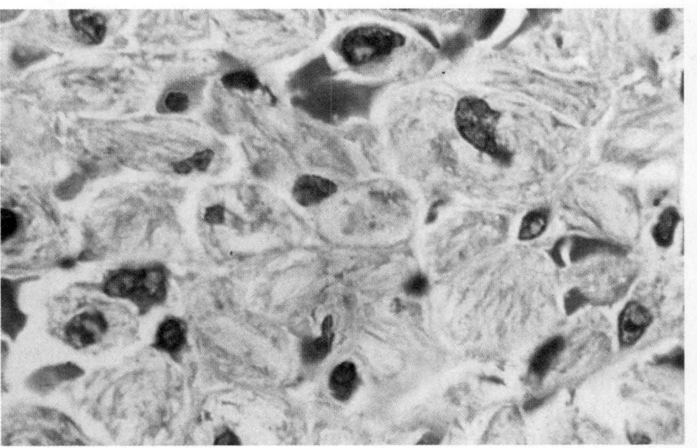

FIGURE 6-25. The spleen in Gaucher disease. Typical Gaucher cells have foamy cytoplasm and eccentrically located nuclei.

gastrointestinal tract and kidneys, although symptoms referable to these organs are uncommon.

When the brain is affected, Gaucher cells are present in Virchow-Robin spaces around blood vessels. In the infantile (neuronopathic) form of Gaucher disease, these cells have also been found in the parenchyma, where they may stimulate gliosis and formation of microglial nodules.

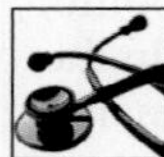

CLINICAL FEATURES: Gaucher disease is classified into three distinct forms, based on the age at onset and degree of neurologic involvement.

- **Type 1 (chronic nonneuronopathic):** This variant is the most common of all lysosomal storage diseases and is found mainly in adult Ashkenazi Jews, among whom the incidence is 1 in 600 to 1 in 2500. Age at onset is highly variable, some cases being diagnosed in infants and others at age 70 years. Similarly, the severity of clinical manifestations varies widely. Most cases are diagnosed as adults and present initially as painless splenomegaly and complications of hypersplenism (i.e., anemia, leukopenia and thrombocytopenia). Hepatomegaly is common, but clinical liver disease is infrequent. Bone involvement, in the form of pain and pathologic fractures, can cause disability severe enough to confine a patient to a wheelchair.
  The life expectancy of most patients with type 1 Gaucher disease is normal, and the disease is now treated by intravenous administration of modified acid glucose cerebrosidase, although its extremely high cost limits its use. Marrow transplantation is also effective but is little used because of the attendant risks. Prenatal diagnosis, based on β-glucosidase activity in amniotic fluid or chorionic villi or on DNA technology, is now routinely available.
- **Type 2 (acute neuronopathic):** Type 2 Gaucher disease is rare and distinctly different from type 1 in age at onset and clinical presentation. It usually presents by age 3 months with hepatosplenomegaly and has no ethnic predilection. Within a few months, infants show neurologic signs, with the classic triad of trismus, strabismus and backward flexion of the neck. Further neurologic deterioration rapidly ensues. Most patients die by the age of 1 year.
- **Type 3 (subacute neuronopathic):** This form is also rare and combines features of types 1 and 2. Neurologic deterioration starts later than in type 2 and progresses more slowly.

Tay-Sachs Disease (GM_2 Gangliosidosis Type 1)

Tay-Sachs disease is a catastrophic infantile form of a class of lysosomal storage diseases known as the GM_2 gangliosidoses, in which this ganglioside is deposited in neurons of the CNS, owing to a failure of lysosomal degradation. The association of a "cherry-red spot" in the retina and profound mental and physical retardation was first pointed out in 1881 by Warren Tay, a British ophthalmologist. Fifteen years later, Bernard Sachs, an American neurologist, described the histologic features of the disorder and coined the term "amaurotic (blind) family idiocy." Tay-Sachs disease is inherited as an autosomal recessive trait and is mainly seen in Ashkenazi Jews, among whom the carrier rate is 1 in 30, with homozygotes seen in 1 in 4000 live newborns. By contrast, the incidence in non–Jewish American populations is less than 1 in 100,000. Screening programs for heterozygotes among Ashkenazi Jews have now reduced the disease incidence by 90%. The other GM_2 gangliosidoses are exceedingly rare.

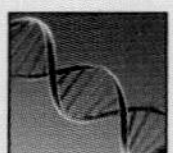

MOLECULAR PATHOGENESIS: Gangliosides are glycosphingolipids with a ceramide and an oligosaccharide chain that contains *N*-acetylneuraminic acid (Fig. 6-24). They are in the outer leaflet of the plasma membrane of animal cells, particularly in brain neurons.

Lysosomal catabolism of 1 of the 12 known gangliosides in the brain, namely, ganglioside GM_2, is through the activity of the β-hexosaminidases (A and B), which have α- and β-subunits and require GM_2-activator protein. Deficiency in any of these components results in clinical disease.

Tay-Sachs disease (also known as hexosaminidase α-subunit deficiency) results from about 50 different mutations in the gene on chromosome 15q23-24 that codes for the α-subunit of hexosaminidase A, with a resulting defect in the synthesis of this enzyme (Table 6-6). An insertion of four nucleotides in exon 11 accounts for over two thirds of the carriers among Ashkenazi Jews (i.e., about 2% of that population). The β-subunits are synthesized normally and associate to form the dimer known as hexosaminidase B, levels of which are normal or even increased in Tay-Sachs disease.

Sandhoff disease is caused by a mutation in the gene for the β-subunit on chromosome 5 and leads to deficiencies of both hexosaminidases A and B.

A third, rare variant is the result of a defect in the synthesis of the GM_2-activator protein (chromosome 5) in the face of normal activities of the hexosaminidases.

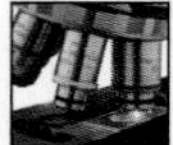

PATHOLOGY: GM_2 ganglioside accumulates in lysosomes of all organs in Tay-Sachs disease, but it is most prominent in brain neurons and cells of the retina. The size of the brain varies with the length of survival of affected infants. Early cases are marked by brain atrophy, but the organ weight may be as much as doubled in those who survive beyond a year. Neurons are markedly distended with storage material that stains positively for lipids. By electron microscopy, neurons are stuffed with "membranous cytoplasmic bodies," composed of concentric whorls of lamellar structures (Fig. 6-26). As disease progresses, neurons are lost and many lipid-laden macrophages are conspicuous in the cortical gray matter. Eventually, gliosis becomes prominent and myelin and axons in the white matter are lost. The pathologies of the other forms of GM_2 gangliosidosis are similar to those of Tay-Sachs disease, although usually less severe.

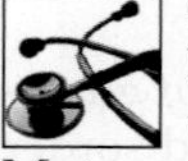

CLINICAL FEATURES: Tay-Sachs disease presents between 6 and 10 months of age with progressive weakness, hypotonia and decreased attentiveness. Motor and mental deterioration, often with generalized seizures, follow rapidly. Vision is seriously impaired. Involvement of retinal ganglion cells is detected by ophthalmoscopy as a **cherry-red spot** in the macula. This feature reflects the pallor of the affected cells, which enhances the prominence of blood vessels underlying the central fovea. Most children with Tay-Sachs disease die before 4 years of age.

Niemann-Pick Disease

In Niemann-Pick disease (NPD), lysosomal storage of **sphingomyelin** is seen in macrophages of many organs, in

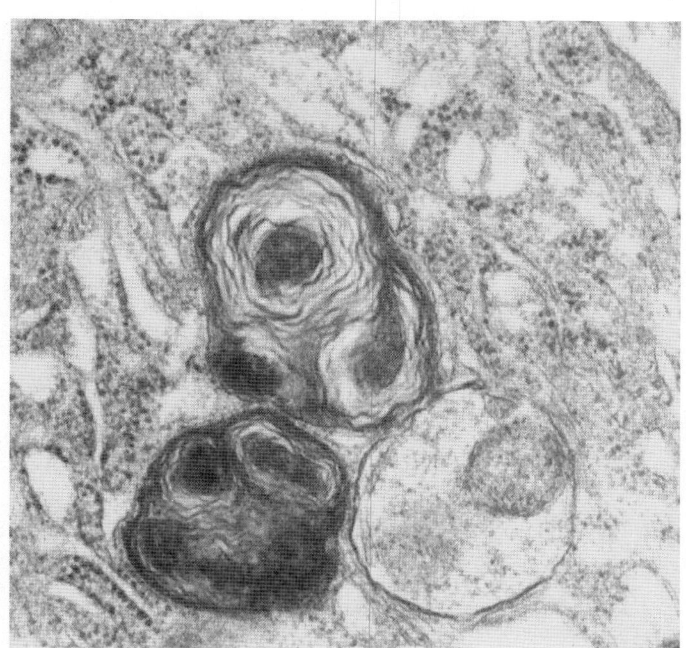

FIGURE 6-26. Tay-Sachs disease. The cytoplasm of the nerve cell contains lysosomes filled with whorled membranes.

hepatocytes and in the brain. There are two variants, **types A and B.** Type A NPD appears in infancy, with hepatosplenomegaly and progressive neurodegeneration. Death occurs by 3 years of age. Type B NPD is more variable, with hepatosplenomegaly, minimal neurologic symptomatology and survival to adulthood. NPD is seen in many ethnic groups but is particularly common among Ashkenazi Jews, among whom the incidence of type A NPD is 1 in 40,000 and of type B 1 in 80,000. The combined heterozygote prevalence is 1 in 100.

MOLECULAR PATHOGENESIS: Sphingomyelin is a membrane phospholipid composed of phosphorylcholine, sphingosine (a long-chain amino alcohol) and a fatty acid. It accounts for up to 14% of all phospholipids of the liver, spleen and brain. The metabolic defect in NPD reflects 12 different mutations in the gene (11p15.1-15.4) for **sphingomyelinase,** the lysosomal enzyme that hydrolyzes sphingomyelin to ceramide and phosphorylcholine. Type A NPD patients have no sphingomyelinase activity; in type B patients up to 10% of normal activity can be detected.

PATHOLOGY: The characteristic storage cell in NPD is a foam cell, that is, an enlarged (20- to 90-μm) macrophage in which the cytoplasm is distended by uniform vacuoles that contain sphingomyelin and cholesterol. By electron microscopy, whorls of concentrically arranged lamellar structures distend the lysosomes.

Foam cells are particularly abundant in the spleen, lymph nodes and bone marrow but are also found in the liver, lungs and gastrointestinal tract. The spleen is enlarged, often massively, and foam cells are diffusely distributed throughout the red pulp. Lymph nodes enlarged by foam cells are seen in many locations. The hematopoietic tissues in the bone marrow may be displaced by aggregates of foam cells. The liver is enlarged by the stored sphingomyelin and cholesterol in lysosomes of both Kupffer cells and hepatocytes.

The brain is the most important organ involved in type A NPD, and neurologic damage is the usual cause of death. At autopsy, the brain is atrophic and in severe cases may be half of normal weight. Neurons are distended by vacuoles with the same stored lipids found elsewhere in the body. In advanced cases neuron loss is severe and may be accompanied by demyelination. Foam cells are noted in many locations. Half of children affected by type A disease have cherry-red retinal spots, as in Tay-Sachs disease.

CLINICAL FEATURES: Type A NPD manifests in early infancy with conspicuous spleen and liver enlargement and psychomotor retardation. Motor and intellectual function are lost over time, and children typically die between the ages of 2 and 3 years. Most type B patients present in childhood with marked hepatosplenomegaly. Pulmonary infiltration with sphingomyelin-laden macrophages eventually impairs respiratory function in many patients with type B disease. However, these patients have few neurologic symptoms and may survive for many years.

Mucopolysaccharidoses

The mucopolysaccharidoses (MPSs) are a group of lysosomal storage diseases in which **glycosaminoglycans (mucopolysaccharides)** accumulate in many organs. All are inherited as autosomal recessive traits, except for Hunter syndrome, which is X-linked recessive. These rare diseases are caused by deficiencies in any 1 of the 10 lysosomal enzymes that catabolize glycosaminoglycans (Fig. 6-27). Six abnormal phenotypes are described, each varying with the specific enzyme deficiency (Table 6-7).

MOLECULAR PATHOGENESIS: Glycosaminoglycans (GAGs) are large polymers of repeating disaccharide units containing *N*-acetylhexosamine and a hexose or hexuronic acid. Either disaccharide may be sulfated. The accumulated GAGs (dermatan sulfate, heparan sulfate, keratan sulfate and chondroitin sulfate) in MPS are all derived from cleavage of proteoglycans, which are important extracellular matrix constituents. GAGs are degraded stepwise by removing sugar residues or sulfate groups. Thus, a deficiency in any one of the glycosidases or sulfatases results in accumulation of undegraded GAGs. A special case is a deficiency of an *N*-acetyltransferase, which leads to deposition of heparan sulfate in Sanfilippo C disease.

PATHOLOGY: Although the severity and location of lesions in MPS vary with the specific enzyme deficiency, most of these syndromes share certain common features. The undegraded GAGs tend to accumulate in connective tissue cells, mononuclear phagocytes (including Kupffer cells), endothelial cells, neurons and hepatocytes. Affected cells are swollen and clear and stains for metachromasia confirm the presence of GAGs. Electron microscopy shows many enlarged lysosomes containing granular or striped material. The most important lesions involve the CNS,

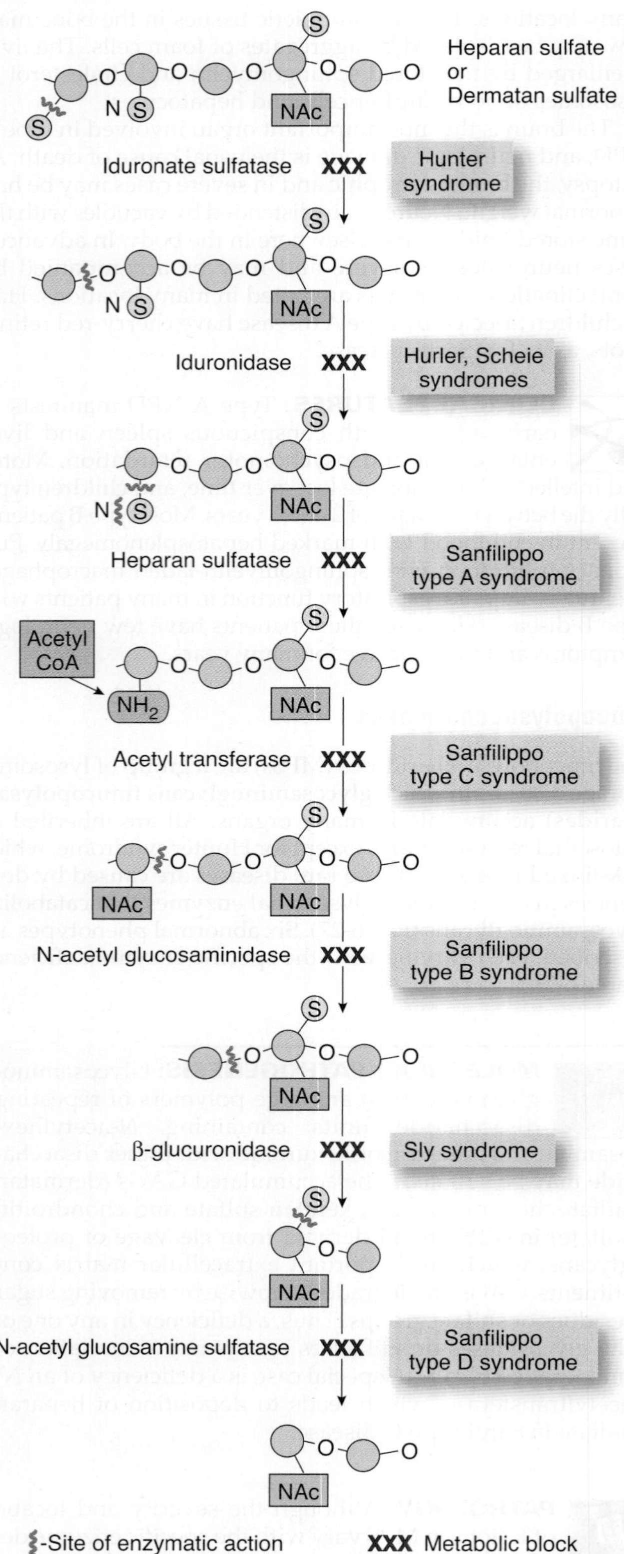

FIGURE 6-27. Metabolic blocks in various mucopolysaccharidoses that affect the degradation of heparan sulfate and dermatan sulfate. Acetyl CoA = acetyl coenzyme A; Nac = *N*-acetyl moiety.

Table 6-7

Mucopolysaccharidoses

Type	Eponym	Location of Gene	Clinical Features
I H	Hurler	4p16.3	Organomegaly, cardiac lesions, dysostosis multiplex, corneal clouding, death in childhood
I S	Scheie	4p16.3	Stiff joints, corneal clouding, normal intelligence, longevity
II	Hunter	X	Organomegaly, dysostosis multiplex, mental retardation, death earlier than 15 years of age
III	Sanfilippo	12q14	Mental retardation
IV	Morquio	16q24	Skeletal deformities, corneal clouding
V	Obsolete	—	—
VI	Maroteaux Lamy	5q13–14	Dysostosis multiplex, corneal clouding, death in second decade
VII	Sly	7q21.1–22	Hepatosplenomegaly, dysostosis multiplex

skeleton and heart, although hepatosplenomegaly and corneal clouding are common.

- Initially, **the CNS** only accumulates GAGs, but as the disease advances, extensive loss of neurons and increasing gliosis occur, leading to cortical atrophy. Communicating hydrocephalus, due to meningeal involvement, is common.
- **Skeletal deformities** result from CAG accumulation in chondrocytes, a process that eventually interferes with normal endochondral ossification. Abnormal foci of osteoid and woven bone are common in the deformed skeleton.
- **Cardiac lesions** are often severe, with thickening and distortion of valves, chordae tendineae and endocardium. The coronary arteries are frequently narrowed by intimal thickening caused by GAG deposits in smooth muscle cells.
- **Hepatosplenomegaly** is secondary to distention of Kupffer cells and hepatocytes in the liver and accumulation of CAG-filled macrophages in the spleen.

CLINICAL FEATURES: Hurler syndrome (MPS IH) is the most severe clinical form of MPS and is the prototype for these syndromes. The clinical features of other varieties of MPS are summarized in Table 6-7. The symptoms of Hurler syndrome appear between 6 months and 2 years of age. Children typically show skeletal deformities, enlarged livers and spleens, a characteristic facies and joint stiffness. The combination of coarse facial features and dwarfism is reminiscent of gargoyle figures that decorate Gothic cathedrals and accounts for the old term, **gargoylism,** for this syndrome.

Children with Hurler syndrome suffer developmental delay, hearing loss, corneal clouding and progressive mental deterioration. Increased intracranial pressure, due to communicating hydrocephalus, can be troublesome. Most patients die from recurrent pulmonary infections and cardiac complications before they reach 10 years.

Detection of heterozygotes is difficult because of the overlap in enzyme activity of cultured cells with the normal population. Prenatal diagnosis is possible for all the MPSs and is routine for Hurler and Hunter syndromes.

Glycogenoses (Glycogen Storage Diseases)

MOLECULAR PATHOGENESIS: The glycogenoses are a group at least 10 inherited disorders characterized by glycogen accumulation, mainly in the liver, skeletal muscle and heart. Each entity reflects a deficiency of one of the enzymes involved in glycogen metabolism (Fig. 6-28). Save for X-linked phosphorylase kinase deficiency, all glycogen storage diseases are autosomal recessive traits. These diseases are rare: they occur in 1 in 100,000 to 1 in 1 million births.

Glycogen is a large glucose polymer (20,000 to 30,000 glucose units per molecule) that is stored in most cells to provide a ready source of energy during the fasting state. Liver and muscle are particularly rich in glycogen, although its function is different in each organ. The liver stores glycogen not for its own use but rather for rapid supply of glucose to the blood, particularly to benefit the brain. By contrast, glycogen in skeletal muscle is used as a local fuel when oxygen or glucose supplies fall. Glycogen is made and degraded by a number of enzymes, deficiency in any of which leads to accumulation of glycogen.

Although each glycogen storage disease causes glycogen accumulation, the significant organ involvement varies with the specific enzyme defect. Some mainly affect the liver, whereas others principally cause cardiac or skeletal muscle dysfunction. ***Symptoms of a glycogenosis may reflect either accumulation of glycogen itself (Pompe disease, Andersen disease) or a lack of the glucose that is normally derived from glycogen degradation (von Gierke disease, McArdle disease).*** We discuss only several representative examples of the known glycogenoses.

VON GIERKE DISEASE (TYPE IA GLYCOGENOSIS): In von Gierke disease glucose-6-phosphatase is lacking. Glycogen accumulates in the liver, and symptoms reflect the inability of the liver to convert glycogen to glucose, leading to hepatomegaly and hypoglycemia. The disorder usually presents in infancy or early childhood. Growth is commonly stunted, but with treatment, the prognosis for normal mental development and longevity are generally good.

POMPE DISEASE (TYPE II GLYCOGENOSIS): Pompe disease is a lysosomal storage disease that involves virtually all organs and results in death from heart failure before the age of 2. Juvenile and adult variants are less common and have a better prognosis. Normally, a small proportion of cytoplasmic glycogen is degraded within lysosomes

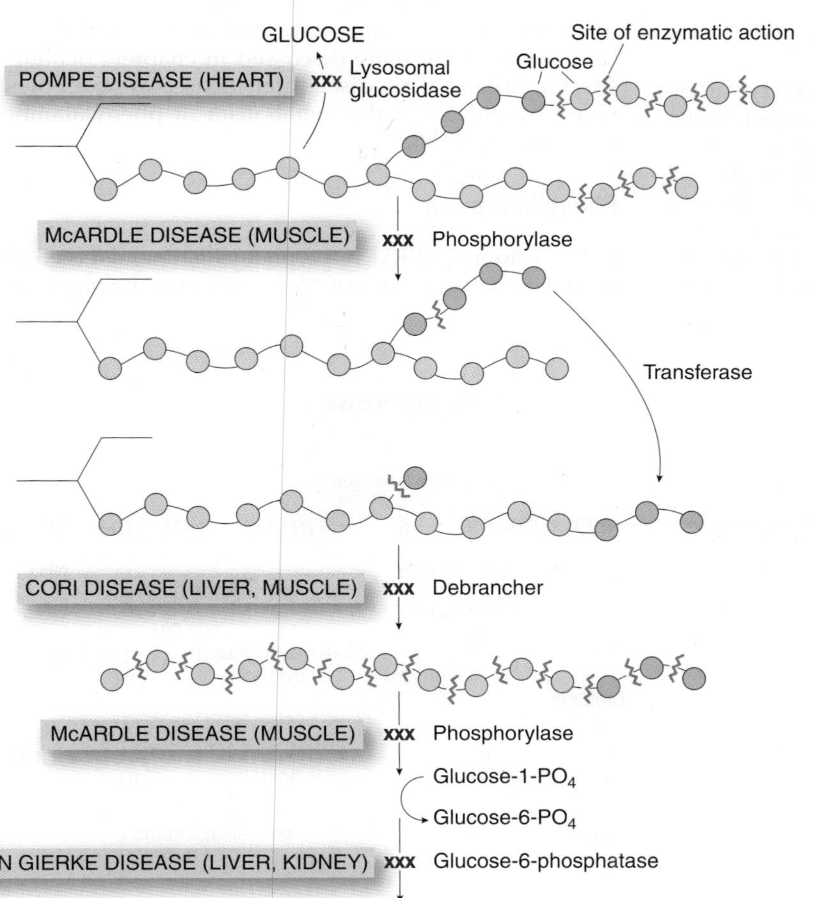

FIGURE 6-28. Sequential catabolism of glycogen and the enzymes that are deficient in various glycogenoses. Glycogen is a long-chain branched polymer of glucose residues, which are connected by α-1,4 linkages, except at branch points, where an α-1,6 linkage is present. Phosphorylase hydrolyzes α-1,4 linkages to a point three glucose residues distal to an α-1,6–linked sugar. These three glucose residues are transferred to the chain linked by α-1,4 bonds, by the bifunctional debrancher enzyme amylo-1,6-glucosidase. Subsequently, the same enzyme removes the α-1,6–linked sugar at the original branch point. This creates a linear α-1,4 chain, which is degraded by phosphorylase to glucose-1-phosphate. Following the conversion to glucose-6-phosphate, glucose is released by the action of glucose-6-phosphatase. A small proportion of glycogen is totally degraded within lysosomes by acid α-glucosidase. Red x's indicate metabolic block.

after an autophagic sequence. Type II glycogenosis is caused by a deficiency in the lysosomal enzyme acid α-glucosidase (17q23), which leads to inexorable accumulation of undegraded glycogen in lysosomes of many different cells. Interestingly, patients do not suffer from hypoglycemia, because the major metabolic pathways of glycogen synthesis and degradation in the cytoplasm are intact.

ANDERSEN DISEASE (TYPE IV GLYCOGENOSIS): Andersen disease is a very rare condition in which the branching enzyme (amyloglucantransferase) (3p12) that creates the branch points in normal glycogen molecules is lacking. The absence of the branching enzyme leads to formation and accumulation of an abnormal, toxic form of glycogen, **amylopectin.** This starch-like material is deposited, mostly in the liver but also in the heart, muscles and nervous system. Children with this disease typically die between 2 and 4 years of age from **cirrhosis of the liver.** Liver transplantation is curative. After a liver transplant, cardiac and other extrahepatic deposits of amylopectin are greatly reduced, although the mechanism for this effect is unknown.

MCARDLE DISEASE (TYPE V GLYCOGENOSIS): In McArdle disease glycogen accumulates in skeletal muscles, owing to a lack of muscle phosphorylase (11q13), the enzyme that releases glucose-1-phosphate from glycogen. Symptoms usually appear in adolescence or early adulthood and consist of muscle cramps and spasms during exercise and sometimes myocytolysis and resulting myoglobinuria. Avoidance of exercise prevents the symptoms.

Cystinosis

Cystinosis is a lysosomal storage disease in which crystalline cystine accrues in lysosomes. **Cystinosin,** a transmembrane cystine transporter, is lacking. The affected gene is at chromosome 17p13. Cystinosis occurs in 1 per 100,000 to 200,000 live births. It is characterized by renal Fanconi syndrome (polydipsia, excretion of large amounts of dilute urine, dehydration, electrolyte imbalances, growth retardation and rickets) beginning between 6 and 12 months of age. Untreated, cystinosis progresses to renal failure, often in childhood. Lung and brain function are often impaired in older patients. Cystine crystals are seen in almost all cells and organs. Renal transplantation can be used to treat the renal failure, and the use of cysteamine to decrease lysosomal cystine greatly slows disease progression and improves survival.

Table 6-8

Representative Inherited Disorders of Amino Acid Metabolism

Representative Inherited Disorders of Amino Acid Metabolism
Phenylketonuria (hyperphenylalaninemia)
Tyrosinemia
Histidinemia
Ornithine transcarbamylase deficiency (ammonia intoxication)
Carbamyl phosphate synthetase deficiency (ammonia intoxication)
Maple syrup urine disease (branched-chain ketoacidemia)
Arginase deficiency
Arginosuccinic acid synthetase deficiency (citrulline accumulation)

Inborn Errors of Amino Acid Metabolism Manifest With Variably Severe Symptoms

Heritable disorders of the metabolism of many amino acids have been described (Table 6-8). Some are lethal in early childhood; others are asymptomatic and are not clinically significant. Some of these are discussed in chapters dealing with specific organs. This discussion focuses on examples provided by defects in the metabolism of phenylalanine and tyrosine (Fig. 6-29).

Phenylketonuria

Phenylketonuria (PKU, hyperphenylalaninemia) is an autosomal recessive deficiency of the hepatic enzyme phenylalanine

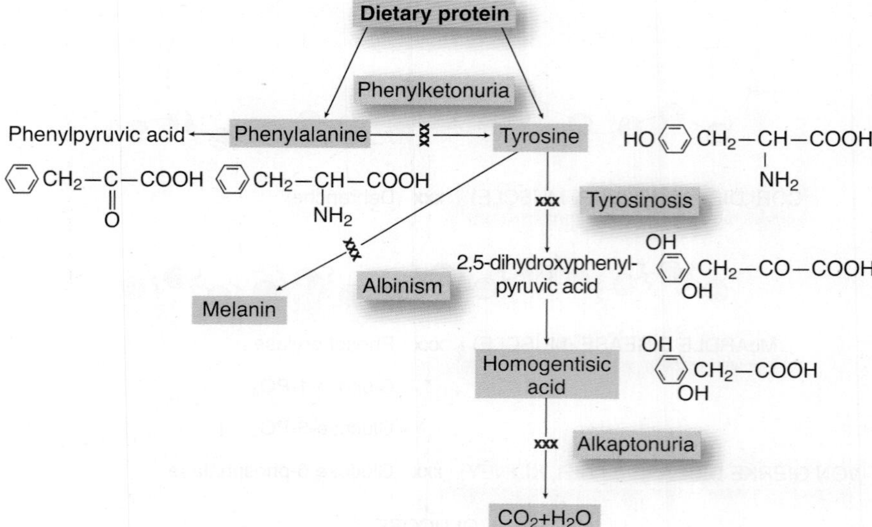

FIGURE 6-29. Diseases caused by disturbances of phenylalanine and tyrosine metabolism.

hydroxylase. In PKU, there are high circulating levels of phenylalanine, which leads to progressive mental deterioration in the first few years of life. The incidence of PKU is 1 per 10,000 in white and Asian populations, but it varies widely across different geographic areas. It is most frequent (1 in 5000) in Ireland and western Scotland and among Yemenite Jews.

MOLECULAR PATHOGENESIS: Phenylalanine is an essential amino acid derived exclusively from the diet. It is oxidized in the liver to tyrosine by phenylalanine hydroxylase (PAH). Deficiency in PAH results in both hyperphenylalaninemia and formation of phenylketones from transamination of phenylalanine. Phenylpyruvic acid and its derivatives are excreted in the urine, but phenylalanine itself, rather than its metabolites, causes the neurologic damage central to this disease. Thus, the term **hyperphenylalaninemia** is actually a more appropriate designation than PKU.

A variety of point mutations in the *PAH* gene, on the long arm of chromosome 12 (12q22-24.1), cause deficiency in PAH in most patients of European origin. By contrast, PKU among Yemenite Jews reflects a single deletion in the *PAH* gene. In the Yemenite Jewish community, this defect began in a common ancestor from Sanà, Yemen, before the 18th century. A different *PAH* gene deletion causes the disease in Scotland.

The mechanism whereby hyperphenylalaninemia is neurotoxic during infancy is not precisely established, but several processes have been implicated: (1) competitive interference with amino acid transport systems in the brain, (2) inhibition of the synthesis of neurotransmitters and (3) disturbance of other metabolic processes. These effects presumably lead to inadequate development of neurons and defective synthesis of myelin.

PAH activity is not always totally lacking, and forms of hyperphenylalaninemia milder than classic PKU are known. In such cases, phenylpyruvic acid is not excreted in the urine. Patients with less than 1% of the normal activity of PAH generally have a PKU phenotype, but those with more than 5% exhibit non-PKU hyperphenylalaninemia, do not suffer neurologic damage and develop normally. It is presumed that non-PKU hyperphenylalaninemia is caused by mutations different from those in classic PKU.

Malignant hyperphenylalaninemia occurs in fewer than 5% of infants with hyperphenylalaninemia. In this case, dietary restriction of phenylalanine does not arrest neurologic deterioration. These patients have a deficiency in tetrahydrobiopterin (BH_4), a cofactor required for hydroxylation of phenylalanine by PAH. In some instances, this defect results from failure to regenerate BH_4, due to a lack of dihydropteridine reductase (DHPR), the enzyme that reduces dihydrobiopterin (BH_2) to the tetrahydro form (BH_4). The mutant *DHPR* gene is on the short arm of chromosome 4, and so is distinct from the *PAH* gene. Alternatively, in some cases synthesis of BH_4 is impaired. Infants with malignant hyperphenylalaninemia are phenotypically indistinguishable from those with classic PKU at first, but BH_4 deficiency also interferes with synthesis of the neurotransmitters dopamine (tyrosine hydroxylase dependent) and serotonin (tryptophan hydroxylase dependent). Thus, the mechanism underlying brain damage in malignant hyperphenylalaninemia most likely involves more than a simple elevation in the levels of phenylalanine.

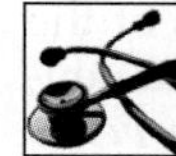

CLINICAL FEATURES: Phenylketonuria illustrates the interaction between "nature and nurture" in the pathogenesis of disease. It is caused by a genetic defect, but its expression requires a dietary constituent. ***Affected infants appear normal at birth, but mental retardation is evident within a few months.*** By 12 months, untreated infants have lost about 50 IQ points, which means that a child who would otherwise demonstrate normal intelligence becomes severely retarded. Infants with PKU tend to have fair skin, blond hair and blue eyes, because the inability to convert phenylalanine to tyrosine leads to reduced melanin synthesis. They exude a "mousy" odor, owing to the phenylacetic acid they make.

Treatment of PKU involves restriction of dietary phenylalanine to 250 to 500 mg/day, which usually requires a semisynthetic formula. How long such restriction is necessary is controversial. At one time it was believed that the dietary regimen could be relaxed after the brain has largely matured (i.e., by 6 years of age). However, recent data suggest that older patients may suffer harm when phenylalanine is reintroduced into the diet. Thus, how long phenylalanine restriction should be maintained is not certain.

In developed countries, the clinical phenotype of classical PKU is now more of historical interest than a significant concern. About 10 million newborns worldwide are screened annually for hyperphenylalaninemia by a simple blood test, and most of the estimated 1000 new cases are promptly treated. The success of newborn PKU screening and the prompt institution of a low-phenylalanine diet allow many PKU homozygotes to live normal lives and to reproduce. Expectant mothers homozygous for PKU (maternal PKU) must restrict phenylalanine intake while pregnant for the fetus to avoid the complications of maternal hyperphenylalaninemia. Infants exposed to high levels of phenylalanine in utero show microcephaly, mental and growth retardation and cardiac anomalies. In other words, high levels of phenylalanine are teratogenic.

Tyrosinemia

Hereditary tyrosinemia (hepatorenal tyrosinemia, tyrosinemia type I) is a rare (1 in 100,000) autosomal recessive inborn error of tyrosine catabolism that manifests as acute liver disease in early infancy or as a more chronic disease of the liver, kidneys and brain in children.

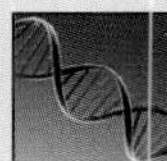

MOLECULAR PATHOGENESIS: Blood levels of tyrosine and its metabolites are elevated. Fumarylacetoacetate hydrolase (15q23-25), the last enzyme in the catabolic pathway that converts tyrosine to fumarate and acetoacetate, is deficient in both forms of the disease. In the acute form there is no enzyme activity, whereas children with chronic disease have variable residual activity. Cell injury in hereditary tyrosinemia is attributed to abnormal toxic metabolites, succinylacetone and succinylacetoacetate.

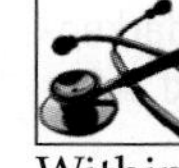

CLINICAL FEATURES: **Acute tyrosinemia** manifests in the first few months of life as hepatomegaly, edema, failure to thrive and a cabbage-like odor. Within a few months, infants die of hepatic failure.

Chronic tyrosinemia is characterized by cirrhosis of the liver, renal tubular dysfunction (Fanconi syndrome) and neurologic abnormalities. ***Hepatocellular carcinoma supervenes in more than a third of patients.*** Most children die before the age of 10 years. Liver transplantation corrects the hepatic metabolic abnormalities and prevents the neurologic crises. Combined liver–kidney transplants have also been performed. Analysis of amniotic fluid for succinylacetone or of cells from amniocentesis or chorionic villus sampling for fumarylacetoacetate hydrolase establishes the diagnosis prenatally.

Alkaptonuria (Ochronosis)

Alkaptonuria is a rare autosomal recessive deficiency of hepatic and renal homogentisic acid oxidase. It features excretion of homogentisic acid in the urine, generalized pigmentation and arthritis. The enzyme deficiency prevents catabolism of homogentisic acid, an intermediate gene product in phenylalanine and tyrosine metabolism. Alkaptonuria has greater historical significance than clinical importance: the reports of Garrod and others 100 years ago of the inheritance of alkaptonuria helped define the idea of hereditary inborn errors of metabolism.

MOLECULAR PATHOGENESIS: Patients with alkaptonuria excrete urine that darkens rapidly on standing, owing to formation of a pigment on the nonenzymatic oxidation of homogentisic acid (Fig. 6-30). In long-standing alkaptonuria, a similar pigment is deposited in numerous tissues, particularly the sclera, cartilage in many areas (ribs, larynx, trachea), tendons and synovial membranes. Although the pigment appears bluish black on gross examination, it is brown under the microscope, accounting for the term **ochronosis** (color of ocher) coined by Virchow. A degenerative and frequently disabling **arthropathy** ("ochronotic arthritis") often develops after years of alkaptonuria. It is tempting to ascribe the joint disease to the pigment deposition, but this has not been proved. Despite affecting many organs, alkaptonuria does not reduce longevity.

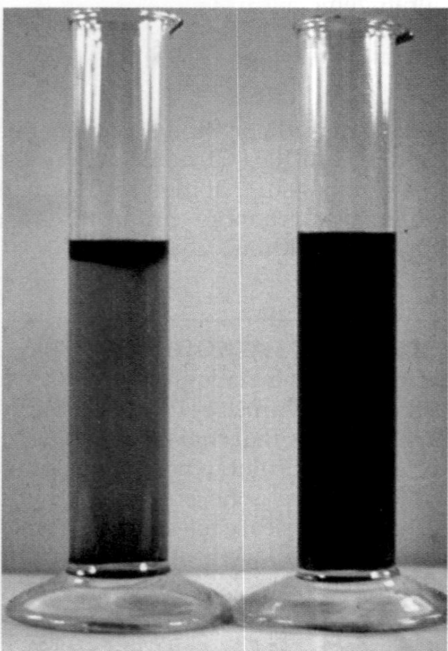

FIGURE 6-30. Urine from a patient with alkaptonuria. The specimen on the left, which has been standing for 15 minutes, shows some darkening at the surface, owing to the oxidation of homogentisic acid. After 2 hours (*right*), the urine is entirely black.

Albinism

Albinism refers to a heterogeneous group of at least 10 inherited disorders in which absent or reduced biosynthesis of melanin causes hypopigmentation. This condition is found throughout the animal kingdom (from insects to humans). The most common type is oculocutaneous albinism (OCA), a family of closely related diseases that (with one rare exception) are autosomal recessive traits (Table 6-6). In OCA melanin pigment is absent or reduced in the skin, hair follicles and eyes. The frequency of OCA in whites is 1 per 18,000 in the United States and 1 in 10,000 in Ireland. American blacks have the same high frequency of OCA as the Irish.

MOLECULAR PATHOGENESIS: Two major forms of OCA are distinguished by the presence or absence of tyrosinase, the first enzyme in the biosynthetic pathway that converts tyrosine to melanin (Fig. 6-29).

Tyrosinase-positive OCA is the most common type of albinism in whites and blacks. Patients typically begin life with complete albinism, but with age, a small amount of clinically detectable pigment accumulates. A defect in the *P* gene (15q11.2-13) prevents melanin synthesis. The *P* gene has been postulated to code for a tyrosine transport protein.

Tyrosinase-negative OCA is the second most common type of albinism and is characterized by complete absence of tyrosinase (11q14-21) and melanin: melanocytes are present but contain unpigmented melanosomes. Affected people have snow-white hair, pale pink skin, blue irides and prominent red pupils, owing to an absence of retinal pigment. They typically have severe ophthalmic problems, including photophobia, strabismus, nystagmus and poor visual acuity.

The skin of all types of albinos is strikingly sensitive to sunlight. Exposed skin areas require strong sunscreen lotions. These patients are at a greatly increased risk for squamous cell carcinomas of sun-exposed skin. In fact, among a group of more than 500 albinos in equatorial Africa, not one survived beyond the age of 40 years, nearly all having succumbed to cancer. Interestingly, albinos seem to have a lower than normal frequency of malignant melanoma.

X-Linked Disorders Feature an Abnormal Gene on the X Chromosome

Expression of an X-linked disorder (Fig. 6-31) is different in males and females. Females, with two X chromosomes, may be homozygous or heterozygous for a given trait. It follows that clinical expression of the trait in a female is variable,

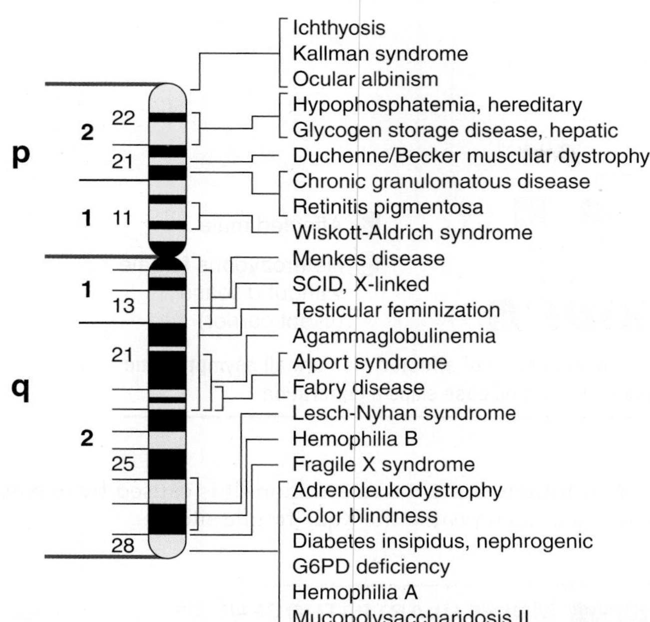

FIGURE 6-31. Localization of representative inherited diseases on the X chromosome. G6PD = glucose-6-phosphate dehydrogenase; SCID = severe combined immunodeficiency (syndrome).

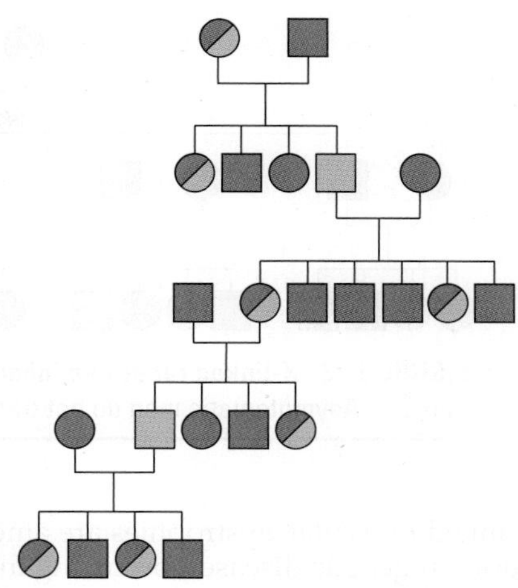

FIGURE 6-32. X-linked dominant inheritance. A heterozygous woman transmits the trait equally to males and females; men transmit the trait only to their daughters. Asymptomatic males and females do not carry the trait.

depending on whether it is dominant or recessive. By contrast, males have only one X chromosome and so are **hemizygous** for that trait. *Thus, regardless of whether the trait is dominant or recessive, it is invariably expressed in the male.*

X-linked traits are not transmitted from father to son: a symptomatic father donates only a normal Y chromosome to his male offspring. By contrast, he always donates his abnormal X chromosome to his daughters, who are therefore obligate carriers of the trait. The disease thus skips a generation in males, as female carriers transmit it to grandsons of a symptomatic male.

X-Linked Dominant Traits

MOLECULAR PATHOGENESIS: X-linked dominance refers to expression of a trait only in the female, since the hemizygous state in the male precludes a distinction between dominant and recessive inheritance (Fig. 6-32). The distinctive features of X-linked dominant disorders are:

- Females are affected twice as frequently as males.
- Heterozygous women transmit the disorder to half their children, whether male or female.
- A man with a dominant X-linked disorder transmits the disease only to his daughters.
- Clinical expression of the disease tends to be less severe and more variable in heterozygous females than in hemizygous males.

Only a few X-linked dominant disorders are known, including familial hypophosphatemic rickets and ornithine transcarbamylase deficiency. Variations in the phenotype of these traits in females may reflect, at least in part, the Lyon effect (i.e., inactivation of one X chromosome), which leads to mosaicism for the mutant allele, and inconstant expression of the trait.

X-Linked Recessive Traits

Most X-linked traits are recessive; that is, heterozygous females do not have clinical disease (Fig. 6-33). The characteristics of this mode of inheritance are:

- Sons of women who are carriers have a 50% chance of inheriting the disease; daughters are not symptomatic. However, 50% of daughters will also be carriers.
- All daughters of affected men are asymptomatic carriers, but the sons of these men do not have the trait and cannot transmit it to their children.
- Symptomatic homozygous females can result from the rare mating of an affected man and an asymptomatic, heterozygous woman. Alternatively, lyonization may preferentially inactivate the normal X chromosome, which, in extreme cases, may lead to an affected heterozygous female.
- The trait tends to occur in maternal uncles and in male cousins descended from the mother's sisters.

Table 6-9 presents a list of representative X-linked recessive disorders.

X-Linked Muscular Dystrophies (Duchenne and Becker Muscular Dystrophies)

The muscular dystrophies are devastating muscle diseases. Most are X linked, although a few are autosomal recessive.

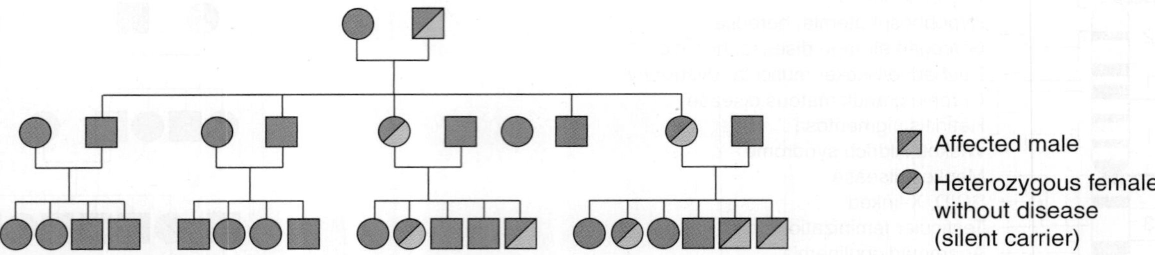

FIGURE 6-33. X-linked recessive inheritance. Only males are affected; daughters of affected men are all asymptomatic carriers. Asymptomatic men do not transmit the trait. Clinical expression of the disease skips a generation.

The X-linked muscular dystrophies are among the most frequent human genetic diseases, occurring in 1 per 3500 boys, the incidence of which approaches that of CF. ***Duchenne muscular dystrophy (DMD),*** the most common variant, is a fatal progressive degeneration of muscle that appears before the age of 4 years. ***Becker muscular dystrophy (BMD)*** is allelic with DMD but is less common and milder (see Chapter 27).

Hemophilia A (Factor VIII Deficiency)

Hemophilia A (see Chapter 20) is an X-linked recessive disorder of blood clotting that results in spontaneous bleeding, particularly into joints, muscles and internal organs.

Fragile X Syndrome

Fragile X syndrome is second only to Down syndrome as a genetic cause of mental retardation. The disease afflicts 1 in 1250 males and 1 in 2500 females and is the most common form of inherited mental retardation. It is caused by expansion of a CGG repeat at the Xq27 fragile site.

MOLECULAR PATHOGENESIS: More males than females are institutionalized for mental retardation, an excess that largely reflects X-linked inheritance of mental retardation. Fully 20% of heritable mental retardation is due to X-linked disorders, and one fifth of these reflect a single genetic defect: an inducible fragile site on the X chromosome (Xq27).

A **fragile site** represents a specific locus, or band, on a chromosome that breaks easily. It is usually detected in cytogenetic preparations as a nonstaining gap or constriction (Fig. 6-34). Importantly, under the routine conditions of preparing cells for karyotypic analysis, most fragile sites are not detected. However, when the same cells in culture are treated so as to impair DNA synthesis (e.g., with methotrexate, floxuridine), fragile sites are revealed. Most people have at least 11, and possibly up to 50, fragile sites, both on autosomes and on the X chromosome. ***However, the locus at Xq27 is associated with mental retardation and other clinical findings that characterize fragile X syndrome.*** As discussed, the fragile site at Xq27 is a distinct kind of mutation characterized by amplification of a CGG repeat.

Within fragile X families, the probability of being affected is related to position in the pedigree; that is, later

Table 6-9

Representative X-Linked Recessive Diseases

Disease	Frequency in Males
Fragile X syndrome	1/2000
Hemophilia A (factor VIII deficiency)	1/10,000
Hemophilia B (factor IX deficiency)	1/70,000
Duchenne-Becker muscular dystrophy	1/3500
Glucose-6-phosphate dehydrogenase deficiency	Up to 30%
Lesch-Nyhan syndrome (HPRT deficiency)	1/10,000
Chronic granulomatous disease	Not rare
X-linked agammaglobulinemia	Not rare
X-linked severe combined immunodeficiency	Rare
Fabry disease	1/40,000
Hunter syndrome	1/70,000
Adrenoleukodystrophy	1/100,000
Menkes disease	1/100,000

HPRT = hypoxanthine-guanine phosphoribosyltransferase.

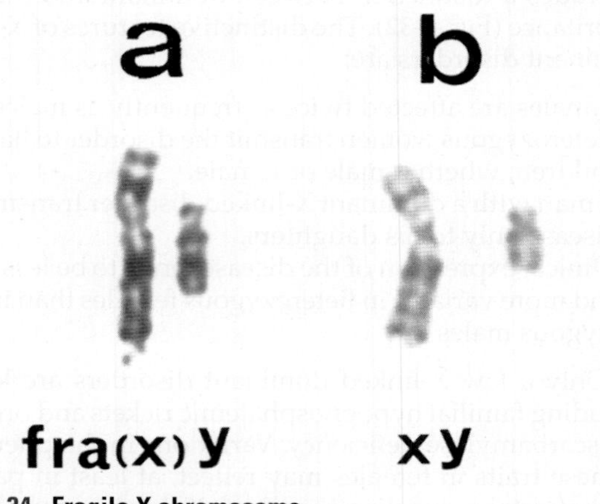

FIGURE 6-34. Fragile X chromosome.

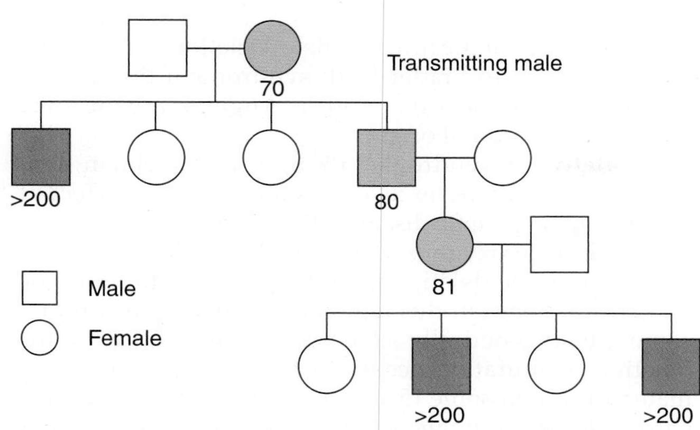

FIGURE 6-35. Inheritance pattern of fragile X syndrome. The number of copies of the trinucleotide repeat (CGG) is shown below selected members in this pedigree. Expansion occurs primarily during meiosis in females. When the number of repeats exceeds ~200, the clinical syndrome is manifested. Individuals shaded orange carry a premutation and are asymptomatic.

generations are more likely than earlier ones to be affected **(Sherman paradox** or **genetic anticipation).** This fact is due to progressive triplet repeat expansion. Chromosomes with more than about 52 repeats can increase the number of repeats—so-called expansion. Small expansions tend to be asymptomatic but can enlarge, particularly during meiosis in females, leading to larger expansions in successive generations. These are known as **premutations.** Expansions with over 200 repeats are associated with mental retardation and are full mutations. Expansion of a premutation to a full mutation during gametogenesis only occurs in females. Thus, daughters of men with premutations (carriers) are never clinically symptomatic, but the sisters of the transmitting males occasionally produce affected daughters. However, the daughters of carrier males always harbor the premutation. The frequency of conversion of a premutation to a full mutation in such women (i.e., the probability that their sons will have fragile X syndrome) varies with the length of the expanded tract. Premutations with more than 90 repeats are almost always converted to full mutations. As fragile X syndrome is recessive, most daughters of carrier males transmit mental retardation to 50% of their sons. These considerations explain the greater risk of the disorder in succeeding generations of fragile X families (Fig. 6-35).

CLINICAL FEATURES: A male newborn with fragile X syndrome appears normal, but during childhood, typical features appear, including increased head circumference, facial coarsening, joint hyperextensibility, enlarged testes and heart valve abnormalities. Mental retardation is profound: IQ scores vary from 20 to 60. ***Interestingly, a significant proportion of autistic boys carry a fragile X chromosome.*** Among mentally handicapped female carriers, the severity of the impairment varies from a learning disability with normal IQ to serious retardation.

About 80% of males with the Xq27 fragile site are mentally retarded; the others are clinically normal but can transmit the trait. They have expansions of less than 200 copies of the trinucleotide repeat. Recently, a new syndrome characterized by tremors, ataxia and declining cognitive abilities was described in elderly men with fragile X premutations. This disorder has some clinical similarities to Parkinson disease and Alzheimer disease and has been called fragile X tremor ataxia syndrome (FTAXS). Two thirds of females who carry a fragile X chromosome (obligate carriers) are intellectually normal, and the fragile site on the X chromosome cannot be demonstrated. By contrast, of the one third of female carriers who are mentally retarded, virtually all display a fragile Xq27 locus. This variability in phenotypic expression in females may relate to the pattern of X chromosome inactivation.

Fabry Disease

Fabry disease is a deficiency of **lysosomal α-galactosidase A.** This X-linked syndrome leads to accumulation of globotriaosylcer-amide and other glycosphingolipids in the endothelium of the brain, heart, skin, kidneys and other organs. A particular type of tumor, angiokeratoma, is a characteristic cutaneous manifestation of Fabry disease. Functionally affected microvasculature becomes increasingly compromised, causing progressive vascular insufficiency with cerebral, renal and cardiac infarcts. Patients die in early adulthood from complications of their vascular disease. Therapy with recombinant α-D-galactosidase A shows promise in arresting the disease.

Mitochondrial Diseases

MOLECULAR PATHOGENESIS: Mitochondrial proteins are encoded by both nuclear and mitochondrial genes. Most mitochondrial respiratory chain proteins are encoded by nuclear genes, although several are products of the mitochondrial genome. A few rare, autosomal recessive (mendelian) disorders that represent defects in nuclear encoded mitochondrial proteins have been described. However, most inherited defects in mitochondrial function result from mutations in the mitochondrial genome itself. To understand these conditions, an explanation of the unique genetics of the mitochondria is needed. These features include:

- **Maternal inheritance:** All vertebrate mitochondria are inherited from the mother via the ovum, which possesses up to 300,000 copies of mitochondrial DNA (mtDNA).
- **Variability of mtDNA copies:** The number of mitochondria and the number of copies of mtDNA per mitochondrion vary in different tissues. Each mitochondrion has 2 to 10 mtDNA copies, and varying tissue needs for ATP correlate with the DNA content per mitochondrion.
- **Threshold effect:** Since any given cell has many mitochondria and thus hundreds or thousands of mtDNA copies, mutations in mtDNA lead to mixed populations of mutant and normal mitochondrial genomes, a situation called **heteroplasmy.** The phenotype of mtDNA mutations reflects the severity of the mutation, the proportion of mutant genomes and the tissue's demand for ATP. Different tissues need different levels of ATP production to sustain their metabolism; the brain, heart and skeletal muscle have particularly great energy demands.

- **High mutation rate:** The rate of mtDNA mutation is much higher than that of nuclear DNA, owing (at least in part) to less DNA repair capacity.

Diseases caused by mutations in the mitochondrial genome principally affect the nervous system, heart and skeletal muscle. Functional deficits in all of these disorders are traced to impaired oxidative phosphorylation (OXPHOS). **OXPHOS diseases** are divided into several classes: I, nuclear mutations; II, mtDNA point mutations; III, mtDNA deletions; and IV, undefined defects.

All inherited mitochondrial diseases are rare and have variable clinical presentations based on the considerations discussed above. The first human mtDNA disease to be discovered was **Leber hereditary optic neuropathy,** which is characterized by progressive loss of vision. Various mitochondrial myopathies and encephalomyopathies are known (see Chapter 27). Hypertrophic cardiomyopathy (see Chapter 11) is also a common manifestation of OXPHOS diseases.

Genetic Imprinting

MOLECULAR PATHOGENESIS: ***Phenotypes associated with some genes differ, depending on whether the allele is inherited from the mother or the father. This phenomenon is called genetic imprinting.*** In the case of imprinted genes, either the maternal or paternal allele is maintained in an inactive state. This normal physiologic process results from methylation of DNA cytosine residues in regulatory regions in the imprinted allele. The nonimprinted allele provides the biological function for that locus. If the nonimprinted allele is disrupted through mutation, the imprinted allele remains inactive and cannot compensate for the missing function. Imprinting occurs in meiosis during gametogenesis, and the pattern of imprinting is maintained to variable degrees in different tissues. It is reset during meiosis in the next generation, so the selection of a given allele for imprinting can vary from one generation to the next.

In extreme cases, experimental embryos that obtain both sets of chromosomes exclusively from either the mother or the father never survive to term. A less severe manifestation of genetic imprinting is seen in **uniparental disomy,** in which both members of a single chromosome pair are inherited from the same parent. The pair of chromosomes may be copies of one parental chromosome (uniparental isodisomy) or may be the same pair found in one parent (uniparental heterodisomy). Uniparental disomy is rare, but is implicated in unexpected inheritance patterns of genetic traits. For instance, a child with uniparental isodisomy may show a recessive disease when only one parent carries the trait, which has been observed in a few cases of cystic fibrosis and hemophilia A. Loss of a chromosome from a trisomy or duplication of a chromosome in the case of a monosomy can lead to uniparental disomy. Interestingly, as many as 1% of viable pregnancies carry uniparental disomy for at least one chromosome.

Genetic imprinting is well illustrated by certain hereditary diseases whose phenotype is determined by the parental source of the mutant allele. Deletion of the 15q11-13 locus results in **Prader-Willi syndrome** if the affected chromosome is maternal, and in **Angelman syndrome** when it is of paternal origin.

Prader-Willi syndrome (PWS) and Angelman syndrome (AS) provide excellent examples of the effect of imprinting on genetic diseases. Both disorders are associated with (heterozygous) deletion in the region of 15(q11-13). In PWS, the deletion is in the paternal chromosome and critical genes in this region of the maternal chromosome are epigenetically silenced. In contrast, in AS, the deletion or mutation occurs in the same region of the maternal chromosome 15 and critical genes in the paternal chromosome are epigenetically silenced. Critical genes silenced by methylation in the maternal 15q11-13 chromosome include *SNRPN* (encoding small nuclear ribonucleoprotein polypeptide), *NDN* (encoding necdin) and a cluster of small nucleolar RNAs (snoRNAs). Deletion of the cluster of 29 copies of SNORD116 in knockout mice is sufficient to induce features similar to PWS observed in humans, and two patients with PWS have been found to have microdeletions in 15(q11-13) limited to the 29 SNORD116 repeats. This species of snoRNAs has been implicated in methylation of specific RNA substrates. In AS, the *UBE3A* gene, which encodes a ubiquitin ligase, is mutated or deleted in the maternal chromosome and epigenetically silenced (in the paternal chromosome).

Genetic diagnosis of these disorders may be done by FISH using probes from the 15(q11-13) region to detect deletions or by methylation studies. Array comparative genomic hybridization determines the DNA copy number using an array with millions of probes that span the genome at regular intervals. Hybridization of small fragments of fluorochrome-labeled patient DNA to the chip is compared with that of a normal control DNA reference labeled with another fluorochrome. Copy number variations, either deletions or increases, are determined from the predominance of a fluorochrome (increased control signal in patient deletions and increased patient signal in amplifications).

The phenotypes of these disorders are remarkably different. PWS features hypotonia, hyperphagia with obesity, hypogonadism, mental retardation and a specific facies. By contrast, AS patients are hyperactive, display inappropriate laughter, have a different facies from that in PWS and suffer from seizures. Thus, Prader-Willi syndrome develops because critical genes in the maternal locus are normally silenced by imprinting, and the same region on the paternal chromosome is deleted, resulting in lack of expression. The converse applies in Angelman syndrome: the paternal gene is normally imprinted and silenced, and the maternal locus is inactivated by mutation or deletion. This pattern is similar to loss of heterozygosity in tumor suppressor genes by aberrant methylation in some cases of cancer (see Chapter 5). The gene responsible for AS appears to be *UBE3A.* The genes responsible for PWS have not been definitively identified.

Genetic imprinting is implicated in a number of other situations relevant to human disease. For example, in some childhood cancers, including Wilms tumor, osteosarcoma, bilateral retinoblastoma and embryonal rhabdomyosarcoma, the maternal allele of a putative tumor suppressor gene is lost and the remaining allele is on a chromosome of paternal origin. In the case of familial glomus tumor, an adult neoplasm, both males and females may carry the trait, but it is transmitted only through the male. Thus, the responsible gene is active only when it is located on the paternal autosome. Finally, as noted above, the premutation of fragile X syndrome is expanded to the full mutation only during female gametogenesis, implying that the trinucleotide repeat is treated differently on passage through the female than in the male.

Multifactorial Inheritance

Multifactorial inheritance describes a process by which a disease results from the effects of a number of abnormal genes and environmental factors. Most normal human traits reflect such complexities and are not inherited as simple dominant nor as recessive mendelian attributes. For example, multifactorial inheritance determines height, skin color and body habitus. Similarly, most of the common chronic disorders of adults—diabetes, atherosclerosis, many forms of cancer, arthritis and hypertension—represent multifactorial genetic diseases and are well known to "run in families." The inheritance of many birth defects is also multifactorial (e.g., cleft lip and palate, pyloric stenosis and congenital heart disease) (Table 6-10).

Multifactorial inheritance entails multiple genes interacting with each other and with environmental factors to produce disease in an individual patient. Such inheritance leads to familial aggregation that does not obey simple mendelian rules. Thus, inheritance of polygenic diseases is studied by population genetics, rather than by analysis of individual families.

The number of involved genes for any polygenic disease is not known. Thus, it is not possible to ascertain accurately the risk of a particular disorder in an individual case. The probability of disease can only be predicted from the numbers of relatives affected, the severity of their disease and statistical projections based on population analyses. Whereas monogenic inheritance implies a specific risk of disease (e.g., 25% or 50%), the probability of symptoms in first-degree relatives of a person affected with a polygenic disease is usually about 5% to 10%.

The basis of polygenic inheritance is that over one fourth of all genes in normal humans have polymorphic alleles. Such genetic heterogeneity leads to wide variability in susceptibility to many diseases and is further compounded by interaction with diverse environmental factors.

- **Expression of symptoms is proportional to the number of mutant genes.** Close relatives of an affected person have more mutant genes than the population at large and a greater chance of expressing the disease. The probability of expressing the same number of mutant genes is highest in identical twins.
- **Environmental factors influence expression of the trait.** Thus, concordance for the disease may occur in only one third of monozygotic twins.
- **The risk in first-degree relatives (parents, siblings, children) is the same (5% to 10%).** The probability of disease is much lower in second-degree relatives.
- **The likelihood of a trait's expression in later offspring is influenced by its expression in earlier siblings.** If one or more children are born with a multifactorial defect, the chance it will recur in later offspring is doubled. For simple mendelian traits, in contrast, the probability is independent of the number of affected siblings.
- **The more severe a defect is, the greater the risk of transmitting it to offspring.** As patients with more severe polygenic defects probably have more mutant genes, their children are more likely to inherit the abnormal genes than offspring of less severely affected relatives.
- **Some diseases that show multifactorial inheritance also show a gender predilection.** Thus, pyloric stenosis is more common in males, while congenital hip dislocation is more common in females. Such differential susceptibility is thought to reflect different thresholds for expression of mutant genes in the two sexes. For example, if the number of mutant genes required for pyloric stenosis in males is A, it may require 4A in the female. Then, a woman who had pyloric stenosis as an infant has more mutant genes to transmit to her children than does a similarly afflicted man. Indeed, the sons of such women actually have a 25% chance of being born with pyloric stenosis, compared with a 4% risk for the son of an affected man. ***As a rule, if there is an altered sex ratio in the incidence of a polygenic defect, a member of the less commonly affected sex has a much greater probability of transmitting the defect.***

Table 6-10

Representative Diseases Associated With Multifactorial Inheritance

Adults	Children
Hypertension	Pyloric stenosis
Atherosclerosis	Cleft lip and palate
Diabetes, type 2	Congenital heart disease
Allergic diathesis	Meningomyelocele
Psoriasis	Anencephaly
Schizophrenia	Hypospadias
Ankylosing spondylitis	Congenital hip dislocation
Gout	Hirschsprung disease

Cleft Lip and Cleft Palate Exemplify Multifactorial Inheritance

At the 35th day of gestation, the frontal prominence fuses with the maxillary process to form the upper lip. This process is under the control of many genes, and disturbances in gene expression (hereditary or environmental) at this time interfere with proper fusion, resulting in cleft lip, with or without cleft palate (Fig. 6-36). This anomaly may also be part of a systemic malformation syndrome caused by teratogens (rubella, anticonvulsants) and is often seen in children with chromosomal abnormalities.

The incidence of cleft lip, with or without cleft palate, is 0.1%. The incidence of cleft palate alone is 1 in 2500. If one child is born with a cleft lip, the chances are 4% that a second child will have the same defect. If the first two children are affected, the risk of cleft lip increases to 9% for the third child. The more severe the defect is, the greater the probability of transmitting cleft lip will be. Whereas 75% of cases of cleft lip occur in boys, the sons of women with cleft lip have a four times higher risk of acquiring the defect than do sons of affected fathers.

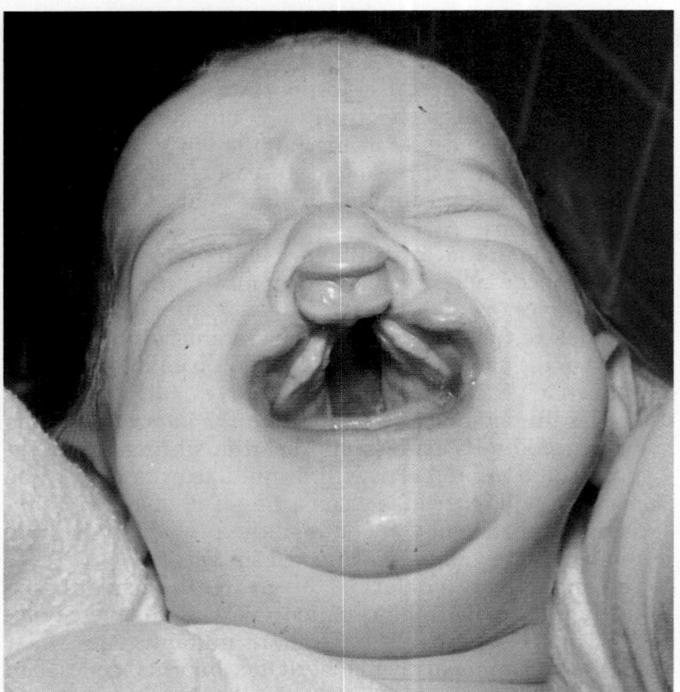

FIGURE 6-36. Cleft lip and palate in an infant.

Screening for Carriers of Genetic Disorders

Until recently, screening for carriers of genetic diseases was not common. Among Ashkenazi Jews, screening to identify carriers of Tay-Sachs disease, an autosomal recessive disease, has been done because of the relatively high frequency of the disease in that group. A number of other inherited conditions are also included in a so-called "Ashkenazi screen." The objective is to identify couples in which both members are heterozygous carriers and who thus have a 25% risk of having an affected offspring with each pregnancy. These couples can be offered prenatal diagnosis to determine the genetic status of their fetus. In vitro fertilization combined with preimplantation genetic diagnosis is available in some centers to ensure that an implanted embryo will not have this disease.

Prenatal screening for carriers of CF has been recommended by national professional organizations for several years, and represents the first large-scale adoption of testing for carriers of genetic diseases. Guidelines are that CF screening be offered to all white and Ashkenazi Jewish women because of the relatively high frequency of CF in these groups. A panel of 25 CF mutations is used for this DNA-based testing. If a woman is a CF carrier, her partner should be tested to see if the couple is at risk of having an affected offspring. Because of the diversity of CF mutations, the recommended panel detects about 80% of known CF mutations in whites, but over 97% among Ashkenazi Jews. Detection rates among other ethnic groups are lower.

Prenatal Diagnosis of Genetic Disorders

Amniocentesis and chorionic villus biopsy are the most important diagnostic tools for genetic or developmental disorders. Both procedures are safe, reliable and easily done, and indications for performing them are:

- **Age 35 years old and over:** The likelihood of having a child with Down syndrome is about 1 in 1200 for a mother age 25, compared with 1 in 300 for a 40-year-old. This risk rises even higher with advanced maternal age.
- **Previous chromosomal abnormality:** The overall risk of recurrence of Down syndrome in a succeeding child of a woman who has already had an infant with trisomy 21 is 1%.
- **Translocation carrier:** Estimates of risks to the offspring of translocation carriers vary from 3% to 15%. ***Carriers of balanced translocations are more likely to produce children with unbalanced karyotypes and resulting phenotypic abnormalities.***
- **History of familial inborn error of metabolism:** Recessive inborn errors of metabolism have a 25% risk for each child if each parent is heterozygous for the trait. Prenatal diagnosis can identify disorders for which a biochemical diagnosis can be made.
- **Identified heterozygotes:** Carrier detection projects (e.g., the Tay-Sachs Disease Prevention Program) identify couples in which both spouses are carriers of the same recessive gene. Each of their pregnancies has a 25% risk of an affected child and diagnosis can be made prenatally.
- **Family history of X-linked disorders:** Fetal sex determination, using amniotic cells, can be offered to women known to be carriers of X-linked disorders. Diagnosis of some of these conditions can be established biochemically by amniotic fluid analysis.

Gene-specific DNA probes have been developed for many genetic diseases, including hemophilia A and B, the hemoglobinopathies, phenylketonuria and α_1-antitrypsin deficiency. Most heterozygous carriers for Duchenne and Becker muscular dystrophies, Huntington chorea and CF can be identified by such techniques.

Diseases of Infancy and Childhood

The period from birth to puberty has been traditionally subdivided into several stages.

- Neonatal age (the first 4 weeks)
- Infancy (the first year)
- Early childhood (1 to 4 years)
- Late childhood (5 to 14 years)

Each of these periods has its own anatomic, physiologic and immunologic characteristics, which determine the nature and form of various pathologic processes. Morbidity and mortality in the neonatal period differ greatly from those in infancy and childhood. Infants and children are not simply "small adults," and they may be afflicted by diseases unique to their particular age group.

Prematurity and Intrauterine Growth Retardation

Human pregnancy normally lasts 40 ± 2 weeks, and most newborns weigh 3300 ± 600 g. The World Health Organization defines prematurity as a gestational age of less than 37 weeks (timed from the first day of the last menstrual period). Traditionally prematurity signified a birth weight below 2500 g, regardless of gestational age. However, since full-term infants may weigh under 2500 g because of intrauterine growth retardation rather than prematurity, **low-birth-weight infants** (<2500 g) are termed (1) appropriate for gestational age (AGA) or (2) small for gestational age (SGA).

In the United States, the frequency of low-birth-weight infants is less than 6% among whites. Two thirds of these infants are premature (AGA). By contrast, when the frequency of low-birth-weight infants exceeds 10%, as it does for blacks (>12%), most of these newborns suffer from intrauterine growth retardation and are considered SGA.

About 1% of infants born in the United States weigh under 1500 g and are classified as **very-low-birth-weight infants.** Such babies account for half of neonatal deaths, and their survival is related to their birth weight. If they are cared for in neonatal intensive care units, 90% of infants over 750 g survive. From 500 g to 750 g, 45% survive, of whom over half develop normally.

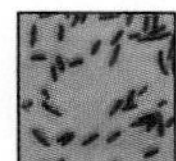

ETIOLOGIC FACTORS: The factors that predispose to premature birth of an infant (AGA) are (1) maternal illness, (2) uterine incompetence, (3) fetal disorders and (4) placental abnormalities. If the life of a fetus is threatened by such conditions, it may be necessary to induce premature delivery to save the infant. In a substantial proportion of AGA infants, the cause of premature birth is unknown. Intrauterine growth retardation and the resulting birth of SGA infants are associated with disorders that (1) impair maternal health and nutrition, (2) interfere with placental circulation or function or (3) disturb fetal growth or development (see Chapter 18).

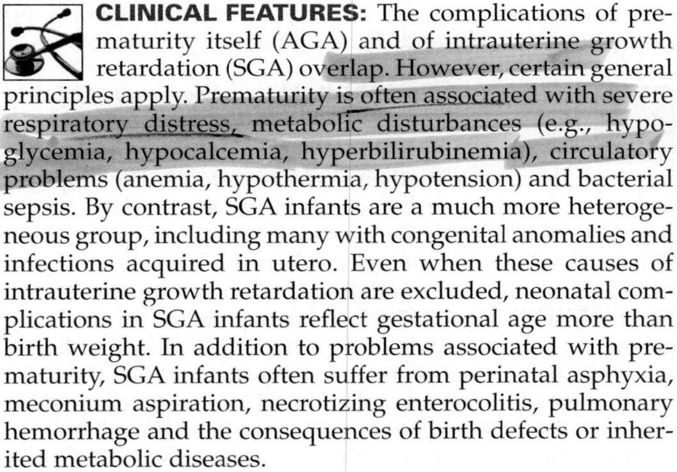

CLINICAL FEATURES: The complications of prematurity itself (AGA) and of intrauterine growth retardation (SGA) overlap. However, certain general principles apply. Prematurity is often associated with severe respiratory distress, metabolic disturbances (e.g., hypoglycemia, hypocalcemia, hyperbilirubinemia), circulatory problems (anemia, hypothermia, hypotension) and bacterial sepsis. By contrast, SGA infants are a much more heterogeneous group, including many with congenital anomalies and infections acquired in utero. Even when these causes of intrauterine growth retardation are excluded, neonatal complications in SGA infants reflect gestational age more than birth weight. In addition to problems associated with prematurity, SGA infants often suffer from perinatal asphyxia, meconium aspiration, necrotizing enterocolitis, pulmonary hemorrhage and the consequences of birth defects or inherited metabolic diseases.

Organ Immaturity Is a Cause of Neonatal Problems

The maturity of the newborn can be defined in both anatomic and physiologic terms. Maturing organs in infants born prematurely differ from those in term infants, although complete maturation of many organs may require days (lungs) to years (brain) after birth.

LUNGS: Pulmonary immaturity is a common and immediate threat to the viability of low-birth-weight infants. The lining cells of the fetal alveoli do not differentiate into type I and type II pneumocytes until late in pregnancy. Amniotic fluid fills fetal alveoli and drains from the lungs at birth.

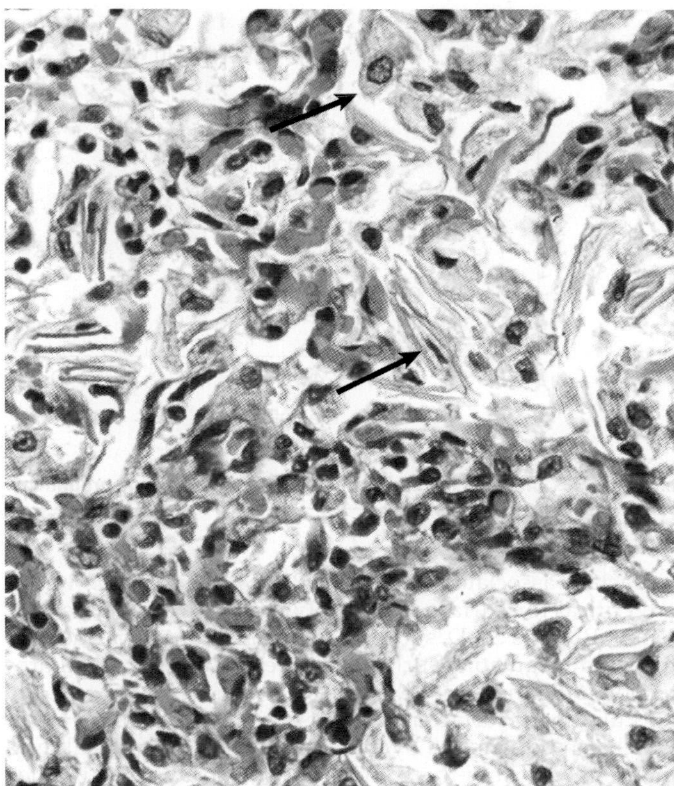

FIGURE 6-37. Retention of amniotic fluid in the lung of a premature newborn. The incompletely expanded lung contains squames (*arrows*) consisting of squamous epithelial cells shed into the amniotic fluid from the fetal skin.

Sometimes immature infants show sluggish respiratory movement that does not fully expel the amniotic fluid from the lungs. Respiratory embarrassment may ensue, a syndrome called **amniotic fluid aspiration,** but that actually represents retained amniotic fluid. Air passages contain desquamated squamous cells **(squames)** and lanugo hair from the fetal skin and protein-rich amniotic fluid (Fig. 6-37; see Chapter 12).

The ability of the alveoli to remain expanded during the respiratory cycle (i.e., not to collapse when one exhales) is largely due to **pulmonary surfactant,** which reduces intra-alveolar surface tension. Surfactant is produced by type II pneumocytes and is a complex mixture of 10% proteins and 90% mixed phospholipids, the latter including 75% phosphatidylcholine (lecithin) and 10% phosphatidylglycerol. Surfactant composition changes as a fetus matures: (1) lecithin increases rapidly at the start of the third trimester and then rises rapidly to peak near term (Fig. 6-38); (2) most lecithin in the mature lung is dipalmitate, but in the immature lung it is a less-surface-active α-palmitate, α-myristate species; (3) phosphatidylglycerol is not present in the lungs before the 36th week of pregnancy; and (4) before the 35th week, the immature surfactant contains a higher proportion of sphingomyelin than adult surfactant.

The protein constituents of surfactant, though they make up a small proportion of its total weight, are important in facilitating the surface activity of the mixture, and serve other functions as well. There are two highly hydrophobic

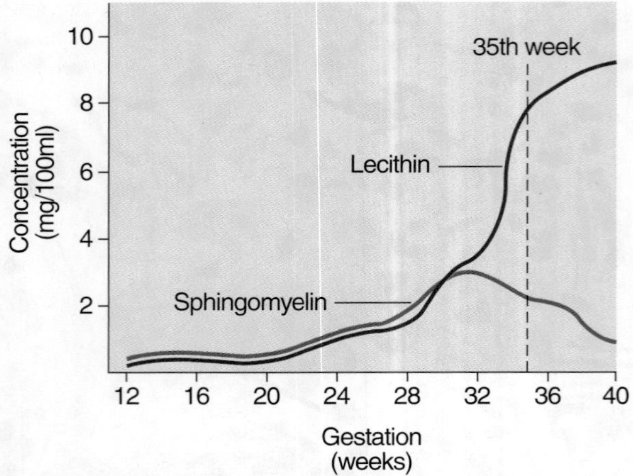

FIGURE 6-38. Changes in amniotic fluid composition during pregnancy.

surfactant-associated proteins (SPs), SP-B and SP-C, which are critical for surface activity. Two more hydrophilic proteins, SP-A and SP-D, subserve additional functions, thought to include regulating surfactant secretion, antimicrobial protection and others.

Pulmonary surfactant is released into the amniotic fluid, which can be sampled by amniocentesis to assess fetal lung maturity. A lecithin-to-sphingomyelin ratio above 2:1 implies that the fetus should survive without developing respiratory distress syndrome. After the 35th week, the appearance of phosphatidylglycerol in the amniotic fluid is the best proof of the maturity of the fetal lungs.

LIVER: The liver of premature infants is morphologically similar to that of the adult organ, except for conspicuous extramedullary hematopoiesis. However, the hepatocytes tend to be functionally immature. Fetal liver is deficient in glucuronyl transferase. The liver's resulting inability to conjugate bilirubin often leads to **neonatal jaundice** (see Chapter 14). This enzyme deficiency is aggravated by the rapid destruction of fetal erythrocytes, a process that results in an increased supply of bilirubin.

BRAIN: The brain of immature newborns differs from that of the adult, morphologically and functionally, but this difference is rarely fatal. On the other hand, incomplete development of the CNS is often reflected in poor vasomotor control, hypothermia, feeding difficulties and recurrent apnea.

The Apgar Score

Clinical assessments of neonatal maturity in general are usually performed 1 minute and 5 minutes after delivery, and certain parameters are scored according to the criteria recommended by Virginia Apgar (Table 6-11). In general, the higher the **Apgar score,** the better the clinical condition of the infant. The score taken at 1 minute is an index of asphyxia and of the need for assisted ventilation. The 5-minute score is a more accurate indication of impending death or the likelihood of persistent neurologic damage. For example, in newborns weighing less than 2000 g who have a 5-minute Apgar score of 9 or 10, the mortality during the first month is less than 5%; it is almost 80% when the Apgar score is reduced to 3 or less.

Table 6-11

Apgar Score*

Sign	0	1	2
Heart rate	Not detectable	Below 100/min	Over 100/min
Respiratory effort	None	Slow, irregular	Good, crying
Muscle tone	Poor	Some flexion of extremities	Active motion
Response to catheter in nostril	No response	Grimace	Cough or sneeze
Color	Blue, pale	Body pink, extremities blue	Completely pink

*Sixty seconds after the completion of birth, these five objective signs are evaluated, and each is given a score of 0, 1, or 2. A maximum score of 10 is assigned to infants in the best possible condition.

Neonatal Respiratory Distress Syndrome Is Due to Deficiency of Surfactant

Neonatal respiratory distress syndrome (RDS) is the leading cause of morbidity and mortality among premature infants. It accounts for half of all neonatal deaths in the United States. Its incidence varies inversely with gestational age and birth weight. Thus, more than half of newborns younger than 28 weeks' gestational age have RDS, but only one fifth of infants between 32 and 36 weeks do. In addition to prematurity, other risk factors for RDS include (1) neonatal asphyxia, (2) maternal diabetes, (3) delivery by cesarean section, (4) precipitous delivery and (5) twin pregnancy.

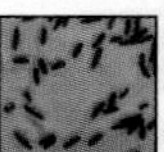

ETIOLOGIC FACTORS: *The pathogenesis of RDS of the newborn is intimately linked to a deficiency of surfactant* (Fig. 6-39). When a newborn starts breathing, type II cells release their surfactant stores. The biophysical role of surfactant is to reduce surface tension (i.e., to decrease the affinity of alveolar surfaces for each other). This allows alveoli to remain open when the baby exhales and reduces resistance to reinflating the lungs with the second breath. If surfactant function is inadequate, as it is in many premature infants with immature lungs, alveoli collapse when the baby exhales and resist expansion when the child tries to take his or her second breath. The energy required for the second breath must then overcome the cell–cell affinity within alveoli. Inspiration therefore requires considerable effort and damages the alveolar lining. The injured alveoli leak plasma into airspaces. Plasma constituents, including fibrinogen and albumin, bind surfactant and impair its function, thus further exacerbating the respiratory insufficiency. Many alveoli are perfused with blood but not ventilated by air, which leads to hypoxia and acidosis and further compromise in the ability of type II pneumocytes to produce surfactant. Resulting hypoxia induces pulmonary arterial vasoconstriction, thereby increasing right-to-left shunting through the ductus arteriosus and foramen ovale and within the lung itself. The resulting pulmonary ischemia further aggravates alveolar epithelial damage and injures the endothelium of the pulmonary capillaries. The leak of

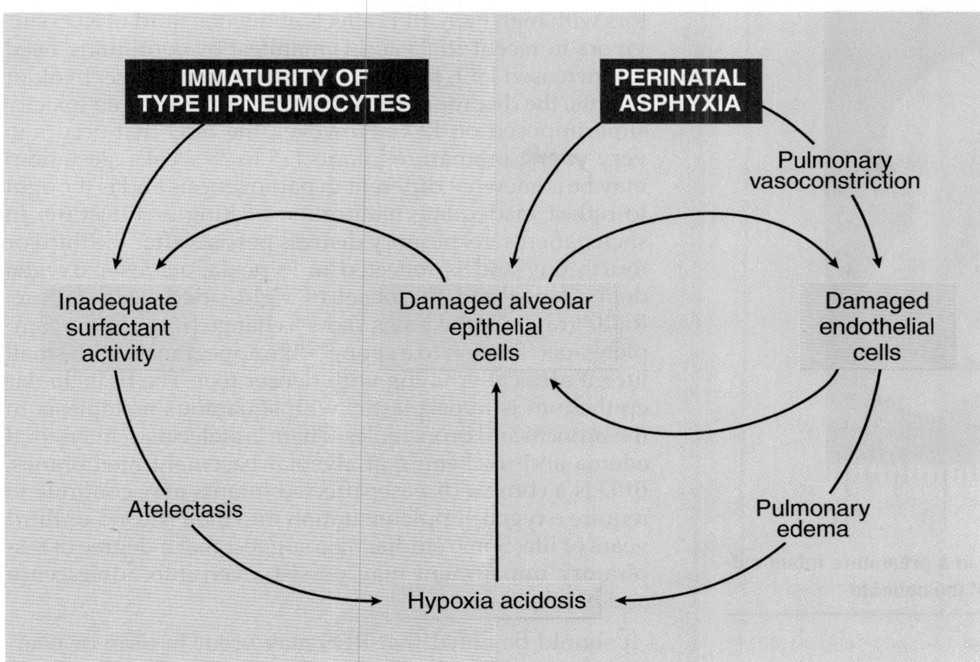

FIGURE 6-39. Pathogenesis of the respiratory distress syndrome of the neonate. Immaturity of the lungs and perinatal asphyxia are the major pathogenetic factors.

protein-rich fluid into the alveoli from the injured vascular bed contributes to the typical clinical and pathologic features of RDS.

The course of RDS is further complicated by the need to expose the infant to high concentrations of inspired oxygen (FiO_2) in order to maintain adequate arterial oxygen levels. Although respiratory support has improved greatly, the damage caused by high FiO_2 levels (see ROS-mediated injury, Chapter 1) adds to the already ongoing lung injury.

PATHOLOGY: The lungs in neonatal RDS are dark red, solid appearing and airless. Alveoli are collapsed. Alveolar ducts and respiratory bronchioles are dilated and contain cellular debris, proteinaceous edema fluid and erythrocytes. The alveolar ducts are lined by conspicuous, eosinophilic, fibrin-rich, amorphous structures, called **hyaline membranes,** hence the original term **hyaline membrane disease** (Fig. 6-40). Walls of collapsed alveoli are thick, capillaries are congested and lymphatics are filled with proteinaceous material.

CLINICAL FEATURES: Most newborns destined to develop RDS appear normal at birth and have high Apgar scores. The first symptom, appearing usually within an hour of birth, is increased respiratory effort, with forceful intercostal retraction and the use of accessory neck muscles. Respiratory rate increases to more than 100 breaths per minute, and the baby becomes cyanotic. Chest radiographs show a characteristic "ground-glass" granularity and in terminal stages the fluid-filled alveoli appear as complete "white-out" of the lungs. In severe cases, the infant becomes progressively obtunded and flaccid. Long periods of apnea ensue and the infant eventually dies of asphyxia.

Therapeutic advances in recent decades have improved the survival of infants with RDS, led to survival of very young premature babies who previously would have had almost no

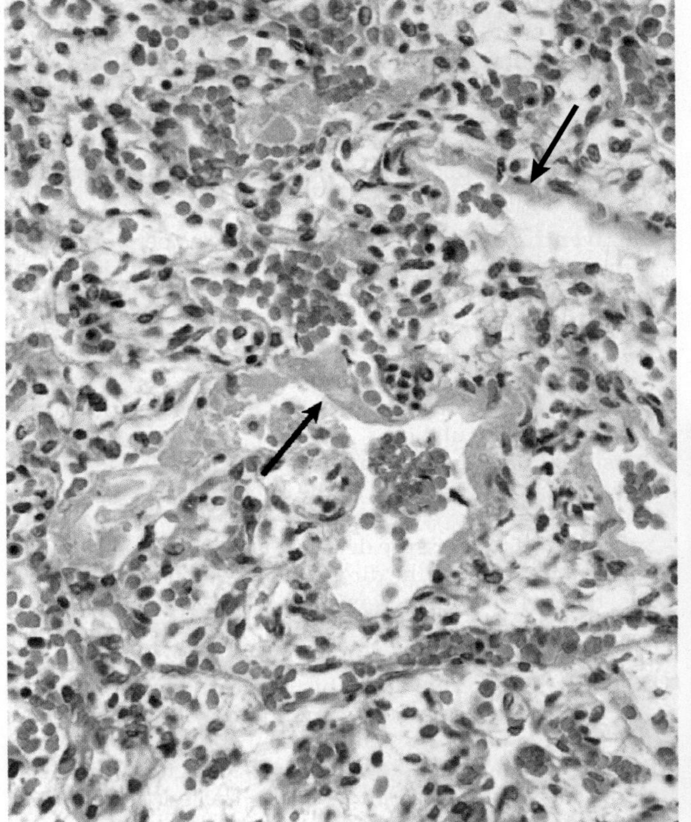

FIGURE 6-40. The lung in respiratory distress syndrome of the neonate. The alveoli are atelectatic, and a dilated alveolar duct is lined by a fibrin-rich hyaline membrane (*arrows*).

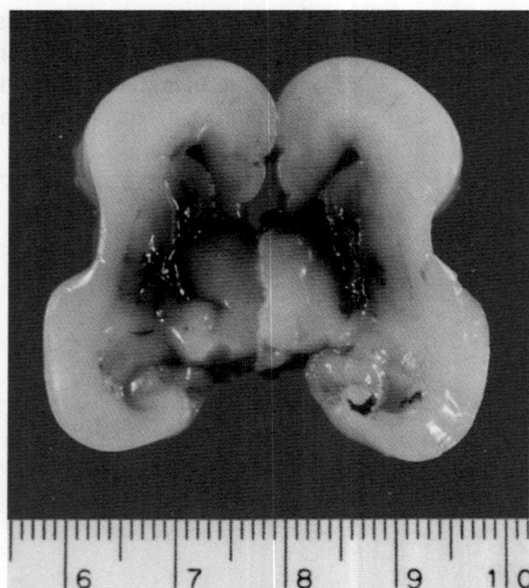

FIGURE 6-41. Intraventricular hemorrhage in a premature infant suffering from respiratory distress syndrome of the neonate.

chance of living and decreased the incidence of many of the complications of RDS (see below). Although studies differ in their test populations and therapeutic approaches used, several general conclusions can be drawn. If labor threatens in a preterm pregnancy, administration of corticosteroids to mothers hastens the maturation of the lung, thereby decreasing the incidence of RDS in preterm babies. Further, the use of animal-derived surfactants (porcine or bovine), combined with improved ventilatory therapy, has dramatically improved the survival of infants with RDS. Currently, even in very small premature infants, 85% to 90% survival is common.

The major complications of RDS relate to anoxia and acidosis and include:

- **Intraventricular cerebral hemorrhage:** The periventricular germinal matrix in the newborn brain is particularly vulnerable to hemorrhage because the dilated, thin-walled veins in this area rupture easily (Fig. 6-41). The pathogenesis of this complication is not fully understood but is believed to reflect anoxic injury to the periventricular capillaries, venous sludging and thrombosis and impaired vascular autoregulation.
- **Persistent patent ductus arteriosus:** In almost one third of newborns who survive RDS, the ductus arteriosus remains patent. With recovery from the pulmonary disease, pulmonary arterial pressure declines, and the higher pressure in the aorta reverses the direction of blood flow in the ductus, thereby creating a persistent left-to-right shunt. Congestive heart failure may ensue and necessitate correction of the patent ductus.
- **Necrotizing enterocolitis:** This intestinal complication of RDS is the most common acquired gastrointestinal emergency in newborns. It is thought to be related to ischemia of the intestinal mucosa, which leads to bacterial colonization, usually with *Clostridium difficile.* The lesions vary from those of typical pseudomembranous enterocolitis to gangrene and perforation of the bowel.
- **Bronchopulmonary dysplasia (BPD):** BPD is a late complication of RDS usually in infants who weigh less than 1500 g and were maintained on positive-pressure respirators with high FiO_2. BPD affects about one third of RDS survivors in recent trials and is manifest by continuing need for increased FiO_2 beyond 1 month postnatal age. In older infants, the disorder probably results from oxygen toxicity superimposed on RDS. However, the BPD that occurs in very young premature infants (25 to 28 weeks' gestation) may be somewhat different in pathogenesis and is thought to reflect inadequate maturation of lung architecture. In such patients, respiratory distress persists after the third or fourth day and is reflected in hypoxia, acidosis, oxygen dependency and the onset of right-sided heart failure. Radiographs of the lungs show a change from almost complete opacification to a sponge-like appearance, with small lucent areas alternating with denser foci. The bronchiolar epithelium is hyperplastic, with squamous metaplasia in the bronchi and bronchioles. There is atelectasis, interstitial edema and thickening of alveolar basement membranes. BPD is a chronic disease; affected infants may continue to require oxygen supplementation into their second or third years of life. Some studies also suggest that a degree of respiratory impairment may persist, even into adolescence and beyond.

It should be noted that RDS may occur in term or near-term infants. Clinically, this syndrome mimics that seen in premature infants who lack adequate surfactant. Recent studies have documented, however, that a high proportion of infants with RDS at term suffer from genetic deficiencies of one of the hydrophobic surfactant proteins (SP-B or SP-C) or that they have mutations in the ATP-binding cassette transporter (ABCA3).

Erythroblastosis Fetalis Is a Hemolytic Disease Caused by Maternal Antibodies Against Fetal Erythrocytes

The disorder was first recognized by Hippocrates but was not fully understood until 1940, when the Rh (Rhesus) antigen on erythrocytes was identified. More than 60 antigens on red blood cell membranes can elicit antibody responses, but only antibodies to Rh D and ABO antigens cause substantial hemolytic disease.

Rh Incompatibility

The distribution of Rh antigens among ethnic groups varies. In American whites, 15% are Rh negative (Rh D−); only 8% of blacks are Rh D−. Japanese, Chinese and Native Americans are essentially all Rh D+. By contrast, 35% of Basque people, among whom the Rh D− phenotype may have arisen, are Rh D−.

MOLECULAR PATHOGENESIS: The Rh blood group system consists of some 25 components, of which only the alleles cde/CDE need be considered here. Antibodies against D cause 90% of erythroblastosis fetalis caused by Rh incompatibility, the remaining cases involving C or E. Rh-positive fetal erythrocytes (>1 mL) enter the circulation of an Rh-negative mother at the time of delivery and elicit maternal antibodies to the fetus' D antigen (Fig. 6-42). As the volume of fetal blood required to sensitize a mother is only introduced into her circulation

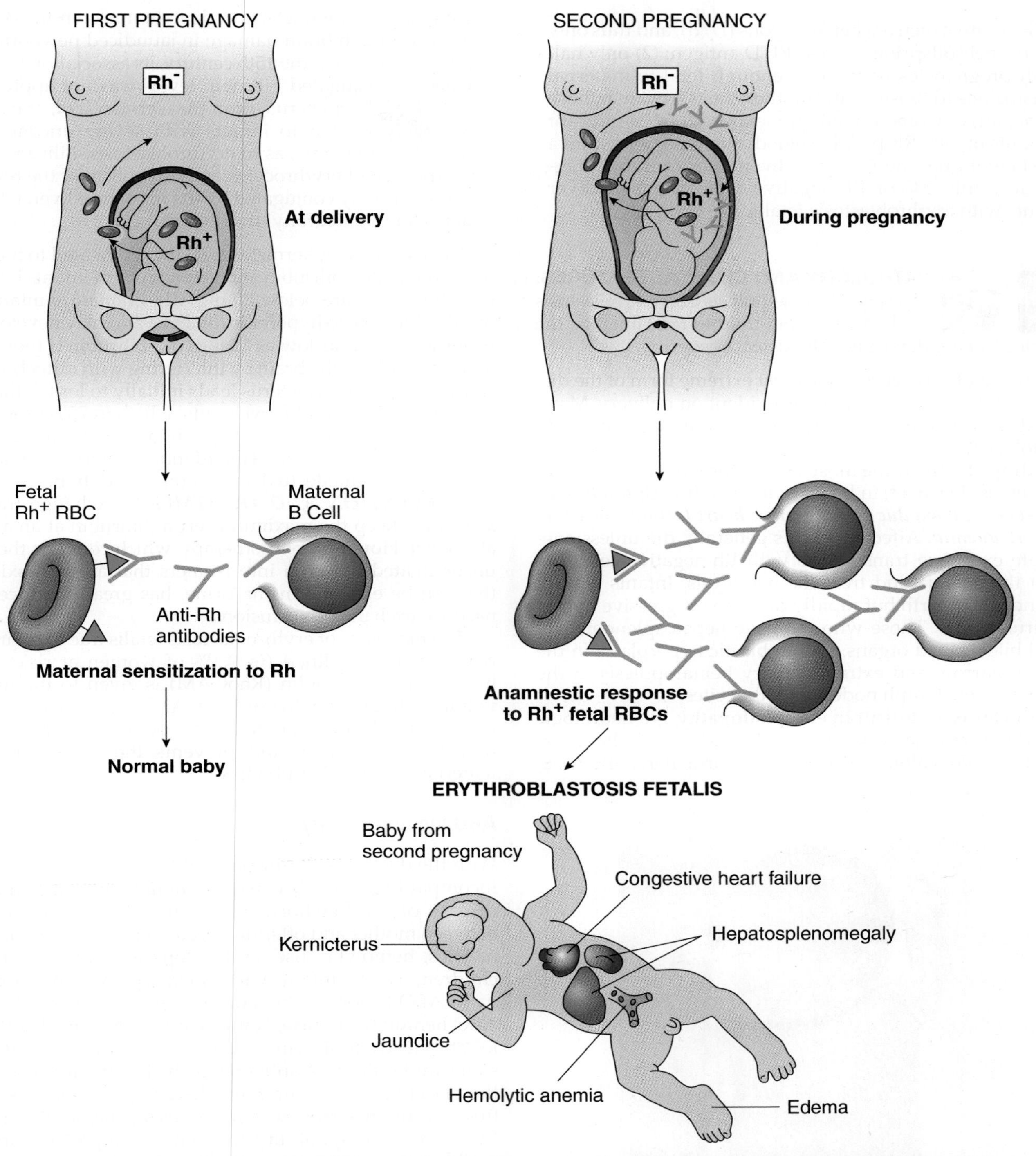

FIGURE 6-42. Pathogenesis of erythroblastosis fetalis due to maternal–fetal Rh incompatibility. Immunization of the Rh-negative mother with Rh-positive erythrocytes in the first pregnancy leads to the formation of anti-Rh antibodies of the immunoglobulin (Ig) G type. These antibodies cross the placenta and damage the Rh-positive fetus in subsequent pregnancies.

at the time of delivery, the disease does not ordinarily affect her first fetus. However, at subsequent pregnancies, when a now sensitized mother again carries an Rh-positive fetus, much smaller quantities of fetal D antigen boost antibody titer. Resulting IgG antibodies cross the placenta and thus cause hemolysis in the fetus. This cycle is magnified in multiparous women, the severity of erythroblastosis increasing progressively with each subsequent pregnancy.

About 15% of white women are Rh D−. Since they have an 85% chance of marrying an Rh D+ man, 13% of marriages are theoretically at risk for maternal–fetal Rh incompatibility. The actual incidence of erythroblastosis fetalis is, however, much lower because (1) more than half of Rh-positive men are heterozygous (D/d), and thus only half of their offspring express Rh D antigen; (2) only half of all pregnancies have large enough fetal-to-maternal transfusions to sensitize the mother; and (3) even in those Rh-negative women who are exposed to significant amounts of fetal Rh-positive blood, many do not mount a substantial immune response. Even after multiple pregnancies, only 5% of Rh-negative women ever deliver infants with erythroblastosis fetalis.

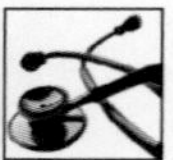

PATHOLOGY AND CLINICAL FEATURES: The severity of hemolysis in erythroblastosis fetalis varies from mild to fatal anemia, the pathology being determined by disease severity.

- **Death in utero** occurs in the most extreme form of the disease, and severe maceration is evident on delivery. Many erythroblasts are seen in organs that are not extensively autolyzed.
- **Hydrops fetalis** is the most serious form of erythroblastosis fetalis (Fig. 6-43) in liveborn infants. ***It is characterized by severe edema due to congestive heart failure caused by severe anemia.*** Affected infants generally die unless adequate exchange transfusions with Rh-negative cells correct the anemia and treat the hemolysis. Infants are not jaundiced at birth but rapidly develop progressive hyperbilirubinemia. Those who die have hepatosplenomegaly and bile-stained organs, erythroblastic hyperplasia in the bone marrow and extramedullary hematopoiesis in the liver, spleen, lymph nodes and other sites.
- **Kernicterus,** or **bilirubin encephalopathy,** is a neurologic condition associated with severe jaundice and characterized by bile staining of the brain, particularly the basal ganglia, pontine nuclei and dentate nuclei in the cerebellum. Although brain damage in jaundiced newborns was first mentioned in the 15th century, its association with elevated unconjugated bilirubin levels was not appreciated until 1952. Kernicterus (from the German *kern,* "nucleus") is largely limited to infants with severe unconjugated hyperbilirubinemia, as in erythroblastosis. Bilirubin from destruction of erythrocytes and catabolism of the released heme is poorly conjugated by the immature liver, which is deficient in glucuronyl transferase.

Development of kernicterus is directly related to the level of unconjugated bilirubin and is rare in term infants if serum bilirubin levels are below 20 mg/dL. Premature infants are more vulnerable to hyperbilirubinemia and may develop kernicterus at levels as low as 12 mg/dL. Bilirubin is thought to injure the cells of the brain by interfering with mitochondrial function. Severe kernicterus leads initially to loss of the startle reflex and athetoid movements, which in 75% progresses to lethargy and death. Most surviving infants have severe choreoathetosis and mental retardation; a minority have varying degrees of intellectual and motor retardation.

PREVENTION AND TREATMENT: Exchange transfusions may keep the maximum serum bilirubin at an acceptable level. However, phototherapy, which converts the toxic unconjugated bilirubin into isomers that are nontoxic and that can be excreted in the urine, has greatly reduced the need for exchange transfusions.

The incidence of erythroblastosis fetalis due to Rh incompatibility has declined (to <1% of women at risk) when human anti-D globulin (RhoGAM) is given to the mother within 72 hours of delivery. RhoGAM neutralizes antigenicity of fetal cells that may have entered the maternal circulation during delivery and prevents the development of maternal anti-Rh D antibodies.

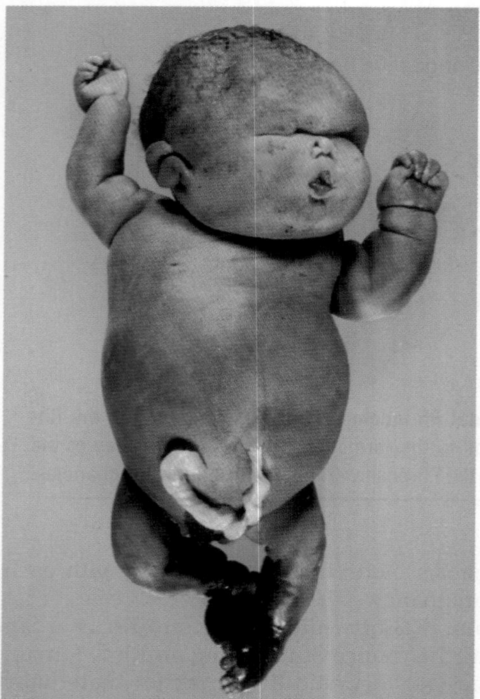

FIGURE 6-43. Hydrops fetalis. The infant shows severe anasarca.

ABO Incompatibility

With the decline in Rh-incompatible erythroblastosis, ABO incompatibility has become the main cause of hemolytic disease of the newborn. Although ABO incompatibility between mother and offspring occurs in one quarter of pregnancies, hemolytic disease develops in only 10% of such children, usually infants with blood type A. Low antigenicity of ABO factors in the fetus accounts for the mildness of ABO hemolytic disease. Natural anti-A and anti-B antibodies are mostly IgM, which does not cross the placenta, but some antibodies to A antigen may be IgG, which does cross the placenta. ABO isoimmune disease may thus be seen in firstborn infants. However, most cases of hemolytic anemia from ABO incompatibility are seen after a previous incompatible pregnancy.

Most infants with ABO incompatibility have mild jaundice as the only clinical feature. The extreme complications of erythroblastosis that is associated with Rh incompatibility are unusual with ABO disease. Nevertheless, kernicterus has occasionally been reported.

Injury at Birth Ranges From Mechanical Trauma to Anoxic Damage

Some birth injuries relate to obstetric manipulation, but many are due to unavoidable events in routine delivery. Birth injuries occur in about 5 per 1000 live births. Predisposing factors include cephalopelvic disproportion, dystocia (difficult labor), prematurity and breech presentation.

Cranial Injury

- **Caput succedaneum** is edema of the scalp caused by trauma to the head during passage through the birth canal. The swelling rapidly disappears and is of little clinical concern.
- **Cephalohematoma** is a subperiosteal hemorrhage of a single cranial bone. It becomes apparent within a few hours after birth and may or may not be associated with a linear fracture of the underlying bone. Most cephalohematomas resolve without complication and require no treatment.
- **Skull fractures** during birth result from the impact of the head on the pelvic bones or pressure from obstetric forceps. Linear fractures, the most common variety, are asymptomatic and do not require treatment. Depressed fractures are usually caused by trauma from forceps. Although many depressed fractures do not initially produce symptoms, they may require mechanical elevation because of the risk of underlying cranial trauma from persistent pressure. In contrast to most fractures, those of the occipital bone often extend through the underlying venous sinuses and produce fatal hemorrhage.
- **Intracranial hemorrhage** is one of the most dangerous birth injuries and may be traumatic, secondary to asphyxia or a result of an underlying bleeding diathesis. Traumatic intracranial hemorrhage occurs in the settings of (1) significant cephalopelvic disproportion, (2) precipitous delivery, (3) breech presentation, (4) prolonged labor or (5) inappropriate use of forceps. These traumas can result in **subdural or subarachnoid hemorrhage,** often due to lacerations of the falx cerebri or tentorium cerebelli that involve the vein of Galen or the venous sinuses. As noted above, anoxic injury from asphyxia, particularly in the premature infant, is often associated with intraventricular hemorrhage.

The prognosis for newborns with intracranial hemorrhage depends on its extent. Massive hemorrhage is often rapidly fatal. Surviving infants may recover completely or may have long-term impairment, usually in the form of cerebral palsy or hydrocephalus. However, many cases of cerebral palsy have been shown by ultrasound studies to relate to brain damage acquired 2 weeks or more prior to birth rather than from birth trauma.

Peripheral Nerve Injury

- **Brachial palsy,** with varying degrees of paralysis of the arm, is caused by excessive traction on the head and neck or shoulders during delivery. If the nerves are severed, impairment may be permanent. Function may return within a few months if the palsy results from edema and hemorrhage.
- **Phrenic nerve paralysis** and associated paralysis of a hemidiaphragm may be associated with brachial palsy and lead to breathing difficulties. The condition generally resolves spontaneously within a few months.
- **Facial nerve palsy** usually presents as a unilateral flaccid paralysis of the face caused by injury to the seventh cranial nerve during labor or delivery, especially with forceps. If severe, the entire affected side of the face is paralyzed and even the eyelid cannot be closed. Prognosis again depends on the extent of nerve injury.

Fractures

The **clavicle** is most vulnerable to fracture during delivery, and there may be associated fracture of the **humerus.** Immobilization of the arm and shoulder usually provides for complete healing. Fractures of other long bones and the nose occasionally occur during birth but heal easily.

Rupture of the Liver

The only internal organ other than the brain that is injured with any frequency during labor and delivery is the liver. Mechanical pressure during difficult or premature births is responsible. Hepatic rupture may cause a hematoma large enough to be palpable and to cause anemia; surgical repair of the laceration may be required.

Sudden Infant Death Syndrome Is an Important Cause of Post-Perinatal Death

Sudden infant death syndrome (SIDS), also known as "crib death" or "cot death," is defined as "sudden death of an infant or young child which is unexpected by history and in which a thorough postmortem examination fails to demonstrate an adequate cause of death."[1] The diagnosis of SIDS is made only after excluding other specific causes of sudden death, such as infection, hemorrhage, aspiration, etc. It is particularly important that homicide be eliminated as a potential cause of SIDS, especially in settings in which more than one sibling has died of apparent SIDS. Descriptions of apparent SIDS date to the Bible, and the syndrome was noted in the American colonies in 1686. However, modern attention to the disorder dates to the late 1960s.

Typically, victims of SIDS are apparently healthy young infants who went to sleep without any hint of the impending calamity but did not wake up. As a number of predisposing factors and environmental, biochemical, structural and genetic contributors are identified, it becomes moot the extent to which the nomenclature SIDS is reserved for the shrinking number of deaths that truly have no identifiable pathogenesis or whether those deaths whose pathogeneses can be traced but do not involve infection, suffocation, etc., may still be included in a more loosely defined diagnostic basket. We choose the latter, more inclusive, definition of this syndrome.

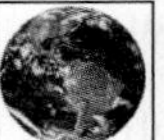

EPIDEMIOLOGY: After the neonatal period, SIDS is the leading cause of death in the first year of life, accounting for more than one third of all deaths in this period. Its incidence in the United States has decreased from 1.2 in 1000 live births in 1992 to 0.5 in 1000 live births in 2006 (see below). Still, SIDS is responsible for over 2000 infant deaths annually in the United States. Most (90%) occur before 6 months of age, although infants up to 12 months are covered by currently accepted diagnostic criteria.

[1]Willinger M, James LS, Catz C. Defining the sudden infant death syndrome (SIDS): deliberations of an expert panel convened by the National Institute of Child Health and Human Development. *Pediatr Pathol* 1991;11:677–684.

The majority of deaths from SIDS occur during the winter months, and a significantly higher percentage of infants dying of SIDS are reported to have experienced upper respiratory infections within the previous 4 weeks. However, deaths involving active infections are by definition excluded. Most deaths occur at night or during periods associated with sleep. It was found that infants who slept prone or on their sides had much higher incidence of SIDS than did those who slept supine. A worldwide "Back to Sleep" campaign that encouraged parents to place infants on their backs for sleeping reduced the incidence of SIDS by about half.

Risk factors for SIDS are difficult to ascertain, and much of what is known is based on retrospective studies. There are both maternal and infant risk factors. The strongest **maternal risk factors** are:

- Low socioeconomic status (poor education, unmarried mother, poor prenatal care)
- Black or Native American parentage (in the United States, and independent of economic status; in other countries indigenous populations, like Maoris in New Zealand and Aborigines in Australia, are also at higher risk)
- Age younger than 20 years at first pregnancy
- Cigarette smoking and/or alcohol consumption during and following pregnancy
- Use of illicit drugs during pregnancy
- Increased parity

The risk factors for the infant are more controversial. The consensus includes:

- Low birth weight
- Prematurity
- An illness, often respiratory, within the last 4 weeks before death
- Subsequent siblings of SIDS victims
- Survivors of an apparent life-threatening event (i.e., an episode of some combination of apnea, color change, marked alteration in muscle tone and choking or gagging). A definite cause, such as seizures or aspiration after vomiting, is established in only half the cases of an apparent life-threatening event.

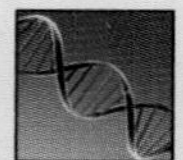
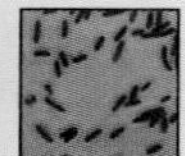

MOLECULAR PATHOGENESIS AND ETIOLOGIC FACTORS: In recent years, studies of the etiology and pathogenesis of SIDS have provided important insight into the factors that contribute to this syndrome and, in some instances, the molecular bases for sudden infant death. As noted above, while the original definition of SIDS excludes from the diagnosis known causes, we use a more expansive definition here because of our improved understanding of both molecular and environmental factors involved.

Channelopathies, inherited abnormalities in cell membrane ion channels (see Chapter 1), are felt to be responsible for about 10% to 12% of cases of SIDS, although this percentage may be higher (up to about 30%) in SIDS deaths between the ages of 6 and 12 months. There are four different cardiac conduction syndromes that are thought to cause sudden infant death. All involve more than one different mutation, producing clustered phenotypes.

The most common of these is long QT syndrome, which is mostly due to loss-of-function mutations in cardiac potassium channels (KCNQ1, KCNH2), but mutations in other ion channel proteins have also been identified in some cases, including sodium channel (SCN5A) and L-type calcium channel (CACNA1C). Long QT syndrome is characterized by prolonged QT intervals on electrocardiography and is seen in about 10% of SIDS deaths.

Other channelopathies associated with SIDS include catecholaminergic polymorphic ventricular tachycardia (CPVT, mostly due to mutation in ryanodine receptor 2), Brugada syndrome (a different mutation in the SCN5A sodium channel, and also mutations in calcium channels) and short QT syndrome (gain-of-function mutations in cardiac potassium channels, causing accelerated repolarization of cardiac muscle). It should be emphasized that these mutations are seen disproportionately in SIDS deaths but are present in many individuals, only a small number of whom die of SIDS. Some manifest much later in life, as sudden death either in adolescence or later. Others may never be symptomatic.

Since SIDS relating to prone sleeping position has largely been removed, **maternal smoking during pregnancy remains probably the most important single etiologic factor in SIDS,** accounting for an estimated 80% or more of SIDS deaths. On the basis of animal studies, and epidemiologic studies of families in which the father smoked but the mother did not, the key factor appears to be exposure to nicotine in utero. A dose-response effect has been reported: the likelihood of an infant developing SIDS is a direct function of the average number of cigarettes smoked by the mother during pregnancy. A baby born to a woman who smoked 20+ cigarettes daily while pregnant has over a fivefold increased risk of SIDS compared to a child of a nonsmoker.

Significant abnormalities have been detected in the brains of infants dying of SIDS, as have significant neurophysiologic abnormalities. These include hypoplasia of the arcuate nucleus, decreased serotonin receptors and decreased muscarinic cholinergic activity in favor of increased, abnormal nicotinic activity. Comparable abnormalities have been seen in experimental animals exposed to nicotine in utero and are associated with depressed ventilatory responses to hypercarbia and hypoxia. Further, prospective studies of babies who later died of SIDS demonstrated abnormal autonomic nervous system physiology, including depressed gasping reflexes and abnormal regulation of heart rhythm.

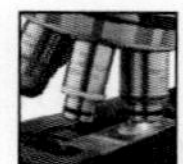

PATHOLOGY: At autopsy, several morphologic alterations are described in victims of SIDS, some of which (see above) may bear on the pathogenesis of this disorder, while the significance of others remains unclear. Thus, arcuate nucleus hypoplasia is seen (see above), as is brainstem gliosis. Medial hypertrophy of small pulmonary arteries, persistence of extramedullary hematopoiesis in the liver, right ventricular hypertrophy and increased periadrenal brown fat suggest a degree of chronic hypoxia. However, except for brainstem pathologies, none of these changes occurs with any regularity. Petechiae on the surfaces of the lungs, heart, pleura and thymus are reported in most infants dying of SIDS, but probably reflect terminal events attributed to negative intrathoracic pressure produced by respiratory efforts.

Neoplasms of Infancy and Childhood

Malignancies between the ages of 1 and 15 years are distinctly uncommon, but cancer remains the leading cause of death from disease in this age group. In children, 10% of deaths are due to cancer, exceeded only by accidental trauma. ***Unlike adults, in whom most cancers are of epithelial origin (e.g., carcinomas of the lung, breast and gastrointestinal tract), most malignant tumors in children arise from hematopoietic, nervous and soft tissues*** (Fig. 6-44). Also, many childhood cancers are part of developmental complexes. Examples include Wilms tumor associated with aniridia, genitourinary malformations and mental retardation (WAGR complex); hemihypertrophy of the body with Wilms tumor, hepatoblastoma and adrenal carcinoma; and tuberous sclerosis with renal tumors and cardiac rhabdomyomas. Some tumors are evident at birth and so obviously developed in utero. In addition, abnormally developed organs, persistent organ primordia and displaced organ rests are all vulnerable to neoplastic transformation.

Individual cancers of childhood are discussed in detail in chapters dealing with the respective organs, and the basic principles of neoplasia and carcinogenesis are discussed in Chapter 5.

Benign Tumors and Tumor-Like Conditions Encompass Diverse Abnormalities

HAMARTOMAS: These lesions are focal, benign overgrowths of one or more mature cellular elements of a normal tissue, often arranged irregularly. Many hamartomas show clonal origin and have defined DNA rearrangements, and so may be classified as true neoplasms.

CHORISTOMAS: Also called **heterotopias,** choristomas are tiny aggregates of normal tissue components in aberrant locations. They are not true tumors. Examples include pancreatic rests in the walls of the gastrointestinal organs, and adrenal tissue in the renal cortex.

HEMANGIOMAS: These lesions, of varying size and in diverse locations, are the most common tumors in childhood. Whether they are true neoplasms is unclear, but half are present at birth and most regress with age. Large, rapidly growing hemangiomas, especially on the head or neck, may occasionally cause serious problems. **Port wine stains** are congenital capillary hemangiomas of the skin of the face and scalp. They are often disfiguring, giving the affected area a dark purple color. Unlike many small hemangiomas, they persist for life.

LYMPHANGIOMAS: Also called **cystic hygromas,** these are poorly circumscribed swellings that are usually present at birth and thereafter rapidly increase in size. Most occur on the head and neck, but the floor of the mouth, mediastinum and buttocks are not uncommon sites. Some researchers consider lymphangiomas to be developmental malformations; others

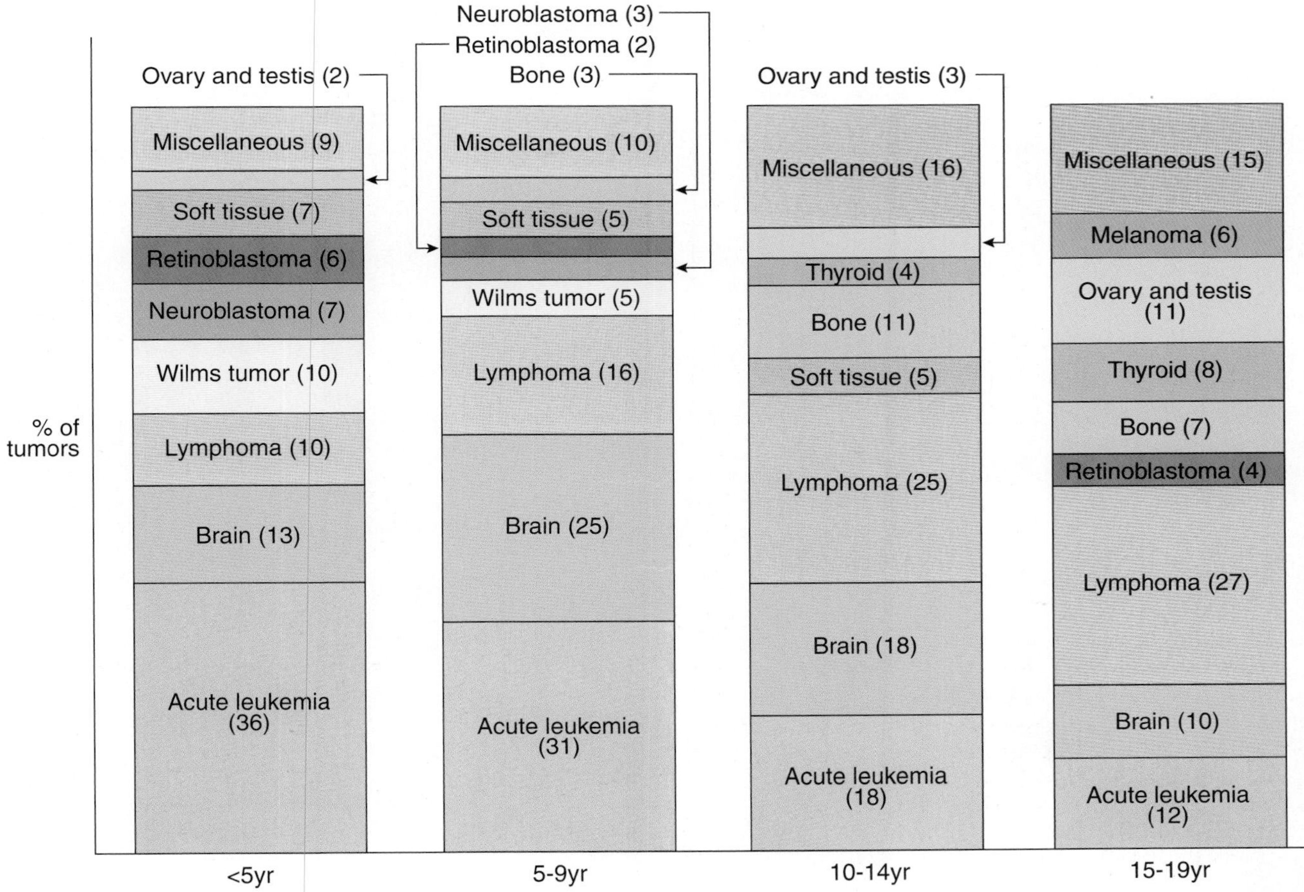

FIGURE 6-44. Distribution of childhood tumors according to age and primary site.

call them neoplasms. They may be unilocular or multilocular and have thin, transparent walls and straw-colored fluid. Myriad dilated lymphatic channels are separated by fibrous septa. Unlike hemangiomas, these lesions do not regress spontaneously and should be resected.

SACROCOCCYGEAL TERATOMAS: These rare germ cell tumors, which occur at 1 in 40,000 live births, are the most common solid neoplasms in the newborn. Over 75% of sacrococcygeal teratomas occur in girls, and a substantial number are seen in twins. They are usually noticed at birth as masses near the sacrum and buttocks. They may be large, lobulated tumors, sometimes as large as the infant's head. One half grow externally and may be connected to the body by a stalk. Some have both external and intrapelvic components, and a few grow entirely in the pelvis. Sacrococcygeal teratomas contain numerous tissues, particularly of neural origin. Most (90%) detected before the age of 2 months are benign, but up to half of those found later in life are malignant. Associated congenital anomalies of vertebrae, the genitourinary system and the anorectum are common. The lesion should be resected promptly.

Malignancies in the Pediatric Age Group Are Uncommon

The incidence of childhood cancer is 1.3 per 10,000 per year in children younger than 15 years. Mortality clearly reflects the intrinsic behavior of the tumor and its response to therapy, but overall, the death rate for childhood cancer is about one third of the incidence. Almost half of all such malignancies are acute leukemias and lymphomas. Leukemias alone, particularly acute lymphoblastic leukemia, represent one third of childhood cancer. Most of the rest are neuroblastomas, brain tumors, Wilms tumors, retinoblastomas, bone cancers and soft tissue sarcomas.

Genetic influences in the development of childhood tumors have been particularly well studied in the case of retinoblastoma, Wilms tumor and osteosarcoma. The interactions of heritable factors and environmental influences in the pathogenesis of malignant tumors in both children and adults are discussed in Chapter 5.

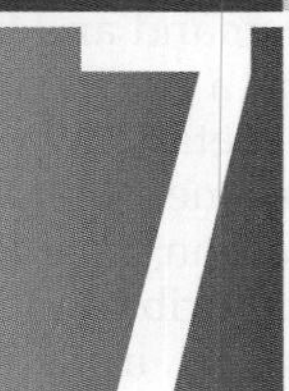

Hemodynamic Disorders

Bruce M. McManus • Michael F. Allard • Robert Yanagawa

Normal Circulation

Normal function and metabolism of organs and cells depend on an intact circulatory system for continuous delivery of oxygen, nutrients, hormones, electrolytes and water, as well as for removal of metabolic waste and carbon dioxide. The circulatory system is a vascular conduit made of a muscular pump connected to tubes (or blood vessels) that deliver blood to organs and tissues and return it to the heart to complete the circuit. Delivery and elimination at the cellular level are controlled by exchanges between the intravascular space, interstitial space, cellular space and lymphatic space, which occur via the smallest-diameter blood vessels in the body (the microcirculation).

The Heart Is a Two-Sided Pump With Vascular Circuits in Series

In this series circuit, the amount of blood handled by the right ventricle, which pumps blood to the lungs (pulmonary circulation), must, over time, exactly equal the amount of blood going through the left ventricle, which distributes blood to the body (systemic circulation). The hemodynamically important parameters are cardiac output, perfusion pressure and peripheral vascular resistance.

- **Cardiac output** is the volume of blood pumped by each ventricle per minute and represents the total blood flow in pulmonary and systemic circuits. Cardiac output is the product of heart rate and stroke volume and, as the **cardiac index**, is often adjusted for body surface area (in square meters) as an indicator of ventricular function.
- **Perfusion pressure** (also called **driving pressure**) is the difference in dynamic pressure between two points along a blood vessel. Blood flow to any segment of the circulation ultimately depends on arterial driving pressure. However, each organ can autoregulate flow and so determine the amount of blood it receives from the circulation. Such local control of perfusion depends on continuous modulation of microvascular beds by hormonal, neural, metabolic and hemodynamic factors.
- **Peripheral vascular resistance** is the sum of the factors that determine regional blood flow in each organ. Two thirds of the resistance in the systemic vasculature is determined by the arterioles.

The sum of all regional flows equals the **venous return**, which in turn determines the cardiac output. Assessment of the heart's response to inflow (preload) and outflow (afterload) relies on cardiac reflexes as well as cardiac muscle integrity and neurohormonal regulation.

The Aorta and Arteries Transport Blood to the Organs

They also convert pulsatile flow into sustained regular flow. The latter function derives from the elastic properties of the aorta and the resistance produced by the arteriolar sphincters.

The Microcirculation Includes Arterioles, Capillaries and Venules

The blood vessels of the microcirculation are less than 100 μM in diameter. Blood from an arteriole enters capillaries, which freely anastomose with each other (Fig. 7-1), either directly or through metarterioles. Capillary length, measured from terminal arteriole to collecting venule, ranges from 0.1 to 3 mm, averaging 1 mm. However, the path length by which blood cells traverse capillaries may actually be longer because of their extensive anastomoses. This fact is probably an important determinant of microvascular exchange of substances such as oxygen because it increases the time available for such exchange to occur. The large aggregate surface area of capillaries means that blood flow is slow, which further enhances microvascular exchange. Capillary density in a tissue also influences microvascular exchange by affecting diffusion distance. For example, in tissues with high oxygen demands, such as the heart, capillary density is very high. Entry into the capillary system is guarded by precapillary sphincters, except for **thoroughfare channels**, which bypass capillaries and are always open. Since not all capillaries are always open, blood flow to a structure can be increased by recruiting additional capillaries. The sum of blood flow through the capillary bed, the thoroughfare channels and the arteriovenous anastomoses determines the regional blood flow.

The exact means by which an organ regulates blood flow according to its metabolic needs are still debated, but there is a link between oxygen demand and blood flow. In the heart, blood flow is adjusted on a second-to-second basis. Factors that mediate and link metabolic vasodilation to cellular metabolism include adenosine, other nucleotides, nitric oxide, certain prostaglandins, carbon dioxide and pH. The microcirculation is an important contributor to all forms of hyperemia and edema, and is a target in septic shock (see below). Vasoregulation in conducting arteries, resistance arteries and veins relies on delicate interactions between blood, endothelium, smooth muscle cells and surrounding stroma.

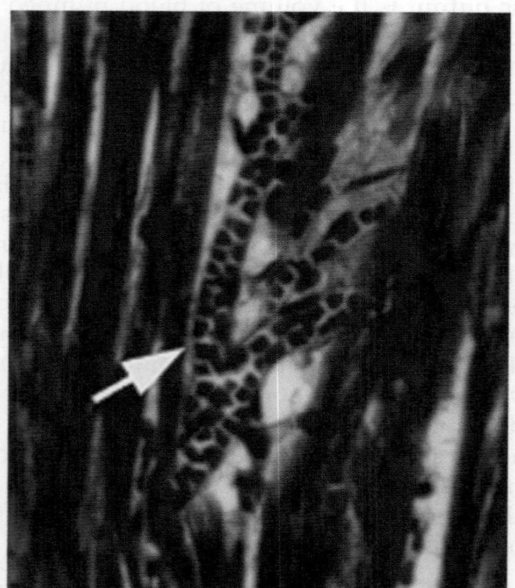

FIGURE 7-1. Microcirculation. Photomicrograph of myocardium showing capillaries and venules (*arrow*).

The Normal Endothelium Provides a Continuous Partition Between Blood and Tissues

Endothelial cells play important roles in anticoagulation, facilitation of migration of substances from blood to tissue and back, regulation of vessel tone (particularly that of resistance arteries) and regulation of vasopermeability (also see Chapters 2 and 10).

Veins and Venules Return Blood to the Heart

Blood from the capillaries enters venules and eventually veins on its route back to the heart. Veins not only serve as a conduit for blood, but also act as a blood reservoir. Roughly 65% of the total blood volume resides in the venous system.

Interstitium Represents 15% of Total Body Volume

The fluid between cells (**interstitial fluid**) helps to deliver nutrients to cells and eliminate cellular wastes. Most interstitial water is bound to a dense network of glycosaminoglycans.

Lymphatics Aid in the Reabsorption of Interstitial Fluid

Most interstitial fluid reenters the circulation at the venous end of capillaries. A small portion is drained by lymphatics. Lymphatic capillaries conduct lymph from the periphery to the central venous system via the thoracic duct. Normal oscillatory constrictions and relaxations of lymphatic vessels contribute to steady return of lymph fluid to the central circulation. Lymph is important for transport of molecules too large to return to the circulation through blood capillaries.

Disorders of Perfusion

Hemodynamic disorders are characterized by disturbed perfusion that may result in organ and cellular injury.

Hyperemia Is an Excess of Blood in an Organ

Hyperemia may be caused either by an increased supply of blood from the arterial system (**active hyperemia**) or by impaired exit of blood through venous pathways (**passive hyperemia** or **congestion**).

Active Hyperemia

Active hyperemia is augmented supply of blood to an organ. It is usually a physiologic response to increased functional

demand, as in the heart and skeletal muscle during exercise. Neurogenic and hormonal influences play a role in active hyperemia (e.g., the blushing bride and the menopausal flush). Although the utility of vasodilation is not always clear, cutaneous hyperemia in febrile states serves to dissipate heat. In addition, skeletal muscle may increase its blood flow (and thus oxygen delivery) 20-fold during exercise. The increased blood supply occurs by arteriolar dilation and recruitment of unperfused capillaries.

The most striking active hyperemia occurs in association with inflammation. Vasoactive materials released by inflammatory cells (see Chapter 2) cause blood vessels to dilate; in the skin this contributes to the classic "tumor, rubor and calor" of inflammation. In pneumonia, for example, alveolar capillaries are engorged with erythrocytes as a hyperemic response to inflammation. Because inflammation can also damage endothelial cells and increase capillary permeability, such hyperemia is often accompanied by edema and local extravasation of erythrocytes.

Reactive hyperemia occurs after temporary interruption of blood supply (ischemia). Removal of the obstruction is followed by active hyperemia, probably due to ischemic tissue injury and release of inflammatory agents such as histamine. The degree and duration of hyperemia is proportional to the period of occlusion until a plateau of hyperemic response is reached.

Passive Hyperemia (Congestion)

Passive hyperemia, or congestion, is engorgement of an organ with venous blood. Acute passive congestion is clinically a consequence of acute left or right ventricular failure. Regarding the former, resultant pulmonary venous engorgement leads to **pulmonary edema,** or accumulation of a transudate within the alveolar space. With acute failure of the right ventricle, the liver can become severely congested.

A generalized increase in venous pressure, typically from chronic heart failure, results in slower blood flow and a consequent increase in blood volume in many organs, including liver, spleen and kidneys. In the past, heart failure from rheumatic mitral stenosis was a common cause of generalized venous congestion, but with the decline in the prevalence of rheumatic fever and the advent of surgical valve replacement, such cases are unusual. Congestive heart failure secondary to coronary artery disease and hypertension and right-sided failure due to pulmonary disease are now more common.

Passive congestion may also be confined to a limb or an organ as a result of more-localized obstruction to venous drainage. Examples include deep thrombosis in the leg veins, resulting in edema of the lower extremity and thrombosis of hepatic veins (Budd-Chiari syndrome) with secondary chronic passive congestion of the liver (see Chapter 14).

LUNGS: Chronic left ventricular failure impedes blood flow out of the lungs and leads to chronic passive pulmonary congestion. As a result, pressure in alveolar capillaries increases and these vessels become engorged with blood. Increased alveolar capillary pressure has four major consequences:

- Microhemorrhages release erythrocytes into alveolar spaces, where they are phagocytosed and degraded by alveolar macrophages. The released iron, in the form of hemosiderin, remains in these macrophages, which are then called "heart failure cells" (Fig. 7-2).

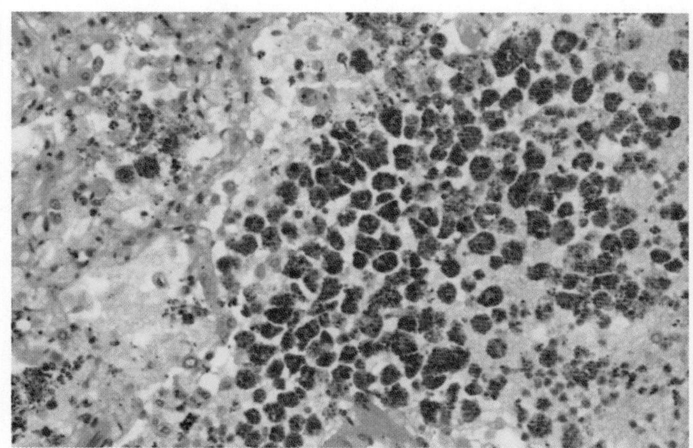

FIGURE 7-2. Passive congestion of lung. Hemosiderin-laden macrophages in the lung of a patient with congestive heart failure.

- Fluid is forced from the blood into the alveolar airspaces. The resulting pulmonary edema (Fig. 7-3) interferes with gas exchange in the lung.
- Fibrosis increases in the interstitium of the lung. The presence of fibrosis and iron is viewed grossly as a firm, brown lung (**brown induration**).
- **Pulmonary hypertension** occurs when the back-pressure from the pulmonary venous circuit is transmitted to the pulmonary arterial system. This may lead to right-sided heart failure and consequent generalized systemic venous congestion.

The morphologic changes associated with chronic passive congestion of the lungs are discussed in Chapter 12.

LIVER: The hepatic veins empty into the vena cava immediately inferior to the heart, so the liver is particularly vulnerable to acute or chronic passive congestion (see Chapter 14). Increased venous pressure causes the central veins of hepatic lobules to dilate and is transmitted to hepatic sinusoids, which dilate, causing centrilobular hepatocytes to undergo pressure atrophy (Fig. 7-4A). Grossly, the cut surface of a chronically congested liver has dark foci of

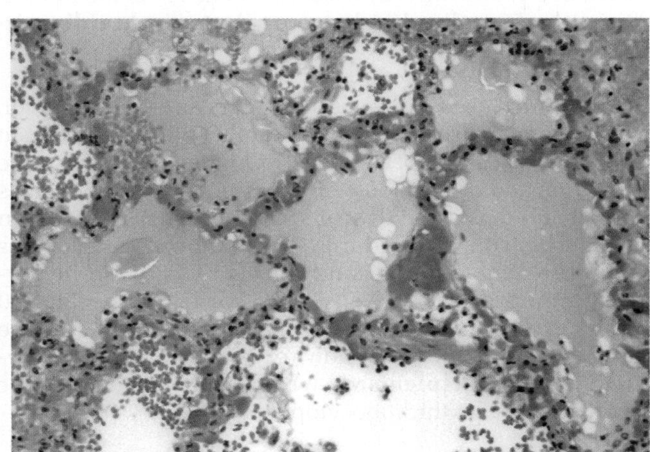

FIGURE 7-3. Pulmonary edema. A patient with congestive heart failure shows pink-staining fluid in the alveoli.

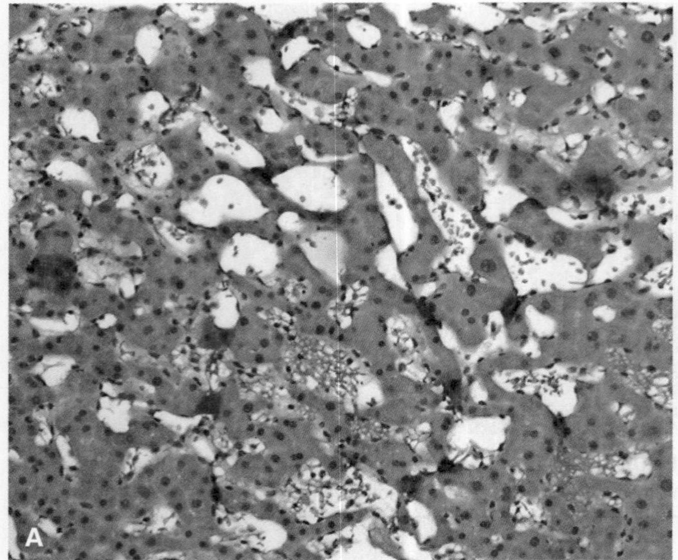

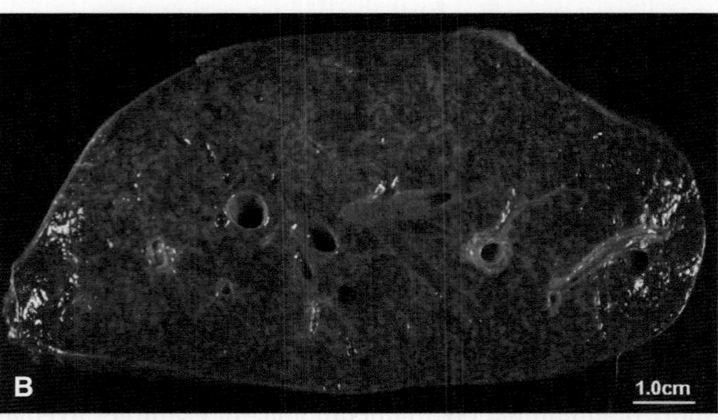

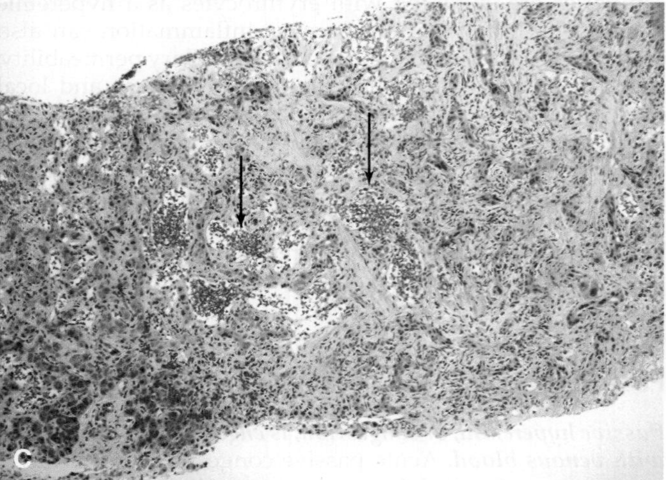

FIGURE 7-4. Passive congestion of liver. A. A photomicrograph of liver shows dilated centrilobular sinusoids. The intervening plates of hepatocytes exhibit pressure atrophy. **B.** A gross photograph of liver shows nutmeg appearance, reflecting congestive failure of the right ventricle. **C.** Late changes in chronic passive congestion characterized by dilated sinusoids (*arrows*) and fibrosis (note the blue staining of collagen in this trichrome stain). Proliferated bile ducts are on the right.

centrilobular congestion surrounded by paler zones of unaffected peripheral portions of the lobules. The result is a reticulated appearance that resembles a cross-section of a nutmeg ("nutmeg liver") (Fig. 7-4B). In severe cases associated with acute right ventricular failure, frank hemorrhagic necrosis of hepatocytes in centrilobular zones is conspicuous. Prolonged hepatic venous congestion eventually leads to thickening of central veins and centrilobular fibrosis. Only in the most extreme cases of venous congestion (e.g., constrictive pericarditis or tricuspid stenosis) is the fibrosis sufficiently generalized and severe to be termed **cardiac cirrhosis** (Fig. 7-4C).

SPLEEN: Increased intravascular pressure in the liver, whether from cardiac failure or an intrahepatic obstruction to blood flow (e.g., cirrhosis), leads to higher pressure in the splenic vein and congestion of the spleen. The organ becomes enlarged and tense, and the cut section oozes dark blood. In long-standing congestion, diffuse splenic fibrosis develops, as do iron-containing, fibrotic and calcified foci of old hemorrhage (Gamna-Gandy bodies). Such a spleen may weigh 250 to 750 g, compared with a normal weight of 150 g. The enlarged spleen sometimes shows excessive functional activity—termed **hypersplenism**—which leads to hematologic abnormalities (e.g., thrombocytopenia).

EDEMA AND ASCITES: Venous congestion impedes capillary blood flow, thereby increasing hydrostatic pressure and promoting edema formation (see below for a discussion of mechanisms of edema formation). Accumulation of edema fluid in heart failure is particularly noticeable in dependent tissues—legs and feet in ambulatory patients and the back in bedridden persons. **Ascites** is accumulation of fluid in the peritoneal space and reflects (among other factors) lack of tissue rigor, a condition in which there is no countervailing external pressure to oppose hydrostatic pressure within the blood vessels.

Hemorrhage Is a Discharge of Blood out of the Vascular Compartment

Blood can be released from the circulation to the exterior of the body or into nonvascular body spaces. The most common and obvious cause is trauma. Severe atherosclerosis may so weaken the wall of the abdominal aorta that it balloons to form an aneurysm, which then may rupture and bleed into the retroperitoneal space (see Chapter 10). In the same way, an aneurysm may complicate a congenitally weak cerebral artery (berry aneurysm) and lead to subarachnoid hemorrhage (see Chapter 28). Certain infections (e.g., pulmonary tuberculosis) and invasive neoplasms may erode blood vessels and lead to hemorrhage.

Hemorrhage also results from damage to capillaries. For instance, rupture of capillaries by blunt trauma leads to a bruise. Increased venous pressure also causes extravasation of blood from pulmonary capillaries. Vitamin C deficiency is associated with capillary fragility and bleeding, due to a defect in the supporting connective tissue structures. The capillary barrier by itself does not suffice to contain blood within the intravascular space. The minor trauma imposed on small vessels and capillaries by normal movement requires an intact coagulation system to prevent hemorrhage. Thus, a severe decrease in the number of platelets (**thrombocytopenia**) or deficiency of a coagulation factor (e.g., factor VIII in hemophilia A or von Willebrand factor in von Willebrand disease) is associated with spontaneous hemorrhage without apparent trauma (see Chapters 10 and 20).

A person may exsanguinate into an internal cavity, as in gastrointestinal hemorrhage from a peptic ulcer (**arterial hemorrhage**) or esophageal varices (**venous hemorrhage**). In such cases, large amounts of fresh blood fill the entire gastrointestinal tract. Bleeding into a serous cavity can result in accumulation of a large amount of blood, even to the point of exsanguination.

A few definitions are in order:

- **Hematoma:** Hemorrhage into soft tissue. Such collections of blood can be merely painful, as in a muscle bruise, or fatal, if located in the brain.
- **Hemothorax:** Hemorrhage into the pleural cavity.
- **Hemopericardium:** Hemorrhage into the pericardial space.
- **Hemoperitoneum:** Bleeding into the peritoneal cavity.
- **Hemarthrosis:** Bleeding into a joint space.
- **Purpura:** Diffuse superficial hemorrhages in the skin, up to 1 cm in diameter.
- **Ecchymosis:** A large superficial hemorrhage in the skin ("black and blue" mark; Fig. 7-5). The initially purple discoloration turns green and then yellow before resolving. This sequence of events reflects progressive oxidation of bilirubin released from the hemoglobin of degraded erythrocytes. A good example of an ecchymosis is a "black eye."
- **Petechiae:** Pinpoint hemorrhages, usually seen in the skin or conjunctiva (Fig. 7-6). This lesion reflects rupture of a capillary or arteriole and occurs in conjunction with coagulopathies or vasculitis. Petechiae may also be produced by microemboli from infected heart valves (bacterial endocarditis).

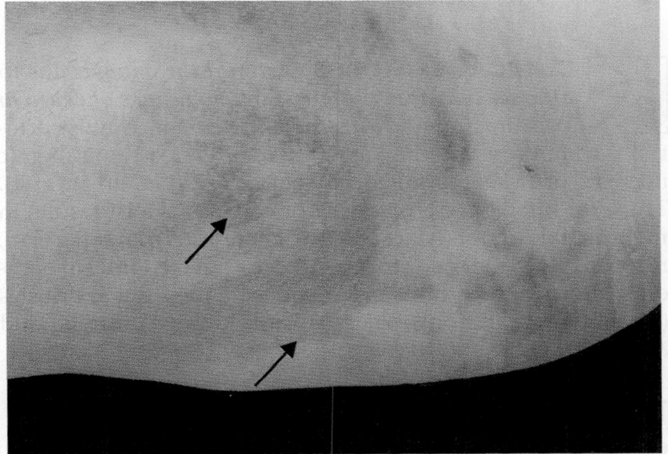

FIGURE 7-5. Ecchymosis. Superficial diffuse hemorrhage (*arrows*) on the thigh caused by blunt force trauma.

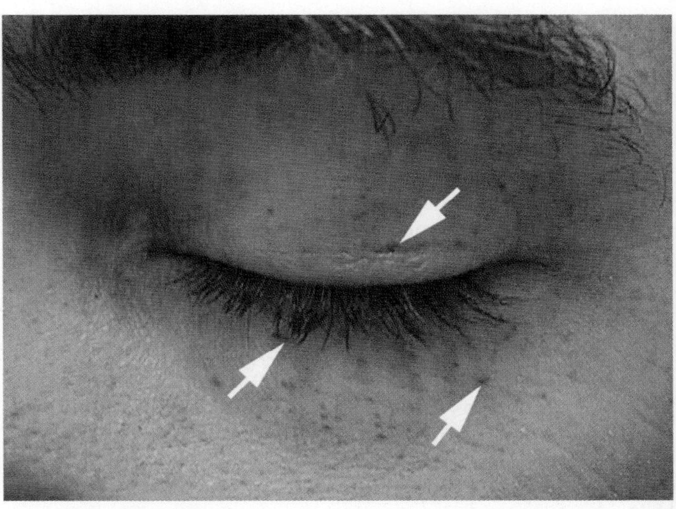

FIGURE 7-6. Petechiae. Periorbital microhemorrhages (*arrows*) appear as punctate red foci.

Thrombosis

A thrombus is an aggregate of coagulated blood containing platelets, fibrin and entrapped cellular elements, within a vascular lumen. Formation of a thrombus is thrombosis. A thrombus by definition adheres to vascular endothelium and should be distinguished from a simple blood clot, which reflects only activation of the coagulation cascade and can form in vitro or even postmortem. Similarly, a thrombus differs from a **hematoma**, which results from hemorrhage and subsequent clotting outside the vascular system. Thrombus formation and the coagulation cascade are discussed in more detail in Chapters 10 and 20. The pathogenesis of venous and arterial thrombosis has classically been considered distinct, but recent epidemiologic evidence demonstrates commonalities in risk factors. Here we present the causes and consequences of thrombosis in these different vascular sites.

Thrombosis in the Arterial System Is Usually Due to Atherosclerosis

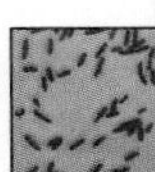

ETIOLOGIC FACTORS: The vessels most commonly involved in arterial thrombosis are coronary, cerebral, mesenteric and renal arteries and arteries of the lower extremities. Less commonly, arterial thrombosis may occur in other disorders, including inflammation of arteries (arteritis), trauma and blood diseases. Thrombi are common in aneurysms (localized dilations of the lumen) of the aorta and its major branches, in which the distortion of blood flow, combined with intrinsic vascular disease, promotes thrombosis.

The pathogenesis of **arterial thrombosis** involves principally three factors:

- **Damage to endothelium,** usually by atherosclerosis, disturbs the anticoagulant properties of the vessel wall and serves as a nidus for platelet aggregation and fibrin formation.
- **Alterations in blood flow,** whether from turbulence in an aneurysm or at sites of arterial bifurcation, is conducive to thrombosis. Slowing of blood flow in narrowed arteries favors thrombosis.

- **Increased coagulability of the blood,** as seen in polycythemia vera or in association with some cancers, leads to an increased risk of thrombosis.

A major risk factor for **venous thrombosis** is immobilization after surgery or after leg casting. Other risk factors include metabolic syndrome, which includes obesity, hyperglycemia, insulin resistance, dyslipidemia and hypertension (see Chapter 22); advanced age; tobacco use; previous thrombosis; and cancer.

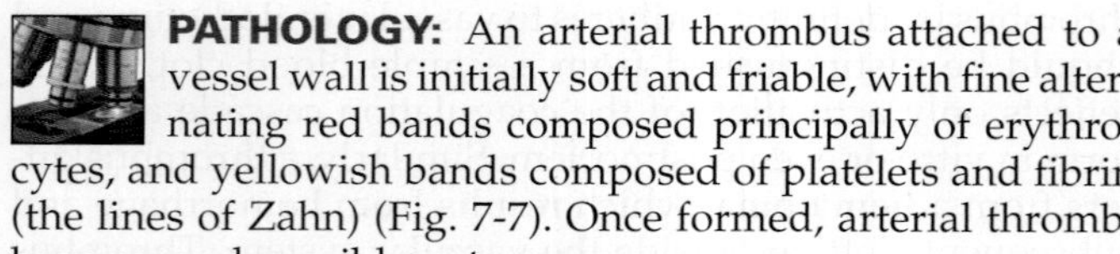

MOLECULAR PATHOGENESIS: Genetic studies of arterial thrombosis have not identified gene mutations that confer risk upon large populations, unlike venous thrombosis, for which mutations in several genes have been identified (see below). This is likely due to the complex polygenetic and multifactorial nature of atherosclerotic plaque formation, erosion or rupture. Weak associations have been shown between certain coagulation factors, fibrinolytic and inflammatory mediators and arterial thrombosis (e.g., factor VII and fibrinogen). Hyperhomocysteinemia is associated with atherosclerotic coronary artery disease and cardiac ischemia. In regards to genetics associated with arterial thrombosis, identification of affected family members may guide screening and treatment.

PATHOLOGY: An arterial thrombus attached to a vessel wall is initially soft and friable, with fine alternating red bands composed principally of erythrocytes, and yellowish bands composed of platelets and fibrin (the lines of Zahn) (Fig. 7-7). Once formed, arterial thrombi have several possible outcomes.

- **Lysis,** owing to the potent thrombolytic activity of the blood
- **Propagation** (i.e., an increase in its size), because a thrombus serves as a focus for further thrombosis
- **Organization**, the eventual invasion of connective tissue elements, which causes a thrombus to become firm and grayish white

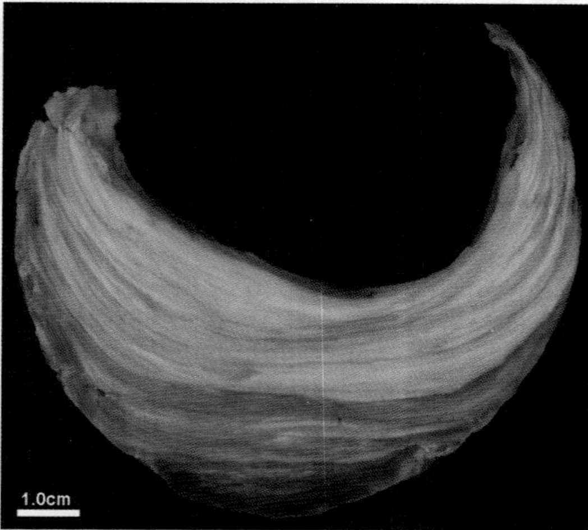

FIGURE 7-7. Arterial thrombus. Gross photograph of a thrombus from an aortic aneurysm shows the laminations of fibrin and platelets known as the lines of Zahn.

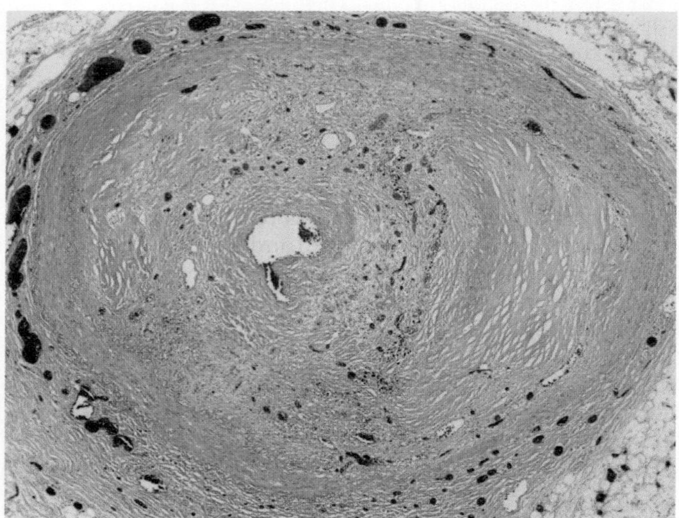

FIGURE 7-8. Canalization of thrombus. Photomicrograph of the left anterior descending coronary artery shows severe atherosclerosis and canalization.

- **Canalization**, by which new lumina lined by endothelial cells form in an organized thrombus (Fig. 7-8)
- **Embolization**, when part or all of the thrombus becomes dislodged, travels through the circulation and lodges in a blood vessel at a distance from the site of thrombus formation (see below for further discussion)

The organized structure of thrombi reflects a tight interaction between platelets and fibrin and differs in appearance from a postmortem clot or one formed in a test tube. Determination of whether a clot formed during life (antemortem clot) or after death (postmortem clot) is often important in a medical autopsy and in forensic pathology. Lines of Zahn stabilize a thrombus formed during life, while a postmortem clot has a more gelatinous structure. Postmortem clots occur in stagnant blood in which gravity fractionates the blood. The part of the clot containing many red blood cells has a reddish, gelatinous appearance, and is referred to as "currant jelly." The overlying clot is firmer and yellow-white, representing coagulated plasma without red blood cells. It is called "chicken fat" because of its color and consistency.

CLINICAL FEATURES: ***Arterial thrombosis due to atherosclerosis is the most common cause of death in Western industrialized countries.*** Since most arterial thrombi occlude the vessel, they often lead to ischemic necrosis of tissue supplied by that artery (i.e., an **infarct**). Thus, thrombosis of a coronary or cerebral artery results in **myocardial infarct** (heart attack) or **cerebral infarct** (stroke), respectively. Other end-arteries that are affected often by atherosclerosis and thrombosis include the mesenteric arteries (**intestinal infarction**), renal arteries (**kidney infarcts**) and arteries of the leg (**gangrene**).

Thrombosis in the Heart Develops on the Endocardium

As in the arterial system, endocardial injury and changes in blood flow in the heart may lead to mural thrombosis (i.e., a

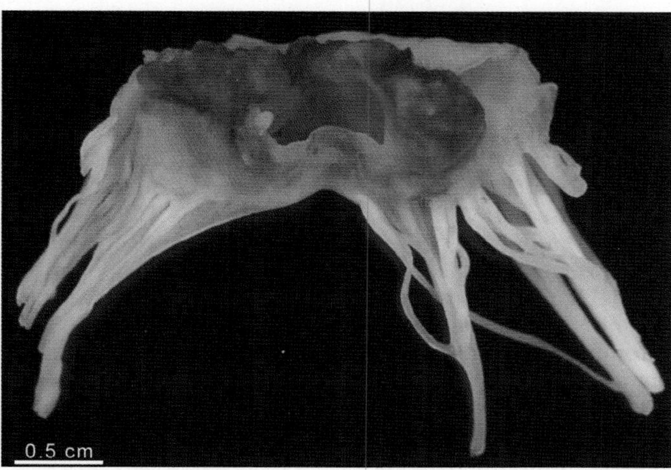

FIGURE 7-9. Endocarditis. The anterior leaflet of the mitral valve is damaged by a friable bacterial vegetation.

thrombus adhering to the underlying wall of the heart). Disorders in which mural thrombi occur include:

- **Myocardial infarction:** Adherent mural thrombi form in the left ventricular cavity over areas of myocardial infarction, owing to damaged endocardium and alterations in blood flow associated with a poorly functional or adynamic segment of the myocardium.
- **Atrial fibrillation:** Disordered atrial rhythm (atrial fibrillation) slows blood flow and impairs left atrial contractility, which predisposes to formation of mural thrombi in atria.
- **Cardiomyopathy:** Primary myocardial diseases are associated with mural thrombi in the left ventricle, presumably because of endocardial injury and altered hemodynamics associated with poor myocardial contractility.
- **Endocarditis:** Small thrombi, **vegetations,** may also develop on cardiac valves, usually mitral or aortic, that are damaged by a bacterial infection (bacterial endocarditis) (Fig. 7-9). Occasionally, vegetations form in the absence of valve infection, on a mitral or tricuspid valve injured by systemic lupus erythematosus (Libman-Sacks endocarditis). In chronic wasting states, as in terminal cancer, large, friable vegetations may appear on cardiac valves (marantic endocarditis), possibly reflecting a hypercoagulable state. ***The major complication of thrombi in any location in the heart is detachment of fragments and their lodging in blood vessels at distant sites* (embolization).**

Thrombosis in the Venous System Is Multifactorial

The term currently used to designate the formation of blood clots in the venous system is **deep venous thrombosis**, which replaces older terminology (phlebothrombosis or, in the absence of inflammation, thrombophlebitis). The most common manifestation of the disorder, namely, thrombosis of the deep venous system of the legs, is aptly described by the current appellation.

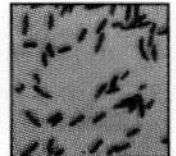

ETIOLOGIC FACTORS: Deep venous thrombosis is caused by the same factors that favor arterial and cardiac thrombosis—endothelial injury, stasis and a hypercoagulable state. Conditions that favor the development of deep venous thrombosis include:

- **Stasis** (heart failure, chronic venous insufficiency, postoperative immobilization, prolonged bed rest, hospitalization and travel, particularly in prolonged airplane trips)
- **Injury and inflammation** (trauma, surgery, childbirth, infection)
- **Hypercoagulability** (oral contraceptives, late pregnancy, cancer, inherited thrombophilic disorders [see Chapter 20])
- **Advanced age** (venous varicosities, phlebosclerosis)
- **Sickle cell disease** (see Chapter 20)

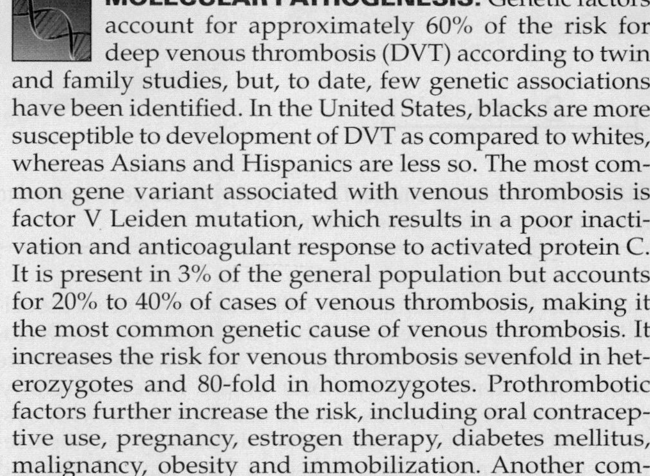

MOLECULAR PATHOGENESIS: Genetic factors account for approximately 60% of the risk for deep venous thrombosis (DVT) according to twin and family studies, but, to date, few genetic associations have been identified. In the United States, blacks are more susceptible to development of DVT as compared to whites, whereas Asians and Hispanics are less so. The most common gene variant associated with venous thrombosis is factor V Leiden mutation, which results in a poor inactivation and anticoagulant response to activated protein C. It is present in 3% of the general population but accounts for 20% to 40% of cases of venous thrombosis, making it the most common genetic cause of venous thrombosis. It increases the risk for venous thrombosis sevenfold in heterozygotes and 80-fold in homozygotes. Prothrombotic factors further increase the risk, including oral contraceptive use, pregnancy, estrogen therapy, diabetes mellitus, malignancy, obesity and immobilization. Another common but mild risk factor for venous thrombosis is the prothrombin G20210A mutation. Deficiencies in proteins C and S and antithrombin are strong risk factors for DVT, but only in 5% to 10% of cases.

Patient genetic profiles may help with risk stratification to identify high-risk prothrombotic groups for postoperative DVT to target use of Doppler ultrasound or prophylactic anticoagulant therapy.

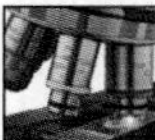

PATHOLOGY: Most (>90%) venous thromboses occur in deep veins of the legs; the rest usually involve pelvic veins. Most venous thrombi begin in the calf veins, frequently in the sinuses above the venous valves. There, venous thrombi have several potential fates:

- **Lysis:** They may remain small and are eventually lysed, posing no further threat to health.
- **Organization:** Many undergo organization similar to those of arterial origin. Small, organized venous thrombi may be incorporated into the vessel wall; larger ones may undergo canalization, with partial restoration of venous drainage.
- **Propagation:** Venous thrombi often serve as a nidus for further thrombosis and thereby propagate proximally to involve the larger iliofemoral veins (Fig. 7-10).
- **Embolization:** Large venous thrombi or those that have propagated proximally represent a significant hazard to life: they may dislodge and be carried to the lungs as pulmonary emboli.

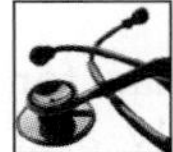

CLINICAL FEATURES: Small thrombi in the calf veins are ordinarily asymptomatic, and even larger thrombi in the iliofemoral system may cause no

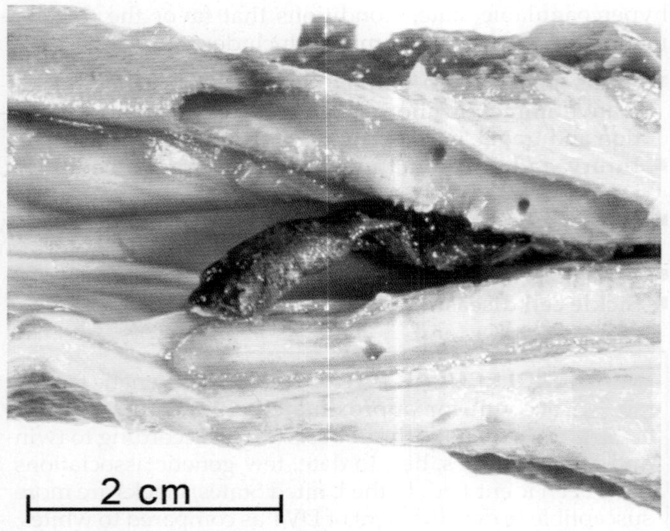

FIGURE 7-10. Venous thrombus. The femoral vein has been opened to reveal a large thrombus within the lumen.

symptoms. Some patients have calf tenderness, often associated with forced dorsiflexion of the foot (**Homan sign**). Occlusive thrombosis of femoral or iliac veins leads to severe congestion, edema and cyanosis of the lower extremity. Symptomatic deep venous thrombosis is treated with systemic anticoagulants, and thrombolytic therapy may be useful in selected cases. In some cases, a filter may be inserted into the vena cava to prevent pulmonary embolization.

The function of venous valves is always impaired in a vein subjected to thrombosis and organization. As a result, chronic deep venous insufficiency (i.e., impaired venous drainage) is virtually inevitable. If a lesion is restricted to a small segment of the deep venous system, the condition may remain asymptomatic. However, more extensive involvement leads to pigmentation, edema and induration of leg skin. Ulceration above the medial malleolus can occur and is often difficult to treat.

Venous thrombi elsewhere may also be dangerous. Thrombosis of mesenteric veins can cause hemorrhagic small-bowel infarction; thrombosis of cerebral veins may be fatal; hepatic vein thrombosis (Budd-Chiari syndrome) may destroy the liver.

Inherited disorders of blood clotting may lead to susceptibility to these types of events. These diseases are covered in detail in Chapter 20.

Embolism

Embolism is passage through venous or arterial circulations of any material that can lodge in a blood vessel and obstruct its lumen. The most common embolus is a thromboembolus—a thrombus formed in one location that detaches from a vessel wall at its point of origin and travels to a distant site.

Pulmonary Arterial Embolism Is Common and Is Potentially Fatal

Pulmonary embolism is estimated to be responsible for 300,000 hospitalizations in the United States yearly and between 50,000 and 100,000 deaths. It represents an important diagnostic and therapeutic challenge. In fact, pulmonary thromboemboli are reported in more than half of all autopsies. Furthermore, this complication occurs in 1% to 2% of postoperative patients over the age of 40. The risk after surgery increases with advancing age, obesity, length of operative procedure, postoperative infection, cancer and preexisting venous disease.

Most pulmonary emboli (90%) arise from deep veins of the lower extremities; most fatal ones form in iliofemoral veins (Fig. 7-11). Only half of patients with pulmonary thromboembolism have signs of deep vein thrombosis. Some thromboemboli arise from the pelvic venous plexus and others from the right side of the heart. Emboli are also derived from thrombi around indwelling lines in the systemic venous system or pulmonary artery. The upper extremities are rarely sources of thromboemboli.

The clinical features of pulmonary embolism are determined by the size of the embolus, the health of the patient and whether embolization occurs acutely or chronically. Acute pulmonary embolism is divided into the following syndromes:

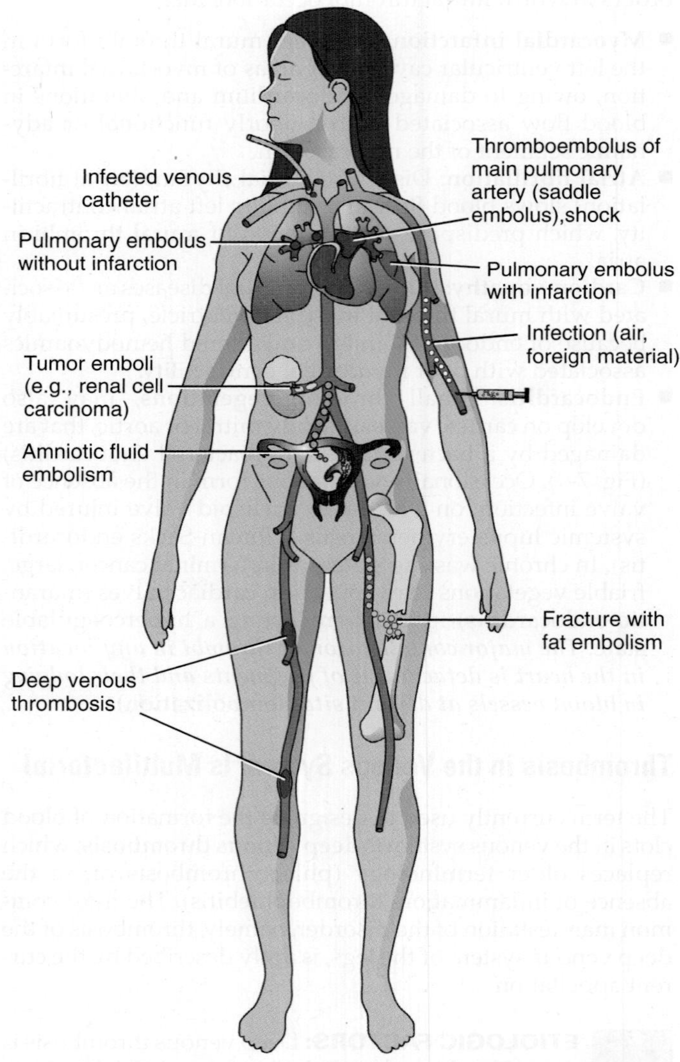

FIGURE 7-11. Sources and effects of venous emboli.

- Asymptomatic small pulmonary emboli
- Transient dyspnea and tachypnea without other symptoms
- Pulmonary infarction, with pleuritic chest pain, hemoptysis and pleural effusion
- Cardiovascular collapse with sudden death

Chronic pulmonary embolism, with numerous (usually asymptomatic) emboli lodged in small arteries of the lung, can lead to pulmonary hypertension and right-sided heart failure (see below).

Massive Pulmonary Embolism

One of the most dramatic calamities complicating hospitalization is the sudden collapse and death of a patient who had appeared to be well on the way to an uneventful recovery. The cause of this catastrophe is often massive pulmonary embolism due to release of a large deep venous thrombus from a lower extremity. Classically, a postoperative patient succumbs upon getting out of bed for the first time. The muscular activity dislodges a thrombus that formed as a result of the stasis from prolonged bed rest. Excluding deaths related to surgery itself, pulmonary embolism is the most common cause of death after major orthopedic surgery and is the most frequent nonobstetric cause of postpartum death. It also is an especially common cause of death in patients who suffer from chronic heart and lung diseases and in those subjected to prolonged immobilization for any reason. Prolonged immobilization associated with air travel can also lead to venous thrombosis and, occasionally, sudden death from a pulmonary embolus.

A large pulmonary embolus may lodge at the bifurcation of the main pulmonary artery (**saddle embolus**), obstructing blood flow to both lungs (Fig. 7-12). Large lethal emboli may also be found in the right or left main pulmonary arteries or their first branches. Multiple smaller emboli may lodge in secondary branches and prove fatal. With acute obstruction of more than half of the pulmonary arterial tree, the patient often experiences immediate severe hypotension (or shock) and may die within minutes.

The hemodynamic consequences of such massive pulmonary embolism are acute right ventricular failure from sudden obstruction of outflow and pronounced reduction in left ventricular cardiac output, secondary to the loss of right ventricular function. The low cardiac output is responsible for the sudden appearance of severe hypotension.

Pulmonary Infarction

Small pulmonary emboli are not ordinarily lethal. They tend to lodge in peripheral pulmonary arteries. Sometimes (15% to 20% of all pulmonary emboli) they produce lung infarcts. Clinically, pulmonary infarction is usually seen in the context of congestive heart failure or chronic lung disease, because the normal dual circulation of the lung ordinarily protects against ischemic necrosis; since the bronchial artery supplies blood to the necrotic area, pulmonary infarcts are typically hemorrhagic. They tend to be pyramidal, with the base of the pyramid on the pleural surface. Patients experience cough, stabbing pleuritic pain, shortness of breath and occasional hemoptysis. Pleural effusion is common and often bloody. With time, the blood in the infarct is resorbed and the center of the infarct becomes pale. Granulation tissue forms at the edge of the infarct, after which it is organized to form a fibrous scar.

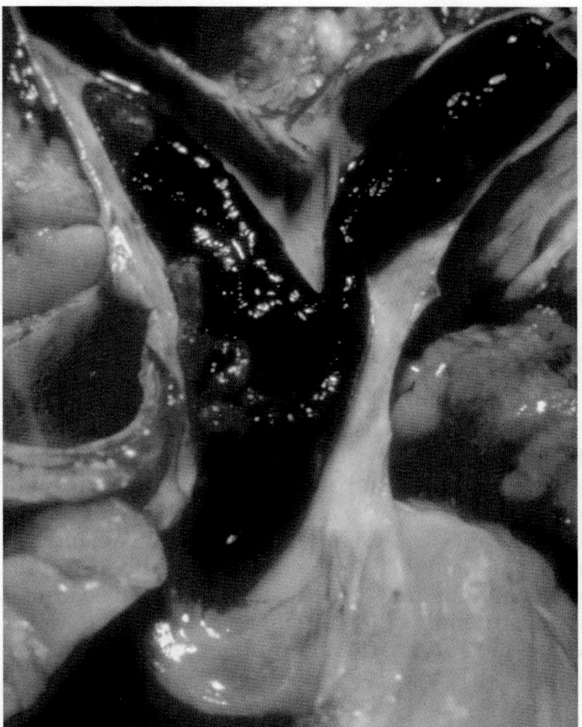

FIGURE 7-12. Pulmonary embolism. The main pulmonary artery and its bifurcation have been opened to reveal a large saddle embolus.

Pulmonary Embolism Without Infarction

Since the lung is supplied by both the bronchial arteries and the pulmonary artery, most (75%) small pulmonary emboli do not produce infarcts. Although most small emboli do not attract clinical attention, a few lead to a syndrome characterized by dyspnea, cough, chest pain and hypotension. Rarely (3%), recurrent pulmonary emboli cause pulmonary hypertension by mechanical blockage of the arterial bed. In this circumstance, reflex vasoconstriction and bronchial constriction, owing to release of vasoactive substances, may contribute to a reduction in size of the functional pulmonary vascular bed.

In the clinical syndrome of "partial infarction," patients have the clinical and radiologic findings of pulmonary infarction due to thromboembolism. However, the lesion resolves instead of contracting to leave a scar. In such cases, hemorrhage and necrosis of the lung tissue in the affected area occur, but the tissue framework remains. Collateral circulation maintains tissue viability and enables its regeneration.

Fate of Pulmonary Thromboemboli

Small pulmonary emboli may completely resolve, depending on (1) the embolic load, (2) the adequacy of the pulmonary vascular reserve, (3) the state of the bronchial collateral circulation and (4) the thrombolytic process. Alternatively, thromboemboli may become organized and leave strings of fibrous tissue attached to a vessel wall in the lumen of pulmonary arteries. Radiologic studies have indicated that half of all pulmonary thromboemboli are resorbed and organized within 8 weeks, with little narrowing of the vessels.

Paradoxical Embolism

Paradoxical embolism refers to emboli that arise in the systemic venous circulation but bypass the lungs by traveling through an incompletely closed foramen ovale, subsequently entering the left side of the heart and blocking flow to the systemic arteries. Since left atrial pressure usually exceeds that in the right, most of these cases occur in the context of a right-to-left shunt (see Chapter 11).

Systemic Arterial Embolism Often Causes Infarcts

Thromboembolism

The heart is the most common source of arterial thromboemboli (Fig. 7-13), which usually arise from mural thrombi (Fig. 7-14) or diseased valves. These emboli tend to lodge at points where vessel lumens narrow abruptly (e.g., at bifurcations or near an atherosclerotic plaque). The viability of tissue supplied by the affected vessel depends on the availability of collateral circulation and on the fate of the embolus itself. The thromboembolus may propagate locally and lead to more severe obstruction, or it may fragment and lyse. Organs that suffer the most from arterial thromboembolism include:

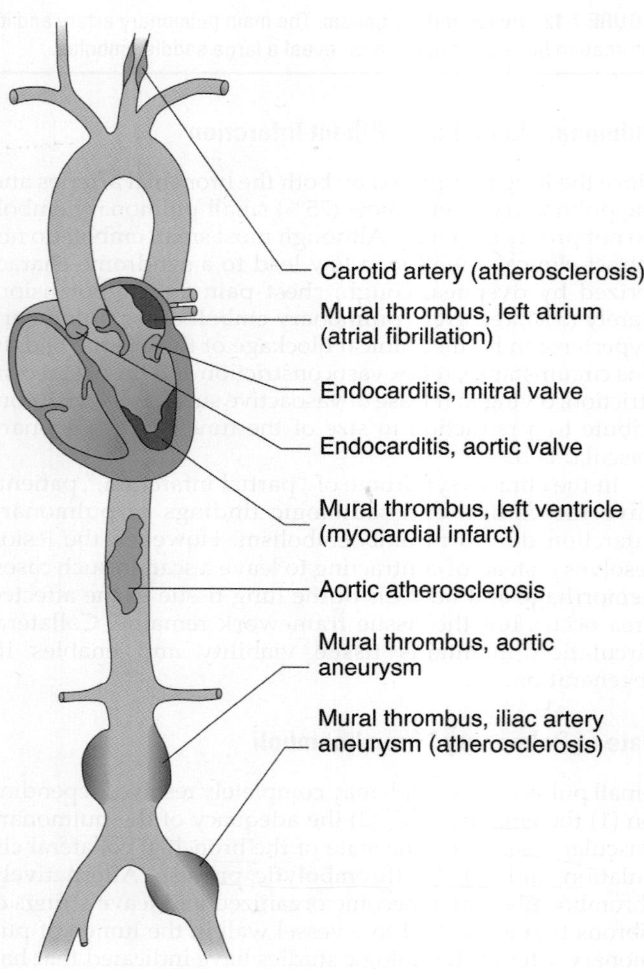

FIGURE 7-13. Sources of arterial emboli.

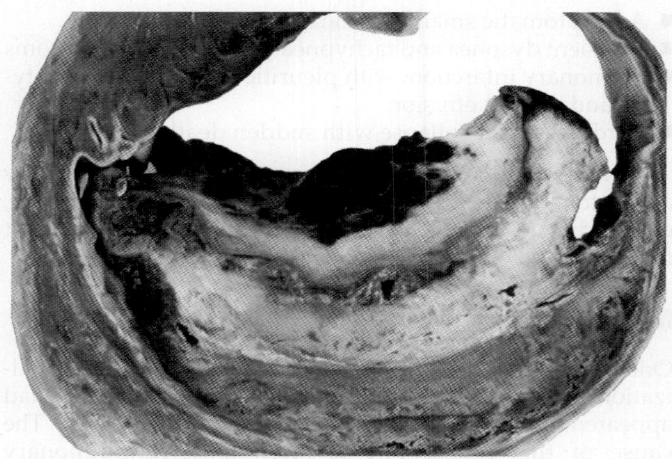

FIGURE 7-14. Mural thrombus of the left ventricle. A laminated thrombus adheres to the endocardium overlying a healed aneurysmal myocardial infarct.

- **Brain:** Arterial emboli to the brain cause ischemic necrosis (strokes).
- **Intestine:** In the mesenteric circulation, emboli cause bowel infarction, which manifests as an acute abdomen and requires immediate surgery.
- **Lower extremity:** Embolism to an artery of the leg leads to sudden pain, absence of pulses and a cold limb. In some cases, the limb must be amputated.
- **Kidney:** Renal artery embolism may infarct an entire kidney but more commonly causes small peripheral infarcts.
- **Heart:** Coronary artery embolism and resulting myocardial infarcts occur but are rare.

The more common sites of infarction from arterial emboli are summarized in Fig. 7-15.

Air Embolism

Air may enter the venous circulation through neck wounds, thoracocentesis or punctures of the great veins during invasive procedures or hemodialysis. Small amounts of circulating air in the form of bubbles are of little consequence, but quantities of 100 mL or more can lead to sudden death. Air bubbles tend to coalesce and physically obstruct blood flow in the right side of the heart, the pulmonary circulation and the brain. Histologically, air bubbles appear as empty spaces in capillaries and small vessels of the lung.

People exposed to increased atmospheric pressure, such as scuba divers and workers in underwater occupations (e.g., tunnels, drilling platform construction), are subject to **decompression sickness,** a unique form of gas embolism. During descent, large amounts of inert gas (nitrogen or helium) dissolve in bodily fluids. When the diver ascends, this gas is released from solution and exhaled. However, if ascent is too rapid, gas bubbles form in the circulation and within tissues, obstructing blood flow and directly injuring cells. Air embolism is the second most common cause of death in sport diving (drowning is the first).

Acute decompression sickness, "the bends," is characterized by temporary muscular and joint pain owing to small vessel obstruction in these tissues. However, severe involvement of cerebral blood vessels may cause coma or even death.

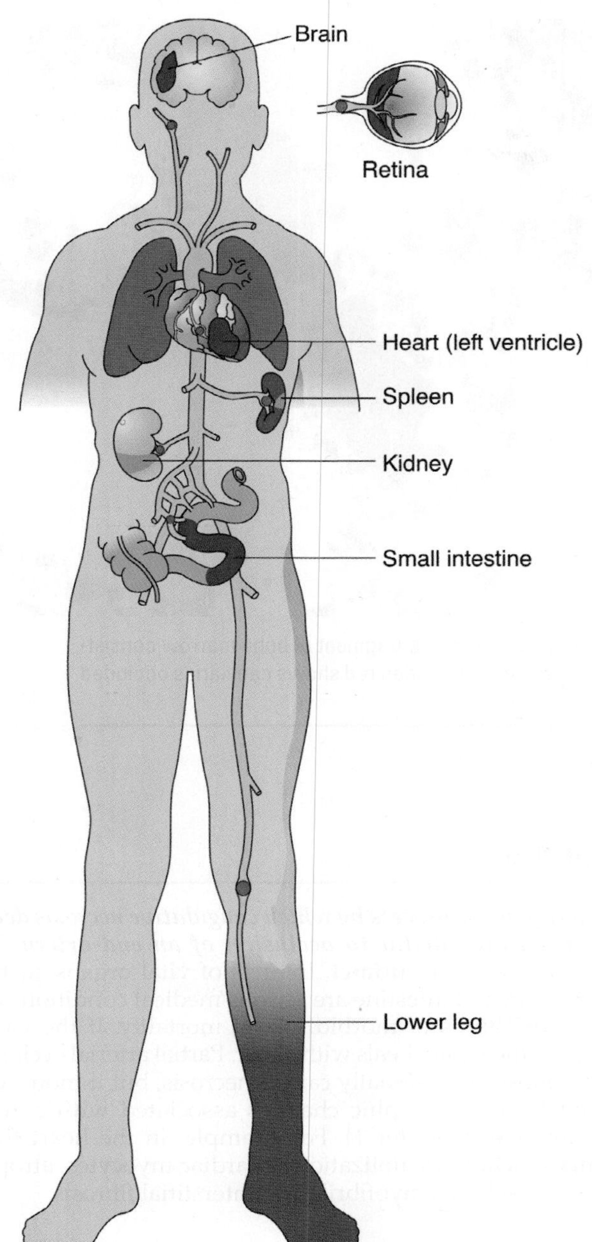

FIGURE 7-15. Common sites of infarction from arterial emboli.

Caisson disease refers to decompression sickness in which vascular obstruction causes multiple foci of ischemic (avascular) necrosis of bone, particularly affecting the head of the femur, tibia and humerus. This complication was originally described in construction workers in diving bells (or caissons).

Amniotic Fluid Embolism

Amniotic fluid containing fetal cells and debris may enter the maternal circulation through open uterine and cervical veins. This rare maternal complication of childbirth usually occurs at the end of labor, and can be catastrophic when it occurs. The emboli are composed of the solid epithelial constituents (squames) contained in the amniotic fluid (Fig. 7-16). The high thromboplastin activity of amniotic fluid may initiate a potentially fatal consumptive coagulopathy.

CLINICAL FEATURES: The clinical presentation of amniotic fluid embolism can be dramatic, with sudden onset of cyanosis and shock, followed by coma and death. If the mother survives this acute episode, she may die of disseminated intravascular coagulation. Should she overcome this complication, she is at substantial risk of developing **acute respiratory distress syndrome** (see Chapter 12). Minor amniotic fluid embolism is probably common and asymptomatic, since autopsies of mothers who have died of other causes in the perinatal period frequently show evidence of this complication.

Fat Embolism

Fat embolism is release of emboli of fatty marrow (Fig. 7-17) into damaged blood vessels after severe trauma to fat-containing tissue, particularly accompanying bone fractures. In most instances, fat embolism is clinically inapparent. However, severe fat embolism leads to **fat embolism syndrome** 1 to 3 days after the injury. In its most severe form, which may be fatal, this syndrome is characterized by respiratory failure, mental changes, thrombocytopenia and widespread petechiae. Chest radiography reveals diffuse opacity of the lungs, which may progress to a "whiteout" typical of acute respiratory distress syndrome. At autopsy, innumerable fat globules are seen in the pulmonary microvasculature (Fig. 7-17B), the brain and sometimes other organs. The lungs typically exhibit the changes of acute respiratory distress syndrome (see Chapter 12). The lesions in the brain include cerebral edema, small hemorrhages and occasionally microinfarcts.

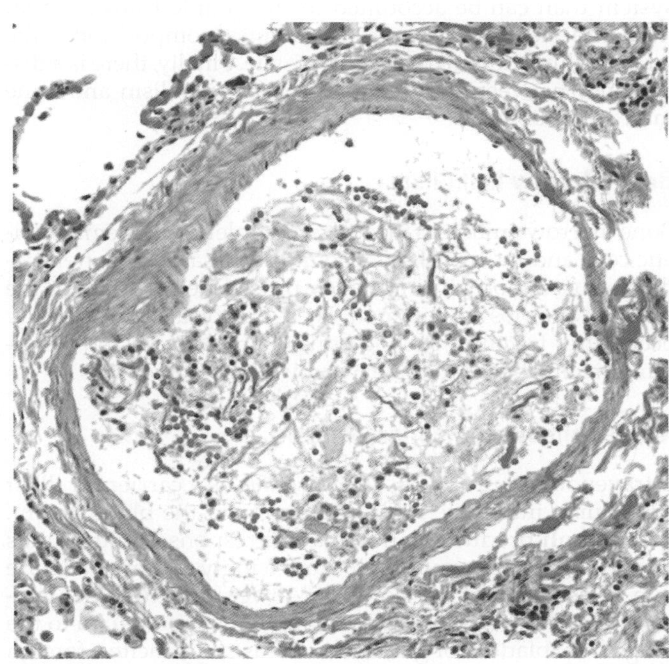

FIGURE 7-16. Amniotic fluid embolism. A section of lung shows a pulmonary artery filled with epithelial squames.

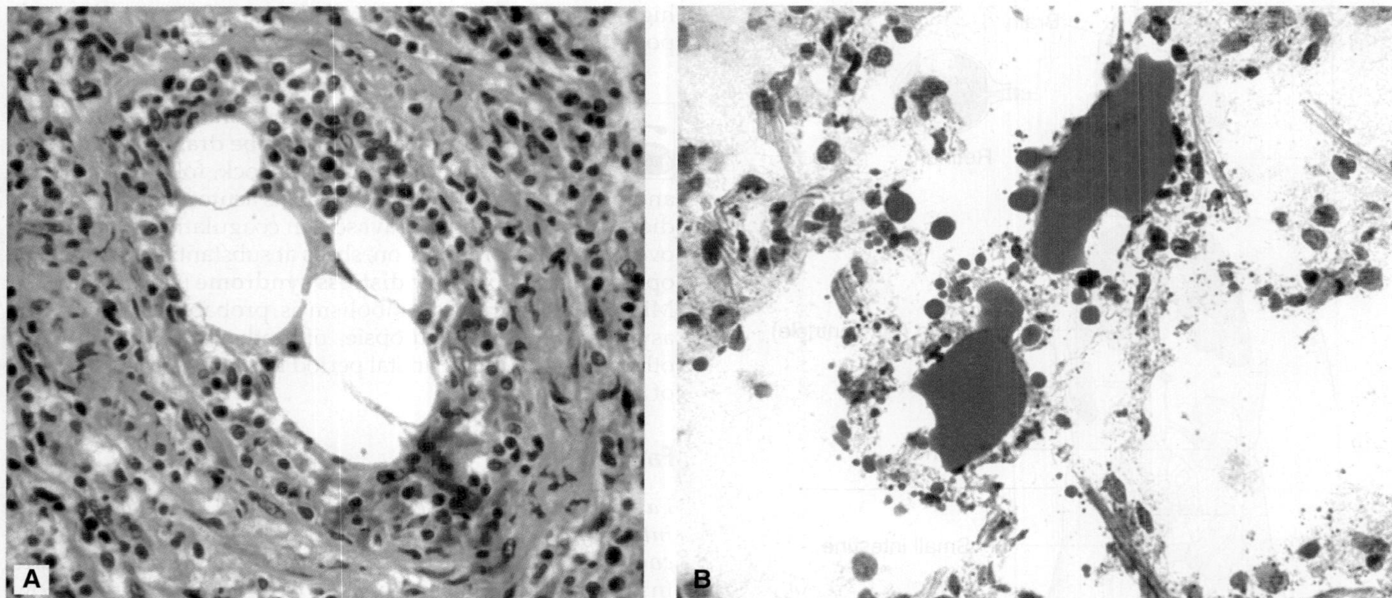

FIGURE 7-17. Fat embolism. A. The lumen of a small pulmonary artery is occluded by a fragment of bone marrow consisting of fat cells and hematopoietic elements. **B.** A frozen section of lung stained with Sudan red shows capillaries occluded by red-staining fat emboli.

Fat embolism is usually considered a direct consequence of trauma, with fat entering ruptured capillaries at the site of the fracture. However, this explanation may be too simplistic. It has been suggested that hemorrhage into the marrow and perhaps also into the subcutaneous fat raises interstitial pressure above capillary pressure, forcing fat into the circulation. Moreover, there is more fat in the pulmonary vascular system than can be accounted for by simple transfer of fat from peripheral depots, and the chemical composition of the fat in the lung differs from that in tissue. Finally, there is a discrepancy between the frequency of fat embolism and bone marrow embolism.

Bone Marrow Embolism

Bone marrow emboli to the lungs, complete with hematopoietic cells and fat, are often encountered at autopsy after cardiac resuscitation, during which procedure fractures of the sternum and ribs are common. These emboli also occasionally occur after fractures of long bones. In most cases no symptoms are attributed to bone marrow embolism.

Miscellaneous Pulmonary Emboli

Intravenous drug abusers who use talc as a carrier for illicit drugs may introduce it into the lung via the bloodstream. **Talc emboli** produce granulomatous responses in the lungs (Fig. 7-18). **Cotton emboli** are surprisingly common and are due to cleansing of the skin prior to venipuncture. **Schistosomiasis** may be associated with embolization of ova to the lungs from bladder or gut, in which case they incite a foreign body granulomatous reaction. **Tumor emboli** are occasionally seen in the lung during hematogenous dissemination of cancer.

Infarction

Infarction is the process by which coagulative necrosis develops in an area distal to occlusion of an end-artery. The necrotic zone is an **infarct**. Infarcts of vital organs such as heart, brain and intestine are serious medical conditions and are major causes of morbidity and mortality. If the victim survives, the infarct heals with a scar. Partial arterial occlusion (i.e., stenosis) occasionally causes necrosis, but it more commonly leads to atrophic changes associated with chronic ischemia (see Chapter 1). For example, in the heart these changes include vacuolization of cardiac myocytes, atrophy, loss of muscle cell myofibrils and interstitial fibrosis.

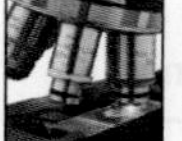

PATHOLOGY: The gross and microscopic appearance of an infarct depends on its location and age. Upon arterial occlusion, the area supplied by the vessel rapidly becomes swollen and deep red. Microscopically, vascular dilation and congestion and occasionally interstitial hemorrhage are noted. Subsequently, several types of infarcts are distinguishable by gross examination.

Pale infarcts are typical in the heart, kidneys and spleen (Fig. 7-19), although certain renal infarcts may be cystic. **Dry gangrene** of the leg due to arterial occlusion (often noted in diabetes) is actually a large pale infarct. On gross examination, 1 or 2 days after the initial hyperemia, an infarct becomes soft, sharply delineated and light yellow (Fig. 7-20). The border tends to be dark red, reflecting hemorrhage into surrounding viable tissue. Microscopically, a pale infarct exhibits uniform coagulative necrosis.

Red infarcts may result from either arterial or venous occlusion and are also characterized by coagulative necrosis.

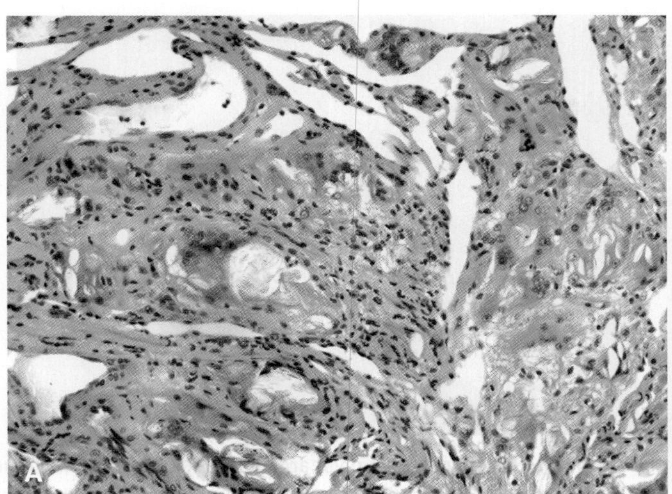

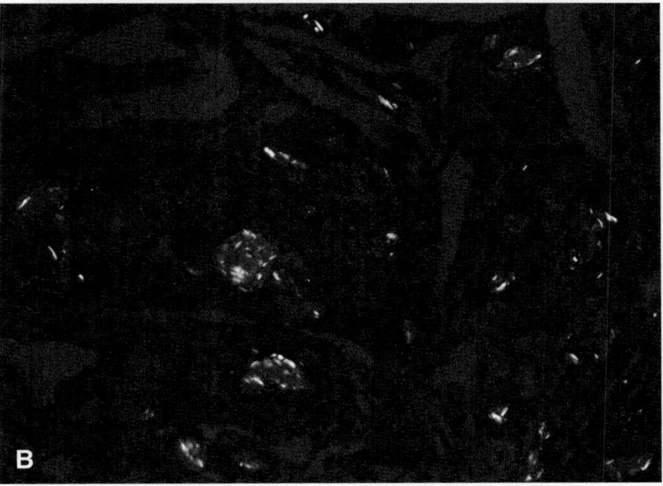

FIGURE 7-18. Talc emboli. A section of lung from an intravenous drug abuser shows talc particles before (**A**) and after (**B**) polarization of light.

However, they are distinguished by bleeding into the necrotic area from adjacent arteries and veins. ***Red infarcts occur principally in organs with a dual blood supply***, such as the lung, or those with extensive collateral circulation, such as the small intestine and brain. In the heart, red infarcts occur when the infarcted area is reperfused, as may occur after spontaneous or therapeutically induced lysis of an occluding thrombus. Grossly, red infarcts are sharply circumscribed, firm and dark red to purple (Fig. 7-21). Over a period of several days, acute inflammatory cells infiltrate the necrotic area from the viable border. The cellular debris is phagocytosed and digested by polymorphonuclear leukocytes and later by macrophages. Granulation tissue eventually forms, to be replaced ultimately by a scar (see Chapter 3). In a large infarct of an organ such as the heart or kidney, the necrotic center may remain inaccessible to inflammatory cells and so persist for months. In the brain, an infarct typically undergoes liquefactive necrosis and may become a fluid-filled cyst, which is referred to as a **cystic infarct** (Fig. 7-22).

Septic infarction results when the necrotic tissue of an infarct is seeded by pyogenic bacteria and becomes infected. Pulmonary infarcts are not uncommonly infected, presumably because the necrotic tissue offers little resistance to

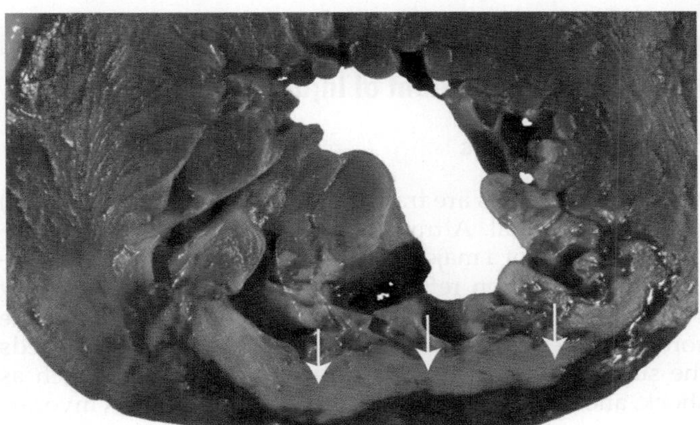

FIGURE 7-20. Acute myocardial infarct. A cross-section of the left ventricle reveals a sharply circumscribed, soft, yellow area of necrosis in the posterior free wall (*arrows*).

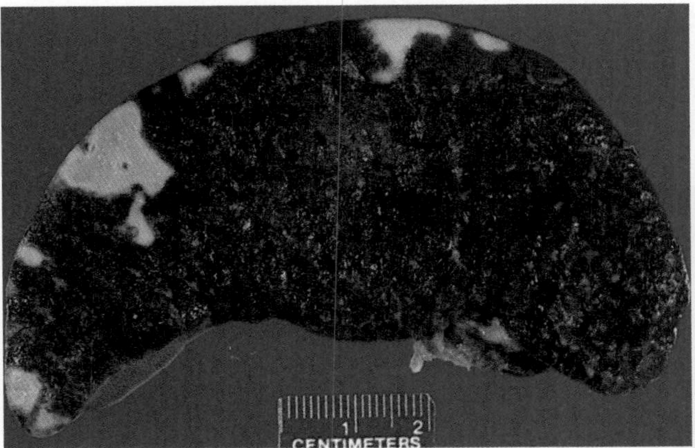

FIGURE 7-19. Spleen infarcts. A cut section of spleen displays multiple pale, wedge-shaped infarcts beneath the capsule.

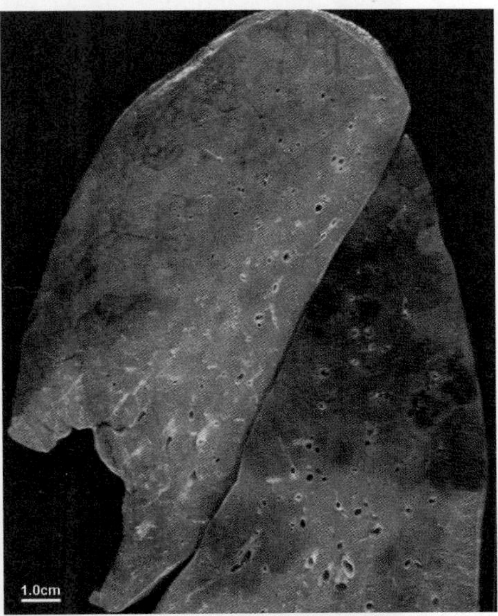

FIGURE 7-21. Red infarct. A sagittal slice of lung shows a hemorrhagic infarct in upper segments of the lower lobe.

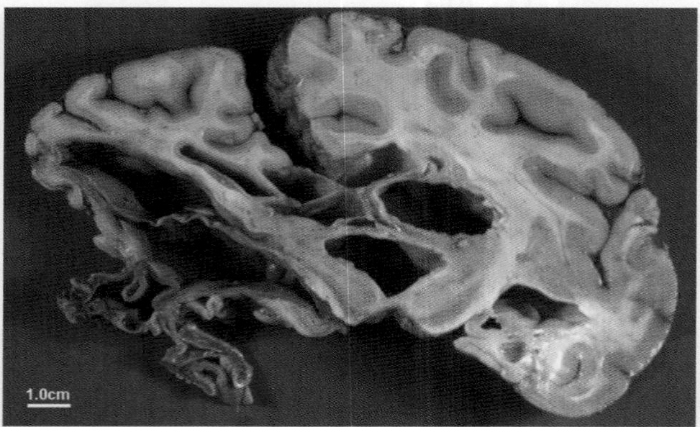

FIGURE 7-22. Cystic infarct. A cross-section of brain in the frontal plane shows a healed cystic infarct.

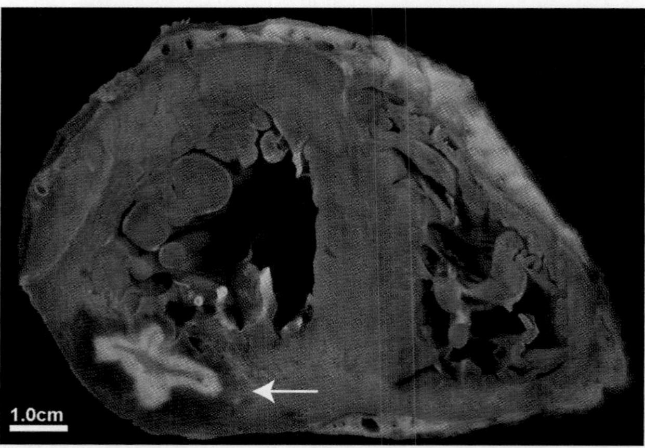

FIGURE 7-23. Septic infarct. A myocardial abscess (*arrow*) within the left ventricular free wall was due to infection with *Staphylococcus aureus.*

inhaled bacteria. In the case of bacterial endocarditis, the emboli themselves are infected and resulting infarcts are often septic. A septic infarct may become an abscess (Fig. 7-23).

The Outcome of Infarction Depends on the Organ Involved and the Extent of Injury

Myocardial Infarcts

Myocardial infarcts are transmural (through the entire wall) or subendocardial. A transmural infarct results from complete occlusion of a major extramural coronary artery. Subendocardial infarction reflects prolonged ischemia caused by partially occluding, atherosclerotic, stenotic lesions of the coronary arteries when the requirement for oxygen exceeds the supply. Such a situation prevails in disorders such as shock, anoxia or severe tachycardia (rapid pulse). A myocardial infarct may be pale or red, depending on the extent of reflow of blood into the infarcted area (Fig. 7-24).

Pulmonary Infarcts

Only about 10% of pulmonary emboli elicit clinical symptoms referable to pulmonary infarction, usually after occlusion of a middle-sized pulmonary artery. Infarction occurs only if circulation from bronchial arteries is inadequate to compensate for supply lost from the pulmonary arteries. This occurs most often in congestive heart failure, although stasis in the pulmonary circulation may contribute. Hemorrhage into the alveolar spaces of the necrotic lining tissue occurs within 48 hours.

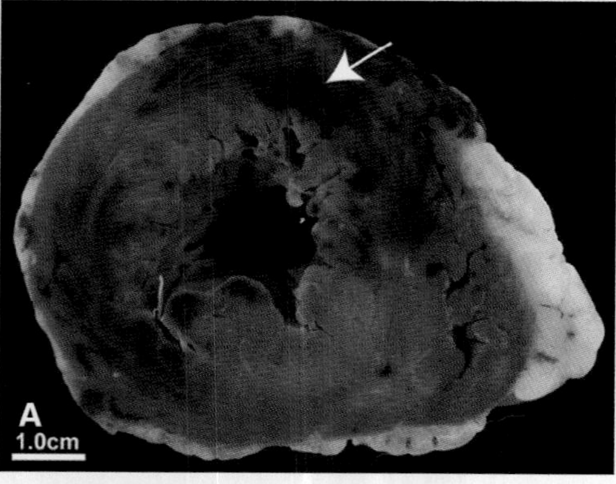

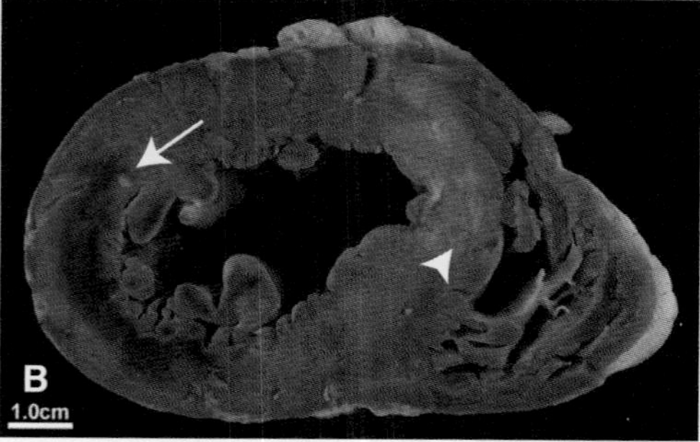

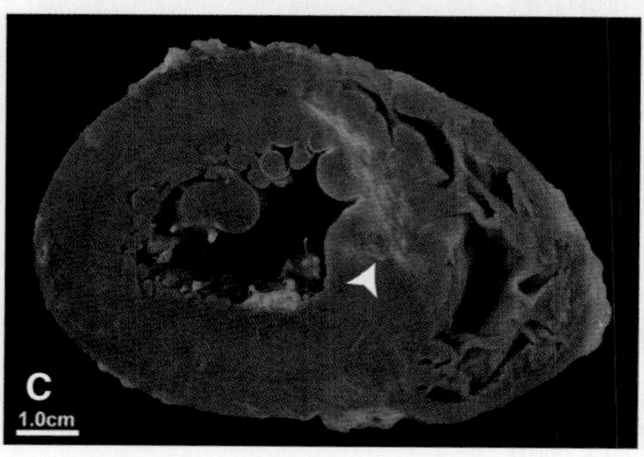

FIGURE 7-24. Myocardial infarct. Transverse sections of ventricular myocardium show (**A**) reperfused, (**B**) acute (*arrow*) and healed (*arrowhead*) together and (**C**) healed infarct. Reperfusion is typically associated with hemorrhage as in A (*arrow*) and B (*arrow*). In C, a white scar (*arrowhead*) is evident in the anterior ventricular septum.

Cerebral Infarcts

Infarction of the brain may result from local ischemia or a generalized reduction in blood flow. The latter often results from systemic hypotension, as in shock, and produces infarction in the border zones between the distributions of the major cerebral arteries (**watershed infarct**). If prolonged, severe hypotension can cause widespread brain necrosis. Occlusion of a single vessel in the brain (e.g., after an embolus has lodged) causes ischemia and necrosis in a well-defined area. This type of cerebral infarct may be pale or red, the latter being common with embolic occlusions. Occlusion of a large artery causes extensive necrosis, which may ultimately resolve as a large fluid-filled cavity in the brain.

Intestinal Infarcts

The earliest tissue changes in intestinal ischemia are necrosis of the tips of the villi in the small intestine and of the superficial mucosa in the large intestine. More severe ischemia leads to hemorrhagic necrosis of the submucosa and muscularis, but not the serosa. Small mucosal infarcts heal within a few days, but more severe injury leads to ulceration. These ulcers can eventually reepithelialize. However, if ulcers are large, they are repaired by scarring, a process that may lead to strictures. Severe transmural necrosis is associated with massive bleeding or bowel perforation, complications that often result in irreversible shock, sepsis and death.

Edema

Edema is excess fluid in interstitial tissue spaces. It may be local or generalized. **Local edema** in most instances occurs with inflammation, the "tumor" of "tumor, rubor and calor." Local edema of a limb, usually the leg, results from venous or lymphatic obstruction. Burns cause prominent local edema by altering the permeability of local vasculature. Local edema may be a prominent component of an immune reaction, like urticaria (hives) or edema of the epiglottis or larynx (angioneurotic edema).

Generalized edema, affecting visceral organs and the skin of the trunk and lower extremities (Fig. 7-25), usually reflects a global disorder of fluid and electrolyte metabolism, most often due to heart failure. Generalized edema is also seen when blood oncotic pressure is reduced, as in renal diseases in which serum proteins are lost in the urine (nephrotic syndrome; see Chapter 16) and in cirrhosis of t production of serum proteins may be impaired. extreme generalized edema, with conspicuous f mulation in subcutaneous tissues, visceral organs an cavities. Edema fluid may also collect in body cavities, as the pleural space (**hydrothorax**), peritoneum (**ascites**) pericardial sac (**hydropericardium**).

Normal Capillary Filtration

Normal formation and retention of interstitial fluid depends on filtration and reabsorption at the level of the capillaries (Starling forces). Internal or hydrostatic pressure in the arteriolar segment of the capillary is 32 mm Hg. At the middle of the capillary, it is 20 mm Hg. Since interstitial hydrostatic pressure is only 3 mm Hg, the pressure differential causes outward fluid filtration at a rate of 14 mL/min. Hydrostatic pressure is opposed by plasma oncotic pressure (26 mm Hg), which results in osmotic reabsorption at 12 mL/min at the venous end of the capillary. Thus, interstitial fluid is formed at the rate of 2 mL/min and is reabsorbed by the lymphatics, so that in equilibrium there is no net fluid gain or loss in the interstitium.

Sodium and Water Metabolism

Water represents 50% to 70% of body weight and is divided between extracellular and intracellular fluid spaces. Extracellular fluid is further divided into interstitial and vascular compartments. Interstitial fluid constitutes about 75% of the latter.

Total body sodium is the principal determinant of extracellular fluid volume because it is the major cation in the extracellular fluid. In other words, increased total body sodium must be balanced by more extracellular water to maintain constant osmolality. Control of extracellular fluid volume depends to a large extent on regulation of renal sodium excretion, which is influenced by (1) atrial natriuretic factor, (2) the renin–angiotensin system of the juxtaglomerular apparatus and (3) sympathetic nervous system activity (see Chapter 10).

Edema Caused by Increased Hydrostatic Pressure

Unopposed increases in hydrostatic pressure result in greater filtration of fluid into the interstitial space and its retention as edema. This happens in decompensated heart disease, in

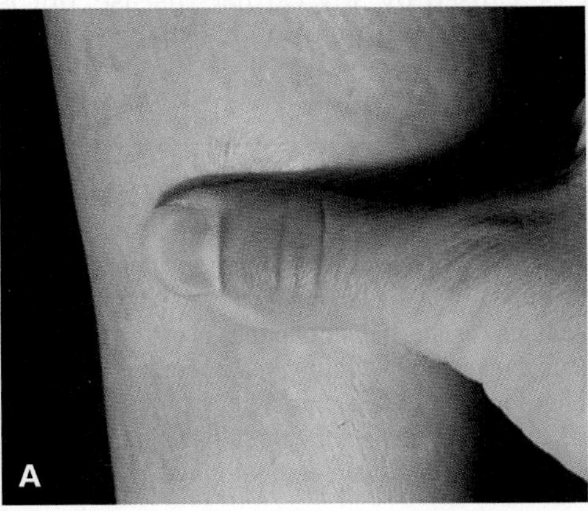

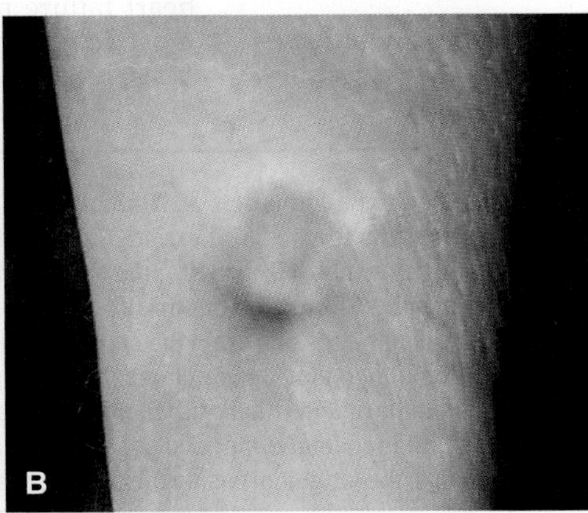

FIGURE 7-25. Pitting edema of the leg. A. In a patient with congestive heart failure, severe edema of the leg is demonstrated by applying pressure with a finger. **B.** The resulting "pitting" reflects the inelasticity of the fluid-filled tissue.

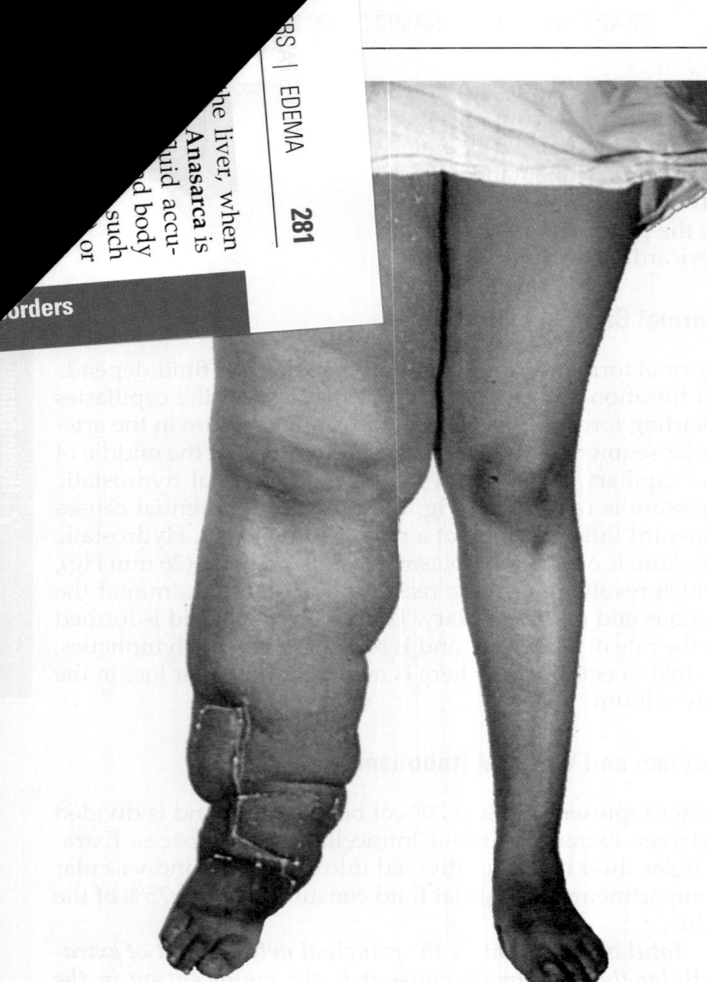

FIGURE 7-26. Edema secondary to lymphatic obstruction. Massive edema of the right lower extremity (elephantiasis) in a patient with obstruction of lymphatic drainage.

which back-pressure in the lungs due to left ventricle failure leads to acute pulmonary edema and right-sided heart failure, and contributes to systemic edema. Similarly, back-pressure caused by venous obstruction in the lower extremity causes edema of the leg. Obstruction to portal blood flow in cirrhosis of the liver contributes to formation of abdominal fluid (**ascites**).

Edema Caused by Decreased Oncotic Pressure

The difference in pressure between intravascular and interstitial compartments is largely determined by the concentration of plasma proteins, especially albumin. Any condition that decreases plasma albumin, whether it is albuminuria in the nephrotic syndrome or reduced albumin synthesis in chronic liver disease or severe malnutrition, promotes generalized edema.

Edema Caused by Lymphatic Obstruction

Under normal circumstances, more fluid is filtered into the interstitial spaces than is reabsorbed into the vascular bed. This excess interstitial fluid is removed by lymphatics. Thus, obstruction to lymphatic flow leads to localized edema. Lymphatic channels can be obstructed by (1) malignant neoplasms, (2) fibrosis resulting from inflammation or irradiation and (3) surgical ablation. For instance, the inflammatory response to filarial worms (Bancroftian and Malayan filariasis; see Chapter 9) can result in lymphatic obstruction that produces massive lymphedema of the scrotum and legs (**elephantiasis**) (Fig. 7-26). Lymphedema of the arm often complicates radical mastectomies for breast cancer, due to removal of axillary lymph nodes and lymphatics.

Lymphatic edema differs from other forms of edema in its high protein content, since lymph returns proteins and interstitial cells to the circulation. The high protein concentration of lymphedema may stimulate dermal fibrosis, which occurs in chronic edema (indurated edema).

The Role of Sodium Retention in Edema

Generalized edema and ascites invariably reflect increased total body sodium, as a consequence of renal sodium retention. By the time peripheral edema is first detectable clinically, the extracellular fluid volume has already expanded by at least 5 L. The most common conditions in which generalized edema is found include congestive heart failure, hepatic cirrhosis, nephrotic syndrome and some cases of chronic renal insufficiency. The mechanisms of edema formation and representative disorders associated with them are summarized in Fig. 7-27 and Table 7-1.

Congestive Heart Failure Is a Consequence of Inadequate Cardiac Output

It is estimated that 2 to 3 million people in the United States have congestive heart failure. Of these, 15% die annually. Half of all patients with congestive heart failure who require admission to the hospital will die within 1 year. Congestive heart failure may be caused by any cardiac disease, but is most commonly associated with chronic cardiac ischemia (see Chapter 11).

FIGURE 7-27. The capillary system and mechanisms of edema formation. A. Normal. The differential between the hydrostatic and oncotic pressures at the arterial end of the capillary system is responsible for the filtration into the interstitial space of approximately 14 mL of fluid per minute. This fluid is reabsorbed at the venous end at the rate of 12 mL/min. It is also drained through the lymphatic capillaries at a rate of 2 mL/min. Proteins are removed by the lymphatics from the interstitial space. **B. Hydrostatic edema.** If the hydrostatic pressure at the venous end of the capillary system is elevated, reabsorption decreases. As long as the lymphatics can drain the surplus fluid, no edema results. If their capacity is exceeded, however, edema fluid accumulates. **C. Oncotic edema.** Edema fluid also accumulates if reabsorption is diminished by decreased oncotic pressure of the vascular bed, owing to a loss of albumin. **D. Inflammatory and traumatic edema.** Edema, either local or systemic, results if the vascular bed becomes leaky following injury to the endothelium. **E. Lymphedema.** Lymphatic obstruction causes the accumulation of interstitial fluid because of insufficient reabsorption and deficient removal of proteins, the latter increasing the oncotic pressure of the fluid in the interstitial space. ►

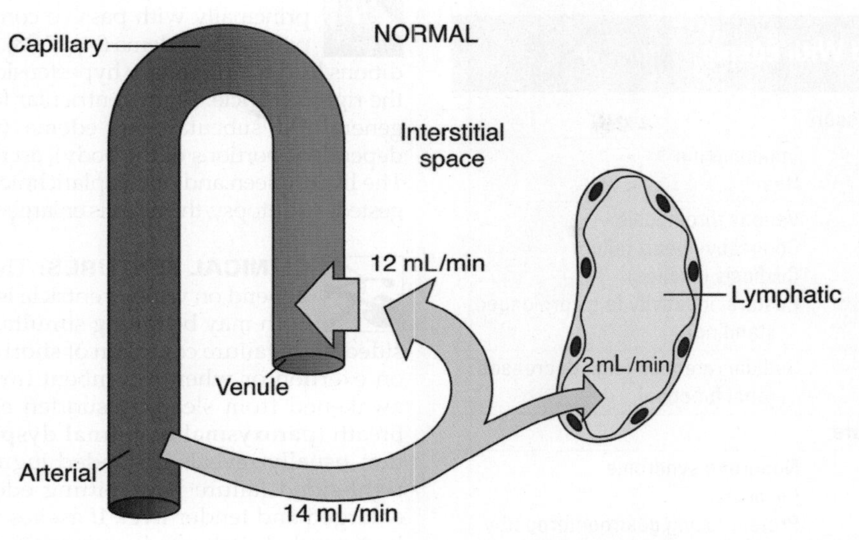
NORMAL
Capillary
Interstitial space
12 mL/min
Lymphatic
2 mL/min
Venule
Arterial
14 mL/min
A
INCREASED HYDROSTATIC PRESSURE
EDEMA
B
DECREASED ONCOTIC PRESSURE
EDEMA
C
INCREASED PERMEABILITY
EDEMA
D
LYMPHATIC OBSTRUCTION
Tumor
EDEMA
E

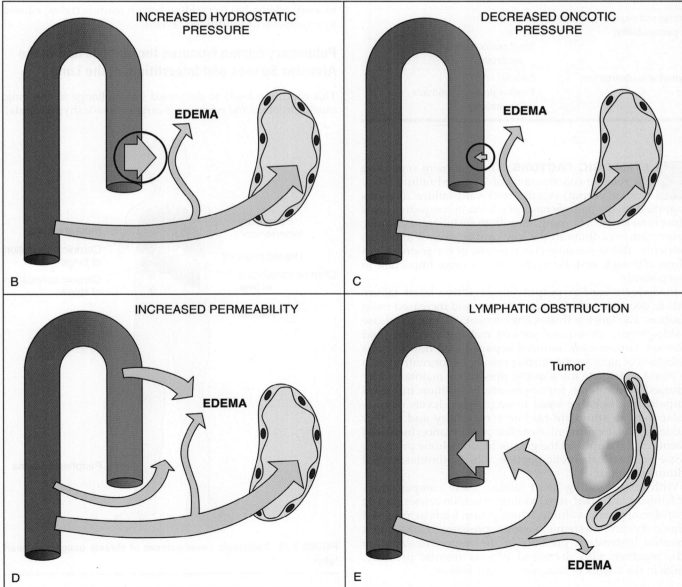

Table 7-1

Disorders Associated With Edema

Increased hydrostatic pressure	
Arteriolar dilation	Inflammation Heat
Increased venous pressure	Venous thrombosis Congestive heart failure Cirrhosis (ascites) Postural inactivity (e.g., prolonged standing)
Hypervolemia	Sodium retention (e.g., decreased renal function)
Decreased oncotic pressure	
Hypoproteinemia	Nephrotic syndrome Cirrhosis Protein-losing gastroenteropathy Malnutrition
Increased capillary permeability	Inflammation Burns Adult respiratory distress syndrome
Lymphatic obstruction	Cancer Postsurgical lymphedema Inflammation

ETIOLOGIC FACTORS: The argument regarding the relative contributions of "forward failure" (low cardiac output) versus "backward failure" (venous congestion) in the pathogenesis of edema in congestive heart failure is no longer a burning issue. Both systolic and diastolic dysfunction contribute to the low cardiac output and high ventricular filling pressure characteristic of congestive heart failure, although systolic dysfunction is more important in most patients.

Inadequate cardiac output in congestive heart failure leads to decreased glomerular filtration and increased renin secretion. The latter activates angiotensin, leading to release of aldosterone, subsequent sodium reabsorption and fluid retention. Furthermore, reduced hepatic blood flow impairs catabolism of aldosterone, further raising its concentration in the blood. Adequate intracardiac pressure is maintained by increased fluid volume, to compensate. In addition, increased sympathetic discharge leads to augmented levels of catecholamines, to stimulate cardiac contractility and further counteract the impairment in cardiac performance. Increased distention of the atria by the greater blood volume promotes release of atrial natriuretic peptide, which stimulates renal sodium excretion.

With long-standing heart failure, these compensatory mechanisms fail. Then, renal sodium retention causes further expansion of plasma volume, which in turn leads to increased pulmonary and systemic venous pressure. Consequent increased hydrostatic pressure in the respective capillary beds, together with decreased plasma oncotic pressure, results in the edema of congestive heart failure.

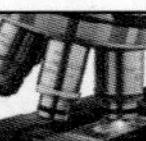

PATHOLOGY: Left ventricular failure is associated principally with passive congestion of the lungs and pulmonary edema (Fig. 7-28). When chronic, these conditions lead to pulmonary hypertension and eventual failure of the right ventricle. Right ventricular failure is characterized by generalized subcutaneous edema (most prominent in the dependent portions of the body), ascites and pleural effusions. The liver, spleen and other splanchnic organs are typically congested. At autopsy, the heart is enlarged and its chambers dilated

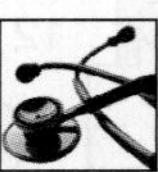

CLINICAL FEATURES: The effects of heart failure depend on which ventricle is failing, recognizing that both may be failing simultaneously. Patients in left-sided heart failure complain of shortness of breath (**dyspnea**) on exertion or when recumbent (**orthopnea**). They may be awakened from sleep by sudden episodes of shortness of breath (**paroxysmal nocturnal dyspnea**). Physical examination usually reveals distended jugular veins. Persons with right-sided failure have pitting edema of the legs and an enlarged and tender liver. If ascites is present, the abdomen is distended. Patients in congestive heart failure with pulmonary edema have crackling breath sounds (**rales**) caused by expansion of fluid-filled alveoli.

Pulmonary Edema Features Increased Fluid in the Alveolar Spaces and Interstitium of the Lung

This condition leads to decreased gas exchange in the lung, causing hypoxia and retention of carbon dioxide (**hypercapnia**).

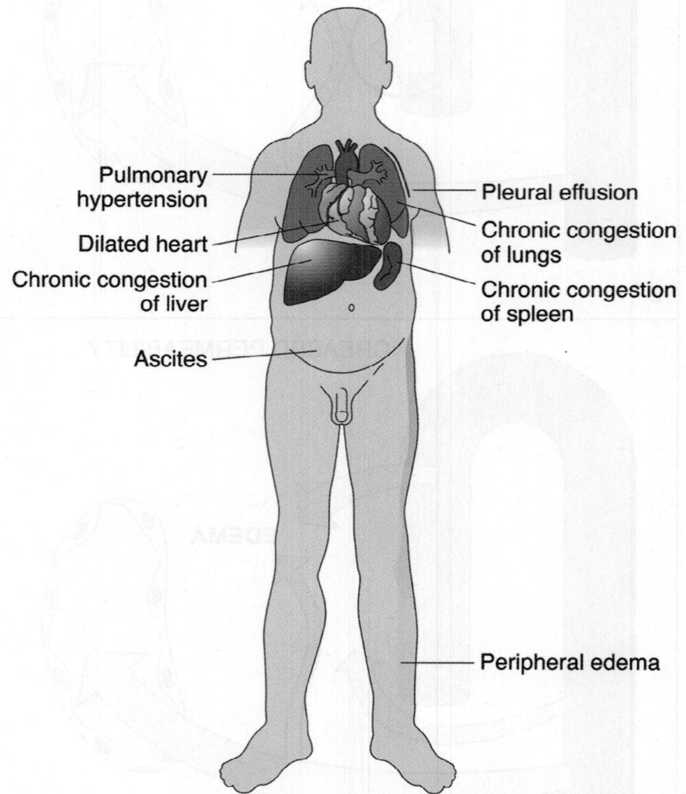

FIGURE 7-28. Pathologic consequences of chronic congestive heart failure.

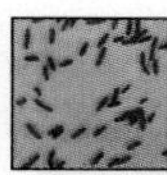
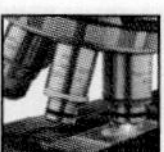

ETIOLOGIC FACTORS AND PATHOLOGY: The lung is a loose tissue without much connective tissue support and, therefore, requires certain conditions to prevent the development of edema. Among these protective devices are:

- Low perfusion pressure in lung capillaries, owing to low right ventricular pressure
- Effective drainage of the interstitial space of the lung by lymphatics, which are under a slightly negative pressure and can accommodate up to 10 times the regular lymph flow
- Tight cellular junctions between endothelial cells, which control capillary permeability

Pulmonary edema results if these protective mechanisms are disturbed. The most common causes of pulmonary edema relate to hemodynamic alterations in the heart that increase perfusion pressure in pulmonary capillaries and block effective lymphatic drainage. These conditions include left ventricular failure (the most common cause), mitral stenosis and mitral insufficiency. Disruption of capillary permeability is the cause of pulmonary edema in acute lung injury associated with adult respiratory distress syndrome, inhalation of toxic gases, aspiration of gastric contents, viral infections and uremia. Acute lung injury entails destruction of endothelial cells or disruption of their tight junctions (see Chapter 12).

Pulmonary edema may be interstitial or alveolar. Interstitial edema is the earliest phase and is an exaggeration of normal fluid filtration. Lymphatics become distended and fluid accumulates in the interstitium of lobular septa and around veins and bronchovascular bundles. Radiologic examination reveals a reticulonodular pattern, more marked at lung bases. Lobular septa become edematous and produce linear shadows ("Kerley B lines") on chest radiographs. Edema results in shunting of blood flow from the bases to the upper lobes. Edema of the bronchovascular tree increases resistance to airflow. Patients are often asymptomatic in this early stage.

When the fluid can no longer be accommodated in the interstitial space, it spills into the alveoli, a condition termed **alveolar edema.** At this stage, a radiologic alveolar pattern is seen, usually worse in central and lower portions of the lung. The patient becomes acutely short of breath and bubbly rales are heard. In extreme cases, frothy fluid is coughed up or wells up out of the trachea.

Microscopic examination of the edematous lung reveals severely congested alveolar capillaries and alveoli filled with a homogeneous, pink-staining fluid permeated by air bubbles (see Fig. 7-3). If pulmonary edema is caused by alveolar damage, cell debris, fibrin and proteins form films of proteinaceous material, called **hyaline membranes**, in the alveoli (Fig. 7-29).

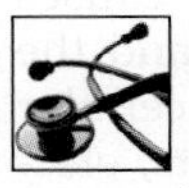

CLINICAL FEATURES: Pulmonary fluid accumulation may go unnoticed at first, but eventually dyspnea and coughing become prominent. If edema is severe, large amounts of frothy pink sputum are expectorated. Hypoxemia is manifested as cyanosis.

Pulmonary function is restricted in severe congestion and in interstitial pulmonary edema because fluid accumulation in the interstitial space reduces pulmonary compliance (i.e., it makes the lung stiffer). Thus, increased respiratory work is required to maintain ventilation. Thickened alveolar walls

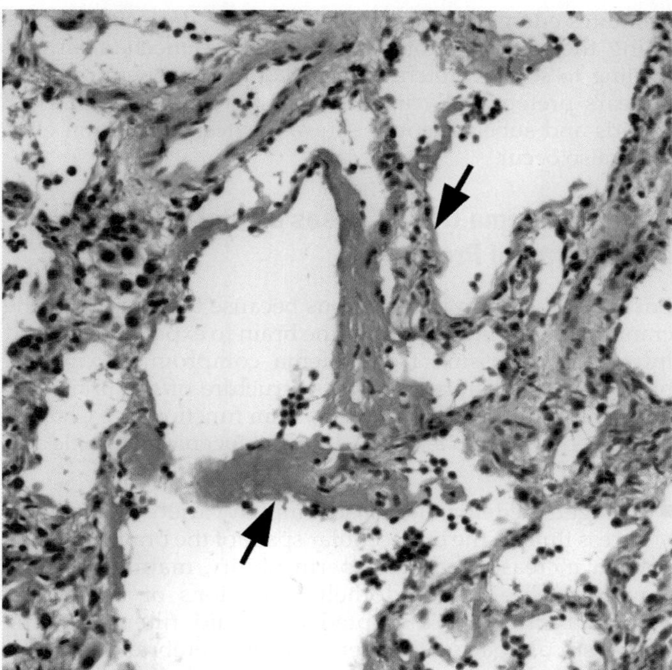

FIGURE 7-29. Pulmonary edema due to diffuse alveolar damage. A section of lung shows hyaline membranes (*arrows*) in alveoli.

represent a greater barrier to oxygen and carbon dioxide exchange. The latter is less affected than the former, resulting in hypoxia with near-normal carbon dioxide levels. Mismatch between ventilation (which is reduced) and perfusion (which persists) leads to hypoxemia in patients with pulmonary edema.

Edema in Cirrhosis of the Liver Is Commonly an End-Stage Condition

Cirrhosis of the liver is often accompanied by ascites and peripheral edema (see Chapter 14). Liver scarring obstructs portal blood flow and leads to portal hypertension and increased hydrostatic pressure in the splanchnic circulation. This situation is compounded by decreased hepatic synthesis of albumin as a result of liver dysfunction. Consequent accumulation of peritoneal fluid decreases effective blood volume, leading to renal sodium retention by mechanisms similar to those operative in congestive heart failure. Alternatively, chronic liver disease itself causes renal sodium retention. Subsequent expansion of extracellular fluid volume further promotes ascites and edema, thus establishing a vicious circle. In addition, increased transudation of lymph from the liver capsule adds to accumulation of fluid in the abdomen.

In Nephrotic Syndrome, the Rate of Protein Loss in the Urine Exceeds the Rate of Protein Replacement by the Liver

The resulting decline in the concentration of plasma proteins, particularly albumin, reduces plasma oncotic pressure and promotes edema. Blood volume therefore decreases, stimulating the renin–angiotensin–aldosterone mechanism and leading to sodium retention. The edema is generalized but appears preferentially in soft connective tissues, the eyes, eyelids and subcutaneous tissues. Ascites and pleural effusions also occur.

Cerebral Edema Often Causes a Fatal Increase in Intracranial Pressure

Edema of the brain is dangerous because the rigidity of the cranium allows little room for the brain to expand. Increased intracranial pressure from edema compromises cerebral blood supply, distorts the gross structure of the brain and interferes with central nervous system function (see Chapter 28). Cerebral edema is divided into vasogenic, cytotoxic and interstitial forms.

- **Vasogenic edema,** the most common variety of edema, is excess fluid in the extracellular space of the brain. It results from increased vascular permeability, mainly in white matter. The tight endothelial junctions of the blood-brain barrier are disrupted and fluid filters into the interstitial space. Disorders causing cerebral vasogenic edema include trauma, neoplasms, encephalitis, abscesses, infarcts, hemorrhage and toxic brain injury (e.g., lead poisoning).
- **Cytotoxic edema** is equivalent to hydropic cell swelling (i.e., accumulation of intracellular water). It is usually a response to cell injury, such as that produced by ischemia. Cytotoxic cerebral edema preferentially affects the gray matter.
- **Interstitial edema** is a consequence of hydrocephalus, in which fluid accumulates in the cerebral ventricles and periventricular white matter.

At autopsy, an edematous brain is soft and heavy. Gyri are flattened and sulci narrowed. Because of alterations in brain function, patients with cerebral edema suffer vomiting, disorientation and convulsions. ***Severe cerebral edema leads to herniation of the cerebellar tonsils, ordinarily a lethal event.***

Fluid Accumulates in Body Cavities as Extensions of the Interstitial Space

The Pleural Space

Pleural effusion (fluid in the pleural space) is a straw-colored transudate of low specific gravity that contains few cells (mainly exfoliated mesothelial cells). Fluid commonly accumulates as an expression of a generalized tendency to form edema in diseases such as the nephrotic syndrome, cirrhosis of the liver and congestive heart failure. Pleural effusions often accompany inflammatory processes or tumors in the lung or on the pleural surface.

The Pericardium

Fluid in the pericardial sac may result from hemorrhage (**hemopericardium**) or injury to the pericardium (**pericardial effusion**). Pericardial effusions occur with pericardial infections, tumors metastatic to the pericardium, uremia and inflammatory conditions such as systemic lupus erythematosus. Pericardial fluid accumulation may also occur after

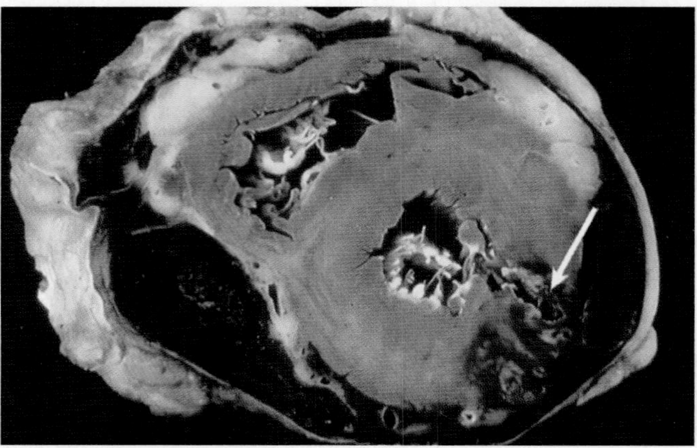

FIGURE 7-30. Cardiac tamponade. A cross-section of the heart shows rupture of a myocardial infarct (*arrow*) with the accumulation of a large quantity of blood in the pericardial cavity.

cardiac operations (**postpericardiotomy syndrome**) or radiation therapy for cancer.

If pericardial fluid accumulates rapidly (e.g., with hemorrhage from a ruptured myocardial infarct, dissecting aortic aneurysm or trauma), the pressure in the pericardial cavity may exceed the filling pressure of the heart. This condition, termed **cardiac tamponade** (Fig. 7-30), leads to a precipitous decline in cardiac output and is often fatal. If pericardial fluid accumulates rapidly, the tolerable limit may be only 90 to 120 mL, but a liter or more of fluid can be accommodated if the process is gradual.

Peritoneum

Peritoneal effusion, also called **ascites**, is caused mainly by hepatic cirrhosis, abdominal tumors, pancreatitis, cardiac failure, the nephrotic syndrome and hepatic venous obstruction (Budd-Chiari syndrome). Obstruction of the thoracic duct by cancer may lead to **chylous ascites**, in which the fluid has a milky appearance and a high fat content. The pathogenesis of ascites in cirrhosis of the liver is discussed above.

Patients with severe ascites accumulate many liters of fluid and have hugely distended abdomens. Complications of ascites reflect increased abdominal pressure and include anorexia and vomiting, reflux esophagitis, dyspnea, ventral hernia and leakage of fluid into the pleural space.

Fluid Loss and Overload

Fluid imbalance, whether excessive loss (dehydration) or overload, has potentially grave consequences. It causes hemodynamic disorders; alterations in osmolality and the quantity of fluid in intravascular, interstitial and cellular spaces may affect perfusion or delivery of nutrients, electrolytes or fluids.

Dehydration Results From Insufficient Fluid Intake, Excessive Fluid Loss or Both

Water loss may exceed intake in cases of vomiting, diarrhea, burns, excessive sweating and diabetes insipidus. When excessive fluid loss occurs, fluid is recruited from the interstitial space to the plasma space. Fluids in cells and within the interstitial and vascular compartments become more concentrated, particularly if there is a preferential loss of water, such as during inappropriate secretion of antidiuretic hormone in diabetes insipidus. Patients suffering from burns, vomiting, excessive sweating or diarrhea both lose fluid and have electrolyte disturbances. As a result, there is insufficient fluid to fill the fluid compartments of the body.

CLINICAL FEATURES: Clinically, only dryness of the skin and mucous membranes is noted initially, but as dehydration progresses, skin turgor is lost. If dehydration persists, **oliguria** (reduced urine output) occurs as a compensation for the fluid loss. More severe fluid loss is accompanied by a shift of water from the intracellular space to the extracellular space, leading to severe cell dysfunction, particularly in the brain. Shrinkage of brain tissue may cause rupture of small vessels and subsequent bleeding. Systemic blood pressure falls with continuous dehydration; declining perfusion eventually leads to death.

In Overhydration, Fluid Intake Exceeds Renal Excretory Capacity

Overhydration is rare, unless injury to the kidneys limits their excretory function or they are prevented from proper counterregulation (e.g., via excessive secretion of antidiuretic hormone). Fluid overload today is mostly caused by administration of excessive amounts of intravenous fluids. The most serious effect of such fluid overload is induction of cerebral edema or congestive heart failure in patients with cardiac dysfunction.

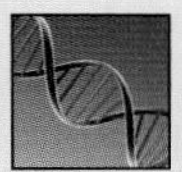

MOLECULAR PATHOGENESIS:

Blood Pressure Control

Twin and family studies suggest that genetics accounts for roughly 30% of blood pressure regulation (see Chapter 10). This may also account for the considerable variation in patient response to antihypertensive medication. Human genetic linkage and whole genome association studies have identified a host of mutations in key blood pressure regulatory processes. Prominent are genes of the renin–angiotensin system, which regulates vasoconstriction and sodium and water balance. Single nucleotide polymorphisms (SNPs) in genes encoding angiotensin, angiotensin-converting enzyme, angiotensin II receptor, renin and renin-binding protein are associated with altered blood pressure control. Hypertension has been associated with SNPs in the vasoconstrictor endothelin and its receptor, the vasodilator nitric oxide synthase and endothelial sodium channel subunits. Polymorphisms of β-adrenergic receptors 1 and 2 are associated with hypertension and altered response to β-agonists. Elucidation of the genetic bases for blood pressure regulation will improve our understanding of how blood pressure is controlled, identify patients at increased risk for development of hypertension and facilitate development of antihypertensive therapies.

Shock

Shock is a profound hemodynamic and metabolic disturbance characterized by failure to maintain an adequate blood supply to the microcirculation, with consequent inadequate perfusion of vital organs. In this often catastrophic circumstance, tissue perfusion and oxygen delivery fall below levels required to meet normal demands, including failure to remove metabolites adequately. The term **shock** encompasses all the reactions that occur in response to such disturbances. During uncompensated shock, rapid circulatory collapse leads to impaired cellular metabolism and death. However, in many cases, compensatory mechanisms sustain the patient, at least for a while. When these adaptations fail, shock becomes irreversible. Shock has been a major cause of morbidity and mortality in intensive care units. Unfortunately, the outcome of shock has not changed appreciably in the past 50 years.

Shock is not synonymous with low blood pressure, although hypotension is often part of the shock syndrome. Hypotension is actually a late sign in shock and indicates failure of compensation. At the same time that peripheral blood flow falls below critical levels, extreme vasoconstriction can maintain arterial blood pressure. The distinction between shock and hypotension is important clinically because rapid restoration of systemic blood flow is the primary goal in treating shock. If blood pressure alone is raised with vasopressive drugs, systemic blood flow may actually be diminished.

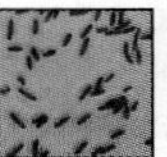

ETIOLOGIC FACTORS: Decreased perfusion in shock most commonly results from decreased cardiac output, due either to the inability of the heart to pump normal venous return or to decreased effective blood volume that leads to decreased venous return. These two mechanisms underlie two of the major types of shock: **cardiogenic** and **hypovolemic** shock. Systemic vasodilation, with or without increased vascular permeability, is responsible for the other categories of shock: septic, anaphylactic and neurogenic shock (Fig. 7-31).

- **Cardiogenic shock** is caused by myocardial pump failure. It usually arises after massive myocardial infarction, but myocarditis may also be responsible. Conditions that prevent left or right heart filling reduce cardiac output, resulting in "obstructive" shock. Such conditions include pulmonary embolism, cardiac tamponade (Fig. 7-30) and (rarely) atrial myxoma.
- **Hypovolemic shock** is secondary to a pronounced decrease in blood or plasma volume, caused by loss of fluid from the vascular compartment. Hemorrhage, fluid loss from severe burns, diarrhea, excessive urine formation, perspiration and trauma are the major causes of fluid loss that can lead to hypovolemic shock. In the case of burns or trauma, direct damage to the microcirculation increases vascular permeability.
- **Septic shock** is caused by severe systemic microbial infections. The pathogenesis of septic shock is complex and is discussed in detail below.
- **Anaphylactic shock** is a consequence of a systemic type I hypersensitivity reaction, which leads to widespread vasodilation and increased vascular permeability.
- **Neurogenic shock** can follow acute injury to the brain or spinal cord, which impairs the neural control of vasomotor tone, causing generalized vasodilation. In the case of both anaphylactic and neurogenic shock, the subsequent

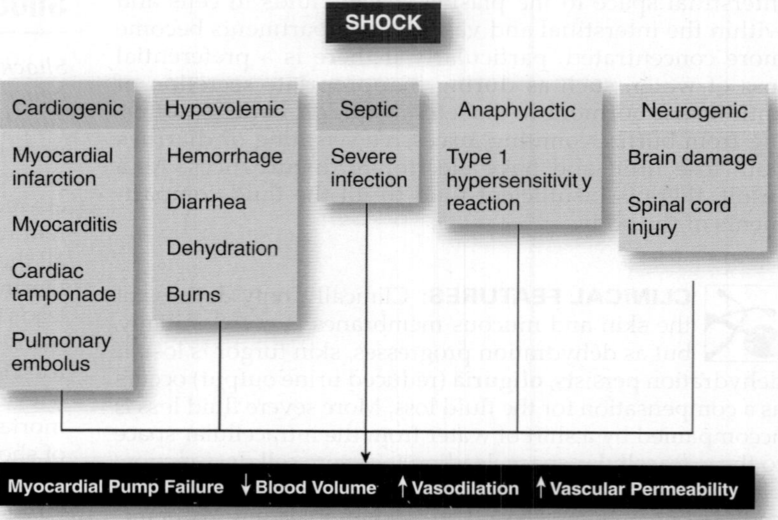

FIGURE 7-31. Classification of shock. Shock results from (1) an inability of the heart to pump adequately (cardiogenic shock), (2) decreased effective blood volume as a consequence of severely reduced blood or plasma volume (hypovolemic shock) or (3) widespread vasodilation (septic, anaphylactic or neurogenic shock). Increased vascular permeability may complicate vasodilation by contributing to reduced effective blood volume.

redistribution of blood to the periphery, with or without increased vascular permeability, reduces the effective circulating blood and plasma volume. This ultimately leads to the same consequences as in hypovolemic shock.

In hypovolemic and cardiogenic shock, lower cardiac output and resultant decreased tissue perfusion are the key steps in the progression from reversible to irreversible shock. Cellular hypoxia is the common consequence of the initial decrease in tissue perfusion. Although such changes do not initially result in irreversible injury, a vicious circle of decreasing tissue perfusion and further cell injury is perpetuated by several mechanisms:

- Injury to endothelial cells, secondary to the hypoxia caused by decreased tissue perfusion and increased vascular permeability, leads to escape of fluid from the vascular compartment.
- Increased exudation of fluid from the circulation reduces (1) blood volume; (2) venous return; and (3) cardiac output, thereby aggravating hypoxic cell injury.
- Decreased perfusion of kidneys and skeletal muscles results in metabolic acidosis, which in turn further decreases cardiac output and tissue perfusion.
- Decreased perfusion of the heart injures myocardial cells and decreases their ability to pump blood, further reducing cardiac output and tissue perfusion.

Systemic Inflammatory Response Syndrome Characterizes Septic Shock

Systemic inflammatory response syndrome (SIRS) is an exaggerated, generalized manifestation of a local immune or inflammatory reaction, and is often fatal. SIRS is a hypermetabolic state characterized by two or more signs of systemic inflammation—such as fever, tachycardia, tachypnea, leukocytosis or leukopenia—in the setting of a known cause of inflammation. **Septic shock** is defined as clinical SIRS so severe that it leads to organ dysfunction and hypotension. The mechanisms responsible for development of septic shock are illustrated in Fig. 7-32. These processes often progress to **multiple organ dysfunction syndrome** (MODS), a term used to describe otherwise unexplained abnormalities of organ function in critically ill patients (see below).

MOLECULAR PATHOGENESIS: ***The massive inflammatory reaction defined by SIRS results from systemic release of cytokines, the most important being tumor necrosis factor (TNF), interleukin-1 (IL-1), IL-6 and platelet-activating factor (PAF).*** Over 30 endogenous mediators of SIRS have been identified. Their interactions may be important in the pathogenesis of SIRS.

Septicemia with gram-negative organisms is the most common cause of septic shock. The invading bacteria release **endotoxin,** a lipopolysaccharide (LPS), whose toxic activity resides in the lipid A component. On entry into the circulation, LPS, via lipid A, binds to LPS-binding protein. This complex binds to CD14 on the surface of monocyte/macrophages, which is part of a recognition complex that also includes the toll-like receptor (TLR) family of proteins and the recently discovered peptidoglycan recognition proteins (PGRP). TLRs are the primary sensors of the innate immune system, which collectively recognize bacteria, fungi and protozoa. Immediately downstream of TLR binding are the myeloid differentiation protein 88 (MyD 88), toll-interleukin-1 (TIR) domain-containing adaptor protein, TIR receptor domain-containing adaptor protein inducing interferon β (TRIF) and TRIF-related adaptor molecule. These mediate signaling through activation of **nuclear factor-κB (NF-κB)** transcription factor and upregulate TNF expression. LPS binding to TLR-4 causes mononuclear phagocytes to secrete large quantities of cytokines, such as TNF, IL-1, IL-6, IL-8, IL-12, macrophage inhibitory factor and others, that mediate a variety of responses. These cytokines, and subsequent production of nitric oxide (NO•) and procoagulant proteins, ultimately cause the overwhelming cardiovascular collapse characteristic of septic shock. In this context activation of inducible NO synthase (iNOS) by TNF upregulates NO• synthesis from L-arginine, an effect that is primarily responsible for the drop in blood pressure that occurs during sepsis. TNF is also central to the pathogenesis of shock that is not associated with endotoxemia (e.g., cardiogenic shock). While LPS is the most potent stimulus, other antigens also promote TNF release. These include toxin-1 of the toxic shock syndrome; enterotoxin; antigens of mycobacteria, fungi, parasites and viruses; and products of complement activation.

When macrophages are exposed to LPS in septic shock, large amounts of TNF are suddenly released, often with lethal consequences. Administering anti-TNF antibody before exposing an animal to endotoxin or to gram-negative bacteria completely protects from septic shock. Unfortunately, comparable studies in humans have not been as successful.

TNF released by monocyte/macrophages exerts a direct toxic effect on endothelial cells by compromising membrane permeability and inducing endothelial cell apoptosis. It also acts indirectly by (1) initiating a cascade of other mediators that amplify its deleterious effects, (2) promoting adhesion of polymorphonuclear leukocytes to endothelial surfaces and (3) activating the extrinsic coagulation pathway. TNF stimulates release of IL-1 and IL-6, PAF and other eicosanoids that may mediate tissue injury. Interestingly, in animal studies, nonlethal doses of TNF may become fatal if administered together with IL-1. TNF also increases expression of adhesion molecules, such as intercellular adhesion molecules (ICAMs), vascular cell adhesion molecules (VCAMs), P-selectin and endothelial-leukocyte adhesion molecules (ELAMs) on endothelial surfaces, thereby promoting leukocyte adhesion and leukostasis. This mechanism presumably plays a role in the respiratory distress syndrome, in which activated neutrophils are sequestered in the pulmonary circulation and damage alveoli. Other vasoactive peptides include the vasodilatory prostacyclins and endothelin (ET)-1, a potent vasoconstrictor (Fig. 7-32). Note that the term **septic syndrome** refers to the physiologic and metabolic response characteristic of sepsis in the absence of an infection.

Recognition of Genetic Polymorphisms in Toll-Like Receptors and Tumor Necrosis Factor Has Helped Elucidate the Pathogenesis of Sepsis

Gene mutations in several cytokines, cell surface receptors and other circulating markers have been associated with variability in susceptibility to sepsis. TLR-pattern recognition receptors recognize pathogen-associated microbial patterns and thus are critical in triggering innate immune responses. Toll-like receptor-4 (TLR4) is critical in recognizing LPS of gram-negative bacteria. A mutation, from aspartic acid to glycine at amino acid 299 of TLR4, leads to reduced inflammatory responses in a variety of clinical settings. Thus, TLR4 appears to be important in magnifying responses to endotoxin and in sepsis. Polymorphisms in TLRs and other pattern recognition receptors may help to explain why patients respond so differently to specific infectious agents.

Similarly, recently discovered mutations in the TNF-α gene have improved our understanding of the role of TNF-α in sepsis. For example, a G to A base change at base 308 of the TNF-α promoter leads to enhanced promoter activity and increased expression of TNF-α and is associated with increased risk of sepsis and shock. Other gene mutations associated with worse prognosis in sepsis are found in IL-1 receptor agonist, CD14 and plasminogen activator inhibitor-1.

Multiple Organ Dysfunction Syndrome Is the End-Result of Shock

Improvements in the early treatment of shock and sepsis have allowed patients to survive long enough to manifest a new problem, progressive deterioration of organ function. Almost all septic shock patients suffer from dysfunction of at least one organ. However, multiple organ dysfunction occurs in one third of patients with septic shock, trauma or burns and in a quarter of those with acute pancreatitis. Whatever the cause, the clinical deterioration of MODS is held to result from common mechanisms of tissue injury subsumed under the rubric of SIRS. ***Mortality of SIRS/MODS exceeds 50%, making it responsible for most deaths in noncoronary intensive care units in the United States.*** In most cases inflammatory reactions and the progression from sepsis to organ dysfunction reflect a balance between proinflammatory and anti-inflammatory factors. As mentioned above, TNF-α, IL-1 and NO• have systemic effects.

Also, reactive oxygen species are important triggers of end-organ dysfunction. The acute response to sepsis is characterized by release of adrenocorticotropic hormone, cortisol, adrenaline and noradrenaline, vasopressin, glucagon and growth hormone. The net result is shutdown of noncritical systems and an overall catabolic state. Although proinflammatory mediators predominate in SIRS, anti-inflammatory factors play an important role in some patients. The result is **compensated anti-inflammatory response syndrome (CARS)**, in which paralysis of the immune system leads to a poor outcome. It is now thought that following bacterial infection, there is an initial response of excessive inflammation and septic shock characteristic of SIRS. Such uncontrolled cytokine induction is preceded by a stage of anergy and immune repression or CARS. Septic patients who cycle between SIRS and CARS are susceptible to increased mortality. Persons with a heterogeneous response are said to have a **"mixed anti-inflammatory response syndrome" (MARS)**.

Vascular Compensatory Mechanisms

Changes in the macrovascular and microvascular circulation are at least partly responsible for variable organ injury in SIRS. Compensatory mechanisms in shock shift blood flow away from the periphery, so as to maintain flow to the heart and the brain. These responses involve the sympathetic nervous system, release of endogenous vasoconstrictors and hormonal substances, and local vasoregulation. The result is increased cardiac output achieved by increasing heart rate and myocardial contractility while constricting arteries and arterioles.

- **Increased sympathetic discharge** augments catecholamine release by the adrenal medulla. Skeletal muscle, splanchnic bed and skin arterioles respond to increased sympathetic discharge; cardiac and cerebral arterioles are less reactive. Thus, increased sympathetic tone shifts blood flow from the periphery to the heart and brain. The marked arteriolar

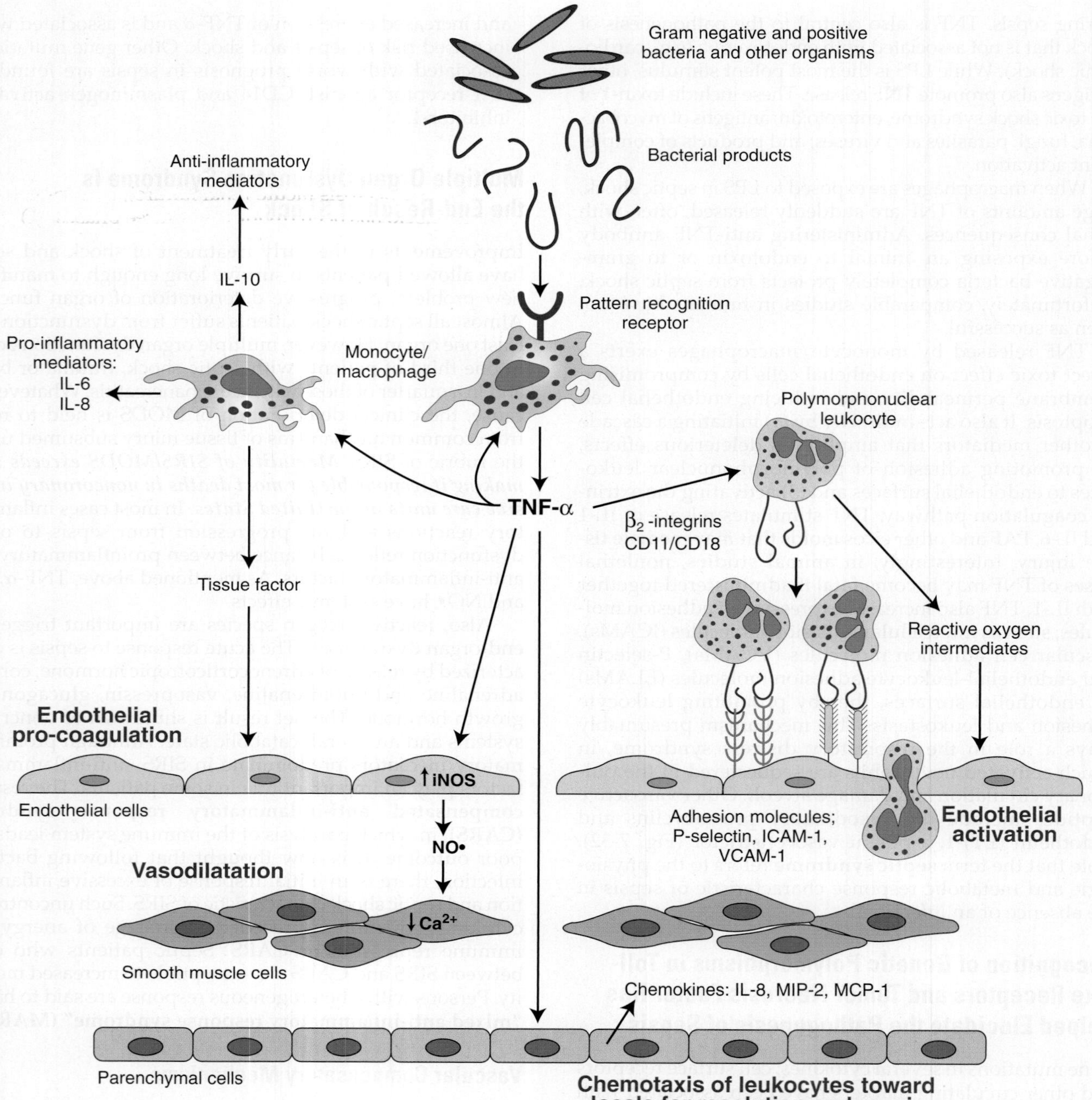

FIGURE 7-32. Pathogenesis of endotoxic shock. Sepsis is caused primarily by gram-negative bacteria and bacterial products such as endotoxin (lipopolysaccharide [LPS]), which is released into the circulation, where it binds to a pattern recognition receptor on the surface of monocyte/macrophages. Such binding stimulates the secretion of substantial quantities of tumor necrosis factor-α (TNF-α). TNF-α mediates septic shock by a number of mechanisms: (1) stimulation of the release of various pro- and anti-inflammatory mediators; (2) induction of endothelial procoagulation by tissue factor, thereby leading to thrombosis and local ischemia; (3) direct cytotoxic damage to endothelial cells; (4) endothelial activation, which enhances the adherence of polymorphonuclear leukocytes; (5) stimulation of endothelial cell nitric oxide production and vasodilation; and (6) release of chemokines to attract leukocytes for resolution and repair of tissue injury. Ca^{2+} = calcium ion; ICAM = intercellular adhesion molecule; IL = interleukin; iNOS = inducible nitric oxide synthetase; MCP-1 = monocyte chemotactic protein-1; MIP-2 = macrophage-inflammatory protein-2; NO• = nitric oxide; VCAM-1 = vascular cell adhesion molecule-1.

vasoconstriction reduces capillary hydrostatic pressure and decreases fluid shifted into the interstitium, facilitating an osmotic fluid shift from the interstitium to the vascular system. This sympathetic–adrenal response can compensate completely for loss of 10% of intravascular blood volume. If more fluid is lost, cardiac output and blood pressure are affected and blood flow to tissues is reduced.

- **The renin–angiotensin–aldosterone system** also helps compensate, by stimulating sodium and water reabsorption, thereby helping to maintain intravascular volume. A similar water-preserving action is provided by pituitary antidiuretic hormone.
- **Vascular autoregulation** preserves regional blood flow to vital organs, particularly the heart and brain, by vasodilation in the coronary and cerebral circulations in response to hypoxia and acidosis. Vasoconstriction mediated largely by α-adrenergic receptors in mesenteric venules and veins helps maintain cardiac filling and arterial pressure. Circulation to organs such as skin and skeletal muscles, which are less sensitive to hypoxia, does not display such tightly controlled autoregulation.

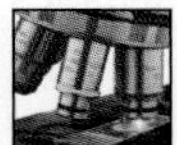

PATHOLOGY: Shock is associated with specific changes in a number of organs (Fig. 7-33), including acute renal tubular necrosis, acute respiratory distress syndrome, liver failure, depression of host defense mechanisms and heart failure. Interestingly, paracrine cross-talk from one injured organ such as proinflammatory mediators from the lung can affect distant organ injury.

Heart

Dysfunction in both systolic and diastolic circuits is associated with sepsis and most likely reflects paracrine injury and possibly hypoperfusion. In sepsis, the heart shows petechial hemorrhages of the epicardium and endocardium. Microscopically, necrotic foci in the myocardium range from loss of single fibers to large areas of necrosis. Prominent contraction bands are visible by light microscopy but are better seen by electron microscopy. Ultrastructurally, flattened areas of the intercalated disk are a sign of cell swelling, and invagination of adjacent cells is considered to be a catecholamine-induced lesion.

Kidney

Acute tubular necrosis (acute renal failure), a major complication of shock, has been divided into three phases: (1) **initiation**, from the onset of injury to the beginning of renal failure; (2) **maintenance**, from the onset of renal failure to a stable, reduced renal function; and (3) **recovery**. In those who survive an episode of shock, the recovery phase begins about 10 days after its onset and may last up to 8 weeks.

Renal blood flow is restricted to one third of normal following the acute ischemic phase. This effect is even more severe in the outer cortex. Constriction of arterioles reduces filtration pressure, thereby reducing the volume of filtrate and contributing to oliguria. Interstitial edema occurs, possibly through a process termed **backflow.** Excessive vasoconstriction is also related to stimulation of the renin–angiotensin system.

During acute renal failure, the kidney is large, swollen and congested, although the cortex may be pale. Cross-section reveals blood pooling in the outer stripe of the medulla. Microscopically, fully developed acute tubular necrosis entails dilation of the proximal tubules and focal necrosis of cells (Fig. 7-34). Frequently, pigmented casts in tubular lumina indicate leakage of hemoglobin or myoglobin. Coarse, "ropy" casts are seen in the distal nephron and distal convoluted tubules. Interstitial edema is prominent in the cortex and mononuclear cells accumulate within tubules and surrounding interstitium. Acute tubular necrosis is discussed in more detail in Chapter 16.

Lung

After the onset of severe and prolonged shock, injury to alveolar walls can result in **shock lung**, which is a cause of **acute**

FIGURE 7-33. Complications of shock.

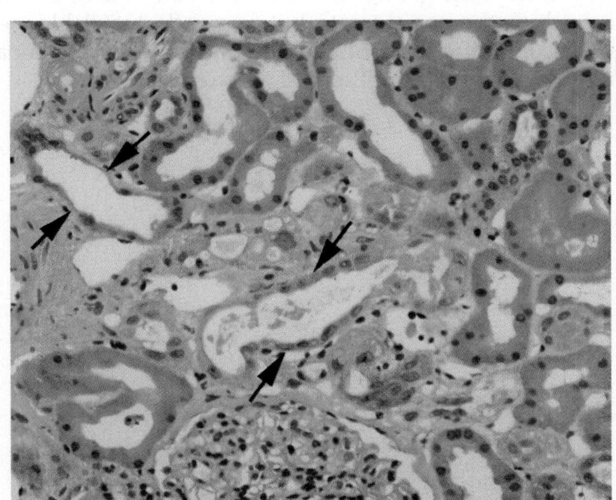

FIGURE 7-34. Acute tubular necrosis. A section of kidney shows swelling and degeneration of tubular epithelium. *Arrows* indicate the thinned and damaged epithelium.

respiratory distress syndrome (ARDS) (see Chapter 12). The sequence of changes is mediated by polymorphonuclear leukocytes and includes interstitial edema, necrosis of endothelial and alveolar epithelial cells and formation of intravascular microthrombi and hyaline membranes lining the alveolar surface.

Macroscopically, the lung is firm and congested and a frothy fluid often exudes from the cut surface. Interstitial edema is first seen around peribronchial connective tissue and lymphatics, subsequently filling the interstitial connective tissue. In this initial period, a large fluid volume drains into the pulmonary lymphatics. Alveolar edema may develop if this fluid is not adequately removed or if the balance of forces that keep the fluid in the interstitial space is disturbed.

Shock-induced lung injury leads to so-called alveolar hyaline membranes (see Fig. 7-29), which also frequently line alveolar ducts and terminal bronchioles. These changes may heal entirely, but in half of patients, repair processes cause thickening of the alveolar wall. Type II pneumocytes proliferate to replace damaged type I pneumocytes and line the alveoli. Fibrous tissue proliferation may lead to organization of the alveolar exudate. These chronic changes may result in persistent respiratory distress and even death. Shock lung and ARDS are more fully discussed in Chapter 12.

Gastrointestinal Tract

Shock often results in diffuse gastrointestinal hemorrhage. Erosions of the gastric mucosa and superficial ischemic necrosis in the intestines are the usual sources of this bleeding. Interruption of the barrier function of the intestine may lead to septicemia. More severe necrotizing lesions contribute to deterioration in the final phase of shock.

Liver

In patients who die in shock, the liver is enlarged and has a mottled cut surface that reflects marked centrilobular pooling of blood. The most prominent histologic lesion is centrilobular congestion and necrosis. The basis for the apparent increased sensitivity of centrilobular hepatocytes to shock may not simply represent their greater distance from the source of blood delivered via the portal tracts, but may reflect variable metabolic susceptibilities among the different zones of the hepatic lobule, a matter that is not settled (see Chapter 14).

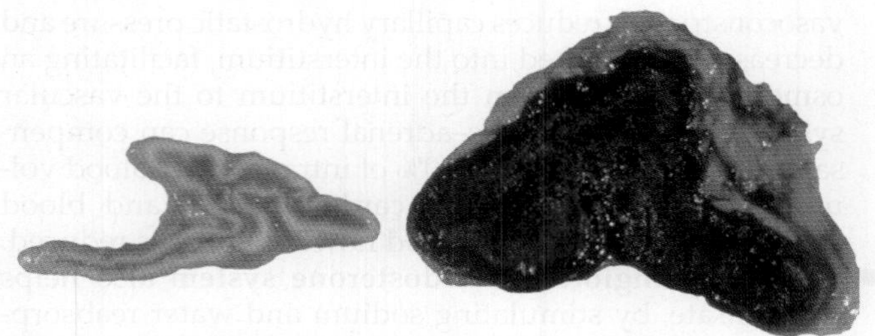

FIGURE 7-35. Waterhouse-Friderichsen syndrome. A normal adrenal gland (*left*) in contrast to an adrenal gland enlarged by extensive hemorrhage (*right*), obtained from a patient who died of meningococcemic shock.

Pancreas

The splanchnic vascular bed, which supplies the pancreas, is particularly affected by impaired circulation during shock. Resulting ischemic damage to the exocrine pancreas unleashes activated catalytic enzymes and causes acute pancreatitis, which further promotes shock.

Brain

Although septic patients often have clinical encephalopathy, discrete brain lesions are rare in SIRS and shock. Microscopic hemorrhages may be seen, but patients who recover do not ordinarily have neurologic deficits. In severe cases, particularly in persons with cerebral atherosclerosis, hemorrhage and necrosis may appear in the overlapping region between the terminal distributions of major arteries, so-called **watershed infarcts** (see Chapter 28).

Adrenals

In severe shock, adrenal glands exhibit conspicuous hemorrhage in the inner cortex. The hemorrhage is often focal. However, it can be massive and accompanied by hemorrhagic necrosis of the entire gland, as seen in **Waterhouse-Friderichsen syndrome** (Fig. 7-35), typically associated with overwhelming meningococcal septicemia.

8 Environmental and Nutritional Pathology

David S. Strayer • Emanuel Rubin

Environmental pathology is the study of diseases caused by exposure to harmful external agents and deficiencies of vital substances. With heightened awareness of the fact that chemical agents may mediate tissue changes and recognition that many of these are environmental contaminants, "occupational pathology" has developed. In this chapter we concentrate on diseases caused by (1) exposure to toxic agents, (2) physical damage and (3) nutritional deficiencies.

Smoking

Smoking tobacco is the single largest preventable cause of death in the United States. ***Some 400,000 deaths per year—about one sixth of the total deaths in the United States—occur prematurely because of smoking.*** Estimates have incriminated tobacco in 11% to 30% of cancer deaths, 17% to 30% of cardiovascular deaths, 30% of deaths from lung diseases and 20% to 30% of the incidence of low–birth-weight infants. Life expectancy is shortened and overall mortality is proportional to the amount and duration of cigarette smoking, commonly quantitated as "pack-years" (Fig. 8-1). For example, a person who smokes two packs of cigarettes a day at the age of 30 years will live an average of 8 years less than a nonsmoker.

The previously increasing adoption of smoking by many women has led to their being afflicted with the same epidemic of smoking-related disease that assaulted men more than a generation earlier. The characteristics of smoking-related illnesses reflect the amount smoked, not the gender of the smoker. In fact, mortality from lung cancer, almost all of which is related to cigarette smoking, exceeds that from cancers of the breast and prostate, which are among the most common cancers in the United States. The excess mortality associated with cigarette smoking declines after one quits smoking: after 15 years of abstinence from cigarettes, the mortality of ex-smokers from all causes approaches that of people who have never smoked. Cancer mortality among those who smoke only cigars or pipes is somewhat greater than that of the nonsmoking population. Use of smokeless

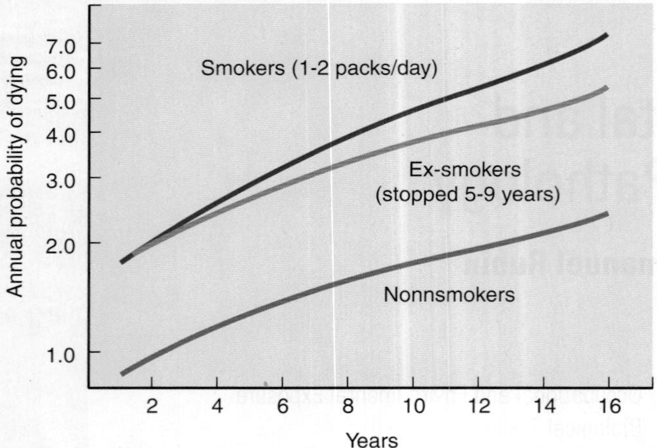

FIGURE 8-1. The risk of dying in smokers and nonsmokers. Note that the annual probability of an individual dying, indicated on the ordinate, is a logarithmic scale. Individuals who have smoked for 1 year have a twofold greater probability of dying than a nonsmoker, whereas those who have smoked for more than 15 years have more than a threefold greater probability of dying.

tobacco (snuff, chewing tobacco) entails little, if any, increased risk of malignancy.

The major diseases responsible for excess mortality reported in cigarette smokers are, in order of frequency, coronary heart disease, lung cancer and chronic obstructive pulmonary disease. Cancers of the oral cavity, larynx, esophagus, pancreas, bladder, kidney, colon and cervix are all more common in smokers than in nonsmokers. Also, smokers show excess mortality from atherosclerotic aortic aneurysms and peptic ulcer disease.

Cardiovascular Disease Is a Major Complication of Smoking

***Cigarette smoking is a major independent risk factor for myocardial infarction. It acts synergistically with other risk factors, such as elevated blood pressure and blood cholesterol levels* (Fig. 8-2).** Smoking precipitates initial myocardial infarction, increases the risk for second heart attacks and diminishes survival after a heart attack among those who continue to smoke. Smoking also increases the incidence of sudden cardiac death: it contributes to development of atherosclerotic plaques and may lead to ischemia and arrhythmias.

Cigarette smoking is an independent risk factor for **ischemic stroke.** The risk correlates with the number of cigarettes smoked and is reduced after cessation of smoking. Tobacco use also increases risk of certain forms of **intracranial hemorrhage.** The combination of smoking and oral contraceptive use in women older than 35 years of age increases the likelihood of **myocardial infarction**. Similarly, use of cigarettes by women who are using oral contraceptives significantly increases their risk of stroke.

Atherosclerosis of the coronary arteries and aorta is more severe and extensive among cigarette smokers than among nonsmokers, and the effect is dose related. As a consequence, cigarette smoking is a strong risk factor for **atherosclerotic aortic aneurysms**. The incidence and severity of **atherosclerotic peripheral vascular disease** are also remarkably increased by smoking. Smoking is also a major risk factor for **coronary vasospasm**. It disturbs regional coronary blood flow in patients with coronary artery disease and lowers the threshold for ventricular fibrillation and cardiac arrest in patients with established ischemic heart disease. The pharmacologic actions of nicotine itself, carbon monoxide (CO) inhalation, reduced plasma high-density lipoprotein levels, increased plasma fibrinogen levels and higher leukocyte

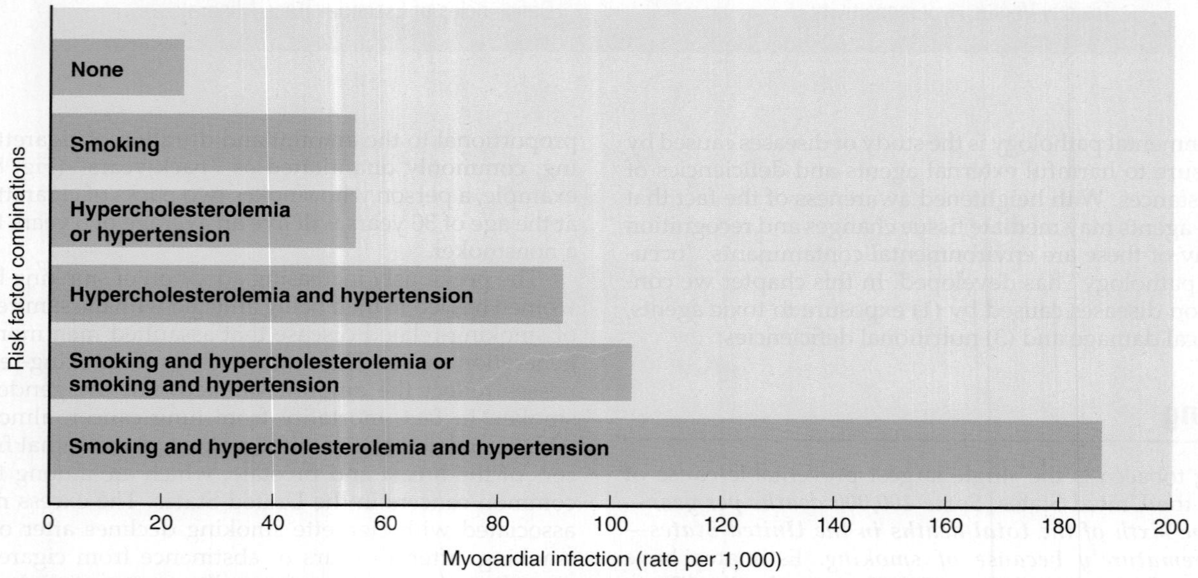

FIGURE 8-2. The risk of myocardial infarction in cigarette smokers. Smoking is an independent risk factor and increases the risk of a myocardial infarction to about the same extent as does hypertension or hypercholesterolemia alone. The effects of smoking are additive to those of these other two risk factors.

counts are all consequences of smoking that may predispose to myocardial infarction.

Buerger disease, a peculiar inflammatory and occlusive disease of the lower leg vasculature, occurs almost only in heavy smokers (see Chapter 10).

Cancer of the Lung Is Largely a Disease of Cigarette Smokers

More than 85% of deaths from lung cancer, the single most common cancer death in both men and women in the United States today, are attributed to cigarette smoking (Fig. 8-3). Although the precise offenders in cigarette smoke have not been identified, clearly cigarette smoke is toxic and carcinogenic to the bronchial mucosa. When cigarette smoke is passed through a filter, it is separated into gas and particulate phases. Cigarette tar, the material that is deposited on the filter, contains more than 3000 compounds, many of which have been identified as carcinogens, mucosal toxins and ciliotoxic agents. Compounds with similar harmful properties are found in the gas phase, but they are fewer. Among smokers, the risk of developing lung cancer is directly related to the number of cigarettes smoked.

Cigarette smoking is also an important factor in the induction of **lung cancer** that is associated with certain occupational exposures. For instance, uranium miners have an increased rate of lung cancer, presumably because of inhalation of radon daughters. The rate of lung cancer among miners who smoke is considerably higher than for nonminers with similar smoking habits. Another example is the case of asbestos workers. Whereas heavy smokers in the general population have a risk of lung cancer some 20 times greater than that of nonsmokers, asbestos workers who manifest pulmonary fibrosis and smoke heavily have a risk that is 40–60 times that of nonsmokers.

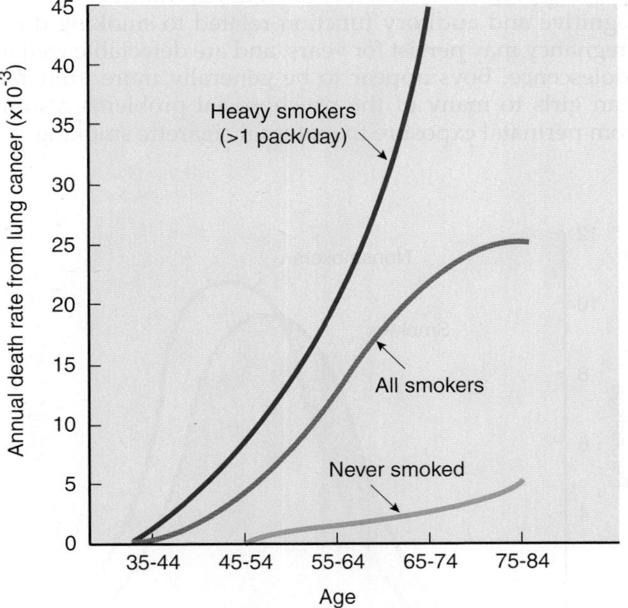

FIGURE 8-3. Death rate from lung cancer among smokers and nonsmokers. Nonsmokers exhibit a small, linear rise in the death rate from lung cancer from the age of 50 onward. By contrast, those who smoke more than one pack per day show an exponential rise in the annual death rate from lung cancer starting at about age 35. By age 70, heavy smokers have about a 20-fold greater death rate from lung cancer than nonsmokers.

- **Cancers of the lip, tongue and buccal mucosa** occur principally (>90%) in tobacco users. All forms of tobacco use—cigarette, cigar and pipe smoking, as well as tobacco chewing—expose the oral cavity to the compounds found in raw tobacco or tobacco smoke.
- **Cancer of the larynx** is similarly related to cigarette smoking. In some large studies, white male smokers have from 6 to 13 times greater a death rate from laryngeal cancer as nonsmokers.
- **Cancer of the esophagus** in the United States and Great Britain is estimated to result from smoking in 80% of cases.
- **Cancer of the bladder** is twice as frequent a cause of death in cigarette smokers as in nonsmokers. In fact, 30% to 40% of all bladder cancers are attributable to smoking. As with most tobacco-related disorders, there is a clear dose-response relationship between incidence of bladder cancer, numbers of cigarettes smoked per day and duration of cigarette smoking.
- **Carcinoma of the kidney** is increased 50% to 100% among smokers. A modest increase in cancer of the renal pelvis has also been documented.
- **Cancer of the pancreas** has shown a steady increase in incidence, which is, at least in part, related to cigarette smoking. The risk ratio in male smokers for adenocarcinoma of the pancreas is 2 to 3, and a dose-response relationship exists. Men who smoke over two packs a day have five times greater risk of developing pancreatic cancer than nonsmokers.
- **Cancer of the uterine cervix** is significantly increased in women smokers. It has been estimated that about 30% of cervical cancer mortality is associated with this habit.
- **Acute myelogenous leukemia (AML)** is associated with smoking: in men, smoking doubles the risk of AML, compared to male nonsmokers.

Smokers Are at Higher Risk for Certain Nonneoplastic Diseases

- **Chronic bronchitis and emphysema** occur primarily in cigarette smokers. The incidence of these diseases is a function of the number of cigarettes smoked (Fig. 8-4; see Chapter 12).
- **Peptic ulcer disease** is 70% more common in male cigarette smokers than in nonsmokers.
- **Osteoporosis** in women is exacerbated by tobacco use. Women who smoke one pack of cigarettes per day during their reproductive period will exhibit a 5% to 10% deficit in bone density at menopause. This deficit is enough to increase the risk of bone fractures.
- **Thyroid diseases** are linked to cigarette smoking. The most conspicuous association is with Graves disease, especially when hyperthyroidism is complicated by exophthalmos.
- **Ocular diseases,** particularly macular degeneration and cataracts, are reportedly more frequent in smokers.

Smoking Impairs Female Reproductive Function

Women who smoke experience an **earlier menopause** than nonsmokers, possibly because of the effects of tobacco on estrogen metabolism.

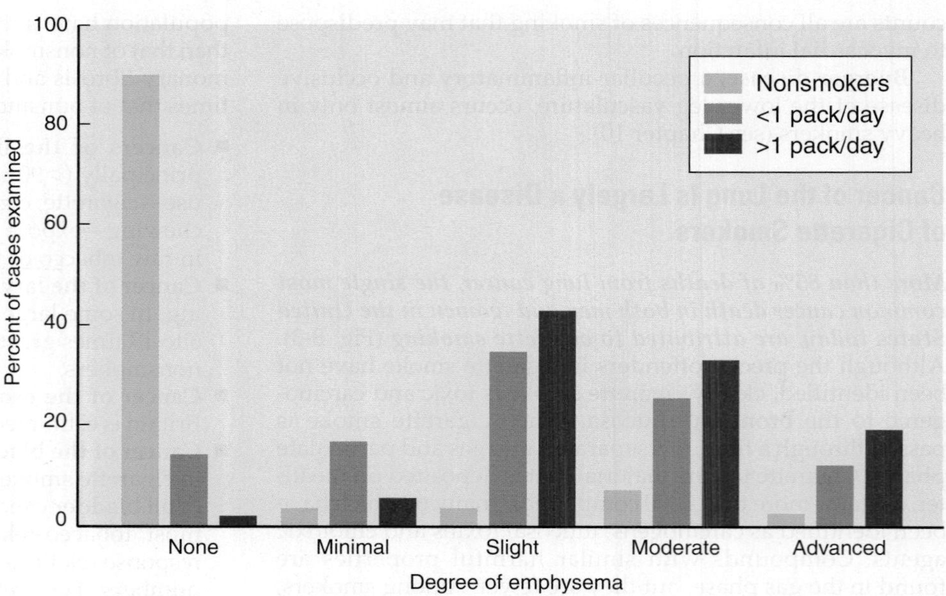

FIGURE 8-4. The association between cigarette smoking and pulmonary emphysema. Some 90% of nonsmokers have no detectable emphysema at autopsy. In contrast, virtually all those who smoke more than one pack per day have morphologic evidence of emphysema at autopsy. Emphysema shows a slight dose dependence on the number of cigarettes smoked. Those who smoke less than one pack per day tend to have less severe emphysema, but 85% to 90% of such smokers have some emphysema at autopsy.

MOLECULAR PATHOGENESIS: In the liver, estradiol is hydroxylated to estrone, which then enters one of two irreversible metabolic pathways. In one, 16-hydroxylation leads to production of estriol, a potent estrogen. In the other, 2-hydroxylation yields methoxyestrone, which has no estrogenic activity. In female smokers, the latter pathway (i.e., the one that leads to the inactive metabolite) is stimulated. Consequently, circulating levels of estriol, the active estrogen, are reduced. The increased incidence of postmenopausal osteoporosis in smokers has been attributed to decreased estriol levels.

Fetal Tobacco Syndrome Produces Smaller Infants

Maternal cigarette smoking impairs the development of the fetus. Infants born to women who smoke during pregnancy are, on average, 200 g lighter than infants born to comparable women who do not smoke. ***These infants are not born preterm but rather are small for gestational age at every stage of pregnancy.*** In fact, 20% to 40% of the incidence of low birth weight can be attributed to maternal cigarette smoking (Fig. 8-5). Thus, this effect of smoking is not idiosyncratic but reflects a direct retardation of fetal growth.

The harmful consequences of maternal cigarette smoking on the fetus are illustrated by its effect on the uteroplacental unit. Perinatal mortality is higher among offspring of smokers, the increases ranging from 20% among progeny of women who smoke less than a pack per day to almost 40% among offspring of those who smoke over one pack per day, with the excess mortality reflecting problems related to the uteroplacental system. Incidences of abruptio placentae, placenta previa, uterine bleeding and premature rupture of membranes are all increased (Fig. 8-6; see Chapter 18). These complications of smoking tend to occur at times when the fetus is not viable or is at great risk (i.e., from 20 to 32 weeks of gestation).

Children born of cigarette-smoking mothers have been reported to be more susceptible to several respiratory diseases, including respiratory infections and otitis media.

Substantial evidence indicates that maternal cigarette smoking inflicts lasting harm on children and impairs physical, cognitive and emotional development. Thus, these children showed measurable deficits in physical growth, intellectual maturation and emotional development. In utero exposure to maternal cigarette smoking has been shown to increase severalfold the risk of certain types of attention deficit hyperactivity disorder (ADHD) in children. Deficits in cognitive and auditory function related to smoking during pregnancy may persist for years, and are detectable well into adolescence. Boys appear to be generally more vulnerable than girls to many of the psychosocial problems resulting from perinatal exposure to maternal cigarette smoking.

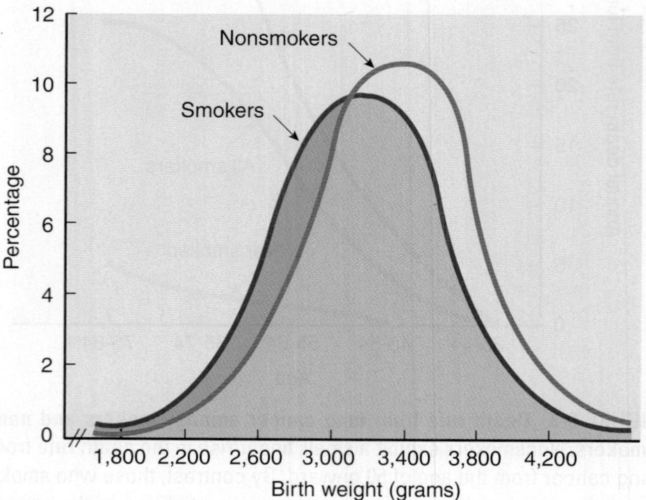

FIGURE 8-5. Effect of smoking on birth weight. Mothers who smoke give birth to smaller infants. In particular, the incidence of babies weighing less than 3000 g is increased significantly by smoking.

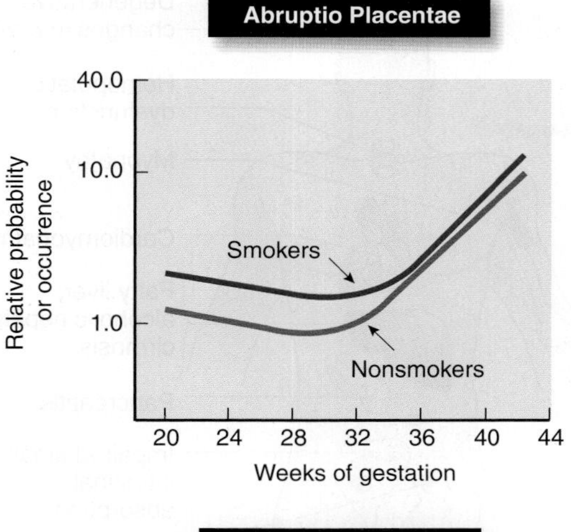

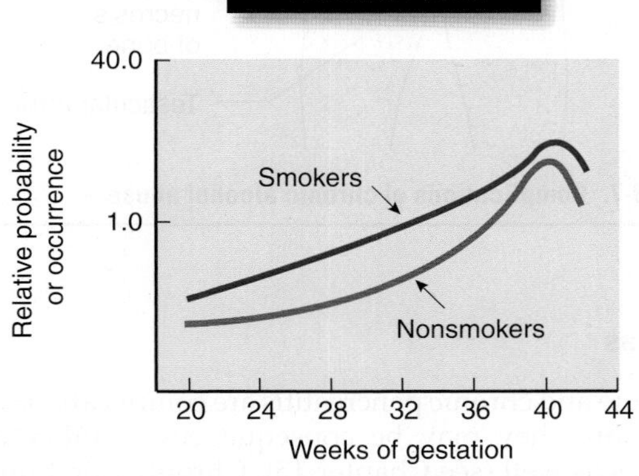

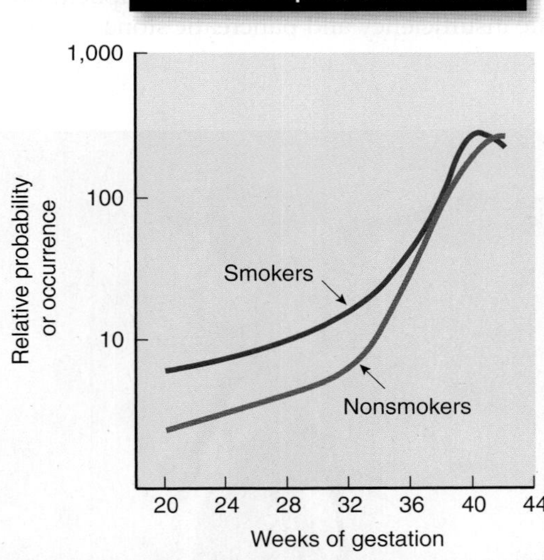

FIGURE 8-6. Effect of smoking on the incidence of abruptio placentae (*top*), placenta previa (*middle*) and the premature rupture of amniotic membranes (*bottom*). In each, the ordinate shows the probability of one of three complications of the third trimester of pregnancy. Note that it is a logarithmic scale. Smoking increases the probability of abruptio placentae and premature rupture of the amniotic membranes prior to 34 weeks of gestation, at which time the fetus is still premature. Smoking increases the risk of placenta previa up to 40 weeks of gestation.

Further, maternal smoking during pregnancy greatly increases (approximately fourfold in a recent study) the risk of sudden infant death syndrome (SIDS; see Chapter 6). This is thought to represent mainly the consequences of prenatal exposure to maternal smoking, since the increase in risk for SIDS if the father, but not the mother, smokes is much less (about 1.5-fold).

In the most comprehensive study to date, 17,000 children born during 1 week in Great Britain were studied at ages 7 and 11 years. Children of mothers who smoked 10 or more cigarettes a day during pregnancy were, on average, 1.0 cm shorter than children of nonsmoking mothers and 3 to 5 months behind in reading, mathematics and general intellectual ability. Moreover, the extent of the deficits was proportional to the number of cigarettes smoked during pregnancy.

Environmental Tobacco Smoke May Produce a Variety of Diseases in Nonsmokers

Involuntary exposure to tobacco smoke in the environment—which is variably termed second-hand smoke, passive smoking or environmental tobacco smoke (ETS)—appears to be a risk factor for some diseases in nonsmokers. ***There is approximately a 20% to 30% increased risk of lung cancer in nonsmoking spouses of smokers.*** The increase in the risk of lung cancer associated with lesser levels of exposure is more difficult to quantify, but the same types of DNA alterations, genotoxicity and carcinogen metabolites have been reported in the urine of people exposed to ETS and of neonates born to smoking mothers as are seen in active smokers.

An increased incidence of respiratory illnesses and hospitalizations has been reported among infants whose parents smoke, and several studies have reported mild impairment of pulmonary function among children of smokers and exacerbation of preexisting asthma. Reduced indices of pulmonary function are also seen in children of smokers. ETS is associated with an increased risk for SIDS as well (see above).

ETS has been linked to an increased risk of both coronary artery disease and sudden death. The magnitude of the risk is dose dependent and disproportionate to the level of smoke exposure as compared to smokers. Nonsmokers are highly sensitive to certain effects of ETS, including increased platelet aggregation, endothelial cell damage, impaired vasodilation, lower blood levels of high-density lipoprotein (HDL), oxidative stress and impaired responsiveness to oxidative stress. In one study, the city of Helena, Montana, banned cigarette smoking in workplaces and public places. This ban was overturned by court order 6 months later. During the interval when the ban was in effect, the number of acute cardiac events leading to hospital admission decreased by about 50%. When the ban on smoking was removed, hospital admissions for acute cardiac events rebounded almost to the levels seen before the ban was instituted. Any number of additional reports have corroborated the basic findings of this study. ETS exposure is associated with acute cardiac events, and decreasing ETS lowers the incidence of such events.

Alcoholism

Chronic alcoholism has been defined as regular intake of sufficient alcohol to injure a person socially, psychologically or physically. It is addiction to ethanol that features dependence and withdrawal symptoms and results in acute and chronic toxic effects of alcohol on the body. There are about 15 to 18 million alcoholics in the United States, approximately one tenth of the population at risk. The proportion has been estimated to be even higher in other countries. Certain ethnic groups, such as Native Americans and Eskimos, have high rates of alcoholism, while others, such as Chinese and Jews, are less afflicted. Although alcoholism is more common in men, the number of female alcoholics has been increasing.

Although there are no firm rules, for most persons, daily consumption of more than 45 g alcohol should probably be discouraged and 100 g or more a day may be dangerous (10 g alcohol = 1 oz, or 30 mL, of 86 proof [43%] spirits).

The short-term effects of alcohol on the brain are familiar to most people, but the mechanism of inebriation is not understood. Like other anesthetic agents, alcohol is a central nervous system (CNS) depressant. However, it is such a weak anesthetic that it must be drunk by the glassful to exert any significant effect. In a normal person, characteristic behavioral changes can be detected at low alcohol concentrations (below 50 mg/dL). Levels above 80 mg/dL are usually associated with slower reaction times and gross incoordination and in American jurisdictions are considered legal evidence of intoxication while driving a motor vehicle. At levels above 300 mg/dL, most people become comatose, and at concentrations above 400 mg/dL, death from respiratory failure is common. In humans, the LD_{50} (median lethal dose) is about 5 g of alcohol per kilogram of body weight.

The situation is somewhat different in chronic alcoholics, who develop CNS tolerance to alcohol. Such persons may easily tolerate blood alcohol levels of 100 to 200 mg/dL; and in fatal automobile accidents, blood levels of 500 to 600 mg/dL or more have been found by medical examiners. The mechanism underlying tolerance has not been established.

Acute alcohol intoxication is hardly a benign condition. Some 40% of all fatalities from motor vehicle accidents involve alcohol—currently about 14,000 deaths annually in the United States. Alcoholism is also a major contributor to fatal home accidents, death in fires and suicide.

Many chronic diseases associated with alcoholism were once attributed to malnutrition, and some alcoholics do suffer from nutritional deficiencies, such as thiamine deficiency (Wernicke encephalopathy) or folic acid deficiency (megaloblastic anemia). ***However, most alcoholics have adequate diets and the great majority of alcohol-related disorders should be attributed to the toxic effects of alcohol alone.*** The diseases associated with alcoholism are discussed in detail in chapters dealing with individual organs, and we restrict this discussion to the spectrum of disease (Fig. 8-7).

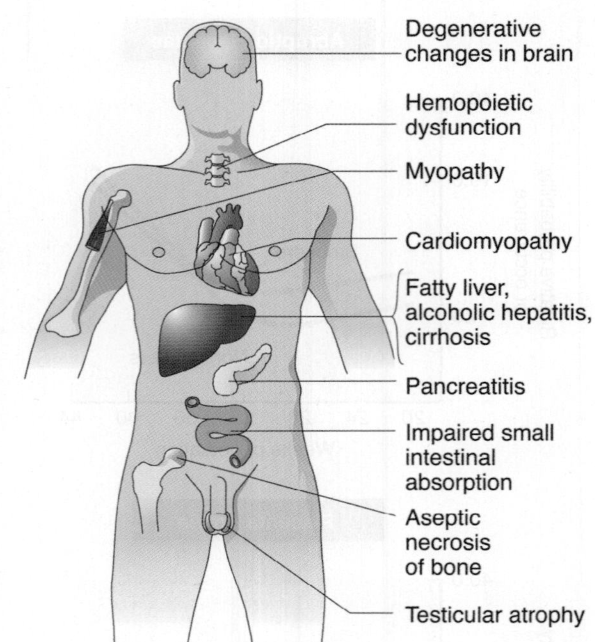

FIGURE 8-7. Complications of chronic alcohol abuse.

Alcohol Ingestion Affects Organs and Tissues

Liver

Alcoholic liver disease, the most common medical complication of alcoholism, has been known for thousands of years and accounts for a large proportion of cases of cirrhosis of the liver (Fig. 8-8) in industrialized countries. The nature of the alcoholic beverage is largely irrelevant; consumed in excess, beer, wine, whiskey, hard cider and so on all produce cirrhosis. Only the total dose of alcohol itself is relevant.

Pancreas

Both acute and chronic pancreatitis are complications of alcoholism, but they may be consequences of other disease processes as well (see Chapter 15). **Chronic calcifying pancreatitis,** on the other hand, is an unquestioned result of alcoholism and an important cause of incapacitating pain, pancreatic insufficiency and pancreatic stones.

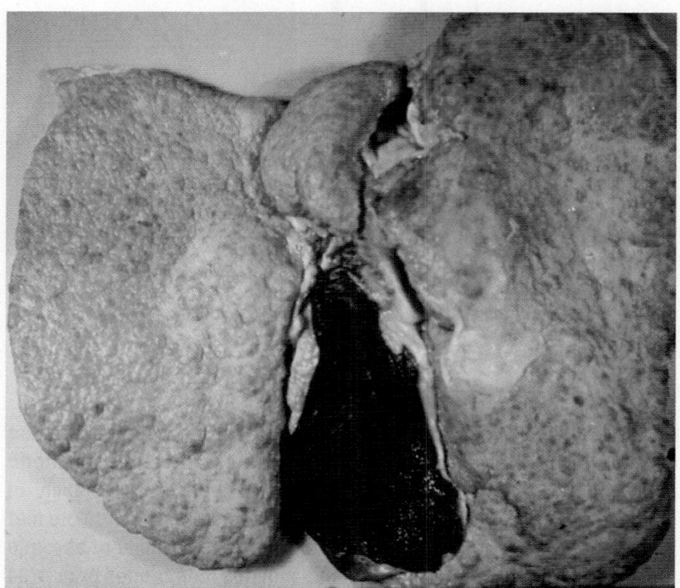

FIGURE 8-8. Cirrhosis of the liver in a chronic alcoholic. The surface displays innumerable small nodules of hepatocytes separated by interconnecting bands of fibrous tissue. The dark structure is the gallbladder.

Heart

Alcohol-related heart disease was recognized over a century ago in Germany, where it was referred to as "beer-drinker's heart." This degenerative disease of the myocardium is a form of dilated cardiomyopathy, termed **alcoholic cardiomyopathy,** and leads to low-output congestive heart failure (see Chapter 11). This cardiomyopathy clearly differs from the heart disease associated with thiamine deficiency (beriberi), a disorder characterized by high-output failure. Alcoholics' hearts seem also to be more susceptible to arrhythmias. Many cases of sudden death in alcoholics are probably caused by sudden, fatal arrhythmias.

In this context, moderate alcohol consumption, or "social drinking" (one to two drinks a day), provides significant protection against coronary artery disease (atherosclerosis) and its consequence, myocardial infarction. Similarly, compared with abstainers, social drinkers have a lower incidence of ischemic stroke.

Skeletal Muscle

Muscle weakness, termed alcoholic myopathy, particularly of the proximal muscles, is common in alcoholics (see Chapter 27). A wide range of changes in skeletal muscle occurs in chronic alcoholics, varying from mild alterations in muscle fibers evident only by electron microscopy to severe, debilitating chronic myopathy, with degeneration of muscle fibers and diffuse fibrosis. Rarely, **acute alcoholic rhabdomyolysis**—necrosis of muscle fibers and release of myoglobin into the circulation—occurs. This sudden event can be fatal because of renal failure secondary to myoglobinuria.

Endocrine System

In male alcoholics, feminization and loss of libido and potency are common. Breasts become enlarged (gynecomastia), body hair is lost and a female distribution of pubic hair (female escutcheon) develops. Some of these changes can be attributed to impaired estrogen metabolism due to chronic liver disease, but many of the changes—particularly atrophy of the testes—occur even if there is no liver disease. Chronic alcoholism leads to lower levels of circulating testosterone because of a complex interference with the pituitary–gonadal axis, possibly complicated by accelerated hepatic metabolism of testosterone. Alcohol has a direct toxic effect on the testes; thus, male sexual impairment is one of the prices exacted by alcoholism.

Gastrointestinal Tract

Since the esophagus and stomach may be exposed to 10 M ethanol, it is not surprising that a direct toxic effect on the mucosa of these organs is common. Injury to the mucosa of both organs is potentiated by hypersecretion of gastric hydrochloric acid stimulated by ethanol. **Reflux esophagitis** may be particularly painful and peptic ulcers are also more common in alcoholics. Violent retching may lead to tears at the esophageal-gastric junction **(Mallory-Weiss syndrome),** sometimes severe enough to cause exsanguinating hemorrhage (see Chapter 13). Small intestine mucosal cells are also exposed to circulating alcohol, and a variety of absorptive abnormalities and ultrastructural changes have been demonstrated. Alcohol inhibits active transport of amino acids, thiamine and vitamin B_{12}.

Blood

Megaloblastic anemia is not uncommon in alcoholics and reflects a combination of dietary deficiency of folic acid and the fact that alcohol is a weak folic acid antagonist in humans. Moreover, folate absorption by the small intestine may be decreased in alcoholics. In addition, chronic ethanol intoxication leads directly to an **increase in mean corpuscular volume of erythrocytes.** In the presence of alcoholic cirrhosis, the spleen is often enlarged by portal hypertension; in such cases, **hypersplenism** often causes **hemolytic anemia.** Transient **thrombocytopenia** is common after acute alcohol intoxication and may result in bleeding. Alcohol also interferes with platelet aggregation, thereby contributing to bleeding.

Bone

Chronic alcoholics, particularly postmenopausal women, are at increased risk for **osteoporosis.** Although it is well established that alcohol, at least in vitro, inhibits osteoblast function, the precise mechanism responsible for accelerated bone loss is not understood. Interestingly, moderate alcohol intake seems to exert a protective effect against osteoporosis. Male alcoholics exhibit an unusually high incidence of **aseptic necrosis of the head of the femur.** The mechanism for this complication is also obscure.

Immune System

Alcoholics seem to be prone to many infections (particularly pneumonias) with organisms that are unusual in the general population, such as *Haemophilus influenzae*. Experimentally, a number of alcohol-induced effects on immune function have been reported.

Nervous System

General cortical atrophy of the brain is common in alcoholics and may reflect a toxic effect of alcohol (see Chapter 28). By contrast, most of the characteristic brain diseases in alcoholics are probably a result of nutritional deficiency.

- **Wernicke encephalopathy** is caused by thiamine deficiency and is characterized by mental confusion, ataxia, abnormal ocular motility and polyneuropathy, reflecting pathologic changes in the diencephalon and brainstem.
- **Korsakoff psychosis** is characterized by retrograde amnesia and confabulatory symptoms. It was once believed to be pathognomonic of chronic alcoholism but has also been seen in several organic mental syndromes and is considered nonspecific.
- **Alcoholic cerebellar degeneration** is differentiated from other acquired or familial cerebellar degeneration by the uniformity of its manifestations. Progressive unsteadiness of gait, ataxia, incoordination and reduced deep tendon reflex activity are present.
- **Central pontine myelinolysis** is another characteristic change in the brain of alcoholics, apparently caused by electrolyte imbalance—usually after electrolyte therapy, after an alcoholic binge or during withdrawal. In this complication, a progressive weakness of bulbar muscles terminates in respiratory paralysis.
- **Amblyopia** (impaired vision) is occasionally seen in alcoholics. It may reflect alcohol-related decreases in tissue

vitamin A, although other vitamin deficiencies may also be involved.

- **Polyneuropathy** is common in chronic alcoholics. It is usually associated with deficiencies of thiamine and other B vitamins, but a direct neurotoxic effect of ethanol may play a role. The most common complaints include numbness, paresthesias, pain, weakness and ataxia.

Fetal Alcohol Syndrome Results From Alcohol Abuse in Pregnancy

Infants born to mothers who consume excess alcohol during pregnancy may show a cluster of abnormalities that together constitute the fetal alcohol syndrome. These include growth retardation, microcephaly, facial dysmorphology, neurologic dysfunction and other congenital anomalies. About 6% of the offspring of alcoholic mothers are afflicted by the full syndrome. More often, exposure of the fetus to high concentrations of ethanol leads to less severe abnormalities, prominent among which are mental retardation, intrauterine growth retardation and minor dysmorphic features. Alcohol acts as an antagonist of *N*-methyl-D-aspartic acid (NMDA) and γ-aminobutyric acid (GABA)-mimetic neurotransmitters and can trigger neuron apoptosis. Fetal alcohol syndrome is discussed in greater detail in Chapter 6.

Alcohol Increases the Risk of Some Cancers

Cancers of the oral cavity, larynx and esophagus occur more often in alcoholics than in the general population. As most alcoholics are also smokers, the differential contributions of ethanol and cigarette smoke to these observed increases are not well defined. The risk of hepatocellular carcinoma is increased in patients with alcoholic cirrhosis. A number of reports have described an increased incidence of breast cancer in alcoholic women, a subject that requires further study.

The Mechanisms by Which Alcohol Injures Tissues Are Not Understood

The pathogenesis of ethanol-induced organ damage remains obscure. In a number of experimental settings, ethanol and its metabolites have been shown to have harmful effects on cells. Among these are changes in redox potential (NAD/NADH ratio). In addition, ethanol may lead to formation of unusual compounds such as the first metabolite of ethanol oxidation, acetaldehyde, protein adducts, fatty acid ethyl esters and phosphatidyl ethanol. It also increases production of reactive oxygen species (ROS; see Chapter 1) and tends to intercalate between phospholipids within biological membranes and thereby disorders them. Moreover, ethanol has pleiotropic effects on cellular signaling and may promote apoptosis under some circumstances. How alcohol-induced perturbations in cell signaling injure cells remains uncertain.

Drug Abuse

Drug abuse has been defined as "the use of any substance in a manner that deviates from the accepted medical, social or legal patterns within a given society." For the most part, drug abuse involves agents that are used to alter mood and perception. These include (1) derivatives of opium (heroin, morphine); (2) depressants (barbiturates, tranquilizers, alcohol); (3) stimulants (cocaine, amphetamines), marijuana and psychedelic drugs (PCP, lysergic acid diethylamide [LSD]); and (4) inhalants (amyl nitrite, organic solvents such as those in glue). Use of illicit drugs is estimated to cause about 17,000 deaths a year in the United States.

Illicit Drugs Are Responsible for Many Pathologic Syndromes

Heroin

Heroin is a common illicit opiate used to induce euphoria. It is often taken intravenously and in the usual dosage is effective for about 5 hours. Overdoses are characterized by hypothermia, bradycardia and respiratory depression. Other opiates that are subject to abuse include morphine and Dilaudid, but these have been largely replaced by oxycodone and fentanyl. Oxycodone, usually combined with acetaminophen, is an opiate alkaloid with both stimulant and analgesic properties. The strongest effect is achieved by intravenous administration. Fentanyl is an opiate similar to morphine but is up to 100 times more potent. Its illicit use involves injection or oral intake, and it is associated with a high risk of addiction.

Cocaine

Cocaine is an alkaloid derived from South American coca leaves. The freebase form of cocaine is hard and is far more potent than coca leaves. It may be taken by sniffing, smoking, intravenous injection or orally. An even more potent form of cocaine ("crack") is generally smoked. It is hard and is then "cracked" into smaller pieces that are smoked. The half-life of cocaine in the blood is about 1 hour.

Cocaine users report extreme euphoria and heightened sensitivity to a variety of stimuli. However, with addiction, paranoid states and conspicuous emotional lability occur. The mechanism of action of cocaine is related to its interference with the reuptake of the neurotransmitter dopamine.

Cocaine overdose leads to anxiety and delirium and occasionally to seizures. Cardiac arrhythmias and other effects on the heart may cause sudden death in otherwise apparently healthy persons. Chronic abuse of cocaine is associated with the occasional development of a characteristic dilated cardiomyopathy, which may be fatal.

Amphetamines

Amphetamines, mainly methamphetamine, are sympathomimetic and resemble cocaine in their effects, although they have a longer duration of action. Methamphetamines are most commonly used as "crystal meth," which is easily produced by hydrogenation of ephedrine or pseudoephedrine. Methamphetamine is often made in home laboratories and is a major public health problem in the United States. The most serious complications of the abuse of amphetamines are seizures, cardiac arrhythmias and hyperthermia. Amphetamine use has been reported to lead to vasculitis of the CNS, and both subarachnoid and intracerebral hemorrhages have been described.

Hallucinogens

Hallucinogens are a group of chemically unrelated drugs that alter perception and sensory experience.

Phencyclidine (PCP) is an anesthetic agent that has psychedelic or hallucinogenic effects. As a recreational drug, it is known as "angel dust" and is taken orally, intranasally or by smoking. The anesthetic properties of phencyclidine cause diminished capacity to perceive pain and, therefore, may lead to self-injury and trauma. Other than its behavioral effects, PCP commonly produces tachycardia and hypertension. High doses result in deep coma, seizures and even decerebrate posturing.

LSD is a hallucinogenic drug whose popularity peaked in the late 1960s and is little used today. It causes perceptual distortion of the senses, interference with logical thought, alteration of time perception and a sense of depersonalization. "Bad trips" are characterized by anxiety and panic and objectively by sympathomimetic effects that include tachycardia, hypertension and hyperthermia. Large overdoses cause coma, convulsions and respiratory arrest.

Organic Solvents

The recreational inhalation of organic solvents is widespread, particularly among adolescents. Various commercial preparations such as fingernail polish, glues, plastic cements and lighter fluid are all sniffed. Among the active ingredients are benzene, carbon tetrachloride, acetone, xylene and toluene. However, many of these compounds are also industrial solvents and reagents and so chronic low-level occupational exposure occurs. These compounds are all CNS depressants, although early effects (e.g., with xylene) may be excitatory. Acute intoxication with organic solvents resembles inebriation with alcohol. Large doses produce nausea and vomiting, hallucinations and eventually coma. Respiratory depression and death may follow. Chronic exposure to, or abuse of, organic solvents may result in damage to the brain, kidneys, liver, lungs and hematopoietic system. Benzene, for example, is a bone marrow toxin and has been associated with the development of acute myelogenous leukemia.

Intravenous Drug Abuse Has Many Medical Complications

Apart from reactions related to pharmacologic or physiologic effects of substance abuse, the most common complications (15% of directly drug-related deaths) are caused by introducing infectious organisms by a parenteral route. Most occur at the site of injection: cutaneous abscesses, cellulitis and ulcers (Fig. 8-9). When these heal, "track marks" persist and these areas may be hypopigmented or hyperpigmented. Thrombophlebitis of the veins draining sites of injection is common. Intravenous introduction of bacteria may lead to septic complications in internal organs. Bacterial endocarditis, often involving *Staphylococcus aureus,* occurs on both sides of the heart (Fig. 8-10) and may lead to pulmonary, renal and intracranial abscesses; meningitis; osteomyelitis; and mycotic aneurysms (Fig. 8-11).

Intravenous drug abusers are at very high risk for acquired immunodeficiency syndrome (AIDS), as well as hepatitis B and C. These people may also suffer from the complications of viral hepatitis, such as chronic active hepatitis, necrotizing angiitis and glomerulonephritis. A focal glomerulosclerosis ("heroin nephropathy") is characterized by immune complexes and has been ascribed to an immune reaction to impurities that contaminate illicit drugs.

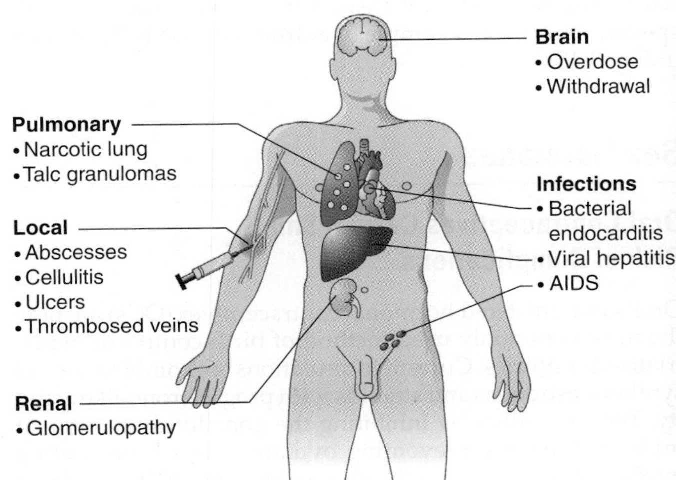

FIGURE 8-9. Complications of intravenous drug abuse.

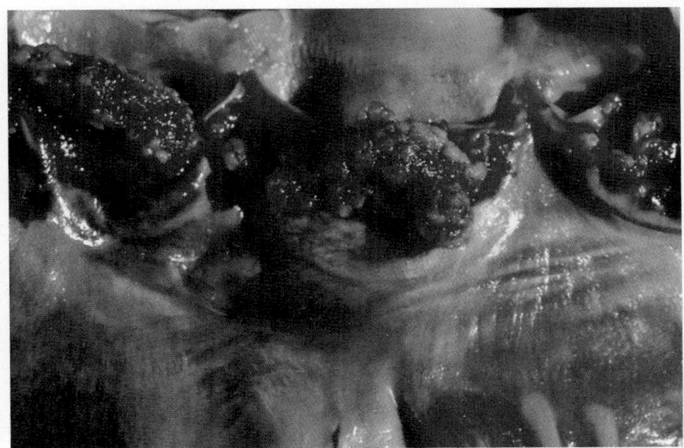

FIGURE 8-10. Bacterial endocarditis. The aortic valve of an intravenous drug abuser displays adherent vegetations.

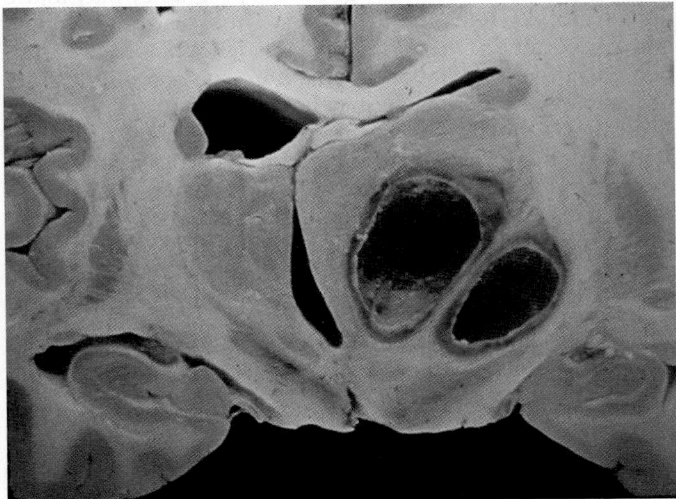

FIGURE 8-11. Brain abscess. Cross-section of the brain from an intravenous drug abuser shows two encapsulated cavities.

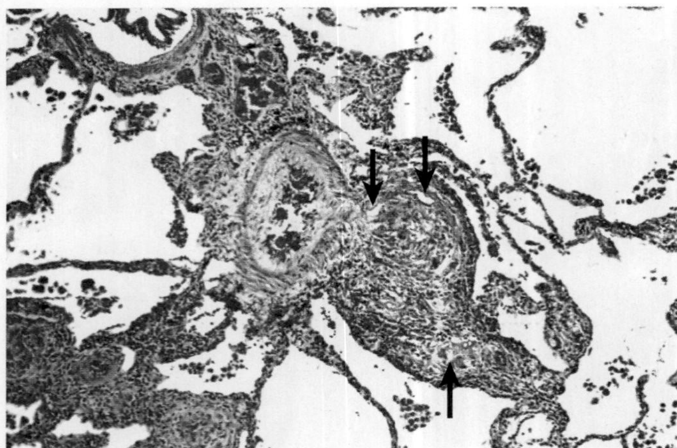

FIGURE 8-12. Talc granulomas in the lung. A section of lung from an intravenous drug abuser viewed under polarized light reveals a granuloma adjacent to a pulmonary artery. The refractile material (*arrows*) is talc that was used to dilute the drug prior to its intravenous injection.

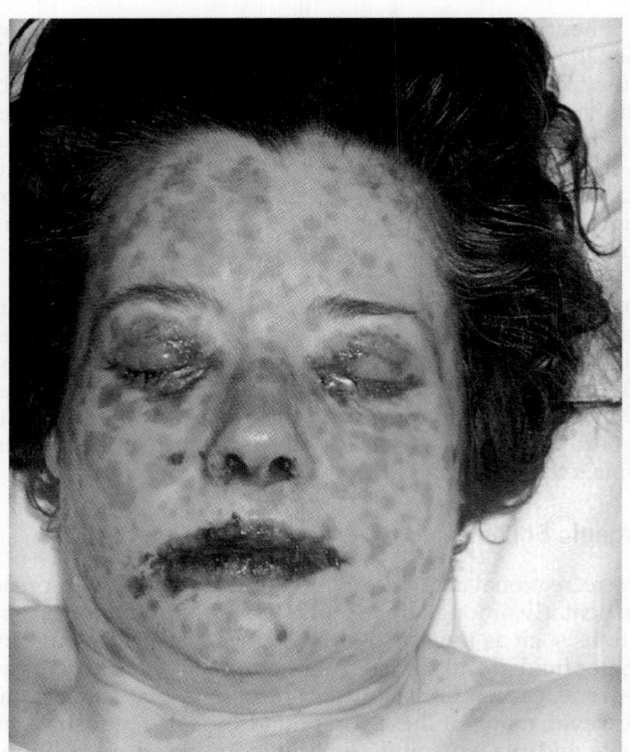

FIGURE 8-13. Erythema multiforme secondary to sulfonamide therapy.

Intravenous injection of talc, which is used to dilute pure drug, is associated with the appearance of foreign body granulomas in the lung (Fig. 8-12). These may be severe enough to lead to interstitial pulmonary fibrosis.

Drug Addiction in Pregnant Women Poses Risks for the Fetus

Maternal drug use may lead to addiction of newborn infants, who often exhibit a full-blown withdrawal syndrome. Moreover, the appearance of the drug withdrawal syndrome in the fetus during labor may result in excessive fetal movements and increased oxygen demand, a situation that increases the risk of intrapartum hypoxia and meconium aspiration. If labor occurs when maternal drug levels are high, the infant is often born with respiratory depression. Mothers who are addicted to drugs experience higher rates of toxemia of pregnancy and premature labor.

Maternal use of illicit drugs during pregnancy may injure the developing fetus in other ways. Thus, pregnant women who use cocaine more commonly experience placental abruption and premature labor. Infants born to such mothers are prone to be low birth weight, to have one of an array of CNS and other anomalies and to show impaired brain function after birth. Maternal addiction to heroin carries a number of risks of abnormalities of pregnancy and premature birth. It is also associated with a large number of postnatal problems (in addition to heroin withdrawal), including SIDS, neonatal respiratory distress syndrome and developmental retardation. Maternal abuse of other substances (e.g., amphetamines and hallucinogens) also leads to variably severe fetal and postnatal disorders.

Iatrogenic Drug Injury

Iatrogenic drug injury refers to the unintended side effects of therapeutic or diagnostic drugs prescribed by physicians. Adverse reactions to pharmaceuticals are surprisingly common. They are seen in 2% to 5% of patients hospitalized on medical services; of these reactions, 2% to 12% are fatal. The typical hospitalized patient is given about 10 different medications and some receive five times as many. The risk of an adverse reaction increases proportionately with the number of different drugs; for example, the risk of injury is at least 40% when more than 15 drugs are administered. Because they are so ubiquitously prescribed, drugs represent a significant environmental hazard. Untoward effects of drugs result from (1) overdose, (2) exaggerated physiologic responses, (3) a genetic predisposition, (4) hypersensitivity, (5) interactions with other drugs and (6) other unknown factors. The characteristic pathologic changes associated with drug reactions are treated in chapters dealing with specific organs. An example of a drug reaction is illustrated in Fig. 8-13.

Sex Hormones

Oral Contraceptives Carry a Small Risk of Complications

Orally administered hormonal contraceptives (OCs) are now the most commonly used method of birth control in industrialized countries. Current formulations are combinations of synthetic estrogens and steroids with progesterone-like activity. They act either by inhibiting the gonadotropin surge at midcycle, thereby preventing ovulation, or by preventing implantation by altering the phase of the endometrium. Most complications of oral contraceptives involve either the vasculature or reproductive organs (Fig. 8-14).

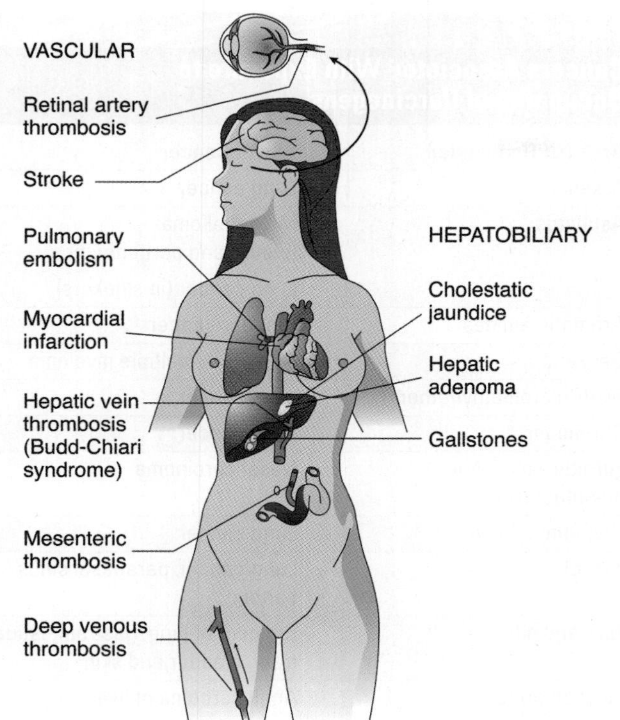

FIGURE 8-14. Complications of oral contraceptives.

Vascular Complications

Deep vein thrombosis is a recognized complication of oral contraceptive use, the risk being increased two to three times. As a consequence, the risk of thromboembolism is correspondingly increased. Obesity and smoking magnify the risk of venous thrombosis attendant to OCs, as do coexisting disorders that increase clotting (thrombophilia).

The risk of arterial thrombotic events in women taking oral contraceptives is also increased. Thus, both myocardial infarction and thrombotic stroke are reported to be increased in some studies.

Neoplastic Complications

Tumors of several of the female reproductive organs, especially ovary, endometrium and breast, are strongly influenced by female hormones. Repeated epidemiologic studies indicate that OC use decreases the risk of ovarian and endometrial cancers by about half, presumably because of suppression of the production of pituitary gonadotropins.

There is a small increase in the frequency of breast cancers in OC users. This observation applies mainly to nonfamilial breast cancers and to women currently taking OCs. The increased risk appears to endure for about 10 years following cessation of OC administration.

Squamous carcinoma of the cervix in women positive for human papilloma virus (HPV) may be somewhat increased in association with long-term (more than 5 years) OC use.

Benign liver adenomas are rare hepatic neoplasms that are significantly increased in incidence among women who use OCs. The risk of these tumors increases conspicuously with the duration of use, particularly after 5 years.

Several small studies have suggested a small increased risk of **hepatocellular carcinoma** among women using OCs. Fortunately, this cancer is rare in young women without chronic viral hepatitis.

Other Complications

For reasons unknown, oral contraceptives may induce an increased pigmentation of the malar eminences, called **chloasma,** which is accentuated by sunlight and persists for a long time after the contraceptives are discontinued.

Cholelithiasis is more frequent (twofold increase) in women who have used OCs for 4 years or less, but its incidence becomes lower than normal after that period of time. Thus, OCs accelerate the process of cholelithiasis but do not increase its overall incidence.

Benefits of Oral Contraceptives

In considering the potential side effects of the use of oral contraceptive agents, it is important to recognize that certain benefits accrue. In addition to a significant reduction in the risk of ovarian and endometrial cancers, the use of these agents decreases the risk of pelvic inflammatory disease, uterine leiomyomas, endometriosis and fibrocystic disease of the breast.

The Risks of Postmenopausal Hormone Replacement Therapy Depend on the Formulation, Age at Which Treatment Begins and Duration of Treatment

Hormone replacement (HR) preparations come in many varieties, the most common being oral estrogen only and oral combined estrogen plus progestogen combinations. These are given to women for diverse reasons, including to alleviate distressing symptoms of menopause, protect from osteoporosis and, more recently, protect from cardiovascular, cerebrovascular and CNS diseases that occur in older women. There is evidence of the effectiveness of these preparations in decreasing the incidence of bone fractures and mitigating many of the problems relating to hormone deficits.

However, there are significant risks associated with hormonal replacement following menopause. Estrogen-only and estrogen–progestogen combinations are associated with a slightly increased risk of venous thromboembolism. This increased risk is most common in the first year of HR and declines thereafter, even with continued HR. With the cessation of treatment, the risk of deep vein thrombosis and embolism declines to that in women who never received hormone replacement.

Because many tumors are hormonally sensitive, it has seemed logical that HR would increase the risk of developing those tumors, particularly those of the breast, endometrium and ovaries. Current data support the conclusion that there is a significantly increased risk of breast cancer in women receiving combined estrogen–progestogen formulations, while there is a slightly increased risk, or none at all, in those receiving estrogens alone. The converse appears to be true for endometrial and ovarian cancers.

There appears to be little overall benefit of either type of preparation in protecting from cardiovascular or cerebrovascular deaths. Women who begin HR more than

6 years after menopause have been reported to have a somewhat higher risk of developing Alzheimer disease, although those who initiate HR during that period appear not to be at risk.

Other Forms of Hormone Replacement

There are scant data regarding the risks of other forms of hormone replacement therapy. Androgen production in men declines with age, resulting in loss of muscle mass, increased adiposity and other problems. However, testosterone replacement therapy for age-related decline in muscular strength, sexual performance and other parameters remains controversial. Although prostate cancer in men is often hormonally sensitive, there are few studies reporting the incidence of prostate or other cancers in men receiving androgen replacement treatments.

Growth hormone (GH) replacement is used in people who lack adequate GH. Although many tumors require GH for their growth, there is no evidence that people who receive GH replacement treatment are more susceptible to developing tumors than other people of their age. GH is being suggested as providing a possible benefit in older people with age-related decreases in skeletal muscle mass. To date, there is little evidence of adverse consequences, although the question of GH-induced insulin resistance remains.

Environmental Chemicals

Awareness of potential hazards posed by harmful chemicals in the environment is not new. In the 12th century Maimonides wrote:

> Comparing the air of cities to the air of deserts is like comparing waters that are befouled and turbid to waters that are fine and pure. In the city, because of the height of its buildings, the narrowness of its streets and all that pours forth from its inhabitants, the air becomes stagnant, turbid, thick, misty and foggy. . . . Wherever the air is altered . . . men develop dullness of understanding, failure of intelligence and defects of memory.

Humans are surrounded by, breathe in and consume many chemicals that are added to, or appear as contaminants in, foods, water and air. Several important mechanisms govern the effect of toxic agents, including the toxin's absorption, distribution, metabolism and excretion. Absorption (whether through pulmonary, gastrointestinal or cutaneous routes) depends largely on the chemical in question. For example, because of their solubility in lipids, the insecticides chlordane and heptachlor are rapidly absorbed and stored in body fat. By contrast, the water-soluble herbicide paraquat is readily eliminated.

The storage, distribution and excretion of chemicals control their concentrations in the organism at any given time. Agents stored in adipose tissue may exert prolonged low-level effects, while more water-soluble materials that are easily excreted by the kidney usually have a shorter duration of action.

Among the most important chemical hazards to which humans are exposed are environmental dusts and carcinogens. Inhalation of mineral and organic dusts occurs primarily in occupational settings (e.g., mining, industrial manufacturing, farming) and occasionally as a result of unusual situations (e.g., bird fanciers, pituitary snuff inhalation). Inhaling mineral dusts leads to pulmonary diseases known as **pneumoconioses**, whereas organic dusts may produce **hypersensitivity pneumonitis.** Pneumoconioses were formerly common, but control of dust exposure in the workplace by modifying manufacturing techniques, improvements in air handling and use of masks has substantially reduced the incidence of these diseases. Because of their importance, pneumoconioses and hypersensitivity pneumonitis are discussed in detail in Chapter 12.

Chemical carcinogens are ubiquitous in the environment. Their potential for causing disease has elicited widespread concern. In particular, exposure to carcinogens in the workplace has been associated epidemiologically with a number of cancers (Table 8-1), which are reviewed in Chapter 5.

Table 8-1

Cancers Associated With Exposure to Occupational Carcinogens

Agent or Occupation	Site of Cancer
Arsenic	Lung cancer
Asbestos	Mesothelioma (pleura and peritoneum) Lung cancer (in smokers)
Aromatic amines	Bladder cancer
Benzene	Leukemia, multiple myeloma
bis-(Chloromethyl)ether	Lung cancer
Chromium	Lung cancer
Furniture and shoe manufacturing	Nasal carcinoma
Hematite mining	Lung cancer
Nickel	Lung cancer, paranasal sinus cancer
Tars and oils	Cancers of lung, gastrointestinal tract, bladder and skin
Vinyl chloride	Angiosarcoma of liver

Toxic Effects Differ From Hypersensitivity Responses

Many substances predictably elicit disease in a variety of animal species in a dose-dependent manner, with a regular time delay and a reproducible pattern of target organ responses. Furthermore, the morphologic changes in injured tissues are constant and reproducible. By contrast, the actions of other agents are unpredictable, showing (1) great variability in their ability to produce disease, (2) irregular lag times before injury is apparent, (3) no dose dependency and (4) lack of reproducibility. Generally, **predictable dose-response reactions** reflect direct actions of a compound or its metabolite on a tissue—a "toxic" effect. The second, **unpredictable type of reaction** is believed to reflect "hypersensitivity," whether involving an immunologic response or other type of idiosyncratic side effect.

Chemical Toxicity May Follow Occupational or Environmental Exposure

Beginning with the industrial revolution, there has been an exponential rise in the number of chemicals manufactured and a corresponding increase in the risk of human exposure. In any consideration of this topic, one must differentiate between acute poisoning and chronic toxicity. One must also distinguish industrial and accidental exposure from that which is likely to occur in the general environment. The lack of adequate quantitative exposure data in humans and the difficulties involved in assessing long-term risks of low-level exposures have led to use of data derived from animal studies to assess toxicities and risks in humans. Such projections can be hazardous because of (1) species differences in sensitivity, (2) differing routes of administration, (3) species-to-species variations in metabolic pathways by which some compounds are modified and (4) extrapolation from very high levels needed to show an effect in a short experimental time frame in animals to low-level exposures over years in humans. These considerations necessarily complicate the need to understand and quantify the potential for human toxicity of a plethora of chemicals.

Except for certain hypersensitivity reactions in susceptible persons, acute poisoning by environmental chemicals does not pose a significant threat to the general population. Concentrations necessary to cause acute functional disorders or structural damage are ordinarily encountered only in the workplace or as a consequence of uncommon accidents.

Accidental mass poisonings with the pesticides endrin and parathion have led to as many as 100 deaths in a single event, but long-term sequelae among the survivors have been difficult to document. The experimental literature dealing with the short- and long-term toxicity of industrial chemicals is voluminous and complicated and often contradictory. For this reason we largely restrict the following discussion to documented effects in humans.

Volatile Organic Solvents and Vapors

Volatile organic solvents and vapors are widely used in industry in many capacities. With few exceptions, exposures to these compounds are industrial or accidental and represent short-term dangers rather than long-term toxicity. For the most part, exposure to solvents is by inhalation rather than by ingestion.

- **Chloroform (CHC_{13}) and carbon tetrachloride (CCl_4):** These solvents exert anesthetic (depressant) effects on the CNS and on the heart and blood vessels, but are better known as hepatotoxins. With both, but classically with carbon tetrachloride, large doses lead to acute hepatic necrosis, fatty liver and liver failure. Long-term exposure to carbon tetrachloride does not pertain to humans, as each exposure to it causes recognizable clinical liver injury, so that continued exposure would not be permitted.
- **Trichloroethylene (C_2HCl_3):** A ubiquitous industrial solvent, trichloroethylene in high concentrations depresses the CNS, but hepatotoxicity is minimal. There is no evidence for chronic sequelae in humans following ordinary long-term industrial exposure.
- **Methanol (CH_3OH):** Because methanol, unlike ethanol, is not taxed, it is used by some impoverished alcoholics as a substitute for ethanol or by unscrupulous merchants as an adulterant of alcoholic beverages, especially in impoverished areas. In methanol poisoning, inebriation similar to that produced by ethanol is succeeded by gastrointestinal symptoms, visual dysfunction, seizures, coma and death. The major toxicity of methanol is believed to arise from its metabolism, first to formaldehyde and then to formic acid. Metabolic acidosis is common after methanol ingestion. The most characteristic lesion of methanol toxicity is necrosis of retinal ganglion cells and subsequent degeneration of the optic nerve, leading to blindness. Severe poisoning may lead to lesions in the putamen and globus pallidus.
- **Ethylene glycol ($HOCH_2CH_2OH$):** Because of its low vapor pressure, toxicity of ethylene glycol chiefly results from ingestion. It is commonly used in antifreeze and has been drunk by chronic alcoholics as a substitute for ethanol for many years. Poisoning with this compound came into prominence when it was used to adulterate wines, owing to its sweet taste and solubility. The toxicity of ethylene glycol is chiefly due to its metabolites, particularly oxalic acid, and occurs within minutes of ingestion. Metabolic acidosis, CNS depression, nausea and vomiting and hypocalcemia-related cardiotoxicity are seen. Oxalate crystals in renal tubules and oxaluria are often noted and may cause renal failure.
- **Gasoline and kerosene:** These fuels are mixtures of aliphatic hydrocarbons and branched, unsaturated and aromatic hydrocarbons. Chronic exposure is by inhalation. Despite prolonged exposure to gasoline by gas station attendants, auto mechanics, and so forth, there is no evidence that inhalation of gasoline over the long term is particularly injurious. Acutely, gasoline is an irritant, but really only causes systemic problems if inhaled in very high concentrations. Increased use of kerosene for home heating has led to accidental poisoning of children.
- **Benzene (C_6H_6):** The prototypic aromatic hydrocarbon is benzene, which must be distinguished from benzine, a mixture of aliphatic hydrocarbons. Benzene is one of the most widely used chemicals in industrial processes, being a starting point for innumerable syntheses and a solvent. It is also a constituent of fuels, accounting for as much as 3% of gasoline. Virtually all cases of acute and chronic benzene toxicity have occurred as industrial exposures (e.g., in shoemakers and workers in shoe manufacturing, occupations that at one time were associated with heavy exposure to benzene-based glues).

Acute benzene poisoning primarily affects the CNS and death results from respiratory failure. However, it is the long-term effects of benzene exposure that have attracted the most attention. In these cases, the bone marrow is the principal target. Patients who develop hematologic abnormalities characteristically exhibit **hypoplasia** or **aplasia of the bone marrow** and **pancytopenia. Aplastic anemia** usually is seen while the workers are still exposed to high concentrations of benzene. In a substantial proportion of cases of benzene-induced anemias, **myelodysplastic syndromes, acute myeloblastic leukemia, erythroleukemia or multiple myeloma** develops during continuing exposure to benzene, or after a variable latent period following removal of the worker from the hazardous environment. Some cases of acute leukemia have occurred without a prior history of aplastic anemia. Although instances of chronic myeloid and chronic lymphocytic leukemia have been reported, a cause-and-effect relationship with benzene exposure is less convincing than that with cases of acute leukemia. Overall, the risk of leukemia is increased 60-fold in workers exposed to the highest atmospheric concentrations of benzene. It deserves mention that both gasoline and tobacco smoke contain benzene, and both contribute to increased benzene levels in the urban atmosphere. The consequent contribution of such benzene concentrations to hematologic diseases is speculative.

The toxic effects of benzene are related to its metabolites, which are the consequence of cytochrome P450 degradation of the parent compound. The closely related compounds toluene and xylenes, also widely used as solvents, have not been incriminated as a cause of hematologic abnormalities, possibly because they are metabolized via different pathways.

Agricultural Chemicals

Pesticides, fungicides, herbicides, fumigants and organic fertilizers are crucial to the success of modern agriculture. Without pesticides, agricultural productivity would be severely compromised. However, many of these chemicals persist in soil and water and may pose a potential long-term hazard. Acute poisoning with very large concentrations of any of these chemicals has already been mentioned above. It is clear that exposure to industrial concentrations or inadvertently contaminated food can cause severe acute illness. Children are particularly susceptible and may ingest home gardening preparations.

Organochlorine pesticides, such as DDT (dichlorodiphenyltrichloroethane), chlordane and others, have caused concern because they accumulate in soils and in human tissues and break down very slowly. High levels of any such pesticide can be harmful to humans in acute exposures, but the side effects of chronic contact with the materials and their buildup are of greatest interest. Many of these compounds function as weak estrogens, but no harmful effects related to this activity have been documented. Some of these compounds, such as aldrin and dieldrin, have been associated with tumor development, but the acute toxicity of most organochlorine insecticides relates to inhibition of CNS GABA responses.

Symptoms of acute toxicity are often related to the mode of action of the toxin. For example, organophosphate insecticides, which have largely replaced organochlorine compounds, are acetylcholinesterase inhibitors that are readily absorbed through the skin. Thus, acute toxicity in humans mainly involves neuromuscular disorders such as visual disturbances, dyspnea, mucous hypersecretion and bronchoconstriction. Death may come from respiratory failure. In the United States, 30 to 40 persons die annually of acute pesticide poisoning. Long-term exposure to substantial concentrations produces symptoms similar to those of acute exposure.

Human exposure to herbicides is not infrequent. Among the best known of these is paraquat. Occupational paraquat exposure is usually via the skin, although toxicity from ingestion and inhalation are documented. The compound is very corrosive and causes burns or ulcers of whatever it contacts. It is transported actively to the lung, where it can damage the pulmonary epithelium, causing edema and even respiratory failure. High-level exposures may lead to death from cardiovascular collapse, while when lower doses are involved, pulmonary fibrosis may ultimately lead to death.

Aromatic Halogenated Hydrocarbons

The halogenated aromatic hydrocarbons that have received considerable attention include (1) the polychlorinated biphenyls (PCBs); (2) chlorophenols (pentachlorophenol, used as a wood preservative); (3) hexachlorophene, previously used as an antibacterial agent in soaps; and (4) the dioxin TCDD (2,3,7,8-tetrachlorodibenzo-p-dioxin), a byproduct of the synthesis of herbicides and hexachlorophene and, therefore, a contaminant of these preparations that has not been produced intentionally. In 1976, an industrial accident in Seveso, Italy, exposed many people to extremely high concentrations of TCDD. As of 2009, small increases in incidences of breast and lymphoid/hematologic cancers are reported, but these results remain inconclusive. Chronic exposure to PCBs and TCDD does not appear to produce demonstrable toxicity. Serious questions have been raised regarding the danger of long-term exposure to dioxin, and there is now a consensus that at the very least this compound is far more carcinogenic in rodents than in humans. The problem of the presence of PCBs in the environment resembles that of agricultural chemicals: long-term animal toxicity is well documented, but there are no significant increases in the incidence of cancer or other diseases in workers exposed to PCBs. The same situation pertains to hexachlorophene and pentachlorophenol.

Cyanide

Prussic acid (HCN) is the classic murderer's tool in detective fiction, where the smell of bitter almonds (*Prunus amygdalus*) betrays the crime. Cyanide blocks cellular respiration by reversibly binding to mitochondrial cytochrome oxidase, the terminal acceptor in the electron transport chain, which is responsible for reducing molecular oxygen to water. The pathologic consequences are similar to those produced by any acute global anoxia.

Air Pollutants

A precise definition of air pollution is elusive, since the meaning of "pure air" is not established. However, for the purposes of this discussion, the most important pollutants are those generated by the combustion of fossil fuels, industrial and agricultural processes and so forth. The most important air pollutants that are implicated as factors in human disease are the irritants sulfur dioxide (SO_2), oxides of nitrogen, CO and ozone, as well as suspended particulates and acid aerosols.

Most common chemical constituents of air pollution are mainly irritants and have been suggested as contributing to development of, or predisposition to, several respiratory illnesses, but are not usually implicated directly as increasing mortality in the developed world. Dissecting the specific effects of these chemicals from the effects of other air pollutants, especially particulates (see below), is difficult. **SO_2** is highly irritative and may be oxidized to sulfuric acid. SO_2 mainly derives from burning fossil fuels. Acute exposure leads to bronchoconstriction and respiratory tract inflammation. Chronic experimental exposure to high levels of SO_2 may lead to a chronic bronchitis-like syndrome, but it is not clear that there are significant sequelae of human exposure to the concentrations of SO_2 normally found in smog.

Nitrogen oxides are generally written NOx, because they are a mixture of several compounds. They, as well, are derived from burning fossil fuels, especially in generating electricity. These gases are oxidants and respiratory irritants that induce airway hyperreactivity in acute exposure settings. Adverse effects attributable to chronic atmospheric levels of NOx have not been demonstrated. Tropospheric **ozone** (i.e., ozone near the ground as opposed to that in the upper atmosphere) is largely produced by the action of sunlight on NO_2, especially on warm, sunny days. It is a strong oxidant that causes both respiratory (cough, dyspnea) and nonrespiratory (nausea, headache) symptoms on acute exposure. Chronic exposure to ozone in smog is reported to lead to deterioration in pulmonary function and is associated with a slight but significant increase in mortality.

Particulates in the air include solid particles and liquid droplets. These vary in size, composition and origin and are generally divided into those between 2.5 μm and 10 μm in aerodynamic diameter and those under 2.5μm. The former (coarse particulates) are mostly deposited in the tracheobronchial tree and are largely derived from natural sources (e.g., windblown soil, dusts). Bioaerosols (e.g., spores, pollens) are included in this group. The fine particulates are mostly from combustion processes. Because of their small size, they penetrate more deeply into the lungs. Even finer particles, (<100 nm) have recently attracted interest as they penetrate very deeply, have a high surface area–to–mass ratio (which allows for greater potential delivery of noxious components) and have been found to pass through the alveolar capillaries into the bloodstream.

Most studies of the effects of air pollution on health have focused on particulates. Such studies have proven to be difficult, and the possible confounding effects of many factors make drawing precise conclusions problematic. Thus, the extent to which chronic exposure to urban air pollution leads to specific effects on morbidity and mortality remains to be established with certainty. Nonetheless, many large short-term and long-term epidemiologic studies suggest that particulate air pollution is associated with increased mortality, both overall and from cardiovascular disease and cancer. Thus, the American Cancer Society estimated that overall, cardiopulmonary and lung tumor deaths were greater, respectively, by 4%, 6% and 8% for every 10 $\mu g/m^3$ increase in average annual exposure to fine particulates. Shorter-term studies showed increases in acute myocardial infarction as a consequence of exposure to higher levels of fine particulates. It has been suggested that residence within 100 meters of a freeway greatly increases the likelihood of cardiovascular death. Furthermore, experimental studies have shown that particulate exposure may lead to higher levels of atherosclerosis, blood pressure, heart rate, coagulability and levels of inflammatory mediators.

There is experimental evidence to support a suggestion that inflammation and oxidative stress are responsible for at least part of the harmful effects of pollutants. Thus, the frequency of exacerbations of asthma is related to levels of fine particulates, especially derived from diesel exhaust and ozone in the air. A cohort of asthmatic children in Mexico City was found to have mutations in glutathione S-transferase, an enzyme that metabolizes a variety of toxins and that can detoxify reactive oxygen species. Treating these children with antioxidant vitamins C and E resulted in clinical improvement.

Carbon Monoxide

CO is an odorless and nonirritating gas that results from the incomplete combustion of organic substances. It combines with hemoglobin with an affinity 240 times greater than that of oxygen to form carboxyhemoglobin. CO binding to hemoglobin also increases the affinity of the remaining heme moieties for oxygen. Oxygen does not dissociate from such hemoglobin in the tissues as readily as it should. The hypoxia that results from CO poisoning is thus far greater than can be attributed to loss of oxygen-carrying capacity alone.

Atmospheric CO is derived principally from automobile exhaust and does not pose a health problem. Carboxyhemoglobin concentrations under 10% are common in smokers and ordinarily do not produce symptoms. Indoor combustion, however, particularly from space heaters, can generate much higher concentrations of CO, which can be hazardous. Concentrations up to 30% usually cause only headache and mild exertional dyspnea. Higher levels of carboxyhemoglobin lead to confusion and lethargy. Above 50%, coma and convulsions ensue. Levels greater than 60% are usually fatal. In fatal CO poisoning, a characteristic cherry-red color is imparted to the skin by the carboxyhemoglobin in the superficial capillaries. Recovery from severe CO poisoning may be associated with brain damage, which may be manifested as subtle intellectual deficits, memory loss or extrapyramidal symptoms (e.g., parkinsonism). Treatment of acute CO poisoning, as in persons who attempt suicide or are trapped in fires, consists principally of the administration of 100% oxygen.

Harmful effects of long-term exposure to low levels of CO have been difficult to substantiate. However, in patients with ischemic heart disease, concentrations of carboxyhemoglobin below 5% to 8% (often found in smokers) may accelerate the onset of exertional angina and cause changes in electrocardiograms.

Metals

Metals are an important group of environmental chemicals that have caused disease in humans from ancient times to the present.

Lead

Lead is a ubiquitous heavy metal that is common in the environment of industrialized countries. Before widespread awareness of chronic exposure to lead in the 1950s and 1960s, the classic symptoms of lead poisoning were commonly encountered in children and adults. In the United States, lead poisoning was primarily a pediatric problem related to pica—the habit of chewing on cribs, toys, furniture and woodwork—and eating painted plaster and fallen paint flakes. Most dwellings built before 1940 had lead-containing paint (up to 40% of dry weight) on interior and exterior walls. Children living in dilapidated older homes heavily coated with flaking paint were at significant risk for chronic lead poisoning. To these sources of lead was added a heavy burden of atmospheric lead in the form of dust derived from the combustion of lead-containing gasoline. Children and adults living near point sources of environmental lead contamination, such as smelters, were exposed to even higher levels of lead.

In adults, occupational exposure to lead occurred primarily among those engaged in lead smelting, which releases metal fumes and deposits lead oxide dust in the area. Lead oxide is a constituent of battery grids and an occupational exposure to lead is a hazard in the manufacture and recycling of automobile batteries. Accidental poisonings occasionally occurred from pottery that had been improperly fired with a lead glaze, renovation of old residences heavily coated with lead paint, "moonshine" whiskey made in lead stills or "sniffing" lead-containing gasoline.

MOLECULAR PATHOGENESIS: Lead is absorbed through the lungs or, less often, the gastrointestinal tract. Once in the blood, it rapidly equilibrates with the plasma and erythrocytes and is excreted by the kidneys. A portion of blood lead remains freely diffusible. Lead crosses the blood-brain barrier readily, and concentrations in the brain, liver, kidneys and bone marrow are directly related to its toxic effects. It binds sulfhydryl groups and interferes with the activities of zinc-dependent enzymes. As well, it interferes with enzymes involved in the synthesis of steroids and cell membranes.

By contrast, bones, teeth, nails and hair represent a tightly bound pool of lead that is not generally regarded as harmful. With chronic exposure, 90% of the total body lead burden is in the bones. During metaphyseal bone formation in children, lead and calcium are deposited to produce the increased bone densities ("lead lines") seen radiographically at the metaphysis, thereby providing a simple method of detecting increased body stores of lead in children.

PATHOLOGY: Classic lead overexposure, which is rarely seen in the United States today, affects many organs, but its major toxicity involves dysfunction in (1) the nervous system, (2) the kidneys and (3) hematopoiesis (Fig. 8-15).

The brain is the target of lead toxicity in children; adults usually present with manifestation of peripheral neuropathy. Children with lead encephalopathy are typically irritable and ataxic. They may convulse or display altered states of consciousness, from drowsiness to frank coma. Children with blood lead levels above 80 μg/dL, but with concentrations lower than those in children with frank encephalopathy (120 μg/dL), exhibit mild CNS symptoms such as clumsiness, irritability and hyperactivity.

Lead encephalopathy is a condition in which the brain is edematous and displays flattened gyri and compressed ventricles. There may be herniation of the uncus and cerebellar tonsils. Microscopically, congestion, petechial hemorrhages and foci of neuronal necrosis are seen. A diffuse astrocytic proliferation in both the gray and white matter may accompany these changes. Vascular lesions in the brain are particularly prominent, with capillary dilation and proliferation.

Peripheral motor neuropathy is the most common manifestation of lead neurotoxicity in the adult, typically affecting the radial and peroneal nerves and resulting in **wristdrop** and **footdrop,** respectively. Lead-induced neuropathy is probably also the basis of the paroxysms of gastrointestinal pain known as **lead colic.**

MOLECULAR PATHOGENESIS: Anemia is a cardinal sign of lead intoxication. Lead disrupts heme synthesis in bone marrow erythroblasts by inhibiting δ-aminolevulinic acid dehydratase, the second enzyme in de novo synthesis of heme. It also inhibits ferrochelatase, which catalyzes the incorporation of ferrous iron into the porphyrin ring. The resulting inability to produce heme adequately is expressed as a microcytic and hypochromic anemia resembling that seen in iron deficiency, in which heme synthesis is also impaired. The anemia of lead intoxication is also characterized by prominent basophilic stippling of erythrocytes, related to clustering of ribosomes. Erythrocyte life span is decreased; thus, the anemia of lead intoxication is due to both ineffective hematopoiesis and accelerated erythrocyte turnover.

Lead nephropathy reflects the toxic effect of the metal on the proximal tubular cells of the kidney. The resulting dysfunction is characterized by aminoaciduria, glycosuria and hyperphosphaturia (Fanconi syndrome). Such functional

FIGURE 8-15. Complications of lead intoxication.

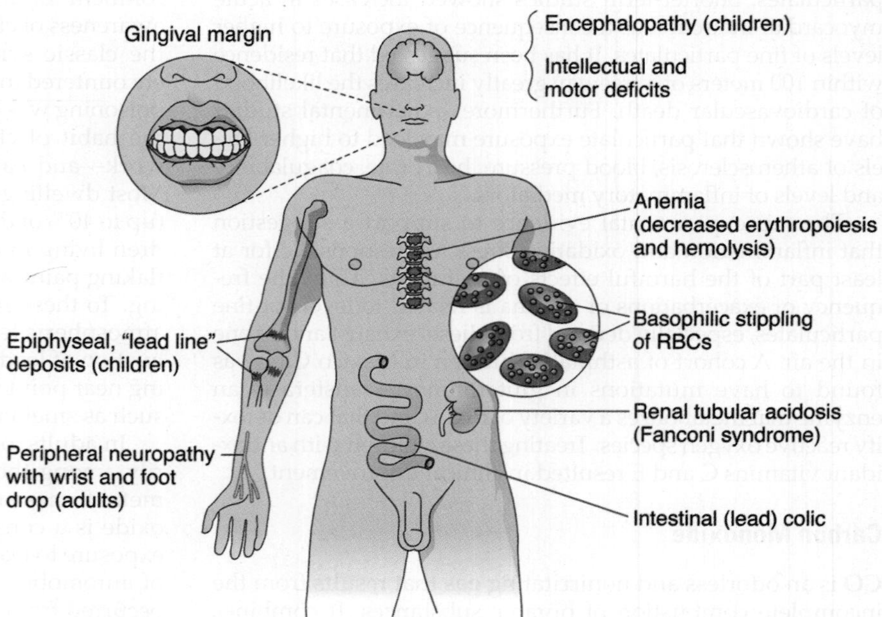

alterations are accompanied by the formation of inclusion bodies in the nuclei of the proximal tubular cells. These inclusions are characteristic of lead nephropathy and are composed of a lead–protein complex containing more than 100 times the concentration of lead in the whole kidney.

Lead poisoning is treated with chelating agents such as ethylene diamine tetra-acetic acid (EDTA), either alone or in combination with dimercaprol (BAL). Both the hematologic and renal manifestations of lead intoxication are usually reversible; alterations in the CNS are generally irreversible.

Laboratory diagnosis is made by demonstrating high blood levels of lead and increased free erythrocyte protoporphyrin. Elevated urinary excretion of δ-aminolevulinic acid and decreased levels of aminolevulinic acid dehydratase in erythrocytes are confirmatory.

EFFECTS OF CHRONIC EXPOSURE TO LOW LEAD LEVELS: Owing to the removal of lead from gasoline, improvements in housing, substitution of titanium for lead in paints and control of industrial point sources, ambient levels of lead have fallen significantly: blood levels in the general population of the United States decreased from an average of 16 μg/dL in 1976 to 1.0 μg/dL in 2000. It has been established that cumulative exposure to lead is best measured in bone, rather than blood. The latter lead levels reflect more ongoing exposure. Thus, elevated bone levels of lead have been correlated with adult hypertension, whereas no relationship has been established with blood levels. The dramatic fall in mean blood lead levels has been accompanied by the near elimination of lead-related childhood fatalities and encephalopathy. However, low lead exposure in children, while not producing recognizable symptoms, may permanently decrease cognitive performance. The regulatory safe threshold for blood levels of lead in children has been progressively reduced and is now thought to be below 10 μg/dL.

Efforts to reduce environmental lead have led to decreases in the percentage of children in the United States with blood levels of 10 μg/dL of lead or more from 88% in the 1970s to 4.4% in the 1990s. However, high blood lead concentrations remain a problem among poor, mainly urban, children and vigorous campaigns to address this situation are justified.

Mercury

Inorganic mercury has been used since prehistoric times and has been known to be an occupation-related hazard at least since the Middle Ages, but in recent years it has become recognized that organic mercury represents a greater risk to human health. Although mercury poisoning still occurs in some occupations, there has been increasing concern over the potential health hazards brought about by the contamination of many ecosystems following several well-known outbreaks of methylmercury poisoning. The most widely publicized episodes occurred in Japan, first in Minamata Bay in the 1950s and then in Niigata. In both cases, local inhabitants developed severe, chronic organic mercury intoxication. This poisoning was traced to the consumption of fish contaminated with mercury that had been discharged into the environment in the effluents from a fertilizer and a plastics factory. Children exposed in utero showed delayed developmental milestones and abnormal reflexes, despite the fact that fetal exposure was estimated to be one-fifth to one-tenth that in adults.

Mercury released into the environment may be bioconcentrated and enter the food chain. Bacteria in bays and oceans can convert inorganic mercury compounds from industrial wastes into highly neurotoxic organomercurials. These compounds are then transferred up the food chain and are eventually concentrated in the large predatory fish (e.g., tuna, pike) that make up a substantial part of the diet in many countries.

Although inorganic mercury is not efficiently absorbed in the gastrointestinal tract, organic mercurial compounds are readily taken up because of their lipid solubility. Both inorganic and organic mercury are preferentially concentrated in the kidney and methylmercury also distributes to the brain. ***The kidney is the principal target of the toxicity of inorganic mercury, but the brain is damaged by organic mercurials.*** Claims that mercuric preservatives in vaccines have led to autism or other neurologic complications have not withstood scientific scrutiny.

NEPHROTOXICITY: At one time, mercuric chloride was widely used as an antiseptic and acute mercuric chloride poisoning was much more common; the compound was ingested by accident or for suicidal purposes. Under such circumstances, **proximal tubular necrosis** was accompanied by oliguric renal failure. Mercurial diuretics were also widely prescribed in the past and chronic mercury nephrotoxicity was a not uncommon complication of their long-term use. Today, chronic mercurial nephrotoxicity is almost always a consequence of long-term industrial exposure. Proteinuria is common in chronic mercurial nephrotoxicity and there may be a nephrotic syndrome with more severe intoxication. Pathologically, there is a membranous glomerulonephritis with subepithelial electron-dense deposits, suggesting immune complex deposition.

NEUROTOXICITY: The neurologic effects of mercury are manifested as a constriction of visual fields, paresthesias, ataxia, dysarthria and hearing loss. Pathologically, there is cerebral and cerebellar atrophy. Microscopically, the cerebellum exhibits atrophy of the granular layer, without loss of Purkinje cells and spongy softenings in the visual cortex and other cortical regions.

Arsenic

The toxic properties of arsenic have been known for centuries. Arsenic-containing compounds have been widely used as insecticides, weed killers and wood preservatives. Arsenicals may also contaminate soil and leach into ground water as a result of naturally occurring arsenic-rich rock formations, from coal burning or from use of arsenical pesticides. As with mercury, there is evidence for the bioaccumulation of arsenic along the food chain.

Acute arsenic poisoning is almost always the result of accidental or homicidal ingestion. Death is due to **CNS toxicity.** Chronic arsenic intoxication affects many organ systems. It is characterized initially by such nonspecific symptoms as malaise and fatigue. Eventually, gastrointestinal, cardiovascular and hematologic dysfunction become evident. Both encephalopathy and peripheral neuropathy develop. The latter is characterized by paresthesias, motor palsies and painful neuritis. On epidemiologic grounds, **cancers of the skin, respiratory tract** and **gastrointestinal tract** have been attributed to industrial and agricultural exposure to arsenic. In some parts of the world, exposure of workers in rice paddies to arsenic in the ground water has been associated with skin cancers. Rare cases of hepatic angiosarcomas have been related to chronic arsenic exposure.

Cadmium

Cadmium is used in ever-increasing quantities in the manufacture of alloys, in the production of rechargeable batteries, in electroplating of other metals (e.g., automobile parts and musical instruments), as a plasticizer and as a pigment. Fumes of cadmium oxide are released in the course of welding steel parts previously plated with a cadmium anticorrosive. It accumulates in the human body, with a half-life of over 20 years, and since it is rarely recycled, the increase in industrial use of the metal is of concern. The main routes of exposure for the general population are ingestion and inhalation. Both plant- and animal-derived foodstuffs may contain substantial levels of cadmium.

Short-term cadmium inhalation irritates the respiratory tract, with pulmonary edema the most dangerous result. The lungs and the kidneys and, to a lesser extent, the skeletal and vascular systems are the principal target organs of chronic cadmium intoxication. Emphysema has been the major finding in the fatal cases of chronic cadmium pneumonitis. Although the confounding effects of smoking complicate interpretation of some of these studies, inhalation of cadmium does appear to lead to lung cancer. Proteinuria, which reflects tubular rather than glomerular damage, has been the most consistent finding in cadmium workers with renal damage.

Chromium

Chromium (Cr) is used extensively in several industries, including metal plating and some types of manufacturing. Although it occurs in any number of oxidation states, only Cr(III) and Cr(VI) are commonly used industrially. Its toxicity is usually a result of inhalation and the consequences of exposure depend on the solubility of the specific salt. Although acute intoxication is known, it is chronic exposure that is most problematic.

Cr(VI) is highly genotoxic. People who chronically inhale salts of hexavalent chromium have an increased risk of lung cancer and possibly other tumors as well. The less soluble chromate salts are generally more potent pulmonary carcinogens, particularly zinc chromate.

Nickel

Nickel is a widely used metal in electronics, coins, steel alloys, batteries and food processing. Dermatitis ("nickel itch"), the most frequent effect of exposure to nickel, may occur from direct contact with metals containing nickel, such as coins and costume jewelry. The dermatitis is a sensitization reaction; the body reacts to nickel-conjugated proteins formed following the penetration of the epidermis by nickel ions. Exposure to nickel, as to arsenic, increases the risk of development of specific types of cancer. Epidemiologic studies have demonstrated that workers who were occupationally exposed to nickel compounds have an increased incidence of lung cancer and cancer of the nasal cavities.

Iron

Iron-deficiency anemia is a common disease, particularly in premenopausal women. Oral iron preparations contain largely ferrous sulfate, the form absorbed by the gastrointestinal mucosa and then converted to the trivalent form. Acute ferrous sulfate poisoning from accidental ingestion occurs, mainly in children between the ages of 1 and 2 years. As little as 1 to 2 g of ferrous sulfate may be lethal, but most fatal cases follow ingestion of 3 to 10 g. Hemorrhagic gastritis and acute liver necrosis have been the most prominent findings at autopsy.

Long-term, excessive dietary intake of iron does not ordinarily lead to abnormal iron accumulation. South African Bantus have a significant incidence of iron overload, which has been attributed to a diet very high in iron, largely derived from iron drums used to prepare homemade beer. The acidic pH of these brews readily solubilizes the iron and their low alcohol content allows large volumes to be consumed. A large proportion of the excess iron is in the liver, and there is a correlation between the degree of siderosis and the presence of cirrhosis. There is also a high incidence of diabetes and heart disease in this "Bantu siderosis."

However, some blacks have shown a similar syndrome, which now is attributed to a mutation in the gene for ferroportin (SLC4A1) that may predispose some people of African descent to iron overload (see Chapter 14).

Cobalt

Acute occupational inhalation of cobalt has led to acute respiratory distress syndrome (see Chapter 12). In addition, excessive intake of cobalt in beer that contained it to enhance foaming qualities was implicated in a degenerative disease of heart muscle (cardiomyopathy; see Chapter 11). When the cobalt was removed from the beer, no further cases of heart disease were reported.

Radioactive Elements

Elements whose radioactive isotopes are potentially hazardous include radium, strontium, uranium, plutonium, thorium and iodine. Chronic toxicities relate principally to radiation-induced carcinogenesis. The individual tumors reflect the organ localization of the elements and are discussed in the chapters that address specific organ pathology.

Biological Toxins Are Organisms and Their Nonviable Components

These toxins are mostly of microbial, algal, plant, protozoan, arthropod or mammalian origin. They include whole organisms, intact particulate or soluble products of those organisms (e.g., exotoxins) and fragments of organisms. Adverse reactions may result from inhalation, ingestion or other contact, and they may reflect infectious, hypersensitivity and toxic effects of those materials. This discussion addresses the latter. Infectious and hypersensitivity reactions to foreign matter are considered in Chapters 9 and 4, respectively, as well as individual organ-specific discussions (e.g., hypersensitivity pneumonitis in Chapter 12).

The toxic effects of microbial products are the best characterized of biological toxicities. **Organic dust toxic syndrome** (ODTS) is a systemic reaction to the direct toxicities of many, mainly fungal, toxins. It consists of flu-like symptoms (fever, malaise, etc.), often with a respiratory component (dyspnea, cough). Unlike hypersensitivity pneumonitis, ODTS appears to reflect cell death and the consequent acute inflammatory reaction. It is usually associated with toxins produced by many common fungi.

Aspergillus, *Stachybotrys*, *Penicillium* and *Fusarium* spp. are the most common culprits. These fungi are particularly abundant in water-damaged buildings and moist warm environments. Their mycotoxins include trichothecenes and β-1,3-glucans, which may elicit disease by ingestion and inhalational routes.

One particular toxin produced by *Aspergillus flavus* and *Aspergillus parasiticus*, called **aflatoxin**, is highly hepatotoxic and is recognized as a potent hepatocarcinogen. There are several known varieties of aflatoxin.

Bacterial endotoxins are lipopolysaccharides derived from gram-negative bacterial cell walls. They are often complexed with proteins and phospholipids. Injected endotoxins are used experimentally to elicit inflammatory and febrile responses characterized by local or systemic macrophage activation. Inhaled, these compounds elicit profuse pulmonary inflammatory responses, involving release of inflammatory mediators (tumor necrosis factor [TNF]-α, interleukin [IL]-1, etc.), causing fever, pneumonitis and pulmonary edema.

The subject of biological toxins is of considerable concern because of possible weaponization for use in biological warfare (see Chapter 9).

Thermal Regulatory Dysfunction

Hypothermia Is a Decrease in Body Temperature Below 35°C (95°F)

Hypothermia can result in systemic or focal injury, the latter exemplified by **trench foot** or **immersion foot.** In localized hypothermia of these types, actual tissue freezing does not occur. **Frostbite,** by contrast, involves the crystallization of tissue water.

Generalized Hypothermia

Hypothermia may occur in a number of settings, including immersion in cold water and exposure to extremely cold air temperatures, especially after taking agents that impair thermoregulation, such as alcohol and some drugs and pharmacologic agents. Perhaps the best studied cause of hypothermia is cold water immersion. Acute immersion in water at 4°C to 10°C (39.2°F to 50°F) reduces central blood flow. Coupled with decreased core body temperature and cooling of the blood perfusing the brain, this results in mental confusion. Tetany makes swimming impossible. Furthermore, increased vagal discharge leads to premature ventricular contractions, ventricular arrhythmias and even fibrillation.

Attempting to increase heat production, the immersed body immediately responds by increasing muscle activity and oxygen consumption. However, there are limits to the sources of energy available for sustained warming. Within 30 minutes, heat loss exceeds heat production because of the combination of high direct conduction of heat from the whole skin surface and altered muscle tone caused by decreased arterial carbon dioxide and exhaustion. Core temperature then begins to fall. Peripheral vasoconstriction is another response to conserve heat. In addition, there is an increased sympathetic neural discharge, resulting in increased heart and basal metabolic rates and shivering. When the core temperature approaches 35°C, this activity may be three to six times above normal. Below 35°C, respiratory rate, heart rate and blood pressure decline because the functional reserve is reduced.

With prolonged cooling, a "cold-induced" diuresis results in increased blood viscosity. As a result, blood flow decreases and oxygen–hemoglobin association is less effective. Cardiac stroke volume decreases and peripheral vascular resistance increases as a direct result of both blood "sludging" and loss of plasma. The most important factor in causing death is cardiac arrhythmia or sudden cardiac arrest. These observations have been confirmed and extended, largely because of the need to induce hypothermia in some patients undergoing open-heart surgery. In fact, with careful pharmacologic control, prolonged periods of lower body temperature can be achieved with no residual harm.

If hypothermia is prolonged, decreased body temperature alters cerebrovascular function. When body core temperature reaches 32°C (89.6°F), the person becomes lethargic, apathetic and withdrawn. A characteristic response is inappropriate behavior, including disrobing, even when cold. If temperature falls further, intermittent "stupor" and eventually coma supervene. If core temperature goes below 28°C (82.4°F), pulse and breathing weaken.

Although there are no specific morphologic changes in those who die from hypothermia, the skin shows red and purple discolorations, ears and hands swell and there is irregular vasoconstriction and vasodilation. Areas of cardiac myocytolysis are seen. Lungs may display pulmonary edema and intra-alveolar, intrabronchial and interstitial hemorrhage.

Focal Thermal Alterations

As discussed above, local reduction in tissue temperature, particularly in the skin, is associated with local vasoconstriction. Tissue water crystallizes if blood circulation is insufficient to counter persistent thermal loss. When freezing occurs slowly, ice crystals form within tissue cells and in the interstitial space. Concomitantly, electrolyte-rich gels are excluded. Injury to cellular organelles reflects the drastic changes in ion concentrations in the excluded volume. Denaturation of macromolecules and physical disruption of cellular membranes by the ice ensue. When freezing is rapid, a gel-like structure forms within the cell that lacks water crystalloids. This water-solid reduces the extent of mechanical and chemical injury. The most significant cellular damage apparently occurs on thawing, when mechanical disruption of membrane structures occurs, perhaps the result of transformation from a gel to a crystal.

The most biologically significant cell injury appears in the endothelial lining of the capillaries and venules, which alters small vessel permeability. This injury initiates extravasation of plasma, formation of localized edema and blisters and an inflammatory reaction. Whereas frostbite results from the actual freezing of water, immersion foot (trench foot) is caused by a prolonged reduction in tissue temperature to a point not low enough to freeze tissue. This cooling causes cellular disruption. Endothelial cell damage leads to local thrombosis and changes caused by altered permeability are prominent. Vascular occlusion often leads to gangrene.

Hyperthermia Means an Increase in Body Temperature

Tissue responses to hyperthermia are similar in some respects to those caused by freezing injuries. In both instances, injury to the vascular endothelium results in altered vascular permeability, edema and blisters. The degree of injury depends on the extent of temperature elevation and how quickly it is reached. Small increases in body temperature increase the metabolic rate. However, above a certain limit, enzymes denature and other proteins precipitate and "melting" of lipid bilayers of cell membranes takes place.

Systemic Hyperthermia

Systemic hyperthermia, or **fever**, is an elevation of body core temperature. It occurs because of (1) increased heat production, (2) decreased elimination of heat from the body (reflecting an aberrant response of the thermal regulatory center) or (3) a disturbance of the thermal regulatory center itself. Hyperthermia can also occur because heat is conducted into the body faster than the system can clear it.

A body temperature above 42.5°C (108.5°F) leads to profound functional disturbances, including general vasodilation, inefficient cardiac function and altered respiration. Isolated heart–lung preparations fail at about the same temperature, suggesting an inherent limitation in the cardiovascular system and perhaps in the myocardial cells themselves. ***In general, systemic temperature elevations above 41°C to 42°C (105°F to 107.6°F) are not compatible with life.***

During infectious and inflammatory responses, several cytokines, including IL-1, IL-6 and TNF-α, interact with a portion of the hypothalamus at the roof of the third ventricle, the organum vasculosum laminae terminalis, and apparently reset the body's "thermostat" to permit a higher body core temperature. There is also evidence that for mild pyrogens, parasympathetic activation may be involved.

Few, if any, defined pathologic changes are associated with fever alone. Physical findings include increased heart and respiratory rates, peripheral vasodilation and diaphoresis, all recognized mechanisms for thermal regulation. The CNS may respond with irritability, restlessness and (particularly in children) convulsions. Nocturnal temperature elevations with "night sweats" are a feature of pulmonary granulomatous infection (especially tuberculosis) and are also observed in lymphoproliferative diseases. Prolonged temperature elevation can produce wasting, principally because of an increased metabolic rate.

Malignant hyperthermia is a thermal alteration, accompanied by a hypermetabolic state and often by rhabdomyolysis (muscle necrosis), that occurs after anesthesia in susceptible persons. This autosomal dominant disorder is associated with at least 70 different mutations in the gene for the sarcoplasmic reticulum ryanodine receptor (RYR1). A less common mutation causing malignant hyperthermia occurs in the gene for the α-subunit of the L-type voltage-gated calcium channel (CACNA1S). Muscle damage is caused by an abnormally high calcium concentration produced by accelerated release of Ca^{2+} through the mutant calcium release channel. After the introduction of treatment with dantrolene, which binds to the ryanodine receptor, mortality from malignant hyperthermia fell from 80% to less than 10%.

Heat stroke is a form of hyperthermia that occurs under conditions of very high ambient temperatures and is not mediated by endogenous pyrogens. It reflects impaired thermal regulatory cooling responses and characteristically occurs in infants, young children and the very aged. Often the disorder is associated with an underlying chronic illness and use of diuretics, tranquilizers that may affect the hypothalamic thermal regulatory center or drugs that inhibit perspiration. Another form of heat stroke is seen in healthy men during unusually vigorous exercise. Lactic acidosis, hypocalcemia and rhabdomyolysis may be severe problems and almost one third of patients with exertional heat stroke develop myoglobinuric acute renal failure. Heat stroke is not amenable to treatment with standard antipyretics and only external cooling and fluid and electrolyte replacement are effective therapy.

Cutaneous Burns

Cutaneous burns are the most common form of localized hyperthermia. Both the elevated temperature and rate of temperature change are important in determining the tissue response. A temperature of 50°C (120°F) may be sustained for 10 minutes or more without cell death, while a temperature 70°C (158°F) or higher for even several seconds causes necrosis of the entire epidermis.

Cutaneous burns have been separated into full-thickness (previously, third-degree) and partial thickness (previously, first- and second-degree) burns (Fig. 8-16).

- **Partial thickness burns,** such as a mild sunburn, are recognized by congestion and pain but are not associated with

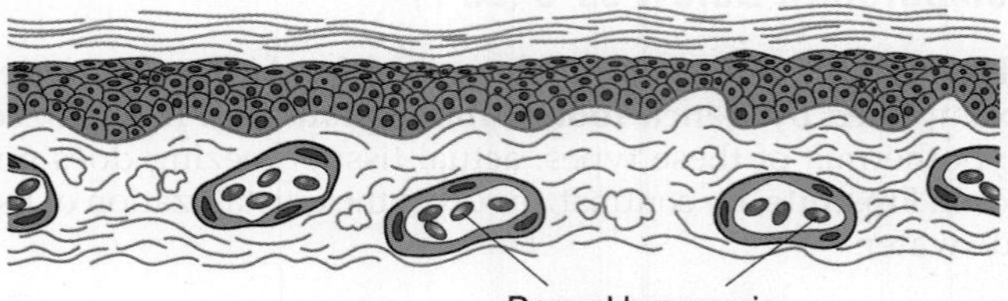

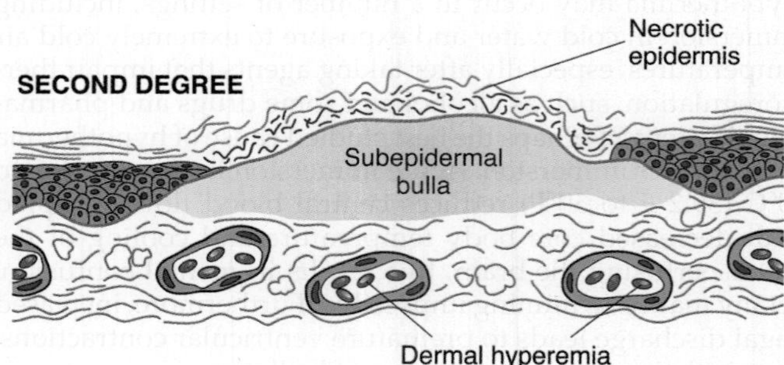

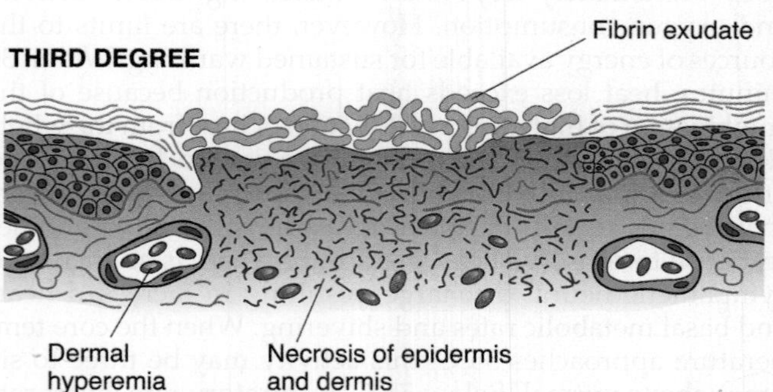

FIGURE 8-16. The pathology of cutaneous burns. A first-degree skin burn exhibits only dilation of the dermal blood vessels. In a second-degree burn, there is necrosis of the epidermis and subepidermal edema collects under the necrotic epidermis to form a bulla. In a third-degree burn, both the epidermis and dermis are necrotic.

necrosis. Mild endothelial injury produces vasodilation, increased vascular permeability and slight edema. More severe partial thickness burns cause epidermal necrosis, but spare the dermis. Clinically, these burns are recognized by blisters, in which the epithelium separates from the dermis.

- **Full-thickness burns** char both epidermis and dermis. Histologically, they are carbonized and cellular structure is lost.

Among the most important functions of the skin are fluid retention and protection from infectious agents. Not surprisingly, then, when skin is severely damaged, its ability to subserve these functions is compromised. One of the most serious systemic disturbances caused by extensive cutaneous burns is fluid loss. Patients with full-thickness burns can lose about 0.3 mL of body water/cm^2 of burned area per day. Resulting hemoconcentration and poor vascular perfusion of the skin and other viscera complicate the recovery of these patients. Many severely burned persons, particularly those with more than 70% of their body surface involved with full-thickness burns, develop shock and acute tubular necrosis of the kidneys and mortality is very high. Severely burned patients who survive longer are at great risk of lethal surface infections and sepsis. Even normal skin saprophytes may cause infection of charred tissue and pose another difficulty for healing.

Healing of cutaneous burns is related to the extent of tissue destruction. Mild partial thickness burns, by definition, have little if any cell loss and healing requires only repair or replacement of injured endothelial cells. More severe partial thickness burns also heal without a scar because epidermal basal cells remain and are a source of regenerating cells for the epithelium. Full-thickness burns, in which the entire thickness of the epidermis is destroyed, pose a separate set of problems. If the skin appendages are spared, reepithelialization can arise from them. Initially, islands of proliferation at the orifices of these glands grow and coalesce to cover the surface. Deeper burns that destroy the skin appendages require new epidermis to be grafted to the débrided area to establish a functional covering. Burned skin that is not replaced by a graft heals with dense scarring. Since this scar tissue lacks the elasticity of normal skin, contractures that limit motion may eventually result.

Inhalation Burns

Persons trapped in burning buildings and vehicles are exposed to air and aerosolized flammable materials heated to very high temperatures. Inhalation of these noxious fumes injures or destroys respiratory tract epithelium from the oral cavity to the alveoli. If a patient survives the acute episode, acute respiratory distress syndrome (ARDS), which itself may be fatal (see Chapter 12), may develop.

Electrical Burns

Electrical injury produces damage through (1) electrical dysfunction of cardiovascular conduction and the nervous system and (2) conversion of electrical energy to heat energy when the current encounters the resistance of the tissues. ***Because electrical energy can potentially disrupt the electrical system within the heart, it frequently causes death through ventricular fibrillation.*** The amount of current necessary for such a disruption depends in part on its pathway through the body and its ease in penetrating the skin. Someone who inadvertently touches a 120-V line in a living room may suffer burns on the hand because the skin that contacts the wire has substantial resistance to the flow of electrical current. If that resistance is decreased, as when a person inadvertently touches the same line in a bathtub, the lower resistance increases transmitted current, leading to disordered cardiac electrical activity.

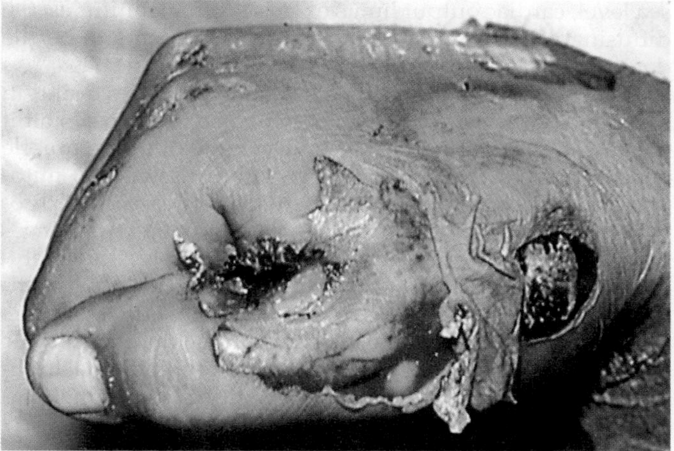

FIGURE 8-17. Electrical burn of the skin. The victim was electrocuted after attempting to stop a fall from a ladder by grasping a high-voltage electrical line.

Electrical burns of the skin reflect the voltage, the area of electrical conductance and the duration of current flow (Fig. 8-17). Very–high-voltage current chars tissue and produces a third-degree burn. On the other hand, broad, moist surfaces exposed to the same flow exhibit less-severe change. With exposure to very–high-voltage currents, the force may be almost "explosive," in which case vaporization of tissue water produces extensive damage.

Altitude-Related Illnesses

High-altitude illness is rare, in large part because mountain climbers tend to acclimate before extreme altitudes are achieved. However, there is an altitude limit beyond which human life cannot be sustained for prolonged periods. Communities in the Andes succeed at 4000 to 4300 meters (13,124 to 14,108 ft). Inhabitants adapt to the decreased pressure and availability of oxygen by developing elevated hematocrits and large "barrel" chests with increased lung volume. Even those who live in this zone do not survive at elevations above 5500 to 6000 meters (18,045 to 19,686 ft). Prolonged stays at this altitude result in weight loss, difficulty in sleeping and lethargy, perhaps because of the redirection of cellular energy simply for survival. For example, 75% to 90% of the oxygen available at 6000 meters is used simply for the effort of inspiration.

The modifications induced by high altitude are related to decreased atmospheric pressure and consequent decreased oxygen availability. Unlike sea level, where activity does not change oxygen saturation, physical activity at these elevations leads to decreased partial pressure of arterial oxygen. At sea level, cardiac output limits exercise; at high altitudes, the diffusing capacity of the lung for oxygen seems to be the determinant.

Acclimation to chronic hypoxia at high altitudes results in a reduced ventilatory drive. Acclimated persons exhibit increases in (1) capillaries per unit volume of brain, muscle and myocardium; (2) myoglobin within tissues; (3) mitochondria per cell; and (4) hematocrit. An increase in erythrocyte levels of 2′3′-diphosphoglycerate, which enhances oxygen delivery to tissues, occurs within hours, but polycythemia takes months. Some of the minor effects of high altitude are systemic edema, retinal hemorrhages and flatulence. The more serious nonfatal diseases are acute and chronic mountain sickness and high-altitude deterioration. Fatal **high-altitude pulmonary edema** and **high-altitude encephalopathy** may ensue.

- **High-altitude systemic edema:** This condition results from asymptomatic increases in vascular permeability, particularly in hands, face and feet and most often at elevations over 3000 meters. It is reflected only in weight gain; on return to lower altitude, diuresis causes the edema to disappear. This disorder may in part reflect endothelial cell responses to hypoxia and is twice as common in women as in men. A calcium channel blocker has been used as treatment.
- **High-altitude retinal hemorrhage:** A critical analysis by funduscopic examination revealed that 30% to 60% of those sleeping above 5000 meters had retinal hemorrhages. The initial effect includes retinal vascular engorgement and tortuousness. Optic disc hyperemia is also noted and multiple flame-shaped hemorrhages subsequently occur. These changes are reversible.
- **High-altitude flatus:** Changes in external pressure and production of intestinal gas provide for expansion of intestinal luminal contents and lead to increased flatus at altitudes above 3500 meters. No medical disease attends these changes, although social problems may ensue.
- **Acute mountain sickness:** This condition is rare below 2500 meters but occurs to some degree in nearly everyone at 3000 to 3600 meters. Initial presentation includes headache, lassitude, anorexia, weakness and difficulty sleeping. The underlying pathophysiology is in part related to hypoxia and shifts in plasma fluid to the interstitial space. Adaptation through increased respiratory rate causes some improvement. Descent to lower altitudes is certainly indicated. Chronic or subacute exacerbation of this disease also occurs, frequently at lower altitudes, and the symptoms may be severe. Prophylaxis with acetazolamide (a carbonic anhydrase inhibitor) or dexamethasone has been successful for acute mountain sickness.
- **High-altitude deterioration:** Generally occurring at very high elevations (5500 meters or more), high-altitude deterioration presents as a decrease in physical and mental performance. The combination of chronic hypoxia, inadequate fluid intake, inadequate nutrition, decreased plasma volume and hemoconcentration are aggravating factors.
- **High-altitude pulmonary edema and cerebral edema:** Serious high-altitude problems, including pulmonary edema and cerebral edema, can occur with a rapid ascent to heights over 2500 meters, particularly in susceptible persons who have difficulty sleeping at higher altitudes. Tachycardia, right ventricular overload and marked reduction in arterial oxygen pressure occur, without changes in pH or carbon dioxide retention. A characteristic patchy pulmonary infiltrate is noted radiographically. Pulmonary hypertension is common in patients with high-altitude pulmonary edema. Hypoxic vasoconstriction and intravascular thrombosis have been proposed as causes of pulmonary hypertension. Eventually, cardiac output is decreased and systemic blood pressure falls. The precapillary arterioles become dilated, increasing capillary bed pressure and inducing interstitial and alveolar edema. Autopsy findings include severe confluent pulmonary edema, proteinaceous alveolar exudates and hyaline membrane formation. Capillary obstruction by thrombi has been noted. A dilated heart and enlarged pulmonary arteries are commonly found.
- **High-altitude encephalopathy** is characterized by confusion, stupor and coma. Autopsies reveal cerebral edema and vascular congestion. A proposed mechanism is severe cerebral hypoxia, with inhibition of the sodium pump and resultant intracellular edema.

Physical Injuries

The effect of mechanical trauma is related to (1) the force transmitted to the tissue, (2) the rate at which the transfer occurs, (3) the surface area to which the force is transferred and (4) the area of the body involved. The compressibility of the tissue adjacent to the transmitted force in part determines its effect. However, transmission of absorbed energy can produce alterations elsewhere in the body. Blows over a hollow viscus can rupture the organ because of compression of the fluid or gas it contains; organs nestled beneath the skin, such as the liver, can be easily ruptured. An impact directly over the heart can even disturb its electrical systems. However, a blow over a large muscle mass, such as the thigh or upper arm, is often less injurious than a direct blow to a poorly shielded bone, such as the anterior tibia. Furthermore, the distribution of the force is important.

A Contusion Is a Localized Mechanical Injury With Focal Hemorrhage

A force with sufficient energy may disrupt capillaries and venules within an organ by physical means alone. The result may be so limited that the only histologic change is hemorrhage in tissue spaces outside the vascular compartment. A discrete extravascular blood pool within the tissue is called a **hematoma.** Initially, the deoxygenated blood renders the area blue to blue-black, as in the classic "black eye." Macrophages ingest the erythrocytes, convert their hemoglobin to bilirubin and so change the color from blue to yellow. Both mobilization of the pigment by macrophages and further metabolism of bilirubin cause the yellow to fade to yellowish green and then to disappear.

An Abrasion Is a Skin Defect Caused by Crushes or Scrapes

The disruptive force may provide a portal of entry for microorganisms. The impact of the agent and its configuration are frequently seen in these wounds and are of special interest to the forensic pathologist.

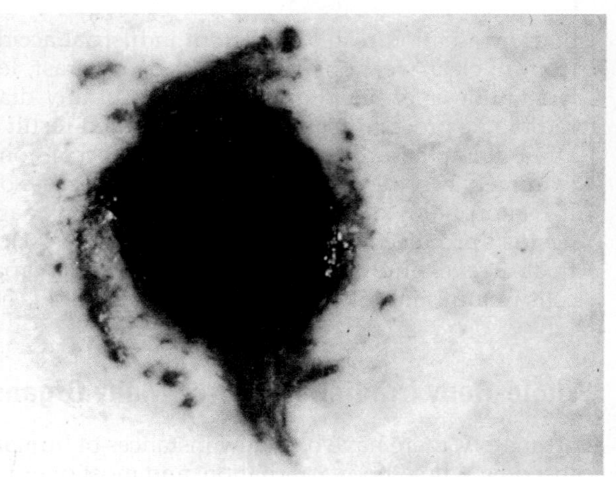

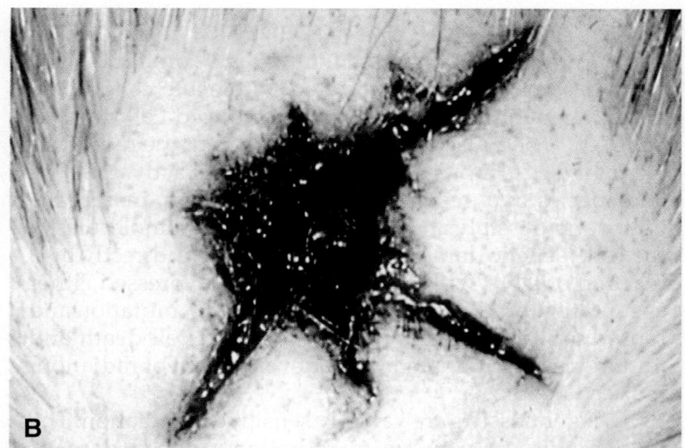

FIGURE 8-18. Bullet wounds. A. The entrance wound is sharply punched out. **B.** The exit wound is irregular with characteristic stellate lacerations.

A Laceration Is a Split or Tear of the Skin

Lacerations result from an impact stronger than that causing an abrasion and are usually the result of unidirectional displacement. When they have crushed margins, they are termed **abraded lacerations.**

Wounds Are Mechanical Disruptions of Tissue Integrity

An incision is a deliberate opening in the skin by a cutting instrument (e.g., a surgeon's scalpel). Incisions have sharp edges and, importantly, spare no tissue to the depth of the wound. **Deep penetrating wounds** made by high-velocity projectiles, such as bullets, are often deceptive, because the energy of the missile as it passes through the body may be released at sites distant from the entrance itself. Bullets, because they rotate, produce a well-defined and usually round entrance wound (Fig. 8-18). Once the projectile enters the flesh, however, it may fragment, tumble, or actually explode, resulting in considerable tissue damage and a large, ragged exit wound.

Ultraviolet Light

Within the large spectrum of electromagnetic radiation emitted by the sun, exposure to ultraviolet (UV) light (100 to 400 nm) has a number of different effects on the human body. It can damage DNA and is a leading cause of cancer of the skin (see Chapter 5).

UV radiation is also absorbed by photoreceptors in the skin, after which substances that suppress cell-mediated immunity may be released. As a consequence, both local and systemic immune functions may be modulated. Recent evidence suggests a beneficial effect of UV light on the severity of some autoimmune diseases, such as multiple sclerosis. Exposure to UV radiation also stimulates endogenous production of vitamin D in the skin (see below). UV wavelengths between 270 nm and 300 nm, termed UVB, result in production of a precursor for vitamin D from a cholesterol derivative. However, the apparent favorable effects of UVB on the level of activity of multiple sclerosis appear to be, at least in part, independent of vitamin D.

Radiation

We can define radiation simply as emission of energy by one body, its transmission through an intervening medium and its absorption by another body. By this definition, radiation encompasses the entire electromagnetic spectrum and certain charged particles emitted by radioactive elements. Alpha particles and the beta particles of elements such as tritium (^{3}H) and carbon 14 (^{14}C) are of immense use scientifically, and pose few hazards for humans. High-energy radiation, in the form of gamma or x-rays, mediates most of the biological effects discussed here. We do not consider the effects of ultraviolet radiation here; they are discussed in Chapters 5 and 24.

Radiation is quantitated in a number of ways:

- **A roentgen** is a measure of the emission of radiant energy from a source. This unit refers to the amount of ionization produced in air.
- **A rad** measures absorption of radiant energy, which is biologically the more important parameter. A rad defines the energy, expressed as ergs, absorbed by a tissue. One rad equals 100 ergs per gram of tissue.
- **A gray** (Gy) corresponds to 100 rads (1 joule/kg of tissue) and a centigray (cGy) is equivalent to 1 rad.
- **The rem** was introduced to describe the biological effect caused by a rad of high-energy radiation, since low-energy particles produce more biological damage than gamma or x-rays.
- **A sievert** (Sv) is the dose in gray multiplied by an appropriate quality factor Q, so that 1 Sv of radiation is roughly equivalent in biological effectiveness to 1 Gy of gamma rays.

For the purposes of this discussion of radiation-induced pathology, the rad, gray, rem and sievert are considered comparable.

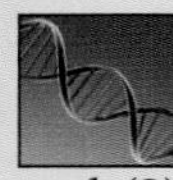

MOLECULAR PATHOGENESIS: At the cellular level, radiation essentially has two effects: (1) a somatic effect, associated with acute cell killing; and (2) genetic damage. Radiation-induced cell death is believed to be caused by the acute effects of the radiolysis of water (see Chapter 1). The production of activated oxygen species may result in lipid peroxidation, membrane injury and possibly an interaction with macromolecules of the cell. Genetic damage to the cell caused indirectly by a reaction of DNA with oxygen radicals is expressed either as mutation or as reproductive failure. Both mutation and reproductive failure may lead to delayed cell death and mutation is incriminated in the development of radiation-induced neoplasia.

Different tissues are variably sensitive to radiation. The vulnerability of a tissue to radiation-induced damage depends on its proliferative rate, which in turn correlates with the natural life span of the constituent cells. For example, the intestine and the hematopoietic bone marrow are far more vulnerable than tissues such as bone and brain. Damage to the DNA of a long-lived, nonproliferating cell does not necessarily impair its function or viability because its reproductive and metabolic functions are separate properties. By contrast, short-lived, proliferating cells, such as intestinal crypt cells or hematopoietic precursors, must be rapidly replaced by division of precursor cells. If radiation-induced DNA damage precludes mitosis of these cells, the mature elements are not replaced and the tissue can no longer function.

It is important to distinguish between whole-body irradiation and localized irradiation. Except for unusual circumstances, as in the high-dose irradiation that precedes bone marrow transplantation, significant levels of whole-body irradiation result only from industrial accidents or from nuclear weapons explosions. By contrast, localized irradiation is an inevitable byproduct of any diagnostic radiologic procedure and it is the intended result of radiation therapy. Rapid somatic cell death occurs only with extremely high doses of radiation, well in excess of 10 Gy. It is morphologically indistinguishable from coagulative necrosis produced by other causes (see Chapter 1). By contrast, irreversible damage to the replicative capacity of cells requires far lower doses, possibly as few as 50 cGy.

Whole-Body Irradiation Injures Many Organs

Fortunately, there have been few instances of human disease caused by whole-body irradiation, and most of our information has been derived from studies of Japanese atom bomb survivors. Further information is now available from the study of the survivors of the much smaller sample of persons exposed in the accident at the Chernobyl nuclear power plant in Ukraine in 1986.

Since comparable doses of radiant energy are transmitted to all organs in whole-body irradiation, development of the different acute radiation syndromes reflects the dissimilarities in vulnerability of the target tissues (Fig. 8-19).

- **300 cGy:** At this dose, a syndrome characterized by **hematopoietic failure** develops within 2 weeks. Following an initial depletion of circulating lymphocytes, a progressive decrease in formed elements of the blood eventually leads to bleeding, anemia and infection. The last is often the cause of death.
- **10 Gy:** In the vicinity of this dose, the main cause of death is related to the **gastrointestinal system.** Although

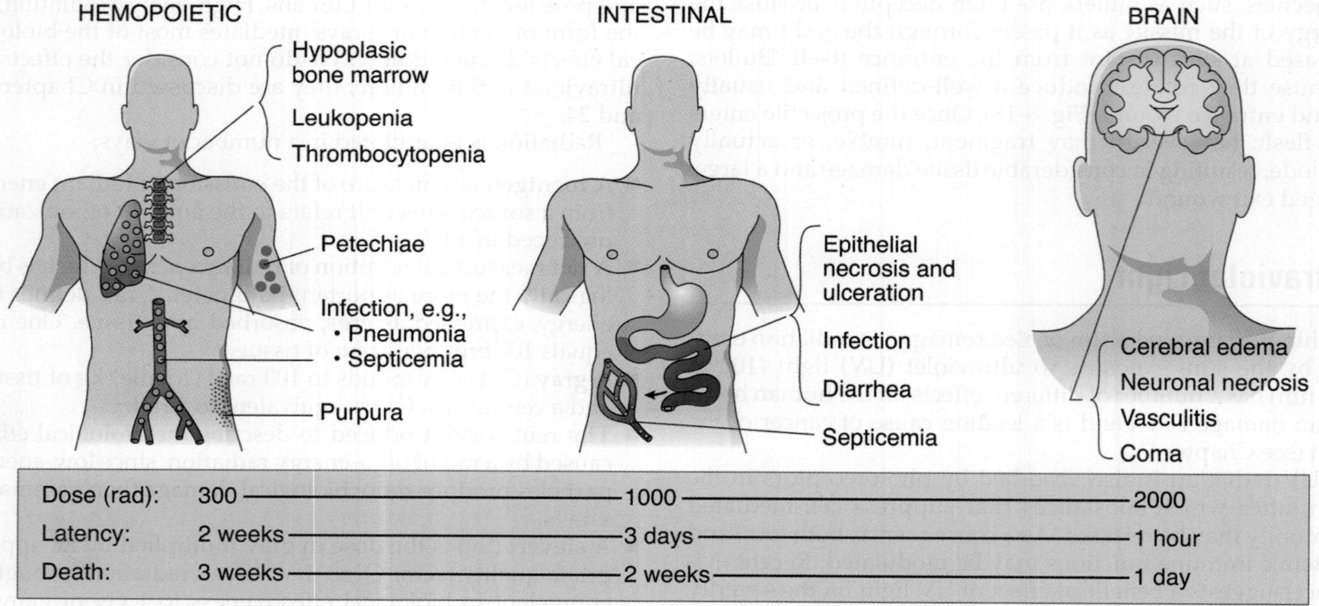

FIGURE 8-19. Acute radiation syndromes. At a dose of approximately 300 rads (cGy) of whole-body radiation, a syndrome characterized by hematopoietic failure develops within 2 weeks. In the vicinity of 1000 rads, a gastrointestinal syndrome with a latency of only 3 days is seen. With doses of 2000 rads or more, disease of the central nervous system appears within 1 hour and death ensues rapidly.

gastrointestinal symptoms occur through the entire dose range of whole-body exposure, at higher levels, the entire epithelium of the gastrointestinal tract is destroyed within 3 days (i.e., the time of the normal life span of villous and crypt cells). As a result, fluid homeostasis of the bowel is disrupted and severe diarrhea and dehydration ensue. Moreover, the epithelial barrier to intestinal bacteria is breached; gut organisms invade and disseminate throughout the body. Septicemia and shock kill the victim.

- **20 Gy:** With whole-body doses of 20 Gy and above, CNS damage causes death within hours. In most cases, cerebral edema and loss of the integrity of the blood-brain barrier, owing to endothelial injury, predominate. With extreme doses, radiation necrosis of neurons can be expected. Convulsions, coma and death follow.

FETAL EFFECTS: The effects of whole-body irradiation on the human fetus have been documented in studies of Hiroshima nuclear bomb survivors. Pregnant women exposed to 25 cGy or more gave birth to infants with reduced head size, diminished overall growth and mental retardation.

In studies of the clinical status of children exposed to therapeutic doses of radiation between the 3rd and 20th weeks of gestation, growth retardation and microcephaly were observed. Other effects of irradiation in utero include hydrocephaly, microphthalmia, chorioretinitis, blindness, spina bifida, cleft palate, clubfeet and genital abnormalities. Data from experimental and human studies strongly suggest that major congenital malformations are highly unlikely at doses below 20 cGy after day 14 of pregnancy. However, lower doses may produce more-subtle effects, such as a decrease in mental capacity. ***To protect against such a possibility, the established maximum permissible dose of radiation to the fetus from exposure of the expectant mother is far below the known teratogenic dose.***

GENETIC EFFECTS: Most data on which predictions of human genetic effects are based are derived from experimental data and analysis of nuclear bomb survivors. ***After long-term follow-up, survivors of the nuclear detonations at Hiroshima and Nagasaki have shown no evidence of genetic damage in the form of either congenital abnormalities or heritable diseases in subsequent offspring or their descendants.*** In experimental animals, the risk of induced mutation per cGy is at most 0.5% to 5% of the risk of spontaneous mutation (the spontaneous risk of mutation in humans is estimated to be 10% of live births). By extension, 20 to 200 cGy of radiation is necessary to double the spontaneous mutation rate. Consequently, the risk of genetic damage to future generations from radiation appears to be small.

AGING: There is to date no evidence that radiation exposure leads to premature aging. A mortality study of survivors of the nuclear bomb explosions in Japan did not show excess mortality beyond that attributable to neoplasia. Nor is there any evidence of acceleration in disease among the survivors in any part of the age range.

Localized Radiation Injury Complicates Radiation Therapy for Tumors

In the course of radiation therapy for malignant neoplasms, some normal tissue is inevitably irradiated. Although almost any organ can be damaged by radiation, the skin, lungs, heart, kidney, bladder and intestine are susceptible and difficult to shield (Fig. 8-20). Localized damage to the bone marrow is clearly of little functional consequence because of the immense reserve capacity of the hematopoietic system.

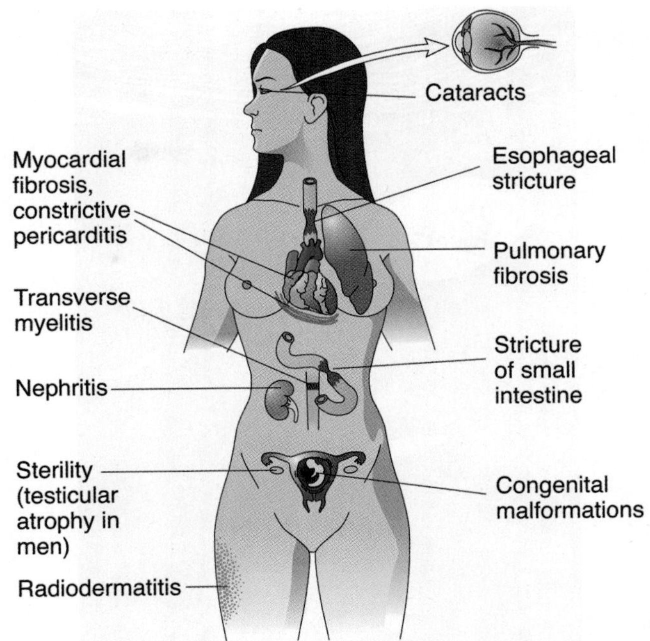

FIGURE 8-20. The nonneoplastic complications of radiation.

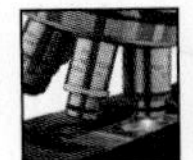

PATHOLOGY: Persistent damage to radiation-exposed tissue can be attributed to (1) compromise of the vascular supply and (2) a fibrotic repair reaction to acute necrosis and chronic ischemia. Radiation-induced tissue injury predominantly affects small arteries and arterioles. The endothelial cells are the most sensitive elements in the blood vessels and in the short term exhibit swelling and necrosis. With time, vascular walls become thickened by endothelial cell proliferation and subintimal deposition of collagen and other connective tissue elements. Striking vacuolization of intimal cells, so-called foam cells, is typical. Fragmentation of the internal elastic lamina, loss of smooth muscle cells, scarring in the media and fibrosis of the adventitia are seen in the small arteries. Bizarre fibroblasts with large hyperchromatic nuclei are common and probably reflect radiation-induced DNA damage.

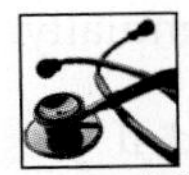

CLINICAL FEATURES: Acute necrosis from radiation is represented by such disorders as **radiation pneumonitis, cystitis, dermatitis** and **diarrhea from enteritis.** Chronic disease is characterized by **interstitial fibrosis** in the heart and lungs, **strictures** in the esophagus and small intestine and **constrictive pericarditis.** Chronic **radiation nephritis,** which simulates malignant nephrosclerosis, is primarily a vascular disease that leads to severe hypertension and progressive renal insufficiency.

As radiation therapy inevitably traverses the skin, it often causes **radiation dermatitis.** The initial damage is evidenced by blood vessel dilation, recognized as **erythema.** Necrosis of the skin may follow and linger as **indolent ulcers** that do not heal because the epithelium is unable to regenerate. Impaired wound healing in irradiated tissues may pose serious problems for surgeons operating in those areas. **Poorly healed** or **dehisced wounds** or **persistent ulcers** often require

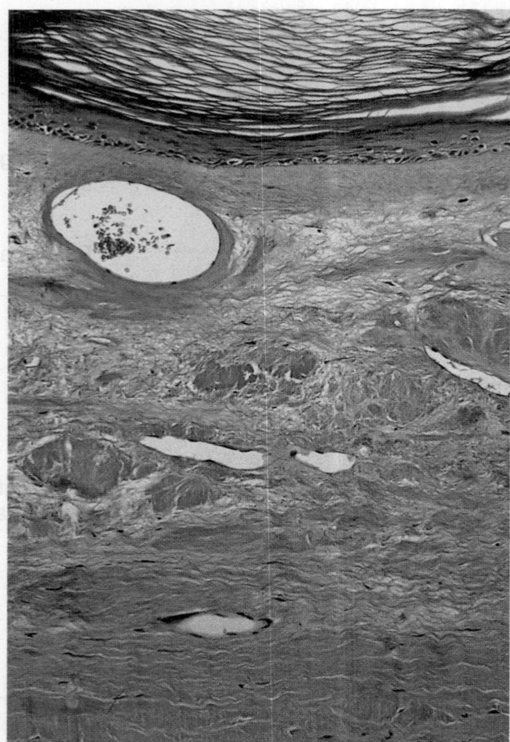

FIGURE 8-21. **Chronic radiation dermatitis.** The epidermis is atrophic. The dermis is densely fibrotic and contains dilated superficial blood vessels.

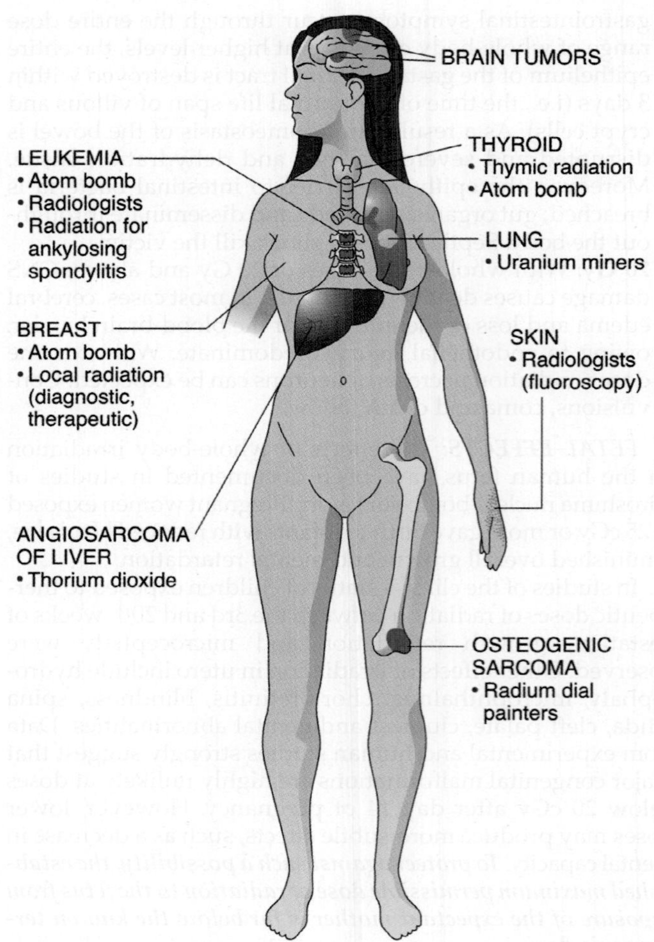

FIGURE 8-22. **Radiation-induced cancers.**

full-thickness skin grafts. **Chronic radiation dermatitis** results from repair and revascularization of the skin and is characterized by atrophy, hyperkeratosis, telangiectasia and hyperpigmentation (Fig. 8-21).

The **gonads,** both testes and ovaries, are similar to other tissues in their dependence on continuous cell cycling and are exquisitely radiosensitive. Acute inhibition of mitosis in the testis results in necrosis of the germinal stem cells, the spermatogonia. The combination of radiation-induced vascular injury and direct damage to the germ cells leads to progressive atrophy of seminiferous tubules, peritubular fibrosis and loss of reproductive function. Interstitial and Sertoli cells do not cycle rapidly and so persist, thereby preserving normal hormonal status. Comparable injury is seen in the irradiated ovary; the follicles become atretic and the organ eventually becomes fibrous and atrophic.

Cataracts (lenticular opacities) may be produced if the eye lies in the path of the radiation beam. **Transverse myelitis** and paraplegia occur when the spinal cord is unavoidably irradiated during treatment of certain thoracic or abdominal tumors. **Vascular damage in the cord** may bring about localized ischemia.

High Doses of Radiation Cause Cancer

The evidence that radiation can lead to cancer is incontrovertible and comes from many sources (Fig. 8-22). In the early part of the 20th century, scientists and radiologists tested their x-ray equipment by placing their hands in the path of the beam. As a result, they developed basal and squamous cell carcinomas of the exposed skin. In addition, early instruments were not properly shielded and the hazards associated with fluoroscopy were not appreciated. The radiologists of that era suffered an unusually high incidence of leukemia. This situation has been rectified with the use of modern shielding and protective equipment.

An unusual occupational exposure to radiation occurred among workers who painted radium-containing material onto watches to create luminous dials. These workers were in the habit of licking their paint brushes to produce a point, which led to their ingesting the radium. Since the body handles radium as it does calcium, it subsequently localized in their bones, so they were exposed to a long-lived isotope that persisted in their bones indefinitely. These people experienced a high incidence of cancer of the bone and of the paranasal sinuses. Another example of occupational exposure to a radioactive element is the high rate of lung cancer in uranium miners who inhaled radioactive dust. Most of these workers also smoked and evidence strongly favors a synergistic effect in lung carcinogenesis.

Iodine is concentrated by the thyroid. If radioactive iodine isotopes are inhaled or ingested, that gland will experience highly concentrated exposure to radioactivity. An explosive increase in the incidence of thyroid cancer among children in geographical areas contaminated by the nuclear catastrophe at Chernobyl in Ukraine in 1986 has been linked to release of radioactive iodine isotopes in that incident.

The risk of **solid tumors,** especially breast cancer, is particularly high among adult women who were treated with thoracic radiation for Hodgkin disease as children. Long-term survivors of childhood Hodgkin disease, who were treated with radiation therapy, have almost a 20-fold increased risk of developing a second neoplasm owing to the radiation. Another example of iatrogenic cancer resulted in Great Britain from widespread use of low-dose spinal irradiation to treat ankylosing spondylitis. These patients later developed aplastic anemia, myelogenous leukemia and other tumors with high frequency. An increase in brain tumors was found in persons who had received cranial irradiation for tinea capitis infection of the scalp in childhood. Thorium dioxide (Thorotrast), a material avidly ingested by phagocytic cells, was used a few decades ago for radionuclide imaging. The persistence in the liver of a long-lived radioisotope resulted in development of hepatic angiosarcomas.

The survivors of the nuclear bomb explosions in Japan suffered from a number of cancers. They exhibited a more than 10-fold increase in the incidence of leukemia, which peaked from 5 to 10 years after exposure, then declined to background rates. Two thirds were cases of acute leukemia; the remainder were of chronic myelogenous leukemia. Chronic lymphocytic leukemia, an uncommon disease in Japan, showed no increase in incidence. The risk of multiple myeloma increased fivefold and there was a small increment in the incidence of lymphoma. The frequency of solid tumors, although not as great as that for leukemia, was clearly increased for the breast, lung, thyroid, gastrointestinal tract and urinary tract. The development of malignant tumors, including leukemia, showed a dose-response relationship.

LOW-LEVEL RADIATION AND CANCER: Few debates have engendered as much heat and as little light as that concerning the potential carcinogenic effect of low levels of radiation. All assumptions are based on extrapolations to zero of the risk of cancer at higher doses or from epidemiologic studies to which valid exception may be taken. The key question that needs to be answered is whether there is a threshold dose of radiation below which there is no increase in the incidence of cancer, or whether any exposure carries a significant risk.

Data currently available from studies of cancer induction in animals, chromosomal damage in human cell cultures, malignant transformation of mammalian cells in vitro and populations exposed to radiation show that the estimates of risk at low radiation doses are very low. The data do not show that the risk of cancer from low-level radiation is zero. There is a general concern that gamma radiation is associated with increased risk of cancer at doses of 5 to 10 cGy. Although DNA damage appears to occur proportionately to the dose of gamma radiation, there is considerable uncertainty as to the extent to which DNA repair mechanisms may be protective at low radiation doses or dose rates.

RADON: The finding that some homes in the United States are contaminated with radon has elicited considerable public concern. Radon is a radioactive noble gas formed from the decay of uranium 238 (^{238}U), which is found in soil and rock formations. Radon is itself inert. Concern about the environmental hazards of radon focus on its radioactive decay products, which are called radon daughters. These include radioactive isotopes of bismuth, lead and polonium, which are chemically active and which bind to particulates and lung tissues. The half-life of the α-emitting isotope, ^{218}Po, is 103 years.

Previously, studies of the risk of radon gas were done in uranium miners and were not well controlled for smoking as an independent risk factor. More recent large-scale studies indicate that people who dwell in homes containing high concentrations of radon gas have an increased risk of developing lung cancer. The relative risk is by far the greatest for smokers and ex-smokers. However, recent studies also indicate that people who never smoked also have increased risk of lung cancer.

Microwave Radiation, Electromagnetic Fields and Ultrasound Are Not Ionizing

Microwaves, produced by ovens, radar and diathermy, are electromagnetic waves that penetrate tissue but do not produce ionization. Unlike x- and gamma radiation, absorption of microwave energy produces only heat. The activation energy of radiofrequency and microwave radiation is too low to modify chemical bonds or alter DNA. Thus, exposure to microwave radiation under ordinary circumstances is highly unlikely to produce any injury. Moreover, a study of 20,000 radar technicians in the Navy who were chronically exposed to high levels of microwave radiation failed to detect any increased incidence of cancer.

Controversy also surrounds possible carcinogenic—especially leukemogenic—effects of exposure to nonionizing electromagnetic fields, such as those encountered in the vicinity of high-voltage electric lines. Recent epidemiologic evidence has led to a consensus that exposure to electromagnetic fields does not raise the incidence of leukemia or other cancers.

Ultrasound, the vibrational waves in air above the audible range, produces mechanical compression but, again, no ionization. Highly focused and energetic ultrasound devices are used to disrupt tissue in vitro for chemical analysis and to clean various surfaces, including teeth. However, there is no reason to believe that diagnostic ultrasound or accidental exposure to any industrial device results in any measurable damage.

Nutritional Disorders

Protein-Calorie Malnutrition Reflects Starvation or Specific Deficiencies

Marasmus is the term used to denote a deficiency of calories from all sources. **Kwashiorkor** is a form of malnutrition in children caused by a diet deficient in protein alone.

Marasmus

Global starvation—that is, a deficiency of all elements of the diet—leads to marasmus. The condition is common throughout the nonindustrialized world, particularly when breast feeding is stopped and a child must subsist on a calorically inadequate diet. Pathologic changes are similar to those in starving adults and include decreased body weight, diminished subcutaneous fat, a protuberant abdomen, muscle wasting and a wrinkled face. In general, the child is a "shrunken old person." Wasting and increased lipofuscin pigment are seen in most visceral organs, especially the heart and the liver. No edema is present. Pulse, blood pressure and temperature are low; diarrhea is common. Since immune responses are impaired, the child suffers from numerous infections. An important consequence of marasmus is **growth failure.** If these children are not provided with adequate food in childhood, they will not reach their full potential stature as adults. Severe marasmus accompanied by iron-deficiency anemia in early childhood, when brain development is under way, may result in permanent intellectual deficits.

Kwashiorkor

Kwashiorkor (Fig. 8-23) results from a **deficiency of protein** in diets relatively high in carbohydrates. It is one of the most common diseases of infancy and childhood in the nonindustrialized world. Like marasmus, it usually occurs after an infant is weaned, when a protein-poor diet, consisting principally of staple carbohydrates, replaces mother's milk. There is generalized growth failure and muscle wasting, as in marasmus, but subcutaneous fat is normal, since caloric intake is adequate. Extreme apathy is notable, in contrast to children with marasmus, who may be alert. Also in contrast to marasmus, severe edema, hepatomegaly, depigmentation of the skin and dermatoses are usual. "Flaky paint" lesions of the skin on the face, extremities and perineum are dry and hyperkeratotic. Hair becomes a sandy or reddish color; a characteristic linear depigmentation of the hair ("flag sign") provides evidence of particularly severe periods of protein deficiency. The abdomen is distended because of flaccid abdominal muscles, hepatomegaly and ascites due to hypoalbuminemia. Along with general atrophy of the viscera, villous atrophy of the intestine may interfere with nutrient absorption. Diarrhea is common. Anemia is the rule, but it is not generally life-threatening. The nonspecific effects on

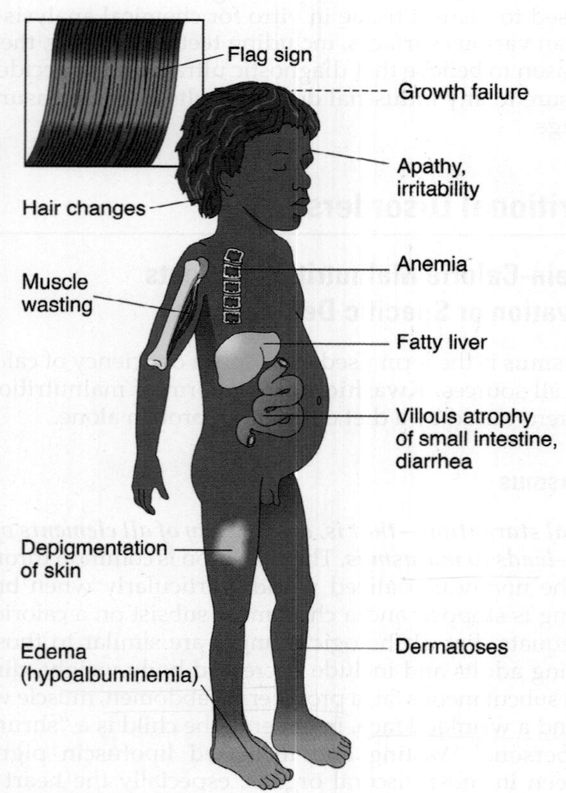

FIGURE 8-23. Complications of kwashiorkor.

growth, pulse, temperature and the immune system are similar to those in marasmus. It has been claimed in some studies that kwashiorkor not only impairs physical development but also stunts later intellectual growth.

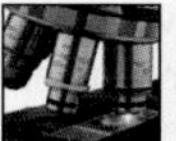

PATHOLOGY: Microscopically, the liver in kwashiorkor is conspicuously fatty. Accumulation of lipid within the cytoplasm of the hepatocyte displaces the nucleus to the periphery of the cell. The adequacy of dietary carbohydrate provides lipid for the hepatocyte, but the inadequate protein stores do not permit synthesis of enough apoprotein carrier to transport the lipid from the liver cell. The changes, with the possible exception of mental retardation, are fully reversible when sufficient protein is made available. In fact, the fatty liver reverts to normal after early childhood, even if the diet remains deficient in protein. In any event, hepatic changes are not progressive and do not lead to chronic liver disease.

Vitamins Are Organic Catalysts That Are Both Required for Normal Metabolism and Available Only From Dietary Sources

Thus, vitamins in one species are not necessarily vitamins in another. For example, humans cannot synthesize ascorbic acid (vitamin C) and so require dietary ascorbate to prevent scurvy, but most lower animals can produce their own vitamin C and do not require it as a vitamin.

Vitamin A

Vitamin A is a fat-soluble substance that is important for skeletal maturation and maintenance of specialized epithelial linings and cell membrane structure. In addition, it is an important constituent of the photosensitive pigments in the retina. Vitamin A occurs naturally as **retinoids** or as a precursor, ***β*-carotene.** The source of the precursor—carotene—is in plants, principally leafy, green vegetables. Fish livers are a particularly rich source of vitamin A itself (retinoids).

Vitamin A appears to be important in immune function and nonimmune defense mechanisms. It has long been known that vitamin A deficiency is associated with poor resistance to infection. However, the effects of vitamin A on specific infectious diseases have been variable, despite the general concern that administration of vitamin A to deficient people reduces overall mortality. In addition, in underdeveloped countries, vitamin A supplementation to pregnant women and their children has reduced infant mortality.

Metabolism

β-Carotene is modified in the intestinal mucosa to retinoids, which are absorbed with chylomicrons. It is stored in the liver, where 90% of the body's vitamin A is located. At times when fat absorption is impaired (e.g., diarrhea), vitamin A absorption decreases.

Vitamin A Deficiency

Although vitamin A deficiency is uncommon in developed countries, it is a significant health problem in poorer regions of the world, including much of Africa, China and Southeast Asia.

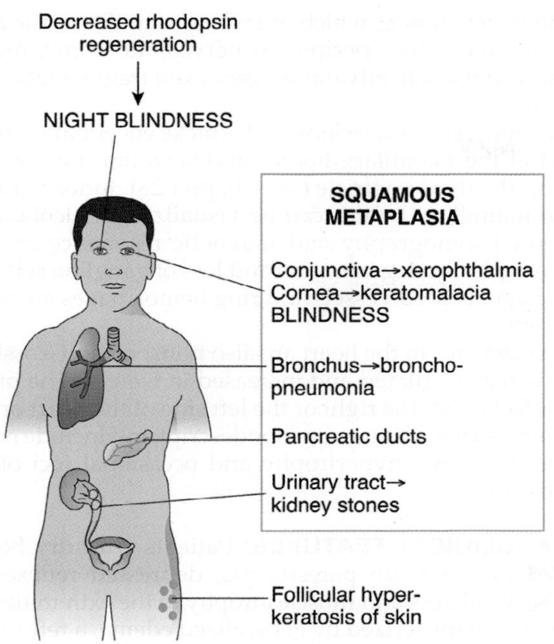

FIGURE 8-24. Complications of vitamin A deficiency.

PATHOLOGY: ***Deficiency of vitamin A results principally in squamous metaplasia, especially in glandular epithelium*** (Fig. 8-24). Thus, keratin debris blocks sweat and tear glands. Squamous metaplasia is common in the trachea and bronchi and bronchopneumonia is a frequent cause of death. The epithelia lining the renal pelvis, pancreatic ducts, uterus and salivary glands are also commonly affected. Epithelial changes in the renal pelvis may be associated with kidney stones. With further diminution of vitamin A stores, squamous metaplasia of conjunctival and tear duct epithelial cells occurs, which leads to **xerophthalmia,** dryness of the cornea and conjunctiva. The cornea becomes softened (**keratomalacia,** Fig. 8-25) and vulnerable to ulceration and bacterial infection, which may lead to blindness. **Follicular hyperkeratosis,** a skin disorder caused by occluded sebaceous glands, is also a feature of this disease.

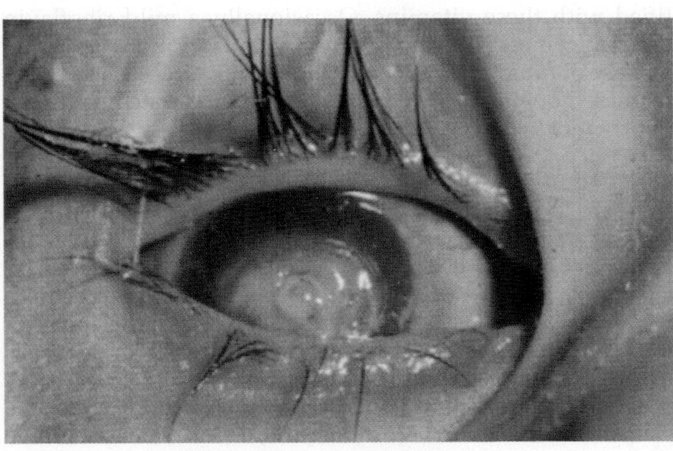

FIGURE 8-25. Keratomalacia in vitamin A deficiency.

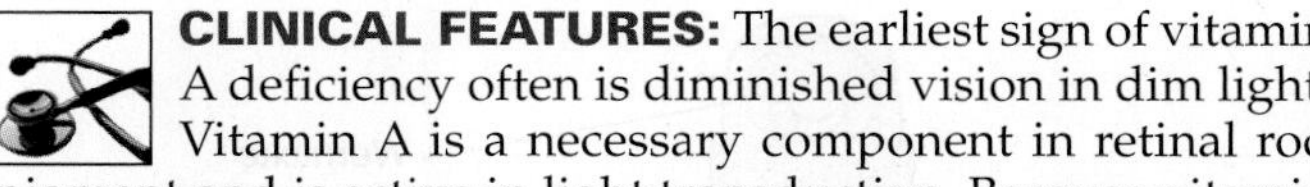

CLINICAL FEATURES: The earliest sign of vitamin A deficiency often is diminished vision in dim light. Vitamin A is a necessary component in retinal rod pigment and is active in light transduction. Because vitamin A aldehyde, retinal, is constantly degraded in generating the light signal, a continuous supply of vitamin A is necessary for night vision.

Vitamin A Toxicity

Vitamin A poisoning is usually caused by overenthusiastic administration of vitamin supplements to children. Early Arctic explorers were said to have experienced vitamin A toxicity because they ate polar bear liver, which is particularly rich in the vitamin. Enlargement of the liver and spleen are common; microscopically, these organs show lipid-laden macrophages. In the liver, vitamin A is also present in hepatocytes, and prolonged hypervitaminosis A has been incriminated in rare cases of cirrhosis. Bone pain and neurologic symptoms, such as hyperexcitability and headache, may be the presenting symptoms. Discontinuing the excess vitamin A consumption reverses all or most of the lesions. Excessive carotene intake is benign and simply stains the skin yellow, which may be mistaken for jaundice.

Synthetic derivatives of retinoic acid are now used pharmacologically to alleviate severe acne. Both retinoic acid and a high dietary intake of preformed vitamin A are particularly dangerous in pregnancy because they are potent teratogens. A number of clinical studies have reported that excess intake of vitamin A leads to reduced bone mineral density and consequently increases the incidence of bone fractures.

Vitamin B Complex

Vitamins in the B group of water-soluble vitamins are numbered 1 through 12, but only eight are distinct vitamins (Table 8-2).

Thiamine (B_1)

Thiamine was the active ingredient in the original description of vitamin B, which was defined as a water-soluble extract in rice polishings that cured beriberi (clinical thiamine deficiency). The vitamin is an essential cofactor in the activity of several enzymes crucial to energy metabolism, mainly in the tricarboxylic acid (Krebs) cycle. Thiamine deficiency was classically seen in the Orient, where the staple food was polished

Table 8-2

B Vitamins

Vitamin	Biochemical Name
B_1	Thiamine
B_2	Riboflavin
B_3	Niacin
B_5	Pantothenic acid
B_6	Pyridoxine
B_7	Biotin
B_9	Folic acid
B_{12}	Cyanocobalamin

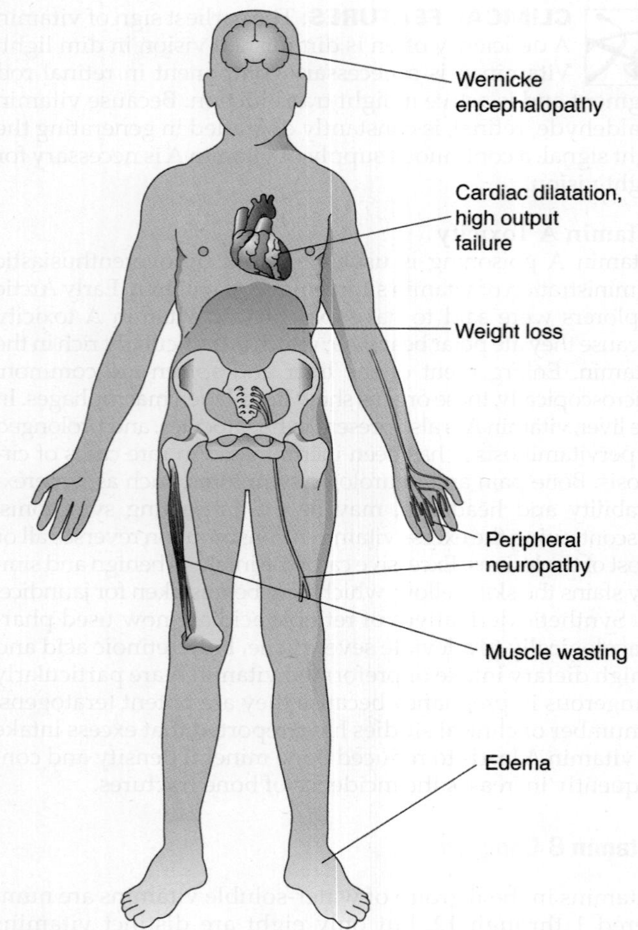

FIGURE 8-26. Complications of thiamine deficiency (beriberi).

rice that had been deprived of its thiamine content by processing. With increased awareness of the disease and improved nutrition in some areas of Asia, the disorder is less common now than in previous generations. In Western countries, the disease occurs in alcoholics, neglected persons with poor overall nutrition and food faddists. ***The cardinal symptoms of thiamine deficiency are polyneuropathy, edema and cardiac failure*** (Fig. 8-26). The deficiency syndrome is classically divided into **dry beriberi,** with symptoms referable to the neuromuscular system, and **wet beriberi,** in which manifestations of cardiac failure predominate.

Thiamine deficiency in chronic alcoholics may be manifested by CNS involvement, in the form of Wernicke syndrome, in which progressive **dementia, ataxia and ophthalmoplegia** (paralysis of the extraocular muscles) are prominent. Korsakoff syndrome, in which a thought disorder is conspicuous, at one time was attributed solely to thiamine deficiency, but is now understood to be seen both in chronic alcoholics and in patients with other organic mental syndromes.

PATHOLOGY: Pathologic examination of the nervous system in thiamine deficiency has not defined a pathognomonic change in the peripheral nerves, given that similar or identical changes can be seen with other peripheral neuropathies. A characteristic alteration is myelin sheath degeneration, which often begins in the sciatic nerve, then involves other peripheral nerves and sometimes the spinal cord itself. In advanced cases, axon fragmentation may be seen.

The most striking lesions in Wernicke encephalopathy are found in the mamillary bodies and surrounding areas that abut on the third ventricle (see Chapter 28). Indeed, atrophy of the mamillary bodies can be visualized in alcoholics by computed tomography and magnetic resonance imaging. Microscopically, degeneration and loss of ganglion cells, rupture of small blood vessels and ring hemorrhages are seen in the brain.

The changes in the heart are also nonspecific. Grossly, the heart is flabby, dilated and increased in weight. The process may affect either the right or the left side of the heart or both. The microscopic changes are nondescript and include edema, inconsistent fiber hypertrophy and occasional foci of fiber degeneration.

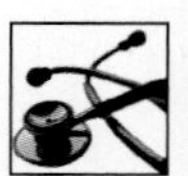

CLINICAL FEATURES: Patients with dry beriberi present with paresthesias, depressed reflexes and weakness and muscle atrophy in the extremities. Wet beriberi is characterized by generalized edema, a reflection of severe congestive failure. The basic lesion is uncontrolled, generalized vasodilation and significant peripheral arteriovenous shunting. This combination leads to a compensatory increase in cardiac output and eventually to a large dilated heart and congestive heart failure. In a patient without documented metabolic disease (e.g., hyperthyroidism), high output failure and generalized edema strongly suggest thiamine deficiency. ***The most reliable diagnostic test for thiamine deficiency is an immediate and dramatic response to parenteral administration of thiamine.*** Measurements of thiamine in the blood and erythrocyte transketolase activity are also useful.

Riboflavin (B_2)

Riboflavin, a vitamin derived from many plant and animal sources, is important for synthesis of flavin nucleotides, which are important in electron transport and other reactions in which energy transfer is crucial. Riboflavin is converted within the body to flavin mononucleotides and dinucleotides. Clinical symptoms of riboflavin deficiency are uncommon; they are usually seen only in debilitated patients with a variety of diseases and in poorly nourished alcoholics.

Deficiencies of thiamine, riboflavin and niacin are unusual in industrialized countries because bread and cereals are fortified with these vitamins. Occasionally, a mild riboflavin deficiency is seen during pregnancy and lactation, or during a phase of rapid growth in childhood and adolescence, when increased demands are combined with moderate nutritional deprivation.

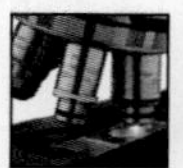
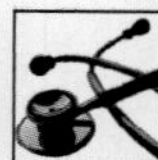

PATHOLOGY AND CLINICAL FEATURES: Riboflavin deficiency, when it occurs, is almost always seen in conjunction with deficiencies of other water-soluble vitamins. It is manifested principally by lesions of the facial skin and corneal epithelium. **Cheilosis,** a term used for fissures in the skin at the angles of the mouth, is a characteristic feature (Fig. 8-27). These cracks in the skin may be painful and often become infected.

Hyperkeratosis and a mild mononuclear infiltrate of the skin are noted. **Seborrheic dermatitis,** an inflammation of the skin that exhibits a greasy, scaling appearance, typically involves the cheeks and the areas behind the ears. The tongue

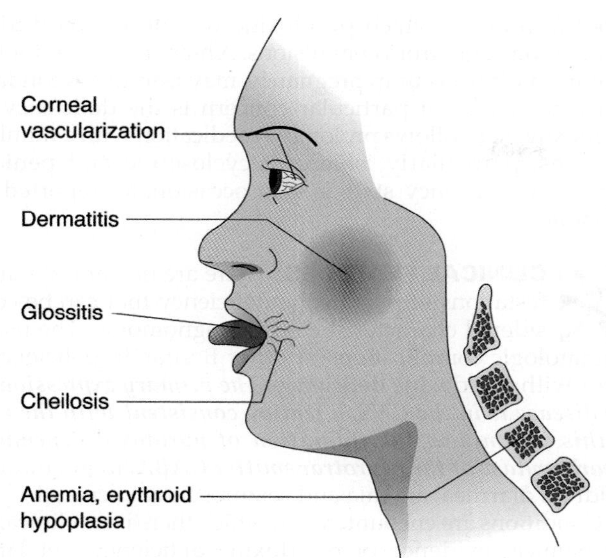

FIGURE 8-27. Complications of riboflavin deficiency.

is smooth and purplish (magenta), owing to mucosal atrophy. The most troubling lesion may be **corneal interstitial keratitis,** which is followed by opacification of the cornea and eventual ulceration. The localization of the lesions in riboflavin deficiency is not explained biochemically. There is no known toxicity from ingesting large amounts of riboflavin.

Niacin (B_3)

Niacin refers to nicotinic acid. Nicotinic acid is derived from dietary sources or biosynthesized from tryptophan. In the body, nicotinic acid is converted to nicotinamide, which plays a major role in formation of NAD. This compound and its phosphorylated derivative, NADP, are important in intermediary metabolism and an extensive variety of oxidation–reduction reactions. Animal protein, as found in meat, eggs and milk, is high in tryptophan and is therefore a good source of endogenously synthesized niacin. Niacin itself is available in many types of grain. **Pellagra** is the term for clinical niacin deficiency. It is uncommon today.

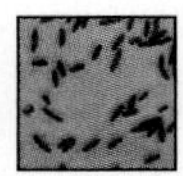

ETIOLOGIC FACTORS: Pellagra is seen principally in patients who have been weakened by other diseases and in malnourished alcoholics. Food faddists who do not eat sufficient protein may suffer a deficiency of tryptophan, which in combination with a lack of exogenous niacin may result in mild pellagra. Malabsorption of tryptophan, as in Hartnup disease, or excessive use of tryptophan for serotonin synthesis in the carcinoid syndrome may also lead to mild symptoms of pellagra. Deficiencies of pyridoxine and riboflavin increase the requirement for dietary niacin because both of these cofactors are required for biosynthesis of niacin from tryptophan. Pellagra is particularly prevalent in areas where corn (maize) is the staple food, because the niacin in corn is chemically bound and thus poorly available. Corn is also a poor source of tryptophan.

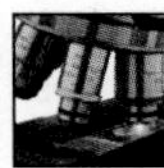

PATHOLOGY: Pellagra (Ital., "rough skin") is characterized by the three "Ds" of niacin deficiency: **dermatitis, diarrhea and dementia** (Fig. 8-28). Areas exposed to light, such as the face and the hands, and those subjected to pressure, such as the knees and the elbows, exhibit a rough, scaly dermatitis (Fig. 8-29). The involvement of the hands leads to so-called glove dermatitis. The lesions are discrete and show areas of pigmentation and of depigmentation. Microscopically, hyperkeratosis, vascularization and chronic inflammation of the skin are characteristic. Subcutaneous

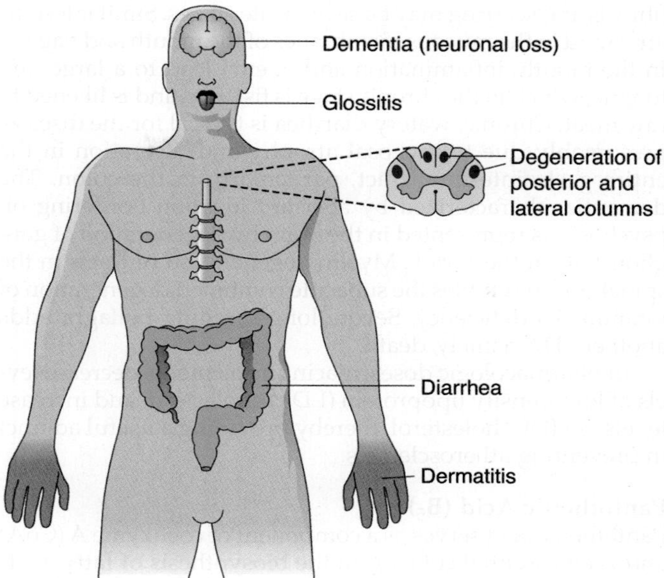

FIGURE 8-28. Complications of niacin deficiency (pellagra).

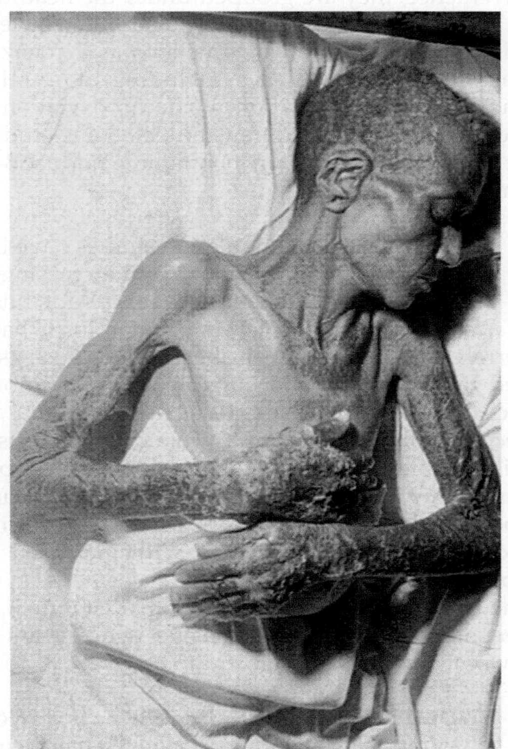

FIGURE 8-29. Pellagra. Dermatitis in sun-exposed areas of the arms and around the neck in this elderly woman is shown.

fibrosis and scarring may be seen in late stages. Similar lesions are found in the mucous membranes of the mouth and vagina. In the mouth, inflammation and edema lead to a large, red tongue, which in the chronic stage is fissured and is likened to raw meat. Chronic, watery diarrhea is typical for the disease, presumably due to mucosal atrophy and ulceration in the entire gastrointestinal tract, particularly in the colon. The dementia, characterized by aberrant ideation bordering on psychosis, is represented in the brain by degeneration of ganglion cells in the cortex. Myelin degeneration of tracts in the spinal cord resembles the subacute combined degeneration of vitamin B_{12} deficiency. Severe long-standing pellagra adds another "**D**," namely, death.

In pharmacologic doses, niacin supplements decrease levels of low-density lipoprotein (LDL) cholesterol and increase levels of HDL cholesterol, thereby providing a useful adjunct in preventing atherosclerosis.

Pantothenic Acid (B_5)

Pantothenic acid serves as a component of coenzyme A (CoA) and is an essential cofactor in the biosynthesis of fatty acids and certain peptides. Major sources of pantothenic acid include beef, chicken, liver, eggs, grains and a number of vegetables.

Deficiency of pantothenic acid is distinctly uncommon, except in severe malnutrition. The syndrome is characterized by behavioral, neurologic and gastrointestinal disturbances.

There are no known adverse effects of overconsumption of pantothenic acid.

Pyridoxine (B_6)

Vitamin B_6 activity is found in three related, naturally occurring compounds: pyridoxine, pyridoxal and pyridoxamine. For convenience, they are grouped under the heading pyridoxine. These compounds are widely distributed in vegetable and animal foods. Vitamin B_6 functions as a coenzyme in numerous metabolic pathways, including those related to amino acids, lipids, methylation and decarboxylation, gluconeogenesis, heme and neurotransmitters. Some studies also suggest a role for vitamin B_6 in maintaining normal B- and T-cell immune function.

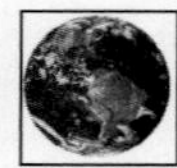

EPIDEMIOLOGY: Population studies have incriminated low levels of pyridoxine in increasing risk of atherosclerosis, but the mechanisms for this effect remain obscure. Low blood levels of vitamin B_6 have also been correlated with a number of conditions such as aging, impaired renal function and inflammatory conditions. The relevance of these correlations merits further study.

A recent analysis of prospective studies suggests a 20% lower risk of colorectal cancer when comparing people with high versus low intake of vitamin B_6. The report found that low blood levels of the active form of vitamin B_6, namely, pyridoxal 5-phosphate, correlated with increased risk of developing colorectal cancer.

In the United States, it is estimated that vitamin B_6 intake is inadequate for about 20% of men over age 50 years and for 40% of women in the same age group.

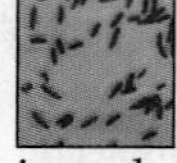

ETIOLOGIC FACTORS: Pyridoxine is converted to pyridoxal phosphate, a coenzyme for many enzymes, including transaminases and carboxylases. Pyridoxine deficiency is rarely caused by an inadequate diet, although infants who have been fed poorly prepared powdered formula in which pyridoxine was destroyed during preparation suffer from convulsions. A higher demand for the vitamin, as may occur in pregnancy, may lead to a secondary deficiency state. Of particular concern is the deficiency of pyridoxine that follows prolonged medication with a number of drugs, particularly isoniazid, cycloserine and penicillamine. A deficiency state is also occasionally reported in alcoholics.

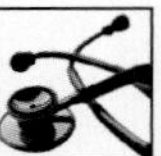

CLINICAL FEATURES: There are no clinical manifestations of pyridoxine deficiency that can be considered characteristic or pathognomonic. The usual dermatologic complications of other B vitamin deficiencies occur with pyridoxine deficiency. ***The primary expression of the disease is in the CNS, a feature consistent with the role of this vitamin in the formation of pyridoxal-dependent decarboxylase of the neurotransmitter GABA.*** In infants and children, diarrhea, anemia and seizures have occurred.

Conditions are encountered in which there is no clinical or biochemical evidence of pyridoxine deficiency, yet large (pharmacologic) doses of the vitamin are useful in treating the disorder. Such diseases are termed pyridoxine-dependency syndromes and include anemia, convulsions and homocystinuria caused by cystathionine synthetase deficiency.

Pyridoxine-responsive anemia is hypochromic and microcytic and therefore can be confused with iron-deficiency anemia. Unlike iron-deficiency anemia, however, pyridoxine-responsive anemia is characterized by saturation of iron stores and increased saturation of transferrin. Thus, administration of iron may simply make pyridoxine-responsive anemia worse. By definition, the anemia responds well to massive doses of pyridoxine.

Biotin (B_7)

Most biotin is found in meats and cereals, where it is largely bound to protein. Biotin is an obligatory cofactor for five carboxylases that participate in intermediary metabolism, including the Krebs cycle.

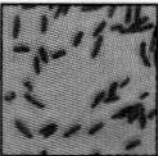

ETIOLOGIC FACTORS: Biotin deficiency is reported in people who consume large amounts of raw eggs, in those with prolonged malabsorption syndrome and in children with severe protein-calorie malnutrition. Chronic administration of anticonvulsant drugs can also lead to biotin depletion.

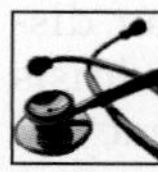

CLINICAL FEATURES: Symptoms of biotin deficiency include seborrheic and eczematous skin rash. In adults, neurologic symptoms include lethargy, hallucinations and paresthesias. In infants, hypotonia and developmental delay have been reported.

There are no known adverse consequences of high-dose biotin administration.

Folic Acid (B_9)

Folic acid is a heterocyclic derivative of glutamic acid and serves as a methyl group donor, especially in nucleotide synthesis. Folate, together with vitamin B_{12} (see below), is a key cofactor in methylation reactions. One of the key reactions in question is the conversion of homocysteine to methionine, which is needed to generate S-adenosylmethionine (SAM). SAM is a key methyl donor in the synthesis of neurotransmitters (norepinephrine to epinephrine), phospholipids (phosphatidylethanolamine to phosphatidylcholine), methylated nucleotides and histones. Folate also is critical in the generation of purine nucleotides and the conversion of uracil to thymidine. The latter reaction is key to understanding the consequences of folate deficiency in causing megaloblastic anemia.

FOLATE DEFICIENCY: Folic acid and vitamin B_{12} (see below) both participate in the pathway to produce methionine (see above), and the extent of the role of SAM in diverse biochemical reactions explains the extent of the overlap between the manifestations of deficiencies of these two vitamins (e.g., megaloblastic anemia; see Chapter 20). The distinction between deficiencies of these two B vitamins was elucidated by Herbert, who, in 1962, developed megaloblastic anemia following a self-imposed experimental diet lacking only folate.

Folate is present in almost all foods, including meat, dairy products, seafood, cereals and vegetables. Deficiency is thus usually a consequence of a generally poor diet, as is seen in some alcoholics, rather than a diet deficient in any single constituent. Malabsorption syndromes may also result in folate deficiency. Because the settings in which folate deficiency occurs affect many nutrients, isolated folate deficiency is rare.

Folate supplements given during early pregnancy have been shown to decrease the incidence of fetal neural tube defects (NTDs). However, maternal folate deficiency rarely causes NTDs and the decreased incidence of these malformations may reflect a pharmacologic effect of folate on a disorder caused by other factors, rather than the rectification of a deficiency state per se. Because neural tube formation occurs before many women know they are pregnant, fortification of cereal and grain products with folic acid has been mandated in the United States since 1998.

Cyanocobalamin (B_{12})

Deficiency of vitamin B_{12} is almost always seen in cases of pernicious anemia and results from the lack of secretion of intrinsic factor in the stomach (see Chapter 15), which prevents absorption of the vitamin in the ileum.

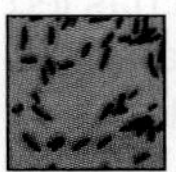

ETIOLOGIC FACTORS: Since vitamin B_{12} is found in almost all animal protein, including meat, milk and eggs, dietary deficiency is seen only in rare cases of extreme vegetarianism and then only after many years of a restricted diet. Parasitization of the small intestine by the fish tapeworm *Diphyllobothrium latum* (from undercooked fish) may lead to vitamin B_{12} deficiency because the parasite absorbs the vitamin in the gut lumen.

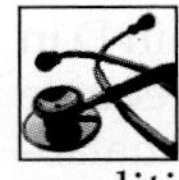

CLINICAL FEATURES: Deficiency of vitamin B_{12} is associated with megaloblastic anemia. In addition, pernicious anemia is complicated by a neurologic condition called subacute combined degeneration of the spinal cord. Comprehensive discussions of vitamin B_{12} deficiency are found in Chapters 20 and 28.

Choline

Choline is an amine that is found in many foods, especially wheat products, peanuts, soybeans, fish and meat. It is incorporated principally into membrane phospholipids and is the major dietary source of methyl groups. Choline is necessary for lipid signaling, transport and metabolism, and for cholinergic neurotransmission. It is also important in reactions involving transfer of methyl groups. Because there is an endogenous pathway for choline biosynthesis, it was not considered to be an essential human nutrient. Recently, however, choline deficiency syndromes have been identified and adequate dietary levels are now established.

Experimentally, a choline-deficient diet led to evidence of liver and muscle damage. Patients maintained on total parenteral nutrition due to short bowel syndrome often develop liver disease, some of which can be prevented by choline supplementation.

Vitamin C (Ascorbic Acid)

The effects of vitamin C deficiency, namely, **scurvy,** were described 5000 years ago in Egyptian hieroglyphs and were mentioned by Hippocrates in 500 BC.

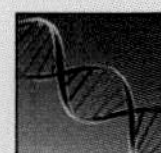

MOLECULAR PATHOGENESIS: Ascorbic acid is a water-soluble vitamin that is a powerful biological reducing agent involved in many oxidation/reduction reactions and in proton transfer. It is important for chondroitin sulfate synthesis and for proline hydroxylation to form the hydroxyproline of collagen. Ascorbic acid serves many other important functions: it prevents oxidation of tetrahydrofolate and augments absorption of iron from the gut. Without vitamin C, biosynthesis of certain neurotransmitters is impaired, leading to, for example, a reduction in dopamine β-hydroxylase activity. Wound healing and immune functions also involve ascorbic acid. The best dietary sources of vitamin C are citrus fruits, green vegetables and tomatoes.

Scurvy is the clinical vitamin C deficiency state. The first demonstration of the need for this vitamin was the remarkable effect of lime in preventing scurvy among 18th-century British sailors. The distribution of limes in the British navy led to the name "limey" for the seamen. Scurvy is uncommon in the Western world, but is often noted in nonindustrialized countries in which other forms of malnutrition are prevalent. In industrialized countries, scurvy is now a disease of people afflicted with chronic diseases who do not eat well, the neglected aged and malnourished alcoholics. The stress of cold, heat, fever or trauma (accidental or surgical) leads to an increased requirement for vitamin C. Children who are fed only milk for the first year of life develop scurvy, as do alcoholics. Mild depression of ascorbic acid levels also occurs in other conditions, including cigarette smoking, tuberculosis, rheumatic fever and many debilitating disorders. Some women who use oral contraceptives may have mildly decreased serum vitamin C levels. About 3% of the body's ascorbic acid is catabolized per day.

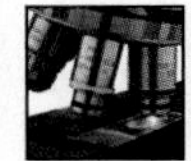

PATHOLOGY: ***Most of the events associated with vitamin C deficiency are caused by formation of abnormal collagen that lacks tensile strength*** (Fig. 8-30). Within 1 to 3 months, subperiosteal hemorrhages lead to pain in bones and joints. Petechial hemorrhages, ecchymoses and purpura are common, particularly after mild trauma or at pressure points. Perifollicular hemorrhages in the skin are particularly typical of scurvy. In advanced cases, swollen, bleeding gums are a classic finding. Alveolar bone resorption results in loss of teeth. Wound healing is poor and dehiscence of previously healed wounds occurs. Anemia may result from prolonged bleeding, impaired iron absorption or associated folic acid deficiency.

In children, vitamin C deficiency leads to growth failure and collagen-rich structures such as teeth, bones and blood vessels

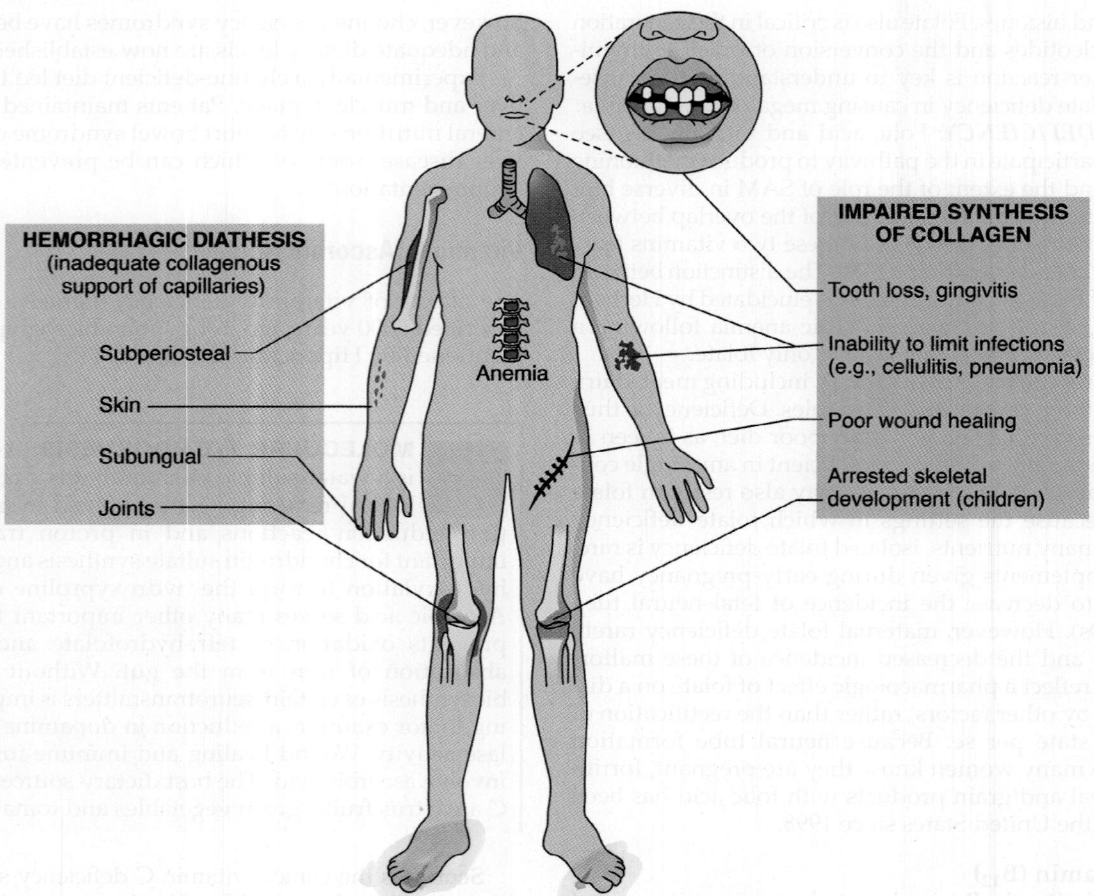

FIGURE 8-30. Complications of vitamin C deficiency (scurvy).

develop abnormally. Effects on developing bone are conspicuous and relate principally to impaired function of osteoblasts (see Chapter 26). In addition to poor wound healing, scorbutic patients have difficulty walling off infections to form abscesses, so that infections spread more easily. The diagnosis of scurvy is confirmed by finding low levels of ascorbic acid in the serum.

While claims that ascorbic acid may help to prevent upper respiratory infections lack substantiation, ingestion of large amounts of vitamin C is not known to be harmful.

Vitamin D

Some 500,000,000 years ago, vitamin D first appeared on Earth in ocean-dwelling phytoplankton, in which it may have functioned to absorb ultraviolet irradiation or act as a photochemical signal. During evolution, terrestrial vertebrates became dependent on vitamin D for the sustenance of their bony skeletons.

Vitamin D is a fat-soluble steroid hormone found in two forms: vitamin D_3 (cholecalciferol) and vitamin D_2 (ergocalciferol), both of which have equal biological potency in humans. Vitamin D_3 is produced in the skin and vitamin D_2 is derived from plant ergosterol. The vitamin is absorbed in the jejunum along with fats and is transported in the blood bound to an α-globulin (vitamin D–binding protein). ***To achieve biological potency, vitamin D must be hydroxylated to active metabolites in the liver and kidney. The active form of the vitamin promotes calcium and phosphate absorption from the small intestine and may directly influence mineralization of bone.***

The discovery of nuclear receptors for 1,25(OH)$_2$-vitamin D in various tissues not related to calcium metabolism has led to a search for pharmacologic applications of this vitamin. It may have uses in the treatment of psoriasis, hypertension, possibly certain cancers and multiple sclerosis.

Vitamin D Deficiency

ETIOLOGIC FACTORS: ***In children, vitamin D deficiency causes rickets; in adults, osteomalacia occurs.*** Vitamin D deficiency results from (1) insufficient dietary vitamin D, (2) insufficient production of vitamin D in the skin because of limited sunlight exposure, (3) inadequate absorption of vitamin D from the diet (as in the fat malabsorption syndromes) or (4) abnormal conversion of vitamin D to its bioactive metabolites. The last occurs in liver disease and chronic renal failure.

CLINICAL FEATURES: The bone lesions of vitamin D deficiency in children (rickets) have been recognized for centuries and were common in the Western industrialized world until recently. It was a disease that affected the urban poor to a much greater extent than their rural counterparts. A partial explanation for this difference lies in the greater exposure of rural residents to sunlight. Addition of vitamin D to milk and many processed foods, administration of vitamin preparations to young children and generally improved levels of nutrition have made rickets a curiosity in industrialized countries. See Chapter 26 for more details.

Hypervitaminosis D

The most common cause of excess vitamin D is the inordinate consumption of vitamin preparations. Abnormal conversion of vitamin D to biologically active metabolites is occasionally seen in granulomatous diseases such as sarcoidosis. In cases of calcium malabsorption, when the underlying disease is corrected, the sensitivity of target tissues to vitamin D may be increased.

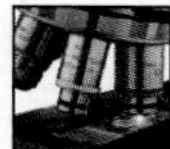

PATHOLOGY: The initial response to excess vitamin D is **hypercalcemia,** which leads to nonspecific symptoms such as weakness and headaches. Increased renal calcium excretion results in **nephrolithiasis** or **nephrocalcinosis. Ectopic calcification** in other organs, such as blood vessels, heart and lungs, may be seen. Infants are particularly susceptible to excess vitamin D, and if the condition is not corrected, they may develop premature arteriosclerosis, supravalvular aortic stenosis and renal acidosis.

Vitamin E

Vitamin E is an antioxidant that (experimentally at least) protects membrane phospholipids against lipid peroxidation by free radicals formed by cellular metabolism. The activity of this fat-soluble vitamin is found in a number of dietary constituents, principally in α-tocopherol. Corn and soy beans are particularly rich in vitamin E.

Dietary deficiency of vitamin E can occur in children as a result of mutations in the α-tocopherol transfer protein, and in adults with various malabsorption syndromes. The deficiency may present clinically as spinocerebellar ataxia, skeletal myopathy and pigmented retinopathy.

In premature infants, hemolytic anemia, thrombocytosis and edema have been associated with vitamin E deficiency. Vitamin E therapy has been reported to improve hemolytic anemia in premature newborns and may reduce the severity, but not the incidence, of retrolental fibroplasia. Vitamin E is reported to retard development of cirrhosis in infants with congenital biliary atresia. A number of interesting experimental effects are produced by vitamin E, such as inhibition of (1) platelet aggregation, (2) conversion of dietary nitrites to carcinogenic nitrosamines and (3) prostaglandin synthesis. Protection against toxins that exert their activity through production of free radical oxygen species has also been shown. The applicability of these results to humans requires further study.

Attempts to use vitamin E as a pharmacologic agent to prevent cancer and coronary artery disease have been unsuccessful.

Vitamin K

Vitamin K, a fat-soluble material, occurs in two forms: vitamin K_1, from plants, and vitamin K_2, which is principally synthesized by the normal intestinal bacteria. Green leafy vegetables are rich in vitamin K and liver and dairy products contain smaller amounts.

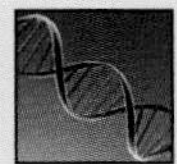

MOLECULAR PATHOGENESIS: Dietary deficiency is very uncommon in the United States; most cases are associated with other disorders. However, inadequate dietary intake of vitamin K does occasionally occur in conjunction with chronic illness associated with anorexia.

Vitamin K deficiency is common in severe fat malabsorption, as seen in sprue and biliary tract obstruction. Destruction of intestinal flora by antibiotics may also result in vitamin K deficiency. Newborn infants frequently exhibit vitamin K deficiency because the vitamin is not transported well across the placenta and the sterile gut of the newborn does not have bacteria to produce it. Vitamin K confers calcium-binding properties to certain proteins and is important for the activity of four clotting factors: prothrombin, factor VII, factor IX and factor X. Deficiency of vitamin K can be serious, because it can lead to catastrophic bleeding. Parenteral vitamin K therapy is rapidly effective.

Amino Acids

Of the 20 amino acids in human proteins, no pathways exist for the synthesis of eight, and possibly nine (the additional amino acid being histidine). These amino acids are required in the diet and are considered to be **essential amino acids.** Another nine amino acids can be synthesized in the human body from simple precursors or from other amino acids. These are termed **nonessential amino acids.** Finally, two amino acids (cysteine, tyrosine) are conditionally dispensable because their synthesis is limited under certain conditions or when adequate quantities of precursors are not available. Table 8-3 lists the 20 amino acids and the extent to which they must be acquired in the diet.

Table 8-3

Amino Acids

Amino Acid	Nature of Requirement
Alanine (A)	Nonessential
Arginine (R)	Nonessential
Asparagine (N)	Nonessential
Aspartic acid (D)	Nonessential
Cysteine (C)	Conditionally essential
Glutamic acid (E)	Nonessential
Glutamine (Q)	Nonessential
Glycine (G)	Nonessential
Histidine (H)	Conditionally essential
Isoleucine (I)	Essential
Leucine (L)	Essential
Lysine (K)	Essential
Methionine (M)	Essential
Phenylalanine (F)	Essential
Proline (P)	Nonessential
Serine (S)	Nonessential
Threonine (T)	Essential
Tryptophan (W)	Essential
Tyrosine (Y)	Conditionally essential
Valine (V)	Essential

Deficiency of essential amino acids is manifest as protein deficiency (kwashiorkor, see above).

Increasing Use of Vitamins

Recent years have witnessed an explosion of interest in potential pharmacologic uses of vitamins, unrelated to treating dietary or other deficiencies. Consequently, many people are consuming certain vitamins in doses that far exceed what is needed to prevent deficiency diseases. It is likely that studies of such people will provide information regarding both the potential beneficial and toxic effects of large doses of vitamins.

Essential Trace Minerals Are Mostly Components of Enzymes and Cofactors

Essential trace minerals include iron, copper, iodine, zinc, cobalt, selenium, manganese, nickel, chromium, tin, molybdenum, vanadium, silicon and fluorine. Dietary deficiencies of these minerals are clinically important in the case of iron and iodine. These are discussed in Chapters 20 and 21, which deal with blood and endocrine diseases, respectively.

Chronic zinc deficiency has been reported in Iran and Egypt to result in hypogonadal dwarfism in boys. The children usually are those who eat clay, a substance that may bind zinc, but a deficiency in dietary protein is usually also present. An inherited disorder of zinc metabolism, acrodermatitis enteropathica, which is a chronic form of zinc deficiency, is characterized by diarrhea, rash, hair loss, muscle wasting and mental irritability. Similar symptoms are seen in acute zinc deficiency associated with total parenteral nutrition. Zinc deficiency is also seen in diseases that cause malabsorption, such as Crohn disease, celiac disease, cirrhosis and alcoholism.

Dietary copper deficiency is rare but may occur in certain inherited disorders, in malabsorption syndromes and during total parenteral nutrition. The most common result is microcytic anemia, although megaloblastic changes have also been described.

Manganese deficiency has been described and causes poor growth, skeletal abnormalities, reproductive impairment, ataxia and convulsions. **Industrial exposure to manganese** causes symptoms closely related to those of parkinsonism.

9 Infectious and Parasitic Diseases

David A. Schwartz

THE TOLL OF INFECTIOUS DISEASES

Perhaps the greatest scourge to humankind, the diverse group of disorders collectively known as the infectious diseases has caused more pain, suffering, disability and premature death than any other group of diseases in history. Bacterial and viral diarrheas, bacterial pneumonias, tuberculosis, measles, malaria, hepatitis B, pertussis and tetanus kill more people each year than all cancers and cardiovascular diseases (Table 9-1). The impact of infectious diseases is greatest in less developed countries, where millions of people, mostly children younger than 5 years of age, die of treatable or preventable infectious diseases. Even in the developed countries of Europe and North America, the mortality, morbidity and loss of economic productivity from infectious diseases is enormous. In the United States each year, infectious diseases cause over 200,000 deaths, more than 50 million days of hospitalization and almost 2 billion days lost from work or school. It is estimated that smallpox claimed between 300 and 500 million human lives during the 20th century alone. Although smallpox has been eradicated from the natural environment, a multitude of other infectious agents continue to claim millions of lives each year. Infectious diseases such as tuberculosis, malaria, childhood diarrhea and human immunodeficiency virus (HIV)/acquired immunodeficiency disease (AIDS) continue to ravage the developing world, taking millions of lives each year. Even in industrialized nations, the morbidity and mortality from infectious disease is still substantial. In the United States, sepsis alone is responsible for an estimated 200,000 deaths per year.

Despite the untold past and present (and, undoubtedly, future) misery for which these diseases are responsible, past accomplishments of individuals great and small illustrate the contributions that can be made in this area to the alleviation of human suffering: Edward Jenner's use of cowpox (vaccinia) virus in 1798 to immunize against smallpox; John Snow's removal of the Broad Street pump handle, which ended the 1854 choleria outbreak in London; and the discovery in 1843 by Oliver Wendell Holmes, Sr., that simply washing hands between patients could dramatically reduce the incidence of puerperal fever. All these discoveries were made before an intelligible theory of causation of these illnesses existed. That theory was to come only with the work of Koch, Pasteur and Lister, who established the field of microbiology, which led directly to identification of agents responsible for many infectious diseases, establishment of effective standards of antisepsis and, eventually, the discovery and development of antibiotics to treat common bacterial, fungal, helminthic and protozoal diseases.

By the 1970s it seemed that infectious diseases would become medical curiosities as a result of the advanced antibiotics, improved sanitation and vaccination. It is instructive that in 1970, the Surgeon General of the United States declared, "the time has come for us to close the book on infectious disease." The fact that we had not conquered infectious diseases and, in fact, that tremendous problems were lurking was illustrated by the discovery of Legionnaires disease in 1976. The end of our naive expectations that infectious diseases were conquered came in 1981, with the first reports of HIV-1/AIDS. Since then, many other infections have emerged, for which we currently have little treatment and no cures: Ebola virus, severe acute respiratory syndrome (SARS), drug-resistant tuberculosis, pandemic strains of influenza virus and others. The recent concern over these and other infectious diseases underscores the facts that the potential for future infectious threats to human existence is real, animal reservoirs of microbes that can be transmitted to humans are bottomless and vigilance can never be relaxed. Finally, the possibility that people may seek to use infectious agents as weapons of warfare should dispel any complacency we have developed that we are safe from these pathogens.

Table 9-1

Sources of Global Deaths

Illness	Annual Deaths
Cardiovascular disease	12×10^6
Diarrheal diseases (rotavirus, Norwalk-like viruses, *Salmonella, Shigella*, diarrheagenic *Escherichia coli*)	5×10^6
Cancer	4.8×10^6
Pneumonia	4.8×10^6
Tuberculosis	3×10^6
Chronic obstructive lung disease	2.7×10^6
Measles	1.5×10^6
Malaria	$1–2 \times 10^6$
Hepatitis B	$1–2 \times 10^6$
Tetanus (neonatal)	775×10^3
Pertussis (whooping cough)	500×10^3
Maternal mortality	500×10^3
AIDS (all) AIDS (children)	200×10^3 28×10^3
Schistosomiasis	200×10^3
Amebiasis	$40–110 \times 10^3$
Hookworm	$50–60 \times 10^3$
Rabies	35×10^3
Typhoid	25×10^3
Yellow fever	25×10^3
African trypanosomiasis (sleeping sickness)	20×10^3
Ascariasis	20×10^3

AIDS = acquired immunodeficiency virus.

Tissue Damage

Infectious diseases represent many of the familiar taxa: bacteria, fungi, protozoa and various parasitic worms. Yet some infectious agents do not qualify as completely independent organisms. Viruses cannot replicate by themselves and are obligate intracellular parasites that hijack the replicative machinery of susceptible cells. Likewise, prions, the class of proteinaceous infectious agents, lack nucleic acids and clearly represent a different infectious disease paradigm.

There is great diversity in how various infectious diseases are acquired. Many of these diseases, such as influenza, syphilis and tuberculosis, are contagious, that is, transmissible from person to person. Yet many infectious diseases, such as legionellosis, histoplasmosis and toxoplasmosis, are not contagious but are rather acquired from the environment. *Legionella* sp. bacteria normally replicate in aquatic amebas but can infect humans via aerosolized water or through microaspiration of contaminated water. Other infectious agents come from many diverse sources, including animals, insects, soil, air, inanimate objects and the endogenous microbial flora of the human body.

Perhaps the greatest paradox is that certain retroviruses have actually been incorporated into the human genome and are passed from generation to generation. Their function is unclear but their possible activation during placentation has led to speculation that such endogenous retroviruses may have allowed placental mammals to evolve.

Infectivity and Virulence

Virulence is the complex of properties that allows an organism to establish infection and to cause disease or death. The organism must (1) gain access to the body, (2) avoid multiple host defenses, (3) accommodate to growth in the human milieu and (4) parasitize human resources. Virulence reflects both the structures inherent to the offending microbe and the interplay of those factors with host defense mechanisms.

Host Defense Mechanisms

The means by which the body prevents or contains infections are known as defense mechanisms (Table 9-2). There are major anatomic barriers to infection—the skin and the aerodynamic filtration system of the upper airway—that prevent most organisms from ever penetrating the body. The mucociliary blanket of the airways is also an essential defense, providing a means of expelling organisms that gain access to the respiratory system. Microbial flora normally resident in the gastrointestinal tract and in various body orifices compete with outside organisms, preventing them from gaining sufficient nutrients or binding sites in the host. The body's orifices are also protected by secretions that possess antimicrobial properties, both nonspecific (e.g., lysozyme and interferon) and specific (usually immunoglobulin A [IgA]). In addition, gastric acid and bile chemically destroy many ingested organisms.

Table 9-2

Host Defenses Against Infection
Skin
Tears
Normal bacterial flora
Gastric acid
Bile
Salivary and pancreatic secretions
Filtration system of nasopharynx
Mucociliary blanket
Bronchial, cervical, urethral and prostatic secretions
Neutrophils
Monocytes
Complement
Stationary mononuclear phagocyte system
Immunoglobulins
Cell-mediated immunity

Heritable Differences in Host Cell Membrane Molecules May Determine Whether an Infection Occurs

The first step in infection is often a highly specific interaction of a binding molecule on an infecting organism with a receptor molecule on the host. If the host lacks a suitable receptor, the organism cannot attach to the target. Thus, *Plasmodium vivax,* one of the organisms that cause human malaria, infects human erythrocytes by using Duffy blood group determinants on the cell surface as receptors. Many persons, particularly blacks, lack these determinants and are not susceptible to infection with *P. vivax*. As a result, *P. vivax* malaria is absent from much of Africa. Similar racial or geographic differences in susceptibility are apparent for many infectious agents, including *Coccidioides immitis* and *Coccidioides posadasii,* which are 14 times more common in blacks and 175 times more frequent in persons of Filipino ancestry than in whites.

Age Is an Important Determinant of Susceptibility to, and Outcome of, Many Infections

The effect of age on the outcome of exposure to many infectious agents is well illustrated by fetal infections. Some organisms produce more severe disease in utero than in children or adults. Infections of the fetus with cytomegalovirus (CMV), rubella virus, parvovirus B19 and *Toxoplasma gondii* interfere with fetal development. Normally, the fetus is protected by maternal IgG (generated by a specific previous infection) that passively crosses the placenta. In acute infection of a pregnant woman who lacks neutralizing antibody, certain pathogens may cross the placenta. These infections are usually subclinical or produce minimal disease in the mother. Depending on the organism and timing of exposure, fetal infection can produce minimal damage, major congenital abnormalities or death.

Age also affects the course of common illnesses, such as the diverse viral and bacterial diarrheas. In older children and adults, these infections cause discomfort and inconvenience, but rarely severe disease. The outcome can be different in children younger than 3 years, who cannot compensate for rapid volume loss resulting from profuse diarrhea. In 2000, the World Health Organization (WHO) estimated that acute diarrheal diseases kill 2.2 million children yearly.

Other examples include infection with *Mycobacterium tuberculosis,* which produces severe, disseminated tuberculosis in children younger than 3 years, probably as a result of the immaturity of their cell-mediated immune systems. By contrast, older persons fare much better.

Maturity, however, is not always an advantage in infections. Epstein-Barr virus (EBV) is more likely to cause symptomatic infections in adolescents and adults than in younger children. Varicella-zoster virus, the cause of chickenpox, produces more severe disease in adults, who are more likely to develop viral pneumonia.

The elderly fare more poorly with almost all infections than younger persons. Common respiratory illnesses such as influenza and pneumococcal pneumonia are more often fatal in those older than 65 years of age.

Human Behavior Plays a Large Role in Exposure to Infectious Agents

The link between behavior and infection is probably most obvious for sexually transmitted diseases. Syphilis, gonorrhea, urogenital chlamydial infections, AIDS and a number of other infectious diseases are transmitted primarily by sexual contact. The type and number of sexual encounters profoundly influence the risk of acquiring sexually transmitted diseases.

Other aspects of behavior also influence the risk of acquiring infections. Humans contract brucellosis and Q fever, which are primarily bacterial diseases of domesticated farm animals, by close contact with infected animals or their secretions. These infections occur in farmers, herders, meat processors and, in the case of brucellosis, in persons who drink unpasteurized milk. Transmission of a number of parasitic diseases is strongly affected by behavior. Schistosomiasis, acquired when water-borne infective parasite larvae penetrate the skin of a susceptible host, is primarily a disease of farmers who work in fields irrigated by infected water. In addition, children who swim in lakes and ponds containing these organisms become infected. The larvae of hookworm and *Strongyloides stercoralis* live in humid soil and penetrate the skin of the feet in people who walk barefoot. The introduction of shoes has probably been the single most important factor in reducing the prevalence of infection with soil-transmitted nematodes. Anisakiasis and diphyllobothriasis are helminthic diseases acquired by eating incompletely cooked fish. Toxoplasmosis is a protozoan infection transmitted from animals to humans by ingestion of incompletely cooked, infected meat or by exposure to infected cat feces. Botulism, a food poisoning caused by a bacterial toxin, is contracted by ingestion of improperly canned food that contains the toxin; by ingestion of spores often via honey by infants; or from inoculation of wounds by spores, which then germinate in devitalized tissue.

As humans change their behavior, they open up new possibilities for infectious diseases. Although the agent of Legionnaires disease is common in the environment, aerosols generated by cooling plants, faucets and humidifiers provide the means for causing human infections. Traditional behaviors are not necessarily health promoting. Hundreds of thousands of cases of neonatal tetanus in less developed countries are linked to coating umbilical stumps with dirt, dung or homemade cheese to stop bleeding. These materials do arrest the bleeding but often contain *Clostridium tetani* spores, which germinate and release the toxin that causes tetanus. In parts of Africa, numerous cases of cysticercosis are caused by ingesting locally prepared potions containing, among other ingredients, the stools of persons infected with *Taenia solium*.

People With Compromised Defenses Are More Likely to Contract Infections and to Have More Severe Infections

Disruption or absence of any of the complex host defenses results in increased numbers and severity of infections. Disruption of epithelial surfaces by trauma or burns can lead to invasive bacterial or fungal infections. Injury to the mucociliary apparatus of the airways, as in smoking or influenza, impairs clearance of inhaled microorganisms and leads to an increased incidence of bacterial pneumonia. Congenital absence of complement components C5, C6, C7 and C8 prevents formation of a fully functional membrane attack complex and permits disseminated, and often recurrent, *Neisseria* infections (see Chapter 2). Diseases such as diabetes mellitus and chemotherapeutic drugs may interfere with neutrophil production or function and increase the likelihood and severity of bacterial infection or invasive fungal infections (see Chapter 20).

Immunologically compromised states create diagnostic and therapeutic challenges and are the consequence of cytotoxic and immunosuppressive therapies, progress in prolonging longevity of debilitated persons and the explosion of the AIDS epidemic. In addition, burn and trauma units, transplantation centers and medical and surgical intensive care facilities are filled with patients whose primary conditions have left them insufficiently able to protect themselves from infections, by lacking the capacity to mount either inflammatory or immune responses. Compromised hosts become infected more easily and they are often attacked by organisms that are innocuous to normal persons. For example, patients deficient in neutrophils frequently develop life-threatening bloodstream infections with commensal microorganisms that normally populate the skin and gastrointestinal tract.

Such organisms that mainly cause disease in hosts with impaired defenses are **opportunistic pathogens.** Many of these are part of normal endogenous human or environmental microbial flora and take advantage of inadequate defenses to attack more violently and concertedly.

VIRAL INFECTIONS: INTRODUCTION

Viruses range from 20 to 300 nm and consist of RNA or DNA contained in a protein shell. Some are also enveloped in lipid membranes. ***Viruses do not engage in metabolism or reproduction independently, and thus are obligate intracellular parasites: they require living cells in order to replicate.*** After invading cells, they divert cells' biosynthetic and metabolic capacities to synthesizing virus-encoded nucleic acids and proteins.

Viruses often cause disease by killing infected cells, but many do not. For example, rotavirus, a common cause of diarrhea, interferes with the function of infected enterocytes without immediately killing them. It prevents enterocytes from synthesizing proteins that transport molecules from the intestinal lumen and thereby causes diarrhea.

Viruses may also promote the release of chemical mediators that elicit inflammatory or immunologic responses. The symptoms of the common cold are due to the release of bradykinin from infected cells. Other viruses cause cells to proliferate and form tumors. Human papillomaviruses (HPVs), for instance, cause squamous cell proliferative lesions, which include common warts and anogenital warts.

Some viruses infect and persist in cells without interfering with cellular functions, a process known as **latency**. Latent viruses can emerge to produce disease years after the primary infection. Opportunistic infections are frequently caused by viruses that have established latent infections. CMV and herpes simplex viruses are among the most frequent opportunistic pathogens because they are commonly present as latent agents and emerge in persons with impaired cell-mediated immunity.

Finally, some viruses may reside within cells, either by integrating into their genomes or by remaining episomal, and cause those cells to generate tumors. Examples of this are Epstein-Barr virus, which causes endemic Burkitt lymphoma in Africa and other tumors in different settings, and human T-cell leukemia virus-1 (HTLV-1, see Chapter 5), which causes a form of T-cell lymphoma.

This section is divided into diseases caused by RNA viruses and those caused by DNA viruses. This division reflects fundamental differences in the biology of these agents. Some viruses with highly organ-specific tropisms are not described here in detail, but are addressed in those chapters that deal with the organs that are principally affected: HIV (Chapter 4), hepatitis B and C (Chapter 14), etc.

VIRAL INFECTIONS: RNA VIRUSES

RNA viruses generally follow different paths to causing disease than do most DNA viruses: the enzymes needed for their infectious cycles may be vastly different, and important aspects of their biology do not have correlates among DNA viruses. Therefore, RNA viruses are treated as a separate category of disease-causing agent.

One of the key differences between some of these viruses and many DNA viruses is that the polymerases of some important pathogenic RNA viruses (e.g., HIV-1, hepatitis C virus [HCV]) do not proofread the strand being synthesized. This has two important consequences. First, the mutation rate—and thus the plasticity of these viruses in circumventing therapies—is very high. Second, a greater percentage of daughter virions are inactive.

Respiratory Viruses

The Common Cold Is the Most Common Viral Disease

The common cold (coryza) is an acute, self-limited upper respiratory tract disorder caused by infection with a variety of RNA viruses, including over 100 distinct rhinoviruses and several coronaviruses. Colds are frequent and worldwide in distribution. They spread from person to person via infected secretions. Infection is more likely during winter months in temperate areas and during the rainy seasons in the tropics, when spread is facilitated by indoor crowding. In the United States, children usually suffer six to eight colds per year and adults two to three.

The viruses infect the nasal respiratory epithelial cells, causing increased mucus production and edema. Rhinoviruses and coronaviruses have a tropism for respiratory epithelium and optimally reproduce at temperatures well below 37°C (98.6°F). Thus, infection remains confined to the cooler passages of the upper airway. Infected cells release chemical mediators, such as bradykinin, which produce most of the symptoms associated with colds: increased mucus production, nasal congestion and eustachian tube obstruction. Resulting stasis may predispose to secondary bacterial infection and lead to bacterial sinusitis and otitis media. Rhinoviruses and coronaviruses do not destroy respiratory epithelium and produce no visible alterations. Clinically, the common cold is characterized by rhinorrhea, pharyngitis, cough and low-grade fever. Symptoms last about a week.

Influenza May Predispose to Bacterial Pneumonia

Influenza is an acute, usually self-limited, infection of the upper and lower airways, caused by influenza virus. These viruses are enveloped and contain single-stranded RNA.

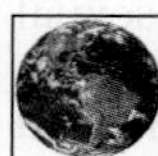

EPIDEMIOLOGY: There are three distinct types of influenza virus—types A, B and C—that cause human disease, but influenza A is by far the most common and causes the most severe disease. Ten to 40 million cases of influenza occur annually in the United States, accounting for over 35,000 deaths. Influenza is highly contagious, and epidemics often spread around the world. New strains emerge regularly, often from animal hosts; infect humans in parts of the world where humans and animals live in close contact; and then disseminate rapidly. Influenza strains are identified by their type (A, B, C) and the serotype of their hemagglutinin (H) and neuraminidase. Thus, the avian influenza virus ("bird flu") strain that emerged in 2003 and still continues to spread around the globe is designated A (H5N1). In 2009, a novel influenza A virus, designated H1N1 ("swine flu"), emerged in Veracruz, Mexico, and swiftly spread globally as a pandemic infection. The potential seriousness and rapidity of the H1N1 strain is evidenced by the occurrence of approximately 10,000 deaths in the United States alone within 7 months of its first being identified. This strain of influenza A virus has produced significant mortality in infected children and pregnant women. Because epidemic influenza virus antigens change so often, host immunity that develops during one epidemic rarely protects against the next one.

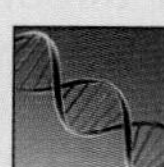

MOLECULAR PATHOGENESIS: Influenza spreads from person to person by virus-containing respiratory droplets and secretions. When it reaches the respiratory epithelial cell surface, the virus binds and enters the cell by fusion with the cell membrane, a process mediated by a viral glycoprotein (hemagglutinin) that binds to sialic acid residues on human respiratory epithelium. Once inside, the virus directs the cell to produce progeny viruses and causes cell death. Infection usually involves both the upper and lower airways. Destruction of ciliated epithelium cripples the mucociliary blanket, predisposing to bacterial pneumonia, especially with *Staphylococcus aureus* and *Streptococcus pneumoniae*.

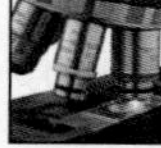

PATHOLOGY: Influenza virus causes necrosis and desquamation of ciliated respiratory tract epithelium, associated with a predominantly lymphocytic inflammatory infiltrate. Extension of the infection to the lungs leads to necrosis and sloughing of alveolar lining cells and the histologic appearance of viral pneumonitis.

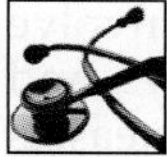
CLINICAL FEATURES: Rapid onset of fever, chills, myalgia, headaches, weakness and nonproductive cough are characteristic. Symptoms may be primarily those of an upper respiratory infection or those of tracheitis, bronchitis and pneumonia. Epidemics are accompanied by deaths from both influenza and its complications, particularly in the elderly and people with underlying cardiopulmonary disease. Killed viral vaccines specific to epidemic strains are 75% effective in preventing influenza.

Parainfluenza Virus Is Associated With Croup

The parainfluenza viruses cause acute upper and lower respiratory tract infections, particularly in young children. These enveloped, single-stranded, negative-sense RNA viruses are the most common cause of croup (laryngotracheobronchitis), which is characterized by stridor on inspiration and a "barking" cough.

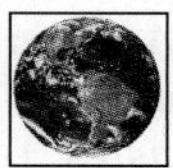
EPIDEMIOLOGY: This condition is common in children under the age of 3 years and is characterized by subglottic swelling, airway compression and respiratory distress. These viruses spread from person to person through infectious respiratory aerosols and secretions. Infection is highly contagious, and disease is present worldwide. The parainfluenza viruses are isolated from 10% of young children with acute respiratory tract illnesses.

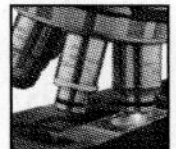
PATHOLOGY: Parainfluenza viruses infect and kill ciliated respiratory epithelial cells and elicit an inflammatory response. In very young children, this process frequently extends into the lower respiratory tract, causing bronchiolitis and pneumonitis. In young children, where the trachea is narrow and the larynx is small, the local edema of laryngotracheitis compresses the upper airway enough to obstruct breathing and cause croup. Parainfluenza infection is associated with fever, hoarseness and cough. A barking cough is characteristic, as is inspiratory stridor. In older children and adults, symptoms are usually mild.

Respiratory Syncytial Virus Causes Bronchiolitis in Infants

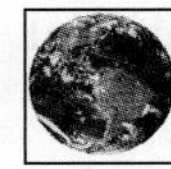
EPIDEMIOLOGY: Respiratory syncytial virus (RSV) belongs to the same family, Paramyxoviridae, as parainfluenza virus. It spreads rapidly from child to child in respiratory aerosols and secretions and is commonly disseminated in daycare centers, hospitals and other settings when small children are confined. The virus, which is present worldwide, is highly contagious, and most children have been infected with RSV by school age.

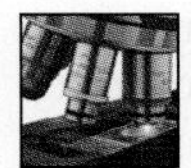
PATHOLOGY: Viral surface proteins interact with specific receptors on host respiratory epithelium to cause viral binding and fusion. RSV produces necrosis and sloughing of bronchial, bronchiolar and alveolar epithelium, associated with a predominantly lymphocytic inflammatory infiltrate. Multinucleated syncytial cells are sometimes seen in infected tissues.

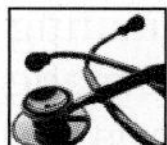
CLINICAL FEATURES: Infants and young children with RSV bronchiolitis or pneumonitis present with wheezing, cough and respiratory distress, sometimes accompanied by fever. The illness is usually self-limited, resolving in 1 to 2 weeks. In older children and adults, RSV produces much milder disease. Among otherwise healthy young children, mortality from RSV infection is very low, but it rises dramatically, up to 20% to 40%, among hospitalized children with congenital heart disease or immunosuppression.

Severe Acute Respiratory Syndrome Is an Emergent Viral Disease Causing Outbreaks of Pneumonia

In early 2002 an epidemic of severe pneumonia was traced to Guangdong Province of China. As outbreaks occurred in Hong Kong, Vietnam and Singapore, the disease swept around the globe via routes of international air travel. This emerging clinical disease, termed SARS, eventually spread to the United States, Canada and Europe. The causative agent is a novel coronavirus, termed the SARS-associated coronavirus (SARS-CoV), which derived from a nonhuman host, now felt most likely to be bats, with civets and other animals as likely intermediate hosts. SARS is a potentially fatal viral respiratory illness with an incubation period of 2 to 7 days, with cases ranging up to 10 days. While this initial pandemic was spreading globally between November 2002 and July 2003, there were over 8,000 known cases and up to 800 deaths, with a case fatality rate of 9.6%. Although the last infected human case occurred in mid-2003, the SARS-associated coronavirus has not been eradicated and has the potential to reemerge.

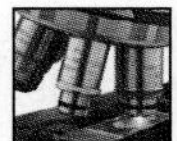
PATHOLOGY: Lungs of patients who died from SARS disclose diffuse alveolar damage (see Chapter 12). Multinucleated syncytial cells without viral inclusions have also been observed.

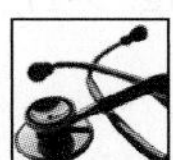
CLINICAL FEATURES: Clinically, SARS begins with fever and headache, followed shortly by cough and dyspnea. Coryza is often absent and diarrhea is quite common. Lymphopenia is common, and aminotransferase levels are modestly increased. Some patients develop acute respiratory distress syndrome (ARDS, see Chapter 12) and are at high risk of complications and death. Most patients recover, but mortality may reach 15% in the elderly and in patients with other respiratory disorders. No specific treatment is available, although corticosteroids may offer some benefit. Unfortunately, no data from controlled clinical trials are available.

Viral Exanthems

Measles (Rubeola) Is a Highly Contagious Virus That May Cause Fatal Infection

Measles virus is an enveloped, single-stranded RNA virus that causes an acute illness, characterized by upper respiratory tract symptoms, fever and rash.

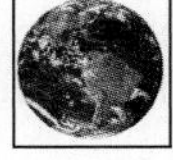
EPIDEMIOLOGY: Measles virus is transmitted to humans in respiratory aerosols and secretions. Among nonimmunized populations, measles is primarily a disease of children. Currently available live attenuated vaccines

are highly effective in preventing measles and in eliminating the spread of the virus. Nationwide immunizations have made measles uncommon in the United States. Similar efforts are under way worldwide to immunize all children.

Measles is a particularly severe disease in the very young, the sick or the malnourished. In impoverished countries, it has a high mortality rate (10% to 25%). It has been estimated to kill 1.5 million children yearly and remains a cause of major vaccine-preventable deaths worldwide. When measles was first introduced to previously unexposed populations (e.g., Native Americans, Pacific Islanders), the resulting widespread infections had devastatingly high mortality rates.

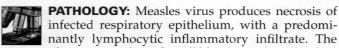

MOLECULAR PATHOGENESIS: The initial site of infection is the mucous membranes of the nasopharynx and bronchi. Two surface glycoproteins, designated "H" and "F" proteins, mediate viral attachment and fusion with respiratory epithelium. The virus then spreads to regional lymph nodes and the bloodstream, leading to widespread dissemination with prominent involvement of the skin and lymphoid tissues. The rash results from the action of T lymphocytes on virally infected vascular endothelium.

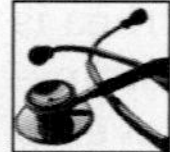

PATHOLOGY: Measles virus produces necrosis of infected respiratory epithelium, with a predominantly lymphocytic inflammatory infiltrate. The virus produces a vasculitis of small blood vessels in the skin. Lymphoid hyperplasia is often prominent in the cervical and mesenteric lymph nodes, spleen and appendix. In lymphoid tissues, the virus sometimes causes fusion of infected cells, producing multinucleated giant cells containing up to 100 nuclei, with both intracytoplasmic and intranuclear inclusions. These cells, **Warthin-Finkeldey giant cells** (Fig. 9-1), are pathognomonic for measles.

CLINICAL FEATURES: Measles first manifests with fever, rhinorrhea, cough and conjunctivitis and progresses to the characteristic mucosal and skin lesions.

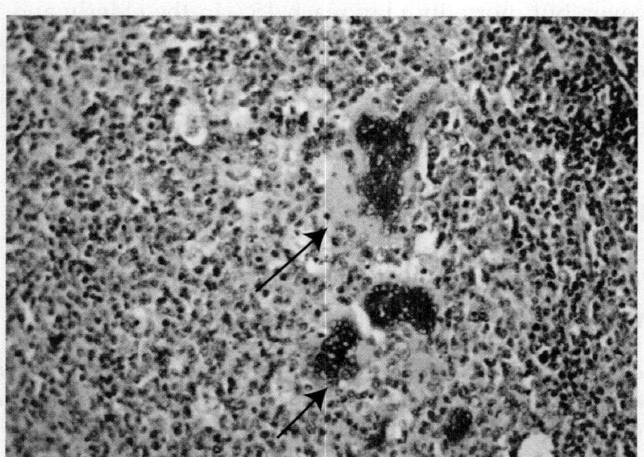

FIGURE 9-1. Warthin-Finkeldey giant cells in measles. A hyperplastic lymph node from a patient with measles shows several multinucleated giant cells (*arrows*).

The mucosal lesions, or "Koplik spots," are minute gray-white dots on a red base that appear on the posterior buccal mucosa. The skin lesions begin on the face as an erythematous maculopapular rash, which usually spreads to involve the trunk and extremities. The rash fades in 3 to 5 days, and symptoms gradually resolve. The clinical course of measles may be much more severe in very young children, malnourished persons or immunocompromised patients. Measles often leads to secondary bacterial infections, especially otitis media and pneumonia. Central nervous system invasion is probably a common event as suggested by changes in electroencephalograph readings. Acute encephalitis is rare but does occur. Uncommonly, patients can develop subacute sclerosing panencephalitis (SSPE), a slow, chronic neurodegenerative disorder that occurs years after a measles infection. The exact pathophysiology of SSPE is unclear, as there is no animal model, but prophylactic vaccination against measles has greatly reduced the incidence of SSPE.

Rubella Infection in Utero Is Associated with Congenital Anomalies

Rubella virus is an enveloped, single-stranded RNA virus that causes a mild, self-limited systemic disease, usually associated with a rash (also known as "German measles"). Many infections are so mild that they go unnoticed. However, in pregnant women, rubella is a destructive fetal pathogen. Infection early in gestation can produce fetal death, premature delivery and congenital anomalies, including deafness, cataracts, glaucoma, heart defects and mental retardation.

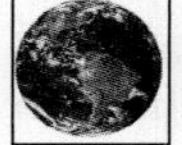

EPIDEMIOLOGY: Rubella virus spreads from person to person, primarily by the respiratory route. Infection occurs worldwide. Rubella is not highly contagious, and in unvaccinated populations, 10% to 15% of young women remain susceptible to infection into their reproductive years. The currently available live attenuated viral vaccine prevents rubella and has largely eliminated the disease from developed countries.

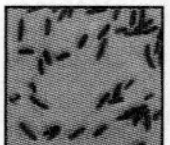

ETIOLOGIC FACTORS: Rubella infects respiratory epithelium, then disseminates through the bloodstream and lymphatics. The rubella rash is believed to result from an immunologic response to the disseminated virus. Fetal infection occurs through the placenta during the viremic phase of maternal illness. A congenitally infected fetus remains persistently infected and sheds large amounts of virus in body fluids, even after birth. Maternal infection after 20 weeks' gestation usually does not cause significant fetal disease.

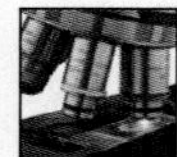

PATHOLOGY: In most patients, rubella is a mild, acute febrile illness, with rhinorrhea, conjunctivitis, postauricular lymphadenopathy and a rash that spreads from face to trunk and extremities. The rash resolves within 3 days; complications are rare. As many as 30% of infections are completely asymptomatic.

In the fetus, the heart, eye and brain are the organs most frequently affected. Cardiac lesions include pulmonary valvular stenosis, pulmonary artery hypoplasia, ventricular septal defects and patent ductus arteriosus. Cataracts, glaucoma and retinal defects may occur. Deafness is a common complication of fetal rubella. Severe brain involvement can produce microcephaly and mental retardation.

Mumps

Mumps virus is an enveloped, single-stranded RNA virus that causes an acute, self-limited systemic illness, characterized by parotid gland swelling and meningoencephalitis.

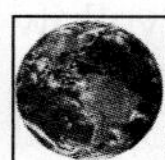

EPIDEMIOLOGY: Mumps is present worldwide and is primarily a disease of childhood. It spreads from person to person via the respiratory route. The virus is highly contagious, and 90% of exposed, susceptible persons become infected, although only 60% to 70% develop symptoms. A live attenuated mumps vaccine prevents mumps, and the disease has been largely eliminated from most developed countries.

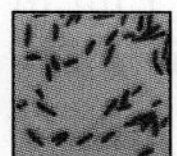

ETIOLOGIC FACTORS: Mumps begins with viral infection of respiratory tract epithelium. The virus then disseminates through the blood and lymphatic systems to other sites, most commonly the salivary glands (especially parotids), central nervous system (CNS), pancreas and testes. Over half of infections involve the CNS, with symptomatic disease in 10%. Epididymoorchitis occurs in 30% of males infected after puberty.

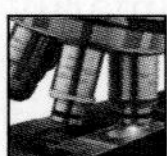

PATHOLOGY: Mumps virus causes necrosis of infected cells, associated with a predominantly lymphocytic inflammatory infiltrate. Affected salivary glands are swollen, their ducts lined by necrotic epithelium and their interstitium infiltrated with lymphocytes. In mumps epididymoorchitis, the testis can be swollen to three times normal size. The swelling of testicular parenchyma, confined within the tunica albuginea, produces focal infarctions. Mumps orchitis is usually unilateral and, thus, rarely causes sterility.

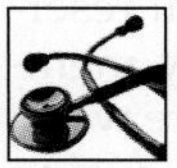

CLINICAL FEATURES: Mumps begins with fever and malaise, followed by painful swelling of the salivary glands, usually one or both parotids. Symptomatic meningeal involvement most often manifests as headache, stiff neck and vomiting. Prior to widespread vaccination, mumps was a leading cause of viral meningitis and encephalitis in the United States. Although severe disease of the pancreas is rare in mumps, most patients exhibit elevated serum amylase activity.

Intestinal Virus Infections

Rotavirus Infection Is the Most Common Cause of Severe Diarrhea Worldwide

Rotavirus produces profuse watery diarrhea that can lead to dehydration and death if untreated. This double-stranded RNA virus usually infects young children.

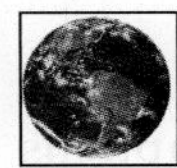

EPIDEMIOLOGY: Rotavirus infection spreads from person to person by the oral–fecal route. Infection is most common among children, who shed huge amounts of virus in the stool. Siblings, playmates, and parents as well as food, water and environmental surfaces are readily contaminated with virus. The peak age of infection is 6 months to 2 years, and virtually all children have been infected by the age of 4 years. In the United States, rotavirus causes about 100 deaths in young children and over 1 million deaths worldwide.

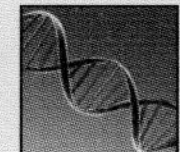

MOLECULAR PATHOGENESIS: Rotavirus infects enterocytes of the upper small intestine, disrupting absorption of sugars, fats and various ions. The resulting osmotic load causes a net loss of fluid into the bowel lumen, producing diarrhea and dehydration. Infected cells are shed from intestinal villi, and the regenerating epithelium initially lacks full absorptive capabilities.

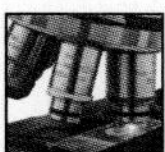

PATHOLOGY: Pathologic changes in rotavirus infection are largely confined to the duodenum and jejunum, where there is shortening of the intestinal villi and a mild infiltrate of neutrophils and lymphocytes.

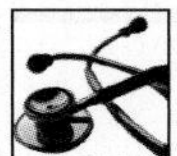

CLINICAL FEATURES: Rotavirus infection manifests as vomiting, fever, abdominal pain and profuse, watery diarrhea. The vomiting usually persists for 2 to 3 days, but diarrhea continues for 5 to 8 days. Without adequate fluid replacement, diarrhea can produce fatal dehydration in young children.

Norwalk Virus and Other Gastrointestinal Viruses Often Cause Outbreaks of Diarrhea

In addition to rotavirus, there are numerous other viral causes of diarrhea. The best understood are the Norwalk family of nonenveloped RNA viruses, a group of caliciviruses whose names derive from the locations of particular outbreaks (e.g., Norwalk virus, Snow Mountain virus, Sapporo virus). Norwalk viruses are responsible for one third of all outbreaks of diarrheal disease. They produce gastroenteritis in children and adults, with self-limited vomiting and diarrhea, similar to that caused by rotavirus. Norwalk viruses infect cells of the upper small bowel and produce changes similar to those that occur with rotavirus.

Viral Hemorrhagic Fevers

Viral hemorrhagic fevers are a group of at least 20 distinct viral infections that cause varying degrees of hemorrhage, shock and sometimes death. There are many similar viral hemorrhagic fevers in different parts of the world, usually named for the area where they were first described. The viral hemorrhagic fevers encompass members of four virus families—the Bunyaviridae, Flaviviridae, Arenaviridae and Filoviridae. On the basis of differences in routes of transmission, vectors and other epidemiologic characteristics, the viral hemorrhagic fevers have been divided into four epidemiologic groups (Table 9-3): mosquito-borne; tick-borne; zoonotic; and the filoviruses, Marburg and Ebola virus, in which the route of transmission is unknown.

Yellow Fever May Lead to Fulminant Hepatic Failure

Yellow fever is an acute hemorrhagic fever, sometimes associated with extensive hepatic necrosis and jaundice. The illness is caused by an insect-borne flavivirus, an enveloped,

Table 9-3

Viral Hemorrhagic Fevers

Vector	Viral Fever
Mosquitoes	Yellow fever Rift valley fever Dengue hemorrhagic fever Chikungunya hemorrhagic fever
Ticks	Omsk hemorrhagic fever Crimean hemorrhagic fever Kyasanur forest disease
Rodents	Lassa fever Bolivian hemorrhagic fever Argentine hemorrhagic fever Korean hemorrhagic fever
Fruit bats	Ebola virus disease

single-stranded RNA virus. Other pathogenic flaviviruses cause Omsk hemorrhagic fever and Kyasanur Forest disease.

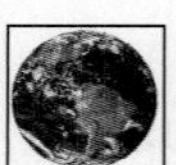

EPIDEMIOLOGY: Yellow fever was first recognized as a nosologic entity in the New World in the 17th century, but its origins probably were in Africa. Today, the virus is restricted to parts of Africa and South America, including both jungle and urban settings. The usual reservoir for the virus is tree-dwelling monkeys, the agent being passed among them in the forest canopy by mosquitoes. These monkeys serve as a reservoir because the virus neither kills them nor makes them ill. Humans acquire jungle yellow fever by entering the forest and being bitten by infected ***Aedes mosquitoes.*** Felling trees increases the risk of infection, because mosquitoes are brought down with the tree. On returning to the village or city, the human victim becomes a reservoir for epidemic yellow fever in the urban setting, where *Aedes aegypti* is the vector.

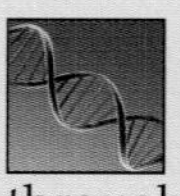

MOLECULAR PATHOGENESIS: On inoculation by the mosquito, the virus multiplies within tissue and vascular endothelium, then disseminates through the bloodstream. It has a tropism for liver cells, where it sometimes produces extensive acute hepatocellular destruction. Extensive damage to the endothelium of small blood vessels may lead to the loss of vascular integrity, hemorrhages and shock.

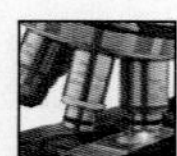

PATHOLOGY: Yellow fever virus causes coagulative necrosis of hepatocytes, which begins among cells in the middle of hepatic lobules and spreads toward the central veins and portal tracts. The infection sometimes produces confluent areas of necrosis in the middle of the hepatic lobules (i.e., midzonal necrosis). In the most severe cases, an entire lobule may be necrotic. Some necrotic hepatocytes lose their nuclei and become intensely eosinophilic. They often dislodge from adjacent hepatocytes, in which case they are known as Councilman bodies (recognized today as apoptotic bodies).

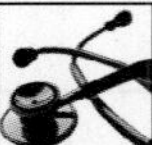

CLINICAL FEATURES: Yellow fever is characterized by abrupt onset of fever, chills, headache, myalgias, nausea and vomiting. After 3 to 5 days, some patients develop the signs of hepatic failure, with jaundice (hence the term "yellow" fever), deficiencies of clotting factors and diffuse hemorrhages. Vomiting of clotted blood ("black vomit") is a classic feature of severe cases of yellow fever. Patients with massive hepatic failure lapse into coma and die, usually within 10 days of onset of illness. Overall mortality of yellow fever is 5%, but among those with jaundice, it rises to 30%.

Ebola Hemorrhagic Fever Is a Fatal African Disease

Ebola virus is an RNA virus belonging to the Filoviridae. It causes a hemorrhagic disease with a high mortality rate in humans in several regions of Africa. The only other filovirus pathogenic to humans is the Marburg virus, which produces Marburg hemorrhagic fever.

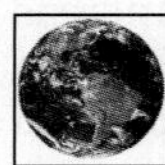

EPIDEMIOLOGY: Ebola virus first emerged in Africa with two major disease outbreaks that occurred almost simultaneously in Zaire and Sudan in 1976. Outbreaks of Ebola hemorrhagic fever have occurred in Africa up to the present time, and are primarily caused by the Ebola Zaire and Ebola Sudan strains. From 2000 to 2003, outbreaks of Ebola hemorrhagic fever caused by the Ebola Zaire strain of the virus occurred in Gabon, Republic of the Congo and Uganda. The case fatality rates ranged from 53% to 89%. In January 2008 a new strain of Ebola virus, the Ebola Bundibugyo strain, emerged in western Uganda.

In the wild, the virus infects humans, gorillas, chimpanzees and monkeys. Recent field evidence from Gabon and the Republic of the Congo area of western Africa has implicated several species of fruit bats as the natural reservoir of Ebola virus. Health care workers and family members have become infected as a result of viral exposure while treating patients with Ebola hemorrhagic fever or during funerary preparation of the bodies of deceased victims. The virus can be transmitted via bodily secretions, blood and used needles.

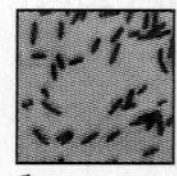
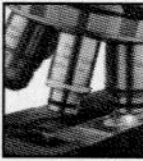

ETIOLOGIC FACTORS AND PATHOLOGY: ***Ebola virus results in the most widespread destructive tissue lesions of all viral hemorrhagic fever agents.*** The virus replicates massively in endothelial cells, mononuclear phagocytes and hepatocytes. Necrosis is most severe in the liver, kidneys, gonads, spleen and lymph nodes. The liver characteristically shows hepatocellular necrosis, Kupffer cell hyperplasia, Councilman bodies and microsteatosis. The lungs are usually hemorrhagic. Petechial hemorrhages are seen in the skin, mucous membranes and internal organs. Injury to the microvasculature and increased endothelial permeability are important causes of shock.

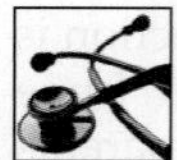

CLINICAL FEATURES: Ebola fever incubates from 2 to 21 days, after which initial symptoms include headache, weakness and fever followed by diarrhea, nausea and vomiting. Some patients develop overt hemorrhage including bleeding from injection sites, petechia, gastrointestinal bleeding and gingival hemorrhage.

West Nile Virus Is Spread by Mosquito Vectors and Birds

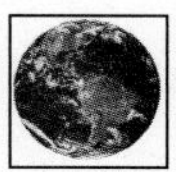

EPIDEMIOLOGY: The virus, a member of the family Flaviviridae, is increasing its geographic distribution as a result of spread by infected migratory birds and among arthropods transported between continents in pooled water in cargo ships. West Nile virus (WNV) was isolated in 1937 from the blood of a febrile woman in the West Nile region of Uganda. It has since spread rapidly through the Mediterranean and temperate parts of Europe. In 1999, WNV was first identified in the Western Hemisphere when it caused an outbreak of meningoencephalitis (West Nile fever) in New York City and the surrounding metropolitan area. In 2009, 663 cases of WNF infection and 30 fatalities were reported in 34 states in the United States. WNV has also emerged as a potential threat to the safety of blood products (109 positive blood donors in 2009).

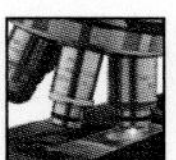

PATHOLOGY: WNV can be recovered from blood for up to 10 days in immunocompetent febrile patients, as late as 22 to 28 days after infection in immunocompromised patients. Laboratory findings include a slightly increased sedimentation rate and a mild leukocytosis; cerebrospinal fluid in patients with CNS involvement is clear, with moderate pleocytosis and elevated protein. Brains show mononuclear meningoencephalitis or encephalitis. The brainstem, particularly the medulla, can be extensively involved, and in some cases the cranial nerve roots had endoneural mononuclear inflammation. There are varying degrees of neuronal necrosis in gray matter, neuronal degeneration and neuronophagia.

CLINICAL FEATURES: Most human WNV infections are subclinical, overt disease occurring in only 1 of 100 infections. The incubation period ranges from 3 to 15 days. Symptoms, if they occur, usually consist of fever, often accompanied by rash, lymphadenopathy and polyarthropathy. Patients with severe illness can develop acute aseptic meningitis or encephalitis, with convulsions and coma. Anterior myelitis, hepatosplenomegaly, hepatitis, pancreatitis and myocarditis may develop. The probability of severe illness increases with increasing age. CNS infection is associated with a 4% to 13% mortality rate and is highest among elderly persons.

VIRAL INFECTIONS: DNA VIRUSES

Adenovirus

Adenoviruses are nonenveloped DNA viruses that are isolated from the respiratory and intestinal tracts of humans and animals. Certain serotypes are common causes of acute respiratory disease and adenovirus pneumonia in military recruits. Some adenoviruses are important causes of chronic pulmonary disease in infants and young children.

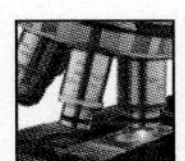

PATHOLOGY: Pathologic changes include necrotizing bronchitis and bronchiolitis, in which sloughed epithelial cells and inflammatory infiltrate may fill the damaged bronchioles. Interstitial pneumonitis is characterized by areas of consolidation with extensive necrosis, hemorrhage and a mononuclear inflammatory infiltrate. Two distinctive types of intranuclear inclusions—smudge cells and Cowdry type A inclusions—involve bronchiolar epithelial cells and alveolar lining cells. Adenoviruses types 40 and 41 infect colonic and small intestinal epithelial cells and may cause diarrhea in both immunocompetent and immunocompromised hosts. Patients with AIDS are particularly susceptible to urinary tract infections caused by adenovirus type 35.

Human Parvovirus B19

Human parvovirus B19 is a single-stranded DNA virus that causes a benign self-limited febrile illness in children known as **erythema infectiosum.** It also causes systemic infections characterized by rash, arthralgias and transient interruption in erythrocyte production in nonimmune adults.

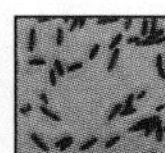

ETIOLOGIC FACTORS: Human parvovirus B19 spreads from person to person by the respiratory route. Infection is common and occurs in outbreaks, mostly among children. It is not known which cells, other than erythroid precursors, support virus replication, but the virus probably replicates in the respiratory tract before it spreads to erythropoietic cells.

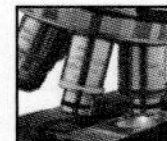

PATHOLOGY: Human parvovirus B19 gains entry to erythroid precursor cells via the P erythrocyte antigen and produces characteristic cytopathic effects in those cells. Nuclei of affected cells are enlarged, with the chromatin displaced peripherally by central glassy eosinophilic material nuclear inclusion bodies (giant pronormoblasts).

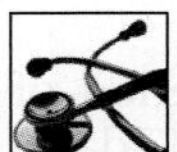

CLINICAL FEATURES: Most persons suffer a mild exanthematous illness, known as **erythema infectiosum ("fifth disease")**, accompanied by an asymptomatic interruption in erythropoiesis. In persons with chronic hemolytic anemias, however, the pause in erythrocyte production causes profound, potentially fatal anemia, known as **transient aplastic crisis** (see Chapter 20). When a fetus is infected by human parvovirus B19, transient cessation of erythropoiesis can lead to severe anemia, hydrops fetalis and death in utero, an outcome that occurs in about 10% of maternal infections.

Smallpox (Variola)

Smallpox is a highly contagious exanthematous viral infection produced by variola virus, a member of the family Poxviridae.

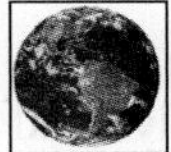

EPIDEMIOLOGY: Smallpox is an ancient disease: a rash resembling smallpox was found in the mummified remains of Egyptian pharaoh Ramses V, who died in 1160 BC. In the 6th century, a Swiss bishop named the etiologic agent of smallpox "variola" from the Latin *varius*, meaning "pimple" or "spot." The infection was common in Europe. It arrived in the New World with Spanish colonists, and often decimated native populations. In 1796, Edward Jenner performed the first successful vaccination when he inoculated a child with lymph from the hand of a milkmaid infected with cowpox. Once the cowpox pustule had regressed, Jenner challenged that child with smallpox and demonstrated that he was protected from the disease. In 1967, the WHO began its uniquely successful campaign to eradicate smallpox. The last occurrence of endemic smallpox was in Somalia in 1977, and the last reported human cases were laboratory-acquired infections in 1978. On May 8, 1980, the WHO declared that smallpox had been eradicated. Two known repositories of variola virus remain: one at the Centers for Disease Control and Prevention (CDC) in the United States and one at the Institute for Virus Preparation in Russia. There has been considerable vigilance to its reemergence, either naturally or as a bioweapon.

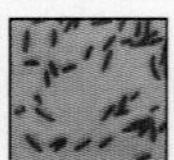

ETIOLOGIC FACTORS: Smallpox was transmitted between smallpox victims and susceptible persons via droplets or aerosol of infected saliva. Viral titers in the saliva were highest in the first week of infection. The virus is highly stable and remains infective for long periods outside its human host. Two types of smallpox have been recognized. *Variola major* was prevalent in Asia and parts of Africa and represented the prototypical form of the infection. *Variola minor* (or alastrim) was found in Africa, South America and Europe and was distinguished by its milder systemic toxicity and smaller pox lesions.

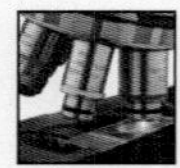

PATHOLOGY: Microscopically, skin vesicles of variola show reticular degeneration and scarce areas of ballooning degeneration. Eosinophilic, intracytoplasmic inclusion bodies (Guarnieri bodies) are seen, but are not specific for smallpox since they occur in most poxviral infections. Vesicles also occur in the palate, pharynx, trachea and esophagus. In severe cases of smallpox there is gastric and intestinal involvement, hepatitis and interstitial nephritis.

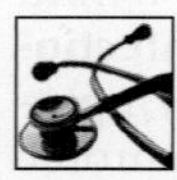

CLINICAL FEATURES: The incubation period of smallpox is approximately 12 days (range, 7 to 17 days) after exposure. After entering the respiratory tract, variola travels to regional lymph nodes, where replication occurs and results in viremia. Clinical manifestations begin abruptly with malaise, fever, vomiting and headache. The characteristic rash, most prominent on the face but also involving the hands and forearms, follows in 2 to 3 days. After subsequent eruptions on the lower extremities, the rash spreads centrally during the next week to the trunk. Lesions progress quickly from macules to papules, then to pustular vesicles (Fig. 9-2), and generally remain synchronous in their stage of development. By 8 to 14 days after onset, the pustules form scabs, which leave depressed scars on healing after 3 to 4 weeks. The case fatality rate is 30% in unvaccinated persons.

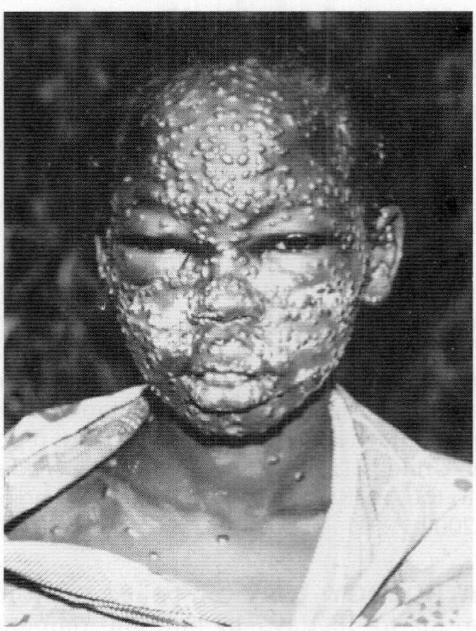

FIGURE 9-2. Child with smallpox, eastern Congo, 1968.

Monkeypox

Monkeypox, a rare viral disease occurring mostly in Central and Western Africa, is the only remaining potentially fatal infection of humans to be caused by a member of the family Poxviridae.

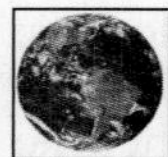

EPIDEMIOLOGY: The virus was first identified from monkeys, giving the agent its name, but it is actually more prevalent in rodents in endemic areas. It is mainly a zoonotic disease occurring in parts of Central and Western Africa. An outbreak occurred in the United States in 2003 in pet owners of prairie dogs that had been exposed to an infected Gambian pouched rat. Dormice and squirrels have also been implicated as natural reservoirs of the virus. Human infection can follow a bite from an infected host or contact with its body fluids. Human-to-human transmission is uncommon.

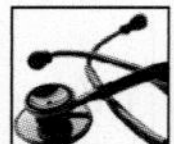

CLINICAL FEATURES: The incubation period in humans is approximately 12 days. Its clinical presentation is similar to smallpox, but milder. Illness begins with fever, headache, lymphadenopathy, malaise, muscle ache and back ache. Within 1 to 3 days after onset of fever, a papular rash occurs in the face or other body parts, which ultimately crusts and falls off. The illness typically lasts for 2 weeks. In Africa, the case fatality is as high as 10%.

Herpesviruses

The virus family Herpesviridae includes a large number of enveloped DNA viruses, many of which infect humans. Almost all herpesviruses express some common antigenic determinants, and many produce type A nuclear inclusions (acidophilic bodies surrounded by a halo). The most important pathogenic human herpesviruses are varicella-zoster, herpes simplex, EBV, human herpesvirus 6 (HHV6, the cause of roseola) and cytomegalovirus. Recently, human herpesvirus 8 (HHV8) was implicated in the pathogenesis of Kaposi sarcoma in HIV-infected patients. ***These viruses are distinguished by their capacity to remain latent for long periods of time.***

Varicella-Zoster Infection Causes Chickenpox and Herpes Zoster

First exposure to varicella-zoster virus (VZV) produces chickenpox, an acute systemic illness characterized by a generalized vesicular skin eruption (Fig. 9-3). The virus then becomes

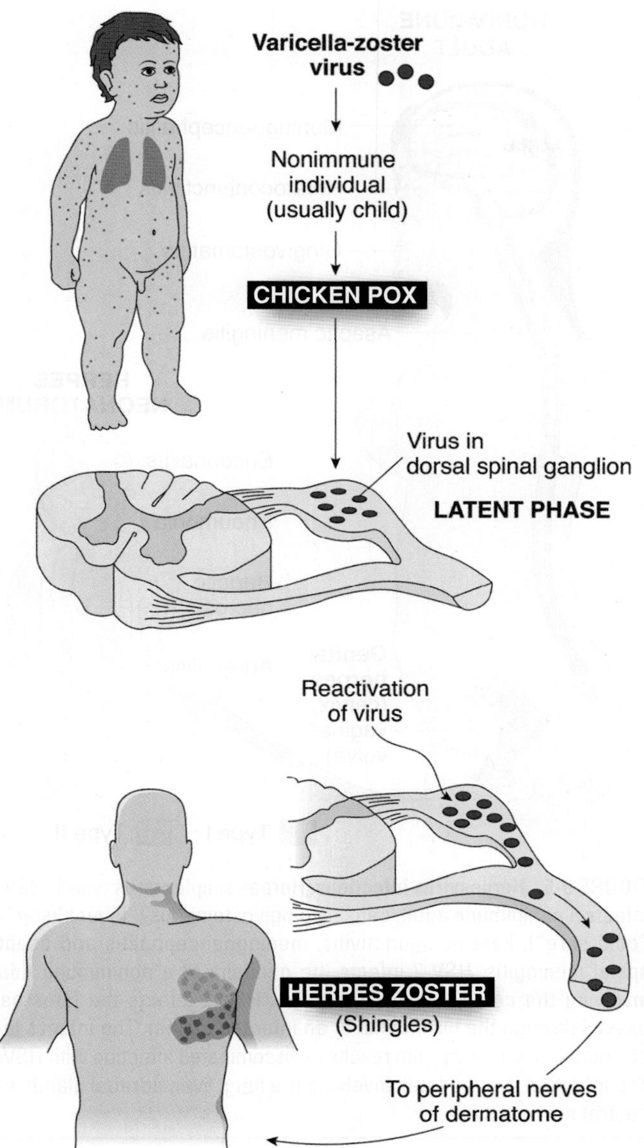

FIGURE 9-3. Varicella (chickenpox) and herpes zoster (shingles). Varicella-zoster virus (VZV) in droplets is inhaled by a nonimmune person (usually a child) and initially causes a "silent" infection of the nasopharynx. This progresses to viremia, seeding of fixed macrophages and dissemination of VZV to skin (chickenpox) and viscera. VZV resides in a dorsal spinal ganglion, where it remains dormant for many years. Latent VZV is reactivated and spreads from ganglia along the sensory nerves to the peripheral nerves of sensory dermatomes, causing shingles.

latent, and its reactivation causes herpes zoster ("shingles"), a localized vesicular skin eruption.

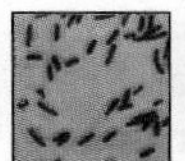 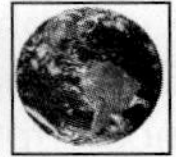

ETIOLOGIC FACTORS AND EPIDEMIOLOGY: VZV is restricted to human hosts and spreads from person to person primarily by the respiratory route. It can also be spread by contact with secretions from skin lesions. The virus is present worldwide and is highly contagious. Most children in the United States are infected by early school age, but an effective vaccine has reduced this incidence.

VZV initially infects cells of the respiratory tract or conjunctival epithelium. There it reproduces and spreads through the blood and lymphatic systems. Many organs are infected during this viremic stage, but skin involvement usually dominates the clinical picture. The virus spreads from the capillary endothelium to the epidermis, where its replication destroys the basal cells. As a result, the upper layers of the epidermis separate from the basal layer to form vesicles.

During primary infection, VZV establishes latent infection in perineuronal satellite cells of the dorsal nerve root ganglia. Transcription of viral genes continues during latency, and viral DNA can be demonstrated years after the initial infection.

Shingles occurs when full virus replication occurs in ganglion cells and the agent travels down the sensory nerve from a single dermatome. It then infects the corresponding epidermis, producing a localized, painful vesicular eruption. The risk of shingles in an infected person increases with age, and most cases occur among the elderly. Impaired cell-mediated immunity also increases the risk of herpes zoster reactivation.

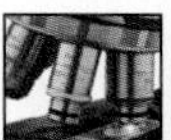

PATHOLOGY: The skin lesions of chickenpox and shingles are identical to each other and also to the lesions of herpes simplex virus (HSV). Vesicles fill with neutrophils and soon erode to become shallow ulcers. In infected cells, VZV produces a characteristic cytopathic effect, with nuclear homogenization and intranuclear inclusions (Cowdry type A). Inclusions are large and eosinophilic and are separated from the nuclear membrane by a clear zone (halo). Multinucleated cells are common (Fig. 9-4). Over several days, vesicles become pustules, then rupture and heal.

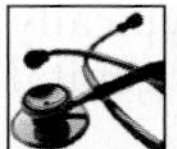

CLINICAL FEATURES: Chickenpox causes fever, malaise and a distinctive pruritic rash that starts on the head and spreads to the trunk and extremities. Skin lesions begin as maculopapules that rapidly evolve into vesicles, then pustules that soon ulcerate and crust. Vesicles may also appear on mucous membranes, especially the mouth. Fever and systemic symptoms resolve in 3 to 5 days; skin lesions heal in several weeks.

Shingles presents with a unilateral, painful, vesicular eruption, similar in appearance to chickenpox but in a dermatomal

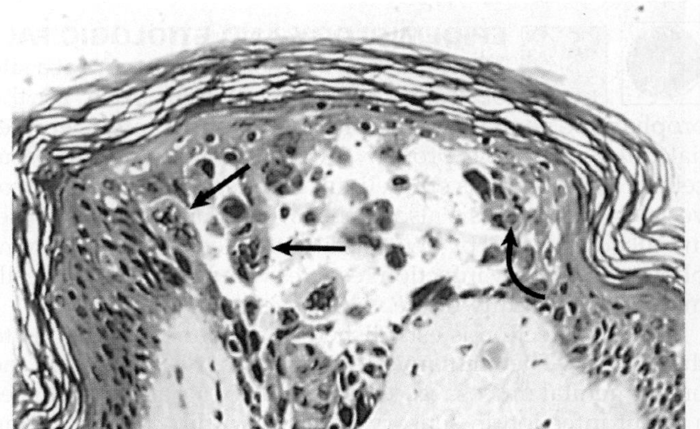

FIGURE 9-4. Varicella. Photomicrograph of the skin from a patient with chickenpox shows an intraepidermal vesicle. Multinucleated giant cells (*straight arrows*) and nuclear inclusions (*curved arrow*) are present.

Table 9-4

Herpes Simplex Viral Diseases

Viral Type	Common Presentations	Infrequent Presentations
HSV-1	Oral–labial herpes	Conjunctivitis, keratitis Encephalitis Herpetic whitlow Esophagitis* Pneumonia* Disseminated infection*
HSV-2	Genital herpes	Perinatal infection Disseminated infection*

*These conditions usually occur in immunocompromised hosts.

pattern, usually localized to a single dermatome. Pain can persist for months after resolution of the skin lesions.

Herpes Simplex Viruses Produce Recurrent Painful Vesicular Eruptions of the Skin and Mucous Membranes

HSVs are common human viral pathogens (Table 9-4). Two antigenically and epidemiologically distinct HSVs cause human disease (Fig. 9-5):

- **HSV-1** is transmitted in oral secretions and typically causes disease "above the waist," including oral, facial and ocular lesions.
- **HSV-2** is transmitted in genital secretions and typically produces disease "below the waist," including genital ulcers and neonatal herpes infection.

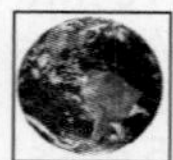

EPIDEMIOLOGY: HSV spreads from person to person, primarily through direct contact with infected secretions or open lesions. HSV-1 spreads in oral secretions, and infection frequently occurs in childhood, most persons (50% to 90%) being infected by adulthood. HSV-2 spreads by contact with genital lesions and is primarily a venereally transmitted pathogen. Neonatal herpes is acquired during birth, when a baby passes through an infected birth canal.

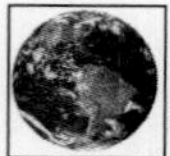

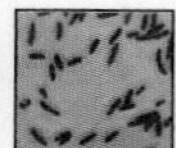

EPIDEMIOLOGY AND ETIOLOGIC FACTORS: Primary HSV disease occurs at a site of initial viral inoculation, such as the oropharynx, genital mucosa or skin. The virus infects epithelial cells, producing progeny viruses and destroying basal cells in the squamous epithelium, with resulting formation of vesicles. Cell necrosis also elicits an inflammatory response, initially dominated by neutrophils and then followed by lymphocytes. Primary infection resolves when humoral and cell-mediated immunity to the virus develop.

Latent infection is established in a manner analogous to that of VZV. The virus invades sensory nerve endings in the oral or genital mucosa, ascends within axons and establishes a latent infection in sensory neurons within corresponding ganglia. From time to time, this latent infection is reactivated, and HSV travels back down the nerve to the epithelial site served by the ganglion, where it again infects epithelial cells. Sometimes this secondary infection produces ulcerating vesicular lesions. At other times, the secondary infection does not cause visible tissue destruction, but contagious progeny viruses are shed from the site of infection. Various factors, usually typical for a given person, can induce reactivation of latent HSV infection. These include intense sunlight, emotional stress, febrile illness and, in women, menstruation. Both HSV-1 and HSV-2 can cause severe protracted and disseminated disease in immunocompromised persons.

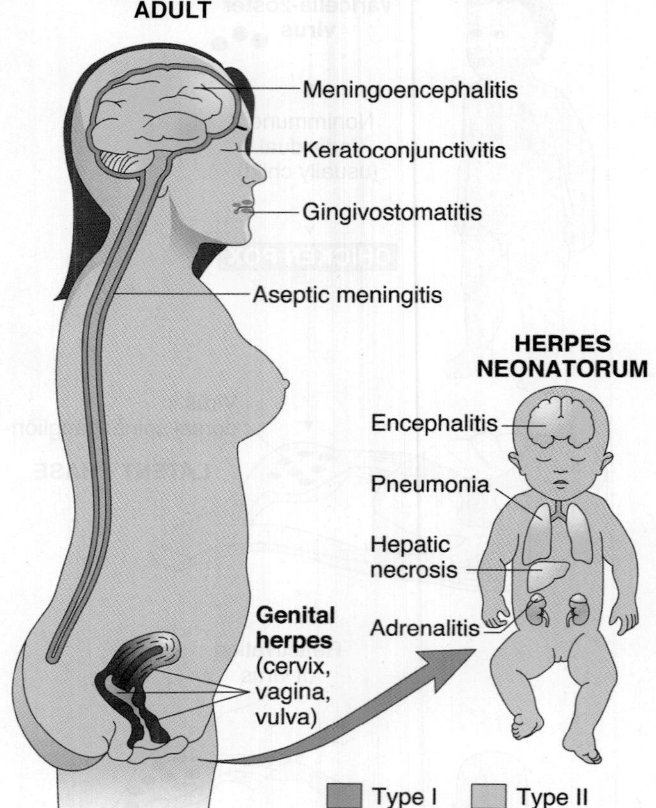

FIGURE 9-5. Herpesvirus infections. Herpes simplex virus type 1 (HSV-1) infects a nonimmune adult, causing gingivostomatitis ("fever blister" or "cold sore"), keratoconjunctivitis, meningoencephalitis and aseptic spinal meningitis. HSV-2 infects the genitalia of a nonimmune adult, involving the cervix, vagina and vulva. HSV-2 infects the fetus as it passes through the birth canal of an infected mother. The infant's lack of a mature immune system results in disseminated infection with HSV-1. The infection is often fatal, involving the lung, liver, adrenal glands and central nervous system.

Herpes encephalitis is a rare (1 in 100,000 HSV infections), but devastating, manifestation of HSV-1 infection. In some instances, it occurs when virus, latent in the trigeminal ganglion, is reactivated and travels retrograde to the brain. However, herpes encephalitis also occurs in persons who have no history of "cold sores," and the pathogenesis of the encephalitis in these cases is poorly understood (see Chapter 28). Equally rare is **herpes hepatitis,** which may occur in immunocompromised patients but is also seen in previously healthy pregnant women.

Neonatal herpes is a serious complication of maternal genital herpes. The virus is transmitted to the fetus from the infected birth canal, often the uterine cervix, and readily disseminates in the unprotected newborn child.

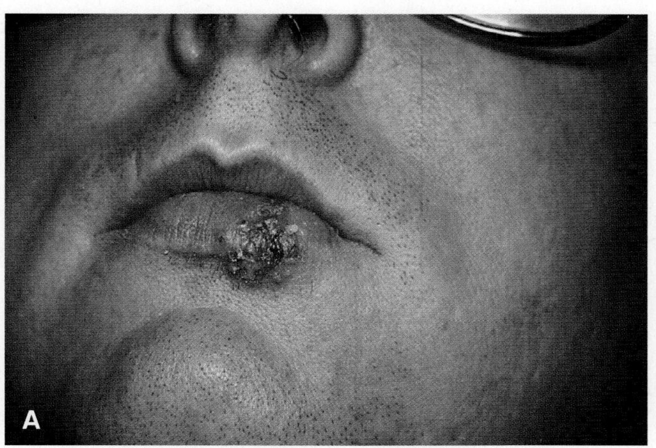

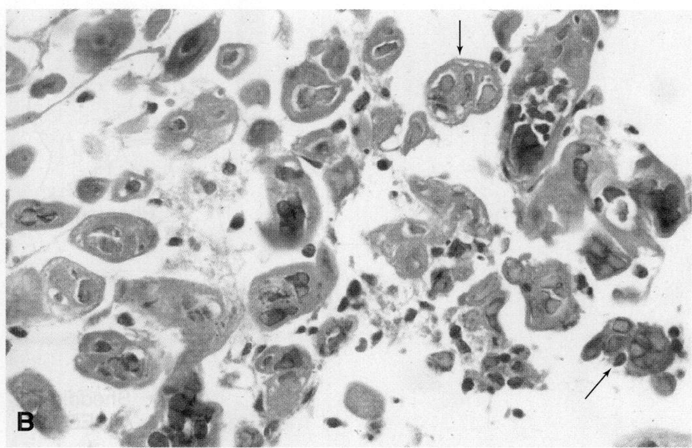

FIGURE 9-6. Herpes simplex, type 1. A. Herpetic vesicles are seen on the surface of the lower lip. **B.** Epithelial cells infected with HSV-1 demonstrate Cowdry type A intranuclear inclusions (*arrows*) and multinucleated giant cells.

Aseptic meningitis without genital involvement may be a manifestation of HSV-2 infection.

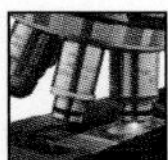

PATHOLOGY: The skin and mucous membranes are the usual sites of HSV infection, but the disease sometimes involves the brain, eye, liver, lungs and other organs. In any location, both HSV-1 and HSV-2 cause necrosis of infected cells, accompanied by a vigorous inflammatory response. Clusters of painful ulcerating vesicular lesions on the skin or mucous membranes are the most frequent manifestation of HSV infection (Fig. 9-6A). These lesions persist for 1 to 2 weeks and then resolve. The cellular alterations include (1) nuclear homogenization, (2) Cowdry type A intranuclear inclusions and (3) multinucleated giant cells (Fig. 9-6B).

CLINICAL FEATURES: Clinical features of HSV infections vary according to host susceptibility (e.g., neonate, normal host, compromised host), viral type and site of infection. A prodromal "tingling" sensation at the site often precedes the appearance of skin lesions. Recurrent lesions appear weeks, months or years later, at the initial site or at a site subserved by the same nerve ganglion. Recurrent herpetic lesions in the mouth or on the lip, commonly called "cold sores" or "fever blisters," frequently appear after sun exposure, trauma or a febrile illness.

Patients with AIDS and other immunocompromised persons are prone to develop herpes esophagitis. Early lesions consist of rounded 1- to 3-mm vesicles located predominantly in the mid- to distal esophagus. As the HSV-infected squamous cells slough from these lesions, sharply demarcated ulcers with elevated margins form and coalesce. This process may result in denudation of the esophageal mucosa. Superimposed *Candida* infection is common at this stage. In immunocompromised patients, HSV may also infect the anal mucosa, where it causes painful blisters and ulcers.

Neonatal herpes begins 5 to 7 days after delivery, with irritability, lethargy and a mucocutaneous vesicular eruption. The infection rapidly spreads to involve multiple organs, including the brain. The infected newborn develops jaundice, bleeding problems, respiratory distress, seizures and coma. Treatment of severe HSV infections with acyclovir is often effective, but neonatal herpes still carries a high mortality.

Epstein-Barr Virus

Infectious mononucleosis is a viral disease characterized by fever, pharyngitis, lymphadenopathy and increased circulating lymphocytes. By adulthood, most people have been infected with EBV. Most EBV infections are asymptomatic, but EBV may cause infectious mononucleosis. It is also associated with several cancers, including African Burkitt lymphoma, B-cell lymphoma in immunosuppressed patients and nasopharyngeal carcinoma. These neoplastic complications are discussed in Chapters 20 and 25.

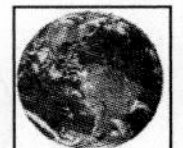

EPIDEMIOLOGY: In areas of the world where children often live in crowded conditions, infection with EBV usually occurs before 3 years of age, and infectious mononucleosis is not encountered. In developed countries, many people remain uninfected into adolescence or early adulthood. Two thirds of those newly infected after childhood develop clinically evident infectious mononucleosis.

EBV spreads from person to person primarily through contact with infected oral secretions (Fig. 9-7). Once it enters the body, EBV remains for life, analogous to latent infections with other herpesviruses. A few people (10% to 20%) shed the virus intermittently. Transmission requires close contact with infected persons. Thus, EBV spreads readily among young children in crowded conditions, where there is considerable "sharing" of oral secretions. Kissing is also an effective mode of transmission, hence the term "kissing disease."

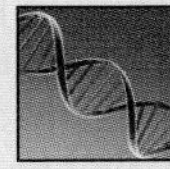

MOLECULAR PATHOGENESIS: The virus first binds to and infects nasopharyngeal cells and then B lymphocytes, which carry the virus throughout the body, producing a generalized infection of lymphoid tissues.

EBV is a polyclonal activator of B cells. In turn, activated B cells stimulate proliferation of specific killer T lymphocytes and suppressor T cells. The former destroy virally infected B cells, whereas suppressor cells inhibit production of immunoglobulins by B cells. The virus is also implicated in Burkitt lymphoma (see Chapters 5 and 20).

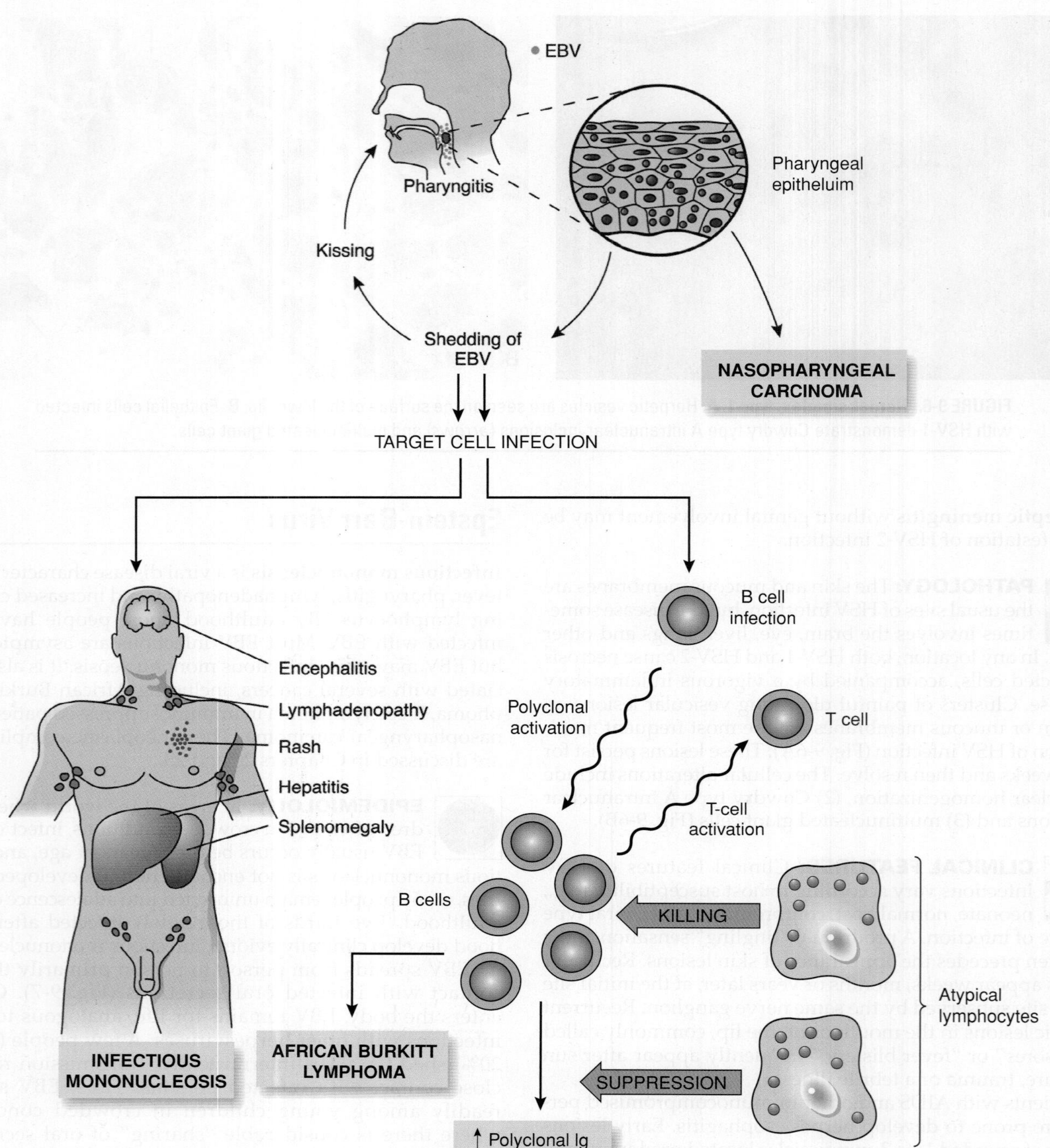

FIGURE 9-7. Role of Epstein-Barr virus (EBV) in infectious mononucleosis, nasopharyngeal carcinoma and Burkitt lymphoma. EBV invades and replicates within the salivary glands or pharyngeal epithelium and is shed into the saliva and respiratory secretions. In some persons, the virus transforms pharyngeal epithelial cells, leading to nasopharyngeal carcinoma. In persons who are not immune from childhood exposure, EBV causes infectious mononucleosis. EBV infects B lymphocytes, which undergo polyclonal activation. These B cells stimulate the production of atypical lymphocytes, which kill virally infected B cells and suppress the production of immunoglobulins. Some infected B cells are transformed into immature malignant lymphocytes of Burkitt lymphoma.

PATHOLOGY: The pathology of infectious mononucleosis involves the lymph nodes and spleen prominently. In most patients, lymphadenopathy is symmetric and most striking in the neck. The nodes are movable, discrete and tender. Microscopically, the general architecture is preserved. Germinal centers are enlarged and have indistinct margins, because of proliferation of immunoblasts. The nodes contain occasional large hyperchromatic cells with polylobular nuclei that resemble Reed-Sternberg cells of Hodgkin disease. Lymph node histology may be difficult to distinguish from Hodgkin disease or other lymphomas (see Chapter 20).

The spleen is large and soft, as a result of hyperplasia of the red pulp, and is susceptible to rupture. Immunoblasts are abundant and infiltrate vessel walls, the trabeculae and the capsule. The liver is almost always involved, with sinusoids and portal tracts containing atypical lymphocytes.

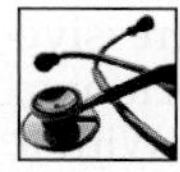

CLINICAL FEATURES: Infectious mononucleosis is characterized by lymphocytosis with **atypical lymphocytes.** These are activated T cells with lobulated, eccentric nuclei and vacuolated cytoplasm, and are involved in suppression and killing of EBV-infected B lymphocytes. Patients with infectious mononucleosis develop a specific **heterophile antibody**—that is, an immunoglobulin produced in one species that reacts with antigens of another species—known as the Paul Bunnell antibody. These antibodies in infectious mononucleosis are detected by their affinity for sheep erythrocytes. This heterophile reaction is a standard diagnostic test for infectious mononucleosis. Specific serologic tests for antibodies against EBV and for EBV antigens are also available.

Infectious mononucleosis manifests as fever, malaise, lymphadenopathy, pharyngitis and splenomegaly. Patients usually have elevated leukocyte counts, with a predominance of lymphocytes and monocytes. Treatment is supportive; symptoms usually resolve in 3 to 4 weeks.

Cytomegalovirus

CMV is a congenital and opportunistic pathogen that usually produces asymptomatic infection. However, the fetus and immunocompromised patients are particularly vulnerable to its destructive effects. CMV infects 0.5% to 2.0% of all fetuses and injures 10% to 20% of those infected, making it the most common congenital pathogen.

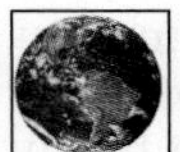

EPIDEMIOLOGY: CMV spreads from person to person by contact with infected secretions and bodily fluids, and is transmitted to the fetus across the placenta. Children spread it in saliva or urine, while transmission among adolescents and adults is primarily through sexual contact.

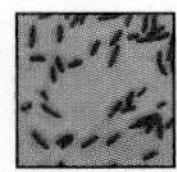

ETIOLOGIC FACTORS: CMV infects various human cells, including epithelial cells, lymphocytes and monocytes, and establishes latency in white blood cells. Normal immune responses rapidly control infection and ill effects are rare. However, virus is shed periodically in body secretions. Like other herpesviruses, CMV may remain latent for life.

When an infected pregnant woman passes CMV to her fetus, the fetus is not protected by maternally derived antibodies and the virus invades fetal cells with little initial immunologic response, causing widespread necrosis and inflammation. The virus produces similar lesions in persons with suppressed cell-mediated immunity.

CMV infection is often symptomatic in immunosuppressed persons, such as organ transplant recipients. In that setting, the CMV infection usually represents reactivation of endogenous latent infection, whether the source is the graft or the recipient. Subsequent dissemination may lead to severe systemic disease.

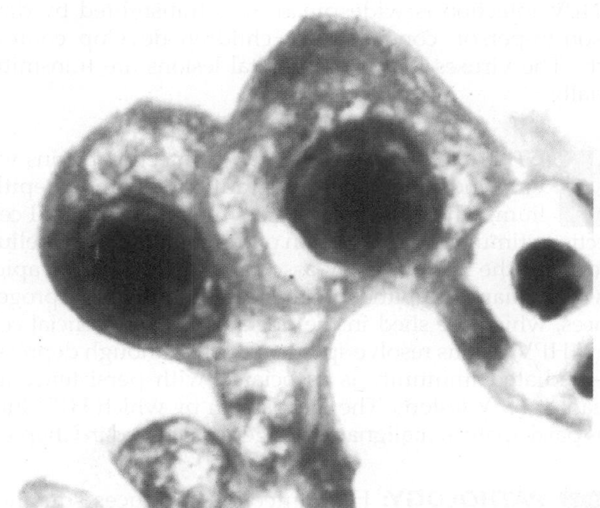

FIGURE 9-8. Cytomegalovirus pneumonitis. Type II pneumocytes display enlarged nuclei containing solitary inclusions surrounded by a clear zone.

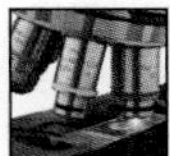

PATHOLOGY: CMV disease of the fetus most commonly involves the brain, inner ears, eyes, liver and bone marrow. Severely affected fetuses may have microcephaly, hydrocephalus, cerebral calcifications, hepatosplenomegaly and jaundice. Microscopically, lesions of fetal CMV disease show cellular necrosis and a characteristic cytopathic effect, consisting of marked cellular and nuclear enlargement, with nuclear and cytoplasmic inclusions. The giant nucleus, which is usually solitary, contains a large central inclusion surrounded by a clear zone (Fig. 9-8). The cytoplasmic inclusions are less prominent.

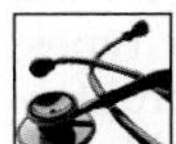

CLINICAL FEATURES: Congenitally acquired CMV has diverse clinical presentations. Severe disease causes fetal death in utero, conspicuous CNS lesions, liver disease and bleeding problems. However, most congenital CMV infections do not produce gross abnormalities, but manifest as subtle neurologic or hearing defects, which may not be detected until later in life.

CMV disease in immunosuppressed patients has a wide range of clinical manifestations. It can manifest as decreased visual acuity (chorioretinitis), diarrhea or gastrointestinal hemorrhage (colonic ulcerations), change in mental status (encephalitis), shortness of breath (pneumonitis) or any number of other symptoms.

Human Papillomavirus

HPVs cause proliferative lesions of squamous epithelium, including common warts, flat warts, plantar warts, and anogenital warts (condyloma acuminatum), as well as laryngeal papillomatosis. Some HPV serotypes cause squamous cell dysplasias and squamous cell carcinomas of the genital tract (see Chapter 18).

HPVs are nonenveloped, double-stranded DNA viruses. Over 100 types of HPV are known, different ones being associated with different lesions. Thus, HPV types 1, 2 and 4 produce common warts and plantar warts. Types 6, 10, 11 and 40 through 45 cause anogenital warts. Types 16, 18 and 31 are associated with squamous carcinomas of the female genital tract.

HPV infection is widespread. It is transmitted by direct person-to-person contact. Most children develop common warts. The viruses that cause genital lesions are transmitted sexually.

ETIOLOGIC FACTORS: HPV infection begins with viral inoculation into a stratified squamous epithelium, where the virus enters the nuclei of basal cells. Infection stimulates proliferation of the squamous epithelium, producing the various HPV-associated lesions. The rapidly growing squamous epithelium replicates innumerable progeny viruses, which are shed in the degenerating superficial cells. Many HPV lesions resolve spontaneously, although depressed cell-mediated immunity is associated with persistence and spread of HPV lesions. The mechanism by which HPV infections participate in malignant change is discussed in Chapter 5.

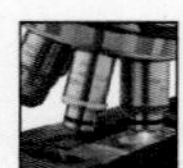

PATHOLOGY: HPV infection produces squamous proliferations, which vary in appearance and biological behavior. Most lesions show thickening of the affected epithelium as a result of enhanced squamous cell proliferation. Some HPV-infected cells display a characteristic cytopathic effect, **koilocytosis,** which features large squamous cells with shrunken nuclei enveloped in large cytoplasmic vacuoles (koilocytes).

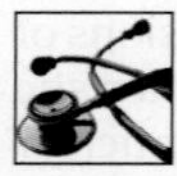

CLINICAL FEATURES: Common warts (verruca vulgaris) are firm, circumscribed, raised, rough-surfaced lesions, which usually appear on surfaces subject to trauma, especially the hands (see Chapter 24). **Plantar warts** are similar squamous proliferative lesions on the soles of the feet but are compressed inward by standing and walking.

Anogenital warts (condyloma acuminatum) are soft, raised, fleshy lesions found on the penis, vulva, vaginal wall, cervix or perianal region. When caused by certain HPV types, flat warts can evolve into malignant squamous cell proliferations. The relationship between HPV, cervical intraepithelial neoplasia (CIN) and invasive squamous carcinoma of the cervix is discussed in Chapter 18.

PRION DISEASES

In the last several decades it has become clear that infection can be transmitted and propagated solely by proteins and without nucleic acids. Despite considerable resistance to this disease paradigm, it is clear that filterable particles that lack nucleic acids can transmit disease. To date, these particles, prions, are only known to cause CNS disease. Prions are essentially misfolded proteins that aggregate in the CNS and cause progressive neurodegeneration that leads to death. The prion protein (PrP) exists in a normal isoform and in a pathogenic form that may be transmissible. These pathogenic isoforms aggregate into prion rods, which are characteristic of these rare disorders. Of particular importance is the uncommon persistence of these infectious agents that are highly resistant to normal methods of sterilization and may be transmitted via surgical instruments or electrodes when implanted in nervous tissue, unless special protocols are followed. The mechanisms of prion-associated diseases are discussed more fully in Chapter 28.

- **Kuru:** The prototypical prion disease for humans is kuru, a progressive neurodegenerative disease that was only found in the South Fore tribe in the remote highlands of Papa New Guinea. *Kuru*, the Fore word for "trembling," was transmitted via cannibalism. Experimental transmission of kuru has been accomplished using tissue from kuru victims to pass the infection to nonhuman primates. Once funerary cannibalism among the Fore was eliminated, kuru disappeared within a generation.
- **Sporadic, familial and iatrogenic Creutzfeldt-Jakob disease** (sCJD, fCJD and iCJD): CJD is a rapidly progressive neurodegenerative disorder characterized by myoclonus, behavior changes and dementia (see Chapter 28). With a frequency of 1/1,000,000, sCJD is probably the most common human prion disease. Rarely, CJD has resulted from transmission through transplanting such tissues as cornea and dural matter. Before the advent of recombinant protein therapeutics, CJD was also transmitted from human growth hormone isolated from human cadaver pituitaries.
- **New Variant Creutzfeldt-Jakob disease** (vCJD): One of the more infamous emerging infectious diseases of the last few decades, both vCJD and the associated bovine spongiform encephalopathy (BSE), also known as "mad cow" disease, underscore the interrelatedness of animal and human infectious agents. The use of certain animal products in feeds for domestic ungulates led to and amplified a prion disease epidemic in cattle herds of the United Kingdom. Nearly 150 persons are known to have been infected with this relentless terminal disease. All patients to date have an uncommon genetic homozygosity: methionine-methionine at codon 129 of the gene (PRNP) that encodes for the prion protein. Presentations have varied from the previously recognized forms of CJD in a number of important ways, with age of onset being most notable. While the mean onset of CJD has been 65 years of age, vCJD has mainly occurred in young adults, with a mean age of 26 years. Psychiatric signs and symptoms have also been predominant in vCJD. Pathologic changes in vCJD are strikingly similar to those seen in BSE and differ somewhat from changes seen in the sporadic form.
- **Fatal familial insomnia:** This is a rare inherited prion disorder that has as its hallmark a progressive course of insomnia that worsens over time until the patient barely sleeps or does not sleep at all. There is also autonomic instability that usually manifests as what appears to be increased sympathetic tone. Altered sensorium may also be present, and signs of motor system degeneration follow. Spongiform changes like those seen in other transmissible spongiform encephalopathies are also seen later in the disease.
- **Gerstmann-Straüssler-Scheinker syndrome:** This is another rare transmissible spongiform encephalopathy that is usually familial, although rare sporadic cases have been described. Patients may present with a variety of symptoms but signs and symptoms of cerebellar degeneration usually predominate. Later in the course dementia may, and often does, become a common feature.

BACTERIAL INFECTIONS

Bacteria, at 0.1 to 10 μm, are the smallest living cells. They have three basic structural components: nuclear body, cytosol and envelope. The **nuclear body** consists of a single, coiled circular molecule of double-stranded DNA with associated RNA and proteins. It is not separated from the cytoplasm by a special membrane, a feature that distinguishes bacteria as prokaryotes instead of eukaryotes. The **cytosol** is densely packed with ribosomes, proteins and carbohydrates and lacks the structured organelles, such as mitochondria and Golgi apparatus, of eukaryotic cells. The **bacterial envelope** is a permeability barrier and is also actively involved in transport, protein synthesis, energy generation, DNA synthesis and cell division.

Bacteria are classified according to the structural features of their envelope. The simplest envelope is only a phospholipid–protein bilayer membrane. Mycoplasmas have such an envelope. Most bacteria, however, have a rigid cell wall that surrounds the cell membrane. Two types of bacterial cell walls are identified by their Gram stain properties:

- **Gram-positive bacteria** retain iodine–crystal violet complexes when decolorized and appear dark blue. Their cell walls contain teichoic acids and a thick peptidoglycan layer.
- **Gram-negative bacteria** lose the iodine–crystal violet stain when decolorized and appear red with a counterstain. Outer membranes of gram-negative bacteria contain a lipopolysaccharide component, known as endotoxin, that is a potent mediator of the shock that complicates infections with these organisms.

Both gram-positive and gram-negative cell walls may be surrounded by an additional layer of polysaccharide or protein gel, a **capsule.** Capsules aid in bacterial attachment and colonization, and may protect bacteria from phagocytosis. Because capsules are important in many infections, bacteria may be classified as **encapsulated** or **unencapsulated.**

The cell wall confers rigidity to bacteria and allows them to be distinguished on the basis of shape and pattern of growth in cultures. Round or oval bacteria are **cocci.** Those that grow in clusters are called **staphylococci,** while those that grow in chains are called **streptococci.** Elongate bacteria are **rods,** or **bacilli,** and curved ones are **vibrios.** Some spiral-shaped bacteria are called **spirochetes.**

Most bacteria can be cultured on chemical media, and so may be described according to their growth requirements on these media. Bacteria that need high levels of oxygen are called **aerobic,** those that grow best without oxygen are **anaerobic** and those that thrive with limited oxygen are **microaerophilic.** Bacteria that grow well with or without oxygen are **facultative anaerobes.**

BACTERIAL EXOTOXINS: Many bacteria secrete toxins (exotoxins) that damage human cells either at the site of bacterial growth or at distant sites. These toxins are often named for the site or mechanism of their activity. Thus, those that act on the nervous system are called **neurotoxins;** those that affect intestinal cells are termed **enterotoxins.** Some toxins that kill target cells, such as diphtheria toxin or some of the *Clostridium perfringens* toxins, are called **cytotoxins.** Others may disturb normal functions of their target cells and damage or kill them, like the diarrheagenic toxin of *Vibrio cholerae* or the neurotoxin of *Clostridium botulinum*. *C. perfringens* produces over 20 toxins that damage the human body in diverse ways.

BACTERIAL ENDOTOXINS: As mentioned above, gram-negative bacteria contain a structural element called **lipopolysaccharide,** or **endotoxin,** in their outer membranes. Lipopolysaccharide activates complement, coagulation, fibrinolysis and bradykinin systems. It also causes release of primary inflammatory mediators, including tumor necrosis factor (TNF) and interleukin-1 (IL-1), and various colony-stimulating factors. Endotoxin may cause shock, complement depletion and disseminated intravascular coagulation.

Many bacteria damage tissues by eliciting inflammatory or immune responses. The capsule of *S. pneumoniae* protects it from phagocytosis while activating a host's inflammatory response. Within the lung, the encapsulated organism causes exudation of fluid and cells that fills alveoli. This inflammation impairs breathing but does not, at least initially, limit the organism's proliferation. *Treponema pallidum,* the spirochete that causes syphilis, persists in the body for years and elicits inflammatory and immune responses that continuously damage host tissues.

Many common bacterial infections (e.g., *S. aureus* skin infections) are characterized by purulent exudates, but tissue responses to bacteria are highly variable. In some cases, such as cholera, botulism and tetanus, there is no inflammatory response at critical sites of cellular injury. Other bacterial infections, including syphilis and Lyme disease, lead to a predominantly lymphocytic and plasma cellular response. Still others (e.g., brucellosis) are characterized by granuloma formation.

Many bacterial diseases are caused by organisms that normally inhabit the human body. The gastrointestinal tract, upper respiratory tract, skin and vagina are all home to diverse bacteria. These microorganisms are normally commensal and cause no harm. However, if they gain access to usually sterile sites or if host defenses are impaired, they can cause extensive destruction. *S. aureus, S. pneumoniae* and *Escherichia coli* are normal flora that are also major human pathogens.

Pyogenic Gram-Positive Cocci

Staphylococcus aureus Produces Suppurative Infections

S. aureus is a gram-positive coccus that typically grows in clusters and is among the most common bacterial pathogens. It normally resides on the skin and is readily inoculated into deeper tissues, where it causes suppurative infections. ***In fact, it is the most common cause of suppurative infections of the skin, joints and bones and is a leading cause of infective endocarditis.*** *S. aureus* is commonly distinguished from other, less virulent staphylococci by the coagulase test. *S. aureus* is coagulase positive; the other staphylococci are coagulase negative.

S. aureus spreads by direct contact with colonized surfaces or persons. Most people are intermittently colonized with *S. aureus* and carry it on the skin, nares or clothing. The organism also survives on inanimate surfaces for long periods.

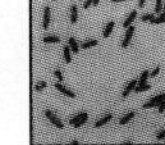

ETIOLOGIC FACTORS: Many *S. aureus* infections begin as localized infections of the skin and skin appendages, producing cellulites and abscesses. The organism, equipped with destructive enzymes and toxins, sometimes invades beyond the initial site, spreading by blood or lymphatics to almost any location in the body. Bones, joints and heart valves are the most common sites of metastatic *S. aureus* infections. *S. aureus* also causes several distinct diseases by elaborating toxins that are carried to distant sites.

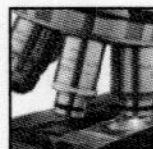

PATHOLOGY: When *S. aureus* is introduced into a previously sterile site, infection usually produces suppuration and abscesses, ranging from microscopic foci to lesions several centimeters in diameter that are filled with pus and bacteria.

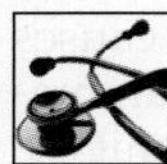

CLINICAL FEATURES: The clinical manifestations of *S. aureus* disease vary according to the sites and types of infection.

- **Furuncles (boils) and styes:** Deep-seated *S. aureus* infections occur in and around hair follicles, often in a nasal carrier. They localize on hairy surfaces, such as the neck, thighs and buttocks of men and the axillae, pubic area and eyelids of both sexes. The boil begins as a nodule at the base of a hair follicle, followed by a pimple that remains painful and red for a few days. A yellow apex forms and the central core becomes necrotic and fluctuant. Rupture or incision of the boil relieves the pain. **Styes** are boils that involve the sebaceous glands around the eyelid. **Paronychias** are staphylococcal infections of nail beds and **felons** are the same infections on the palmar side of the fingertips.
- **Carbuncles:** These lesions, mostly on the neck, result from coalescing infections with *S. aureus* around hair follicles and produce draining sinuses (Fig. 9-9).
- **Scalded skin syndrome:** This disease affects infants and children younger than 3 years who present with a sunburn-like rash that begins on the face and spreads over the body. Bullae begin to form and even gentle rubbing causes skin to desquamate. The disease begins to resolve in 1 to 2 weeks, as the skin regenerates. Desquamation is due to systemic effects of a specific exotoxin and the site of *S. aureus* proliferation is often occult.
- **Osteomyelitis:** Acute staphylococcal osteomyelitis, usually in the bones of the legs, most commonly afflicts boys between 3 and 10 years old. There is usually a history of infection or trauma. Osteomyelitis may become chronic if not properly treated. Adults older than 50 years are more frequently afflicted with vertebral osteomyelitis, which may follow staphylococcal infections of the skin or urinary tract, prostatic surgery or pinning of a fracture.

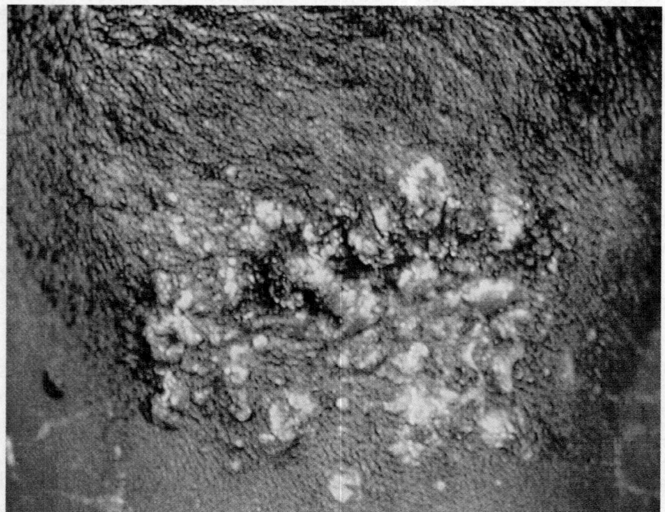

FIGURE 9-9. Staphylococcal carbuncle. The posterior neck is indurated and shows multiple follicular abscesses discharging purulent material.

- **Infections of burns or surgical wounds:** These sites often become infected with *S. aureus* from the patient's own nasal carriage or from medical personnel. Newborns and elderly, malnourished, diabetic and obese persons all have increased susceptibility.
- **Respiratory tract infections:** Staphylococcal respiratory tract infections occur mostly in infants younger than 2 years, and especially younger than 2 months. The infection is characterized by ulcers of the upper airway, scattered foci of pneumonia, pleural effusion, empyema and pneumothorax. In adults, staphylococcal pneumonia may follow viral influenza, which destroys the ciliated surface epithelium and leaves the bronchial surface vulnerable to secondary infection.
- **Bacterial arthritis:** *S. aureus* is the causative organism in half of all cases of septic arthritis, mostly in patients 50 to 70 years old. Rheumatoid arthritis and corticosteroid therapy are common predisposing conditions.
- **Septicemia:** Septicemia with *S. aureus* afflicts patients with lowered resistance who are in the hospital for other diseases. Some have underlying staphylococcal infections (e.g., septic arthritis, osteomyelitis), some have had surgery (e.g., transurethral prostate resection) and some have infections from an indwelling intravenous catheter. Miliary abscesses and endocarditis are serious complications.
- **Bacterial endocarditis:** Bacterial endocarditis is a common complication of *S. aureus* septicemia. It may develop spontaneously on normal valves, on valves damaged by rheumatic fever or on prosthetic valves. Intravenous drug abuse predisposes to staphylococcal endocarditis.
- **Toxic shock syndrome:** This disorder most commonly afflicts menstruating women, who present with high fever, nausea, vomiting, diarrhea and myalgias. Subsequently, they develop shock and within several days a sunburn-like rash. Toxic shock syndrome is associated with use of tampons, particularly hyperabsorbent tampons, which provide a site for *S. aureus* replication and toxin elaboration. Toxic shock syndrome occurs rarely in children and men and is then usually associated with an occult *S. aureus* infection.
- **Staphylococcal food poisoning:** Staphylococcal food poisoning typically begins less than 6 hours after a meal. Nausea and vomiting begin abruptly and usually resolve within 12 hours. This disease is caused by preformed toxin present in the food at the time it is eaten.
- **Antibiotic-resistant *S. aureus*.** One of the most important clinical issues concerning *S. aureus* is the relentless increase in its antibiotic resistance since penicillin was introduced in the early 1940s. *S. aureus* was one of the first important pathogens to become completely resistant to penicillin and, with time, to each subsequent generation of penicillin derivatives. Today, methicillin-resistant *S. aureus* (MRSA) infections are usually acquired in the hospital, in an environment that selects for antibiotic-resistant bacteria. MRSA represents one of the most dreaded of nosocomial infections. According to the CDC, between 1995 and 2004 in patients in intensive care units, the percentage of *S. aureus* infections due to MRSA approximately doubled, to almost two thirds. As of 2007, approximately 0.8% of the U.S. population is colonized with MRSA, and serious MRSA infections are associated with approximately 19,000 deaths annually. The most worrisome feature of MRSA infection is the difficulty in treatment when it becomes invasive and imperils health. The recent increase in community-acquired

MRSA (CA-MRSA) raises concerns of dissemination of antibiotic resistance among *Staphylococcus* and other bacteria. CA-MRSA appears to be a different strain of MRSA from that normally associated with hospital-acquired MRSA infections and displays enhanced virulence characteristics and different susceptibility profiles to antibiotics. It may spread in schools and gymnasiums and mostly causes skin and soft tissue infections.

Coagulase-Negative Staphylococci Infect Prosthetic Devices

Coagulase-negative staphylococci are the major cause of infections involving medical devices, including intravenous catheters, prosthetic heart valves, heart pacemakers, orthopedic prostheses, cerebrospinal fluid shunts and peritoneal catheters.

Disease caused by coagulase-negative staphylococci usually derives from the normal bacterial flora. Of the more than 20 known species of coagulase-negative staphylococci, 10 are normal residents of human skin and mucosal surfaces. Staphylococcus epidermidis *is the most frequent cause of infections associated with medical devices*. Another species, *Staphylococcus saprophyticus*, causes 10% to 20% of acute urinary tract infections in young women.

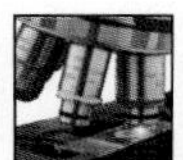

MOLECULAR PATHOGENESIS: Coagulase-negative staphylococci readily contaminate foreign bodies, on which they proliferate slowly, inducing inflammatory responses that damage adjacent tissue. Bacteria present on an intravascular surface, such as the tip of an intravascular catheter, can spread through the bloodstream to cause metastatic infections. Coagulase-negative staphylococci lack the enzymes and toxins that permit *S. aureus* to cause extensive local tissue destruction. Some strains of coagulase-negative staphylococci produce a polysaccharide gel biofilm, which enhances their adherence to foreign objects and protects them from host antimicrobial defenses and from many antibiotics.

PATHOLOGY: Medical devices infected with coagulase-negative staphylococci are usually thinly coated with tan, fibrinous material. Unlike infections caused by *S. aureus*, coagulase-negative staphylococcal infections usually do not produce extensive local tissue necrosis or large quantities of pus. Microscopic examination of infected devices shows clusters of gram-positive bacteria embedded in fibrin and cellular debris, with an associated acute inflammatory infiltrate.

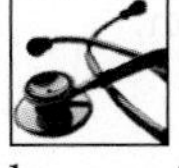

CLINICAL FEATURES: Coagulase-negative staphylococcal infections usually have subtle clinical presentations, and the only symptom of infection may be persistent low-grade fever. Infection of orthopedic prostheses frequently causes progressive loosening and dysfunction of the devices. These infections are usually indolent, but in compromised hosts, they may be fatal. Treatment usually requires replacement of any infected foreign object and appropriate antibiotic therapy. Nosocomial strains of coagulase-negative *Staphylococcus* are often multidrug resistant. Close to 80% of such hospital-acquired isolates have the *mecA* gene, which encodes resistance to all classes of β-lactam antibiotics. Thus, treatment should be with non–β-lactam antibiotics.

Streptococcus pyogenes Causes Suppurative, Toxin-Related and Immunologic Reactions

S. pyogenes, ***also known as group A Streptococcus, is one of the most common human bacterial pathogens, causing many diseases of diverse organ systems, from acute self-limited pharyngitis to major illnesses such as rheumatic fever*** (Fig. 9-10). *S. pyogenes* is a gram-positive coccus that is frequently part of the endogenous flora of the skin and oropharynx.

Diseases caused by *S. pyogenes* may be suppurative or nonsuppurative. The former occur at sites of bacterial invasion and consequent tissue necrosis and usually involve acute inflammatory responses. Suppurative *S. pyogenes* infections include pharyngitis, impetigo, cellulitis, myositis, pneumonia and puerperal sepsis. By contrast, the locations of nonsuppurative diseases caused by *S. pyogenes* are remote from the site of bacterial invasion. The two major nonsuppurative complications of *S. pyogenes* are rheumatic fever and acute poststreptococcal glomerulonephritis. These involve (1) organs far from the sites of streptococcal invasion, (2) a time delay after the acute infection and (3) immune reactions. Rheumatic fever is discussed in Chapter 11 and poststreptococcal glomerulonephritis in Chapter 16.

S. pyogenes elaborates several exotoxins, including erythrogenic toxins and cytolytic toxins (**streptolysins S and O**). Erythrogenic toxins cause the rash of scarlet fever. Streptolysin S lyses bacterial protoplasts (L forms) and probably destroys neutrophils after they ingest *S. pyogenes*. Streptolysin O induces a persistently high antibody titer, an effect that provides a useful marker for the diagnosis of *S. pyogenes* infections and their nonsuppurative complications.

Streptococcal Pharyngitis ("Strep Throat")

S. pyogenes, the common bacterial cause of pharyngitis, spreads from person to person by direct contact with oral or respiratory secretions. "Strep throat" occurs worldwide, predominantly affecting children and adolescents.

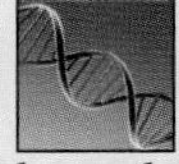

MOLECULAR PATHOGENESIS: *S. pyogenes* attaches to epithelial cells by binding to fibronectin on their surface. The bacterium produces hemolysins, DNAase, hyaluronidase and streptokinase, which allow it to damage and invade human tissues. *S. pyogenes* also has cell wall components that protect it from the inflammatory response. One of these, **M protein,** protrudes from cell walls of virulent strains and prevents complement deposition, thereby protecting bacteria from phagocytosis. Another surface protein destroys C5a, blocking its opsonizing effect and inhibiting phagocytosis. The invading organism elicits acute inflammation, often producing an exudate of neutrophils in the tonsillar fossae.

CLINICAL FEATURES: "**Strep throat**" is a sore throat with fever, malaise, headache and elevated leukocyte count. It usually lasts 3 to 5 days. ***In a few cases, streptococcal pharyngitis leads to rheumatic fever or acute poststreptococcal glomerulonephritis.*** Penicillin treatment shortens the course of strep throat and, more importantly, prevents nonsuppurative sequelae.

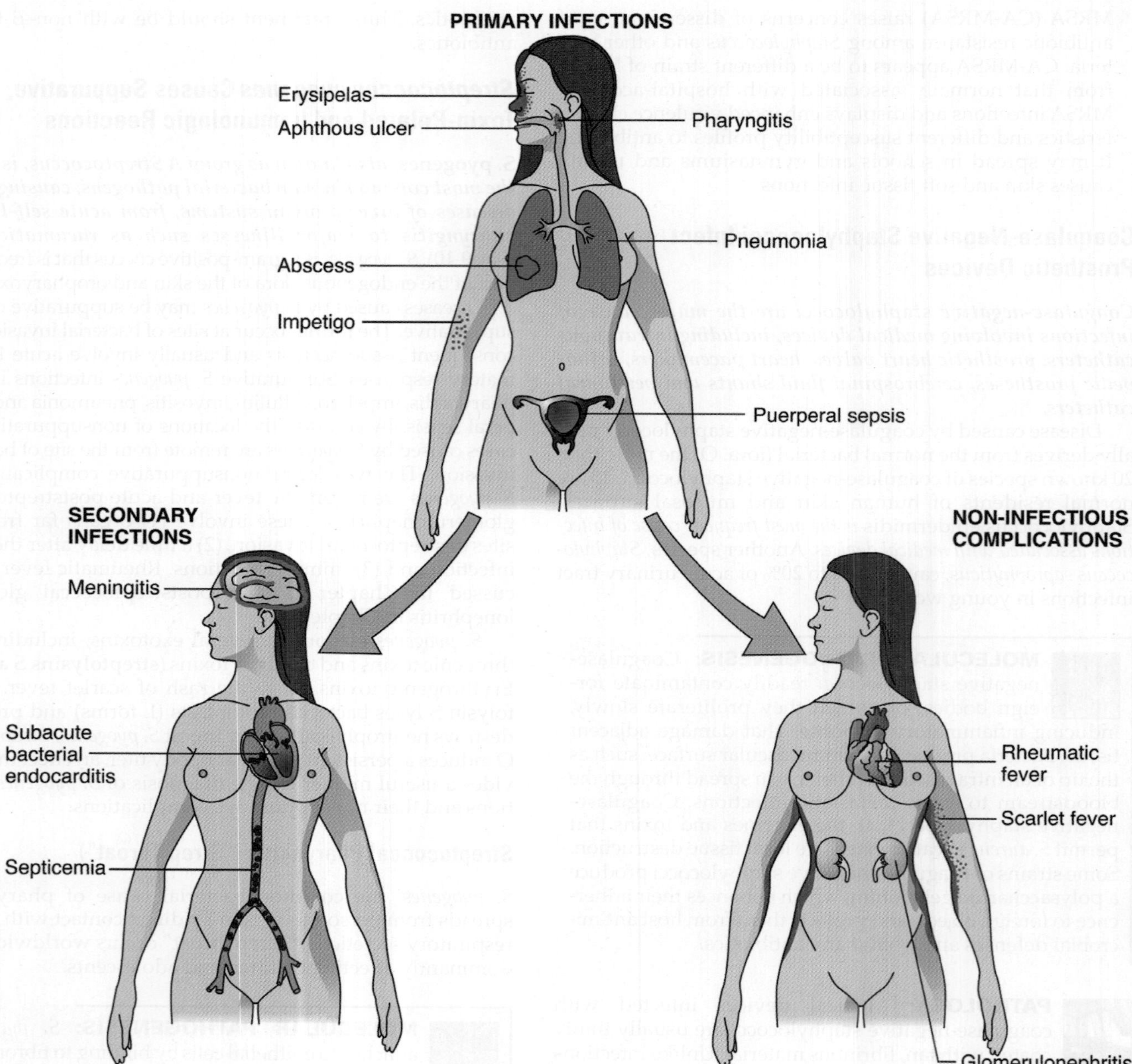

FIGURE 9-10. Streptococcal diseases.

Scarlet Fever

Scarlet fever (**scarlatina**) describes a punctate red rash on skin and mucous membranes in some suppurative *S. pyogenes* infections, most commonly pharyngitis. It usually begins on the chest and spreads to the extremities. The tongue may develop a yellow-white coating, which sheds to reveal a "beefy-red" surface. Scarlet fever is caused by an erythrogenic toxin.

Erysipelas

Erysipelas is an erythematous swelling of the skin caused chiefly by *S. pyogenes* (Fig. 9-11). Erysipelas is common in warm climates but is not often seen before the age of 20 years. It usually begins on the face and spreads rapidly. A diffuse, edematous, acute inflammatory reaction in the epidermis and dermis extends into subcutaneous tissues. The inflammatory infiltrate is principally composed of neutrophils and is most intense around vessels and adnexa of the skin. Cutaneous microabscesses and small foci of necrosis are common.

Impetigo

Impetigo (**pyoderma**) is a localized, intraepidermal infection caused by *S. pyogenes* or *S. aureus*. Strains of *S. pyogenes* that cause impetigo are antigenically and epidemiologically distinct from those that cause pharyngitis.

Impetigo spreads from person to person by direct contact and most commonly affects children aged 2 to 5 years. Infection begins with skin colonization with the causative organism. Minor trauma or an insect bite then inoculates the

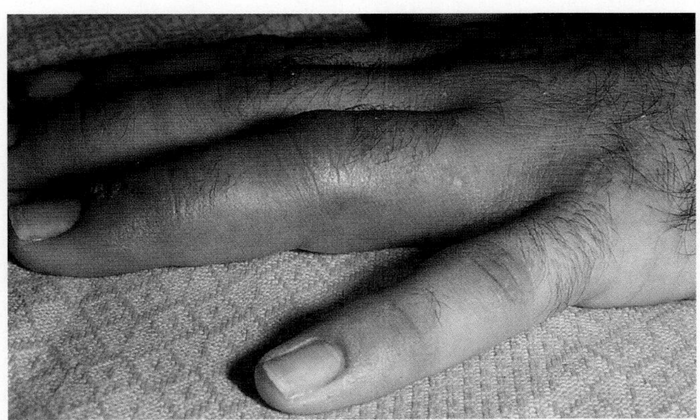

FIGURE 9-11. Erysipelas. Streptoccocal infection of the skin has resulted in an erythematous and swollen finger.

bacteria into the skin, where they form an intraepidermal pustule, which ruptures and leaks a purulent exudate.

Lesions begin on exposed body surfaces as localized erythematous papules (Fig. 9-12). These become pustules, which erode within a few days to form a thick honey-colored crust. Impetigo sometimes leads to poststreptococcal glomerulonephritis, but it does not lead to rheumatic fever.

Streptococcal Cellulitis

S. pyogenes causes an acute spreading infection of the loose connective tissue of the deeper layers of the dermis. This suppurative infection results from traumatic inoculation of microorganisms into the skin and frequently occurs on the extremities in the context of impaired lymphatic drainage. Cellulitis usually begins at sites of unnoticed injury and appears as spreading areas of redness, warmth and swelling.

Puerperal Sepsis

Puerperal sepsis is postpartum infection of the uterine cavity by *S. pyogenes*. The disease was once common but is now rare in developed countries. It is spread by the contaminated hands of attendants at delivery.

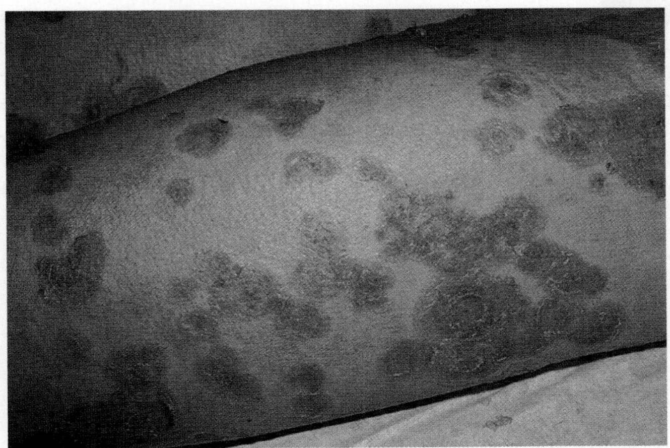

FIGURE 9-12. Streptococcal impetigo. The lower extremities exhibit numerous erythematous papules, with central ulceration and the formation of crusts.

Streptococcus pneumoniae Infection Is a Major Cause of Lobar Pneumonia

S. pneumoniae, often simply called **pneumococcus,** causes pyogenic infections, primarily of the lungs (**pneumonia**), middle ear (**otitis media**), sinuses (**sinusitis**) and meninges (**meningitis**). ***It is one of the most common human bacterial pathogens. Most children in the world have had at least one episode of pneumococcal disease (usually otitis media) by age 5.***

S. pneumoniae is an aerobic, gram-positive diplococcus. Most strains that cause clinical disease have a capsule, although nonserotypeable isolates are a known cause of epidemic conjunctivitis. There are over 80 antigenically distinct serotypes of pneumococcus; antibody to one does not protect from infection with another. *S. pneumoniae* is a commensal organism in the oropharynx and virtually everyone has been colonized at some time.

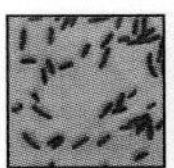 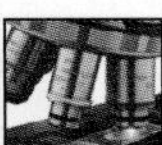

ETIOLOGIC FACTORS AND PATHOLOGY: Pneumococcal disease begins when the organism gains access to sterile sites, usually those in proximity to its normal residence in the oropharynx. Pneumococcal sinusitis and otitis media are usually preceded by a viral illness, such as the common cold, which injures the protective ciliated epithelium and fills affected air spaces with fluid. Pneumococci then thrive in the nutrient-rich tissue fluid. Infection of the sinuses or middle ear can spread to the adjacent meninges.

Pneumococcal pneumonia arises in a similar fashion. The lower respiratory tract is protected by the mucociliary blanket and cough response, which normally expel organisms that reach the lower airways. Insults that interfere with respiratory defenses, including influenza, other viral respiratory illness, smoking and alcoholism, allow *S. pneumoniae* to reach the alveoli. Once there, the organisms proliferate and elicit an acute inflammatory response. As the bacteria multiply and fill alveoli, they spread to other alveoli. Their polysaccharide capsule prevents activation of the alternate complement pathway, thereby blocking production of the opsonin C3b. Consequently, the organism can proliferate and spread unimpeded by phagocytes until antibody is produced. In the lungs, *S. pneumoniae* spreads rapidly to involve an entire lobe or several lobes (lobar pneumonia).

Alveoli fill with proteinaceous fluid, neutrophils and bacteria. The clinical features of pneumococcal infections are discussed in Chapter 12. Pneumonia caused by *S. pneumoniae* often resolves completely, unlike that caused by *S. aureus,* which can cause permanent lung damage. If there is an underlying problem, such as chronic aspiration, diabetes, or alcohol abuse, or if bacterial opsonization is compromised, as in multiple myeloma, hypogammaglobinemia or sickle cell disease, pneumococcal disease may spread. Patients with prior splenectomies are at high risk of rapid, fulminant septic shock and death.

Group B Streptococci Are the Leading Cause of Neonatal Pneumonia, Meningitis and Sepsis

Group B streptococci are gram-positive bacteria that grow in short chains. Several thousand neonatal infections with group B streptococci occur in the United States each year; about 30% of infected infants die. Group B streptococci are part of the normal vaginal flora in 10% to 30% of women. Most babies born to colonized women acquire the organisms as they pass through the birth canal. Group B streptococci may also cause pyogenic infections in adults infrequently.

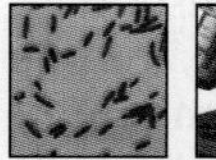
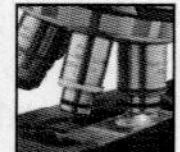

ETIOLOGIC FACTORS AND PATHOLOGY: Particular risk factors associated with development of neonatal group B streptococcal infections include premature delivery and low levels of maternally derived IgG antibodies against the organism. Newborns have little functional reserve for granulocyte production, so once the bacterial infection is established, it rapidly overwhelms the body's defenses. Group B streptococcal infection may be limited to the lungs or CNS or may be widely disseminated. Histopathologically, the involved tissues show a pyogenic response, often with overwhelming numbers of gram-positive cocci.

Bacterial Infections of Childhood

Diphtheria Is a Necrotizing Upper Respiratory Tract Infection

Infection with *Corynebacterium diphtheriae*—an aerobic, pleomorphic, gram-positive rod—may lead to cardiac and neurologic disturbances due to toxin production. The disease is preventable by vaccination with inactivated *C. diphtheriae* toxin (toxoid).

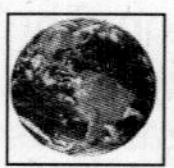

EPIDEMIOLOGY: Humans are the only known reservoir for *C. diphtheriae,* and most people are asymptomatic carriers. The organism spreads from person to person in respiratory droplets or oral secretions. Diphtheria was once a leading cause of death in children 2 to 15 years of age. Immunization programs have largely eliminated the disease in the Western world, but diphtheria persists as a major health problem in less developed countries.

MOLECULAR PATHOGENESIS: *C. diphtheriae* enters the pharynx and proliferates, often on the tonsils. Diphtheria toxin is absorbed systemically and acts on many tissues, with the heart, nerves and kidneys being most susceptible to damage. Diphtheria toxin has A and B subunits. The B subunit binds glycolipid receptors on target cells, and the A subunit acts within the cytoplasm on elongation factor 2 to interrupt protein synthesis. The toxin is one of the most potent known: one molecule suffices to kill a cell. Not all strains of *C. diphtheriae* produce exotoxin. The exotoxin is encoded by a lysogenic β-bacteriophage.

PATHOLOGY: The characteristic lesions of diphtheria are the thick, gray, leathery membranes composed of sloughed epithelium, necrotic debris, neutrophils, fibrin and bacteria that line affected respiratory passages (from the Greek *diphtheria,* "leather"). The epithelial surface beneath the membranes is denuded, and the submucosa is acutely inflamed and hemorrhagic. The inflammation often causes swelling in surrounding soft tissues, which can be severe enough to cause respiratory compromise. When the heart is affected, the myocardium displays fat droplets in the myocytes and focal necrosis (Fig. 9-13). In the case of neural involvement, affected peripheral nerves show demyelination.

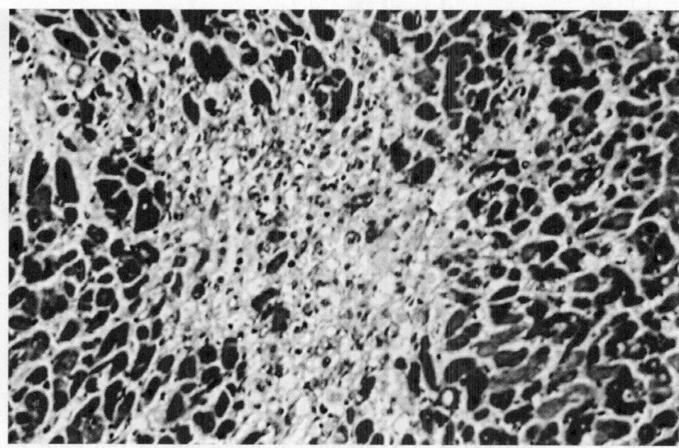

FIGURE 9-13. Diphtheric myocarditis. Focal degeneration of cardiac myocytes is evident.

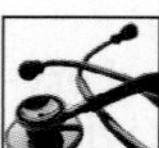

CLINICAL FEATURES: Diphtheria begins with fever, sore throat and malaise. The dirty gray membrane usually develops first on the tonsils and may spread throughout the posterior oropharynx. The membrane is firmly adherent, and an attempt to strip it from the underlying mucosa produces bleeding. Cardiac and neurologic symptoms develop in a minority of those infected, usually people with the most severe local disease.

Cutaneous diphtheria results from inoculation of the organism into a break in the skin and manifests as a pustule or ulcer; it rarely leads to cardiac or neurologic complications. Diphtheria is treated by prompt administration of antitoxin and antibiotics.

Pertussis Is Characterized by Debilitating Paroxysmal Coughing

The paroxysm is followed by a long, high-pitched inspiration, the "whoop," which gives the disease its name, "whooping cough." The causative organism is *Bordetella pertussis,* a small, gram-negative coccobacillus.

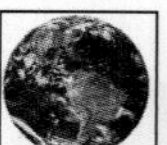

EPIDEMIOLOGY: *B. pertussis* is highly contagious and spreads from person to person, primarily by respiratory aerosols. Humans are the only reservoir of infection. In susceptible populations, pertussis is primarily a disease of children under 5 years, but infection incidence is increasing among adults. Vaccination is protective, but there are some 50 million cases of pertussis each year worldwide, and almost 1 million deaths, particularly in infants.

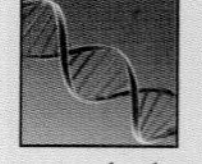

MOLECULAR PATHOGENESIS: *B. pertussis* initiates infection by attaching to the cilia of respiratory epithelial cells. The organism then elaborates a cytotoxin that kills ciliated cells. The progressive destruction of ciliated respiratory epithelium and ensuing inflammatory response cause the local respiratory symptoms. Several other toxins include "pertussis toxin," an agent that causes the pronounced lymphocytosis often associated with whooping cough. Another toxin inhibits adenylyl cyclase, an effect that blocks bacterial phagocytosis.

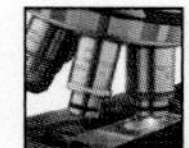

PATHOLOGY: *B. pertussis* causes an extensive tracheobronchitis, with necrosis of ciliated respiratory epithelium and an acute inflammatory response. With the loss of the protective mucociliary blanket, there is increased risk of pneumonia from aspirated oral bacteria. Coughing paroxysms and vomiting make aspiration likely. Secondary bacterial pneumonia commonly causes death.

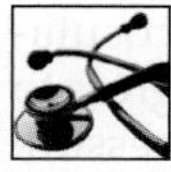

CLINICAL FEATURES: Whooping cough is a prolonged upper respiratory tract illness, lasting 4 to 5 weeks and passing through three stages:

- The **catarrhal stage** resembles a common viral upper respiratory tract illness, with low-grade fever, runny nose, conjunctivitis and cough.
- The **paroxysmal stage** occurs 1 week into the illness. Cough worsens and becomes paroxysmal, with 5 to 15 consecutive coughs, often followed by an inspiratory whoop. The patient develops a marked lymphocytosis: total leukocyte counts often exceed 40,000 cells/μL. The paroxysms persist for 2 to 3 weeks.
- The **convalescent phase** usually lasts for several weeks.

Haemophilus influenzae Causes Pyogenic Infections in Young Children

Haemophilus influenzae infections involve the middle ear, sinuses, facial skin, epiglottis, meninges, lungs and joints. The organism is a major pediatric bacterial pathogen and a leading cause of bacterial meningitis worldwide. It is an aerobic, pleomorphic gram-negative coccobacillus that may be either encapsulated or not. Nonencapsulated strains (type a) usually produce localized infections; encapsulated strains, type b, are more virulent and cause over 95% of the invasive bacteremic infections.

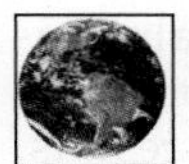

EPIDEMIOLOGY: *H. influenzae* only infects humans and spreads from person to person, mainly in respiratory droplets and secretions. It normally resides in the human nasopharynx of 20% to 50% of healthy adults. Most colonizing strains are nonencapsulated, but 3% to 5% are *H. influenzae* type b.

Most severe *H. influenzae* type b infections occur in children under the age of 6 years. The incidence of serious disease peaks at 6 to 18 months of age, corresponding to the period between the loss of maternally acquired immunity and the acquisition of native immunity. The *H. influenzae* type b vaccine has been credited with greatly reducing the complications of invasive *H. influenzae* type b disease, particularly meningitis, in children. However, as vaccination also reduces *H. influenzae* type b carriage and the repeated immunologic boosting effect that carriage provides, continued vigilance is important.

MOLECULAR PATHOGENESIS: Unencapsulated *H. influenzae* strains produce disease by spreading locally from their normal sites of residence to adjoining sterile locations, such as the sinuses or middle ear. This is facilitated by injury to normal defense mechanisms, as with a viral upper respiratory tract illness. At these previously sterile sites, unencapsulated organisms proliferate and elicit acute inflammatory responses, which injure local tissue but eventually contain the infection. Unencapsulated strains do not usually produce bacteremia.

In contrast, encapsulated H. influenzae type b is capable of tissue invasion. The capsular polysaccharide of type b organisms allows them to evade phagocytosis, and bacteremic infections are common. Epiglottitis, facial cellulitis, septic arthritis and meningitis result from invasive bacteremic infections. *H. influenzae* type b also elaborates an IgA protease, which facilitates local survival of the organism in the respiratory tract.

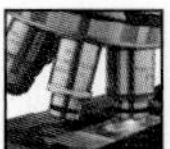

PATHOLOGY: *H. influenzae* elicits strong acute inflammatory responses. Specific pathologic features vary according to the sites affected. *H. influenzae* meningitis resembles other acute bacterial meningitides, with a predominantly acute inflammatory leptomeningeal infiltrate, sometimes involving the subarachnoid space.

H. influenzae pneumonia usually complicates chronic lung disease. In half of patients it follows a viral infection of the respiratory tract. Alveoli are filled with neutrophils, macrophages containing bacilli and fibrin. The bronchiolar epithelium is necrotic and infiltrated by macrophages.

Epiglottitis is swelling and acute inflammation of the epiglottis, aryepiglottic fold and pyriform sinuses. It may sometimes completely obstruct the upper airway. In **facial cellulitis**, the site of infection and inflammation is the dermis, usually of the cheek or periorbital region.

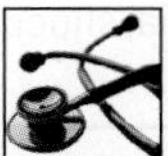

CLINICAL FEATURES: Most bacteremic *H. influenzae* infections afflict young children. ***H. influenzae is the most common cause of meningitis in children younger than the age of 2 years,* although vaccination has reduced its frequency.** Onset is insidious and may follow an otherwise unremarkable upper respiratory tract infection or otitis media.

- **Bronchopneumonia or lobar pneumonia** is characterized by fever, cough, purulent sputum and dyspnea.
- **Epiglottitis** affects primarily children aged 2 to 7 years but also occurs in adults. Death may occur from obstruction of the upper respiratory tract.
- **Septic arthritis** is secondary to bacteremic seeding of large weight-bearing joints. Symptoms include fever, heat, erythema, swelling and pain on movement.
- **Facial cellulitis** or periorbital cellulitis is another severe bacteremic infection affecting primarily young children. Patients present with fever, profound malaise, and a raised, hot, red-blue discolored area of the face, usually involving the cheek or an area about the eye. There is often concomitant meningitis or septic arthritis.

Neisseria meningitides Causes Pyogenic Meningitis and Overwhelming Shock

Neisseria meningitidis, or **meningococcus,** produces disseminated blood-borne infections, often accompanied by shock and profound disturbances in coagulation (Fig. 9-14). The organism is aerobic and appears as paired, bean-shaped, gram-negative cocci. There are eight major serogroups, of which A, B and C are most important.

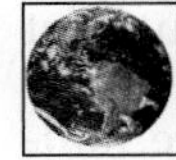

EPIDEMIOLOGY: Meningococci spread from person to person, primarily by respiratory droplets. About 5% to 15% of the population carries them as commensals in the nasopharynx. Carriers develop antibodies to their colonizing strain of *N. meningitidis* and are not susceptible to disease caused by that strain.

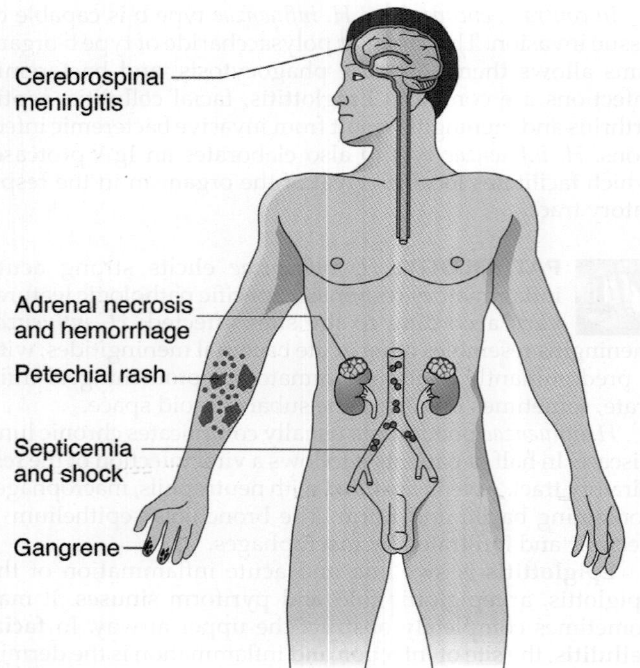

FIGURE 9-14. Meningococcemia. Meningococcal infections have a variety of clinical manifestations including meningitis, septicemia, shock and associated complications.

Meningococcal diseases appear as sporadic cases, clusters of cases and epidemics. Most infections in industrialized countries are sporadic and afflict children under the age of 5. Epidemic disease occurs mostly in crowded quarters, such as among military recruits in barracks. There are over 6000 cases of meningococcal meningitis each year in the United States, and over 600 deaths. Fatal meningococcal disease is more common in less developed countries.

MOLECULAR PATHOGENESIS: Upon colonizing the upper respiratory tract, *N. meningitidis* attaches to nonciliated respiratory epithelium by means of its pili. Most exposed persons then develop protective bactericidal antibodies over the following weeks, and some become carriers. If the organism spreads to the bloodstream before protective immunity develops, it can proliferate rapidly and cause fulminant meningococcal disease.

Many of the systemic effects of meningococcal disease are due to the endotoxin of the bacterial outer membrane lipopolysaccharide. Endotoxin promotes a conspicuous increase in TNF production and simultaneous activation of complement and coagulation cascades. Disseminated intravascular coagulation, fibrinolysis and shock follow.

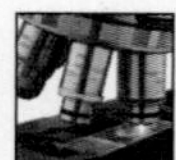

PATHOLOGY: Meningococcal disease can be confined to the CNS or may be disseminated throughout the body in the form of septicemia. In the former case, the leptomeninges and subarachnoid space are infiltrated with neutrophils and underlying brain parenchyma is swollen and congested. Meningococcal septicemia is characterized by diffuse damage to the endothelium of small blood vessels, with widespread petechiae and purpura in the skin and viscera.

Rarely (3% to 4% of all cases), vasculitis and thrombosis produce hemorrhagic necrosis of both adrenals, called the **Waterhouse-Friderichsen syndrome.**

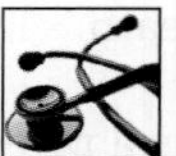

CLINICAL FEATURES: Meningitis begins with rapid onset of fever, stiff neck and headache. In meningococcal sepsis, fever, shock and mucocutaneous hemorrhages appear abruptly. Patients may progress to shock within minutes, and treatment requires blood pressure support and antibiotics. Meningococcal disease was once almost invariably fatal, but antibiotic treatment has reduced mortality to less than 15%. Some patients who survive the early phase of meningococcemia develop late immunologic complications such as polyarthritis, cutaneous vasculitis and pericarditis. Severe vasculitis may be associated with extensive cutaneous ulceration and even gangrene of the distal extremities.

Sexually Transmitted Bacterial Diseases

Gonorrhea Remains a Common Infection That Causes Sterility

Neisseria gonorrhoeae, also termed **gonococcus,** causes gonorrhea, an acute suppurative genital tract infection, that manifests as urethritis in men and endocervicitis in women. It is one of the oldest and still one of the most common sexually transmitted diseases. *N. gonorrhoeae* is an aerobic, bean-shaped, gram-negative diplococcus.

Gonococcal pharyngitis and proctitis are not uncommon and are also sexually transmitted. In women, infection often ascends the genital tract, producing endometritis, salpingitis and pelvic inflammatory disease. Ascending spread in men is less common, but if it occurs, epididymitis results. Gonococcal infection may rarely be bacteremic, in which case septic arthritis and skin lesions develop. Neonatal infections derived from the birth canal of a mother with gonorrhea usually manifest as conjunctivitis, although disseminated infections are occasionally seen. Neonatal gonococcal conjunctivitis is still a major cause of blindness in much of Africa and Asia but is largely eliminated in developed countries by routine instillation of antibiotics into the conjunctiva at birth.

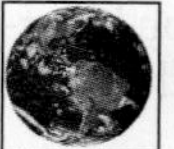

EPIDEMIOLOGY: This common infection is spread directly from person to person. Except for perinatal transmission, spread is almost always by sexual intercourse. Infected persons who are asymptomatic are a significant reservoir of infection.

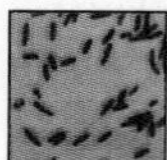

ETIOLOGIC FACTORS: Gonorrhea begins in the mucous membranes of the urogenital tract (Fig. 9-15). Bacteria attach to surface cells, after which they invade superficially and provoke acute inflammation. Gonococcus lacks a true polysaccharide capsule, but hair-like extensions, termed "pili," project from the cell wall. The pili contain a protease that digests IgA on the mucous membrane, thereby facilitating bacterial attachment to the columnar and transitional epithelium of the urogenital tract.

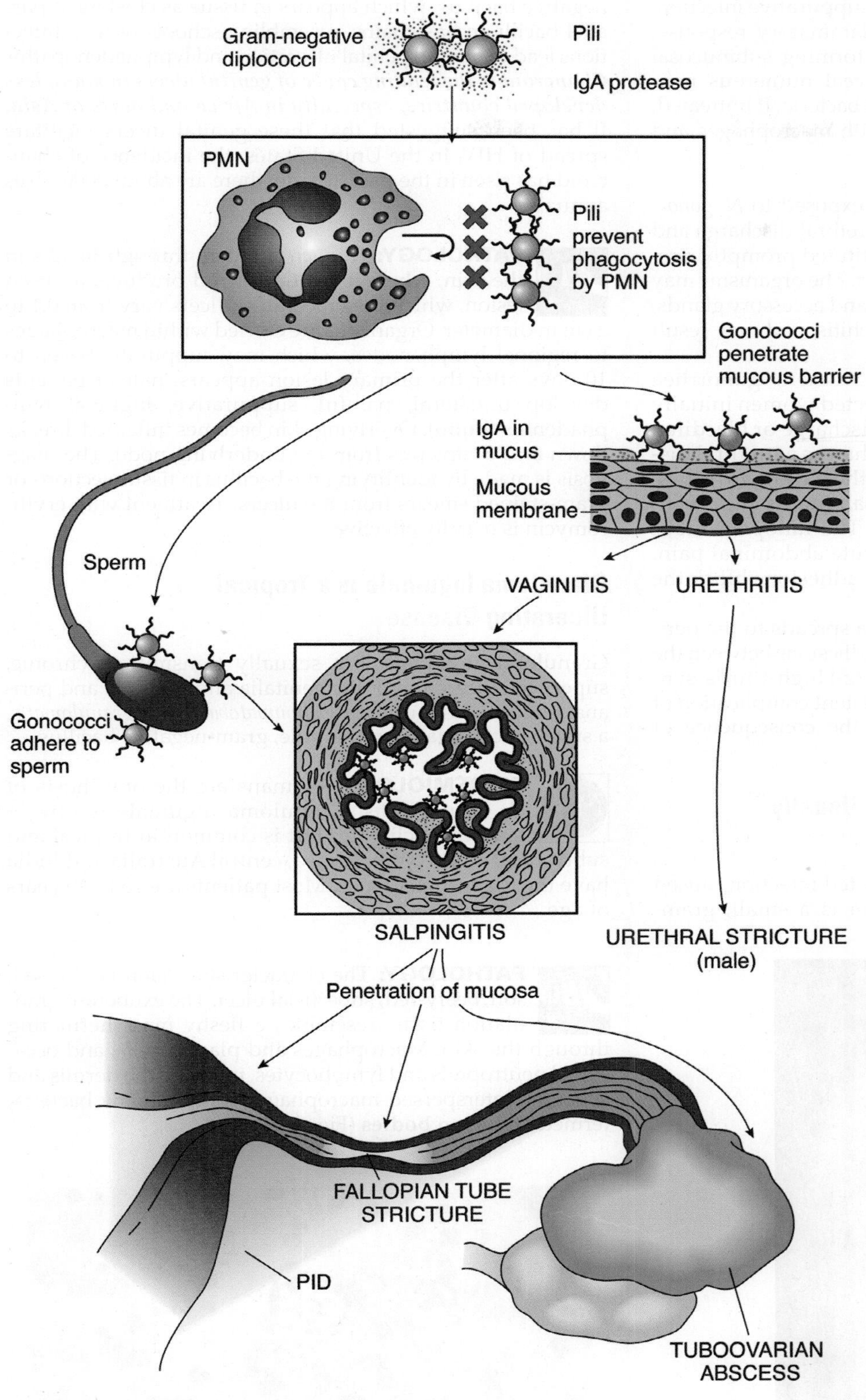

FIGURE 9-15. Pathogenesis of gonococcal infections. *Neisseria gonorrhoeae* is a gram-negative diplococcus whose surface pili form a barrier against phagocytosis by neutrophils. The pili contain an immunoglobulin A (IgA) protease that digests IgA on the luminal surface of the mucous membranes of the urethra, endocervix and fallopian tube, thereby facilitating attachment of gonococci. Gonococci cause endocervicitis, vaginitis and salpingitis. In men, gonococci attached to the mucous membrane of the urethra cause urethritis and, sometimes, urethral stricture. Gonococci may also attach to sperm heads and be carried into the fallopian tube. Penetration of the mucous membrane by gonococci leads to stricture of the fallopian tube, pelvic inflammatory disease (PID) or tuboovarian abscess.

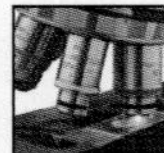

PATHOLOGY: Gonorrhea is a suppurative infection, eliciting a vigorous acute inflammatory response, with copious pus, and often forming submucosal abscesses. Stained smears of pus reveal numerous neutrophils, often containing phagocytosed bacteria. If untreated, the inflammation becomes chronic, with macrophages and lymphocytes predominant.

CLINICAL FEATURES: Men exposed to *N. gonorrhoeae* present with purulent urethral discharge and dysuria. If treatment is not instituted promptly, urethral stricture is a common complication. The organisms may also extend to the prostate, epididymis and accessory glands, where they cause epididymitis and orchitis, and may result in infertility.

In about one half of infected women, gonorrhea remains asymptomatic. The other infected women initially exhibit endocervicitis, with vaginal discharge or bleeding. Urethritis presents as dysuria rather than as a urethral discharge. Infection often extends to the fallopian tubes, where it produces acute and chronic salpingitis and, eventually, pelvic inflammatory disease. The fallopian tubes swell with pus (Fig. 9-16), causing acute abdominal pain. Infertility occurs when inflammatory adhesions block the tubes.

From the fallopian tubes, gonorrhea spreads to the peritoneum, healing as fine "violin string" adhesions between the liver and the parietal peritoneum (Fitz-Hugh-Curtis syndrome). Chronic endometritis is a persistent complication of gonococcal infection and is usually the consequence of chronic gonococcal salpingitis.

Chancroid Causes Genital Ulcers, Usually in Less Developed Regions

Chancroid is an acute sexually transmitted infection caused by *Haemophilus ducreyi*. The organism is a small, gram-negative bacillus, which appears in tissue as clusters of parallel bacilli and as chains, resembling schools of fish. Infections lead to painful genital ulceration and lymphadenopathy. ***Chancroid is the leading cause of genital ulcers in many less developed countries, especially in Africa and parts of Asia.*** It has been suggested that these genital ulcers facilitate spread of HIV. In the United States, the incidence of chancroid has risen in the past decade: there are about 5000 cases annually.

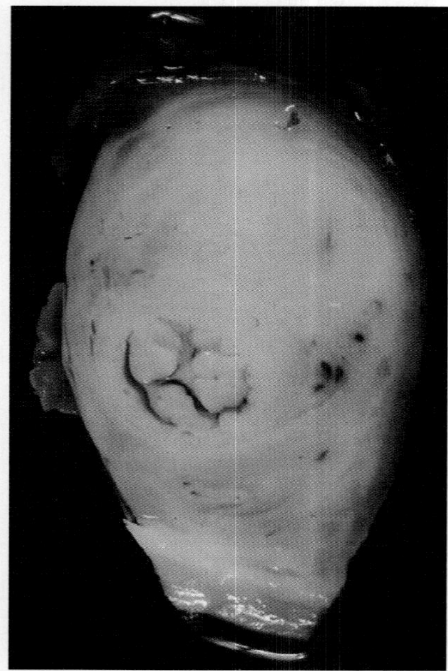

FIGURE 9-16. **Gonorrhea of the fallopian tube.** Cross-section of a "pus tube" shows thickening of the wall and a lumen swollen with pus.

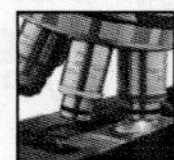

PATHOLOGY: *H. ducreyi* enters through breaks in the skin, where it multiplies and produces a raised lesion, which then ulcerates. Ulcers vary from 0.1 to 2 cm in diameter. Organisms are carried within macrophages to regional lymph nodes, which may suppurate. Seven to 10 days after the primary lesion appears, half of patients develop unilateral, painful, suppurative, inguinal lymphadenitis (**bubo**). Overlying skin becomes inflamed, breaks down and drains pus from the underlying node. The diagnosis is made by identifying the bacillus in tissue sections or gram-stained smears from the ulcers. Treatment with erythromycin is usually effective.

Granuloma Inguinale Is a Tropical Ulcerating Disease

Granuloma inguinale is a sexually transmitted, chronic, superficial ulceration of the genitalia and inguinal and perianal regions. It is caused by *Calymmatobacterium granulomatis*, a small, encapsulated, nonmotile, gram-negative bacillus.

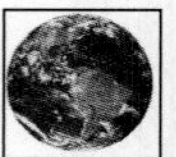

EPIDEMIOLOGY: Humans are the only hosts of *C. granulomatis*. Granuloma inguinale is rare in temperate climates but is common in tropical and subtropical areas. New Guinea, central Australia and India have the highest incidence. Most patients are 15 to 40 years of age.

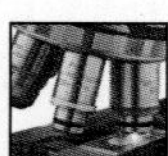

PATHOLOGY: The characteristic lesion is a raised, soft, beefy-red, superficial ulcer. The exuberant granulation tissue resembles a fleshy mass herniating through the skin. Macrophages and plasma cells, and occasional neutrophils and lymphocytes, infiltrate the dermis and subcutis. Interspersed macrophages contain many bacteria, termed **Donovan bodies** (Fig. 9-17).

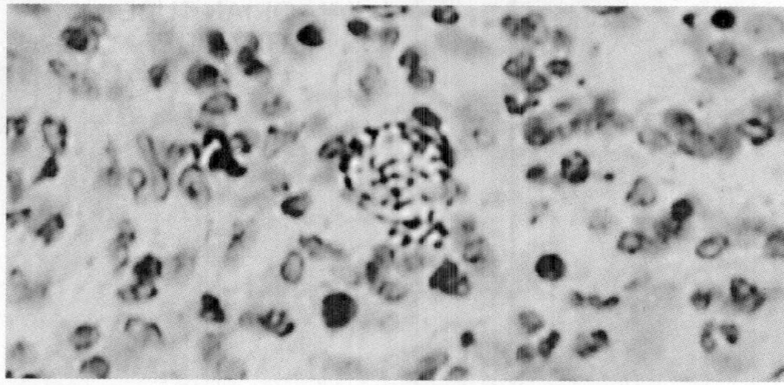

FIGURE 9-17. **Granuloma inguinale.** A photomicrograph of a skin lesion shows *Calymmatobacterium granulomatis* (Donovan bodies) clustered in a large macrophage. Intense silver staining by Warthin-Starry technique makes the organisms large, black and easily seen.

CLINICAL FEATURES: Untreated granuloma inguinale follows an indolent, relapsing course, often healing with an atrophic scar. Secondary fusospirochetal infection may cause ulceration, mutilation or amputation of the genitalia. Massive scarring of the dermis and subcutis may obstruct lymphatics and cause genital **elephantiasis.** Antibiotic therapy is effective in early cases.

Enteropathogenic Bacterial Infections

Escherichia coli Is a Common Cause of Diarrhea and Urinary Tract Infections

***E. coli* is among the most frequent and important human bacterial pathogens, causing over 90% of all urinary tract infections and many cases of diarrheal illness worldwide.** It is also a major opportunistic pathogen, frequently causing pneumonia and sepsis in immunocompromised hosts and meningitis and sepsis in newborns.

E. coli are a group of antigenically and biologically diverse, aerobic (facultatively anaerobic), gram-negative bacteria. Most strains are intestinal commensals, well adapted to growth in the human colon without harming the host. However, *E. coli* can be aggressive when it gains access to usually sterile body sites, such as the urinary tract, meninges or peritoneum. Strains of *E. coli* that produce diarrhea possess specialized virulence properties, usually plasmid-borne, that cause intestinal disease.

Escherichia coli Diarrhea

There are four distinct strains of *E. coli* that cause diarrhea:

ENTEROTOXIGENIC E. coli: *Enterotoxigenic* E. coli *is a major cause of diarrhea in poor tropical areas and probably causes most "traveler's diarrhea" among visitors to such regions.* It is acquired from contaminated water and food. Many people in Latin America, Africa and Asia are asymptomatic carriers of the infection.

MOLECULAR PATHOGENESIS: Nonimmune persons (local children or travelers from abroad) develop diarrhea when they encounter the organism. Enterotoxigenic strains produce diarrhea by adhering to the intestinal mucosa and elaborating one or more of at least three enterotoxins that cause secretory dysfunction of the small bowel. One of the enterotoxins is structurally and functionally similar to cholera toxin, and another acts on guanylyl cyclase. Enterotoxigenic *E. coli* produces no distinctive macroscopic or light-microscopic alterations in the intestine.

Enterotoxigenic *E. coli* causes an acute, self-limited diarrheal illness with watery stools lacking neutrophils and erythrocytes. In severe cases, fluid and electrolyte loss can cause extreme dehydration and even death.

ENTEROPATHOGENIC E. coli: Historically, enteropathogenic *E. coli* was the first group of this genus to be identified as a causal agent of diarrhea. The organism is a major cause of diarrheal illness in poor tropical areas, especially in infants and young children. Although it has virtually disappeared from developed countries, it still causes sporadic outbreaks of diarrhea, particularly among hospitalized infants younger than 2 years. Enteropathogenic *E. coli* is acquired by ingesting contaminated food or water. The organism is not invasive and causes disease by adhering to and deforming the microvilli of the intestinal epithelial cells (Fig. 9-18A). Enteropathogenic *E. coli* produces diarrhea, vomiting, fever and malaise.

ENTEROHEMORRHAGIC E. coli: Enterohemorrhagic *E. coli* (serotype 0157:H7) causes a bloody diarrhea, which occasionally is followed by the **hemolytic–uremic syndrome** (see Chapter 16). The source of infection is usually ingestion of contaminated meat or milk. Enterohemorrhagic *E. coli* adheres to colonic mucosa and elaborates an enterotoxin, virtually identical to Shigatoxin (see below), that destroys the epithelial cells. Patients infected with *E. coli* 0157:H7 present with cramping abdominal pain, low-grade fever and sometimes bloody diarrhea. Microscopic examination of stool shows both leukocytes and erythrocytes.

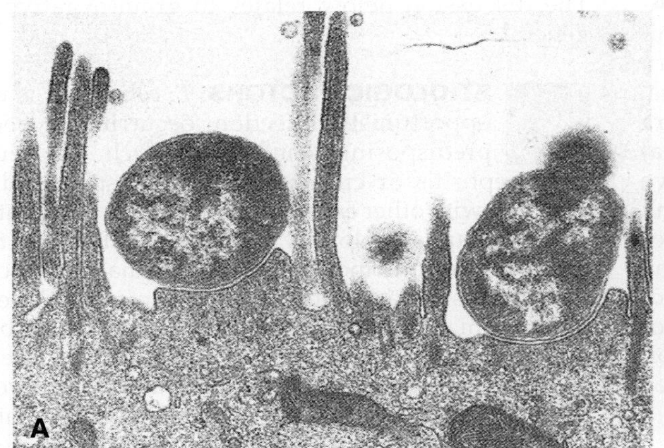

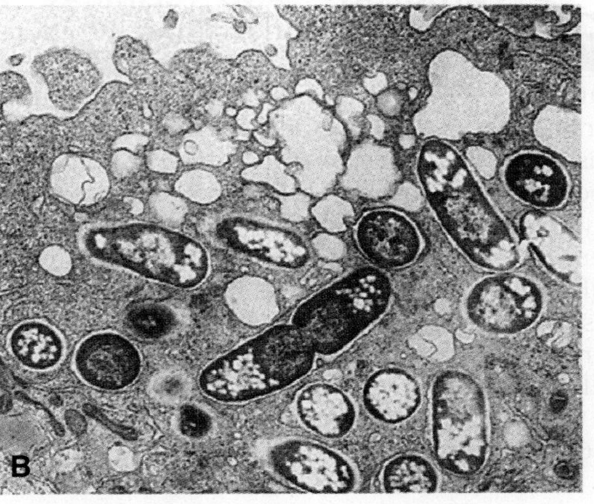

FIGURE 9-18. Enteric *Escherichia coli* infections. A. Enteropathogenic *E. coli* infection. An electron micrograph shows adherence of the bacteria to the intestinal mucosal cells and localized destruction of microvilli. **B.** Enteroinvasive *E. coli* infection. An electron micrograph shows organisms within a cell.

ENTEROINVASIVE E. coli: Enteroinvasive *E. coli* causes food-borne dysentery, which is clinically and pathologically indistinguishable from that caused by Shigella. The agent shares extensive DNA homology and antigenic and biochemical characteristics with *Shigella*. It invades and destroys mucosal cells of the distal ileum and colon (Fig. 9-18B). As in shigellosis, the mucosae of the distal ileum and colon are acutely inflamed and focally eroded and are sometimes covered by an inflammatory pseudomembrane. Patients have abdominal pain, fever, tenesmus and bloody diarrhea, usually for about a week. Antibiotic treatment is similar to that for shigellosis.

Escherichia coli Urinary Tract Infection

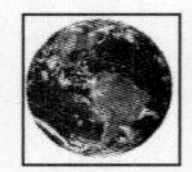

EPIDEMIOLOGY: Urinary tract infections with *E. coli* are most common in sexually active women and in persons of both sexes who have structural or functional abnormalities of the urinary tract. ***Such infections are extremely common, afflicting more than 10% of the human population, often repeatedly.*** *E. coli* in the urinary tract usually derive from resident flora of the perineum and periurethral areas, reflecting fecal contamination of these regions.

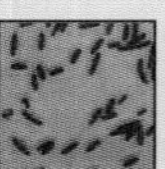 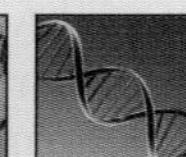

ETIOLOGIC FACTORS AND MOLECULAR PATHOGENESIS: *E. coli* gain access to the sterile proximal urinary tract by ascending from the distal urethra. Because the shorter female urethra provides a less effective mechanical barrier to infection, women are much more prone to urinary tract infections. Sexual intercourse can suffice to propel organisms into the female urethra. Uropathogenic *E. coli* organisms have specialized adherence factors (Gal-Gal) on the pili, which enable them to bind to galactopyranosyl-galactopyranoside residues on the uroepithelium. Structural abnormalities of the urinary tract (e.g., congenital deformities, prostatic hyperplasia, strictures) and instrumentation (catheterization) overwhelm normal host defenses and facilitate the establishment of urinary tract infections. These conditions account for most urinary tract infections in men.

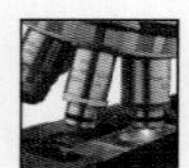 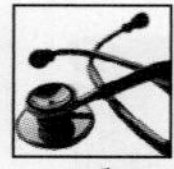

PATHOLOGY AND CLINICAL FEATURES: *E. coli* urinary tract infections initially produce an acute inflammatory infiltrate at the site of infection, usually the bladder mucosa. Urinary tract infections involving the bladder or urethra manifest as urinary urgency, burning on urination (**dysuria**) and leukocytes in the urine. If infection ascends to involve the kidney (**pyelonephritis**), patients develop acute flank pain, fever and elevated leukocyte counts. An infiltrate of neutrophils spills from the mucosa into the urine, and the blood vessels of the submucosa are dilated and congested. Chronic infections exhibit an inflammatory infiltrate of neutrophils and mononuclear cells. Chronic renal infection may lead to chronic pyelonephritis and renal failure (see Chapter 16).

Escherichia coli Pneumonia

Pneumonia caused by enteric gram-negative bacteria is considered opportunistic, occurring mostly in debilitated persons. *E. coli* is the most common cause, but other normal bowel flora, such as *Klebsiella*, *Serratia* and *Enterobacter* spp., produce similar disease. *The discussion below applies to all opportunistic gram-negative pneumonias.*

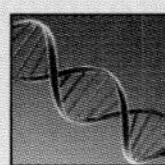

MOLECULAR PATHOGENESIS: Enteric gram-negative bacteria are transiently introduced into the oral cavity of healthy people but cannot compete successfully with the predominant gram-positive flora, which adhere to the fibronectin that coats mucosal cell surfaces. Chronically ill or severely stressed persons elaborate a salivary protease that degrades fibronectin, allowing gram-negative enteric bacteria to overcome the normal gram-positive flora and colonize the oropharynx.

Inevitably, droplets of the resident oral flora are aspirated into the respiratory tract. Debilitated patients often have weak local defenses and cannot destroy these organisms. Decreased gag and cough reflexes, abnormal neutrophil chemotaxis, injured respiratory epithelium and foreign bodies, such as endotracheal tubes, all facilitate entry and survival of the aspirated organisms.

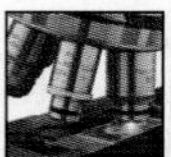

PATHOLOGY: *E. coli* pneumonia results from proliferation of aspirated organisms in terminal airways, usually at multiple sites in the lung. Multifocal areas of consolidation result and terminal airways and alveoli are filled with proteinaceous fluid, fibrin, neutrophils and macrophages.

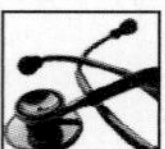

CLINICAL FEATURES: Because pneumonia caused by *E. coli* and other enteric gram-negative organisms afflicts patients who are often already severely ill, symptoms of pneumonia may be less obvious than in healthy persons. Increased malaise, fever and labored breathing are often the first signs of pneumonia. If *E. coli* pneumonia remains untreated, the organisms may invade the blood to produce fatal septicemia. Treatment requires parenteral antibiotics.

Escherichia coli Sepsis (Gram-Negative Sepsis)

E. coli is the most common cause of enteric gram-negative sepsis, but other gram-negative rods, including *Pseudomonas*, *Klebsiella* and *Enterobacter* spp., produce identical disease. The discussion below relates to gram-negative sepsis in general.

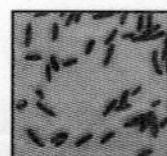

ETIOLOGIC FACTORS: *E. coli* sepsis is usually an opportunistic infection, occurring in people with predisposing conditions, such as neutropenia, pyelonephritis or cirrhosis, and in hospitalized patients. Together with other enteric gram-negative rods that normally reside in human colon, *E. coli* occasionally seeds the bloodstream. In healthy individuals, macrophages and circulating neutrophils phagocytose these bacteria. Patients with neutropenia or cirrhosis develop *E. coli* sepsis because of impaired ability to eliminate even low-level bacteremias. Persons with ruptured abdominal organs or acute pyelonephritis suffer gram-negative sepsis because the large numbers of organisms that gain access to the circulation overwhelm the normal defenses.

The presence of *E. coli* in the bloodstream causes septic shock through the effects of TNF (among other factors), whose release from macrophages is stimulated by bacterial endotoxin. Septic shock is discussed in Chapters 7 and 20.

Neonatal *Escherichia coli* Meningitis and Sepsis

E. coli and group B streptococci are the main causes of meningitis and sepsis in the first month after birth. Both colonize the vagina, and newborns acquire them on passage through the birth canal. *E. coli* then colonize the infant's gastrointestinal tract. It is postulated that the organisms spread to the bloodstream from the gastrointestinal tract, then seed the meninges. The pathology of *E. coli* meningitis is identical to that of other bacterial meningitides. Although antibiotic treatment for neonatal *E. coli* meningitis and sepsis is often effective, the mortality rate is still 15% to 50%. Almost half of survivors suffer neurologic sequelae.

Salmonella Enterocolitis and Typhoid Fever Are Both Intestinal Infections

The bacterial genus *Salmonella* contains over 1500 antigenically distinct but biochemically and genetically related gram-negative rods, which cause two important human diseases: *Salmonella* enterocolitis and typhoid fever.

Salmonella Enterocolitis

Salmonella enterocolitis is an acute self-limited (1 to 3 days) gastrointestinal illness that presents as nausea, vomiting, diarrhea and fever. Infection is typically acquired by eating food containing nontyphoidal *Salmonella* strains and is commonly called **Salmonella food poisoning.**

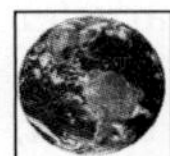

EPIDEMIOLOGY: Nontyphoidal *Salmonella* infect diverse animal species, including amphibians, reptiles, birds and mammals. They also readily contaminate foodstuffs derived from infected animals (e.g., meat, poultry, eggs, dairy products). If these foods are not cooked, pasteurized or irradiated, the bacteria persist and proliferate, particularly at warm temperatures. Once a person is infected, the organism can spread from person to person by the fecal–oral route, which is infrequent among adults but common among small children in day-care settings or within families. *Salmonella* enterocolitis remains a major cause of childhood mortality in less developed countries.

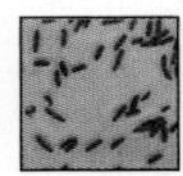 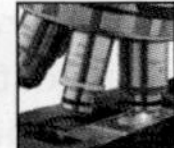

ETIOLOGIC FACTORS AND PATHOLOGY: *Salmonella* proliferate in the small intestine and invade enterocytes in the distal small bowel and colon. The nontyphoidal *Salmonella* spp. elaborate several toxins that injure intestinal cells. The mucosae of the ileum and colon are acutely inflamed and sometimes superficially ulcerated.

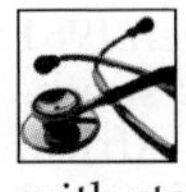

CLINICAL FEATURES: *Salmonella* enterocolitis typically manifests as diarrhea, within 12 to 48 hours after consuming contaminated food. This contrasts with staphylococcal food poisoning, which is caused by a preformed toxin and begins 1 to 6 hours after eating. The diarrhea of *Salmonella* food poisoning is self-limited. It lasts 1 to 3 days and is often accompanied by nausea, vomiting, cramping abdominal pain and fever. Treatment is supportive: antibiotics rarely improve the clinical course.

Typhoid Fever

Typhoid fever is an acute systemic illness caused by infection with *Salmonella typhi*. **Paratyphoid fever** is a clinically similar but milder disease that results from infection with other species of *Salmonella*, including *Salmonella paratyphi*. The term **enteric fever** includes both typhoid and paratyphoid fever.

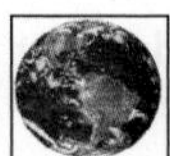

EPIDEMIOLOGY: Humans are the only natural reservoir for *S. typhi* and typhoid fever is acquired from infected patients or chronic carriers. The latter tend to be older women with gallstones or biliary scarring: *S. typhi* colonizes their gallbladder or biliary tree. The disease is spread primarily by ingestion of contaminated water and food, especially dairy products and shellfish. Less commonly, the organisms are disseminated by direct finger-to-mouth contact with feces, urine or other secretions. Infected food handlers with poor personal hygiene and urine from patients with typhoid pyelonephritis can be a significant source of infection. Typhoid fever accounts for over 25,000 annual deaths worldwide but is uncommon in the United States.

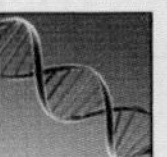

MOLECULAR PATHOGENESIS: *S. typhi* attaches to and invades small-bowel mucosa without causing clinical enterocolitis. Invasion tends to be most prominent in the ileum in areas overlying Peyer patches. The organisms are engulfed by macrophages, then block the respiratory burst of the phagocytes and multiply within these cells. Infected cells spread first to regional lymph nodes, then throughout the body via lymphatics and bloodstream, infecting mononuclear macrophages in lymph nodes, bone marrow, liver and spleen. Infection of macrophages stimulates IL-1 and TNF production, thereby causing the prolonged fever, malaise and wasting characteristic of typhoid fever.

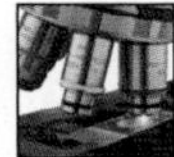

PATHOLOGY: The earliest pathologic change in typhoid fever is degeneration of the intestinal epithelium brush border. As bacteria invade, Peyer patches become hypertrophic. In some cases, intestinal lymphoid hyperplasia progresses to capillary thrombosis, causing necrosis of overlying mucosa and the characteristic ulcers oriented along the long axis of the bowel (Fig. 9-19). These

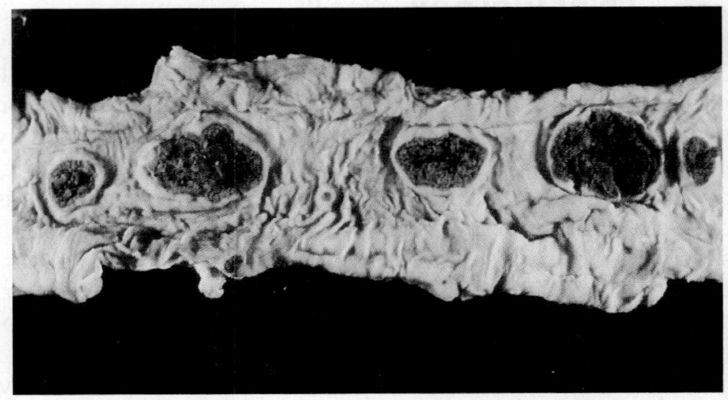

FIGURE 9-19. Ulcers of the terminal ileum in fatal typhoid fever. The ulcers have a longitudinal orientation because they are located over hyperplastic and necrotic Peyer patches.

ulcers frequently bleed and occasionally perforate, producing infectious peritonitis. Systemic dissemination of the organisms leads to focal granulomas in the liver, spleen and other organs, termed **typhoid nodules.** These are composed of aggregates of macrophages ("typhoid cells") containing ingested bacteria, erythrocytes and degenerated lymphocytes.

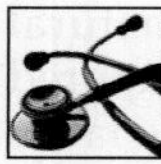

CLINICAL FEATURES: Untreated typhoid fever was classically divided into five stages (Fig. 9-20):

- **Incubation:** 10 to 14 days.
- **Active invasion/bacteremia:** The patient suffers for about a week with a variety of nonspecific symptoms, including daily stepwise elevation in temperature (up to 41°C [105.8°F]), malaise, headache, arthralgias and abdominal pain.
- **Fastigium:** Fever and malaise increase over several days until the infected person is prostrate. Patients may become toxic from the release of endotoxins from dead bacteria. Hepatomegaly is accompanied by derangement in liver function. The spleen is conspicuously enlarged.
- **Lysis:** In patients destined to survive, fever and toxic symptoms gradually diminish. Gastrointestinal bleeding and intestinal perforation at sites of ulceration may occur in any stage but are most common during lysis, which commonly lasts a week.
- **Convalescence:** Fever abates and patients gradually recover over several weeks to months. Some relapse or have metastatic foci of infection.

The treatment of typhoid fever entails antibiotics and supportive care. Ten to 20% of untreated patients die, usually of secondary complications, such as pneumonia. However, treatment within 3 days of the onset of fever is generally curative.

Shigellosis Is a Necrotizing Infection of the Distal Small Bowel and Colon

It is caused by any of four species of *Shigella (Shigella boydii, Shigella dysenteriae, Shigella flexneri* and *Shigella sonnei),* which are aerobic, gram-negative rods. Of these species, *S. dysenteriae* is the most virulent. Shigellosis is a self-limited disease that typically presents with abdominal pain and bloody, mucoid stools.

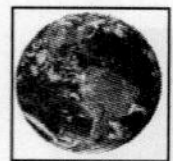

EPIDEMIOLOGY: *Shigella* organisms are spread from person to person by the fecal–oral route. They have no animal reservoir and do not survive well outside the stool. Infection usually occurs through ingestion of fecally contaminated food or water, but can be acquired by oral contact with any contaminated surface (e.g., clothing, towels or skin surfaces). As a result, endemic shigellosis is more common in areas with poor hygiene and sanitation. It is also spread in closed communities, such as hospitals, barracks and households. In developed countries, *S. flexneri* and *S. sonnei* are more common, and infection tends to be sporadic.

In the United States, about 300,000 cases occur annually, but the incidence of the disease is much higher in countries lacking sanitary systems for human waste disposal. Like other diarrheal illnesses, shigellosis is a significant cause of childhood mortality in developing countries.

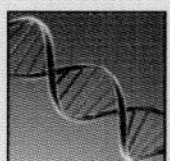
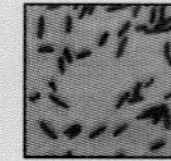

MOLECULAR PATHOGENESIS AND ETIOLOGIC FACTORS: Shigellae are among the most virulent enteropathogens. Disease is produced by ingesting as few as 10 to 100 organisms, and there are few asymptomatic carriers. The agent proliferates rapidly in the small bowel and attaches to enterocytes, where it replicates within the cytoplasm. Endocytosis is essential for virulence and the virulence factor is encoded by a plasmid. Replicating shigellae kill infected cells and then spread to adjacent cells and into the lamina propria.

Shigellae also produce a potent exotoxin, known as **Shiga toxin,** that is like the verotoxin of *E. coli* O157:H7. This toxin interferes with 60S ribosomal subunits and inhibits protein synthesis. It also causes watery diarrhea, probably by interfering with fluid absorption in the colon. Although shigellae extensively damage the epithelium of the ileum and colon, they rarely invade beyond the intestinal lamina propria, and bacteremia is uncommon.

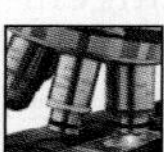

PATHOLOGY: The distal colon is almost always affected, although the entire colon and distal ileum can be involved. The affected mucosa is edematous, acutely inflamed and focally eroded. Ulcers appear first on the edges of mucosal folds, perpendicular to the long axis of the colon. A patchy inflammatory **pseudomembrane,** composed of neutrophils, fibrin and necrotic epithelium, is commonly found on the most severely affected areas. Regeneration of infected colonic epithelium occurs rapidly, and healing is usually complete within 10 to 14 days.

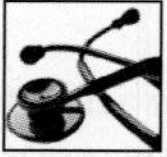

CLINICAL FEATURES: Shigellosis often begins with watery diarrhea, which changes in character within 1 to 2 days to the classic dysenteric stools. These are small-volume stools that contain gross blood, sloughed pseudomembranes and mucus. Cramping abdominal pain, tenesmus and urgency at stool typically accompany the diarrhea. Symptoms persist for 3 to 8 days, if the disease is untreated. Treatment with antibiotics shortens the course of the illness.

Cholera Is an Epidemic Enteritis Usually Acquired From Contaminated Water

Cholera is a severe diarrheal illness caused by the enterotoxin of* V. cholerae, *an aerobic, curved gram-negative rod. The organism proliferates in the lumen of the small intestine and causes profuse watery diarrhea, rapid dehydration and (if fluids are not restored) shock and death within 24 hours of the onset of symptoms.

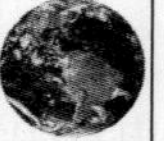

EPIDEMIOLOGY: Cholera is common in most parts of the world, but it periodically "disappears" spontaneously. A major pandemic occurred between 1961 and 1974, extending throughout Asia, the Middle East, southern Russia, the Mediterranean basin and parts of Africa. Cholera remains endemic in the river deltas of India and Bangladesh, where it may cause up to a half-million deaths annually.

It is acquired by ingesting *V. cholerae,* mainly in contaminated food or water. Epidemics spread readily in areas where human feces pollute the water supply. Shellfish and plankton

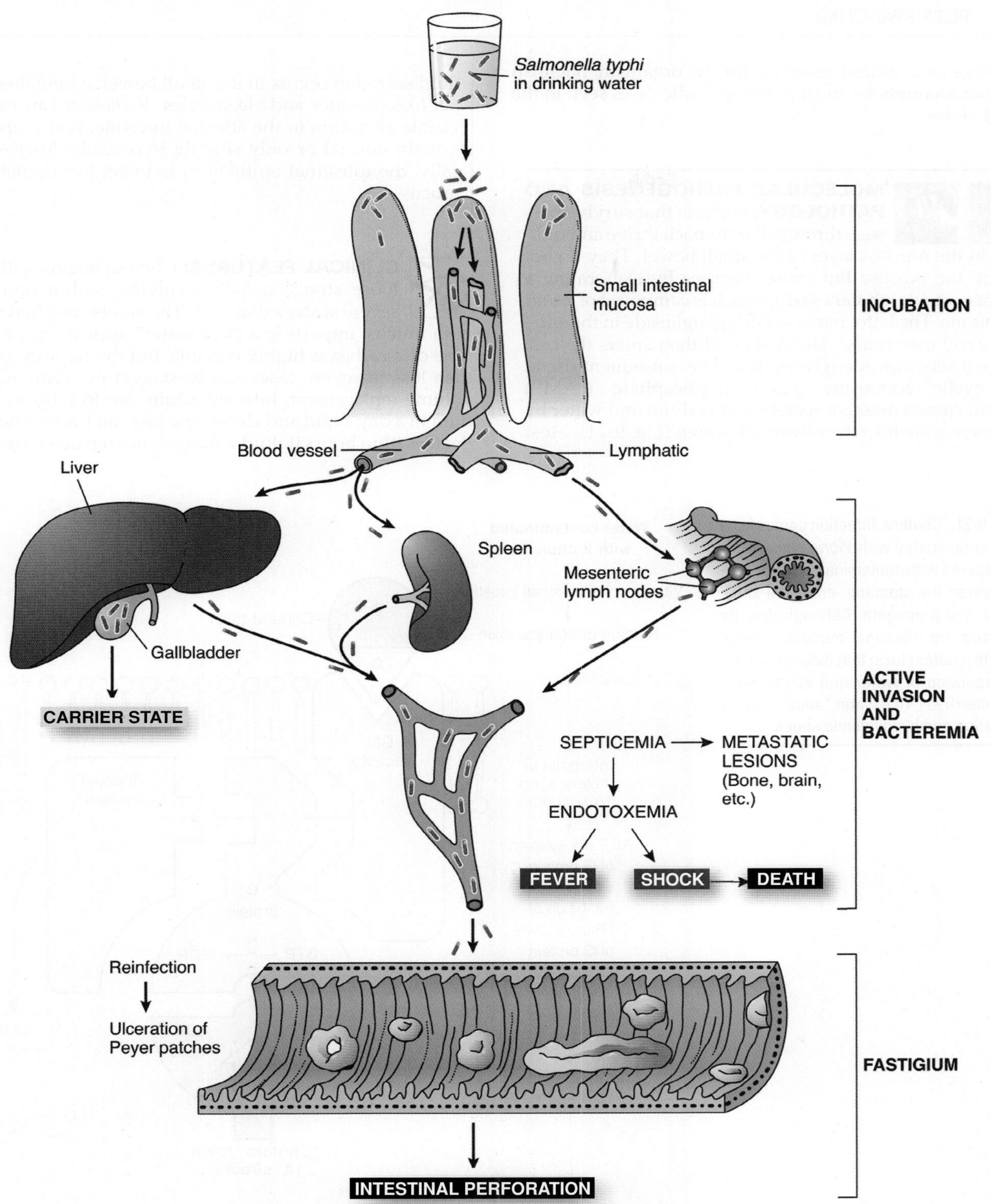

FIGURE 9-20. Stages of typhoid fever.
Incubation (10–14 days). Water or food contaminated with *Salmonella typhi* is ingested. Bacilli attach to the villi in the small intestine, invade the mucosa and pass to the intestinal lymphoid follicles and draining mesenteric lymph nodes. The organisms proliferate further within mononuclear phagocytic cells of the lymphoid follicles, lymph nodes, liver and spleen. Bacilli are sequestered intracellularly in the intestinal and mesenteric lymphatic system.
Active invasion/bacteremia (1 week). Organisms are released and produce a transient bacteremia. The intestinal mucosa becomes enlarged and necrotic, forming characteristic mucosal lesions. The intestinal lymphoid tissues become hyperplastic and contain "typhoid nodules"—aggregates of macrophages ("typhoid cells") that phagocytose bacteria, erythrocytes and degenerated lymphocytes. Bacilli proliferate in several organs, reappear in the intestine, are excreted in stool and may invade through the intestinal wall.
Fastigium (1 week). Dying bacilli release endotoxins that cause systemic toxemia.
Lysis (1 week). Necrotic intestinal mucosa sloughs, producing ulcers, which hemorrhage or perforate into the peritoneal cavity.

may serve as a natural reservoir for the organism. Shellfish ingestion accounts for most of the sporadic cases seen in the United States.

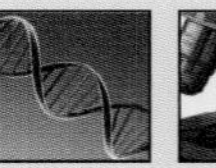
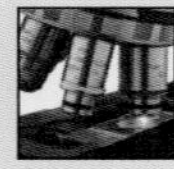

MOLECULAR PATHOGENESIS AND PATHOLOGY: Bacteria that survive passage through the stomach thrive and multiply in the mucous layer of the small bowel. They do not invade the mucosa but cause diarrhea by elaborating a potent exotoxin, **cholera toxin,** which is composed of A and B subunits. The latter binds to GM_1 ganglioside in the enterocyte cell membrane. The A subunit then enters the cell, where it activates adenylyl cyclase. The consequent rise in cell cyclic adenosine 3′,5′-monophosphate (cAMP) content causes massive secretion of sodium and water by the enterocyte into the intestinal lumen (Fig. 9-21). Most fluid secretion occurs in the small bowel, where there is a net loss of water and electrolytes. *V. cholerae* causes little visible alteration in the affected intestine, which appears grossly normal or only slightly hyperemic. Microscopically, the intestinal epithelium is intact but depleted of mucus.

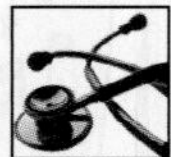

CLINICAL FEATURES: Cholera begins with a few loose stools, usually evolving within hours into severe watery diarrhea. The stools are often flecked with mucus, imparting a "rice water" appearance. The volume of diarrhea is highly variable, but the rapidity and volume loss in severe cases can be staggering. With adequate volume replacement, infected adults can lose up to 20 L of fluid in a day. Fluid and electrolyte loss can lead to shock and death within hours if fluid volume is not replaced. Untreated

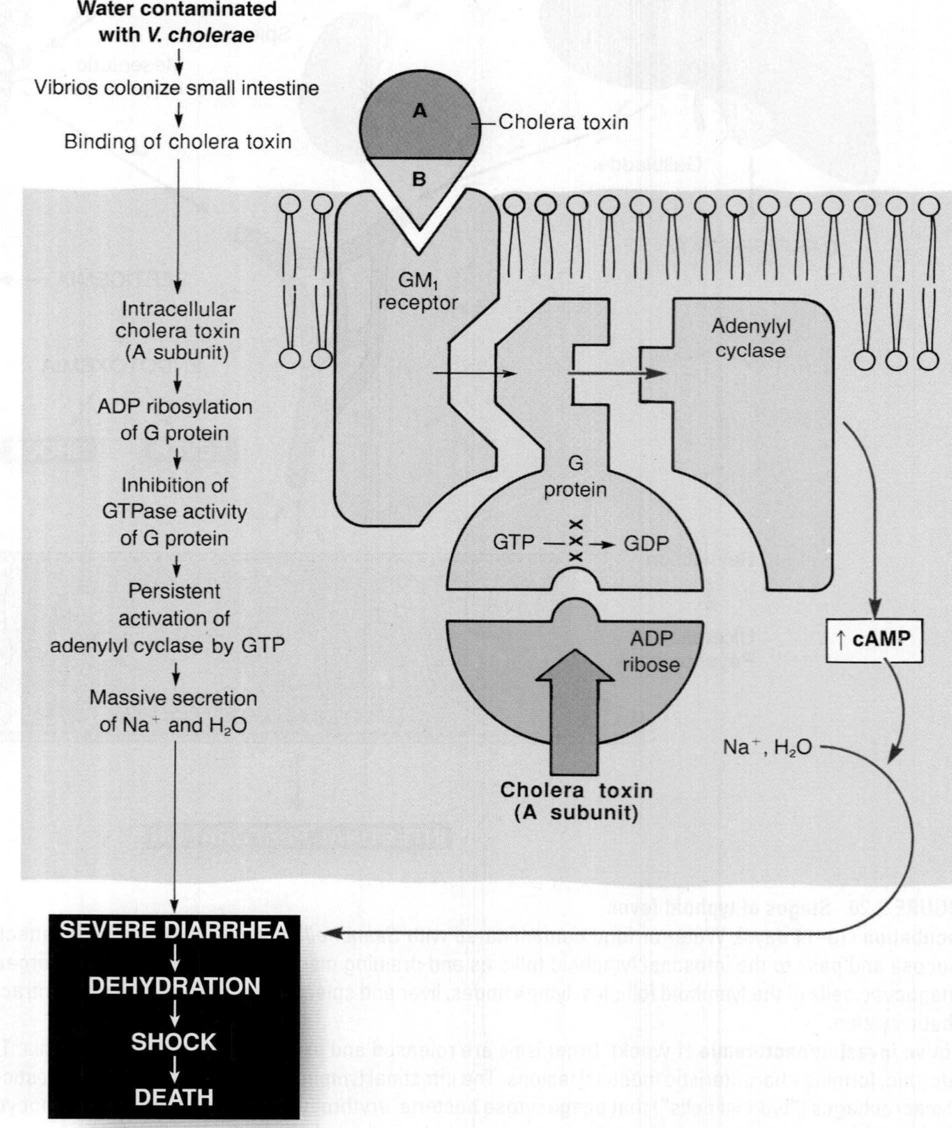

FIGURE 9-21. Cholera. Infection comes from water contaminated with *Vibrio cholerae* or food prepared with contaminated water. Vibrios traverse the stomach, enter the small intestine and propagate. Although they do not invade the intestinal mucosa, vibrios elaborate a potent toxin that induces a massive outpouring of water and electrolytes. Severe diarrhea ("rice water" stool) leads to dehydration and hypovolemic shock.

cholera has a 50% mortality rate. Replacing lost salts and water is a simple, effective treatment, which can often be accomplished by oral rehydration with preparations of salt, glucose and water. The illness subsides spontaneously in 3 to 6 days, which can be shortened by antibiotic therapy. Infection with *V. cholerae* confers long-term protection from recurrent illness, but available vaccines have limited effectiveness.

Vibrio parahaemolyticus

There are several "noncholera" vibrios, of which *Vibrio parahaemolyticus* is the most common. This organism is a gram-negative bacillus that causes acute gastroenteritis. It is found in marine life and coastal waters around the world in temperate climates, causing outbreaks in the summer. Its range may be expanding, whether due to global warming or other factors, as confirmed cases have occurred in Alaska, more than 1000 miles north of any previous outbreaks. Gastroenteritis is associated with consumption of inadequately cooked or poorly refrigerated seafood. The clinical syndrome resembles *Salmonella* enteritis. No deaths have been reported.

Campylobacter jejuni Is the Most Common Cause of Bacterial Diarrhea in the Developed World

Campylobacter jejuni is the major human pathogen in the genus *Campylobacter*. It causes an acute, self-limited inflammatory diarrheal illness. The organism is distributed worldwide and is responsible for over 2 million cases annually in the United States. *C. jejuni* is a microaerophilic, curved gram-negative rod, morphologically similar to the vibrios.

EPIDEMIOLOGY: *C. jejuni* infection is acquired through contaminated food or water. The bacteria inhabit gastrointestinal tracts of many animal species, including cows, sheep, chickens and dogs, which are a significant animal reservoir for infection. In fact, *Campylobacter* infections cause serious economic losses to farmers because of abortions and infertility of infected cattle and sheep. Raw milk and inadequately cooked poultry and meat are frequent sources of disease. *C. jejuni* can also spread from person to person by fecal–oral contact. The organism is a major cause of childhood mortality in developing countries and causes many cases of "travelers' diarrhea."

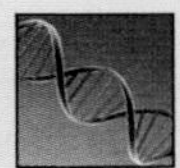

MOLECULAR PATHOGENESIS: Ingested *C. jejuni* that survive gastric acidity multiply in the alkaline environment of the upper small intestine. The agent elaborates several toxic proteins that correlate with the severity of the symptoms.

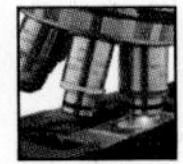

PATHOLOGY: *C. jejuni* causes a superficial enterocolitis, primarily involving the terminal ileum and colon, with focal necrosis of intestinal epithelium and acute inflammation. In severe cases, it progresses to small ulcers and patchy inflammatory exudates (pseudomembranes) composed of necrotic cells, neutrophils, fibrin and debris. Colon epithelial crypts often fill with neutrophils, forming so-called crypt abscesses. These pathologic changes resolve in 7 to 14 days.

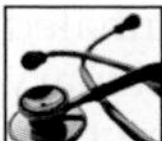

CLINICAL FEATURES: Patients with *C. jejuni* usually produce more than 10 stools per day, varying from profuse watery stools to small-volume stools containing gross blood and mucus. Symptoms resolve in 5 to 7 days. Treatment with antibiotics is probably of marginal benefit. A few patients develop a more severe, protracted illness resembling acute ulcerative colitis. Gastrointestinal infections with *C. jejuni* have been associated with Guillain-Barré syndrome.

Yersinia Infections Produce Painful Diarrhea

Yesinia enterocolitica and *Yersinia pseudotuberculosis* are gram-negative coccoid or rod-shaped bacteria.

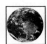

EPIDEMIOLOGY: These organisms are facultative anaerobes found in feces of wild and domestic animals, including rodents, sheep, cattle, dogs, cats and horses. *Y. pseudotuberculosis* is also often seen in domestic birds, including turkeys, ducks, geese and canaries. Both organisms have been isolated from drinking water and milk. *Y. enterocolitica* is more likely to be acquired from contaminated meat, and *Y. pseudotuberculosis* from contact with infected animals.

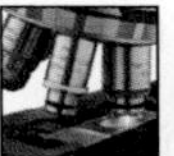
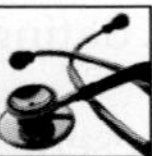

PATHOLOGY AND CLINICAL FEATURES: *Y. enterocolitica* proliferates in the ileum and invades the mucosa, causing ulceration and necrosis of Peyer patches. It migrates by way of lymphatics to mesenteric lymph nodes. Fever, diarrhea (sometimes bloody) and abdominal pain begin 4 to 10 days after mucosal penetration. Abdominal pain in the right lower quadrant has led to an incorrect diagnosis of appendicitis. Arthralgia, arthritis and erythema nodosum are complications. Septicemia is uncommon, but kills about one half of those in whom it occurs.

Y. pseudotuberculosis penetrates ileal mucosa, localizes in ileal–cecal lymph nodes and produces abscesses and granulomas in the lymph nodes, spleen and liver. Fever, diarrhea and abdominal pain may also suggest appendicitis.

Pulmonary Infections With Gram-Negative Bacteria

Klebsiella and *Enterobacter* Produce Nosocomial Infections That Cause Necrotizing Lobar Pneumonia

Klebsiella and *Enterobacter* spp. are short, encapsulated, gram-negative bacilli.

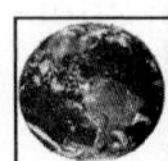

EPIDEMIOLOGY: These organisms cause 10% of all hospital-acquired (nosocomial) infections, including pneumonia and infections of the urinary tract, biliary tract and surgical wounds. Person-to-person transmission by hospital personnel is a special hazard. Predisposing factors are obstructive pulmonary disease in endotracheal tubes, indwelling catheters, debilitating conditions and immunosuppression. Secondary pneumonia caused by these bacteria may complicate influenza or other respiratory viral infections.

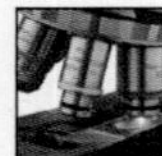

PATHOLOGY: *Klebsiella* and *Enterobacter* are inhaled and multiply in the alveolar spaces. The pulmonary parenchyma becomes consolidated, and a mucoid exudate of macrophages, fibrin and edema fluid fills the alveoli. As the exudate accumulates, alveolar walls become compressed and then necrotic. Numerous small abscesses may coalesce and lead to cavitation.

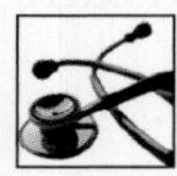

CLINICAL FEATURES: The onset of pneumonia is sudden, with fever, pleuritic pain, cough and a characteristic **thick mucoid sputum.** When infection is severe, these symptoms progress to dyspnea, cyanosis and death in 2 to 3 days. *Klebsiella* and *Enterobacter* infections may be complicated by fulminating, often fatal, septicemia and aggressive antibiotic therapy is required.

Legionella Cause Pneumonia That Ranges From Mild to Life-Threatening

Legionella pneumophila is a minute aerobic bacillus that has the cell wall structure of a gram-negative organism but reacts poorly with Gram stains. It was first identified 6 months after an outbreak of a severe respiratory disease of unknown cause at the 1976 American Legion convention in Philadelphia. Subsequently, retrospective studies demonstrated antibodies in sera from previously unexplained epidemics, dating to 1957.

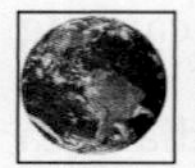

EPIDEMIOLOGY: *Legionella* are present in small numbers in natural bodies of fresh water. They survive chlorination and proliferate in devices such as cooling towers, water heaters, humidifiers and evaporative condensers. Infection occurs when people inhale aerosols from contaminated sources. The disease is not contagious, and the organism is not normal human oropharyngeal flora. An estimated 75,000 cases of *Legionella* infection occur in the United States annually.

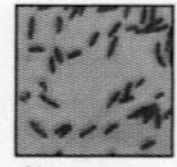

ETIOLOGIC FACTORS: *Legionella* cause two distinct diseases, namely, **pneumonia** and **Pontiac fever.** The pathogenesis of *Legionella* pneumonia (Legionnaires disease) is understood in some detail, whereas that of Pontiac fever remains largely a mystery. *Legionella* pneumonia begins when the organisms arrive in the terminal bronchioles or alveoli, where they are phagocytosed by alveolar macrophages. The bacteria replicate within phagosomes and protect themselves by blocking fusion of lysosomes with the phagosomes. The multiplying *Legionella* are released and infect freshly arriving macrophages. When immunity develops, macrophages are activated and cease to support intracellular growth of the organisms.

The native respiratory tract defenses, such as the mucociliary blanket of the airway, provide a first line of defense against *Legionella* infection in the lower respiratory tract. Smoking, alcoholism and chronic lung diseases, which interfere with respiratory defenses, also increase the risk of developing *Legionella* pneumonia.

PATHOLOGY: Legionnaires disease is an acute bronchopneumonia. It is usually patchy but may show a lobar pattern of infiltration. Affected alveoli and bronchioles are filled with an exudate composed of proteinaceous fluid, fibrin, macrophages and neutrophils (Fig. 9-22) and microabscesses. Alveolar walls become necrotic and are destroyed. Many macrophages show eccentric nuclei, pushed aside by cytoplasmic vacuoles containing *L. pneumophila.* As the pneumonia resolves, the lungs heal with little permanent damage.

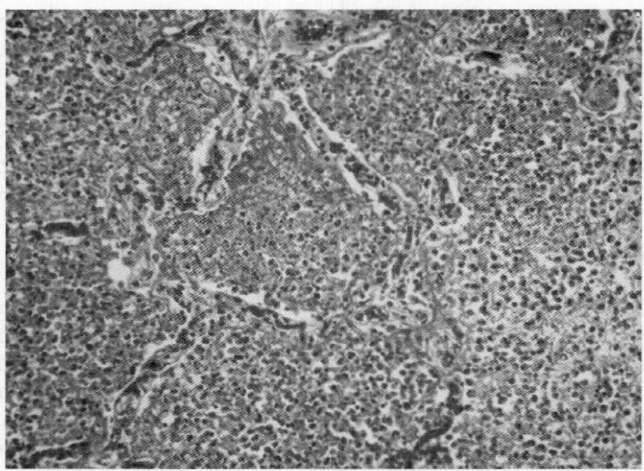

FIGURE 9-22. Legionnaires pneumonia. The alveoli are packed with an exudate composed of fibrin, macrophages and neutrophils.

CLINICAL FEATURES: After incubating 2 to 10 days, clinical onset is characterized by a rapidly progressive pneumonia, fever, nonproductive cough and myalgia. Chest radiographs reveal unilateral, diffuse, patchy consolidation, progressing to widespread nodular consolidation. Toxic symptoms, hypoxia and obtundation may be prominent, and death may follow within a few days. In those who survive, convalescence is prolonged. The mortality rate among hospitalized patients averages 15%, although there is a much greater risk of death if there is a serious underlying illness. Infection is amenable to treatment with macrolide antibiotics.

Pontiac fever is a self-limited, flu-like illness with fever, malaise, myalgias and headache. It differs from Legionnaires disease in showing no evidence of pulmonary consolidation. The disease resolves spontaneously in 3 to 5 days.

Pseudomonas aeruginosa Is a Highly Antibiotic-Resistant Opportunistic Pathogen

The organism only infrequently infects humans. However, it causes disease, particularly in hospital environments, where it is associated with pneumonia, wound infections, urinary tract disease and sepsis in debilitated or immunosuppressed persons. Burns, urinary catheterization, cystic fibrosis, diabetes and neutropenia all predispose to infection with *P. aeruginosa.*

It is a ubiquitous aerobic, gram-negative rod that requires moisture and only minimal nutrients. It thrives in soil and water, on animals and on moist environmental surfaces. Antibiotic use selects for *P. aeruginosa* infection, as the organism is resistant to most antibiotics.

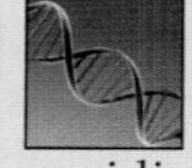

MOLECULAR PATHOGENESIS: *P. aeruginosa* elaborates an array of proteins that allow it to attach to, invade and destroy host tissues while avoiding host inflammatory and immune defenses. Injury to epithelial cells uncovers surface molecules that serve as binding sites for the pili of *P. aeruginosa*. Many strains of *P. aeruginosa* produce a proteoglycan that surrounds and protects them from mucociliary action, complement and phagocytes. The organism releases extracellular enzymes—including an elastase, an alkaline protease and a cytotoxin—which facilitate tissue invasion and are partially responsible for the necrotizing lesions of *Pseudomonas* infections. The elastase probably determines the distinctive ability of *P. aeruginosa* to invade blood vessel walls. The organism also causes systemic pathologic effects through endotoxin and several systemically active exotoxins.

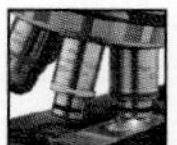

PATHOLOGY: *Pseudomonas* infection produces an acute inflammatory response. The organism often invades small arteries and veins, producing vascular thrombosis and hemorrhagic necrosis, particularly in the lungs and skin. Blood vessel invasion predisposes to dissemination and sepsis and leads to the development of multiple nodular lesions in the lungs. Gram stains of necrotic tissue infected with *Pseudomonas* commonly show blood vessel walls densely infiltrated with organisms. Sometimes disseminated infections are marked by skin lesions called **ecthyma gangrenosum.** These nodular, necrotic lesions represent sites where the organism has disseminated to the skin, invaded blood vessels and produced localized hemorrhagic infarcts.

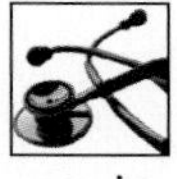

CLINICAL FEATURES: *Pseudomonas* infections are among the most aggressive human bacterial diseases, often progressing rapidly to sepsis. They require immediate medical intervention and are associated with high mortality.

Melioidosis Is Characterized by Abscesses in Many Organs

Melioidosis (Rangoon beggars disease) is an uncommon disease caused by *Burkholderia* (formerly *Pseudomonas*) *pseudomallei*, a small gram-negative bacillus in the soil and surface water of Southeast Asia and other tropical areas. During the conflict in Vietnam, several hundred American servicemen acquired melioidosis. The organism flourishes in wet environments, such as rice paddies and marshes. The skin is the usual portal of entry: organisms enter preexisting lesions, including penetrating wounds and burns. Humans may also be infected by inhaling contaminated dust or aerosolized droplets. The incubation period may last months to years, and the clinical course is variable.

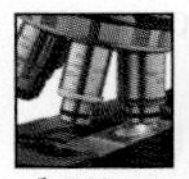
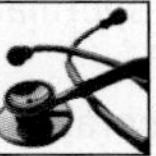

PATHOLOGY AND CLINICAL FEATURES: **Acute melioidosis** is a pulmonary infection, ranging from a mild tracheobronchitis to an overwhelming cavitary pneumonia (Fig. 9-23). Patients with severe cases present with the sudden onset of high fever, constitutional symptoms and a cough that may produce blood-stained sputum. Splenomegaly, hepatomegaly and jaundice are sometimes present. Diarrhea may be as severe as in cholera. Fulminating septicemia, shock, coma and death may develop in spite of antibiotic therapy. Acute septicemic melioidosis causes discrete abscesses throughout the body, especially in the lungs, liver, spleen and lymph nodes.

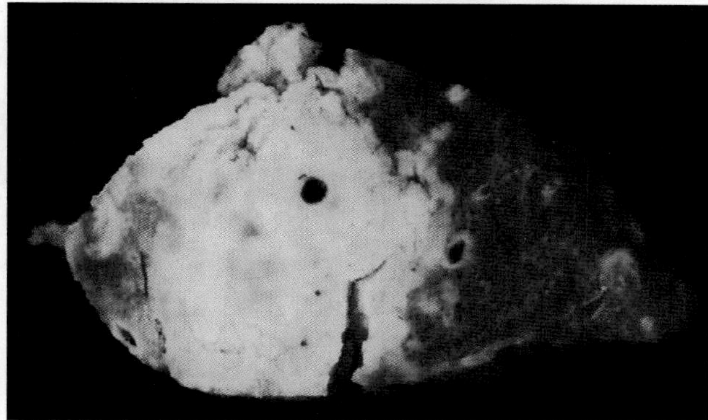

FIGURE 9-23. Acute melioidosis. The lung is consolidated and necrotic.

Chronic melioidosis is a persistent localized infection of the lungs, skin, bones or other organs. Lesions are suppurative or granulomatous abscesses and in the lung may be mistaken for tuberculosis. Chronic melioidosis may lie dormant for months or years, only to appear suddenly.

Clostridial Diseases

Clostridia are gram-positive, spore-forming, obligate anaerobic bacilli. The vegetative bacilli are found in the gastrointestinal tract of herbivorous animals and humans. Anaerobic conditions promote vegetative division, whereas aerobic ones lead to sporulation. Spores pass in animal feces and contaminate soil and plants, where they can survive well in unfavorable environments. Under anaerobic conditions, spores revert to vegetative cells, thereby completing the cycle. During sporulation, vegetative cells degenerate and their plasmids produce a variety of specific toxins that cause widely differing diseases, depending on the species (Fig. 9-24).

- **Food poisoning and necrotizing enteritis (pigbel)** are caused by enterotoxins of *C. perfringens*.
- **Gas gangrene** is produced by myotoxins of *C. perfringens*, *Clostridium novyi*, *Clostridium septicum* and other species.
- **Tetanus** is due to *C. tetani* neurotoxin.
- **Botulism** results from neurotoxins of *C. botulinum*.
- **Pseudomembranous enterocolitis** is caused by exotoxins made by *Clostridium difficile*.

Clostridial Food Poisoning Is Common and Is Self-Limited

C. perfringens is one of the most common causes of bacterial food poisoning in the world, causing an acute, generally benign, diarrheal disease, usually lasting less than 24 hours. It is omnipresent in the environment, contaminating soil, water, air samples, clothing, dust and meat.

Its spores survive cooking temperatures and germinate to yield vegetative forms, which proliferate when food is allowed to stand without refrigeration. Cooking drives out enough air to make the food anaerobic, a condition that is conducive to growth but not to sporulation. As a result, contaminated food contains vegetative clostridia but little preformed enterotoxin. The vegetative bacteria sporulate in the small

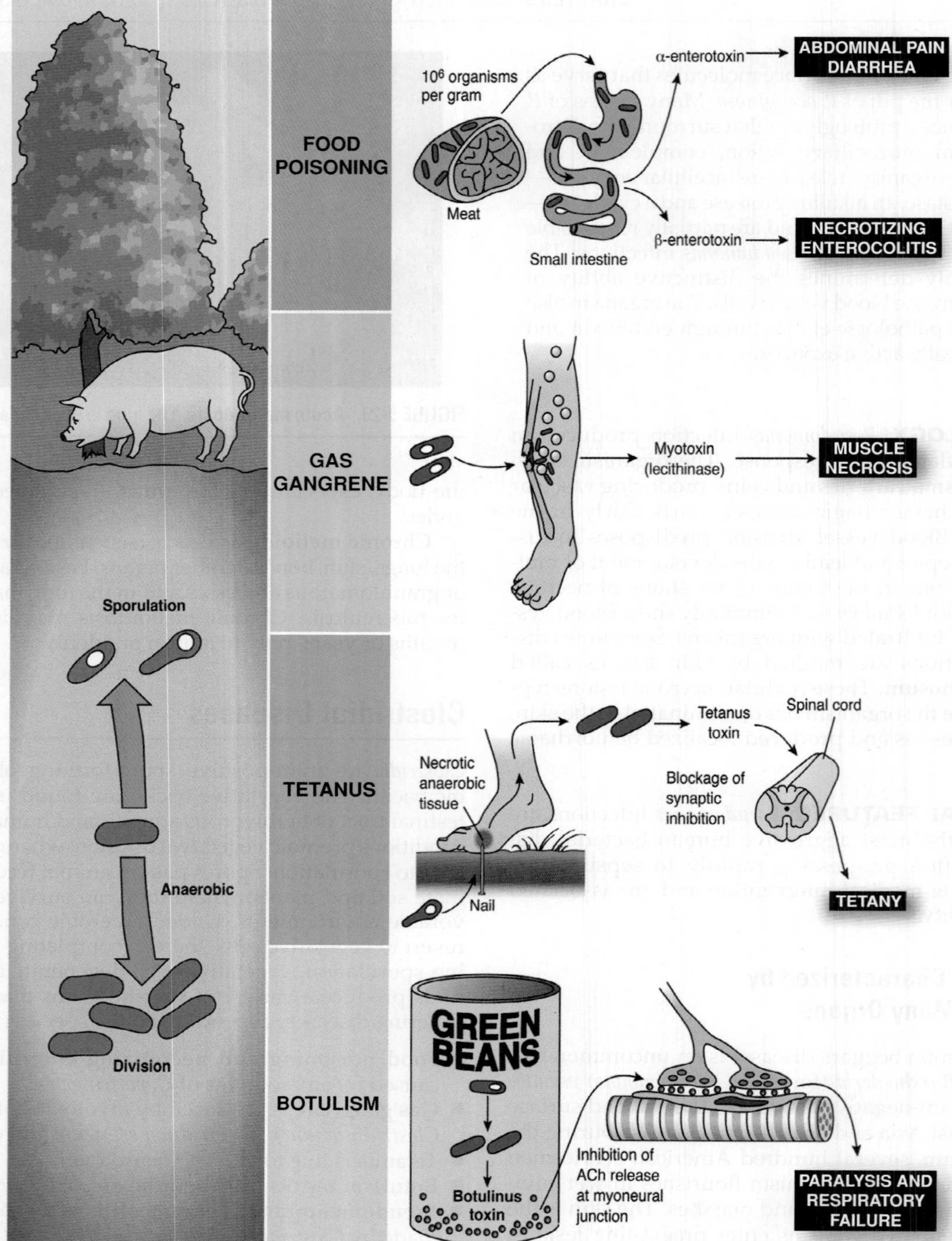

FIGURE 9-24. Clostridial diseases. *Clostridia* in the vegetative form (bacilli) inhabit the gastrointestinal tract of humans and animals. Spores pass in the feces, contaminate soil and plant materials and are ingested or enter sites of penetrating wounds. Under anaerobic conditions, they revert to vegetative forms. Plasmids in the vegetative forms elaborate toxins that cause several clostridial diseases.

Food poisoning and necrotizing enteritis. Meat dishes left to cool at room temperature grow large numbers of clostridia ($>10^6$ organisms per gram). When contaminated meat is ingested, *Clostridium perfringens* types A and C produce α enterotoxin in the small intestine during sporulation, causing abdominal pain and diarrhea. Type C also produces β enterotoxin.

Gas gangrene. Clostridia are widespread and may contaminate a traumatic wound or surgical operation. *C. perfringens* type A elaborates a myotoxin (α toxin), an α lecithinase that destroys cell membranes, alters capillary permeability and causes severe hemolysis following intravenous injection. The toxin causes necrosis of previously healthy skeletal muscle.

Tetanus. Spores of *Clostridium tetani* are in soil and enter the site of an accidental wound. Necrotic tissue at the wound site causes spores to revert to the vegetative form (bacilli). Autolysis of vegetative forms releases tetanus toxin. The toxin is transported in peripheral nerves and (retrograde) through axons to the anterior horn cells of the spinal cord. The toxin blocks synaptic inhibition and the accumulation of acetylcholine in damaged synapses leads to rigidity and spasms of the skeletal musculature (tetany).

Botulism. Improperly canned food is contaminated by the vegetative form of *Clostridium botulinum,* which proliferates under aerobic conditions and elaborates a neurotoxin. After the food is ingested, the neurotoxin is absorbed from the small intestine and eventually reaches the myoneural junction, where it inhibits the release of acetylcholine (ACh). The result is a symmetric descending paralysis of cranial nerves, trunk and limbs, with eventual respiratory paralysis and death.

bowel, where they elaborate a variety of exotoxins, which are cytotoxic to enterocytes and cause loss of intracellular ions and fluid. Certain types of food, including meats, gravies and sauces, are ideal substrates for *C. perfringens*. Clostridial food poisoning presents as abdominal cramping and watery diarrhea. Symptoms begin 8 to 24 hours after ingestion of contaminated food and usually resolve within 24 hours.

Necrotizing Enteritis Is a Catastrophic Childhood Infection in New Guinea

C. perfringens type C also produces an enterotoxin that causes necrotizing enterocolitis. The illness is rare in the industrialized world but remains endemic in parts of New Guinea, especially in children who have participated in pig feasts (hence the pidgin term *pigbel*). Adults, because they have circulating antibodies, tend not to develop the disease, which is segmental and may be restricted to a few centimeters or may involve the entire small intestine. Green, necrotic pseudomembranes are seen in areas of necrosis and peritonitis. More-advanced lesions perforate the bowel wall. Histologic sections reveal infarction of intestinal mucosa, with edema, hemorrhage and a suppurative transmural infiltrate.

Gas Gangrene May Complicate Penetrating Wounds

Gas gangrene (clostridial myonecrosis) is a necrotizing, gas-forming infection that begins in contaminated wounds and spreads rapidly to adjacent tissues. The disease can be fatal within hours of onset. *C. perfringens* is the most common cause of gas gangrene, but other clostridial species occasionally produce the disease.

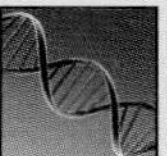

MOLECULAR PATHOGENESIS: Gas gangrene follows anaerobic deposition of *C. perfringens* into tissue. Clostridial growth requires extensive devitalized tissue, as in severe penetrating trauma, wartime injuries and septic abortions. Clostridial myonecrosis is rare if wounds are débrided promptly.

Necrosis of previously healthy muscle is caused by myotoxins elaborated by a few species of clostridia. *C. perfringens* type A is the source of the myotoxin in 80% to 90% of cases, but *C. novyi* and *C. septicum* may also produce myotoxin. Clostridial myotoxin is a phospholipase that destroys the membranes of muscle cells, leukocytes and erythrocytes.

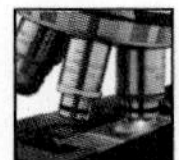

PATHOLOGY: Affected tissues rapidly become mottled and then frankly necrotic. Tissues such as muscle may even liquefy. The overlying skin becomes tense, as edema and gas expand underlying soft tissues. Microscopic examination shows extensive tissue necrosis with dissolution of the cells. A striking feature is the paucity of neutrophils, which are apparently destroyed by the myotoxin. Affected tissues often show typical, lozenge-shaped, gram-positive rods.

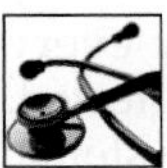

CLINICAL FEATURES: The incubation period of gas gangrene is commonly 2 to 4 days after injury. Sudden, severe pain occurs at the wound site, which is tender and edematous. Skin darkens, because of hemorrhage and cutaneous necrosis. The lesion develops a thick, serosanguineous discharge, which has a fragrant odor and may contain gas bubbles. Hemolytic anemia, hypotension and renal failure may develop; in the terminal stages, coma, jaundice and shock supervene.

Tetanus Is Spastic Skeletal Muscle Contractions Caused by *Clostridium tetani* Neurotoxin

It is also known as "lockjaw" because of early involvement of the muscles of mastication.

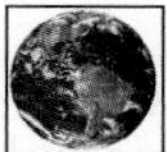

EPIDEMIOLOGY: *C. tetani* is present in the soil and lower intestine of many animals. Tetanus occurs when the organism contaminates wounds and proliferates in tissue, releasing its exotoxin. Using a vaccine composed of inactivated tetanus toxin, immunization programs have largely eliminated the disease from developed countries. Nonetheless, tetanus remains a frequent and lethal disease in developing countries. Many deaths occur in newborns in primitive societies as a result of the custom of coating umbilical stumps with dirt or dung to prevent bleeding.

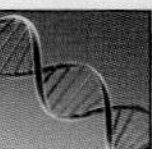

MOLECULAR PATHOGENESIS: Necrotic tissue and suppuration create a fertile anaerobic environment for the spores to revert to vegetative bacteria. Tetanus toxin is released from autolyzed vegetative cells. Although infection remains localized, the potent neurotoxin (**tetanospasmin**) is transported retrograde through the ventral roots of peripheral nerves to the anterior horn cells of the spinal cord. It crosses the synapse and binds to ganglioside receptors on presynaptic terminals of motor neurons in the ventral horns. After it is internalized, its endopeptidase activity selectively cleaves a protein that mediates exocytosis of synaptic vesicles. Thus, release of inhibitory neurotransmitters is blocked, permitting unopposed neural stimulation and sustained contraction of skeletal muscles (**tetany**). The loss of inhibitory neurotransmitters also accelerates heart rate and leads to hypertension and cardiovascular instability.

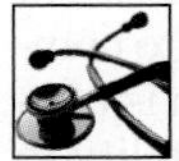

CLINICAL FEATURES: Tetanus incubates for 1 to 3 weeks, then begins subtly with fatigue, weakness and muscle cramping that progresses to rigidity. Spastic rigidity often begins in the muscles of the face, hence **"lockjaw,"** which extends to several facial muscles, causing a fixed grin (**risus sardonicus**). Rigidity of the muscles of the back produces a backward arching (**opisthotonos**) (Fig. 9-25). Abrupt stimuli, including noise, light or touch, can precipitate painful generalized muscle spasms. Prolonged spasm of respiratory and laryngeal musculature may lead to death. Infants and persons older than 50 years of age have the highest mortality.

Botulism Is a Paralyzing Disease Due to *Clostridium botulinum* Neurotoxin

The disease entails symmetric descending paralysis of cranial nerves, limbs and trunk.

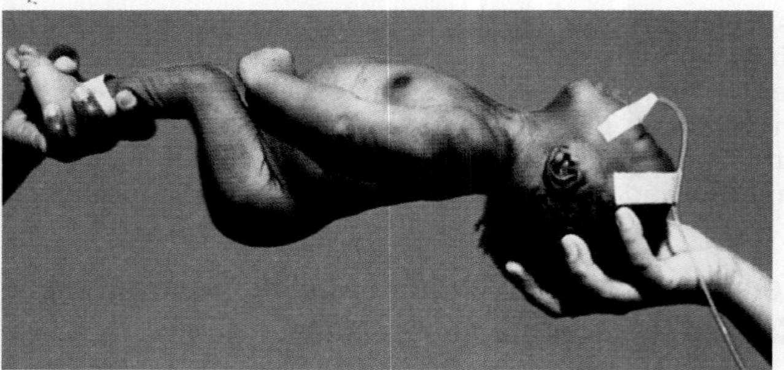

FIGURE 9-25. Tetanus. Opisthotonus (backward arching) in an infant due to intense contraction of the paravertebral muscles.

EPIDEMIOLOGY: *C. botulinum* spores are widely distributed and are especially resistant to drying and boiling. In the United States, the toxin is most often present in foods that have been improperly home canned and stored without refrigeration. These circumstances provide suitable anaerobic conditions for growth of the vegetative cells that elaborate the neurotoxin. Botulism can also be contracted from home-cured ham and other meats left unrefrigerated for several days, and from raw, smoked and fermented fish products. It is also caused by absorption of toxin from organisms proliferating in infants' intestines (**infantile botulism**) or rarely by absorption of toxin from organisms growing in contaminated wounds (**wound botulism**).

MOLECULAR PATHOGENESIS: Ingested botulinum neurotoxin resists gastric digestion and is readily absorbed into the blood from the proximal small intestine. Circulating toxin reaches the cholinergic nerve endings at the myoneural junction. There are seven serotypes of neurotoxin (A to G), with diverse mechanisms of action. The most common serotype, A, binds gangliosides at presynaptic nerve terminals and inhibits acetylcholine release.

CLINICAL FEATURES: Botulism is characterized by a descending paralysis, first affecting cranial nerves and causing blurred vision, photophobia, dry mouth and dysarthria. Weakness progresses to involve neck muscles, extremities, the diaphragm and accessory muscles of breathing. Respiratory weakness can progress rapidly to complete respiratory arrest and death. Untreated botulism is usually lethal, but treatment with antitoxin reduces mortality to 25%. Botulinum toxin is often used as treatment for many forms of dystonia, and has recently found popularity as a cosmetic vehicle to erase frown lines transiently (Botox).

Clostridium difficile Colitis Follows Antibiotic Treatment

C. difficile *colitis is an acute necrotizing infection of the terminal small bowel and colon. It is responsible for a large fraction (25% to 50%) of antibiotic-associated diarrheas and is potentially lethal.*

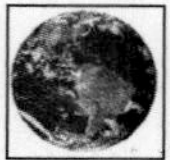

EPIDEMIOLOGY: *C. difficile* resides in the colon in some healthy persons. A change in intestinal flora, often due to antibiotic administration (e.g., clindamycin), allows it to flourish, produce toxin and damage the colonic mucosa. Such colitis can also be precipitated by other insults to the colonic flora, such as bowel surgery, dietary changes and chemotherapeutic agents. In hospitals where many patients receive antibiotics, fecal shedding of *C. difficile* results in person-to-person spread.

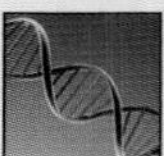

MOLECULAR PATHOGENESIS: As mentioned above, colonic bacteria ordinarily limit the growth of *C. difficile,* but alterations in the normal flora permit the organism to proliferate, elaborate toxins and destroy mucosal cells. The bacterium does not invade the colonic mucosa but rather produces two exotoxins. Toxin A causes fluid secretion; toxin B is directly cytopathic.

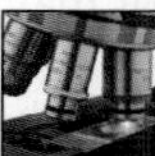

PATHOLOGY: *C. difficile* destroys colonic mucosal cells and incites an acute inflammatory infiltrate. Lesions range from focal colitis limited to a few crypts and only detectable on biopsy to massive confluent mucosal ulceration. Inflammation initially involves only the mucosa, but if the disease progresses, it can extend into the submucosa and muscularis propria. An inflammatory exudate, called a "pseudomembrane," of cellular debris, neutrophils and fibrin often forms over affected areas of the colon. *C. difficile* colitis is often called **pseudomembranous colitis,** even though that condition may have many etiologies.

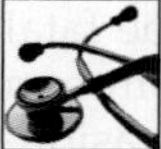

CLINICAL FEATURES: *C. difficile* colitis may start with very mild symptoms, or with diarrhea, fever and abdominal pain. Stools may be profuse and often contain neutrophils. The symptoms and signs are not specific and do not distinguish *C. difficile* colitis from other acute inflammatory diarrheal illnesses. Mild cases can often be treated simply by discontinuing the precipitating antibiotic. More-severe cases require an antibiotic effective against *C. difficile.*

Bacterial Infections With Animal Reservoirs or Insect Vectors

Brucellosis Is a Chronic Febrile Disease Acquired From Domestic Animals

Human brucellosis may manifest as an acute systemic disease or as a chronic infection with waxing and waning febrile episodes, weight loss and fatigue. *Brucella* are small, aerobic, gram-negative rods. In humans they primarily infect monocytes/macrophages.

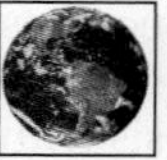

EPIDEMIOLOGY: Brucellosis is a zoonotic disease caused by one of four *Brucella* spp. Each species of *Brucella* has its own animal reservoir:

- *Brucella melitensis:* sheep and goats
- *Brucella abortus:* cattle
- *Brucella suis:* swine
- *Brucella canis:* dogs

Brucellosis is encountered worldwide. Virtually every type of domesticated animal and many wild ones are affected. The organisms reside in the animals' genitourinary systems, and infection is often endemic in animal herds. Humans acquire the bacteria by several mechanisms, including (1) contact with infected blood or tissue, (2) ingesting contaminated meat or milk or (3) inhaling contaminated aerosols. Brucellosis is an occupational hazard among ranchers, herders, veterinarians and slaughterhouse workers.

Elimination of infected animals and vaccination of herds have reduced the incidence of brucellosis in many countries, including the United States, where only about 200 cases are reported annually. Yet, the disease remains prevalent throughout Central and South America, Africa, Asia and Southern Europe. Unpasteurized milk and cheese remain a major source of infection in these areas. In the arctic and subarctic regions, humans acquire brucellosis by eating raw bone marrow of infected reindeer.

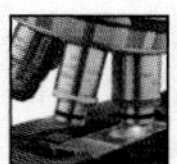

PATHOLOGY: Bacteria enter the circulation through skin abrasions, the lungs, the conjunctiva or the oropharynx. They then spread in the bloodstream to the liver, spleen, lymph nodes and bone marrow, where they multiply in macrophages. Generalized hyperplasia of these cells may ensue, causing lymphadenopathy and hepatosplenomegaly in 15% of patients infected with *B. melitensis* and in 40% of those infected with *B. abortus*. Patients infected with *B. abortus* develop conspicuous noncaseating granulomas in the liver, spleen, lymph nodes and bone marrow. By contrast, classic granulomas are not present in patients infected with *B. melitensis,* who may have only small aggregates of mononuclear inflammatory cells scattered throughout the liver. *B. suis* infection may cause suppurative liver abscesses rather than granulomas. The organisms usually cannot be demonstrated histologically. Periodic release of organisms from infected phagocytic cells may be responsible for the febrile episodes of the illness.

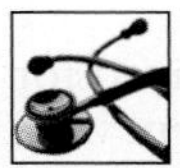

CLINICAL FEATURES: Brucellosis is a systemic infection that can involve any organ or organ system, with an insidious onset in half of cases. It is characterized by a multitude of somatic complaints, such as fever, sweats, anorexia, fatigue, weight loss and depression. Fever occurs in all patients at some time during the illness, but it can wax and wane (hence the term **undulant fever**) over a period of weeks to months if untreated. The mortality rate from brucellosis is less than 1%; death is usually caused by endocarditis.

The most common complications of brucellosis involve the bones and joints and include spondylitis of the lumbar spine and suppuration in large joints. Peripheral neuritis, meningitis, orchitis, endocarditis, myocarditis and pulmonary lesions are described. Prolonged treatment with tetracycline is usually effective; the relapse rate is dramatically reduced if rifampin or an aminoglycoside antibiotic is used.

Yersinia pestis Causes Bubonic Plague

Plague is a bacteremic, often fatal, infection that is usually accompanied by enlarged, painful regional lymph nodes (**buboes**). Historically, plague caused massive epidemics that killed much of the then civilized world. *Yersinia pestis* is a short gram-negative rod that stains more heavily at the ends (i.e., bipolar staining), particularly with Giemsa stains.

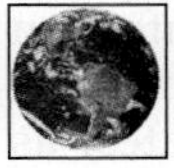

EPIDEMIOLOGY: *Y. pestis* infection is an endemic zoonosis in many parts of the world, including the Americas, Africa and Asia. The organisms are found in wild rodents, such as rats, squirrels and prairie dogs. Fleas transmit it from animal to animal, and most human infections result from bites of infected fleas. Some infected humans develop plague pneumonia and shed large numbers of organisms in aerosolized respiratory secretions, which allows disease transmission from person to person.

Major plague epidemics have occurred when *Y. pestis* was introduced into large urban rat populations in crowded, squalid cities. Infection spread first among rats; then, as they died, infected fleas fed on the human population, causing widespread disease. The Black Death pandemic in mid–14th-century (1347–1350) Europe killed about a third of Europe's population, perhaps 34 million people. In the United States, 30 to 40 cases of plague occur annually, mostly in the desert Southwest.

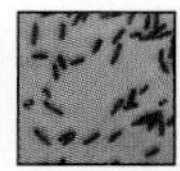
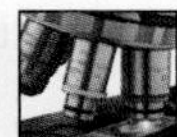

ETIOLOGIC FACTORS AND PATHOLOGY: After inoculation into the skin, *Y. pestis* is phagocytosed by neutrophils and macrophages. Organisms ingested by neutrophils are killed, but those engulfed by macrophages survive and replicate intracellularly. The bacteria are carried to regional lymph nodes, where they continue to multiply, producing extensive hemorrhagic necrosis. From regional lymph nodes, they disseminate via the bloodstream and lymphatics. In the lungs, *Y. pestis* produces a necrotizing pneumonitis that releases organisms into the alveoli and airways. These are expelled by coughing, enabling pneumonic spread of the disease. Affected lymph nodes, known as "buboes," are frequently enlarged and fluctuant, owing to extensive hemorrhagic necrosis. Infected patients often develop necrotic, hemorrhagic skin lesions, hence the name "black death" for this disease.

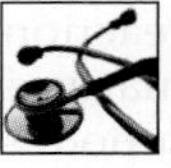

CLINICAL FEATURES: There are three clinical presentations of *Y. pestis* infection, although they often overlap.

- **Bubonic plague** begins within 2 to 8 days of the flea bite, with headache, fever and myalgias and with painful enlargement of regional lymph nodes, mostly in the groin, because flea bites usually occur in the lower extremities. Disease progresses to septic shock within hours to days after appearance of the bubo.
- **Septicemic plague** (10% of cases) occurs when bacteria are inoculated directly into the blood and do not produce buboes. Patients die of overwhelming bacterial growth in the bloodstream. Fever, prostration and meningitis occur suddenly, and death ensues within 48 hours. All blood vessels contain bacilli, and fibrin casts surround the organisms in renal glomeruli and dermal vessels.
- **Pneumonic plague** results from inhalation of air-borne particles from carcasses of animals or the cough of infected persons. Within 2 to 5 days after infection, high fever, cough and dyspnea begin suddenly. The sputum teems with bacilli. Respiratory insufficiency and endotoxic shock kill the patient within 1 to 2 days.

All types of plague carry a high mortality rate (50% to 75%) if untreated. Tetracycline, combined with streptomycin, is the recommended therapy.

Tularemia Is an Acute Febrile Disease Usually Acquired From Rabbits

Tularemia is caused by *Francisella tularensis,* a small gram-negative coccobacillus.

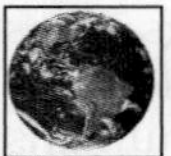

EPIDEMIOLOGY: Tularemia is a zoonosis whose most important reservoirs are rabbits and rodents, although other wild and domestic animals may harbor the organisms. Human infection with *F. tularensis* results from contact with infected animals or from the bites of infected insects, including ticks, deerflies and mosquitoes. Ticks and rabbits are responsible for most human infections. Bacteria may enter the body when blood-sucking insects inoculate them through the skin or via unnoticed breaks in the skin if there is direct contact with an infected animal. Tularemia can also result from inhalation of infected aerosols, ingestion of contaminated food and water or inoculation into the eye. It is found in temperate zones of the Northern Hemisphere. The incidence of tularemia has declined dramatically in the United States in the past five decades, to about 250 cases annually, presumably related to a decline in hunting and trapping.

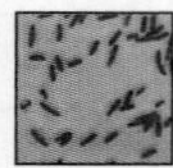

ETIOLOGIC FACTORS: *F. tularensis* multiplies at the site of inoculation, producing a focal ulcer there. The bacteria then spread to regional lymph nodes. Dissemination in the bloodstream leads to metastatic infections that involve the monocyte/macrophage system and sometimes the lungs, heart and kidneys. *F. tularensis* survives within macrophages until these cells are activated by a cell-mediated immune response to the infection.

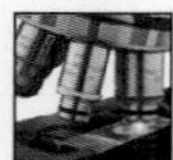

PATHOLOGY: Lesions of tularemia occur at the inoculation site and in the lymph nodes, spleen, liver, bone marrow, lungs (Fig. 9-26), heart and kidneys. Initial skin lesions are exudative, pyogenic ulcers. Later, disseminated lesions undergo central necrosis and are surrounded by a perimeter of granulomatous reaction resembling the lesions of tuberculosis. Hyperemia and abundant macrophages in the sinuses make lymph nodes large and firm; they later soften as necrosis and suppuration develop. Pulmonary lesions resemble those of primary tuberculosis.

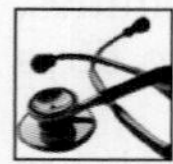

CLINICAL FEATURES: The incubation period of tularemia is from 1 to 14 days, depending on the dose and route of transmission, with a mean of 3 to 4 days. There are four distinct clinical presentations:

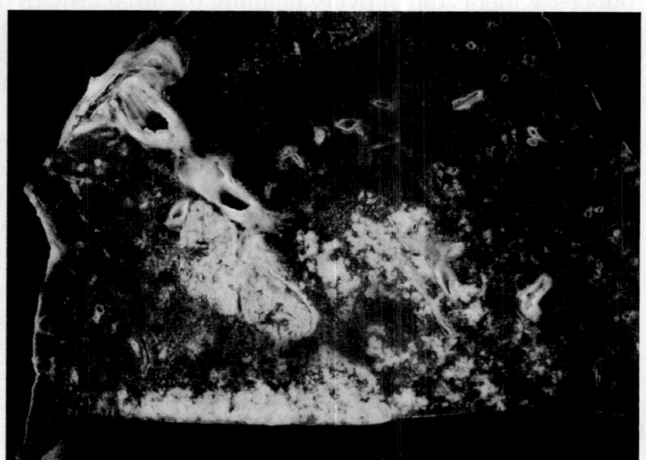

FIGURE 9-26. Tularemia. The lung shows firm, consolidated and necrotic areas.

- **Ulceroglandular tularemia** is the most common form of the disease (80% to 90% of cases) and begins as a tender, erythematous papule at the site of inoculation, usually on a limb. This develops into a pustule, which then ulcerates. Regional lymph nodes become large and tender and may suppurate and drain through sinus tracts. In some instances, generalized lymphadenopathy (**glandular tularemia**) is the first manifestation of infection.

  Initial bacteremia is accompanied by fever, headache, myalgias and occasionally prostration. Within a week, generalized lymphadenopathy and splenomegaly develop. The most serious infections are complicated by secondary pneumonia and endotoxic shock, in which case the prognosis is grave. Some patients develop meningitis, endocarditis, pericarditis or osteomyelitis.
- **Oculoglandular tularemia** is rare (<2% of cases) and is characterized by a primary conjunctival papule, which forms a pustule and ulcerates. Lymphadenopathy of the head and neck become prominent. Severe ulceration may cause blindness, if infection penetrates the sclera and reaches the optic nerve.
- **Typhoidal tularemia** is diagnosed when fever, hepatosplenomegaly and toxemia are the presenting signs and symptoms.
- **Pneumonic tularemia**, in which pneumonia is a major feature, may complicate any of the other types.

The illness lasts 1 week to 3 months, but this may be shortened by prompt treatment with streptomycin.

Anthrax Is Rapidly Fatal When It Disseminates

Anthrax is a necrotizing disease caused by *Bacillus anthracis*, which is a large spore-forming, gram-positive rod.

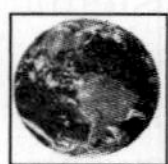

EPIDEMIOLOGY: Anthrax has been recognized for centuries, and descriptions of disease consistent with anthrax were reported in early Hebrew, Roman and Greek records. The major reservoirs are goats, sheep, cattle, horses, pigs and dogs. Spores form in the soil and dead animals, resisting heat, desiccation and chemical disinfection for years. Humans are infected when spores enter the body through breaks in the skin, by inhalation or by ingestion. Human disease may also result from exposure to contaminated animal byproducts, such as hides, wool, brushes or bone meal.

Anthrax has been a persistent problem in Iran, Turkey, Pakistan and Sudan. One of the largest recorded naturally occurring outbreaks of anthrax occurred in Zimbabwe, when an estimated 10,000 persons became infected in 1978 to 1980. In North America, human infection is extremely rare (one case per year for the past few years) and usually results from exposure to imported animal products. However, increased vigilance for anthrax has emerged following a recent bioterrorism episode involving transport of organisms by the postal system (see below).

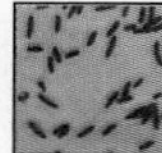

ETIOLOGIC FACTORS: The spores of *B. anthracis* germinate in the human body to yield vegetative bacteria that multiply and release a potent necrotizing toxin. In 80% of cases of cutaneous anthrax, infection remains localized and host immune responses eventually eliminate the organism. If the infection disseminates, as occurs when the organisms are inhaled or ingested, the resulting widespread tissue destruction is usually fatal.

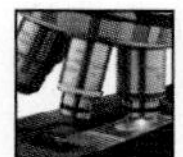

PATHOLOGY: *B. anthracis* produces extensive tissue necrosis at the sites of infection, associated with only a mild infiltrate of neutrophils. Cutaneous lesions are ulcerated, contain numerous organisms and are covered by a black scab. Pulmonary infection produces a necrotizing, hemorrhagic pneumonia, associated with hemorrhagic necrosis of mediastinal lymph nodes and widespread dissemination of the organism.

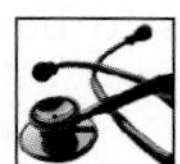

CLINICAL FEATURES: Anthrax mode of presentation depends on the site of inoculation.

- **Malignant pustule** is the cutaneous form, accounting for 95% of all anthrax. The patient presents with an elevated skin papule that enlarges and erodes into an ulcer. Bloody purulent exudate accumulates and gradually darkens to purple or black. The ulcer is often surrounded by a zone of brawny edema, which is disproportionately large for the size of the ulcer. Regional lymphadenitis portends a poor prognosis, since lymphatic invasion precedes septicemia. If infection does not disseminate, cutaneous lesions heal without sequelae.
- **Pulmonary, or inhalational, anthrax,** sometimes called "woolsorters' disease," is a hazard of handling raw wool and develops after inhalation of the spores of *B. anthracis*. It begins as a flu-like illness that rapidly progresses to respiratory failure and shock. Death often ensues within 24 to 48 hours. Only 18 cases of inhalational anthrax were reported in the United States from 1900 to 1980. As a result of the anthrax bioterror attack in the United States in 2001, 11 cases of inhalational anthrax occurred. The only hope is early antibiotic therapy.
- **Septicemic anthrax** more commonly follows pulmonary anthrax than malignant pustule. Disseminated intravascular coagulation is a common complication. Moreover, a bacterial toxin depresses the respiratory center, which explains why death can occur even when antibiotic therapy has cured the infection.
- **Gastrointestinal anthrax** is rare and is acquired by eating contaminated meat. Stomach or bowel ulceration and invasion of regional lymphatics are common. Death is caused by fulminant diarrhea and massive ascites.

Listeriosis Is a Systemic Multiorgan Infection With a High Mortality

It is caused by *Listeria monocytogenes*, a small, motile, gram-positive coccobacillus.

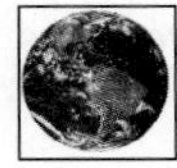

EPIDEMIOLOGY: Listeriosis is usually sporadic but may be epidemic. The organism has been isolated worldwide from surface water, soil, vegetation, feces of healthy persons, many species of wild and domestic mammals and several species of birds. However, spread of infection from animals to humans is rare. Most human infections occur in urban rather than rural environments, usually in the summer. *L. monocytogenes* grows at refrigerator temperatures, and outbreaks have been traced to unpasteurized milk, cheese and dairy products.

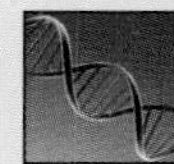

MOLECULAR PATHOGENESIS: *L. monocytogenes* has an unusual life cycle, which accounts for its ability to evade intracellular and extracellular host antibacterial defenses. After phagocytosis by host cells, the organisms enter phagolysosomes, where acidic pH activates *listeriolysin O*, an exotoxin that disrupts the vesicular membrane and allows bacteria to escape into the cytoplasm. After replicating, bacteria usurp host cytoskeleton contractile elements to form elongated protrusions that are engulfed by adjacent cells. Thus, *Listeria* spread from one cell to another without exposure to the extracellular environment.

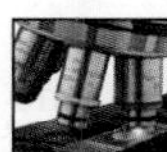
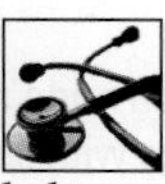

PATHOLOGY AND CLINICAL FEATURES: **Listeriosis of pregnancy** includes prenatal and postnatal infections. Listeriosis of the adult population is most commonly characterized by meningoencephalitis and septicemia, but may be localized to skin, eyes, lymph nodes, endocardium or bone.

Maternal infection early in pregnancy may lead to abortion or premature delivery. Infected infants rapidly develop respiratory distress, hepatosplenomegaly, cutaneous and mucosal papules, leukopenia and thrombocytopenia. Intrauterine infections involve many organs and tissues, including amniotic fluid, the placenta and the umbilical cord. Abscesses are found in many organs. Microscopically, foci of necrosis and suppuration contain many bacteria. Older lesions tend to be granulomatous. Neurologic sequelae are common, and the mortality of neonatal listeriosis is high even with prompt antibiotic therapy. Neonatal listeriosis may also be acquired during delivery, in which case the onset of clinical disease is 3 days to 2 weeks after birth.

Chronic alcoholics, patients with cancer or receiving immunosuppressive therapy and patients with AIDS are far more susceptible to infection than is the general population. Meningitis is the most common form of the disease in adults and resembles other bacterial meningitides.

Septicemic listeriosis is a severe febrile illness most common in immunodeficient patients. It may lead to shock and disseminated intravascular coagulation, leading to misdiagnosis as gram-negative sepsis. Prolonged treatment with antimicrobials is usually required because patients tend to experience relapse if therapy is administered for less than 3 weeks. The mortality from systemic listeriosis remains at 25%.

Cat-Scratch Disease Is a Self-Limited Granulomatous Lymphadenitis

Cat-scratch disease is a self-limited infection usually caused by *Bartonella henselae* and more rarely by *Bartonella quintana*. The bacteria are small (0.2 to 0.6 μm) gram-negative rods. They are difficult to culture but are easily seen in tissue sections of the skin, lymph nodes and conjunctiva when stained with a silver impregnation technique (Fig. 9-27).

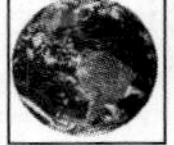

EPIDEMIOLOGY: The animal reservoir is thought to be cats; surveys have shown that up to 30% of cats are bacteremic. Infection begins when the bacillus is inoculated into the skin by the claws of cats (or, rarely, other animals) or by thorns or splinters. Sometimes the conjunctiva is contaminated by close contact with a cat, possibly by licking around the eye. Infections are more common in children

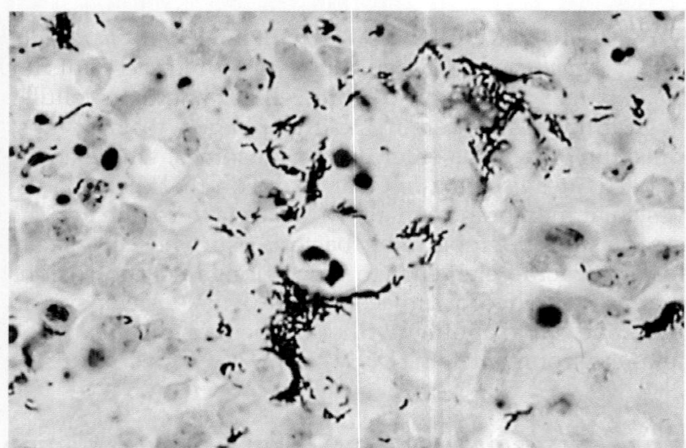

FIGURE 9-27. Cat-scratch disease. Section of a lymph node shows the bacilli, which are gram negative but difficult to visualize with tissue Gram stains. They are blackened by the Warthin-Starry silver impregnation technique.

(80%) than adults, and they may cluster when a stray cat joins a family.

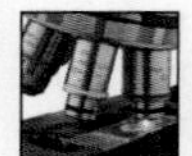 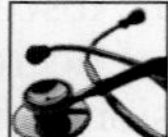

PATHOLOGY AND CLINICAL FEATURES: Bacteria multiply in the walls of small vessels and about collagen fibers at the site of inoculation. The organisms are then carried to regional lymph nodes, where they cause a **suppurative** and **granulomatous lymphadenitis.** In early lesions, clusters of bacteria fill and expand lumina of small blood vessels. However, bacteria are rare in late lesions. A papule develops at the site of inoculation, followed by tenderness and enlargement of regional lymph nodes. Nodes remain enlarged for 3 to 4 months and may drain through the skin. About half of patients have other symptoms, including fever and malaise, rash, a brief encephalitis and erythema nodosum. **Parinaud oculoglandular syndrome** (preauricular adenopathy secondary to conjunctival infection) is common. Antibiotics are not known to help.

Glanders Is a Granulomatous Infection Acquired From Horses

Glanders is an infection of equine species (horses, mules, donkeys) that is only rarely transmitted to humans, in whom it causes acute or chronic granulomatous disease. It is caused by *Pseudomonas mallei*, a small gram-negative, nonmotile bacillus. Although uncommon, the infection remains endemic in South America, Asia and Africa. Humans acquire the disease by contact with infected equines through broken skin or inhalation of contaminated aerosols.

- **Acute glanders** is characterized by bacteremia, severe prostration and fever. Granulomatous abscesses may form in subcutaneous tissues and many other organs, including the lung, liver, spleen, muscles and joints. Acute glanders is almost always fatal.
- **Chronic glanders** features low-grade fever, draining abscesses of the skin, lymphadenopathy and hepatosplenomegaly. Granulomas in many organs mimic tuberculosis. The mortality in chronic glanders exceeds 50%.

Bartonellosis Causes Acute Anemia and Chronic Skin Disease

Bartonellosis is an infection by *Bartonella bacilliformis*, a small, multiflagellated, gram- negative coccobacillus.

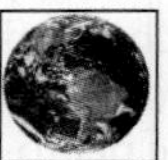

EPIDEMIOLOGY: Bartonellosis occurs only in Peru, Ecuador and Colombia in river valleys of the Andes and is transmitted by sandflies. Humans are the only reservoir and acquire the infection at sunrise and sunset, when sandflies are most active. In endemic areas, 10% to 15% of the population have latent infections. Newcomers are susceptible, whereas the indigenous population tends to be resistant.

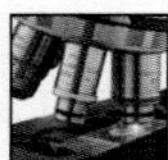 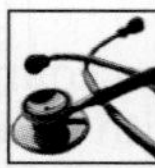

PATHOLOGY AND CLINICAL FEATURES: Bartonellosis presents a biphasic pattern, with acute hemolytic anemia (**Oroya fever**) first, followed some months later by a chronic dermal phase (**verruga peruana**). Either phase may occur by itself.

The most severe consequence of bartonellosis is hemolytic anemia. After *B. bacilliformis* is inoculated into the skin by a sandfly, bacteria proliferate in the vascular endothelium and then invade erythrocytes, leading to profound hemolysis.

The **acute anemic phase** follows 3 weeks of incubation and is characterized by abrupt onset of fever, skeletal pains and severe, hemolytic anemia. If untreated, 40% of patients in the anemic phase die. Secondary *Salmonella* sepsis is frequent and contributes to the high mortality.

The **dermal eruptive phase** of bartonellosis may coexist with the anemic phase but is usually separated by an interval of 3 to 6 months. Many small hemangioma-like lesions stud the dermis, and bacteria may be identified in endothelial cells. Nodular lesions may be prominent on extensor surfaces of the arms and legs. Large deep-seated lesions, which tend to ulcerate, develop near joints and limit motion. The dermal eruptive phase is often prolonged but eventually heals spontaneously. The mortality in this phase is less than 5%.

Infections Caused by Branching Filamentous Organisms

Actinomycosis Is Characterized by Abscesses and Sinus Tracts

Actinomycosis is a slowly progressive, suppurative, fibrosing infection involving the jaw, thorax or abdomen. The disease is caused by a number of anaerobic and microaerophilic bacteria termed *Actinomyces*. These are branching, filamentous, gram-positive rods that normally reside in the oropharynx, gastrointestinal tract and vagina. Several *Actinomyces* spp. cause human disease, the most common being *Actinomyces israelii*.

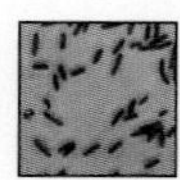 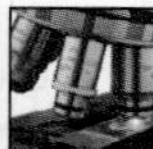

ETIOLOGIC FACTORS AND PATHOLOGY: *Actinomyces* is not ordinarily virulent: the organisms reside as saprophytes in the body without producing disease. Two uncommon conditions must occur for *Actinomyces* to cause disease. First, it must be inoculated into deeper tissues, since it cannot invade. Second, an anaerobic atmosphere is necessary for bacterial proliferation.

Trauma can produce tissue necrosis, providing an excellent anaerobic medium for growth of *Actinomyces*, and can inoculate the organism into normally sterile tissue. Actinomycosis occurs at four distinct sites:

- **Cervicofacial actinomycosis** results from jaw injury, dental extraction or dental manipulation.
- **Thoracic actinomycosis** is due to aspiration of organisms contaminating dental debris.
- **Abdominal actinomycosis** follows traumatic or surgical disruption of the bowel, especially the appendix.
- **Pelvic actinomycosis** is associated with the prolonged use of intrauterine devices (IUDs).

Actinomycosis begins as a nidus of proliferating organisms that attract an acute inflammatory infiltrate. The small abscess grows slowly, becoming a series of abscesses connected by sinus tracts. Tracts burrow across normal tissue boundaries and into adjacent organs. Eventually, a tract may reach an external surface or mucosal membrane and produce a draining sinus. The walls of abscesses and tracts are composed of granulation tissue, often thick, densely fibrotic and chronically inflamed. Within abscesses and sinuses are pus and colonies of organisms.

The colonies of *Actinomyces* within these lesions can grow to several millimeters in diameter and be visible to the naked eye. They appear as hard, yellow grains known as **sulfur granules**, because of their resemblance to elemental sulfur. Sulfur granules consist of tangled masses of narrow, branching filaments, embedded in a polysaccharide–protein matrix (**Splendore-Hoeppli material**). Histologically, the colonies appear as rounded, basophilic grains with scalloped eosinophilic borders (Fig. 9-28A). Individual filaments of *Actinomyces* cannot be discerned with hematoxylin and eosin stain but are readily visible on Gram staining or silver impregnation (Fig. 9-28B).

CLINICAL FEATURES: The signs and symptoms of actinomycosis depend on the site of infection. If infection originates in a tooth socket or the tonsils, it is characterized by swelling of the jaw ("lumpy jaw"), face and neck, at first painless and fluctuant but later painful. In pulmonary infections, sinus tracts may penetrate from lobe to lobe, through the pleura and into ribs and vertebrae. Abdominal or pelvic disease may present as an expanding mass, suggesting a locally spreading tumor. Actinomycosis responds to prolonged antibiotic therapy, and penicillin is highly effective.

Nocardiosis Is a Suppurative Respiratory Infection in Immunocompromised Hosts

Nocardia are aerobic, gram-positive filamentous, branching bacteria. They are weakly acid fast, a characteristic used to distinguish them from the morphologically similar actinomycetes. From the lungs, infection often spreads to the brain and skin.

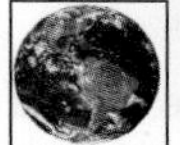

EPIDEMIOLOGY: *Nocardia* spp. are widely distributed in soil. Human disease is caused by inhaling or inoculating soil-borne organisms. It is not transmitted from person to person. *Nocardia asteroides* is the species most often involved in human disease. Nocardiosis is most common in patients with impaired immunity, particularly cell-mediated immunity. Organ transplantation, long-term corticosteroid therapy, lymphomas, leukemias and other debilitating diseases are predisposing factors.

Two other pathogenic species of *Nocardia*, *Nocardia brasiliensis* and *Nocardia caviae*, may cause pulmonary nocardiosis resembling that produced by *N. asteroides*. They are usually encountered in underdeveloped countries as a cause of mycetomas.

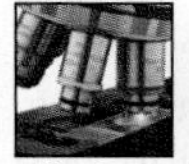

PATHOLOGY AND CLINICAL FEATURES: The respiratory tract is the usual portal of entry for *Nocardia*. The organism elicits a brisk infiltrate of neutrophils, and disease begins as a slowly progressive, pyogenic pneumonia. If an infected person mounts a vigorous cell-mediated immune response, the infection may be eliminated. In immunocompromised people, however, *Nocardia* produces pulmonary abscesses, which are frequently multiple and confluent. Direct extension to the pleura, trachea and heart and blood-borne metastases to the brain or skin carry a grave prognosis. Nocardial abscesses are filled with neutrophils, necrotic debris and scattered organisms. Bacteria can be demonstrated by silver

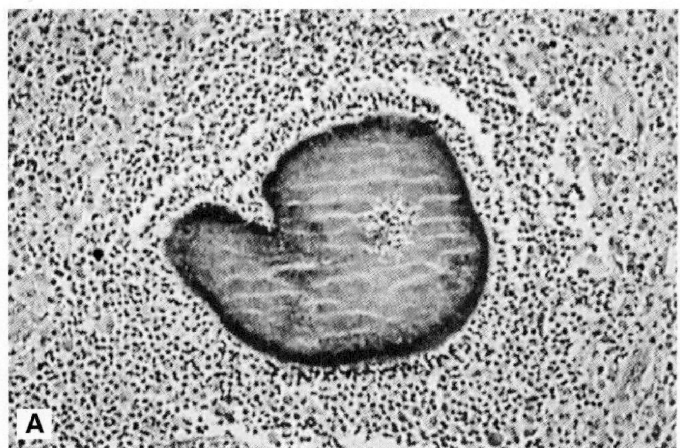

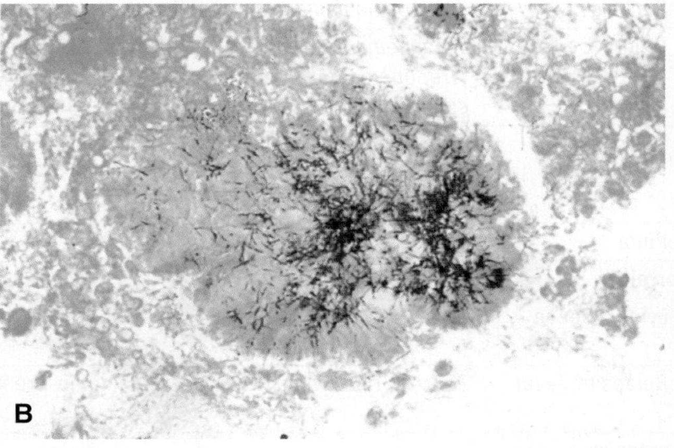

FIGURE 9-28. Actinomycosis. A. A typical sulfur granule lies within an abscess. **B.** The individual filaments of *Actinomyces israeli* are readily visible with the silver impregnation technique.

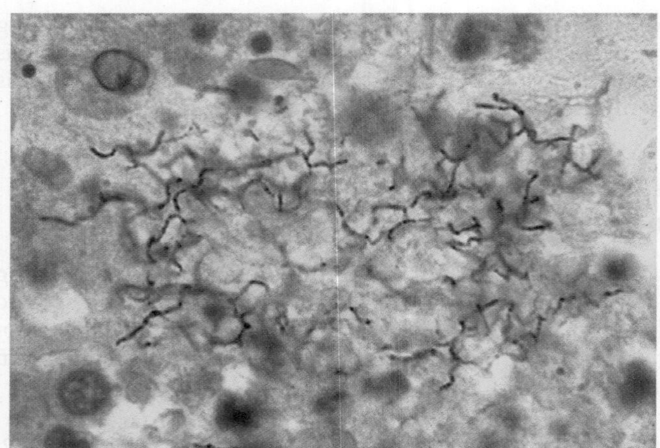

FIGURE 9-29. Nocardiosis. A silver stain of a necrotic exudate reveals the branching, filamentous rods of *Nocardia asteroides*.

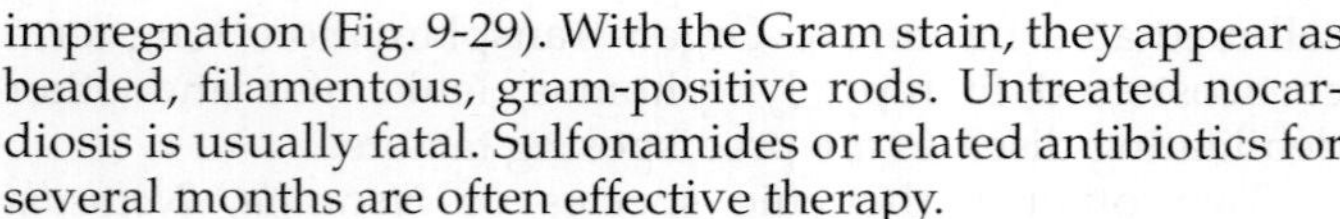

impregnation (Fig. 9-29). With the Gram stain, they appear as beaded, filamentous, gram-positive rods. Untreated nocardiosis is usually fatal. Sulfonamides or related antibiotics for several months are often effective therapy.

SPIROCHETAL INFECTIONS

Spirochetes are long, slender, helical bacteria with specialized cell envelopes that permit them to move by flexion and rotation. The thinner organisms are below the resolving power of routine light microscopy. Specialized techniques, such as darkfield microscopy or silver impregnation, are needed to visualize them. Although spirochetes have the basic cell wall structure of gram-negative bacteria, they stain poorly with the Gram stain.

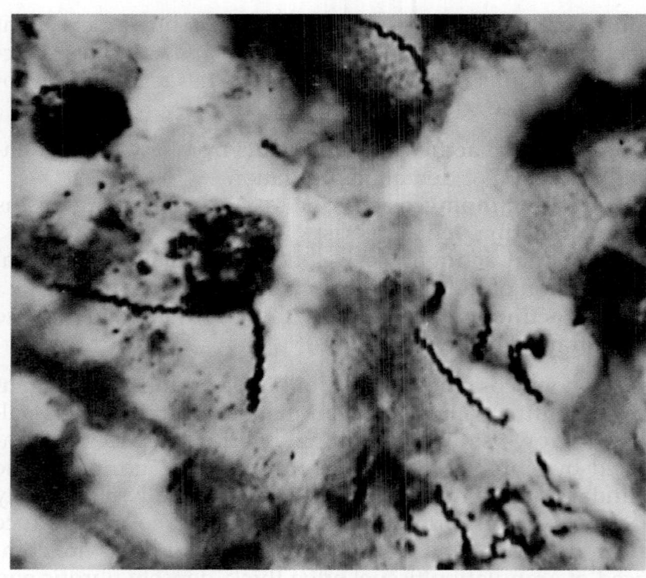

FIGURE 9-30. Syphilis. Spirochetes of *Treponema pallidum*, visualized by silver impregnation, in the eye of a child with congenital syphilis.

Three genera of spirochetes, *Treponema, Borrelia* and *Leptospira,* cause human disease (Table 9-5). They are adept at evading host inflammatory and immunologic defenses, and diseases caused by these organisms are all chronic or relapsing.

Syphilis

Syphilis (lues) is a chronic, sexually transmitted, systemic infection caused by *T. pallidum. T. pallidum* is a thin, long spirochete (Fig. 9-30) that cannot be grown in artificial media.

Table 9-5

Spirochete Infections

Disease	Organism	Clinical Manifestation	Distribution	Mode of Transmission
Treponemes				
Syphilis	*Treponema pallidum*	See text	Common worldwide	Sexual contact, congenital
Bejel	*Treponema endemicum (Treponema pallidum,* subsp. *endemicum)*	Mucosal, skin and bone lesions	Middle East	Mouth-to-mouth contact
Yaws	*Treponema pertenue (Treponema pallidum* subsp. *pertenue)*	Skin and bone	Tropics	Skin-to-skin contact
Pinta	*Treponema carateum*	Skin lesions	Latin America	Skin-to-skin contact
Borrelia				
Lyme disease	*Borrelia burgdorferi*	See text	North America, Europe, Russia, Asia, Africa, Australia	Tick bite
Relapsing fever	*Borrelia recurrentis*	Relapsing flu-like illness	Worldwide	Tick bite, louse bite and related species
Leptospira				
Leptospirosis	*Leptospira interrogans*	Flu-like illness, meningitis	Worldwide	Contact with animal urine

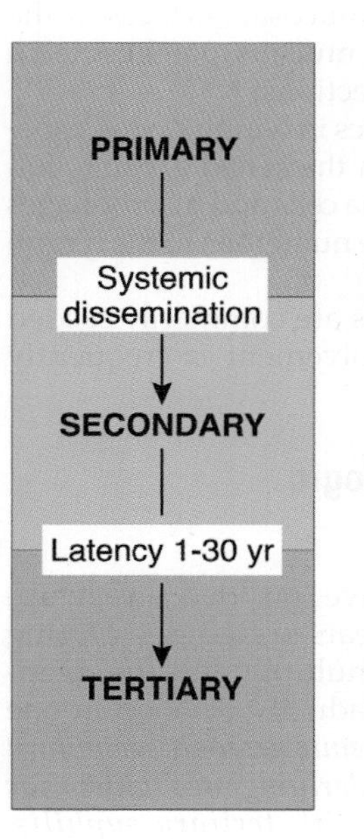

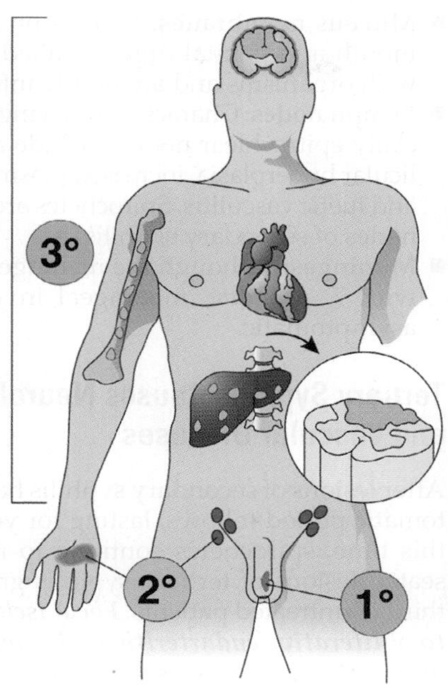

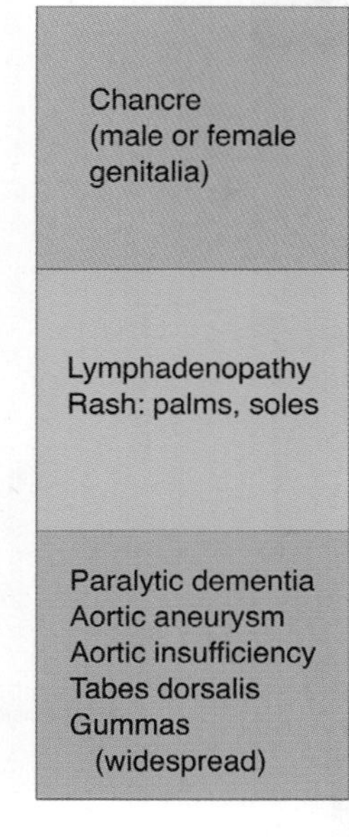

FIGURE 9-31. Clinical characteristics of the various stages of syphilis.

The disease was first recognized in Europe in the 1490s and has been related to Columbus's return from the New World. Urbanization and mass movements of people caused by war contributed to its rapid spread. Originally, syphilis was an acute disease that caused destructive skin lesions and early death, but it has become milder, with a more protracted and insidious clinical course.

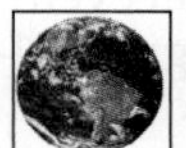

EPIDEMIOLOGY: Syphilis is a worldwide disease that is transmitted almost exclusively by sexual contact. Infection may also spread from an infected mother to her fetus (**congenital syphilis**). The incidence of primary and secondary syphilis has declined since the introduction of penicillin therapy at the end of World War II.

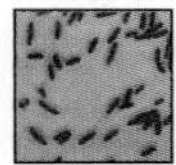

ETIOLOGIC FACTORS: *T. pallidum* is very fragile and is killed by soap, antiseptics, drying and cold. Person-to-person transmission requires direct contact between a rich source of spirochetes (e.g., an open lesion) and mucous membranes or abraded skin of the genital organs, rectum, mouth, fingers or nipples. The organisms reproduce at the site of inoculation, pass to regional lymph nodes, gain access to systemic circulation and disseminate throughout the body. Although *T. pallidum* induces an inflammatory response and is taken up by phagocytic cells, it persists and proliferates. Chronic infection and inflammation cause tissue destruction, sometimes for decades. The course of syphilis is classically divided into three stages (Fig. 9-31).

The Classical Lesion of Primary Syphilis Is the Chancre

Chancres (Fig. 9-32) are characteristic ulcers at sites of *T. pallidum* entry, usually the penis, vulva, anus or mouth. They appear 1 week to 3 months after exposure, with an average of 3 weeks, and tend to be solitary, with firm, raised borders. Spirochetes tend to concentrate in vessel walls and in the epidermis around the ulcer. Chancres, as well as the lesions of the other stages of syphilis, show a characteristic "**luetic vasculitis**," with endothelial cell proliferation and swelling, and vessel walls becoming thickened by lymphocytes and fibrosis.

Chancres quickly erode to a characteristic ulcer. They are painless and can go unnoticed in some locations, such as the uterine cervix, anal canal and mouth. They last 3 to 12 weeks, are frequently accompanied by inguinal lymphadenopathy and heal without scarring.

Secondary Syphilis Reflects Dissemination of Spirochetes

In secondary syphilis *T. pallidum* spreads systemically and proliferates to cause lesions in the skin, mucous membranes, lymph nodes, meninges, stomach and liver. Lesions show perivascular lymphocytic infiltration and obliterative endarteritis.

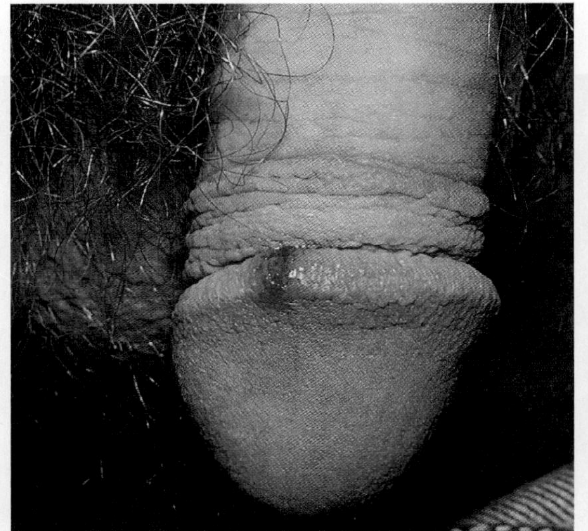

FIGURE 9-32. Syphilitic chancre. A patient with primary syphilis displays a raised, erythematous penile lesion.

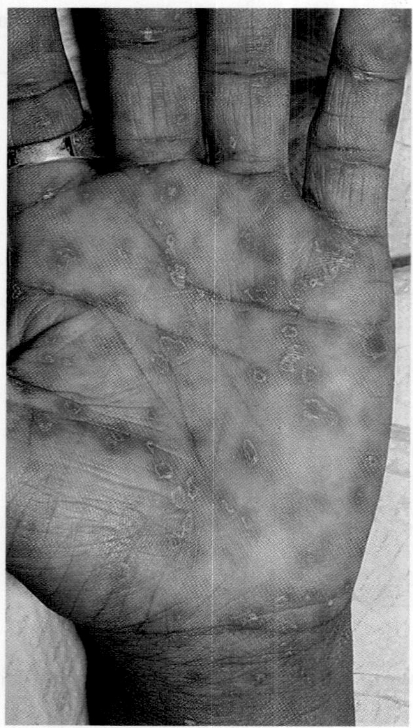

FIGURE 9-33. Secondary syphilis. A maculopapular rash is present on the palm.

- **Skin:** Secondary syphilis most often appears as an erythematous and maculopapular rash of the trunk and extremities, often including the palms (Fig. 9-33) and soles. The rash appears 2 weeks to 3 months after the chancre heals. Other skin lesions in secondary syphilis include **condylomata lata** (exudative plaques in the perineum, vulva or scrotum, which abound in spirochetes) (Fig. 9-34), **follicular syphilids** (small papular lesions around hair follicles that cause loss of hair) and **nummular syphilids** (coin-like lesions of the face and perineum).
- **Mucous membranes:** Lesions on mucosal surfaces of the mouth and genital organs, called **mucous patches**, teem with organisms and are highly infectious.
- **Lymph nodes:** Characteristic changes in lymph nodes, especially epitrochlear nodes, include a thickened capsule, follicular hyperplasia, increased plasma cells and macrophages and luetic vasculitis. Spirochetes are numerous in the lymph nodes of secondary syphilis.
- **Meninges:** Although the meninges are commonly seeded with *T. pallidum*, meningeal involvement is frequently asymptomatic.

Tertiary Syphilis Causes Neurologic and Vascular Diseases

After lesions of secondary syphilis have subsided, an asymptomatic period follows, lasting for years or decades. During this time, spirochetes continue to multiply and the deep-seated lesions of tertiary syphilis gradually develop in one third of untreated patients. ***Focal ischemic necrosis secondary to obliterative endarteritis is the underlying mechanism for many of the processes associated with tertiary syphilis.*** *T. pallidum* elicits mononuclear inflammation, mainly of lymphocytes and plasma cells. These cells infiltrate small arteries and arterioles, producing a characteristic obstructive vascular lesion (**endarteritis obliterans**). Small arteries are inflamed and their endothelial cells are swollen. They are surrounded by concentric layers of proliferating fibroblasts, giving the vascular lesions an "onion skin" appearance.

- **Syphilitic aortitis:** This lesion results from a slowly progressive endarteritis obliterans of vasa vasorum that eventually leads to necrosis of the aortic media, gradual weakening and stretching of the aortic wall, and aortic aneurysm. Syphilitic aneurysms are saccular and involve the ascending aorta, which is an unusual site for the much more common atherosclerotic aneurysms. On gross examination, the aortic intima is rough and pitted (**tree-bark appearance**) (Fig. 9-35) (see Chapter 10). The aortic media is gradually replaced by scar tissue, after which the aorta loses its strength and resilience. The aorta stretches, becoming progressively thinner to the point of rupture, massive

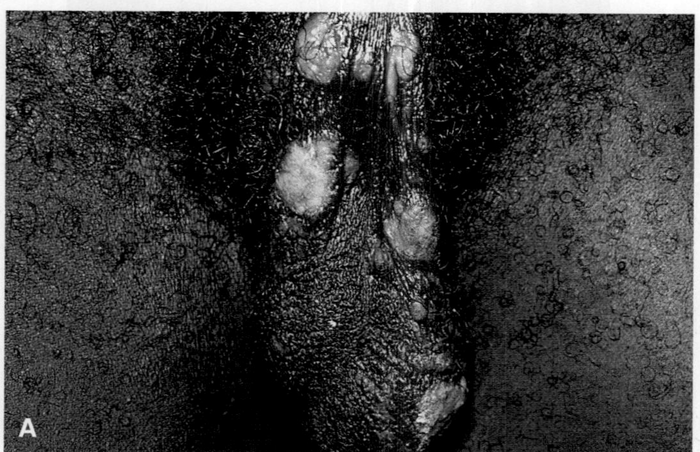

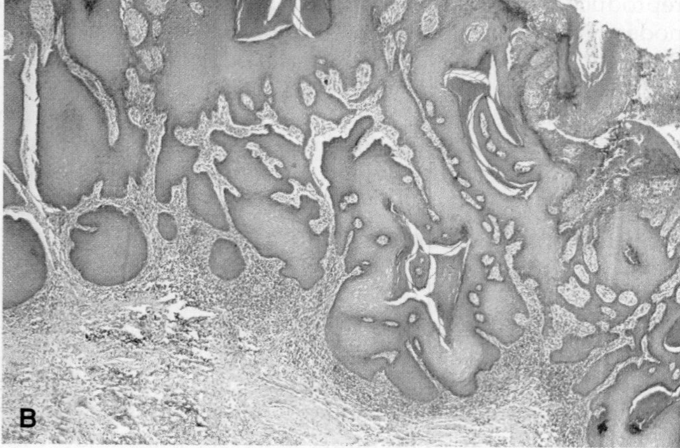

FIGURE 9-34. Condylomata lata in secondary syphilis. A. Whitish plaques are seen on the vulva and perineum. **B.** A photomicrograph shows papillomatous hyperplasia of the epidermis with underlying chronic inflammation.

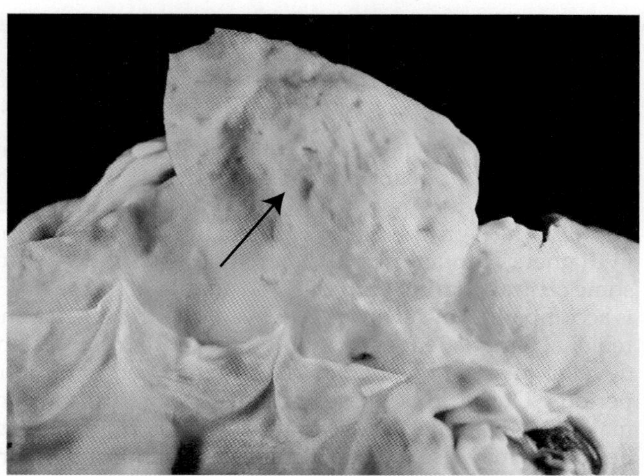

FIGURE 9-35. Syphilitic aortitis. The ascending aorta exhibits a roughened intima (*arrow*, "tree bark" appearance), owing to destruction of the media.

hemorrhage and sudden death. ***Damage to and scarring of the ascending aorta also commonly lead to dilation of the aortic ring, separation of the valve cusps and regurgitation of blood through the aortic valve (aortic insufficiency).*** Luetic vasculitis may narrow or occlude the coronary arteries and cause myocardial infarction.

- **Neurosyphilis:** The slowly progressive infection damages the meninges, cerebral cortex, spinal cord, cranial nerves or eyes. Tertiary syphilis of the CNS is subclassified according to the predominant tissue affected. Thus, there are **meningovascular syphilis** (meninges), **tabes dorsalis** (spinal cord) and **general paresis** (cerebral cortex) (see Chapter 28).
- **Benign tertiary syphilis:** The appearance of a gumma (Fig. 9-36) in any organ or tissue is the hallmark of benign tertiary syphilis. Gummas are most common in the skin, bone and joints, although they can occur anywhere. These granulomatous lesions have a central area of coagulative necrosis, epithelioid macrophages, occasional giant cells and peripheral fibrous tissue. Gummas are usually localized lesions that do not significantly damage the patient.

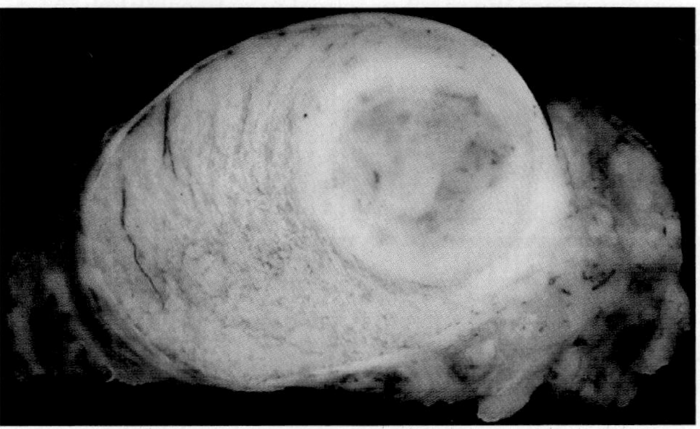

FIGURE 9-36. Syphilitic gumma. A patient with tertiary syphilis shows a sharply circumscribed gumma in the testis, characterized by a fibrogranulomatous wall and a necrotic center.

Congenital Syphilis Is Transmitted From an Infected Mother to the Fetus

In this setting, the organism disseminates in fetal tissues, which are injured by the proliferating organisms and accompanying inflammatory response. Fetal infection produces stillbirth, neonatal illness or death or progressive postnatal disease.

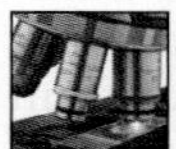

PATHOLOGY: Histopathologically, lesions of congenital syphilis are identical to those of adult disease. Infected tissues show a chronic inflammatory infiltrate of lymphocytes and plasma cells and endarteritis obliterans. Virtually any tissue can be affected, but the skin, bones, teeth, joints, liver and CNS are characteristically involved (see Chapter 6).

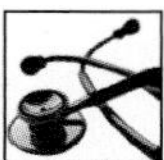

CLINICAL FEATURES: The presentation of congenital syphilis is variable, and infected newborns are often asymptomatic. Early signs of infection include a rhinitis (**snuffles**) and a desquamative rash. Infection of the periosteum, bone, cartilage and dental pulp produce deformities of bones and teeth, including **saddle nose,** anterior bowing of the legs (**saber shins**) and peg-shaped upper incisor teeth (**Hutchinson teeth**). The progression of congenital syphilis can be arrested by penicillin.

Nonvenereal Treponematoses

In tropical and subtropical climes, there are nonvenereal, chronic diseases caused by treponemes indistinguishable from *T. pallidum*. Like syphilis, they result from inoculation of the organism into mucocutaneous surfaces. They also pass through clearly defined clinical and pathologic stages, including a primary lesion at the site of inoculation; secondary skin eruptions; a latent period; and a tertiary, late stage.

Yaws is a Tropical Disease Caused by *Treponema pertenue*

Yaws occurs among poor rural populations in warm, humid areas of tropical Africa, South America, Southeast Asia and Oceania. Children and adolescents in impoverished tropical regions are at risk. Transmission is by skin-to-skin contact and is facilitated by breaks or abrasions. Two to 5 weeks after exposure, a single "mother yaw" appears at the site of inoculation, usually on an exposed part. The lesion evolves from a papule to a 2- to 5-cm "raspberry-like" papilloma. The secondary or disseminated stage begins with the eruption of similar, but smaller, yaws on other parts of the skin. Microscopically, the mother yaw and secondary lesions show hyperkeratosis, papillary acanthosis and an intense neutrophilic infiltrate of the epidermis. The epidermis at the apex of the papilloma lyses to form a shallow ulcer, and plasma cells invade the upper dermis. Spirochetes are numerous in the dermal papillae.

Painful papillomas on the soles of the feet lead patients to walk on the side of their feet like a crab, a condition called "**crab yaw.**" Treponemes are borne by the blood to bones, lymph nodes and skin, where they grow during a latent period of 5 or more years. The lesions in the late stage include cutaneous gummas, which are destructive to the face and upper airway. Periostitis of the tibia causes "saber shins" or "boomerang legs." One dose of long-acting penicillin cures yaws.

Bejel Is Characterized by Gummas of the Skin, Airways and Bone

Bejel (also known as "endemic syphilis") has a focal distribution in Africa, western Asia and Australia. Bejel is transmitted by nonvenereal routes, such as from an infected infant to the breast of the mother; from mouth to mouth; or from utensils to the mouth and is caused by *T. pallidum* subsp. *endemicum*. Other than on the nursing breast, primary lesions are rare. Secondary lesions in the mouth are identical to the mucosal lesions of syphilis and may spread from the upper airway to the larynx. Lesions of the perineum and bone are encountered, and gummas of the breast occur.

Pinta Is a Tropical Skin Disease Caused by *Treponema carateum*

Pinta (from the Spanish for "painted" or "blemish") is a treponematosis characterized by variably colored spots on the skin. It is prevalent in remote, arid, inland regions and river valleys of the American tropics. The lesions of the three stages of pinta are limited to the skin and tend to merge. Transmission is by skin-to-skin inoculation, usually after long intimate contact with an infected person.

Lyme Disease

Lyme disease is a chronic systemic infection that begins with a characteristic skin lesion and later manifests as cardiac, neurologic or joint disturbances. The causative agent is *Borrelia burgdorferi*, a large, microaerophilic spirochete.

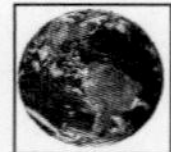

EPIDEMIOLOGY: Lyme disease was first described in patients from Lyme, Connecticut, but has since been recognized in many other areas. *B. burgdorferi* is transmitted from its animal reservoir to humans by the bite of the minute *Ixodes* tick. This pinhead-sized insect is found in wooded areas, where it usually feeds on mice and deer. Transmission to humans is most likely from May through July, when nymph forms of the tick feed.

Lyme disease is a growing problem in the United States, where it is the most common tick-borne illness, causing an estimated 15,000 to 20,000 cases annually. It is concentrated along the eastern seaboard from Maryland to Massachusetts, in the Midwest in Minnesota and Wisconsin and in the West in California and Oregon. The disease is also seen in Europe, Australia and Asia.

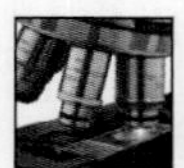 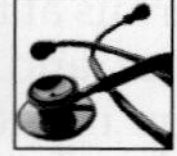

PATHOLOGY AND CLINICAL FEATURES: *B. burgdorferi* reproduces locally at the site of inoculation, spreads to regional lymph nodes and disseminates throughout the body via the bloodstream. Like other spirochetal diseases, Lyme disease is chronic, occurring in stages, with remissions and exacerbations. Studies of skin and synovium have shown that *B. burgdorferi* elicits a chronic inflammatory infiltrate, composed of lymphocytes and plasma cells. In patients who died of the disease, organisms have been seen at autopsy in virtually every organ affected, including the skin, myocardium, liver, CNS and musculoskeletal system.

Lyme disease is a prolonged illness in which three clinical stages are described:

- **Stage 1:** The characteristic skin lesion, **erythema chronicum migrans,** appears at the site of the tick bite. It begins 3 to 35 days after the bite as an erythematous macule or papule, which grows into an erythematous patch 3 to 7 cm in diameter. It often is intensely red at its periphery, with some central clearing, imparting an annular appearance. It is accompanied by fever, fatigue, headache, arthralgias and regional lymphadenopathy. Secondary annular skin lesions develop in about half of patients and may persist for long periods. During this phase, patients experience constant malaise and fatigue, headache and fever. Intermittent manifestations may also include meningeal irritation, migratory myalgia, cough, generalized lymphadenopathy and testicular swelling.
- **Stage 2:** The second stage begins several weeks to months after the skin lesion and is characterized by exacerbation of migratory musculoskeletal pains and cardiac and neurologic abnormalities. In 10% of cases, conduction abnormalities, particularly atrioventricular block, result from myocarditis. Neurologic abnormalities, most commonly meningitis and facial nerve palsies, occur in 15% of patients.
- **Stage 3:** The third stage of Lyme disease begins months to years afterwards, with joint, skin and neurologic abnormalities. Over half of these patients have arthralgia, with severe arthritis of the large joints, especially the knee. The histopathology of affected joints is virtually indistinguishable from that of rheumatoid arthritis, with villous hypertrophy and a conspicuous mononuclear infiltrate in the subsynovial lining area.

Neurologic manifestations may begin months to years after the disease begins. They range from intermittent tingling paresthesias without demonstrable neurologic deficits to slowly progressive encephalomyelitis, transverse myelitis, organic brain syndromes and dementia.

Distinctive late skin manifestations of Lyme disease include acrodermatitis chronica atrophicans. This occurs years after erythema chronicum migrans and presents as patchy atrophy and sclerosis of the skin.

The diagnosis of Lyme disease is established by culturing *B. burgdorferi* from infected patients, but the yield is low. Therefore, antibody titers (initially IgM and later IgG) against the organism are the most practical way to establish the diagnosis. Treatment with tetracycline or erythromycin is effective in eliminating early Lyme disease. In later stages and when there are extensive extracutaneous manifestations, high doses of intravenous penicillin G or other combinations of antibiotic regimens for long periods are necessary.

LEPTOSPIROSIS

Leptospirosis is an infection with spirochetes of the genus *Leptospira*. For the most part (90% of patients) leptospirosis is a mild, self-limited, febrile disease. More-severe infections may entail hepatic and renal failure, which may prove fatal.

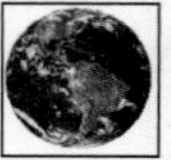

EPIDEMIOLOGY: Leptospirosis is a zoonosis of worldwide distribution. Leptospires penetrate abraded skin or mucous membranes following contact with infected rats, contaminated water or mud. Since warm, moist environments favor survival of the spirochetes, the incidence is higher in the tropics. Between 30 and 100 cases are reported annually in the United States, some of them in slaughterhouse workers and trappers, but recently some cases were reported among destitute persons in urban areas.

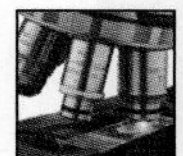
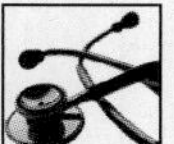

PATHOLOGY AND CLINICAL FEATURES: The symptoms of leptospirosis begin 4 days to 3 weeks after exposure to *Leptospira interrogans*. In most cases, the disease resolves within a week without sequelae. In more severe infections, leptospirosis is a biphasic disease.

- In the **leptospiremic phase** leptospires are present in the blood and cerebrospinal fluid. There is an abrupt onset of fever, shaking chills, headache and myalgias. Symptoms abate after 1 to 2 weeks, as the leptospires disappear from the blood and bodily fluids.
- The **immune phase** begins within 3 days of the end of the leptospiremic phase and is accompanied by the production of IgM antibodies. The earlier symptoms recur, and signs of meningeal irritation become apparent. At this time, the cerebrospinal fluid shows a prominent pleocytosis. In severe cases, jaundice appears and may be followed by hepatic and renal failure and the appearance of widespread hemorrhages and shock. This severe form of leptospirosis has historically been referred to as **Weil disease.**

Untreated Weil disease has a mortality rate of 5% to 30%. At autopsy tissues are bile stained, and hemorrhages are seen in many organs. Microscopically, the principal lesion is a diffuse vasculitis with capillary injury. Livers show dissociation of liver cell plates, erythrophagocytosis by Kupffer cells, minimal necrosis of hepatocytes, neutrophils in the sinusoids and a mixed inflammatory cell infiltrate in portal tracts. Renal tubules are swollen and necrotic. Spirochetes are numerous in tubular lumina, and particularly in bile-stained casts (Fig. 9-37).

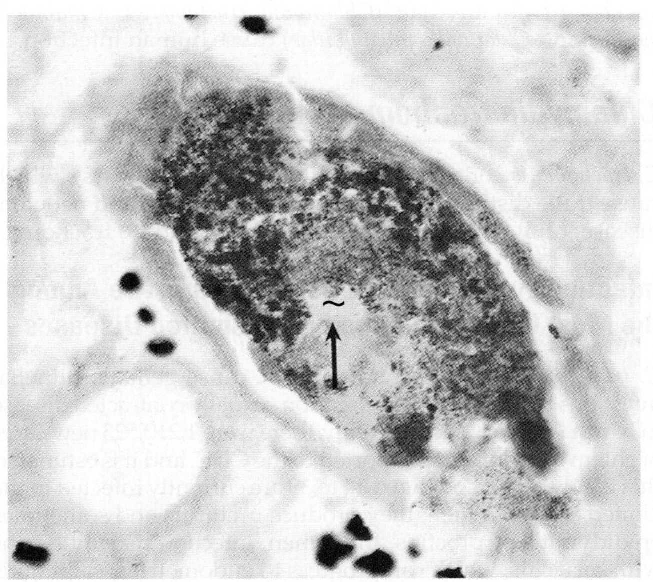

FIGURE 9-37. Leptospirosis. A distal renal tubule is obstructed by a bile-stained mass of hemoglobin and cellular debris. A leptospire (*arrow*) is in the center of this mass.

Relapsing Fever

Relapsing fever is an acute, febrile, septicemic illness caused by spirochetes of the genus *Borrelia*. There are two main types of relapsing fever:

- **Epidemic relapsing fever** is caused by *Borrelia recurrentis* and is transmitted by the bite of an infected louse. Humans are the only reservoir.
- **Endemic relapsing fever** is produced by a number of *Borrelia* spp. and is transmitted from rodents and other animals by the bite of an infected tick.

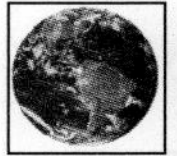
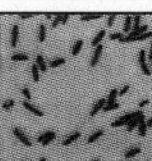

EPIDEMIOLOGY AND ETIOLOGIC FACTORS: The human body louse, *Pediculus humanus humanus,* becomes infected with *B. recurrentis* when it feeds on an infected person. The spirochetes cross the gut wall of the louse into the hemolymph, where they multiply. Here they remain, unless the louse is crushed when feeding. If this occurs, the borrelliae escape and penetrate at the site of the bite or even through the intact skin. War, crowded migrant worker camps and heavy clothing during cold weather all favor mobilization of lice and the spread of relapsing fever. Furthermore, lice dislike the higher temperatures of the feverish victims and seek new hosts, another factor in the rapid spread of relapsing fever during epidemics. Louse-borne relapsing fever is currently seen in several African countries, especially Ethiopia and Sudan and also in the South American Andes.

In endemic, tick-borne relapsing fever, ticks are infected while biting rats and other hosts. The borrelliae grow in the hemocoelom of the tick and invade other tissues, including the salivary glands. Humans are infected by saliva or coxal fluid of the tick. Ticks have a considerably longer life span than lice and may harbor spirochetes for 12 to 15 years without a blood meal. Tick-borne relapsing fever occurs sporadically worldwide.

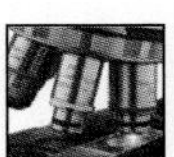

PATHOLOGY: In fatal infections, the spleen is enlarged and contains miliary microabscesses. Spirochetes form tangled aggregates around the necrotic centers. Lymphocytes and neutrophils infiltrate central and midzonal areas of the liver, where spirochetes lie free in the sinusoids. Focal hemorrhages involve many organs.

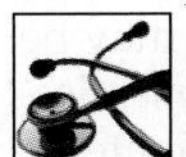

CLINICAL FEATURES: Arthralgias and lethargy with fever, headache and myalgias appear within 1 to 2 weeks of a bite of an infected arthropod. The liver and spleen enlarge, and there are petechiae of the skin, conjunctival hemorrhages and abdominal tenderness. The fever ends abruptly within 3 to 9 days, only to begin 7 to 10 days later. During the afebrile period, spirochetes disappear from the blood and change their antigenic coats. With each relapse, symptoms are milder and the illness is shorter. In severe cases, the initial episode may be characterized by a rash, meningitis, myocarditis, liver failure and coma. Tetracycline is an effective treatment for both types of relapsing fever.

Fusospirochetal Infections

Tropical Phagedenic Ulcer Is a Painful Lesion of the Leg

Tropical phagedenic (rapid spreading and sloughing) ulcer, also known as **tropical foot,** is a painful, necrotizing lesion of

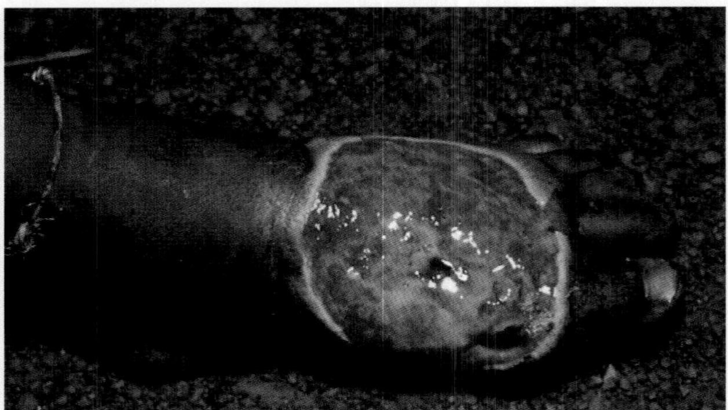

FIGURE 9-38. Tropical phagedenic ulcer caused by infection by fusospirochetal organisms, following penetrating trauma.

the skin and subcutaneous tissues of the leg that afflicts persons in tropical climates. Although flora in the ulcers are often mixed, bacteriologic studies indicate *Bacillus fusiformis* and *Treponema vincentii* to be causal. Malnutrition may predispose to infection.

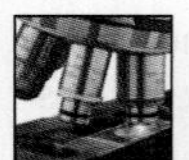 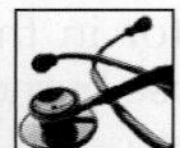

PATHOLOGY AND CLINICAL FEATURES: The lesion usually starts on the skin at a point of trauma and develops rapidly. The surface sloughs to form an ulcer with raised borders and a cup-shaped crater, which contains gray, putrid exudates (Fig. 9-38). The ulcer may be so deep that the underlying bone and tendons are exposed. The margin becomes fibrotic, but complete healing may be delayed for years. In addition to secondary infection, tibial osteomyelitis and squamous cell carcinoma may be late complications. Antibiotics may be effective, but reconstructive plastic surgery is often necessary to close the defect.

Noma Is a Destructive Lesion of the Face

Noma (gangrenous stomatitis, cancrum oris) is a rapidly progressive necrosis of soft tissues and bones of the mouth and face and, less commonly, of such other sites as the chest, limbs and genitalia. It afflicts malnourished children in the tropics, many of whom are further debilitated by recent infections (e.g., measles, malaria, leishmaniasis). A variety of bacteria may be recovered from these lesions, but *T. vincentii, B. fusiformis, Bacteroides* spp. and *Corynebacterium* spp. tend to predominate.

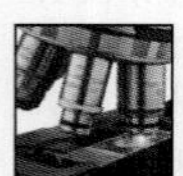 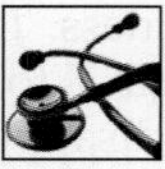

PATHOLOGY AND CLINICAL FEATURES: The ulcer is destructive, disfiguring and usually unilateral (Fig. 9-39). Initially it is a small papule, often on the cheek opposite the molars or premolars. Large malodorous defects quickly develop. The lesions are painful and advanced lesions reveal necrosis of skin, muscle and adipose tissue, with exposure of underlying bone. Without treatment, patients usually die. Antibiotics are helpful, but reconstructive surgery is often required.

CHLAMYDIAL INFECTIONS

Chlamydiae are obligate intracellular parasites that are smaller than most other bacteria. They cannot generate adenosine triphosphate (ATP), and so must parasitize the metabolic machinery of a host cell to reproduce. The chlamydial life cycle involves two distinct morphologic forms. The

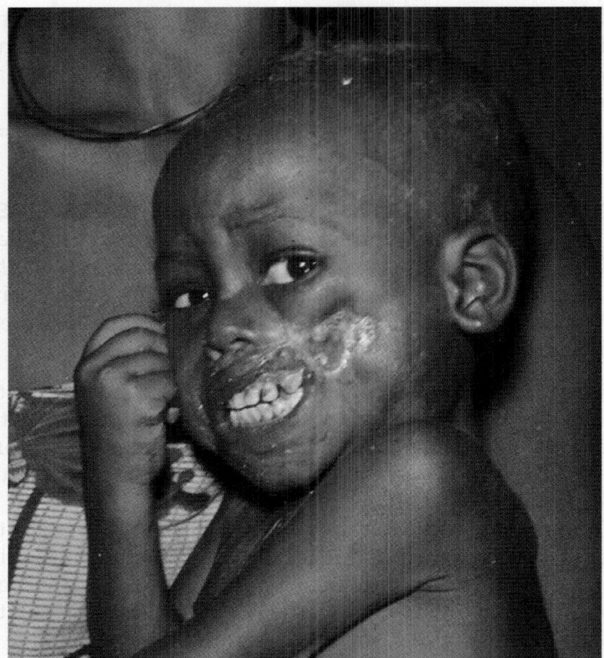

FIGURE 9-39. Noma. There is massive destruction of the soft tissues and bones of the mouth and cheek.

elementary body is the smaller, metabolically inactive form, which survives extracellularly. It attaches to the appropriate host cell and induces endocytosis, forming a vacuole. It then transforms into the larger, metabolically active form, the **reticulate body,** which commandeers host cell metabolism to fuel chlamydial replication. The reticulate body divides repeatedly, forming daughter elementary bodies and destroying the host cell. Necrotic debris elicits inflammatory and immunologic responses that further damage infected tissue.

Chlamydial infections are widespread among birds and mammals and as many as 20% of humans are infected. Three species of chlamydiae (*Chlamydia trachomatis, Chlamydia psittaci* and *Chlamydia pneumoniae*) cause human infection.

Chlamydia trachomatis Infection

C. trachomatis contains a variety of strains (serovars), which cause three distinct types of disease: (1) genital and neonatal disease, (2) lymphogranuloma venereum and (3) trachoma.

Infections with *Chlamydia trachomatis* Are Among the Most Common Sexually Transmitted Diseases

C. trachomatis serovars D through K cause genital epithelial infections that are the most common sexually contracted disease in North America. Most recently, there were 1,210,523 new cases of chlamydial infection reported to the CDC, and it is estimated that 2,291,000 persons aged 14 to 39 are currently infected in the United States. In men, they produce urethritis and sometimes epididymitis or proctitis. In women, infection usually begins with cervicitis, which can progress to endometritis, salpingitis and generalized infection of the pelvic adnexal organs (pelvic inflammatory disease). Repeated episodes of salpingitis are associated with scarring, which can lead to infertility or ectopic pregnancy. Perinatal transmission of *C. trachomatis* causes neonatal conjunctivitis and pneumonia.

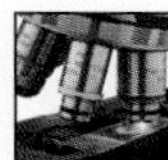

EPIDEMIOLOGY: The organism spreads in genital secretions. Infection is chronic and frequently asymptomatic, providing an enormous reservoir for transmission. As with all sexually transmitted diseases, people with the largest number of sexual partners are at greatest risk of infection. Newborns acquire the organism by contact with infected endocervical secretions on passage through the birth canal. Two thirds of exposed newborns develop *C. trachomatis* conjunctivitis.

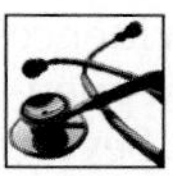

PATHOLOGY: Chlamydial infection elicits an infiltrate of neutrophils and lymphocytes. Lymphoid aggregates, with or without germinal centers, may appear at the site of infection. In newborns, the conjunctival epithelium often contains characteristic vacuolar cytoplasmic inclusions and the disease is frequently called **inclusion conjunctivitis.**

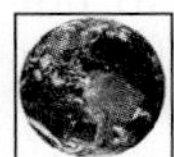

CLINICAL FEATURES: Most genital infections are asymptomatic. In men, clinically apparent infection presents as a purulent penile discharge, with dysuria and urinary urgency. Chlamydial cervicitis causes a mucopurulent drainage from the cervical os. Chlamydial disease in the newborn presents as reddened conjunctivae with a watery or purulent discharge. Untreated neonatal conjunctivitis is potentially serious, although it may resolve without sequelae. Chlamydial pneumonia manifests in the second or third month with tachypnea and paroxysmal cough, usually without fever. Inclusion conjunctivitis is treated with systemic or topical antibiotics.

Lymphogranuloma Venereum Is a Sexually Transmitted Disease That Causes Necrotizing Lymphadenitis

Lymphogranuloma venereum begins as a genital ulcer, spreads to lymph nodes (Fig. 9-40A) and may cause local scarring. It is caused by *C. trachomatis* serovars L1 to L3.

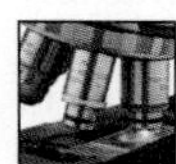

EPIDEMIOLOGY: Lymphogranuloma venereum is uncommon in developed countries but is endemic in the tropics and subtropics. It accounts for 5% of sexually transmitted disease in Africa, India, parts of southeast Asia, South America and the Caribbean. In North America and Europe, it is primarily a disease of homosexual men.

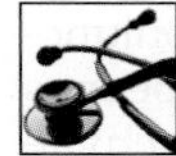

PATHOLOGY: The organism is introduced through a break in the skin. After incubation for 4 to 21 days, an ulcer appears, usually on the penis, vagina or cervix, although the lips, tongue and fingers may also be primary sites. The organisms are transported by lymphatics to regional lymph nodes, where a **necrotizing lymphadenitis** erupts 1 to 3 weeks after the primary lesion. Abscesses develop within involved lymph nodes, often extending to adjacent lymph nodes. Over the next few weeks, the nodes become tender and fluctuant and frequently ulcerate and discharge pus. The intense inflammatory process can result in severe scarring, which may produce chronic lymphatic obstruction, ischemic necrosis of overlying structures or strictures and adhesions. The necrotizing process produces enlarged and matted lymph nodes, containing multiple, coalescing abscesses, which often develop a stellate shape (Fig. 9-40B). Abscesses resemble granulomas, with neutrophils and necrotic debris in the center, surrounded by palisading epithelioid cells, macrophages and occasional giant cells. There is a rim of lymphocytes, plasma cells and fibrous tissue. Nodal architecture is eventually effaced by fibrosis.

CLINICAL FEATURES: Patients with lymphogranuloma venereum present with lymphadenopathy. Most infections resolve completely, even without antimicrobial therapy. However, progressive ulceration of the penis, urethra or scrotum, with fistulas and urethral stricture, develop in 5% of men. Women and homosexual men often present with hemorrhagic proctitis, and most late complications, such as rectal stricture, rectovaginal fistulas and genital elephantiasis, occur in women.

Trachoma Is a Leading Cause of Blindness in Many Developing Countries

Trachoma is a chronic infection that causes progressive scars of the conjunctiva and cornea. *C. trachomatis* serovars A, B, Ba and C cause the disease.

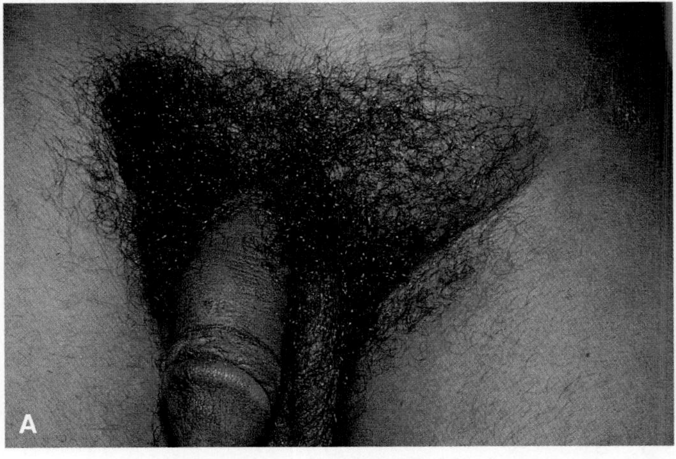

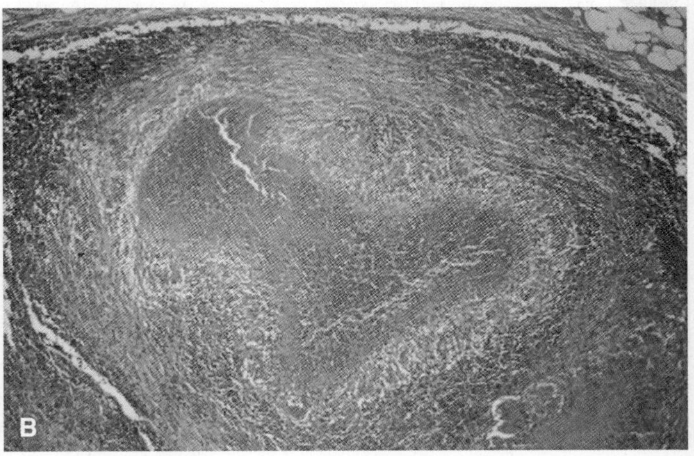

FIGURE 9-40. Lymphogranuloma venereum. A. Painful inguinal lymphadenopathy in a man infected with *Chlamydia trachomatis*. **B.** Microscopic section of a lymph node shows a necrotic central area surrounded by a granulomatous zone.

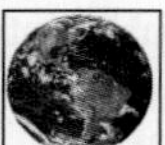

EPIDEMIOLOGY: Trachoma is worldwide, associated with poverty and most prevalent in dry or sandy regions. Only humans are naturally infected, and poor personal hygiene and inadequate public sanitation are common factors. Trachoma remains a major problem in parts of Africa, India and the Middle East. The infection is spread mostly by direct contact, but may also be transmitted by fomites, contaminated water and probably flies. Subclinical infections are an important reservoir. In endemic areas, infection is acquired early in childhood, becomes chronic and eventually progresses to blindness.

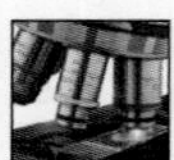

PATHOLOGY: When *C. trachomatis* is inoculated into the eye, it reproduces in the conjunctival epithelium, inciting a mixed acute and chronic inflammatory infiltrate. Histologic examination of early lesions shows chronic inflammation, lymphoid aggregates, focal degeneration and chlamydial inclusions in the conjunctiva. As trachoma progresses, lymphoid aggregates enlarge and the conjunctiva becomes scarred and focally hypertrophic. The cornea is invaded by blood vessels and fibroblasts, forming a scar reminiscent of a cloth ("pannus" in Latin), and is eventually opacified (see Chapter 29).

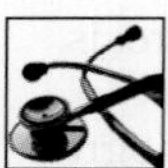

CLINICAL FEATURES: Early trachoma is characterized by abrupt onset of palpebral and conjunctival inflammation, leading to tearing, purulent conjunctivitis and photophobia. The lymphoid aggregates appear as small yellow grains beneath the palpebral conjunctivae within 3 to 4 weeks. After months or years, eyelid deformities eventually interfere with normal ocular function and secondary bacterial infections and corneal ulcers are common. Blindness is a common endpoint.

Psittacosis (Ornithosis)

Psittacosis is a self-limited pneumonia transmitted to humans from birds. The causative agent, *C. psittaci*, is spread by infected birds. The resulting disease is known as both psittacosis (association with parrots) or ornithosis (contact with birds in general).

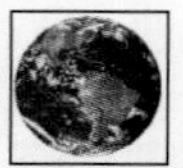

EPIDEMIOLOGY: *C. psittaci* is present in the blood, tissues, excreta and feathers of infected birds. Humans inhale infectious excreta or dust from feathers. Although infection is endemic in tropical birds, *C. psittaci* can infect almost any species and can spread to humans from many bird species, including parrots, parakeets, canaries, pigeons, sea gulls, ducks, chickens and turkeys. Use of tetracycline-containing bird feeds and quarantine of imported tropical birds limits the spread of disease, and fewer than 50 cases are reported annually in the United States.

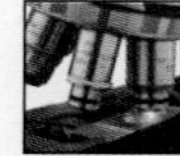

PATHOLOGY: *C. psittaci* first infects pulmonary macrophages, which carry the organism to the phagocytes of the liver and spleen, where it reproduces. The organism is then distributed by the bloodstream, producing systemic infection, particularly diffuse involvement of the lungs. *C. psittaci* reproduces in alveolar lining cells, whose destruction elicits an inflammatory response. The pneumonia is predominantly interstitial, with an interstitial lymphocytic inflammatory infiltrate. Dissemination of the infection is characterized by foci of necrosis in the liver and spleen and diffuse mononuclear cell infiltrates in the heart, kidneys and brain.

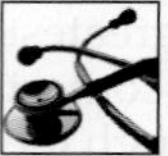

CLINICAL FEATURES: The spectrum of clinical illness varies widely. There is usually a persistent dry cough, with constitutional symptoms of high fever, headache, malaise, myalgias and arthralgias. Untreated, fever persists for 2 to 3 weeks and then subsides as the pulmonary disease regresses. With tetracycline therapy, the disease is rarely fatal.

Chlamydia pneumoniae

C. pneumoniae causes acute, self-limited, usually mild respiratory tract infections, including pneumonia. It is transmitted from person to person, and infection appears to be very common. In the developed world, half of all adults show evidence of past exposure, but only 10% of infections cause clinical pneumonia. Symptoms include fever, sore throat and cough. Severe pneumonia occurs only if there is an underlying pulmonary condition. Untreated disease usually resolves in 2 to 4 weeks.

RICKETTSIAL INFECTIONS

The rickettsiae are small, gram-negative coccobacillary bacteria that are obligate intracellular pathogens and cannot replicate outside a host but, unlike chlamydiae, replicate by binary fission. They can synthesize their own ATP via a proton-translocating ATPase and can also obtain ATP from the host using ATP/adenosine diphosphate (ADP) translocase. The organisms induce endocytosis by target cells and replicate in the cytoplasm of host cells. Rickettsiae have cell wall structures like gram-negative bacteria. However, they do not stain well with Gram stain and are best demonstrated by the Gimenez method or with acridine orange.

Humans are accidental hosts for most species of *Rickettsia*. The organisms reside in animals and insects and do not require humans for perpetuation. Human rickettsial infection results from insect bites. Several species of *Rickettsia* cause different human diseases (Table 9-6), but these infections share many common features. ***In humans, the target cell for all rickettsiae is the endothelial cell of capillaries and other small blood vessels.*** The organisms reproduce within these cells, killing them in the process and producing a necrotizing vasculitis. Human rickettsial infections are traditionally divided into the **"spotted fever group"** and the **"typhus group."**

Rocky Mountain Spotted Fever

Rocky Mountain spotted fever is an acute, potentially fatal, systemic vasculitis that is usually attended by headache, fever and rash. The causative organism, *Rickettsia rickettsii*, is transmitted to humans by tick bites.

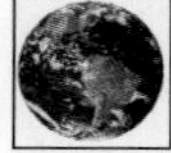

EPIDEMIOLOGY: Rocky Mountain spotted fever is acquired by bites of infected ticks, which are the vectors for *R. rickettsii*. The organism passes from mother to progeny ticks without killing them, thereby maintaining a natural reservoir for human infection. Rocky Mountain spotted fever occurs in various areas throughout North,

Table 9-6

Rickettsial Infections

Disease	Organism	Distribution	Transmission
Spotted-fever Group (genus *Rickettsia*)			
Rocky Mountain spotted fever	*R. rickettsii*	Americas	Ticks
Queensland tick fever	*R. australis*	Australia	Ticks
Boutonneuse fever, Kenya tick fever	*R. conorii*	Mediterranean, Africa, India	Ticks
Siberian tick fever	*R. sibirica*	Siberia, Mongolia	Ticks
Rickettsialpox	*R. akari*	United States, Russia, Central Asia, Korea, Africa	Mites
Typhus Group			
Louse-borne typhus (epidemic typhus)	*R. prowazekii*	Latin America, Africa, Asia	Lice
Murine typhus (endemic typhus)	*R. typhi*	Worldwide	Fleas
Scrub typhus	*R. tsutsugamushi*	South Pacific, Asia	Mites
Q fever	*Coxiella brunetti*	Worldwide	Inhalation

Central and South America. About 500 cases occur annually in the United States, mostly from the eastern seaboard (Georgia to New York) westward to Texas, Oklahoma and Kansas. Its name derives from its discovery in Idaho, but the disease is uncommon in the Rocky Mountain region.

ETIOLOGIC FACTORS: *R. rickettsii* in salivary glands of ticks are introduced into the skin as the ticks feed. Organisms spread via lymphatics and small blood vessels to the systemic and pulmonary circulation. They attach to vascular endothelial cells, are engulfed and reproduce in the cytoplasm and are then shed into the vascular and lymphatic systems. Further infection and destruction of vascular endothelium causes a systemic vasculitis. The rash, produced by inflammatory damage to cutaneous vessels, is the most visible manifestation of the generalized vascular injury. Whereas other rickettsiae infect only capillary endothelial cells, *R. rickettsii* spreads to vascular smooth muscle and endothelium of larger vessels. Extensive damage to blood vessel walls causes loss of vascular integrity, exudation of fluid and disseminated intravascular coagulation. Fluid loss can be so extensive as to lead to shock. Damage to pulmonary capillaries can produce pulmonary edema and acute alveolar injury.

PATHOLOGY: The vascular lesions of Rocky Mountain spotted fever are seen throughout the body, affecting capillaries, venules, arterioles and sometimes larger vessels. Necrosis and reactive hyperplasia of vascular endothelium are often associated with thrombosis of small-caliber vessels. Vessel walls are infiltrated, initially with neutrophils and macrophages and later with lymphocytes and plasma cells. Microscopic infarctions and extravasation of blood into surrounding tissues are common. The orientation of the intracellular bacilli in parallel rows and in an end-to-end pattern gives them the appearance of a "flotilla at anchor facing the wind."

CLINICAL FEATURES: Rocky Mountain spotted fever manifests with fever, headache and myalgias, followed by a rash. Skin lesions begin as a maculopapular eruption but rapidly become petechial, spreading centripetally from the distal extremities to the trunk (Fig. 9-41). Cutaneous lesions usually appear on the palms and soles, a

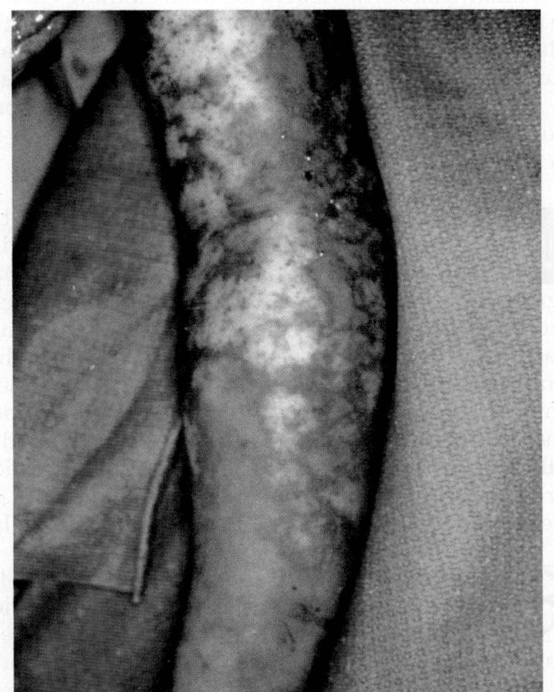

FIGURE 9-41. Rocky mountain spotted fever. A severe petechial and purpuric eruption is noted on the arm in this fatal case.

distinctive feature of the disease. If untreated, more than 20% to 50% of infected persons die within 8 to 15 days. Prompt diagnosis and antibiotic treatment (chloramphenicol and tetracycline) is lifesaving: mortality in the United States is less than 5%.

Epidemic (Louse-Borne) Typhus

Epidemic typhus is a severe systemic vasculitis transmitted by bites of infected lice. It is caused by *Rickettsia prowazekii*, an organism that has a human–louse–human life cycle (Fig. 9-42).

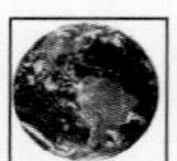

EPIDEMIOLOGY: The disease is widely distributed in some regions of Africa, Asia, Europe and the Western Hemisphere. Devastating epidemics of typhus were associated with cold climates, poor sanitation and crowding during natural disasters, famine or war. Infrequent bathing and lack of changes of clothing lead to louse infestation of human populations and consequently epidemics of typhus. Mass displacements of populations in Eastern Europe in World War I led to epidemic typhus affecting over 30 million people and killing over 3 million. Epidemic louse-borne typhus last occurred in the United States in 1921.

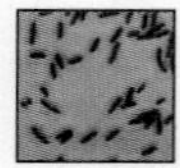

ETIOLOGIC FACTORS: After a louse takes blood from someone infected with *R. prowazekii*, the organisms enter the epithelial cells of the midgut, multiply there and rupture the cells within 3 to 5 days. Large numbers of rickettsiae are released into the lumen of the louse intestine. Contaminated louse feces on the skin or clothing of a second host may remain infectious for more than 3 months. Human infection begins when contaminated louse feces penetrate an abrasion or scratch, or when the person inhales airborne rickettsiae from clothing containing louse feces. Epidemic typhus begins as localized infection of capillary endothelium and progresses to a systemic vasculitis. Louse-borne typhus differs from other rickettsial diseases in that *R. prowazekii* can establish latent infection and produce recrudescent disease (Brill-Zinsser disease) many years after primary infection.

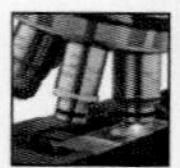

PATHOLOGY: The pathology produced by *R. prowazekii* is similar to Rocky Mountain spotted fever and other rickettsial diseases. At autopsy, there are few gross findings except for splenomegaly and occasional areas of necrosis. Microscopically, collections of mononuclear cells are found in various organs (e.g., skin, brain and heart). The infiltrate includes mast cells, lymphocytes, plasma cells and macrophages, frequently arranged as **typhus nodules** around arterioles and capillaries. Throughout the body, the endothelium of small blood vessels is focally necrotic and hyperplastic and the walls contain inflammatory cells. Rickettsiae can be demonstrated within the endothelial cells.

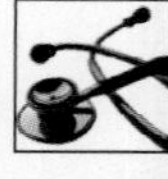

CLINICAL FEATURES: Symptoms of louse-borne typhus are fever, headache and myalgias, followed by a rash. Macular lesions, which become petechial, appear on the upper trunk and axillary folds and spread centrifugally to the extremities. In fatal cases, the rash commonly becomes confluent and purpuric. Mild rickettsial pneumonia may precede a bacterial pneumonia. Dying patients may exhibit the symptoms of encephalitis, myocarditis, interstitial pneumonia, interstitial nephritis and shock. Fatalities usually occur during the second or third week of illness. In patients who recover, the symptoms abate after about 3 weeks.

Epidemic typhus can be controlled by large-scale delousing of the population, steam sterilization of clothing and use of insecticides.

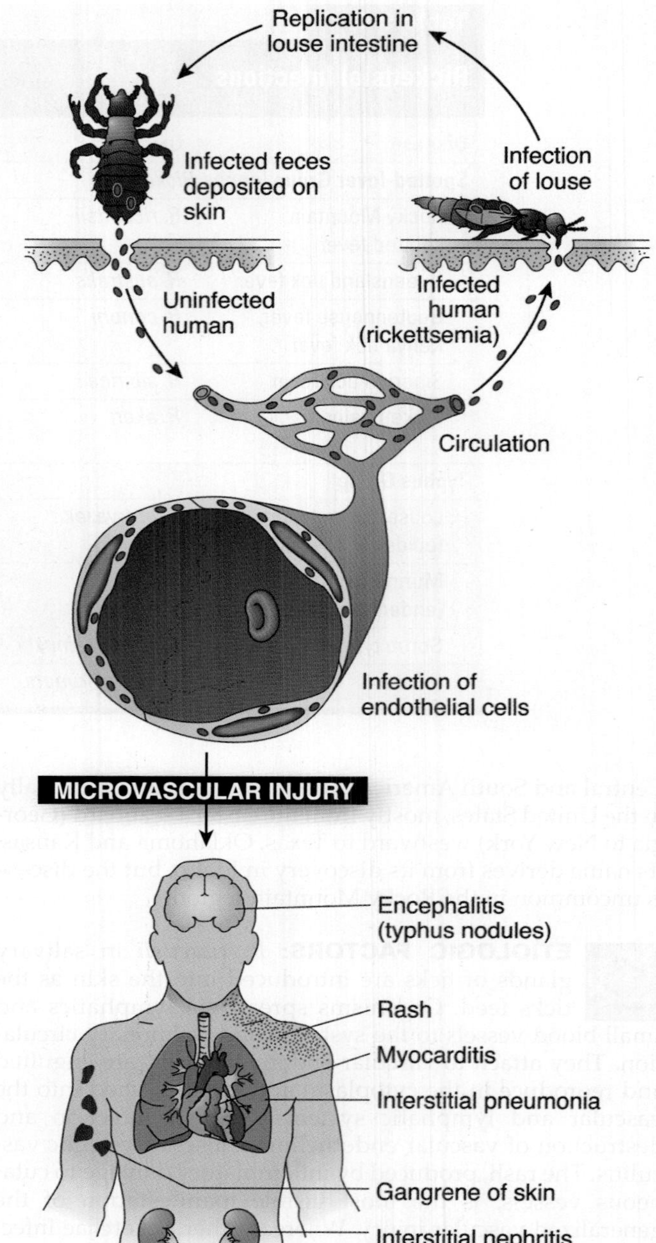

FIGURE 9-42. Epidemic typhus (louse-borne typhus). *Rickettsia prowazekii* has a man–louse–man life cycle. The organism multiplies in endothelial cells, which detach, rupture and release organisms into the circulation (rickettsemia). A louse taking a blood meal becomes infected with rickettsiae, which enter the epithelial cells of its midgut, multiply and rupture the cells, thereby releasing rickettsiae into the lumen of the louse intestine. Contaminated feces are deposited on the skin or clothing of a second host, penetrate an abrasion or are inhaled. The rickettsiae then enter endothelial cells, multiply and rupture the cells, thus completing the cycle.

Endemic (Murine) Typhus

Endemic typhus is similar to epidemic typhus but tends to be milder. Humans are infected with *Rickettsia typhi,* interrupting the rat–flea–rat cycle of transmission. Contaminated flea feces on the skin may enter the body via the small wound made by the bite. *R. typhi* may also contaminate clothes and become airborne. If inhaled, they cause pulmonary infection. Outbreaks of murine typhus are associated with an exploding population of rats, although sporadic infections occur in the southwestern United States. These are associated with rat-infested dwellings and with occupations that bring humans into contact with rats, such as the handling and storage of grain.

Scrub Typhus

Scrub typhus **(Tsutsugamushi fever)** is an acute, febrile illness of humans caused by *Rickettsia tsutsugamushi.* Rodents are the natural mammalian reservoir, from which the organism is passed to trombiculid mites known as chiggers. These insects transmit the infection to their larvae, which crawl to the tips of vegetation and attach to passersby. While feeding, mites inoculate the organisms into the skin. Rickettsemia and lymphadenopathy follow shortly. Scrub typhus is widely distributed in eastern and southern Asia and the islands of the southern and western Pacific, including Japan. Endemic infection is unknown in the Western world.

A multiloculated vesicle forms at the inoculation site and ulcerates, followed by an eschar. As the lesion heals, headache and fever appear suddenly, followed by pneumonia, a macular rash, lymphadenopathy and hepatosplenomegaly. Severe infections are complicated by myocarditis, meningoencephalitis and shock. Mortality rates in untreated patients have ranged up to 30%.

Q Fever

Q fever is a self-limited, systemic infection, usually manifesting as headache, fever and myalgias. The disease is caused by *Coxiella burnetii,* a small pleomorphic coccobacillus with a gram-negative cell wall. Unlike true rickettsiae, *C. burnetii* enters cells passively upon phagocytosis by macrophages. *C. burnetii* infection does not produce a vasculitis, and thus there is no associated rash.

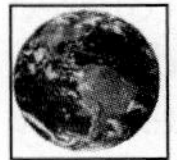

EPIDEMIOLOGY: Humans acquire Q fever by exposure to infected animals or animal products. Infection is endemic in many wild and domesticated animals, but cattle, sheep and goats are the usual sources of human infection. These animals shed large numbers of organisms in urine, feces, milk, bodily fluids and birth products. Q fever is most often seen in herders, slaughterhouse workers, veterinarians, dairy workers and others with occupational exposure to infected domesticated animals. Aerosol droplets may spread infection from person to person. Q fever is rare in the United States.

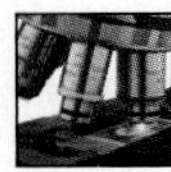

PATHOLOGY: Q fever begins with inhalation of organisms, which are phagocytosed by alveolar macrophages and replicate in phagolysosomes. Recruitment of neutrophils and macrophages produces a focal bronchopneumonia. The nonactivated phagocytes fail to kill *C. burnetii,* and the organism disseminates through the body, primarily infecting monocytes and macrophages. Most infections resolve with the onset of specific cell-mediated immunity, but occasional cases persist as chronic infections.

The lungs and liver are most prominently involved in Q fever. The lungs show single or multiple irregular areas of consolidation, in which the pulmonary parenchyma is infiltrated by neutrophils and macrophages. Organisms may be demonstrated in macrophages by the Giemsa stain. In the liver, Q fever is usually characterized by multiple microscopic granulomas with a distinctive "fibrin ring." In these granulomas, epithelioid macrophages encircle a ring of fibrin, sometimes containing a lipid vacuole.

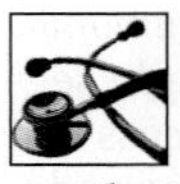

CLINICAL FEATURES: Q fever is usually a self-limited mildly symptomatic febrile disease. More-severe cases may present with headache, fever, fatigue and myalgias, with no rash. Pulmonary infection is virtually always present, but it may appear as an atypical pneumonia with dry cough, a rapidly progressive pneumonia or chest roentgenographic abnormalities without significant respiratory symptoms. Many patients have some hepatosplenomegaly. Q fever usually resolves spontaneously in 2 to 14 days.

MYCOPLASMAL INFECTIONS

At less than 0.3 μm in greatest dimension, mycoplasmas are the smallest free-living **prokaryotes.** They lack the rigid cell walls of more complex bacteria. Mycoplasmas are widespread, geographically and ecologically, as saprophytes and as parasites of many animals and plants. Numerous *Mycoplasma* spp. inhabit the human body, but only three are pathogenic: *Mycoplasma pneumoniae, Mycoplasma hominis* and *Ureaplasma urealyticum*. The diseases associated with these organisms are shown in Table 9-7.

M. pneumoniae *produces acute, self-limited lower respiratory tract infections, affecting mostly children and young adults.* It can also cause pharyngitis and otitis media.

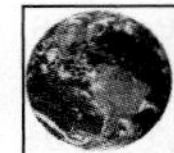

EPIDEMIOLOGY: Most infections occur in small groups of persons who have frequent close contact (e.g., families, college fraternities, military units and residents of closed institutions). The organism is spread by aerosol transmission from person to person over a period of

Table 9-7

Mycoplasmal Infections

Organism	Disease
Mycoplasma pneumoniae	Tracheobronchitis Pneumonia Pharyngitis Otitis media
Ureaplasma urealyticum	Urethritis Chorioamnionitis Postpartum fever
Mycoplasma hominis	Postpartum fever

several months, with an attack rate exceeding 50% within the group. *M. pneumoniae* infection occurs worldwide, and in developed countries, the organism causes 15% to 20% of all pneumonias.

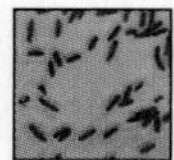

ETIOLOGIC FACTORS: *M. pneumoniae* initiates infection by attaching to a glycolipid on the surface of the respiratory epithelium. The organism remains outside the cells, where it reproduces and causes progressive dysfunction and eventual death of host cells. Because *M. pneumoniae* infection rarely produces symptomatic disease in children younger than the age of 5 years, it is thought that the host immune response plays a role in tissue injury.

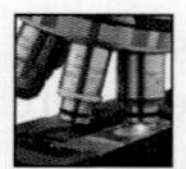

PATHOLOGY: Pneumonia caused by *M. pneumoniae* usually shows patchy consolidation of a single segment of a lower lung lobe, although the process can be more widespread. The mucosa of affected airways is edematous and infiltrated by a mostly mononuclear inflammatory infiltrate. Alveoli show a largely interstitial process, with reactive alveolar lining cells and mononuclear infiltration. Pulmonary changes are often complicated by bacterial superinfection. The organism itself is too small to be seen by routine light microscopy.

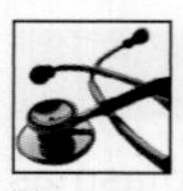

CLINICAL FEATURES: *Mycoplasma* pneumonia tends to be milder than other bacterial pneumonias, and is sometimes called "walking pneumonia." Fever rarely lasts more than 2 weeks, although cough may linger for 6 weeks or more. Death from *M. pneumoniae* infection is rare. However, life-threatening cases of Stevens-Johnson syndrome have been linked to mycoplasma infection.

MYCOBACTERIAL INFECTIONS

Mycobacteria are distinctive organisms, 2 to 10 μm in length, with cell wall architecture like that of gram-positive bacteria, but also containing large amounts of lipid. The high lipid content interferes with staining by aniline dyes, including crystal violet used in the Gram stain. Thus, although mycobacteria are structurally gram positive, this property is difficult to demonstrate by routine staining. ***The waxy lipids of the cell wall make the mycobacteria "acid fast" (i.e., they retain carbolfuchsin after rinsing with acid alcohol).***

Mycobacteria grow more slowly than other pathogenic bacteria, and their diseases are chronic, slowly progressive illnesses. The organisms produce no known toxins. They damage human tissues by inducing inflammatory and immune responses. Most mycobacterial pathogens replicate within cells of the monocyte/macrophage lineage and elicit granulomatous inflammation. The outcome of mycobacterial infection is largely determined by the host's capacity to contain the organism through delayed-type hypersensitivity mechanisms and cell-mediated immune responses.

The two main mycobacterial pathogens, *Mycobacterium tuberculosis* and *Mycobacterium leprae,* only infect humans and have no environmental reservoir. Other pathogenic mycobacteria are environmental organisms that only occasionally cause human disease.

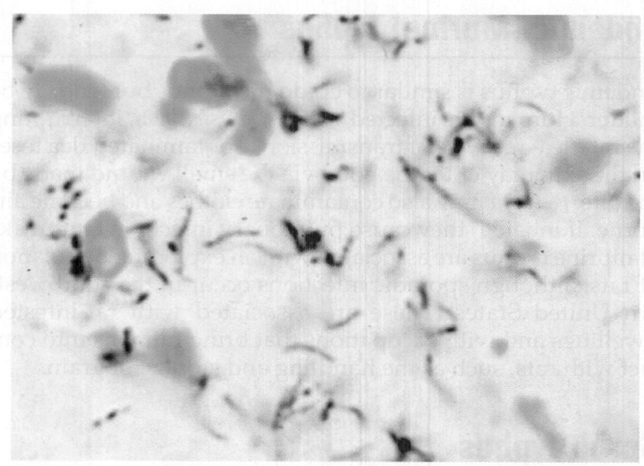

FIGURE 9-43. Mycobacterium tuberculosis. A smear of a pulmonary lesion shows slender, beaded, acid-fast bacilli.

Tuberculosis

Tuberculosis is a chronic, communicable disease in which the lungs are the prime target, although any organ may be infected. Disease is mainly caused by* M. tuberculosis hominis *(Koch bacillus) but also occasionally by* M. tuberculosis bovis. *The characteristic lesion is a spherical granuloma with central caseous necrosis.

M. tuberculosis is an obligate aerobe, a slender, beaded, nonmotile, acid-fast bacillus (Fig. 9-43). It grows slowly in culture, with a doubling time of 24 hours, and 3 to 6 weeks are commonly required to produce visible growth in culture.

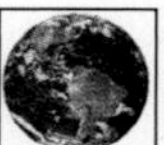

EPIDEMIOLOGY: Tuberculosis is worldwide and is one of the most important human bacterial diseases. Although rates of infection are now low in developed countries, HIV-infected, homeless and malnourished people are highly susceptible, as are immigrants from areas where the disease is endemic. In the United States, the annual incidence of tuberculosis is 12 per 100,000 and mortality is 1 to 2 per 100,000. In some developing countries, the incidence reaches 450 per 100,000, with a high fatality rate. There are also racial and ethnic differences—Africans, Native Americans and Eskimos are more susceptible than are Caucasians. In the United States, tuberculosis is most common among the elderly, possibly reflecting reactivation of infections acquired early in life before the decline in the prevalence of the disease.

M. tuberculosis is transmitted from person to person by aerosolized droplets. Coughing, sneezing and talking all create aerosolized respiratory droplets; usually, droplets evaporate, leaving an organism (droplet nucleus) that is readily carried in the air. Tuberculosis can also be caused by the closely related *M. tuberculosis bovis*, which is acquired by drinking nonpasteurized milk from infected cows.

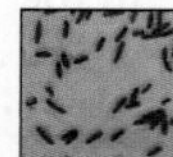

ETIOLOGIC FACTORS: The course of tuberculosis depends on age and immune competence, as well as total burden of organisms. Some patients have only an indolent, asymptomatic infection, while in others, tuberculosis is a destructive, disseminated disease. Many more people are infected with *M. tuberculosis* than develop clinical symptoms. Thus, one must distinguish between infection and active tuberculosis. **Tuberculous infection** means that the organism is growing in a person, whether or not there is symptomatic disease. **Active tuberculosis** denotes the subset of tuberculous infections manifested by destructive, symptomatic disease.

Primary tuberculosis occurs on first exposure to the organism and can pursue either an indolent or aggressive course (Fig. 9-44). **Secondary tuberculosis** develops long after a primary infection, mostly due to reactivation of a primary infection. Secondary tuberculosis can also be produced by exposure to exogenous organisms and is always an active disease.

Primary Tuberculosis Occurs Upon First Exposure to the Tubercle Bacillus

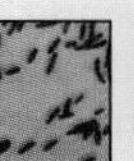
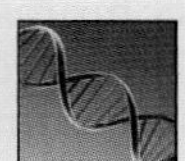

ETIOLOGIC FACTORS AND MOLECULAR PATHOGENESIS: Inhaled *M. tuberculosis* is deposited in alveoli, usually in the lower segments of the lower and middle lobes and the anterior segments of the upper lobes. The organisms are phagocytosed by alveolar macrophages but resist killing; cell wall lipids of *M. tuberculosis* apparently block fusion of phagosomes and lysosomes and allow the bacilli to proliferate within macrophages. As bacilli multiply, the macrophages degrade some and present antigens to T lymphocytes. Some macrophages carry organisms from the lung to regional (hilar and mediastinal) lymph nodes, from which they may disseminate by the bloodstream. Bacilli continue to proliferate at the primary site in the lungs and elsewhere, including lymph nodes, kidneys, meninges, epiphyseal plates of long bones and vertebrae and apical areas of the lungs.

Although the macrophages that first ingest *M. tuberculosis* cannot kill it, they initiate hypersensitivity and cell-mediated immunologic responses that eventually contain the infection. Infected macrophages present mycobacterial antigens to T cells. Clones of sensitized T cells proliferate, produce interferon-γ and activate macrophages, thereby increasing their concentrations of lytic enzymes and augmenting their capacity to kill mycobacteria. The lytic enzymes of these activated macrophages may, if released, also damage host tissues.

Development of activated lymphocytes responsive to *M. tuberculosis* antigen is the hypersensitivity response to the organism. The emergence of activated macrophages that can ingest and destroy the bacilli comprises the cell-mediated immune response. These responses together combat the organisms, a process that requires 3 to 6 weeks to come into play.

If an infected person is immunologically competent and the burden of organisms is small, a vigorous granulomatous reaction is produced. Tubercle bacilli are ingested and killed by activated macrophages, surrounded by fibrous tissue, and successfully contained. When the number of organisms is high, the hypersensitivity reaction produces significant tissue necrosis, which has a characteristic cheese-like (caseous) consistency. Although not invariably caused by *M. tuberculosis*, caseous necrosis is so strongly associated with tuberculosis that its discovery in tissue must raise a suspicion of this disease.

In immunologically immature or compromised subjects (young children or immunosuppressed patients),

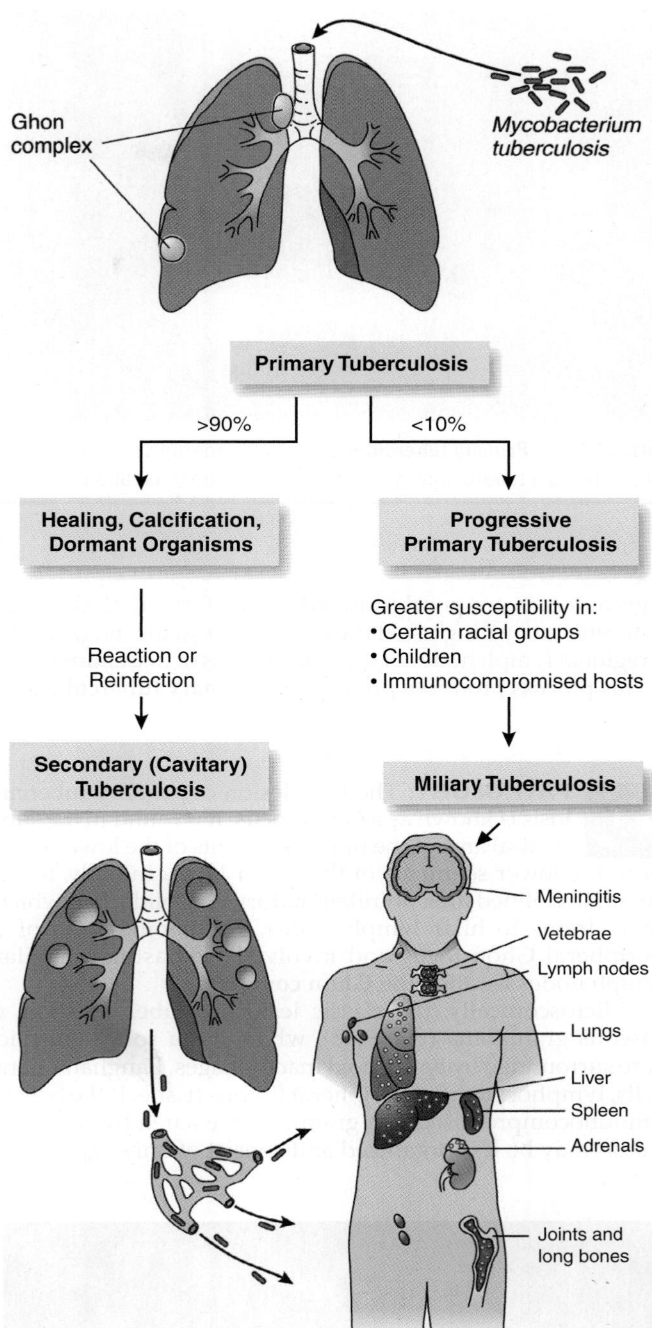

FIGURE 9-44. Stages of tuberculosis. Primary tuberculosis develops in a person lacking previous contact or immune responsiveness. **Progressive primary** tuberculosis develops in less than 10% of infected normal adults, but more frequently in children and immunosuppressed patients.
Secondary (cavitary) tuberculosis results from reactivation of dormant endogenous bacilli or reinfection with exogenous bacilli. **Miliary** tuberculosis is caused by dissemination of tubercle bacilli to produce numerous, minute, yellow-white lesions (resembling millet seeds) in distant organs.

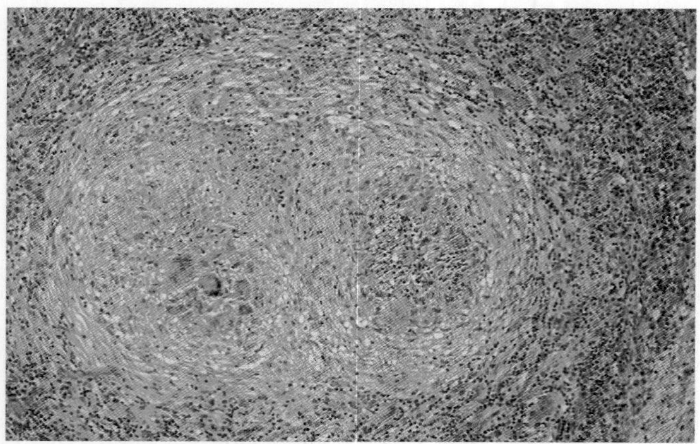

FIGURE 9-45. Primary tuberculosis. Photomicrograph of a hilar lymph node shows a tuberculous granuloma with central caseation.

granulomas are poorly formed or not formed at all, and infection may progress at the primary site in the lung, in the regional lymph nodes or in multiple sites of dissemination. This process produces **progressive primary tuberculosis**.

PATHOLOGY: The lung lesion of primary tuberculosis is known as a **Ghon focus.** It is found in the subpleural area of the upper segments of the lower lobes or in the lower segments of the upper lobes. Initially, it is a small, ill-defined area of inflammatory consolidation, which then drains to hilar lymph nodes. The combination of a peripheral Ghon focus and involved mediastinal or hilar lymph nodes is called the **Ghon complex.**

Microscopically, the classic lesion of tuberculosis is a caseous granuloma (Fig. 9-45), which has a soft, semisolid core surrounded by epithelioid macrophages, Langhans giant cells, lymphocytes and peripheral fibrous tissue. If the host is immunocompromised, the granulomas elicited by *M. tuberculosis* may be less organized and consist of only aggregates of macrophages, without the architecture or Langhans giant cells of the classic granuloma.

In over 90% of normal adults, tuberculous infection is self-limited. In both lungs and lymph nodes, the Ghon complex heals, undergoing shrinkage, fibrous scarring and calcification, the latter visible radiographically. Small numbers of organisms may remain viable for years. Later, if immune mechanisms wane or fail, resting bacilli may proliferate and break out, causing serious secondary tuberculosis.

In **progressive primary tuberculosis** the host immune response fails to control the tubercle bacilli. This happens in fewer than 10% of normal adults, but it is common in children younger than 5 years and in patients with suppressed or defective immunity. The Ghon focus enlarges and may even erode into the bronchial tree. Affected hilar and mediastinal lymph nodes also enlarge, sometimes compressing the bronchi to produce atelectasis of the distal lung; collapse of the middle lobe (**middle lobe syndrome**) is a common result of this compression. In some instances, the infected lymph nodes erode into an airway to spread organisms throughout the lungs.

Miliary tuberculosis occurs when infection disseminates to produce multiple, small, yellow, nodular lesions in several organs (Fig. 9-46). The term "miliary" refers to the resemblance of these lesions to millet seeds. The lungs, lymph nodes, kidneys, adrenals, bone marrow, spleen and liver are common sites of miliary lesions. Progressive disease may involve the meninges and cause tuberculous meningitis.

CLINICAL FEATURES: Most people contain primary infection successfully, and primary tuberculosis is generally asymptomatic. In those who develop progressive primary disease, symptoms are usually insidious and nonspecific, with fever, weight loss, fatigue and night sweats. Sometimes onset of symptoms is abrupt, with high fever, pleurisy, pleural effusion and lymphadenitis. Cough and hemoptysis develop only when active pulmonary disease is well established. In miliary tuberculosis, symptoms vary according to the organs affected and tend to occur late in the course of disease.

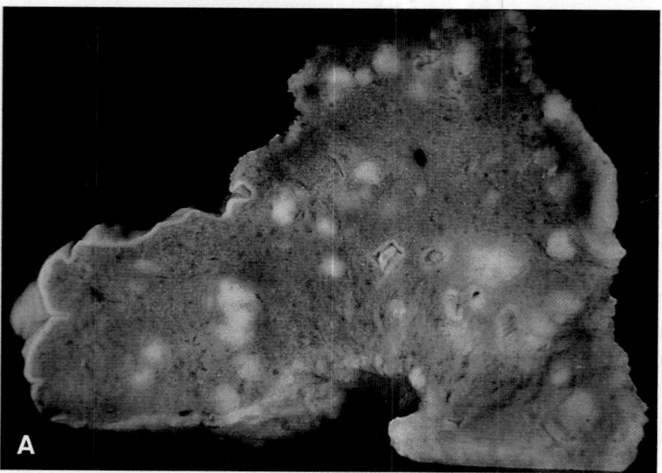

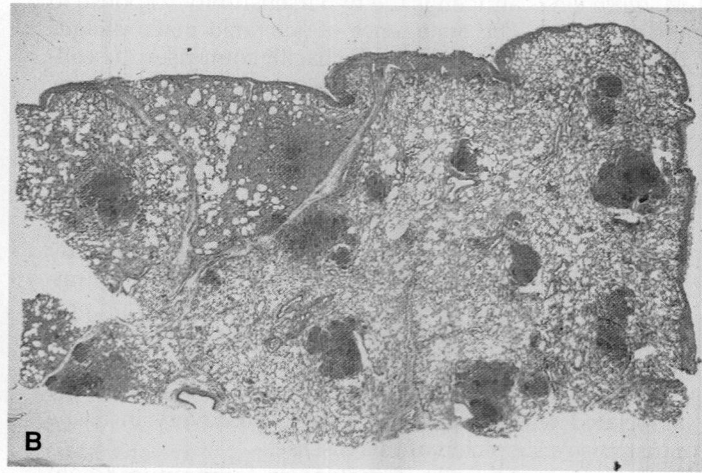

FIGURE 9-46. Miliary tuberculosis. A. The cut surface of the lung reveals numerous uniform, white nodules. **B.** A low-power photomicrograph discloses many foci of granulomatous inflammation.

Secondary (Cavitary) Tuberculosis Results From Proliferation of *Mycobacterium tuberculosis* in Someone Who Has Previously Contained the Infection

The mycobacteria in secondary tuberculosis may be either dormant organisms from old granulomas (which is usually the case) or newly acquired bacilli. Various conditions, including cancer, antineoplastic chemotherapy, immunosuppressive therapy, AIDS and old age, predispose to reemergence of endogenous dormant *M. tuberculosis*. Secondary tuberculosis may develop even decades after primary infection.

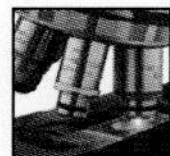

PATHOLOGY: Any location may be involved but the lungs are by far the most common site for secondary tuberculosis. In the lungs, secondary tuberculosis usually begins in apical–posterior segments of the upper lobes, where organisms are commonly seeded during primary infection. There, the bacilli proliferate and elicit an inflammatory response, causing localized consolidation. ***Ensuing T-cell–mediated immune responses to the now familiar tuberculous antigens lead to tissue necrosis and production of tuberculous cavities*** (Fig. 9-47). Apical cavities are optimal sites for multiplication of *M. tuberculosis*, and large numbers of organisms are produced in this environment. Cavities are typically 2 to 4 cm in diameter when first detected clinically but can exceed 10 cm. They contain necrotic material teeming with mycobacteria and are surrounded by a granulomatous response.

Lung lesions in secondary tuberculosis may be complicated by secondary effects:

- Scarring and calcification
- Spread to other areas
- Pleural fibrosis and adhesions
- Rupture of a caseous lesion, spilling bacilli into the pleural cavity
- Erosion into a bronchus, which seeds bronchioles, bronchi and trachea
- Implantation of bacilli in the larynx, causing hoarseness and pain on swallowing

Tubercle bacilli may also spread throughout the body through the lymphatics and bloodstream to cause miliary tuberculosis.

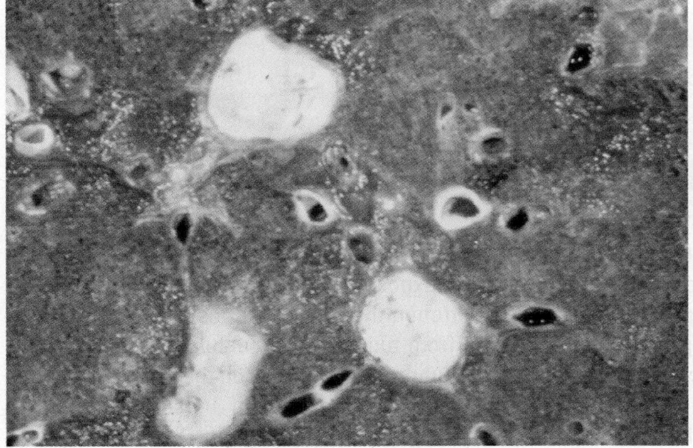

FIGURE 9-47. Secondary pulmonary tuberculosis. A cross-section of lung shows several tuberculous cavities filled with necrotic, caseous material.

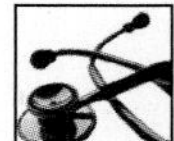

CLINICAL FEATURES: Cough (which may be mistakenly attributed to smoking or a cold), low-grade fever, general malaise, fatigue, anorexia, weight loss and often night sweats are the usual manifestations. Cavitation may be accompanied by hemoptysis, on occasion severe enough to cause exsanguination. Chest radiographs that show unilateral or bilateral apical cavities suggest the diagnosis of secondary tuberculosis. If disease is disseminated, the signs and symptoms reflect the particular organs involved.

Untreated secondary tuberculosis is a wasting disease that is eventually fatal, and at one time chronic cavitary tuberculosis was a most common cause of secondary amyloidosis. Tuberculosis is now treated with prolonged courses of antituberculous antibiotics, including isoniazid, pyrazinamide, rifampin and ethambutol. Strains of *M. tuberculosis* resistant to these antibiotics have recently emerged, usually as a consequence of poor compliance with the full regimen of antibiotic therapy.

Leprosy

Leprosy (Hansen disease) is a chronic, slowly progressive, destructive process involving peripheral nerves, skin and mucous membranes, caused by *Mycobacterium leprae*. This agent is a slender, weakly acid-fast rod, which cannot be cultured on artificial media or in cell culture.

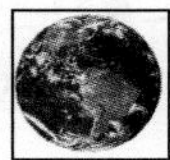

EPIDEMIOLOGY: Leprosy is one of the oldest recognized human diseases. Lepers were isolated from the community in the Old Testament. For centuries, leprosy was widespread in Europe, including England. In 1873, Hansen first documented the causative agent (leprosy is also called "Hansen disease").

Lepra bacilli multiply in experimental animals at sites with temperatures below that of the internal organs, such as foot pads of mice and ear lobes of hamsters, rats and other rodents. Naturally acquired leprosy has been recognized in armadillos in Louisiana and Texas. Lepra bacilli have been experimentally transmitted to armadillos, whose susceptibility is related, at least in part, to their low body temperature (32°C to 35°C [89.6°C to 95°F]).

Leprosy is transmitted from person to person, after years of intimate contact. *M. leprae* is present in nasal secretions or ulcerated lesions of infected persons. The mode of infection is unclear but probably involves inoculation of bacilli into the respiratory tract or open wounds. Leprosy is now rare in developed countries, but worldwide 15 million people are infected, mainly in tropical areas such as India, Papua-New Guinea, Southeast Asia and tropical Africa. Fewer than 400 cases are diagnosed yearly in the United States, mostly in immigrants from endemic areas.

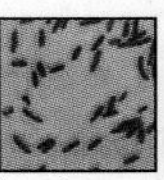

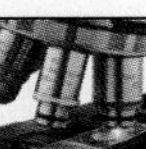

ETIOLOGIC FACTORS AND PATHOLOGY: *M. leprae* multiplies best at temperatures below core human body temperature and lesions tend to occur in cooler parts of the body (e.g., hands and face). Leprosy exhibits a bewildering variety of clinical and pathologic features. Lesions vary from the small, insignificant and self-healing macules of tuberculoid leprosy to the diffuse, disfiguring and sometimes fatal lesions of lepromatous leprosy (Fig. 9-48). This extreme variation in disease presentation probably reflects differences in immune reactivity.

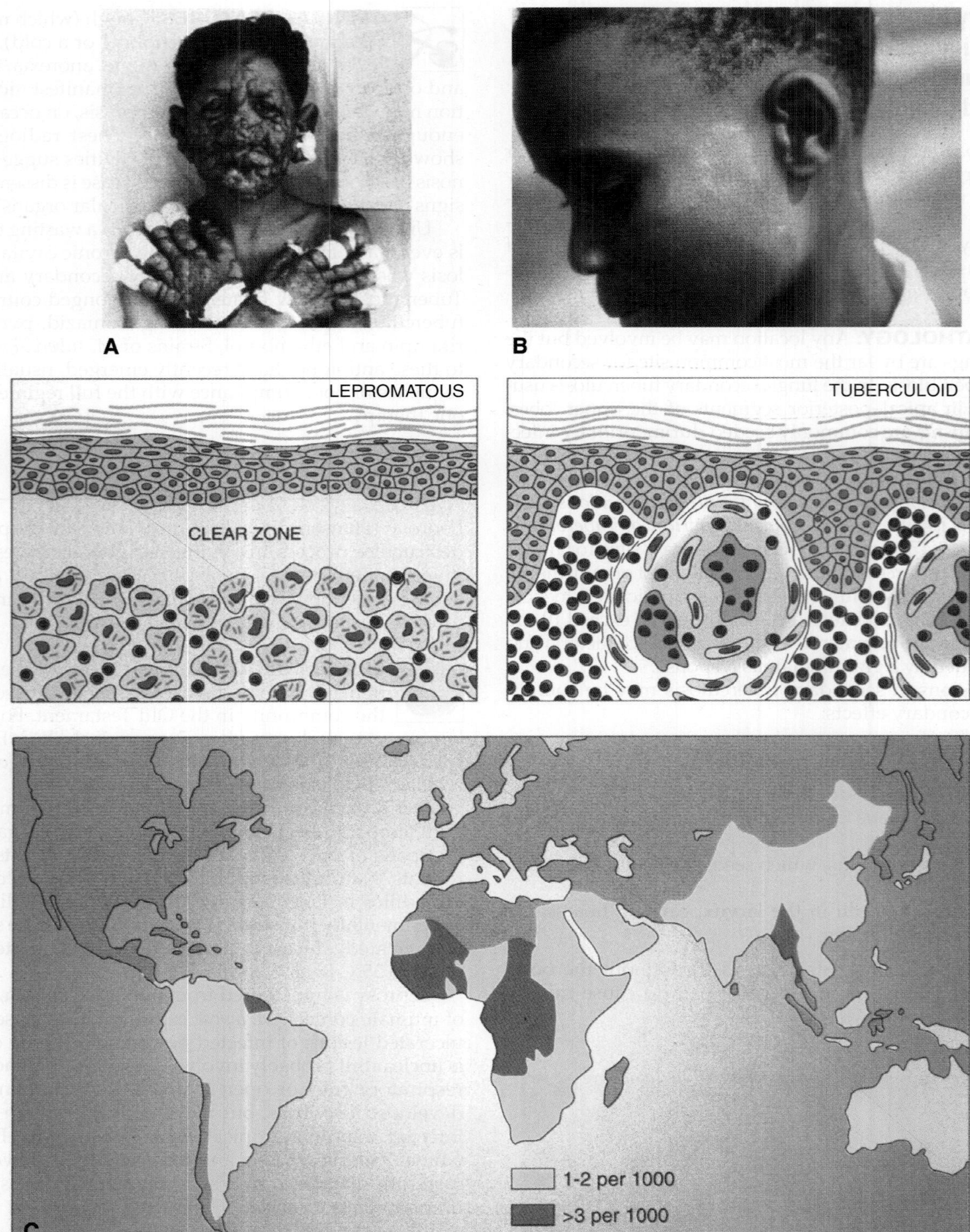

FIGURE 9-48. A. (*Top*) **Lepromatous leprosy**. There is diffuse involvement, including a leonine face, loss of eyebrows and eyelashes and nodular distortions, especially on the face, ears, forearms and hands—the exposed (cool) parts of the body. (*Bottom*) The nodular skin lesions of advanced lepromatous leprosy. Swelling has flattened the epidermis (loss of rete ridges). A characteristic "clear zone" of uninvolved dermis separates the epidermis from tumor-like accumulations of macrophages, each containing numerous lepra bacilli (*Mycobacterium leprae*). **B.** (*Top*) **Tuberculoid leprosy** on the cheek, showing a hypopigmented macule with a raised, infiltrated border. The central portion may be hypesthetic or anesthetic. (*Bottom*) Macular skin lesion of tuberculoid leprosy. Skin from the raised "infiltrated" margin of the plaque contains discrete granulomas that extend to the basal layer of the epidermis (without a clear zone). The granulomas are composed of epithelioid cells and Langhans giant cells and are associated with lymphocytes and plasma cells. Lepra bacilli are rare. **C. Distribution of leprosy**. Prevalence is greatest in tropical regions of Africa, Asia and Latin America.

Most (95%) persons have a natural protective immunity to *M. leprae* and are not infected, despite intimate and prolonged exposure. Susceptible individuals (5%) span a broad spectrum of immune function from anergy to hyperergy and may develop symptomatic infection. At one end of the spectrum, anergic patients have little or no resistance and develop **lepromatous leprosy,** while hyperergic patients with high resistance contract **tuberculoid leprosy**. Most patients, in between these extremes, have **borderline leprosy.**

TUBERCULOID LEPROSY: This is characterized by a single lesion or very few lesions of the skin, usually on the face, extremities or trunk. Microscopically, lesions show well-formed, circumscribed dermal granulomas with epithelioid macrophages, Langhans giant cells and lymphocytes. Nerve fibers are almost invariably swollen and infiltrated with lymphocytes. Destruction of small dermal nerve twigs accounts for the sensory deficit associated with tuberculoid leprosy. Bacilli are rare and often not found with acid-fast stains. The term "tuberculoid leprosy" is used because the granulomas vaguely resemble those of tuberculosis. However, leprous granulomas lack caseation. The lesions of tuberculoid leprosy cause minimal disfigurement and are not infectious.

LEPROMATOUS LEPROSY: This form exhibits multiple, tumor-like lesions of the skin, eyes, testes, nerves, lymph nodes and spleen. Nodular or diffuse infiltrates of foamy macrophages contain myriad bacilli (Fig. 9-49). The epidermis is stretched thinly over the nodules, and beneath it is a narrow, uninvolved "clear zone" of the dermis. Rather than destroying the bacilli, macrophages seem to act as microincubators. When subjected to acid-fast stains, the numerous organisms within the foamy macrophages appear as aggregates of acid-fast material, called "globi." The dermal infiltrates expand slowly to distort and disfigure the face, ears, and upper airway and to destroy the eyes, eyebrows and eyelashes, nerves and testes. The nodular skin lesions of lepromatous leprosy may ulcerate. Claw-shaped hands, hammertoes, saddle nose and pendulous ear lobes are common. Nodular lesions of the face may coalesce to produce a lion-like appearance ("leonine facies"). Involvement of the upper airways leads to chronic nasal discharge and voice change. Infection of the eyes may cause blindness.

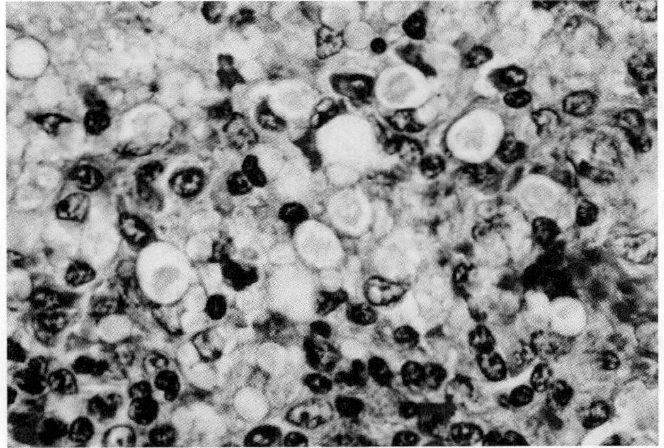

FIGURE 9-49. Lepromatous leprosy. A section of skin shows a tumor-like mass of foamy macrophages. The faint masses within the vacuolated macrophages are enormous numbers of lepra bacilli.

Mycobacterium avium-intracellulare Complex

Mycobacterium avium and *Mycobacterium intracellulare* are similar species that cause identical diseases and are grouped as *M. avium-intracellulare* (MAI) complex, or simply MAI. MAI causes two types of disease: (1) a rare, slowly progressive granulomatous pulmonary disease in immunocompetent persons and (2) a progressive systemic disease in patients with AIDS. ***MAI infection is the third most common opportunistic infection in AIDS patients in the United States.***

MAI is found in soil, water and foodstuffs worldwide. Humans probably acquire it from the environment by inhaling aerosols from infected water sources. Colonization by the organisms is common. As many as 70% of the population shows immunologic responsiveness to MAI, indicating prior exposure.

Granulomatous *Mycobacterium avium-intracellulare* Disease Occurs in Immunocompetent Persons

Most immunocompetent persons with granulomatous pulmonary disease caused by MAI are older (50 to 70 years), and many suffer from preexisting pulmonary disease. ***Clinically and pathologically, MAI disease resembles tuberculosis but progresses much more slowly. It causes pulmonary nodules and cavities and caseating granulomas.***

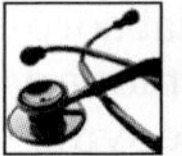

CLINICAL FEATURES: The most common antecedent illnesses predisposing to pulmonary MAI infection are chronic obstructive pulmonary disease, treated tuberculosis, pneumoconioses and bronchiectasis. Cough is a common symptom, but the fever, night sweats, fatigue and weight loss that characterize tuberculosis are lacking. MAI lung disease is indolent or only slowly progressive, causing lung function to decline gradually over years or decades. The organism is quite resistant to first-line antituberculous drugs, and combination therapies often yield disappointing results.

Mycobacterium avium-intracellulare Causes Disseminated Infection in AIDS

One third of AIDS patients in the United States develop overt MAI infection; as many as one half have evidence of infection at autopsy.

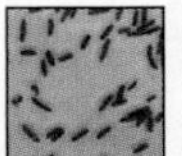

ETIOLOGIC FACTORS: In patients with AIDS, progressive depletion of helper T cells cripples immune responses that normally prevent MAI disease. Although macrophages phagocytose the organisms, they cannot kill them. The bacilli replicate, fill the cells and spread first to other macrophages and then throughout the body via the lymphatics and bloodstream.

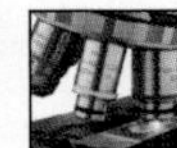

PATHOLOGY: Infected macrophages are found in many organs. Proliferation of the organisms leads to recruitment of additional macrophages, causing expanding nodular lesions that range from structured epithelioid granulomas with few organisms to loose aggregates of foamy macrophages packed with acid-fast bacilli (Fig. 9-50).

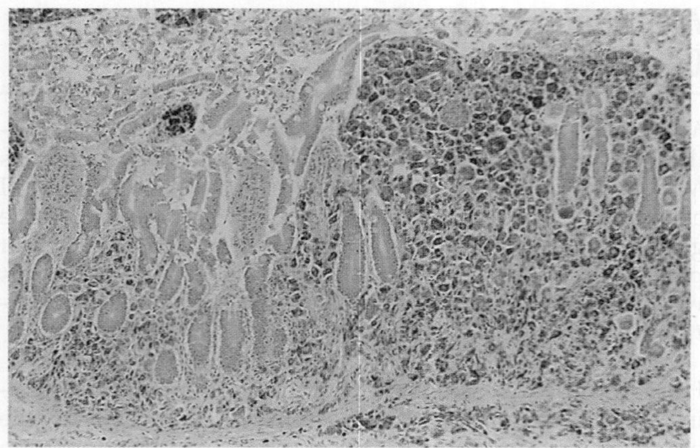

FIGURE 9-50. *Mycobacterium avium-intracellulare* (MAI). A section of small bowel from a patient with acquired immunodeficiency syndrome (AIDS) reveals the presence of numerous macrophages stuffed with acid-fast bacilli in the lamina propria.

Eventually, lymph nodes, spleen and bone marrow may be almost completely replaced by aggregates of macrophages and lesions in the bowel erode into the lumen of the gut.

CLINICAL FEATURES: Early, constitutional symptoms of MAI disease in AIDS resemble those of tuberculosis: fever, night sweats, fatigue and weight loss. Progressive small-bowel involvement produces malabsorption and diarrhea, often with abdominal pain. Pulmonary involvement is common but does not usually produce symptoms. Combinations of five or more different antibiotics, including clarithromycin, may control, but rarely cure, widespread MAI infection in AIDS patients.

Atypical Mycobacteria

Several other species of environmental mycobacteria occasionally produce human disease. These organisms are also present in surface waters, dust and dirt and people acquire infection by inhalation, inoculation or ingestion of environmental material.

These bacteria, including MAI, are often lumped together as the "atypical mycobacteria" (in contrast to *M. tuberculosis*, regarded as the "typical" mycobacterium). The atypical mycobacteria are biologically diverse and the uncommon diseases that they produce in humans differ in circumstances of acquisition, pathology, clinical presentations and therapies. The features of these diseases are compared in Table 9-8.

- ***Mycobacterium kansasii*** causes a chronic, slowly progressive granulomatous pulmonary disease in people older than 50 years, similar to that produced by MAI in immunocompetent patients.
- ***Mycobacterium scrofulaceum***, a common soil inhabitant, causes a draining, granulomatous, cervical lymphadenitis in young children (aged 1 to 5 years). The infection affects the submandibular lymph nodes and probably results from inoculation or ingestion of organisms by toddlers playing in soil. The disease is localized, and surgical excision of affected lymph nodes is curative.
- ***Mycobacterium marinum***, commonly found on underwater surfaces, produces a localized nodular skin lesion

Table 9-8

Atypical Mycobacterial Infections

Organism	Disease	Ages Affected	Pathology	Source	Distribution
Mycobacterium kansasii	Chronic granulomatous pulmonary disease (similar to that caused by *Mycobacterium avium-intracellulare*)	50–70	Granulomatous inflammation	Inhaled organisms from soil, dust or water	Worldwide
Mycobacterium scrofulaceum	Cervical lymphadenitis	1–5	Granulomatous inflammation	Probably ingested organisms from soil or dust	Worldwide
Mycobacterium marinum	Localized skin lesions	All	Granulomatous inflammation	Direct inoculation of organisms from fish or underwater surfaces (swimming pools, fish tanks)	Worldwide
Mycobacterium ulcerans	Large, solitary, severe ulcer of skin and subcutaneous tissue	Usually 5–25	Coagulative necrosis	Probably inoculation of environmental organisms	Australia, Africa
Mycobacterium fortuitum and *Mycobacterium chelonae*	Infections associated with traumatic or iatrogenic inoculations	All	Pyogenic inflammation	Inoculation of environmental organisms	Worldwide

("swimming pool granuloma"), sometimes with lymphatic involvement. Infection is acquired by traumatic inoculation, such as abrading an elbow on a swimming pool ladder or cutting a finger on a fish spine. Tissue reactions may be pyogenic or granulomatous.

- ***Mycobacterium ulcerans*** leads to a severe ulcerating skin disease in Australia, Africa and New Guinea. Infection presents as a solitary, undermining, deep ulcer of the skin and subcutaneous fat of the extremities.
- ***Mycobacterium chelonae* and *Mycobacterium fortuitum*** are closely related organisms that are ubiquitous in the environment. Infection is associated with traumatic or iatrogenic inoculation of material contaminated with organisms. Painless, fluctuant abscesses appear at the site of inoculation, ulcerate and gradually heal spontaneously. The tissue reaction can be pyogenic or granulomatous.

FUNGAL INFECTIONS

Of more than 100,000 known fungi, only a few cause human disease. Of these, most are "opportunists": they only infect people with impaired immune mechanisms. ***Thus, corticosteroid administration, antineoplastic therapy and congenital or acquired T-cell deficiencies all predispose to mycotic infections.***

Fungi are larger and more complex than bacteria. They vary from 2 to 100 μm and are eukaryotes. Thus, they possess nuclear membranes and cytoplasmic organelles, such as mitochondria and endoplasmic reticulum.

There are two basic morphologic types of fungi: yeasts and molds.

- **Yeasts** are unicellular forms of fungi. They are round or oval cells that reproduce by budding, by which process daughter organisms pinch off from a parent. Some yeasts produce buds that do not detach but instead produce **pseudohyphae** (i.e., chains of elongated yeast cells that resemble hyphae).
- **Molds** are multicellular filamentous fungal colonies with branching tubules, or **hyphae**, 2 to 10 μm in diameter. The mass of tangled hyphae in the mold form is called a **mycelium**. Some hyphae are separated by septa that are located at regular intervals; others are nonseptate.
- **Dimorphic fungi** may grow as yeasts or molds, depending on their environment.

Most fungi are visible on tissue sections stained with hematoxylin and eosin. The periodic acid–Schiff (PAS) and Gomori methenamine silver (GMS) stains outline fungal cell walls and are commonly used to detect fungal infection in tissues.

Pneumocystis jiroveci Pneumonia

Pneumocystis jiroveci (formerly, carinii) causes progressive, often fatal, pneumonia in people with impaired cell-mediated immunity and is commonly seen as an opportunistic pathogen in AIDS. The organism has recently been reclassified with the fungi.

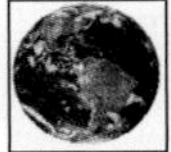

EPIDEMIOLOGY: *P. jiroveci* is distributed worldwide. Since 75% of the population have antibodies by 5 years of age, it is likely that the organisms are inhaled by all. If cell-mediated immunity is intact, infection is rapidly contained without producing symptoms.

In the 1960s and 1970s, 100 to 200 cases of active *Pneumocystis* disease were reported annually in the United States, mainly in people with hematologic malignancies, transplant recipients or those treated with corticosteroids or cytotoxic therapy. *Pneumocystis* became a common pathogen with the AIDS pandemic: before the use of highly active antiretroviral therapy (see Chapter 4), 80% of AIDS patients developed *Pneumocystis* pneumonia.

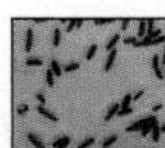

ETIOLOGIC FACTORS: *P. jiroveci* reproduces in association with alveolar type 1 lining cells and active disease is confined to the lungs. Infection begins with attachment of *Pneumocystis* trophozoites to alveolar lining cells. Trophozoites feed on host cells, enlarge and transform into the cyst form, which contains daughter organisms. The cyst ruptures to release new trophozoites, which attach to additional alveolar lining cells. If the process is not checked by the host immune system or antibiotics, infected alveoli eventually fill with organisms and proteinaceous fluid. The progressive filling of alveoli prevents adequate gas exchange and the patient slowly suffocates.

It is assumed, but not proven, that most cases of pneumocystosis derive from latent endogenous infection. Outbreaks of *Pneumocystis* pneumonia have also occurred among severely malnourished (and thus immunosuppressed) infants in nurseries; these are believed to represent primary infection with the organism.

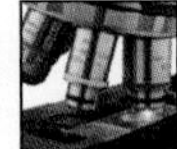

PATHOLOGY: *P. jiroveci* causes progressive consolidation of the lungs. Microscopically, alveoli contain a frothy eosinophilic material, composed of alveolar macrophages and cysts and *P. jiroveci* trophozoites (Fig. 9-51). There are hyaline membranes and prominent type 2 pneumocytes. In newborns, alveolar septa are thickened by lymphoid cells and macrophages. The prominent plasma cells in the infantile disease led to the now obsolete term *plasma cell pneumonia*.

The various forms of *P. jiroveci* are best visualized with methenamine silver stains. The cyst form measures about 60 μm in diameter (Fig. 9-51B); extracellular trophozoites and intracystic forms of the organism appear as irregularly shaped cells, 1 to 3 μm across, with punctate violet nuclei by Giemsa staining.

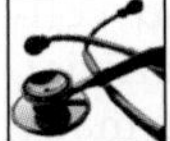

CLINICAL FEATURES: *P. jiroveci* pneumonia features fever and progressive shortness of breath, often exacerbated by exertion and accompanied by a nonproductive cough. Dyspnea may be subtle in onset and slowly progressive over many weeks. Chest radiographs show a diffuse pulmonary process. The diagnosis requires recovery of alveolar material (by bronchoscopy, endobronchial washing or sputum induction) for staining. The disease is fatal if untreated. Therapy is with trimethoprim-sulfamethoxazole or pentamidine.

Candida

The genus *Candida,* composed of over 20 species of yeasts, includes the most common opportunistic pathogens. Many *Candida* spp. are endogenous human flora, well adapted to life on or in the human body, but they can cause disease when host defenses are compromised. Although the various forms

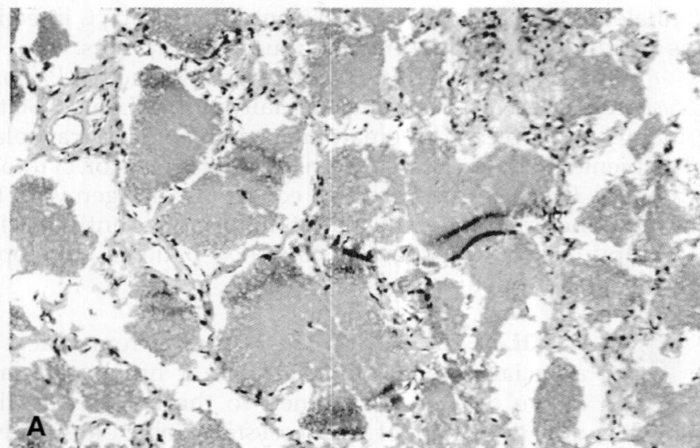

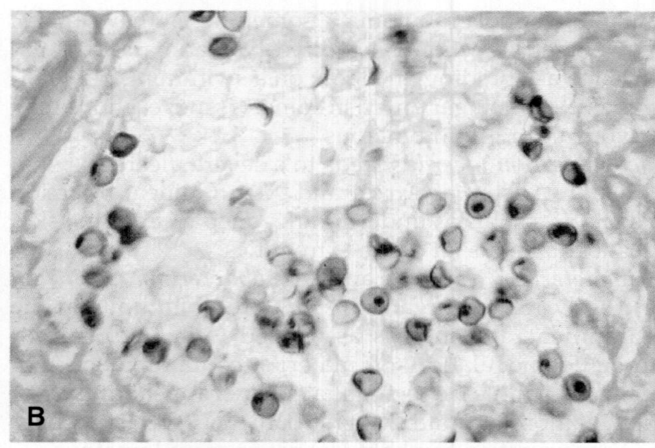

FIGURE 9-51. *Pneumocystis jiroveci* pneumonia. A. The alveoli contain a frothy eosinophilic material that is composed of alveolar macrophages and cysts and trophozoites of *P. jiroveci*. **B.** A silver stain shows crescent-shaped organisms, which are collapsed and degenerated. Some have a characteristic dark spot in their walls.

of candidiasis vary in clinical severity, most are localized, superficial diseases, limited to a particular mucocutaneous site, including:

- **Intertrigo:** infection of opposed skin surfaces
- **Paronychia:** infection of the nail bed
- **Diaper rash**
- **Vulvovaginitis**
- **Thrush:** oral infection
- **Esophagitis**

Candidal infections of deep tissues are much less common than superficial infections but can be life-threatening. The most common deep sites affected are the brain, eye, kidney and heart. Deep infections, with candidal sepsis and disseminated candidiasis, occur only in immunologically compromised persons and are often fatal.

Most candidal infections derive from endogenous flora. *Candida albicans* resides in small numbers in the oropharynx, gastrointestinal tract and vagina and is the most frequent candidal pathogen, being responsible for more than 95% of these infections.

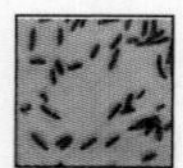

ETIOLOGIC FACTORS: Mechanical barriers, inflammatory cells, humoral immunity and cell-mediated immunity relegate *Candida* to superficial, nonsterile sites. In turn, the resident bacterial flora normally limit the number of fungal organisms. Bacteria (1) block candidal attachment to epithelial cells, (2) compete with them for nutrients and (3) prevent conversion of the fungus to tissue-invasive forms. When any of the above defenses is compromised, candidal infections can occur (Table 9-9). ***Antibiotic use suppresses competing bacterial flora and is the most common precipitating factor for candidiasis.*** Under conditions of unopposed growth, the yeast converts to its invasive form (hyphae or pseudohyphae), invades superficially and elicits an inflammatory or immunologic response.

Although *Candida* inhabits skin surfaces, it does not cause cutaneous disease without a predisposing skin lesion. The most common such factor is maceration, or softening and destruction of the skin. Chronically warm and moist areas, such as between fingers and toes, between skin folds and under diapers, are prone to maceration and superficial candidal disease.

The incidence of invasive candidal infections is increasing. Frequent use of potent broad-spectrum antibiotics eliminates bacteria that otherwise limit *Candida* colonization. Expanded use of medical devices, such as intravascular catheters, monitoring devices, endotracheal tubes and urinary catheters, provides access to sterile sites. AIDS and iatrogenic neutropenias render individuals less capable of defending themselves from even weak pathogens, such as *Candida*. Finally, intravenous drug users develop deep candidal infections because of inoculation of the fungi into the bloodstream.

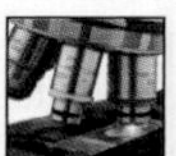 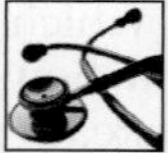

PATHOLOGY AND CLINICAL FEATURES: Superficial infections of the skin, oropharynx (Fig. 9-52A) and esophagus show invasive organisms in the most superficial epithelial layers and are associated with acute inflammatory infiltrates. Yeast,

Table 9-9

Candidal Infections

Disease	Predisposing Conditions
Superficial Infections	
Intertrigo (opposed skin surfaces)	Maceration
Paronychia (nail beds)	Maceration
Diaper rash	Maceration
Vulvovaginitis	Alteration in normal flora
Thrush (oral)	Decreased cell-mediated immunity
Esophagitis	Decreased cell-mediated immunity
Deep Infections	
Urinary tract infections	Indwelling urinary catheters
Sepsis and disseminated infection	Neutropenia, indwelling vascular catheters and change in normal flora

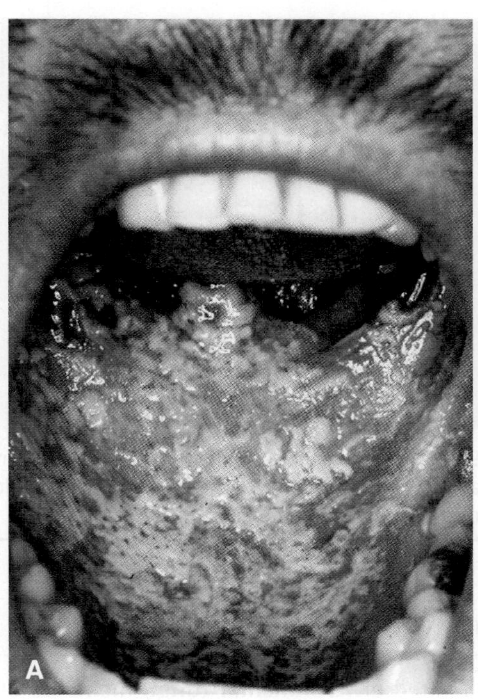

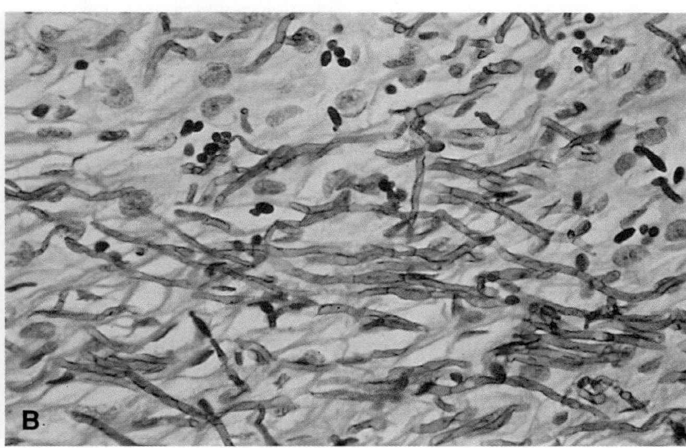

FIGURE 9-52. Candidiasis. A. The oral cavity of a patient with acquired immunodeficiency syndrome (AIDS) is covered by a white, curd-like exudate containing numerous fungal organisms. **B.** A periodic acid–Schiff (PAS) stain shows numerous septate hyphae and yeast forms.

pseudohyphae and hyphae are present (Fig. 9-52B). The yeasts are round and 3 to 4 μm in diameter and the hyphae are septate. Candidal vaginitis is characterized by superficial invasion of the squamous epithelium, but inflammation is usually scanty. Deep infections consist of multiple microscopic abscesses with yeast, hyphae, necrotic debris and neutrophils. Rarely, *Candida* elicit granulomatous responses.

The various superficial cutaneous infections manifest as tender, erythematous papules, which expand to form confluent erythematous areas.

- **Thrush:** This lesion involves the tongue and mucous membranes of the mouth. Early in life, it is the most common form of mucocutaneous candidiasis. Candidal vaginitis during pregnancy predisposes newborns to infection. There are friable, white, curd-like membranes adherent to affected surfaces. These patches contain fungi, necrotic debris, neutrophils and bacteria, and can be dislodged by scraping. Removal of the membranes leaves a painful, bleeding surface.
- **Candidal vulvovaginitis:** This condition causes a thick, white vaginal discharge with vaginal and vulvar itching. Involved areas of the vulva are erythematous and tender. Candidal vaginitis is most intense when vaginal pH is low. Antibiotics, pregnancy, diabetes and corticosteroids predispose to this form of vaginitis.
- **Candidal sepsis and disseminated candidiasis:** Systemic candidiasis is rare and is ordinarily a terminal event in someone with altered immunity or neutropenia. Several candidal species can produce invasive disease in this context. Organisms may enter through ulcerated skin or mucous membrane lesions or may be introduced iatrogenically (e.g., peritoneal dialysis, intravenous lines or urinary catheters). The urinary tract is most commonly involved, and the incidence in women is four times that in men. Renal lesions may be blood-borne or may arise from an ascending pyelonephritis.
- **Candidal endocarditis:** This infection is characterized by large vegetations on the heart valves and a high incidence of embolization to large arteries. In most patients with candidal endocarditis, the cause is not immunosuppression but unusual vulnerability. Drug addicts who use unsterilized needles and persons with preexisting valvular disease who have had prolonged antibacterial therapy or indwelling vascular catheters are at risk for endocarditis. One of the most serious complications of invasive candidiasis is septic embolism to the brain.

Aspergillosis

Aspergillus spp. are common environmental fungi that cause opportunistic infections, usually involving the lungs. There are three types of pulmonary aspergillosis: (1) **allergic bronchopulmonary aspergillosis,** (2) **colonization of a preexisting pulmonary cavity** (**aspergilloma** or **fungus ball**) and (3) **invasive aspergillosis** (see Chapter 12). Of the over 200 identified species of *Aspergillus,* approximately 20 cause human disease. *Aspergillus fumigatus* is by far the most frequent human pathogen.

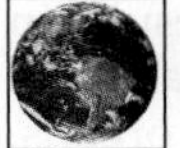

EPIDEMIOLOGY: *Aspergillus* is a saprophyte found worldwide in soil, decaying plant matter and dung. Pulmonary aspergillosis is acquired by inhaling small (2 to 3 μm) spores, **conidia,** that are in the air in almost every human environment. The spores are small enough to reach the alveoli when inhaled. Exposure is greatest when the fungus's habitat is disturbed, as during soil excavations or handling decaying organic matter.

In tissues, *Aspergillus* show septate hyphae, 2 to 7 μm in diameter, branching progressively at acute angles. The multiple dichotomous branching led to the name *Aspergillus* (from the Latin *aspergere,* "to sprinkle"). It derives from a fancied resemblance to the aspergillum, a device used to sprinkle holy water during Catholic religious ceremonies.

Allergic Bronchopulmonary Aspergillosis May Complicate Asthma

Inhalation of *Aspergillus* spores delivers fungal antigens to airways and alveoli; contact subsequently initiates an allergic response in susceptible persons. The situation is aggravated if spores can germinate and grow in the airways, thereby causing long-term exposure to the antigen. Allergic bronchopulmonary aspergillosis is virtually restricted to asthmatics, 20% of whom eventually develop this disorder (see Chapter 12).

Bronchi and bronchioles show infiltrates of lymphocytes, plasma cells and variable numbers of eosinophils. Sometimes airways are impacted with mucus and fungal hyphae. Patients experience exacerbations of asthma, often accompanied by pulmonary infiltrates and eosinophilia.

Aspergillomas Occur in Patients With Pulmonary Cavities or Bronchiectasis

Inhaled spores germinate in the warm humid atmosphere provided by these hollows and fill them with masses of hyphae. The organisms do not invade (see Chapter 12).

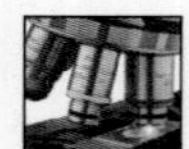

PATHOLOGY: An aspergilloma is a dense, roundish mass of tangled hyphae, 1 to 7 cm in diameter, within a fibrous cavity. The cavity wall is collagenous connective tissue, with lymphocytes and plasma cells. The hyphae do not invade adjacent tissues.

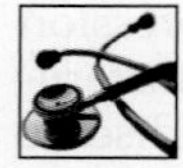

CLINICAL FEATURES: Aspergillomas occur most commonly in old tuberculous cavities. Symptoms reflect the underlying disease. The radiologic appearance of a dense round ball in a cavity is characteristic. Aspergillomas are usually best left untreated, but surgical excision may be indicated in some cases.

Invasive Aspergillosis Generally Afflicts Neutropenic Patients

Whenever neutrophil number or activity is compromised, invasive aspergillosis may occur. The most common settings are high-dose steroid or cytotoxic therapy or acute leukemia. In profoundly neutropenic patients, inhaled spores germinate to produce hyphae, which invade through bronchi into the lung parenchyma, from where the fungi may spread widely.

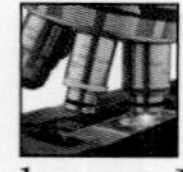

PATHOLOGY: *Aspergillus* readily invades blood vessels and produces thrombosis (Fig. 9-53). As a result, multiple nodular infarcts are seen throughout both lungs. Involvement of larger pulmonary arteries results in large, wedge-shaped, pleural-based infarcts. Vascular invasion also leads to fungus dissemination to other organs. Microscopically, *Aspergillus* hyphae are arranged radially around blood vessels and extend through their walls. Acute aspergillosis may also start in a nasal sinus and spread to the face, orbit and brain.

CLINICAL FEATURES: Invasive aspergillosis presents as fever and multifocal pulmonary infiltrates in a compromised patient. Because of frequent thrombosis and bloodstream dissemination, the disease is often fatal. Antifungal therapy with amphotericin B may be successful but must be initiated early and given in high doses.

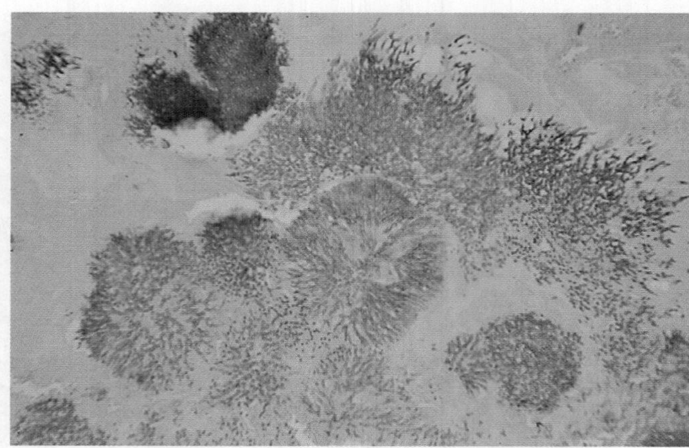

FIGURE 9-53. Invasive aspergillosis. A section of lung impregnated with silver shows branching fungal hyphae surrounding blood vessels and invading the adjacent parenchyma.

Mucormycosis (Zygomycosis)

Several related environmental fungi, members of the class Zygomycetes—namely, *Rhizopus, Mucor, Rhizomucor* and *Absidia*—produce severe, necrotizing, invasive, opportunistic infections that begin in the nasal sinuses or lungs. The infections they produce are usually called **mucormycoses** or **zygomycoses.**

In tissues, zygomycetes have large (8 to 15 μm across) hyphae that branch at right angles, have thin walls, and lack septa. In tissue sections, they appear as hollow tubes. Lacking cross-walls, their liquid contents flow, leaving long empty segments. They also may resemble "twisted ribbons," which represent collapsed hyphae.

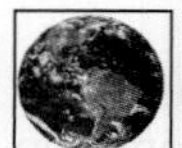

EPIDEMIOLOGY: *Rhizopus, Rhizomucor, Mucor,* and *Absidia* are ubiquitous in the environment, inhabiting soil, food and decaying vegetable matter. Their spores are inhaled, and in susceptible persons, disease begins in the lungs. Mucormycosis occurs almost exclusively in the setting of compromised defenses. Common causes include severe neutropenia (e.g., after treatment for leukemia), high-dose glucocorticoid therapy and, particularly, severe diabetes.

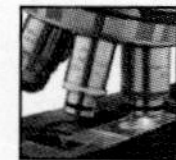
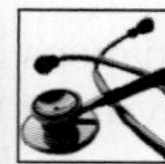

PATHOLOGY AND CLINICAL FEATURES: The three predominant forms of mucormycosis are rhinocerebral, pulmonary, and subcutaneous.

- **Rhinocerebral mucormycosis:** Fungi proliferate in nasal sinuses, invade surrounding tissues and extend into facial soft tissues, nerves, blood vessels and the brain. The palate or nasal turbinates are covered by a black crust and underlying tissue is friable and hemorrhagic. Fungal hyphae grow into the arteries and cause devastating, rapidly progressive, septic infarction of affected tissues. Extension into the brain leads to fatal, necrotizing, hemorrhagic encephalitis. Therapy requires surgical excision of involved tissues, amphotericin B and correction of the predisposing abnormality.
- **Pulmonary mucormycosis:** This infection resembles invasive pulmonary aspergillosis, including vascular invasion

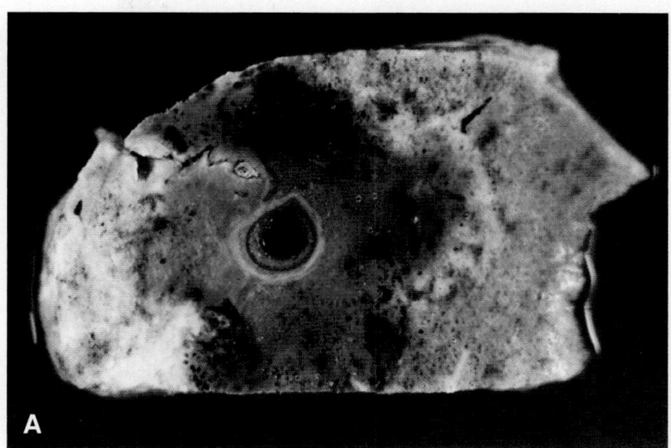

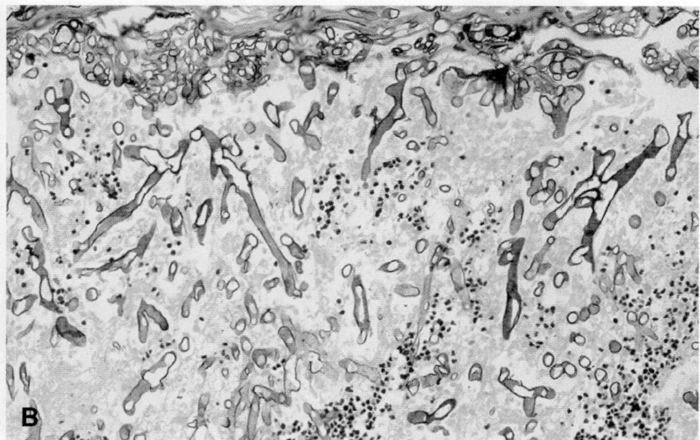

FIGURE 9-54. Pulmonary mucormycosis. A. A cross-section of the lung shows the vessel in the center of the field to be invaded by mucormycetes and occluded by a septic thrombus. The surrounding tissue is infarcted. **B.** Invasive mucormycosis, stained with Gomori-methamine silver.

and multiple areas of septic infarction (Fig. 9-54). Both rhinocerebral and pulmonary mucormycosis are usually fatal.

- **Subcutaneous zygomycosis:** This infection is limited to the tropics and is caused by *Basidiobolus haptosporus*. The fungus grows slowly in the panniculus, producing a gradually enlarging, hard inflammatory mass, usually on the shoulder, trunk, buttock or thigh.

Cryptococcosis

Cryptococcosis is a systemic mycosis caused by *Cryptococcus neoformans*, which principally affects the meninges and lungs (Fig. 9-55). *C. neoformans* has a worldwide distribution. Its main reservoir is pigeon droppings, which are alkaline and hyperosmolar. These conditions keep cryptococci small, allowing inhaled organisms to reach the terminal bronchioles. *C. neoformans* is unique among pathogenic fungi in having a proteoglycan capsule, which is essential for pathogenicity. The organisms appear as faintly basophilic yeasts with a clear 3- to 5-μm-thick mucinous capsule.

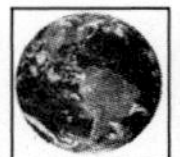

EPIDEMIOLOGY: Cryptococcus ***almost exclusively affects persons with impaired cell-mediated immunity.*** Although the organism is ubiquitous and exposure is common, cryptococcosis is rare in the absence of predisposing illness. Disease is uncommon even among persons such as pigeon fanciers, who are exposed to high concentrations of the organism. Cryptococcosis occurs in patients with AIDS, lymphomas (particularly Hodgkin disease), leukemias and sarcoidosis, and in those treated with high doses of corticosteroids.

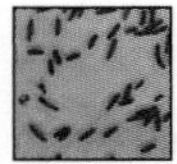

ETIOLOGIC FACTORS: In immunologically intact persons, neutrophils and alveolar macrophages kill *C. neoformans* and no clinical disease develops. By contrast, in a patient with defective cell-mediated immunity, the cryptococci survive, reproduce locally and then disseminate. Although the lung is the portal of entry, the CNS is the most common site of disease, owing to the excellent environment provided by the cerebrospinal fluid.

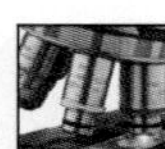

PATHOLOGY: Over 95% of cryptococcal infections involve the meninges and brain. Lesions in the lungs can be demonstrated in half of patients. In a small minority skin, liver and other involvement occurs. In cryptococcal meningoencephalitis, the entire brain is swollen and soft, and leptomeninges are thickened and gelatinous from infiltration by the thickly encapsulated organisms. Inflammatory responses are variable but are often minimal, with large numbers of cryptococci infiltrating tissue with no inflammatory response. If present, inflammation may be neutrophilic, lymphocytic or granulomatous.

Cryptococcosis in the lung may appear as diffuse disease or as isolated areas of consolidation. Affected alveoli are distended by clusters of organisms, usually with minimal inflammation.

Because of its thick capsule, *C. neoformans* stains poorly with routine hematoxylin and eosin and appears as bubbles or holes in tissue sections (Fig. 9-56A). Fungal stains (PAS and GMS) show the yeasts well but do not stain the polysaccharide capsule. The organism thus appears to be surrounded by a halo. The capsule can be highlighted by mucicarmine stain (Fig. 9-56B).

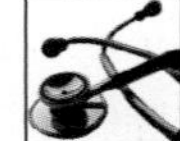

CLINICAL FEATURES: Cryptococcal CNS disease often begins insidiously with nonfocal symptoms, including headache, dizziness, sleepiness and loss of coordination. Untreated cryptococcal meningitis is invariably fatal. Therapy requires prolonged systemic administration of antifungal agents. Cryptococcal pneumonia presents as diffuse progressive pulmonary disease.

Histoplasmosis

Histoplasmosis is caused by *Histoplasma capsulatum*. ***Infection is usually self-limited but may lead to a systemic granulomatous disease.*** Most cases of histoplasmosis are asymptomatic, but progressive disseminated infections occur in people with impaired cell-mediated immunity. *H. capsulatum* is a dimorphic fungus of worldwide distribution that grows as a mold at ambient temperatures and as a yeast in the body (37°C [98.6°F]). The yeast cell is round and has a central

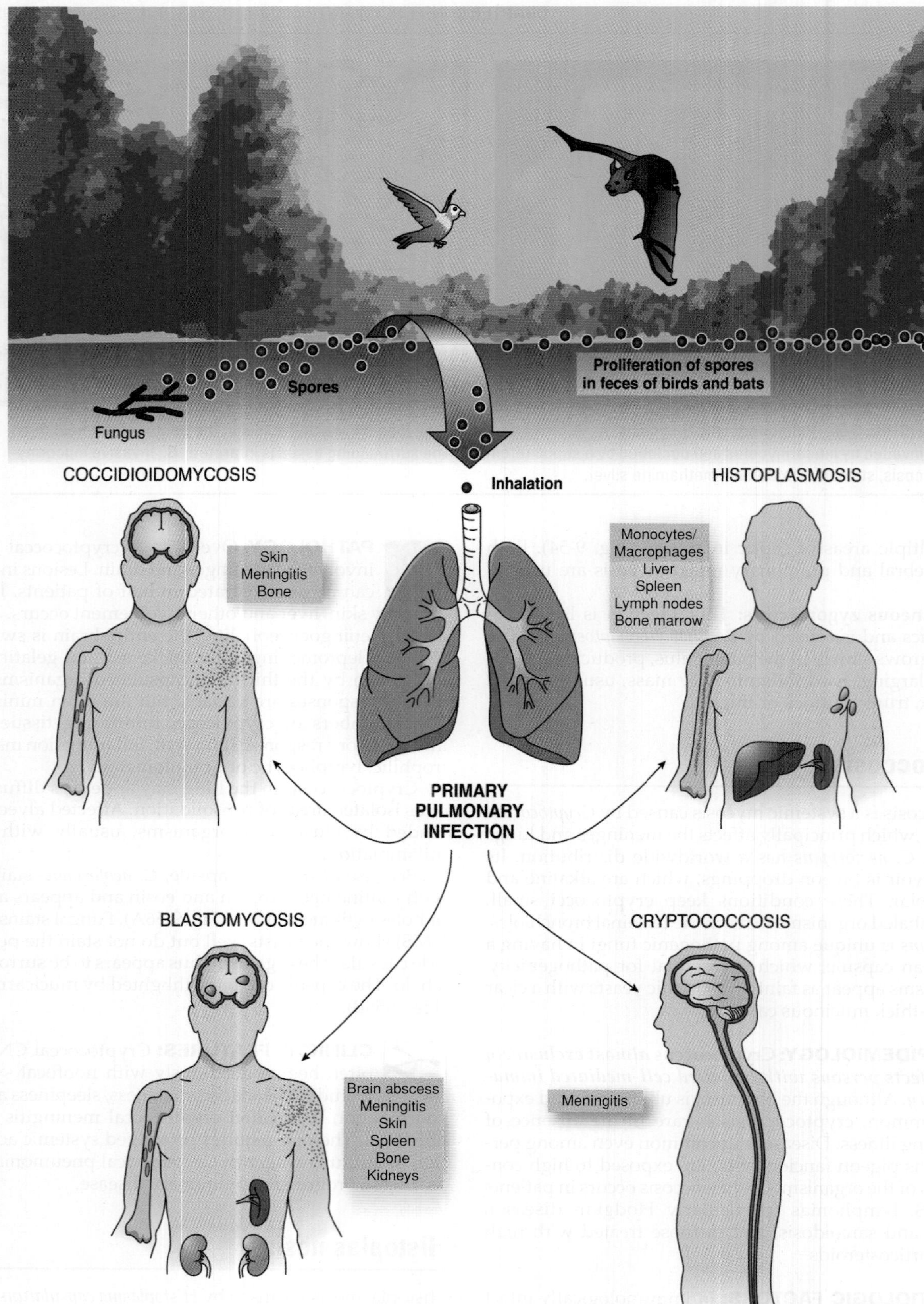

FIGURE 9-55. Pulmonary and disseminated fungal infection. Fungi grow in soil and air and in the feces of birds and bats; they produce spores, some of which are infectious. When inhaled, spores cause primary pulmonary infection. In a few patients, the infection disseminates.
Histoplasmosis. Primary infection is in the lung. In susceptible patients, the fungus disseminates to target organs, namely, the monocyte/macrophage system (liver, spleen, lymph nodes and bone marrow) and the tongue, mucous membranes of the mouth and the adrenals.
Cryptococcosis. Primary infection of the lung disseminates to the meninges.
Blastomycosis. Primary infection of the lung disseminates widely. The principal targets are the brain, meninges, skin, spleen, bone and kidney.
Coccidioidomycosis. Primary infection of the lung may disseminate widely. The skin, meninges and bone are common targets.

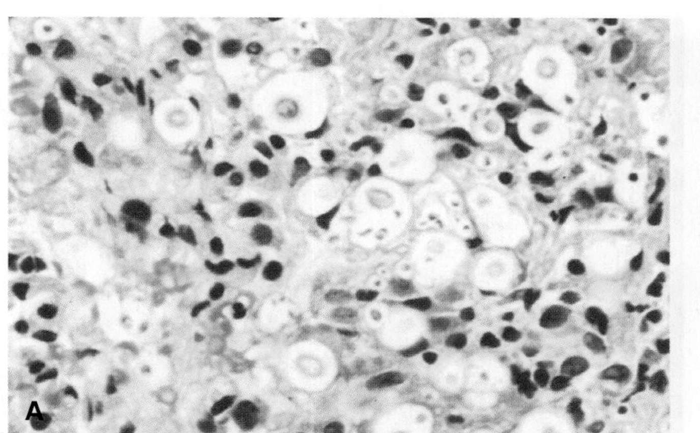

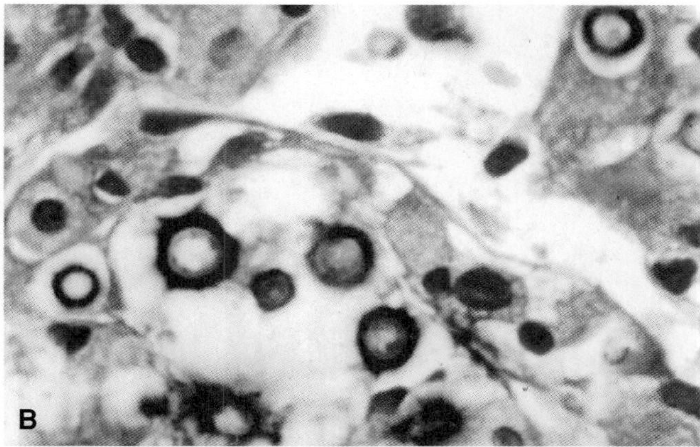

FIGURE 9-56. Cryptococcosis. A. In a section of the lung stained with hematoxylin and eosin, *Cryptococcus neoformans* appears as holes or bubbles. **B.** The same section stained with mucicarmine illustrates the capsule of the organism.

basophilic body surrounded by a clear zone or halo, which in turn is encircled by a rigid cell wall 2 to 4 μm in diameter. In caseous lesions, silver impregnation identifies the remains of degenerating yeast forms.

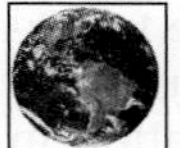

EPIDEMIOLOGY: Histoplasmosis is acquired by inhalation of infectious spores of *H. capsulatum* (Fig. 9-55). The reservoir for the fungus is bird droppings and soil. In the Americas, hyperendemic areas are the eastern and central United States, western Mexico, Central America, the northern countries of South America and Argentina. In the tropics, bat nests, caves and soil beneath trees are foci of exposure.

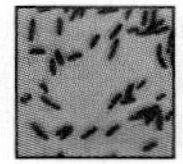

ETIOLOGIC FACTORS: The disease resembles tuberculosis in many ways. Primary infection begins with phagocytosis of microconidia by alveolar macrophages. Like *M. tuberculosis, H. capsulatum* reproduces in immunologically naïve macrophages. As organisms grow, additional macrophages are recruited to the site of infection, producing an area of pulmonary consolidation. A few macrophages carry organisms first to hilar and mediastinal lymph nodes and then throughout the body, where fungi further infect monocytes/macrophages. The organisms proliferate within these cells until the onset of hypersensitivity and cell-mediated immune responses, usually within 1 to 3 weeks. Normal immune responses usually limit the infection. Activated macrophages destroy the phagocytosed yeasts, forming necrotizing granulomas at sites of infection.

The course of infection varies with the size of the infecting inoculum and the immunologic competence of the host. Most infections (95%) involve small inocula of organisms in immunologically competent persons. They affect small areas of the lung and regional lymph nodes and invariably remain unnoticed. On the other hand, exposure to a large inoculum, as occurs in an excavated bird roost, may lead to rapidly evolving pulmonary disease, with large areas of consolidation, prominent mediastinal and hilar nodal involvement and extension of the infection to the liver, spleen and bone marrow.

Disseminated histoplasmosis develops in people who do not mount an effective immune response to *H. capsulatum.* Infants, people with AIDS and patients treated with corticosteroids are at particular risk. In addition, some individuals with no known underlying illness also develop disseminated histoplasmosis.

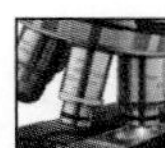

PATHOLOGY: Acute self-limited histoplasmosis is characterized by necrotizing granulomas in the lung, mediastinal and hilar lymph nodes, spleen and liver. Early in infection, the caseous material is surrounded by macrophages, Langhans giant cells, lymphocytes and plasma cells. Yeast forms of *H. capsulatum* can be demonstrated within macrophages and in the caseous material. Eventually, the cellular components of the granuloma largely disappear and the caseous material calcifies, forming a "fibrocaseous nodule" (Fig. 9-57A).

Disseminated histoplasmosis is characterized by progressive organ infiltration with macrophages carrying *H. capsulatum* (Fig. 9-57B). In mild cases, immune responses can control the organism, but not eliminate it. For long periods, disease is largely confined to macrophages in infected organs. If the patient is immunocompromised, clusters of macrophages filled with *H. capsulatum* infiltrate the liver, spleen, lungs, intestine, adrenals and meninges.

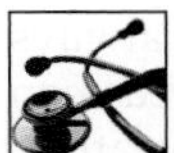

CLINICAL FEATURES: Most infections are asymptomatic, but with extensive disease, patients present with fever, headache and cough. The symptoms persist for a few days to a few weeks, but the disease requires no therapy.

Disseminated histoplasmosis features weight loss, intermittent fever and weakness. In cases of subtle immunodeficiency, the disease may persist and progress for years, even decades. With more-profound immunodeficiency, dissemination progresses rapidly, often with high fever, cough, pancytopenia and changes in mental status. Disseminated histoplasmosis is treated with systemic antifungal agents.

Coccidioidomycosis

Coccidioidomycosis is a chronic, necrotizing mycotic infection that clinically and pathologically resembles tuberculosis. The disease, caused by *Coccidioides immitis,* includes a spectrum of infections that begin as focal pneumonitis. Most are mild and asymptomatic and are limited to the lungs and regional lymph nodes. Occasionally, *C. immitis* infections spread outside the lungs to produce life-threatening disease.

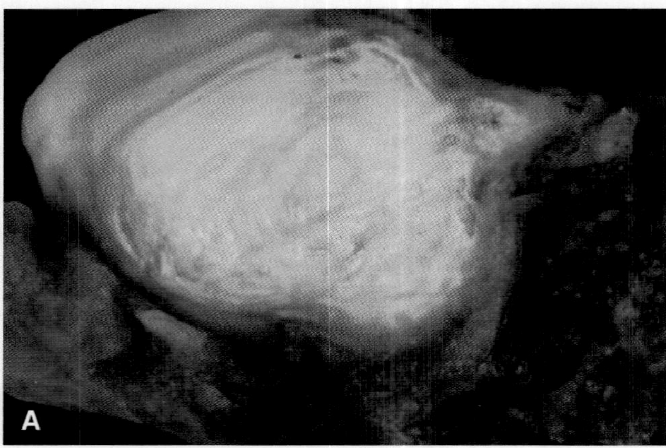

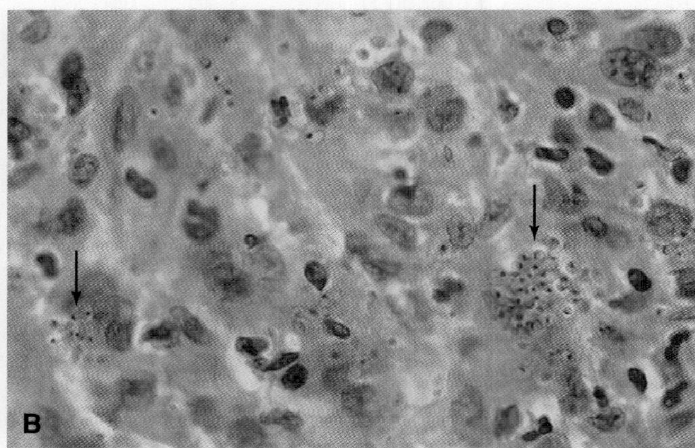

FIGURE 9-57. Histoplasmosis. A. A section of lung shows an encapsulated, subpleural, fibrocaseous nodule. **B.** A section of liver from a patient with disseminated histoplasmosis reveals Kupffer cells containing numerous yeasts of *Histoplasma capsulatum* (*arrows*) (periodic acid–Schiff [PAS] stain).

EPIDEMIOLOGY: *C. immitis* is a dimorphic fungus that grows as a mold in the soil, where it forms spores. Inhaled spores reach the alveoli and terminal bronchioles (Fig. 9-55), enlarge into spherules and then mature to form sporangia, 30 to 60 μm across. These gradually fill with 1 to 5 μm endospores, which accumulate by endosporulation, a process unique among pathogenic fungi. The sporangia eventually rupture and release endospores, which then repeat the cycle.

C. immitis is found in the soil in restricted climatic regions, particularly the Lower Sonoran life zones of the Western Hemisphere. These are areas with sparse rainfall, hot summers and mild winters. In the United States, large portions of California, Arizona, New Mexico and Texas are natural habitats for *C. immitis*. The disease is particularly common in California's San Joaquin Valley, where it is called "**valley fever**." It also occurs in Mexico and parts of South America.

Long-term residents of endemic regions are almost always infected with *C. immitis.* Even brief visits to these areas can cause infection (usually asymptomatic). Dry, windy weather, which lifts spores into the air, favors infection. The disease is not contagious.

ETIOLOGIC FACTORS: Coccidioidomycosis begins with focal bronchopneumonia where the spores are deposited. These elicit mixed inflammatory infiltrates of neutrophils and macrophages, but the spores survive these immunologically naïve inflammatory cells. As in tuberculosis and histoplasmosis, the host controls *C. immitis* infection only when inflammatory cells become immunologically activated. Necrotizing granulomas form with the onset of specific hypersensitivity and cell-mediated immune responses, which kills or contains the fungi.

The course of coccidioidomycosis varies from acute, self-limited disease to disseminated infection, depending on the size of the infecting dose and the immune status of the host. Coccidioidomycosis begins with focal bronchopneumonia. Most infections are produced by small inocula of organisms in immunologically competent hosts and are acute and self-limited. Extensive pulmonary involvement and fulminant disease may occur in persons from a nonendemic region exposed to large numbers of organisms.

Disseminated coccidioidomycosis occurs in immunocompromised persons, from a primary infection or reactivation of old disease. Immunologically compromised patients are at greatest risk. Certain racial groups, including Filipinos, other Asians and blacks, are particularly susceptible to dissemination of coccidioidomycosis, probably because of a specific immunologic defect. The risk of dissemination in Filipinos is 175 times that in whites. Pregnant women are also unusually susceptible to spread of the disease if they develop primary infection during the latter half of pregnancy.

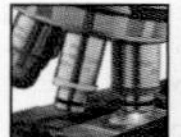

PATHOLOGY: Acute self-limited coccidioidomycosis causes solitary lesions or patchy pulmonary consolidation, in which affected alveoli are infiltrated by neutrophils and macrophages (Fig. 9-58). *C. immitis* spherules elicit an infiltrate of macrophages, whereas endospores predominantly attract neutrophils. Once an immune reaction begins, necrotizing, caseous granulomas develop. Successful immune responses cause the granuloma to heal, sometimes leaving a fibrocaseous nodule composed of caseous material and rimmed by residual macrophages and a thin capsule. In contrast to histoplasmosis, old granulomas of coccidioidomycosis rarely calcify.

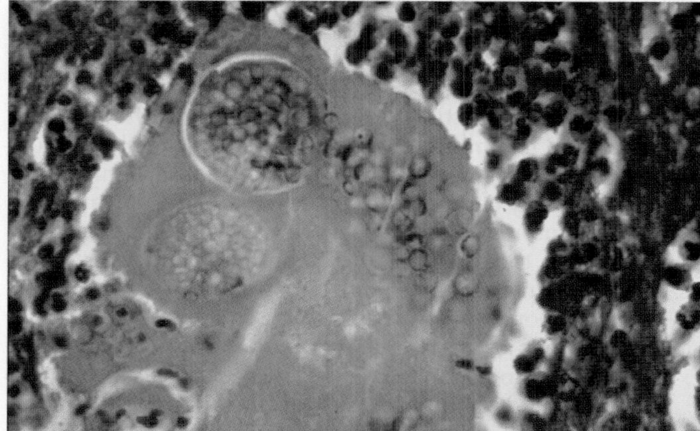

FIGURE 9-58. Coccidioidomycosis. A photomicrograph of the lung from a patient with acute coccidioidal pneumonia shows an acute inflammatory infiltrate surrounding spherules and endospores of *Coccidioides immitis.*

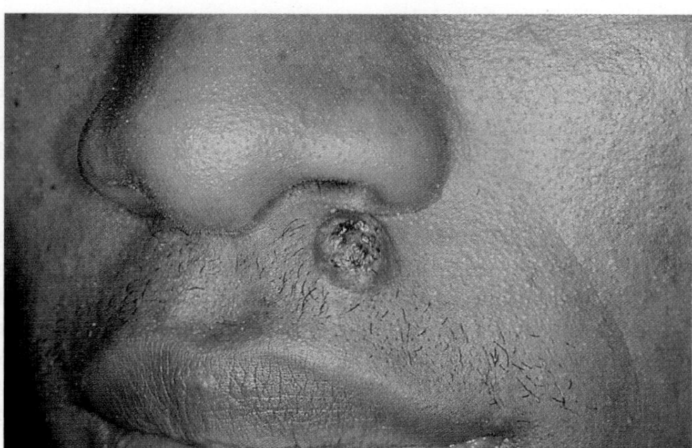

FIGURE 9-59. Disseminated coccidioidomycosis. A single raised, central ulcerated lesion is present on the face.

The spherules and endospores of *C. immitis* stain with hematoxylin and eosin. Spherules in various stages of development appear as basophilic rings. Mature spherules (sporangia) contain endospores that appear as smaller basophilic rings. As in other fungal infections, PAS and GMS stains can be used to enhance the staining of *C. immitis*.

Disseminated coccidioidomycosis may involve almost any body site and may manifest as a single extrathoracic site or as widespread disease, involving the skin (Fig. 9-59), bones, meninges, liver, spleen and genitourinary tract. Inflammatory responses at sites of dissemination are highly variable, ranging from infiltrates of neutrophils to granulomas.

CLINICAL FEATURES: Coccidioidomycosis is a disease of protean manifestations, which vary from a subclinical respiratory infection to one that disseminates and is rapidly fatal. Like syphilis and typhoid fever, this disease is a great imitator: almost any complaint or syndrome may be its initial presentation.

Most people with coccidioidomycosis (>60%) are asymptomatic. The others develop a flu-like syndrome, with fever, cough, chest pain and malaise. Infection usually resolves spontaneously. Cavitation is the most frequent complication of pulmonary coccidioidomycosis, although it fortunately occurs in only few patients (<5%). The cavity, which may be mistaken for tuberculosis, is usually solitary and may persist for years. Progression or reactivation may lead to destructive lesions in the lungs, or more seriously, to disseminated lesions.

The signs and symptoms of disseminated coccidioidomycosis vary according to the site affected. Coccidioidal meningitis manifests with headache, fever, alteration in mental status or seizures and is fatal if untreated. Skin lesions in disseminated disease often have a warty appearance (Fig. 9-59). Even with prolonged amphotericin B therapy, the prognosis is poor in acute disseminated coccidioidomycosis, although the response rate can be quite good with some of the newer azole antifungal agents.

Blastomycosis

Blastomycosis is a chronic granulomatous and suppurative pulmonary disease, which is often followed by dissemination to other body sites, principally the skin and bone. The causative organism, *Blastomyces dermatitidis,* is a dimorphic fungus that grows as a mold in warm moist soil rich in decaying vegetable matter.

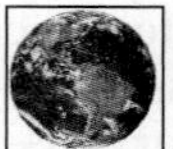

EPIDEMIOLOGY: Blastomycosis is acquired by inhalation of infectious spores from the soil (Fig. 9-55). The infection occurs within restricted geographic regions of the Americas, Africa and possibly the Middle East. In North America, the fungus is endemic along the distributions of the Mississippi and Ohio Rivers, the Great Lakes and the St. Lawrence River. Disturbance of the soil, either by construction or by leisure activities such as hunting or camping, leads to formation of aerosols containing fungal spores.

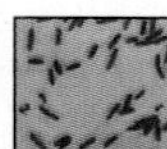

ETIOLOGIC FACTORS: Inhaled spores of *B. dermatitidis* germinate to form yeasts, which reproduce by budding. The host responds to the proliferating organisms with neutrophils and macrophages, producing a focal bronchopneumonia. However, organisms persist until the onset of specific hypersensitivity and cell-mediated immunity, when activated neutrophils and macrophages kill them.

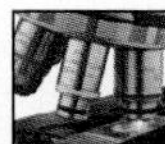

PATHOLOGY: Blastomycosis is usually confined to the lungs, where infection mostly produces small areas of consolidation. *B. dermatitidis* incites a mixed suppurative and granulomatous inflammatory response and even in the same patient, lesions may range from neutrophilic abscesses to epithelioid granulomas. Pulmonary disease usually resolves by scarring, but some patients develop progressive miliary lesions or cavities. The skin (>50%) and bones (>10%) are the most common sites of extrapulmonary involvement. Skin infection often elicits a marked pseudoepitheliomatous hyperplasia, imparting a warty appearance to the lesions.

Infected areas contain numerous yeasts of *B. dermatitidis,* which are spherical and 8 to 14 μm across, with broad-based buds and multiple nuclei in a central body (Fig. 9-60). With hematoxylin and eosin stains, the yeasts are rings with thick, sharply defined cell walls. They may be found in epithelioid

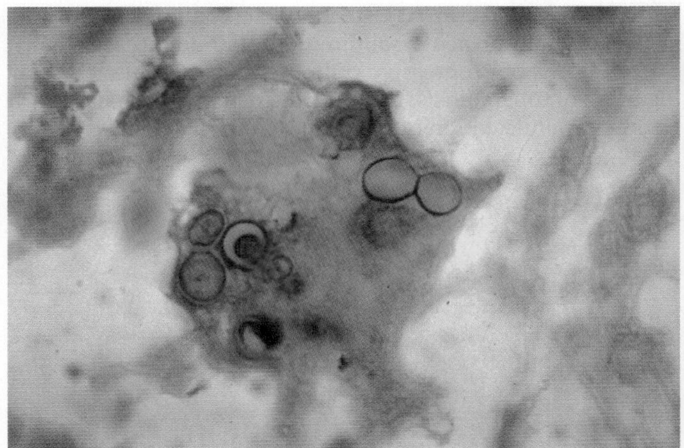

FIGURE 9-60. Blastomycosis. The yeasts of *Blastomyces dermatitidis* have a doubly contoured wall and nuclei in the central body. The buds have broad-based attachments.

cells, macrophages or giant cells, or they may lie free in microabscesses.

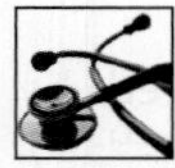

CLINICAL FEATURES: Pulmonary blastomycosis is self-limited in one third of cases. Symptomatic acute infection presents as a flu-like illness, with fever, arthralgias and myalgias. Progressive pulmonary disease is characterized by low-grade fever, weight loss, cough and predominantly upper lobe infiltrates on the chest radiograph. Skin lesions often resemble squamous cell carcinomas of the skin and are the most common signs of extrapulmonary dissemination. Although the lung infection may appear to resolve totally, in some patients, blastomycosis may appear at distant sites months to years later.

Paracoccidioidomycosis (South American Blastomycosis)

Paracoccidioidomycosis is a chronic granulomatous infection that begins with lung involvement and disseminates to involve the skin, oropharynx, adrenals and macrophages of the liver, spleen and lymph nodes. The causative organism is *Paracoccidioides brasiliensis*, a dimorphic fungus, whose mold form is thought to reside in the soil.

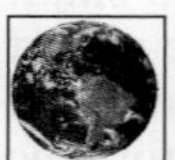

EPIDEMIOLOGY: Paracoccidioidomycosis is acquired by inhaling spores from the environment in restricted regions of Central and South America. Most infections are asymptomatic. Reactivation of latent infection occurs and active disease can develop many years after someone leaves an endemic region. Interestingly, men develop symptomatic infections 15 times more often than women, perhaps because of hormonal influences on conversion of the organism to its yeast phase.

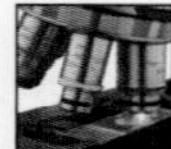

PATHOLOGY: Paracoccidioidomycosis can involve the lungs alone (Fig. 9-61) or multiple extrapulmonary sites, most commonly skin, mucosal surfaces and lymph nodes. *P. brasiliensis* elicits a mixed suppurative and granulomatous response, producing lesions similar to those seen in blastomycosis and coccidioidomycosis.

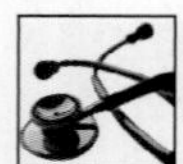

CLINICAL FEATURES: Paracoccidioidomycosis is usually an acute, self-limited and mild disease. Symptoms of progressive pulmonary involvement resemble those of tuberculosis. Chronic mucocutaneous ulcers are a frequent manifestation of extrapulmonary disease.

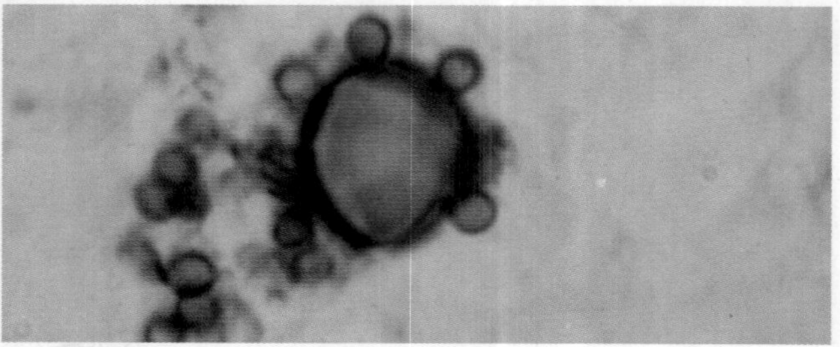

FIGURE 9-61. Paracoccidioidomycosis. The lung contains *Paracoccidioides braziliensis,* which displays many external buds arising circumferentially from the mother organism.

Sporotrichosis

Sporotrichosis is a chronic infection of the skin, subcutaneous tissues and regional lymph nodes caused by *Sporothrix schenckii*. This dimorphic fungus grows as a mold in soil and decaying plant matter and as yeast in the body.

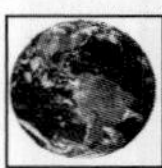

EPIDEMIOLOGY: Sporotrichosis is endemic in parts of the Americas and southern Africa. Most cases are cutaneous, resulting from accidental inoculation of the fungus from thorns (especially rose thorns) or splinters or by handling reeds or grasses. Cutaneous sporotrichosis is particularly common among gardeners, botanical nursery workers and others who suffer abrasions while working with soil, moss, hay or timbers. Infected animals, particularly cats, can also transmit the disease.

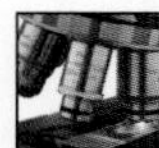

PATHOLOGY: On entry into the skin, *S. schenckii* proliferates locally, eliciting an inflammatory response that produces an ulceronodular lesion. The infection frequently spreads along subcutaneous lymphatic channels, resulting in a chain of similar nodular skin lesions (Fig. 9-62A). Extracutaneous disease is much less common than skin disease. Joint and bone involvement is the commonest form of extracutaneous disease and infections of the wrist, elbow, ankle or knee account for most (80%) of the cases.

The lesions of cutaneous sporotrichosis are usually in the dermis or subcutaneous tissue. The periphery of the nodules is granulomatous and the center is suppurative. Surrounding skin shows exuberant pseudoepitheliomatous hyperplasia. Some yeasts are surrounded by an eosinophilic, spiculated zone and are termed "asteroid bodies" (Fig. 9-62B). The material surrounding the yeasts ("Splendore-Hoeppli substance") probably consists of antigen–antibody complexes.

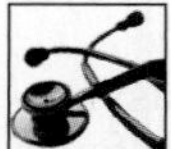

CLINICAL FEATURES: Cutaneous sporotrichosis begins as a solitary nodular lesion at the site of inoculation, typically on a hand, arm or leg. Weeks afterwards, additional nodules may appear along the lymphatic drainage of the primary lesion. Nodules often ulcerate and drain serosanguineous fluid. Joint involvement appears as pain and swelling of the affected joint, without involving overlying skin. Untreated cutaneous sporotrichosis continues to spread along the skin. The skin infection responds to systemic iodine therapy, but extracutaneous sporotrichosis requires systemic antifungal therapy.

Chromomycosis

Chromomycosis is a chronic skin infection caused by several species of fungi that live as saprophytes in soil and decaying vegetable matter. The fungi are brown, round, thick walled and 8 μm across and have been likened to "copper pennies" (Fig. 9-63). The infection is most common in barefooted agricultural workers in the tropics, in whom the fungus is implanted by trauma, usually below the knee. The lesions begin as papules and over the years become verrucous, crusted and sometimes ulcerated. The infection spreads by contiguous growth and through lymphatics and eventually may involve an entire limb.

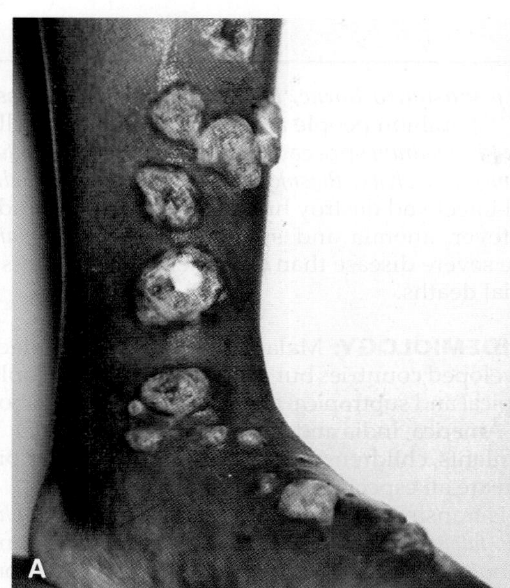

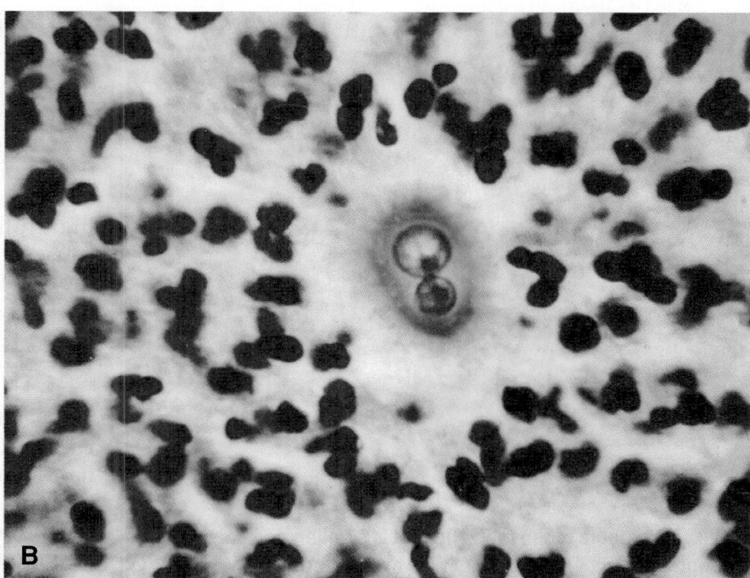

FIGURE 9-62. Sporotrichosis. A. The leg shows typical lymphocutaneous spread. **B.** A section of the lesion in (A) shows an asteroid body, composed of a pair of budding yeasts of *Sporothrix schenckii* surrounded by a layer of Splendore-Hoeppli substance, with radiating projections.

Dermatophyte Infections

Dermatophytes are fungi that cause localized superficial infections of keratinized tissues, including skin, hair and nails. There are about 40 species of dermatophytes in three genera: *Trichophyton, Microsporum* and *Epidermophyton*. ***Dermatophyte infections are minor illnesses, but are among the most common skin diseases for which medical help is sought.*** They are resident in soil, on animals and on humans. Most dermatophyte infections in temperate countries are acquired by direct contact with persons who have infected hairs or skin scales.

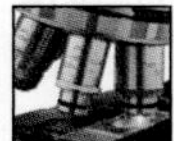

PATHOLOGY: Dermatophytes proliferate within the superficial keratinized tissues. They spread centrifugally from the initial site, producing round, expanding lesions with sharp margins. The appearance once suggested that a worm was responsible for the disease, hence the names **ringworm** and **tinea** (from the Latin *tinea*, "worm").

Dermatophyte infections produce thickening of the squamous epithelium, with increased numbers of keratinized cells. Lesions severe enough to be biopsied show a mild lymphocytic inflammatory infiltrate in the dermis. Hyphae and spores of the infecting dermatophytes are confined to the nonviable portions of skin, hair and nails.

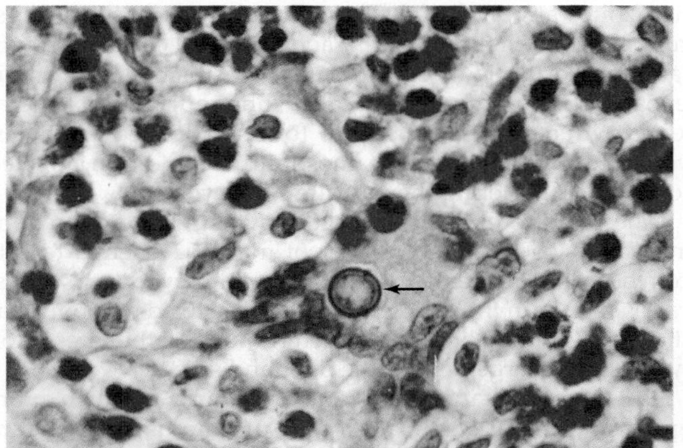

FIGURE 9-63. Chromomycosis. A section of skin shows a giant cell in the center, which contains a thick-walled, brown, sclerotic body (copper penny, *arrow*), representing the fungus.

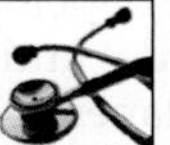

CLINICAL FEATURES: Dermatophyte infections are named according to the sites of involvement (e.g., scalp, tinea capitis; feet, tinea pedis, "athlete's foot"; nails, tinea unguium; intertriginous areas of the groin, tinea cruris, "jock itch"). These infections range from asymptomatic disease to chronic, fiercely pruritic eruptions and are treated with topical antifungal agents.

Mycetoma

A mycetoma is a slowly progressive, localized, and often disfiguring infection of the skin, soft tissues and bone produced by inoculation of various soil-dwelling fungi and filamentous bacteria. Responsible organisms include *Madurella mycetomatis, Petrilidium boydii, Actinomadura madurae and Nocardia brasiliensis*.

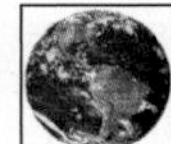

EPIDEMIOLOGY: Mycetoma usually occurs in the tropics among farmers and outdoor laborers whose skin is exposed to trauma. The foot is a common site of infection in locales where persons walk barefoot on soggy ground, and the disease is also known as **Madura foot.** Frequent immersion of the foot macerates the skin and facilitates deep inoculation with soil organisms.

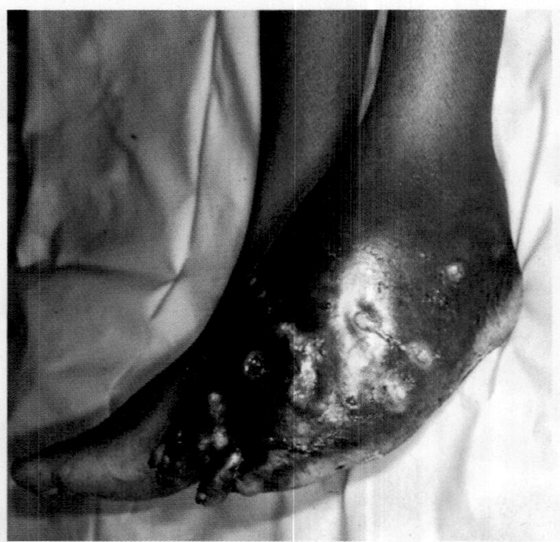

FIGURE 9-64. Mycetoma of the foot. The foot is swollen and painful and drains through the skin. The extremity was amputated.

PATHOLOGY: The organisms proliferate in the subcutis and spread to adjacent tissues, including bone. This incites a mixed suppurative and granulomatous inflammatory infiltrate that fails to eliminate the infecting organism. Surrounding granulation tissue and scarring produce progressive disfigurement of the affected sites.

A mycetoma begins as a solitary subcutaneous abscess and slowly expands to form multiple abscesses interconnected by sinus tracts (Fig. 9-64). Sinus tracts eventually drain to the skin surface. Abscesses contain colonies of compact bacteria or fungi surrounded by neutrophils and an outer layer of granulomatous inflammation. The colonies of organisms, called "grains," resemble the "sulfur granules" of actinomycosis.

CLINICAL FEATURES: A mycetoma initially manifests as a painless, localized swelling at a site of penetrating injury. The lesion slowly expands and produces sinus tracts that tend to follow fascial planes in their lateral and deep spread through connective tissue, muscle and bone. Treatment is usually wide excision of the affected area.

PROTOZOAL INFECTIONS

Protozoa are single-celled eukaryotes that fall into three general classes: **amebae, flagellates** and **sporozoites.** Amebae move by projection of cytoplasmic extensions termed **pseudopods.** Flagellates move through thread-like structures, flagella, which extend out from the cell membrane. Sporozoites do not have organelles of locomotion and also differ from amebae and flagellates in their mode of replication.

Protozoa cause human disease by diverse mechanisms. Some, such as *Entamoeba histolytica,* are extracellular parasites that digest and invade human tissues. Others, such as plasmodia, are obligate intracellular parasites that replicate in and kill human cells. Still others, such as trypanosomes, damage human tissue largely by inflammatory and immunologic responses they elicit. Some protozoa (e.g., *T. gondii*) can establish latent infections and cause reactivation disease in immunocompromised hosts.

Malaria

Malaria is a mosquito-borne, hemolytic, febrile illness. It affects over 200 million people and kills more than 1 million yearly. Four *Plasmodium* spp. cause malaria: *Plasmodium falciparum, Plasmodium vivax, Plasmodium ovale* and *Plasmodium malariae*. All infect and destroy human erythrocytes, producing chills, fever, anemia and splenomegaly. *P. falciparum* causes more severe disease than the others and accounts for most malarial deaths.

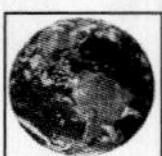

EPIDEMIOLOGY: Malaria has been eradicated in developed countries but continues to afflict people in tropical and subtropical areas, especially Africa, South and Central America, India and Southeast Asia (Fig. 9-65). The rural poor, infants, children, malnourished persons and pregnant women are all especially susceptible to infection.

Malaria is transmitted by the bite of the female *Anopheles* mosquito. *P. falciparum* and *P. vivax* are the most common pathogens, but there is considerable geographic variation in species distribution. *P. vivax* is rare in Africa, where much of the black population lacks the erythrocyte cell surface receptors required for infection. *P. falciparum* and *P. ovale* are the predominant species in Africa. *P. malariae* is the least common and mildest form of malaria, although it has a broad geographic distribution.

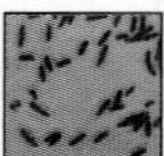

ETIOLOGIC FACTORS: The life cycle of the *Plasmodium* sp. responsible for human malaria requires both human and mosquito hosts (Fig. 9-66). Infected humans produce forms of the organism (gametocytes) that mosquitoes acquire upon feeding. Within these insects, the organism reproduces sexually, producing plasmodial forms (sporozoites), which the mosquito transmits to humans when it feeds.

The anopheline mosquito inoculates the sporozoites into a human's bloodstream. There, they undergo asexual division ("schizogony"). Circulating sporozoites rapidly invade hepatocytes and reproduce in the liver, yielding numerous daughter organisms, "merozoites" (exoerythrocytic phase). Within 2 to 3 weeks of hepatic infection, these rupture host hepatocytes exit into the bloodstream and invade erythrocytes.

Merozoites feed on hemoglobin, grow and reproduce inside erythrocytes. Within 2 to 4 days, mature progeny merozoites are produced. These daughter merozoites burst from infected erythrocytes, invade naïve red cells and so initiate another cycle of erythrocytic parasitism. This cycle is repeated many times. Eventually, subpopulations of merozoites differentiate into sexual forms called gametocytes, which are ingested when a mosquito feeds on an infected host, thus completing the parasite's life cycle.

The rupture of infected erythrocytes releases pyrogens and causes the chills and fever of malaria. Anemia results from both loss of circulating infected erythrocytes and sequestration of cells in the enlarging spleen. The fixed mononuclear phagocytes of the liver and spleen respond to the infestation by causing enlargement of the liver and spleen.

P. falciparum causes **malignant malaria,** a much more aggressive disease than the other plasmodia. It is distinguished from other malarial parasites in four respects:

- It has no secondary exoerythrocytic (hepatic) stage.
- It parasitizes erythrocytes of any age, causing marked parasitemia and anemia. In other types of malaria, only

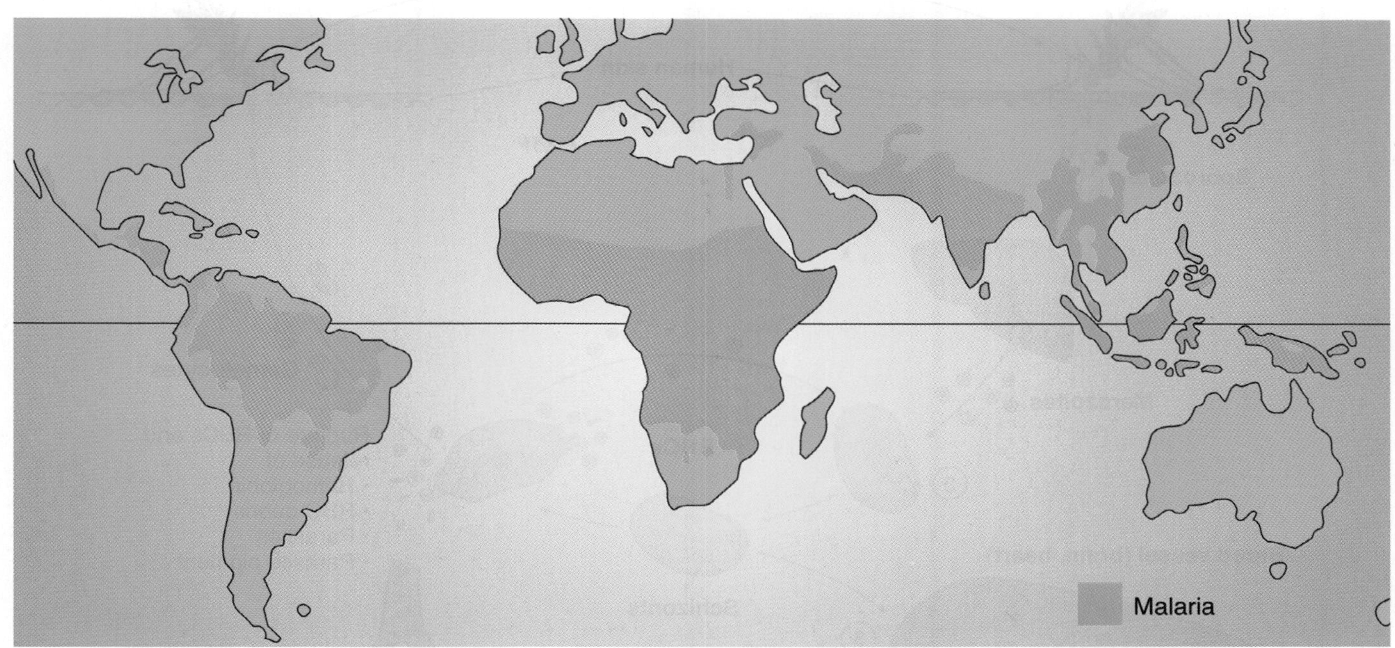

FIGURE 9-65. The geographic distribution of malaria.

subpopulations of erythrocytes (e.g., only young or old forms) are parasitized, leading to lower-level parasitemias and more modest anemias.

- There may be several parasites in a single red cell.
- *P. falciparum* alters flow characteristics and adhesive properties of infected erythrocytes, so they adhere to endothelial cells of small blood vessels. Obstruction of small blood vessels frequently produces severe tissue ischemia, which is probably the most important factor in the organism's virulence.

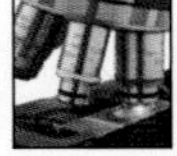

PATHOLOGY: All forms of malaria display hepatosplenomegaly as red blood cells are sequestered by fixed mononuclear phagocytes. The organs of this system (liver, spleen, lymph nodes) are darkened ("slate gray") by macrophages filled with hemosiderin and malarial pigment, the end-product of parasitic digestion of hemoglobin.

Adherence of infected red cells to microvascular endothelium in falciparum malaria has two consequences. First, parasitized erythrocytes attached to endothelial cells do not circulate, so patients with severe falciparum malaria have few circulating parasites. Second, capillaries of deep organs, especially the brain, become obstructed, leading to ischemia of the brain, kidneys and lungs. Brains of patients who die of cerebral malaria show congestion and thrombosis of small blood vessels in the white matter, which are rimmed with edema and hemorrhage ("ring hemorrhages") (Fig. 9-67). Obstruction of renal blood flow produces acute renal failure, whereas intravascular hemolysis leads to hemoglobinuric nephrosis **(blackwater fever).** In the lung, damage to alveolar capillaries produces pulmonary edema and acute alveolar damage.

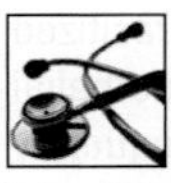

CLINICAL FEATURES: Malaria is characterized by recurrent **paroxysms** of chills and high fever. They begin with chills and sometimes headache, followed by a high, spiking fever with tachycardia, often accompanied by nausea, vomiting and abdominal pain. The high fever produces marked vasodilation and often associated orthostatic hypotension. The patient defervesces after several hours and is usually exhausted and drenched in sweat.

A period of 2 to 3 days follows, during which the patient feels well, only to be followed by a new paroxysm. Paroxysms recur for weeks, eventually subsiding as an immune response is mounted. Each paroxysm reflects the rupture of infected erythrocytes and release of daughter merozoites. As the mononuclear macrophage system responds to the infection, patients develop hepatosplenomegaly. Splenic enlargement can be dramatic. Indeed, some of the largest spleens on record are due to chronic malaria. Hypersplenism can exacerbate the anemia of malarial infection. *P. falciparum* infection produces a graver disease than do other plasmodia. As the level of parasitemia grows, fever may become virtually continuous. Ischemic brain injury causes symptoms from somnolence, hallucinations and behavioral changes to seizures and coma. CNS disease has a mortality of 20% to 50%.

Malaria is diagnosed by demonstrating the organisms on Giemsa-stained blood smears. The several species are distinguished by their appearance in infected erythrocytes. Malarias other than falciparum malaria are treated with oral chloroquine, sometimes with primaquine. Therapy for falciparum malaria varies, as widespread chloroquine resistance requires new treatments.

Babesiosis

Babesiosis is a malaria-like infection caused by protozoa of the genus *Babesia*, which is transmitted by hard-bodied ticks.

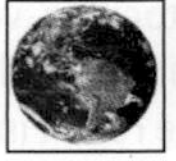

EPIDEMIOLOGY: *Babesia* infections are common in animals and in some locations are responsible for serious economic losses to the livestock industry. By contrast, human babesiosis is almost a medical curiosity, with

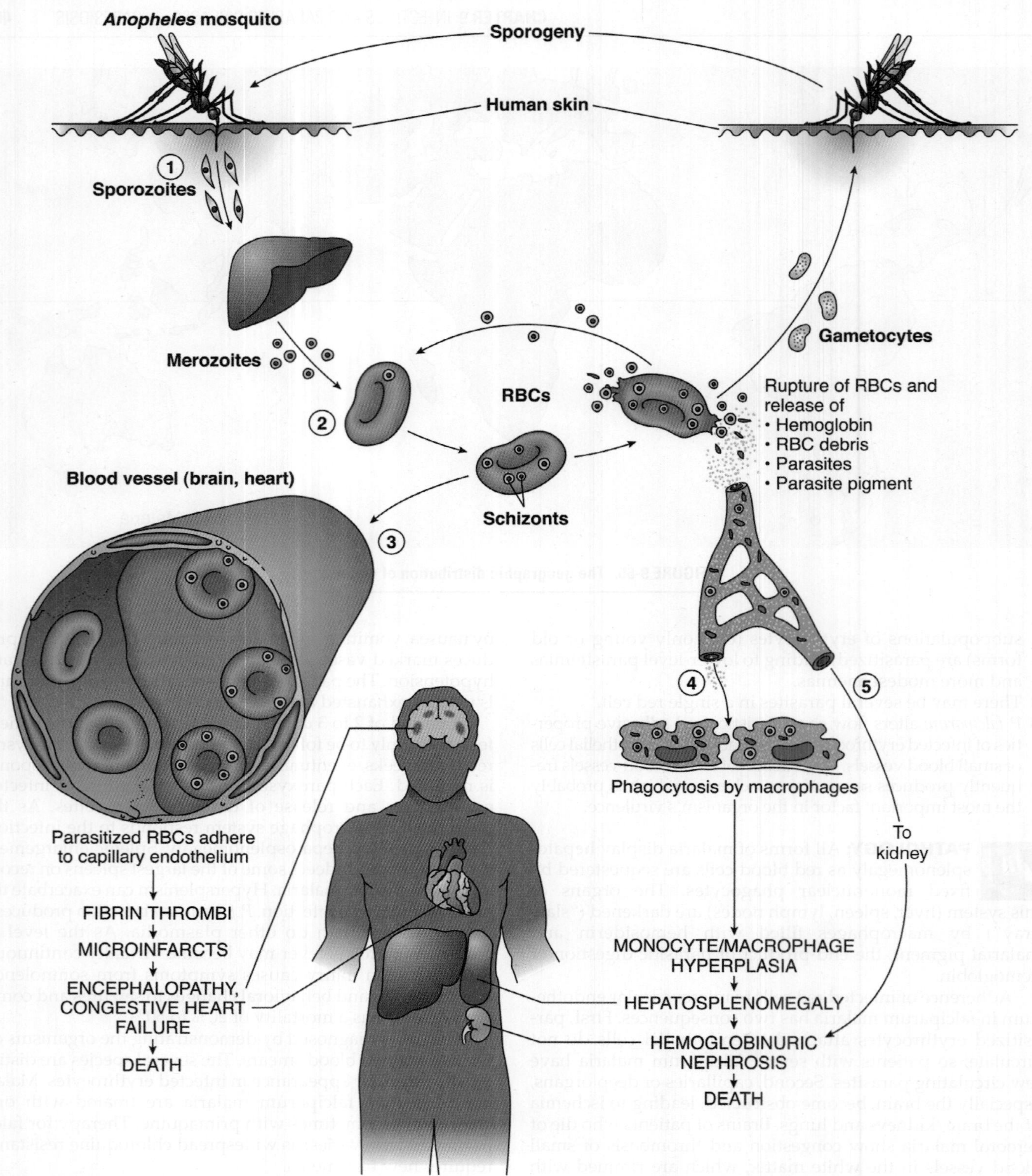

FIGURE 9-66. Life cycle of malaria. An *Anopheles* mosquito bites an infected person, taking blood that contains micro- and macrogametocytes (sexual forms). In the mosquito, sexual multiplication (sporogony) produces infective sporozoites in the salivary glands. **(1)** During the mosquito bite, sporozoites are inoculated into the bloodstream of the vertebrate host. Some sporozoites leave the blood and enter the hepatocytes, where they multiply asexually (exoerythrocytic schizogony) and form thousands of uninucleated merozoites. **(2)** Rupture of hepatocytes releases merozoites, which penetrate erythrocytes and become trophozoites, which then divide to form numerous schizonts (intraerythrocytic schizogony). Schizonts divide to form more merozoites, which are released on the rupture of erythrocytes and reenter other erythrocytes to begin a new cycle. After several cycles, subpopulations of merozoites develop into micro- and macrogametocytes, which are taken up by another mosquito to complete the cycle. **(3)** Parasitized erythrocytes obstruct capillaries of the brain, heart, kidney and other deep organs. Adherence of parasitized erythrocytes to capillary endothelial cells causes fibrin thrombi, which produce microinfarcts. These result in encephalopathy, congestive heart failure, pulmonary edema and frequently death. Ruptured erythrocytes release hemoglobin, erythrocyte debris and malarial pigment. **(4)** Phagocytosis leads to monocyte/macrophage hyperplasia and hepatosplenomegaly. **(5)** Released hemoglobin produces hemoglobinuric nephrosis, which may be fatal. RBCs = red blood cells.

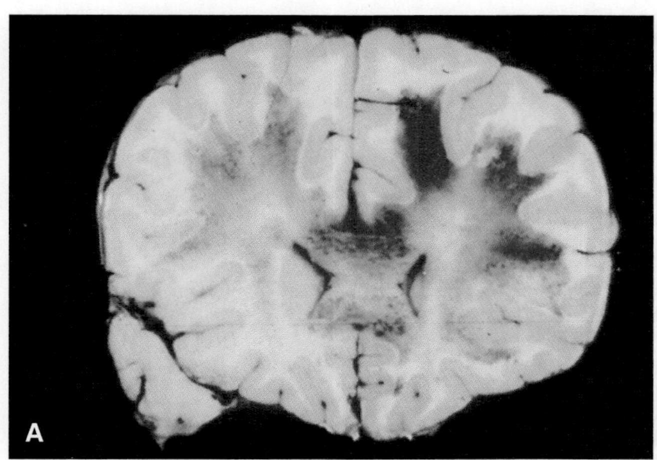

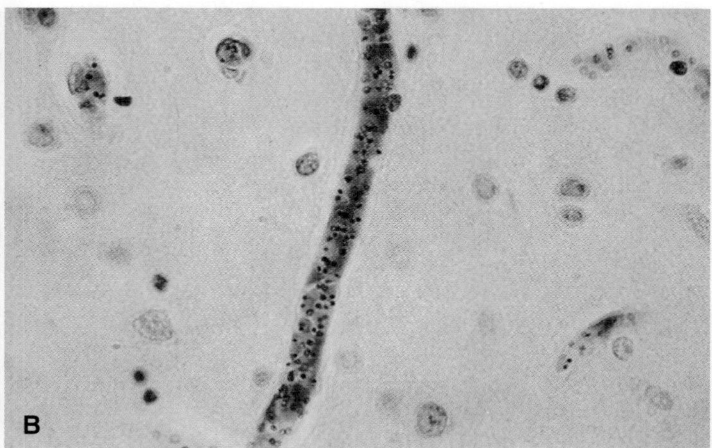

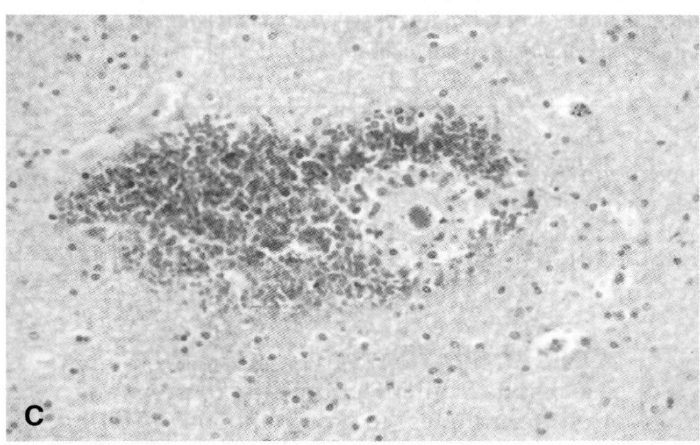

FIGURE 9-67. Acute falciparum malaria of the brain. A. There is severe diffuse congestion of the white matter and focal hemorrhages. **B.** A section of (A) shows a capillary packed with parasitized erythrocytes. **C.** Another section of (A) displays a ring hemorrhage around a thrombosed capillary, which contains parasitized erythrocytes in a fibrin thrombus.

the parasites infecting humans only when people intrude into the zoonotic cycle between the tick vector and its vertebrate host. Human babesiosis is reported only in Europe and North America. Infections in the United States have been concentrated in islands off the New England coast. The organisms invade and destroy erythrocytes, causing hemoglobinemia, hemoglobinuria and renal failure. The disease is usually self-limited, but uncontrolled infections can be fatal. *Babesia* spp. are resistant to most antiprotozoal drugs.

Toxoplasmosis

Toxoplasmosis is a worldwide infectious disease caused by a protozoan, *T. gondii.* Most infections are asymptomatic, but if they occur in a fetus or immunocompromised host, devastating necrotizing disease may result.

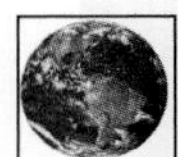 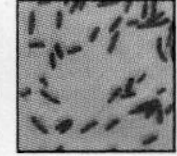

EPIDEMIOLOGY AND ETIOLOGIC FACTORS: In some areas (e.g., France), the prevalence of *T. gondii* infection exceeds 80% of adults; in other regions (e.g., the southwestern United States), few people are affected. *T. gondii* infects many mammals and birds as intermediate hosts. The only final host is the cat, which becomes infected by ingesting toxoplasma cysts in tissues of an infected mouse or other intermediate host. In the cat's intestinal epithelium, five multiplicative stages end with shedding of oocysts. Oocysts sporulate in feces and soil and differentiate into sporocysts, which contain sporozoites. These are ingested by intermediate hosts, such as birds, mice or humans, and develop in the intermediate host to complete the life cycle.

T. gondii has two stages in tissue, tachyzoites and bradyzoites, both crescent shaped and 2×6 μm. In acute infection, tachyzoites multiply rapidly to form "groups" within intracellular vacuoles of parasitized cells, eventually causing the cells to rupture. Tachyzoites spread from the gut through lymphatics to regional lymph nodes, and through the blood to the liver, lungs, heart, brain and other organs. During chronic infection, the organisms, now called "bradyzoites," multiply slowly. The bradyzoites store PAS-positive material and hundreds of organisms are tightly packed in "cysts," which originate in intracellular vacuoles, enlarge beyond the usual size of the cell and push the nucleus to the periphery.

Except for congenital infection, toxoplasmosis is acquired by eating infectious forms of the organism. In the tropics, where infection is generally acquired in childhood, oocysts in contaminated soil are the main source of infection. In developed countries, the major mechanism of infection is eating incompletely cooked meat (lamb and pork) that carries *Toxoplasma* tissue cysts. Another source of infection is cat feces: oocysts contaminate the hands and food of people who live in close proximity to cats. **Congenital infection** is acquired by transplacental transmission of infectious forms from an acutely infected (usually asymptomatic) mother to the fetus.

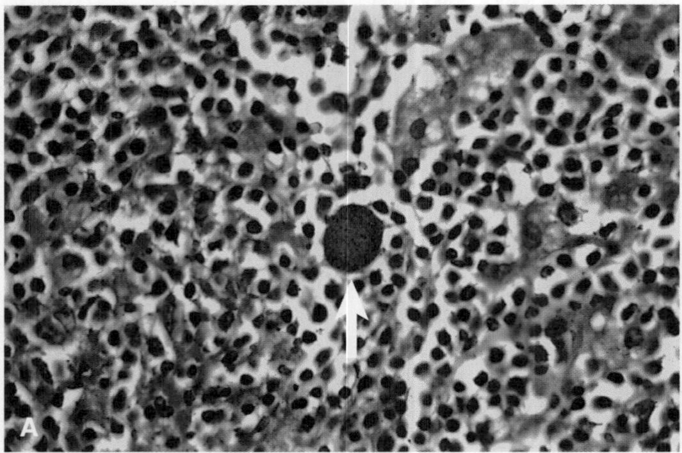

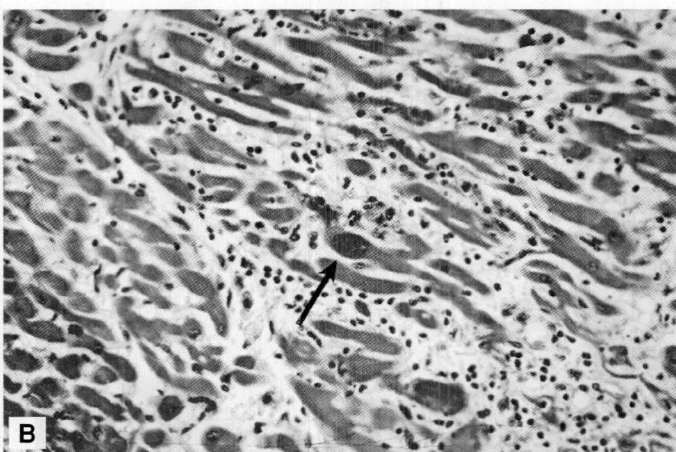

FIGURE 9-68. Toxoplasmosis. A. A photomicrograph of an enlarged lymph node reveals bradyzoites of *Toxoplasma gondii* within a cyst (*arrow*). **B.** A section of heart shows a cyst of bradyzoites of *T. gondii* within a myofiber (*arrow*), with edema and inflammatory cells in the adjacent tissue.

The active infection is usually terminated by the development of cell-mediated immune responses. In most *T. gondii* infections, little significant tissue destruction occurs before the immune response brings the active phase of the infection under control, and those infected suffer few clinical effects. *T. gondii* establishes latent infection, however, by forming dormant tissue cysts in some infected cells. These survive for decades in host cells. If an infected person loses cell-mediated immunity, the organism can emerge from its encysted form and reestablish a destructive infection.

Toxoplasma Lymphadenopathy Occurs in Immunocompetent Persons

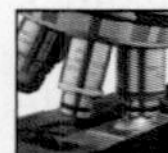

PATHOLOGY: The most common manifestation of *T. gondii* infection in immunocompetent hosts is lymphadenopathy (see Chapter 20). Virtually any lymph node group may be involved, but enlarged cervical nodes are most readily apparent. The histology of affected lymph nodes is distinctive, with numerous epithelioid macrophages surrounding and encroaching on reactive germinal centers.

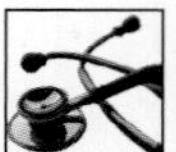

CLINICAL FEATURES: In *Toxoplasma* lymphadenitis (Fig. 9-68A), patients present with nontender regional lymph node enlargement, sometimes accompanied by fever, sore throat, hepatosplenomegaly and circulating atypical lymphocytes. Hepatitis, myocarditis (Fig. 9-68B) and myositis have been documented. Lymphadenopathy usually resolves spontaneously in several weeks to several months and therapy is seldom required.

Congenital *Toxoplasma* Infections Principally Affect the Brain

T. gondii infection in a fetus is far more destructive than is postnatal infection (see Chapter 6).

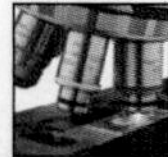

PATHOLOGY: The fetus lacks the immunologic capacity to contain the infection. The developing brain and eye are readily infected, leading to a necrotizing meningoencephalitis, which in the most severe cases leads to loss of brain parenchyma, cerebral calcifications (Fig. 9-69) and marked hydrocephalus. Ocular infection causes chorioretinitis (i.e., necrosis and inflammation of the choroid and retina).

CLINICAL FEATURES: The most severe fetal disease results from infection early in pregnancy and often terminates in spontaneous abortion. In infants born with congenital toxoplasmosis, the effects of brain involvement range from severe mental retardation and seizures to subtle psychomotor defects. Ocular involvement may cause congenital visual impairment. Latent ocular infection established in utero may recrudesce later in life to produce visual loss. Some newborns have *Toxoplasma* hepatitis, with large areas of necrosis and giant cells. Adrenal necrosis is also occasionally observed. Congenital toxoplasmosis requires therapy with antiprotozoal agents.

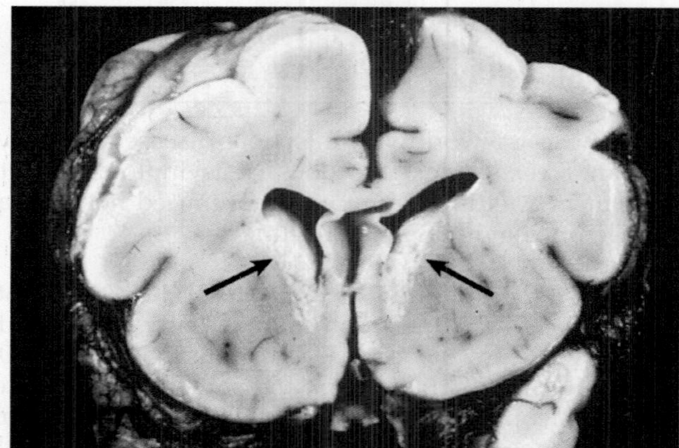

FIGURE 9-69. Congenital toxoplasmosis. The brain of a premature infant reveals subependymal necrosis with calcification appearing as bilaterally symmetric areas of whitish discoloration (*arrows*).

Toxoplasmosis in Immunocompromised Hosts Produces Encephalitis

Devastating *T. gondii* infections occur in people with impaired cell-mediated immunity (e.g., patients with AIDS or receiving immunosuppressive therapy). In most cases, the disease reflects reactivation of a latent infection. The brain is most commonly affected, and infection with *T. gondii* produces a multifocal necrotizing encephalitis. Patients with encephalitis present with paresis, seizures, alterations in visual acuity and changes in mentation. *Toxoplasma* encephalitis in immunocompromised patients is fatal if not treated with effective antiprotozoal agents.

Amebiasis

Amebiasis is infection with *Entamoeba histolytica*, which principally involves the colon and occasionally the liver. *E. histolytica* is named for its lytic actions on tissue. Intestinal infection ranges from asymptomatic colonization to severe invasive infection with bloody diarrhea. On occasion, parasites spread beyond the colon to involve other organs. The most common site of extraintestinal disease is the liver, where *E. histolytica* causes slowly expanding, necrotizing abscesses.

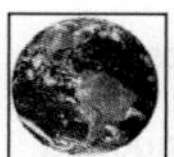

EPIDEMIOLOGY: Humans are the only known reservoir for *E. histolytica,* which reproduces in the colon and passes in the feces. Although amebiasis is found worldwide, it is more common and more severe in tropical and subtropical areas, where poor sanitation prevails. ***Amebiasis is acquired by ingestion of materials contaminated with human feces.***

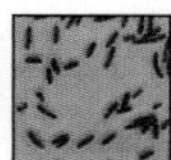

ETIOLOGIC FACTORS: *E. histolytica* has three distinct stages: the trophozoite, the precyst and the cyst.

Amebic trophozoites, 10 to 60 μm across, are found in stools of patients with acute symptoms. They are spherical or oval and have a thin cell membrane, a single nucleus, condensed chromatin on the interior of the nuclear membrane and a central karyosome. The trophozoites sometimes contain phagocytosed erythrocytes. PAS stains the cytoplasm of the trophozoites and makes them stand out in tissue sections. In the colon, trophozoites develop into cysts through an intermediate form termed the **precyst,** during which process trophozoites stop feeding, become round and nonmotile, lose some digestive vacuoles and form glycogen masses and chromatoidal bodies.

Amebic cysts are the infecting stage and are found only in stools, since they do not invade tissue. They are spherical, have thick walls, measure 5 to 25 μm across and usually have four nuclei. From the stools, the cysts contaminate water, food or fingers (Fig. 9-70). On ingestion, cysts traverse the stomach and excyst in the lower ileum. A metacystic ameba containing four nuclei divides to form four small, immature trophozoites, which then grow to full size. These thrive in the colon and feed on bacteria and human cells. They may colonize any part of the large bowel, but the cecum is most affected. Patients with symptomatic amebic colitis pass both cysts and trophozoites. The latter survive only briefly outside the body and are also destroyed by gastric secretions. Host factors, such as nutritional status, coexistent colonic flora and immunologic status, also affect the course of *E. histolytica* infection. Invasion begins with attachment of a trophozoite to a colonic epithelial cell. The organism kills target cells by elaborating a lytic protein that breaches the cell membrane. Progressive death of mucosal cells produces a superficial ulcer.

Intestinal Amebiasis Is an Ulcerating Disease of the Colon

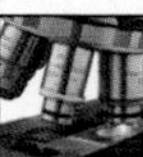

PATHOLOGY: Amebic lesions begin as small foci of necrosis that progress to ulcers (Fig. 9-71A). Undermining of the ulcer margin and confluence of expanding ulcers lead to irregular sloughing of the mucosa. The ulcer bed is gray and necrotic, with fibrin and cellular debris. The exudate raises the undermined mucosa, producing chronic amebic ulcers whose shape has been described as resembling a flask or a bottle neck.

Trophozoites are found on the ulcer surface, in the exudate and in the crater (Fig. 9-71B). They are also frequent in the submucosa, muscularis propria, serosa and small veins of the submucosa. There is little inflammatory response in early amebic ulcers. However, as the ulcers enlarge, acute and chronic inflammatory cells accumulate.

An **ameboma** is an infrequent complication of amebiasis, occurring when amebae invade through the intestinal wall. It is an inflammatory thickening of the bowel wall that resembles colon cancer and tends to form a "napkin-ring constriction." It consists of granulation tissue, fibrosis and clusters of trophozoites.

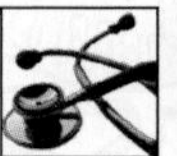

CLINICAL FEATURES: Intestinal amebiasis ranges from completely asymptomatic to a severe dysenteric disease. The incubation period for acute amebic colitis is 8 to 10 days. Gradually increasing abdominal discomfort, tenderness and cramps are accompanied by chills and fever. Nausea, vomiting, malodorous flatus and intermittent constipation are typical features. Liquid stools (up to 25 a day) contain bloody mucus, but diarrhea is rarely prolonged enough to cause dehydration. Amebic colitis often persists for months or years and patients may become emaciated and anemic. Clinical features may be bizarre and sometimes must be differentiated from those of appendicitis, cholecystitis, intestinal obstruction or diverticulitis. In severe amebic colitis, massive destruction of colonic mucosa may lead to fatal hemorrhage, perforation or peritonitis. Therapy for intestinal amebiasis includes metronidazole, which acts against trophozoites, and diloxanide, which is effective against cysts.

Amebic Liver Abscess Is a Major Complication of Intestinal Amebiasis

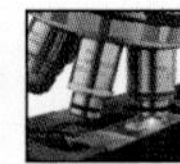

PATHOLOGY: *E. histolytica* trophozoites that have invaded submucosal veins of the colon enter the portal circulation and reach the liver. Here the organisms kill hepatocytes, producing a slowly expanding necrotic cavity, filled with a dark brown, odorless, semisolid material, reported to resemble "anchovy paste" in color and consistency (Fig. 9-72). Neutrophils are rare within the cavity and trophozoites are found along the edges adjacent to hepatocytes.

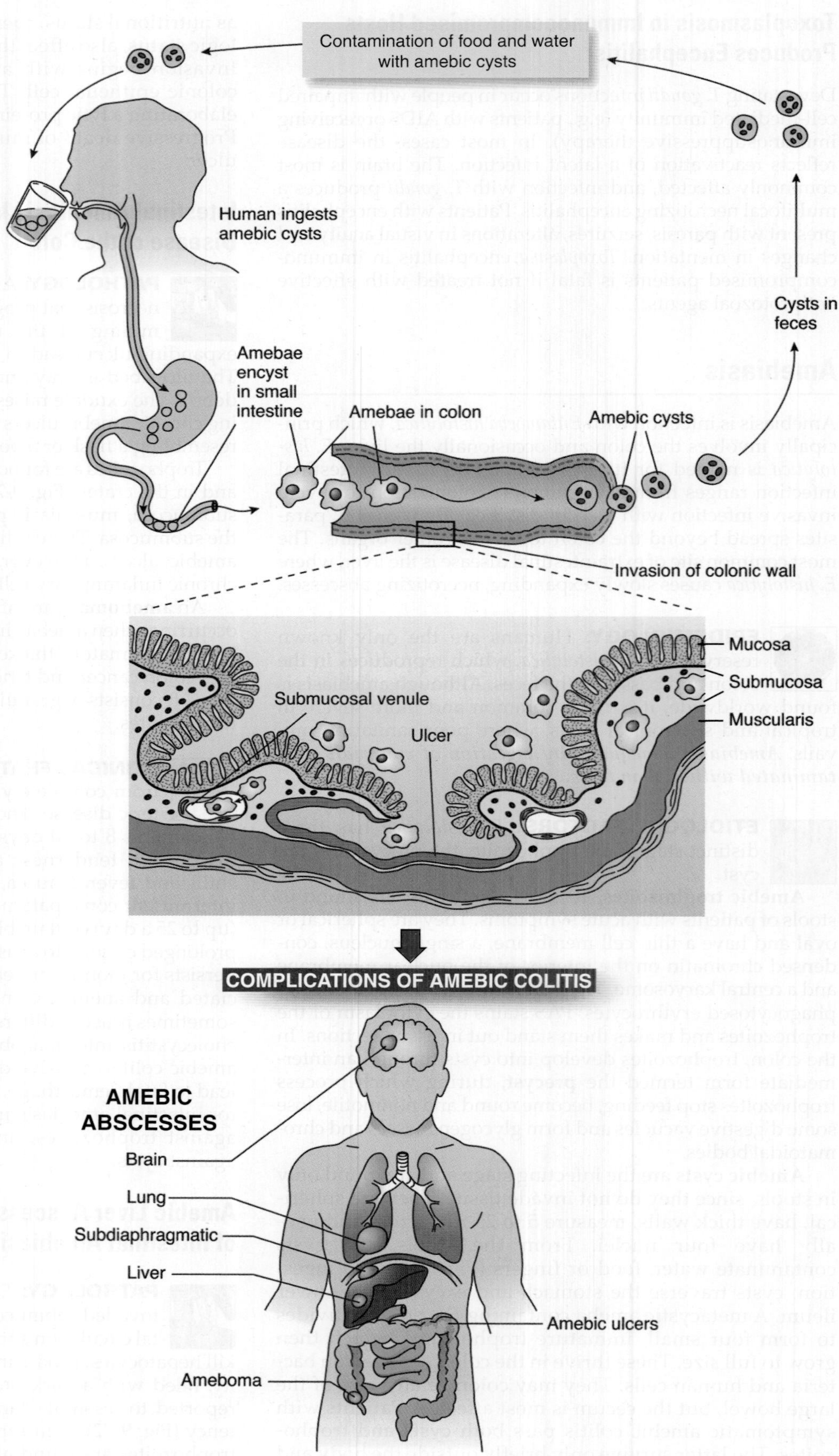

FIGURE 9-70. Amebic colitis and its complications. Amebiasis results from the ingestion of food or water contaminated with amebic cysts. In the colon, the amebae penetrate the mucosa and produce flask-shaped ulcers of the mucosa and submucosa. The organisms may invade submucosal venules, thereby disseminating the infection to the liver and other organs. The liver abscess can expand to involve adjacent structures.

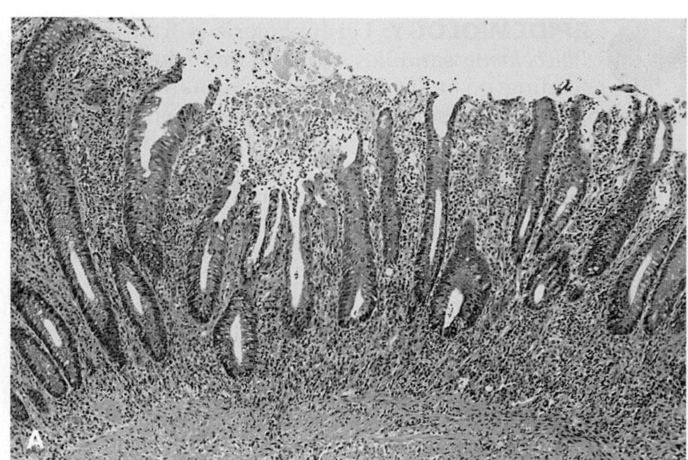

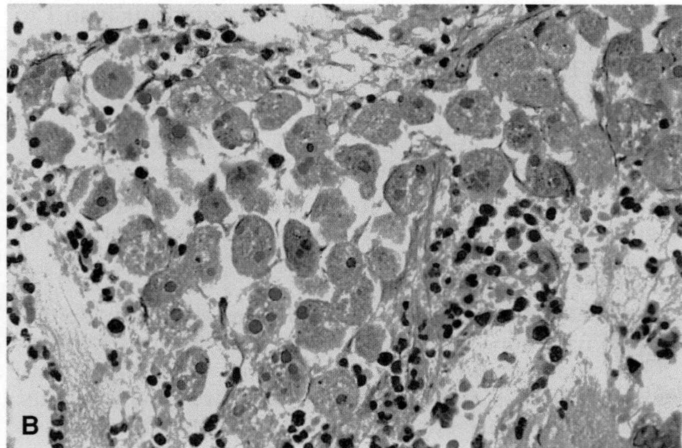

FIGURE 9-71. Intestinal amebiasis. A. The colonic mucosa shows superficial ulceration beneath a cluster of trophozoites of *Entamoeba histolytica*. The lamina propria contains excess acute and chronic inflammatory cells, including eosinophils. **B.** Higher-power view shows numerous trophozoites in the luminal exudate.

Amebic liver abscesses may expand, rupture through the capsule and extend into the peritoneum, diaphragm, pleural cavity, lungs or pericardium. Rarely, a liver abscess, or even a lesion in the colon, may spread amebae to the brain by a hematogenous route to form large necrotic lesions.

CLINICAL FEATURES: Patients with amebic liver abscess present with severe right upper quadrant pain, low-grade fever and weight loss. Only a minority of patients give a history of an antecedent diarrheal illness and *E. histolytica* is demonstrated in the feces of less than one third of patients with extraintestinal disease. The diagnosis is usually made by radiologic or ultrasound demonstration of the abscess, in conjunction with serologic testing for antibodies to *E. histolytica*. Amebic abscess is treated by percutaneous or surgical drainage and antiamebic drugs.

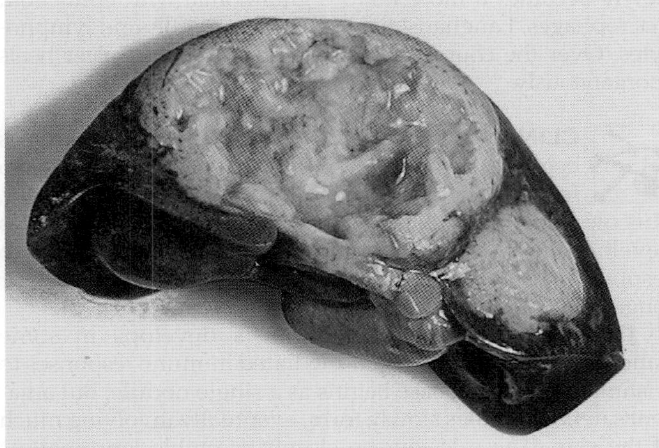

FIGURE 9-72. Amebic abscesses of the liver. The cut surface of the liver shows multiple abscesses containing "anchovy paste" material.

Cryptosporidiosis

Cryptosporidiosis is an enteric infection with protozoa of the genus *Cryptosporidium* that cause diarrhea in persons with compromised immunity. The infection varies from a self-limited gastrointestinal infection to a potentially life-threatening illness. It is acquired by ingesting *Cryptosporidium* oocysts, which are shed in feces of infected humans and animals. Most infections probably result from person-to-person transmission, but many domesticated animals harbor the parasite and are a reservoir for human infection.

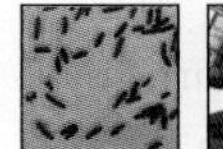
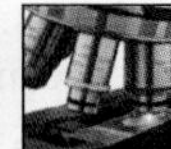

ETIOLOGIC FACTORS AND PATHOLOGY: *Cryptosporidium* oocysts survive passage through the stomach and release forms that attach to the microvillous surface of the small bowel. Unlike *Toxoplasma* and other coccidia, *Cryptosporidia* remain extracellular. They reproduce on the luminal surface of the gut, from stomach to rectum, forming progeny that also attach to the epithelium.

In immunocompetent people, infection is terminated by unknown immune responses. Patients with AIDS and some congenital immunodeficiencies cannot contain the parasite and develop chronic infections, which may spread from the bowel to involve the gallbladder and intrahepatic bile ducts.

Cryptosporidiosis produces no grossly visible alterations. The organisms are visible microscopically as round, 2- to 4-μm blebs attached to the luminal surface of the epithelium. In the small intestine, there may be moderate or severe chronic inflammation in the lamina propria and some villous atrophy directly related to the density of the parasites. The colon has a chronic active colitis, with minimal architectural disruption.

CLINICAL FEATURES: Cryptosporidiosis presents as a profuse, watery diarrhea, sometimes accompanied by cramping abdominal pain or low-grade fever. Extraordinary volumes of fluid can be lost as diarrhea and intensive fluid replacement is required. In immunologically competent patients, diarrhea resolves spontaneously in 1 to 2 weeks. In immunocompromised patients, diarrhea persists indefinitely and may contribute to death.

Giardiasis

Giardiasis is an infection of the small intestine caused by the flagellated protozoan *Giardia lamblia* and characterized by abdominal cramping and diarrhea.

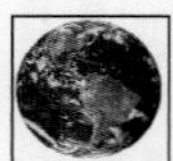

EPIDEMIOLOGY: *G. lamblia* has a worldwide distribution, with a prevalence of infection from less than 1% to more than 25% in some areas with warmer climates and crowded, unsanitary environments. Children are more susceptible than adults. Giardiasis is acquired by ingesting infectious cyst forms of the organism, which are shed in the feces of infected humans and animals. Infection spreads directly from person to person and also in contaminated water or food. *Giardia* can be acquired from wilderness water sources, where infected animals, such as beavers and bears, serve as the reservoir of infection. Infection may be epidemic, and outbreaks have occurred in orphanages and institutions.

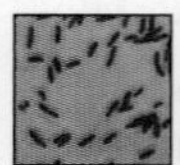
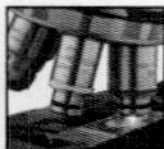

ETIOLOGIC FACTORS AND PATHOLOGY: *G. lamblia* has two stages: trophozoites and cysts. The former are flat, pear-shaped, binucleate organisms with four pairs of flagella. They are most numerous in the duodenum and proximal small intestine. A curved, disk-like "sucker plate" on their ventral surface aids mucosal attachment. Ingested cysts contain two or four nuclei and revert to trophozoites on reaching the intestine. The stools usually contain only cysts, but trophozoites may also be present in patients with diarrhea.

Giardia cysts survive gastric acidity and rupture in the duodenum and jejunum to release trophozoites. These attach to small-bowel epithelial microvilli and reproduce. Giardiasis produces no grossly visible alterations. Microscopic examination shows minimal associated mucosal changes, with *Giardia* trophozoites on villous surfaces and within crypts.

CLINICAL FEATURES: *G. lamblia* is usually a harmless commensal, but can cause acute or chronic symptoms. Acute giardiasis occurs with abrupt onset of abdominal cramping and frequent, foul-smelling stools. The infection is highly variable. In some patients, symptoms resolve spontaneously in 1 to 4 weeks. Others complain of persistent abdominal cramping and poorly formed stools for months. In children, chronic giardiasis may cause malabsorption, weight loss and retarded growth. The infection is treated effectively with various antibiotics, including metronidazole.

Leishmaniasis

Leishmaniae are protozoans that are transmitted to humans by insect bites and cause a spectrum of clinical syndromes from indolent, self-resolving cutaneous ulcers to fatal disseminated disease. There are numerous *Leishmania* spp., which differ in their natural habitats and the types of disease that they produce.

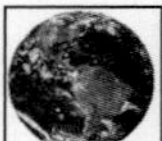

EPIDEMIOLOGY: Leishmaniasis is transmitted by *Phlebotomus* sandflies, which acquire the infection by feeding on infected animals. In many subtropical and tropical areas, leishmanial infection is endemic in animal populations: dogs, ground squirrels, foxes and jackals are reservoirs and potential sources for transmission to humans. It is mainly a disease of less-developed countries where humans live in close proximity to animal hosts and the fly vector. There are estimated to be 20 million persons infected worldwide.

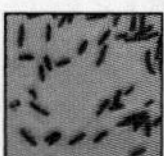

ETIOLOGIC FACTORS: Infection begins when the organisms are inoculated into human skin by a sandfly bite. Shortly thereafter, leishmaniae are phagocytosed by mononuclear phagocytes and transformed into amastigotes, which reproduce within the macrophage. Daughter amastigotes eventually rupture from the cell and spread to other macrophages. Reproduction continues in this way and eventually a cluster of infected macrophages forms at the site of inoculation.

From this initial local infection, the disease may take widely divergent courses depending on two factors: the immunologic status of the host and the infecting species of *Leishmania*. Three distinct clinical entities are recognized: (1) localized cutaneous leishmaniasis, (2) mucocutaneous leishmaniasis and (3) visceral leishmaniasis.

Localized Cutaneous Leishmaniasis Is an Ulcerating Disorder

Several *Leishmania* spp. in Central and South America, Northern Africa, the Middle East, India and China cause a localized skin disease, also known as "oriental sore" or "tropical sore."

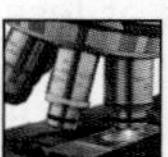

PATHOLOGY: Localized cutaneous leishmaniasis begins as a collection of amastigote-filled macrophages that ulcerates the overlying epidermis. In tissue sections, the oval amastigotes measure 2 μm and contain two internal structures, a nucleus and a kinetoplast. Under low power, amastigotes in macrophages appear as multiple regular cytoplasmic dots, **Leishman-Donovan bodies.** With progressive development of cell-mediated immunity, macrophages are activated and kill the intracellular parasites. The lesion slowly becomes a more mature granuloma, with epithelioid macrophages, Langhans giant cells, plasma cells and lymphocytes. Over the course of months, the cutaneous ulcer heals spontaneously.

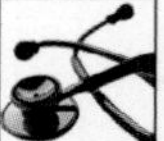

CLINICAL FEATURES: Cutaneous leishmaniasis begins as an itching, solitary papule, which erodes to form a shallow ulcer with a sharp, raised border. This ulcer can grow to 6 to 8 cm in diameter. Satellite lesions develop along draining lymphatics. The ulcers begin to resolve at 3 to 6 months, but healing may take a year or longer.

Diffuse cutaneous leishmaniasis develops in some patients who lack specific cell-mediated immune responses to leishmaniae. The disease begins as a single nodule, but adjacent satellite nodules slowly form, eventually involving much of the skin. These lesions so closely resemble lepromatous leprosy that some patients have been cared for in leprosaria. The nodule of anergic leishmaniasis is caused by enormous numbers of macrophages replete with leishmaniae.

Mucocutaneous Leishmaniasis Is a Late Complication of Cutaneous Leishmaniasis

Mucocutaneous leishmaniasis is caused by infection with *Leishmania braziliensis*. Most cases occur in Central and South America, where rodents and sloths are reservoirs.

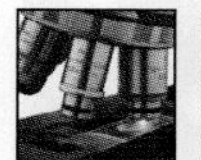
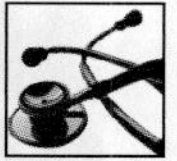

PATHOLOGY AND CLINICAL FEATURES: The early course and pathologic changes of mucocutaneous leishmaniasis are like those of localized cutaneous leishmaniasis. A solitary ulcer appears, expands and resolves. Years afterward, an ulcer develops at a mucocutaneous junction, such as the larynx, nasal septum, anus or vulva. The mucosal lesion progresses slowly, is highly destructive and disfiguring and erodes mucosal surfaces and cartilage. Destruction of the nasal septum sometimes produces a "tapir nose" deformity. The patient may die if the ulcers obstruct the airways. Mucocutaneous leishmaniasis requires treatment with systemic antiprotozoal agents.

Visceral Leishmaniasis (Kala Azar) Is a Potentially Fatal Infection of the Monocyte/Macrophage System

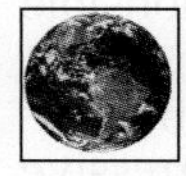

EPIDEMIOLOGY: Kala azar is produced by several subspecies of *Leishmania donovani*. Reservoirs of the agent and susceptible age groups vary in different parts of the world. Humans are the reservoir in India, and foxes in, for instance, southern France and central Italy. Other canine and rodent species are reservoirs elsewhere in the world.

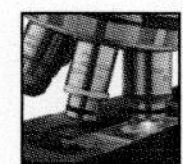

PATHOLOGY: Infection with *L. donovani* begins with localized collections of infected macrophages at the site of a sandfly bite (Fig. 9-73); these spread the organisms throughout the mononuclear phagocyte system. *L. donovani* are mostly destroyed by cell-mediated immune responses, but 5% of patients develop visceral leishmaniasis. Children and malnourished people are especially susceptible. The liver (Fig. 9-74A), spleen and lymph nodes become massively enlarged, as macrophages in these organs fill with proliferating leishmanial amastigotes. Normal organ architecture is gradually replaced by sheets of parasitized macrophages (Fig. 9-74B). Eventually, these cells accumulate in other organs, including the heart and kidney.

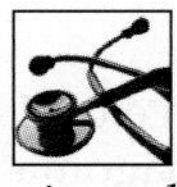

CLINICAL FEATURES: Patients with visceral leishmaniasis have persistent fever, progressive weight loss, hepatosplenomegaly, anemia, thrombocytopenia and leukopenia. Light-skinned persons develop darkening of the skin; the Hindi name for leishmaniasis, *kala azar,* means "black sickness." Over the course of months, a patient with visceral leishmaniasis becomes profoundly cachectic with massive splenomegaly. The untreated disease is invariably fatal. Treatment entails systemic antiprotozoal therapy.

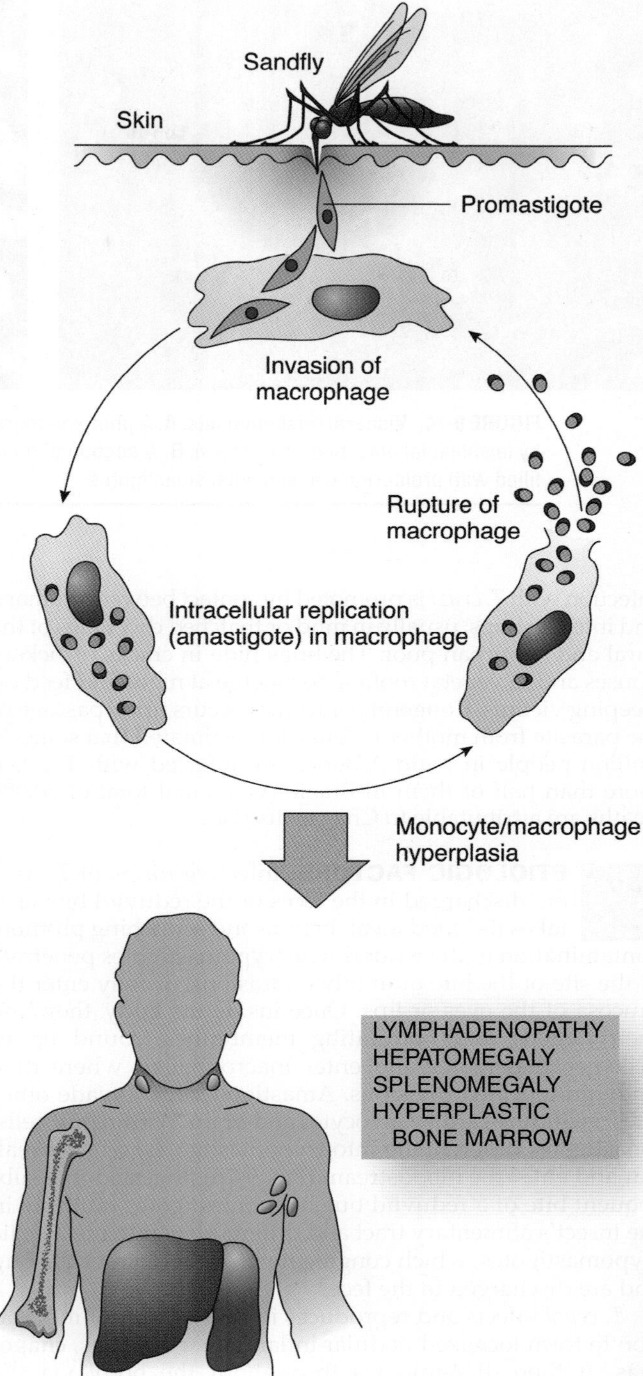

FIGURE 9-73. Leishmaniasis. Blood-sucking sandflies ingest amastigotes from an infected host. These are transformed in the sandfly gut into promastigotes, which multiply and are injected into the next vertebrate host. There they invade macrophages, revert to the amastigote form and multiply, eventually rupturing the cell. They then invade other macrophages, thus completing the cycle.

Chagas Disease (American Trypanosomiasis)

Chagas disease is an insect-borne, zoonotic infection by the protozoan *Trypanosoma cruzi*, which causes a systemic infection of humans. Acute manifestations and long-term sequelae occur in the heart and gastrointestinal tract.

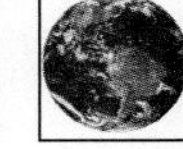

EPIDEMIOLOGY: *T. cruzi* infection is endemic in wild and domesticated animals (e.g., rats, dogs, goats, cats, armadillos) in Central and South America, where it is transmitted by the reduviid ("kissing") bug.

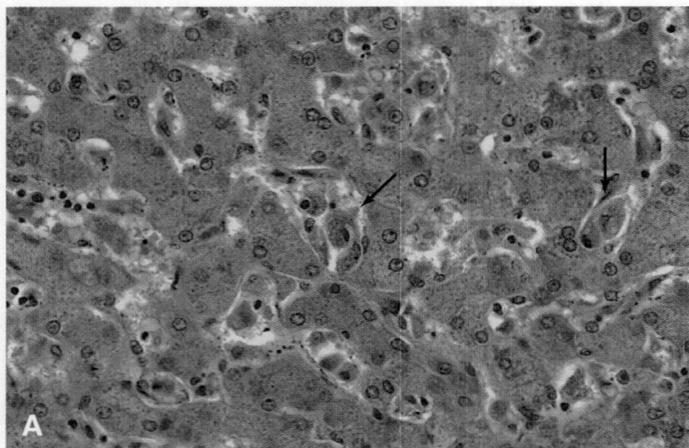

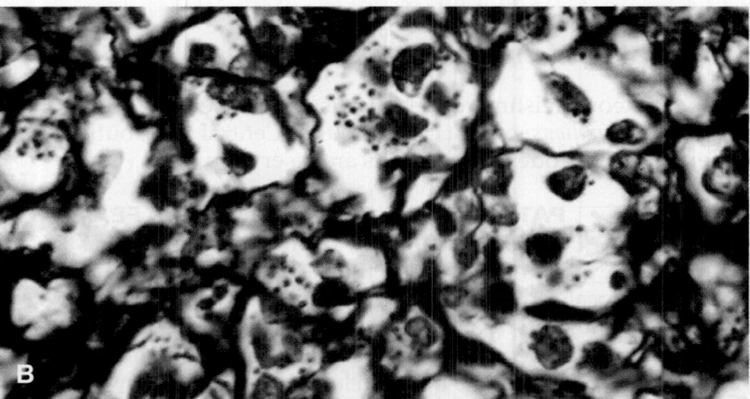

FIGURE 9-74. Visceral leishmaniasis. A. A photomicrograph of an enlarged liver shows prominent Kupffer cells distended by leishmanial amastigotes (*arrows*). **B.** A section of bone marrow subjected to silver impregnation shows macrophages filled with proliferating leishmanial amastigotes.

Infection with *T. cruzi* is promoted by contact between humans and infected bugs, usually in mud or thatched dwellings of the rural and suburban poor. The bugs hide in cracks of rickety houses and in vegetal roofing, to emerge at night and feed on sleeping victims. Congenital infection occurs upon passage of the parasite from mother to fetus. It is estimated that some 20 million people in Latin America are infected with *T. cruzi,* more than half of them in Brazil. An annual total of 50,000 deaths are attributable to Chagas disease.

ETIOLOGIC FACTORS: Infective forms of *T. cruzi* are discharged in the feces of the reduviid bug as it takes its blood meal. Itching and scratching promote contamination of the wound. The trypomastigotes penetrate at the site of the bite or at other abrasions, or may enter the mucosa of the eyes or lips. Once inside the body, they lose their flagella and undulating membranes, round up to become amastigotes and enter macrophages, where they undergo repeated divisions. Amastigotes also invade other sites, including cardiac myocytes and brain. Within host cells, amastigotes differentiate into trypomastigotes, which break out and enter the bloodstream (Fig. 9-75). Ingested in a subsequent bite of a reduviid bug, trypomastigotes multiply in the insect's alimentary tract and differentiate into metacyclic trypomastigotes, which congregate in the rectum of the bug and are discharged in the feces.

T. cruzi infects and reproduces in cells at sites of inoculation to form localized nodular inflammatory lesions, **chagomas.** It then disseminates throughout the body via the bloodstream. Strains of *T. cruzi* differ in their predominant target cells; infections of cardiac myocytes, gastrointestinal ganglion cells and meninges cause the most significant disease. Parasitemia and widespread cellular infection are responsible for the systemic symptoms of acute Chagas disease. The onset of cell-mediated immunity eliminates the acute manifestations, but chronic tissue damage may continue. Progressive destruction of cells at sites of infection—particularly the heart, esophagus and colon—causes organ dysfunction, manifested decades after the acute infection.

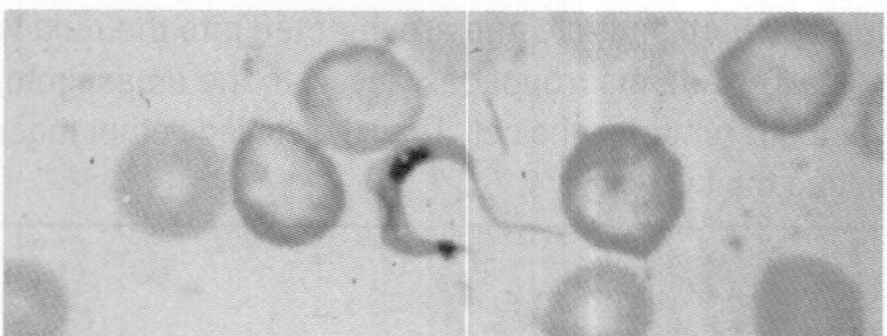

FIGURE 9-75. Chagas disease. A blood smear demonstrates a trypomastigote of *Trypanosoma cruzi* with its characteristic "C" shape, flagellum, nucleus and terminal kinetoplast.

Acute Chagas Disease May Cause Fatal Myocarditis

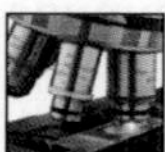

PATHOLOGY: *T. cruzi* circulates in the blood as a 20-μm-long, curved flagellate that is easily recognized on blood films. Within infected cells, it reproduces as a nonflagellated amastigote, 2 to 4 μm in diameter. In fatal cases, the heart is enlarged and dilated, with a pale, focally hemorrhagic myocardium. Microscopically, numerous parasites are seen in the heart and amastigotes are evident within pseudocysts in myofibers (Fig. 9-76). There is extensive chronic inflammation and phagocytosis of parasites is conspicuous.

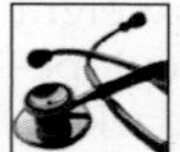

CLINICAL FEATURES: Acute symptoms develop 1 to 2 weeks after inoculation with *T. cruzi*. A chagoma (see above) develops at the site. Parasitemia appears 2 to 3 weeks after inoculation, usually associated with a mild illness characterized by fever, malaise, lymphadenopathy and hepatosplenomegaly. However, the disease can be lethal when there is extensive myocardial or meningeal involvement.

Chronic Chagas Disease May Lead to Cardiac Failure and Gastrointestinal Disease

The most frequent and most serious consequences of *T. cruzi* infection develop years or decades after acute infection. It is estimated that 10% to 40% of those acutely infected eventually develop chronic disease. In this phase of the illness,

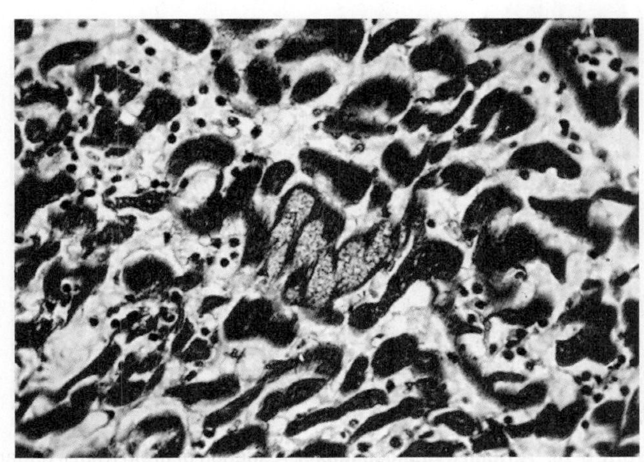

FIGURE 9-76. Acute Chagas myocarditis. The myofibers in the center contain numerous amastigotes of *Trypanosoma cruzi* and are surrounded by edema and chronic inflammation.

T. cruzi is no longer present in blood or tissue. Infected organs have been damaged, however, by chronic, progressive inflammation.

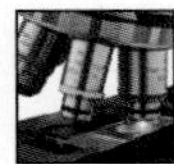 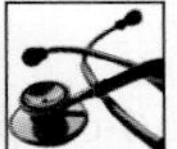

PATHOLOGY AND CLINICAL FEATURES: Chronic myocarditis is characterized by a dilated heart, prominent right ventricular outflow tract and dilation of the valve rings. The interventricular septum is often deviated to the right and may immobilize the adjacent tricuspid leaflet. Microscopically, there is extensive interstitial fibrosis, hypertrophied myofibers and focal lymphocytic inflammation, often involving the cardiac conduction system. Progressive cardiac fibrosis causes dysrhythmia or congestive heart failure. In endemic regions, chronic Chagas disease is a leading cause of heart failure in young adults.

Megaesophagus, dilation of the esophagus caused by failure of the lower esophageal sphincter (achalasia), is common in chronic Chagas disease. It results from destruction of parasympathetic ganglia in the wall of the lower esophagus and leads to difficulty in swallowing, which may be so severe that the patient can consume only liquids.

Megacolon, massive dilation of the large bowel, is similar to megaesophagus in that the myenteric plexus of the colon is destroyed. The progressive aganglionosis of the colon causes severe constipation.

Congenital Chagas disease occurs in some pregnant women with parasitemia. Infection of the placenta and fetus leads to spontaneous abortion. In the infrequent live births, the infants die of encephalitis within a few days or weeks.

Antiprotozoal chemotherapy is effective for acute Chagas disease but not for its chronic sequelae. Cardiac transplantation has been effective in a number of patients.

African Trypanosomiasis

African trypanosomiasis, popularly termed **sleeping sickness,** is an infection with *Trypanosoma brucei gambiense* or *Trypanosoma brucei rhodesiense*, leading to life-threatening meningoencephalitis. Gambian trypanosomiasis is a chronic infection often lasting more than a year. By contrast, East African (Rhodesian) trypanosomiasis is a rapidly progressive infection that kills the patient in 3 to 6 months. The organisms are curved flagellates, 15 to 30 μm in length. Although they can be demonstrated in blood or cerebrospinal fluid, they are difficult to find in infected tissues.

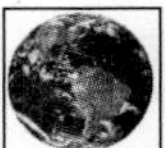

EPIDEMIOLOGY: *T. brucei gambiense* and *T. brucei rhodesiense* are hemoflagellate protozoa transmitted by several species of blood-sucking tsetse flies of the genus *Glossina*. The patchy distribution of African trypanosomiasis is related to the habitats of these flies. In Gambian trypanosomiasis, *T. brucei gambiense* is transmitted by tsetse flies of the riverine bush, mainly in endemic pockets of West and Central Africa. ***Humans are the only important reservoir for this trypanosome.***

In East African trypanosomiasis, *T. brucei rhodesiense* is spread by tsetse flies of the woodland savanna of East Africa. Antelope, other game animals and domestic cattle are natural reservoirs of *T. brucei rhodesiense*. Infection of humans is an occupational hazard of game wardens, fishermen and cattle herders.

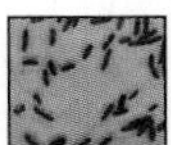

ETIOLOGIC FACTORS: While biting an infected animal or human, the tsetse fly ingests trypomastigotes with the blood (Fig. 9-77). These (1) lose their coat of surface antigen, (2) multiply in the midgut of the fly, (3) migrate to the salivary gland, (4) develop for 3 weeks through the epimastigote stage and (5) multiply in the fly's saliva as infective metacyclic trypomastigotes. During another bite, metacyclic trypomastigotes are injected into the lymphatics and blood vessels of a new host. They disseminate to the bone marrow and tissue fluids and some eventually invade the CNS. After replicating by binary fission in blood, lymph and spinal fluid, trypomastigotes are ingested by another fly to complete the cycle.

African trypanosomiasis involves immune complex formation by variable trypanosomal antigens and antibodies. Autoantibodies reacting with galactocerebrosides, the major components of myelin, and with neurofilaments, the intermediate filaments of neurons, have been reported and possibly contribute to the central nervous system damage caused by this parasite. The trypanosome evades immune attack in mammals by periodically altering its glycoprotein antigen coat, which occurs in a genetically determined pattern, not by mutation. Thus, each wave of circulating trypomastigotes includes different antigenic variants that are a step ahead of the immune response.

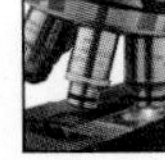

PATHOLOGY: *T. brucei* multiplies at sites of inoculation, occasionally producing localized nodular lesions: "primary chancres." Generalized involvement of lymph nodes and spleen is prominent early in the disease. Microscopic changes in affected nodes and spleen include foci of lymphocyte and macrophage hyperplasia. Infection eventually localizes to small blood vessels of the CNS, where replicating organisms elicit a destructive vasculitis, producing the progressive decrease in mentation characteristic of sleeping sickness. In *T. brucei rhodesiense* infection, the organisms also localize to blood vessels in the heart, sometimes causing a fulminant myocarditis.

Lesions in the lymph nodes, brain, heart and various other sites (including the inoculation site) show vasculitis of small blood vessels, with endothelial cell hyperplasia and dense perivascular infiltrates of lymphocytes, macrophages and plasma cells. The CNS vasculitis causes destruction of

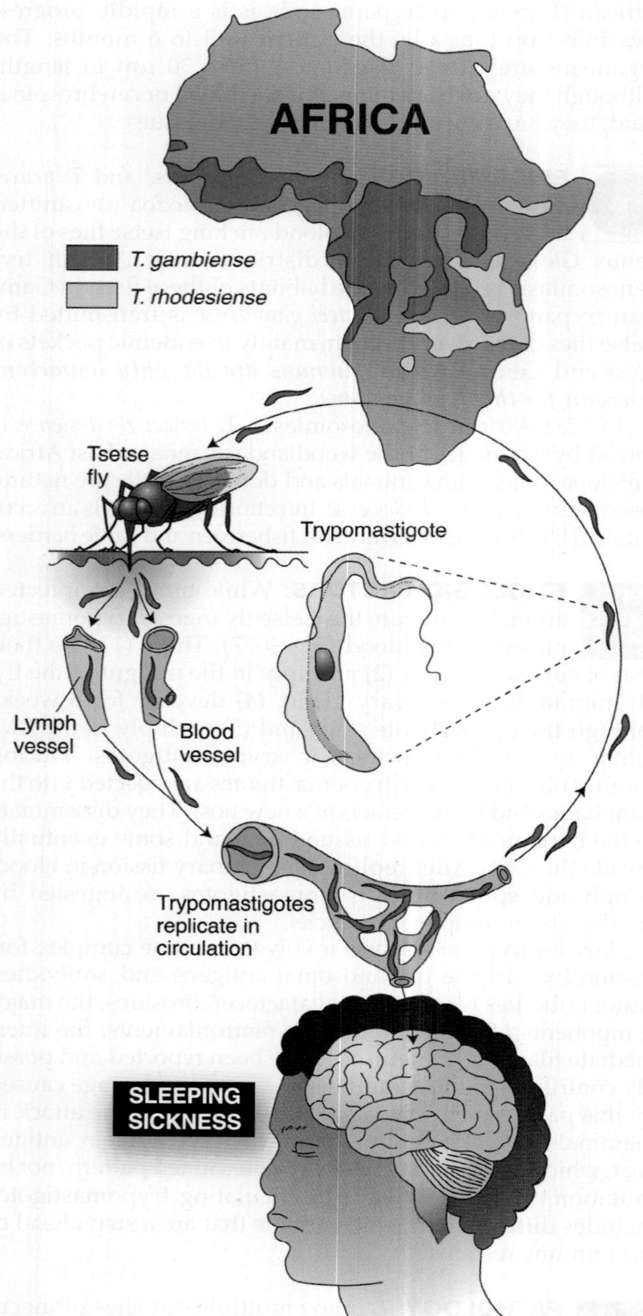

FIGURE 9-77. African trypanosomiasis (sleeping sickness). The distribution of Gambian and Rhodesian trypanosomiasis is related to the habitats of the vector tsetse flies (*Glossina* spp.). A tsetse fly bites an infected animal or human and ingests trypomastigotes, which multiply into infective, metacyclic trypomastigotes. During another fly bite, these are injected into lymphatic and blood vessels of a new host. A primary chancre develops at the site of the bite (stage 1a). Trypomastigotes replicate further in the blood and lymph, causing a systemic infection (stage 1b). Another fly ingests hypomastigotes to complete the cycle. In stage 2, invasion of the central nervous system by trypomastigotes leads to meningoencephalomyelitis and associated symptoms, including lethargy and daytime somnolence. Patients with Rhodesian trypanosomiasis may die within a few months. *T. gambiense* = *Trypanosoma brucei gambiense; T. rhodesiense* = *Trypanosoma brucei rhodesiense.*

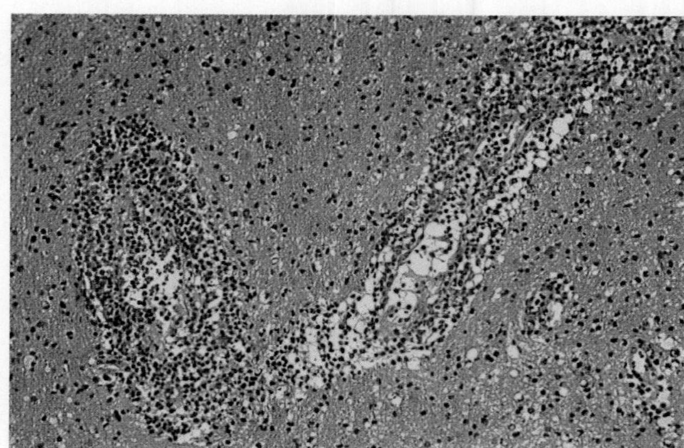

FIGURE 9-78. African trypanosomiasis. A section of brain from a patient who died from infection with *Trypanosoma brucei rhodesiense* shows a perivascular mononuclear cell infiltrate.

neurons, demyelination and gliosis. The perivascular infiltrate thickens the leptomeninges and involves the Virchow-Robin spaces (Fig. 9-78).

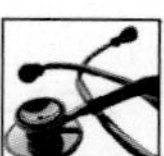

CLINICAL FEATURES: African trypanosomiasis is divided into three clinical stages:

1. **Primary chancre:** After 5 to 15 days, a 3- to 4-cm papillary swelling topped by a central red spot appears at the inoculation site. It subsides spontaneously within 3 weeks.
2. **Systemic infection:** Shortly after the appearance of the chancre (if any) and within 3 weeks of a bite, bloodstream invasion is marked by intermittent fever, for up to a week, often with splenomegaly and local and generalized lymphadenopathy. Enlargement of posterior cervical lymph nodes, "Winterbottom sign," is characteristic of Gambian trypanosomiasis. The evolving illness is marked by remitting irregular fevers, headache, joint pains, lethargy and muscle wasting. Myocarditis may be a complication and is more common and severe in Rhodesian trypanosomiasis. Dysfunction of the lungs, kidneys, liver and endocrine system occurs commonly in both forms of the disease.
3. **Brain invasion:** The two forms of sleeping sickness primarily differ in the timing of CNS invasion, which occurs early (weeks or months) in Rhodesian trypanosomiasis and late (months or years) in the Gambian form. Brain invasion is marked by apathy, daytime somnolence and sometimes coma. A diffuse meningoencephalitis is characterized by tremors of the tongue and fingers; fasciculations of the muscles of the limbs, face, lips and tongue; oscillatory movements of the arms, head, neck and trunk; indistinct speech; and cerebellar ataxia, causing problems in walking.

Primary Amebic Meningoencephalitis

Amebic meningoencephalitis is fatal and is caused by *Naegleria fowleri*.

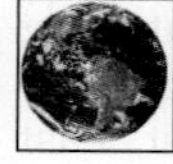

EPIDEMIOLOGY: *N. fowleri* is a free-living, soil ameba that inhabits ponds and lakes throughout tropical and subtropical regions, but it is reported in temperate areas, including the United States. Primary amebic meningoencephalitis is rare (fewer than 300 reported cases), affecting people who swim or bathe in these waters.

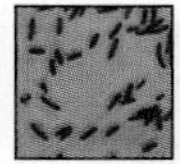
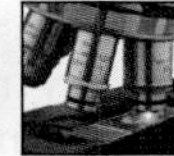

ETIOLOGIC FACTORS AND PATHOLOGY: *N. fowleri* is inoculated into nasal mucosa near the cribriform plate when a person swims in or dives into water containing high concentrations of the organism. Amebae invade the olfactory nerves, migrate into the olfactory bulbs, then proliferate in the meninges and brain.

In tissue sections, the trophozoites are 8 to 15 μm across, with sharply outlined nuclei that stain deeply with hematoxylin. Grossly, the brain is swollen and soft, with vascular congestion and a purulent meningeal exudate, most prominent over the lateral and basal areas. The amebae invade the brain along the Virchow-Robin spaces and cause massive tissue damage. Thrombosis and destruction of blood vessels are associated with extensive hemorrhage. The olfactory tract and bulbs are enveloped and destroyed, and there is an exudate between the bulb and the inferior surface of the temporal lobe. Proliferation of *Naegleria* in the brain may produce solid masses of amebae (amebomas). Meningitis can extend the full length of the spinal cord.

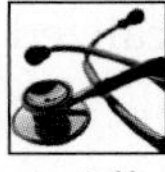

CLINICAL FEATURES: Primary amebic meningoencephalitis due to *N. fowleri* begins suddenly with fever, nausea, vomiting and headache. Disease progresses rapidly. Within hours the patient suffers profound deterioration in mental status. Cerebrospinal fluid contains numerous neutrophils, blood and amebae. The disease is rapidly fatal.

HELMINTHIC INFECTION

Helminths, or worms, are among the most common human pathogens. At any given time, 25% to 50% of the world's population carries at least one helminth species. Although most do little harm, some cause significant disease. Schistosomiasis, for instance, is among the leading global causes of morbidity and mortality.

Helminths are the largest and most complex organisms capable of living within the human body. Their adult forms range from 0.5 mm to over 1 m in length. Most are visible to the naked eye. They are multicellular animals with differentiated tissues, including specialized nervous tissues, digestive tissues and reproductive systems. Their maturation from eggs or larvae to adult worms is complex, often involving multiple morphologic transformations (molts). Some undergo these metamorphoses in different hosts before attaining adulthood, and the human host may be only one in a series that supports this maturation process. Within the human body, the helminths frequently migrate from the port of entry through several organs to a site of final infection.

Most helminths that infect humans are well adapted to human parasitism, causing limited or no host tissue damage. They gain entry by ingestion, skin penetration or insect bites. With two exceptions, they do not multiply in the human body, so a single organism cannot become an overwhelming infection. The exceptions are *Strongyloides stercoralis* and *Capillaria philippinensis*, which can complete their life cycle and multiply within the human body.

Helminths cause disease in various ways. A few compete with their human host for certain nutrients. Some grow to block vital structures, producing disease by mass effect. Most, however, cause dysfunction through the destructive inflammatory and immunologic responses that they elicit. For example, morbidity in schistosomiasis, the most destructive helminthic infection, results from granulomatous responses to schistosome eggs deposited in tissue.

Eosinophils contain basic proteins toxic to some helminths and are a major component of inflammatory responses to these organisms. Parasitic helminths are categorized based on overall morphology and the structure of digestive tissues:

- **Roundworms (nematodes)** are elongate cylindrical organisms with tubular digestive tracts.
- **Flatworms (trematodes)** are dorsoventrally flattened organisms with digestive tracts that end in blind loops.
- **Tapeworms (cestodes)** are segmented organisms with separate head and body parts; they lack a digestive tract and absorb nutrients through their outer walls.

Filarial Nematodes

Lymphatic Filariasis Results in Massive Lymphedema (Elephantiasis)

Lymphatic filariasis (bancroftian and Malayan filariasis) is an inflammatory parasitic infection of lymphatic vessels caused by the roundworms *Wuchereria bancrofti* and *Brugia malayi*. Adult worms inhabit the lymphatics, most frequently in inguinal, epitrochlear and axillary lymph nodes; testis; and epididymis. There they cause acute lymphangitis and, in a minority of infected subjects, lymphatic obstruction, leading to severe lymphedema (Fig. 9-79). These and similar organisms are known as filarial worms, because of their thread-like appearance (from the Latin *filum*, meaning "thread").

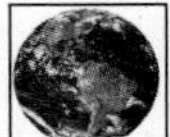

EPIDEMIOLOGY: The elephantiasis characteristic of lymphatic filariasis was familiar to Hindi and Persian physicians as early as 600 BC. Humans, the only definitive host of these filarial nematodes, acquire infection from the bites of at least 80 species of mosquitoes of the genera *Culex, Aedes, Anopheles* and *Mansonia*. *W. bancrofti* infection

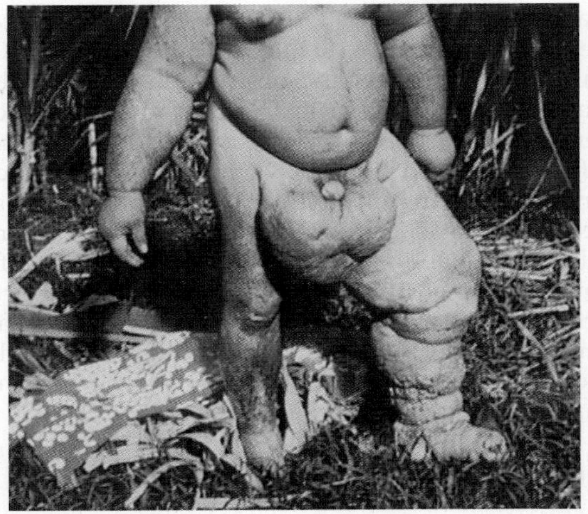

FIGURE 9-79. Bancroftian filariasis. Massive lymphedema (elephantiasis) of the scrotum and left lower extremity are present.

9 | Infectious and Parasitic Diseases

is widespread in southern Asia, the Pacific, Africa and parts of South America. *B. malayi* is localized to coastal southern Asia and western Pacific islands. Worldwide, 100 to 200 million people are estimated to be infected.

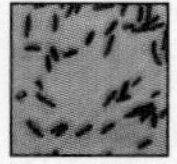

ETIOLOGIC FACTORS: Mosquito bites transmit infectious larvae that migrate to lymphatics and lymph nodes. After maturing into adult forms over several months, worms mate and the female releases microfilariae into lymphatics and the bloodstream. The manifestations of filariasis result from inflammatory responses to degenerating adult worms in the lymphatics. Repeated infections are common in endemic regions and produce numerous bouts of lymphangitis (filarial fevers), which cause extensive scarring and obstruction of lymphatics over years. This blockage causes localized dependent edema, most commonly affecting the legs, arms, genitalia and breasts. In its most severe form (less than 5% of the infected population), this is known as **elephantiasis.**

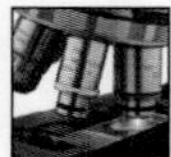

PATHOLOGY: The adult nematode is a white, thread-like worm that is very convoluted within lymph nodes. Females are 80 to 100 mm in length and 0.20 to 0.3 mm in width, twice the size of males. In blood films stained with Giemsa, the microfilariae appear as gracefully curved worms, measuring about 300 μm in length.

Lymphatic vessels harboring adult worms are dilated. Their endothelial lining is thickened. In adjacent tissues, worms are surrounded by chronic inflammation, including eosinophils. A granulomatous reaction may develop and degenerating worms can provoke acute inflammation. Microfilariae are seen in blood vessels and lymphatics and degenerating microfilariae also provoke a chronic inflammatory reaction. After repeated bouts of lymphangitis, lymph nodes and lymphatics become densely fibrotic, often containing calcified remnants of the worms.

CLINICAL FEATURES: In endemic areas, most of the infected population either has antifilarial antibodies with no detectable infection or asymptomatic microfilaremia. A smaller number develop recurrent episodes of filarial fevers, with malaise, lymphadenopathy and lymphangitis, which persist for 1 to 2 weeks and then resolve spontaneously. In a small subset of these, late manifestations of disease appear after two to three decades of recurrent bouts of filarial fevers. Lymphatic obstruction leads to chronic edema of dependent tissues. The overlying skin becomes thickened and warty. The diagnosis is made by identifying microfilariae in blood samples. Diethylcarbamazine and ivermectin are the agents effective against lymphatic filariasis.

Occult filariasis, characterized by indirect evidence of filarial infection (antifilarial antibodies), is the cause of **tropical pulmonary eosinophilia.** This condition is virtually restricted to southern India and some Pacific Islands. Patients present with cough, wheezing diffuse pulmonary infiltrates and peripheral eosinophilia. The severity ranges from mild asthma to fatal pneumonia.

Onchocerciasis Causes Blindness

Onchocerciasis ("**river blindness**") is a chronic inflammatory disease of the skin, eyes and lymphatics caused by the filarial nematode *Onchocerca volvulus*.

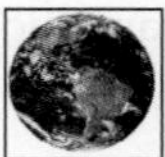

EPIDEMIOLOGY: Onchocerciasis is one of the world's major endemic diseases, afflicting an estimated 40 million people, of whom 2 million are blind. The disease is transmitted by bites of *Simulium damnosum* blackflies, which transmit infectious larvae to humans, who are the only definitive hosts. The flies require rapidly running water for breeding. Onchocerciasis is thus endemic along rivers and streams (hence, "river blindness") in parts of tropical Africa, southern Mexico, Central America and South America.

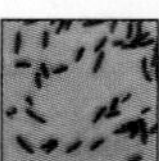

ETIOLOGIC FACTORS: Adult worms live as coiled tangled masses in deep fasciae and subcutaneous tissues. They do not cause tissue damage or elicit inflammatory responses, but gravid females release millions of microfilariae, which migrate into the skin, eyes, lymph nodes and deep organs, producing corresponding onchocercal lesions. Ocular onchocerciasis results from migration of microfilariae into all regions of the eye, from the cornea to the optic nerve head.

When microfilariae die, they incite vigorous inflammatory and immune responses. Inflammatory damage to the cornea, choroids or retina leads to partial or total loss of vision. Cutaneous inflammation causes microabscess formation and chronic degenerative changes in the epidermis and dermis. In lymph nodes and lymphatics, responses to dying microfilariae cause chronic lymphatic obstruction and localized dependent edema.

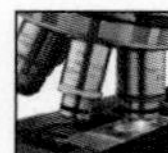

PATHOLOGY: *Onchocerca volvulus* is a thin, very long nematode; the female is 400 × 0.3 mm and the male 30 × 0.2 mm. Masses of adult worms become encapsulated by a fibrous scar, forming discrete, 1- to 3-cm, **onchocercal nodules** in the deep dermis and subcutis. Nodules form over bony prominences of the skull, scapula, ribs, iliac crest, trochanter, sacrum and knee. Microscopically, these nodules have an outer fibrous layer and a central inflammatory infiltrate, which varies from suppurative to granulomatous. Active lesions in the eyes and lymphatics all show degenerating microfilariae surrounded by chronic inflammation, including eosinophils. Ocular involvement leads to sclerosing keratitis, iridocyclitis, chorioretinitis and optic atrophy. The femoral inguinal nodes become enlarged and then fibrotic.

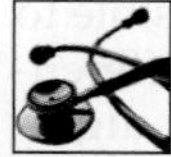

CLINICAL FEATURES: Symptoms of onchocerciasis result from inflammatory responses to degenerating microfilariae. Skin manifestations begin with generalized pruritus that becomes so intense that it can interfere with sleeping. Continuing damage produces areas of depigmentation, hypertrophy or atrophy of the skin. Progressive destruction of the cornea, choroid or uvea leads to loss of vision. Chronic lymphadenitis leads to localized edema that may cause chronic swelling (elephantiasis) of the legs, scrotum or other dependent portions of the body. Systemic antihelminthic therapy, particularly with ivermectin, is effective.

Loiasis Principally Affects the Eyes and Skin

Loiasis is infection by the filarial nematode *Loa loa*, the African "eyeworm."

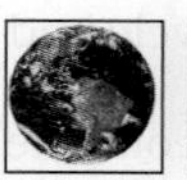 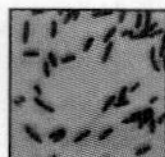

EPIDEMIOLOGY AND ETIOLOGIC FACTORS: Loiasis is prevalent in the rain forests of Central and West Africa. Humans and baboons are the definitive hosts and infection is transmitted

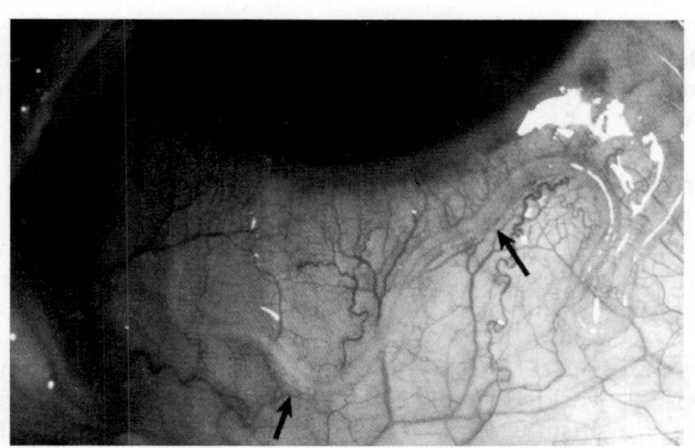

FIGURE 9-80. Loiasis. A thread-like *Loa loa* (*arrows*) is migrating in the subconjunctival tissues.

by mango flies. Adult worms (4 cm long) migrate in the skin and occasionally cross the eye beneath the conjunctiva, making the patient acutely aware of this infection (Fig. 9-80). Gravid worms discharge microfilariae, which circulate in the blood during the day but reside in capillaries of the skin, lungs and other organs at night.

PATHOLOGY: Migrating worms cause no inflammation, but static ones are surrounded by eosinophils, other inflammatory cells and a foreign body giant cell reaction. Rarely, those infected may develop acute generalized loiasis, characterized by obstructive fibrin thrombi, containing degenerating microfilariae in small vessels of most organs. Brain involvement, with obstruction of vessels by filarial thrombi, may cause lethal sudden and diffuse cerebral ischemia.

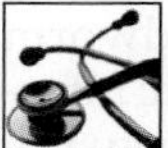

CLINICAL FEATURES: Most infections are asymptomatic but persist for years. Some patients have pruritic, red, subcutaneous "Calabar" swellings, which may be a reaction to migrating adult worms or to microfilariae in the skin. Ocular symptoms include swelling of the eyelids, itching and pain. Worms may be extracted during their migration beneath the conjunctiva. Systemic reactions include fever, pain, itching, urticaria and eosinophilia. Dead worms in or near major nerves may cause paresthesia or paralysis. Treatment with microfilariacides may cause massive death of microfilariae and provoke fever, meningoencephalitis and death.

Intestinal Nematodes

The adult forms of several nematode species (Table 9-10) reside in the human bowel but rarely cause symptomatic disease. Clinical symptoms occur almost exclusively in patients with very large numbers of worms or who are immunocompromised. Humans are the exclusive or primary host for all of intestinal nematodes and infection spreads from person to person via eggs or larvae passed in the stool or deposited in the perianal region. Infection is most prevalent in settings where hand washing and hygienic disposal of feces are lacking (e.g., less developed countries). Warm, moist climates are required for the infectious forms of many intestinal nematodes to survive outside the body. These worms are, thus, endemic in tropical and subtropical climates.

Table 9-10

Intestinal Nematodes

Species	Common Name	Site of Adult Worm	Clinical Manifestations
Ascaris lumbricoides	Roundworm	Small bowel	Allergic reactions to lung migration; intestinal obstruction
Ancylostoma duodenale	Hookworm	Small bowel	Allergic reactions to cutaneous inoculation and lung migration; intestinal blood loss
Necator americanus	Hookworm	Small bowel	Allergic reactions to cutaneous inoculation and lung migration; intestinal blood loss
Trichuris trichiura	Whipworm	Large bowel	Abdominal pain and diarrhea; rectal prolapse (rare)
Strongyloides stercoralis	Threadworm	Small bowel	Abdominal pain and diarrhea; dissemination to extraintestinal sites in immunocompromised persons
Enterobius vermicularis	Pinworm	Cecum, appendix	Perianal and perineal itching

Ascariasis Is Usually an Asymptomatic Infestation of the Small Bowel

Ascariasis refers to infection by the large roundworm *Ascaris lumbricoides*. It is the most common helminthic infection of humans, affecting at least 1 billion people, usually without causing symptoms. Infection is worldwide, but is most common in areas with warm climates and poor sanitation.

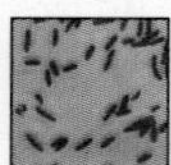

ETIOLOGIC FACTORS: Adult worms live in the small intestine, where gravid females discharge eggs that pass in the feces. These eggs hatch when ingested. *Ascaris* larvae emerge in the small intestine, penetrate the bowel wall and reach the lungs through the venous circulation. They leave the pulmonary capillaries, enter the alveoli, then migrate up the trachea to the glottis, where they are swallowed and again reach the small bowel. There, they mature and live as adult worms within the lumen for 1 to 2 years.

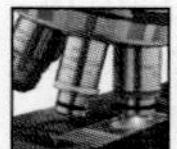
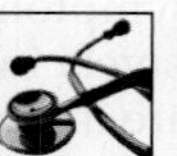

PATHOLOGY AND CLINICAL FEATURES: Adult worms (15 to 35 cm long) usually cause no pathologic changes. Heavy infections may cause vomiting, malnutrition and sometimes intestinal obstruction (Fig. 9-81). On rare occasions, worms enter the ampulla of Vater or pancreatic or biliary ducts, where they may cause obstruction, acute pancreatitis, suppurative cholangitis and liver abscesses. Eggs deposited in the liver or other tissues may produce necrosis, granulomatous inflammation and fibrosis. *Ascaris* pneumonia, which may be fatal, develops when large numbers of larvae migrate within the air spaces.

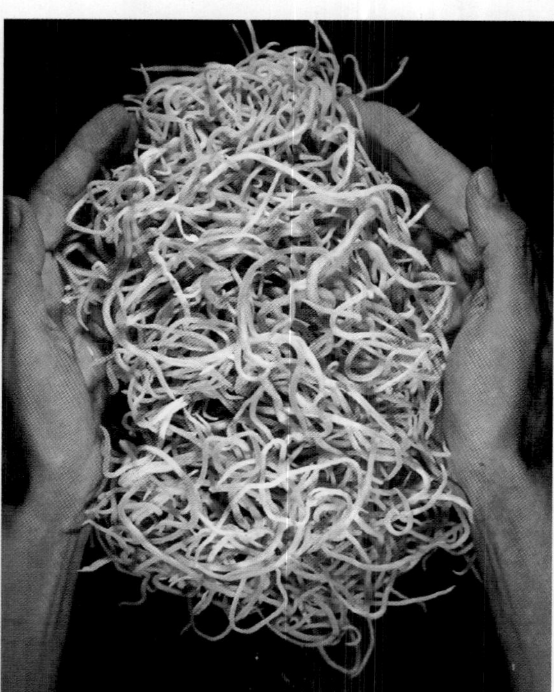

FIGURE 9-81. Ascariasis. This mass of over 800 worms of *Ascaris lumbricoides* obstructed and infarcted the ileum of a 2-year-old girl in South Africa.

Ascariasis is diagnosed by identifying eggs in the feces. Occasionally, adult worms may pass with the stools or even emerge from the nose or mouth. Ascaricidal drugs are effective.

Trichuriasis Is a Superficially Invasive Infection of the Large Bowel

Trichuriasis is caused by the intestinal nematode *Trichuris trichiura* **("whipworm").**

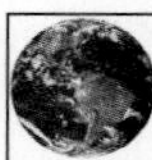

EPIDEMIOLOGY: Whipworm infection is found worldwide, affecting over 800 million people. Parasitism is most common in warm, moist places with poor sanitation, but over 2 million persons in the United States are infected. Children are especially susceptible. Adult worms live in the cecum and upper colon, where females produce eggs that pass in the feces. Eggs embryonate in moist soil and become infective in 3 weeks. Humans are infected by ingesting eggs in contaminated soil, food or drink.

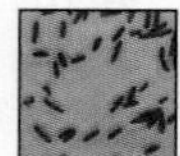
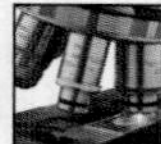

ETIOLOGIC FACTORS AND PATHOLOGY: Larvae emerge from ingested eggs in the small bowel and migrate to the cecum and colon, where adult worms burrow their anterior portions into the superficial mucosa (Fig. 9-82). This invasion causes small erosions, focal active inflammation and continuous loss of small quantities of blood. *T. trichiura* measures 3 to 5 cm in length, with a long, slender anterior portion and a short, blunt posterior.

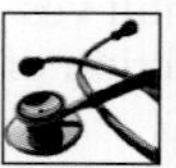

CLINICAL FEATURES: Most *T. trichiura* infections are asymptomatic. Heavy infestation may produce cramping abdominal pain, bloody diarrhea, weight loss and anemia. The diagnosis is made by finding the characteristic eggs in the stool. Mebendazole is effective therapy.

Hookworms Cause Intestinal Blood Loss and Anemia

Necator americanus and *Ancylostoma duodenale* ("hookworms") are intestinal nematodes that infect the human small bowel. They lacerate the bowel mucosa, causing intestinal blood loss, which can produce symptomatic disease in heavy infestations.

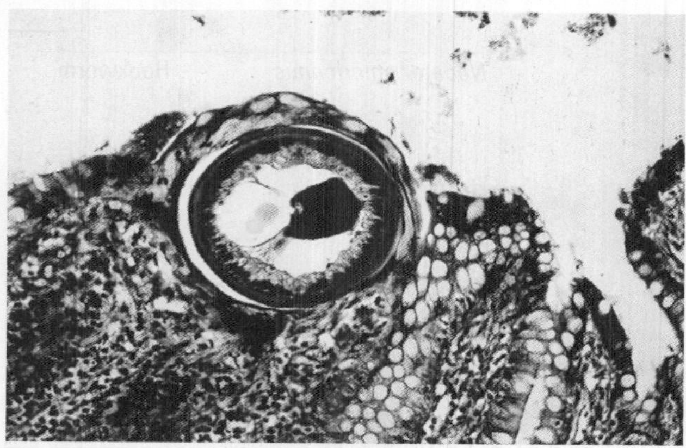

FIGURE 9-82. Trichuriasis. The anterior "whip" end of *Trichuris trichiura* is threaded into the mucosa of the colon.

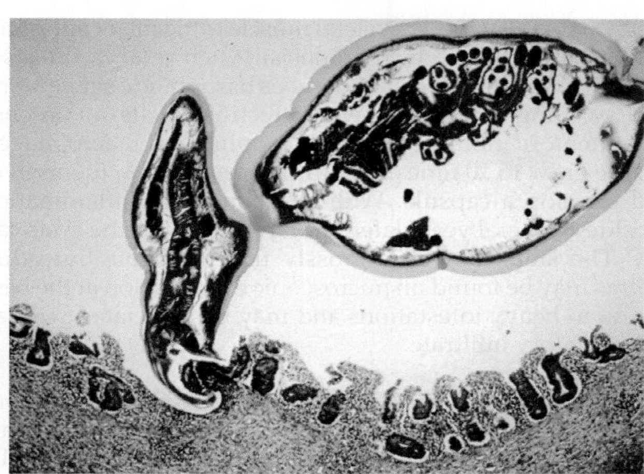

FIGURE 9-83. Ancylostomiasis. Section of the ileum shows two portions of a single adult worm, *Ancylostoma duodenale.* A plug of mucosa is in the buccal cavity of the hookworm.

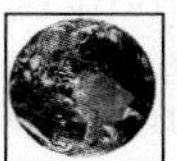

EPIDEMIOLOGY: Hookworm infections are found in moist, warm, temperate and tropical areas and cause serious public health problems worldwide. In fact, both *A. duodenale* ("Old World" hookworm) and *N. americanus* ("American" hookworm) prevail on most continents and have overlapping epidemiologic boundaries. More than 700 million persons are infected with hookworms, including a half-million persons in the United States.

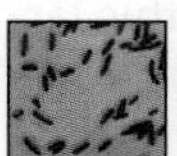 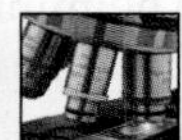

ETIOLOGIC FACTORS AND PATHOLOGY: Filariform larvae directly penetrate the human epidermis on contact and enter the venous circulation. They travel to the lungs and lodge in alveolar capillaries. After rupturing into the alveoli, larvae migrate up the trachea to the glottis and are then swallowed. They molt in the duodenum, attach to the mucosal wall with tooth-like buckle plates and clamp off a section of a villus and ingest it (Fig. 9-83). In extensive infestations, particularly with *A. duodenale,* blood loss can be sufficient to cause anemia. Hookworms are about 1 cm in length. They are grossly visible attached to the small bowel mucosa alongside punctate areas of hemorrhages. There is no attendant inflammation.

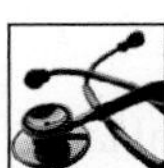

CLINICAL FEATURES: ***Although most people with hookworm infection have no symptoms, this parasite is the most important cause of chronic anemia worldwide.*** In people with heavy worm burdens (particularly women who consume a diet low in iron) and in populations with inadequate iron intake, chronic intestinal blood loss can produce severe iron deficiency anemia. Skin penetration is sometimes associated with a pruritic eruption ("ground itch"), and the phase of larval migration through the lungs occasionally causes asthma-like symptoms.

Strongyloidiasis Is Disseminated in Immunocompromised Hosts

Strongyloidiasis is a small intestinal infection with a nematode, *Strongyloides stercoralis* ("threadworm"). ***Although most cases are asymptomatic, the infection can progress to lethal disseminated disease in immunocompromised persons.*** Infection is most frequent in areas with warm, moist climates and poor sanitation. Endemic pockets of strongyloidiasis still exist in the United States, particularly in the Appalachian region and in institutions where personal hygiene is poor, such as hospitals for the mentally ill.

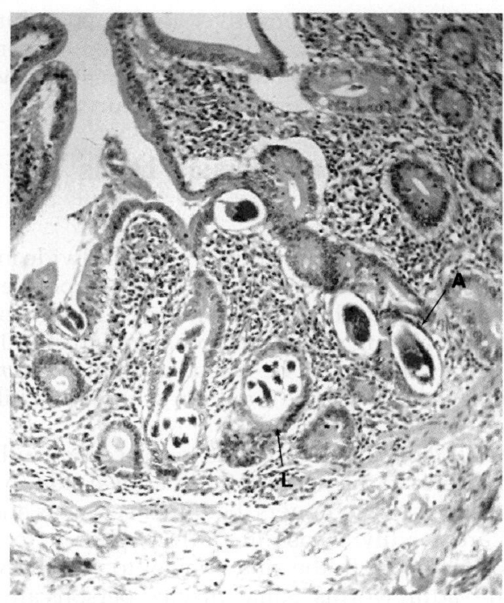

FIGURE 9-84. Strongyloidiasis. A section of jejunum shows adult (A) worms and larvae (L).

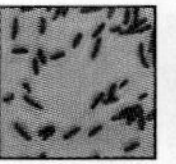 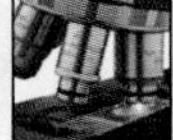

ETIOLOGIC FACTORS AND PATHOLOGY: *S. stercoralis* is the smallest of the intestinal nematodes, measuring 0.2 to 0.3 cm in length. Adult females are buried in the crypts of the duodenum or jejunum but produce no visible alterations. Microscopically, the coiled females, along with eggs and developing larvae, lie within the mucosa, usually with no associated inflammation (Fig. 9-84).

Parasitic females live in the mucosa of the small intestine, where they lay eggs that hatch quickly and release rhabditiform larvae. These are passed in the feces, and in the soil become filariform, the infective stage that penetrates human skin. On entering the skin, *S. stercoralis* larvae pass in the bloodstream to the lungs and then to the small bowel, similarly to hookworms. The worms mature in the small bowel. Unlike other intestinal nematodes, *S. stercoralis* may reproduce in human hosts by a mechanism known as **autoinfection.** This occurs when rhabditiform larvae become infective (filariform) within a host's intestine and repenetrate either the intestinal wall or the perianal skin, thereby starting a new parasitic cycle within a single host.

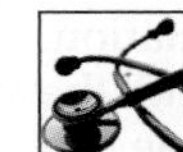

CLINICAL FEATURES: Most infected people are asymptomatic, but moderate eosinophilia is common. **Disseminated strongyloidiasis** or **hyperinfection syndrome** occurs in patients with suppressed immunity, particularly those receiving corticosteroids. In such patients, internal autoinfection is greatly increased, and extraordinary numbers of filariform larvae penetrate intestinal walls and disseminate to distant organs. In disseminated strongyloidiasis, the gut may show ulceration, edema and severe inflammation.

Sepsis, usually with gram-negative organisms, and infection of parenchymal organs eventuate. Untreated, disseminated strongyloidiasis is fatal; even with prompt treatment with thiabendazole or ivermectin, only one third survive.

Pinworm Infection (Enterobiasis) Leads to Perianal Itching

Enterobius vermicularis ("pinworm") is a worldwide intestinal nematode, most often encountered in temperate zones. Although people can be infected at any age, parasitism is most common among young children. More than 200 million persons are estimated to be infected with *E. vermicularis* worldwide, including some 5 million school-age children in the United States.

The adult female worm resides in the cecum and appendix but migrates to the perianal and perineal skin to deposit eggs. The eggs stick to fingers, bed linens, towels and clothing and are readily transmitted from person to person. Ingested eggs hatch in the small bowel to yield larvae that mature into adult worms. Some infected persons are asymptomatic, but most complain of perineal pruritus, caused by migrating worms depositing eggs. Several agents, including mebendazole, are effective against pinworms.

Tissue Nematodes

Trichinosis Is Myositis Acquired by Eating Pork

Trichinosis is produced by the roundworm *Trichinella spiralis*.

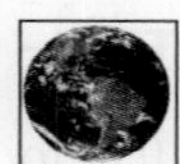

EPIDEMIOLOGY: Infection with *T. spiralis* occurs worldwide. Humans acquire trichinosis by eating inadequately cooked meat with encysted *T. spiralis* larvae. The larvae are found in the skeletal muscles of various carnivorous or omnivorous wild and domesticated animals, including pigs, rats, bears and walruses. Pork is the most common source of human trichinosis (Fig. 9-85).

Animals acquire trichinosis by feeding on the flesh of other infected animals. Infection is common among some wild animal populations and can be readily introduced into domesticated animals, such as pigs, when they feed on garbage or uncooked meat. Meat inspection programs and restriction of feeding practices have largely eliminated *T. spiralis* from domesticated pigs in many developed countries. Only about 100 cases of trichinosis are reported in the United States annually, but these represent only the most severely symptomatic cases and infection is probably much more common.

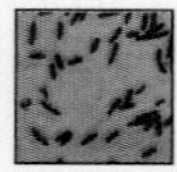

ETIOLOGIC FACTORS: In the small bowel, *T. spiralis* larvae emerge from the ingested tissue cysts and burrow into the intestinal mucosa, where they develop into adult worms. The adults mate, and the female liberates larvae that invade the intestinal wall and enter the circulation. Production of larvae may continue for 1 to 4 months, until the worms are finally expelled from the intestine. The larvae can invade nearly any tissue but can survive only in striated skeletal muscle, where they encyst and remain viable for years. The resulting myositis is especially prominent in the diaphragm, extrinsic ocular muscles, tongue, intercostal muscles, gastrocnemius and deltoids. Sometimes the CNS or heart is also inflamed, causing meningoencephalitis or myocarditis.

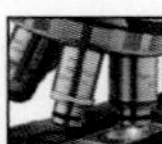

PATHOLOGY: Skeletal muscle is the major site of tissue damage in trichinosis. When a larva infects a myocyte, the cell undergoes basophilic degeneration and swelling. Early myocyte infection elicits an intense inflammatory infiltrate rich in eosinophils and macrophages. Larvae grow to 10 times their initial size, fold on themselves and develop a capsule. With encapsulation, inflammation subsides. Several years later, the larvae die and the cysts calcify. The small bowel is grossly unremarkable but adult worms may be found on microscopic examination at the base of villi in heavy infestations and may be associated with an inflammatory infiltrate.

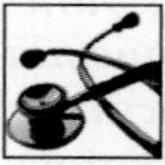

CLINICAL FEATURES: Most human infections with *T. spiralis* involve small numbers of cysts and are asymptomatic. Symptomatic trichinosis is usually self-limited and patients recover in a few months. If large numbers of cysts are eaten, abdominal pain and diarrhea may result from small-bowel invasion by the worms. Major symptoms, in the form of fever, weakness and severe pain and tenderness of affected muscles, usually develop several days later. **Eosinophilia may be extreme (over 50% of all leukocytes)**. Involvement of extraocular muscles produces periorbital edema. Infection of the brain or myocardium can be fatal. Severe trichinosis is treated with corticosteroids to attenuate the inflammation. Antihelminthic drugs are required to remove adult worms from the intestine.

Visceral Larva Migrans (Toxocariasis) Is Transmitted by Cats and Dogs

Toxocariasis is an infection of deep organs by helminthic larvae migrating in aberrant hosts.

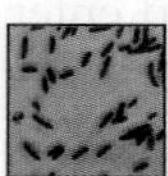
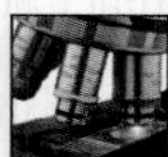

ETIOLOGIC FACTORS AND PATHOLOGY: The infestation is a sporadic disease, mainly of young children, typically in the setting of overcrowded dwellings, living with dogs and cats. The most common causes of visceral larva migrans are *Toxocara* spp., especially *Toxocara canis* and *Toxocara cati*. These roundworms live in the intestines of dogs and cats, and infection is transmitted to humans by ingestion of embryonated ova. Eggs hatch and larvae invade the intestinal wall. They are carried to the liver, from where a few emerge to reach the systemic circulation and may be carried to any part of the body. In tissues, larvae die and elicit small granulomas, which eventually heal by scarring.

CLINICAL FEATURES: Many cases of visceral larva migrans are asymptomatic, but any infection can potentially cause severe disease. The typical symptomatic patient is a child with hypereosinophilia, pneumonitis and hypergammaglobulinemia. In these patients, ocular manifestations are common, and the chief complaint is often loss of vision in one eye. In fact, eyes with toxocaral endophthalmitis have been mistakenly enucleated for retinoblastoma. The infection is generally self-limited and symptoms disappear within a year. It is treated with diethylcarbamazine and thiabendazole.

Cutaneous Larva Migrans Is a Pruritic Eruption

Cutaneous larva migrans is caused by larval nematodes migrating through the skin, where they provoke severe

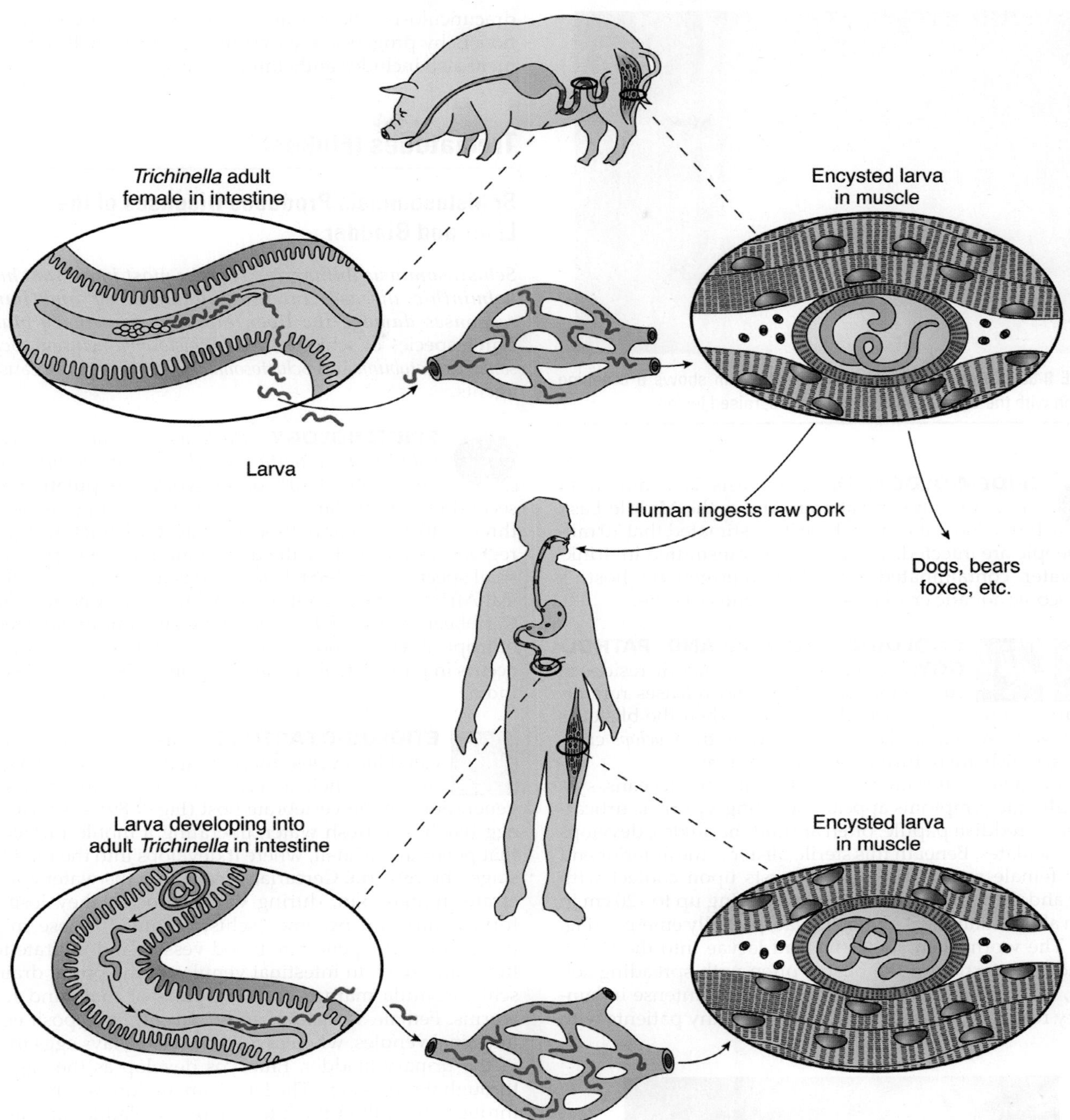

FIGURE 9-85. Trichinosis. After being ingested by the pig, cysts of *Trichinella* are digested in the gastrointestinal tract, liberating larvae that mature to adult worms. Female worms release larvae that penetrate the intestinal wall, enter the circulation and lodge in striated muscle, where they encyst. When humans ingest inadequately cooked pork, the cycle is repeated, resulting in the muscle disease characteristic of trichinosis.

inflammation that appears as serpiginous urticarial trails (Fig. 9-86). The names applied to cutaneous larva migrans are as varied as the organisms that cause it and include creeping eruptions, sand worm, plumber's itch, duck hunter's itch and epidermis linearis migrans. The more common larval nematodes include *Strongyloides stercoralis, Ancylostoma braziliensis* and *Necator americanus*. Dogs and cats infected with hookworms are the major source of the disease. Outbreaks of cutaneous larva migrans occur at subtropical and tropical beaches. Plumbers who crawl under houses and animal caretakers are frequently infected. Thiabendazole is the treatment of choice.

Dracunculiasis Features Long Adult Worms Beneath the Skin

Dracunculiasis (guinea worm) is an infection of connective and subcutaneous tissues with the guinea worm, *Dracunculus medinensis*.

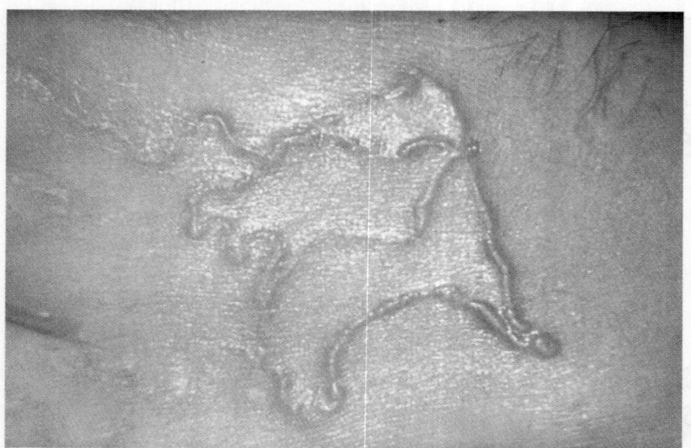

FIGURE 9-86. Cutaneous larva migrans. The skin shows a creeping eruption with the characteristic serpiginous, raised lesion.

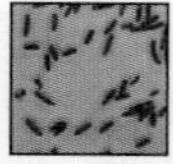

EPIDEMIOLOGY: Dracunculiasis is common in rural areas of sub-Saharan Africa, the Middle East, India and Pakistan, where it is estimated that 10 million people are infected. The disease is transmitted in drinking water contaminated with the intermediate host, a microscopic aquatic crustacean of the genus *Cyclops*.

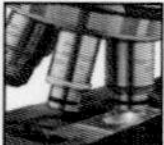

ETIOLOGIC FACTORS AND PATHOLOGY: The adult female nematode resides in subcutaneous tissues and releases numerous larvae through an ulcerated blister. When the blister is immersed in water, larvae are ingested by the *Cyclops* crustaceans, which are in turn ingested by humans.

About a year after ingestion of infected crustaceans, systemic allergic symptoms appear, including a pruritic urticarial rash. A reddish papule, often around the ankles, develops and vesiculates. Beneath this sterile blister is the anterior end of the female worm. The blister bursts upon contact with water and the female worm, now measuring up to 120 cm in length and containing 3 million larvae, partially emerges (Fig. 9-87). The worm then spews myriad larvae into the water. Secondary infection of the blister, often with spreading cellulitis, is common. Dead worms provoke an intense inflammatory response, causing debilitation in many patients with dracunculosis. The worm is often extracted by local practitioners by progressively twisting it onto a small stick. Treatment also includes anthelminthic drugs.

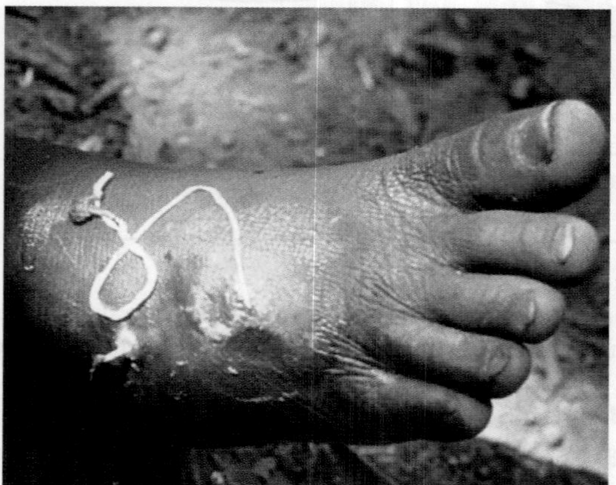

FIGURE 9-87. Dracunculiasis. A female guinea worm is seen emerging from the foot, which is swollen because of secondary bacterial infection.

Trematodes (Flukes)

Schistosomiasis Produces Diseases of the Liver and Bladder

Schistosomiasis (bilharziasis) is the most important human helminthic disease. Intense inflammatory and immune responses damage the liver, intestine or urinary bladder. Three species of schistosomes, *Schistosoma mansoni, Schistosoma haematobium* and *Schistosoma japonicum,* are the causative agents.

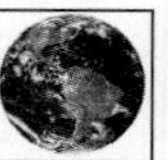

EPIDEMIOLOGY: *Schistosomiasis causes greater morbidity and mortality than all other worm infections.* It affects about 10% of the world's population and is second only to malaria as a cause of disabling disease. The three schistosomal pathogens affect distinct geographic regions, as dictated by the distribution of their specific host snail species (Fig. 9-88). *S. mansoni* is found in much of tropical Africa, parts of southwest Asia, South America and the Caribbean islands. *S. haematobium* is endemic in large regions of tropical Africa and parts of the Middle East. *S. japonicum* occurs in parts of China, the Philippines, Southeast Asia and India.

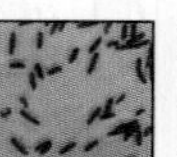

ETIOLOGIC FACTORS: Schistosomes have complicated life cycles, alternating between asexual generations in their invertebrate host (snail) and sexual generations in the vertebrate host (Fig. 9-89). A schistosome egg hatches in fresh water, liberating a motile **miracidium** that penetrates a snail, where it develops into the final larval stage, the **cercaria.** Cercariae escape into the water and penetrate human skin, during which process they lose their forked tails and become "schistosomula." These migrate through tissues, penetrate blood vessels and migrate to the lungs and liver. In intestinal venules of the portal drainage, schistosomula mature, forming pairs of male and female worms. Female *S. mansoni* and *S. japonicum* deposit eggs in intestinal venules, whereas *S. haematobium* lays eggs in those of the urinary bladder. Embryos develop as the eggs pass through these tissues. The larvae are mature when eggs pass through the wall of the intestine or the bladder and are discharged in feces or urine. They hatch in fresh water, liberating miracidia and completing the life cycle.

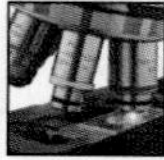

PATHOLOGY: ***The basic lesion is a circumscribed granuloma or a cellular infiltrate of eosinophils and neutrophils around an egg.*** Adult schistosomes provoke no inflammation while alive in the veins. Granulomas that form about the eggs also obstruct microvascular blood flow and produce ischemic damage to adjacent tissue. The result is progressive scarring and dysfunction in affected organs.

Female worms deposit hundreds or thousands of eggs daily for 5 to 35 years. Most infected people harbor fewer than 10 adult females. However, if the worm burden is large, the granulomatous response to the enormous number of eggs poses significant problems. The site of involvement is determined by the tropism of the particular schistosome species.

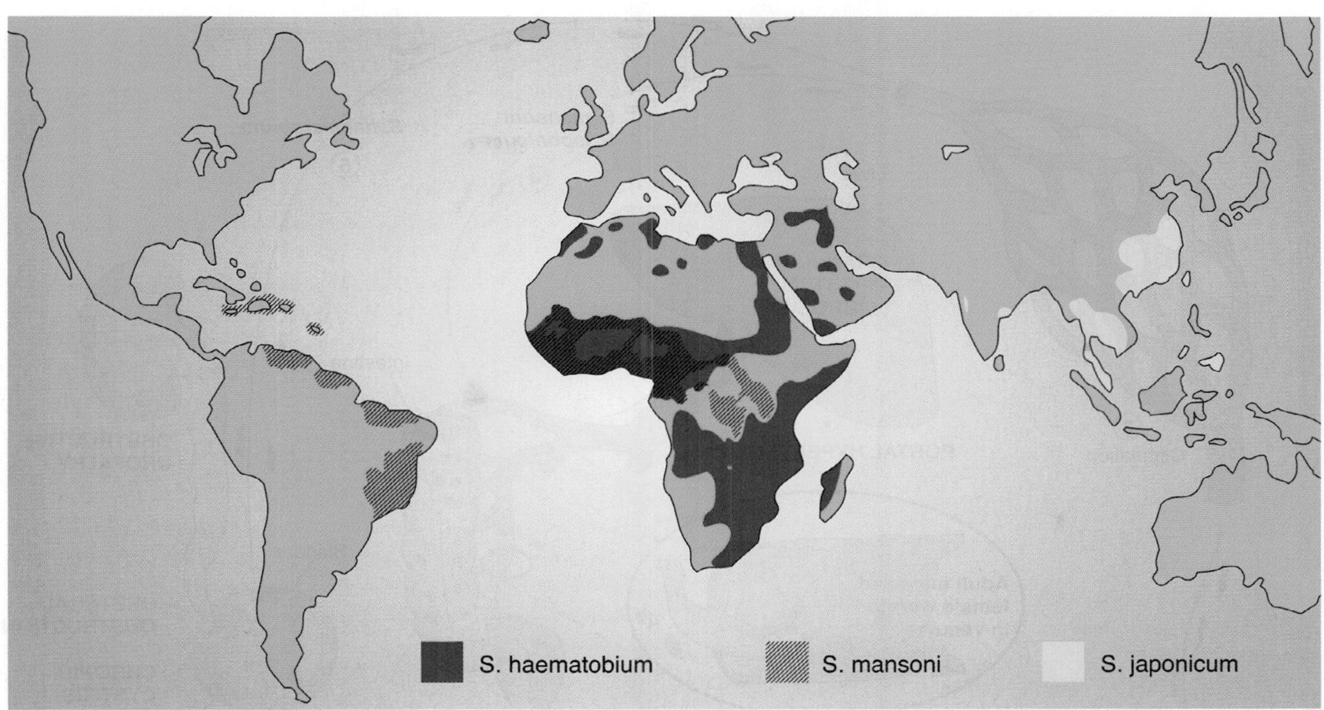

FIGURE 9-88. Distribution of schistosomiasis caused by *Schistosoma mansoni, Schistosoma haematobium* and *Schistosoma japonicum*.

- *S. mansoni* inhabits the branches of the inferior mesenteric vein, thereby affecting the distal colon and liver.
- *S. haematobium* winds its way to the veins serving the rectum, bladder and pelvic organs.
- *S. japonicum* deposits eggs predominantly in the branches of the superior mesenteric vein, thereby damaging the small bowel, ascending colon and liver.

Liver disease caused by *S. mansoni* or *S. japonicum* begins as periportal granulomatous inflammation (Fig. 9-90) and progresses to dense periportal fibrosis (**pipestem fibrosis**) (Fig. 9-91). In severe hepatic schistosomiasis, this causes obstruction of portal blood flow and portal hypertension. *S. mansoni* and *S. japonicum* also damage the intestine, where granulomatous responses produce inflammatory polyps and foci of mucosal and submucosal fibrosis.

In **urogenital schistosomiasis,** caused by *S. haematobium*, eggs are most numerous in the bladder, ureter and seminal vesicles, although they may also reach the lungs, colon and appendix. Eggs in the bladder and ureters lead to a granulomatous reaction, inflammatory protuberances and patches of mucosal and mural fibrosis. These may obstruct urine flow, and so cause secondary inflammatory damage to the bladder, ureters and kidneys. Bladder disease produced by *S. haematobium* may lead to **squamous cell carcinoma of the bladder.** In areas where *S. Haematobium* is prevalent, this is the most common form of carcinoma.

The granulomas of schistosomiasis surround schistosome eggs. Eosinophils often predominate in early granulomas. In older granulomas, epithelioid macrophages and giant cells are prominent and the oldest granulomas are densely fibrotic. The eggs of the various schistosomal species are identified on the basis of their size and shape.

CLINICAL FEATURES: Skin penetration by the schistosome larvae is sometimes associated with a self-limited, intensely pruritic rash. Most cases are dominated by the manifestations of chronic granulomatous tissue damage. Hepatic involvement leads to portal hypertension, splenomegaly, ascites and bleeding esophageal varices. Intestinal disease is usually only minimally symptomatic, but some patients have abdominal pain and bloody stools. Schistosomiasis of the bladder causes hematuria, recurrent urinary tract infections and sometimes progressive obstruction leading to renal failure. Identification of schistosome eggs in the urine or feces establishes the diagnosis. Schistosomes are effectively killed by systemic antihelminthic agents, but structural changes due to extensive scarring are irreversible.

Clonorchiasis Leads to Biliary Obstruction

Clonorchiasis is an infection of the hepatic biliary system by the Chinese liver fluke, *Clonorchis sinensis*. Although the fluke usually causes only mild symptoms, it is sometimes associated with bile duct stones, cholangitis and bile duct cancer.

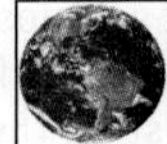

EPIDEMIOLOGY: Clonorchiasis is endemic in east Asia, from Vietnam to Korea, where uncooked freshwater fish is common fare. In parts of Vietnam, China and Japan, over 50% of the adult population is infected. Human infection is acquired by ingesting inadequately cooked freshwater fish containing *C. sinensis* larvae.

Adult worms are flat and transparent, live in human bile ducts and pass eggs to the intestine and feces. After ingestion by a specific snail, the egg hatches into a miracidium.

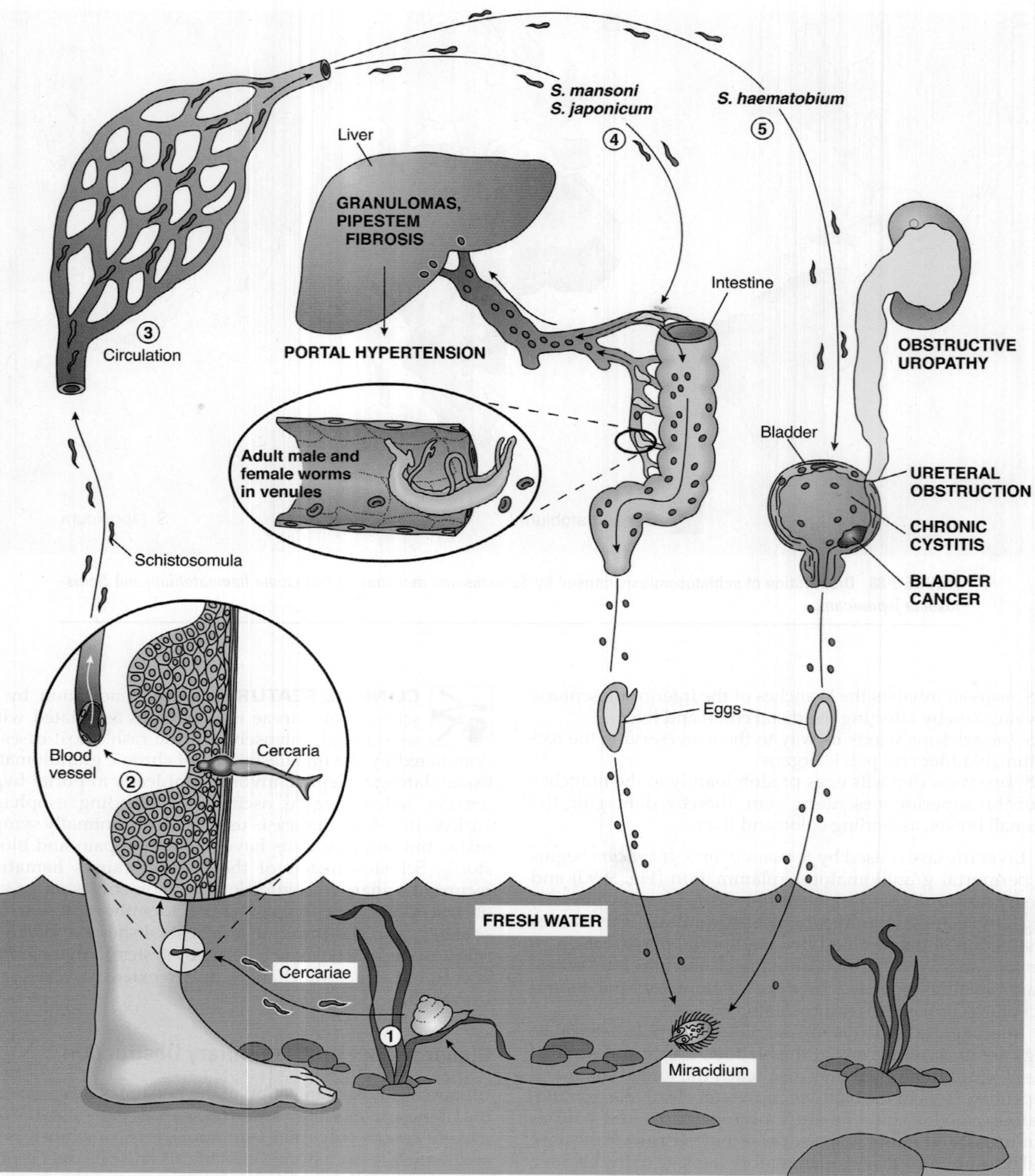

FIGURE 9-89. Life cycle of *Schistosoma* and clinical features of schistosomiasis. The schistosome egg hatches in water, liberates a miracidium that penetrates a snail and develops through two stages to a sporocyst to form the final larval stage, the cercaria. **(1)** The cercaria escapes from the snail into water, "swims" and penetrates the skin of a human host. **(2)** The cercaria loses its forked tail to become a schistosomulum, which migrates through tissues, penetrates a blood vessel and **(3)** is carried to the lung and later to the liver. In hepatic portal venules, the schistosomula become sexually mature and form pairs, each with a male and a female worm, the female worm lying in the gynecophoral canal of the male worm. The organism causes lesions in the liver, including granulomas, portal ("pipestem") fibrosis and portal hypertension. **(4)** The female worm deposits immature eggs in small venules of the intestine and rectum (*Schistosoma mansoni* and *Schistosoma japonicum*) or **(5)** of the urinary bladder (*Schistosoma haematobium*). The bladder infestation leads to obstructive uropathy, ureteral obstruction, chronic cystitis and bladder cancer. Embryos develop during passage of the eggs through tissues, and larvae are mature when eggs pass through the wall of the intestine or urinary bladder. Eggs hatch in water and liberate miracidia to complete the cycle.

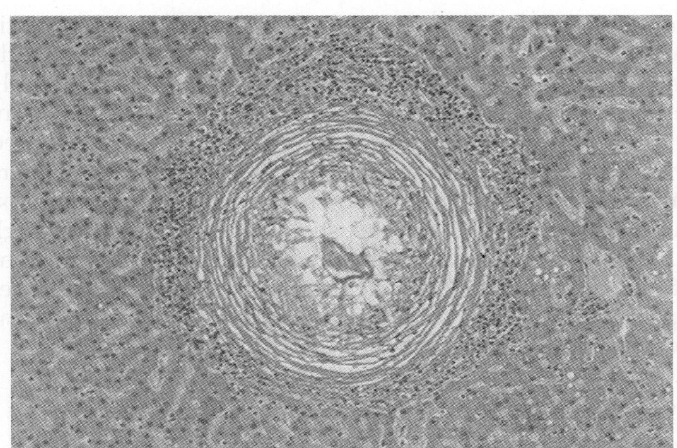

FIGURE 9-90. Hepatic schistosomiasis. A hepatic granuloma surrounds a degenerating egg of *Schistosoma mansoni.*

Cercariae escape from the snail and seek out certain fish, which they penetrate and in which they encyst. When humans eat the fish, cercariae emerge in the duodenum, enter the common bile duct through the ampulla of Vater and mature in the distal bile ducts to adult flukes.

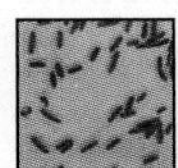
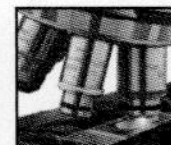

ETIOLOGIC FACTORS AND PATHOLOGY: The presence of *Clonorchis* in the bile ducts elicits an inflammatory response that does not eliminate the worm but causes dilation and fibrosis of the ducts. Sometimes the worms cause calculus formation in the hepatic bile ducts, leading to ductal obstruction. The adult *Clonorchis* persists in the ducts for decades, and long-standing infection is associated with an increased incidence of bile duct carcinoma **(cholangiocarcinoma).**

In heavy *Clonorchis* infections, the liver may be up to three times the normal size. Dilated bile ducts are seen through the capsule, and the cut surface is punctuated with thick-walled dilated bile ducts (Fig. 9-92). Flukes (up to 2.5 cm in length), sometimes in the thousands, can be expressed from the bile ducts. Microscopically, the epithelial duct lining is initially hyperplastic and then metaplastic. Surrounding stroma is fibrotic. Secondary bacterial infection is common and may be associated with suppurative cholangitis. Eggs deposited in the liver parenchyma elicit a fibrous and granulomatous reaction. Masses of eggs may lodge in the bile ducts and cause cholangitis. Pancreatic ducts may also be invaded, dilated and thickened, lined by metaplastic epithelium and eventually surrounded by fibrosis.

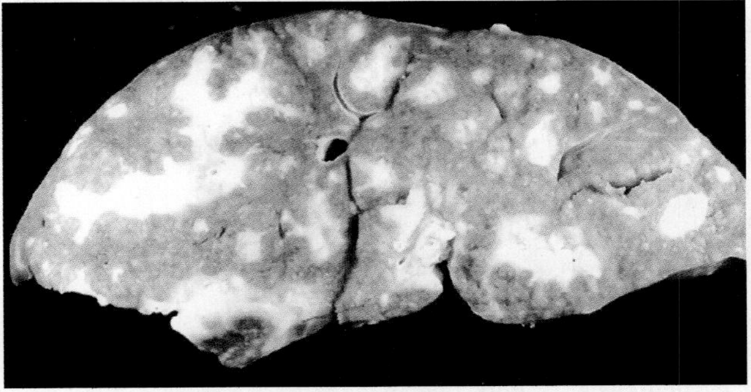

FIGURE 9-91. Hepatic schistosomiasis. Chronic infection of the liver with *Schistosoma japonicum* has led to the characteristic "pipestem" fibrosis.

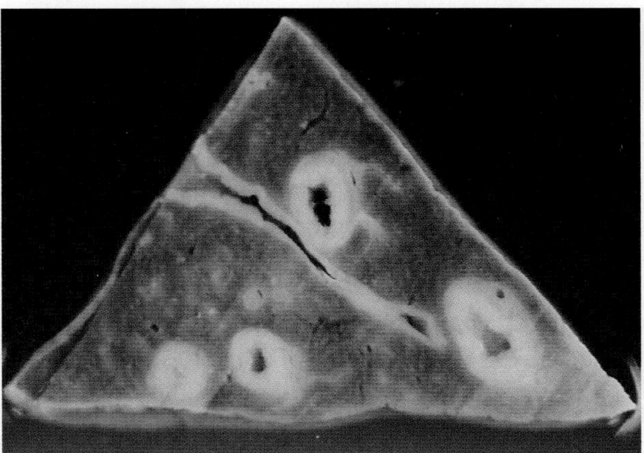

FIGURE 9-92. Clonorchiasis of the liver. The bile ducts are greatly thickened and dilated because of the presence of adult flukes (*Clonorchis sinensis*).

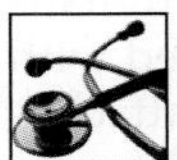

CLINICAL FEATURES: Migration of *C. sinensis* into the bile ducts causes transient fever and chills, but most infected persons are asymptomatic. Patients with clonorchiasis may die of a variety of complications, including biliary obstruction, bacterial cholangitis, pancreatitis and cholangiocarcinoma. The diagnosis is made by identifying eggs of *C. sinensis* in stools or duodenal aspirates. The infestation is treated effectively with systemic anti-helminthic agents.

Paragonimiasis Is a Lung Disease

Paragonimiasis is a pulmonary infection by several species of the genus *Paragonimus,* the oriental lung fluke. The most common human pathogen is *Paragonimus westermani*, which is common in Asian countries (Korea, the Philippines, Taiwan and China) where uncooked, lightly salted or wine-soaked fresh crabs are delicacies. Use of raw crab juices as medicines or seasonings also has been associated with the infection.

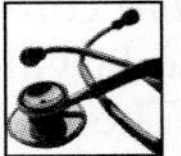

CLINICAL FEATURES: Pulmonary paragonimiasis is frequently misdiagnosed as tuberculosis. It manifests as fever, malaise, night sweats, chest pain and cough. However, unlike tuberculosis, peripheral eosinophilia is common. The sputum is sometimes blood tinged and chest radiographs reveal transient diffuse pulmonary infiltrates. The prognosis in pulmonary paragonimiasis is good, but ectopic lesions of the brain may be fatal. Eggs in the sputum or stools provide the definitive diagnosis.

Fascioliasis Is a Biliary Disease Acquired From Sheep

Fascioliasis is an infection of the liver by the sheep liver fluke, *Fasciola hepatica*. Humans may acquire the infection wherever sheep are raised. People become infected by eating vegetation, such as watercress, that is contaminated with the cysts passed by sheep.

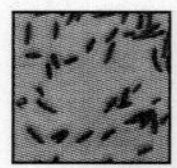

ETIOLOGIC FACTORS: After reaching the duodenum, cysts liberate metacercariae that pass into the peritoneal cavity, penetrate the liver and migrate through the hepatic parenchyma into the bile ducts. The larvae mature to adults and live in both the intrahepatic and extrahepatic bile ducts. Later, the adult flukes penetrate the wall of the bile ducts and wander back into the liver parenchyma, where they feed on liver cells and deposit their eggs.

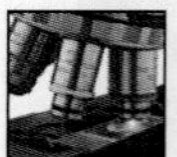 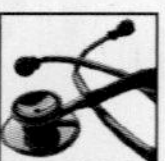

PATHOLOGY AND CLINICAL FEATURES: Eggs of *F. hepatica* lead to hepatic abscesses and granulomas. The worms induce hyperplasia of bile duct epithelium, portal and periductal fibrosis, proliferation of bile ductules and varying degrees of biliary obstruction. Eosinophilia, vomiting and acute gastric pain are characteristic. Severe untreated infections may be fatal. The diagnosis is made by recovering eggs from the stools or biliary tract.

Fasciolopsiasis Is an Infestation of the Small Intestine

Fasciolopsiasis is caused by the giant intestinal fluke, *Fasciolopsis buski*. The disease is common in the Orient. Humans are infected by eating aquatic vegetables contaminated with encysted cercariae. The worm is large (3 × 7 cm). It attaches to the duodenal or jejunal wall, which may ulcerate, become infected and cause pain like that of a peptic ulcer. Acute symptoms may also be due to intestinal obstruction or by toxins released by large numbers of worms. The diagnosis is made by identifying *F. buski* eggs in the stool. Treatment is with systemic antihelminthic agents.

Cestodes: Intestinal Tapeworms

Taenia saginata, Taenia solium and *Diphyllobothrium latum* are tapeworms that infect humans, growing to their adult forms within the intestine (Table 9-11). Presence of these adult worms rarely damages the human host.

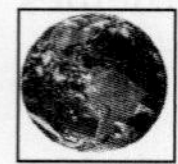

EPIDEMIOLOGY: Intestinal tapeworm infections are acquired by eating inadequately cooked beef (*T. saginata*), pork (*T. solium*) or fish (*D. latum*) containing larvae. Tapeworm life cycles involve cystic larval stages in animals and worm stages in the human. The life cycles of beef and pork tapeworms require that the animals ingest material tainted with infected human feces. The cystic larval forms develop in the animals' muscles. Modern cattle and pig farming practices, plus meat inspection, have largely eliminated beef and pork tapeworms in industrialized countries, but infection remains common in the underdeveloped world. Fish tapeworm infection is prevalent in areas where raw, pickled or partly cooked freshwater fish are common fare. Tapeworm infections are usually asymptomatic, although it may be distressing when an infected person passes portions of the worm in the stool. The fish tapeworm (*D. latum*) takes up vitamin B_{12} and a small number (<2%) of infected persons develop pernicious anemia (see Chapter 20).

Cysticercosis Is a Systemic Infection by the Larvae of the Pork Tapeworm

Adult *T. solium* is acquired by eating undercooked pork infected with cysticerci (measly pork).

ETIOLOGIC FACTORS: Pigs acquire cysticerci by ingesting eggs of *T. solium* in human feces. This cycle, although a public health concern, is essentially benign for both humans and pigs. However, when humans accidentally ingest tapeworm eggs from human feces and become infected with cysticerci, the consequences may be catastrophic. The eggs release oncospheres, which penetrate the gut wall, enter the bloodstream, lodge in tissue, encyst and differentiate to cysticerci.

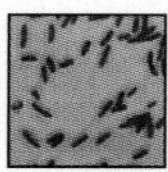

PATHOLOGY: The cysticercus is a spherical, milky white cyst about 1 cm in diameter containing fluid and an invaginated scolex (head of the worm) with birefringent hooklets. Cysts can remain viable for an indefinite period and provoke no inflammation; rather, as they grow they compress adjacent tissues. Degenerating cysts are the ones usually responsible for symptoms. They attach to tissue and are densely inflamed with eosinophils, neutrophils, lymphocytes and plasma cells. Multiple cysticerci in the brain may impart a "Swiss cheese" appearance to the tissue (Fig. 9-93).

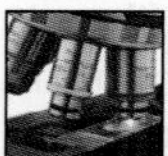

CLINICAL FEATURES: Cysticercosis of the brain manifests as headaches or seizures and symptoms depend on the sites affected. Massive cerebral cysticercosis causes convulsions and death. Cysticerci in the retina blind the patient. In the heart, they may cause arrhythmias and sudden death. Depending on the site involved, cysticercosis is treated with surgery or antihelminthic therapy.

Table 9-11

Tapeworm Infections

Species	Human Disease	Source of Human Infection
Taenia saginata	Adult tapeworm in intestine	Beef
Taenia solium	Adult tapeworm in intestine; cysticercosis	Pork; human feces
Diphyllobothrium latum	Adult tapeworm in intestine	Fish
Echinococcus granulosus	Hydatid cyst disease	Dog feces

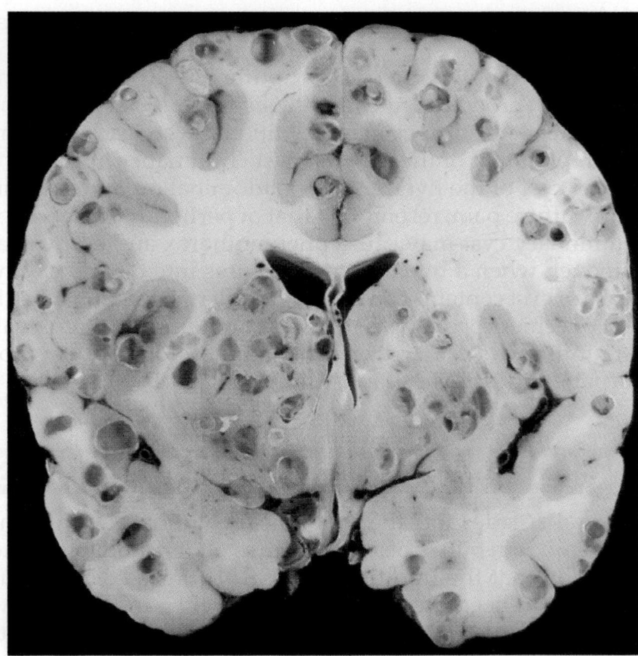

FIGURE 9-93. Cysticercosis. A cross-section of the brain from a patient infected with the larvae of *Taenia solium* shows many cysticerci in the gray matter, imparting a "Swiss cheese" appearance.

Echinococcosis Features Cysts of the Liver and Lungs

Echinococcosis (hydatid disease) is a zoonotic infection caused by larval cestodes of the genus *Echinococcus*. The most common offender is *Echinococcus granulosus,* which causes cystic hydatid disease. Rarely, *Echinococcus multilocularis* and *Echinococcus vogeli* infect humans.

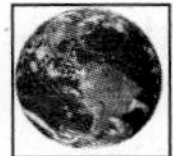

EPIDEMIOLOGY: Infestation with the tapeworm *E. granulosus* is endemic in sheep, goats and cattle as well as their attendant dogs. Dogs contaminate their habitats (and their human keepers) with infectious eggs. Humans become infected when they inadvertently ingest the tapeworm eggs. The resulting hydatid disease is present worldwide among herding populations who live in close proximity to dogs and herd animals, especially Australia, New Zealand, Argentina, Greece and herding countries of Africa and the Middle East. In the United States, hydatid cyst disease is seen among immigrants and among the indigenous sheep-herding populations of the southwest.

E. multilocularis causes alveolar hydatid disease in humans. Dogs and cats are domestic definitive hosts; the domestic intermediate host is the house mouse. Rare infections by *E. multilocularis* have been reported in Germany, Switzerland, China and the republics of the former Soviet Union.

Dogs are definitive hosts for *E. vogeli*. Humans may become accidental intermediate hosts for *E. vogeli* by ingesting eggs shed by domestic dogs. Polycystic hydatid disease caused by *E. vogeli* has been reported in Central and South America.

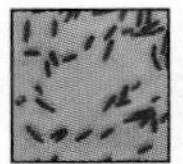

ETIOLOGIC FACTORS: The adult tapeworms (2 to 6 mm long) live in the small intestines of carnivorous hosts (e.g., wolves, foxes, etc.; Fig. 9-94). *E. granulosus* has a scolex with suckers and numerous hooklets to attach to

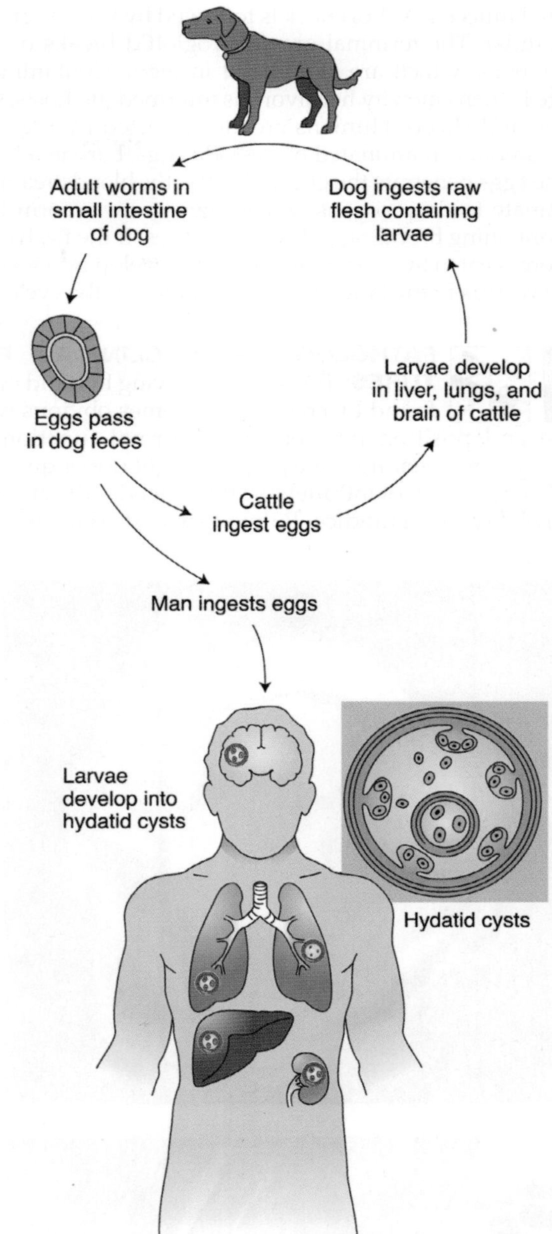

FIGURE 9-94. Life cycle of *Echinococcus granulosus* and cystic hydatid disease. The adult cestode lives in the small intestine of a dog (the definitive host). A gravid proglottid ruptures, releasing cestode eggs into the dog's feces. Cestode eggs are ingested by cattle or sheep (the intermediate hosts), hatch in the intestine and release oncospheres that penetrate the wall of the gut, enter the bloodstream, disseminate to various deep organs and grow to form hydatid cysts, containing brood capsules and scolices. When another dog ingests raw flesh from the cattle or sheep, the scolices are ingested and develop into mature worms in the dog's intestine to complete the cycle. A person who ingests cestode eggs in contaminated plant material becomes an accidental intermediate host. The larvae increase in size, but the parasite reaches a "dead end" without developing into an adult tapeworm. Hydatid cysts in humans occur predominantly in the liver but may also involve lung, kidney, brain and other organs.

intestinal mucosa. A short neck is followed by three segments (proglottids). The terminal gravid proglottid breaks off and releases eggs, which are eliminated in feces. Contaminated herbage is then eaten by herbivorous intermediate hosts, such as cattle and sheep. Humans are also infected by ingesting plant material contaminated by cestode eggs. Larvae released from the eggs penetrate the gut wall, enter the bloodstream and disseminate to deep organs, where they grow to form large cysts containing brood capsules and scolices. If the flesh of the herbivore is eaten by a carnivore, scolices develop into sexually mature worms in the latter, thereby completing the cycle.

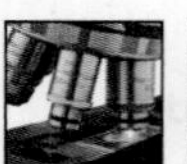
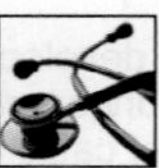

PATHOLOGY AND CLINICAL FEATURES: The slowly growing hydatid cyst is found by chance or becomes obvious when its size and position interfere with normal functions. A hepatic cyst may manifest as a palpable right upper quadrant mass. Compression of intrahepatic bile ducts by the cyst may lead to obstructive jaundice. Pulmonary cysts (Fig. 9-95) are often asymptomatic and discovered incidentally on a chest radiograph.

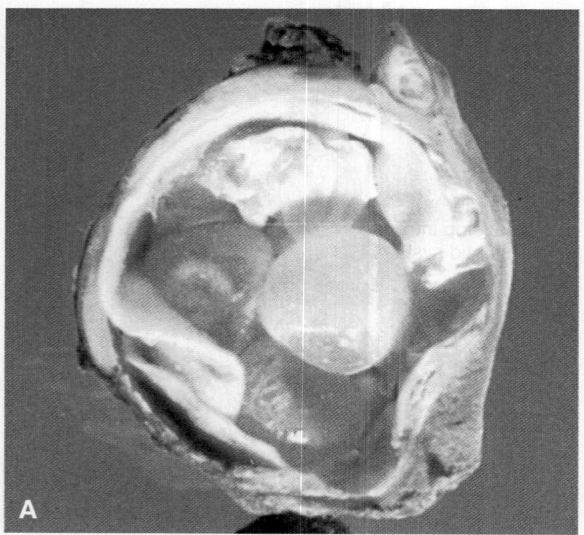

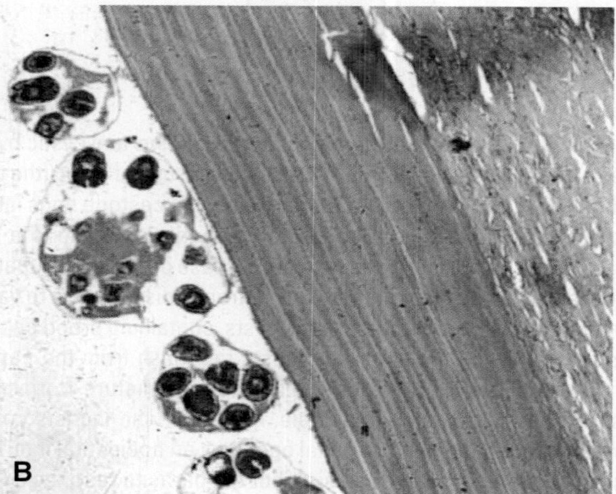

FIGURE 9-95. Echinococcal cyst. A. An echinococcal cyst showing daughter cysts was resected from the liver of a patient infected with *Echinococcus granulosus.* **B.** A photomicrograph of the cyst wall shows (*from right to left*) a laminated, nonnuclear layer, a nucleated germinal layer with brood capsules attached and numerous scolices in the cyst cavity.

A major complication of cyst rupture is seeding of adjacent tissues with brood capsules and scolices. When these "seeds" germinate, they produce many additional cysts, each with the growth potential of the original cyst. Traumatic rupture of a hydatid cyst of the liver or other abdominal organ results in severe diffuse pain, resembling that of peritonitis. Rupture of a pulmonary cyst may cause pneumothorax and empyema. Moreover, when a hydatid cyst ruptures into a body cavity, release of cyst contents can cause fatal allergic reactions. Treatment of echinococcal cysts requires careful surgical removal: cysts must be sterilized with formalin before drainage or extirpation to prevent intraoperative anaphylactic shock.

EMERGING AND REEMERGING INFECTIONS

Several decades ago, the antibiotic revolution, vaccinations and modern public health measures understandably led to the notion that the traditional global scourges of infectious diseases had been brought to bay. However, in the last few decades we have witnessed reemergence of microbial threats including resurgent well-known agents (e.g., cholera, dengue fever, influenza, anthrax), as well as previously unknown pathogens. Antibiotic resistance among organisms, particularly communicable ones, such as tuberculosis, presents a new set of challenges.

Equally important has been the discovery of new pathogens belonging to all classes: viruses, bacteria, parasites and fungi. AIDS and hepatitis C were unknown in the 1970s and alone have caused millions of deaths, despite therapeutic advances. The resilience of influenza virus as a pathogen is underscored by the global influenza pandemics (e.g., H1N1, H5N1).

Table 9-12 is a partial list of newly recognized human infections. It should serve as a reminder that the equilibrium between humans and the pathogens that confront them is a dynamic one: continuous vigilance is obligatory, and complacency invites disaster. The reader is referred to other sources for those infections not discussed above.

Agents of Biowarfare

Biological agents have been used as weapons since ancient times. The earliest documentation of use of biological weapons is described in Hittite texts from 1500 to 2000 BC, in which victims of plague were driven into enemy lands. The great Carthaginian warrior Hannibal first delivered bioweapons in 184 BC when, in preparing for a naval battle against King Eumenes of Pergamum, his army filled earthenware pots with serpents and hurled them to the decks of the Pergamene ships. In 1346, the Tatars lay siege to the Genoese-controlled seaport of Caffa (modern-day Feodosiya, Ukraine). During the siege, the Tatars were ravaged by plague. The Tatar leader catapulted his own dead soldiers, victims of the disease, into the besieged town to spread the epidemic, and forced the Genoese army to flee to Italy. Similar tactics were used at Karlstein in Bohemia in 1422 and by Russian troops in fighting Swedish forces in Reval in 1710.

Smallpox was used as a biological weapon by Francisco Pizarro in his conquest of South America in the 15th century when he presented variola-contaminated clothing as gifts.

Table 9-12

Examples of Recently Discovered and Emerging Infections

Year	Agent	Human Disease/Association
2010	*Listeria ivanovii*	Gastroenteritis and bacteremia
2009	*H1N1 "swine" influenza virus*	Pneumonia
2009	Human rhinovirus C (HRV-C)	Repiratory disease, pericarditis
2008	*Human parvovirus 4 (PARV4)*	Unknown
2008	*Merkel cell polyomavirus (MC PyV)*	Identified in Merkel cell carcinoma tissue
2007	*Segniliparus rugosus*	Respiratory disease
2007	*Mycobacterium massiliense*	Sepsis
2007	*Schineria larvae*	Human myiasis
2007	*Saffold virus*	Acute gastroenteritis
2007	*KI virus (KI PyV)*	Respiratory
2007	*WU virus (WU PyV)*	Respiratory
2006	*Rickettsia massiliae*	Rickettsial spotted fever
2006	*Mycobacterium tilburgii*	Multiorgan disease
2005	Coronavirus HCoV-HKU-1	Pneumonia
2005	*Rickettsia mongolotimonae*	Lymphangitis
2004	H5N1 "avian" influenza	Pneumonia
2004	Arcobacter spp.	Intestinal infection
2004	*Rickettsia parkeri*	Rickettsial spotted fever
2002	SARS-associated coronavirus	Severe atypical pneumonia (SARS-CoV)
2002	*Rickettsia aeschlimannii*	Rickettsial spotted fever
2000	*Rickettsia felis*	Rickettsial spotted fever
2000	Human metapneumovirus (hMPV)	Respiratory tract infection
1999	Nipah virus	Acute respiratory syndrome
1997	Alkhurma hemorrhagic fever virus	Saudi Arabian hemorrhagic fever
1997	*Rickettsia slovaca* (tickborne lymphadenopathy); TIBOLA	Lymph node enlargement
1996	*Rickettsia africae*	African tick bite fever
1995	New variant Creutzfeldt-Jakob Disease	Spongiform encephalopathy ("mad cow")
1994	Hendra virus	Acute respiratory syndrome
1994	Sabia virus	Brazilian hemorrhagic fever
1994	Human herpesvirus 8 (HHV8)	Kaposi sarcoma, body cavity lymphomas
1994	*Ehrlichia phagocytophilia*-like agent	Human granulocytic ehrlichiosis
1993	*Balamuthia mandrillaris*	Amebic meningoencephalitis
1993	*Cyclospora cayetanensis*	Coccidian diarrhea
1993	Sin nombre virus	Hantavirus pulmonary syndrome
1993	*Septata intestinalis* (now *Encephalitozoon intestinalis*)	Intestinal and disseminated microsporidiosis
1992	Vibrio cholerae 0139	Epidemic cholera
1992	*Bartonella henselae*	Bacillary angiomatosis, cat-scratch fever
1991	*Ehrlichia chaffeensis*	Human ehrlichiosis
1991	Guanarito virus	Venezuelan hemorrhagic fever
1991	*Encephalitozoon hellem*	Disseminated microsporidiosis
1990	*Anaplasma phagocytophilum*	Human granulocytic anaplasmosis
1990	*Haemophilus influenzae* biotype *aegyptius*	Brazilian purpuric fever

(*continued*)

Table 9-12

Examples of Recently Discovered and Emerging Infections (*Continued*)

Year	Agent	Human Disease/Association
1990	Human herpesvirus 7 (HHV7)	Aseptic meningitis
1989	*Pythium insidiosum*	Cutaneous and deep fungal infections
1989	*Chlamydia pneumoniae* (TWAR)	Respiratory infection
1989	Hepatitis C virus	Chronic hepatitis, cirrhosis, liver cancer
1989	Barmah Forest virus	Polyarthritis
1986	Human herpesvirus 6 (HHV6)	Roseola (Exanthema subitum)
1986	Porogia virus	Hemorrhagic fever/renal syndrome (HFRS)
1986	HIV-2	AIDS-like illness
1985	*Enterocytozoon bieneusi*	Intestinal and hepatobiliary microsporidiosis
1983	HIV-1	AIDS
1983	*Helicobacter pylori*	Gastric and duodenal infection, ulcers
1983	Hepatitis E virus	"Epidemic" non-A non-B hepatitis
1983	*Borrelia burgdorferi*	Lyme disease

AIDS = acquired immunodeficiency syndrome; HIV = human immunodeficiency virus; SARS = severe acute respiratory syndrome; SARS-CoV = severe acute respiratory syndrome-associated corona virus.

The English used a similar tactic in the French-Indian War in 1763, when Sir Jeffrey Amherst presented smallpox-laden blankets to the Delaware Indians loyal to the French. American colonists during the Revolutionary War also delivered smallpox to their adversaries. The colonists were immune to smallpox, as General George Washington had ordered mandatory vaccination. (Interestingly, this vaccination was achieved by variolation, in which smallpox pustules were inoculated into naive recipients, and differs from Jenner's vaccination.)

Allegations of biowarfare surfaced in World War I. The Germans were reported to spread cholera to Italy, plague to St. Petersburg and anthrax and glanders to the United States and elsewhere. Although the League of Nations following the war found no definite proof of any of these actions by Germany, the psychological impact of the potential use of biological weaponry in inducing terror was firmly established in modern times. The United States established Camp Detrick in Maryland in 1942–1943 to investigate biological weapons.

The 20th century has unfortunately witnessed many national bioweapons programs, mainly covert, and a few notorious for human experimentation. During the Sino-Japanese War, 1937 to 1945, Japanese Army Unit 731 conducted bioweapons experimentation on many thousands of Chinese civilians, as well as Russian and American prisoners of war. The Japanese Army used bioweapons during military campaigns against Chinese soldiers and civilians. In 1940, Japanese planes bombed Ningbo with ceramic bombs containing plague-infested fleas. It is estimated that 400,000 Chinese died as a direct result of this use of biological weapons.

Accidental biological contamination has also occurred. In 1942, Gruinard Island off the northwest coast of Scotland was rendered uninhabitable for almost 50 years after British field trials of anthrax. In 1979, accidental release of anthrax from a Sverdlovsk (now Yekaterinburg) military facility, Compound 19, was perhaps the largest biological weapons accident known; sheep developed anthrax 200 km from the release point and over 60 people died.

There is legitimate fear in modern times over the use of bioweapons as a terrorist tool. In September 1984, an outbreak of *Salmonella* gastroenteritis was caused by followers of the Indian guru Bagwan Shree Rajneesh in Oregon, infecting over 700 people. In 1993, an apocalyptic Japanese cult group sprayed anthrax spores from a high-rise building in Tokyo, but no one was injured. The same cult group was found to be preparing vast quantities of *C. difficile* spores for terrorist use. In 1995, the American Type Culture Collection (ATCC), a nonprofit organization that supplies biological specimens to scientists, shipped a package containing three vials of *Y. pestis* to the home of a political extremist in Ohio. A search of his home revealed a variety of explosive devices, detonating fuses and triggers. Most recently, dried anthrax was mailed in letters through the U.S. postal system, causing five deaths.

Only a few biological agents have been considered or proven to be effective as weapons of biowarfare or bioterrorism (Table 9-13). Key factors that make an infectious agent suitable for large-scale biowarfare include (1) ease of large-scale production; (2) ability to cause death or incapacity of humans at doses that are deliverable; (3) appropriate particle size as an aerosol; (4) ease of dissemination; (5) stability during storage, in the environment or placement into a delivery system; and (6) susceptibility of intended victims, but nonsusceptibility of friendly forces. Some biological weapons are potentially extremely lethal: 1 g of purified botulinum toxin could kill 10 million people.

Extraterrestrial Microbial Organisms

An important concern since the early years of space programs has been the possibility of introducing extraterrestrial infectious agents when an astronaut or space vehicle returns

Table 9-13

Potential Biological Agents of Warfare and Bioterror

Bacteria
Bacillus anthracis
Brucella abortus, Brucella suis, Brucella melitensis
Listeria monocytogenes
Vibrio cholerae
Rickettsia prowazekii, Rickettsia rickettsii
Burkholderia mallei, Burkholderia pseudomallei
Coxiella burnetii, Francisella tularensis, Yersinia pestis
Clostridium botulinum and botulinum neurotoxin-producing species of *Clostridium*
Viruses
Arenaviruses—Lassa, Machupo, Sabia, Junin, Guanarito
Bunyaviruses—Rift Valley fever virus, Congo-Crimean hemorrhagic fever virus
Filoviruses—Ebolavirus, Marburg virus
Flaviviruses—Kyasanur forest disease
Influenza
Kumlinge, Omsk hemorrhagic fever, Russian spring-summer encephalitis, tick-borne encephalitis
Poxviruses—smallpox (Variola) and monkeypox
Togaviruses—Eastern equine encephalitis virus
Venezuelan equine encephalitis virus
Biological Toxins
Botulinum, *Clostridium perfringens* ε toxin
Staphylococcal enterotoxin B
Shigatoxin
Conotoxins
Abrin
Ricin
Tetrodotoxin
Saxitoxin
T-2 toxin
Diacetoxyscirpenol
Microcystins
Aflatoxins
Satratoxin H
Palytoxin
Anatoxin A

to Earth. As a result, lunar samples brought back to Earth by Apollo astronauts in 1969 and subsequent missions were quarantined, as were the astronauts themselves. A NASA Lunar Receiving Laboratory was developed for that purpose. Quarantine is being planned by U.S., European and Russian space agencies for a manned mission to Mars to occur in the next few decades. In addition, Mars must be protected from contamination by Earth microbes (**forward contamination**) in order to preserve its indigenous martian life forms, if any, for future study as well as to protect the indigenous extraterrestrial biosphere from devastation by Earth's bacteria. Another danger is that extraterrestrial microbes accidentally brought back from Mars in the martian samples might be introduced into the Earth's biosphere (**back-contamination**). The purpose of quarantine upon return from a voyage to Mars is the protection of the Earth from microbial back-contamination. A number of organisms living on Earth under extreme environmental conditions, "extremophiles," are being studied as possible analogues of microbes that could live in the harsh lunar and martian environments. Of course, extraterrestrial microbes may have originated on Earth, flung into space by ancient meteoric impacts. Given their possible pre-evolutionary origin, their pathogenicity for modern-day terrestrials cannot be dismissed.

10 Blood Vessels

Avrum I. Gotlieb • Amber Liu

Structure of Blood Vessels

Arteries Include Conducting and Resistance Vessels

The vascular portion of the circulatory system is composed of a variety of blood vessel compartments that are categorized by size, structure and function. These include arteries, which are conducting and resistance vessels; capillaries; and veins (Fig. 10-1).

Elastic Arteries

The largest blood vessels in the body, the aorta and the elastic arteries, are conduits for blood flow to smaller arterial branches and are composed of three layers:

- **Tunica intima:** This consists of a single layer of endothelial cells, a subendothelial compartment containing a few smooth muscle cells and connective tissue extending to the luminal side of the internal elastic lamina. The aortic intima is thicker than the other elastic arteries and contains

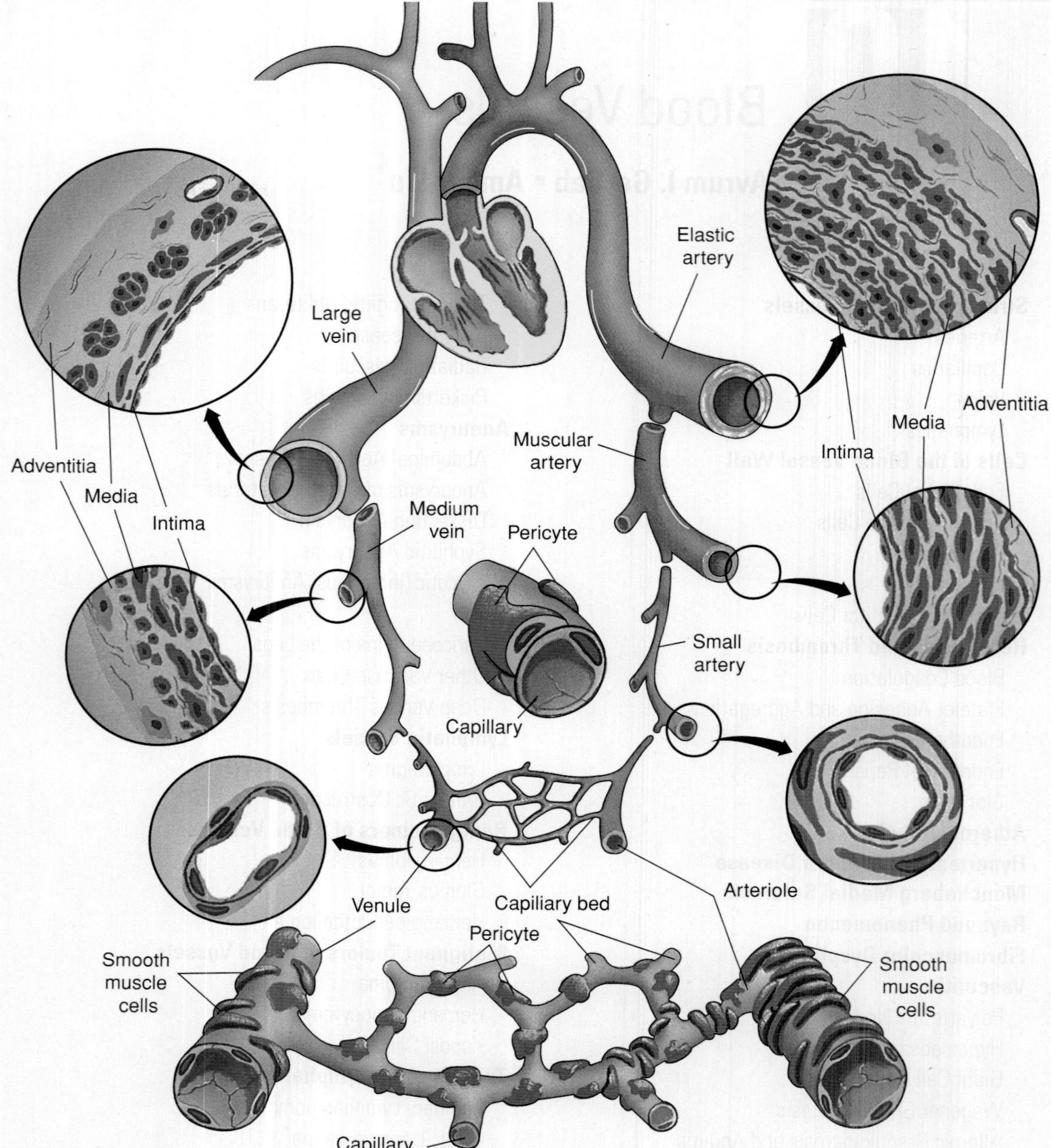

FIGURE 10-1. Subdivisions and histologic structure of the vascular system. Each subdivision is subject to a set of pathologic changes conditioned by the structure–function relationship of that part of the system. For example, the aorta, an elastic artery subject to great pressure, frequently shows a pathologic dilation (aneurysm) if the supporting elastic media is damaged. Muscular arteries are the most significant sites of atherosclerosis. Small arteries, particularly arterioles, are sites of hypertensive changes. Capillary beds, venules and veins each display their own types of pathologic changes.

matrix proteins including collagen, proteoglycans and small amounts of elastin. Occasional resident lymphocytes, macrophages and other blood-derived inflammatory cells are also normally present.

- **Tunica media:** The next layer outward is the tunica media, the thickest tunica. It is bounded by internal and external elastic laminae and itself displays numerous elastic laminae and smooth muscle cells within an extracellular connective tissue matrix. In the aorta, the media is organized into lamellar units each consisting of two concentric elastic laminae with smooth muscle cells and their associated matrix in between the laminae. The media of the thoracic aorta contains more elastin and the abdominal aorta more collagen. In elastic arteries, elastic fibers are interposed between smooth muscle cells and serve to minimize energy loss during the pressure changes between systole and diastole.

In smaller elastic arteries nutrition for the media is provided by diffusion from the blood vessel lumen. Nutrients traverse the endothelium and the layers of smooth muscle. However, blood vessels with more than 28 layers of smooth muscle cells have a vasculature of their own, the **vasa vasorum.** These small vessels arise from the visceral and parietal branches of the aorta and both form a superficial plexus at the adventitia–media border and penetrate into the outer two thirds of the media. The tunica media also contains autonomic nerve fibers that influence vascular contractility.

- **Tunica adventitia:** The most external vessel wall layer contains fibroblasts, connective tissue, nerves and small vessels that give rise to the vasa vasorum. Occasional inflammatory cells, including collections of lymphocytes, may also be present in the adventitia.

Muscular Arteries

Blood conducted by the elastic arteries is distributed to individual organs through large muscular arteries (Figs. 10-1 and 10-2). The tunica media of a muscular artery consists of layers of smooth muscle cells without prominent bands of elastin, although a prominent internal elastic lamina and usually an external elastic lamina are present. Fenestrae interrupt the continuity of the internal elastic lamina, permitting smooth muscle cells to migrate from the media into the intima. Lacking heavy elastin layers, muscular arteries contract more efficiently. The intima of muscular arteries, like that of the aorta, also contains small numbers of smooth muscle cells, connective tissue and occasional inflammatory cells. Vasa vasorum are present in the outer wall of the thicker muscular arteries but are not seen in the smaller ones. As the vascular tree branches further, the tunica media becomes thinner, and except for the endothelium, the tunica intima disappears.

The small muscular arteries are important regulators of blood flow. Their narrow lumens increase resistance, thereby reducing blood pressure to levels appropriate for exchange of water and plasma constituents across downstream thin-walled capillaries. The small muscular arteries, sometimes called **resistance vessels**, also maintain systemic pressure by regulating total peripheral resistance.

Arterioles

Arterioles are the smallest elements of the arterial system. They have an endothelial lining surrounded by one or two layers of smooth muscle cells. No elastic layers are evident. The smallest arterioles provide dynamic regulation of blood flow by vasomotion (change in the caliber of an artery), thus controlling the distribution of blood in the capillary tree.

Capillaries Permit Transport From the Blood to the Interstitium

In these smallest blood vessels, the endothelium is supported only by sparse smooth muscle cells. The capillary endothelium provides for exchange of solutes and cells between blood and extracellular fluid. A necessary feature of this exchange is a marked lowering of pressure, which prevents intravascular fluid from shifting into the extracellular space.

The capillary endothelium is a semipermeable membrane, in which exchange of plasma solutes with extracellular fluid is controlled by molecular size and charge. The permeability of capillaries depends on their endothelial cells. Brain capillaries are highly impermeable because junctions between endothelial cells are tightly sealed, preventing exchange of proteins across the vessel wall. Transport in other capillary beds is mediated either by passage of molecules through incomplete cell junctions or by pinocytosis, a process by which molecules traverse the cytoplasm through vesicular transport. Some investigators have suggested that vesicles are connected with each other to provide a channel for direct transport of plasma proteins across the cytoplasm. In some locations, the capillary endothelium itself may have permanent channels through endothelial cells or discontinuous gaps between them. Fenestrated capillaries in renal glomeruli are specifically adapted to filter plasma. Liver sinusoids, which are not true capillaries, also show a fenestrated endothelium, which permits free access of plasma to liver cells.

Veins Return Blood to the Heart

Venules are the first vessels to collect blood from capillaries. Their thin media is appropriate for a vessel that does not face high intraluminal pressures. Venules merge into small and medium-sized veins, which in turn converge into large veins. The walls of large veins do not display the characteristic elastic lamellae of elastic arteries; even the internal elastic lamina is well developed only in the largest veins. The media is thin and is virtually absent in the smaller tributaries. Many veins, particularly in the extremities, have valves, made of endothelial-lined folds of the tunica intima, that prevent backflow and help to move blood under the low pressure of the venous circulation. Postcapillary venules are the site of leukocyte transmigration into tissue in inflammatory reactions (see Chapter 2).

Lymphatics Drain Interstitial Fluid

Lymphatic circulation is composed of blind-ended lymphatic capillaries, consisting of (1) endothelium with no pericytes; (2) precollecting lymphatics; and (3) collecting lymphatics, which pump lymph toward the lymph nodes, lymphatic trunks and finally thoracic and right lymphatic ducts, which return lymph back to the blood. Filtrate from capillaries and venules enters the lymphatics, which act as a pathway to regional lymph nodes for cells, foreign material and microorganisms. The collecting lymphatics have an intrinsically contractile layer of smooth muscle cells that propel lymph forward. Intraluminal valves, as in veins, prevent backflow. Embryonic development and postnatal growth of lymphatics are regulated by vascular endothelial growth factors (VEGFs), platelet-derived growth factors (PDGFs) and angiopoietin 1 and 2.

Cells of the Blood Vessel Wall

The cells of the blood vessel wall have unique properties that are critical for a normal physiologic function and for the pathogenesis of vascular diseases.

A Single Layer of Endothelial Cells Comprises a Confluent Macromolecular Barrier

Endothelial cells are highly metabolically active and are intimately involved in several biological functions, including coagulation, platelet regulation, fibrinolysis, inflammation, immunoregulation and repair. They also modulate vascular smooth muscle cell function through paracrine pathways.

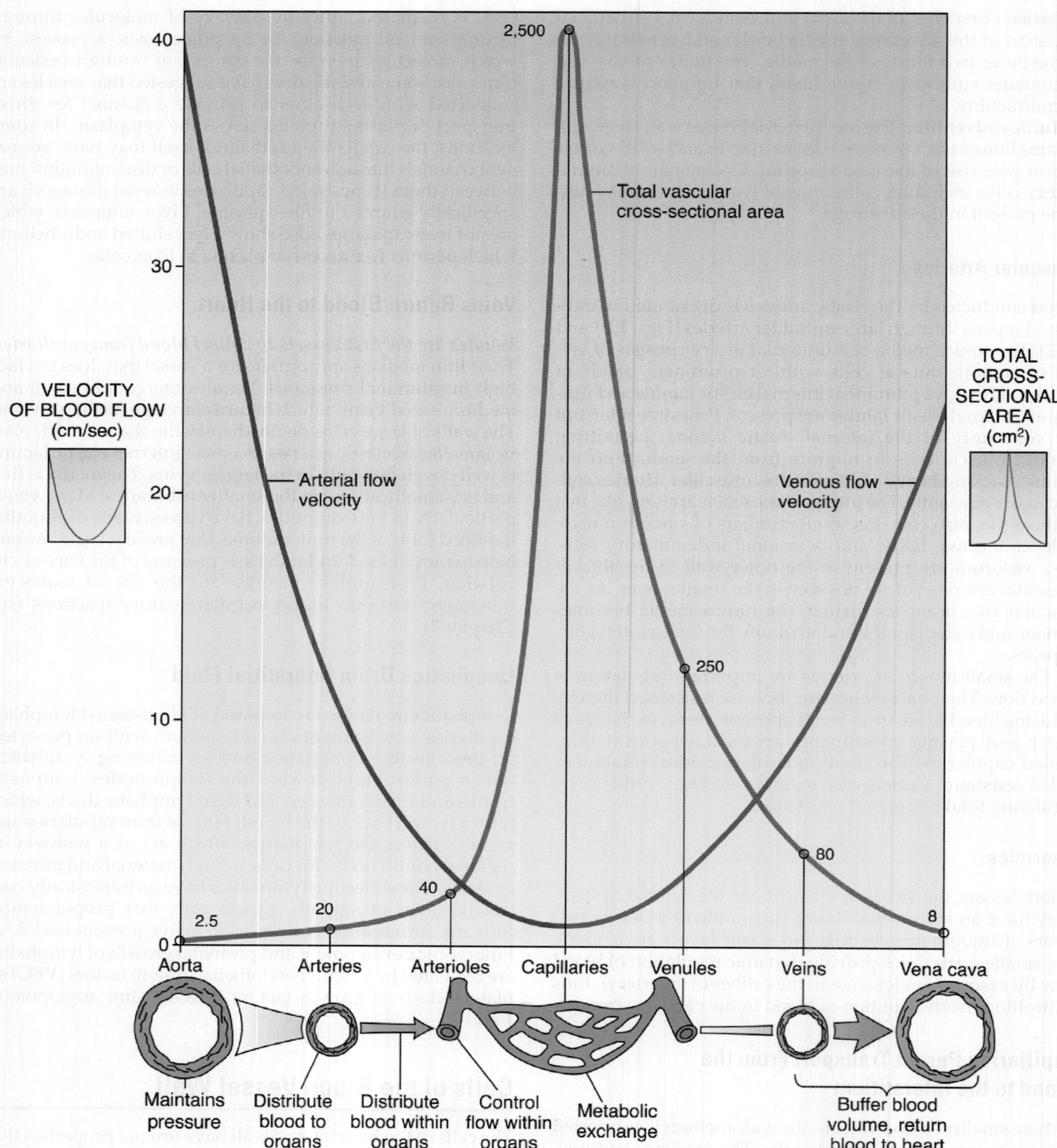

FIGURE 10-2. Relationship between velocity of blood flow and cross-sectional area in the vasculature. The vascular tree is a circuit that conducts blood from the heart through large-diameter, low-resistance conducting vessels to small arteries and arterioles, which lower blood pressure and protect the capillaries. The capillaries are thin walled and allow the exchange of nutrients and waste products between tissue and blood, a process that requires a very large surface area. The circuit back to the heart is completed by the veins, which are distensible and provide a volume buffer that acts as a capacitance for the vascular circuit.

Endothelial cells also form a unique mechanotransduction structure that modulates the effects of hemodynamic shear stress on the vessel wall. By virtue of mechanical sensing, endothelial cell membranes may deform, activating biochemical signaling and leading to expression of vasoactive compounds, growth factors, coagulation/fibrinolytic/complement factors, matrix degradation enzymes, inflammatory mediators and adhesion molecules.

Endothelium integrity depends on several types of adhesion complexes that promote cell–substratum and cell–cell adhesions (see Chapter 2).

- **Cell–substrate adhesion molecules** attach endothelial cells to their substratum (e.g., basal lamina). They complex with intracellular cytoskeleton, which participates in intracellular signal transduction. For example, integrins are heterodimeric transmembrane molecules that bind endothelial cells to extracellular matrix adhesive molecules, including laminin, fibronectin, fibrinogen, von Willebrand factor and thrombospondin. The cytoplasmic tails of the integrins bind the complex of proteins that regulate adhesion at focal contact sites and associate with actin microfilaments and microtubules of the cytoskeleton (Fig. 10-3).
- **Cell–cell adhesion molecules** attach one endothelial cell to its neighbor. Thus, cadherin is located at intercellular adhesion junctions and occludin at intercellular tight junctions. The cadherins are linked to the actin cytoskeleton by catenins.

Endothelial cells carry out a large variety of important metabolic functions (Table 10-1). Many of these functions are regulated by serum and hemodynamic factors, which activate surface receptors and signal transduction pathways and/or regulate gene transcription. Endothelial cells do not normally proliferate, but after vascular injury and loss of endothelial cells, they spread, migrate and proliferate rapidly to reestablish the structural integrity of the endothelium, and thus protect the wall from disease (Fig. 10-4).

Table 10-1

Functions of Endothelial Cells of the Blood Vessels

Functions of Endothelial Cells of the Blood Vessels
Permeability barrier
Vasoactive factors: Nitric oxide (EDRF), endothelin
Antithrombotic agent production: Prostacyclin (PGI_2), adenine metabolites
Anticoagulant production: Thrombomodulin, other proteins
Fibrinolytic agent production: Tissue plasminogen activator, urokinase-like factor, tissue factor pathway inhibitor
Procoagulant production: Tissue factor, plasminogen activator/inhibitor, factor V, factor VIIIa (von Willebrand factor)
Inflammatory mediator production: Interleukin-1, cell adhesion molecules
Receptors for factor IX, factor X, low-density lipoproteins, modified low-density lipoproteins, thrombin
Growth factor production: Blood cell colony-stimulating factors, insulin-like growth factors, fibroblast growth factor, platelet-derived growth factor
Growth inhibitor: Heparin
Replication

EDRF = endothelium-derived relaxing factor.

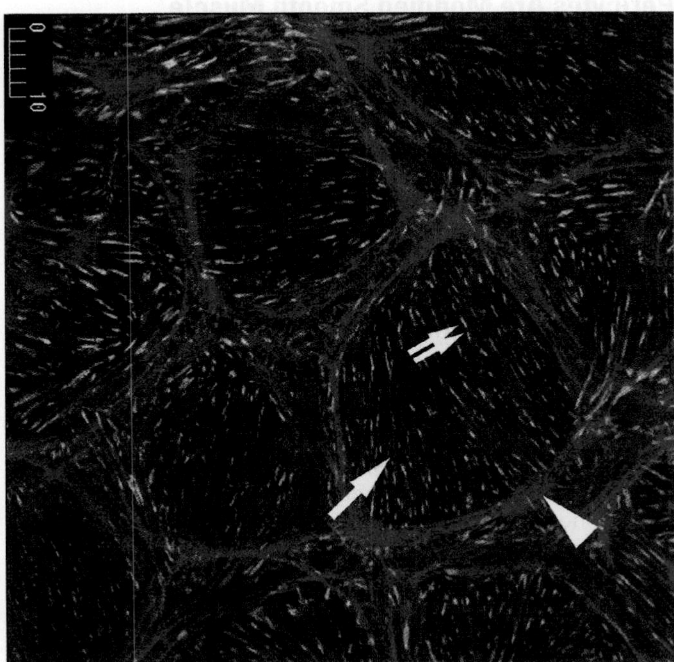

FIGURE 10-3. Focal adhesion protein, vinculin. Porcine aortic endothelial cells were grown to confluency and double-stained for actin/vinculin. Endothelial cells in confluent monolayers contain a dense peripheral band of actin microfilament bundles (*arrowhead*) and central microfilament or "stress fibers" (*single arrow*). Vinculin in confluent monolayer localizes to the tips of stress fibers (*double arrow*).

Endothelial cells release a number of biologically active factors when they are activated. Some of these potent bioactive molecules are released locally, act at short distances and are rapidly inactivated. For example, prostacyclin (PGI_2), derived from the cyclooxygenase (COX) pathway, relaxes smooth muscle and inhibits platelet aggregation. Endothelial nitric oxide synthase (NOS) converts L-arginine and O_2 to L-citrulline and nitric oxide (NO•). NO• inhibits platelet adhesion and aggregation. It also modulates vascular tone and vascular smooth muscle cell proliferation by increasing cyclic guanosine 3′,5′-monophosphate (cGMP), in turn activating cGMP-dependent protein kinase. NO• likely helps to control the muscular tone of large arteries and resistance vessels. After stimulation of endothelial cell receptors by agonists, prostacyclin and NO• are released and together inhibit platelet aggregation. Compounds that promote NO• release include acetylcholine, bradykinin and adenosine diphosphate (ADP). NO• is even more labile than prostacyclin, with a half-life of 6 seconds.

Vascular tone is also affected by a number of bioactive peptides. The **endothelins** are a family of potent vasoconstrictive proteins synthesized by endothelial cells. They bind two distinct receptor subtypes; both are found on smooth muscle cells, but only one on endothelial cells. The endothelial enzyme angiotensin-converting enzyme (ACE) converts angiotensin I to angiotensin II, a potent vasoconstrictor that is important in the pathogenesis of hypertension.

Endothelial cell–derived factors also control some immune responses. Like macrophages, endothelial cells express

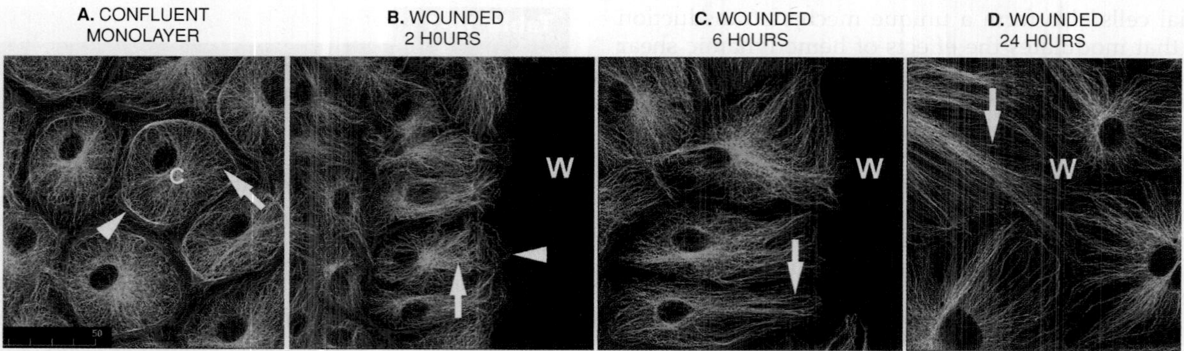

FIGURE 10-4. Remodeling in response to loss of endothelial integrity. Porcine aortic endothelial cells were grown to confluency, and a 1-mm wound was created using a scraper. Cells were fixed and double-stained for actin/tublin at 2, 6, and 24 hours after wounding. **A.** Endothelial cells in confluent monolayers contain a dense peripheral band (DPB) of actin microfilament bundles (*arrowhead*) and centrosomes (C) toward the cell periphery. **B.** Two hours after wounding, there is formation of lamellipodia (*arrowhead*), and stress fibers (*arrow*) rearrange to become parallel to the wound edge (W). Centrosomes migrate around the nucleus toward the wound edge, and the microtubules begin emanating toward the wound (W). **C.** By 6 hours, changes in microtubules and microfilaments are more prominent, the microtubule/microfilaments are more prominent, and the microtubule–microfilament networks (*arrow*) begin to reorganize perpendicular to the wound edge (W) as the cells begin to spread. **D.** 24 hours after wounding, the microtubule–microfilament networks (*arrow*) are aligned perpendicular to the wound edge (W) as the cells migrate into the wound.

class II histocompatibility antigens when stimulated. They may thus work with monocytes—or even replace them—in activating lymphocytes. Immune responses to endothelial cells are a major part of organ rejection following transplantation and play a role in the pathogenesis of graft arteriosclerosis.

Smooth Muscle Cells Maintain Blood Vessel Integrity

Vascular smooth muscle cells are derived from local mesoderm after endothelial tubes are formed (Fig. 10-5). However, the smooth muscle cells of major arteries in the upper part of the body are derived from neural crest. Thus, vascular smooth muscle cell structural and functional diversity has a developmental basis and may have pathogenetic implications for diseases of the adult vascular system.

Smooth muscle cells maintain blood vessel integrity and provide support for endothelium. They control blood flow by contracting or dilating in response to specific stimuli. Smooth muscle cells synthesize the connective tissue matrix of the vessel wall, which includes elastin, collagen and proteoglycans as well as proteolytic enzymes and their inhibitors for tissue remodeling and repair. In normal arteries, smooth muscle cells rarely divide. Rather, like endothelial cells, they proliferate in response to injury, and are important in the pathogenesis of atherosclerotic plaques. Smooth muscle cells are major producers of the growth factors, cytokines and chemokines involved in atherogenesis.

Leukocytes Enter Vessel Walls and Are Important in Atherosclerosis

Macrophages and lymphocytes, in particular, promote vascular disease. Atherosclerosis (see below) may be considered to be an inflammatory disease in which monocyte-derived macrophages are very important. T lymphocytes are present in the adventitia in normal arteries and are increased in number in atherosclerotic plaques. Dendritic cells are found in intimal atherosclerotic lesions and adventitial leukocytes are organized into clusters similar to lymphoid tissue in areas beneath plaques. Polymorphonuclear leukocytes are important in acute vasculitis, and T cells in acute and chronic vasculitis.

Pericytes Are Modified Smooth Muscle Cells That Surround Capillaries

They are in close contact with endothelial cells, and both share the same basement membrane. The functions of pericytes are largely unknown. They may be contractile or regulate the function and proliferation of adjacent endothelial cells. The capillary adventitia merges with, and is indistinguishable from, the surrounding connective tissue.

Vacular Progenitor/Stem Cells Regulate Vasculogenesis

The discovery of vascular progenitor/stem cells has aided our understanding of blood vessel injury and repair. Several types of progenitor/stem cells have been identified. **Endothelial progenitor cells** (EPCs) are bone marrow–derived cells arising from perinatal hemangioblasts, and are present in adult bone marrow and peripheral circulation. EPCs are identified by their expression of CD133, CD34, c-kit, VEGFR-2, CD144 and Sca-1. They are multipotent immature cells that can proliferate, migrate and differentiate into endothelial cells. Unlike mature endothelial cells, they express CD133, but not endothelial cadherin or von Willebrand factor. The presence of circulating EPCs in adults suggests that new blood vessel growth in adults occurs by **vasculogenesis**, not only by **angiogenesis** as previously thought (angiogenesis refers to the sprouting of new capillaries from existing blood vessels, whereas vasculogenesis is the differentiation of angioblasts [precursor cells] into endothelial cells that form a vascular network de novo). Vasculogenesis, present in the developing

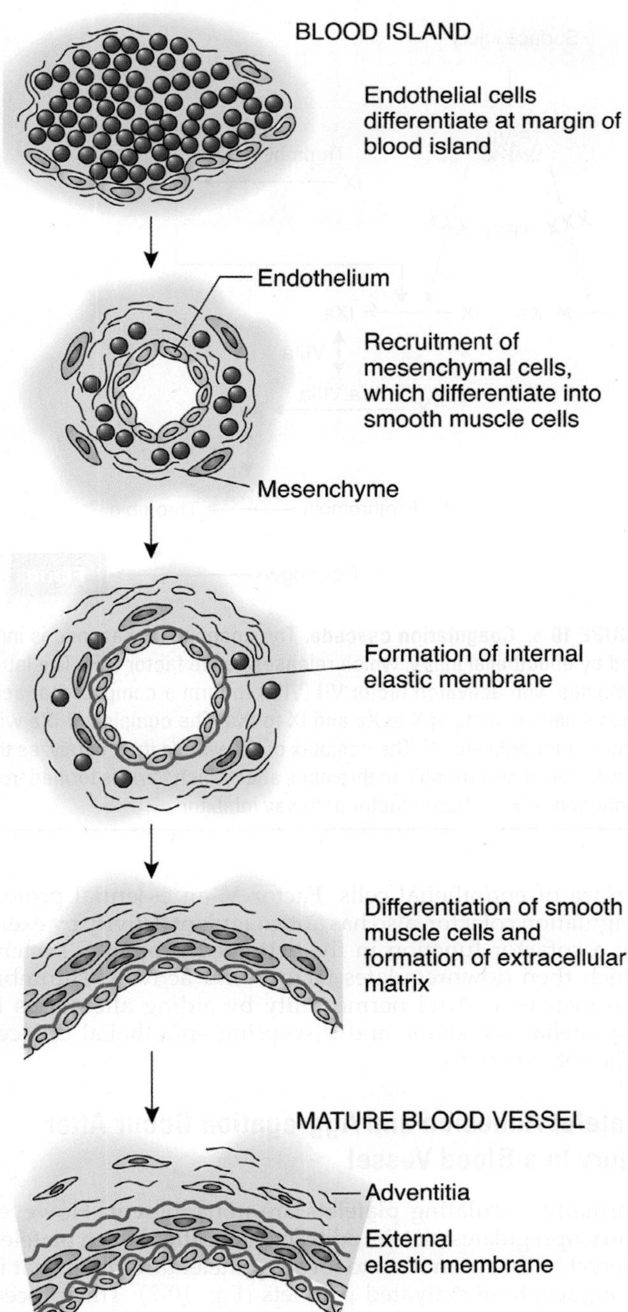

FIGURE 10-5. Differentiation of vessels in early embryos. The course of events from the development of blood islands on the chorioallantoic membrane starts with differentiation of endothelium and proceeds to fully developed arteries and veins.

embryo, reappears in adults when EPCs are mobilized and recruited to regions of new blood vessel formation. Embryonic and adult vasculogenesis show many similarities, suggesting that initiating stimuli and regulatory pathways for both are similar.

The number and migratory activity of circulating EPCs are decreased in patients with stable coronary artery disease and are inversely correlated with the number of risk factors in coronary artery disease patients. EPC proliferation in patients with type 2 diabetes mellitus is significantly less than in controls, and EPCs from subjects at high risk for cardiovascular events senesce in culture more readily than do cells from subjects at low risk. These findings suggest that EPCs may be sensitive indicators of increased risk of vascular disease, especially atherosclerosis.

EPCs have been the subject of intense experimental and clinical investigation due to their therapeutic potential in cardiovascular regeneration. EPC transplantation to promote collateral circulation is an innovative therapy to treat tissue ischemia. Blood EPCs from healthy humans can differentiate into endothelial cells and improve blood supply in experimentally injured limbs, and contribute to neovascularization following experimental myocardial infarction. EPC therapy also inhibited left ventricular fibrosis and preserved left ventricular function.

In addition, EPCs can contribute to maintaining patency of blood vessels after therapeutic stenting. Technologies designed to capture EPCs, such as incorporating anti-CD34 antibody into stents, has shown promise in delaying or preventing restenosis of implanted stents. Therefore, the discovery of adult circulating EPCs may both improve our understanding of blood vessel injury and repair and contribute to the treatment of vascular compromise.

Hemostasis and Thrombosis

Hemostasis is an exquisitely controlled physiologic process initiated to arrest hemorrhage by forming a blood clot. It is a response to vascular injury and involves local vasoconstriction, tissue swelling, coagulation, platelet adhesion, aggregation and activation, resulting in a hemostatic plug extending intravascularly and extravascularly at sites of injury.

Thrombosis is a pathologic process leading to formation of a blood clot, or thrombus, within the circulation. A thrombus is an aggregate of coagulated blood that contains platelets, fibrin, leukocytes and red blood cells. Its formation involves a "tug of war" between those factors that favor clotting and those that inhibit it. ***Thrombi are formed when antithrombotic systems fail to balance prothrombotic processes.*** Thrombosis involves (1) activation of platelets, (2) activation of coagulation pathways, (3) participation of the monocyte/macrophage system and (4) active involvement of the endothelial cells of the vessel wall.

Coagulation can be induced in vitro in a test tube by activation of the coagulation cascade. In vivo hemostasis involves the coagulation network of activating and inactivating enzymes, and cofactors derived from different cells and tissues, some circulating and some locally produced (Table 10-2). Disorders of hemostasis are discussed in detail in Chapters 7 and 20.

Blood Coagulation Occurs When Fibrinogen Is Converted to Fibrin

The endpoint of coagulation of blood is the conversion of soluble plasma fibrinogen to an insoluble fibrillar polymer–fibrin, a reaction catalyzed by the serine protease enzyme thrombin. This process must be carefully controlled to prevent a massive activation of the system and extensive clotting throughout the entire circulation. A series of finely tuned steps is mediated by a number of coagulation factors (Table 10-2), many of which are restricted by specific inhibitors. This

Table 10-2

Coagulation Factor Designations

Factor	Standard Name
I	Fibrinogen
II	Prothrombin
III	Tissue factor
IV	Calcium ions
V	Proaccelerin
VII	Proconvertin
VIII	Antihemophilic factor (AHF)
IX	Plasma thromboplastin (PTC)
X	Stuart factor
XI	Plasma thromboplastin antecedent (PTA)
XII	Hageman factor
XIII	Fibrin-stabilizing factor (FSF)
–	Prekallikrein
–	High-molecular-weight kininogen

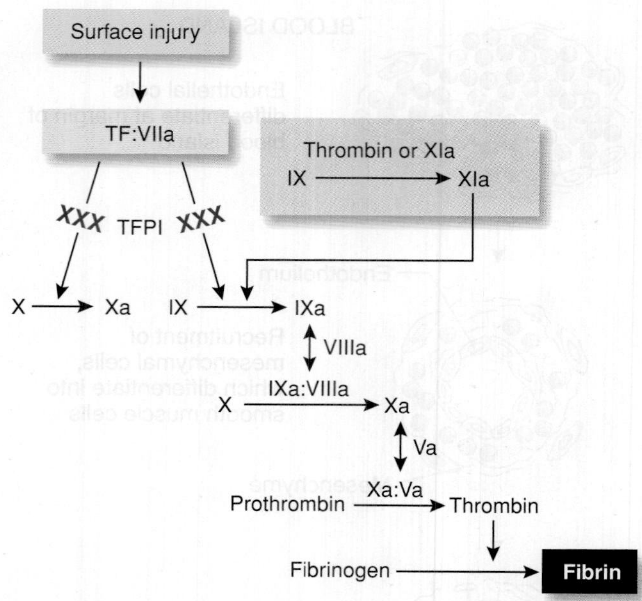

FIGURE 10-6. Coagulation cascade. The coagulation cascade is initiated by endothelial injury, which releases tissue factor (TF). The latter combines with activated factor VII (VIIa) to form a complex that activates small amounts of X to Xa and IX to IXa. The complex of IXa with VIIIa further activates X. The complex of Xa with Va then catalyzes the conversion of prothrombin to thrombin, after which fibrin is formed from fibrinogen. TFPI = tissue factor pathway inhibitor.

coagulation cascade amplifies an initial signal into the eventual generation of thrombin, production of which is key to progression and stabilization of a thrombus. For example, one molecule of an upstream coagulation factor, factor Xa, generates about 1000 molecules of thrombin.

Historically, the coagulation cascade was divided into the "intrinsic" pathway, now called the **contact activation pathway**, and the "extrinsic" pathway, now called **the tissue factor pathway**. However, this dichotomy does not accurately reflect the primary mechanisms of clotting, and the intrinsic contact activation pathway plays a minor role in coagulation.

The current view of coagulation (Fig. 10-6) highlights the importance of **tissue factor** (TF), a membrane-bound glycoprotein. The dynamic association of factor VIIa–TF complexes with TF pathway inhibitor (TFPI) is crucial to thrombosis. TFPI inhibits initiation of coagulation by binding TF–FXa–FVIIa complex. A major pool of TFPI on the surface of endothelial cells thus probably regulates coagulation. Hemostasis starts when activated factor VII (VIIa) encounters TF at a site of injury, forming the TF–VIIa complex. This complex activates small amounts of factors IX and X to IXa and Xa. Activation of larger amounts of X to Xa is promoted by factors VIIIa and IXa. Xa converts small amounts of prothrombin to thrombin, and these traces of thrombin catalyze activation of factor XI, which in turn augments conversion of factor IX to IXa. The IXa and VIIIa complex generates more factor Xa from X. In the presence of calcium, this Xa binds Va to form the **prothrombinase complex** on phospholipids from platelet membranes. This complex then catalyzes activation of the inactive zymogen prothrombin to thrombin. Thrombin converts fibrinogen to fibrin monomers, which form polymers. Thrombin also activates factor XIII to factor XIIIa, forming cross-linked fibrin strands to stabilize the clot.

Besides its important role in coagulation and platelet aggregation, thrombin participates in production of fibrinolytic molecules and regulation of growth factors and leukocyte adhesion molecules. It also mediates the protein C anticoagulant pathway by binding thrombomodulin at the surface of endothelial cells. Factor V, an essential protein coagulation cofactor, also has anticoagulant activity by exerting a cofactor function in the activated protein C system, which then downregulates factor VIIIa activity. Thrombin also increases vessel permeability by aiding alterations in endothelial cell shape and disrupting endothelial cell–cell adhesion junctions.

Platelet Adhesion and Aggregation Occur After Injury to a Blood Vessel

Normally, circulating platelets are nonadherent. However, injury upregulates platelet adhesiveness, after which platelets interact with one another to form a platelet thrombus, that is, an aggregate of activated platelets (Fig. 10-7). This process requires changes in platelet shape that reflect reorganization of actin microfilaments. Several molecules may promote platelet aggregation including thrombin, collagen, ADP, epinephrine, thromboxane A_2, platelet-activating factor (PAF) and vasopressin. Platelet aggregates occlude injured small vessels and prevent leakage of blood.

Once platelets are stimulated to adhere to a vessel wall, their granular contents are released, in part by contraction of the platelet cytoskeleton. These granules promote aggregation of other platelets. Platelet adhesion is enhanced by release of subendothelial von Willebrand factor, which is adhesive for glycoprotein (Gp) Ib platelet membrane protein and for fibrinogen. Activated platelets also release ADP and thromboxane A_2, a product of arachidonic acid metabolism, which recruit additional platelets to the process. The platelet membrane protein complex GpIIb–IIIa binds fibrinogen to form fibrinogen bridges between platelets, enhance aggregation and

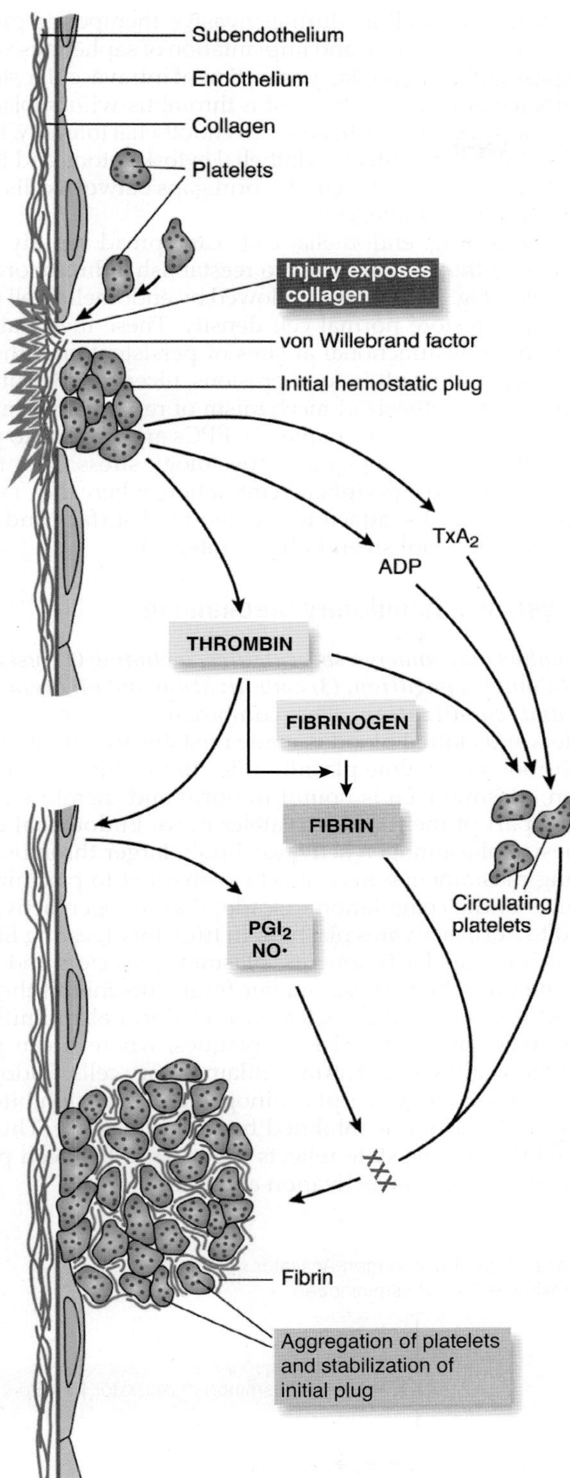

FIGURE 10-7. The role of platelets in thrombosis. Following vessel wall injury and alteration in flow, platelets adhere and then aggregate. Adenosine diphosphate (ADP) and thromboxane A_2 (TxA_2) are released and, along with locally generated thrombin, recruit additional platelets, causing the mass to enlarge. The growing platelet thrombus is stabilized by fibrin. Other elements, including leukocytes and red blood cells, are also incorporated into the thrombus. The release of prostacyclin (PGI_2) and nitric oxide (NO•) by endothelial cells regulates the process by inhibiting platelet aggregation.

stabilize the nascent thrombus. Activated platelets in turn release factors that initiate coagulation, thus forming a complex thrombus on the vessel wall. Thrombin itself stimulates further release of platelet granules and subsequent recruitment of new platelets.

Endothelial Cells Make Factors That Regulate Procoagulant and Anticoagulant Processes

Endothelium-derived modulators of coagulation are listed in Table 10-3. Endothelial cells produce and secrete **PGI_2**, which inhibits platelet aggregation. Endothelial NO• strongly inhibits platelet aggregation and adhesion to the vessel wall. Endothelial cells metabolize ADP, a strong promoter of thrombogenesis, to antithrombogenic metabolites. The luminal surface of the endothelium is coated with heparan sulfate, which binds a number of clotting factors, including the antiprotease β_2-macroglobulin. Endothelial heparan sulfate activates antithrombin, which binds to several coagulation factors, IIa, IXa, Xa, Xia and XIIa, which are free and not

Table 10-3

Regulation of Coagulation at the Endothelial Cell Surface

Downregulation

1. Thrombin inactivators
   a. Antithrombin III
   b. Thrombomodulin
2. Activated protein C pathway
   a. Synthesis and expression of thrombomodulin
   b. Synthesis and expression of protein S
   c. Thrombomodulin-mediated activation of protein C
   d. Inactivation of factor V_a and factor VIII_a by APC–protein S complex
3. Tissue factor pathway inhibition
4. Fibrinolysis
   a. Synthesis of tissue plasminogen activator, urokinase plasminogen activator, and plasminogen activator inhibitor-1
   b. Conversion of Glu-plasminogen to Lys-plasminogen
   c. APC-mediated potentiation
5. Synthesis of unsaturated fatty acid metabolites
   a. Lipoxygenase metabolites—13-HODE
   b. Cyclooxygenase metabolites—PGI_2 and PGE_2

Procoagulant Pathways

1. Synthesis and expression of:
   a. Tissue factor (thromboplastin)
   b. Factor V
   c. Platelet-activating factor (PAF)
2. Binding of clotting factors IX/IX_a, X (prothrombinase complex)
3. Downregulation of APC pathway
4. Increased synthesis of plasminogen activator inhibitor
5. Synthesis of 15-HPETE

APC = adenomatous polyposis coli; 13-HODE = 13-hydroxy-octadeca-dienoic acid; HPETE = hydroperoxyeicosatetraenoic acid; PGE_2 = prostaglandin E_2, PGI_2 = prostacyclin.

10 | Blood Vessels

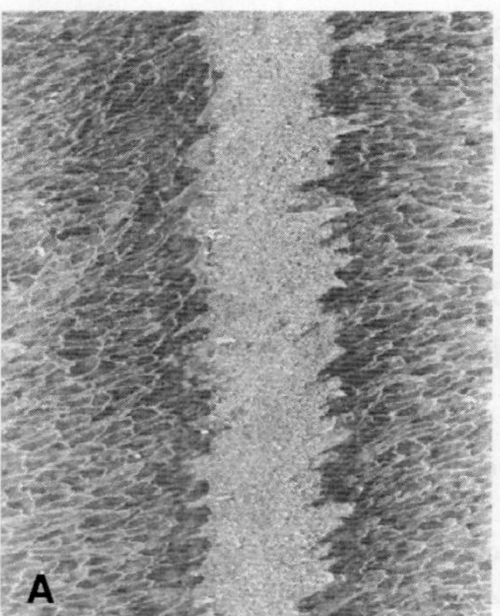

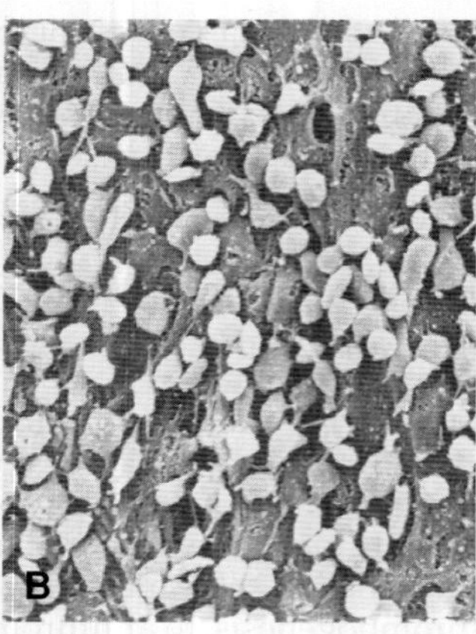

FIGURE 10-8. Scanning electron micrograph of the endothelial surface of a rat aorta 1 hour after the endothelial cells were removed by scraping with a nylon filament. A. Intact endothelium and scratched portion. **B.** Higher-power view of the scratched area shows a pavement of intact platelets that adheres to the underlying connective tissue in the high-velocity arterial stream.

bound in complexes or in the clot. Endothelial cells may also lyse some clots as they form through the **plasminogen/plasminogen activator/plasmin system**.

Endothelial cells have several other anticoagulant activities. A cofactor on the endothelial cell surface inactivates thrombin by forming a complex with thrombin and antithrombin III (a plasma antiprotease). Thrombin itself activates protein C by binding its receptor, **thrombomodulin**, at endothelial cell surfaces. Both protein C and thrombomodulin are synthesized by endothelial cells. Activated protein C destroys coagulation factors V and VIII. TFPI generated during coagulation is bound to endothelium, where it inhibits the TF–VIIa complex (Fig. 10-6). TF and TFPI are synthesized and secreted by endothelial cells as well as other vascular cells.

The endothelium is also intimately involved in initiating and propagating thrombosis. The event that triggers most thrombosis is endothelial injury, which imparts a prothrombotic property to endothelium (Fig. 10-7). Endothelial cells synthesize von Willebrand factor, which promotes platelet adherence and activates clotting factor V. Endothelial cells also bind factors IX and X, a process that favors coagulation at the endothelial surface. Finally, inflammatory agents, including cytokines released from monocytes, activate procoagulants on the surface of intact endothelium. Interleukin-1 and tumor necrosis factor cause endothelial cells to present thromboplastin to the plasma, thus potentially triggering the extrinsic coagulation pathway.

Thus, thrombi may form when endothelial function is altered, when endothelial continuity is lost or when blood flow in a vessel becomes abnormal, such as turbulent or static. Simple loss of endothelial cells or injury to a vessel with good flow produces platelet pavementing but not thrombosis (Fig. 10-8).

Endothelial Cells Repair Defects by Spreading and Migrating Into Affected Areas

The most common denuding injury is progressive endothelial disruption by atherosclerotic plaque. Denuding endothelial injury is also described in homocystinuria, hypoxia and endotoxemia, as well as during invasive therapeutic procedures such as harvesting and implantation of saphenous veins for bypass grafts, angioplasty, insertion of intravascular stents and atherectomy. Interactions of a thrombus with subjacent endothelial cells may further disturb endothelial integrity. Both fibrin and thrombin affect endothelial cytoskeletons and initiate endothelial shape changes to form gaps between cells that disrupt endothelial integrity.

In that setting, endothelial cells can spread rapidly and migrate into the denuded area to reestablish a thromboresistant barrier (Fig. 10-4). This is followed by endothelial cell proliferation to restore normal cell density. These mechanisms may become dysfunctional at sites of persistent endothelial cell damage and result in focal erosions, ulcers and fissures.

Another hypothesized mechanism of repair is migration of EPCs (see above and Chapter 3). EPCs are thought to proliferate after vascular injury and physiologic stress. They then are released into the peripheral circulation, where they target injured vessel walls, attach to the denuded surface and differentiate to reestablish endothelial integrity.

Clot Lysis Is a Regulatory Mechanism

A thrombus may undergo several fates, including (1) lysis, (2) growth and propagation, (3) embolization and (4) organization and canalization. The combination of aggregated platelets and clotted blood is made unstable by activation of the fibrinolytic enzyme plasmin (Fig. 10-9). During clot formation, plasminogen is bound to fibrin and therefore is an integral part of the forming platelet mass. Endothelial cells synthesize plasminogen activator, but in larger thrombi, circulating plasminogen may also be converted to plasmin by products of the coagulation cascade. Plasminogen activator bound to fibrin activates plasmin. In turn, by digesting fibrin strands into smaller fragments, plasmin lyses clots and disrupts the thrombus. These smaller fragments inhibit thrombin and fibrin formation. Clearance of fibrin also limits its accumulation in atherosclerotic plaques, where it can promote plaque growth and attract inflammatory cells. Endothelial cells also synthesize plasminogen activator inhibitor-1 (PAI-1) and plasmin is inhibited by α_2-antiplasmin. Thus, a regional fibrinolytic state reflects the balance between plasminogen and plasmin activation and inhibition.

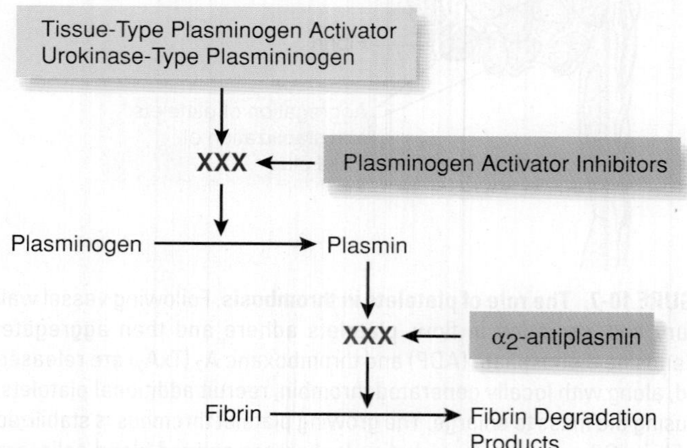

FIGURE 10-9. Mechanisms of fibrinolysis. Plasmin formed from plasminogen lyses fibrin. The conversion of plasminogen to plasmin and the activity of plasmin itself are suppressed by specific inhibitors.

Table 10-4

Atherogenesis

• Initiation and growth of fibroinflammatory lipid atheroma is a slowly evolving dynamic process with superimposed acute events.
• Risk factors accelerate progression.
• The pathogenesis is multifactorial and thus the relative importance of specific genetic and environmental factors may vary in individuals.
• Interactions between cellular and matrix components of the vessel wall and serum constituents, leukocytes, platelets and physical forces regulate the formation of the fibroinflammatory lipid atheroma.

Thrombi may undergo organization and become incorporated into vessel walls. Arterial smooth muscle cells or venous fibroblasts migrate into the thrombus meshwork of cross-linked fibrin and produce matrix. The matrix proteolytic enzymes and their inhibitors remodel the thrombus, digest the fibrin and form a fibrous structure with its own new blood vessels formed by angiogenic factors present in the thrombus. This revascularization is called **recanalization**. Macrophages also likely participate in this remodeling by releasing proteolytic enzymes.

Atherosclerosis

In atherosclerosis, inflammatory and immune cells, smooth muscle cells, lipid and connective tissue progressively accumulate in the intima of large and medium-sized elastic and muscular arteries. The classic atherosclerotic lesion is best described as a fibroinflammatory lipid plaque **(atheroma)**. These plaques develop over several decades (Tables 10-4 and 10-5). Their continued growth encroaches on the media of the arterial wall and into the lumen of the vessel, narrowing the lumen. Atherosclerotic lesions are also called atherosclerotic plaques, atheromas, fibrous plaques or fibrofatty lesions.

Table 10-5

Important Components of Fibroinflammatory Lipid Atheroma

Cells	– Endothelial cells	Lipids and lipoproteins
	– Foam cells	Serum proteins
	– Giant cells	Platelet and leukocyte products
	– Lymphocytes	Necrotic debris
	– Mast cells	New microvessels
	– Macrophages	Hydroxyapatite crystals
Matrix	– Collagen	Growth factors
	– Elastin	Oxidants/antioxidants
	– Glycoproteins	Proteolytic enzymes
	– Proteoglycans	Procoagulant factors

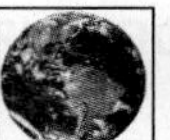

EPIDEMIOLOGY: The major complications of atherosclerosis, including ischemic heart disease (coronary artery disease), myocardial infarction, stroke and gangrene of the extremities, account for more than half of the annual mortality in the United States, with ischemic heart disease being the leading cause of death. The incidence of death from ischemic heart disease in Western countries peaked in the late 1960s, then declined by more than 30%. There are wide geographic and racial variations in the incidence of ischemic heart disease and their progression to clinically significant disease.

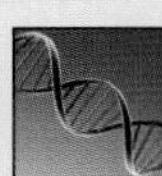
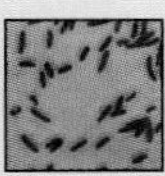

MOLECULAR PATHOGENESIS AND ETIOLOGIC FACTORS: Over the years, many theories have been proposed to explain the origins of atherosclerotic plaques. With the new knowledge from experimental and clinical observations, a comprehensive description of the pathogenesis of atherosclerosis is now possible, with the caveat that the formation, growth and clinical presentation of each plaque may vary from patient to patient. This is because genetic and environmental risk factors do vary from patient to patient.

A Unifying Theory of Atherogenesis

The sequence of events in atherogenesis (Figs. 10-10 to 10-13) may find its origins in fetal life, with the formation of intimal cell masses, or perhaps shortly after birth, when fatty streaks begin to evolve. However, the characteristic atherosclerotic lesion, which is not initially clinically significant, normally requires 20 to 30 years to form. An exception is homozygous familial hypercholesterolemia where lesions develop in the first decade of life. Once formed, serious acute complications may occur or complicated lesions may emerge after several more years of development.

The life of a plaque can be divided into three stages: (1) initiation and formation, (2) adaptation and (3) clinical. Biologically active molecules regulate several dynamic cellular functions. Identification of a single "master" atherogenic gene responsible for most atherosclerosis is unlikely. Rather, one should consider that multiple gene defects and/or polymorphisms interact with the environment and with each other. When an imbalance between proatherogenic and antiatherogenic factors and processes favors atherogenesis, atherosclerotic plaques begin and grow.

Initiation and Formation Stage

1. Intimal lesions initially occur at sites that appear to be predisposed to lesion formation due to structural features (intimal cell mass, bifurcations and curvatures in the artery) and endothelial dysfunction, which may be secondary to hemodynamic shear stress or may be constitutive in association with vessel wall structure. Atherosclerotic lesions tend to arise where shear stresses are low but fluctuate rapidly (e.g., branch points and bifurcations). Subendothelial smooth muscle cells accumulate in an intimal cell mass at branch and other points in certain vessels. This cell mass predisposes to plaque formation. The coronary arteries are particularly affected in this regard.

FIBROINFLAMMATORY LIPID ATHEROMA

LESION-PRONE AREA OF ARTERY → PRECURSOR LESIONS ← NONPRONE AREA OF ARTERY

PRECURSOR LESIONS (fatty streak, intimal hyperplasia)

ATHEROGENIC INJURY ← RISK FACTORS ← GENETIC PREDISPOSITION

REGRESSION ← ? – FIBROINFLAMMATORY LIPID ATHEROMA

INITIATION/ FORMATION STAGE (Subclinical)

ATHEROMA AND WALL REMODELING

REGRESSION ← ? — ATHEROMA → DESTABILIZED

GROWTH OF CELLS AND MATRIX; MURAL THROMBUS

ADAPTATION STAGE (Subclinical)

PLAQUE ENLARGEMENT → ACUTE COMPLICATIONS
- PLAQUE RUPTURE
- PLAQUE HEMORRHAGE
- THROMBOSIS (± EMBOLI)

LUMEN STENOSIS

REGRESSION ← ? DESTABILIZED

COMPLICATED PLAQUE

THROMBOSIS

LUMEN STENOSIS

OCCLUSION

CLINICAL STAGE

FIGURE 10-10. A unifying hypothesis for the pathogenesis of atherosclerosis.

At sites prone to plaque development, expression of proinflammatory genes, vascular cell adhesion molecule-1 (VCAM-1) and intercellular adhesion molecule-1 (ICAM-1) by endothelial cells increases. These molecules are important for recruitment of monocytes into vessel walls. Monocyte/macrophage recruitment is one of the early events in atherogenesis and is orchestrated through a multistep process involving adhesion and transmigration. Adhesion is regulated by cell surface adhesion molecules including P-selectin, E-selectin, VCAM-1, ICAM-1 and several chemokines. Transmigration involves platelet endothelial cell adhesion molecule-1 (PECAM-1).

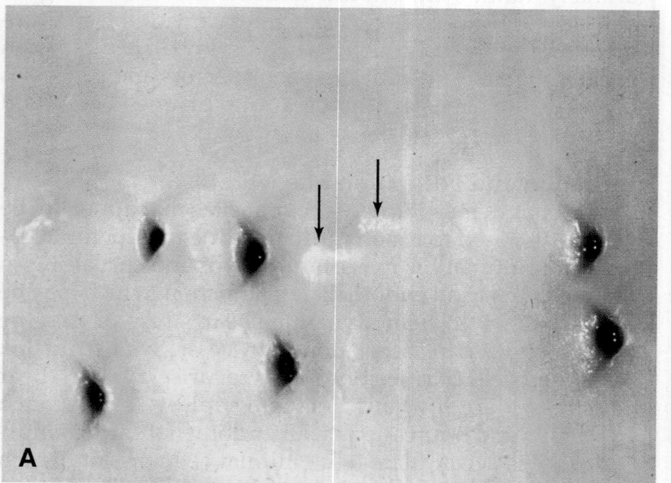

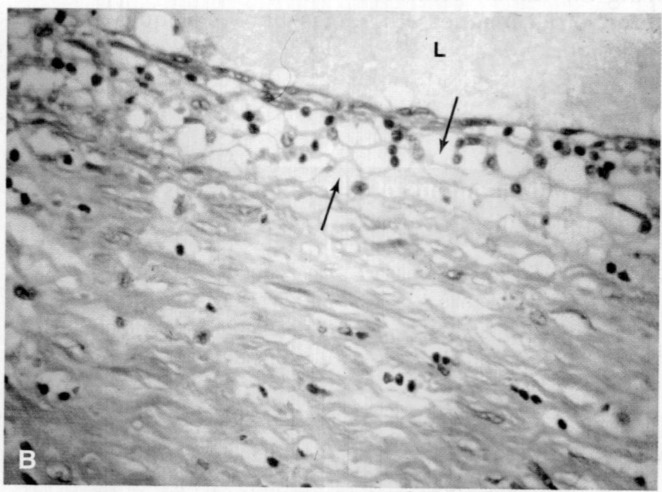

FIGURE 10-11. Fatty streak and atherosclerosis. A. Fatty streak. Gross photo of yellow fatty streaks (*arrows*) in the thoracic aorta. **B.** Fatty streak. Microscopic features of fatty streak in artery wall with intimal foam cells (*arrows*). (*continued*)

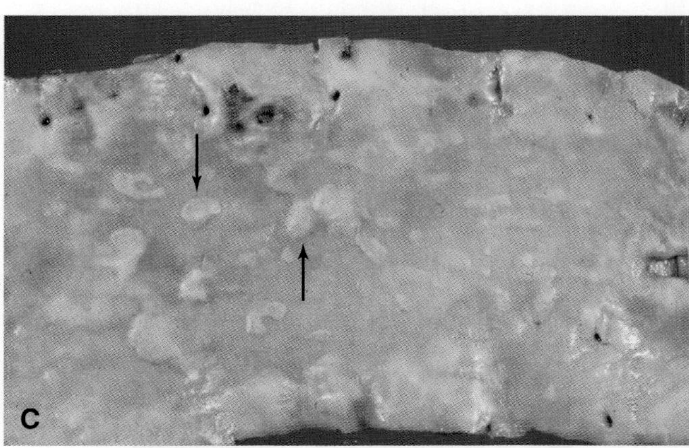

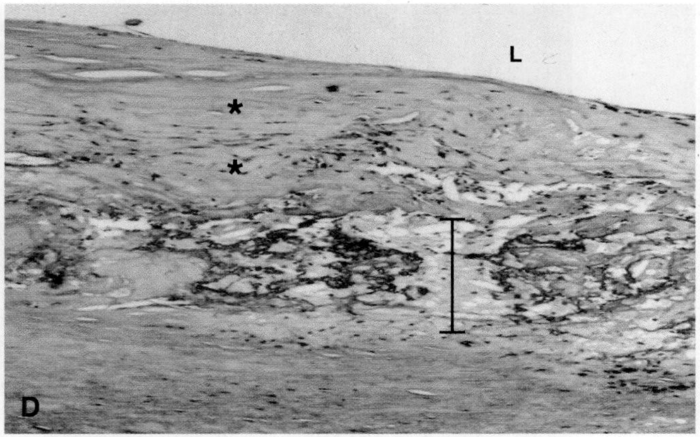

FIGURE 10-11. (*Continued*) **C.** Fibroinflammatory lipid plaques. Focal elevated plaques in thoracic aorta. L, lumen. **D.** Fibroinflammatory lipid plaques. Fibrous cap (astericks) separating lumen (L) from central necrotic core (bracket).

The distribution of atherosclerotic lesions in large vessels and differences in location and frequency of lesions in different vascular beds encourage a belief in the role of hemodynamic factors. The fact that hypertension enhances the severity of atherosclerotic lesions (e.g., in the pulmonary artery in pulmonary hypertension) further supports a role for hemodynamic factors in atherosclerogenesis. Hemodynamic forces induce unique gene expression patterns including several factors in endothelial cells that are likely to promote atherosclerosis, including fibroblast growth factor 2 (FGF-2), TF, plasminogen activator, endothelin and PECAM. However, shear stress also induces gene expression of agents that may be antiatherogenic, including NOS and PAI-1. In people at increased risk of atherosclerosis, lesions also occur in areas that are not predisposed to the disease.

2. Lipid accumulation depends on disruption of the integrity of the endothelial barrier through cell loss and/or cell dysfunction. Oxidative stress in endothelial cells and macrophages leads to cellular dysfunction and damage. Low-density lipoproteins (LDLs) carry lipids into the intima. Since oxidized LDL activates cell adhesion molecules, macrophages can adhere to activated endothelial cells and transmigrate into the intima, bringing lipids with them. Some of these "foamy" macrophages undergo necrosis and release lipids. Alterations in types of matrix proteoglycans synthesized by the smooth muscle cells in the intima also render these sites prone to lipid accumulation by binding lipids and trapping them in the intima. ***Reduced egress of lipids out of the artery wall also promotes lipid accumulation.***

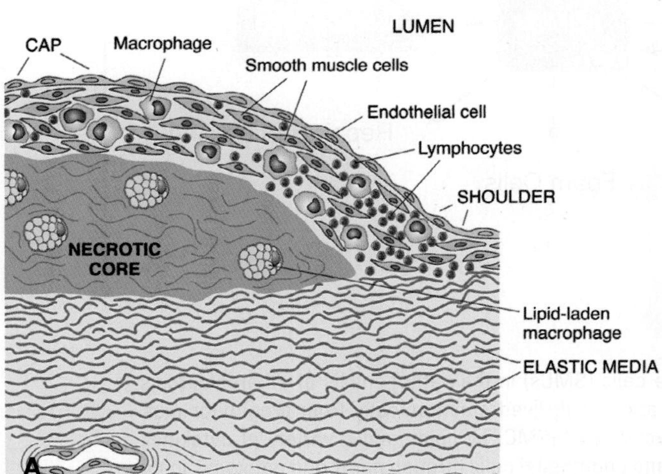

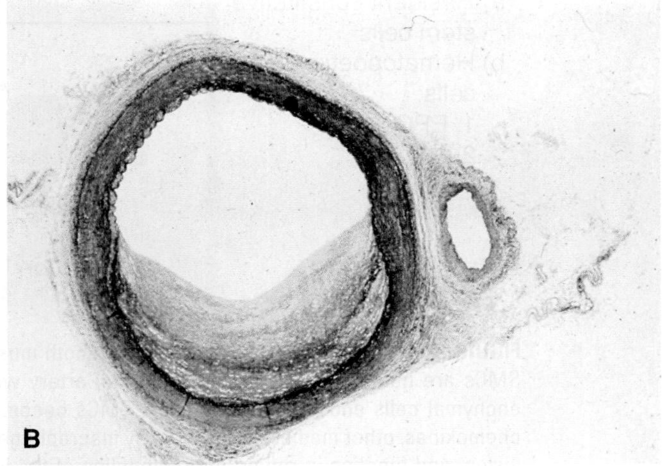

FIGURE 10-12. Fibrofatty plaque of atherosclerosis. A. In this fully developed fibrous plaque, the core contains lipid-filled macrophages and necrotic smooth muscle cell debris. The "fibrous" cap is composed largely of smooth muscle cells, which produce collagen, small amounts of elastin, and glycosaminoglycans. Also shown are infiltrating macrophages and lymphocytes. Note that the endothelium over the surface of the fibrous cap frequently appears intact. **B.** Adaptive stage with atherosclerotic plaque and vessel wall dilatation to maintain the normal size of the lumen. Normal artery wall is at the top. (*continued*)

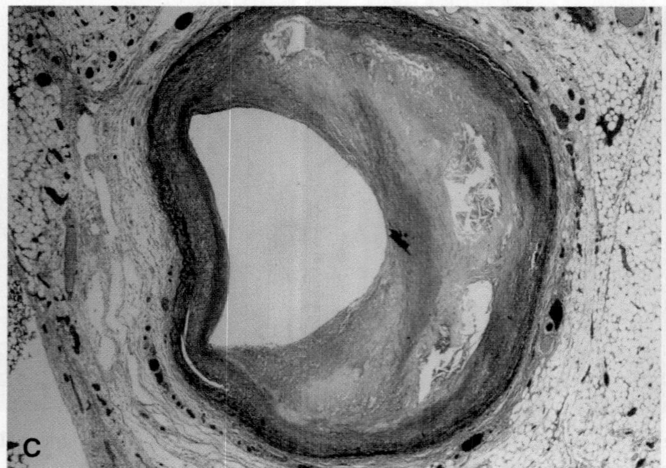

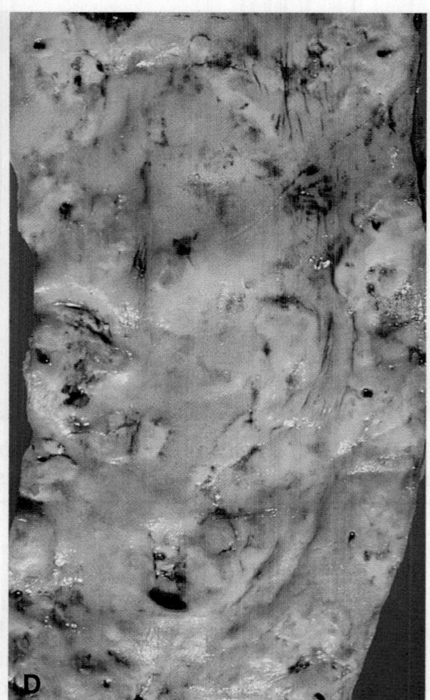

FIGURE 10-12. (*Continued*) **C.** Stenotic coronary artery with atherosclerotic plaque. **D.** The aorta shows discrete, raised, tan plaques. Focal plaque ulcerations are also evident.

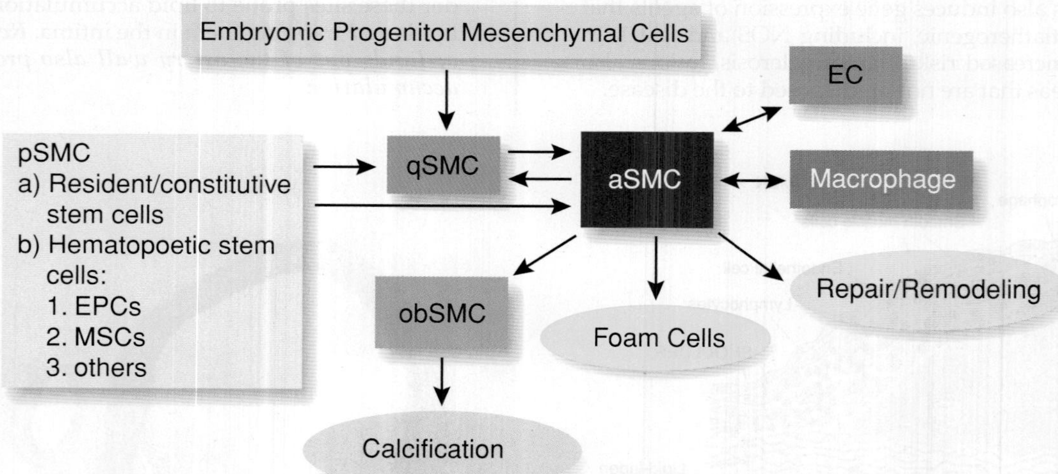

FIGURE 10-13. The hypothesized roles of smooth muscle cells (SMCs) in the pathogenesis of atherosclerosis. SMCs are quiescent (qSMC) in the normal artery wall and are derived embryonically from progenitor mesenchymal cells and neural crest cells. SMCs become activated (aSMC) by lipids and a variety of cytokines, chemokines, other mediators secreted by macrophages and endothelial cells through paracrine pathways in the lesion, and function in repair and remodeling of the lesion. aSMCs migrate, proliferate and secrete prominent extracellular matrix, while qSMCs exhibit a differentiated and contractile phenotype. aSMCs can accumulate lipids and become foam cells in the lesion. aSMCs can also undergo a change in phenotype to show osteoblastic functions (obSMC) promoting calcification in the atherosclerotic lesion. Progenitor SMCs (pSMCs) such as resident stem cells, bone marrow–derived hematopoietic stem cells, endothelial progenitor cells (EPCs) and bone marrow–derived mesenchymal stem cells (MSCs) may replenish SMCs in the vasculature, especially during a response to injury. aSMCs interact with endothelial cells (ECs) and macrophages directly or indirectly to regulate atherosclerotic plaque growth.

3. Mononuclear macrophages, in addition to being central to atherogenesis by participating in lipid accumulation, also release growth factors that stimulate further accumulation of smooth muscle cells. **Oxidized lipoproteins** induce tissue damage and recruit macrophages. Monocytes/macrophages synthesize PDGF, FGF, tumor necrosis factor (TNF), interleukin (IL)-1, interferon-α (IFN-α) and transforming-growth factor-β (TGF-β), each of which can stimulate or inhibit growth of smooth muscle or endothelial cells. For example, IFN-γ and TGF-γ limit cell proliferation and could account for the failure of endothelial cells to maintain continuity over the lesion. Alternatively, they could inhibit growth-stimulatory peptides. IL-1 and TNF stimulate endothelial cells to produce PAF, TF and PAI. Thus, the combination of macrophages and endothelial cells may transform the normal anticoagulant vascular surface to a procoagulant one.
4. As a lesion progresses, mural thrombi may form on the damaged intimal surface. This stimulates PDGF release, accelerating smooth muscle proliferation and secretion of matrix components. The thrombus may grow, lyse or become organized and incorporated into the plaque.
5. The deeper parts of the thickened intima are poorly nourished because of a distance limitation that nutrients can diffuse. This tissue undergoes ischemic necrosis, which is augmented by proteolytic enzymes released by macrophages (i.e., cathepsins) and tissue damage caused by oxidized LDL, reactive oxygen species and other agents. This, along with specific platelet and macrophage-derived angiogenic factors, initiates angiogenesis, with new vasa vasorum forming in the plaque.
6. The fibroinflammatory lipid plaque is formed, with a central necrotic core and a fibrous cap, which separates the core from the blood in the lumen. Inflammatory and immune cells infiltrate, mingling with smooth muscle cells, deposited lipids and variably organized matrix. TGF-β, a key regulator of extracellular matrix deposition, induces formation of several types of collagen, fibronectin and proteoglycans. It also enhances expression of inhibitors of proteolytic enzymes that promote matrix degradation. TGF-β also has anti-inflammatory properties and has been reported to promote PDGF-dependent and -independent growth of smooth muscle cells. Since its effects depend on the environment, TGF-β may be both atherogenic and antiatherogenic.
7. The immune system participates in atherogenesis. Expression of human leukocyte antigen (HLA)-DR antigens on the endothelial and smooth muscle cells of plaques implies that these cells may have undergone immunologic activation, perhaps in response to IFN-γ released by activated T cells in the plaque. In this scenario, the presence of T cells reflects an autoimmune response (e.g., against oxidized LDL that is important for progression of atherosclerotic lesions). Dendritic cells and T lymphocytes also increase in the plaque.

Adaptation Stage

8. As the plaque protrudes into the lumen (e.g., in coronary arteries), the wall of the artery remodels to maintain lumen size. When a plaque occupies about half of the lumen, such remodeling can no longer compensate, and the arterial lumen becomes narrowed **(stenosis).** Hemodynamic shear stress, an important regulator of vessel wall remodeling, acts through the mechanotransduction properties of endothelial cells. Smooth muscle cell turnover, proliferation, apoptosis and matrix synthesis and degradation modulate remodeling of the vessel and the plaque in the face of atherosclerosis. Matrix metalloproteinases (MMPs) and their inhibitors (TIMPs) are important in this process (see Chapter 3). Just as remodeling maintains vessel patency, it also allows a plaque to be "clinically silent." Even a small plaque at this stage can rupture, with catastrophic results, as noted below.

Clinical Stage

9. As a plaque encroaches on the lumen, hemorrhage into it may increase its size without rupture. This hemorrhage occurs when fragile new vessels are formed in the plaques, which may rupture locally. Macrophages clean up the hemorrhagic material.
10. Complications develop in the plaque, including surface ulceration, fissure formation, calcification and aneurysm formation. Activated mast cells at sites of erosion may release proinflammatory mediators and cytokines. Continued plaque growth leads to severe stenosis or occlusion of the lumen. Plaque rupture, involving the fibrous cap, and ensuing thrombosis and occlusion may precipitate catastrophic events in these advanced plaques (e.g., acute myocardial infarction). However, recent angiographic studies suggest that even plaques causing less than 50% stenosis may suddenly rupture. There are several conditions that appear to favor rupture, as noted in Fig. 10-10.

Fig. 10-10 shows how these hypothetical mechanisms may operate in atherogenesis.

The Initial Lesion of Atherosclerosis

PATHOLOGY: Two distinct lesions have been seen as precursors of atherosclerotic plaques.

FATTY STREAK: Fatty streaks are flat or slightly elevated lesions in the intima in which intracellular and extracellular lipids accumulate. They are seen in young children as well as in adults. Cells filled with lipid droplets ("foam cells") congregate (Fig. 10-11). Macrophages contain the most lipid, but smooth muscle cells contain fat as well.

In children who die accidentally, significant fatty streaks may be evident in many parts of the arterial tree. However, these do not correspond to the distribution of atherosclerotic lesions in adults: fatty spots are common in the thoracic aorta in children, but atherosclerosis in adults is far more prominent in the abdominal aorta. Nonetheless, many believe that fatty infiltration is a precursor lesion of atherosclerosis and that other factors control the transition from fatty streak to clinically significant atherosclerotic plaque.

INTIMAL CELL MASS: The intimal cell mass is another candidate for a precursor lesion of atherosclerosis. Intimal cell masses are white, thickened areas at branch points in the arterial tree. Microscopically, they contain smooth muscle cells and connective tissue but no lipid. The location of these

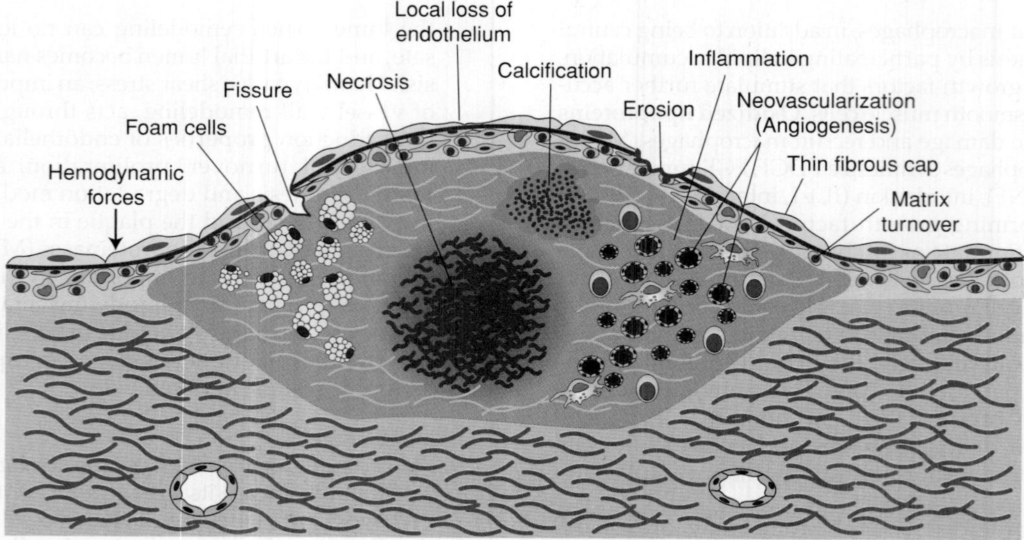

FIGURE 10-14. Complicated lesions of atherosclerosis. The luminal surface of the abdominal aorta and the common iliac arteries shows numerous fibrous plaques and raised, ulcerated lesions containing friable, atheromatous debris. The distal portion of the aorta displays a small aneurysmal dilation.

lesions, also known as "cushions," at arterial branch sites correlates well with the locations of later atherosclerotic lesions.

THE CHARACTERISTIC LESION OF ATHEROSCLEROSIS: The characteristic lesion of atherosclerosis is the fibroinflammatory lipid plaque. Simple plaques are focal, elevated, pale yellow, smooth-surfaced lesions, irregular in shape but with well-defined borders. Fibrofatty plaques (Fig. 10-12) represent more-advanced lesions and tend to be oval, with diameters of up to 12 cm. In smaller vessels, such as the coronary or cerebral arteries, a plaque is often eccentric; that is, it occupies only part of the circumference of the lumen. In later stages, fusion of plaques in muscular arteries can give rise to larger lesions, which occupy several square centimeters.

Microscopically, atherosclerotic plaques are initially covered by endothelium and tend to involve the intima and very little of the upper media (see Fig. 10-12B). The area between the lumen and the necrotic core—the **fibrous cap**—contains smooth muscle cells, macrophages, lymphocytes, lipid-laden cells (foam cells) and connective tissue components. The central core contains necrotic debris. Cholesterol crystals and foreign body giant cells may be present within the fibrous tissue and necrotic areas. Foam cells represent both macrophages and smooth muscle cells that have taken up lipids. Numerous inflammatory and immune cells, especially T cells, are present within a plaque.

Neovascularization is an important contributor to plaque growth and its subsequent complication (Fig. 10-13). It is postulated that vessels grow inward from the vasa vasorum. They are rare in healthy coronary arteries but plentiful in atherosclerotic plaques. Newly formed vessels are fragile and may rupture, resulting in acute expansion of the plaque from intraplaque hemorrhage. Foci of hemosiderin-laden macrophages are often present in plaques, indicating a remote intraplaque hemorrhage.

COMPLICATED ATHEROSCLEROTIC PLAQUES: A **complicated** plaque may reflect several conditions: erosion, ulceration or fissuring of the plaque surface; plaque hemorrhage; mural thrombosis; calcification; and aneurysm (Figs. 10-12C and D, 10-14, and 10-15). Progression from a simple fibrofatty atherosclerotic plaque to a complicated lesion may occur in the third decade of life, but most affected people are 50 or 60 years of age.

Cellular interactions in progression of atherosclerotic lesions are summarized in Fig. 10-16.

- **Calcification** occurs in areas of necrosis and elsewhere in the plaque. Calcification in the artery is thought to depend on mineral deposition and resorption, which are regulated by osteoblast-like and osteoclast-like cells in the vessel wall. These cells are considered to be rare precursor cells in the artery wall, derived from smooth muscle–type cells that have undergone a phenotypic transformation and/or possibly circulating stem/precursor cells derived from bone marrow. Calcification may also reflect changes in the physical-chemical properties of a diseased vessel wall to lead to hydroxyapatite crystal formation.
- **Mural thrombosis** results from abnormal blood flow around the plaque, where it protrudes into the lumen creating turbulence, reduced luminal flow or stasis. The disturbance in flow also causes damage to the endothelial lining, which may become dysfunctional or locally denuded and no longer present a thromboresistant surface. Thrombi often form at sites of erosion and fissuring on the surface of the fibrous cap. Mural thrombi in the proximal region of a coronary artery may embolize to more distal sites.
- **The vulnerable atheroma** has structural and functional alterations that predispose to plaque destabilization. There is much investigation to identify patients with vulnerable plaques, especially by serum biomarkers.
- **Atheroma destabilization**, often resulting in acute coronary syndromes, may occur whenever the dynamic balance of opposing biological and physical processes is disrupted, leading to mural thrombosis, fibrous cap rupture or intraplaque hemorrhage. Clinically silent ruptures occur and can heal. In a ruptured plaque, the necrotic material

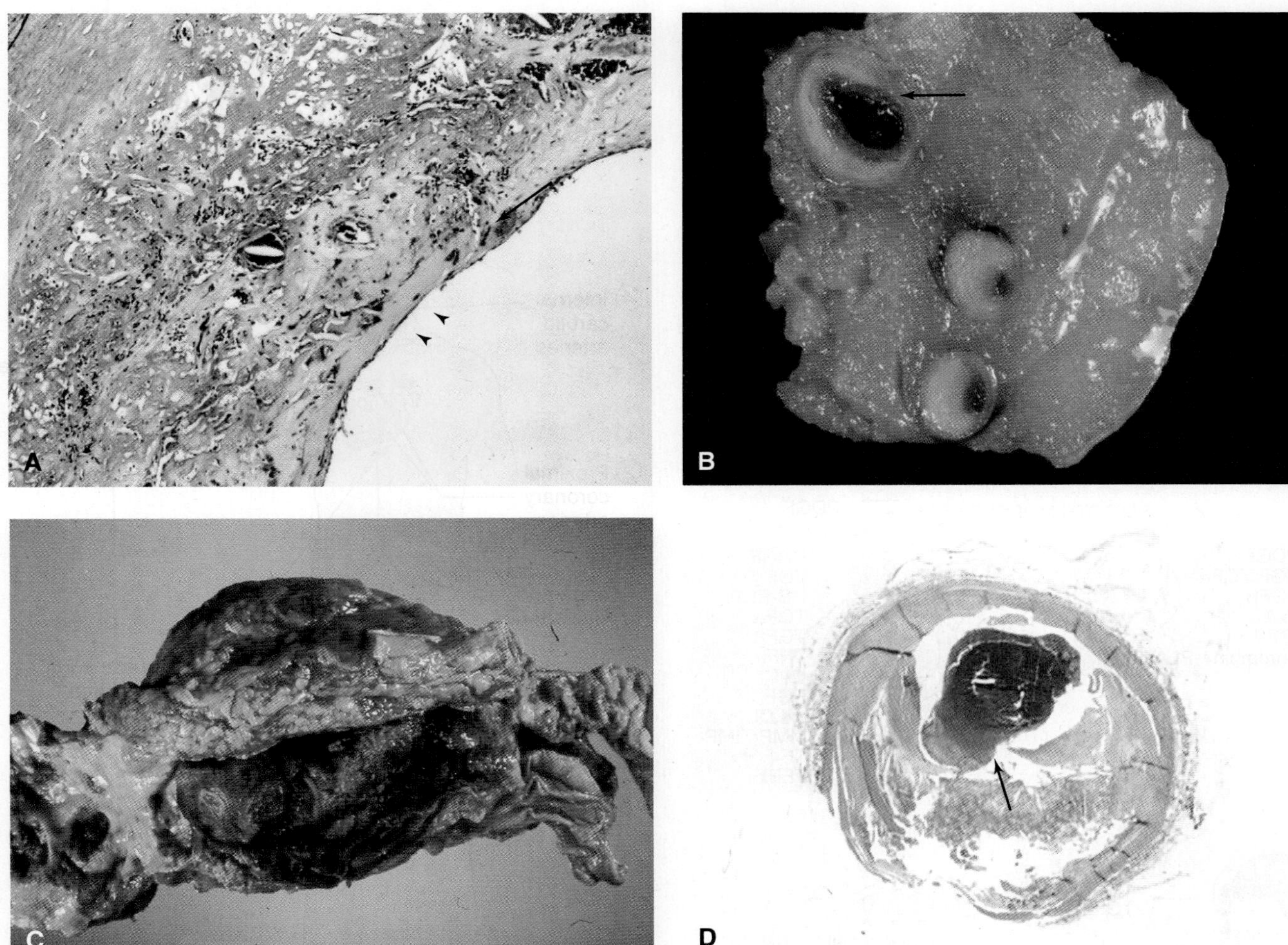

FIGURE 10-15. Complications of atherosclerosis. A. Fibroinflammatory lipid plaque. Microscopic features of plaque erosion (*arrowheads*) and fissure formation (*arrow*). **B. Fibroinflammatory lipid plaque** with occlusive luminal thrombosis (*arrow*). **C. Abdominal aortic aneurysm with thrombus. D.** Rupture of fibrous cap and occlusive luminal thrombosis (*arrow*) in atherosclerotic coronary artery.

that comes in contact with the blood contains TF and is very thrombogenic. Adjacent endothelium has reduced TFPI levels and lower antiplatelet and fibrinolytic activities, all favoring coagulation. The presence of circulating markers of inflammation suggests that procoagulant inflammatory mediators may also participate.

Once a plaque **ruptures**, the exposed thrombogenic material promotes clot formation in the lumen, causing an occlusive thrombus. Plaque rupture may also heal without clinical complications. Plaque hemorrhage due to rupture of thin, newly formed vessels may occur within a plaque with or without a subsequent rupture of the fibrous cap. In the latter case hemorrhage may expand the plaque, and so narrow the lumen further. The hemorrhage will be resorbed over time within the plaque, leaving telltale residual hemosiderin-laden macrophages.

Most plaques that rupture show less than 50% luminal stenosis, and over 95% are less than 70% stenosed. Plaque rupture often occurs at the shoulder of the plaque, suggesting that hemodynamic shear stress weakens and tears the fibrous cap. If not repaired, endothelial loss leads to plaque erosion, weakening the fibrous cap and exposing the plaque to blood constituents. Plaque rupture has been associated with (1) areas of inflammation, (2) large lipid core size, (3) thin fibrous cap ($<65\ \mu$M), (4) decreased smooth muscle cells owing to apoptosis, (5) imbalance of proteolytic enzymes and their inhibitors in the fibrous cap, (6) calcification in the plaque and (7) intraplaque hemorrhage leading to inside-out rupture of the fibrous cap.

Several circulating markers have been associated with plaque burden, including C-reactive protein (CRP), fibrinogen, soluble VCAM, IL-1, IL-6 and TNF.

Complications of Atherosclerosis

The complications of atherosclerosis depend on the location and size of the affected vessel (Fig. 10-17) and the chronicity of the process.

- **Acute occlusion:** Thrombosis on an atherosclerotic plaque may abruptly occlude the lumen of a muscular artery (Fig. 10-18). The result is ischemic necrosis (infarction) of the tissue supplied by that vessel, manifested clinically as

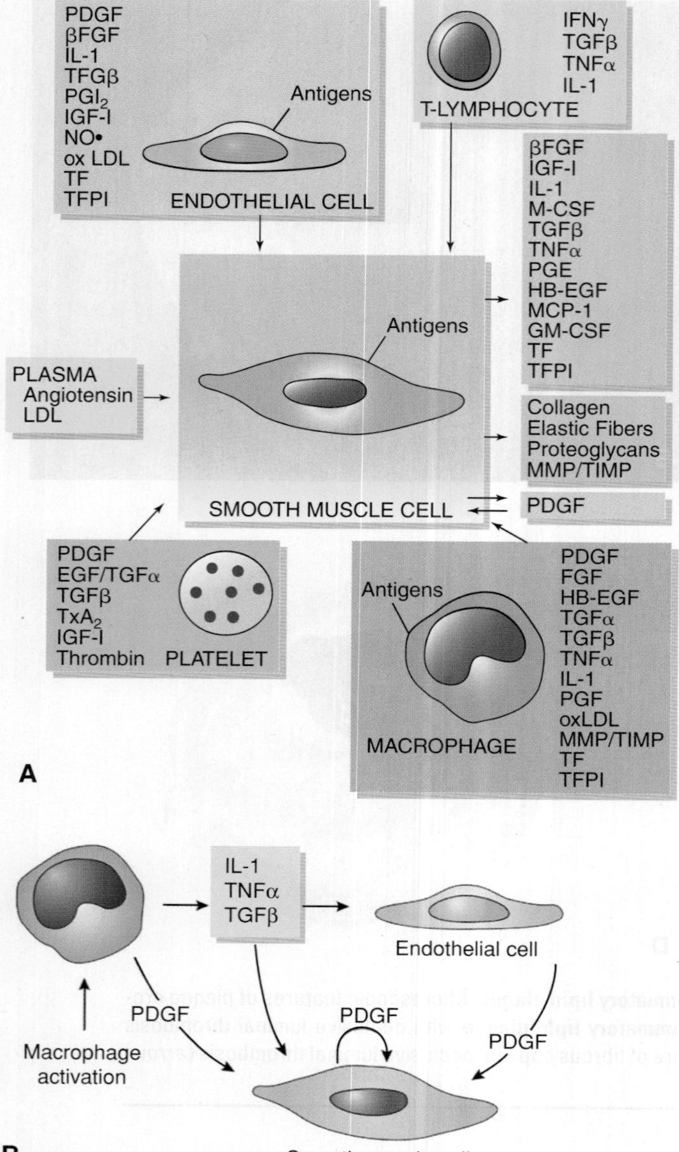

FIGURE 10-16. Cellular interactions in the progression of the atherosclerotic plaque. A. Endothelium, platelets, macrophages, T lymphocytes and smooth muscle cells elaborate a variety of cytokines, growth factors and other substances. The scheme illustrated here emphasizes their influence on smooth muscle cells. **B. The cellular interactions that promote the proliferation of smooth cells.** FGF = fibroblast growth factor; EGF = endothelial growth factor; HB-EGF = heparin-binding epidermal growth factor; IFN = interferon; IGF-I = insulin-like growth factor I; IL = interleukin; MCP-1 = monocyte chemotactic protein-1; M-CSF = macrophage colony-stimulating factor; MMP = matrix metalloproteinase; NO• = nitric oxide; oxLDL = oxidated low-density lipoprotein; PDGF = platelet-derived growth factor; PGE = prostaglandin; PGI_2 = prostacyclin; TF = tissue factor; TGF = tumor growth factor; TFPI = tissue factor pathway inhibitor; TNF = tumor necrosis factor; TIMP = inhibitors of MMPs; TxA_2 = thromboxane A_2.

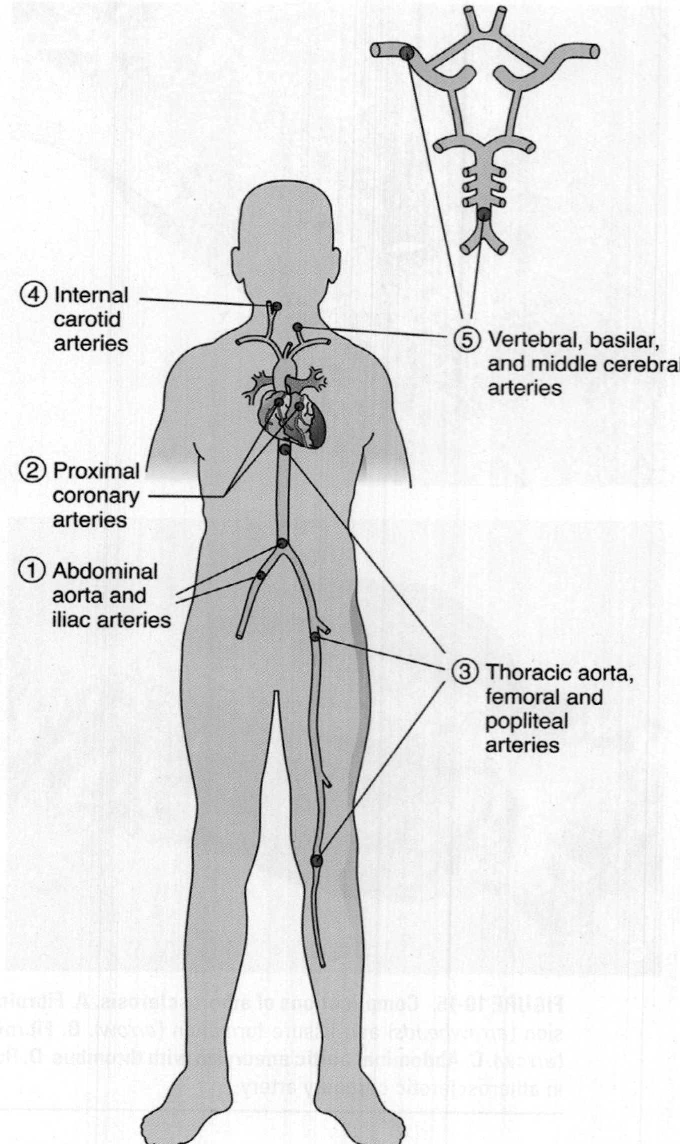

FIGURE 10-17. Sites of severe atherosclerosis in order of frequency.

myocardial infarction, stroke or gangrene of the intestine or lower extremities. Some occlusive thrombi can be dissolved by enzymes that activate plasma fibrinolytic activity, including streptokinase and tissue plasminogen activator.

- **Chronic narrowing of the vessel lumen:** As an atherosclerotic plaque grows, it may impinge on the lumen, progressively reducing blood flow to the tissue served by that artery. Chronic ischemia of the affected tissue causes atrophy of the organ, as exemplified by (1) unilateral renal artery stenosis leading to renal atrophy, (2) mesenteric artery atherosclerosis causing intestinal stricture or (3) ischemic atrophy of the skin occurring in a diabetic with severe peripheral vascular disease.
- **Aneurysm formation:** The complicated lesions of atherosclerosis may extend into the media of elastic arteries and weaken their walls, so as to allow aneurysm formation, typically in the abdominal aorta. Sudden rupture of these aneurysms may precipitate a vascular catastrophe.

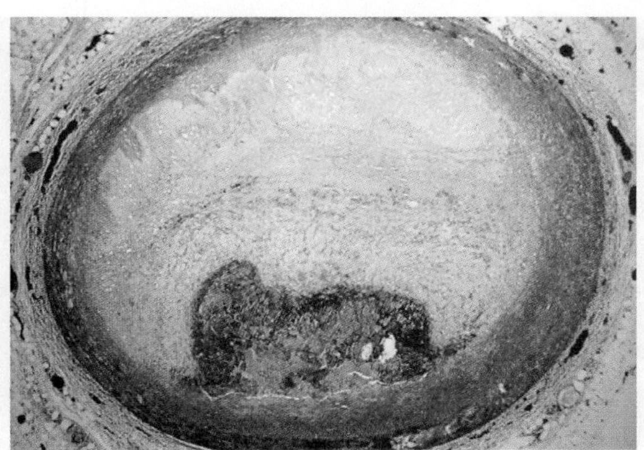

FIGURE 10-18. Coronary artery thrombosis. A microscopic section of a coronary artery shows severe atherosclerosis and a recent thrombus in the narrowed lumen.

- **Embolism:** A thrombus formed over an atherosclerotic plaque may detach and lodge in a distal vessel. For example, embolization from a thrombus in an abdominal aortic aneurysm may acutely occlude the popliteal artery, with subsequent gangrene of the leg. Ulceration of an atherosclerotic plaque may also dislodge atheromatous debris and produce so-called "cholesterol crystal emboli," which appear as needle-shaped spaces in affected tissues (Fig. 10-19), most commonly in the kidney.

Restenosis

Percutaneous transluminal coronary angioplasty is an important treatment for stenotic atherosclerotic vascular disease, especially that of the epicardial coronary arteries. With a catheter-based approach, coronary arteries are revascularized by inflating a balloon catheter to dilate the stenotic portion of the artery. The balloon causes endothelial damage and tears in the plaque and the media. In 30% to 40% of cases in which the vessel lumen is satisfactorily dilated, restenosis occurs within 3 to 6 months.

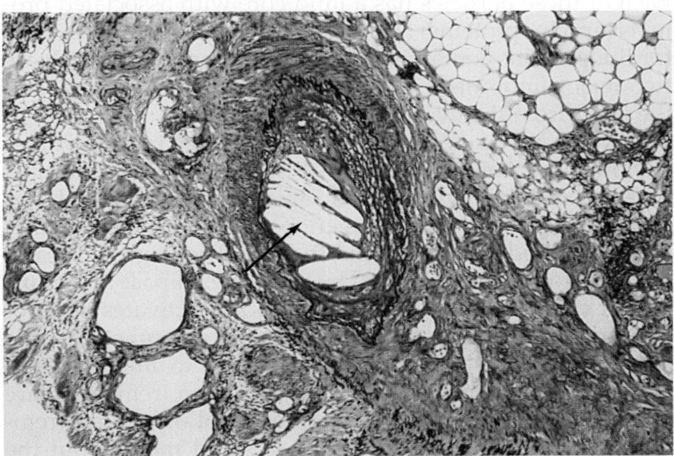

FIGURE 10-19. Cholesterol crystal embolus. Needle-shaped clefts (*arrow*) are seen in an atherosclerotic embolus that has occluded a small artery.

Intimal hyperplasia due to smooth muscle cell proliferation and matrix deposition, with or without an organized mural thrombus on the luminal surface, leads to restenosis. In addition, vascular wall remodeling, induced in part by trauma to the vessel wall and involving the adventitia, also results in luminal narrowing through contraction of the vessel wall.

Restenosis is reduced when a stent, a tubular scaffold device, is deployed to keep the diseased atherosclerotic artery open. Originally, bare metal stents were used, but because of frequent restenosis, these have been replaced by stents coated with biocompatible polymers and biologically active agents, with much less restenosis. For example, drug-eluting stents with antiproliferative agents block cell cycle progression and thus inhibit overgrowth of smooth muscle cells in the vessel wall. Although long-term complications are not fully known, especially as they relate to thrombosis, drug-eluting stents are used extensively.

Transplanted saphenous veins used as autografts in coronary artery bypass operations undergo a series of adaptive and reparative changes. These include (1) intimal thickening associated with phlebosclerosis, (2) occasional medial calcification, (3) focal muscle cell hypertrophy and, eventually, (4) adventitial scarring. However, venous grafts in place for a few years develop atherosclerotic plaques indistinguishable from those found in native coronary arteries (Fig. 10-20). Half of bypass grafts occlude within 5 to 10 years as a result of neointimal hyperplasia and atherosclerosis.

Risk Factors for Atherosclerosis

Factors associated with a twofold or greater risk of ischemic heart disease include:

- **Hypertension:** High blood pressure is consistently associated with greater risk of myocardial infarction. Recent evidence indicates that both diastolic and systolic hypertension contribute equally to this increased risk. Men with systolic blood pressures over 160 mm Hg have almost triple the incidence of myocardial infarction as those with systolic pressures under 120 mm Hg. Control of hypertension has significantly reduced myocardial infarction and stroke.
- **Blood cholesterol level:** Serum cholesterol levels correlate directly with development of ischemic heart disease and accounts for much of the observed geographic variation in the incidence of coronary artery disease. In the absence of genetic disorders of lipid metabolism (see below), the amount of cholesterol in the blood correlates strongly with dietary intake of saturated fat. Use of cholesterol-lowering drugs lowers risk of myocardial infarction. Total serum cholesterol does not necessarily predict a patient's risk of ischemic heart disease since cholesterol is transported by atherogenic and antiatherogenic lipoproteins. Thus, therapeutic decisions are based on LDL cholesterol values.
- **Cigarette smoking:** Coronary and aortic atherosclerosis are more severe and extensive in cigarette smokers than in nonsmokers, and the effect is dose related (see Chapter 8). Thus, smoking markedly increases risk of myocardial infarction, ischemic stroke and abdominal aortic aneurysms.
- **Diabetes:** Diabetics are at greater risk for occlusive atherosclerotic vascular disease in many organs. However, the relative contributions of carbohydrate intolerance alone, as opposed to hypertension and hyperlipidemias common in diabetics, are not well defined (see Chapter 22).

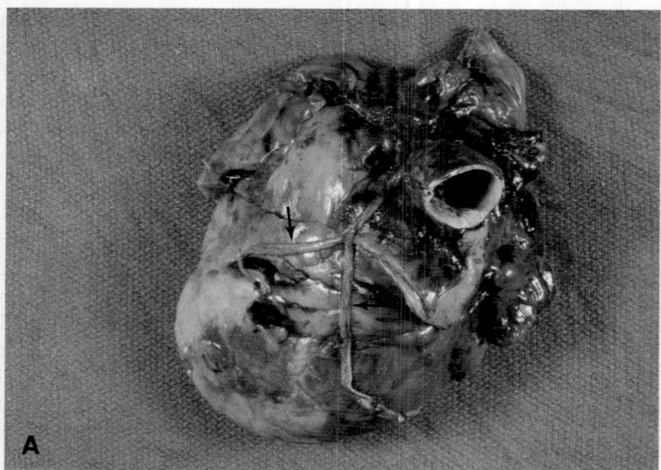

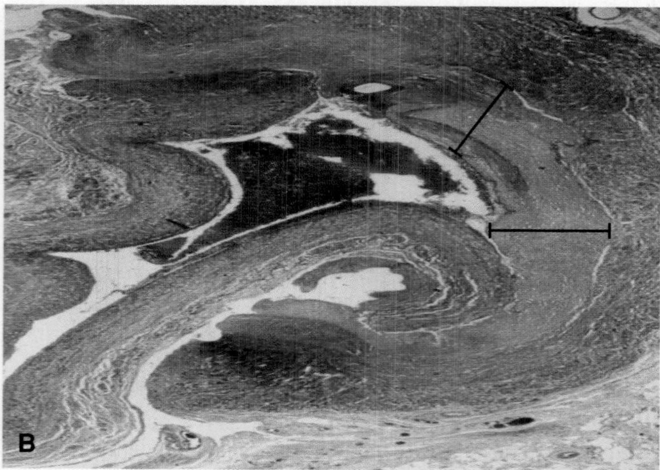

FIGURE 10-20. Saphenous vein aortocoronary bypass. A. Saphenous vein aortocoronary bypass on the surface of the heart (epicardium) (*arrows*). **B.** Distal anastomosis site with atherosclerotic coronary artery (*brackets*).

- **Increasing age and male sex:** These factors are strongly correlated with risk of myocardial infarction, but both probably reflect the accumulated effects of other risk factors.
- **Physical inactivity and stressful life patterns:** Both of these factors correlate with increased risk of ischemic heart disease, but their role in the evolution of atherosclerosis is not clear.
- **Homocysteine:** Homocystinuria is a rare autosomal recessive disease caused by mutations in the gene encoding cystathionine synthase. The disorder causes premature and severe atherosclerosis. Mild elevations of plasma homocysteine in people who do not have this disease are common, and are an independent risk factor for atherosclerosis of coronary arteries and other large vessels. The increased risk associated with high plasma homocysteine is similar in magnitude to those of smoking and hyperlipidemia. Homocysteine is toxic to endothelial cells and impairs several anticoagulant mechanisms in endothelial cells. It inhibits thrombomodulin on the endothelial cell surface, antithrombin III–binding activity of heparan sulfate proteoglycan, binding of tissue plasminogen activator and ecto-adenosine diphosphatase (ADPase) activity on the endothelial cell surface, which promotes platelet aggregation. In addition, oxidative interactions between homocysteine, lipoproteins and cholesterol have been shown. Low dietary folate intake may aggravate genetic predispositions to hyperhomocysteinemia, but it is not known whether folic acid treatment protects from atherosclerotic vascular disease.
- **C-reactive protein:** CRP is an acute phase reactant mainly produced by hepatocytes. It is a serum marker for systemic inflammation, and has been linked to increased risk of myocardial infarction and ischemic stroke. This observation, and the presence of CRP in atherosclerotic plaques, suggests that systemic inflammation may contribute to atherogenesis.

Infection and Atherosclerosis

Seroepidemiologic studies suggest that some infectious agents may contribute to atherosclerosis. *Chlamydia pneumoniae* and cytomegalovirus have been the most studied, although there is also interest in *Helicobacter pylori*, herpesvirus and others. DNA from these agents has been found in human atherosclerotic lesions, but the nature of this association is not known.

Lipid Metabolism

Since Rudolf Virchow in the 19th century first identified cholesterol crystals in atherosclerotic lesions, considerable information has accumulated on lipoproteins and their roles in lipid transport and metabolism in atherosclerosis. Since cholesterol and other lipids (mainly triglycerides) are insoluble, the system of lipoprotein particles functions as a special transport system (Table 10-6; Fig. 10-21). These particles differ in protein and lipid composition, size and density. They are categorized according to density:

- Chylomicrons
- Very-low-density lipoproteins (VLDLs)
- LDLs
- High-density lipoproteins (HDLs)

Each of these particles has a lipid core with associated proteins (apolipoproteins) (Table 10-6). The metabolic pathways for lipoproteins containing the B apolipoproteins (apoB) are two major lipoprotein cascades, one from the intestine and the other from the liver (Fig. 10-22).

EXOGENOUS PATHWAY: This metabolic route involves chylomicrons containing apoB-48 secreted by the intestine. After secretion, chylomicrons rapidly acquire apoCII and apoE from HDL. These triglyceride-rich lipoproteins mainly transport lipid from intestine to liver. The triglycerides in chylomicrons are hydrolyzed by lipoprotein lipase at the surface of capillary endothelial cells. ApoCII activates lipoprotein lipase and causes removal of triglycerides, converting chylomicrons to "remnants" and finally to intermediate-density lipoproteins (IDLs). Chylomicron remnants are removed by hepatocytes through an apoE-mediated (remnant) receptor process. As we understand more about the nature of lipoprotein particles, additional therapeutic targets will undoubtedly be identified.

ENDOGENOUS PATHWAY: This network of reactions involves triglyceride-rich lipoproteins containing apoB-100

Table 10-6

The Apolipoproteins

Apolipoprotein	Approximate Molecular Weight	Major Density Class	Major Sites of Synthesis in Humans	Major Function in Lipoprotein Metabolism
AI	28,000	HDL	Liver, intestine	Activates lecithin: cholesterol acyltransferase
AII	18,000	HDL	Liver, intestine	
AIV	45,000	Chylomicrons	Intestine	
B-100	250,000	VLDL, IDL, LDL	Liver	Binds to LDL receptor
B-48	125,000	Chylomicrons, VLDL, IDL	Intestine	
CI	6500	Chylomicrons, VLDL, HDL	Liver	Activates lecithin: cholesterol acyltransferase
CII	10,000	Chylomicrons, VLDL, HDL	Liver	Activates lipoprotein lipase
CIII	10,000	Chylomicrons	Liver	Inhibits lipoprotein uptake by the liver
D	20,000	HDL		Cholesteryl ester exchange protein
E	40,000	Chylomicrons, VLDL, HDL	Liver, macrophage	Binds to E receptor system

HDL = high-density lipoprotein; IDL = intermediate-density lipoprotein; LDL = low-density lipoprotein; VLDL = very-low-density lipoprotein.

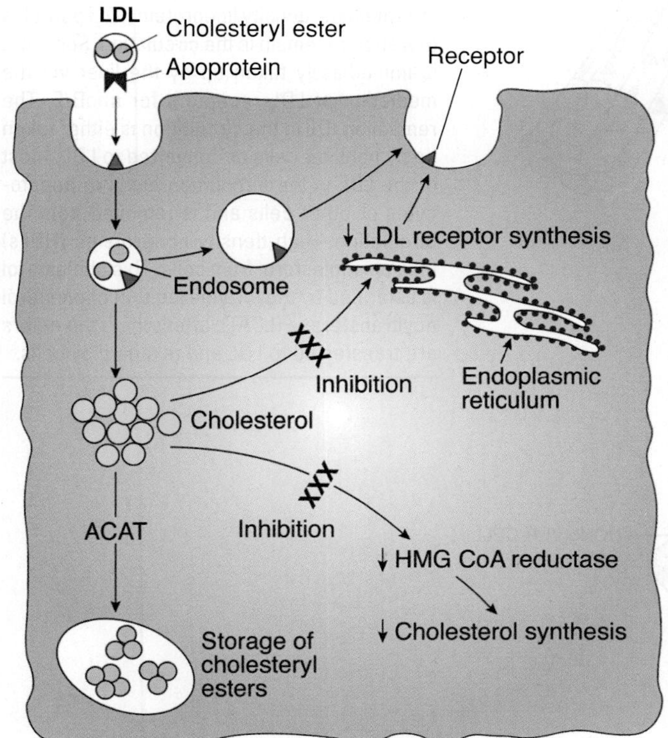

FIGURE 10-21. The relationship between circulating low-density lipoprotein (LDL) cholesterol, LDL receptors, and the synthesis of cholesterol. LDL, which contains cholesteryl esters, is taken up by cells into vesicles by a receptor-mediated pathway to form an endosome. The receptor and lipids are dissociated, and the receptor is returned to the cell surface. The exogenous cholesterol, now in the cytoplasm, causes a reduction in receptor synthesis in the endoplasmic reticulum and inhibits the activity of hydroxymethylglutaryl–coenzyme A (HMG–CoA) reductase in the cholesterol-synthesizing pathway. Excess cholesterol in the cell is esterified to cholesteryl esters and stored in vacuoles. ACAT = acyl-CoA:cholesterol acyltransferase.

secreted by the liver. Liver VLDL particles acquire apoCII and apoE from HDL shortly after their secretion. The triglycerides on VLDL are hydrolyzed by lipoprotein lipase. The particles containing apoB-100 are initially converted to IDLs, then to LDLs. Hepatic lipoprotein lipase converts, at least in part, IDL to LDL, at which point most apoCII and apoE dissociates from the particles and reassociates with HDL. Lipoprotein lipase acts both as a triglyceride hydrolase and, more importantly, as a phospholipase. LDL, which contains apoB-100, interacts with high-affinity receptors on hepatocytes and other cells, including smooth muscle cells, fibroblasts and adrenal cells (Fig. 10-22). Interaction of LDL with its receptor initiates receptor-mediated endocytosis, leading to catabolism of LDL.

HIGH-DENSITY LIPOPROTEIN: HDL containing apoAI and apoAII, is synthesized by several pathways. These include direct secretion of HDL by intestine and liver and transfer of lipid and apolipoprotein constituents released during lipolysis of lipoproteins that contain apoB. Two major functions have been proposed for HDL: (1) a reservoir for apolipoproteins, mainly apoCII and apoE, and (2) interaction with cells in the transport system to carry extrahepatic cholesterol, including that in the arterial wall, to the liver for ultimate removal from the body. The latter function has been termed **reverse cholesterol transport**. The cholesterol removed from cells is principally free cholesterol, which is rapidly esterified to cholesteryl esters. Cholesteryl esters are transferred to the cores of lipoprotein particles or are exchanged to VLDL and LDL. These transfers are mediated by specific transfer proteins (e.g., cholesterol ester transfer protein). Defects in cholesteryl ester transfer and exchange lead to dyslipoproteinemia, increased intracellular cholesteryl ester concentrations and premature atherosclerosis.

HDL is referred to as the "good" cholesterol. ***An inverse correlation between ischemic heart disease and HDL cholesterol levels has been established.*** Factors that increase HDL levels include female gender, estrogens, vigorous exercise and moderate alcohol consumption. Decreased HDL occurs with diets low in fat or high in polyunsaturated fats, truncal obesity, diabetes, smoking and androgen administration.

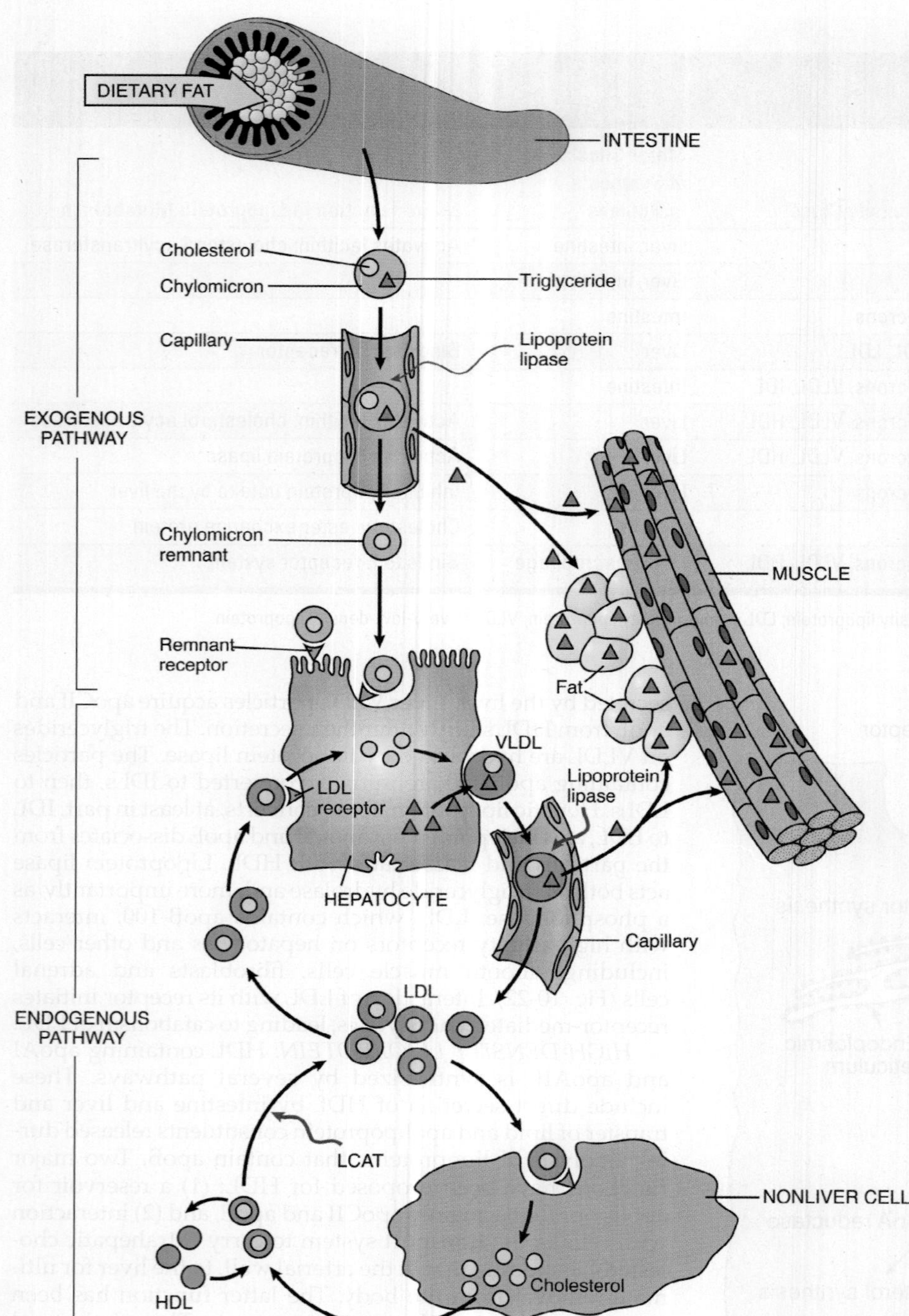

FIGURE 10-22. Exogenous and endogenous cholesterol transport pathway. In the exogenous pathway, cholesterol and fatty acids from food are absorbed through the intestinal mucosa. Fatty acid chains are linked to glycerol to form triglycerides. Triglycerides and cholesterol are packaged into chylomicrons that are returned via the lymph to the blood. The lipids are coupled to proteins by enzymes such as the microsomal transfer protein complex. In the capillaries (mainly of fat tissue and muscle, but also other tissues), the ester bonds holding the fatty acids in triglycerides are split by lipoprotein lipase. Fatty acids are removed, leaving cholesterol-rich lipoprotein remnants. These bind to special remnant receptors and are taken up by liver cells. The cholesterol of the remnant is either secreted into the intestine, largely as bile acids, or packaged as very-low-density lipoprotein (VLDL) particles, which are then secreted into the circulation. This is the first step in the endogenous cycle. In fat or muscle tissue the triglyceride is removed from the VLDL with the aid of lipoprotein lipase. The intermediate-density lipoprotein (IDL) particles (not shown) remain in the circulation. Some IDL is immediately taken up by the liver via the mediation of LDL receptors for apoB/E. The remaining IDL in the circulation is either taken up by nonliver cells or converted to LDL. Most of the LDL in the circulation binds to hepatocytes or other cells and is removed from the circulation. High-density lipoproteins (HDLs) take up cholesterol from cells. This cholesterol is esterified by the enzyme lecithin:cholesterol acyltransferase (LCAT), after which the esters are transferred to LDL and taken up by cells.

LOW-DENSITY LIPOPROTEIN: LDL contains apoB-100 and cholesterol esters as its main lipid entity. LDLs are heterogeneous in particle density, which correlates with differences in atherogenicity. Macrophages, endothelial cells and smooth muscle cells in atherosclerotic lesions can oxidize LDL, increasing LDL atherogenicity, facilitating LDL recognition by the macrophage scavenger receptor and leading to massive cholesterol uptake by macrophages. Oxidized lipoproteins also affect other processes that may contribute to atherogenesis, including regulation of vascular tone, activation of inflammatory and immune responses and coagulation. Autoantibodies to oxidized LDL are detected in both plasma and plaques in patients with atherosclerosis, and may be important in plaque development. Oxidized LDLs are toxic to vascular wall cells, may disrupt endothelial integrity and lead to accumulation of cell debris within atheromas. They are also chemotactic for macrophages, thereby increasing their accumulation in atheromas even more. Nonetheless, clinical trials of antioxidants to prevent ischemic heart disease have not demonstrated protection.

Heritable Dyslipoproteinemias

Familial clustering of ischemic heart diseases is well documented (Table 10-7).

Table 10-7

Molecular Defects in Dyslipoproteinemias

Disease	Genetic Defect	Clinical Features
Apolipoprotein Defects		
ApoAI deficiency	ApoA1 truncations or rearrangements (11q23)	Absent HDL, severe atherosclerosis
ApoAI variants	ApoA1 point mutations (11q23)	Reduced HDL, variable atherosclerosis
Abetalipoproteinemia (absence of both apoB-100 defects, absence of atherosclerosis and apoB-48)	Microsomal triglyceride protein mutations (4q22–24)	Ataxia, malabsorption, hemolytic anemia, visual
ApoB-100 absence	Unknown (2p24)	Mild ataxia, malabsorption, absence of atherosclerosis
ApoCII deficiency	ApoCII mutations (19q13.2)	Type I hyperlipidemia: severe hypertriglyceridemia, variable atherosclerosis
ApoE variants	ApoE mutations (19q13.2)	Type III hyperlipidemia: elevated triglycerides, premature atherosclerosis
Enzyme Defects		
Lipoprotein lipase deficiency	Lipoprotein lipase mutations (8p22)	Type I hyperlipidemia: hypertriglyceridemia; minimal atherosclerosis
Hepatic lipase deficiency	Hepatic lipase mutations (15q21–23)	Elevations of IDL and HDL; severe atherosclerosis
Lecithin:cholesterol acyltransferase (LCAT) deficiency	LCAT mutations (16q22.1)	Mild hypertriglyceridemia; reduced HDL; corneal opacities; variable atherosclerosis
Receptor Defect		
Familial hypercholesterolemia	LDL receptor mutations (19p13.2)	Type II hyperlipidemia: severe elevation of LDL; premature atherosclerosis

Apo = apoprotein; HDL = high-density lipoprotein; IDL = intermediate-density lipoprotein; LDL = low-density lipoprotein.

FAMILIAL HYPERCHOLESTEROLEMIA: The Nobel Prize in Physiology or Medicine was awarded in 1985 to Michael S. Brown and Joseph L. Goldstein for the discovery of the LDL receptor. Their work identified the pathways regulating cholesterol homeostasis (Fig. 10-21) and provided an essential foundation to our understanding of receptor-mediated endocytosis and regulation of cell membrane receptors. The LDL receptor is a cell surface glycoprotein that regulates plasma cholesterol by mediating endocytosis and recycling of apoE, the major plasma cholesterol transport protein. Mutations in the LDL receptor gene, on the short arm of chromosome 19, lead to familial hypercholesterolemia (FH), an autosomal dominant disease for which about 1 in 500 people are heterozygotes and 1 in 1,000,000 are homozygotes.

Most untreated homozygotes die from coronary artery disease before the age of 20. The prevalence of familial hypercholesterolemia may approach 6% in people who have had myocardial infarctions associated with hyperlipidemia. Among people under 60 years of age who had a myocardial infarction, 5% are heterozygous for FH. Such heterozygotes have plasma LDL levels that are twice normal, while homozygotes have a 6- to 10-fold increase in plasma LDL. Heterozygote patients also suffer from premature myocardial infarction but at a later age than do homozygotes (40 to 45 years of age in men).

More than 400 mutant alleles for familial hypercholesterolemia are known, including point mutations, insertions and deletions. These mutations fall into five main classes, based on their effects on receptor protein function (Fig. 10-23). Genetic issues in familial hypercholesterolemia are discussed more fully in Chapter 6.

In addition to accelerated accumulation of cholesterol in arteries (premature atherosclerosis), LDL cholesterol also deposits in skin and tendons to form xanthomas (Fig. 10-24). In some cases (before age 10 in homozygotes), an arcus lipoides is present in the cornea.

APOLIPOPROTEIN E: Genetic variations in various apoproteins are also accompanied by alterations in LDL levels. Polymorphisms in apoE and variants of apolipoprotein AI and AII have been observed. Apolipoprotein E is one of the main protein constituents of VLDL and of a subclass of HDL. The gene locus that codes for apoE is polymorphic; three common alleles, E2, E3 and E4, code for three major apoE isoforms and determine the six apoE phenotypes. Some 20% of the variability in serum cholesterol has been attributed to apoE polymorphism. In men, the apoE 3/2 phenotype is associated with a 20% lower LDL level than the most common phenotype, apoE 3/3. By contrast, the E4 allele is associated with elevated serum cholesterol. Interestingly, E2 allele is increased, and E4 decreased, among male octogenarians. The E4 allele is a major risk factor for late-onset Alzheimer disease. Patients who are E2/2 clear chylomicron remnants and IDLs poorly and have familial type III hyperlipoproteinemia with premature atherosclerosis.

HIGH-DENSITY LIPOPROTEIN: The genes for apolipoproteins AI and CIII are on chromosome 11 and are physically

tions of the low-density lipopro- familial hypercholesterolemia.

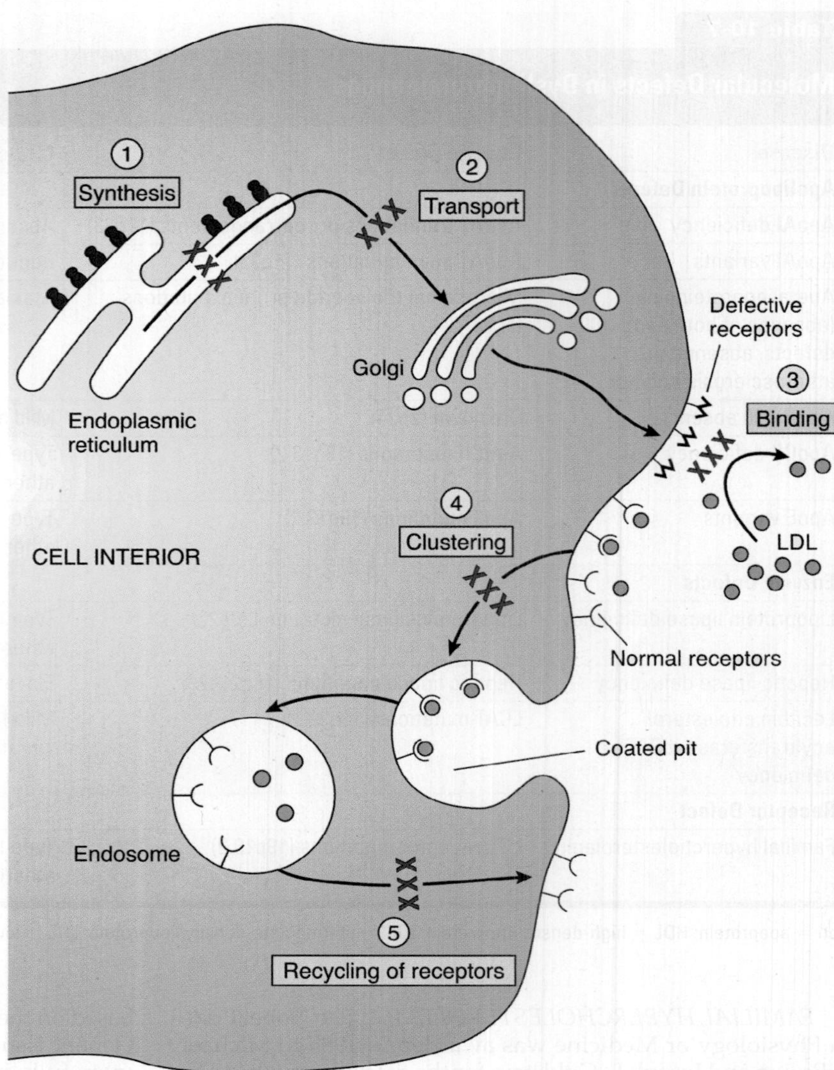

linked, whereas the gene for AII is on chromosome 1. Polymorphisms of apoAI are associated with premature atherosclerosis, as are rare cases of hereditary apoAI deficiency. Hypertriglyceridemia is often associated with low HDL cholesterol.

LIPOPROTEIN (a): Lipoprotein (a) (Lp[a]) is an LDL-like particle to which the glycoprotein apo(a) is attached through a disulfide bridge with apoB-100. High circulating levels of Lp(a) are associated with an increased risk of atherosclerosis of the coronary arteries and larger cerebral vessels in both men and women. Plasma levels of this cholesterol-rich lipoprotein vary greatly (<1 to >140 mg/dL) and appear to be independent of LDL levels. The Lp(a)-specific protein, apo(a), has been detected in atherosclerotic lesions, and high Lp(a) levels correlate with target organ damage in hypertensive patients.

Apo(a) is encoded by a gene on chromosome 6 (6q2.7), close to the gene for plasminogen, to which apo(a) is highly homologous. Apo(a) and plasminogen display similar domains that mediate interactions with fibrin and cell surface receptors. Lp(a) enhances cholesterol delivery to injured blood vessels, suppresses generation of plasmin and promotes smooth muscle proliferation. Thus, it may be an important link between atherosclerosis and thrombosis.

Lp(a) plasma levels are heritable and not altered by most cholesterol-lowering drugs, although they are reduced by nicotinic acid. Taken together, this information distinguishes a risk factor that appears superficially to be related to serum cholesterol but the effect of which may actually be linked to an alteration in clot lysis.

Hypertensive Vascular Disease

There has been a significant increase in the prevalence of hypertension worldwide, with dramatic increases since the beginning of the 20th century. Hypertension affects over 30% of the population of the United States. It is present in more than half of cases of myocardial infarction, stroke and chronic renal disease. It is included in the "metabolic syndrome" (see Chapter 22) along with hyperglycemia, insulin resistance, dyslipidemia and obesity. Hypertension is present in 95% or greater of ascending aortic dissections and/or rupture. Blacks are particularly plagued by hypertension, and are more likely

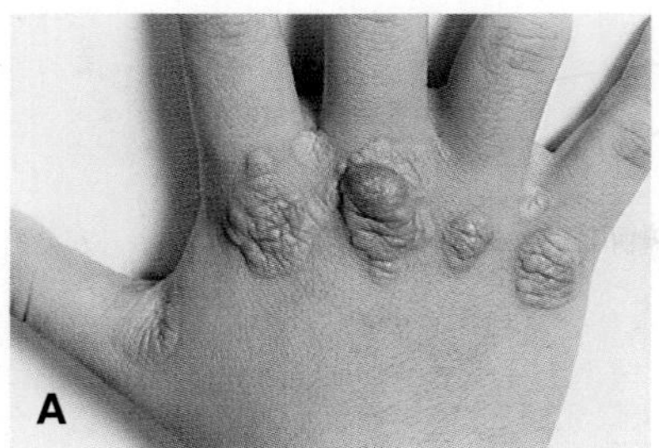

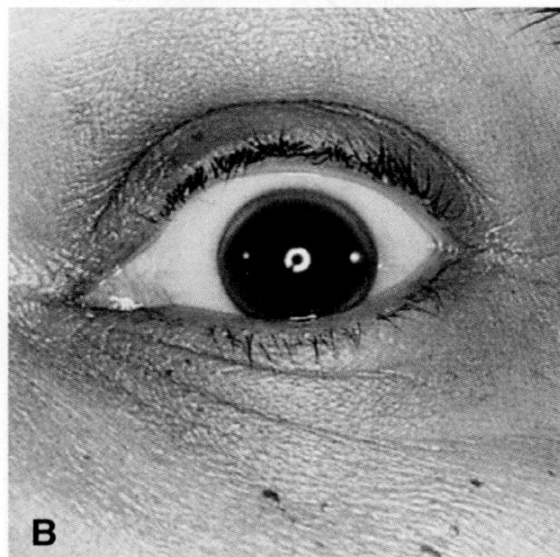

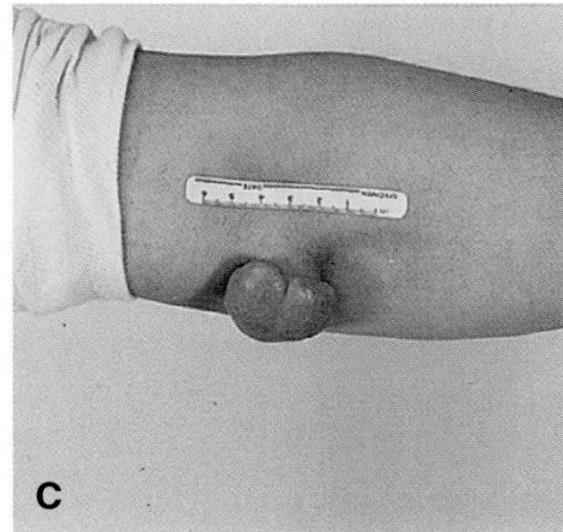

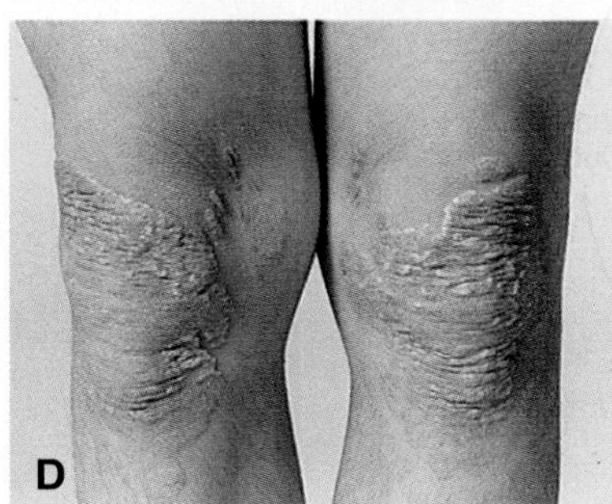

FIGURE 10-24. Xanthomas in familial hypercholesterolemia. A. Dorsum of the hand. **B.** Arcus lipoides represents the deposition of lipids in the peripheral cornea. **C.** Extensor surface of the elbow. **D.** Knees.

than are whites to experience severe complications. At least three fourths of patients with dissecting aortic aneurysm, intracerebral hemorrhage or myocardial wall rupture also have elevated blood pressure.

In 95% of patients, hypertension occurs without an identifiable cause. This is referred to as **essential** or **primary** hypertension. As the pathophysiology and molecular pathogenesis of hypertension became better understood in the past decade, the term *essential hypertension* has significantly contracted and has become less clinically applicable. A number of diseases contribute to the development of hypertension, including renal artery stenosis, most forms of chronic renal disease, diabetes mellitus, primary elevation of aldosterone levels, Cushing syndrome, pheochromocytoma, hyperthyroidism, coarctation of the aorta and renin-secreting tumors. In addition, patients with severe atherosclerosis may have high systolic pressure because a sclerotic aorta cannot properly absorb the kinetic energy of the pulse wave. Whatever the etiology, effective treatment of hypertension prolongs life.

The definition of hypertension depends on a statistical estimate of the distribution of systolic and diastolic blood pressures in the general population. Both systolic and diastolic pressures are important in determining the risk of cardiovascular disease, especially atherosclerosis. Over the course of the day, blood pressure varies widely, depending on exertion, emotional state and other poorly understood factors. It also exhibits a circadian rhythm falling at night or during sleep, as sympathetic nervous system tone declines. Blood pressure also varies with age. Diagnosis and treatment of hypertension hinges on correct and timely measurement of blood pressure. Diagnosis of hypertension should ideally be based on several blood pressure measurements taken on separate days. Home blood pressure readings, done correctly, may be more accurate reflections of blood pressure than measurements in the doctor's office. The mean systolic blood pressure in 20-year-old men is about 130 mm Hg, but 95% confidence limits range from 105 to 150 mm Hg. Average systolic blood pressure increases with age, so that in 80-year-olds, it reaches 170 mm Hg, with 95% confidence limits from 125 to 220. The World Health Organization (WHO) defines hypertension as systolic pressure above 160 mm Hg and/or diastolic pressure above 90. Patients with some diseases, such as diabetes mellitus, are managed to achieve blood pressures lower than the WHO criteria.

ETIOLOGIC FACTORS: Blood pressure is the product of cardiac output and systemic vascular resistance to blood flow. The most widespread hypothesis holds that primary hypertension results from an imbalance in the interactions between these mechanisms (Fig. 10-25). However, both of these functions are critically influenced by renal function and sodium homeostasis. Frequency of hypertension increases as the glomerular filtration rate (GFR) falls even with mild renal dysfunction. Reduced GFR in renal dysfunction causes sodium retention and volume expansion, which should be compensated by reduced tubular sodium reabsorption. Impaired renal tubular sodium handling plus reduced GFR are likely be important in the hypertension seen in patients with chronic kidney disease due to diabetes and with aging.

A complex endocrine axis centers on the renin–angiotensin system. Renal artery occlusion or dietary salt restriction leads to increased renal secretion of renin. Renin is a protease that cleaves angiotensinogen to a decapeptide, angiotensin I. In turn, angiotensin I is converted to angiotensin II by the endothelial surface protein ACE. Angiotensin II causes vasoconstriction and also affects the central nervous system (CNS) centers that control sympathetic outflow and stimulate adrenal aldosterone release. Aldosterone increases sodium reabsorption by the renal tubules. The net effect of all these actions is increased total body fluid. Thus, the **renin–angiotensin** system elevates blood pressure by three mechanisms:

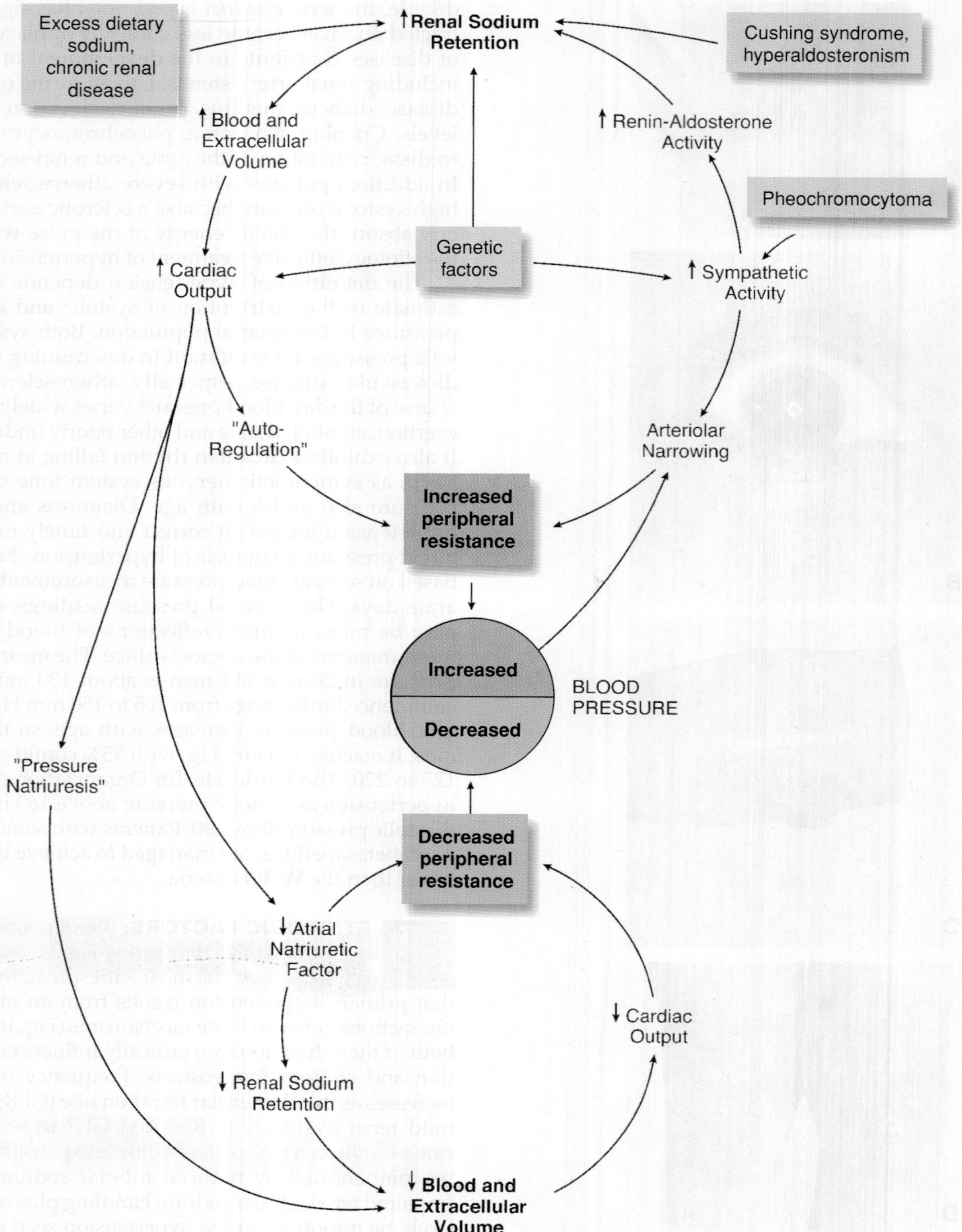

FIGURE 10-25. Factors contributing to hypertension and the counterregulatory factors that lower blood pressure. An imbalance in these factors results in the increased peripheral resistance that is responsible for most cases of essential (primary) hypertension. Note the central role of peripheral resistance.

- Increased sympathetic output
- Increased mineralocorticoid secretion
- Direct vasoconstriction

This axis is antagonized by atrial natriuretic factor (ANF), a hormone secreted by specialized cells in the cardiac atria. ANF binds specific receptors in kidney and increases urinary sodium excretion, thus opposing angiotensin II–induced vasoconstriction. Secretion of ANF may be controlled by atrial distention, a consequence of increased volume, or by as-yet undefined endocrine interactions.

The importance of this hormonal axis in regulating blood pressure in hypertension is demonstrated by the therapeutic success of sympathetic antagonists (β-adrenergic blockers), diuretics and inhibitors of ACE. Nonetheless, no central defect in the renin–angiotensin axis has been identified, in part because the vasculature responds quickly to hemodynamic changes in the tissues by autoregulation (Fig. 10-26).

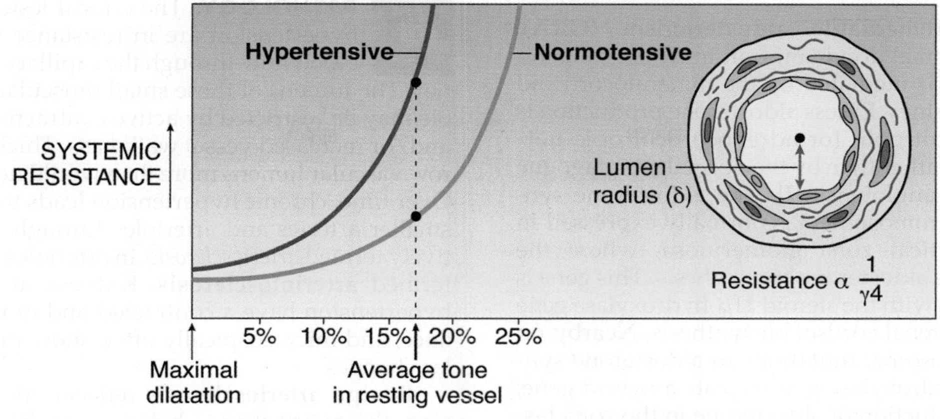

FIGURE 10-26. Structural autoregulation of blood pressure. Hypertension, regardless of its primary cause, increases the ability of the resistance vessel walls to respond to vasoactive stimuli. Resistance is increased even in maximally dilated vessels because the lumen size is decreased in the hypertensive vascular bed. As the smooth muscle cells contract, the increase in vessel wall thickness increases the resistance, which is inversely proportional to the fourth power of the radius of the lumen. Note that at the average resting muscular tone, the resistance in hypertensive persons is considerably higher than normal.

There are extensive mechanisms for regulating renal sodium excretion. The final segment of the nephron, the collecting ducts, is important in maintaining sodium balance when alterations in more proximal parts of the nephron occur. Thus, dysregulation of sodium transport at the collecting duct can lead to the greatest deficit in sodium handling. Genetic mutations involving sodium reabsorption at this final segment are strongly associated with hypertension. Defects in the epithelial sodium channel in the renal distal tubule and collecting duct, or defects in signaling pathways regulating its expression, are responsible for several rare genetic forms of hypertension including mutations in WNK protein kinases and increased expression of epithelial sodium channels.

In the case of hypertension, the end result of autoregulation is always increased peripheral resistance. For example, hypertension can be induced experimentally by surgically removing large amounts of renal tissue, followed by administering excess sodium and water. Cardiac output, and therefore blood pressure, increases rapidly as a result of the rapid change in blood volume. However, within a few days, pressure-induced diuresis restores near-normal cardiac output and plasma volume. At that point, blood pressure is maintained by increased peripheral resistance. Thus, although the blood pressure elevation is initially due to increased volume, compensatory mechanisms successfully mask the volume changes and cause apparent essential hypertension. Many cases of human hypertension may also result from a process that begins with altered cardiac output, salt metabolism or ANF release.

The Prothrombotic Paradox

Hypertension is a hemodynamic disorder and exposes the arterial tree to increased pulsatile stress. However, paradoxically, most major complications of chronic hypertension such as heart attack and stroke are thrombotic, rather than hemorrhagic. This is known as the prothrombotic paradox of hypertension. Virchow's triad of thrombosis is seen in hypertensive individuals with abnormalities in blood flow, endothelial damage or dysfunction and a hypercoagulable state. This prothrombotic state can result from chronic shear stress and low-grade inflammation. Endothelial dysfunction may be multifactorial and include decreased activity of vasodilator agents and increased activity of, or increased sensitivity to, vasoconstrictor agents. Enhanced activity of the renin–angiotensin system and kallikrein–kinin system has opposite effects via angiotensin II–converting enzyme, causing vasoconstriction and vasodilation, respectively. Increased activity of these systems also leads to a hypercoagulable state. Thus, there is an increased load on the myocardium, which gives rise to left ventricular hypertrophy and ventricular and atrial arrhythmias and impairs coronary circulation.

Acquired Causes of Hypertension

Causes of hypertension are identifiable in a small proportion of cases. These include renal artery stenosis, most forms of chronic renal disease, diabetes mellitus, primary elevation of aldosterone levels (Conn syndrome), Cushing syndrome, pheochromocytoma, hyperthyroidism, coarctation of the aorta and renin-secreting tumors. In addition, people with severe atherosclerosis may have high systolic pressure, because a sclerotic aorta cannot properly absorb the kinetic energy of pulse waves, and because they have renovascular hypertension more often.

MOLECULAR PATHOGENESIS: We know from family and twin studies that genetic factors are likely to be important in the pathogenesis of essential hypertension. Although essential hypertension probably involves interactions of many gene products, the study of rare inherited forms of hypertension has helped identify genes that may contribute to control of blood pressure. A number of monogenic forms of hypertension have been defined:

- **Glucocorticoid-remediable aldosteronism (GRA):** GRA is an autosomal dominant trait in which congenital hypertension is mediated by the mineralocorticoid receptor in the kidney. Excess aldosterone production is caused by corticotropin (or adrenocorticotropic hormone [ACTH]), rather than by the normal secretagogue for aldosterone, angiotensin II. The aldosterone synthase gene on chromosome 8 is normally expressed in the adrenal cortical zona glomerulosa, where the enzyme catalyzes aldosterone biosynthesis. This gene is 95% homologous with the steroid 11β-hydroxylase gene that regulates adrenal cortisol biosynthesis. Nearby, on the same chromosome, mutations in aldosterone synthase and 11β-hydroxylase genes create a hybrid gene, with ectopic production of aldosterone in the zona fasciculata under the control of ACTH. In turn, unrestrained secretion of mineralocorticoids leads to prolonged volume expansion and hypertension.
- **Syndrome of apparent mineralocorticoid excess (AME):** In this autosomal recessive form of early-onset hypertension, the mineralocorticoid receptor is stimulated, despite very low levels of aldosterone. Normally, the mineralocorticoid receptor responds both to aldosterone and to cortisol, albeit much more weakly. The aldosterone-like activity of cortisol is suppressed when 11β-hydroxysteroid dehydrogenase in renal tubular epithelial cells converts it to cortisone. In AME, inactivating mutations in the gene for this enzyme allow cortisol to accumulate and constitutively stimulate the mineralocorticoid receptor. Interestingly, consumption of large quantities of licorice can produce a similar syndrome, because glycyrrhetinic acid in licorice inhibits 11β-hydroxysteroid dehydrogenase.
- **Liddle syndrome:** This rare autosomal dominant form of hypertension stems from a gain-of-function mutation in a gene on chromosome 16 that codes for the amiloride-sensitive epithelial sodium channel. Mutations are almost always in the cytoplasmic C terminus of either the β- or γ-subunit of the epithelial sodium channel. Patients have constitutively activated renal tubule sodium channels but low mineralocorticoid levels. Sustained channel activation due to lack of the repressor activity that normally promotes internalization and degradation of the cell surface channel causes kidneys to resorb too much salt and water, independently of mineralocorticoids, leading to volume expansion and hypertension.

All mutations that cause hereditary hypertension result in constitutively increased renal sodium reabsorption. Conversely, mutations that result in sodium-losing syndromes, for example, pseudohypoaldosteronism type I and Gitelman syndrome (with inactivating mutations in the SLC12A3 gene encoding the thiazide-sensitive sodium chloride cotransporter), are associated with profound hypotension. ***Thus, these Mendelian disorders illustrate the central role of sodium homeostasis in determining blood pressure.***

Increasing evidence indicates that common polymorphisms of the angiotensinogen gene contribute to essential hypertension: (1) the angiotensinogen locus is linked to elevated blood pressure in sibling pairs, (2) specific angiotensinogen variants have been tied to hypertension in case-control studies and (3) the same variants are associated with increased plasma angiotensinogen.

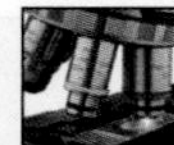

PATHOLOGY: The critical lesions in most cases of hypertension are in resistance vessels that control blood flow through the capillary beds and in the kidney. The lumens of these small muscular arteries and arteriole may be restricted by active contraction of the vessel wall and/or increased vessel wall mass. Thicker vessel walls narrow vascular lumens more than would normal, thinner walls. Over time, chronic hypertension leads to reactive changes in smaller arteries and arterioles throughout the body, collectively termed *arteriosclerosis.* In arterioles, such alterations are termed **arteriolosclerosis**. Kidneys affected with chronic hypertension have a contracted and granular gross appearance, and microscopically often show tubular and glomerular changes.

Benign arteriosclerosis reflects mild chronic hypertension, the major change being a variable increase in arterial wall thickness (Fig. 10-27A). In the smallest arteries and arterioles, these lesions are referred to as **hyaline arteriosclerosis** and **arteriolosclerosis.** "Hyaline" refers to the glassy scarred appearance of the blood vessel walls on light microscopy. Arteriolar walls are thickened by deposition of basement membrane material and accumulation of plasma proteins (Fig. 10-27B). The small muscular arteries have new layers of elastin, manifesting as reduplication of the intimal elastic lamina and increased connective tissue. The vascular lesions of benign arteriosclerosis are particularly evident where they result in loss of renal parenchyma, termed **benign nephrosclerosis**. The presence of benign arteriosclerosis is not diagnostic of hypertension since similar morphologic alterations are common with aging. In addition, hyaline arteriosclerosis may be present in diabetes.

In **malignant hypertension**, elevated blood pressure causes rapidly progressive vascular compromise with the onset of symptomatic disease of the brain, heart or kidney. Although malignant hypertension cannot be defined strictly by the degree of blood pressure elevation, blood pressures usually exceed 160/110 mm Hg. Modern antihypertensive therapy has made malignant hypertension a rare disorder. Malignant hypertension produces dramatic microvascular pathologic changes. Segmental constriction and dilation of retinal arterioles in severely hypertensive persons are sufficiently prominent to allow one to make the diagnosis by

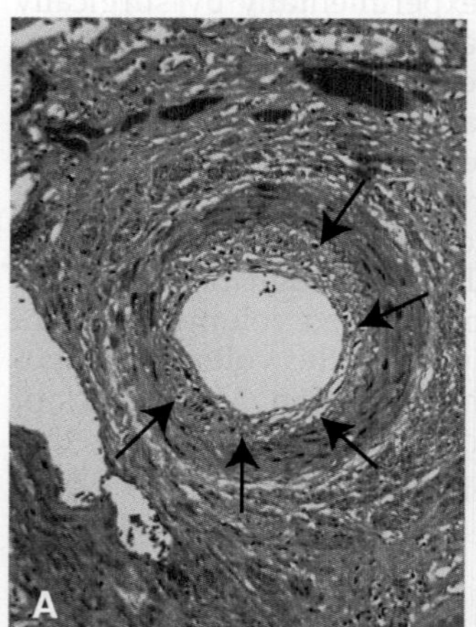

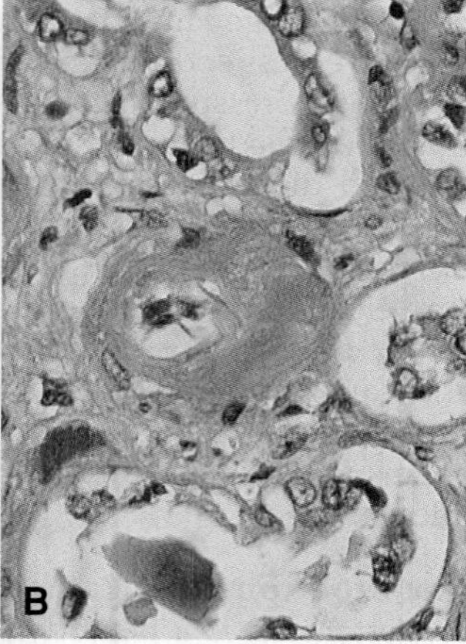

FIGURE 10-27. Benign arteriosclerosis. A. A cross-section of a renal intralobular artery shows irregular thickening of the intima (*arrows*). **B.** A renal arteriole exhibits hyaline arteriolosclerosis (*center*).

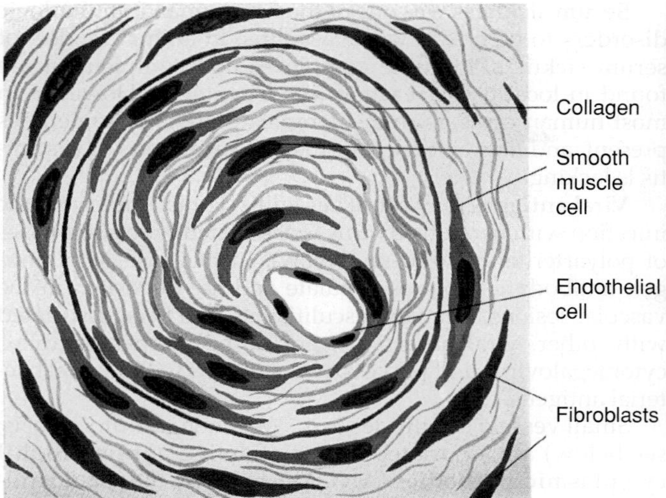

FIGURE 10-28. Arteriolosclerosis. In cases of hypertension, the arterioles exhibit smooth muscle cell proliferation and increased amounts of intercellular collagen and glycosaminoglycans, resulting in an "onion-skin" appearance. The mass of smooth muscle and associated elements tends to fix the size of the lumen and restrict the arteriole's capacity to dilate.

ophthalmoscopy (see Chapter 29). If blood pressure rises rapidly, retinal arterioles show microaneurysms, focal hemorrhages and retinal scarring. Ischemic necrosis and edema of the retina appear as "cotton wool spots" with the ophthalmoscope. These retinal changes are typical of those in other resistance vessels when pressure rises rapidly.

In malignant hypertension, small muscular arteries show segmental dilation due to necrosis of smooth muscle cells. Endothelial integrity is lost in these regions and increased vascular permeability leads to entry of plasma proteins into the vessel wall, deposition of fibrin and an appearance termed **fibrinoid necrosis** (see Chapter 1). Acute injury is rapidly followed by smooth muscle proliferation and a striking concentric increase in the number of layers of smooth muscle cells, producing an "onion-skin" appearance (Fig. 10-28). This form of smooth muscle proliferation may be a response to release of growth factors from platelets and other cells at sites of vascular injury. Together, these changes are labeled **malignant arteriosclerosis** or **arteriolosclerosis**, depending on the size of the vessels affected. In the kidney, lesions of malignant hypertension are known are malignant **nephrosclerosis**.

Mönckeberg Medial Sclerosis

Mönckeberg medial sclerosis refers to degenerative calcification of the media of large and medium-sized muscular arteries. The disorder occurs principally in older persons and most often involves arteries of the upper and lower extremities. It is also common in advanced chronic kidney disease.

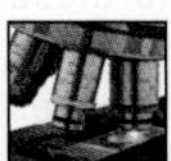

PATHOLOGY: Involved arteries are hard and dilated. Microscopically, the smooth muscle of the media is focally replaced by pale-staining, acellular, hyalinized fibrous tissue, with concentric dystrophic calcification. In most cases the internal elastic lamina shows focal calcification. Osseous metaplasia in calcified areas is occasionally observed. Mönckeberg medial sclerosis is distinct from atherosclerosis and ordinarily does not entail any clinically significant impairment. Some feel that in patients with chronic renal disease the features of Mönckeberg medial sclerosis in arteries should be considered to be a form of accelerated atherosclerosis.

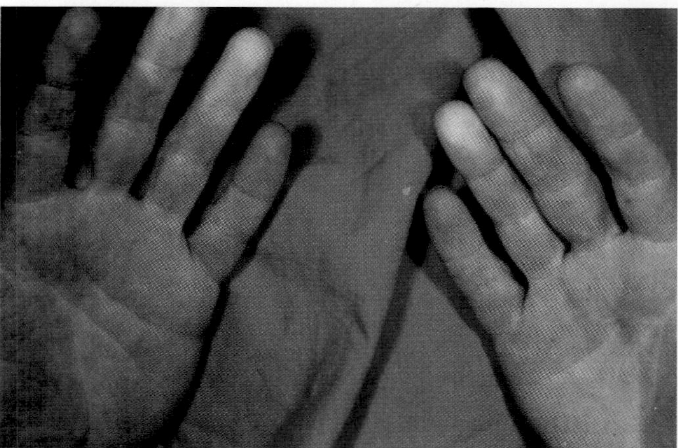

FIGURE 10-29. Raynaud phenomenon. The tips of the fingers show marked pallor.

Raynaud Phenomenon

Raynaud phenomenon refers to intermittent, bilateral attacks of ischemia of the fingers or toes, and sometimes the ears or nose. It is characterized by severe pallor (Fig. 10-29) and is often accompanied by paresthesias and pain. Symptoms are precipitated by cold or emotional stimuli and relieved by heat. Primary cold sensitivity of the Raynaud type is more common in women, and it often starts in the late teens. It is bilateral and symmetric and, on rare occasions, may lead to ulcers or gangrene of the tips of digits. The hands are more commonly affected than feet.

The Raynaud phenomenon may occur as an isolated disorder or as a part of a number of systemic diseases of connective tissue (collagen vascular disorders), particularly scleroderma and systemic lupus erythematosus. It includes primary and secondary cold sensitivity, livedo reticularis and acrocyanosis. Whatever its cause, Raynaud phenomenon reflects vasospasm of the arteries and the arterioles in the skin. Dysregulation of vascular tone by sympathetic nerve activity and by neurohumoral factors may play a role in the pathogenesis of this phenomenon.

Fibromuscular Dysplasia

Fibromuscular dysplasia is a rare, noninflammatory thickening of large and medium-sized muscular arteries, which is distinct from atherosclerosis and arteriosclerosis. The cause is unknown; however, it may be developmental in nature. Renal artery stenosis due to this condition is an important cause of renovascular hypertension, although fibromuscular dysplasia may affect almost any other vessel, including carotid, vertebral and splanchnic arteries. It is typically a disease of women during their reproductive years, but may appear at any age, even in childhood.

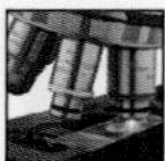

PATHOLOGY: In most cases, the distal two thirds of the renal artery and its primary branches have several segmental stenoses, which represent fibrous and muscular ridges that project into the lumen. Microscopically, these segments show disorderly arrangement and proliferation of the cellular elements of the vessel wall, without necrosis or inflammation. Smooth muscle is replaced by fibrous tissue and myofibroblasts. The media may be thinned. In some cases, intimal fibroplasia predominates, and in unusual instances, connective tissue encircles the adventitia. Other than renal hypertension, the major complication of fibromuscular dysplasia is dissecting aneurysm due to thinning of the media of affected arteries.

Vasculitis

Vasculitis is inflammation and necrosis of blood vessels. It may affect arteries, veins and capillaries (Table 10-8). Arteries or veins may be damaged by immune mechanisms, infectious agents, mechanical trauma, radiation or toxins. However, in many cases, no specific cause is determined.

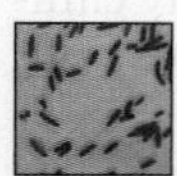

ETIOLOGIC FACTORS: Vasculitic syndromes are thought to involve immune mechanisms, including (1) **deposition of immune complexes,** (2) **direct attack on vessels by circulating antibodies** and (3) **various forms of cell-mediated immunity**. Although the agents that incite these reactions are largely unknown, vasculitis is associated with viral infection in some instances.

Table 10-8

Inflammatory Disorders of Blood Vessels

Polyarteritis Nodosa Group of Systemic Necrotizing Vasculitis
Classic polyarteritis nodosa
Allergic angiitis and granulomatosis (Churg-Strauss variant)
"Overlap syndrome" of systemic angiitis
Hypersensitivity Vasculitis
Serum sickness and similar reactions
Henoch-Schönlein purpura
Vasculitis associated with connective tissue disorders
Vasculitis in cases of essential mixed cryoglobulinemia
Vasculitis associated with other primary disorders
Wegener Granulomatosis
Lymphomatoid Granulomatosis
Giant Cell Arteritis
Temporal arteritis
Takayasu arteritis
Central Nervous System Vasculitis
Vasculitis Associated with Cancer
Mucocutaneous Lymph Node Syndrome (Kawasaki Disease)
Thromboangiitis Obliterans (Buerger Disease)
Behçet Disease
Miscellaneous Vasculitis Syndromes

Serum sickness was one of the first human immunologic disorders to be linked with vasculitis. In animal models of serum sickness, immune complexes and complement are found in local tissue reaction (see Chapter 4). However, in most human cases, immune complexes are only sometimes present, and firm evidence for them in most cases of vasculitis is lacking.

Viral antigens may cause vasculitis. For example, chronic infection with hepatitis B virus is associated with some cases of polyarteritis nodosa (see below). In this case, viral antigen–antibody complexes circulate and are deposited in the vascular lesions. Human vasculitis has also been associated with other viral infections, including herpes simplex, cytomegalovirus and parvovirus, as well as with several bacterial antigens.

Small vessel vasculitides (e.g., Wegener granulomatosis; see below) are associated with circulating **antineutrophil cytoplasmic antibodies (ANCAs)**, but why these autoantibodies appear and how they lead to vasculitis are not known. Some studies suggest that infection plays a role in the development of ANCAs. ANCA may cause endothelial damage by activating neutrophils, and antibody titers correlate with disease activity in some cases. ANCA is detected by indirect immunofluorescence assays using patients' sera and ethanol-fixed neutrophils. Common patterns include a **perinuclear immunofluorescence (P-ANCA,** mainly against myeloperoxidase [MPO]) and a more general **cytoplasmic immunofluorescence (C-ANCA,** mainly against proteinase 3 [PR3]).

The significance of ANCA requires further study, but neutrophils that are activated by, for example, TNF to degranulate express myeloperoxidase and proteinase-3 at their surfaces. ANCA, present as part of the response to infection, can then bind and activate the neutrophils. Other autoantibodies that activate neutrophils and injure endothelial cells have also been identified in vasculitides (Fig. 10-30).

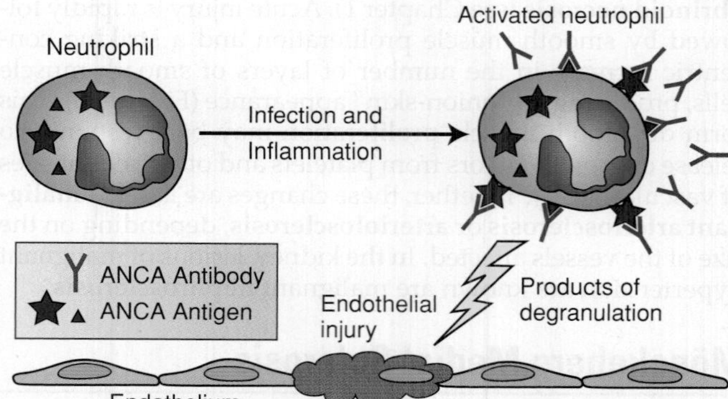

FIGURE 10-30. Model of the pathogenesis of antineutrophil cytoplasmic antibodies (ANCA) vasculitis. ANCA antigens are normally found in the neutrophil cytoplasm with very little surface expression. In inflammation and infection, increased cell surface expression of ANCA antigens is induced in the neutrophils. ANCA present in the circulation due to previous formation through unknown mechanisms binds to these ANCA antigens on the surface, leading to neutrophil activation and interaction with endothelial cells. Neutrophil degranulation releases toxic factors including reactive oxygen species, PR3 and MPO, and other granule enzymes cause endothelial cell apoptosis and necrosis, leading to endothelial injury.

Polyarteritis Nodosa Is an Acute, Necrotizing Vasculitis

Polyarteritis nodosa affects medium-sized and smaller muscular arteries and, occasionally, larger arteries. It is more common in men than in women. The disease was rare until the 1940s, when there was a striking rise in its incidence. The increased frequency of polyarteritis nodosa at that time seemed to be associated with the widespread use of antisera to bacteria and toxins produced in animals, and with use of sulfonamides. The incidence of polyarteritis nodosa now seems to be subsiding.

PATHOLOGY: The characteristic lesions of polyarteritis nodosa are found in small to medium-sized muscular arteries and are distributed in a patchy pattern. However, on occasion they extend into larger arteries, such as the renal, splenic or coronary arteries. Each lesion is no more than a millimeter long and may involve part or all of the circumference of the vessel. The most prominent morphologic feature of an affected artery is an area of fibrinoid necrosis, in which the medial muscle and adjacent tissues are fused into a structureless eosinophilic mass that stains for fibrin. A vigorous acute inflammatory response envelops the area of necrosis, usually involving the entire adventitia (periarteritis), and extends through the other coats of the vessel (Fig. 10-31). Neutrophils, lymphocytes, plasma cells and macrophages are present in varying proportions, and eosinophils are often conspicuous.

As a result of thrombosis in an affected segment of an artery, infarcts are commonly found in involved organs.

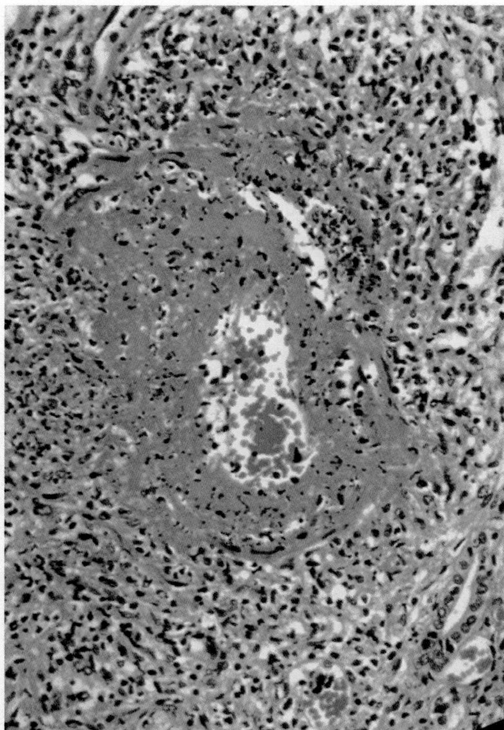

FIGURE 10-31. Polyarteritis nodosa. The intense inflammatory cell infiltrate in the arterial wall and surrounding connective tissue is associated with fibrinoid necrosis and disruption of the vessel wall.

Injury to larger arteries may cause small aneurysms (<0.5 cm in diameter), particularly in branches of the renal, coronary and cerebral arteries. An aneurysm may rupture and, if located in a critical area, may result in fatal hemorrhage.

Over time, many vascular lesions will show evidence of healing, especially if corticosteroids have been administered. Necrotic tissue and inflammatory exudate are resorbed, and the vessel is left with fibrosis of the media and conspicuous gaps in the elastic laminae.

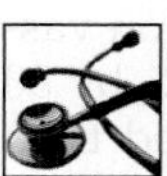

CLINICAL FEATURES: Clinical manifestations of polyarteritis nodosa are highly variable and depend on the chance locations of lesions in different organs. Kidneys, heart, skeletal muscle, skin and mesentery are most frequently involved, but lesions may occur in almost any organ, including the bowel, pancreas, lungs, liver and brain. Constitutional symptoms such as fever and weight loss are common. Polyarteritis nodosa–like lesions may occur in viral infections including hepatitis B and C and human immunodeficiency virus (HIV).

Without treatment, polyarteritis nodosa is usually fatal, but anti-inflammatory and immunosuppressive therapy, in the form of corticosteroids and cyclophosphamide, leads to remissions or cures in most patients.

Hypersensitivity Angiitis Is a Response to Exogenous Substances

Hypersensitivity angiitis refers to a broad category of inflammatory vascular lesions that are thought to represent a reaction to foreign materials (e.g., bacterial products or drugs). In the case of vascular lesions confined predominantly to skin, the terms **leukocytoclastic vasculitis** (referring to nuclear debris from disintegrating neutrophils), **cutaneous vasculitis** or **cutaneous necrotizing venulitis** (emphasizing the predominant involvement of the venules) are applied. **Systemic hypersensitivity angiitis**, also referred to as **microscopic polyangiitis**, affects many of the same organs as polyarteritis nodosa but is restricted to the smallest arteries and arterioles.

CLINICAL FEATURES: Cutaneous vasculitis may follow administration of many drugs, including aspirin, penicillin and thiazide diuretics. It is also commonly related to such disparate infections as streptococcal and staphylococcal illnesses, viral hepatitis, tuberculosis and bacterial endocarditis. The disease typically presents as palpable purpura, principally on the lower extremities. Microscopically, superficial cutaneous venules show fibrinoid necrosis with acute inflammation. Cutaneous vasculitis is generally self-limited (see Chapter 24).

Systemic hypersensitivity angiitis may be an isolated entity or a feature of other conditions, including collagen vascular diseases (lupus erythematosus, rheumatoid arthritis, Sjögren syndrome), Henoch-Schönlein purpura, dysproteinemias and a variety of malignancies. Patients with systemic hypersensitivity angiitis may also have cutaneous purpuric lesions. The most feared complication of microscopic polyangiitis is renal involvement, characterized by rapidly progressive glomerulonephritis and renal failure (see Chapter 16). *Microscopic polyarteritis is strongly associated with P-ANCA.*

Giant Cell Arteritis (Temporal Arteritis, Granulomatous Arteritis) Is a Focal, Chronic, Granulomatous Inflammation, Mainly of the Temporal Arteries

Although it most often affects the temporal artery, it may also involve other cranial arteries, the aorta (giant cell aortitis) and its branches and occasionally other arteries. Aortic aneurysms and dissection occur. The average age at onset is 70 years; it is rare before age 50. It is the most common vasculitis; its incidence rises with age and may reach 1% by 80 years of age. Women are slightly more often affected than men. The age at onset helps differentiate it from other vasculitides that may involve the same vessels in younger people, such as Takayasu disease.

MOLECULAR PATHOGENESIS: The etiology of giant cell arteritis is obscure. Its association with HLA-DR4 and its occurrence in first-degree relatives support a genetic component in its pathogenesis. The morphologic alterations, including the presence of activated CD4$^+$ T-helper cells and macrophages and association of giant cell arteritis with a specific polymorphism of the leukocyte adhesion molecule ICAM-1, suggest an immune reaction. B lymphocytes are lacking. Macrophages at the border of the intima and media produce matrix metalloproteinases that digest tissue matrix. ANCA is absent in giant cell arteritis. Generalized muscle aching and widespread distribution of its manifestations are consistent with a relationship to rheumatoid diseases.

PATHOLOGY: Affected vessels are cord-like with nodular thickening. Lumens are reduced to slits or may be obliterated by a thrombus (Fig. 10-32A). Microscopically, the media and intima show granulomatous inflammation; aggregates of macrophages, lymphocytes and plasma cells are admixed with variable numbers of eosinophils and neutrophils. Giant cells tend to be distributed at the internal elastic lamina (Fig. 10-32B) but vary widely in number. Foreign body giant cells and Langhans giant cells are both seen. Foci of necrosis are characterized by changes in the internal elastica, which becomes swollen, irregular and fragmented, and in advanced lesions may completely disappear. Fragments of the elastica occasionally appear in the giant cells. In the late stages, the intima is conspicuously thickened and the media is fibrotic. Thrombi may obliterate the lumen, after which organization and canalization occur.

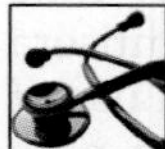

CLINICAL FEATURES: Giant cell arteritis tends to be benign and self-limited, and symptoms subside in 6 to 12 months. Patients present with headache and throbbing temporal pain. In some instances, there are early constitutional symptoms, including malaise, fever and weight loss, plus generalized muscular aching or stiffness in the shoulders and hips. Throbbing and pain over the temporal artery are accompanied by swelling, tenderness and redness in overlying skin. Almost half of patients have visual symptoms, which may proceed from transient to permanent blindness in one or both eyes, sometimes rapidly. Occasionally, the disease causes myocardial, CNS or gastrointestinal infarcts, which may be fatal. Because the inflammatory process is patchy, biopsy of the temporal artery may not be diagnostic in as many as 40% of patients with otherwise classic manifestations. Response to corticosteroids is usually dramatic; symptoms subside within days.

Wegener Granulomatosis Is a Vasculitis of the Respiratory Tract and Kidney

Wegener granulomatosis is a systemic necrotizing vasculitis of unknown etiology, characterized by granulomatous lesions of the nose, sinuses and lungs and renal glomerular disease. Men are affected more often than women, usually in the fifth and sixth decades. The etiology is unknown. More than 90% of patients with Wegener granulomatosis are positive for ANCA, of whom 75% have C-ANCA. It has been suggested that these antibodies activate circulating neutrophils to attack blood vessels. The response to immunosuppressive therapy supports an immunologic basis for the disease.

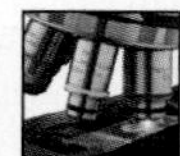

PATHOLOGY: Lesions of Wegener granulomatosis feature parenchymal necrosis, vasculitis and granulomatous inflammation composed of neutrophils,

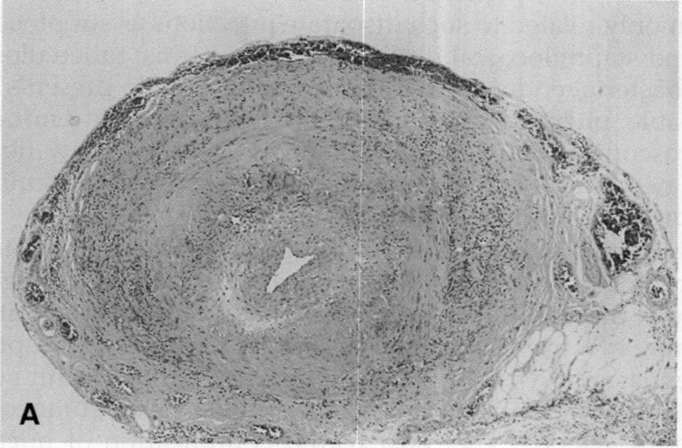

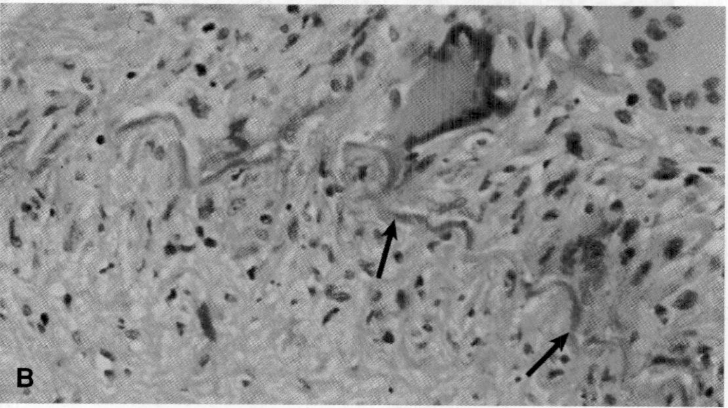

FIGURE 10-32. Temporal arteritis. A. A photomicrograph of a temporal artery shows chronic inflammation throughout the wall and a lumen severely narrowed by intimal thickening. **B.** A high-power view shows giant cells adjacent to the fragmented internal elastic lamina (*arrows*).

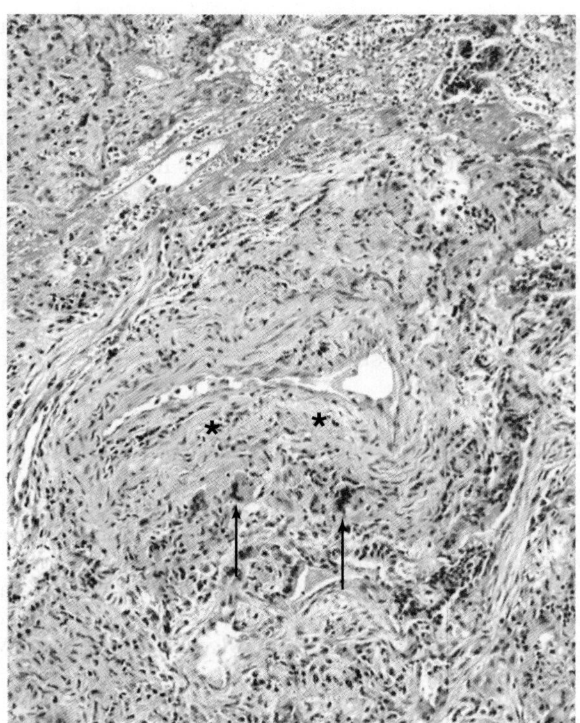

FIGURE 10-33. Wegener granulomatosis. A photomicrograph of the lung shows vasculitis of a pulmonary artery. There are chronic inflammatory cells and Langerhans giant cells (*arrows*) in the wall, together with thickening of the intima (*asterisks*).

lymphocytes, plasma cells, macrophages and eosinophils. Individual lesions in the lung may be as large as 5 cm across and must be distinguished from tuberculosis. Vasculitis involving small arteries and veins may be seen anywhere but occurs most frequently in the respiratory tract (Fig. 10-33), kidney and spleen. Arteritis is characterized principally by chronic inflammation, although acute inflammation, necrotizing and nonnecrotizing granulomatous inflammation and fibrinoid necrosis are frequently present. Medial thickening and intimal proliferation are common and often lead to narrowing or obliteration of the lumen.

The most prominent pulmonary feature is persistent bilateral pneumonitis, with nodular infiltrates that undergo cavitation similarly to tuberculous lesions (although the mechanisms are clearly different). Chronic sinusitis and nasopharyngeal mucosal ulcers are common. The kidney at first shows focal necrotizing glomerulonephritis, which progresses to crescentic glomerulonephritis (see Chapter 17).

CLINICAL FEATURES: Most patients present with symptoms referable to the respiratory tract, particularly pneumonitis and sinusitis. In fact, the lung is eventually involved in over 90% of patients. Radiologically, multiple pulmonary infiltrates are prominent, which are often cavitary. Hematuria and proteinuria are common, and glomerular disease can progress to renal failure. Rash, muscular pains, joint involvement and neurologic symptoms occur. Most patients (80%) die within a year if untreated, with a mean survival of 5 to 6 months. Treatment with cyclophosphamide produces both complete remissions and substantial disease-free intervals in most patients. Interestingly, antimicrobial sulfa drugs significantly reduce the incidence of relapses, suggesting a relationship of the disease to bacterial infection.

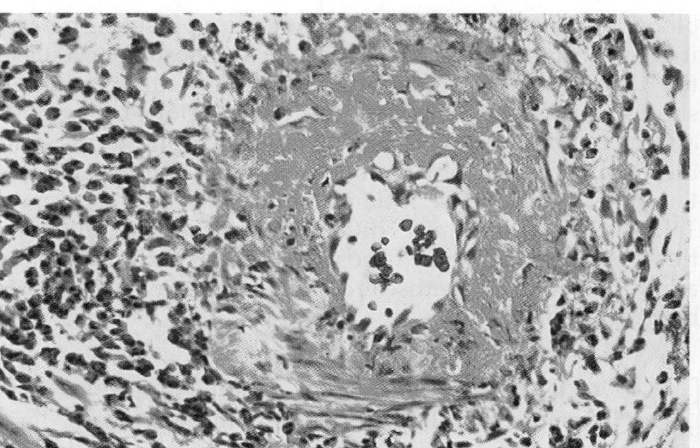

FIGURE 10-34. Churg-Strauss syndrome. A medium-sized artery shows fibrinoid necrosis and a surrounding eosinophilic infiltrate.

Allergic Granulomatosis and Angiitis (Churg-Strauss Syndrome) Is a Systemic Vasculitis of Young Patients with Asthma

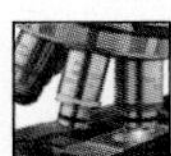

PATHOLOGY: Two thirds of patients with Churg-Strauss syndrome have P-ANCA. Widespread necrotizing lesions of small and medium-sized arteries (Fig. 10-34), arterioles and veins are found in the lungs, spleen, kidney, heart, liver, CNS and other organs. These lesions are granulomas and intense eosinophilic infiltrates in and around blood vessels. The resulting fibrinoid necrosis, thrombosis and aneurysm formation may simulate polyarteritis nodosa, although Churg-Strauss syndrome seems to be a distinct entity. It must also be distinguished from other eosinophilic syndromes, such as parasitic and fungal infestations, Wegener granulomatosis, eosinophilic pneumonia (Loeffler syndrome) and drug vasculitis.

Untreated, these patients have a poor prognosis, but corticosteroid therapy is almost always effective.

Takayasu Arteritis Is an Inflammatory Disease Affecting the Aorta and Its Major Branches

This form of arteritis is seen worldwide. It mainly affects women (90%), most of whom are under 30 years of age. The cause of Takayasu arteritis is unknown, but an autoimmune basis has been proposed.

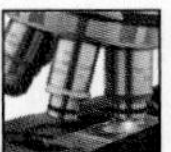

PATHOLOGY: Takayasu arteritis is classified according to the extent of aortic involvement: (1) disease restricted to the aortic arch and its branches, (2) arteritis only affecting the descending thoracic and abdominal aorta and its branches and (3) combined involvement of the arch and descending aorta. The pulmonary artery is also occasionally affected and involvement of the retinal vasculature is often a prominent feature.

On gross examination, the aorta is thickened. The intima exhibits focal, raised plaques. Branches of the aorta often have localized stenosis or occlusion, which interferes with blood flow and accounts for the synonym **pulseless disease** if the subclavian arteries are affected. The aorta, particularly the distal thoracic and abdominal segments, commonly shows variably sized aneurysms. Early lesions of the aorta and its main branches consist of an acute panarteritis, with infiltrates of neutrophils, mononuclear cells and occasional Langhans giant cells. Inflammation of vasa vasorum in Takayasu arteritis requires differentiation from syphilitic aortitis. Late lesions display fibrosis and severe intimal proliferation. Secondary atherosclerotic changes may obscure the basic disease.

CLINICAL FEATURES: Patients with early Takayasu arteritis complain of constitutional symptoms, dizziness, visual disturbances, dyspnea and, occasionally, syncope. As the disease progresses, cardiac symptoms become more severe with intermittent claudication of the arms or legs. Asymmetric differences in blood pressure may develop and pulses in one extremity may actually disappear. Hypertension may reflect coarctation of the aorta or renal artery stenosis. Most patients eventually develop congestive heart failure. Loss of visual acuity may range from field defects to total blindness. Early Takayasu arteritis responds to corticosteroids, but the later lesions require surgical reconstruction.

Kawasaki Disease (Mucocutaneous Lymph Node Syndrome) Is a Childhood Vasculitis That Targets Coronary Arteries

It is an acute necrotizing vasculitis of infancy and early childhood characterized by high fever, rash, conjunctival and oral lesions and lymphadenitis. In 70% of patients, vasculitis affects the coronary arteries and leads to coronary artery aneurysms (Fig. 10-35), which may cause death in 1% to 2% of cases.

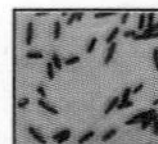

ETIOLOGIC FACTORS: Kawasaki disease is usually self-limited. Although an infectious cause has been sought, none has been conclusively demonstrated. Infection with *parvovirus B19* or with *New Haven coronavirus* has been implicated in some cases, and there is evidence for various bacterial infections including *Staphylococcus*, *Streptococcus* and *Chlamydia* in others. The common theme seems to be viral or bacterial production of superantigens (i.e., molecules that bind to major histocompatability complex [MHC] class II receptors and the V-beta region of the T-cell receptor, thereby massively activating immune responses in an antigen-nonspecific manner). Autoantibodies to endothelial and smooth muscle cells have been identified in some patients.

Thromboangiitis Obliterans (Buerger Disease) Is a Peripheral Vascular Disease of Smokers

It is an occlusive inflammatory disease of medium and small arteries in the distal arms and legs. At one time Buerger disease occurred almost exclusively in young and middle-aged men who smoked heavily, but it is now also described in women. It is more common in the Mediterranean area, Middle East and Asia.

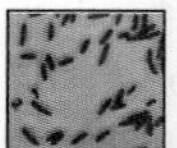

ETIOLOGIC FACTORS: The etiologic role of smoking in Buerger disease is underscored by the fact that cessation of smoking may lead to remission, and resumption of smoking to exacerbation. Yet, how tobacco smoke produces Buerger disease is obscure. Certain polyphenols from tobacco elicit antibodies and can induce inflammation. Smokers show a higher incidence of such sensitivity to tobacco than do nonsmokers. Cell-mediated hypersensitivity to collagen types II and III has also been observed. Endothelium-dependent vasodilatory responses in nondiseased blood vessels are dysfunctional in some patients, suggesting that there may be a generalized impairment of

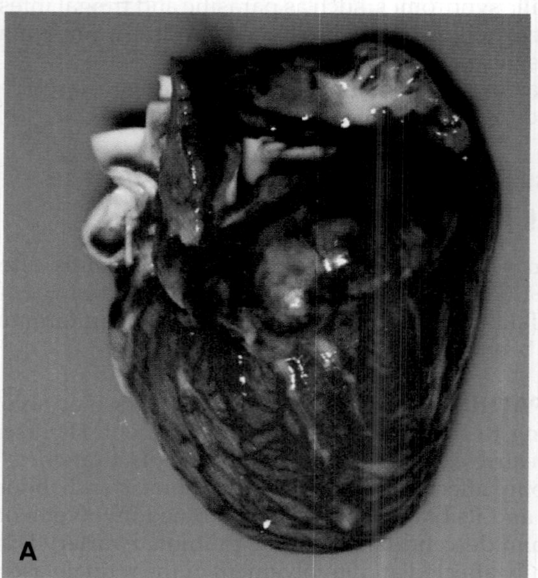

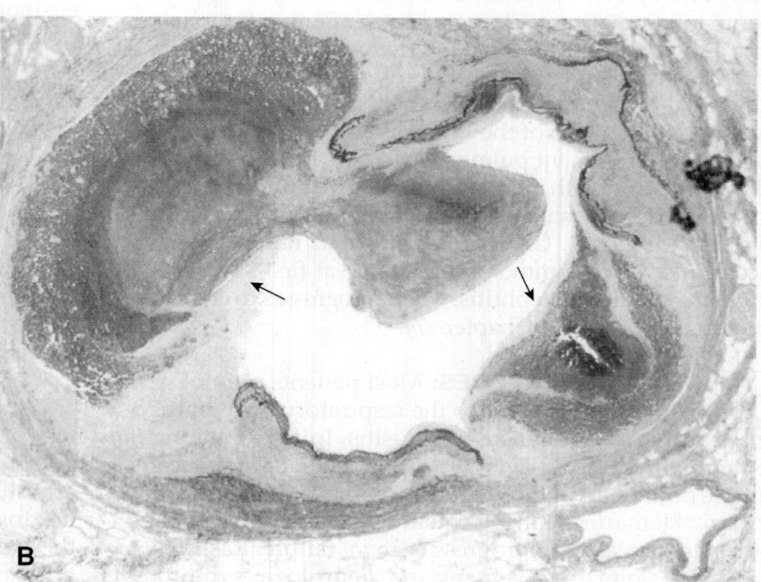

FIGURE 10-35. Kawasaki disease. A. The heart of a child who died from Kawasaki disease shows conspicuous coronary artery aneurysms. **B.** A microscopic section of a coronary artery from the same patient shows two large defects (*arrows*) in the internal elastic lamina, with two small aneurysms filled with thrombus.

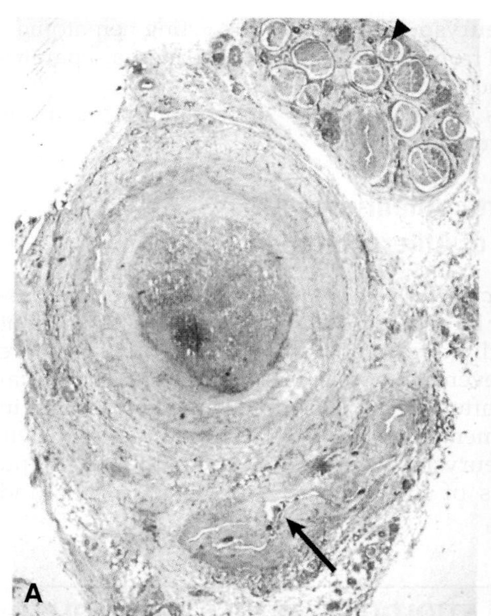

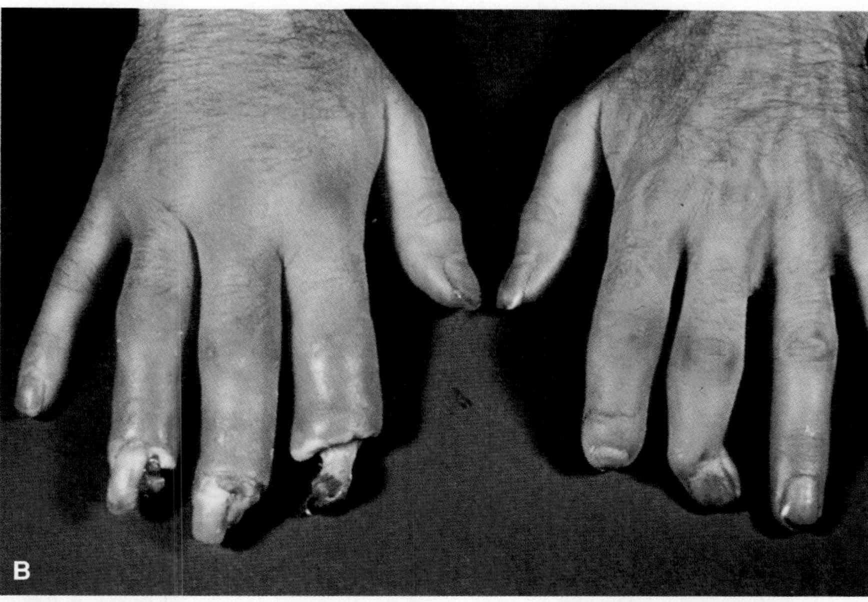

FIGURE 10-36. Buerger disease. A. Section of the upper extremity shows an organized arterial thrombus that has occluded the lumen. Some inflammatory cells are evident in the adventitial fat. In this instance, the vein (*arrow*) and the adjacent nerve (*arrowhead*) show foci of chronic inflammation. **B.** The hand shows necrosis of the tips of the fingers.

endothelial function. HLA-A9 and HLA-B5 haplotypes are more common among Buerger patients, further suggesting that a genetically controlled hypersensitivity to tobacco is involved in the pathogenesis of disease.

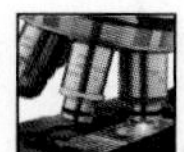

PATHOLOGY: The earliest change in Buerger disease is acute inflammation of medium-sized and small arteries. Neutrophil infiltrates extend to involve neighboring veins and nerves. Involvement of the endothelium in inflamed areas leads to thrombosis and obliteration of the lumen (Fig. 10-36A). Small microabscesses of the vessel wall, with a central area of neutrophils surrounded by fibroblasts and Langhans giant cells, distinguish this process from thrombosis associated with atherosclerosis. Early lesions often become severe enough to cause gangrene of the extremity, leading to amputation. Late in the course of the disease, thrombi are completely organized and partly canalized.

CLINICAL FEATURES: Symptoms of Buerger disease usually start between the ages of 25 and 40 as intermittent claudication (cramping pains in muscles after exercise, quickly relieved by rest). Patients often present with painful ulceration of a digit, which progresses to destruction of the tips of the involved digits (Fig. 10-36B). Persons with Buerger disease who continue to smoke may slowly lose both hands and feet.

Behçet Disease Is a Vasculitis Mainly Involving Mucous Membranes of Many Organs

Behçet disease is a systemic vasculitis characterized by oral aphthous ulcers, genital ulcers and ocular inflammation. Occasionally, there are lesions in the CNS, gastrointestinal tract and cardiovascular system. Both large and small vessels show vasculitis. The mucocutaneous lesions exhibit nonspecific vasculitis of arterioles, capillaries and venules, with infiltration of vessel walls and perivascular tissue by lymphocytes and plasma cells. Occasional endothelial cells are proliferated and swollen. Medium and large arteries show destructive arteritis, with fibrinoid necrosis, mononuclear infiltration, thrombosis, aneurysms and hemorrhage. The cause is unknown, but the effectiveness of corticosteroid treatment and an association with specific HLA subtypes suggest an immune basis.

Radiation Vasculitis Has Acute and Chronic Phases

The acute phase of radiation vasculitis shows endothelial injury and denudation, ballooning degeneration of intimal smooth muscle cells and macrophages and medial smooth muscle cell necrosis, which may be fibrinoid. Thrombi may be seen in small arteries and arterioles. In the chronic phase, intimal hyperplasia and fibrosis of the vessel wall are noted. Occasionally, vessels show complete fibrous occlusion. Radiation damage predisposes to accelerated atherosclerosis.

Rickettsial Vasculitis Is Caused by Intracellular Parasites

Rickettsiae are obligate intracellular parasites that produce a characteristic vasculitis (see Chapter 9). Each different rickettsial disease affects different types of small vessels and its extent and severity varies. The organisms usually disseminate from the entry site into the blood and invade endothelial cells, smooth muscle cells of the media of small vessels and capillaries.

Aneurysms

Arterial aneurysms are localized dilations of blood vessels caused by a congenital or acquired weakness of the media. They are not rare, and their incidence tends to rise with age.

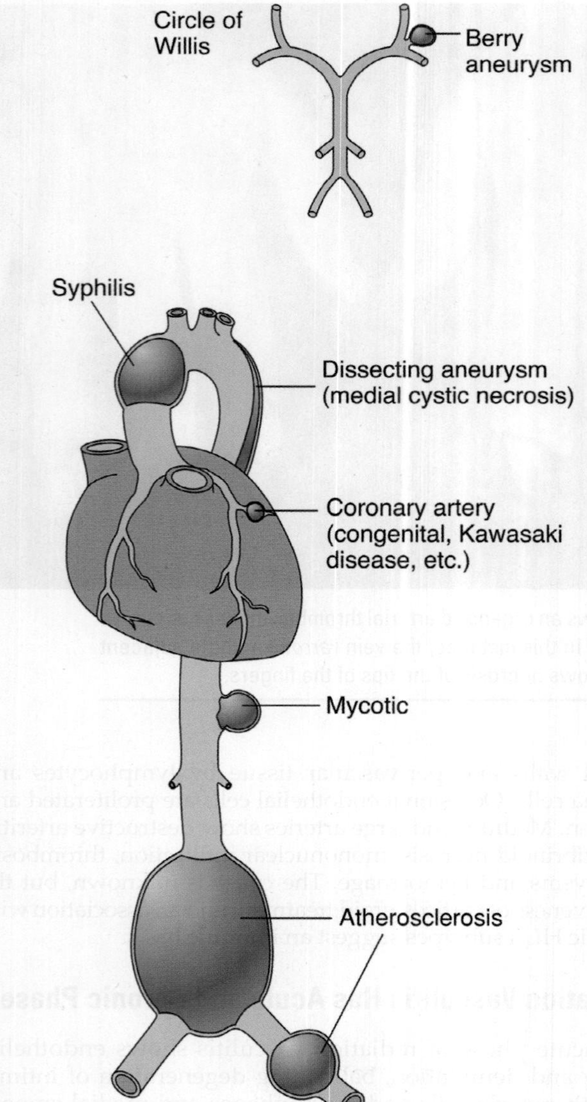

FIGURE 10-37. The locations of aneurysms. Syphilitic aneurysms are the common variety in the ascending aorta, which is usually spared by the atherosclerotic process. Atherosclerotic aneurysms can occur in the abdominal aorta or muscular arteries, including the coronary and popliteal arteries and other vessels. Berry aneurysms are seen in the circle of Willis, mainly at branch points; their rupture leads to subarachnoid hemorrhage. Mycotic aneurysms occur almost anywhere that bacteria can deposit on vessel walls.

Aneurysms of the aorta and other arteries are found in as many as 10% of autopsies. The wall of an aneurysm is formed by stretched remnants of the arterial wall.

Aneurysms are classified by location, configuration and etiology (Fig. 10-37). The location refers to the type of vessel involved—artery or vein—and the specific vessel affected, such as the aorta or popliteal artery. There are several categories of aneurysms:

- **Fusiform aneurysms** are ovoid swellings parallel to the long axis of the vessel.
- **Saccular aneurysms** are bubble-like arterial wall outpouchings at a site of weakened media.
- **Dissecting aneurysms** are actually dissecting hematomas, in which blood from hemorrhage into the media separates the layers of the vascular wall.
- **Arteriovenous aneurysms** are direct communications between an artery and a vein.

Abdominal Aortic Aneurysms Are Complications of Atherosclerosis

Abdominal aortic aneurysms are dilations that increase vessel wall diameter by at least 50%. They are the most frequent aneurysms, usually developing after the age of 50, and are associated with severe atherosclerosis of the artery. The prevalence rises to 6% after age 80. They occur much more often in men than in women, and half of patients are hypertensive. Occasionally, aneurysms are found in ascending, arch and descending parts of the thoracic aorta, and in iliac and popliteal arteries.

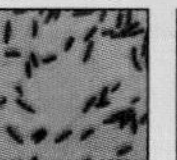
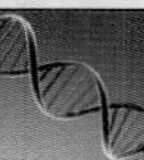

ETIOLOGIC FACTORS AND MOLECULAR PATHOGENESIS: Abdominal aortic aneurysms invariably occur in the context of atherosclerosis. However, it is thought that the disease is actually multifactorial, involving inflammation and dysregulation of matrix remodeling and repair. The growth of the aneurysm is regulated in part by hemodynamic forces that occur in the aneurysm, and as the radius of the vessel increases, so does circumferential wall stress. Enzymes important in the proteolysis of medial and adventitial type I/III fibrillar collagen promote the growth of abdominal aneurysms, including matrix metalloproteinase 8; cysteine proteases cathepsins K, L and S; and osteoclastic proton pump vH$^+$-adenosine triphosphatase (ATPase). IL-1β, TNF-α, monocyte chemotactin protein-1 (MCP-1), IL-8 and other proinflammatory cytokines have been linked to the pathogenesis of abdominal aneurysms. Aneurysm walls show increases in chemokines and growth factors that regulate remodeling, such as granulocyte colony-stimulating factor (G-CSF), macrophage colony-stimulating factor (M-CSF), IL-13, insulin-like growth factor-1 (IGF-1), TGF-β, macrophage inflammatory protein-1α (MIP-1α) and MIP-1β, MMP-2 and MMP-9. Familial clustering suggests a genetic predisposition, although this is poorly understood.

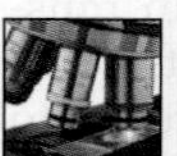

PATHOLOGY: Most abdominal aortic aneurysms occur distal to the renal arteries and proximal to the aortic bifurcation (Fig. 10-38). They are usually fusiform, but saccular varieties are occasionally seen. The lesions may be of almost any size, but most of the symptomatic ones are over 5 to 6 cm in diameter. Some extend into the iliac arteries, which occasionally exhibit distinct aneurysms distal to the one in the aorta. Aneurysms that extend above the renal arteries may occlude the origin of the superior mesenteric artery and the celiac axis.

Most abdominal aortic aneurysms are lined by raised, ulcerated and calcified (complicated) atherosclerotic lesions. Most contain mural thrombi of varying degrees of organization, portions of which may embolize to peripheral arteries. Infrequently, a thrombus itself may enlarge enough to compromise the lumen of the aorta.

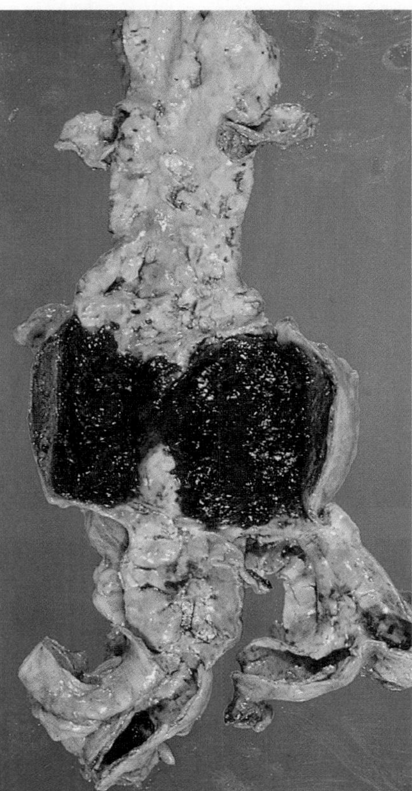

FIGURE 10-38. Atherosclerotic aneurysm of the abdominal aorta. The aneurysm has been opened longitudinally to reveal a large mural thrombus in the lumen. The aorta and common iliac arteries display complicated lesions of atherosclerosis.

Microscopically, arterial walls of complicated atherosclerotic lesions are destroyed and replaced by fibrous tissue. Remnants of normal media are seen focally, and atheromatous lesions extend to variable depths. The adventitia is thickened and focally inflamed as a response to severe atherosclerosis.

CLINICAL FEATURES: Many abdominal aortic aneurysms are asymptomatic and are discovered only by palpating a mass in the abdomen or on radiologic examination for some other reason. In some cases the condition is brought to medical attention by the onset of abdominal pain, which often reflects aneurysm expansion. Abrupt occlusion of a peripheral artery by an embolus from a mural thrombus presents as sudden ischemia of a lower limb. The most dreaded complication of aortic aneurysms is rupture and exsanguination into the retroperitoneum (or chest), in which case the patient presents with pain, shock and a pulsatile mass in the abdomen. This is an acute emergency, and half of patients die, even with prompt surgical intervention. Therefore, even asymptomatic large aneurysms are often replaced by or bypassed with prosthetic grafts.

The risk of rupture of an abdominal aortic aneurysm is a function of its size. Aneurysms under 4 cm in diameter rarely rupture (2%), while 25% to 40% of those larger than 5 cm rupture within 5 years of their discovery.

Aneurysms of Cerebral Arteries Lead to Subarachnoid Hemorrhage

The most common type of cerebral aneurysm is saccular and is called a **berry aneurysm**, because it resembles a berry attached to a twig of the arterial tree. Berry aneurysms occur due to congenital defects at branch points in arterial walls and tend to arise at branches in the circle of Willis or one of the arterial junctions. The most common sites are (1) between the anterior cerebral and anterior communicating arteries, (2) between the internal carotid and posterior communicating arteries and (3) between the first main divisions of the middle cerebral artery and the bifurcation of the internal carotid artery. These aneurysms are also discussed Chapter 28.

In a Dissecting Aneurysm Blood Enters the Arterial Wall and Separates Its Layers

The dissection occurs on a path along the length of the vessel (Fig. 10-39) and represents essentially a false lumen within the wall of the artery. Although the lesion is usually termed an aneurysm, it is actually a form of hematoma. Dissecting aneurysms most often affect the aorta, especially the ascending aorta, and major branches of the aorta. Thoracic dissections may involve the ascending aorta alone (type A) or the distal aorta sparing the ascending aorta (type B). Their frequency has been estimated to be as high as 1 in 400 autopsies, with men affected three times as frequently as women. They may occur at almost any age, but are most common in the sixth and seventh decades. Almost all patients have a history of hypertension and associated conditions include atherosclerosis, bicuspid aortic valve and idiopathic aortic root dilatation.

MOLECULAR PATHOGENESIS: The basis of dissecting aneurysms is usually weakening of the aortic media. The changes were originally described as **cystic medial necrosis (of Erdheim)**, because focal loss of elastic and muscle fibers in the media leads to "cystic" spaces filled with a metachromatic myxoid material. These spaces are not true cysts but are rather pools of matrix collected between the cells and tissues of the media. The mechanisms of medial degeneration are not well understood. However, genetic studies have linked some cases to specific syndromes including Marfan, Ehlers-Danlos and Loeys-Dietz syndromes, and to filamin mutations. In Marfan syndrome, a systemic connective tissue disorder, specific mutations in the gene encoding the extracellular matrix protein fibrillin have been identified (see Chapter 6). In addition, in some patients, mutations have been identified in other genes including TGF-β receptors 1 and 2, smooth muscle cell–specific β-myosin (MYH11) and α-actin (ACTA2). Aging also results in mild degenerative changes in the aorta, with focal elastin loss and medial fibrosis. Patients with dissection of the thoracic aorta show decreased expression of fibulin-5, an extracellular protein that regulates elastic fiber assembly. Abnormal release of MMP-2 and its inhibitor by smooth muscle cells has been implicated in aortic aneurysms. In animals, defective cross-linking of collagen induced by a copper-deficient diet (lysyl oxidase is a copper-dependent enzyme) causes

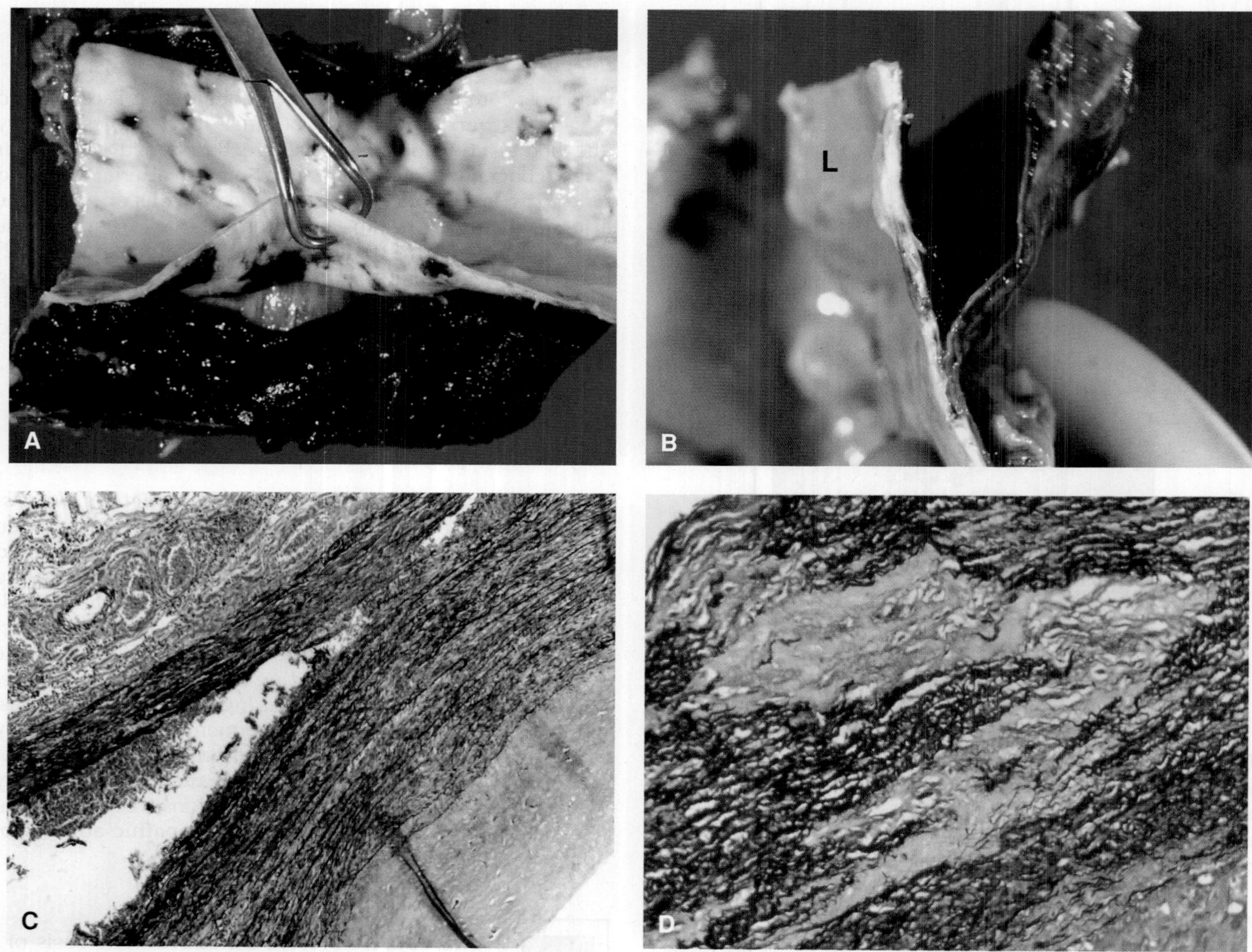

FIGURE 10-39. Dissecting aortic aneurysm. A. Thoracic aorta with metal clamps revealing the dissection and hematoma in the wall with old blood clot. **B.** The thoracic aorta has been opened longitudinally and reveals clotted blood dissecting the media of the vessel. L, lumen. **C.** Atherosclerotic aorta with dissection along the outer third of the media (elastic stain). **D.** A section of the aortic wall stained with aldehyde fuchsin shows pools of metachromatic material characteristic of the degenerative process known as cystic medial necrosis.

dissecting aneurysm of the aorta. The same lesion is produced by feeding β-aminopropionitrile, an inhibitor of lysyl oxidase. Persons with Wilson disease who are treated with penicillamine, a copper chelator, also may develop medial necrosis of the aorta. Taken together, these data suggest that the common factor in these several situations is a molecular defect that leads to weakness of aortic connective tissue.

PATHOLOGY: The initial event that triggers medial dissection is controversial. Over 95% of cases have a transverse tear in the intima and internal media, and it is widely held that spontaneous laceration of the intima allows blood from the lumen to enter and dissect the media. Alternatively, it has been proposed that hemorrhage from vasa vasorum into a media weakened by cystic medial necrosis initiates stress on the intima, which in turn leads to the ubiquitous intimal tear.

Most intimal tears are in the ascending aorta, 1 or 2 cm above the aortic ring. Dissection in the media occurs within seconds and separates the inner two thirds of the aorta from the outer third. It can also involve coronary arteries, great vessels of the neck and renal, mesenteric or iliac arteries. Since the outer wall of the false channel of the dissecting aneurysm is thin, hemorrhage into the extravascular space—including the pericardium, mediastinum, pleural space and retroperitoneum—frequently causes death. In 5% to 10% of cases, the blood within the dissection reenters the lumen via a second distal tear to form a "double-barreled aorta." In a comparable proportion, a reentry site leads to communication of the aorta with a major artery, most often the iliac artery.

CLINICAL FEATURES: Typically patients present with acute onset of severe, "tearing" pain in the anterior chest, which is sometimes misdiagnosed as myocardial infarction. Loss of one or more arterial pulses is common, as is a murmur of aortic regurgitation. Hypertension

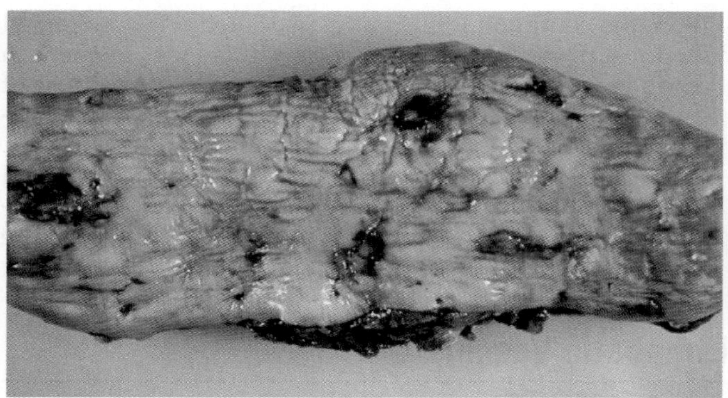

FIGURE 10-40. Syphilitic aortitis. The thoracic aorta is dilated, and its inner surface shows the typical "tree bark" appearance.

is a frequent finding, but hypotension is an ominous sign and suggests aortic rupture. Cardiac tamponade or congestive heart failure is diagnosed by the usual criteria.

Before antihypertensive and surgical treatment became available, more than a third of patients with aortic dissection died within 24 hours, and 80% succumbed by 2 weeks. Half of the survivors died within 3 months. Surgical intervention and control of hypertension have reduced overall mortality to less than 20%.

Syphilitic Aneurysms Are Due to Inflammation of Aortic Vasa Vasorum

Syphilis was once the most common cause of aortic aneurysms, but as syphilis has become less common, so has syphilitic vascular disease, including aortitis and aneurysms. Syphilitic aneurysms mainly affect the ascending aorta, which shows endarteritis and periarteritis of vasa vasorum. These vessels ramify in the adventitia and penetrate the outer and middle thirds of the aorta, where they become encircled by lymphocytes, plasma cells and macrophages. Obliterative changes in the vasa vasorum cause focal medial necrosis and scarring and disruption and disorganization of elastic lamellae. The depressed medial scars lead to a roughened intimal surface, a "tree bark" appearance (Fig. 10-40). The relentless pressure of the blood eventually forces the weakened wall of the ascending aorta and aortic arch to form a fusiform aneurysm.

Mycotic (Infectious) Aneurysms Result From Weakening of a Vessel Wall by a Microbial Infection

Mycotic aneurysms have a tendency to rupture and hemorrhage. They may develop in the aortic wall or in cerebral vessels during septicemia, most commonly due to bacterial endocarditis. Mesenteric, splenic or renal arteries are also commonly affected. Mycotic aneurysms may also occur adjacent to a focus of tuberculous or a bacterial abscess.

Veins

Varicose Veins Are Enlarged, Tortuous Veins

Superficial varicosities of leg veins are usually in the saphenous system, and are very common. They vary from a trivial knot of dilated veins to painful and disabling distention of the whole venous system of the leg, with secondary trophic disturbances. It is estimated that as much as 10% to 20% of the population has some varicosities in the leg veins, but only a fraction of these develop symptoms.

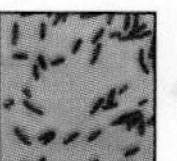

ETIOLOGIC FACTORS: There are a number of risk factors for varicose veins:

- **Age:** Varicose veins increase in frequency with age and may reach 50% in persons over 50. This increase in incidence may reflect age-related degenerative changes in connective tissues of vein walls, loss of supporting fat and connective tissues, more flaccid muscle tone and inactivity.
- **Sex:** Among 30- to 50-year-olds, women are more often affected by varicose veins than men, particularly women who have experienced increased venous pressure from the pressure of a pregnant uterus on the iliac veins.
- **Heredity:** There is a strong familial predisposition to varicose veins, possibly owing to inherited configurations or structural weaknesses of the walls or valves of the veins.
- **Posture:** Leg vein pressure is 5 to 10 times higher when someone is erect rather than recumbent. As a result, the incidence of varicose veins and its complications are greater in people whose occupations require them to stand in one place for long periods.
- **Obesity:** Excessive body weight increases the incidence of varicose veins, possibly because of increased intra-abdominal pressure or poor support provided by subcutaneous fat to vessel walls.

Other factors that raise venous pressure in the legs can cause varicose veins, including pelvic tumors, congestive heart failure and thrombotic obstruction of the main venous trunks of the thigh or pelvis.

In the pathogenesis of varicose veins, it is not clear whether incompetence of the valves or dilation of the vessels comes first. Whatever the case, the two reinforce each other. As the vein increases in length and diameter, tortuousities develop. Once the process begins, the varicosity extends progressively throughout the length of the affected vein. As each valve becomes incompetent, increasing strain is put on the vessel and valve below. The role of inflammation is not well studied, although elevated expression of leukocyte-endothelial adhesion molecules is reported in affected veins.

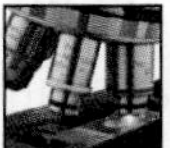

PATHOLOGY: Microscopically, varicose veins show variations in wall thickness. Some areas are thin, due to dilation, while others are thickened by smooth muscle hypertrophy, subintimal fibrosis and incorporation of mural thrombi into the wall. Patchy calcification is frequently seen. Valvular deformities consist of thickening, shortening and rolling of the cusps.

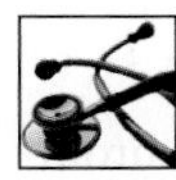

CLINICAL FEATURES: Visual inspection makes the diagnosis of varicose veins of the leg. Most varicose veins have little clinical effect and are mainly cosmetic problems. The principal symptoms are aching in the legs, aggravated by standing and relieved by elevation. Severe varicosities (Fig. 10-41) may lead to trophic changes in the skin drained by the affected veins, termed **stasis dermatitis.** Surgery is mandated if the overlying skin has ulcerated or if spontaneous bleeding or extensive thrombosis (which may lead to pulmonary embolism) occurs.

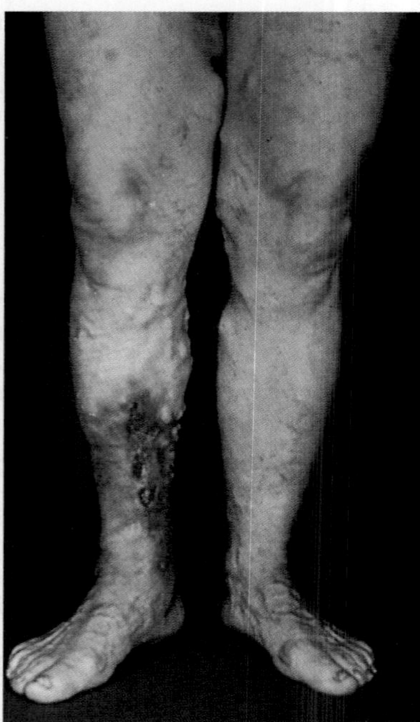

FIGURE 10-41. Varicose veins of the legs. Severe varicosities of the superficial leg veins have led to stasis dermatitis and secondary ulcerations.

Varicose Veins Also Occur at Other Sites

HEMORRHOIDS: These are dilations of the veins of the rectum and anal canal, and may occur inside or outside the anal sphincter (see Chapter 13). Although there may be a hereditary predisposition, the condition is aggravated by factors that increase intra-abdominal pressure, such as constipation and pregnancy, or venous obstruction by rectal tumors. Hemorrhoids often bleed, which may be confused with bleeding rectal cancers. Thrombosed hemorrhoids are exquisitely painful.

ESOPHAGEAL VARICES: This complication of portal hypertension is caused mainly by cirrhosis of the liver (see Chapter 14). High portal pressure distends the anastomoses between portal and systemic venous circulations at the lower end of the esophagus. Although they may be prominent radiologically, esophageal varices are usually unimpressive at autopsy. After their collapse at death, bluish streaks in the esophageal mucosa may be all that is evident. Hemorrhage from esophageal varices is a common cause of death in cirrhosis.

VARICOCELE: This palpable scrotal mass represents varicosities of the pampiniform plexus (see Chapter 17).

Deep Venous Thrombosis Principally Affects Leg Veins

- **Thrombophlebitis** is inflammation and secondary thrombosis of small veins and sometimes larger ones, commonly as part of a local reaction to bacterial infection.
- **Phlebothrombosis** is the term for venous thrombosis that occurs without an initiating infection or inflammation.
- **Deep venous thrombosis** now refers to both phlebothrombosis and thrombophlebitis. Since most cases of venous thrombosis are not associated with inflammation or infection, the condition is currently associated with prolonged bed rest or reduced cardiac output. It is most frequent in deep leg veins and can be a major threat to life because of pulmonary embolization (witness the well-known phenomenon of sudden death with ambulation after surgery). Deficiencies of anticoagulants, such as protein C and antithrombin, increase the incidence of venous thromboembolism. Deep venous thrombosis is discussed more fully in Chapter 7.

Lymphatic Vessels

The lymphatic vessels are thin-walled low-pressure channels. They are important for normal tissue fluid balance, providing drainage of plasma filtrates, cells and foreign material from the interstitial spaces. They are also important in fat digestion, through lacteals in the intestinal villi, and in immune surveillance. Lymphatic vessels are more permeable than blood vessels, in part because the former have fewer tight junctions. NO• may act as a mediator of several growth factors that are lymphangiogenic and may be important in lymphatic function. For example, NO• may inhibit pumping in collecting lymphatics. Inflammation and tumors may spread via lymphatics.

MOLECULAR PATHOGENESIS: Understanding the complex steps of lymphatic development is likely to help to treat diseases involving the lymphatics. Fox2, the forkhead transcription factor, regulates lymphatic valve morphogenesis and maintains the lymphatic capillary phenotype late in development. The VEGF-C/VEGFR-3 pathway mediates lymphatic endothelial cell migration, proliferation and survival. Missense mutations in VEGFR-3 result in lymphedema and lymphatic hypoplasia. PROX-1 is essential for early steps in lymphatic formation, such as budding from the anterior cardinal vein and forming lymph sacs. It also contributes, along with podoplanin, VEGFR-3 and neuropilin-2 to primary lymphatic plexus development. In inflammatory conditions, VEGF-C is upregulated by cytokines, and macrophages express VEGFR-3 and secrete VEGF-C. In experimental studies, tumor metastasis and lymphangiogenesis can be blocked by inhibiting VEGF-C/VEGFR-3. In some patients, primary lymphedema is associated with mutations in VEGFR-3, FOXC2 and SOX18.

Lymphangitis Reflects Infection and Inflammation in Lymphatic Vessels

Transport of infectious material to regional lymph nodes incites **lymphadenitis**. The periphery of a focus of inflammation reveals dilated lymphatics filled with fluid exudate, cells, cellular debris and bacteria. When tissues are expanded by exudate, there is comparable distention of lymphatic channels and an opening of intercellular channels between endothelial cells.

Almost any pathogen can cause acute lymphangitis, but β-hemolytic streptococci (pyogenes) are notorious offenders. The process may extend beyond these channels into surrounding tissues. Draining lymph nc[illegible]re regularly enlarged and inflamed. Painful subcutaneous red streaks, often accompanied by painful regional lymph nodes, characterize acute lymphangitis.

Lymphatic Obstruction Causes Lymphedema

Lymphatics may be obstructed by scar tissue, intraluminal tumor cells, pressure from surrounding tumor tissue or plugging with parasites. As collateral lymphatic routes are abundant, lymphedema (distention of tissue by lymph) usually occurs only when major trunks are obstructed, especially in the axilla or groin. For example, when radical mastectomy for breast cancer was routine, axillary lymph node dissection frequently disrupted lymphatic channels and led to lymphedema of the arm. Prolonged lymphatic obstruction causes progressive dilation of lymphatic vessels, termed **lymphangiectasia**, and overgrowth of fibrous tissue. The term **elephantiasis** describes a lymphedematous limb that is grossly enlarged. In the tropics, filariasis, in which a parasitic worm invades lymphatics (see Chapter 9), is a common cause of elephantiasis.

Milroy disease is an inherited type of lymphedema that is present at birth. It usually affects only one limb, but it may be more extensive and involve the eyelids and lips. Affected tissues show hugely dilated lymphatic channels, and the entire area appears honeycombed or spongy. This lesion is more properly considered lymphangiectasia rather than simply lymphedema.

Benign Tumors of Blood Vessels

Tumors of the vascular system are common. Many are hamartomas, that is, masses of mature but disorganized cells and tissues characteristic of the particular organ, rather than true neoplasms. Some mutations have been linked to vascular anomalies. For example, endoglin and ALK-1 mutations have been identified in hereditary hemorrhagic telangiectasia and several gene mutations have been identified in familial cerebral cavernous malformation.

Hemangiomas Are Common Benign Tumors of Vascular Channels

Hemangiomas usually occur in the skin but may also be found in internal organs.

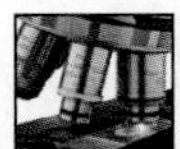

PATHOLOGY:

CAPILLARY HEMANGIOMA: ***This lesion is composed of vascular channels with the size and structure of normal capillaries.*** Capillary hemangiomas may occur in any tissue. The most common sites are skin; subcutaneous tissues; mucous membranes of the lips and mouth; and internal viscera, including spleen, kidneys and liver. Capillary hemangiomas vary from a few millimeters to several centimeters in diameter. They are bright red to blue, depending on the degree of oxygenation of the blood. In the skin, capillary hemangiomas are known as **birthmarks** or **ruby spots.** The only disability is cosmetic disfiguration.

JUVENILE HEMANGIOMA: Also called **strawberry hemangiomas**, these lesions are found on the skin of newborns. They grow rapidly in the first months of life, begin to fade at 1 to 3 years of age and completely regress in most

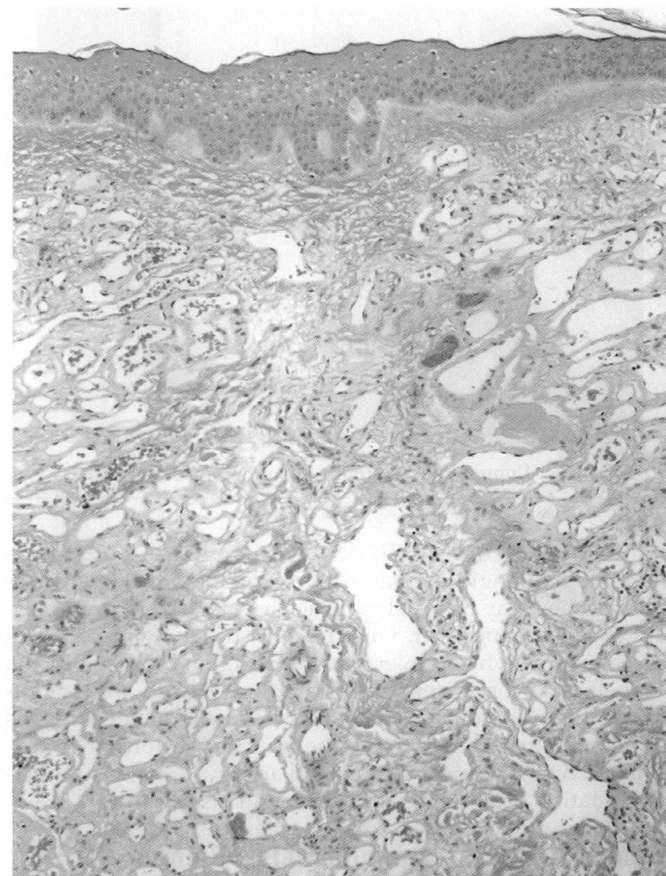

FIGURE 10-42. Juvenile hemangioma. A network of delicate, anastomosing vessels is present subcutaneously.

(80%) cases by 5 years of age. Juvenile hemangiomas contain packed masses of capillaries separated by connective tissue stroma (Fig. 10-42). The endothelium-lined channels are usually filled with blood. Thromboses, sometimes organized, are common. Occasionally, the vascular channels rupture, causing scarring and accumulation of hemosiderin. Juvenile hemangiomas are usually well demarcated despite lacking capsules. Although finger-like projections of the vascular tissue may give the impression of invasion, these growths are benign; they do not invade or metastasize.

CAVERNOUS HEMANGIOMA: ***This term is reserved for lesions made of large vascular channels, often interspersed with small, capillary-type vessels.*** When cavernous hemangiomas occur in the skin (Fig. 10-43), they are termed **port wine stains**. They also appear on mucosal surfaces and visceral organs, including the spleen, liver and pancreas. If they occur in the brain, they may enlarge slowly and cause neurologic symptoms after long quiescent periods.

A cavernous hemangioma is a red-blue, soft, spongy mass, with a diameter of up to several centimeters. Unlike capillary hemangiomas, cavernous hemangiomas do not regress spontaneously. Although the lesion is demarcated by a sharp border, it is not encapsulated. Large endothelial-lined, blood-containing spaces are separated by sparse connective tissue. Cavernous hemangiomas can undergo a variety of changes, including thrombosis and fibrosis, cystic cavitation and intracystic hemorrhage.

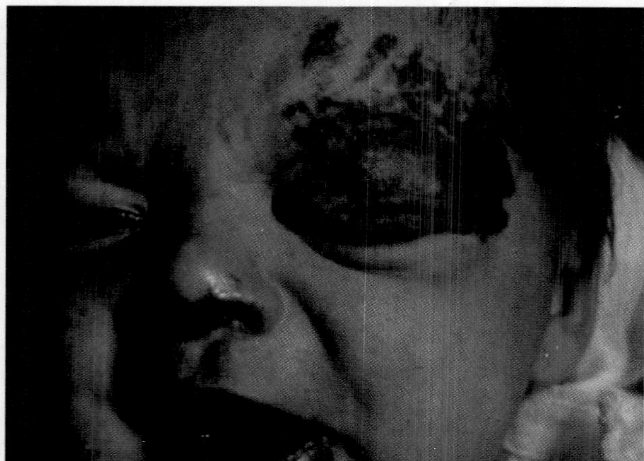

FIGURE 10-43. Congenital cavernous hemangioma of the skin.

MULTIPLE HEMANGIOMATOUS SYNDROMES: More than one hemangioma may occur in a single tissue. Two or more tissues may be involved, such as skin and nervous system or spleen and liver. **von Hippel-Lindau syndrome** is a rare entity in which cavernous hemangiomas occur in the cerebellum or brainstem and the retina. **Sturge-Weber syndrome** involves a developmental disturbance of blood vessels in the brain and skin. Other closely related lesions are plexiform or racemose angiomas, cirsoid aneurysms and angiomatous dilation of vessels of the brain and elsewhere.

Glomus Tumor (Glomangioma) Is a Painful Tumor of the Glomus Body

Glomus bodies are normal neuromyoarterial receptors that are sensitive to temperature and regulate arteriolar flow. Glomus tumors are widely distributed in the skin, mostly in the distal regions of fingers and toes. This pattern is reflected in the location of glomus tumors at these sites, typically in a subungual location.

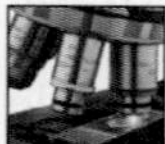

PATHOLOGY: The lesions are usually under 1 cm in diameter; many are smaller than a few millimeters. In the skin, they are slightly elevated, rounded, red-blue and firm (Fig. 10-44). The two main histologic components are branching vascular channels in a connective tissue stroma and aggregates or nests of specialized glomus cells. The latter are regular, round to cuboidal cells that reveal typical smooth muscle cell features by electron microscopy.

Hemangioendothelioma Is a Vascular Tumor of Endothelial Cells That is Intermediate Between Benign Hemangiomas and Frankly Malignant Angiosarcomas

The epithelioid or histiocytoid hemangioendothelioma displays endothelial cells with considerable eosinophilic, often vacuolated, cytoplasm. Vascular lumina are evident, as are a few mitoses. These tumors occur in almost all locations. Surgical removal is generally curative, but about one fifth of patients develop metastases.

Spindle cell hemangioendothelioma occurs principally in males of any age, usually in the dermis and subcutaneous tissue of distal extremities. It features vascular, endothelial-lined spaces into which papillary projections extend. Although the lesion may recur locally after excision, it rarely metastasizes.

Malignant Tumors of Blood Vessels

Malignant vascular neoplasms are rare. Only rarely do they arise in preexisting benign tumors.

Angiosarcoma Is a Rare, Highly Malignant Tumor of Endothelial Cells

These tumors occur in either sex and at any age. They begin as small, painless, sharply demarcated, red nodules. The most common locations are skin, soft tissue, breast, bone, liver and spleen. Eventually, most enlarge to become pale gray, fleshy masses without a capsule. These tumors often undergo central necrosis, with softening and hemorrhage.

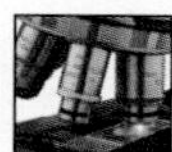

PATHOLOGY: Angiosarcomas exhibit varying degrees of differentiation, ranging from those composed mainly of distinct vascular elements to undif-

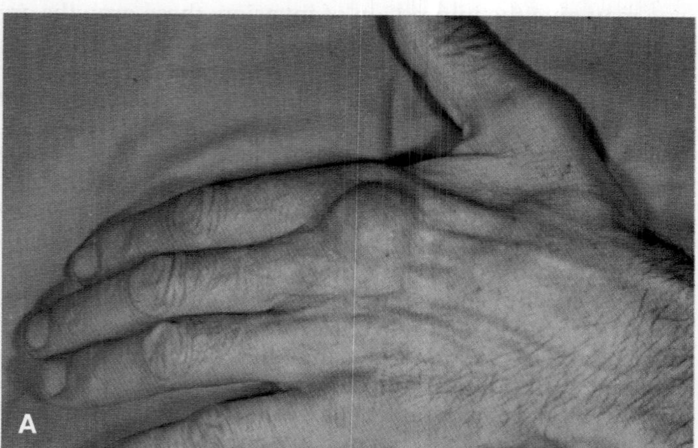

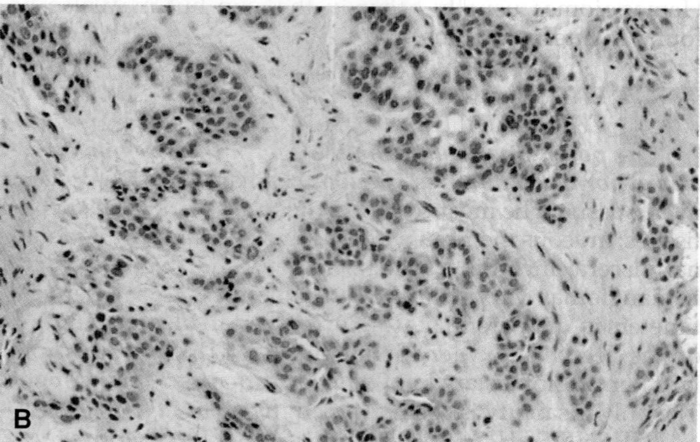

FIGURE 10-44. Glomus tumor. A. The dorsal surface of the hand displays a prominent tumor nodule on the proximal third finger. **B.** A photomicrograph of (A) reveals nests of glomus tumor cells embedded in a fibrovascular stroma.

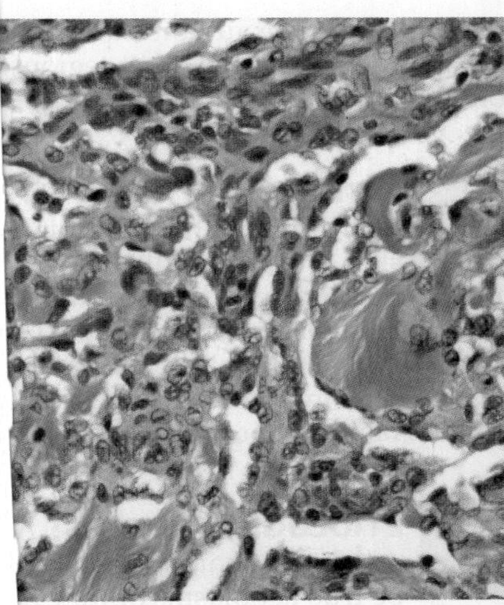

a. Malignant spindly cells line vague chan- CD31, an endothelial marker.

few recognizable blood channels splay frequent mitoses, pleomor- end to be more malignant. Almost arcoma die of the disease.

of the liver is of special interest; it is asso- environmental carcinogens, particularly arsenic (a component of pesticides) and vinyl chloride (used in production of plastics). Hepatic angiosarcoma was observed after administration of thorium dioxide, a radioactive contrast medium (Thorotrast) used by radiologists prior to 1950. Thorotrast is engulfed by macrophages of the liver sinusoids, where it remains for life.

There is a long latent period between exposure to the chemicals or radionuclide and development of hepatic angiosarcoma. The earliest detectable changes are atypia and diffuse hyperplasia of the cells lining the hepatic sinusoids. The tumors are frequently multicentric and may arise in the spleen as well. Hepatic angiosarcomas are highly malignant and spread by both local invasion and metastasis.

Hemangiopericytoma

Hemangiopericytoma is a rare neoplasm previously thought to arise from pericytes, modified smooth muscle cells outside the walls of capillaries and arterioles. However, it is not clear that the neoplasm actually derives from these cells. These tumors present as small masses of capillary-like channels surrounded by, and frequently enclosed within, nests and masses of round to spindle-shaped cells. The tumor cells are characteristically invested by a basement membrane.

Hemangiopericytomas can occur anywhere, but are most common in the retroperitoneum and lower extremities. Most are removed surgically without having invaded or metastasized. Malignant hemangiopericytomas metastasize to lungs, bone, liver and lymph nodes.

Kaposi Sarcoma Is a Common Complication of Acquired Immunodeficiency Syndrome

Kaposi sarcoma is a malignant angioproliferative tumor derived from endothelial cells.

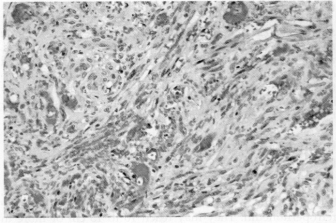

FIGURE 10-46. Kaposi sarcoma. A photomicrograph of a vascular lesion from a patient with acquired immune deficiency syndrome shows numerous poorly differentiated, spindle-shaped neoplastic cells and a vascular lesion filled with red blood cells.

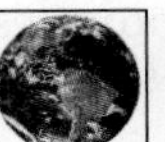

EPIDEMIOLOGY: Kaposi sarcoma was originally described in the 19th century by Moritz Kaposi as a sporadic tumor endemic in parts of central Africa, but otherwise an oddity that occurred mainly in men in the sixth and seventh decades. However, Kaposi sarcoma is now seen in epidemic form in immunosuppressed patients, especially with acquired immunodeficiency syndrome (AIDS). A member of the herpesvirus family, human herpesvirus 8 (HHV8) (Kaposi sarcoma–associated herpes virus [KSHV]), is responsible for this tumor. Only a small faction of KSHV-infected individuals develop Kaposi sarcoma. Cofactors that influence the risk of Kaposi sarcoma among individuals who are not infected with HIV are not well understood.

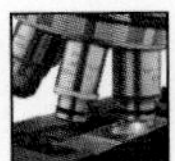

PATHOLOGY: Kaposi sarcoma begins as painful purple or brown cutaneous nodules, 1 mm to 1 cm in diameter. They appear most often on the hands or feet but may occur anywhere. Their histology is highly variable. One form resembles a simple hemangioma, with tightly packed clusters of capillaries and scattered hemosiderin-laden macrophages. Other forms are highly cellular and the vascular spaces are less prominent (Fig. 10-46). The lesions may be difficult to distinguish from fibrosarcomas, but their origin from endothelial cells is demonstrable by immunochemistry and by electron microscopy. Kaposi sarcoma is considered a malignant lesion and may be widely disseminated in the body, but is only exceptionally a cause of death.

Tumors of the Lymphatic System

Many histologic and clinical variants of local enlargements of the lymphatics have been described. It is difficult to distinguish among anomalies, proliferations due to stasis and true neoplasms. In general, lymphatic tumors are distinguished by their size and location. The spaces may be small, as in capillary lymphangiomas, or large and dilated, as in cystic or cavernous lesions. Lymphangiomatous lesions can arise at almost any site, including skin, mediastinum, retroperitoneum, spleen and elsewhere.

Capillary Lymphangioma

Sometimes called "simple lymphangiomas," these benign tumors are small, circumscribed, grayish pink, fleshy nodules, which can be single or multiple. They are subcutaneous and occur in the skin of the face, lips, chest, genitalia or extremities. Capillary lymphangiomas are composed of variably sized, thin-walled spaces lined by endothelial cells, and contain lymph and occasional leukocytes.

Cystic Lymphangioma (Cystic Hygroma, Cavernous Lymphangioma)

These benign lesions are most common in the neck and axilla, but also occur in the mediastinum and occasionally in the retroperitoneum. They may reach 10 to 15 cm or more in diameter and fill the axilla or distort structures of the neck.

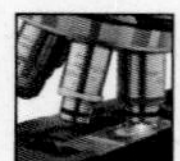

PATHOLOGY: Cystic lymphangiomas are soft, spongy and pink. Watery fluid exudes from their cut surfaces. Microscopically, they contain endothelial-lined spaces with a protein-rich fluid. These spaces are distinguished from blood vessels because they lack erythrocytes and leukocytes. Abundant irregularly distributed smooth muscle and connective tissue cells may be present.

Lymphangiosarcoma May Occur Following Lymphedema or Radiation

These are rare malignant tumors that develop in 0.1% to 0.5% of patients with lymphedema of the arm after radical mastectomy. Distinction between this tumor and angiosarcoma is difficult, and some authors equate the two. Lymphangiosarcoma may also occur in other regions, for example, in the leg following radiation therapy for uterine cervical carcinoma.

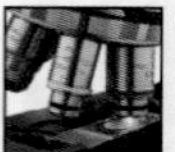

PATHOLOGY: Lymphangiosarcomas present as purplish, frequently multiple, nodules in edematous skin. Histologically, the nodules are composed of cells resembling capillary endothelial cells and showing zonulae adherentes between cells. The walls of tumor vessels have a rudimentary form of basal basement membrane. Lymphangiosarcomas are highly malignant and, despite radical surgery, have a poor prognosis.

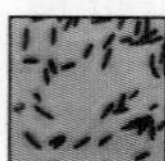

ETIOLOGIC FACTORS: Although hemangiomas are clearly benign, their origin is uncertain; they may be true neoplasms or they may be hamartomas. The evidence favoring hamartoma (i.e., a malformation) includes (1) the lesion is present at birth; (2) it grows only as the rest of the body grows, and remains limited in size; and (3) after growth ceases, it usually remains unchanged indefinitely absent trauma, thrombosis or hemorrhage.

The development of these vascular malformations recalls the embryology of the vascular system. A network of endothelial channels undergoes remodeling, acquiring a muscular coat and adventitia. In this view, vascular malformations reflect the persistence of the original or modified channels and mixtures of connective tissue elements derived from the mesenchyme. At present, hemangiomas are classified by histologic type and location, although molecular characterization will likely lead to new classifications and better understanding of the prognosis of given lesions.

11 The Heart

Jeffrey E. Saffitz

The heart is a fist-sized muscular pump that has the remarkable capacity to work unceasingly for the 90 or more years of a human lifetime. As demand requires, it can increase its output manyfold, in part because the coronary circulation can augment its blood flow to over 10 times normal. The ventricles also respond to short-term increases in workload by dilating, in accordance with Starling's law of the heart. When an increased workload is imposed for a longer period (e.g., in cases of systemic hypertension), the left ventricle hypertrophies, an adaptation that increases its work capacity. However, this compensatory mechanism has its limits, and a point is reached when the heart can no longer supply blood adequately to peripheral tissues; the result is congestive heart failure. Damage to the myocardium, caused most commonly by ischemic heart disease, also limits the capacity of the left ventricle to pump blood and similarly results in heart failure.

Anatomy of the Heart

The heart of an adult man weighs 280 to 340 g, and that of a woman, 230 to 280 g. The organ is a two-sided pump. Blood enters each side through a thin-walled atrium, from which it is propelled forward by thicker muscular ventricles. The right ventricle is considerably thinner (<0.5 cm) than the left ventricle (1.3 to 1.5 cm) owing to the low venous pressure and relatively low afterload on the right side. Blood enters the ventricles across the atrioventricular valves, the mitral valve on the left and the tricuspid valve on the right. The leaflets of these valves are held in place by chordae tendineae, strong fibrous cords attached to the inner surface of the ventricular wall via papillary muscles. The entrances to the aorta and pulmonary arteries are guarded respectively by the aortic and pulmonary valves, each consisting of three semilunar cusps.

The heart wall has three layers: outer epicardium, middle myocardium and inner endocardium. The heart is surrounded and enclosed by visceral and parietal pericardia, which are separated by the pericardial cavity.

Cardiac Myocytes Generate Contractile Force

The myocardium is composed of a network of individual myocytes, each of which normally has a single nucleus and is separated from adjacent cells by intercalated disks that contain cell–cell adhesion and electrical junctions. Electron microscopy reveals the structure and distribution of the sarcolemma, sarcoplasmic reticulum (SR), T system of tubules, nucleus and numerous mitochondria (Fig. 11-1A). The contractile elements of the myocyte, the myofilaments, are arranged in bundles referred to as myofibrils, which are separated by mitochondria and SR. Myofibrils are organized into repeating units termed **sarcomeres.**

The sarcomere is the basic functional unit of the contractile apparatus. It consists of a Z disk on each end and interdigitated thick and thin filaments, oriented perpendicular to the Z disk (Fig. 11-1). The thick filaments contain myosin heavy chains, myosin-binding protein C and myosin light chains. The thick filaments, which are limited to the A band, interact with the giant sarcomeric protein, titin (~27,000

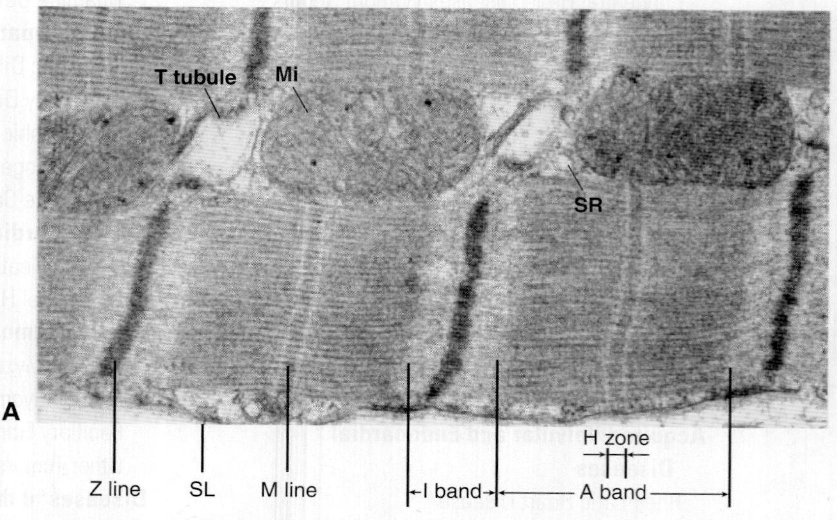

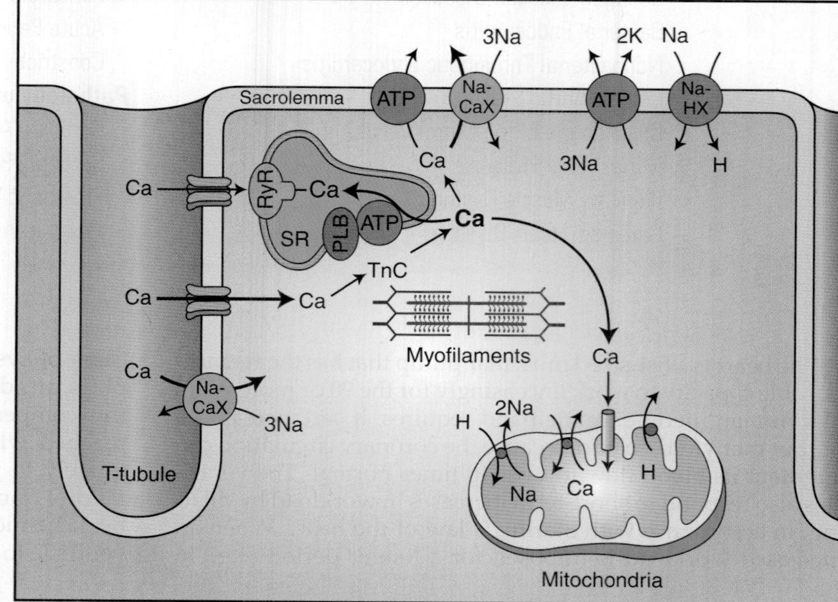

FIGURE 11-1. Ultrastructure of the myocardium. **A.** Electron micrograph of left ventricle in the longitudinal plane, showing the sarcolemma (SL); the sarcomeres of the myofibrils, delimited by Z lines; A bands; I bands; H zones; and M lines. Also present are mitochondria (Mi), sarcoplasmic reticulum (SR) and T tubules. The I bands and H zones are absent when the myofibrils are shortened. The structural basis for the banding is shown in the electron micrograph. The fine threads that extend at right angles to the thick (myosin) filaments are the cross-bridges that form the force-generating cross-links with actin. The amount of force that can be generated is proportional to the length of the adjoining myofilaments and is at a maximum when the sarcomeres are between 2 and 2.2 μm in length. When the sarcomeres are less than 2 μm in length, the thin filaments slide across each other and overlap, decreasing the potential for force-generating cross-links; similarly, when the sarcomeres are stretched beyond 2.2 μm, there is a decrease in force that is proportional to the widening of the H zone. This mechanism can be invoked as the basis for Starling's law of the heart. **B.** Pathways regulating Ca^{2+} homeostasis and excitation–contraction coupling in cardiac myocytes. The cardiac action potential brings depolarizing current into T tubules where voltage-gated L-type Ca^{2+} channels reside in high concentrations (green channel structures). Influx of Ca^{2+} through these channels (ICa) stimulates release of Ca^{2+} from the SR (located in immediate proximity to the T tubule) via RyR2. The transient increase in cytosolic Ca^{2+} promotes contraction through interactions with cardiac troponin T (TnC). Resting diastolic Ca^{2+} levels are restored by reuptake into the SR and extrusion via sodium–calcium exchange (Na-CaX) and an adenosine triphosphate (ATP) pump.

amino acids long), which spans from the Z disk to the M line, thereby forming a third filament system of the sarcomere. Titin helps maintain precise assembly of myofibrillar proteins and contributes to the viscoelastic properties of cardiac muscle. The thin filaments contain actin and regulatory proteins, including **α-tropomyosin-1** and the **troponin complex** (cardiac troponins I, C and T), and extend from the Z disk through the I band and into the A band. The interaction of these myofilaments generates the force for contraction. The amount of force that can be generated is proportional to the extent of overlap between adjoining thick and thin filaments, and is maximum when sarcomeres are 2.0 to 2.2 μm in length.

When sarcomere length is under 2 μm, the thin filaments slide across each other and overlap, decreasing the potential for force-generating cross-links. When it is stretched beyond 2.2 μm, force decreases in proportion to the widening of the H zone. ***This mechanism is the basis for Starling law of the heart, which states that the contractile force of the heart is a function of fiber length during diastole.*** Average sarcomere length is about 2.2 μm when left ventricular end-diastolic pressure is at the upper limit of normal.

Contraction of cardiac muscle is initiated by increases in cytosolic free calcium. In a normal myocyte, an action potential triggers entry of calcium ions into the myocyte through voltage-gated L-type calcium channels in T tubules. These invaginations of the sarcolemma bring depolarizing current and resultant voltage-gated Ca^{2+} entry into intimate proximity to intracellular organelles regulating calcium homeostasis (lateral cisterns of the SR) and the contractile apparatus itself (Fig. 11-1B). The entering calcium stimulates release of Ca^{2+} sequestered in the SR (Ca^{2+}-induced Ca^{2+} release) via the cardiac ryanodine receptor (RyR2). The increase in cytosolic Ca^{2+} produces a conformational change in the regulatory myofilament proteins, in particular troponin, which permits cross-bridges between actin and myosin to break and reform repetitively. As a result, the filaments slide over one another, causing myocardial contraction. ***The number of contractile sites activated and the resulting force generated are directly proportional to the concentration of Ca^{2+} nearby the myofibrils.***

The myocardium relaxes when cytosolic Ca^{2+} returns to its normal low (diastolic) concentration of 10^{-7} M. This process depends on calcium adenosine triphosphatase (ATPase) of the SR, which pumps Ca^{2+} from the cytosol into the SR. Cytosolic Ca^{2+} also is lowered to the normal resting diastolic concentration by its outward transport through sodium–calcium exchange and sarcolemmal calcium pumps (Fig. 11-1B). ***Thus, myocardial relaxation is an active, energy-requiring event.***

The Conduction System Consists of Specialized Myocytes

These myocytes have two major functions: (1) they initiate heartbeats by generating electric current through their automatic rhythmicity, which is more rapid in the sinoatrial node than in more distal parts of the system; and (2) they distribute electric current to activate atrial and ventricular myocardium in an appropriate temporal–spatial pattern. Fibers of the atrioventricular conduction system generally conduct impulses at a faster rate (~1 to 2 m/sec) than do working (contractile) atrial and ventricular fibers (~0.5 to 1 m/sec). By contrast, conduction through the atrioventricular node is exceptionally slow (~0.1 m/sec). Slow conduction through the atrioventricular junction delays ventricular activation, and thereby facilitates ventricular filling.

The heartbeat normally originates in the sinoatrial node, located near the junction of the superior vena cava and the roof of the right atrium. If the node is diseased or otherwise prevented from functioning as the pacemaker, more distal components of the conduction system or even the ventricular muscle itself assume the role of pacemaker. ***As a rule, the more distal the pacemaker site, the slower the heart rate.*** On leaving the sinoatrial node, an electrical impulse activates the atria. Atrial wavefronts converge on the atrioventricular node, which conducts the impulse through the common bundle (bundle of His) to the left and right bundle branches of the Purkinje system. Purkinje fibers run within the endocardium on either side of the interventricular septum and distribute current to the overlying ventricular muscle. During each cycle, ventricular contraction begins along the interventricular septum and at the apex. It progresses from apex to base, resulting in smooth and efficient ejection of blood into the great vessels.

The His bundle in the normal adult heart is the only electrical connection between the atria and ventricles. However, additional abnormal connections may occasionally arise as small bundles or tracts of cardiac myocytes. Such "bypass tracts" can activate ventricular muscle before the normal impulse arrives via the conduction system. They are found in patients with the **Wolff-Parkinson-White syndrome** and are responsible for establishing circuits that promote **supraventricular tachycardia.** Congenital discontinuities in the conduction system may be caused by placentally transmitted autoantibodies in mothers with connective tissue diseases such as systemic lupus erythematosus (SLE). Acquired defects may arise because of infarction, inflammatory or infiltrative disease, cardiac surgery or cardiac catheterization.

Coronary Arteries Supply Blood to the Heart

The right and left main coronary arteries originate in, or immediately above, the sinuses of Valsalva of the aortic valve. The left main coronary artery bifurcates within 1 cm of its origin into the left anterior descending (LAD) and left circumflex coronary arteries. The left circumflex coronary artery rests in the left atrioventricular groove and supplies the lateral wall of the left ventricle (Fig. 11-2). The LAD coronary artery lies in the anterior interventricular groove and provides blood to the (1) anterior left ventricle, (2) adjacent anterior right ventricle and (3) anterior half to two thirds of the interventricular septum. In the apical region, the LAD artery supplies the ventricles circumferentially (Fig. 11-2).

The right coronary artery travels along the right atrioventricular groove and nourishes the bulk of the right ventricle and posteroseptal left ventricle (Fig. 11-2), including the posterior third to half of the interventricular septum at the base of the heart (also referred to as the "inferior" or "diaphragmatic" wall). From these distributions, one can predict the location of infarcts that result from occlusion of any of the three major epicardial coronary arteries.

The epicardial coronary arteries are usually arranged in a so-called right coronary–dominant distribution. The pattern of dominance is determined by the coronary artery that contributes most of the blood to the posterior descending coronary artery. Five to 10% of human hearts display a left-dominant pattern, with the left circumflex coronary artery supplying the posterior descending coronary artery.

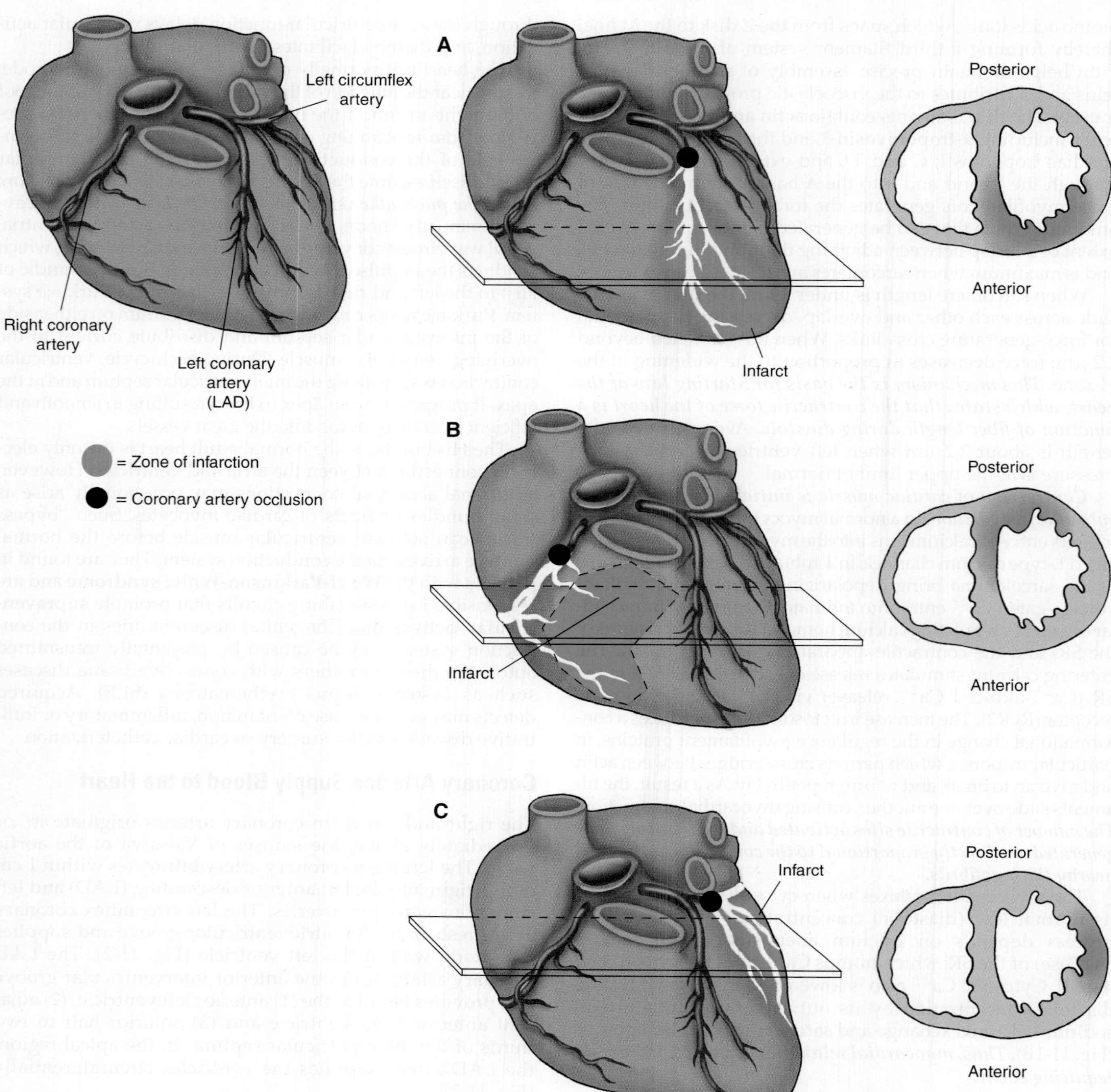

FIGURE 11-2. Position of left ventricular infarcts resulting from occlusion of each of the three main coronary arteries. A. Anterior infarct, which follows occlusion of the anterior descending branch (left anterior descending, LAD) of the left coronary artery. The infarct is located in the anterior wall and adjacent two thirds of the septum. It involves the entire circumference of the wall near the apex. **B. A posterior ("inferior" or "diaphragmatic") infarct** results from occlusion of the right coronary artery and involves the posterior wall, including the posterior third of the interventricular septum and the posterior papillary muscle in the basal half of the ventricle. **C. Posterolateral infarct,** which follows occlusion of the left circumflex artery and is present in the posterolateral wall.

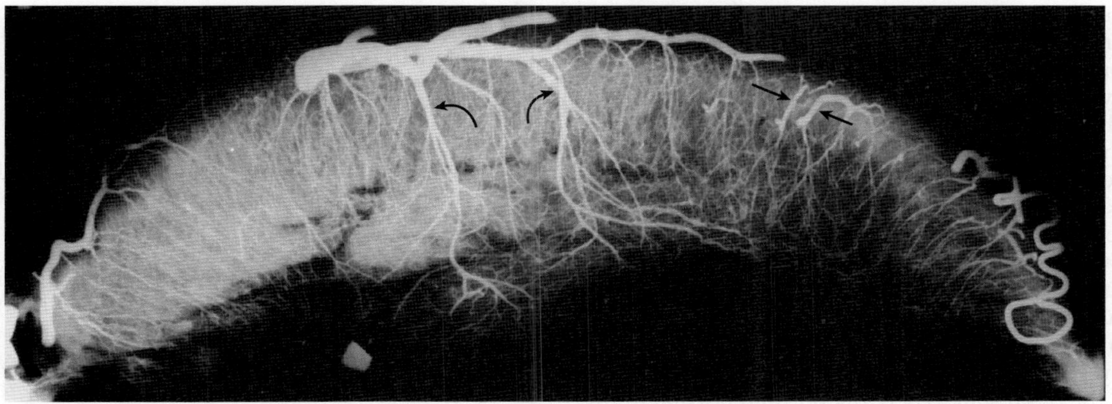

FIGURE 11-3. Arteriogram of a longitudinal segment of the posterior wall of the left ventricle including the posterior papillary muscle. Note the two types of branches passing into the myocardium at right angles to the epicardial artery (*top*): class A, which quickly divide into a fine network (*straight arrows*), and class B, which maintain a large diameter and pass with little branching into the subendocardial region and the papillary muscle (*curved arrows*).

Blood flow in the myocardium occurs inward from epicardium to endocardium. Thus, as a general rule, endocardium is most vulnerable to ischemia when flow through a major epicardial coronary artery is compromised. Some of the small intramyocardial coronary arteries branch as they course through the ventricular wall; others maintain a large diameter and pass to the endocardial surface without branching (Fig. 11-3). Because capillary networks arising from penetrating arteries do not interconnect, the borders between viable and infarcted myocardium after coronary artery occlusion are distinct.

The epicardial portion of each coronary artery fills and expands during systole and empties and narrows during diastole. The intramyocardial arteries have the opposite action and are compressed by the systolic muscular pressure. As a result, blood flow within myocardium, especially in the subendocardial ventricular regions, is decreased or absent during systole. Nevertheless, blood flow is roughly equal throughout the myocardium because of autoregulation.

Myocardial Hypertrophy and Heart Failure

The ventricles are compliant in a normal heart, and diastolic filling occurs at low atrial pressures. During systole, ventricles contract vigorously and eject about 60% of the blood present in them at the end of diastole (**ejection fraction**). When a heart is injured, the clinical consequences are similar, regardless of the cause of cardiac dysfunction. ***If the initial impairment is severe, cardiac output is not maintained despite compensatory changes and the result is acute, life-threatening,*** **cardiogenic shock.** When the functional impairment is less, compensatory mechanisms (see below) maintain cardiac output by increasing diastolic ventricular filling pressure and end-diastolic volume. This situation results in the characteristic signs and symptoms of congestive heart failure. Because of the heart's capacity to compensate, congestive heart failure is often tolerated for years.

The ability of the heart to adapt to injury is based on the same mechanisms that allow cardiac output to increase in response to stress. ***The fundamental compensatory mechanism is the Frank-Starling mechanism: cardiac stroke volume is a function of diastolic fiber length; within certain limits, a normal heart will pump whatever volume is brought to it by the venous circulation*** (Fig. 11-4). Stroke volume, a measure of ventricular function, is enhanced by increasing ventricular end-diastolic volume secondary to an increase in atrial filling pressure.

The increased contractile force in response to ventricular dilation is a result of myofibrillar organization, in which

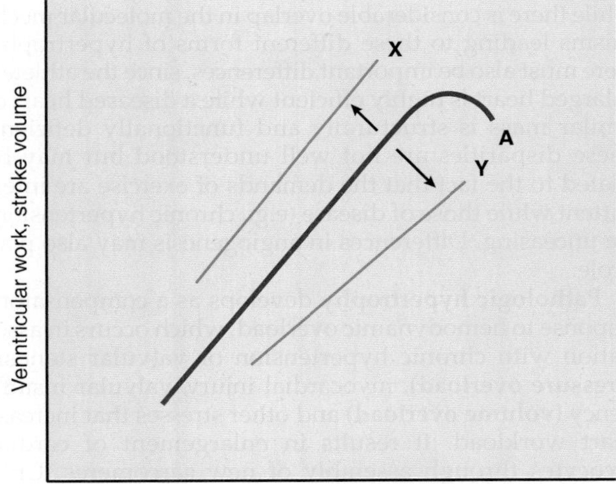

FIGURE 11-4. Relation between the work of the heart (or stroke volume) and the level of venous inflow, as measured by atrial pressure, ventricular end-diastolic volume (EDV) or end-diastolic pressure (EDP). *Curve A* indicates that as ventricular EDV, EDP or left atrial pressure increases, the amount of work done by the heart increases linearly up to a point. Beyond this point, the work done decreases, and the heart fails. However, the downslope of this curve is reached only at very high left atrial pressures. The curve may shift upward to position *X* or downward to position *Y*, depending on whether contractility has increased (e.g., because of the action of norepinephrine) or decreased (i.e., in failure), respectively. The failing heart usually functions on the ascending limb of a depressed curve.

stretching of sarcomeres results in a greater potential for overlap of thick and thin filaments during contraction. This allows enhanced force generation, provided the sarcomere is not stretched beyond 2.2 μm. When there is a sudden need to increase cardiac output in a normal heart, as during exercise, catecholamine stimulation increases both heart rate and contractility. The latter is mainly mediated by modulating the activities of key proteins that regulate Ca^{2+} transients during excitation–contraction coupling. As a result, the normal relationship between end-diastolic volume and stroke volume is shifted upward (from curve A to curve X in Fig. 11-4). End-diastolic volume may also increase, causing a large increase in cardiac output.

If the heart is injured, overall cardiac function tends to be depressed in the basal state. Then, higher than normal filling pressures are required to maintain cardiac output (curve Y in Fig. 11-4). Moreover, in cardiac failure, catecholamine stimulation is often present in the basal state. A comparable increase in cardiac output thus requires a greater increase in atrial pressure in a failing heart than in a normal one. ***The most prominent feature of heart failure is the abnormally high atrial filling pressure relative to stroke volume.*** However, the absolute values of stroke volume and cardiac output are generally well maintained.

MOLECULAR PATHOGENESIS: Myocardial hypertrophy is an adaptive response that augments myocyte contractile strength. There is a distinction between **physiologic hypertrophy,** which develops in highly trained athletes, and **pathologic hypertrophy,** which occurs in response to injury or disease. While there is considerable overlap in the molecular mechanisms leading to these different forms of hypertrophy, there must also be important differences, since the athlete's enlarged heart is highly efficient while a diseased heart of similar mass is structurally and functionally deficient. These disparities are not well understood but may be related to the fact that the demands of exercise are intermittent while those of disease (e.g., chronic hypertension) are unceasing. Differences in angiogenesis may also play a role.

Pathologic hypertrophy develops as a compensatory response to hemodynamic overload, which occurs in association with chronic hypertension or valvular stenosis (**pressure overload**), myocardial injury, valvular insufficiency (**volume overload**) and other stresses that increase heart workload. It results in enlargement of cardiac myocytes through assembly of new sarcomeres. Until recently, this had been thought to occur without an increase in the number of cardiac myocytes, but it is now known that cardiac progenitor cells exist with at least the potential to contribute to hyperplastic growth (see below).

Hypertrophy initially reflects compensatory and potentially reversible mechanisms, but in the face of persistent stress, the myocardium becomes irreversibly enlarged and dilated.

Receptor-mediated myocardial events that are triggered by a stimulus promote the hypertrophic response by autocrine and paracrine mechanisms. Contractile cells respond to mechanical stimuli, such as stretching or pressure overload, by releasing ligands that activate receptor-mediated signaling pathways to produce hypertrophy (Fig. 11-5). Among the most important ligands are (1) angiotensin II (AngII), (2) endothelin-1 (ET-1), (3) norepinephrine (NE) and (4) various growth factors, including insulin-like growth factor-I (IGF-I) and transforming growth factor-β (TGF-β). Some of these mediators may also act on interstitial fibroblasts in the heart to promote synthesis and deposition of extracellular matrix. These ligands bind to and activate G-protein–coupled receptors and receptor tyrosine kinases, which initiate intracellular signaling cascades, the most important of which include (1) mitogen-activated protein kinases (MAPKs), phosphoinositide-3-kinases (PI3Ks), β-adrenergic (protein kinase A) pathways and protein kinase C (PKC) pathways, which are all activated by G-protein–coupled receptors; and (2) Ca^{2+}/calmodulin-dependent protein kinase (CaMK) pathways, which are regulated by calcium. Events mediated by β-adrenergic receptors are implicated in the transition from compensatory hypertrophy to heart failure. The following is a brief description of ligands, signaling cascades, downstream targets and mechanisms involved in the hypertrophic response (see also Chapter 1).

ANGIOTENSIN II: All components of the renin–angiotensin system (renin, angiotensinogen, angiotensin-converting enzyme [ACE] and AngII receptors) are present in both cardiac myocytes and interstitial fibroblasts of the myocardium. AngII is released locally in response to load or stress stimuli and acts by autocrine and paracrine mechanisms to promote myocyte protein synthesis and hypertrophy and stimulate fibroblast proliferation and secretion of extracellular matrix. AngII interacts with two different classes of receptors to activate, either directly or indirectly, multiple signaling cascades including those involving MAPKs and CaMK. Treatment with an ACE inhibitor tends to reverse cardiac hypertrophy and to normalize heart size. ACE inhibitors also prevent cardiac hypertrophy induced by experimental hypertension, without reducing the elevated arterial pressure.

ENDOTHELIN-1: ET-1 is a powerful vasoconstrictor produced by many cells, including endothelial cells and cardiac myocytes. It is also a potent growth factor for cardiac myocytes. Like AngII, ET-1 activates MAPK cascades upon binding to its receptor, to promote cardiac hypertrophy.

INSULIN-LIKE GROWTH FACTOR-I: IGF-I is a growth-promoting peptide synthesized in most tissues. As a growth factor for cardiac myocytes, IGF-I acts through PI3K pathways to promote cardiac hypertrophy.

EXTRACELLULAR MATRIX: Short-term heart overload leads to a prompt increase in collagen synthesis. Interstitial fibrosis, which occurs in virtually all forms of heart failure, is an obligatory feature of the hypertrophic response. Deposition of matrix proteins results, at least in part, from stimulation of cardiac fibroblasts by TGF-β and AngII. After myocardial infarction, fibrosis is important in replacing necrotic myocytes and preventing cardiac rupture. However, when it occurs diffusely, myocardial fibrosis can interfere with diastolic relaxation and impair diffusion of oxygen and nutrients. It can also lead to remodeling of electrical conduction pathways in the heart, which is a major factor in the pathogenesis of atrial fibrillation and ventricular tachycardia.

MITOGEN-ACTIVATED PROTEIN KINASE PATHWAYS: MAPK cascades modulate the hypertrophic response to pressure overload. Activation of the ERK1/2

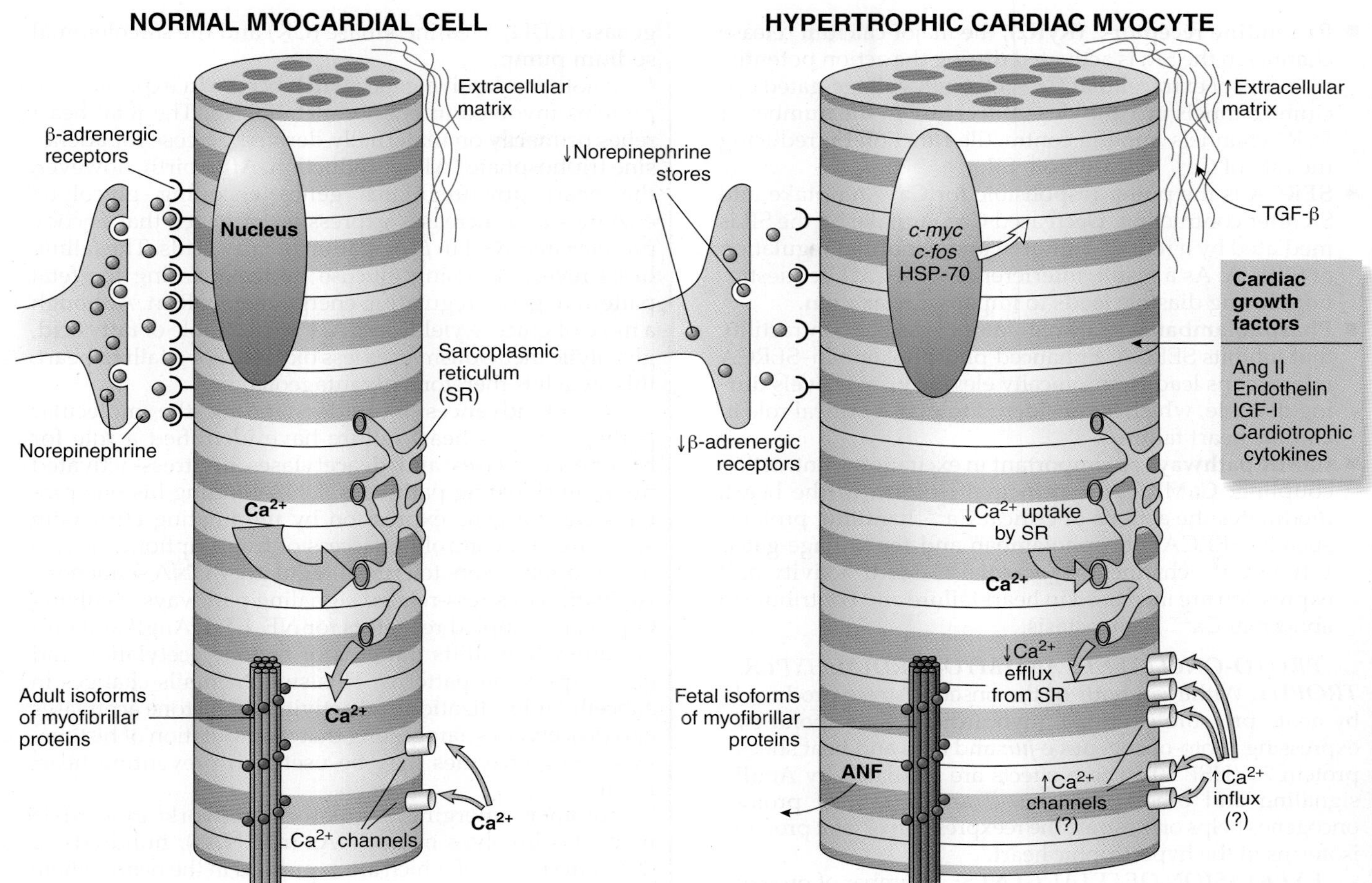

FIGURE 11-5. Biochemical characteristics of myocardial hypertrophy and congestive heart failure. ANF = atrial natriuretic factor; ANG II = angiotensin II; HSP-70 = heat shock protein 70; IGF = insulin-like growth factor; TGF = transforming growth factor.

(extracellular receptor kinase 1/2) cascade promotes growth and survival of cardiac myocytes, whereas activation of JNK (c-Jun N-terminal kinase) and p38 MAPK cascades is involved in pathologic remodeling and apoptosis of cardiac myocytes.

PHOSPHATIDYLINOSITOL-3-KINASE PATHWAYS: Activation of PI3K leads to phosphorylation of membrane lipids and generation of second messengers such as phosphatidylinositol-3,4,5-trisphosphate. The p110α isoform of PI3K is activated by receptor tyrosine kinases such as IGF-I receptor. This isoform of PI3K helps mediate physiologic hypertrophy in response to exercise training, promotes cell survival, inhibits cardiac fibrosis and attenuates pathologic hypertrophy. By contrast, activation of the p110γ isoform of PI3K exerts detrimental effects by promoting internalization of β-adrenergic receptors and inhibiting sarco/endoplasmic reticulum Ca^{2+}-ATPase (SERCA) activity.

β-ADRENERGIC SIGNALING AND DESENSITIZATION: Stimulation of β-adrenergic receptors by norepinephrine (NE) turns on the stimulatory G protein G_S and activates adenylyl cyclase. The latter produces cyclic adenosine 3′,5′-monophosphate (cAMP) as a second messenger, activating protein kinase A to enhance contractility. The poor responses to catecholamines by chronically failing hearts presumably reflect adaptive responses to increases in circulating NE in heart failure. Desensitization of β-adrenergic receptors contributes to sluggish responses of a failing heart to exercise. Chronic overstimulation leads to decreases in the number and responsiveness of β-adrenergic receptors and a defect in coupling to adenylyl cyclase. The failing heart also stores less norepinephrine in autonomic nerve endings. Although β_1-adrenergic receptors are desensitized in heart failure, treatment with blockers of this receptor class reduces mortality and improves contractile function in patients with advanced heart failure. Seemingly paradoxical, this response is consistent with abundant evidence that β_1-adrenergic receptors mediate cardiotoxic effects of NE in the failing heart including maladaptive cardiac myocyte hypertrophy and apoptosis, interstitial fibrosis, contractile dysfunction and sudden death.

CALCIUM HOMEOSTASIS: A variety of defects in calcium homeostasis occur in hypertrophy and heart failure. Expression and function of important calcium-regulating proteins in cardiac myocytes are altered, including (1) RyR2, (2) SERCA and (3) phospholamban (see Fig. 11-1B).

- **Ryanodine receptor-2 (RyR2),** the major calcium release channel in the SR, is activated during the action potential by influx of extracellular Ca^{2+} through voltage-gated calcium channels in T tubules. A decrease in the number of RyR2 channels impairs contractile function by reducing the rate of Ca^{2+} release from SR.
- **SERCA** is the pump responsible for Ca^{2+} reuptake into SR after contraction. Decreased Ca^{2+} uptake by the SR is mediated by a reduced amount and abnormal regulation of SERCA. As a result, interference with Ca^{2+} sequestration during diastole leads to impaired relaxation.
- **Phospholamban** is a key regulator of cardiac contractility that inhibits SERCA. Enhanced phospholamban–SERCA interactions lead to chronically elevated Ca^{2+} levels during diastole, which is considered to play a critical role in chronic heart failure.
- **CaMK pathways** are important in excitation–contraction coupling. CaMKII, the principal isoform in the heart, modulates the actions of critical Ca^{2+} handling proteins such as SERCA, phospholamban and the voltage-gated L-type Ca^{2+} channel. Myocardial CaMKII activity and expression are increased in heart failure and contribute to abnormal Ca^{2+} homeostasis.

PROTO-ONCOGENES AND MYOCARDIAL HYPERTROPHY: Within an hour of the onset of stress produced by acute pressure overload, myocardial cells respond by expressing proto-oncogenes *c-jun* and *c-fos* and heat shock protein 70 (HSP 70). These effects are mediated by AngII signaling and other pathways. Transcription of proto-oncogenes helps orchestrate the reexpression of fetal protein isoforms in the hypertrophic heart.

EXPRESSION OF FETAL GENES: A number of protein isoforms are expressed in fetal hearts, but not after birth. In cardiac hypertrophy induced by hemodynamic overload, many of these genes are reexpressed. For example, atrial natriuretic factor (ANF) is expressed in the fetal ventricle and atrium, but after birth, its production is restricted to the atrium. In a hypertrophic ventricle, however, ANF and brain natriuretic protein (now called B-type natriuretic protein or BNP) are abundantly reexpressed and reduce hemodynamic overload through effects on salt and water metabolism (see Chapter 7). BNP levels in the blood are a useful biomarker of the severity of heart failure.

Cardiac hypertrophy is also accompanied by reexpression of fetal isoforms of several contractile proteins. In the rat, the normal adult isoform is a β-myosin that has high ATPase activity and a rapid shortening velocity. By contrast, the fetal type is a β-myosin that has lower ATPase activity and a slower shortening velocity. In experimental cardiac hypertrophy, "fast" β-myosin is replaced by "slow" β-myosin, leading to impaired myocardial contractility. However, this change in myosin gene expression is also adaptive, since it increases the tension generated during systole and improves contraction efficiency, thus conserving energy. Hypertrophied hearts exhibit similar, but not identical, changes in myosin isoforms. The ventricle contains only slow myosin, and the hypertrophic heart changes from fast to slow myosin only in the atrium. However, fetal isoforms of other myofibrillar proteins appear in ventricular myocardium, including fetal forms of actin and tropomyosin. The hypertrophied heart also contains abnormal varieties of lactic dehydrogenase (LDH), creatine kinase (CK) and the sarcolemmal sodium pump.

Another adaptive gene switch occurs in expression of proteins involved in energy metabolism. The fetal heart relies primarily on maternally derived glucose for adenosine triphosphate (ATP) production. After birth, however, the heart downregulates genes encoding glycolytic enzymes and increases expression of genes that encode proteins involved in β-oxidation of fatty acids. The failing heart reverts to using glucose by reexpressing the fetal pattern of genes regulating energy metabolism. Although a mole of glucose yields less ATP than a mole of fatty acid, glycolytic metabolism uses less oxygen. For a failing heart, this switch is therefore advantageous.

Recent advances in understanding the molecular pathogenesis of heart failure have identified a role for histone acetylases and deacetylases in stress-activated myocyte signaling pathways. DNA-binding histone proteins control gene expression by modulating chromatin structure and controlling access of transcriptional activators and repressors to critical regulatory DNA sequences. Activation of stress-related signaling pathways involving G-protein–coupled receptors for NE, ET-1, AngII and others ultimately shifts patterns of histone acetylation and gene expression patterns. This switch entails changes in subcellular localization and activities of histone acetylases and deacetylases, suggesting that manipulation of histone-modifying enzymes may be useful in preventing heart failure.

Another emerging regulatory network in cardiac myocytes involves microRNAs (miRNAs), hundreds of different species of which are expressed in the heart, where they may help to orchestrate expression of large groups of genes important in development and phenotypic specification. miRNAs do not encode proteins but rather bind to target mRNAs in a sequence-specific manner, to promote their degradation or inhibit their translation. Specific patterns of miRNAs are upregulated in response to stress and have been implicated in mediating the hypertrophic response.

Apoptosis of cardiac myocytes may be an important factor in heart failure. A fivefold increase in the number of cardiac myocytes undergoing apoptosis has been observed in animal models of heart disease, and senescent rats have 30% fewer cardiac myocytes than young ones. Pathologic hypertrophy is generally associated with greater cardiac myocyte apoptosis, which may contribute to the transition from compensated hypertrophy to heart failure. Signaling by agonists such as AngII and ET-1 increases expression of proapoptotic genes via JNK and p38 MAPK pathways, and signaling by adrenergic agonists increases the sensitivity of cardiac myocytes to apoptotic stimuli. In contrast, p110α PI3K signaling via IGF-1 receptor enhances survival. Thus, various signaling pathways in cardiac hypertrophy may exert both proapoptotic and antiapoptotic influences, the final outcome depending on the balance between them.

CARDIAC STEM CELLS AND MYOCARDIAL REGENERATION: The heart has traditionally been thought of as a static organ incapable of growing new myocytes to regenerate or repair damage owing to a lack of cardiac stem cells. There is now compelling evidence that cardiac stem cells exist in adults and that they are probably important in maintaining cardiac function in health and disease (see Chapter 1). For example, male transplant recipients who have received female hearts exhibit fully differentiated cardiac myocytes bearing the Y chromosome. Embryonic stem cells and adult bone marrow–derived cells can repopulate areas of experimental myocardial injury and improve clinical outcomes, although whether they can differentiate into fully functional cardiac myocytes remains controversial.

PATHOLOGY: Anything that increases cardiac workload for a prolonged period or produces structural damage may eventuate in myocardial failure. ***Ischemic heart disease is by far the most common condition responsible for cardiac failure, accounting for more than 80% of deaths from heart disease.*** Most of the remaining deaths are caused by nonischemic forms of heart muscle disease (cardiomyopathies) and congenital heart disease. Virtually all body organs suffer when the heart fails. The subject is discussed in detail in Chapter 7, and only the salient features are reviewed here.

Other than changes characteristic of specific disease entities (e.g., ischemic heart disease or cardiac amyloidosis), the morphology of failing hearts is nonspecific. ***Ventricular hypertrophy is seen in virtually all conditions associated with chronic heart failure.*** Initially, only the left ventricle may be hypertrophied, as in compensated hypertensive heart disease. But when the left ventricle fails, some right ventricular hypertrophy usually follows, owing to the increased workload imposed on the right ventricle by the failing left ventricle. ***In most cases of clinically apparent systolic heart failure, the ventricles are conspicuously dilated.*** The distribution of end-organ involvement depends on whether the heart failure is predominantly left sided or right sided.

Left-sided heart failure is more common, because the most frequent causes of cardiac injury (e.g., ischemic heart disease and hypertension) primarily affect the left ventricle. To compensate for left ventricular failure, left atrial and pulmonary venous pressures increase, resulting in passive pulmonary congestion. The capillaries in the alveolar septa fill with blood and small ruptures allow erythrocytes to escape. As a result, alveoli contain many hemosiderin-laden macrophages (so-called heart failure cells). Moreover, if capillary hydrostatic pressure exceeds plasma osmotic pressure, fluid leaks from capillaries into alveoli. Resultant **pulmonary edema** (see Chapter 10) may be massive, with alveoli being "drowned" in a transudate. Interstitial pulmonary fibrosis results when congestion is present over an extended period.

Right-sided heart failure commonly complicates left-sided failure, or it can develop independently secondary to intrinsic pulmonary disease or pulmonary hypertension, which creates resistance to blood flow through the lungs. As a consequence, right atrial pressure and systemic venous pressure both increase, resulting in jugular venous distention, edema of lower extremities and congestion of liver and spleen. Hepatic congestion in heart failure is characterized by distended central veins, which stand out on the cut surface of the liver as dark red foci against the yellow of the cells in the lobular periphery. This gives the liver a gross appearance that has been compared to the cut surface of a nutmeg (hence, "nutmeg liver"; see Chapter 14).

Chronically injured cardiac myocytes exhibit loss of myofibrils. Regardless of the type of injury, dysfunctional myocytes lose sarcomeres and correspondingly increase cytosol and glycogen. This process (**myocytolysis**) causes the cells to appear vacuolated (a dramatic example is shown in Fig. 11-6). These changes are apparently reversible and likely result from perturbations in myocyte metabolism. Myocytolysis may be an adaptive response to enhance myocyte survival in the face of chronic injury. Such histopathology is especially prominent in "hibernating myocardium," a condition in which contractile function is impaired at rest in the setting of reduced coronary blood flow.

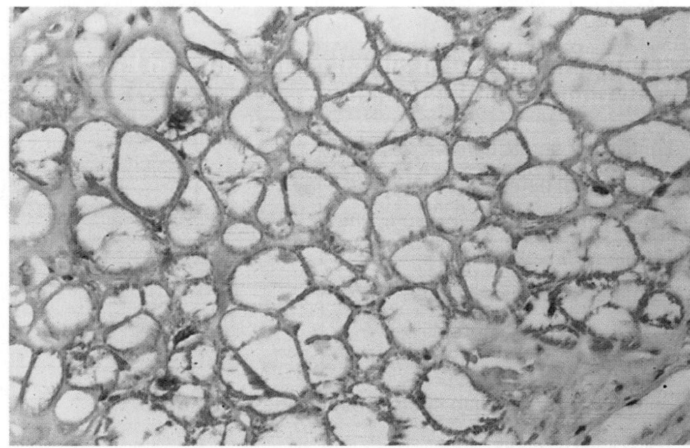

FIGURE 11-6. Severe myocytolysis in a patient with end-stage heart failure. Chronically injured myocytes show dramatic loss of myofibrils, giving the cells a marked vacuolated appearance. Only a thin rim of contractile cytoplasm is present, immediately beneath the sarcolemma.

Diastolic heart failure is often seen in elderly patients. Ventricles become progressively stiffer with advancing age, and require greater filling (diastolic) pressures. Some patients exhibit signs and symptoms of heart failure even though their hearts are normal in size and have normal systolic contractile function. These patients do not tolerate increases in blood volume well and are susceptible to developing pulmonary edema in response to a fluid challenge. Microscopically, these hearts typically exhibit interstitial fibrosis, which may contribute to the decreased compliance of ventricular myocardium.

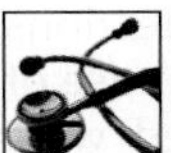

CLINICAL FEATURES: Symptoms of left-sided failure include **dyspnea on exertion, orthopnea** (dyspnea when lying down) and **paroxysmal nocturnal dyspnea** (respiratory distress that awakens patients from sleep). Dyspnea on exertion reflects the increasing pulmonary congestion that accompanies a higher end-diastolic pressure in the left atrium and ventricle. Orthopnea and paroxysmal nocturnal dyspnea result when lung blood volume increases, owing to reduced blood volume in the lower extremities during recumbency.

Although much of the clinical presentation of heart failure can be explained by venous congestion (**backward failure**), important aspects of congestive failure involve inadequate perfusion of vital organs (**forward failure**). Most patients with left-sided heart failure retain sodium and water (edema) due to poor renal perfusion, decreased glomerular filtration rate and activation of the renin–angiotensin–aldosterone system (see Chapter 7). Inadequate cerebral perfusion can lead to confusion, memory loss and disorientation. Reduced perfusion of skeletal muscle leads to fatigue and weakness.

Table 11-1

Relative Incidence of Specific Anomalies in Patients With Congenital Heart Disease

Ventricular septal defects: 25%–30%
Atrial septal defects: 10%–15%
Patent ductus arteriosus: 10%–20%
Tetralogy of Fallot: 4%–9%
Pulmonary stenosis: 5%–7%
Coarctation of the aorta: 5%–7%
Aortic stenosis: 4%–6%
Complete transposition of the great arteries: 4%–10%
Truncus arteriosus: 2%
Tricuspid atresia: 1%

Congenital Heart Disease

Congenital heart disease (CHD) results from faulty embryonic development, expressed either as misplaced structures (e.g., transposition of the great vessels) or arrested progression of a normal structure from an early stage to a more advanced one (e.g., atrial septal defect).

Significant CHD occurs in almost 1% of all live births. This does not include certain common defects that are not functionally important (e.g., an anatomically patent foramen ovale that is functionally closed by the left atrial flap that covers it). In this circumstance, the foramen ovale remains closed as long as left atrial pressure exceeds that in the right atrium. A bicuspid aortic valve is also common and is usually asymptomatic until adulthood. Estimates of the incidence of particular cardiovascular anomalies vary, depending on many factors. A range derived from several sources is shown in Table 11-1.

ETIOLOGIC FACTORS: The best evidence for intrauterine influence in the occurrence of congenital cardiac defects relates to maternal rubella infection during the first trimester, especially during the first 4 weeks of gestation. An association with other viral infections is suspected but is not as well documented. Maternal use of certain drugs in early pregnancy is also associated with increased numbers of cardiac defects in offspring. For example, in the thalidomide syndrome (phocomelia) there was a 10% incidence of CHD (see Chapter 6). Other drugs implicated in CHD include alcohol, phenytoin, amphetamines, lithium and estrogenic steroids. Maternal diabetes is also associated with increased incidence of CHD.

MOLECULAR PATHOGENESIS: The causes of CHD are usually not ascertained. However, it is worthwhile to determine whether a defect in any one case can be recognized as being mainly of genetic origin or primarily acquired, as this issue is important to parents in planning future pregnancies. Most congenital heart defects reflect both multifactorial genetic, epigenetic and environmental influences. As in other diseases with multifactorial inheritance (see Chapter 6), the risk of recurrence is greater among siblings of an affected child: CHD occurs in 1% of the general population, which increases to 2% to 15% for a pregnancy following the birth of a child with a heart defect. The risk of a third affected child may be as high as 30%. Moreover, an infant born to a mother with CHD is at increased risk for CHD.

Chromosomal abnormalities may cause CHD, most prominently Down syndrome (trisomy 21), other trisomies, Turner syndrome and DiGeorge syndrome. Together, these account for no more than 5% of all cases of CHD.

Much has been learned recently about genes encoding transcription factors that regulate cardiogenesis. The best studied is *Csx/NKX2.5*, a member of the evolutionarily conserved *NK* homeobox gene family. *Csx/NKX2.5* is a mammalian homolog of the *Drosophila* gene *NK4*, also known as *tinman* (from the *Wizard of Oz*) because deletion of this gene leads to failure of cardiac myocyte fate specification and lack of formation of a heart. Cardiac myocytes are formed when *Csx/NKX2.5* is deleted in mammals, but certain features of morphogenesis are arrested and growth of the heart tube is retarded. Expression of several cardiac genes is also reduced, including genes encoding myosin light chain 2v, ANF, cardiac ankyrin repeat protein and various transcription factors such as dHAND and eHAND, which are expressed in chamber-specific patterns and exert important regulatory influences over the development of the right and left ventricles. Various mutations in *Csx/NKX2.5* in humans have been associated with a spectrum of congenital cardiac malformations including atrial and ventricular septal defects, tetralogy of Fallot, double-outlet right ventricle, tricuspid valve abnormalities and hypoplastic left heart syndrome.

Classifications of Congenital Heart Disease Reflect Cyanosis and Shunting

There are several ways to categorize congenital heart defects. One of the earliest clinically useful schemes put cases into three groups based on the presence or absence of cyanosis:

- **The acyanotic group** does not have an abnormal communication between the systemic and pulmonary circuits. Examples of the acyanotic group include coarctation of the aorta, right-sided aortic arch and Ebstein malformation.
- **The cyanose tardive group** is defined as an initial left-to-right shunt with late reversal of flow, including patent ductus arteriosus (PDA), patent foramen ovale and ventricular septal defect. In patients with these anomalies, cyanosis supervenes later (i.e., tardive). Although the shunt is initially left to right, it later becomes right to left (**Eisenmenger complex**) because progressive increases in pulmonary vascular resistance cause the right ventricular pressure to rise to the point where it exceeds that in the left ventricle (see below).
- **The cyanotic group** describes a permanent right-to-left shunt. This category of CHD includes tetralogy of Fallot, truncus arteriosus, tricuspid atresia and complete transposition of the great vessels.

Additional classification schemes have been developed to provide the detail necessary to meet clinical requirements,

Table 11-2

Classification of Congenital Heart Disease

Classification of Congenital Heart Disease
Initial Left-to-Right Shunt
Ventricular septal defect
Atrial septal defect
Patent ductus arteriosus
Persistent truncus arteriosus
Anomalous pulmonary venous drainage
Hypoplastic left heart syndrome
Right-to-Left Shunt
Tetralogy of Fallot
Tricuspid atresia
No Shunt
Complete transposition of the great vessels
Coarctation of the aorta
Pulmonary stenosis
Aortic stenosis
Coronary artery origin from pulmonary artery
Ebstein malformation
Complete heart block
Endocardial fibroelastosis

especially those of the cardiac surgeon. **A more contemporary classification divides the cases into the groups shown in Table 11-2.**

Early Left-to-Right Shunt Reflects the Higher Pressure on the Left Side of the Heart

Ventricular Septal Defect

Ventricular septal defects (VSDs) are among the most common congenital heart lesions (Table 11-1). They occur as isolated lesions or in combination with other malformations.

ETIOLOGIC FACTORS: The fetal heart consists of a single chamber until the fifth week of gestation, after which it is divided by the development of interatrial and interventricular septa and by formation of atrioventricular valves from endocardial cushions. A muscular interventricular septum grows upward from the apex toward the base of the heart (Fig. 11-7). It is joined by the downward-growing membranous septum, separating right and left ventricles. ***The most common VSD is related to partial or complete formation of the membranous portion of the septum.***

PATHOLOGY: VSDs occur as (1) a small hole in the membranous septum; (2) a large defect involving more than the membranous region (perimembranous defects); (3) defects in the muscular portion, which are more common anteriorly but can occur anywhere in the muscular septum and are often multiple; or (4) complete absence of the muscular septum (leaving a single ventricle).

VSDs are most common in the superior portion of the septum below the pulmonary artery outflow tract (below the crista supraventricularis, i.e., infracristal) and behind the septal leaflet of the tricuspid valve. The common bundle (bundle of His) is located immediately below the defect (inlet type). Less commonly, the defect is above the crista supraventricularis (supracristal) and just below the pulmonary valve (infra-arterial). The supracristal variety of septal defect is often associated with other defects, such as an overriding pulmonary artery (the **Taussig-Bing** type of double-outlet right ventricle), transposition of the great vessels or persistent truncus arteriosus.

CLINICAL FEATURES: *A small septal defect may have little functional significance and may close spontaneously as the child matures.* Closure is accomplished by either hypertrophy of adjacent muscle or adherence of tricuspid valve leaflets to the margins of the defect. In infants with large septal defects, higher left ventricular pressure creates initially a left-to-right shunt. Left ventricular dilation and congestive heart failure are common complications of such shunts. If a defect is small enough to permit prolonged survival, augmented pulmonary blood flow caused by shunting of blood into the right ventricle eventually results in thickening of pulmonary arteries and increased pulmonary vascular resistance. This increased vascular resistance may be so great that the direction of the shunt is then reversed, and goes from right to left (**Eisenmenger complex**). A patient with this condition displays late onset of cyanosis (i.e., tardive cyanosis), right ventricular hypertrophy and right-sided heart failure.

Additional complications of ventricular septal defects include (1) infective endocarditis at the lesional site, (2) paradoxical emboli and (3) prolapse of an aortic valve cusp (with resulting aortic insufficiency). Large ventricular septal defects are repaired surgically, usually in infancy.

Atrial Septal Defects

Atrial septal defects (ASDs) range in severity from clinically insignificant and asymptomatic anomalies to chronic, life-threatening conditions. They arise embryologically by defects in the formation of atrial septum. Embryologic development of the atrial septum occurs in a sequence that permits continued passage of oxygenated placental blood from the right to the left atrium through the patent foramen. The developing atrial septum permits this right-to-left shunt to continue until birth. Beginning at the fifth week of intrauterine life, the septum primum extends downward from the roof of the common atrium to join with the endocardial cushions, thereby closing the incomplete segment, or "ostium primum" (Fig. 11-7A). Before this closure is complete, the midportion of the septum primum develops a defect, or "ostium secundum," so that right-to-left flow continues. During the sixth week, a second septum (septum secundum) develops to the right of the septum primum, passing from the roof of the atrium toward the endocardial cushions (Fig. 11-7B). This process leaves a patent foramen, the **foramen ovale,** in the position of the original ostium secundum. The defect persists until it is sealed off after birth by fusion of the septum primum and septum secundum, whereupon it is termed the **fossa ovalis.**

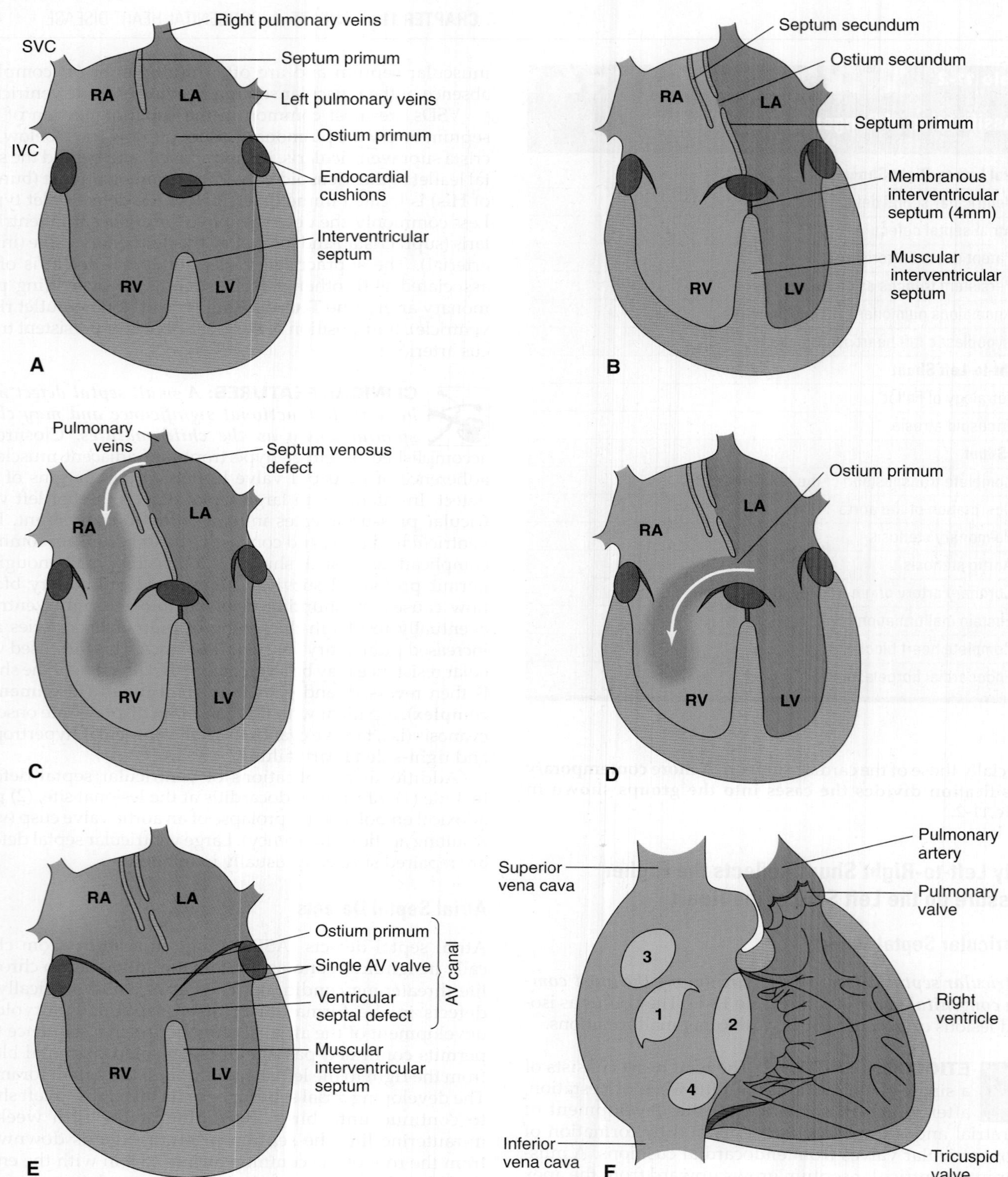

FIGURE 11-7. Pathogenesis of ventricular and atrial septal defects. A. The common atrial chamber is being separated into the right and left atria (RA and LA) by the septum primum. Because the septum primum has not yet joined the endocardial cushions, there is an open ostium primum. The ventricular cavity is being divided by a muscular interventricular septum into right and left chambers (right and left ventricles, RV and LV). SVC = superior vena cava; IVC = inferior vena cava. **B.** The septum primum has joined the endocardial cushions but at the same time has developed an opening in its midportion (the ostium secundum). This opening is partly overlaid by the septum secundum, which has grown down to cover, in part, the foramen ovale. Simultaneously, the membranous septum joins the muscular interventricular septum to the base of the heart, completely separating the ventricles. **C.** The **sinus venosus type of atrial septal** defect is located in the most cephalad region and is adjacent to the inflow of the right pulmonary veins, which thus tend to open into the RA. **D.** The **ostium primum defect** occurs just above the atrioventricular (AV) valve ring, sometimes in the presence of an intact valve ring. It may also, in conjunction with a defect of the valve ring and ventricular septum, form an AV canal, as shown in panel **E**. This common opening allows free communication between the atria and the ventricles. **F. Location of atrial septal defects.** In decreasing order of frequency: 1. Ostium secundum; 2. Ostium primum; 3. Sinus venosus; and 4. Coronary sinus type.

MOLECULAR PATHOGENESIS: The cause of most ASDs is not determined, but a minority occur as a component of certain genetic syndromes. Approximately 15% of familial ASDs and 3% of sporadic ASDs are associated with coding errors in *NKX2.5*. Deletion of the T-box gene *TBX1* in the DiGeorge syndrome (chromosome 22Q11 deletion) has been implicated in ASD formation. Mutations in a related T-box gene, *TBX5*, cause the Holt-Oram syndrome in which large secundum-type ASDs typically occur.

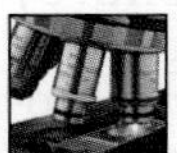

PATHOLOGY: ASDs occur at a number of sites (see Fig. 11-7).

- **Patent foramen ovale:** Tissue derived from the septum primum situated on the left side of the foramen ovale functions as a flap valve that normally fuses with the margins of the foramen ovale, thereby sealing the opening. An incomplete seal of the foramen ovale, which can be traversed with a probe (**probe patent foramen ovale**), is found in 25% of normal adults and is not normally problematic. However, it may become a true shunt if circumstances increase right atrial pressure, as can occur with recurrent pulmonary thromboemboli. In this case, a right-to-left shunt will be produced, and thromboemboli from the right-sided circulation will pass directly into the systemic circulation. Such **paradoxical emboli** may cause infarcts in many parts of the arterial circulation, most commonly in the brain, heart, spleen, intestines, kidneys and lower extremities. A widely patent foramen ovale is occasionally encountered and is actually an acquired atrial septal defect caused by a disproportion between the size of the foramen ovale and the length of the valve covering it.
- **Atrial septal defect, ostium secundum type:** This defect accounts for 90% of all cases of ASDs. It is a true deficiency of the atrial septum and should not be confused with a patent foramen ovale. An ostium secundum defect occurs in the middle portion of the septum and varies from a trivial opening to a large defect of the entire fossa ovalis region. A small defect is usually not problematic, but a larger one may allow sufficient blood to shunt from left to right to cause dilation and hypertrophy of the right atrium and ventricle. In this setting, pulmonary artery diameter may exceed that of the aorta.

  Lutembacher syndrome, a variant of ostium secundum atrial septal defect, combines mitral stenosis and an ostium secundum atrial septal defect. Mitral stenosis may be due to a congenital malformation or rheumatic fever. It is thought that increased left atrial pressure secondary to mitral valve obstruction keeps the atrial septum patent.
- **Sinus venosus defect:** This anomaly, accounting for 5% of ASDs, occurs in the upper portion of the atrial septum, above the fossa ovalis, near the entry of the superior vena cava (Fig. 11-7C). It is usually accompanied by drainage of right pulmonary veins into the right atrium or superior vena cava.
- **Atrial septal defect, ostium primum type:** This condition involves the region adjacent to the endocardial cushions (Fig. 11-7D) and comprises 7% of all atrial septal defects. There are usually clefts in the anterior leaflet of the mitral valve and the septal leaflet of the tricuspid valve, which may be accompanied by a defect in the adjacent interventricular septum.

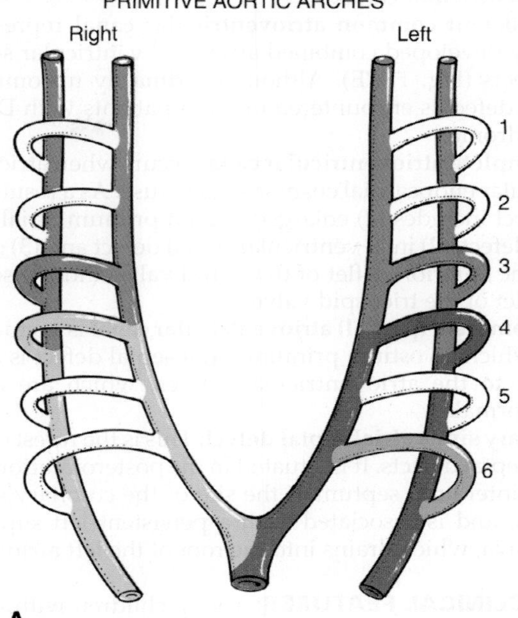

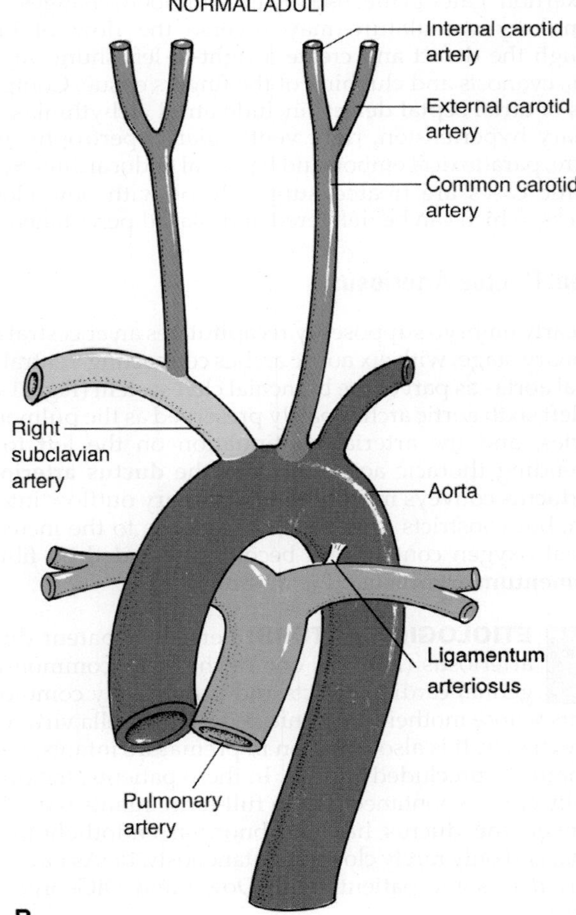

FIGURE 11-8. Derivatives of the aortic arches. A. Complete primitive aortic arch system. **B.** In the normal adult, the left fourth aortic arch is preserved as the arch of the adult aorta, and the left sixth arch gives rise to the pulmonary artery and ligamentum arteriosus (closed ductus arteriosus).

- **Atrioventricular canal:**
  - **Persistent common atrioventricular canal** represents fully developed combined atrial and ventricular septal defects (Fig. 11-7E). Although ordinarily uncommon, this defect is encountered often in patients with Down syndrome.
  - **Complete atrioventricular canal** occurs when atrioventricular endocardial cushions fail to fuse. As a result, the defect includes (1) enlarged ostium primum atrial septal defect, (2) inlet ventricular septal defect and (3) clefts in the anterior leaflet of the mitral valve and the septal leaflet of the tricuspid valve.
  - **Incomplete (partial) atrioventricular canal** is a situation in which an ostium primum atrial septal defect is adjacent to the atrioventricular valves, which are often abnormal.
- **Coronary sinus atrial septal defect:** This is the rarest of the atrial septal defects. It is situated in the posteroinferior part of the interatrial septum at the site of the coronary sinus ostium, and is associated with a persistent left superior vena cava, which drains into the roof of the left atrium.

CLINICAL FEATURES: Young children with atrial septal defects are ordinarily asymptomatic, although they may complain of easy fatigability and dyspnea on exertion. Later in life, usually in adulthood, changes in the pulmonary vasculature may reverse the flow of blood through the defect and create a right-to-left shunt. In such cases, cyanosis and clubbing of the fingers ensue. Complications of atrial septal defects include atrial arrhythmias, pulmonary hypertension, right ventricular hypertrophy, heart failure, paradoxical emboli and bacterial endocarditis. Symptomatic cases are treated surgically or with new closure devices, which can be delivered and placed percutaneously.

Patent Ductus Arteriosus

The early embryo supposedly recapitulates an ancestral evolutionary stage, with six aortic arches connecting ventral and dorsal aortas as part of the branchial cleft system (Fig. 11-8A). The left sixth aortic arch is partly preserved as the pulmonary arteries, and the arterial continuation on the left to the descending thoracic aorta becomes the **ductus arteriosus.** The ductus conveys most of the pulmonary outflow into the aorta, but constricts after birth in response to the increased arterial oxygen content and becomes occluded by fibrosis (**ligamentum arteriosus**) (Fig. 11-8B).

ETIOLOGIC FACTORS: Persistent patent ductus arteriosus (PDA) is one of the most common congenital cardiac defects and is especially common in infants whose mothers were infected with rubella virus early in pregnancy. It is also common in premature infants, whose prematurity precluded closure. In these patients, the ductus usually closes spontaneously. In full-term infants with PDA, however, the ductus has an abnormal endothelium and media, and only rarely closes spontaneously. PDAs have been reported in some patients with Down and DiGeorge syndromes.

CLINICAL FEATURES: Luminal diameters of PDAs vary greatly. A small shunt has little effect on the heart, but a large one causes considerable diversion of blood from the aorta to the low-pressure pulmonary artery. In severe cases, more than half of the left ventricular output may be shunted into the pulmonary circulation. Left ventricular hypertrophy and heart failure ensue due to increased demand for cardiac output. In patients with a large PDA, the increased volume and pressure of blood in the pulmonary circulation eventually lead to pulmonary hypertension and its cardiac complications. Infective endarteritis involving the pulmonary artery side of the ductus is a frequent complication of untreated PDA.

PDA can be corrected surgically or by interventional cardiac catheterization. It can be caused to contract and then close by instilling prostaglandin synthesis inhibitors (e.g., indomethacin). Conversely, it can be kept open after birth by administering prostaglandins (PGE_2) if survival of patients born with a cardiac defect requires a left-to-right or right-to-left shunt. Examples include patients with isolated pulmonary stenosis, complete transposition of the great vessels or hypoplastic left heart syndrome.

Aortopulmonary window is a defect between the base of the aorta and the pulmonary artery. It is a rare condition that is functionally similar to PDA and is clinically difficult to differentiate from it.

Other abnormalities of the aortic arch system can be predicted by visualizing the variations that could occur in the development of the complete aortic arch system (Fig. 11-8). For example, the right side of the aortic arch system rather than the left may be retained, resulting in the condition known as a **right aortic arch.** This variant is seen in about 25% of patients with tetralogy of Fallot and in 50% of patients with truncus arteriosus. A right aortic arch is innocuous unless it creates a vascular ring that compresses the esophagus and trachea.

Persistent Truncus Arteriosus

The truncus arteriosus is the embryonic arterial trunk that initially opens from both ventricles and is later separated into the aorta and the pulmonary trunk by the spiral septum. ***Persistent truncus arteriosus is a common trunk of origin for the aorta, pulmonary arteries and coronary arteries, resulting from absent or incomplete partitioning of the truncus arteriosus by the spiral septum. Truncus arteriosus always overrides a VSD and receives blood from both ventricles.*** The valve of the truncus usually has three or four semilunar cusps but may have as few as two or as many as six. The coronary arteries arise from the base of the valve.

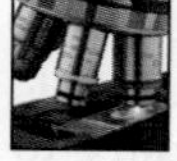

PATHOLOGY: There are several variants of truncus arteriosus:

- **Type 1** is most common, and consists of a single trunk that gives rise to a common pulmonary artery and ascending aorta.
- **Type 2** displays right and left pulmonary arteries that originate from a common site in the posterior midline of the truncus.
- **Type 3** has separate pulmonary arteries arising laterally from a common trunk.
- **Type 4** consists of other rare variants in which there is no pulmonary trunk at all and in which the pulmonary circulation is supplied from the aorta by enlarged bronchial arteries. This type is difficult to differentiate from tetralogy of Fallot with pulmonary artery atresia.

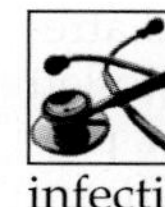

CLINICAL FEATURES: Most infants with truncus arteriosus have torrential pulmonary blood flow, causing heart failure, recurrent respiratory tract infections and often early death. Pulmonary vascular disease develops in children with prolonged survival, in which case cyanosis, polycythemia and clubbing of the fingers appear. Open-heart surgery before significant pulmonary vascular changes develop is an effective treatment.

Hypoplastic Left Heart Syndrome

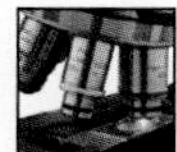

PATHOLOGY: This usually profound malformation is characterized by hypoplasia of the left ventricle and ascending aorta and hypoplasia or atresia of the left-sided valves. Severe aortic valvular stenosis or aortic atresia is often the main defect. Some mitral valve structures are usually present, although the mitral valve may also be atretic. If the mitral valve is atretic rather than hypoplastic, the left ventricle may consist of only a thin slit lined by endocardium.

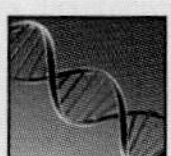

MOLECULAR PATHOGENESIS: No specific mutations have been implicated in this complex malformation, but there is a 2% to 4% risk of recurrence in future pregnancies. In families with two affected children, the risk increases to 25%. Maternal chromosome abnormalities have been linked to the syndrome in about 10% of cases. The most common of these is terminal 11q deletion (Jacobsen syndrome) in which 10% of all children have hypoplastic left heart syndrome.

CLINICAL FEATURES: Atresia of the aortic valve precludes left ventricular outflow into the aorta. There is an obligate left-to-right shunt through a patent foramen ovale. Cardiac output is entirely via the right ventricle and pulmonary artery. Systemic blood flow depends on flow from the pulmonary trunk to the aorta through a PDA. Coronary blood flow depends on retrograde flow from a hypoplastic ascending aorta to the sinuses of Valsalva. Because pulmonary vascular resistance is high at birth and both the foramen ovale and ductus arteriosus are patent, newborns with hypoplastic left heart syndrome may appear well initially. However, as pulmonary vascular resistance falls and systemic blood flow (and especially coronary blood flow) decreases, infants become symptomatic. Over 95% die within the first month of life without surgical intervention. Treatment includes surgical approaches or cardiac transplantation.

Anomalous Pulmonary Vein Drainage

The pulmonary veins form a network in the dorsal mesoderm. A bud from the region of the atrium joins the pulmonary venous confluence, and eventually all four pulmonary veins drain into the left atrium. Failure of these tissues to join correctly results in various venous anomalies.

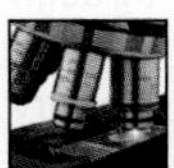

PATHOLOGY: **Total anomalous pulmonary vein drainage** may occur as an isolated defect or as part of the asplenia syndrome (splenic agenesis, congenital heart defects and situs inversus of abdominal organs). Most commonly, the pulmonary veins drain into a common pulmonary venous chamber and then through a persistent left superior vena cava (the persistent left pericardial vein) into the innominate vein or the right superior vena cava. Alternate routes for common pulmonary vein drainage may lead into the coronary sinus or entail persistent posterior and subcardinal veins. The latter form a middorsal trunk that crosses the diaphragm and enters the portal vein or ductus venosus, and may be associated with some pulmonary venous obstruction.

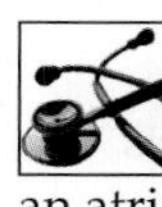

CLINICAL FEATURES: In total anomalous pulmonary drainage, there is no direct venous return to the left side of the heart and life is sustained only by an atrial septal defect or patent foramen ovale. Heart failure, severe hypoxemia and pulmonary venous obstruction result from total anomalous pulmonary vein drainage. Good results have been obtained with surgical correction.

Partial anomalous pulmonary venous drainage may result from less severe circulatory impairment. This anomaly may involve one or two pulmonary veins, especially in association with a sinus venosus type of atrial septal defect. The prognosis is excellent, similar to that for atrial septal defects.

Right-to-Left Shunt Is the Most Common Cyanotic Congenital Heart Disease

Tetralogy of Fallot

Tetralogy of Fallot represents 10% of all cases of CHD. It has a familial recurrence rate of 2% to 3% but little is known of its potential genetic and epigenetic causes.

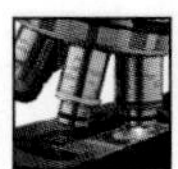

PATHOLOGY: The four anatomic changes that define the tetralogy of Fallot are (Fig. 11-9):

- **Pulmonary stenosis**
- **Ventricular septal defect**
- **Dextroposition of the aorta so that it overrides the ventricular septal defect**
- **Right ventricular hypertrophy**

The ventricular septal defect, which may be as large as the aortic orifice, results from incomplete closure of the membranous septum, and affects both the muscular septum and the endocardial cushions. In addition, development of the spiral septum, which normally divides the common truncus region into an aorta and a pulmonary artery, is abnormal. As a result, the aorta is displaced to the right and overlies the septal defect. The ventricular septal defect is immediately below the overriding aorta. Pulmonary stenosis is often due to subpulmonary muscular hypertrophy, with an enlarged infundibular muscle obstructing blood flow into the pulmonary artery. In about one third of these hearts, the valve itself is the main cause of stenosis; in such cases, the valve is usually funnel shaped, with the narrow part more distal.

The heart is hypertrophied so as to give it a boot shape. Almost half of patients with tetralogy of Fallot have other cardiac anomalies, including ostium secundum atrial septal defects, PDA, left superior vena cava and endocardial cushion defects. The aortic arch is on the right side in about 25% of cases of tetralogy of Fallot. The surgeon must remember that a large branch of the right coronary artery may cross the pulmonary conus region, which is the site of the cardiotomy made to enlarge the outflow tract. Patency of the ductus arteriosus is actually protective, because it provides a source of blood to the otherwise deprived pulmonary vascular bed.

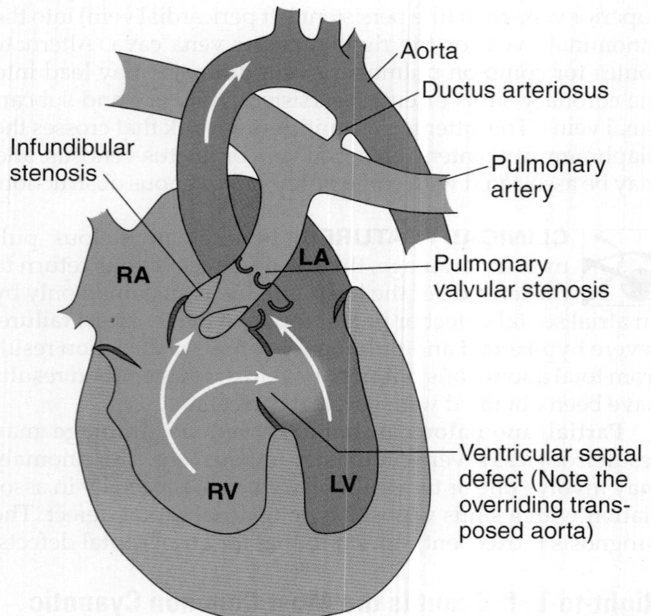

FIGURE 11-9. Tetralogy of Fallot. Note the pulmonary stenosis, which is due to infundibular hypertrophy as well as pulmonary valvular stenosis. The ventricular septal defect involves the membranous septum region. Dextroposition of the aorta and right ventricular hypertrophy are shown. Because of the pulmonary obstruction, the shunt is from right to left, and the patient is cyanotic. LA = left atrium; LV = left ventricle; RA = right atrium; RV = right ventricle.

CLINICAL FEATURES: In the face of severe pulmonary stenosis, right ventricular blood is shunted through the ventricular septal defect into the aorta, resulting in arterial desaturation and cyanosis. Surgical correction is typically done in the first 2 years of life. Otherwise, the affected child complains of dyspnea on exertion, and often assumes a squatting position to relieve the shortness of breath. Physical development is characteristically retarded. Cerebral thromboses owing to marked polycythemia may complicate the disease. Patients are also at risk for bacterial endocarditis and brain abscesses. Increasing cyanosis and shortness of breath may indicate that a beneficial PDA has closed spontaneously. Left-sided heart failure is not common.

Without surgical intervention, the prognosis of tetralogy of Fallot is dismal. However, total correction is possible with open-heart surgery, which carries less than 10% mortality. After successful surgery, patients become asymptomatic and have excellent long-term prognoses.

Tricuspid Atresia

PATHOLOGY: ***Tricuspid atresia, a congenital absence of the tricuspid valve, results in an obligate right-to-left shunt through the patent foramen ovale.*** This defect usually occurs with a VSD through which blood gains access to the pulmonary artery. **Type I** tricuspid atresia (75% of patients with tricuspid atresia) is associated with normally related great arteries. **Type II** is associated with D-transposition of the great arteries, and the rare **type III** features L-malposition (see below).

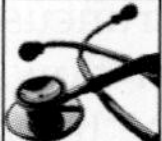

CLINICAL FEATURES: Infants with tricuspid atresia present with cyanosis due to the atrial right-to-left shunt. If the VSD is small, the limitation of pulmonary blood flow can result in even more significant cyanosis. In this scenario, a prominent cardiac murmur is typically noted. Surgical intervention is aimed at bypassing the atretic tricuspid valve and small right ventricle. Staged surgical palliation is the goal of current therapy.

Congenital Heart Diseases Without Shunts Involve Various Cardiovascular Sites

Transposition of the Great Arteries

In transposition of the great arteries (TGA), the aorta arises from the right ventricle and the pulmonary artery from the left ventricle. The condition shows a male predominance and is more common if mothers are diabetic. TGA causes over half of deaths from cyanotic heart disease in the first year of life.

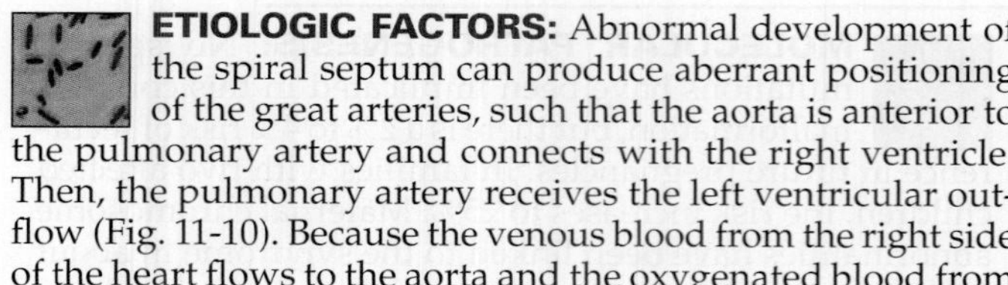

ETIOLOGIC FACTORS: Abnormal development of the spiral septum can produce aberrant positioning of the great arteries, such that the aorta is anterior to the pulmonary artery and connects with the right ventricle. Then, the pulmonary artery receives the left ventricular outflow (Fig. 11-10). Because the venous blood from the right side of the heart flows to the aorta and the oxygenated blood from

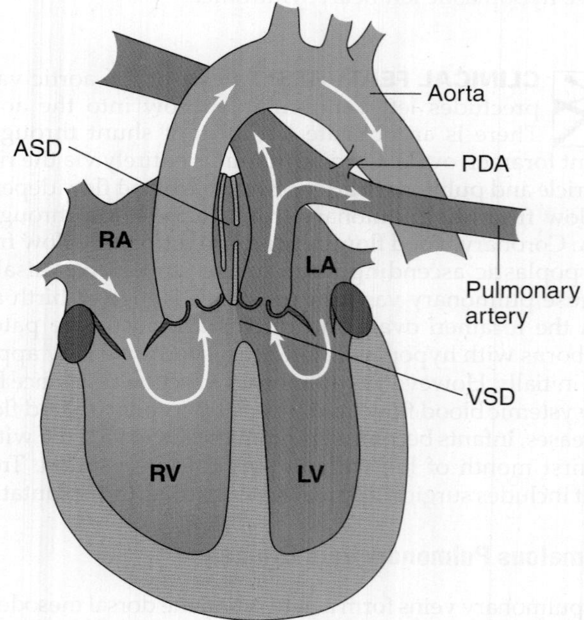

FIGURE 11-10. Complete transposition of great arteries, regular type. The aorta is anterior to, and to the right of, the pulmonary artery ("D-transposition") and arises from the right ventricle. In the absence of interatrial or interventricular connections or patent ductus arteriosus, this anomaly is incompatible with life. The volume and direction of blood flow through intracardiac communications and patent ductus arteriosus, if present, depend on pressure gradients across the communications which can vary during early stages of extrauterine life. LA = left atrium; LV = left ventricle; RA = right atrium; RV = right ventricle; PDA = patent ductus arteriosus; ASD = atrial septal defect; VSD = ventricular septal defect.

the lungs returns to the pulmonary artery, there are in effect two independent and parallel blood circuits for the systemic and pulmonary circulations. Survival is possible only if there is a communication between the circuits. Virtually all such infants have an ASD, one half have a VSD and two thirds have a PDA.

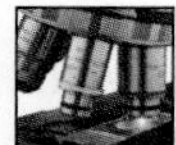

PATHOLOGY: The aorta normally arises posterior and to the left of the pulmonary artery. In its ascending portion, it courses behind and to the right of the pulmonary artery. In TGA, the aorta is anterior to the pulmonary artery and to its right **("D" or dextrotransposition)** all the way from its origin.

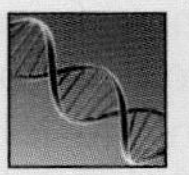

CLINICAL FEATURES: Before cardiac surgery, the outlook for infants with TGA was dismal: 90% died in their first year. It is now possible to correct the malformation within the first 2 weeks of life using an arterial-switch operation, with overall survival of 90%.

Congenitally corrected transposition is a condition in which the aorta is anterior to, but passes to the left of, the pulmonary artery **("L" transposition).** Although the great arteries are thus abnormally related to each other and arise from discordant ventricles, the circulatory pattern is functionally corrected because of coexistent atrioventricular discordance. Patients in whom corrected TGA is the only malformation are clinically entirely normal. Unfortunately, many cases are complicated by other cardiac anomalies, which require their own specific interventions.

The **Taussig-Bing malformation** is a double-outlet right ventricle (both great vessels arise from the right ventricle) in which a VSD is above the crista supraventricularis and directly beneath an overriding pulmonary artery. This condition is functionally and clinically similar to TGA with a VSD and pulmonary hypertension.

MOLECULAR PATHOGENESIS: Various types of double-outlet right ventricle have been observed in patients with autosomal trisomies (13, 18, 21) and 22q11 deletions. Mutations in *NKX2.5* and maternal exposure to teratogens that influence neural crest development have also been implicated in a few cases.

Coarctation of the Aorta

Coarctation of the aorta is a local constriction that almost always occurs immediately below the origin of the left subclavian artery at the site of the ductus arteriosus. Rare coarctations can occur at any point from the aortic arch to the abdominal bifurcation. The condition is two to five times more frequent in males than females and is associated with a bicuspid aortic valve in two thirds of cases. Mitral valve malformations, VSDs and subaortic stenosis may also accompany coarctation of the aorta. There is a particular association of coarctation with Turner syndrome, and berry aneurysms in the brain are also more common.

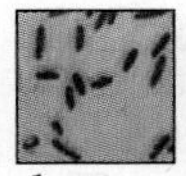
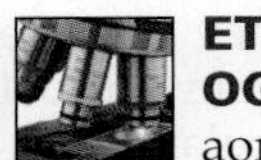

ETIOLOGIC FACTORS AND PATHOLOGY: The pathogenesis of coarctation of the aorta is related to the pattern of flow in the ductus arteriosus during fetal life (Fig. 11-11). In utero blood flow through the ductus is considerably greater than that across the aortic valve. The blood leaving the ductus is diverted into two streams by a posterior aortic shelf opposite the orifice of the ductus. One stream passes cephalad into the relatively hypoplastic aortic isthmus to supply the head and upper extremities; the other enters the descending thoracic aorta. In late fetal life, increasing left ventricular output dilates the isthmus, and the increased blood flow bypasses the obstruction (represented by the posterior shelf) through the wide ductal orifice. After birth, the ductal orifice is obliterated and the posterior shelf normally involutes, thereby removing the obstruction. The shelf may not involute because of inadequate antegrade flow in the aortic arch in utero due to anomalies that limit left ventricular output (e.g., bicuspid aortic valve). Often the obstructing shelf fails to involute for unknown reasons. In any event, the result is the most common type of coarctation of the aorta, a **juxtaductal constriction.**

The **infantile (preductal) type of coarctation** results when the aortic isthmus remains narrow (hypoplastic) into late fetal life and after birth. This lesion is usually accompanied by a PDA and a right-to-left shunt through a VSD.

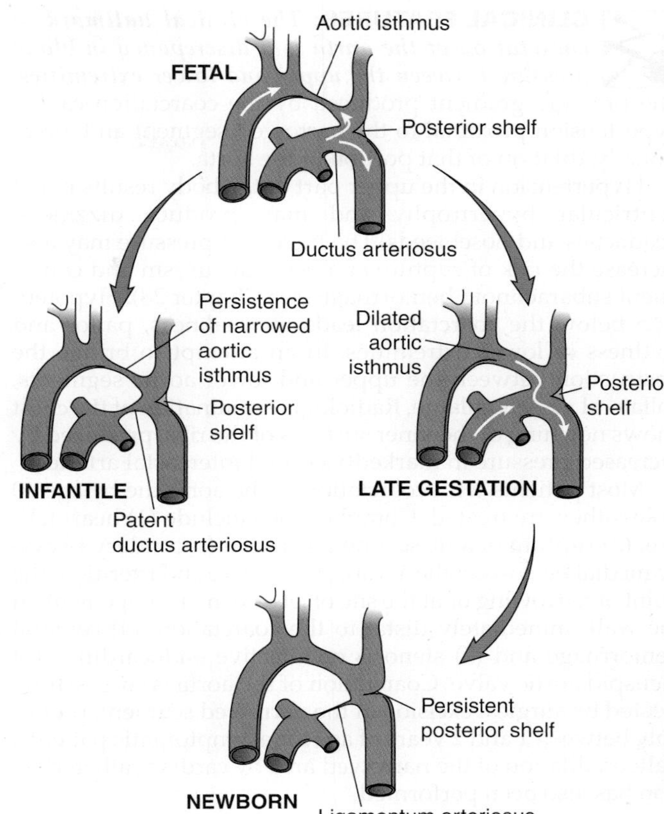

FIGURE 11-11. Pathogenesis of coarctation of the aorta. In the fetus, ductal blood is diverted into cephalad and descending streams by the posterior aortic shelf. In late fetal life, the isthmus dilates and the increased descending blood flow is accommodated by the ductal orifice. After birth, if the shelf does not undergo the normal involution, obliteration of the ductal orifice does not permit free flow around the persistent posterior shelf, thereby creating a juxtaductal obstruction of blood flow to the distal aorta. If the aortic isthmus does not dilate during late fetal life, it remains narrow, resulting in an infantile or preductal coarctation. In this circumstance, the ductus arteriosus usually remains patent.

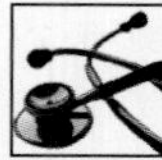

CLINICAL FEATURES: ***The clinical hallmark of coarctation of the aorta is a discrepancy in blood pressure between the upper and lower extremities.*** The pressure gradient produced by the coarctation causes hypertension proximal to the narrowed segment and, occasionally, dilation of that portion of the aorta.

Hypertension in the upper part of the body results in left ventricular hypertrophy and may produce dizziness, headaches and nosebleeds. The increased pressure may also increase the risk of rupture of a berry aneurysm and consequent subarachnoid hemorrhage (see Chapter 28). Hypotension below the coarctation leads to weakness, pallor and coldness of lower extremities. In an attempt to bridge the obstruction between the upper and lower aortic segments, collateral vessels enlarge. Radiologic examination of the chest shows notching of the inner surfaces of the ribs, produced by increased pressure in markedly dilated intercostal arteries.

Most patients with coarctation of the aorta die by age 40 unless they are treated. Complications include (1) heart failure, (2) rupture of a dissecting aneurysm (secondary to cystic medial necrosis of the aorta), (3) infective endarteritis at the point of narrowing or at the site of jet-stream impingement on the wall immediately distal to the coarctation, (4) cerebral hemorrhage and (5) stenosis or infective endocarditis of a bicuspid aortic valve. Coarctation of the aorta is successfully treated by surgical excision of the narrowed segment, preferably between 1 and 2 years of age for asymptomatic patients. Balloon dilation of the narrowed area by cardiac catheterization has also been performed.

Pulmonary Stenosis

Pulmonary stenosis results from (1) developmental deformities arising from the endocardial cushion region of the heart (with involvement of the pulmonary valves), (2) an abnormality of the right ventricular infundibular muscle (subvalvular or infundibular stenosis, especially as part of tetralogy of Fallot) or (3) abnormal development of the more distal parts of the pulmonary artery tree (peripheral pulmonary stenosis). Peripheral pulmonary stenosis, which is much less common than the other two, may produce "coarctation" of the pulmonary arteries at one or several sites. This anomaly is more common in newborns with **Williams syndrome,** a disorder often associated with deletion mutations in the gene encoding elastin.

Isolated pulmonary stenosis ordinarily involves the valve cusps, which are fused to form an inverted cone or funnel type of constriction. The artery distal to the valve may develop poststenotic dilation after several years. In severe cases, infants exhibit right ventricular and atrial hypertrophy. If the foramen ovale is patent, there is a right-to-left shunt with cyanosis, secondary polycythemia and clubbing of the fingers. Good results have been obtained with balloon dilation of the stenotic valve by cardiac catheterization.

Congenital Aortic Stenosis

Three types of congenital aortic stenosis are recognized: valvular, subvalvular and supravalvular.

VALVULAR AORTIC STENOSIS: The most common congenital aortic stenosis, bicuspid valve, arises through abnormal development of the endocardial cushions. A congenitally bicuspid aortic valve is much more frequent (4:1) in males than females and is associated with other cardiac anomalies (e.g., coarctation of the aorta) in 20% of cases. Typically, two of the three semilunar cusps (the right coronary cusp with one of the adjacent two cusps) are fused.

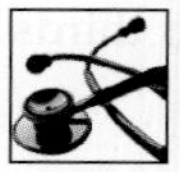

CLINICAL FEATURES: Many children with bicuspid aortic stenosis are asymptomatic. Over the years, the resulting bicuspid valve tends to become thickened and calcified, generally causing symptoms in adulthood. More severe forms of congenital aortic stenosis result in a unicommissural valve or one without any commissures. These malformations cause symptoms in early life. Exertional dyspnea and angina pectoris may be prominent. Sudden death, principally owing to ventricular arrhythmias, is a distinct threat for patients with severe obstruction. Bacterial endocarditis sometimes complicates the disease. Valve replacement may be indicated.

SUBVALVULAR AORTIC STENOSIS: This defect accounts for 10% of all cases of congenital aortic stenosis and is caused by abnormal development of a band of subvalvular fibroelastic tissue or a muscular ridge. Stenosis results from a membranous diaphragm or fibrous ring that surrounds the left ventricular outflow tract immediately below the aortic valve. It is twice as common in males as in females.

Many people with subvalvular aortic stenosis develop thickening and immobility of the aortic cusps, with mild aortic regurgitation. Bacterial endocarditis carries its own risks and may also aggravate the regurgitation. Surgical treatment of subvalvular aortic stenosis involves excising the membrane or fibrous ridge.

SUPRAVALVULAR AORTIC STENOSIS: This type of stenosis is much less common than the other two, and is often associated with idiopathic infantile hypercalcemia **(Williams syndrome)** characterized by mental retardation and multiple system disorders.

Origin of a Coronary Artery From the Pulmonary Artery

A single coronary artery or, rarely, both may originate from the pulmonary artery rather than the aorta. When one coronary artery has an anomalous origin (most often the left coronary), anastomoses develop between the right and left coronary arteries. This produces an arterial–arterial shunt through which blood flows from the artery originating from the aorta to that arising from the pulmonary artery. The myocardium supplied by the anomalous artery is vulnerable to episodes of ischemia. The result may be myocardial infarction, fibrosis and calcification and endocardial fibroelastosis.

Ebstein Malformation

Ebstein malformation results from downward displacement of an abnormal tricuspid valve into an underdeveloped right ventricle. One or more tricuspid valve leaflets are plastered to the right ventricular wall for a variable distance below the right atrioventricular annulus.

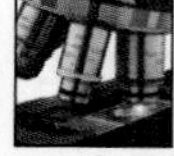

PATHOLOGY: Septal and posterior tricuspid valve leaflets are usually affected. They are irregularly elongated and adherent to the right ventricular wall, so that the upper part of the right ventricular cavity (inflow region) functions separately from the distal chamber. The anterior leaflet is usually the least involved, and may be normal. The valve ring may or may not be displaced downward from its usual position. In any event, the effective tricuspid valve orifice is displaced downward into the ventricle, thus dividing it into two separate parts: the "atrialized" ventricle (proximal ventricle) and the functional right ventricle (distal ventricle). In two thirds of cases, conspicuous dilation of the functional ventricle hinders its ability to pump blood efficiently through the pulmonary arteries. The degree of tricuspid valve insufficiency depends on the severity and configuration of the defect in the leaflets.

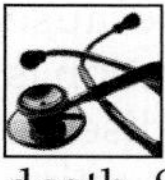

CLINICAL FEATURES: Ebstein malformation leads to heart failure, massive right atrial dilation, arrhythmias with palpitations and tachycardia and sudden death. Surgical treatment has met with variable success.

Congenital Heart Block

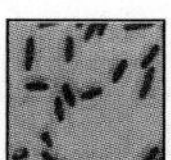

ETIOLOGIC FACTORS: Congenital complete heart block is usually associated with other cardiac anomalies. In such cases, disruption in the continuity of the conduction system is probably caused by the accompanying cardiac abnormality. However, in cases of isolated complete heart block, failure of the atrioventricular conduction system is believed to result from lack of regression of the sulcus tissue, which entirely encloses the conducting tissue during early development. Congenital heart block without structural heart disease has been linked to maternal connective tissue disease, especially systemic lupus erythematosus. If maternal SS-A/Ro or SS-B/La autoantibodies are transmitted to the fetus transplacentally, the incidence of congenital complete heart block approaches 100%.

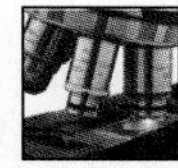 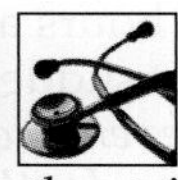

PATHOLOGY AND CLINICAL FEATURES: Hearts of patients with congenital heart block tend to show a lack of continuity between the atrial myocardium and the atrioventricular node. Alternatively, the defect may consist of a fibrous separation of the atrioventricular node from the ventricular conducting tissue. Although the heart rate is abnormally slow, patients with isolated heart block often have little functional difficulty. Later in life, cardiac hypertrophy, attacks of Stokes–Adams syncope (dizziness and unexpected fainting), arrhythmias and heart failure may develop.

Endocardial Fibroelastosis

Endocardial fibroelastosis (EFE) is characterized by fibroelastotic thickening of the left ventricular endocardium, and may also affect the valves. The disorder may be primary or secondary, the latter being far more common.

SECONDARY ENDOCARDIAL FIBROELASTOSIS: This occurs in association with underlying cardiovascular anomalies that lead to left ventricular hypertrophy in the face of an inability to meet the increased myocardial oxygen demands. Thus, secondary EFE is a frequent complication of congenital aortic stenosis (including hypoplastic left ventricle syndrome) and coarctation of the aorta. Some type of endocardial injury is likely involved in its pathogenesis.

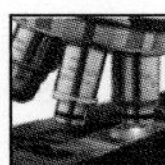

PATHOLOGY: On gross examination, the left ventricle endocardium displays irregular, opaque, gray-white patches, which also may be present on the cardiac valves. Microscopically, these plaques are areas of endocardial fibroelastotic thickening, frequently accompanied by degeneration of adjacent subendocardial myocytes. Valves may show collagenous thickening.

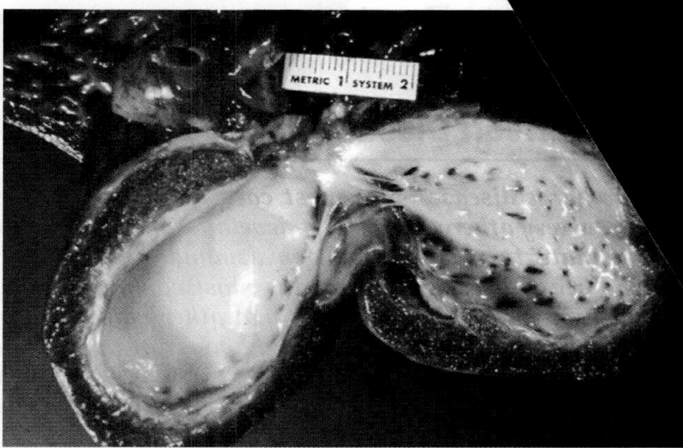

FIGURE 11-12. Endocardial fibroelastosis. The left ventricle of an infant who died of endocardial fibroelastosis has been opened to reveal a thickened endocardium lining most of the cavity and virtually obliterating the trabeculae carneae.

PRIMARY ENDOCARDIAL FIBROELASTOSIS: Defined as fibroelastosis in the absence of any associated lesion, this disorder is now quite rare. It afflicts infants, usually 4 to 10 months of age. Although it has occurred in siblings, no specific mode of inheritance has been established. Some evidence links primary EFE to mumps infection, which may explain why this condition is now seen so infrequently.

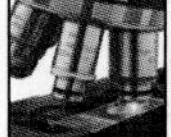

PATHOLOGY: The left ventricle is usually conspicuously dilated but occasionally contracted and hypertrophic. Diffuse endocardial thickening involves most of the left ventricle (Fig. 11-12) and aortic and mitral valve leaflets. The thickened endocardium tends to obscure the trabecular pattern of the underlying myocardium, and papillary muscles and chordae tendineae are thick and short. Mural thrombi may complicate the situation.

Infants with primary EFE develop progressive heart failure. The prognosis is dismal, and cardiac transplantation offers the only hope for a cure.

Dextrocardia

Dextrocardia is rightward orientation of the base–apex axis of the heart. It is often associated with a mirror image of the normal left-sided location and configuration. The position of the ventricles is determined by the direction of the embryonic cardiac loop. If the loop protrudes to the right, the future right ventricle develops on the right, and the left ventricle comes to occupy its proper position. If the loop protrudes to the left, the opposite occurs.

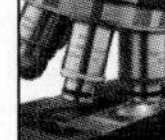

PATHOLOGY: If dextrocardia occurs without abnormal positioning of the visceral organs (**situs inversus**), it is invariably associated with severe cardiovascular anomalies. These include transposition of the great arteries, a variety of atrial and ventricular septal defects, anomalous pulmonary venous drainage and many others. If dextrocardia

… heart is functionally normal, … common.

…ses, a consequence of … develops when blood flow … oxygen demands of the heart. …s by far the most common type of … United States and other industrialized … it remains the leading cause of death. It is …e for at least 80% of all deaths attributable to heart …se.* By contrast, atherosclerotic heart disease is far less frequent in underdeveloped countries. The principal effects of ischemic heart disease are angina pectoris, myocardial infarction, chronic congestive heart failure and sudden death.

ANGINA PECTORIS: This term refers to the pain of myocardial ischemia. It typically produces a severe crushing or burning sensation in the substernal portion of the chest and may radiate to the left arm, jaw or epigastrium. It is the most common symptom of ischemic heart disease. Coronary atherosclerosis usually becomes symptomatic only when the luminal cross-sectional area of the affected vessel is reduced by more than 75%. A patient with typical angina pectoris exhibits recurrent episodes of chest pain, usually brought on by increased physical activity or emotional excitement. The pain is of limited duration (1 to 15 minutes) and is relieved by reducing physical activity or by treatment with sublingual nitroglycerin (a potent vasodilator).

Although the most common cause of angina pectoris is severe coronary atherosclerosis, decreased coronary blood flow can result from other conditions, including coronary vasospasm, aortic stenosis or aortic insufficiency. Angina pectoris is not usually associated with anatomic changes in the myocardium as long as the duration and severity of ischemic episodes are insufficient to cause myocardial necrosis. However, repetitive bouts of angina may eventually contribute to myocytolytic degeneration of the myocardium (Fig. 11-6).

Prinzmetal angina (variant angina) *is an atypical form of angina that occurs at rest and is caused by coronary artery spasm.* The responsible mechanisms are not fully understood but endothelial dysfunction plays a major role. Patients typically exhibit vasoconstrictor responses to acetylcholine reflecting abnormal nitric oxide production. Thromboxane derived from platelet activation may also be involved. Spasm in structurally normal coronary arteries may be part of a systemic syndrome of abnormal arterial vasomotor reactivity, which includes migraine headache and Raynaud phenomenon. Usually, however, it develops in atherosclerotic coronary arteries, often in a portion of a vessel nearby an atherosclerotic plaque. In this case, coronary artery spasm may contribute to acute myocardial infarction or affect the size of an infarct, but is generally not the principal cause of infarction.

Unstable angina, *a variety of chest pain that has a less predictable relationship to exercise than does stable angina and may occur during rest or sleep, is associated with development of nonocclusive thrombi over atherosclerotic plaques.* In some cases of unstable angina, episodes of chest pain become progressively more frequent and longer over a 3- to 4-day period. Electrocardiographic changes are not characteristic of infarction and serum levels of cardiac-specific intracellular proteins, such as the MB isoform of CK (MB-CK) or cardiac troponins T or I (evidence of myocardial necrosis), remain normal. Unstable angina is also termed **preinfarction angina, accelerated angina** or **"crescendo" angina.** Without pharmacologic or mechanical intervention to "open up" the coronary narrowing, many such patients progress to myocardial infarction.

MYOCARDIAL INFARCT: A myocardial infarct is a discrete focus of ischemic muscle necrosis in the heart. This definition excludes patchy foci of necrosis caused by drugs, toxins or viruses. The development of an infarct is related to the duration of ischemia and the metabolic rate of the ischemic tissue. In experimental coronary artery ligation, foci of necrosis form after 20 minutes of ischemia and become more extensive as the period of ischemia lengthens.

CHRONIC CONGESTIVE HEART FAILURE: Because early mortality associated with acute myocardial infarction is now less than 5%, many patients with ischemic heart disease survive longer and eventually develop chronic congestive heart failure. Coronary artery disease is responsible for heart failure in more than 75% of all patients with heart failure. Contractile impairment in these patients is due to irreversible loss of myocardium (previous infarcts) and hypoperfusion of surviving muscle, which leads to chronic ventricular dysfunction ("hibernating" myocardium; Fig. 11-6). Many of these patients die suddenly, especially those in whom contractile impairment is not severe. Others develop progressive pump failure and die of multiorgan failure. Because coronary artery disease is often so extensive in these patients and many have already undergone coronary artery bypass surgery, the only treatments available are cardiac transplantation or the use of artificial pumps (ventricular assist devices).

SUDDEN DEATH: In some patients, the first and only clinical manifestation of ischemic heart disease is sudden death due to spontaneous ventricular tachycardia that degenerates into ventricular fibrillation. Some authorities consider death to be sudden only if it occurs within 1 hour of the onset of symptoms. Others regard death within 24 hours after the onset of symptoms to be sudden or require that sudden death be diagnosed only if it is unexpected. *In any event, coronary atherosclerosis underlies most cases of cardiac death occurring during the first hour after the onset of symptoms.*

Experimental animals subjected to acute coronary occlusion show a high incidence of ventricular fibrillation within 1 hour. Sudden cardiac death due to ventricular fibrillation also occurs in humans as a result of acute coronary artery thrombosis. On the other hand, such an arrhythmia also appears in patients with marked coronary artery disease and no detectable thrombosis. Clinical studies of patients who have been defibrillated and survived an arrhythmia have shown that most have not suffered acute myocardial infarction: serum markers and electrocardiographic changes characteristic of infarction do not develop. *Thus, in many cases, lethal arrhythmia is likely triggered by acute ischemia without overt myocardial infarction.* The presence of a healed infarct or ventricular hypertrophy increases the risk that an episode of acute ischemia will initiate life-threatening ventricular arrhythmia.

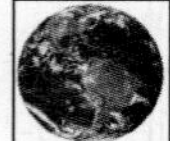

EPIDEMIOLOGY: *The major risk factors that predispose to coronary artery disease are (1) systemic hypertension, (2) cigarette smoking, (3) diabetes mellitus and (4) elevated blood cholesterol.* Any one of these factors significantly increases the risk of myocardial infarction, but a combination of multiple factors augments that risk more than sevenfold (see Chapter 8).

During the 20th century, the United States experienced first a dramatic increase and then a dramatic reversal in mortality from ischemic heart disease. In 1950, the age-adjusted death rate from myocardial infarction was 226 per 100,000 cases; 40 years later it was 108. This shift reflects many factors, including reduced smoking, lower dietary saturated fat and new drugs that control hypertension, reduce cholesterol and dissolve coronary thrombi. Important advances in medical technology include construction of coronary care units, coronary revascularization procedures and use of defibrillators and ventricular assist devices. Concurrently, the role of hyperlipidemia in the pathogenesis of coronary artery atherosclerosis attracted much more attention. This was driven initially by epidemiologic evidence showing that populations in which men have high mean serum cholesterol values had higher rates of coronary artery disease. Since then, multiple studies established that elevated serum low-density lipoproteins (LDLs) increase risk of myocardial infarction, whereas high levels of high-density lipoproteins (HDLs) decrease that risk. The total cholesterol–to–HDL cholesterol ratio appears to be a better predictor of coronary artery disease than serum cholesterol level alone.

Although blood lipid profile is an important indicator of the risk of atherogenesis, other risk factors exert powerful independent effects. A person with a blood pressure of 160/95 mm Hg has twice the risk of ischemic heart disease as one whose blood pressure is 140/75 mm Hg or less. The risk of ischemic heart disease increases in proportion to the number of cigarettes smoked. Serum factors involved in thrombosis or thrombolysis or that contribute to endothelial injury have also been implicated in atherogenesis. For example, plasma fibrinogen levels directly correlate with risk of ischemic heart disease, presumably because of the role of fibrinogen in atherogenesis and coronary artery thrombosis. Other factors reported to contribute to increased risk of myocardial infarction include factor VII, plasminogen activator inhibitor-1 (PAI-1), homocysteine and decreased fibrinolytic activity. Levels of selected serum markers of inflammation such as C-reactive protein also predict ischemic heart disease risk.

During the past several years, there has been a remarkable increase in the incidence of type 2 diabetes in the United States, which mirrors a similar increase in obesity (see Chapter 22). Ischemic heart disease is a consequence of both type 1 and type 2 diabetes, the risk being twofold to threefold greater than in nondiabetic persons. Conversely, atherosclerotic cardiovascular disease (myocardial infarction, stroke, peripheral vascular disease) accounts for 80% of all deaths in patients with diabetes.

Other risk factors for ischemic heart disease include:

- **Obesity:** In a major, longitudinal study of one population (Framingham Heart Study), obesity was an independent risk factor for cardiovascular disease, with an increased risk for obese persons over lean ones of 2 to 2.5.
- **Age:** The risk of infarction is greater with increasing age, up to age 80 years.
- **Sex:** Sixty percent of coronary events occur in men. Angina pectoris is considerably more frequent in men than in women; the ratio at ages younger than 50 years is 4:1, and is 2:1 after age 60.
- **Family history:** In one study that controlled for other risk factors, relatives of patients with ischemic heart disease had a twofold to fourfold increased risk for coronary artery disease. The genetic basis for this familial risk may interact with the other risk factors.
- **Use of oral contraceptives:** Women over 35 years who smoke cigarettes and use oral contraceptives have a modestly increased incidence of myocardial infarction.
- **Sedentary life habits:** Regular exercise reduces risk of myocardial infarction, perhaps by increasing HDL levels. In one study, the least-fit quartile of persons subjected to exercise testing had six times the risk of myocardial infarction than persons in the fittest quartile.
- **Personality features:** Early studies suggested that aggressive, time-conscious, executive-type individuals ("type A" personality) have more heart disease than do easygoing, relaxed persons ("type B" personality). "Coronary-prone" subjects, those of the type A behavior pattern, differ from type B individuals in having higher plasma triglyceride and cholesterol levels and greater urinary catecholamine excretion. However, the relationship between coronary artery disease and type A personality is controversial. Recent studies have failed to show the strong association previously reported.

Many Conditions Limit the Supply of Blood to the Heart

The heart is an aerobic organ, requiring oxidative phosphorylation to provide energy for contraction. The anaerobic glycolysis used by skeletal muscle under conditions of extreme physical exertion is insufficient to sustain cardiac contraction. Ischemic heart disease is caused by an imbalance between myocardial oxygen requirements and the supply of oxygenated blood (Table 11-3).

Table 11-3

Causes of Ischemic Heart Disease

Decreased Supply of Oxygen
Conditions that influence the supply of blood
Atherosclerosis and thrombosis
Thromboemboli
Coronary artery spasm
Collateral blood vessels
Blood pressure, cardiac output, and heart rate
Miscellaneous: arteritis (e.g., periarteritis nodosa), dissecting aneurysm, luetic aortitis, anomalous origin of coronary artery, muscular bridging of coronary artery
Conditions that influence the availability of oxygen in the blood
Anemia
Shift in the hemoglobin–oxygen dissociation curve
Carbon monoxide
Cyanide
Increased Oxygen Demand (i.e., Increased Cardiac Work)
Hypertension
Valvular stenosis or insufficiency
Hyperthyroidism
Fever
Thiamine deficiency
Catecholamines

Atherosclerosis and Thrombosis

The pathogenesis of atherosclerosis is detailed in Chapter 10. Here we discuss only briefly the features of special importance to ischemic heart disease. The coronary arteries are conductance vessels, small muscular arteries with a prominent internal elastic lamina. Their principal role is to deliver blood to the regulatory vasculature (small intramural arteries and arterioles), which controls nutritive myocardial blood flow. A healthy person has substantial coronary flow reserve and myocardial perfusion can be increased to four to eight times the resting blood flow. In a normal heart, the large coronary arteries provide almost no resistance to blood flow and myocardial circulation is mainly controlled by constriction and dilation of small, intramyocardial branches less than 400 μm in diameter. In advanced atherosclerosis of the main epicardial coronary arteries, luminal stenosis decreases blood pressure distal to the narrowed zone. To compensate for reduced perfusion pressure, microvessels dilate, thereby maintaining normal resting blood flow. Thus, most patients with coronary atherosclerosis do not have ischemia or angina at rest. However, with exercise, the capacity of the microcirculation to dilate further is limited, myocardial oxygen demand exceeds the supply and the result is ischemia and angina.

Maximal blood flow to the myocardium is not impaired until about 75% of the cross-sectional area of an epicardial coronary artery (~50% of the diameter as assessed during coronary angiography) is compromised by atherosclerosis. However, resting blood flow is not reduced until more than 90% of the lumen is occluded. In patients with long-standing angina pectoris, the extent and distribution of collateral circulation exerts an important influence on the risk of acute myocardial infarction. In some conditions (e.g., hypotension or tachycardia) demand for oxygen and perfusion pressure may be so out of balance that myocardial infarction ensues even when a coronary artery is not ordinarily sufficiently narrowed to produce ischemia.

Although myocardial infarction often occurs during physically demanding activities such as running or shoveling snow, many infarcts occur at rest or even during sleep. Thus, for most persons, the conversion of clinically silent coronary atherosclerosis to the catastrophic event of myocardial infarction involves a sudden, marked decrease in myocardial blood flow, with or without an increase in myocardial oxygen demand. ***It is now well established that coronary artery thrombosis is the event that usually precipitates an acute myocardial infarction. Thrombosis typically results from spontaneous rupture of an atherosclerotic plaque, usually in a region that contains numerous inflammatory cells and a thin fibrous cap.*** The initiating event may be hemorrhage into or beneath the plaque.

Thromboemboli

Thromboembolism is a rare cause of myocardial infarction. The coronary embolus is usually traced to the heart itself, usually valvular vegetations caused by infective or nonbacterial endocarditis. Coronary emboli occur in patients with atrial fibrillation and mitral valve disease who have mural thrombi in the left atrial appendage (Fig. 11-13). Thromboembolic occlusion of a coronary artery is also seen in patients with left ventricular mural thrombi secondary to infarction, aneurysm or dilated cardiomyopathy.

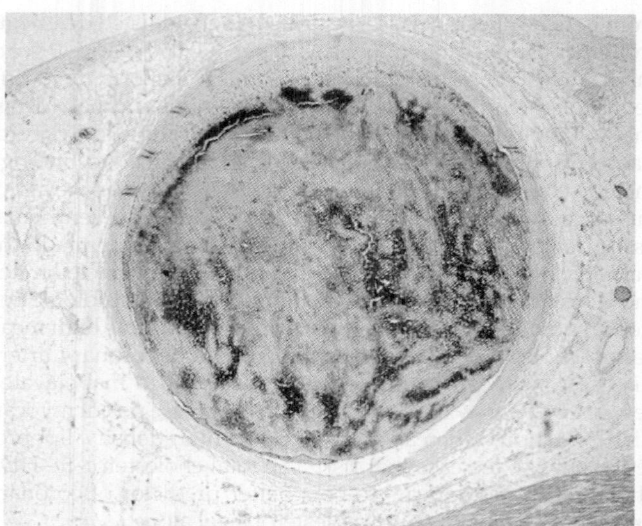

FIGURE 11-13. Thromboembolus in the left anterior descending coronary artery of a man who had old rheumatic heart disease, mitral stenosis and a mural thrombus in the left atrial appendage.

Coronary Collateral Circulation

Normal coronary arteries function as endarteries. Although most normal hearts have anastomoses 20 to 200 μm in diameter between coronary vessels, these collateral vessels do not function under normal circumstances because there is no pressure gradient between the arteries that they connect. However, the pressure differential resulting from abrupt occlusion of a coronary artery allows blood to flow from the patent coronary artery to the ischemic area. Extensive collateral connections develop in hearts with severe coronary atherosclerosis. These collaterals may actually provide enough arterial flow to prevent infarction completely or to limit infarct size when a major epicardial coronary artery is acutely occluded.

Well-developed coronary collaterals can explain certain unusual situations, such as anterior infarction after recent thrombotic occlusion of the right coronary artery (so-called *infarction at a distance*). This circumstance reflects the presence of collaterals between the LAD and right coronary arteries that formed (e.g., in response to gradual atherosclerotic narrowing of the LAD). As a result, myocardium normally supplied by the LAD distal to the occlusion now depends on blood flow from the right coronary artery via collaterals. Under these conditions, acute thrombosis of the right coronary artery may cause paradoxical infarction of the anterior wall of the left ventricle.

Other Conditions That Limit Coronary Blood Flow

- **Coronary arteritis** is caused by various vasculitides such as polyarteritis nodosa or Kawasaki disease. It may produce luminal narrowing due to vessel wall thickening. It can also create local aneurysms that may become occluded by thrombus.
- **Dissecting aneurysm of the aorta** occasionally extends into and obstructs coronary arteries. Occasionally, medial necrosis and dissecting aneurysms are confined to a coronary artery.

- **Syphilitic aortitis** characteristically involves the ascending aorta, where it may obliterate a coronary artery orifice.
- **Congenital anomalous origin of a coronary artery** (origin of a coronary artery from the pulmonary trunk or passage of an anomalous coronary artery between the aorta and pulmonary artery) has been associated with sudden death in young, otherwise healthy individuals.
- **An intramural course of the LAD coronary artery** may cause myocardial ischemia and sudden death. The artery normally runs in the epicardial fat. However, in some hearts it dips into the myocardium for a short distance. The muscular bridge over the LAD coronary artery may compress the vessel during systole or predispose to coronary spasm.

If the Ability of the Blood to Deliver Oxygen Is Limited, the Myocardium Is at Risk for Ischemia

Anemia is a common cause of decreased oxygen delivery to the myocardium. Although a heart with normal circulation can survive severe anemia, severe coronary atherosclerosis may limit any compensatory increases in coronary blood flow so much that cardiac necrosis results. Anemia also increases cardiac workload because increased output is required to oxygenate vital organs adequately.

Carbon monoxide (CO) poisoning (see Chapter 8) decreases oxygen delivery to the tissues. The high affinity of hemoglobin for CO displaces oxygen, thereby depriving tissues of oxygen. In this regard it should be noted that cigarette smoking produces significant levels of carboxyhemoglobin (a measure of CO) in the blood.

Increased Oxygen Demand May Cause Cardiac Ischemia

Any increase in cardiac workload increases the heart's need for oxygen. Conditions that raise blood pressure or cardiac output, such as exercise or pregnancy, augment oxygen demand by the myocardium, which may lead to angina pectoris or myocardial infarction. Disorders in this category include valvular disease (mitral or aortic insufficiency, aortic stenosis), infection and conditions such as hypertension, coarctation of the aorta and hypertrophic cardiomyopathy (HCM) (Table 11-3).

The increased metabolic rate and tachycardia seen in patients with hyperthyroidism are accompanied by increased oxygen demand and greater cardiac workload. Treatment of the underlying thyroid disease is the best therapy for a hyperthyroid patient with symptoms of ischemic heart disease. Fever also increases basal metabolic rate, cardiac output and heart rate.

Myocardial Infarcts Are Mainly Subendocardial or Transmural

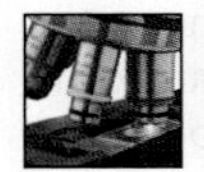

PATHOLOGY:

Location of Infarcts

There are important differences between these two types of infarction (Table 11-4).

A **subendocardial infarct** affects the inner one third to one half of the left ventricle. It may arise within the territory of one of the major epicardial coronary arteries or it may be circumferential, involving subendocardial distributions of multiple coronary arteries. ***Subendocardial infarction generally results from hypoperfusion of the heart.*** It may be due to atherosclerosis in a specific coronary artery, or it may develop in disorders that limit myocardial blood flow globally, such as aortic stenosis, hemorrhagic shock or hypoperfusion during cardiopulmonary bypass. Most subendocardial infarcts do not arise as a consequence of occlusive coronary thrombi, although small particles of platelet–fibrin thrombus may be seen in the epicardial coronary artery that supplies the region of infarction. For circumferential subendocardial infarction caused by global hypoperfusion of the myocardium, coronary artery stenosis need not be present. Because necrosis is limited to the inner layers of the heart, complications arising in transmural infarcts (e.g., pericarditis and ventricular rupture) do not follow subendocardial infarction.

Table 11-4

Differences Between Subendocardial and Transmural Infarcts

Subendocardial Infarcts	Transmural Infarcts
Multifocal	Unifocal
Patchy	Solid
May be circumferential	In distribution of a specific coronary artery
Coronary thrombosis rare	Coronary thrombosis common
Often result from hypotension or shock	Often cause shock
No epicarditis	Epicarditis common
Do not form aneurysms or lead to ventricular rupture	May result in aneurysm or ventricular rupture

A **transmural infarct** involves the full left ventricular wall thickness, usually after occlusion of a coronary artery. As a result, transmural infarcts typically conform to the distribution of one of the three major coronary arteries (Fig. 11-2).

- **Right coronary artery:** Occlusion of the proximal portion of this vessel results in an infarct of the posterior basal region of the left ventricle and the posterior third to half of the interventricular septum ("inferior" infarct).
- **LAD coronary artery:** Blockage of this artery produces an infarct of the apical, anterior and anteroseptal walls of the left ventricle.
- **Left circumflex coronary artery:** Obstruction of this vessel is the least common cause of myocardial infarction and leads to an infarct of the lateral wall of the left ventricle.

Myocardial infarction does not occur instantaneously. Rather, it first develops in the subendocardium and progresses as a wavefront of necrosis from subendocardium to subepicardium over the course of several hours. Transient coronary occlusion may cause only subendocardial necrosis, whereas persistent occlusion eventually leads to transmural necrosis. The goal of acute coronary interventions (pharmacologic or mechanical thrombolysis) is to interrupt this wavefront and limit myocardial necrosis.

The volume of arterial collateral flow is the chief determinant of transmural progression of an infarct. In chronic cardiac hypoperfusion, extensive collateral circulation, which preferentially supplies the outer or subepicardial layer, often limits an infarct to subendocardial myocardium. However, in fatal cases of acute myocardial infarction, transmural infarcts are more common than those restricted to the subendocardium.

Infarcts involve the left ventricle much more commonly and extensively than the right ventricle. This difference may be partly explained by the greater workload imposed on the left ventricle by systemic vascular resistance and the greater thickness of the left ventricular wall. Right ventricular hypertrophy (e.g., in pulmonary hypertension) increases the incidence of right ventricular infarction. Infarction of the posterior right ventricle occurs in about a third of left ventricular posteroseptal infarcts (right coronary artery territory), but infarcts limited to the right ventricle are rare.

Macroscopic Characteristics of Myocardial Infarcts

The early stages of myocardial infarction have been characterized most thoroughly in experimental animals. Within 10 seconds after ligation of a coronary artery, the affected myocardium becomes cyanotic and, rather than contracting, bulges outward during systole. If the obstruction is promptly relieved, myocardial contractions resume and no anatomic damage ensues, although contractility may be depressed in the postischemic tissue for many hours (**stunned myocardium**) as a result of the deleterious effects of reactive oxygen species formed upon reperfusion of acutely ischemic myocardium. This reversible stage continues for 20 to 30 minutes of total ischemia, beyond which time damaged myocytes progressively die.

On gross examination, an acute myocardial infarct is not identifiable within the first 12 hours. By 24 hours, it can be recognized by its pallor on the cut surface of the involved ventricle. After 3 to 5 days, it becomes mottled and more sharply outlined, with a central pale, yellowish, necrotic region bordered by a hyperemic zone (Fig. 11-14). By 2 to 3 weeks, the infarcted region is depressed and soft, with a refractile, gelatinous appearance. Older, healed infarcts are firm and contracted and have the pale gray appearance of scar tissue (Fig. 11-15).

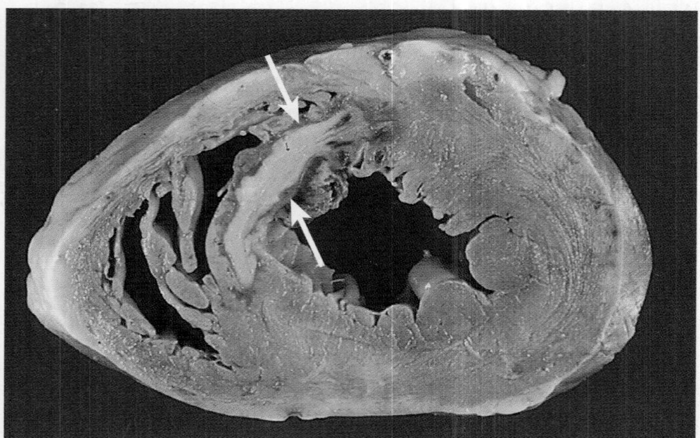

FIGURE 11-14. Acute myocardial infarct. A transverse section of the heart of a patient who died a few days after the onset of severe chest pain shows a transmural infarct in the anteroseptal region of the left ventricle (left anterior descending [LAD] coronary artery territory). The necrotic myocardium is soft, yellowish and sharply demarcated (*arrows*).

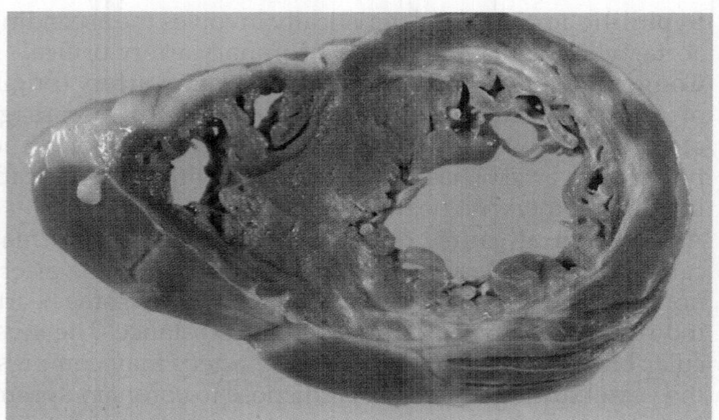

FIGURE 11-15. Healed myocardial infarct. A cross-section of the heart from a man who died after a long history of angina pectoris and several myocardial infarctions shows near-circumferential scarring of the left ventricle.

Microscopic Characteristics of Myocardial Infarcts

THE FIRST 24 HOURS: Electron microscopy is required to discern the earliest morphologic features of ischemic injury (Fig. 11-16). Reversibly injured myocytes show subtle changes of sarcoplasmic edema, mild mitochondrial swelling and loss of glycogen (the ultrastructural correlates of stunned myocardium). After 30 to 60 minutes of ischemia, when myocyte injury has become irreversible, mitochondria are greatly swollen with disorganized cristae and amorphous matrix densities composed of calcium phosphate salts formed by massive Ca^{2+} overload in severely injured cells. The nucleus shows clumping and margination of chromatin and the sarcolemma is focally disrupted.

Loss of sarcolemmal integrity leads to release of intracellular proteins, such as myoglobin, LDH, CK and troponins I and T. Ion gradients are also dissipated, and tissue potassium decreases as sodium, chloride and calcium increase.

The noncontractile ischemic myocytes are stretched with each systole and become **"wavy fibers."** By 24 hours, myocytes are deeply eosinophilic (Fig. 11-17) and show the characteristic changes of coagulative necrosis (see Chapter 1). However, it takes several days for the myocyte nucleus to disappear totally.

TWO TO 3 DAYS: Polymorphonuclear leukocytes are attracted to necrotic myocytes, but they gain access only at the periphery of the infarct, where blood flow is maintained. Hence, they accumulate at infarct borders and reach maximal concentration after 2 to 3 days (Figs. 11-17 and 11-18). Interstitial edema and microscopic areas of hemorrhage may also appear. By 2 to 3 days, muscle cells are more clearly necrotic, nuclei disappear and striations become less prominent. Some of the neutrophils that were attracted to the area begin to undergo karyorrhexis.

FIVE TO 7 DAYS: By this time, few, if any, polymorphonuclear leukocytes remain. The periphery of the infarcted region shows phagocytosis of dead muscle by macrophages. Fibroblasts begin to proliferate, and new collagen is

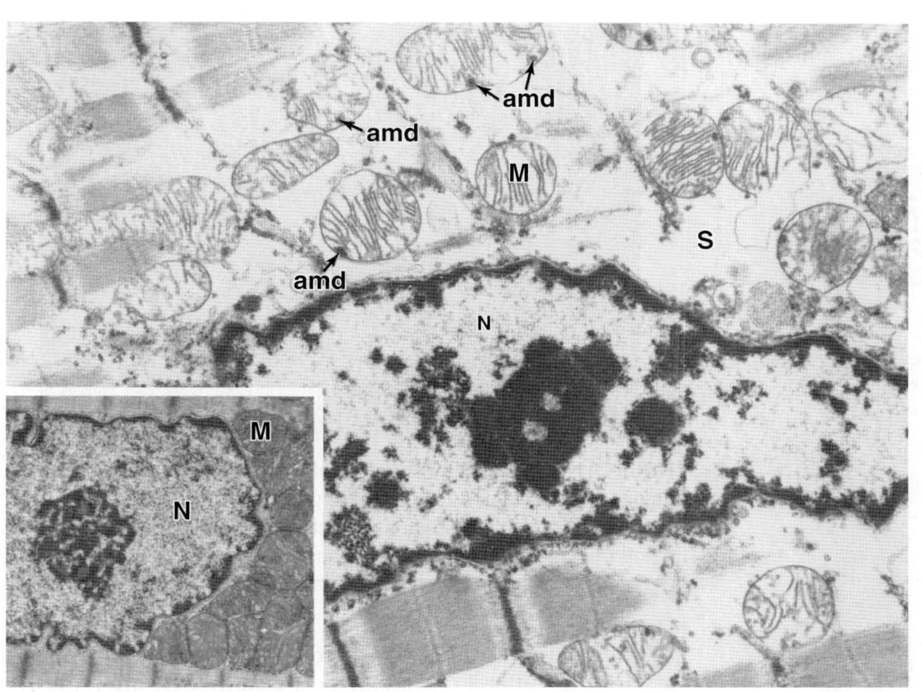

FIGURE 11-16. Ultrastructure of myocardial ischemia. Electron micrograph of an irreversibly injured myocyte from a canine heart subjected to 40 minutes of low-flow ischemia induced by proximal occlusion of the circumflex branch of the left coronary artery. (*Inset* shows a nonischemic control myocyte from the same heart. N = nucleus.) The affected myocyte is swollen and has abundant clear sarcoplasm (S). The mitochondria (M) are also swollen and contain amorphous matrix densities (amd), which are characteristic of lethal cell injury. The sarcolemma of this myocyte (*not shown*) exhibited small areas of disruption. The chromatin of the nucleus (N) is aggregated peripherally, in contrast to the uniformly distributed chromatin in normal tissue.

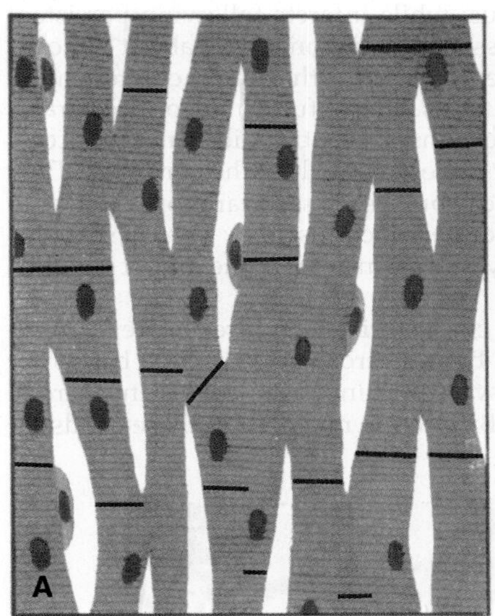

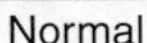

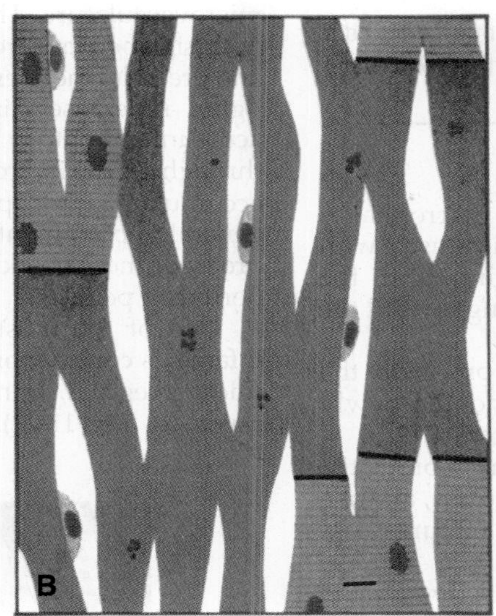

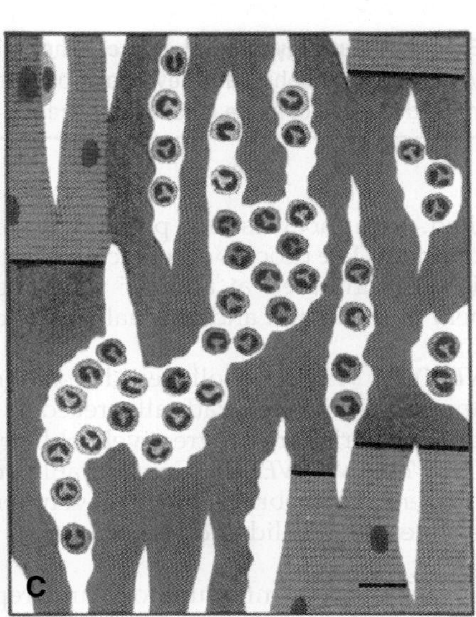

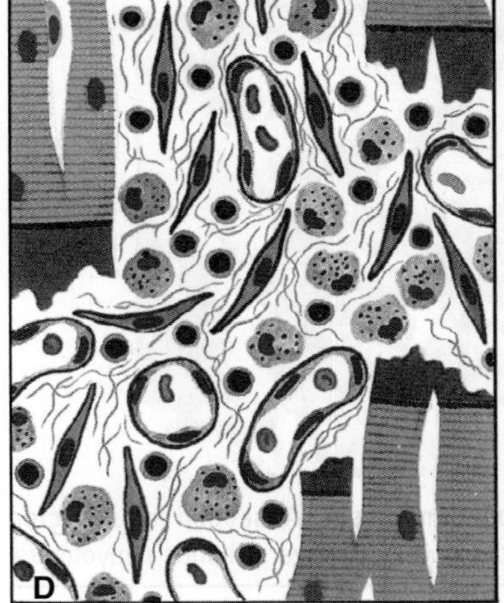

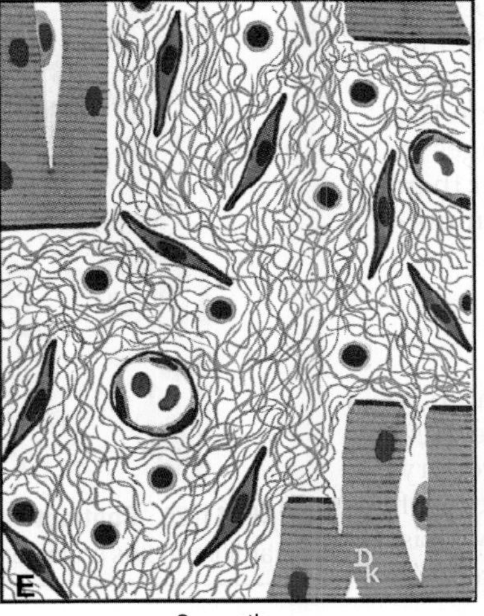

FIGURE 11-17. Development of a myocardial infarct. A. Normal myocardium. **B.** After about 12 to 18 hours, the infarcted myocardium shows eosinophilia (*red staining*) in sections of the heart stained with hematoxylin and eosin. **C.** About 24 hours after the onset of infarction, polymorphonuclear neutrophils infiltrate necrotic myocytes at the periphery of the infarct. **D.** After about 3 weeks, peripheral portions of the infarct are composed of granulation tissue with prominent capillaries, fibroblasts, lymphoid cells and macrophages. The necrotic debris has been largely removed from this area, and a small amount of collagen has been laid down. **E.** After 3 months or more, the infarcted region has been replaced by scar tissue.

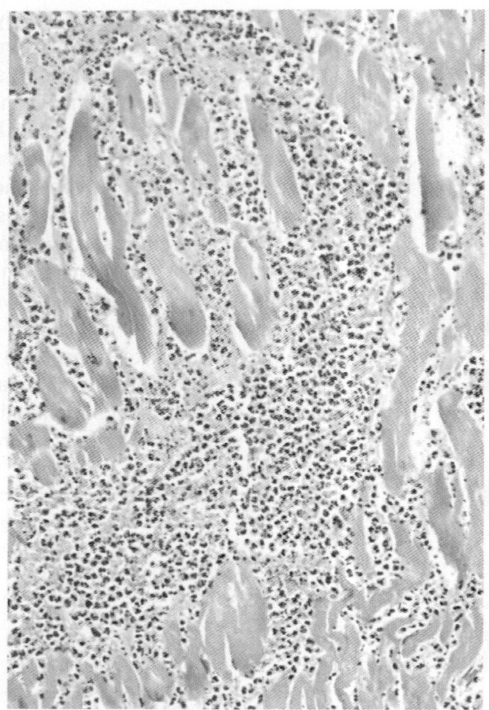

FIGURE 11-18. Acute myocardial infarct. The necrotic myocardial fibers, which are eosinophilic and devoid of cross-striations and nuclei, are immersed in a sea of acute inflammatory cells.

deposited. Lymphocytes and pigment-laden macrophages are prominent. The process of replacing necrotic muscle with scar tissue is initiated at about 5 days, beginning at the periphery of the infarct and gradually extending toward the center.

ONE TO 3 WEEKS: Collagen deposition proceeds, the inflammatory infiltrate gradually recedes and the newly sprouted capillaries are progressively obliterated.

MORE THAN 4 WEEKS: Considerable dense fibrous tissue is present. The debris is progressively removed, and the scar becomes more solid and less cellular as it matures (Fig. 11-19).

This sequence of inflammatory and reparative events can be altered by local or systemic factors. For example, immediate extension of an infarct into a region that previously had patchy necrosis may not show the expected changes. A large infarct tends not to mature in its center as rapidly as a smaller one. In estimating the age of a large infarct, it is more accurate to base the interpretation on the outer border where repair begins, rather than on changes in the central region. In fact, in some large infarcts, rather than being removed, dead myocytes remain indefinitely "mummified."

Reperfusion of Ischemic Myocardium

The foregoing descriptions pertain to healing of infarcts caused by persistent coronary occlusion, such as those arising from thrombotic occlusion of an epicardial coronary artery. However, blood flow may be restored to regions of evolving infarcts either because of spontaneous thrombolysis or in response to therapeutic opening of occluded coronary

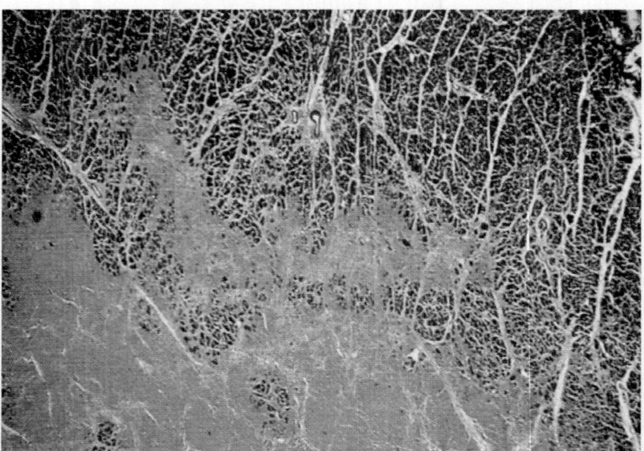

FIGURE 11-19. Healed myocardial infarct. A section at the edge of a healed infarct stained for collagen, which appears blue-green here, shows dense, acellular regions of collagenous matrix sharply demarcated from the adjacent viable myocardium.

arteries. When that happens, gross and microscopic appearances of the infarct change. Reperfused infarcts are typically hemorrhagic, owing to blood flow through damaged microvasculature. Thus, while infarcts following persistent occlusion become grossly apparent only after about 12 hours and are pale, the presence of hemorrhage immediately highlights reperfused infarcts. Reperfusion also accelerates acute inflammatory responses. Neutrophils can gain access throughout the infarct rather than only at the periphery. They accumulate more rapidly but also disappear more rapidly. In general, replacement of necrotic muscle by fibrous scar also proceeds more quickly, at least in areas of the infarct in which perfusion persists.

One of the most characteristic features of reperfused infarcts is **contraction band necrosis.** Contraction bands are thick, irregular, transverse eosinophilic bands in necrotic myocytes (Fig. 11-20). By electron microscopy, these bands are

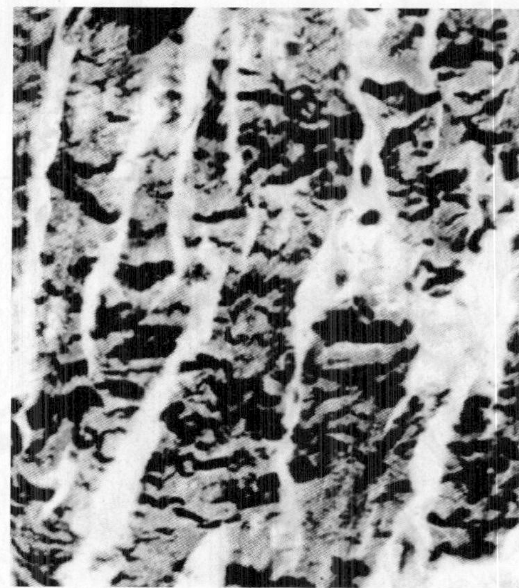

FIGURE 11-20. Contraction band necrosis. A section of infarcted myocardium shows prominent, thick, wavy, transverse bands in myofibers.

small groups of hypercontracted and disorganized sarcomeres with thickened Z lines. The sarcolemma is disrupted and mitochondria located between the contraction bands swell. They may contain deposits of calcium phosphate in the matrix, as well as amorphous matrix densities. Contraction bands occur whenever there is a massive influx of Ca^{2+} into cardiac myocytes. Reperfusion of ischemic myocardium causes extensive sarcolemmal damage mediated largely by reactive oxygen species, which permits unrestrained entry of extracellular Ca^{2+} into myocytes. The massive Ca^{2+} influx leads to hypercontraction in cells still able to contract. Influx of Ca^{2+} into more severely injured cells that can no longer contract still produces dense deposits in mitochondria as shown in Fig. 11-16. Contraction band necrosis is most prominent when ischemic myocardium is reperfused (e.g., after thrombolytic therapy or following prolonged cardiopulmonary bypass in which the myocardium has sustained irreversible injury). In infarcts arising from persistent coronary occlusion, microscopic foci of contraction band necrosis are often seen at the margins, where dynamic ebb and flow of blood creates conditions that favor Ca^{2+} influx. Other conditions associated with contraction band injury include massive catecholamine release in patients with pheochromocytoma or head injuries, or patients in shock treated with large doses of pressors.

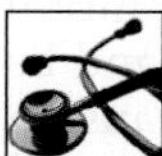

CLINICAL FEATURES:

Clinical Diagnosis

The onset of acute myocardial infarction is often sudden and associated with severe, crushing substernal or precordial pain. The pain may be experienced as epigastric burning (simulating indigestion) or it may extend into the jaw or down the inside of either arm. It is often accompanied by sweating, nausea, vomiting and shortness of breath. In some cases an acute myocardial infarction is preceded by unstable angina of several days' duration. ***One fourth to one half of all nonfatal myocardial infarctions occur without any symptoms and infarcts are identified only later by electrocardiographic changes or at autopsy.*** These "clinically silent" infarcts are particularly common among diabetic patients with autonomic dysfunction and also in cardiac transplant patients whose hearts are denervated.

The diagnosis of acute myocardial infarction is confirmed by electrocardiography and the appearance of increased levels of certain enzymes or proteins in the serum. The electrocardiogram exhibits new Q waves and changes in the ST segment and the conformation of the T wave. There is a reasonable correlation between the pathologic distinction of transmural versus subendocardial infarcts and the electrocardiographic distinction of STEMI (ST elevation myocardial infarction) versus non-STEMI events. Identification in serum of cardiac proteins such as MB-CK or cardiac troponins T and I is evidence of myocardial necrosis.

Complications of Myocardial Infarction

Early mortality in acute myocardial infarction (within 30 days) has dropped from 30% in the 1950s to less than 5% today. Nevertheless, the clinical course after acute infarction may be dominated by functional or mechanical complications of the infarct.

ARRHYTHMIAS: Virtually all patients who have a myocardial infarct have abnormal cardiac rhythm at some time during their illness. Arrhythmias still account for half of all deaths caused by ischemic heart disease, although the advent of coronary care units and defibrillators has greatly reduced early mortality. Acute infarction is often associated with premature ventricular beats, sinus bradycardia, ventricular tachycardia, ventricular fibrillation and paroxysmal atrial tachycardia. Partial or complete heart block can also occur. The causes of these arrhythmias are often multifactorial. Acute ischemia alters conduction, increases automaticity and promotes triggered activity related to after-depolarizations. Enhanced sympathetic activity mediated by increased levels of local or circulating catecholamines plays an important role.

LEFT VENTRICULAR FAILURE AND CARDIOGENIC SHOCK: Development of left ventricular failure soon after myocardial infarction is an ominous sign that generally indicates massive loss of muscle. Fortunately, cardiogenic shock occurs in fewer than 5% of cases, owing to the development of techniques that limit the extent of infarction (thrombolytic therapy, angioplasty) or assist damaged myocardium (intra-aortic balloon pump). Cardiogenic shock tends to develop early after infarction when 40% or more of the left ventricle has been lost; mortality is as high as 90%.

EXTENSION OF THE INFARCT: Clinically recognizable extension of an acute myocardial infarct occurs in the first 1 to 2 weeks in up to 10% of patients. In careful echocardiographic studies, half of all patients with anterior myocardial infarction showed some extension of the infarct during the first 2 weeks, indicating that many episodes of infarct extension are not recognized. Clinically significant infarct extension is associated with a doubling of mortality.

RUPTURE OF THE FREE WALL OF THE MYOCARDIUM: Myocardial rupture (Fig. 11-21) may occur at almost any time during the 3 weeks following acute myocardial infarction but is most common between the first and fourth days, when the infarcted wall is weakest. During this vulnerable period, the infarct is composed of soft, necrotic tissue in which the extracellular matrix has been degraded by proteases released by inflammatory cells but new matrix deposition has not yet occurred. Once scar tissue begins to form, rupture is less likely. Rupture of the free wall is a complication of transmural

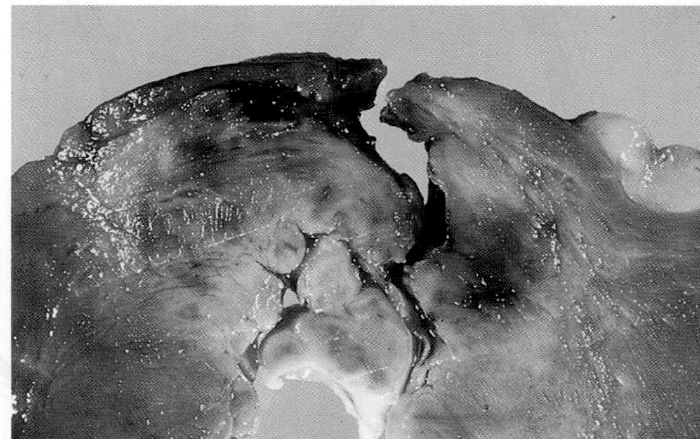

FIGURE 11-21. Rupture of an acute myocardial infarct. An elderly woman with a recent myocardial infarct died of cardiac tamponade. The pericardium was filled with blood, and the cut surface of the left ventricle shows a linear rupture of the necrotic myocardium.

infarcts; surviving muscle overlying subendocardial infarcts prevents rupture. However, rupture usually occurs in relatively small transmural infarcts. The remaining viable, contractile myocardium produces mechanical forces that can initiate and propagate tearing along the lateral border of the infarct where neutrophils accumulate.

Rupture of the free wall of the left ventricle most often leads to hemopericardium and death from pericardial tamponade. Myocardial rupture accounts for 10% of deaths after acute myocardial infarction in hospitalized patients. This complication is more common in elderly patients who have sustained a first infarct (most of whom are women). Rarely, a ruptured ventricle may become walled off and the patient survives with a false aneurysm (Fig. 11-22).

OTHER FORMS OF MYOCARDIAL RUPTURE: A few patients in whom a myocardial infarct involves the interventricular septum develop **septal perforation,** varying in length from 1 cm or more. The magnitude of the resulting left-to-right shunt and, therefore, the prognosis depend on the size of the rupture.

Rupture of a portion of a papillary muscle results in mitral regurgitation. In some cases, an entire papillary muscle is transected, in which case, massive mitral valve incompetence may be fatal.

ANEURYSMS: Left ventricular aneurysms complicate 10% to 15% of transmural myocardial infarcts. After acute transmural infarction, the affected ventricular wall tends to bulge outward during systole in one third of patients. As the infarct heals, the newly deposited collagenous matrix is susceptible to further stretching, although eventually the scar tissue becomes nondistensible. Localized thinning and stretching of the ventricular wall in the region of a healing myocardial infarct has been termed "infarct expansion" but is actually an early aneurysm. Such an aneurysm is composed of a thin layer of necrotic myocardium and collagenous tissue, which expands with each contraction of the heart. As the evolving aneurysm becomes more fibrotic, its tensile strength increases. However, the aneurysm continues to dilate with each beat, thereby "stealing" some of the left ventricular output and increasing the workload of the heart. Patients with left ventricular aneurysms are at increased risk of developing ventricular tachycardia owing to increased opportunities for reentry along the periphery of the aneurysm. Mural thrombi often develop within aneurysms and are a source of systemic emboli.

A distinction should be made between **"true"** and **"false" aneurysms** (Fig. 11-22). True aneurysms are much more common than false aneurysms, and are caused by bulging of an intact, but weakened, left ventricular wall (Fig. 11-23). By contrast, false aneurysms result from rupture of a portion of the left ventricle that has been walled off by pericardial scar tissue. Thus, the wall of a false aneurysm is composed of pericardium and scar tissue, not left ventricular myocardium.

MURAL THROMBOSIS AND EMBOLISM: One third to one half of patients who die after myocardial infarction have mural thrombi overlying the infarct at autopsy (Fig. 11-24). This occurs particularly often when the infarct involves the apex of the heart. In turn, half of these patients have some evidence of systemic embolization. Inflammation of the endocardium lining an infarct promotes platelet adhesion and fibrin deposition. Also, the poor contractile function of the underlying myocardium allows the fibrin–platelet mural thrombus to grow. Particles of thrombus can detach and be swept along with the arterial blood, potentially causing strokes or myocardial or visceral infarcts. Documented mural thrombosis justifies anticoagulant therapy and antiplatelet medications.

PERICARDITIS: A transmural myocardial infarct involves the epicardium and leads to inflammation of the pericardium in 10% to 20% of patients. Pericarditis is manifested clinically as chest pain and may produce a pericardial friction rub. One quarter of patients with acute myocardial infarction, particularly those with larger infarcts and congestive heart failure,

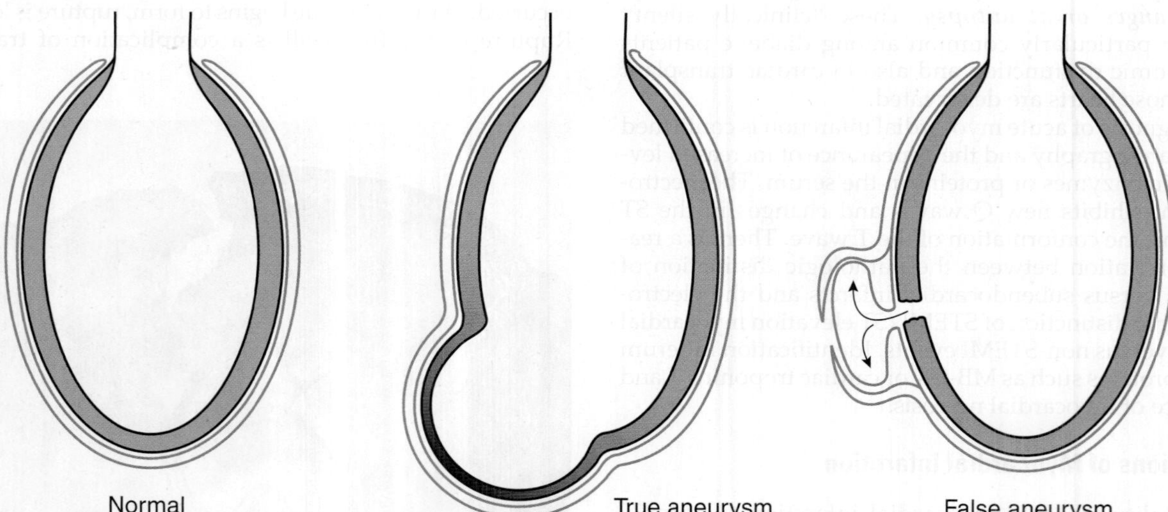

FIGURE 11-22. True and false aneurysms of the left ventricle. Left. Normal heart. The left ventricular wall (*shaded*) is enclosed by the pericardial sac. **Center.** True aneurysm shows an intact wall (*black*), which bulges outward. **Right.** False aneurysm shows a ruptured infarct that is walled off externally by adherent pericardium. Note that the mouth of the true aneurysm is wider than that of the false aneurysm.

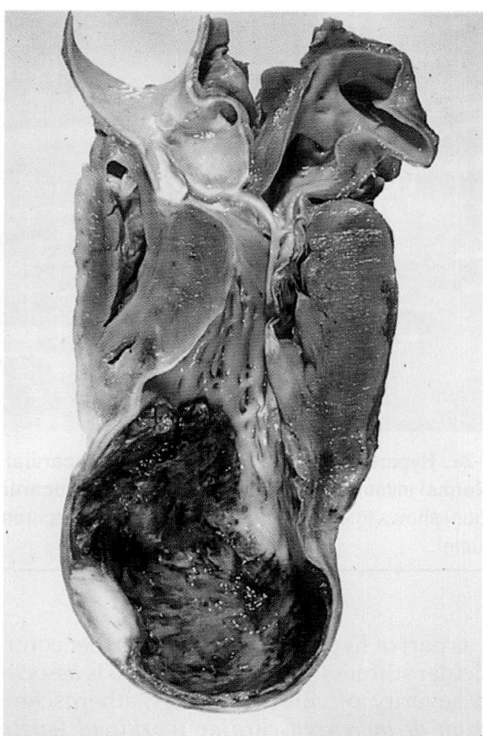

FIGURE 11-23. Ventricular aneurysm. The heart of a patient with a history of an anteroapical myocardial infarct who developed a massive ventricular aneurysm. The apex of the heart shows marked thinning and aneurysmal dilation.

develop a pericardial effusion, with or without pericarditis. Less frequently, anticoagulant therapy has been associated with hemorrhagic pericardial effusions and even with cardiac tamponade.

Postmyocardial infarction syndrome (Dressler syndrome) refers to a delayed form of pericarditis that develops 2 to 10 weeks after infarction. A similar disorder may occur after cardiac surgery. Antibodies to heart muscle appear in these patients. The condition improves with corticosteroid therapy, suggesting that Dressler syndrome may have an immunologic basis.

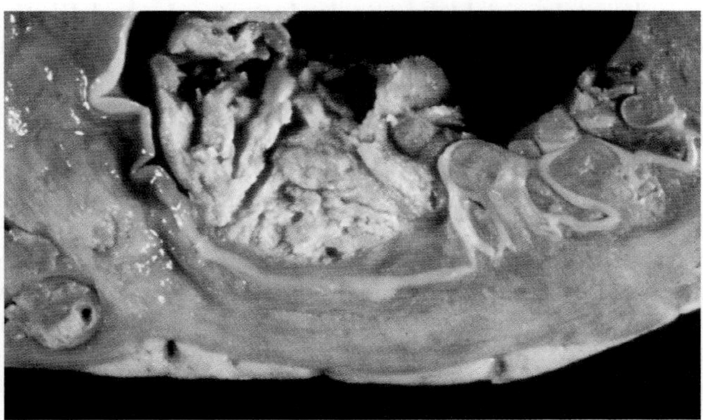

FIGURE 11-24. Mural thrombus overlying a healed myocardial infarct. In this cross-section of a fixed heart, an organized, friable, grayish white mural thrombus overlies a thickened endocardium situated over scarred myocardium.

Therapeutic Interventions Can Limit Infarct Size

Because the amount of myocardium that undergoes necrosis is an important predictor of morbidity and mortality, any therapy that limits infarct size should be beneficial. By definition, such therapy is directed at preventing death of reversibly injured, ischemic myocytes and limiting infarct extension. Damaged myocytes can be salvaged for some time after the onset of ischemia if the tissue can be reperfused with arterial blood.

- **Restoration of arterial blood flow** remains the only way to salvage ischemic myocytes permanently, although a number of interventions can delay ischemic injury. The most notable is hypothermia, which is used during cardiac surgery to minimize myocardial injury during cardiopulmonary bypass. Several methods have been developed to restore blood flow to the area of myocardium supplied by an obstructed coronary artery.
- **Thrombolytic enzymes** such as tissue plasminogen activator or streptokinase can be infused intravenously to dissolve the clot causing the obstruction.
- **Percutaneous coronary intervention (PCI)** is dilation of a narrowed coronary artery by inflation with a balloon catheter. This can be done as a primary procedure immediately after onset of ischemia or as a rescue procedure if thrombolytic agents fail to restore arterial blood flow. PCI nearly always includes placement of a stent in the coronary artery to maintain its patency.
- **Coronary artery bypass grafting** can restore blood flow to the distal segment of a coronary artery with a proximal occlusion.

Procedures that restore blood flow must be performed as quickly as possible, preferably within the first few hours after the onset of symptoms. Beyond 6 hours, it is unlikely that much salvageable ischemic myocardium remains, although infarct healing may be enhanced by reperfusion at this point with the potential to limit maladaptive postinfarct remodeling.

Chronic Ischemic Heart Disease Can Lead to Cardiomyopathy

In a minority of patients with severe coronary atherosclerosis, myocardial contractility is impaired globally without discrete infarcts, as in dilated cardiomyopathy. This situation usually reflects a combination of ischemic myocardial dysfunction, diffuse fibrosis and multiple small healed infarcts. However, there is a group of patients with left ventricular failure in whom cardiac dysfunction occurs without obvious infarction. These patients are said to have **ischemic cardiomyopathy**. In some patients, the dysfunctional myocardium has been subjected to repetitive episodes of ischemic injury, which causes degenerative changes in myocytes, characterized principally by loss of myofibrils (hibernating myocardium) (Fig. 11-6). The contractile function of hibernating myocardium is restored when affected tissue is revascularized. Thus, to the extent that hibernation plays a role in ischemic cardiomyopathy, surgical revascularization is potentially beneficial.

Hypertensive Heart Disease

Effects of Hypertension on the Heart

Hypertension has been defined by the World Health Organization as a persistent increase of systemic blood pressure above 140 mm Hg systolic or 90 mm Hg diastolic, or both (see Chapter 10). Systemic hypertension is one of the most prevalent and serious causes of coronary artery and myocardial disease in the United States. Chronic hypertension leads to pressure overload resulting first in compensatory left ventricular hypertrophy and, eventually, cardiac failure. The term **hypertensive heart disease** is used when the heart is enlarged in the absence of a cause other than hypertension.

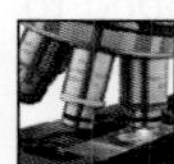

PATHOLOGY: Hypertension causes compensatory left ventricular hypertrophy as a result of the increased cardiac workload. The left ventricular free walls and interventricular septum become thickened uniformly and concentrically (Fig. 11-25), and heart weight increases, exceeding 375 g in men and 350 g in women. Microscopically, hypertrophic myocardial cells have an increased diameter, with enlarged, hyperchromatic, and rectangular ("boxcar") nuclei (Fig. 11-26).

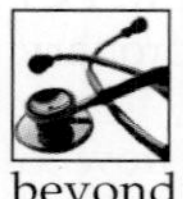

CLINICAL FEATURES: Myocardial hypertrophy clearly adds to the ability of the heart to handle increased workload. However, there is a limit beyond which additional hypertrophy no longer compensates. This upper limit to useful hypertrophy may reflect increasing diffusion distance between the interstitium and the center of each myofiber; if that distance becomes too great, oxygen supply to the myofiber will be impaired.

Diastolic dysfunction is the most common functional abnormality caused by hypertension and by itself can lead to congestive heart failure. Some interstitial fibrosis typically develops as part of hypertrophy, which further contributes to left ventricular stiffness. Hypertension also is associated with increased severity of coronary artery atherosclerosis. ***The combination of increased cardiac workload (systolic dysfunction), diastolic dysfunction and narrowed coronary arteries leads to greater risk of myocardial ischemia, infarction and heart failure.***

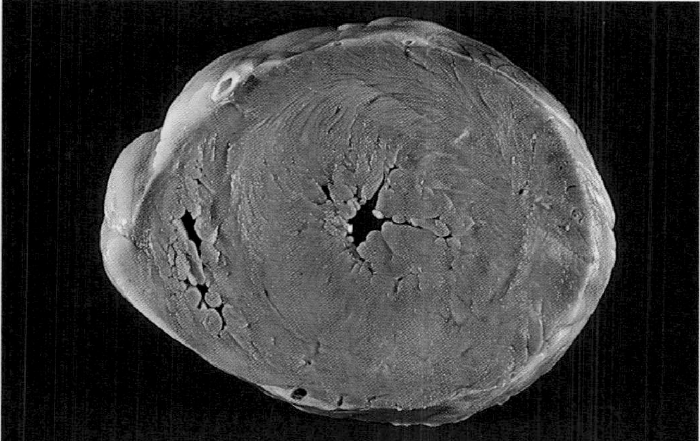

FIGURE 11-25. Hypertensive heart disease. A transverse section of the heart shows marked hypertrophy of the left ventricular myocardium without dilation of the chamber. The right ventricle is of normal dimensions.

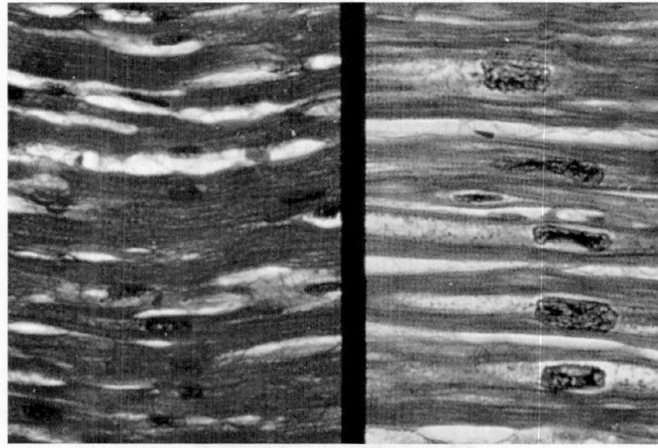

FIGURE 11-26. Hypertensive heart disease with myocardial hypertrophy. Left. Normal myocardium. Right. Hypertrophic myocardium (same magnification) shows thicker fibers and enlarged, hyperchromatic, rectangular nuclei.

Congestive Heart Failure Is the Major Cause of Death in Patients With Untreated Hypertension

Fatal intracerebral hemorrhage is also common. Death may also result from coronary atherosclerosis and myocardial infarction, dissecting aneurysm of the aorta or ruptured berry aneurysm of the cerebral circulation. Renal failure may supervene when nephrosclerosis induced by hypertension becomes severe.

Cor Pulmonale

Cor pulmonale is right ventricular hypertrophy and dilation due to pulmonary hypertension. Increased pressure in the pulmonary circulation may reflect a disorder of lung parenchyma or, more rarely, a primary disease of the vasculature (e.g., primary pulmonary hypertension, recurrent small pulmonary emboli).

Acute cor pulmonale is the sudden occurrence of pulmonary hypertension, most commonly as a result of sudden, massive pulmonary embolization. This condition causes acute right-sided heart failure and is a medical emergency. At autopsy, the only cardiac findings are severe dilation of the right ventricle and sometimes the right atrium.

Chronic cor pulmonale is a common heart disease, accounting for 30% to 40% of all cases of heart failure in an English study and 10% to 30% in a series in the United States. This frequency reflects the prevalence of chronic pulmonary disease in these countries, especially chronic bronchitis and emphysema. In many cases of chronic lung disease, the severity of pulmonary hypertension correlates more closely

Table 11-5

Causes of Cor Pulmonale

Causes of Cor Pulmonale
Parenchymal Diseases of the Lung
Chronic bronchitis and emphysema
Pulmonary fibrosis (from any cause)
Cystic fibrosis
Pulmonary Vascular Diseases
Recurrent pulmonary emboli
Primary pulmonary hypertension
Peripheral pulmonary stenosis
Intravenous drug abuse
Residence at high altitude
Schistosomiasis
Congenital Heart Diseases
Impaired Movement of the Thoracic Cage
Kyphoscoliosis
Pickwickian syndrome
Pleural fibrosis
Neuromuscular disorders
Idiopathic hypoventilation

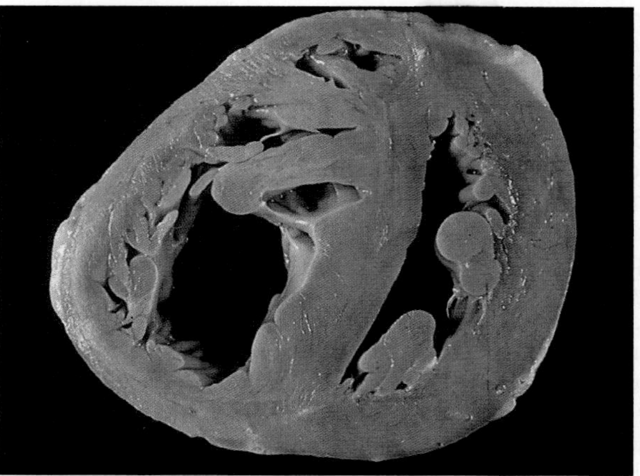

FIGURE 11-27. Cor pulmonale. A transverse section of the heart from a patient with primary (idiopathic) pulmonary hypertension shows a markedly hypertrophied right ventricle (on the left in this image). The right ventricular free wall has a thickness nearly equal to the left ventricular wall. The right ventricle is dilated. The straightened interventricular septum has lost its normal curvature toward the left ventricle as part of the remodeling process in cor pulmonale.

with survival than any other variable. In fact, fewer than 10% of patients with pulmonary artery pressures exceeding 45 mm Hg survive 5 years.

ETIOLOGIC FACTORS: Chronic cor pulmonale may be caused by any pulmonary disease that interferes with ventilatory mechanics or gas exchange or obstructs the pulmonary vasculature (Table 11-5). ***The most common causes of chronic cor pulmonale are chronic obstructive pulmonary disease and pulmonary fibrosis.*** Severe kyphoscoliosis may deform the chest wall and interfere with its function as a bellows, resulting in hypoxemia and pulmonary vasoconstriction. A few cases of cor pulmonale are attributed to **primary pulmonary hypertension,** a disorder of unknown etiology. As discussed above, some congenital heart diseases associated with increased pulmonary blood flow are complicated by pulmonary hypertension and cor pulmonale.

The pathogenesis of pulmonary hypertension secondary to recurrent pulmonary emboli is related clearly to progressive mechanical obstruction of blood flow. However, mechanisms of pulmonary hypertension in chronic parenchymal diseases of the lungs are more complicated. In addition to the obliteration of blood vessels in the lung, these disorders also lead to pulmonary arteriolar vasoconstriction, which reduces the effective cross-sectional area of the pulmonary vascular bed without destroying the vessels. Hypoxia, acidosis and hypercapnia directly cause pulmonary vasoconstriction. Hypoxia also increases pulmonary vascular resistance indirectly by leading to polycythemia, which increases blood viscosity. Persons living at very high altitude, for instance, natives of the Andes mountain range, often develop cor pulmonale secondary to the effects of chronic hypoxemia.

MOLECULAR PATHOGENESIS: Some individuals with primary pulmonary hypertension have a familial disease with dominant inheritance and incomplete penetrance. Many of these individuals have mutations in the gene encoding the bone morphogenic protein receptor type 2 (*BMPR2*), which participates in signaling pathways that regulate gene expression and intersect with other signaling cascades (e.g., MAPK pathway).

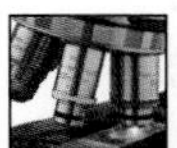

PATHOLOGY: Chronic cor pulmonale is characterized by conspicuous right ventricular hypertrophy (Fig. 11-27), which may exceed 1.0 cm in thickness (normal range, 0.3 to 0.5 cm). Dilation of the right ventricle and right atrium is often present. Normally, the interventricular septum is concave to the left (i.e., it is part of the left ventricle). With development of severe right ventricular hypertrophy, the interventricular septum remodels by straightening or even becoming concave to the right.

Acquired Valvular and Endocardial Diseases

A variety of inflammatory, infectious and degenerative diseases damage cardiac valves and impair their function. The valves normally consist of thin flexible membranes, which close tightly to prevent backward blood flow. When they become damaged, leaflets or cusps may be thickened and fused enough to narrow the aperture and obstruct blood flow, a condition labeled **valvular stenosis.** Diseases that destroy valve tissue may also allow retrograde blood flow, termed **valvular regurgitation** or **insufficiency.** Diseases of the cardiac valves may produce both stenosis and insufficiency, but one or the other generally predominates.

Stenosis of a cardiac valve results in **pressure overload** hypertrophy of the myocardium proximal (i.e., upstream, in terms of blood flow) to the obstruction. Once compensatory mechanisms are exhausted, dilation and failure of the chamber proximal to the valve eventually occur. Thus, mitral stenosis leads to left atrial hypertrophy and dilation. As the left atrium decompensates and can no longer force the pulmonary venous return through the stenotic mitral valve, signs of pulmonary congestion develop, followed by right ventricular hypertrophy and even cor pulmonale. Similarly, aortic stenosis causes left ventricular hypertrophy and eventually left heart failure.

Valvular regurgitation or insufficiency also results in hypertrophy and dilation of the chamber proximal to the valve, owing to **volume overload.** In aortic insufficiency, the left ventricle first hypertrophies. Then, when it can no longer accommodate the regurgitant volume and provide adequate cardiac output, it dilates. On the other hand, an incompetent mitral valve leads to hypertrophy and dilation of both the left atrium and left ventricle, because both are subjected to volume overload. Marked left ventricular dilation from any condition in which cardiac contractility is inadequate (e.g., congestive failure after a large myocardial infarct) also may widen the mitral valve ring and splay the left ventricular papillary muscles. These effects may be so severe that the valve leaflets do not close properly, leading to mitral regurgitation.

The semilunar valves are structurally and functionally simple compared with the atrioventricular valves. The latter consist of the valve leaflets, muscular valve annuli and subvalvular apparatus (chordae tendineae and papillary muscles). In general, valvular stenosis involves pathologic changes of leaflets themselves, but regurgitation can be caused by abnormalities of valve leaflets, annulus or subvalvular apparatus.

Rheumatic Heart Disease Encompasses Acute Myocarditis and Residual Valvular Deformities

Acute Rheumatic Fever

Rheumatic fever (RF) is a multisystem childhood disease that follows a streptococcal infection and is characterized by an inflammatory reaction involving the heart, joints and central nervous system.

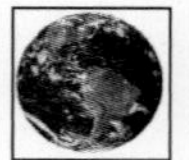

EPIDEMIOLOGY: RF is a complication of an acute streptococcal infection, almost always pharyngitis (i.e., "strep" throat) (see Chapter 9). The offending agent is *Streptococcus pyogenes*, also known as group A β-hemolytic *Streptococcus*. In some epidemics of streptococcal pharyngitis, the incidence of RF has been as high as 3%. RF is principally a disease of childhood, the median age being 9 to 11 years, although it can occur in adults.

In the first half of the 20th century, RF reached almost epidemic proportions in the United States, but its incidence has decreased dramatically. Between 1950 and 1972, the death rate fell from 14.5 to 6.8 per 100,000, and has decreased further since then. Although this decline may have been partly the result of widespread antibiotic treatment, such therapy cannot account for the entire reduction, because the death rate had begun to decrease well before antibiotics were generally available. Improved socioeconomic conditions, in particular less crowded living circumstances, probably contributed to the decrease. ***Despite its declining importance in industrialized countries, RF is a leading cause of death of heart disease in persons 5 to 25 years old in less-developed regions.***

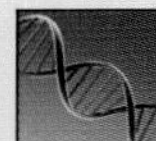

MOLECULAR PATHOGENESIS: The pathogenesis of acute RF involves the triad of (1) a genetically susceptible host, (2) a rheumatogenic strain of group A *Streptococcus* and (3) an abnormal host immune response. It remains unclear why only a small number of individuals infected with the offending microorganism go on to develop RF. Human leukocyte antigen (HLA) class II molecules appear to have a close association with disease susceptibility. The mechanism underlying HLA association is unknown but may involve defective presentation by the HLA molecule related to similarities between some HLA class II alleles and streptococcal antigens. This is thought to lead to aberrant cytokine production and antibody formation against proteins on valves and other host tissues. Alternatively, structural similarities may cause streptococcal antigens to mimic HLA molecules, which initiates an aberrant immune response. These mechanisms suggest the possibility of an autoimmune etiology (Fig. 11-28).

Streptococcal antigens structurally similar to those in the heart include hyaluronate in the bacterial capsule, cell wall polysaccharides similar to the carbohydrate moiety of heart valve glycoproteins and bacterial membrane antigens that share epitopes with sarcolemma and smooth muscle constituents. Although antibodies to these antigens are found in patients with RF, it has not been proved that they are cytotoxic or that they are directly involved in the pathogenesis of the disease. A direct toxic effect of some streptococcal product on the myocardium has not yet been excluded.

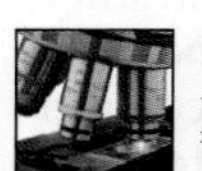

PATHOLOGY: Acute rheumatic heart disease is a pancarditis; that is, it involves all three layers of the heart (endocardium, myocardium and pericardium).

MYOCARDITIS: In severe cases of RF, a few patients may die during the earliest acute phase of the illness before the characteristic granulomatous inflammation has developed. At this early stage, the heart tends to be dilated and exhibits a nonspecific myocarditis, in which lymphocytes and macrophages predominate, although a few neutrophils and eosinophils may be evident. Fibrinoid degeneration of collagen, in which fibers become swollen, fragmented and eosinophilic, is characteristic of this early phase.

The **Aschoff body** is the characteristic granulomatous lesion of rheumatic myocarditis (Fig. 11-29), developing several weeks after symptoms begin. This structure initially consists of a perivascular focus of swollen eosinophilic collagen surrounded by lymphocytes, plasma cells and macrophages. With time, the Aschoff body assumes a granulomatous appearance, with a central fibrinoid focus associated with a perimeter of lymphocytes, plasma cells, macrophages and giant cells. Eventually, the Aschoff body is replaced by a nodule of scar tissue.

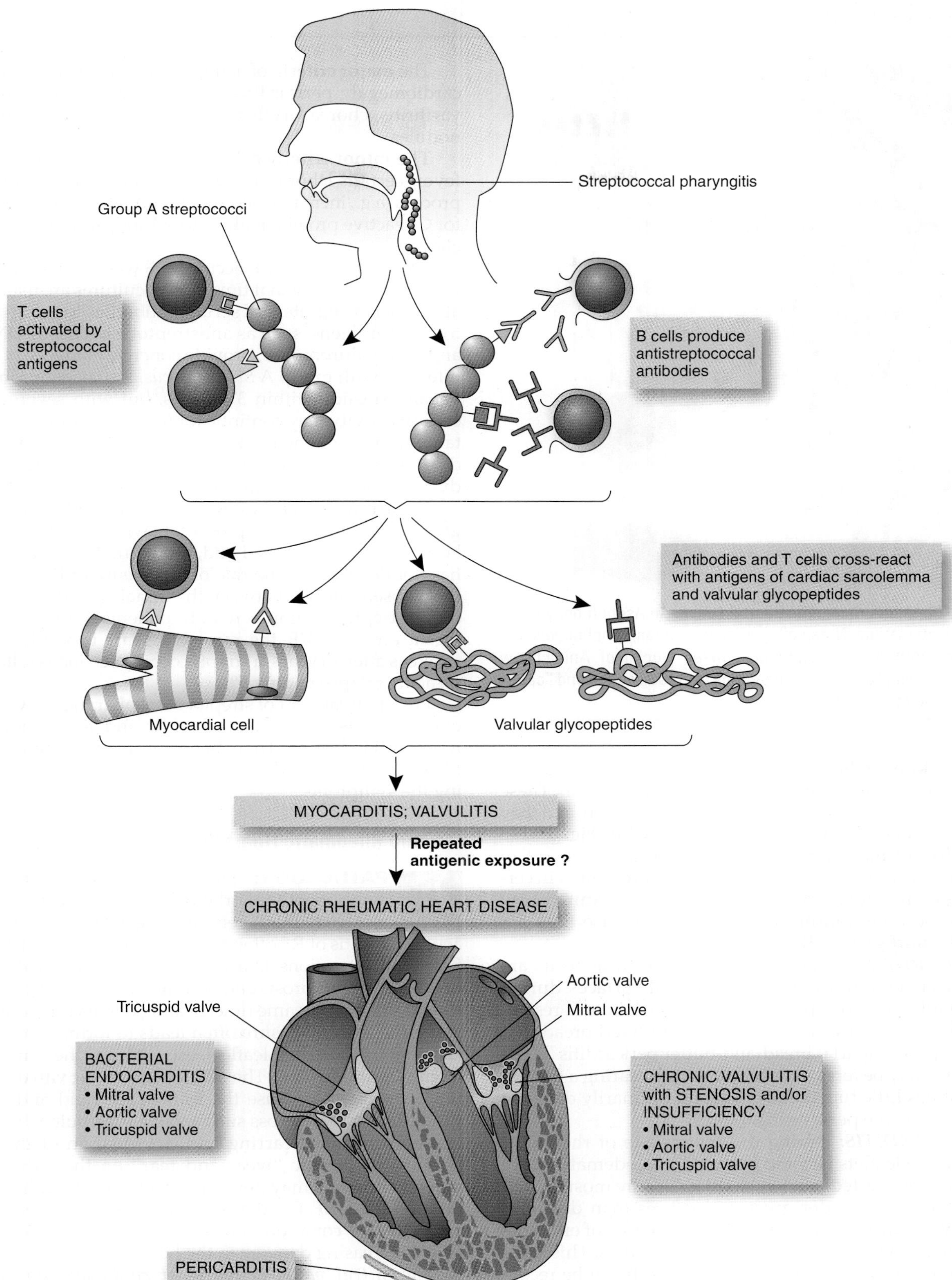

FIGURE 11-28. Biological factors in rheumatic heart disease. The upper portion illustrates the initiating β-hemolytic streptococcal infection of the throat, which introduces the streptococcal antigens into the body and may also activate cytotoxic T cells. These antigens lead to the production of antibodies against various antigenic components of the streptococcus, which can cross-react with certain cardiac antigens, including those from the myocyte sarcolemma and glycoproteins of the valves. This may be the mechanism for inflammation of the heart in acute rheumatic fever, which involves all cardiac layers (endocarditis, myocarditis and pericarditis). This inflammation becomes apparent after a latent period of 2 to 3 weeks. Active inflammation of the valves may eventually lead to chronic valvular stenosis or insufficiency. These lesions involve the mitral, aortic and tricuspid valves, in that order of frequency.

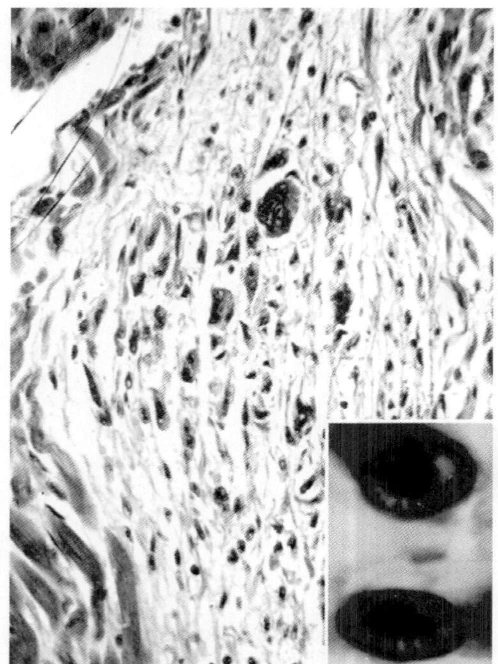

FIGURE 11-29. Acute rheumatic heart disease. An Aschoff body in the myocardial interstitium. Note collagen degeneration, lymphocytes and a multinucleated Aschoff giant cell. *Inset.* Nuclei of Anitschkow myocytes, showing "owl-eye" appearance in cross-section and "caterpillar" shape longitudinally.

Anitschkow cells are unusual cells within the Aschoff body, whose nuclei contain a central band of chromatin. These nuclei have an "owl eye" appearance in cross-section, and they resemble a caterpillar when cut longitudinally (Fig. 11-29). These cells are macrophages that are normally present in small numbers but accumulate and become prominent in certain types of inflammatory diseases of the heart. Anitschkow cells may become multinucleated, in which case they are termed **Aschoff giant cells.**

PERICARDITIS: Tenacious irregular fibrin deposits are found on visceral and parietal pericardial surfaces during the acute inflammatory phase of RF. These exudates resemble the shaggy surfaces of two slices of buttered bread that have been pulled apart ("bread-and-butter pericarditis"). The pericarditis may be recognized clinically by hearing a friction rub, but it has little functional effect and ordinarily does not lead to constrictive pericarditis.

ENDOCARDITIS: During the acute stage of rheumatic carditis, valve leaflets become inflamed and edematous. All four valves are affected, but left-sided valves are most injured because they close under greater pressures than do right-sided valves. The result is damage and focal loss of endothelium along the lines of closure of the valve leaflets. This leads to deposition of tiny nodules of fibrin, which can be recognized grossly as "verrucae" along the leaflets (so-called verrucous endocarditis of acute RF).

CLINICAL FEATURES: There is no specific test for RF. The clinical diagnosis is made when two major—or one major and two minor—criteria (**the Jones criteria**) are met. If there is evidence of recent streptococcal infection, the probability of RF is high.

The **major criteria** of acute RF include carditis (murmurs, cardiomegaly, pericarditis and congestive heart failure), polyarthritis, chorea, erythema marginatum and subcutaneous nodules.

The minor criteria are previous history of RF, arthralgia, fever, certain laboratory tests indicating an inflammatory process (e.g., increased sedimentation rate, positive test result for C-reactive protein, leukocytosis) and electrocardiographic changes.

The symptoms of RF occur 2 to 3 weeks after an infection with *S. pyogenes*. By that time, throat cultures are usually negative. Increasing titers of serum antibodies to group A streptococcal antigens, such as antistreptolysin O, anti-DNAase B and antihyaluronidase, provide concrete evidence of a recent infection with group A *Streptococcus*. Acute symptoms of RF usually subside within 3 months, but with severe carditis, clinical activity may continue for 6 months or more. The mortality from acute rheumatic carditis is low. The main cause of death is heart failure due to myocarditis, although valvular dysfunction may also play a role.

Recurrent attacks of RF are associated with types of group A β-hemolytic streptococci to which the patient has not been previously exposed and, therefore, to which immunity has not developed. The rate of recurrence of RF is related to the elapsed interval between the initial episode and a subsequent streptococcal infection. In patients with a history of a recent attack of RF, the recurrence rate is as high as 65%, whereas after 10 years, a streptococcal infection is followed by an acute relapse in only 5%.

Prompt treatment of streptococcal pharyngitis with antibiotics prevents an initial attack of RF and, less often, a recurrence of the disease. There is no specific treatment for acute RF, but corticosteroids and salicylates are helpful in managing the symptoms.

Chronic Rheumatic Heart Disease

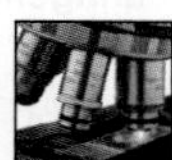

PATHOLOGY: The myocardial and pericardial components of rheumatic pancarditis typically resolve without permanent sequelae. By contrast, the acute valvulitis of RF often results in long-term structural and functional alterations. During the healing phase, valve leaflets develop diffuse fibrosis and become thickened, shrunken and less pliable. At the same time, healing of the verrucous lesions along the lines of closure often leads to formation of fibrous "adhesions" between leaflets, especially at the commissures (commissural fusion). The result is a stenotic valve that does not open freely because the leaflets are rigid and partially fused. Blood flow across such a valve is turbulent, which can cause even more scarring and deformation of the leaflets because of chronic "wear and tear" on the valve. Severe valvular scarring may develop months or years after a single bout of acute RF. On the other hand, recurrent episodes of acute RF are common and result in repeated and progressively increasing damage to the heart valves.

The mitral valve is the most commonly and severely affected valve in chronic rheumatic disease. It snaps shut under systolic pressure and, thus, bears the greatest mechanical burden of all cardiac valves. Chronic mitral valvulitis is characterized by conspicuous, irregular thickening and calcification of the leaflets, often with fusion of the commissures and chordae tendineae (Fig. 11-30). In severe chronic rheumatic mitral valve disease, the valve orifice becomes reduced to a fixed narrow opening with the appearance of a "fish mouth" when viewed

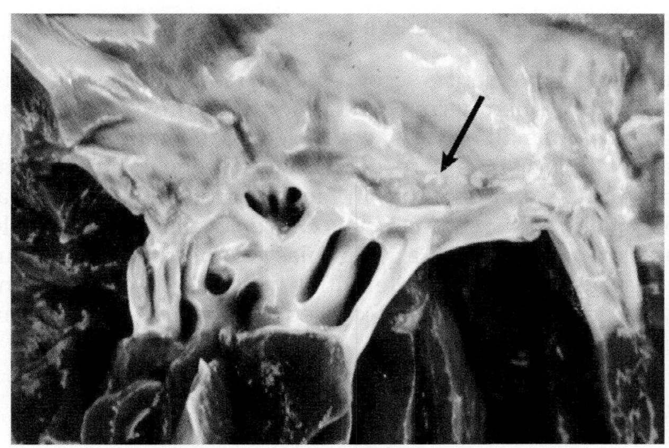

FIGURE 11-30. Chronic rheumatic valvulitis. The mitral valve leaflets are thickened and focally calcified (*arrow*), and the commissures are partially fused. The chordae tendineae are also short, thick and fused.

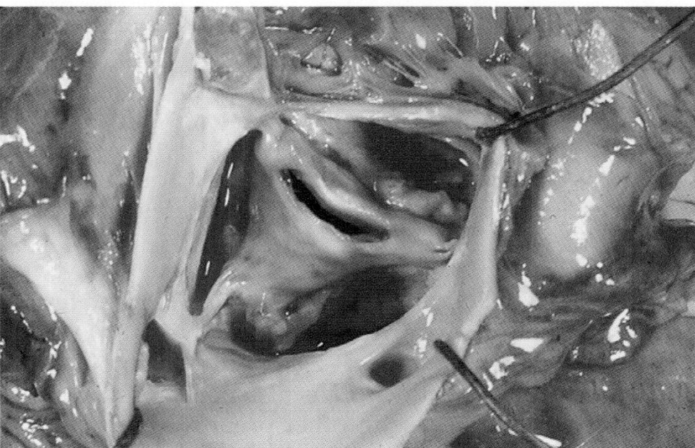

FIGURE 11-32. Chronic rheumatic aortic valvulitis. An example of severe rheumatic aortic stenosis. Three sinuses of Valsalva are recognizable, but the cusps are rigidly fibrotic and calcified, and extensive fusion of the commissures has narrowed the orifice into a fixed slit-like configuration that does not change during the cardiac cycle.

from the ventricular aspect (Fig. 11-31). Mitral stenosis is the predominant functional lesion, but such a valve is also regurgitant. Chronic regurgitation produces a "jet" of blood directed at the posterior aspect of the left atrium, which damages the atrial endocardium and produces a discrete focus of rough, wrinkled endocardium referred to as a "MacCallum patch."

The aortic valve, which snaps shut under diastolic pressure, is the valve second most commonly involved in rheumatic heart disease. Diffuse fibrous thickening of the cusps and fusion of the commissures cause aortic stenosis, which may be mild initially but which progresses because of the chronic effects of turbulent blood flow across the valve. Often, cusps become rigidly calcified as the patient ages, resulting in stenosis and insufficiency, although either lesion may predominate (Fig. 11-32). The lower pressures experienced by the right-sided valves are usually protective. In cases of recurrent RF, however, the tricuspid valve may become deformed, virtually always in association with mitral and aortic lesions. The pulmonic valve is rarely affected.

Complications of Chronic Rheumatic Heart Disease

- **Bacterial endocarditis** follows episodes of bacteremia (e.g., during dental procedures). The scarred valves of rheumatic heart disease provide an attractive environment for bacteria that would bypass a normal valve.
- **Mural thrombi** form in atrial or ventricular chambers in 40% of patients with rheumatic valvular disease. They give rise to thromboemboli, which can produce infarcts in various organs. Rarely, a large thrombus in the left atrial appendage develops a stalk and acts as a ball valve that obstructs the mitral valve orifice.
- **Congestive heart failure** is associated with rheumatic disease of both mitral and aortic valves.
- **Adhesive pericarditis** commonly follows the fibrinous pericarditis of the acute attack, but almost never results in constrictive pericarditis.

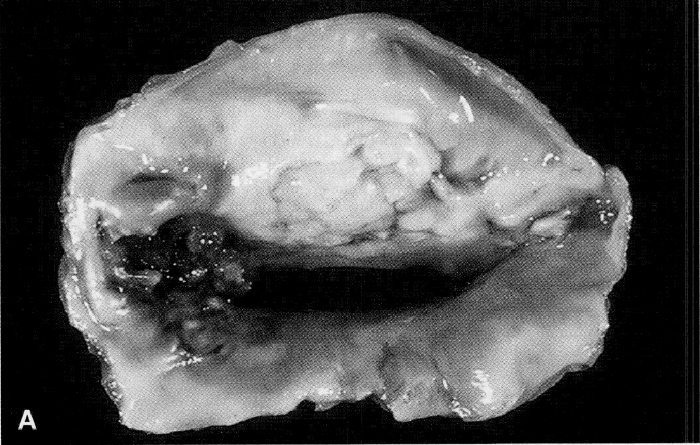

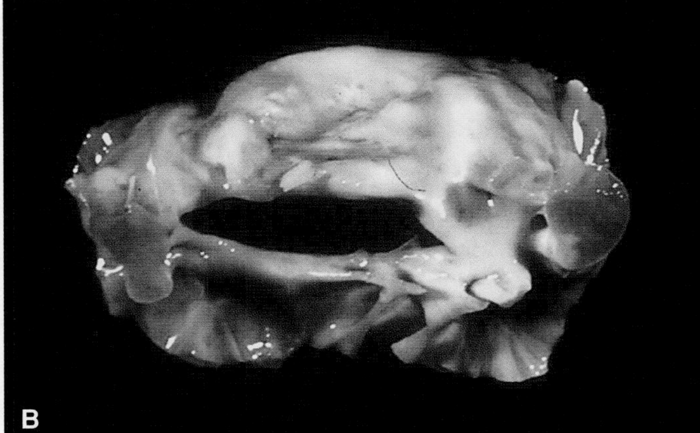

FIGURE 11-31. Chronic rheumatic valvulitis. A view of a surgically excised rheumatic mitral valve from the left atrium **(A)** and left ventricle **(B)** shows rigid, thickened and fused leaflets with a narrow orifice, creating the characteristic "fish mouth" appearance of rheumatic mitral stenosis. Note that the tips of the papillary muscles (shown in B) are directly attached to the underside of the valve leaflets, reflecting marked shortening and fusion of the chordae tendineae.

Collagen Vascular Diseases Affect Both Cardiac Valves and Myocardium

Systemic Lupus Erythematosus

The heart is often involved in SLE, but cardiac symptoms are usually less prominent than are other manifestations of the disease.

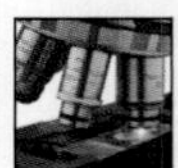

PATHOLOGY: The most common cardiac lesion is **fibrinous pericarditis,** usually with an effusion. **Myocarditis** in SLE, at least in the form of subclinical left ventricular dysfunction, is also common and reflects the severity of the disease in other organs. Microscopically, fibrinoid necrosis of small vessels and focal degeneration of interstitial tissue are seen.

Endocarditis is the most striking cardiac lesion of SLE. Verrucous vegetations, up to 4 mm across, occur on endocardial surfaces and are termed **Libman-Sacks endocarditis.** They are most common on the mitral valve (Fig. 11-33), characteristically on the atrial surface, close to the origin of the leaflets from the valve ring. Aortic valve involvement is described rarely, and the verrucae may extend onto the chordae tendineae and the papillary muscles. Ordinarily, Libman-Sacks endocarditis heals without scarring and does not produce a functional deficit.

Rheumatoid Arthritis

The heart is rarely involved in patients with rheumatoid arthritis. Characteristic rheumatoid granulomatous inflammation, with fibrinoid necrosis and palisaded lymphocytes and macrophages, may occur in the pericardium, myocardium or valves. Involvement of the heart in rheumatoid arthritis does not compromise function.

Ankylosing Spondylitis

A characteristic aortic valve lesion develops in as many as 10% of patients with long-standing ankylosing spondylitis. The aortic valve ring is dilated and its cusps are scarred and shortened. Focal inflammatory lesions occur in all layers of the aortic wall, particularly near the valve ring. Aortic regurgitation is the principal functional consequence.

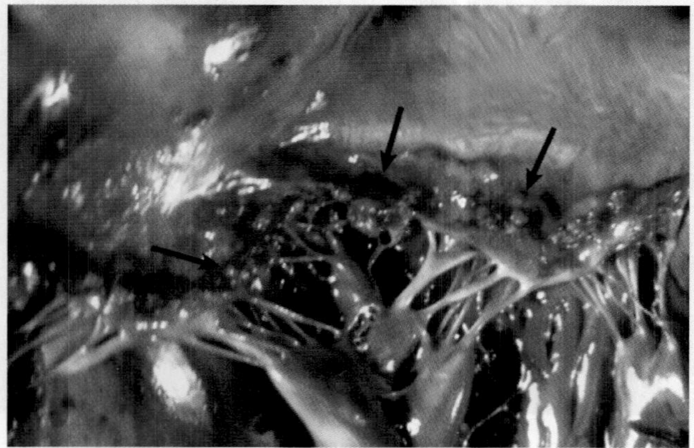

FIGURE 11-33. Libman-Sacks endocarditis. The heart of a patient who died of complications of systemic lupus erythematosus displays verrucous vegetations (*arrows*) on the leaflets of the mitral valve.

Scleroderma (Progressive Systemic Sclerosis)

Cardiac involvement is second only to renal disease as a cause of death in scleroderma. The myocardium exhibits intimal sclerosis of small arteries, which leads to small infarcts and patchy fibrosis. As a result, congestive heart failure and arrhythmias are common. In fact, electrocardiography may show ventricular ectopy in two thirds of patients with scleroderma, and serious arrhythmias in one fourth. Cor pulmonale secondary to interstitial fibrosis of the lungs and hypertensive heart disease (caused by renal involvement) are also seen.

Polyarteritis Nodosa

The heart is involved in up to 75% of cases of polyarteritis nodosa. Necrotizing lesions in branches of the coronary arteries result in myocardial infarction, arrhythmias or heart block. Cardiac hypertrophy and failure secondary to renal vascular hypertension are common.

Bacterial Endocarditis Is Infection of the Cardiac Valves

Fungi, chlamydia and rickettsiae may also cause infective endocarditis, but such cases are uncommon. Before the antibiotic era, bacterial endocarditis was untreatable and almost invariably fatal. The infection was classified according to its clinical course as either acute or subacute endocarditis. **Acute bacterial endocarditis** was described as an infection of a normal cardiac valve by highly virulent suppurative organisms, typically *Staphylococcus aureus* and *S. pyogenes*. The affected valve was rapidly destroyed, and the patient died within 6 weeks, owing to acute heart failure or overwhelming sepsis.

Subacute bacterial endocarditis was a less fulminant disease in which less virulent organisms (e.g., *Streptococcus viridans* or *Staphylococcus epidermidis*) infected a structurally abnormal valve, which typically had been deformed by rheumatic heart disease. These patients typically survived for 6 months or more, and infectious complications were uncommon.

Antimicrobial therapy changed the clinical patterns of bacterial endocarditis, and classical presentations described earlier are today unusual. The disease is now classified according to the anatomic location and the offending organism (Table 11-6).

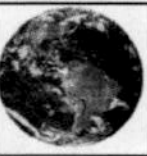

EPIDEMIOLOGY: Most children with bacterial endocarditis have an underlying cardiac lesion. In the past, rheumatic heart disease accounted for a third of such cases. However, as incidence of RF has declined, fewer than 10% of cases of bacterial endocarditis in children are now attributable to this disease. ***The most common predisposing condition for bacterial endocarditis in children currently is congenital heart disease.***

The epidemiology of bacterial endocarditis has also changed in adults. Rheumatic heart disease once comprised three fourths of the cases, but now underlies only a few. Most adults with bacterial endocarditis have no predisposing cardiac lesion. ***Mitral valve prolapse (MVP) and congenital heart disease are today the most frequent bases for bacterial endocarditis in adults.***

- In **rheumatic heart disease,** the mitral valve is affected in over 85% of cases of bacterial endocarditis, and the aortic

Table 11-6

Etiologic Factors in Bacterial Endocarditis

	Children (%)		Adults (%)	
	Newborns	<15 y	15–60 y	>60 y
Underlying Disease				
Congenital heart disease	30	80	10	2
Rheumatic heart disease	—	5	25	8
Mitral valve prolapse	—	10	10	10
Valvular calcification	—	—	5	30
Intravenous drug abuse	—	—	15	10
Other	—	—	10	10
None	70	5	25	30
Microorganisms*				
Staphylococcus aureus	45	25	35	30
Coagulase-negative staphylococci	10	5	5	10
Streptococci	15	45	45	35
Enterococci	—	5	5	15
Gram-negative bacteria	10	5	5	5
Fungi	10	Rare	Rare	Rare
Negative culture	5	10	5	5

*Five percent of neonatal infections are polymicrobial.

valve is involved in 50%. Involvement of a single valve occurs more often in women (2:1) in the case of mitral valve disease, whereas the male-to-female ratio in isolated aortic endocarditis is 4:1.

- **Intravenous drug abusers** inject pathogenic organisms along with their illicit drugs, and bacterial endocarditis is a notorious complication. In such patients, 80% have no underlying cardiac lesion, and the tricuspid valve is infected in half of cases. The most common source of bacteria in intravenous drug abusers is the skin, with *S. aureus* causing more than half of the infections.
- **Prosthetic valves** are sites of infection in 15% of all cases of endocarditis in adults, and 4% of patients with prosthetic valves have this complication. Staphylococci are again responsible for half of these infections, and most of the rest are caused by gram-negative aerobic organisms, streptococci, enterococci and fungi. Another iatrogenic form of endocarditis originates from bacterial colonization of indwelling vascular catheters.
- **Transient bacteremia** from any procedure may lead to infective endocarditis. Examples include dental procedures, urinary catheterization, gastrointestinal endoscopy and obstetric procedures. Antibiotic prophylaxis is recommended during such maneuvers for patients at increased risk for bacterial endocarditis (e.g., those with a history of RF or a cardiac murmur).
- **The elderly** also have an increasing tendency to develop endocarditis. A number of degenerative changes in heart valves, including calcific aortic stenosis and calcification of the mitral annulus, predispose to endocarditis.
- **Diabetes** and **pregnancy** are also associated with increased incidence of bacterial endocarditis.

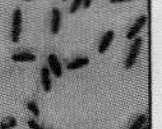

ETIOLOGIC FACTORS AND MOLECULAR PATHOGENESIS: Virulent organisms, such as *S. aureus*, can infect apparently normal valves, but the mechanism of such bacterial colonization is poorly understood. The pathogenesis of the infection of a damaged valve by less virulent organisms has been related to (1) hemodynamic factors, (2) the formation of an initially sterile platelet–fibrin thrombus and (3) the adherence properties of the microorganisms. A key feature is abnormal blood flow across a damaged valve. Lesions form on the inflow portions of valves where high pulsatile shear stresses occur. The pressure gradient formed across a narrow orifice (valve or congenital defect) produces turbulent flow at the periphery and a high-velocity jet stream at the center, both of which tend to denude valve endothelial surfaces. This leads to focal deposition of platelets and fibrin, creating small sterile vegetations that are hospitable sites for bacterial colonization and growth. Indeed, platelet adhesion is enhanced at high shear rates, which occur at the leaflet free edge. The surrounding endothelium becomes activated by the presence of the platelet–fibrin thrombus and upregulates expression of adhesion molecules (vascular cell adhesion molecule-1 [VCAM-1], intracellular adhesion molecule-1 [ICAM-1] and E-selectin), which attract inflammatory cells. Microorganisms that gain access to the circulation, as a result of a dental procedure for example, can be deposited within the vegetations. In this protected environment, colony counts upon culture may reach 10^{10} organisms per gram of tissue. Bacterial matrix metalloproteinases begin to destroy valves, facilitating formation of adjacent vegetations.

Factors that promote bacterial adherence to the sterile vegetations are believed to be important in the pathogenesis of endocarditis. Cell-associated and circulating fibronectin both bind to surface molecules of the bacteria, facilitating adhesion of fibrin, collagen and cells. Some microorganisms produce extracellular polysaccharides, which also function as adhesion factors.

PATHOLOGY: Bacterial endocarditis most commonly involves the left-sided heart valves (mitral or aortic valves, or both). The most common congenital heart lesions that underlie bacterial endocarditis are PDA, tetralogy of Fallot, VSD and bicuspid aortic valve, which is an increasingly recognized risk factor, especially in men older than 60 years. ***As a rule, vegetations in bacterial endocarditis form on the atrial side of atrioventricular valves and on the ventricular side of semilunar valves, often at points where leaflets or cusps close (i.e., the inflow surfaces)*** (Fig. 11-34). Vegetations are composed of platelets, fibrin, cell debris and masses of organisms. Underlying valve tissue is edematous and inflamed, and may eventually become so damaged that a leaflet perforates, causing regurgitation. Lesions vary in size from a small, superficial deposit to bulky, exuberant vegetations. The infective process may spread locally to involve the valve ring or adjacent mural endocardium and chordae tendineae.

Infected thromboemboli travel to multiple systemic sites, causing infarcts or abscesses in many organs, including the brain, kidneys, intestine and spleen.

Focal segmental glomerulonephritis may complicate infective endocarditis (see Chapter 16). It is the result of immune complex deposition in glomeruli, producing a patchy hemorrhagic appearance of the kidneys referred to as "flea-bitten kidneys."

CLINICAL FEATURES: Many patients show early symptoms of bacterial endocarditis within a week of the bacteremic episode, and almost all are symptomatic within 2 weeks. The disease begins with nonspecific symptoms of low-grade fever, fatigue, anorexia and weight loss. Heart murmurs develop almost invariably, and often change during the course of the disease. In cases of more than 6 weeks' duration, splenomegaly, petechiae and clubbing of the fingers are frequent. In one third of patients, systemic emboli are recognized at some time during the illness. Pulmonary emboli characterize tricuspid valve endocarditis in drug addicts. One third of the victims of bacterial endocarditis show some evidence of neurologic dysfunction, owing to the frequency of embolization to the brain. Mycotic aneurysms of cerebral vessels, brain abscesses and intracerebral bleeding are observed.

Antibacterial therapy is effective in limiting the morbidity and mortality of bacterial endocarditis. Most patients defervesce within a week of instituting such therapy. However, the prognosis depends to some extent on the offending organism and the stage at which the infection is treated. ***A third of cases of* S. aureus *endocarditis are still fatal.*** Surgical replacement of a valve destroyed by endocarditis is risky and carries high surgical mortality unless the infection is fully cleared. ***The most common serious complication of bacterial endocarditis is congestive heart failure, usually due to destruction of a valve.*** Myocardial abscesses and infarction secondary to coronary artery emboli occasionally contribute to heart failure. At this stage the prognosis is grim.

Nonbacterial Thrombotic Endocarditis Is a Complication of Wasting Diseases

Nonbacterial thrombotic endocarditis (NBTE), also known as marantic endocarditis, refers to sterile vegetations on apparently normal cardiac valves, almost always in association with cancer or some other wasting disease. NBTE affects mitral (Fig. 11-35) and aortic valves with equal frequency. Its gross appearance is similar to that of infective endocarditis, but it does not destroy the affected valve, and microscopic examination shows neither inflammation nor microorganisms.

The cause of NBTE is poorly understood. It is seen commonly as a paraneoplastic condition, usually complicating adenocarcinomas (particularly of pancreas and lung) and hematologic malignancies. NBTE may also occur in disseminated intravascular coagulation or accompany a variety of

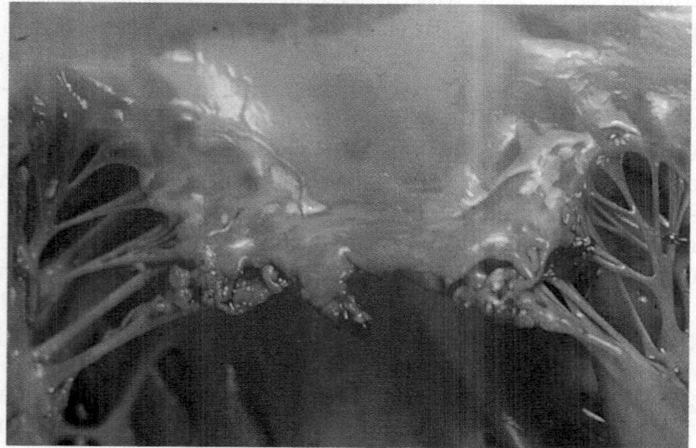

FIGURE 11-34. Bacterial endocarditis. The mitral valve shows destructive vegetations, which have eroded through the free margins of the valve leaflets.

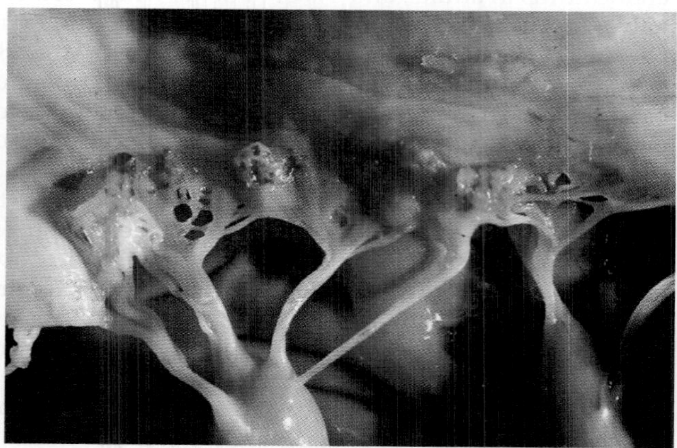

FIGURE 11-35. Marantic endocarditis. Sterile platelet–fibrin vegetations are seen on the leaflets of a structurally normal mitral valve.

debilitating nonneoplastic diseases, accounting for the term "marantic endocarditis" (from the Greek, *marantikos,* "wasting away"). It has been attributed to increased blood coagulability or immune complex deposition. In the absence of bacteria, the vegetations remain small and there is no valve destruction. The main danger posed by NBTE is embolization to distant organs, clinically manifested as infarcts of many organs, but this is unusual and NBTE is often identified as an incidental finding at autopsy.

Calcific Aortic Stenosis Reflects Chronic Damage to the Valve

Calcific aortic stenosis refers to narrowing of the aortic valve orifice due to calcium deposition in the valve cusps and ring.

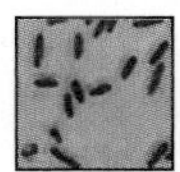
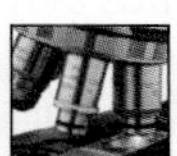

ETIOLOGIC FACTORS AND PATHOLOGY: Calcific aortic stenosis has three main causes.

- **Rheumatic aortic valve disease** is characterized by diffuse fibrous thickening and scarring of the cusps, commissural fusion and deposition of calcium, all of which reduce the valve orifice and limit valve mobility (Fig. 11-32). Rheumatic aortic stenosis virtually never occurs in isolation; there is nearly always evidence of rheumatic mitral valve disease as well. Now that acute RF has become so rare in the United States and most elderly patients with rheumatic valve disease have either undergone valve replacement or died, calcific aortic stenosis is usually attributed to other causes.
- **Degenerative (senile) calcific stenosis** develops in elderly patients as a degenerative process involving a tricuspid aortic valve. Valve cusps become rigidly calcified, but commissural fusion (Fig. 11-36), a hallmark of rheumatic aortic valves, is not seen. The mitral valve is usually normal in patients with senile calcific aortic stenosis, although the mitral annulus may also be calcified.
- **Congenital bicuspid aortic stenosis** often develops with age (Fig. 11-37).
- **Calcific aortic stenosis** in both congenitally malformed valves and normal ones is probably related to the cumulative effect of years of trauma, owing to turbulent blood flow around the valve. For example, although a bicuspid valve is not inherently stenotic, its orifice is elliptical rather than round, and flow across the valve is somewhat turbulent. Increasing rigidity of the cusps eventually produces functional derangements, typically in patients beyond the age of 60.

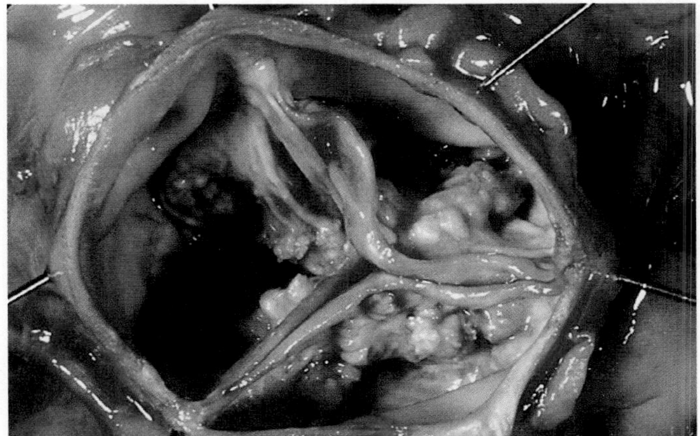

FIGURE 11-36. Calcific aortic stenosis in a three-cuspid aortic valve in an elderly person. The leaflets are heavily calcified, but there is no commissural fusion (compare with Fig. 11-32).

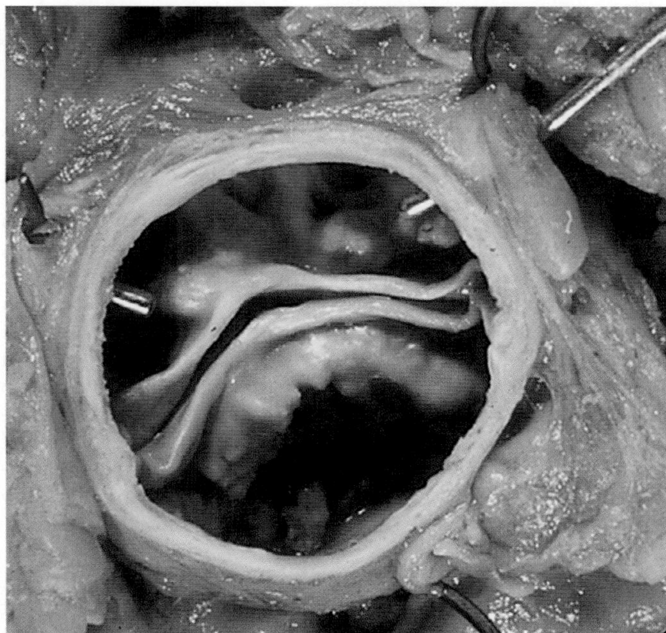

FIGURE 11-37. Calcific aortic stenosis of a congenitally bicuspid aortic valve. The two leaflets are heavily calcified, but there is no commissural fusion.

In any of the forms of calcific aortic stenosis, calcification produces nodules restricted to the base and lower half of the cusps, and rarely involves the free margins. Without rheumatic scarring, the commissures are not fused and three distinct cusps are evident.

Aortic valve calcification is not a purely passive process in which devitalized tissue becomes mineralized, as the term "dystrophic calcification" seems to imply. In fact, valvular calcification is an active process involving modulation of valvular interstitial cells to an osteoblastic phenotype and new gene expression resulting in cell-mediated mineralization of the extracellular matrix. Many of the mechanisms and risk factors associated with valvular calcification are the same for atherosclerosis. Mechanical forces promote accumulation of LDL particles and other factors, which results in inflammation, activation and transformation of valvular interstitial cells, remodeling of extracellular matrix and secretion of osteogenic proteins such as bone morphogenic protein-2 and other noncollagenous matrix proteins. However, despite these similarities, effective approaches to preventing atherosclerosis, such as statins, do not prevent valvular calcification.

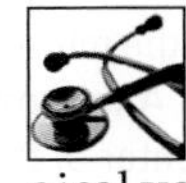

CLINICAL FEATURES: Severe aortic stenosis causes striking concentric left ventricular hypertrophy. Eventually, the ventricle dilates and fails. Surgical valve replacement is highly successful treatment (5-year survival rate of 85%), provided it is done before ventricular dysfunction is irreversible. The hypertrophic left ventricle then returns to normal size.

Calcification of the Mitral Valve Annulus Is Usually Asymptomatic

Calcification of the mitral valve annulus occurs commonly in the elderly and is usually without functional significance, although it often produces a murmur. However, if it is severe enough to interfere with posterior mitral leaflet excursion during systole, mitral regurgitation occurs. Calcification of the mitral valve annulus in the elderly differs from that in rheumatic mitral valve disease. The former entails little or no deformation of valve leaflets, and calcification is most prominent in the annulus rather than the leaflets. About 40% of women older than 90 years have this lesion, whereas the incidence is only 15% in men. Calcification of the mitral valve annulus is aggravated by the presence of aortic stenosis, hypertension and diabetes.

Calcific deposits transform the mitral ring into a rigid, curved bar up to 2 cm in diameter, which may be evident radiologically. Amorphous masses of calcified material first develop in the connective tissue of the valve ring. However, with time, the calcification extends into the base of the leaflets and eventually to the ventricular septum.

Mitral Valve Prolapse Is the Most Common Indication for Valve Repair or Replacement

MVP is a condition in which mitral valve leaflets become enlarged and redundant. Chordae tendineae become thinned and elongated, such that the billowed leaflets prolapse into the left atrium during systole (Fig. 11-38A). Also referred to as "floppy mitral valve syndrome," MVP is the most frequent cause of mitral regurgitation that requires surgical valve repair or replacement. As much as 5% of the adult population may show echocardiographic evidence of MVP, although most will not have regurgitation severe enough to warrant surgical intervention.

MOLECULAR PATHOGENESIS: MVP has an important hereditary component and many cases appear to be transmitted as an autosomal dominant trait. Three different loci on chromosomes 16, 11 and 13 have been linked to the disease, but no specific gene mutations have been identified. Prolapsed mitral valves accumulate striking amounts of myxomatous connective tissue in the center of the valve leaflet (Fig. 11-38B). Proteoglycans in the valve are increased, and electron microscopy shows fragmentation of collagen fibrils. Presumably, these changes reflect a molecular defect in the extracellular matrix that allows the leaflets and chordae to enlarge and stretch under the high-pressure conditions they experience during the cardiac cycle. MVP is usually an isolated finding, but it is particularly prevalent in patients with Marfan syndrome, Ehlers-Danlos syndrome, osteogenic imperfecta and other collagen-related disorders. This association with inherited connective tissue disorders suggests an abnormality of connective tissue in the pathogenesis of myxomatous degeneration, but thus far, no abnormalities in fibrillar collagen genes or TGF-β signaling have been identified. Pectus excavatum, scoliosis and loss of kyphosis of the thoracic spine are common in patients with MVP, but it is not known if these bony abnormalities are genetically linked to MVP. The risk of sudden death in patients with MVP, presumably due to ventricular tachyarrhythmias, is twice that expected in the general population. Repair of a regurgitant floppy mitral valve appears to lower this risk. The mechanisms are not well understood, but the risk appears to depend primarily on the degree of mitral regurgitation, perhaps related to ventricular remodeling associated with volume overload.

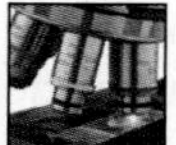

PATHOLOGY: On gross examination, mitral valve leaflets are redundant and deformed (Fig. 11-38A). On cross-section they have a gelatinous appearance and slippery texture, due to accumulation of acid mucopolysaccharides (proteoglycans). The myxomatous degenerative process also affects the annulus and chordae tendineae, increasing the

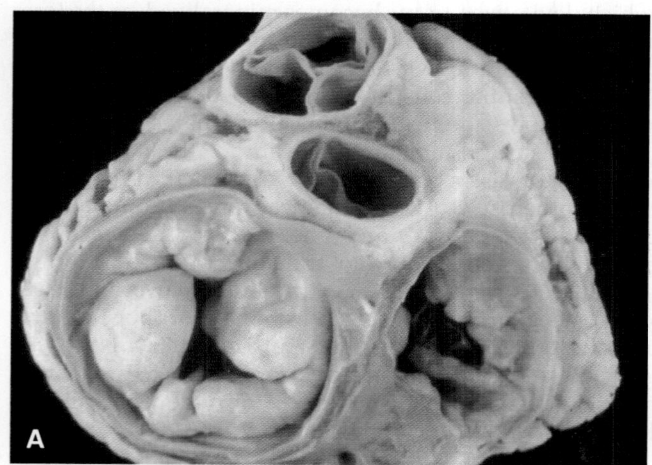

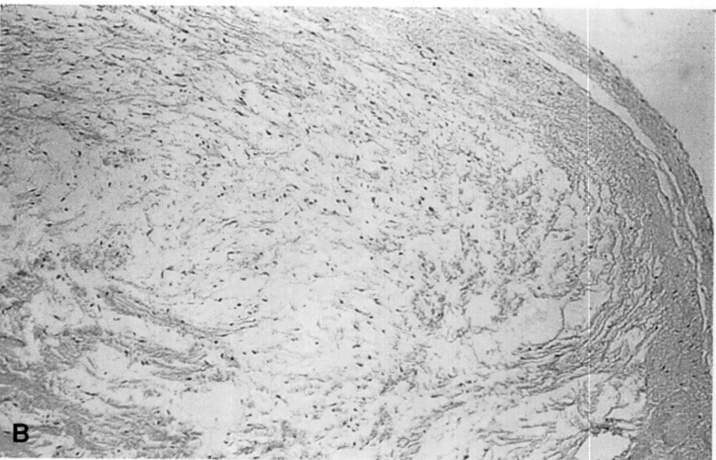

FIGURE 11-38. Mitral valve prolapse. A. A view of the mitral valve (*left*) from the left atrium shows redundant and deformed leaflets, which billow into the left atrial cavity. **B.** A microscopic section of one of the mitral valve leaflets reveals conspicuous myxomatous connective tissue in the center of the leaflet.

degree of prolapse and regurgitation. Damage to the chordae may be so severe that they rupture. Rupture of multiple chordae can produce a flail mitral valve that is totally incompetent. Although the mitral valve is usually the only valve affected, myxomatous degeneration can develop in the other heart valves, especially in patients with Marfan syndrome, 90% of whom have some clinical evidence of MVP.

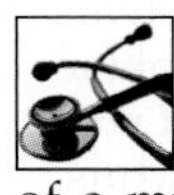

CLINICAL FEATURES: Most patients with MVP are asymptomatic. Clinical recognition of MVP is based on recognition of the classical auscultatory findings of a mid- to late systolic click, caused by the snap of the redundant leaflets as they prolapse into the left atrium. A late systolic murmur is present if mitral regurgitation is significant. Endocarditis, both infective and nonbacterial, is sometimes a serious complication, and cerebral emboli are common. Significant mitral regurgitation develops in 15% of patients after 10 to 15 years of MVP, after which mitral valve repair or replacement is indicated.

Papillary Muscle Dysfunction May Produce Mitral Regurgitation

Dysfunction of the left ventricular papillary muscles is most often caused by ischemia. The papillary muscles are especially vulnerable to ischemic injury because they are supplied by the terminal branches of the intramyocardial coronary arteries. Thus, any reduction in coronary blood flow may preferentially interfere with papillary muscle function. Brief periods of ischemia (e.g., during episodes of angina pectoris) can result in transient papillary muscle dysfunction (stunning) and temporary mitral regurgitation. By contrast, myocardial infarction and subsequent scarring of papillary muscles can lead to permanent mitral regurgitation. In fact, one third of all patients being evaluated for coronary artery bypass surgery have some evidence of "ischemic mitral regurgitation." Papillary muscle dysfunction may also be associated with a healed myocardial infarct, in which impaired myocardial contractility at the base of the papillary muscle interferes with its function. Rarely, patients may suddenly develop life-threatening mitral regurgitation after rupture of an acutely infarcted papillary muscle.

Carcinoid Heart Disease Affects Right-Sided Valves

Carcinoid heart disease is an unusual condition that uniquely affects the right side of the heart, leading to tricuspid regurgitation and pulmonary stenosis. It arises in patients with carcinoid tumors, usually of the small intestine, that have metastasized to the liver.

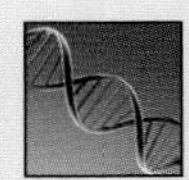

MOLECULAR PATHOGENESIS: The pathogenesis of carcinoid heart disease is not fully understood, but the valvular and endocardial lesions are thought to be caused by high concentrations of serotonin or other vasoactive amines and peptides produced by the tumor in the liver. Because these moieties are metabolized in the lung, carcinoid heart disease affects the right side of the heart almost exclusively. There are reports of left-sided involvement in patients with atrial or ventricular septal defects.

During the 1990s, reports surfaced of mitral and aortic valve disease in patients taking the appetite-suppressing drugs fenfluramine-phentermine ("fen-phen"). Gross and microscopic features of the valve lesions were strikingly similar to those seen in carcinoid heart disease, except that they developed on the left-sided valves. Since then, other anorexigenic drugs and ergot alkaloid drugs such as methysergide and ergotamine used to treat migraine headaches have also been linked to this type of valve disease. Because these drugs interfere with serotonin metabolism and signaling, it has been suggested that the pathogenesis of drug-related and carcinoid valve disease is similar.

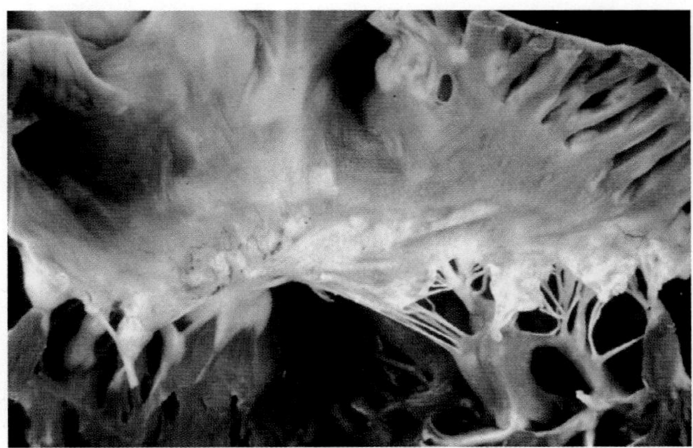

FIGURE 11-39. Carcinoid heart disease. Pearly white deposits are seen on the tricuspid valve leaflets and adjacent endocardium. Although the valve leaflets have not been destroyed, they have become deformed and "stuck down" on the ventricular endocardium, which usually produces tricuspid regurgitation.

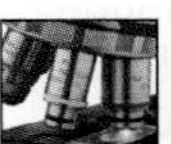

PATHOLOGY: The cardiac lesions are plaque-like deposits of dense, pearly gray, fibrous tissue on the tricuspid (Fig. 11-39) and pulmonary valves, and on the endocardial surface of the right ventricle. Microscopically, these patches appear "tacked on" to valve leaflets, without associated inflammation or apparent damage to underlying valve structures. However, leaflets become deformed, and their surface area reduced. As a result, tricuspid leaflets become "stuck down" onto adjacent right ventricular mural endocardium, resulting in tricuspid insufficiency or stenosis. Shrinkage of the pulmonary valve and its annulus leads to pulmonary stenosis.

Myocarditis

Myocarditis is inflammation of the myocardium associated with myocyte necrosis and degeneration. This definition specifically excludes ischemic heart disease. The true incidence of myocarditis is difficult to establish because many cases are asymptomatic. It can occur at any age but is most common in children between the ages of 1 and 10. It is one of the few heart diseases that can produce acute heart failure in previously healthy children, adolescents or young adults. Severe myocarditis can cause arrhythmias and even sudden cardiac death.

Most Cases of Viral Myocarditis Are Without an Easily Demonstrable Cause

Viral etiology is generally suspected to be responsible, although the evidence is usually circumstantial unless polymerase chain

Table 11-7

Causes of Myocarditis

Idiopathic
Infectious
• Viral: Coxsackievirus, adenovirus, echovirus, influenza virus, human immunodeficiency virus and many others
• Rickettsial: Typhus, Rocky Mountain spotted fever
• Bacterial: Diphtheria, staphylococcal, streptococcal, meningococcal, *Borrelia* (Lyme disease) and leptospiral infection
• Fungi and protozoan parasites: Chagas disease, toxoplasmosis, aspergillosis, cryptococcal and candidal infection
• Metazoan parasites: *Echinococcus, Trichina*
Noninfectious
• Hypersensitivity and immunologically related diseases: Rheumatic fever, systemic lupus erythematosus, scleroderma, drug reaction (e.g., to penicillin or sulfonamide) and rheumatoid arthritis
• Radiation
• Miscellaneous: Sarcoidosis, uremia

reaction (PCR) studies identify viral genomes in heart biopsies. The most common viral causes of myocarditis are listed in Table 11-7.

MOLECULAR PATHOGENESIS: The pathogenesis of viral myocarditis involves direct viral cytotoxicity and cell-mediated immune reactions against infected myocytes. In animal models, inoculation of a cardiotropic virus is followed shortly by viral replication in the myocardium. Microscopically, there are only small isolated foci of acute myocyte necrosis with little, if any, inflammatory cell infiltration, and there is little evidence of functional impairment. Over the next few days, mononuclear cells, principally T lymphocytes and macrophages, infiltrate the myocardium extensively. At the point of maximum inflammation, signs of heart failure develop, although viral cultures of blood and myocardium are negative. This finding is consistent with the observation that patients with symptomatic myocarditis generally have negative viral cultures, although viral nucleic acid sequences can still be detected by PCR.

The two most common viruses to infect the heart, coxsackievirus and adenovirus, both enter cardiac myocytes after binding to the same cell surface receptor, the coxsackie-adenovirus receptor (CAR). Deletion of this molecule in mice prevents viral infection. CAR belongs to the family of intercellular adhesion molecules. It is especially abundant in children, which may explain why viral myocarditis is so common in this age group. Once within a myocyte, coxsackieviruses produce proteases, such as protease 2A, which play a role in viral replication. These proteases cleave important myocyte proteins such as dystrophin, which may be involved in release of virus from the myocyte (intracellular viral load is increased in the absence of dystrophin). Proteases could also contribute to myocardial dysfunction in viral myocarditis.

Cardiac myocytes contain a powerful innate antiviral defense mechanism mediated by Janus kinase (JAK) and signal transducers and activators of transcription (STAT) pathways activated by interferon-α/β, interferon-γ and interleukin-6 (IL-6). However, these actions can be inhibited by suppressors of cytokine signaling (SOCS), proteins that limit the potentially deleterious actions of cytokine signaling in cardiac myocytes. Levels of SOCS affect susceptibility to coxsackievirus infection profoundly. Thus, the highly variable clinical and pathologic manifestations of viral myocarditis depend on the dynamic interplay between mechanisms that determine viral entry, replication and release, and immune mechanisms (innate and T-cell mediated) of host responsiveness.

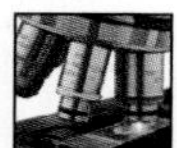

PATHOLOGY: The hearts of patients with myocarditis who develop clinical heart failure during the active inflammatory phase show biventricular dilation and generalized myocardial hypokinesis. At autopsy, these hearts are flabby and dilated. The histologic changes of viral myocarditis vary with the clinical severity of the disease, but with few exceptions, microscopic features are nonspecific and indistinguishable from toxic myocarditis. Most cases show a patchy or diffuse interstitial, predominantly mononuclear, inflammatory infiltrate composed principally of T lymphocytes and macrophages (Fig. 11-40). Multinucleated giant cells may also be present. The inflammatory cells often surround individual myocytes, and focal myocyte necrosis is seen. During the resolving phase, fibroblast proliferation and

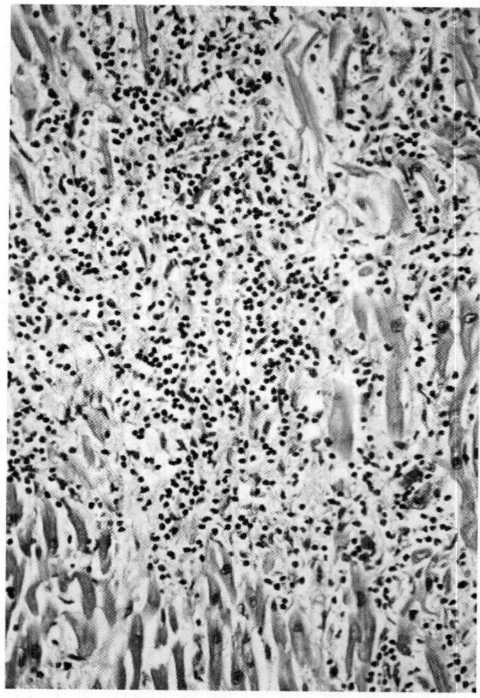

FIGURE 11-40. Viral myocarditis. The myocardial fibers are disrupted by a prominent interstitial infiltrate of lymphocytes and macrophages.

interstitial collagen deposition predominate. Neutrophils are not usually seen in viral myocarditis. However, if necrosis is extensive, the histology may resemble that seen in an infarct, namely, a neutrophilic infiltrate followed by organization and repair. Most viruses that cause myocarditis also cause pericarditis.

CLINICAL FEATURES: Many persons who develop viral myocarditis may be asymptomatic. When symptoms do occur, they usually begin a few weeks after infection. Most patients recover from acute myocarditis, although a few die of congestive heart failure or arrhythmias. The disease may be unusually severe in infants and pregnant women. Despite resolution of the active inflammatory phase of viral myocarditis, subtle functional impairment may persist for years and progression to overt cardiomyopathy is well documented. There is no specific treatment for viral myocarditis, and supportive measures are the rule. Antiviral and immunomodulatory therapies shown to be effective in animal models are not of proven utility in humans.

MYOCARDITIS IN ACQUIRED IMMUNODEFICIENCY SYNDROME: A significant proportion of symptomatic patients with acquired immunodeficiency syndrome (AIDS) have some clinical or pathologic evidence of cardiac disease (pericardial effusions, myocarditis, endocarditis or cardiomyopathy). An unusually high incidence of viral myocarditis due to cardiotropic viruses, such as coxsackievirus and adenovirus, is documented in AIDS. Human immunodeficiency virus type 1 (HIV-1) infection of cardiac myocytes appears to play a minor role.

Other Transmissible Agents in Addition to Viruses May Cause Infectious Myocarditis

Thus, other microorganisms that gain access to the bloodstream can infect the heart. Among these, brucellosis, meningococcemia and psittacosis often lead to infectious myocarditis. Some bacteria (e.g., diphtheria) produce cardiotoxins, which may produce a fatal myocarditis. The most common cause of myocarditis in South America is the protozoan *Trypanosoma cruzi,* the agent of Chagas disease (see Chapter 9).

- **Bacterial infection** of the myocardium is characterized by multiple foci of a mixed inflammatory cell infiltrate, with neutrophils as the major component. Microabscesses can occur when septic emboli lodge in the coronary circulation, often as a consequence of infective endocarditis.
- **Rickettsial diseases** commonly cause widespread vasculitis, which affects small coronary blood vessels.
- **Fungal infection** of the myocardium typically occurs in immunocompromised patients, although the heart is relatively resistant to fungal infection.
- **Toxoplasmosis** can involve the myocardium in immunosuppressed patients; the intracellular parasites proliferate within cardiac myocytes and elicit a focal mixed inflammatory response, with neutrophils and eosinophils.
- **Chagas disease** is associated with proliferation of parasites within cardiac myocytes and a mixed inflammatory cell infiltrate, composed principally of lymphocytes, plasma cells and macrophages.

Granulomatous Myocarditis May Be Caused by Microorganisms or Immunologically Mediated Injury

Granulomatous inflammation of the myocardium associated with myocyte necrosis is seen in a variety of diseases. Microorganisms associated with granulomatous myocarditis include *Mycobacteria* and some types of fungi. Immunologically mediated injury of the myocardium may also produce granulomatous myocarditis. Examples include rheumatic myocarditis (Fig. 11-29) and sarcoidosis (see Fig. 11-46).

Hypersensitivity Myocarditis Is a Reaction to Drugs

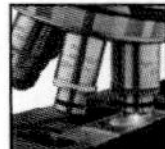

PATHOLOGY: The inflammation consists of an interstitial and perivascular infiltrate, which is often confined to the myocardium and does not affect other organs. The inflammatory infiltrate in hypersensitivity myocarditis resembles that seen in viral myocarditis, but the former displays numerous eosinophils, as well as lymphocytes and plasma cells. Another typical feature is the virtual absence of myocyte necrosis, even when the infiltrate is intense.

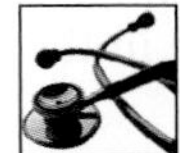

CLINICAL FEATURES: Hypersensitivity myocarditis is usually clinically silent. The diagnosis is often made as an incidental finding at autopsy. However, it may produce chest pain and electrocardiographic changes that resemble acute myocardial ischemia. Occasionally, it is responsible for fatal ventricular arrhythmias. When the disease causes symptoms, treatment consists of discontinuing the offending drug and administering corticosteroids or immunosuppressive agents.

Giant Cell Myocarditis Is Usually Fatal

Giant cell myocarditis is a rare, highly aggressive disease of the heart characterized by intense inflammation, extensive areas of myocyte necrosis and numerous multinucleated giant cells of macrophage origin. The cause is unknown, but it sometimes occurs in patients with SLE, hyperthyroidism or thymoma. An autoimmune etiology has been suggested, but there is no persuasive evidence for this theory.

Giant cell myocarditis is usually a rapidly fatal disease of adults in the third to fifth decades of life, although it also occurs in adolescents. Patients die of congestive heart failure or sudden death from arrhythmias. At autopsy, the heart is flabby and dilated, and may contain mural thrombi. Microscopically, prominent giant cells, lymphoid cells and macrophages are seen at the margins of serpiginous areas of myocardial necrosis. Although giant cells are numerous, granulomas do not form. The only effective treatment is cardiac transplantation, although giant cell myocarditis recurs in transplanted hearts in one fourth of cases.

Metabolic Diseases of the Heart

Hyperthyroidism Causes High-Output Failure

Thyroid hormone has direct inotropic and chronotropic effects on the heart: (1) it increases the activity of the sarcolemmal sodium pump; (2) it enhances the synthesis of a myosin isoform with rapid ATPase activity and reduces production of a slower isoform; and (3) it upregulates expression of slow calcium channels in the sarcolemma, thereby facilitating contractility. Hyperthyroidism thus causes conspicuous tachycardia and an increased cardiac workload, owing to decreased peripheral resistance and increased cardiac output. It may eventually lead to angina pectoris and high-output failure.

Hypothyroid Heart Disease Diminishes Cardiac Output

Patients with severe hypothyroidism (**myxedema**) have decreased cardiac output, reduced heart rate and impaired myocardial contractility—changes that are the opposite of those seen in hyperthyroidism. There may be a pericardial effusion created by increased capillary permeability and leakage of fluid and protein into the pericardial cavity. Pulse pressure is decreased because of higher peripheral resistance and lower blood volume.

The hearts of patients with myxedema are flabby and dilated, and the myocardium exhibits myofiber swelling. Basophilic (mucinous) degeneration is common. Interstitial fibrosis may also be present. Despite these changes, myxedema does not produce congestive heart failure in the absence of other cardiac disorders.

Thiamine Deficiency (Beriberi) Heart Disease Is Similar to Hyperthyroidism

Beriberi heart disease develops in patients who consume a diet inadequate in vitamin B_1 (thiamine) for at least 3 months (see Chapter 8). It is seen in parts of Asia where the diet consists largely of shelled rice. In the United States, thiamine deficiency is occasionally seen in alcoholics or neglected persons. Beriberi heart disease results in decreased peripheral vascular resistance and increased cardiac output, a combination similar to that produced by hyperthyroidism. The result is high-output failure. Interestingly, heart failure may develop so suddenly that patients die within 2 days of the onset of symptoms. At autopsy, the heart is dilated and shows only nonspecific microscopic changes.

Cardiomyopathy

Cardiomyopathy refers to a primary disease of the myocardium. Strictly defined, it excludes damage caused by extrinsic factors. There are various classification schemes including some based primarily on increasingly recognized genetic causes. Usually, the primary cardiomyopathies are divided into the major clinicopathologic groups of **dilated cardiomyopathy** (DCM), **hypertrophic cardiomyopathy** (HCM), **arrhythmogenic right ventricular cardiomyopathy** (ARVC) and **restrictive cardiomyopathy** (RCM). DCM is the most common type of cardiomyopathy and is a leading indication for heart transplantation. It is characterized by biventricular dilation, impaired contractility and eventually congestive heart failure. DCM can develop in response to a large number of known insults that directly injure cardiac myocytes (**secondary DCM**), or it may be idiopathic (**primary DCM**).

Idiopathic Dilated Cardiomyopathy Is Characterized by Impaired Contractility

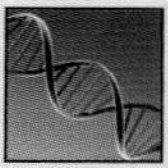

MOLECULAR PATHOGENESIS: Numerous etiologies have been implicated in idiopathic DCM and most cases are probably related to the interplay between genetic, epigenetic and environmental factors.

Genetic factors are now recognized as playing an important role in the pathpgenesis of DCM. Among patients with idiopathic DCM, at least a third have a familial disease. The proportion may be even greater because incomplete penetrance often makes it difficult to identify early or latent disease in family members. Most familial cases seem to be transmitted as an autosomal dominant trait, but autosomal recessive, X-linked recessive and mitochondrial inheritance patterns have all been described (Table 11-8).

Several mutations implicated in DCM occur in genes encoding cytoskeletal proteins such as lamin A/C, desmin and metavinculin. Others occur in genes such as δ-sarcoglycan and dystrophin, which are involved in anchoring the cytoskeleton and the sarcolemma to the extracellular matrix (Table 11-8). ***This has given rise to the hypothesis that defects in force transmission lead to development of a dilated, poorly contracting heart*** (Fig. 11-41). Interestingly, mutations in genes encoding proteins such as actin, titin, troponin T and β- or α-myosin heavy chain may produce either DCM or HCM phenotypes, perhaps depending on whether they produce a defect in force generation (HCM) or force transmission. For example, actin mutations associated with HCM have been localized to a portion of the molecule near a myosin-binding site, which could impair sarcomeric function. By contrast, DCM-associated mutations in actin are within the region that binds to the dystrophin–sarcoglycan complex (Fig. 11-41). While the force transmission hypothesis is appealing, it may not account for other mutations linked to DCM such as those involving the cardiac sodium channel or presenilin, both of which have also been implicated in others types of diseases (Table 11-8). As the list of genetic factors expands, so too does the breadth of potential molecular mechanisms.

Viral myocarditis may eventually lead to DCM, but how this would develop is not clear. Once they have infected cardiac myocytes, viruses can harness the host ubiquitin/proteasomal system and the autophagy machinery to facilitate their replication. Ongoing interactions between the virus and these host systems can impair normal host protein turnover kinetics and promote oxidative stress. This could, in turn, lead to abnormal regulation of contractile proteins and promote apoptosis and autophagic cell death with the eventual emergence of a clinical phenotype of ventricular remodeling and failure. Indeed, persistence of viral genomes in the heart detected by PCR is associated with progressive impairment of left ventricular function, whereas spontaneous viral elimination is associated with improved function.

Immunologic abnormalities involving both cellular and humoral effects have been recognized in both myocarditis and idiopathic DCM. Autoantibodies have been identified against a number of cardiac antigens including a variety of mitochondrial antigens, cardiac myosin and β-adrenergic receptors. However, as in many cases of

Table 11-8

Gene Defects Associated with Dilated Cardiomyopathy (DCM)

Gene	Chromosome Locus	OMIM*	Gene Product	Frequency	Related Disorders
Autosomal Dominant					
LMNA	1q21.2	150330	Lamin A/C	4%–8%	Lipodystrophy, Charcot-Marie-Tooth, Emery-Dreifuss muscular dystrophy, Hutchinson-Gilford progeria syndrome, limb girdle muscular dystrophy (LGMD)
MYH7	14q12	160760	β-myosin heavy chain	4%–6%	Laing distal myopathy, hypertrophic cardiomyopathy (HCM)
TNNT2	1q32	191045	Cardiac troponin T	3%	HCM
SCN5A	3p21	600163	Sodium channel	2%–3%	Long QT syndrome, Brugada syndrome, idiopathic ventricular fibrillation, sick sinus syndrome, cardiac conduction system disease
MYH6	14q12	160710	α-myosin heavy chain	? 2%–3%	HCM, dominantly inherited atrial septal defect
DES	2q35	125660	Desmin	<1%–1%	Desminopathy
VCL	10q22.1-23	193065	Metavinculin	<1%–1%	HCM
LDB3	10q22.2-23.3	605906	LIM domain-binding 3	<1%–1%	HCM
TCAP	17q12	604488	Titin-cap or telethonin	<1%–1%	LGMD, HCM
PSEN1/PSEN2	14q24.3/1q31-q42	104311/600759	Presenilin 1/2	<1%–1%	Alzheimer disease
ACTC	15q14	102540	Cardiac actin	<1%	HCM
TPM1	15q22.1	191010	α-Tropomyosin 1	<1%	HCM
SGCD	5q33–34	601411	δ-Sarcoglycan	<1%	Delta sarcoglycanopathy (LGMD)
CSRP3	11p15.1	600824	Muscle LIM protein	<1%	HCM
ACTN2	1q42-q43	102573	α-actinin-2	<1%	HCM
ABCC9	12p12.1	601439	SUR2A	<1%	NA
TNNC1	3p21.3-p14.3	191040	Cardiac troponin C	<1%	NA
X-linked FDC					
DMD	Xp21.2	300377	Dystrophin	?	Dystrophinopathies (Duchenne muscular dystrophy, Becker muscular dystrophy)
TAZ/G4.5	Xq28	300394	Tafazzin	?	Barth syndrome, endocardial fibroelastosis, familial isolated noncompaction of the left ventricular myocardium
Autosomal Recessive					
TNNI3	19q13.4	191044	Cardiac troponin I	<1%	HCM, restrictive cardiomyopathy

*OMIM is Online Mendelian Inheritance in Man, http://www.ncbi.nlm.nih.gov/sites/entrez?db=omim, where additional information for each gene can be found.

autoimmune disease, a pathogenic role for immune mechanisms remains to be proved: circulating autoantibodies may be the result of myocardial injury, rather than its cause.

PATHOLOGY: The pathology of DCM is generally nonspecific, and is similar whether the disorder is idiopathic or secondary to a known injurious agent. At autopsy, the heart is invariably enlarged, with conspicuous left and right ventricular hypertrophy. The weight of the heart may be as much as tripled (>900 g). As a rule, all chambers of the heart are dilated, though the ventricles are more severely affected than are the atria (Fig. 11-42). At end-stage, left ventricular dilation is usually so severe that the left ventricle wall appears to be of normal thickness or even thinned. The myocardium is flabby and pale, and small subendocardial scars are occasionally evident. The left ventricle endocardium, especially at the apex, tends to be thickened. Adherent mural thrombi are often present in this area.

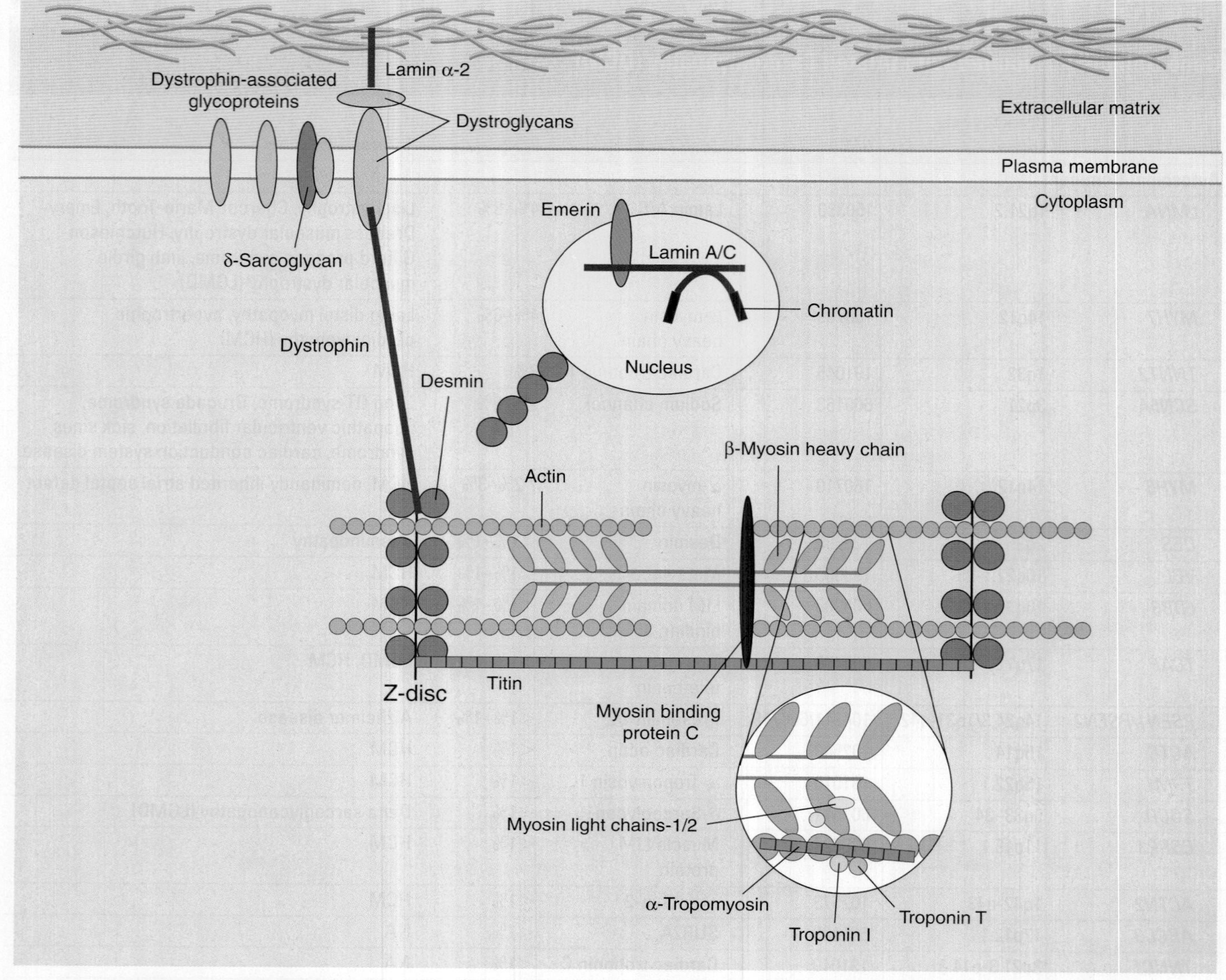

FIGURE 11-41. Subcellular distribution and molecular interactions of mutant proteins implicated in the pathogenesis of dilated and hypertrophic cardiomyopathy. The specific mutations responsible for each type are provided in Tables 11-8 and 11-9.

Microscopically, DCM is characterized by atrophic and hypertrophic myocardial fibers. Cardiac myocytes, especially in the subendocardium, often show advanced degenerative changes characterized by myofibrillar loss (myocytolysis), an effect that gives cells a vacant, vacuolated appearance. Interstitial and perivascular fibrosis of myocardium is evident, also most prominently in the subendocardial zone. Scattered chronic inflammatory cells may be present, but are not conspicuous. Electron microscopy typically shows loss of sarcomeres and an apparent increase in mitochondria.

CLINICAL FEATURES: The clinical courses of idiopathic and secondary DCM are comparable. Both begin insidiously with compensatory ventricular hypertrophy and asymptomatic left ventricular dilation. Exercise intolerance usually progresses relentlessly to frank congestive heart failure and 75% of patients die within 5 years of the onset of symptoms. Half of all deaths in DCM patients are sudden, and are attributed to ventricular arrhythmias. Abnormalities in intracellular Ca^{2+} handling and certain repolarizing (K^+) currents are common features in all forms of heart failure. They tend to prolong the QT interval and increase the likelihood of arrhythmias initiated by triggered activity. Supportive treatment is useful, but cardiac transplantation or a ventricular assist device is eventually necessary.

Over 100 Diseases May Cause Clinical Features of Secondary Dilated Cardiomyopathy

Thus, secondary DCM is best viewed as a final common pathway for the effects of virtually any toxic, metabolic or infectious disorder that directly injures cardiac myocytes. In this context, alcohol abuse, hypertension, pregnancy and viral myocarditis predispose to secondary DCM. Diabetes mellitus and cigarette smoking are also associated with an increased incidence of DCM.

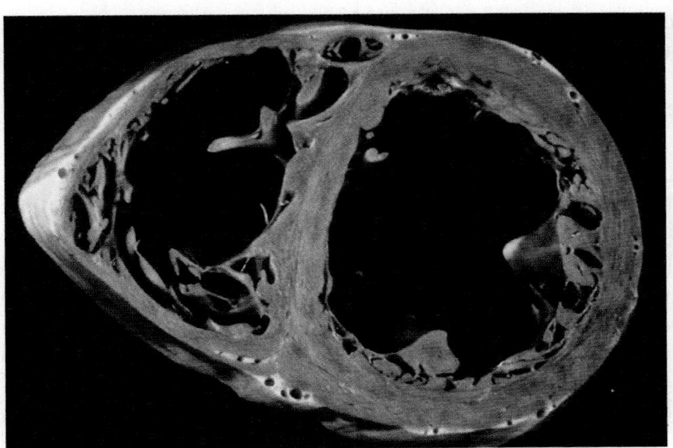

FIGURE 11-42. Idiopathic dilated cardiomyopathy. A transverse section of the enlarged heart reveals conspicuous dilation of both ventricles. Although the ventricular wall appears thinned, the increased mass of the heart indicates considerable hypertrophy.

Toxic Cardiomyopathy

Numerous chemicals and drugs cause myocardial injury, but only a few of the more important chemicals are discussed here.

ETHANOL: Alcoholic cardiomyopathy is the single most common identifiable cause of DCM in the United States and Europe. Ethanol abuse can lead to chronic, progressive cardiac dysfunction, which may be fatal. The disorder is more common in men, because alcoholism is more frequent in men. The typical patient is between 30 and 55 years of age and has been drinking heavily for at least 10 years.

MOLECULAR PATHOGENESIS: The pathogenesis of alcoholic cardiomyopathy remains obscure. In experimental animals the presence of ethanol exerts a negative inotropic effect (decreased contractile strength) on cardiac muscle, impairs calcium flux, inhibits protein synthesis and produces oxidative stress. Moreover, adducts of ethanol, metabolic products such as acetaldehyde and fatty acid ethyl esters, have been reported to impair the function of cardiac myocytes. Yet all of these effects are entirely reversible upon discontinuation of ethanol consumption. Since the development of human alcoholic cardiomyopathy requires more than 10 years of alcohol abuse and is related to the total lifetime dose of alcohol, the role of reversible changes is questionable. It has recently been demonstrated that alcohol abuse increases the rate of apoptosis in human cardiac myocytes, and inhibitory effects on certain types of progenitor cells have been shown. Whether alcoholic cardiomyopathy represents an imbalance between apoptosis and replacement of cardiac myocytes, as has been claimed for biological aging, is a subject for further study.

COBALT: The cardiac toxicity of cobalt is discussed in Chapter 8.

CATECHOLAMINES: In high concentrations, catecholamines can cause focal myocyte necrosis (contraction band necrosis). Toxic myocarditis may occur in patients with pheochromocytomas or who require high doses of inotropic drugs to maintain blood pressure and in accident victims who sustain massive head trauma. Multiple mechanisms contribute to myocardial injury, but the most important is enhanced calcium flux into myocytes. Focal ischemia caused by platelet aggregation and microvascular constriction may also contribute.

ANTHRACYCLINES: Doxorubicin (Adriamycin) and other anthracycline drugs are potent chemotherapeutic agents whose usefulness is limited by cumulative, dose-dependent, cardiac toxicity. The clinical major effect is poor myocyte contractility due to chronic, irreversible degeneration of cardiac myocytes. The histopathology of this disorder includes vacuolization and loss of myofibrils. Myocyte necrosis is rare, but once severe degeneration occurs, intractable congestive heart failure develops and the prognosis is grim.

MOLECULAR PATHOGENESIS: DCM begins to appear in patients who receive a cumulative dose of more than 500 mg doxorubicin per m^2, and 35% of those receiving more than 550 mg/m^2 develop cardiomyopathy. The mechanism by which anthracyclines damage the heart appears related mainly to formation of reactive oxygen species through redox cycling of aglycone metabolites and anthracycline–iron complexes. Although the heart is relatively resistant to radiation injury, anthracyclines and radiation act synergistically. Thus, a patient who has received radiotherapy to the mediastinum is at risk of developing anthracycline toxicity at a lower dose than someone who was not irradiated.

CYCLOPHOSPHAMIDE: This alkylating agent is often used in high doses before bone marrow transplantation. Although it does not cause classical DCM, it can cause pericarditis and occasionally massive hemorrhagic myocarditis. The latter is thought to be secondary to endothelial injury and thrombocytopenia.

COCAINE: Cocaine use is frequently associated with chest pain and palpitations. True DCM is an unusual complication of cocaine abuse, but myocarditis, focal necrosis and thickening of intramyocardial coronary arteries have been reported. Myocardial ischemia or infarction associated with cocaine use has been attributed to coronary vasoconstriction in the face of increased myocardial oxygen demand. Sudden death due to spontaneous ventricular tachyarrhythmias is well documented. Cocaine-induced arrhythmias may be due to drug-related vasoconstriction, sympathomimetic activity, hypersensitivity responses and direct toxicity.

Cardiomyopathy of Pregnancy

A unique form of DCM develops in the last trimester of pregnancy or the first 6 months after delivery. The disorder is relatively uncommon in the United States, but in some regions of Africa, it is seen in as many as 1% of pregnant women. The risk of cardiomyopathy of pregnancy is greatest in black, multiparous women, older than 30 years. Some patients exhibit inflammatory cells in heart biopsies taken during the symptomatic phase of the illness, consistent with the hypothesis that disordered immunity may underlie development of DCM in this setting.

Unlike most other varieties of DCM, half of women with cardiomyopathy of pregnancy spontaneously recover normal cardiac function. The other half are left with persistent left ventricular dysfunction or proceed to overt congestive heart failure and early death. In patients who survive, subsequent pregnancies pose a high risk of recurrence and maternal mortality.

MOLECULAR PATHOGENESIS: Overproduction of prolactin has been implicated in cardiomyopathy of pregnancy. In normal pregnancy, prolactin increases blood volume, decreases blood pressure and diminishes renal excretion of water, sodium and potassium. Patients with peripartum cardiomyopathy exhibit increased blood levels of a biologically active proteolytic fragment of prolactin. Small clinical studies using the prolactin secretion inhibitor bromocriptine have shown promising results.

In Hypertrophic Cardiomyopathy Cardiac Hypertrophy Is out of Proportion to the Hemodynamic Load

HCM develops for no apparent physiologic reason, is probably genetically determined in most patients and is an autosomal dominant trait in half of patients. Many people without a family history probably have spontaneous mutations or a mild form of disease that is difficult to detect. The prevalence of HCM in the United States is about 1 in 500.

MOLECULAR PATHOGENESIS: The clinical picture of HCM is typically caused by dominant mutations in genes encoding proteins of the sarcomere (Table 11-9). Unlike DCM in which no single mutant gene accounts for many cases, 80% of HCM cases for which a genetic basis can be identified involve mutations in only two genes: those encoding β-myosin heavy chain and myosin-binding protein C. Mutations in genes for cardiac troponin T, cardiac troponin I and α-tropomyosin-1 (components of the troponin complex) account for most of the remaining cases. However, like DCM, there is marked allelic heterogeneity in HCM such that most mutations occur "privately" or at frequencies of less than 1%. Thus, hundreds of different mutations, mostly missense, have been identified. In addition, mutations in several nonsarcomeric protein genes have rarely been linked to the clinical phenotype of HCM. As noted in the discussion of DCM, different mutations in the same gene can give rise to diverse clinical phenotypes of DCM or HCM.

Table 11-9

Genetic Causes of Hypertrophic Cardiomyopathy

Gene	Locus	OMIM*	Gene Product	Frequency	Related Disorders
Autosomal Dominant					
MYH7	14q12	160760	β-myosin heavy chain	30%–40%	Dilated cardiomyopathy (DCM)
MYBPC3	11p11.2	600958	Myosin-binding protein C	30%–40%	DCM
TNNT2	1q32	191045	Cardiac troponin T	5%	DCM
TNNI3	19q13.4	191044	Cardiac troponin I	5%	DCM, restrictive cardiomyopathy
TPM1	15q22.1	191010	α-tropomyosin 1	≈1%–2%	DCM
MYL2	12q23-q24.3	160781	Cardiac myosin light chain 2	?	
MYL3	3p	160790	Myosin light chain 3	≈1%	
ACTC	15q14	102540	Cardiac actin	≈1%	DCM
TTN	2q31	188840	Titin	Rare	DCM
MYH6	14q12	160710	α-myosin heavy chain	<1%	DCM, dominantly inherited atrial septal defect
TCAP	17q12	604488	Titin cap or telethonin	<1%	DCM, limb girdle muscular dystrophy (LGMD)
MYOZ2	4q26-q27	605602	Myozenin 2	<1%	
CSRP3	11p15.1	600824	Muscle LIM protein	Rare	DCM
MYLK2	20q13.3	606566	Myosin light chain kinase 2	Rare	
LDB3	10q22.2-q23.3	605906	LIM domain-binding 3	Rare	DCM
VCL	10q22.1-q23	193065	Metavinculin	Rare	DCM
ACTN2	1q42-q43	102573	α-actinin 2	Rare	DCM
PLN	6q22.1	172405	Phospholamban	Rare	DCM
JPH2	20q12	605267	Junctophilin 2	Rare	
CAV3	3p25	601253	Caveolin 3	Rare	Long QT syndrome, LGMD
CALR3	19p13.12	611414	Calreticulin 3	Rare	

*OMIM is Online Mendelian Inheritance in Man, http://www.ncbi.nlm.nih.gov/sites/entrez?db=omim.

The mechanistic link between the mutations and the resultant clinical and pathologic phenotypes of HCM is poorly understood. In general, it is thought that the mutant protein is incorporated into the sarcomere, where it acts in a dominant-negative fashion to cause a loss of sarcomeric function. ***This proposed mechanism has led to the hypothesis that HCM is related to defects in force generation due to altered sarcomeric function.*** Hypertrophy may then occur as a compensatory response. Other mutations, such as those involving myosin light chain and α-tropomyosin-1 genes, may actually enhance contractility and, thereby, lead to hypertrophy. Still others (e.g., mutations in the myosin-binding protein C gene) may produce proteins that do not become incorporated into sarcomeres. These might lead to hypertrophy because a functional protein is missing, rather than by a dominant-negative effect.

Because of the risk of sudden death in HCM, there have been many attempts to use genetics to help stratify risk. Overall, the results have been disappointing, although some correlations have been recognized. For example, selected mutations in β-myosin heavy-chain and troponin T genes involve a high likelihood of sudden death. In the case of the β-myosin heavy-chain mutations, the risk of sudden death correlates with the amount of hypertrophy, whereas troponin T mutations, which are also linked to sudden death, produce minimal or no hypertrophy. HCM in patients with myosin-binding protein C mutations is usually benign clinically, and is associated with slowly progressive hypertrophy developing late in life. A few patients (2% to 5%) have mutations in two genes. This is generally associated with earlier onset and a more severe clinical phenotype.

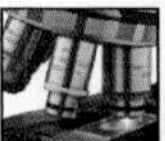

PATHOLOGY: The heart in HCM is always enlarged, but the degree of hypertrophy is different in different genetic forms. The left ventricular wall is thick, and its cavity is small, sometimes being reduced to a slit. Papillary muscles and trabeculae carneae are prominent and encroach on the lumen. More than half of cases exhibit asymmetric hypertrophy of the interventricular septum, with a ratio of the thickness of the septum to that of the left ventricular free wall greater than 1.5 (Fig. 11-43A). There are some rare genetic forms of HCM in which only the apical portion of the left ventricle or the papillary muscles are selectively hypertrophied. Often, the thickened, hypertrophied interventricular septum bulges into the left ventricular outflow tract early in ventricular systole, causing subvalvular obstruction of the aortic outflow tract. In this situation, an endocardial mural plaque is typically seen in the outflow tract, corresponding to the contact point where the anterior mitral valve leaflet impinges on the septal wall of the outflow tract during systole. Both atria are commonly dilated.

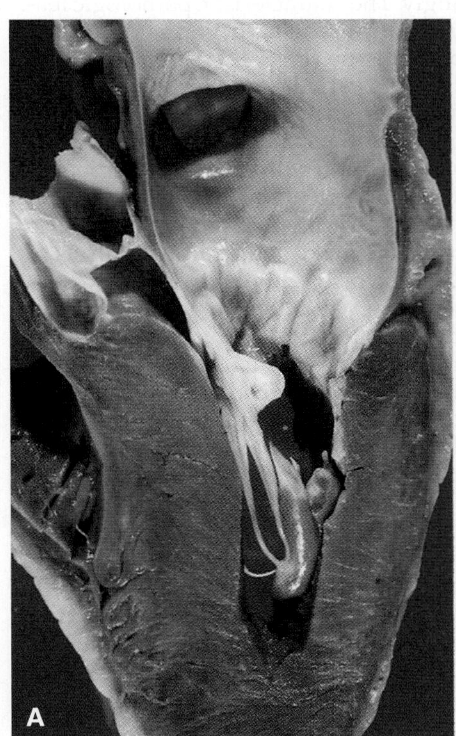

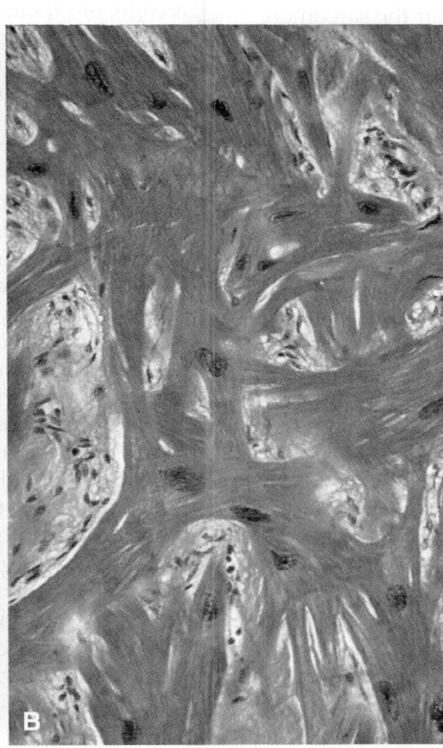

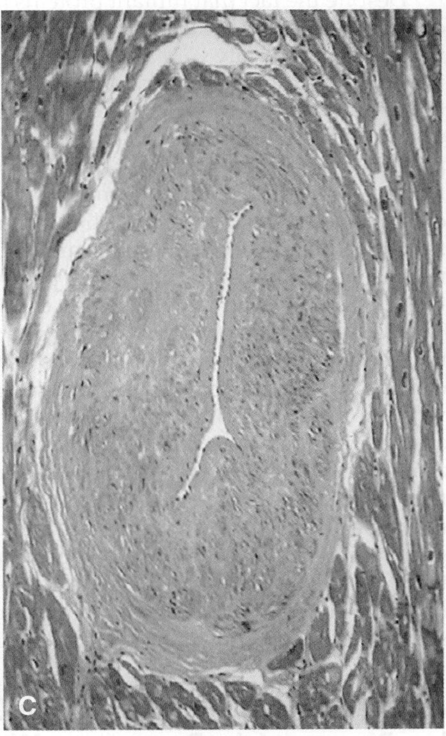

FIGURE 11-43. Hypertrophic cardiomyopathy (HCM). A. The heart has been opened to show striking asymmetric left ventricular hypertrophy. The interventricular septum is thicker than the free wall of the left ventricle and impinges on the outflow tract such that it contacts the underside of the anterior mitral valve leaflet. The left atrium is markedly enlarged. **B.** A section of the myocardium shows the characteristic myofiber disarray and hyperplasia of interstitial cells. **C.** A small intramural coronary artery shows a thickened, hypercellular media. This type of remodeling of coronary vessels could contribute to development of angina-like symptoms in some patients with HCM.

The most notable histologic feature of HCM is **myofiber disarray,** which is most extensive in the interventricular septum. Instead of the usual parallel arrangement of myocytes into muscle bundles, myofiber disarray is characterized by oblique and often perpendicular orientations of adjacent hypertrophic myocytes (Fig. 11-43B). By electron microscopy, myofibrils and myofilaments within individual myocytes are also disorganized. Such structural disarrangements are also frequently present in infants with congenital heart defects and can be observed under a variety of circumstances. However, they are always extensive in HCM and are not as widespread in other situations. There is usually hyperplasia of interstitial cells, and intramural coronary arteries may become thick and cellular (Fig. 11-43C).

CLINICAL FEATURES: Many patients with HCM have few, if any, symptoms, and the diagnosis is commonly made during screening of the family with an affected member. Despite a lack of symptoms, such persons may be at risk for sudden death, particularly during severe exertion. In fact, unsuspected HCM is commonly found at autopsy in young competitive athletes who die suddenly (see Fig. 11-47). Clinical recognition of HCM can occur at any age, often in the third, fourth or fifth decade of life, but the disorder also is encountered in the elderly (mainly in patients with myosin-binding protein C mutations). Some patients with HCM become incapacitated by cardiac symptoms, of which dyspnea, angina pectoris and syncope are most common. The clinical course tends to remain stable for many years, although eventually the disease can progress to congestive heart failure. In 10% of patients, DCM supervenes.

Despite the fact that mutant proteins impair the sarcomere, contractile function in HCM tends to be hyperdynamic. Ejection fractions are typically very high and most of the stroke volume is ejected during early systole. The most prominent dysfunctional aspect of HCM is decreased left ventricular compliance (diastolic dysfunction), which results in increased end-diastolic pressure. Mitral regurgitation is also seen in many such patients, leading to the atrial dilation commonly seen in HCM (note the enlarged left atrium in Fig. 11-43). In one fourth of patients, functional obstruction of the left ventricular outflow tract occurs near the end of systole, resulting in a pressure gradient between the apex and the subvalvular region of the left ventricle.

HCM responds paradoxically to pharmacologic interventions. Heart failure from other causes is typically treated with cardiac glycosides to increase myocardial contractility and with diuretics to reduce intravascular volume. These drugs aggravate symptoms of HCM. Rather, HCM is treated with β-adrenergic blockers and calcium channel blockers, which reduce contractility, decrease outflow tract obstruction and may improve left ventricular relaxation during diastole. Surgical removal of a portion of the hypertrophic septum or injection of ethanol into a septal artery to cause localized infarction has been successful in relieving symptoms of obstruction but seems to have no impact on the risk of sudden death.

Arrhythmogenic Right Ventricular Cardiomyopathy Is a Disease of the Desmosome With a High Risk of Sudden Death

ARVC affects roughly 1 in 5000 individuals. It occurs most commonly in Mediterranean countries where it is a leading cause of sudden death in young people (younger than 35 years of age).

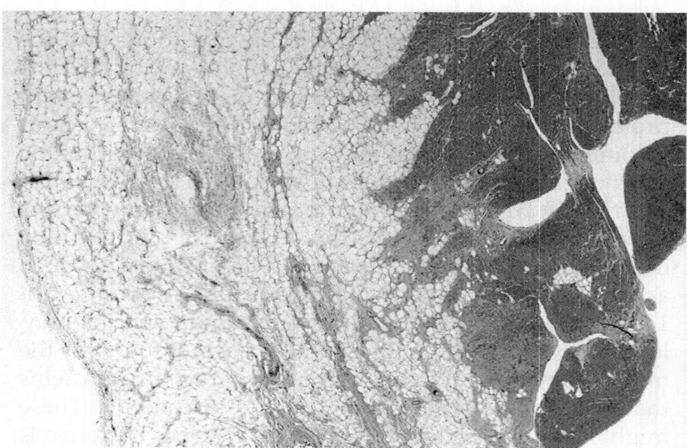

FIGURE 11-44. Arrhythmogenic right ventricular cardiomyopathy. This section of the right ventricular free wall shows that much of the myocardium has been replaced by mature adipose tissue and fibrosis such that only subendocardial muscle bundles remain.

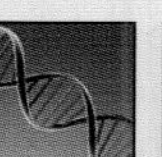
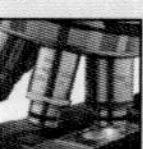

MOLECULAR PATHOGENESIS AND PATHOLOGY: ARVC is a associated with serious arrhythmias and/or sudden death, which may occur early in the disease before significant structural remodeling and contractile dysfunction develop. It typically affects the right ventricular free wall, although left dominant and biventricular forms are being recognized increasingly. The characteristic pathologic features are degeneration of cardiac myocytes and replacement by fat and fibrous tissue (Fig. 11-44), but the extent of this change can be quite variable and it is not necessarily conspicuous in patients who die suddenly.

ARVC is a familial disease, usually inherited in an autosomal dominant pattern. Its true incidence is probably underestimated because of very variable penetrance, age-related progression and large phenotypic variation. The diagnosis can be difficult to make and requires analysis of various clinical criteria, which, although relatively specific, are not very sensitive. Mutations in genes encoding proteins in desmosomes, cell–cell adhesion organelles, can be identified in nearly half of individuals who fulfill these criteria. These include genes for desmosomal adhesion molecules such as desmoglein-2 and intracellular desmosomal proteins including plakoglobin, desmoplakin and plakophilin-2, which form a complex that links the adhesion molecules to the desmin cytoskeleton in cardiac myocytes. Desmosomes are particularly abundant in heart and skin, two organs that experience the greatest mechanical burden, and mutations in desmosomal genes generally give rise to cutaneous and/or cardiac disease depending on the tissue-specific expression pattern of the mutant isoform. Ultimately, the mechanism by which desmosome mutations causes ARVC is unresolved.

Restrictive Cardiomyopathy Impairs Diastolic Function

Restrictive cardiomyopathy describes a group of diseases in which myocardial or endocardial abnormalities limit diastolic filling while contractile function remains normal. It is the least common category of cardiomyopathy in Western countries, although in some less developed regions (e.g., parts of equatorial Africa, South America and Asia), endomyocardial disease related to parasitic infections leads to many cases of restrictive cardiomyopathy.

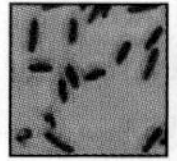
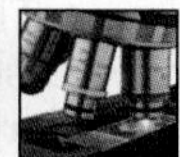

ETIOLOGIC FACTORS AND PATHOLOGY: Restrictive cardiomyopathy is caused by (1) interstitial infiltration of amyloid, metastatic carcinoma or sarcoid granulomas; (2) endomyocardial disease characterized by marked fibrotic thickening of the endocardium; (3) genetic and storage diseases, including hemochromatosis and desmin-related cardiomyopathies; and (4) markedly increased interstitial fibrous tissue. The pathophysiologic consequence is a preload-dependent state, characterized by defective diastolic compliance, restricted ventricular filling, increased end-diastolic pressure, atrial dilation and venous congestion. In many respects, these hemodynamic changes are similar to the consequences of constrictive pericarditis. Many cases of restrictive cardiomyopathy are classified as idiopathic, with interstitial fibrosis as the only histologic abnormality.

The disease almost invariably progresses to congestive heart failure, and only 10% of the patients survive for 10 years.

Amyloidosis

The heart is affected in most forms of generalized amyloidosis (see Chapter 23). In fact, restrictive cardiomyopathy is the most common cause of death in AL amyloidosis of plasma cell dyscrasias.

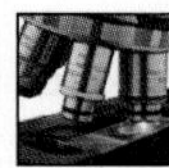

PATHOLOGY: Amyloid infiltration of the heart results in cardiac enlargement without ventricular dilation. The gross appearance of the heart may resemble that seen in hypertrophic cardiomyopathy. Ventricular walls are typically thickened, firm and rubbery. Microscopically, amyloid accumulation is most prominent in interstitial, perivascular and endocardial regions (Fig. 11-45). Endocardial involvement is common in the atria, where nodular endocardial deposits often impart a granular appearance and gritty texture to the endocardial surface. Amyloid deposits also can cause thickening of cardiac valves. In rare cases, amyloid deposition within the walls of intramural coronary arteries narrows the lumens and causes ischemic injury.

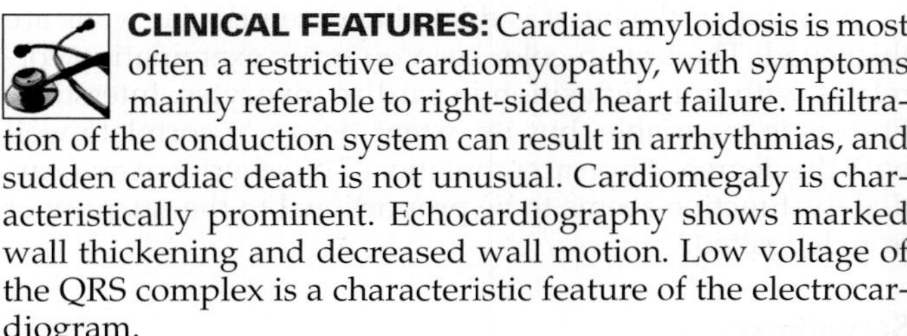

CLINICAL FEATURES: Cardiac amyloidosis is most often a restrictive cardiomyopathy, with symptoms mainly referable to right-sided heart failure. Infiltration of the conduction system can result in arrhythmias, and sudden cardiac death is not unusual. Cardiomegaly is characteristically prominent. Echocardiography shows marked wall thickening and decreased wall motion. Low voltage of the QRS complex is a characteristic feature of the electrocardiogram.

Some patients with cardiac amyloidosis initially present with congestive heart failure secondary to impaired systolic or contractile function. In these patients, diastolic dysfunction is often inconspicuous. As in patients with a restrictive presentation, the prognosis is grim: most survive less than 1 year once the disease becomes symptomatic.

SENILE CARDIAC AMYLOIDOSIS: In senile cardiac amyloidosis a protein closely related to prealbumin (transthyretin) is deposited in the hearts of elderly persons

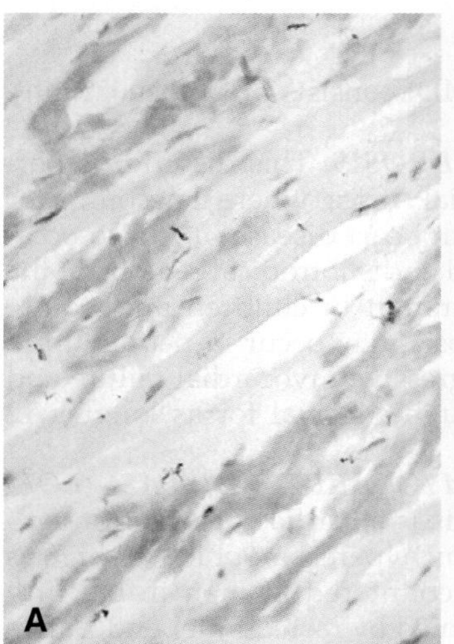

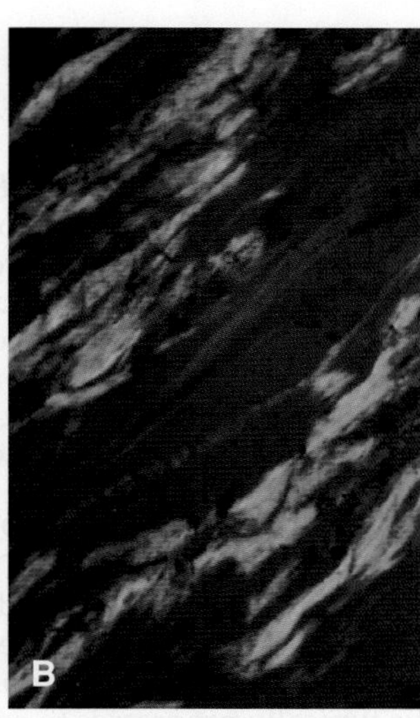

FIGURE 11-45. Cardiac amyloidosis. A. A section of myocardium stained with Congo red shows interstitial, pink-staining deposits of amyloid. **B.** Under polarized light, the same section displays the characteristic green birefringence of amyloid fibrils.

(see Chapter 23). The disorder may be present to some extent in up to 25% of patients 80 years old or older. It not only involves the heart (atria and ventricles) but, in many cases, the lungs and rectum as well. Amyloid deposits also may be found in blood vessel walls in many organs, but virtually never in renal glomeruli. The functional significance of senile cardiac amyloidosis is often minimal: it is usually an incidental finding at autopsy. Even when amyloid deposition is extensive and is associated with symptoms of congestive heart failure, progression of the disease is much slower than that in AL amyloidosis.

Two additional forms of isolated cardiovascular amyloidosis are common in the elderly: **senile aortic amyloidosis** and **isolated atrial amyloidosis.** Neither of these forms of amyloid contains prealbumin or closely related proteins.

Desmin-Related Cardiomyopathies

Desmin is the intermediate filament protein in cardiac, striated and smooth muscle. Desmin filaments bind to desmosomes at intercalated disks and span the length of the cardiac myocyte by binding to Z disks of sarcomeres and other intracellular organelles.

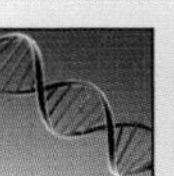
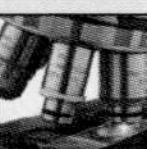

MOLECULAR PATHOGENESIS AND PATHOLOGY: Numerous mutations in desmin have been described in patients with skeletal and cardiomyopathies; most are inherited as autosomal dominant traits. The heart disease usually falls in the clinicopathologic spectrum of restrictive cardiomyopathies characterized by ventricular wall thickening, loss of ventricular compliance and diastolic dysfunction. In many forms, the mutant protein is expressed and presumably interferes with normal desmin filament production. Large intracellular aggregates of refractile material can be seen by light microscopy, which are tangled masses of misfolded desmin filaments.

Endomyocardial Disease

Endomyocardial disease (EMD) consists of two geographically separate disorders.

ENDOMYOCARDIAL FIBROSIS: This disorder is particularly common in equatorial Africa, where it accounts for 10% to 20% of all deaths from heart disease. It is also occasionally seen in other tropical and subtropical regions of the world. While it is most common in children and young adults, endomyocardial fibrosis may occur in people up to age 70 years. It leads to progressive myocardial failure and has a poor prognosis, although survival for as long as 12 years has been reported.

EOSINOPHILIC ENDOMYOCARDIAL DISEASE (LÖFFLER ENDOCARDITIS): This is a cardiac disorder of temperate regions characterized by hypereosinophilia (as high as 50,000/μL). It is usually encountered in men in the fifth decade and is often accompanied by rash. Löffler endocarditis typically progresses to congestive heart failure and death, although corticosteroids may improve survival.

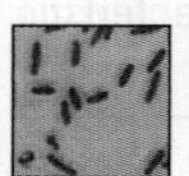

ETIOLOGIC FACTORS: Endomyocardial fibrosis and Löffler endocarditis were once considered distinct entities, but there is a growing consensus that they represent variants of the same underlying disease. ***EMD is suspected to result from myocardial injury produced by eosinophils, possibly mediated by cardiotoxic granule components.*** In the tropics, transient high blood eosinophil counts often result from parasitic infestations; in temperate climates, idiopathic hypereosinophilia is often persistent.

EMD can be divided into three stages:

1. The necrotic stage occurs within the first few months of the illness and is characterized by an intense eosinophilic infiltrate involving the inner layers of the myocardium, usually of both ventricles. The infiltrate is perivascular and interstitial, and there is evidence of vascular injury and myocyte necrosis. The necrotic stage lasts for several months, but significant functional impairment is rare.
2. The thrombotic stage develops about a year later, with mural thrombi attached to the injured and slightly thickened endocardium. At this time, the myocardium is no longer inflamed but shows early hypertrophy. Embolization is a common complication.
3. The fibrotic stage is the chronic phase of EMD and features conspicuous fibrotic thickening of the endocardium. Marked endocardial fibrosis results in decreased compliance and abnormal diastolic function. Adherence of the posterior mitral valve leaflet to the endocardium results in mitral regurgitation or, on the right side, tricuspid regurgitation.

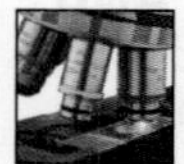

PATHOLOGY: At autopsy, a grayish white layer of thickened endocardium extends from the apex of the left ventricle over the posterior papillary muscle to the posterior leaflet of the mitral valve and for a short distance into the left outflow tract. On cut section, endocardial fibrosis spreads into the inner one third to one half of the ventricle wall. Mural thrombi in various stages of organization may be present. When the right ventricle is involved, the entire cavity may exhibit endocardial thickening, which may penetrate as far as the epicardium. Microscopically, the fibrotic endocardium contains only a few elastic fibers. Myofibers trapped within the collagenous tissue display nonspecific degenerative changes.

Storage Diseases

Lysosomal storage diseases are discussed in detail in Chapter 6. Only the cardiac manifestations are reviewed here.

GLYCOGEN STORAGE DISEASES: Of the various forms of glycogen storage disease, types II (Pompe disease), III (Cori disease) and IV (Andersen disease) affect the heart. The most common and severe involvement is with Pompe disease. In infants with this condition, the heart is markedly enlarged (up to seven times normal), with 20% of patients having endocardial fibroelastosis. Myocytes are vacuolated owing to large amounts of stored glycogen. Functionally, patients show a restrictive type of cardiomyopathy, and usually die from cardiac failure.

MUCOPOLYSACCHARIDOSES: Several of the mucopolysaccharidoses involve the heart. Cardiac disease results from lysosomal accumulation of mucopolysaccharides (glycosaminoglycans) in various cells. In general, pseudohypertrophy of the ventricles develops and contractility gradually diminishes. The coronary arteries may be narrowed by intimal and medial thickening. In Hurler and Hunter syndromes, myocardial infarction is common. Valve leaflets may be thickened, thereby producing progressive valvular dysfunction, manifested as aortic stenosis (Scheie syndrome) or mitral regurgitation (Hurler, Morquio syndromes). Cor pulmonale may result from pulmonary hypertension related to narrowing of the airways.

SPHINGOLIPIDOSES: **Fabry disease** may result in glycosphingolipid accumulation in the heart, with functional and pathologic changes similar to those that complicate the mucopolysaccharidoses. Fabry disease typically produces gross and microscopic changes that mimic HCM, but the characteristic vacuolated appearance of cardiac myocytes is an important clue of an underlying storage disease. **Gaucher disease,** which only rarely involves the heart, may feature interstitial infiltration of the left ventricle by cerebroside-laden macrophages, with impairment of left ventricular compliance and cardiac output.

HEMOCHROMATOSIS: This multiorgan disease is associated with excessive iron deposition in many tissues (see Chapter 14). The degree of iron deposition in the heart varies and only roughly correlates with that in other organs. Cardiac involvement has features of both dilated and restrictive cardiomyopathy, with systolic and diastolic impairment. ***Congestive heart failure occurs in as many as one third of patients with hemochromatosis.***

At autopsy, the heart is dilated and ventricular walls are thickened. The brown color seen on gross examination correlates with iron deposition in cardiac myocytes. Interstitial fibrosis is invariable, but its extent does not correlate well with the degree of iron accumulation. The severity of myocardial dysfunction seems to be proportional to the quantity of iron deposited.

Sarcoidosis

Sarcoidosis is a generalized granulomatous disease that may involve the heart (see Chapter 12). One quarter of cases of sarcoidosis show some granulomas in the heart at autopsy, but fewer than 5% of patients with this condition have clinical symptoms. Sarcoid heart disease is seen clinically as a mixed pattern of dilated and restrictive cardiomyopathy. Sarcoid granulomas often produce large areas of myocardial damage. The base of the interventricular

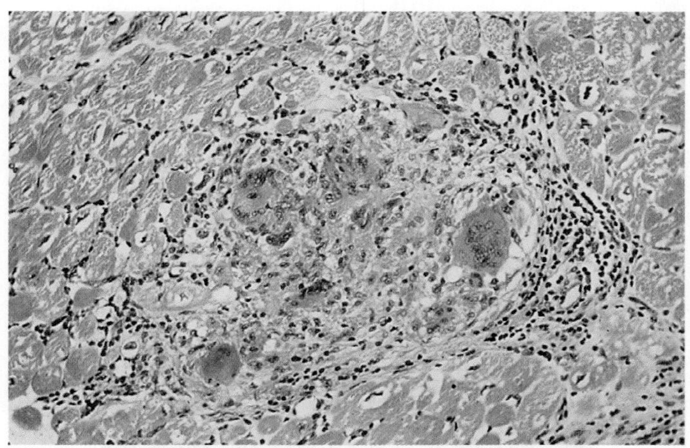

FIGURE 11-46. Cardiac sarcoidosis. The myocardium is infiltrated by noncaseating granulomas, with prominent giant cells. There is considerable destruction of cardiac myocytes with fibrosis.

septum is preferentially involved. Because this region contains major components of the atrioventricular conduction system, bundle branch blocks or complete heart block is often seen. More serious life-threatening arrhythmias and sudden death are common. Microscopic examination of the heart in severe cases of sarcoid heart disease reveals infiltration of the myocardium by noncaseating granulomas, massive destruction of myocytes and replacement by interstitial fibrosis (Fig. 11-46).

Sudden Cardiac Death

More than 300,000 people in the United States die suddenly each year. Most of these deaths are caused by spontaneous lethal ventricular tachyarrhythmias—ventricular tachycardia and ventricular fibrillation—in patients with some type of heart disease. Many sudden deaths occur out of hospital in apparently healthy individuals who exhibit coronary artery disease at autopsy but may have had little clinical evidence of heart disease during life.

Common causes of sudden cardiac death differ in young and old individuals. This has been studied most thoroughly in competitive athletes (Fig. 11-47). In subjects younger than 35 years of age, HCM, idiopathic left ventricular hypertrophy (presumably reflecting genetic forms of heart muscle disease in at least some) and congenital coronary anomalies account for over 75% of sudden deaths. In Italy and other Mediterranean countries, ARVC is a leading cause of sudden death in young people. ***However, in economically developed nations, coronary artery disease is responsible for most sudden deaths in middle-aged and older adults.***

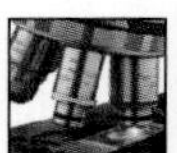

PATHOLOGY: The surface electrocardiogram (ECG) may occasionally indicate a specific pathologic structure that can be implicated in causing sudden death such as an accessory atrioventricular connection in Wolff-Parkinson-White syndrome or a lesion that disrupts a discrete component of the ventricular conduction system causing new bundle branch block. ***However, lethal arrhythmias usually arise from pathologic changes affecting conduction properties of the working ventricular myocardium.*** At autopsy, the heart of a sudden death victim typically exhibits structural alterations of myocardium that create "anatomic substrates of arrhythmias." These changes may be localized (e.g., healed myocardial infarcts or left ventricular aneurysms) or diffuse (e.g., variable degrees of cardiac myocyte hypertrophy and interstitial fibrosis). Spontaneous development of a lethal cardiac arrhythmia may be regarded as a stochastic event arising from complex interactions between relatively fixed anatomic substrates and acute, transient triggering events such as acute ischemia, neurohormonal activation, changes in electrolytes or other stresses. Many patients have potential arrhythmia substrates in their hearts. In most cases, they may be necessary but are not sufficient for arrhythmogenesis. An arrhythmia is most likely when acute electrophysiologic changes (triggers) are superimposed on an existing substrate of remodeled myocardium with characteristic conduction

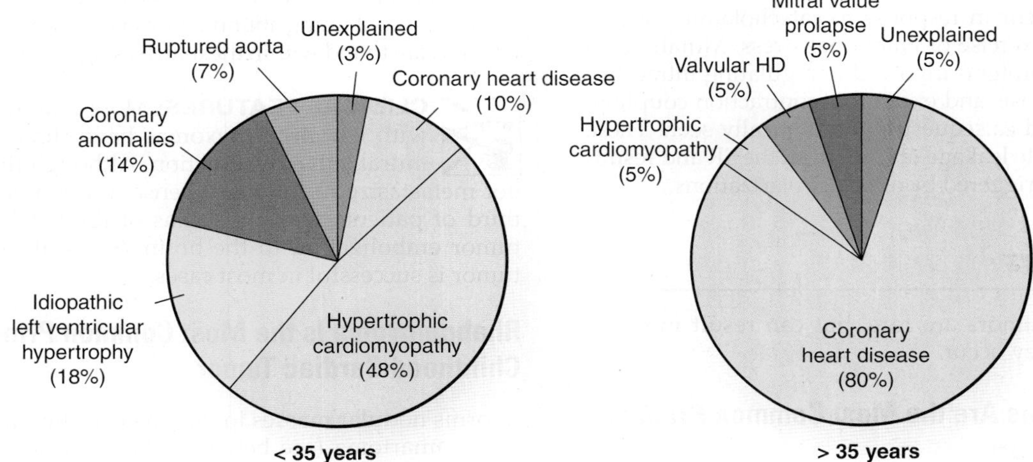

FIGURE 11-47. Different causes of sudden cardiac death in young and older adult competitive athletes. HD = heart disease.

abnormalities. Indeed, the most frequent clinicopathologic scenario in which sudden death occurs involves acute ischemia (a transient triggering event) in an area of the heart containing a healed infarct (a common anatomic substrate).

Sudden Cardiac Death Occurs in Patients With Structurally Normal Hearts, but This Is Rare

Some (perhaps many) of these patients have "channelopathies," genetic diseases in which mutations in genes for Na^+, K^+ and Ca^{2+} channel proteins are responsible for sudden death syndromes (see Chapter 1). Although these syndromes are rare, they have provided valuable insights into molecular mechanisms of lethal arrhythmias.

MOLECULAR PATHOGENESIS: *LONG QT SYNDROME:* This condition is defined by prolongation of the QT interval and T-wave abnormalities on the surface ECG along with a history of syncope, ventricular arrhythmias or sudden, unexpected death. More than 10 different types of congenital long QT syndrome have been defined. Most are caused by loss-of-function mutations in genes encoding proteins that form various K^+ channels. The loss of function prolongs repolarization of the cardiac action potential (thereby increasing the QT interval on the surface ECG) and promotes arrhythmias by increasing the likelihood of after-depolarizations. The long QT syndrome can also be caused by gain-of-function mutations in *SCN5A*, the gene encoding the cardiac Na^+ channel protein. These mutations prolong QT intervals by allowing leakage of depolarizing current during repolarization. Mutations in proteins responsible for ion channel trafficking or scaffolding, such as ankyrin B and caveolin-3, are also implicated in long QT syndrome.

BRUGADA SYNDROME: This is an autosomal dominant disease in a structurally normal heart with characteristic ST-segment elevation in the right precordial leads, right bundle branch block and susceptibility to life-threatening arrhythmias. Loss-of-function mutations in *SCN5A* are identified in approximately 25% of cases.

CATECHOLAMINERGIC POLYMORPHIC VENTRICULAR TACHYCARDIA: In this condition, arrhythmias and sudden death occur in response to catecholamine surges associated with exercise or emotional stress. Mutations in genes encoding proteins involved in regulating intracellular Ca^{2+} homeostasis and excitation–contraction coupling, such as RyR2 and calsequestrin, are typically seen. These mutations promote leakage of Ca^{2+} from the SR and resultant arrhythmias triggered by after-depolarizations.

Cardiac Tumors

Primary cardiac tumors are rare, but can result in serious problems when they occur.

Cardiac Myxomas Are the Most Common Primary Tumors of the Heart

Cardiac myxomas account for 30% to 50% of all primary cardiac tumors. They are usually sporadic, but are occasionally associated with familial autosomal dominant syndromes.

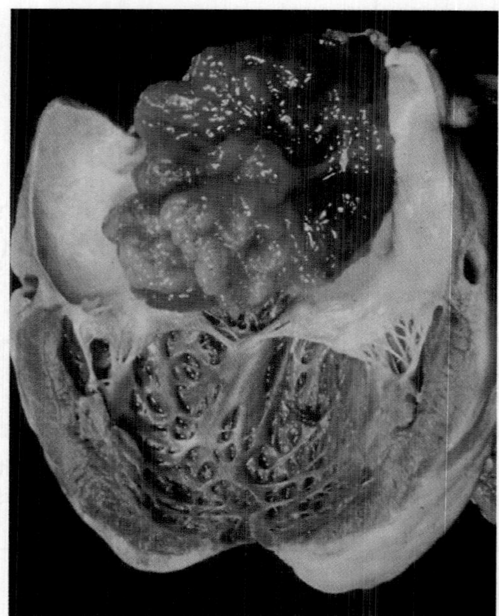

FIGURE 11-48. Cardiac myxoma. The left atrium contains a large, polypoid tumor that protrudes into the mitral valve orifice.

MOLECULAR PATHOGENESIS: Most cardiac myxomas appear sporadically, but about 7% are part of a familial autosomal dominant syndrome that also includes pigmented lesions of the skin and adrenocortical hyperplasia. These cases have been linked to mutations in the gene encoding a regulatory subunit of cAMP-dependent protein kinase (protein kinase A), which, among other actions, appears to be a tumor suppressor gene that controls cell proliferation.

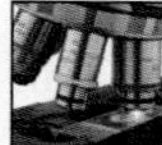

PATHOLOGY: Myxomas can occur in any cardiac chamber or on a valve, but most (75%) arise in the left atrium. The tumors appear as glistening, gelatinous, polypoid masses, usually 5 to 6 cm in diameter, with a short stalk (Fig. 11-48). They may be sufficiently mobile to obstruct the mitral valve orifice. Microscopically, they show loose myxoid stroma containing abundant proteoglycans. Polygonal stellate cells are found within the matrix, singly or in small clusters.

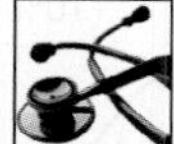

CLINICAL FEATURES: More than half of patients with left atrial myxomas have clinical evidence of mitral valve dysfunction. Although the tumor does not metastasize in the usual sense, it often embolizes. One third of patients with myxomas of the left heart die from tumor embolization to the brain. Surgical removal of the tumor is successful in most cases.

Rhabdomyoma Is the Most Common Primary Childhood Cardiac Tumor

It forms nodular masses in the myocardium. It may actually be a hamartoma (see below) rather than a true neoplasm, although the issue is still debated. Almost all are multiple and involve both ventricles and, in one third of cases, the atria as well. In half of cases, the tumor projects into a cardiac chamber and obstructs the lumen or valve orifices.

MOLECULAR PATHOGENESIS: Rhabdomyomas occur in one third of patients with tuberous sclerosis, the familial form of which is caused by mutations in *TSC1* and *TSC2*, genes that encode hamartin and tuberin, respectively. Both genes function as tumor suppressors and regulate embryonic and neonatal growth and differentiation of cardiac myocytes.

PATHOLOGY: On gross examination, cardiac rhabdomyomas are pale masses, 1 mm to several centimeters in diameter. Microscopically, tumor cells show small central nuclei and abundant glycogen-rich clear cytoplasm, in which fibrillar processes containing sarcomeres radiate to the margin of the cell ("spider cell"). These tumors often occur in association with tuberous sclerosis (one third to one half of cases). A few cardiac rhabdomyomas have been successfully excised.

Papillary Fibroelastoma Involves the Valves

Papillary fronds resembling a sea anemone and measuring up to 3 to 4 cm in diameter may grow on the heart valves. These tumors are not neoplasms and are more appropriately termed **hamartomas.** The fronds have a central dense core of collagen and elastic fibers surrounded by looser connective tissue. They are covered by a continuation of valvular endothelial cells on which the tumor originates. In most instances, papillary fibroelastomas pose no clinical problem, but they can fragment and embolize to other organs or occlude a coronary artery orifice and produce myocardial ischemia.

Other Tumors in the Heart Are Rare

Other primary tumors of the heart include angiomas, fibromas, lymphangiomas, neurofibromas and their sarcomatous counterparts. Lipomatous hypertrophy of the interatrial septum and encapsulated lipomas have been reported.

Metastatic tumors to the heart are seen most frequently in patients with the most prevalent forms of carcinomas—that is, lung, breast and gastrointestinal tract. Still, only a minority of patients with these tumors will show cardiac metastases. Lymphomas and leukemia also may involve the heart. Of all tumors, the one most likely to metastasize to the heart is malignant melanoma (Fig. 11-49). Metastatic cancer involving the myocardium can result in clinical manifestations of restrictive cardiomyopathy, particularly if the cardiac tumors are associated with extensive fibrosis.

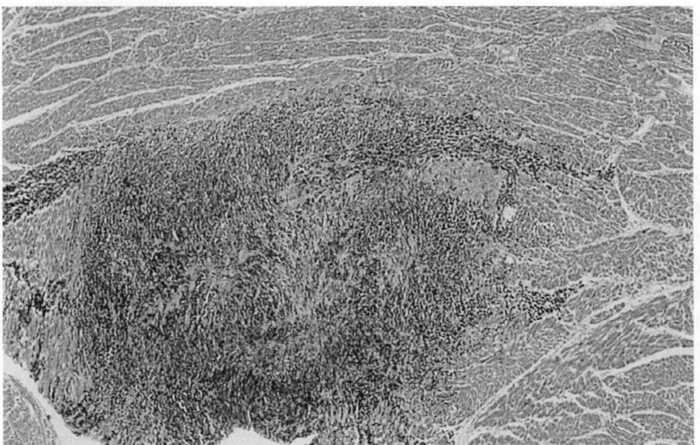

FIGURE 11-49. Malignant melanoma metastatic to the heart. The myocardium contains a heavily pigmented tumor metastasis.

Diseases of the Pericardium

Pericardial Effusion Can Cause Cardiac Tamponade

Pericardial effusion is accumulation of excess fluid within the pericardial cavity, as either a transudate or an exudate. The pericardial sac normally contains no more than 50 mL of lubricating fluid. If the pericardium is slowly distended, it can accommodate up to 2 L of fluid without notable hemodynamic consequences. However, rapid accumulation of as little as 150 to 200 mL of pericardial fluid or blood may significantly increase intrapericardial pressure and restrict diastolic filling, especially of the right ventricle.

- **Serous pericardial effusion** is often a complication of an increase in extracellular fluid volume, as occurs in congestive heart failure or the nephrotic syndrome. The fluid has a low protein content and few cellular elements.
- **Chylous effusion** (fluid containing chylomicrons) results from a communication of the thoracic duct with the pericardial space due to lymphatic obstruction by tumor or infection.
- **Serosanguineous pericardial effusion** may develop after chest trauma, either accidentally or caused by cardiopulmonary resuscitation.
- **Hemopericardium** is bleeding directly into the pericardial cavity (Fig. 11-50). The most common cause is ventricular

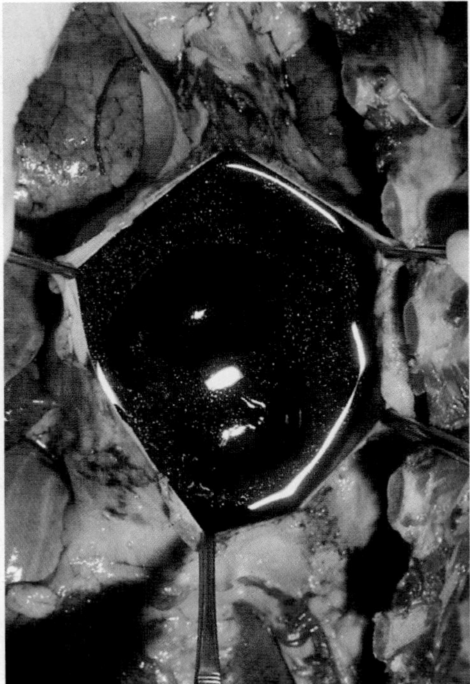

FIGURE 11-50. Hemopericardium. The parietal pericardium has been opened to reveal the pericardial cavity distended with fresh blood. The patient sustained a rupture of a myocardial infarct.

free wall rupture at a myocardial infarct. Less frequent causes are penetrating cardiac trauma, rupture of a dissecting aneurysm of the aorta, infiltration of a vessel by tumor or a bleeding diathesis.

Cardiac tamponade *is the syndrome produced by rapid accumulation of pericardial fluid, which restricts the filling of the heart.* The hemodynamic consequences range from a minimally symptomatic condition to abrupt cardiovascular collapse and death. As pericardial pressure increases, it reaches and then exceeds central venous pressure, thereby limiting return of blood to the heart. Cardiac output and blood pressure decrease, and **pulsus paradoxus** (an abnormal decrease in systolic pressure with inspiration) occurs in almost all patients. Acute cardiac tamponade is almost invariably fatal unless the pressure is relieved by removing pericardial fluid, by either needle pericardiocentesis or surgical procedures.

Acute Pericarditis May Follow Viral Infections

Pericarditis refers to inflammation of the visceral or parietal pericardium.

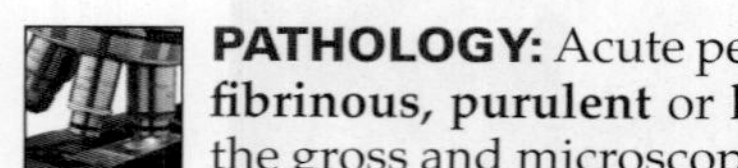

ETIOLOGIC FACTORS: The causes of pericarditis are similar to those for myocarditis (Table 11-7). In most cases, the cause of acute pericarditis is obscure and (as in myocarditis) is attributed to undiagnosed viral infection. Bacterial pericarditis is unusual in the antibiotic era. Metastatic tumors may induce serofibrinous or hemorrhagic exudative and inflammatory reactions when they involve the pericardium. The most common tumors to involve the pericardium and cause a malignant pericardial effusion are breast and lung carcinomas. Pericarditis associated with myocardial infarction and rheumatic fever is discussed above.

PATHOLOGY: Acute pericarditis can be classified as **fibrinous, purulent** or **hemorrhagic,** depending on the gross and microscopic characteristics of the pericardial surfaces and fluid. The most common form is fibrinous pericarditis, in which the normal smooth, glistening pericardial surfaces are replaced by a dull, granular fibrin-rich exudate (Fig. 11-51). The rough texture of inflamed pericardial surfaces produces the characteristic friction rub heard by auscultation. Effusion fluid in fibrinous pericarditis is usually rich in protein, and the pericardium contains primarily mononuclear inflammatory cells. Uremia can cause fibrinous pericarditis (Fig. 11-52), although with the widespread availability of renal dialysis, uremic pericarditis is now unusual in the United States. The most common causes are viral infection and pericarditis following myocardial infarcts.

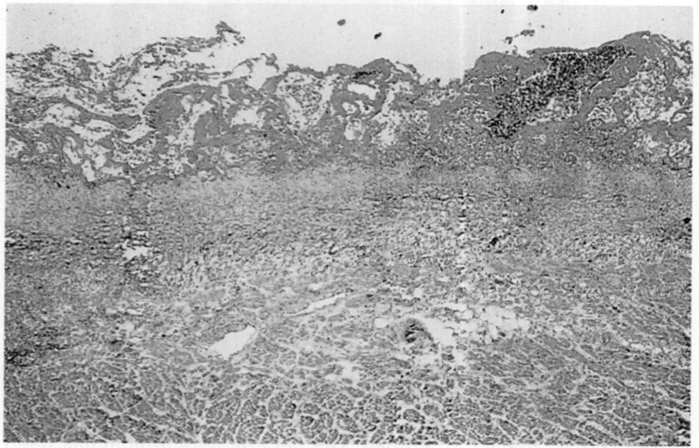

FIGURE 11-51. Fibrinous pericardial exudate. The epicardial surface is edematous, inflamed and covered with tentacles of fibrin.

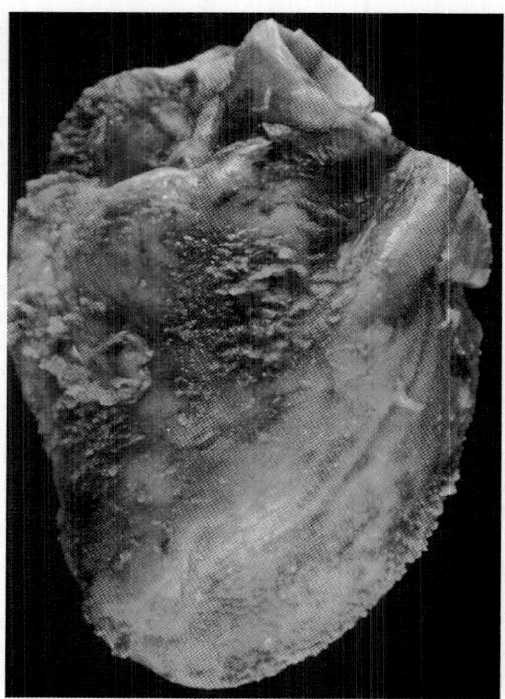

FIGURE 11-52. Fibrinous pericarditis. The heart of a patient who died in uremia displays a shaggy, fibrinous exudate covering the visceral pericardium.

Bacterial infection leads to a purulent pericarditis, in which the pericardial exudate resembles pus and contains many neutrophils. Bleeding into the pericardial space caused by aggressive infectious or neoplastic processes or coagulation defects leads to hemorrhagic pericarditis.

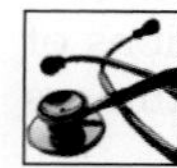

CLINICAL FEATURES: The initial manifestation of acute pericarditis is sudden, severe, substernal chest pain, sometimes referred to the back, shoulder or neck. It is distinguished from the pain of angina pectoris or myocardial infarction by its failure to radiate down the left arm. A characteristic pericardial friction rub is easily heard. Electrocardiographic changes reflect repolarization abnormalities of the myocardium.

Idiopathic or viral pericarditis is a self-limited disorder, although it may infrequently lead to constrictive pericarditis. Corticosteroids are the treatment of choice. Therapy for other specific forms of acute pericarditis varies with the cause.

Constrictive Pericarditis May Mimic Right Heart Failure

Constrictive pericarditis is a chronic fibrosing disease of the pericardium that compresses the heart and restricts inflow.

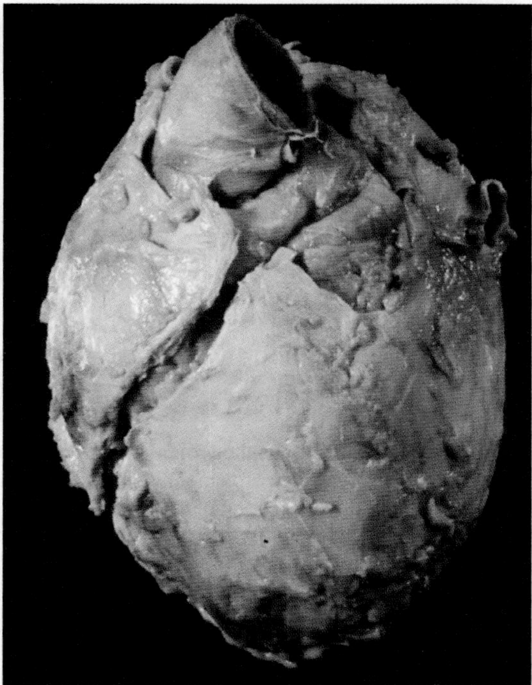

FIGURE 11-53. Constrictive pericarditis. The pericardial space has been obliterated, and the heart is encased in a fibrotic, thickened pericardium.

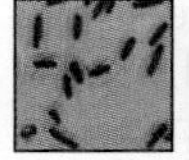
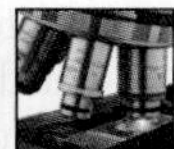

ETIOLOGIC FACTORS AND PATHOLOGY: Constrictive pericarditis is not an active inflammatory condition. Rather, it results from an exuberant healing response after acute pericardial injury. The pericardial space becomes obliterated and visceral and parietal layers become fused in a dense, rigid mass of fibrous tissue. The scarred pericardium may be so thick (up to 3 cm) that it narrows the orifices of the venae cavae (Fig. 11-53). The fibrous envelope may contain calcium deposits. The condition is infrequent today and, in developed countries, is predominantly idiopathic. Prior radiation therapy to the mediastinum and cardiac surgery account for more than one third of cases. In others, constrictive pericarditis follows a purulent or tuberculous infection. Although tuberculosis today accounts for fewer than 15% of cases of constrictive pericarditis in industrialized countries, it is still the major cause in underdeveloped regions.

CLINICAL FEATURES: Patients with constrictive pericarditis have a small, quiet heart in which venous inflow is restricted, as the rigid pericardium determines the diastolic volume of the heart. These patients have high venous pressure, low cardiac output, small pulse pressure and fluid retention with ascites and peripheral edema. Total pericardiectomy is the treatment of choice.

Adhesive pericarditis is a much milder form of healing of an inflamed pericardium. Commonly seen as an incidental finding at autopsy, it is the outcome of many different types of pericarditis that have healed and left only minor fibrous adhesions between the visceral and parietal surfaces.

Pathology of Interventional Therapies

Percutaneous Coronary Interventions Are Used to Treat Atherosclerotic Coronary Disease

PCI is used to mechanically dilate an artery narrowed by atherosclerosis and keep the lumen open. A catheter with a deflated balloon covered by a collapsed cylindrical metallic mesh (**stent**) is positioned in the stenotic segment. Inflating the balloon fractures the plaque and stretches the vessel wall. As the stent deploys, it holds the fragmented wall open and keeps the vessel lumen patent. Acute complications of PCI such as coronary artery dissection, acute thrombotic occlusion and perforation are uncommon. Most patients receive drug-eluting stents, which slowly release antiproliferative agents such as sirolimus or paclitaxel. Their use has dramatically reduced the incidence of restenosis.

Coronary Bypass Grafts Circumvent Obstructed Segments

Coronary bypass grafting, using a saphenous vein or left internal mammary artery to direct blood around a blockage, is common treatment for proximal coronary stenosis. Although operative mortality is low and early symptomatic relief occurs in most patients, myocardial perfusion is not permanently improved, owing to several complications: (1) early thrombosis, (2) intimal hyperplasia and (3) atherosclerosis of vein grafts. Moreover, progressive atherosclerosis of the native coronary arteries is not affected by the grafting procedure.

Internal mammary artery grafts develop fewer pathologic changes and so last longer than vein grafts. Excised saphenous vein segments used as grafts are subjected to unavoidable surgical manipulation and an interval of ischemia during harvesting, which results in endothelial cell injury. Grafted veins are also exposed to arterial pressures that are much higher than those in its native location. Finally, the caliber of the vein, which is expanded by arterial blood pressure, is usually much greater than that of the distal coronary artery at the graft anastomosis, and this mismatch promotes blood stasis. In the immediate postoperative period, these factors enhance the probability of thrombosis and probably play a role in the eventual development of intimal hyperplasia. Intimal hyperplasia is characterized by a concentric proliferation of smooth muscle cells and fibroblasts and collagen deposition in the intima of the vein. After several years, lipids may deposit and atherosclerotic plaques may form in the thickened intima of vein grafts. Atherosclerosis is the most frequent cause of vein graft failure in patients who have had good graft function for several years after surgery.

Because arteries are better suited than veins to serve as aortocoronary bypass conduits, some surgeons have developed total arterial bypass procedures that use internal mammary, radial and selected abdominal arteries that can be harvested without causing significant end-organ damage.

There Are Two Types of Valve Replacements: Tissue Xenografts and Mechanical Valves

In most patients with severe valve dysfunction, valve replacement is the best prospect for long-term symptomatic improvement. Operative mortality is low, especially for patients with good preoperative myocardial function. Half of all patients with prosthetic valves are free of complications after 10 years.

TISSUE VALVES: The most commonly used tissue-valve prostheses use a mechanical frame to which glutaraldehyde-fixed porcine aortic valve cusps or pieces of bovine pericardium are attached. These valves have good hemodynamic characteristics, cause little obstruction and resist thromboembolic complications. Unfortunately, they are not very durable. The most common cause of failure of tissue-valve prostheses is tissue degeneration with severe calcification and fragmentation of the prosthetic valve cusps. This complication developed in virtually all early-generation porcine aortic valves within 5 years of implantation and led to valve failure in 20% to 30% of patients within 10 years. However, improved understanding of prosthetic tissue valve calcification has led to development of anticalcification treatments that improve valve longevity and performance. Tissue valve calcification occurs mainly within residual cells devitalized by glutaraldehyde treatment. Strategies to prevent or delay valve calcification include removal of residual cells, binding of calcification inhibitors to the glutaraldehyde-fixed tissue and use of other tissue cross-linking and preservation reagents.

MECHANICAL VALVES: The most widely used mechanical prostheses involve single or bileaflet tilting disk designs that do not obstruct blood flow across the valve and have excellent durability. However, the risk of thromboembolism makes long-term anticoagulant therapy imperative.

Heart Transplantation May Cure Many End-Stage Heart Diseases but Is Subject to Host Rejection Processes

The development of effective immunosuppressive drugs and surveillance endomyocardial biopsy protocols has made cardiac transplantation an effective treatment for end-stage heart disease. Allograft rejection (see Chapter 4), however, is a major complication of cardiac transplantation.

Hyperacute rejection occurs if there are blood-group incompatibility or major histocompatibility differences. In these situations, preformed antibodies cause immediate vascular injury to the donor heart, with diffuse hemorrhage, edema, intracapillary platelet–fibrin thrombi, vascular necrosis and infiltration of neutrophils. Screening for blood-group incompatibility has rendered this complication rare.

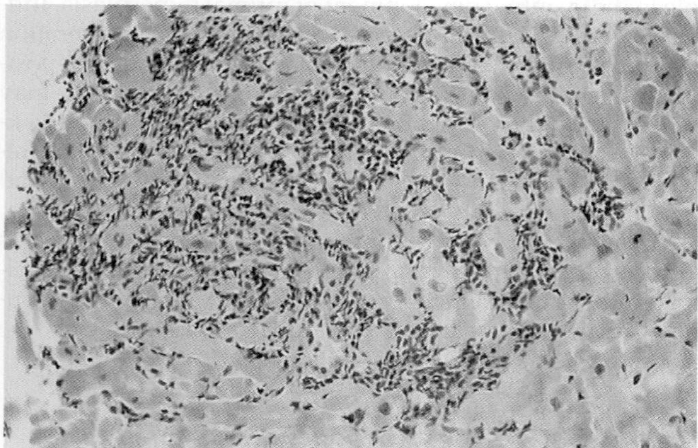

FIGURE 11-54. Cardiac transplant rejection. An endomyocardial biopsy shows lymphocytes surrounding individual myocytes and expanding the interstitium.

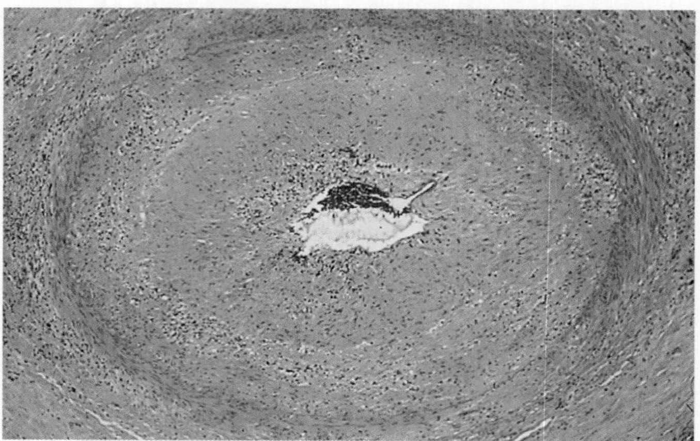

FIGURE 11-55. Chronic cardiac transplant rejection. An intramyocardial branch of a coronary artery shows prominent intimal proliferation and inflammation with concentric narrowing of the lumen.

Acute humoral rejection is characterized by vascular deposition of antibody and complement, endothelial cell swelling and edema. This unusual form of rejection has a worse prognosis than acute cellular rejection.

Acute cellular rejection, the most common form of allograft rejection, usually occurs in the first few months after transplantation. It begins as perivascular T-cell infiltration, which is focal and is not associated with acute myocyte necrosis. This reaction often resolves spontaneously and, therefore, does not necessitate a change in the immunosuppressive regimen. Moderate cellular rejection is characterized by T-cell infiltration into adjacent interstitial spaces, where lymphocytes surround individual myocytes and expand the interstitium (Fig. 11-54). In this instance, focal acute myocyte necrosis is also present. Moderate cellular rejection usually does not produce detectable functional impairment and tends to resolve within a few days to a week after treatment. However, additional immunosuppressive therapy is instituted because moderate cellular rejection can progress to severe rejection. The latter is characterized by vascular damage, widespread myocyte necrosis, neutrophil infiltration, interstitial hemorrhage and functional impairment, which is difficult to reverse.

The early stage of cellular allograft rejection is typically asymptomatic. Once symptoms develop, rejection is usually much more advanced and has caused irrecoverable loss of cardiac myocytes. The most reliable screening procedure is endomyocardial biopsy of the right side of the interventricular septum, performed by cardiac catheterization.

Chronic vascular rejection, also referred to as **accelerated coronary artery disease,** is the most common cause of death in heart transplant patients beyond the first year after transplantation. It affects proximal and distal epicardial coronary arteries, the penetrating coronary artery branches and even the arterioles. Microscopically, accelerated coronary artery disease is characterized by concentric intimal proliferation (Fig. 11-55), which can lead to coronary occlusion and myocardial infarction. This complication is silent because the transplanted heart is denervated. Thus, extensive myocardial damage can develop before the transplant patient is aware that ischemic injury has occurred.

12 The Respiratory System

Mary Beth Beasley • William D. Travis • Emanuel Rubin

THE NORMAL RESPIRATORY SYSTEM

Embryology

The respiratory system includes the larynx, trachea, bronchi, bronchioles and alveoli. During the fourth week of gestation, the laryngotracheal groove develops as a ventral outpouching of the foregut.

1. **Embryonic period:** Between 4 and 6 weeks' gestation, the tracheobronchial bud divides to form proximal airways to the level of segmental bronchi.
2. **Pseudoglandular period:** From 6 to 16 weeks' gestation, the distal airways are formed up to the level of the terminal bronchioles.
3. **Acinar or canalicular development:** During weeks 17 to 28, (a) the framework of the gas-exchanging unit of the lung develops, (b) acini are formed, (c) the vascular system develops, (d) capillaries reach the epithelium and (e) gas exchange can occur. At this point extrauterine life becomes possible.
4. **Saccular period:** At 28 to 34 weeks of gestation, primary saccules become subdivided by secondary crests, a process that results in greater complexity of the gas-exchanging surface and thinning of airspace walls.
5. **Alveolar period:** The last step in lung development corresponds to 34 to 36 weeks of gestation and is the time when alveoli develop. At birth, the number of alveoli is highly variable, ranging from 20 to 150 million. Most alveoli develop in the first 2 years of life.

Anatomy

TRACHEA AND BRONCHI: The trachea is a hollow tube up to 25 cm in length and up to 2.5 cm in diameter. The right bronchus diverges at a lesser angle from the trachea than does the left, which is why foreign material is more frequently aspirated on the right side. On entering the lung, the main bronchi divide into lobar bronchi, then into segmental bronchi, which supply the 19 lung segments. Because the segments are individual units with their own bronchovascular supply, they can be resected individually.

The tracheobronchial tree contains cartilage and submucosal mucous glands in the wall (Fig. 12-1). The latter are compound tubular glands, which contain **mucous cells** (pale) and **serous cells** (granular, more basophilic). The pseudostratified epithelium appears as layers, although all cells reach the basement membrane. Most cells are ciliated, but there are also mucus-secreting **(goblet)** cells and basal cells. The **basal cells**, which do not reach the surface, are precursors that differentiate into more specialized tracheobronchial epithelial cells. There are also nonciliated columnar cells, or **Clara cells**, which accumulate and detoxify many inhaled toxic agents (e.g., nitrogen dioxide [NO_2]). **Neuroendocrine cells** are scattered in the tracheobronchial mucosa and contain a variety of hormonally active polypeptides and vasoactive amines.

BRONCHIOLES: Distal to the bronchi are the bronchioles, which differ from bronchi in that they lack cartilage and mucus-secreting glands (Fig. 12-1). Bronchiolar epithelium becomes thinner with progressive branching, until only one cell layer is present. The last purely conducting structure free of alveoli is the **terminal bronchiole,** which exhibits pseudostratified ciliated respiratory epithelium and a smooth muscle wall. Mucous cells gradually disappear from the lining of the bronchioles until they are entirely replaced in the small bronchioles by the nonciliated, columnar Clara cells. The terminal bronchioles divide into **respiratory bronchioles,** which merge into **alveolar ducts** and **alveoli. Acini** are the gas exchange units of the lung and consist of respiratory bronchioles, alveolar ducts and alveoli.

ALVEOLI: Alveoli are lined by two types of epithelium (Fig. 12-1). **Type I cells** cover 95% of the alveolar surface, but constitute only 40% of alveolar epithelial cells. They are thin and have a large surface area, a combination that facilitates gas exchange. **Type II cells** produce surfactant and make up 60% of the alveolar lining cells. As they are more cuboidal than type I cells, they represent only 5% of the alveolar surface. Type I cells are particularly vulnerable to injury. When they are lost, type II pneumocytes multiply and differentiate to form new type I cells, restoring the integrity of the alveolar surface.

Alveolar epithelial and endothelial cells are arranged ideally for gas exchange. The cytoplasm of epithelial and endothelial cells is spread very thinly on either side of a fused basement membrane, allowing efficient exchange of oxygen and carbon dioxide. An extensive capillary network supplies 85% to 95% of the alveolar surface. Away from the site of gas exchange, interstitial connective tissue is more abundant, consisting of collagen, elastin and proteoglycans. Fibroblasts and myofibroblasts may also be present. This expanded region forms the interstitial space of the alveolar wall, where significant fluid and molecular exchange occurs.

PULMONARY VASCULATURE: The lung has a **dual blood supply** from the pulmonary and the bronchial systems. Pulmonary arteries accompany airways in a sheath of connective tissue, the **bronchovascular bundle.** The more proximal arteries are elastic and are succeeded by muscular arteries, pulmonary arterioles and eventually pulmonary capillaries.

The smallest veins, which resemble the smallest arteries, join other veins and drain into lobular septa, connective tissue partitions that subdivide the lung into small respiratory units. In these septa, the veins form a network separate from the bronchovascular bundles.

Bronchial arteries arise from the thoracic aorta and nourish the bronchial tree as far as the respiratory bronchioles. These arteries are accompanied by their respective veins, which drain into the azygous or hemiazygous veins.

There are no lymphatics in most alveolar walls. These vessels begin in alveoli at the periphery of acini, which lie along lobular septa, bronchovascular bundles or the pleura. The lymphatics of the lobular septa and bronchovascular bundle accompany these structures, and the pleural lymphatics drain toward the hilus through the bronchovascular lymphatics.

Defense Mechanisms

The respiratory system has effective defense mechanisms to cope with the numerous particulates and infectious agents inhaled on inspiration.

The **nose and trachea** warm and humidify air entering the lung. The nose traps almost all particles over 10 μm in diameter and about half of all particles of 3 μm aerodynamic diameter (Fig. 12-2). (Aerodynamic diameter refers to the way particles behave in air rather than to their actual size.)

The **mucociliary blanket** of the airway epithelium disposes of particles 2 to 10 μm in diameter. The ciliary beat drives the mucous blanket toward the trachea. Particles that land on it are thus removed from the lungs and swallowed or coughed up.

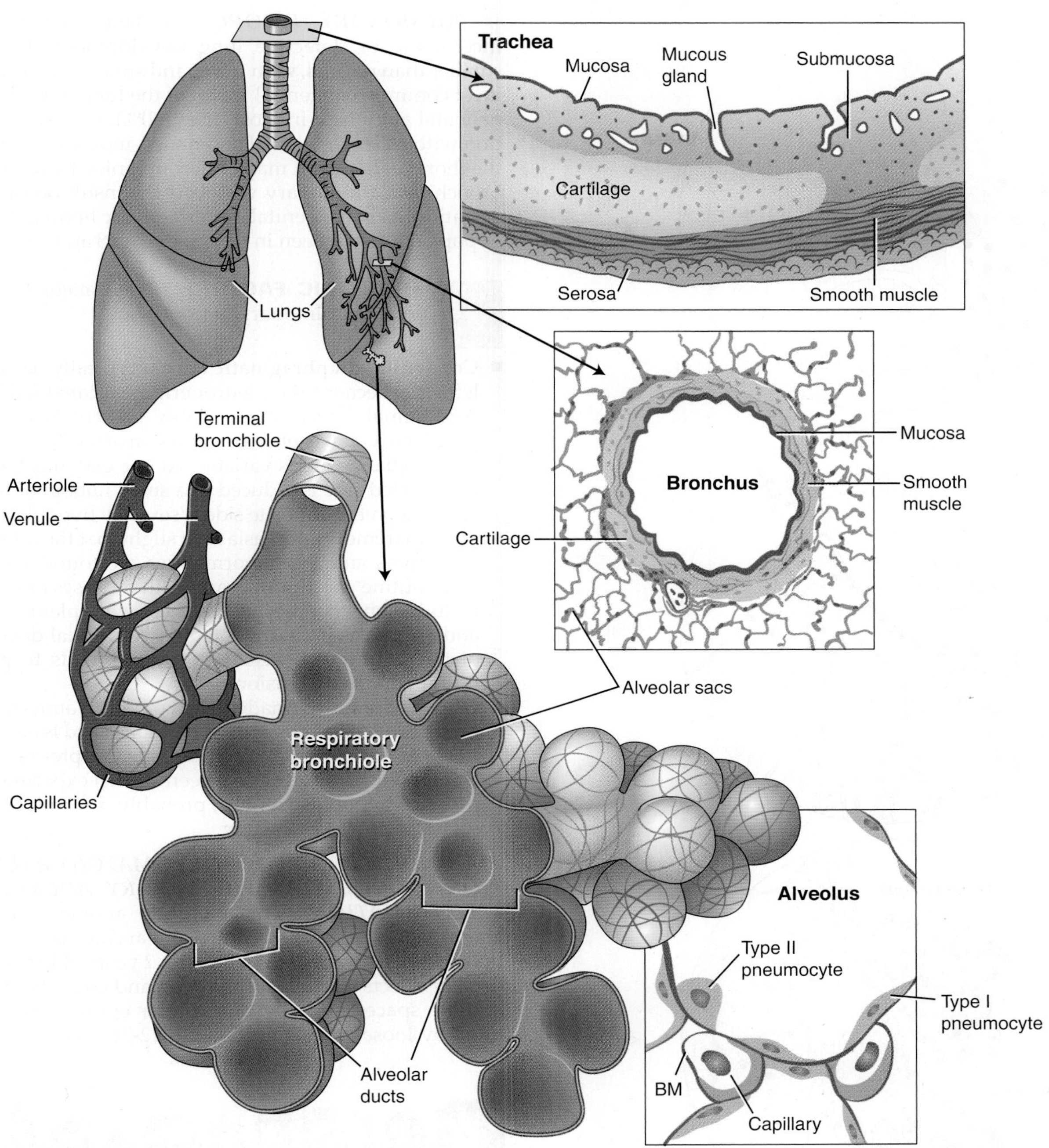

FIGURE 12-1. Anatomy of the lung. The conducting structures of the lung include (1) the trachea, which has horseshoe-shaped cartilages; (2) the bronchi, which have plates of cartilage in their walls (both the trachea and bronchi have mucus-secreting glands in their walls); and (3) the bronchioles, which do not have cartilage in their walls and terminate in the terminal bronchioles. The gas-exchanging components compose the unit distal to the terminal bronchiole, namely, the acinus. Alveoli are lined by type I cells, which are large, flat cells that cover most of the alveolar wall, and by type II cells, which secrete surfactant and are the progenitor cells of the alveolar epithelium. Gas exchange occurs at the level of the alveolar wall.

Alveolar macrophages protect the alveolar space. These cells are derived from the bone marrow, probably undergo a maturation division in the interstitium of the lung and then enter the alveolar space. They are particularly effective in dealing with particles with aerodynamic diameters under 2 μm. Very small particles are not phagocytosed and are exhaled.

THE LUNGS

Congenital Anomalies

BRONCHIAL ATRESIA: This abnormality most often involves the bronchus to the apical posterior segment of the

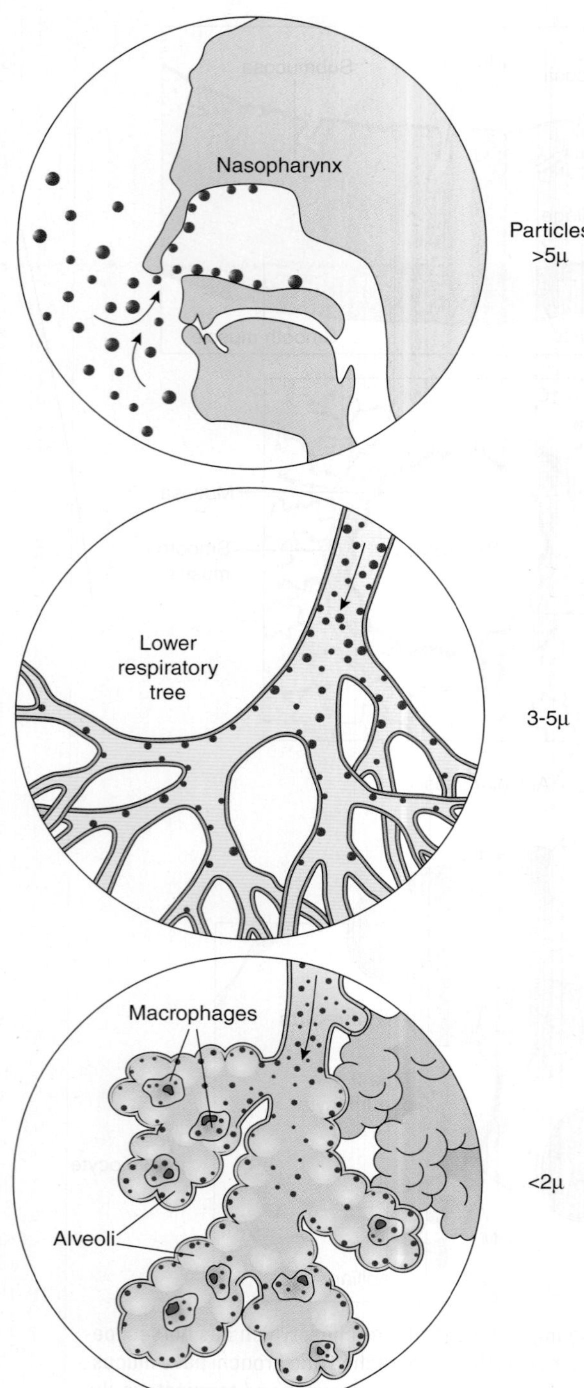

FIGURE 12-2. Deposition of particles in the respiratory tract. Large particles are trapped in the nose. Intermediate-sized particles deposit on the bronchi and bronchioles and are removed by the mucociliary blanket. Smaller particles terminate in the airspaces and are removed by macrophages. Very small particles behave as a gas and are breathed out.

left upper lobe. In infants the lesion may result in an overexpanded part of the lung. In later life the overexpanded lobe may also be emphysematous. Bronchial mucus accumulating distal to the atretic region may appear on radiologic examination as a mass.

PULMONARY HYPOPLASIA: This condition reflects incomplete or defective lung development. The lung is smaller than normal, with fewer and smaller acini. This is the most common congenital lesion of the lung, found in 10% of neonatal autopsies. In most cases (90%), it occurs in association with other congenital anomalies, most of which involve the thorax. The lesion may be accompanied by hypoplasia of bronchi and pulmonary vessels if the insult occurs early in gestation, as in congenital diaphragmatic hernia. Pulmonary hypoplasia also is seen in trisomies 13, 18 and 21.

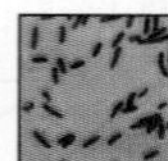

ETIOLOGIC FACTORS: Three major factors may lead to pulmonary hypoplasia:

- **Congenital diaphragmatic hernia** typically occurs on the left side, because the pleuroperitoneal canal fails to close. Abdominal viscera are variably present in the affected hemithorax and result in compression of the lung. The degree of hypoplasia is thus variable. At one extreme, the lung on the affected side is reduced to a small nubbin of tissue and the lung on the opposite side is severely hypoplastic. At the other extreme, hypoplasia is so slight that the infant has no symptoms and the abnormalities are found incidentally on a routine chest radiograph. Other causes of hypoplasia include abnormalities of the chest wall, pleural effusions and ascites, as in hydrops fetalis. Abnormal development of the pulmonary vasculature often leads to persistent pulmonary hypertension.
- **Oligohydramnios** (inadequate volume of amniotic fluid) is usually due to genitourinary anomalies and is an important cause of pulmonary hypoplasia (see Chapter 6).
- **Decreased respiration** has been shown experimentally to produce hypoplastic lungs, probably due to lack of repetitive stretching of the lung.

CONGENITAL CYSTIC ADENOMATOID MALFORMATION (CONGENITAL PULMONARY ADENOMATOID MALFORMATION): This common anomaly consists of abnormal bronchiolar structures of varying sizes or distribution. Most cases are seen in the first 2 years of life. The lesion usually affects one lobe of the lung and consists of multiple cystlike spaces lined by bronchiolar epithelium and separated by loose fibrous tissue (Fig. 12-3). Some patients will

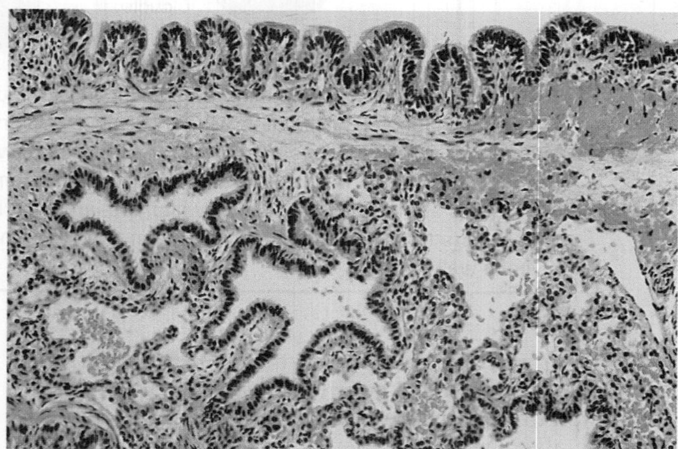

FIGURE 12-3. Congenital cystic adenomatoid malformation. Multiple glandlike spaces are lined by bronchiolar epithelium.

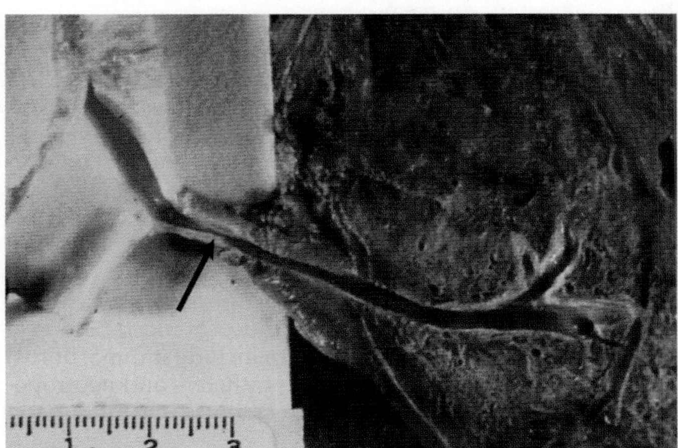

FIGURE 12-4. Extralobar sequestration. The sequestered pulmonary tissue is situated outside the lung parenchyma. It is supplied by an aberrant artery (*arrow*) from the aorta and is not connected to the bronchial tree.

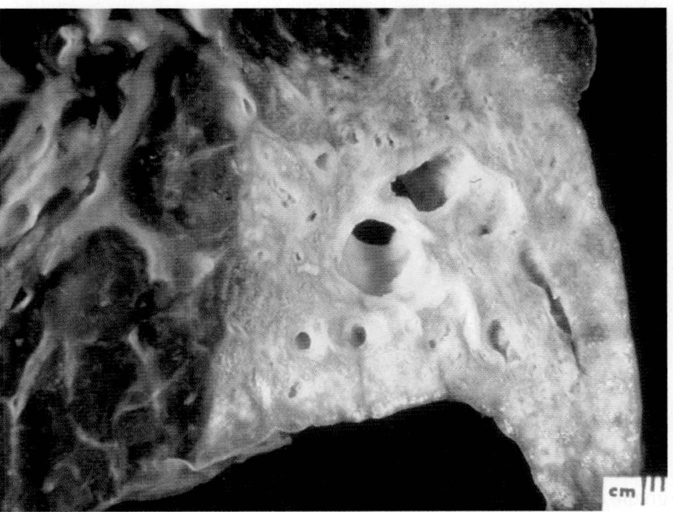

FIGURE 12-5. Intralobar sequestration. The sequestered tissue lies within the visceral pleura and exhibits cystic change and dense fibrosis. An aberrant arterial supply to this lesion was identified (not shown).

have other congenital anomalies. The most common presenting symptoms are respiratory distress and cyanosis. Surgical resection is the treatment of choice.

BRONCHOGENIC CYST: This lesion is a discrete, extrapulmonary, fluid-filled mass lined by respiratory epithelium and limited by walls that contain muscle and cartilage. It is most commonly found in the middle mediastinum. In newborns, a bronchogenic cyst may compress a major airway and cause respiratory distress. Secondary infection of the cyst in older patients may lead to hemorrhage and perforation. Many bronchogenic cysts are asymptomatic and are found on routine chest radiographs.

EXTRALOBAR SEQUESTRATION: Extralobar sequestration is a mass of lung tissue that is not connected to the bronchial tree and is located outside the visceral pleura. An abnormal artery, usually arising from the aorta, supplies the sequestered tissue (Fig. 12-4).

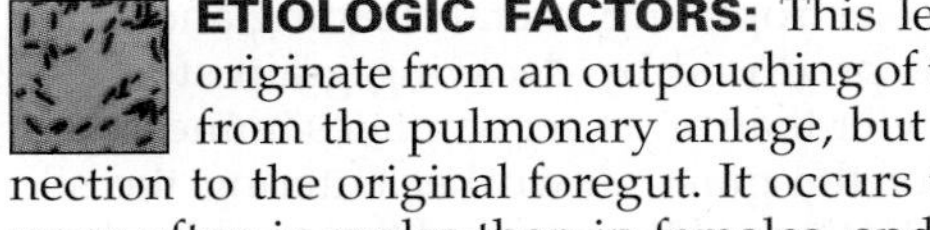

ETIOLOGIC FACTORS: This lesion is thought to originate from an outpouching of the foregut, distinct from the pulmonary anlage, but later loses its connection to the original foregut. It occurs three to four times more often in males than in females, and is associated with other anomalies in two thirds of patients.

PATHOLOGY: On gross examination, extralobar sequestrations are pyramidal or round masses, 1 to 15 cm in size, covered by pleura. Microscopically, dilated bronchioles, alveolar ducts and alveoli are noted. Infection or infarction may alter the histologic appearance.

CLINICAL FEATURES: In half of cases, extralobar sequestration is detected before 1 month of age, and is recognized by 2 years of age in 75% of patients. In many cases the condition is associated with congenital cystic adenomatoid malformation. In the neonatal period, extralobar sequestration may cause dyspnea and cyanosis, often in the first day of life. In older children, recurrent bronchopulmonary infections may bring it to medical attention. Surgical excision is curative.

INTRALOBAR SEQUESTRATION: Intralobar sequestration is a mass of lung tissue within the visceral pleura, isolated from the tracheobronchial tree and supplied by a systemic artery (Fig. 12-5). Previously considered a congenital malformation, it is now felt to be acquired.

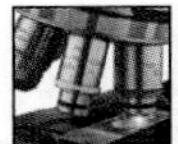

PATHOLOGY: Intralobar sequestrations are almost always found in a lower lobe. Bilateral involvement is distinctly unusual. On gross examination, the sequestered tissue shows the result of chronic recurrent pneumonia, with end-stage fibrosis and honeycomb cystic changes. These cysts range up to 5 cm in diameter, and lie in a dense fibrous stroma. Microscopically, the cystic spaces are mostly lined by cuboidal or columnar epithelium and the lumen contains foamy macrophages and eosinophilic material. Interstitial chronic inflammation and follicular lymphoid hyperplasia are often prominent. Acute and organizing pneumonia may be seen.

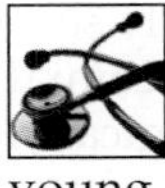

CLINICAL FEATURES: Cough, sputum production and recurrent pneumonia are seen in almost all patients. Most cases are discovered in adolescents or young adults. Only one fourth of patients are in the first decade of life, and the lesion is rarely identified in infants. Surgical resection is often indicated.

Diseases of the Bronchi and Bronchioles

Most bronchial and bronchiolar diseases are acute conditions and their sequelae. We discuss chronic bronchitis later, in the section on chronic obstructive pulmonary disease (COPD).

Airway Infections Are Caused by Diverse Organisms

Here, we distinguish between infections of the airways and parenchyma for convenience and reasons of classification, but this division should not be thought of as rigid. Agents causing these infections are discussed in detail in Chapter 9.

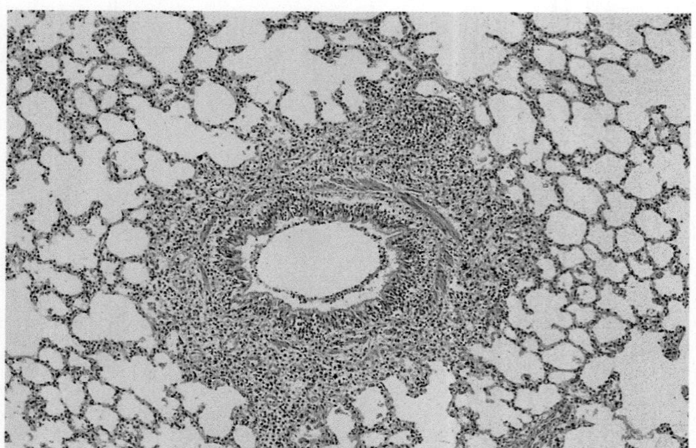

FIGURE 12-6. Bronchiolitis due to adenovirus. The wall of this bronchiole shows an intense chronic inflammatory infiltrate with local extension into the surrounding peribronchial tissue.

Many infectious agents that involve the intrapulmonary airways tend to affect the more peripheral airways **(bronchiolitis),** for example, adenovirus, respiratory syncytial virus (RSV) and measles. All are more serious in malnourished children and populations not ordinarily exposed to these agents. Severe symptomatic infections are more common in infants and children, and recovery is the rule. Symptoms include cough, a feeling of tightness in the chest and, in extreme cases, shortness of breath and even cyanosis.

INFLUENZA: This is a characteristic example of tracheobronchitis, and in the occasional patient who dies with this infection, the appearance of the bronchi is dramatic. The surface of the airway is fiery red, reflecting acute inflammation and congestion of the mucosa.

ADENOVIRUS: Infection with adenovirus produces the most serious sequelae, with extensive inflammation of bronchioles (Fig. 12-6) and then healing by fibrosis. Bronchioles may become obliterated or occluded by loose fibrous tissue **(obliterative bronchiolitis).**

RESPIRATORY SYNCYTIAL VIRUS (RSV): RSV infection often occurs in epidemics in nurseries. It is usually self-limited, but rare fatal cases do occur. It can cause nosocomial infection in children and (rarely) in adults. Histologically, peribronchiolar inflammation and disorganization of the epithelium are evident. Severe overdistention may be found without obvious bronchiolar obstruction, possibly due to displacement of surfactant from the bronchiolar surface.

MEASLES: At one time a major cause of bronchiolitis, measles is rarely a problem in developed countries since the advent of the measles vaccine. However, measles-induced bronchiolitis remains a serious problem particularly in populations seldom exposed to the virus. Similar to adenovirus, it may cause bronchiolar obliteration and bronchiectasis.

BORDETELLA PERTUSSIS: This bacterium commonly infects the airways and is the cause of whooping cough. With widespread use of a pertussis vaccine, the disease became rare in the United States. Unfortunately, vaccination is no longer compulsory in England, and the incidence of pertussis is rising. Clinically, whooping cough is typified by fever and severe prolonged bouts of coughing, followed by a characteristic deep whooping inspiration. Severe bronchial and bronchiolar inflammation are found in fatal cases. Before immunization was available, whooping cough commonly led to the development of bronchiectasis.

HAEMOPHILUS INFLUENZAE AND STREPTOCOCCUS PNEUMONIAE: In addition to pneumonia, these organisms have been implicated in exacerbations of chronic bronchitis. Such episodes contribute to the morbidity of chronic bronchitis and are treated with antibiotics.

CANDIDA ALBICANS: This fungus is a normal commensal organism in the oral cavity, gut and vagina, and is best known for infections in those regions. It may also affect the lungs, usually as a noninvasive growth on airway surface epithelium, where it may produce mucosal ulceration. Predisposing factors for invasive growth include trauma, burns, gastrointestinal surgery, indwelling catheters and neutropenia, such as may be associated with cytotoxic chemotherapy for acute leukemia.

Irritant Gases Derive From Air Pollution and Industrial Accidents

The most important irritant gases in the atmosphere are oxidants (ozone, nitrogen oxides) and sulfur dioxide (SO_2). Oxidants derive from the action of sunlight on automobile exhaust fumes and are important in major urban areas that have temperature inversions. SO_2 is produced mainly by burning fossil fuels. The effects of low concentrations of these agents alone are not certain, but they may compound the adverse effects of tobacco smoke. Indeed, inhabitants of urban and more polluted areas have worse pulmonary function (e.g., reduced expiratory flow rates) than do those who reside in cleaner environments. Respiratory infections are also more common in young children who live in regions of high pollution. However, these effects are small in the healthy population.

In persons with chronic pulmonary disease, the situation is different: experimentally, ozone makes airways more reactive, an effect related to airway inflammation. ***Thus, air pollution may exacerbate symptoms in asthmatic persons and in those with established respiratory disease. In high concentrations, irritant gases produce serious morphologic and functional effects.***

NO_2: NO_2 is often encountered in industrial settings, including welding, electroplating, metal cleaning and blasting. The gas is also produced by decaying grain stored in silos. As NO_2 is heavier than air, it accumulates immediately above the surface of the grain. A worker entering the silo inhales high concentrations of the gas, and the resulting lung injury is known as **silo-filler disease.** Respiratory symptoms in such cases may be delayed for up to 30 hours, after which cough and dyspnea develop. Most patients recover but some develop progressive bronchiolitis obliterans and may die of respiratory failure.

SO_2: This highly soluble gas, when inhaled chronically by experimental animals, produces lesions in the more central airways that resemble chronic bronchitis and that may progress to squamous metaplasia. In humans, exposure to very high concentrations of SO_2 has been associated with severe inflammation and bronchiolitis.

CHLORINE AND AMMONIA: These gases are released in high concentrations in industrial accidents. On inhalation, they produce extensive bronchial and bronchiolar mucosal injury. Secondary inflammation may lead to extensive bronchiectasis, in part from bronchiolar obliteration and in part from direct damage to the bronchi.

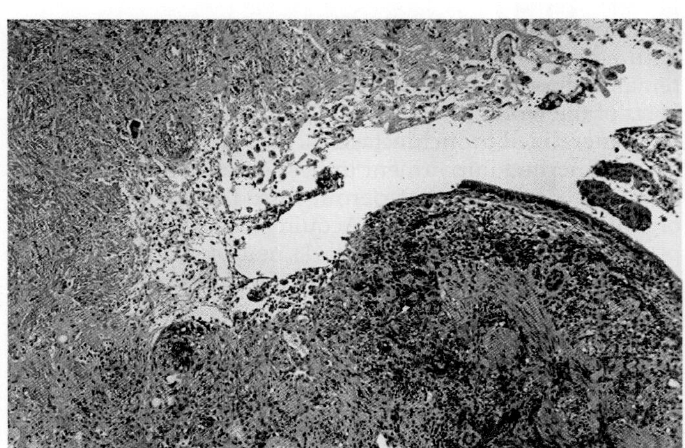

FIGURE 12-7. Bronchocentric granulomatosis. This bronchiole shows ulceration and necrosis of the mucosa and submucosa with granulomatous inflammation. The patient had Wegener granulomatosis with lung involvement in the pattern of bronchocentric granulomatosis.

Bronchocentric Granulomatosis Usually Reflects Allergic Responses to Infection

Bronchocentric granulomatosis is a nonspecific granulomatous inflammation centered on bronchi or bronchioles (Fig. 12-7). The condition can be the predominant pulmonary pathologic finding in two groups of patients, namely, asthmatics and nonasthmatics. ***The histologic pattern can be seen in a number of clinical settings and is not a distinct clinical entity.***

Asthmatic patients, for the most part, have allergic bronchopulmonary aspergillosis (see below). In addition to bronchocentric granulomatosis, such persons have bronchial mucous plugs, bronchiectasis and bronchiolectasis and eosinophilic pneumonia. Irregular, fragmented *Aspergillus* hyphae may be seen in the mucous plugs. A nonspecific secondary vasculitis is centered on the airways rather than the vessels.

Nonasthmatic patients with bronchocentric granulomatosis are likely to have an infection, especially tuberculosis or fungi such as *Histoplasma capsulatum*. The disorder can also be a manifestation of immune problems, such as rheumatoid arthritis, ankylosing spondylitis and Wegener granulomatosis. Patients with bronchocentric granulomatosis of either allergic or nonallergic type generally respond well to corticosteroid therapy.

Constrictive Bronchiolitis May Obliterate an Airway

In constrictive bronchiolitis, an initial inflammatory bronchiolitis is followed by bronchiolar scarring and fibrosis, with progressive narrowing and, eventually, complete destruction of the airway lumen (Fig. 12-8). **Obliterative bronchiolitis** is a synonym.

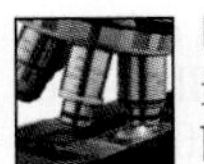

PATHOLOGY: Bronchioles show chronic mural inflammation and varying amounts of fibrosis between the epithelium and smooth muscle, with resultant narrowing of the lumen. These lesions are often focal and may be difficult to identify. Elastic stains may help in recognizing the scarred bronchioles. Bronchiolectasis and mucous plugs may be seen in adjacent airways. The surrounding lung is usually normal.

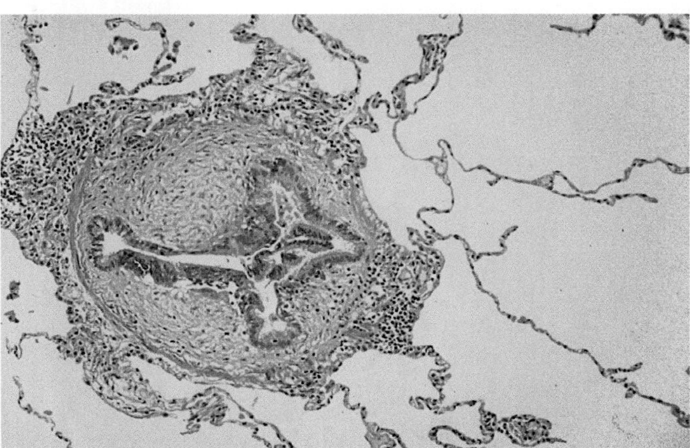

FIGURE 12-8. Constrictive bronchiolitis. The lumen of a bronchiole is markedly narrowed, owing to marked submucosal fibrosis.

CLINICAL FEATURES: Patients may have dyspnea and wheezing due to severe obstructive pulmonary function. Chest radiographs and computed tomography (CT) scans may be normal, or they may show overinflation, caused by air trapping distal to the obliterated bronchioles. This pattern of fibrosis is seen in several situations, including (1) bone marrow transplantation (graft-versus-host disease), (2) lung transplantation (chronic rejection), (3) collagen vascular diseases (especially rheumatoid arthritis), (4) postinfectious disorders (especially viral infections), (5) after inhalation of toxins (SO_2, ammonia, phosgene) and (6) ingestion of certain drugs (penicillamine). It may also be idiopathic. Most patients have a relentless progressive clinical course. Although many patients are treated with steroids, no therapy is effective for this disease.

Bronchial Obstruction Leads to Atelectasis

Bronchial obstruction in adults occurs mostly because of endobronchial extension of primary lung tumors, although mucous plugs, aspirated gastric contents or foreign bodies may also be responsible, especially in children. If obstruction is partial, trapped air may cause overdistention of the distal affected segment; complete obstruction results in atelectasis. Areas distal to the obstruction may also develop pneumonia, abscesses and bronchiectasis (see below).

Atelectasis refers to the collapse of expanded lung tissue (Fig. 12-9). If the air supply is obstructed, gas transfers from the alveoli to the blood, causing the affected region to collapse. Atelectasis occurs as an important postoperative complication of abdominal surgery, because of (1) mucous obstruction of a bronchus and (2) diminished respiratory movement resulting from postoperative pain. It is often asymptomatic, but when severe, it results in hypoxemia and a shift of the mediastinum *toward* the affected side.

Atelectasis is usually caused by bronchial obstruction, but may also result from direct compression of the lung (e.g., hydrothorax or pneumothorax). If the compression is severe

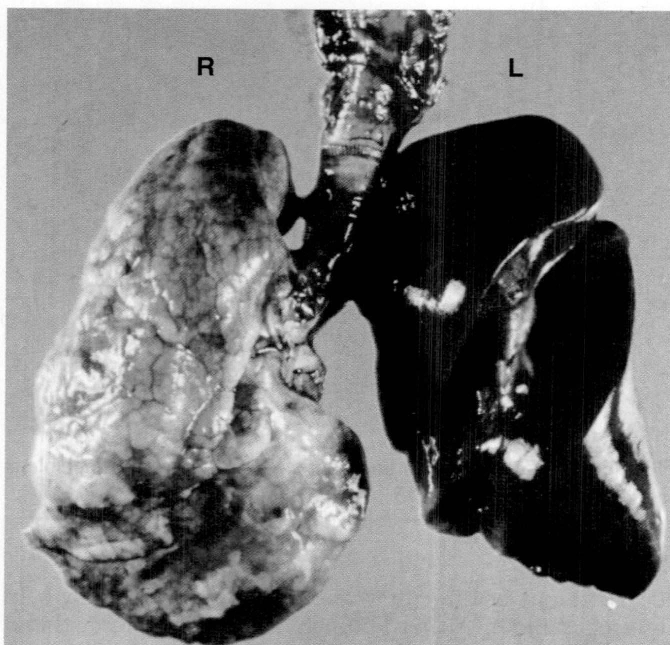

FIGURE 12-9. Atelectasis. The right lung of an infant is pale and expanded by air; the left lung is collapsed.

enough, the function of the affected lung may be jeopardized and the mediastinum may shift *away* from the affected side.

In long-standing atelectasis, the area of collapsed lung becomes fibrotic and bronchi dilate, in part due to infection distal to the obstruction. Permanent bronchial dilation (bronchiectasis) results.

Right middle lobe syndrome refers to atelectasis due to obstruction of the bronchus to the right middle lobe, usually from external compression by hilar lymph nodes. This bronchus is particularly susceptible to external compression because it is long and slender and surrounded by lymph nodes. Histologically, the lung shows bronchiectasis, chronic bronchitis and bronchiolitis, lymphoid hyperplasia, abscess formation and dense fibrosis. Acute and organizing pneumonia may both be present. Tuberculous lymphadenitis or metastatic lung cancer may cause the lymph node enlargement, but the cause of the obstruction is often undetermined.

Bronchiectasis Is Irreversible Dilation of Bronchi Caused by Destruction of Bronchial Wall Muscle and Elastic Elements

ETIOLOGIC FACTORS: Bronchiectasis may be obstructive or nonobstructive.

Obstructive bronchiectasis is localized and occurs distal to a mechanical obstruction of a central bronchus by, for example, tumors, inhaled foreign bodies, mucous plugs in asthma or lymph node enlargement. **Nonobstructive bronchiectasis** usually follows respiratory infections or defects in airway defenses from infection. It may be localized or generalized.

Localized nonobstructive bronchiectasis was once common, usually following childhood bronchopulmonary infections with measles, pertussis or other bacteria. Vaccines and antibiotics have reduced the incidence of bronchiectasis, but most cases still follow bronchopulmonary infection, usually with adenovirus or RSV. Childhood respiratory infections remain important causes of bronchiectasis in less developed parts of the world.

Generalized bronchiectasis is, for the most part, secondary to inherited impairment in host defense mechanisms or acquired conditions that permit introduction of infectious organisms into the airways. Acquired disorders that predispose to bronchiectasis include (1) neurologic diseases that impair consciousness, swallowing, respiratory excursions and the cough reflex; (2) incompetence of the lower esophageal sphincter; (3) nasogastric intubation; and (4) chronic bronchitis. The main **inherited conditions** associated with generalized bronchiectasis are cystic fibrosis, dyskinetic ciliary syndromes, hypogammaglobulinemias and deficiencies of specific immunoglobulin (Ig) G subclasses.

Kartagener syndrome is one of the immotile cilia syndromes (ciliary dyskinesia) and consists of the triad of dextrocardia (with or without situs inversus), bronchiectasis and sinusitis. It is caused by defects in the outer or inner dynein arms of cilia, which generate or regulate cilia beats, respectively. Other dyskinetic ciliary syndromes include **radial spoke deficiency** ("Sturgess syndrome") and absence of the central doublet of cilia. In these diseases cilia are deficient throughout the body. Both men and women are sterile, because of impaired ciliary mobility in the vas deferens and the fallopian tube. In the respiratory tract, ciliary defects lead to repeated upper and lower respiratory tract infections and, thus, to bronchiectasis.

Immunodeficiency may also predispose to repeated pulmonary infection and bronchiectasis. In hypogammaglobulinemias the lack of IgAs or IgGs that protect against viruses or bacteria can result in recurrent lung infections. Acquired and inherited disorders of neutrophils also lead to a greater risk of respiratory infections and bronchiectasis.

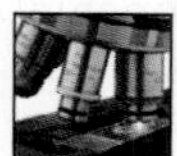

PATHOLOGY: On gross examination, bronchial dilation is saccular, varicose or cylindrical.

- **Saccular bronchiectasis** affects the proximal third to fourth bronchial branches (Fig. 12-10). These bronchi are severely dilated and end blindly in dilated sacs, with collapse and fibrosis of the distal lung parenchyma.
- **Cylindrical bronchiectasis** involves the sixth to the eighth bronchial branchings, which show uniform, moderate dilation. It is a milder disease than saccular bronchiectasis and leads to fewer clinical symptoms.
- **Varicose bronchiectasis** results in bronchi that resemble varicose veins when visualized by radiologic bronchography, with irregular dilations and constrictions. Two to eight branchings of bronchi are recognized grossly. Bronchiolar obliteration is not as severe, and parenchymal abnormalities are variable.

Generalized bronchiectasis is usually bilateral and is most common in the lower lobes, the left more than the right. Localized bronchiectasis may occur wherever there was obstruction or infection. Bronchi are dilated, with white or yellow thickened walls. Bronchial lumens often contain thick, mucopurulent secretions. Microscopically, severe inflammation of bronchi and bronchioles results in destruction of all components of the bronchial wall. With the consequent collapse of distal lung parenchyma, damaged bronchi dilate. Inflammation of central airways leads to mucus hypersecretion and abnormalities of the surface epithelium, including squamous

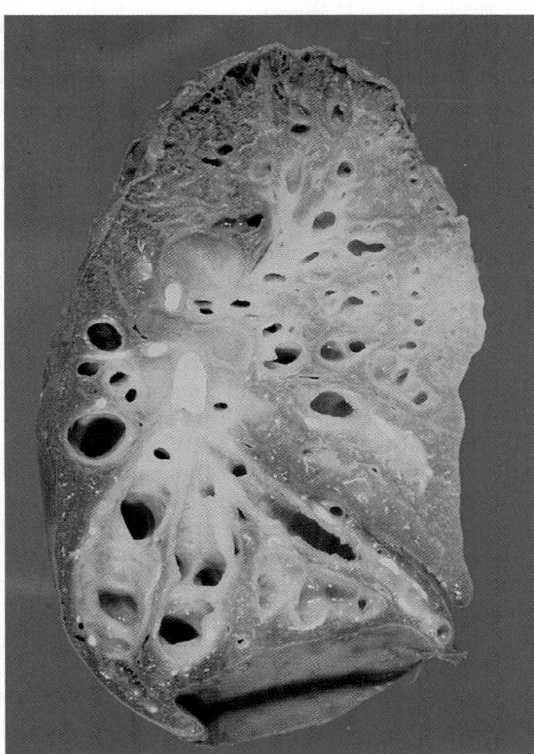

FIGURE 12-10. Bronchiectasis. The resected upper lobe shows widely dilated bronchi, with thickening of the bronchial walls and collapse and fibrosis of the pulmonary parenchyma.

metaplasia and increased goblet cells. Lymphoid follicles are often seen in bronchial walls, and distal bronchi and bronchioles are scarred and often obliterated. The bronchial arteries increase in size to supply the inflamed bronchial wall and fibrous tissue. A vicious circle may be established, because a pool of mucus is liable to further infection, which leads to progressive destruction of the bronchial walls.

CLINICAL FEATURES: Patients with bronchiectasis have chronic productive cough, often with several hundred milliliters of mucopurulent sputum a day. Hemoptysis is common, as bronchial inflammation erodes through the walls of adjacent bronchial arteries. Dyspnea and wheezing are variable, depending on the extent of the disease. Pneumonia is common, and patients with long-standing cases are at risk of chronic hypoxia and pulmonary hypertension. Radiologically, the bronchi appear dilated and have thickened walls. The definitive diagnosis is made by CT scan of the lung. Surgical treatment of localized bronchiectasis may be necessary, especially if complications such as severe hemoptysis or pneumonia arise. However, in the generalized disease, surgical resection is more palliative than curative.

Acute, reversible bronchial dilation may follow bacterial or viral bronchopulmonary infection, and it may take months before the bronchi return to normal size.

Infections

Pulmonary infections are discussed in detail in Chapter 9. The major pulmonary entities are described below, with particular emphasis on pathologic features.

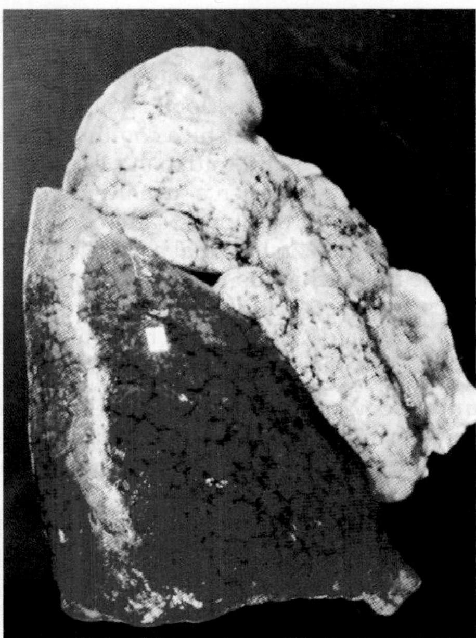

FIGURE 12-11. Lobar pneumonia. The entire left lower lobe is consolidated and in the stage of red hepatization. The upper lobe is normally expanded.

Bacterial Pneumonia Is Inflammation and Consolidation of Lung Parenchyma

Bacterial pneumonia has been historically divided into lobar pneumonia or bronchopneumonia, but these terms have little clinical relevance today. In **lobar pneumonia** an entire lobe is consolidated (Fig. 12-11), whereas **bronchopneumonia** refers to scattered solid foci in the same or several lobes (Fig. 12-12).

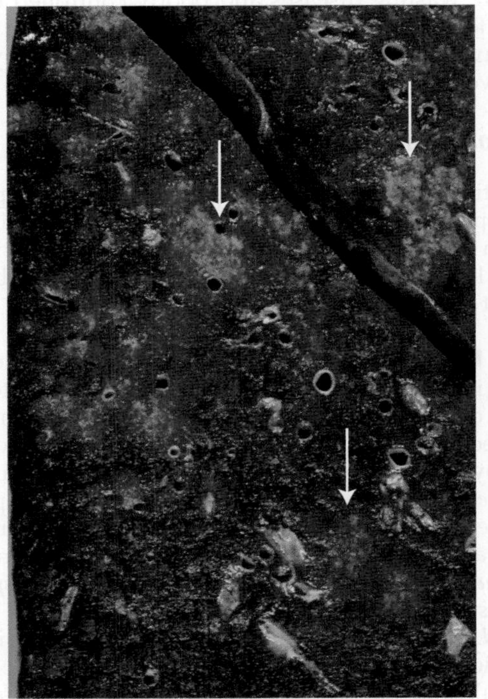

FIGURE 12-12. Bronchopneumonia. Scattered foci of consolidation (*arrows*) are centered on bronchi and bronchioles.

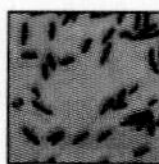

ETIOLOGIC FACTORS: *Streptococcus pneumoniae* was the classic cause of lobar pneumonia, but with antibiotic therapy, involvement of a lobe tends to be incomplete, and more than one lobe is usually affected. By contrast, bronchopneumonia is still a common cause of death and has been referred to as "the old man's friend." It typically develops in terminally ill patients, usually in the dependent and posterior portions of the lung. Scattered irregular foci of pneumonia are centered on terminal bronchioles and respiratory bronchioles. Bronchiolitis is seen, with polymorphonuclear exudates in adjacent alveoli. Large contiguous areas of alveolar involvement do not occur in bronchopneumonia.

Bacterial pneumonias occur in three settings:

- **Community-acquired pneumonia** arises outside the hospital in persons with no primary disorder of the immune system. The term may be used loosely to denote lobar pneumonia.
- **Nosocomial pneumonia** is infection that develops in hospital environments and tends to affect compromised patients.
- **Opportunistic pneumonia** afflicts persons whose immune status is defective.

Bacterial pneumonias should be classified on the basis of the etiologic agent, because clinical and morphologic features, and thus therapies, often vary with the causative organism.

Most bacteria that cause pneumonia are normal inhabitants of the oropharynx and nasopharynx that reach alveoli by aspiration of secretions. Other routes of infection include inhalation from the environment, hematogenous dissemination from an infectious focus elsewhere and (rarely) spread of bacteria from an adjacent site. A change in oropharyngeal flora from the normal commensals to a virulent organism often precedes the development of pneumonia. Predisposing conditions usually entail depressed host defenses and include cigarette smoking, chronic bronchitis, alcoholism, severe malnutrition, wasting diseases and poorly controlled diabetes. Debilitated or immunosuppressed patients in the hospital often have altered oropharyngeal flora and as many as 25% may develop nosocomial pneumonia.

Pneumococcal Pneumonia

Antibiotic therapy notwithstanding, *S. pneumoniae* (pneumococcus) pneumonia remains a significant problem. It is principally a disease of young to middle-aged adults. It is rare in infants, less common in the elderly and considerably more frequent in men than in women.

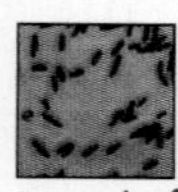

ETIOLOGIC FACTORS: Pneumococcal pneumonia is mostly a consequence of altered respiratory tract defenses. Frequently it follows a viral upper respiratory infection (e.g., influenza). The bronchial secretions stimulated by a viral infection provide a hospitable environment for *S. pneumoniae,* which are normal flora of the nasopharynx, to proliferate. The thin, watery secretions carry the organisms into the alveoli, thereby initiating an inflammatory response. ***The remarkably severe acute inflammation with spreading edema suggests that immunologic mechanisms may be involved.*** Aspiration of pneumococci may also follow impaired epiglottic reflexes, as occurs with exposure to cold, anesthesia and alcohol intoxication. Lung injury caused by, for example, congestive heart failure and irritant gases also increases susceptibility to pneumococcal pneumonia.

The capsule of the pneumococcus provides a defense against phagocytosis by alveolar macrophages. The organisms must therefore be opsonized before they can be ingested and killed. In an immune-competent person, antipneumococcal antibodies act as opsonins, but a host not previously exposed to the specific infecting strain of *S. pneumoniae* must use the alternative complement pathway to opsonize the bacteria.

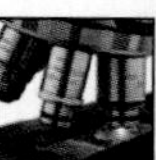

PATHOLOGY: In the earliest stage of pneumococcal pneumonia, protein-rich edema fluid containing numerous organisms fills the alveoli (Fig. 12-13). Marked capillary congestion leads to massive outpouring of polymorphonuclear leukocytes and intra-alveolar hemorrhage (Fig. 12-14). Because the firm consistency of the affected lung is reminiscent of the liver, this stage has been aptly named "**red hepatization**" (Fig. 12-13).

The next phase, occurring after 2 or more days, depending on the success of treatment, involves lysis of polymorphonuclear leukocytes and appearance of macrophages, which phagocytose the fragmented neutrophils and other inflammatory debris. At this stage, the congestion has diminished, but the lung is still firm ("**gray hepatization**") (Fig. 12-13). The alveolar exudate is then removed and the lung gradually returns to normal.

A number of complications may follow pneumococcal pneumonia:

- **Pleuritis,** often painful, is common, because the pneumonia readily extends to the pleura.
- **Pleural effusion** occurs frequently, but usually resolves.
- **Pyothorax** results from infection of a pleural effusion, and may heal with extensive fibrosis.
- **Empyema** (loculated collection of pus with fibrous walls) results from persistent pyothorax.
- **Bacteremia** occurs in the early stages of pneumococcal pneumonia in more than 25% of patients, and may lead to endocarditis or meningitis. Patients whose spleens have been removed often die of this bacteremia.
- **Pulmonary fibrosis** is a rare complication of pneumococcal pneumonia. The intra-alveolar exudate organizes to form intra-alveolar plugs of granulation tissue, known as **organizing pneumonia.** Gradually, increasing alveolar fibrosis leads to a shrunken and firm lobe, a rare complication known as **carnification.**
- **Lung abscess** is an unusual complication of pneumococcal pneumonia.

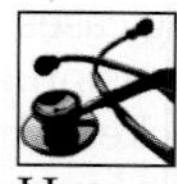

CLINICAL FEATURES: Pneumococcal pneumonia begins abruptly, with fever and chills. Chest pain secondary to pleural involvement is common. Hemoptysis is frequent and is characteristically "rusty," because it is derived from altered blood in alveolar spaces. Radiologic examination shows alveolar filling in large areas of lung, producing a solid appearance that extends to entire lobes or segments. Before antibiotic therapy, severe fever, dyspnea, debility and even loss of consciousness were common. Such symptoms were followed by **crisis** after 5 to 10 days, when a moribund patient would suddenly become afebrile and return from death's door. Satisfactory resolution of a crisis reflected effective immune responses to the infection. Unfortunately, about one third of patients died. Currently, pneumococcal pneumonia treatment is effective, and although symptoms respond rapidly, the radiographic lesion still takes several days to resolve.

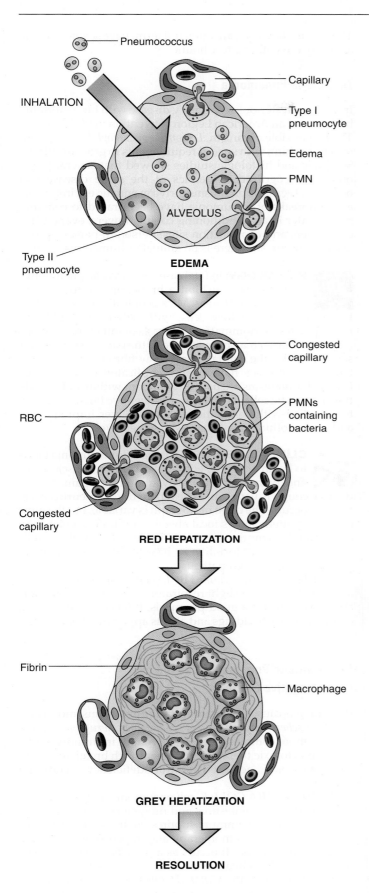

Pneumococcus
INHALATION
Capillary
Type I pneumocyte
Edema
PMN
ALVEOLUS
Type II pneumocyte
EDEMA
Congested capillary
PMNs containing bacteria
RBC
Congested capillary
RED HEPATIZATION
Fibrin
Macrophage
GREY HEPATIZATION
RESOLUTION

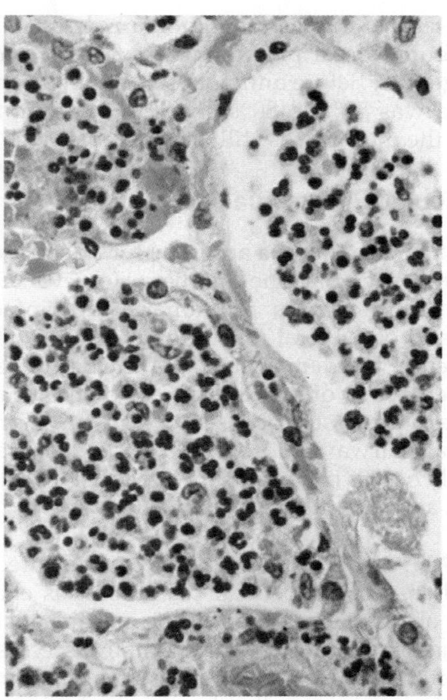

FIGURE 12-14. Pneumococcal pneumonia. The alveoli are packed with an exudate composed of polymorphonuclear leukocytes and occasional macrophages.

Klebsiella Pneumonia

Other than *S. pneumoniae, Klebsiella pneumoniae* is the only organism that causes lobar pneumonia with any frequency. However, *K. pneumoniae* accounts for only about 1% of all community-acquired pneumonias. The disease is commonly associated with alcoholism and is seen mostly in middle-aged men, although diabetes and chronic lung disease also increase the risk.

PATHOLOGY: The stages of *Klebsiella* pneumonia are not as well described as those in pneumococcal pneumonia, but acute phase congestion and hemorrhage are less pronounced. *K. pneumoniae* has a thick, gelatinous capsule, giving the cut lung surface a characteristic mucoid appearance. Another distinctive feature of *Klebsiella* pneumonia is that the affected lobe increases in size, so that the fissure "bulges" toward the unaffected region. There is a tendency toward tissue necrosis and abscess formation. A serious complication is **bronchopleural fistula** (i.e., a communication between the bronchial airway and the pleural space).

FIGURE 12-13. Pathogenesis of pneumococcal lobar pneumonia. Pneumococci, characteristically in pairs (diplococci), multiply rapidly in the alveolar spaces and produce extensive edema. They incite an acute inflammatory response in which polymorphonuclear leukocytes and congestion are prominent (red hepatization). As the inflammatory process progresses, macrophages replace the polymorphonuclear leukocytes and ingest debris (gray hepatization). The process usually resolves, but complications may ensue. PMN = polymorphonuclear neutrophil; RBC = red blood cell.

The onset of *Klebsiella* pneumonia is less dramatic than that of pneumococcal pneumonia, but the disease may be more dangerous. Before antibiotics, mortality from *Klebsiella* pneumonia was 50% to 80%. Even with prompt antibiotic treatment, the mortality is still considerable.

Staphylococcal Pneumonia

Staphylococcal pneumonia accounts for only 1% of community-acquired bacterial pneumonias. However, *Staphylococcus aureus* is a common pulmonary superinfection after influenza and other viral respiratory tract infections. In the 1918 influenza pandemic, it was a major cause of death. Repeated episodes of staphylococcal pneumonia are seen in patients with cystic fibrosis, owing to colonization of bronchiectatic airways. Nosocomial staphylococcal pneumonia typically occurs in chronically ill people who are prone to aspiration, and in intubated patients.

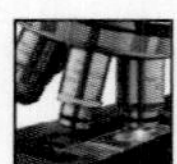

PATHOLOGY: Like staphylococcal infections elsewhere, staphylococcal pneumonia is characterized by abscess development. The multiple foci of staphylococcal pneumonia produce many small abscesses. In infants and, less often, in adults, these may lead to **pneumatoceles,** thin-walled cystic spaces lined primarily by respiratory tissue. Pneumatoceles may expand rapidly and compress surrounding lung or rupture into the pleural cavity and cause a tension pneumothorax. A pneumatocele develops when an abscess breaks into an airway, allowing expansion of the former by the pressure of inspired air. Cavitation and pleural effusions are common complications of staphylococcal pneumonia, but empyema is infrequent. Staphylococcal pneumonia requires aggressive therapy, particularly because *S. aureus* is often antibiotic resistant.

Other Streptococcal Pneumonias

Pulmonary infection with group A *Streptococcus pyogenes* was identified among soldiers as early as the 19th century. Its pathologic features were described during World War I. Streptococcal pneumonia typically follows viral respiratory tract infections and was a common superinfection in the 1918–1919 influenza pandemic. It is distinctly unusual in a community setting but is occasionally encountered in debilitated patients.

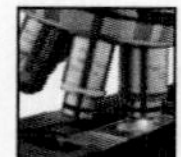

PATHOLOGY: On gross examination, the lungs of patients who die of streptococcal pneumonia are heavy, with bloody edema. Dry consolidation (hepatization) is not a feature of this disease. Microscopically, alveoli are filled with fibrin-containing fluid, but neutrophils are few. Alveolar necrosis may follow prolonged pneumonia. Empyema is a common complication.

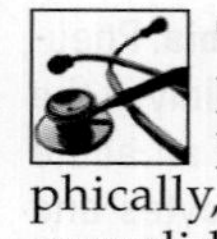

CLINICAL FEATURES: Patients with streptococcal pneumonia have abrupt fever, dyspnea, cough, chest pain, hemoptysis and often cyanosis. Radiographically, a bronchopneumonia pattern is observed; lobar consolidation is not seen. Intensive antibiotic therapy is indicated.

Streptococcal pneumonia in the newborn is usually caused by group B streptococci (*Streptococcus agalactiae*), a normal resident of the female genital tract. Symptoms are similar to those of the infantile respiratory distress syndrome. The infants, however, are often full term, have severe toxemia and may die within a few hours.

Legionella Pneumonia

In 1976, a mysterious respiratory disease with high mortality broke out at an American Legion convention in Philadelphia. The responsible organism, *Legionella pneumophila*, is a fastidious bacterium, with special requirements to grow in culture. Serologic and histologic studies showed that several previously unrecognized epidemics of the same disease had occurred. *Legionella* organisms thrive in aquatic environments and outbreaks of pneumonia have been traced to contaminated water in air-conditioning cooling towers, evaporative condensers and construction sites. Person-to-person spread does not occur, and there is no animal or human reservoir.

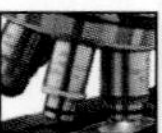

PATHOLOGY: In fatal cases of *Legionella* pneumonia, multiple lobes exhibit a bronchopneumonia, with large confluent areas. Microscopically, alveoli contain fibrin and inflammatory cells, with either neutrophils or macrophages predominating. Necrosis of inflammatory cells (leukocytoclasis) may be extensive. If the patient survives for several weeks, the exudate may show fibrous organization. One third of cases have been complicated by empyema. *Legionella* organisms are usually abundant within and outside the phagocytic cells. They are gram-negative but are difficult to visualize with conventional stains. Silver impregnation and immunofluorescent stains show them well.

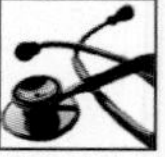

CLINICAL FEATURES: *Legionella* pneumonia tends to begin abruptly, with malaise, fever, muscle aches and pains and, curiously, abdominal pain. A productive cough is usual, and chest pain due to pleuritis occasionally occurs. The chest radiograph is variable, but the most common pattern shows focal alveolar infiltrates, which may be bilateral. Symptoms are usually less severe than radiographs suggest. Mortality is 10% to 20%, especially in immunocompromised patients.

Pontiac fever, also caused by *Legionella* species, is mainly a febrile illness with slight respiratory symptoms, radiologic abnormalities and a good prognosis. It has occurred in epidemics in office buildings and affects apparently healthy persons.

Opportunistic Pneumonia Caused by Gram-Negative Bacteria

Pneumonias caused by gram-negative organisms, most commonly *Escherichia coli* and *Pseudomonas aeruginosa*, have become more common with the advent of immunosuppressive and cytotoxic therapies, treatment with broad-spectrum antibiotics and acquired immunodeficiency syndrome (AIDS).

ESCHERICHIA COLI: *E. coli* pneumonia may follow bacteremia after gastrointestinal and urogenital surgery, even in patients who are not immunosuppressed. It also is seen in cancer patients given chemotherapy and in people with chronic lung or heart disease. It occurs as a bronchopneumonia and responds poorly to treatment.

PSEUDOMONAS AERUGINOSA: *Pseudomonas* pneumonia is most often seen in patients who are immunocompromised or have burns or cystic fibrosis. A history of antibiotic treatment of another infection is common. Often an infectious vasculitis, in which large numbers of organisms can be seen in blood vessel walls, results in pulmonary infarction. Antibiotic treatment of *Pseudomonas* pneumonia is often unsatisfactory.

Pneumonia Caused by Anaerobic Organisms

Many anaerobic organisms are normal commensals of the oral cavity, especially in people with poor dental hygiene. These include certain streptococci, fusobacteria and *Bacteroides* sp. Swallowing disorders, as in stuporous alcoholics, anesthetized patients and people subject to seizures, predispose to aspirating anaerobic bacteria. Resulting pulmonary infections cause necrotizing pneumonias, which often lead to lung abscesses. The most dramatic complication is gangrene of the lung, a result of thrombosis of a branch of the pulmonary artery and consequent infarction. This is a medical emergency and requires resection of the affected lung.

Psittacosis

Psittacosis is a lung infection due to inhalation of **Chlamydia psittaci** in dust contaminated with excreta from birds, usually pets and often parrots. It is characterized by severe systemic symptoms, with fever, malaise, and muscle aches, but surprisingly few respiratory symptoms other than cough. Chest radiographs may be negative, and when abnormal, they show irregular consolidation and an interstitial pattern. The morphologic patterns in most cases are unknown, but the disease is likely to be an interstitial pneumonia. In fatal cases, varying degrees of diffuse alveolar damage are present, together with edema, intra-alveolar pneumonia and necrosis.

Anthrax Pneumonia and Pneumonic Plague

Recent world events have focused considerable attention on infectious agents that could be used as weapons of bioterrorism. Chief among these are *Bacillus anthracis* and *Yersinia pestis*.

B. anthracis is the causative agent of anthrax, a gram-positive, spore-forming bacillus. Anthrax occurs in many species of domestic animals, but human infection occurs infrequently or in sporadic outbreaks. Transmission is via direct contact with the spores, and person-to-person transmission is uncommon. Cutaneous anthrax is rarely fatal, but inhalational anthrax has a high mortality. Anthrax spores are highly resistant to drying, and when inhaled they are transported to mediastinal lymph nodes. From there, bacilli emerge and rapidly disseminate through the bloodstream to other organs, including the lungs. Hemorrhagic necrosis of infected organs ensues, the most pronounced of which is a hemorrhagic mediastinal mass. In the lungs, the disease is manifested by hemorrhagic bronchitis and confluent areas of hemorrhagic pneumonia.

Y. pestis, the causative agent of *plague,* produces two forms of infection, a bubonic form and a pneumonic form. In pneumonic plague the organisms are inhaled directly without transmission by an arthropod vector, and disease may be spread from person to person. The lungs typically show extensive hemorrhagic bronchopneumonia, pleuritis and enlargement of mediastinal lymph nodes. The untreated disease progresses rapidly and is highly fatal.

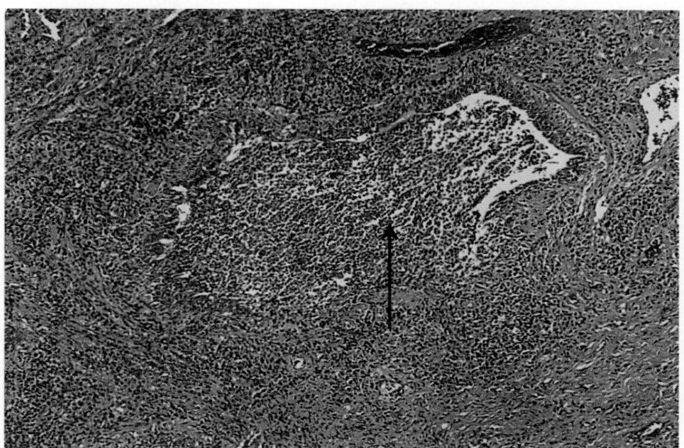

FIGURE 12-15. Mycoplasma pneumonia. Chronic bronchiolitis with a neutrophilic luminal exudate (*arrow*).

Mycoplasma Pneumoniae Causes Atypical Pneumonia

Unlike lobar pneumonia, atypical pneumonia begins insidiously. Leukocytosis is absent or slight and the course is prolonged. Respiratory symptoms may be minimal or severe, and the chest radiograph shows a patchy intra-alveolar pneumonia or an interstitial infiltrate. The infection characteristically causes a bronchiolitis with a neutrophilic intraluminal exudate and an intense lymphoplasmacytic infiltrate in bronchiolar walls (Fig. 12-15). *Mycoplasma* lack the rigid cell wall that most bacteria possess. They are slow growing and often difficult to culture by traditional methods. The diagnosis is often established by serologic detection of *M. pneumoniae* antibodies or cold agglutinins. Erythromycin is effective, and the infection is only rarely fatal.

Tuberculosis Is the Classic Granulomatous Infection

Known since ancient Egypt, tuberculosis was the scourge of 19th-century Europe and North America. Its prevalence declined exponentially in the 20th century, and the introduction of antituberculosis drugs further diminished the impact of the disease. However, tuberculosis has recently reemerged, particularly drug-resistant strains and among patients with AIDS. The infection is discussed in detail in Chapter 9. Here we consider only the pulmonary pathology.

Tuberculosis represents infection with *Mycobacterium tuberculosis,* although atypical mycobacterial infections may mimic tuberculosis. The disease is divided into primary and secondary (or reactivation) tuberculosis.

PRIMARY TUBERCULOSIS: The disease is acquired from the initial exposure to *M. tuberculosis,* most commonly as a result of inhaling infected aerosols generated when a person with cavitary tuberculosis coughs. The inhaled organisms multiply in the alveoli because the alveolar macrophages cannot readily kill the bacteria.

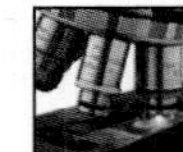

PATHOLOGY: The **Ghon lesion** is the first lesion of primary tuberculosis and consists of a peripheral parenchymal granuloma, often in the upper lobes.

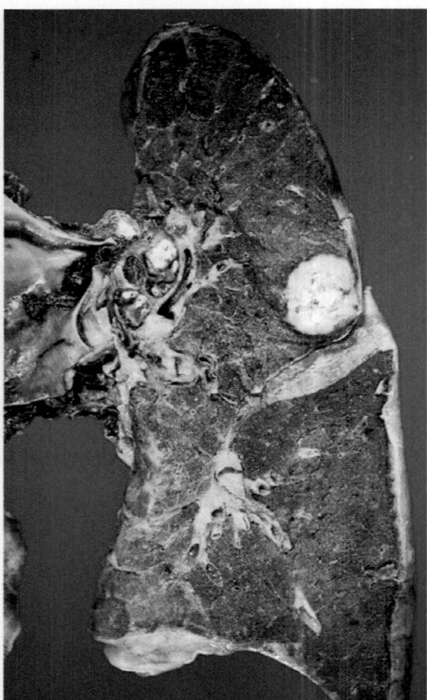

FIGURE 12-16. Primary tuberculosis. A healed Ghon complex is represented by a subpleural nodule and involved hilar lymph nodes.

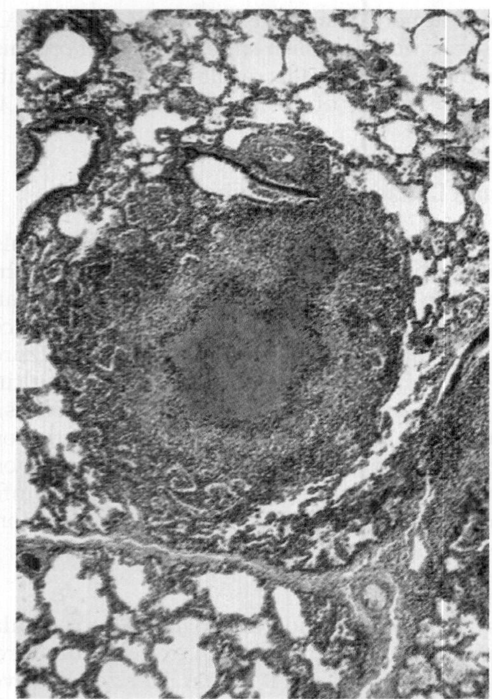

FIGURE 12-17. Necrotizing granuloma due to *Mycobacterium tuberculosis.* A small tuberculous granuloma with conspicuous central caseation is present in the pulmonary parenchyma. The necrotic center is surrounded by histiocytes, giant cells and fibrous tissue.

When this lesion is associated with an enlarged mediastinal lymph node, a **Ghon complex** is formed (Fig. 12-16). On gross examination, the healed, subpleural Ghon nodule is 1 to 2 cm in diameter, well circumscribed and centrally necrotic. In later stages, it is fibrotic and calcified. Microscopically, a granuloma with central caseous necrosis (Fig. 12-17) shows varying degrees of fibrosis. The microscopic features of draining hilar lymph nodes are similar to those of the peripheral parenchymal lesion.

Most (90% or more) primary tuberculous infections are asymptomatic; lesions remain localized and heal. In some instances there is self-limited extension to the pleura, with secondary pleural effusion. Less often, primary tuberculosis is not limited but spreads to other parts of the lung **(progressive primary tuberculosis).** This usually happens in young children or immunosuppressed adults. In this situation, the initial lesion enlarges, producing necrotic areas up to 6 cm or more in greatest dimension. Central liquefaction results in cavities, which may expand to occupy most of the lower lobe. At the same time, draining lymph nodes display similar histologic changes. Erosion of a bronchus by the necrotizing process leads to further pulmonary dissemination of the disease.

SECONDARY TUBERCULOSIS: This stage represents either reactivation of primary pulmonary tuberculosis or new infection in a host previously sensitized by primary tuberculosis.

PATHOLOGY: The initial reaction to *M. tuberculosis* is different in secondary tuberculosis. A cellular immune response occurs after a latent interval and leads to formation of many granulomas and extensive tissue necrosis. Apical and posterior segments of the upper lobes are most commonly involved, but the superior segment of the lower lobe is also often affected, and no part of the lung can be excluded. A diffuse, fibrotic, poorly defined lesion develops, with focal areas of caseous necrosis. Often these foci heal and calcify, but some may erode into bronchi, after which drainage of infectious material creates a tuberculous cavity.

Tuberculous cavities range from under 1 cm in diameter to large, cystic areas occupying almost the entire lung. Most measure 3 to 10 cm in diameter and tend to be situated in the apices of the upper lobes (Fig. 12-18), although they may occur anywhere in the lung. The wall of the cavity is composed of

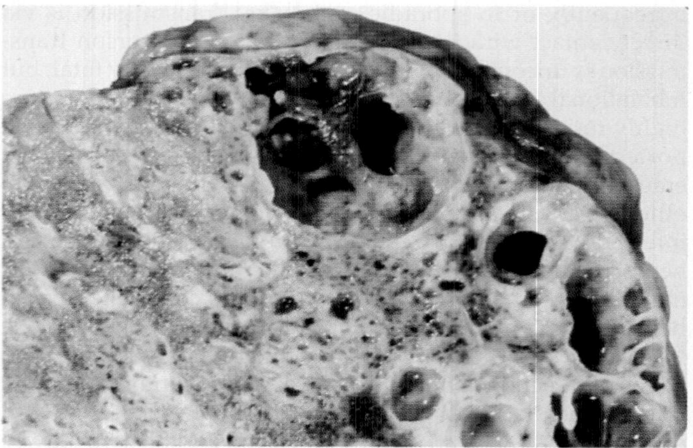

FIGURE 12-18. Cavitary tuberculosis. The apex of the left upper lobe shows tuberculous cavities surrounded by consolidated and fibrotic pulmonary parenchyma that contains small tubercles.

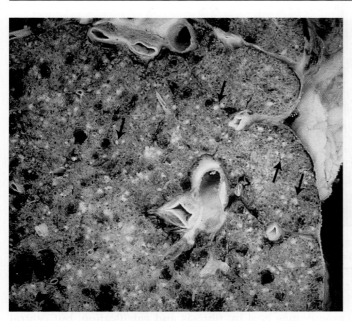

FIGURE 12-19. Miliary tuberculosis. Multiple millimeter-sized nodules (*arrows*) are scattered throughout the lung parenchyma.

an inner, thin, gray membrane encompassing soft necrotic nodules; a middle zone of granulation tissue; and an outer collagenous border. The lumen is filled with caseous material containing acid-fast bacilli. Cavities often communicate freely with a bronchus, and the release of infectious material into airways spreads infection within the lung. The walls of healed tuberculous cavities eventually become fibrotic and calcified.

Secondary tuberculosis is associated with a number of complications:

- **Miliary tuberculosis** is the presence of multiple, small (size of millet seeds), tuberculous granulomas (Fig. 12-19) in many organs. The organisms disseminate from the lung or other sites via the blood, usually during secondary tuberculosis, but occasionally in primary disease.
- **Hemoptysis** is caused by erosion of small pulmonary arteries in the wall of a cavity. It may be severe enough to drown patients in their own blood.
- **Bronchopleural fistula** occurs when a subpleural cavity ruptures into the pleural space. In turn, tuberculous empyema and pneumothorax result.
- **Tuberculous laryngitis** is a consequence of coughing up infectious material.
- **Intestinal tuberculosis** may follow swallowing of the same tuberculous material.
- **Aspergilloma** is a fungal mass that follows superinfection of a persistent open cavity with *Aspergillus;* the fungi may fill the entire cavity.

MYCOBACTERIUM AVIUM-INTRACELLULARE (MAI): In patients with AIDS, whose ability to mount a granulomatous reaction may be impaired, MAI pneumonia is characterized by an extensive infiltrate of macrophages and innumerable acid-fast organisms (Fig. 12-20). MAI may colonize airways of older, immunocompetent individuals with underlying pulmonary disorders such as bronchiectasis, or it may produce granulomatous inflammation with or without cavitation. *Mycobacterium kansasii* produces a spectrum of disease similar to that of MAI but is not as frequently encountered, owing to a more restricted geographic distribution.

Actinomycosis Features Multiple Lung Abscesses

Actinomycosis is caused by infection with actinomycetes, and the usual pulmonary organism is *Actinomyces israelii.* Although actinomycetes resemble fungi in appearance, they are anaerobic filamentous bacteria. These gram-positive organisms normally inhabit the mouth and nose, and infect the lung by aspiration of oropharyngeal contents or by extension from an actinomycotic subdiaphragmatic abscess or liver abscess.

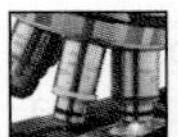

PATHOLOGY: Lung lesions of actinomycosis consist of multiple, interconnecting, small lung abscesses. The abscess margins are granulomatous, but central necrotic areas are purulent and contain colonies of organisms,

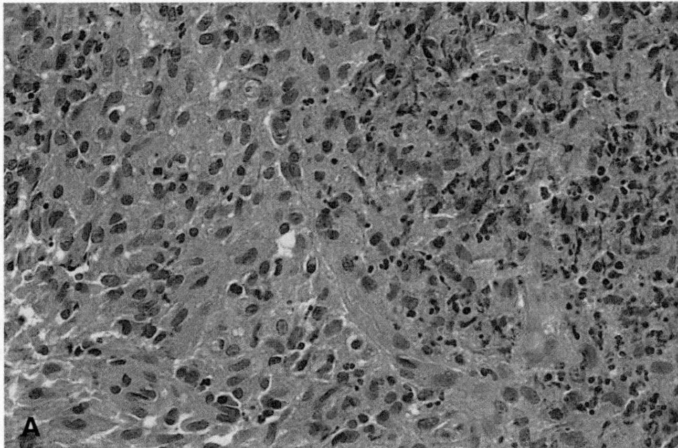

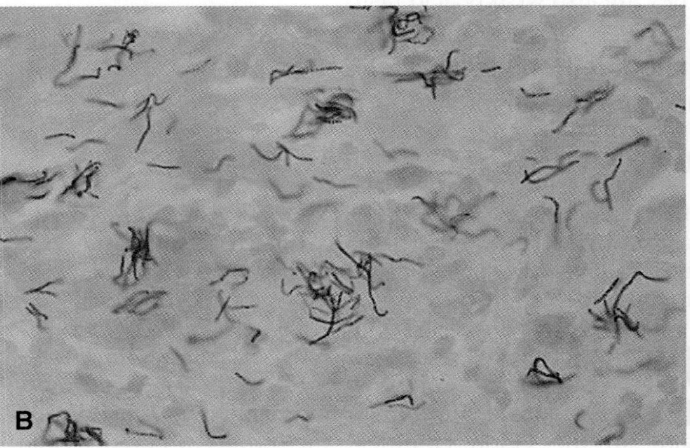

FIGURE 12-20. *Mycobacterium avium-intracellulare* pneumonia in acquired immunodeficiency syndrome (AIDS). **A.** The pneumonia is characterized by an extensive infiltrate of macrophages. **B.** The Ziehl-Neelsen stain shows numerous acid-fast organisms.

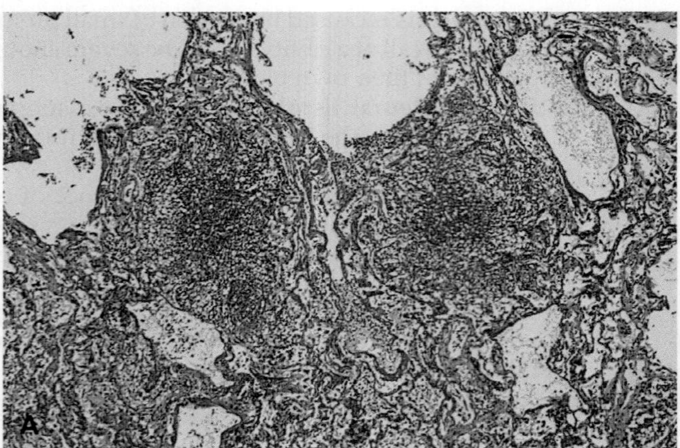

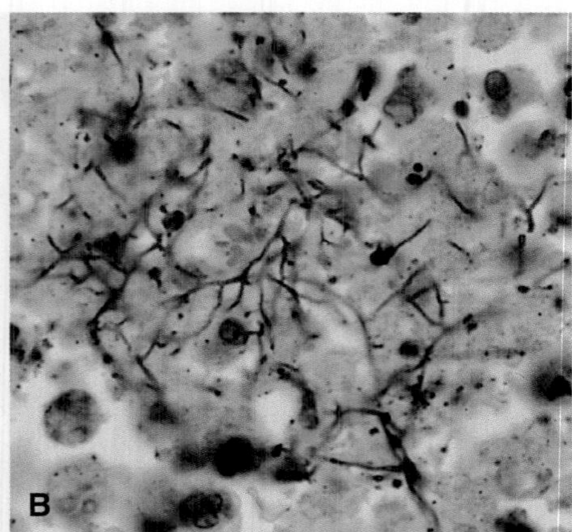

FIGURE 12-21. Nocardiosis. A. This lung shows abscesses consisting of focal collections of acute inflammation. **B.** The organisms are thin, filamentous, branching bacteria (Gomori methenamine silver).

which are thin, branching, filamentous, gram-positive bacteria. Clubbed basophilic filaments are noted at the margins of the colonies, which are visible to the naked eye as small yellow particles (**"sulfur granules"**). The abscesses may invade the pleura and produce bronchopulmonary fistulas and empyema. They may also invade the chest wall.

Nocardia Is Usually an Opportunistic Organism

Nocardia is a gram-positive filamentous bacterium that causes an acute progressive or chronic bacterial pneumonia. Infection is mostly seen in immunocompromised patients, particularly those with lymphomas, neutropenia, chronic granulomatous disease of childhood and pulmonary alveolar proteinosis. *Nocardia asteroides* is the most common *Nocardia* sp. to cause pneumonia.

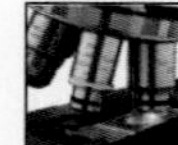

PATHOLOGY: Histologically, lungs show abscesses (Fig. 12-21A), which may have granulomatous features in chronic infections. The organisms are delicate, beaded, thin filaments, which branch mostly at right angles (Fig. 12-21B). In tissue sections, they are best seen with a Gram stain or Gomori methenamine silver stain (Fig. 12-21B). They are also weakly acid fast.

Fungal Infections May be Geographic or Opportunistic

Histoplasmosis

Histoplasmosis is a disease of the midwestern and southeastern United States, particularly the Mississippi and Ohio river valleys. It is caused by inhalation of *Histoplasma capsulatum* in infected dust, commonly from bird droppings.

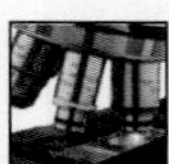

PATHOLOGY: Histoplasmosis has many clinical and pathologic similarities to tuberculosis. Most infections are asymptomatic and result in lesions comparable to the Ghon complex, including a parenchymal granuloma and similar lesions in the draining lymph nodes. The granulomas are particularly prone to calcify, often with a concentric laminar pattern. In the acute phase, numerous organisms are seen within macrophages. Granulomatous inflammation follows, often with central areas of necrosis. The granulomas heal by fibrosis and calcification, but central necrotic areas may persist. The spherical organisms are best seen with a silver stain as 2 to 4 μm in diameter with narrow-based budding.

In a few cases, pulmonary lesions progress or reactivate, leading to a progressive fibrotic and necrotic lesion that closely resembles that of reactivation tuberculosis. However, lesions of histoplasmosis are more fibrotic than those of tuberculosis, and cavitation is less common. The reason for progression is not known, although large infective doses and poor host responses are usually considered to be responsible. Immunocompromised patients are at particular risk for the dissemination of *Histoplasma* within the lungs and spread to other organs.

Coccidioidomycosis

Coccidioidomycosis, caused by inhalation of spores of *Coccidioides immitis,* was originally known as San Joaquin Valley fever, after the location where the disease has been endemic for many years. However, the infection is widespread throughout the southwestern part of the United States and shares many of the clinical and pathologic features of histoplasmosis and tuberculosis. In histologic sections the organism is a spherule, 30 to 100 μm in diameter, with a thick refractile wall. The spherules contain innumerable endospores, 2 to 5 μm in diameter. Empty spherules or endospores that have been released into the tissue may also be visible.

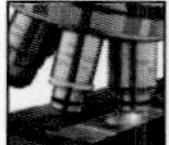

PATHOLOGY: In most instances lesions are limited to a peripheral parenchymal granuloma, with or without lymph node granulomas. Sometimes, the lesion may be slowly progressive. In immunocompromised persons the disease may progress rapidly, with release of endospores into the lung, in which case the tissue reaction may be purulent as well as granulomatous.

Cryptococcosis

Cryptococcosis results from the inhalation of spores of *Cryptococcus neoformans,* which is often found in pigeon droppings. Lung lesions range from small parenchymal granulomas to several large granulomatous nodules, pneumonic consolidation and even cavitation. Most serious cases of pulmonary cryptococcosis occur in immunocompromised patients, in whom the organisms proliferate extensively within alveolar spaces, with little tissue reaction. The organisms are 4 to 6 μm in diameter, but may be larger, with narrow-based budding and a thick mucoid capsule.

North American Blastomycosis

Blastomycosis is an uncommon condition caused by *Blastomyces dermatitidis*. It is concentrated in the basins of the Missouri, Mississippi and Ohio rivers in the United States, and in southern Manitoba and northwestern Ontario in Canada. Clinical and pathologic features resemble those of the fungi mentioned above. Initial infection produces a lesion resembling a Ghon complex or progressive pneumonitis. Unlike tuberculous Ghon complexes, the focal lesions of blastomycosis show central necrosis with a purulent reaction, surrounded by granulomatous inflammation. The organisms are 8 to 15 μm in diameter, have a thick refractile wall and exhibit broad-based budding.

Aspergillosis

Infection of the lungs by *Aspergillus* spp., usually *Aspergillus niger* or *Aspergillus fumigatus,* can occur under a number of circumstances.

- **Invasive aspergillosis:** This is the most serious form of *Aspergillus* infection, occurring almost exclusively as an opportunistic infection in people with compromised immunity, usually due to cytotoxic therapy or AIDS. The lungs show patchy, multifocal consolidation and, occasionally, cavities. Extensive blood vessel invasion (usually arterial [Fig. 12-22]) results in occlusion, thrombosis and infarction of lung tissue. Invasive aspergillosis is a fulminant pulmonary infection that is not amenable to therapy.
- **Aspergilloma ("fungus ball" or mycetoma):** *Aspergillus* spp. may grow in preexisting cavities, such as those caused by tuberculosis or bronchiectasis, where they proliferate to form fungus balls (Fig. 12-23). Radiographs show a large mass within an air-filled cavity. Fungus balls are usually clinically inapparent and merely represent an interesting radiologic finding. However, if they become clinically evident, they most often present with hemoptysis, owing to either the underlying condition or, less commonly, fungal infection of the cavity wall.
- **Allergic bronchopulmonary aspergillosis (ABPA):** Certain asthmatics have an unusual immunologic reaction to *Aspergillus* that is characterized by (1) transient pulmonary infiltrates on chest radiographs, (2) eosinophilia of blood and sputum, (3) skin sensitivity and serum precipitins to *A. fumigatus* and (4) increased serum IgE. Computed tomography shows thickened bronchial walls and mucous plugs in the bronchi.

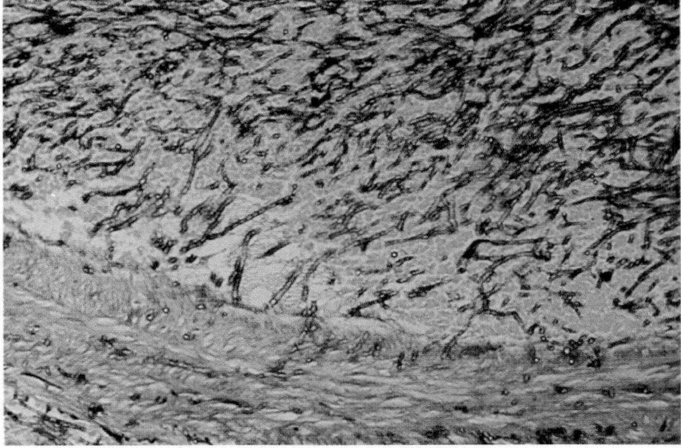

FIGURE 12-22. Invasive pulmonary aspergillosis. A branch of the pulmonary artery shows fungal hyphae in the wall and within the lumen (Gomori methenamine silver stain).

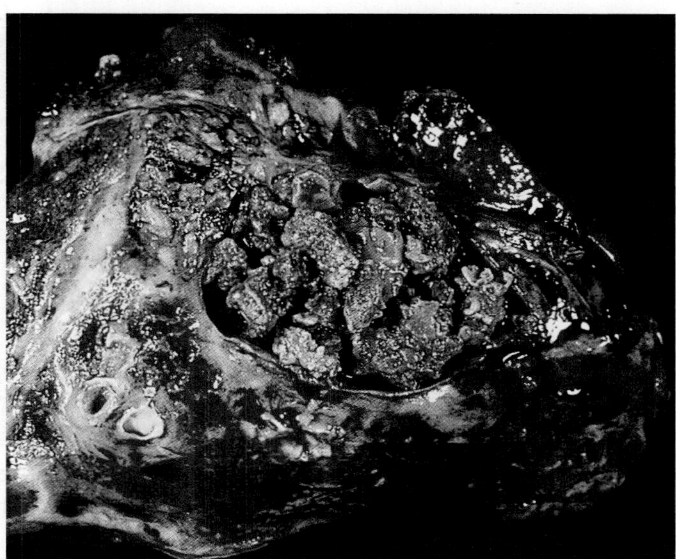

FIGURE 12-23. ***Aspergillus* fungus ball.** The lung contains a cavity filled with a fungus ball.

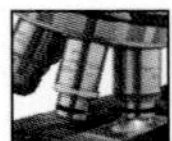

PATHOLOGY: ABPA is invariably associated with proximal (central) bronchiectasis, involving segmental bronchi and the next two to four orders of subsegmental bronchi. The lungs show bronchial and bronchiolar mucous plugs, infiltrates of eosinophils and Charcot-Leyden crystals (Fig. 12-24A,B). Bronchocentric granulomatosis and eosinophilic pneumonia may be present. The bronchial mucus may contain septate, fungal hyphae, with 45° branching. Interestingly, the peripheral bronchial tree is spared.

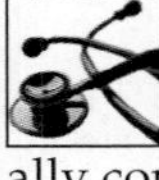

CLINICAL FEATURES: Patients with ABPA have wheezing, chest pain and cough, and often produce thick mucous plugs. Systemic corticosteroids usually control the acute episode.

Pneumocystis jiroveci

First described as "plasma cell pneumonia," pulmonary infection with *Pneumocystis jiroveci* (formerly *Pneumocystis carinii*) was identified in malnourished infants at the end of World War II. It was increasingly recognized as use of immunosuppression for renal transplantation and in the chemotherapy for malignant disease became common. It also frequently causes infectious pneumonia in patients with AIDS. Once

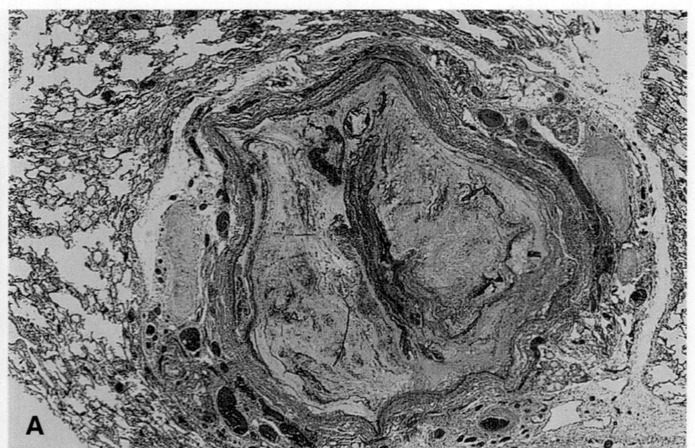

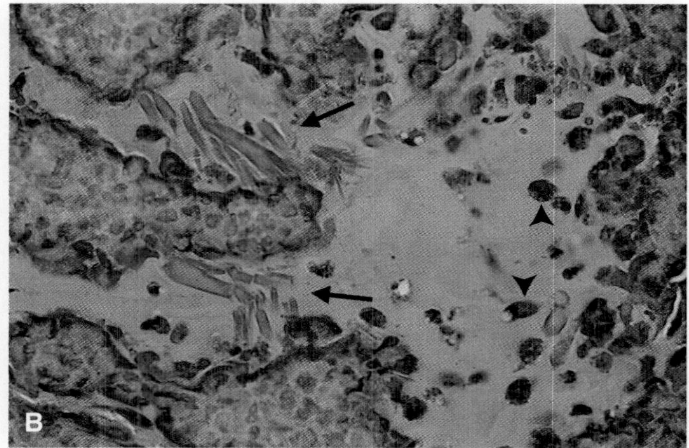

FIGURE 12-24. Allergic bronchopulmonary aspergillosis. A. A dilated bronchus is filled with a mucous plug that has dense layers of eosinophilic infiltrates. **B.** Higher magnification shows numerous eosinophils (*arrowheads*) and Charcot-Leyden crystals (*arrows*).

considered a protozoan, *Pneumocystis* has been reclassified as a fungus.

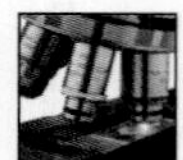

PATHOLOGY: The classic lesion of *Pneumocystis* pneumonia is an interstitial infiltrate of plasma cells and lymphocytes and hyperplasia of type II pneumocytes. Alveoli are filled with a characteristic foamy exudate, in which the organisms appear as small bubbles in a background of proteinaceous exudate (Fig. 12-25A). With silver impregnation, cysts appear as round or indented ("crescent moon") bodies, 5 μm in diameter (Fig. 12-25B). A darkly stained focus represents focal thickening of the capsule. After sporozoites develop within the cyst, it ruptures and assumes an indented shape. Sporozoites develop into trophozoites, which may be seen with stains such as Giemsa in cytology specimens, but are very difficult to see in routine histologic sections. Granulomatous inflammation in *Pneumocystis* pneumonia is rare but occurs in up to 5% of lung biopsies from human immunodeficiency virus (HIV)-infected patients. In some cases, *Pneumocystis* also produces diffuse alveolar damage (see below).

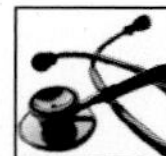

CLINICAL FEATURES: Clinically and radiologically, *Pneumocystis* pneumonia presents *a* variable picture. At one extreme, symptoms may be minimal, while at the other, there is rapidly progressive respiratory failure. In HIV-infected patients, thin-walled cysts may develop and predispose to pneumothorax. The diagnosis is made by identifying the organism using sputum examination, bronchoalveolar lavage, transbronchial biopsy, needle aspiration of the lung or open lung biopsy. Treatment is with trimethoprim–sulfamethoxazole or pentamidine.

Viral Infections of the Lung Produce Diffuse Alveolar Damage or Interstitial Pneumonia

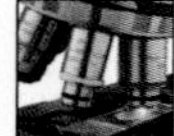

PATHOLOGY: Viral infections initially affect the alveolar epithelium and result in a mononuclear infiltrate in the interstitium of the lung (Fig. 12-26). Hyaline membranes and necrosis of type I epithelial cells lead to an appearance indistinguishable from diffuse alveolar damage from other causes. In some instances, alveolar

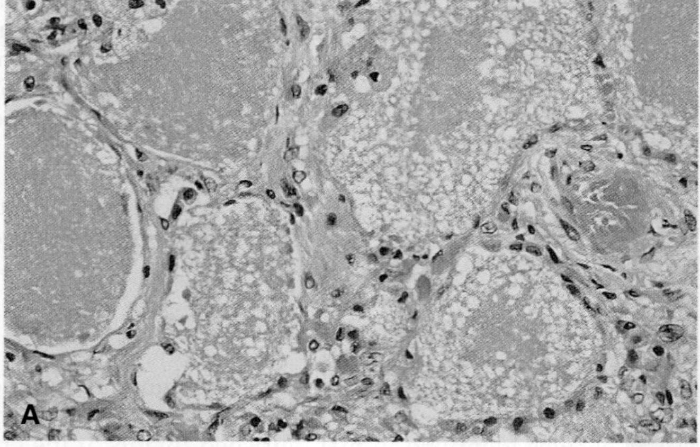

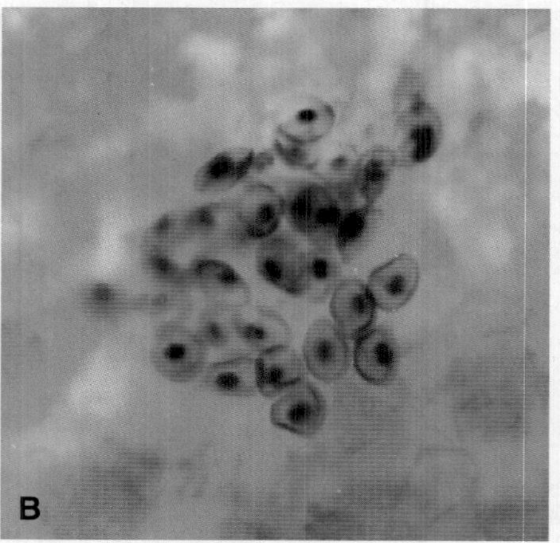

FIGURE 12-25. *Pneumocystis jiroveci* pneumonia. A. The alveoli are filled with a foamy exudate, and the interstitium is thickened and contains a chronic inflammatory infiltrate. **B.** A centrifuged bronchoalveolar lavage specimen impregnated with silver shows a cluster of *Pneumocystis* cysts.

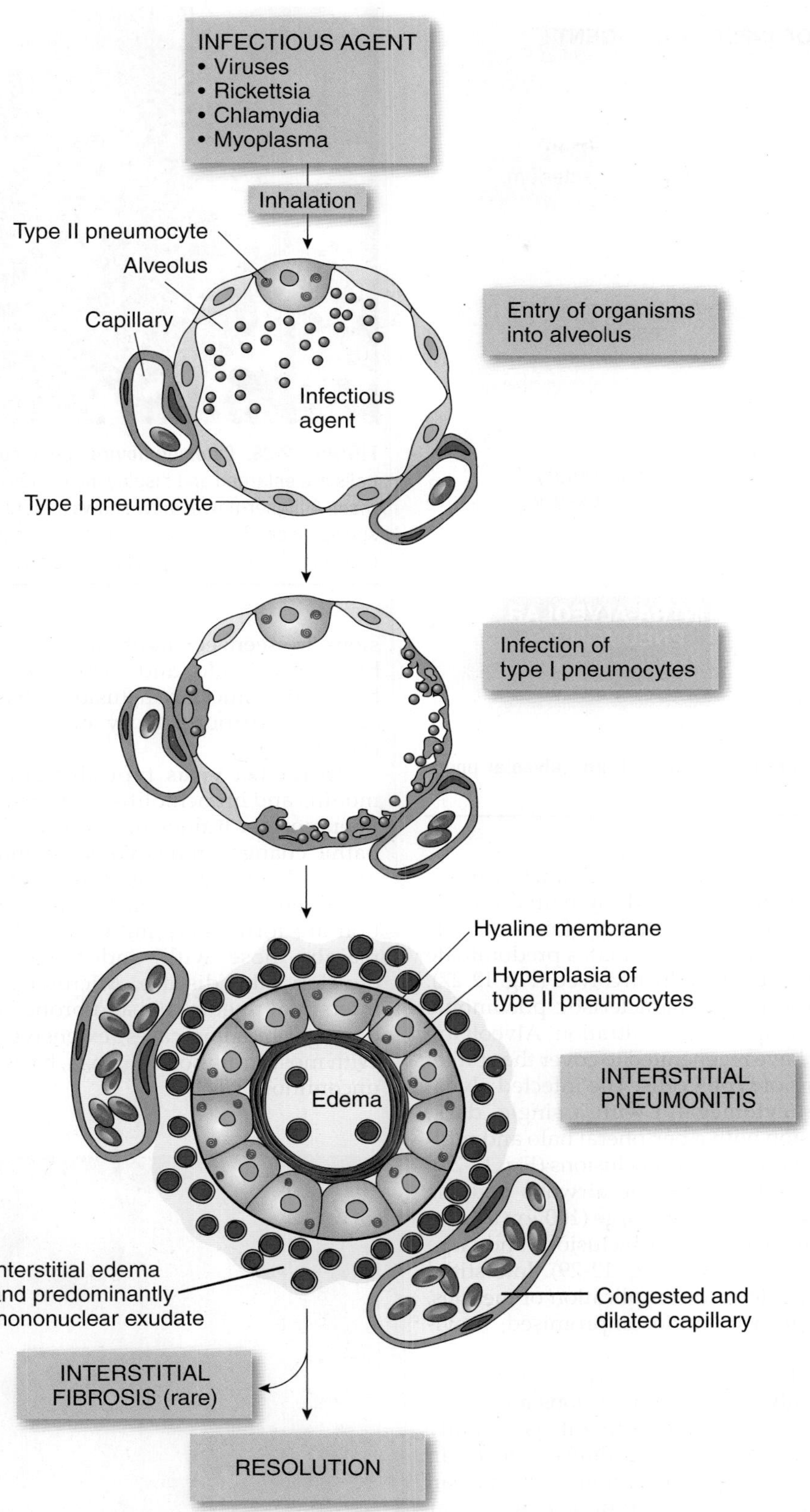

FIGURE 12-26. Pathogenesis of interstitial pneumonia. Although interstitial pneumonia is most commonly caused by viruses, other organisms also may cause significant interstitial inflammation. Type I cells are the most sensitive to damage, and loss of their integrity leads to intra-alveolar edema. The proteinaceous exudate and cell debris form hyaline membranes, and type II cells multiply to line the alveoli. Interstitial inflammation is characterized mainly by mononuclear cells. The disease generally resolves completely but occasionally progresses to interstitial fibrosis.

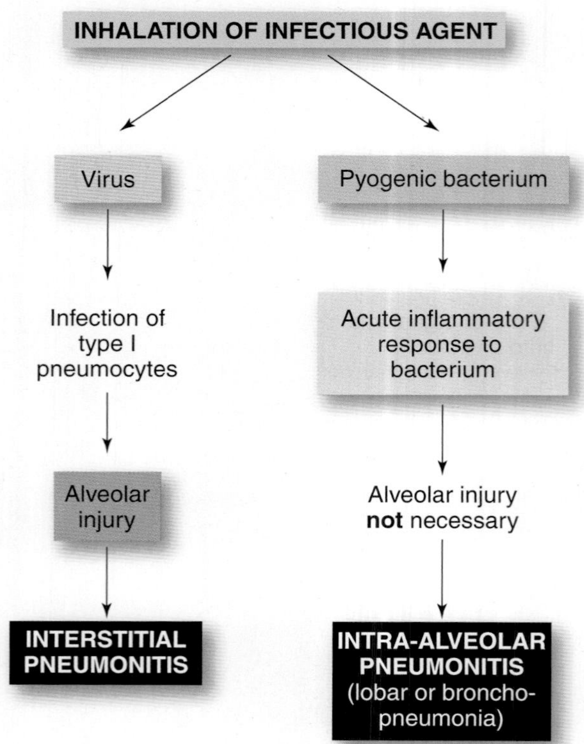

FIGURE 12-27. Pathogenesis of interstitial and intra-alveolar pneumonitis.

damage may be indolent, and the disease is characterized by hyperplasia of type II pneumocytes and interstitial inflammation. This appearance contrasts with that of most bacterial infections, in which intra-alveolar exudates predominate and the interstitium is only incidentally involved (Fig. 12-27).

Cytomegalovirus produces a characteristic pneumonia with intense interstitial lymphocytic infiltration. Alveoli are lined by type II cells that have regenerated to cover the epithelial defect left by necrosis of type I cells. The infected alveolar cells are very large (cytomegaly) with a single, dark, basophilic nuclear inclusion with a peripheral halo and multiple, indistinct cytoplasmic, basophilic inclusions (Fig. 12-28).

Measles infection involves both the airways and the parenchyma. It is characterized by very large (100 μm across) multinucleated giant cells with nuclear inclusions and large eosinophilic cytoplasmic inclusions (Fig. 12-29). Interstitial pneumonia is a well-characterized complication of measles, but is rarely fatal, except in immunocompromised, previously unexposed persons.

Varicella infection (chickenpox and herpes zoster) produces disseminated, focally necrotic lung lesions and interstitial pneumonia. Pulmonary involvement is usually asymptomatic, except in immunocompromised hosts, in whom it may be fatal. The viral inclusions are nuclear, eosinophilic and refractile and are surrounded by a clear halo. Multinucleation can occur.

Herpes simplex can cause a necrotizing tracheobronchitis as well as diffuse alveolar damage. Viral inclusions are identical to those seen in varicella infection.

Adenovirus pneumonia causes necrotizing bronchiolitis and bronchopneumonia. Two types of nuclear inclusions are seen: eosinophilic nuclear inclusions surrounded by a clear halo and "smudge cells," with indistinct, basophilic, nuclear inclusions that fill the entire nucleus and are surrounded by only a thin rim of chromatin (Fig. 12-30).

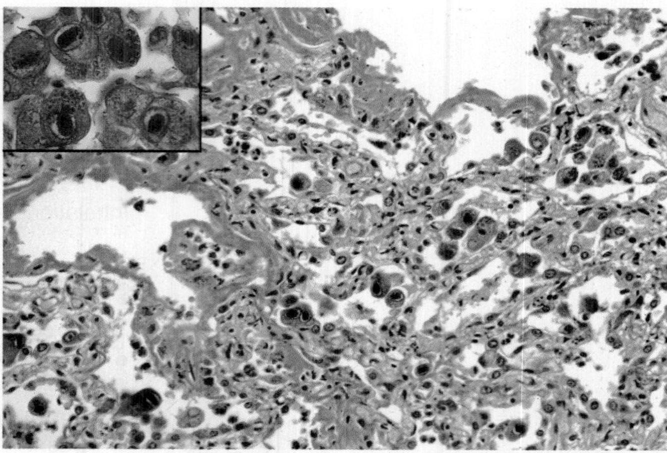

FIGURE 12-28. Cytomegalovirus pneumonitis. The infected alveolar cells are enlarged and display the typical dark blue nuclear inclusions. *Inset.* A higher-power view shows infected alveolar cells that display a single basophilic nuclear inclusion with a perinuclear halo and multiple, indistinct, basophilic, cytoplasmic inclusions.

Influenza virus typically produces interstitial pneumonitis and bronchiolitis similar to those seen in other viral pneumonias. It does not produce characteristic viral cytopathic changes in histologic sections. The recent pandemic of H1N1 influenza has drawn attention to the pathology of influenza pneumonia. Whereas most cases of H1N1 infection are fortunately mild and self-limited, some patients, mainly those with underlying health problems, may develop fatal disease. Microscopic findings range from interstitial pneumonia and bronchiolitis to diffuse alveolar damage. In some cases, extensive hemorrhage is present. With most strains of influenza, bacterial superinfection is not uncommon.

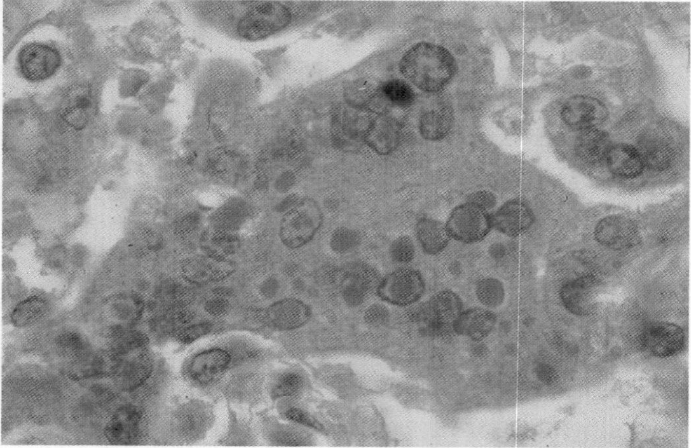

FIGURE 12-29. Measles pneumonitis. This multinucleated giant cell shows single, eosinophilic, refractile inclusions within each of the nuclei, as well as multiple, irregular, eosinophilic, cytoplasmic inclusions.

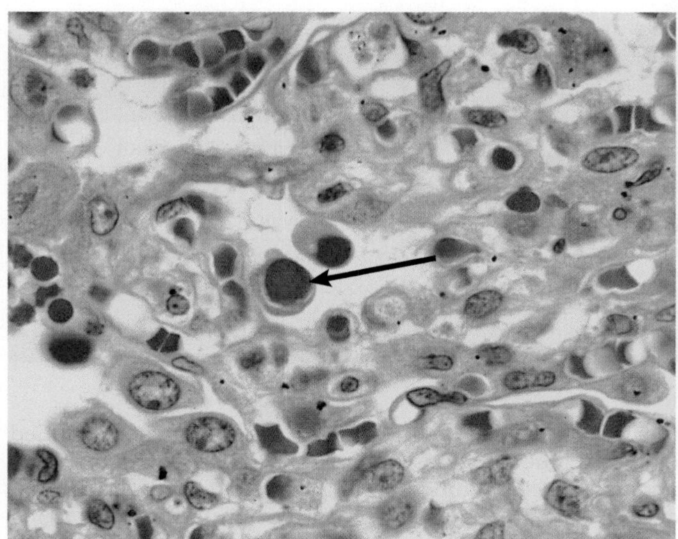

FIGURE 12-30. Adenovirus pneumonia. The "smudge" cell in the center (*arrow*) consists of a smudgy basophilic nuclear inclusion.

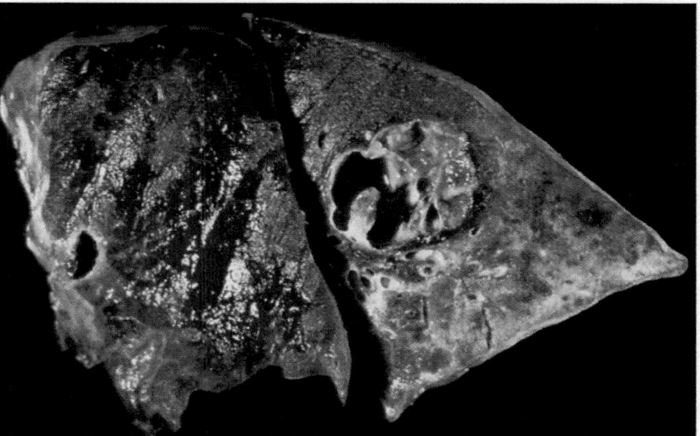

FIGURE 12-31. Pulmonary abscess. A large cystic abscess contains a purulent exudate and is contained by a fibrous wall. Pneumonia is present in the surrounding pulmonary parenchyma.

The Most Common Cause of Lung Abscess Is Aspiration

Lung abscesses are localized accumulations of pus accompanied by destruction of pulmonary parenchyma, including alveoli, airways and blood vessels.

A state of depressed consciousness often predisposes to the aspiration that causes lung abscesses, and aspirated oropharyngeal anaerobic bacteria produce over 90% of cases. Infections are typically polymicrobial, often with fusiform bacteria and *Bacteroides* spp. Other organisms encountered in lung abscesses caused by aspiration include *S. aureus, K. pneumoniae, S. pneumoniae* and *Nocardia*.

Aspiration of enough bacteria to produce a lung abscess requires that a large number of anaerobic bacteria are present in the oral flora, as in people with poor oral hygiene or periodontal disease. The cough reflex or tracheobronchial clearance must also be impaired. Not surprisingly, alcoholism is the most common condition predisposing to lung abscess. Drug overdoses, epilepsy and neurologic impairment also increase the risk. Other causes of lung abscess include necrotizing pneumonias, bronchial obstruction, infected pulmonary emboli, penetrating trauma and extension of infection from tissues adjacent to the lung.

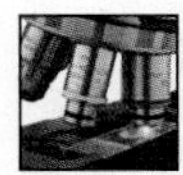

PATHOLOGY: Lung abscesses mostly range from 2 to 6 cm in diameter; 10% to 20% have multiple cavities, usually after a necrotizing pneumonia or a shower of septic pulmonary emboli. The right side of the lung is more often involved than the left, because the right main bronchus follows the direction of the trachea more closely at its bifurcation. Acute lung abscesses are not well separated from the surrounding lung parenchyma. They show abundant polymorphonuclear leukocytes and, depending on the age of the lesion, variable numbers of macrophages and debris from necrotic tissue. Abscesses are surrounded by hemorrhage, fibrin and inflammation. As they age, a fibrous wall forms around the margin. Lung abscesses differ from abscesses elsewhere in that they may drain spontaneously. The cavity thus formed contains air, necrotic debris and inflammatory exudate (Fig. 12-31), creating a fluid level that is easily seen radiographically. The cavity lining becomes covered with regenerating squamous epithelium. Walls of old abscesses may be lined by ciliated respiratory epithelium, making a distinction from bronchiectasis difficult.

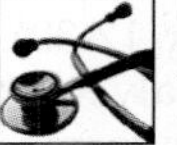

CLINICAL FEATURES: Almost all patients with lung abscess present with fever and cough, characteristically producing large amounts of foul-smelling sputum. Many patients complain of pleuritic chest pain, and 20% develop hemoptysis.

The differential diagnosis of lung abscess includes lung cancer and cavitary tuberculosis. Indeed, cancer is a more common cause of cavitation than is lung abscess. Cavitation due to cancer reflects necrosis of the tumor half the time, with the other half following bronchial obstruction with subsequent infection. Tuberculous cavities only rarely show the air–fluid levels characteristic of lung abscesses.

Complications of lung abscess include rupture into the pleural space, with resulting empyema, and severe hemoptysis. The abscess may drain into a bronchus, with subsequent spread of infection to other parts of the lung. Despite vigorous antimicrobial therapy, principally directed against anaerobic bacteria, the mortality of lung abscess remains 5% to 10%.

Diffuse Alveolar Damage (Acute Respiratory Distress Syndrome)

Diffuse alveolar damage (DAD) refers to a pattern of reaction on the part of alveolar epithelial and endothelial cells to a variety of acute insults (Table 12-1). The clinical counterpart of severe DAD is **acute respiratory distress syndrome** (ARDS). In ARDS, apparently normal lungs sustain damage that progresses rapidly to respiratory failure. Lung compliance is decreased (usually requiring mechanical ventilation), with hypoxemia and extensive radiologic opacities in both lungs ("white-out"). The mortality of ARDS is more than 50%, and in patients older than 60 years, it is as high as 90%.

Table 12-1

Important Causes of the Acute Respiratory Distress Syndrome

Nonthoracic Trauma	Infection	Aspiration	Drugs and Therapeutic Agents
Shock due to any cause	Gram-negative septicemia	Near-drowning	Heroin
Fat embolism	Other bacterial infections	Aspiration of gastric contents	Oxygen
	Viral infections		Radiation
			Paraquat
			Cytotoxic drugs

ETIOLOGIC FACTORS: DAD is a final common pathology caused by a large variety of insults (Table 12-1), including respiratory infections, sepsis, shock, aspiration of gastric contents, inhalation of toxic gases, near-drowning, radiation pneumonitis and many drugs and other chemicals. These conditions are linked by the fact that they can all injure alveolar epithelial and endothelial cells, thereby producing DAD. ***Importantly, unless a specific infectious agent is identified, the precise cause of DAD cannot be determined from the morphology of the lung alone.*** In some patients, no cause can be found. Such idiopathic DAD is referred to clinically as **acute interstitial pneumonia** (AIP) and also includes cases historically referred to as **Hamman-Rich disease.** Injury to endothelial cells allows the leakage of protein-rich fluid from alveolar capillaries into the interstitial space (Fig. 12-32). Loss of type I pneumocytes permits fluid to enter alveolar spaces, where deposition of plasma proteins results in formation of fibrin-containing precipitates (hyaline membranes) on the injured alveolar walls (Fig. 12-33). Although it is denuded of type I pneumocytes, the alveolar basement membrane remains intact and functions as a scaffold for type II pneumocytes, whose proliferation replaces the normal epithelial lining of the alveoli. In response to the cell injury of DAD, inflammatory cells accumulate in the interstitial space.

If the patient survives the acute phase of ARDS, fibroblasts proliferate in the interstitial space and deposit collagen in the alveolar walls (Fig. 12-34). In patients who recover completely, lesions may heal, the alveolar exudate and hyaline membranes are resorbed and the normal alveolar epithelium is restored. Fibroblast proliferation ceases, and the extra collagen is metabolized. Patients who recover from ARDS regain normal lung function. In patients who do not recover, DAD can progress to end-stage fibrosis in which remodeling of lung architecture produces many cystlike spaces throughout the lung **(honeycomb lung).** These spaces are separated by fibrous tissue, and are lined by type II pneumocytes, bronchiolar epithelium or squamous cells.

The mechanisms underlying DAD are not entirely clear. It is thought that activation of complement (e.g., by endotoxin in the case of gram-negative septicemia) leads to sequestration of neutrophils in the marginating pool. Only a small proportion, perhaps one third, of neutrophils actively circulate in the blood; most of the remainder are in the lung. Normally, these neutrophils cause no damage, but after activation by complement, they release oxygen radicals and hydrolytic

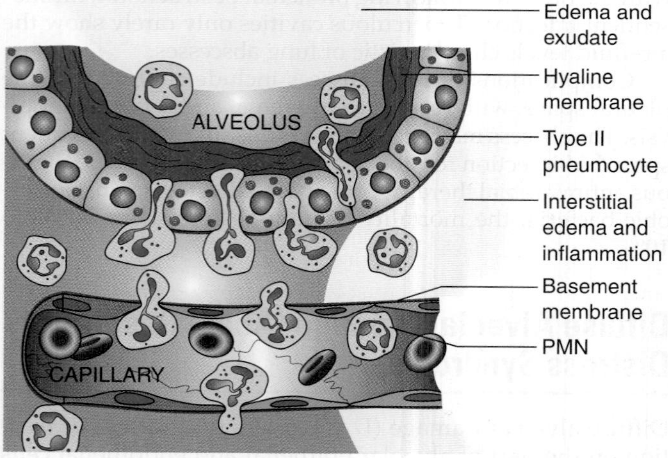

FIGURE 12-32. Diffuse alveolar damage (acute respiratory distress syndrome, ARDS). In ARDS, type I cells die as a result of diffuse alveolar damage. Intra-alveolar edema follows, after which there is formation of hyaline membranes composed of proteinaceous exudate and cell debris. In the acute phase, the lungs are markedly congested and heavy. Type II cells multiply to line the alveolar surface. Interstitial inflammation is characteristic. The lesion may heal completely or progress to interstitial fibrosis. PMN = polymorphonuclear neutrophil.

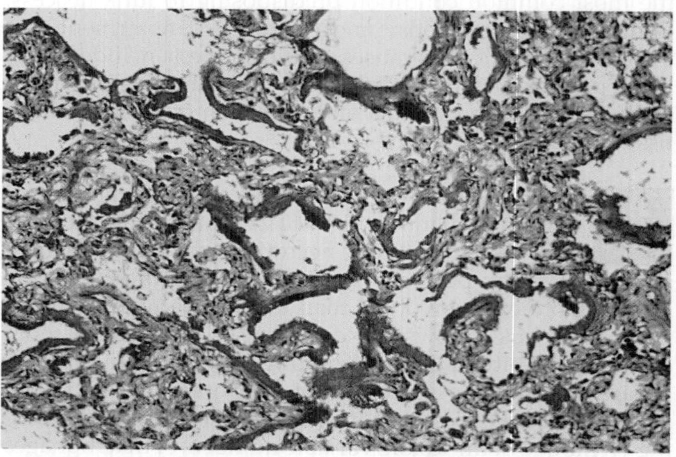

FIGURE 12-33. Diffuse alveolar damage, acute (exudative) phase. The alveolar septa are thickened by edema and a sparse inflammatory infiltrate. The alveoli are lined by eosinophilic hyaline membranes.

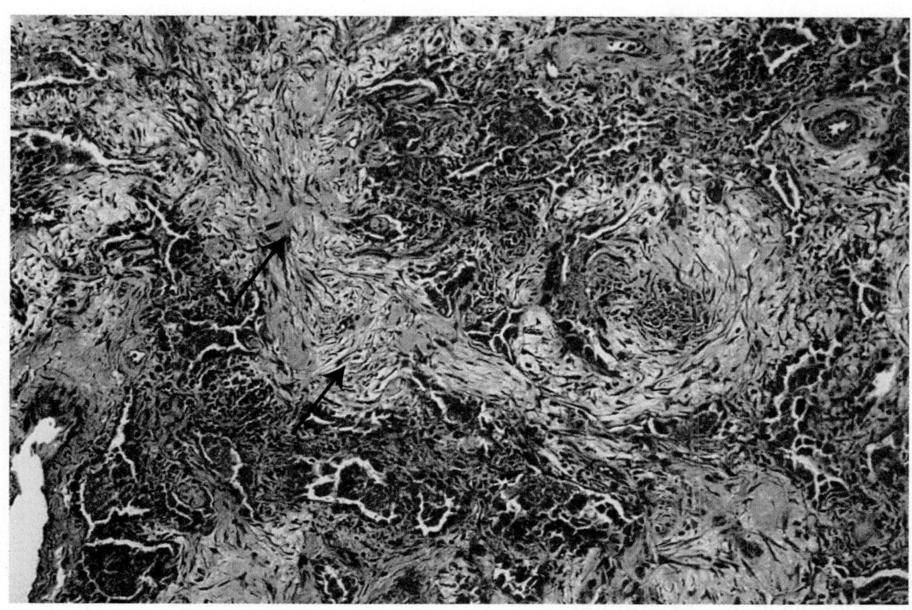

FIGURE 12-34. Diffuse alveolar damage, acute and organizing phase. The alveolar walls are thickened by fibroblasts and loose connective tissue (*arrows*).

enzymes, which damage pulmonary capillary endothelium. The role of neutrophils in the pathogenesis of DAD is still debated because ARDS has been reported in severely neutropenic patients.

In DAD following the inhalation of toxic gases or near-drowning, the damage is primarily at the alveolar epithelial surface. Alveolar epithelial junctions are usually very tight; damage to the epithelium disrupts these junctions, permitting exudation of fluid and proteins from the interstitium into the alveolar spaces.

PATHOLOGY: An initial exudative phase of DAD is followed by an organizing phase.

The exudative phase of DAD develops in the first week after pulmonary insult, with edema, hyaline membranes, leakage of plasma proteins and accumulation of inflammatory cells (Fig. 12-33). Alveolar injury is first detected by electron microscopy as degenerative changes in endothelial cells and type I pneumocytes. This is followed by sloughing of type I cells, thereby denuding basement membranes. Interstitial and alveolar edema is prominent by the first day but soon recedes. "**Hyaline membranes**" begin to appear by the second day and are the most conspicuous morphologic feature of the exudative phase after 4 to 5 days. They are eosinophilic and glassy, consisting of precipitated plasma proteins and cytoplasmic and nuclear debris from sloughed epithelial cells. Interstitial inflammation, with lymphocytes, plasma cells and macrophages, is apparent early and peaks in about a week. Toward the end of the first week and persisting during the subsequent organizing stage, regularly spaced, cuboidal type II pneumocytes become arrayed along the denuded alveolar septa. Alveolar capillaries and pulmonary arterioles may contain fibrin thrombi. In fatal cases of DAD, the lungs are heavy, edematous and virtually airless.

The organizing phase of DAD, beginning about a week after the initial injury, is marked by the proliferation of fibroblasts within alveolar walls (Fig. 12-34). Interstitial inflammation and proliferated type II pneumocytes persist, but hyaline membranes are no longer formed. Alveolar macrophages digest the remnants of hyaline membranes and other cellular debris. Alveolar septa are thickened by loose fibrosis, which resolves in mild cases. In severe DAD, fibrosis progresses to restructuring of the pulmonary parenchyma.

CLINICAL FEATURES: Patients destined to develop ARDS have a symptom-free interval for a few hours after the initial insult. Then, tachypnea and dyspnea mark the onset of the syndrome. Blood gas analyses show arterial hypoxemia and decreased pCO_2. As ARDS progresses, dyspnea worsens and the patient becomes cyanotic. Diffuse, bilateral, interstitial and alveolar infiltrates are noted radiologically. Increasing oxygen tension in the inspired air does not suffice to restore adequate blood oxygenation, and mechanical ventilation becomes necessary. In fatal cases the combination of increasing tachypnea and decreasing tidal volume eventuates in alveolar hypoventilation, progressive hypoxemia and increasing pCO_2.

Patients who survive ARDS may recover normal pulmonary function but, in severe cases, they are left with scarred lungs, respiratory dysfunction and, in some instances, pulmonary hypertension.

Diffuse Alveolar Damage Has Diverse Causes

Oxygen Toxicity

During World War II, aviators at high altitude were required to breathe increased concentrations of oxygen. Animal experiments had shown harmful effects of oxygen on the lung, and patients who received high levels of oxygen for respiratory problems were found to develop DAD. Lung lesions have been noted to follow long-term exposure to as little as 28% oxygen, but it is usually safe to breathe 40% to 60% oxygen for long periods. Oxygen toxicity is thought to be caused by increased production of activated oxygen species in the lung (see Chapter 1).

Shock

ARDS often follows shock from any cause, including gram-negative sepsis, trauma or blood loss, in which case the pulmonary condition is colloquially referred to as "shock lung." The pathogenesis of DAD associated with shock is poorly understood, but is likely multifactorial. Tissue necrosis in organs damaged by trauma or ischemia may lead to release of vasoactive peptides into the circulation. These enhance vascular permeability in the lung. Disseminated intravascular coagulation may damage alveolar capillaries, and fat emboli from bone fractures may obstruct the distal capillary bed of the lung. The pathogenesis of endothelial cell injury in endotoxic shock is discussed in Chapter 7.

Aspiration

Aspiration of gastric contents introduces acid with a pH less than 3.0 into the alveoli. The severe chemical injury to the alveolar lining cells leads to DAD. In near-drowning, aspiration of water produces pulmonary injury and ARDS.

Drug-Induced Diffuse Alveolar Damage

Many drugs cause DAD, especially cytotoxic chemotherapeutic agents. The best known is bleomycin, but others include 1,3-bis-(2-chloroethyl)-1-nitrosourea (BCNU), methotrexate, 5-fluorouracil, busulfan and cyclophosphamide. With bleomycin, an imprecise dose-dependent relation has been demonstrated, but such an effect is not apparent with most other drugs.

Bizarre, atypical, hyperchromatic nuclei in type II cells are particularly common when alveolar damage is due to chemotherapy (Fig. 12-35). Damage progresses even when the offending agent is discontinued, although it may be modified by administration of corticosteroids. Progressive interstitial fibrosis occurs, usually with retention of lung structure. Methotrexate differs from the other chemotherapeutic agents in that it may sometimes cause a hypersensitivity reaction in the lung, in which case the DAD is reversible after the drug is discontinued. The lesions that reflect hypersensitivity are characterized by granulomatous inflammation and occasionally vasculitis. Drugs other than chemotherapeutic agents that may cause DAD include nitrofurantoin, amiodarone and penicillamine.

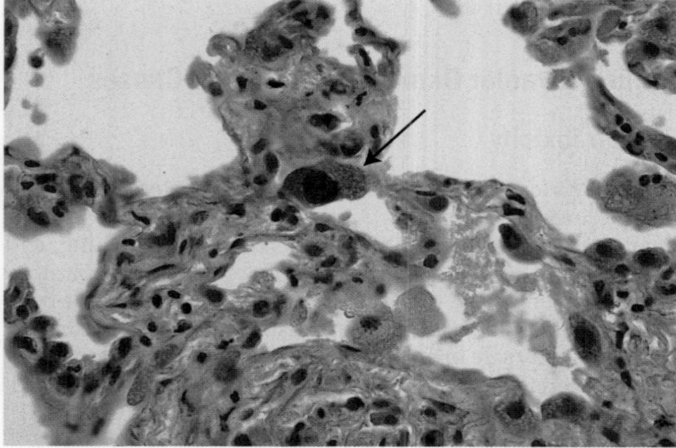

FIGURE 12-35. Diffuse alveolar damage (DAD) associated with busulfan treatment. An atypical pneumocyte (*arrow*) was encountered in a case of organizing DAD associated with busulfan therapy.

Radiation Pneumonitis

There are two forms of radiation pneumonitis: acute DAD and chronic pulmonary fibrosis. Alveolar injury is believed to be caused by oxygen radicals generated by the radiolysis of water (see Chapter 1).

Acute radiation pneumonitis occurs in as many as 10% of patients irradiated for lung or breast cancer, or for mediastinal lymphoma. DAD caused by radiation is mostly dose related and appears 1 to 6 months after radiation therapy, when patients develop fever, cough and dyspnea. Pathologically, the lungs show atypical alveolar lining cells, with enlarged hyperchromatic nuclei and multinucleated cells. Most patients recover from acute radiation pneumonitis.

In **chronic radiation pneumonitis,** interstitial fibrosis may follow acute DAD or may develop insidiously. Lung biopsy demonstrates interstitial fibrosis, radiation-induced vascular changes and atypical type II pneumocytes. The disease is asymptomatic unless a substantial volume of the lung is affected.

Paraquat

Exposure to paraquat, a common herbicide, may cause DAD. Pulmonary disease becomes apparent 4 to 7 days after ingestion, as ARDS develops. Patients rarely recover once pulmonary complications have evolved. A curious intra-alveolar exudate and organization occur, as well as the more usual interstitial fibrosis. The intra-alveolar exudate organizes in such a way that the alveolar framework persists and the airspaces are filled with loose granulation tissue.

Respiratory Distress Syndrome of the Newborn Is a Counterpart of Acute Respiratory Distress Syndrome

Neonatal respiratory distress syndrome (NRDS) results from immaturity of the surfactant system at birth, usually because of severe prematurity. The advent of surfactant replacement therapy and improvements in ventilatory techniques have improved survival and decreased the frequency of complications of NRDS in older premature infants, but very premature infants may still develop **bronchopulmonary dysplasia (BPD).** BPD originally reflected damage to lung acini and subsequent repair, which led to atelectasis, fibrosis and destruction of clusters of acini. With the advent of surfactant replacement therapy, the necrotizing bronchiolitis and alveolar septal fibrosis of BPD have largely disappeared, and decreased alveolarization is the main finding now. NRDS and BPD are discussed in further detail in Chapter 6.

Rare Alveolar Diseases

Alveolar Proteinosis Features Excess Intra-Alveolar Lipid-Rich Material

Alveolar proteinosis, also termed **lipoproteinosis,** is a rare condition in which alveoli are filled with a granular eosinophilic material, which has a very high surfactant content. Initially described as idiopathic, alveolar proteinosis is now associated with (1) compromised immunity; (2) a number of cancers, particularly leukemia and lymphoma; (3) respiratory infections; and (4) exposure to environmental inorganic dusts. It is also a rare congenital disease caused by a point mutation in the gene for the granulocyte-macrophage colony-stimulating factor (GM-CSF) receptor.

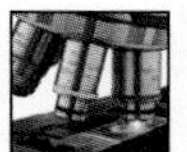

MOLECULAR PATHOGENESIS: Alveolar proteinosis is thought to be related to defective surfactant clearance by macrophages. It has recently been attributed to defective activity, or deficiency, of GM-CSF. Anti–GM-CSF autoantibodies are detected in most patients with the idiopathic form of the disease, suggesting an autoimmune etiology. The pathogenesis of secondary alveolar proteinosis is less clear, but appears related to defective macrophage function via altered GM-CSF activity.

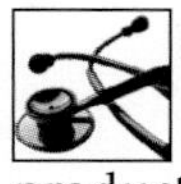

PATHOLOGY: On gross examination, the lungs are very heavy and viscid, and yellow fluid leaks from the cut surface. Scattered, firm, yellow-white nodules vary in size from a few millimeters to 2 cm in diameter. Microscopically, granular material is seen in alveoli, respiratory bronchioles and alveolar ducts (Fig. 12-36). Cell debris, foamy macrophages, ghosts of degenerated cells and detached type II pneumocytes are seen in the eosinophilic material, which contains high concentrations of surfactant, demonstrable by immunostaining. Electron microscopy shows characteristic surfactant tubular myelin structures. Importantly, the interstitial architecture of the lung is intact, and little inflammation is present.

CLINICAL FEATURES: Although a few cases have been reported in infants and children, alveolar proteinosis is a disease of adults. Patients have fever, productive cough and dyspnea. Chest radiographs show diffuse, bilateral, symmetric, alveolar infiltrates, which may radiate from the hilar regions. Repeated respiratory tract infections, often with fungi or *Nocardia,* are common, perhaps due to altered neutrophil and macrophage activity. Interestingly, infections occur at both pulmonary and extrapulmonary sites, indicating that the predisposition to infections is systemic. Before treatment became available, alveolar proteinosis gradually progressed to respiratory failure in one third of patients. Today, bronchoalveolar lavage can remove the alveolar material, and repeated lavage (sometimes for years) cures or arrests the disease. GM-CSF reconstitution is being investigated.

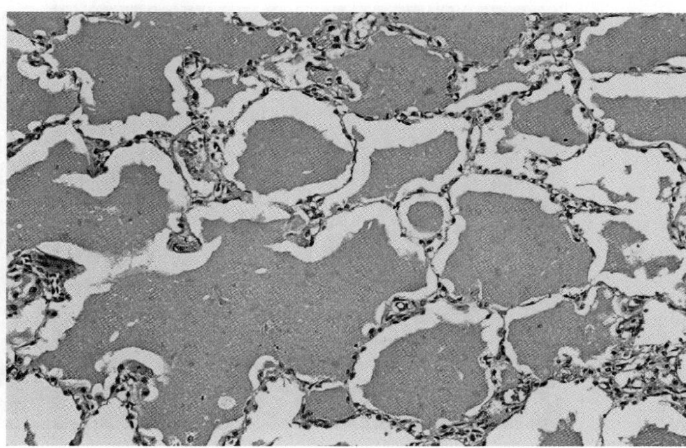

FIGURE 12-36. Alveolar proteinosis. The alveoli and alveolar ducts contain a granular, eosinophilic material.

Diffuse Pulmonary Hemorrhage Syndromes Are Mainly Immunologic Disorders

Diffuse alveolar hemorrhage can occur in diverse clinical settings (Table 12-2). Histologically, the diseases are characterized by acute hemorrhage (numerous intra-alveolar red blood cells) or chronic hemorrhage (hemosiderosis). In virtually all of these disorders, neutrophils infiltrate the alveolar walls **(neutrophilic capillaritis),** reminiscent of leukocytoclastic vasculitis seen in other organs such as the skin. This lesion tends to be most prominent in hemorrhagic syndromes associated with Wegener granulomatosis or systemic lupus erythematosus.

Some diffuse pulmonary hemorrhage syndromes are associated with characteristic immunofluorescence patterns. Linear fluorescence along alveolar walls is seen in antibasement membrane antibody disease, or Goodpasture syndrome. A

Table 12-2

Conditions of Pulmonary Hemorrhage

Disease	Immunologic Mechanism	Immunofluorescence Pattern
Goodpasture syndrome	Antibasement membrane antibody	Linear
Microscopic polyangiitis	Antineutrophilic cytoplasmic antibody (ANCA)	Negative/pauci-immune
Systemic lupus erythematosus	Immune complexes	Granular
Mixed cryoglobulinemia		
Henoch-Schönlein purpura		
Immunoglobulin A (IgA) disease		
Wegener granulomatosis	Antineutrophil cytoplasmic antibody (ANCA)	Negative or pauci-immune
Idiopathic glomerulonephritis		
Idiopathic pulmonary hemorrhage	No immunologic marker	

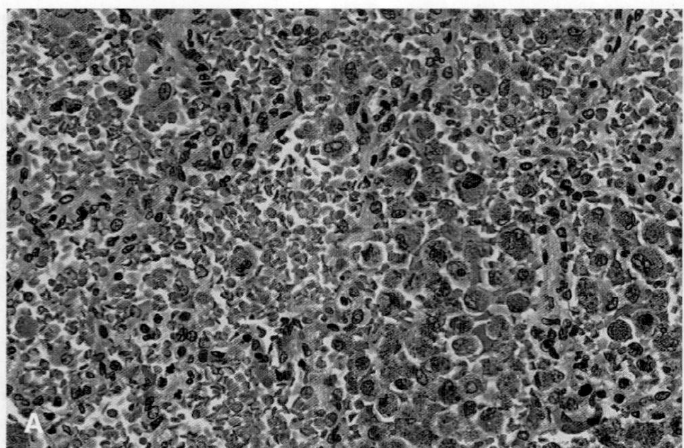

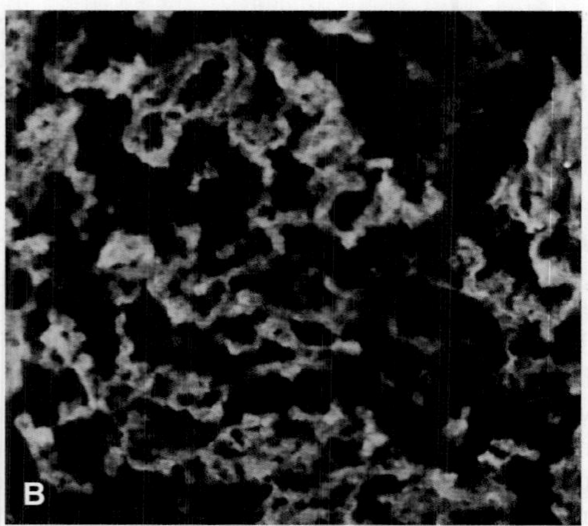

FIGURE 12-37. Goodpasture syndrome. A. A section of lung shows extensive intra-alveolar hemorrhage (*left*) and collections of hemosiderin-laden macrophages (*right*). The alveolar septa are thickened, and the alveoli are lined by hyperplastic type II pneumocytes. **B.** Linear deposition of immunoglobulin G (IgG) within the alveolar septa is demonstrated by immunofluorescence.

granular pattern occurs in immune complex–associated diseases, such as systemic lupus erythematosus. Pauci-immune disorders consist of antineutrophil cytoplasm antibody (ANCA)-associated diseases (e.g., Wegener granulomatosis, microscopic polyangiitis or idiopathic pulmonary hemorrhage syndromes), in which no etiology or immunologic mechanism can be determined (Table 12-2).

Goodpasture Syndrome (Antiglomerular Basement Membrane Antibody Disease)

Goodpasture syndrome refers to a triad of diffuse alveolar hemorrhage, glomerulonephritis and a circulating cytotoxic autoantibody to a component of basement membranes. Cross-reactivity between alveolar and glomerular basement membranes accounts for the simultaneous attack on the lung and kidney. The pathogenesis of this syndrome is detailed in Chapter 16.

PATHOLOGY: Patients with Goodpasture syndrome have extensive intra-alveolar hemorrhage (Fig. 12-37A). Grossly, the lungs are dark red and heavy in the acute phase and rusty brown later, when the erythrocytes have been phagocytosed. Histologically, erythrocytes and hemosiderin-laden macrophages fill the airspaces. The presence of neutrophils in and around alveolar capillaries may suggest an "alveolitis," but this reaction may be transient. Alveolar septa are mildly thickened by interstitial fibrosis and type II pneumocyte hyperplasia is seen. By immunofluorescence, IgG and complement are deposited in the basement membranes of alveoli and glomeruli (Fig. 12-37B).

CLINICAL FEATURES: Goodpasture syndrome may affect adults of either sex and any age, but it occurs mostly in young men. Most (95%) patients are seen initially with hemoptysis, often accompanied by dyspnea, weakness and mild anemia. Evidence of glomerulonephritis follows pulmonary manifestations within about 3 months (1 week to 1 year), although some patients do not develop renal disease. Radiographic examination reveals diffuse, bilateral alveolar infiltrates, which may resolve rapidly in a matter of days as erythrocytes lyse and are phagocytosed. Hypoxemia and respiratory alkalosis are common, but respiratory function returns to normal as the hemorrhage resolves. The diagnosis is made on the basis of a renal or pulmonary biopsy.

Goodpasture syndrome is treated with corticosteroids, cytotoxic drugs and plasmapheresis. Before such aggressive treatment was used, the mortality of Goodpasture syndrome was 80%. Even with current therapy, the 2-year survival is now only 50%, and the outlook is worse if renal failure is present.

Microscopic Polyangiitis

Microscopic polyangiitis is a pauci-immune vasculitis involving arterioles, venules and capillaries. Almost all patients also show evidence of glomerulonephritis, and microscopic polyangiitis has emerged as one of the more common causes of "pulmonary-renal syndrome." Joints and muscle, upper respiratory tract and skin may also be involved. Over 80% of patients have a positive ANCA, most often of the "perinuclear" type (P-ANCA), adirected against myeloperoxidase. Microscopic polyangiitis may occur at any age and is of equal incidence in both males and females. Lung biopsies show alveolar hemorrhage with neutrophilic capillaritis. Immunoglobulin deposition is not seen.

Idiopathic Pulmonary Hemorrhage

This rare disease (also known as **idiopathic pulmonary hemosiderosis**) is characterized by diffuse alveolar bleeding similar to that of Goodpasture syndrome but lacking renal involvement or antibasement membrane antibodies. It is microscopically indistinguishable from the lung of Goodpasture syndrome.

CLINICAL FEATURES: Idiopathic pulmonary hemosiderosis mainly affects children, but 20% of patients are adults, usually younger than 30 years. There is a 2:1 male predominance in adults, but an equal sex distribution in children. The patients complain of cough (with or without hemoptysis), dyspnea, substernal chest pain, fatigue and iron-deficiency anemia. Pulmonary hemorrhages are recurrent and intermittent. The course is more protracted than that of Goodpasture syndrome.

The response to corticosteroids is variable, and mean survival is 3 to 5 years. One fourth of patients die rapidly of massive hemorrhage. Another quarter have persistent, active disease; repeated episodes of hemoptysis result in interstitial fibrosis and cor pulmonale. In another fourth of patients, the disease remains inactive, but dyspnea and anemia may persist. The remaining patients recover completely without recurrence.

Hypersensitivity to cow's milk in infants and children generally younger than 2 years can result in diffuse pulmonary hemorrhage similar to that seen in idiopathic pulmonary hemorrhage. Removal of milk from the diet ameliorates the condition.

Eosinophilic Pneumonia Is Largely an Allergic or Hypersensitivity Reaction

Eosinophilic pneumonia refers to the accumulation of eosinophils in alveolar spaces. The disease is classified as **idiopathic** or **secondary** to an underlying illness (Table 12-3).

Idiopathic Eosinophilic Pneumonia

SIMPLE EOSINOPHILIC PNEUMONIA: Simple eosinophilic pneumonia (Löffler syndrome) is a mild condition characterized by fleeting pulmonary infiltrates, which usually resolve within a month. Patients typically have peripheral blood eosinophilia but are often asymptomatic. Histologically, the lung shows eosinophilic pneumonia, but the diagnosis is usually established clinically, and lung biopsy is rarely performed.

ACUTE EOSINOPHILIC PNEUMONIA: In this disorder, patients are first seen with fewer than 7 days of symptoms, which include fever, hypoxemia and diffuse interstitial and alveolar infiltrates on chest radiograph. The etiology is not known, but it is thought to be a type of hypersensitivity reaction. Although peripheral blood eosinophilia is frequently absent, bronchoalveolar lavage consistently demonstrates increased eosinophils. Histologically, the lung shows eosinophilic pneumonia accompanied by features of diffuse alveolar damage (i.e., hyaline membranes). Patients respond dramatically to corticosteroids, and unlike chronic eosinophilic pneumonia, acute eosinophilic pneumonia does not recur.

CHRONIC EOSINOPHILIC PNEUMONIA: The etiology of chronic eosinophilic pneumonia is unknown, but an allergic diathesis is noted in some patients.

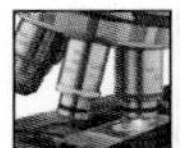

PATHOLOGY: Alveolar spaces are flooded with eosinophils, alveolar macrophages and a proteinaceous exudate (Fig. 12-38). Some cases may also show an eosinophilic interstitial pneumonia. Hyperplasia of type II pneumocytes may be prominent. Eosinophilic abscesses, with central masses of necrotic eosinophils surrounded by palisaded macrophages, are sometimes found. A mild eosinophilic vasculitis may be seen. An organizing pneumonia pattern is also occasionally described (see below).

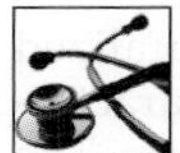

CLINICAL FEATURES: Patients have fever, night sweats, weight loss, cough productive of eosinophils and dyspnea. Asthma is present in many patients, and circulating eosinophilia may be conspicuous. The chest radiograph is diagnostic and has been described as "the photographic negative of pulmonary edema," characterized by peripheral alveolar infiltrates with sparing of the hilum. The response to corticosteroids is dramatic and helps to confirm the diagnosis.

Table 12-3

Types of Eosinophilic Pneumonia

Idiopathic
Chronic eosinophilic pneumonia
Acute eosinophilic pneumonia
Simple eosinophilic pneumonia (Löffler syndrome)
Secondary Eosinophilic Pneumonia
Infection
Parasitic
Tropical eosinophilic pneumonia
Ascaris lumbricoides, Toxocara canis, filaria
Dirofilaria
Fungal
Aspergillus
Drug induced
Antibiotics
Cytotoxic drugs
Anti-inflammatory agents
Antihypertensive drugs
L-Tryptophan (eosinophilic fasciitis)
Immunologic or systemic diseases
Allergic bronchopulmonary aspergillosis
Churg-Strauss syndrome
Hypereosinophilic syndrome

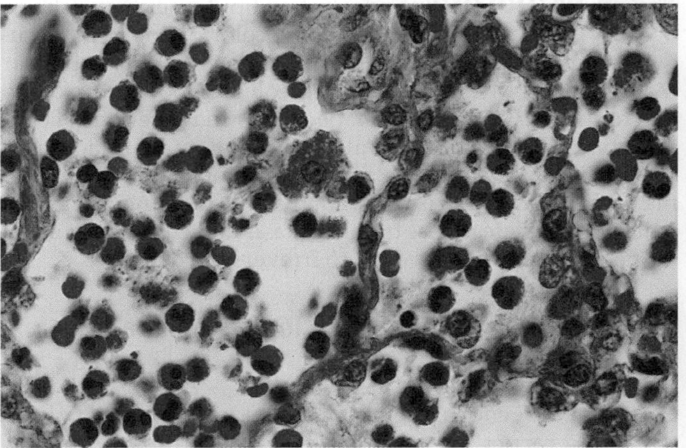

FIGURE 12-38. Eosinophilic pneumonia. The alveolar spaces are filled with an inflammatory exudate composed of eosinophils and macrophages. The alveolar septa are thickened by the presence of numerous eosinophils.

Secondary Eosinophilic Pneumonia

Eosinophilic pneumonia can occur in a variety of known clinical settings, including parasitic or fungal infection, drug toxicity and systemic disorders such as Churg-Strauss syndrome (Table 12-3). In industrialized countries, the most frequent cause of eosinophilic pneumonia is drug hypersensitivity, including reactions to antibiotics, anti-inflammatory agents, cytotoxic drugs and antihypertensive agents. The pulmonary disease resolves without long-term sequelae. The clinical presentations and histologic findings are the same as described above.

The classic form of **infectious eosinophilic pneumonia** associated with parasitic infection is **tropical eosinophilic pneumonia.** The migration of parasites through the lung is often accompanied by an acute, self-limited, respiratory illness, characterized clinically by (1) fever, (2) a cough productive of sputum containing eosinophils and (3) transient pulmonary infiltrates.

In temperate zones, *Ascaris lumbricoides* is the usual inciting organism. Hypersensitivity to *Toxocara canis* is also occasionally encountered. However, the most distinctive infection associated with eosinophilic pneumonia is allergic bronchopulmonary aspergillosis (see discussion above on aspergillosis).

In tropical regions, eosinophilic pneumonia is most commonly a response to infestation with the filarial nematodes *Wuchereria bancrofti* and *Brugia malayi,* although other parasites may also be responsible.

Endogenous Lipid Pneumonia Reflects Bronchial Obstruction

This disease, also termed "golden pneumonia," is a localized condition distal to an obstructed airway, which is characterized by lipid-laden macrophages in the alveolar spaces. The size of the affected area corresponds to the caliber of the involved bronchus. Bronchial obstruction leads to retention of secretions and breakdown products of inflammatory and epithelial cells. Although the protein component is readily digested, lipids are phagocytosed by macrophages, which fill alveoli distal to the obstruction.

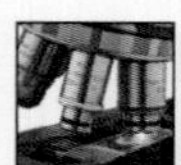

PATHOLOGY: Endogenous lipid pneumonia has a characteristic golden-yellow color, owing to the accumulation of fine lipid droplets within alveolar macrophages. Microscopically, alveoli are flooded by foamy macrophages with needle-shaped clefts characteristic of cholesterol crystals. Alveolar walls typically remain intact. Mild chronic inflammation and fibrosis accompany the pneumonia. If the obstruction is relieved, the affected lung can return to its normal state unless bronchiectasis and chronic recurrent bronchopneumonia have led to irreversible damage.

Exogenous Lipid Pneumonia Is a Response to Aspirated Oils

Causes of exogenous pneumonia include mineral oil (a laxative and a carrier for medications in nose drops), vegetable oils used in cooking and animal oils ingested in the form of cod-liver oil and other vitamin preparations. Oil-based contrast media used for radiologic bronchography have also been associated with the disorder. Exogenous lipid pneumonia is most common in older persons, who take nose drops or laxatives at bedtime and aspirate during sleep. Computed tomography may reveal a spiculated mass that appears worrisome for malignancy. Children may aspirate oily medications while vigorously resisting the dosing.

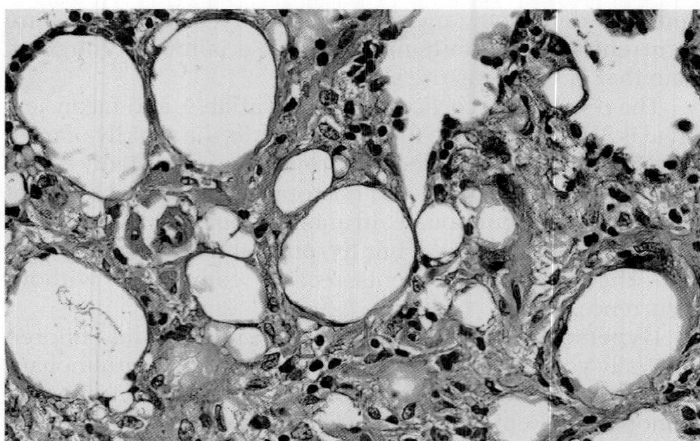

FIGURE 12-39. Exogenous lipoid pneumonia (mineral oil aspiration). The cystic spaces are empty because the lipid was washed out during paraffin processing. A giant cell reaction is also present.

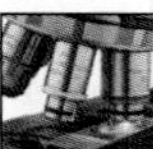

PATHOLOGY: On gross examination, exogenous lipid pneumonia is gray, greasy and poorly demarcated. Foamy macrophages are seen in alveolar and interstitial spaces (Fig. 12-39). Large oil droplets in both locations are surrounded by a foreign body granulomatous response. Because most of the oil is removed by processing for paraffin embedding, empty vacuolar spaces are noted in histologic sections. In chronic cases, affected areas may become densely fibrotic.

Patients with exogenous lipid pneumonia are usually asymptomatic; the condition comes to medical attention when a mass simulating an infection or a tumor is seen on a chest radiograph.

Obstructive Pulmonary Diseases

Several different diseases, including chronic bronchitis, emphysema, asthma and in some classifications bronchiectasis and cystic fibrosis, are grouped together because they have in common an obstruction to airflow in the lungs.

COPD applies to chronic bronchitis and emphysema, in which forced expiratory volume, measured by spirometry, is decreased.

Airflow has a hydraulic basis and can be reduced by increasing resistance to airflow or by reducing outflow pressure. In the lung, narrowed airways produce increased resistance, whereas loss of elastic recoil results in diminished pressure. Airway narrowing occurs in chronic bronchitis or asthma, and emphysema causes loss of recoil.

Chronic Bronchitis Is the Presence of a Chronic Productive Cough Without a Discernible Cause for More Than Half of the Time Over 2 Years

The pathologic definition of the disease is less satisfactory, as its morphologic alterations are a continuum; milder chronic bronchitis may overlap morphologic features seen in ostensibly normal people.

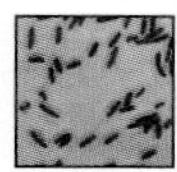

ETIOLOGIC FACTORS: ***Since 90% of chronic bronchitis cases are smokers, the disease mainly reflects the consequences of cigarette smoke (see Chapter 8).*** Chronic bronchitis occurs in less than 5% of nonsmokers, 10% to 15% of moderate smokers and over 25% of heavy smokers. The frequency and severity of acute respiratory tract infections are increased in patients with chronic bronchitis; conversely, infections have been incriminated in its etiology and progression. Chronic bronchitis is more common among urban dwellers in areas of substantial air pollution and in workers exposed to toxic industrial inhalants, but the effects of cigarette smoking far outweigh other contributing factors.

How cigarette smoke and other pollutants injure bronchi is not well understood. Experimentally, rodents that inhale cigarette smoke or SO_2, or are given dilute acids by instillation, exhibit squamous metaplasia of the bronchial epithelium. A similar change occurs when certain proteases are introduced into the bronchi, the effect of which is prevented by pretreating with antiproteases. Bronchial epithelial metaplasia also occurs in rodents given adrenergic and cholinergic agonists, suggesting that autonomic stimulation may play a role in the pathogenesis of chronic bronchitis.

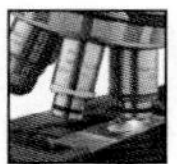

PATHOLOGY: The main morphologic finding in chronic bronchitis is an increased bronchial mucus-secreting apparatus (Fig. 12-40). Two types of cells line the mucous glands: pale mucous cells, which are more common, and serous cells, which are more basophilic and contain granules. **In *chronic bronchitis mucous cells undergo hyperplasia and hypertrophy, and are increased relative to serous cells.*** Thus, both individual acini and glands enlarge (Fig. 12-41).

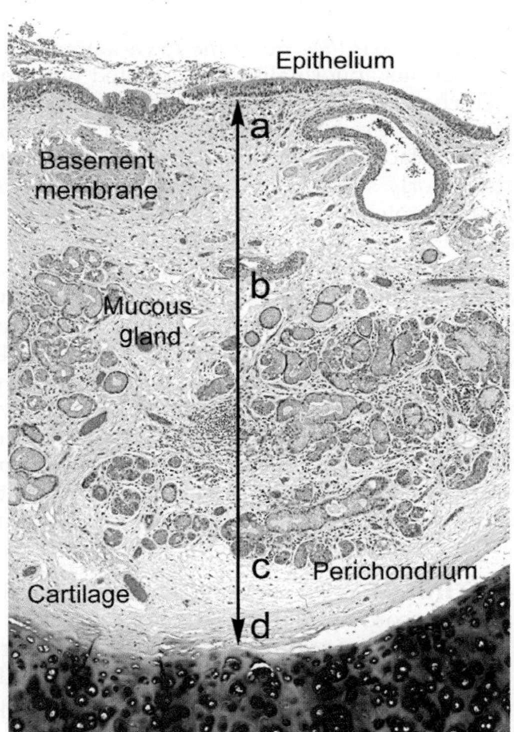

FIGURE 12-40. Chronic bronchitis. The bronchial submucosa is greatly expanded by hyperplastic submucosal glands that compose well over 50% of the thickness of the bronchial wall. The Reid index equals the maximum thickness of the bronchial mucous glands internal to the cartilage (*b to c*) divided by the bronchial wall thickness (*a to d*).

The Reid index measures the size of the mucous glands (Fig. 12-40): the area occupied by the glands in the plane vertical to the cartilage and epithelium as a proportion of the thickness of the entire bronchial wall (basement membrane to inner perichondrium). A normal Reid index is 0.4 or less; in chronic bronchitis it is more than 0.5.

Other morphologic changes in chronic bronchitis are variable and include:

- Excess mucus in central and peripheral airways
- "Pits" on the surface of the bronchial epithelium, which represent dilated bronchial gland ducts into which several glands open
- Thickening of the bronchial wall by mucous gland enlargement and edema, encroaching on the bronchial lumen
- Increased numbers of goblet cells (hyperplasia) in the bronchial epithelium
- Increased smooth muscle, which may indicate bronchial hyperreactivity
- Squamous metaplasia of the bronchial epithelium, reflecting epithelial damage from tobacco smoke, an effect that is probably independent of the other changes seen in chronic bronchitis

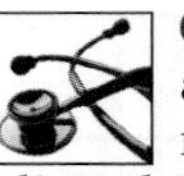

CLINICAL FEATURES: Chronic bronchitis is often accompanied by emphysema (see below), and separating the relative contributions of each to a patient's clinical presentation may be difficult. In general, patients with predominantly chronic bronchitis have had a productive cough for many years. Cough and sputum production are initially more severe in the winter, but they progress over time from hibernal to perennial. Exertional dyspnea and cyanosis supervene, and cor pulmonale may ensue. The combination of cyanosis and edema due to cor pulmonale has led to the label "blue bloater" for such patients.

In patients with advanced chronic bronchitis, pulmonary infections, thromboembolism, left ventricular failure and major episodes of air pollution may precipitate acute respiratory failure, with progressive hypoxemia and hypercapnia. Because of retained mucous secretions, people with chronic bronchitis are at increased risk for pulmonary bacterial infections, particularly with *Haemophilus influenzae* and *S. pneumoniae*.

People with chronic bronchitis must be warned to stop smoking. Prompt antibiotic treatment of pulmonary infections, use of bronchodilator drugs and occasionally bronchopulmonary drainage are the mainstays of treatment.

Emphysema Causes Overinflation of the Lungs in Smokers

Emphysema is a chronic lung disease characterized by enlargement of airspaces distal to the terminal bronchioles, with destruction of their walls but without fibrosis. Although it is classified in anatomic terms, the severity of emphysema is more important than the type. In practical terms, as emphysema becomes more severe, it becomes more difficult to classify. Moreover, several anatomic patterns may be present in the same lung.

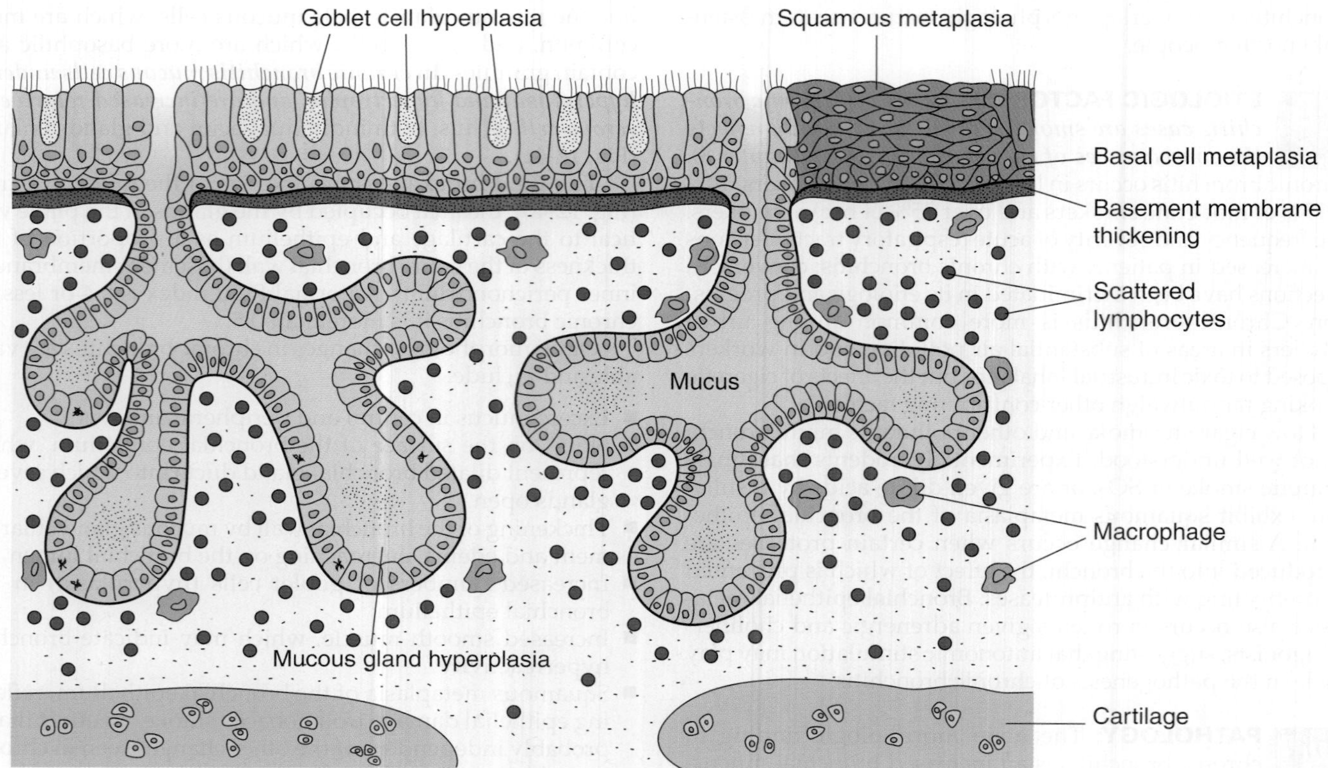

FIGURE 12-41. Chronic bronchitis. Morphologic changes in chronic bronchitis.

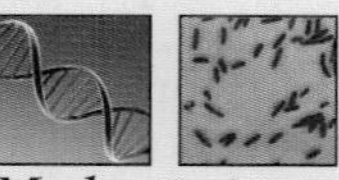

MOLECULAR PATHOGENESIS AND ETIOLOGIC FACTORS: *The major cause of emphysema is cigarette smoking. Moderate to severe emphysema is rare in nonsmokers* (see Chapter 8). In considering the pathogenesis of emphysema, it is thought that a balance exists between elastin synthesis and catabolism in the lung (Fig. 12-42). In other words, emphysema results when elastolytic activity increases or antielastolytic activity is reduced.

Increased numbers of neutrophils, which contain serine elastase and other proteases, are found in the bronchoalveolar lavage fluid of smokers. Smoking also interferes with α_1-antitrypsin (α_1-AT) activity, by oxidizing methionine residues in α_1-antitrypsin. In this way, unopposed and increased elastolytic activity leads to destruction of elastic tissue in the walls of distal airspaces, thereby impairing elastic recoil. At the same time, other cellular proteases may be involved in injury to the airspace walls. This theory, although attractive, awaits further confirmation.

α1-ANTITRYPSIN DEFICIENCY: Hereditary deficiency in α_1-AT accounts for about 1% of patients with COPD and is much more common in young people with severe emphysema. α_1-AT is a circulating glycoprotein produced in the liver and is a key inhibitor of many proteases, including elastase, trypsin, chymotrypsin, thrombin and bacterial proteases. α_1-AT represents 90% of antiproteinase activity in the blood. In the lung, it inhibits neutrophil elastase, an enzyme that digests elastin and other structural components of alveolar septa.

The amount and type of α_1-AT is determined by a pair of codominant *Pi* (protease inhibitor) alleles. The most common genotype is *PiM*, but some 75 variants are known. The most serious abnormality is associated with the *PiZ* allele, which occurs in some 5% of the population. It is more common in people of Scandinavian origin, and is rare in Jews, blacks, and Japanese. Because the abnormal protein is poorly secreted by the liver, plasma α_1-AT in *PiZZ* homozygotes is only 15% to 20% of normal. These persons are at risk for both cirrhosis of the liver (see Chapter 14) and emphysema. **In fact, most patients with clinically diagnosed emphysema under age 40 have α_1-AT deficiency (PiZ).** The mean age of onset of emphysema in PiZZ homozygotes who do not smoke is between 45 and 50 years; those who smoke develop it at about age 35 years. Importantly, two thirds of nonsmoking *PiZZ* homozygotes show no evidence of emphysema. The association of α_1-AT deficiency with emphysema supports the concept that cigarette smoking by itself causes emphysema by altering the balance of proteases and antiproteases in the lung.

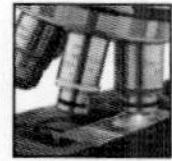

PATHOLOGY: Emphysema is morphologically classified according to the location of the lesions within the pulmonary acinus (Fig. 12-43). Only the proximal acinus (the respiratory bronchiole) is affected in centrilobular emphysema, whereas the entire acinus is destroyed in panacinar emphysema.

CENTRILOBULAR EMPHYSEMA: This form of emphysema is most common, and is usually associated with cigarette smoking and with clinical symptoms. It is characterized by destruction of the cluster of terminal bronchioles near the end of the bronchiolar tree in the central part of the pulmonary lobule (Fig. 12-44A). This is the smallest portion of the lung

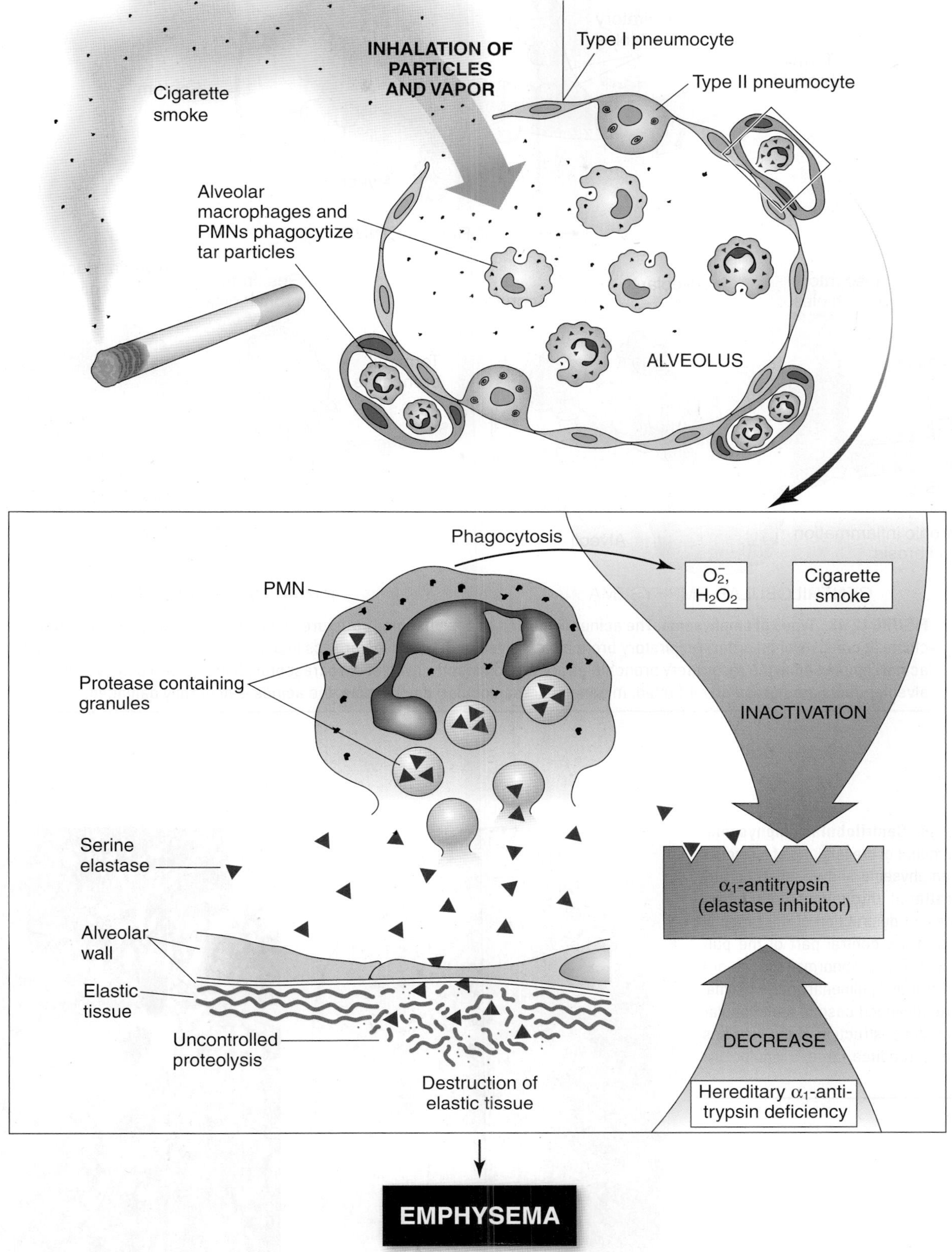

FIGURE 12-42. The proteolysis–antiproteolysis theory of the pathogenesis of emphysema. Cigarette (tobacco) smoking is closely related to the development of emphysema. Some product in tobacco smoke induces an inflammatory reaction. The serine elastase in polymorphonuclear leukocytes, which is a particularly potent elastolytic agent, injures the elastic tissue of the lung. Normally, this enzyme activity is inhibited by α_1-antitrypsin, but tobacco smoke, directly or through the generation of free radicals, inactivates α_1-antitrypsin (protease inhibitor). H_2O_2 = hydrogen peroxide; O_2^- = superoxide ion; PMN = polymorphonuclear neutrophil.

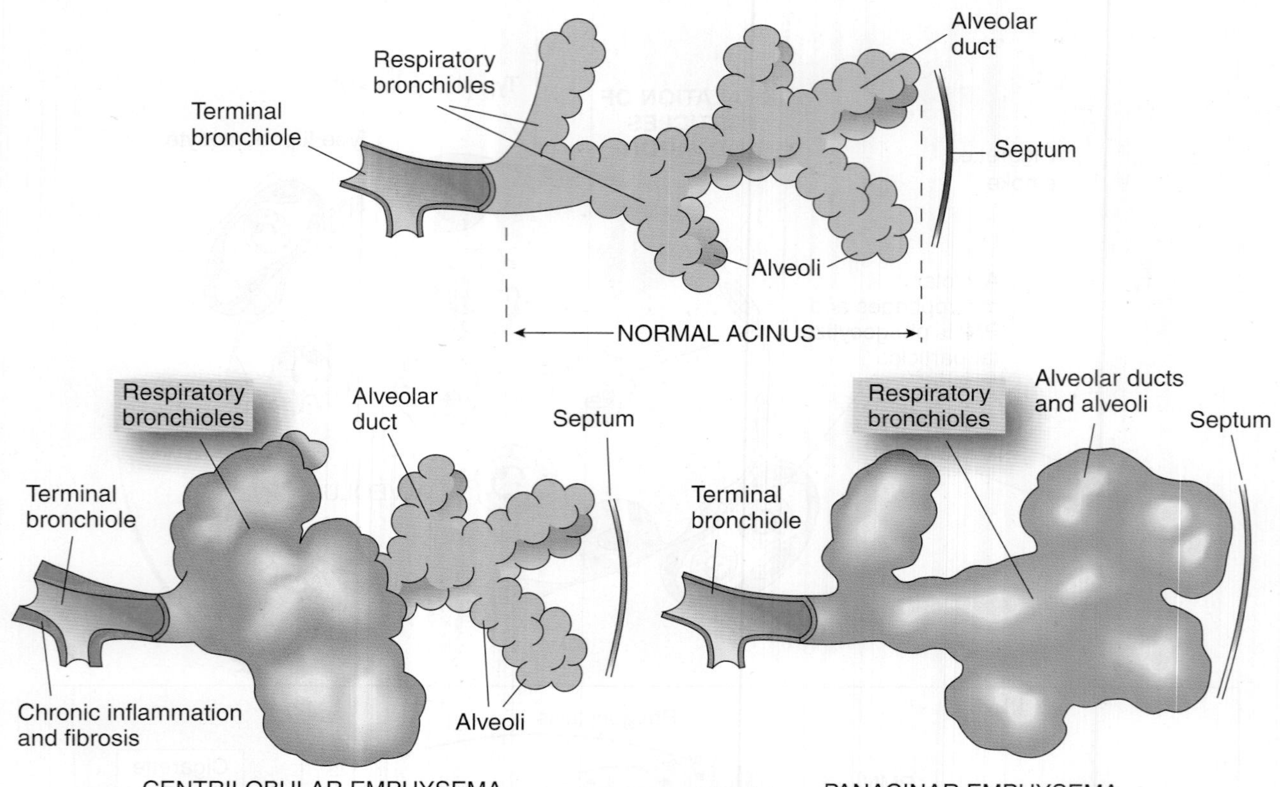

FIGURE 12-43. Types of emphysema. The acinus is the unit gas-exchanging structure of the lung distal to the terminal bronchiole. It consists of (in order) respiratory bronchioles, alveolar ducts, alveolar sacs and alveoli. In centrilobular (proximal acinar) emphysema, the respiratory bronchioles are predominantly involved. In paraseptal (distal acinar) emphysema, the alveolar ducts are particularly affected. In panacinar (panlobular) emphysema, the acinus is uniformly damaged.

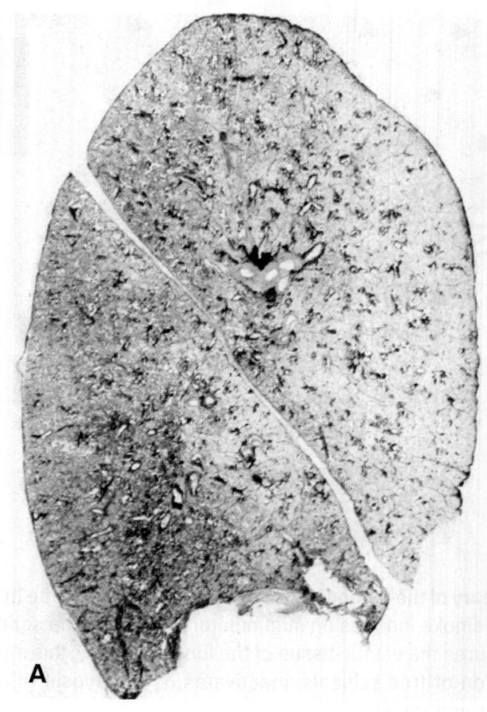

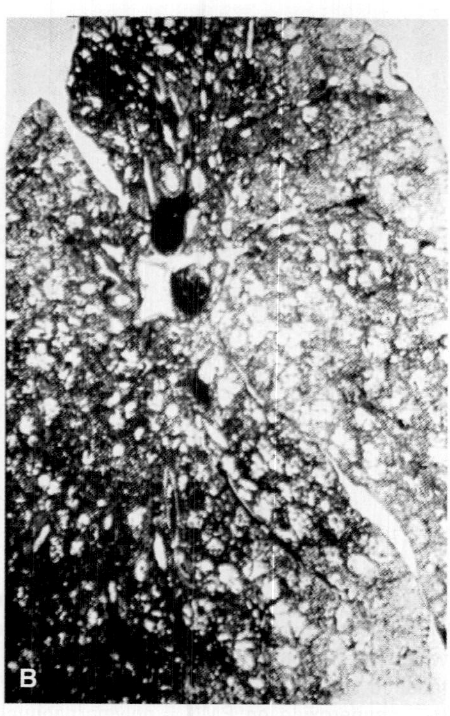

FIGURE 12-44. Centrilobular emphysema. A. A whole mount of the left lung of a smoker with mild emphysema shows enlarged airspaces scattered throughout both lobes, which represent destruction of the terminal bronchioles in the central part of the pulmonary lobule. These abnormal spaces are surrounded by intact pulmonary parenchyma. **B.** In a more advanced case of centrilobular emphysema, the destruction of the lung has progressed to produce large, irregular airspaces.

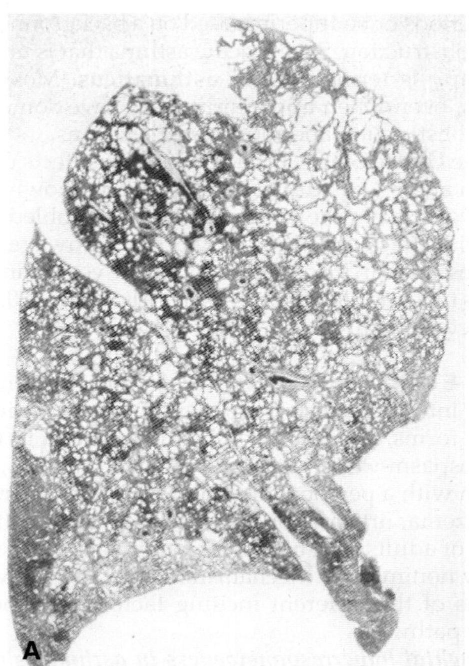

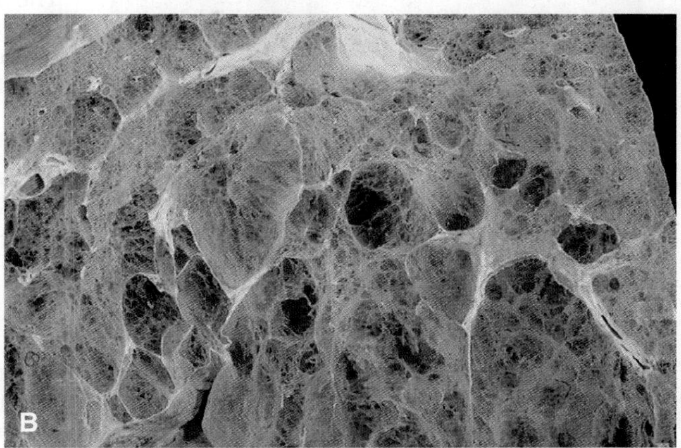

FIGURE 12-45. Panacinar emphysema. A. A whole mount of the left lung from a patient with severe emphysema reveals widespread destruction of the pulmonary parenchyma, which in some areas leaves behind only a lacy network of supporting tissue. **B.** The lung from this patient with α_1-antitrypsin deficiency shows a panacinar pattern of emphysema. The loss of alveolar walls has resulted in markedly enlarged airspaces.

bounded by septa, which includes several acini. Dilated respiratory bronchioles form enlarged airspaces that are separated from each other and from lobular septa by normal alveolar ducts and alveoli. As centrilobular emphysema progresses, these distal structures may also be involved (Fig. 12-44B). Bronchioles proximal to emphysematous spaces are inflamed and narrowed. Centrilobular emphysema is most severe in the upper lobes and the superior segment of the lower lobes.

Focal dust emphysema, a disease of coal miners, resembles centrilobular emphysema but differs in that the affected spaces are smaller and more regular and inflammation of the bronchioles is not apparent. Importantly, the lesion is primarily distensive rather than destructive. Focal dust emphysema is discussed below in the section on coal worker's pneumoconiosis.

PANACINAR EMPHYSEMA: In panacinar emphysema, acini are uniformly involved, with destruction of alveolar septa from the center to the periphery of acini (Fig. 12-45A,B). The loss of alveolar septa is illustrated by histologic comparison of normal lungs with those affected by α_1-AT deficiency (Fig. 12-46). In the final stage, panacinar emphysema leaves behind a lacy network of supporting tissue ("cotton-candy lung"). Diffuse

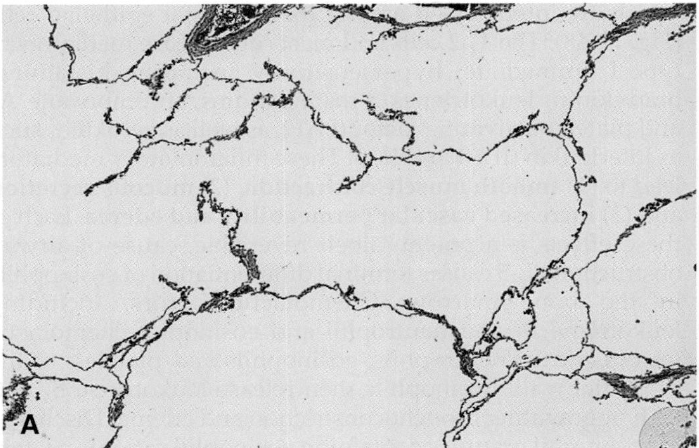

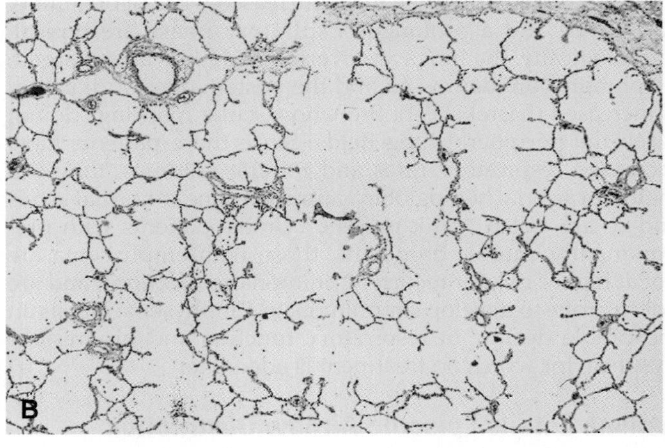

FIGURE 12-46. Panacinar emphysema. A. This lung, from a patient with α_1-antitrypsin deficiency, shows large, irregular airspaces and a markedly reduced number of alveolar walls. **B.** The extensive loss of alveolar walls in A is emphasized by comparison with this section of normal lung at the same magnification.

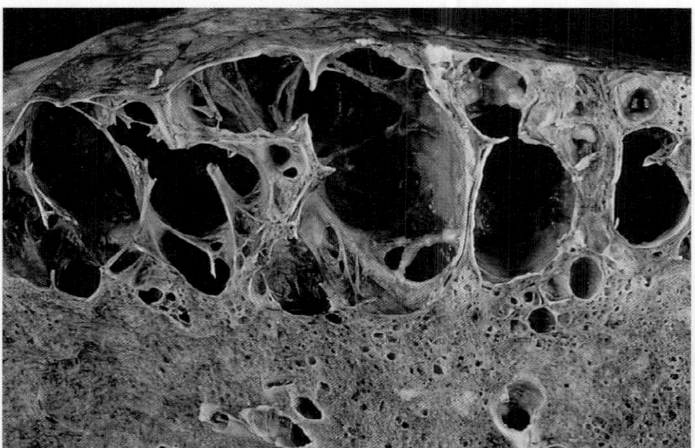

FIGURE 12-47. Localized emphysema. The subpleural parenchyma shows markedly enlarged airspaces owing to the loss of alveolar tissue.

panacinar emphysema is typically associated with α_1-AT deficiency, but it may also occur in cigarette smokers in association with centrilobular emphysema. In such cases, the panacinar pattern tends to occur in the lower zones of the lung, whereas centrilobular emphysema is seen in the upper regions.

LOCALIZED EMPHYSEMA: This condition, previously known as "paraseptal emphysema," is characterized by destruction of alveoli and results in emphysema at only one or at most a few locations. The remainder of the lungs is normal. The lesion is usually found at the apex of an upper lobe in a subpleural location, although it may occur anywhere (Fig. 12-47). Although it is of no clinical significance itself, rupture of an area of localized emphysema may produce spontaneous pneumothorax (see below). Progression of localized emphysema can result in a large area of destruction, termed a **bulla,** which ranges in size from as small as 2 cm to a large lesion that occupies an entire hemithorax.

CLINICAL FEATURES: Most patients with emphysema present at age 60 years or older, with long histories of exertional dyspnea, but a minimal, nonproductive cough. They have lost weight and use accessory muscles of respiration to breathe. Weight loss is probably due less to lack of calories than to the increased work of breathing. Tachypnea and a prolonged expiratory phase are typical. Radiologically, the lungs are overinflated: they are enlarged, diaphragms are depressed and the posteroanterior diameter is increased (barrel chest). Bronchovascular markings do not reach the peripheral lung fields. Since these patients have increased respiratory rates and minute volumes, they can maintain arterial hemoglobin saturation at near-normal levels and so are called "pink puffers." Unlike patients with predominantly chronic bronchitis, those with emphysema are not at higher risk for recurrent pulmonary infections, and are not so prone to develop cor pulmonale. Emphysema entails an inexorable decline in respiratory function and progressive dyspnea, for which no treatment is adequate.

Asthma Entails Episodic Airflow Obstruction in Response to a Number of Stimuli

Asthmatic patients typically have paroxysms of wheezing, dyspnea and cough. Attacks may alternate with asymptomatic periods or be superimposed on a background of chronic airway obstruction. Severe acute asthma that is unresponsive to therapy is termed **status asthmaticus.** Most asthmatic patients, even when apparently well, have some persistent airflow obstruction and morphologic lesions.

In the United States, bronchial asthma affects up to 10% of children and 5% of adults. For reasons unknown, the prevalence of asthma in the United States has doubled since 1980. The initial attack of asthma may occur at any age, but half of the cases appear in patients under 10 years, and the incidence is twice as high in boys as in girls. By age 30, both sexes are affected equally.

ETIOLOGIC FACTORS: Asthma was once divided into **extrinsic (allergic)** and **intrinsic (idiosyncratic)** forms, depending on inciting factors. In the former, bronchospasm was induced by inhaled antigens, usually in children with a personal or family history of allergic disease (e.g., eczema, urticaria or hay fever). Intrinsic asthma was a disease of adults, and bronchial hyperreactivity was precipitated by nonimmune mechanisms. Asthma is now described in terms of the different inciting factors and the common effector pathways.

Bronchial hyperresponsiveness in asthma is now generally attributed to inflammatory reactions to diverse stimuli. After exposure to an inciting factor (e.g., allergens, drugs, cold, exercise), inflammatory mediators released by activated macrophages, mast cells, eosinophils and basophils induce bronchoconstriction, increased vascular permeability and mucous secretion. Resident inflammatory cells may be activated to release chemotactic factors, which in turn recruit more effector cells and amplify the response of the airways. Inflammation of the bronchial walls also may injure the epithelium, stimulating nerve endings and initiating neural reflexes that further aggravate and propagate the bronchospasm.

Many inflammatory mediators and chemotactic factors have been implicated in the bronchospasm and mucous hypersecretion of asthma. The relative contributions of the different substances probably vary with the inciting stimulus. The best-studied situation associated with the induction of asthma is inhaled allergens.

In a sensitized person, an inhaled allergen interacts with T_H2 cells and IgE antibody bound to the surface of mast cells, which are interspersed among the bronchial epithelial cells (Fig. 12-48). The T_H2 cells and mast cells release mediators of type I (immediate) hypersensitivity, including histamine, bradykinin, leukotrienes, prostaglandins, thromboxane A_2 and platelet-activating factor (PAF), as well as cytokines such as interleukin (IL)-4 and IL-5. These inflammatory mediators lead to (1) **smooth muscle contraction,** (2) **mucous secretion** and (3) **increased vascular permeability and edema.** Each of these effects is a potent, albeit reversible, cause of airway obstruction. IL-5 causes terminal differentiation of eosinophils in the bone marrow. Chemotactic factors, including leukotriene B_4 and neutrophil and eosinophil chemotactic factors, attract neutrophils, eosinophils and platelets to the bronchial wall. Eosinophils then release leukotriene B_4 and PAF, aggravating bronchoconstriction and edema. Discharge of eosinophil granules containing eosinophil cationic protein and major basic protein into the bronchial lumen further impairs mucociliary function and damages epithelial cells. Epithelial cell injury is suspected to stimulate nerve endings in the mucosa, an initiating autonomic discharge that

A IMMEDIATE RESPONSE

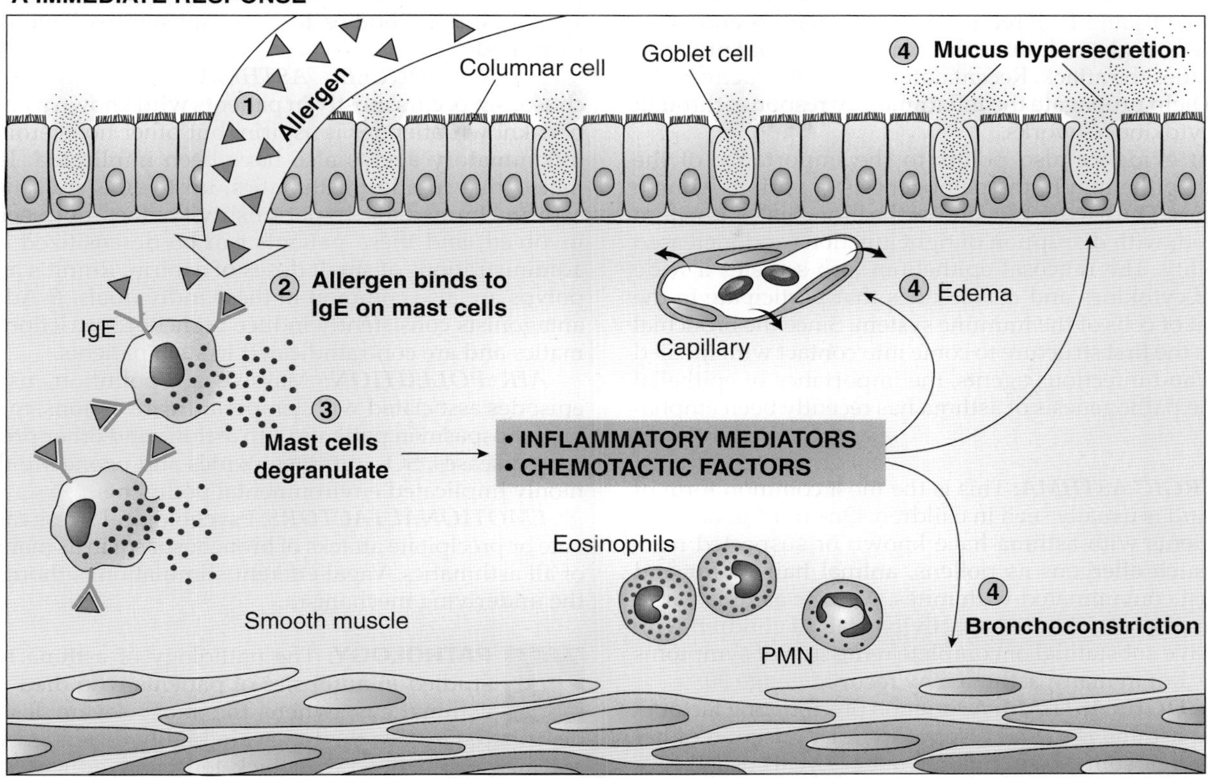

B DELAYED RESPONSE

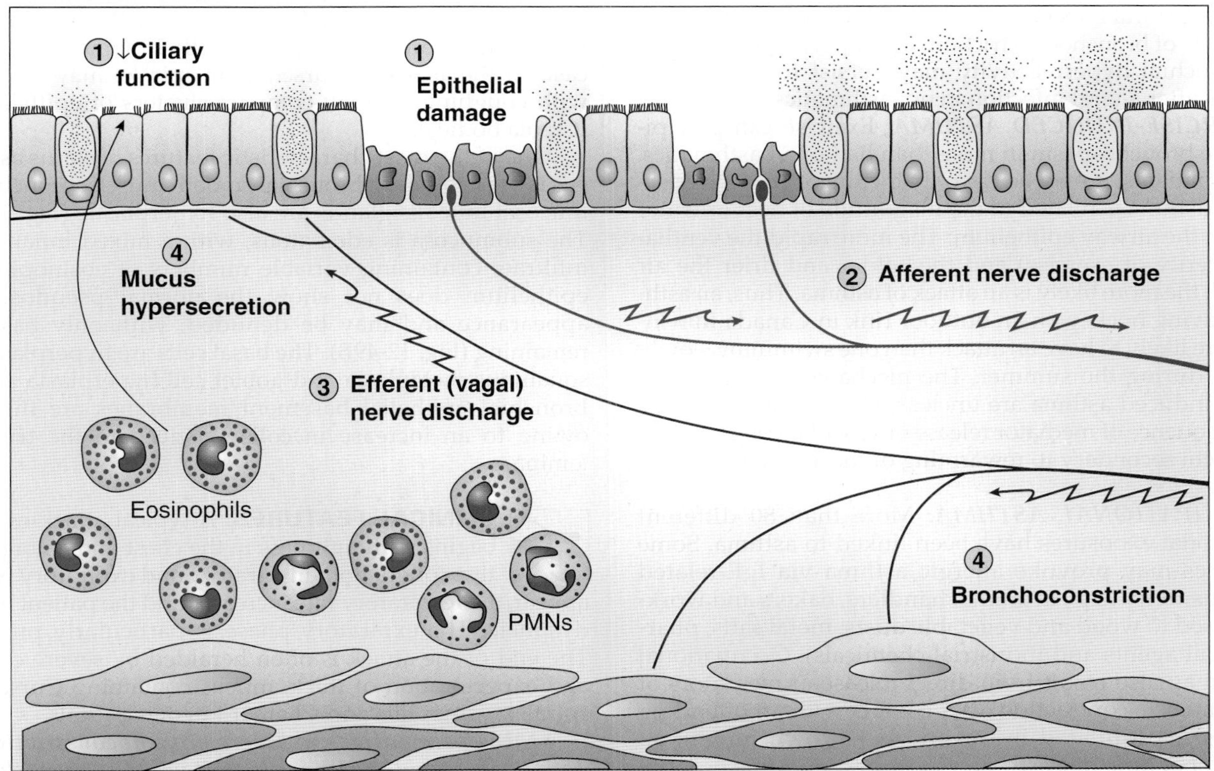

FIGURE 12-48. Pathogenesis of asthma. A. Immunologically mediated asthma. Allergens interact with immunoglobulin E (IgE) on mast cells, either on the surface of the epithelium or, when there is abnormal permeability of the epithelium, in the submucosa. Mediators are released and may react locally or by reflexes mediated through the vagus. **B.** The discharge of eosinophilic granules further impairs mucociliary function and damages epithelial cells. Epithelial cell injury stimulates nerve endings (in red) in the mucosa, thereby initiating an autonomic discharge that contributes to airway narrowing and mucus secretion. PMNs = polymorphonuclear neutrophils.

contributes to airway narrowing and mucous secretion. Leukotriene B_4 and PAF recruit more eosinophils and other effector cells, and so continue the vicious circle that prolongs and amplifies the attack. Recent data suggest that activated T cells also help propagate the inflammatory response through various cytokine networks.

Recent evidence also points to the importance of the bronchial epithelium in the pathogenesis of various asthma phenotypes. The barrier function of the bronchial epithelium is impaired, with disruption of tight junctions and increased permeability. The mucosal epithelium also secretes a wide variety of cytokines and chemokines that participate in the regulation of cells of the immune system. Since the bronchial mucosa is the first structure to come into contact with inhaled allergens and infectious agents, the importance of epithelial cells in the pathogenesis of asthma has recently been emphasized.

ALLERGIC ASTHMA: This is the most common form of asthma, and is usually seen in children. One third to one half of all patients with asthma have known or suspected reactions to such allergens as pollens, animal hair or fur and house dust contaminated with mites. Allergic asthma correlates strongly with skin-test reactivity. Half of children with asthma have substantial or complete remission of symptoms by age 20, but in many, asthma may recur after age 30.

INFECTIOUS ASTHMA: A common precipitating factor in childhood asthma is a viral respiratory tract infection rather than an allergic stimulus. In children under 2 years of age, RSV is the usual agent; in older children, rhinovirus, influenza and parainfluenza are common inciting organisms. Inflammatory responses to viral infection in susceptible people may trigger the episode of bronchoconstriction. In support of this hypothesis, bronchial hyperreactivity may persist for as long as 2 months after a viral infection in nonasthmatics.

EXERCISE-INDUCED ASTHMA: Exercise can precipitate some bronchospasm in more than half of all asthmatics. In some patients, it may be the only inciting factor. Exercise-induced asthma is related to the magnitude of heat or water loss from the airway epithelium. The more rapid the ventilation (severity of exercise) and the colder and drier the air breathed, the more likely is an attack of asthma. Thus, an asthmatic playing hockey on an outdoor rink in Canada in winter is more likely to have an attack than one swimming slowly in Texas during the summer. The mechanisms underlying exercise-induced asthma are unclear. The condition may be the consequence of mediator release or vascular congestion in the bronchi secondary to rewarming of the airways after the exertion.

OCCUPATIONAL ASTHMA: More than 80 different occupational exposures have been linked to asthma. Some substances may provoke allergic asthma via IgE-related hypersensitivity (e.g., in animal handlers, bakers and workers exposed to wood and vegetable dusts, metal salts, pharmaceutical agents and industrial chemicals). Occupational asthma may also result from direct release of mediators of smooth muscle contraction after contact with an offending agent, as is postulated in byssinosis ("brown lung"), an occupational lung disease of cotton workers. Some occupational exposures affect the autonomic nervous system directly. For instance, organic phosphorus insecticides act as anticholinesterases and produce overactivity of the parasympathetic nervous system. Substances such as toluene diisocyanate and western red cedar dust are thought to operate through hypersensitivity mechanisms, although specific IgE antibodies to these substances have not been identified.

DRUG-INDUCED ASTHMA: Drug-induced bronchospasm occurs mostly in patients with known asthma. The best-known offender is aspirin, but other nonsteroidal anti-inflammatory agents also have been implicated. It is estimated that in adult asthmatics, up to 10% are sensitive to aspirin. Immediate hypersensitivity does not seem to be involved, and these patients can be desensitized by daily administrations of small doses of aspirin. Rhinitis and nasal polyps are also common in these individuals. β-Adrenergic antagonists consistently induce bronchoconstriction in asthmatics and are contraindicated in such patients.

AIR POLLUTION: Massive air pollution, usually in episodes associated with temperature inversions, may cause bronchospasm in patients with asthma and other preexisting lung diseases. SO_2, nitrogen oxides and ozone are the commonly implicated environmental pollutants.

EMOTIONAL FACTORS: Psychological stress can aggravate or precipitate attacks of bronchospasm in as many as half of all asthmatics. Vagal efferent stimulation is thought to be the underlying mechanism.

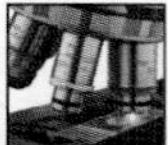

PATHOLOGY: The pathology of asthma has been studied in autopsies of patients who died in status asthmaticus, where the most severe lesions are described. Grossly, the lungs are highly distended with air, and airways are filled with thick, tenacious, adherent mucous plugs. Microscopically, these plugs (Fig. 12-49A) contain strips of epithelium and many eosinophils. Charcot-Leyden crystals, derived from phospholipids of the eosinophil cell membrane, are also seen (Fig. 12-24B). In some cases, mucoid casts of the airways (Curschmann spirals) may be expelled with coughing, as may compact clusters of epithelial cells (Creola bodies).

One of the most characteristic features of status asthmaticus is hyperplasia of bronchial smooth muscle. Bronchial submucosal mucous glands are also hyperplastic (Fig. 12-49A). The submucosa is edematous, with a mixed inflammatory infiltrate containing variable numbers of eosinophils. The epithelium does not show the normal pseudostratified appearance and may be denuded, with only basal cells remaining (Fig. 12-49B). The basal cells are hyperplastic, and squamous metaplasia and goblet cell hyperplasia are seen. Bronchial epithelial basement membranes are thickened, owing to an increase in collagen deep to the true basal lamina.

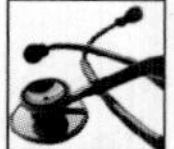

CLINICAL FEATURES: A typical attack of asthma begins with tightness in the chest and a nonproductive cough. Both inspiratory and expiratory wheezes appear, the respiratory rate increases and the patient becomes dyspneic. The expiratory phase is particularly prolonged. The end of the attack is often heralded by severe coughing and expectoration of thick, mucus-containing Curschmann spirals, eosinophils and Charcot-Leyden crystals.

Status asthmaticus is severe bronchoconstriction that does not respond to the drugs that usually abort the acute attack. This situation is potentially serious and requires hospitalization. Patients in status asthmaticus have hypoxemia and often hypercapnia. In particularly severe episodes, they may die. Patients require oxygen and other pharmacologic interventions.

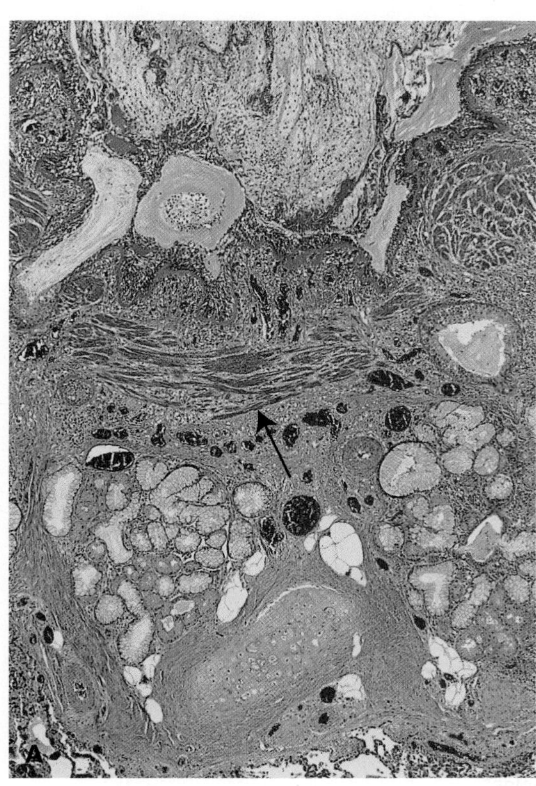

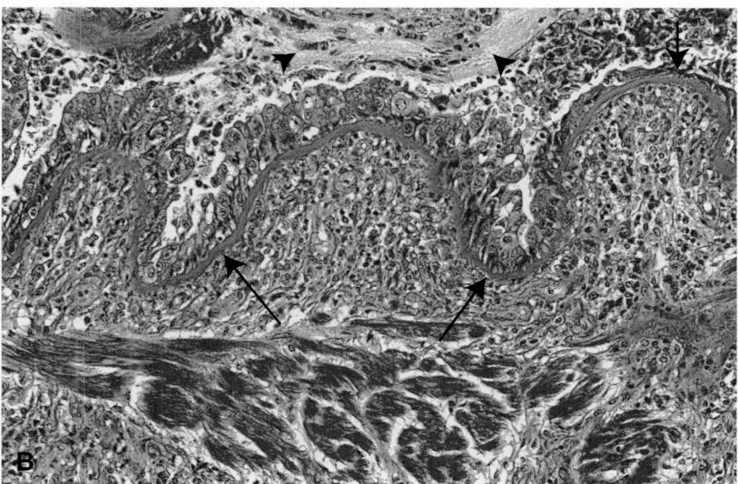

FIGURE 12-49. Asthma. A. A section of lung from a patient who died in status asthmaticus reveals a bronchus containing a luminal mucous plug, submucosal gland hyperplasia and smooth muscle hyperplasia (*arrow*). **B.** Higher magnification shows hyaline thickening of the subepithelial basement membrane (*long arrows*) and marked inflammation of the bronchiolar wall, with numerous eosinophils. The mucosa exhibits an inflamed and metaplastic epithelium (*arrowheads*). The epithelium is focally denuded (*short arrow*).

The cornerstone of asthma treatment includes administration of β-adrenergic agonists, inhaled corticosteroids, cromolyn sodium, methylxanthines and anticholinergic agents. Systemic corticosteroids are reserved for status asthmaticus or resistant chronic asthma. The inhalation of bronchodilators often provides dramatic relief.

Pneumoconioses

Pneumoconioses are pulmonary diseases caused by mineral dust inhalation. Over 40 inhaled minerals cause lung lesions and radiographic abnormalities. Most, like tin, barium and iron, are innocuous and simply accumulate in the lung. However, some lead to crippling pulmonary diseases. The specific types of pneumoconioses are named by the substance inhaled (e.g., silicosis, asbestosis, talcosis). Sometimes, the offending agent is uncertain, and the occupation is simply cited (e.g., "arc welder's lung"). Historically, occupations were known to predispose to lung disease before an etiology was recognized. Thus, "knife grinder's lung" was used before the disease was recognized as silicosis.

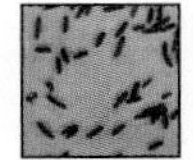

ETIOLOGIC FACTORS: *The key factor in the genesis of symptomatic pneumoconioses is the capacity of inhaled dusts to stimulate fibrosis* (Fig. 12-50). Thus, small amounts of silica or asbestos produce extensive fibrosis, whereas coal and iron are only weakly fibrogenic.

In general, lung lesions produced by inorganic dusts reflect the dose and size of the particles that reach the lung. The dose is a function of the concentration of dust in the air and the duration of exposure. As inhaled particles are often irregular, their size should be expressed as aerodynamic particle diameter, a parameter that describes the particle's motion in inspired air and that determines where inhaled dusts deposit in the lung (Fig. 12-2). The most dangerous particles are those that reach the peripheral zones (i.e., the smallest bronchioles and the acini). Particles over 10 μm in diameter deposit on bronchi and bronchioles, and are removed by the mucociliary escalator. Smaller particles reach the acini, and the smallest ones behave as a gas and are exhaled.

Alveolar macrophages ingest inhaled particles and are the main defenders of the alveolar space. Most phagocytosed particles ascend to the mucociliary carpet, to be coughed up or swallowed. Others migrate into the lung interstitium, and thence into lymphatics. Many ingested particles accumulate in and about respiratory bronchioles and terminal bronchioles. Others are not phagocytosed but migrate through epithelial cells into the interstitium.

Silicosis Is Caused by Inhalation of Silicon Dioxide (Silica)

The earth's crust is composed largely of silicon and its oxides, and silicosis is one of the oldest recorded diseases, possibly having begun in the Paleolithic period when humans began to fashion flint instruments. Dyspnea in metal diggers was reported by Hippocrates, and early Dutch pathologists wrote that the lungs of stone cutters sectioned like a mass of sand. The 19th-century English literature provided numerous descriptions of silicosis, and the disease remained the major cause of death in workers exposed to silica dust for the first half of the 20th century.

Silicosis was described historically as a disease of sandblasters, but exposure to silica occurs in numerous other occupations, including mining, stone cutting, polishing and sharpening of metals, ceramic manufacturing, foundry work and cleaning of boilers. The use of air-handling equipment

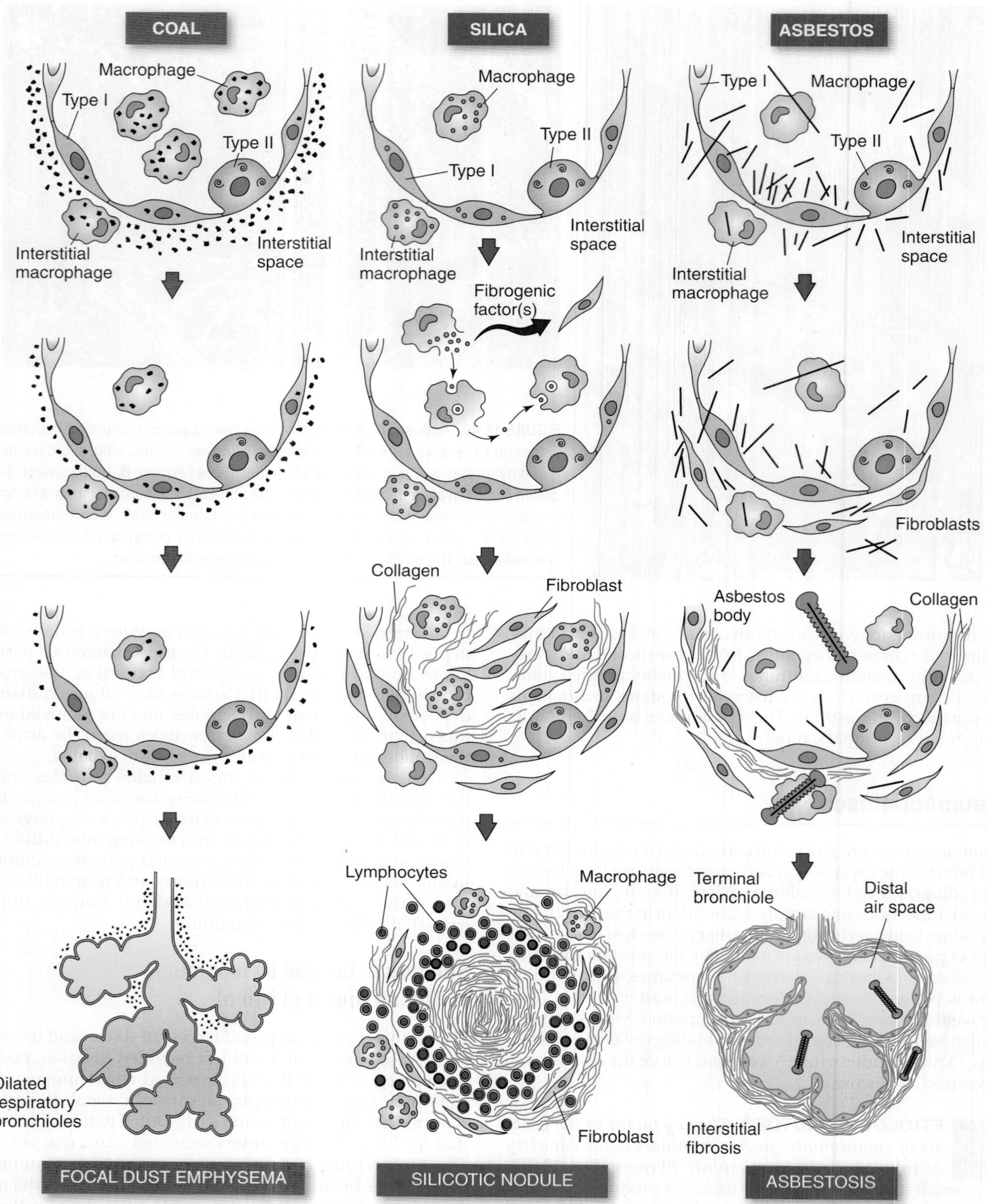

FIGURE 12-50. Pathogenesis of pneumoconioses. The three most important pneumoconioses are illustrated. In simple coal workers' pneumoconiosis, massive amounts of dust are inhaled and engulfed by macrophages. The macrophages pass into the interstitium of the lung and aggregate around the respiratory bronchioles. Subsequently, the bronchioles dilate. In silicosis, the silica particles are toxic to macrophages, which die and release a fibrogenic factor. In turn, the released silica is again phagocytosed by other macrophages. The result is a dense fibrotic nodule, the silicotic nodule. Asbestosis is characterized by little dust and much interstitial fibrosis. Asbestos bodies are the classic features.

and face masks has substantially reduced the incidence of silicosis.

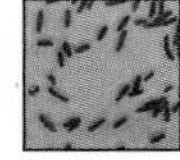

ETIOLOGIC FACTORS: The biological effects of silica particles depend on a number of factors, some involving the particle itself and others related to the host response. Crystalline silica (quartz) is more toxic than amorphous forms, and its biological activity is related to its surface properties. Particles of 0.2 to 2.0 μm are the most dangerous. Removal of the soluble surface layer by acid washing or creation of new surfaces by sandblasting enhances the biological activity of silica particles.

After their inhalation, silica particles are ingested by alveolar macrophages. Silicon hydroxide groups on the surface of the particles form hydrogen bonds with phospholipids and proteins, an interaction that is presumed to damage cellular membranes and thereby kill the macrophages. The dead cells release free silica particles and fibrogenic factors. The released silica is then reingested by macrophages and the process is amplified.

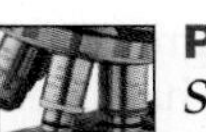

PATHOLOGY:

SIMPLE NODULAR SILICOSIS: This is the most common form of silicosis and is almost inevitable in any worker with long-term exposure to silica. Twenty to 40 years (but sometimes only 10 years) after initial exposure to silica, the lungs contain silicotic nodules less than 1 cm in diameter (usually 2 to 4 mm). Histologically, they have a characteristic whorled appearance, with concentrically arranged collagen forming the largest part of the nodule (Fig. 12-51). At the periphery are aggregates of mononuclear cells, mostly lymphocytes and fibroblasts. Polarized light reveals doubly refractile needle-shaped silicates within the nodule.

Hilar nodes may become enlarged and calcified, often at the edge of the node ("eggshell calcification"). Simple silicosis does not usually lead to significant respiratory dysfunction.

PROGRESSIVE MASSIVE FIBROSIS: Radiographically, progressive massive fibrosis signifies nodular masses greater than 2 cm diameter, in a background of simple silicosis. These larger lesions, most of which are 5 to 10 cm across, represent coalescence of smaller nodules, and are usually in the upper zones of the lungs bilaterally (Fig. 12-52). The lesions often exhibit central cavitation. Progressive massive fibrosis is related to the amount of silica in the lung. Disability is caused by destruction of lung tissue that was incorporated into the nodules.

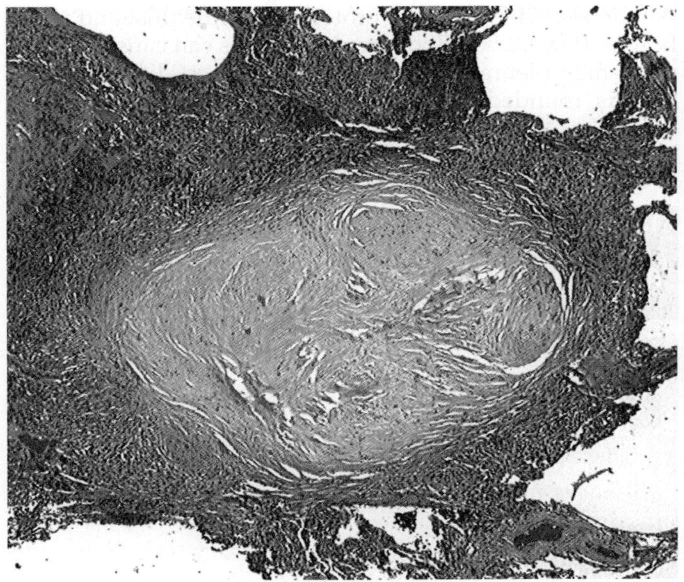

FIGURE 12-51. Silicosis. A silicotic nodule is composed of concentric whorls of dense, sparsely cellular collagen.

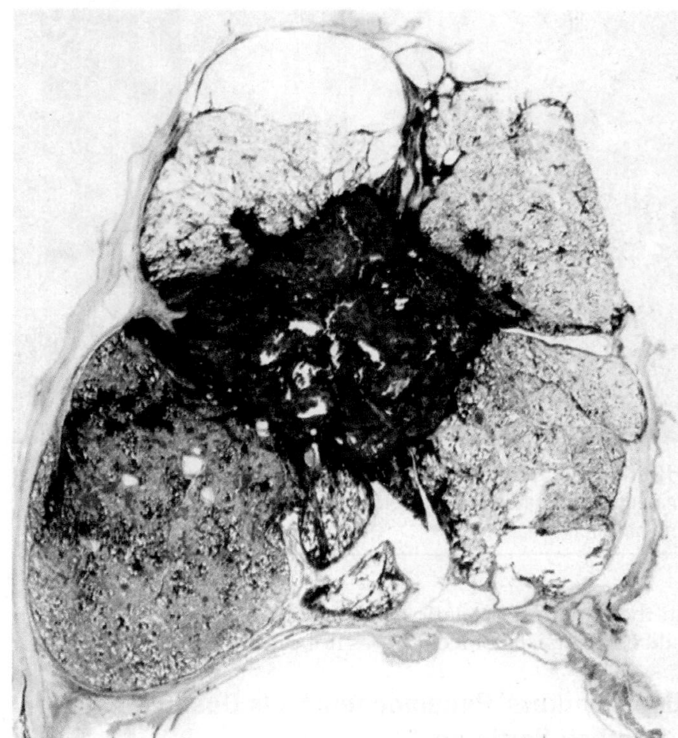

FIGURE 12-52. Progressive massive fibrosis. A whole mount of a silicotic lung from a coal miner shows a large area of dense fibrosis containing entrapped carbon particles.

ACUTE SILICOSIS: Now uncommon, acute silicosis results from heavy exposure to finely particulate silica during sandblasting or boiler scaling. It is associated with diffuse fibrosis of the lung. Silicotic nodules are not found. Dense eosinophilic material accumulates in alveolar spaces to produce an appearance resembling alveolar lipoproteinosis **(silicoproteinosis).** The disease progresses rapidly over a few years, unlike other forms of silicosis in which progression is measured in decades. On radiologic examination, acute silicosis shows diffuse linear fibrosis and reduced lung volume. Clinically, there is a severe restrictive defect.

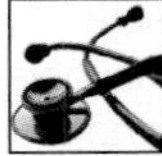

CLINICAL FEATURES: Simple silicosis is usually a radiologic diagnosis without significant symptoms. Dyspnea on exertion and later at rest suggests progressive massive fibrosis or other complications of silicosis. In acute silicosis, dyspnea may become rapidly disabling, after which respiratory failure ensues.

It is well recognized that **tuberculosis** is much more common in patients with silicosis than in the general population. The incidence of tuberculosis in patients with silicosis is higher in acute silicosis and among populations with a high prevalence of tuberculosis. Although the incidence of tuberculosis

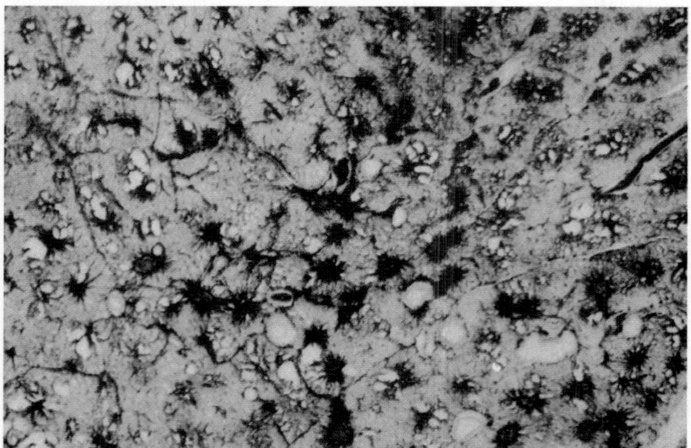

FIGURE 12-53. Anthracosilicosis. A whole mount of the lung of a coal miner demonstrates scattered, irregular, pigmented nodules throughout the parenchyma.

in the general population has declined, the association with silicosis persists. Silicosis does not predispose to lung cancer.

Coal Workers' Pneumoconiosis Is Due to Inhalation of Carbon Particles

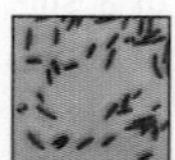

ETIOLOGIC FACTORS: Coal dust is composed of amorphous carbon and other constituents of the earth's surface, including variable amounts of silica. Anthracite (hard) coal contains significantly more quartz than does bituminous (soft) coal. Workers who inhale large amounts of quartz particles, such as those who work within mines, are at greater risk than those working above ground or loading coal for transport. In this context, amorphous carbon by itself is not fibrogenic. It does not kill alveolar macrophages, but is simply a nuisance dust that causes an innocuous anthracosis. By contrast, silica is highly fibrogenic, and inhaled anthracotic particles may thus lead to **anthracosilicosis** (Fig. 12-53).

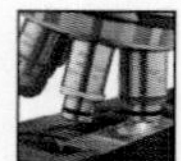

PATHOLOGY: Coal workers' pneumoconiosis (CWP) is typically divided into **simple CWP** and **complicated CWP** (a.k.a. progressive massive fibrosis). The typical lung lesions of simple CWP include nonpalpable **coal-dust macules** and palpable **coal-dust nodules,** both of which are multiple and scattered throughout the lung as 1- to 4-mm black foci. Microscopically, coal-dust macules contain many carbon-laden macrophages, which surround distal respiratory bronchioles, extend to fill adjacent alveolar spaces and infiltrate peribronchiolar interstitial spaces. Respiratory bronchioles may be mildly dilated (focal dust emphysema), probably due to atrophy of smooth muscle.

Nodules are round or irregular, may or may not be associated with bronchioles and consist of dust-laden macrophages associated with a fibrotic stroma. They occur when coal is admixed with fibrogenic dusts such as silica, and are more properly classified as anthracosilicosis (Fig. 12-53). Coal-dust macules and nodules appear on chest radiographs as small nodular densities. Simple CWP was once thought to cause severe disability, but it is now clear that at worst it causes minor impairment of lung function. If coal miners have severe airflow obstruction, it is usually due to smoking.

Complicated CWP occurs on a background of simple CWP and is defined as a lesion 2.0 cm or greater in size, and may cause significant respiratory impairment.

Caplan syndrome was first described as rheumatoid nodules **(Caplan nodules)** in the lungs of coal miners with rheumatoid arthritis. However, the term is now also used to refer to the association of pulmonary rheumatoid nodules with other pneumoconioses, such as silicosis or asbestosis. The nodular lesions are large (1 to 10 cm in diameter), multiple, bilateral and usually peripheral, and microscopically resemble rheumatoid nodules associated with inhaled dust deposits. Rheumatoid nodules are large, central, necrotic areas with a border of chronic inflammation and palisading macrophages (see Chapter 26). Caplan nodules are not identical to rheumatoid nodules, and may represent a combination of silicotic and rheumatoid nodules.

Asbestos-Related Diseases May Be Reactive or Neoplastic

Asbestos (Greek, "unquenchable") includes a group of fibrous silicate minerals that occur as thin fibers. It has been used for diverse purposes for over 4000 years, since early Finns fashioned pottery from it. Roman vestal virgins used it to manufacture oil-lamp wicks, and Marco Polo remarked that asbestos-containing Chinese cloth resisted fire. More recently, asbestos has been used in insulation, construction materials and automative brake linings. Asbestos mining proceeded exponentially in the 20th century until its deleterious effects eventually elicited alarm.

There are six natural types of asbestos, which can be divided into two mineralogic groups. **Chrysotile** accounts for the bulk of commercially used asbestos. The **amphiboles** include amosite, crocidolite, tremolite, actinolite and anthophyllite. Of the amphiboles, only amosite and crocidolite have been used commercially to any significant extent. Another form of asbestos is termed erionite and is mined in Turkey and adjacent areas. It is similar to the amphiboles in pathogenicity. If coal is a classic example of much dust and little fibrosis, asbestos is the prototype of little dust and much fibrosis (Fig. 12-50). Exposure to asbestos can cause asbestosis, benign pleural effusion, pleural plaques, diffuse pleural fibrosis, rounded atelectasis and mesothelioma (Table 12-4).

Table 12-4

Asbestos-Related Lung Disease

Pleural Lesions
Benign pleural effusion
Parietal pleural plaques
Diffuse pleural fibrosis
Rounded atelectasis
Interstitial Lung Disease
Asbestosis
Malignant Mesothelioma
Carcinoma of the lung (in smokers)

All commercially used forms of asbestos are associated with lung diseases, but the amphiboles, and crocidolite in particular, have a much greater propensity to produce disease than does chrysotile.

ASBESTOSIS: Asbestosis is diffuse interstitial fibrosis resulting from inhalation of asbestos fibers. Development of asbestosis requires heavy exposure to asbestos of the type historically seen in asbestos miners, millers and insulators.

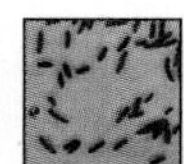

ETIOLOGIC FACTORS: Asbestos fibers may be long (up to 100 μm) but thin (0.5 to 1 μm), so their aerodynamic particle diameter is small. They deposit in distal airways and alveoli, particularly at bifurcations of alveolar ducts. The smallest particles are engulfed by macrophages, but many larger fibers penetrate into the interstitial space. The first lesion is an alveolitis that is directly related to asbestos exposure. Release of inflammatory mediators by activated macrophages and the fibrogenic character of the free asbestos fibers in the interstitium promote interstitial pulmonary fibrosis.

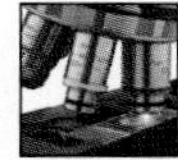

PATHOLOGY: Asbestosis is characterized by bilateral, diffuse interstitial fibrosis and asbestos bodies in the lung (Figs. 12-54 and 12-55). In the early stages, fibrosis occurs in and around alveolar ducts and respiratory bronchioles, and in the periphery of the acinus. When the fibers deposit in bronchioles and respiratory bronchioles, they incite a fibrogenic response that leads to mild chronic airflow obstruction. Thus, asbestos may produce obstructive as well as restrictive defects. As the disease progresses, fibrosis spreads beyond the peribronchiolar location and eventually results in an end-stage or "honeycomb" lung. Asbestosis is usually more severe in the lower zones of the lung.

Asbestos bodies are found in the walls of bronchioles or within alveolar spaces, often engulfed by alveolar macrophages. The particles have a distinctive morphology, consisting of a clear, thin asbestos fiber (10 to 50 μm long) surrounded by a beaded iron–protein coat. By light microscopy, they are golden brown (Fig. 12-55) and react strongly with the Prussian blue stain for iron. The fibers are only partly engulfed by macrophages because they are too large for a single cell. The macrophages coat the asbestos fiber with protein, proteoglycans and ferritin.

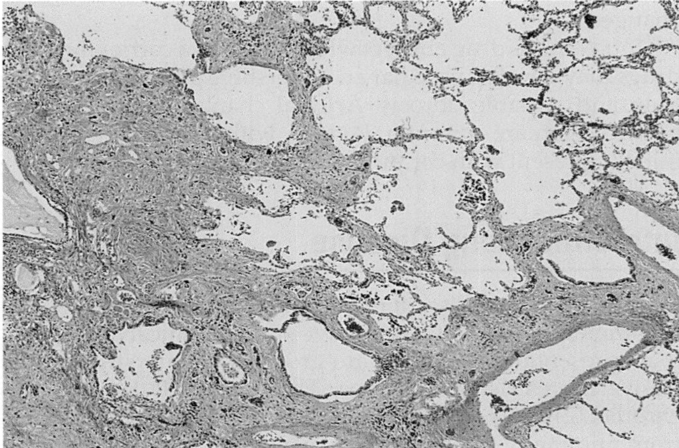

FIGURE 12-54. Asbestosis. The lung shows patchy, dense, interstitial fibrosis.

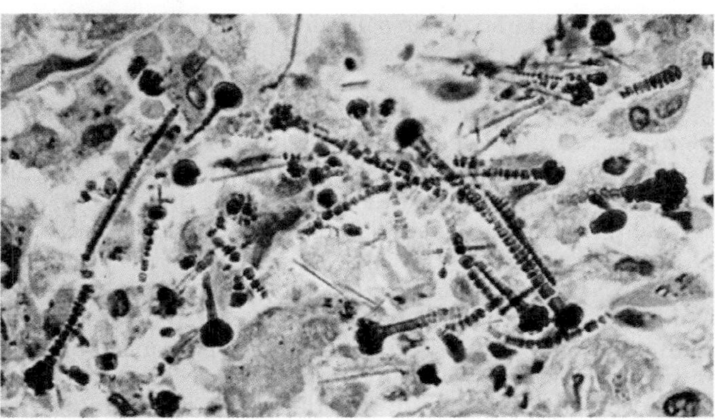

FIGURE 12-55. Asbestos bodies. These ferruginous bodies are golden brown and beaded, with a central, colorless, nonbirefringent core fiber. Asbestos bodies are encrusted with protein and iron.

Finding asbestos bodies incidentally at autopsy does not warrant a diagnosis of asbestosis; the lungs must also show diffuse interstitial fibrosis. Digests and concentrates of autopsy lungs demonstrate asbestos bodies to varying degrees in the lungs of virtually all adults.

BENIGN PLEURAL EFFUSION: Benign pleural effusion associated with asbestos inhalation is diagnosed by (1) a history of asbestos exposure, (2) identification of a pleural effusion with radiographs or thoracentesis, (3) absence of other diseases that could cause effusion and (4) no malignant tumor after 3 years of follow-up. Pleural effusions often occur within 10 years of initial exposure and are seen in about 3% of workers exposed to asbestos.

PLEURAL PLAQUES: Pleural plaques typically occur on parietal and diaphragmatic pleura, often 10 to 20 years after exposure to asbestos. They may be found in up to 15% of the general population and half of all patients with plaques at autopsy may not have a history of asbestos exposure. Plaques occur most often on the parietal pleura, in the posterolateral regions of the lower thorax and on the domes of the diaphragm.

Grossly, pleural plaques are pearly white and have a smooth or nodular surface (Fig. 12-56). They are usually bilateral, but not necessarily symmetric. Plaques may measure over 10 cm in diameter and become calcified. Histologically, they consist of acellular, dense, hyalinized fibrous tissue, with

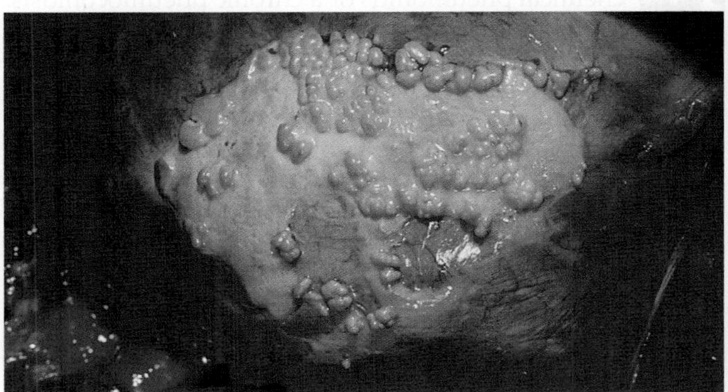

FIGURE 12-56. Pleural plaque. The dome of the diaphragm is covered by a smooth, pearly white, nodular plaque.

numerous slitlike spaces in a parallel fashion ("basket-weave pattern"). Pleural plaques are not predictors of asbestosis, nor do they evolve into mesotheliomas.

DIFFUSE PLEURAL FIBROSIS: Fibrosis limited to the pleura is usually detected at least 10 years after the initial exposure, and should be distinguished from asbestosis, in which fibrosis affects the interstitium of the underlying lung diffusely. Plaques and pleural fibrosis can occur in association with all types of asbestos.

ROUNDED ATELECTASIS: Asbestosis exposure occasionally leads to pleural fibrosis and adhesions associated with atelectasis, which has a rounded appearance on chest radiograph. Radiographically, rounded atelectasis is characterized by a pleural-based, rounded or oval, 2.5- to 5.0-cm shadow, which usually lies along the posterior surface of a lower lobe. Pathologically, the lung shows pleural fibrosis or plaques, with curved pleural invaginations extending several centimeters into the underlying parenchyma. The condition is clinically benign.

MESOTHELIOMA: ***The relation between asbestos exposure and malignant mesothelioma is firmly established.*** Sometimes exposure is indirect and slight (e.g., wives of asbestos workers who wash their husbands' clothes). More often, mesothelioma is seen in workers heavily exposed to asbestos, mainly crocidolite and amosite. This malignancy is discussed below with diseases of the pleura.

CARCINOMA OF THE LUNG: There are reports that lung cancer is more common in nonsmoking asbestos workers than in similar workers not exposed to asbestos, but data are limited and no firm conclusion is possible at this point. However, in asbestos workers who smoke, the incidence of carcinoma of the lung is vastly increased: up to 40 to 60 times that of the general nonsmoking population. The link between asbestos and lung cancer is most convincingly supported in the presence of asbestosis (diffuse interstitial fibrosis).

Berylliosis Is Characterized by Noncaseating Granulomas

Berylliosis refers to the pulmonary disease that follows the inhalation of beryllium. Today this metal is used principally in structural materials in aerospace, industrial ceramics and nuclear industries. Exposure to beryllium may also occur in those who mine and extract beryllium ores.

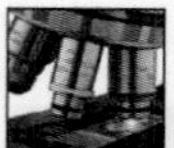

PATHOLOGY: Berylliosis may occur as an acute chemical pneumonitis or a chronic pneumoconiosis. In the acute form, symptoms begin within hours or days after inhalation of metal particles and manifest pathologically as diffuse alveolar damage. Of all patients with acute beryllium pneumonitis, 10% progress to chronic disease, although chronic berylliosis is often observed in workers without any history of an acute illness.

Chronic berylliosis differs from other pneumoconioses in that the amount and duration of exposure may be small. The lesion is thus suspected to be a hypersensitivity reaction. Pulmonary lesions are indistinguishable from those of sarcoidosis (see below). Multiple noncaseating granulomas are distributed along the pleura, septa and bronchovascular bundles (Fig. 12-57). The beryllium lymphocyte proliferation test may aid in separating these two entities. The disease may progress to end-stage fibrosis and **honeycomb lung** (see below). Patients with chronic berylliosis have an insidious onset of dyspnea 15 or more years after the initial exposure. The disease appears to be associated with an increased risk of lung cancer.

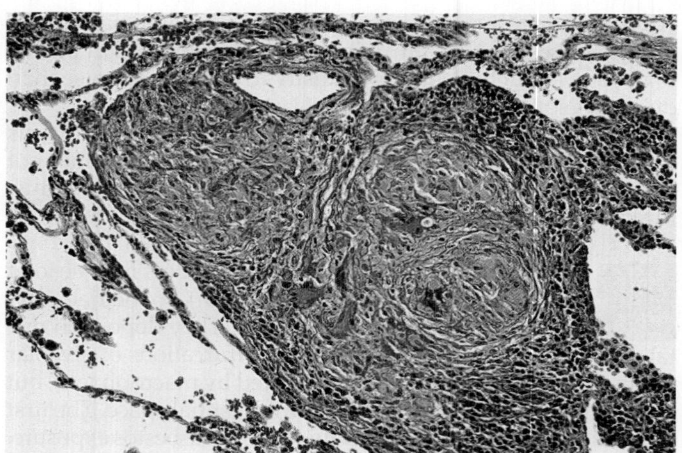

FIGURE 12-57. Berylliosis. A noncaseating granuloma consists of a nodular collection of epithelioid macrophages and multinucleated giant cells.

Talcosis Results From Prolonged and Heavy Exposure to Talc Dust

Talc consists of magnesium silicates that are used in a number of industries for their lubricant properties, and in cosmetics and pharmaceuticals. Occupational exposure to talc occurs among workers engaged in mining and milling the mineral and in the leather, rubber, paper and textile industries. Industrial talcs may include other minerals such as tremolite or silica. Cosmetic talc is more than 90% pure and rarely causes lung disease.

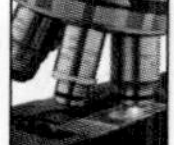

PATHOLOGY: Grossly, talcosis lesions vary from tiny nodules to severe fibrosis. Microscopically, foreign body granulomas associated with birefringent platelike talc particles are scattered throughout the parenchyma, which displays fibrotic nodules and interstitial fibrosis. Associated minerals such as silica may contribute to the fibrotic changes.

Intravenous drug abusers who use talc as a carrier for illicit drugs may develop vascular and interstitial granulomas in the lung and variable fibrosis. Arterial changes of pulmonary hypertension are common. Persons with these changes may initially present with cor pulmonale.

Interstitial Lung Disease

Many pulmonary disorders are characterized by interstitial inflammatory infiltrates and have similar clinical and radiologic presentations, and so are grouped as interstitial, infiltrative or restrictive diseases. These may (1) be acute or chronic, (2) be of known or unknown etiology and (3) vary from minimally symptomatic to severely incapacitating and lethal interstitial fibrosis. Restrictive lung diseases are characterized by decreased lung volume and decreased oxygen-diffusing capacity on pulmonary function studies.

Hypersensitivity Pneumonitis (Extrinsic Allergic Alveolitis) Is a Response to Inhaled Antigens

Inhalation of many antigens leads to hypersensitivity pneumonitis, with acute or chronic interstitial inflammation in the lung. Most of these antigens are encountered in occupational settings, and the resulting diseases are often labeled accordingly. Thus, **farmer's lung** occurs in persons exposed to *Micropolyspora faeni* from moldy hay, **bagassosis** results from exposure to *Thermoactinomyces sacchari* in moldy sugar cane, **maple bark–stripper's disease** follows exposure to the fungus *Cryptostroma corticale* in moldy maple bark and **bird fancier's lung** affects bird keepers with long-term exposure to proteins from bird feathers, blood and excrement. Other causes of hypersensitivity pneumonitis include inhalation of pituitary snuff **(pituitary snuff taker's disease),** moldy cork **(suberosis)** and moldy compost **(mushroom worker's disease).** Hypersensitivity pneumonitis may also be caused by fungi that grow in stagnant water in air conditioners, swimming pools, hot tubs and central heating units. Skin tests and serum precipitating antibodies are often used to confirm the diagnosis. Often, especially in chronic hypersensitivity pneumonitis, an inciting antigen is never identified. In acute cases, the diagnosis is usually established clinically, so lung biopsies are performed only in chronic cases.

MOLECULAR PATHOGENESIS: Acute hypersensitivity pneumonitis is characterized by neutrophilic infiltrates in alveoli and respiratory bronchioles; chronic lesions show mononuclear cells and granulomas, typical of delayed hypersensitivity. Most cases have serum IgG precipitating antibodies against the offending agent. Hypersensitivity pneumonitis represents a combination of immune complex–mediated (type III) and cell-mediated (type IV) hypersensitivity reactions, although the precise contribution of each is still debated (Fig. 12-58). Importantly, most people who have serum precipitins to inhaled antigens do not develop hypersensitivity pneumonitis, suggesting a genetic component in host susceptibility.

PATHOLOGY: The histology in florid cases of chronic hypersensitivity pneumonitis is virtually diagnostic. However, in subtle cases, the diagnosis may require careful clinical and radiologic correlation, and even then it may remain tentative. Microscopic features of chronic hypersensitivity pneumonitis are bronchiolocentric cellular interstitial pneumonia, noncaseating granulomas and organizing pneumonia (Fig. 12-59A,B). The bronchiolocentric cellular interstitial infiltrate consists of lymphocytes, plasma cells and macrophages and varies from severe to subtle; eosinophils are uncommon. Poorly formed noncaseating granulomas are seen in two thirds of cases (Fig. 12-59B), as is organizing pneumonia (Fig. 12-59A). In the end stage, interstitial inflammation recedes, leaving pulmonary fibrosis, which may resemble usual interstitial pneumonia.

CLINICAL FEATURES: Hypersensitivity pneumonitis may present as acute, subacute or chronic pulmonary disease, depending on the frequency and intensity of exposure to the offending antigen. Farmer's lung is the prototype of hypersensitivity pneumonitis, caused by inhaling thermophilic actinomycetes from moldy hay. Typically, a farm worker enters a barn where hay has been stored for winter feeding. After a lag period of 4 to 6 hours, he rapidly develops dyspnea, cough and mild fever. Symptoms remit within 24 to 48 hours but return on reexposure; with time, the disorder becomes chronic. Patients with chronic hypersensitivity pneumonitis have a more nonspecific presentation, with a gradual onset of dyspnea and cor pulmonale.

Pulmonary function studies show a restrictive pattern, characterized by decreased compliance, reduced diffusion capacity and hypoxemia. In the chronic stage, airway obstruction may be troublesome. Bronchoalveolar lavage shows T lymphocytosis, mostly $CD8^+$ suppressor/cytotoxic cells. Removing the offending antigen is the only adequate treatment for hypersensitivity pneumonitis. Steroid therapy may be effective in acute forms and for some chronically affected patients.

Sarcoidosis Is a Granulomatous Disease of Unknown Etiology

In sarcoidosis the lung is the organ most often involved, but lymph nodes, skin, eye and other organs are also common targets (Fig. 12-60).

EPIDEMIOLOGY: Sarcoidosis is a worldwide disease, affecting all races and both sexes, but with strong racial and ethnic predilections. In North America, it is much more common in blacks than in whites, the ratio being about 15:1. However, it is uncommon in tropical Africa. In Scandinavian countries, the prevalence is 64/100,000, but is 10/100,000 in France and 3/100,000 in Poland. The reported prevalence of sarcoidosis in Irish women in London is an astonishing 200/100,000. The disease is distinctly uncommon in China.

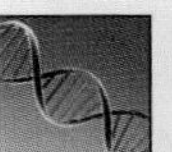

MOLECULAR PATHOGENESIS: The exact pathogenesis of sarcoidosis remains obscure, but there is a consensus that it reflects exaggerated helper/inducer T-lymphocyte responses to exogenous or autologous antigens. These cells accumulate in affected organs, where they secrete lymphokines and recruit macrophages, which participate in forming noncaseating granulomas. $CD4^+$:$CD8^+$ T-cell ratios are 10:1 in organs with sarcoid granulomas, but are 2:1 in uninvolved tissues. The basis for this abnormal accumulation of helper/inducer T lymphocytes is unclear. A defect in suppressor cell function may permit unopposed helper cell proliferation. Inherited or acquired differences in immune response genes may favor one type of T-cell response over another. Nonspecific polyclonal activation of B cells by T-helper cells leads to hyperglobulinemia, a characteristic feature of active sarcoidosis.

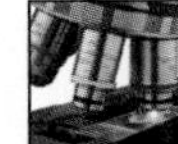

PATHOLOGY: Pulmonary sarcoidosis most often affects the lungs and hilar lymph nodes, although either involvement may occur separately. Radiologically, a diffuse reticulonodular infiltrate is typical, but occasional cases may show larger nodules. Histologically, multiple sarcoid granulomas are scattered in the interstitium

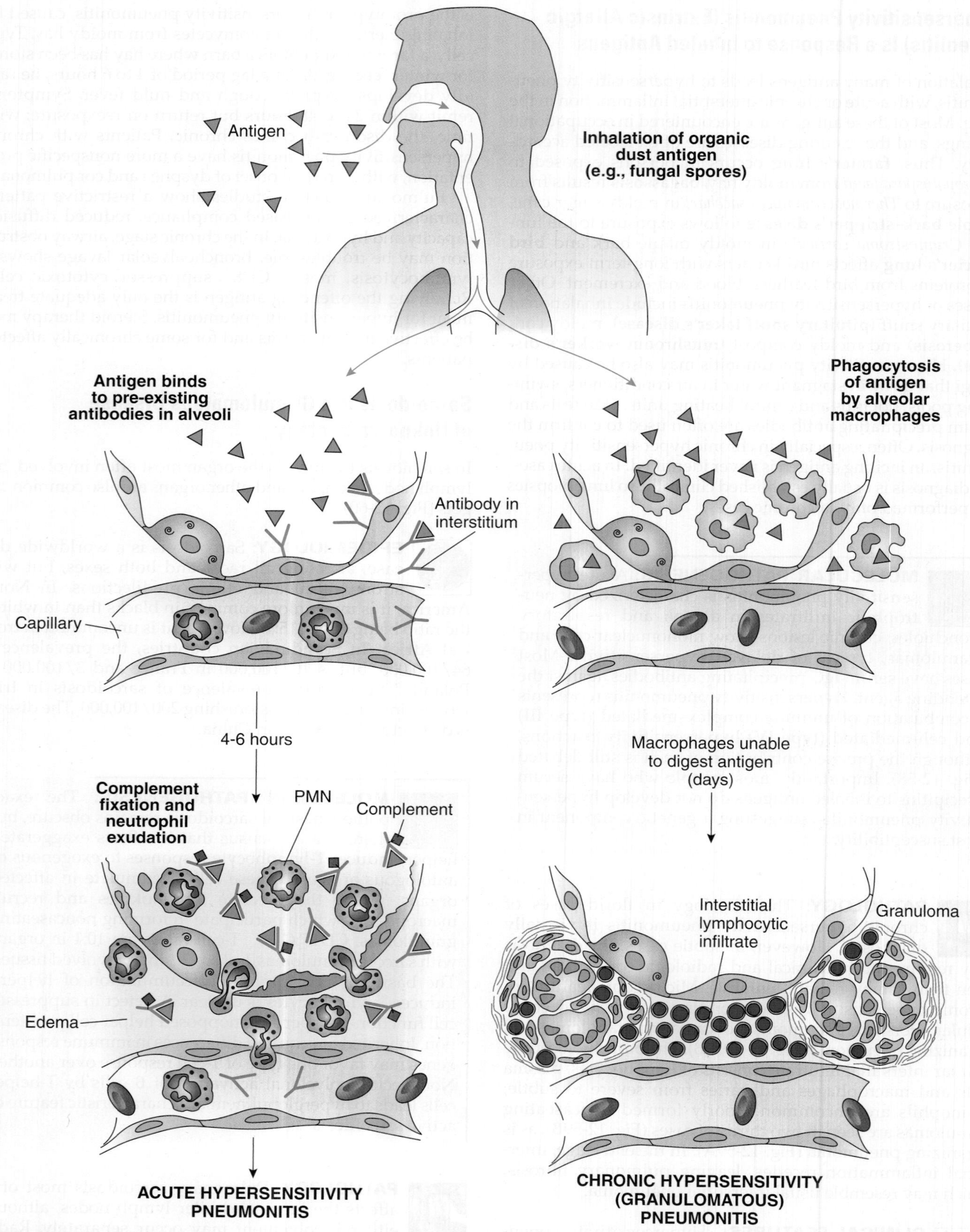

FIGURE 12-58. Hypersensitivity pneumonitis. An antigen–antibody reaction occurs in the acute phase and leads to acute hypersensitivity pneumonitis. If exposure is continued, this is followed by a cellular or subacute phase, with the formation of granulomas and chronic interstitial pneumonitis. PMN = polymorphonuclear neutrophil.

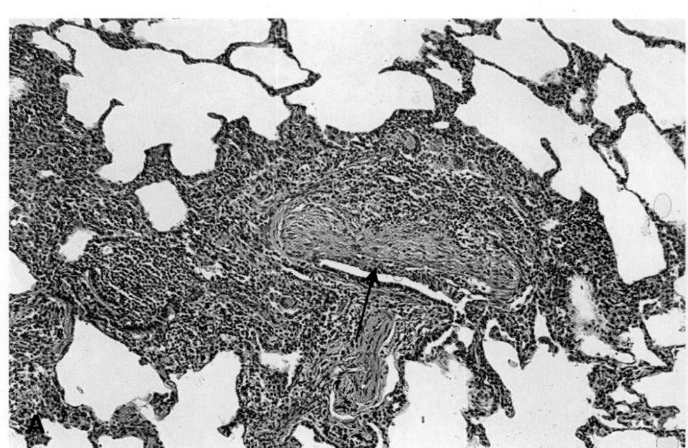

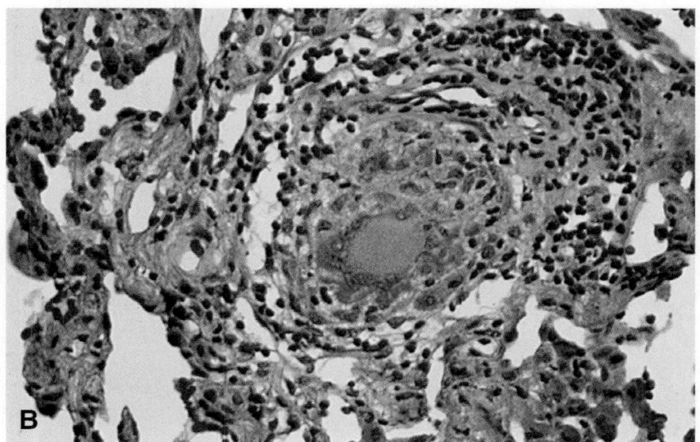

FIGURE 12-59. Hypersensitivity pneumonitis. A. A lung biopsy specimen shows a mild peribronchiolar chronic inflammatory interstitial infiltrate, with a focus of intraluminal organizing fibrosis (*arrow*). **B.** Focal poorly formed granulomas were scattered in the lung biopsy specimen.

of the lung (Fig. 12-61). The distribution is distinctive—along the pleura and interlobular septa and around bronchovascular bundles (Fig. 12-61A). Frequent bronchial or bronchiolar submucosal infiltration by sarcoid granulomas accounts for the high diagnostic yield (≅90%) on bronchoscopic biopsy. Granulomas in airways may occasionally be so prominent as to lead to airway obstruction (endobronchial sarcoid).

The granulomatous phase of sarcoidosis can progress to a fibrotic phase. Fibrosis often begins at the periphery of a granuloma and may show an onion-skin pattern of lamellar fibrosis around the giant cells. Significant necrosis is uncommon, but one third of open lung biopsies show small foci of necrosis. Interstitial chronic inflammation tends to be inconspicuous. Granulomatous vasculitis is seen in two thirds of open lung biopsies from patients with sarcoidosis. Although **asteroid bodies** (star-shaped crystals) (Fig. 12-61B) and **Schaumann bodies** (small lamellar calcifications) are commonly encountered, they are not specific for sarcoidosis and may be seen in most granulomatous processes.

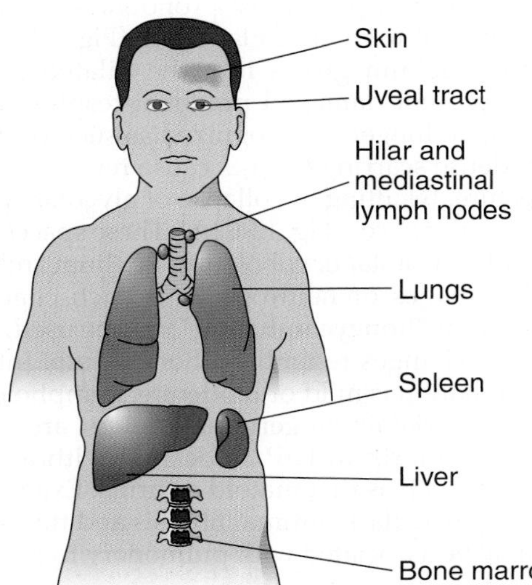

FIGURE 12-60. Organs commonly affected by sarcoidosis. Sarcoidosis involves many organs, most commonly the lymph nodes and lung.

Interstitial fibrosis is not prominent in pulmonary sarcoidosis. However, progressive pulmonary fibrosis leads to a honeycomb lung, respiratory insufficiency and cor pulmonale.

CLINICAL FEATURES: Sarcoidosis is most common in young adults of both sexes. **Acute sarcoidosis** has an abrupt onset, usually followed by spontaneous remission within 2 years and an excellent response to steroids. **Chronic sarcoidosis** begins insidiously, and patients are more likely to have persistent or progressive disease. Sarcoidosis causes several chest radiographic patterns, the most classic of which is bilateral hilar adenopathy, with or without interstitial pulmonary infiltrates. It may also affect the skin (erythema nodosum), mostly in women. Black patients tend to have more severe uveitis, skin disease and lacrimal gland involvement. Cough and dyspnea are the major respiratory complaints. However, the disease can be mild and may be discovered as an incidental finding on a chest radiograph in an asymptomatic patient.

No laboratory test is specific for the diagnosis of sarcoidosis. Transbronchial lung biopsy via a fiberoptic bronchoscope often reveals granulomas. Occasionally, the diagnosis is made by mediastinoscopy, identifying multiple noncaseating granulomas in a mediastinal lymph node. Bronchoalveolar lavage often shows an increase in the proportion of $CD4^+$ T lymphocytes. Increased uptake of gallium-67, a material phagocytosed by activated macrophages, can demonstrate granulomatous areas. Serum angiotensin-converting enzyme (ACE) levels are elevated in two thirds of patients with active sarcoidosis, and 24-hour urine calcium is frequently increased. These laboratory data, together with supportive clinical and radiologic findings, allow the diagnosis of sarcoidosis to be made with a high probability.

Other organs commonly involved include the skin, eye (uveal tract), heart, central nervous system, extrathoracic lymph nodes, spleen and liver (Fig. 12-60). These are discussed separately in individual chapters.

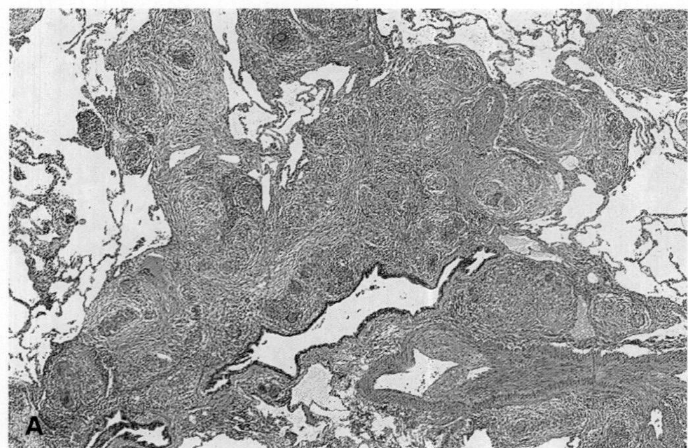

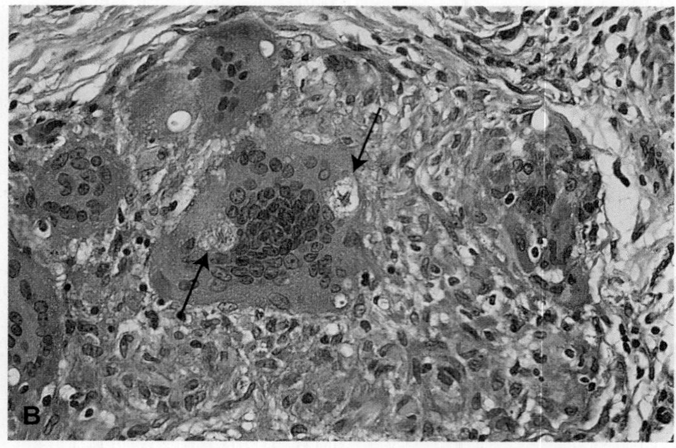

FIGURE 12-61. Sarcoidosis. A. Multiple noncaseating granulomas are present along the bronchovascular interstitium. **B.** Noncaseating granulomas consist of tight clusters of epithelioid macrophages and multinucleated giant cells. Several asteroid bodies are present (*arrows*).

The prognosis in pulmonary sarcoidosis is favorable; most patients do not develop clinically significant sequelae. In 60% of patients pulmonary sarcoidosis resolves, but this is less likely in older patients and those with extrathoracic disease, particularly in the bone and skin. In up to 20% of cases, sarcoidosis does not remit or recurs at intervals, but it leads to death in only 10% of cases. Corticosteroid therapy is effective for active sarcoidosis.

Usual Interstitial Pneumonia Is the Histologic Pattern Seen in Clinical Idiopathic Pulmonary Fibrosis

Usual interstitial pneumonia (UIP) is one of the most common types of interstitial pneumonia, with an annual incidence of 6 to 14 cases per 100,000 people. It has a slight male predominance and a mean age at onset of 50 to 60 years. The clinical term **idiopathic pulmonary fibrosis** (IPF) is applied when the disease is determined to be of unknown origin.

ETIOLOGIC FACTORS: The etiology of IPF is unknown, but immunologic, viral and genetic factors are thought to play a role. A history of flulike illness favors viral origin in some patients. A genetic role is suggested by cases of familial IPF and the association of UIP-like diseases in patients with inherited disorders such as neurofibromatosis and Hermansky-Pudlak syndrome. An association with collagen vascular diseases in about 20% of cases, including rheumatoid arthritis, systemic lupus erythematosus and progressive systemic sclerosis, suggests immune system involvement. UIP also occurs with such autoimmune disorders as Hashimoto thyroiditis, primary biliary cirrhosis, autoimmune hepatitis, idiopathic thrombocytopenic purpura and myasthenia gravis. Circulating autoantibodies are often found (e.g., antinuclear antibodies and rheumatoid factor), and immune complexes have been demonstrated in the circulation, inflamed alveolar walls and bronchoalveolar lavage fluids. No antigen has yet been identified. It has been postulated that alveolar macrophages become activated upon phagocytosis of immune complexes, after which they release cytokines that recruit neutrophils. These in turn damage alveolar walls, setting in motion a series of events that culminates in interstitial fibrosis.

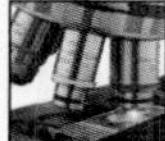

PATHOLOGY: UIP is a histologic pattern that occurs in a variety of clinical settings, including collagen vascular disease, chronic hypersensitivity pneumonitis, drug toxicity and asbestosis. Many cases lack an identifiable etiology and are thus considered idiopathic (IPF). The lungs are small in UIP, and fibrosis tends to be worse in the lower lobes, in the subpleural regions and along interlobular septa. Retraction of the scars, especially of lobular septa, gives the external surface of the lung a hobnail appearance, reminiscent of cirrhosis of the liver. Fibrosis is often patchy, with areas of dense scarring and honeycomb cystic change (Fig. 12-62A).

The histologic hallmark of UIP is patchy interstitial fibrosis, with areas of normal lung adjacent to fibrotic areas (Fig. 12-62B). The fibrosis is of different ages, which has been termed "**temporal heterogeneity.**" Areas of loose fibroblastic tissue **(fibroblast foci)** may be adjacent to dense collagen (Fig. 12-62C). The fibrosis is most pronounced beneath the pleura and adjacent to interlobular septa (Fig. 12-62B). The bronchiolar epithelium grows into the dilated airspaces, which may represent damaged proximal respiratory bronchioles but can no longer be recognized as such (Fig. 12-63). The areas of dense scarring fibrosis cause remodeling of the lung architecture, resulting in collapse of alveolar walls and formation of cystic spaces (Fig. 12-62A). These spaces are typically lined by bronchiolar or cuboidal epithelium and contain mucus, macrophages or neutrophils. If such changes are extensive, the term **"honeycomb lung"** may be used, because the gross cystic changes resemble a honeycomb. Interstitial chronic inflammation is mild or moderate. Lymphoid aggregates, sometimes containing germinal centers, are occasionally noted, particularly in UIP associated with a collagen vascular disease such as rheumatoid arthritis. Extensive vascular changes, particularly intimal fibrosis and thickening of the media, may be associated with pulmonary hypertension.

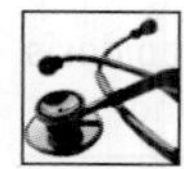

CLINICAL FEATURES: UIP begins insidiously, with the gradual onset of dyspnea on exertion and dry cough, usually over 1 to 3 years. Patients have

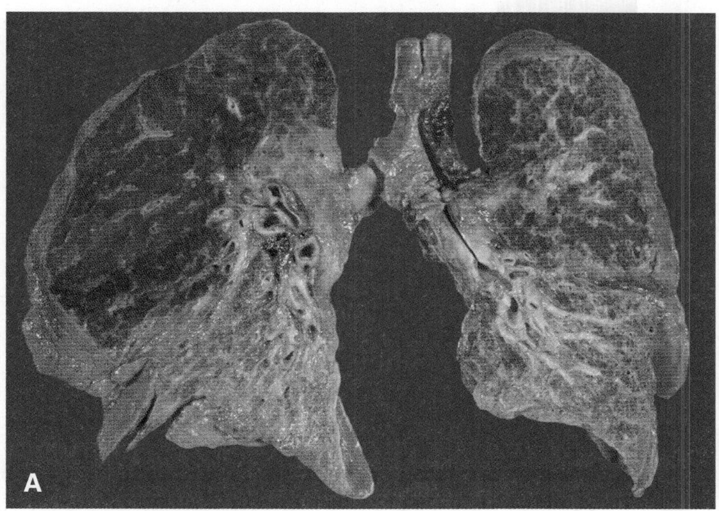

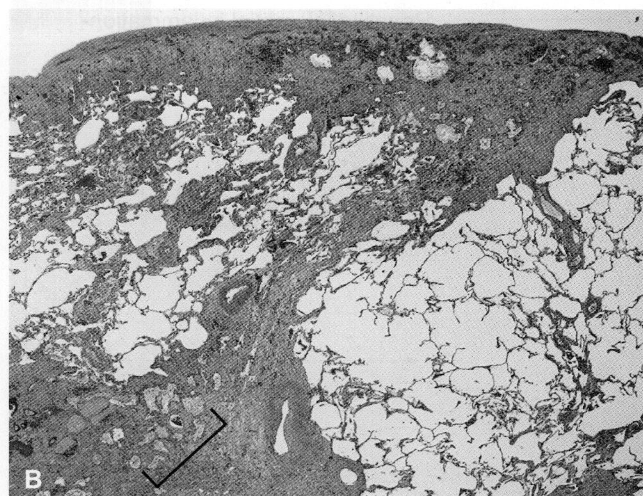

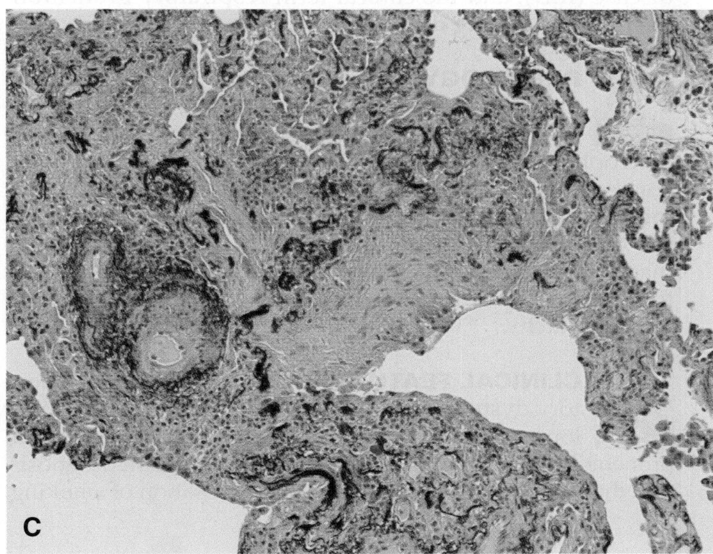

FIGURE 12-62. Usual interstitial pneumonitis. A. A gross specimen of the lung shows patchy dense scarring with extensive areas of honeycomb cystic change, predominantly affecting the lower lobes. This patient also had polymyositis. **B.** A microscopic view shows patchy subpleural fibrosis with microscopic honeycomb fibrosis (*bracket*). The areas of dense fibrosis display remodeling, with loss of the normal lung architecture. **C.** Elastin stain highlights the fibroblastic focus in green, which contrasts with the adjacent area of yellow staining of dense collagen and black staining of collapsed elastic fibers.

restrictive lung disease by pulmonary function testing. Clubbing of the fingers is common, especially late in the disease. In about 50% of patients, CT scans show distinctive findings: peripheral, subpleural reticular opacities, traction bronchiectasis and honeycombing, mostly in the posterior lower lobes.

The classic auscultatory finding is late inspiratory crackles and fine ("Velcro") rales at the lung bases. Tachypnea at rest, cyanosis and cor pulmonale eventually follow. The prognosis is bleak, with a mean survival of 4 to 6 years. Patients are treated with corticosteroids and sometimes cyclophosphamide, but lung transplantation generally offers the only hope of a cure.

Nonspecific Interstitial Pneumonia Has Multiple Etiologies

Nonspecific interstitial pneumonia (NSIP) is a histologic pattern of disease that may reflect diverse potential etiologies (infection, collagen vascular disease, hypersensitivity pneumonitis, drug reaction and others) or it may be idiopathic.

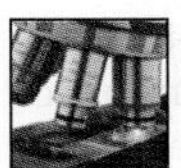

PATHOLOGY: NSIP shows a spectrum of **cellular** and **fibrosing patterns.** Unlike the patchy distribution and temporal heterogeneity of UIP, lung changes in NSIP are diffuse and uniform. In the **cellular form,** alveolar septa are diffusely involved by a mild to moderate lymphocytic infiltrate. In the **fibrosing form,** septa show diffuse fibrosis, with or without significant associated inflammation. Honeycombing and fibroblastic foci are inconspicuous or absent.

CLINICAL FEATURES: In NSIP, shortness of breath and cough develop over several months to years. Computed tomography findings are variable but most frequently show bilateral lower lobe "ground glass" changes or reticulation with traction bronchiectasis. The prognosis of idiopathic NSIP is favorable compared to IPF; overall 5-year survival is 80%.

Desquamative Interstitial Pneumonia Is a Diffuse Lung Disease of Cigarette Smokers Characterized by Marked Accumulation of Intra-Alveolar Macrophages

Interstitial fibrosis is minimal in desquamative interstitial pneumonia (DIP; Fig. 12-64A,B). The term "desquamative"

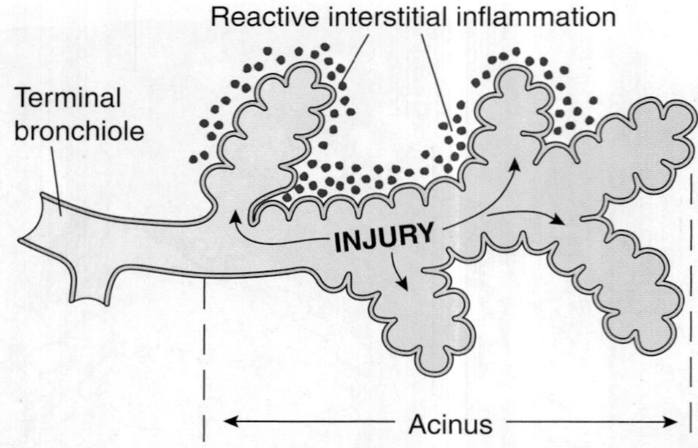

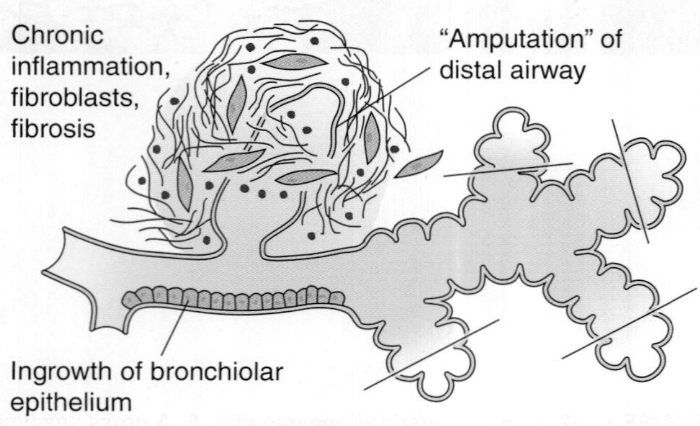

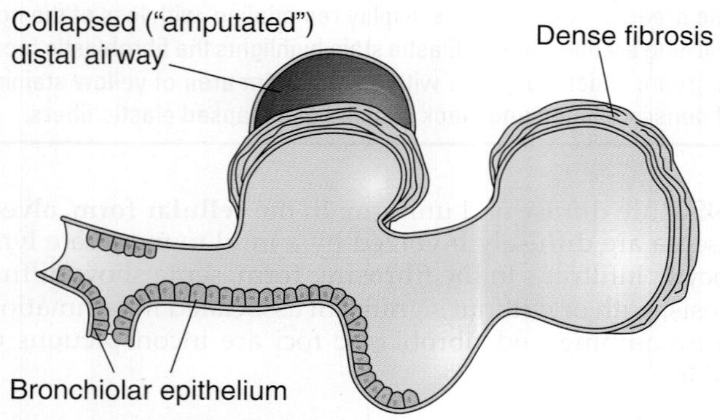

FIGURE 12-63. Pathogenesis of honeycomb lung. Honeycomb lung is the result of a variety of injuries. Interstitial and alveolar inflammation destroys ("amputates") the distal part of the acinus. The proximal parts dilate and become lined by bronchiolar epithelium.

reflected the misconception that the intra-alveolar cells were desquamated epithelial cells, whereas they are now recognized as macrophages. Unlike UIP, the alveolar architecture is preserved in DIP, and the disorder lacks the patchy scarring and remodeling of lung parenchyma of UIP. The macrophages contain a fine golden-brown pigment. Alveolar walls in DIP may, however, be mildly thickened by chronic inflammation and interstitial fibrosis (Fig. 12-64B). Scattered lymphoid aggregates also may be present. Hyperplasia of type II pneumocytes is often prominent.

DIP is seen almost exclusively in cigarette smokers, typically in the fourth or fifth decade, and occurs twice as often in men as in women. The prevailing opinion is that DIP and respiratory bronchiolitis–interstitial lung disease (see below) represent a spectrum of disease related to cigarette smoking, although the mechanism is unclear. The radiographic picture of DIP is not specific but is most frequently described as bilateral ground glass infiltrates with a lower lobe predominance. DIP has a much better prognosis than UIP, with an overall 10-year survival between 70% and 100%. Most patients respond well to steroid therapy and smoking cessation.

Respiratory Bronchiolitis–Interstitial Lung Disease Is a Malady of Smokers

Respiratory bronchiolitis (RB) is a histologic lesion that occurs in cigarette smokers. It is most often an incidental histologic finding, but it may rarely be the sole cause of interstitial lung disease (ILD), and the clinical term **respiratory bronchiolitis–interstitial lung disease** (RB-ILD) is appropriate.

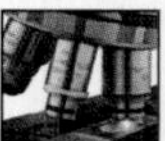

PATHOLOGY: Histologically, RB is a patchy accumulation of pigmented macrophages in the airspaces, centered on bronchioles (Fig. 12-65). These macrophages are present within lumina of bronchioles and adjacent alveolar spaces. Bronchiolar walls show mild chronic inflammation and fibrosis. However, interstitial fibrosis does not extend into the surrounding lung. The pigment in the macrophages is usually brown and finely granular. In contrast to DIP, which is diffuse, the lesions in RB are bronchiolocentric and patchy.

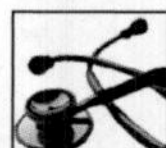

CLINICAL FEATURES: Patients have mild respiratory dysfunction. Radiographically, there is an upper lobe predominance, with thickening of the peripheral bronchioles. Patients with RB-ILD have an excellent prognosis, and the symptoms usually resolve after cessation of smoking.

In Organizing Pneumonia Pattern (Cryptogenic Organizing Pneumonia) Polypoid Plugs of Tissue Fill the Bronchiolar Lumen and Surrounding Alveolar Spaces

Organizing pneumonia pattern was previously referred to as "bronchiolitis obliterans–organizing pneumonia" (BOOP). ***It is not specific for any particular etiologic agent, and the cause cannot be determined from the morphologic appearance.*** Thus, it is seen in many settings, including in respiratory tract infections (particularly viral bronchiolitis), in inhalation of toxic materials, after administration of a number of drugs and in several inflammatory processes (e.g., collagen vascular diseases). ***A substantial number of cases are idiopathic, and are referred to as cryptogenic organizing pneumonia (or idiopathic BOOP).***

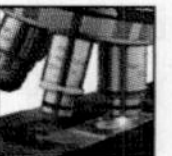

PATHOLOGY: Histologically, organizing pneumonia pattern features patchy areas of loose organizing fibrosis and chronic inflammatory cells in the distal airways adjacent to normal lung. Plugs of organizing fibroblastic tissue occlude bronchioles (bronchiolitis obliterans), alveolar ducts and surrounding alveoli (organizing pneumonia; Fig. 12-66). The pattern is mainly one of patchy alveolar

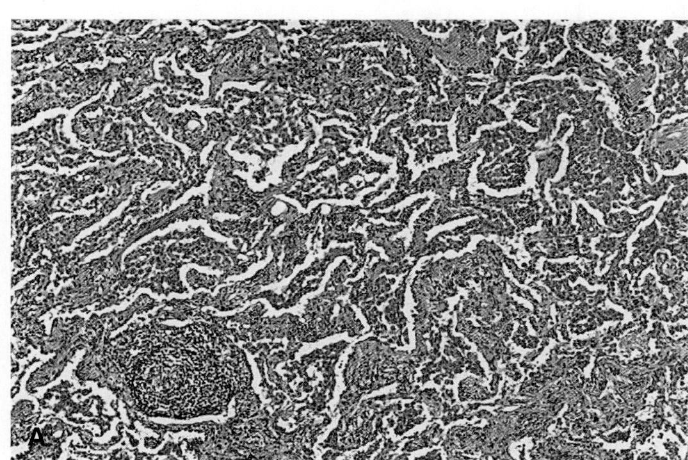

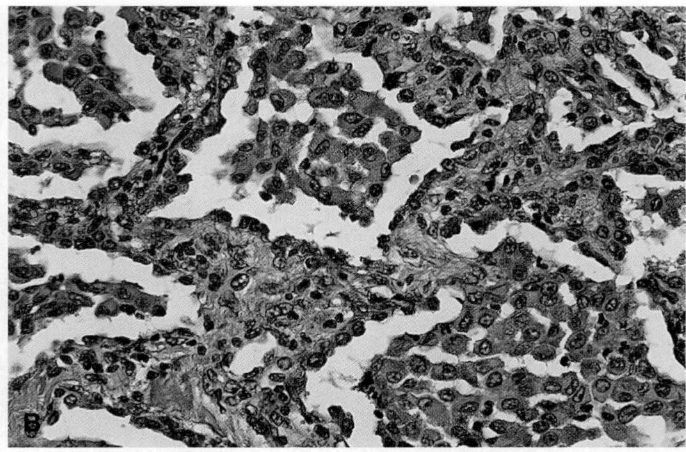

FIGURE 12-64. Desquamative interstitial pneumonia (DIP). A. A diffuse process in the lungs is characterized by the accumulation of alveolar macrophages, preservation of the alveolar architecture and a lymphoid aggregate. **B.** In addition to alveolar macrophage accumulation, there is mild alveolar septal fibrosis, type II pneumocyte hyperplasia and mild interstitial chronic inflammation.

organizing pneumonia, and bronchiolitis obliterans may not be seen in all cases. The lung architecture is preserved and the remodeling or honeycomb changes seen in UIP are absent. Obstructive or endogenous lipid pneumonia may develop if there is significant bronchiolitis obliterans owing to occlusion of the distal airways. The alveolar septa are only slightly thickened with chronic inflammatory cells, and type II pneumocyte hyperplasia is mild.

CLINICAL FEATURES: Cryptogenic organizing pneumonia pattern presents at a mean age of 55 years. The onset is acute, with fever, cough and dyspnea, often with a history of a flulike illness 4 to 6 weeks previously. As noted above, some patients may have predisposing conditions. Chest radiographs reveal localized opacities or bilateral interstitial infiltrates, which may migrate over time. Pulmonary function studies demonstrate a restrictive ventilatory pattern. Corticosteroid therapy is effective, and some patients recover within weeks to months even without therapy.

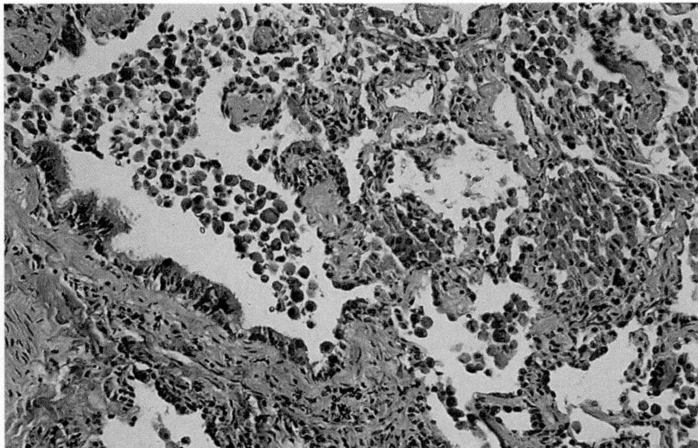

FIGURE 12-65. Respiratory bronchiolitis. There is marked accumulation of macrophages within the bronchioles and surrounding airspaces. Mild fibrotic thickening and chronic inflammation of the bronchiolar wall are present.

Lymphoid Interstitial Pneumonia Occurs in the Setting of Autoimmune Diseases

Lymphoid interstitial pneumonia (LIP) is a rare disease in which lymphoid infiltrates are distributed diffusely in the interstitial spaces of the lung.

PATHOLOGY: The hallmark of LIP is diffuse infiltration of alveolar septa and peribronchiolar spaces by lymphocytes, plasma cells and macrophages (Fig. 12-67). The alveolar architecture is preserved without scarring or remodeling of the lung. Hyperplasia of type II pneumocytes may be conspicuous, and inconspicuous foci of organizing interstitial fibrosis are occasionally present. Sarcoidlike, noncaseating granulomas are often seen. Alveolar spaces tend to contain a proteinaceous exudate. Occasionally, scattered lymphoid aggregates are present, some containing germinal centers. Hyperplasia of peribronchiolar lymphoid tissue may be prominent.

CLINICAL FEATURES: LIP may be idiopathic, but often occurs in patients with collagen vascular disease (especially Sjögren syndrome), dysproteinemia and HIV infection (Table 12-5). It is largely a disease of adults, but pediatric cases are recorded. In children, LIP is a defining criterion for the diagnosis of AIDS. Associated autoimmune manifestations include increased or reduced serum γ-globulins, a variety of dysproteinemias and increased circulating autoantibodies, such as rheumatoid factor and antinuclear antibodies. Lymphoma may rarely develop in patients with LIP, particularly in patients with Sjögren syndrome and AIDS.

Symptoms of LIP include cough and progressive dyspnea. The disease varies from an indolent condition to one that progresses to end-stage lung and respiratory failure. Corticosteroids and cytotoxic agents have been of some benefit.

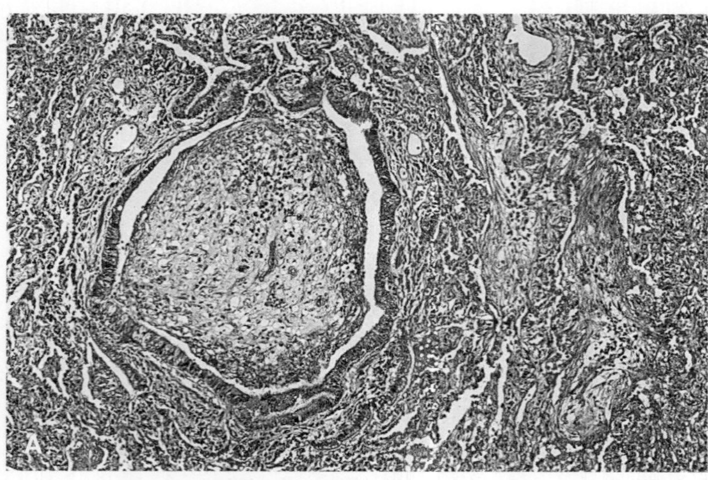
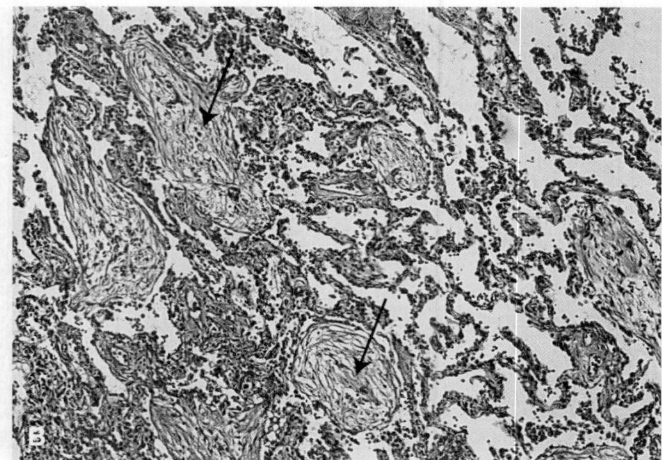

FIGURE 12-66. Organizing pneumonia pattern. A. Polypoid plugs of loose fibrous tissue are present in a bronchiole and the adjacent alveolar ducts and alveoli. **B.** The alveolar spaces contain similar plugs of loose organizing connective tissue (*arrows*).

Langerhans Cell Histiocytosis (Histiocytosis X) Encompasses a Spectrum of Localized and Systemic Cell Proliferations

Different presentations of Langerhans cell histiocytosis (LCH) have been called **eosinophilic granuloma, Hand-Schüller-Christian disease** and **Letterer-Siwe disease** (see Chapter 20). LCH can affect the lung as a distinctive form of interstitial lung disease. In adults it is most often an isolated lesion (previously termed **pulmonary eosinophilic granuloma**), with extrapulmonary manifestations such as bone lesions or diabetes insipidus occurring in 10% to 15% of cases. ***Virtually all of these patients are cigarette smokers.*** In children, lung involvement may occur in association with Letterer-Siwe disease or Hand-Schüller-Christian disease.

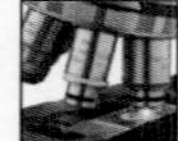

PATHOLOGY: Histologically, pulmonary LCH appears as scattered nodular infiltrates with a stellate border extending into the surrounding interstitium (Fig. 12-68A). These lesions are frequently centered on bronchioles or subpleurally. The cellular lesions contain varying proportions of Langerhans cells admixed with lymphocytes, eosinophils and macrophages. Langerhans cells are round to oval, with a moderate amount of eosinophilic cytoplasm and prominently grooved nuclei with small inconspicuous nucleoli (Fig. 12-68B). As the disease progresses, lesions cavitate and become fibrotic, and honeycomb fibrosis may result. Lung parenchyma adjacent to the nodular lesions may show marked accumulation of intra-alveolar macrophages, owing to respiratory bronchiolitis caused by smoking.

Langerhans cells have distinctive characteristics, including (1) cytoplasmic Birbeck granules (on electron microscopy); (2) C3, IgG-F_c receptors, CD1a and human leukocyte antigen (HLA)-DR; and (3) S-100 protein expression. Whether pulmonary LCH is a neoplastic proliferation or an abnormal immunologic response to antigens within cigarette smoke is unknown.

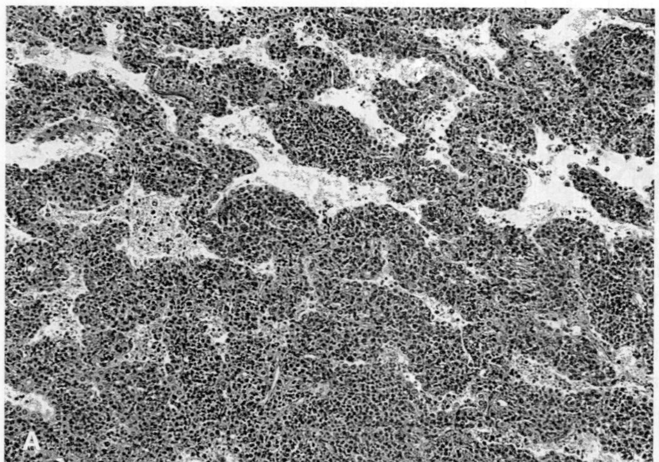
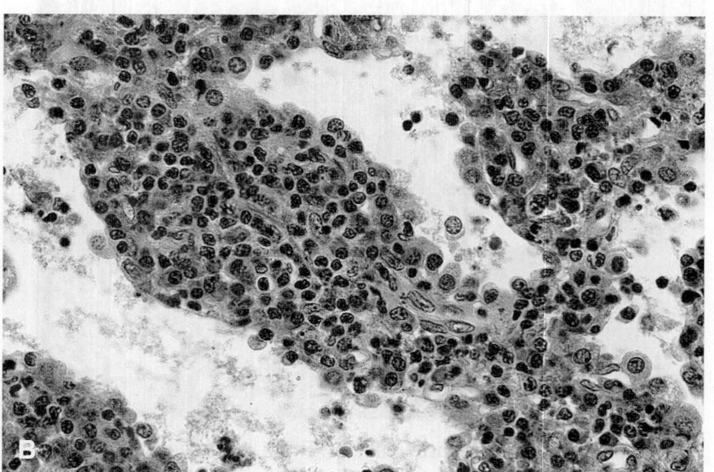

FIGURE 12-67. Lymphocytic interstitial pneumonia (LIP). A. The walls of the alveolar septa are diffusely infiltrated by chronic inflammation. **B.** The inflammatory infiltrate is composed of lymphocytes and plasma cells.

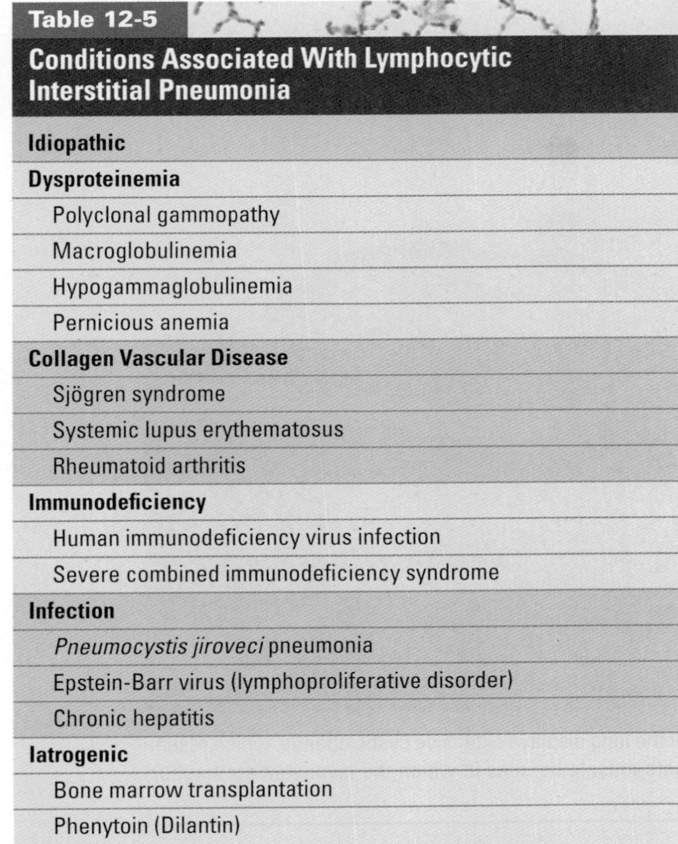

Table 12-5

Conditions Associated With Lymphocytic Interstitial Pneumonia

Idiopathic
Dysproteinemia
Polyclonal gammopathy
Macroglobulinemia
Hypogammaglobulinemia
Pernicious anemia
Collagen Vascular Disease
Sjögren syndrome
Systemic lupus erythematosus
Rheumatoid arthritis
Immunodeficiency
Human immunodeficiency virus infection
Severe combined immunodeficiency syndrome
Infection
Pneumocystis jiroveci pneumonia
Epstein-Barr virus (lymphoproliferative disorder)
Chronic hepatitis
Iatrogenic
Bone marrow transplantation
Phenytoin (Dilantin)

CLINICAL FEATURES: Pulmonary LCH usually affects patients in their third and fourth decades. The most common presenting symptoms are nonproductive cough, dyspnea on exertion and spontaneous pneumothorax, but 25% of patients are asymptomatic at the time of diagnosis. Chest radiographs show diffuse, bilateral, reticulonodular lesions, usually in the upper lobes. The lesions frequently undergo cavitation. Although most patients have a good prognosis, some develop chronic pulmonary dysfunction. In a small subset of cases, progressive pulmonary fibrosis can lead to death. Cessation of smoking is beneficial in the early stages of the disease.

Lymphangioleiomyomatosis Features Abnormal Smooth Muscle Proliferation in the Lung and Lymphatics

Lymphangioleiomyomatosis (LAM) is a rare interstitial lung disease that occurs almost exclusively in women of childbearing age and is characterized by widespread abnormal proliferation of smooth muscle in the lung, mediastinal and retroperitoneal lymph nodes and major lymphatic ducts. Its etiology is unknown, but clinical responses to oophorectomy and progesterone therapy suggest that the smooth muscle proliferation is under hormonal control. Its occurrence in patients with tuberous sclerosis and its association with renal angiomyolipomas suggest that LAM may be a forme fruste of **tuberous sclerosis**. Additionally, LAM is associated with mutations in the tuberous sclerosis gene complex, whether or not the patient has fully developed tuberous sclerosis. LAM cells are thought to be derived from perivascular epithelioid cells similar to other lesions associated with tuberous sclerosis, such as angiomyolipoma and clear cell tumor.

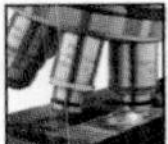

PATHOLOGY: Grossly, the lungs show bilateral, diffuse enlargement, with extensive cystic changes resembling those of emphysema (Fig. 12-69A). Histologically, numerous cystic spaces are lined by focal nodules or bundles of abnormal smooth muscle cells. These round or spindle-shaped cells (LAM cells) resemble immature smooth muscle cells but lack the parallel orientation of normal smooth muscle around airways and blood vessels (Fig. 12-69B). The smooth muscle proliferation typically follows a lymphatic distribution in the lung, around blood vessels and bronchioles and along the pleura and interlobular septa. Blood vessel walls, especially in small pulmonary veins, may also be infiltrated, resulting in microscopic hemorrhage and hemosiderin accumulation in alveolar macrophages. Immunostaining for HMB-45 (a melanoma antigen)

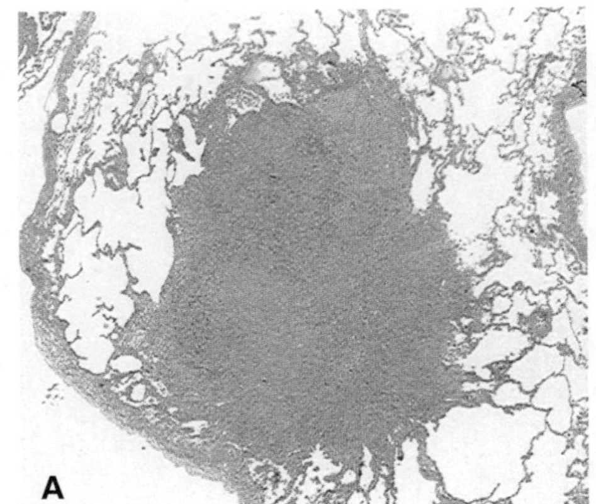

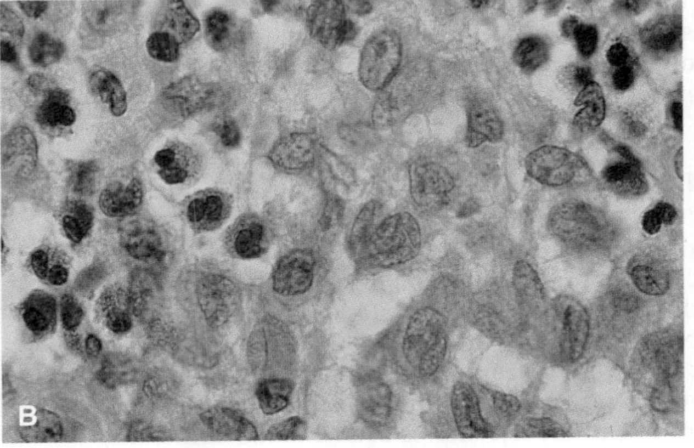

FIGURE 12-68. Langerhans cell histiocytosis. A. The interstitial nodular infiltrate has a stellate shape, with extension of the cells into the adjacent alveolar septa. **B.** Higher-power view shows Langerhans cells with moderate amount of eosinophilic cytoplasm and prominently grooved nuclei. Eosinophils are present.

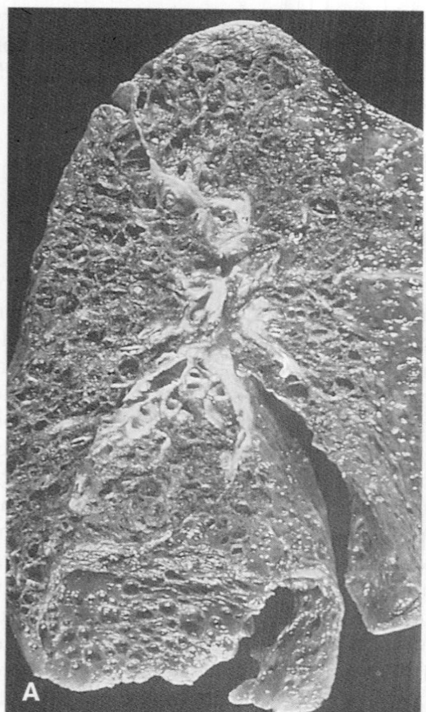

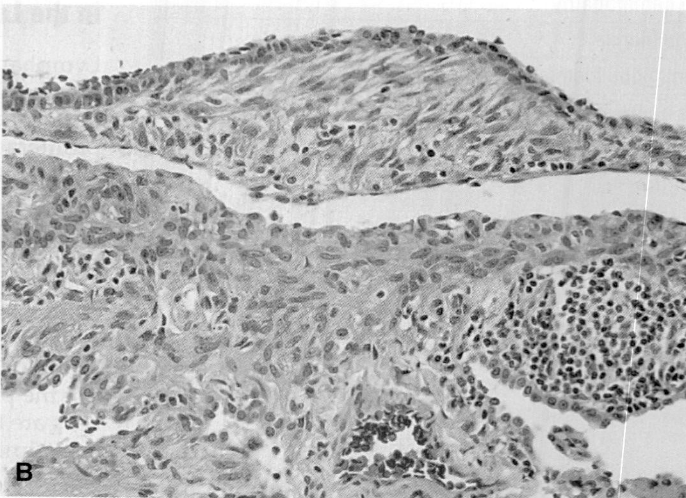

FIGURE 12-69. Lymphangioleiomyomatosis. A. The cut surface of the lung displays extensive cystic change, which resembles emphysema. **B.** An abnormal cystic space is lined by smooth muscle bundles in which the myocytes are haphazardly arranged.

specifically identifies LAM cells but not other lung smooth muscle cells. LAM cells usually express estrogen or progesterone receptors.

CLINICAL FEATURES: Patients with LAM have shortness of breath, spontaneous pneumothorax, hemoptysis, cough and chylous effusions. In early stages, the chest radiograph may be normal, but may show a diffuse interstitial reticular or cystic pattern as the disease progresses. Pleural effusions, marked hyperinflation of the lungs and pneumothorax may ensue. Pulmonary function tests show markedly increased total lung capacity, decreased diffusing capacity and obstructive or restrictive features. Some patients have an indolent clinical course, but many die of progressive respiratory failure. Hormonal ablation through oophorectomy, as well as antiestrogen (tamoxifen) and progesterone therapy, have shown some promise.

Lung Transplantation

Patients who undergo lung transplantation are prone to acute and chronic rejection and infection. The histology of acute rejection includes perivascular infiltrates of small round lymphocytes, plasmacytoid lymphocytes, macrophages and eosinophils. In severe cases the inflammation may involve adjacent alveoli, and hyaline membranes may be seen. The major pattern of chronic rejection is bronchiolitis obliterans, characterized by bronchiolar inflammation and varying degrees of fibrosis. The latter can take the form of polypoid plugs of intraluminal granulation tissue or concentric mural fibrosis, with the pattern of constrictive bronchiolitis (Fig. 12-70).

Bronchiectasis is common in long-term survivors of lung transplants, which may reflect poor perfusion of the airways, denervation and recurrent airway infection.

Opportunistic infections, including bacteria, fungi, viruses and *Pneumocystis,* are common in transplant patients. The most common fungal pneumonias are due to *Candida* and *Aspergillus* spp. Cytomegalovirus is the most common cause of viral pneumonia. Of lung transplant patients who survive more than 30 days, 3% to 8% develop **lymphoproliferative disorders,** owing to uncontrolled proliferation of Epstein-Barr

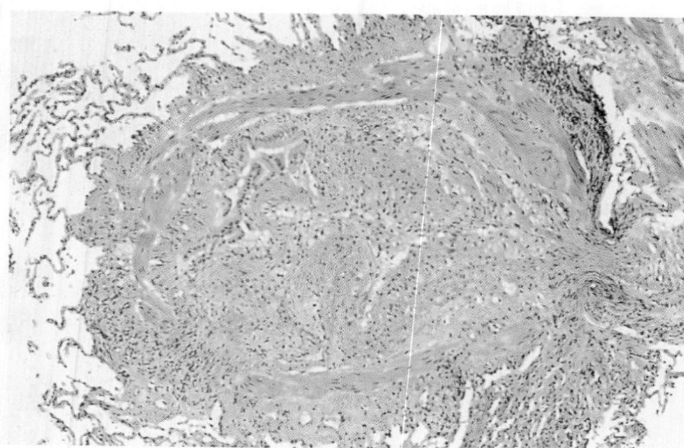

FIGURE 12-70. Obliterative bronchiolitis, chronic rejection in lung transplantation. The lumen of this bronchiole is virtually entirely obliterated by concentric fibrosis.

virus (EBV)-infected B lymphocytes as a result of immunosuppression by cyclosporine.

Vasculitis and Granulomatosis

Many pulmonary conditions result in vasculitis, most of which are secondary to other inflammatory processes, such as necrotizing granulomatous infections. Only a few primary idiopathic vasculitis syndromes affect the lung, the most important of which are Wegener granulomatosis (WG), Churg-Strauss granulomatosis and necrotizing sarcoid granulomatosis.

Wegener Granulomatosis Affects the Respiratory Tract and Kidneys

WG is a disease of unknown cause characterized by aseptic, necrotizing, granulomatous inflammation and vasculitis of small and medium-sized vessels. It chiefly affects the upper and lower respiratory tracts and the kidneys (see Chapter 10), although many cases also involve the eyes, joints, skin and peripheral nerves. WG glomerulonephritis is discussed in Chapter 16, and the upper respiratory tract lesions are described in Chapter 25. Here, we deal only with pulmonary manifestations of WG.

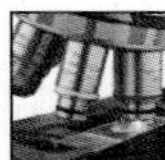

PATHOLOGY: In the lung WG is characterized by necrotizing granulomatous inflammation, parenchymal necrosis and vasculitis. In most cases of pulmonary WG, multiple bilateral nodules, averaging 2 to 3 cm in diameter, are seen. The nodules have irregular edges, tan-brown or hemorrhagic cut surfaces and frequent central cavitation.

Nodules of parenchymal consolidation show (1) tissue necrosis; (2) granulomatous inflammation with a mixed inflammatory infiltrate of lymphocytes, plasma cells, neutrophils, eosinophils, macrophages and giant cells; and (3) fibrosis. Necrosis may feature neutrophilic microabscesses or large basophilic zones of "geographical" necrosis with irregular serpiginous borders (Fig. 12-71A). Patterns of WG granulomas include palisading macrophages along the border of the large necrotic zones, loosely clustered multinucleated giant cells and scattered giant cells. Vasculitis may affect arteries (Fig. 12-71B), veins or capillaries, and may show acute, chronic or granulomatous inflammation. Organizing pneumonia is common at the edges of the nodules of inflammatory consolidation. The lungs often show acute or chronic alveolar hemorrhage. "Neutrophilic capillaritis," with neutrophils in alveolar walls, is often present.

CLINICAL FEATURES: WG mostly affects the head and neck, then the lung, kidney and eye. Respiratory manifestations include cough, hemoptysis and pleuritis. Chest radiographs often show multiple intrapulmonary nodules, although single nodules may also be seen. Head and neck manifestations consist of sinusitis, nasal disease, otitis media, hearing loss, subglottic stenosis, ear pain, cough and oral lesions. Systemic symptoms include arthralgias, fever, skin lesions, weight loss, peripheral neuropathy, central nervous system abnormalities and pericarditis.

Diffuse pulmonary hemorrhage, an important complication of WG, is a fulminant life-threatening crisis with severe respiratory failure. It is usually accompanied by acute renal failure.

It is currently thought that ANCAs are responsible for the inflammation in WG. Serum ANCA is a useful marker for WG and other vasculitis syndromes. This test yields two major immunofluorescence patterns: cytoplasmic or classical (C-ANCA) and perinuclear (P-ANCA). C-ANCAs reacting with proteinase 3 occur in more than 85% of patients with active generalized WG. Most P-ANCAs are specific for myeloperoxidase and are seen with idiopathic necrotizing and crescentic glomerulonephritis, polyarteritis nodosa or Churg-Strauss syndrome.

Most patients with WG are treated effectively with corticosteroids and cyclophosphamide, and 5-year survival is now almost 90%. Some patients respond to trimethoprim-sulfamethoxazole, suggesting a possible bacterial infection. Because of Dr. Wegener's close association with the genocidal machinery of the Nazi regime, it has been suggested that the disease be termed "ANCA-associated granulomatous vasculitis."

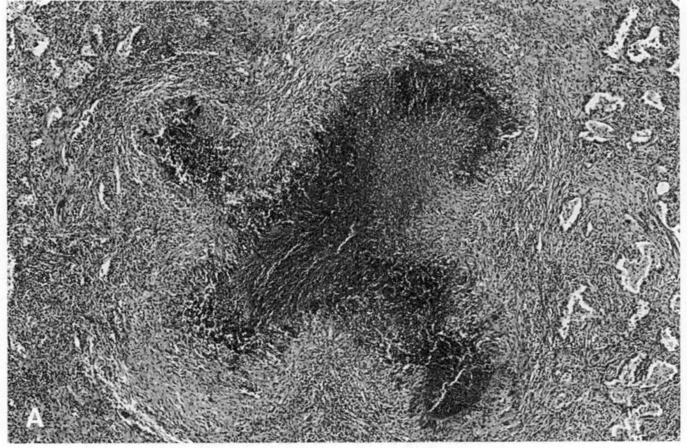

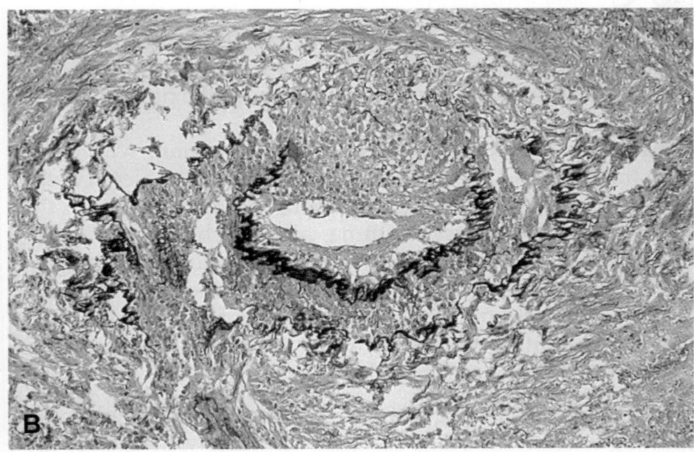

FIGURE 12-71. Wegener granulomatosis. A. This large area of necrosis has a "geographical" pattern with serpiginous borders and a basophilic center. **B.** Vasculitis in this artery is characterized by a focal, eccentric, transmural chronic inflammatory infiltrate that destroys the inner and outer elastic laminae (elastic stain).

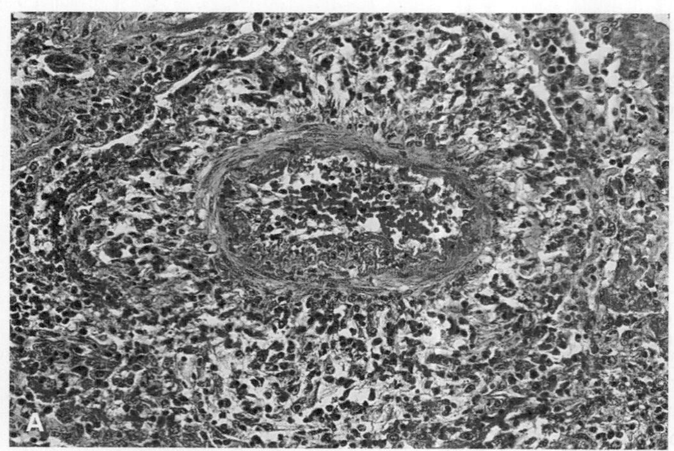
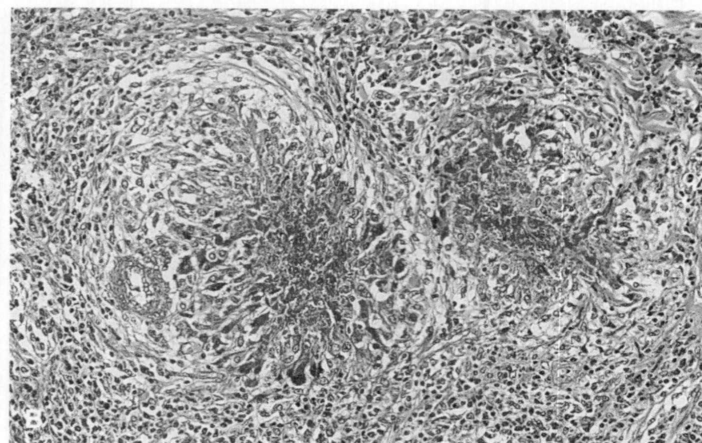

FIGURE 12-72. Churg-Strauss syndrome. A. An artery shows severe vasculitis consisting of a dense infiltrate of chronic inflammatory cells and eosinophils. **B.** A necrotic ("allergic") granuloma has a central eosinophilic area of necrosis surrounded by palisading macrophages and giant cells.

Churg-Strauss Syndrome (Allergic Angiitis and Granulomatosis) Is a Disorder of Unknown Etiology, Defined by Asthma, Eosinophilia and Vasculitis

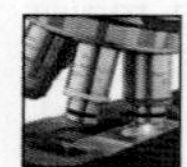

PATHOLOGY: The lungs of patients with Churg-Strauss syndrome show changes of asthmatic bronchitis or bronchiolitis (see above discussion of asthma), including eosinophilic pneumonia, vasculitis (Fig. 12-72A), parenchymal necrosis (Fig. 12-72B) and granulomatous inflammation. Infiltrates of eosinophils may be seen in any anatomic compartment of the lung. Involvement of blood vessel walls causes vasculitis and damage to airway walls and results in bronchitis or bronchiolitis. The vasculitis includes diverse inflammatory cells: eosinophils, lymphocytes, plasma cells, macrophages, giant cells and neutrophils (Fig. 12-72A). Necrotic foci have eosinophilic centers owing to accumulation of dead eosinophils (Fig. 12-72B).

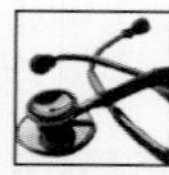

CLINICAL FEATURES: Churg-Strauss syndrome has three clinical phases.

- **Prodrome:** Patients have one or more of the following: allergic rhinitis, asthma, peripheral eosinophilia and eosinophilic infiltrative disease (eosinophilic pneumonia or eosinophilic enteritis).
- **Systemic vasculitic phase:** Extrapulmonary vasculitic manifestations are present, such as cutaneous leukocytoclastic vasculitis or peripheral neuropathy.
- **Postvasculitic phase:** Asthma, allergic rhinitis and complications of neuropathy and hypertension may persist. Cardiovascular manifestations are common and include pericarditis, hypertension and cardiac failure. Renal disease and sinus involvement are usually less severe than those in WG.

The cause of Churg-Strauss syndrome remains obscure, although an autoimmune mechanism is likely, in view of the presence of hypergammaglobulinemia, increased IgE, rheumatoid factor and ANCA.

Patients with Churg-Strauss syndrome usually are positive for P-ANCA in the vasculitic phase. Most patients respond to corticosteroid therapy, but cyclophosphamide may be needed in severe cases. With treatment the 5-year survival is 60%.

Necrotizing Sarcoid Granulomatosis Shows Large Zones of Necrosis and Vasculitis

Necrotizing sarcoid granulomatosis is a rare condition featuring nodular confluent sarcoidal granulomas (Fig. 12-73). This is not a systemic vasculitis, but is usually limited to the lung. Giant cells and necrotizing granulomas (Fig. 12-73B) are seen, as is chronic inflammation with lymphocytes and plasma cells. Most patients are asymptomatic, and chest radiographs typically show multiple, well-circumscribed, pulmonary nodules. Extrapulmonary disease is uncommon, and localized lesions may be treated effectively by surgical removal. Corticosteroids are usually effective for patients with multiple lesions. The prognosis is excellent.

Pulmonary Hypertension

In fetal life, pulmonary arterial walls are thick, reflecting high pulmonary arterial pressure. Blood is oxygenated through the placenta, not the lungs. Thus, high fetal pulmonary arterial pressure helps to shunt right ventricular output through the ductus arteriosus into the systemic circulation, effectively bypassing the lungs. After birth, the ductus arteriosus closes and the lungs must oxygenate venous blood. The lungs must thus adapt to accept the entire cardiac output, which demands the high-volume and low-pressure system of the mature lung. By the third day of life, pulmonary arteries dilate, their walls become thin and pulmonary arterial pressure declines.

Elevated pulmonary arterial pressure is defined as a mean pressure over 25 mm Hg at rest. Increased pulmonary blood flow or vascular resistance may lead to higher pulmonary arterial pressure. Whatever the cause, increased pulmonary artery pressure alters pulmonary artery histology (Fig. 12-74). The Heath and Edwards grading system was devised to

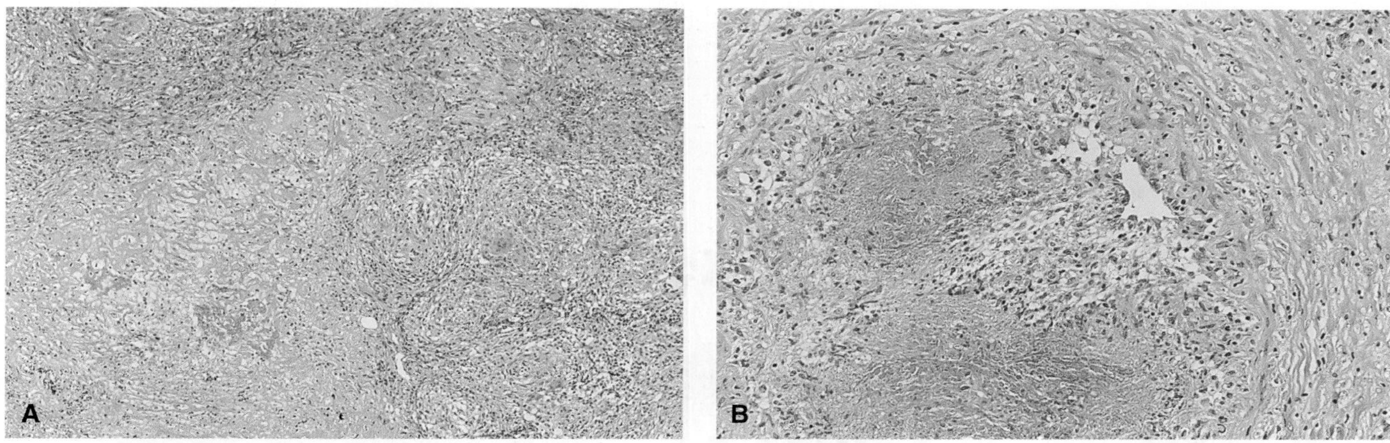

FIGURE 12-73. Necrotizing sarcoid granulomatosis. A. A large area of necrosis is surrounded by confluent sarcoidal granulomas. **B.** The vasculitis consists of a necrotizing granuloma in the wall of an artery.

determine if the arterial changes of pulmonary hypertension could be reversed with corrective cardiac surgery. Grades 1, 2, and 3 are generally reversible; grades 4 and above are generally not.

- **Grade 1:** Medial hypertrophy of muscular pulmonary arteries and appearance of smooth muscle in pulmonary arterioles.
- **Grade 2:** Intimal proliferation with increasing medial hypertrophy.
- **Grade 3:** Intimal fibrosis of muscular pulmonary arteries and arterioles, which may be occlusive (Fig. 12-75A).
- **Grade 4:** Plexiform lesions, dilation and thinning of pulmonary arteries. These nodular lesions are composed of irregular interlacing blood channels and further obstruct pulmonary blood flow (Fig. 12-75B).
- **Grade 5:** Plexiform lesions in combination with dilation or angiomatoid lesions. Rupture of dilated thin walled vessel, with parenchymal hemorrhage and hemosiderosis, is also present.
- **Grade 6:** Fibrinoid necrosis of arteries and arterioles.

Even mild atherosclerosis of the pulmonary vasculature is uncommon if pulmonary arterial pressure is normal. However, with all grades of pulmonary hypertension, atherosclerosis is seen in the largest pulmonary arteries. Increased pressure in the lesser circulation leads to hypertrophy of the right ventricle **(cor pulmonale).**

Pulmonary Hypertension May Be Precapillary or Postcapillary in Origin

The primary source of increased flow or resistance, whether proximal or distal to the pulmonary capillary bed, may be used to understand the pathophysiology of pulmonary hypertension. Precapillary hypertension includes left-to-right cardiac shunts, primary pulmonary hypertension, thromboembolic pulmonary hypertension and hypertension due to fibrotic lung disease and hypoxia. Postcapillary hypertension includes pulmonary veno-occlusive disease and hypertension secondary to left-sided cardiac disorders, such as mitral stenosis and aortic coarctation.

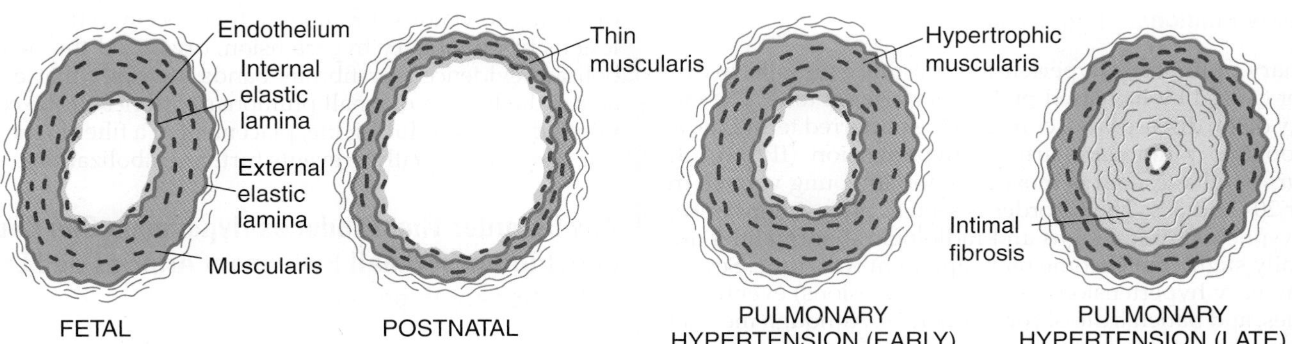

FIGURE 12-74. Histopathology of pulmonary hypertension. In late gestation, the pulmonary arteries have thick walls. After birth, the vessels dilate, and the walls become thin. Mild pulmonary hypertension is characterized by thickening of the media. As pulmonary hypertension becomes more severe, there is extensive intimal fibrosis and muscle thickening.

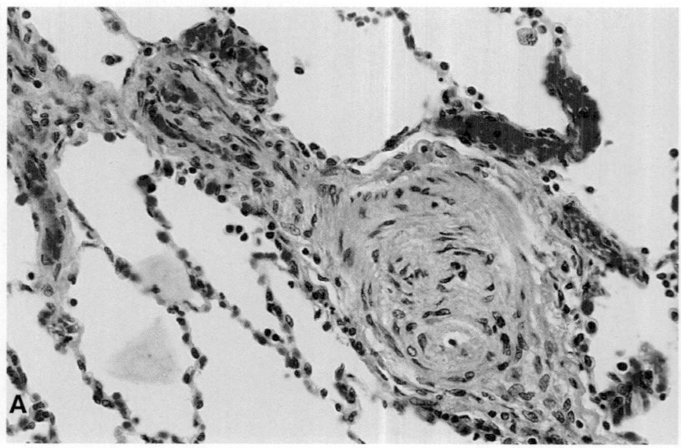

FIGURE 12-75. Pulmonary arterial hypertension. A. A small pulmonary artery is virtually occluded by concentric intimal fibrosis and thickening of the media. **B.** A plexiform lesion (*arrow*) is characterized by a glomeruloid proliferation of thin-walled vessels adjacent to a parent artery, which shows marked hypertensive changes of intimal fibrosis and medial thickening (*curved arrows*).

Left-to-Right Shunts

Shunts from the systemic to the pulmonary circuit increase blood flow to the lungs. Most cases represent congenital left-to-right shunts (see Chapter 11). At birth, the pulmonary artery and the aorta have about the same number of elastic lamellae in their media. Normally, elastic lamellae in the pulmonary artery are lost after birth, but if pulmonary hypertension is present, the fetal pattern of elastic lamellation persists.

Primary Pulmonary Hypertension

Primary pulmonary hypertension is a rare precapillary disorder caused by increased pulmonary arterial tone. The etiology of the disease is obscure, and the preferred term is now "idiopathic pulmonary arterial hypertension (IPAH)." It occurs at all ages, but is most common in young women in their 20s and 30s. The disorder is seen as an insidious onset of dyspnea. Physical signs and radiologic abnormalities are initially slight, but become more apparent with time. Severe pulmonary hypertension (i.e., plexiform lesions) eventually ensues, and patients die of cor pulmonale. Although medical treatment is mostly ineffective, recent use of prostacyclin analogues, endothelin receptor antagonists and phosphodiesterase-5 inhibitors have led to a 5-year survival of about 30%. Heart–lung transplantation is often indicated. Some patients with collagen vascular diseases and certain drug reactions (such as those reported with the diet drug "phen-phen"), have identical clinical and morphologic findings.

Recurrent Pulmonary Emboli

Multiple thromboemboli in the smaller pulmonary vessels often result from asymptomatic, episodic showers of small emboli from the periphery. They gradually restrict the pulmonary circulation and lead to pulmonary hypertension. Some patients have evidence of peripheral venous thrombosis, usually in the leg veins, or a history of circumstances predisposing to venous thrombosis. In addition to the vascular lesions of pulmonary hypertension, organized thromboemboli are evidenced by fibrous bands ("webs") that extend across the lumina of small pulmonary arteries. If the condition is diagnosed during life, placement of a filter in the inferior vena cava usually prevents further embolization.

Any Disorder That Produces Hypoxemia Can Cause Constriction of Small Pulmonary Arteries and Lead to Pulmonary Hypertension

Predisposing conditions include chronic airflow obstruction (chronic bronchitis), interstitial lung disease and living at high altitude. Severe kyphoscoliosis or extreme obesity **(Pickwickian syndrome)** may impede ventilation and lead to hypoxemia and pulmonary hypertension.

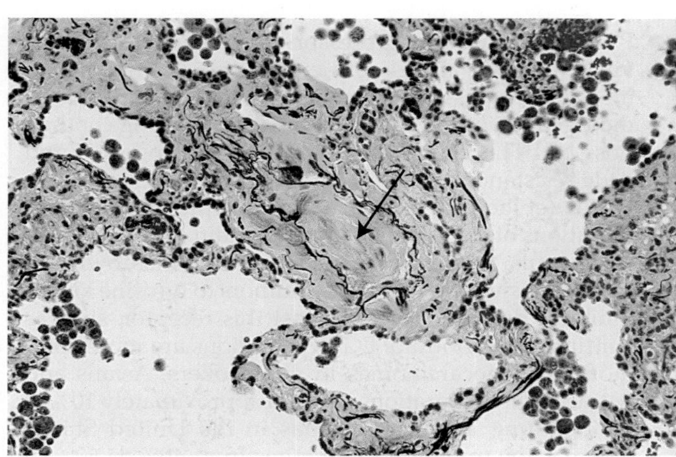

FIGURE 12-76. Veno-occlusive disease of the lung. This pulmonary vein is occluded by intimal fibrosis (*arrow*; Movat stain).

Left Ventricular Failure Increases Pulmonary Venous Pressure and Secondarily Pulmonary Arterial Pressure

Both mitral stenosis and insufficiency produce severe venous hypertension and significant pulmonary artery hypertension. In such cases, the lungs exhibit lesions of both pulmonary hypertension and chronic passive congestion (see Chapter 7).

Pulmonary Veno-Occlusive Disease Involves Fibrotic Obstruction of Small Veins

Pulmonary veno-occlusive disease is a rare condition of uncertain etiology in which the small pulmonary veins and venules are occluded by loose, sparsely cellular, intimal fibrosis (Fig. 12-76). Some large veins may also be involved, and in half of cases, similar but less severe lesions involve the pulmonary arteries. Canalization of the obstructive lesions suggests that they represent organized thrombi, possibly reflecting endothelial damage. The disease has been reported to follow viral infections, exposure to toxic agents and chemotherapy. More than half of cases occur in the first three decades of life. In children, girls and boys are affected similarly, but after age 15, it is more common in men.

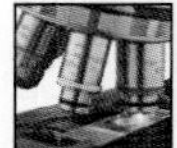

PATHOLOGY: Pulmonary veno-occlusive disease produces severe pulmonary hypertension. Grossly, the lung shows brown induration and atherosclerosis of large pulmonary arteries. Microscopically, small veins and venules are partly or totally occluded and larger veins show eccentric intimal thickening. Moderate alveolar wall fibrosis and foci of hemosiderosis are common. Pulmonary arteries show recent thrombi and lesions of severe pulmonary hypertension.

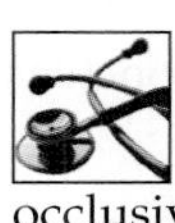

CLINICAL FEATURES: The clinical presentation of progressive dyspnea is similar to that of primary pulmonary hypertension, but pulmonary veno-occlusive disease has a more fulminant course. Radiologic examination reveals scattered infiltrates in the lung, representing hemorrhage and hemosiderosis, which increase as the disease progresses. There is no effective therapy, and heart–lung transplantation should be contemplated.

Pulmonary Hamartoma

Although the term *hamartoma* implies a malformation, hamartomas are true tumors. They typically occur in adults, with a peak in the sixth decade of life, and account for some 10% of "coin" lesions discovered incidentally on chest radiographs. A characteristic ("popcorn") pattern of calcification is often seen by x-ray.

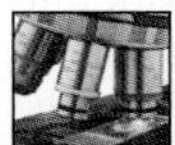

PATHOLOGY: Grossly, pulmonary hamartomas are solitary, circumscribed, lobulated masses, averaging 2 cm in diameter, with a white or gray, cartilaginous cut surface (Fig. 12-77A). The tumor consists of elements usually present in the lung: cartilage, fibromyxoid connective tissue, fat, bone and occasionally smooth muscle (Fig. 12-77B). These are interspersed with clefts lined by respiratory epithelium. Hamartomas are benign and well circumscribed and shell out from the surrounding lung parenchyma. Most are seen in the periphery, but 10% occur in a central endobronchial

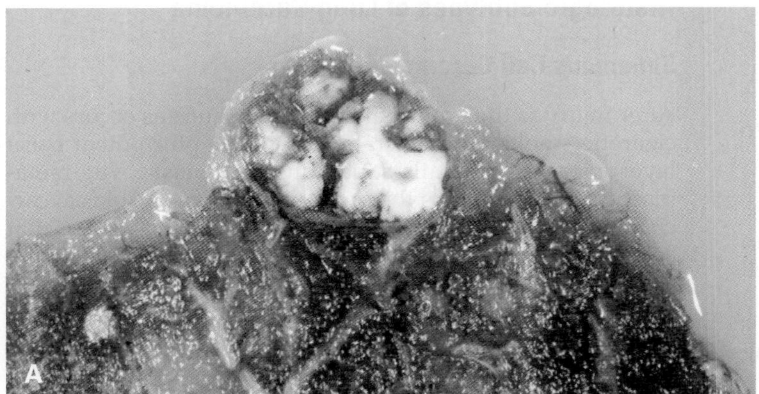

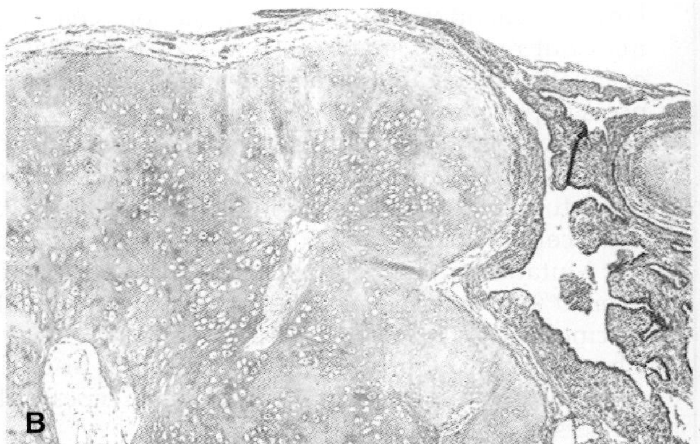

FIGURE 12-77. Pulmonary hamartoma. A. The cut surface of a sharply circumscribed, peripheral pulmonary nodule shows a lobulated structure. **B.** A photomicrograph reveals nodules of hyaline cartilage separated by connective tissue lined by respiratory epithelium.

Table 12-6
Distribution of Non–Small Cell Lung Carcinoma by Subtypes

Subtype	Smokers	Never-Smokers
Squamous cell carcinoma	42	33
Adenocarcinoma	39	35
Bronchioloalveolar carcinoma	4	10
Carcinoid	7	16
Other	8	6

location. The latter may cause symptoms due to bronchial obstruction.

Carcinoma of the Lung

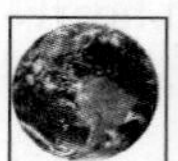

EPIDEMIOLOGY: Regarded as a rare tumor as late as 1945, lung cancer is currently the most common cause of cancer mortality worldwide, including the United States, where it is the leading cause of cancer death in both men and women. Some 85% to 90% of lung cancers occur in cigarette smokers (see Chapter 8), but, conversely, among smokers, the lifetime risk of developing lung cancer is about 12% to 17%. Smokers are at risk for both non–small cell (NSCLC) and small cell (SCLC) lung carcinoma, whereas the majority of never-smokers who develop lung cancer usually have an adenocarcinoma. In general, some 80% of lung cancers are NSCLC and about 17% are SCLC. The distribution of subtypes of NSCLC is shown in Table 12-6. The peak age for lung cancer is between 60 and 70 years, with most patients between 50 and 80 years old. The former male predominance is decreasing as smoking increases among women.

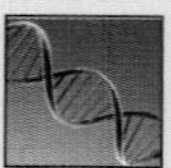

MOLECULAR PATHOGENESIS: No simple mutation is responsible for the development of lung cancer, but a number are common and may present opportunities for targeted chemotherapy.

- **K-*ras*:** Mutations in this oncogene, particularly codons 12 and 13, are seen in 25% of adenocarcinomas, 20% of large cell carcinomas and 5% of squamous cell carcinomas, but rarely in small cell tumors. These mutations correlate with cigarette smoking and with a poor prognosis in patients with adenocarcinoma.
- ***Myc:*** Overexpression of this oncogene occurs in 10% to 40% of small cell carcinomas but is rare in other types.
- ***p53:*** Mutations of *p53* are identified in more than 80% of small cell carcinomas and 50% of non–small cell tumors.
- **Rb*:*** Mutations in the retinoblastoma (Rb) gene occur in over 80% of small cell cancers and 25% of non–small cell carcinomas.
- **Chromosome 3 (3p)*:*** Deletions in the short arm of this chromosome are frequently found in all types of lung cancers.
- ***bcl-2:*** This protooncogene, which encodes a protein that inhibits programmed cell death (apoptosis), is expressed in 25% of squamous cell carcinomas and 10% of adenocarcinomas.
- **PTEN:** This tumor suppressor gene regulates cell survival signaling and is deficient by one of a number of mechanisms (loss of heterozygosity, mutation, promoter methylation, etc.) in many non–small cell lung cancers. Loss of PTEN is associated with poor prognosis and drug resistance.
- **EGFR** (epidermal growth factor receptor): Activating mutations of the tyrosine kinase domain of this gene are of particular interest in lung adenocarcinomas, owing to the responsiveness of mutated tumors to tyrosine kinase inhibitor drugs targeted against this receptor, such as gefitinib and erlotinib. EGFR mutations are more common in adenocarcinomas in nonsmokers, Asians and women. These mutations occur in approximately 10% to 15% of lung adenocarcinomas in the United States, whereas the mutation rate ranges from 40% to 60% in East Asian studies.
- **Human papillomavirus (HPV):** Evidence for HPV infection in NSCLC has now been described in many regions, although the statistics are highly variable. The reported frequency in the United States averages 15%, whereas it has been reported to be much higher in East Asia. Interestingly, survivors of HPV-positive cancer of the uterine cervix are at an increased risk of developing NSCLC.

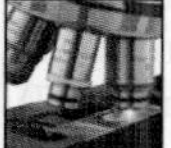

PATHOLOGY: Squamous cell carcinoma, adenocarcinoma, large cell carcinoma and small cell carcinoma are the major forms of lung cancer. Although the term **bronchogenic** carcinoma was once used, about one fourth of primary lung cancers do not have an obvious bronchial origin.

Histologic subtyping of lung cancer is based on the best-differentiated component, unless an area of small cell carcinoma is present. However, the degree of differentiation is graded according to the worst-differentiated component. If a tumor is mostly poorly differentiated large cells but has foci of squamous cells or adenocarcinoma, it is classified as a poorly differentiated squamous cell carcinoma or adenocarcinoma, respectively. Any cancer with a component of small cell carcinoma is regarded as a subtype of that tumor (see below).

Histologic Subtypes of Lung Carcinoma

Squamous Cell Carcinoma

After injury to the bronchial epithelium, such as occurs with cigarette smoking, regeneration from the pluripotent basal layer commonly entails squamous metaplasia. The metaplastic mucosa follows the same sequence of dysplasia, carcinoma in situ and invasive tumor as is observed in sites that are normally lined by squamous epithelium, such as the cervix or skin.

Most squamous cell carcinomas arise in the central portion of the lung from major or segmental bronchi, although 10% originate in the periphery. They tend to be firm, gray-white, 3- to 5-cm ulcerated lesions that extend through the bronchial wall into the adjacent lung parenchyma (Fig. 12-78A). Central cavitation is frequent. On occasion, a central squamous carcinoma occurs as an endobronchial tumor.

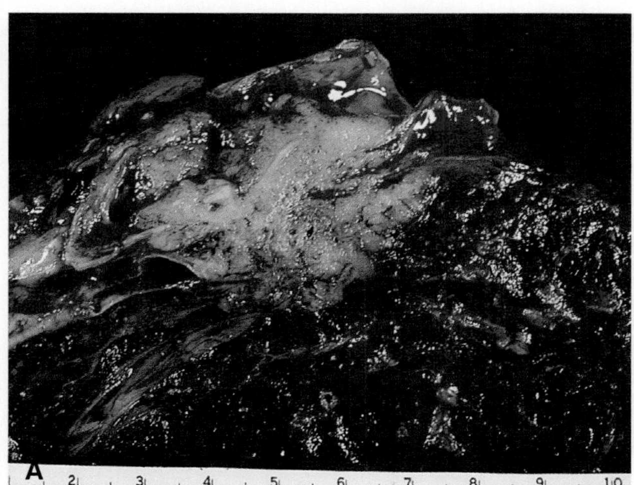

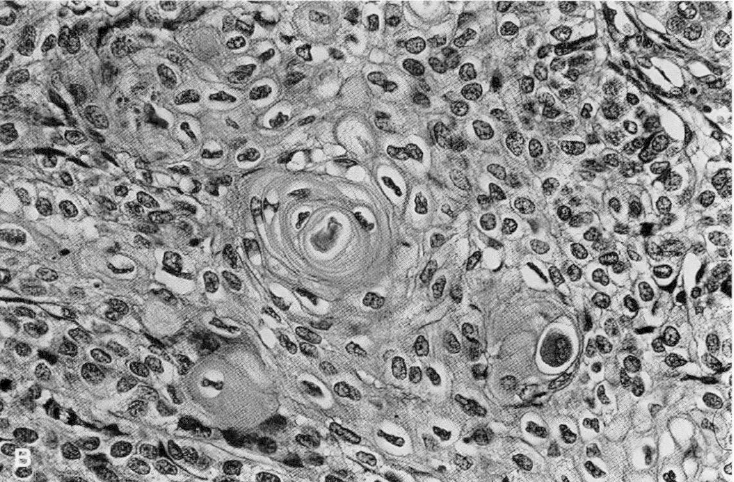

FIGURE 12-78. Squamous cell carcinoma of the lung. A. The tumor grows within the lumen of a bronchus and invades the adjacent intrapulmonary lymph node. **B.** A photomicrograph shows well-differentiated squamous cell carcinoma with a keratin pearl composed of cells with brightly eosinophilic cytoplasm.

Microscopically, squamous cell carcinomas are highly variable. Well-differentiated tumors have keratin "pearls," which are small round nests of brightly eosinophilic aggregates of keratin surrounded by concentric ("onion skin") layers of squamous cells (Fig. 12-78B). Individual cell keratinization also occurs, in which a cell's cytoplasm becomes glassy and intensely eosinophilic. Intercellular bridges are identified in some well-differentiated squamous cancers as slender gaps between adjacent cells, which are traversed by fine strands of cytoplasm. By contrast, some squamous tumors are so poorly differentiated that they lack keratinization and are difficult to distinguish from large cell, small cell or spindle cell carcinomas. Tumor cells may be readily found in the sputum, in which case the diagnosis is made by exfoliative cytology.

Adenocarcinoma

In many countries, including the United States, adenocarcinoma has overtaken squamous cell carcinoma as the most common subtype of lung cancer and is the most common type in women. It tends to arise in the periphery and is often associated with pleural fibrosis and subpleural scars, which can lead to pleural puckering (Fig. 12-79). These cancers were once thought to arise in scars left by old tuberculosis or healed infarcts, but it is now recognized that most of these scars represent a desmoplastic response to the tumor.

Atypical adenomatous hyperplasia (AAH) is recognized as a putative precursor lesion for adenocarcinomas. AAH is a well-demarcated lesion, usually less than 5 mm, with atypical proliferation of epithelial cells along alveolar septa. In a sequence similar to the "adenoma-carcinoma" sequence in colon cancers, lung adenocarcinomas are thought potentially to originate as AAH and progress to bronchioloalveolar carcinomas and then to more aggressive mixed-type adenocarcinomas. The finding of progressive accumulation of mutations as the lesions advance supports this hypothesis. It is currently unclear if all foci of AAH will progress to carcinoma or if all adenocarcinomas arise via this sequence of events.

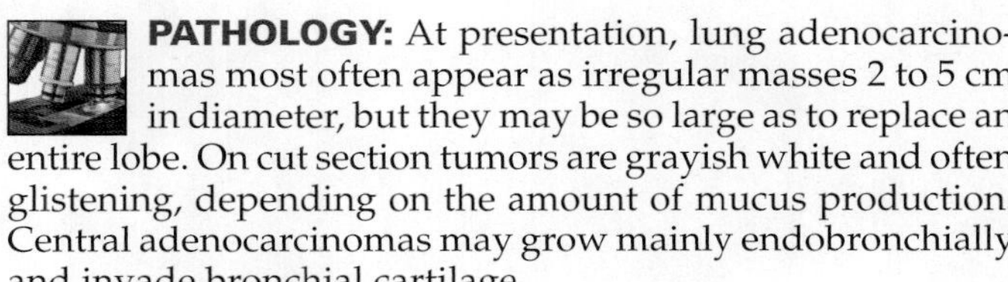

PATHOLOGY: At presentation, lung adenocarcinomas most often appear as irregular masses 2 to 5 cm in diameter, but they may be so large as to replace an entire lobe. On cut section tumors are grayish white and often glistening, depending on the amount of mucus production. Central adenocarcinomas may grow mainly endobronchially and invade bronchial cartilage.

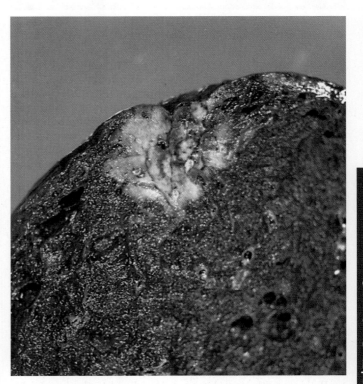

FIGURE 12-79. Adenocarcinoma of the lung. A peripheral tumor of the right upper lobe has an irregular border and a tan or gray cut surface and causes puckering of the overlying pleura.

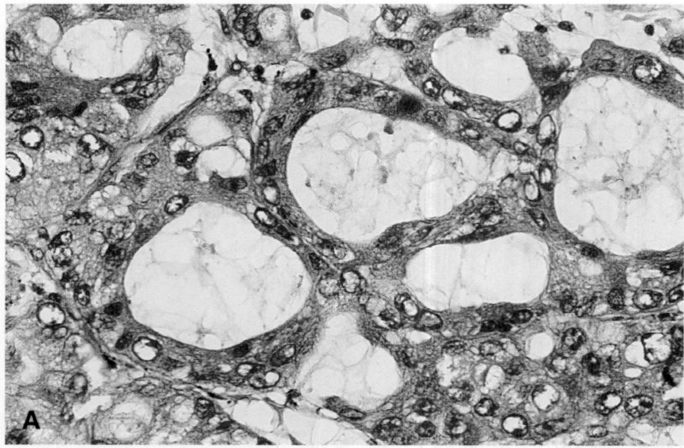

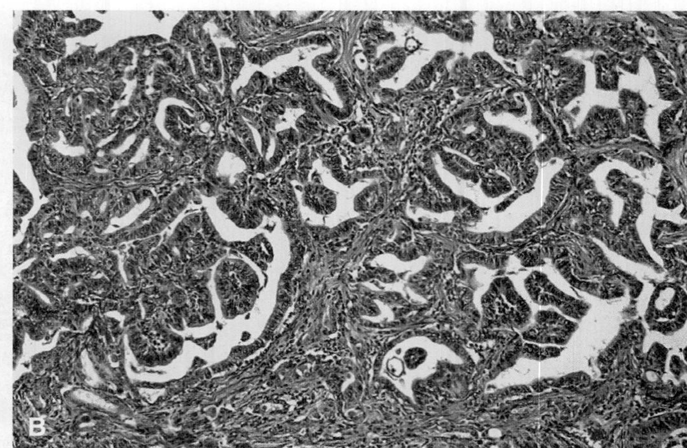

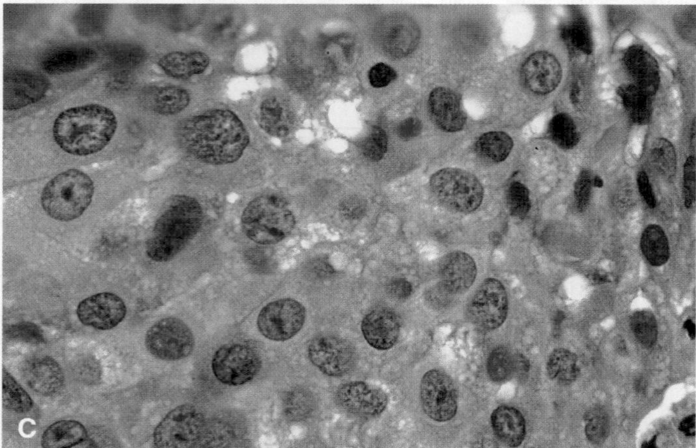

FIGURE 12-80. Adenocarcinoma of the lung. A. The malignant epithelial cells of an acinar adenocarcinoma form glands. **B.** A papillary adenocarcinoma consists of malignant epithelial cells growing along thin fibrovascular cores. **C.** A tumor grows in the pattern of solid adenocarcinoma with mucin formation. Several red intracytoplasmic mucin droplets stain positively with the mucicarmine stain.

There are four major subtypes of adenocarcinoma, as defined by the World Health Organization (Fig. 12-80, and see Figs. 12-81 and 12-82): (1) acinar, (2) papillary, (3) solid with mucus formation and (4) bronchioloalveolar. Although some adenocarcinomas consist purely of one of these patterns, it is common to encounter a mixture of these histologic subtypes. Bronchioloalveolar carcinoma is distinctive enough to merit special attention (see below).

Pulmonary adenocarcinoma may reflect the architecture and cell population of any part of the respiratory mucosa, from the large bronchi to the smallest bronchioles. The neoplastic cells may resemble ciliated or nonciliated columnar epithelial cells, goblet cells, cells of bronchial glands or Clara cells. The most common histologic type of adenocarcinoma features the acinar pattern, which is distinguished by regular glands lined by cuboidal or columnar cells (Fig. 12-80A). Papillary adenocarcinomas exhibit a single cell layer on a core of fibrovascular connective tissue (Fig. 12-80B). Solid adenocarcinomas with mucus formation are poorly differentiated tumors, which are distinguishable from large cell carcinomas by demonstrating mucin with mucicarmine or periodic acid–Schiff (PAS) stains (Fig. 12-80C).

Patients with stage I cancers (localized to the lung) who undergo complete surgical removal have a 5-year survival of 50% to 80%.

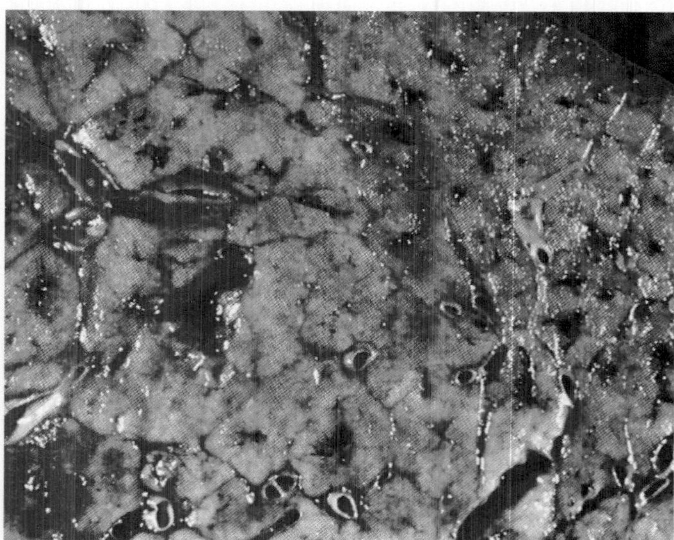

FIGURE 12-81. Bronchioloalveolar carcinoma. The cut surface of the lung is solid, glistening and mucoid, an appearance that reflects a diffusely infiltrating tumor.

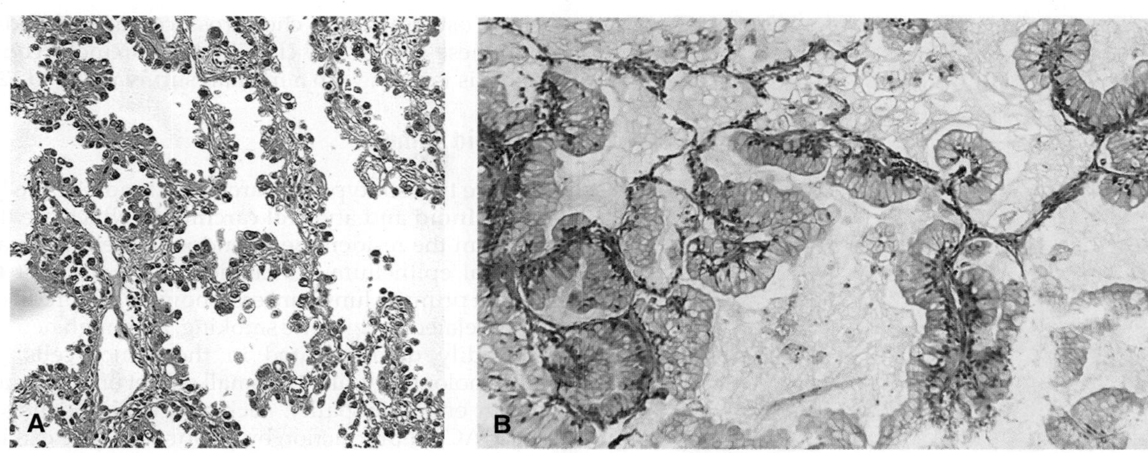

FIGURE 12-82. Bronchioloalveolar carcinoma. A. Nonmucinous bronchioloalveolar carcinomas consist of atypical cuboidal to low columnar cells proliferating along the existing alveolar walls. **B.** Mucinous bronchioloalveolar carcinoma consists of tall columnar cells filled with apical cytoplasmic mucin that grow along the existing alveolar walls.

Bronchioloalveolar Carcinoma

Bronchioloalveolar carcinoma is a distinctive subtype of adenocarcinoma that grows purely along preexisting alveolar walls (lepidic growth) and accounts for 1% to 5% of all lung adenocarcinomas. It has not been definitively linked to smoking. Copious mucin in the sputum (bronchorrhea) is a distinctive sign of bronchioloalveolar carcinoma, particularly the mucinous subtype, but is seen in fewer than 10% of patients.

Grossly, bronchioloalveolar carcinomas may be single peripheral nodules with a "ground glass" appearance radiographically, multiple nodules or a diffuse infiltrate indistinguishable from a pneumonia (Fig. 12-81). Two thirds of tumors are nonmucinous, consisting of Clara cells and type II pneumocytes (Fig. 12-82A); the others are mucinous, featuring goblet cells (Fig. 12-82B). In nonmucinous tumors cuboidal cells grow along the alveolar walls. Mucinous tumors are composed of columnar cells with abundant apical cytoplasm filled with mucus. Particularly for mucinous tumors, the possibility that the tumor is metastatic from another site must be excluded.

Patients with stage I nonmucinous bronchioloalveolar carcinomas have a good prognosis, approaching 100% 5-year survival in many studies. It should be stressed that this improved prognosis applies only to tumors with pure lepidic growth. Lepidic growth is very commonly admixed with other patterns of lung carcinoma (acinar, papillary, solid, etc.), and these tumors do not have the same good prognosis. Similarly, those who have multiple nodules or diffuse lung involvement are more likely to have a poor outcome.

Large Cell Carcinoma

Large cell carcinoma is a diagnosis of exclusion: a poorly differentiated tumor that does not show squamous or glandular differentiation and is not a small cell carcinoma (Fig. 12-83). This tumor type accounts for 10% of all invasive lung tumors. The cells are large and exhibit ample cytoplasm. The nuclei frequently show prominent nucleoli and vesicular chromatin.

Some large cell carcinomas called **large cell neuroendocrine carcinoma** grow similarly to carcinoid tumors, described below (organoid growth, trabecular growth, peripheral palisading of cells, rosette formation) and show immunohistochemical or ultrastructural evidence of neuroendocrine differentiation. Mitotic rates are high and necrosis is frequent. These are aggressive tumors with 5-year survival rates similar to small cell carcinoma.

Small Cell Carcinoma

Small cell carcinoma (formerly "oat cell" carcinoma) is a highly malignant epithelial tumor of the lung with neuroendocrine features. It accounts for 20% of all lung cancers and is strongly associated with cigarette smoking. The male-to-female ratio is 2:1. These tumors grow and metastasize rapidly, and 70% of patients are first seen at advanced stages. Small cell carcinomas are often responsible for paraneoplastic syndromes, including **diabetes insipidus, ectopic adrenocorticotropic hormone (ACTH; corticotropin) syndrome** and **Eaton-Lambert syndrome.**

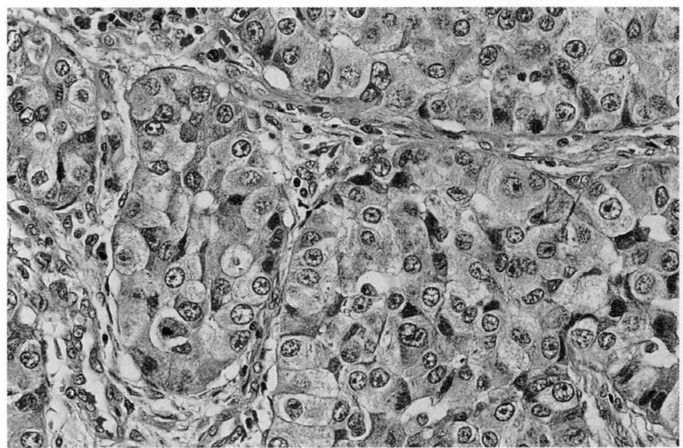

FIGURE 12-83. Large cell carcinoma of the lung. This poorly differentiated tumor is growing in sheets. The tumor cells are large and contain ample cytoplasm and prominent nucleoli.

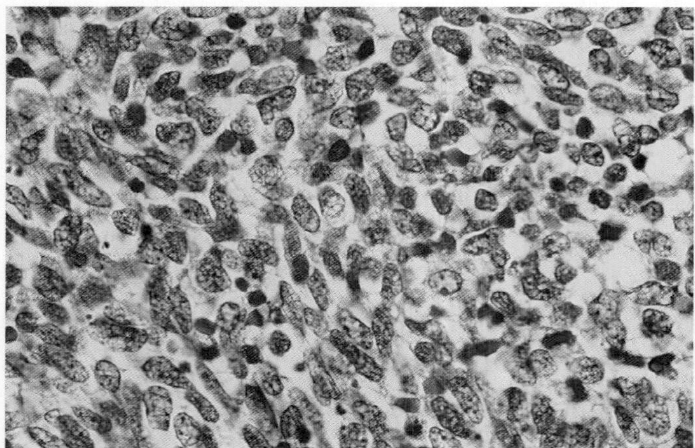

FIGURE 12-84. Small cell carcinoma of the lung. This tumor consists of small oval to spindle-shaped cells with scant cytoplasm, finely granular nuclear chromatin and conspicuous mitoses.

PATHOLOGY: Small cell carcinomas are usually perihilar masses, often with extensive lymph node metastases. On cut section, they are soft and white, often with extensive hemorrhage and necrosis. The tumor typically spreads along bronchi in a submucosal and circumferential fashion.

Histologically, small cell carcinomas consist of sheets of small, round, oval or spindle-shaped cells with scant cytoplasm. Their nuclei are distinctive, with finely granular nuclear chromatin and absent or inconspicuous nucleoli (Fig. 12-84). By immunohistochemistry, most tumors express neuroendocrine markers such as CD56, chromogranin or synaptophysin. Mitotic rates are very high, averaging 60 to 70 mitoses per 2-mm^2 area of tumor (10 high-power fields). Necrosis is frequent and extensive. Although there is no absolute measure for the size of the tumor cells, a useful rule of thumb in small cell carcinoma is the diameter of three small resting lymphocytes. Rarely, a small cell carcinoma may be combined with a "non–small cell carcinoma" such as adenocarcinoma or squamous cell carcinoma. In such cases, the behavior and clinical outcome reflects the small cell component, so they are classified as combined small cell carcinoma with mention of the non–small cell histologic type (i.e., combined small cell carcinoma and adenocarcinoma). Unlike other lung cancers, small cell tumors, at least initially, are very sensitive to chemotherapy, which is the mainstay of treatment for this tumor type.

Lung Carcinomas With Histologic Heterogeneity

Lung carcinomas may contain a combination of histologic subtypes within one tumor: small cell carcinomas may occur in combination with non–small cell carcinomas, or several non–small cell subtypes may also occur in the same tumor. Of lung cancers classified as adenosquamous, 1% to 2% may contain at least 10% of both adenocarcinoma and squamous cell carcinoma.

Sarcomatoid tumors are less than 1% of lung cancers. Most are pleomorphic carcinomas with at least 10% spindle and/or giant cell carcinoma in addition to other non–small cell carcinoma patterns such as adenocarcinoma or squamous cell carcinoma. If true sarcomatous components are present such as osteosarcoma, chondrosarcoma or rhabdomyosarcoma, these tumors are classified as carcinosarcomas. Their prognosis is poor, with a median survival of 9 to 12 months.

Carcinoid Tumors

There are two subtypes of carcinoid tumors of the lung **(typical carcinoid and atypical carcinoid)**, which are thought to arise from the resident neuroendocrine cells normally in the bronchial epithelium. Carcinoid tumors account for 1% to 2% of all primary lung cancers, show no sex predilection and are not related to cigarette smoking. Although neuropeptides are readily demonstrated in the tumor cells, most are endocrinologically silent. A small subset of cases is associated with an endocrinopathy, such as Cushing syndrome with ectopic ACTH production by tumor cells. The carcinoid syndrome (see Chapter 13) occurs in 1% of cases, usually in the setting of hepatic metastases. Nodular neuroendocrine proliferations less than 0.5 cm are called as tumorlets, can be found in the setting of interstitial fibrosis or small airway disorders and usually represent incidental findings of no known clinical significance.

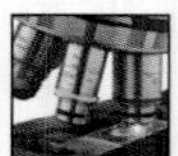

PATHOLOGY: One third of carcinoid tumors are central, one third are peripheral (subpleural) and one third are in the midportion of the lung. Central carcinoid tumors tend to have a large endobronchial component, with fleshy, smooth, polypoid masses protruding into bronchial lumens (Fig. 12-85A). The tumors average 3.0 cm in diameter, but range from 0.5 to 10 cm.

Carcinoid tumors are characterized histologically by an organoid growth pattern and uniform cytologic features: eosinophilic, finely granular cytoplasm and nuclei with finely granular chromatin (Fig. 12-85B). A variety of neuroendocrine patterns may be seen, including trabecular growth, peripheral palisading and rosettes.

Atypical carcinoid tumors differ from typical carcinoids by (1) increased mitoses, with 2 to 10 mitoses per 2 mm^2 of tumor; (2) tumor necrosis (Fig. 12-86); (3) areas of increased cellularity and disorganization of the architecture; and (4) nuclear pleomorphism, hyperchromatism and high nuclear: cytoplasmic ratio.

CLINICAL FEATURES: Carcinoid tumors grow slowly, so half of patients are asymptomatic at presentation. Such tumors are often discovered as a mass in a chest radiograph. If a patient is symptomatic, the most common pulmonary manifestations are hemoptysis, postobstructive pneumonitis and dyspnea. There is a slight female predominance. The mean age at diagnosis is 55 years, but carcinoid tumors can occur at any age. In fact, bronchial carcinoids are the most common lung tumor in childhood. Atypical carcinoid tumors tend to be more aggressive than typical ones. Regional lymph node metastases are seen in 15% of patients with typical carcinoids and 50% of those with atypical carcinoids. Patients with typical carcinoids have an excellent prognosis, with 90% 5-year survival after surgery, compared with 60% for atypical carcinoids.

Rare Pulmonary Tumors

INFLAMMATORY PSEUDOTUMOR/INFLAMMATORY MYOFIBROBLASTIC TUMOR: Inflammatory pseudotumor of the lung is an uncommon lesion that consists of variable

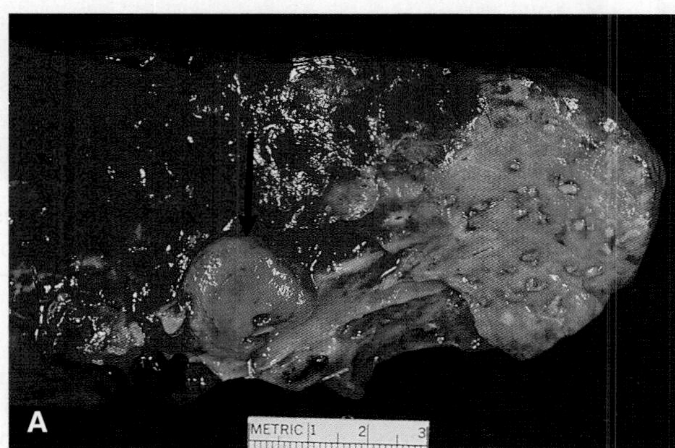

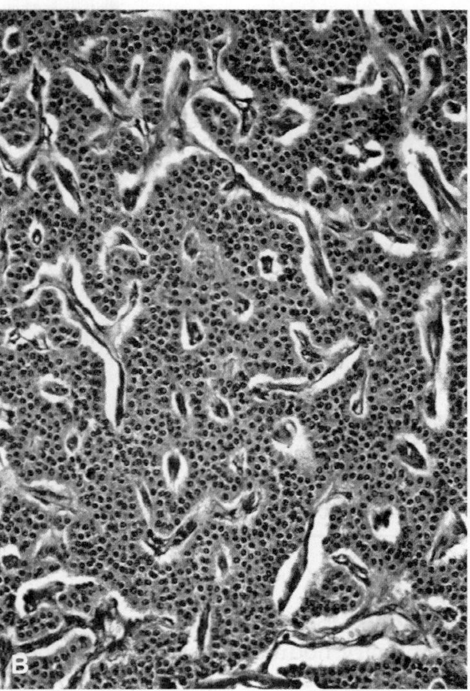

FIGURE 12-85. Carcinoid tumor of the lung. A. A central carcinoid tumor (*arrow*) is circumscribed and protrudes into the lumen of the main bronchus. The compression of the bronchus by the tumor caused the postobstructive pneumonia seen in the distal lung parenchyma (*right*). **B.** A microscopic view shows ribbons of tumor cells embedded in a vascular stroma.

amounts of inflammatory cells, foamy macrophages and fibroblasts. Most of these masses are within the lung, although the pleura may be involved. In 5% of cases, tumors invade structures outside the lung, such as the esophagus, mediastinum, chest wall, diaphragm or pericardium.

Inflammatory pseudotumors encompass a spectrum of lesions with a range of histologic findings as described below; as knowledge expands, some of these lesions may be better classified as other entities. Some of these tumors, which had been regarded as inflammatory, nonneoplastic process, are now known to be inflammatory myofibroblastic tumors, a lesion originally described in the soft tissue. However, demonstrations of mutations of the *ALK* gene suggest that at least some of these represent true neoplasms. Other lesions previously categorized as so-called "plasma cell granuloma" variants of inflammatory pseudotumor may be pulmonary manifestations of immune-related processes such as IgG4-related systemic sclerosing disease.

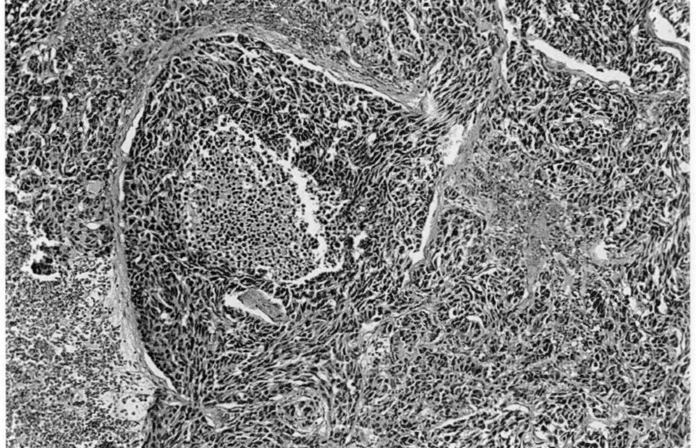

FIGURE 12-86. Atypical carcinoid tumor of the lung. A cellular tumor shows central necrosis and a disorganized architecture.

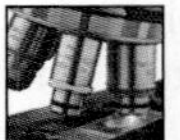

PATHOLOGY: The tumors are solitary circumscribed, with a mean size of 4 cm. Virtually any inflammatory cells may be present, including lymphocytes, plasma cells, macrophages, giant cells, mast cells and eosinophils. Inflammatory pseudotumor causes consolidation of the lung parenchyma and loss of architecture. Two major histologic patterns are fibrohistiocytic (Fig. 12-87) and plasma cell granuloma, depending on the predominant component. In some cases, foamy macrophages impart a xanthomatous pattern.

CLINICAL FEATURES: Most patients are younger than 40 years, although inflammatory pseudotumor can occur at any age and is one of the most common lung tumors of childhood. Half of patients are asymptomatic at presentation. A previous history of a pulmonary infection can be elicited in one third of patients. Most inflammatory pseudotumors are cured by surgical excision, but 5% recur within the chest.

PULMONARY EPITHELIOID HEMANGIOENDOTHELIOMA: Pulmonary epithelioid hemangioendotheliomas are rare low- to intermediate-grade vascular sarcomas. Most patients are young adults and 80% are women. Half of patients are asymptomatic.

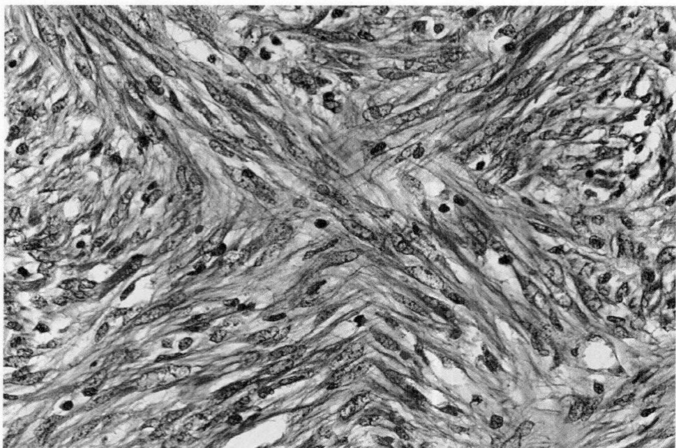

FIGURE 12-87. Inflammatory pseudotumor. A photomicrograph shows intersecting spindle cells and scattered lymphocytes and macrophages.

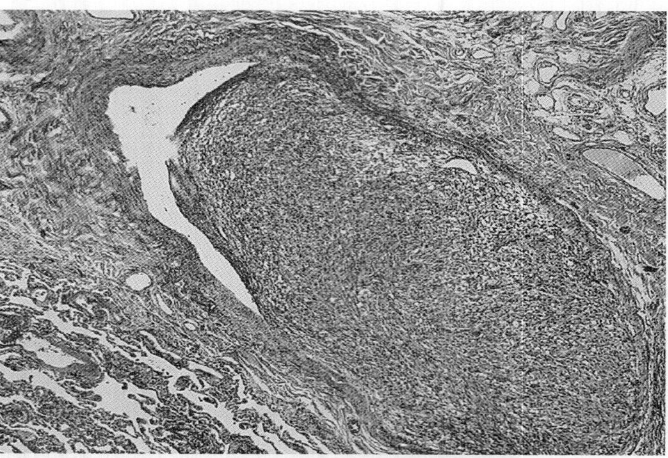

FIGURE 12-89. Pulmonary artery sarcoma. A polypoid mass of malignant spindle cells is spreading within the lumen of this pulmonary artery.

PATHOLOGY: Most patients are first seen with multiple pulmonary nodules. Histologically, the tumor consists of oval-shaped nodules with central, sclerotic, hypocellular zones and cellular peripheral zones. The tumors spread within alveolar spaces (Fig. 12-88). Tumor cells have abundant cytoplasm, with frequent intracytoplasmic vascular lumina, which may contain red blood cells. The tumor matrix is abundant and eosinophilic. The tumors express vascular markers, such as factor VIII. Epithelioid hemangioendotheliomas with a histologic pattern similar to that seen in the lung may occur in the liver, bone and soft tissue. Pulmonary epithelioid hemangioendothelioma has a variable clinical course, with a mean survival of 5 years.

PULMONARY BLASTOMA: This malignant tumor resembles embryonal lung, with a glandular component consisting of poorly differentiated columnar cells arranged in tubules, without mucus secretion. The intervening tumor contains spindle cells that resemble embryonal mesoderm. There is a histologic overlap between pulmonary blastoma and carcinosarcoma, including heterologous elements, and the clinical features are similar.

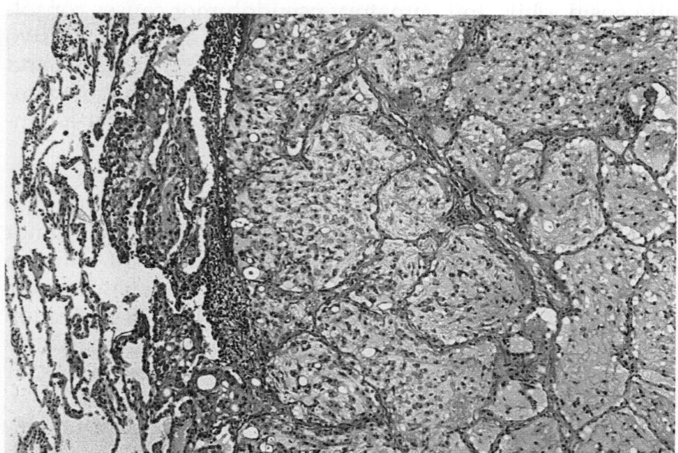

FIGURE 12-88. Epithelioid hemangioendothelioma. A nodule of tumor has spread within alveolar spaces.

Despite its embryonal appearance, pulmonary blastomas occur primarily in adults (median age range, 35 to 43 years), and most patients are cigarette smokers. The prognosis for patients with biphasic tumors is poor and comparable to that for carcinoma of the lung.

MUCOEPIDERMOID CARCINOMA AND ADENOID CYSTIC CARCINOMA: These neoplasms resemble their namesakes in the salivary glands. They are derived from the tracheobronchial mucous glands and are seen in the trachea or proximal bronchus as a luminal mass, often associated with obstructive symptoms. Adenoid cystic carcinomas are difficult to resect locally and often metastasize.

PULMONARY ARTERY SARCOMA: Pulmonary artery sarcoma is a rare tumor of connective tissue (Fig. 12-89), which has a broad histologic spectrum, including fibrosarcoma, leiomyosarcoma, osteosarcoma, rhabdomyosarcoma, angiosarcoma or unclassifiable sarcoma. These tumors are rarely diagnosed during life and may be discovered because of pulmonary hypertension. They often grow in an intraluminal fashion, within proximal arteries, and may extend, wormlike, to peripheral pulmonary artery branches, causing peripheral infarcts.

Pulmonary Lymphomas

All lymphomas, both Hodgkin and non-Hodgkin types, may involve the lung (see also Chapter 20). Most lymphomas involving the lung are metastatic. Primary pulmonary lymphomas are rare, the most common being **extranodal marginal zone B-cell lymphoma.** These tumors are thought to arise from mucosa-associated lymphoid tissue of the lung and are sometimes termed "MALT" lymphomas. They are low-grade tumors, generally with a favorable prognosis.

Diffuse large B-cell lymphoma may also arise as a primary pulmonary lymphoma (see Chapter 20). **Lymphomatoid granulomatosis,** a subtype of diffuse large B-cell lymphoma, is characterized by pulmonary nodular lymphoid infiltrates with frequent central necrosis and vascular permeation (Fig. 12-90). It affects middle-aged people and is more common in immunosuppressed people. The lung is the major location, but kidney, skin and upper respiratory tract may also be involved. The lymphoid infiltrate is angiocentric and angioinvasive, with polymorphous, small to medium-sized lymphocytes,

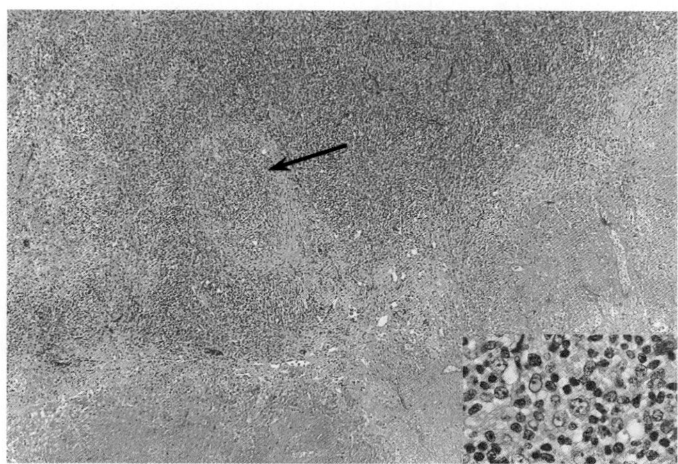

FIGURE 12-90. Lymphomatoid granulomatosis. This extensively necrotic nodular mass consists of a cellular lymphoid infiltrate that penetrates a blood vessel (*arrow*) at the edge of the lesion. *Inset.* The lymphoid infiltrate is composed of a polymorphous population of small, medium-sized and large atypical lymphoid cells.

mainly T cells, admixed with variable numbers of large atypical B cells. The latter typically express EBV, which is thought to drive the proliferation. Lymphomatoid granulomatosis is typically divided into grades depending on the percentage of atypical B cells present. Previously, only the highest grade was considered a "true" lymphoma, the lower grades being considered as less aggressive lesions; however, all grades are now considered as subtypes of diffuse large B-cell lymphoma for treatment purposes. Despite remissions with chemotherapy, half of all patients eventually develop large cell lymphoma. Even with aggressive treatment, the prognosis is poor.

General Features of Lung Cancer

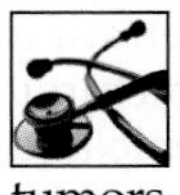

CLINICAL FEATURES: Clinically, squamous cell carcinoma, adenocarcinoma and large cell carcinoma are grouped as "non–small cell carcinoma" because these tumors are all treated similarly, and therapy differs from that used for small cell carcinoma. Historically, non–small cell carcinomas have been treated surgically, if possible, and do not respond consistently to chemotherapy, whereas small cell tumors do respond, at least initially, to chemotherapy. As targeted therapies become more available, chemotherapy is now more effective in treating non–small cell carcinomas. Thus, the distinction between adenocarcinoma and squamous cell carcinoma has become increasingly important, since EGFR mutations are more common in adenocarcinomas than in squamous cell carcinomas, and mutated tumors are more likely to respond to certain agents, such as the EGFR tyrosine kinase inhibitors. Overall 5-year survival for all patients with NSCLC has remained 15% for the past two decades, and is similar for adenocarcinoma and squamous cell carcinoma, with the exception of pure bronchioloalveolar carcinomas as discussed below. Small cell carcinomas have a dismal prognosis with 5% or less 5-year survival. ***Tumor stage remains the single most important predictor of prognosis.*** The staging system for lung carcinoma is primarily based on tumor size, extent and location of involvement, presence of lymph node involvement and presence of distant metastases or malignancy involving the pleural fluid. The staging system for lung cancer is summarized in Table 12-7.

Table 12-7

American Joint Commission on Cancer Lung Cancer Staging System

T1	Tumor <3 cm surrounded by lung or visceral pleura and not involving the mainstem bronchus T1a: <2 cm T1b: 2–3 cm
T2	Tumor >3 cm but ≤7 cm OR tumor with any of the following features: Involves main bronchus, ≥2 cm distal to the carina Invades visceral pleura Associated with atelectasis or obstructive pneumonitis that extends to the hilar region but does not involve the entire lung T2a: >3 cm but ≤5 cm T2b: >5 cm but ≤7 cm
T3	Tumor >7 cm OR a tumor with involvement of any of the following: chest wall (including superior sulcus tumors), diaphragm, mediastinal pleura, pericardium or main stem bronchus 2 cm from carina OR entire lung atelectasis OR separate tumor nodules in the same lobe
T4	Tumor with invasion of mediastinum, heart, great vessels, trachea, esophagus, vertebral body or carina OR separate tumor nodules in a different ipsilateral lobe
N0	No demonstrable metastasis to regional lymph nodes
N1	Ipsilateral hilar or peribronchial nodal involvement
N2	Metastasis to ipsilateral mediastinal or subcarinal lymph nodes
N3	Metastasis to contralateral mediastinal or hilar lymph nodes, ipsilateral or contralateral scalene or supraclavicular lymph nodes
M0	No distant metastasis
M1	Distant metastasis M1a: separate tumor nodule in contralateral lobe or separate pleural nodules or malignant pleural effusion M1b: distant metastasis

Lung Cancer Stage Groupings

Stage Ia	T1	N0	M0
Stage Ib	T2	N0	M0
Stage IIa	T1	N1	M0
Stage IIb	T2	N1	M0
	T3	N0	M0
Stage IIIa	T1–3	N2	M0
	T3	N1	M0
Stage IIIb	Any T	N3	M0
	T3	N2	M0
	T4	Any N	M0
Stage IV	Any T	Any N	M1

Data from Edge SB, Byrd DR, Compton CC, et al., eds. AJCC Cancer Staging Manual. 7th Ed. New York: Springer, 2010.

LOCAL EFFECTS: Lung cancer can produce cough, dyspnea, hemoptysis, chest pain, obstructive pneumonia and pleural effusion. A lung cancer (usually squamous) in the apex of the lung **(Pancoast tumor)** may extend to involve the eighth cervical and first and second thoracic nerves, leading to shoulder pain that radiates down the arm in an ulnar distribution **(Pancoast syndrome).** A Pancoast tumor also may paralyze cervical sympathetic nerves and cause **Horner syndrome** on the affected side with (1) depression of the eyeball (enophthalmos), (2) ptosis of the upper eyelid, (3) constriction of the pupil (miosis) and (4) absence of sweating (anhidrosis).

Most central endobronchial tumors produce symptoms related to bronchial obstruction: persistent cough, hemoptysis and obstructive pneumonia, or atelectasis. Effusions can result from tumor extension into the pleura or pericardium. Lymphangitic spread of the tumor within the lung may interfere with oxygenation. Tumors arising peripherally are more likely to be discovered on routine chest radiographs or after they have become advanced. The latter circumstance features invasion of the chest wall with resulting chest pain, superior vena cava syndrome and nerve entrapment syndromes.

MEDIASTINAL SPREAD: Tumor growth within the mediastinum can cause superior vena cava syndrome (due to tumorous obstruction of this vein) and nerve entrapment syndromes.

METASTASES: Lung carcinomas metastasize most frequently to regional lymph nodes, particularly hilar and mediastinal nodes, and to the brain, bone and liver. Extranodal metastases often involve the adrenal gland, but adrenal insufficiency is uncommon.

PARANEOPLASTIC SYNDROMES: Disorders associated with lung cancer include acanthosis nigricans, dermatomyositis/polymyositis, clubbing of the fingers and myasthenic syndromes, such as Eaton-Lambert syndrome and progressive multifocal encephalopathy. Endocrine syndromes are also seen, for example, Cushing syndrome or the syndrome of inappropriate release of antidiuretic hormone (SIADH) in small cell carcinomas, and hypercalcemia (secretion of a parathormone-like substance) with squamous cell carcinomas. Small cell carcinomas may also be associated with a syndrome of paraneoplastic encephalomyelitis and sensory neuropathy associated with circulating anti-Hu antibodies.

Extrapulmonary Tumors Frequently Metastasize to the Lung

In one third of all fatal cancers, pulmonary metastases are evident at autopsy. In fact, metastatic tumors are the most common lung malignancy. Metastatic tumors in the lung are typically multiple and circumscribed. When large nodules are seen in the lungs radiologically, they are called "cannon ball" metastases (Fig. 12-91). The histologic appearance of most metastases resembles that of the primary tumor. Rarely, metastatic tumors may mimic bronchioloalveolar carcinoma, in which cases the usual primary site is the pancreas or stomach.

In **lymphangitic carcinoma** a metastatic tumor spreads widely through pulmonary lymphatic channels to form a sheath of tumor around the bronchovascular tree and veins. Clinically, patients suffer from cough and shortness of breath and display a diffuse reticulonodular pattern on the chest radiograph. The common primary sites are the breast, stomach, pancreas and colon.

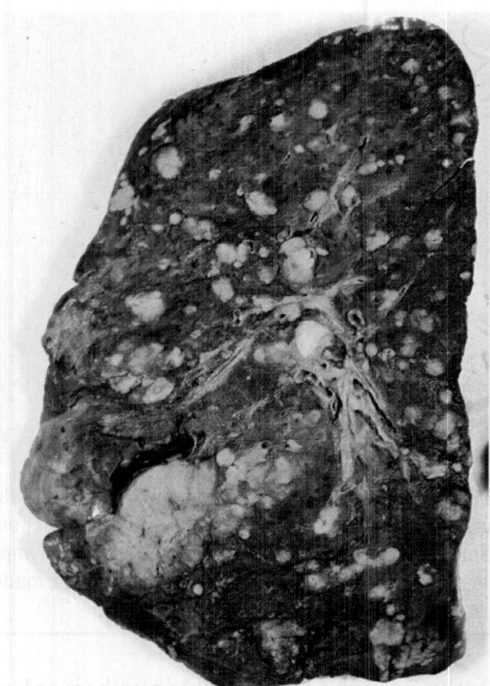

FIGURE 12-91. Metastatic carcinoma of the lung. A section through the lung shows numerous nodules of metastatic carcinoma corresponding to "cannon ball" metastases seen radiologically.

THE PLEURA

Pneumothorax

Pneumothorax is the presence of air in the pleural cavity. It may occur with traumatic perforation of the pleura or may be "spontaneous." Traumatic causes include penetrating wounds of the chest wall (e.g., a stab wound or a rib fracture). Traumatic pneumothorax is most commonly iatrogenic and is seen after aspiration of fluid from the pleura (thoracentesis), pleural or lung biopsies, transbronchial biopsies and positive pressure–assisted ventilation.

Spontaneous pneumothorax is typically seen in young adults. For example, a young man may develop acute chest pain and shortness of breath during vigorous exercise. A chest radiograph shows collapse of the lung on the side of the pain and a large collection of air in the pleural space. The cause is rupture, usually of a subpleural emphysematous bleb. In most cases, spontaneous pneumothorax subsides by itself, but some patients require withdrawal of the air.

Tension pneumothorax refers to unilateral pneumothorax extensive enough to shift the mediastinum to the opposite side, with compression of the opposite lung. The condition may be life-threatening and must be relieved by immediate drainage.

Bronchopleural fistula is a serious condition in which there is free communication between the airway and pleura. It is usually iatrogenic, caused by the interruption of bronchial continuity by biopsy or surgery. It may also be due to extensive infection and necrosis of lung tissue, in which case the infection is more important than the air.

Pleural Effusion

Pleural effusion is accumulation of excess fluid in the pleural cavity. Only a small amount of fluid in the pleural cavity lubricates the space between the lungs and chest wall. Fluid is secreted into the pleural space by the parietal pleura and absorbed by the visceral pleura. These effusions vary from a few milliliters, detectable only radiologically as obliteration of the costophrenic angle, to massive accumulations that shift the mediastinum and the trachea to the opposite side.

HYDROTHORAX: Hydrothorax is an effusion that resembles water and would be regarded as edema elsewhere. It may be due to increased capillary hydrostatic pressure, as occurs in patients with heart failure or in any condition that produces systemic or pulmonary edema. Hydrothorax also occurs in patients with low serum osmotic pressure, as in nephrotic syndrome, cirrhosis of the liver or severe starvation. Other important causes of hydrothorax are collagen vascular diseases (notably systemic lupus erythematosus and rheumatoid arthritis) and asbestos exposure.

PYOTHORAX: A turbid effusion containing many polymorphonuclear leukocytes (pyothorax) results from infections of the pleura. It may occasionally be caused by an external penetrating wound that introduces pyogenic organisms into the pleural space, but more commonly is a complication of bacterial pneumonia that extends to the pleural surface, the classic example of which is pneumococcal pneumonia. Pyothorax is a rare complication of medical procedures involving the pleural cavity.

EMPYEMA: This disorder is a variant of pyothorax in which thick pus accumulates within the pleural cavity, often with loculation and fibrosis.

HEMOTHORAX: Blood in the pleural cavity as a result of trauma or rupture of a vessel (e.g., dissecting aneurysm of the aorta) is hemothorax. A pleural effusion may be blood stained in tuberculosis, cancers involving the pleura and pulmonary infarction.

CHYLOTHORAX: Chylothorax is accumulation of milky, lipid-rich fluid (chyle) in the pleural cavity due to lymphatic obstruction. It has an ominous portent, because lymphatic obstruction suggests disease of the lymph nodes in the posterior mediastinum. Chylothorax is thus a rare complication of mediastinal tumors, such as lymphoma. In tropical countries, it may result from nematode infestations. It can also be seen in pulmonary lymphangioleiomyomatosis.

Pleuritis

Pleuritis, or inflammation of the pleura, may result from extension of any pulmonary infection to the visceral pleura, bacterial infections within the pleural cavity, viral infections, collagen vascular disease or pulmonary infarction that involves the lung surface. The most striking symptom is sharp, stabbing chest pain on inspiration. It is often associated with pleural effusions.

Tumors of the Pleura

Localized (Solitary) Fibrous Tumors of the Pleura Are Usually Benign

Solitary fibrous tumor of the pleura is an uncommon localized neoplasm arising in the pleura. Most are benign, but a small percentage are malignant. Some 80% arise on the visceral pleura, the remainder being from the parietal pleura. Similar tumors can develop on any mesothelial surface, including the mediastinum, peritoneum, pericardium, liver and tunica vaginalis. They arise from submesothelial connective tissue, not mesothelium, and are unrelated to asbestos.

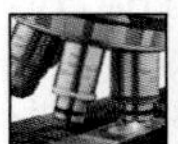

PATHOLOGY: The tumors are usually pedunculated. More than 60% are over 10 cm in diameter and some reach 40 cm and may weigh up to 3800 g. The cut surface is gray-white, with a nodular, whorled or lobulated appearance (Fig. 12-92A). Cysts are occasionally present, especially at the base near the pleural attachment.

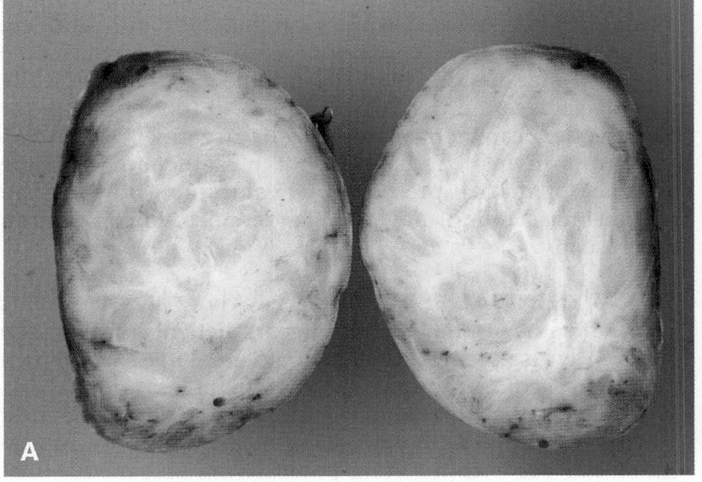

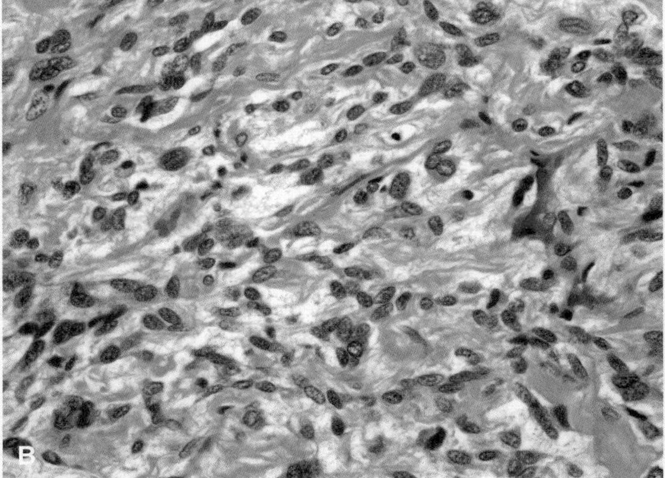

FIGURE 12-92. Pleural localized (solitary) fibrous tumor. A. The tumor is circumscribed with a whorled, tan cut surface. **B.** The tumor cells are round to oval and spindle shaped, with a dense eosinophilic or "ropy" collagen stroma and slitlike blood vessels.

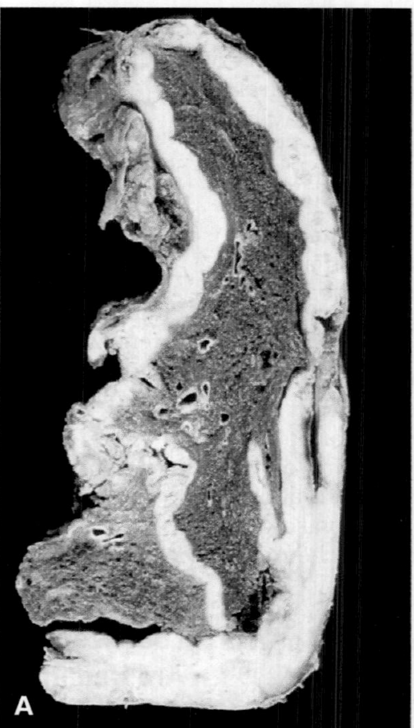

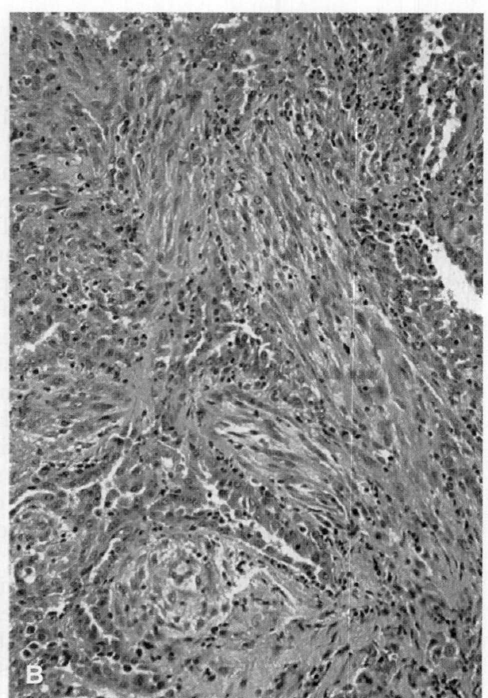

FIGURE 12-93. Pleural malignant mesothelioma. **A.** The lung is encased by a dense pleural tumor that extends along the interlobar fissures but does not involve the underlying lung parenchyma. **B.** This mesothelioma is composed of a biphasic pattern of epithelial and sarcomatous elements.

The most common histologic appearance is the "patternless pattern" of disorderly or randomly arranged mixtures of fibroblast-like cells and connective tissue. Other arrangements include hemangiopericytoma-like, storiform (starlike, or spiral), herringbone, leiomyoma-like, or neurofibroma-like arrangements (Fig. 12-92B). The tumor cells are spindle to oval shaped, often with a fibroblast-like appearance. The collagen is compressed between the cells in a lacy network or it may form dense, wirelike bands. Histologic features suggesting malignancy include increased cellularity, pleomorphism, necrosis and more than four mitoses per 10 high-power fields. Most tumors are immunopositive for CD34 and *bcl*-2.

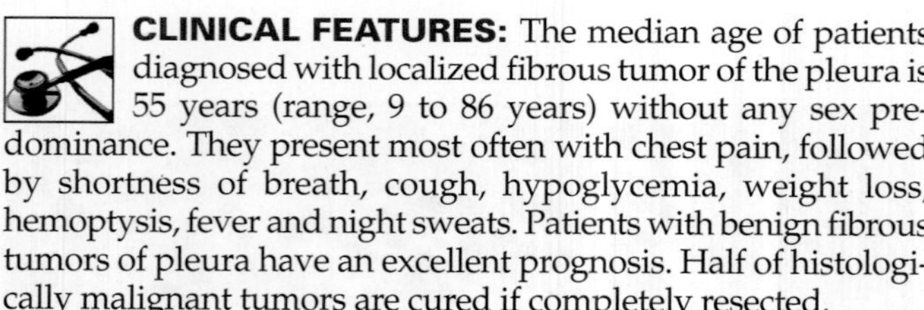

CLINICAL FEATURES: The median age of patients diagnosed with localized fibrous tumor of the pleura is 55 years (range, 9 to 86 years) without any sex predominance. They present most often with chest pain, followed by shortness of breath, cough, hypoglycemia, weight loss, hemoptysis, fever and night sweats. Patients with benign fibrous tumors of pleura have an excellent prognosis. Half of histologically malignant tumors are cured if completely resected.

Malignant Mesothelioma Is a Complication of Asbestos Exposure

Malignant mesothelioma is a neoplasm of mesothelial cells. It is most common in the pleura but also occurs in the peritoneum, pericardium and tunica vaginalis of the testis.

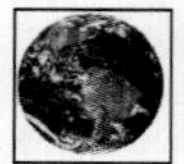

EPIDEMIOLOGY: Some 2000 new cases of malignant mesothelioma develop yearly in the United States. In the United States, Great Britain and South Africa, 80% of patients report exposure to asbestos. The latency period between asbestos exposure and the appearance of malignant mesothelioma is usually to 40 years, with a range of 12 to 60 years.

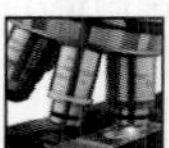

PATHOLOGY: Grossly, pleural mesotheliomas often encase and compress the lung, extending into fissures and interlobar septa, a distribution often referred to as a "pleural rind" (Fig. 12-93A). Invasion of pulmonary parenchyma is generally limited to the periphery adjacent to the tumor. Lymph nodes tend to be spared. Microscopically, classic mesotheliomas show both epithelial and sarcomatous patterns (Fig. 12-93B). Glands and tubules that resemble adenocarcinoma are admixed with sheets of spindle cells that are similar to a fibrosarcoma. In some instances, only one or the other component is present: if it is epithelial, the tumor may be difficult to distinguish from adenocarcinoma. Less commonly, only a sarcomatous component is present.

Immunohistochemistry is essential for differentiating mesothelioma from adenocarcinoma (see Chapter 5). Both are positive for cytokeratins; however, adenocarcinomas often, but not always, express carcinoembryonic antigen, Leu-M1, B72.3 and BER-EP4, but mesotheliomas are negative for these markers. In contrast, mesotheliomas are typically positive for calretinin, WT-1 and D2-40 (podoplanin), for which adenocarcinomas are typically negative. Other criteria supportive of a diagnosis of mesothelioma include absence of mucin, presence of hyaluronic acid (positive Alcian blue staining) and long, slender microvilli on electron microscopy.

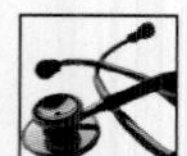

CLINICAL FEATURES: The average age of patients with mesothelioma is 60 years. Patients are first seen with a pleural effusion or a pleural mass, chest pain and nonspecific symptoms, such as weight loss and malaise. Pleural mesotheliomas tend to spread locally within the chest cavity, invading and compressing major structures. Metastases can occur to the lung parenchyma and mediastinal lymph nodes, as well as to extrathoracic sites such as liver, bones, peritoneum and adrenals. Treatment is largely ineffective and prognosis is poor: few patients survive longer than 18 months after diagnosis.

13 The Gastrointestinal Tract

Raphael Rubin

THE ESOPHAGUS

Anatomy

The gut and respiratory tract arise embryologically from the same anlage and constitute a single tube. This structure divides into two separate tubes, the dorsal esophagus and, ventrally, the future respiratory tract. The adult esophagus is a 25-cm conduit for the passage of food and liquid into the stomach. It contains striated and smooth muscle in its upper portion and smooth muscle alone in its lower portion. The organ is fixed superiorly at the cricopharyngeus muscle, which is considered the upper esophageal sphincter. It courses inferiorly through the posterior mediastinum behind the trachea and heart and exits the thorax through the diaphragm. Tonic muscular contraction at its lower end creates the so-called **lower esophageal sphincter,** which is not a true anatomic sphincter but rather a functional one.

As for the entire gastrointestinal tract, the esophagus has a mucosa, submucosa, muscularis propria and adventitia. The mucosa is lined by a nonkeratinizing, stratified squamous epithelium. The transition to gastric mucosa at the **esophagogastric junction** occurs abruptly at the level of the diaphragm. The esophageal submucosa contains mucous glands, a rich lymphatic plexus and nerve fibers. The lymphatics of the upper third of the esophagus drain to cervical lymph nodes, those of the middle third to the mediastinal nodes and those of the lower third to the celiac and gastric lymph nodes. These anatomic features are significant in the spread of esophageal cancer.

The venous drainage of the esophagus is important, because the veins can form varices if there is portal hypertension. These varices are invariably found in the lower third of the esophagus, as the veins of the upper third drain into the superior vena cava and those of the middle third empty into the azygous system. Only the veins of the lower third of the esophagus drain into the portal vein via the gastric veins.

Congenital Disorders

Tracheoesophageal Fistula Leads to Aspiration Pneumonia

Congenital **atresias** and **stenoses** may occur at any gastrointestinal site. Esophageal atresia occurs in about 1 in 3000 births and stenosis in about 1 in 50,000 births. Atresia is usually associated with polyhydramnios (see Chapter 18).

Tracheoesophageal fistula is the most common esophageal anomaly (Fig. 13-1). It is usually combined with some form of esophageal atresia. Atresia of the proximal esophagus without a fistula occurs in only about 10% of cases. It may be associated with VATER syndrome (vertebral defects, anal atresia, tracheoesophageal fistula and renal dysplasia). Maternal hydramnios has been recorded in some cases of esophageal atresia and, less often, in cases of tracheoesophageal fistula. Esophageal

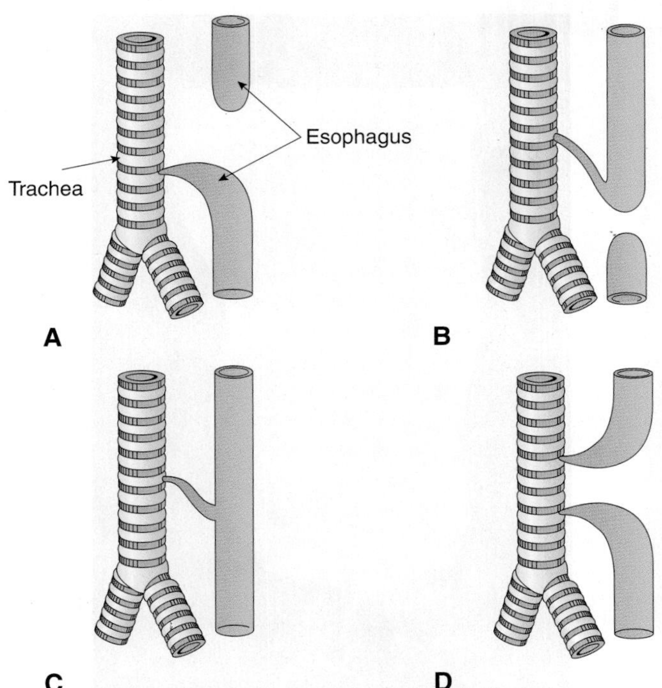

FIGURE 13-1. Congenital tracheoesophageal fistulas. A. The most common type (85% of cases) is a communication between the trachea and the lower portion of the esophagus. The upper segment of the esophagus ends in a blind sac. **B.** In a few cases, the proximal esophagus communicates with the trachea. **C.** H-type fistula without esophageal atresia. **D.** Tracheal fistulas to both a proximal esophageal pouch and distal esophagus.

atresia and fistulas are frequently associated with congenital heart disease.

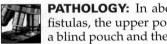

PATHOLOGY: In about 85% of tracheoesophageal fistulas, the upper portion of the esophagus ends in a blind pouch and the superior end of the lower segment communicates with the trachea (Fig. 13-1). ***In this type of atresia, the upper blind sac soon fills with mucus, which the infant then aspirates.*** Surgical correction is feasible but difficult.

The most common of the other fistulas is a communication between the proximal esophagus and the trachea; the lower esophageal pouch communicates with the stomach. ***Infants with this condition develop aspiration immediately after birth.*** In another variant, an **H-type fistula,** a communication exists between an intact esophagus and an intact trachea. In some cases, the lesion becomes symptomatic only in adulthood, with the onset of repeated pulmonary infections.

Duplication Cysts Replicate the Normal Anatomy of the Affected Bowel

Cystic or tubular remnants of a segment of the gut are termed duplications, which may occur at any gastrointestinal site. The small bowel is the most common site for duplications (50%), followed by the esophagus (20%). They are usually continuous with the segment of bowel from which they arise, although ectopic sites may occur. They may form expanding, intramural masses, which can obstruct the affected bowel, either partially or completely.

Rings and Webs Cause Dysphagia

ESOPHAGEAL WEBS: Occasionally, a thin mucosal membrane projects into the esophageal lumen. Webs are usually single and thin (2 to 5 mm) and can occur anywhere in the esophagus. They have a core of fibrovascular tissue lined by normal esophageal epithelium. Middle-aged women are most commonly affected; they report difficulty swallowing (dysphagia). They are often successfully treated by dilation with large rubber bougies; occasionally, they can be excised with biopsy forceps during endoscopy.

PLUMMER-VINSON (PATERSON-KELLY) SYNDROME: This disorder is characterized by (1) a cervical esophageal web, (2) mucosal lesions of the mouth and pharynx and (3) iron-deficiency anemia. Dysphagia, often associated with aspiration of swallowed food, is the most common clinical manifestation. Ninety percent of cases occur in women. ***Carcinoma of the oropharynx and upper esophagus is a complication of the Plummer-Vinson syndrome.***

SCHATZKI RING: This lower esophageal narrowing is usually seen at the gastroesophageal junction (Fig. 13-2). The upper surface of the mucosal ring has stratified squamous epithelium; the lower, columnar epithelium. Although they are seen in up to 14% of barium meal examinations, Schatzki rings are usually asymptomatic. Patients with narrow Schatzki rings, however, may complain of intermittent dysphagia.

Esophageal Diverticula Often Reflect Motor Dysfunction

A **true esophageal diverticulum** is an outpouching of the wall that contains all layers of the esophagus. If a sac has no muscular layer, it is a **false diverticulum.** Esophageal diverticula occur in the hypopharyngeal area above the upper

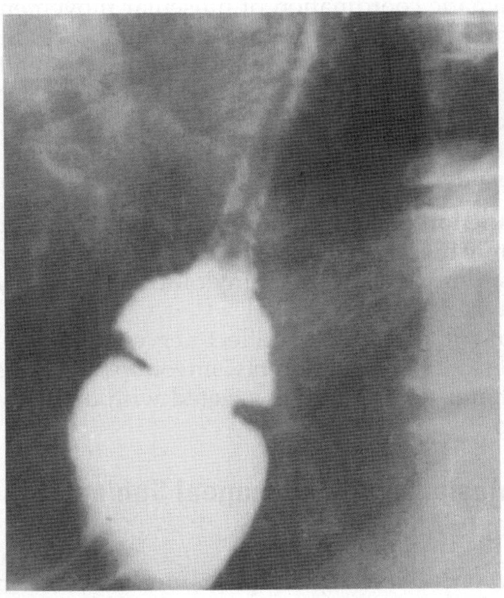

FIGURE 13-2. Schatzki mucosal ring. A contrast radiograph illustrates the lower esophageal narrowing.

esophageal sphincter, in the middle esophagus and immediately proximal to the lower esophageal sphincter.

ZENKER DIVERTICULUM: Zenker diverticulum is an uncommon lesion that appears high in the esophagus and affects men more than women. The cause of this false diverticulum is probably disordered function of cricopharyngeal musculature. Most affected people who come to medical attention are older than 60, suggesting that Zenker diverticula are acquired.

These diverticula can enlarge conspicuously and accumulate a large amount of food. The typical symptom is regurgitation of food eaten some time previously (occasionally days), in the absence of dysphagia. Recurrent aspiration pneumonia may be a serious complication. When symptoms are severe, surgical intervention is the rule.

TRACTION DIVERTICULA: Traction diverticula are outpouchings that occur mainly in the middle of the esophagus. They were so named because they attach to adjacent mediastinal lymph nodes and are usually associated with tuberculous lymphadenitis. Such adhesions are uncommon today, and these pouches often reflect a disturbance in the motor function of the esophagus. A diverticulum in the midesophagus ordinarily has a wide stoma and the pouch is usually higher than its orifice. Thus, it does not retain food or secretions and remains asymptomatic, with only rare complications.

EPIPHRENIC DIVERTICULA: These diverticula are located immediately above the diaphragm. Motor disturbances of the esophagus (e.g., achalasia, diffuse esophageal spasm) are found in two thirds of patients with this true diverticulum. In addition, reflux esophagitis may play a role in the pathogenesis of epiphrenic diverticula.

Unlike other diverticula, epiphrenic diverticula are encountered in young people. Nocturnal regurgitation of large amounts of fluid stored in the diverticulum during the day is typical. When symptoms are severe, surgery to correct the motor abnormality (e.g., myotomy) is appropriate.

Motor Disorders

The automatic coordination of muscular movement during swallowing is termed a **motor function** and results in free passage of food through the esophagus. The hallmark of motor disorders is difficulty in swallowing, or **dysphagia.** Dysphagia is often an awareness that a bolus of food is not moving downward and in itself is not painful. Pain on swallowing is **odynophagia.** Motor disorders can be caused by:

- **Dysfunction of striated muscle** in the upper esophagus
- **Systemic diseases of skeletal muscle** such as myasthenia gravis, dermatomyositis, amyloidosis, hyperthyroidism and myxedema
- **Neurologic diseases** that affect nerves to skeletal muscle (e.g., cerebrovascular accidents, amyotrophic lateral sclerosis)
- **Peripheral neuropathy** associated with diabetes or alcoholism

In Achalasia Lower Esophageal Sphincter Function Is Abnormal

Achalasia, once termed **cardiospasm,** is characterized by failure of the lower esophageal sphincter to relax with swallowing and absence of peristalsis in the body of the esophagus. As a result of these defects in both the outflow tract and the pumping mechanisms of the esophagus, food is retained in the esophagus, and the organ hypertrophies and dilates (Fig. 13-3).

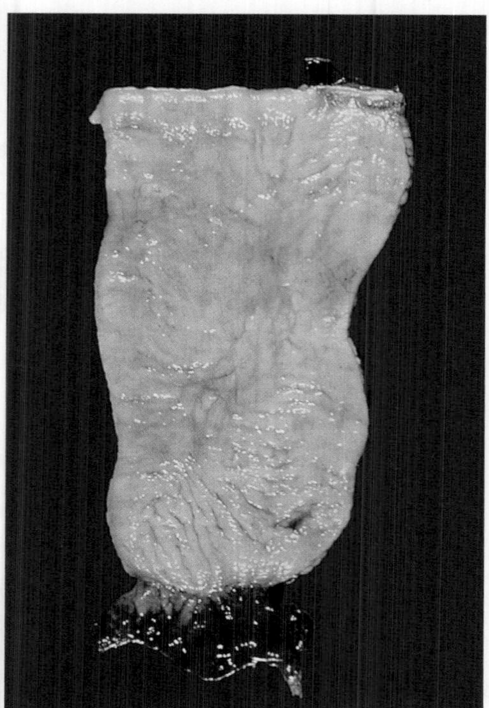

FIGURE 13-3. Esophagus and upper stomach of a patient with advanced achalasia. The esophagus is markedly dilated above the esophagogastric junction, where the lower esophageal sphincter is located. The esophageal mucosa is redundant and has hyperplastic squamous epithelium.

Achalasia is associated with loss or absence of myenteric ganglion cells. Chronic inflammation may be observed around myenteric nerves and residual ganglion cells. The cause of the inflammation is unknown, but genetic, viral and autoimmune factors have been suggested. Degenerative changes in the dorsal motor nucleus of the vagus and extraesophageal vagus nerves have also been described. In Latin America, secondary achalasia is a common complication of **Chagas disease,** in which the ganglion cells are destroyed by the protozoan *Trypanosoma cruzi.* Symptoms of achalasia may arise in amyloidosis, sarcoidosis and infiltrative malignancies.

Dysphagia, occasionally odynophagia and regurgitation of material retained in the esophagus are common symptoms of achalasia. Squamous carcinoma may develop in longstanding cases. Treatment is pneumatic dilation or surgical myotomy of the lower esophageal sphincter, which can lead to gastroesophageal reflux.

Scleroderma Causes Fibrosis of the Esophageal Wall

Scleroderma (progressive systemic sclerosis) causes fibrosis in many organs and produces a severe abnormality of esophageal muscle function (see Chapter 4). The lower esophageal sphincter may become so impaired that the lower esophagus and upper stomach are no longer distinct functional entities and are visualized as a common cavity. In addition, there may be a lack of peristalsis in the entire esophagus.

Microscopically, fibrosis of esophageal smooth muscle (especially the inner layer of the muscularis propria) and nonspecific inflammatory changes are seen. Intimal fibrosis of small arteries and arterioles is common and may play a role in the pathogenesis of the fibrosis. Clinically, patients have dysphagia and heartburn caused by peptic esophagitis, owing to reflux of acid from the stomach. Severe reflux changes may occur (see below).

Hiatal Hernia

Hiatal hernia is a herniation of the stomach through an enlarged diaphragmatic opening. Two basic types of hiatal hernia are observed (Fig. 13-4).

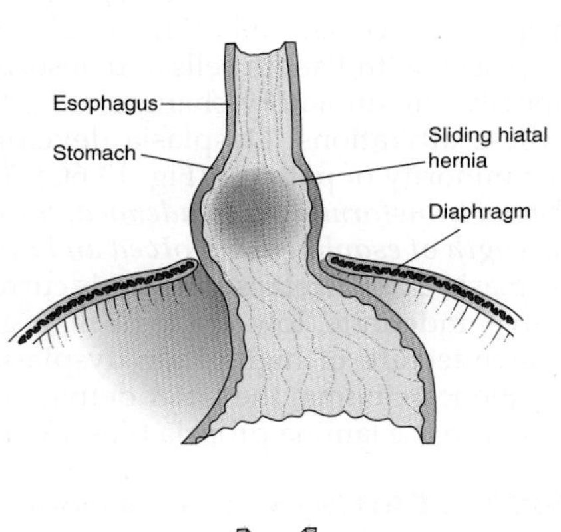

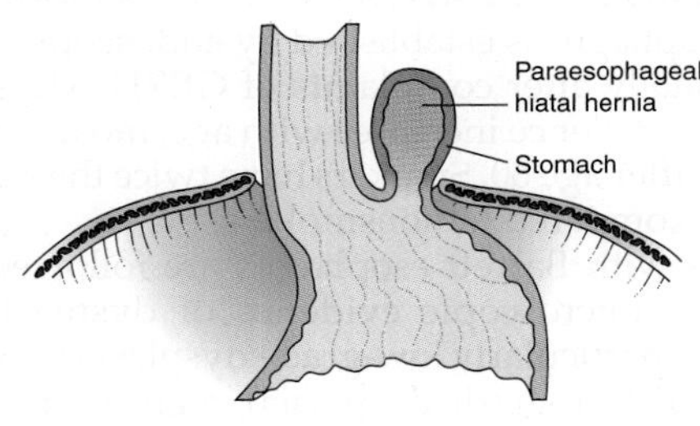

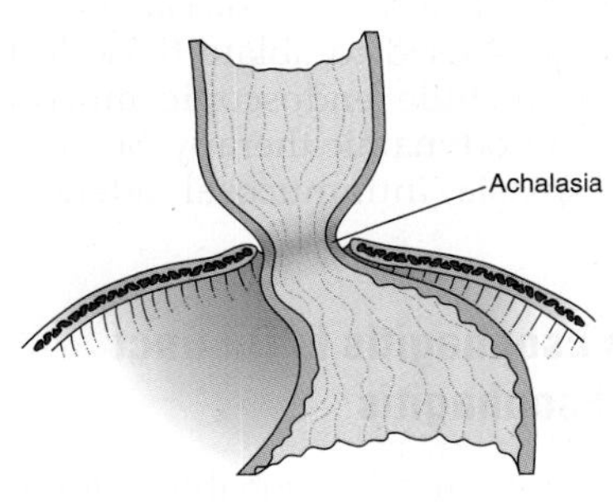

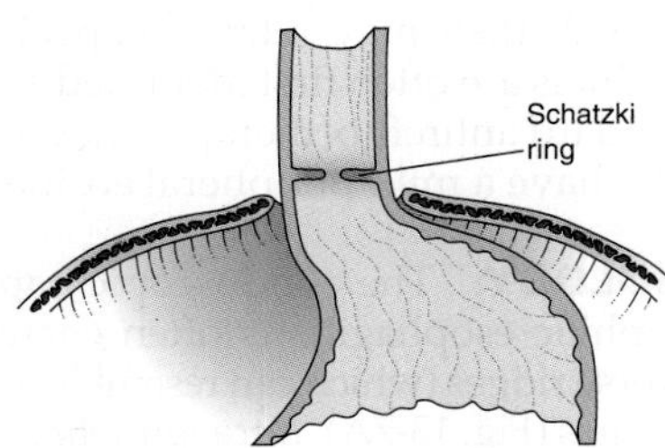

FIGURE 13-4. Disorders of the esophageal outlet.

SLIDING HERNIA: Enlargement of the diaphragmatic hiatus and laxity of the circumferential connective tissue allow a cap of gastric mucosa to move upward, above the diaphragm. This condition is common and is asymptomatic in most patients. Only 5% of patients diagnosed radiologically complain of symptoms of gastroesophageal reflux.

PARAESOPHAGEAL HERNIA: In this uncommon form of hiatal hernia, a portion of gastric fundus herniates through a defect in the diaphragmatic connective tissue that defines the esophageal hiatus and lies beside the esophagus. The hernia progressively enlarges, and the hiatus grows increasingly wide. In extreme cases, most of the stomach herniates into the thorax.

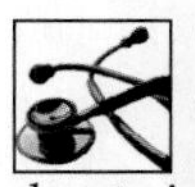

CLINICAL FEATURES: Symptoms of hiatal hernia, mostly heartburn and regurgitation, are attributed to reflux of gastric contents into the esophagus, primarily due to incompetence of the lower esophageal sphincter. Classically, symptoms are worse when subjects are recumbent, which facilitates acid reflux. Dysphagia, painful swallowing and occasionally bleeding may also be troublesome. Large herniations carry a risk of gastric volvulus or intrathoracic gastric dilation.

Sliding hiatal hernias generally do not require surgery and symptoms are treated medically. An enlarging paraesophageal hernia should be corrected surgically, even if it is asymptomatic.

Esophagitis

Reflux Esophagitis Is Caused by Reflux of Gastric Juice (Gastroesophageal Reflux Disease)

This is by far the most common type of esophagitis. It is often seen together with sliding hiatal hernias, but may occur through an incompetent lower esophageal sphincter with no anatomic lesion.

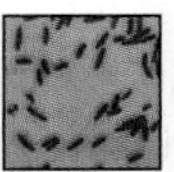

ETIOLOGIC FACTORS: The main barrier to reflux of gastric contents into the esophagus is the lower esophageal sphincter. Transient reflux is normal, particularly after a meal. The mucosa is partially protected by alkaline secretions from submucosal glands. Esophagitis results when these episodes are more frequent and prolonged. Agents that decrease the pressure of the lower esophageal sphincter (e.g., alcohol, chocolate, fatty foods, cigarette smoking) also cause reflux, as may certain central nervous system depressants (e.g., morphine, diazepam), pregnancy, estrogen therapy and the presence of a nasogastric tube. Although acid damages the esophageal mucosa, the combination of acid and pepsin may be particularly injurious. Moreover, gastric fluid often contains refluxed bile from the duodenum, which is harmful to the esophageal mucosa. Alcohol, hot beverages and spicy foods also may injure the mucosa directly.

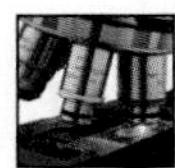

PATHOLOGY: The first grossly evident change caused by gastroesophageal reflux is hyperemia. Affected areas are susceptible to superficial mucosal erosions and ulcers, which often appear as vertical linear streaks. Mild injury to the squamous epithelium

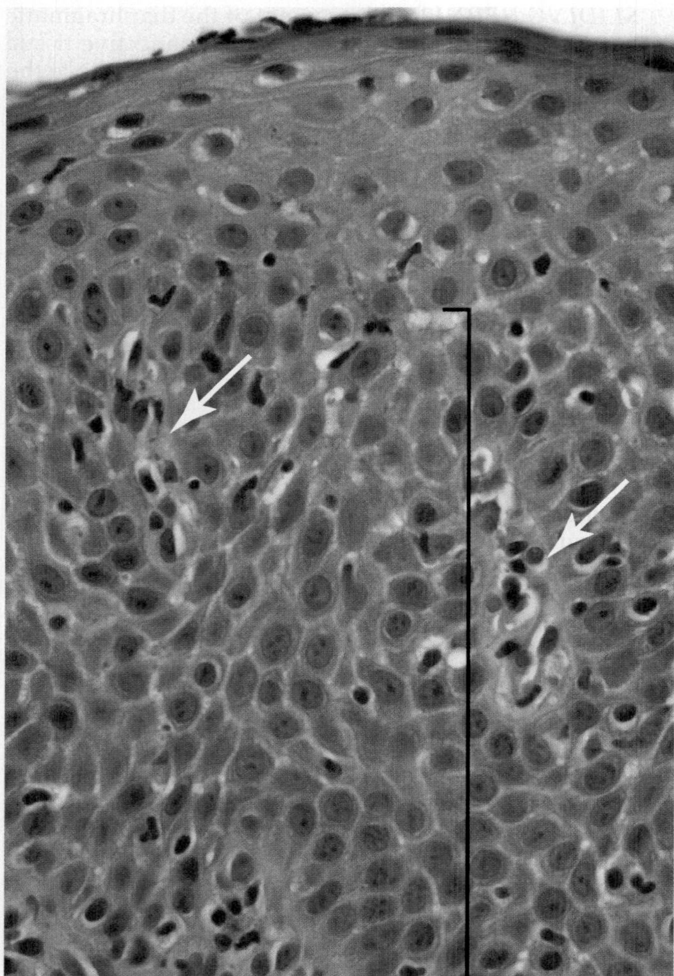

FIGURE 13-5. Reflux esophagitis. Biopsy from a patient with longstanding heartburn. Note the basal hyperplasia (*bracket*) and papillae (*arrows*), squamous hyperplasia and inflammation.

is manifested by cell swelling (hydropic change). With chronic injury, squamous hyperplasia develops, in which the basal epithelium is thickened, and the papillae of the lamina propria are elongated and extend toward the surface because of reactive proliferation (Fig. 13-5). Capillary vessels in the papillae are often dilated. An increase in mucosal lymphocytes, neutrophils and eosinophils is usually present. Mucosal ulceration develops in severe cases. Esophageal stricture may eventuate in those patients in whom the ulcer persists and damages the esophageal wall deep to the lamina propria. In this circumstance, reactive fibrosis can narrow the esophageal lumen.

CLINICAL FEATURES: Gastroesophageal reflux disease (GERD) generally occurs after age 30 and can be nonerosive, erosive or involved by Barrett esophagus (see below). Heartburn and dysphagia are the usual presenting symptoms and can usually be controlled by agents that reduce gastric acidity (histamine-2 [H_2] receptor antagonists or proton pump inhibitors). In cases of erosive GERD, ulceration, hematemesis and stricture may occur.

Barrett Esophagus Is Replacement of Esophageal Squamous Epithelium by Columnar Epithelium (Intestinal Metaplasia)

Barrett esophagus is a result of chronic GERD. For reasons unknown, its incidence has been increasing in recent years, particularly among white men. This disorder occurs in the lower third of the esophagus but may extend higher.

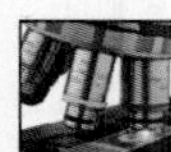

PATHOLOGY: Metaplastic Barrett epithelium may partially involve the circumference of short segments or may line the entire lower esophagus (Fig. 13-6A). The sine qua non of Barrett esophagus is the presence of a distinctive type of "specialized epithelium." By endoscopy, it has a characteristically salmon-pink color and is an admixture of intestine-like epithelium with well-formed goblet cells interspersed with gastric foveolar cells (Fig. 13-6B). Complete intestinal metaplasia, with Paneth cells and absorptive cells, occurs occasionally. Inflammatory changes are often superimposed on these alterations. Dysplasia develops in this epithelium in a minority of patients (Fig. 13-6C). ***The risk of Barrett esophagus transforming into adenocarcinoma correlates with the length of esophagus involved and the degree of dysplasia.*** Dysplasia in a Barrett esophagus is currently classified as negative, indefinite, low grade or high grade. The cytology and architecture of high-grade dysplasia overlap intramucosal adenocarcinoma, the latter definitively identified by invasion into the lamina propria (Fig. 13-6D).

CLINICAL FEATURES: The diagnosis of Barrett esophagus is established by endoscopy with biopsy, usually after complaints of GERD. Males predominate (3:1). Prevalence increases with age, most patients being diagnosed after age 60. Smokers have twice the risk of Barrett esophagus compared to nonsmokers.

Patients with Barrett esophagus are followed closely to detect early microscopic evidence of dysplastic mucosa. Many cases, particularly low-grade dysplasia (or even microscopic foci of high-grade dysplasia), regress after pharmacologic reduction in gastric acidity. However, high-grade dysplasia and certainly intramucosal carcinoma require intervention. Techniques used to ablate these lesions (short of esophagectomy) include endoscopic mucosectomy, laser treatment and photodynamic therapy. Standards of care for high-grade dysplasia/intramucosal adenocarcinoma are evolving.

Eosinophilic Esophagitis Is Distinct From Reflux Esophagitis

Eosinophilic esophagitis is probably allergic in etiology. Patients often complain of a sensation of food "sticking" upon swallowing, which they may relate to specific foodstuffs. Affected individuals are often first identified after they fail to improve on standard antireflux therapy. They are also usually atopic and often have a mild peripheral eosinophilia.

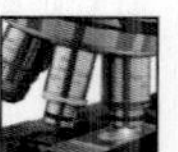

PATHOLOGY: The endoscopic appearance of eosinophilic esophagitis is often characteristic with transverse ridges (which can resemble the trachea) and small white plaques (Fig. 13-7A). Intraepithelial eosinophils are abundant, typically 20 or more per high-power field, and tend to cluster superficially (Fig. 13-7B).

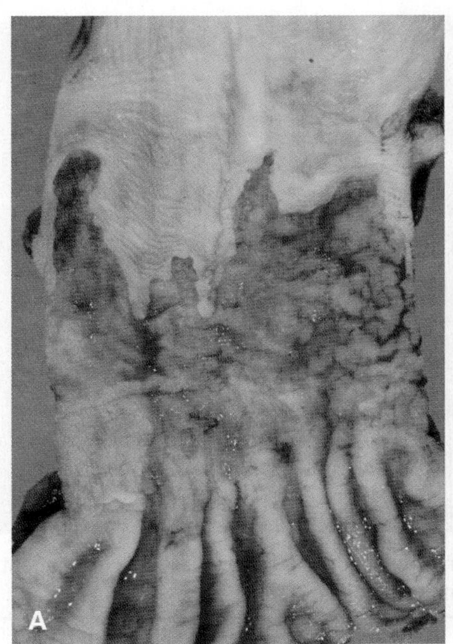

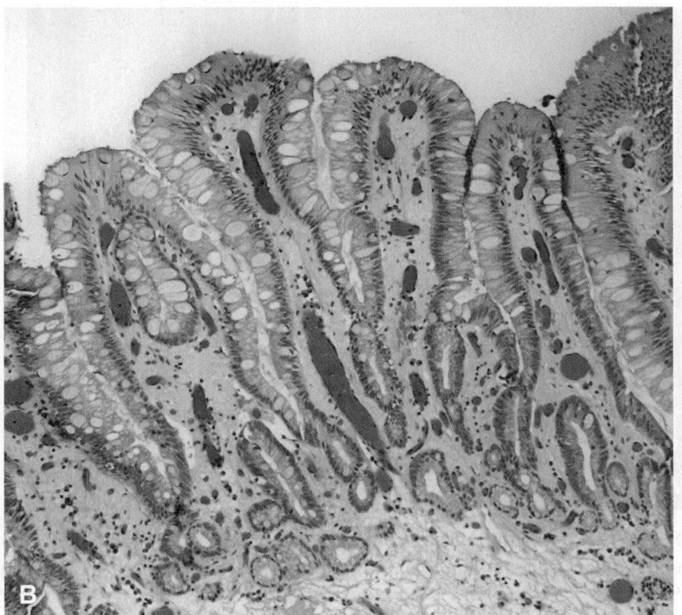

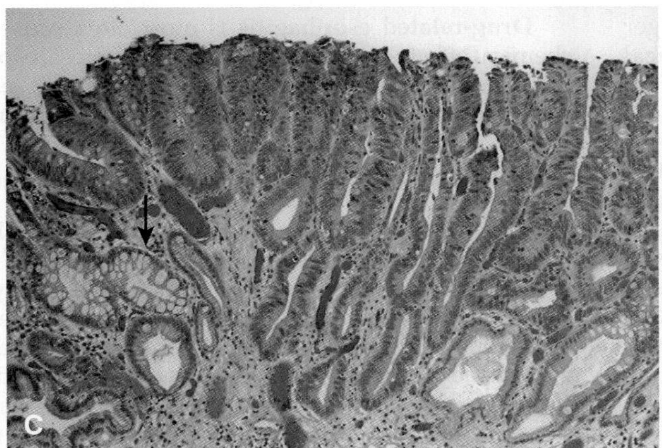

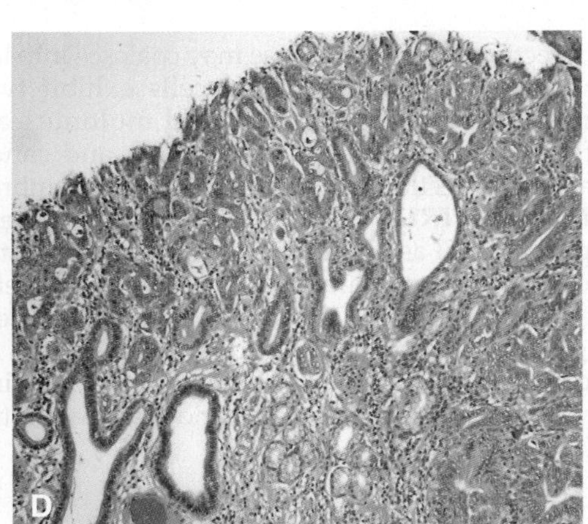

FIGURE 13-6. Barrett esophagus. A. The presence of the tan tongues of epithelium interdigitating with the more proximal squamous epithelium is typical of Barrett esophagus. **B.** The specialized epithelium has a villiform architecture and is lined by cells that are foveolar gastric-type cells and intestinal goblet-type cells. **C. High-grade dysplasia.** Markedly dysplastic glands predominate with hyperchromatic nuclei and early architectural distortion. Intestinalized, nondysplastic glands persist (*arrow*). **D. Intramucosal adenocarcinoma.** Malignant glands are restricted to the mucosa, and there is no evidence of invasion.

Infective Esophagitis Is Associated With Immunosuppression

CANDIDA ESOPHAGITIS: This fungal infection has become common as an increasing number of patients are immunocompromised owing to chemotherapy for malignant disease, immunosuppression after organ transplantation or acquired immunodeficiency syndrome (AIDS). Esophageal candidiasis also occurs in patients with diabetes and those receiving antibiotic therapy. It is uncommon in the absence of known predisposing factors. Dysphagia and severe pain on swallowing are the usual symptoms.

PATHOLOGY: In mild cases, a few small, elevated white mucosal plaques are surrounded by a hyperemic zone in the middle or lower third of the esophagus. In severe cases, confluent pseudomembranes lie on a hyperemic and edematous mucosa. The candidal pseudomembrane contains fungal mycelia, necrotic debris and fibrin. *Candida* sometimes involves only the superficial epithelium, but involvement of deeper layers of the esophageal wall can lead to disseminated candidiasis or fibrosis, sometimes severe enough to create a stricture.

HERPETIC ESOPHAGITIS: Esophageal infection with herpesvirus type I is mostly associated with lymphomas and leukemias and is often manifested by odynophagia (see Chapter 9). However, it may occur on occasion in otherwise healthy individuals.

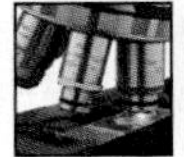

PATHOLOGY: The well-developed lesions of herpetic esophagitis grossly resemble those of candidiasis. In early cases, vesicles, small erosions or plaques

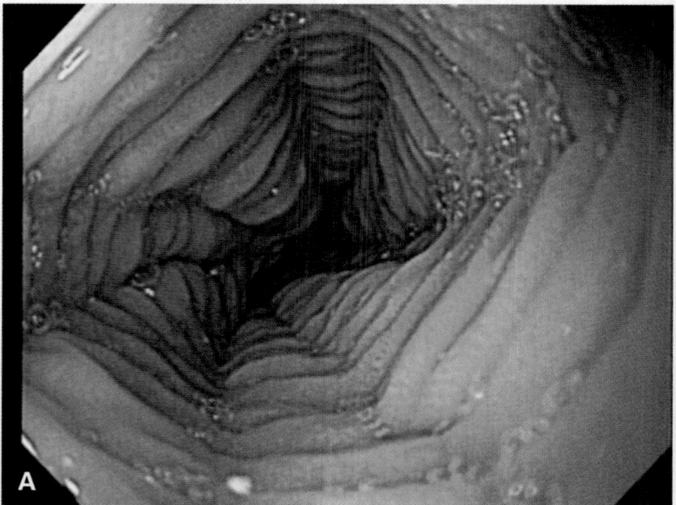

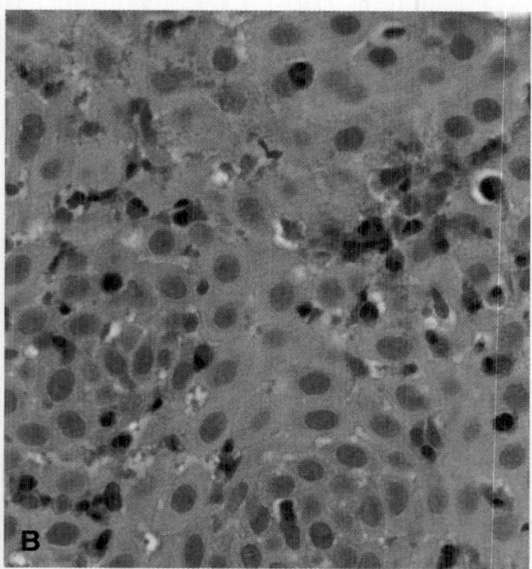

FIGURE 13-7. Eosinophilic esophagitis. A. Endoscopic view of a deeply furrowed mucosa ("trachealization") in a patient with eosinophilic esophagitis. **B.** Intense eosinophilic infiltrate within squamous mucosa.

are seen; as infection progresses, these may coalesce into larger lesions. In herpetic lesions epithelial cells exhibit typical nuclear herpetic inclusions and occasional multinucleation. Necrosis of infected cells leads to ulceration, and candidal and bacterial superinfection may generate pseudomembranes.

CYTOMEGALOVIRUS ESOPHAGITIS: Involvement of the esophagus, as well as all other segments of the gastrointestinal tract, with cytomegalovirus (CMV) usually reflects systemic viral disease in severely immunosuppressed patients (e.g., people with AIDS). Mucosal ulceration, as in herpetic esophagitis, is common. Characteristic CMV inclusion bodies are seen in endothelial cells and granulation tissue fibroblasts.

Chemical Esophagitis Results From Ingestion of Corrosive Agents

Chemical injury to the esophagus usually reflects accidental poisoning in children, attempted suicide in adults or contact with medication ("pill esophagitis"). Ingestion of strong alkaline agents (e.g., lye) or strong acids (e.g., sulfuric or hydrochloric acid), both of which are used in various cleaning solutions, can produce chemical esophagitis. The former are particularly insidious, because they are generally odorless and tasteless and so easily swallowed before protective reflexes come into play.

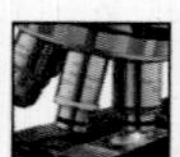

PATHOLOGY: Alkaline agents cause liquefactive necrosis with conspicuous inflammation and saponification of membrane lipids in the epithelium, submucosa and muscularis propria of the esophagus and stomach. Thrombosis of small vessels adds ischemic necrosis to the injury. Severe injury is the rule with liquid alkali, but less than 25% of those who ingest granular preparations have pronounced complications.

Strong acids produce immediate coagulative necrosis, which results in a protective eschar that limits injury and penetration. Nevertheless, half of patients who ingest concentrated hydrochloric or sulfuric acid develop severe esophageal injury.

Drug-related esophagitis is most often caused by direct chemical effects on the squamous-lined mucosa, especially with capsules; esophageal dysmotility and cardiac enlargement (which impinges on the esophagus) may be contributing factors.

Esophagitis May Complicate Systemic Illnesses

Esophageal squamous mucosa resembles, and shares some reactions with, the epidermis.

The **dermolytic (dystrophic) form of epidermolysis bullosa** (see Chapter 24) involves all organs lined by, or derived from, squamous epithelium, including skin, nails, teeth and esophagus. Bullae occur episodically and evolve from fluid-filled vesicles to weeping ulcers. Dysphagia and painful swallowing are the rule. Stricture, usually in the upper esophagus, may occur.

Bullous pemphigoid produces subepithelial bullae in the skin and esophagus but does not lead to scarring. Other dermatologic disorders associated with esophagitis include pemphigus, dermatitis herpetiformis, Behçet syndrome and erythema multiforme.

Graft-versus-host disease in recipients of bone marrow transplants can cause esophageal lesions and dysphagia, odynophagia and gastroesophageal reflux. The upper and middle thirds of the esophageal mucosa appear friable and esophageal motor function may be impaired.

Esophagitis May Be Iatrogenic

External irradiation for treatment of thoracic cancers may include portions of the esophagus and lead to esophagitis and even stricture. **Nasogastric tubes** may cause pressure ulcers when they are in place for prolonged periods, although acid reflux also plays a role in these cases.

Esophageal Varices

Esophageal varices are dilated veins immediately beneath the mucosa* (Fig. 13-8) *that are prone to rupture and hemorrhage (also see Chapter 14). They arise in the lower third of

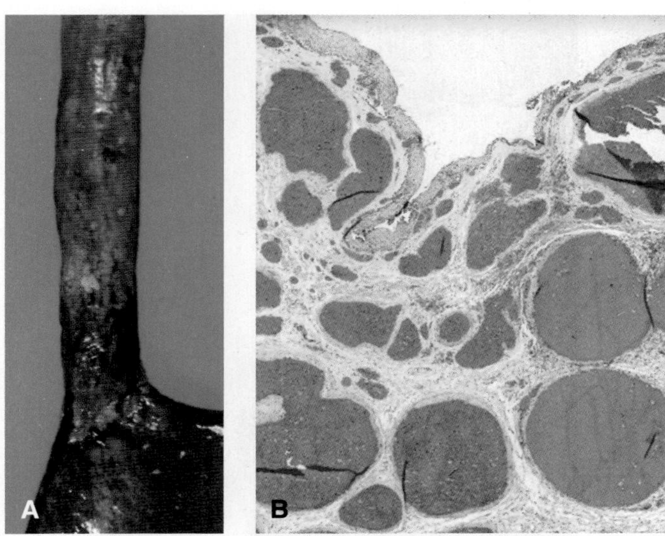

FIGURE 13-8. Esophageal varices. A. Numerous prominent blue venous channels are seen beneath the mucosa of the everted esophagus, particularly above the gastroesophageal junction. **B.** Section of the esophagus reveals numerous dilated submucosal veins.

the esophagus, virtually always in patients with cirrhosis and portal hypertension. Lower esophageal veins are linked to the portal system via gastroesophageal anastomoses. If portal system pressure exceeds a critical level, these anastomoses become prominent in the upper stomach and lower esophagus. If varices exceed 5 mm in diameter, they tend to rupture, leading to life-threatening hemorrhage. Reflux injury or infective esophagitis can contribute to variceal bleeding.

Lacerations and Perforations

Lacerations of the esophagus result from external trauma, such as automobile accidents, as well as from medical instrumentation. However, the most common cause is severe vomiting, during which intraesophageal pressure may reach 300 mm Hg. The diaphragm descends rapidly, and part of the upper stomach is forced up through the hiatus. Thus, forceful retching may cause mucosal tears, at first in the gastric epithelium and extending into the esophagus.

Mallory-Weiss syndrome refers to severe retching, often associated with alcoholism, that leads to mucosal lacerations of the upper stomach and lower esophagus. These tears result in the patient vomiting bright red blood. Bleeding may be so severe as to require transfusion of many units of blood. The lacerations may also cause perforation into the mediastinum. Esophageal rupture owing to vomiting is called **Boerhaave syndrome.**

Esophageal perforation, whether from trauma or vomiting, can be catastrophic. It is a well-known occurrence in newborns, in whom it is caused occasionally by suctioning or feeding with a nasogastric tube. However, it may also occur spontaneously.

The major nonneoplastic disorders of the esophagus are summarized in Fig. 13-9.

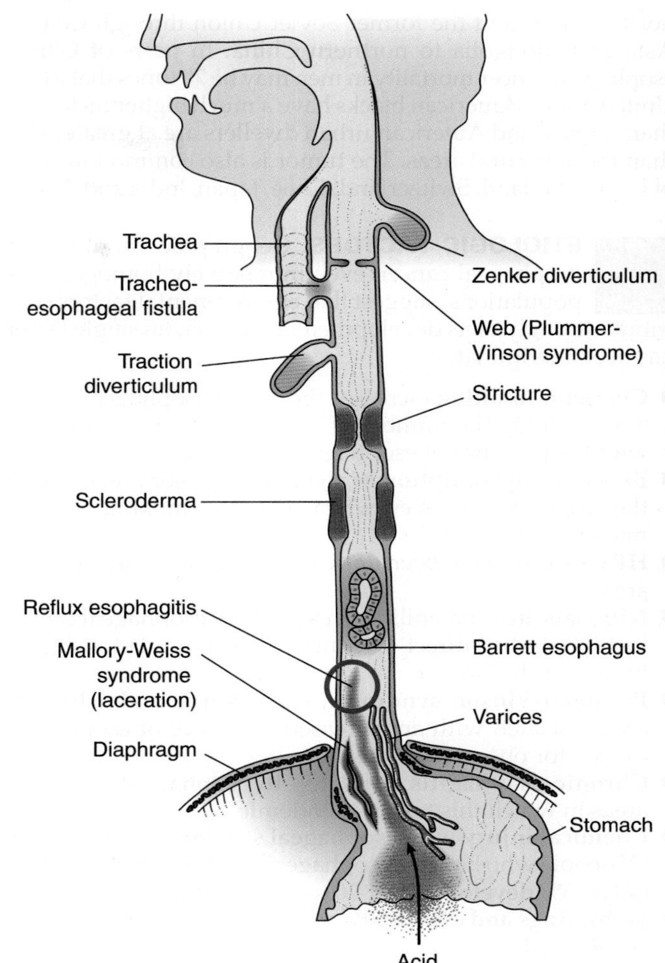

FIGURE 13-9. Nonneoplastic disorders of the esophagus.

Neoplasms

Benign Tumors of the Esophagus Are Uncommon

Unlike the remainder of the gastrointestinal tract, most spindle cell submucosal tumors of the esophagus derive from smooth muscle **(leiomyoma)** rather than from interstitial cells of Cajal (gastrointestinal stromal tumors [GISTs]; see below). They are almost always benign. **Squamous papilloma** of the esophagus is rare and may be related to human papilloma virus (HPV) infection.

Esophageal Squamous Cell Carcinoma Varies Geographically and Histologically

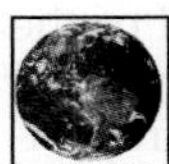

EPIDEMIOLOGY: Worldwide, most esophageal cancers are squamous cell carcinomas, but in the United States, adenocarcinoma is now more common (see below). Esophageal cancer accounts for about 2% of cancer deaths in the United States.

Worldwide geographic variations in the incidence of esophageal carcinoma are striking, and areas of high incidence are adjacent to areas of low incidence. An esophageal cancer belt extends across Asia from the Caspian Sea region of northern Iran and the former Soviet Union through Central Asia and Mongolia to northern China. In parts of China, esophageal cancer mortality in men may be 70 times that in the United States. American blacks have a much higher incidence than whites, and American urban dwellers are at greater risk than those in rural areas. The tumor is also common in parts of France, Finland, Switzerland, Chile, Japan, India and Africa.

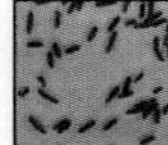

ETIOLOGIC FACTORS: Geographic variations in esophageal cancer, even in relatively homogeneous populations, suggest that environmental factors contribute strongly to its development. However, no single factor has been incriminated.

- **Cigarette smoking** increases the risk of esophageal cancer 5- to 10-fold. The number of cigarettes smoked correlates with the presence of esophageal dysplasia.
- **Excessive consumption of alcohol** is a major risk factor in the United States, even when cigarette smoking is taken into account.
- **HPV infection** has been detected in some cases in high-risk areas.
- **Nitrosamines** and aniline dyes produce esophageal cancer in animals, but direct evidence for such a relationship in humans is lacking.
- **Plummer-Vinson syndrome, celiac sprue and achalasia** are associated with an increased incidence of esophageal cancer, for obscure reasons.
- **Chronic esophagitis** is related to esophageal cancer in areas in which this tumor is endemic.
- **Chemical injury with esophageal stricture** is a risk factor. Of people who have an esophageal stricture after ingestion of lye, 5% develop cancer 20 to 40 years later.
- **Webs, rings and diverticula** are sometimes associated with esophageal cancer.

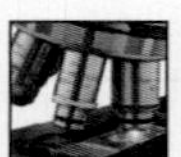

PATHOLOGY: About half of cases of esophageal squamous cell carcinoma involve the middle and upper thirds of the esophagus. Grossly, tumors may be endophytic or exophytic (Fig. 13-10). They can also be infiltrating, in which case the principal plane of growth is in the wall. Bulky polypoid tumors tend to obstruct early, but ulcerated ones are more likely to bleed. Infiltrating tumors gradually narrow the lumen by circumferential compression. Local extension of tumor into mediastinal structures is commonly a major problem.

Neoplastic squamous cells range from well differentiated, with epithelial "pearls," to poorly differentiated, without evidence of squamous differentiation. Some tumors have a predominant spindle cell population of tumor cells (metaplastic carcinoma).

The rich lymphatic drainage of the esophagus provides a route for most metastases. Accordingly, tumors of the upper third metastasize to cervical, internal jugular and supraclavicular nodes. Cancer of the middle third spreads to paratracheal and hilar lymph nodes and to nodes in the aortic, cardiac and paraesophageal regions. Because the lower third of the esophagus is fed by the left gastric artery, lower esophageal tumors spread via accompanying lymphatics to retroperitoneal, celiac and left gastric nodes. Metastases to liver and lung are common, but almost any organ may be affected.

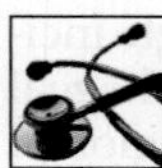

CLINICAL FEATURES: The most common presenting complaint is dysphagia, but by the time a patient complains of dysphagia, most tumors are unresectable. Patients with esophageal cancer are almost invariably cachectic owing to anorexia, difficulty in swallowing and the remote effects of a malignancy. Odynophagia occurs in half of patients, and persistent pain suggests mediastinal extension of the tumor or involvement of spinal nerves. Compression of the recurrent laryngeal nerve causes hoarseness, and tracheoesophageal fistula is manifested clinically by a chronic cough. Surgery and radiation therapy are palliative, but the prognosis remains dismal. Many patients are inoperable, and of those who undergo surgery, only 20% survive for 5 years.

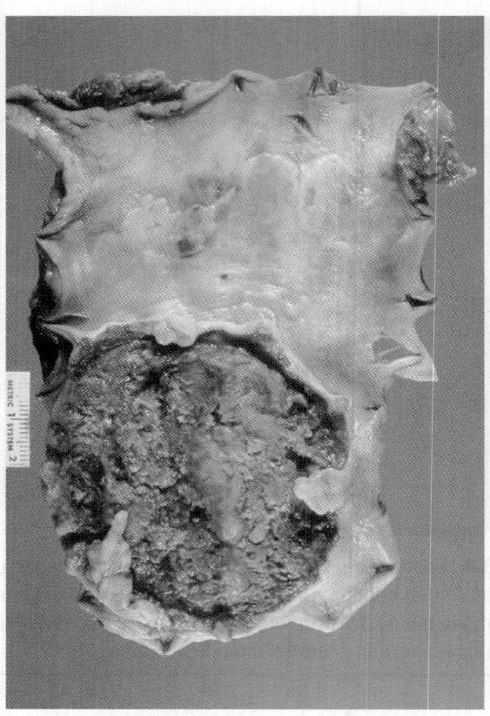

FIGURE 13-10. Esophageal squamous cell carcinoma. There is a large ulcerated mass present in the squamous mucosa with normal squamous mucosa intervening between the carcinoma and the stomach.

Adenocarcinoma of the Esophagus Arises in a Background of Barrett Esophagus

Adenocarcinoma of the esophagus is now more common (60%) in the United States than is squamous carcinoma. The vast majority of these adenocarcinomas arise in the context of Barrett esophagus (Fig. 13-11), although some originate in submucosal mucous glands. Men are more often affected than women. Numerous molecular events attend conversion of Barrett epithelium to adenocarcinoma, the most common being inactivation of the *INK4A/CDKN* tumor suppressor gene *p16* (see Chapter 5). Other features include *p53* loss, inactivation of *RB*, aneuploidy and amplification of cell cycle–related genes.

Endoscopic surveillance for adenocarcinoma is now commonly done in patients with Barrett esophagus, particularly in those with dysplasia (see above). The symptoms and clinical course of esophageal adenocarcinoma are similar to those of squamous cell carcinoma.

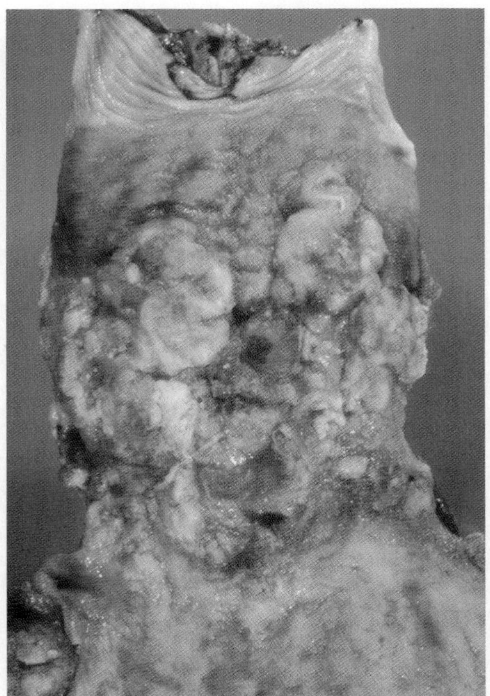

FIGURE 13-11. Esophageal adenocarcinoma. There is a large exophytic ulcerated mass lesion just proximal to the gastroesophageal junction. This well-differentiated adenocarcinoma was separated from the most proximal squamous epithelium by a tan area representing Barrett esophagus.

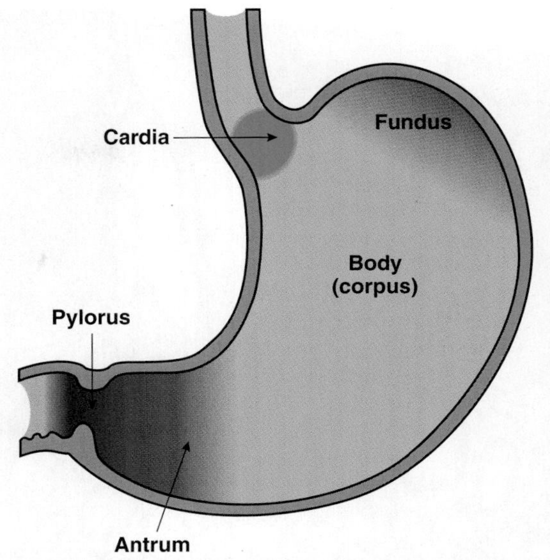

FIGURE 13-12. Anatomic regions of the stomach.

THE STOMACH

Anatomy

The stomach, a J-shaped saccular organ with a volume of 1200 to 1500 mL, arises as a dilation of the primitive foregut. It is continuous with the esophagus superiorly and the duodenum inferiorly. Situated in the upper abdomen, the stomach extends from the left hypochondrium across the epigastrium. The gastric convexity, extending leftward from the gastroesophageal junction, is the **greater curvature.** The concavity of the right side of the stomach, called the **lesser curvature,** is about one fourth as long as the greater curvature. The entire stomach is invested in peritoneum, which descends from the greater curvature as the **greater omentum.**

The stomach is divided into five regions, superiorly to inferiorly (Fig. 13-12):

1. The **cardia** is a small, grossly indistinct zone that extends a short distance from the gastroesophageal junction.
2. The **fundus** is the dome-shaped part of the stomach to the left of the cardia, extending superiorly above the level of the gastroesophageal junction.
3. **The body, or corpus,** is two thirds of the stomach. It descends from the fundus to the most inferior region, where the organ turns right to form the bottom of the J.
4. **The antrum,** the distal third of the stomach, is positioned horizontally and extends from the body to the pyloric sphincter.
5. **The pyloric sphincter** is the most distal tubular segment of the stomach. It is entirely surrounded by the thick muscular layer that controls passage of food into the duodenum.

The wall of the stomach is composed of a mucosa, submucosa, muscularis and serosa. The lining of the fundus and body has prominent folds, the gastric rugae.

Branches of the celiac, hepatic and splenic arteries supply blood to the stomach. Gastric veins drain directly into the portal system or indirectly through splenic and superior mesenteric veins. A rich plexus of lymphatic channels empties into gastric and other regional lymph nodes. Both vagal nerves supply parasympathetic innervation to the stomach and the celiac plexus provides sympathetic innervation.

The histology of the gastric mucosa varies by anatomic region. Surface mucus-secreting, columnar epithelium extends into numerous foveolae, or pits. These are the orifices of millions of branched, tubular glands. There are three types of glands (Fig. 13-13):

- **Cardiac glands** are located in the cardia.
- **Parietal (oxyntic) glands** are found in the body and fundus of the stomach.
- **Pyloric glands** are situated in the antrum and the pyloric canal.

Gastric glands, the principal secretory elements of the stomach, are densely arranged perpendicular to the mucosa and enter the base of the foveola through a narrowed segment called the **neck of the gland.** Gastric glands have five cell types:

- **Zymogen, or chief, cells:** These are primarily in the lower half of glands. They are pyramidal, basophilic cells with zymogen granules that contain pepsinogen.
- **Parietal, or oxyntic, cells:** These oval or pyramidal eosinophilic cells occupy the upper half of the gastric gland and secrete hydrochloric acid. They contain numerous mitochondria to provide energy for the ion transport needed for acid secretion. Ultrastructurally, parietal cells have many surface membrane invaginations, **secretory canaliculi,** which vastly expand the surface area for acid secretion. Parietal cells also produce intrinsic factor, which is necessary for intestinal absorption of vitamin B_{12}.

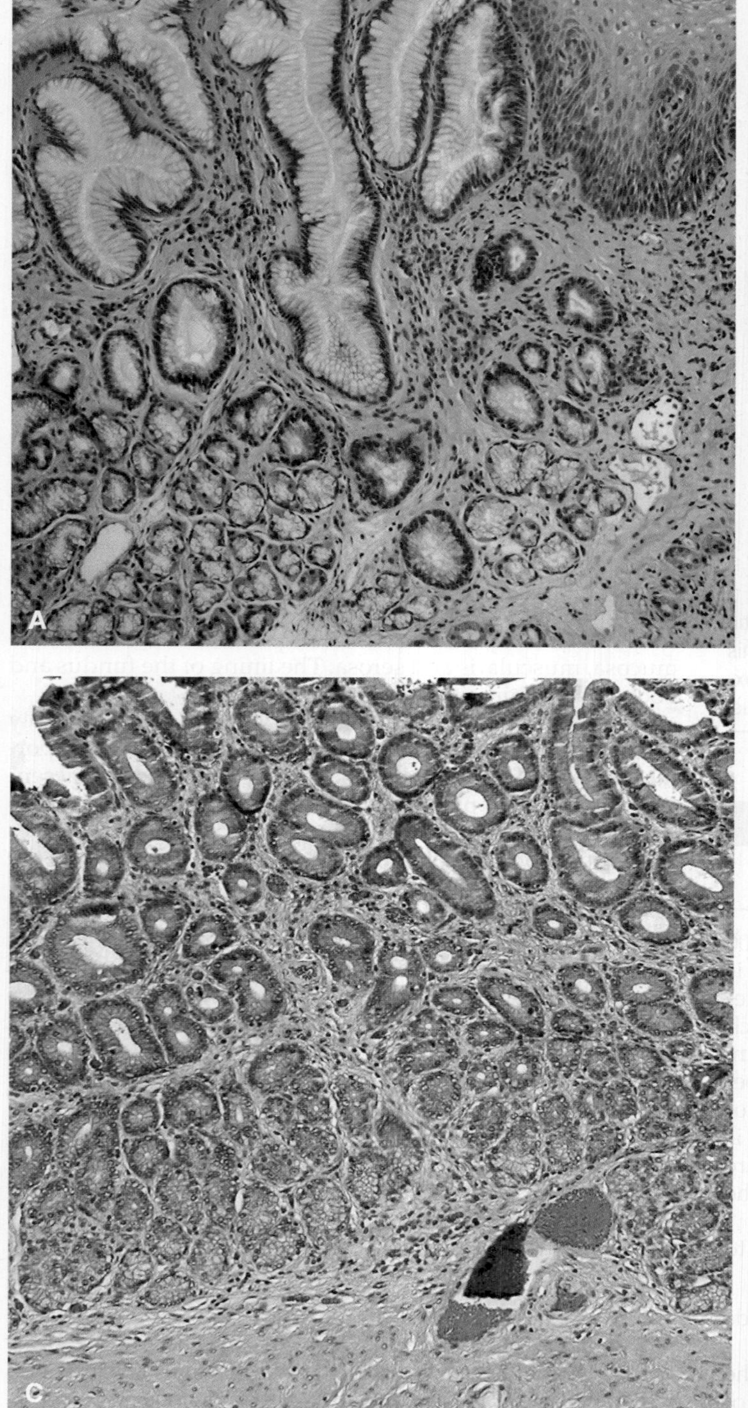

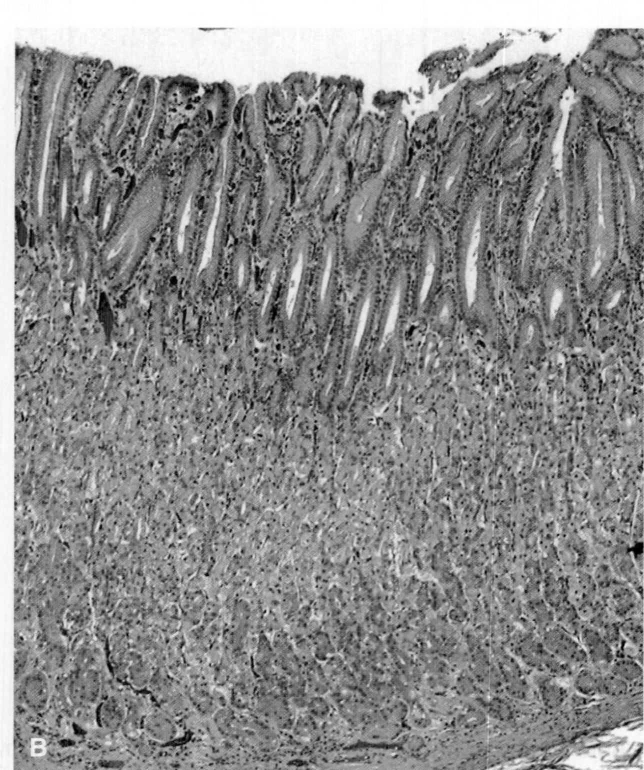

FIGURE 13-13. Histology of the mucosa of the stomach. A. Cardiac. B. Fundus. C. Antrum. See text for details.

- **Mucous neck cells:** These mucus-secreting, basophilic components are interspersed among the parietal cells in the neck of the gastric gland.
- **Endocrine cells:** These are scattered, mostly between the zymogen cells and the basement membrane. They are small, round or pyramidal cells filled with granules. These cells contain biogenic amines such as serotonin and polypeptide hormones (e.g., gastrin and somatostatin). Gastric endocrine cells include gastrin-secreting cells (G cells). Vasoactive intestinal peptide (VIP) is found in neural elements of the mucosa but not within endocrine cells. Endocrine cells are best visualized by immunostaining, for more generic markers such as chromogranin or synaptophysin, or with antibodies directed against specific peptides, such as gastrin.

- **Pyloric glands** are branched and quite coiled, and empty into foveolae that are much deeper than those elsewhere in the stomach. The glands are lined by pale cells that resemble mucous neck cells and cells of Brunner glands in the duodenum. G cells are also present.
- **Cardiac glands** are lined by cells that are similar to mucous neck cells and those of the pyloric glands but lack G cells.

Congenital Disorders

Congenital Pyloric Stenosis Causes Projectile Vomiting in Infancy

Congenital pyloric stenosis is concentric enlargement of the pyloric sphincter and narrowing of the pyloric canal that obstructs the gastric outlet. ***This is the most common indication for abdominal surgery in the first 6 months of life.*** It is four times more common in boys than girls and affects first-born children more than subsequent ones. It occurs in 1 in 250 white infants but is rare in blacks and Asians.

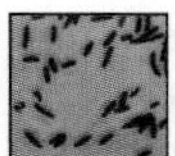

ETIOLOGIC FACTORS: Congenital pyloric stenosis may have a genetic basis; there is a familial tendency, and the condition is more common in identical twins than in fraternal ones. It also may occur together with other developmental abnormalities, such as Turner syndrome, trisomy 18 and esophageal atresia. Embryopathies due to rubella infection and maternal intake of thalidomide have also been associated with congenital pyloric stenosis. Congenital pyloric stenosis may occur with a deficiency of nitric oxide synthase in the nerves of pyloric smooth muscle (nitric oxide mediates relaxation of smooth muscle).

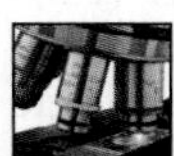

PATHOLOGY: The stomach shows concentric pyloric enlargement and narrowing of the pyloric canal. There is extreme hypertrophy of the circular muscle coat. After pyloromyotomy, the lesion disappears, although occasionally a small mass remains.

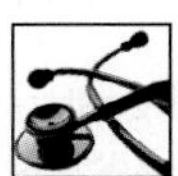

CLINICAL FEATURES: Projectile vomiting is the main symptom and is usually seen in the first month of life. Consequent loss of hydrochloric acid leads to hypochloremic alkalosis in one third of affected infants. A palpable pyloric lesion and visible peristalsis are common. Surgical incision of hypertrophied pyloric muscle is curative.

Congenital Diaphragmatic Hernia

Congenital diaphragmatic hernias of variable size and location are related to incomplete closure of embryologic foramina or abnormalities of the esophageal hiatus. Congenital malrotations of the intestine may occur simultaneously. The stomach, plus other abdominal organs, may eventrate into the thoracic cavity.

Congenital Abnormalities of the Stomach Are Rare

DUPLICATIONS, DIVERTICULA AND CYSTS: These lesions are usually lined by normal gastric mucosa and are distinctly uncommon. Whereas all layers of the stomach wall tend to be present in congenital duplications, muscle coats are often deficient in diverticula and cysts. Patients with these disorders are generally asymptomatic.

SITUS INVERSUS: This causes the stomach to be to the right of the midline, as is the esophageal hiatus. Correspondingly, the duodenum is on the left.

ECTOPIC PANCREATIC TISSUE: Nodules of pancreatic tissue are common in the wall of the antrum and pylorus. These embryonic rests are identical to normal pancreatic tissue, except that islets are rare. Heterotopic pancreatic tissue is usually asymptomatic, but pyloric obstruction and epigastric pain have been reported.

PARTIAL GASTRIC ATRESIAS: Lack of development of the body, antrum and pylorus has been described, as have cases in which the stomach ends blindly.

CONGENITAL PYLORIC AND ANTRAL MEMBRANES: These lesions are presumably caused by failure of the stomach to canalize during embryogenesis. They may cause obstruction in the neonatal period but more commonly become symptomatic in adults.

Acute Gastritis

Acute hemorrhagic erosive gastritis is characterized by mucosal necrosis, which may extend into the deeper tissues to form an ulcer. The necrosis is accompanied by an acute inflammatory response and hemorrhage, which may be severe enough to result in exsanguination.

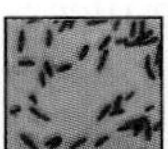

ETIOLOGIC FACTORS: All forms of acute hemorrhagic gastritis break down the mucosal barrier, permitting acid-induced injury. Acute hemorrhagic gastritis is most often associated with ingestion of aspirin, other nonsteroidal anti-inflammatory drugs (NSAIDs) or excess alcohol, or with ischemic injury. Oral corticosteroid use may also lead to acute hemorrhagic gastritis. Uncommonly, accidental or suicidal ingestion of corrosive substances, such as those that produce erosive esophagitis, causes acute gastric injury. Any serious illness (e.g., shock, uremia) that is accompanied by profound physiologic alterations renders the gastric mucosa more vulnerable to acute hemorrhagic gastritis because of mucosal ischemia.

Stress ulcers and erosions occur in severely burned persons **(Curling ulcer)** and commonly result in bleeding. Ulcers may be deep enough to cause perforation of the stomach. Patients occasionally have both gastric and duodenal ulcers.

Central nervous system trauma, accidental or surgical **(Cushing ulcer),** may also cause stress ulcers. These ulcers, which also may occur in the esophagus or duodenum, are characteristically deep and carry a substantial risk of perforation. Injury to the brain, particularly if it results in a decerebrate state, often increases gastric acid secretion, most likely due to increased vagal tone. **Severe trauma,** especially if accompanied by **shock, prolonged sepsis and incapacitation** from many debilitating chronic diseases, also predisposes to development of acute hemorrhagic gastritis.

Hypersecretion of gastric acid is often, but not always, at the root of acute hemorrhagic gastritis. Acid secretion is sometimes increased, as in neurologic trauma, but not with stress ulcers. Still, gastric acid secretion is felt to play a role, if not an obligatory one, in stress ulceration as blocking it (e.g., with histamine-receptor antagonists) is protective.

Microcirculatory changes in the stomach induced by shock or sepsis suggest that ischemic injury may contribute to development of acute hemorrhagic gastritis.

Each of these defensive factors of the gastric mucosa has been individually investigated:

- **Corticosteroids and aspirin** decrease mucus production and cause gastric ulcers after experimental administration.
- **Prostaglandin deficiency,** caused by nonsteroidal anti-inflammatory agents that inhibit prostaglandin synthesis, may decrease mucosal resistance to gastric contents. By contrast, certain prostaglandins that stimulate mucus secretion also protect against gastric erosions.
- **Renewal of gastric epithelium** is clearly necessary for healing erosions of any etiology. Chemotherapeutic agents that reduce cellular renewal may damage the gastric lining.
- **Increased intramural pH of the gastric mucosa** protects from gastric erosions in hemorrhagic shock. Thus, acid-induced damage to the gastric mucosa is important in the pathogenesis of certain erosions.

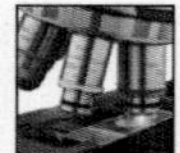

PATHOLOGY: Widespread petechial hemorrhages anywhere in the stomach, or regions of confluent mucosal or submucosal bleeding, are seen (Fig. 13-14). Lesions vary from 1 to 25 mm across and appear occasionally as sharply punched-out ulcers. Patchy mucosal necrosis, which can extend to the submucosa, occurs next to normal mucosa. Fibrinous exudate, hemorrhage and edema in the lamina propria are present in early lesions. Necrotic epithelium is eventually sloughed, but deeper erosions and hemorrhage may be present. In extreme cases, penetrating ulcers may reach the serosa.

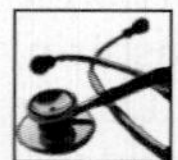

CLINICAL FEATURES: Symptoms of acute hemorrhagic gastritis range from vague abdominal discomfort to massive, life-threatening hemorrhage, or clinical manifestations of gastric perforation. Patients with gastritis due to aspirin and other nonsteroidal anti-inflammatory agents may be seen with hypochromic, microcytic anemia caused by undetected chronic bleeding. However, in patients with a severe underlying illness, the first sign of stress ulcers may be exsanguinating hemorrhage. Antacids and histamine-receptor antagonists may be effective.

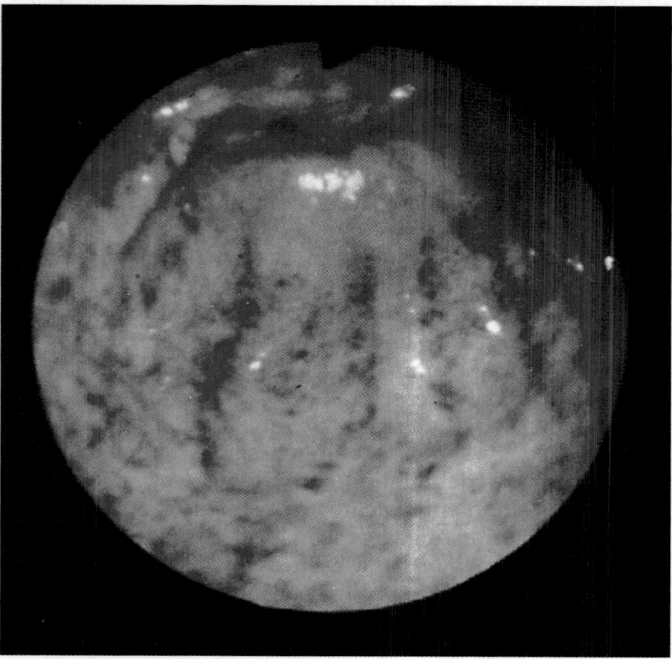

FIGURE 13-14. Erosive gastritis. This endoscopic view of the stomach in a patient who was ingesting aspirin reveals acute hemorrhagic lesions.

Chronic Gastritis

Chronic gastritis refers to chronic inflammatory diseases of the stomach, which range from mild superficial involvement of gastric mucosa to severe atrophy. This is a heterogeneous group of disorders with distinct anatomic distributions within the stomach, varying etiologies and characteristic complications. The predominant symptom is dyspepsia. The diseases are also commonly discovered in asymptomatic persons undergoing routine endoscopic screening.

Helicobacter pylori Is the Most Common Cause of Chronic Gastritis in the United States

Helicobacter pylori ***gastritis is a chronic inflammatory disease of the gastric body and antrum.*** *H. pylori* or, occasionally, *Helicobacter heilmannii,* are implicated. The organism affects nearly 70% of the world's population, in some regions approaching 90%, including children and adults. *H. pylori* is also strongly associated with atrophic gastritis, peptic ulcer disease of the stomach and duodenum, mucosa-associated lymphoid tissue (MALT) lymphoma and gastric carcinoma.

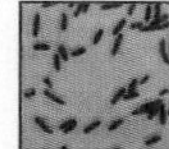

ETIOLOGIC FACTORS: *Helicobacter* are widely distributed, small, curved, gram-negative rods with polar flagella and a corkscrew-like motion (Proteobacteria). The prevalence of *H. pylori* infection increases with age: by age 60 years, half the population has serologic evidence of infection. Twin studies have shown genetic influences in susceptibility to *H. pylori* infection. Intrafamilial clustering suggests person-to-person spread. ***Two thirds of those infected with*** **H. pylori** ***show histologic evidence of chronic gastritis.***

H. pylori is felt to be responsible for chronic antral gastritis, rather than a commensal that colonizes injured gastric mucosa, because (1) gastritis develops in healthy people after they ingest the organism, (2) *H. pylori* attaches to the epithelium in areas of chronic gastritis and is absent from uninvolved areas of the gastric mucosa, (3) eradicating the infection with bismuth or antibiotics cures the gastritis, (4) antibodies against *H. pylori* are routinely found in people with chronic gastritis and (5) the increasing prevalence of *H. pylori* infection with age parallels that of chronic gastritis.

H. pylori is found only on the epithelial surface and does not invade. Its pathogenicity is related to the *cag* pathogenicity island in its genome—a horizontally acquired locus of 40 kb that contains 31 genes. This virulence marker is putatively associated with duodenal ulcer and gastric cancer. A separate region of the genome contains the gene for vacuolating cytotoxin (*vac A*), which is also associated with duodenal ulcer disease.

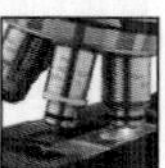

PATHOLOGY: In chronic active gastritis, polymorphonuclear leukocytes are seen in glands and their lumina and increased numbers of plasma cells and

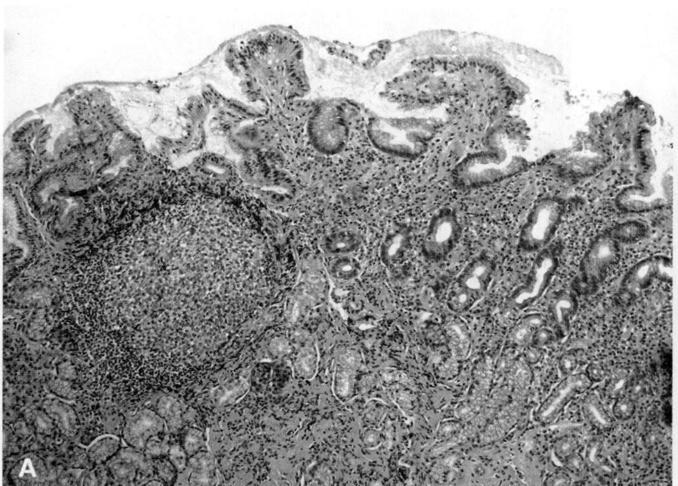
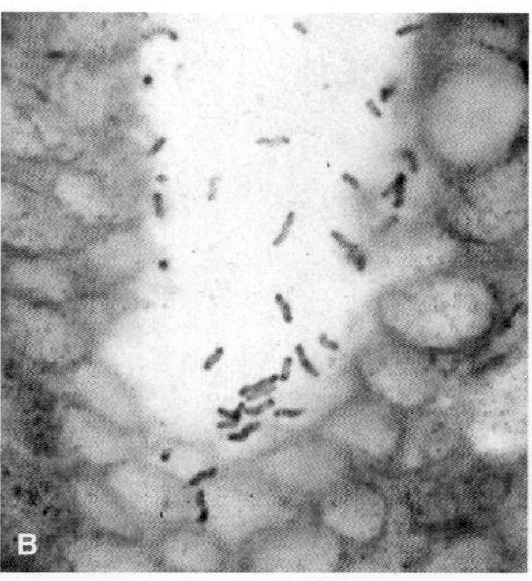

FIGURE 13-15. *Helicobacter pylori*–associated gastritis. A. The antrum shows an intense lymphocytic and plasma cell infiltrate, which tends to be heaviest in the superficial portions of the lamina propria. **B.** The microorganisms appear on silver staining as small, curved rods on the surface of the gastric mucosa.

lymphocytes are seen in the lamina propria (Fig. 13-15A). Lymphoid hyperplasia with germinal centers is frequent. The curved rods of *H. pylori* are found in the surface mucus of epithelial cells and in gastric foveolae (Fig. 13-15B). The less common *H. heilmannii* is long and has tight spirals, resembling a spirochete.

Nonatrophic and **atrophic** patterns of *H. pylori*–associated chronic gastritis are recognized, the most common being **nonatrophic antral-predominant gastritis,** which involves the antrum and spares the corpus. **Nonatrophic corpus-predominant gastritis** may follow long-term proton pump inhibitor use. **Nonatrophic pangastritis** is frequent in geographic areas of poor hygiene.

Atrophic forms of chronic gastritis feature reduction in the number of glands and intestinal metaplasia and include **antrum-restricted atrophic gastritis** and **multifocal atrophic gastritis (MAG),** although antral and multifocal forms of the disease may be different stages of the same disease. The factors that determine whether *H. pylori* gastritis is nonatrophic or atrophic are not clear, but the duration of the disease may play a role.

Multifocal Atrophic Gastritis (Environmental Metaplastic Atrophic Gastritis)

Multifocal atrophic gastritis typically involves the antrum and adjacent areas of the body.

- It is considerably more common than autoimmune atrophic gastritis (see below) and is four times as frequent among whites as in other races.
- It is not linked to autoimmune phenomena.
- Like autoimmune gastritis, it is associated with reduced acid secretion (hypochlorhydria).
- Complete absence of gastric secretion (achlorhydria) and pernicious anemia are uncommon.

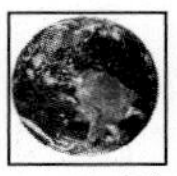

EPIDEMIOLOGY: The age and geographic distribution of environmental metaplastic atrophic gastritis parallel those of gastric carcinoma, and this type of gastritis seems to be a precursor of stomach cancer. Certain populations, particularly in Asia, Scandinavia and parts of Europe and Latin America, are disproportionately affected. It also increases in incidence with age in all populations in which it is prevalent. Offspring of emigrants from areas of high risk for stomach cancer to areas of low risk lose their predisposition to this tumor. Environmental etiologic factors include *H. pylori* and diet.

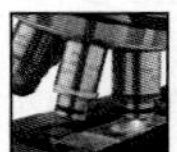

PATHOLOGY: *The pathology of autoimmune (see below) and multifocal atrophic gastritis is similar, except for the restricted localization of the autoimmune type to the fundus and body and of the multifocal variety mainly to the antrum and corpus.*

ATROPHIC GASTRITIS: This condition is characterized by chronic inflammation in the lamina propria. Occasionally, lymphoid cell follicles are misdiagnosed as lymphoma, especially in patients with *H. pylori* infection. Involvement of gastric glands leads to degenerative changes in their epithelial cells and ultimately to conspicuous reduction in the number of glands (thus the name **atrophic gastritis;** Fig. 13-16A). Eventually, inflammation may abate, leaving only thin atrophic mucosa, to which the term **gastric atrophy** is applied.

INTESTINAL METAPLASIA: This lesion is a common and important feature of both autoimmune and multifocal types of atrophic gastritis. In response to gastric mucosal injury, normal epithelium is replaced by intestinal-type cells (Fig. 13-16B). Many mucin-containing goblet cells and enterocytes line crypt-like glands. Paneth cells, which are not normal in the stomach, are present. Intestine-like villi may form. The metaplastic cells also contain enzymes characteristic of the intestine but not the stomach (e.g., alkaline phosphatase, aminopeptidase).

Atrophic Gastritis and Stomach Cancer

Patients with autoimmune (see below) or multifocal atrophic gastritis have greater risk of carcinoma of the stomach. Atrophic gastritis is usually asymptomatic and so does not ordinarily come under medical scrutiny, so this relationship is hard to quantify. However, patients with pernicious anemia, who invariably have atrophic gastritis, have a threefold higher

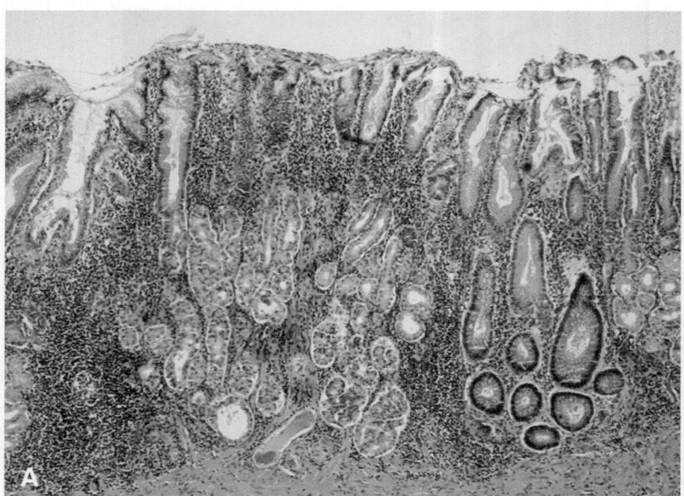

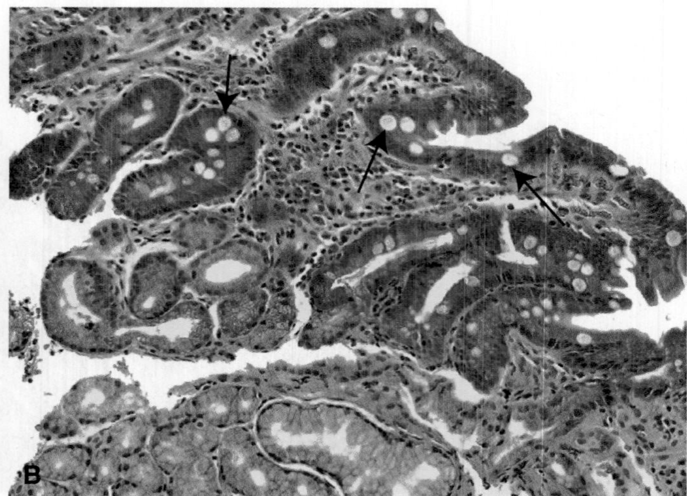

FIGURE 13-16. Multifocal atrophic gastritis. A. The gastric mucosa shows chronic inflammation within the lamina propria. The diminished number of antral glands indicates atrophy. **B.** The atrophic glands show goblet cells (*arrows*), and there is chronic inflammation in the lamina propria.

risk of gastric adenocarcinoma and a 13-fold higher risk of carcinoid (neuroendocrine) tumors. Cancer arises in the antrum several times more often than in the body of the stomach, suggesting that antral gastritis is related to gastric carcinogenesis.

Intestinal metaplasia of the stomach is a preneoplastic lesion because (1) gastric cancer arises in areas of such metaplasia, (2) half of all stomach cancers are of the intestinal cell type and (3) many gastric cancers show aminopeptidase activity like that seen in areas of intestinal metaplasia. Dysplasia, from low grade to carcinoma in situ, may be seen in metaplastic intestinal epithelium and is felt to be a precursor of invasive gastric cancer.

The Stomach Is the Most Common Extranodal Site of Lymphoma

Most gastric lymphomas are low-grade B-cell tumors of the mucosa-associated lymphoid tissue lymphoma **(MALToma)** type that arise in the setting of chronic *H. pylori* gastritis with lymphoid hyperplasia. Some MALTomas actually regress after the *H. pylori* infection is eradicated. Primary lymphoma of the stomach accounts for about 5% of all gastric malignancies and 20% of all extranodal lymphomas. Clinically and radiologically, it mimics gastric adenocarcinoma. Presenting symptoms, as with the latter, are usually weight loss, dyspepsia and abdominal pain. Age at diagnosis is usually 40 to 65 years and there is no sex predominance. The tumors, like carcinomas, may be polypoid, ulcerating or diffuse (Fig. 13-17A). Other histopathologic types resemble comparable primary nodal lymphomas. Molecular characteristics of MALT lymphomas are discussed in Chapter 20.

Autoimmune Atrophic Gastritis Is Related to Pernicious Anemia

Autoimmune atrophic gastritis is a chronic, diffuse inflammatory disease of the body and fundus of the stomach associated with autoimmunity. This disorder typically exhibits:

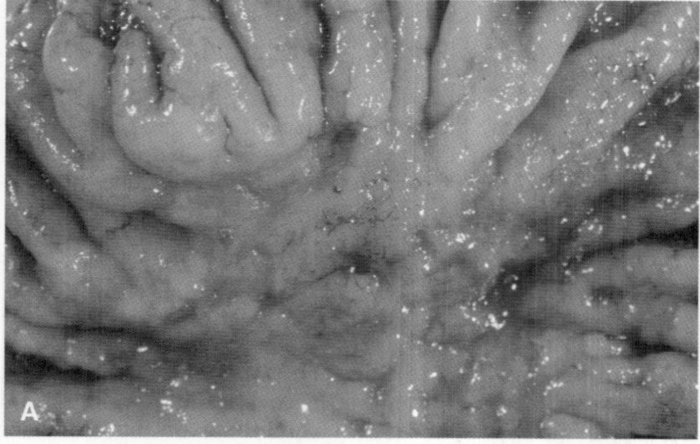

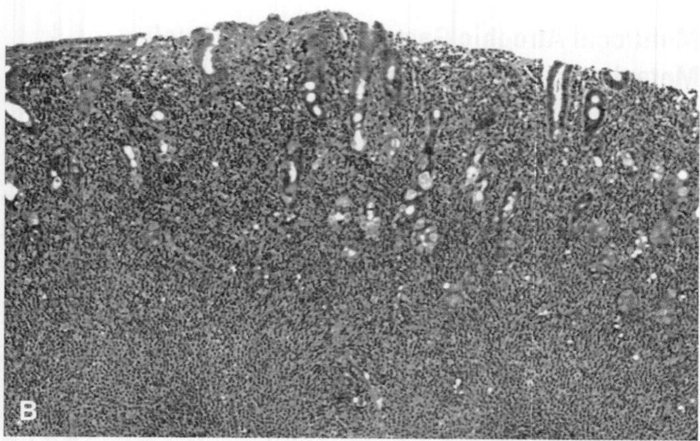

FIGURE 13-17. Mucosa-associated lymphoid tissue (MALT) lymphoma. A. There is loss of detail within the gastric mucosa as a MALT lymphoma infiltrates the mucosa over a large surface area, although a discrete mass was not formed. **B.** Microscopically, a monotonous population of lymphoid cells expands the lamina propria.

- Diffuse atrophic gastritis in the body and fundus of the stomach, with lack of, or minimal involvement of, the antrum
- Antibodies to parietal cells and intrinsic factor
- Significant reduction in or absence of gastric secretion, including acid (achlorhydria)
- Increased serum gastrin, owing to G-cell hyperplasia of the antral mucosa
- Enterochromaffin-like (ECL) cell hyperplasia in atrophic oxyntic mucosa, because of gastrin stimulation

Pernicious anemia ***is a megaloblastic anemia caused by malabsorption of vitamin B_{12} owing to a deficiency of intrinsic factor. It is usually a complication of autoimmune gastritis.*** The latter disorder is also associated with other autoimmune diseases such as chronic thyroiditis, Graves disease, Addison disease, vitiligo, diabetes mellitus type I and myasthenia gravis.

Like multifocal atrophic gastritis, autoimmune gastritis is a risk factor for development of dysplasia and adenocarcinoma. Up to 40% of patients with pernicious anemia have multiple sessile polyps, a minority of which show dysplasia. Achlorhydria leads to hypergastrinemia, which stimulates enterochromaffin cell proliferation, thus increasing the risk for malignant carcinoid tumors.

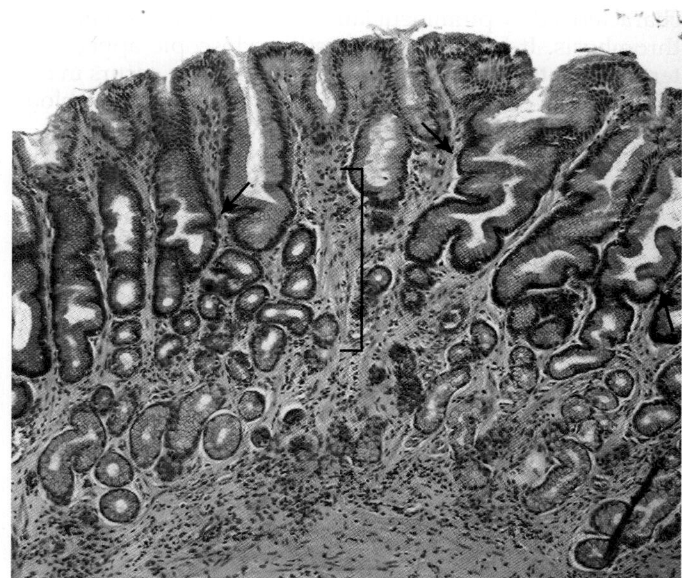

FIGURE 13-18. Reactive gastropathy. The antral mucosa shows serration of the fundic glands (*arrows*), mild acute and chronic inflammation and increased smooth muscle in the lamina propria (*bracket*).

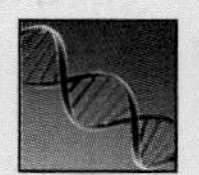

MOLECULAR PATHOGENESIS: Autoimmune gastritis reflects the presence of autoantibodies and is associated with other autoantibody-mediated diseases.

CYTOTOXIC ANTIBODIES: Circulating antibodies to parietal cells, some of which are cytotoxic in the presence of complement, occur in 90% of patients with pernicious anemia. Parietal cell autoantibodies react with α and β subunits of the proton pump (H^+/K^+-ATPase). This enzyme is the major protein of the secretory canaliculi of parietal cells and mediates secretion of H^+ in exchange for K^+. Importantly, some 20% of persons over 60 years of age have parietal cell antibodies, but few have pernicious anemia.

INTRINSIC FACTOR ANTIBODIES: Two additional types of autoantibodies to intrinsic factor are common in pernicious anemia. Two thirds of patients have an antibody to intrinsic factor that impedes its binding to vitamin B_{12}, preventing formation of the complex that is absorbed in the ileum. About half of patients with this antibody also have an antibody against the intrinsic factor–vitamin B_{12} complex that interferes with its absorption.

OTHER ANTIBODIES: Half of patients with pernicious anemia have circulating antibodies to thyroid tissue. Conversely, about one third of patients with chronic thyroiditis possess gastric autoantibodies.

Reactive (Chemical) Gastropathy Is Usually Due to Ingestion of Nonsteroidal Anti-Inflammatory Drugs (NSAIDs)

This disorder was first recognized in patients with bile reflux but is increasingly recognized with increasing frequency in association with chronic NSAID use. Bile reflux commonly occurs after a gastroduodenostomy or gastrojejunostomy, but can be seen in intact stomachs. Reactive gastropathy may be a manifestation of prolapse with mucosal trauma.

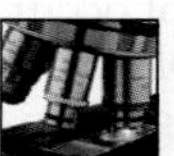

PATHOLOGY: The normal flat mucosal surface is replaced by villiform projections with fibromuscular proliferation in the lamina propria (Fig. 13-18). Surface foveolar cells show prominent reactive nuclear atypia out of proportion to the sparse inflammatory infiltrate. Unlike *H. pylori* gastritis, inflammation is minimal.

Other Forms of Chronic Gastritis Reflect Diverse Etiologies

Granulomatous gastritis may be caused by infection (e.g., *Mycobacterium tuberculosis,* fungus) or it may be a manifestation of systemic illness (e.g., sarcoidosis, Crohn disease). However, most cases of granulomatous gastritis are idiopathic.

In **eosinophilic gastritis,** which is often seen together with eosinophilic enteritis, eosinophils involve all layers of the stomach wall or are selectively localized in a single layer. Classically, the antrum and pylorus are mainly affected: diffuse thickening of the wall, presumably by muscular hypertrophy, may narrow the pylorus and cause symptoms of obstruction. These are occasionally severe enough as to require surgical relief. In some cases, ulceration in an affected area leads to chronic blood loss and anemia. Peripheral eosinophilia and a history of food allergies are common, but many patients have neither. Corticosteroid therapy is often effective.

Lymphocytic gastritis is characterized by prominent intraepithelial lymphocytes (>20 per 100 epithelial nuclei). It can be associated with celiac disease, but in most cases the etiology is unknown. Some cases may be related to prior *H. pylori* infection.

Vascular gastropathies include gastric antral vascular ectasia (GAVE) and portal hypertensive gastropathy. GAVE is characterized by prominent lamina propria vessels with focal thrombosis. It has a characteristic endoscopic appearance termed "watermelon stomach." GAVE mostly occurs in elderly patients and may be associated with significant blood loss.

Ménétrier Disease Causes Protein Loss

This disease (hyperplastic hypersecretory gastropathy) is an uncommon disorder characterized by enlarged gastric rugae. It is often accompanied by severe loss of plasma proteins (including albumin) from the altered gastric mucosa. A childhood form is due to cytomegalovirus infection; an adult form is attributed to overexpression of transforming growth factor-α (TGF-α).

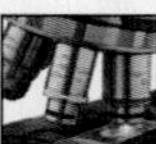

PATHOLOGY: The stomach in Ménétrier disease is enlarged. The folds of the greater curvature in the fundus and body of the stomach, and occasionally in the antrum, are taller and thicker, forming a convoluted brainlike surface (Fig. 13-19). Ménétrier disease is restricted to the oxyntic mucosa. Hyperplasia of the gastric pits results in a conspicuous increase in their depth and a tortuous (corkscrew) structure. Mucus-secreting cells of the surface or neck type line the foveolae. The glands are elongated. Many appear cystic and are lined by superficial-type, mucus-secreting epithelial cells rather than parietal and chief cells. The glands may penetrate the muscularis mucosae, like the sinuses of Rokitansky-Aschoff in the gallbladder. Pseudopyloric metaplasia may be seen, but intestinal metaplasia does not occur. Lymphocytes, plasma cells and occasional neutrophils are seen in the lamina propria. Concurrent lymphocytic gastritis is often present.

CLINICAL FEATURES: Ménétrier disease is four times more common in men than women and affects all ages. The presenting symptom is usually postprandial pain, relieved by antacids. Weight loss, sometimes of rapid onset, occurs occasionally. Peripheral edema is common. In some cases, ascites and cachexia, which are related to a loss of plasma proteins from the gastric mucosa, may suggest a malignancy. The cause of the enormous protein loss into the lumen of the stomach is unclear, but treatment with anticholinergic agents or an inhibitor of acid secretion may be successful. Gastric acidity is usually low, but severe peptic ulceration associated with hyperacidity is occasionally observed.

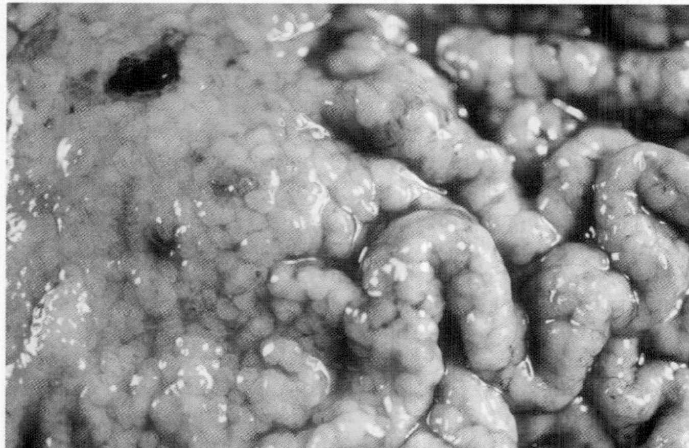

FIGURE 13-19. Ménétrier disease. The folds of the stomach are increased in height and thickness, forming a convoluted surface that has been likened to those of the cerebrum.

The disease does not usually resolve spontaneously in adults, and partial gastrectomy is necessary in intractable cases. ***It is considered a precancerous condition, and regular endoscopy is recommended.***

Peptic Ulcer Disease

"Peptic ulcer disease" refers to focal destruction of gastric mucosa and small intestine, mainly the proximal duodenum, caused by gastric secretions. About 10% of people in Western industrialized countries may develop such ulcers at some time during their lives. However, both the incidence and prevalence of duodenal ulcers have declined greatly during the past 30 years.

Although peptic ulceration can occur as high as Barrett esophagus and as low as Meckel diverticulum with gastric heterotopia, ***for practical purposes, the disease affects the distal stomach and proximal duodenum.*** Many clinical and epidemiologic features distinguish gastric from duodenal ulcers; ***the common factors that unite them are gastric hydrochloric acid secretion and* H. pylori *infection.***

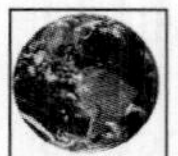

EPIDEMIOLOGY: The peak age for peptic ulcer disease has progressively increased in the past 50 years, and for duodenal ulcer disease it is now between 30 and 60 years of age, although it may occur at any age, even infancy. Gastric ulcers mainly afflict the middle-aged and elderly. Duodenal ulcers are more common in males, but gastric ulcers affect the sexes equally.

Racial differences in the incidence of peptic ulcers have been noted, but studies of different ethnic populations are confounded by variations in many other environmental factors. For example, in Africa, duodenal ulcers are rare among blacks, but in the United States the incidence is similar in blacks and whites. Most data suggest that all ethnic groups are susceptible in an urban Western setting. Surveys in the United States and Great Britain suggest a trend toward an inverse relation between duodenal ulcers and socioeconomic status and education.

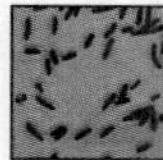

ETIOLOGIC FACTORS: Many etiologies have been suggested in the pathogenesis of peptic ulcers in the duodenum and stomach, but no single agent seems to be responsible.

HELICOBACTER PYLORI INFECTION: H. pylori *is isolated from the gastric antrum of virtually all patients with duodenal ulcers.* The converse is not true; that is, only a small minority of those carrying the bacterium have duodenal ulcer disease. Thus, *H. pylori* infection may be necessary, but not sufficient, for development of peptic duodenal ulcers. ***Such ulcers heal more quickly after treatment for* H. pylori *infection and recur less.***

Just how *H. pylori* infection predisposes to duodenal ulcers is not completely known, but several mechanisms have been proposed. Cytokines produced by inflammatory cells that respond to the infection stimulate gastrin release and suppress somatostatin secretion. Interleukin (IL)-1β, an acid inhibitor, has also emerged as an important mediator of inflammation in *H. pylori*–infected gastric mucosa. These effects, together with release of histamine metabolites from the organism itself, may stimulate basal gastric acid secretion. In addition, luminal cytokines from the stomach may enter and injure duodenal epithelium. There is evidence that *H. pylori* infection blocks inhibitory signals from the antrum to the G cells and the parietal cell region, increasing gastrin release and impairing inhibition of gastric acid secretion. Such an effect might increase acid load in the duodenum, thereby contributing to duodenal ulceration. ***Acidification of the duodenal bulb leads to islands of metaplastic gastric mucosa in the duodenum in many patients with peptic ulcers.*** Such gastric epithelium in the duodenum is sometimes colonized with *H. pylori,* like the gastric mucosa, and infection of the metaplastic epithelium by *H. pylori* may render the mucosa more susceptible to peptic injury (Fig. 13-20).

H. pylori ***infection is probably also important in the pathogenesis of gastric ulcers, because the organism is responsible for most cases of the chronic gastritis that underlies this disease.*** About 75% of patients with gastric ulcers harbor *H. pylori.* The remaining 25% of cases may represent an association with other types of chronic gastritis. The various gastric and duodenal factors that have been implicated as possible mechanisms in the pathogenesis of duodenal ulcers are summarized in Fig. 13-21.

HYDROCHLORIC ACID SECRETION: ***Hyperacidity owing to increased hydrochloric acid secretion is necessary for formation and persistence of peptic ulcers in the stomach and duodenum.*** This is evidenced principally by (1) all patients with duodenal ulcers and almost all with gastric ulcers are gastric acid secretors; (2) experimental ulcer production in animals requires acid; (3) hypersecretion of acid is present in many, but not all, patients with duodenal ulcers (there is no evidence that acid overproduction alone explains duodenal ulceration); and (4) surgical or medical treatment that reduces acid production results in the healing of peptic ulcers. Gastric secretion of pepsin, which may also play a role in peptic ulceration, parallels that of hydrochloric acid.

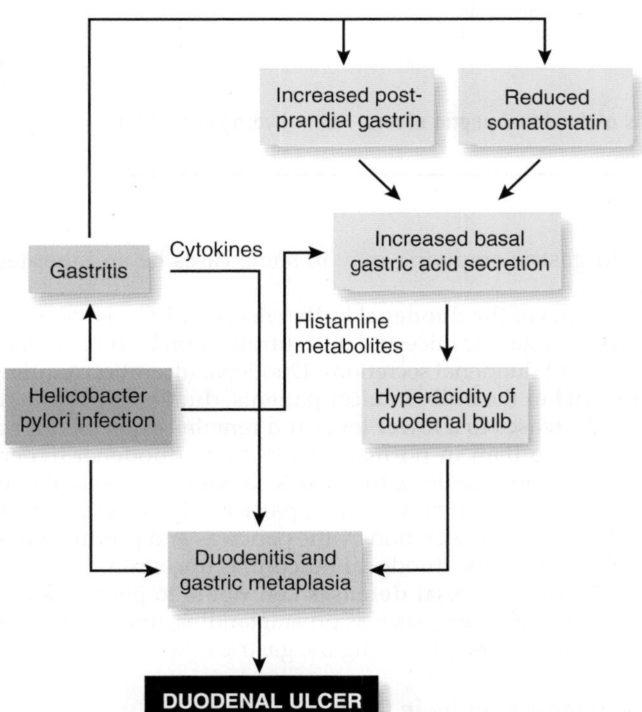

FIGURE 13-20. Possible mechanisms in the pathogenesis of duodenal ulcer disease associated with *Helicobacter pylori* infection.

DIET: Despite the folk wisdom that spicy food and caffeine are ulcerogenic, there is little evidence that any food or beverage, including coffee and alcohol, contributes to the development or persistence of peptic ulcers.

DRUGS: **Aspirin** is an important contributor to duodenal, and especially gastric, ulcers. **Other nonsteroidal anti-inflammatory agents and analgesics** have been incriminated in production of peptic ulcers. Prolonged treatment with high doses of corticosteroids may also increase the risk of peptic ulceration slightly.

CIGARETTE SMOKING: Smoking is a definite risk factor for duodenal and gastric ulcers, particularly gastric ulcers.

GENETIC FACTORS: First-degree relatives of people with duodenal or gastric ulcers have a threefold higher risk of developing an ulcer, but only at the same site. Monozygotic twins show much higher concordance for these ulcers than do dizygotic twins, but even that 50% concordance indicates that environmental factors must also be involved.

The role of genetic factors is further supported by the fact that **blood-group antigens** correlate with peptic ulcer disease. Duodenal ulcers are 30% more likely in people with type O blood than in those with other types. This does not hold for gastric ulcers. People who do not secrete blood-group antigens in saliva or gastric juice have a 50% greater risk of duodenal ulcers. Those who are both blood group O and nonsecretors (10% of white people) have a 2.5-fold increase in duodenal ulcers.

Pepsinogen I is secreted by gastric chief and mucous neck cells and appears in gastric juice, blood and urine. Serum levels of this proenzyme correlate with the capacity for gastric acid secretion and are a measure of parietal cell mass. ***Someone with high blood pepsinogen I levels has five times the normal risk of developing a duodenal ulcer.*** Hyperpepsinogenemia I occurs in half of children of ulcer patients with hyperpepsinogenemia and has been attributed to autosomal dominant inheritance. Thus, hyperpepsinogenemia may reflect an inherited tendency to have increased parietal cell mass.

Familial tendencies for other features are reported in ulcer patients. Many such patients have normal pepsinogen I secretion and still show familial aggregation. Family clustering of duodenal ulcers and rapid gastric emptying have been noted, as has familial hyperfunction of antral G cells. Patients with a childhood duodenal ulcer are much more likely to have a family history of ulcers than persons in whom the disease begins when they are adults.

Physiologic Factors in Duodenal Ulcers

Maximal capacity for gastric acid production is a function of total parietal cell mass. Patients with duodenal ulcers may have up to double normal parietal cell mass and maximal acid secretion. ***However, there is a large overlap with normal values, and only one third of ulcer patients secrete excess acid.*** Increased chief cell mass often accompanies increased parietal cells, reflecting the prevalence of hyperpepsinogenemia in patients with ulcers.

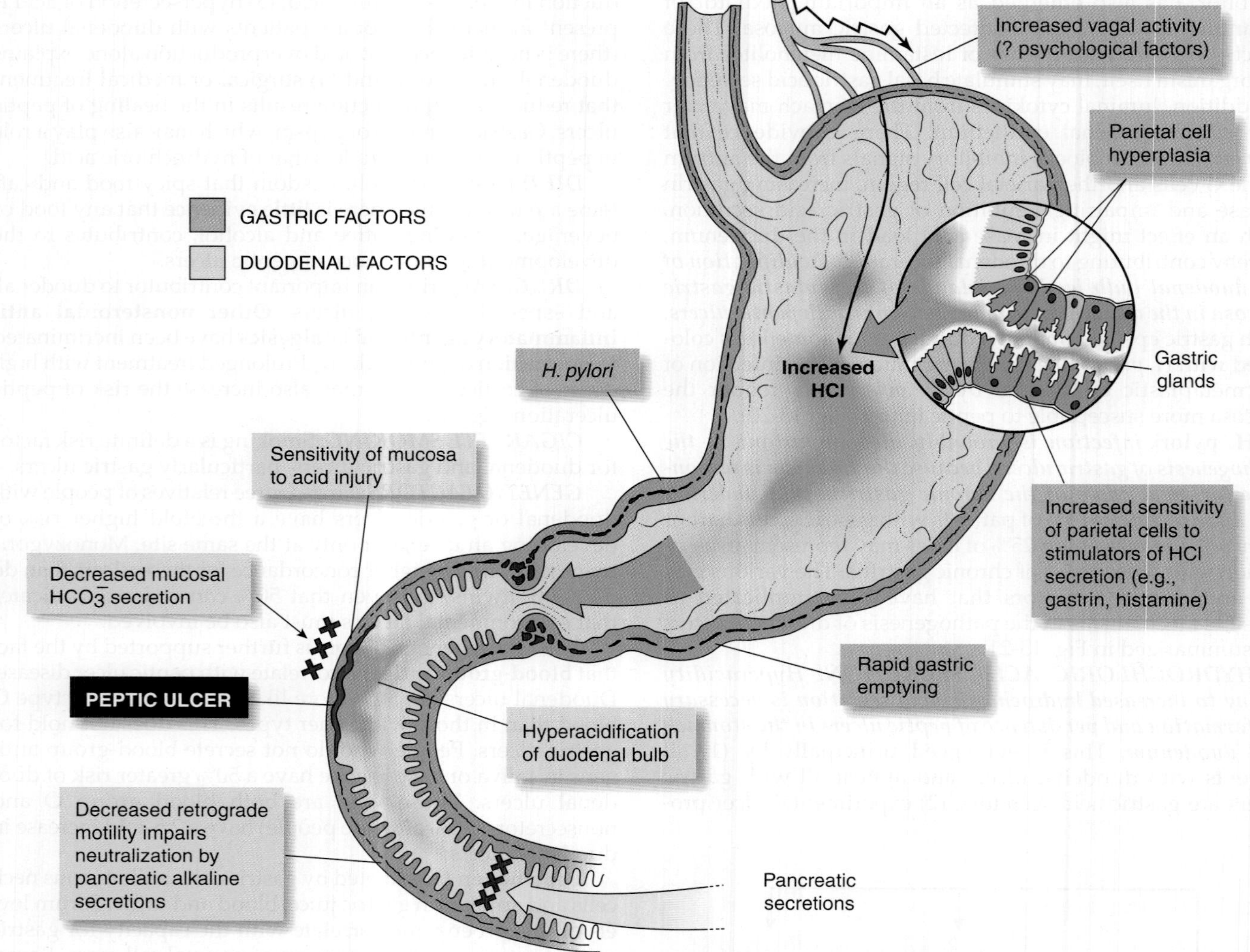

FIGURE 13-21. Gastric and duodenal factors in the pathogenesis of duodenal peptic ulcers. HCl = hydrochloric acid; HCO_3 = bicarbonate.

Food-stimulated gastric acid secretion is increased in magnitude and duration in people with duodenal ulcers, but here, too, there is significant overlap with normal values. This may involve, at least in part, altered G-cell responses to meals. Such patients show postprandial hypergastrinemia and increased numbers of antral G cells. Most people with duodenal ulcers, however, show no evidence of G-cell hyperfunction.

Acid secretion in people with duodenal ulcers may also be more sensitive than normal to gastric secretagogues such as gastrin, possibly owing to increased vagal tone or increased affinity of parietal cells for gastrin. It is further possible that brisk secretion of acid after a meal is stimulated by increased vagal tone.

Accelerated gastric emptying has been noted in patients with duodenal ulcers. This might lead to excessive acidification of the duodenum. However, as with other factors, there is overlap with normal rates. Normally, duodenal bulb acidification inhibits further gastric emptying, but not in most patients with duodenal ulcer. In them, duodenal acidification leads to continued, rather than delayed, gastric emptying. Rapid gastric emptying may in some cases be an inherited trait.

The pH of the duodenal bulb reflects the balance between delivery of gastric juice and its neutralization by biliary, pancreatic and duodenal secretions. Duodenal ulceration requires acidic pH in the bulb. In ulcer patients, duodenal pH after a meal decreases to a lower level and remains depressed for a longer time than in normal people. Such duodenal hyperacidity certainly reflects the gastric factors discussed above. The role of neutralizing factors, particularly secretin-stimulated bicarbonate secretion by the pancreas and production of bicarbonate by the duodenal mucosa, is uncertain.

Impaired mucosal defenses contribute to peptic ulceration. Mucosal factors, such as prostaglandins, may or may not be similar to those protecting the gastric mucosa (see above).

Physiologic Factors in Gastric Ulcers

Gastric ulcers almost invariably arise in the setting of epithelial injury by **H. pylori** *or chemical gastritis.* Just how chronic gastritis predisposes to gastric ulceration is obscure. *Most*

patients with gastric ulcers secrete less acid than do those with duodenal ulcers and even less than normal people. Factors implicated include (1) back-diffusion of acid into the mucosa, (2) decreased parietal cell mass and (3) abnormalities of parietal cells themselves. A few gastric ulcer patients produce excess acid. Their ulcers are usually near the pylorus and are considered variants of duodenal ulcers. Interestingly, intense gastric hypersecretion such as occurs in the Zollinger-Ellison syndrome (see below) is associated with severe ulceration of the duodenum and even the jejunum but rarely of the stomach.

The concurrence of gastric ulcers and gastric hyposecretion implies (1) the gastric mucosa may in some way be particularly sensitive to low concentrations of acid, (2) something other than acid may damage the mucosa (e.g., NSAIDs) or (3) the gastric mucosa may be exposed to potentially injurious agents for unusually long periods. As discussed above, the mucosal barrier to the action of acid and perhaps to other contents of the stomach may be impaired in some patients with gastric ulcers, although evidence is not conclusive. Bile reflux (particularly deoxycholic acid and lysolecithin) and pancreatic secretions have been suggested as causes of gastric ulcers.

Diseases Associated With Peptic Ulcers

CIRRHOSIS: Duodenal ulcers occur 10 times more frequently in patients with cirrhosis than in normal individuals.

CHRONIC RENAL FAILURE: End-stage renal disease with hemodialysis increases the risk of peptic ulceration. Patients with kidney transplants also show a much higher incidence of peptic ulceration and its complications, such as bleeding and perforation.

HEREDITARY ENDOCRINE SYNDROMES: There is an increased frequency of peptic ulcers in people with **multiple endocrine neoplasia type I** (see Chapter 21). **Zollinger-Ellison syndrome,** a cause of severe peptic ulceration, is characterized by gastric hypersecretion caused by a gastrin-producing islet cell adenoma of the pancreas.

α_1-ANTITRYPSIN DEFICIENCY: Almost one third of patients with this disease have peptic ulcers, and the incidence is even higher if they also have lung disease. Moreover, peptic ulcer is increased in people heterozygous for mutant α_1-antitrypsin.

CHRONIC LUNG DISEASE: Long-standing pulmonary dysfunction significantly raises the risk of ulcers. One fourth of those with such disorders have peptic ulcer disease. Conversely, chronic lung disease is increased two- to three-fold in people with peptic ulcers.

PATHOLOGY: Most peptic ulcers arise in the lesser gastric curvature, in the antral and prepyloric regions and in the first part of the duodenum.

Gastric ulcers (Fig. 13-22) are usually single and smaller than 2 cm in diameter. Ulcers on the lesser curvature are often associated with chronic gastritis; those on the greater curvature are commonly related to NSAIDs. Edges tend to be sharply punched out, with overhanging margins. Deeply penetrating ulcers produce a serosal exudate that may cause the stomach to adhere to nearby structures. Scarring of ulcers in the prepyloric region may be severe enough to produce pyloric stenosis. ***Grossly, chronic peptic ulcers may resemble ulcerated gastric carcinomas.*** The endoscopist must therefore take multiple biopsies from the edges and bed of any gastric ulcer because the centers of the lesions usually show only necrotic tissue.

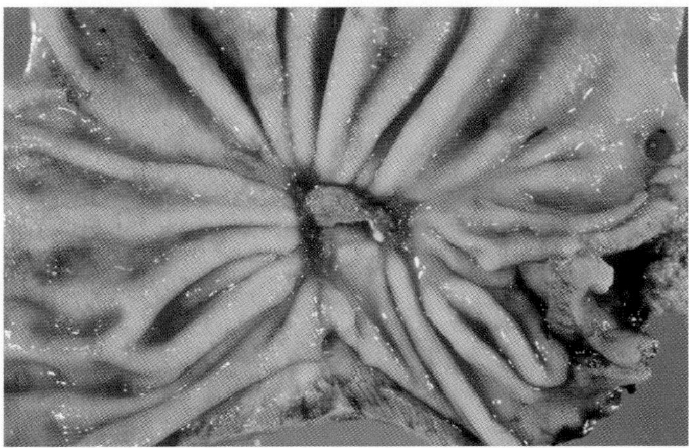

FIGURE 13-22. Gastric ulcer. There is a characteristic sharp demarcation from the surrounding mucosa, with radiating gastric folds. The base of the ulcer is gray owing to fibrin deposition.

Duodenal ulcers (Fig. 13-23) are ordinarily on the anterior or posterior wall of the first part of the duodenum, close to the pylorus. Lesions are usually solitary, but it is not uncommon to find paired ulcers on both walls, so-called kissing ulcers.

Gastric and duodenal ulcers are histologically similar (Fig. 13-24). From the lumen outward, there are (1) a superficial zone of fibrinopurulent exudate, (2) necrotic tissue, (3) granulation tissue and (4) fibrotic tissue with variable degrees of chronic inflammation at the ulcer's base. Ulceration may penetrate muscle layers, interrupting them with scar tissue after healing. Blood vessels at the margins of the ulcer are often thrombosed. The mucosa at the margins tends to be hyperplastic. With healing, it grows over the ulcerated area as a single epithelial layer. Duodenal ulcers are usually accompanied by peptic duodenitis, with Brunner gland hyperplasia and gastric mucin cell metaplasia.

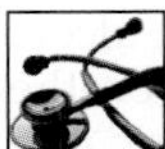

CLINICAL FEATURES: The symptoms of gastric and duodenal ulcers are so similar that the two conditions are generally not distinguishable by history

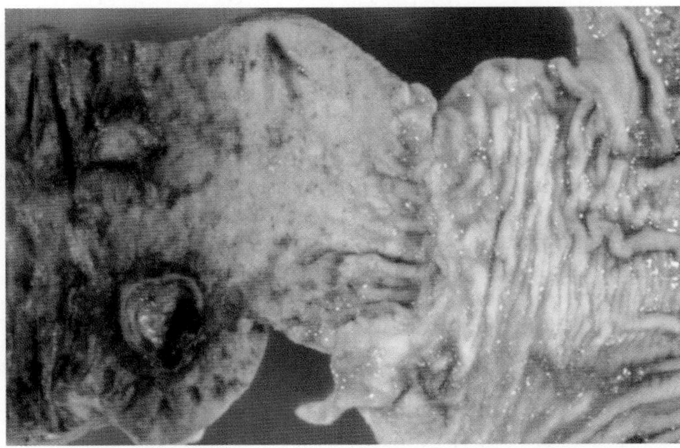

FIGURE 13-23. Duodenal ulcers. There are two sharply demarcated duodenal ulcers surrounded by inflamed duodenal mucosa. The gastroduodenal junction is in the midportion of the photograph.

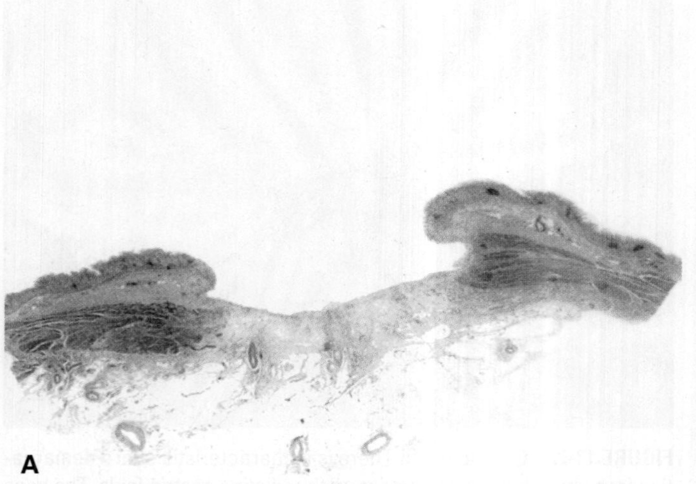

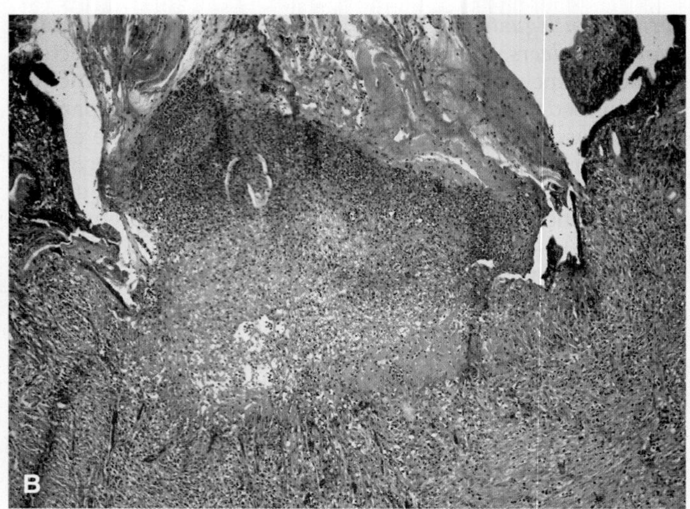

FIGURE 13-24. Gastric ulcer. A. There is full-thickness replacement of the gastric muscularis with connective tissue. **B.** Photomicrograph of a peptic ulcer with superficial exudate over necrosis, granulation tissue and fibrosis.

or physical examination. The classic duodenal ulcer is characterized by epigastric pain 1 to 3 hours after a meal, or that awakens a patient at night. Alkali and food relieve these symptoms. Dyspeptic symptoms commonly associated with gallbladder disease, including fatty food intolerance, distention and belching, occur in half of patients with peptic ulcers. The major complications of peptic ulcer disease are hemorrhage, perforation with peritonitis and obstruction.

HEMORRHAGE: The most common complication of peptic ulcers, occurring in up to 20% of patients, is bleeding. It is often occult and, if there are no other symptoms, may manifest as iron-deficiency anemia or occult blood in stools. ***Massive life-threatening bleeding is a well-known complication of active peptic ulcers.***

PERFORATION: Perforation is a serious complication that occurs in 5% of patients; in one third of cases, there are no antecedent symptoms of a peptic ulcer. Duodenal ulcers perforate more often than do gastric ulcers, mostly on the anterior wall of the duodenum. As the anterior gastric and duodenal walls are undefended by contiguous tissue, perforations there are more likely to lead to generalized peritonitis and accumulation of air in the abdominal cavity, called **pneumoperitoneum.** Posterior gastric ulcers perforate into the lesser peritoneal sac, where inflammation may be contained. An ulcer that penetrates the pancreas, liver or greater omentum can cause intractable symptoms. Ulcers may also penetrate the biliary tract and fill it with air.

Perforation carries a high mortality rate, which is 10% to 40% for gastric ulcers, two to four times more than for duodenal ulcers (10%). Perforations may be complicated by hemorrhage. Shock, abdominal distention, and pain are common symptoms, but perforations are occasionally diagnosed for the first time at autopsy, particularly in institutionalized, elderly patients.

PYLORIC OBSTRUCTION (GASTRIC OUTLET OBSTRUCTION): Pyloric obstruction occurs in up to 10% of ulcer patients, and peptic ulcer disease is its most common cause in adults. Narrowing of the pyloric lumen by an adjacent peptic ulcer may be caused by muscular spasm, edema, muscular hypertrophy or contraction of scar tissue, or, most commonly, a combination of these. Eventually obstruction may ensue.

DEVELOPMENT OF COMBINED ULCERS: Gastric and duodenal ulcers may occur together in the same patient far more often than can be accounted for by chance alone. Patients with either one have a much greater risk of developing the other later.

MALIGNANT TRANSFORMATION OF BENIGN GASTRIC ULCERS: It is very difficult to distinguish a cancer arising in a preexisting gastric ulcer from an ulcerated primary carcinoma. In contrast, ***malignant transformation of a duodenal ulcer is very uncommon.*** Still, gastric cancers originating in benign peptic ulcers are well known but are infrequent, probably representing fewer than 1% of all malignant tumors in the stomach.

TREATMENT: Peptic ulcers are now cured using antibiotics to eliminate *H. pylori* and blocking gastric acid secretion with histamine-receptor blockers and proton pump inhibitors.

Benign Neoplasms

Gastrointestinal Stromal Tumors (GISTs) in the Stomach Tend to Be Nonaggressive

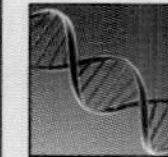

MOLECULAR PATHOGENESIS: GISTs occur in the stomach, small and large intestines and, rarely, extragastrointestinal sites. Nearly all such tumors are derived from the **pacemaker cells of Cajal.** GISTs are the vast majority of mesenchymal-derived stromal tumors of the entire gastrointestinal tract. Pacemaker cells and the tumor cells express c-*kit* oncogene (CD117) that encodes a tyrosine kinase that regulates cell proliferation and apoptosis. About 80% of GISTs have a gain-of-function mutation in c-*kit*. About 10% of GISTs have an activating mutation of the platelet-derived growth factor receptor-α (PDGFRα).

The criteria for assessing aggressive behavior in all GISTs include size, necrosis and mitotic activity. Interestingly, many

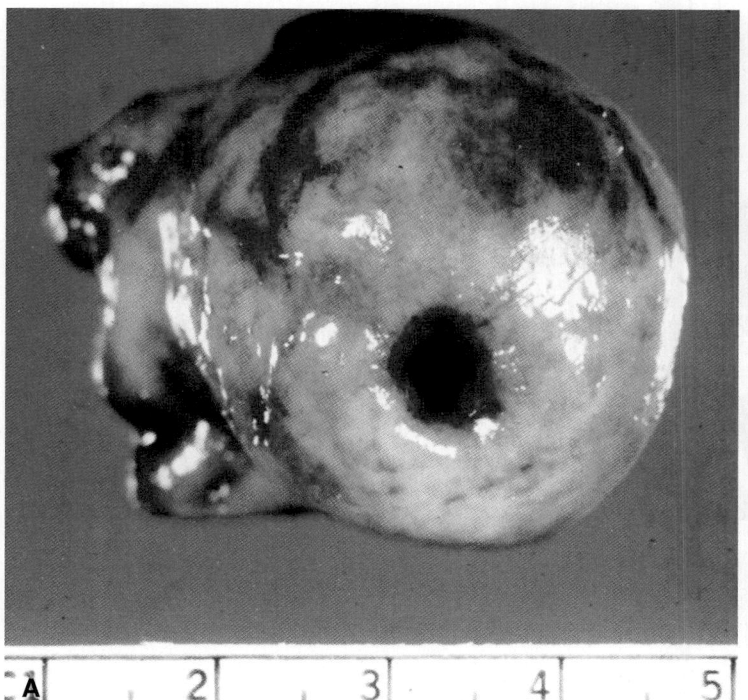

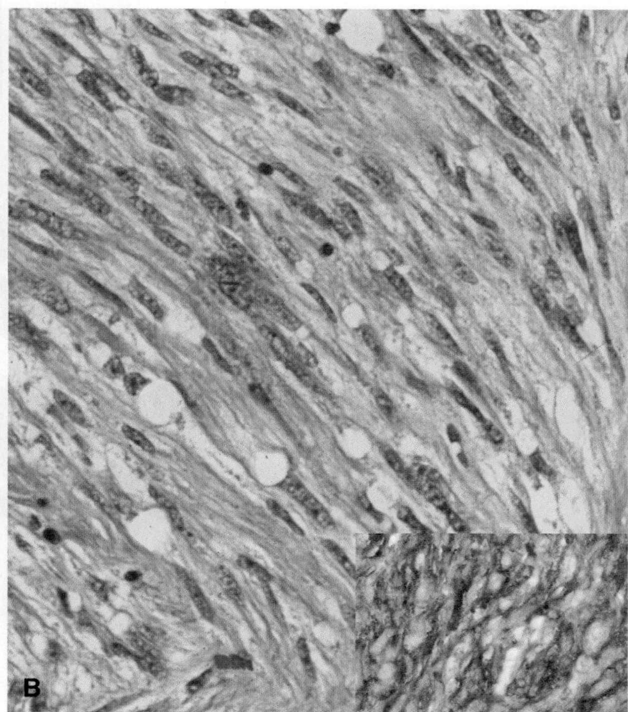

FIGURE 13-25. A. Gastrointestinal stromal tumor of the stomach. The resected tumor is submucosal and covered by a focally ulcerated mucosa. **B.** Microscopic examination of the tumor shows spindle cells with vacuolated cytoplasms. *Inset.* Immunohistochemical staining for c-*kit*.

gastric GISTs, independent of size, tend to behave in an indolent fashion, whereas those of the small and large bowel are more commonly aggressive.

Gastric GISTs are usually submucosal (Fig. 13-25A) and covered by intact mucosa or, when they project externally, by peritoneum. The cut surface is whorled. They are variably cellular. Spindle-shaped cells in whorls and interlacing bundles and with cytoplasmic vacuoles are embedded in a collagenous stroma (Fig. 13-25B). Bizarre and giant nuclei are common in benign tumors. GISTs can also appear more epithelioid, with polygonal cells that have eosinophilic cytoplasm. In most cases, immunostaining showing overexpression of c-*kit* is diagnostic.

With few exceptions, gastric GISTs are tumors of low malignant potential. Treatment consists mainly of surgical resection and treatment with imatinib, which inhibits the tyrosine kinase activity of c-*kit* and PDGFRA.

Gastric Epithelial Polyps Are Usually Benign

HYPERPLASTIC POLYPS: These most common of gastric polyps may be single or multiple, pedunculated or sessile lesions of variable sizes. Hyperplastic polyps are common in the atrophic oxyntic mucosa of the body and fundus of patients with autoimmune metaplastic atrophic gastritis, but also occur in the antrum of patients with *H. pylori* gastritis. These polyps show elongated, branched crypts lined by foveolar epithelium, beneath which pyloric or gastric glands are present (Fig. 13-26A). ***They appear to represent a response to injury. Their epithelium is not dysplastic, and gastric hyperplastic polyps have no malignant potential.***

TUBULAR ADENOMAS (ADENOMATOUS POLYPS): These are true neoplasms that occur mostly in the antrum (Fig. 13-26B). They vary from less than 1 cm to a considerable size. Many are about 4 cm. Most are sessile and solitary. Tubular adenomas show tubular structures or a combination of tubular and villous structures. Glands are usually lined by dysplastic epithelium, which is sometimes intestinalized. ***Adenomatous polyps may become malignant, variably reported at 5% to 75%.*** This risk increases with the size of the polyp and is greatest for lesions over 2 cm. Dysplasia can also occur in flat gastric mucosa. ***Patients with familial adenomatous polyposis with multiple tubular adenomas are at greatly increased risk of adenocarcinoma.***

FUNDIC GLAND POLYPS: Fundic gland polyps contain dilated oxyntic glands lined by parietal and chief cells and by mucous cell metaplasia (Fig. 13-26C). They were first noted in patients with familial polyposis but now are mostly seen in patients treated with proton pump inhibitors. The carry no increased risk of gastric carcinoma.

Malignant Tumors

Carcinoma of the Stomach Relates to Many Environmental Factors

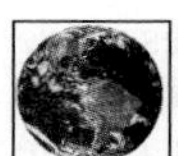

EPIDEMIOLOGY: As recently as the mid-20th century, gastric carcinoma was the most common cause of cancer death in men in the United States, but now accounts for only about 3% of cancer deaths in the United States. It remains exceedingly common in such countries as Japan and Chile, where rates are seven to eight times that in the United States. The incidence of cancer of the stomach declines in emigrants from high-risk to low-risk areas (see Chapter 5),

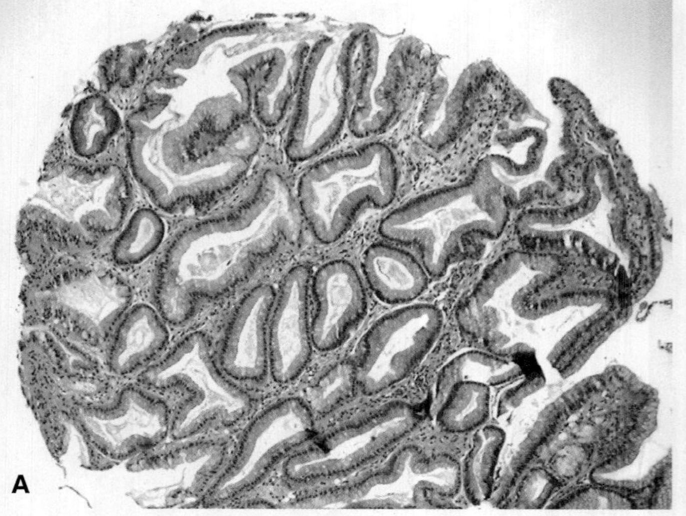

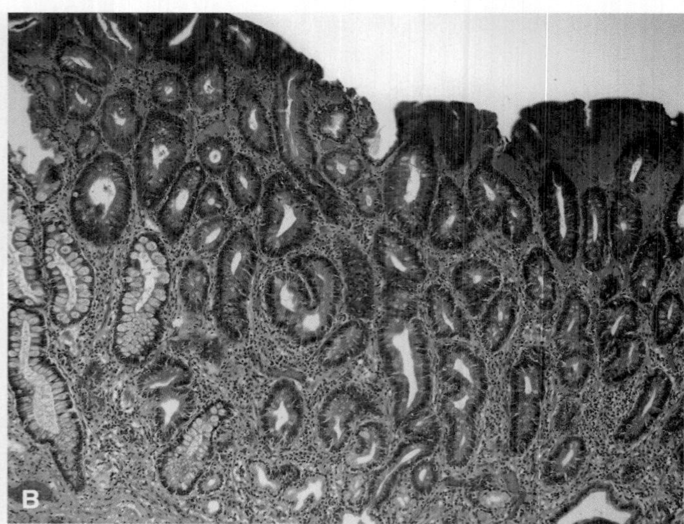

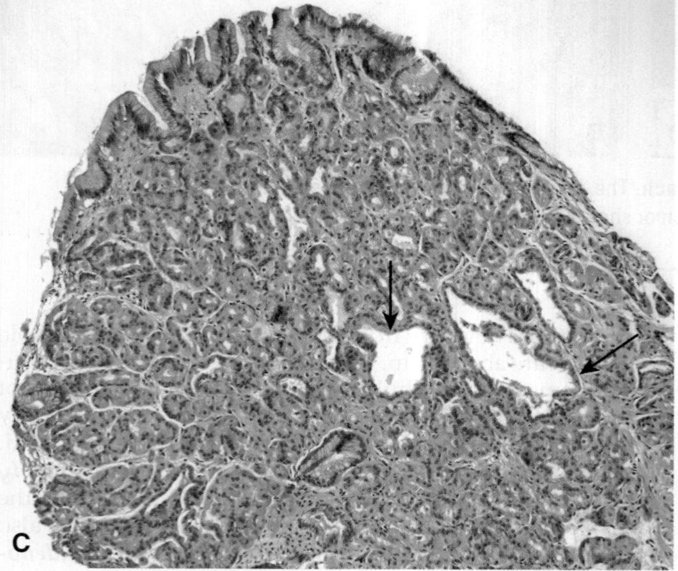

FIGURE 13-26. Gastric polyps. A. Hyperplastic polyp. Tortuous and hyperplastic foveolar glands form the polyp. There is mild inflammation between the glands. **B. Tubular adenoma.** Dysplastic glands predominate. Note the background of intestinal metaplasia (*left*). Adenomas provide fertile soil for the development of adenocarcinoma. **C. Fundic gland polyp.** These polyps display a marked increase in the number of oxyntic glands and atrophic foveolar epithelium, with occasional cystic dilation (*arrows*).

which strongly implicates environmental factors in its gastric carcinogenesis. Worldwide, gastric cancer is the fourth most common cancer and is the second most frequent cause of cancer deaths. About 800,000 people die yearly from this tumor.

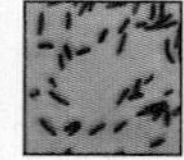

ETIOLOGIC FACTORS: No single factor explains gastric cancer, but important associations are evident.

HELICOBACTER PYLORI: **H. pylori infection is probably the most important causative agent for stomach cancer and is implicated in about two thirds of cases.** ***Serologic studies show a high prevalence of gastric infection with*** **H. pylori** ***many years before a stomach cancer is detected.*** People who are seropositive for *H. pylori* are three times more likely than are seronegative persons to develop gastric adenocarcinoma in the ensuing 1 to 24 years. In view of the observation that risk of stomach cancer is determined largely by environmental factors in the first decades of life (see below), it is noteworthy that populations at high risk for this tumor show a high prevalence of childhood *H. pylori* infection, while those at low risk do not. However, gastric cancer develops in only a small proportion of persons infected with *H. pylori,* and some tumors occur in uninfected people.

SMOKING: Cigarette smoking is a risk factor for gastric carcinoma. The relative risk for developing the tumor increases with the amount of cigarettes smoked and the duration of the habit. The magnitude of the increase in risk is about 50% and is more pronounced for tumors of the cardia than for tumors of the more distal stomach.

DIETARY FACTORS AND NITROSAMINES: Gastric cancer is more common among people who eat large amounts of starch, smoked or cured fish and meat and pickled vegetables. In particular, a possible role of nitrosamines, which are powerful carcinogens in animals but are of uncertain carcinogenicity in humans, has been suggested. Dietary nitrites and nitrates (which are converted to nitrates both enzymatically by *H. pylori* and other bacteria and nonenzymatically) are converted to nitrosamines. The role of these compounds in human gastric cancer remains unclear.

Consumption of whole milk and fresh vegetables rich in vitamin C and other antioxidants is inversely related to the occurrence of stomach cancer.

GENETIC FACTORS: Gastric cancer occurs with higher frequency in hereditary nonpolyposis colorectal cancer (HNPCC) syndrome, a disorder caused by germline mutations of genes responsible for DNA nucleotide mismatch repair. Rare familial cases of diffuse gastric cancer and lobular carcinoma of the breast are attributed to a germline mutation in the gene for E-cadherin (*CDH1*).

AGE AND SEX: Gastric cancer is uncommon under 30 years of age and shows a sharp peak in incidence over age 50. The age at onset is somewhat lower in Japan, where the disease is endemic. In the United States, there is only a slight male predominance, but in countries with a high incidence of this tumor, the male-to-female ratio is about 2:1.

LOW SOCIOECONOMIC SETTINGS: These situations pose an increased risk of gastric cancer, an observation that has been used to explain the higher frequency of the tumor among American blacks and the fact that the incidence of the disease in that population has not declined as rapidly as it has among whites.

Atrophic gastritis, autoimmune gastritis, pernicious anemia, subtotal gastrectomy and **gastric adenomatous polyps** are discussed above as factors associated with a high risk of stomach cancer.

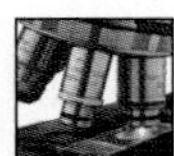

PATHOLOGY: Gastric adenocarcinoma accounts for over 95% of malignant gastric tumors, with two major but overlapping types: **diffuse** and **intestinal.** Cancers occur most often in the distal stomach, the lesser curvature of the antrum and the prepyloric region. Adenocarcinoma may occur anywhere but is rare in the fundus.

ADVANCED GASTRIC CANCER: By the time most gastric cancers in the Western world are detected, they are advanced; that is, they have penetrated beyond the submucosa into the muscularis propria and may extend through the serosa. The gross appearance of advanced stomach cancers is of great importance to radiologists and endoscopists, who may need to distinguish carcinomas from benign lesions. There are three major macroscopic types:

- **Polypoid (fungating) adenocarcinoma** accounts for one third of advanced cancers. It is a solid mass, often several centimeters in diameter, that projects into the stomach lumen. The surface may be partly ulcerated, and deeper tissues may or may not be infiltrated.
- **Ulcerating adenocarcinomas** make up another third of all gastric cancers. They have shallow ulcers of variable size (Fig. 13-27). Surrounding tissues are firm, raised and nodular. Usually, the ulcer's lateral margins are irregular and its base is ragged. This appearance differs from that of typical benign peptic ulcers, which have punched-out margins and a smooth base. Still, radiologic differentiation of ulcerating cancer from peptic ulcer may be very difficult.
- **Diffuse or infiltrating adenocarcinoma** accounts for one tenth of all stomach cancers. No true tumor mass is seen; instead, the stomach wall is thickened and firm (Fig. 13-28). If the entire stomach is involved, it is called a **linitis plastica** tumor. In the diffuse type of gastric carcinoma, invading tumor cells induce extensive fibrosis in the submucosa and muscularis. Thus, the stomach wall is stiff and may be more than 2 cm thick.

The histology of advanced gastric cancers varies from well-differentiated adenocarcinoma with gland formation (intestinal type) to poorly differentiated tumors without glands. The polypoid variant typically contains well-differentiated glands, and linitis plastica is most often poorly differentiated. Particularly in the ulcerated type of cancer, tumor cells may be arranged in cords or small foci. They may contain cytoplasmic mucin that displaces the nucleus to the periphery of the cell, resulting in the so-called signet ring cell (Fig. 13-29). Extracellular mucinous material may be so prominent that the malignant cells seem to float in a gelatinous matrix, in which case it is called a **mucinous (colloid) carcinoma.**

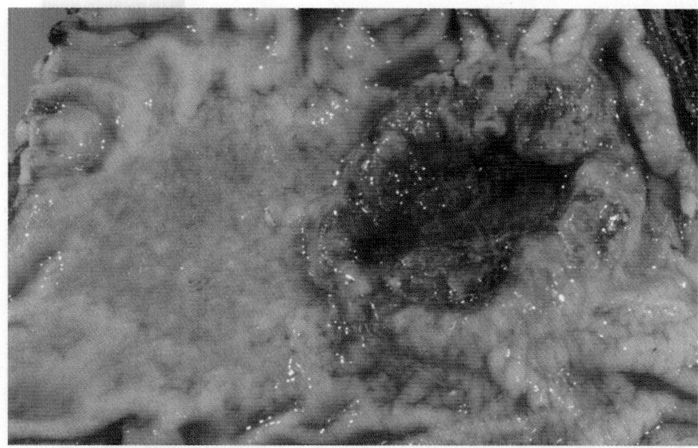

FIGURE 13-27. Ulcerating gastric carcinoma. In contrast to the benign peptic ulcer, the edges of this lesion are raised and firm. Note the atrophy of the surrounding mucosa (*left of ulceration*).

EARLY GASTRIC CANCER: Early gastric cancer is a tumor limited to the mucosa or submucosa (Fig. 13-30). The older term, **superficial spreading carcinoma,** is a synonym. In Japan, early gastric cancer accounts for one third of all stomach cancers, but only 5% in the United States and Europe.

Early gastric cancer is strictly a pathologic diagnosis based on depth of invasion; the term does not refer to the duration of the disease, its size, presence of symptoms, absence of metastases or curability. Up to 20% of early gastric cancers have already metastasized to lymph nodes at the time of detection.

Like advanced cancer, most early gastric cancers are in the distal stomach and are classified by macroscopic appearance:

- **Type I** protrudes into the lumen as a polypoid or nodular mass.
- **Type II** is a superficial, flat lesion that may be slightly elevated or depressed.

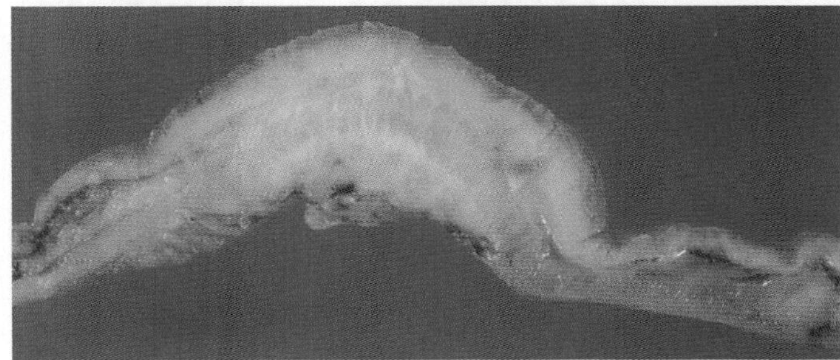

FIGURE 13-28. Infiltrating gastric carcinoma (linitis plastica). Cross-section of gastric wall thickened by tumor and fibrosis.

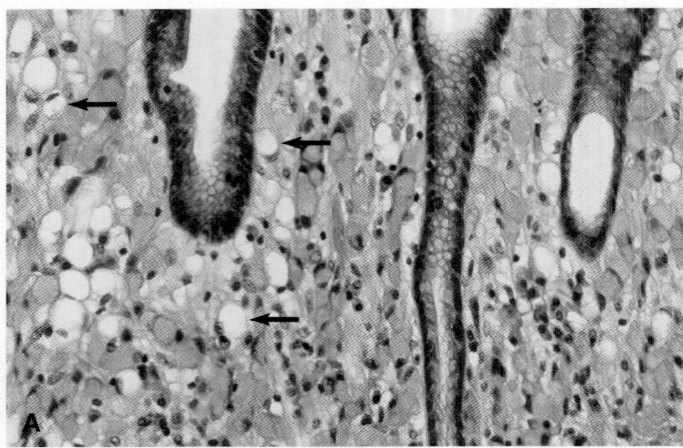

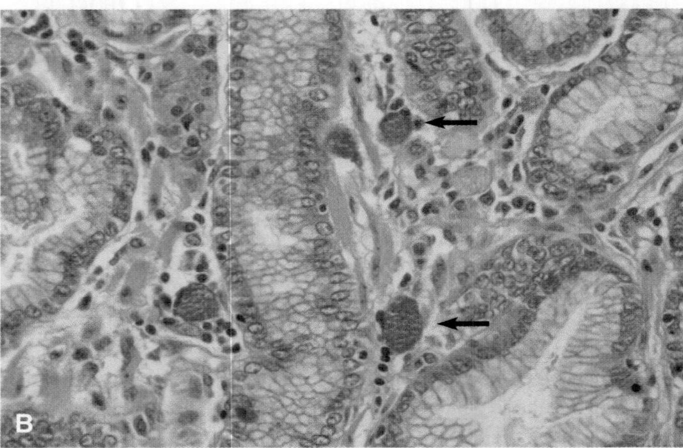

FIGURE 13-29. Infiltrating gastric carcinoma. A. Numerous signet ring cells (*arrows*) infiltrate the lamina propria between intact crypts. **B.** Mucin stains highlight the presence of mucin within the neoplastic cells (*arrows*).

- **Type III** is an excavated malignant ulcer that does not ordinarily occur alone but rather represents ulceration of type I or type II tumors.

Polypoid and superficial elevated early gastric cancers are typically well-differentiated intestinal-type adenocarcinomas. Flattened or depressed superficial early cancers range from well to poorly differentiated. Type III tumors are more often undifferentiated tumors.

Most intestinal-type gastric cancers originate from areas of intestinal metaplasia. Less differentiated and anaplastic diffuse-type tumors are more likely to derive from the necks of gastric glands without intestinal metaplasia.

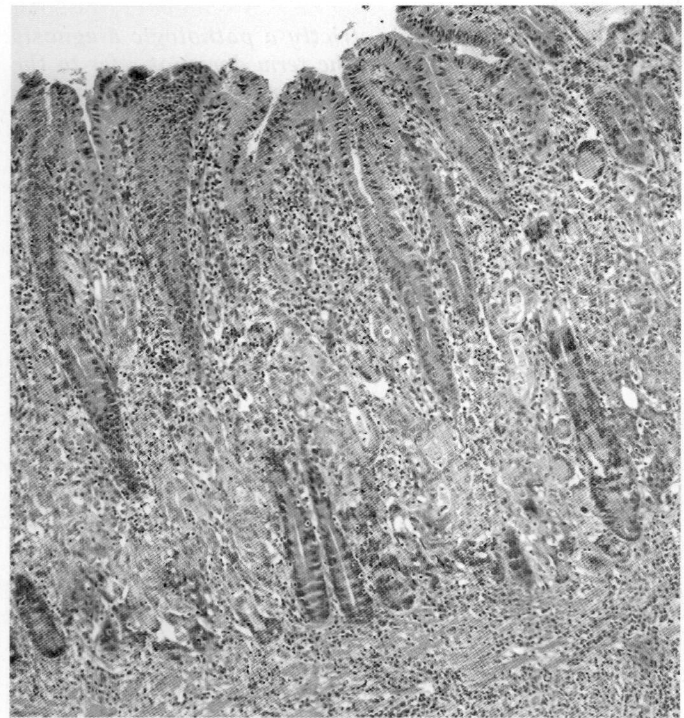

FIGURE 13-30. Early gastric cancer. Gastric adenocarcinoma showing infiltrating malignant glands restricted to the submucosa.

Intuitively, one would suppose that early gastric cancer would be the precursor of advanced gastric cancer, but this is not always the case. Early gastric cancer may sometimes be a different disease from advanced cancer, more benign and more curable because it is inherently less invasive. This biological difference may reflect differences between intestinal and gastric cell types. For example, even with lymph node metastases, early gastric cancer has a much better prognosis than does advanced cancer. Ten-year survival for surgically treated advanced gastric cancer is about 20%, compared with 95% for early gastric cancer. Moreover, the mean age at onset of early gastric cancer is uniformly younger than that of advanced cancer, and the early variety shows a striking geographic distribution.

Gastric cancers metastasize mainly via lymphatics to regional lymph nodes of the lesser and greater curvature, porta hepatis and subpyloric region. Distant lymphatic metastases also occur, the most common being an enlarged supraclavicular node, called **Virchow node.** Hematogenous spread may seed any organ, including liver, lung or brain. Direct extension to nearby organs is common. Ovarian spread, as a **Krukenberg tumor,** usually elicits a desmoplastic response.

Fig. 13-31 schematically depicts the major types of gastric cancer.

CLINICAL FEATURES: In the United States and Europe, most patients with gastric cancer have metastases when they first present. Thus, the symptoms and course are usually those of advanced cancer. The most frequent initial symptom is weight loss, usually with anorexia and nausea. Most patients complain of epigastric or back pain, mimicking a benign gastric ulcer. Antacids or H_2-receptor antagonists may be useful at first but provide little relief for more advanced disease.

Gastric outlet obstruction may occur with large tumors of the antrum or prepyloric region. Massive bleeding is uncommon, but chronic bleeding often leads to anemia and finding occult blood in the stools. Tumors involving the esophagogastric junction cause dysphagia and may mimic achalasia and esophageal adenocarcinoma.

Patients with early gastric cancer may be asymptomatic but usually complain of dyspepsia or epigastric pain. Weight loss, melena and anemia are present in a minority.

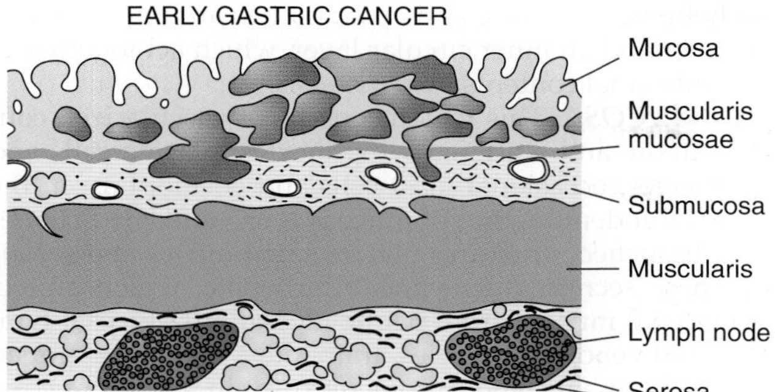

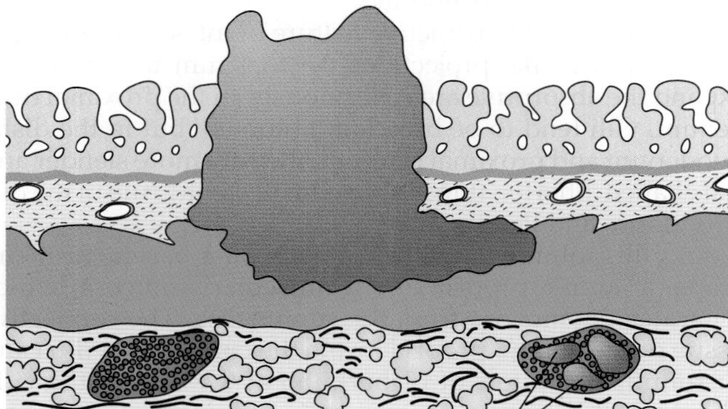

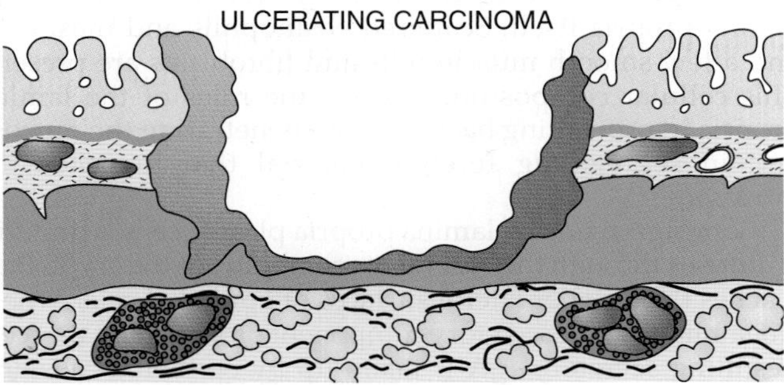

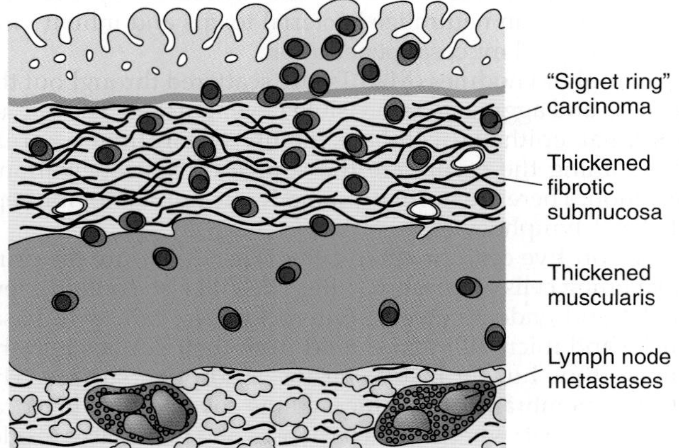

FIGURE 13-31. The major types of gastric cancer.

Gastric Neuroendocrine (Carcinoid) Tumors Are Low-Grade Malignancies

Endocrine cells in the gastric mucosa may give rise to neoplasms, collectively termed carcinoid tumor (neuroendocrine tumors; NETs). These may recur locally and metastasize. Metastasis reflects more tumor size than histopathology. Gastric NETs are not usually hormonally active but sometimes secrete serotonin, and metastases can cause **carcinoid syndrome.**

Gastric NETs may arise in the setting of hypergastrinemia associated with autoimmune gastritis. In this context, NETs derive from hyperplastic neuroendocrine cells in the proximal stomach (ECL cells) in response to hypergastrinemia that follows loss of parietal cells. Sporadic gastric NETs tend to be more aggressive.

Bezoars

Bezoars are foreign bodies made of food or hair altered by digestion.

PHYTOBEZOAR: These vegetable concretions are unusual, except in people who eat many persimmons or swallow unchewed bubble gum. Phytobezoars are usually seen in patients with delayed gastric emptying, as in the peripheral neuropathy of diabetes or gastric cancer, and in people undergoing therapy with anticholinergic agents. Additional causes of delayed gastric emptying include hypochlorhydria after partial gastrectomy, particularly when surgery includes vagotomy. Plant bezoars contain vegetable or fruit fibers. Most patients with persimmon bezoars have bleeding from an associated gastric ulcer.

The preferred treatment of phytobezoars is chemical attack with cellulase; in some cases, endoscopic manual disruption, including with jets of water, has been successful. However, enzymatic therapy is usually not effective for persimmon bezoars, and surgery is required.

TRICHOBEZOAR: This mass is a hairball within a gelatinous matrix, usually seen in long-haired girls or young women who eat their own hair as a nervous habit. Trichobezoars may grow by accretion to form a complete cast of the stomach, potentially reaching 3 kg (Fig. 13-32).

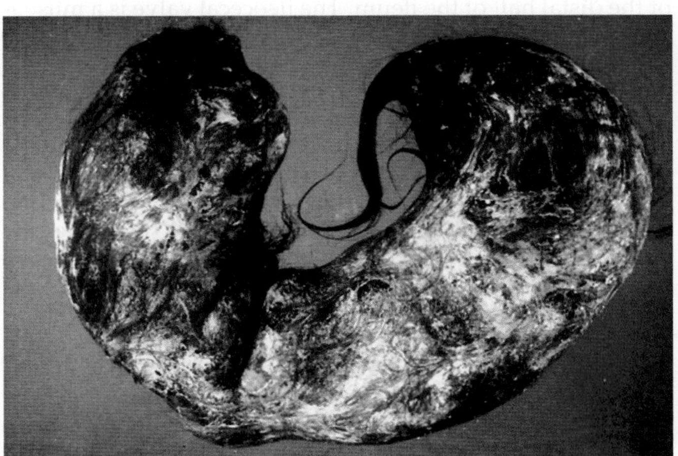

FIGURE 13-32. Trichobezoar (hairball). A mass of hair in a gelatinous matrix forms a cast of the stomach.

THE SMALL INTESTINE

Anatomy

The intestinal tract develops as a tube from the stomach to the cloaca. This tube progressively elongates and its cephalic portion becomes the segment that extends from the distal duodenum to the proximal ileum. The more caudal portion develops into distal ileum and the proximal two thirds of transverse colon. The vitelline duct, which connects the primitive duct with the yolk sac, may persist as a Meckel diverticulum (see below). To achieve the final position of the intestine, the fetal gut undergoes a complex series of rotations.

The small intestine extends from the pylorus to the ileocecal valve and, depending on its muscle tone, is from 3.5 to 6.5 m long. It is divided into three regions:

1. **The duodenum** extends to the ligament of Treitz.
2. **The jejunum** is the proximal 40% of the remainder of the small intestine.
3. **The ileum** is the distal 60%.

The duodenum is almost entirely retroperitoneal and therefore fixed. The remainder of small intestine, which is disposed in redundant loops, is movable.

The C-shaped duodenum surrounds the head of the pancreas. It receives biliary drainage of the liver and pancreatic secretions through the common bile duct at the ampulla of Vater. The distal duodenum becomes invested by mesentery and merges with the jejunum at the ligament of Treitz. The proximity of the duodenum to its neighbors means that it may be affected by disorders such as cancer of the pancreas and cholecystoduodenal fistulas. Conversely, duodenal ulcers may penetrate into the pancreas, liver and aorta, the latter leading to catastrophic bleeding. There is no demarcation between jejunum and ileum, which merge gradually. The wall of the jejunum is thicker and its lumen wider than that of the ileum.

The plicae circularis, spiral folds that consist of mucosa and submucosa, are most prominent in the distal duodenum and proximal jejunum, usually disappearing in the terminal ileum. **Peyer patches** are lymphoid aggregates in the submucosa up to 3 cm in diameter, in the antimesenteric aspect of the distal half of the ileum. The ileocecal valve is a muscular sphincter that regulates the flow of intestinal contents into the cecum.

The duodenum is served by the pancreaticoduodenal branch of the hepatic artery, which arises from the celiac artery. The jejunum and ileum are supplied by the superior mesenteric artery (a branch of the aorta), which is arranged in arcades in the mesentery, thereby providing abundant collateral circulation in its distal reaches. Venous flow from the small intestine empties into the portal venous system. Duodenal lymphatic channels drain into portal and pyloric lymph nodes; those of the jejunum and ileum communicate with mesenteric lymph nodes. The lymphatics of terminal ileum empty into ileocolic nodes. Sympathetic innervation is from the celiac plexus and ganglia, and parasympathetic fibers from the vagus nerve. The small intestinal wall has four layers: mucosa, submucosa, muscularis and serosa. In the retroperitoneal duodenum, however, only the anterior wall is covered by a serosa.

SEROSA AND MUSCULARIS PROPRIA: The serosa contains loose connective tissue bounded by a single layer of mesothelium. The muscularis propria has an outer longitudinal layer and an inner circular layer, which act together to propel intestinal contents by peristalsis.

SUBMUCOSA: This region consists of vascularized connective tissue and scattered lymphocytes, plasma cells and macrophages, occasional mast cells and eosinophils. In the proximal duodenum, the submucosa is occupied by Brunner glands, branched structures that contain mucous and serous cells. These secrete mucus and bicarbonate, which protect the duodenal mucosa from peptic ulceration. Mucosal lymphatics and venous capillaries drain into a highly developed system of lymphatic and venous plexuses in the submucosa. The **myenteric nerve plexus of Auerbach,** which lies between the two layers of the muscularis, and **Meissner plexus** in the submucosa are interconnected.

MUCOSA: The distinctive feature of intestinal mucosa is its villi, finger-like projections 0.5 to 1 mm in length that expand the absorptive area enormously. In the proximal duodenum, villi tend to be broad and blunted, but in the distal duodenum and proximal jejunum, they are more slender and leaf shaped. Shorter, finger-shaped villi are the rule in the distal jejunum and ileum.

In villi, columnar epithelium sits on a basement membrane, a lamina propria and a muscularis mucosa, which separates the mucosa from the submucosa. The connective tissue of the lamina propria forms the core of the villus and surrounds the crypts of Lieberkühn at the base of the villi. The normal lamina propria contains lymphocytes, plasma cells and macrophages. Plasma cells here mainly secrete immunoglobulin A (IgA) into the intestinal lumen or the lamina propria itself. Scattered eosinophils and mast cells and a few smooth muscle cells and fibroblasts are present. This cellular composition reflects the roles of the lamina propria in preventing bacteria from penetrating the mucosa and in segregating foreign material that breaches the mucosa.

Some IgA made by lamina propria plasma cells is dimeric. It diffuses through the basement membrane of the crypt, then reaches the basal or lateral surfaces of epithelial cells, where it combines with a secretory component produced by that cell. Resulting **secretory IgA** is taken up by epithelial cells and secreted into the lumen. Secretory IgA is more resistant to proteolysis than is serum IgA. It binds food antigens and prevents bacterial adherence to the intestinal epithelium. Moreover, it can neutralize bacterial toxins and inhibit viral replication and mucosal penetration.

Lymphoid nodules (MALTs) are scattered throughout the mucosa and aggregate into visible Peyer patches. The villous columnar epithelial cells are mainly absorptive, whereas those lining the crypts are the source of cell renewal and secretion. There are normally a moderate number of intraepithelial T lymphocytes.

Absorptive cells, or enterocytes (Fig. 13-33), are the principal lining cells of intestinal villi. The villi also contain a few goblet and endocrine cells. Enterocytes are tall, with basal nuclei and microvilli that extend from their surface into the lumen, thus hugely increasing the absorptive surface. The plasma membrane of the microvilli is covered by a glycocalyx (fuzzy coat) where disaccharidases and peptidases reside. Certain receptors, such as that for the intrinsic factor–vitamin B_{12} complex in the ileum, are also present in the membrane–glycocalyx complex.

The cytosol just under the microvilli has a network of actin microfilaments, the **terminal web.** These filaments are

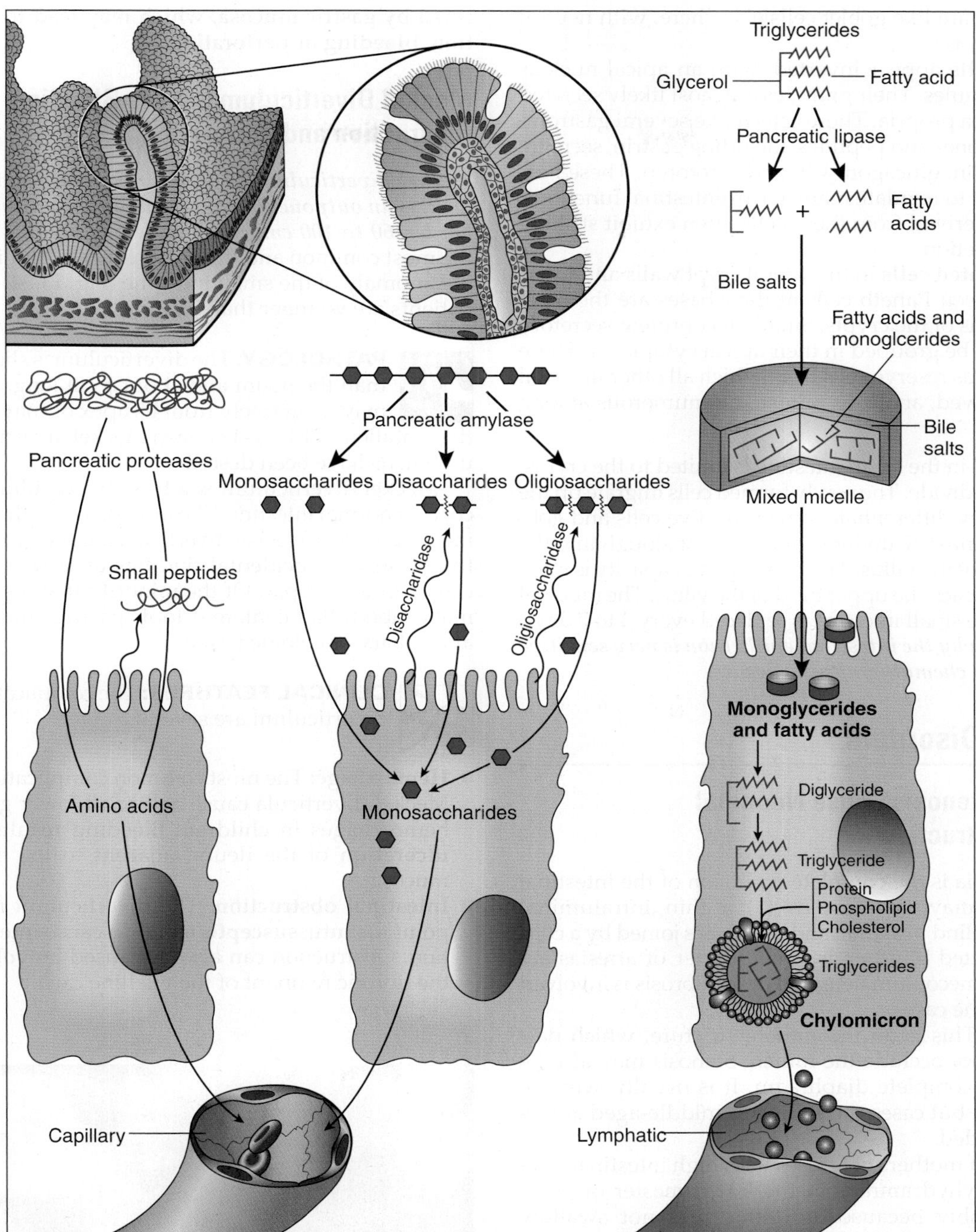

FIGURE 13-33. Mechanisms of nutrient absorption in the small intestine.

also associated with myosin and other contractile proteins, insert into the core of the microvilli and presumably serve as a contractile apparatus. The sides of adjacent plasma membranes form tight junctions that are impermeable to macromolecules but permit passive transport of small molecules by the paracellular route. Absorbed material is transported from epithelial cells to the intercellular space between absorptive cells, through lateral or basal plasma membranes. It then penetrates the basement membrane, traverses the lamina propria and enters a capillary or a lymphatic channel.

There are four cell types in the crypts:

- **Paneth cells** at the base of the crypts resemble zymogen cells of the pancreas and salivary glands that are active in exocrine secretion. Their eosinophilic secretory granules fill a basophilic cytoplasm. Paneth cells function in **mucosal defense,** as evidenced by the presence of lysozyme; antimicrobial products, including peptides called **crypt defensins** (cryptdins); and **CD95 ligand,** which is a member of the tumor necrosis factor (TNF) family of cytokines.
- **Goblet cells** of the lateral walls of the crypts are flask shaped and filled with mucus granules. In structure and

function they are like goblet cells elsewhere, with neutral and acid mucins.

- **Endocrine cells** appear inverted, with an apical nucleus and basal granules. Their granules are most likely secreted into the lamina propria. These cells make several gastrointestinal hormones and peptides, including gastrin, secretin, cholecystokinin, glucagon, VIP and serotonin. These hormones are felt to regulate many gastrointestinal functions, and tumors derived from these cells often exhibit striking hormone secretion.
- **Undifferentiated cells** in the lateral crypt walls and interspersed between Paneth cells at their bases are the most numerous cells of the crypts. Small glycoprotein secretory granules may be grouped in their apical cytoplasm. These cells function as reserve cells from which all other mucosal cells are renewed, and thus mitoses are numerous among them.

Cell renewal in the small intestine is limited to the crypts, where stem cells divide. The newly formed cells migrate up the villus, where they differentiate into absorptive cells and goblet cells, and eventually undergo apoptosis or slough into the lumen at the tip of the villus. Their absorptive capacity is maximal when they reach the upper third of the villus. The mucosal epithelium of the small intestine is replaced every 4 to 7 days, which ***explains why the intestinal epithelium is very sensitive to radiation and chemotherapeutic agents.***

Congenital Disorders

Atresia and Stenosis Cause Neonatal Intestinal Obstruction

ATRESIA: Atresia is the complete occlusion of the intestinal lumen, which may manifest as (1) a thin intraluminal diaphragm, (2) blind proximal and distal sacs joined by a cord or (3) disconnected blind ends. One quarter of atresias are associated with meconium ileus and cystic fibrosis is involved in one tenth of the cases.

STENOSIS: This is an incomplete stricture, which narrows but does not occlude the lumen. Stenosis may also be caused by an incomplete diaphragm. It is usually symptomatic in infancy, but cases presenting in middle-aged adults have been recorded.

One fourth of mothers of fetuses with high intestinal atresia develop polyhydramnios in the last trimester of pregnancy, presumably because the fetus does not swallow amniotic fluid. Intestinal atresia or stenosis is diagnosed on the basis of persistent vomiting of bile-containing fluid in the first day of life. Meconium is not passed. The obstructed fetal intestine is dilated and filled with fluid, which can be detected radiologically. Surgical correction is usually successful, but there are often other complicating anomalies.

Duplications (Enteric Cysts) May Occur From the Esophagus to the Anus

These cysts are spherical or tubular structures attached to the alimentary tract. They may be isolated cystic structures or may communicate with the gut lumen. Intestinal duplications are most common in the ileum and less so in the jejunum. They have smooth muscle walls and gastrointestinal-type epithelium. **Communicating duplications are often lined by gastric mucosa, which may lead to peptic ulceration, bleeding or perforation.**

Meckel Diverticulum Causes Bleeding, Obstruction and Perforation

Meckel diverticulum, caused by persistence of the vitelline duct, is an outpouching of the gut on the antimesenteric ileal border, 60 to 100 cm from the ileocecal valve in adults. It is the most common and the most clinically significant congenital anomaly of the small intestine (Fig. 13-34). Two thirds of patients are younger than 2 years.

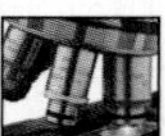

PATHOLOGY: The diverticulum is slightly narrower than the ileum and about 5 cm long. A fibrous cord may hang freely from its apex or may be attached to the umbilicus. Fistulas between Meckel diverticulum and the umbilicus have been described.

Meckel diverticulum is a true diverticulum, with all the coats of normal intestine. The mucosa is like that of the adjoining ileum. Most Meckel diverticula are asymptomatic and are found only as incidental findings at laparotomy for other causes or at autopsy. Of the minority that becomes symptomatic, about half contain ectopic gastric, duodenal, pancreatic, biliary or colonic tissue.

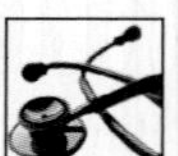

CLINICAL FEATURES: The complications of Meckel diverticulum are several.

- **Hemorrhage:** The most common complication is bleeding. Meckel diverticula cause half of all lower gastrointestinal hemorrhages in children. Bleeding results from **peptic ulceration** of the ileum adjacent to the ectopic gastric mucosa.
- **Intestinal obstruction:** The diverticulum may be a lead point for **intussusception** and so cause intestinal obstruction. Obstruction can also be caused by **volvulus** around the fibrotic remnant of the vitelline duct.

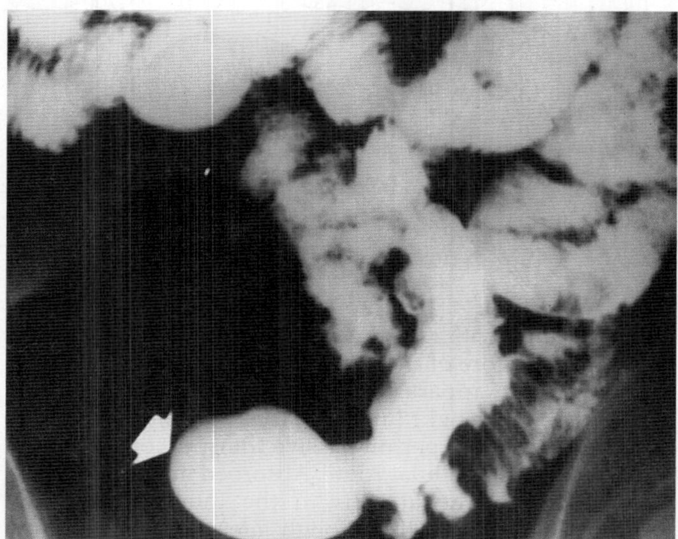

FIGURE 13-34. Meckel diverticulum. A contrast radiograph of the small intestine shows a barium-filled diverticulum of the ileum (*arrow*).

- **Diverticulitis:** Inflammation of a Meckel diverticulum (i.e., diverticulitis) leads to symptoms indistinguishable from those of appendicitis. Thus, a surgeon suspecting acute appendicitis who encounters a normal appendix is well advised to search for a Meckel diverticulum.
- **Perforation:** Peptic ulceration, either in the diverticulum or the ileum, may cause perforation and lead to rapidly spreading peritonitis.
- **Fistula:** A fecal discharge from the umbilicus may be observed.

Malrotation May Lead to Bowel Obstruction

Defective intestinal rotation in fetal life leads to abnormal positions of the small intestine and colon, anomalous attachments and bands. The clinical importance of such rotational anomalies lies in their propensity to cause catastrophic volvulus of the small and large intestine and incarceration of bowel in an internal hernia.

Meconium Ileus Is an Early Complication of Cystic Fibrosis

In cystic fibrosis highly viscous mucous (see Chapters 6 and 12) may block the pancreatic duct and thicken intestinal contents. In the neonatal period, tenacious meconium may accumulate and obstruct the small intestine. Beyond the obstruction, the distal ileum is usually contracted, and the midileum proximal to the inspissated meconium is dilated. In half of affected infants, meconium ileus is complicated by (1) volvulus, (2) perforation with meconium peritonitis or (3) intestinal atresia. Meconium ileus must be differentiated from distal intestinal obstruction associated with cystic fibrosis, in which a small plug of meconium in the distal colon may eventually be passed, thereby relieving the obstruction.

Infections of the Small Intestine

Bacterial Diarrhea Is a Major Cause of Death Worldwide

Infectious diarrhea is particularly lethal in underdeveloped countries and in infants. In countries with poor sanitation, the death toll from childhood diarrhea is staggering: 1.5 million children under 5 years succumb annually to diarrhea, over 80% of them in Africa and south Asia.

The small bowel normally has few bacteria (usually $<10^4$/mL), mostly anaerobic bacilli such as lactobacilli. These organisms travel in the food stream and ordinarily do not colonize the small intestine. Infectious diarrhea is caused by bacterial colonization (e.g., with toxigenic strains of *Escherichia coli* and *Vibrio cholerae*). The most significant factor in infectious diarrhea is increased intestinal secretion, stimulated by bacterial toxins and enteric hormones. Decreased absorption and increased peristaltic activity contribute less to the diarrhea.

The colon harbors an abundant bacterial flora, at concentrations seven orders of magnitude greater than in the small intestine. Anaerobic bacteria in the colon (e.g., *Bacteroides* and *Clostridium* spp.) outnumber aerobic organisms 1000-fold. With the more rapid transit of intestinal contents during diarrhea, flora are shifted to more aerobic populations, including *E. coli, Klebsiella* and *Proteus.* Moreover, offending organisms themselves become conspicuous and pathogens of the small intestine such as *V. cholerae* may be the major isolate in the stool.

Several factors limit the numbers of bacteria in the stomach and small bowel: (1) gastric acid inhibits bacterial growth, which explains bacterial overgrowth in the stomach in achlorhydria; (2) bile has antimicrobial activity; (3) peristalsis propels intestinal contents, limiting bacterial accumulation; (4) normal flora secrete their own antimicrobial substances to maintain an ecologic balance (indeed, treatment with broad-spectrum antibiotics alters the natural flora and allows overgrowth of ordinarily harmless organisms); and (5) plasma cells of the lamina propria secrete IgA into the intestinal lumen.

Individual agents responsible for infectious diarrhea are discussed in Chapter 9. Here we review the major entities only briefly. Agents of infectious diarrhea are classified as **toxigenic** (i.e., producing diarrhea by elaborating toxins) or as **adherent** or **invasive bacteria.**

Toxigenic Diarrhea

The prototypical organisms that cause diarrhea by secreting toxins are ***V. cholerae*** and **toxigenic strains of *E. coli.***

The characteristics of toxigenic diarrhea are:

- Damage to the intestinal mucosa is minimal or absent.
- The organism remains on the mucosal surface, where it secretes its toxin.
- Fluid secreted into the small intestine causes watery diarrhea, which can lead to dehydration, particularly in the case of cholera.

Many organisms have been isolated in so-called travelers' diarrhea, but toxigenic *E. coli is* the most common in almost all studies.

Invasive Bacteria Cause Diarrhea by Directly Injuring the Intestinal Mucosa

Among these organisms, *Shigella, Salmonella,* and certain strains of *E. coli, Yersinia* and *Campylobacter* are the most widely recognized. Invasive organisms tend to infect the distal ileum and colon, while toxigenic bacteria mainly involve the upper intestinal tract. The mechanism by which invasive bacteria produce diarrhea is uncertain. Enterotoxins have been identified, but their role in causing diarrhea is not established. Mucosal invasion by bacteria increases synthesis of prostaglandins in the affected tissue and inhibitors of prostaglandin synthesis seem to block fluid secretion. It also may be that damaged mucosa cannot absorb fluid from the lumen.

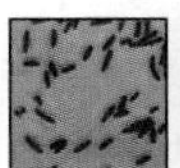
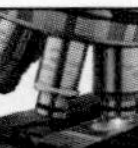

ETIOLOGIC FACTORS AND PATHOLOGY: *SHIGELLOSIS:* Shigellosis mainly affects the colon, but the terminal ileum is occasionally involved. A granular and hemorrhagic mucosa has many shallow serpiginous ulcers. Inflammation is especially severe in the sigmoid colon and rectum but is usually superficial. In the early stage, neutrophils accumulate in damaged crypts (crypt abscesses), similar to ulcerative colitis (see below), and the lymphoid follicles of the mucosa break down to form ulcers. As infection recedes, ulcers heal and the mucosa returns to normal.

TYPHOID FEVER: Typhoid fever (*Salmonella* enteritis) is uncommon today in the industrialized world but is still a problem in underdeveloped countries. Necrosis of lymphoid tissue, principally in the terminal ileum, leads to scattered ulcers. Infection of Peyer patches results in oval ulcers, in which the longer dimension is in the long axis of the intestine. Occasionally, lymphoid follicles in the large bowel or the appendix are ulcerated. The base of the ulcer contains black necrotic tissue mixed with fibrin.

The early lesions of typhoid fever show large basophilic macrophages filled with typhoid bacilli, erythrocytes and necrotic debris. Necrosis of lymphoid follicles becomes confluent and mucosal ulceration follows. Similar lymphoid hyperplasia and necrosis are seen in regional lymph nodes. Within a week of the acute symptoms, ulcers heal completely, leaving little fibrosis or other sequelae. **Intestinal hemorrhage and perforation,** principally in the ileum, are the most feared complications of typhoid fever and tend to occur in the third week and during convalescence.

NONTYPHOIDAL SALMONELLOSIS: Formerly known as **paratyphoid fever,** this enteritis is caused by *Salmonella* strains other than *S. typhi* and is generally far less serious than typhoid fever. The principal target is the ileum, but minor involvement of the colon may also occur. Organisms invade the mucosa, which shows mild ulceration, edema and infiltration with neutrophils. Hematogenous dissemination from the intestine may carry infection to bones, joints and meninges. Interestingly, people with sickle cell anemia tend to develop *Salmonella* osteomyelitis, presumably because phagocytosis of the products of hemolysis prevents further cellular ingestion of the organisms and allows their dissemination through the bloodstream.

***ENTEROINVASIVE, ENTEROADHERENT AND ENTEROHEMORRHAGIC STRAINS OF* ESCHERICHIA COLI:** These organisms may uncommonly cause bloody diarrhea similar to shigellosis and are a prominent cause of travelers' diarrhea. Certain strains of *E. coli,* particularly serotype 0157:H7, produce *Shigella*-like toxins, but the role of these proteins in the pathogenesis of the enterocolitis is not understood. Serotype 0157:H7 has also been implicated in the hemolytic–uremic syndrome in children.

YERSINIA *ENTEROCOLITIS:* *Yersinia enterocolitica* and *Yersinia pseudotuberculosis* are transmitted by pets or contaminated food, and infection is most common in young children. *Yersinia* infection causes diarrhea, cramps and fever and lasts 1 to 3 weeks. Peyer patches are hyperplastic, with acute ulceration of overlying mucosa. A fibrinopurulent exudate covers the ulcers and often contains many organisms.

In addition to causing enterocolitis, *Yersinia* causes acute mesenteric adenitis and right lower quadrant pain. Infected children have undergone laparotomy as a result of the disease being mistaken for appendicitis. Microscopically, lymph nodes show epithelioid granulomas with central necrosis in the case of *Y. pseudotuberculosis.* The ileum and appendix may contain similar granulomas, causing an appearance that has been mistaken for Crohn disease.

Adults, who are less susceptible to *Yersinia* infection than are children, have acute diarrhea, often followed within a few weeks by erythema nodosum, erythema multiforme or polyarthritis. Patients with chronic debilitating diseases may develop fatal *Yersinia* bacteremia, resistant to antibiotic treatment. Interestingly, people with thalassemia have a propensity for *Y. enterocolitica* infection.

Table 13-1

Histologic Patterns of Bacterial Infections of the Gastrointestinal Tract

Minimal inflammatory changes	*Vibrio cholerae* Toxigenic *Escherichia coli* *Neisseria* sp.
Acute self-limited colitis	*Shigella* *Campylobacter jejuni* *Aeromonas* *Salmonella* *Clostridium difficile*
Pseudomembranous pattern	*C. difficile* *Shigella* Enterohemorrhagic *E. coli*
Granulomas	*Yersinia* sp. *Mycobacterium bovis* *Mycobacterium avium-intracellulare* *Actinomycosis*
Macrophages	Whipple disease (*Tropheryma whippelii*) *M. avium-intracellulare*
Lymphocytes, macrophages	*Lymphogranuloma venereum*
Architectural distortion	*Salmonella typhimurium* Shigella

CAMPYLOBACTER JEJUNI: *Campylobacter jejuni* is one of the most common causes of bacterial diarrhea, with a higher incidence of nontyphoidal *Salmonella* and *Shigella* in some U.S. studies. In a report from Great Britain, *Campylobacter* caused half of bacterial diarrhea. Humans contract the disease mainly by contact with infected domestic animals or by eating poorly cooked or contaminated food. Adults usually recover in less than 1 week.

The basic pathology of gastrointestinal bacterial infections is listed in Table 13-1.

Food Poisoning

Infectious agents can produce diarrhea by elaborating enterotoxins in contaminated food that is then ingested.

STAPHYLOCOCCUS AUREUS: *Staphylococcus aureus* is a common cause of food poisoning. Symptoms result from ingesting food contaminated with *Staphylococcus* strains that produce an exotoxin that damages the gastrointestinal epithelium. Severe vomiting and abdominal cramps occur within 6 hours, often followed by diarrhea. Most patients recover in 1 to 2 days.

CLOSTRIDIUM PERFRINGENS: This bacterium elaborates an enterotoxin that causes vomiting and diarrhea. The organism is anaerobic, but tolerates exposure to air for up to 3 days. Enterotoxin activity is maximal in the ileum. In most cases, watery diarrhea and severe abdominal pain begin 8 to 24 hours after ingestion of contaminated food and last about 1 day.

Rotavirus and Norwalk Virus Are the Most Common Causes of Viral Gastroenteritis in the United States

ROTAVIRUS: Rotavirus infection is a common cause of infantile diarrhea. It accounts for about half of acute diarrhea in hospitalized children under 2 years. Rotavirus has been demonstrated in duodenal biopsy specimens and is associated with injury to the surface epithelium and impaired intestinal absorption for periods of up to 2 months.

NORWALK VIRUSES: These agents account for one third of the epidemics of viral gastroenteritis in the United States. The virus targets the upper small intestine, causing patchy mucosal lesions and malabsorption. Vomiting and diarrhea are usual, but symptoms resolve within 2 days.

Other viruses implicated as etiologic agents of infective diarrhea include echovirus, coxsackievirus, cytomegalovirus, adenovirus and coronavirus.

Intestinal Tuberculosis Occurs After Ingesting *Mycobacterium Bovis*

Once an important disease, gastrointestinal tuberculosis is now uncommon in industrialized countries, but it is still a problem in underdeveloped areas of the world. Intestinal tuberculosis usually involves infection with *Mycobacterium bovis,* which was mainly transmitted by contaminated milk. However, control of tuberculosis in dairy herds and pasteurization of milk have made infection with *M. bovis* a curiosity.

Intestinal tuberculosis is mostly caused by ingesting the bacteria in food or by swallowing infectious sputum. The tubercle bacillus is protected from digestion by its waxy capsule and passes into the small bowel. It then establishes a locus of infection, usually (90% of patients) in the ileocecal region, where lymphoid tissue is abundant. Infection also occurs in the colon, jejunum, appendix, rectum and duodenum, in that order of frequency.

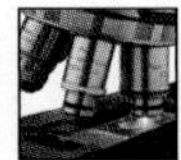

PATHOLOGY: Intestinal tuberculosis may present with circular ulcers of varying size in the transverse plane of the bowel. As the ulcers heal, reactive fibrosis may cause a circumferential ("napkin ring") stricture of the bowel lumen. Mesenteric lymph nodes are typically enlarged, with caseous necrosis.

Granulomas may be found in all layers of the bowel wall, particularly in Peyer patches and lymphoid follicles. Tuberculous strictures are difficult to distinguish from other causes of stricture, such as ischemic enterocolitis or Crohn disease.

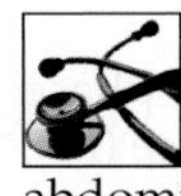

CLINICAL FEATURES: Almost all patients with intestinal tuberculosis complain of chronic abdominal pain and about two thirds have a palpable abdominal mass, usually in the right lower quadrant. Malnutrition, weight loss, fever and weakness are common. Complications include obstruction, fistulas, perforation and abscess.

Intestinal Fungal Infections Occur Mainly in Immunocompromised Patients

The gastrointestinal tract is not a hospitable environment for fungi, and there are few commensal fungi (mostly yeasts and anaerobic actinomycetes); ***fungal infections of the gut are usually opportunistic.*** Suppression of normal bacterial flora by antibiotics also favors fungal growth. Under these circumstances, the most common mycosis is caused by *Candida.* Other fungi, including *Histoplasma* and *Mucor,* are occasionally found.

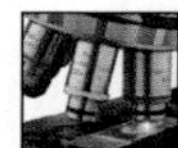

PATHOLOGY: Candidiasis and mucormycosis typically cause mucosal erosions, which may progress to larger ulcers surrounded by hemorrhage and necrosis. The inflammatory reaction is usually acute but reflects the extent of immunosuppression. Mucormycosis often invades blood vessels, with thrombosis and infarction, but hematogenous dissemination from the intestine is rare. Disseminated histoplasmosis may involve the bowel, where it causes elevated plaques that ulcerate and may even perforate.

Small Intestinal Parasites Include Both Protozoan and Metazoan Species

Parasitic diseases of the small bowel are detailed in Chapter 9 and include (1) **protozoa,** such as *Giardia lamblia, Coccidia* sp. and cryptosporidia; (2) **nematodes (roundworms),** such as *Ascaris, Strongyloides* and hookworms; and (3) **flatworms.** The latter may be tapeworms (cestodes), such as *Diphyllobothrium latum, Taenia solium, Taenia saginata* and *Hymenolepis nana.* Flukes (trematodes) include schistosomes and the giant intestinal fluke *Fasciolopsis buski.* In addition, trichinosis has an intestinal phase during which vomiting, diarrhea and colic mimic acute food poisoning or bacterial enteritis.

Vascular Diseases of the Small Intestine

Impaired intestinal blood flow for any reason can cause **ischemic bowel disease.** Manifestations of intestinal ischemia are diverse. The most common type of ischemic bowel disease is acute intestinal ischemia, which causes injury ranging from mucosal necrosis to transmural bowel infarction. Chronic intestinal ischemia syndromes are less common and generally require the severe compromise of two or more major arteries, usually by atherosclerosis.

Superior Mesenteric Artery Occlusion Is the Most Common Cause of Acute Intestinal Ischemia

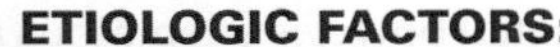

ETIOLOGIC FACTORS:

ARTERIAL OCCLUSION: Sudden occlusion of a large artery by thrombosis or embolization leads to small bowel infarction before collateral circulation can compensate. Depending on the size of the artery, infarction may be segmental or may lead to gangrene of virtually the entire small bowel (Fig. 13-35). Occlusive intestinal infarction is most often caused by embolic or thrombotic occlusion of the superior mesenteric artery. A lesser number are the result of vasculitis, which often involves small arteries. In addition to intrinsic vascular lesions, volvulus, intussusception and incarceration of the intestine in a hernial sac may all lead to arterial as well as venous occlusion.

NONOCCLUSIVE INTESTINAL ISCHEMIA: Intestinal ischemic necrosis without any acute vascular occlusion is more common than the occlusive type and may be just as extensive. It is seen in hypoxic patients with reduced cardiac output from shock of a variety of causes including hemorrhage, sepsis and acute myocardial infarction. In shock, blood flow redistributes to favor the brain and other vital organs, and patients often receive α-adrenergic agents, which further shunt blood away from the intestine. Drastically lowered perfusion pressure leads to arteriolar collapse, aggravating the ischemia.

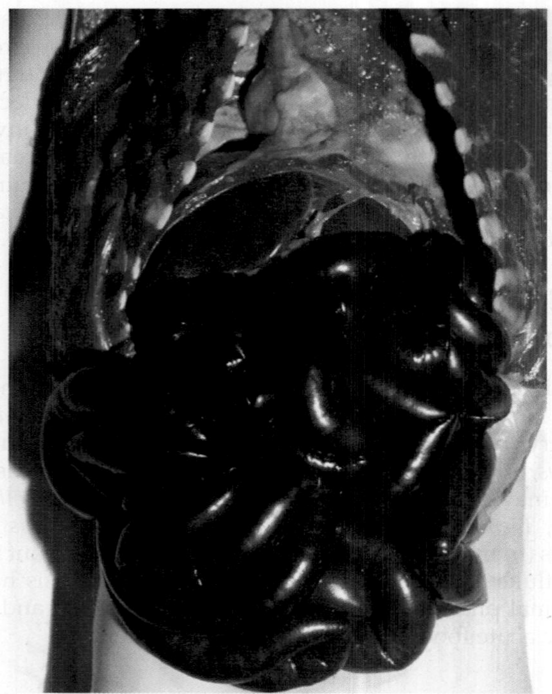

FIGURE 13-35. Infarct of the small bowel. This infant died after an episode of intense abdominal pain and shock. Autopsy demonstrated volvulus of the small bowel that had occluded the superior mesenteric artery. The entire small bowel is dilated, gangrenous and hemorrhagic.

MESENTERIC VEIN THROMBOSIS: Causes of mesenteric vein thrombosis include hypercoagulable states, stasis and inflammation (pylephlebitis). Almost all thromboses affect the superior mesenteric vein; only 5% involve the inferior mesenteric vein. The collateral flow in the distribution of the superior mesenteric vein usually suffices to preclude infarction of the intestine.

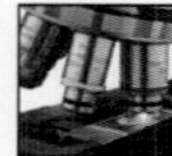

PATHOLOGY: Infarcted bowel is edematous and diffusely purple. The demarcation between the infarcted bowel and normal tissue is usually sharp, although venous occlusion may lead to a more diffuse appearance. Hemorrhage is prominent in the mucosa and submucosa, especially in venous occlusion (e.g., mesenteric vein thrombosis). The mucosal surface shows irregular white sloughs, and the wall becomes thin and distended. Bubbles of gas (pneumatosis) may be present in the bowel wall and mesenteric veins. The serosal surface is cloudy and covered by an inflammatory exudate.

Dysfunction of smooth muscle interferes with peristalsis and leads to **adynamic ileus,** in which the bowel proximal to the lesion is dilated and filled with fluid. Intestinal organisms may pass through the damaged wall and cause **peritonitis** or **septicemia.**

In nonocclusive intestinal ischemia, the principal lesion is restricted initially to the mucosa. Mucosal changes range from foci of dilated capillaries with a few extravasated erythrocytes to severe hemorrhagic necrosis and bleeding into the lumen. If the patient survives the episode of hypoperfusion, the bowel may be completely repaired, or it may heal with granulation tissue and fibrosis, with eventual **stricture formation.**

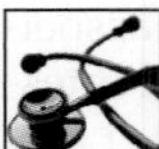

CLINICAL FEATURES: Abdominal pain begins abruptly, often with bloody diarrhea, hematemesis and shock. In untreated cases, perforation is frequent. ***As infarction progresses, systemic manifestations become more severe (multiple organ dysfunction syndrome).*** In extensive infarction that is a result of occlusion in the proximal superior mesenteric artery, almost the entire small bowel must be resected, a situation not compatible with ultimate survival.

Chronic Intestinal Ischemia Leads to Recurrent Abdominal Pain

Atherosclerotic narrowing of major splanchnic arteries leads to chronic intestinal ischemia. As in the heart, it causes intermittent abdominal pain, termed **intestinal (abdominal) angina.** The pain usually starts within a half hour of eating and lasts for a few hours. Frank intestinal infarction may be heralded by abdominal angina. Recurrent abdominal pain may also reflect pressure on the celiac axis from surrounding structures, called the **celiac compression syndrome.**

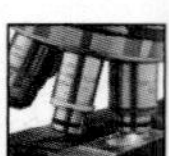

PATHOLOGY: Chronic small bowel ischemia may lead to fibrosis and stricture formation. Ischemic strictures of the small bowel may be single or multiple and produce intestinal obstruction or, occasionally, malabsorption due to stasis and bacterial overgrowth. These strictures are concentric, and the mucosa of this region is atrophic, often with one or more small ulcers. The submucosa is thickened and fibrotic with granulation tissue, which may involve the muscular layers. Hemosiderin deposition may be seen, particularly near the muscularis mucosae.

Malabsorption

Malabsorption is a general term that describes a number of clinical conditions in which important nutrients are inadequately absorbed by the gastrointestinal tract. Some nutrient absorption occurs in the stomach and colon, but only absorption from the small intestine, mainly in the proximal portion, is clinically important. Two substances are preferentially absorbed by the distal small intestine: **bile salts** and **vitamin B_{12}.**

In normal intestinal absorption there is a luminal phase and an intestinal phase (Fig. 13-36). The **luminal phase** (i.e., those processes that occur within the small intestine lumen) alters the physicochemical state of nutrients so that they can be taken up by absorptive cells. The **intestinal phase** includes processes occurring in cells and transport channels of the intestinal wall. Each phase has several critical components; derangement of one or more leads to impaired absorption.

In the luminal phase, **pancreatic enzymes** and **bile acids** must be secreted into the duodenal lumen in adequate amounts and in a normal physicochemical condition. In addition, a normal and regulated flow of gastric contents into the duodenum and an appropriately high duodenal pH must be present. Normal pancreatic enzyme excretion into the duodenum requires adequate pancreatic exocrine function and unobstructed flow of pancreatic juice.

Supply of bile in normal quantity and quality to the duodenum entails (1) adequate liver function, (2) unobstructed

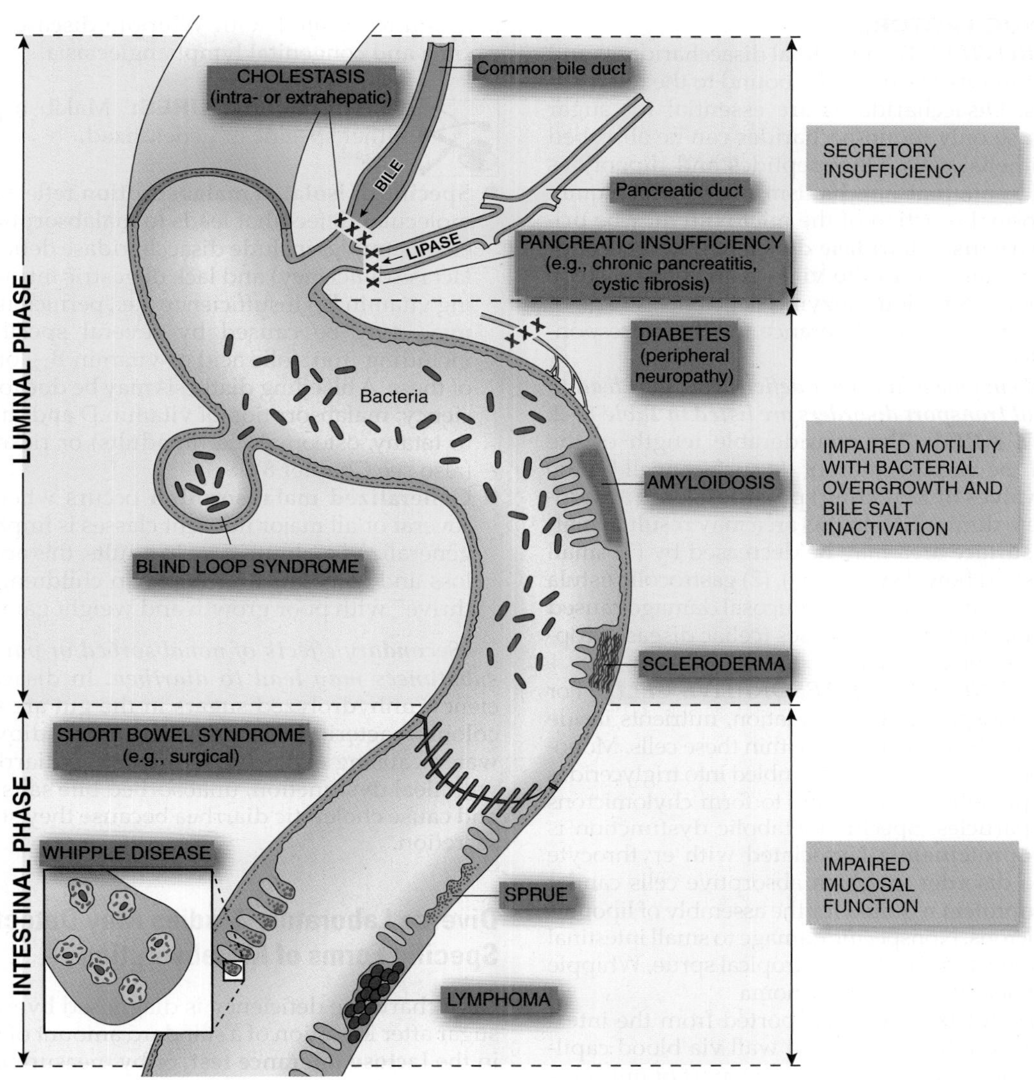

FIGURE 13-36. Causes of malabsorption.

bile flow and (3) intact enterohepatic bile salt circulation. The enterohepatic circulation of bile begins with absorption of most intestinal bile salts from the distal ileum and ends with their excretion into the duodenum through the bile ducts. Normally, 95% of intestinal bile salts are recycled through this circuit; 5% are excreted in the stool. Normal functioning of the enterohepatic circulation requires (1) normal intestinal microflora, (2) normal ileal absorptive function and (3) an unobstructed biliary system.

Luminal-Phase Malabsorption Often Reflects Insufficient Bile Acids

- **Interruption of the normal continuity of the distal stomach and duodenum** occurs after gastroduodenal surgery (gastrectomy, antrectomy, pyloroplasty).
- **Pancreatic dysfunction** can be due to chronic pancreatitis, pancreatic carcinoma or cystic fibrosis.
- **Deficient or ineffective bile salts** may result from three possible causes:
  1. **Impaired excretion of bile** resulting from liver disease.
  2. **Bacterial overgrowth** from impaired gut motility, as in blind-loop syndrome, multiple diverticula of the small bowel and muscular or neurogenic defects of the intestinal wall (e.g., amyloidosis, scleroderma, diabetic enteropathy). When gastrointestinal motility is defective, bile salts are deconjugated by the excess bacterial flora and cannot form micelles, which are essential for normal absorption of monoglycerides and free fatty acids.
  3. **Deficient bile salts** due to the absence or bypass of the distal ileum caused by surgical excision, surgical anastomoses, fistulas or ileal disease (e.g., Crohn disease, lymphoma).

Intestinal-Phase Malabsorption Frequently Reflects Specific Enzyme Defects or Impaired Transport

Although abnormalities in any one of the four components of the intestinal phase may cause malabsorption, some diseases affect more than one of these components. Fig. 13-36 summarizes the major causes of malabsorption.

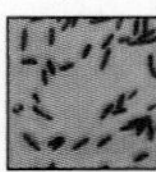

ETIOLOGIC FACTORS:

MICROVILLI: The intestinal disaccharidases and oligopeptidases are integrally bound to the microvillous membranes. Disaccharidases are essential for sugar absorption, because only monosaccharides can be absorbed by intestinal epithelial cells. Oligopeptides and dipeptides may be absorbed by alternate mechanisms that do not require peptidases. Abnormal function of the microvilli may be primary, as in **primary disaccharidase deficiencies**, or secondary, when there is damage to the villi, as in celiac disease (sprue; see below). The various enzyme deficiencies (e.g., of lactase) are characterized by intolerance for the corresponding disaccharides.

Rare inherited enzyme and carrier deficiencies that lead to selective intestinal transport disorders are listed in Table 13-2.

ABSORPTIVE AREA: The considerable length of the small bowel and the amplification of its surface wall by the intestinal folds (valves of Kerckring) provide a large absorptive surface. Severe diminution in this area may result in malabsorption. The surface area may be decreased by (1) small bowel resection (short bowel syndrome), (2) gastrocolic fistula (bypassing the small intestine) or (3) mucosal damage caused by a number of small intestinal diseases (celiac disease, tropical sprue and Whipple disease).

METABOLIC FUNCTION OF ABSORPTIVE CELLS: For their subsequent transport to the circulation, nutrients inside absorptive cells must be metabolized within these cells. Monoglycerides and free fatty acids are reassembled into triglycerides and coated with proteins (apoproteins) to form chylomicrons and lipoprotein particles. Specific metabolic dysfunction is seen in **abetalipoproteinemia** (associated with erythrocyte acanthocytosis), a disorder in which absorptive cells cannot synthesize the apoprotein required for the assembly of lipoproteins and chylomicrons. Nonspecific damage to small intestinal epithelial cells occurs in celiac disease, tropical sprue, Whipple disease and hyperacidity due to gastrinoma.

TRANSPORT: Nutrients are transported from the intestinal epithelium through the intestinal wall via blood capillaries and lymphatic vessels. Impaired transport of nutrients through these conduits is probably important in the malabsorption associated with Whipple disease, intestinal lymphoma and congenital lymphangiectasia.

Table 13-2

Congenital Intestinal Transport Diseases

Fat	Cystic fibrosis
	Abetalipoproteinemia and hypobetalipoproteinemia
	Chylomicron retention disease
Carbohydrates	Glucose-galactose malabsorption
	Disaccharidase deficiencies
	Congenital lactase deficiency
	Sucrase-isomaltase deficiency
Amino acids	Hartnup disease
	Lysinuric protein intolerance
Electrolytes	Congenital Cl^- and congenital Na^+ diarrhea
Vitamins	Transcobalamin II deficiency
	Cobalamin C deficiency

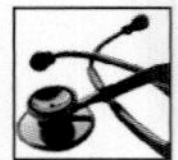

CLINICAL FEATURES: Malabsorption may be either specific or generalized.

- **Specific or isolated malabsorption** reflects an identifiable molecular defect that leads to malabsorption of one nutrient. Examples include disaccharidase deficiencies (notably lactase deficiency) and lack of gastric intrinsic factor, causing vitamin B_{12} insufficiency (i.e., pernicious anemia). Anemias may be caused by several specific deficiencies, including iron, folic acid or vitamin B_{12}, or a combination of these. A bleeding diathesis may be due to vitamin K deficiency; malabsorption of vitamin D and calcium may lead to tetany, osteomalacia (in adults) or rickets (in children) (also see Chapter 8).
- **Generalized malabsorption** occurs when absorption of several or all major nutrient classes is impaired. It leads to generalized malnutrition. In adults, this appears as weight loss and sometimes cachexia; in children, it is "failure to thrive" with poor growth and weight gain.

Secondary effects of nonabsorbed or partially absorbed substances may lead to diarrhea. In disaccharidase deficiency, unhydrolyzed sugars in the gut are metabolized by colonic bacteria to lactic acid, carbon dioxide (CO_2) and water, causing explosive fermentative diarrhea. In patients with ileal dysfunction, unabsorbed bile salts enter the colon and cause choleretic diarrhea because they stimulate colonic secretion.

Diverse Laboratory Studies May Detect Specific Forms of Malabsorption

Disaccharidase deficiency is diagnosed by measuring blood sugar after ingestion of a standard amount of disaccharide, as in the **lactose tolerance test,** or by measuring enzyme activity in small bowel biopsies. In the **Schilling test,** isotopically labeled vitamin B_{12} is given orally and its blood level then determined. This helps to distinguish between malabsorption resulting from intrinsic factor deficiency and other causes of vitamin B_{12} malabsorption.

In generalized malabsorption, there is almost always impaired absorption of dietary fat. Quantitative fecal fat analysis is the most reliable and sensitive test of overall digestive and absorptive function and is a standard for all other tests for malabsorption. Steatorrhea (fat in the stools) is the hallmark of generalized malabsorption.

A few tests currently in use to evaluate various causes of malabsorption merit mention.

- **D-Xylose Absorption:** Xylose is a five-carbon sugar whose absorption does not require any component of the luminal phase. Blood levels and urinary excretion of this compound after ingestion of a defined amount thus are useful to test the intestinal phase of absorption.
- **$^{14}CO_2$-cholyl-glycine breath test:** Measuring $^{14}CO_2$ in exhaled air after oral administration of $^{14}CO_2$-cholylglycine is a test of bile salt absorption by the ileum. It is used in the diagnosis of the blind- or stagnant-loop syndrome (caused by bacterial overgrowth) and of ileal absorptive function. A newer test to detect bacterial overgrowth is the ^{14}C-xylose breath test.

- **Schilling test:** Originally devised to diagnose pernicious anemia, this test has been modified to test ileal absorption, bacterial overgrowth and pancreatic function.

Lactase Deficiency Causes Intolerance to Milk Products

The intestinal brush border contains disaccharidases that are important for absorption of carbohydrates. As a prominent constituent of milk and many other dairy products, lactose is one of the most common disaccharides in the diet. Before milk-producing animals were domesticated about 9000 years ago, human milk was probably the only milk consumed by babies and young children. Dairy products were nonexistent. The availability of nonhuman milk favored lactase production, perhaps leading cattle-herding societies (e.g., Europeans) to be lactose tolerant, whereas non–cattle herders (e.g., Native Americans, Asians) tend to be lactose intolerant.

Acquired lactase deficiency is widespread, with symptoms typically beginning in adolescence. Patients complain of abdominal distention, flatulence and diarrhea after consuming dairy products. Removing milk and its products from the diet relieves these symptoms. Diseases that injure the intestinal mucosa (e.g., celiac disease or radiation enteritis) may also lead to acquired lactase deficiency. Congenital lactase deficiency is rare but may be lethal if not recognized.

Celiac Disease Reflects an Immune Response to Gluten in Cereals

Celiac disease (celiac sprue, gluten-sensitive enteropathy) is characterized by (1) generalized malabsorption, (2) small intestinal mucosal lesions and (3) prompt clinical and histopathologic response to withdrawal of gluten-containing foods from the diet.

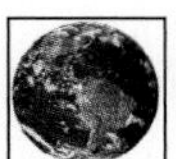

EPIDEMIOLOGY: Celiac disease is worldwide and affects all ethnic groups, including perhaps 1% of whites. There is a slight female predominance, 1.3:1. It may be seen any time after cereals are introduced into the diet. Most cases are diagnosed during childhood, but the disease may first become clinically apparent as late as the seventh decade of life.

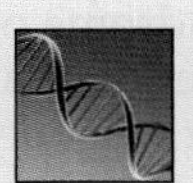

MOLECULAR PATHOGENESIS: Genetic predisposition and gliadin exposure are crucial factors in the development of celiac disease.

ROLE OF CEREAL PROTEINS: If successfully treated, asymptomatic patients with celiac disease consume wheat, barley or rye flour, the clinical and histopathologic features of celiac sprue follow. Other grains, such as rice and corn flour, do not have such an effect. Both the water-insoluble portion of wheat flour, **gluten**, and an alcoholic extract, called **gliadin**, have the same effect.

GENETIC FACTORS: Celiac sprue is caused by an interplay of complex genetic factors plus an abnormal immune response to ingested cereal antigens. Overt and latent celiac disease run in families. Concordance for celiac disease in first-degree relatives is between 8% and 18% and reaches 70% in monozygotic twins. About 90% of patients with celiac disease carry the histocompatibility antigen HLA B8 and a comparable frequency has been reported for HLA DR8 and DQ2.

IMMUNOLOGIC FACTORS: Celiac disease is characterized by damage to intestinal epithelial cells and a marked increase in $CD8^+$ T lymphocytes in the epithelium and of plasma cells in the lamina propria. Gliadin challenge of people with treated celiac sprue stimulates local immunoglobulin synthesis.

Most (90%) untreated patients with celiac disease have serologic evidence of prior infection with serotype 12 adenovirus. This virus infects the human gastrointestinal tract, and one of its proteins has a region of amino acid sequence homology to α-gliadin. Exposure of a genetically susceptible person to gluten-containing cereals might then stimulate an immune reaction to gliadin at the intestinal epithelial cell surface.

Serum antigliadin and antiendomysial antibodies are present in almost all patients, but their role in the pathogenesis of the disease remains to be established.

ASSOCIATION WITH DERMATITIS HERPETIFORMIS: Celiac disease is occasionally associated with dermatitis herpetiformis (DH), a vesicular skin disease that typically affects extensor surfaces and exposed parts of the body. In DH, subepidermal neutrophil infiltration leads to local edema and blister formation. Basement membrane IgA deposits are detected. Almost all patients with DH have a small bowel mucosal lesion like that of celiac disease, although only 10% have overt malabsorption. Treatment with a gluten-free diet leads to improvement in both gastrointestinal symptoms and skin lesions. HLA-B8 is much more common in patients with dermatitis herpetiformis than in others.

Malabsorption in celiac disease probably results from multiple factors, including reduced intestinal mucosal surface area (due to blunting of villi and microvilli) and impaired intracellular metabolism in damaged epithelial cells. Secondary disaccharidase deficiency, due to damage to microvilli, may play a role as well. A hypothetical mechanism for the pathogenesis of celiac disease is presented in Fig. 13-37.

PATHOLOGY: Small bowel biopsies taken very early in the disease may show intraepithelial lymphocytic infiltration of the crypts and surface epithelium in normal-appearing villi. Fully developed celiac disease shows a flat mucosa, with (1) blunting or total disappearance of villi, (2) damaged mucosal surface epithelial cells with numerous intraepithelial lymphocytes (T cells) and (3) increased plasma cells in the lamina propria but not in deeper layers (Fig. 13-38). The most severe histologic abnormalities in untreated celiac disease usually occur in the duodenum and proximal jejunum. There is a progressive decrease in severity distally and in some cases the ileal mucosa looks virtually normal. The clinical severity of the disease is related to the length of intestine affected. Lymphocytic gastritis and lymphocytic colitis often occur with celiac disease.

In the small bowel, the total mucosal thickness may not be decreased, because lengthening of the crypts compensates for villous shortening. Absorptive cells are flattened and more basophilic than normal, and the basal polarity of their nuclei

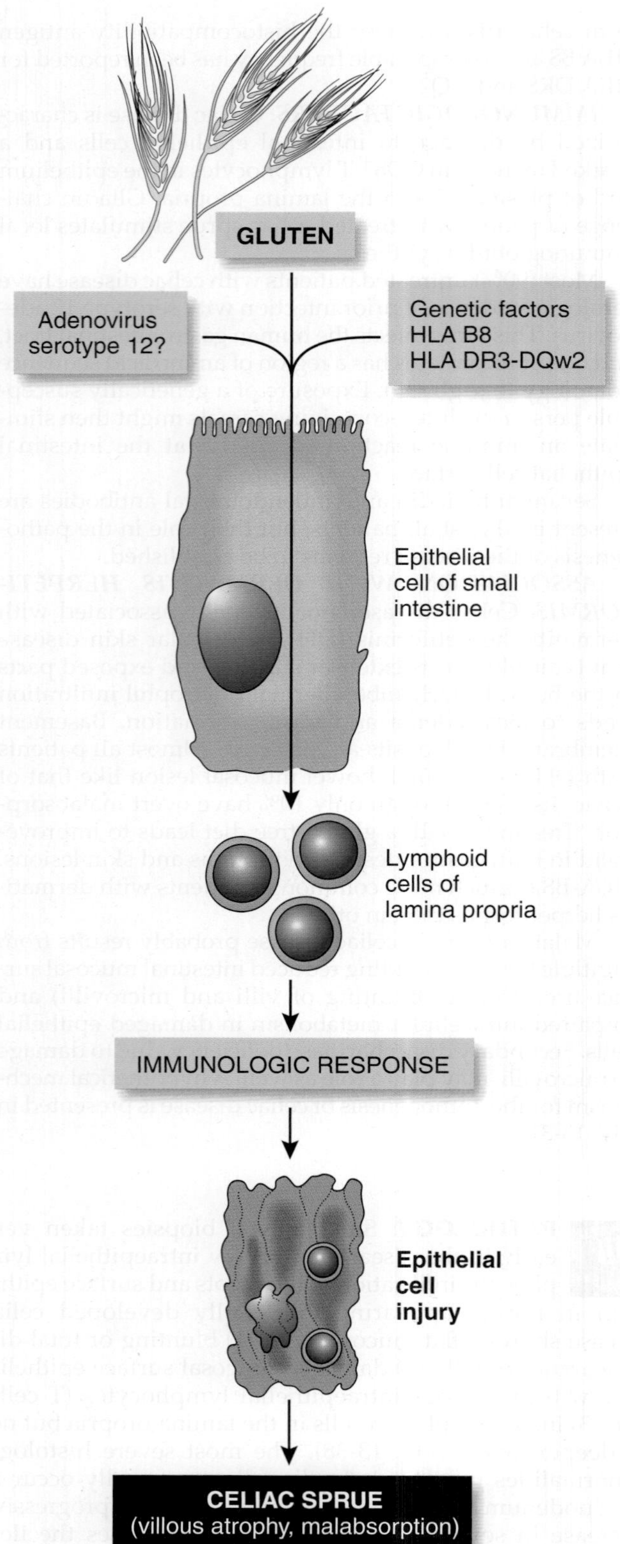

FIGURE 13-37. Hypothetical mechanisms in the pathogenesis of celiac disease. HLA = human leukocyte antigen.

is lost. Lymphocytes and plasma cells in the lamina propria are markedly increased. Polymorphonuclear leukocytes and eosinophils may also be increased in the epithelium and lamina propria.

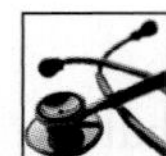

CLINICAL FEATURES: ***Generalized malabsorption characterizes fully developed celiac disease.*** Overt signs of malabsorption in children are often lacking, and the disease is suspected only because of growth retardation. In adults, iron-deficiency anemia resistant to oral therapy often suggests celiac disease. Signs of generalized malabsorption may first appear in older children, adolescents and adults. Testing for **IgA antiendomysial** and **anti-tissue transglutaminase antibodies** shows that celiac disease is more common than previously thought.

Treatment with a strict gluten-free diet usually leads to complete and prolonged clinical and histopathologic remission. Some patients who do not respond to a gluten-free diet, partly or completely, may have **refractory sprue** and require corticosteroids. In this case, T cells may lose surface CD4 and CD8 and show monoclonal *T-cell receptor-γ* gene rearrangements. Thus, some cases of refractory sprue may represent monoclonal T-cell proliferations.

The systemic manifestations of celiac disease are related to the various deficiency states that result from generalized malabsorption. Late complications in some cases include **ulcerative jejunitis** and **small bowel T-cell lymphoma**. Adenocarcinoma of the small bowel and squamous cancers of the oropharynx and esophagus also occur. Increased risk for colorectal carcinoma is also reported. Other extraintestinal manifestations include follicular keratosis, peripheral neuropathy and infertility.

Collagenous sprue is a rare disorder characterized by deposition of collagen in the lamina propria of the small bowel. The disorder initially mimics celiac disease but does not respond to a gluten-free diet. The prognosis in collagenous sprue is grave: no reported patients have survived.

Autoimmune Enteropathy Features Autoantibodies to Gut Epithelium

Autoimmune enteropathy (AIE) is one of the common forms of severe, intractable diarrhea in infants and children. There is a strong male predominance and a tendency to occur in siblings. AIE is often associated with the X-linked syndrome of immunodysregulation, polyendocrinopathy and enteropathy (IPEX syndrome) due to mutation in the *FoxP3* gene, which encodes the scurfin protein that is critical for development of $CD4^+$ regulatory T cells. The signature of AIE is autoantibodies, particularly against enterocytes, which deposit along the apex and basolateral border of those cells. The mucosa shows villus atrophy. An inflammatory infiltrate in the lamina propria, in contrast to celiac disease, tends to be modest. The stomach and colon are often involved. Extragastrointestinal sites are often involved, including the thyroid (thyroiditis), kidney (glomerulonephritis), liver (autoimmune hepatitis) and erythrocytes (autoimmune hemolytic anemia). Antibody-mediated destruction of islets and insulin-dependent diabetes may occur. Mortality approaches 30%. Immunosuppression is useful in many cases, as is bone marrow transplantation.

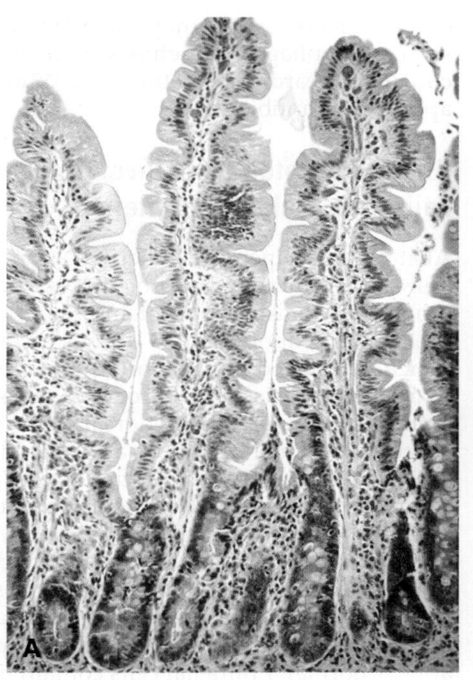

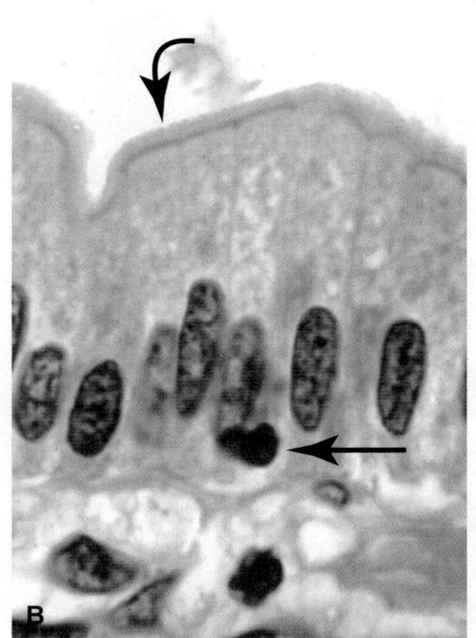

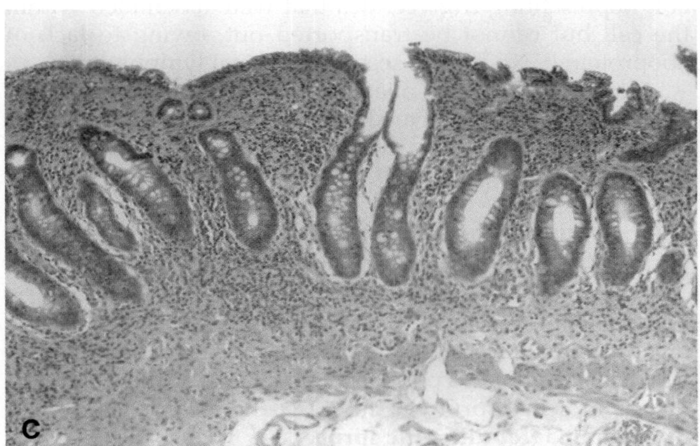

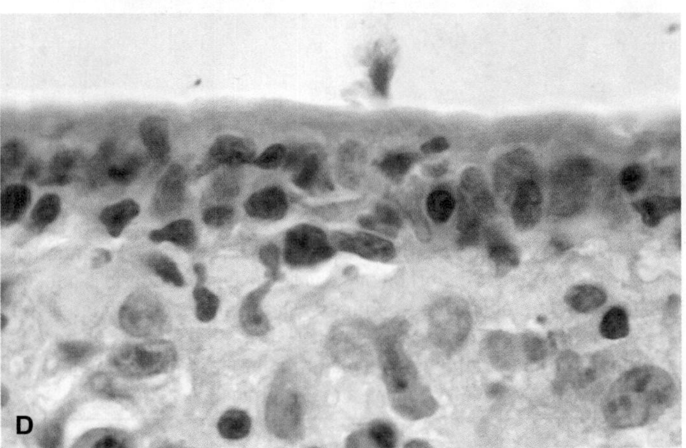

FIGURE 13-38. Celiac disease. A. Normal proximal small intestine shows tall slender villi with crypts present at the base. **B.** Normal surface epithelium shows an occasional intraepithelial lymphocyte (*straight arrow*) as well as an intact brush border (*curved arrow*). **C.** A mucosal biopsy from a patient with advanced celiac disease shows complete loss of the villi with infiltration of the lamina propria by lymphocytes and plasma cells. The crypts are increased in height. **D.** At higher power the surface epithelium is severely damaged with large numbers of intraepithelial lymphocytes and loss of the brush border.

In Whipple Disease the Small Bowel Is Filled With Macrophages Packed with Small Rod-Shaped Bacteria

Malabsorption is the most prominent feature of Whipple disease. White men in their 30s and 40s are most affected. The disease is systemic, and other clinical findings include fever, increased skin pigmentation, anemia, lymphadenopathy, arthritis, pericarditis, pleurisy, endocarditis and central nervous system involvement.

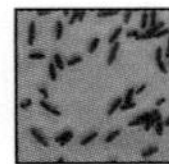

ETIOLOGIC FACTORS: The causative organism is one of the gram-positive actinomycetes, *Tropheryma whippelii.* Interestingly, *T. whippelii* is distantly related to mycobacteria such as *Mycobacterium avium-intracellulare* and *Mycobacterium paratuberculosis,* both of which have been associated with illnesses resembling Whipple disease. Several studies suggest that host susceptibility factors, possibly defective T-cell function, may predispose to the disease. Macrophages from patients with Whipple disease show impaired ability to degrade intracellular microorganisms. Circulating cells expressing CD11b, a cell-adhesion and complement-receptor molecule on macrophages, are reduced. CD11b is involved in activating macrophages to kill intracellular pathogens. Dramatic clinical remissions occur with antibiotic therapy.

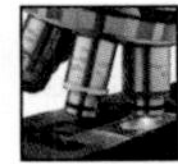

PATHOLOGY: The bowel wall is thickened and edematous; mesenteric lymph nodes are usually enlarged. Villi are flat and their lamina propria is extensively

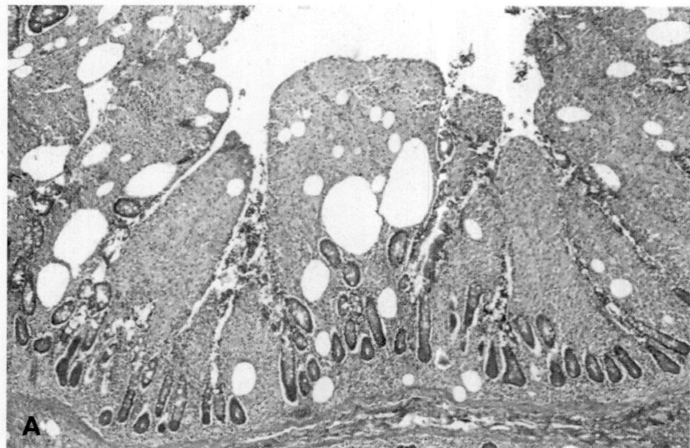

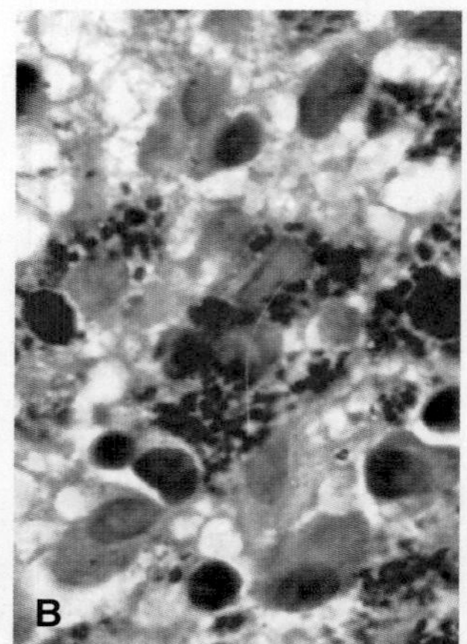

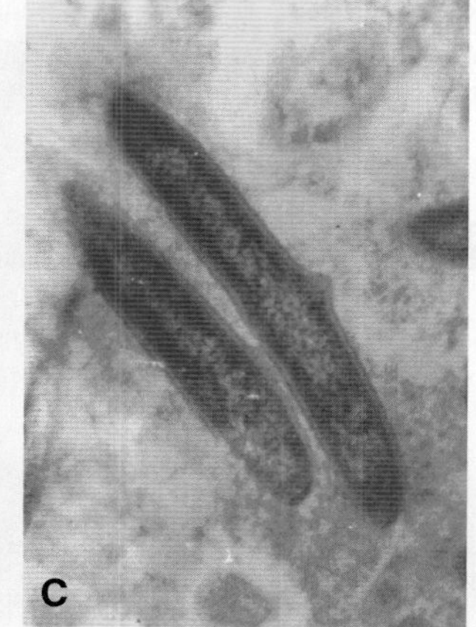

FIGURE 13-39. Whipple disease. A. A photomicrograph of a section of jejunal mucosa shows distortion of the villi. The lamina propria is packed with large, pale-staining macrophages. Dilated mucosal lymphatics are prominent. **B.** A periodic acid–Schiff (PAS) reaction shows numerous macrophages filled with cytoplasmic granular material. **C.** An electron micrograph shows small bacilli in a macrophage.

infiltrated with large foamy macrophages (Fig. 13-39A) whose cytoplasm is filled with large glycoprotein granules that stain strongly with periodic acid–Schiff (PAS) (Fig. 13-39B). The other normal cellular components of the lamina propria (i.e., plasma cells and lymphocytes) are depleted. Lymphatic vessels in the mucosa and submucosa are dilated and large lipid droplets abound within lymphatics and in extracellular spaces, suggesting lymphatic obstruction. In contrast to the striking distortion of villous architecture, epithelial cells show only patchy abnormalities, including attenuation of microvilli and accumulation of lipid droplets within the cytoplasm.

Electron microscopy reveals numerous small bacilli within macrophages and free in the lamina propria (Fig. 13-39C). The PAS-positive granules seen by light microscopy are lysosomes engorged with bacilli in various stages of degeneration. Many bacilli cluster just beneath the epithelial basement membrane.

Mesenteric lymph nodes draining affected segments of small bowel show similar microscopic changes. Macrophages containing bacilli may also be found infiltrating most other organs. Heart lesions may include valve vegetations with such macrophages, sometimes with superimposed streptococcal endocarditis. Treatment of Whipple disease is with appropriate antibiotics.

Abetalipoproteinemia Involves Failure to Make Apoprotein B

Abetalipoproteinemia is inherited as an autosomal recessive disease. The missing apoprotein B is a part of the membrane coat of low-density lipoproteins. Small intestinal absorptive cells lacking apoprotein B do not assemble chylomicrons, which are needed to transport lipid out of the cell. This leads to **acanthocytosis in erythrocytes** and **selective demyelinization,** particularly of the dorsal spinal cord columns. Typical neurologic manifestations are loss of deep tendon reflexes, sensory ataxia and a mild form of retinitis pigmentosa. The serum contains no chylomicrons, very-low-density lipoproteins or low-density lipoproteins. Blood levels of cholesterol and triglycerides are low, and serum lipids are mostly carried in high-density lipoprotein particles. Absorption of fat-soluble vitamins (A, D, E, K) is severely impaired.

Microscopically, the villi, lamina propria and submucosa appear normal. Epithelial cells contain lipid vacuoles, probably representing triglycerides that were assembled within the cell but cannot be transported out, owing to lack of apoprotein B. No lipid is seen in intestinal lymphatics.

Malabsorption in abetalipoproteinemia is partially reversed by ingestion of medium-chain (rather than the usual long-chain) triglycerides; these lipids are transported through the absorptive cells without an apoprotein coat.

Hypogammaglobulinemia May Lead to Malabsorption

The small intestine in hypogammaglobulinemia contains few or no plasma cells in the lamina propria and often shows nodular lymphoid hyperplasia. Occasionally, the mucosa is flat, as in celiac sprue; in this case, the disorder is termed **hypogammaglobulinemic sprue.**

Most hypogammaglobulinemic patients with malabsorption have small intestinal infection with *G. lamblia.* Treatment with metronidazole improves intestinal absorption.

Congenital Lymphangiectasia Is a Generalized Malformation That Causes Malabsorption

Congenital lymphangiectasia is a poorly understood disease that usually begins in childhood. Patients have steatorrhea caused by impaired transport of chylomicrons by intestinal lymphatics and a **protein-losing enteropathy** (i.e., they lose large amounts of plasma proteins into the gut). Combined intestinal lymphangiectasia and peripheral lymphedema is known as **Milroy disease.**

Other important features of congenital lymphangiectasia are lymphopenia and impaired cell-mediated immunity, caused by loss of small lymphocytes into the bowel lumen. Chylous ascites (milky, lipid-containing peritoneal fluid) due to leakage of lymph from the mesenteric or serosal lymphatic vessels into the peritoneal cavity may occur.

Opalescent white mucosal spots represent **dilated lymphatics (lacteals)** in the lamina propria. Submucosal lymphatics also tend to be dilated. The epithelium is normal, but villi may be blunted or even absent in areas overlying severe lymphatic dilation.

Acquired intestinal lymphangiectasia, with all or some of the clinical features described above, may be a secondary manifestation of small intestinal or retroperitoneal lymphoma, other retroperitoneal tumors, tuberculosis, sarcoidosis, chronic pancreatitis and retroperitoneal fibrosis.

Tropical Sprue Is a Disease of Unknown Etiology That Causes Folate Deficiency

The disease is endemic in some tropical areas and is characterized by progressively severe malabsorption and nutritional deficiency. Symptoms usually improve after treatment with oral tetracycline and folic acid. The cause of tropical sprue is not known. Some studies suggest that **long-term contamination of the bowel with bacteria,** perhaps toxigenic *E. coli,* may be involved and that resultant **folate deficiency** may play a role in perpetuating the intestinal lesion.

Histologic findings vary from mild widening and blunting of villi to a completely flat mucosa like that seen in celiac sprue. The morphologic injury in the epithelium and the inflammation of the lamina propria usually parallel the severity of the alterations in the villi.

Typically, steatorrhea, anemia and weight loss precede progressively severe manifestations of folic acid and vitamin B_{12} deficiencies and hypoalbuminemia. Laboratory findings include increased fecal fat, impaired D-xylose absorption, megaloblastic anemia and decreased intestinal mucosa disaccharidase activity.

Radiation Enteritis Results From Abdominal Radiotherapy

Transient damage to the small intestinal mucosa is seen. Anorexia, abdominal cramps and changes in bowel habits are common during abdominal radiation treatments, and laboratory studies in such patients indicate malabsorption of bile salts and disaccharides. Transient histologic changes include shortening of small bowel villi, increased cellularity in the lamina propria and submucosal edema.

Occasionally, subacute or chronic radiation damage occurs, especially if (1) the radiation dose is very high, (2) parts of small bowel become fixed as a result of postoperative or inflammatory adhesions, (3) the bowel's blood supply is impaired or (4) radiation is combined with chemotherapeutic agents that may augment radiation damage.

Subacute and chronic radiation damage to the small intestine and elsewhere in the gastrointestinal tract leads to (1) mucosal ulceration, (2) swelling and detachment of endothelial cells of small arterioles in the submucosa, (3) obliteration by fibrin plugs of arteriolar lumina and (4) large foam cells beneath the intima. Thickening and fibrosis of the submucosa ensue, together with signs of progressive ischemia, to produce stricture.

Mechanical Obstruction

Mechanical obstruction to the passage of intestinal contents can be caused by (1) a luminal mass, (2) an intrinsic lesion of the bowel wall or (3) extrinsic compression.

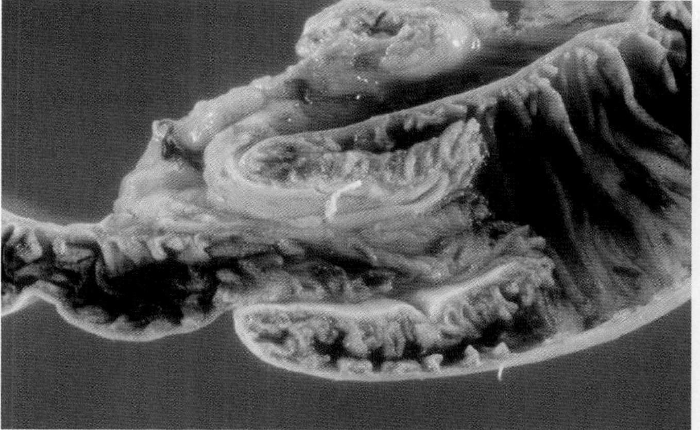

FIGURE 13-40. Intussusception. A cross-section through the area of the obstruction shows "telescoped" small intestine surrounded by dilated small intestine.

INTUSSUSCEPTION: In this form of intraluminal small bowel obstruction a segment of bowel (intussusceptum) telescopes distally into a surrounding outer portion (intussuscipiens) (Fig. 13-40). Intussusception usually occurs in infants or young children, in whom it occurs without a known cause. In adults, the leading point of an intussusception is usually a lesion in the bowel wall, such as Meckel diverticulum or a tumor. Once the leading point is entrapped in the intussuscipiens, peristalsis drives the intussusceptum forward. In addition to acute intestinal obstruction, intussusception compresses the blood supply to the intussusceptum, which may become infarcted. If the obstruction is not relieved spontaneously, treatment requires surgery.

VOLVULUS: This is an example of intestinal obstruction causing an acute abdomen, in which a segment of gut twists on its mesentery, kinking the bowel and usually interrupting its blood supply. Volvulus is almost always a sign of a congenital malformation. Malrotation of the bowel permits undue mobility of bowel loops and predisposes to **midgut volvulus.** If the cecum or right colon is invested with a mesentery, rather than being retroperitoneal, **cecal volvulus** may result. An unusually long sigmoid colon, as sometimes occurs in patients with idiopathic chronic constipation, permits the development of **sigmoid volvulus.**

ADHESIONS: Fibrous scars caused by previous surgery or peritonitis cause obstruction by kinking or angulating the bowel or directly compressing the lumen.

HERNIAS: Loops of small bowel may be incarcerated in an inguinal or femoral hernia, in which case the lumen may become obstructed and the vascular supply compromised. Similarly, portions of the bowel may be trapped internally by hernias that represent congenital or surgically acquired defects in the mesentery.

PSEUDO-OBSTRUCTION: Patients with signs and symptoms of intestinal obstruction but without a mechanical cause are said to have pseudo-obstruction. The process may be familial or sporadic. There may be an underlying myopathy or neuropathy, but often, no anatomic lesion is found. The myopathies feature fibrosis around muscle cells in the lamina propria.

A common form of pseudo-obstruction is limited to the colon in which no morphologic lesion is found, referred to as severe idiopathic constipation. Pseudo-obstruction may be secondary to intestinal involvement by diseases such as scleroderma, amyloidosis, hypothyroidism or adverse drug effect. Such cases are often referred to as secondary pseudo-obstruction.

Neoplasms

Fewer than 5% of all gastrointestinal tumors arise in the small intestine.

Benign Tumors Include Adenomas, Peutz-Jeghers Polyps and Stromal Tumors

Adenomas

Small bowel adenomas resemble those of the colon. Depending on the predominant component, adenomatous polyps of the small intestine may be tubular, villous or tubulovillous. Villous adenomas are rare in the small intestine. If they occur, it is usually in the periampullary region of the duodenum. ***Adenomas, especially the villous type, may undergo malignant transformation.*** Benign adenomas are often asymptomatic, but bleeding and intussusception are occasional complications.

Peutz-Jeghers Syndrome

Peutz-Jeghers syndrome is an autosomal dominant hereditary disorder of intestinal hamartomatous polyps and mucocutaneous melanin pigmentation, particularly on the face, buccal mucosa, hands, feet and perianal and genital areas. Except for the buccal pigmentation, the freckle-like macular lesions usually fade at puberty. The polyps occur mostly in the proximal small intestine but are sometimes seen in the stomach and colon. Patients usually have symptoms of obstruction or intussusception; in as many as one fourth of cases, however, the diagnosis is suggested by pigmentation in an otherwise asymptomatic person.

Peutz-Jeghers syndrome is associated with inactivating mutations of a gene (*LKB1*) on chromosome 19p that encodes a protein kinase. Carriers of the defective gene are also at increased risk for cancers of many organs including breast, lung, pancreas, gonads and thyroid.

Peutz-Jeghers polyps are hamartomas, with branching networks of smooth muscle fibers continuous with the muscularis mucosae supporting the glandular epithelium of the polyp (Fig. 13-41). They are generally considered benign, but 3% of patients develop adenocarcinoma, although not necessarily in the hamartomatous polyps.

Gastrointestinal Stromal Tumors (GISTs)

GISTs occur throughout the small intestine but mostly in the jejunum. They grow as intramural masses covered by intact mucosa and are similar to those in other locations. Intestinal obstruction is uncommon, but volvulus may be a complication. Small intestinal GISTs are more likely to behave aggressively than their gastric counterparts.

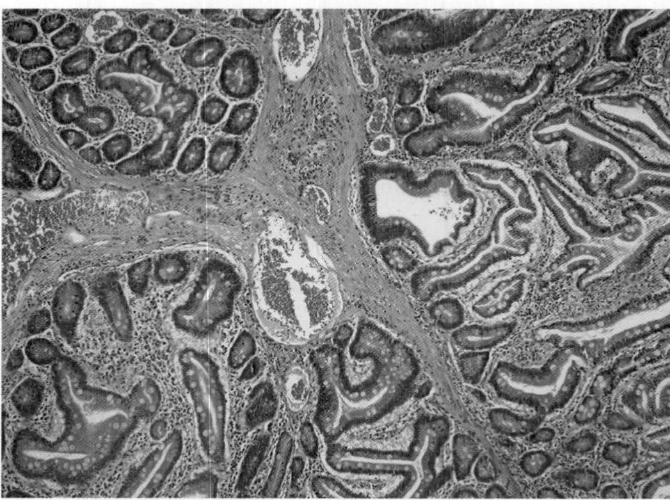

FIGURE 13-41. Peutz-Jeghers polyps. The intestinal epithelium has peculiar shapes but unremarkable nuclear and cytoplasmic features. Arborizing large bundles of smooth muscle are characteristic.

Malignant Tumors of the Small Bowel Are Uncommon

Adenocarcinoma

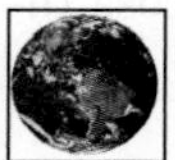

EPIDEMIOLOGY: Although small bowel adenocarcinomas are a tiny proportion of all gastrointestinal tumors, they account for half of small bowel malignant tumors. Most occur in the duodenum and jejunum, usually in middle-aged people, with a moderate male predominance. Interestingly, the geographic variation in the incidence of small bowel adenocarcinoma correlates with that of colon—but not stomach—cancer.

Crohn disease of the small bowel is a risk factor for adenocarcinoma. Such patients develop these tumors on average 10 years younger than other patients. In Crohn disease patients, the tumors tend to occur near inflammatory lesions (i.e., mostly in the ileum). Familial adenomatous polyposis, HNPCC syndrome (Lynch syndrome) and celiac disease are additional risk factors.

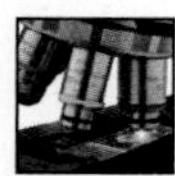

PATHOLOGY AND CLINICAL FEATURES: Adenocarcinoma of the small intestine may be polypoid, ulcerative or simply annular and stenosing. In addition to causing intestinal obstruction directly, a polypoid tumor may be the lead point of an intussusception. ***Adenocarcinomas begin in crypt epithelium, rather than the villi, and, therefore, resemble colorectal cancers.***

The symptoms of small bowel adenocarcinoma commonly relate to progressive intestinal obstruction. Occult bleeding is common and often leads to iron-deficiency anemia. If duodenal adenocarcinomas involve the papilla of Vater, they are termed **ampullary carcinomas.** These tumors cause obstructive jaundice or pancreatitis. By the time patients become symptomatic, most of these tumors have spread to local lymph nodes and 5-year survival is less than 20%. This tumor is the second most common cause of death in familial adenomatous polyposis.

Primary Intestinal Lymphoma

Lymphomas are the second most common malignancies of the small intestine in industrialized countries, accounting for about 15% of small bowel cancers. Many of these arise from MALT and are termed **Western-type lymphomas** (see below).

A different primary small intestinal lymphoma arises in the context of celiac disease and is called **enteropathy-type intestinal T-cell lymphoma (EITCL).** As their name implies, these tumors often complicate celiac disease, particularly refractory sprue (see above), which does not respond to gluten restriction. EITCLs are also known to complicate ulcerative jejunoileitis. These tumors are often widespread at the time of diagnosis and are associated with aberrant expression of CD130, but lack of CD4 or CD8.

The risk of intestinal lymphoma is also increased in settings that favor development of nodal lymphoma, particularly immunodeficiency following treatment with immunosuppressive drugs.

MEDITERRANEAN LYMPHOMA: Mediterranean lymphoma typically occurs in poor countries in young men of low socioeconomic status; it is therefore thought by some to have an environmental cause. It is associated with α-heavy-chain disease, a disorder of intestinal B lymphocytes that secrete the heavy chain of IgA without light chains. Mediterranean lymphoma and α-chain disease are often grouped as **immunoproliferative small intestinal disease.**

Mediterranean intestinal lymphoma predominantly involves the duodenum and proximal jejunum. A long segment of small intestine, or even the entire small bowel, is characteristically affected. Typically a diffuse infiltrate of plasmacytoid lymphocytes or plasma cells is seen in the mucosa and submucosa (Fig. 13-42). Lymphomatous infiltration of the mucosa leads to mucosal atrophy and severe malabsorption.

WESTERN-TYPE INTESTINAL LYMPHOMA: This disorder usually affects adults over 40 and children under 10. It is most often seen in the ileum as (1) a fungating mass that projects into the lumen, (2) an elevated ulcerated lesion, (3) a diffuse segmental thickening of the bowel wall or (4) plaque-like mucosal nodules. Intestinal obstruction, intussusception and perforation are important complications. Occult bleeding is common, although massive acute hemorrhage may also occur. All varieties of malignant lymphoma are encountered. When extraintestinal spread is present, the 5-year survival rate is less than 10%.

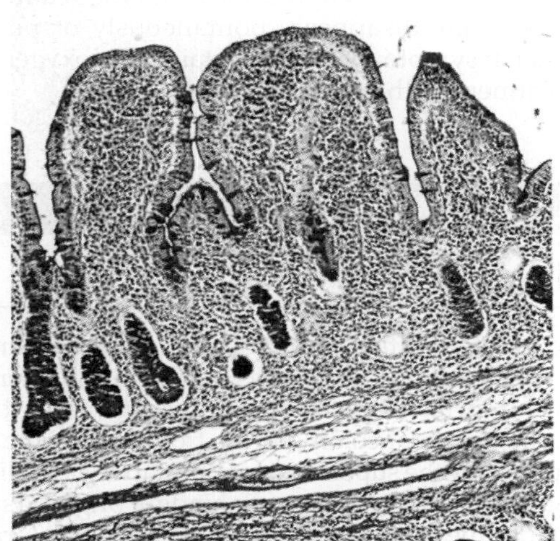

FIGURE 13-42. Mediterranean intestinal lymphoma. The villi are short and blunted, and the lamina propria is filled with lymphoid cells.

Chronic abdominal pain, diarrhea and clubbing of fingers are the most frequent clinical signs of intestinal lymphoma. Diarrhea and weight loss reflect the underlying malabsorption.

Neuroendocrine Tumors (Carcinoid Tumors)

The term **neuroendocrine tumors** (NETs) has largely replaced the term **carcinoid tumors.** All these tumors are considered malignant, but usually with low metastatic potential. The gut is the most common site for NETs (the bronchus being the next most common site). The site of origin is a major determinant of behavior. Other important considerations include size, depth of invasion, hormonal responsiveness and presence or absence of function.

The appendix is the most common gastrointestinal site of origin, followed by the rectum. Tumors of these sites are usually small and rarely aggressive. The next most common site is the ileum, where they are often multiple and more aggressive. ***NETs account for about 20% of all small intestinal malignancies.*** They are also seen in the multiple endocrine neoplasia (MEN) syndromes, particularly MEN type 1 (see Chapter 21).

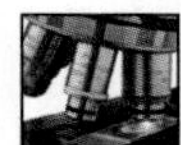

PATHOLOGY: Small NETs present as submucosal nodules covered by intact mucosa. Larger tumors may grow in a polypoid, intramural or annular pattern (Fig. 13-43A) and often undergo secondary ulceration. Cut surfaces are firm and white to yellow. As they enlarge, the tumors invade the muscular coat and penetrate the serosa, often causing a conspicuous desmoplastic reaction leading to peritoneal adhesions and kinking of the bowel, with possible intestinal obstruction.

Small, round cells in NETs form nests, cords and rosettes (Fig. 13-43B). Occasional gland-like structures are also seen (hence the term "carcinoid"). Nuclei are remarkably regular and mitoses are rare. The abundant eosinophilic cytoplasm contains granules, typically of the neurosecretory type. Goblet cell carcinoids or adenocarcinoid tumors have glandular differentiation. These tumors have a higher rate of aggressive behavior than do typical NETs.

These tumors metastasize first to regional lymph nodes. Subsequently, hematogenous spread produces metastases at distant sites, particularly the liver. Patients may occasionally present with an extraordinary volume of metastatic NET in the liver due to a small, clinically silent primary tumor in the small intestine.

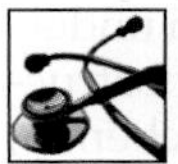

CLINICAL FEATURES: **Carcinoid syndrome** marks a small percentage of NETs and is a unique but uncommon clinical condition caused by release of active tumor products. Most NETs are to some extent functional, but this syndrome mainly occurs in patients with extensive hepatic metastases. ***Classic symptoms include diarrhea (often the most distressing symptom), episodic flushing, bronchospasm, cyanosis, telangiectasia and skin lesions.*** Half of patients also have right-sided cardiac valvular disease. Diarrhea is thought to be caused by serotonin.

After its release into the blood, serotonin is metabolized to 5-hydroxyindoleacetic acid (5-HIAA) by monoamine oxidase

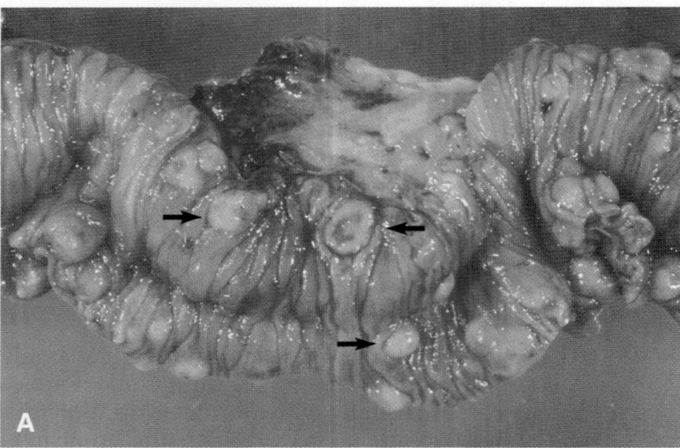

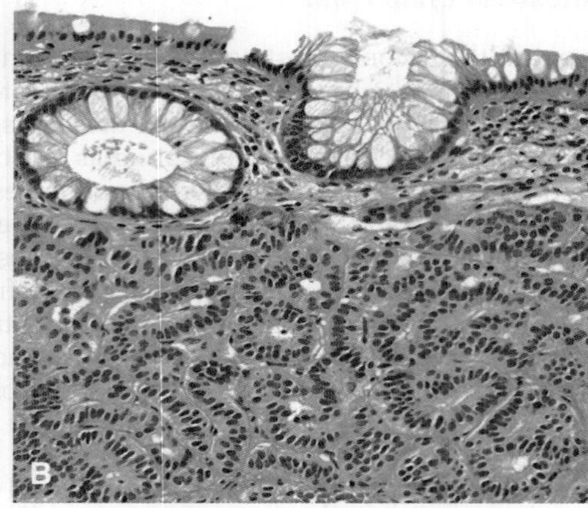

FIGURE 13-43. Neuroendocrine tumor of small intestine. A. A resected segment of distal ileum shows multiple neuroendocrine tumors (*arrows*). **B.** A photomicrograph of the lesion in A demonstrates cords of uniform small, round cells.

(MAO) in the tumor or in other tissues. The urine 5-HIAA test is diagnostic for the carcinoid syndrome. Whereas liver, lung and brain all have high levels of activity of MAO and (presumably) of enzymes that inactivate other tumor secretions, the right side of the heart is exposed to the full effects of tumor products that are released into the vena cava from hepatic metastases. **Endocardial fibrosis** results (see carcinoid heart disease, Chapter 11), probably from endothelial damage. Fibrous plaques form on tricuspid and pulmonic valves, the endocardium of the right-sided cardiac chambers, the vena cava, the coronary sinus and the pulmonary artery. ***Valvular distortion leads to pulmonic stenosis and tricuspid regurgitation.***

Metastatic Tumors

The most common malignant tumors in the small intestine are metastatic. Cancer of adjacent organs (e.g., stomach, pancreas, colon) may spread to the small intestine by direct extension. Lung and female genital organs and skin (melanomas) are the most frequent primary sites of small intestinal metastases. Secondary involvement of the small intestine with systemic lymphoma may simulate metastatic carcinoma. Solitary, submucosal metastatic tumors may easily be mistaken for a primary cancer, and the symptoms may be indistinguishable.

Pneumatosis Cystoides Intestinalis

Pneumatosis cystoides intestinalis is an uncommon disorder in which numerous pockets of gas are found in the gut wall anywhere in the gut. Most cases are associated with an underlying gastrointestinal disease, including intestinal obstruction, peptic ulcer, Crohn disease, mesenteric ischemia, volvulus and neonatal necrotizing enterocolitis. Some occur in patients with chronic obstructive pulmonary disease or who are treated with mechanical ventilation. Pneumatosis in adults is ordinarily benign, depending on the underlying disease. However, intestinal pneumatosis associated with neonatal necrotizing enteritis has a high mortality.

The cause of intestinal pneumatosis depends on the associated conditions. A mechanical break in mucosal continuity allows air from the lumen to enter the submucosa. Or, the gas can be a product of bacterial action, particularly in neonatal necrotizing enterocolitis. Dissection of air bubbles along the mesentery is common in patients with obstructive lung disease or mechanical ventilation.

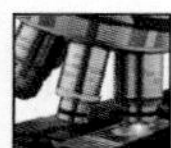

PATHOLOGY: Macroscopically, cysts appear as bubbles under the serosa of the intestine, and the bowel wall feels spongy. In some cases, air cysts are principally in the submucosa, in which case the cut surface of the bowel wall may appear honeycombed. The cysts vary from a few millimeters to several centimeters. Cysts may also occur in the stomach and the mesentery. Microscopic examination reveals cystic spaces in the submucosa or beneath the serosa, which are often lined by large macrophages and multinucleated giant cells.

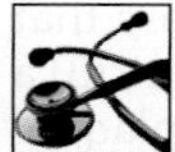

CLINICAL FEATURES: Many cases are found during investigation of symptoms unrelated to the pneumatosis. Some patients have episodic diarrhea. There is often blood in the stools, and rectal bleeding may be brisk. When intestinal pneumatosis is a complication of neonatal necrotizing enterocolitis, bowel perforation and peritonitis are frequent, but these complications are rare in adults.

Gas cysts may disappear spontaneously or persist for years. Relief of symptoms may be obtained by oxygen inhalation or treatment with metronidazole.

THE LARGE INTESTINE

Anatomy

The large intestine is that portion of the gastrointestinal tract from the ileocecal valve to the anus. It is 90 to 125 cm in length in adults and includes the colon and rectum. As in the small intestine, the proximal colon derives from embryonic midgut and is supplied by the superior mesenteric artery. The distal half of the large intestine is of embryonic hindgut origin, is supplied by the inferior mesenteric artery and is mainly for storage.

MACROSCOPIC FEATURES: The large intestine has six regions, distally from the ileocecal valve: (1) cecum, (2) ascending colon, (3) transverse colon, (4) descending colon,

(5) sigmoid colon and (6) rectum. The bend between the ascending and transverse colon in the right upper quadrant is the **hepatic flexure,** and that between the transverse and descending segments in the left upper quadrant is the **splenic flexure.** The caliber of the lumen progressively diminishes from the cecum to the sigmoid colon.

Like the small intestine, the colon has outer longitudinal and inner circular muscle coats. However, in the colon, the longitudinal muscle has three separate bundles, the **taeniae coli.** Evaginations of the colonic wall between the taeniae, the **haustra,** appear as external sacculations. The appendices epiploicae are small serosal masses of fat, invested by peritoneum. The vermiform appendix arises at the apex of the cecum and terminates as a blind tube; it averages about 8 cm in length but occasionally measures up to 20 cm.

The ileocecal valve is a sphincter that regulates the flow of intestinal contents into the cecum. However, it is an incompetent sphincter, and reflux of cecal contents into the ileum is usual. The internal sphincter of the anal canal is continuous with colonic smooth muscle. The external anal sphincter is the major mechanism by which bowel continence is maintained. It surrounds the anal canal with a layer of skeletal muscle. The mucosal surface of the large bowel has prominent folds, which are less pronounced in the rectum.

MICROSCOPIC FEATURES: Colonic mucosa is flat and is punctuated by numerous pits, the **crypts of Lieberkühn.** Both are lined by tall columnar epithelium. The surface epithelium is primarily simple columnar cells with occasional goblet cells. The crypts mostly contain goblet cells, except at their bases, where a few stem cells and a variety of neuroendocrine cells are located. The basal undifferentiated cells are the mucosa reserve cells and divide continuously. Mucosal cells migrate from the crypt bases toward the luminal surface. Mucosal cell apoptosis (see Chapter 1) and sloughing balance proliferation, thus maintaining an equilibrium in the crypt epithelial cell population.

The lamina propria contains lymphocytes, plasma cells, macrophages and fibroblasts, plus occasional eosinophils. Lymphoid aggregates traverse the muscularis mucosae and extend into the submucosa. The submucosa is similar to that in the small intestine, but lymphatic channels are far less prominent. These lymphatics drain into paracolic nodes in the serosal fat, intermediate nodes along the colic blood vessels and central nodes near the aorta. Parasympathetic and sympathetic innervations terminate in Meissner submucosal and Auerbach myenteric plexuses.

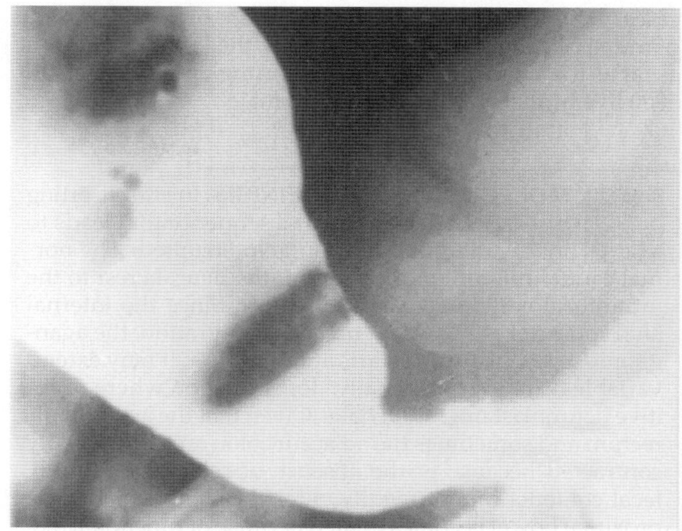

FIGURE 13-44. Hirschsprung disease. A contrast radiograph shows marked dilation of the rectosigmoid colon proximal to the narrowed rectum.

Congenital Disorders

Congenital Megacolon (Hirschsprung Disease) Is Due to Segmental Absence of Ganglion Cells

That is, in Hirschsprung disease colon dilation (Fig. 13-44) is due to defective colorectal innervation: ganglion cells are absent in part of the colon, beginning in the wall of the rectum and extending variably proximally (Fig. 13-45). In 25% of

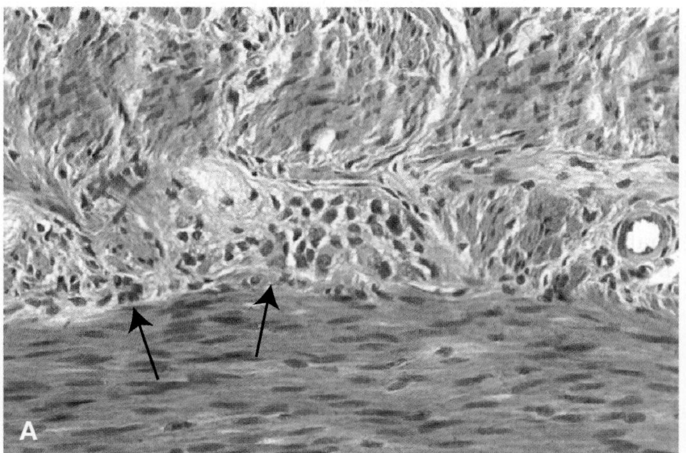

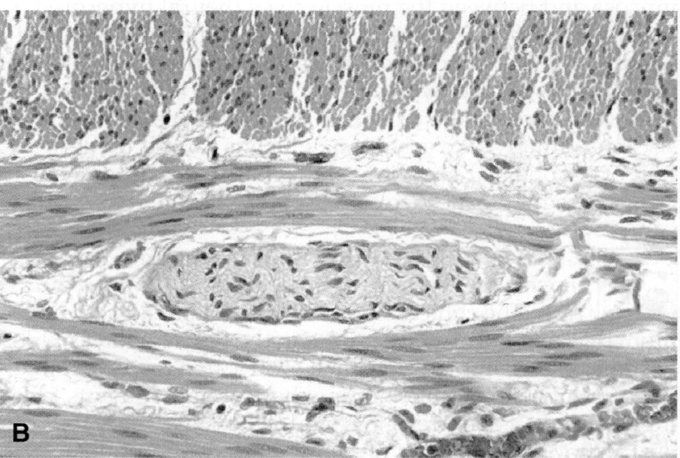

FIGURE 13-45. Hirschsprung disease. A. A photomicrograph of ganglion cells in the wall of the rectum (*arrows*). **B.** A rectal biopsy specimen from a patient with Hirschsprung disease shows a nonmyelinated nerve in the mesenteric plexus and an absence of ganglion cells.

13 | The Gastrointestinal Tract

cases, ganglion cells are deficient in more proximal portions of the colon, and in unusual instances, the lesion may extend as far as the small intestine. Hirschsprung disease affects 1 in 5000 live births; 80% of patients are male.

MOLECULAR PATHOGENESIS: In Hirschsprung disease the developmental sequence that leads to innervation of the colon is interrupted. The normal caudal migration of cells from the neural crest to the intramural ganglion cells is cut short. Since the internal anal sphincter is at the far end of this migration, the aganglionic segment always starts at the rectum. It may extend variable distances proximally, depending on where primitive neuroblast migration halts. Given that the aganglionic rectum and sometimes the adjacent colon are permanently contracted because of the absence of relaxation stimuli, fecal contents cannot readily enter the stenotic area. The proximal bowel becomes dilated because of functional distal obstruction.

Most cases of Hirschsprung disease are sporadic, but 10% of cases are familial. Half of familial cases and 15% of sporadic ones reflect inactivating mutations of the RET receptor tyrosine kinase gene on chromosome 10q (see MEN2 syndrome, Chapter 21). Some cases involve mutations in the endothelin-B receptor or in genes that encode ligands of the RET receptor and endothelin-B receptor.

The incidence of congenital megacolon is 10 times higher than normal in infants with **Down syndrome;** 2% of Down syndrome infants are born with Hirschsprung disease. Most cases are uncomplicated by other lesions, but congenital anomalies, including those of the kidneys and lower urinary tract, imperforate anus and ventricular septal defect, are reported.

PATHOLOGY: The large intestine in Hirschsprung disease has a constricted and spastic aganglionic segment. Proximal to this, the bowel is very dilated. Definitive diagnosis depends on the absence of ganglion cells upon rectal biopsy (Fig. 13-45B). There is also a striking increase in nonmyelinated cholinergic nerve fibers in the submucosa and between the muscle coats (neural hyperplasia). The absence of ganglion cells leads to accumulation of acetylcholine and acetylcholinesterase. Histochemical demonstration of this enzyme, which is not detected in normal rectal mucosa, improves the reliability of rectal biopsy for diagnosis. Interestingly, like achalasia, which is caused by destruction of esophageal ganglion cells, Chagas disease may also cause aganglionic megacolon.

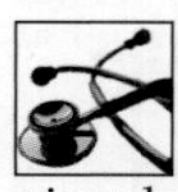

CLINICAL FEATURES: *Hirschsprung disease is the most common cause of congenital intestinal obstruction.* The clinical signs are delayed passage of meconium by a newborn and vomiting in the first few days of life. In some cases, complete intestinal obstruction requires immediate surgical relief. In children whose rectal segments lacking ganglion cells are short and who have only partial obstruction, constipation, abdominal distention and recurrent fecal impactions are characteristic.

The most serious complication is an enterocolitis, in which necrosis and ulceration affect the dilated proximal segment of the colon and may extend into the small intestine. Hirschsprung disease is treated by removal of the aganglionic segment and reconstruction.

Acquired Megacolon Often Reflects Laxative Use

Acquired megacolon sometimes occurs in children and often has a psychogenic background. It may be associated with chronic constipation and prolonged laxative use ("cathartic colon"). If, in infancy, ganglion cells are seen by rectal biopsy, fecal incontinence should be suspected. The cause is not well understood, but it is thought to represent a functional abnormality of colonic motility. Acquired megacolon in adults can result from disorders that interfere with bowel innervation or smooth muscle function, such as diabetic neuropathy, parkinsonism, myotonic dystrophy, scleroderma, amyloidosis and hypothyroidism.

Anorectal Malformations Are Common Developmental Defects

These malformations vary from minor narrowing to serious and complex defects. They result from arrested development of the caudal region of the gut in the first 6 months of fetal life. These anomalies are classified by the relation of the terminal bowel to the levator ani muscle. The deformity may be (1) high or supralevator, if the bowel ends above the pelvic floor; (2) intermediate; or (3) low or translevator, if the bowel ends below the pelvic floor.

- **Anorectal agenesis and rectal atresia** are supralevator deformities.
- **Anal agenesis and anorectal stenosis** are classified as intermediate deformities.
- **Imperforate anus** is a low or translevator deformity in which the anal opening is covered by a cutaneous membrane behind which meconium is visible. **Anal stenosis** is a variant of imperforate anus.
- **Fistulas** between the malformation and the bladder, urethra, vagina or skin may occur in all types of anorectal anomalies.

Infections of the Large Intestine

The principal infections of the colon, including tuberculosis and amebiasis, are discussed in Chapter 9 or above in the context of small intestine infectious diarrhea. Most of the remaining infectious diseases are transmitted sexually and involve the anorectal region, often in male homosexuals, including gonorrhea, syphilis, lymphogranuloma venereum, anorectal herpes and venereal warts (condylomata acuminata). Immunosuppressed people have a high incidence of colonic infections (e.g., amebiasis and shigellosis). Bone marrow transplant recipients often contract cytomegalovirus and herpes infection of the gastrointestinal tract.

Pseudomembranous Colitis Usually Follows Antibiotic Treatment

Pseudomembranous colitis is a generic term for an inflammatory disease of the colon that is characterized by **exudative plaques** on the mucosa.

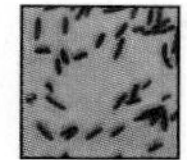

ETIOLOGIC FACTORS: After the introduction of antibiotics in the early 1950s, it was found that these drugs, mainly tetracycline and chloramphenicol, often led to pseudomembranous colitis. Today, most antibiotics may cause the disease. *Clostridium difficile,* which is also implicated in neonatal necrotizing enterocolitis, is usually the culprit. ***It is not invasive, but produces toxins that damage the colonic mucosa.***

Other conditions that can produce pseudomembranes include various diseases of the colon, shock, burns, uremia and chemotherapy. Simply being hospitalized leads to a 30% colonization rate with *C. difficile.*

Just how *C. difficile* becomes pathogenic is not entirely clear. Alteration of fecal flora by antibiotics contributes. Only 2% to 3% of healthy adults harbor the organism, but 10% to 20% of patients recently treated with antibiotics are infected. However, it can be isolated from the stool in 95% of patients with antibiotic-associated pseudomembranous colitis.

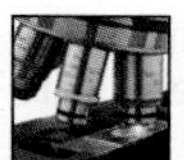

PATHOLOGY: The colon, particularly the rectosigmoid region, shows raised yellowish plaques up to 2 cm that adhere to the underlying mucosa (Fig. 13-46). Intervening mucosa is congested and edematous but is not ulcerated. In severe cases, plaques coalesce into extensive pseudomembranes. Necrosis of the superficial epithelium is believed to be the initial pathologic event. Subsequently, colonic crypts become disrupted and expanded by mucin and neutrophils. The pseudomembrane consists of the debris of necrotic epithelial cells, mucus, fibrin and neutrophils. In milder cases, well-formed pseudomembranes may be absent, and the pathology is more subtle, with focal damage to the surface epithelium.

If both small and large bowel are affected, the condition is **pseudomembranous enterocolitis.** Pseudomembranes occur occasionally in other enteric infections involving *S. aureus, Candida,* invasive bacteria and verotoxin-producing *E. coli.* Ischemic bowel disease may also show pseudomembranes.

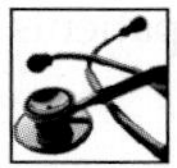

CLINICAL FEATURES: Antibiotic-associated *C. difficile* infections are virtually always accompanied by diarrhea, but in most cases the disorder does not progress to colitis. In patients with pseudomembranous colitis, fever, leukocytosis and abdominal cramps are superimposed on the diarrhea. Before antibiotics, many patients with this form of colitis died within hours or days from ileus and irreversible shock. Today, pseudomembranous colitis, although still serious, is usually controlled with antibiotics and supportive fluid and electrolyte therapy. Milder cases can be confused with an array of diarrheal diseases.

Neonatal Necrotizing Enterocolitis Complicates Prematurity

Necrotizing enterocolitis is one of the most common acquired surgical emergencies in newborns. It is particularly common in premature infants after oral feeding and is likely related principally to an ischemic event involving the intestinal mucosa, which is followed by bacterial colonization, usually with *C. difficile.* Lesions vary from those of typical pseudomembranous enterocolitis to gangrene and perforation of the bowel.

Diverticular Disease

Diverticular disease refers to two entities: **diverticulosis** and an inflammatory complication called **diverticulitis.**

Diverticulosis Reflects Environmental and Structural Factors

Diverticulosis is an acquired herniation (diverticulum) of the mucosa and submucosa through the muscular layers of the colon.

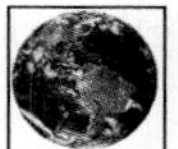

EPIDEMIOLOGY: Diverticulosis shows striking geographic variability. It is common in Western societies and infrequent in Asia, Africa and underdeveloped countries. Diverticulosis increases in frequency with age. Some 10% of persons in Western countries are afflicted.

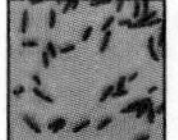

ETIOLOGIC FACTORS: The striking variation in the prevalence of diverticulosis implies that environmental factors are primarily responsible. Western populations consume a diet in which refined carbohydrates

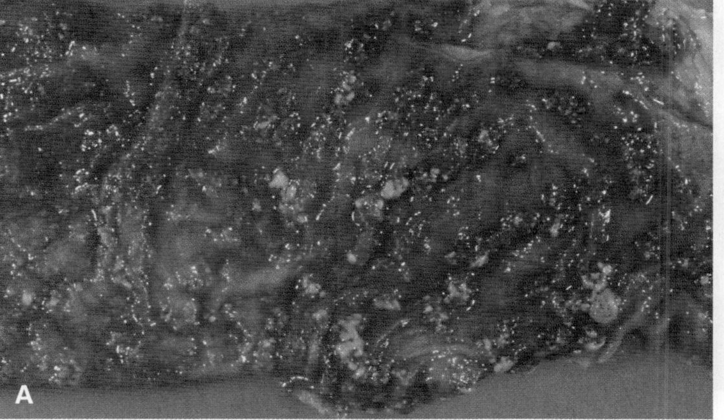

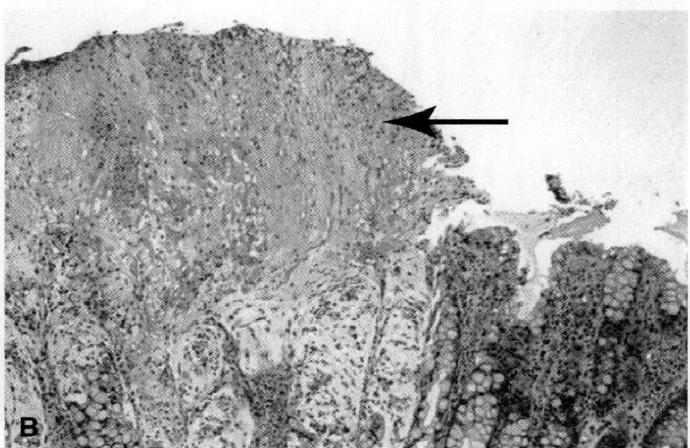

FIGURE 13-46. Pseudomembranous colitis. A. The colon shows variable involvement ranging from erythema to yellow-green areas of pseudomembrane. **B.** Microscopically, the pseudomembrane (*arrow*) consists of fibrin, mucin and inflammatory cells (largely neutrophils).

and meat have replaced crude cereal grains, and it is widely assumed that the lack of indigestible fibers in some way facilitates formation of diverticula in susceptible people. In this respect, the larger fecal mass in those who ingest a high-fiber diet diminishes spontaneous motility and intraluminal pressure in the colon.

INCREASED INTRALUMINAL PRESSURE: According to the fiber theory, Western diets lack dietary residue, leading to sustained bowel contractions and consequently increased intraluminal pressure. Such prolonged increased pressure is believed to lead to herniation of the superficial coats of the colon through the muscular layers into the serosa.

DEFECTS IN THE WALL OF THE COLON: In addition to pressure, defects in the colon wall are required. The circular muscle of the colon is interrupted by connective tissue clefts at the sites of penetration by the nutrient vessels that supply the submucosa and mucosa. In older people, this connective tissue loses its resilience and thus its resistance to the effects of increased intraluminal pressure. This concept is supported by the fact that people with heritable connective tissue disorders (e.g., Marfan syndrome, Ehlers-Danlos syndrome) acquire precocious diverticulosis, primarily of the small bowel.

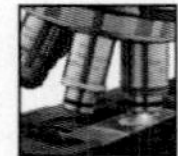

PATHOLOGY: True diverticula involve all layers of the intestinal wall. In diverticulosis the structures are actually pseudodiverticula, in which only the mucosa and submucosa are herniated through the muscle layers. The sigmoid colon is affected in 95% of cases, but diverticulosis can affect any segment of the colon, including the cecum. Diverticula vary in number from a few to hundreds. Most appear in parallel rows between the mesenteric and lateral taeniae. They measure up to 1 cm and are connected to the intestinal lumen by necks of varying length and caliber. The muscular wall of the affected colon is consistently thickened.

Diverticula are characteristically seen as flask-like structures that extend from the lumen through the muscle layers (Fig. 13-47). Their walls are continuous with the surface mucosa and thus have epithelium *and* a submucosa. The outer base is formed by serosal connective tissue.

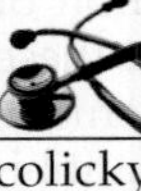

CLINICAL FEATURES: ***Diverticulosis is generally asymptomatic, and 80% of affected individuals are symptom free.*** Many patients complain of episodic colicky abdominal pain. Both constipation and diarrhea, sometimes alternating, may occur, and flatulence is common. Sudden, painless and severe bleeding from colonic diverticula is a cause of serious lower gastrointestinal hemorrhage in the elderly, occurring in as many as 5% of persons with diverticulosis. Chronic blood loss may lead to anemia.

Diverticulitis Is Inflammation at the Base of a Diverticulum

Diverticulitis presumably results from irritation caused by retained fecal material. In 10% to 20% of patients with diverticulosis, diverticulitis develops at some point.

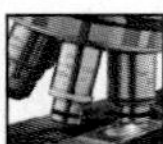

PATHOLOGY: Diverticulitis produces inflammation of the wall of the diverticulum, an event that may lead to perforation and release of fecal bacteria into the peridiverticular tissues. The resulting abscess is usually contained by the appendices epiploicae and the pericolonic tissue. Infrequently, free perforation leads to generalized peritonitis. Fibrosis in response to repeated episodes of diverticulitis may constrict the bowel lumen, causing obstruction. Fistulas may form between the colon and adjacent organs, including the bladder, vagina, small intestine and skin of the abdomen. Additional complications include pylephlebitis and liver abscesses.

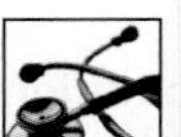

CLINICAL FEATURES: The most common symptoms of diverticulitis, usually following microscopic or gross perforation of the diverticulum, are persistent lower abdominal pain and fever. Changes in bowel habits, from diarrhea to constipation, are frequent and dysuria indicates bladder irritation. Most patients have left lower quadrant tenderness and, often, a palpable mass in that area. Leukocytosis is the rule. Antibiotics and supportive measures usually alleviate acute diverticulitis, but about 20% of patients eventually require surgery.

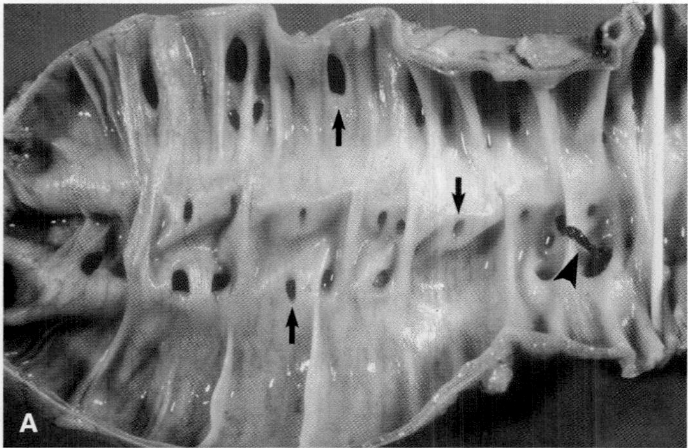

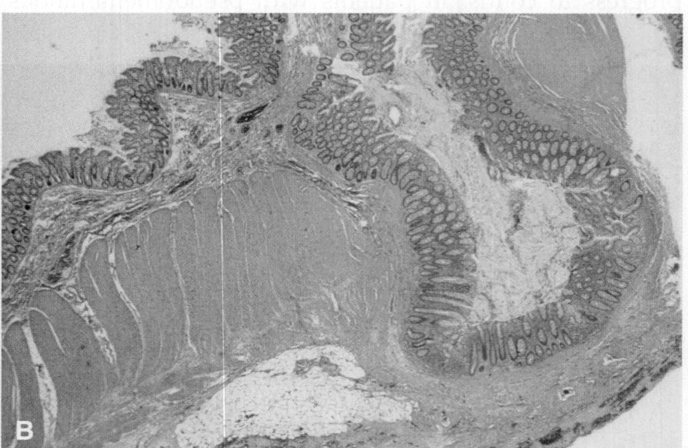

FIGURE 13-47. Diverticulosis of the colon. A. The colon was inflated with formalin. The mouths of numerous diverticula are seen between the taenia (*arrows*). There is a blood clot seen protruding from the mouth of one of the diverticula (*arrowhead*). This was the source of massive gastrointestinal bleeding. **B.** Sections show mucosa including muscularis mucosa, which has herniated through a defect in the bowel wall, producing a diverticulum.

Inflammatory Bowel Disease

The term **inflammatory bowel disease** encompasses **Crohn disease** and **ulcerative colitis.** Although these two disorders usually differ enough to be clearly distinguishable, they have certain common features. Similarities apart, they have different clinical courses and natural histories. Their causes are unknown. However, epidemiologic, clinical and animal studies suggest that mucosal injury accrues from altered immune responses and abnormal interactions of bacteria with intestinal epithelia.

Crohn Disease Is Chronic Segmental Transmural Inflammation of the Intestine

Crohn disease occurs principally in the distal small intestine but may involve any part of the digestive tract and even extraintestinal tissues. The colon, particularly the right colon, may be affected. Crohn disease has variously been referred to as **terminal ileitis** and **regional enteritis** when it involves mainly the ileum, and **granulomatous colitis** and **transmural colitis** when it principally affects the colon.

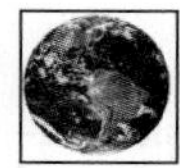

EPIDEMIOLOGY: Crohn disease is worldwide, with an annual incidence of 0.5 to 5 per 100,000. Its incidence has increased dramatically over the past 30 years. Crohn disease usually appears in adolescents or young adults and is most common in people of European origin, with a considerably higher frequency among Jews. There is a slight female predominance (1.6:1).

MOLECULAR PATHOGENESIS: Epidemiologic studies, particularly concordance rates in twin pairs and siblings, indicate a genetic predisposition to Crohn disease. A family history of inflammatory bowel disease is more common for Crohn disease than for ulcerative colitis. A putative susceptibility locus for Crohn disease has been assigned to the centromeric region of chromosome 16, at least in non-Jewish patients. Other susceptibility loci may reside on chromosomes 3, 7 and 12. *NOD2* and *CARD15* mutations determine ileal disease, and the clinical pattern of Crohn disease has been linked to specific genotypes. *NOD2* expresses a protein that binds bacterial peptidoglycans, and as such, mutants may be less able to ward off bacterial entry into the lamina propria.

Crohn disease has only rarely been described in both a husband and a wife. Thus, environmental factors alone do not suffice to cause the disease. Interestingly, smoking is associated with Crohn disease, but ulcerative colitis is uncommon in smokers. Several infectious agents have been suggested as possible causative agents, but definitive links are lacking. Several studies report impaired cell-mediated immunity in patients with Crohn disease, increased suppressor T-cell activity and depressed phagocytic function.

The chronic and recurrent nature of the inflammation and the association with systemic manifestations often linked to autoimmune diseases suggest an immune origin, possibly related to cell-mediated cytotoxicity. Some studies suggest that cytotoxic T cells sensitized to bacterial or other antigens damage the intestinal wall. In this respect, cyclosporine, a potent inhibitor of cell-mediated immunity that is widely used to prevent transplant rejection, has been reported to ameliorate symptoms of Crohn disease.

TNF-α production is increased in vitro in mucosal cells from patients with Crohn disease, as is a shift in the mucosal balance of T-cell–mediated cytokine production toward TNF-α. Administration of anti–TNF-α antibodies to patients with Crohn disease provides effective short-term symptom remission.

A role of fecal stream in the pathogenesis of Crohn disease is suggested by (1) the beneficial effects of surgical bypass, (2) the pattern of preanastomotic recurrence in patients with side-to-end anastomotic sites and (3) the frequency of early inflammatory lesions (aphthoid erosions) in the epithelium in association with mucosal lymphoid tissue.

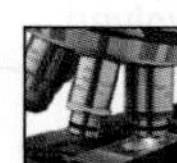

PATHOLOGY: Two key features of Crohn disease differentiate it from other gastrointestinal inflammatory diseases. First, inflammation usually involves all layers of the bowel wall and is thus referred to as **transmural inflammatory disease.** Second, involvement of the intestine is discontinuous; that is, segments of inflamed tissue are separated by apparently normal intestine.

Crohn disease may follow four general patterns, although many patients do not fit any one of them precisely. The disease involves (1) mainly the ileum and cecum in about half of cases, (2) only the small intestine in 15%, (3) only the colon in 20% and (4) mainly the anorectal region in 15%. Ileal and cecal involvement is more frequent in young patients; colitis is common in older patients. The disease is occasionally seen in the duodenum, stomach and esophagus as focal acute inflammation with or without granulomas. In women with anorectal Crohn disease, the inflammation may spread to involve the external genitalia.

The pathology of Crohn disease is highly variable. The bowel and adjacent mesentery are thickened and edematous. Mesenteric fat often surrounds the bowel ("creeping fat"). Mesenteric lymph nodes are frequently enlarged, firm and matted together. The intestinal lumen is narrowed by edema in early cases and by a combination of edema and fibrosis in long-standing disease. Nodular swelling, fibrosis and mucosal ulceration lead to a "cobblestone" appearance (Fig. 13-48A). In early cases, ulcers have either an aphthous or a serpiginous appearance; later they become deeper and appear as linear clefts or fissures (Fig. 13-48B).

The appearance of the bowel wall underscores the transmural nature of the disease, with thickening, edema and fibrosis of all layers. Involved loops of bowel are often adherent and fistulas between such segments are frequent. These fistulas, presumably a late result of the deep mural ulcers, may also penetrate from the bowel into other organs, including the bladder, uterus, vagina and skin. Most fistulas end blindly, forming abscess cavities in the peritoneal cavity, mesentery or retroperitoneal structures. Lesions in the distal rectum and anus may create perianal fistulas, a well-known presenting feature.

Crohn disease histologically is a chronic inflammatory process. Early in the disease, inflammation may be confined to the mucosa and submucosa. Small, superficial mucosal ulcers (aphthous ulcers) are seen, as are mucosal and submucosal

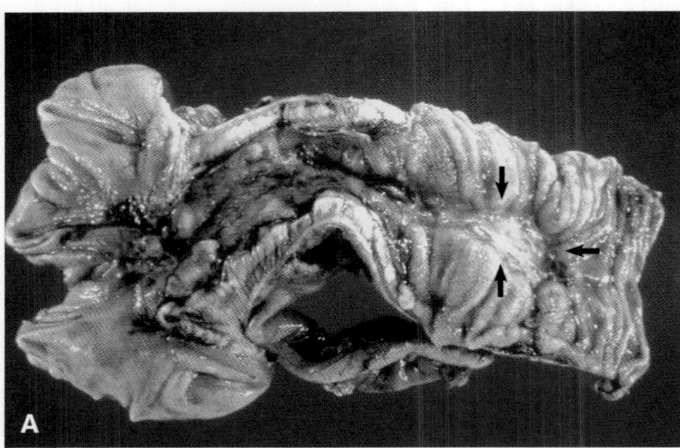

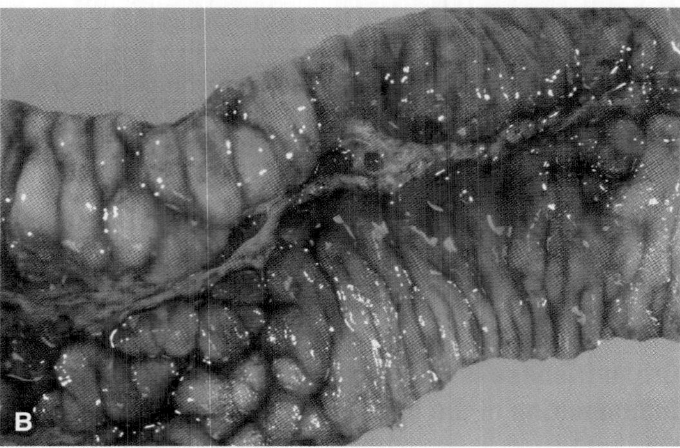

FIGURE 13-48. Crohn disease. A. The terminal ileum shows striking thickening of the wall of the distal portion with distortion of the ileocecal valve. A longitudinal ulcer is present (*arrows*). **B.** Another longitudinal ulcer is seen in this segment of ileum. The large rounded areas of edematous damaged mucosa give a "cobblestone" appearance to the involved mucosa. A portion of the mucosa to the lower right is uninvolved.

edema and increased numbers of lymphocytes, plasma cells and macrophages. Destruction of mucosal architecture, with regenerative changes in crypts and villous distortion, is frequent. Pyloric metaplasia and Paneth cell hyperplasia is common in the small intestine and colorectum. Later, long, deep, fissure-like ulcers are seen, and vascular hyalinization and fibrosis become apparent.

Transmural nodular lymphoid aggregates, with proliferative changes of the muscularis mucosae and nerves of submucosal and myenteric plexuses, are characteristic (Fig. 13-49A). ***Discrete, noncaseating granulomas, mostly in the submucosa, may be present*** (Fig. 13-49B). These resemble those of sarcoidosis, with focal aggregates of epithelioid cells, vaguely limited by a rim of lymphocytes. Multinucleated giant cells may be present. The centers of the granulomas usually display hyaline material and only very rarely necrosis.

The presence of discrete granulomas strongly suggests Crohn disease, but their absence does not exclude the

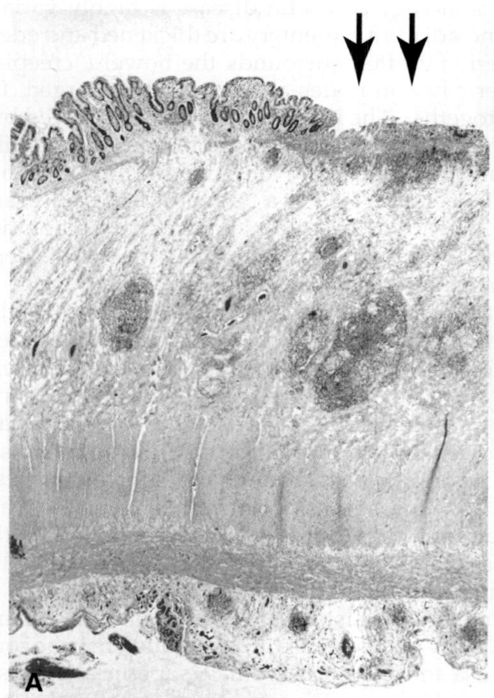

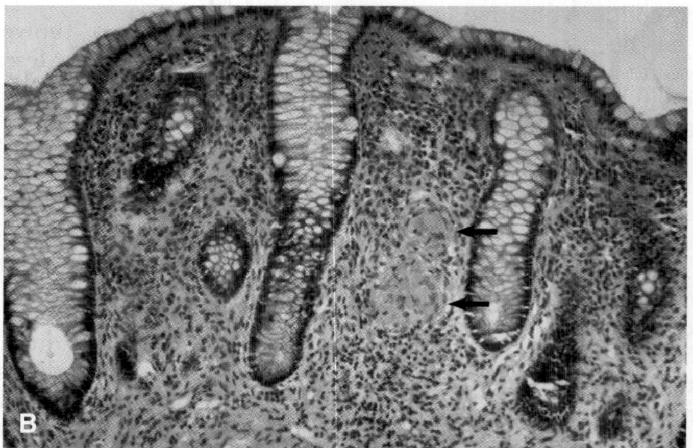

FIGURE 13-49. Crohn disease. A. The colon involved with Crohn disease shows an area of mucosal ulceration (*arrows*), an expanded submucosa with lymphoid aggregates and numerous lymphoid aggregates in the subserosal tissues immediately adjacent to the muscularis externa. **B.** This mucosal biopsy in Crohn disease shows a small epithelioid granuloma (*arrows*) between two intact crypts.

diagnosis, as less than half the cases show the typical granulomas.

The pathologic features of Crohn disease are summarized in Fig. 13-50.

CLINICAL FEATURES: The clinical manifestations and natural history of Crohn disease are highly variable and reflect the range of anatomic sites involved by the disease. The most common symptoms, which are seen in over 75% of patients, are **abdominal pain** and **diarrhea.** Recurrent **fever** is evident in 50%. When it mainly involves the ileum and cecum, a sudden onset may mimic appendicitis, and the diagnosis may first be made at the time of abdominal surgery. If ilial disease predominates, right lower quadrant pain, intermittent diarrhea and fever and a tender mass in the right lower quadrant are often seen. When the small intestine is diffusely involved, **malabsorption** and malnutrition may be major features. Lipid malabsorption may also result from interruption of the enterohepatic cycle of bile salts because of ileal disease. Colonic involvement leads to **diarrhea** and sometimes **colonic bleeding.** In a few patients, the major site of involvement is the anorectal region and recurrent anorectal fistulas may be presenting signs.

Intestinal obstruction and **fistulas** are the most common intestinal complications of Crohn disease. Occasionally, free perforation of the bowel occurs. **Small bowel cancer** is at least threefold more common in patients with Crohn disease, and the disease also predisposes to **colorectal cancer.** When it begins in childhood, it may cause slowing of growth and physical development. **Systemic complications** also include liver disease (sclerosing cholangitis), cholelithiasis, renal oxalate stones and amyloidosis. The most frequent extraintestinal inflammatory features are in the eye (episcleritis or uveitis), medium-sized joints (arthritis) and skin (erythema nodosum).

There is currently no cure. Several medications suppress the inflammatory reaction, including corticosteroids, sulfasalazine, metronidazole, 6-mercaptopurine, cyclosporine

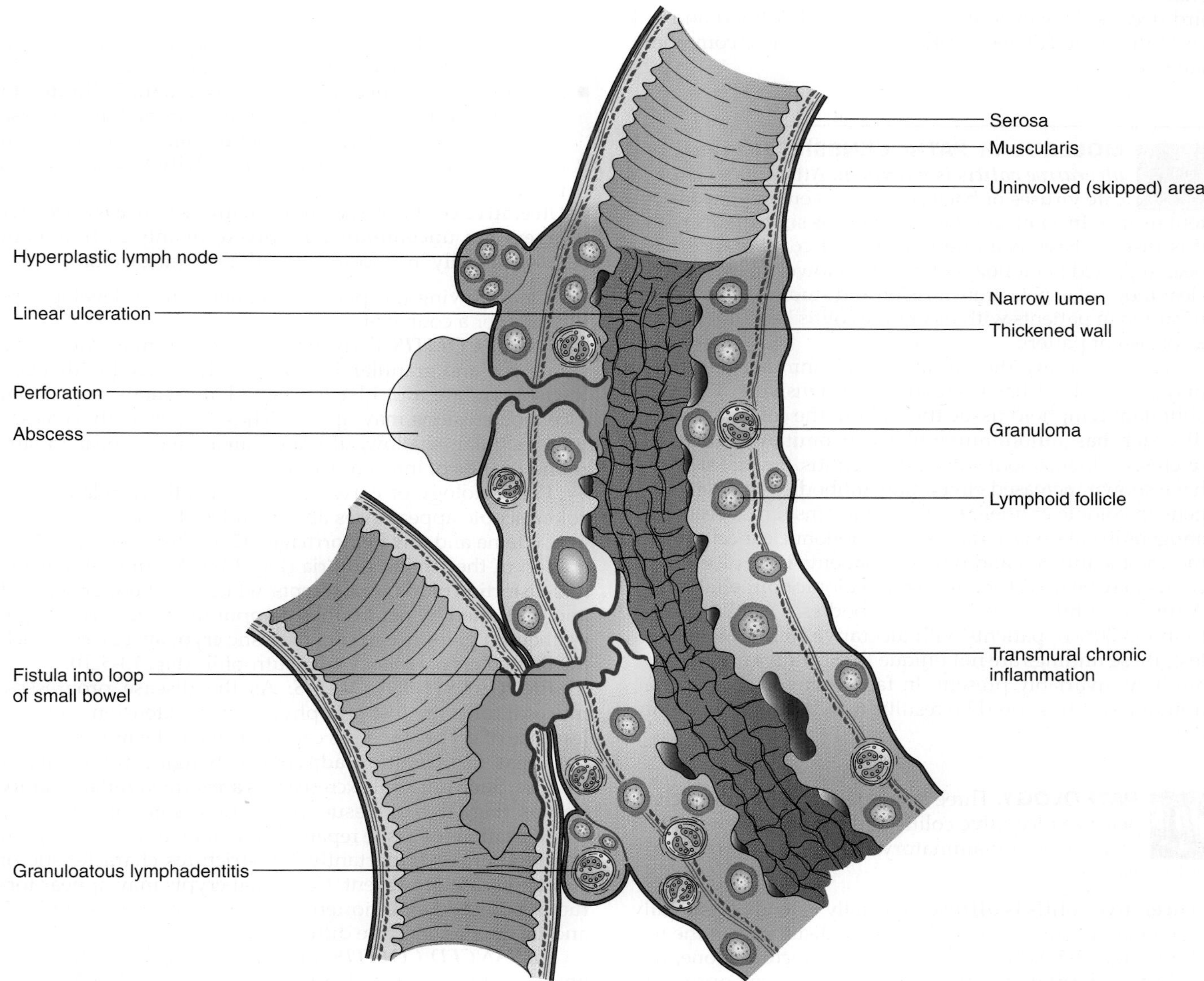

FIGURE 13-50. Crohn disease. A schematic representation of the major features of Crohn disease in the small intestine.

and anti-TNF antibodies. Surgical resection of obstructed areas or of severely involved portions of intestine and drainage of abscesses caused by fistulas are required in some cases. Preanastomotic or prestomal recurrences after construction of an enterostomy occur commonly, making clinical management difficult. The need for repeated resections can lead to short-bowel syndrome in some patients.

Ulcerative Colitis Is a Chronic Superficial Inflammation of the Colon and Rectum

Ulcerative colitis is characterized by chronic diarrhea and rectal bleeding, with a pattern of exacerbations and remissions and with the possibility of serious local and systemic complications. The disorder occurs mainly, but not solely, in young adults.

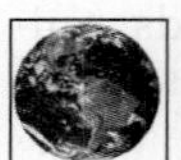

EPIDEMIOLOGY: In Europe and North America, the incidence of ulcerative colitis is 4 to 7 per 100,000 population; its prevalence is 40 to 80 per 100,000. It usually begins in early adult life, with a peak incidence in the third decade. However, it also occurs in childhood and old age. In the United States, whites are affected more commonly than blacks.

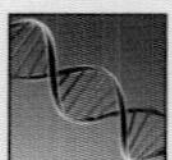

MOLECULAR PATHOGENESIS: ***The cause of ulcerative colitis is unknown.*** Attempts to implicate viruses or bacteria have given only inconsistent results. In some families, as many as six patients with this disease have been described, and concordance has been reported in monozygotic twins. However, there is no clear mode of genetic transmission and studies of HLA distribution in patients with ulcerative colitis have not found a consistent pattern.

The possibility that an abnormal immune response may be involved has been studied extensively. There is abundant lymphoid tissue throughout the colon, and this disorder has autoimmune-like concomitants, such as uveitis, erythema nodosum and vasculitis. Several studies have shown increased circulating antibodies against antigens in colonic epithelial cells and against cross-reacting antigens in enterobacteria. As well, mononuclear cells from the colonic mucosa and blood of patients with ulcerative colitis may be toxic for autologous colonic epithelial cells. Antineutrophil cytoplasmic antibodies (ANCAs) are found in 80% of patients with ulcerative colitis. Nonetheless, these findings are not unique to ulcerative colitis, nor are they invariably present. In fact, some or all of these immune features could be results, not causes, of mucosal damage.

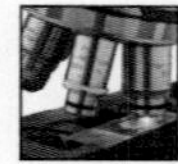

PATHOLOGY: Three major pathologic features characterize ulcerative colitis and help to differentiate it from other inflammatory conditions, particularly Crohn disease:

- **Ulcerative colitis is diffuse.** It usually extends proximally for a variable distance from the most distal part of the rectum (Fig. 13-51). When it involves the rectum alone, it is called **ulcerative proctitis.** When the process approaches the splenic flexure, the terms **proctosigmoiditis** and **left-sided colitis** are used. Sparing of the rectum or involvement of the right side of the colon alone is rare and should suggest a different disorder, like Crohn disease.

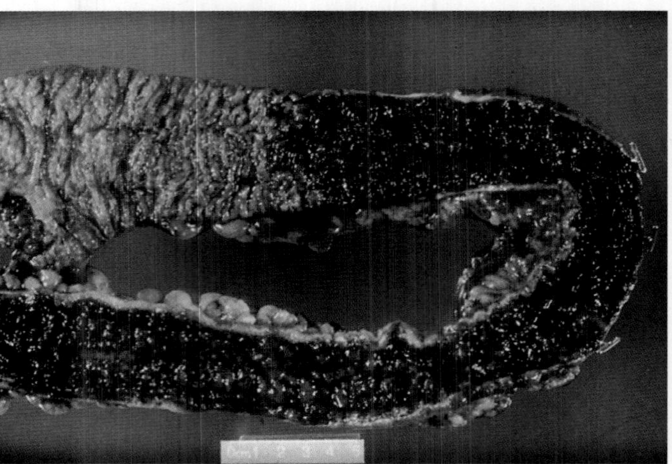

FIGURE 13-51. Ulcerative colitis. Prominent erythema and ulceration of the colon begin in the ascending colon and are most severe in the rectosigmoid area.

- **Inflammation in ulcerative colitis is generally limited to the colon and rectum.** If the cecum is affected, the disease ends at the ileocecal valve, although minor inflammation of the adjacent ileum **(backwash ileitis)** is sometimes noted.
- **Ulcerative colitis is essentially a mucosal disease. Deeper layers are uncommonly involved,** mainly in fulminant cases, usually in association with toxic megacolon.

The following morphologic sequence may develop rapidly or over a course of years.

EARLY COLITIS: Early in the disease, the mucosal surface is raw, red and granular. It is frequently covered with a yellowish exudate and bleeds easily. Later small, superficial ulcers or erosions may appear. These occasionally coalesce into irregular, shallow, ulcerated areas that appear to surround islands of intact mucosa.

The histology of early ulcerative colitis correlates with colonoscopic appearances and includes (1) mucosal congestion, edema and tiny hemorrhages; (2) diffuse chronic inflammation in the lamina propria (Fig. 13-52A); and (3) damage and distortion of colorectal crypts, which are often surrounded and infiltrated by neutrophils. Suppurative necrosis of crypt epithelium gives rise to characteristic **crypt abscesses,** which are dilated crypts filled with neutrophils (Fig. 13-52B).

PROGRESSIVE COLITIS: As the disease progresses, mucosal folds are lost (atrophy). Lateral extension and coalescence of crypt abscesses can undermine the mucosa, leaving areas of ulceration adjacent to hanging fragments of mucosa. Such mucosal excrescences are termed **inflammatory polyps** (Fig. 13-53). Tissue destruction is accompanied by manifestations of tissue repair. Granulation tissue develops in denuded areas. Importantly, the strictures characteristic of Crohn disease are absent. Colorectal crypts may appear tortuous, branched and shortened in the late stages (Fig. 13-52C) and the mucosa may be diffusely atrophic.

ADVANCED COLITIS: In long-standing cases, the large bowel is often shortened, especially in the left side. Mucosal folds are indistinct and are replaced by a granular or smooth mucosal pattern. Advanced ulcerative colitis shows mucosal

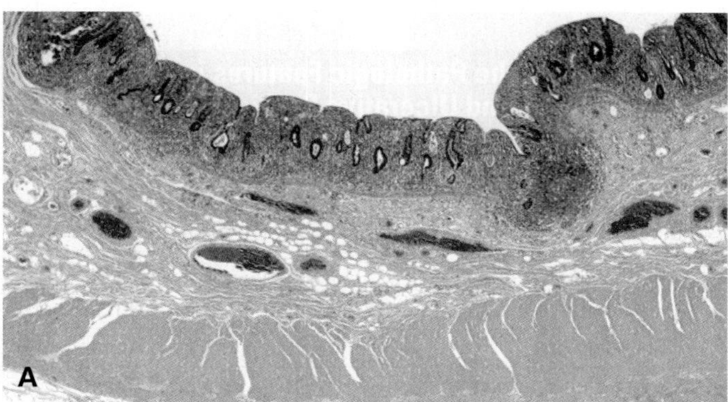

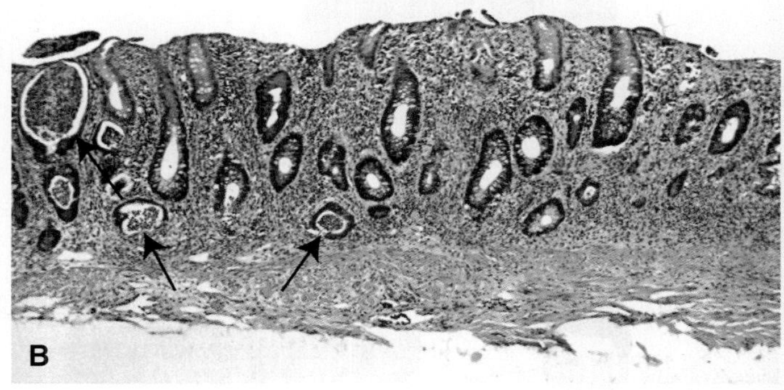

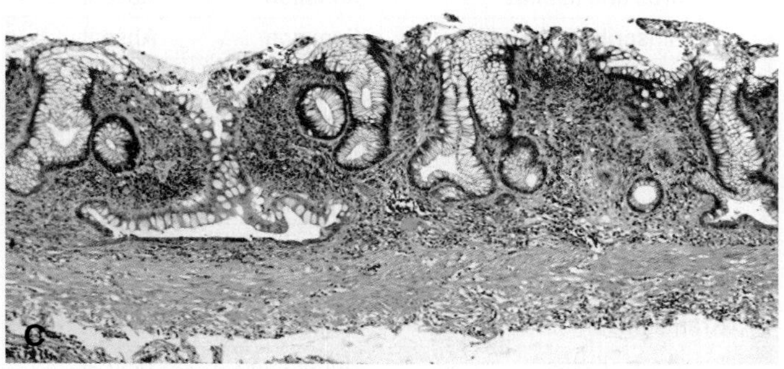

FIGURE 13-52. Ulcerative colitis. A. A full-thickness section of colon resected for ulcerative colitis shows inflammation affecting the mucosa with sparing of the submucosa and muscularis propria. **B.** Sections of a mucosal biopsy from a patient with active ulcerative colitis show expansion of the lamina propria and several crypt abscesses (*arrows*). **C.** Chronic ulcerative colitis shows significant crypt distortion and atrophy.

atrophy and a chronic inflammatory infiltrate in the mucosa and superficial submucosa. Paneth metaplasia is common.

CLINICAL FEATURES: The clinical course and manifestations are very variable. Most patients (70%) have intermittent attacks, with partial or complete remission in between. A few (<10%) have a very long remission (several years) after their first attack. The remaining 20% have continuous symptoms without remission.

MILD COLITIS: Half of patients with ulcerative colitis have mild disease. Their major symptom is rectal bleeding, sometimes with tenesmus (rectal pressure and discomfort). In these patients the disease is usually limited to the rectum but may extend to the distal sigmoid colon. Extraintestinal complications are uncommon, and in most patients in this category, disease remains mild throughout their lives.

MODERATE COLITIS: About 40% of patients have moderate ulcerative colitis. They usually have episodic loose bloody stools, crampy abdominal pain and often low-grade fever, lasting days or weeks. Moderate anemia is commonly due to chronic fecal blood loss.

SEVERE COLITIS: About 10% of patients have severe or fulminant disease, sometimes from its onset but often during a flare of activity. They may have more than 6, and sometimes more than 20, bloody bowel movements daily, often with fever and other systemic symptoms. Blood and fluid loss rapidly leads to anemia, dehydration and electrolyte depletion. Massive hemorrhage may be life-threatening. A particularly dangerous complication is **toxic megacolon,** an extreme dilation of the colon that carries a high risk for perforation of the colon. Fulminant ulcerative colitis is a medical emergency requiring immediate, intensive medical therapy and, in some cases, prompt colectomy. About 15% of patients with fulminant courses die of the disease.

The medical treatment of ulcerative colitis depends on the sites involved and the severity of the inflammation. The 5-aminosalicylate–based compounds are the mainstays of treatment for patients with mild to moderate ulcerative colitis. Corticosteroids and immunosuppressive and immunoregulatory agents (azathioprine or mercaptopurine) are used in patients who have severe and refractory disease.

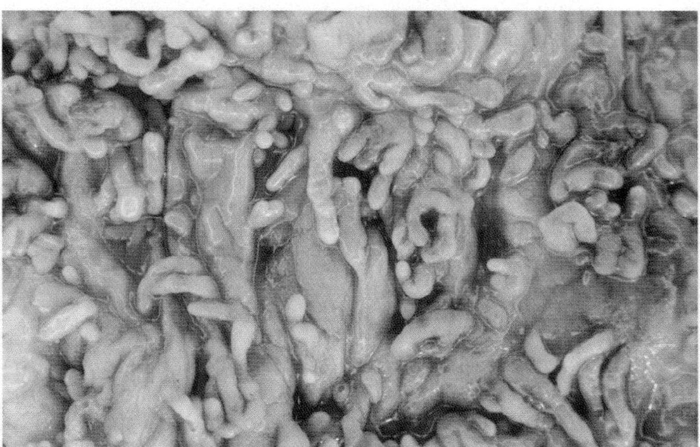

FIGURE 13-53. Inflammatory polyps of the colon in ulcerative colitis. Nodules of regenerative mucosa and inflammation surrounded by denuded areas provide a diffuse polypoid appearance of the mucosa.

Extraintestinal Manifestations

Arthritis is seen in 25% of patients with ulcerative colitis. Eye inflammation (mostly **uveitis**) and skin lesions develop in about 10%. The most common cutaneous lesions are

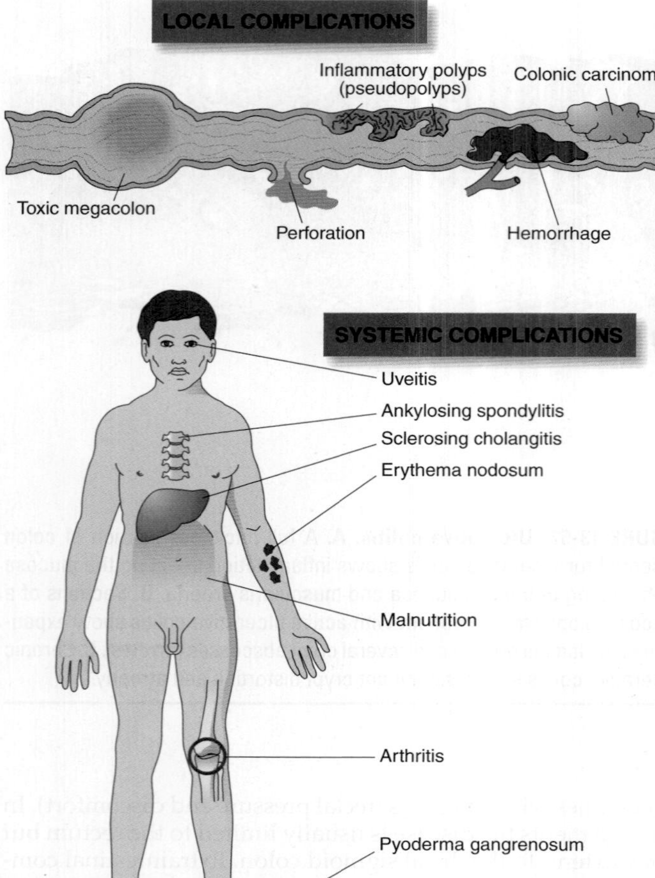

FIGURE 13-54. Complications of ulcerative colitis.

erythema nodosum and **pyoderma gangrenosum,** the latter a serious, noninfective disorder with deep, purulent, necrotic ulcers in the skin.

Liver disease occurs in about 4% of patients, mostly **primary sclerosing cholangitis,** which carries a risk for development of **cholangiocarcinoma.** Thromboembolic phenomena, mostly deep vein thromboses of the lower extremities, occur in 6% of ulcerative colitis patients.

The various complications of ulcerative colitis are shown in Fig. 13-54.

Differential Diagnosis

The most important conditions to be distinguished from ulcerative colitis are other forms of chronic colitis due to specifically treatable causes, and Crohn disease. Other conditions that should be considered in the differential diagnosis of ulcerative colitis are bacterial infections and amebic colitis, especially in areas where it is endemic. When inflammation is limited to the rectum, other infectious agents, including viruses, *Chlamydia,* fungi and other parasites, merit consideration. Proctitis due to these agents is common in male homosexuals and a variety of opportunistic infections of the bowel are seen in patients with AIDS. Other conditions that may mimic ulcerative colitis are ischemic colitis, antibiotic-associated colitis, radiation injury and solitary rectal ulcer syndrome.

Table 13-3

Comparison of the Pathologic Features in the Colon of Crohn Disease and Ulcerative Colitis

Lesion	Crohn Disease	Ulcerative Colitis
Macroscopic		
Thickened bowel wall	Typical	Uncommon
Luminal narrowing	Typical	Uncommon
"Skip" lesions	Common	Absent
Right colon predominance	Typical	Absent
Fissures and fistulas	Common	Absent
Circumscribed ulcers	Common	Absent
Confluent linear ulcers	Common	Absent
Pseudopolyps	Absent	Common
Microscopic		
Transmural inflammation	Typical	Uncommon
Submucosal fibrosis	Typical	Absent
Fissures	Typical	Rare
Granulomas	Common	Absent
Crypt abscesses	Uncommon	Typical

The distinction between ulcerative colitis and Crohn colitis is based on different anatomic localization and histopathology (Table 13-3). Ulcerative colitis is a diffuse process, usually more severe distally, whereas Crohn colitis is patchy or segmental and often spares the rectum. The inflammation in ulcerative colitis is superficial (i.e., usually limited to the mucosa) and is largely an acute inflammatory infiltrate, with neutrophils and crypt abscesses. By contrast, Crohn colitis is transmural and involves all layers, with granulomas in some of the specimens.

If disease stops at the ileocecal valve, or is limited to the distal colon, ulcerative colitis is more likely. Involvement of the terminal ileum suggests Crohn colitis.

In 10% of cases, definitive discrimination is not possible. This occurs mostly in fulminant colitis; the inflammatory bowel disease is then termed **indeterminate colitis.** Distinguishing between ulcerative colitis and Crohn colitis is important because of (1) different surgical therapy (Crohn disease often recurs, so continent ileostomy and ileoanal pouch procedures may be contraindicated), (2) a higher risk of cancer in ulcerative colitis and (3) different medical therapy.

Ulcerative Colitis and Colorectal Cancer

Patients with long-standing ulcerative colitis have a considerably higher risk of colorectal cancer than the general population. This risk is related to the extent and duration of the disease. If the entire colon is involved, the risk of developing colorectal cancer is greater. If the inflammatory disease is limited to the rectum, the risk of colorectal cancer is like that of the general population. The incidence of colorectal cancer in the United States is estimated to be between 5% and 10%

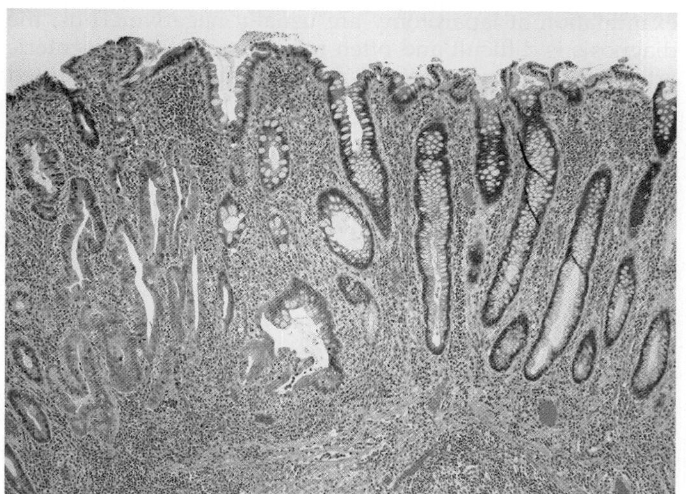

FIGURE 13-55. Dysplasia in ulcerative colitis. The colonic mucosa shows the chronic changes of ulcerative colitis (see Fig. 13-52C). The crypts to the left are dysplastic, showing architectural distortion, hyperchromatic nuclei and lack of glandular maturation.

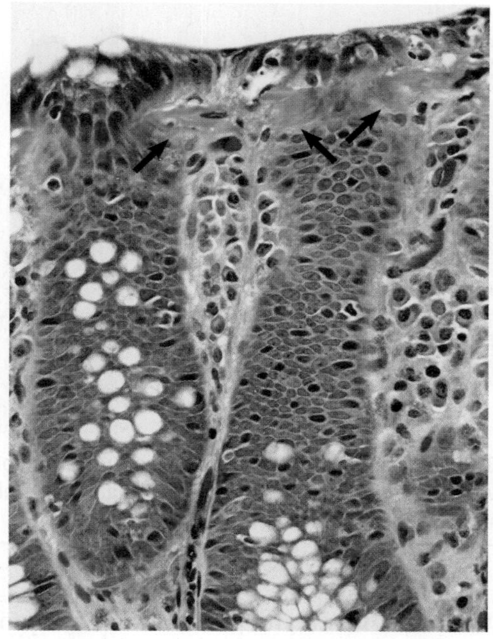

FIGURE 13-56. Collagenous colitis. A trichrome stain highlights the characteristic thickening of the collagen table (blue, note *arrows*) with entrapment of capillaries. The intercryptal surface epithelium is flattened and contains an increased number of intraepithelial lymphocytes.

for each decade of pancolitis. Young age at the onset of ulcerative colitis is not an independent risk factor, but since patients in whom the disease develops at a young age have it longer, they also have a higher cumulative incidence of cancer.

Colorectal **epithelial dysplasia** is a neoplastic epithelial proliferation and precursor to colorectal carcinoma in patients with long-term ulcerative colitis (Fig. 13-55). The histologic criteria include (1) altered mucosal architecture, (2) epithelial abnormalities (hypercellularity and stratification of nuclei) and (3) epithelial dysplasia (variation in nuclear size, shape and staining qualities). Dysplasia may be **low grade** or **high grade.** The latter carries a high risk for development of colorectal cancer and, when identified in a biopsy, is a strong indication for colectomy. Routine colonoscopic surveillance and biopsy of all patients with ulcerative colitis are therefore recommended.

Collagenous Colitis and Lymphocytic Colitis Cause Chronic Diarrhea

Collagenous colitis is an inflammatory disorder of the colon characterized clinically by chronic watery diarrhea and pathologically by a thickened subepithelial collagen band. The disorder mainly afflicts middle-aged and elderly women.

The colonic mucosa appears grossly normal. Indeed, the term *microscopic colitis* has been applied to the condition. The diagnosis of collagenous colitis is made by demonstrating a chronic inflammatory cell infiltrate in the mucosa and a band of collagen up to 80 μm in width immediately beneath the surface epithelium (Fig. 13-56). The surface epithelium shows flattened or cuboidal cells and even separation of epithelial cells from underlying structures. Intraepithelial lymphocytes are common. The lamina propria contains increased chronic inflammatory cells, and neutrophils are also found in some patients.

Lymphocytic colitis also features prominent infiltration of the damaged colonic epithelium by lymphocytes but lacks the collagen table and has an equal sex distribution. Patients with lymphocytic colitis have more than 10 lymphocytes for every 100 epithelial cells.

MOLECULAR PATHOGENESIS: The etiologies of collagenous colitis and lymphocytic colitis are unknown. The fibrosis of collagenous colitis may result from persistent inflammation. Although the diseases are not consistently linked to other systemic disorders, an autoimmune etiology also has been suggested, based on putative association with rheumatoid arthritis and thyroid dysfunction. Compared with patients with collagenous colitis, those with lymphocytic colitis have an increased frequency of HLA-A1 and decreased HLA-A3. Many patients with these diseases have taken nonsteroidal anti-inflammatory drugs. Lymphocytic colitis is common in patients with celiac disease.

Vascular Diseases

The Colon Is Subject to the Same Types of Ischemic Injury as the Small Intestine

Unlike the small bowel, extensive infarction of the colon is uncommon; chronic segmental disease is the rule. ***The most vulnerable areas are those between adjacent arterial distributions, so-called watershed areas.*** For example, the splenic flexure lies between the regions supplied by the superior and inferior mesenteric arteries, and the rectosigmoid area shares blood from the inferior mesenteric and internal iliac arteries. However, the rectum itself is usually spared in ischemic colitis. Most cases of ischemic colitis are caused by atherosclerosis of major intestinal arteries, and the disease usually occurs in people older than 50 years. Recurrent bouts of abdominal pain due to ischemic colitis are called "intestinal angina."

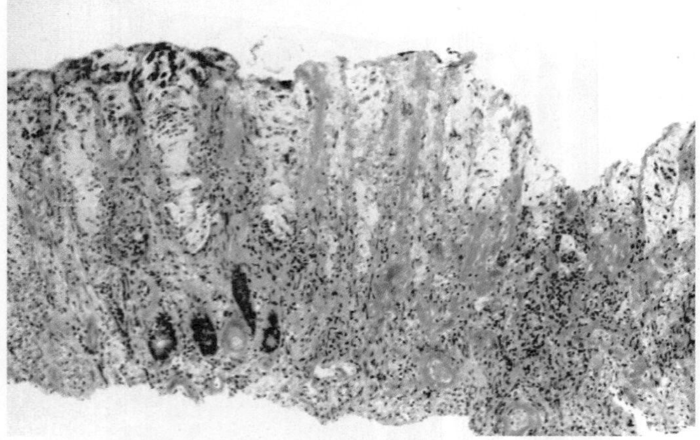

FIGURE 13-57. Ischemic colitis. A mucosal biopsy shows coagulative necrosis with "ghostly" outlines of the preexisting crypts. Only a small portion of the base of several crypts remains.

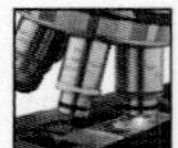

PATHOLOGY: Some patients with symptoms and complications of bowel infarction require immediate surgery. However, in most patients, the acute signs stabilize, and radiography shows only patterns of intramural hemorrhage and edema. On endoscopy, multiple ulcers, hemorrhagic nodular lesions or a pseudomembrane is seen. Biopsy reveals ischemic necrosis of the bowel: mucosal ulceration, crypt abscesses, edema and hemorrhage (Fig. 13-57). Patients may recover completely or develop a colonic stricture, in which case surgical removal of the obstructed segment is necessary. Segments of ischemic stricture show variable mucosal ulceration and inflammation, as well as submucosal widening by granulation tissue and fibrosis. Hemosiderin-laden macrophages and patchy fibrosis of the muscular coats may be noted.

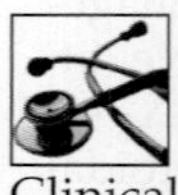

CLINICAL FEATURES: Ischemic disease of the rectosigmoid area typically manifests as abdominal pain, rectal bleeding and a change in bowel habits. Clinically, ischemic colitis often cannot be distinguished from some forms of infective colitis, ulcerative colitis and Crohn colitis. Prognosis and treatment depend on the primary cause and extent of involvement. The goal is to improve blood supply to the colon by treating patients' overall cardiovascular status. Acute interruption of blood supply to the colon can be fatal in neonates and the elderly.

Angiodysplasia (Vascular Ectasia) May Cause Intestinal Bleeding

Angiodysplasia (vascular ectasia) is localized arteriovenous malformations, mainly in the cecum and ascending colon, that cause lower intestinal bleeding. The mean age at presentation is 60 years. Younger people usually have lesions at other sites, including the rectum, stomach and small bowel. Interestingly, angiodysplasia is associated with aortic valve disease in some patients. It has been suggested that it may result from chronic intestinal circulatory insufficiency, intestinal muscle hypertrophy and consequent venous obstruction. Patients complain of multiple bleeding episodes, but chronic bleeding may also be occult. Radiologic studies and examination at laparotomy are usually negative. Thus, the diagnosis is difficult and often requires selective mesenteric arteriography or colonoscopy. Surgical removal of the affected segment is curative.

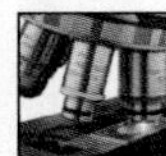

PATHOLOGY: The resected specimen often has multiple vascular lesions, usually less than 0.5 cm. The submucosal veins and capillaries are tortuous, thin walled and dilated. The attenuated walls of these vessels are presumably responsible for their propensity to bleed.

Hemorrhoids Are Dilated Venous Channels of the Hemorrhoidal Plexuses

They result from downward displacement of the anal cushions. Internal hemorrhoids arise from the superior hemorrhoidal plexus above the pectinate line. External hemorrhoids originate from the inferior hemorrhoidal plexus below that line. ***Hemorrhoids are common in Western countries, to some degree afflicting at least half the population over age 50.*** They are common in pregnancy, presumably because of the increased abdominal pressure.

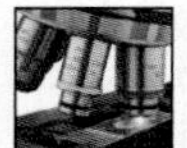

PATHOLOGY: Hemorrhoids are dilated vascular spaces with excess smooth muscle in their walls. Hemorrhage and thrombosis of varying severity are common.

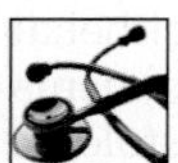

CLINICAL FEATURES: The key clinical feature of hemorrhoids is bleeding. Chronic blood loss may lead to **iron-deficiency anemia. Rectal prolapse** is common. Prolapsed hemorrhoids may become irreducible and lead to painful strangulated hemorrhoids. **Thrombosis** of external hemorrhoids is exquisitely painful and requires evacuation of the intravascular clot.

Radiation Enterocolitis

Radiation therapy for malignant disease of the pelvis or abdomen may be complicated by injury to the small intestine and colon.

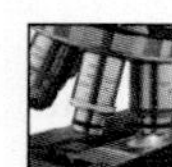

PATHOLOGY: Clinically significant radiation colitis is most common in the rectum (radiation proctitis). The lesions vary from reversible intestinal mucosal injury to chronic inflammation, ulceration and fibrosis of the intestine. In the short term, radiation damages epithelium and endothelium, causing decreased mitoses and, in the small bowel, villous shortening. Mucosal inflammation is conspicuous and abscesses may be seen in the colorectal crypts. Failure of epithelial renewal may lead to ulceration. Subacute changes occur 2 to 12 months after radiation therapy, after the mucosa has healed. Damage to submucosal vessels leads to thrombosis. The submucosa becomes fibrotic and often contains bizarre fibroblasts. As a result of radiation vascular injury, progressive ischemia further damages the bowel.

Complications of radiation enterocolitis include perforation and subsequent development of internal fistulas, hemorrhage and stricture, sometimes severe enough to obstruct the intestines.

Solitary Rectal Ulcer Syndrome

Internal mucosal prolapse of the rectum can produce mucosal changes that are easily mistaken clinically and pathologically for chronic inflammatory disease or a tumor. The hallmark of solitary rectal ulcer syndrome is smooth muscle proliferation from the muscularis mucosae into the lamina propria. Despite the name, some patients have no ulcers, whereas others display multiple erosions, ulcers, or even polypoid lesions. Mucosal abnormalities often appear as a mass that can simulate a neoplasm. Dilated glands can be entrapped in the rectal wall, a condition termed **colitis cystica profunda.**

Polyps of the Colon and Rectum

A gastrointestinal polyp is a mass that protrudes into the lumen of the gut. Polyps are classified by their attachment to the bowel wall (e.g., sessile, or pedunculated with a discrete stalk), their histology (e.g., hyperplastic or adenomatous) and their neoplastic potential (i.e., benign or malignant). By themselves, polyps are infrequently symptomatic and their clinical importance lies in their potential for malignant transformation.

Adenomatous Polyps Are Potentially Premalignant

Adenomatous polyps (tubular adenomas) are neoplasms that arise from colonic epithelium. They are composed of neoplastic epithelial cells that migrated to the surface and accumulated beyond the needs for replacement of the cells sloughed into the lumen.

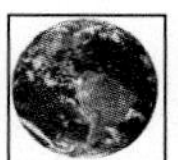

EPIDEMIOLOGY: The prevalence of adenomatous colon polyps is highest in industrialized countries. As with diverticular disease, the only known consistent environmental difference between high-risk and low-risk populations is diet. In the United States, at least one adenomatous polyp is present in half of the adult population, a figure that increases to more than two thirds among those older than 65. There is a modest male predominance (1.4:1). Blacks have a higher proportion of right-sided adenomas and cancers. Polyps are multiple 25% of the time.

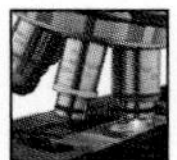

PATHOLOGY: ***Almost half of all adenomatous polyps of the colon in the United States are in the rectosigmoid region and thus are detectable by digital examination or by sigmoidoscopy.*** The remaining half are evenly distributed throughout the rest of the colon. Adenomas vary from barely visible nodules or small, pedunculated adenomas to large, sessile (flat) lesions. They are classified by architecture into tubular, villous and tubulovillous types. They are the usual precursors to colon carcinoma, and their epithelium is often dysplastic.

TUBULAR ADENOMAS: These represent two thirds of benign large bowel adenomas. They are typically smooth-surfaced lesions, less than 2 cm, which often have a stalk (Fig. 13-58). Some tubular adenomas, particularly the smaller ones, are sessile.

Tubular adenomas show closely packed epithelial tubules, which may be uniform or irregular and excessively branched (Fig. 13-58C). The tubules are embedded in a fibrovascular stroma similar to normal lamina propria. Most tubular adenomas show little epithelial dysplasia, but 20% (particularly larger tumors) may have dysplastic features, which vary from mild nuclear pleomorphism to frank invasive carcinoma (Fig. 13-59). In high-grade dysplasia, glands are crowded and highly irregular in size and shape. Papillary or cribriform (sieve-like or perforated) growth patterns are common. ***As long as the dysplastic focus is confined to the mucosa, the lesion is almost always cured by resection of the polyp.***

The risk of invasive carcinoma correlates with the size of the tubular adenoma. Only 1% of tubular adenomas under 1 cm have invasive cancer at the time of resection; among those 1 to 2 cm, 10% harbor malignancy; and of those over 2 cm, 35% are cancerous. Small flat adenomas may be missed during conventional endoscopy and have a high malignant potential.

VILLOUS ADENOMAS: These polyps constitute one tenth of colonic adenomas and are found predominantly in the rectosigmoid region. They are typically large, broad-based, elevated lesions with shaggy, cauliflower-like surfaces (Fig. 13-60A), but they can be small and pedunculated. Most exceed 2 cm, and they may reach 10 to 15 cm. Villous adenomas are composed of thin, tall, finger-like processes that superficially resemble the villi of the small intestine. They are lined externally by neoplastic epithelial cells and are supported by a core of fibrovascular connective tissue like the normal lamina propria (Fig. 13-60B).

Features of dysplasia in villous adenomas are similar to those in tubular adenomas. ***However, villous adenomas contain foci of carcinoma more often than tubular adenomas.*** In polyps less than 1 cm across, the risk is 10 times higher than that for comparably sized tubular adenomas. ***Of greater importance is the fact that 50% of villous adenomas larger than 2 cm harbor invasive carcinoma. Given that most villous adenomas measure more than 2 cm, more than one third of all resected villous adenomas contain invasive cancer.***

TUBULOVILLOUS ADENOMAS: Many adenomatous polyps have both tubular and villous features. Polyps with between 25% and 75% villous architecture are termed "tubulovillous." These tend to be intermediate in distribution and size between the tubular and villous forms, one fourth to one third being larger than 2 cm across. Tubulovillous polyps are also intermediate between tubular and villous adenomas in the risk of invasive carcinoma.

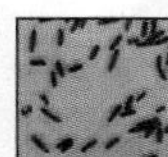

ETIOLOGIC FACTORS: The precursor to colorectal carcinoma is dysplasia, usually in the form of an adenoma. The pathogenesis of adenomas of the colon and rectum involves neoplastic alteration of crypt epithelial homeostasis with (1) diminished apoptosis, (2) persistent cell replication and (3) failure of epithelial cells to mature and differentiate as they migrate toward the surface of the crypts (Fig. 13-61). Normally, DNA synthesis ceases when cells reach the upper third of the crypts, after which they mature, migrate to the surface and then undergo apoptosis or are sloughed into the lumen. Adenomas represent focal disruption of this orderly sequence, in that epithelial cells may proliferate throughout the entire depth of the crypt: mitotic figures are present both along the entire length of the crypt and on the mucosal surface. As the lesion evolves, the rate of proliferation exceeds that of apoptosis and sloughing, and cells accumulate in upper crypts and on the surface. Accumulated cells on the mucosal surface then form tubules or villous structures, in concert with stromal elements.

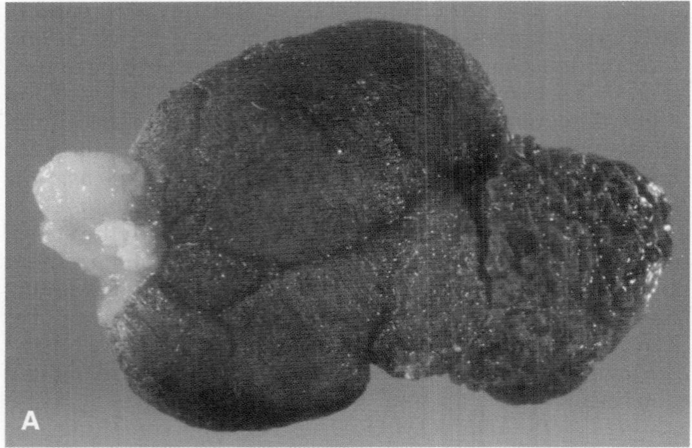

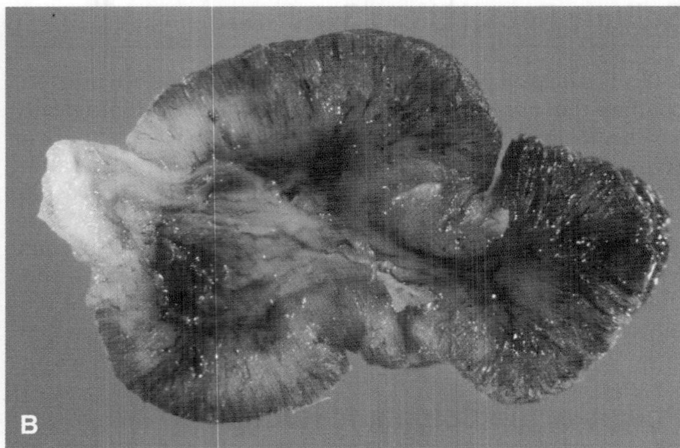

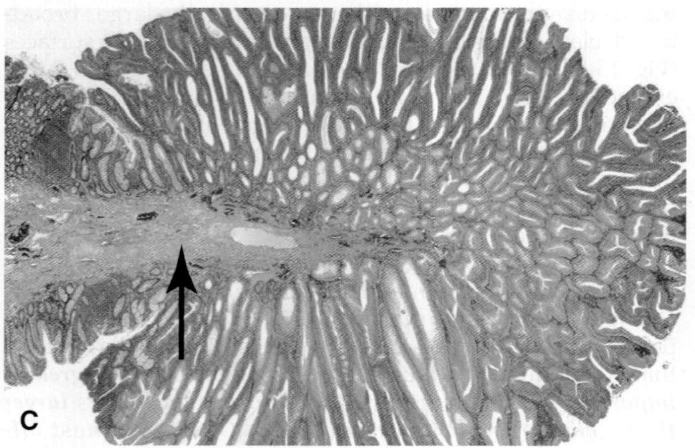

FIGURE 13-58. **Tubular adenoma of the colon. A.** The adenoma shows a characteristic stalk and bosselated surface. **B.** The bisected adenoma shows the stalk covered by the adenomatous epithelium. The ashen white color is cautery at the polypectomy resection margin from the polypectomy. **C.** Microscopically, the adenoma shows a repetitive pattern that is largely tubular. The stalk (*arrow*) is in continuity with the submucosa of the colon, is not involved and is lined by normal colonic epithelium.

ADENOMATOUS POLYPS AND COLORECTAL CANCER: The origin of colon cancer in adenomatous polyps is supported by the following:

- **There is geographic coincidence** in the incidence of adenomatous polyps and colorectal cancer. In regions at high risk for colorectal cancer, adenomatous polyps tend to be larger, are more often villous and display more high-grade dysplasia than do those in low-risk areas. Both adenomas and carcinomas occur most frequently in the sigmoid colon in Western countries.

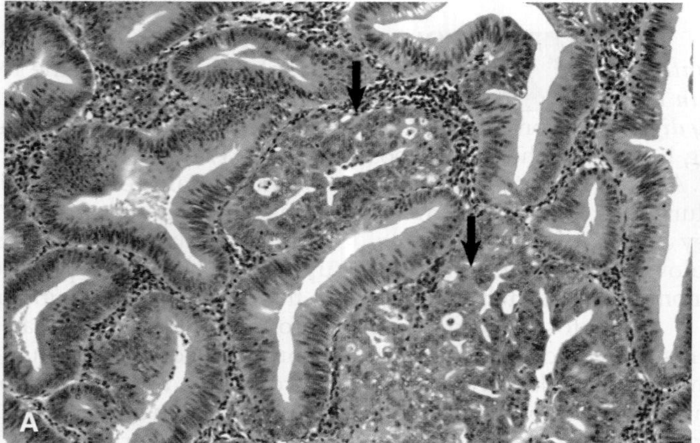

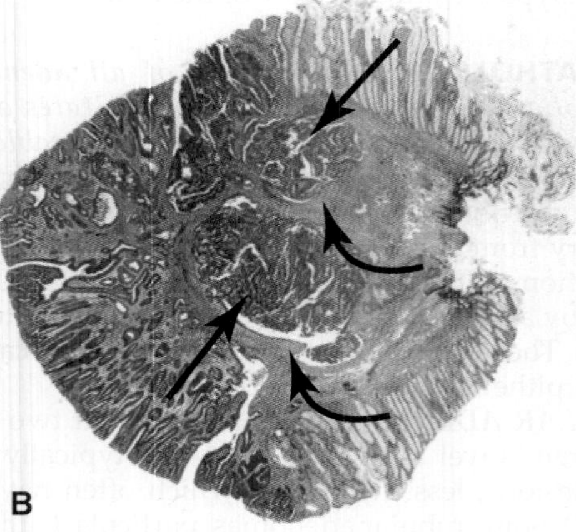

FIGURE 13-59. Adenocarcinoma arising in a pedunculated adenomatous polyp. A. Both low-grade dysplasia and high-grade dysplasia are present. The latter is characterized by a cribriform pattern and increased nuclear pleomorphism (*arrows*). **B.** Trichrome stain showing tumor invading (*straight arrows*) the stalk (blue, *curved arrows*). Since there was a margin of resection of over 1 mm, polypectomy was sufficient therapy.

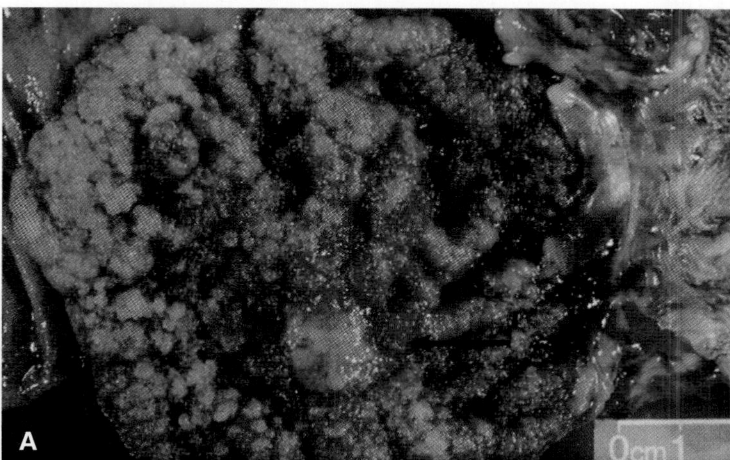

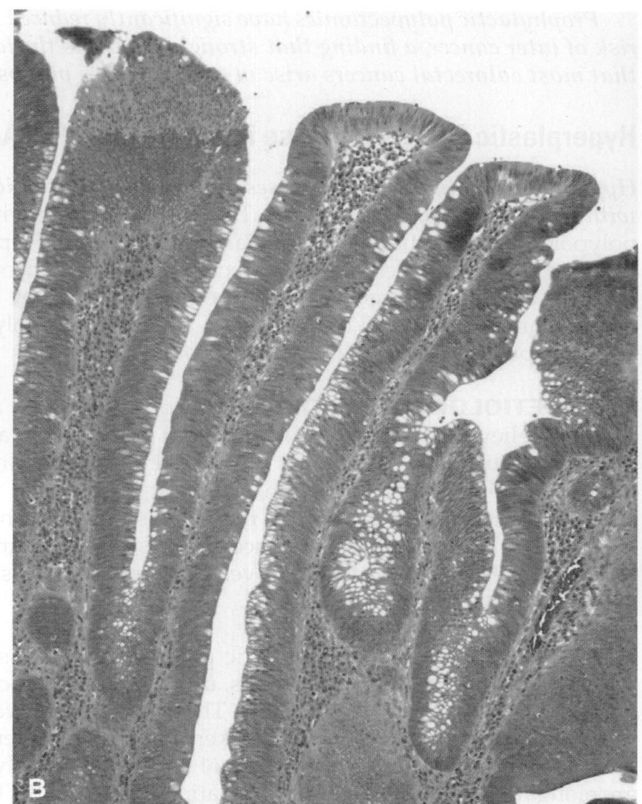

FIGURE 13-60. Villous adenoma of the colon. A. The colon contains a large, broad-based, elevated lesion that has a cauliflower-like surface. A firm area near the center of the lesion proved on histologic examination to be an adenocarcinoma. **B.** Microscopic examination shows finger-like processes with fibrovascular cores lined by hyperchromatic nuclei.

- **Adenomatous polyps tend to antedate colon cancer by 10 to 15 years,** suggesting that the latter follows the former.
- **Carcinomas are found in adenomas,** and some carcinomas have adenomatous remnants at their periphery.
- **An associated carcinoma** is commonly found in colons that harbor adenomas. Also, one third of colons resected for cancer contain an adenomatous polyp. Moreover, the presence of an adenomatous polyp in a colon partly resected for cancer doubles the risk that another carcinoma will develop in the remaining colon.
- **In familial adenomatosis polyposis** (see below), the innumerable adenomatous polyps are initially benign, but colorectal cancer invariably develops at a later age.

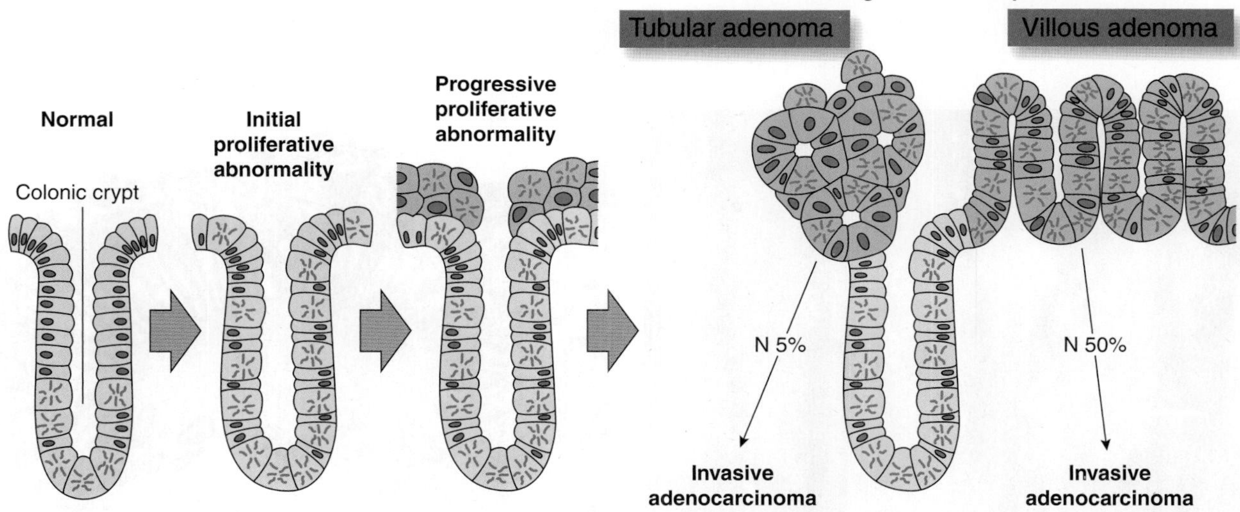

FIGURE 13-61. The histogenesis of adenomatous polyps of the colon. The initial proliferative abnormality of the colonic mucosa, the extension of the mitotic zone in the crypts, leads to the accumulation of mucosal cells. Adenocarcinoma arises in adenomatous polyps (see text).

Prophylactic polypectomies have significantly reduced the risk of later cancer, a finding that strongly supports the idea that most colorectal cancers arise in adenomatous polyps.

Hyperplastic Polyps Increase in Incidence With Age

Hyperplastic polyps are small, sessile mucosal protrusions with exaggerated crypt architecture. They are the most common polypoid lesions of the colon, especially in the rectum. Hyperplastic polyps are present in 40% of rectal specimens in people younger than 40 years and in 75% of older people. They are more common than usual in colons with adenomatous polyps and in populations with higher rates of colorectal cancer.

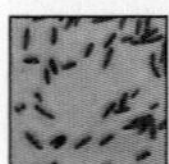

ETIOLOGIC FACTORS: Hyperplastic polyps are believed to arise due to a defect in proliferation and maturation of normal mucosal epithelium. In a hyperplastic polyp, proliferation occurs at the base of the crypt, and upward migration of the cells is slowed. Thus, epithelial cells differentiate and acquire absorptive characteristics lower in the crypts. Moreover, cells persist at the surface longer than do normal cells.

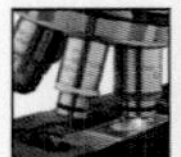

PATHOLOGY: Hyperplastic polyps are small, sessile, raised mucosal nodules, up to 0.5 cm, but occasionally larger (Fig. 13-62A). They are almost always multiple and have even been mistaken for familial adenomatous polyposis (FAP). The crypts of hyperplastic polyps are elongated and may show cystic dilation (Fig. 13-62B). The epithelium contains goblet cells and absorptive cells, with no dysplasia. The surface cells are elongated giving a tufted appearance; this accounts for the serrated contour of the glands near the surface.

There Are Several Variants of Hyperplastic Polyps (Serrated Adenomas)

The nomenclature of these variants is unsettled. One form, termed **serrated adenoma,** has a serrated arrangement like that of hyperplastic polyps but with nuclear features of adenomas (Fig. 13-63A). Another type, a **sessile serrated adenoma,** resembles classic hyperplastic polyps, but does not show adenomatous features, and often appears as a large deformed mucosal fold (Fig. 13-63B, C). These lesions have a high incidence of microsatellite instability. The carcinomas that arise from them tend to be bulky, mucinous and right sided. Some investigators simply refer to the latter entities as **serrated polyps.** In yet a third variant areas of hyperplastic polyp and adenoma are juxtaposed. These are **mixed hyperplastic adenomatous polyps** (Fig. 13-63D). ***Unlike classic hyperplastic polyps, patients with these variants have increased risk for the development of adenocarcinoma.***

Familial Adenomatous Polyposis (FAP) Is an Autosomal Dominant Trait That Invariably Leads to Cancer

Also termed **adenomatous polyposis coli** (APC), FAP accounts for less than 1% of colorectal cancers. It is caused by a mutation of the *APC* gene on the long arm of chromosome 5 (5q21–22) (see below). Most cases are familial, but 30% to 50% reflect new mutations. In FAP there are hundreds to thousands of adenomas carpeting the colorectal mucosa, sometimes throughout its length, but particularly in the rectosigmoid (Fig. 13-64). These are mostly tubular adenomas, but tubulovillous and villous adenomas may also be present. Microscopic adenomas, sometimes involving a single crypt, are numerous. A few polyps are usually present by age 10, but the mean age for occurrence of symptoms is 36 years, by which time cancer is often already present. ***Carcinoma of the colon and rectum is inevitable, the mean age of onset being 40 years.*** Total colectomy before the onset of cancer is curative, but some patients also have tubular adenomas in the small intestine and stomach that have the same malignant potential as those in the colon.

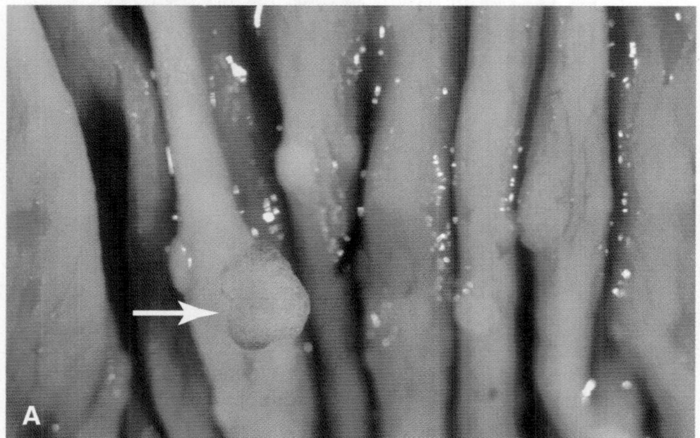

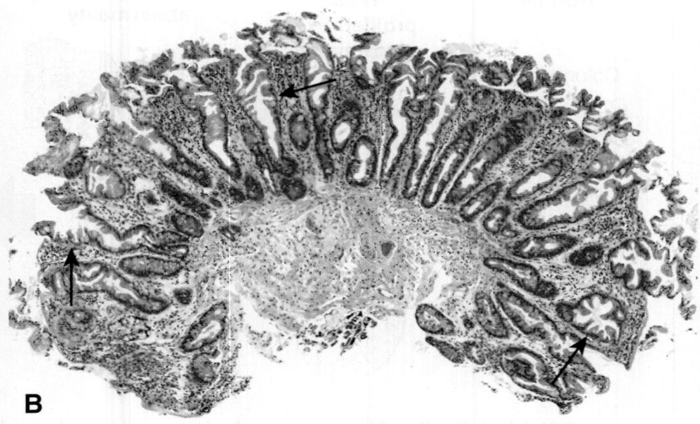

FIGURE 13-62. Hyperplastic polyp. A. This hyperplastic polyp (*arrow*) is small, sessile and pale. There are smaller adjacent hyperplastic polyps. **B.** Microscopically, there is a "sawtooth" appearance to the surface (*arrows*).

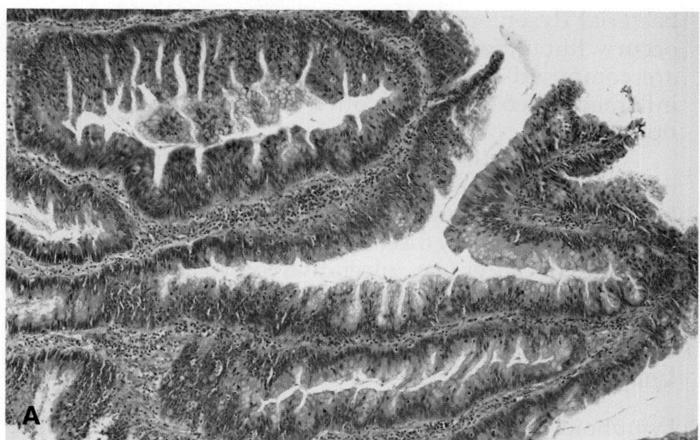

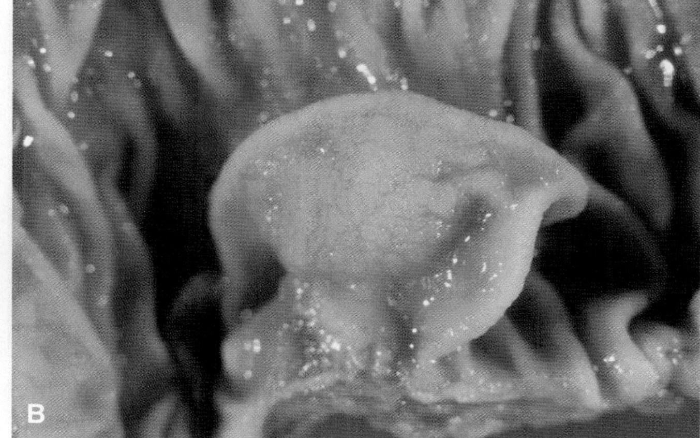

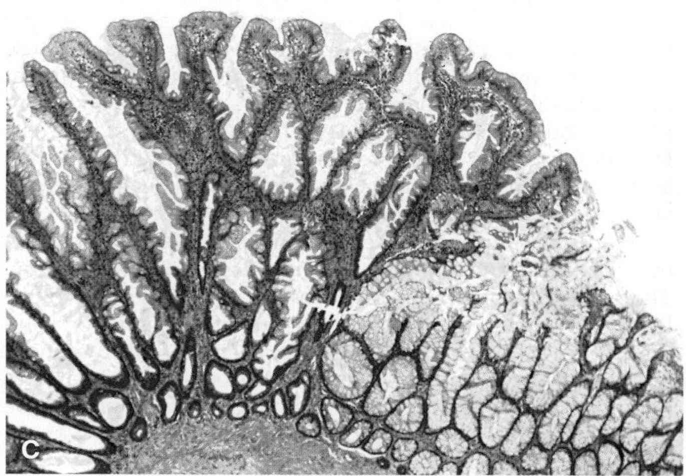

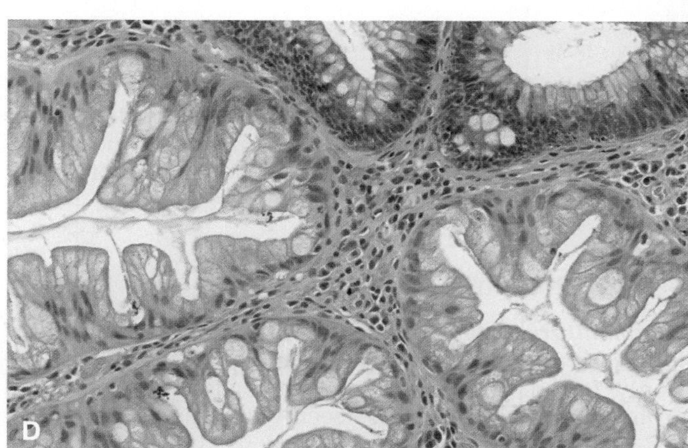

FIGURE 13-63. Variants of hyperplastic polyps. A. Serrated adenoma. The epithelium shows contours typical of hyperplastic polyps with adenomatous nuclear features. **B. Sessile serrated adenoma.** A polypoid lesion appears to be an enlarged flattened fold. **C. Sessile serrated adenoma** features irregular, asymmetric crypts that are often dilated by mucin. **D. Mixed hyperplastic adenomatous polyp.** Two adenomatous crypts in the upper right contrast with the three hyperplastic crypts.

Genetic testing for FAP is available, but mutations are found in only 75% of familial cases. Subtypes of FAP include:

- **Attenuated FAP:** In this condition adenomas in the colon number less than 100.
- **Gardner syndrome:** This variant features extracolonic lesions including osteomas of the skull, mandible and long bones; epidermoid cysts; desmoid tumors; and congenital hypertrophy of retinal pigment epithelium. *APC* gene mutations do not predict this phenotype.
- **Turcot syndrome:** This rare disorder combines FAP with malignant tumors of the central nervous system. Many cases, especially those with medulloblastoma, are due to germline mutation of the *APC* gene. Some cases, especially those with glioblastoma multiforme, are part of the spectrum of the HNPCC syndrome (see below).

Nonneoplastic Polyps Are Acquired Lesions

Nonneoplastic polyps are entirely different entities and are grouped together solely because of their gross appearance as raised lesions of the colonic mucosa.

Juvenile Polyps (Retention Polyps)

Juvenile polyps are **hamartomatous proliferations** of the colonic mucosa. They are most common in children younger than 10 years, although one third occur in adults.

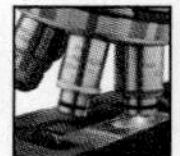

PATHOLOGY: Juvenile polyps are single or (rarely) multiple. They mostly occur in the rectum, but may be anywhere in the small or large bowel. Most are pedunculated lesions up to 2 cm in diameter, with smooth, rounded surfaces, unlike fissured surfaces of adenomatous polyps. Dilated and cystic epithelial tubules are filled with mucus (hence the name "retention polyp") and are embedded in a fibrovascular lamina propria (Fig. 13-65). Surface epithelial erosion is common, and reactive epithelial proliferation is evident, but the epithelium usually lacks dysplasia.

Patients with five or more juvenile polyps, or with juvenile polyps outside the colon, plus a family history of juvenile polyps are likely to have the syndrome of familial juvenile polyposis. This syndrome is caused by mutation of *SMAD4*, which encodes an intracellular signaling protein in the

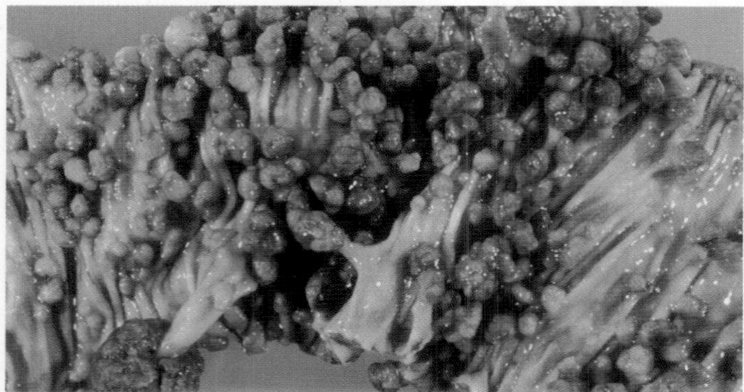

FIGURE 13-64. Familial polyposis. The colon contains thousands of adenomatous polyps with only several exceeding 1 cm in diameter.

TGF-β pathway. Other TGF-β signaling pathway mutations have also been identified (e.g., *BMPR1A*). These patients have an increased risk for gastrointestinal carcinoma, not necessarily arising from the polyps or even the segment of the gut where they are located.

Inflammatory Polyps

Inflammatory polyps are not neoplasms but are elevated nodules of inflamed, regenerating epithelium. They are commonly found in association with ulcerative colitis and Crohn disease; they are also seen with amebic colitis and bacterial dysentery. However, inflammatory polyps often occur without demonstrable colonic disease. These polyps are composed of a variable component of distorted and inflamed mucosal glands, often intermixed with granulation tissue.

As healing proceeds, epithelial regeneration characterized by large, basophilic epithelial cells restores mucosal architecture. These lesions are not precancerous, but occur in chronic inflammatory diseases that are associated with a high incidence of cancer (e.g., ulcerative colitis) and must thus be distinguished from adenomatous polyps.

Lymphoid Polyps

Lymphoid polyps are single, sessile submucosal accumulations of lymphoid tissue, almost invariably in the rectum, from pinpoint size to as large as 5 cm. On occasion, multiple lesions impart a cobblestone appearance to the mucosa. These polyps are covered by intact mucosa and contain prominent lymphoid follicles with germinal centers. In this context, lymphoid tissue is normally present in the colorectal mucosa. Lymphoid polyps are more common in women than men and occur at any age, including childhood. They are benign and usually asymptomatic.

Nodular lymphoid hyperplasia is seen mainly in children or with **common variable immunodeficiency syndrome.** There is excessive accumulation of the normal lymphoid follicles of the colon. There are numerous small sessile or polypoid nodules up to 0.5 cm in diameter that resemble lymphoid polyps microscopically. The condition is only rarely related to malignant lymphoma, but the radiologic appearance can be mistaken for FAP.

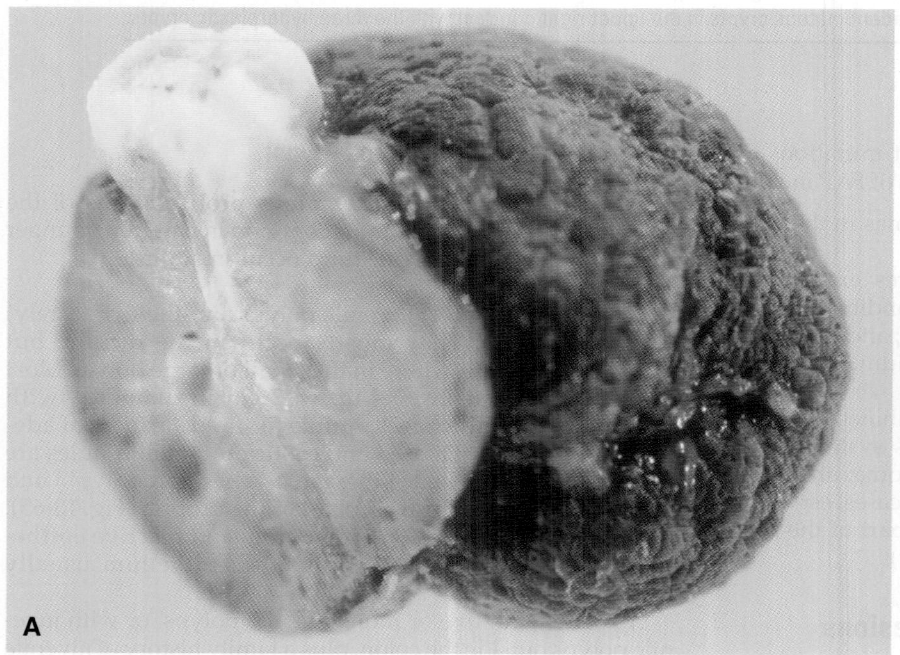

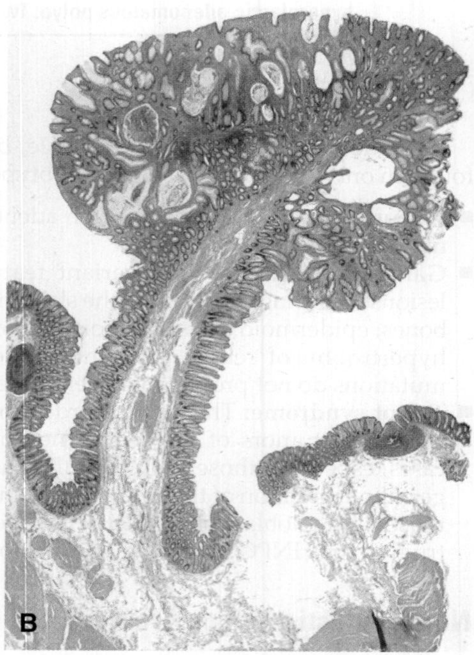

FIGURE 13-65. Juvenile polyp. A. The resected specimen shows a rounded surface. The cut surface (*left*) is cystic. **B.** Microscopically, the polyp displays cystically dilated glands.

Malignant Tumors

Colorectal Adenocarcinomas Mostly Arise in Adenomatous Polyps

In Western societies, colorectal cancer is the most common cause of cancer deaths that are not directly attributable to tobacco use. Some 5% of Americans develop this cancer during their lives. Although the widely used term **colorectal** implies a common biology, differences between cancers of the colon and rectum seem to be more fundamental than just location. For instance, colon cancer is much more common in the United States than in Japan, but the incidence of rectal cancer in the two populations is nearly the same. Rectosigmoid carcinoma accounts for a much higher proportion of large bowel cancers in populations at high risk for this tumor (including the United States) than in low-risk populations. Also, colon cancer shows a slight female preponderance, but rectal cancer is somewhat more common in men. The proportion of cancers in the distal colorectum has been declining in recent decades.

ETIOLOGIC FACTORS: Most cancers of the colon and rectum arise in adenomatous polyps; thus, factors related to the development of such polyps may favor colorectal cancer as well. The possible role of environmental factors is suggested by the high incidence of the disease in industrialized countries and among emigrants from low-risk to high-risk regions. However, most attempts to identify specific dietary contributors to colon carcinogenesis have been unsuccessful, so considerable skepticism is probably appropriate in this area.

DIETARY FAT: Consumption of animal fats parallels incidence of colorectal cancer. Moreover, certain ethnic groups in the United States whose diets are lower in animal fat have less colorectal cancer. Ingestion of fat elicits bile secretion into the intestine, and some bile acids may augment the tumorigenicity of experimental intestinal carcinogens. However, the relationship between dietary fat, or different types of dietary fat, and development of colorectal cancer remains conjectural.

ANAEROBIC BACTERIA: The feces of people in high-risk populations have more anaerobic bacteria than do those in low-risk populations. It is speculated that *Bacteroides* sp. may produce potentially mutagenic compounds and that their replacement with *Lactobacillus* protects experimental animals from chemically induced colon cancer.

DIETARY FIBER: Diets low in indigestible fiber and high in animal fat have been implicated in other colonic diseases, including diverticulosis and appendicitis. Attempts have been made for years to link low dietary fiber to colon cancer. However, data now show that no unambiguous link between dietary fiber and colon cancer can be drawn.

OTHER DIETARY FACTORS: A low prevalence of colorectal cancer has been related to high selenium levels in soil and plants in certain geographic areas. The endogenous antioxidant enzyme glutathione peroxidase contains selenium. Diets rich in cruciferous vegetables (e.g., cauliflower, Brussels sprouts, cabbage) and vitamin A may be associated with a lower incidence of colorectal cancer, but this hypothesis is so far is unproven.

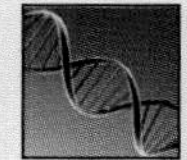

MOLECULAR PATHOGENESIS: In 85% of cases of colorectal carcinoma, it is estimated that at least 8 to 10 mutational events must accumulate before an invasive cancer with metastatic potential develops. This process is initiated in histologically normal mucosa, proceeds through an adenomatous precursor stage and ends as invasive adenocarcinoma (see also Chapter 5).

The most important mutational events are illustrated in Fig. 13-66 and involve:

- ***APC* gene:** As noted above, germline mutations in *APC* (adenomatous polyposis coli), a putative tumor suppressor gene, lead to familial adenomatous polyposis. Normal APC is a negative regulator of β-catenin: normal APC binding causes phosphorylation, followed by ubiquitination and eventual proteasomal degradation of β-catenin. Mutant APC allows β-catenin to accumulate in the nucleus, where it acts as a transcription factor to activate key proliferation genes (e.g., *cyclin D1* and *MYC*). ***APC is mutated in most sporadic colorectal cancers.*** Some tumors with normal *APC* have mutations in the **β-catenin gene.** A specific *APC* mutation (isoleucine → lysine at codon 1307) is found in 6% of Ashkenazi Jews and seems to render surrounding regions of the gene susceptible to inactivating frame-shift mutations and increases risk of colon cancer 10% to 20%. *APC* mutations are seen in normal colonic mucosa preceding development of sporadic adenomas. These data suggest

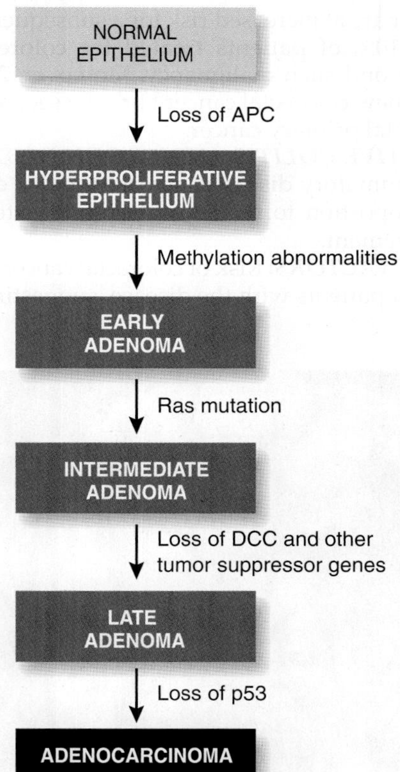

FIGURE 13-66. Model of some of the genetic alterations involved in colonic carcinogenesis. APC = adenomatous polyposis coli; DCC = "deleted in colon cancer."

13 | The Gastrointestinal Tract

an important role for *APC* in the early development of most colorectal neoplasms.

- ***Ras* oncogene:** Activating mutations of the *ras* protooncogene occur early in tubular adenomas of the colon.
- ***DCC* gene:** A putative tumor suppressor gene, *DCC* ("deleted in colon cancer") is located on chromosome 18 and is often missing in colorectal cancers.
- ***p53* tumor suppressor gene:** Mutation of *p53* facilitates the transition from adenoma to the most common type of adenocarcinoma and is a late event in the carcinogenic pathway.

In 15% of colorectal cancers, **DNA mismatch repair** (MMR) is impaired, leading to deficient repair of spontaneous replication errors, particularly in simple repetitive sequences (microsatellites). MMR deficiencies can occur through two mechanisms. In a hereditary form (HNPCC, Lynch syndrome; see below), a germline mutation in one of the MMR genes is followed by a somatic mutation of the other allele ("second hit") later in life. In a sporadic form, hypermethylation of the promoter of the *MLH1* gene, encoding a MMR protein, inactivates transcription of the gene.

Risk Factors for Colorectal Carcinoma

AGE: Increasing age is probably the single most important risk factor for colorectal cancer in the general population. The risk is low before age 40. It increases steadily to age 50, after which it doubles with each decade.

PRIOR COLORECTAL CANCER: Patients with one colorectal cancer are at increased risk for a subsequent tumor. In fact, 5% to 10% of patients treated for colorectal cancer develop a second such malignancy. Moreover, 2% to 5% of those with a new colorectal cancer harbor a second (synchronous) colorectal primary cancer.

ULCERATIVE COLITIS AND CROHN DISEASE: These chronic inflammatory diseases increase the risk of colorectal cancer in proportion to their duration and extent of large bowel involvement.

GENETIC FACTORS: Risk of colorectal cancer is increased in relatives of patients with the disease, suggesting a genetic contribution to tumorigenesis. People with two or more first- or second-degree relatives with colorectal cancer constitute 20% of all patients with this tumor. Some 5% to 10% of all colorectal cancers are inherited as autosomal dominant traits. A history of cancer at other sites, particularly breast or genital cancer in women, is associated with a higher than normal frequency of colorectal cancer.

DIET: As previously noted, prospective studies involving large populations in various countries have reported that the daily consumption of red meat and animal fat leads to a higher risk of colorectal cancer than that in persons who eat little or no meat.

PATHOLOGY: Grossly, colorectal cancers resemble adenocarcinomas elsewhere in the gut. They tend to be polypoid and ulcerating or infiltrative, and may be annular and constrictive (Fig. 13-67A). Polypoid cancers are more common in the right colon, particularly in the cecum, where the large lumen allows unimpeded intraluminal growth. Annular constricting tumors are more common in the distal colon. Tumors often ulcerate, regardless of growth pattern.

The vast majority of colorectal cancers are adenocarcinomas microscopically similar to their counterparts elsewhere in the digestive tract (Fig. 13-67B). Some 10% to 15% secrete abundant mucin and are called **mucinous** adenocarcinomas. The degree of differentiation influences prognosis; better-differentiated tumors tend to have a more favorable outlook.

These tumors spread by direct extension or vascular invasion. The former is common in resected specimens. Serosal connective tissue offers little resistance to tumor spread, and cancer cells are often seen in the fat and serosa far from the primary tumor. The peritoneum is occasionally involved, in which case there may be multiple deposits throughout the abdomen.

Colorectal cancer invades lymphatic channels and initially involves lymph nodes just below the tumor. In most patients with metastatic disease the liver is involved, but the tumor may metastasize widely. The prognosis of colorectal cancer is more closely related to tumor extension through the large bowel wall than to its size or histopathology.

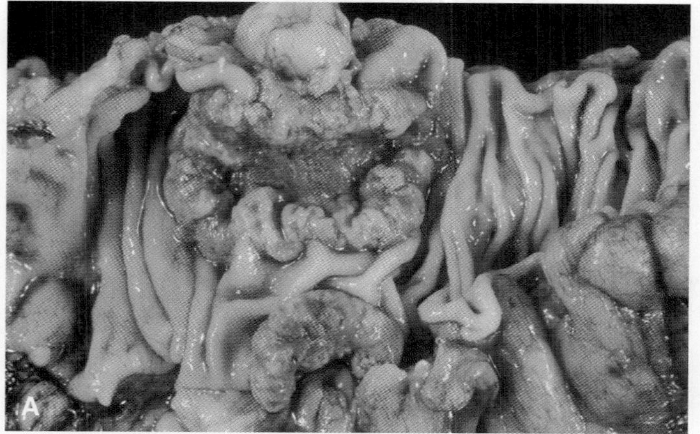

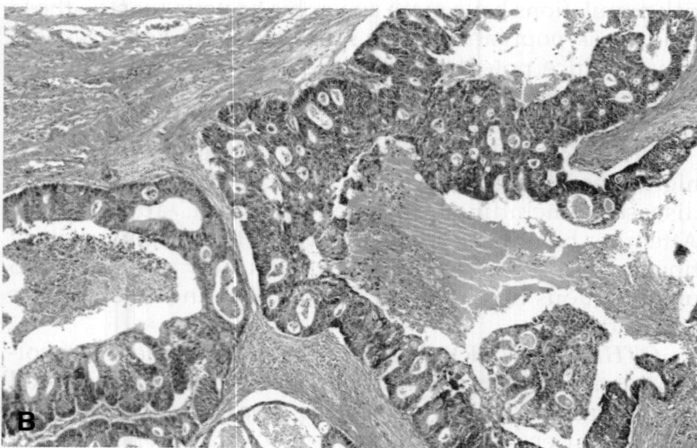

FIGURE 13-67. Adenocarcinoma of the colon. A. A resected colon shows an ulcerated mass with enlarged, firm, rolled borders. **B.** Microscopically, this colon adenocarcinoma consists of moderately differentiated glands with a prominent cribriform pattern and frequent central necrosis.

Current staging of these tumors uses the TNM system (tumor, lymph nodes, metastasis). T1 tumors invade the submucosa; T2 tumors infiltrate into, but not through, the muscularis propria; T3 tumors invade into the subserosal tissue; and T4 tumors penetrate the serosa or involve adjacent organs. N refers to the presence or absence of nodal metastases, and M to the presence or absence of extranodal metastases.

CLINICAL FEATURES: Initially, colorectal cancer is clinically silent. As the tumor grows, the most common sign is **fecal occult blood** when the tumor is in the proximal colon. Both occult blood and **bright red blood** in the feces may occur if a lesion is in the distal colorectum.

Cancers on the left side of the colon, where the lumen is narrow and the fecal contents more solid, often constrict the lumen, producing **obstructive symptoms.** These include changes in bowel habits and abdominal pain. Colorectal cancers may **perforate** early and cause peritonitis. By contrast, right-sided cancers can grow to large size without causing obstruction, particularly in the cecum where the lumen is large and fecal contents are liquid. In this setting, asymptomatic chronic bleeding may cause **iron-deficiency anemia** as the first indication of colorectal cancer. A tumor that extends beyond the colorectum may produce enterocutaneous and rectovaginal **fistulas,** tumor masses in the abdominal wall, bladder symptoms and sciatic nerve pain. Spread within the abdomen may cause **small intestinal obstruction** and malignant **ascites.**

A positive test for fecal occult blood predicts the presence of a cancer or an adenoma in 50% of cases. Periodic fiberoptic colonoscopy and testing for occult blood in feces improves the prognosis of colorectal cancer, as these methods can often detect the tumor at an early stage.

Resection is the only curative treatment for colorectal cancer. Small polyps are easily removed endoscopically; large lesions require segmental resection. Tumors near the anal verge often necessitate abdominal-perineal resection and colostomy, although newer surgical techniques may preserve sphincter function. In rectal cancers, preoperative chemotherapy and radiotherapy may improve the prognosis.

Hereditary Nonpolyposis Colorectal Cancer (HNPCC)

HNPCC, or Warthin-Lynch syndrome, is an autosomal dominant inherited disease that accounts for 3% to 5% of all colorectal cancers.

MOLECULAR PATHOGENESIS: HNPCC is caused by germline mutations in DNA mismatch repair genes. Usually, *hMSH2* (human MutS homolog 2) on chromosome 2p and *hMLH1* (human MutL homolog 1) on chromosome 3p are affected. Some mutations involve *hMSH6* (human MutS homolog 6) or *hPMS2* (human postmeiotic segregation 2) on chromosomes 2p and 7p, respectively. In HNPCC there is a germline mutation in one allele of one of the mismatch repair genes and the second allele is deleted in a somatic "second hit." Thus, spontaneous replication errors are not repaired effectively. This leads to widespread genomic instability, particularly in simple repetitive sequences (microsatellites), which are particularly prone to replication errors. Thus, genes that regulate growth and differentiation, and other mismatch repair genes, are disabled by unrepaired mutations.

Mismatch repair deficiency can be assessed by testing for microsatellite instability and for loss of expression of mismatch repair proteins in a tumor. If suspicion of HNPCC persists, mutation analysis of mismatch repair genes is available.

Histologically, HNPCC tumors are characterized by a high frequency of mucinous, signet ring cell and solid (medullary) histologies and frequent intratumoral lymphocytes. Clinically, HNPCC patients tend to (1) develop cancer at a young age (Table 13-4); (2) have few adenomas (hence "nonpolyposis"); (3) show tumors proximal to the splenic flexure (70%); (4) have multiple synchronous or metachronous colorectal cancers; and (5) develop extracolonic cancers, especially of the endometrium, ovary, stomach, small intestine and hepatobiliary tract, as well as transitional cell carcinomas of the renal pelvis and ureter. Patients with HNPCC may also have sebaceous adenomas and carcinomas and multiple keratoacanthomas (see Chapter 24).

Neuroendocrine Colon Tumors Resemble Their Counterparts of the Small Intestine

These tumors are also called carcinoid tumors. Half of colorectal carcinoid tumors have metastasized at the time they are discovered.

Large Bowel Lymphoma Is Usually B-Cell Malignancy

Primary lymphoma of the colorectum is uncommon. It may be seen with (1) segmental mucosal involvement, (2) diffuse polypoid lesions or (3) a mass extending beyond the colorectum.

Table 13-4

Hereditary Nonpolyposis Colorectal Cancer (HNPCC)

Hereditary Nonpolyposis Colorectal Cancer (HNPCC)
Amsterdam Criteria
At least three relatives must have histologically verified colorectal cancer
One must be a first-degree relative of the other two
At least two successive generations must be affected
At least one of the relatives with colorectal cancer must have received the diagnosis before the age of 50 years
Familial adenomatous polyposis must have been excluded
Bethesda Guidelines
Amsterdam I criteria met
Individuals with more than one HNPCC
Colorectal cancer (CRC) and first-degree relative with CRC/HNPCC, one cancer at younger than age 45 years or one adenoma at younger than age 40 years
CRC/endometrial cancer at younger than age 45 years
Right-sided CRC, undifferentiated, at younger than age 45 years
Signet-ring CRC at younger than age 45 years
Adenomas at younger than age 40 years

The symptoms are like those of other intestinal cancers, but the diffuse polypoid form may resemble inflammatory polyps or adenomatous polyps. Most colonic lymphomas are tumors of B cells.

Cancers of the Anal Canal Are Mostly Epidermoid Carcinomas

These cancers constitute 2% of cancers of the large bowel and may arise at or above the dentate line. They occur in both sexes but are more common in women and in blacks.

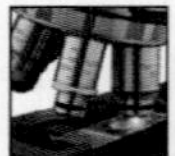

PATHOLOGY: Anal cancers have various histologic patterns, such as squamous, basaloid (cloacogenic) or mucoepidermoid, but these different tumor types tend to behave similarly and so are all classed as **epidermoid carcinomas. Bowen disease of the anus** is squamous carcinoma in situ, while **extramammary Paget disease** at this site is an intraepithelial adenocarcinoma (either primary of the mucosa or metastatic). Malignant melanoma and cloacogenic carcinoma may also arise in the anus. Anal carcinomas spread directly into surrounding tissues, including internal and external sphincters, perianal soft tissues, prostate and vagina.

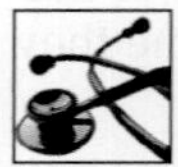

CLINICAL FEATURES: Human papilloma virus (HPV) and chronic inflammatory disease of the anus (e.g., venereal disease), fissures and trauma predispose to anal cancer. Factors associated with genital carcinoma (cancer of the penis, scrotum, cervix or vulva), poor hygiene and having many sexual partners are also noted in patients with anal cancer.

The usual symptoms of anal cancers include bleeding, pain and an anal or rectal mass. Often a tumor is not first recognized as malignant and may be discovered only in a hemorrhoidectomy specimen. Combined chemotherapy and radiation therapy is the customary treatment, although abdominal-perineal resection is sometimes used. Most patients survive for at least 5 years.

Miscellaneous Disorders

Endometriosis Involves the Colon and Rectum in 15% to 20% of Cases

Colorectal endometriosis is mostly asymptomatic and discovered incidentally during laparotomy for other reasons. When symptoms occur (abdominal pain, constipation, intestinal obstruction), they may be mistaken for those of colorectal cancer. **Endometriomas** are indurated tumors of up to 5 cm in the serosa and muscularis propria of the bowel, although they may penetrate the submucosa. As a result of repeated hemorrhage, the lesions are surrounded by reactive fibrosis.

Melanosis Coli Is Usually the Result of Chronic Use of Anthracene Laxatives

The cathartics include cascara sagrada, rhubarb, senna and aloe, and the finding can indicate surreptitious laxative abuse. In melanosis coli the mucosa is dark brown. Despite its name, the pigment is lipofuscin-like, is derived from the breakdown of cellular membranes and is unrelated to melanin. Macrophages in the lamina propria have brown pigment granules in their lysosomes.

Table 13-5

Gastrointestinal Pathogens Associated With AIDS

Bacteria	
	Mycobacterium avium-intracellulare
	Shigella
	Salmonella
	Clostridium difficile
Viruses	
	Cytomegalovirus
	Herpes simplex
Fungi	
	Candida
	Aspergillus
Protozoa	
	Cryptosporidium
	Toxoplasma
	Giardia
	Entameba histolytica
	Microsporidia
	Isospora belli
Helminths	
	Strongyloides
	Enterobius

Gastrointestinal Infections Are Common Complications of AIDS

The AIDS epidemic has resulted in many gastrointestinal infections once considered rare. Most patients with AIDS (50% to 90%) have chronic diarrhea. Virtually all forms of infectious agents—including bacteria, fungi, protozoa and viruses—afflict patients with AIDS (Table 13-5).

Kaposi sarcoma of the gut is almost exclusively seen in patients with AIDS. One third to one half of AIDS patients with cutaneous Kaposi sarcoma also show digestive tract involvement. In most, intestinal Kaposi sarcoma does not lead to symptoms, although gastrointestinal bleeding, obstruction and malabsorption have been reported.

A common presentation of lymphoma in AIDS patients is involvement of the gastrointestinal tract. Any portion may be affected. The histology and prognosis of these tumors in AIDS patients are similar to those elsewhere.

THE APPENDIX

Anatomy

The vermiform appendix is usually 8 to 10 cm long and is attached to the gut retrocecally. Its tip is generally not fixed and can move freely. It is invested with a mesentery, the **mesoappendix.** The wall of the appendix has the same layers as the rest of the intestine. The most prominent microscopic feature is the predominance of submucosal lymphoid tissue, which develops in early infancy, reaches its largest size during adolescence and then progressively atrophies.

Appendicitis

Acute appendicitis is inflammation of the wall of the appendix that may become transmural and lead to perforation and peritonitis. This condition is by far the most common disease of the appendix and is the most frequent abdominal emergency. Although incidence peaks in the second and third decades, acute appendicitis may occur at any age.

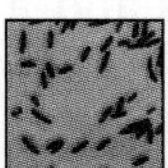

ETIOLOGIC FACTORS: ***Acute appendicitis relates to obstruction of its orifice, with secondary distention of the lumen and bacterial invasion of the wall.*** In one third of cases mechanical obstruction by fecaliths or solid fecal material in the cecum is found. Sometimes tumors, parasites (e.g., *Enterobius vermicularis*) or foreign bodies are responsible. Lymphoid hyperplasia due to bacterial or viral infection (e.g., by *Salmonella* or measles) may obstruct the lumen and lead to appendicitis. ***However, no obstruction is seen in up to half of patients with appendicitis,*** and the factor that precipitates the disease in these patients is unknown.

As secretions distend an obstructed appendix, intraluminal pressure increases until it exceeds the venous pressure. This causes venous stasis and ischemia and leads to mucosal ulceration and invasion by intestinal bacteria. Neutrophils accumulate to form microabscesses. Interestingly, appendectomy protects from development of ulcerative colitis but not Crohn disease.

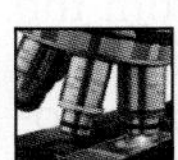

PATHOLOGY: The appendix is congested, tense and covered by a fibrinous exudate. Its lumen often contains purulent material. A fecalith may be evident (Fig. 13-68). Early cases show mucosal microabscesses and a purulent exudate in the lumen. As infection progresses, the entire wall is infiltrated with neutrophils, which eventually reach the serosa. Mural perforation releases luminal contents into the peritoneal cavity.

The complications of appendicitis are principally related to perforation, which occurs in one third of children and young adults. Appendices in almost all children under 2 years with the disease have perforated at the time of operation, as do three fourths of patients over 60 years.

- **Periappendiceal abscesses** are common, but abscesses may occur throughout the abdomen.
- **Fistulous tracts** may appear between the perforated appendix and adjacent structures, including the small and large bowel, bladder, vagina or abdominal wall.
- **Pylephlebitis** (thrombophlebitis of the intrahepatic portal vein radicals) and **secondary hepatic abscesses** may occur, because venous blood from the appendix drains into the superior mesenteric vein.
- **Diffuse peritonitis and septicemia** are dangerous sequelae.
- **Wound infection** is the most common complication of acute appendicitis after surgery; it occurs in one fourth of patients with perforation and in one third of cases of periappendiceal abscesses.

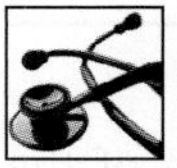

CLINICAL FEATURES: Cramping epigastric or periumbilical pain is typical, but the pain may be diffuse or initially restricted to the right lower quadrant. Nausea and vomiting soon follow, and the patient develops a low-grade fever and moderate leukocytosis. The pain shifts to the right lower quadrant, where point tenderness (McBurney point) is the rule. A diseased retrocecal appendix is shielded from the anterior abdominal wall by the cecum and ileum; atypical symptoms are thus easily misinterpreted because of their poor localization. In the elderly, appendicitis may produce only vague symptoms, and the diagnosis is often not made until perforation occurs. Several conditions that do not require surgery may be misdiagnosed as appendicitis, especially mesenteric adenitis in children, Meckel diverticulitis, rupture of an ovarian follicle during ovulation and acute salpingitis.

Treatment is surgical in the vast majority of cases. As perforation carries a much higher risk of death than does laparoscopic surgery, early surgical intervention is warranted, even if the diagnosis of acute appendicitis is not entirely secure.

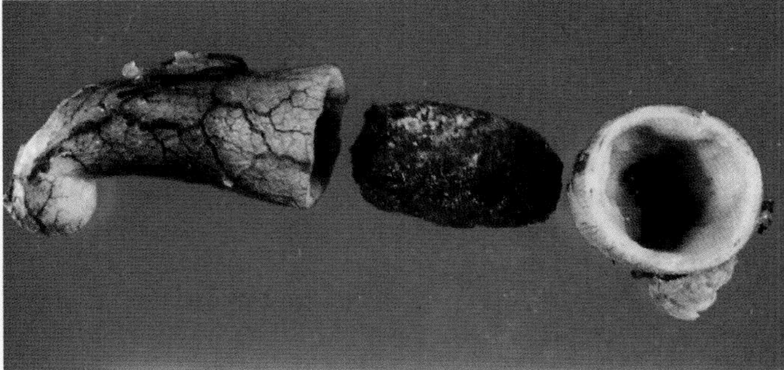

FIGURE 13-68. Acute appendicitis. The lumen of this acutely inflamed appendix is dilated and contains a large fecalith.

Neoplasms

HYPERPLASTIC POLYPS: Appendiceal hyperplastic polyps are rare. More common is diffuse hyperplasia, which are likely sessile serrated adenomas (see above).

MUCOCELE: ***A mucocele is a gross term denoting a dilated mucus-filled appendix*** (Fig. 13-69) and may be due to both neoplastic and nonneoplastic disease processes. In the nonneoplastic variety, chronic obstruction leads to retention of mucus in the appendiceal lumen.

Most mucoceles are associated with neoplastic epithelium. The dilated appendix is lined by villous, adenomatous mucosa or with epithelium of sessile serrated adenoma. The amount of mucin within the lumen varies greatly. Noninvasive, low-grade lesions are commonly termed **mucinous cystadenomas;** frankly malignant lining with or without invasion is **mucinous cystadenocarcinoma.** Invasive, appendiceal adenocarcinomas resemble their colonic counterparts histologically.

A mucocele may become secondarily infected and rupture, discharging mucin and debris into the peritoneum. This material may be mistaken at laparotomy for peritoneal tumor implants. However, when a mucocele results from mucus

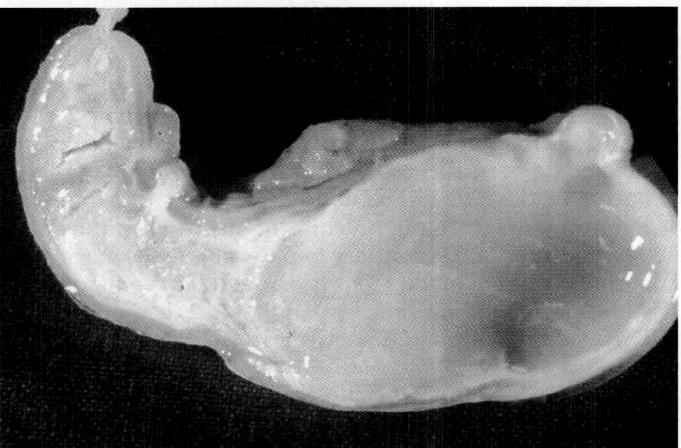

FIGURE 13-69. Mucocele of the appendix. The appendix is conspicuously dilated by mucinous material secreted by a cystadenoma.

secretion by a cystadenoma or cystadenocarcinoma of the appendix, perforation may lead to **pseudomyxoma peritonei,** or seeding of the peritoneum by mucus-secreting tumor cells (Fig. 13-70). As appendiceal adenocarcinoma resembles ovarian mucinous adenocarcinoma, it is difficult to estimate the proportions of each responsible for pseudomyxoma peritonei. However, most probably arise in the appendix, and many malignant ovarian mucinous tumors are seeded from the appendix.

Low-grade appendiceal adenomas (either traditional adenomas or sessile serrated adenomas) occasionally invade or rupture the appendix, seed the peritoneum and induce pseudomyxoma peritonei. However, if epithelial cells are seen in the mucus, even the lowest-grade tumors must be considered malignant (well-differentiated appendiceal adenocarcinomas), the nomenclature for which is unsettled. Some investigators have applied the term *low-grade appendiceal mucinous neoplasm* to distinguish these lesions from frank *invasive adenocarcinoma.*

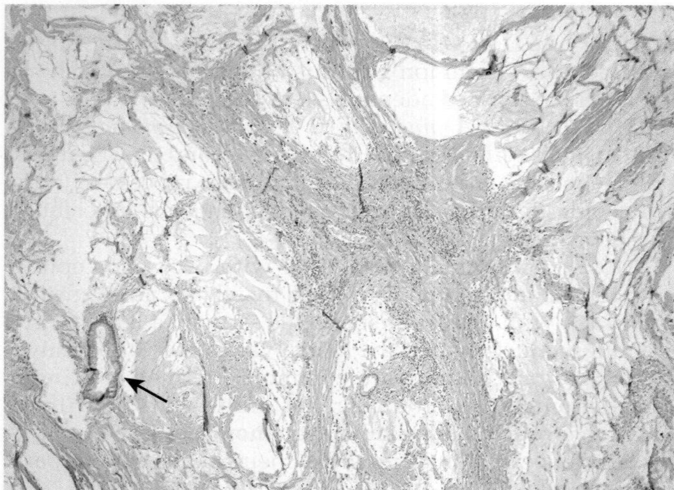

FIGURE 13-70. Pseudomyxoma peritonei. Pools of acellular mucin accumulate on the peritoneal surface. A malignant gland is identified (*arrow*), metastatic from an appendiceal adenocarcinoma.

Carcinoid tumors of the appendix are common and are unlikely to metastasize unless they are over 1.5 cm, which is very rare.

Figs. 13-71 through 13-74 summarize the causes of gastrointestinal bleeding and obstruction and the major benign and malignant tumors of the gastrointestinal tract.

THE PERITONEUM

The peritoneum is the mesothelial lining of the abdominal cavity and its viscera. The visceral peritoneum invests the gastrointestinal tract from stomach to rectum and encircles the liver. The parietal peritoneum lines the abdominal wall and retroperitoneal space. The omentum, which has a double layer of peritoneum, encloses blood vessels and a variable amount of fat.

Peritonitis

Bacterial Peritonitis Is Usually Caused by Intestinal Organisms

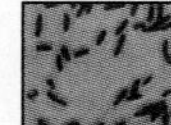

ETIOLOGIC FACTORS:

PERFORATION: ***The most common cause of bacterial peritonitis is perforation of an abdominal viscus*** (e.g., an inflamed appendix, peptic ulcer or colonic diverticulum). Peritonitis results in an acute abdomen, with severe abdominal pain and tenderness. Nausea, vomiting and a high fever are usual, and in severe cases, generalized peritonitis, paralytic ileus and septic shock ensue. Often the perforation becomes "walled off," in which case a peritoneal abscess results.

The bacteria released into the peritoneal cavity from the gastrointestinal tract vary according to the site of perforation and the duration of the peritonitis. Commonly, several aerobic and anaerobic species are cultured, including *E. coli, Bacteroides* sp., various *Streptococcus* spp. and *Clostridium.* Despite antibiotic treatment, surgical drainage and débridement and supportive measures, generalized peritonitis still carries substantial mortality and is especially dangerous in the elderly.

PERITONEAL DIALYSIS: Chronic peritoneal dialysis is today a frequent cause of bacterial peritonitis, owing to contamination of instruments or dialysate. The clinical course is usually milder than that noted with a perforated viscus and *Staphylococcus* and *Streptococcus* spp. are most often responsible. One fourth of cases of peritonitis that occur with chronic dialysis are aseptic, presumably caused by some chemical in the dialysate to which the peritoneum is sensitive.

SPONTANEOUS BACTERIAL PERITONITIS: This term refers to a peritoneal infection lacking a clear precipitating circumstance, such as a perforated viscus. ***The most common setting for spontaneous bacterial peritonitis in adults is cirrhosis complicated by portal hypertension and ascites*** (see Chapter 14). The pathogenesis appears to involve movement of enteric organisms, mainly gram-negative bacilli, from the gut to mesenteric lymph nodes. Seeding of ascitic fluid then ensues, with depressed phagocytic activity and low antibacterial activity in ascitic fluid.

In children, spontaneous bacterial peritonitis can complicate the **nephrotic syndrome.** Most cases of spontaneous peritonitis in children are due to gram-negative organisms,

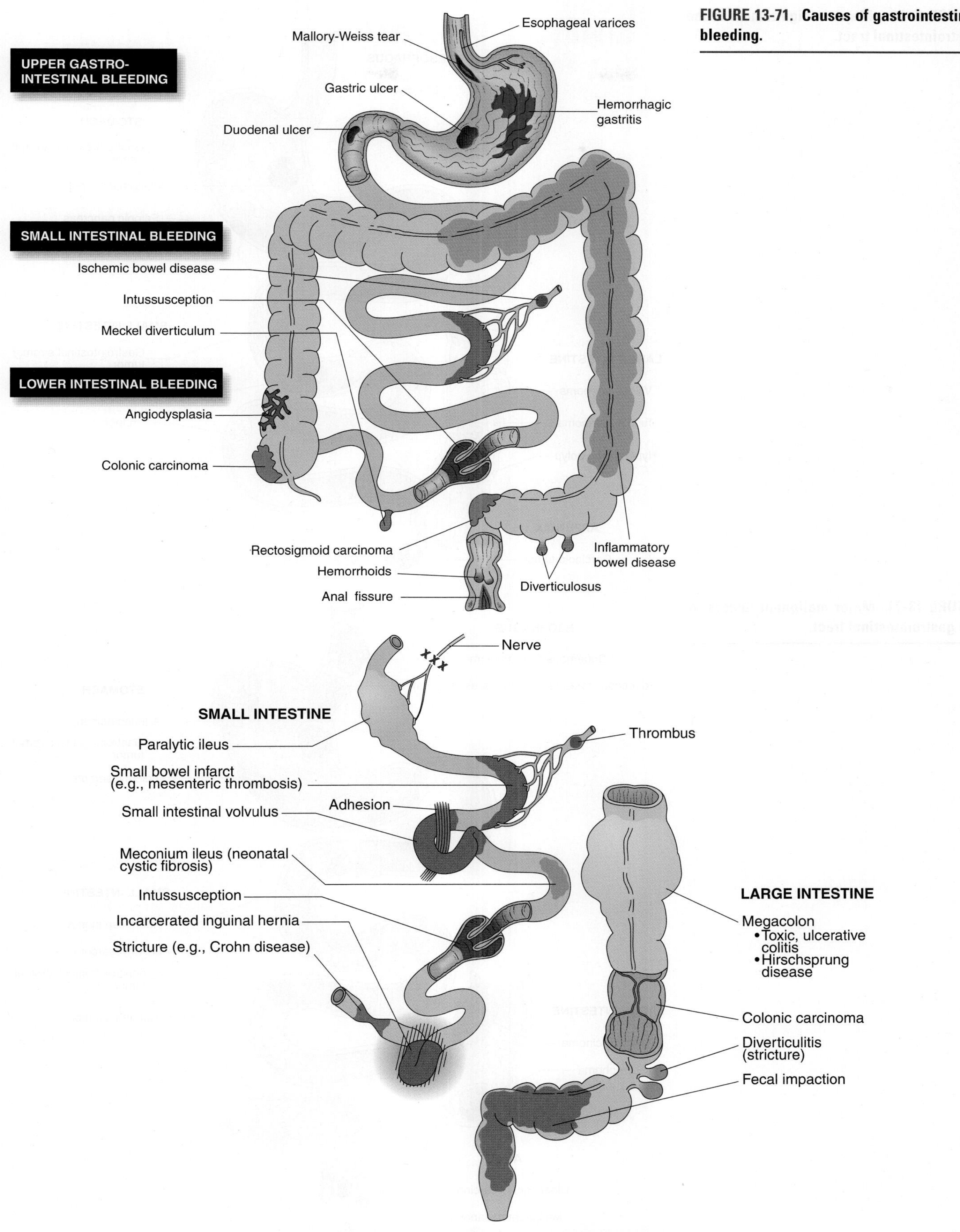

FIGURE 13-71. Causes of gastrointestinal bleeding.

FIGURE 13-72. Causes of gastrointestinal obstruction.

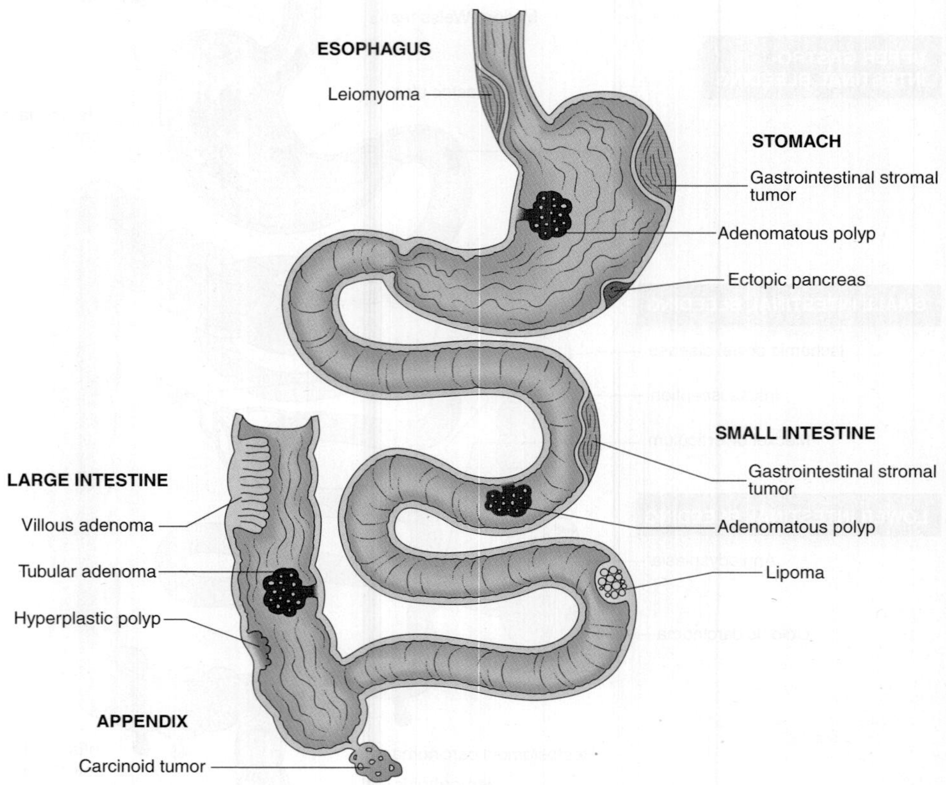

FIGURE 13-73. Major benign tumors of the gastrointestinal tract.

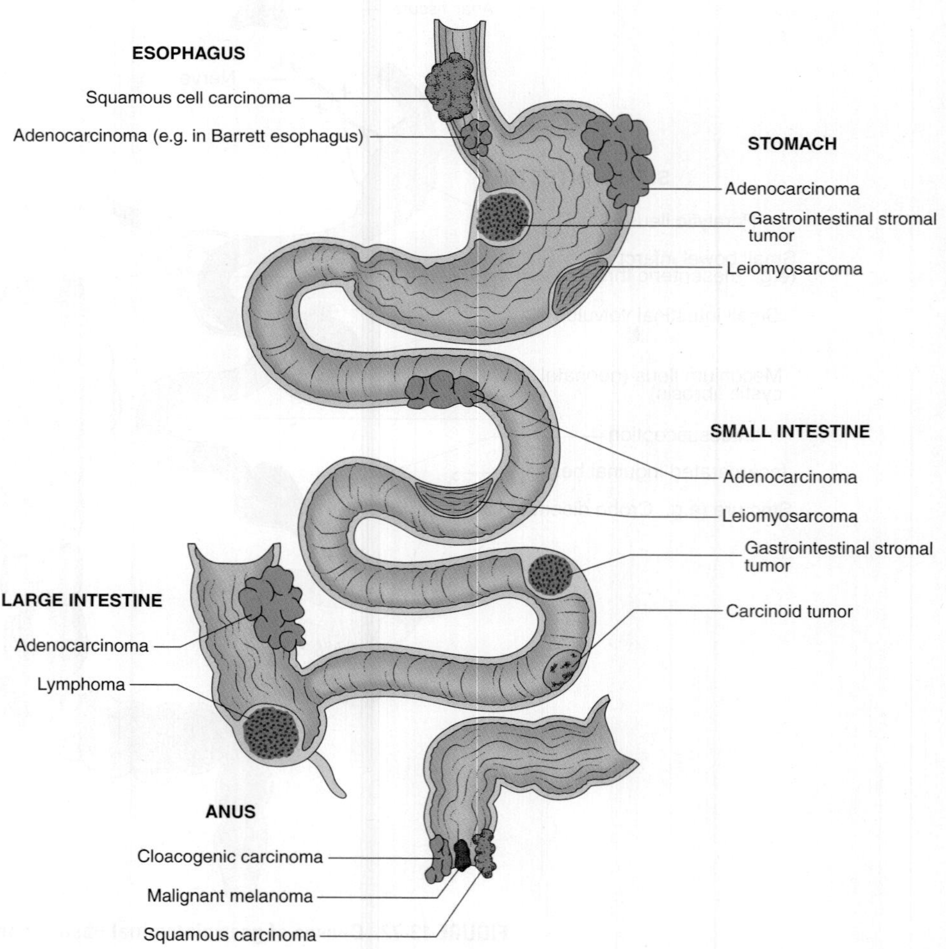

FIGURE 13-74. Major malignant tumors of the gastrointestinal tract.

usually from urinary tract infections. The disease causes symptoms of an acute abdomen and ordinarily leads to surgical intervention, unless the child is known to have nephrotic syndrome. Even with antibiotic treatment, mortality is 5% to 10%.

TUBERCULOUS PERITONITIS: This infection is rarely seen in industrialized countries anymore, but it may complicate tuberculosis in developing countries. Many patients with tuberculous peritonitis do not have apparent pulmonary or miliary disease, an observation that suggests activation of latent tuberculous foci in the peritoneum derived from previous hematogenous dissemination.

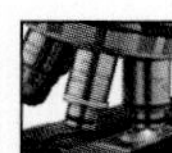

PATHOLOGY: Grossly, bacterial peritonitis resembles purulent infection elsewhere. A fibrinopurulent exudate covers the surface of the intestines. When it organizes, fibrinous and fibrous adhesions form between loops of bowel, which become joined to each other. Such adhesions may eventually be lysed, or they may lead to **volvulus** and **intestinal obstruction.** Bacterial salpingitis, usually gonococcal, may lead to pelvic peritonitis and adhesions, which define **pelvic inflammatory disease.**

Chemical Peritonitis Usually Results From Endogenous Sources

- **Bile peritonitis** occurs when bile enters the peritoneum, usually from a perforated gallbladder but sometimes from needle biopsy of the liver. This abrupt insult may lead to shock.
- **Hydrochloric acid or hemorrhage** from a perforated peptic ulcer of the stomach or duodenum may elicit an inflammatory reaction in the peritoneum.
- In **acute pancreatitis** activated lipolytic and proteolytic enzymes are released and lead to severe peritonitis with fat necrosis. Shock is common and may be lethal unless it is adequately treated.
- **Foreign materials** introduced by surgery (e.g., talc) or by trauma are unusual causes of chemical peritonitis.
- **Leakage of urine** can produce ascites.

Familial Paroxysmal Polyserositis (Familial Mediterranean Fever) Leads to Peritonitis and Amyloidosis

Familial Mediterranean fever (FMF) is an inherited autosomal recessive disorder with recurrent episodes of aseptic peritonitis with fever and abdominal pain. It is caused by mutations in a gene on the short arm of chromosome 16. FMF presents first as peritonitis in half of cases, as arthritis in 25% and as pleuritis in 5%. However, almost all affected people eventually have peritonitis, and more than half develop arthritis and pleuritis at some time. The disease predominates in Sephardic Jews and other Mediterranean populations, such as Armenians, Turks and Arabs. The pathogenesis of FMF remains obscure, but in the absence of complications, the prognosis is good. Unfortunately, **amyloidosis** is a frequent complication (see Chapter 23).

Retroperitoneal Fibrosis

Idiopathic retroperitoneal fibrosis, an uncommon fibrosing condition of the abdomen, becomes symptomatic when it causes obstruction of the ureters. No cause is known in most cases, but it has been linked to treatment of migraine headaches with methysergide. A similar idiopathic fibrosis also has been described in the mediastinum (fibrosing mediastinitis). The disease may affect the mesentery, causing secondary intestinal obstruction.

Neoplasms of the Peritoneum

Mesenteric and Omental Cysts Are Usually of Lymphatic Origin

They may also derive from other embryonic tissues. Usually a slowly enlarging, painless mass is discovered in a child older than 10 years. The cyst may come to medical attention because of rupture, bleeding, torsion or intestinal obstruction. Surgical excision is curative.

Mesotheliomas Are the Most Common Primary Peritoneal Tumor

One fourth of all mesotheliomas arise in the peritoneum. ***Like pleural mesotheliomas, most of these malignant tumors are associated with exposure to asbestos.*** The pathologic characteristics of peritoneal mesotheliomas are identical to those of their pleural counterparts (see Chapter 12).

Primary Peritoneal Carcinoma Resembles Ovarian Carcinoma

Primary peritoneal carcinoma presents as tumor masses involving the omentum and peritoneum. It is morphologically identical to ovarian serous carcinoma of the ovary, except that the ovaries are normal.

Metastatic Carcinoma Is the Most Common Malignancy of the Peritoneum

Ovarian, gastric and pancreatic carcinomas are particularly likely to seed the peritoneum, but any intra-abdominal carcinoma can spread to the peritoneum.

14 The Liver and Biliary System

Steven K. Herrine • Victor J. Navarro • Raphael Rubin

THE LIVER

Anatomy

The liver arises from the embryonic foregut as an entodermal bud that differentiates into the hepatic diverticulum. Strands of entodermal cells mingle with proliferating mesenchymal cells to form all the structures of the adult liver, gallbladder and extrahepatic biliary ducts.

The liver weighs about 1500 g in the average adult man and is in the right upper quadrant of the abdomen. Just below the diaphragm, it has two lobes, a larger **right lobe** and a smaller **left lobe,** which meet at the level of the gallbladder bed. Inferiorly, the right lobe has lesser segments, the **caudate** and **quadrate lobes.** The **gallbladder** is inferior, in a fossa of the right hepatic lobe, and normally extends slightly beyond the inferior margin of the liver.

The liver has a dual blood supply: (1) **the hepatic artery,** a branch of the celiac axis, and (2) **the portal vein,** formed by the convergence of the splenic and superior mesenteric veins. **The hepatic veins** empty into the inferior vena cava, which is partly surrounded by the posterior surface of the liver. Hepatic lymphatics drain mainly into porta hepatis and celiac lymph nodes.

The common hepatic duct is formed by the union of the right and left hepatic ducts and joins the cystic duct from the gallbladder to form the common bile duct. The common bile duct meets with the pancreatic duct just before emptying into the duodenum. It terminates in the ampulla of Vater, where its lumen is guarded by the sphincter of Oddi.

The Liver Lobule Is the Basic Unit of the Liver

Liver lobules are polyhedral (Figs. 14-1 and 14-2), classically depicted as hexagons. **Portal triads** (or portal tracts) are peripheral, at the angles of the polygon, and contain intrahepatic branches of the (1) **bile ducts,** (2) **hepatic artery** and (3) **portal vein.** The collagenous portal tracts are surrounded by an adjacent circumferential layer of hepatocytes, **the limiting plate.** The **central vein** (also known as the **terminal hepatic venule**) is at the center of the lobule. Radiating from it are **one-cell-thick plates of hepatocytes,** which extend to the edge of the lobule, where they are continuous with plates of other lobules. Between plates of hepatocytes are **hepatic sinusoids,** which are lined by endothelial cells, Kupffer cells and stellate cells.

The large blood vessels that enter the liver at the porta hepatis eventually divide into the small interlobular branches of the hepatic artery and portal vein in the portal triads. From the portal triads, the interlobular vessels distribute blood to hepatic sinusoids, where it flows centripetally toward the central vein. Central veins coalesce to form sublobular veins, which eventually merge into the hepatic veins.

Bile flows in a direction opposite to that of the blood. Bile is secreted by hepatocytes into **bile canaliculi,** formed by apposed lateral surfaces of contiguous hepatocytes. Contraction of the bile canaliculus is mediated by the pericanalicular cytoskeleton of the hepatocytes and propels bile toward the portal tract. From the canaliculi, the bile flows into **bile ductules (canals of Hering** or **cholangioles)** at the border of the portal tract and then enters a branch of the **intrahepatic bile ducts.** Within each liver lobe, smaller bile ducts progressively merge, eventually forming the right and left hepatic ducts.

The Liver Acinus Is the Functional Interpretation of the Lobule

The structural lobule described above is arranged around the central vein and reflects the liver's histologic appearance. ***However, functionally, a lobule can be conceptualized with the portal tract at the center*** (Fig. 14-2). Such a construct reflects

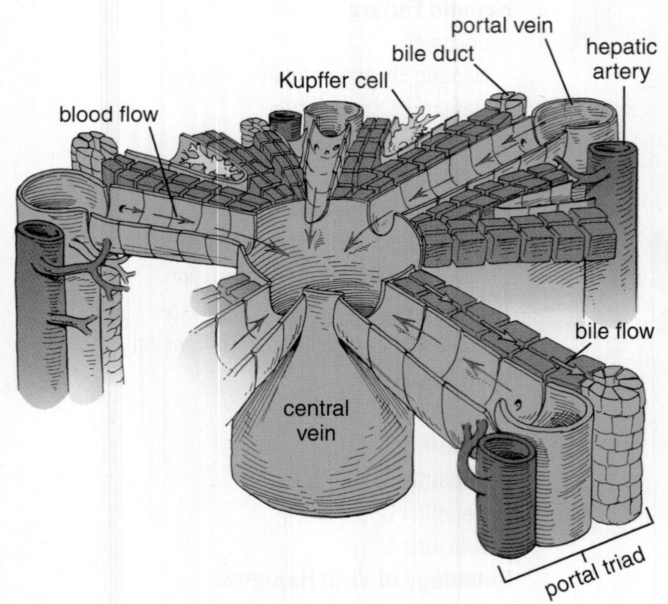

FIGURE 14-1. Microanatomy of the liver. The classic lobule is composed of portal triads, hepatic sinuses, a terminal hepatic venule (central vein) and associated plates of hepatocytes. *Red arrows* indicate the direction of sinusoidal blood flow. *Green arrows* show the direction of bile flow.

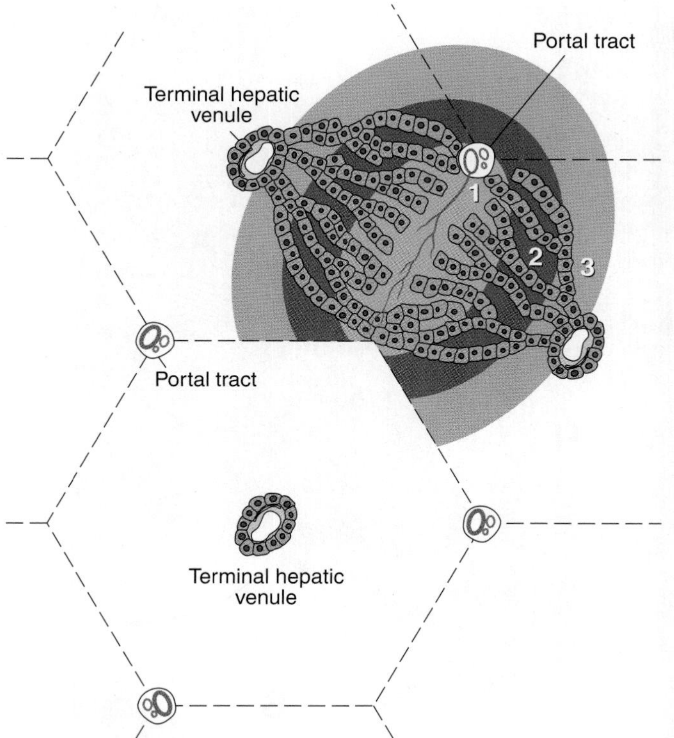

FIGURE 14-2. Morphologic and functional concepts of the liver lobule. In the classic *morphologic* liver lobule, the periphery of the hexagonal lobule is anchored in the portal tracts, and the terminal hepatic venule is in the center. The *functional* liver lobule is an acinus derived from the gradients of oxygen and nutrients in the sinusoidal blood. In this scheme, the portal tract, with the richest content of oxygen and nutrients, is in the center (zone 1). The region most distant from the portal tract (zone 3) is poor in oxygen and nutrients and surrounds the terminal hepatic venule.

the functional gradients within lobules. That is, oxygen, nutrients and hormones delivered by the blood are most concentrated by the portal tracts, then decline progressively as hepatocytes extract these materials from the blood as it goes through the sinusoids toward the central vein. Such a construct allows for concentric functional zones. **Zone 1** is the most highly oxygenated zone, around portal tracts, while **zone 3,** which surrounds central veins, is oxygen poor. Ischemic injury usually affects zone 3 before other zones. The intermediate or midlobular area is **zone 2.** Differences in hepatocytes are not restricted to blood flow. The acinus is also heterogeneous with respect to metabolism, independent of oxygenation. In particular, toxic injury is often prominent in zone 3, owing to enrichment in hepatocyte enzymes involved in drug detoxification and biotransformation. For convenience, pathologic changes in the liver are usually designated in relation to the classic histologic lobule. For example, centrilobular necrosis refers to a lesion around the central veins, whereas periportal fibrosis is seen at the periphery of the classic lobule.

The Hepatocyte Performs the Major Functions of the Liver

Hepatocytes make up 60% of liver cells, and about 90% of the organ's volume. They are roughly 30 μm across and have three specialized surfaces: **sinusoidal, lateral and canalicular.** Each cell has two sinusoidal surfaces, with numerous slender microvilli. The sinusoidal surface is separated from the endothelial cells that line the sinusoids by the **space of Disse** (Fig. 14-3). Canalicular surfaces of adjacent hepatocytes form the **bile canaliculus,** a collecting structure that is actually an intercellular space without a separate and distinct wall. Along this surface, microvilli extend into the lumen. A tight junctional complex between adjacent hepatocytes prevents bile leakage from the canaliculus. Lateral, or intercellular, surfaces of adjacent hepatocytes are in close contact and contain gap junctions.

Hepatocyte nuclei are occasionally multiple and are centrally placed and spherical, with one or more nucleoli. Most are diploid, but tetraploid and octaploid nuclei are common. The cytoplasm is rich in organelles, with prominent rough and smooth endoplasmic reticulum, Golgi complexes, mitochondria, lysosomes and peroxisomes. In addition, in the fed state, abundant glycogen and occasional fat droplets are evident.

Hepatic Sinusoids Are the Channels Through Which Blood Traverses the Liver

Sinusoids contain three cell types: endothelial, Kupffer and stellate cells.

ENDOTHELIAL CELLS: Endothelial cells, which are penetrated by numerous holes called **fenestrae** (Fig. 14-3), line sinusoids. In contrast to other tissues, adjacent endothelial cells do not form junctions, and there are many gaps between them. The result is a sieve-like structure that affords free communication between the sinusoidal lumen and the space of Disse. The absence of a basement membrane between the endothelial cells and liver cells further facilitates access of sinusoidal plasma to hepatocytes.

KUPFFER CELLS: Kupffer cells are bone marrow–derived phagocytes, located either in the gaps between adjacent endothelial cells or on their surfaces (Fig. 14-1). Because of their origin, the Kupffer cells that repopulate transplanted livers are from the recipient rather than the donor. Like other macrophages, they protect against infection and circulating toxins (e.g., endotoxin). Activated Kupffer cells also release cytokines, such as tumor necrosis factor (TNF), interleukins (ILs), interferons and transforming growth factors (TGFs)-α and -β.

STELLATE CELLS: Stellate cells (also known as Ito cells) are occasionally seen beneath endothelial cells in the space of Disse and have specialized storage capacities. They contain fat, vitamin A and other lipid-soluble vitamins. These cells also secrete extracellular matrix components, including various collagens, laminin and proteoglycans. In some diseases, these are made in great excess, leading to the hepatic fibrosis characteristic of cirrhosis.

The most abundant extracellular matrix component in the space of Disse is fibronectin. Occasional bundles of type I collagen fibers provide a scaffold for liver lobules.

Functions of the Liver

The Hepatocyte Serves Myriad Functions

Hepatocyte functions can be classified as metabolic, synthetic, storage, catabolic and excretory.

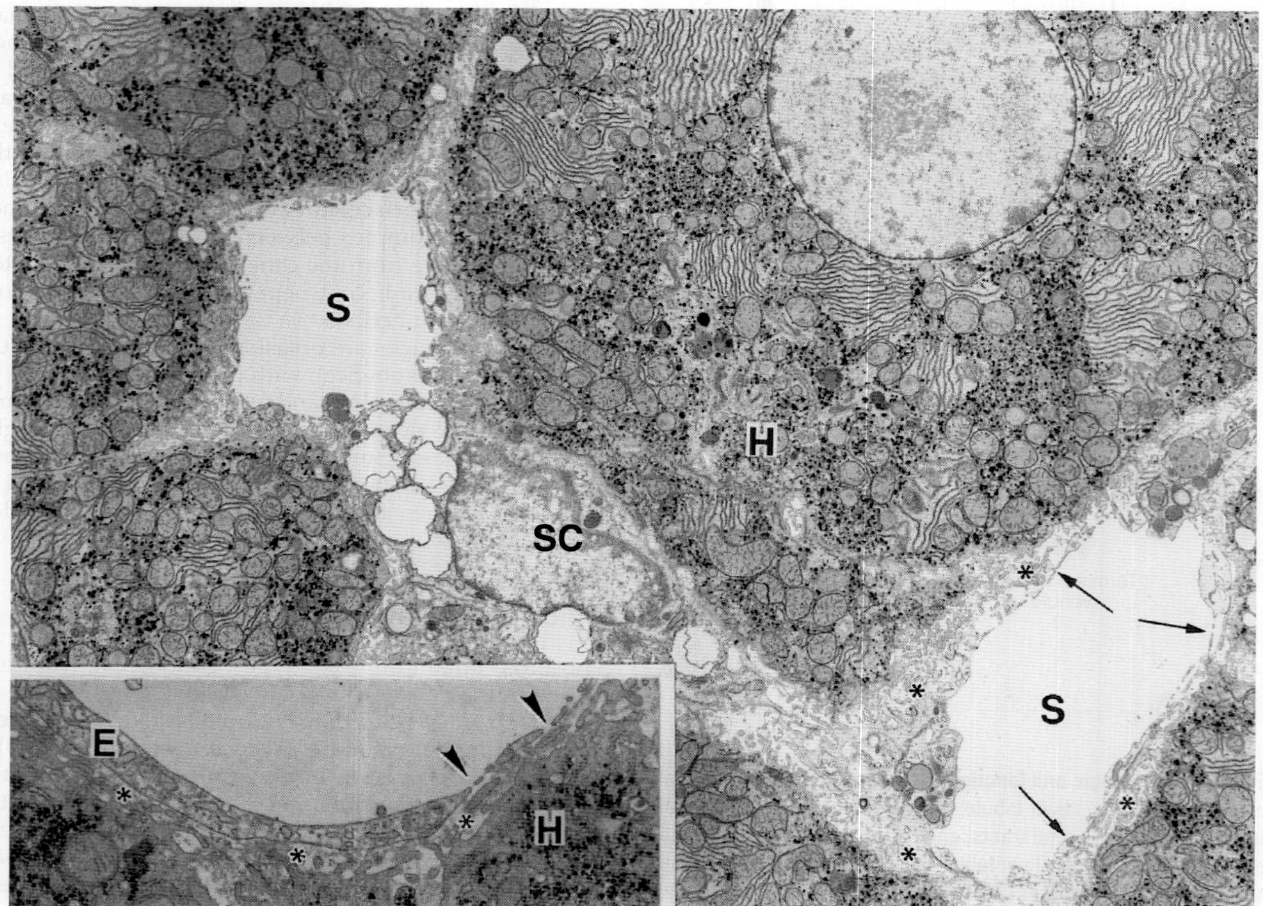

FIGURE 14-3. Hepatic sinusoids and space of Disse. An electron micrograph illustrates the relationship between hepatocytes, sinusoids, the space of Disse and hepatic stellate cells (Ito cells, fat-storing cells). The *arrow* indicates the endothelial cell, and the *asterisk* indicates the space of Disse. H = hepatocyte; S = sinusoid; SC = stellate cell. *Inset.* The relationship between hepatocytes (*H*) and endothelial cells (*E*). The *arrowheads* indicate fenestrae in the endothelial cells; the *asterisks* are in the space of Disse.

METABOLIC FUNCTIONS: The liver is the central organ of **glucose homeostasis** and responds rapidly to fluctuations in blood glucose levels. In the fed state, excess blood glucose is shunted to the liver to be stored as glycogen; during fasting, blood glucose levels are stabilized by hepatic **glycogenolysis** and **gluconeogenesis.** For gluconeogenesis, the liver uses amino acids, lactate and glycerol. The nitrogenous portion of amino acids is converted to urea. Free fatty acids are taken up by the liver, where they are oxidized to produce energy. Alternatively, they are converted to triglycerides and secreted as **lipoproteins** to be used elsewhere.

SYNTHETIC FUNCTIONS: Most serum proteins are synthesized in the liver. **Albumin** is the main source of plasma oncotic pressure; decreased albumin in chronic liver disease leads to edema and ascites. Blood coagulation requires ongoing production of **clotting factors,** most of which, including prothrombin and fibrinogen, are produced by hepatocytes. Liver failure may thus be characterized by severe and often life-threatening bleeding. Endothelial cells of the liver manufacture **factor VIII,** and hemophilia is ameliorated by liver transplantation. **Complement** and other "acute phase reactants" are also secreted by the liver, as are numerous specific **binding proteins** (e.g., those for iron, copper and vitamin A).

STORAGE FUNCTIONS: The liver is an important storage site for glycogen, triglycerides, iron, copper and lipid-soluble vitamins. Severe liver disease can result from excessive storage—for instance, abnormal glycogen in type IV glycogenosis and excess iron in hemochromatosis.

CATABOLIC FUNCTIONS: Endogenous substances, including hormones and serum proteins, are catabolized by the liver to balance their production and elimination. As a result, in chronic liver disease, impaired catabolism of estrogens contributes to feminization in men. The liver is also the principal site for **detoxification of foreign compounds** (xenobiotics), such as drugs, industrial chemicals, environmental contaminants and perhaps products of bacterial metabolism in the intestine. Ammonia, a product of amino acid metabolism, is mainly removed by the liver. Serum ammonia increases in liver failure and is used as a marker for this condition.

EXCRETORY FUNCTIONS: The principal excretory product of the liver is **bile,** an aqueous mixture of conjugated bilirubin, bile acids, phospholipids, cholesterol and electrolytes. Bile is a repository for the products of heme catabolism and is vital for fat absorption in the small intestine. Normal bile formation is critical for eliminating environmental toxins, carcinogens and drugs and their metabolites.

Regeneration Is a Unique Characteristic of the Liver

Liver size is normally maintained within narrow limits, relative to body size. When liver tissue is damaged (e.g., after mechanical, toxic or viral challenge that causes substantial loss of functional tissue), it recovers by regrowth of the undamaged tissue in a process called **liver regeneration.** Hepatocytes, which normally are in a fully differentiated, quiescent state (G_0), reenter the cell cycle for one or more synchronized rounds of replication to recover the organ's original size. Uniquely, this process takes place while maintaining the differentiated functions of the liver. Little is known about the factors that guide this part of the process or how the liver recognizes the recovery of its normal size and architecture. ***Conditions that interfere with regeneration may cause permanent liver dysfunction and lead to fibrosis and cirrhosis.***

Several phases are distinguished in liver regeneration:

- **Priming:** Liver tissue has to recognize that damage has occurred and that the remaining functional parenchymal cells must make the transition from the quiescent G_0 state to the G_1 phase of the cell cycle. This phase is often referred to as "priming." It is associated with expression of immediate-early genes, many of which are transcription factors required for production of cell cycle proteins. The priming phase depends on release of different cytokines, notably TNF-α and IL-6.
- **Progression to mitosis:** The second phase involves progression through the G_1 phase of the cell cycle and transition into the S phase, where DNA synthesis occurs. This sequence is followed by the G_2 and M phases, where cell division takes place. A number of growth factors promote this part of the process, including hepatocyte growth factor, also known as scatter factor (HGF/SF), epidermal growth factor (EGF), TGF-α and others. Several growth factors (e.g., HGF, IL-6) promote hepatoprotection and survival in various models of liver injury. After one or two rounds of cell division (depending on need) are completed, the cells become quiescent again and resume normal function.
- **Nonparenchymal cells:** In the third phase of liver regeneration, nonparenchymal cells (sinusoidal endothelial cells, Kupffer cells, stellate cells and biliary epithelial cells) replicate and tissue remodels to recover the original structure of liver cell plates. Hepatic progenitor cells ("oval cells") that exist within the terminal branches of the bile ductules and canals of Hering contribute to ductular proliferation after hepatic necrosis. However, controversy remains over the importance of these cells to hepatic regeneration, as well as the potential contribution of bone marrow–derived stem cells (see Chapter 3).

Bilirubin Metabolism and Mechanisms of Jaundice

Bilirubin Is the End Product of Heme Catabolism

About 80% of bilirubin is derived from senescent erythrocytes, which are removed from the circulation by mononuclear phagocytes of the spleen, bone marrow and liver. The rest comes from degradation of heme produced from other sources, including cytochrome P450 isoenzymes, myoglobin and premature breakdown of hemoglobin in erythroid progenitors in the bone marrow. Beyond this, no specific physiologic role for bilirubin is known.

Bilirubin is poorly soluble in water. After its release into the circulation, it is bound to albumin and transported to the liver. The albumin in the blood and extracellular space is a large binding reservoir for bilirubin and ensures a low extracellular concentration of free (unbound) bilirubin. Free bilirubin, unlike that bound to albumin or conjugated to glucuronic acid, is toxic to the brain in newborns and in high concentrations causes irreversible brain injury, **kernicterus.**

Transfer of bilirubin from the blood to the bile involves four steps:

1. **Uptake:** On reaching the sinusoidal plasma membrane of the hepatocyte, the albumin–bilirubin complex is dissociated, and bilirubin is transported across the plasma membrane. Uptake by hepatocytes appears to be partly passive, but also dependent on a variety of organic transporter proteins.
2. **Binding:** Within hepatocytes, bilirubin is bound to a group of cytosolic proteins known collectively as **glutathione S-transferases** (also termed ligandin).
3. **Conjugation:** To be excreted, bilirubin must be converted to a water-soluble form, which is done by conjugating it to glucuronic acid in the endoplasmic reticulum (ER). The ER contains the uridine diphosphate-glucuronyl transferase (UGT) system that attaches glucuronic acid to bilirubin. Water-soluble bilirubin diglucuronide and a little (<10%) monoglucuronide result.
4. **Excretion:** Conjugated bilirubin diffuses through the cytosol to the bile canaliculus and is excreted into the bile against a concentration gradient by an energy-dependent carrier-mediated process, which is the rate-limiting step for overall transhepatic transport of bilirubin.

Conjugated bilirubin enters the small intestine as part of mixed micelles, but is not absorbed there. It remains intact until it reaches the distal small bowel and colon, where it is hydrolyzed by bacterial flora to free bilirubin (now unconjugated), which is reduced to a mixture of pyrroles, known collectively as **urobilinogen.** Most urobilinogen is excreted in feces, but a small amount is absorbed in the terminal ileum and colon, returned to the liver and reexcreted into the bile. Bile acids are also reabsorbed in the terminal ileum and salvaged by the liver. The recycling of bile constituents is referred to as the **enterohepatic circulation of bile.** Some urobilinogen escapes reabsorption by the liver, reaches the systemic circulation and is excreted in the urine.

- **Hyperbilirubinemia** denotes increased blood levels of bilirubin (>1.0 mg/dL).
- **Jaundice** or **icterus** means yellow skin and sclerae (Fig. 14-4), whose color becomes apparent when the circulating bilirubin concentration exceeds 2.5 to 3.0 mg/dL.
- **Cholestasis** is the presence of plugs of inspissated bile in dilated bile canaliculi and visible bile pigment in hepatocytes.
- **Cholestatic jaundice** is characterized by histologic cholestasis and hyperbilirubinemia.

As shown in Fig. 14-5, many conditions are associated with hyperbilirubinemia.

Overproduction of bilirubin, interference with hepatic uptake or intracellular metabolism of bilirubin and impairment of bile excretion are all causes of jaundice (Fig. 14-5).

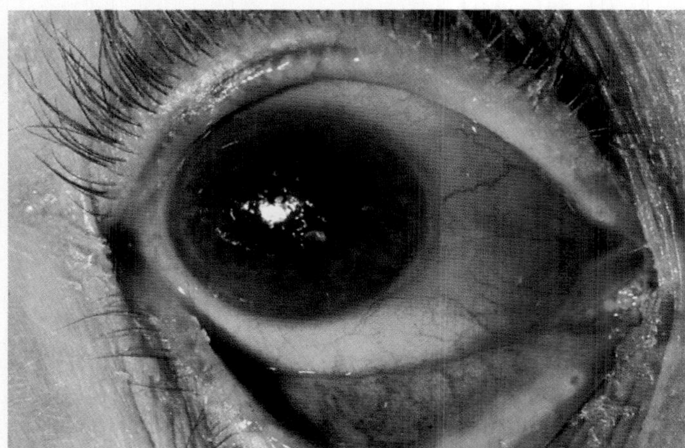

FIGURE 14-4. Jaundice. A patient in hepatic failure displays yellow sclera.

Overproduction of Bilirubin Can Lead to Unconjugated Hyperbilirubinemia

Increased production of bilirubin results from increased destruction of erythrocytes (e.g., hemolytic anemia) or ineffective erythropoiesis. In unusual circumstances, breakdown of erythrocytes in a large hematoma (e.g., after trauma) may also generate excess bilirubin.

In adults, even severe hemolytic anemia does not cause a sustained increase in serum bilirubin beyond 4.0 mg/dL if hepatic bilirubin clearance is normal. However, prolonged hemolysis, as in sickle cell anemia, in the context of intrinsic liver disease, such as viral hepatitis, leads to extremely high blood bilirubin levels (up to 100 mg/dL) and pronounced jaundice.

Hyperbilirubinemia due to uncomplicated hemolytic disease mainly reflects unconjugated bilirubin, whereas parenchymal liver disease causes both conjugated and unconjugated bilirubin. Although the unconjugated hyperbilirubinemia of hemolytic disease is of little clinical significance in adults, it may be catastrophic in newborns. In hemolytic disease of the newborn concentrations of unconjugated bilirubin may be high enough to cause **kernicterus** (see Chapter 6). Kernicterus generally occurs if bilirubin concentrations exceed 20 mg/dL, but subtle psychomotor retardation may follow considerably lower bilirubin concentrations.

In disorders of ineffective erythropoiesis (e.g., megaloblastic or sideroblastic anemias), the fraction of bilirubin derived from the bone marrow may be increased to the point that hyperbilirubinemia develops. In a rare hereditary disease of unknown etiology, "primary shunt hyperbilirubinemia" or "idiopathic dyserythropoietic jaundice," massive overproduction of bone marrow–derived bilirubin is associated with chronic unconjugated hyperbilirubinemia.

Decreased Hepatic Uptake of Bilirubin Is a Common Cause of Jaundice

Hyperbilirubinemia can result from impaired hepatic uptake of unconjugated bilirubin. This occurs in generalized liver cell injury (e.g., viral hepatitis). Certain drugs (e.g., rifampin and probenecid) interfere with the net uptake of bilirubin by liver cells and may produce a mild unconjugated hyperbilirubinemia.

Decreased Bilirubin Conjugation Occurs in Several Hereditary Syndromes

Crigler-Najjar Syndrome

Crigler-Najjar syndrome type I is a rare, recessively inherited condition characterized by chronic, severe, unconjugated hyperbilirubinemia, due to the complete absence of hepatic UGT activity. Several mutations in this gene lead to synthesis of a completely inactive enzyme. Phenobarbital, which induces microsomal enzymes (including UGT), is without effect.

Liver morphology is normal. However, Crigler-Najjar syndrome type I was invariably lethal until phototherapy and liver transplantation greatly improved quality of life and survival.

Crigler-Najjar syndrome type II is similar but is less severe and entails only a partial decrease in UGT activity. Almost all patients with type II syndrome develop normally, but some show neurologic changes resembling kernicterus.

Gilbert Syndrome

Gilbert syndrome is an inherited, mild, chronic unconjugated hyperbilirubinemia (<6 mg/dL) that is caused by **impaired clearance of bilirubin** in the absence of detectable functional or structural liver disease. Both autosomal dominant and recessive inheritance have been suggested, although the latter is favored today. Mutations in the promotor region of the *UGT* gene lead to reduced transcription of the gene and, consequently, inadequate synthesis of the enzyme. In a few patients the *UGT* promotor is normal, but missense mutations in the coding region have been described. Factors that elevate serum bilirubin concentrations in normal persons, such as fasting or an intercurrent illness, produce an exaggerated increase in persons with Gilbert syndrome. Mild hemolysis, which also tends to increase bilirubin levels, is believed to occur in more than half of persons with Gilbert syndrome, but the mechanism is unclear.

Gilbert syndrome is exceptionally common, occurring in 5% to 10% of the population. It is seen more often in men than in women and is usually recognized after puberty. The sex differences and the age at onset suggest that hormones influence the modulation of bilirubin metabolism in the liver. Gilbert syndrome is generally without clinical import, except for the possibility that drug metabolism may be altered.

Decreased Transport of Conjugated Bilirubin Often Involves Mutations in the Multidrug Resistance Protein Family

Multidrug resistance proteins (MRPs) mediate transmembrane transport of organic ions, including conjugated bilirubin, bile acids and phospholipids. Mutations in these proteins, as well as an array of other canalicular transporters, impair hepatocellular secretion of bilirubin glucuronides and other organic anions into canaliculi. These diseases are heterogeneous, varying from innocuous to lethal.

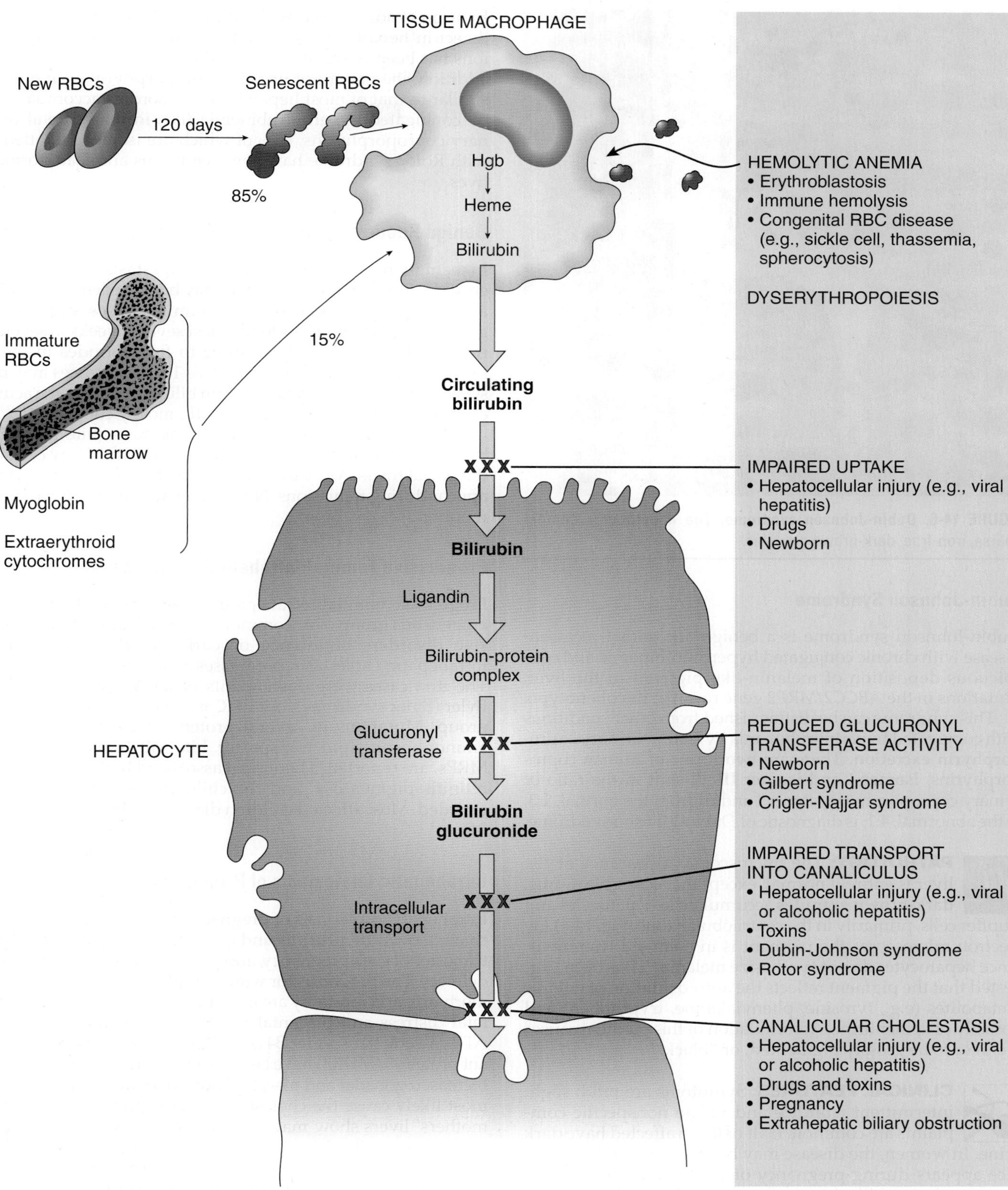

FIGURE 14-5. Mechanisms of hyperbilirubinemia at the level of the hepatocyte. Bilirubin is derived principally from the senescence of circulating red blood cells (RBCs), with a smaller contribution from the degradation of erythropoietic elements in the bone marrow, myoglobin and extraerythroid cytochromes. Hyperbilirubinemia and jaundice result from overproduction of bilirubin (hemolytic anemia), dyserythropoiesis, impaired bilirubin uptake or defects in its hepatic metabolism. The locations of specific blocks in the metabolic pathway of bilirubin in the hepatocyte are illustrated. Hgb = hemoglobin.

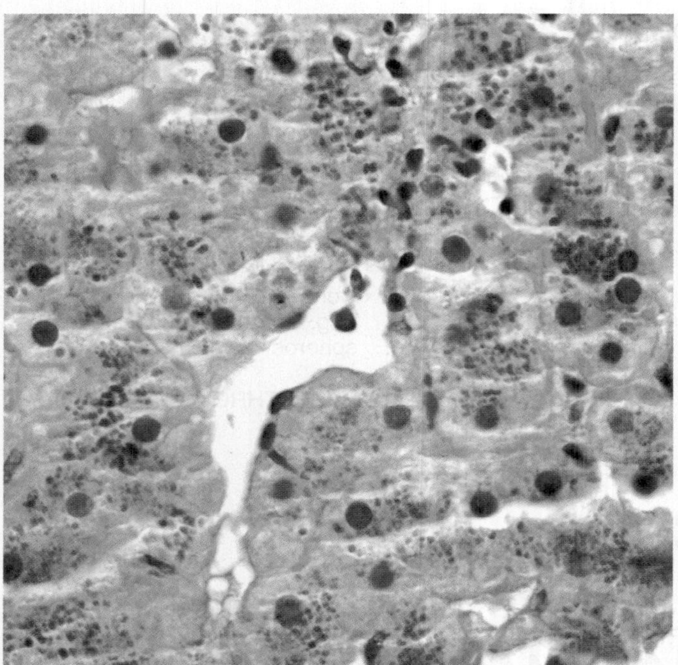

FIGURE 14-6. Dubin-Johnson syndrome. The hepatocytes contain coarse, iron-free, dark-brown granules.

Dubin-Johnson Syndrome

Dubin-Johnson syndrome is a benign autosomal recessive disease with chronic conjugated hyperbilirubinemia and conspicuous deposition of melanin-like pigment in the liver. Mutations in the *ABCC2/MRP2* gene result in the phenotype.

This syndrome can be distinguished from other conditions with conjugated hyperbilirubinemia by testing **urinary coproporphyrin excretion.** There are two forms of human coproporphyrins, **isomer I** and **isomer III.** A shift in the ratio of urinary coproporphyrin isomer I and III from the normal, 1:3, to the abnormal, 4:1, is diagnostic of Dubin-Johnson syndrome.

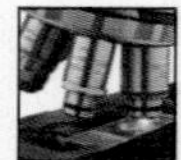

PATHOLOGY: The microscopic appearance of the liver is entirely normal, except that coarse, iron-free, **dark-brown granules** accumulate in hepatocytes and Kupffer cells, primarily in the centrilobular zone (Fig. 14-6). By electron microscopy, the pigment is in enlarged lysosomes. Since hepatocytes do not synthesize melanin, it has been suggested that the pigment reflects the auto-oxidation of anionic metabolites (e.g., tyrosine, phenylalanine, tryptophan) and possibly of epinephrine. Accumulation of this pigment causes the liver to be grossly pigmented, or "black."

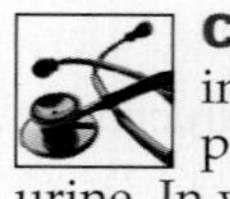

CLINICAL FEATURES: Symptoms are mild: slight intermittent jaundice and vague nonspecific complaints are common. Half of those affected have dark urine. In women, the disease may be discovered when jaundice appears during pregnancy or with use of oral contraceptives. Serum bilirubin levels are 2 to 5 mg/dL, but may transiently be much higher.

Rotor Syndrome

Rotor syndrome is an autosomal recessive, familial conjugated hyperbilirubinemia that is clinically similar to Dubin-Johnson syndrome but without pigmentation of the liver. A defect in hepatic uptake or intracellular binding of organic ions has been postulated as the basis of Rotor syndrome. In addition, the pattern of urinary coproporphyrin excretion is similar to that of most hepatobiliary disorders accompanied by conjugated hyperbilirubinemia (i.e., increased total urinary coproporphyrins, 65% of which are isomer I). Patients with Rotor syndrome have few symptoms and lead normal lives.

Benign Recurrent Intrahepatic Cholestasis

In benign recurrent intrahepatic cholestasis, self-limited, episodic intrahepatic cholestasis may be preceded by malaise and itching. The occurrence of familial cases suggests a genetic origin. Symptoms tend to last several weeks to several months. Patients may have three to five episodes in their lives, but some may have as many as 10. Recurrences may be separated by weeks to years. Serum bilirubin during the acute episodes range from 10 to 20 mg/dL, mostly conjugated.

The liver shows centrilobular cholestasis (bile plugs in bile canaliculi) and a few mononuclear inflammatory cells in the portal tracts. All structural and functional alterations disappear during remissions. No permanent sequelae have been reported.

Progressive Familial Intrahepatic Cholestasis

Progressive familial intrahepatic cholestasis (PFIC) is a heterogeneous group of uncommon, inherited, autosomal recessive disorders of infancy or early childhood in which intrahepatic cholestasis progresses relentlessly to cirrhosis. The first cases were descendents of an Amish man, Jacob Byler (Byler syndrome), but PFIC is not limited to that ethnic group. Mutations in several proteins, including FIC1, an aminophospholipid transporter, bile salt transporters and MRPs, are reported. There is an associated high incidence of retinitis pigmentosa, and the children are often mentally retarded. Most affected children die within the first 2 years of life.

Intrahepatic Cholestasis of Pregnancy

Intrahepatic cholestasis of pregnancy (ICP) is a rare disorder characterized by pruritus and cholestasis, usually in the last trimester of each pregnancy, and promptly disappearing after delivery. The prognosis for women with ICP is good, but fetal morbidity and mortality are increased, as are premature labor, fetal distress and placental insufficiency. Mutations in the ATP-cassette transporter B4 (ABCB4) and the multidrug resistant protein-3 (MDR3) have been described in women with ICP. Increased gonadal and placental hormones during pregnancy most likely cause the cholestasis in susceptible women. The mothers' livers show mainly centrilobular cholestasis. Diagnosis is generally clinical and is confirmed by the markedly increased maternal total bile acid levels. Therapy with ursodeoxycholic acid provides some relief of pruritus.

Sepsis Can Cause Jaundice

Severe conjugated hyperbilirubinemia may be associated with septicemia involving both gram-positive and gram-negative bacteria, although the latter infections are more common. In these situations, serum alkaline phosphatase activity and cholesterol levels are usually low, suggesting an isolated defect in excretion of conjugated bilirubin. In jaundice associated with sepsis, liver pathology is nonspecific and includes mild canalicular cholestasis and slight fat accumulation. Portal tracts may contain excess inflammatory cells and variable bile ductule proliferation. Occasionally, dilated ductules are filled with inspissated bile.

Neonatal (Physiologic) Jaundice Occurs in Most Newborns

Neonatal hyperbilirubinemia occurs in the absence of any specific disorder. Transhepatic clearance of bilirubin in the fetus is negligible; hepatic uptake, conjugation and biliary excretion are all much lower than in children and adults. Hepatic UGT activity is less than 1% of that in adults, and ligandin levels are low. Fetal bilirubin levels are low because bilirubin traverses the placenta and is conjugated and excreted by the maternal liver.

The liver of the newborn assumes the responsibility for bilirubin clearance before its conjugating and excretory capacities are fully developed. Moreover, the demands on the liver in the newborn are actually increased because of augmented destruction of circulating erythrocytes during this period. ***As a consequence, 70% of normal newborns have transient unconjugated hyperbilirubinemia.*** This physiologic jaundice is more pronounced in premature infants, both because hepatic clearance of bilirubin is less developed and because turnover of erythrocytes is greater than in term infants. The hepatic bilirubin-conjugating capacity reaches adult levels about 2 weeks after birth; ligandin takes somewhat longer to reach adult levels. As a result of this hepatic maturation, serum bilirubin levels rapidly decline to adult values shortly after birth. Absorption of light by unconjugated bilirubin generates water-soluble bilirubin isomers. ***Thus, phototherapy is now routinely used to treat neonatal jaundice.***

Maternal–fetal blood group incompatibilities may lead to erythroblastosis fetalis (see Chapter 6), in which striking bilirubin overproduction in the fetus is due to immune-mediated hemolysis. Although newborns with erythroblastosis fetalis display increased bilirubin levels in cord blood, jaundice becomes severe only after birth, because maternal metabolism of bilirubin no longer compensates for the immaturity of the neonatal liver.

Impaired Canalicular Bile Flow Accompanied by Visible Biliary Pigment (Cholestasis) Reflects Either Extrahepatic or Intrahepatic Biliary Obstruction

Functionally, cholestasis represents decreased bile flow through the canaliculus and reduced secretion of water, bilirubin and bile acids by hepatocytes. The clinical diagnosis is based on the accumulation in the blood of materials normally transferred to the bile, including bilirubin, cholesterol and bile acids, and the presence in the blood of elevated activities of certain enzymes, typically alkaline phosphatase. Cholestasis due to intrinsic liver disease is termed **intrahepatic cholestasis** (Fig. 14-5), while that caused by obstruction of large bile ducts is **extrahepatic cholestasis.** ***In any event, cholestasis is caused by a defect in the transport of bile across the canalicular membrane.***

The inability to excrete bile acids into canaliculi raises serum and hepatocellular bile acid concentrations. Bile acids injure cells by their detergent action and by direct activation of apoptosis. These hydrophobic molecules are thus potent hepatotoxins, and their accumulation within hepatocytes causes much of the hepatic injury and progression to cirrhosis associated with cholestasis. Elevation of serum bile acids is the likely cause of severe itching **(pruritus).**

The extrahepatic biliary system may be obstructed by a number of lesions. These include gallstones that lodge in the common bile duct, cancer of the bile duct or surrounding tissues (pancreas or ampulla of Vater), external compression by enlarged neoplastic lymph nodes in the porta hepatis (as in Hodgkin disease), benign strictures (postoperative scarring or primary sclerosing cholangitis) and congenital biliary atresia (Fig. 14-7).

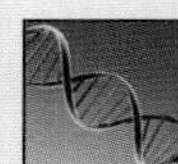
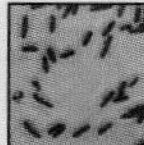

MOLECULAR PATHOGENESIS AND ETIOLOGIC FACTORS: Bile secretion into canaliculi and passage into the biliary collecting system are active processes that depend on (1) functional and structural characteristics of canalicular microvilli, (2) permeability of the canalicular plasma membrane, (3) intracellular contractile systems around canaliculi (microfilaments, microtubules) and (4) interactions of bile acids with the secretory apparatus.

The biochemical basis of cholestasis is not entirely clear, but a number of abnormalities in the formation and movement of bile are described. For extrahepatic biliary obstruction, the effects clearly begin with increased pressure in the bile ducts. However, for the early stages, the biochemistry and morphology at the canalicular level are similar to those in intrahepatic cholestasis, including initial centrilobular appearance of canalicular bile plugs (Fig. 14-8).

The invariable presence of bile constituents in the blood of people with cholestasis implies regurgitation of conjugated bilirubin from hepatocytes into the blood. Hepatic clearance of unconjugated bilirubin in cholestasis is normal. Even if bile duct obstruction is complete, serum bilirubin levels rise only to 30 to 35 mg/dL because renal excretion of bilirubin prevents further accumulation.

Both intrahepatic and extrahepatic cholestasis are characterized initially by preferential centrilobular localization of visible bile pigment. Fluid secretion into the canalicular bile is normally divided into two components: one dependent on secretion of bile acids and the other independent of bile acid secretion. Since periportal hepatocytes secrete most of the bile acids, the fluid content in the periportal zone of the canaliculus exceeds that in the central zone, thus keeping bilirubin in solution. Also, the bile acids themselves act as detergents in the intestine and solubilize aggregates of bilirubin in the periportal areas. Add to the above factors the higher activity of microsomal mixed-function oxidases in the central zone, which predisposes central hepatocytes to injury by a variety of drugs and toxins. Such an effect may favor deposition of bile in the centrilobular areas in cholestatic disorders.

Several mechanisms of cholestasis have been proposed:

DAMAGE TO THE CANALICULAR PLASMA MEMBRANE: The canalicular plasma membrane is the site of sodium (and therefore fluid) secretion into the bile. In addition, this membrane participates in secretion of bile

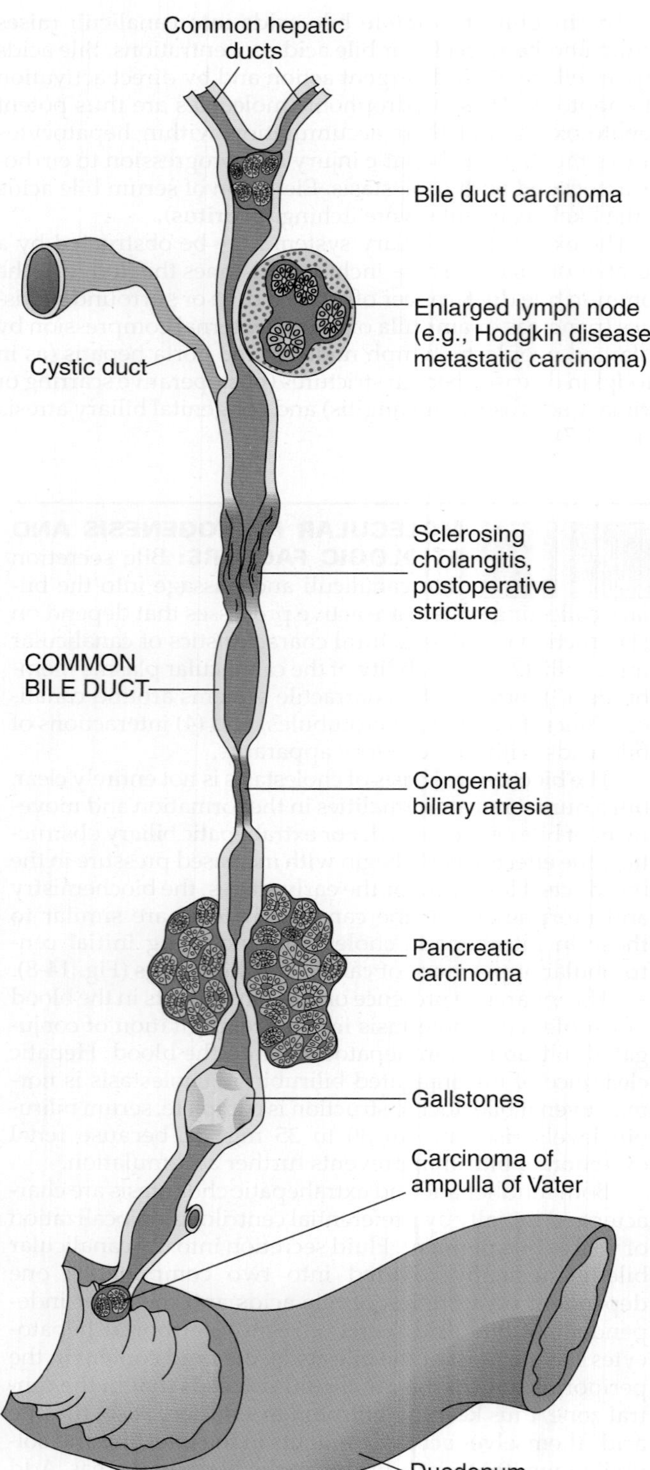

FIGURE 14-7. Major causes of extrahepatic biliary obstruction.

acids and bilirubin. The secretion of fluid is controlled by the Na^+/K^+-ATPase of the canalicular membrane. Alterations in the canalicular membrane by a number of drugs and other agents capable of perturbing its structure inhibit Na^+/K^+-ATPase, decrease bile flow or produce morphologic alterations.

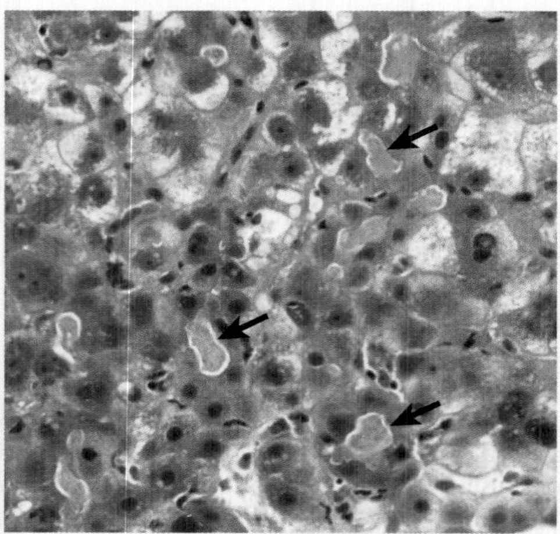

FIGURE 14-8. Bile stasis. A photomicrograph of the liver from a patient with drug-induced cholestasis shows prominent bile plugs in dilated bile canaliculi (*arrows*). In the absence of inflammation, this lesion may be termed "pure cholestasis."

ALTERATION IN THE CONTRACTILE PROPERTIES OF THE CANALICULUS: Bile is propelled along the canaliculus by a peristalsis-like contractile activity of the hepatocytes. Agents that interact with the pericanalicular actin microfilaments (e.g., cytochalasin, phalloidin) inhibit this peristalsis and may cause cholestasis.

ALTERATIONS IN THE PERMEABILITY OF THE CANALICULAR MEMBRANE: It has been suggested that certain agents that produce cholestasis, including estrogens and taurolithocholate, permit back-diffusion of bile components by making canalicular membranes more permeable, or "leaky."

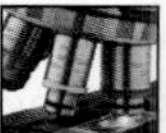

PATHOLOGY: ***Cholestasis is characterized by the presence of brownish bile pigment within dilated canaliculi and in hepatocytes*** (Figs. 14-8, 14-9 and 14-10). Canaliculi are enlarged. By electron microscopy, the microvilli are blunted and fewer in number or even absent. Bile stasis in hepatocytes is reflected in the presence of large, bile-laden lysosomes.

When cholestasis persists, secondary morphologic abnormalities develop. Scattered necrotic hepatocytes probably reflect the toxicity of excess intracellular bile. Intrasinusoidal macrophages and Kupffer cells contain bile pigment and cellular debris. Whereas early cholestasis is restricted almost exclusively to the central zone, chronic cholestasis is also marked by the appearance of bile plugs in the periphery of the lobule.

In **extrahepatic biliary obstruction,** the liver is swollen and bile stained. With prolonged obstruction, the bile becomes almost colorless ("white bile") because bilirubin secretion is suppressed, although the liver remains green. Initially, centrilobular cholestasis is accompanied by edema of the portal tracts. As obstruction proceeds, mononuclear inflammatory cells infiltrate the portal tracts. Tortuous and distended bile ductules proliferate (Fig. 14-9). Damaged hepatocytes with large amounts of bile manifest (1) hydropic swelling, (2) diffuse impregnation with bile pigment and (3) a reticulated appearance. This triad is termed **feathery degeneration**

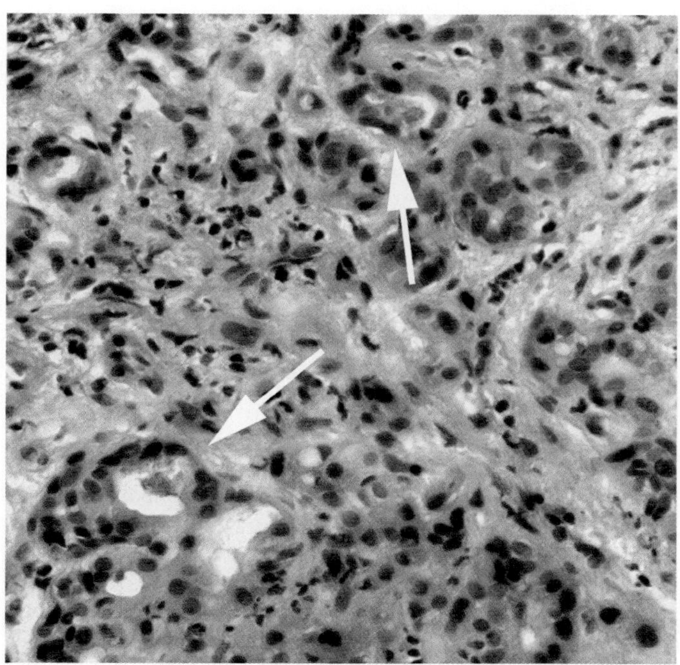

FIGURE 14-9. Extrahepatic biliary obstruction. A portal tract is expanded by proliferated bile ducts and acute and chronic inflammation. Several ducts are plugged with bile (*arrows*).

(Fig. 14-10). The cholestasis eventually extends to the periphery of the lobule. Dilated bile ducts may rupture, leading to **bile lakes** (Fig. 14-11), which appear as focal, golden-yellow deposits surrounded by degenerating hepatocytes. Infection of the obstructed biliary passages often leads to a superimposed suppurative cholangitis, intraluminal pus and even intrahepatic abscesses. Within bile ducts and proliferated ductules, biliary concretions may be conspicuous.

In time, the portal tracts become enlarged and fibrotic (Fig. 14-12). If extrahepatic biliary obstruction is untreated, septa eventually extend between the portal tracts of contiguous lobules to form **micronodular cirrhosis** (discussed below).

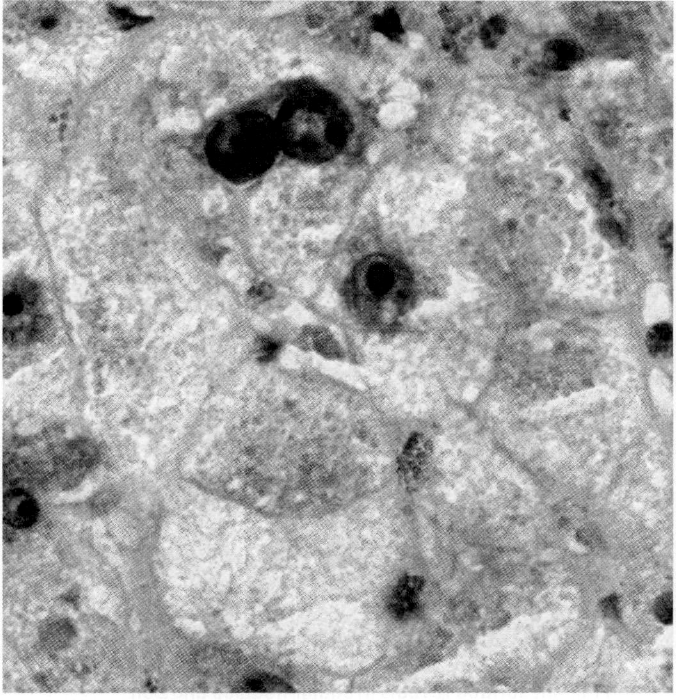

FIGURE 14-10. Cholestasis. Hepatocytes are swollen and bile stained (feathery degeneration).

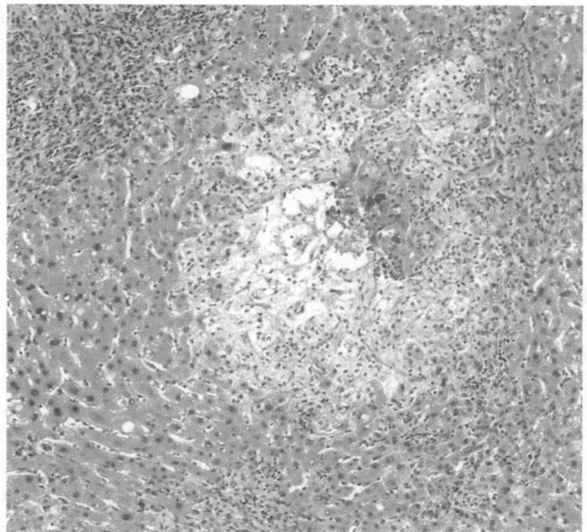

FIGURE 14-11. Bile infarct (bile lake). A photomicrograph of the liver in a patient with extrahepatic biliary obstruction shows an area of necrosis and the accumulation of extravasated bile.

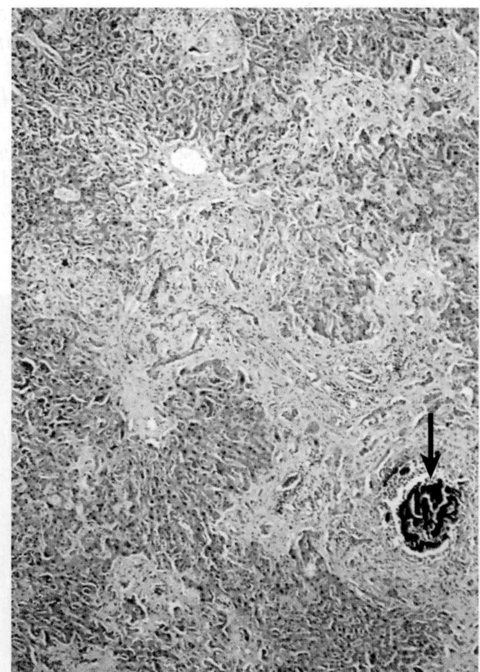

FIGURE 14-12. Secondary biliary cirrhosis. A photomicrograph of the liver from a patient with a carcinoma of the pancreas that obstructed the common bile duct. Irregular fibrous septa extend from enlarged portal tracts containing a dilated interlobular bile duct that encloses a dense biliary concretion (*arrow*). Proliferated bile ductules are seen within the septa.

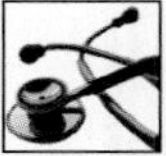

CLINICAL FEATURES: Cholestasis usually presents with jaundice, irrespective of its underlying cause. **Pruritus** (itching) is common and can be severe and intractable. It may be caused by deposition of bile acids within the skin, but other components of bile may play a role. Cholesterol accumulates in the skin in the form of **xanthomas. Malabsorption** may develop in cases of protracted cholestasis (see Chapter 13).

Cirrhosis

Cirrhosis is the destruction of the normal liver architecture by fibrous septa that encompass regenerative nodules of hepatocytes. This morphologic pattern invariably results from persistent liver cell necrosis. Advanced cases of cirrhosis all tend to have a similar appearance, and often the cause can no longer be ascertained by morphologic examination alone. During earlier stages, on the other hand, features characteristic of the inciting pathogenic insult may be evident. For example, fat and Mallory bodies are typical of alcoholic liver injury, whereas chronic inflammation and periportal necrosis are prominent in chronic hepatitis.

Many terms are applied to the different forms of cirrhosis, rivaling the number of etiologies incriminated in chronic liver disease, but some patterns emerge. At one end of this spectrum, usually early in the evolution of cirrhosis, is the **micronodular** type (Fig. 14-13), characterized by small, uniform nodules separated by thin fibrous septa. At the other end, ordinarily late in the disease, is **macronodular cirrhosis** (Fig. 14-14). This pattern consists of grossly visible, coarse, irregular nodules, which are mirrored histologically by large nodules of varying size and shape that are encircled by bands of connective tissue. These collagenous septa also vary conspicuously in width. ***Between these extremes are many cases with features of both types. In practice, the different appearances of cirrhosis are less important than their etiologies.***

Historically, cirrhosis has been considered to be irreversible. Recent observations suggest that collagen resorption and hepatic remodeling can occur over years to decades, if the underlying cause of cirrhosis is removed. However, despite functional and structural improvement in the cirrhotic liver, it is unlikely that complete regression ever occurs.

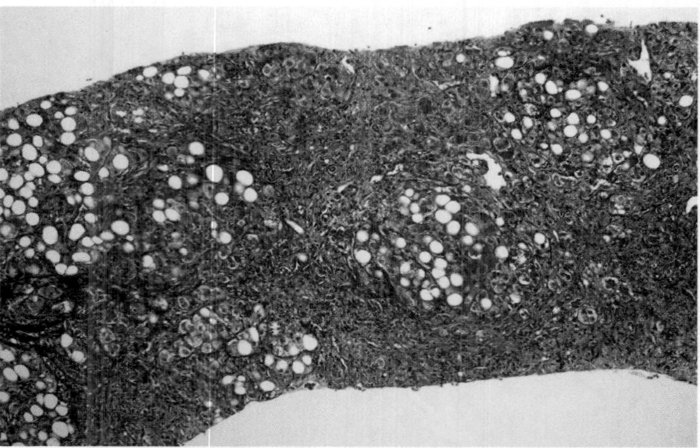

FIGURE 14-13. Micronodular cirrhosis. A photomicrograph of the cirrhotic liver of a chronic alcoholic. Note the small, regenerative nodules of parenchyma and fatty change.

MICRONODULAR CIRRHOSIS: This form of liver disease was previously termed **Laennec cirrhosis,** which honors the early 19th-century French physician who provided the first accurate description of it (Laennec also invented the stethoscope). In micronodular cirrhosis, the nodules are scarcely larger than a lobule, usually less than 3 mm in diameter (Fig. 14-13). The micronodules show no landmarks of lobular architecture in the form of portal tracts or central venules. Connective tissue septa separating the nodules are usually thin, but irregular focal collapse of parenchyma may lead to wider septa. In the active stages of cirrhosis, mononuclear inflammatory cells and proliferated bile ductules inhabit the septa. ***The prototypical cause of micronodular cirrhosis is alcoholic injury, but other etiologies may also be responsible.***

MACRONODULAR CIRRHOSIS: Macronodular cirrhosis is classically associated with chronic hepatitis. Connective tissue septa in macronodular cirrhosis are broad (Fig. 14-14), showing elements of preexisting portal tracts, mononuclear

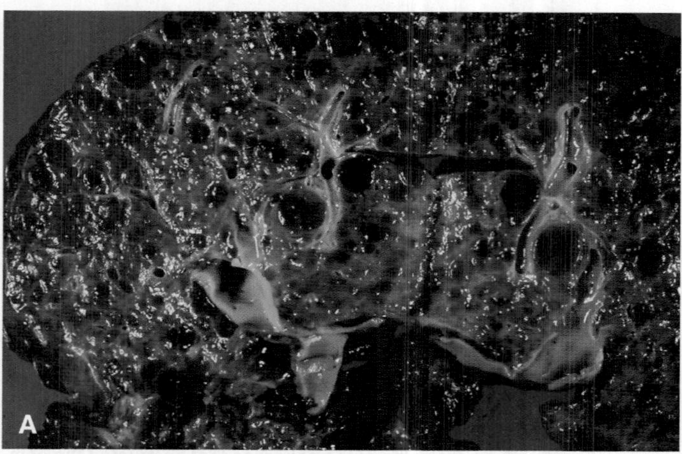

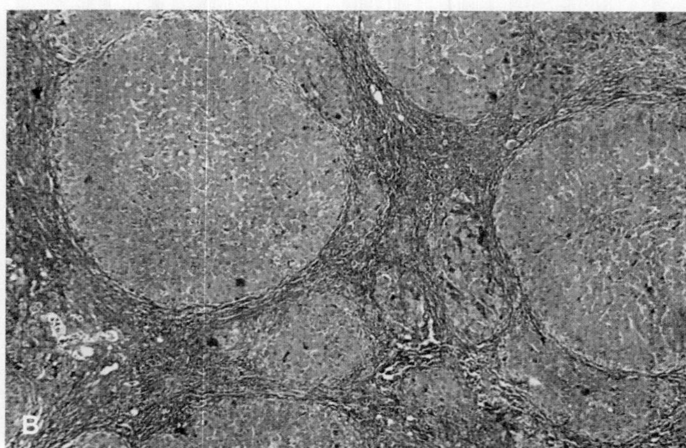

FIGURE 14-14. Macronodular cirrhosis. A. The liver is misshapen, and the cut surface reveals irregular nodules and connective tissue septa of varying width. **B.** A photomicrograph shows nodules of varying size and irregular fibrous septa.

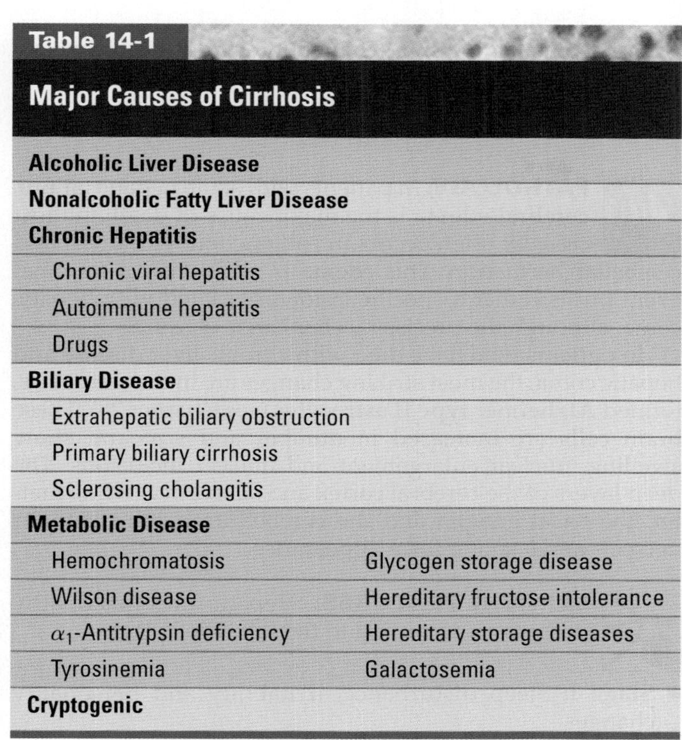

Table 14-1

Major Causes of Cirrhosis

Alcoholic Liver Disease	
Nonalcoholic Fatty Liver Disease	
Chronic Hepatitis	
Chronic viral hepatitis	
Autoimmune hepatitis	
Drugs	
Biliary Disease	
Extrahepatic biliary obstruction	
Primary biliary cirrhosis	
Sclerosing cholangitis	
Metabolic Disease	
Hemochromatosis	Glycogen storage disease
Wilson disease	Hereditary fructose intolerance
α_1-Antitrypsin deficiency	Hereditary storage diseases
Tyrosinemia	Galactosemia
Cryptogenic	

inflammatory cells and proliferated bile ductules. Micronodular cirrhosis can convert to a macronodular pattern by continued regeneration and expansion of existing nodules, especially in alcoholics who stop drinking.

The diseases associated with cirrhosis are listed in Table 14-1. They have little in common except that they all entail persistent liver cell necrosis. Most cases of cirrhosis are attributable to alcoholism and chronic viral hepatitis. Despite advances in diagnostic modalities, 15% of are of unknown origin and are classified as **cryptogenic cirrhosis.** Nonalcoholic steatohepatitis is now thought to account for a significant proportion of cryptogenic cirrhosis (see below).

Hepatic Failure

Hepatic failure is the clinical syndrome that occurs when the mass of liver cells or their function cannot sustain the vital activities of the liver. Liver failure may develop acutely, mostly due to viral hepatitis or toxic liver injury. By contrast, chronic liver diseases, such as chronic viral hepatitis or cirrhosis, may lead to an insidious onset of hepatic failure. Cirrhosis also causes portal hypertension and its complications (see below). Although advances in supportive care have improved survival in acute hepatic failure, the mortality for this condition exceeds 50%. The consequences of hepatic failure are depicted in Fig. 14-15.

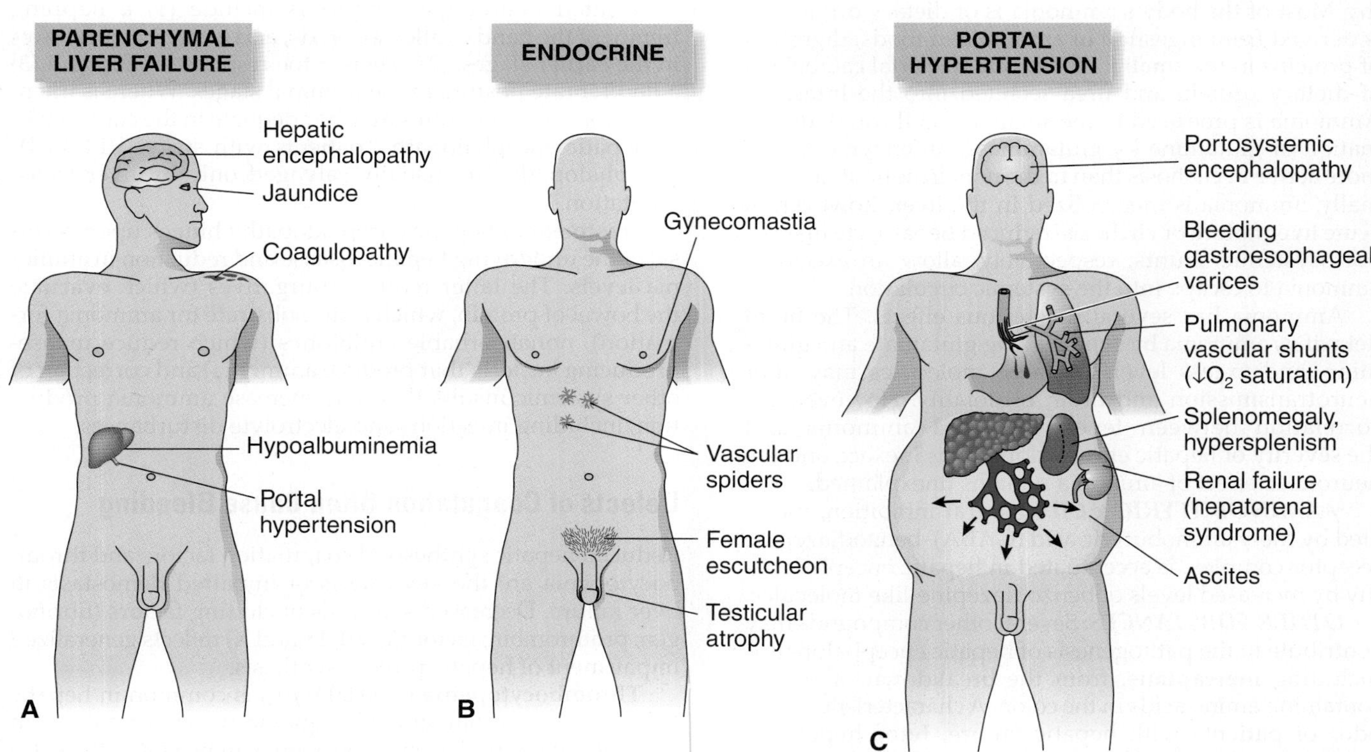

FIGURE 14-15. Complications of cirrhosis and hepatic failure. Clinical features related to **(A) parenchymal liver failure, (B) endocrine disturbances** and **(C) portal hypertension.** There is considerable overlap of these clinical features as regards their pathogeneses.

Jaundice Is Caused by Inadequate Clearance of Bilirubin by the Liver

Hyperbilirubinemia associated with hepatic failure is for the most part conjugated, although the level of unconjugated bilirubin also tends to increase. On occasion, increased erythrocyte turnover may add to unconjugated hyperbilirubinemia, thereby aggravating the jaundice.

Hepatic Encephalopathy Refers to Neurologic Signs and Symptoms of Liver Failure

Alterations in mental status are common in patients with acute liver failure and portal hypertension (see below).

MOLECULAR PATHOGENESIS: The pathogenesis of hepatic encephalopathy is unclear. No single factor explains the clinical syndrome. Harmful compounds absorbed from the intestine are inculpated, at least in part. Because of hepatocyte dysfunction or the existence of structural or functional vascular shunts, these compounds escape hepatic detoxification. The latter mechanism is particularly evident after the surgical construction of a portal–systemic anastomosis (portal vein to inferior vena cava or its equivalent) for the relief of portal hypertension (see below), which accounts for the synonym **portosystemic encephalopathy.**

AMMONIA: Ammonia levels are usually increased in the blood and brain of patients with hepatic encephalopathy. Most of the body's ammonia is of dietary origin and is derived from ingestion of ammonia in foods, digestion of proteins in the small intestine and bacterial catabolism of dietary protein and urea secreted into the intestine. Ammonia is produced in the small bowel through deamination of glutamine by glutaminase, an enzyme that is more active in cirrhosis than in the noncirrhotic state. Normally, ammonia is metabolized in the liver; however, in acute liver failure or cirrhosis, reduced hepatocyte mass or portosystemic shunts, respectively, allow an excess of ammonia to escape into the systemic circulation.

Ammonia has several deleterious effects. The brain detoxifies ammonia by synthesizing glutamate and glutamine, and excess levels of these molecules may alter neurotransmission and brain osmolality. However, the correlation between levels of blood ammonia and the severity of hepatic encephalopathy is inexact, and the neurotoxic effect of ammonia remains unexplained.

γ-AMINOBUTYRIC ACID: Neural inhibition, mediated by the γ-aminobutyric acid (GABA)–benzodiazepine receptor complex, is accentuated in hepatic encephalopathy by increased levels of benzodiazepine-like molecules.

OTHER SUBSTANCES: Several other compounds may contribute to the pathogenesis of hepatic encephalopathy, including **mercaptans,** from the breakdown of sulfur-containing amino acids in the colon. A characteristic breath odor of patients with hepatic failure, **fetor hepaticus,** reflects the presence of these mercaptans in saliva. Blood levels of aromatic amino acids are increased in hepatic failure and in turn impair synthesis of normal neurotransmitters such as norepinephrine but increase production of **false neurotransmitters** (e.g., octopamine). A toxic effect of **phenols** and **short-chain fatty acids** on the brain has also been postulated. Finally, the blood-brain barrier may be incompletely effective in patients with hepatic failure.

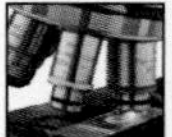

PATHOLOGY: In patients with acute hepatic failure, **cerebral edema** is the major cause of death in most cases. It often occurs in conjunction with uncal and cerebellar herniation. This edema is not simply a terminal event but is rather a specific lesion associated with hepatic coma, although the precise mechanism is obscure.

In patients who have died with chronic liver disease and hepatic coma, the most striking changes are in the astrocytes, termed **Alzheimer type II astrocytes** (see Chapter 28). These brain cells are increased in number and size and show swelling, nuclear enlargement and nuclear inclusions. The deep layers of the cerebral cortex and subcortical white matter, the basal ganglia and the cerebellum exhibit laminar necrosis and a spongiform appearance.

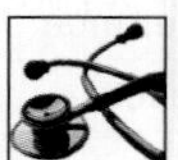

CLINICAL FEATURES: Hepatic encephalopathy progresses according to the following stages:

- **Stage I:** Sleep disturbance, irritability and personality changes
- **Stage II:** Lethargy and disorientation
- **Stage III:** Deep somnolence
- **Stage IV:** Coma

This sequence may progress over many months, or it may evolve rapidly in days or weeks in cases of acute liver failure. Associated neurologic symptoms include (1) a flapping tremor of the hands, called **asterixis,** and hyperactive reflexes in the earlier stages; (2) extensor toe responses later; and (3) a decerebrate posture in the terminal stages. Whereas intensive supportive measures may be adequate in the early stages of hepatic encephalopathy, patients with stages III and IV encephalopathy are usually salvaged only by liver transplantation.

Treatment of hepatic encephalopathy hinges upon reversal of the underlying hepatic disease and reduction in ammonia levels. The latter requires purgatives (which evacuate the bowel of protein, which is the substrate for ammonia formation), nonabsorbable antibiotics (which reduce urease-producing bacteria that produce ammonia) and correction of other systemic insults that may increase ammonia production, including infections and electrolyte disturbances.

Defects of Coagulation Often Cause Bleeding

Reduced hepatic synthesis of coagulation factors and thrombocytopenia are the key causes of impaired hemostasis in liver failure. Decreased synthesis of clotting factors (fibrinogen; prothrombin; factors V, VII, IX and X) reflects generalized impairment of hepatic protein synthesis.

Thrombocytopenia ($<$80,000/μL) is common in hepatic failure and is accompanied by qualitative abnormalities in platelet function. Thrombocytopenia may result from (1) hypersplenism, (2) bone marrow depression or (3) consumption of circulating platelets by intravascular coagulation.

Disseminated intravascular coagulation (DIC) occurs frequently in liver failure. It may be stimulated by liver cell necrosis, activation of factor XII (Hageman factor) by endotoxin or inadequate hepatic clearance of activated clotting factors from the circulation.

Hypoalbuminemia Complicates Hepatic Failure

Decreased circulating albumin is due to impaired hepatic synthesis and is an important factor in the pathogenesis of the edema that often complicates chronic liver disease.

Cirrhosis Leads to Feminization in Men and Gonadal Failure in Women

Hyperestrogenism in chronic liver failure in men leads to **gynecomastia,** a female body habitus and female distribution of pubic hair (female escutcheon). Vascular manifestations of hyperestrogenism are common and include **spider angiomas** in the territory drained by the superior vena cava (upper trunk and face) and **palmar erythema.**

Feminization is attributed to reduced hepatic catabolism of estrogens and weak androgens. The weak androgens (androstenedione and dehydroepiandrosterone) are converted to estrogens in peripheral tissues, thereby increasing circulating estrogen levels. Extrahepatic portal–systemic shunts secondary to portal hypertension in cirrhosis permit these hormones to bypass the liver.

Men with alcoholic liver disease are more likely to be feminized than those with liver disease from other causes, and the feminization is usually more severe. Chronic alcoholics also suffer hypogonadism, with testicular atrophy, impotence and loss of libido. Alcoholic women also have gonadal failure, which presents as oligomenorrhea, amenorrhea, infertility, ovarian atrophy and loss of secondary sex characteristics. These effects in both sexes reflect a direct toxic action of alcohol on gonadal function and are independent of chronic liver disease.

Portal Hypertension

Arising at the junction of the superior mesenteric vein with the splenic vein, the hepatic portal vein carries the major venous drainage from the gastrointestinal tract, pancreas and spleen to the liver. It delivers two thirds of the hepatic blood flow but accounts for less than half of the total oxygen supply, the remainder being supplied by the hepatic artery. ***Portal hypertension is defined by either an absolute increase in portal venous pressure, usually above 8 mm Hg, or an increase in the pressure gradient between the portal vein and the hepatic vein of 5 mm Hg or more.*** Portal hypertension results from obstruction to blood flow somewhere in the portal circuit. Increased portal pressure causes opening of collateral channels, bleeding from gastroesophageal varices, ascites, splenomegaly and renal and pulmonary disease (Fig. 14-15).

The presence of portal hypertension is most accurately determined by direct measurement of hepatic vein pressure: a balloon-tipped catheter is inserted into the internal jugular vein and advanced to a terminal hepatic vein. In this position, the **free hepatic vein pressure** (FHVP) is obtained. The **wedged hepatic vein pressure** (WHVP) is determined after balloon inflation. The WHVP is an indirect measure of the portal vein pressure. The difference between WHVP and FHVP is the **hepatic vein pressure gradient** (HVPG); that is, WHVP − FHVP = HVPG.

Increased resistance to blood outflow from the portal circulation is the basis for the diagnosis of portal hypertension (Fig. 14-16). The increase in resistance can originate in one of three areas:

1. **Sinusoidal** or **intrahepatic.** Injury to the sinusoids leads to sinusoidal, or intrahepatic, portal hypertension. In the Western world cirrhosis is the most common cause of intrahepatic portal hypertension and, in fact, the most common cause of portal hypertension in any form. In cirrhosis, fibrosis leads to obstruction of the intrahepatic sinusoids, which, in turn, impedes the inflow of portal blood. The result is increased pressure within the portal vein, relative to the hepatic vein. In sinusoidal portal hypertension, the pressure difference between the WHVP and FHVP (HVPG) usually is 5 mm Hg or more.
2. **Presinusoidal.** If the resistance to blood flow is in the extrahepatic portal vein or intrahepatic portal veins or venules (e.g., thrombotic occlusion), it is **presinusoidal portal hypertension.** If the point of resistance is within portal venules (i.e., within the liver), the HVPG may be increased. However, if the point of resistance is more distal, allowing for a zone of normal pressure in the portal vein, between the occlusion and the sinusoids, the HVPG can be normal.
3. **Postsinusoidal.** If the point of resistance is in the hepatic veins, venules or cardiac circulation, **postsinusoidal portal hypertension** may result. This scenario can arise in obstruction of the hepatic veins, as in the Budd-Chiari syndrome, or congestive heart failure. The HVPG usually is normal in this situation. That is, if the hepatic vein pressure is measured distal to the point of postsinusoidal obstruction, the FHVP will be increased, and the HVPG can be expected to be normal, as the sinusoids are normal and pose no significant resistance to the flow of blood into the liver. However, under constant high pressure due to outflow resistance, the sinusoids may become progressively injured, leading to an eventual elevation in the HVPG.

Intrahepatic Portal Hypertension Is Usually Caused by Cirrhosis

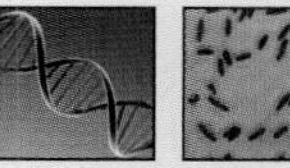

MOLECULAR PATHOGENESIS AND ETIOLOGIC FACTORS: Intrahepatic portal hypertension as occurs in cirrhosis offers the best paradigm for understanding the pathogenesis of portal hypertension. Even before fibrosis distorts sinusoidal architecture, active contraction of vascular smooth muscle and stellate cells initiates the resistance to the flow of blood into the liver from the portal vein. The trigger for this event is not clear, but is likely related to factors that incite inflammation, such as alcohol hepatitis and viral hepatitis. As fibrosis develops, sinusoids become increasingly disordered. Regenerative nodules in the cirrhotic liver impinge on the hepatic veins, thereby obstructing blood flow distal to the lobules. The small portal veins and venules are trapped, narrowed and often obliterated by scarring of the portal tracts. Blood flow through the hepatic artery is increased and small arteriovenous communications become functional. In this way, portal hypertension due to obstruction of blood flow distal to the sinusoid is augmented by increased arterial blood flow.

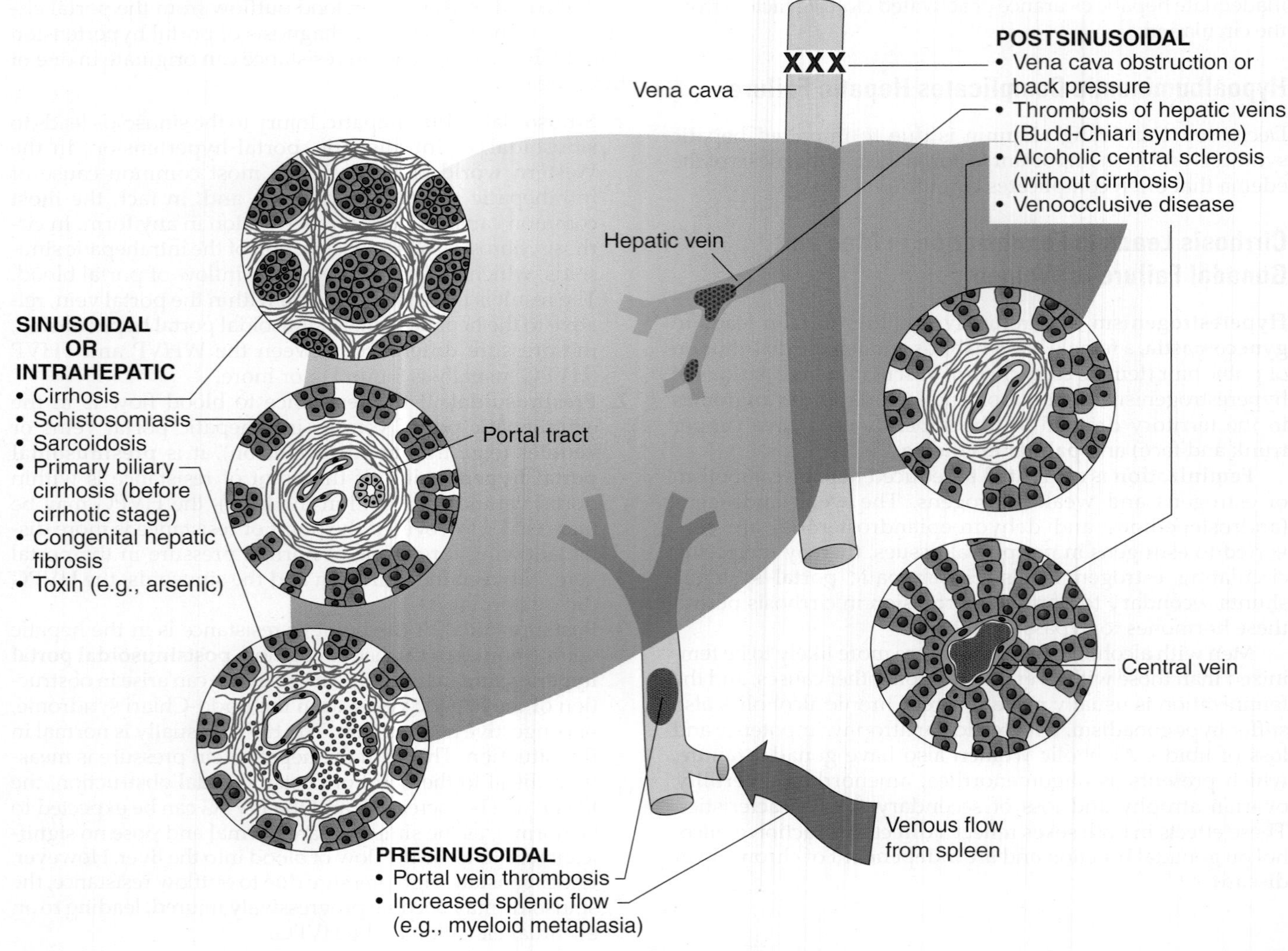

FIGURE 14-16. Causes of portal hypertension.

In cirrhosis, **endothelial cell dysfunction** occurs in the liver and in the systemic circulation, increasing hepatic vascular tone and intrahepatic vasoconstriction. Reduced endothelial nitric oxide synthetase (eNOS) activity is followed by decreased hepatic nitric oxide (NO•) production, leading to vasoconstriction and thus increased resistance to portal blood flow into the liver. Several factors trigger the reduced eNOS activity, including impaired eNOS phosphorylation, reduced NO• availability due to oxidative stress and an excess of vasoconstrictive factors such as angiotensinogen, endothelin and eicosanoids.

Just as resistance to blood flow to the liver increases, **mesenteric arterial vasodilation** increases in the volume of blood flowing into the portal vein. This vasodilation results from increased NO• caused by greater sheer forces upon the mesenteric vessels due to increased resistance to portal blood flow into the liver, increased vascular endothelial growth factor (VEGF) and inflammatory mediators such as TNF-α. ***Progressive portal hypertension parallels mesenteric arterial vasodilation, leading to dysfunctional systemic circulation, with systemic arterial vasodilation and reduced effective arterial blood volume.***

The reduction in effective arterial blood volume, owing to systemic arteriolar vasodilation, leads to clinical manifestations of advanced portal hypertension, including **ascites, hepatorenal syndrome** and **hepatopulmonary syndrome.** The increased portal pressure also opens vascular shunts that decompress the portal circuit. Although ostensibly valuable, these shunts may lead to further clinical complications, particularly bleeding varices and encephalopathy (see above).

***Worldwide, hepatic schistosomiasis* (Schistosoma mansoni *and* Schistosoma japonicum) *is a major cause of intrahepatic portal hypertension* (see Chapter 9).** Ova released from the intestinal veins traverse the portal system and lodge in intrahepatic portal venules, where they elicit a granulomatous reaction that heals by scarring. Because the obstruction within the liver occurs mainly before the portal blood enters the hepatic sinusoids, hepatic schistosomiasis is functionally similar to prehepatic portal hypertension. Thus, liver function is well maintained, but the intrahepatic presinusoidal vascular obstruction leads to severe portal hypertension.

Idiopathic portal hypertension refers to occasional cases of intrahepatic portal hypertension with splenomegaly that occur in the absence of any demonstrable intrahepatic or extrahepatic disease. In some countries (England, Japan), idiopathic portal hypertension accounts for 15% to 35% of all cases that require surgery to decompress the portal circulation.

Intrahepatic portal hypertension can be caused by other conditions that interfere with blood flow through the liver, including (1) cystic disease of the liver (see Chapter 16, which includes a discussion of cystic disease of the kidney), (2) partial nodular transformation of the liver in the region of the porta hepatis and (3) nodular regenerative hyperplasia (small regenerative nodules without fibrosis that compress the intervening hepatic parenchyma).

Presinusoidal Portal Hypertension Is Often Caused by Portal Vein Thrombosis

ETIOLOGIC FACTORS: Portal vein thrombosis occurs most often in the setting of cirrhosis. Other causes include tumors, infections, hypercoagulability states, pancreatitis and surgical trauma. Some cases are of unknown etiology. Primary hepatocellular carcinoma generally invades branches of the portal vein and may occlude the main portal vein. When the portal vein is obstructed by a septic thrombus, bacteria may seed the intrahepatic branches of the portal vein (suppurative pylephlebitis) and cause multiple hepatic abscesses.

Portal vein occlusion (Fig. 14-17) may occur in the neonatal period or in early childhood. In some cases, umbilical sepsis is an important cause, but other local and systemic infections may also play a role. Sometimes the thrombosed portal or splenic vein is replaced by a fibrous cord or interlacing vascular channels, a condition termed **cavernous transformation.**

The liver normally offers little resistance to the outflow of blood through the sinusoids and so can accommodate substantial increases in blood flow without a secondary increase in pressure. However, increased portal venous blood flow can lead to prehepatic portal hypertension on occasion. Arteriovenous fistulas (i.e., abnormal communications between an artery and the portal vein) may lead to prehepatic portal hypertension. These generally arise from trauma or rupture of an aneurysm of the splenic or hepatic artery. They may also develop in patients with hereditary hemorrhagic telangiectasia (Osler-Weber-Rendu syndrome). Splenomegaly due to, for example, polycythemia vera, myeloid metaplasia and chronic myelogenous leukemia may lead to portal hypertension. The splenomegaly that accompanies cirrhosis may aggravate portal hypertension.

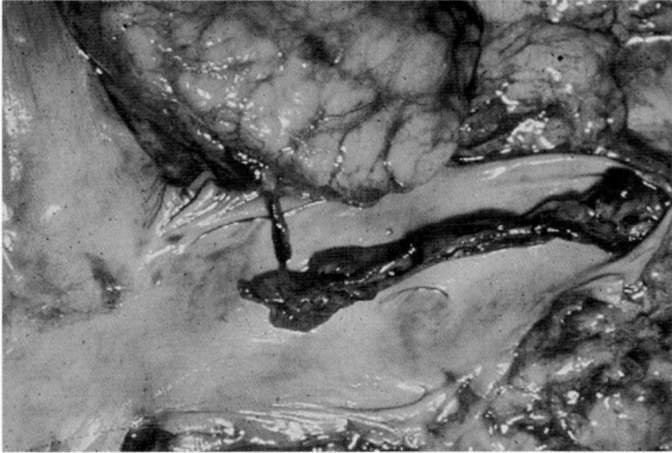

FIGURE 14-17. Portal vein thrombosis.

Postsinusoidal Portal Hypertension Refers to Obstruction to Blood Flow Beyond the Liver Lobules

Budd-Chiari Syndrome

Budd-Chiari syndrome is a congestive disease of the liver caused by occlusion of the hepatic veins and their tributaries.

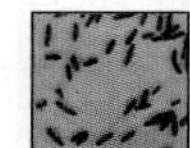

ETIOLOGIC FACTORS: The principal cause of Budd-Chiari syndrome is thrombosis of the hepatic veins, which may occur in such diverse conditions as polycythemia vera (10% to 40% of cases) and other myeloproliferative disorders, hypercoagulable states associated with malignant tumors, use of oral contraceptives, pregnancy, bacterial infections, paroxysmal nocturnal hemoglobinuria, metastatic and primary tumors in the liver and surgical trauma. In 20% of cases, there is no clear cause. Thrombi form most often in the large hepatic veins, close to their exit from the liver and in the intrahepatic portion of the inferior vena cava. In parts of Africa and Asia, membranous webs of unknown cause, presumably congenital, compromise the vena cava above the orifices of the hepatic veins and commonly cause Budd-Chiari syndrome. Increased venous back-pressure due to severe congestive heart failure, tricuspid stenosis or regurgitation or constrictive pericarditis may mimic Budd-Chiari syndrome.

Hepatic veno-occlusive disease is a variant of the Budd-Chiari syndrome and is caused by occlusion of the central venules and small branches of the hepatic veins. This disorder is most often traced to ingestion of toxic pyrrolizidine alkaloids in plants of the *Crotalaria* and *Senecio* genera, which are used in "bush teas". It is also seen in patients treated with certain antineoplastic chemotherapeutic agents, after hepatic irradiation and in association with bone marrow transplantation, possibly as a manifestation of graft-versus-host disease.

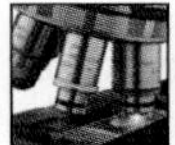

PATHOLOGY: In the acute stage of **hepatic vein thrombosis,** the liver is swollen and tense. The cut surface is mottled and oozes blood (Fig. 14-18A). In the chronic stage, the cut surface is paler, and the liver is firm, owing to an increase in connective tissue. The hepatic veins have thrombi in varying stages of evolution, from recent clots to well-organized thrombi that have been recanalized.

In the acute stage of both Budd-Chiari syndrome and veno-occlusive disease, the sinusoids of the central zone are dilated and packed with erythrocytes (Fig. 14-18B). Liver cell plates are compressed, with necrosis of centrilobular hepatocytes and hemorrhage. In long-standing venous congestion, fibrosis of the central zone radiating into the more peripheral portions of the lobules is conspicuous (Fig. 14-18C). The

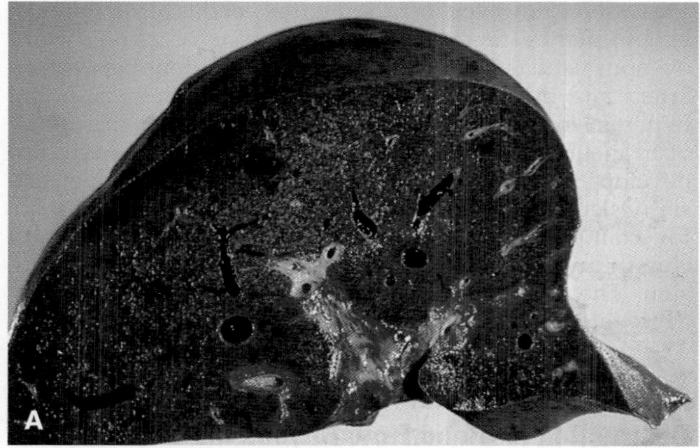

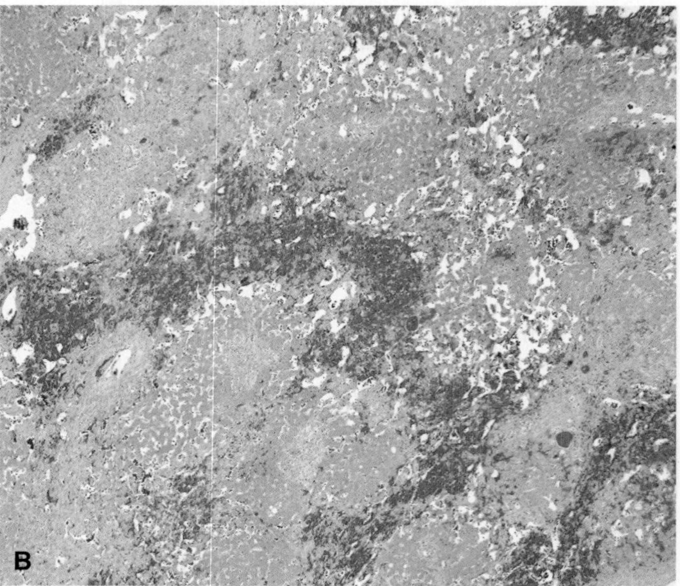

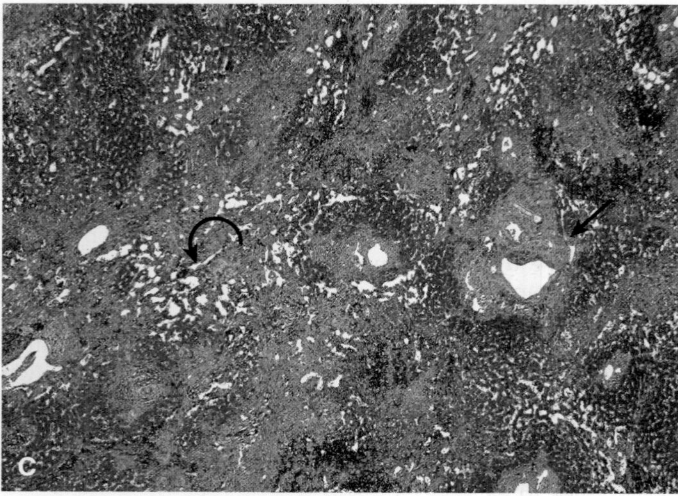

FIGURE 14-18. Budd-Chiari syndrome. A. The cut surface of the liver from a patient who died from Budd-Chiari syndrome shows thrombosis of the hepatic veins and diffuse congestion of the parenchyma. **B.** A needle biopsy of the liver from a patient with **acute Budd-Chiari syndrome** reveals centrilobular necrosis and hemorrhage and expanded sinusoids (e.g., *lower left*). **C. Chronic Budd-Chiari syndrome.** Cirrhosis has developed with bridging fibrosis emanating from the central veins rather than the portal tracts. Note the dilated sinusoids (*curved arrow*) and intact portal tract (*arrow*).

sinusoids are dilated, and the central to midzonal hepatocytes show pressure atrophy. Eventually, connective tissue septa link adjacent central zones to form nodules with a single central portal tract, a process known as reverse lobulation. This fibrosis is usually not severe enough to justify a label of cirrhosis.

CLINICAL FEATURES: Complete thrombosis of the hepatic veins presents as an acute illness with abdominal pain, enlargement of the liver, ascites and mild jaundice. Acute hepatic failure and death often occur rapidly. Most often, the obstruction of the hepatic venous circulation is incomplete, and similar symptoms persist for periods from a month to a few years. More than 90% of patients with Budd-Chiari syndrome develop ascites, usually severe, and splenomegaly is seen in over 30%. Typically, serum bilirubin and aminotransferase activities increase only modestly. Most patients eventually die in hepatic failure or from the complications of portal hypertension. Liver transplantation has been successful in curing the disease.

Portal Hypertension Has Systemic Complications Affecting Many Organ Systems

Esophageal Varices

Esophageal varices are the most important complication of portal hypertension and arise from the opening of portal–systemic collateral vascular channels to relieve pressure in the portal venous system. One of the most common causes of death in patients with cirrhosis and other disorders associated with portal hypertension is exsanguinating upper gastrointestinal tract hemorrhage from **bleeding esophageal varices** (see Chapter 13).

ETIOLOGIC FACTORS: The collaterals of most clinical significance are in the submucosa of the lower esophagus and upper stomach and are the result of communications between the portal vein and the gastric coronary vein. Because of the increased blood flow and higher pressures that follow the opening of these collaterals, the submucosal veins in the vicinity of the esophagogastric junction become dilated and protrude into the lumen. There is no simple correlation between portal venous pressure and the risk of variceal bleeding, although the risk does rise with increasing size of the varices.

CLINICAL FEATURES: The prognosis in patients with bleeding esophageal varices is poor, and acute mortality may be as high as 40%. In patients with cirrhosis who survive an initial episode of variceal bleeding, long-term survival is unlikely because of a high risk of rebleeding or worsening liver failure. By contrast, patients in whom portal hypertension is caused by a presinusoidal block without underlying hepatic dysfunction, as in hepatic schistosomiasis, have a much better prognosis than those with cirrhosis. Importantly, death associated with bleeding esophageal varices is frequently not attributable directly to exsanguination and shock. Rather, it is the result of hepatic failure precipitated by stress, ischemic necrosis of the liver and the encephalopathy caused by the acute nitrogenous load imposed by blood in the intestinal tract.

Initial treatment of acute variceal hemorrhage focuses on stopping the bleeding: by endoscopic variceal ligation, injection of varices with a sclerosing agent during endoscopy or direct tamponade with an inflatable balloon. In addition, intravenous administration of the somatostatin analog octreotide inhibits splanchnic vasodilation and, in turn, reduces splanchnic blood flow and portal venous pressure. If these measures fail and variceal bleeding recurs, permanent decompression of the portal circulation can be achieved by angiographic insertion of a small stent, or shunt, to join the portal and systemic circulations (transjugular intrahepatic portosystemic shunt [TIPS]). This, in addition to surgically constructed portasystemic shunts, diverts blood from the high-pressure portal circulation to the lower-pressure systemic venous circulation. In some cases, liver transplantation is an alternative to shunt surgery.

Back-pressure in the portal vein is also transmitted to its tributaries, including the inferior hemorrhoidal veins, which become dilated and tortuous **(anorectal varices).** Collateral veins radiating about the umbilicus produce a pattern known as **caput medusae.**

Splenomegaly

The spleen in portal hypertension enlarges progressively and often gives rise to the syndrome of **hypersplenism,** which is a decrease in the life span of all of the formed elements of the blood and, therefore, a reduction in their circulating numbers (pancytopenia). Hypersplenism is attributed to an increased rate of removal of erythrocytes, leukocytes and platelets because of the prolonged transit time through the hyperplastic spleen.

On gross examination, the spleen is firm and enlarged, up to 1000 g, and its cut surface is uniformly deep red, with inapparent white pulp. Splenic sinusoids are dilated. Their walls are thickened by fibrous tissue and lined by hyperplastic endothelial cells and macrophages. Focal hemorrhages cause fibrotic, iron-laden nodules, known as **Gamna-Gandy bodies.**

Ascites

Ascites is the accumulation of fluid in the peritoneal cavity. It often accompanies portal hypertension, and the amount of fluid may be so great (frequently many liters) that it not only distends the abdomen but also interferes with breathing. The onset of ascites in cirrhosis is associated with a poor prognosis.

ETIOLOGIC FACTORS: Reduced effective arterial blood volume and mean arterial pressure lead to predictable homeostatic responses. Early in portal hypertension, heart rate and cardiac output increase, thus preserving arterial pressure. However, as peripheral arterial vasodilation worsens, circulatory dysfunction becomes more pronounced: cardiac output cannot keep pace with homeostatic demand, and endogenous vasoactive mechanisms become engaged. In order to preserve arterial pressure, the

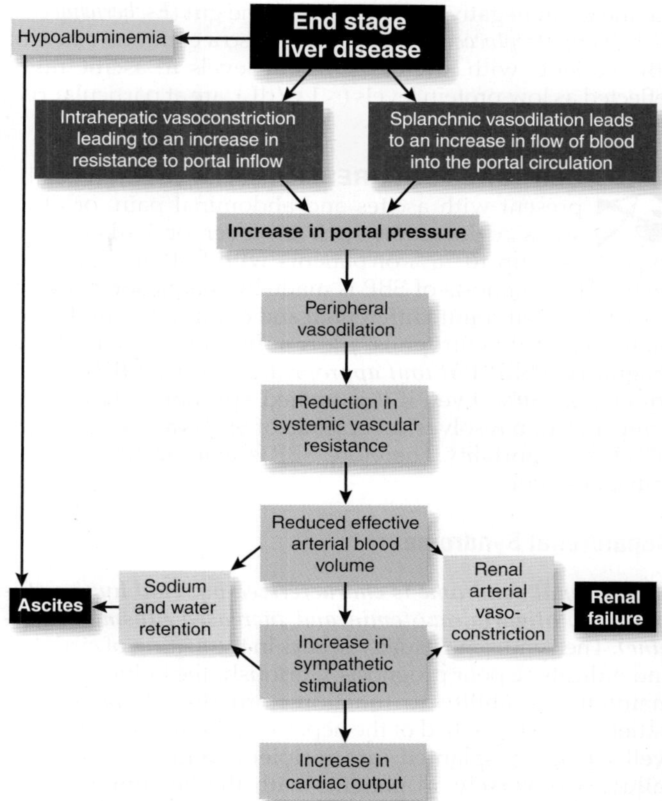

FIGURE 14-19. Pathogenesis of ascites.

activities of the renin–angiotensin system and sympathetic nervous system increase. This leads to renal sodium and water retention. Vasodilation also activates antidiuretic hormone secretion, leading to additional water retention and dilutional hyponatremia.

Ascites results from sodium and water retention, compounded by increased liver sinusoidal pressure leading to hydrostatic movement of fluid and lymph from the sinusoids into the space of Disse. These fluids spill into the peritoneal cavity as ascites. Decreased albumin synthesis lowers intravascular oncotic pressure and facilitates movement of fluid into the peritoneal space.

In cirrhosis, accumulation of fibrosis leads to an increasingly impervious sinusoidal endothelium. As its permeability falls, less protein and albumin spill into the ascites fluid. This leads to an increase in the ratio of serum to ascites albumin; an increase in the serum–to–ascites albumin gradient, or SAAG, of greater than 1.1 is associated with the ascites due to portal hypertension from cirrhosis.

The pathogenesis of ascites is illustrated in Fig. 14-19.

Spontaneous Bacterial Peritonitis

Spontaneous bacterial peritonitis (SBP) is an important complication in patients with both cirrhosis and ascites.

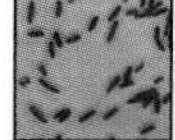

ETIOLOGIC FACTORS: SBP is thought to be due to translocation of intestinal bacteria into the systemic circulation, with secondary infection of ascites fluid. This correlates with the fact that the most common bacteria are the gram negatives that populate the gut (*Escherichia coli, Klebsiella*); *Streptococcus pneumonia* is also a common cause of SBP. Patients with low complement levels in ascitic fluid, reflected as low protein levels (<1 g/dL), are at particular risk for SBP.

CLINICAL FEATURES: Patients with SBP typically present with ascites and abdominal pain, or other signs of infection such as fever or leukocytosis. Importantly, up to 20% of patients with SBP are asymptomatic. The diagnosis of SBP is made by diagnostic paracentesis, white cell count, differential and culture. The finding of more than 250 neutrophils/μL is sufficient to establish the diagnosis of SBP. ***Without appropriate therapy, SBP mortality exceeds 80%.*** Even if it is treated appropriately and the acute infection resolves, an episode of SBP is associated with 70% 1-year mortality. Therefore, SBP is an indication for liver transplantation.

Hepatorenal Syndrome

Hepatorenal syndrome is characterized by renal hypoperfusion (i.e., oliguria, azotemia and increased plasma creatinine). The syndrome usually occurs in the setting of cirrhosis and indicates a poor prognosis. Curiously, the kidneys clearly maintain the ability to function normally. Kidneys from patients who have died of the hepatorenal syndrome function well when transplanted into recipients with chronic renal failure. Conversely, in patients with the hepatorenal syndrome, liver transplantation can restore renal function.

ETIOLOGIC FACTORS: In the early stages of portal hypertension, renal glomerular filtration pressure is protected from systemic arteriolar vasodilation by intrarenal prostaglandins. With increasingly severe arteriolar vasodilation, these intrarenal factors become ineffective, renal arterial vasoconstriction intensifies and glomerular perfusion and filtration decline. Eventually, this leads to clinically evident renal dysfunction, or hepatorenal syndrome (HRS). The diagnosis of HRS also requires serum creatinine levels greater than 1.5 mg/dL that do not improve after diuretic withdrawal and volume expansion.

There are two types of HRS. Type I HRS is rapidly and inexorably progressive. Liver transplantation is the only definitive therapy for type I HRS. Type II HRS is more slowly progressive and usually seen in the setting of severe ascites that is unresponsive to conventional therapies with salt restriction and diuretics. This form of HRS may be mitigated by volume expansion or diuretic withdrawal. However, type II ultimately progresses to type I HRS if portal hypertension is not reversed.

Pulmonary Complications of Portal Hypertension

The pulmonary complications of portal hypertension and cirrhosis include **hepatopulmonary syndrome (HPS), portopulmonary hypertension** and **hepatic hydrothorax.** Directly or indirectly, these result from the circulatory and vascular disturbances of advanced liver disease.

HPS results from creation of shunts of various sizes within the pulmonary vascular bed in the setting of portal hypertension. Up to one third of patients with cirrhosis may show signs of HPS, which is associated with reduced survival, particularly if arterial oxygen is less than 50 mm Hg. Patients with HPS are treated with supplemental oxygen, but liver transplantation is the only effective therapy, leading to reversal of the intrapulmonary shunting in most. Clinically, patients with HPS present with progressive shortness of breath due to hypoxemia and orthodeoxia, which refers to dyspnea and hypoxemia that is more severe in the upright position. Chest radiography and pulmonary hemodynamics (pulmonary arterial pressures) are typically normal.

Portopulmonary hypertension (PPHTN) results from increased pulmonary vascular resistance in the setting of portal hypertension. Usually, this is associated with increased mean pulmonary arterial pressure, to more than 25 mm Hg. Approximately 2% of patients with portal hypertension have PPHTN. The pathophysiology of PPHTN is speculative and may relate to features common to the hyperdynamic circulation typical of portal hypertension: shear stress, endothelial injury, vasoconstriction and liberation of vasoactive factors. Proliferative pulmonary arteriopathy develops. PPHTN is inexorably progressive and usually does not reverse following liver transplantation. In fact, severe PPHTN is a risk factor for intraoperative death due to acute heart failure and represents a contraindication to liver transplantation.

Hepatic hydrothorax refers to the presence of a pleural effusion attributed to portal hypertension. Most such effusions occur in the right chest and result from transdiaphragmatic movement of fluid from the abdomen. Typically, fluid has the same characteristics (protein content) as ascites and, like ascites, can develop spontaneous infection.

Viral Hepatitis

Viral hepatitis is an infection of hepatocytes that produces necrosis and inflammation of the liver. The disease has been recognized as "epidemic jaundice" for millennia. Worldwide, over 500 million people are infected with hepatotropic viruses and are at considerable risk of developing hepatocellular carcinoma. Many viruses and other infectious agents can produce hepatitis and jaundice (Table 14-2), but in the industrialized world, more than 95% of cases of viral hepatitis involve a limited number of hepatotropic viruses, named from A to G. Hepatitis F virus seems to be a variant of hepatitis B. Hepatitis G virus is 25% homologous with hepatitis C virus, but it does not lead to acute or chronic hepatitis.

Table 14-2

Infectious Agents That Cause Hepatitis

Hepatitis A virus (HAV)	Herpes simplex virus
Hepatitis B virus (HBV)	Cytomegalovirus
Hepatitis C virus (HCV)	Enteroviruses other than HAV
Hepatitis E virus Yellow fever virus	Leptospires (leptospirosis)
Epstein-Barr virus (infectious mononucleosis)	*Entamoeba histolytica* (amebic hepatitis)
Lassa, Marburg, and Ebola viruses	

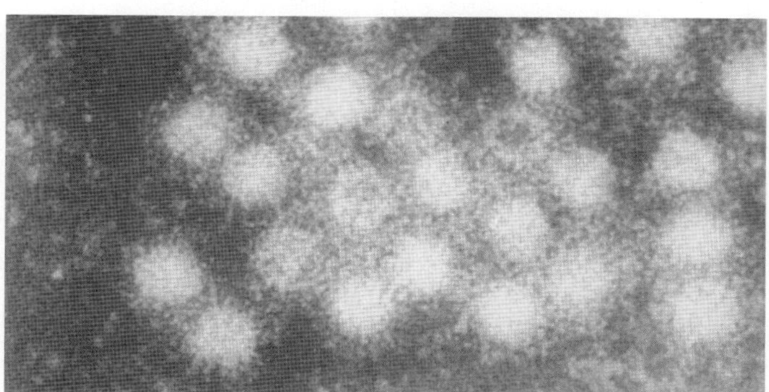

FIGURE 14-20. Electron micrograph of hepatitis A virus (HAV). A fecal extract was treated with convalescent serum containing anti-HAV.

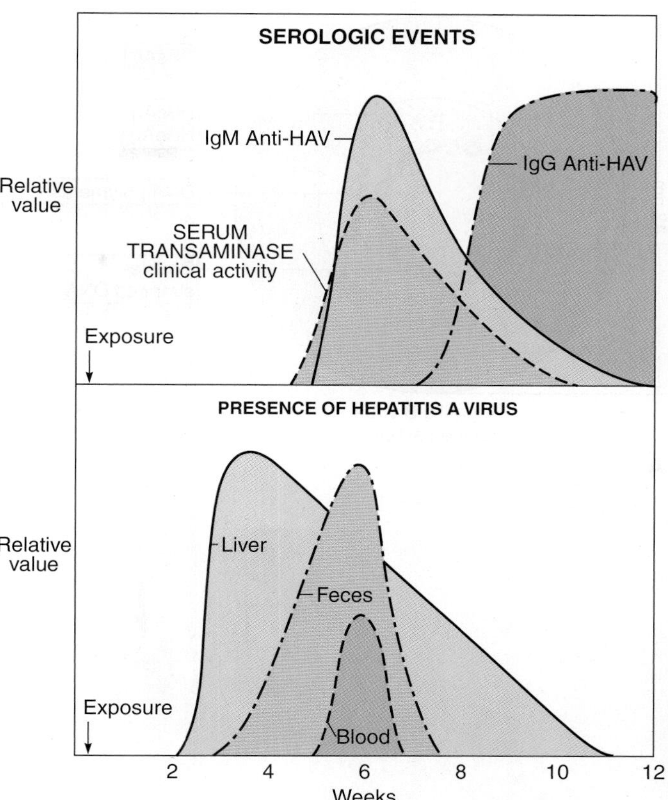

FIGURE 14-21. Typical serologic events associated with hepatitis A (HAV).

The following discussion emphasizes the illnesses commonly termed **viral hepatitis.** The reader is referred to Chapter 9 for consideration of the other agents.

Hepatitis A Virus Is the Most Common Cause of Acute Hepatitis

Hepatitis A virus (HAV) is a small RNA-containing enterovirus of the picornavirus group (which includes the polio virus) (Fig. 14-20). The virus mainly replicates in hepatocytes, although gastrointestinal epithelial cells may also be infected. Infectious virus progeny are shed into the bile and are found in the feces. HAV is not directly cytopathic, and hepatic injury has been attributed to an immunologic reaction to virally infected hepatocytes.

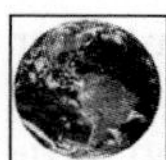

EPIDEMIOLOGY: The only reservoir for HAV is acutely infected people, so transmission depends primarily on serial transmission from person to person by the fecal–oral route. Epidemics of hepatitis A occur under crowded and unsanitary conditions, such as exist in warfare, or by fecal contamination of water and food. Edible shellfish in contaminated waters concentrate the virus and may transmit infection if they are not adequately cooked.

In the industrialized countries, which have low rates of infection, most cases of hepatitis A are seen in older children and adults. By contrast, in less developed regions, where the disease is endemic, most of the population is infected before 10 years of age.

In the United States, about 10% of the population under 20 years show serologic evidence of previous HAV infection. ***This observation indicates that most HAV infections are anicteric.*** Hepatitis A is common in day care centers, international travelers and men who have sex with men. However, no source can be identified in about half of cases. Hepatitis A vaccination confers long-term protection against the disease. Universal vaccination programs have significantly reduced acute hepatitis A infection in the United States.

CLINICAL FEATURES: After an incubation period of 3 to 6 weeks (mean, about 4 weeks), HAV-infected patients develop nonspecific symptoms, including fever, malaise and anorexia. Concomitantly, liver injury is evidenced by a rise in serum aminotransferases (Fig. 14-21). As aminotransferases begin to decline, usually 5 to 10 days later, jaundice may appear. It remains evident for an average of 10 days but may persist for more than a month. Aminotransferase levels generally return to normal by the time jaundice has disappeared. ***Hepatitis A never becomes chronic. There is no carrier state, and infection provides lifelong immunity.*** Fulminant hepatitis is rarely seen, and virtually all patients recover without sequelae.

HAV is detectable in the liver about 2 weeks after infection, peaks in another 2 weeks and disappears shortly thereafter (Fig. 14-21). Fecal shedding of HAV follows its appearance in the liver by about a week and lasts for only a brief time. The period of viremia is also short, occurring early in the course of the disease.

IgM anti-HAV is the first detectable immune response to HAV and appears in the blood during the acute illness. Antibody titers begin to decline within a few weeks and generally disappear by 3 to 5 months. IgG anti-HAV appears as patients recover and persists for life. Finding IgM anti-HAV in the serum of a patient with acute hepatitis confirms HAV as the cause.

Hepatitis B Virus Is a Major Cause of Acute and Chronic Liver Disease

Hepatitis B virus (HBV) is a hepatotropic DNA virus that was the first of the so-called hepadnaviruses. The genomes of hepadnaviruses are among the smallest of all known viruses. The genome of HBV is one circular predominantly double-stranded DNA containing the entire genome, and a shorter complementary strand that varies from 50% to 85% of the length of the longer strand (Fig. 14-22). The virus particle is a

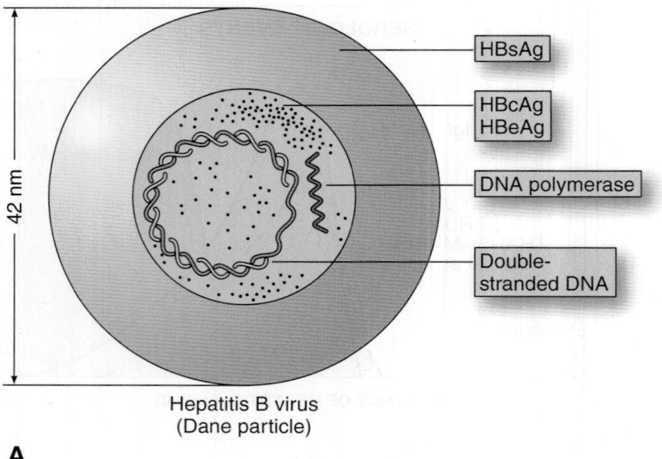

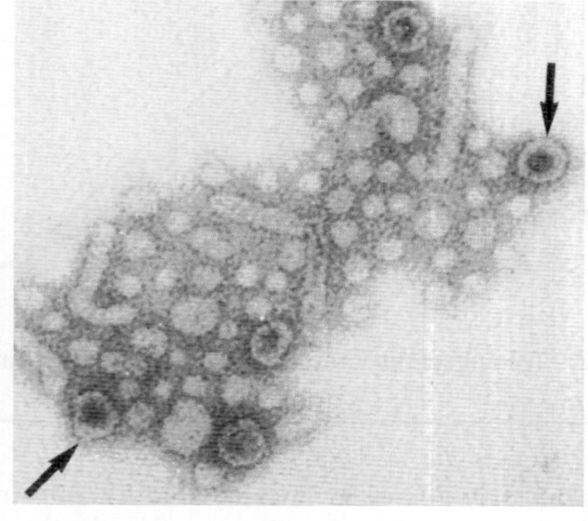

FIGURE 14-22. Hepatitis B virus. A. Schematic representation of the hepatitis B virus (HBV) and serum particles associated with HBV infection. (Antigens [Ag] for hepatitis B are indicated by their letters: c = core, e, and s = surface.) **B.** Electron micrograph of particles from centrifuged serum in a case of hepatitis. Rod-like and spherical particles containing HBsAg are evident. The complete virion, composed of the viral core and its surrounding envelope, is represented by Dane particles (*arrows*).

42-nm sphere (*Dane particle*) that contains the viral DNA. The HBV genome contains four genes:

- **Core (*C*) gene:** The core of the virus contains the **core antigen (HBcAg)** and the **e antigen (HBeAg),** both products of the *C* gene. The *C* gene includes two consecutive open reading frames, the precore and core regions. Transcription of the core frame alone yields HBcAg, whereas HBeAg is derived by proteolysis of the translation product of the entire *C* gene.
- **Surface gene:** The outer HBV coat contains **hepatitis B surface antigen (HBsAg).** HBsAg is synthesized by infected hepatocytes independently of the viral core, and vast amounts are secreted into the blood. This material is visualized by electron microscopy of centrifuged serum as two distinct particles (Fig. 14-22), one a 22-nm sphere and the other a tubular structure 22 nm in diameter and 40 to 400 nm in length. These particles are immunogenic but not infectious.
- **Polymerase gene:** The *P* gene encodes the viral DNA polymerase.
- ***X* gene:** The small X protein activates viral transcription and probably plays a role in the pathogenesis of hepatocellular carcinoma associated with chronic HBV infection.

The HBV replication cycle begins with attachment to host hepatocytes, followed by viral entry, uncoating and entry into the nucleus. Within the hepatocyte nucleus, the viral genome is converted into covalently closed circular DNA (cccDNA), which serves as a template for transcription of viral messenger RNA (mRNA). The persistent presence of cccDNA appears to inhibit HBV viral clearance from the host, even in the setting of potent antiviral pharmacotherapy.

There are six distinct serotypes (A through F) of HBV. Mutations are common, both in native infection and under the influence of pharmacotherapy. ***Precore mutant HBV results in a virus that does not express HBeAg, but whether this mutant has implications regarding prognosis is unclear.*** Antiviral treatment selects for HBV mutants at rates approaching 50% after 4 years of therapy. Newer nucleoside and nucleotide analogs are associated with lower rates of HBV mutation.

EPIDEMIOLOGY: It is estimated that there are more than 350 million chronic carriers of HBV in the world, constituting an enormous reservoir of infection (Fig. 14-23). Depending on the incidence of primary infection with HBV, the carrier rates of chronic infection vary from 0.3% (United States and western Europe) to 20% (Southeast Asia, sub-Saharan Africa, Oceania and the Pacific and Amazon basins). In endemic areas, high carrier rates are sustained by vertical transmission of the virus from a carrier mother to her newborn.

In the United States, between 500,000 and 1.5 million individuals are thought to be chronically infected HBV carriers, and 200,000 to 300,000 newly diagnosed cases of HBV occur annually. The availability of a protective vaccine has lowered the incidence of HBV in the United States from 10.7/100,000 in 1983 to 1.6/100,000 in 2006. Only one fourth of new cases present with jaundice. Fulminant hepatitis B causes 250 to 300 deaths per year in the United States. At one time, chronic HBV carriers were commonly sources of posttransfusion hepatitis, but routine screening for HBsAg has eliminated this threat.

The incidence of HBV chronicity is inversely proportional to the age at viral acquisition. In countries with high endemicity, the high chronicity rate is a result of vertical transmission and unsafe injection practices. In areas with lower endemicity, such as the United States, HBV transmission is most frequently horizontal. Whereas no more than 10% of adults infected with HBV become carriers, neonatal hepatitis B leads to persistent infection, as a rule. Males become carriers more often than females. In the United States, chronic HBV carriers are particularly common among male homosexuals and intravenous drug users.

Humans are the only significant reservoir of HBV. Unlike hepatitis A, HBV is not transmitted by the fecal–oral route, nor does it contaminate food and water supplies. ***Although HBsAg is found in most secretions, infectious virus has been demonstrated only in blood, saliva and semen.*** While direct transfer of blood products, by transfusion or sharing contaminated needles, was once thought to be the major route of

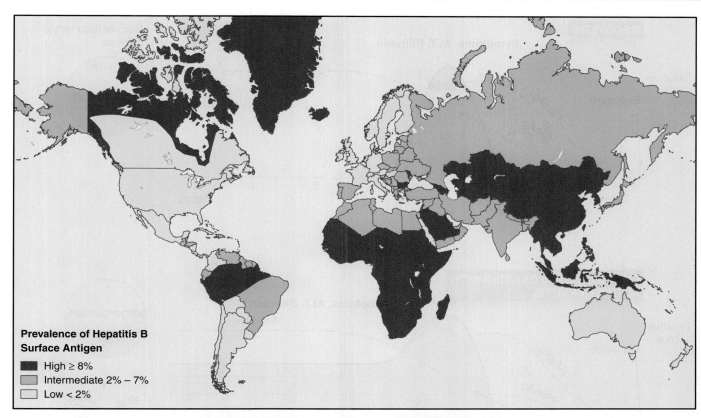

Prevalence of Hepatitis B Surface Antigen

High ≥ 8%

Intermediate 2% – 7%

Low < 2%

FIGURE 14-23. Geographic prevalence of hepatitis B infection.

transmission, it is now clear that most cases of hepatitis B are transmitted by intimate contact. Such contact transmission probably involves direct transfer of the virus through breaks in the skin or mucous membranes. In this respect, anal sexual contact is an important mode of transmission.

Synthetic vaccines for hepatitis B, composed of recombinant HBsAg or its immunogenic epitopes, are highly effective and confer lifelong immunity. In some regions where hepatitis B is endemic, vaccination has significantly reduced the prevalence of the disease. It is now routine in the United States. to administer the vaccine. Vaccination of infants is common in most nations (currently 177 of 193 countries).

MOLECULAR PATHOGENESIS: HBV is not directly cytopathic, as reflected in the fact that asymptomatic chronic carriers of the virus maintain a large burden of infectious virus in the liver for years without functional or biochemical evidence of liver cell injury. Cytotoxic ($CD8^+$) T lymphocytes (CTLs) that target multiple HBV epitopes cause most of the destruction of hepatocytes and consequent clinical liver disease. In conjunction with human leukocyte antigen (HLA) class I molecules, the target viral antigens are expressed on the surface of infected hepatocytes. In that location, they are recognized by $CD8^+$ CTLs, which in turn kill the infected hepatocytes.

The infectivity of blood from patients with chronic hepatitis B tends to decline with the duration of the disease. This is largely due to a decline in episomal (extrachromosomal) replication of infectious virions. The intact viral genome does not integrate into host DNA, but genomic fragments are progressively integrated, after which they produce several viral antigens. Thus, despite declining infectivity of the blood, chronic hepatitis tends to persist.

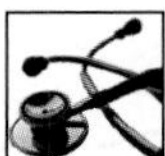

CLINICAL FEATURES: There are three well-recognized clinical courses associated with HBV infection (Fig. 14-24):

- Acute hepatitis
- Fulminant hepatitis
- Chronic hepatitis

ACUTE HEPATITIS B: Most adult patients have acute, self-limited hepatitis similar to that produced by HAV, usually followed by complete recovery and lifelong immunity. Symptoms of hepatitis B are, for the most part, similar to those of hepatitis A, although acute hepatitis B tends to be somewhat more severe and the incubation period is considerably longer. Typically, symptoms appear 2 to 3 months after exposure, but incubation periods may vary from under 6 weeks to 6 months. As in hepatitis A, many cases, including virtually all infections in infants and children, are anicteric and, therefore, not clinically apparent.

HBsAg is the first marker to appear in the serum of patients with acute hepatitis B. It is detected 1 week to 2 months after exposure (Fig. 14-24) and disappears from the blood during the convalescent phase in patients who recover rapidly. Simultaneously with, or shortly after, the disappearance of HBsAg,

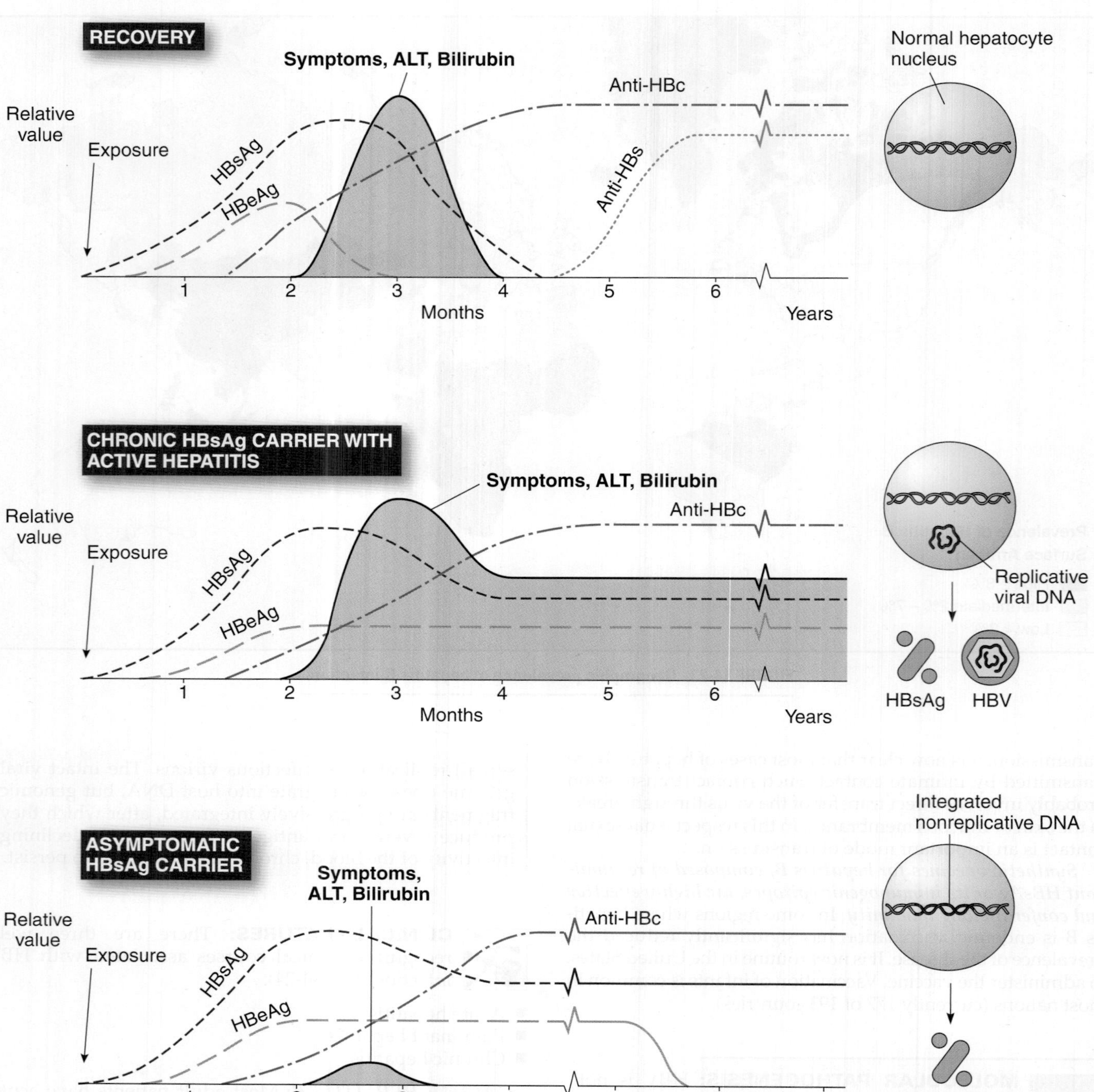

FIGURE 14-24. Typical serologic events in three distinct outcomes of hepatitis B. Top panel. In most cases, the appearance of antibody to hepatitis B surface antigen (HBsAg; anti-HBs) ensures complete recovery. Viral DNA disappears from the nucleus of the hepatocyte. **Middle panel.** In about 10% of cases of hepatitis B, HBs antigenemia is sustained for longer than 6 months, owing to the absence of anti-HBs. Patients in whom viral replication remains active, as evidenced by sustained high levels of HBeAg in the blood, develop active hepatitis. In such cases, the viral genome persists in the nucleus but is not integrated into host DNA. **Lower panel.** Patients in whom active viral replication ceases or is attenuated, as reflected in the disappearance of HBeAg from the blood, become asymptomatic carriers. In these individuals, fragments of the hepatitis B virus (HBV) genome are integrated into the host DNA, but episomal DNA is absent.

serum antibody to HBsAg (anti-HBs) is detectable. Its appearance heralds complete recovery, and its presence provides lifelong immunity.

HBcAg (core antigen) does not circulate in the serum of persons with acute hepatitis B, but antibody to HBcAg (anti-HBc) appears shortly after HBsAg. Antibody to HBcAg does not clear the virus or protect against reinfection, although it is a marker of a previous HBV infection.

HBeAg, the second circulating antigen to appear in hepatitis B, is seen before the onset of clinical disease and after the appearance of HBsAg. It generally disappears within about 2 weeks, while HBsAg is still present. The presence of HBeAg in the serum correlates with a period of intense viral replication and, hence, maximal infectivity of the patient. Anti-HBe appears shortly after the antigen disappears and is detectable for up to 2 or more years after the hepatitis resolves. A minor subset of patients who seroconvert to anti-HBe antibody and lose serum HBeAg have persistent HBV replication. The HBV viruses in these cases are replication competent but are unable to produce HBeAg because of mutations either in the precore region ("precore mutants") or the basic core promoter region of the HBV genome.

FULMINANT HEPATITIS B: More often than hepatitis A, but still only rarely, acute hepatitis B is a fulminant disease, with massive liver cell necrosis, hepatic failure and high mortality. Nucleoside and nucleotide analogs have improved outcomes for patients with fulminant hepatitis B, compared to historical controls. Individuals with fulminant acute hepatitis B can decompensate rapidly, with death caused primarily by cerebral edema, cardiopulmonary collapse or sepsis. Liver transplantation, when available, gives excellent patient survival.

CHRONIC HEPATITIS B: Chronic hepatitis is continued necrosis and inflammation in the liver for more than 6 months. Individuals with chronic HBV infection are at increased risk for cirrhosis and hepatocellular carcinoma. Men are at a higher risk than women. Other risk factors include age over 40 years, high levels of HBV viremia and certain viral determinants, such as genotypes C and F or a precore promoter mutation.

MOLECULAR PATHOGENESIS: Three phases of chronic HBV infection are widely accepted: (1) immune tolerant phase, (2) immune active phase and (3) inactive phase. A fourth, recovery, phase is not yet generally accepted. People chronically infected with HBV often progress temporally through these phases, but can revert backward as well.

1. **Immune tolerant phase:** Patients in the HBV immune tolerant phase are HBeAg positive, with very high HBV DNA levels (>20,000 IU/mL) and little significant hepatocellular inflammation or necrosis, as demonstrated by normal serum aminotransferase levels. This phase can persist for decades and is commonly seen in those people who acquired HBV infection vertically. Since HBV integrates into hepatocyte DNA, even patients in the immune tolerant phase are at increased risk of hepatocellular carcinoma.
2. **Immune active phase:** This phase is characterized by HBV viremia and liver cell necrosis (i.e., elevated serum aminotransferases). Portal-based inflammatory infiltrates and hepatocyte necrosis are seen. Those infected patients with detectable HBe tend to have higher levels of viremia than those who are HBe negative/anti-HBe positive. It is the immune active phase that provides the highest risk of significant liver injury, development of cirrhosis and hepatocellular carcinoma. This phase is the most frequent setting for initiation of pharmacologic antiviral therapy.
3. **Inactive phase:** In the inactive phase of chronic HBV infection, blood anti-HBe is seen but HBeAg is not, serum aminotransferases are normal and circulating HBV DNA (<2000 IU/mL) is low. This group, sometimes referred to as "healthy carriers," appear to have a very low risk of progression to cirrhosis or hepatocellular carcinoma. However, they may revert to the immune active phase, and so require long-term follow-up.

In some chronic HBV carriers, HBsAg–anti-HBs complexes circulate in the blood. Although these patients produce antibody, they do not clear the virus from the circulation. These immune complexes may lead to a variety of **extrahepatic** ailments, including a serum sickness–like syndrome (fever, rash, urticaria, acute arthritis), polyarteritis, glomerulonephritis and cryoglobulinemia. In fact, one third to one half of patients with polyarteritis nodosa are HBV carriers. As is discussed in detail under the heading of hepatocellular carcinoma, chronic hepatitis B is associated with a significant risk of liver cancer. ***The possible outcomes of infection with HBV are summarized in Figs. 14-24 and 14-25.***

Hepatitis D Virus Is a Defective RNA Virus

Assembly of hepatitis D virus (HDV) in the liver requires HBsAg to be present. Therefore, infection with HDV is limited to people who are also infected with HBV. The two

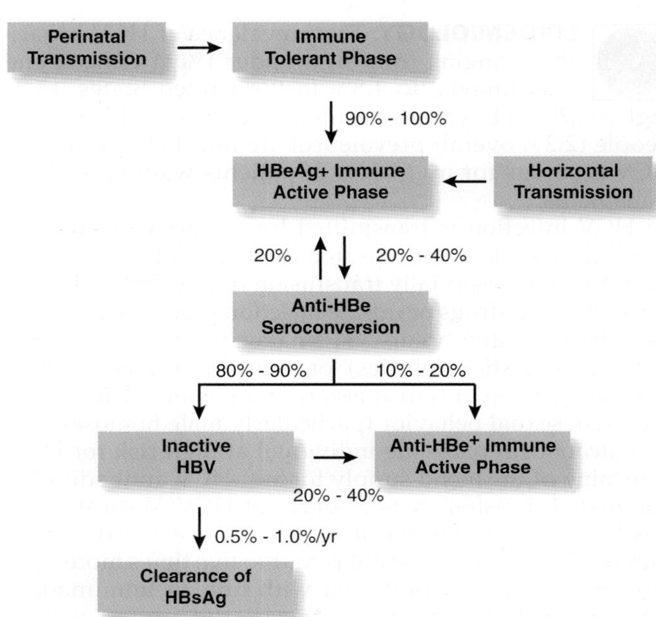

FIGURE 14-25. Possible outcomes of infection with the hepatitis B virus (HBV).

infections may be simultaneous (coinfection) or HDV infection may follow HBV infection (superinfection). HDV and HBsAg are cleared together, and the clinical course is usually similar to that for the usual acute hepatitis B. However, in some patients, coinfection with HDV leads to severe, fulminant and often fatal hepatitis, particularly in intravenous drug abusers. ***Superinfection of an HBV carrier with HDV typically increases the severity of an existing chronic hepatitis.*** In fact, 70% to 80% of HBsAg carriers superinfected with HDV develop chronic hepatitis. Since the discovery of HDV in Turin, Italy, in 1979, recognition of its natural history has led to a significant drop in HDV transmission. The virus remains a clinical problem especially in developing nations endemic for HBV.

Hepatitis C Virus Is a Common Cause of Chronic Hepatitis and Cirrhosis

Hepatitis C virus (HCV) is an enveloped flavivirus. Its single-stranded RNA genome of about 9600 bp encodes one mRNA. This mRNA is translated into a polyprotein of about 3000 amino acids, which is cleaved into three structural proteins (one core and two envelope proteins) and six nonstructural proteins. Short untranslated regions at the end of the genome are required for replication.

The virus is genetically unstable, which leads to multiple genotypes and subtypes. Six different but related HCV genotypes are recognized. Types 1, 2 and 3 are the most common (about 75% in the United States and western Europe). Genotypes 2 and 3 respond better to antiviral therapy than type 1. In an individual patient, many mutant HCV strains arise, which likely accounts for several features of infection, including (1) the inability of anti-HCV IgG antibodies to clear the infection, (2) persistent and relapsing infection in the chronic hepatitis phase and (3) lack of progress in developing a vaccine.

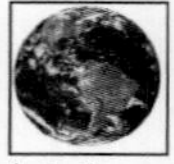

EPIDEMIOLOGY: The prevalence of HCV is variable, ranging from well under 1% in Canada and Scandinavia, to 1.8% in the United States, to as high as 22% in Egypt. It is estimated that some 170 million people (2.2% overall prevalence) are infected worldwide. HCV accounts for up to 50% of patients waiting for liver transplants.

HCV infection is transmitted by contact with infected blood through large or repeated direct percutaneous exposures to blood, especially transfusion from infected donors, use of injected drugs or unsafe injection practices. Less-efficient transmission occurs via smaller percutaneous exposures (needlestick injuries) or mucosal routes such as vertical and sexual transmission. Intravenous drug abuse, high-risk sexual behavior (particularly male homosexuals) and alcoholism place the individual at high risk for HCV. Screening of the blood supply for anti-HCV antibodies has eliminated transfusion as a source of HCV. Vertical transmission, from an infected mother to her newborn baby, is infrequent (2.7% to 8.4%) but is four to five times more common if women are coinfected with human immunodeficiency virus (HIV). Unsafe injection practices are recognized as a significant cause of HCV transmission in some countries. A minority of cases occur in the absence of known risk factors.

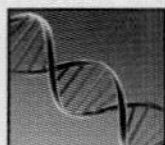

MOLECULAR PATHOGENESIS: HCV is not directly cytopathic, and many chronic HCV carriers have no evidence of liver cell injury. Despite active humoral and cellular immune responses against all viral proteins, most patients show persistent viremia. ***Liver cell injury has been attributed to cytotoxic T-cell responses to virus-infected hepatocytes.*** The mechanisms by which HCV persists are unknown. In addition to mutational escape, defects in HCV-specific cellular immunity have been described.

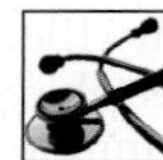

CLINICAL FEATURES: The incubation period of hepatitis C is similar to that of hepatitis B, and serum aminotransferases (Fig. 14-26) usually rise within 4 to 12 weeks of exposure (range, 2 to 26 weeks). HCV RNA can be detected in the serum by polymerase chain reaction (PCR) within 1 to 3 weeks of infection. Anti-HCV antibodies usually appear 7 to 8 weeks after HCV infection and persist during the chronic phase of infection. Acute hepatitis C is surprisingly mild, or asymptomatic, in the large majority of infected individuals: only about 10% to 20% of patients develop jaundice. Around 20% of these patients clear the virus spontaneously. Persistent viremia is lower in patients who present with jaundice and higher in those who acquire the virus as a

ACUTE RESOLVING HEPATITIS C

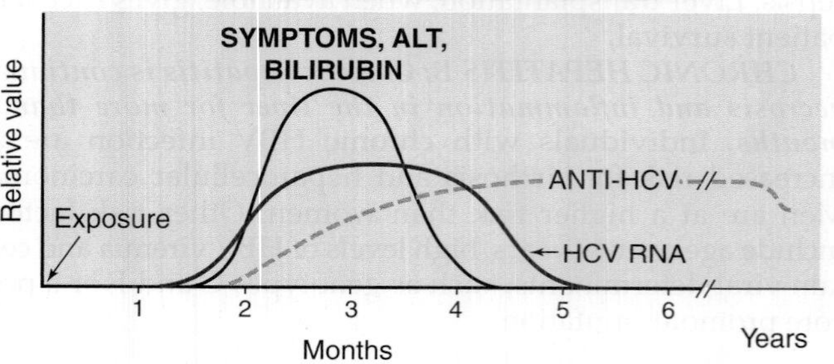

CHRONIC HEPATITIS C

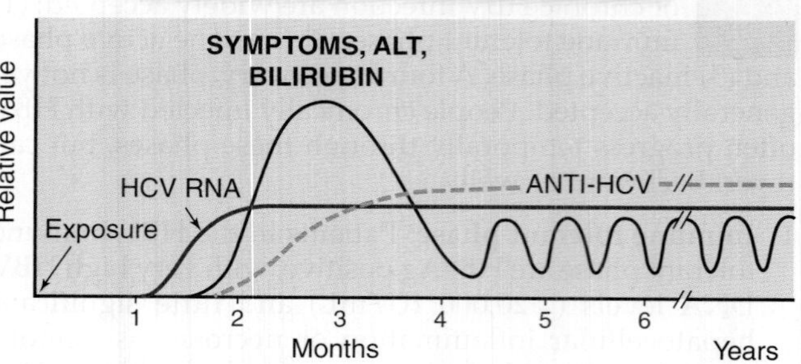

FIGURE 14-26. Clinical course of hepatitis C. Typical serologic events in two distinct outcomes. **Top panel.** About 20% of the patients with acute hepatitis C have a self-limited infection that resolves in a few months. Anti-HCV appears at the end of the clinical course and persists. **Bottom panel.** The remaining patients with hepatitis C develop chronic illness, with exacerbations and remissions of clinical symptoms. The development of anti-HCV does not affect the clinical outcome. Chronic hepatitis often eventuates in cirrhosis. ALT = alanine aminotransferase.

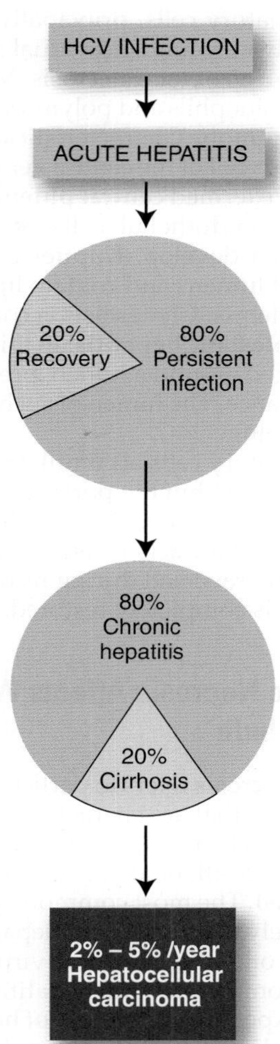

FIGURE 14-27. Possible outcomes of infection with the hepatitis C virus (HCV).

result of intravenous drug use. Fulminant hepatitis, if it occurs at all, is rare.

The most important consequences of infection with HCV relate to chronic disease. Despite complete recovery from clinical and biochemical acute liver disease, at least 80% or more patients develop chronic disease (Fig. 14-27). Cirrhosis develops in 15% to 20% of patients chronically infected with HCV for 10 to 30 years. The risk of cirrhosis is greater in males, older people, alcoholics and those who are also infected with HIV or HBV. Even in the absence of elevated aminotransferases or significant risk factors for progression, patients can present with significant fibrosis and even cirrhosis. Liver biopsy remains an important method of estimating the risk of clinical progression.

Chronic hepatitis ensues in 50% to 80% of infected people. The disease in most patients is mild for at least 10 years, and in many cases for 20 or more years. Importantly, some 20% of patients with chronic hepatitis C eventually develop cirrhosis. ***In patients with well-established cirrhosis, up to 5% develop primary hepatocellular carcinoma per year.***

Liver disease in patients with chronic HCV infection tends to be more severe in the face of concurrent hepatitis B, alcoholic liver disease, hemochromatosis or α_1-antitrypsin deficiency. About 25% of patients with advanced alcoholic liver disease have antibodies to HCV, although rates vary in different locales. The relationship is unexplained, and it is possible that HCV actually accounts for a proportion of cases otherwise classified as alcoholic cirrhosis.

Extrahepatic manifestations of hepatitis C are well recognized. The strongest association is for mixed cryoglobulinemia, a systemic vasculitis caused by deposition of circulating immune complexes in the microvasculature. Organs that can be involved by cryoglobulinemia include the skin (leukocytoclastic vasculitis), salivary glands (sicca syndrome), nervous system (mononeuritis multiplex) and kidney (membranoproliferative glomerulonephritis). B-cell non-Hodgkin lymphomas are more common in patients with chronic hepatitis C.

Because it is largely asymptomatic, acute HCV does not often come to medical attention. For patients who are treated for acute HCV, success rates are higher than in chronic cases. Chronic hepatitis C is generally treated with a combination of injected interferon-α and oral ribavirin. Using such a regimen, 40% to 50% of patients with genotype 1 and 75% to 80% with genotypes 2 or 3 achieve sustained clearance of HCV viremia.

Table 14-3 compares the major features of the common forms of viral hepatitis.

Table 14-3

Comparative Features of the Common Forms of Viral Hepatitis

	Hepatitis A	Hepatitis B	Hepatitis C
Genome	RNA	DNA	RNA
Incubation period	3–6 weeks	6 weeks–6 months	7–8 weeks
Transmission	Oral	Parenteral	Parenteral
Blood	No	Yes	Yes
Feces	Yes	No	No
Vertical	No	Yes	5%
Fulminant	Very rare	Yes	Rare hepatic necrosis
Chronic hepatitis	No	10%	80%
Carrier state	No	Yes	Yes
Liver cancer	No	Yes	Yes

Hepatitis E Virus Is a Major Cause of Epidemic Hepatitis in Poor Countries

Hepatitis E is a self-limited, acute, icteric disease similar to hepatitis A. Hepatitis E virus (HEV) is an enteric RNA virus of the Hepeviridae family, four genotypes of which are now known. HEV accounts for more than half of cases of acute viral hepatitis in young to middle-aged people in poor regions of the world. Large outbreaks have been reported in India, Nepal, Burma, Pakistan, the former Soviet Union, Africa and Mexico. Most of these epidemics have followed heavy rains in areas with inadequate sewage disposal. HEV infection may be transmitted via several routes: waterborne, zoonotic (especially consumption of raw or undercooked meat of infected wild animals such as pig, boar or deer), parenteral and vertical transmission. HEV closely resembles a swine virus, suggesting that the latter may represent a reservoir of infection.

The average incubation period for HEV is 35 to 40 days. Jaundice, hepatomegaly, fever and arthralgias are common and usually resolve within 6 weeks. Mortality ranges from 1% to 12%. Like hepatitis A, clinical illness from hepatitis E is far more common in adults than in children, suggesting that the latter infection is often subclinical. The disease is especially dangerous in pregnant women, where reported mortality may be as high as 20% to 40%. No chronic disease or carrier state has been identified in immunocompetent patients, but chronic hepatitis has been reported in solid organ transplant recipients. A successful vaccine against HEV infection has been developed and tested in Nepal, but is not yet licensed in the United States.

Pathology of Viral Hepatitis

All Forms of Acute Viral Hepatitis Are Pathologically Similar

The hallmark of acute viral hepatitis is liver cell death (Fig. 14-28). Within the hepatic lobule, scattered necrosis of single cells or of small clusters of hepatocytes is seen. A few apoptotic liver cells appear as small, deeply eosinophilic bodies **(Councilman or acidophilic bodies),** sometimes with pyknotic nuclei (apoptotic cells). Although acidophilic bodies are characteristic of viral hepatitis, they are also seen in many other liver diseases. In acute viral hepatitis, many liver cells show varying degrees of hydropic swelling and differences in size, shape and staining. Concomitantly, regenerative liver cells that display a larger nucleus and expanded basophilic cytoplasm are also seen. Resulting irregular liver cell plates are described as **lobular disarray.**

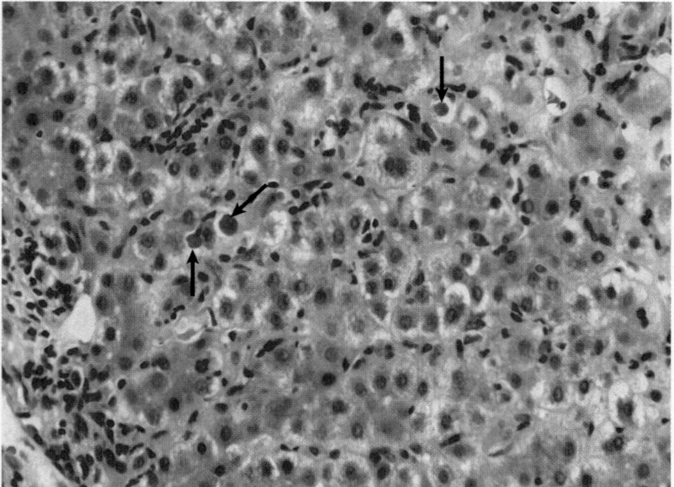

FIGURE 14-28. Acute viral hepatitis. A photomicrograph shows disarray of liver cell plates, swollen (ballooned) hepatocytes and an infiltrate of lymphocytes and scattered mononuclear inflammatory cells. The remnants of necrotic hepatocytes have been extruded into the sinusoids, where they appear as acidophilic, or Councilman, bodies (*arrows*).

Chronic inflammatory cells, principally lymphoid, infiltrate lobules diffusely, surround individual necrotic liver cells and accumulate in areas of focal necrosis. Macrophages may be prominent and eosinophils and polymorphonuclear leukocytes are not uncommon. Characteristically, lymphocytes infiltrate between the wall of the central vein and the liver cell plates, an appearance termed **central phlebitis.** Swelling and proliferation of the endothelial cells of the central vein **(endophlebitis)** often develop. Kupffer cells are enlarged, project into sinusoid lumens and contain lipofuscin pigment and phagocytosed debris. Cholestasis is common and when severe is termed **cholestatic hepatitis.** In this situation, many liver cells are arranged around a lumen, presenting an acinar or glandular appearance. The lumen of such an "acinus" may contain a large bile plug.

Chronic inflammatory cells accumulate within the portal tracts. Lymphoid cells within the portal tracts may form follicles, particularly in hepatitis C. The limiting plate of hepatocytes around the portal tracts is usually intact. Pathologic changes are gradually reversed during recovery, and normal hepatic architecture is completely restored.

Confluent Hepatic Necrosis Affects Whole Regions of the Lobule

Confluent hepatic necrosis refers to particularly severe forms of acute viral hepatitis that are characterized by the death of numerous hepatocytes in a geographical distribution and, in extreme cases, by the death of almost all the liver cells **(massive hepatic necrosis).** The most common viral cause is acute hepatitis B; only rarely does confluent hepatic necrosis result from infection with other hepatotropic viruses. Importantly, the lesions are not confined to viral hepatitis but may also be encountered after exposure to a variety of hepatotoxic agents and in autoimmune hepatitis (see below). Unlike most common forms of acute viral hepatitis, in which liver cell necrosis appears to be random and patchy, confluent hepatic necrosis typically affects whole regions of the lobule. The lesions of confluent hepatic necrosis, in order of increasing severity, are bridging necrosis, submassive necrosis and massive necrosis.

BRIDGING NECROSIS: At the milder end of the spectrum of lesions that constitute confluent hepatic necrosis are bands of necrosis (bridging necrosis) that stretch between adjacent portal tracts, between adjacent central veins and between portal tracts and central veins (Fig. 14-29). The death of adjacent plates of hepatocytes results in collapse of the collagenous stroma to form bands of connective tissue, best visualized with a reticulin stain. When such bands encircle an area of liver cells, a nodular pattern, similar to that seen in cirrhosis, may be apparent.

SUBMASSIVE HEPATIC NECROSIS: This form of acute hepatitis defines an even more severe injury involving necrosis of entire lobules or groups of adjacent lobules. Clinically, these patients manifest severe hepatitis, which may rapidly proceed to hepatic failure, in which case the disease is classed clinically as **fulminant hepatitis.**

MASSIVE HEPATIC NECROSIS (ACUTE YELLOW ATROPHY): Massive hepatic necrosis, the most feared variant of acute viral hepatitis, is fortunately uncommon. It is a form of fulminant hepatitis that is almost invariably fatal. Grossly, the liver is shrunken to as little as 500 g (one third of normal weight). The capsule is wrinkled, and the mottled,

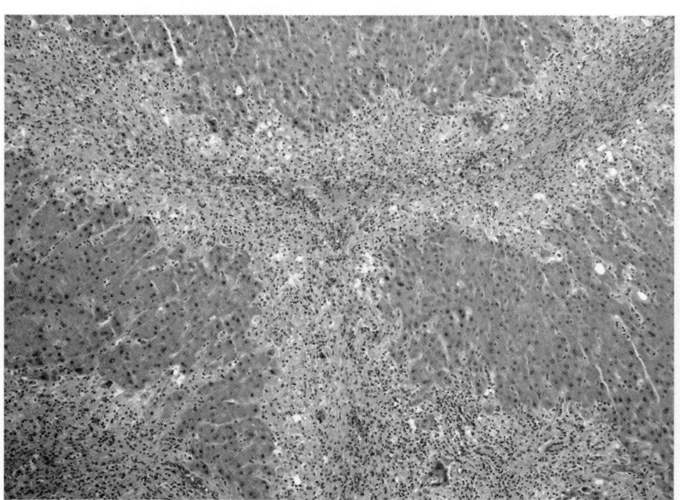

FIGURE 14-29. Confluent hepatic necrosis. Hemorrhagic zones of necrosis bridge adjacent central veins and portal tracts (bridging necrosis).

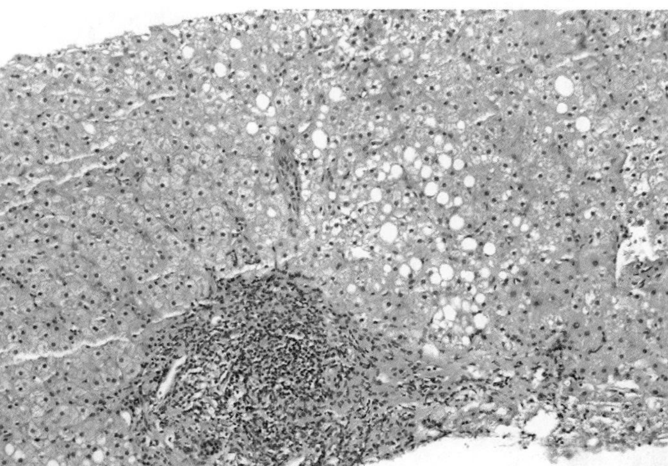

FIGURE 14-31. Mild chronic hepatitis. A photomicrograph shows a portal tract infiltrated by mononuclear inflammatory cells. The lobular parenchyma is intact. Mild fatty change often accompanies hepatitis C.

red-tan parenchyma is soft and flabby. Virtually all the hepatocytes are dead (Fig. 14-30), the hepatic lobules being represented only by the collagenous framework, which in many areas has collapsed. Macrophages, erythrocytes and necrotic debris fill sinusoids. For unknown reasons, the massive necrosis does not elicit a vigorous inflammatory response in either the parenchyma or the portal tracts. Liver transplantation is a mainstay of therapy.

Chronic Hepatitis May Be a Complication of Hepatitis B and C, As Well As Several Metabolic and Immune Disorders

The morphologic spectrum of chronic hepatitis ranges from mild, portal inflammation with little or no evidence of liver cell necrosis (Fig. 14-31) to a widespread inflammatory, necrotizing and fibrosing condition that often eventuates in cirrhosis (Fig. 14-32).

PORTAL TRACT LESIONS: In chronic hepatitis portal tracts are variably infiltrated by lymphocytes, plasma cells and macrophages (Figs. 14-31 and 14-32). These expanded portal tracts often display mild to severe proliferation of bile ductules, which is a nonspecific response to chronic liver injury. In the case of chronic hepatitis C, lymphoid aggregates or follicles with reactive centers are often present.

PIECEMEAL NECROSIS: This term refers to focal inflammatory destruction of the limiting plate of hepatocytes. A periportal chronic inflammatory infiltrate creates an irregular border between the portal tracts and the lobular parenchyma (Fig. 14-32A).

INTRALOBULAR LESIONS: Focal necrosis and inflammation within the parenchyma are typical of chronic hepatitis. Scattered acidophilic bodies, and enlarged Kupffer cells within sinusoids, are common (Fig. 14-28). In chronic hepatitis B, scattered hepatocytes may show large granular cytoplasm with abundant HBsAg **(ground-glass hepatocytes)** (Fig. 14-33).

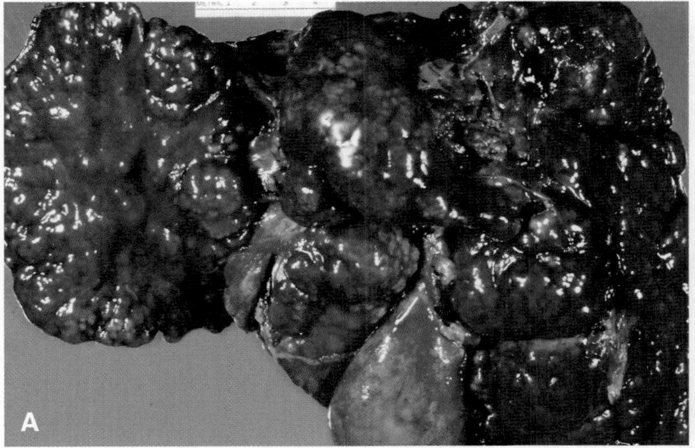

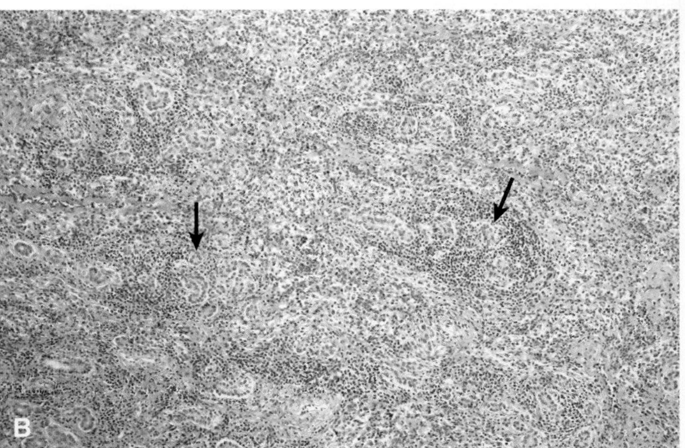

FIGURE 14-30. Massive hepatic necrosis. A. The liver is soft and reduced in size and shows a mottled, yellowish surface ("acute yellow atrophy"). **B.** A photomicrograph shows complete loss of the hepatocytes. The framework of the lobule has collapsed. The portal tracts (*arrows*) are expanded and contain proliferated bile ducts.

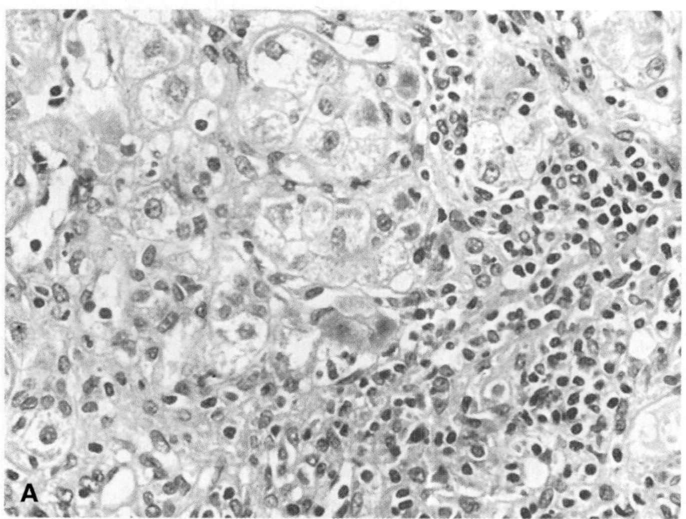

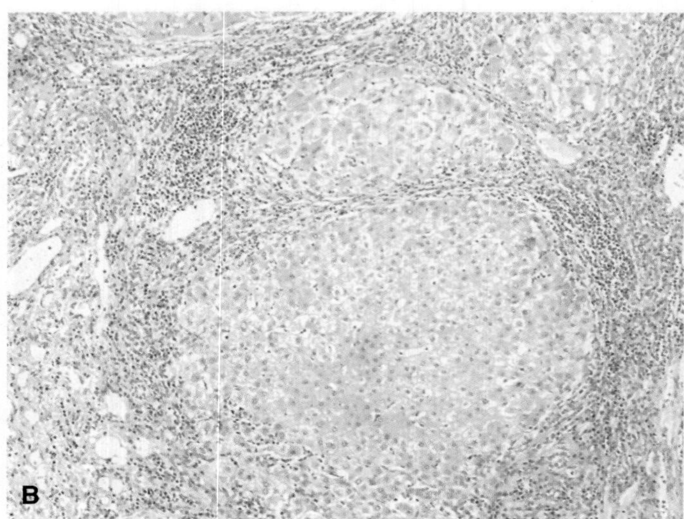

FIGURE 14-32. Severe chronic hepatitis. A. A photomicrograph discloses a mononuclear inflammatory infiltrate in an expanded portal tract (*lower right*). The inflammation penetrates the limiting plate and surrounds groups of hepatocytes at the border of the portal tract. **B. Chronic hepatitis with cirrhosis.** A photomicrograph of a liver biopsy from a patient with long-standing chronic hepatitis C shows bridging fibrosis and nodular transformation.

PERIPORTAL FIBROSIS: Progressive loss of periportal hepatocytes by piecemeal necrosis leads to deposition of collagen, which gives portal tracts a stellate (star-shaped) appearance. In time, the fibrosis may bridge to adjacent portal tracts or into the lobule itself toward the central vein, ultimately developing into cirrhosis (Fig. 14-32B).

Autoimmune Hepatitis

Autoimmune hepatitis is a severe type of chronic hepatitis of unknown cause that is associated with circulating autoantibodies and high levels of serum immunoglobulins. The disorder may appear at any age but occurs mainly in young women. Up to one third of patients are men, however. In the United States, autoimmune hepatitis affects up to 200,000 persons and accounts for 6% of liver transplants.

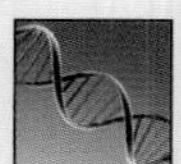

MOLECULAR PATHOGENESIS: Two types of autoimmune hepatitis are identified:

- **Type I** autoimmune hepatitis is the most common form of the disease (80% of cases) and features antinuclear and anti–smooth muscle antibodies. Some 70% of cases occur in women younger than 40 years, among whom one third have other autoimmune diseases, including thyroiditis, rheumatoid arthritis and ulcerative colitis. Importantly, a quarter of patients with type I autoimmune hepatitis

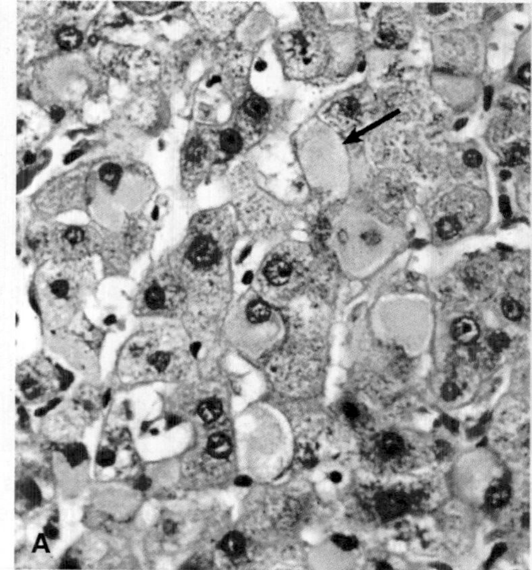

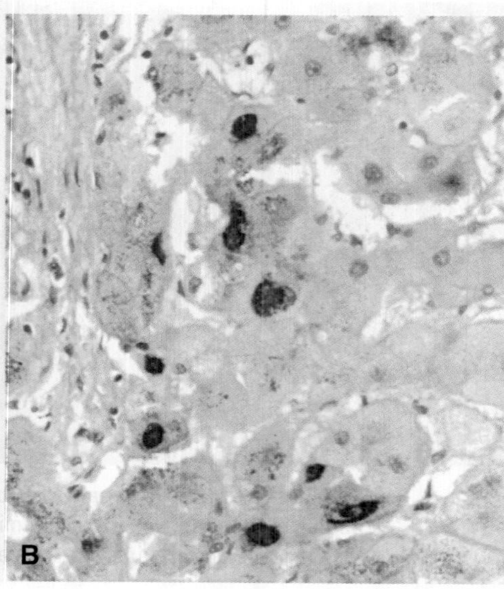

FIGURE 14-33. "Ground-glass" hepatocytes. A. A photomicrograph of liver from a patient with chronic hepatitis B shows scattered hepatocytes (*arrow*) with an abundant granular cytoplasm containing hepatitis B surface antigen (HBsAg). **B.** The same specimen has been stained for HBsAg by the immunoperoxidase method. The abundant cytoplasmic HBsAg appears brown.

present with cirrhosis, indicating that the disease usually has a prolonged asymptomatic course. Antibodies to numerous cytosolic enzymes are described, but the hepatocyte membrane asialoglycoprotein receptor is the leading candidate target for antibody-dependent cell-mediated cytotoxicity. Susceptibility to type I autoimmune hepatitis resides mainly within the HLA-*DRB1* gene. A minority of patients present with a poorly characterized "overlap syndrome" with mixed clinical and histologic features of autoimmune hepatitis and either primary biliary cirrhosis or primary sclerosing cholangitis.

- **Type II** autoimmune hepatitis occurs principally in children aged 2 to 14 years and is recognized by the presence of antibody to liver and kidney microsomes (anti-LKM). However, the target autoantigen is a P450-type drug-metabolizing enzyme (CYP 2D6). Patients often have other autoimmune diseases, especially type I diabetes and thyroiditis. The genetic background for type II autoimmune hepatitis is less well defined than for type I.

PATHOLOGY: Autoimmune hepatitis basically resembles acute and chronic viral hepatitis histologically, although lobular inflammation and necrosis tend to be more pronounced. An inflammatory infiltrate rich in plasma cells is an important diagnostic feature. Confluent hepatic necrosis may be seen in severe acute cases.

CLINICAL FEATURES: Autoimmune hepatitis is more common in women and can present insidiously. A personal or family history of autoimmunity is often elicited. Fatigue and mild right upper quadrant abdominal discomfort are common. Eventually, serum aminotransferase levels (e.g., aspartate aminotransferase [AST], alanine aminotransferase [ALT]) can become markedly elevated, occasionally exceeding 1000 IU/mL. Pronounced hyperglobulinemia is characteristic. In severe cases, jaundice, hepatic synthetic dysfunction and even liver failure may ensue. A fulminant presentation is occasionally observed. If the syndrome remains untreated, autoimmune hepatitis often progresses to cirrhosis.

Autoimmune hepatitis usually responds to therapy with corticosteroids, particularly when combined with immunosuppressive drugs, usually azathioprine. Liver transplantation is an option for patients whose disease progresses to end-stage cirrhosis. The disease recurs in up to 20% of patients after liver transplantation. De novo autoimmune hepatitis occurs rarely in patients having undergone liver transplantation for other diseases.

Alcoholic Liver Disease

The harmful effects of excess alcohol (ethanol, ethyl alcohol) consumption have been recognized since the early days of recorded history. The prophet Isaiah warned, "Woe to him that is mighty to drink wine." Although early investigators confused alcoholic liver injury with the effects of malnutrition, ethanol per se is now seen as a hepatotoxin that acts both directly and indirectly.

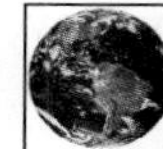

EPIDEMIOLOGY: ***The cirrhosis is most prevalent in countries with the highest per capita consumption of alcohol***, regardless of the specific preferred beverage (e.g., wine in France, beer in Australia, spirits in Scandinavia). Although only a minority of chronic alcoholics develop cirrhosis, a dose-response relationship between lifetime dose of alcohol (duration of exposure and daily amount of alcohol consumed) and the appearance of cirrhosis has been established.

About 10% of the adult male population in the United States abuse alcohol. In some other countries, this figure is considerably higher. ***About 15% of alcoholics develop cirrhosis, and many of these people die in hepatic failure or from extrahepatic complications of cirrhosis.*** In fact, in many urban areas of the United States with high alcoholism rates, cirrhosis of the liver is the third or fourth leading cause of death in men younger than 45 years.

The amount of alcohol required to produce chronic liver disease depends on body size, age, gender and ethnicity, but the lower range seems to be about 20 g/day (approximately 2 ounces of 86 proof [43%] whiskey, two glasses of wine, or two 12-ounce bottles of beer daily) for women and 40 g/day in men; in general, over 10 years of alcohol use at this level is required to produce cirrhosis, although a few cirrhotic patients give shorter histories of heavy alcohol use.

Women are predisposed to the deleterious effects of alcohol. The reasons for the greater sensitivity in women are unknown but may relate to their different rates of ethanol metabolism compared to men and lower body mass index.

The epidemiology of alcoholic liver disease has recently been complicated by the discovery of its association with hepatotropic viruses. The prevalence of serum HBV markers is two- to fourfold higher in alcoholics than in control populations. The prevalence of anti-HCV antibodies is up to 10% among alcoholics, and is considerably higher among alcoholics with chronic liver disease. As noted above, patients who consume alcohol and also have hepatitis C are more likely to develop liver disease than their counterparts not infected with hepatitis C.

Ethanol Is Mainly Metabolized in the Liver

Ethanol is rapidly absorbed from the stomach and eventually distributed in body water space. Between 5% and 10% is excreted unchanged, mostly in the urine and expired breath. The remainder, over 90% of that consumed, is metabolized by the liver to acetaldehyde and acetate, largely by cytosolic **alcohol dehydrogenase (ADH).** The **microsomal ethanol-oxidizing system** in the smooth endoplasmic reticulum, which is a mixed-function oxidase, is a minor metabolic pathway for alcohol. Unlike most drugs, clearance of alcohol from the body is linear—that is, a fixed quantity is metabolized per unit time. Roughly, for the average man, 7 to 10 g of alcohol is eliminated per hour. However, as the microsomal pathway of ethanol metabolism is upregulated in chronic alcoholics, these people metabolize ethanol more rapidly, provided that they do not suffer from active liver disease.

Alcohol Consumption Causes a Spectrum of Liver Diseases

Alcoholic liver disease spans three major morphologic and clinical entities: **fatty liver, acute alcoholic hepatitis** and **cirrhosis.**

Although these lesions usually occur sequentially, they may coexist in any combination and may actually be independent entities.

Fatty Liver

MOLECULAR PATHOGENESIS: Virtually all chronic alcoholics, regardless of their pattern of drinking, accumulate fat in hepatocytes **(steatosis).** The pathogenesis of fatty liver is not precisely understood, and relative contributions of different pathways may depend on the amount of alcohol consumed, dietary lipid content, body stores of fat, hormonal status and other variables. ***Nevertheless, accumulation of fat clearly depends on alcohol intake, since it is fully and rapidly reversible if alcohol ingestion stops.***

Dietary fat, in the form of chylomicrons and free fatty acids, is transported to the liver, where it is taken up by hepatocytes. Triglycerides are then hydrolyzed to free fatty acids. These, in turn, undergo β-oxidation in the mitochondria or are converted to triglycerides in the endoplasmic reticulum. The newly synthesized triglycerides are secreted as lipoproteins or are retained for storage.

Most of the fat deposited in the liver after chronic alcohol consumption is derived from the diet. Ethanol increases lipolysis and thus delivery of free fatty acids to the liver. Within hepatocytes, ethanol (1) increases fatty acid synthesis, (2) decreases mitochondrial oxidation of fatty acids, (3) increases production of triglycerides and (4) impairs release of lipoproteins. Collectively, these metabolic consequences produce a fatty liver.

PATHOLOGY: In the setting of high alcohol intake, the liver becomes yellow and enlarged, sometimes massively, to as much as three times normal weight. The increased weight does not reflect fat accumulation alone, since protein and water content also increase. Microscopically, the extent of visible fat accumulation varies from minute droplets scattered in the cytoplasm of a few hepatocytes to distention of the entire cytoplasm of most cells by coalesced droplets (Fig. 14-34). In the latter situation, liver cells are barely recognizable as such and resemble adipocytes with their cytoplasm distended by a clear area and their nuclei flattened and displaced to the periphery of the cell.

The ultrastructural appearance of hepatocytes in alcohol-induced fatty liver reflects the cytotoxicity of ethanol rather than an effect of fat per se. Mitochondria are enlarged, with occasional bizarre giant forms. The smooth endoplasmic reticulum is hyperplastic, resembling that produced by other inducers of microsomal drug-metabolizing enzymes (see Chapter 1).

The ultrastructural changes in mitochondria and endoplasmic reticulum produced by chronic ethanol ingestion are paralleled by functional alterations. Hepatic mitochondria show decreased rates of substrate oxidation (e.g., of fatty acids) and impaired adenosine triphosphate (ATP) formation. Hyperplasia of the smooth endoplasmic reticulum is accompanied by increased activity of the cytochrome P450–dependent mixed-function oxidases. Not only is the microsomal ethanol-oxidizing system induced, but the metabolism of a variety of drugs is also enhanced. ***The increased microsomal function also augments metabolism of hepatic toxins, thus exaggerating the danger of agents such as acetaminophen.*** In contrast to chronic alcohol consumption, which promotes microsomal functions, the presence of ethanol after acute alcohol ingestion inhibits mixed-function oxidases and acutely reduces the rate of clearance of drugs from the body.

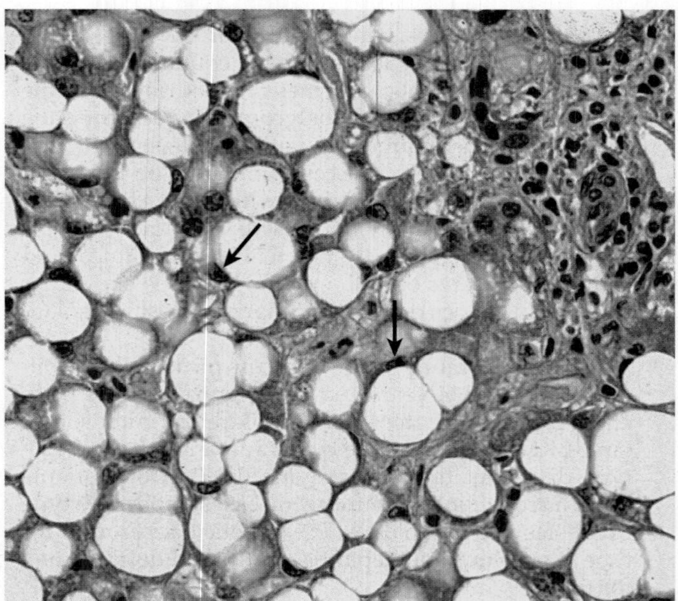

FIGURE 14-34. Alcoholic fatty liver. A photomicrograph shows the cytoplasm of almost all the hepatocytes distended by fat that displaces the nucleus to the periphery (*arrows*).

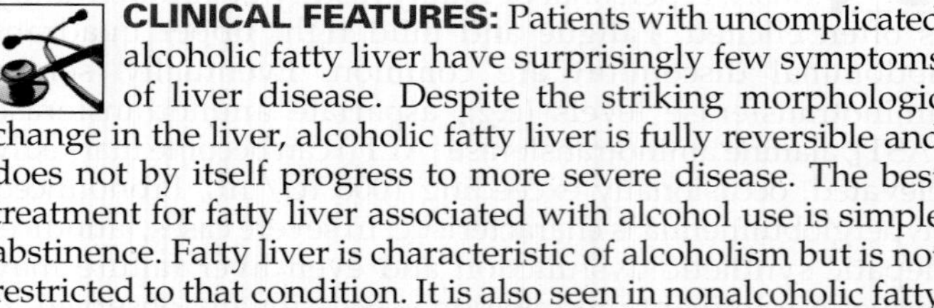

CLINICAL FEATURES: Patients with uncomplicated alcoholic fatty liver have surprisingly few symptoms of liver disease. Despite the striking morphologic change in the liver, alcoholic fatty liver is fully reversible and does not by itself progress to more severe disease. The best treatment for fatty liver associated with alcohol use is simple abstinence. Fatty liver is characteristic of alcoholism but is not restricted to that condition. It is also seen in nonalcoholic fatty liver disease (see below), in hepatitis C, following administration of certain drugs and in many other conditions.

Alcoholic Hepatitis

Alcoholic hepatitis is characterized by (1) necrosis of hepatocytes, predominantly in the central zone; (2) cytoplasmic hyaline inclusions within hepatocytes (Mallory bodies); (3) a neutrophilic inflammatory infiltrate in the lobule; and (4) perivenular fibrosis (Fig. 14-35). **The pathogenesis of alcoholic hepatitis is a mystery.** Alcoholics may have mild fatty liver for many years and, without any change in drinking habits, suddenly develop acute alcoholic hepatitis. It may be that long-standing, subclinical alcoholic hepatitis precedes clinically overt hepatitis. Nevertheless, the often explosive presentation of alcoholic hepatitis suggests that an environmental or physiologic cofactor may be involved, although none has been forthcoming.

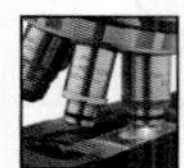

PATHOLOGY: Typically, hepatic architecture is intact, with portal tracts situated normally with relation to central venules. Hepatocytes show variable hydropic swelling, which gives them a heterogeneous appearance. Isolated necrotic liver cells or clusters of them have pyknotic nuclei and show karyorrhexis. Scattered hepatocytes contain **Mallory bodies (alcoholic hyaline)** (Fig. 14-35). These cytoplasmic inclusions are more common in visibly damaged, swollen hepatocytes and appear as irregular skeins of eosinophilic material or as solid eosinophilic masses, often perinuclearly. Ultrastructurally, they are aggregates of intermediate (cytokeratin) filaments (Fig. 14-35C). The damaged, ballooned hepatocytes, particularly those with Mallory bodies, are surrounded by neutrophils, and a more diffuse, intralobular inflammatory infiltrate is also present. Mild to severe cholestasis is present in up to one third of cases. Alcoholic hepatitis is usually superimposed on an existing fatty liver, although there is no evidence that fat accumulation predisposes or contributes to development of alcoholic hepatitis.

Collagen deposition is always seen in alcoholic hepatitis, especially around central veins (terminal hepatic venules). Chronic alcohol exposure activates hepatic stellate cells (Ito cells) to deposit intrasinusoidal collagen. In severe cases, the venule and perivenular sinusoids are obliterated and surrounded by dense fibrous tissue to yield **central hyaline sclerosis** (Figs. 14-35 and 14-36). Central hyaline sclerosis is often associated with noncirrhotic portal hypertension.

Portal tracts in alcoholic hepatitis are highly variable. Some are virtually normal, whereas others are enlarged and contain a mononuclear infiltrate and proliferated bile ductules. The altered portal tracts often display spurs of fibrous tissue that penetrate the lobules.

CLINICAL FEATURES: Patients with alcoholic hepatitis have malaise and anorexia, fever, right upper quadrant abdominal pain and jaundice. Leukocytosis is common. Levels of serum aminotransferases, particularly aspartate aminotransferase, are moderately elevated, but not to the levels often noted in viral hepatitis. Accordingly, AST usually remains under 400; the AST:ALT ratio is typically 2:1. Serum alkaline phosphatase is usually increased. In severe cases, the prothrombin time may be prolonged, which is associated with an ominous prognosis.

The prognosis in patients with alcoholic hepatitis reflects the severity of liver cell injury. In some patients, the disease progresses rapidly to hepatic failure and death. The mortality in the acute stage of alcoholic hepatitis is about 10%. Among those who abstain from alcohol after recovery from

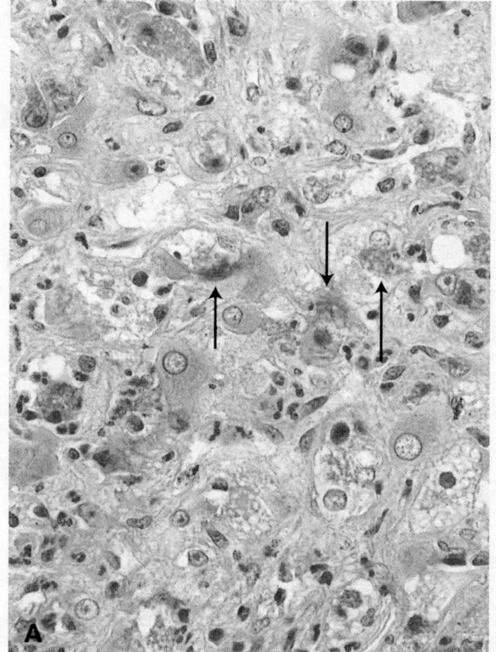

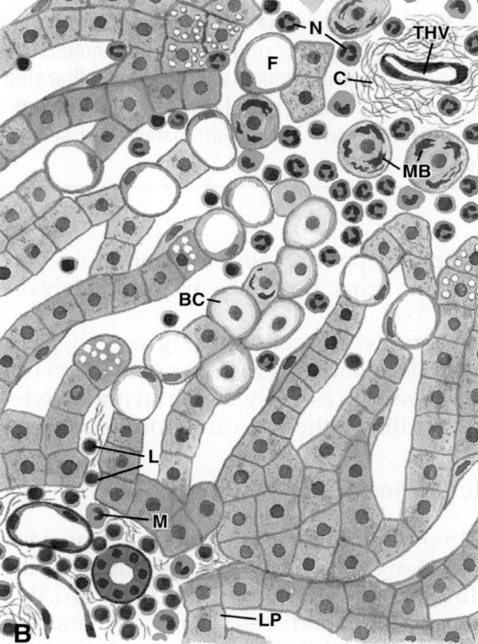

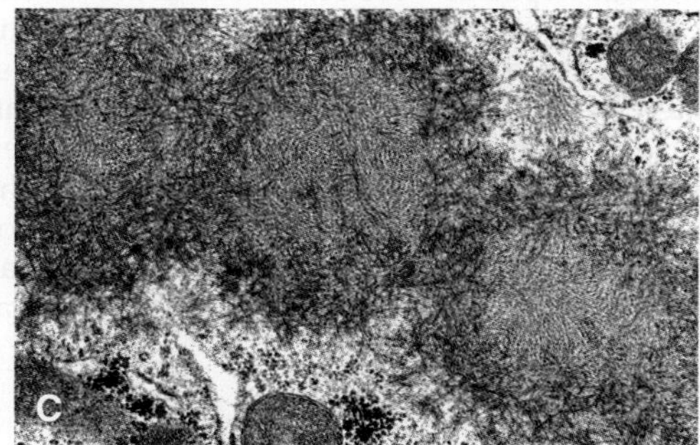

FIGURE 14-35. Alcoholic hepatitis. A. A photomicrograph shows necrosis and degeneration of hepatocytes, Mallory bodies (eosinophilic inclusions) in the cytoplasm of injured hepatocytes (*arrows*) and infiltration by neutrophils. **B. Schematic representation of the major pathologic features of alcoholic hepatitis.** The lesions are predominantly centrilobular and include necrosis and loss of hepatocytes, ballooned cells (*BC*) and Mallory bodies (*MB*) in the cytoplasm of damaged hepatocytes. The inflammatory infiltrate consists predominantly of neutrophils (*N*), although a few lymphocytes (*L*) and macrophages (*M*) are also present. The central vein, or terminal hepatic venule (*THV*), is encased in connective tissue (*C*) (central sclerosis; also see Fig. 14-36). Fat-laden hepatocytes (*F*) are evident in the lobule. The portal tract displays moderate chronic inflammation, and the limiting plate (*LP*) is focally breached. **C. Ultrastructure of Mallory bodies.** Dense, interwoven bundles of cytokeratin filaments are in the cytoplasm of hepatocytes.

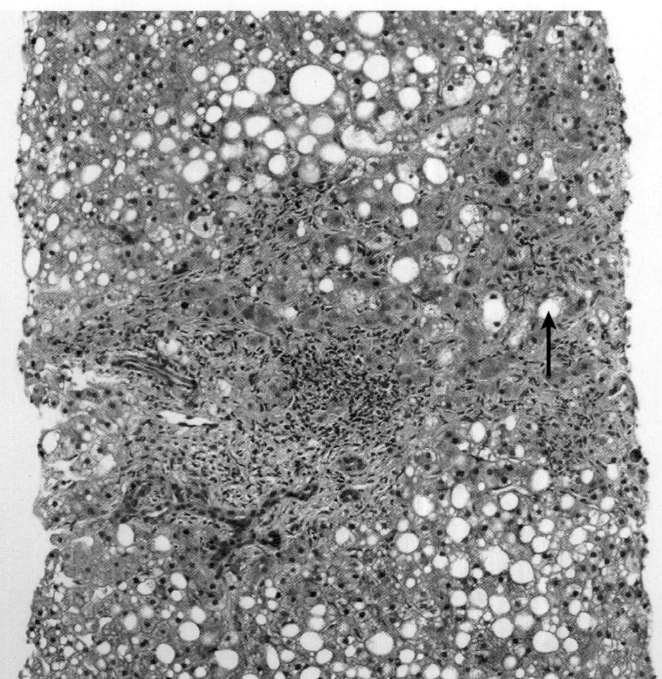

FIGURE 14-36. Central hyaline sclerosis. This photomicrograph (trichrome stain) from the liver of a patient with nonalcoholic steatohepatitis shows the central terminal venule to be obliterated by fibrous tissue (*blue*). An expanded portal tract is on the left. Note the macrovesicular fat (*arrow*). This lesion mimics that seen in alcoholic liver disease.

acute alcoholic hepatitis, most recover. However, of those who continue to drink, up to 70% may ultimately develop cirrhosis.

Corticosteroids are commonly given to patients with severe alcoholic hepatitis, if there is no infection or renal failure, as they have been associated with an improved short-term mortality. Nutritional therapy can improve patient outcome.

Alcoholic Cirrhosis

In about 15% of alcoholics, hepatocellular necrosis, fibrosis and regeneration eventually lead to formation of fibrous septa surrounding hepatocellular nodules (Fig. 14-13). The other lesions of alcoholic liver disease—fatty liver and acute or persistent alcoholic hepatitis—are often seen in conjunction with cirrhosis, and some believe that progression to alcoholic cirrhosis requires at least subclinical alcoholic hepatitis. A role for activated hepatic stellate cells as producers of intrasinusoidal collagen probably contributes to the pathogenesis of cirrhosis. The prognosis in cases of established alcoholic cirrhosis is considerably better in those who abstain from alcohol. Nevertheless, many patients progress to end-stage liver disease, and alcoholic liver disease is a common indication for liver transplantation.

Nonalcoholic Fatty Liver Disease

Nonalcoholic fatty liver disease (NAFLD) is so named because of its close resemblance to alcoholic liver disease. It represents a spectrum of liver injuries that start with simple steatosis, with or without associated hepatitis (nonalcoholic steatohepatitis [NASH]), and progress to bridging fibrosis and cirrhosis. Risk factors for NAFLD include obesity, type 2 diabetes mellitus and hyperlipidemia (see Chapter 22). About half of people with both severe obesity and diabetes have NASH, and as many as one fifth of this population seem to develop cirrhosis.

Histologic features of NAFLD overlap those of alcoholic liver disease and include steatosis, lobular and portal inflammation, hepatocyte necrosis, Mallory bodies and fibrosis. As in alcoholic liver disease, centrilobular fibrosis is commonly observed (Fig. 14-36). With the development of cirrhosis, steatosis often disappears. ***Thus, NAFLD is the likely cause of many cases of so-called cryptogenic cirrhosis.***

NAFLD may result from oxidant injury to the liver. In this respect, the pathogenesis of NAFLD and NASH might overlap that of alcoholic hepatitis. Insulin resistance is associated with increased hepatic mitochondrial oxidation of free fatty acids, increased oxidative stress and lipid peroxidation, and appears to be the strongest risk factor for NAFLD and NASH. Progression to cirrhosis in NAFLD is often insidious, and many patients remain asymptomatic, with only moderate increases in serum liver enzymes.

Weight reduction, including via bariatric surgery, tends to improve NAFLD and NASH, but no definitive treatment is yet available. Several drugs used to treat the inflammatory component of NASH, including antioxidants, and drugs used to treat insulin resistance (e.g., metformin, thiazolidinediones) can give rise to fibrosis. They are not routine therapy of NASH, however.

Primary Biliary Cirrhosis

Primary biliary cirrhosis (PBC) is an immune-mediated chronic progressive cholestatic liver disease with destruction of intrahepatic bile ducts **(nonsuppurative destructive cholangitis).** The loss of bile ducts leads to impaired bile secretion, cholestasis and hepatic damage. PBC occurs mainly in middle-aged women (10:1 female predominance). The term *cirrhosis* in this context is somewhat misleading: cirrhosis is actually a late complication of the disease.

PBC accounts for up to 2% of deaths from cirrhosis. Cases are sporadic, although familial clusters of the disease have been reported. The prevalence in families of patients with PBC is considerably higher than that in the general population, suggesting a hereditary predisposition.

MOLECULAR PATHOGENESIS: PBC is associated with many immune abnormalities and so is widely held to be an autoimmune disease. Most (85%) patients have at least one other disease usually classified as autoimmune, and almost half (40%) have two or more such ailments. Among these disorders are chronic thyroiditis, rheumatoid arthritis, scleroderma, Sjögren syndrome and systemic lupus erythematosus. Molecular mimicry to certain bacteria and environmental agents has been proposed as a mechanism for the initiation of autoimmunity in PBC, but definitive evidence is lacking.

The DRB1*008 family of major histocompatibility complex–encoded genes is associated with PBC, while the disease is less common in people carrying DRB1*11 and DRB1*13. Polymorphisms of key immune regulatory genes, such as those encoding tumor necrosis factor and cytotoxic T-lymphocyte antigen 4, have been detected in patients with a variety of autoimmune diseases, including PBC. Increased X chromosome monosomy may explain the strong female predominance of PBC.

Both humoral and cellular immunity appear to be altered. Serum immunoglobulin levels are increased, especially the level of IgM. ***Over 95% of patients have circulating antimitochondrial antibodies (AMAs), a finding commonly used in the diagnosis of PBC.*** Autoantibodies bind epitopes associated with the mitochondrial pyruvate dehydrogenase complex. Despite their specificity, AMAs do not affect mitochondrial function and play no known role in the pathogenesis or progression of the disease. Other circulating autoantibodies are antinuclear, antithyroid, antiplatelet, antiacetylcholine receptor and antiribonucleoprotein antibodies. The complement system is also chronically activated.

The cells surrounding and infiltrating the sites of bile duct damage are predominantly suppressor/cytotoxic ($CD8^+$) lymphocytes, suggesting that they mediate the destruction of the ductal epithelium.

PATHOLOGY: Pathologic stages of PBC entail ductal lesions, scarring and cirrhosis.

STAGE I: THE DUCT LESION: Early PBC features a unique lesion, a **chronic destructive cholangitis** affecting small and medium-sized intrahepatic bile ducts (Fig. 14-37). The injury to the bile ducts is segmental and so appears focal in histologic sections. Bile ducts are mainly surrounded by lymphocytes, but plasma cells and macrophages are also seen. The bile duct epithelium is irregular and hyperplastic, with stratification and occasional papillary ingrowths of epithelial cells. Discrete epithelioid granulomas often occur in the portal tracts and may impinge on the bile ducts. In stage I PBC, lobular parenchyma tends to be normal.

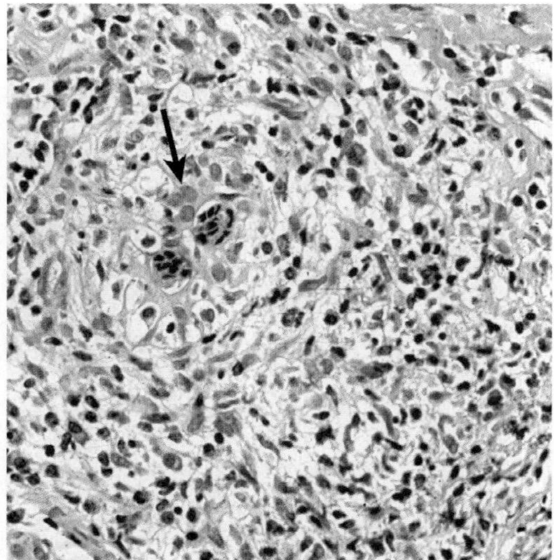

FIGURE 14-37. Primary biliary cirrhosis (PBC), stage I. A photomicrograph shows a portal tract expanded by an inflammatory infiltrate consisting of lymphocytes, plasma cells, eosinophils and macrophages. A bile duct (*arrow*) is damaged by the inflammation.

STAGE II: SCARRING: As a result of the destructive inflammation in stage I PBC, small bile ducts virtually disappear, and scarring of medium-sized bile ducts is common. Proliferation of bile ductules within portal tracts is usual and may be florid. Collagenous septa extend from the portal tracts into the lobular parenchyma and begin to encircle some lobules. Cholestasis, when present, may be severe and is located at the periphery of the portal tracts.

STAGE III: CIRRHOSIS: The end stage of PBC is cirrhosis, characterized by a dark green bile-stained liver that exhibits fine nodularity. Microscopically, small bile ducts are scarce and medium-sized ducts are conspicuously fewer in number. There is little inflammation within either the fibrous septa or the parenchymal nodules.

CLINICAL FEATURES: ***Some 90% to 95% of those afflicted with PBC are women, usually 30 to 65 years of age.*** Fatigue and pruritus are the most common initial symptoms, but many patients have no symptoms during the early stage of PBC. Some remain asymptomatic and appear to have an excellent prognosis; others ultimately develop advanced cirrhosis and its complications. The diagnosis of PBC is confirmed when a patient meets two of three currently internationally recognized criteria: (1) AMA titer greater than or equal to 1:40, (2) biochemical cholestasis as indicated by elevated serum alkaline phosphatase for at least 6 months and (3) typical liver histology. The unusual diagnosis of so-called AMA-negative PBC rests on characteristic histologic and clinical findings (criteria 2 and 3).

Typically in PBC, serum alkaline phosphatase is high but bilirubin is normal or only slightly elevated. The patient may suffer from severe pruritus. As the disease advances, serum bilirubin progressively increases in most patients. Serum AST and ALT are only moderately elevated. Serum cholesterol levels increase strikingly, and an abnormal lipoprotein (lipoprotein-X) appears that is found in many forms of chronic cholestasis. Cholesterol-laden macrophages accumulate in subcutaneous tissues, where they form localized lesions termed **xanthomas.** Impaired bile excretion into the intestine often leads to severe **steatorrhea,** due to fat malabsorption. Because of associated malabsorption of vitamin D and calcium, **osteomalacia** and **osteoporosis** are important complications of PBC. About one third of patients develop gallstones. Patients who eventually develop cirrhosis die of liver failure or complications of portal hypertension. PBC is treated with ursodeoxycholic acid (UDCA). UDCA increases transplant-free survival and leads to biochemical remission in about 40% of patients. The course of PBC is usually indolent, and may be as long as 20 to 30 years. Liver transplantation is highly effective in end-stage PBC.

Primary Sclerosing Cholangitis

Primary sclerosing cholangitis (PSC) is a chronic cholestatic liver disease of unknown cause, in which inflammation and fibrosis narrow and eventually obstruct intrahepatic and extrahepatic bile ducts. Up to 70% of patients are men with a mean age of 40 years and a prevalence of 14 cases per 100,000 population. Progressive biliary obstruction typically leads to persistent obstructive jaundice and eventually to secondary biliary cirrhosis.

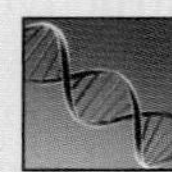

MOLECULAR PATHOGENESIS: ***Although the cause of PSC is unknown, two thirds of patients also have ulcerative colitis.*** A few cases have been described in patients with Crohn disease of the colon. Associations with retroperitoneal fibrosis, lymphoma and the fibrosing variant of chronic thyroiditis (Riedel struma) are also reported. In one fourth of cases, there is no associated disease. Increased colonic permeability to bacteria associated with ulcerative colitis may be a source of antigen for PSC, but this hypothesis remains unproved.

Genetic and immunologic factors contribute to the pathogenesis of PSC. The disease can occur in families and is associated with certain HLA haplotypes, including HLA B8. Hypergammaglobulinemia is common, as are circulating antineutrophil cytoplasmic antibodies (perinuclear or P-ANCAs), circulating immune complexes and complement activation by the classic pathway. The portal tracts exhibit an increased number of T cells.

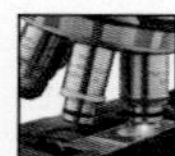

PATHOLOGY: The histopathology of PSC liver disease can be divided into three stages:

- **Stage I:** Initially, there is periductal inflammation and fibrosis in the portal tracts (Fig. 14-38A).
- **Stage II:** Many bile ducts become obliterated (Fig. 14-38B), and fibrous septa extend into the parenchyma.
- **Stage III:** Secondary biliary cirrhosis eventually develops (Fig. 14-38B).

Similar inflammatory and fibrotic changes may be seen in large intrahepatic and extrahepatic bile ducts, in both of which they can cause obstruction. Since the disease tends to be segmental, contrast radiography shows a characteristic beaded appearance of the intrahepatic biliary tree, which, in the proper clinical setting, is diagnostic. The same inflammatory process affects the gallbladder wall. Some patients with typical clinical features of PSC have normal-appearing bile ducts on cholangiography, in which case the condition is termed "small duct PSC."

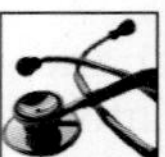

CLINICAL FEATURES: The median survival in symptomatic patients with PSC is 8 to 9 years. Asymptomatic patients have a better prognosis. The clinical presentation of PSC ranges from the discovery of asymptomatic elevations in cholestatic liver tests to symptoms of biliary obstruction and evidence of end-stage liver disease. Infection may culminate in abscess formation. ***Cholangiocarcinoma develops in up to 20% of patients with PSC.*** Liver transplantation is curative, but recurrence of PSC is not uncommon.

Iron Overload Syndromes

Several conditions are characterized by excessive accumulation of iron in the body (siderosis). Iron overload syndromes are divided into two major categories on the basis of the cause of the excess iron. **Hereditary hemochromatosis** (HH) is caused by a common genetic alteration in control of intestinal iron absorption. **Secondary iron overload** (1) complicates certain hematologic disorders; (2) entails parenteral iron overload, in which the iron is obtained from multiple blood transfusions or parenteral administration of iron itself; or (3) is caused by an enormous dietary intake of iron. Secondary iron overload alone rarely causes liver disease.

Hereditary Hemochromatosis Is a Common Disorder of Iron Metabolism

In HH too much iron is absorbed, causing its toxic accumulation in parenchymal cells, particularly of the liver, heart and pancreas. In this disease, 20 to 40 g of iron may accumulate. The excess iron in HH is only within body storage compartments. ***The clinical hallmarks of advanced HH are cirrhosis, diabetes, skin pigmentation and cardiac failure*** (Fig. 14-39). The disease most often manifests clinically in patients aged 40 to 60. Men are afflicted 10 times more often as women, probably due to the increased loss of iron in women in menstruation. However, postmenopausal women may also develop the disease. As maximum daily iron

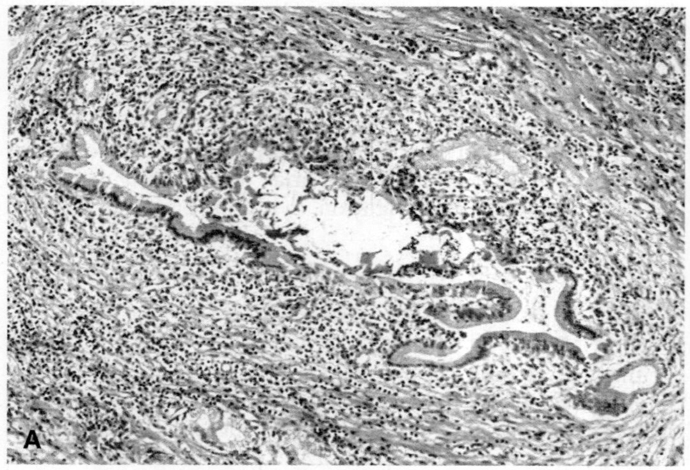

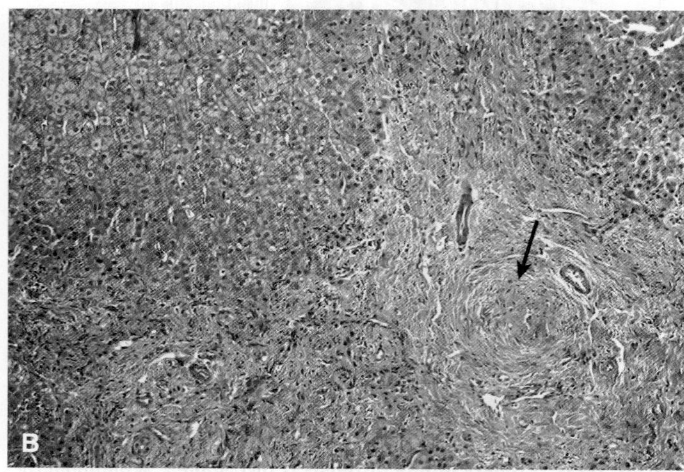

FIGURE 14-38. Primary sclerosing cholangitis (PSC). A. A photomicrograph of a liver removed for hepatic transplantation shows an edematous, fibrotic and inflamed portal tract. Inflammatory debris is present within the lumen of the bile duct. **B.** In another patient with PSC, there is bridging fibrosis. The bile ducts have been destroyed (*arrow*).

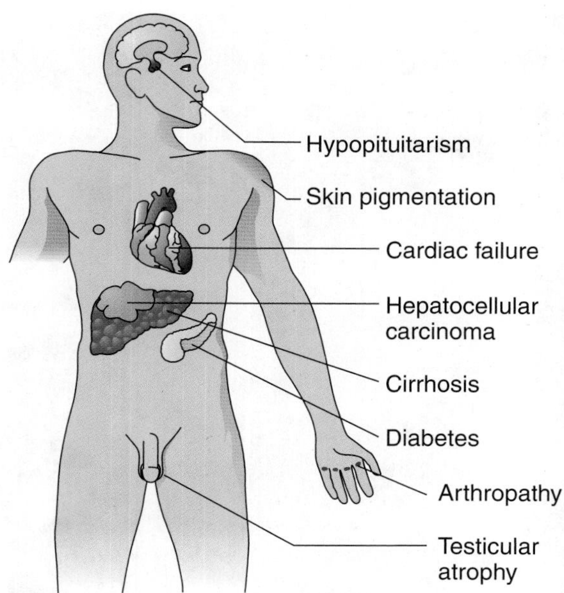

FIGURE 14-39. Complications of hemochromatosis.

absorption is about 4 mg, hemochromatosis develops over years.

MOLECULAR PATHOGENESIS: HH follows **autosomal recessive** inheritance. Lesser degrees of iron overload are often seen in relatives of those with the disease. As noted in Chapter 1, iron is a key participant in cell injury mediated by activated oxygen species. Their excess cellular iron probably renders HH patients more susceptible to oxidative injury.

Normal Iron Metabolism

A normal 70-kg man's body contains 3 to 5 g of iron, two thirds of which is in hemoglobin, myoglobin and iron-containing enzymes. Erythrocytes contain 2500 mg, 1000 mg is stored in the liver, 300 mg is part of myoglobin and respiratory enzymes and about 4 mg is bound to transfer proteins (e.g., transferrin) in plasma. Obligatory daily iron loss in urine and desquamated cells of the gut and skin is about 1 mg in men. Women lose more during menstruation and pregnancy. Daily iron use is about 20 mg, largely for erythropoiesis. Most of this comes from reutilized iron from senescent red cells. Thus, only 1 to 2 mg of daily dietary iron is required.

Total body iron content is controlled at the level of intestinal absorption and storage utilization, not excretion. Daily iron absorption may range from less than 0.5 mg in people with normal iron balance to as much as 4 mg in those with iron deficiency. If the body's stores of iron are adequate, iron absorption is relatively constant.

Dietary iron is digested by gastric acid and absorbed mainly in the duodenum. This is an active process that is closely regulated. Dietary ascorbate is important for iron absorption because ferric iron in the diet is reduced by ascorbic acid to ferrous iron, in which form it can be absorbed by the small intestine. Without dietary vitamin C, much less iron can be absorbed. Thus, enterocytes absorb ferrous iron. This process requires a divalent metal transporter (DMT-1) on the luminal surface of mucosal cells in the duodenum, which binds dietary ferrous iron and transfers it to the intracellular compartment, from which it is absorbed into the circulation. Cellular iron transport is facilitated by **ferroportin.** Export requires a carrier protein, **hephastin,** which also oxidizes ferrous iron to ferric iron, which complexes in the serum to **transferrin.**

Serum iron is mostly bound to transferrin. Upon binding to cells that bear the transferrin receptor (TfR1), transferrin releases it into cells, which internalize it. Iron is thus transferred to all cells of the body via TfR1 and, to a lesser extent, by the uptake of non–transferrin-bound iron. Liver cells express a second transferrin receptor, **TfR2.** About 20 mg of iron from phagocytosed, senescent erythrocytes are complexed with **ferritin.** Export from phagocytic cells is regulated by the action of ferroportin and hepcidin, among other proteins (see below).

Ferritin, the primary iron storage protein, is present in the cytoplasm of all cells and, in small amounts, in the circulation. **Hemosiderin** is a product of ferritin degradation. It is seen by light microscopy as golden-yellow granules that stain with the Prussian blue reaction. The liver and bone marrow are the main sites of iron storage in the body.

The most important regulator of plasma iron is **hepcidin,** a peptide hormone that is produced in the liver and that controls iron levels by binding to **ferroportin.** The latter is a transmembrane protein on duodenal enterocytes, liver cells and macrophages. Ferroportin transports iron from within those cells to the extracellular fluid. Upon binding hepcidin, ferroportin—and thus the iron bound to it—is retained within cells. Hepcidin levels are increased by iron and by inflammatory states and decreased by iron deficiency and hypoxia. Hepcidin synthesis is controlled by TfR2, hemojuvelin (HJV) and HFE, the product of the hemochromatosis gene. Most hereditary hemochromatosis is due to the effects of mutations in these proteins on hepcidin production.

Iron Metabolism in Hereditary Hemochromatosis

The gene involved in most forms of HH, *HFE,* is on the short arm of chromosome 6. It encodes a transmembrane protein that resembles MHC class I molecules. Mutations in other genes that control iron metabolism less commonly lead to iron overload and syndromes like hemochromatosis. The most common form of HH, accounting for 90% of patients, is due to homozygosity for a mutation (C282Y) in the *HFE* gene. A less common HFE mutation is H63D. Among Europeans, 10% are heterozygous for C282Y, and 1 of 200 to 400 people is homozygous. Interestingly, some homozygotes do not develop HH or iron overload. Thus, only 1 in 400 people develops clinically apparent hemochromatosis. A rare form of adult hemochromatosis is caused by mutations in TfR2.

HFE protein regulates iron delivery to the cytoplasm, most likely by binding TfR1 and controlling its interaction with transferrin. HFE is present in most tissues, including the gut, and binds duodenal crypt cells with high affinity. ***A current hypothesis holds that mutant HFE protein, including that of duodenal enterocytes, cannot promote***

iron uptake. As a result, duodenal crypt cells sense an iron deficiency and upregulate DMT-1 and ferroportin expression, which then increases absorption of dietary iron. The accelerated transfer of iron across the mucosal cell leads to increased concentration of non–transferrin-bound iron in the blood and its subsequent accumulation in parenchymal organs.

A competing hypothesis invokes a role for the protein hepcidin, which is thought to downregulate iron release by enterocytes and macrophages. Hepcidin levels are depressed in persons with HFE-related disease and in Hfe-knockout mice. In this hypothesis, HFE senses circulating iron levels. Further support for this hypothesis is drawn from the finding in juvenile hemochromatosis related to mutations in the hepcidin gene *HAMP*. However, the relationship between HFE activity and hepcidin expression, as well as the specific role of hepcidin in HH, has not been clarified.

In **juvenile hemochromatosis** a mutation in hemojuvelin (HJV) causes rapid and severe progression of tissue damage. Recent data suggest that hemojuvelin binds bone morphogenic protein (BMP) to signal hepcidin production. Consistent with this, hepcidin production is diminished in patients with HJV mutations. Other mutations associated with juvenile hemochromatosis involve the gene *HAMP*, which encodes hepcidin. ***In summary, hepcidin appears to play a central role in many forms of hemochromatosis, including those caused by mutations in HFE, hepcidin itself (HAMP), HJV and TfR2.***

The causes of iron overload are summarized in Table 14-4.

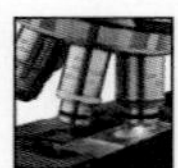

PATHOLOGY: In HH very large amounts of iron accumulate in the parenchymal cells of a variety of organs and tissues.

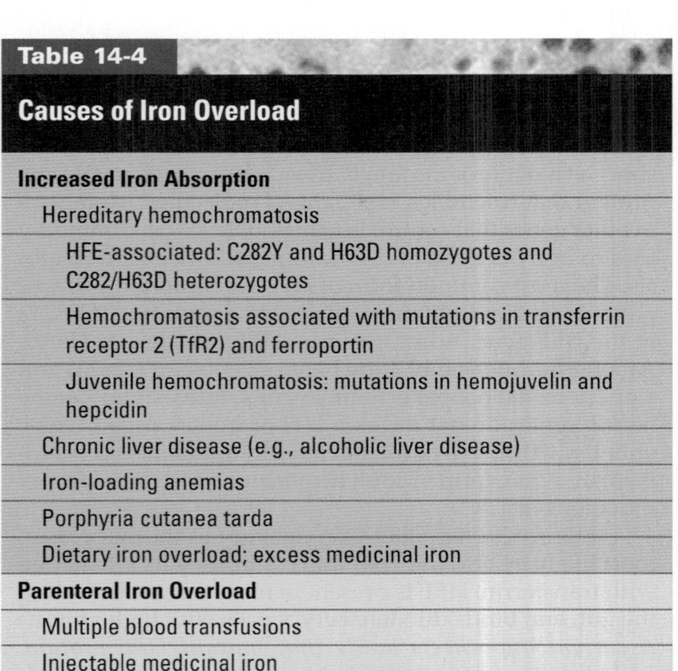

Table 14-4

Causes of Iron Overload

Increased Iron Absorption
Hereditary hemochromatosis
HFE-associated: C282Y and H63D homozygotes and C282/H63D heterozygotes
Hemochromatosis associated with mutations in transferrin receptor 2 (TfR2) and ferroportin
Juvenile hemochromatosis: mutations in hemojuvelin and hepcidin
Chronic liver disease (e.g., alcoholic liver disease)
Iron-loading anemias
Porphyria cutanea tarda
Dietary iron overload; excess medicinal iron
Parenteral Iron Overload
Multiple blood transfusions
Injectable medicinal iron

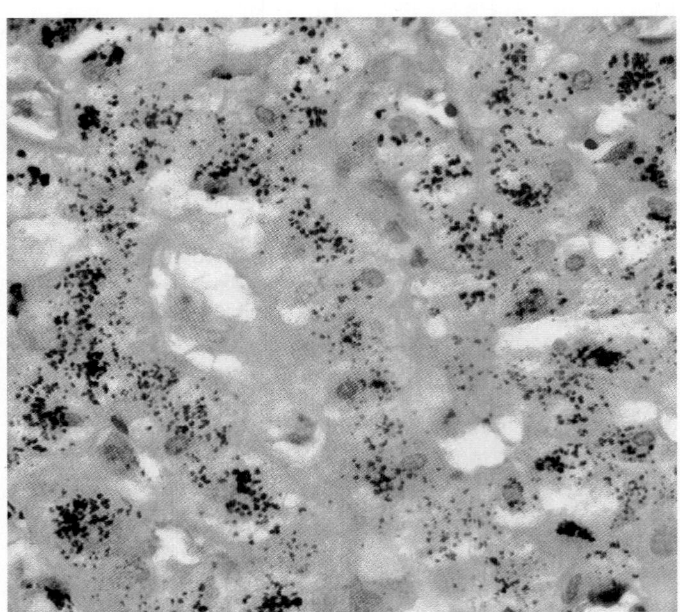

FIGURE 14-40. Hemochromatosis. Prussian blue stain demonstrates considerable iron in hepatocytes.

LIVER: The liver is always affected in HH, and has more than 0.5 g iron per 100 g wet weight in the late stages. The organ is enlarged and reddish brown, with micronodular cirrhosis. Hepatocytes and bile duct epithelium are filled with iron granules (Fig. 14-40). The excess cellular iron is stored predominantly in lysosomes as ferric iron. Late in the disease, iron deposits conspicuously in Kupffer cells, reflecting phagocytosis of necrotic hepatocytes. Within the fibrous septa, iron is prominent in proliferated bile ductules and macrophages. Eventually, as with other forms of micronodular cirrhosis, macronodular cirrhosis supervenes.

SKIN: The skin in patients with HH is typically pigmented, but iron deposits in the skin in only half of patients. Most patients display increased melanin in the basal melanocytes.

PANCREAS: Diabetes is a common complication of HH and results from deposition of iron in the pancreas. Grossly, the organ appears rust colored and fibrotic. Exocrine and endocrine cells contain excess iron, and there is loss of both acinar cells and islets of Langerhans. The combination of pigmented skin and glucose intolerance in patients with HH is referred to as **bronze diabetes.**

HEART: Congestive heart failure is a common cause of death in patients with HH. The myocardial fibers contain iron pigment, which is more extensive in the ventricles than in the atria. Necrosis of cardiac myocytes and accompanying interstitial fibrosis are common.

ENDOCRINE SYSTEM: Numerous endocrine glands are affected in HH, including the pituitary, adrenal, thyroid and parathyroid glands. However, tissue damage is not a usual feature in these organs, except for the pituitary, in which release of gonadotropins is impaired. As a result, testicular atrophy is seen in one fourth of male patients, even without iron deposition in the testes. The disturbance in the pituitary–gonadal axis is characterized by loss of libido and amenorrhea in women and impotence and sparse body hair in men.

JOINTS: About half of HH patients show arthropathy, most severe in the fingers and hands. HH arthritis affecting larger joints, like the knee, may be severe enough to be disabling.

CLINICAL FEATURES: HH generally becomes symptomatic in midlife. Liver disease usually pursues an indolent and prolonged course, but one fourth of untreated patients eventually die in hepatic coma or from gastrointestinal hemorrhage. Cirrhosis in HH may lead to hepatocellular carcinoma, and in this setting the 10-year cumulative probability of liver cancer is as high as 30%. By contrast, noncirrhotic patients with HH have much lower risk of liver malignancy.

Normal plasma iron ranges from 80 to 100 g/dL, and transferrin is ordinarily about one-third saturated. HH patients show serum iron levels more than twice normal, with 100% saturation of transferrin. Blood ferritin, which parallels the amount of storage iron, is greatly increased in HH.

Treatment of HH is to remove iron from the body, most effectively by repeated phlebotomy. Weekly phlebotomies for 2 to 3 years can remove 20 to 40 g of iron, after which phlebotomies every 2 to 3 months maintain iron balance. The beneficial effect of repeated phlebotomy is impressive. In homozygotes without cirrhosis or diabetes, iron depletion allows a life expectancy identical to that of the general population. Without treatment, 10-year survival with HH is 6%.

Secondary Iron Overload Occurs in People Without Hereditary Hemochromatosis Mutations

ETIOLOGIC FACTORS: Within certain limits, the amount of iron absorbed is a function of the amount ingested. For example, hemochromatosis is unlikely to develop in someone with a diet low in iron. Many patients with secondary iron overload (up to 40%) have a long history of alcohol abuse; it is thought that alcohol may enhance both the accumulation of iron and its associated cell injury.

Iron accumulation among blacks of sub-Saharan Africa, commonly misnamed "Bantu siderosis," is an example of secondary iron overload. This occurs because these populations consume large amounts of iron-containing alcoholic beverages. As such "home-brewed" beverages (low alcohol, high iron) are replaced by Western spirits (high alcohol, low iron), siderosis has become less common while alcoholic cirrhosis has increased.

Massive iron overload occurs in patients with certain hemolytic anemias, such as sickle cell anemia, thalassemia major and other anemias with ineffective erythropoiesis. The excess iron derives from patients' diets or transfused blood. Increased iron absorption occurs despite transferrin saturation; release of iron by intravascular hemolysis adds a further burden of iron. Patients with thalassemia often develop secondary iron overload whether or not they have received blood transfusions. On the other hand, multiple blood transfusions alone are generally insufficient to produce secondary iron overload, even in patients with hypoplastic anemia given many transfusions (250 mg iron/500 mL unit of blood). In these patients, iron is concentrated principally in mononuclear phagocytes, and cirrhosis is rare.

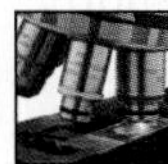

PATHOLOGY: Transfusional and other types of siderosis are characterized by the uniform, initial deposition of iron in Kupffer cells, with eventual spillover into the hepatocytes. Cirrhosis with secondary iron overload shows varying degrees of iron accumulation, but hepatic iron deposition is generally less than that in HH and is often restricted to the periphery of the nodules.

Heritable Disorders Associated With Cirrhosis

Wilson Disease (Hepatolenticular Degeneration) Is a Rare Disorder of Copper Metabolism

Wilson disease (WD) is an autosomal recessive disease in which excess copper may be deposited in the liver and brain. One in 150 to 180 people is a carrier, and 1 in 30,000 children develop clinical disease.

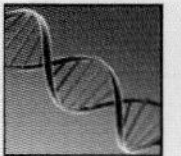

MOLECULAR PATHOGENESIS: Dietary copper intake usually exceeds the body's needs, the excess copper being excreted by the liver into the bile. In addition to biliary secretion, copper is normally bound to ceruloplasmin in hepatocytes, and the complex is secreted into the blood. The gene for WD, namely, *ATP7B* on chromosome 13, codes for an ATP-dependent transmembrane cation channel that transports copper within hepatocytes before it is excreted. ***Mutations in ATP7B impair copper transport, and both biliary excretion and incorporation into ceruloplasmin are deficient.*** Some 200 different mutations in the WD gene are known. In European and North American populations, a single mutation, H1069Q, accounts for 70% of WD, but this mutation is rare in India and Asia. Most patients are compound heterozygotes and possess two different mutant alleles.

In Wilson disease serum ceruloplasmin levels are very low, but this deficiency is thought to be due to hepatic copper overload. Excess copper causes the death of hepatocytes, copper from which is released into the blood and subsequently deposits in extrahepatic tissues. The primacy of the liver as the seat of WD is attested to by its cure with liver transplantation.

The mechanism by which excess copper injures cells is unclear. Like iron, copper catalyzes formation of potent oxidizing species from the superoxide anions and hydrogen peroxide byproducts of normal oxygen metabolism. Copper can replace iron in the Fenton reaction, to convert hydrogen peroxide into hydroxyl radicals (see Chapter 1).

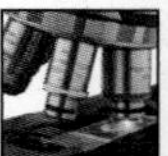

PATHOLOGY: ***In WD, the liver progresses from mild to severe chronic hepatitis. Cirrhosis may develop rapidly, even in childhood*** (Fig. 14-41). Features of severe hepatocyte injury (e.g., severe hydropic change) may be seen. Periportal hepatocytes often contain Mallory bodies, and cholestasis is common. Initially, cirrhosis is micronodular, but in time, it becomes macronodular. Chemical measurement of liver copper in unfixed tissue from livers of patients with WD reveals more than 250 μg of copper per gram of dry weight.

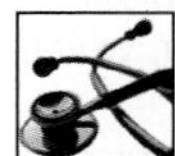

CLINICAL FEATURES: Half of patients with WD show some symptoms by adolescence. The remainder usually become ill early in adulthood, but later

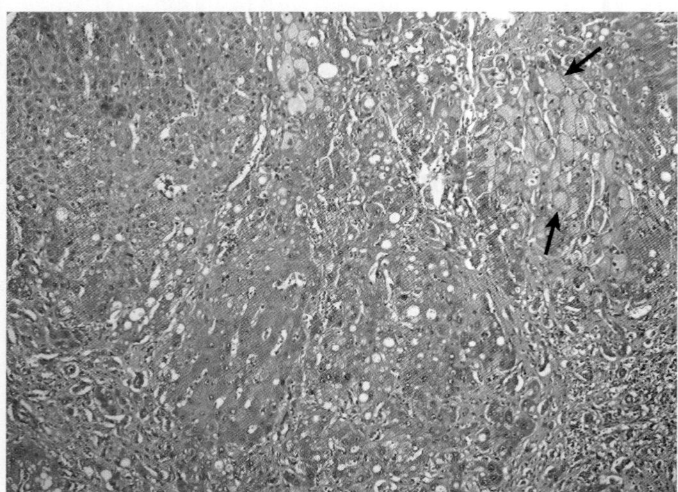

FIGURE 14-41. Wilson disease. The liver shows cirrhosis. There is severe hepatocyte injury with hydropic change (*arrows*).

presentations can occur. Initial symptoms reflect chronic liver disease in about half of patients; one third initially present with neurologic complaints; and about one tenth present with psychiatric illnesses.

LIVER: Liver-related symptoms are nonspecific at first and may progress to chronic liver disease indistinguishable from that of other forms of chronic hepatitis. Eventually, chronic hepatitis and cirrhosis result in jaundice, portal hypertension and hepatic failure. WD can present rarely as acute liver failure. Unlike hemochromatosis, there is no increased risk of liver cancer.

BRAIN: Neurologic disease begins with mild incoordination and tremors. In untreated patients, dysarthria and dysphagia appear, and later, disabling dystonia and spasticity occur.

EYE: Ophthalmic manifestations invariably accompany neurologic disease. **Kayser-Fleischer rings** are golden-brown, bilateral corneal discolorations that encircle the periphery of the iris and obscure its muscular pattern (Fig. 14-42). They represent deposition of copper in Descemet membrane. In some patients, Kayser-Fleischer rings are accompanied by "sunflower cataracts," which are green discs of copper deposition in the anterior capsule of the lens.

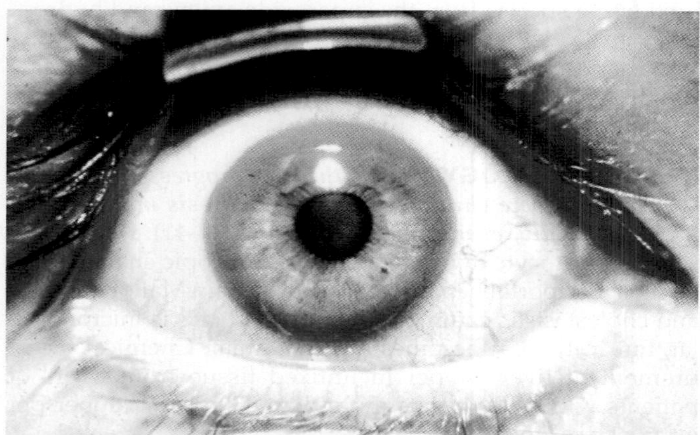

FIGURE 14-42. Kayser-Fleischer ring. The deposition of copper in Descemet membrane is reflected in a peripheral brown color, which obstructs the view of the underlying iris.

BONES: Skeletal lesions are common and include osteomalacia, osteoporosis, spontaneous fractures and various arthropathies.

KIDNEY: Renal glomerular and tubular dysfunction, manifested by proteinuria, lowered glomerular filtration, aminoaciduria and phosphaturia, is common in WD. These abnormalities are due to copper deposition in renal tubules.

BLOOD: Transient acute hemolytic episodes, presumably related to a sudden release of free copper from the liver, occur in as many as 15% of patients with WD.

Treatment of WD not only prevents copper accumulation in tissues but also extracts copper that has already been deposited. Trientine and D-penicillamine, copper-chelating agents, augment copper excretion in the urine. Both central nervous system (CNS) dysfunction and symptoms of liver disease are often reversed by treatment. For presymptomatic patients, maintenance treatment is with zinc, which blocks intestinal absorption of copper. Liver transplantation is curative for WD.

Cystic Fibrosis May Cause Biliary Obstruction

Mutated cystic fibrosis transmembrane regulator (CFTR; see Chapter 6) is expressed in biliary epithelial cells and leads to biliary obstruction from accumulation of tenacious mucous plugs in the intrahepatic biliary tree. This may present in the first few weeks of life. The most common hepatic lesion seen in cystic fibrosis (CF) is focal or diffuse biliary cirrhosis. Some infants die in hepatic failure. In patients who survive to adolescence, liver involvement becomes clinically symptomatic in some 15%. Secondary biliary cirrhosis is found in 10% of patients who survive beyond 25 years. Liver disease accounts for 2.5% of deaths in CF, making it the most common nonpulmonary cause of death from the disease. Ursodeoxycholic acid (UDCA) therapy improves liver chemistry and histology, but not survival.

α_1-Antitrypsin Deficiency Leads to Cirrhosis

α_1-Antitrypsin (α_1-AT) deficiency is an autosomal recessive disease that was initially described as a cause of emphysema (see Chapter 12). Later, cases of liver disease without lung involvement were reported, and disease of both organs is recognized. It is the most common genetic cause of liver disease and the most frequent genetic disease treated by liver transplantation. Although α_1-AT deficiency occurs in 1 of 2000 live births, only 10% to 15% of those affected develop liver disease.

MOLECULAR PATHOGENESIS: α_1-AT is a serine protease inhibitor (serpin) produced primarily in the liver that mainly deactivates neutrophil elastase. Both pulmonary and hepatic disorders reflect a defect in the secretion of a mutant variant by the liver. The α_1-AT gene locus is termed *Pi;* over 75 isoforms are known. PiZ is the most common mutant α_1-AT protein, substituting a lysine for a glutamate at position 342 (95% of all cases). The mutant protein is retained within the lumen of the endoplasmic reticulum, where it folds abnormally and forms an insoluble protein aggregate, thereby damaging that cell.

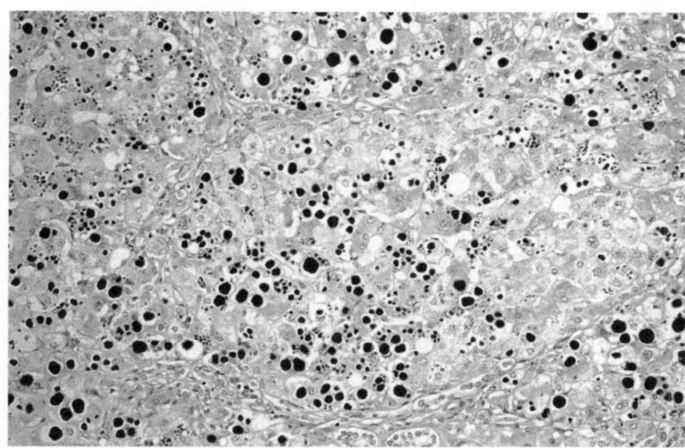

FIGURE 14-43. α_1-Antitrypsin deficiency. A photomicrograph of a section of cirrhotic liver stained by the periodic acid–Schiff (PAS) reaction with diastase digestion to remove glycogen reveals numerous cytoplasmic globules in the hepatocytes.

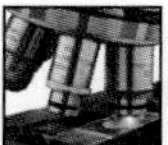

PATHOLOGY: Hepatocytes in patients with α_1-AT deficiency contain faintly eosinophilic, periodic acid–Schiff (PAS)-positive cytoplasmic droplets (Fig. 14-43), which, by electron microscopy contain amorphous material within dilated endoplasmic reticulum cisternae. The disease often presents with chronic hepatitis, which terminates in cirrhosis.

α_1-AT deficiency is a cause of hepatitis in the newborn (see below). Micronodular cirrhosis develops by the age of 2 to 3 years in these children and may ultimately become macronodular.

CLINICAL FEATURES: Liver disease in α_1-AT deficiency is highly variable. It ranges from rapidly fatal neonatal hepatitis to absence of any hepatic dysfunction. ***Of those infants with the ZZ genotype—that is, those who are susceptible to the development of clinical disease—10% develop neonatal cholestatic jaundice (conjugated hyperbilirubinemia).*** α_1-AT deficiency accounts for up to 30% of cases of neonatal conjugated hyperbilirubinemia. Most infants recover within 6 months, but 10% to 20% develop permanent liver disease. Children with cirrhosis usually die before the age of 10 years from hepatic failure or other complications of the disease. However, liver transplantation is curative.

Some patients are asymptomatic until early adulthood, when they may present with symptoms of cirrhosis as the initial complaint. ***The cirrhosis of α_1-AT deficiency is complicated by a high incidence of hepatocellular carcinoma.***

Inborn Errors of Carbohydrate Metabolism Affect the Liver

Glycogen Storage Diseases

The biochemical basis of the glycogen storage diseases is discussed in Chapter 6. ***Only glycogenosis type IV (Brancher deficiency, Andersen disease) is usually complicated by cirrhosis.*** A slowly developing cirrhosis may occur in glycogenosis type III (Debrancher deficiency, Cori disease) but is not inevitable. Glycogenosis type I (glucose-6-phosphatase deficiency, von Gierke disease) is associated with striking hepatomegaly, and type II (acid-glucosidase deficiency, Pompe disease) features mild hepatomegaly. Neither type I nor type II is complicated by cirrhosis.

GLYCOGENOSIS TYPE I: Hepatocytes are distended by large amounts of glycogen, which appears pale in sections stained with hematoxylin and eosin and red with PAS. Fat accumulation varies from mild to severe, but fibrosis is usually absent. Hepatic adenomas often develop in adolescence but regress with dietary therapy.

GLYCOGENOSIS TYPE III: Infants with Cori disease show severe hepatomegaly, and the liver morphologically resembles that seen in type I. Fat is less conspicuous, but fibrosis is present and may progress to cirrhosis.

GLYCOGENOSIS TYPE IV: Infants present with severe hepatomegaly and usually die of cirrhosis by age 4 years. Sharply circumscribed, PAS-positive inclusions are present in enlarged hepatocytes. By electron microscopy, these inclusions consist of fibrillar material that represents abnormal glycogen. Deposits of mutant glycogen are also found in the heart, skeletal muscle and brain. Liver transplantation is curative for glycogenosis type IV.

Galactosemia

Galactosemia is inherited as an autosomal recessive trait in which galactose-1-phosphate uridyl transferase is lacking. This enzyme catalyzes the second step in the conversion of galactose to glucose. As a result, galactose and its metabolites accumulate in the liver and other organs. Infants with this disorder who are fed milk rapidly develop hepatosplenomegaly, jaundice and hypoglycemia. Cataracts and mental retardation are common.

Within 2 weeks of birth, the liver shows extensive and uniform fat accumulation and striking bile ductule proliferation in and around portal tracts. Cholestasis is often seen in canaliculi and bile ductules. Bile plugs fill many of these pseudoacini. At about 6 weeks of age, fibrosis begins to extend from portal tracts into the lobules and progresses to cirrhosis by 6 months. Institution of a galactose-free diet improves the disease and reverses many of the morphologic alterations.

Hereditary Fructose Intolerance

Hereditary fructose intolerance is an autosomal recessive disease due to deficiency of fructose-1-phosphate aldolase. Fructose feeding in early infancy causes hepatomegaly, jaundice and ascites. However, if initial exposure to fructose occurs after 6 months, resulting disease is far less severe, the only clinical impairment being spontaneous hypoglycemia. Infants with liver disease show many of the changes of neonatal hepatitis. Fat accumulation may be marked, in which case the appearance resembles that of galactosemia. Progressive fibrosis culminates in cirrhosis.

Tyrosinemia

Tyrosinemia is an autosomal recessive trait in which tyrosine catabolism to fumarate and acetoacetate is impaired. The enzyme that is lacking is fumarylacetoacetate hydrolase (FAH), and over 30 different mutations in the *FAH* gene are responsible. Accumulation of succinyl acetone and succinyl acetoacetate, both of which are potent electrophiles that can react with the sulfhydryl groups of glutathione and proteins, damages the liver and kidneys.

Acute tyrosinemia begins within a few weeks or months of birth and is characterized by hepatosplenomegaly with liver failure and death, usually before 1 year of age. The appearance of the liver is remarkably like that in galactosemia, including progression to cirrhosis.

Chronic tyrosinemia begins in the first year of life, with growth retardation, renal disease and hepatic failure. Death usually supervenes before the age of 10 years. ***The incidence of hepatocellular carcinoma in chronic tyrosinemia is extraordinarily high.*** Tyrosinemia is treated by liver transplantation.

Miscellaneous Inherited Causes of Cirrhosis

A number of inborn errors of metabolism have been associated with cirrhosis, including storage diseases, such as Gaucher disease, Niemann-Pick disease, mucopolysaccharidoses, neonatal adrenoleukodystrophy, Wolman disease and Zellweger syndrome.

Indian Childhood Cirrhosis

Indian childhood cirrhosis (ICC) is a fatal disorder largely restricted to preschool children in India. Similar cases are occasionally described elsewhere. ICC predominantly affects boys 1 to 4 years old. The liver displays micronodular cirrhosis and abundant Mallory bodies, similar to alcoholic liver disease.

The etiology and pathogenesis of ICC are not well understood. Familial cases have been reported, but no hereditary pattern has been established. Interestingly, children with this disease display a marked excess of copper and copper-binding protein in the liver, but the significance of these findings remains obscure.

Drug-Induced Liver Injury

Drug-induced liver injury can mimic nearly any type of liver disease, with severity ranging from asymptomatic elevations of transaminases to acute liver failure. ***In fact, drugs are the most common cause of acute liver failure in the United States.*** Chapter 1 includes a discussion of possible mechanisms by which toxin may produce liver necrosis. See Chapter 4 for a review of immune-mediated mechanisms of injury.

Conventionally, drugs cause injury in either **predictable** or **unpredictable** patterns. The former refers to drugs that cause liver injury in a dose-dependent manner (e.g., carbon tetrachloride, the mushroom poison phalloidin, the analgesic acetaminophen), whereas the latter refers to injury that can occur with low frequency, irrespective of dose and without obvious predisposition **(idiosyncratic reaction).**

The defining characteristics of predictable drug-induced hepatoxicity are:

- The agent, in sufficiently high doses, always produces liver cell damage.
- The extent of hepatic injury is dose dependent.
- The same lesions are seen in different animal species.
- Liver necrosis is characteristically zonal—often, but not exclusively, centrilobular.
- The time between exposure and development of liver cell necrosis is short.

Most drug reactions are unpredictable and seem to represent idiosyncratic events. This type of hepatotoxicity occurs in people with metabolic or genetic predispositions, and injury usually reflects unusual sensitivity to a dose-related side effect. That is, individuals may be predisposed to idiosyncratic reactions because their metabolic pathways differ from those of the general population (*metabolic idiosyncrasy*) or because they possess genetic variations in systems of biotransformation or detoxification of reactive metabolites. Furthermore, some drugs may trigger an immunologic reaction in the liver (autoimmune hepatitis).

There is no specific diagnostic test to predict or to diagnose drug-induced hepatotoxicity. Thus, a close history of medications, drugs and dietary supplements must be elicited from patients with elevated liver enzymes or jaundice. Other liver diseases must be ruled out (e.g., viral hepatitis, genetic disease, autoimmune hepatitis, alcoholic hepatitis). Liver biopsy is often of limited value in a strict diagnosis of drug injury, since histologic patterns of acute or chronic drug-induced liver disease overlap with non–drug-related diseases.

Histologic Patterns of Drug-Induced Liver Disease Are Exceedingly Diverse

Drugs can cause nearly the entire range of pathologies seen in non–drug-induced liver disease. However, individual drugs usually have characteristic patterns of liver toxicity.

Zonal Hepatocellular Necrosis

Toxic doses of acetaminophen *predictably* cause centrilobular necrosis (Fig. 14-44A), but very high doses can cause panlobular necrosis (see Chapter 1). The zonal nature of this injury presumably reflects the greater activity of drug-metabolizing enzymes in the central zones. Classic agents that produce such injury are carbon tetrachloride and the toxin of the mushroom *Amanita phalloides*. In the affected zones, hepatocytes show coagulative necrosis, hydropic swelling and variable amounts of fat. Inflammation tends to be sparse. Patients either die in acute hepatic failure or recover without sequelae. ***Acetaminophen-induced hepatotoxicity is the most common cause of acute liver failure in the United States and is frequently seen in suicidal gestures. Patients usually present soon after an ingestion.***

Chronic exposure to some hepatotoxins that cause zonal necrosis (e.g., carbon tetrachloride) produces cirrhosis experimentally. However, this is generally not a problem in humans; once acute toxic injury is recognized, reexposure to the offending agent is rare.

Cholestasis

Injury to intralobular and interlobular bile ducts is a common, unpredictable reaction to drugs. When it occurs, bile accumulates in hepatocytes and canaliculi. Without lobular inflammation, this is termed "pure cholestasis" (Fig. 14-8). Drugs that cause pure cholestasis include the estrogens and several antibiotics (e.g., sulfamethoxazole). If cholestasis is accompanied by inflammation, the term **cholestatic hepatitis** is used.

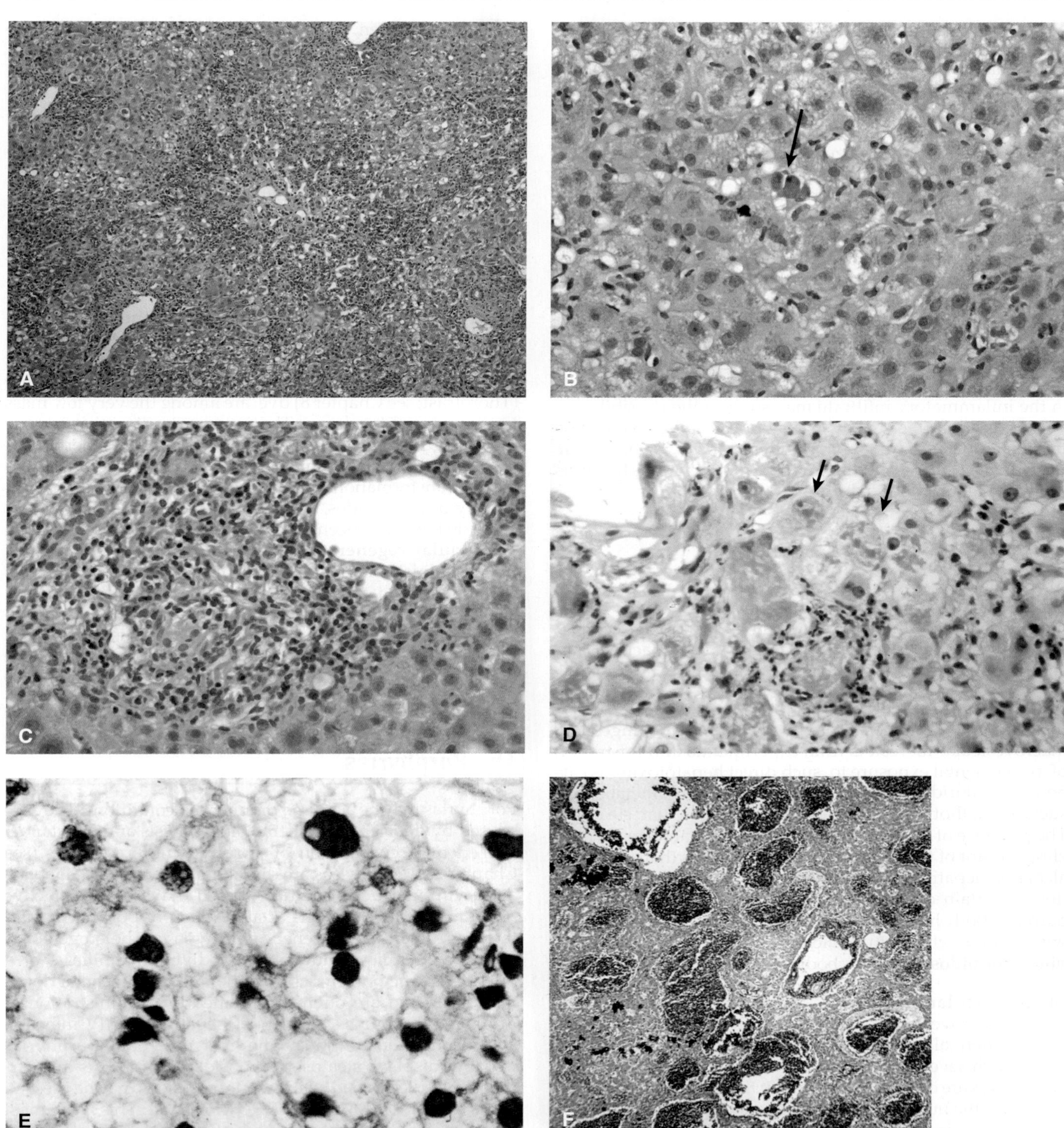

FIGURE 14-44. Drug-induced hepatotoxicity. A. Toxic centrilobular necrosis. This liver biopsy was obtained from a 20-year-old man who attempted suicide with an overdose of acetaminophen. There is centrilobular, hemorrhagic necrosis. Note that the surviving hepatocytes are markedly swollen. **B. Acute hepatitis.** The patient was started on isoniazid for treatment of tuberculosis. After 3 weeks, the aspartate aminotransferase (AST) and alanine aminotransferase (ALT) were elevated. The liver biopsy shows features of acute hepatitis including lobular disarray, inflammation, acidophil bodies (*arrow*) and focal necrosis. **C. Eosinophilic portal inflammatory infiltrate.** A 33-year-old woman developed fatigue 2 weeks after initiating therapy with a nonsteroidal anti-inflammatory agent. The AST was 250 U/L. Portal tracts show expansion by acute and chronic inflammation with eosinophils. **D. Phospholipidosis**. Liver biopsy from a patient treated with amiodarone. The hepatocytes are swollen and display ample Mallory bodies (*arrows*). **E. Reye syndrome.** A liver biopsy specimen shows small-droplet fat in hepatocytes and centrally located nuclei. **F. Peliosis hepatis.** The patient was a 44-year-old weight lifter who used anabolic steroids. The liver contains numerous large, irregular, blood-filled spaces.

Acute and Chronic Hepatitis

Inflammatory reactions are common in many *unpredictable* hepatotoxic drug reactions. All the features of acute viral hepatitis can occur after exposure to a wide variety of drugs (e.g., isoniazid, antibiotics). The causes of inflammation are diverse, and it usually is a general response to cell injury and necrosis, similar to a wide variety of etiologies (e.g., viral hepatitis and autoimmune hepatitis) (Fig. 14-44B). ***The entire range of acute liver injury, from mild anicteric hepatitis to rapidly fatal massive hepatic necrosis, is encountered.*** Typically, drug-induced hepatitis and the liver enzyme elevations associated with it resolve when the offending drug is withdrawn. If exposure continues, chronic hepatitis and even cirrhosis may develop. Sometimes, inflammation may reflect **drug-induced autoimmune hepatitis** (e.g., nitrofurantoin) either as an immune response to the drug or by unmasking classical autoimmune hepatitis. The presence of eosinophils in the inflammatory infiltrate may suggest the possibility of a drug reaction (Fig. 14-44C). ***The presence of an inflammatory infiltrate, no matter what its composition, is not specific for drug-associated hepatotoxicity.*** Granulomatous hepatitis is also a rare reaction to drugs.

Fatty Liver

Accumulation of triglycerides within hepatocytes (i.e., hepatic steatosis or fatty liver) generally occurs in a predictable fashion. Although there may be substantial overlap, two morphologic patterns are recognized (i.e., macrovesicular and microvesicular steatosis).

Macrovesicular Steatosis

In addition to its association with chronic ethanol ingestion, macrovesicular fat results from experimental administration of, or accidental exposure to, such direct hepatotoxins as carbon tetrachloride. Corticosteroids and some antimetabolites, such as methotrexate, also cause macrovesicular steatosis. The presence of fat per se does not injure hepatocytes. A puzzling variant of toxic macrovesicular steatosis that resembles alcoholic hepatitis **(steatohepatitis)** occurs after administration of certain drugs (e.g., the antiarrhythmic agent amiodarone). Both hepatocytes and Kupffer cells are enlarged, with foamy cytoplasm, which represents accumulation of **phospholipidosis.** Mallory bodies are abundant (Fig. 14-44D).

Microvesicular Steatosis

Unlike macrovesicular steatosis, which by itself is clinically inconsequential, microvesicular fatty liver is commonly associated with severe, and sometimes fatal, liver disease. Small fat vacuoles are dispersed throughout the cytoplasm of hepatocytes, and the nucleus retains its central position (Fig. 14-44E). The microvesicular fat is important, not in and of itself, but as a manifestation of metabolic severe injury to subcellular structures, mainly mitochondria.

REYE SYNDROME: This rare acute disease of children is characterized by microvesicular steatosis, hepatic failure and encephalopathy. Edema and fat accumulation are reported in the brain. Symptoms usually begin after a febrile illness, commonly influenza or varicella infection, and may correlate with aspirin administration. However, the doses of aspirin involved were far too low to cause liver injury, and Reye syndrome is more complex than simple aspirin toxicity. In any event, as the use of aspirin and the incidence of influenza decline in children, Reye syndrome has fortunately become distinctly uncommon.

Vascular Lesions

Occlusion of the hepatic veins **(Budd-Chiari syndrome;** Fig. 14-18) may follow use of oral contraceptive agents, perhaps reflecting hypercoagulability associated with use of these steroids.

Peliosis hepatis is a peculiar hepatic lesion, characterized by cystic, blood-filled cavities that are not lined by endothelial cells (Fig. 14-44F). Anabolic sex steroids, contraceptive steroids and the antiestrogen compound tamoxifen sometimes produce this lesion.

Mass Lesions and Altered Hepatic Morphology

Hepatic adenomas, induced by exogenous steroids (estrogens and anabolic steroids), and **hepatic angiosarcoma,** caused by intravenous administration of thorium dioxide (Thorotrast; see Chapter 8) dye, are among the very few mass lesions caused by drugs. Thorium is a radioactive isotope that is engulfed by Kupffer cells, where it remains inert indefinitely, emits local radiant energy and thereby produces neoplastic transformation. Chronic exposure to inorganic arsenic, usually in insecticides, and occupational inhalation of vinyl chloride have also been linked to hepatic angiosarcomas.

Nodular regenerative hyperplasia has been observed after administration of antimetabolites (e.g., 6-thioguanine), previously used to treat inflammatory bowel disease, and azathioprine. The liver appears nodular, grossly, with nodularity on microscopical examination. There is no fibrosis. Patients typically present with portal hypertension because the architectural distortion impairs flow of portal blood into the liver.

The Porphyrias

Porphyrias may be acquired or inherited conditions. They are caused by deficiencies in heme biosynthesis and are characterized by accumulation of porphyrin intermediates (see Chapter 20). Porphyrias are divided into two types—hepatic and erythropoietic porphyrias—based on where the defective heme metabolism and the accumulation of porphyrins and their precursors occur. Genetic porphyrias are heterogeneous, usually with unique mutations in individual families.

The hepatic porphyrias are inherited as autosomal dominant traits and are often precipitated by administration of drugs, sex hormones, starvation, hepatitis C, HIV infection and alcohol consumption. The liver in hepatic porphyrias variably displays steatosis, hemosiderosis, fibrosis and cirrhosis. Needle-shaped cytoplasmic inclusions may be present.

ACUTE INTERMITTENT PORPHYRIA: This is the most common genetic porphyria and reflects a deficiency of porphobilinogen deaminase activity in the liver. Only 10% of gene carriers show clinical symptoms, which generally affect young adults. Colicky abdominal pain and neuropsychiatric symptoms predominate.

PORPHYRIA CUTANEA TARDA: This chronic hepatic porphyria is the most frequent porphyria and is either acquired or inherited as an autosomal dominant trait. Uroporphyrinogen decarboxylase activity in the liver is deficient. Typical patients are middle-aged or elderly, with cutaneous photosensitivity and liver disease with hepatic iron overload.

Other inherited porphyrias, termed **erythropoietic porphyrias** and **congenital erythropoietic porphyrias,** are caused by enzyme deficiencies in cells of erythrocytic lineage. They are characterized by cutaneous photosensitivity and occasionally liver disease.

Vascular Disorders

Congestive Heart Failure Is the Major Cause of Liver Congestion

Acute Passive Congestion

At autopsy, the liver is often acutely congested, presumably because of a terminal failing heart (see Chapter 7). On cut section, the liver is diffusely speckled with small red foci, which represent centrilobular zones with dilated and congested sinusoids and terminal venules. These changes are not clinically significant.

Chronic Passive Congestion

In persistent congestive heart failure, pressure in the peripheral venous circulation increases, thereby impeding venous outflow from the liver and producing chronic passive hepatic congestion. Chronically congested livers are often reduced in size and show an accentuated lobular pattern, with alternating light and dark areas (Fig. 14-45A), termed **nutmeg liver.** In severe cases, the centrilobular terminal venules and adjacent sinusoids are markedly dilated and filled with erythrocytes (Fig. 14-45B), and liver cell plates in this zone are thinned by pressure atrophy.

If **right-sided heart failure** is severe and long-standing (e.g., tricuspid valvular disease or constrictive pericarditis), chronic passive congestion may progress to hepatic fibrosis (Fig. 14-45C). Delicate fibrous strands envelop terminal venules, and septa radiate from the centrilobular zones. Fibrous septa may link adjacent central veins, thereby producing a "reverse lobulation." Pressure atrophy of centrilobular hepatocytes is prominent. This is not "cardiac cirrhosis," since complete septa and regenerative nodules, as are seen in true cirrhosis, are rarely encountered.

Chronic passive congestion of the liver usually has little effect on hepatic function. Infrequently, features of portal hypertension, such as splenomegaly and ascites, may develop.

Shock Results in Decreased Perfusion of the Liver

Shock from any cause may cause ischemic necrosis of centrilobular hepatocytes. The centrilobular zone, zone 3 in the functional concept of hepatic acini (Fig. 14-2), is farthest from the blood that originates in the portal tracts, and so is the area most vulnerable to ischemic insult, leading to coagulative necrosis of centrilobular hepatocytes and frank hemorrhage.

Liver Infarction Is Uncommon Because of Its Dual Blood Supply and the Anastomotic Structure of the Hepatic Sinusoids

Acute occlusion of the hepatic artery or its branches can occur, rarely, as a result of embolism, polyarteritis nodosa or accidental ligation during surgery. Under such circumstances,

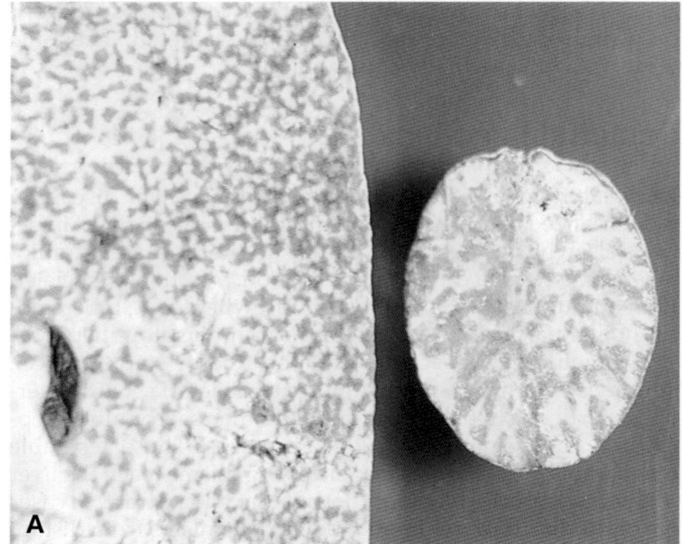

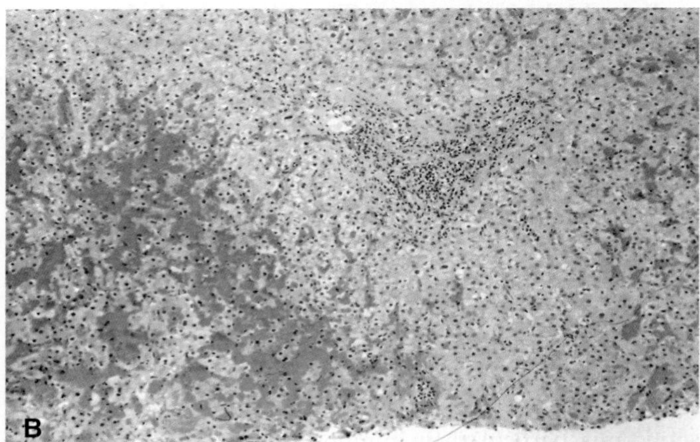

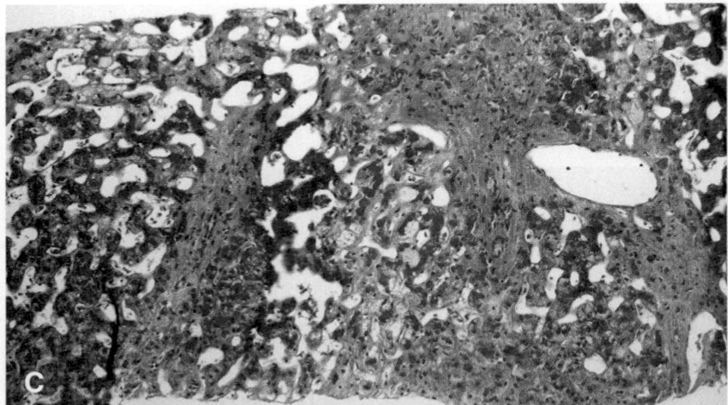

FIGURE 14-45. Chronic passive congestion of the liver. A. The surface of this fixed liver exhibits an accentuated lobular pattern, an appearance resembling that of a nutmeg (*right*). **B.** There is congestion and widening of central sinusoids. **C.** A Masson-trichrome stain shows fibrosis (*blue*) emanating out of central veins.

irregular pale areas, often surrounded by a hyperemic zone, reflect the underlying ischemic necrosis.

Acute occlusion of intrahepatic branches of the portal vein, generally in the setting of elevated hepatic venous pressure, classically produces the **Zahn infarct,** a dark-red, triangular area with its base on the surface of the liver. Microscopically, only sinusoid dilation and congestion are noted. Thus, the term "infarct" is actually a misnomer.

Bacterial Infections

Bacterial infections are uncommon causes of liver disease in industrialized countries and are mostly complications of infections elsewhere. The main reactions in the liver are granulomas, abscesses and diffuse inflammation. Infections associated with granulomatous inflammation elsewhere (e.g., tuberculosis, tularemia, brucellosis) also cause granulomatous hepatitis.

Pyogenic liver abscesses are produced by staphylococci, streptococci and gram-negative enterobacteria. Gut anaerobes, particularly *Bacteroides* spp. and microaerophilic streptococci, commonly cause liver abscesses. These resemble comparable abscesses in other sites. Organisms reach the liver in arterial or portal blood or through the biliary tract. In cases of septicemia, the liver is seeded with organisms from distant sites through the arterial blood.

Pylephlebitic abscesses (Fig. 14-46) result from intra-abdominal suppuration, as in peritonitis or diverticulitis, with the organisms being transmitted to the liver in portal blood. Pylephlebitis was once the most common cause of hepatic abscesses, but with antibiotic control of abdominal sepsis, this has become an uncommon route of infection.

Cholangitic abscesses in the liver are the most common form of hepatic abscess in Western countries today. Biliary obstruction from any cause is often complicated by bacterial infection of the biliary tree, called **ascending cholangitis.** Retrograde biliary dissemination of organisms (usually *E. coli*) then leads to cholangitic abscesses.

Hepatic abscesses occur more commonly in the right lobe of the liver. Diffuse inflammation of the liver from bacterial infection is distinctly uncommon today but may be encountered in septicemia, particularly in immunocompromised patients. The source of infection is unknown in about half of cases.

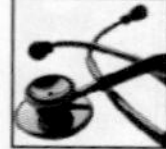

CLINICAL FEATURES: A patient with a hepatic abscess typically presents with high fever, rapid weight loss, right upper quadrant abdominal pain and hepatomegaly. Jaundice occurs in one fourth of cases; serum alkaline phosphatase is almost always elevated. Solitary abscesses are treated with percutaneous or surgical drainage and antibiotics, but if abscesses are multiple, treatment is more problematic. The main complications of hepatic abscesses are rupture and direct spread of the infection. Pleuropulmonary fistulas, from rupture of an abscess through the diaphragm, and peritonitis, from leakage into the abdominal cavity, occur. Dissemination of organisms in the blood may lead to septicemia and metastatic abscesses elsewhere in the body. The mortality from hepatic abscess, even when treated, is high, ranging from 40% to 80%.

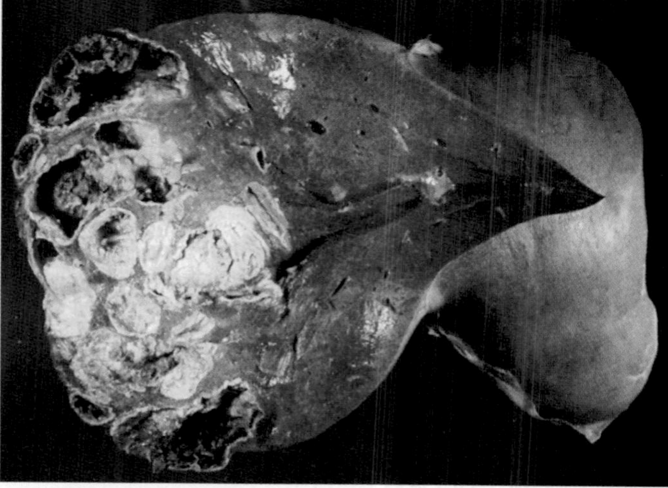

FIGURE 14-46. Pylephlebitic abscesses of the liver. The cut surface of the liver shows large, confluent, irregular abscess cavities.

Parasitic Infestations

Parasitic infestations of the liver are a serious public health problem worldwide but are uncommon in industrialized countries. These diseases are discussed in Chapter 9. Here we summarize the major parasitic diseases that affect the liver.

Protozoal Diseases Frequently Involve the Liver

AMEBIASIS: In the United States, the carrier rate for *Entamoeba histolytica* is probably less than 5%, but a prevalence of up to 35% has been reported in homosexual men. Amebiasis of the liver, the most common extraintestinal complication, leads to amebic abscesses, which are multiple in about half of cases (Fig. 14-47).

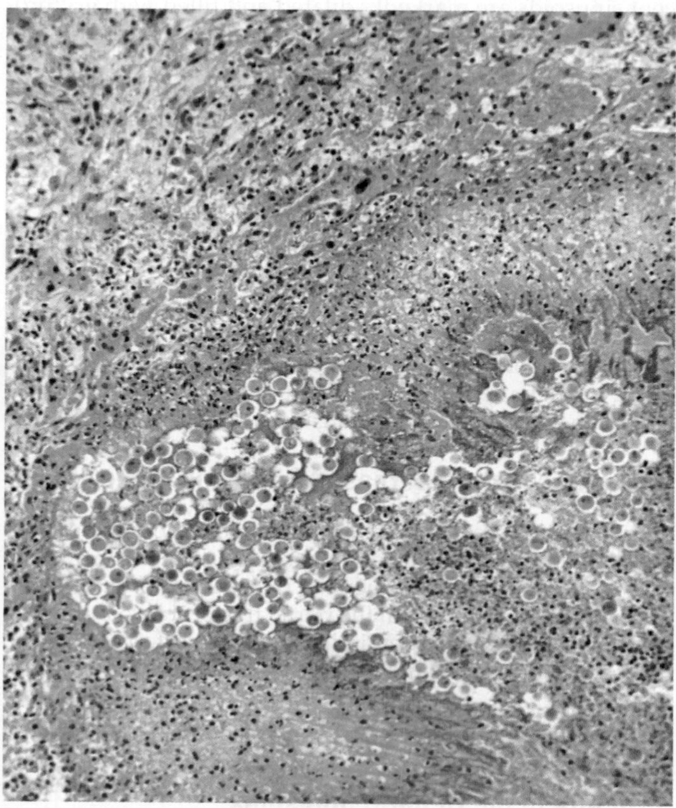

FIGURE 14-47. Amebic abscess of the liver. A photomicrograph of the margin of an amebic abscess shows fibroblastic proliferation surrounding the cavity and amebic trophozoites in the lumen.

Grossly, amebic abscesses are from 8 to 12 cm in diameter, well circumscribed and filled with thick, dark pasty material. Trophozoites can usually be seen by the edge of the necrotic debris.

The symptoms associated with amebic abscesses are similar to those of pyogenic abscesses. With appropriate treatment (tissue amebicides), the abscess may heal with only a residual scar remaining. Percutaneous or surgical drainage of large abscesses is important. If an amebic abscess continues to grow, it may rupture into the peritoneum and produce peritonitis, which carries a mortality rate as high as 40%. Amebae may also invade the blood and cause abscesses of the brain and lung.

MALARIA: Hepatic involvement in malaria is a frequent cause of hepatomegaly in endemic areas. It reflects Kupffer cell hypertrophy and hyperplasia secondary to phagocytosis of debris from the rupture of parasitized erythrocytes. Liver function is not compromised.

VISCERAL LEISHMANIASIS (KALA-AZAR): As in malaria, chronic visceral leishmaniasis causes hyperplasia of mononuclear phagocytes in the liver. Unlike malaria, however, the Kupffer cells ingest the parasitic organisms themselves, which appear as **Donovan bodies.** Clinically, there is little evidence of hepatic dysfunction.

Helminthic Diseases Are Problems of Underdeveloped Areas

Diseases caused by helminths are described in Chapter 9, and **hepatic schistosomiasis** is discussed above in the context of portal hypertension.

ASCARIASIS: From the duodenum, the worms of *Ascaris lumbricoides* enter the biliary tree, where they may produce acute biliary colic. Worms lodge in the intrahepatic biliary passages, where their disintegration liberates innumerable eggs, which cause severe, suppurative cholangitis. Resulting cholangitic abscesses may rupture into the peritoneal cavity or pleural space. Spread of the infection into the hepatic or portal veins causes pylephlebitis, a highly dangerous complication. The liver is enlarged, with numerous irregular cavities containing foul-smelling material in which the remnants of degenerated parasites are found.

LIVER FLUKES: The major parasitic flukes of the human liver are *Clonorchis sinensis* and *Fasciola hepatica*. Humans are the definitive host for *C. sinensis*, but sheep and cattle are the main reservoir of *F. hepatica*. Both parasites lodge in the intrahepatic biliary tree, where they provoke hyperplasia of the biliary epithelium, particularly severely in clonorchiasis (Fig. 14-48). In high-grade infestations with *C. sinensis*, accumulation of material from degenerated worms, parasite eggs and viscid mucus (secreted by metaplastic goblet cells in the biliary epithelium) obstructs intrahepatic bile flow and leads to intrahepatic pigment gallstones. Secondary infection of the bile with *E. coli* causes cholangitis and cholangitic abscesses, which are common causes of surgical emergencies in some Asian countries. ***Biliary* C. sinensis *infestation is associated with development of cholangiocarcinoma.***

ECHINOCOCCOSIS (CYSTIC HYDATID DISEASE): Infection with the tapeworms of the genus *Echinococcus*, principally *Echinococcus granulosus*, is an important zoonosis of the human liver. Echinococcal cysts expand slowly and produce symptoms only after many years. Within the liver, cysts behave as space-occupying lesions. Systemic manifestations reflect toxic or allergic reactions to the absorption of constituents of the organisms.

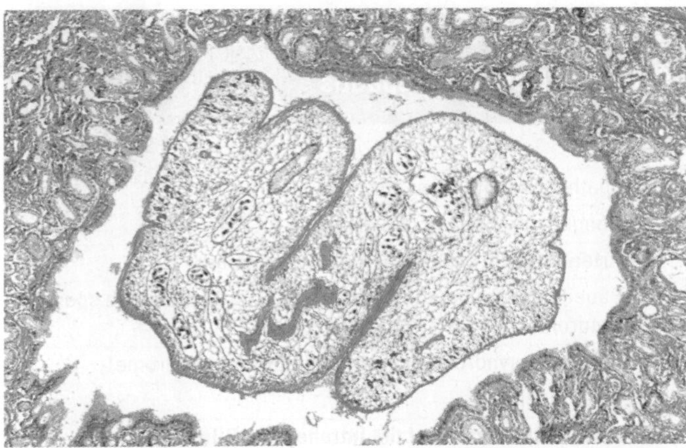

FIGURE 14-48. Infection of the liver by *Clonorchis sinensis*. The lumen of a bile duct contains an adult liver fluke, and the mucosa is hyperplastic.

Leptospirosis (Weil Disease) Is an Accidental Infection From a Zoonosis

Leptospira spirochetes infect many animal species. Despite the animal reservoir of leptospira, fewer than one fifth of patients who contract leptospirosis give a history of direct contact with animals. **Weil syndrome** refers to leptospirosis complicated by prolonged fever and jaundice and in severe cases by azotemia, hemorrhages and altered consciousness. Weil syndrome occurs in only 1% to 6% of all cases of leptospirosis. Liver pathology in fatal cases is nonspecific: focal necrosis, enlarged Kupffer cells and centrilobular cholestasis. The organisms are generally not demonstrable in the liver.

Liver Lesions May Complicate Congenital Syphilis or Tertiary Syphilis

Congenital syphilis causes neonatal hepatitis, with diffuse fibrosis in the portal tracts and around individual liver cells or groups of hepatocytes. **Tertiary syphilis** is characterized by hepatic gummas (i.e., focal lesions resembling granulomas), which heal with dense scars. Retraction produces deep clefts and a gross pseudolobation of the liver, termed **hepar lobatum,** a condition that should not be confused with cirrhosis.

Cholestatic Syndromes of Infancy

Diseases characterized by prolonged cholestasis and jaundice in infants represent either diseases primarily affecting hepatocytes or biliary obstruction.

Neonatal Hepatitis Is an Entity of Multiple Causes

Neonatal hepatitis features prolonged cholestasis, morphologic evidence of liver cell injury and inflammation.

Table 14-5

Causes of Neonatal Hepatitis

Idiopathic
Idiopathic neonatal hepatitis
Prolonged intrahepatic cholestasis
Arteriohepatic dysplasia (Alagille syndrome)
Paucity of intrahepatic bile ducts not associated with specific syndromes
Zellweger syndrome (cerebrohepatorenal syndrome)
Byler disease
Mechanical Obstruction of the Intrahepatic Bile Ducts
Congenital hepatic fibrosis
Caroli disease (cystic dilation of intrahepatic ducts)
Metabolic Disorders
Defects of carbohydrate metabolism
Galactosemia
Hereditary fructose intolerance
Glycogenosis type IV
Defects in lipid metabolism
Gaucher disease
Niemann-Pick disease
Wolman disease
Tyrosinemia (defect of amino acid metabolism)
α_1-Antitrypsin deficiency
Cystic fibrosis
Parenteral nutrition
Hepatitis
Hepatitis B
TORCH agents (toxoplasmosis, "other", rubella, cytomegalovirus, and herpes simplex)
Varicella
Syphilis
ECHO (enteric cytopathic human orphan) viruses
Neonatal sepsis
Chromosomal Abnormalities
Down syndrome
Trisomy 18
Extrahepatic biliary obstruction

ETIOLOGIC FACTORS: In about half of cases of neonatal hepatitis, the cause is known (Table 14-5). About 30% are due to α_1-antitrypsin deficiency alone. Most other cases with known causes are due to congenital infections with viral hepatitis B, toxoplasmosis, rubella, cytomegalovirus, herpes simplex virus or other agents. Hepatic injury caused by metabolic defects (e.g., galactosemia or fructose intolerance) account for some cases, and occasional cases are seen with Down syndrome and other chromosomal disorders. The other half of cases of neonatal hepatitis are unexplained.

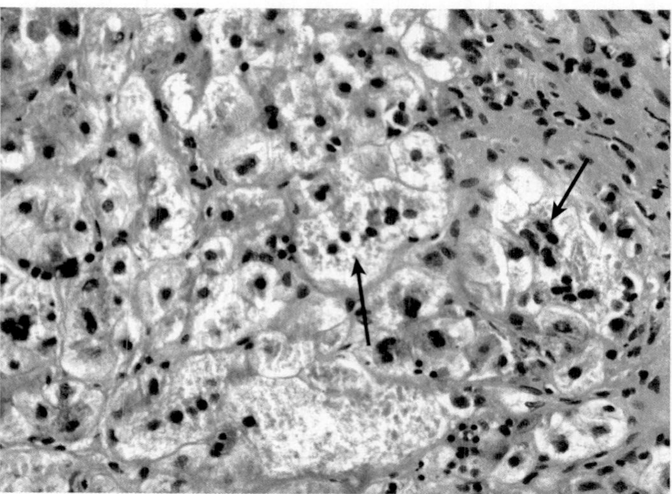

FIGURE 14-49. Neonatal hepatitis. A photomicrograph shows severe hepatocyte swelling (hydropic change), multinucleated giant hepatocytes (*arrows*), a mild chronic inflammatory infiltrate and fibrosis (*upper right*).

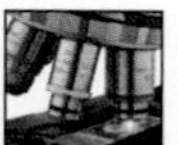

PATHOLOGY: The characteristic lesion of neonatal hepatitis is giant cell transformation of hepatocytes, hence the former term **giant cell hepatitis** (Fig. 14-49). These giant cells contain as many as 40 nuclei and may appear detached from other cells in the liver plate. Their pale, distended cytoplasm contains large amounts of glycogen and iron. Numbers of these cells decline with time, and they are rare in children older than 1 year of age. Bile pigment is often prominent within canaliculi and hepatocytes. Ballooned hepatocytes, acinar transformation of hepatocytes and acidophilic bodies are also typical of neonatal hepatitis. Extramedullary hematopoiesis is often conspicuous. Chronic inflammatory infiltrates are seen in the portal tracts as well as in the lobular parenchyma. Pericellular fibrosis around degenerating hepatocytes, singly or in groups, is common, and fibrous tissue septa extend from the portal tracts.

Biliary Atresia Refers to the Lack of a Lumen in the Biliary Tree

Both extrahepatic and intrahepatic biliary atresias are often associated with the morphologic features of neonatal hepatitis.

Extrahepatic Biliary Atresia

Extrahepatic biliary atresia (EXBA) is a cholestatic disease with inflammatory obliteration of the lumen of all or part of the biliary tree outside the liver, not associated with calculi, tumor or rupture. EXBA is rare, with an estimated incidence of 1 in 5,000 to 19,000 live births, the higher frequency being in East Asia. Biliary atresia is the most common indication for liver transplantation in children. EXBA is thought to represent the end result of heterogeneous conditions during gestational and perinatal development. Other organs, including the heart, intestine and spleen, show anomalies in 20% of cases. Other associations include known causes of neonatal hepatitis, such as chromosomal abnormalities (notably trisomy 18 and 21) and a number of viral infections. Cholangiograms in

EXBA show no bile flow into the duodenum or liver, depending on the site of the affected segment of the biliary tract.

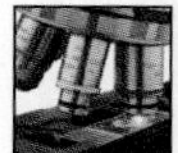

PATHOLOGY: EXBA may involve all extrahepatic bile ducts or may be limited to parts of the proximal or distal biliary tree. The gallbladder is often atretic. At one extreme, acute and chronic periluminal inflammation is prominent, with epithelial necrosis, and cellular debris within the obstructed or narrowed lumen. At the other extreme, the original lumen is completely replaced by mature connective tissue, and little or no inflammation is seen. Histologically, cholestasis and periportal bile ductular proliferation in the liver are evident. Some cases display multinucleated giant hepatocytes, like those seen in neonatal hepatitis. Although the intrahepatic bile ducts may initially appear normal, they are gradually obliterated with the persistence of cholestasis. Eventually, secondary biliary cirrhosis supervenes.

Intrahepatic Biliary Atresia

In intrahepatic biliary atresia there are few bile ducts within the liver. This occurs under three different circumstances:

- In association with known causes of neonatal hepatitis (e.g., α_1-AT deficiency, various chromosomal anomalies and metabolic derangements)
- **Alagille syndrome** (syndromic bile duct paucity), an autosomal dominant disease, also characterized by congenital abnormalities of the heart, eye, skeleton, kidneys and central nervous system, which involves mutations in the Notch signaling pathway
- Unassociated with other conditions (idiopathic)

Many observations support the concept that neonatal hepatitis, intrahepatic biliary atresia, EXBA and possibly choledochal cyst all result from a common inflammatory process ("infantile obstructive cholangiopathy").

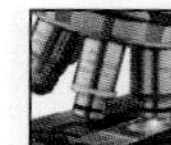

PATHOLOGY: In intrahepatic biliary atresia there are very few bile ducts in the liver. Giant cell transformation, cholestasis and bile ductular proliferation are common; cirrhosis is not.

CLINICAL FEATURES: Most patients with uncomplicated neonatal hepatitis recover without sequelae. Intrahepatic biliary atresia associated with neonatal hepatitis carries a grave prognosis, and many of these children progress to biliary cirrhosis. By contrast, the outlook in Alagille syndrome is good. Uncorrected EXBA invariably leads to progressive secondary biliary cirrhosis and is incompatible with survival. Surgical correction may cure in some anatomically favorable cases, but transplantation is the best treatment for both extrahepatic and intrahepatic biliary atresia.

Benign Tumors and Tumor-Like Lesions

Hepatic Adenomas Are Benign Tumors That Occur Principally in Women

Once rare, these tumors are more common since the advent of oral contraceptives. Use of newer estrogen and progesterone combinations has reduced the incidence of liver adenomas.

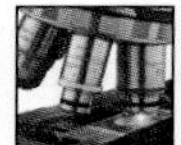

PATHOLOGY: Hepatic adenomas are usually solitary, sharply demarcated masses, up to 40 cm in diameter and 3 kg in weight (Fig. 14-50A). In one fourth of cases, multiple smaller adenomas are present. These tumors are encapsulated and paler than surrounding liver parenchyma. ***The neoplastic hepatocytes resemble their normal counterparts, except that they are not arrayed in a lobular architecture.*** Portal tracts and central venules are absent (Fig. 14-50B). The cells of the adenoma may be very large and

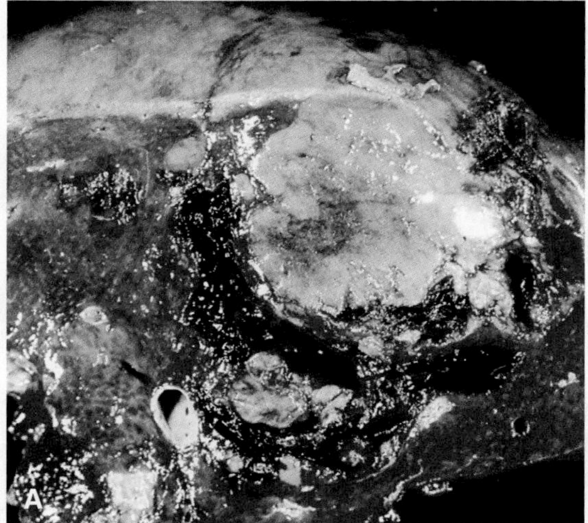

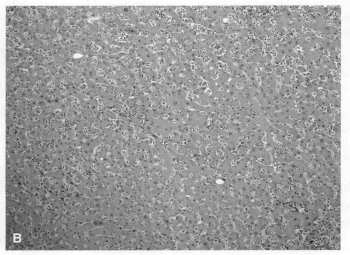

FIGURE 14-50. Hepatic adenoma. A. A surgically resected portion of liver shows a tan, lobulated mass beneath the liver capsule. The tumor has ruptured, resulting in intraparenchymal and intraperitoneal hemorrhage. The patient was a woman who had taken birth control pills for a number of years and presented with sudden intraperitoneal bleeding. **B.** Microscopically, the adenomatous hepatocytes do not differ from normal hepatocytes and are arranged without discernible lobular architecture. Note the absence of portal tracts.

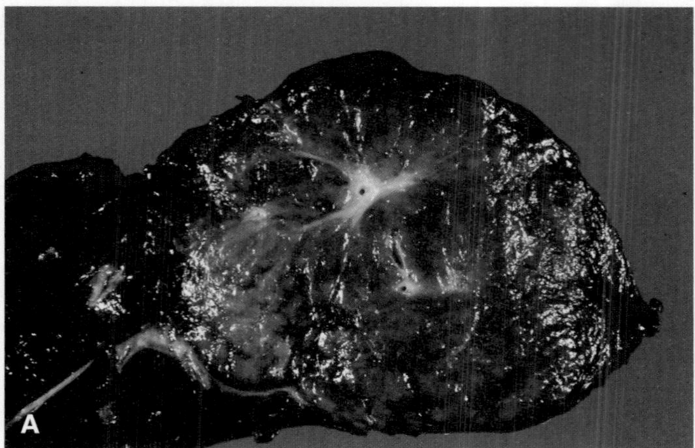

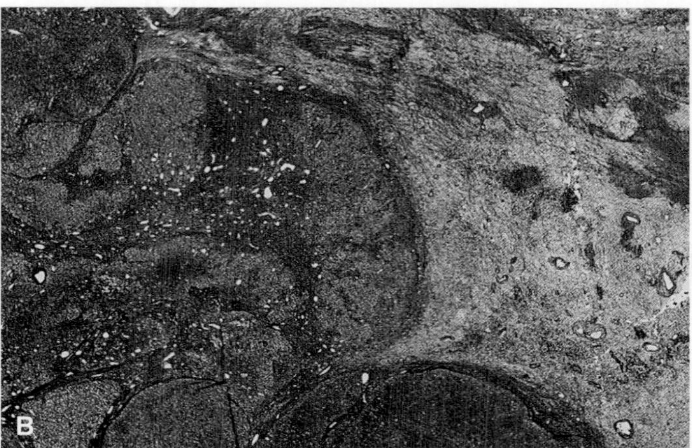

FIGURE 14-51. Focal nodular hyperplasia. A. A resected mass shows nodules with central scarring. **B.** A photomicrograph of a surgically resected mass from the liver shows a vascular central scar and irregular fibrous septa dissecting hepatic parenchyma, accounting for the resemblance to cirrhosis.

eosinophilic or filled with glycogen, which makes the cytoplasm appear clear. The presence of small arteries within the parenchyma may serve as a clue to adenoma versus normal parenchyma.

CLINICAL FEATURES: In about one third of patients with hepatic adenomas (particularly in pregnant women who have used oral contraceptives), the tumors bleed into the peritoneal cavity and require immediate surgery. Even large adenomas may disappear if oral contraceptives are discontinued. A few adenomas have been reported in men who use anabolic steroids.

Focal Nodular Hyperplasia Is a Nodular Lesion That Resembles Cirrhosis

Focal nodular hyperplasia (FNH) is characterized by multiple fibrous septa and regenerative nodules (Fig. 14-51A). It measures up to 15 cm in diameter and weighs as much as 700 g. On occasion, FNH protrudes from the surface of the liver, and it may even be pedunculated. The cut surface has a central scar from which fibrous septa radiate. Hepatocytic nodules are circumscribed by fibrous septa (Fig. 14-51B), with many tortuous bile ducts and mononuclear inflammatory cells. Lobular architecture is absent within nodules. Large arteries and veins, but little hemorrhage, are seen in the septa.

Focal nodular hyperplasia occurs in both sexes and at all ages but most often in young women. It is not a neoplasm and is not associated with the use of oral contraceptives.

Nodular Regenerative Hyperplasia (Nodular Transformation of the Liver, Partial Nodular Transformation) Causes Portal Hypertension

Nodular regenerative hyperplasia is characterized by small, hyperplastic nodules without fibrosis in an otherwise normal liver. The lesion may be partial and located predominantly in the perihilar region or may be diffuse throughout the liver. Nodules are composed of liver cells in plates two and three cells thick, compressing the surrounding parenchyma.

Nodular regenerative hyperplasia is associated with portal hypertension and was once called **noncirrhotic portal hypertension.** Its etiology is unknown, but it has been associated with use of oral contraceptives or anabolic steroids, extrahepatic infections, neoplasms and chronic inflammatory and autoimmune diseases. Nodular regenerative hyperplasia is not preneoplastic.

Hemangiomas Are the Most Common Tumors of the Liver

Benign hemangiomas in the liver occur at all ages and in both sexes and are found in up to 7% of autopsy specimens (Fig. 14-52). They are ordinarily small and asymptomatic, although larger tumors have been reported to cause abdominal symptoms and even hemorrhage into the peritoneal cavity. Grossly, the tumor is usually solitary and less than 5 cm in diameter, but multiple hemangiomas and giant forms have

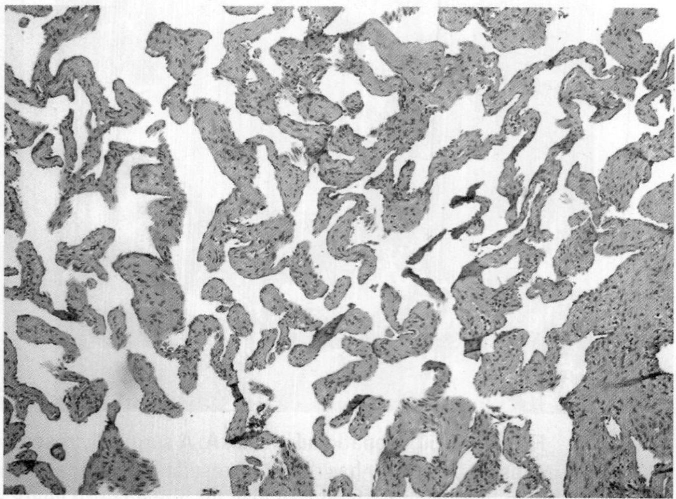

FIGURE 14-52. Cavernous hemangioma.

been described. Microscopically, the tumor is similar to cavernous hemangiomas found elsewhere.

Cystic Disease of the Liver Represents a Spectrum of Lesions

BILE DUCT MICROHAMARTOMAS (VON MEYENBURG COMPLEXES): These clinically inapparent lesions consist of anomalous, small cystic bile ducts embedded in a fibrous stroma. They are usually multiple and vary from barely visible grayish white foci to nodules 1 cm in diameter. The cysts are lined by bile duct epithelium and sometimes have inspissated bile.

SOLITARY AND MULTIPLE SIMPLE CYSTS: Simple liver cysts are lined by cuboidal to columnar epithelium and may be associated with adult polycystic kidney disease (see Chapter 16). They are not infrequently seen in livers containing von Meyenburg complexes.

CONGENITAL HEPATIC FIBROSIS: This recessively inherited disorder is marked by enlarged portal tracts with extensive fibrosis and numerous bile ductules. It is seen mainly in children and adolescents. Bile ductules may be so dilated as to resemble microcysts, but even in these cases, they still communicate with the biliary system. Regenerative nodules are absent, which distinguishes this condition from cirrhosis. The origin of the lesion is unknown, but it has been postulated that it may result from abnormal differentiation of primitive duct structures. The principal complication of congenital hepatic fibrosis is severe portal hypertension with recurrent bleeding from esophageal varices. **Infantile polycystic disease** of the liver resembles congenital hepatic fibrosis and is also inherited as an autosomal recessive trait.

Malignant Tumors of the Liver

Hepatocellular Carcinoma Is a Malignant Tumor of Hepatocytes or Their Precursors

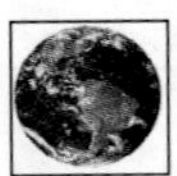

EPIDEMIOLOGY: Hepatocellular carcinoma (HCC) is probably the most common human cancer. It occurs in all parts of the world but shows a striking geographical variability. In Western industrialized countries, HCC is uncommon, but its incidence has nearly doubled in the last 20 years. In sub-Saharan Africa, Southeast Asia and Japan, HCC incidence may be up to 50 times greater. For example, in Mozambique, which seems to have the highest incidence in the world, two thirds of all cancers in men and one third in women are HCC. The incidence of HCC in the United States is rising due to the increased prevalence of HCV infection.

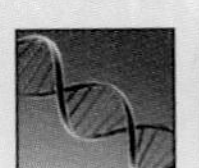

MOLECULAR PATHOGENESIS AND ETIOLOGIC FACTORS:

HEPATITIS B: HBV and HCC are closely intertwined. Over 85% of cases of HCC occur in countries with a high prevalence of chronic HBV infection. Most patients have chronic hepatitis B for years, the disease often being transmitted from an infected mother to her newborn child perinatally. Persistent HBV infection is indeed dangerous and carries as much as a 200-fold increased risk for developing HCC. One fourth of those with chronic hepatitis B acquired at or near birth ultimately develop HCC. The risk of HCC in men who are positive for HBsAg and HBeAg is about four times as great as in those only positive for HBsAg. Most (>80%) cases of HCC associated with HBV infection occur in patients with cirrhosis, although numerous instances are reported in noncirrhotic chronic hepatitis B.

Although cirrhosis has been blamed for the emergence of HCC in HBV-infected livers, the fact is that many HBV-associated HCCs occur in patients without cirrhosis. It is more likely that HBV genome integration into cell DNA and expression of HBV genes are the key factors. Thus, the *X* gene of HBV encodes a viral protein (HBxAg) that inactivates tumor suppressor proteins and transactivates certain oncogenes. It is hoped that vaccination to prevent HBV will significantly decrease occurrences of HBV-related HCC.

HEPATITIS C: HCV is less common than HBV worldwide, but most cases of HCC in Europe and North America are associated with hepatitis C. In the United States, HCV infection is present in about 50% of HCC. As with HCC in hepatitis B, most patients with HCV who develop HCC have underlying cirrhosis, and the cumulative occurrence of HCC in HCV-induced cirrhosis is as high as 70% after 15 years.

Coinfection with HBV and HCV entails a risk of liver cancer threefold higher than infection with either virus alone. Carcinogenesis by HCV is poorly understood, but the interaction of HCV core protein with a variety of cellular proteins is considered by some to be critical.

OTHER CAUSES OF HEPATOCELLULAR CARCINOMA: **Alcoholic cirrhosis** predisposes to HCC, but the risk is not large, and the mechanism is unknown. Because many alcoholics are infected with HBV and HCV, the role of alcohol alone in HCC is difficult to determine. Alcoholics with chronic hepatitis C have double the risk for HCC, compared with HCV infection alone.

Hemochromatosis and **α_1-AT deficiency** carry substantial risk of HCC: about 10% of patients with hemochromatosis may be expected to develop the tumor. On the other hand, HCC is not increased in patients with "autoimmune" chronic hepatitis and cirrhosis, Wilson disease and PBC. ***These data, like those above with HBV-related HCC in the absence of cirrhosis, further suggest that cirrhosis itself does not lead to liver cancer.***

Aflatoxin B_1 is a fungal contaminant of many foods, mostly in less developed countries, and causes HCC in a number of mammalian species. Incidence of liver cancer in humans correlates roughly with dietary content of aflatoxin. Presence of urinary metabolites of aflatoxin B_1 is associated with a threefold increased risk of HCC. Aflatoxin and HBV infection are synergistic: combined exposure increases the risk of HCC 60-fold.

Half of DNA samples from HCCs occurring in areas endemic for aflatoxin had mutations in the *p53* gene. Most of these mutations were G-to-T substitutions in one particular codon (249), a change known to be produced experimentally by aflatoxin B_1.

14 | The Liver and Biliary System

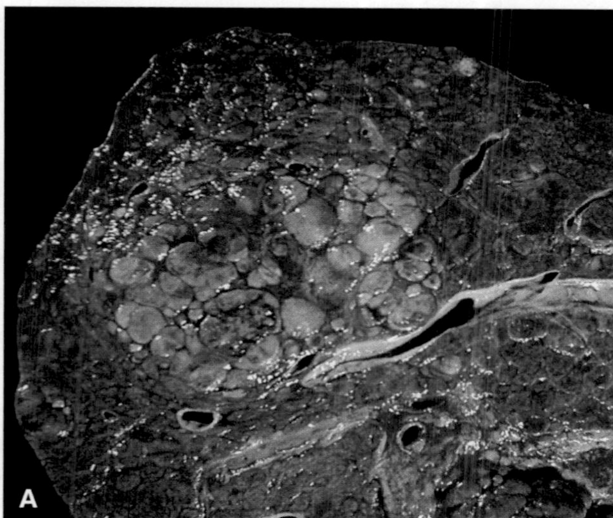

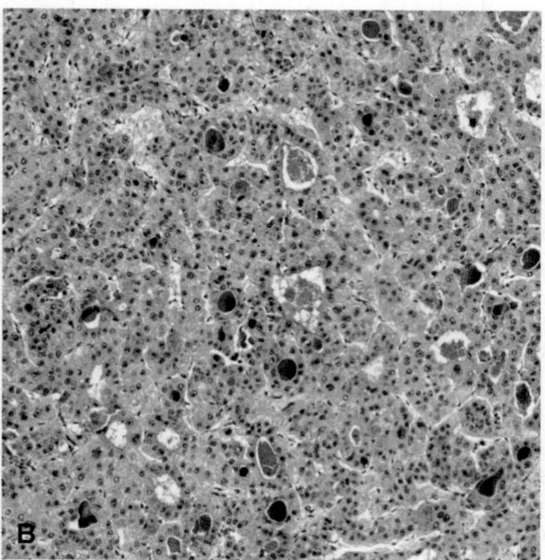

FIGURE 14-53. Hepatocellular carcinoma. A. Cross-section of a cirrhotic liver shows a poorly circumscribed, nodular area of yellow, partially hemorrhagic hepatocellular carcinoma. **B.** In this moderately differentiated tumor, hepatocellular carcinoma cells are arranged in an acinar pattern and surround concretions of inspissated bile.

PATHOLOGY: HCCs are solitary or multiple soft, hemorrhagic tan masses (Fig. 14-53A). Occasionally, a green color indicates bile staining. Multiplicity of lesions may indicate multiple origins, but intrahepatic metastases of one HCC cannot be excluded. HCCs tend to grow into the portal and hepatic veins. Tumor may extend from the latter into the vena cava and even the right atrium. Tumor may spread widely, but metastases favor the lungs and portal lymph nodes.

HCCs range from well-differentiated tumors, difficult to distinguish from normal liver, to anaplastic or undifferentiated. In most HCCs the tumor cells are arranged in trabeculae or plates similar to normal liver ("trabecular pattern"). The plates are separated by endothelium-lined sinusoids. In the "pseudoglandular (adenoid, acinar) pattern," malignant hepatocytes are arranged around a lumen, which may contain bile (Fig. 14-53B). Despite their resemblance to glands, these are not true glands, and the lesion should not be confused with adenocarcinoma. Neither histologic pattern carries a particular prognostic significance.

Fibrolamellar HCC is an uncommon variant, with a distinctive histologic appearance. It arises in an apparently normal liver, mostly in adolescents and young adults. The tumor is composed of large, eosinophilic, neoplastic hepatocytes arranged in clusters and surrounded by delicate collagen fibers (Fig. 14-54). Fibrolamellar HCC was once thought to carry a better prognosis than other forms of HCC, but recent data make this conclusion doubtful.

CLINICAL FEATURES: HCC usually presents as a painful and enlarging mass. If discovered at an advanced stage, the prognosis is dismal, and patients die of malignant cachexia, rupture of the tumor with catastrophic bleeding into the peritoneal cavity or complications of cirrhosis.

HCC may cause several paraneoplastic manifestations (e.g., polycythemia, hypoglycemia, hypercalcemia) due to hormone production by the tumor. α-Fetoprotein (AFP) levels are often elevated (as in other benign and malignant liver diseases and some extrahepatic disorders).

If a small tumor is confined to one hepatic lobe, segmental resection can provide acceptable tumor-free survival rates. Ablative therapies (e.g., absolute alcohol injection, radiofrequency ablation, cryotherapy and transarterial embolization) can slow tumor progression. In patients with cirrhosis and limited tumor burden, liver transplantation gives the best tumor-free survival.

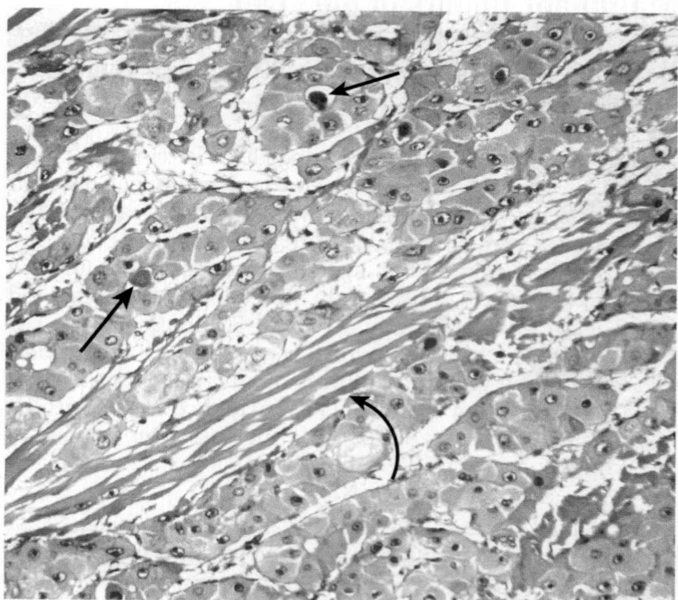

FIGURE 14-54. Fibrolamellar hepatocellular carcinoma. Eosinophilic tumor cells show a lamellar pattern. A fibrous band (*curved arrow*) traverses the tumor. Bile casts (*straight arrows*) are seen within neoplastic acini.

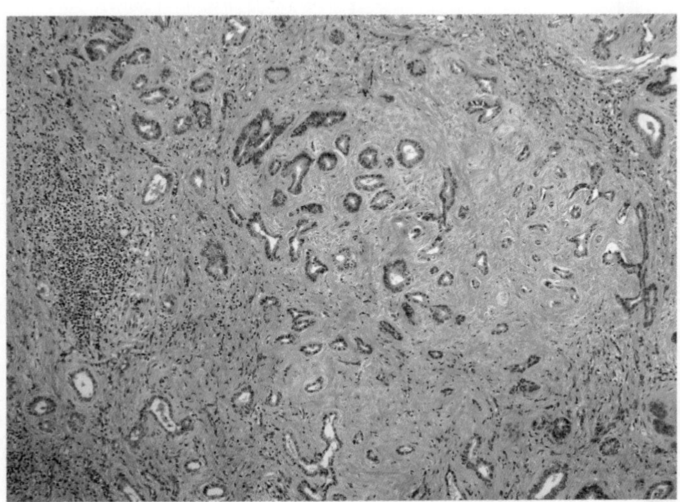

FIGURE 14-55. Cholangiocarcinoma. Well-differentiated neoplastic glands are embedded in a dense fibrous stroma.

Cholangiocarcinoma (Bile Duct Carcinoma) Arises From Biliary Epithelium

Cholangiocarcinoma originates anywhere in the biliary tree, from large intrahepatic bile ducts at the porta hepatis to the smallest bile ductules at the periphery of hepatic lobules. It occurs mainly in older people of both sexes, with an average age at presentation of 60 years. This cancer is particularly common in parts of Asia where the liver fluke (*C. sinensis*) is endemic, but the tumor occurs throughout the world. Primary sclerosing cholangitis predisposes strongly to cholangiocarcinoma. One quarter of livers with PSC removed for transplantation have cholangiocarcinoma. Choledochal cysts and Caroli disease (see below) are also risk factors.

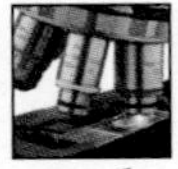

PATHOLOGY: Peripheral tumors contain small cuboidal cells in ductular or glandular patterns (Fig. 14-55). They often show substantial fibrosis, and so may be confused with metastatic breast or pancreas carcinomas on liver biopsy. Combined HCC and peripheral cholangiocarcinoma has been labeled **cholangiohepatocellular carcinoma.**

Hilar cholangiocarcinomas are extrahepatic tumors that arise at the convergence of the right and left hepatic ducts. They present as (1) small sclerosing tumors that obliterate the duct, (2) tumors that spread within the duct wall and (3) a rare intraductal papillary variant. All produce symptoms of extrahepatic biliary obstruction.

Cholangiocarcinomas invade portal and hepatic veins less than HCCs. They metastasize throughout the body, particularly to portal lymph nodes. Liver transplantation is rarely successful in eradicating the tumor. Cholangiocarcinomas in livers explanted for PSC carry a dismal prognosis.

Hepatoblastoma Is a Rare Malignant Tumor of Children

Hepatoblastoma is usually discovered at birth or before the age of 3 years.

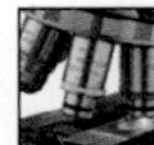

PATHOLOGY: Hepatoblastomas are circumscribed masses up to 25 cm that are partially necrotic and hemorrhagic, with epithelial- and mesenchymal-appearing cells. Occasionally the latter are not seen. The former resemble embryonic and fetal cells. "Embryonal" cells are small and fusiform and are arranged in ribbons or rosettes. The "fetal" cells resemble hepatocytes, contain glycogen and fat and are arranged in trabeculae with intervening sinusoids. Foci of squamous epithelium are occasionally encountered. The mesenchymal elements include connective tissue, cartilage and osteoid.

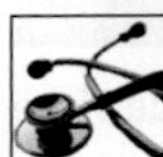

CLINICAL FEATURES: Abdominal enlargement, vomiting and failure to thrive are common presenting symptoms. Serum α-fetoprotein is almost always elevated, and occasionally secretion of ectopic gonadotropin leads to sexual precocity. Congenital anomalies may be present, including cardiac and renal malformations, hemihypertrophy and macroglossia. Untreated, these tumors are fatal, but liver transplantation or partial hepatectomy may often be curative.

Hemangiosarcoma May Result From Exposure to Chemicals

Hemangiosarcoma is the only significant sarcoma of the liver. It often results from exposure to thorium dioxide, vinyl chloride or inorganic arsenic. It has become distinctly uncommon.

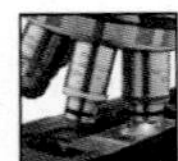

PATHOLOGY: This is a characteristically multicentric tumor, originating as multiple hemorrhagic nodules that may coalesce. Spindle-shaped, neoplastic, endothelial cells line sinusoids and compress the liver cell plates (Fig. 14-56). Cavernous blood spaces and solid masses of neoplastic cells are common. Widespread metastases are usual.

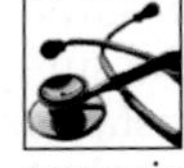

CLINICAL FEATURES: These patients present with hepatomegaly, jaundice and ascites. Hematologic abnormalities, including pancytopenia and hemolytic anemia, are often prominent and in many cases reflect

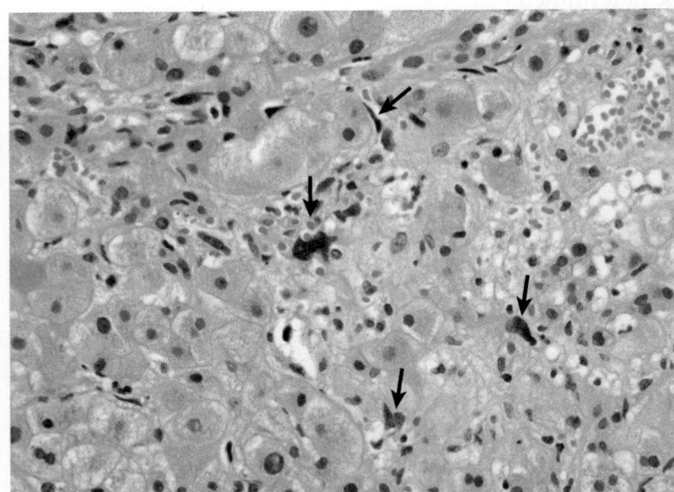

FIGURE 14-56. Angiosarcoma. Bizarre nuclei of angiosarcoma line the sinusoids (*arrows*).

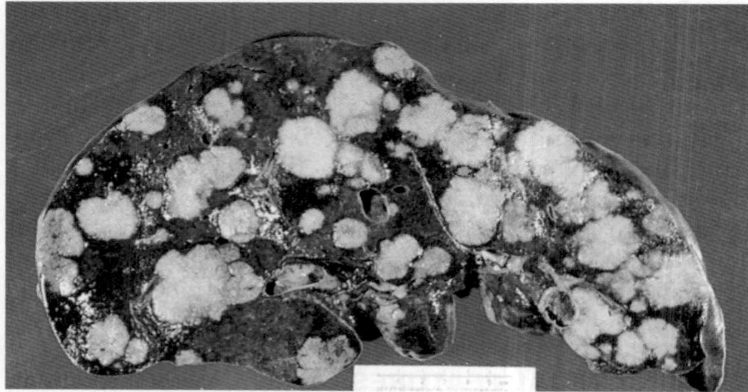

FIGURE 14-57. Metastatic carcinoma in the liver. The cut surface of the liver shows many firm, pale masses of metastatic colon cancer.

splenomegaly from noncirrhotic portal hypertension. Tumor rupture with vigorous intra-abdominal hemorrhage is common. The prognosis is dismal.

Metastatic Cancer Is the Most Common Malignant Tumor of the Liver

One third of all metastatic cancers affect the liver, including half of cancers of the gastrointestinal tract, breast and lung. Pancreatic carcinoma, malignant melanoma and hematologic malignancies also often involve the liver, but any tumor may do so.

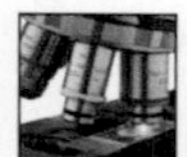

PATHOLOGY: The liver may contain a single metastatic nodule or may be virtually replaced by metastases (Fig. 14-57), and may weigh 5 kg or more. ***Liver metastases are the most common cause of massive hepatomegaly.*** Metastatic carcinomas can appear on the surface of the liver as umbilicated masses. Hepatic metastases tend to be histologically similar to the primary tumor, but may be so poorly differentiated that the primary site cannot be determined.

CLINICAL FEATURES: Weight loss is a common presentation of metastatic cancer in the liver. Portal hypertension with splenomegaly, ascites and gastrointestinal bleeding may occur. Obstruction of the major bile ducts or replacement of most of the liver parenchyma leads to jaundice. If the patient lives long enough, hepatic failure may ensue. Often the first indication of a metastatic tumor is an unexplained increase in serum alkaline phosphatase. Most patients die within a year of diagnosis, but surgical resection of a solitary metastasis may be curative.

Liver Transplantation

The increasing use of hepatic transplantation and the accompanying problems related to allograft rejection have focused attention on the morphologic criteria by which the outcome can be assessed and therapy recommended. Despite immunosuppressive therapy, some patients subjected to hepatic transplantation develop graft rejection.

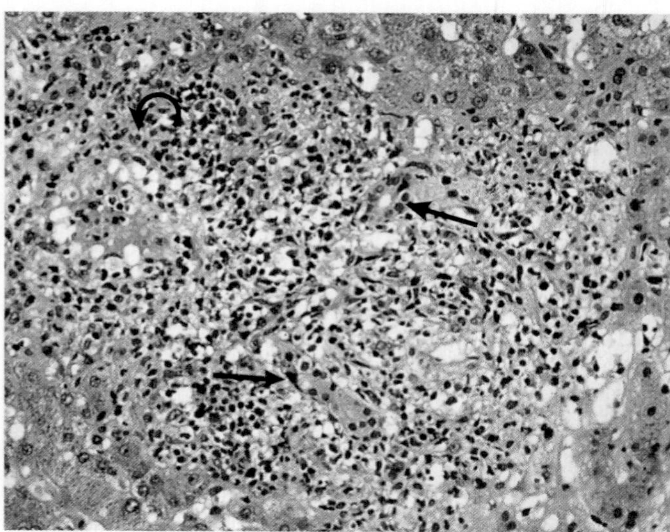

FIGURE 14-58. Acute rejection of a liver transplant. A portal tract is expanded by a polymorphous inflammatory infiltrate consisting of large and small lymphocytes, plasma cells, macrophages and neutrophils. The bile ducts (*arrows*) are damaged. A vein (*curved arrow*) is also inflamed (endophlebitis).

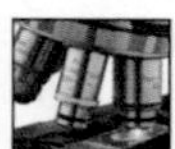

PATHOLOGY: In acute rejection, bile ducts are distorted by portal inflammation that may involve the ductal epithelium itself. Epithelial atypia may be seen (Fig. 14-58). Lymphocytes often adhere to the endothelium of terminal venules and small branches of the portal veins, with or without subendothelial inflammation (endothelialitis).

In allograft rejection lasting over 2 months there is damage to interlobular bile ducts. These small bile ducts are progressively destroyed, leading to persistent cholestasis, the end stage of which is called **chronic ductopenic rejection** or **vanishing bile duct syndrome** (Fig. 14-59). Subintimal foam cells, intimal sclerosis and myointimal hyperplasia may cause arterial narrowing or occlusion (Fig. 14-60).

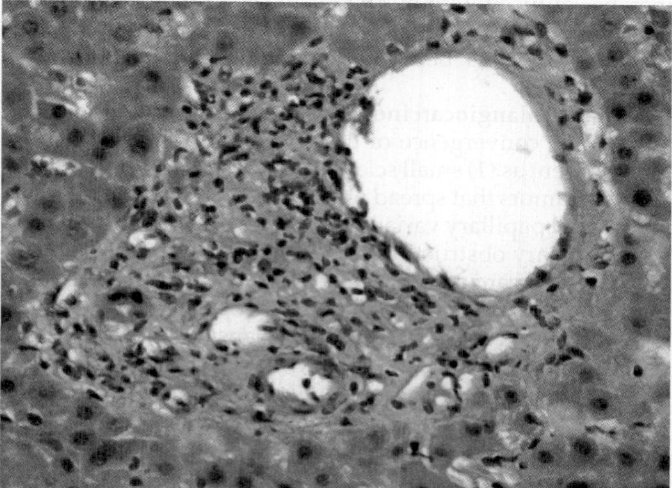

FIGURE 14-59. Chronic ductopenic rejection (vanishing bile duct syndrome). A portal tract shows mild chronic inflammation and absence of the bile duct.

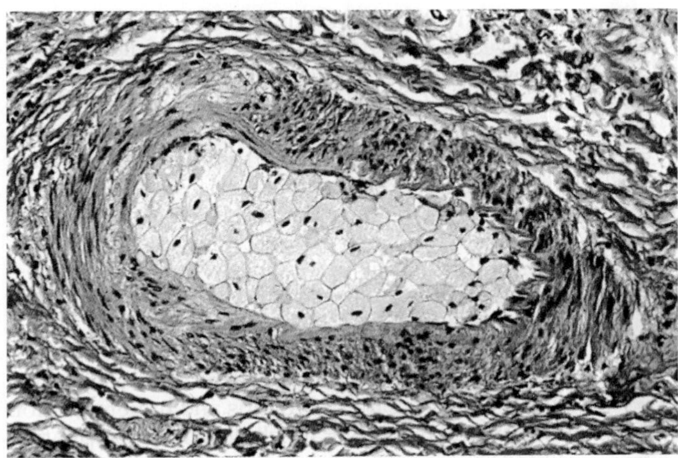

FIGURE 14-60. Arterial lesions in chronic rejection of a liver transplant. Subintimal foam cells, intimal sclerosis and myointimal hyperplasia virtually obliterate the lumen of a hepatic artery.

THE GALLBLADDER AND EXTRAHEPATIC BILE DUCTS

Anatomy

The gallbladder originates from the same foregut diverticulum that gives rise to the liver. It is a thin elongated sac about 8 cm long and about 50 mL in volume that occupies a fossa on the inferior surface of the liver between the right and the quadrate lobes. Its primary function is storage, concentration and release of bile. The cystic duct is about 3 cm long and drains the gallbladder into the hepatic duct. It conducts dilute bile from the hepatic duct into the gallbladder, where it is concentrated and subsequently discharged into the common bile duct.

The wall of the gallbladder is composed of a mucous membrane, a muscularis and an adventitia. It is covered by a reflection of the visceral peritoneum. The mucosa is thrown into folds and consists of a columnar epithelium and a lamina propria of loose connective tissue. Dipping into the wall of the gallbladder are mucosal diverticula **(Rokitansky-Aschoff sinuses).**

Congenital Anomalies

Developmental anomalies of the gallbladder are rare and of little clinical significance except for surgeons. Anomalies of the bile duct include **duplication** and **accessory bile ducts**. Congenital bile duct dilations are **choledochal cysts** (85% of all cases), **choledochal diverticula** or **choledochoceles** (Fig. 14-61). Multiple cysts may occur as segmental dilations in the entire extrahepatic biliary tree. Similar multiple dilations in the intrahepatic portion of the biliary tree, termed **Caroli disease,** predispose to bacterial cholangitis. It has been suggested that choledochal cysts form part of the same complex as neonatal hepatitis and biliary atresia.

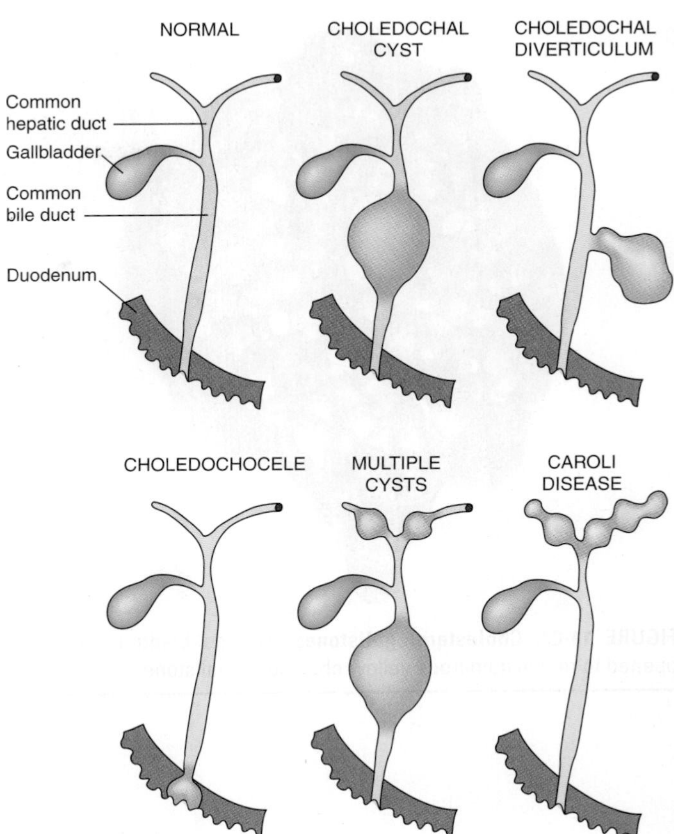

FIGURE 14-61. Congenital dilations of the bile ducts.

Cholelithiasis

In cholelithiasis there are stones within the gallbladder lumen or in the extrahepatic biliary tree. Three fourths of gallstones in the industrialized countries are mainly **cholesterol;** the remainder are composed of **calcium bilirubinate and other calcium salts (pigment gallstones).** However, pigment stones predominate in the tropics and Asia. Most gallstones are not radiopaque but are readily detected by ultrasonography. Gallstones are often asymptomatic but may cause mild to severe pain **(biliary colic)** by impacting in the cystic or common bile ducts.

Cholesterol Stones Are the Most Common Gallstones

Cholesterol stones measure up to 4 cm and may be round or faceted, yellow to tan, and single or multiple (Fig. 14-62). They are over 50% cholesterol, the rest being calcium salts and mucin.

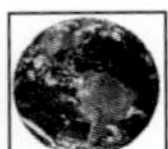

EPIDEMIOLOGY: Some 20% of American men and 35% of women over 75 years have gallstones at autopsy. ***However, women of reproductive age develop cholesterol gallstones three times more than do men, the incidence being higher in users of oral contraceptives and in women with several pregnancies.*** Cholesterol gallstones are very common in Pima Indian women of the American Southwest: 75% are affected by age 25 and 90% by the age of 60 years.

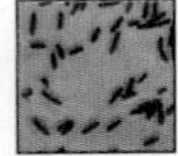

ETIOLOGIC FACTORS: Formation of cholesterol gallstones reflects the physicochemical qualities of bile and local factors in the gallbladder itself (Fig. 14-63):

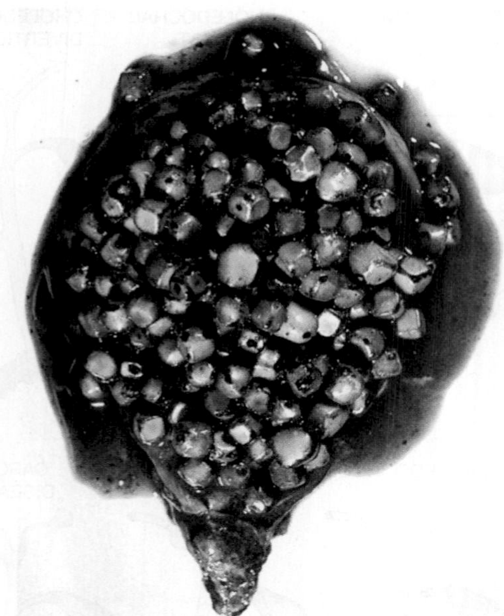

FIGURE 14-62. Cholesterol gallstones. The gallbladder has been opened to reveal numerous yellow cholesterol gallstones.

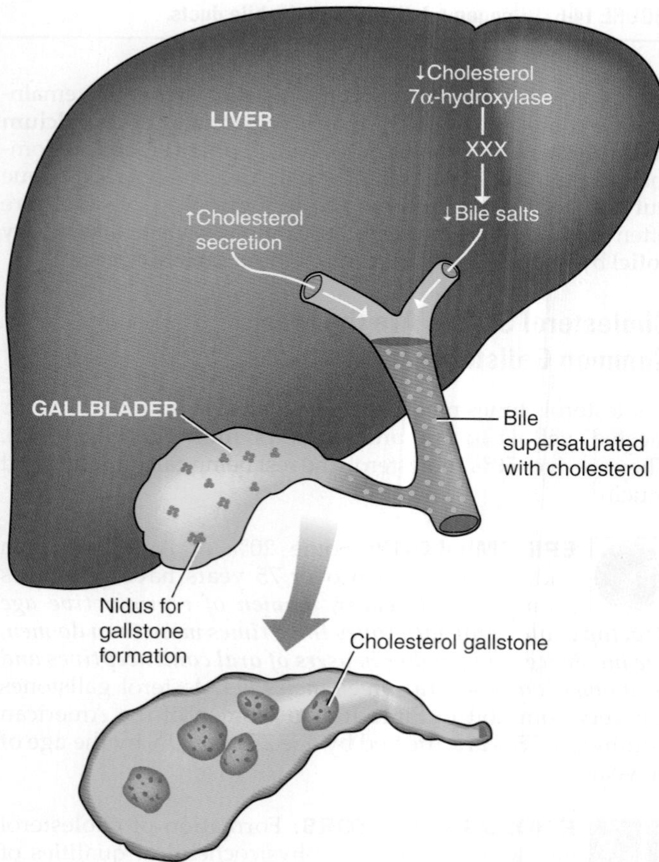

FIGURE 14-63. Pathogenesis of cholesterol gallstones.

- **Bile formation in the liver:** Cholesterol is insoluble in water. When secreted by hepatocytes into the bile, it is held in solution by the combined action of bile acids and lecithin and is carried in the form of mixed lipid micelles. If bile has too much cholesterol or is deficient in bile acids, it becomes supersaturated in cholesterol. Bile from people who have cholesterol gallstones contains more cholesterol and fewer bile salts as it leaves the liver than bile of normal persons. The supersaturated cholesterol precipitates as solid crystals to form stones **(lithogenic bile).** Obesity increases cholesterol secretion by the liver still further, augmenting the supersaturation of the bile with cholesterol.
- **Local factors in the gallbladder:** Bile in the gallbladder from patients with gallstones crystallizes more easily than normal. Pronucleating biliary proteins and hypersecretion of gallbladder mucus accelerate cholesterol precipitation from gallbladder bile.
- **Gallbladder motility:** Impaired gallbladder motor function leads to bile stasis and permits biliary sludge to form. This sludge progresses to macroscopic stones.

Estrogens increase hepatic secretion of cholesterol and decrease secretion of bile acids, perhaps explaining the increased susceptibility of women to cholesterol gallstone formation. Pregnancy magnifies these effects. Progesterone, the predominant hormone of pregnancy, inhibits discharge of bile from the gallbladder. Thus, the gallbladder empties more slowly, causing stasis and increasing the opportunity for cholesterol crystals to precipitate. These mechanisms may also explain the increase in gallstones due to oral contraceptive use.

Other major risk factors for cholesterol gallstones entail increased biliary cholesterol secretion, decreased secretion of bile salts and lecithin or a combination of the two.

Factors associated with **increased biliary cholesterol secretion** include:

- Increasing age
- Obesity
- Ethnicity (e.g., Chilean women, some northern European groups)
- Familial predisposition
- Diet high in calories and cholesterol
- Certain metabolic abnormalities associated with high blood cholesterol levels (e.g., diabetes, some genetic hyperlipoproteinemias, and PBC)

The risk of symptomatic gallstones is a direct function of body weight. In obese people, the relative risk of gallstones may be fivefold that of nonobese people. Hepatic cholesterol synthesis is stimulated by insulin, and the hyperinsulinism that accompanies increased body fat may explain the increased biliary excretion of cholesterol associated with obesity.

Decreased secretion of bile salts and lecithin occurs in nonobese whites who develop gallstones. Disorders that interfere with enterohepatic circulation of bile acids (e.g., pancreatic insufficiency in cystic fibrosis or Crohn disease) also decrease bile acid secretion and favor gallstone formation.

Cholesterol synthesis is above normal, and bile salts and lecithin are lower in American Pima Indians and in people taking certain drugs (e.g., clofibrate). Moderate alcohol intake decreases the risk of gallstones, probably because it lowers biliary cholesterol concentration.

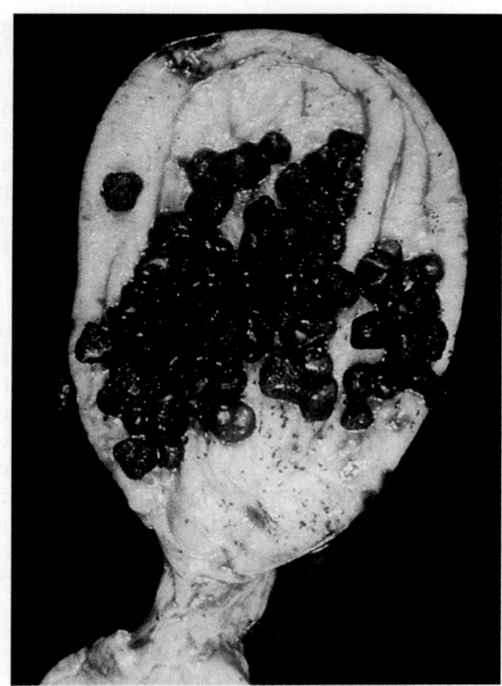

FIGURE 14-64. Pigment gallstones. The gallbladder has been opened to reveal numerous small, dark stones composed of calcium bilirubinate.

Pigment Stones Are Classed As Black or Brown Stones

Black Pigment Stones

Black pigment stones are under 1 cm, irregular and glassy (Fig. 14-64). They contain calcium bilirubinate, bilirubin polymers, calcium salts and mucin.

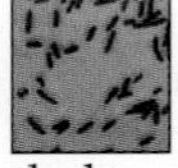

ETIOLOGIC FACTORS: Black stones occur more in older or undernourished people of both sexes and all races. Chronic hemolysis, as in sickle cell anemia or thalassemia, predisposes to development of black pigment stones. Cirrhosis, either because it increases hemolysis or because of damage to liver cells, is also associated with a high incidence of black stones. However, usually no cause for formation of black pigment stones is evident.

Unconjugated bilirubin is insoluble in bile and is usually present in only trace amounts. When increased amounts are secreted by the hepatocyte, the unconjugated bilirubin precipitates as calcium bilirubinate, probably around a nidus of mucinous glycoproteins. For unexplained reasons, patients without known predisposing factors who develop black pigment stones have increased concentrations of unconjugated bilirubin in the bile.

Brown Pigment Stones

Brown pigment stones are spongy and laminated and contain principally calcium bilirubinate mixed with cholesterol and calcium soaps of fatty acids. Unlike other types of gallstones, they are more common in intrahepatic and extrahepatic bile ducts than in the gallbladder.

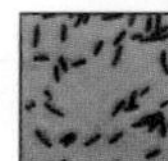

ETIOLOGIC FACTORS: Brown stones are almost always associated with bacterial cholangitis, for which *E. coli* is the main cause. They are uncommon in Western countries but are not infrequent in Asia, where they are almost entirely seen in people infested with *A. lumbricoides* or *C. sinensis*, helminths that may invade the biliary tract. The rare cases in Western countries are seen in patients with chronic mechanical obstruction to bile flow, as in sclerosing cholangitis or the presence of a catheter in the common bile duct after common bile duct surgery.

Bacterial β-glucuronidase or other hydrolytic enzymes hydrolyze conjugated bilirubin to its unconjugated form. Increased unconjugated bilirubin favors formation of brown stones.

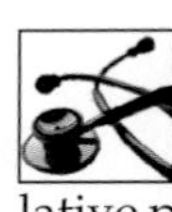

CLINICAL FEATURES: Gallstones in the gallbladder may remain "silent" for many years, and few patients die of cholelithiasis itself. The 15-year cumulative probability that asymptomatic stones will lead to biliary pain or other complications is less than 20%. Laparoscopic cholecystectomy is the treatment of choice.

Most complications of cholelithiasis relate to obstruction of the cystic or common bile ducts by gallstones. Passage of a stone into the cystic duct often, but not always, causes severe biliary colic and may lead to acute cholecystitis. Repeated bouts of acute cholecystitis lead to chronic cholecystitis. The latter condition may also result from the presence of stones alone. Gallstones may enter the common duct **(choledocholithiasis)** and cause obstructive jaundice, cholangitis and pancreatitis. Gallstones are the most common cause of acute pancreatitis in people who do not drink alcohol. Passage of a large gallstone into the small intestine may even cause intestinal obstruction, a condition called **gallstone ileus.** In obstruction of the cystic duct, with or without acute cholecystitis, bile in the gallbladder is reabsorbed and replaced by a clear mucinous fluid secreted by gallbladder epithelium. **Hydrops of the gallbladder (mucocele)** (Fig. 14-65) describes a distended and palpable gallbladder, which may become secondarily infected.

Acute Cholecystitis

Acute cholecystitis is diffuse inflammation of the gallbladder, usually secondary to obstruction of the gallbladder outlet.

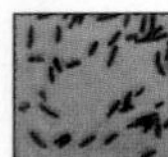

ETIOLOGIC FACTORS: ***Some 90% of cases of acute cholecystitis occur in people with gallstones.*** The remaining cases **(acalculous cholecystitis)** are linked to sepsis, severe trauma, infection of the gallbladder with *Salmonella typhosa* and polyarteritis nodosa. Bacterial infection is usually secondary to biliary obstruction, rather than a primary event.

Obstruction of the cystic duct by a gallstone may lead to release of phospholipase from the gallbladder epithelium. This enzyme may then hydrolyze lecithin to release lysolecithin, a membrane-active toxin. The mucous coat of the epithelium is disrupted, exposing the mucosal cells to the detergent action of concentrated bile salts. Bile supersaturated with cholesterol may be toxic to the epithelium.

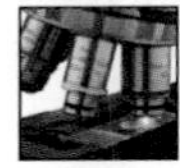

PATHOLOGY: In acute cholecystitis, the external surface of the gallbladder is congested and layered with a fibrinous exudate. The wall is thickened by

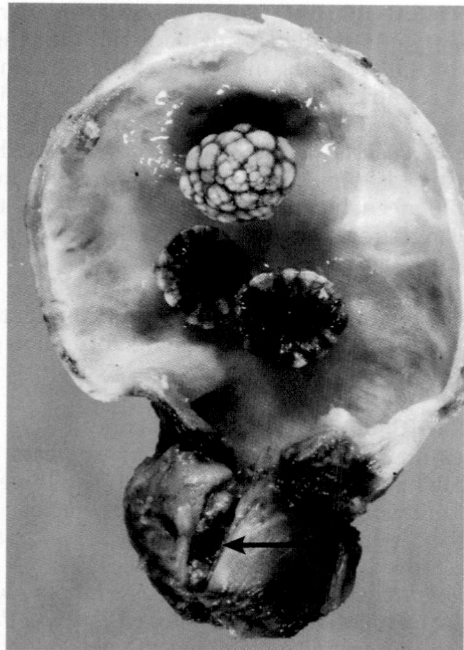

FIGURE 14-65. Hydrops of the gallbladder. The lumen of the dilated gallbladder is filled with clear mucus and contains cholesterol stones. Note the stone (*arrow*) obstructing the cystic duct.

edema, and the mucosa is fiery red or purple. Gallstones are usually found in the lumen, and one is often seen obstructing the cystic duct. Rarely, in **empyema of the gallbladder,** the cystic duct is completely obstructed, allowing bacteria to invade the gallbladder, and the cavity may be distended by cloudy, purulent fluid.

In the gallbladder wall, edema and hemorrhage are striking, with accompanying acute and chronic inflammation (Fig. 14-66). Suppuration in the gallbladder wall may follow bacterial invasion. The mucosa shows focal ulcers or, in severe cases, widespread necrosis, to which case the term **gangrenous cholecystitis** is applied.

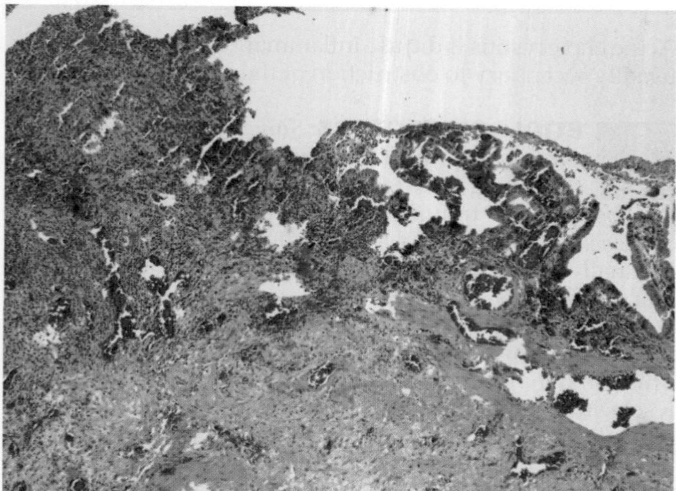

FIGURE 14-66. Acute cholecystitis. Gallbladder removed from a patient with acute cholecystitis demonstrates ulceration of the mucosa (*left*) and acute and chronic inflammation.

Gallbladder perforation is a dreaded complication that may follow secondary bacterial infection, most commonly of the fundus. Bile discharged into the abdominal cavity results in **bile peritonitis.** More often, inflammatory adhesions form a **pericholecystic abscess** and limit spread of gallbladder contents after perforation. Erosion of gallbladder contents into a viscus may create, for example, a **cholecystenteric fistula.**

CLINICAL FEATURES: Right upper quadrant abdominal pain is usually the presenting symptom. Most patients have already had episodes of biliary colic. Mild jaundice, caused by stones in, or edema of, the common bile duct, is seen in 20% of patients. The acute illness generally subsides within a week, but persistent pain, fever, leukocytosis and shaking chills herald progression of the acute cholecystitis and the need for cholecystectomy. As inflammation resolves, the gallbladder wall becomes fibrotic and the mucosa heals. However, the function of the gallbladder usually remains impaired.

Chronic Cholecystitis

Chronic cholecystitis (i.e., persistent chronic inflammation) is the most common disease of the gallbladder. It is almost always associated with gallstones but may also result from repeated attacks of acute cholecystitis. In the latter case, the pathogenesis probably relates to chronic irritation and chemical injury to the gallbladder epithelium.

PATHOLOGY: Grossly, the wall of the chronically inflamed gallbladder is thickened and firm (Fig. 14-67A), and the serosal surface may show fibrous adhesions to surrounding structures as a result of previous episodes of acute cholecystitis. Gallstones are usually found within the lumen. The bile often contains gravel or sludge (i.e., fine precipitates of calculous material) and carries coliform organisms in about half of cases. The mucosa may be focally ulcerated and atrophic or may appear intact. The fibrotic wall is chronically inflamed throughout and is often penetrated by sinuses of Rokitansky-Aschoff (Fig. 14-67B). Long-standing inflammation may lead to calcification **(porcelain gallbladder).**

CLINICAL FEATURES: Many patients with chronic cholecystitis complain of nonspecific abdominal symptoms, although it is not at all clear that these are necessarily related to the gallbladder disease. On the other hand, pain in the right hypochondrium is typical and often episodic. The diagnosis is best made by ultrasound examination, which demonstrates gallstones in a thick, contracted gallbladder. Cholecystectomy is the definitive treatment.

Cholesterolosis

Cholesterolosis of the gallbladder is the accumulation of cholesterol-laden macrophages within the submucosa. It reflects supersaturation of bile with cholesterol and does not ordinarily cause symptoms. The mucosa shows scattered, yellow flecks and mucosal folds are swollen with large, foamy

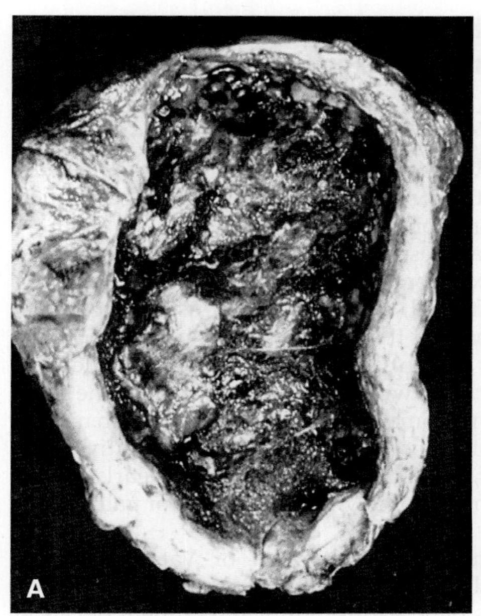

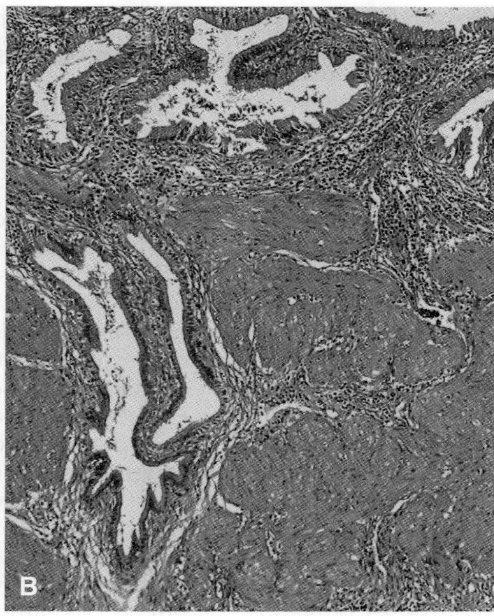

FIGURE 14-67. Chronic cholecystitis. A. The gallbladder is thickened and fibrotic. The lumen had contained several gallstones. **B.** A photomicrograph of A shows chronic inflammation of the gallbladder and a sinus of Rokitansky-Aschoff extending into the muscularis.

macrophages, in which a small nucleus is displaced to the periphery.

Tumors

Benign Tumors of the Gallbladder and Extrahepatic Biliary Ducts Are Rare

Papillomas are the most common benign tumors of the gallbladder and may be single or multiple. They are associated with gallstones in 75% of cases. A combined proliferation of smooth muscle with an adenoma is an **adenomyoma.** Fibromas, lipomas, leiomyomas and myxomas have also been recorded. Similar benign tumors may occur in the bile ducts, where they may obstruct biliary flow and cause jaundice, and so come to clinical attention.

Adenocarcinoma Is the Most Common Tumor of the Gallbladder

Adenocarcinoma of the gallbladder is not rare. It is found incidentally in 2% of patients who undergo gallbladder surgery. Since this cancer is usually associated with cholelithiasis

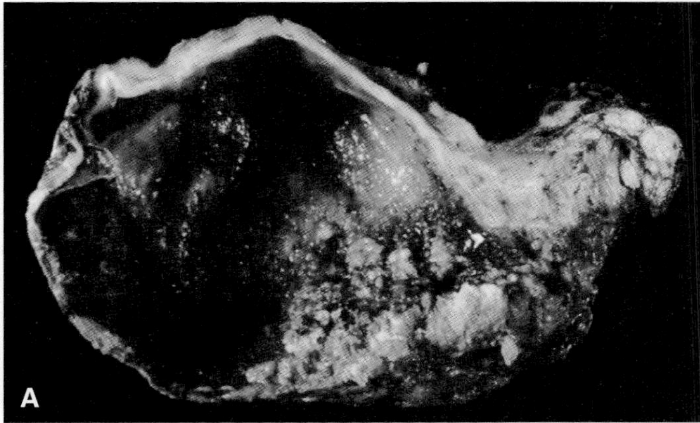

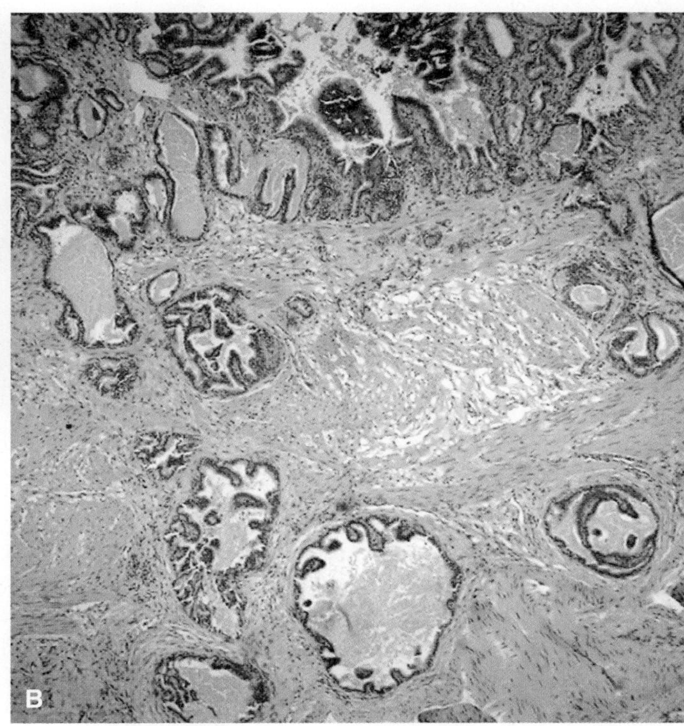

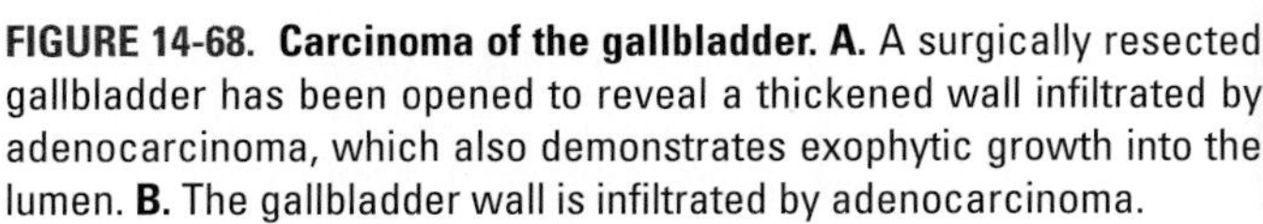

FIGURE 14-68. Carcinoma of the gallbladder. A. A surgically resected gallbladder has been opened to reveal a thickened wall infiltrated by adenocarcinoma, which also demonstrates exophytic growth into the lumen. **B.** The gallbladder wall is infiltrated by adenocarcinoma.

and chronic cholecystitis, it is much more common in women and in populations with a high incidence of cholelithiasis, such as Native Americans. Calcified (porcelain) gallbladders (see above) are particularly prone to developing gallbladder cancer.

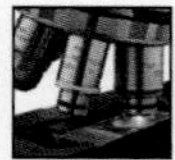

PATHOLOGY: Gallbladder carcinoma may occur anywhere in the gallbladder but appears most often in the fundus. The tumor is characteristically an infiltrative, well-differentiated adenocarcinoma. It is usually desmoplastic, and thus the gallbladder wall becomes thickened and leathery (Fig. 14-68). Anaplastic, giant cell and spindle cell forms of gallbladder carcinoma are reported. The organ's rich lymphatic plexus provides the most common route of metastasis, but vascular dissemination and direct spread into the liver and contiguous structures also occur.

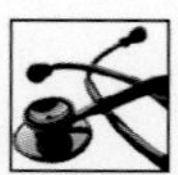

CLINICAL FEATURES: The symptoms of carcinoma of the gallbladder are similar to those of gallstone disease. However, by the time these tumors become symptomatic, they are almost invariably incurable: 5-year survival is under 3%. For practical purposes, only those patients whose tumors are discovered incidentally during cholecystectomy may be cured.

Carcinomas of the Bile Duct and Ampulla of Vater Present as Obstructive Jaundice

Cancer of the extrahepatic bile ducts (extrahepatic cholangiocarcinoma; see above) is almost always adenocarcinoma. It may occur anywhere along the length of the bile duct, including the location where the right and left hepatic ducts join to form the common hepatic duct.

These tumors are less common than gallbladder cancer and affect both sexes comparably. Gallstones are frequently found in those affected, and there is an association with inflammatory disease of the colon. The tumor may occur in choledochal cysts and in Caroli disease. In Asia, bile duct carcinoma is associated with biliary infestation by the fluke *C. sinensis*. As in carcinoma of the gallbladder, growth may be endophytic (into the lumen) or diffusely infiltrative. The prognosis is poor, but since symptoms arise early in the disease, the outcome is somewhat better than for gallbladder carcinoma.

Adenocarcinoma of the ampulla of Vater may also obstruct bile flow. It usually presents as obstructive jaundice, but occasionally as pancreatitis. Surgical treatment of cancer of the ampulla of Vater provides a 5-year survival rate of about 35%.

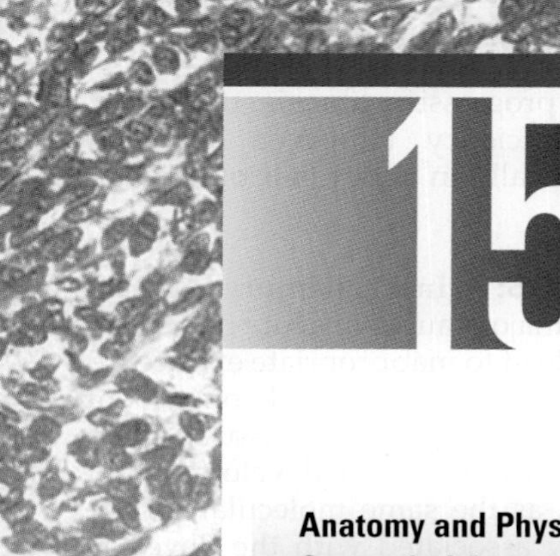

The Pancreas

David S. Klimstra • Edward B. Stelow

Anatomy and Physiology

Pancreatic development begins at 4 weeks as two endodermal outpouchings on the dorsal and ventral sides of the embryonic duodenal tube. The ventral pancreas and the common bile duct migrate posteriorly around the duodenum. The ductal systems of the two embryonic pancreatic anlagen merge at 7 weeks, giving rise to a main pancreatic duct **(duct of Wirsung)** composed of the ventral pancreatic duct that extends from the ampulla of Vater at the duodenum into the distal portion of the dorsal pancreatic duct. The proximal remnant of the dorsal duct becomes the **duct of Santorini,** which may remain patent through the minor papilla into the duodenum, but this connection usually is obliterated. The ducts branch progressively into smaller ducts and ductules that extend into the pancreatic lobules. Acinar cells arise from ductules and acquire their distinctive zymogen granules. The enzymatic secretions of the acinar cells drain into the smallest ductules between the centroacinar cells, which bridge the acinar lumina into the ductal system. Islet cells are also derived from ducts and acquire different small, dense, secretory granules, corresponding to the different peptides they produce.

The pancreas is a mixed exocrine/endocrine gland, 10 to 15 cm long and weighing 60 to 150 g, that lies transversely in the upper abdomen, cradled between the loop of the duodenum and the hilum of the spleen. It is retroperitoneal, behind the lesser omental sac and the stomach, although the anterior surface is covered by peritoneum. It is thus inaccessible to physical examination. It has three anatomic subdivisions: (1) the **head** is in the concavity of the duodenum and extends to the superior mesenteric vessels, which pass through a groove immediately behind the organ, (2) the **neck** connects the head to the distal portion of the gland and (3) the **tail** constitutes the distal two thirds of the pancreas and extends to the hilum of the spleen.

Exocrine pancreatic secretions drain into the major ducts of Wirsung and Santorini, which join the common bile duct and empty into the duodenum through the papilla of Vater. These pancreatic and biliary ducts usually merge a variable distance (1 to 5 mm) below the duodenal mucosa in a common channel that is the prototypical ampulla of Vater. In a significant minority of individuals, these ducts remain separated by a septum and enter the duodenum independently. The ampulla is surrounded by a circular complex of smooth muscle fibers, the **sphincter of Oddi,** that controls passage of pancreatic juice and bile into the duodenum.

Exocrine tissue makes up 80% to 85% of the pancreas and consists of acini with a single layer of pyramidal cells, whose basal cytoplasm is basophilic due to abundant rough endoplasmic reticulum. The apical cytoplasm contains eosinophilic zymogen granules. Acinar cells synthesize some 20 different digestive enzymes, mostly in the form of inactive proenzymes. Upon neural and hormonal stimulation, these enzymes, including trypsin, chymotrypsin, amylase, lipase and elastase, are secreted and subsequently activated in the duodenum. Amylase and lipase are secreted in their active forms. The daily secretion of 1.5 to 3 liters of pancreatic juice attests to the remarkable synthetic and secretory capacity of the exocrine pancreas.

The endocrine pancreas is organized into **islets of Langerhans.** These are present throughout the organ but comprise only 1% to 2% of the total pancreatic mass. Most islets consist of circumscribed lobules of cells derived from the dorsal embryonic pancreas. These **compact islets** contain several cell types, principally alpha and beta cells that produce glucagon and insulin, respectively; somatostatin-producing delta cells and pancreatic polypeptide cells are present in small numbers. Islets derived from the ventral embryonic pancreas mainly contain beta and pancreatic polypeptide cells. These **diffuse islets** are arranged in cords interspersed between acinar cells. Each islet cell makes only one peptide hormone, which is secreted directly into the blood (see below). The major endocrine disease of the pancreas, diabetes mellitus, is discussed in Chapter 22.

Congenital Anomalies

There are many anatomic variations in the configuration of the major pancreatic ducts and their relationship to the common bile duct. Most of these variations are considered normal and are rarely of clinical significance. Other developmental variations have clinical consequences and are therefore regarded as developmental defects.

PANCREAS DIVISUM: Pancreas divisum, the most common congenital anomaly, results from failure of the two embryonic pancreatic ducts to fuse, leading to retention of two separate ductal systems, each draining into the duodenum through the major and minor papillae, respectively. Thus, the major portion of the pancreas is drained by the duct of Santorini through the minor papilla. Chronic pancreatitis develops in up to 25% of people with pancreas divisum.

HETEROTOPIC PANCREAS: Pancreatic tissue occurring outside its normal location, mostly in the walls of the duodenum, stomach and jejunum, is an incidental finding in 2% to 15% of autopsies. Such heterotopic tissue may contain all components of normal pancreas, but some cases contain only ducts, whereas coexisting acini and islets are not always found. Smooth muscle is usually abundant in pancreatic heterotopia involving the tubular gastrointestinal tract. Pancreatic tumors may arise in heterotopic tissue, most often infiltrating ductal adenocarcinoma.

ANNULAR PANCREAS: In this uncommon condition, the pancreatic head partly or completely surrounds the second portion of the duodenum. Infants with annular pancreas often have other congenital anomalies, including trisomy 21 (Down syndrome). Some affected patients also have duodenal atresia, which requires surgery immediately after birth. About half of patients with annular pancreas do not develop symptoms until 60 or 70 years of age.

CYSTS: True cysts of the pancreas are believed to arise from faulty development of pancreatic ducts. There is an association with other anatomic anomalies, including renal tubular dysplasia, anorectal malformations, polydactyly and thoracic dystrophy.

PARTIAL OR COMPLETE PANCREATIC AGENESIS: Homozygous mutations of homeodomain transcription factor IPF1 (PDX1) are reported in these rare conditions.

Acute Pancreatitis

Acute pancreatitis results from aberrant release of pancreatic exocrine enzymes. It is not truly an inflammatory condition, but instead reflects myriad locoregional and systemic changes seen with release of these enzymes. The devastation of acute pancreatitis was justly described by Lord Moynihan in 1925 as the "most terrible of all calamities [of] the abdominal viscera. The suddenness of its onset, the illimitable agony which accompanies it and the mortality attendant upon it render it a formidable disease." For unknown reasons, the incidence of acute pancreatitis has increased 10-fold in the past few decades.

The severity of acute pancreatitis varies greatly from case to case. At one end of the spectrum is a mild, self-limited disease, with acute inflammation and stromal edema, and little or no acinar cell necrosis. This is usually not associated with systemic manifestations of disease. At the other extreme is a severe, sometimes fatal, acute hemorrhagic pancreatitis with massive necrosis, in which systemic manifestations such as shock, acute respiratory distress, acute renal failure and disseminated intravascular coagulation may develop.

Repeated bouts of acute pancreatitis may lead to chronic pancreatitis, which is characterized by recurrent attacks of severe abdominal pain and progressive fibrosis, ultimately leading to pancreatic insufficiency. However, no acute episodes are recognized clinically in about half of cases of chronic pancreatitis.

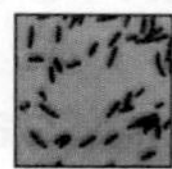

ETIOLOGIC FACTORS: Acinar cell injury and **duct obstruction** are the major causes of acute pancreatitis. These processes lead to inappropriate extracellular leakage of activated digestive enzymes and consequent autodigestion of pancreatic and extrapancreatic tissues. There may be some genetic predispositions to the development of acute pancreatitis; however, as the same molecular pathogenetic factors are generally associated with the development of chronic pancreatitis, they are discussed in that section.

ACTIVATED PANCREATIC ENZYMES: Inappropriate activation of pancreatic proenzymes occurs in all forms of pancreatitis. Acinar cells are shielded from the potentially destructive action of their digestive enzymes (proteases, nucleases, amylase, lipase and phospholipase A) by three mechanisms:

1. Enzymes are physically isolated from the cytosol by an intricate, intracellular, cavitary system of endoplasmic reticulum, Golgi complex and zymogen granule membranes.
2. Many digestive enzymes are synthesized as inactive forms (e.g., chymotrypsinogen, proelastase, prophospholipase and trypsinogen).
3. Specific enzyme inhibitors tend to protect the pancreas.

Inhibitors of proteolytic enzymes defend against inappropriate activation of pancreatic proenzymes and are present in many body fluids and tissues. The plasma protease inhibitors are α_1-antitrypsin, α_2-macroglobulin, C_1 esterase inhibitor and pancreatic secretory trypsin inhibitor. Several trypsin inhibitors are described in different body compartments, but they protect only incompletely from trypsin activation. Trypsin does not produce cell necrosis. However, it activates other pancreatic proenzymes, such as prophospholipase A_2 and proelastase, and so is central to the pathogenesis of acute pancreatitis.

SECRETION AGAINST OBSTRUCTION AND DUCT INSUFFICIENCY: Most enzymes secreted by acinar cells are discharged into the ductal system and enter the duodenum. A small amount diffuses back into periductular extracellular fluid and eventually into plasma. Whenever lumina of pancreatic ducts are narrowed or easy outflow of exocrine secretions is impaired, intraductal pressure and back-diffusion across the ducts increase. This is suspected to cause inappropriate activation of digestive proenzymes. Heavy meals may lead to release of pancreatic secretagogues, and so augment production of pancreatic enzymes.

Gallstones sometimes obstruct pancreatic ducts, and 45% of patients with acute pancreatitis also have cholelithiasis. Conversely, the risk of acute pancreatitis in patients with gallstones is 25 times higher than in the general population, and about 5% of patients with gallstones develop acute pancreatitis. Also, if gallstones are not eliminated after one attack, pancreatitis recurs in half the cases. The reason for the association between pancreatitis and cholelithiasis remains obscure since fewer than 5% of patients with acute pancreatitis have impacted stones at the ampulla of Vater. Neither ligation of the pancreatic duct nor its occlusion by tumor generally leads to severe acute pancreatitis. It may be that the reflux of bile or duodenal contents into the pancreatic duct may lead to pancreatitis, but there is little evidence to support this theory.

Anatomic anomalies (e.g., pancreas divisum) and **neoplasms** (ampullary and pancreatic neoplasms, including intraductal processes) can also lead to acute pancreatitis due to duct insufficiency or obstruction, respectively.

ETHANOL: ***Chronic alcohol abuse accounts for a third of cases of acute pancreatitis, although only 5% to 10% of chronic alcoholics develop this complication.*** The pathogenesis of ethanol-induced pancreatitis (acute and chronic) is not well understood (see below). Ethanol does not cause significant injury to pancreatic acinar or duct cells.

Alcohol consumption may cause spasm or acute edema of the sphincter of Oddi, especially after an alcoholic binge. It also stimulates secretion from the small intestine, which triggers the exocrine pancreas to release pancreatic juice.

OTHER CAUSES OF ACUTE PANCREATITIS: Rare causes of acute pancreatitis are:

- **Viruses,** such as mumps, coxsackievirus and cytomegalovirus. The incidence of acute pancreatitis is particularly high in patients with acquired immunodeficiency syndrome (AIDS) due to human immunodeficiency virus type 1 (HIV-1) itself, or, most commonly, cytomegalovirus infection.
- **Therapeutic drugs** may cause acute pancreatitis. These include immunosuppressive drugs (e.g., azathioprine), antineoplastic agents, estrogens, sulfonamides and diuretics. The mechanisms of pancreatic injury by these compounds are unclear.
- **Blunt trauma** to the upper abdomen with contusive injury to the pancreas and leakage of digestive enzymes into the pancreas and peripancreatic tissues is another cause. Patients undergoing endoscopic retrograde cholangiopancreatography (ERCP), fine needle aspiration biopsy and surgical manipulation occasionally develop acute pancreatitis.
- **Acute ischemia** due to shock, vasculitis and thrombosis may cause acute pancreatitis.
- **Hyperlipidemia.** Hydrolysis of triglycerides in the extracellular space by inappropriate leakage of pancreatic lipase may be responsible. Released free fatty acids are cytotoxic.
- **Hypercalcemia,** regardless of cause, is associated with acute pancreatitis.
- **Obesity.** Obese people are at greater risk for severe pancreatitis. Increased peripancreatic fat may predispose them to greater fat necrosis after local release of pancreatic lipase.
- **Idiopathic pancreatitis** is the third most common form of the disease, accounting for 10% to 20% of all cases.
- **Parasites** (e.g., *Ascariasis*), bacteria (e.g., *Mycoplasma* spp.) and **pregnancy** are rare causes of acute pancreatitis.

Factors implicated in acute hemorrhagic pancreatitis are shown in Fig. 15-1.

PATHOLOGY: In acute hemorrhagic pancreatitis, the pancreas is initially edematous and hyperemic. Within a day, pale, gray foci appear, rapidly becoming friable and hemorrhagic (Fig. 15-2A). In severe cases, these foci enlarge so that most of the pancreas is converted into a large retroperitoneal hematoma, in which pancreatic tissue is barely recognizable. Yellow-white areas of fat necrosis appear around the pancreas, including the adjacent mesentery (Fig. 15-2B). These nodules of necrotic fat have a pasty consistency that becomes firmer and chalklike as more calcium and magnesium soaps are produced. Saponification reflects the interaction of cations with free fatty acids released by the action of activated lipase on triglycerides in fat cells. As a result, blood calcium may be depressed, sometimes to the point of causing neuromuscular irritability.

The most prominent microscopic findings in acute pancreatitis are acinar cell and fat necrosis, often with some degree of acute inflammation (Fig. 15-3). Necrosis is usually patchy, and rarely involves the entire gland. Irregular fibrosis of the pancreas and occasionally calcification (i.e., chronic pancreatitis) result from healed acute pancreatitis.

PANCREATIC PSEUDOCYST: As many as half of patients surviving acute pancreatitis may develop pancreatic pseudocysts (Fig. 15-4). These are delimited by connective tissue and contain degraded blood, inflammatory cells, debris and fluid rich in pancreatic enzymes. Pseudocysts may enlarge to compress and even obstruct the duodenum or other structures. They may become secondarily infected and form abscesses. Rupture is a rare complication that may lead to chemical or septic peritonitis, or both.

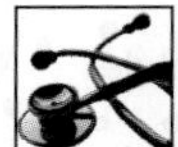

CLINICAL FEATURES: Patients with acute pancreatitis present with severe epigastric pain that is referred to the upper back, nausea and vomiting. Within hours, catastrophic peripheral vascular collapse and shock may ensue. With sustained, profound shock, **acute respiratory distress syndrome** and **acute renal failure** may occur within the first week. Early in the disease, pancreatic digestive enzymes from injured acinar cells enter the blood and retroperitoneal area. ***Elevated serum amylase and lipase within 24 to 72 hours is diagnostic for acute pancreatitis.*** Infection of the pancreas with gram-negative bacteria from the intestinal tract greatly increases mortality.

Chronic Pancreatitis

Chronic pancreatitis results from progressive destruction of pancreatic parenchyma and its replacement with fibrosis. Since its original description and its association with stones two centuries ago, the pathogenesis, clinical course and treatment of chronic pancreatitis remain enigmatic. Its symptoms include recurrent or persisting abdominal pain, or simply evidence of pancreatic exocrine or endocrine insufficiency.

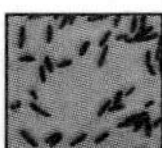

ETIOLOGIC FACTORS: Most factors that cause acute pancreatitis also cause chronic pancreatitis. The fact that chronic pancreatitis is often characterized by intermittent "acute" attacks with periods of quiescence suggests that it may evolve from repeated episodes of acute pancreatitis, with scarring. However, half of patients give no history of acute pancreatitis.

- **Chronic alcoholism** is the major cause of chronic pancreatitis, accounting for nearly 80% of adult cases. Even among alcoholics without symptoms of chronic pancreatitis, autopsy reveals evidence of this disease in about half. A comparable proportion of asymptomatic alcoholics show abnormal results for pancreatic exocrine function tests. The role of alcohol is undisputed, but the mechanism by which it causes chronic pancreatitis is still debated.

  The link between alcohol and pancreatitis rests on the fact that alcohol is a pancreatic secretagogue. Hypersecretion of enzymes by acinar cells without increased fluid

Reflux bile
+
Intraductal phospholipase
Lysolecithin
Cell injury

Bile
Common bile duct
Gallstone

Oxygen free radicals due to inflammation
O_2^-, H_2O_2, OH•, NO

PANCREATIC ACINUS

Secretagogue effect

OBSTRUCTION
- Gallstone in common bile duct
- Cystic fibrosis pancreatic duct
- Tumors
- ?Edema or spasm of sphincter of Oddi

Ductule

Leakage of enzymes through injured ductule

Release of enzymes from damaged acinar cells

ACINAR CELL INJURY

EXOGENOUS
- Alcohol
- Viruses (e.g., mumps)
- Drugs (e.g., thiazide diuretics)
- Trauma

ENDOGENOUS
- Hypercalcemia
- Hyperlipidemia
- Obesity

Pancreatic enzymes

Increased Serum Amylase
Lipase
Proteases

DIAGNOSTIC TEST
FAT NECROSIS
VASCULAR DESTRUCTION

ACUTE PANCREATITIS

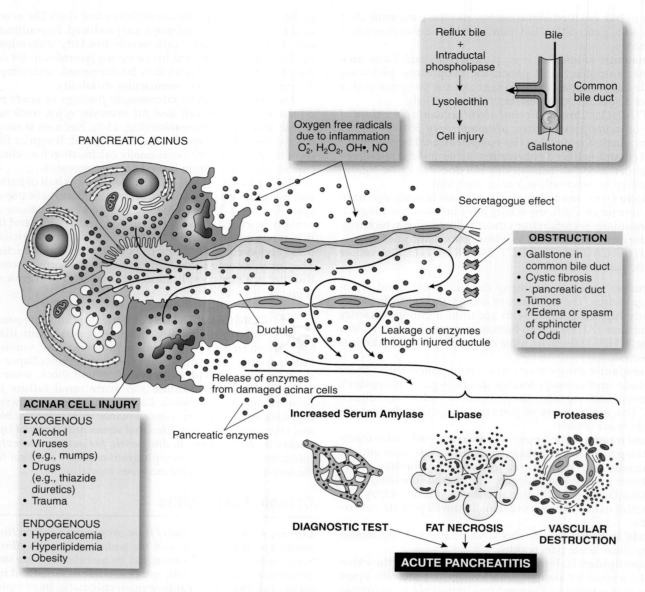

FIGURE 15-1. The pathogenesis of acute pancreatitis. Injury to the ductules or the acinar cells leads to the release of pancreatic enzymes. Lipase and proteases destroy tissue, thereby causing acute pancreatitis. The release of amylase is the basis of a test for acute pancreatitis. H_2O_2 = hydrogen peroxide; NO• = nitric acid; O_2^- = superoxide ion; OH• = hydroxyl radical.

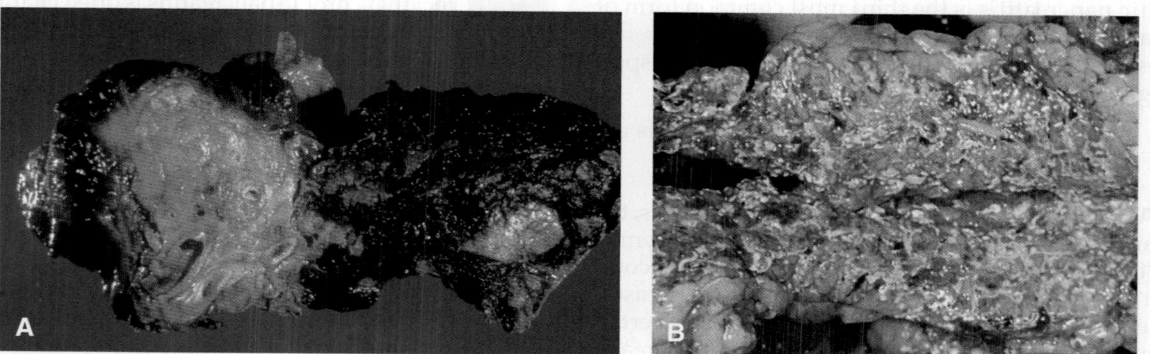

FIGURE 15-2. Acute hemorrhagic pancreatitis. A. Large areas of the pancreas are intensely hemorrhagic. **B.** The cut surface of the pancreas in a less severe case of acute pancreatitis, and at a somewhat later stage than in (A), shows numerous yellow-white foci of fat necrosis.

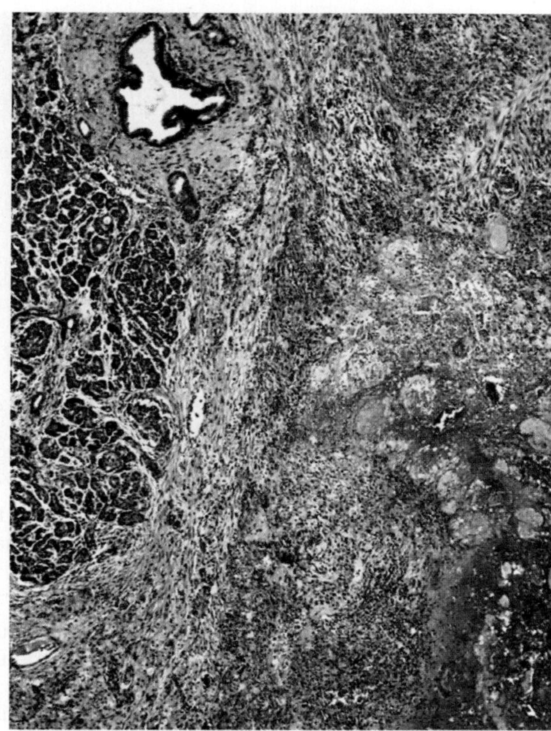

FIGURE 15-3. Acute hemorrhagic pancreatitis. A photomicrograph of the pancreas shows areas of acinar cell necrosis, hemorrhage and fat necrosis (*lower right*). An intact lobule is seen on the left.

leads to precipitation of "protein plugs" in small pancreatic ducts. These deposits obstruct the small ducts, at first, causing only mild acute pancreatitis. Resolution with fibrosis facilitates development of more plugs (that grow and lead to calcium carbonate stones) in a vicious cycle that increases the risk of developing more and worse acute pancreatitis. Since only a minority of severe alcoholics develop clinical chronic pancreatitis, other factors may also play a role. Malformations (e.g., pancreatic divisum) or mutations (e.g., in the cystic fibrosis gene) may predispose some alcoholics to developing chronic pancreatitis.

- **Obstruction or insufficiency of the pancreatic duct** sometimes leads to chronic pancreatitis. However, acute obstruction by gallstones may cause acute pancreatitis but not progression to chronic pancreatitis.

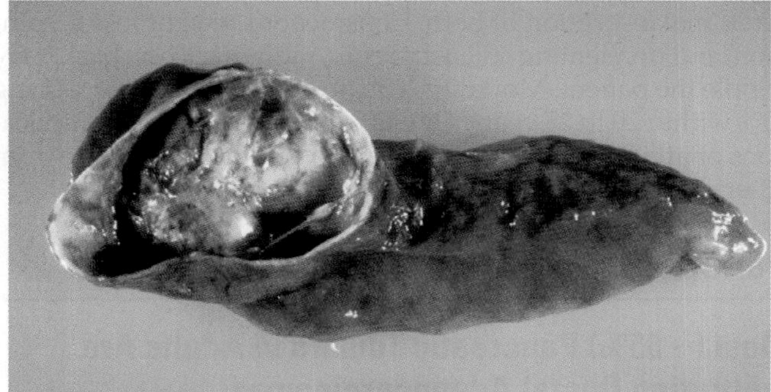

FIGURE 15-4. Pancreatic pseudocyst. A cystic cavity arises from the head of the pancreas.

Groove or **paraduodenal pancreatitis** is a particular form of chronic pancreatitis that develops within the "groove" between the head of the pancreas, the common bile duct and the duodenum. Its etiology is not entirely clear; however, the disease usually develops in alcoholics, and some have suggested that certain anatomic variations in the region of the minor papilla predispose these people to develop disease here. Because of the location of the disease, patients frequently develop jaundice (secondary to bile duct obstruction) or duodenal obstruction. Cystic changes are also common in this condition. Thus, patients are often brought to surgery for expected pancreatic ductal adenocarcinoma or other neoplasm.

- **Chronic injury to acinar cells** (e.g., in hemochromatosis) is associated with pancreatic fibrosis and atrophy.
- **Chronic renal failure** increases the incidence of acute and chronic pancreatitis.
- **Autoimmune chronic pancreatitis (lymphoplasmacytic sclerosing pancreatitis, duct-destructive chronic pancreatitis, etc.)** often occurs in association with other autoimmune and sclerosing disorders (e.g., chronic sclerosing sialadenitis and retroperitoneal fibrosis). The disorder affects both sexes, often in early adulthood. Symptoms vary from abdominal pain to painless jaundice. Imaging studies may suggest a masslike lesion (mimicking carcinoma) or irregular beading of the pancreatic or bile ducts.

MOLECULAR PATHOGENESIS: The pathogenesis of autoimmune pancreatitis is unknown, and multiple forms of the disease may exist. Serum immunoglobulin IgG4 is often elevated and IgG4-positive plasma cells are present in the parenchyma. Immunoglobulin deposits within basement membranes are described. The presence of hypergammaglobulinemia and autoantibodies, including antinuclear antibody (ANA), rheumatoid factor, antilactoferrin and anti–carbonic anhydrase, suggest possible autoimmune etiology.

- **Cystic fibrosis** (CF; see Chapter 6) may manifest as chronic pancreatitis. In patients with CF, intraductal secretions are abnormally viscid, accounting for the older name, **mucoviscidosis.** Plugs of inspissated mucus obstruct cystically distended pancreatic ducts, leading to chronic pancreatitis and eventually to exocrine pancreatic insufficiency. In late stages of CF, the entire organ is replaced by adipose tissue. Malabsorption is common in CF, causing bulky, fatty stools (steatorrhea). However, death in CF usually reflects pulmonary disease.
- **Hereditary pancreatitis** is a rare autosomal dominant disease with 80% penetrance. It is characterized by recurring severe abdominal pain that often manifests in childhood.

MOLECULAR PATHOGENESIS: Most disease develops because of point mutations that increase trypsin levels within the pancreas, largely due to autoactivation of trypsinogen. Point mutations in the **cationic trypsinogen gene (protease serine 1,** ***PRSS1***; chromosome 7q) and in the **serine protease inhibitor gene** (*SPINK 1*) are associated with the disease, and most forms of hereditary pancreatitis are caused by one of three point mutations in the **cationic trypsinogen** gene.

Hereditary pancreatitis is occasionally accompanied by aminoaciduria, although the two conditions are not necessarily linked etiologically. Some patients exhibit hypercalcemia secondary to parathyroid hyperplasia or adenomas. ***About 40% of patients with hereditary pancreatitis later develop pancreatic ductal carcinomas.*** Clinically and pathologically, the features of hereditary pancreatitis are indistinguishable from those of other forms of chronic pancreatitis, including ductal stones and the late complications.

- **Idiopathic chronic pancreatitis** has a bimodal distribution: a juvenile form with a mean age of 25 years and a second form in older patients with a peak at age 60.

MOLECULAR PATHOGENESIS: Mutations in the cystic fibrosis transmembrane conductance regulator (*CFTR*) gene are seen in 10% to 30% of patients with idiopathic chronic pancreatitis. Somatic mutations in the gene for pancreatic secretory trypsin inhibitor (*SPINK1*) are also associated with chronic pancreatitis. Thus, many cases of chronic idiopathic pancreatitis may be related to cystic fibrosis or hereditary pancreatitis but lack other clinical signs of the diseases.

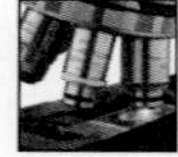

PATHOLOGY: By the time chronic pancreatitis is clinically evident, it is usually advanced. The pathology may vary somewhat, based on the etiology. Chronic calcifying pancreatitis is the most common type of the disease and is associated with chronic alcoholism in over 90% of cases.

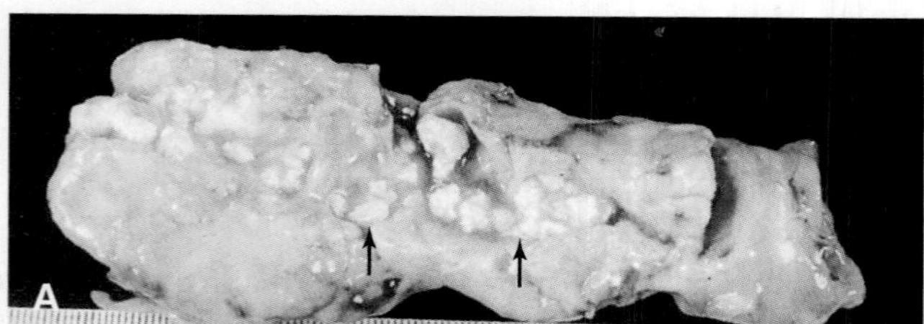

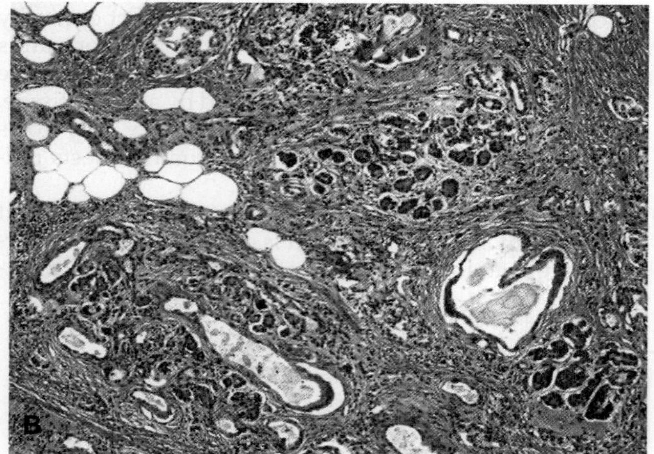

FIGURE 15-5. Chronic calcifying pancreatitis. A. The pancreas is shrunken and fibrotic, and the dilated duct contains numerous stones (*arrows*). **B.** Atrophic lobules of acinar cells are surrounded by dense fibrous tissue infiltrated by lymphocytes. The pancreatic ducts are dilated and contain inspissated proteinaceous material.

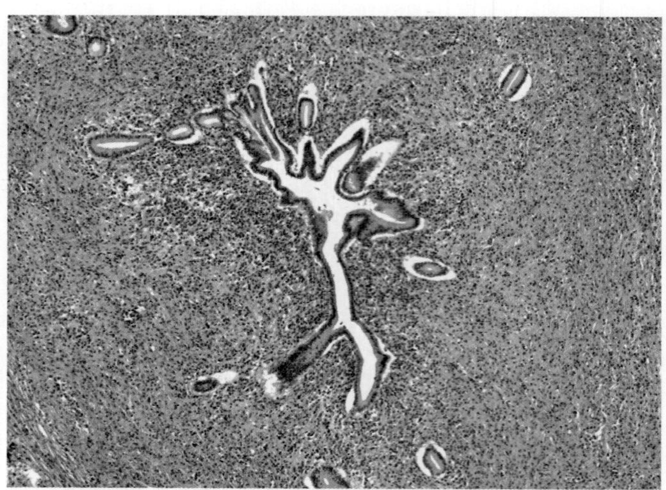

FIGURE 15-6. Autoimmune pancreatitis. There is loss of acinar tissue and the pancreatic duct is surrounded by a dense lymphoplasmacytic inflammatory infiltrate.

The pancreas can be affected focally, segmentally or diffusely. The parenchyma is firm, and the cut surface lacks the usual lobular appearance (Fig. 15-5A). The main pancreatic duct and its tributaries are commonly dilated, owing to obstruction by thick proteinaceous plugs, intraductal stones or strictures. Pseudocysts or abscess formation is common.

Microscopically, large regions of the gland show irregular areas of fibrosis with loss of acinar and, eventually, endocrine parenchyma (Fig. 15-5B). Remaining pancreatic islets are embedded in the sclerotic tissue, and may appear fused and enlarged until they, too, disappear. Fibrotic areas show myofibroblasts and variable amounts of lymphocytes, plasma cells and macrophages. Pancreatic ducts of all sizes contain variably calcified proteinaceous material, a finding more commonly associated with alcoholism. Ductal epithelium may be atrophic or hyperplastic, and may show squamous metaplasia.

In autoimmune pancreatitis, a dense lymphoplasmacytic inflammatory infiltrate and fibrosis surround the ductal epithelium (Fig. 15-6). Intraepithelial acute inflammation and obliterative venulitis may be seen with some forms of the disease.

CLINICAL FEATURES: Half of patients with chronic pancreatitis suffer repeated episodes of acute pancreatitis. One third of cases present with gradual onset of continuous or intermittent pain, with no acute attacks (Fig. 15-7). In some patients, chronic pancreatitis is initially painless but presents with diabetes or malabsorption. Once pancreatic calcifications are visible radiologically, most patients have diabetes, malabsorption or both. Conspicuous weight loss is common, and unrelenting epigastric pain, radiating to the back, may cripple the patient. Mortality is 3% to 4% per year, approaching 50% within 20 to 25 years. One fifth of patients die of complications of attacks of acute pancreatitis. The other deaths are from other causes, particularly alcohol-related disorders.

Pancreatic Exocrine Neoplasia

Most (~85%) Pancreatic Tumors in Adults Are Infiltrating Ductal Adenocarcinomas

Due to its preponderance, pancreatic adenocarcinoma is often synonymous with "pancreatic cancer." It is the fourth most

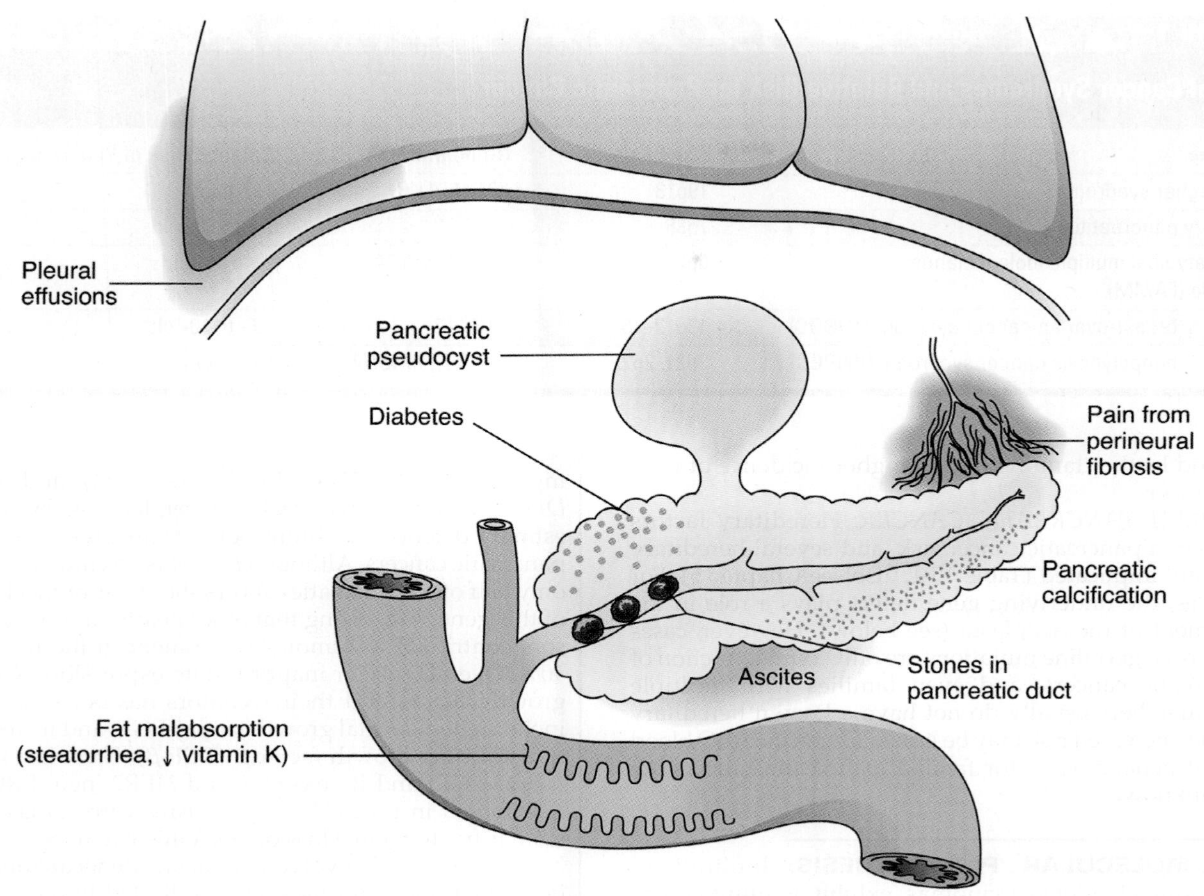

FIGURE 15-7. Complications of chronic pancreatitis.

common cause of cancer death in American men and the fifth in women. The prognosis is dismal: 5-year survival is less than 5%. Pancreatic cancer is increasing in many countries, and has tripled in the United States over the past 50 years.

EPIDEMIOLOGY: Pancreatic cancer occurs worldwide. The highest incidence (twice that in the United States) is among male Maoris, Polynesian aborigines of New Zealand and female natives of Hawaii. Over 32,000 new cases occur yearly in the United States, where it is 50% more common in Native Americans and blacks than in whites. Pancreatic cancer is a disease of late life, with peak incidence in people over 60 years of age, although it may occur as early as the third decade. It shows a significant male predominance (up to 3:1) in younger age groups but almost equal sex distribution in old age.

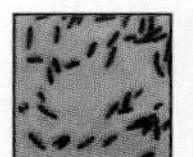

ETIOLOGIC FACTORS: The pathogenesis of pancreatic cancer is obscure. Epidemiologic studies implicate host and environmental factors.

SMOKING: About 25% of pancreatic cancers are attributable to cigarette smoking; cigarette smoking increases the risk of pancreatic cancer two- to threefold, correlating with the number of cigarettes smoked per day. Smokers may show proliferative lesions in the pancreatic ducts at autopsy. However, as only a small fraction of smokers develop pancreatic cancer, additional genetic and environmental factors are undoubtedly important.

BODY MASS INDEX AND DIETARY FACTORS: Diets high in meat, fat and nitrates may increase the risk of pancreatic cancer. However, confounding factors such as methods of cooking (i.e., frying, boiling, barbecuing) may play a role. Increased body mass index (BMI) raises the risk of pancreatic cancer. Diets high in fruits, vegetables, fiber and vitamin C seem to protect against pancreatic cancer. There is no clear link to coffee or alcohol consumption.

DIABETES MELLITUS: Diabetics are at greater risk for carcinoma of the pancreas. Up to 80% of patients with pancreatic cancer have evidence of diabetes mellitus at the time of cancer diagnosis. In some patients, the diabetes may be caused by the pancreatic cancer, rather than the reverse. However, patients with diabetes mellitus for 5 or more years have double the risk for pancreatic cancer.

CHRONIC PANCREATITIS: Chronic pancreatitis is a risk factor for pancreatic cancer, although conventional types (such as alcoholic pancreatitis) likely account for few cases. Hereditary pancreatitis and tropical calcifying pancreatis are more clearly linked to cancer. Since chronic pancreatitis may be mild and clinically silent, its role in development of pancreatic carcinoma may be underestimated. On the other hand, pancreatic cancers may cause obstructive chronic pancreatitis since they invade pancreatic ducts and obstruct the distal gland. Thus, the relationship of pancreatitis and cancer has been difficult to unravel.

ADDITIONAL FACTORS: Other environmental factors are suggested by increased risk linked to specific occupations. Workers exposed to coal gas, metal, dry cleaning

Table 15-1

Familial Cancer Syndromes and Relative Risk for Pancreatic Cancer

Syndrome	Chromosome	Gene Mutation	Relative Risk of Pancreatic Cancer
Peutz-Jegher syndrome	19p13	*STK11/LKB1*	132-fold
Hereditary pancreatitis	7q35	*PRSS1*	50- to 80-fold
Familial atypical multiple mole melanoma syndrome (FAMM)	9p21	*P16 (CDKN2A)*	9- to 38-fold
Hereditary breast-ovarian cancer syndrome (HBOC)	13q12–13	*BRCA2*	3.5- to 10-fold
Hereditary nonpolyposis cancer syndrome (HNPCC)	3p21, 2p22	*hMLH1, hMSH2*	Unknown

agents and leather tanning have a higher incidence of pancreatic cancer.

FAMILIAL PANCREATIC CANCER: Hereditary factors play a role in pancreatic cancer risk, and several hereditary diseases are implicated (Table 15-1; also see Chapter 5). For these cases, the underlying gene defect plays a role in the development of the neoplasm (see below). However, cases due to known germline mutations are only a small fraction of all pancreatic cancers, and even families with multiple affected members usually do not have a known hereditary syndrome. Increased risk may be linked to specific ABO blood types, but genetic bases for familial pancreatic cancers are largely unknown.

MOLECULAR PATHOGENESIS: Infiltrating ductal adenocarcinomas exhibit a number of genetic alterations, some of which occur in most cases and others of which are infrequent. A genetic tumor progression model is supported by morphologic findings of preneoplastic ductal proliferative lesions, termed **pancreatic intraductal neoplasia (PanIN),** the more recent nomenclature for dysplasia of the ducts. PanINs are characterized by mucinous epithelium replacing the normal lining of the ducts. PanINs are separated into three grades with increasing cytoarchitectural and genetic abnormalities. Early events, PanIN1, include telomere shortening and mutational activation of the *KRAS* oncogene, which is mutated in up to 95% of ductal adenocarcinomas. Later in the sequence of neoplastic progression, there is mutational inactivation or deletion of tumor suppressor genes, including *p53* (50% to 75%), *p16/CDKN2A* (95%) and *MAD4/DPC-4* (deleted in pancreatic cancer, locus 4; 55%). Interestingly, deletions in chromosome 18 are present in 90% of pancreatic cancers. Although *DPC-4* is on chromosome 18, only half of all pancreatic cancers show loss or inactivation of this gene, suggesting that other nearby tumor suppressors contribute to tumor development in the remaining 40%. Overactivity or inappropriate expression of several growth factors and their receptors has been described, including epidermal growth factor (EGF) and its receptor, transforming growth factor-β (TGF-β), fibroblast growth factor (FGF) and its receptor and HER2/neu. BRCA1 is inactivated in up to 7% of pancreatic carcinomas, and a similar fraction have loss of DNA mismatch repair genes. Many other genes involved in ductal adenocarcinoma are being identified, but most are implicated in only a small proportion of cases. The timing of abnormalities of the most commonly involved genes in the progression of PanIN to invasive carcinoma is shown in Fig. 15-8.

PATHOLOGY: Ductal adenocarcinoma may arise anywhere in the pancreas, but is most common in the head (60% to 70%), followed by the body (10%) and tail (10% to 15%). In some cases, the pancreas is diffusely involved. Tumors of the head of the pancreas may cause biliary obstruction by compressing the intrapancreatic common bile duct or ampulla of Vater. Classically, both the bile duct and the pancreatic duct are dilated. Carcinomas of the head tend to be smaller at the time of diagnosis than those elsewhere, with less spread to regional lymph nodes or distant sites.

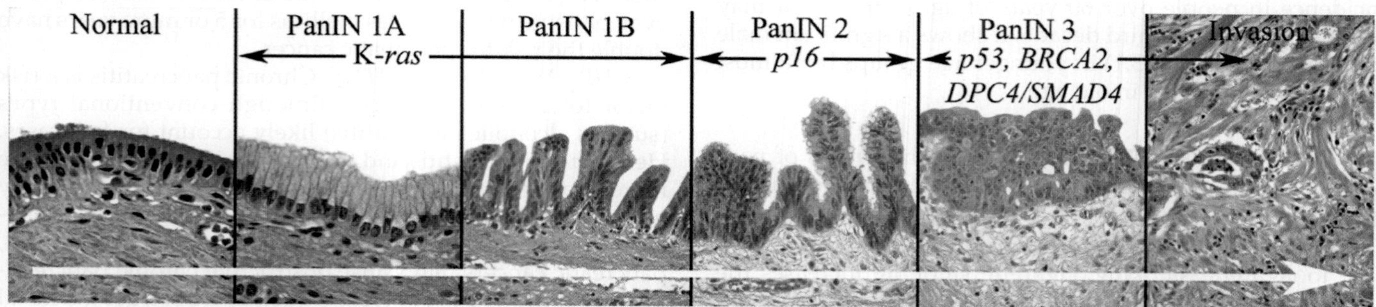

FIGURE 15-8. Pancreatic intraepithelial neoplasia (PanIN). From the left to the right, one proceeds from normal ductal epithelium to invasive carcinoma. Frequently mutated genes are shown when they are typically mutated within the spectrum of PanIN.

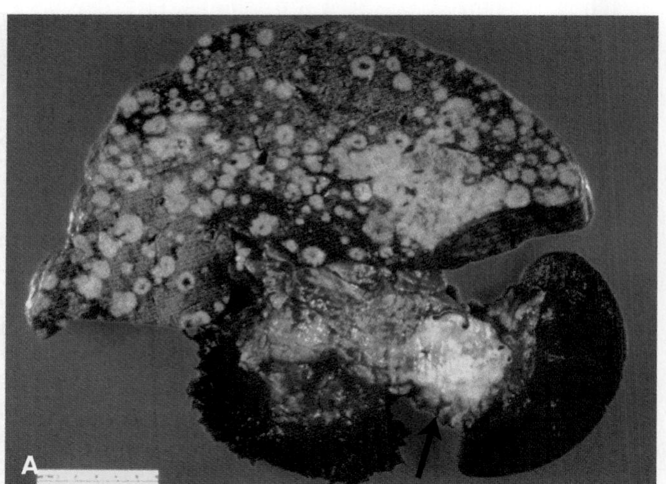

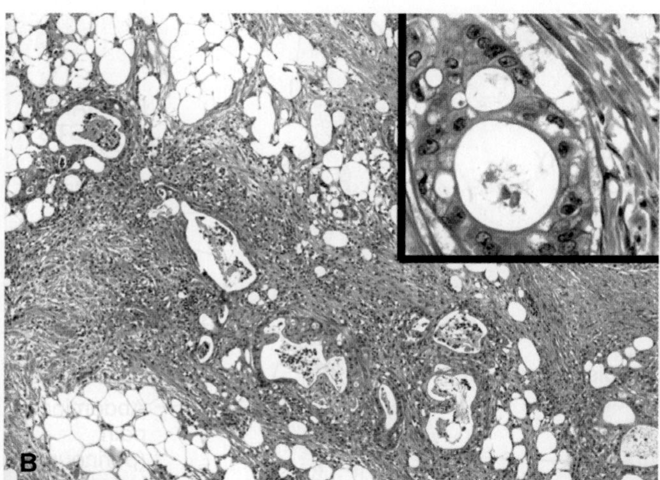

FIGURE 15-9. Infiltrating ductal adenocarcinoma of the pancreas. A. An autopsy specimen shows a large tumor in the tail of the pancreas (*arrow*) and extensive metastases in the liver. **B.** A section of the tumor reveals malignant glands infiltrating into adipose tissue with surrounding fibrous stroma. *Inset.* High-power image of a malignant gland.

On gross examination, ductal adenocarcinoma is usually a very firm, gray, poorly demarcated mass (Fig. 15-9A) that can be difficult to distinguish from surrounding areas of fibrosing chronic pancreatitis. Invasion of peripancreatic tissues and other local structures is common. Tumors of the head of the pancreas may invade the common bile duct and duodenal wall. They may also obstruct the main pancreatic duct and cause atrophy of the body and tail. Carcinomas of the tail of the gland may extend into the spleen, transverse colon or stomach. Metastases in regional lymph nodes and liver are common. Other frequent metastatic sites include the peritoneum, lungs, adrenals and bones; distant metastases render most cases unresectable.

Microscopically, over 75% of infiltrating ductal adenocarcinomas are well to moderately differentiated (Fig. 15-9B), characterized by well-formed individual tubular glands containing mucin-producing epithelial cells. Nuclear atypia may be marked, but malignant glands may be so bland as to be difficult to distinguish from nonneoplastic ducts. Striking desmoplasia around the neoplastic glands is the rule. The tumors are highly infiltrative and poorly circumscribed. Microscopic extension well beyond the gross limits of the tumor is common. Perineural invasion is a characteristic of these tumors, and accounts for the early and persistent pain associated with them. Of the 25% of ductal adenocarcinomas that are poorly differentiated, sheets of cells or individual cells are seen. Additional variants include colloid carcinoma, medullary carcinoma, adenosquamous carcinoma and various undifferentiated carcinomas, including undifferentiated carcinoma with osteoclast-like giant cells.

Some ductal adenocarcinomas and variants arise in association with preinvasive neoplasms such as mucinous cystic neoplasms and intraductal papillary mucinous neoplasms (see below).

CLINICAL FEATURES: Patients with pancreatic cancer present with anorexia, conspicuous weight loss and gnawing epigastric pain that often radiates to the back. Painless jaundice is seen in about half of all patients with cancer localized to the head of the pancreas, but is uncommon in tumors of the body or tail. Depression often occurs, out of proportion to the severity of the disease. Serum levels of cancer antigen (CA) 19-9, a Lewis blood group antigen, are usually increased, but this finding is not specific. Early diagnosis of pancreatic cancer is unusual because the tumor is rarely symptomatic until it is well advanced. Most have already metastasized at the time of diagnosis, and curative surgery is uncommon. Progressive deterioration almost invariably ensues, with intractable pain, cachexia and death. Half of patients die within 6 months of diagnosis, and the overall 5-year survival rate is less than 5%.

Courvoisier sign is acute, painless gallbladder dilation accompanied by jaundice, owing to common bile duct obstruction by tumor. In about one third of patients it may be the first sign of pancreatic cancer, but it does not identify potentially curable tumors.

Migratory thrombophlebitis (**Trousseau syndrome,** deep venous thrombosis) develops in 10% of patients with pancreatic cancer, especially when the tumor involves the body and tail of the pancreas. It is not uncommon for migratory thrombophlebitis to be the first evidence of an underlying pancreatic malignancy, although it may be seen with other cancers also. Unexplained thrombophlebitis in an otherwise healthy person demands a careful search for occult malignancy. The mechanisms underlying the hypercoagulable state that leads to migratory thrombophlebitis are not completely understood, but (1) a serine protease synthesized and released by malignant tumor cells directly activates plasma factor X; (2) tumor cells shed plasma membrane vesicles, which have procoagulant activity; and (3) necrotic tumor releases tissue thromboplastins.

The complications of pancreatic ductal carcinoma are shown in Fig. 15-10.

Acinar Cell Carcinoma Is an Uncommon Tumor of Older Adults

Acinar cell carcinomas are rare (1% to 2% of pancreatic carcinomas) and recapitulate normal pancreatic acini, including production of exocrine enzymes by tumor cells. These

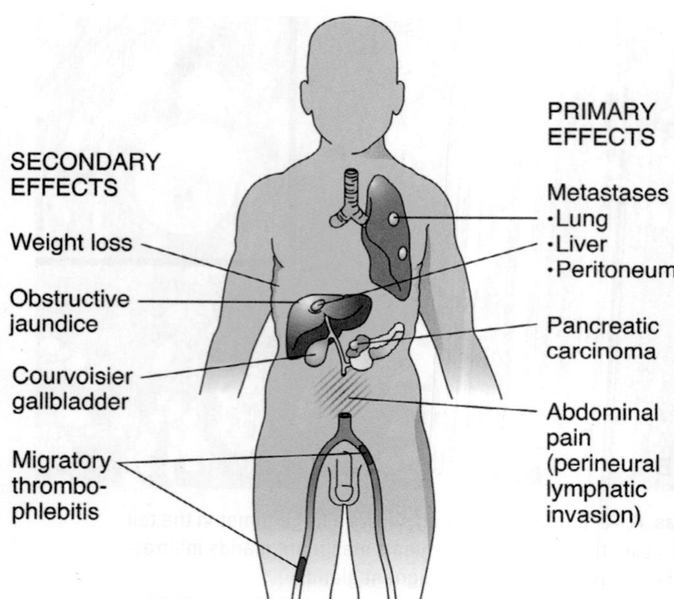

FIGURE 15-10. Complications of pancreatic ductal adenocarcinoma.

carcinomas usually develop in the seventh decade of life, although they do occur in children. Some patients show a characteristic paraneoplastic syndrome of subcutaneous fat necrosis, polyarthralgia and peripheral eosinophilia attributable to hypersecretion of massive amounts of lipase into serum. The prognosis of acinar cell carcinoma is poor, but it is less rapidly fatal than ductal adenocarcinoma. Acinar cell carcinomas are large and circumscribed and lack the desmoplastic stroma of ductal cancers. Microscopically, they are composed of uniform cells arranged in small acini and nests (Fig. 15-11). Immunohistochemistry demonstrates production of exocrine enzymes. The molecular pathogenesis of acinar cell carcinoma is very different from that of ductal adenocarcinoma. Some cases have abnormalities in the adenomatous polyposis coli (APC)/β-catenin pathway, but the

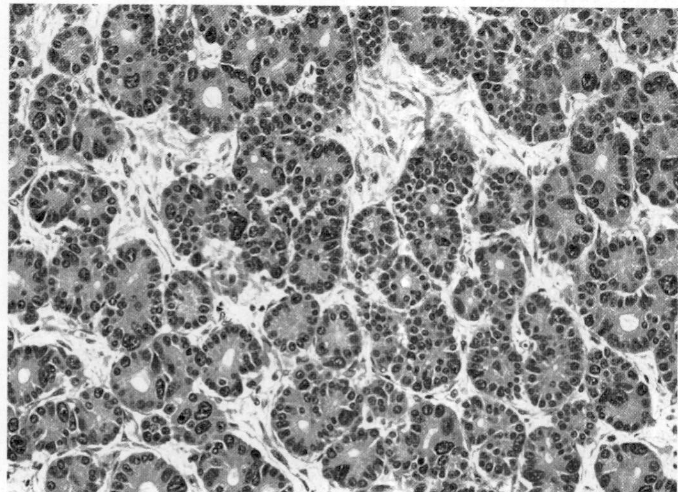

FIGURE 15-11. Acinar cell carcinoma. This malignant tumor is characterized by acinar formations reminiscent of normal pancreatic parenchyma.

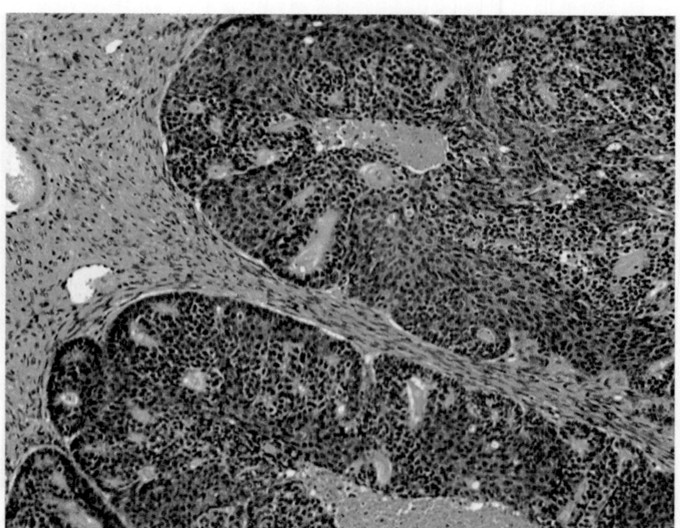

FIGURE 15-12. Pancreatoblastoma. Epithelial islands containing acinar structures and squamoid nests are separated by cellular stromal bands.

genes typically abnormal in ductal adenocarcinoma are not altered.

Pancreatoblastoma Is a Tumor of Childhood

These tumors are usually seen in the first decade of life, and may occur in the setting of Beckwith-Wiedemann syndrome. Serum α-fetoprotein levels may be elevated. Microscopically, tumors are composed of polygonal cells in solid islands and acinar structures, with interspersed squamoid nests (Fig. 15-12). Acinar differentiation, with production of exocrine enzymes, is consistently present, and some cases also have ductal or endocrine differentiation. Lymph node or hepatic metastases occur in a third of patients, and are associated with a poor prognosis. Surgery and chemotherapy can be curative in patients without metastatic disease.

Serous Cystic Neoplasms of the Pancreas Are Nearly Always Benign

Serous cystic neoplasms are composed of cystic structures uniformly lined by glycogen-rich cuboidal epithelium (Fig. 15-13). They usually occur in adults, in the pancreatic body or tail. There is a 3:1 female predominance, and patients with von Hippel-Lindau (VHL) syndrome are at increased risk for its development. It is not surprising, then, that tumors are often associated with inactivation of the *VHL* gene. Serous cystadenomas range from 1 to 25 cm in diameter. Most patients present with nonspecific symptoms related to local mass effects, but many are asymptomatic. There is often a large, stellate central scar, sometimes with microcalcifications giving a "sunburst" pattern on imaging studies. The tumors are sometimes removed because of clinical concern for malignancy or because of symptoms.

Intraductal Papillary Mucinous Tumors May Be Associated With Invasive Carcinoma

Intraductal papillary mucin-producing neoplasms (IPMNs) are composed of dilated pancreatic ducts (>1 cm) lined by

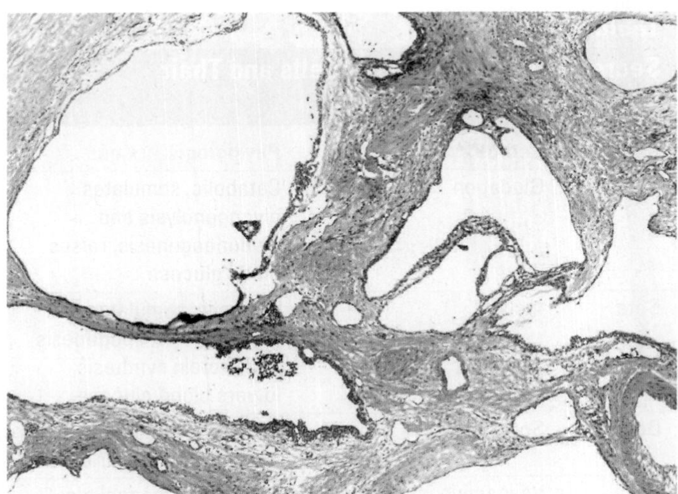

FIGURE 15-13. Serous cystadenoma. Cysts are embedded in a dense, fibrous stroma. The epithelial lining is composed of a single layer of glycogen-rich clear cells.

neoplastic mucinous epithelium and filled with mucus. Numerous papillary proliferations extend into the duct lumen (Fig. 15-14). IPMNs arise in the head of the pancreas and are usually diagnosed in late adulthood, after being found incidentally, or in patients with chronic pancreatitis. Duct involvement may be unifocal, multifocal or diffuse.

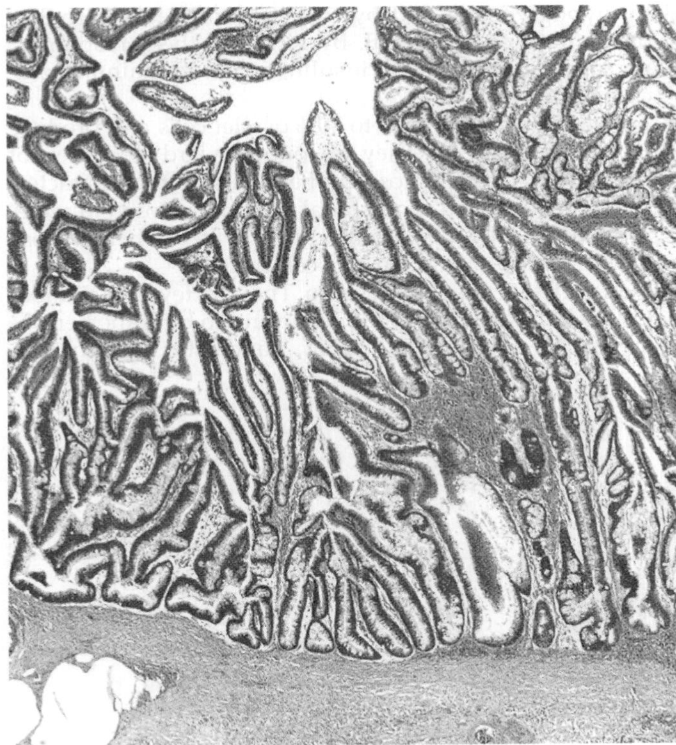

FIGURE 15-14. Intraductal papillary mucinous neoplasm. An exuberant papillary proliferation of tall mucin-secreting epithelium fills the pancreatic duct.

Some IPMNs involve the main pancreatic ducts, whereas others are in peripheral (branch) ducts and mimic cystic lesions on imaging studies. IPMNs exhibit varying degrees of epithelial dysplasia, which is graded as low grade, intermediate grade or high grade. A focus of invasive adenocarcinoma is found in up to one third of cases. Because they may harbor invasive carcinomas, larger tumors or those with atypical radiographic features are often resected. The molecular pathogenesis of many of these tumors is like that of typical PanIN and pancreatic ductal adenocarcinoma. However, some develop via alternative molecular pathways, perhaps explaining the diverse phenotypes of these tumors compared to PanIN.

Mucinous Cystic Neoplasms Are Most Often Found in the Pancreatic Tail of Middle-Aged Women

Mucinous cystic neoplasm (MCN) is a unilocular or multilocular cystic neoplasm lined by mucin-secreting epithelium with underlying cellular stroma (ovarian-type stroma) (Fig. 15-15). MCNs occur almost exclusively in middle-aged women. Tumors may reach 10 cm in diameter and do not communicate with the pancreatic duct system. MCNs have a predilection for the body and tail of the pancreas. Like IPMNs, these tumors may have varying degrees of epithelial dysplasia and are sometimes associated with invasive carcinoma. The prognosis of MCN (noninvasive) is excellent if it is completely removed. Molecular changes in MCNs are similar to those in PanIN and invasive pancreatic ductal adenocarcinoma.

Solid Pseudopapillary Neoplasms Are Very Low-Grade Malignancies in Girls and Young Women

Solid pseudopapillary neoplasms (SPNs) are solid and circumscribed, often with large cystically degenerated areas filled with blood and necrotic debris. Tumors are composed of monomorphic cells forming loose solid sheets and

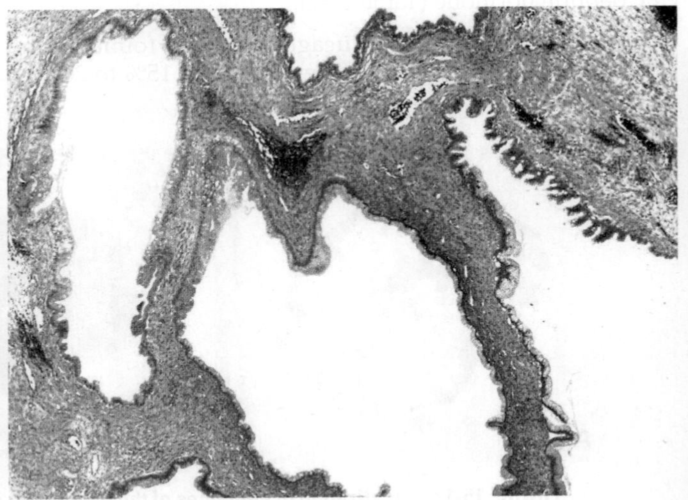

FIGURE 15-15. Mucinous cystic neoplasm. A mucin-rich epithelial lining of this cystic lesion rests on an ovarian-type stroma.

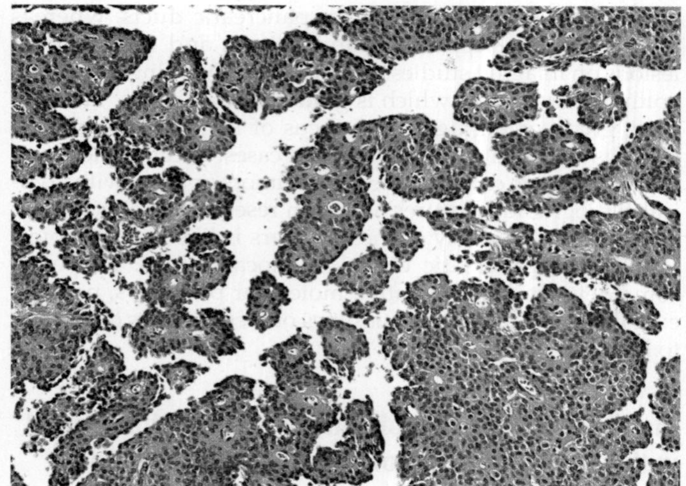

FIGURE 15-16. Solid pseudopapillary neoplasm. The tumor is composed of pseudopapillae with vascular cores.

pseudopapillary structures (Fig. 15-16). Most SPNs are very indolent and curable by complete surgical resection. Metastases, usually to the liver, occur in about 10% of cases, and even those patients usually live for many years, underscoring the slow-growing nature of this neoplasm. These tumors are treated by resection. Clinically they may mimic other malignancies of the pancreas. Most SPNs have mutations of the *β-catenin* gene.

The Endocrine Pancreas

The Islets of Langerhans Form the Endocrine Pancreas

These islets are irregularly scattered throughout the pancreas and consist of richly vascularized spherical or lobulated aggregates of endocrine cells. Four major distinct cell types are present in the islets, and each cell produces only one specific peptide hormone (Table 15-2).

Table 15-2

Secretory Products of Islet Cells and Their Physiologic Actions

Cell	Secretory Product	Physiologic Actions
Alpha	Glucagon	Catabolic, stimulates glycogenolysis and gluconeogenesis, raises blood glucose
Beta	Insulin	Anabolic; stimulates glycogenesis, lipogenesis and protein synthesis; lowers blood glucose
Delta	Somatostatin	Inhibits secretion of alpha, beta, D_1 and acinar cells
D_1	Vasoactive intestinal polypeptide (VIP)	Same as glucagon; also regulates tone and motility of the gastrointestinal tract and activates 3′,5′ cyclic adenosine monophosphate (cAMP) of intestinal epithelium
PP	Human pancreatic polypeptide (hPP)	Stimulates gastric enzyme secretion, inhibits intestinal motility and bile secretion

- **Alpha cells** synthesize glucagon and are found at the periphery of islet lobules. They make up 15% to 20% of the total islet cell population (Fig. 15-17A). Glucagon induces glycogenolysis and gluconeogenesis in the liver, thereby raising blood glucose. Its secretion is stimulated by hypoglycemia and by ingestion of a low-carbohydrate, high-protein meal. By virtue of these responses, glucagon, together with insulin, serves to maintain glucose homeostasis.
- **Beta cells** comprise 60% to 70% of islet cells and produce insulin (Fig. 15-17B). They are found toward the centers of islets. By electron microscopy, beta cells contain characteristic polygonal and rhomboidal crystals enclosed in secretory vesicles. Insulin secretion is activated when glucose binds to receptors on the beta cell surface.
- **Delta cells** secrete somatostatin. They are fewer in number (5% to 10%) and, like alpha cells, tend to be at the periphery of the islets (Fig. 15-17C). Pancreatic somatostatin

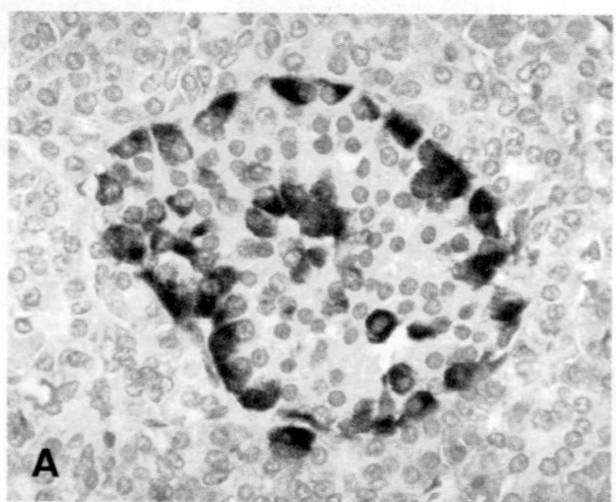

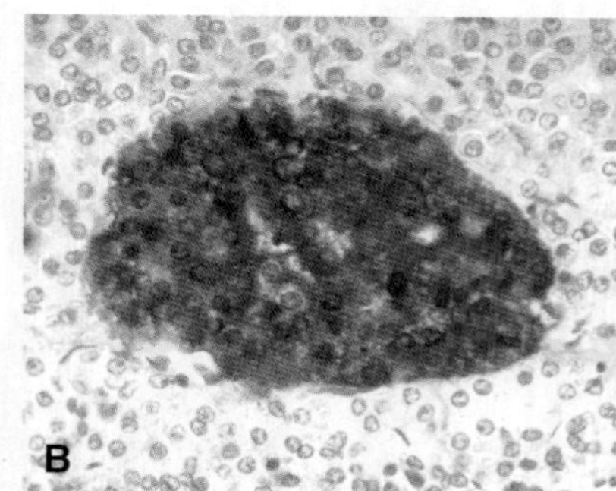

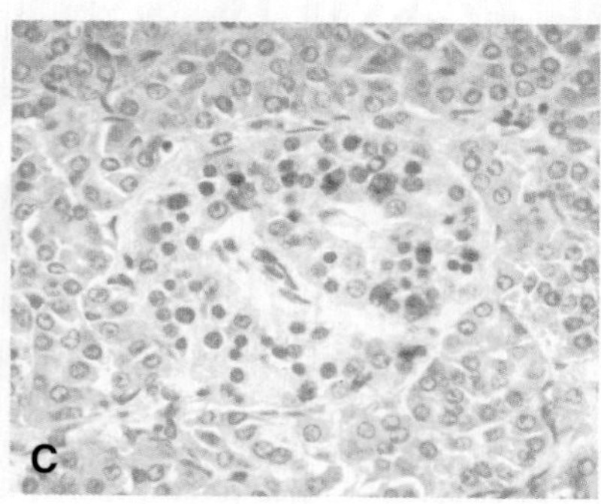

FIGURE 15-17. Localization of hormones of the pancreatic islet by specific antibodies. The immunoperoxidase technique reveals **(A)** glucagon in alpha cells at the periphery of the islet; **(B)** insulin in beta cells distributed throughout the islet; and **(C)** somatostatin in sparsely distributed delta cells.

inhibits pituitary release of growth hormone; secretion by alpha, beta and acinar cells of the pancreas; and certain hormone-secreting cells in the gastrointestinal tract. These hormonal interactions suggest that somatostatin plays a regulatory role in glucose homeostasis.

- **Pancreatic polypeptide-secreting cells** are primarily in the islets of that part of the head of the pancreas derived from the embryonic ventral pancreas. They synthesize a polypeptide that appears to have diverse functions, including stimulating enzyme secretion by the gastric mucosa and inhibiting smooth muscle contraction in intestine and gallbladder, production of gastric acid and secretion by the exocrine pancreas and biliary system.

Pancreatic Neuroendocrine Tumors Are About 5% of Pancreatic Tumors

Pancreatic neuroendocrine tumors (PanNETs) have distinctive morphologic features: they resemble normal islet cells and other well-differentiated neuroendocrine tumors of the body, such as carcinoid tumors. Previously known as "islet cell tumors," PanNETs may secrete hormones that cause dramatic paraneoplastic syndromes, or they may be nonfunctioning. Functioning PanNETs include insulinoma, glucagonoma, somatostatinoma, gastrinoma, VIPoma and other rare types. PanNETs exhibit a range of clinical aggressiveness; when small, they are easily cured by surgical resection, but larger examples may develop incurable metastases. Predicting the likely clinical behavior of PanNETs is difficult, although features such as large size, high proliferative activity and more extensive invasion increase the likelihood of recurrence. Even in the presence of distant metastases, PanNETs often grow relatively slowly, and survival for years or even decades can occur. If functioning PanNETs cannot be completely removed by surgery, the hormonal syndromes they cause may be highly morbid. Very small PanNETs (<0.5 cm) are common incidental findings designated pancreatic endocrine microadenomas.

Most PanNETs are nonfunctioning, but among functioning PanNETs, insulinomas are most common. PanNETs may be seen at any age but most occur between 40 and 60 years, affecting men and women equally. The distinctive clinical syndromes of the more common functioning types are shown in Fig. 15-18 and discussed further below. Nonfunctioning PanNETs are detected incidentally by imaging studies and attract attention by local effects or metastases (e.g., in the liver).

MOLECULAR PATHOGENESIS: PanNETs are a component of multiple endocrine neoplasia syndrome type 1 (MEN1), which also involves pituitary and parathyroid adenomas and, less commonly, endocrine tumors of other organs. Affected patients usually have multiple pancreatic endocrine microadenomas and PanNETs, at least one of which is functioning. Patients with von Hippel-Lindau syndrome also develop nonfunctioning PanNETs that may be histologically distinguished by their clear cytoplasm.

The genes involved in the MEN1 and VHL syndromes have been identified (*MEN1* and *VHL* tumor suppressor genes, respectively) and show biallelic inactivation in the hereditary PanNETs in these patients. The molecular pathogenesis of sporadic PanNETs is not well established. Losses at the chromosomal locus of the *MEN1* gene, chromosome 11q, are common, but the *MEN1* gene itself is usually not involved. PanNETs do not usually have mutations in the genes involved in the development of ductal adenocarcinoma (*KRAS*, *p53*, *p16/CDKN2A* and *MAD4/DP-4*).

Functioning Pancreatic Neuroendocrine Tumors Produce Dramatic Paraneoplastic Syndromes

- **Insulinomas,** the most common functioning PanNETs, secrete sufficient insulin to cause hypoglycemia. Insulin secretion by the tumor cells is not regulated by blood glucose levels, so the tumors secrete insulin continuously. Although these tumors are usually small (75% are <2 cm), the symptoms may be profound, and include both the direct central nervous system effects of hypoglycemia and the secondary effects of the resulting catecholamine response. Patients complain of sweating, visual changes, confusion, nervousness and hunger, which may progress to confusion, lethargy and even seizures or coma. Their abnormal behavior may falsely suggest a psychiatric disorder. Insulinomas occur somewhat more often in the tail of the pancreas (Fig. 15-19). Although 30% of the functioning PanNETs in patients with MEN1 are insulinomas, only 5% of insulinomas arise in the setting of MEN1. Compared to other PanNETs, insulinomas have a benign clinical course, perhaps because they are usually very small when detected. Surgical removal, even by enucleation, is usually curative.
- **Glucagonomas** are associated with a syndrome of (1) mild diabetes; (2) a necrotizing, migratory, erythematous rash; (3) anemia; (4) diarrhea; and (5) deep vein thromboses. Psychiatric disturbances also occur. Glucagonomas constitute 8% to 13% of functioning PanNETs and occur between the ages of 40 and 70 years, with a slight female predominance. In patients with alpha cell tumors, plasma glucagon levels may be up to 30 times above normal. Like other functioning PanNETs (except insulinomas) and nonfunctioning PanNETs, glucagonomas exhibit malignant behavior in 50% to 70% of cases.
- **Somatostatinomas** are rare and produce a syndrome of mild diabetes, gallstones, steatorrhea, hypochlorhydria, anemia and weight loss, due to the inhibitory actions of somatostatin on other cells of the pancreatic islets and on neuroendocrine cells of the gastrointestinal tract. Consequently, blood levels of insulin and glucagon are low.
- **Pancreatic gastrinoma** is a functioning PanNET composed of so-called G cells, which produce gastrin, a potent hormonal stimulus for gastric acid secretion. The location of this tumor in the pancreas is curious, because gastrin-producing cells do not normally occur in the islets. Pancreatic gastrinoma causes Zollinger-Ellison syndrome, a disorder showing (1) intractable gastric hypersecretion, (2) severe peptic ulceration of the duodenum and jejunum and (3) high blood gastrin levels. Among functioning PanNETs, gastrinomas are second in frequency to insulinomas, and they are the most common functioning tumor in MEN1 patients. However, the pancreas is a less common location for gastrinomas than is the duodenum, especially in cases not associated with MEN1. Gastrinomas of the pancreas are usually over 2 cm, whereas duodenal gastrinomas can measure only a few millimeters. Sometimes, only lymph node metastases are found, with no evidence of a primary gastrinoma. Gastrinomas are most common between the

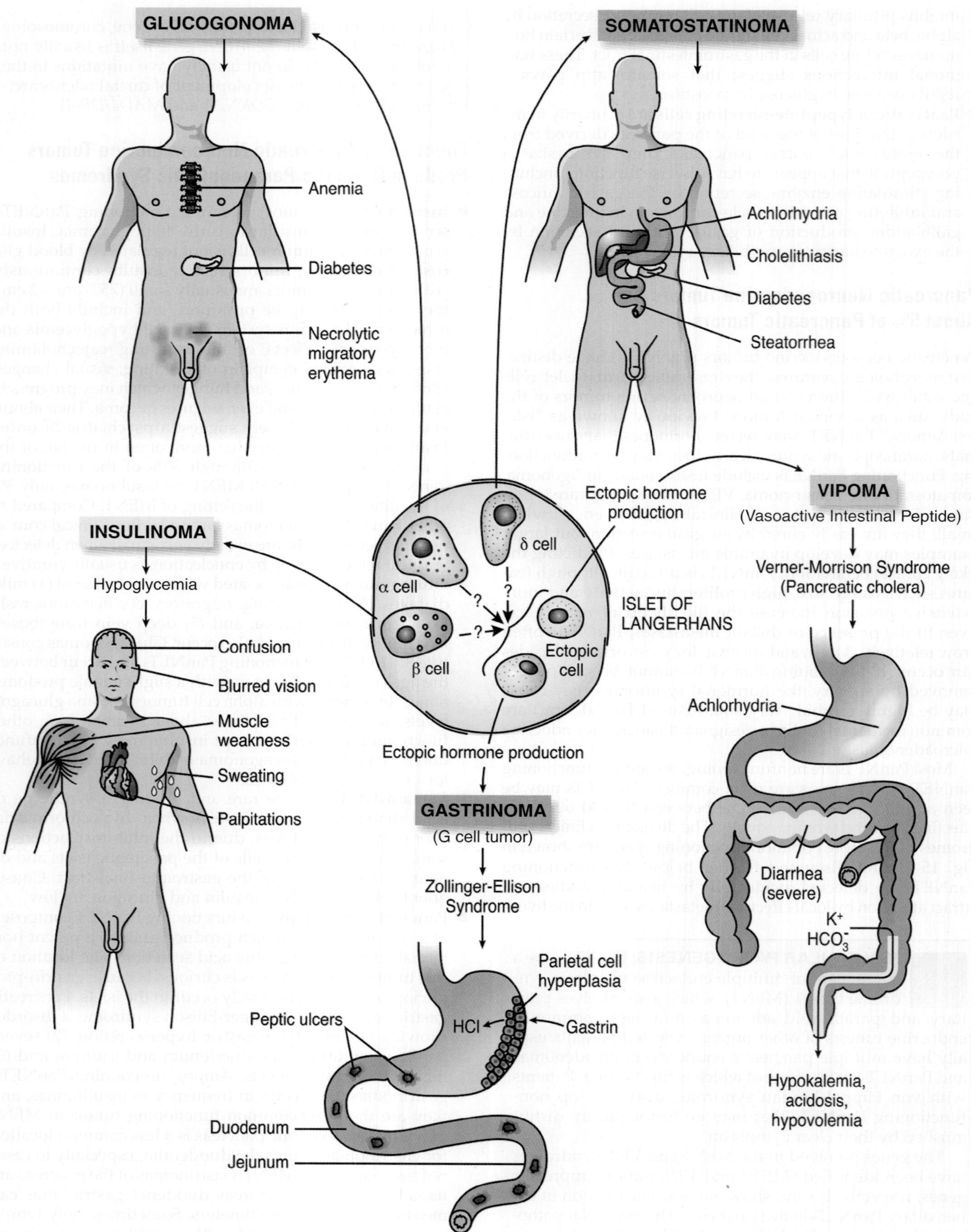

FIGURE 15-18. Syndromes associated with pancreatic neuroendocrine tumors.

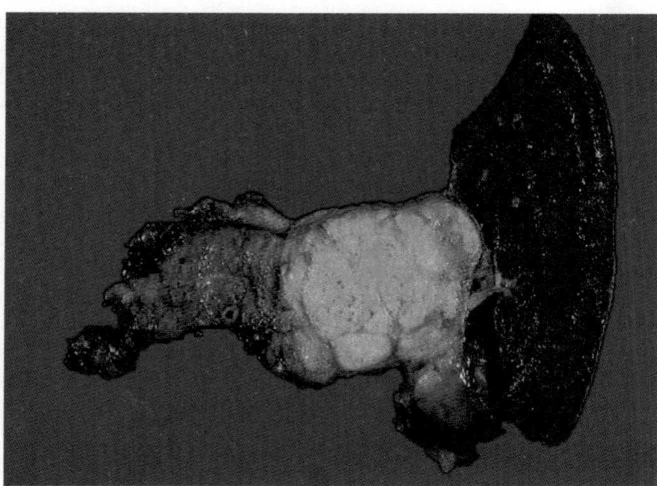

FIGURE 15-19. Pancreatic neuroendocrine tumor. This well-circumscribed, somewhat nodular tumor was located in the tail of the pancreas near the spleen.

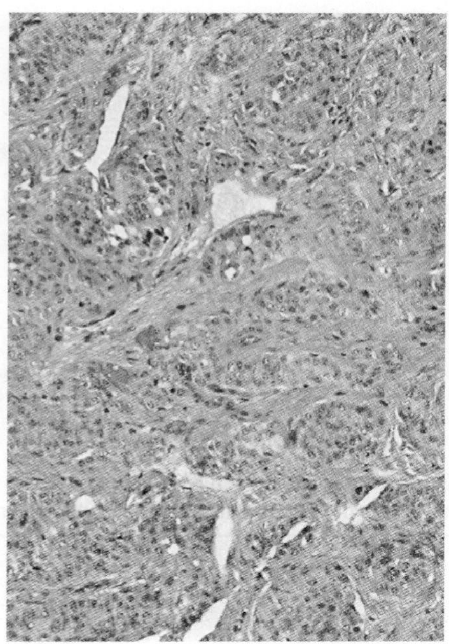

FIGURE 15-21. Insulinoma. Nests of tumor cells are surrounded by numerous capillaries.

ages of 30 and 50, with a slight male predominance. Most pancreatic examples arise in the head of the gland. Pancreatic gastrinomas are aggressive, although those arising in the duodenum usually remain localized, even when lymph node metastases are present.

- **VIPomas** are functioning PanNETs that produce vasoactive intestinal polypeptide (VIP). Like gastrin, VIP is not normally found in nonneoplastic islet cells but rather is made in ganglion cells and nerve fibers of the pancreas, gut and brain. VIP induces glycogenolysis and hyperglycemia and regulates ion and water secretion by the gastrointestinal epithelium. VIPomas induce Verner-Morrison syndrome, which is characterized by explosive and profuse watery diarrhea, hypokalemia and achlorhydria (also known as WDHA syndrome or pancreatic cholera). VIPomas are rare (3% to 8% of all PanNETs and 10% of functioning PanNETs) and are usually large and solitary.
- PanNETs may rarely secrete **other hormones not ordinarily produced by the pancreas (ectopic hormones),** including adrenocorticotropic hormone (ACTH), parathyroid hormone, calcitonin and vasopressin. These ectopic hormones may be produced either alone or in combination with normally occurring pancreatic hormones. Pancreatic polypeptide can also be secreted by some PanNETs, dubbed "PPomas," but no specific clinical syndrome is attributed to this hormone, so technically PPomas are clinically nonfunctioning.

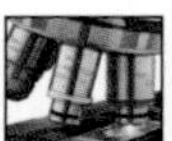

PATHOLOGY: Other than the smaller size for insulinomas, functioning and nonfunctioning PanNETs are grossly similar. They are usually solitary, circumscribed masses of pink to tan, soft tissue (Fig. 15-19). Larger tumors are multinodular and have areas of hemorrhage. Cystic degeneration can occur, and some cases are firm and fibrotic. Microscopically, PanNETs have uniform cells arranged in so-called organoid patterns, including nests, ribbons, glands and festoons (Figs. 15-20 and 15-21). Nuclei are uniform and coarsely stippled, and the proliferative rate is low. Sometimes the stroma contains amyloid, or it may be

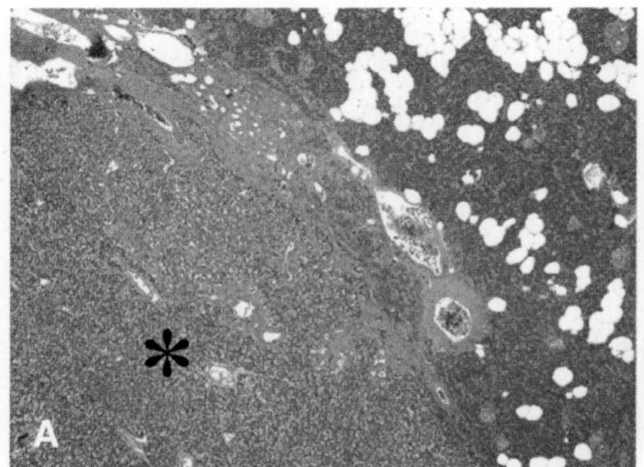

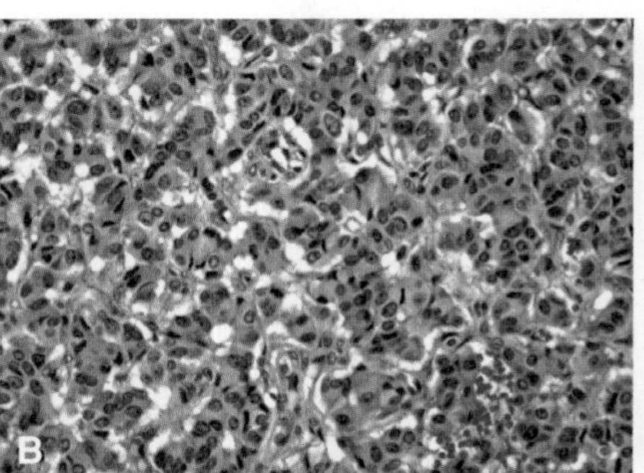

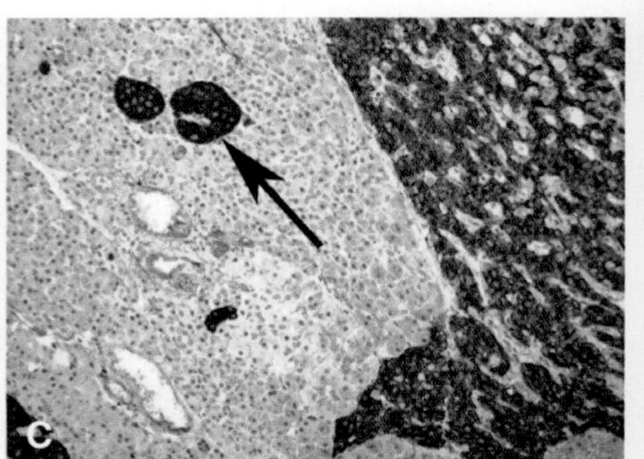

FIGURE 15-20. Pancreatic neuroendocrine tumor. A. The well-circumscribed nature of the tumor (*asterisk*) can be appreciated at low power. **B.** A higher-power image showed the uniform neoplastic epithelioid cells to be arranged in cords. **C.** An immunohistochemical stain for chromogranin highlights tumor and the islets (*arrow*) within the adjacent pancreas.

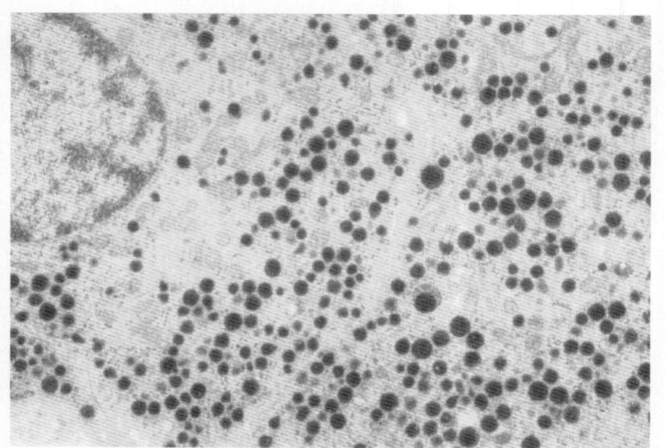

FIGURE 15-22. Alpha cells in a functional glucagonoma. The granules are indistinguishable from those of normal alpha cells (electron micrograph).

sclerotic. Certain histologic patterns have been attributed to the various functioning types of PanNETs, but this relationship is loose at best and cannot be used to determine the cell type of the PanNET. The endocrine nature of the tumor is demonstrated using immunohistochemistry with antibodies against chromogranin A (Fig. 15-20) and synaptophysin. Often, functioning PanNETs can be shown to produce the hormone responsible for the clinical syndrome using immunohistochemistry, but production of a number of different hormones in minor cell populations is not uncommon, even in clinically nonfunctioning PanNETs. Electron microscopy will also demonstrate characteristic neurosecretory granules (Fig. 15-22), and in some functioning PanNETs the granule morphology matches that of the specific granules in the nonneoplastic islet cell counterparts.

16 The Kidney

J. Charles Jennette

Anatomy

The kidneys are paired, bean-shaped organs located on both sides of the vertebral column in the retroperitoneal space. Adult kidneys average 150 g and are approximately 11 cm long, 6 cm wide and 3 cm thick. Each kidney consists of an outer cortex and an inner medulla (Fig. 16-1). When a kidney is bisected, the medulla has approximately 12 pyramids, with their bases at the corticomedullary junction. A medullary pyramid and its overlying cortex constitute a renal lobe. A pyramid has an inner and an outer zone. The inner zone, the **papilla,** empties into a calyx, a funnel-shaped structure that conducts urine into the renal pelvis, which empties into the ureter.

Blood Vessels

The kidney is one of the most vascular organs in the body and receives about one fifth to one fourth of the cardiac output. The blood supply usually derives from a single main renal artery, although a quarter of kidneys have one or more accessory renal arteries. Before entering the renal parenchyma, the renal artery divides into anterior and posterior branches, which in turn give rise to interlobar arteries

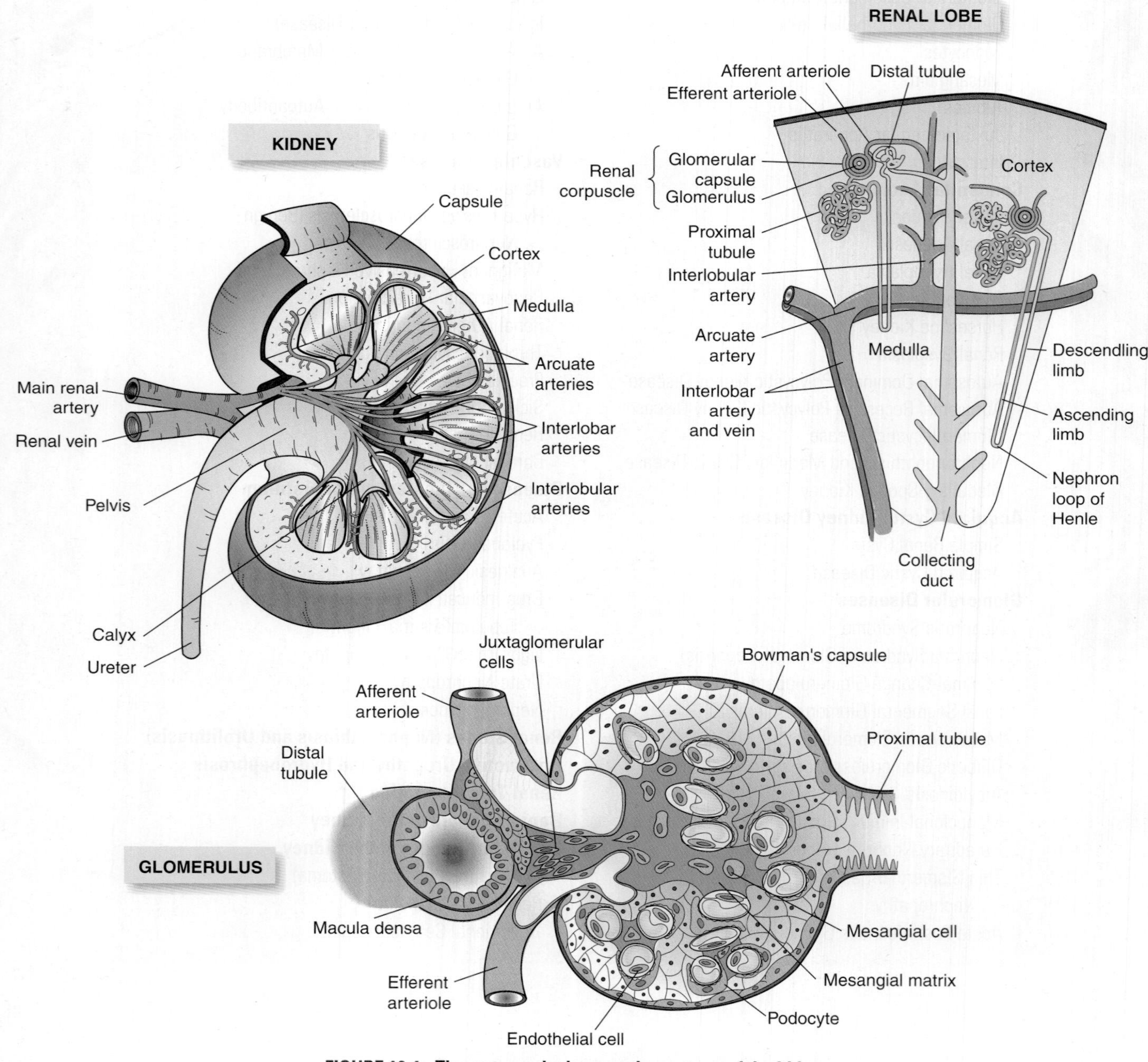

FIGURE 16-1. The gross and microscopic anatomy of the kidney.

(Fig. 16-1). The latter branch into the arcuate arteries, which run parallel to the renal surface near the corticomedullary junction. The interlobular arteries arise from the arcuate arteries and extend toward the renal surface, giving off afferent arterioles, each of which supplies a single glomerulus. Efferent arterioles drain the glomeruli and then branch into capillaries. Those in the outer cortex give rise to capillaries that supply blood to the cortical parenchyma, and those in the deep cortex, adjacent to the medulla, provide vessels that extend into the medulla to become the medullary peritubular vessels, namely, the **vasa recta.**

The Glomerulus Is the Renal Filter

The **nephron** is the functional unit of the kidney and includes the glomerulus and its tubule, the latter terminating at a common collecting system (Fig. 16-1). The glomerulus is a specialized network of capillaries covered by epithelial cells called **podocytes** and supported by modified smooth muscle cells called **mesangial cells** (Figs. 16-1, 16-2, 16-3 and 16-4). As it enters the glomerulus the afferent arteriole branches into capillaries, which form the convoluted glomerular tuft and eventually coalesce into the efferent arteriole that exits the glomerulus. Glomerular capillaries are lined by fenestrated endothelial cells lying on a basement membrane. The outer surface of this basement membrane is covered by **podocytes.** The Bowman space lies between the podocytes and the epithelial cells that line the Bowman capsule.

Glomerular Basement Membrane

The glomerular basement membrane (GBM) (Figs. 16-3, 16-4 and 16-5) separates endothelial cells from podocytes in peripheral capillary walls and also podocytes from the mesangium. Since the GBM does not completely surround each capillary lumen, but rather splays out over the mesangium as the paramesangial GBM, substances in the blood may potentially enter the mesangium without crossing the GBM.

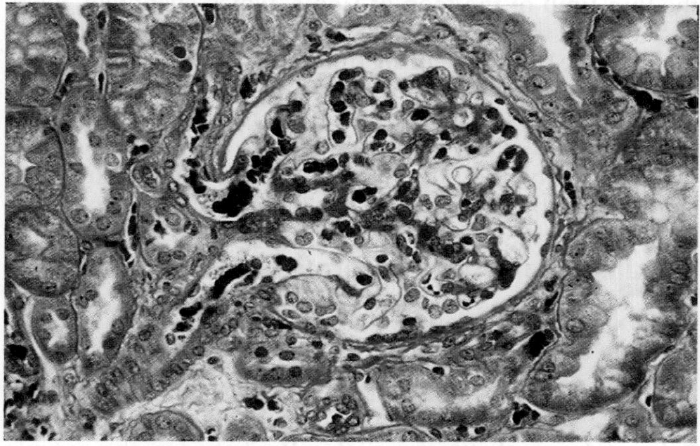

FIGURE 16-2. Normal glomerulus, light microscopy. The Masson trichrome stain shows a glomerular tuft with delicate blue capillary wall basement membranes, small amounts of blue matrix surrounding mesangial cells, and the hilum on the left. The afferent arteriole enters below and the efferent arteriole exits above.

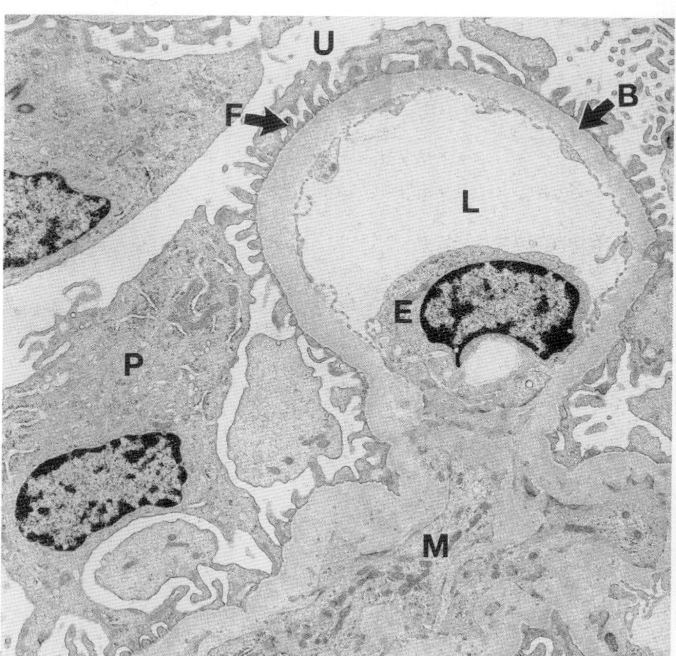

FIGURE 16-3. Normal glomerulus. In this electron micrograph of a single capillary loop and adjacent mesangium, the capillary wall portion of the lumen (L) is lined by a thin layer of fenestrated endothelial cytoplasm that extends out from the endothelial cell body (E). The endothelial cell body is in direct contact with the mesangium, which includes the mesangial cell (M) and adjacent matrix. The outer aspect of the basement membrane (B) is covered by foot processes (F) from the podocyte (P) that line the urinary space (U). Compare this figure with Figure 16-4.

Although morphologically similar to many other basement membranes, the GBM is functionally and chemically distinct. Ultrastructurally, it is approximately 350 nm thick and has three definable layers (Fig. 16-5):

- **Lamina densa:** A central electron-dense zone
- **Lamina rara interna:** A thin inner electron-lucent zone
- **Lamina rara externa:** A thin outer electron-lucent zone

The GBM is composed mainly of type IV collagen, which provides its major scaffolding. Genetic abnormalities in type IV collagen and autoantibodies directed against type IV collagen cause glomerular disease. Other constituents include glycosaminoglycans, laminin, entactin and fibronectin. The polyanionic glycosaminoglycans, which are rich in heparan sulfate, impart a strong negative charge to the GBM. This charged property allows charge-selective filtration of electrically neutral and cationic molecules and relative exclusion of negatively charged molecules such as albumin. The GBM also discriminates among molecules on the basis of size.

Glomerular Endothelial Cells

The glomerular endothelial cell layer is 50 nm thick and contains numerous 60- to 100-nm pores (Fig. 16-5), which are not a major filtration barrier to plasma constituents. Endothelial surface membrane proteins (e.g., adhesion molecules) and endothelial secretory products (e.g., prostaglandins and nitric oxide) play important roles in the pathogenesis of inflammatory and thrombotic glomerular diseases.

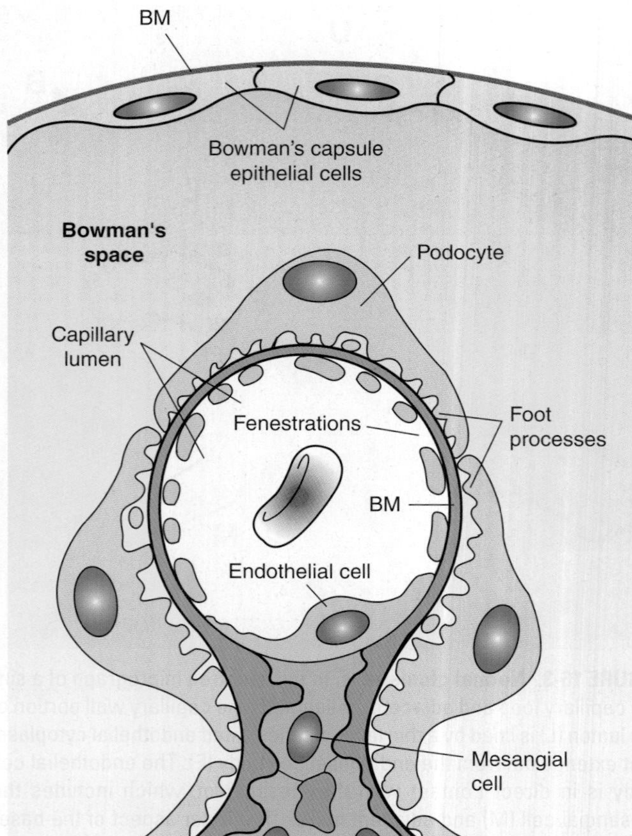

FIGURE 16-4. Normal glomerulus. The relationship of the different glomerular cell types to the basement membrane and mesangial matrix is illustrated using a single glomerular loop. The entire outer aspect of the glomerular basement membrane (BM) (peripheral loop and stalk) is covered by the visceral epithelial cell (podocyte) foot processes. The outer portions of the fenestrated endothelial cell are in contact with the inner surface of the basement membrane, whereas the central part is in contact with the mesangial cell and adjacent mesangial matrix. Compare this figure with Figure 16-3.

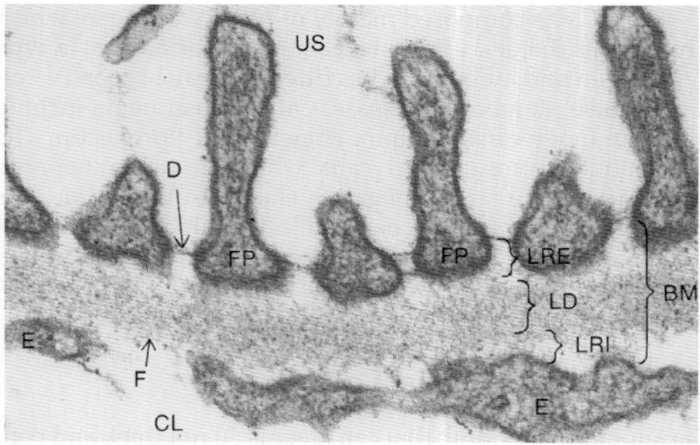

FIGURE 16-5. The glomerular filter. An electron micrograph illustrates the structures of the glomerular filter. Molecules that pass from the capillary lumen (CL) to the urinary space (US) traverse the fenestrations (F) of the endothelial cell (E), the trilaminar basement membrane (BM) (lamina rara interna [LRI], lamina densa [LD] and lamina rara externa [LRE]) and the slit pore diaphragm (D) that connects podocyte foot processes (FP).

Podocytes

Podocytes rest on the outer aspect of the GBM and send cytoplasmic projections, **foot processes,** onto the lamina rara externa of the GBM (Fig. 16-5). Between adjacent foot processes is a thin membrane called the **slit diaphragm,** which is a modified adherens junction. The podocytes are the major glomerular barrier to protein loss in the urine. Mutations in the proteins in podocytes and the slit diaphragm (e.g., **nephrin, podocin, α-actinin-4 and transient receptor potential cation channel 6 [TRPC6])** can result in abnormal protein loss into the urine (proteinuria).

Mesangium

The mesangium is a cellular and matrix network that supports the glomerulus. Mesangial cells are modified smooth muscle cells situated in the center of the glomerular tuft between capillary loops. Important functions of the mesangium are:

- Mechanical support for the glomerulus
- Endocytosis and processing of plasma proteins, including immune complexes
- Maintenance of basement membrane and matrix elements
- Modulation of glomerular filtration by the contractility of mesangial cells
- Generation of molecular mediators (e.g., prostaglandins and cytokines)

The Tubules Comprise Most of the Nephron

The major segments of the tubule that arises from each glomerulus are the proximal tubule, loop of Henle and distal tubule, which empties into the collecting duct. At the origin of the proximal tubule from the glomerulus, the flat epithelium of the Bowman capsule abruptly transforms into tall columnar cells of the **proximal tubule,** which have numerous tall microvilli that form a brush border. The initial segment is very tortuous and is called the **proximal convoluted tubule.** As it descends into the medulla, the proximal tubule straightens into the thick **descending limb of the loop of Henle.** Further into the medulla, the thick descending limb thins into the **thin limb of the loop of Henle,** which eventually loops back toward the cortex. Approaching the cortex, the thin limb becomes the **thick ascending limb.** This abuts the glomerulus from which it arose, contributes to that glomerulus' juxtaglomerular apparatus, then becomes the **distal convoluted tubule.** Several distal tubules unite to form a **collecting duct,** which ultimately empties into the ducts of Bellini, which discharge urine through the papillae into the calyces.

The Juxtaglomerular Apparatus Secretes Hormones

The juxtaglomerular apparatus is at the hilus of the glomerulus and consists of:

- **Macula densa,** a region of the thick ascending limb of the loop of Henle that has closely packed nuclei
- **Extraglomerular mesangial cells,** between the macula densa and the hilar arterioles
- **Terminal afferent arteriole and proximal efferent arteriole**

The wall of the afferent arteriole contains characteristic granular cells involved in the synthesis and secretion of renin and angiotensin.

The Interstitium Offers Structural Support

The renal interstitium is composed of interstitial cells that resemble fibroblasts and surrounding collagenous matrix. The interstitium occupies only 10% of cortical volume but constitutes 20% to 30% of medullary volume. In addition to providing structural support, some cortical interstitial cells secrete erythropoietin and some medullary cells elaborate prostaglandins.

Congenital Anomalies

Potter Sequence Results From Insufficient Amniotic Fluid

Potter sequence (oligohydramnios sequence) is the syndrome of pathologic abnormalities that are caused by markedly reduced intrauterine urine production (also see Chapter 6). Reduced urine production results in less amniotic fluid (oligohydramnios). The amniotic fluid normally cushions the fetus. With less fluid, the fetus is compressed by the uterus; this causes low-set ears, small receding chin, beak-like nose and abnormally bent lower extremities. The most life-threatening component of Potter sequence is pulmonary hypoplasia, which is caused by inadequate maturational stimuli from amniotic fluid and by compression of the chest wall by the uterus. Because even neonates can be dialyzed, severe respiratory insufficiency secondary to Potter sequence (rather than renal insufficiency) may be the cause of death in infants with severe congenital renal anomalies.

Renal Agenesis Is the Complete Absence of Renal Tissue

Most infants born with bilateral renal agenesis are stillborn and have Potter sequence. Bilateral agenesis is often associated with other anomalies, especially elsewhere in the urinary tract or lower extremities. Unilateral renal agenesis is not serious if there are no associated anomalies, since the contralateral kidney hypertrophies sufficiently to maintain normal renal function. Later in life, however, there is an increased risk for developing progressive glomerular sclerosis (secondary focal segmental glomerulosclerosis [FSGS]) due to overwork of the nephron.

Renal Hypoplasia Refers to a Congenital Reduction in Renal Mass

The kidney is histologically normal, and is formed by six or fewer renal lobes (medullary pyramids with overlying cortex). Renal hypoplasia must be differentiated from small kidneys secondary to atrophy or scarring. A frequent variant of hypoplasia features enlargement of the too few glomeruli and thus is termed **oligomeganephronia.**

Renal Ectopia Is a Normal Kidney in an Abnormal Location

The misplaced kidney is usually in the pelvis, due to failure of the fetal kidney to migrate from the pelvis to the flank. One or both kidneys may be affected. In **simple ectopia,** the ureters drain into the appropriate side of the bladder. In **crossed ectopia,** the ectopic kidney is on the same side as its normal mate; the ectopic ureter crosses the midline and drains into the contralateral side of the bladder.

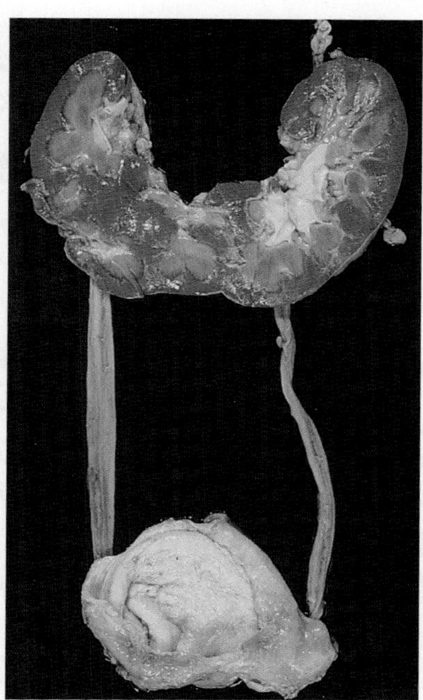

FIGURE 16-6. Horseshoe kidney. The kidneys are fused at the lower pole.

Horseshoe Kidney Is a Single, Large, Midline Organ

The kidneys are fused, usually at the lower poles (Fig. 16-6). This anomaly increases the risk for obstruction and renal infection (pyelonephritis) because the ureters must cross over the junction between the two kidneys when the organ is fused at the lower pole.

Renal Dysplasia Is a Developmental Disorder

It is characterized by undifferentiated tubular structures surrounded by primitive mesenchyme, sometimes with heterotopic tissue such as cartilage. Cysts often form from the abnormal tubules.

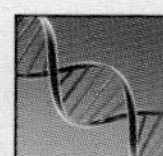

MOLECULAR PATHOGENESIS: Renal dysplasia results from abnormal metanephric differentiation and has multiple genetic and somatic causes. Some familial forms of dysplasia probably result from abnormal differentiation signals that affect the inductive interactions between the ureteric bud and the metanephric blastema. Many forms of dysplasia are accompanied by other urinary tract abnormalities, especially ones that cause obstruction of urine flow. This association suggests that obstruction to urine flow in utero can cause dysplasia. Frequent associated anomalies include:

- Ureteral agenesis
- Ureteral atresia
- Ureteropelvic junction obstruction
- Ureterovesical stenosis or posterior urethral valves

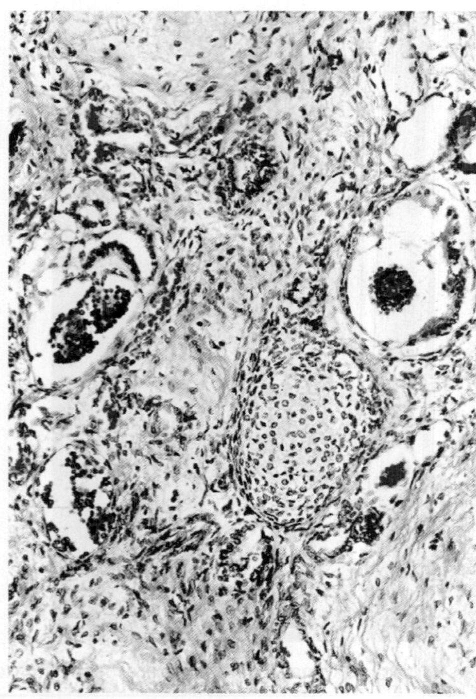

FIGURE 16-7. Renal dysplasia. Immature glomeruli, tubules and cartilage are surrounded by loose, undifferentiated mesenchymal tissue.

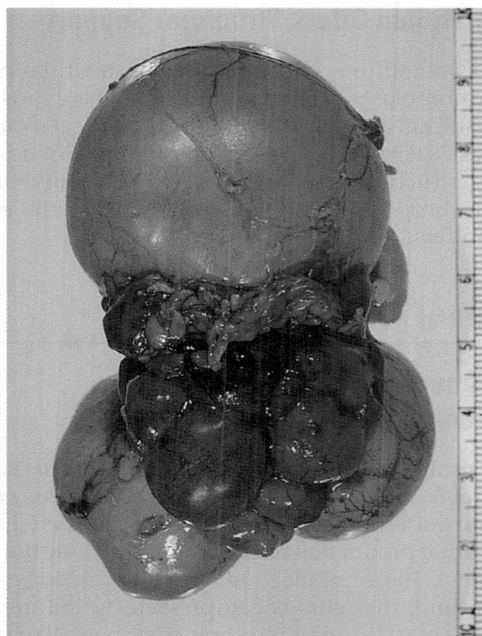

FIGURE 16-8. Multicystic renal dysplasia. An irregular mass of variably sized cysts does not have a reniform shape.

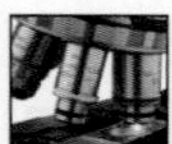

PATHOLOGY: The histologic hallmark of renal dysplasia is undifferentiated tubules and ducts lined by cuboidal or columnar epithelium. These structures are surrounded by mantles of undifferentiated mesenchyme that may contain smooth muscle and islands of cartilage (Fig. 16-7). Rudimentary glomeruli may be seen, and tubules and ducts may be cystically dilated. Renal dysplasia can be unilateral or bilateral, and the affected kidney may be quite large or very small.

- **Aplastic renal dysplasia** results in very small misshapen dysplastic kidneys, which may be difficult to identify by gross examination.
- **Multicystic renal dysplasia** is usually unilateral and is characterized by renal enlargement by multiple cysts, ranging from microscopic to several centimeters in diameter. The kidney does not have the usual kidney shape, but is rather an irregular mass of cysts (Fig. 16-8).
- **Diffuse cystic renal dysplasia** features more uniformly sized cysts and preservation of a kidney shape.
- **Obstructive renal dysplasia,** focal or diffuse, unilateral or bilateral, is caused by intrauterine obstruction to urine flow, such as posterior urethral valves or ureteropelvic junction stenosis.

CLINICAL FEATURES: In most patients with multicystic renal dysplasia, a palpable flank mass is discovered shortly after birth, although small multicystic kidneys may not be apparent until years later. ***Unilateral multicystic renal dysplasia is the most common cause of an abdominal mass in newborns,*** and is adequately treated by removing the affected kidney. Bilateral aplastic dysplasia and diffuse cystic dysplasia cause oligohydramnios and the resultant Potter sequence and life-threatening pulmonary hypoplasia. Aplastic renal dysplasia and diffuse cystic dysplasia are more often hereditary than multicystic dysplasia, especially if they are associated with multiple anomalies in other organs, as in Meckel-Gruber syndrome.

In Autosomal Dominant Polycystic Kidney Disease Kidneys Are Enlarged and Multicystic

Autosomal Dominant Polycystic Kidney Disease (ADPKD) is the most common of a group of congenital diseases characterized by numerous cysts in the renal parenchyma (Fig. 16-9). It affects 1:400 to 1:1000 people in the United States; half of these patients eventually develop end-stage renal failure. ADPKD is responsible for 5% of all cases of renal disease that require dialysis or transplantation. Only diabetes and hypertension cause more end-stage renal disease than does ADPKD.

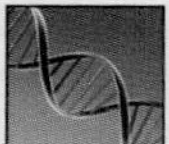

MOLECULAR PATHOGENESIS: Some 85% of ADPKD is caused by mutations in the polycystic kidney disease 1 gene (*PKD1*) and 15% by mutations in *PKD2*. The products of these genes, polycystin-1 and polycystin-2, are in the primary cilia of tubular epithelial cells and in cell–cell adhesion complexes that sense the extracellular environment including urine flow, resulting in regulation of intracellular calcium and of tubule epithelial proliferation and apoptosis. Defects in these proteins disrupt calcium signaling from cilia that normally inhibits renal tubule growth.

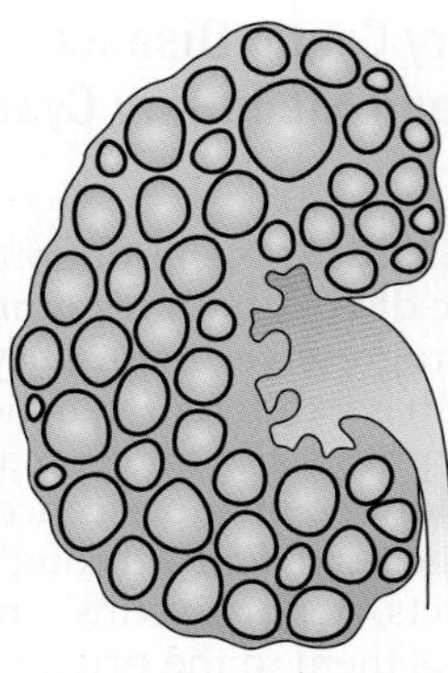

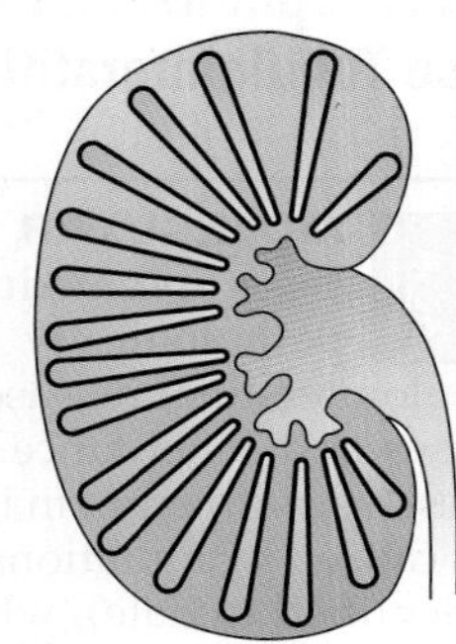

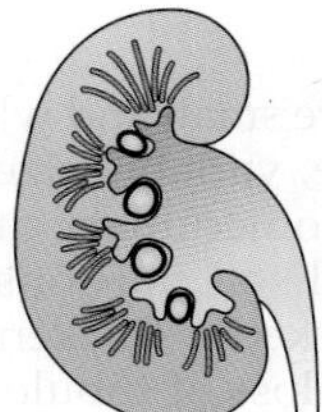

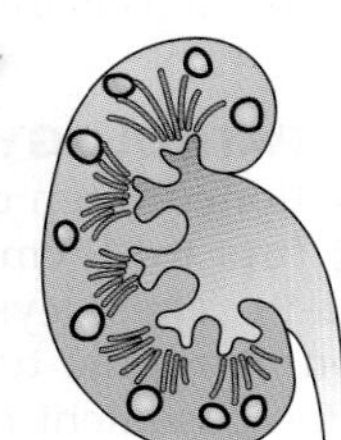

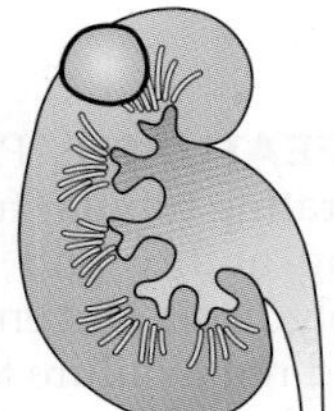

FIGURE 16-9. Cystic diseases of the kidney.

Although the precise pathogenesis of ADPKD remains unclear, it is held that cysts arise in segments of renal tubules from a few cells that proliferate abnormally. The tubule wall becomes covered by undifferentiated cells with a high nucleus-to-cytoplasm ratio and only few microvilli. Concomitantly, a defective basement membrane just below the abnormal epithelium allows the affected tubule portion to dilate. Cyst fluid is initially derived from the glomerular filtrate, but eventually most cysts lose connection with the tubules, in which case fluid accumulates by transepithelial secretion. Although end-stage renal disease in ADPKD was attributed to the pressure exerted by the dilating cysts on the surrounding normal parenchyma, it is now appreciated that cysts originate in less than 2% of nephrons and that factors other than crowding of normal tissue by expanding cysts likely contribute to the loss of functioning renal tissue. Apoptotic loss of renal tubules and accumulation of inflammatory mediators have been incriminated in the destruction of normal renal mass.

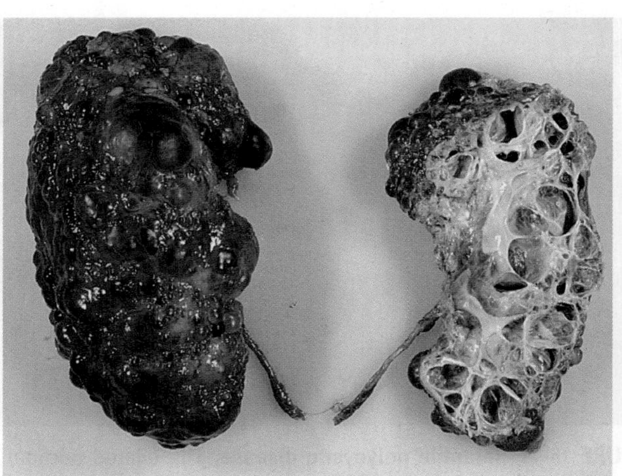

FIGURE 16-10. Adult polycystic disease. The kidneys are enlarged, and the parenchyma is almost entirely replaced by cysts of varying size.

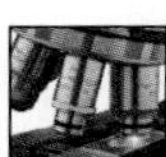

PATHOLOGY: The kidneys in ADPKD are markedly enlarged bilaterally, up to 4500 g (Fig. 16-10). The external contours of the kidneys are distorted by numerous cysts, as large as 5 cm in diameter, filled with a straw-colored fluid. Microscopically, these cysts are lined by cuboidal and columnar epithelium. Cysts arise from any point along the nephron, including glomeruli, proximal tubules, distal tubules and collecting ducts. Areas of normal renal parenchyma between the cysts undergo progressive atrophy and fibrosis as the disease advances with age.

One third of patients with ADPKD also have **hepatic cysts,** whose lining resembles bile duct epithelium. Cysts occur in the spleen (10% of patients) and pancreas (5%). One fifth of patients have **cerebral aneurysms,** and intracranial hemorrhage is the cause of death in 15% of patients with ADPKD. Interestingly, many patients with ADPKD also develop colonic diverticula.

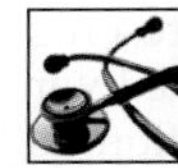

CLINICAL FEATURES: Most patients with ADPKD do not manifest clinically until the fourth decade of life, which is why this condition was once called *adult* polycystic kidney disease. A small minority of patients develop symptoms during childhood, and rarely are symptomatic at birth. Symptoms include a sense of heaviness in the loins, bilateral flank and abdominal pain and masses. Hypertension is one of the earliest and most common manifestations. Eventually, hematuria, low-level proteinuria and progressive renal insufficiency develop.

Autosomal Recessive Polycystic Kidney Disease Occurs in Infants

Autosomal recessive polycystic disease (ARPKD) is characterized by cystic transformation of collecting ducts. It is rare compared with ADPKD, occurring in about 1 in 6000 to 40,000 live births. One quarter of these infants die in the neonatal period, often because of pulmonary hypoplasia caused by oligohydramnios (Potter sequence) and because the large size of the kidneys impairs lung development and function. Children who survive the neonatal period have varying onset and rate of progression of renal insufficiency as well as hepatic fibrosis with portal hypertension.

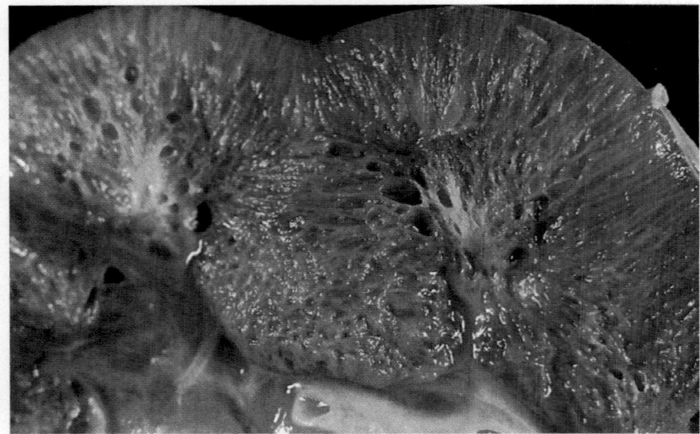

FIGURE 16-11. Infantile polycystic disease. The dilated cortical and medullary collecting ducts are arranged radially, and the external surface is smooth.

MOLECULAR PATHOGENESIS: ARPKD is caused by mutations in the *PKHD1* gene. The gene product, **fibrocystin,** is found in the primary cilia of the collecting ducts of the kidney, biliary ducts of the liver and exocrine ducts of the pancreas, and appears to be involved in regulation of cell differentiation, proliferation and adhesion. Mutations of *PKHD1* also cause pancreatic cysts and hepatic biliary dysgenesis and fibrosis.

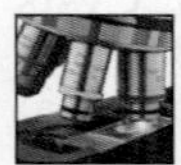

PATHOLOGY: Unlike ADPKD, the external kidney surface in ARPKD is smooth. The disease is invariably bilateral. The kidneys are often so large that delivery of the infant is impeded. The cysts are fusiform dilations of cortical and medullary collecting ducts and have a striking radial arrangement, perpendicular to the renal capsule (Fig. 16-11). Interstitial fibrosis and tubular atrophy are common, particularly in children in whom disease presents later. As in ADPKD, the calyceal system is normal. The liver usually is affected by **congenital hepatic fibrosis,** with fibrous expansion of portal tracts with bile duct proliferation (see Chapter 14).

In Glomerulocystic Disease the Bowman Capsule Is Dilated in Many Glomeruli

The disorder occurs as an isolated process or as a component of other cystic disease, such as ADPKD, nephronophthisis–medullary cystic disease complex and diffuse cystic dysplasia. Thus, there are multiple causes for glomerulocystic disease. One form is autosomal dominant, caused by mutations in the gene for hepatocyte nuclear factor-1β (HNF-1β).

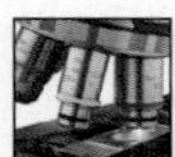

PATHOLOGY: The kidneys may be large or small. The cut surface reveals numerous small round cysts rarely more than 1 cm in diameter. Light microscopy shows dilation of the Bowman capsule in many glomeruli. The residual glomerular tuft is often distorted or appears immature.

Nephronophthisis and Medullary Cystic Disease Cause Tubulointerstitial Injury and Medullary Cysts

MOLECULAR PATHOGENESIS: Nephronophthisis and medullary cystic disease both result in pathologically similar progressive medullary tubulointerstitial disease, but they have different genetic causes and inheritance. Nephronophthisis is autosomal recessive, with onset in infancy, childhood or adolescence. It is caused by mutations in *NPHP* genes (*NPHP1* through *9* identified to date), whose products, nephrocystins, are located in primary cilia, which links them to the primary cilia location of the *PKD* and *PKHD* gene products. Medullary cystic disease is autosomal dominant with onset in adolescence and renal failure in adulthood that is caused by defects in the *MCKD1* or *2* genes.

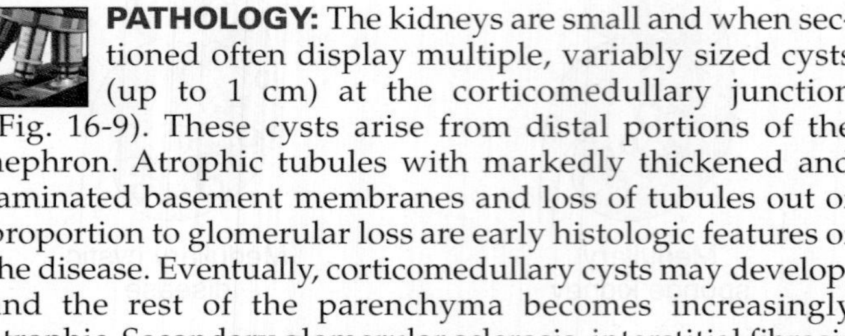

PATHOLOGY: The kidneys are small and when sectioned often display multiple, variably sized cysts (up to 1 cm) at the corticomedullary junction (Fig. 16-9). These cysts arise from distal portions of the nephron. Atrophic tubules with markedly thickened and laminated basement membranes and loss of tubules out of proportion to glomerular loss are early histologic features of the disease. Eventually, corticomedullary cysts may develop, and the rest of the parenchyma becomes increasingly atrophic. Secondary glomerular sclerosis, interstitial fibrosis and nonspecific inflammatory infiltrates dominate the late histologic picture.

CLINICAL FEATURES: Patients present initially with deteriorating tubular function, such as impaired concentrating ability and sodium wasting, manifested as polyuria, polydipsia and enuresis (bed wetting). Progressive azotemia and renal failure follow. Nephronophthisis is seen in three clinical variants: infantile, juvenile and adolescent. The juvenile form is most common and accounts for 5% to 10% of end-stage renal disease (ESRD) in children. Symptoms begin between 4 and 6 years of age, and ESRD usually develops within 10 years. The onset and progression to ESRD of adolescent nephronophthisis overlap with the juvenile form, but the adolescent form results from defects in *NEPH3* and more often causes ESRD at 10 and 20 years of age. Defects in *NPHP2* are most common in the infantile form, which progresses to ESRD before 2 years of age. Among all patients with nephronophthisis, the *NEPH1* mutation is most common.

Medullary cystic disease is characterized by onset of renal failure after the fourth decade and usually presents with polyuria. Hyperuricemia and gout may be accompanying findings.

Medullary Sponge Kidney Is Distinguished by Cysts in the Papillae

The papillary cysts are multiple and small (<5 mm in diameter) (Fig. 16-9), arise from collecting ducts in the renal papillae and are lined by cuboidal or columnar epithelium. The disease is bilateral in 75% of patients. A few familial cases have been described.

Medullary sponge kidney is asymptomatic in young adults. Symptomatic cases are usually discovered between the ages of 30 and 60, presenting with flank pain, dysuria, hematuria or "gravel" in the urine caused by stone formation in the cysts. Although the disease itself does not pose a threat to health, the cysts may predispose to secondary pyelonephritis.

Acquired Cystic Kidney Disease

Simple Renal Cysts Are Seen in Half of People Over 50 Years Old

Simple cysts are usually incidental findings at autopsy and are rarely clinically symptomatic unless they are very large. They may be solitary or multiple, and are usually found in the outer cortex, where they bulge the capsule. Simple cysts occur less commonly in the medulla. Microscopically, they are lined by flat epithelium.

Long-Term Dialysis Leads to Acquired Cystic Disease

Multiple cortical and medullary cysts may form in kidneys of patients with ESRD who are maintained on dialysis. After 5 years of dialysis, over 75% of patients show bilateral cystic kidneys. The cysts are initially lined by flat-to-cuboidal epithelium, but hyperplastic and neoplastic epithelial proliferation may develop within 10 years of initiating dialysis. **Renal cell carcinoma** develops in approximately 5% of patients with acquired cystic disease.

Glomerular Diseases

Many renal disorders are caused by injury to the glomerulus. Glomeruli may be the only major site of disease (primary glomerular disease; e.g., immunoglobulin [Ig]A nephropathy) or part of a disease affecting several organs (secondary glomerular disease; e.g., lupus glomerulonephritis). Signs and symptoms of glomerular disease fall into one of the following categories:

- Asymptomatic proteinuria
- Nephrotic syndrome
- Asymptomatic hematuria
- Acute nephritic syndrome
- Rapidly progressive nephritic syndrome
- Chronic kidney injury
- ESRD

Nephrotic Syndrome Features Severe Proteinuria (>3.5 g/day)

It is also characterized by hypoalbuminemia, edema, hyperlipidemia and lipiduria. Increased glomerular capillary permeability allows loss of protein from plasma into the urine (proteinuria). Proteinuria is caused by many different glomerular diseases and by a variety of mechanisms.

Severe proteinuria causes the nephrotic syndrome (Fig. 16-12), but lower levels of proteinuria may be asymptomatic. Nephrotic syndrome results from **primary** glomerular

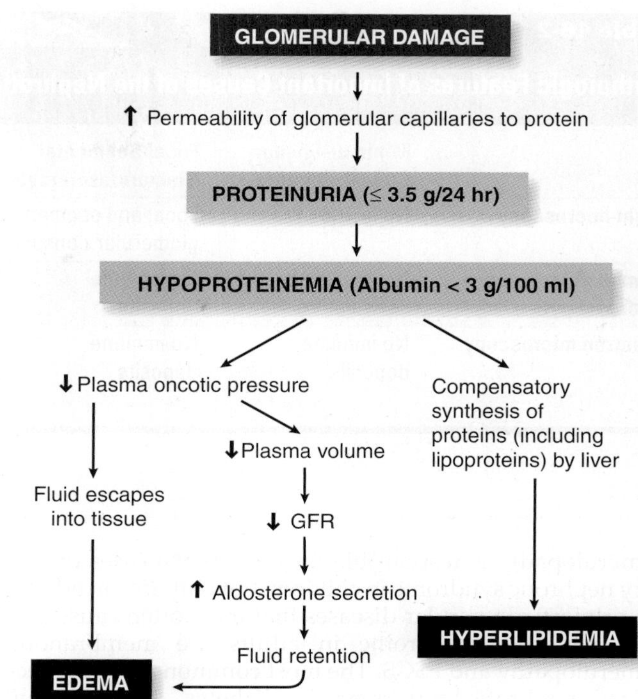

FIGURE 16-12. Pathophysiology of the nephrotic syndrome. GFR = glomerular filtration rate.

diseases unrelated to a systemic disease, or may be **secondary** to a systemic disease that affects other organs as well as the kidneys. Diabetic glomerulosclerosis is the most common cause for secondary nephrotic syndrome in adults. Table 16-1 lists the major causes and approximate frequency of the primary nephrotic syndrome in adults and children. Table 16-2 details selected pathologic features of some of these diseases (discussed below).

There are important differences in the rates of specific glomerular diseases that cause nephrotic syndrome in adults versus those in children. For example, minimal-change

Table 16-1

Frequency of Causes for the Nephrotic Syndrome Induced by Primary Glomerular Diseases in Children and Adults

Cause	Children (%)	Adults (%)
Minimal-change glomerulopathy	75	15
Membranous glomerulopathy	5	30
Focal segmental glomerulosclerosis	10	30
Type I membranoproliferative glomerulonephritis	5	5
Other glomerular diseases*	5	20

*Includes many forms of mesangioproliferative and proliferative glomerulonephritis, such as immunoglobulin A nephropathy, which often also cause nephritic features.

Table 16-2

Pathologic Features of Important Causes of the Nephrotic Syndrome

	Minimal-Change Glomerulopathy	Focal Segmental Glomerulosclerosis	Membranous Glomerulopathy	Membranoproliferative Glomerulonephritis
Light microscopy	No lesion	Focal and segmental glomerular consolidation	Diffuse global capillary wall thickening	Capillary wall thickening and endocapillary hypercellularity
Immunofluorescence microscopy	No immune deposits	No immune deposits	Diffuse capillary wall immunoglobulin	Diffuse capillary wall complement
Electron microscopy	No immune deposits	No immune deposits	Diffuse subepithelial dense deposits	Subendothelial (type I) dense deposits; intramembranous (type II) dense deposits

glomerulopathy is responsible for most (70%) cases of primary nephrotic syndrome in children, but only 15% in adults. The primary glomerular diseases that most often cause primary nephrotic syndrome in adults are membranous glomerulopathy and FSGS. The most common cause for secondary nephrotic syndrome is diabetes. Membranous glomerulopathy is the most frequent cause in whites and Asians, whereas FSGS is the most common etiology in American blacks. The incidence of FSGS has been increasing over the past decade. Systemic diseases that involve the kidney, such as diabetes, amyloidosis and systemic lupus erythematosus (SLE), account for many cases of nephrotic syndrome in adults. In third world countries where chronic infectious diseases are common, type I membranoproliferative glomerulonephritis is a much more frequent reason for nephrotic syndrome.

Nephritic Syndrome (Glomerulonephritis) Is an Inflammatory Disease

Nephritic syndrome is characterized by hematuria (microscopic or grossly visible), variable degrees of proteinuria and decreased glomerular filtration rate. It results in elevated blood urea nitrogen and serum creatinine, oliguria, salt and water retention, hypertension and edema. Glomerular diseases associated with the nephritic syndrome are caused by inflammatory changes in glomeruli (e.g., infiltration by leukocytes, hyperplasia of glomerular cells and, in severe lesions, necrosis). Sufficient injury to glomerular capillaries results in spillage of protein and blood cells into the urine (proteinuria and hematuria). The inflammatory damage may also impair glomerular flow and filtration, resulting in renal insufficiency, fluid retention and hypertension. Nephritic manifestations may (1) develop rapidly and result in reversible renal insufficiency (acute glomerulonephritis); (2) progress rapidly, with renal failure that resolves only with aggressive treatment (rapidly progressive glomerulonephritis); or (3) persist for years continuously or intermittently and proceed slowly to renal failure (chronic glomerulonephritis).

Some glomerular diseases tend to cause the nephrotic syndrome, whereas others lead to the nephritic syndrome (Table 16-3). However, except for minimal-change glomerulopathy (which almost always causes nephrotic syndrome), all glomerular diseases may occasionally cause mixed nephritic and nephrotic manifestations that confound clinical diagnosis. ***Renal biopsy evaluation is the only means of definitive diagnosis for most glomerular diseases, although clinical and laboratory data may provide presumptive evidence for a specific disease.***

MOLECULAR PATHOGENESIS: Glomerulonephritis is often caused by immunologic mechanisms. Antibody- and cell-mediated immunity may both lead to glomerular inflammation, but three types of antibody-induced inflammation have been incriminated as the major pathogenetic processes in most forms of glomerulonephritis (Fig. 16-13):

- In situ immune complex formation
- Deposition of circulating immune complexes
- Antineutrophil cytoplasmic autoantibodies (ANCAs)

Immune complex formation in situ involves circulating antibodies binding to intrinsic antigens or foreign antigens within glomeruli. For example, anti-GBM autoantibodies

Table 16-3

Tendencies of Glomerular Diseases to Manifest Nephrotic and Nephritic Features

Disease	Nephrotic	Nephritic
Minimal-change glomerulopathy	++++	–
Membranous glomerulopathy	+++	++
Focal segmental glomerulosclerosis	+++	++
Mesangioproliferative glomerulonephritis*	++	++
Membranoproliferative glomerulonephritis	++	++
Proliferative glomerulonephritis*	+	+++
Crescentic glomerulonephritis*	+	++++

*These histologic phenotypes can be caused by many categories of glomerular disease, including immunoglobulin A nephropathy, postinfectious glomerulonephritis, lupus glomerulonephritis, antineutrophil cytoplasmic autoantibody glomerulonephritis and antiglomerular basement membrane glomerulonephritis.

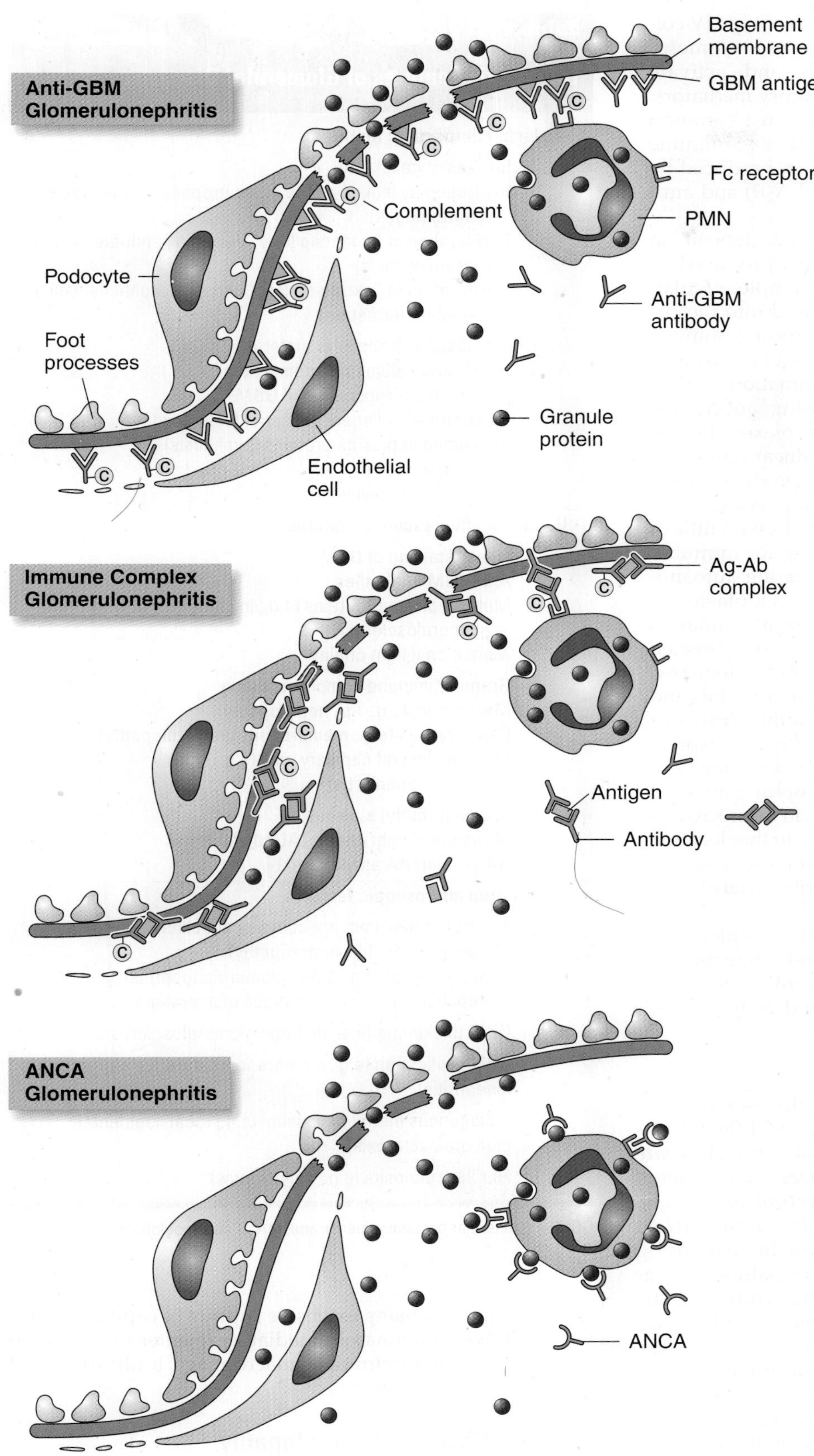

FIGURE 16-13. Antibody-mediated glomerulonephritis. Top panel. Anti–glomerular basement membrane (GBM) antibodies cause glomerulonephritis by binding in situ to basement membrane antigens. This activates complement and recruits inflammatory cells. PMN = polymorphonuclear neutrophil. **Middle panel.** Immune complexes that deposit from the circulation also activate complement and recruit inflammatory cells. Ag-Ab complex = antigen–antibody complex. **Bottom panel.** Antineutrophil cytoplasmic antibodies (ANCAs) cause inflammation by activating leukocytes by direct binding of the antibodies to the leukocytes and by Fc receptor engagement of ANCA bound to antigen.

bind a very specific epitope on the $\alpha 4$ chain of type IV collagen in GBMs. Resultant immune complexes in glomerular capillary walls attract leukocytes and activate complement and other humoral inflammatory mediators, resulting in inflammatory injury. In the most common form of primary membranous glomerulopathy, immune complexes form in situ between an antigen produced by podocytes, phospholipase A_2 receptor (PLA_2R) and anti-PLA_2R antibodies from the circulation.

Circulating immune complexes may deposit in glomeruli and incite inflammation like that produced by immune complex formation in situ. For example, circulating antibodies can bind to antigens released into the circulation by bacterial or viral infection to produce immune complexes. If these complexes escape phagocytosis, they can deposit in glomeruli and incite inflammation.

Immunofluorescence microscopy using antihuman antibodies detects such immune complexes in the glomeruli. Anti-GBM antibodies produce linear staining of GBMs, whereas other immune complexes produce granular staining in capillary walls, mesangium or both.

ANCAs cause a severe glomerulonephritis with little or no glomerular immunofluorescent staining for immunoglobulins. Such patients often have circulating autoantibodies specific for antigens in the cytoplasm of neutrophils, which can mediate glomerular inflammation by activating neutrophils. Most ANCAs are directed against myeloperoxidase (MPO-ANCA) or proteinase-3 (PR3-ANCA). Even minor stimulation of neutrophils and monocytes, such as by increased circulating levels of cytokines during viral infection, causes them to express surface MPO and PR3, which then can interact with ANCAs. This interaction leads to neutrophil activation and results in adhesion to endothelial cells in the microvasculature, especially glomerular capillaries. In that location they release injurious products that promote vascular inflammation, including glomerulonephritis, arteritis and venulitis.

The formation of glomerular immune complexes in situ, deposition of immune complexes and interaction of ANCAs with leukocytes all initiate glomerular inflammatory injury, which involves attraction and activation of leukocytes (Fig. 16-13).

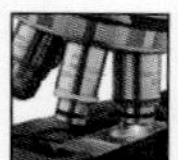

PATHOLOGY: Specific glomerular diseases have distinctive pathologic features, as well as different natural histories and appropriate treatments. ***Accurate pathologic diagnosis of glomerular diseases requires renal tissue by light, immunofluorescence and electron microscopy, and integrating those findings with clinical information.*** Table 16-4 lists pathologic features useful in diagnosing glomerular diseases. Table 16-2 summarizes pathologic features of important causes for the nephrotic syndrome. The algorithm in Fig. 16-14 shows how pathologic and clinical data are integrated to diagnose specific glomerular diseases.

In general, pathologic features of acute inflammation, such as endocapillary and extracapillary hypercellularity, leukocyte infiltration and necrosis, are more common in disorders characterized mainly as nephritic than in those that are more typically nephrotic. **Glomerular crescent formation** (extracapillary proliferation) correlates with a more rapidly progressive course. Crescents are not specific for a particular cause of glomerular inflammation. They are, rather, markers of severe injury causing extensive rupture of capillary walls, which allows inflammatory mediators to enter the Bowman space, where they stimulate macrophage infiltration and epithelial proliferation.

Table 16-4

Diagnostic Features of Glomerular Diseases

I. Light microscopic features

- A. Increased cellularity
  - Infiltration by leukocytes (e.g., neutrophils, monocytes, macrophages)
  - Proliferation of "endocapillary" cells (i.e., endothelial and mesangial cells)
  - Proliferation of "extracapillary" cells (i.e., epithelial cells) (crescent formation)
- B. Increased extracellular material
  - Localization of immune complexes
  - Thickening or replication of GBM
  - Increases in collagenous matrix (sclerosis)
  - Insudation of plasma proteins (hyalinosis)
  - Fibrinoid necrosis
  - Deposition of amyloid

II. Immunofluorescence features

- A. Linear staining of GBM
  - Anti-GBM antibodies
  - Multiple plasma proteins (e.g., in diabetic glomerulosclerosis)
  - Monoclonal light chains
- B. Granular immune complex staining
  - Mesangium (e.g., IgA nephropathy)
  - Capillary wall (e.g., membranous glomerulopathy)
  - Mesangium and capillary wall (e.g., lupus glomerulonephritis)
- C. Irregular (fluffy) staining
  - Monoclonal light chains (AL amyloidosis)
  - AA protein (AA amyloidosis)

III. Electron microscopic features

- A. Electron-dense immune complex deposits
  - Mesangial (e.g., IgA nephropathy)
  - Subendothelial (e.g., lupus glomerulonephritis)
  - Subepithelial (e.g., membranous glomerulopathy)
- B. GBM thickening (e.g., diabetic glomerulosclerosis)
- C. GBM replication (e.g., membranoproliferative glomerulonephritis)
- D. Collagenous matrix expansion (e.g., focal segmental glomerulosclerosis)
- E. Fibrillary deposits (e.g., amyloidosis)

GBM = glomerular basement membrane; IgA = immunoglobulin A.

Minimal-Change Glomerulopathy Causes Nephrotic Syndrome

Pathologically, the disease is characterized by effacement of podocyte foot processes.

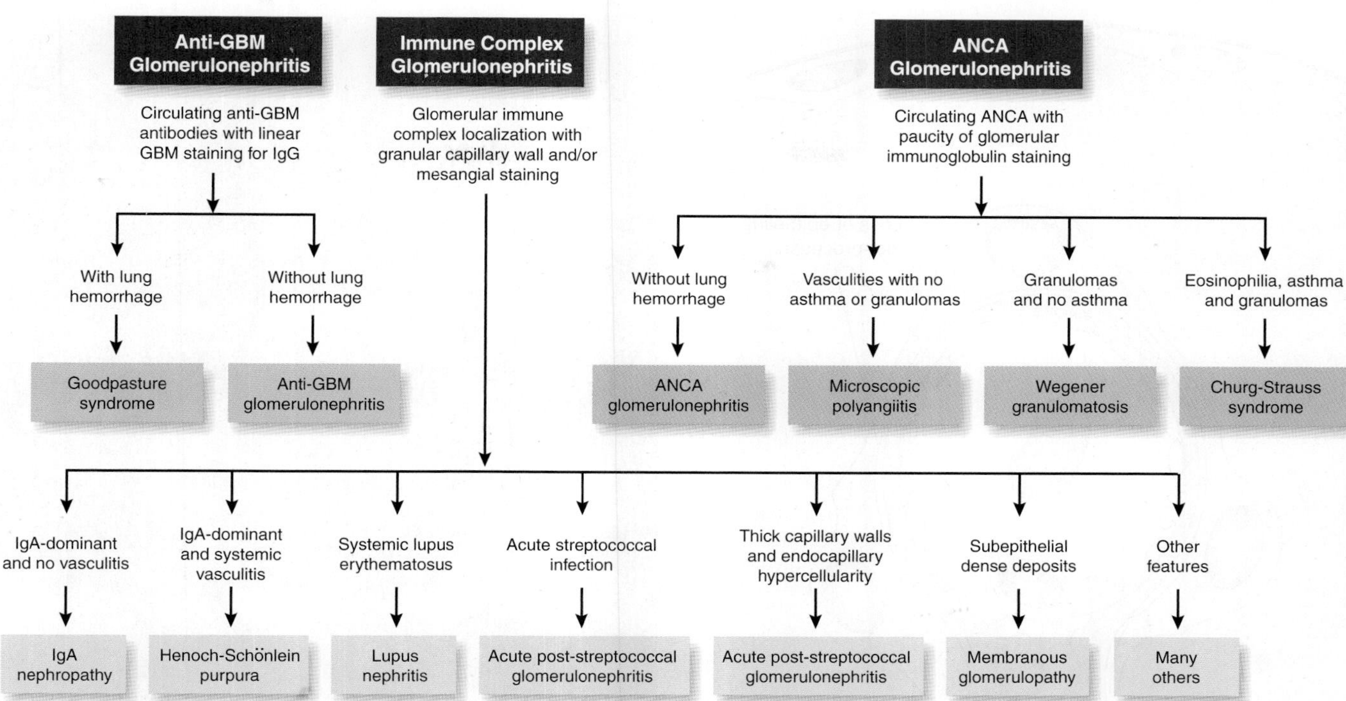

FIGURE 16-14. Algorithm demonstrating the integration of pathologic findings with clinical data to make a diagnosis of a specific form of primary or secondary glomerulonephritis. Note that an important initial categorization is as anti–glomerular basement membrane (GBM), immune complex or antineutrophil cytoplasmic autoantibody (ANCA) glomerulonephritis. Once this determination is made, more specific diagnoses depend on additional clinical or pathologic observations.

MOLECULAR PATHOGENESIS: The pathogenesis of minimal-change glomerulopathy is unknown. Involvement of the immune system has been postulated because the disease frequently enters remission when treated with corticosteroids and because it may occur in association with an allergic disease or a lymphoid neoplasm. The occasional association with Hodgkin disease (a condition associated with T-cell dysfunction) and with T-cell lymphomas has led to speculation that minimal-change glomerulopathy may be caused by a disorder of T lymphocytes, possibly by their producing a cytokine that increases glomerular permeability, probably by effects on podocytes. The heavy proteinuria of minimal-change glomerulopathy is accompanied by a loss of polyanionic sites on the GBM and podocytes, which allows anionic proteins, particularly albumin, to pass more easily across capillary walls.

PATHOLOGY: *By light microscopy, glomeruli in minimal-change glomerulopathy are essentially normal* (Fig. 16-15). Electron microscopy shows diffuse obliteration of podocyte foot processes. Loss of protein in the urine leads to hypoalbuminemia, and compensatory increase in lipoprotein secretion by the liver results in hyperlipidemia. The loss of lipoproteins through the glomeruli causes lipids to accumulate in proximal tubular cells, which is reflected histologically as glassy (hyaline) droplets in tubular epithelial cytoplasm. Such droplets are not specific for minimal-change disease but are seen in any glomerular disease causing nephrotic syndrome.

Electron microscopy reveals extensive **effacement of podocyte cell foot processes** (Figs. 16-16 and 16-17). This occurs in almost all cases of proteinuria in the nephrotic range; it is not specific for minimal-change glomerulopathy. Immunofluorescence studies for immunoglobulins and complement are most often negative, but there is occasional weak mesangial staining for IgM and the complement component C3.

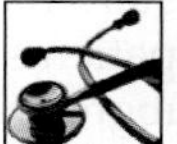

CLINICAL FEATURES: *Minimal-change glomerulopathy causes 90% of primary nephrotic syndrome cases in young children, 50% in older children and*

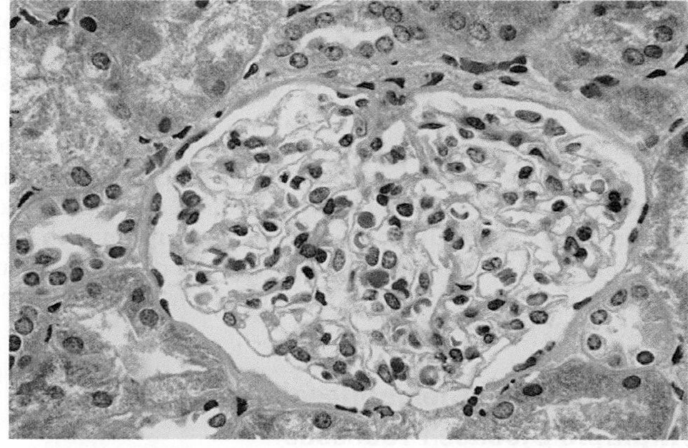

FIGURE 16-15. Minimal-change glomerulopathy. A light micrograph shows no abnormality.

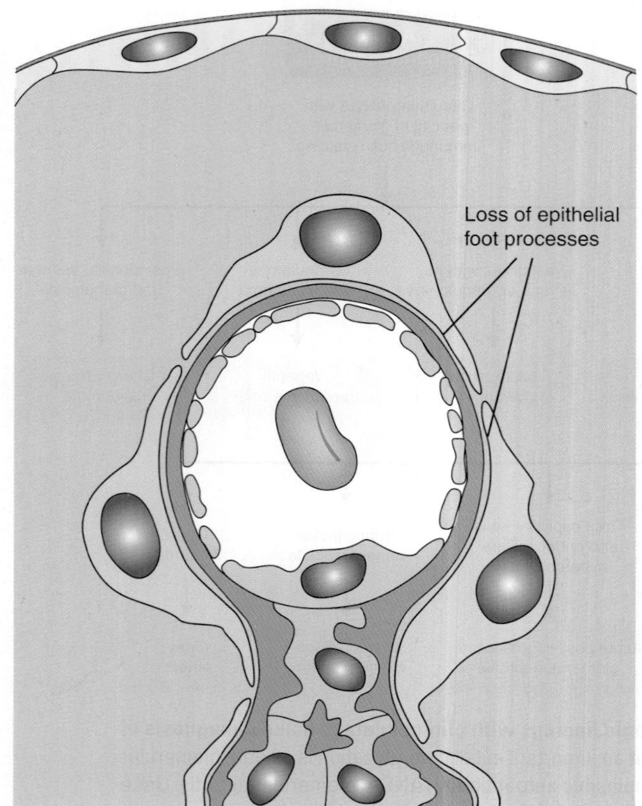

FIGURE 16-16. Minimal-change glomerulopathy. This condition is characterized predominantly by epithelial cell changes, particularly the effacement of the foot processes. All other glomerular structures appear intact.

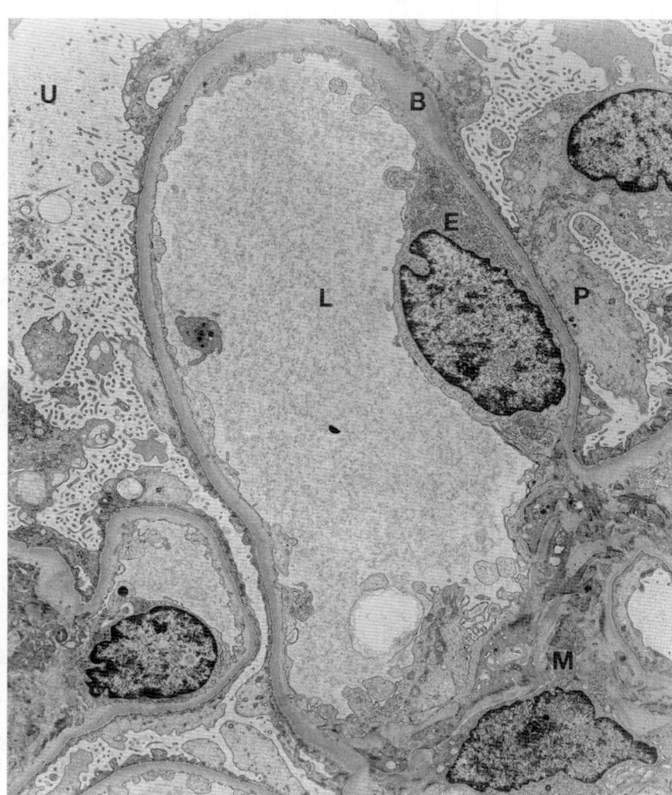

FIGURE 16-17. Minimal-change glomerulopathy. In this electron micrograph, the podocyte (P) displays extensive effacement of foot processes and numerous microvilli projecting into the urinary space (U). B = basement membrane; E = endothelial cell; L = lumen; M = mesangial cell.

15% in adults. Proteinuria is generally more selective (albumin > globulins) than in the nephrotic syndrome caused by other diseases, but there is too much overlap for this selectivity to be used as a diagnostic criterion. In over 90% of children and in fewer adults with minimal-change glomerulopathy, proteinuria remits completely within 8 weeks of initiating corticosteroid therapy. Adults often require a longer course of steroids for remission. If corticosteroids are withdrawn, most patients have intermittent relapses for up to 10 years. A small subgroup of patients has only partial remission with corticosteroid therapy and continues to lose protein in the urine. In an even smaller group that is totally resistant to corticosteroid therapy, the diagnosis of minimal-change glomerulopathy may not be accurate and FSGS that was not sampled in the initial biopsy specimen may be present.

In the absence of complications, the long-term outlook for patients with minimal-change glomerulopathy is no different from that of the general population. Development of azotemia in a patient diagnosed as having minimal-change glomerulopathy should suggest an incorrect diagnosis, usually FSGS or perhaps a complication such as drug-induced interstitial nephritis.

Focal Segmental Glomerulosclerosis Is Seen in Multiple Disease Processes

In FSGS glomerular consolidation affects some (focal), but not all, glomeruli and initially involves only part of an affected glomerular tuft (segmental). Consolidated segments often show increased collagenous matrix (sclerosis; Fig. 16-18). There are primary and secondary forms of FSGS.

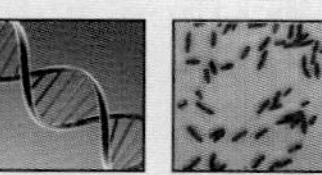
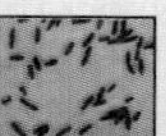

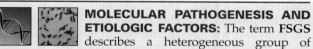

MOLECULAR PATHOGENESIS AND ETIOLOGIC FACTORS: The term **FSGS** describes a heterogeneous group of glomerular diseases with different causes, pathologies,

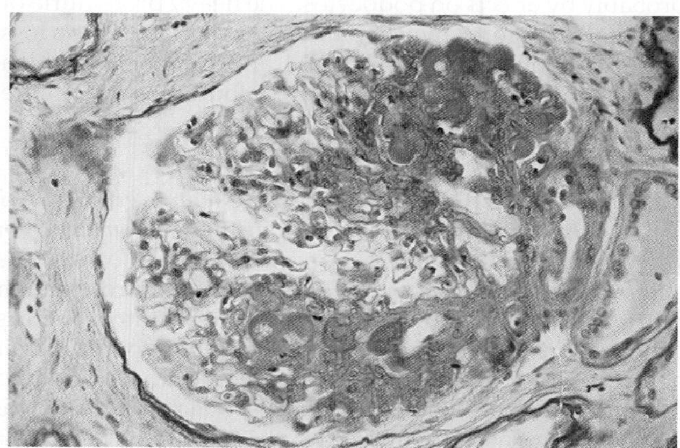

FIGURE 16-18. Focal segmental glomerulosclerosis. Periodic acid–Schiff (PAS) staining shows perihilar areas of segmental sclerosis and adjacent adhesions to the Bowman capsule.

Table 16-5

Categories of Focal Segmental Glomerulosclerosis

Idiopathic (primary) focal segmental glomerulosclerosis
Perihilar variant
Collapsing variant
Tip lesion variant
Cellular variant
Secondary focal segmental glomerulosclerosis
Hereditary/genetic
Obesity (perihilar variant)
Reduced renal mass (perihilar variant)
Cyanotic congenital heart disease (usually perihilar variant)
Sickle cell nephropathy (usually perihilar variant)
Human immunodeficiency virus (collapsing variant)
Pamidronate (collapsing variant)
Intravenous drug abuse (usually collapsing variant)

responses to treatment and outcomes. It may be idiopathic (primary) or secondary to several conditions (Table 16-5). Multiple factors probably lead to a final common pathway of injury. Pathologic features and genetic evidence suggest that injury to podocytes may be common to all types of FSGS.

Several hereditary forms of FSGS reflect genetic abnormalities in podocyte proteins (e.g., podocin, nephrin, α-actinin-4 and transient receptor potential cation channel 6 [TRPC6]). This supports the hypothesis that injury to, or dysfunction of, podocytes causes FSGS.

Congenital (e.g., unilateral agenesis) and acquired (e.g., reflux nephropathy) reductions in renal mass place adaptive stress on the reduced number of nephrons. In turn, this strain appears to cause FSGS from overwork, with increased glomerular capillary pressure and filtration, and glomerular enlargement. A normal amount of renal tissue can also be stressed by excessive body mass (obesity), resulting in FSGS. Reduced blood oxygen (e.g., as in sickle cell disease or cyanotic congenital heart disease) also causes a similar pattern of glomerular injury. In all of these settings, glomerular enlargement reflects functional overwork, placing undue stress on podocytes because of their limited proliferative capacity.

Viruses, drugs and serum factors are implicated as causes of FSGS. Infection with human immunodeficiency virus (HIV), especially in blacks, is associated with a variant of FSGS with a collapsing pattern of sclerosis (Fig. 16-19). Such an appearance may also occur in idiopathic FSGS. Collapsing FSGS may also be caused by viral infection of podocytes. Pamidronate, a drug used to treat osteolytic bone disease in patients with cancer, causes collapsing FSGS in some patients. The drug probably causes FSGS by injuring podocytes. A serum permeability factor has been detected in some patients with FSGS, which suggests a systemic cause for the glomerular injury. This is further supported by the recurrence of FSGS in renal transplants, especially in patients who have the permeability factor.

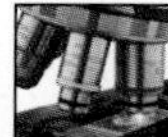

PATHOLOGY: By light microscopy, varying numbers of glomeruli show segmental obliteration of capillary loops by increased matrix or accumulation of cells, or both. Insudation of plasma proteins and lipid gives lesions a glassy appearance, called **hyalinosis.** Adhesions to the Bowman capsule occur adjacent to sclerotic lesions. Uninvolved glomeruli may look entirely normal, although mild mesangial hypercellularity is occasionally present. Because uninvolved glomeruli usually appear normal, FSGS can be mistaken for minimal-change glomerulopathy in small biopsy specimens that contain only nonsclerotic glomeruli.

Several histologic variants of focal segmental glomerulosclerosis are recognized. Particularly in patients with reduced renal mass or obesity, the sclerosis localizes **perihilar** segments within glomeruli and in deep cortical (juxtamedullary) glomeruli (Fig. 16-18). A **collapsing** pattern of sclerosis with hypertrophied and hyperplastic podocytes adjacent to sclerotic segments is typical of HIV-associated nephropathy and also occurs with intravenous drug abuse, with pamidronate-induced disease and as an idiopathic process. This collapsing variant has a poor prognosis, and half of patients reach end-stage disease within 2 years. Sclerosis limited to glomerular segments by the origin of the proximal tubule has been designated **tip lesion** and is more likely to respond to steroid therapy than other forms of FSGS. A **cellular variant** of FSGS has prominent lipid-laden cells within the sites of glomerular consolidation.

By electron microscopy, epithelial cell foot processes are diffusely effaced in FSGS, with occasional focal detachment or loss of podocytes from the GBM. Sclerotic segments show increased matrix material, wrinkling and thickening of basement membranes and capillary collapse. Accumulation of electron-dense material in sclerotic segments represents insudative trapping of plasma proteins and corresponds to hyalinosis seen by light microscopy. ***Immune complexes are absent.***

Immunofluorescence microscopy shows irregular trapping of IgM and C3 in the segmental areas of sclerosis and hyalinosis. IgG, C4, and C1q are less often found in sclerotic segments. Nonsclerotic segments do not stain or do so weakly, usually for IgM and C3 in the mesangium.

CLINICAL FEATURES: FSGS causes 30% of primary nephrotic syndrome in adults and 10% in children. It is more common in blacks than in whites and is the leading cause of primary nephrotic syndrome in American blacks. Its frequency has been increasing over the past few decades for unknown reasons. Clinical presentations and outcomes vary among the different patterns of injury. Most often asymptomatic proteinuria begins insidiously and progresses to the nephrotic syndrome. Many patients are hypertensive. Microscopic hematuria is frequent.

Most people with FSGS show persistent proteinuria and progressive decline in renal function. Many progress to end-stage renal disease after 5 to 20 years. Some, but not all, patients improve with corticosteroid therapy. Although renal transplantation is the preferred treatment for end-stage renal disease, FSGS recurs in half of transplanted kidneys.

Patients with FSGS due to obesity or reduced renal mass usually have a more indolent course that benefits from treatment with angiotensin-converting enzyme (ACE) inhibitors or angiotensin receptor blockers (ARBs). Patients with the tip lesion variant often present with severe nephrotic syndrome but respond better to corticosteroids than those with other forms of FSGS. HIV-associated and idiopathic collapsing FSGS have the worst prognoses. They typically have severe

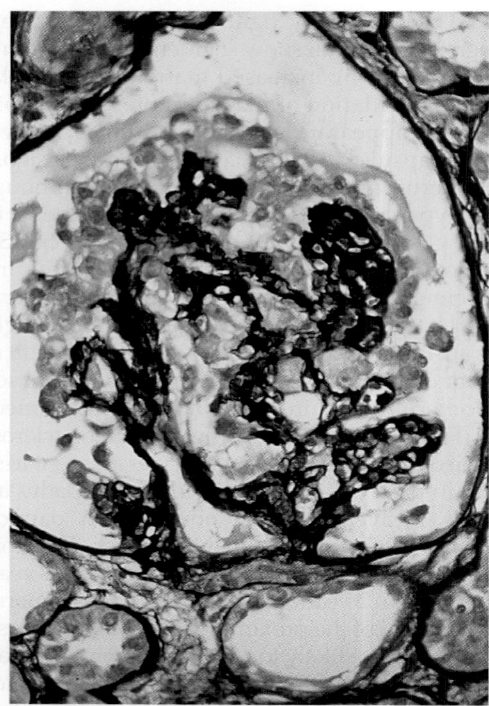

FIGURE 16-19. Human immunodeficiency virus (HIV)-associated nephropathy. Silver staining shows a collapsing pattern of focal segmental glomerulosclerosis (FSGS), with collapse of glomerular capillaries, increased matrix material (sclerosis) and hypertrophy of podocytes.

nephrotic syndrome and renal failure, often progressing to end-stage renal disease within a year.

HIV-1–Associated Nephropathy

HIV-1-associated nephropathy is a severe, rapidly progressive collapsing form of focal segmental glomerulosclerosis.

ETIOLOGIC FACTORS: The occurrence of nephropathy in patients with HIV-1 infection has raised the possibility that it is caused by HIV-1 within the renal parenchyma. A different hypothesis proposes that the nephropathy is caused by another virus that has infected the kidney of an immunocompromised person.

PATHOLOGY: HIV-1–associated nephropathy shows a segmental or global collapsing pattern of focal sclerosis (Fig. 16-19). Sclerotic segments display collapse of capillaries, frequently with adjacent swollen podocytes that have numerous protein droplets. Interstitial fibrosis and infiltration by mononuclear leukocytes are common. Tubular epithelial atrophy and degeneration are conspicuous; cystically dilated tubules contain proteinaceous casts. By electron microscopy, many tubuloreticular inclusions are seen in endothelial cells, similar to those in lupus nephritis.

CLINICAL FEATURES: Some 5% of HIV-positive patients, of whom over 90% are black, develop nephropathy. Idiopathic collapsing FSGS also occurs predominantly in blacks. The disease presents with severe proteinuria (often >10 g/day) and renal insufficiency. More than half of patients progress to end-stage renal disease in less than a year.

Membranous Glomerulopathy Is an Immune Complex Disease

Membranous glomerulopathy is a common cause of nephrotic syndrome in adults. It is caused by accumulation of immune complexes in the subepithelial zone of glomerular capillaries.

MOLECULAR PATHOGENESIS: Immune complexes localize in the **subepithelial zone** (between the podocyte and the GBM) as a result of immune complex formation in situ or deposition of circulating immune complexes. Formation in situ occurs in the animal model of membranous glomerulopathy called **Heymann nephritis** in which rats are immunized with a renal epithelial antigen and develop autoantibodies. The antibodies cross GBMs and bind to antigens on podocytes. Resultant immune complexes are shed into the adjacent subepithelial zone and produce membranous glomerulopathy. A rare form of neonatal membranous glomerulopathy is caused by transplacental passage of antibodies that react with an alloantigen on neonatal podocytes (neutral endopeptidase) that is not shared by the mother. Most patients with primary membranous glomerulopathy have circulating autoantibodies against a podocyte transmembrane receptor, PLA_2R. PLA_2R and anti-PLA_2R can be isolated from the immune complexes, supporting in situ subepithelial immune complex formation.

Membranous glomerulopathy is also induced in animals by repeated injection of foreign proteins, leading to formation of circulating immune complexes. In some circumstances, free antigens and antibodies can form immune complexes in situ. The result is a chronic serum sickness, which may be analogous to some forms of secondary membranous glomerulopathy in which antibodies and antigens form immune complexes in the circulation, with a subpopulation of these complexes depositing in glomerular capillary walls.

The following are general causes of membranous glomerulopathy:

- Primary membranous glomerulopathy
  Anti-PLA_2R autoantibodies
  Anti–neutral endopeptidase alloantibodies
- Secondary membranous glomerulopathy
  Autoimmune disease (SLE, autoimmune thyroid disease)
  Infectious disease (hepatitis B, malaria, syphilis, schistosomiasis)
  Therapeutic agents (penicillamine, gold salts)
  Neoplasms (lung, prostate and gastrointestinal cancer)

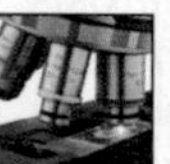

PATHOLOGY: Glomeruli usually are normocellular. Depending on the duration of the disease, capillary walls are normal or thickened (Fig. 16-20). In intermediate disease stages, silver stains (which highlight basement membranes) reveal multiple projections or "spikes" of argyrophilic material on the epithelial side of the basement membrane (Fig. 16-21). These spikes are projections of basement membrane material deposited around subepithelial immune complexes, which do not stain with silver. As disease progresses, capillary lumina narrow, and glomerular sclerosis eventually ensues. Advanced membranous glomerulopathy

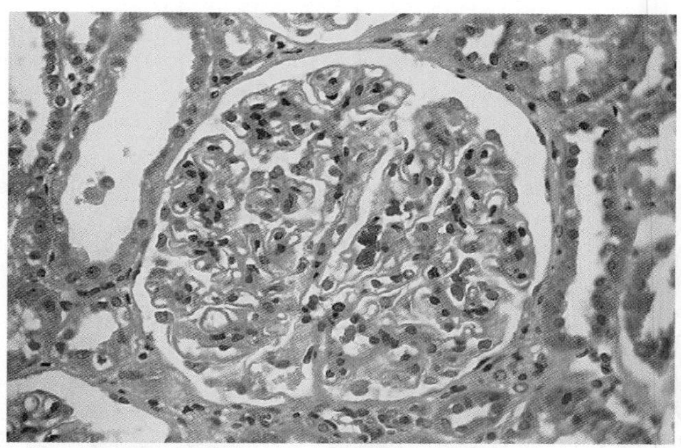

FIGURE 16-20. Membranous glomerulopathy. The glomerulus is slightly enlarged and shows diffuse thickening of the capillary walls. There is no hypercellularity. Compare capillary walls to those shown in Figure 16-15.

cannot be distinguished from other forms of chronic glomerular disease. Atrophy of tubules and interstitial fibrosis parallel the degree of glomerular sclerosis.

By electron microscopy, immune complexes appear in capillary walls as electron-dense deposits (Figs. 16-22 and 16-23). The progressive ultrastructural alterations that are induced by the subepithelial immune complexes are divided into stages:

- **Stage I:** Subepithelial dense deposits without adjacent projections of GBM material
- **Stage II:** Projections of GBM material adjacent to the dense deposits (Fig. 16-23)
- **Stage III:** Enclosure of the dense deposits within GBM material
- **Stage IV:** Rarefaction of the deposits within a thickened GBM

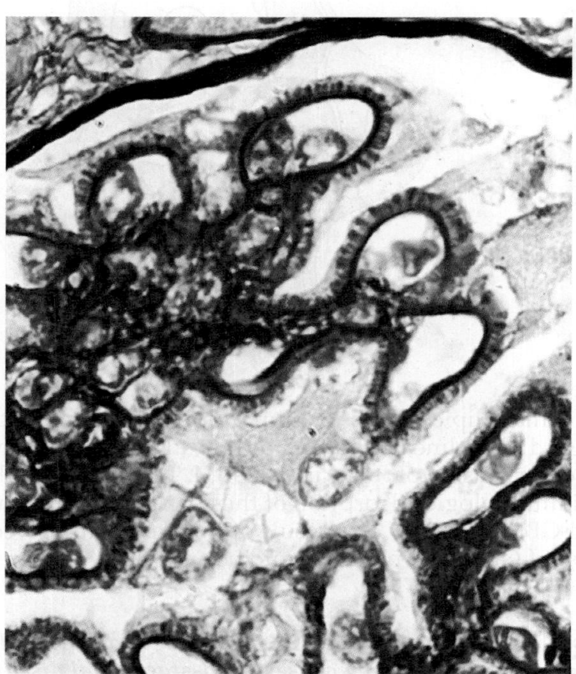

FIGURE 16-21. Membranous glomerulopathy. Silver staining reveals multiple "spikes" diffusely distributed in the glomerular capillary basement membranes. This pattern corresponds to the stage II lesion illustrated in Figure 16-22. The appearance is produced by the deposition of silver-positive basement membrane material around silver-negative immune complex deposits.

Mesangial electron-dense deposits are rare in primary membranous glomerulopathy but common in secondary disease (e.g., in lupus nephropathy). This difference may reflect the fact that primary disease is caused by antigens normally present in the subepithelial zone (e.g., podocyte phospholipase A_2 receptor and neutral endopeptidase), whereas the secondary type is produced by circulating antigens (e.g., hepatitis B virus antigens) in complexes with circulating antibodies that can localize in mesangial as well as subepithelial locations.

Immunofluorescence reveals diffuse granular staining of capillary walls for IgG and C3 (Fig. 16-24). There is intense staining for terminal complement components, including the membrane attack complex, which participate in inducing glomerular injury, especially to podocytes.

CLINICAL FEATURES: Membranous glomerulopathy is the most common primary glomerular cause of the nephrotic syndrome in white and Asian adults in the United States (the most common secondary glomerular cause is diabetic glomerulosclerosis). The course of membranous glomerulopathy is highly variable. Approximately 25% of patients remit spontaneously within 20 years, and the 10-year renal survival rate is greater than 65%. Lower survival rates are associated with male gender, age older than 50 years, proteinuria greater than 6 g/day and extensive glomerular sclerosis and chronic tubulointerstitial disease. Treatment is controversial. Patients with progressive renal failure receive corticosteroids or immunosuppressive drugs, or both. The prognosis is better in children because of a higher rate of permanent spontaneous remission.

Diabetic Glomerulosclerosis Results in Proteinuria and Progressive Renal Failure

MOLECULAR PATHOGENESIS: Glomerulosclerosis is a part of diabetic vasculopathy that involves small vessels throughout the body in patients with diabetes mellitus (see Chapter 22). Diabetes is complicated by generalized increases in synthesis of basement membrane material in the microvasculature, resulting from the abnormal metabolic state. One hypothesis proposes that increased **oxidative injury** and abnormal **nonenzymatic glycosylation** of serum and matrix proteins, including those of the GBM and mesangial matrix, induce excessive matrix production and podocyte injury.

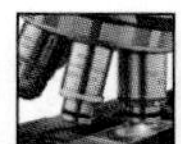

PATHOLOGY: The earliest lesions of diabetic glomerulosclerosis are glomerular enlargement, GBM thickening and mesangial matrix expansion (Fig. 16-25). Numbers of podocytes decline. Mild mesangial hypercellularity may be present along with the increase in mesangial matrix. In patients who develop symptomatic disease, GBM thickening and especially mesangial matrix

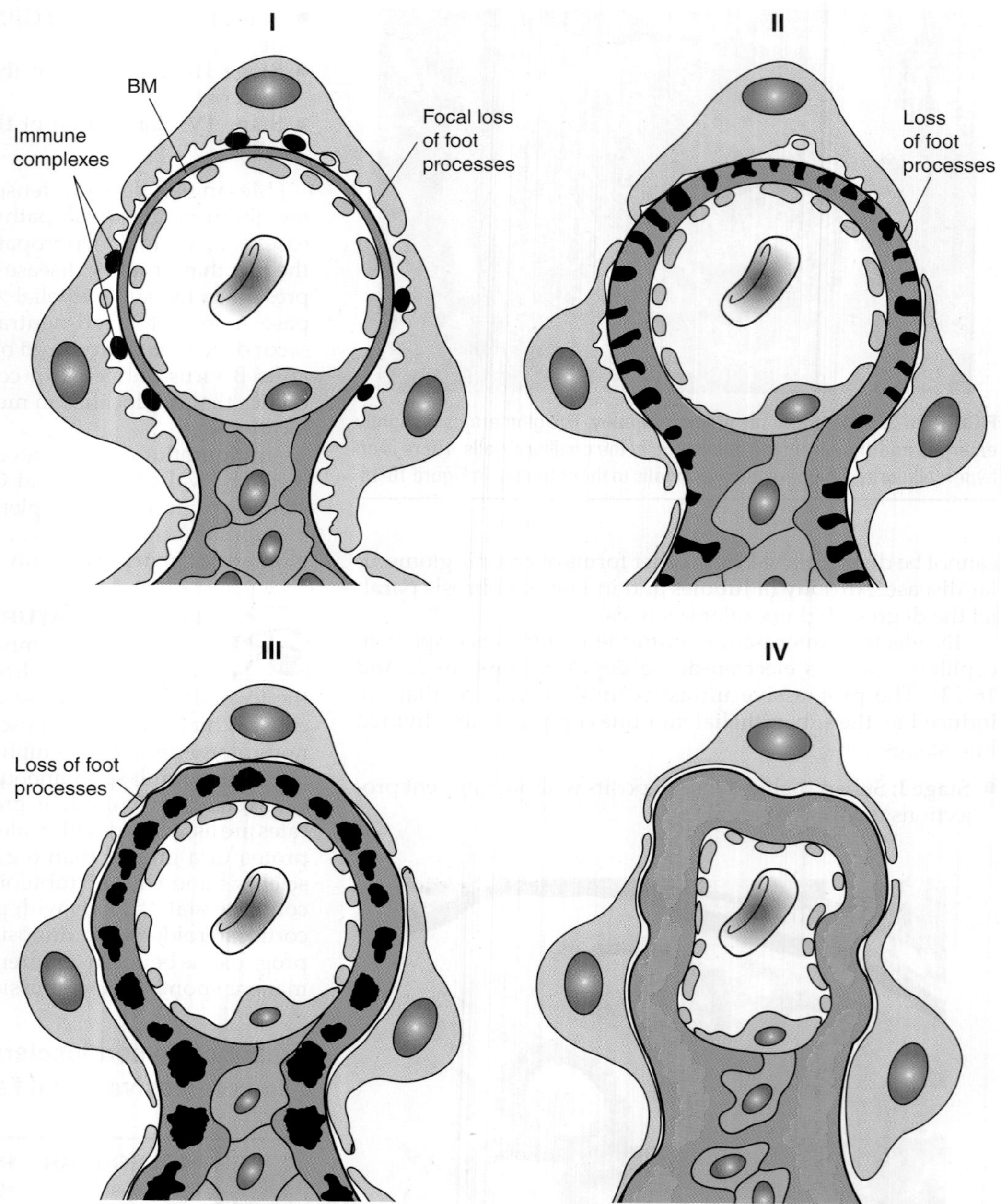

FIGURE 16-22. Membranous glomerulopathy. This disease is caused by the subepithelial accumulation of immune complexes and the accompanying changes in the basement membrane (BM). Stage I exhibits scattered subepithelial deposits. The outer contour of the basement membrane remains smooth. Stage II disease has projections (spikes) of basement membrane material adjacent to the deposits. In stage III disease, newly formed basement membrane has surrounded the deposits. With stage IV disease, the immune complex deposits lose their electron density, resulting in an irregularly thickened basement membrane with irregular electron-lucent areas.

expansion result in changes visible on light microscopy. In diabetic glomerulosclerosis, diffuse global GBM thickening and diffuse mesangial matrix expansion are accompanied by sclerotic **Kimmelstiel-Wilson nodules** (Fig. 16-26). Insudated proteins form rounded nodules between the Bowman capsule and the parietal epithelium ("capsular drops") or subendothelial accumulations along capillary loops ("hyaline caps"). Tubular basement membranes are thickened. Sclerosing and insudative changes in afferent and efferent arterioles cause hyaline arteriolosclerosis. Generalized renal arteriosclerosis is usually present. Vascular narrowing and reduced blood flow to the medulla predispose to papillary necrosis and pyelonephritis.

Electron microscopy shows up to 5- to 10-fold thickening of the basement membrane lamina densa. Mesangial matrix is increased, particularly in nodular lesions (Fig. 16-27). The hyaline insudative lesions appear as electron-dense masses that contain lipid debris. Immunofluorescence microscopy shows diffuse linear trapping of IgG, albumin, fibrinogen and other plasma proteins in the GBM. This finding reflects nonimmunologic adsorption of these proteins to the thickened GBM, possibly as a result of nonenzymatic glycosylation of GBM and plasma proteins.

CLINICAL FEATURES: ***Diabetic glomerulosclerosis is the leading cause of end-stage renal disease in the United States, accounting for a third of all chronic renal failure.*** It occurs in type 1 and type 2 diabetes mellitus. The earliest manifestation is microalbuminuria (slightly increased proteinuria). Overt proteinuria occurs between 10 and 15 years after the onset of diabetes and often becomes severe enough to cause nephrotic syndrome. In time, diabetic glomerulosclerosis progresses to renal failure. Strict

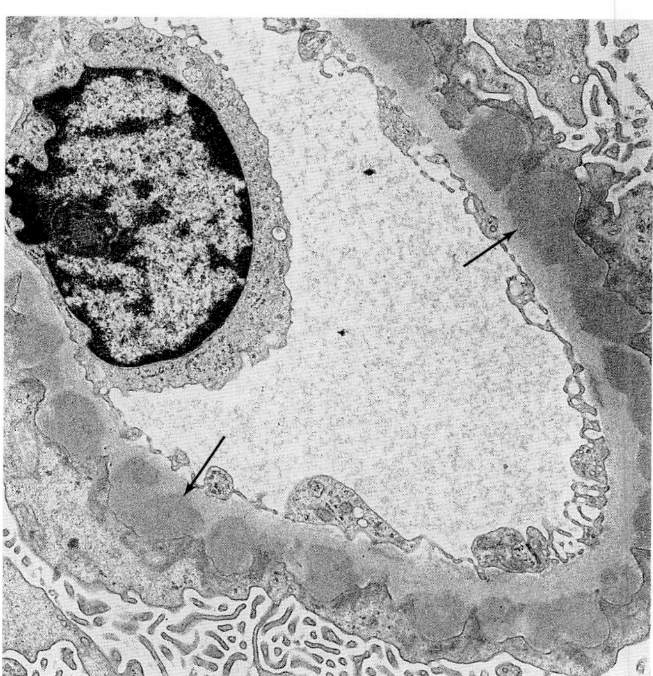

FIGURE 16-23. **Stage II membranous glomerulopathy.** An electron micrograph shows deposits of electron-dense material (*arrows*), with intervening delicate projections of basement membrane material.

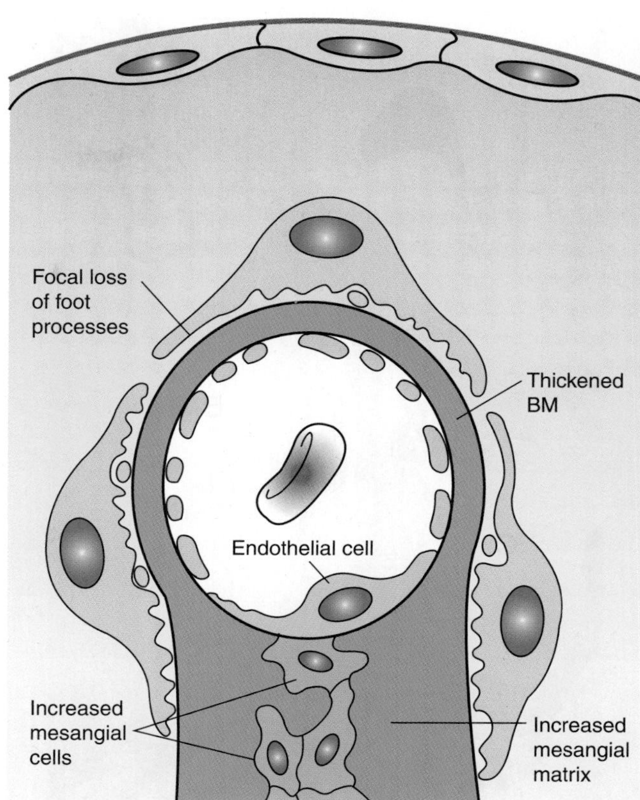

FIGURE 16-25. **Diabetic glomerulosclerosis.** The lamina densa of the glomerular basement membrane (BM) is thickened, and there is an increase in mesangial matrix material.

control of blood glucose reduces the incidence of diabetic glomerulosclerosis and retards progression once it develops. Control of hypertension and dietary protein restriction also slow progression of the disease.

Amyloidosis Leads to Nephrotic Syndrome and Renal Failure

Renal disease is a frequent complication of AA and AL amyloidosis (see Chapter 23).

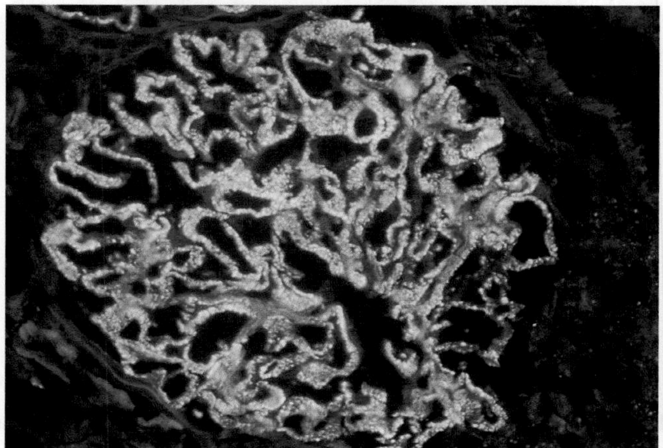

FIGURE 16-24. **Membranous glomerulopathy.** Immunofluorescence microscopy shows granular deposits of immunoglobulin G (IgG) outlining the glomerular capillary loops.

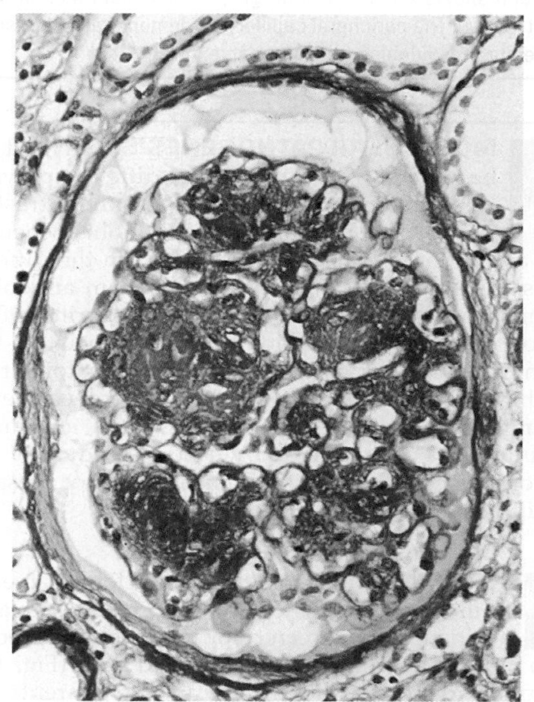

FIGURE 16-26. **Diabetic glomerulosclerosis.** Periodic acid–Schiff (PAS) staining reveals a prominent increase in the mesangial matrix, forming several nodular lesions. Dilation of glomerular capillaries is evident, and some capillary basement membranes are thickened.

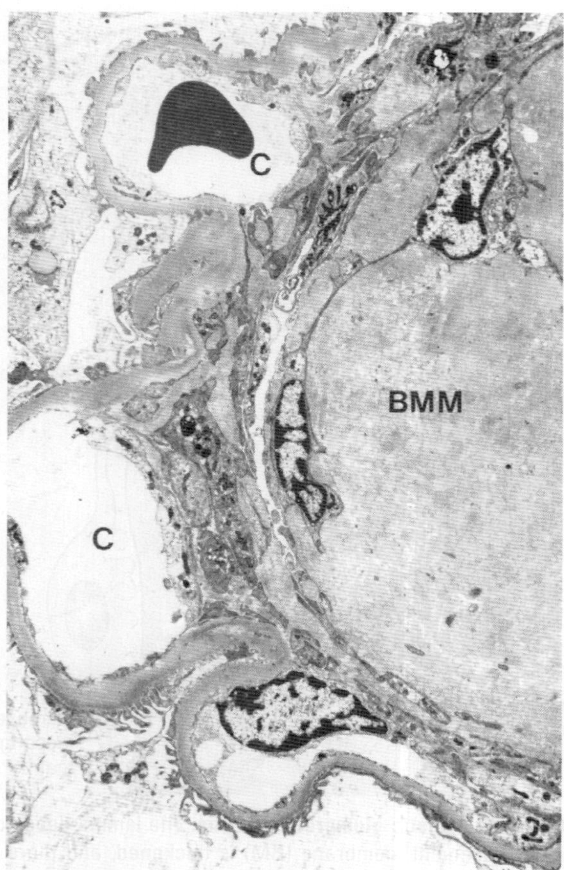

FIGURE 16-27. Advanced diabetic glomerulosclerosis. An electron micrograph shows a nodular aggregate of basement membrane–like material (BMM). The peripheral capillary (C) demonstrates diffuse basement membrane widening but a normal texture.

MOLECULAR PATHOGENESIS: Amyloid may be formed from a number of different polypeptides. In each case, the histologic and ultrastructural appearance is similar, and immunohistochemical tests are required to differentiate between the different forms. **AA amyloid** is derived from serum amyloid A protein (SAA), which increases markedly during inflammation. Thus, AA amyloid is often associated with chronic inflammatory disorders (e.g., rheumatoid arthritis, chronic tuberculosis, familial Mediterranean fever). **AL amyloid** is derived from λ or, less often, κ immunoglobulin light chains made by a neoplastic clone of B cells or plasma cells. Thus, it often occurs in, or presages, multiple myeloma.

PATHOLOGY: Histologically, amyloid is an eosinophilic, amorphous material (Fig. 16-28) with a characteristic apple-green color in sections stained with Congo red and examined with polarized light (Fig. 16-29). Acidophilic deposits initially are most apparent in the mesangium but later extend into capillary walls and may obliterate capillary lumens (Figs. 16-28 and 16-30). Glomerular structure is completely obliterated in advanced amyloidosis, and glomeruli appear as large eosinophilic spheres.

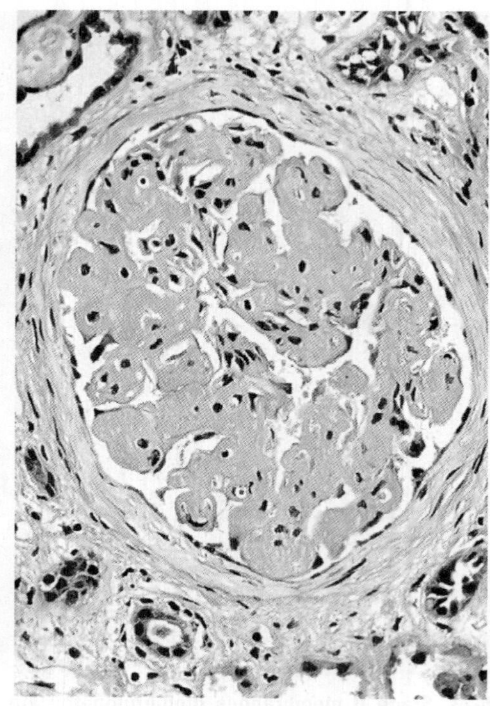

FIGURE 16-28. Amyloid nephropathy. Amorphous acellular material expands the mesangial areas and obstructs the glomerular capillaries. The deposits of amyloid may take on a nodular appearance, somewhat resembling those of diabetic glomerulosclerosis (see Fig. 16-26). However, amyloid deposits are not periodic acid–Schiff positive and are identifiable by Congo red staining.

Amyloid is composed of nonbranching fibrils, approximately 10 nm in diameter. These are initially most prominent in the mesangium, but often extend into capillary walls, especially in advanced cases (Figs. 16-30 and 16-31). Podocyte foot processes overlying the GBM are effaced.

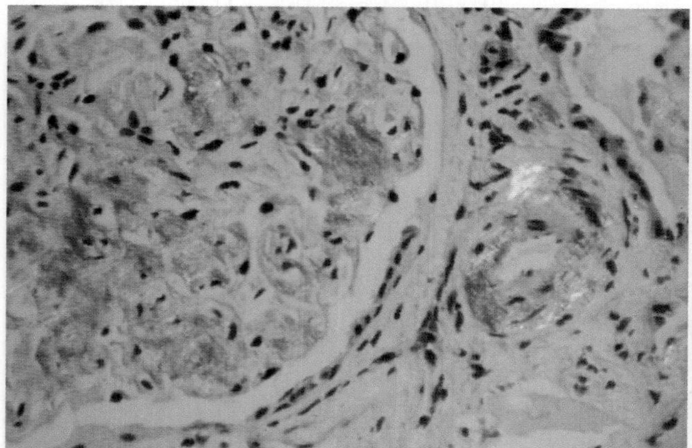

FIGURE 16-29. Amyloid nephropathy. In a section stained with Congo red and examined under polarized light, the amyloid deposits in the glomerulus and the adjacent arteriole show a characteristic apple-green birefringence.

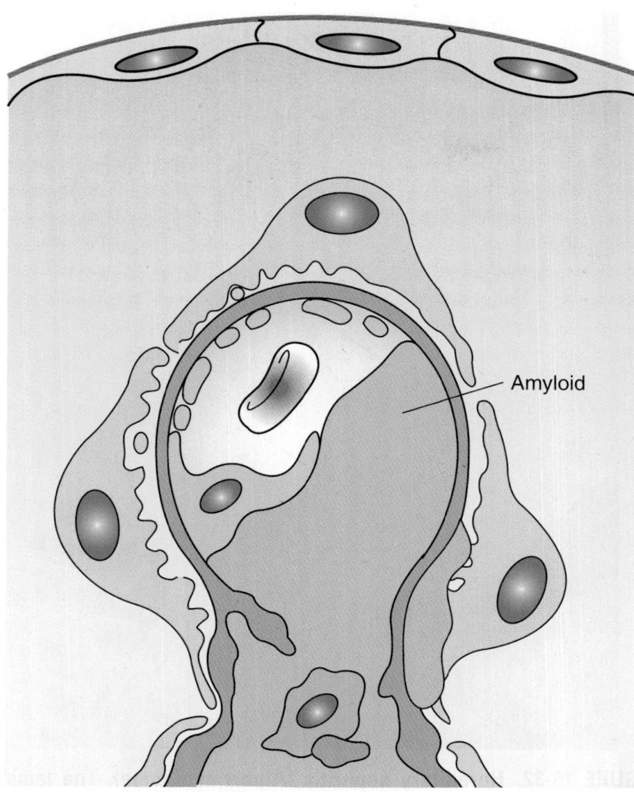

FIGURE 16-30. Amyloid nephropathy. This disorder is initially associated with the accumulation of characteristic fibrillar deposits in the mesangium. These inert masses, which are fibrillar by electron microscopy, extend along the inner surface of the basement membrane, frequently obstructing the capillary lumen. Focal extension of amyloid through the basement membrane may elevate the epithelial cell, in which case irregular spikes are seen along the outer surface of the basement membrane.

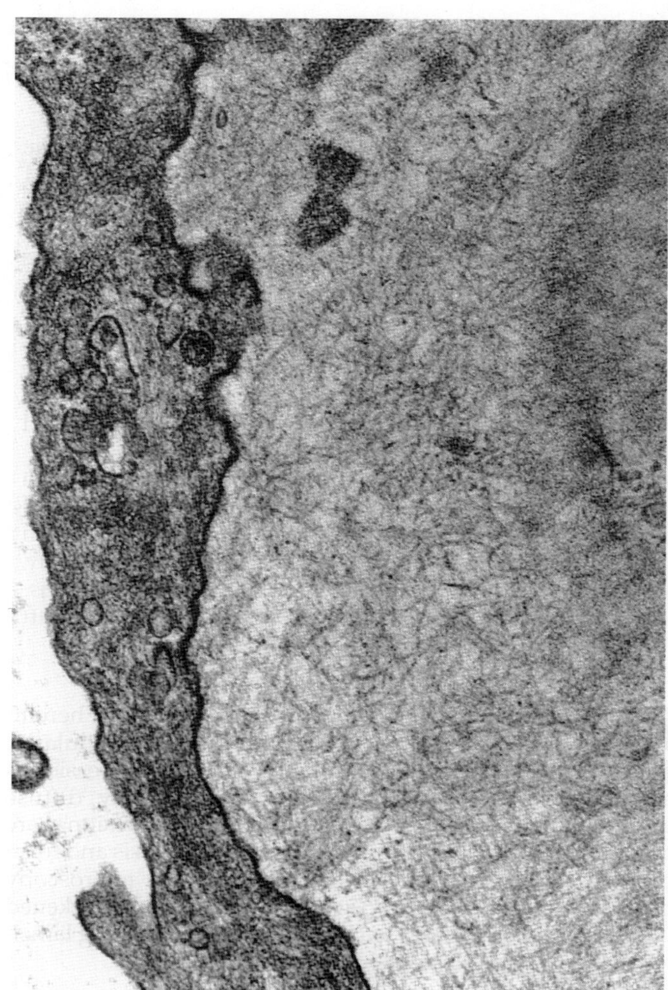

FIGURE 16-31. Amyloid nephropathy. Deposits of fibrils (10 nm diameter) in a glomerulus adjacent to podocyte cytoplasm with effaced foot processes.

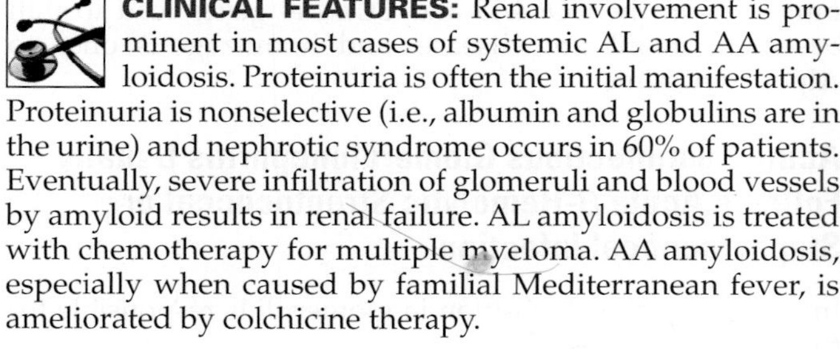

CLINICAL FEATURES: Renal involvement is prominent in most cases of systemic AL and AA amyloidosis. Proteinuria is often the initial manifestation. Proteinuria is nonselective (i.e., albumin and globulins are in the urine) and nephrotic syndrome occurs in 60% of patients. Eventually, severe infiltration of glomeruli and blood vessels by amyloid results in renal failure. AL amyloidosis is treated with chemotherapy for multiple myeloma. AA amyloidosis, especially when caused by familial Mediterranean fever, is ameliorated by colchicine therapy.

Monoclonal Immunoglobulin Deposition Disease Occurs in B-Cell Neoplasia and Results From Deposition of Immunoglobulin Components

Such deposition may be in GBMs, glomerular mesangial matrix and tubular basement membranes. The underlying B-cell neoplasm may be occult or there may be overt multiple myeloma or lymphoma. The most common offender in light-chain disease is κ light chains. The immunoglobulin heavy chains that cause this pattern of injury have deleted domains, so they resemble light chains. Monoclonal immunoglobulin deposition stimulates increased matrix production in basement membranes, causing thickening of glomerular and tubular basement membranes. Nodular expansion of mesangial regions resembles diabetic glomerulosclerosis. Importantly, the increased extracellular material does not stain with Congo red, which distinguishes monoclonal immunoglobulin deposition disease from amyloidosis. Electron microscopy reveals a uniform, finely granular, electron-dense material along the glomerular and tubular basement membranes and within the mesangial matrix. Amyloid fibrils are not present. Immunofluorescence microscopy demonstrates linear staining for monoclonal immunoglobulin chains along the involved basement membranes. Light-chain and heavy-chain deposition disease usually manifest clinically as nephrotic syndrome and renal failure.

Hereditary Nephritis (Alport Syndrome) Reflects Abnormal Glomerular Basement Membrane Type IV Collagen

Hereditary nephritis is a proliferative and sclerosing glomerular disease, often accompanied by defects of the ears or the eyes. It is caused by mutations in type IV collagen. In

Alport syndrome hereditary nephritis is accompanied by a hearing deficit.

MOLECULAR PATHOGENESIS: Several genetic mutations cause molecular defects in the GBM that lead to the renal lesions of hereditary nephritis. The most common, accounting for 85% of hereditary nephritis, is X linked and is caused by a mutation in the gene for the $\alpha 5$ chain of type IV collagen (*COL4A5* gene). A deletion at the 5′ end of *COL4A5* that extends into the *COL4A6* gene, which codes for the $\alpha 6$ chain of type IV collagen, causes hereditary nephritis and multiple leiomyomas in the gastrointestinal and genital tracts. An autosomal recessive form of hereditary nephritis is caused by mutations in *COL4A3* and *COL4A4.*

Because of disturbed basement membrane structure in hereditary nephritis, serum from patients with anti-GBM disease (e.g., Goodpasture syndrome) fails to react with GBMs from patients with hereditary nephritis. Conversely, patients with hereditary nephritis who have renal transplants are at risk for developing antibodies to allograft GBMs.

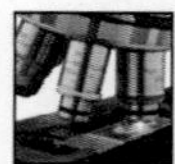

PATHOLOGY: Early glomerular lesions of hereditary nephritis show mild mesangial hypercellularity and matrix expansion. Renal disease progression is associated with increasing focal and eventually diffuse glomerular sclerosis. Advanced glomerular lesions are accompanied by tubular atrophy, interstitial fibrosis and foam cells in the tubules and interstitium. Electron microscopy makes the diagnosis, demonstrating an irregularly thickened GBM with splitting of the lamina densa into interlacing lamellae that surround electron-lucent areas (Fig. 16-32).

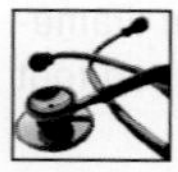

CLINICAL FEATURES: Hematuria develops early in boys with X-linked hereditary nephritis, and proteinuria and progressive renal failure usually follow in the second to fourth decades of life. In females, the X-linked disease is generally milder, the rate of progression varying substantially among patients, possibly due to the degree of random inactivation (lyonization) of the mutated X chromosome. Autosomal recessive hereditary nephritis resembles X-linked disease except that males and females are affected equally. Autosomal dominant hereditary nephritis with progressive renal failure is rare and difficult to distinguish from severe thin basement membrane disease (see below). Sensorineural, high-frequency hearing loss affects half of males with X-linked disease and a higher proportion of males and females with autosomal disease. A quarter to a third of patients have ocular defects, most often involving the lens.

Thin Glomerular Basement Membrane Nephropathy Is a Benign Cause of Hematuria

Thin basement membrane nephropathy, also termed **benign familial hematuria,** is a common hereditary GBM disorder that typically manifests as asymptomatic microscopic hematuria, and occasionally with intermittent gross hematuria. This disease and IgA nephropathy are common diagnostic considerations in patients with asymptomatic glomerular hematuria. Patients with thin basement membrane nephropathy usually do not develop renal failure or substantial proteinuria. By light microscopy, glomeruli are unremarkable. Electron microscopy shows reduced thickness of the GBM (150 to 300 nm; normal is 350 to 450 nm). The most common mode of inheritance is autosomal dominant. Heterozygous mutations in the *COL4A3* and *COL4A4* genes lead to thin basement membrane disease, and homozygous ones to Alport syndrome.

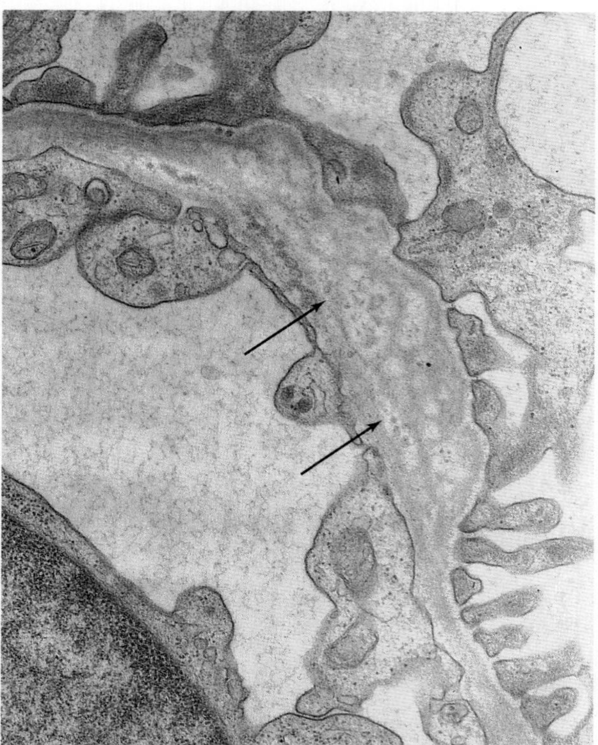

FIGURE 16-32. Hereditary nephritis (Alport syndrome). The lamina densa of the glomerular basement membrane is laminated (*arrows*) rather than forming a single dense band (compare this electron micrograph with Fig. 16-5).

Acute Postinfectious Glomerulonephritis Usually Follows Acute β-Hemolytic Streptococcal or Staphylococcal Infection

Immune complex deposition in glomeruli is responsible for this disease.

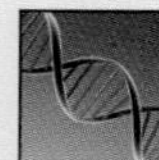

MOLECULAR PATHOGENESIS: Acute postinfectious glomerulonephritis is mostly caused by nephritogenic strains of group A (β-hemolytic) streptococci. The proportion of cases caused by staphylococcal infection (e.g., acute staphylococcal endocarditis, staphylococcal abscess) is increasing. Rare cases result from viral (e.g., hepatitis B) or parasitic (e.g., malaria) infections. The exact mechanism by which infection causes the characteristic inflammatory changes in glomeruli is not completely understood. Similarities to experimental acute serum sickness suggest that postinfectious glomerulonephritis is caused by deposition of immune complexes of antibody plus bacterial antigens in glomeruli. Both poststreptococcal glomerulonephritis in patients and acute serum sickness caused by injecting foreign proteins into animals are similar in the latent period between antigen exposure and glomerulonephritis (9 to 14 days), immunofluorescence pattern of immune complexes (granular) and ultrastructural appearance (dense deposits) (see below). Immune complexes could form in the circulation and deposit glomeruli or form in situ as bacterial antigens trapped in glomeruli bind circulating antibodies. The responsible streptococcal antigens have not been conclusively identified, but possibilities include streptococcal glyceraldehyde phosphate dehydrogenase and streptococcal cationic proteinase exotoxin B, which can localize in glomerular capillary walls and activate complement even without antibodies.

Immune complexes within glomeruli initiate inflammation by activating complement, as well as other humoral and cellular inflammatory mediators. Complement activation is so extensive that over 90% of patients develop hypocomplementemia. The inflammatory mediators attract and activate neutrophils and monocytes, and stimulate mesangial and endothelial cell proliferation. These effects result in marked glomerular hypercellularity, which defines acute diffuse proliferative glomerulonephritis.

PATHOLOGY: In the acute phase of postinfectious glomerulonephritis glomeruli are diffusely enlarged and hypercellular (Fig. 16-33). The latter reflects proliferation of both endothelial and mesangial cells (Fig. 16-34), and infiltration by neutrophils and monocytes. Crescents are uncommon. Interstitial edema and mild mononuclear infiltration parallel the glomerular changes.

The acute phase begins 1 or 2 weeks after the onset of the nephritogenic infection and resolves in over 90% of patients after several weeks. Neutrophils and endothelial hypercellularity disappear first. Mesangial hypercellularity and matrix expansion remain, but all histologic changes resolve completely in most patients after several months.

Ultrastructurally, acute postinfectious glomerulonephritis shows distinctive **subepithelial dense deposits** shaped like **"humps"** (Figs. 16-34 and 16-35). These are invariably accompanied by mesangial and subendothelial deposits, which may be more difficult to find but are probably more important in pathogenesis due to their proximity to the inflammatory mediator systems in the blood. The variably sized, dome-shaped humps are on the epithelial side of the GBM. They are not as widely distributed as the deposits of membranous glomerulopathy (compare Figs. 16-22 and 16-34). In the first weeks of disease, immunofluorescence microscopy typically reveals granular deposits of IgG and C3 along the basement membrane, corresponding to the humps. Later in the disease, C3 is present without IgG, possibly since immune complexes containing IgG no longer accumulate in glomeruli after the infection clears (Fig. 16-36).

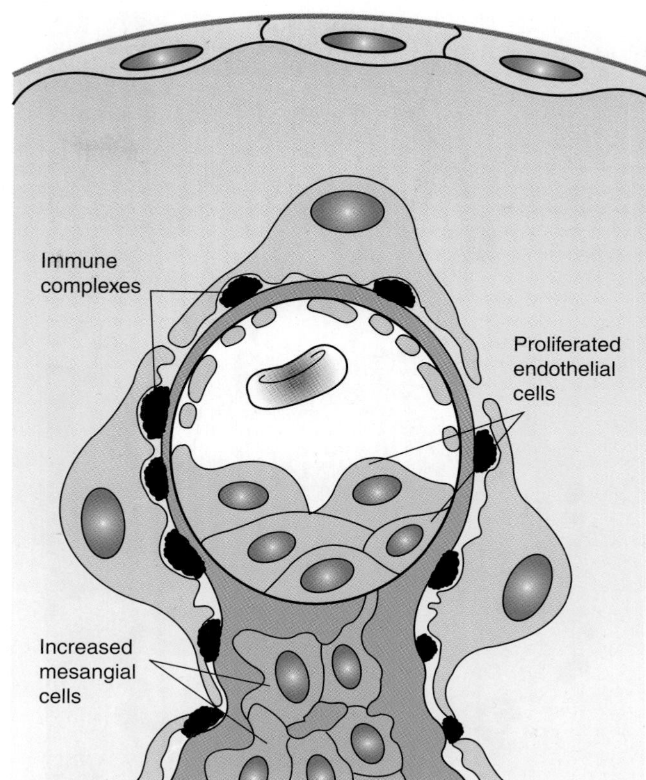

FIGURE 16-34. Postinfectious glomerulonephritis. Accumulation of numerous subepithelial immune complexes as hump-like structures is a characteristic feature. Less prominent subendothelial immune complexes are associated with endothelial cell proliferation and are related to increased capillary permeability and narrowing of the lumen. Frequently, proliferation of mesangial cells and a thickened mesangial matrix result in widening of the stalk.

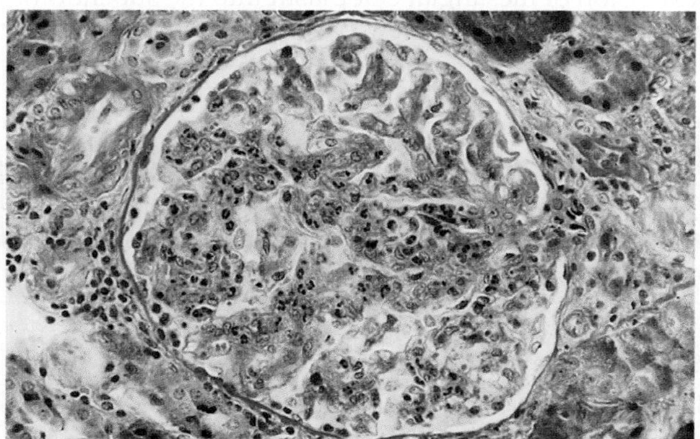

FIGURE 16-33. Acute poststreptococcal glomerulonephritis. The glomerulus of a patient who developed glomerulonephritis after a streptococcal infection contains numerous neutrophils (Masson trichrome stain).

CLINICAL FEATURES: The incidence of acute postinfectious glomerulonephritis is declining in most developed countries but remains high in developing countries because of higher rates of nephritogenic infections. It is still one of the most common childhood renal diseases. Primary infection involves the pharynx (pharyngitis) or, in hot and humid environments, the skin (pyoderma). In recent years, the proportion of cases following staphylococcal infection has been increasing. Because organisms may

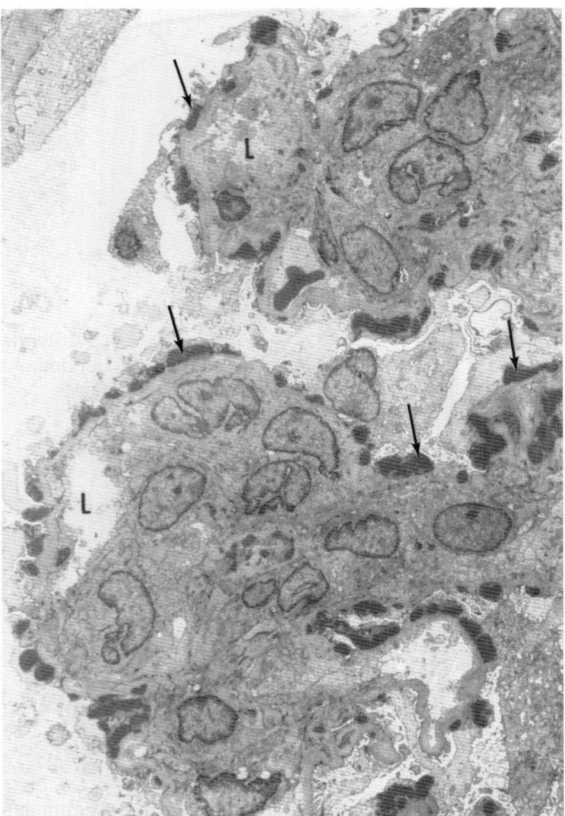

FIGURE 16-35. Acute postinfectious glomerulonephritis. An electron micrograph demonstrates numerous subepithelial humps (*arrows*). The capillary lumina (L) are markedly narrowed.

not be recoverable at the time nephritis develops, the diagnosis depends on serologic evidence of increasing antibody titers to streptococcal antigens. The nephritic syndrome begins abruptly with oliguria, hematuria, facial edema and hypertension. Serum C3 levels are lower during the acute syndrome, but return to

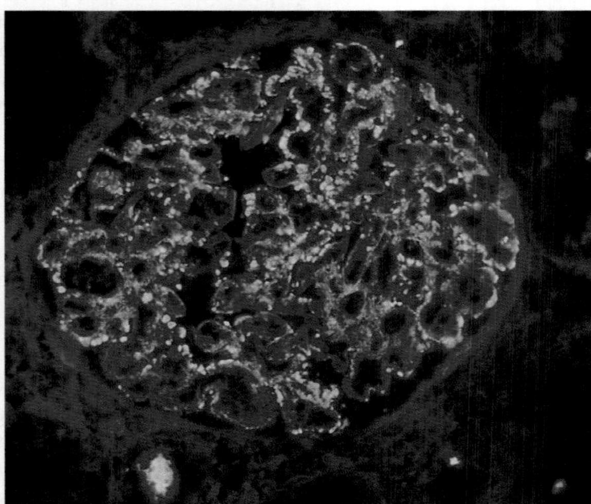

FIGURE 16-36. Acute postinfectious glomerulonephritis. An immunofluorescence micrograph demonstrates granular staining for C3 in capillary walls and the mesangium.

normal within 1 to 2 weeks. Overt nephritis resolves after several weeks, but hematuria and especially proteinuria may persist for several months. A few patients have abnormal urinary sediment for years after the acute episode, and rare patients (particularly adults) develop progressive renal failure.

Type I Membranoproliferative Glomerulonephritis Is a Chronic Immune Complex Disease

Type I membranoproliferative glomerulonephritis (MPGN) is characterized by hypercellularity and capillary wall thickening; deposition of mesangial and subendothelial immune complexes causes mesangial proliferation and extension into the subendothelial zone.

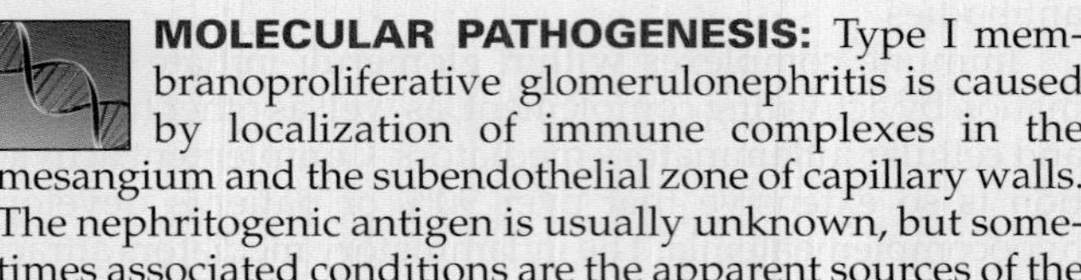

MOLECULAR PATHOGENESIS: Type I membranoproliferative glomerulonephritis is caused by localization of immune complexes in the mesangium and the subendothelial zone of capillary walls. The nephritogenic antigen is usually unknown, but sometimes associated conditions are the apparent sources of the antigen (Table 16-6).

Eliminating the associated condition (e.g., bacterial endocarditis or osteomyelitis) may cause the glomerulonephritis to resolve, thus suggesting a causal relationship between the two. Unlike the pathogens of acute postinfectious glomerulonephritis, those associated with type I MPGN cause persistent, indolent infections with chronic antigenemia. This condition leads to chronic localization of immune complexes in glomeruli and resultant hypercellularity and matrix remodeling.

PATHOLOGY: Glomeruli in type I MPGN are diffusely enlarged, with florid mesangial cell proliferation and infiltration of monocytes/macrophages. Consequent glomerular lobular distortion ("hypersegmentation"; Fig. 16-37) was once called **lobular glomerulonephritis.** Of these patients, 20% have crescents, usually involving only a minority of glomeruli. Capillary walls are thickened, and silver stains show a doubling or complex replication of GBMs.

Electron microscopy reveals thickening and replication of GBMs probably caused by endothelial cell activation as well as extension of mesangial cytoplasm into the subendothelial zone and deposition of new basement membrane material

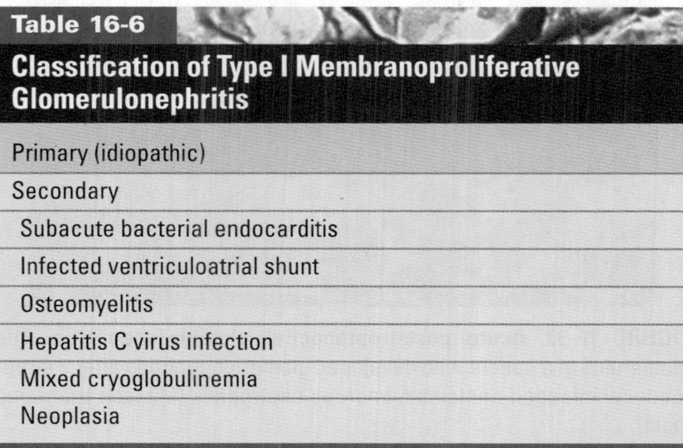

Table 16-6

Classification of Type I Membranoproliferative Glomerulonephritis

Primary (idiopathic)
Secondary
Subacute bacterial endocarditis
Infected ventriculoatrial shunt
Osteomyelitis
Hepatitis C virus infection
Mixed cryoglobulinemia
Neoplasia

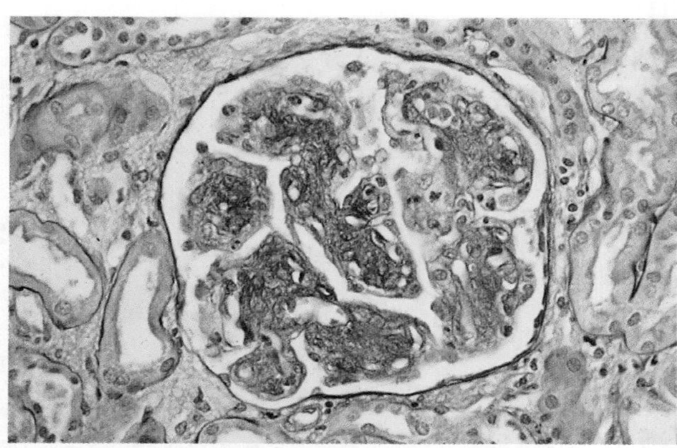

FIGURE 16-37. Type I membranoproliferative glomerulonephritis. The glomerular lobulation is accentuated. Increased cells and matrix in the mesangium and thickening of capillary walls are noted.

between the mesangial cytoplasm and endothelial cell (Figs. 16-38 and 16-39). Subendothelial and mesangial electron-dense deposits, corresponding to immune complexes, are the likely stimuli for the endothelial and mesangial response. Variable numbers of subepithelial dense deposits may also be seen. Immunofluorescence microscopy shows granular deposition of immunoglobulins and complement in glomerular capillary loops and mesangium (Fig. 16-40).

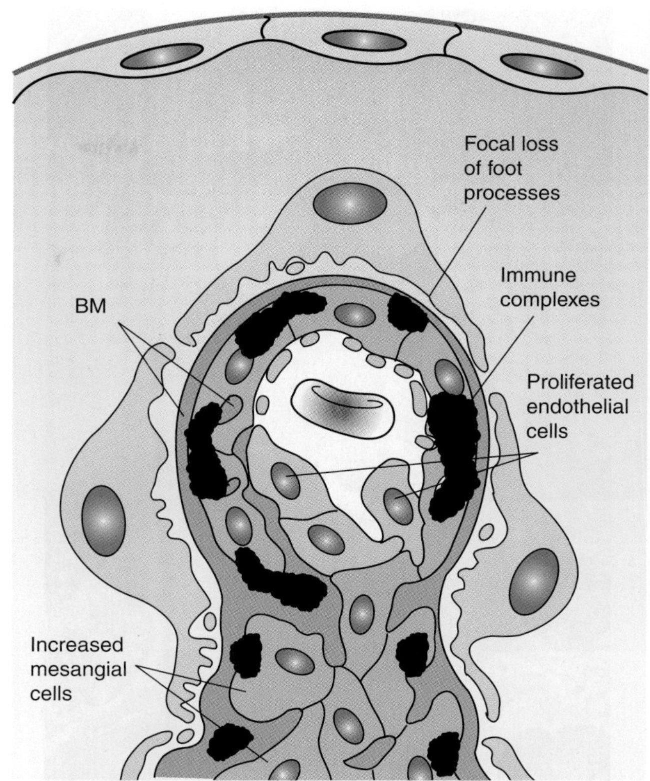

FIGURE 16-38. Membranoproliferative glomerulonephritis, type I. In this disease, the glomeruli are enlarged. Hypercellular tufts and narrowing or obstruction of the capillary lumen are seen. Large subendothelial deposits of immune complexes extend along the inner border of the basement membrane. The mesangial cells proliferate and migrate peripherally into the capillary. Basement membrane (BM) material accumulates in a linear fashion parallel to the basement membrane in a subendothelial position. The interposition of mesangial cells and basement membrane between the endothelial cells and the original basement membrane creates a double-contour effect. The accumulation of mesangial cells and stroma in the tufts narrows the capillary lumen. The proliferation of mesangial cells and the accumulation of basement membrane material also widen the mesangium. The entire process leads progressively to lobulation of the glomerulus. Note the proliferation of endothelial cells and focal effacement of foot processes.

CLINICAL FEATURES: Type I MPGN can occur at any age, but is most frequent in older children and young adults. It may manifest as nephrotic or nephritic syndromes, or a combination of both. Type I disease accounts for 5% of primary nephrotic syndrome in children and adults in the United States. It is much more common in underdeveloped countries where chronic infections are more prevalent. Patients often have low C3 levels. The differential diagnosis includes acute postinfectious glomerulonephritis and lupus glomerulonephritis, both of which can cause nephritis with hypocomplementemia. Type I MPGN is usually a persistent, slowly progressive disease. Half of patients reach end-stage renal disease after 10 years.

Type II Membranoproliferative Glomerulonephritis Is Characterized by Electron-Dense Deposits in the Glomerular Basement Membrane

In type II MPGN (dense deposit disease), there is a pathognomonic electron-dense transformation of GBMs and extensive complement deposition.

MOLECULAR PATHOGENESIS: The extensive localization of complement in the GBMs and mesangial matrix in type II MPGN indicates that complement activation is a major mediator of the structural and functional abnormalities. The basis for complement activation in dense deposit disease is unknown. Immunoglobulins are absent in glomeruli, indicating that immune complexes are not involved. Deficiency of, and mutations in, alternative pathway complement regulatory factors (e.g., factor H) are associated with dense deposit disease, implicating dysregulation of the alternative pathway. Most patients have a serum IgG autoantibody, **C3 nephritic factor,** which stabilizes activated C3 convertase (C3bBb) of the alternative complement pathway. The result is prolongation of C3 cleaving activity. A similar C3 nephritic factor is also present in a minority of patients with type I membranoproliferative glomerulonephritis and lupus nephritis. The role of this factor, if any, in dense deposit disease is unclear. However, dense deposit disease often recurs in renal transplants, suggesting that a humoral factor mediates glomerular injury.

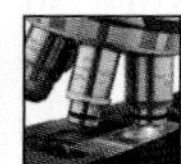

PATHOLOGY: The histology of dense deposit disease may be similar to that of type I MPGN, with capillary wall thickening and hypercellularity (Fig. 16-41).

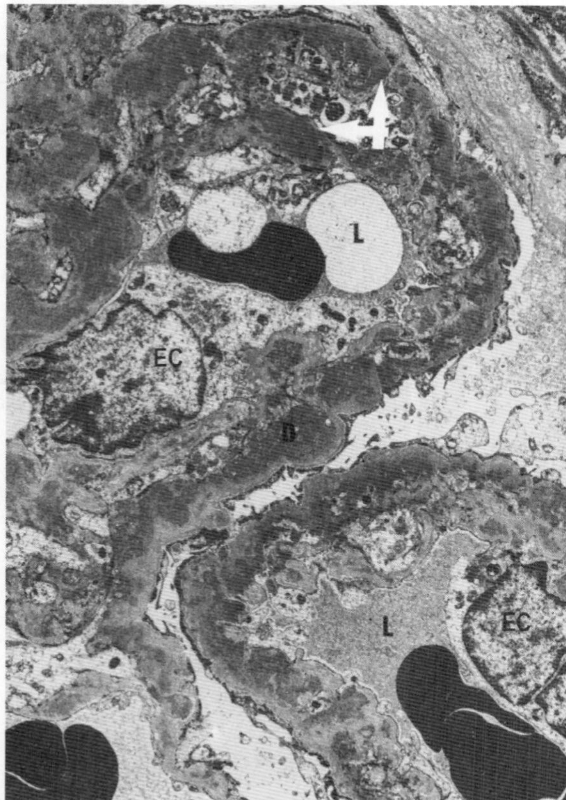

FIGURE 16-39. Type I membranoproliferative glomerulonephritis. An electron micrograph demonstrates a double-contour basement membrane, with mesangial interposition and prominent subendothelial deposits. EC = endothelial cell; L = capillary lumen ; D = immune complex deposit.

However, in many patients hypercellularity may be less pronounced or absent, making the term "proliferative" problematic. The distinctive ribbon-like zone of increased density in the center of a thickened GBM and in the mesangial matrix (Fig. 16-42) justifies the alternative name, **dense deposit disease.** Areas of density are found in the membranes of peritubular capillaries and arteriolar elastic laminae. Linear

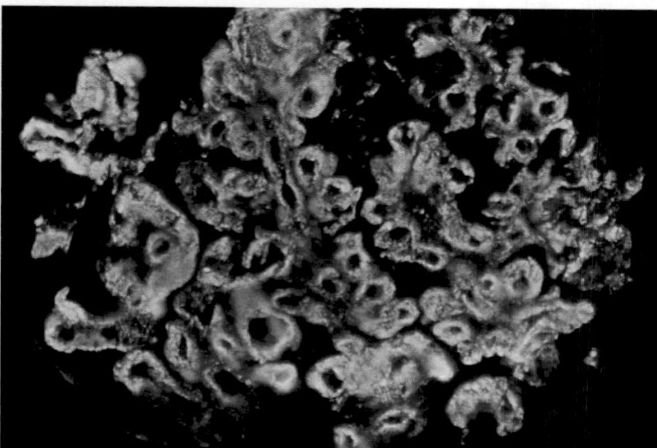

FIGURE 16-40. Type I membranoproliferative glomerulonephritis. An immunofluorescence micrograph demonstrates granular to band-like staining for C3 in the capillary walls and mesangium.

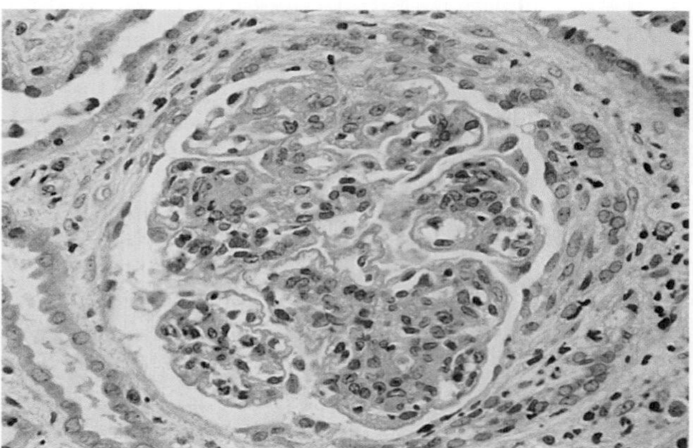

FIGURE 16-41. Type II membranoproliferative glomerulonephritis (dense deposit disease). Capillary wall thickening, hypercellularity and a small crescent are evident.

deposition of C3 in capillary walls is seen, with little or no immunoglobulin (Fig. 16-43).

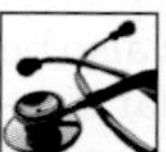

CLINICAL FEATURES: Dense deposit disease is rare (2:1,000,000). It resembles type I membranoproliferative glomerulonephritis in clinical presentation

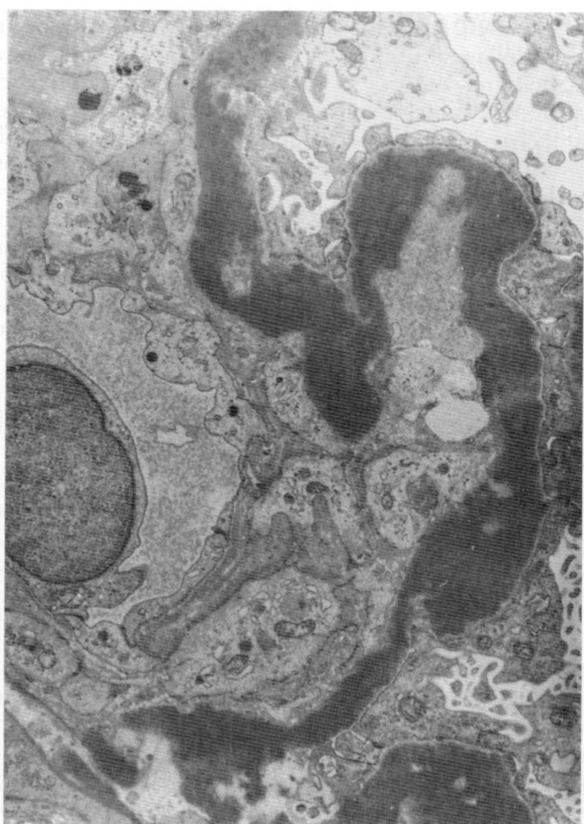

FIGURE 16-42. Type II membranoproliferative glomerulonephritis (dense deposit disease). An electron micrograph demonstrates thickening of the basement membrane and intramembranous dense deposits.

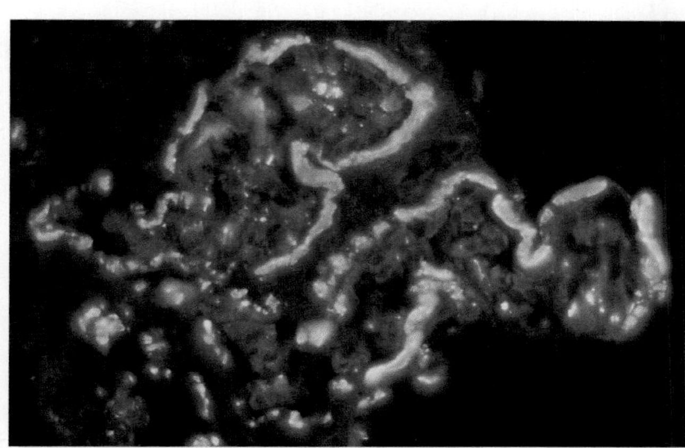

FIGURE 16-43. Type II membranoproliferative glomerulonephritis (dense deposit disease). An immunofluorescence micrograph demonstrates bands of capillary wall staining and coarsely granular mesangial staining for C3.

Table 16-7

Pathologic and Clinical Features of Lupus Nephritis

Class	Location of Immune Complexes	Clinical Manifestations
I: No lesion by light microscopy	Mesangial	Mild hematuria and proteinuria
II: Mesangial proliferative	Mesangial	Mild hematuria and proteinuria
III: Focal proliferative	Mesangial and subendothelial	Moderate nephritis
IV: Diffuse proliferative	Mesangial and subendothelial	Severe nephritis
V: Membranous	Subepithelial	Nephrotic syndrome
VI: Chronic sclerosing	Variable	Chronic renal failure

and course, save that hypocomplementemia is more common and the prognosis is slightly worse.

Lupus Glomerulonephritis Includes Diverse Patterns of Immune Complex Deposition

SLE is an autoimmune disease with generalized dysregulation and hyperactivity of B cells, and production of autoantibodies to many nuclear and nonnuclear antigens, including DNA, RNA, nucleoproteins and phospholipids. SLE is most common in women, especially of childbearing age. Blacks, Asians and Hispanics have more severe disease than whites. Nephritis is one of the most common complications of SLE.

Immune complexes in the mesangium cause less inflammation than subendothelial immune complexes. The latter are more exposed to cellular and humoral inflammatory mediator systems in blood and are, therefore, more likely to initiate inflammation. Subepithelial localization of immune complexes causes proteinuria but does not stimulate overt glomerular inflammation.

MOLECULAR PATHOGENESIS: Defective apoptosis and impaired clearance of chromatin fragments may contribute to the genesis of antinuclear autoimmune responses and provide target antigens for nephritogenic immune complex formation. Immune complexes may localize in glomeruli by deposition from the circulation, formation in situ or both. Circulating immune complexes formed by high-avidity antibodies deposit in subendothelial and mesangial zones; low-affinity antibodies form immune complexes in situ in the subepithelial zone. Immune complexes formed in situ may involve antigens such as double-stranded DNA and nucleosomes that have been planted on GBMs or mesangial matrix by charge interactions. Glomerular immune complexes activate complement and initiate inflammatory injury. Complement activation in the kidneys and elsewhere often causes hypocomplementemia. Immune complexes also localize in the renal interstitium, walls of interstitial vessels and tubular basement membranes, where they may be involved in the tubulointerstitial inflammation seen in patients with lupus nephritis.

PATHOLOGY: The pathologic and clinical manifestations of lupus nephritis are highly variable because of variable patterns of immune complex accumulation in different patients (Table 16-7) and in the same patient over time.

- **Class I (minimal mesangial lupus glomerulonephritis):** Immune complexes are confined to mesangium and cause no changes by light microscopy.
- **Class II (mesangial proliferative lupus glomerulonephritis):** Immune complexes are confined to mesangium and cause varying degrees of mesangial hypercellularity and matrix expansion.
- **Class III (focal lupus glomerulonephritis):** Immune complexes accumulate in the subendothelial zone, which is always accompanied by mesangial immune complexes, and stimulate inflammation, proliferation of mesangial and endothelial cells and influx of neutrophils and monocytes (Fig. 16-44).

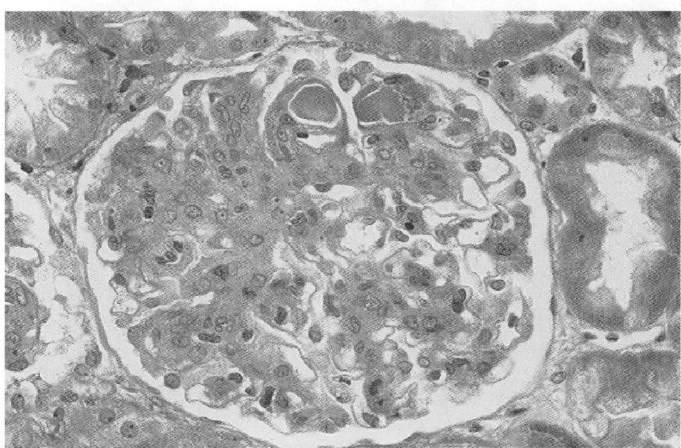

FIGURE 16-44. Proliferative lupus glomerulonephritis. Segmental endocapillary hypercellularity and thickening of capillary walls are present.

This overt glomerular inflammation is termed **focal proliferative lupus glomerulonephritis** if it involves less than 50% of glomeruli.

- **Class IV (diffuse lupus glomerulonephritis):** This type is similar to class III but involves more than 50% of glomeruli. Glomerular involvement may be predominantly global (IV-G) or predominantly segmental (IV-S).
- **Class V (membranous lupus glomerulonephritis):** Immune complexes are mostly in the subepithelial zone. Some patients have a background of class V injury and a concurrent class III or IV injury. Even pure class V lupus nephritis has mesangial immune complexes that can be detected by electron microscopy.
- **Class VI (advanced sclerosing lupus glomerulonephritis):** Advanced chronic disease.

By electron microscopy, immune complex dense deposits occur in mesangial, subendothelial and subepithelial locations. Class I and II lesions primarily have mesangial deposits. Classes III and IV-G have mesangial and subendothelial deposits, and usually scattered subepithelial deposits (Fig. 16-45). Class IV-S tends to have fewer glomerular immune complexes and more segmental necrosis. Class V lesions have numerous subepithelial dense deposits. Some 80% of specimens have **tubuloreticular inclusions** in endothelial cells, which are induced by high interferon levels. Lupus nephritis and HIV-associated nephropathy are the only renal diseases with a high frequency of these structures.

By immunofluorescence, the subepithelial complexes are granular and the subendothelial deposits may be granular or band-like (Fig. 16-46). The immune complexes often stain most intensely for IgG, but IgA and IgM are also almost always present, as are C3, C1q and other complement components. Granular staining along tubular basement membranes and interstitial vessels is seen in over half of patients.

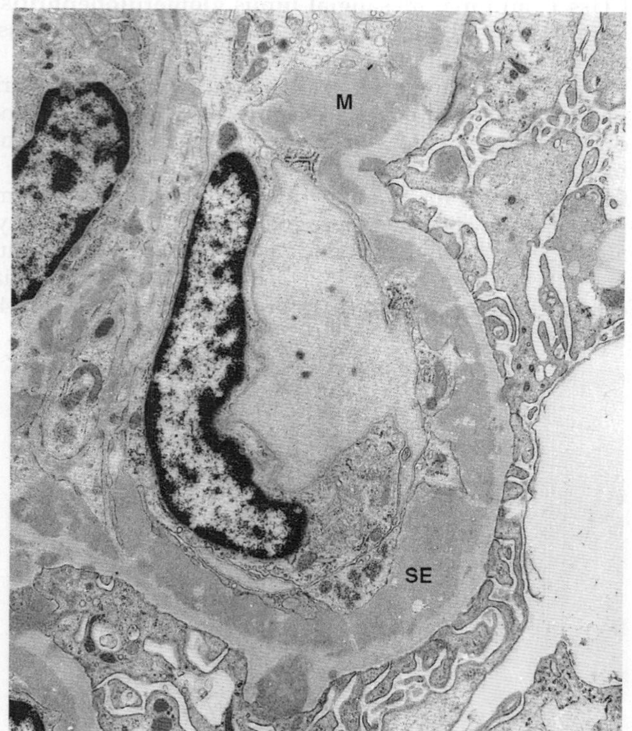

FIGURE 16-45. Diffuse proliferative class IV-G lupus glomerulonephritis. An electron micrograph reveals large subendothelial (SE) and mesangial (M) dense deposits and a few subepithelial deposits.

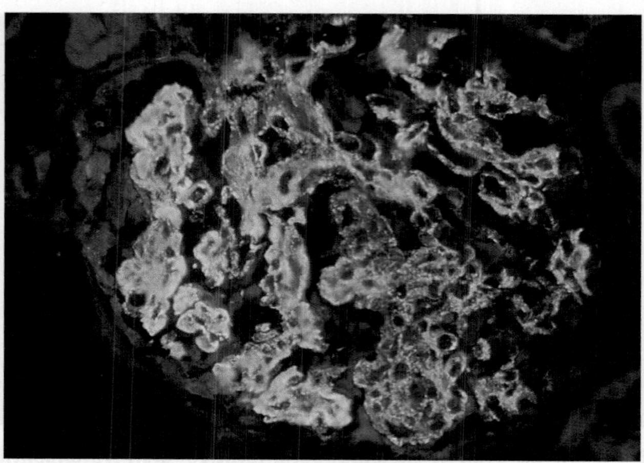

FIGURE 16-46. Diffuse proliferative lupus glomerulonephritis. An immunofluorescence micrograph demonstrates segmental staining for immunoglobulin G in the capillary walls and mesangium.

CLINICAL FEATURES: Renal disease develops in 70% of patients with SLE, and is often the major cause of morbidity and mortality. As noted in Table 16-7, the clinical manifestations and prognosis of renal dysfunction are varied and depend on the pathologic nature of the underlying renal disease. It is most common and more severe in black women. ***Renal biopsy specimens from patients with lupus are used to assess disease category, activity and chronicity, as well as to diagnose lupus glomerulonephritis.*** Class III and class IV lupus nephritis have the poorest prognosis and are treated most aggressively, usually with high doses of corticosteroids and immunosuppressive drugs. Over time, sometimes due to treatment, lupus nephritis may change from one type to another, with the corresponding changes in clinical manifestations. Less than 20% of patients with class IV disease reach end-stage renal failure within 5 years.

IgA Nephropathy (Berger Disease) Is Caused by IgA Immune Complexes

MOLECULAR PATHOGENESIS: Although deposition of IgA-dominant immune complexes is the cause of IgA nephropathy, the constituent antigens and mechanism of accumulation (deposition versus formation in situ) are not known. Patients with IgA nephropathy often have aberrant IgA molecules, elevated blood levels of IgA and circulating IgA-containing immune complexes or aggregated IgA. ***Exacerbations of IgA nephropathy are often initiated by respiratory or gastrointestinal infections.*** Mucosal exposure to viral, bacterial or dietary antigens stimulates an IgA-dominant immune response that results in the glomerular immune complex accumulation. Abnormal glycosylation of the hinge region of IgA1 appears to be an important predisposing factor in many patients with IgA nephropathy. The immune deposits contain predominantly IgA1 rather than IgA2. IgA1, but not IgA2, has a hinge region with O-linked glycan chains. In IgA nephropathy, serum IgA1 has less terminal galactosylation of these chains. Autoantibodies against these abnormal chains may develop. This abnormality in IgA1 galactosylation may lead to lack of receptor engagement by the abnormal IgA, reducing clearance of IgA complexes from the circulation, increasing aggregation of IgA in the circulation and resulting in mesangial trapping, formation of immune complexes between the abnormal IgA1 and IgG autoantibodies against the abnormal IgA or combinations of these processes.

IgA-containing immune complexes in the mesangium most likely activate complement by the alternative pathway. The demonstration of C3 and properdin, but not C1q and C4, in the IgA deposits supports this hypothesis.

PATHOLOGY: Immunofluorescence microscopy is essential for diagnosis of IgA nephropathy. The diagnostic finding is mesangial immunostaining for IgA more intense than, or equivalent to, staining for IgG or IgM (Fig. 16-47). This is almost always accompanied by staining for C3. IgA deposited in the glomerular capillary wall (in addition to the mesangium) may be present in more severe cases and suggests a less favorable prognosis.

Depending on the severity and duration of the disease, a continuum of histologies is seen in IgA nephropathy, from (1) no discernible light microscopic changes, to (2) focal or diffuse mesangial hypercellularity, to (3) focal or diffuse proliferative glomerulonephritis (Fig. 16-48) to (4) chronic sclerosing glomerulonephritis. At the time of initial renal biopsy diagnosis, focal proliferative glomerulonephritis is the most frequent manifestation. Crescents are not common, save in unusually severe cases. This spectrum of pathologic changes is analogous to that seen with lupus nephritis but tends to be less severe.

Ultrastructural examination reveals mesangial electron-dense deposits (Figs. 16-49 and 16-50). Dense deposits in capillary walls are usually seen in patients with severe disease.

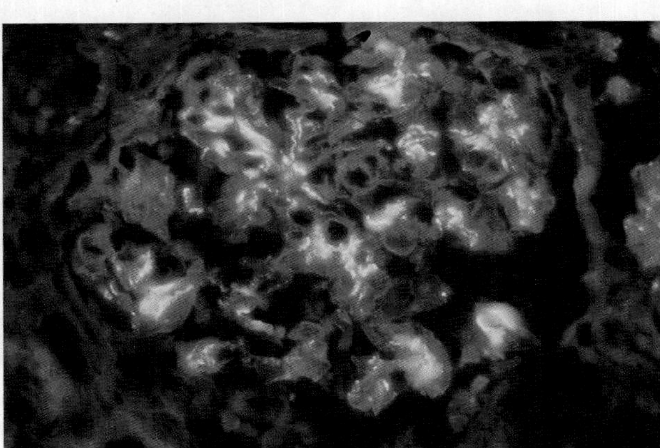

FIGURE 16-47. Immunoglobulin A (IgA) nephropathy. An immunofluorescence micrograph shows deposits of IgA in the mesangial areas.

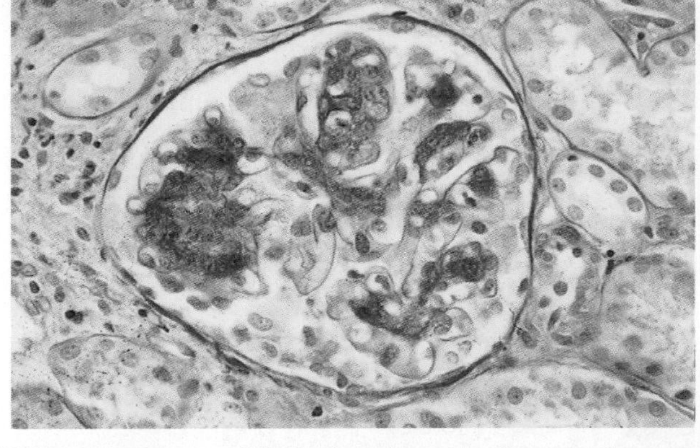

FIGURE 16-48. Immunoglobulin A nephropathy. Segmental mesangial hypercellularity and matrix expansion caused by the mesangial immune deposits (periodic acid–Schiff stain).

CLINICAL FEATURES: ***IgA nephropathy (Berger disease) is the most common form of glomerulonephritis in developed countries.*** It accounts for 10% of cases in the United States, 20% in Europe and 40% in Asia. IgA nephropathy is common in Native Americans and is rare in blacks. It occurs most often in young men, with a peak age of 15 to 30 years at diagnosis. Clinical presentations are varied, which reflects the varied pathologic severity: 40%

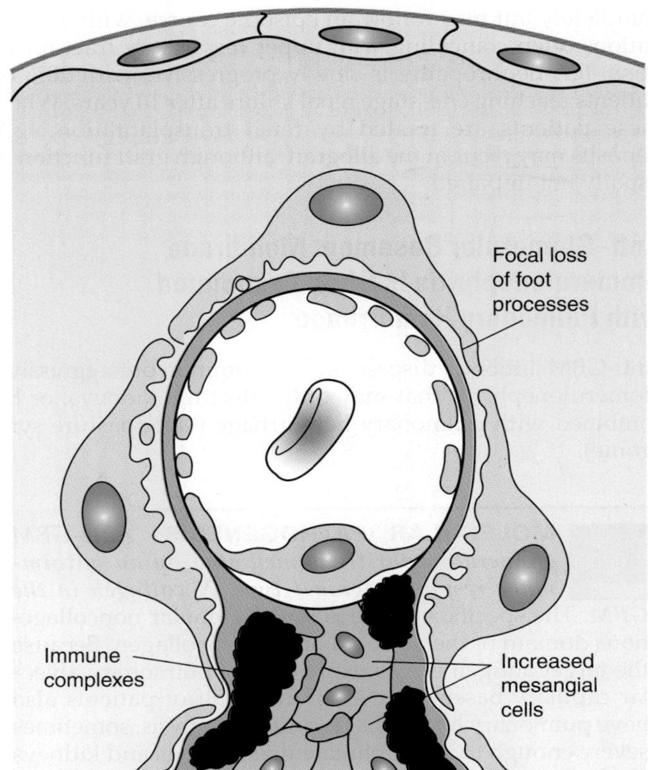

FIGURE 16-49. Immunoglobulin A (IgA) nephropathy. Significant accumulation of IgA is seen in the mesangium, most commonly between the mesangial cells and the basement membrane.

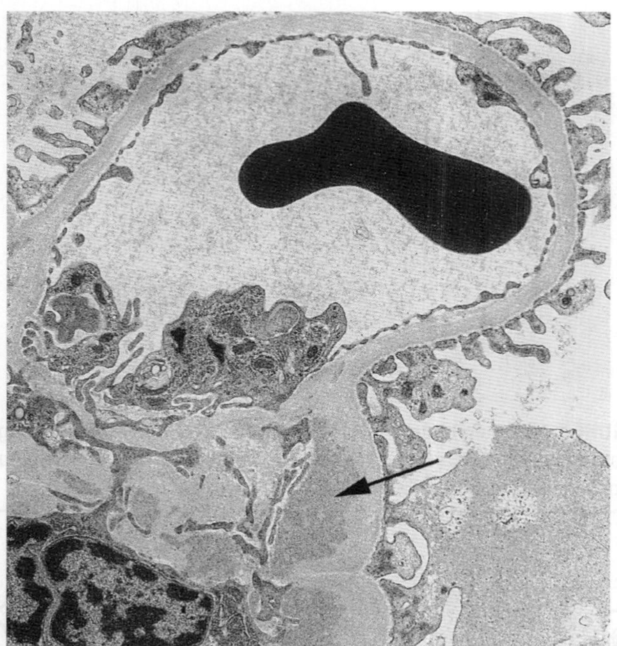

FIGURE 16-50. Immunoglobulin A nephropathy. An electron micrograph demonstrates prominent dense deposits in the mesangial matrix (*arrow*).

of patients have asymptomatic microscopic hematuria, 40% have intermittent gross hematuria, 10% have nephrotic syndrome and 10% have renal failure. The disease rarely resolves completely but may follow an episodic course, with exacerbations often coinciding with upper respiratory tract infections. IgA nephropathy is slowly progressive, with 20% of patients reaching end-stage renal failure after 10 years. When these patients are treated by renal transplantation, IgA deposits may recur in the allograft, although graft function is usually not impaired.

Anti–Glomerular Basement Membrane Glomerulonephritis Is Often Associated with Pulmonary Hemorrhage

Anti-GBM antibody disease is an uncommon but aggressive glomerulonephritis that may only affect the kidneys, or be combined with pulmonary hemorrhage (Goodpasture syndrome).

MOLECULAR PATHOGENESIS: *Anti-GBM glomerulonephritis is mediated by an autoimmune response against type IV collagen in the GBM.* The specific epitope is in the globular noncollagenous domain of the $\alpha3$ chain of type IV collagen. Because the target antigen is also expressed on pulmonary alveolar capillary basement membranes, half of patients also have pulmonary hemorrhages and hemoptysis, sometimes severe enough to be life-threatening. If lungs and kidneys are both involved, the eponym **Goodpasture syndrome** is used (Fig. 16-14). Anti-GBM antibodies, anti-GBM T cells or both may mediate the injury. The antibodies bind the autoantigens in situ, initiating acute inflammation by activating mediator systems, such as complement. Experimental studies suggest that T cells specific for GBM antigens may mediate the vascular injury. Genetic susceptibility to anti-GBM disease is strongly associated with human leukocyte antigen (HLA)-DRB1. Disease onset often follows viral upper respiratory tract infections, and pulmonary involvement appears to require synergistic injurious agents, such as cigarette smoke.

PATHOLOGY: *The pathologic hallmark of anti-GBM glomerulonephritis is diffuse linear GBM immunostaining for IgG, indicating autoantibodies bound to the basement membrane* (Fig. 16-51). This finding is not, however, entirely specific. Thus, nonimmune binding of IgG to basement membranes occurs in diabetic glomerulosclerosis and monoclonal immunoglobulin deposition disease. Over 90% of patients with anti-GBM glomerulonephritis have glomerular crescents **(crescentic glomerulonephritis)** (Figs. 16-52 and 16-53), usually involving over 50% of glomeruli. Focal glomerular fibrinoid necrosis is common. Involved lungs have marked intra-alveolar hemorrhage. By electron microscopy, GBMs show focal breaks in, but no immune complex–type electron-dense deposits.

CLINICAL FEATURES: Anti-GBM glomerulonephritis typically presents with rapidly progressive renal failure and nephritic signs and symptoms. *It accounts for 10% to 20% of rapidly progressive (crescentic) glomerulonephritis* (Table 16-8). Anti-GBM antibodies are serologically detectable in approximately 90% of patients. Treatment consists of high-dose immunosuppressive therapy and plasma exchange, which are most effective at an early stage of the disease, before severe renal failure supervenes. If end-stage renal failure develops, renal transplantation is successful with little risk of losing the allograft to recurrent glomerulonephritis if transplantation is done after anti–GBM antibodies have disappeared.

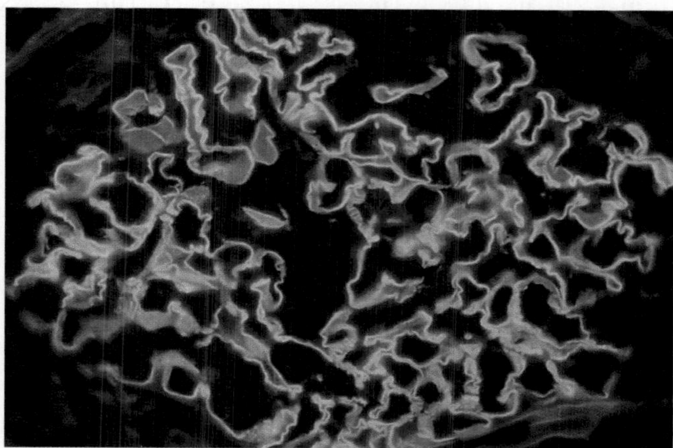

FIGURE 16-51. Anti–glomerular basement membrane (GBM) glomerulonephritis. Linear immunofluorescence for immunoglobulin G is seen along the GBM. Contrast this linear pattern of staining with the granular pattern of immunofluorescence typical for most types of immune complex deposition within capillary walls (see Fig. 16-36).

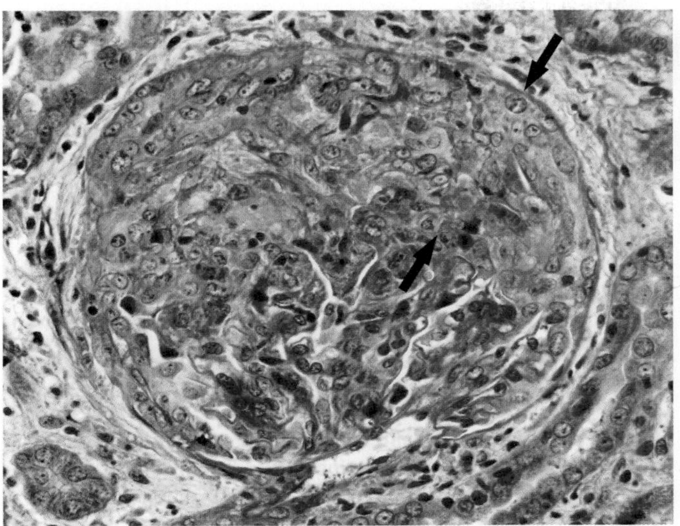

FIGURE 16-52. Crescentic anti–glomerular basement membrane glomerulonephritis. The Bowman space is filled by a cellular crescent (*between arrows*). The injured glomerular tuft is at the bottom (Masson trichrome stain).

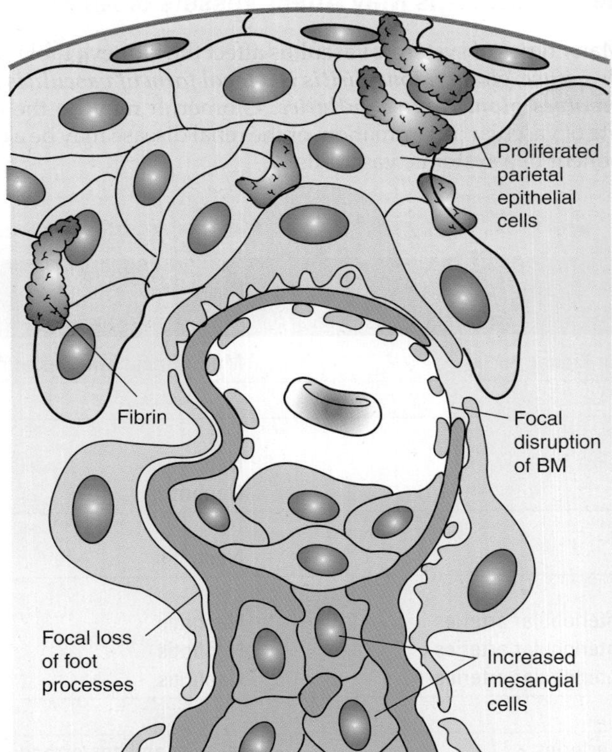

FIGURE 16-53. Crescentic (rapidly progressive) glomerulonephritis. A variety of different pathogenic mechanisms cause crescent formation by disrupting glomerular capillary walls. This allows plasma constituents into the Bowman space, including coagulation factors and inflammatory mediators. Fibrin forms, and there is proliferation of parietal epithelial cells and influx of macrophages, resulting in crescent formation.

Table 16-8

Frequency (%) of Immunopathologic Categories of Crescentic Glomerulonephritis* in Different Age Groups

	Age (years)		
Category	<20	20–64	>65
Anti–glomerular basement membrane	10	10	10
Immune complex	55	40	10
Antineutrophil cytoplasmic autoantibody (ANCA)	30	45	75
No evidence for the three categories above	5	5	5

*Glomerulonephritis with crescents in >50% of glomeruli.

Antineutrophil Cytoplasmic Autoantibody Glomerulonephritis Is an Aggressive Disease Mediated by Neutrophils

ANCA glomerulonephritis is characterized by glomerular necrosis and crescents.

MOLECULAR PATHOGENESIS: ANCA glomerulonephritis was once called *idiopathic crescentic glomerulonephritis* because there was no evidence of glomerular deposition of anti-GBM antibodies or immune complexes. The discovery that 90% of patients with this pattern of glomerular injury have circulating ANCAs led to the demonstration that these autoantibodies cause the disease. ***ANCAs are specific for proteins in the cytoplasm of neutrophils and monocytes, usually myeloperoxidase (MPO-ANCA) or proteinase 3 (PR3-ANCA).*** The autoantibodies activate neutrophils to adhere to endothelial cells, release toxic oxygen metabolites, degranulate and kill endothelial cells. Neutrophils activated by ANCAs also activate the alternative complement pathway, which further amplifies the inflammation. Transplacental transfer of MPO-ANCA can cause neonatal glomerulonephritis and pulmonary hemorrhage, which supports the pathogenic potential of ANCA.

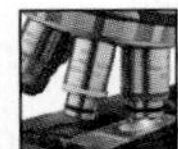

PATHOLOGY: Over 90% of patients with ANCA glomerulonephritis have glomerular necrosis (Fig. 16-54) and crescent formation (Fig. 16-55). In many cases, over 50% of glomeruli exhibit crescents. Nonnecrotic segments may appear normal or have slight neutrophil infiltration or mild endocapillary hypercellularity. Immunofluorescence microscopy shows no or little staining for immunoglobulins and complement, which distinguishes ANCA glomerulonephritis from anti-GBM glomerulonephritis and immune complex glomerulonephritis. A minority of patients with crescentic glomerulonephritis have serologic and pathologic evidence of glomerulonephritis involving ANCA and anti-GBM antibody or immune complexes. Electron microscopy does not demonstrate immune complex–type dense deposits in ANCA glomerulonephritis.

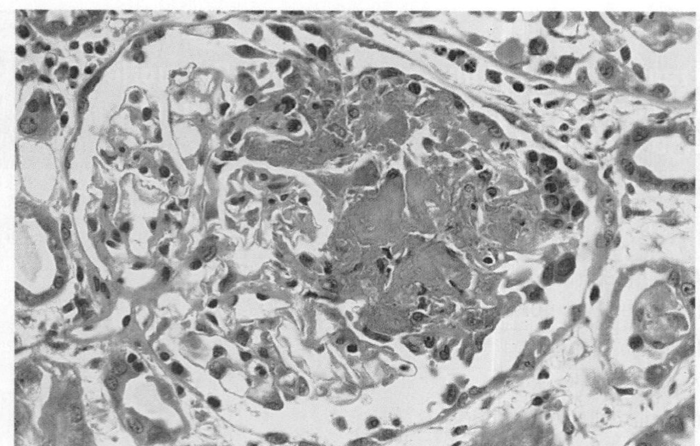

FIGURE 16-54. Antineutrophil cytoplasmic autoantibody glomerulonephritis. Segmental fibrinoid necrosis is illustrated. In time, this lesion stimulates crescent formation.

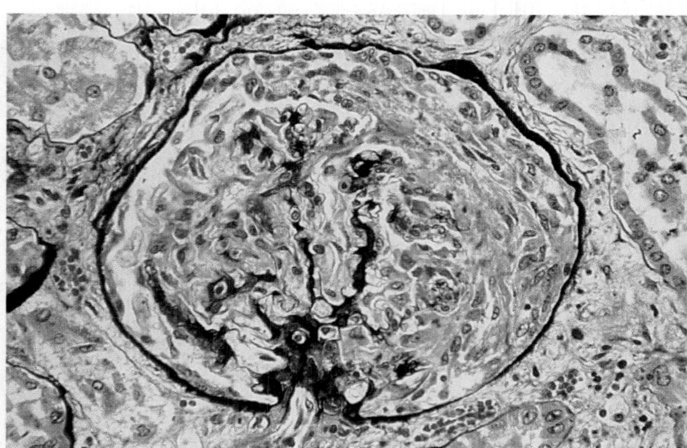

FIGURE 16-55. Antineutrophil cytoplasmic autoantibody glomerulonephritis. Silver staining shows focal disruption of glomerular basement membranes and crescent formation within the Bowman space.

CLINICAL FEATURES: ANCA glomerulonephritis most commonly presents with rapidly progressive renal failure, with nephritic signs and symptoms. The disease accounts for 75% of rapidly progressive (crescentic) glomerulonephritis in patients over 60 years old, 45% in middle-aged adults and 30% in young adults and children (Table 16-8). ***Three quarters of patients with ANCA glomerulonephritis have systemic small vessel vasculitis (see below), which has many systemic manifestations, including pulmonary hemorrhage.*** ANCA glomerulonephritis with pulmonary vasculitis causes **pulmonary–renal vasculitic syndrome** much more often than does Goodpasture syndrome. Over 80% of patients with ANCA glomerulonephritis develop end-stage renal disease within 5 years if untreated. Immunosuppressive therapy reduces this figure to less than 20%. Once remission of disease is induced with high-dose immunosuppressive treatment, patients are at risk for recurrent disease. ANCA glomerulonephritis recurs in 15% of patients who receive renal transplants.

Vascular Diseases

Renal Vasculitis May Affect Vessels of All Sizes

Many types of systemic vasculitis affect the kidney (Table 16-9). ***In a sense, glomerulonephritis is a local form of vasculitis that involves glomerular capillaries.*** Glomeruli may be the only site of vascular inflammation, or the renal disease may be a component of a systemic vasculitis.

Table 16-9

Types of Vasculitis That Involve the Kidneys

Type of Vasculitis	Major Target Vessels in Kidney	Major Renal Manifestations
Small Vessel Vasculitis		
Immune complex vasculitis		
Henoch-Schönlein purpura	Glomeruli	Nephritis
Cryoglobulinemic vasculitis	Glomeruli	Nephritis
Anti-GBM vasculitis		
Goodpasture syndrome	Glomeruli	Nephritis
ANCA vasculitis		
Wegener granulomatosis	Glomeruli, arterioles, interlobular arteries	Nephritis
Microscopic polyangiitis	Glomeruli, arterioles, interlobular arteries	Nephritis
Churg-Strauss syndrome	Glomeruli, arterioles, interlobular arteries	Nephritis
Medium-Sized Vessel Vasculitis		
Polyarteritis nodosa	Interlobar and arcuate arteries	Infarcts and hemorrhage
Kawasaki disease	Interlobar and arcuate arteries	Infarcts and hemorrhage
Large Vessel Vasculitis		
Giant cell arteritis	Main renal artery	Renovascular hypertension
Takayasu arteritis	Main renal artery	Renovascular hypertension

ANCA = antineutrophil cytoplasmic autoantibody; GBM = glomerular basement membrane.

Small Vessel Vasculitis

Small vessel vasculitis affects small arteries, arterioles, capillaries and venules, and any of these may lead to glomerulonephritis. Other common manifestations include purpura, arthralgias, myalgias, peripheral neuropathy and pulmonary hemorrhage. Immune complexes, anti–basement membrane antibodies or ANCAs (Table 16-9) can cause small vessel vasculitides.

Henoch-Schönlein purpura is the most common childhood vasculitis. It is caused by vascular localization of immune complexes containing mostly IgA. The glomerular lesion is identical with that of IgA nephropathy.

Cryoglobulinemic vasculitis causes proliferative glomerulonephritis, usually type I MPGN. By light microscopy, aggregates of cryoglobulins ("hyaline thrombi") are often seen within capillary lumina (Fig. 16-56).

ANCA vasculitis involves vessels outside the kidneys in 75% of patients with ANCA glomerulonephritis. Based on clinical and pathologic features, patients with systemic ANCA vasculitis are classified as follows (Fig. 16-14):

- **Wegener granulomatosis,** if there is necrotizing granulomatous inflammation, usually in the respiratory tract
- **Churg-Strauss syndrome,** if there is eosinophilia and asthma
- **Microscopic polyangiitis,** if there is no asthma or granulomatous inflammation

In addition to causing necrotizing and crescentic glomerulonephritis, ANCA vasculitides often display necrotizing inflammation in other renal vessels, such as arteries (Fig. 16-57), arterioles and medullary peritubular capillaries.

Medium-Sized Vessel Vasculitis

Medium-sized vessel vasculitides affect arteries, but not arterioles, capillaries or venules (see Chapter 10). The necrotizing arteritides, such as **polyarteritis nodosa,** which occurs mainly in adults, and **Kawasaki disease,** which principally afflicts young children, rarely cause renal dysfunction. However, they may involve renal arteries and cause pseudoaneurysm formation and renal thrombosis, infarction and hemorrhage.

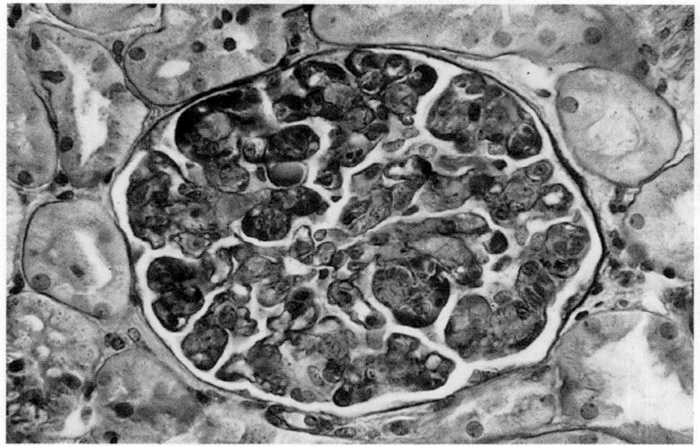

FIGURE 16-56. Cryoglobulinemic glomerulonephritis. The pattern of glomerular inflammation is similar to that of type I membranoproliferative glomerulonephritis. However, as in this specimen, there typically are conspicuous glassy aggregates ("hyaline thrombi") in the capillary lumina and subendothelial spaces. These are not true thrombi but rather are large aggregates of cryoglobulins (periodic acid–Schiff stain).

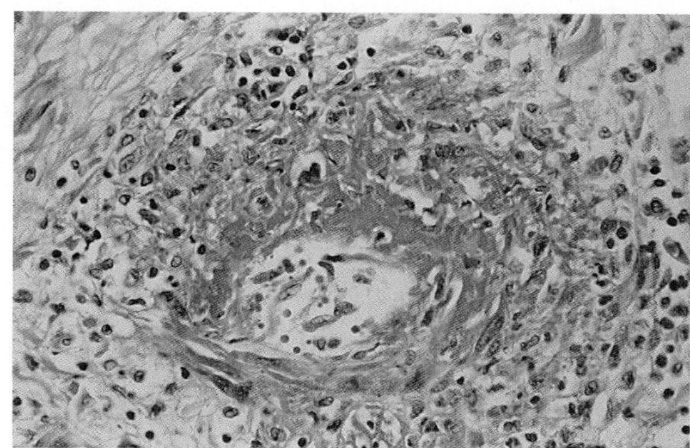

FIGURE 16-57. Antineutrophil cytoplasmic autoantibody necrotizing arteritis. Fibrinoid necrosis and inflammation involve an interlobular artery in the renal cortex.

Large Vessel Vasculitis

Large vessel vasculitides, such as **giant cell arteritis** and **Takayasu arteritis,** affect the aorta and its major branches. These disorders may cause renovascular hypertension by involving the main renal arteries or the aorta at the origin of the renal arteries (see Chapter 10). Narrowing or obstruction of these vessels results in renal ischemia, which stimulates increased renin production and consequent hypertension (Table 16-9).

Hypertensive Nephrosclerosis (Benign Nephrosclerosis) May Obliterate Glomeruli

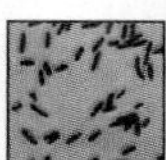

ETIOLOGIC FACTORS: Sustained systolic pressures over 140 mm Hg and diastolic pressures over 90 mm are generally felt to represent hypertension (see Chapter 10). Mild to moderate hypertension causes typical hypertensive nephrosclerosis and thus is not truly benign. In fact, hypertensive nephrosclerosis is identified in about 15% of patients with "benign hypertension." Changes like those in hypertensive nephrosclerosis may occur in older individuals who have never had hypertension, and are attributed to aging itself.

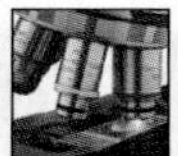

PATHOLOGY: The kidneys are smaller than normal (atrophic) and are usually affected bilaterally. Renal cortical surfaces are finely granular (Fig. 16-58), but coarser scars are occasionally present. On cut section, the cortex is thinned. Microscopically, many glomeruli appear normal; others show varying degrees of ischemic change. Initially, glomerular capillaries are thickened because of thickening, wrinkling and collapse of GBMs. Cells of the glomerular tuft are progressively lost, and collagen and matrix material are deposited within the Bowman space. Eventually, glomerular tufts are obliterated by a dense, eosinophilic globular scar, all inside the Bowman capsule. Tubular atrophy, due to glomerular obsolescence, is associated with interstitial fibrosis and chronic inflammation. Globally, sclerotic glomeruli and

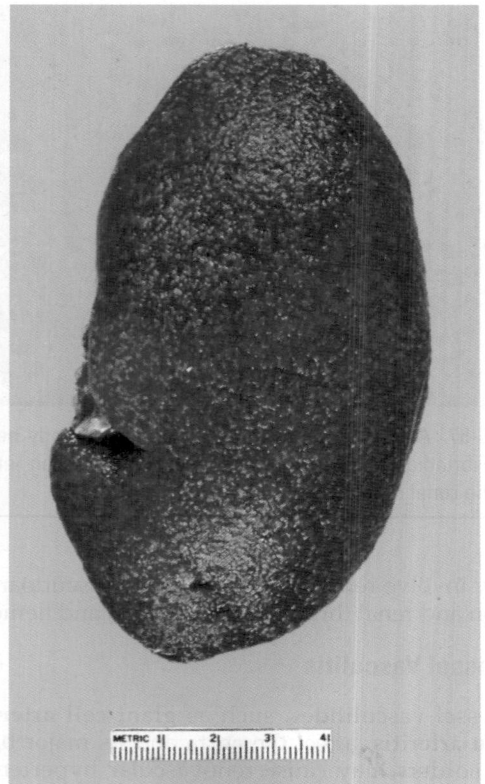

FIGURE 16-58. **Hypertensive nephrosclerosis.** The kidney is reduced in size, and the cortical surface exhibits fine granularity.

surrounding atrophic tubules are often clustered in focal subcapsular zones, with adjacent areas of preserved glomeruli and tubules (Fig. 16-59), which accounts for the granular surfaces of nephrosclerotic kidneys.

The pattern of change in renal blood vessels depends on vessel size. Intimas of arteries down to the size of arcuate arteries have fibrotic thickening, replication of the elastica-like lamina and partial replacement of the muscularis with fibrous tissue. Interlobular arteries and arterioles may develop medial hyperplasia. Arterioles exhibit concentric hyaline thickening of the wall, often with the loss of smooth muscle cells or their displacement to the periphery. This arteriolar change is termed **hyaline arteriolosclerosis.**

CLINICAL FEATURES: Although hypertensive nephrosclerosis does not usually impair renal function, some people with "benign" hypertension develop progressive renal failure, which may lead to end-stage renal disease. Since "benign" hypertension is so common, the small proportion of these patients who develop renal insufficiency amounts to one third of all patients with end-stage renal disease. Benign nephrosclerosis is most prevalent and aggressive among blacks. ***In fact, among blacks, hypertension with no malignant phase is the leading cause of end-stage renal disease.***

Malignant Hypertensive Nephropathy Is a Potentially Fatal Renal Disease

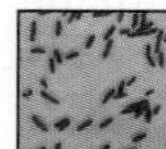

ETIOLOGIC FACTORS: No specific blood pressure defines malignant hypertension, but diastolic pressures over 130 mm Hg, retinal vascular changes,

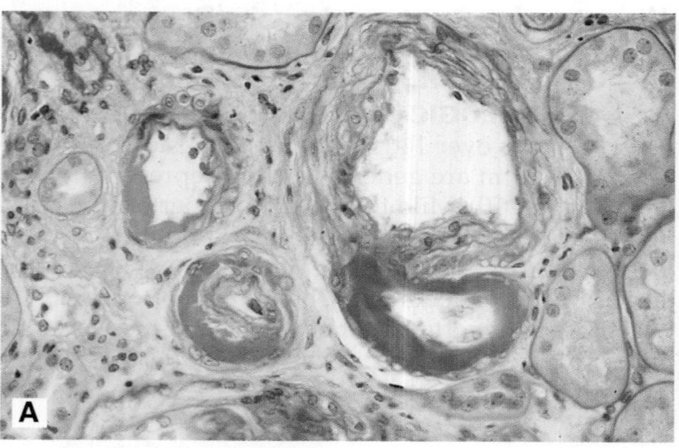

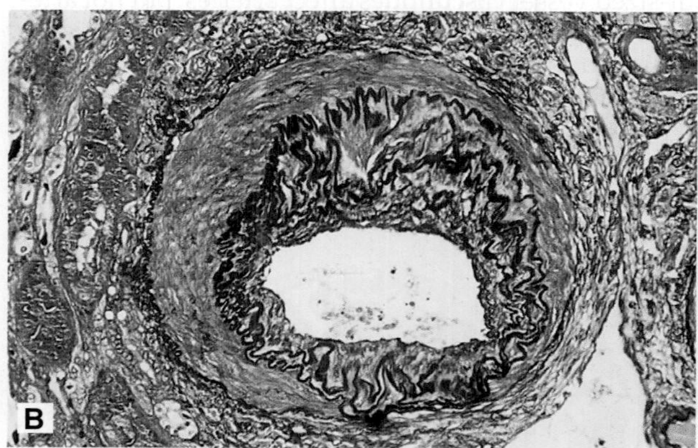

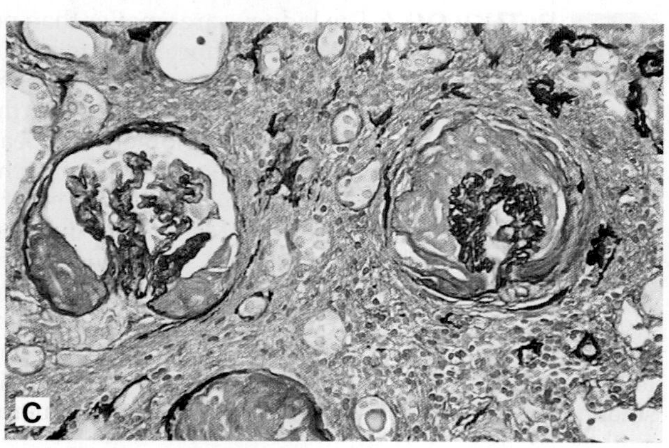

FIGURE 16-59. **Hypertensive nephrosclerosis. A.** Three arterioles with hyaline sclerosis (periodic acid–Schiff stain). **B.** Arcuate artery with fibrotic intimal thickening causing narrowing of the lumen (silver stain). **C.** One glomerulus with global sclerosis and one with segmental sclerosis. Note also the tubular atrophy, interstitial fibrosis and chronic inflammation (silver stain).

papilledema and renal functional impairment are usual criteria. About half of patients have prior histories of benign hypertension, and many others have a background of chronic renal injury caused by many different diseases. Occasionally, malignant hypertension arises de novo in apparently healthy people, particularly young black men. The pathogenesis of the vascular injury in malignant hypertension is not entirely clear. One hypothesis proposes that very high blood pressures, combined with microvascular vasoconstriction, cause endothelial injury as blood slams into narrowed small vessels. At such sites, plasma constituents leak into injured arteriolar walls (causing fibrinoid necrosis), into arterial intimas (inducing edematous intimal thickening) and into the subendothelial zone of glomerular capillaries (consolidating glomeruli). At these sites of vascular injury, thrombosis can result in focal renal cortical necrosis (infarcts).

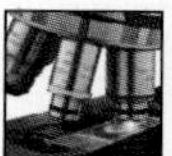

PATHOLOGY: The size of the kidneys in malignant hypertensive nephropathy varies from small to enlarged, depending on the duration of preexisting benign hypertension. The cut surface is mottled red and yellow, with occasional small cortical infarcts. Microscopically, malignant hypertensive nephropathy is often superimposed on hypertensive nephrosclerosis, with edematous (myxoid, mucoid) intimal expansion in arteries and fibrinoid necrosis of arterioles. Glomerular changes vary from capillary congestion to consolidation to necrosis (Fig. 16-60). Severe cases show thrombosis and focal ischemic cortical necrosis (infarction). By electron microscopy, electron-lucent material expands glomerular subendothelial zones. Fluorescence microscopy documents focal insudation of plasma proteins into injured vessel walls. These changes are identical to those seen in other forms of thrombotic microangiopathy (see below).

CLINICAL FEATURES: Malignant hypertension is more common in men than in women, typically around the age of 40 years. Patients suffer headache, dizziness and visual disturbances and may develop overt encephalopathy. Hematuria and proteinuria are frequent. Progressive renal deterioration develops if the condition persists. Aggressive antihypertensive therapy often controls the disease.

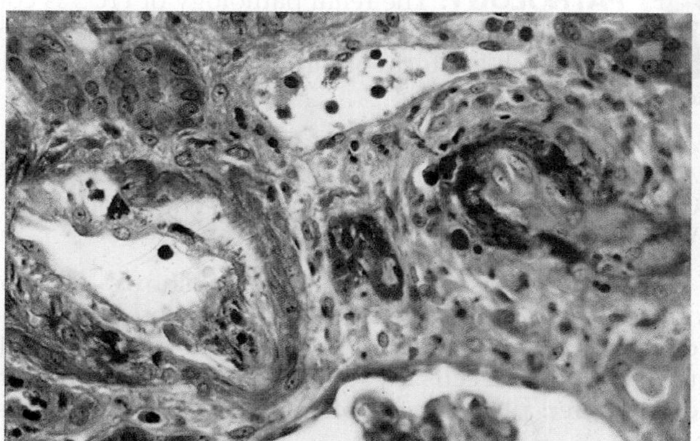

FIGURE 16-60. Malignant hypertensive nephropathy. Red fibrinoid necrosis in the wall of the arteriole on the right and clear edematous expansion in the intima of the interlobular artery on the left from a patient with malignant hypertension (Masson trichrome stain).

Renovascular Hypertension Follows Narrowing of a Renal Artery

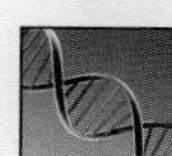

MOLECULAR PATHOGENESIS: Stenosis or total occlusion of a main renal artery produces hypertension that is potentially curable if the arterial lumen is restored. Harry Goldblatt carried out the initial study of this syndrome in dogs more than a half century ago. Since that time, a kidney deprived of vascular supply has been known as a **Goldblatt kidney.** In patients with renal artery stenosis, hypertension reflects increased production of renin, angiotensin II and aldosterone. Renal vein renin from an ischemic kidney is elevated, but it is normal in the contralateral kidney. Most (95%) cases are caused by atherosclerosis, which explains why this disorder is twice as common in men as in women and is primarily seen at older ages (average age, 55 years). Fibromuscular dysplasia and vasculitis are less common causes overall but are the most frequent causes in children.

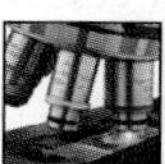

PATHOLOGY: Regardless of the cause of renal artery stenosis, renal parenchymal changes are the same. The size of the involved kidney is reduced. Glomeruli appear normal but are closer to each other than normal, because intervening tubules show marked ischemic atrophy without extensive interstitial fibrosis. Many glomeruli lose their attachment to the proximal tubule. The juxtaglomerular apparatus is prominent, hyperplastic and with increased granularity.

When atherosclerotic plaques cause the vascular stenosis, they impinge on the aortic ostium or narrow the renal artery lumen, more frequently on the left than on the right. Occasionally, an abdominal aortic aneurysm compromises the origin of the renal arteries. Takayasu arteritis and giant cell arteritis cause renal artery stenosis by producing inflammatory and sclerotic thickening of the artery wall with resultant narrowing of the lumen.

Fibromuscular dysplasia is characterized by fibrous and muscular stenosis of the renal artery. There are several patterns of renal artery involvement. The major categories are intimal fibroplasia, medial fibroplasia, perimedial fibroplasia and periarterial fibroplasia. As the names imply, these disorders affect different layers of the artery, from the intima to the adventitia. Medial fibroplasia is the most common and accounts for two thirds of all fibromuscular dysplasia. This process creates areas of medial thickening alternating with areas of atrophy, producing a "string of beads" pattern in angiograms.

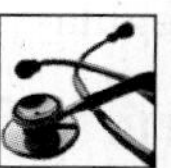

CLINICAL FEATURES: Renovascular hypertension is characterized by mild to moderate blood pressure elevations. A bruit may be heard over the renal artery. The diagnosis requires some type of imaging, such as angiography. In over half of patients, surgical revascularization, angioplasty or nephrectomy cures hypertension. When there is long-standing renovascular hypertension, the uninvolved kidney may become damaged by hypertensive nephrosclerosis.

Renal Atheroembolism May Complicate Aortic Atherosclerosis

In patients with severe aortic atherosclerosis, atheromatous debris may embolize into the renal arteries and vascular tree as far as glomerular capillaries and cause acute renal failure. This

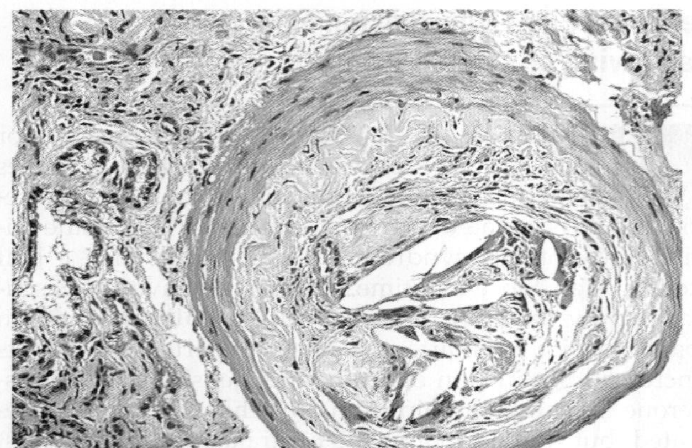

FIGURE 16-61. Atheroembolus. An atheroembolus obstructs an arcuate artery. Note the cholesterol clefts.

may occur spontaneously or be initiated by trauma, such as angiographic procedures. **Cholesterol clefts** are seen in vessel lumina (Fig. 16-61). Early lesions are surrounded by atheromatous material or thrombus. They may later elicit a foreign body reaction and may stimulate fibrosis in the adjacent vessel wall.

Thrombotic Microangiopathies Cause Microangiopathic Hemolytic Anemia and Renal Failure

MOLECULAR PATHOGENESIS: Thrombotic microangiopathy has a variety of causes and at least two distinct pathogenic pathways. One pathogenic pathway that causes typical and atypical **hemolytic–uremic syndrome (HUS)** produces endothelial damage that allows plasma constituents to enter the intima of arteries, walls of arterioles and subendothelial zone of glomerular capillaries, narrowing vessel lumina and causing ischemia. The injured endothelial surfaces promote thrombosis, which worsens ischemia and may cause focal ischemic necrosis. Typical HUS follows diarrhea due to toxin-producing bacteria, most often *Escherichia coli* (usually O157:H7 strain), in contaminated food. The toxin injures endothelial cells in glomerular capillaries, initiating the sequence described above. Atypical HUS is unrelated to diarrhea and is caused by different mechanisms, including genetic abnormalities in complement regulatory proteins (mostly factor H but also factor I and membrane cofactor protein), autoantibodies to complement regulatory proteins (anti–factor H) or both.

Thrombotic thrombocytopenic purpura (TTP) is caused by a genetic or acquired deficiency of a protease that cleaves multimers of von Willebrand factor on the surface of endothelial cells (see Chapter 20). The large uncleaved multimers promote platelet aggregation and microvascular thrombosis. Passage of blood through vessels injured by either HUS or TTP leads to a nonimmune (Coombs-negative) hemolytic anemia, with misshapen and disrupted erythrocytes (schistocytes) and thrombocytopenia. This hematologic syndrome is termed **microangiopathic hemolytic anemia (MAHA).** Thus, HUS and TTP can be very difficult to distinguish clinically because they both present with MAHA. Thrombotic microangiopathies that resemble HUS and TTP also can occur secondary to drugs, autoimmune diseases and malignant hypertension (Table 16-10).

Table 16-10

Causes of Thrombotic Microangiopathy

Thrombotic Thrombocytopenic Purpura
Autoantibodies against ADAMTS13
Inherited deficiency in ADAMTS13
Infections Typical of Hemolytic–Uremic Syndrome
Escherichia coli
Shigella spp.
Pseudomonas spp.
Atypical Hemolytic–Uremic Syndrome
Genetic mutation (factor H, factor I, membrane cofactor protein)
Anti–factor H
Drug-Induced Thrombotic Microangiopathies
Mitomycin
Cisplatin
Cyclosporin
Tacrolimus
Anti-VEGF therapy
Autoimmune Diseases
Systemic sclerosis (scleroderma) Systemic lupus erythematosus Antiphospholipid antibody syndrome
Acute Postpartum Renal Failure
Malignant Hypertension
Pregnancy and Postpartum Factors

VEGF = vascular endothelial growth factor.

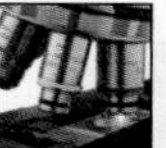

PATHOLOGY: The renal pathology of HUS is comparable to that of malignant hypertensive nephropathy, which is a form of thrombotic microangiopathy. The basic renal lesions are:

- Arteriolar fibrinoid necrosis
- Arterial edematous intimal expansion
- Glomerular consolidation, necrosis or congestion
- Vascular platelet-rich thrombosis

Electron microscopy of glomeruli shows electron-lucent expansion of the subendothelial zone (Figs. 16-62 and 16-63), due to insudation of plasma proteins under injured endothelial cells. By fluorescence microscopy, fibrin and insudated plasma proteins are seen in injured vessel walls.

TTP may have vascular lesions that resemble HUS, but is characterized by more numerous platelet-rich thrombi in glomerular capillaries as well as in capillaries, arterioles and small arteries in many tissues of the body.

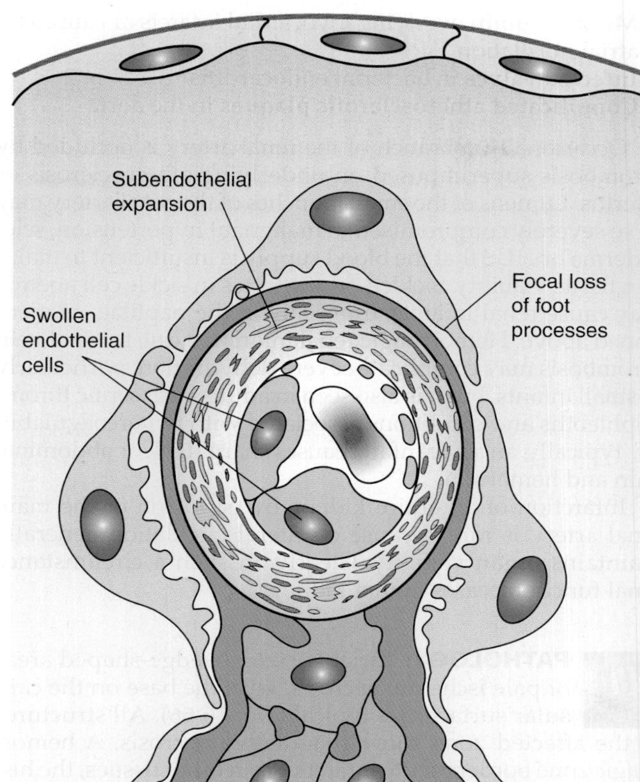

FIGURE 16-62. Hemolytic–uremic syndrome. A wide band of subendothelial electron-lucent material causes narrowing of the capillary lumen. Endothelial cell swelling also contributes to narrowing of the lumen.

CLINICAL FEATURES: Various clinical presentations and causes allow recognition of different categories of thrombotic microangiopathy. The various clinical disorders share microangiopathic hemolytic anemia, thrombocytopenia, hypertension and renal failure, although these features are present to different degrees. In a patient with MAHA, an accompanying diseases process (e.g., bloody diarrhea, SLE, systemic sclerosis) or treatment (e.g., mitomycin, cisplatin, vascular endothelial growth factor [VEGF] inhibitor) may point to the cause of the thrombotic microangiopathy.

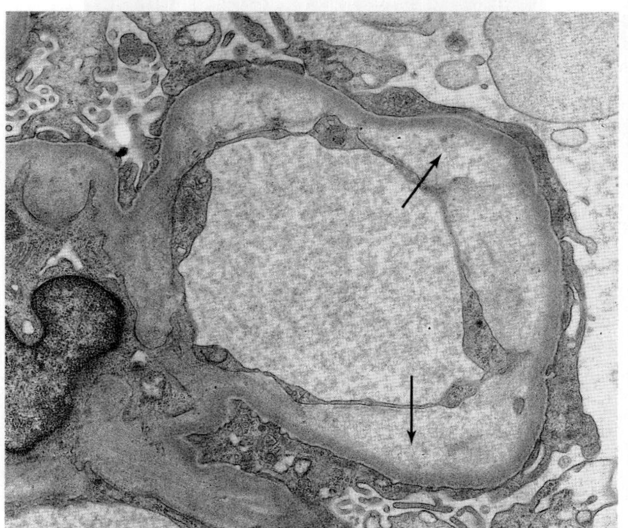

FIGURE 16-63. Thrombotic microangiopathy. An electron micrograph shows a wide band of lucent material in the subendothelial zone (*arrows*), which causes marked narrowing of the lumen.

Hemolytic–Uremic Syndrome

Typical postdiarrheal HUS features microangiopathic hemolytic anemia and acute renal failure, with little or no significant vascular disease outside the kidneys. ***Typical HUS is one of the most common causes of acute renal failure in children.*** It is less common in adults. HUS occurs as isolated cases or in epidemics caused by food contaminated with enterohemorrhagic *E. coli*. Patients present with hemorrhagic diarrhea and rapidly progressive renal failure. Even when dialysis is required, normal renal function usually returns within several weeks. However, impaired renal function may eventually reemerge after 15 to 25 years in over half of patients. Atypical HUS is more frequent in adults and is not preceded by diarrhea. Its prognosis is worse than for typical HUS, often with multiple recurrences and more chance of progression to ESRD.

Thrombotic Thrombocytopenic Purpura

In TTP systemic microvascular thrombosis is characterized clinically by thrombocytopenia, purpura, fever and changes in mental status. Unlike HUS, renal involvement is often absent or less important than other organ disease. Bleeding, caused by the consumptive thrombocytopenia, is also more severe in TTP than it is in HUS. TTP is more common in adults than children. Plasmapheresis and plasma infusion improve outcomes by removal of anti-ADAMTS13 or replacing genetically deficient ADAMTS13, respectively (see Chapter 20).

In Preeclampsia, Hypertension, Proteinuria and Edema Occur in the Third Trimester of Pregnancy

If these features are complicated by **convulsions**, the term **eclampsia** is used (see Chapter 18). Glomeruli in preeclampsia are uniformly enlarged and endothelial cells are swollen, resulting in apparently bloodless glomerular tufts (Figs. 16-64 and 16-65). These endothelial changes may be induced by elevated levels in the maternal circulation of antiangiogenic factors released by the placenta. By electron microscopy, the swollen endothelial cells contain large, irregular vacuoles. Vacuoles are also present in podocytes. Mild and moderate disease can be controlled with bed rest and antihypertensive agents. Severe cases may require induction of delivery. Hypertension and proteinuria typically disappear 1 to 2 weeks after delivery.

Nephropathy Is the Most Common Organ Manifestation of Sickle Cell Disease

The interstitial tissue in which the vasa recta course is hypertonic and has a low oxygen tension. As a result, erythrocytes in the vasa recta in sickle cell patients tend to sickle and occlude the lumen. Infarcts in the medulla and papilla ensue, sometimes severe enough to cause papillary necrosis. Ischemic scarring of the medulla leads to focal tubular loss and atrophy. Glomeruli are conspicuously congested with sickle cells. FSGS or, less often, MPGN occurs in a minority of patients and may cause the nephrotic syndrome.

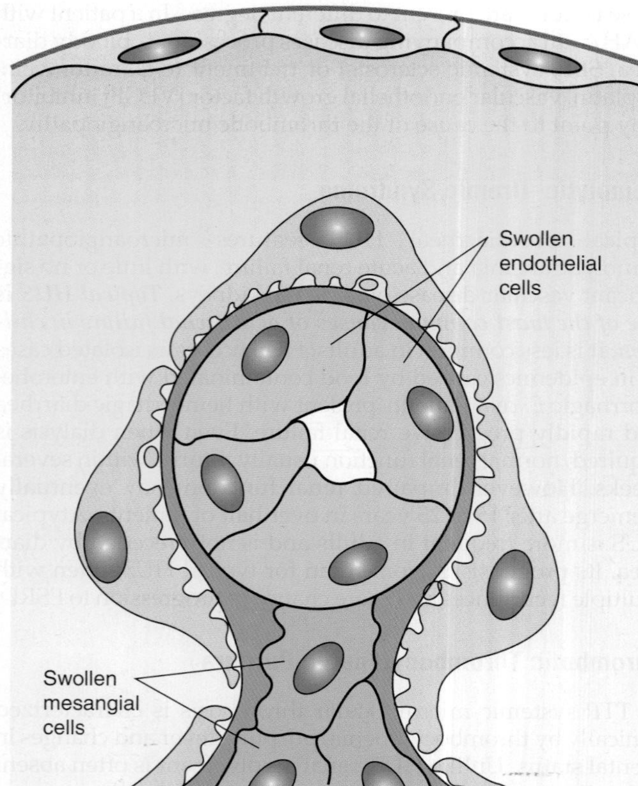

FIGURE 16-64. Preeclamptic nephropathy. Preeclamptic nephropathy, or pregnancy-induced nephropathy, exhibits marked swelling of endothelial cells with narrowing of the lumina. Both endothelial and mesangial cells are enlarged and have multiple vacuoles and vesicular structures.

Renal Infarcts Usually Result From Embolization to Interlobar or Arcuate Arteries

Renal infarcts are mostly caused by embolic arterial obstruction.

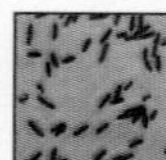

ETIOLOGIC FACTORS: The size of the infarct varies with the size of the occluded vessel. Common sources of emboli include:

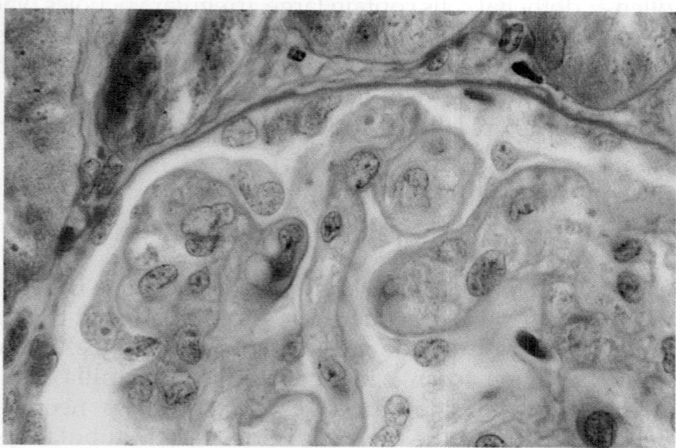

FIGURE 16-65. Preeclampsia. Capillary lumens are obliterated by swollen endothelial cells (Masson trichrome stain).

- **Mural thrombi** overlying myocardial infarcts or caused by atrial fibrillation
- **Infected valves** in bacterial endocarditis
- **Complicated atherosclerotic plaques** in the aorta

Occasionally, a branch of the renal artery is occluded by thrombosis superimposed on underlying atherosclerosis or arteritis. Lumens of the small branches of the renal artery may be so severely compromised in malignant hypertension, scleroderma or HUS that the blood supply is insufficient to maintain tissue viability. Sickled erythrocytes in sickle cell anemia may cause renal infarcts, especially in the papillae, as mentioned above. Hemorrhagic renal infarction due to renal vein thrombosis may complicate severe dehydration, particularly in small infants, but it is also seen in adults with septic thrombophlebitis and conditions associated with hypercoagulability. Typically, an acute infarct causes sharp flank or abdominal pain and hematuria.

Infarction of an entire kidney by occlusion of the main renal artery is rare because collateral circulation generally maintains organ viability. Clearly, in such a circumstance renal function ceases in that kidney.

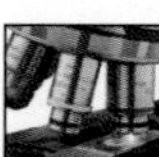

PATHOLOGY: Variably sized, wedge-shaped areas of pale ischemic necrosis, with the base on the capsular surface, are typical (Fig. 16-66). All structures in the affected zone show coagulative necrosis. A hemorrhagic zone borders acute infarcts. As in other tissues, the histologic response to the infarct progresses through phases of acute inflammation, granulation tissue and fibrosis. Healed infarcts are sharply circumscribed and depressed cortical scars containing ghosts of obliterated glomeruli, atrophic tubules, interstitial fibrosis and a mild chronic inflammatory infiltrate. Dystrophic calcification is occasionally encountered

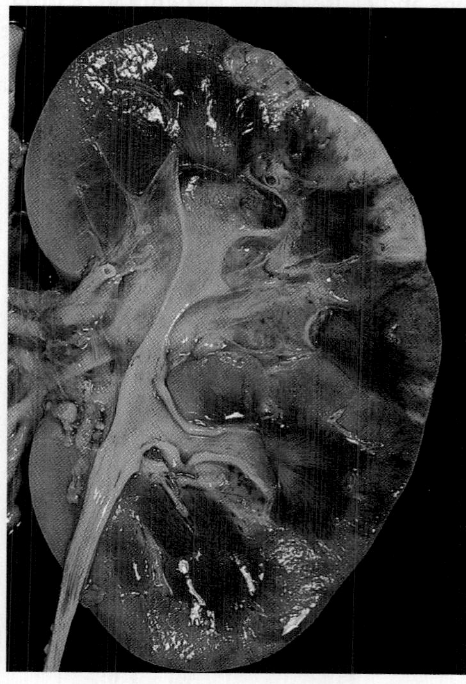

FIGURE 16-66. Renal infarct. A cross-section of the kidney shows multiple areas of infarction characterized by marked pallor, which extends to the subcapsular surface.

in old infarcts. At the margins of a healed infarct, the viable tissue resembles that seen in chronic ischemia, with tubular atrophy, interstitial fibrosis and infiltration by chronic inflammatory cells.

Cortical Necrosis Is Secondary Severe Ischemia and Spares the Medulla

Cortical necrosis affects part or all of the renal cortex. The term **infarct** is used when there is one area (or a few areas) of necrosis caused by occlusion of arteries, whereas **cortical necrosis** implies more-widespread ischemic necrosis.

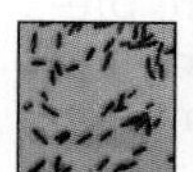

ETIOLOGIC FACTORS: Renal cortical necrosis can complicate any condition associated with hypovolemic or endotoxic shock, the classical situation being premature placental separation late in pregnancy (see Chapter 18). All forms of shock can result in reversible prerenal or intrarenal ischemia, which can precede irreversible cortical necrosis.

Vasa recta that supply arterial blood to the medulla arise from juxtamedullary efferent arterioles, proximal to vessels supplying the outer cortex. Thus, occlusion of outer cortical vessels (e.g., by vasospasm, thrombi or thrombotic microangiopathy) leads to cortical necrosis and spares the medulla. Experimentally, renal cortical necrosis may be caused by vasoconstrictors such as vasopressin and serotonin, or by eliciting disseminated intravascular coagulation (see Chapter 20).

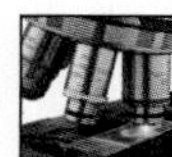

PATHOLOGY: Cortical necrosis may vary from patchy to confluent (Fig. 16-67). In the most severely involved areas, all parenchymal elements exhibit coagulative necrosis. The proximal convoluted tubules are invariably necrotic, as are most of the distal tubules. In adjacent viable portions of the cortex, glomeruli and distal convoluted tubules are usually unaffected, but many proximal convoluted tubules may show ischemic injury, such as epithelial flattening or necrosis.

With extensive necrosis, the cortex is pale and diffusely necrotic, save for thin rims of viable tissue just beneath the capsule and at the corticomedullary junction. These are supplied by capsular and medullary collateral blood vessels, respectively. Patients who survive cortical necrosis may develop striking dystrophic calcification of the necrotic areas.

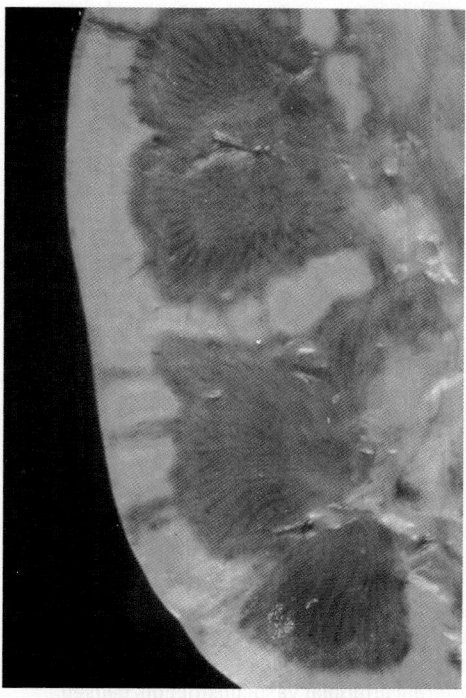

FIGURE 16-67. Renal cortical necrosis. The cortex of the kidney is pale yellow and soft owing to diffuse cortical necrosis.

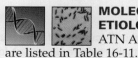

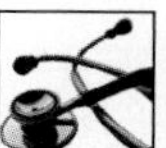

CLINICAL FEATURES: Severe cortical necrosis manifests as acute renal failure, which initially may be indistinguishable from that produced by acute tubular necrosis (ATN). However, the former is more often irreversible. A renal arteriogram or biopsy may be required for diagnosis. Recovery is determined by the extent of the disease, but hypertension is common among survivors.

Diseases of Tubules and Interstitium

An acute rise in serum creatinine has been called acute renal failure (ARF). It is classified as **prerenal** ARF if caused by reduced blood flow to the kidneys, **intrarenal** ARF if caused by injury to the renal parenchyma and **postrenal** ARF if caused by urinary tract obstruction. Intrarenal ARF is now called **acute kidney injury** (AKI). AKI is categorized by the portion of the kidney that is primarily injured: **glomeruli** (e.g., acute glomerulonephritis), **vessels** (e.g., vasculitis), **tubules** (e.g., ischemic acute tubular injury) or **interstitium** (acute interstitial nephritis). ***The most common cause for intrarenal AKI is ischemic acute tubular injury.***

Acute Ischemic and Nephrotoxic Acute Tubular Necrosis Are Frequent Causes of Acute Renal Failure

ATN is severe, but potentially reversible, renal failure due to impaired tubular epithelial function caused by ischemia or toxic injury. Because necrosis often is not a prominent feature of ATN, this process also is called acute renal injury (ARI). Ischemia and toxins can cause injury to tubules that results in ARF. Ischemic prerenal ARF is reversible pathophysiologic ARF with no structural tubular epithelial changes. ***If ischemia is severe enough to cause histologic tubular epithelial injury, it is considered intrarenal ARF or ischemic AKI.*** Extensive ischemia can cause overt necrosis of tubular epithelial cells and has been called **ATN.** However, most ischemic acute tubular injury does not have widespread tubular epithelial necrosis and thus in this setting the term ATN would be a misnomer.

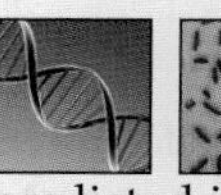
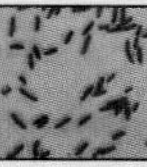

MOLECULAR PATHOGENESIS AND ETIOLOGIC FACTORS: Some causes of ATN AKI caused by acute tubular injury are listed in Table 16-11.

Ischemic ATN acute tubular injury results from reduced renal perfusion, usually associated with hypotension. Tubular epithelial cells, with their high rate of energy-consuming

Table 16-11

Causes of Acute Tubular Necrosis and Acute Tubular Injury

Cause
Ischemic Prerenal Acute Renal Failure or Ischemic Acute Tubular Injury
Massive hemorrhage
Septic shock
Severe burns
Dehydration
Prolonged diarrhea
Congestive heart failure
Volume redistribution (e.g., pancreatitis, peritonitis)
Nephrotoxin Acute Tubular Injury
Antibiotics (e.g., aminoglycosides, amphotericin B)
Radiographic contrast agents
Heavy metals (e.g., mercury, lead, cisplatin)
Organic solvents (e.g., ethylene glycol, carbon tetrachloride)
Poisons (e.g., paraquat)
Heme Protein Cast Nephropathies
Myoglobin (from rhabdomyolysis, e.g., with crush injury)
Hemoglobin (from hemolysis, e.g., with transfusion reaction)

metabolic activity and numerous organelles, are particularly sensitive to hypoxia and anoxia, which cause rapid depletion of intracellular adenosine triphosphate (ATP) in tubular epithelium. The most frequent histologic abnormality is flattening (simplification) of tubular epithelial cells resulting from sloughing of the apical cytoplasm into the urine (which leads to formation of granular pigmented casts that can be seen in the urine and detected by urinalysis). Tubular epithelial cells may be simplified (flattened) but not necrotic in some patients with typical clinical ATN. Overt necrosis is less frequent.

Nephrotoxic ATN is caused by chemically induced injury to epithelial cells. Tubular epithelial cells are preferred targets for certain toxins because they absorb and concentrate toxins. The high rate of energy consumption by epithelial cells also makes them susceptible to injury by toxins that perturb oxidative or other metabolic pathways. Hemoglobin and myoglobin can be considered endogenous toxins that can induce ATN acute tubular injury **(pigment nephropathy)** when they are present in the urine in high concentrations.

The pathophysiology of ATN AKI in acute tubular injury involves decreased glomerular filtration and tubular epithelial dysfunction due to some or all of the following (Fig. 16-68):

- Intrarenal vasoconstriction
- Alteration of arteriolar tone by tubuloglomerular feedback
- Decreased glomerular hydrostatic pressure

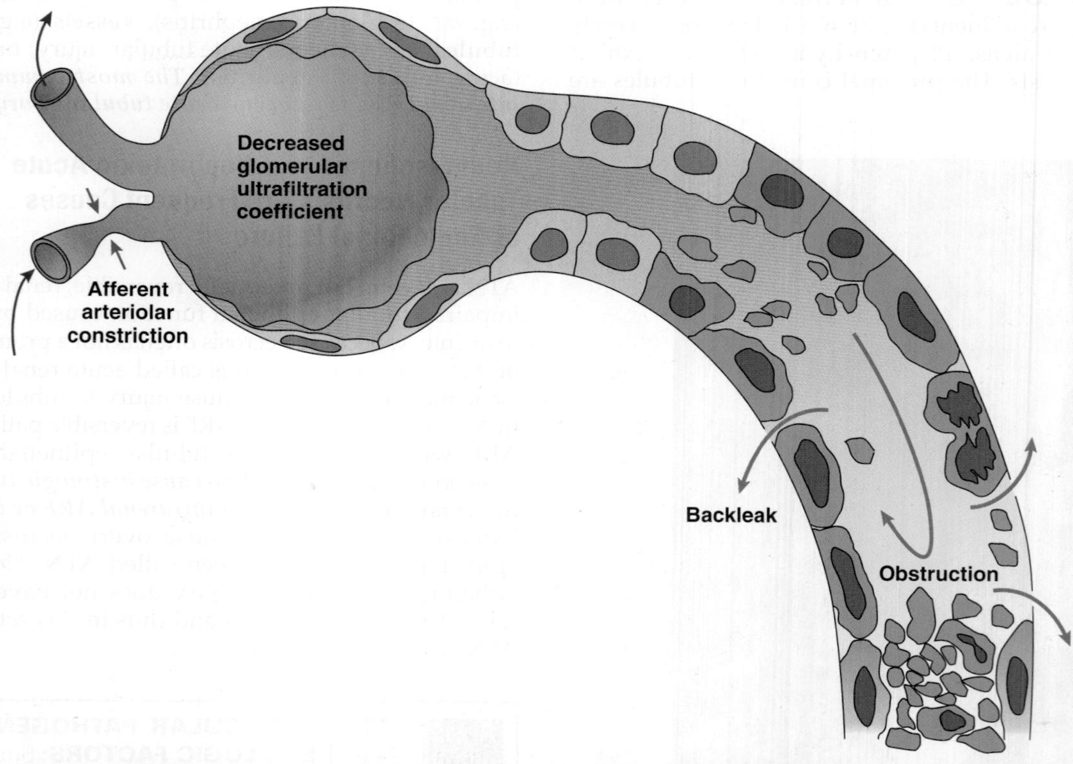

FIGURE 16-68. Pathogenesis of acute renal failure caused by acute tubular injury (acute tubular necrosis). Sloughing and necrosis of epithelial cells result in cast formation. The presence of casts leads to obstruction and increased intraluminal pressure, which reduces glomerular filtration. Afferent arteriolar vasoconstriction, caused in part by tubuloglomerular feedback, results in decreased glomerular capillary filtration pressure. Tubular injury and increased intraluminal pressure cause fluid back-leakage from the lumen into the interstitium.

- Decreased glomerular capillary permeability (K_f)
- Tubular obstruction by cellular debris, with increased hydrostatic pressure
- Back-leakage of glomerular filtrate into the interstitium through damaged tubular epithelium

PATHOLOGY: In ischemic ATN acute tubular injury kidneys are swollen, with a pale cortex and a congested medulla. Glomeruli and blood vessels are normal. Tubule injury is focal and is most pronounced in the proximal tubules and thick limbs of the loop of Henle of the outer medulla. The epithelium is flattened, lumina are dilated and brush borders are lost (epithelial simplification), due in part to sloughing of apical cytoplasm, which appears in distal tubular lumina and urine as brown granular casts. (The color reflects renal cytochrome pigments.) Electron microscopy shows decreased infoldings at the basolateral membranes of proximal tubular epithelial cells. Widespread necrosis of tubular epithelial cells is not generally seen, but simplification may be evident. Instead, "necrosis" is subtle, and is observed in individual necrotic cells within some proximal or distal tubules. These single necrotic cells, plus a few viable cells, are shed into the tubular lumen, resulting in focal denudation of tubular basement membrane (Fig. 16-69). Interstitial edema is common. The vasa recta of the outer medulla are congested and often contain nucleated cells, which are predominantly mononuclear leukocytes.

Toxic ATN acute tubular injury shows more-extensive necrosis of tubular epithelium than is usually seen in ischemic ATN acute tubular injury (compare Figs. 16-69 and 16-70).

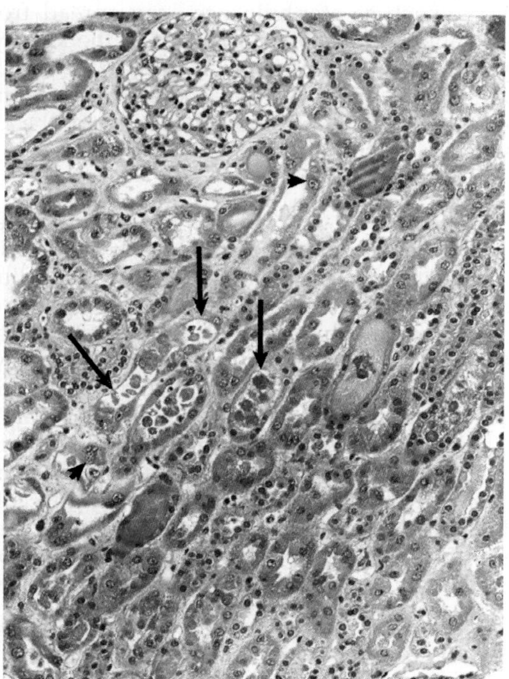

FIGURE 16-69. Ischemic acute tubular injury (acute tubular necrosis). Necrosis of individual tubular epithelial cells is evident both from focal denudation of the tubular basement membrane (*arrows*) and from the individual necrotic epithelial cells present in some tubular lumina. Some enlarged, regenerative-appearing epithelial cells are also present (*arrowheads*). Note the lack of significant interstitial inflammation.

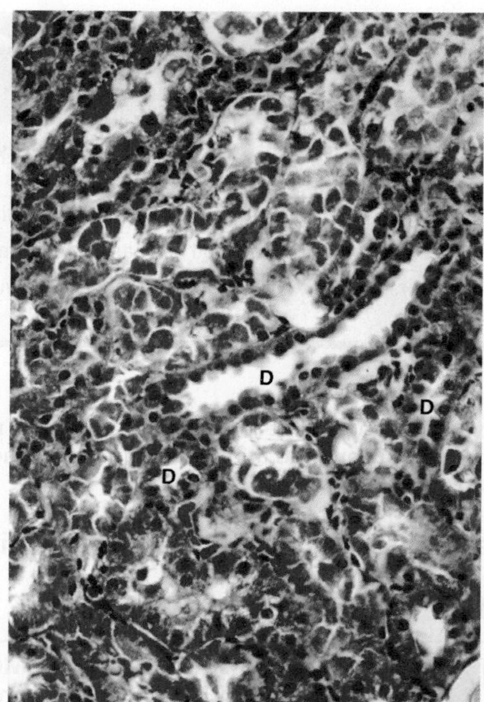

FIGURE 16-70. Toxic acute tubular necrosis due to mercury poisoning. There is widespread necrosis of proximal tubular epithelial cells, with sparing of distal and collecting tubules (D). Interstitial inflammation is minimal.

However, toxic necrosis is largely limited to the tubular segments that are most sensitive to the particular toxin, most often the proximal tubule. ATN acute tubular injury due to hemoglobinuria or myoglobinuria also has many red-brown tubular casts that are colored by heme pigments.

During the recovery phase of ATN acute tubular injury that has caused necrosis, tubular epithelium regenerates, with mitoses, increased size of cells and nuclei, and cell crowding. Survivors eventually display complete restoration of normal renal architecture.

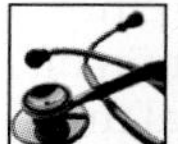

CLINICAL FEATURES: ***ATN ischemia is the leading cause of acute renal failure.*** Rapidly rising serum creatinine level, usually with decreased urine output **(oliguria),** is characteristic. **Nonoliguric** acute renal failure is less common. Urinalysis shows degenerating epithelial cells and **"dirty brown" granular casts** (acute renal failure casts) with cell debris rich in cytochrome pigments. Urinalysis may help to differentiate among the three major intrinsic renal diseases that cause acute renal failure (Table 16-12). Prerenal ischemic acute tubular injury typically has a less than 1.0% fractional excretion of sodium, whereas intrarenal acute tubular injury has a fractional excretion of sodium greater than 2.0%, which is a marker of overt tubular epithelial damage.

The duration of renal failure in patients with ATN ischemic acute tubular injury depends on many factors, especially the nature and reversibility of the cause. Many patients develop uremia (azotemia, fluid retention, metabolic acidosis, hyperkalemia), at least transiently, and may require dialysis. If the insult is immediately removed after the start of the injury, renal function often recovers within

Table 16-12

Urinalysis in Acute Renal Failure

Causes of Acute Renal Failure	Urinalysis Sediment Findings
Acute tubular injury	Dirty brown casts and epithelial cells
Acute glomerulonephritis	Red blood cell casts and proteinuria
Acute tubulointerstitial nephritis	White blood cell casts and pyuria

1 to 2 weeks, although it may be delayed for months. Increased urine output and a fall in serum creatinine herald the recovery phase.

Pyelonephritis Is Bacterial Infection of the Kidney

Acute Pyelonephritis

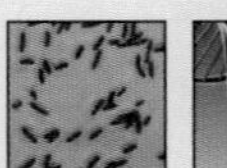
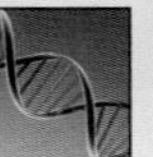

ETIOLOGIC FACTORS AND MOLECULAR PATHOGENESIS: Gram-negative bacteria from the feces, mostly *E. coli*, cause 80% of acute pyelonephritis. *E. coli* that cause urinary tract infections **(uropathogenic *E. coli*)** have virulence factors that enhance their ability to cause not only urinary tract infections but also pyelonephritis. The best studied of these are adhesins on fimbria (pili) encoded by *pyelonephritis-associated pili* (*PAP*) genes. Uropathogenic *E. coli* pili attach to adhesin-binding sites on urothelial cells as well as epithelial cells of the kidney. Infection reaches the kidney by ascending through the urinary tract, a process that depends on several factors:

- Bacterial urinary infection
- Reflux of infected urine up the ureters into the renal pelvis and calyces
- Bacterial entry through the papillae into the renal parenchyma

Bladder infections, which precede acute pyelonephritis, are more common in females because of a short urethra, lack of antibacterial prostatic secretions and facilitation of bacterial migration by sexual intercourse. The normal urethral commensal flora are replaced by fecal organisms in some women who are unusually vulnerable to recurrent urinary tract infections. This change in flora may reflect poor hygiene, hormonal effects and genetic predisposition (e.g., increased numbers of receptors for *E. coli* on urothelial cells).

Pregnancy predisposes to acute pyelonephritis for several reasons, including a high frequency of asymptomatic bacteriuria (10%), one fourth of which develops into acute pyelonephritis. Other causes include increased residual urine volume because high levels of progesterone make bladder musculature flaccid and less able to expel urine.

The bladder normally empties all but 2 to 3 mL of residual urine. Subsequent addition of sterile urine from the kidneys dilutes any bacteria that may have gotten into the bladder. However, if residual urine volume is increased (e.g., with prostatic obstruction or bladder atony due to neurogenic disorders such as paraplegia or diabetic neuropathy), sterile urine from the kidneys is insufficient to dilute residual bladder urine to prevent bacterial accumulation. Diabetic glycosuria also facilitates infection by providing a rich bacterial growth medium.

Bacteria in bladder urine usually do not ascend to the kidneys. The ureter commonly inserts into the bladder wall at a steep angle (Fig. 16-71) and its most distal portion courses parallel to the bladder wall, between the mucosa and muscularis. Increased intravesicular pressure during micturition occludes the distal ureteral lumen and prevents urinary reflux. An anatomic abnormality, a short passage of the ureter within the bladder wall, leads the ureter to insert more perpendicularly to the mucosal surface of the bladder. As a result, rather than occluding the lumen, on micturition intravesicular pressure forces urine into the patent ureter. This reflux can force the urine into the renal pelvis and calyces.

Even if reflux pressure delivers bacteria to the calyces, the renal parenchyma is not necessarily contaminated. The convexity of the simple papillae of central calyces blocks reflux urine from entering (Fig. 16-71), but the concavity of peripheral compound papillae allows easier access to the collecting system. ***However, if pressure is prolonged, as in obstructive uropathy, even simple papillae are eventually vulnerable to retrograde entry of urine.*** From the collecting tubules, bacteria access the renal interstitium and tubules.

In addition to ascending through urine, bacteria and other pathogens can gain access to renal parenchyma through blood, causing **hematogenous pyelonephritis.** For example, in bacterial endocarditis gram-positive organisms, such as staphylococci, can spread from an infected valve and establish infection in the kidney. The kidney is commonly involved in miliary tuberculosis. Fungi, such as *Aspergillus*, can seed kidneys in an immunosuppressed host. Hematogenous infections of the kidney preferentially affect the cortex.

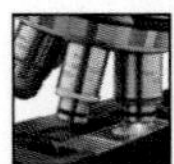

PATHOLOGY: The kidneys in acute pyelonephritis have small white abscesses on subcapsular surfaces and cut surfaces. Pelvic and calyceal urothelium may be hyperemic and covered by purulent exudate. The disease is often focal, and much of the kidney may appear normal.

Most infections involve only a few papillary systems. Microscopically, the parenchyma, particularly the cortex, typically shows extensive focal destruction by the inflammatory process, although vessels and glomeruli often are preferentially preserved. Inflammatory infiltrates mainly contain neutrophils, which often fill tubules and especially collecting ducts (Fig. 16-72). In severe cases of acute pyelonephritis, necrosis of the papillary tips may occur (Fig. 16-73) or infection may extend beyond the renal capsule to cause a perinephric abscess.

CLINICAL FEATURES: Symptoms of acute pyelonephritis include fever, chills, sweats, malaise, flank pain and costovertebral angle tenderness. Leukocytosis with neutrophilia is common. Differentiating upper from lower urinary tract infection clinically is often difficult, but the finding of **leukocyte casts** in the urine supports a diagnosis of pyelonephritis.

FIGURE 16-71. Anatomic features of the bladder and kidney in pyelonephritis caused by ureterovesical reflux. In the normal bladder, the distal portion of the intravesical ureter courses between the mucosa and the muscularis, forming a mucosal flap. On micturition, the elevated intravesicular pressure compresses the flap against the bladder wall, thereby occluding the lumen. Persons with a congenitally short intravesical ureter have no mucosal flap, because the angle of entry of the ureter into the bladder approaches a right angle. Thus, micturition forces urine into the ureter. In the renal pelvis, simple papillae of the central calyces are convex and do not readily allow reflux of urine. By contrast, the peripheral compound papillae are concave and permit entry of refluxed urine.

Chronic Pyelonephritis

ETIOLOGIC FACTORS: Chronic pyelonephritis is caused by recurrent and persistent bacterial infection due to urinary tract obstruction, urine reflux or both (Fig. 16-74). Whether reflux without infection can produce chronic pyelonephritis is controversial.

In chronic pyelonephritis caused by reflux or obstruction, medullary tissue and overlying cortex are preferentially injured by recurrent acute and chronic inflammation. Progressive atrophy and scarring ensue, with resultant contraction of the involved papillary tip (or sloughing if there is papillary necrosis) and thinning of the overlying cortex. This process results in the distinctive gross appearance of a broad depressed area of cortical fibrosis and atrophy overlying a dilated calyx **(caliectasis)** (Fig. 16-75).

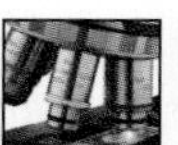

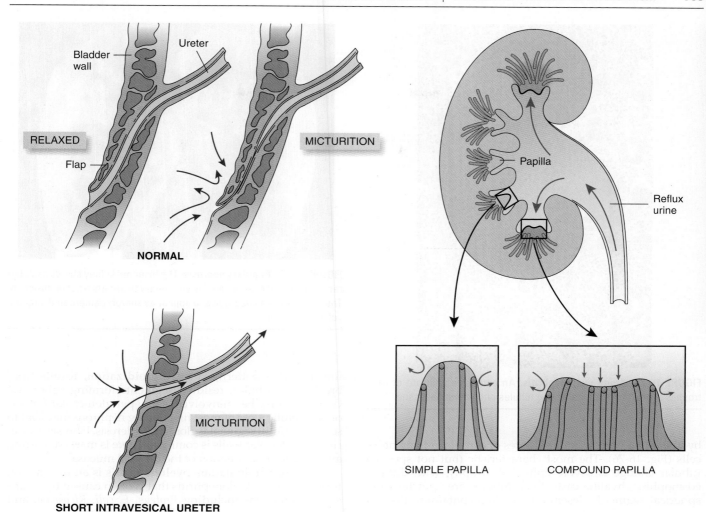

PATHOLOGY: The histology of chronic pyelonephritis is nonspecific. Many diseases cause chronic injury to the tubulointerstitial compartment and induce chronic interstitial inflammation, interstitial fibrosis and tubular atrophy. Thus, chronic pyelonephritis is one of many causes of a pattern of injury termed **chronic tubulointerstitial nephritis.** The gross appearance of chronic pyelonephritis is more distinctive. Only chronic pyelonephritis and analgesic nephropathy produce both caliectasis and overlying corticomedullary scarring. In obstructive uropathy, all of the calyces and the renal pelvis are dilated, and the parenchyma is uniformly thinned (Fig. 16-75). In cases associated with vesicoureteral reflux, the calyces at the poles of the kidney are preferentially expanded and are associated with overlying discrete, coarse scars that indent the renal surface. Microscopically, the scars have atrophic dilated tubules surrounded

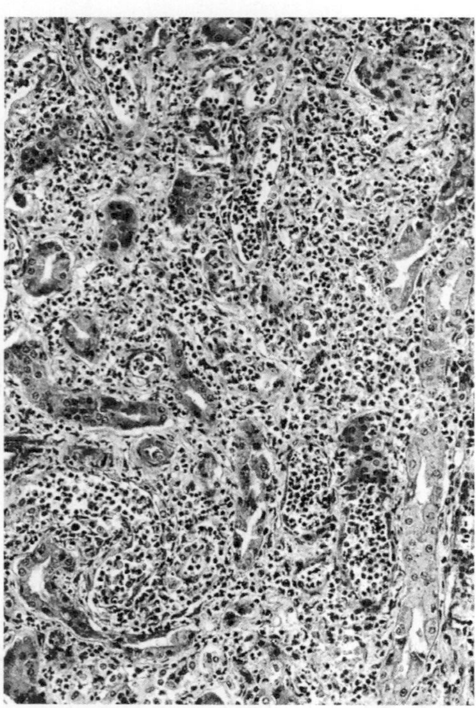

FIGURE 16-72. Acute pyelonephritis. An extensive infiltrate of neutrophils is present in the collecting tubules and interstitial tissue.

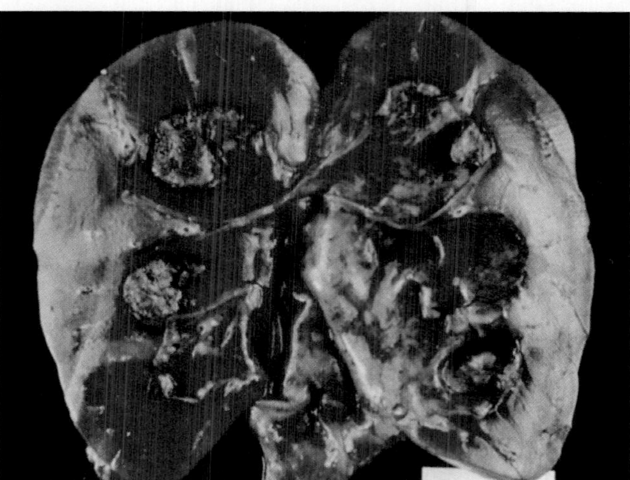

FIGURE 16-73. Papillary necrosis. The bisected kidney shows a dilated renal pelvis and dilated calyces secondary to urinary tract obstruction. The papillae are all necrotic and appear as sharply demarcated, ragged, yellowish areas.

by interstitial fibrosis and infiltrates of chronic inflammatory cells (Fig. 16-76). The most characteristic (but not specific) tubular change is severe epithelial atrophy, with diffuse, eosinophilic, hyaline casts. Such tubules are "pinched-off" spherical segments, resembling colloid-containing thyroid follicles. This pattern, called **thyroidization,** results from breakup of tubules, residual segments forming spherules. Glomeruli may be uninvolved, show periglomerular fibrosis or be sclerotic. Loss of most functioning nephrons may lead to secondary focal segmental glomerulosclerosis. Fibrosis of arterial and arteriolar walls is common. There is marked scarring and chronic inflammation of the calyceal mucosa.

Xanthogranulomatous pyelonephritis is an uncommon form of chronic pyelonephritis that is often caused by a variety of pathogens including *Proteus, E. coli, Klebsiella,* and

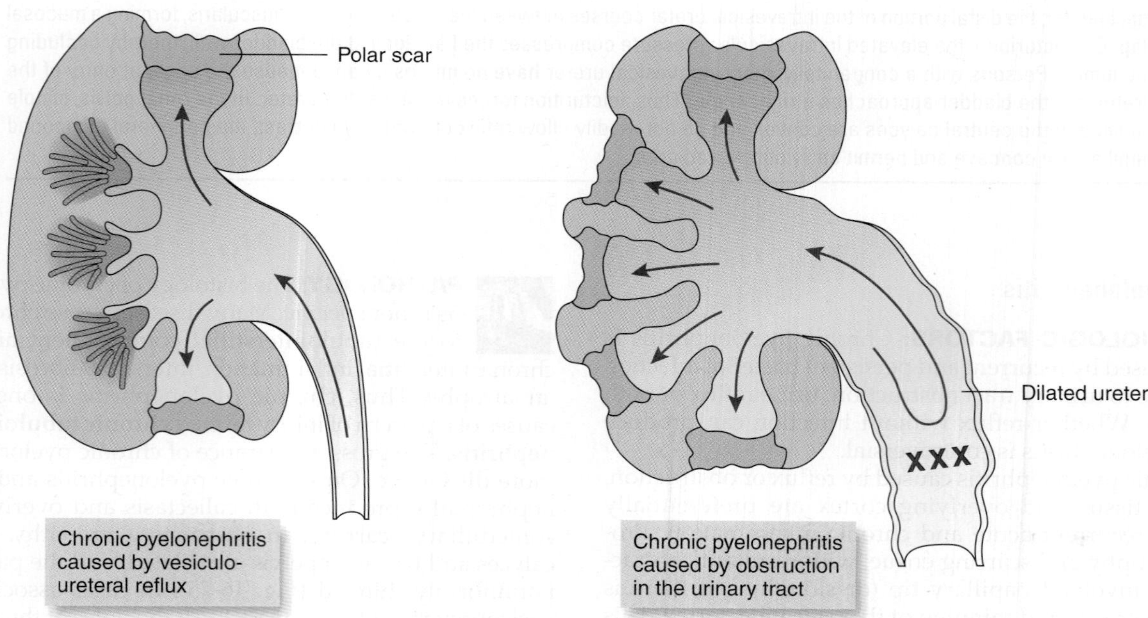

FIGURE 16-74. The two major types of chronic pyelonephritis. Left. Vesicoureteral reflux causes infection of the peripheral compound papillae and, therefore, scars in the poles of the kidney. **Right.** Obstruction of the urinary tract leads to high-pressure backflow of urine, which causes infection of all papillae, diffuse scarring of the kidney and thinning of the cortex.

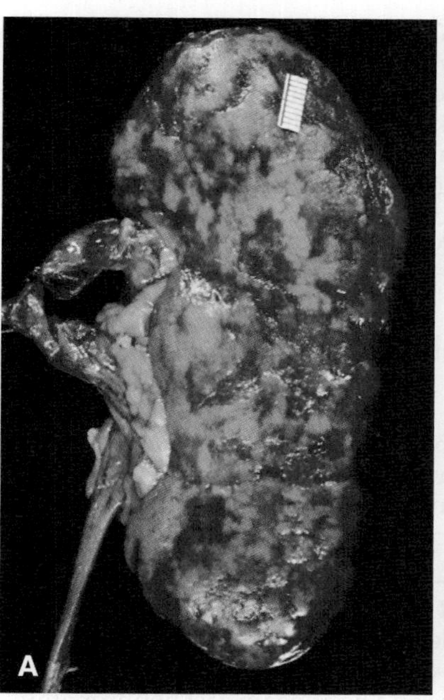

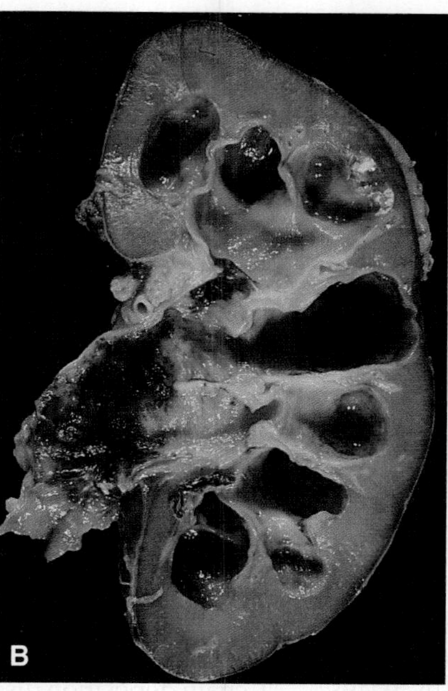

FIGURE 16-75. Chronic pyelonephritis. A. The cortical surface contains many irregular, depressed scars (reddish areas). **B.** There is marked dilation of calyces (caliectasis) caused by inflammatory destruction of papillae, with atrophy and scarring of the overlying cortex.

Pseudomonas. The name derives from the yellow gross appearance of the nodular renal lesions, caused by numerous lipid-laden foamy macrophages **(xanthoma cells).** The disease is usually unilateral. The clinical and pathologic features can be confused with renal cell carcinoma (RCC).

CLINICAL FEATURES: Most patients with chronic pyelonephritis have episodic symptoms of urinary tract infection or acute pyelonephritis, such as recurrent fever and flank pain. Some have a silent course until end-stage renal disease develops. Urinalysis shows leukocytes, and imaging studies reveal caliectasis and cortical scarring.

Analgesic Nephropathy Results From Chronic Overconsumption of Painkillers

Patients with analgesic nephropathy typically have taken over 2 kg of analgesics, often in combinations, such as aspirin and phenacetin, or aspirin and acetaminophen. Phenacetin most often leads to nephropathy and is banned in many countries, including the United States. Acetaminophen induces nephropathy more readily than do aspirin or nonsteroidal anti-inflammatory drugs (NSAIDs). The basis for analgesic nephropathy is not clear. Possibilities include direct nephrotoxicity, ischemic damage due to drug-induced vascular changes or both.

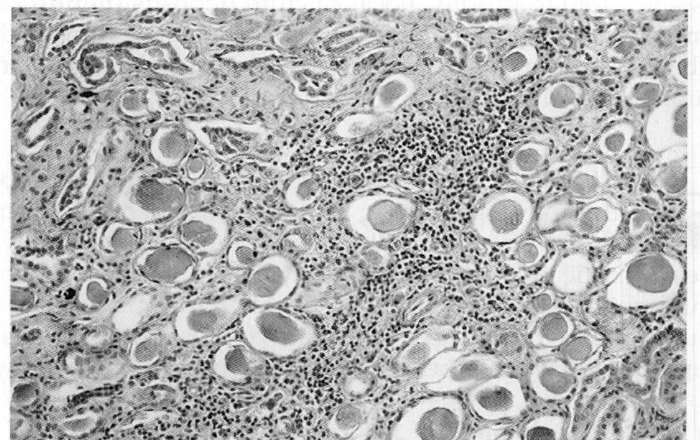

FIGURE 16-76. A light micrograph shows tubular dilation and atrophy, with many tubules containing eosinophilic hyaline casts resembling the colloid of thyroid follicles (so-called thyroidization). The interstitium is scarred and contains a chronic inflammatory cell infiltrate.

PATHOLOGY: Medullary injury with papillary necrosis appears to be the earliest event in analgesic nephropathy, followed by atrophy, chronic inflammation and scarring of the overlying cortex. The earliest histologic abnormality is a distinctive homogeneous thickening of capillary walls just beneath the transitional epithelium of the urinary tract. Early parenchymal changes are confined to papillae and the inner medulla, and consist of focal basement membrane thickening of tubules and capillaries, interstitial fibrosis and focal coagulative necrosis. Necrotic areas eventually become confluent and extend to the corticomedullary junction, after which the collecting ducts become involved. Few inflammatory cells are found around the necrotic foci. Eventually, the entire papilla becomes necrotic **(papillary necrosis),** often remaining in place as a structureless mass. Dystrophic calcification of such necrotic papillae is common. Papillae may remain partly attached at the demarcation zone or be completely sloughed. There is secondary tubular atrophy, interstitial fibrosis and chronic inflammation in the overlying cortex.

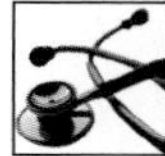

CLINICAL FEATURES: Signs and symptoms occur only late in analgesic nephropathy and include an inability to concentrate the urine, distal tubular acidosis, hematuria, hypertension and anemia. Sloughing of necrotic papillary tips into the renal pelvis may result in colic as they pass through the ureters. Progressive renal failure often develops and leads to end-stage renal disease.

Drug-Induced (Hypersensitivity) Acute Tubulointerstitial Nephritis Is a Cell-Mediated Immune Response

MOLECULAR PATHOGENESIS: Acute drug-induced tubulointerstitial nephritis is characterized histologically by infiltrates of activated T cells and eosinophils, a pattern that indicates a type IV cell-mediated immune reaction. The immunogen could be the drug itself, the drug bound to certain tissue components, a drug metabolite or a tissue component altered due to the drug. Drugs most commonly implicated include NSAIDs, diuretics and certain antibiotics, especially β-lactam antibiotics, such as synthetic penicillins and cephalosporins.

PATHOLOGY: Microscopically, there is patchy infiltration of cortex and (to a much lesser extent) medulla by lymphocytes and occasional eosinophils (5% to 10% of the total leukocytes in the tissue) (Fig. 16-77). Eosinophils tend to concentrate in small foci and may be seen within tubular lumina and in the urine. Neutrophils are rare; their presence should raise suspicion of pyelonephritis or hematogenous bacterial infection. Granulomatous foci may be seen, especially later in the disease. Proximal and distal tubules are focally invaded by white blood cells ("tubulitis"). Glomeruli and vessels are not inflamed, but drug-induced tubulointerstitial nephritis caused by NSAIDs may show minimal-change glomerulopathy.

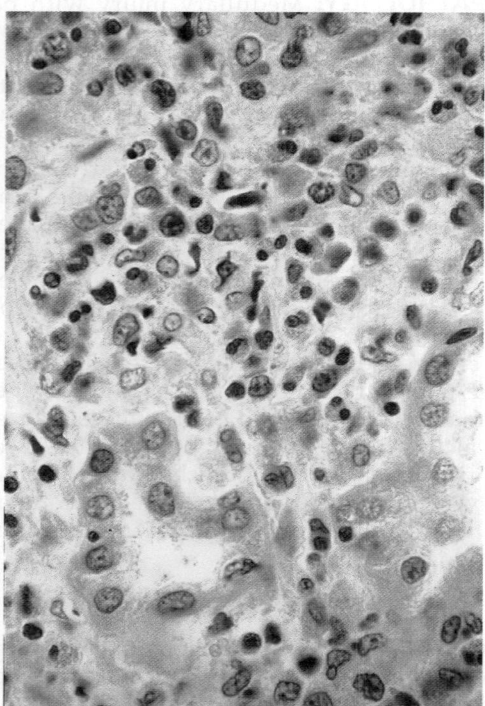

FIGURE 16-77. Hypersensitivity tubulointerstitial nephritis. There is interstitial edema and infiltration by mononuclear leukocytes, with admixed eosinophils.

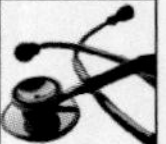

CLINICAL FEATURES: Acute tubulointerstitial nephritis usually presents as acute renal failure, typically about 2 weeks after a drug is started. Urinalysis shows erythrocytes, leukocytes (including eosinophils) and sometimes leukocyte casts. Tubular defects are common, including sodium wasting, glucosuria, aminoaciduria and renal tubular acidosis. Systemic allergic symptoms such as fever and rash may also be present. Most patients recover fully within several weeks or months if the offending drug is discontinued.

Light-Chain Cast Nephropathy May Complicate Multiple Myeloma

Light-chain cast nephropathy is renal injury caused by monoclonal immunoglobulin light chains in the urine, which produce tubular epithelial injury and numerous tubular casts.

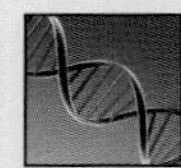

MOLECULAR PATHOGENESIS: As discussed above, multiple myeloma may produce AL amyloidosis, light-chain deposition disease, heavy-chain deposition disease and light-chain cast nephropathy. The latter is the most common renal disease associated with multiple myeloma, and is caused by glomerular filtering of circulating light chains. At the acidic pH typical of urine, the light chains bind to Tamm-Horsfall glycoproteins secreted by distal tubular epithelial cells and form casts. Renal dysfunction results from the toxicity of free light chains for tubular epithelium and obstruction by the casts. Light chain structure determines whether they will induce light-chain cast nephropathy, AL amyloidosis or light-chain deposition disease. Occasional patients show several of these renal diseases.

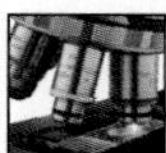

PATHOLOGY: Tubular lesions show many dense, brightly eosinophilic and glassy (hyaline) casts in the distal tubules and collecting ducts (Fig. 16-78). Casts often have fractures, angular borders and a crystalline appearance. They may elicit foreign body reactions, with macrophages and multinucleated giant cells. Interstitial chronic inflammation and edema typically accompany the tubular lesions. More chronic lesions show interstitial fibrosis and tubular atrophy. Focal calcium deposits **(nephrocalcinosis)** are often noted in the fibrotic interstitium of the tubules. By immunostaining, casts contain light chains and Tamm-Horsfall proteins.

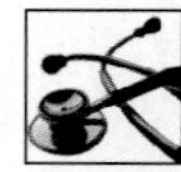

CLINICAL FEATURES: Light-chain cast nephropathy may manifest as acute or chronic renal failure. Proteinuria is usually present, but not necessarily in the nephrotic range, and most often consists predominantly of immunoglobulin light chains. Nephrotic-range proteinuria in multiple myeloma suggests AL amyloidosis or light-chain deposition disease rather than light-chain cast nephropathy.

In Urate Nephropathy, Urate Crystals Deposit in the Tubules and Interstitium

Any condition with elevated blood levels of uric acid may cause urate nephropathy. The classic chronic disease in this category is primary gout (see Chapter 26).

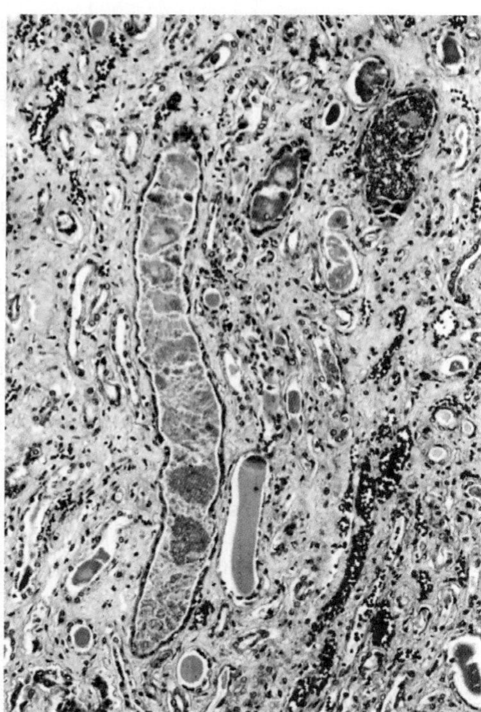

FIGURE 16-78. Light-chain cast nephropathy. A light micrograph shows numerous casts within tubular lumina.

MOLECULAR PATHOGENESIS: In **chronic urate nephropathy** due to gout, crystalline monosodium urate is deposited in tubules and interstitium. **Acute urate nephropathy** can be caused by increased cell turnover (e.g., leukemia or polycythemia). For example, chemotherapy for malignant neoplasms results in **tumor lysis syndrome,** a sudden increase in blood uric acid due to massive necrosis of cancer cells. Hepatic catabolism of large amounts of purines released from the DNA of necrotic cells leads to hyperuricemia. Uric acid crystals precipitate in the acidic pH of collecting ducts, leading to obstruction and acute renal failure. Interference with uric acid excretion (e.g., chronic intake of certain diuretics) can also cause hyperuricemia. Chronic lead intoxication interferes with uric acid secretion by proximal tubules and leads to **saturnine gout.**

PATHOLOGY: In acute urate nephropathy, uric acid precipitated in collecting ducts is seen grossly as yellow streaks in the papillae. Histologically, the tubular deposits appear amorphous, but in frozen sections, birefringent crystals are apparent (Fig. 16-79). Proximal to the obstruction tubules are dilated. Uric acid crystals in collecting ducts may also elicit foreign body reactions.

The basic disease process of chronic urate nephropathy is similar to that of the acute form, but the prolonged course results in greater deposition of urate crystals in the interstitium, interstitial fibrosis and cortical atrophy. The diagnostic feature is the **gouty tophus,** a focal accumulation of urate crystals surrounded by inflammatory cells, which may appear granulomatous and include multinucleated giant cells. Uric acid stones account for 10% of all cases of urolithiasis, and occur in 20% of patients with chronic gout and 40% of those with acute hyperuricemia.

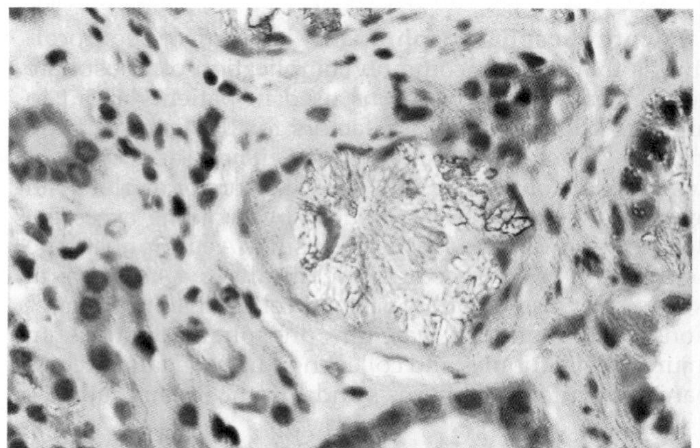

FIGURE 16-79. Urate nephropathy. A frozen section demonstrates tubular deposits of uric acid crystals.

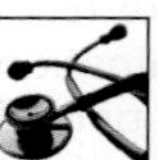

CLINICAL FEATURES: Acute urate nephropathy manifests as acute renal failure; chronic urate nephropathy causes chronic renal tubular defects. Although histologic renal lesions are seen in most patients with chronic gout, less than half have significant renal functional impairment.

Nephrocalcinosis Is Deposition of Calcium in the Renal Parenchyma

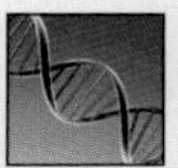

MOLECULAR PATHOGENESIS: Hypercalciuria may result in nephrocalcinosis (Table 16-13), formation of calcium-containing stones **(nephrolithiasis)** or both. Nephrocalcinosis may impair renal function, especially tubular defects such as poor concentrating ability, salt wasting and renal tubular acidosis. If nephrocalcinosis is caused by hypercalcemia, it is categorized as **metastatic calcification,** while calcification at sites of renal parenchymal injury (e.g., infarcts or cortical necrosis) is representative of **dystrophic calcification.**

Table 16-13

Causes of Hypercalcemia That Lead to Nephrocalcinosis

Increased Resorption of Calcium From Bone
Renal osteodystrophy
Primary hyperparathyroidism
Neoplasms producing parathormone or parathormone-like protein
Osteolytic neoplasms and metastases
Increased Intestinal Absorption of Calcium
Idiopathic hypercalcemia
Vitamin D excess
Milk-alkali syndrome
Sarcoidosis

Acute phosphate nephropathy is a form of nephrocalcinosis that is an uncommon complication of phosphate bowel cleansing preparations used in patients about to undergo colonoscopy. Risk factors for this complication include older age, renal insufficiency and use of angiotensin-converting enzyme inhibitors or angiotensin receptor blockers. Risk is reduced by avoiding excessive dehydration during bowel cleansing. Acute phosphate nephropathy is characterized clinically by AKI several weeks after use of phosphate bowel cleansing preparations. Pathologically, calcium phosphate deposits in injured distal tubules and collecting ducts, usually accompanied by interstitial fibrosis and chronic inflammation.

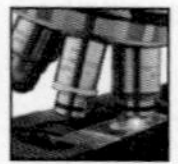

PATHOLOGY: At autopsy, 20% of kidneys have small calcium deposits that have no functional significance or recognized association with hypercalcemia. In patients with nephrocalcinosis caused by hypercalcemia, the extent of calcification varies from microscopic deposits to marked calcium accumulation visible grossly and radiologically. If hypercalcemia is severe (e.g., caused by primary hyperparathyroidism), gross examination characteristically reveals wedge-shaped scars interspersed with relatively normal renal tissue. These scars reflect parenchymal atrophy and interstitial fibrosis caused by the calcification. Histologically, there is striking calcification of renal tubular basement membranes, particularly in proximal convoluted tubules. The interstitial tissue also contains calcium deposits. Such deposits also accumulate in the cytoplasm of tubular epithelial cells, which eventually degenerate and are sloughed into the lumina to aggregate as calcified casts. Scattered glomeruli show calcification of the Bowman capsule. Intrarenal arteries may also be calcified. Calcium deposits stain deeply blue with hematoxylin. They are black with the more specific von Kossa stain. By electron microscopy, the mitochondria of renal tubular epithelial cells contain abundant calcium deposits.

Renal Stones (Nephrolithiasis and Urolithiasis)

Nephrolithiasis and urolithiasis are stones within the renal collecting system **(nephrolithiasis)** or elsewhere in the collecting system of the urinary tract **(urolithiasis).** Calculi often form and accumulate in the renal pelvis and calyces. Stones vary in composition, depending on individual factors, geography, metabolic alterations and the presence of infection.

For unknown reasons, renal stones are more common in men than in women. They vary in size from gravel (<1 mm in diameter) to large stones that dilate the entire renal pelvis. While they may be well tolerated, in some cases, they lead to severe hydronephrosis and pyelonephritis. They can also erode the mucosa and cause hematuria. Passage of a stone into the ureter causes excruciating flank pain, **renal colic.** Until recently, most kidney stones required surgical removal, but ultrasonic disintegration (lithotripsy) and endoscopic removal are now effective.

A urinary stone is usually associated with increased blood levels and urinary excretion of its principal component. This is the case with uric acid and cystine stones. However, many patients with calcium stones have hypercalciuria without hypercalcemia. Mixed urate and calcium stones are common with hyperuricemia, as urate crystals act as a nidus for calcium salts to precipitate.

- **Calcium stones:** Most (75%) renal stones are calcium complexed with oxalate or phosphate, or a mixture of these anions. Calcium oxalate is more common in the United States, whereas in England, calcium phosphate predominates. Calcium oxalate stones are hard and occasionally dark, because they are covered by hemorrhage from the mucosa of the renal pelvis injured by the sharp calcium oxalate crystals. Calcium phosphate stones tend to be softer and paler.
- **Infection stones:** Infection, often with urea-splitting bacteria like *Proteus* or *Providencia* spp., cause about 15% of stones. Resulting alkaline urine favors magnesium ammonium phosphate **(struvite)** and calcium phosphate **(apatite)** precipitation. Such stones may be hard, or soft and friable. Infection stones occasionally fill the pelvis and calyces to form a cast of these spaces, a **staghorn calculus** (Fig. 16-80). Infection stones cause frequent complications, such as intractable urinary tract infection, pain, bleeding, perinephric abscess and urosepsis.
- **Uric acid stones:** These stones occur in 25% of patients with hyperuricemia and gout, but most patients with uric acid stones have neither condition **(idiopathic urate lithiasis).** Urate stones are smooth, hard and yellow, and are usually less than 2 cm in diameter. Importantly, and in contrast to calcium-containing stones, pure uric acid stones are radiolucent.
- **Cystine stones:** These stones account for only 1% of total stones but are a significant fraction of childhood calculi, and occur exclusively in hereditary cystinuria. Although the stones are composed entirely of cystine, they may be enveloped by a layer of calcium phosphate.

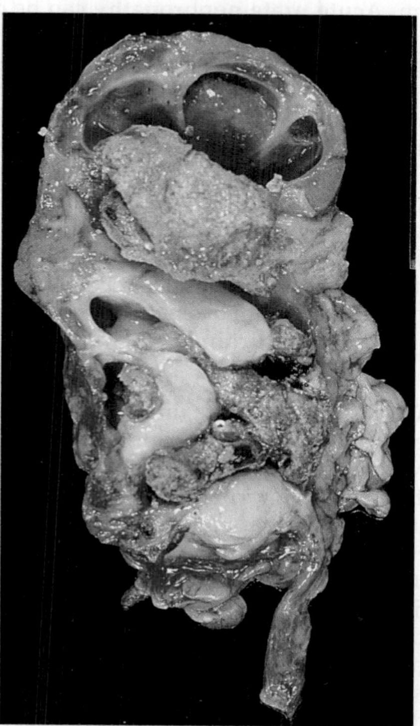

FIGURE 16-80. Staghorn calculi. The kidney shows hydronephrosis and stones that are casts of the dilated calyces.

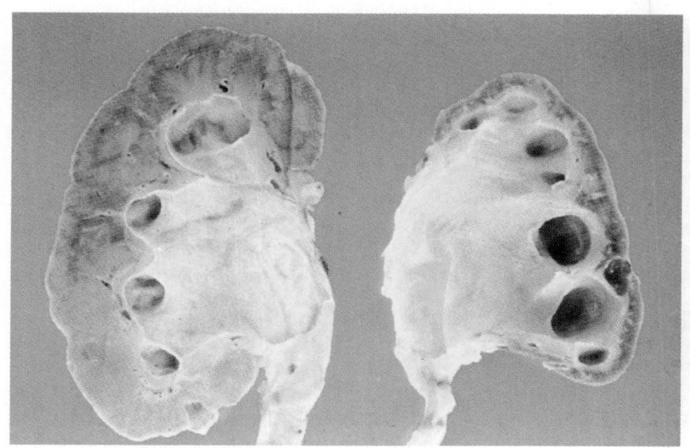

FIGURE 16-81. Hydronephrosis. Bilateral urinary tract obstruction has led to conspicuous dilation of the ureters, pelves and calyces. The kidney on the right shows severe parenchymal atrophy.

Table 16-14

Categories of Renal Allograft Rejection

Category	Most Characteristic Lesion
Hyperacute humoral rejection	Neutrophils in peritubular capillaries, hemorrhage and necrosis
Acute cellular rejection	
Acute tubulointerstitial rejection	Tubulitis (mononuclear leukocytes in tubules)
Acute cellular vascular rejection	Endarteritis (mononuclear leukocytes in intima)
Acute humoral rejection	
Acute humoral capillary rejection	Neutrophils and C4d in capillaries
Acute necrotizing vascular rejection	Arterial fibrinoid necrosis
Chronic rejection	Arterial intimal thickening, interstitial fibrosis and tubular atrophy Glomerular capillary wall thickening C4d in glomerular and peritubular capillaries

Obstructive Uropathy and Hydronephrosis

Obstructive uropathy is caused by structural or functional abnormalities in the urinary tract that impede urine flow, which may cause renal dysfunction (obstructive nephropathy) and dilation of the collecting system (hydronephrosis). Urinary tract obstruction is detailed in Chapter 17.

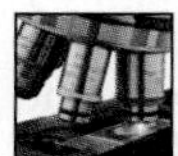

PATHOLOGY: The most prominent microscopic finding in early hydronephrosis is dilation of collecting ducts, followed by dilation of proximal and distal convoluted tubules. Eventually, the proximal tubules become widely dilated, and loss of tubules is common. Glomeruli are usually spared. Grossly, progressive dilation of the renal pelvis and calyces occurs, and atrophy of the renal parenchyma ensues (Fig. 16-81). A hydronephrotic kidney is more susceptible to pyelonephritis, which adds injury to insult.

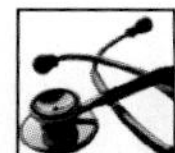

CLINICAL FEATURES: Bilateral acute urinary tract obstruction causes acute renal failure **(postrenal acute renal failure).** Unilateral obstruction is often asymptomatic. As many causes of acute obstruction are reversible, prompt recognition is important. Left untreated, an obstructed kidney undergoes atrophy. If obstruction is bilateral, chronic renal failure ensues.

Renal Transplantation

Renal transplantation is the treatment of choice for most patients with end-stage renal disease. The major obstacle is immunologic rejection, but the disease that destroyed the native kidneys and nephrotoxicity from immunosuppressive drugs may both injure the renal allograft. Table 16-14 lists distinct, but often coexisting, patterns of humoral and cellular renal allograft rejection.

ABO blood group antigens and **HLA antigens** are the two main antigenic targets on a transplanted kidney. ABO antigens are expressed on endothelial cells and erythrocytes, and are the most problematic barriers to transplantation. Because anti-ABO antibodies are preformed, they bind to graft endothelial cells and cause immediate (hyperacute) rejection. ***The more commonly encountered (and more gradual) patterns of acute and chronic rejection are caused primarily by recipient reactivity against donor HLA antigens. HLA are several closely related loci on chromosome 6, whose products are expressed on most cells, including endothelial cells.*** Sensitization of kidney allograft recipients to HLAs produces both cell-mediated and antibody-mediated reactions (see Chapter 4). Renal allograft rejection can be classified on the basis of its clinical course, pathologic features and presumed pathogenesis (Table 16-14). However, an allograft may be subject to more than one type of rejection at the same time.

HYPERACUTE HUMORAL REJECTION: Hyperacute rejection is rare (fewer than 0.5% of grafts) because of current compatibility testing. If recipient blood with antibodies to major alloantigens (usually ABO or class I HLAs) enters allograft vessels, those antibodies immediately bind endothelial cells and cause prompt and irreversible injury within minutes. Intraoperatively, the graft may become mottled, cyanotic and flaccid. Antibody binding to endothelial alloantigens activates complement, thereby attracting neutrophils. The cytotoxic effects of complement and neutrophil activation cause endothelial cell swelling, vacuolization and lysis. Accumulation of neutrophils in glomerular capillaries is a sign of impending rejection. Endothelial cell changes are followed by platelet thrombi and later by fibrin thrombi. Interstitial edema, hemorrhage and cortical necrosis develop over the next 12 to 24 hours.

ACUTE HUMORAL REJECTION: The most common type of acute humoral rejection is directed primarily at capillaries and may cause only subtle or no pathologic changes by light microscopy. Neutrophils or mononuclear leukocytes are

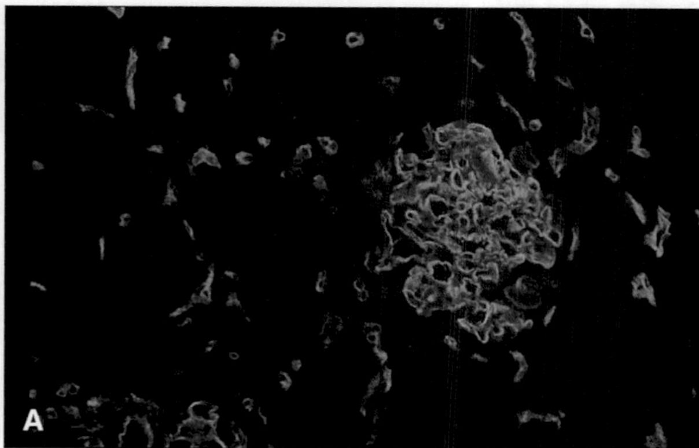

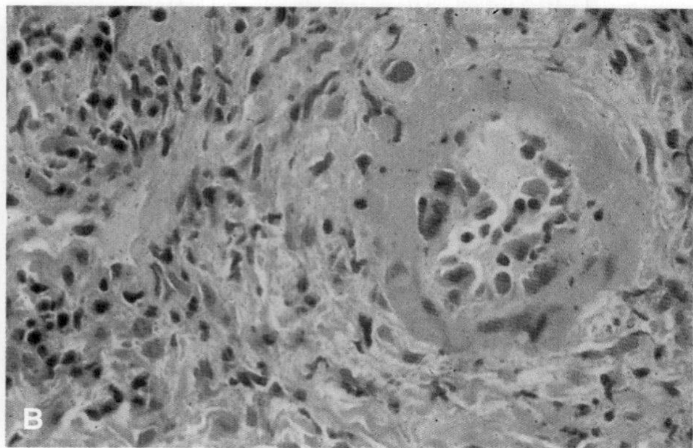

FIGURE 16-82. Acute humoral allograft rejection. A. Staining of peritubular and glomerular capillaries with a fluoresceinated anti-C4d antibody showing evidence of complement activation by antibodies directed against donor antigens on endothelial cells. **B.** Acute humoral necrotizing acute vasculitis in an interlobular artery with extensive fibrinoid necrosis of the muscularis. The vascular and interstitial infiltrates of mononuclear leukocytes indicate concurrent acute cellular rejection.

increased in peritubular and glomerular capillaries, and in tubules. Complement activation products, especially C4d, localize to the walls of peritubular and glomerular capillaries (Fig. 16-82A) consistently. The most severe, but least common, pattern of acute humoral rejection involves **necrotizing arteritis** with fibrinoid necrosis of the media (Fig. 16-82B). It occurs in less than 1% of allografts in patients whose immunosuppression includes a calcineurin inhibitor, although before these agents were introduced it occurred in 5% of renal allografts. If necrotizing arteritis develops, fewer than 30% of grafts survive 1 year, even with aggressive immunosuppression.

ACUTE CELLULAR REJECTION: ***This is the most common form of acute rejection.*** It is characterized by infiltration of the interstitium, tubules, arteries, arterioles or glomeruli by T lymphocytes and macrophages. Nuclei of infiltrating lymphocytes vary in size and shape because the cells are at various stages of activation. Immunoblasts may be seen. Usually, interstitial infiltrates are patchy, rather than diffuse. Involvement of tubules **(tubulitis)** is manifested by lymphocytes crossing tubular basement membranes and lying between tubular epithelial cells (Fig. 16-83A). Arterial involvement by cellular rejection leads to penetration of T lymphocytes and monocytes across the endothelium, expanding the intima with mononuclear leukocytes **(intimal arteritis, or endarteritis)** (Fig. 16-83B). Arterioles are occasionally similarly affected. Glomerular infiltration by mononuclear leukocytes with obliteration of capillary lumens **(acute transplant glomerulitis)** is uncommon in acute cellular rejection. Renal transplants with tubulitis but not endarteritis have an 80% chance for 1-year graft survival, compared with 60% for allografts with end-arteritis.

CHRONIC HUMORAL REJECTION: The pathology of this type of rejection includes **chronic transplant arteriopathy** and **chronic transplant glomerulopathy** (Table 16-15).

Chronic rejection affects arteries of all sizes, up to the main renal artery. In chronic transplant arteriopathy the intima is thickened by stromal cell proliferation and matrix deposition (Fig. 16-84), but without the dense fibrosis and elastic lamination seen in nonspecific arteriosclerosis. Inflammation is absent, or much less prominent than in active acute cell-mediated intimal arteritis (Fig. 16-83B). Foam cells may be conspicuous and the internal elastic lamina may be interrupted. Peritubular capillaries show basement membrane thickening and replication.

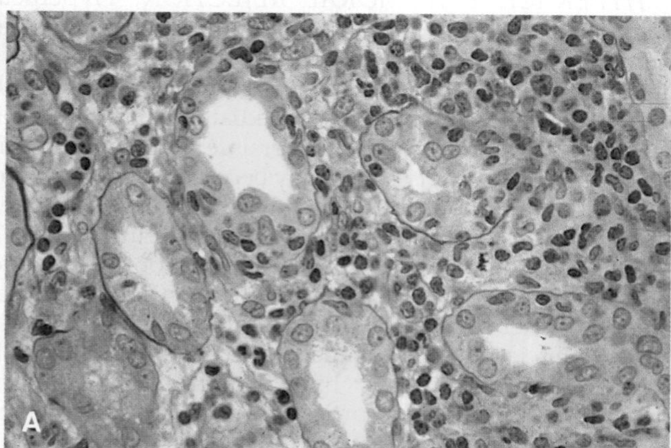

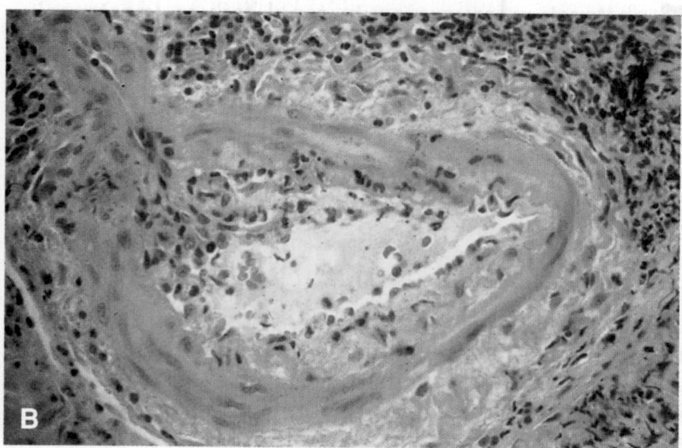

FIGURE 16-83. Acute cellular allograft rejection. A. Acute tubulointerstitial cellular rejection with tubulitis indicated by the lymphocytes on the epithelial side of the basement membrane (period acid–Schiff stain). **B.** Acute cellular vascular rejection with endarteritis indicated by the mononuclear leukocytes infiltrating into the intima of an arcuate artery.

Table 16-15

Histologic Features of Chronic Renal Allograft Rejection

Fibrotic intimal thickening of arteries
Tubular atrophy
Interstitial fibrosis
Interstitial mononuclear leukocytes
Glomerular capillary wall thickening and mesangial expansion
Glomerular sclerosis

In chronic transplant glomerulopathy, the walls of glomerular capillaries are thickened, owing to expansion of the glomerular capillary subendothelial zone and replication of glomerular basement membranes. This also occurs in peritubular capillaries. The mesangium is widened. These changes apparently result from persistent, low-level, immune injury to the vascular endothelium because donor-specific, antiendothelial antibodies usually are detected in serum and C4d is often present in peritubular and glomerular capillary walls. Ischemia due to narrowing of arteries and peritubular capillaries leads, in part, to tubular atrophy and interstitial fibrosis. Tubulointerstitial injury may also result from indolent tubulitis.

RECURRENCE OF KIDNEY DISEASE: The same disease that led to renal failure in native kidneys may recur in a transplanted kidney. The frequency and significance of recurrence vary among different types of glomerular disease (Table 16-16).

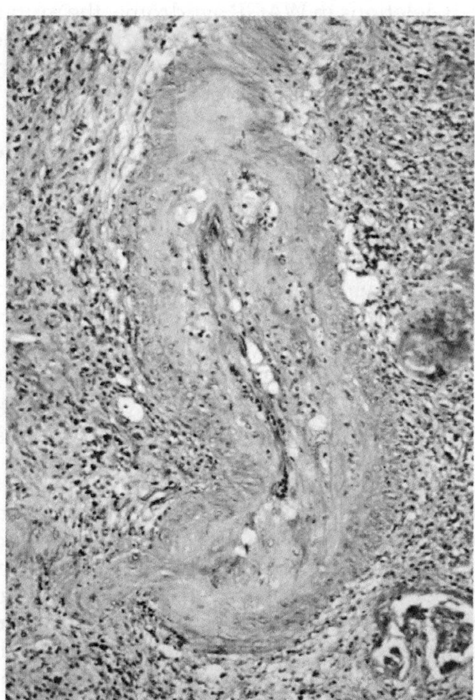

FIGURE 16-84. Chronic humoral allograft rejection. The lumen of this medium-sized artery is occluded by a thickened intima, which contains a few inflammatory cells.

Table 16-16

Recurrence of Disease in Renal Allografts

Disease	Recurrence Rate (%)	Rate of Graft Loss (%)
Type II membranoproliferative glomerulonephritis	>90	15
Diabetic glomerulosclerosis	>90	<5
IgA nephropathy	40	<10
Focal segmental glomerulosclerosis	35	30
Type I membranoproliferative glomerulonephritis	30	<10
Membranous glomerulopathy	20	<5
ANCA glomerulonephritis	15	<5
Anti-GBM glomerulonephritis	5	<5
Lupus glomerulonephritis	5	<5

ANCA = antineutrophil cytoplasmic autoantibody; GBM = glomerular basement membrane; IgA = immunoglobulin A.

CALCINEURIN INHIBITOR NEPHROTOXICITY OF CYCLOSPORINE AND TACROLIMUS (FK506): Cyclosporine and tacrolimus are immunosuppressive inhibitors of calcineurin that have dramatically improved allograft survival for kidneys and other organs (e.g., liver, heart, lungs). Unfortunately, both drugs are nephrotoxic and can injure both kidney allografts and native kidneys of patients given these drugs for other reasons. Acute or chronic renal failure can result.

The most characteristic renal lesion is an **arteriolopathy** that begins with smooth muscle cell degeneration and necrosis. The destroyed arteriolar muscle cells are replaced by acidophilic hyaline material (Fig. 16-85). In fulminant cases, vascular lesions take on the appearance of a full-blown thrombotic microangiopathy, with circumferential fibrinoid necrosis of arterioles. In chronic toxicity there are zones of interstitial fibrosis and tubular atrophy ("striped fibrosis").

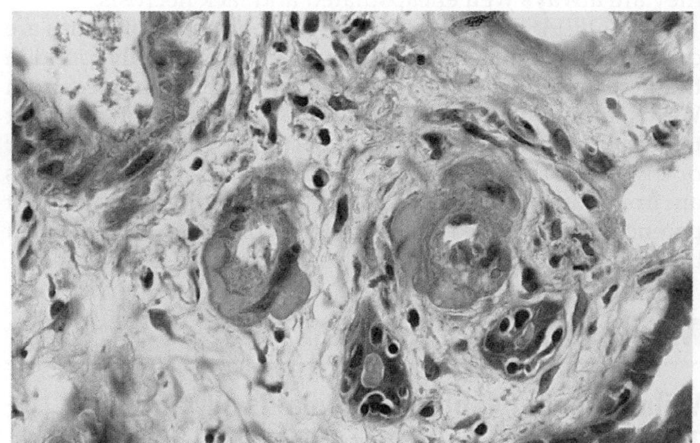

FIGURE 16-85. Cyclosporine nephrotoxicity with arteriolopathy. Marked destructive hyalinosis of arterioles is present.

BK POLYOMAVIRUS INFECTION: Reactivation of latent BK virus infection in a transplant can be caused by immunosuppression, and can result in acute tubular injury and tubulointerstitial nephritis. Intranuclear viral inclusions in tubular cells may suggest this possibility, which can be confirmed by immunohistochemistry.

Benign Tumors of the Kidney

PAPILLARY RENAL ADENOMA: There is controversy as to whether any epithelial renal cell tumor should be considered benign. Tumor size, which has been used to separate adenomas from carcinomas, is problematic because all carcinomas start out as small lesions. Renal epithelial neoplasms less than 3 cm in diameter rarely metastasize, but "rarely" is not "never." Tumors composed of cells resembling clear cell, chromophobe or collecting duct RCCs should not be called adenomas even if they are small. Neoplasms under 5 mm with papillary or tubulopapillary growth patterns can be considered adenomas. Papillary renal adenomas occur more often with advancing age, and are incidental autopsy findings in 40% of patients over 70.

RENAL ONCOCYTOMA: This benign neoplasm accounts for 5% to 10% of primary renal neoplasms removed surgically. The neoplastic cells derive from collecting duct intercalated cells. They are plump, with abundant, finely granular, acidophilic cytoplasm and round nuclei that lack atypia. The distinctive appearance of the tumor is due to abundant mitochondria in the cytoplasm. Grossly, oncocytomas are characteristically mahogany-brown owing to mitochondrial lipochrome pigments. Renal oncocytomas rarely metastasize.

MEDULLARY FIBROMA: Medullary fibromas (renomedullary interstitial cell tumors) are typically small (<0.5 cm in diameter), pale gray, well-circumscribed tumors, usually in the midportion of medullary pyramids. They are composed of small stellate to polygonal cells in a loose stroma. Renal medullary fibromas are incidental findings in half of all adult autopsies.

ANGIOMYOLIPOMA: ***These tumors are strongly associated with tuberous sclerosis.*** Of patients with tuberous sclerosis, 80% have angiomyolipomas, but fewer than 50% of patients with angiomyolipomas have tuberous sclerosis. These lesions are mixtures of well-differentiated adipose tissue, smooth muscle and thick-walled vessels. Grossly, they are yellow and bosselated, and may resemble RCC. However, they are always well encapsulated and lack necrosis.

MESOBLASTIC NEPHROMA: Mesoblastic nephromas are congenital benign neoplasms or hamartomas usually found in the first 3 months of life. They must be differentiated from Wilms tumors. The lesions range from under 1 cm in diameter to over 15 cm, and are composed of spindle cells of fibroblastic or myofibroblastic lineage. Characteristically, tumor margins are irregular, with bands of cells interdigitating with adjacent parenchyma. If some of these tongues of tumor tissue are left behind after surgical resection, local recurrence is possible.

Malignant Tumors of the Kidney

Wilms Tumor (Nephroblastoma) Is a Malignant Tumor of Embryonal Renal Elements

Component nephrogenic elements include mixtures of blastemal, stromal and epithelial tissue. With a prevalence of 1 in 10,000, this is the most common abdominal solid tumor of children.

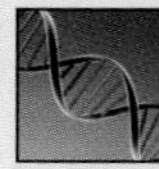

MOLECULAR PATHOGENESIS: In most (90%) cases the Wilms tumor is sporadic and unilateral. In 5% of cases, however, it arises as part of three different congenital syndromes, all of which increase risk for development of this cancer at an early age and often bilaterally:

- **WAGR syndrome**—*W*ilms tumor, *a*niridia, *g*enitourinary anomalies, mental *r*etardation
- **Denys-Drash syndrome (DDS)**—Wilms tumor, intersexual disorders, glomerular mesangial sclerosis
- **Beckwith-Wiedemann syndrome (BWS)**—Wilms tumor, overgrowth ranging from gigantism to hemihypertrophy, visceromegaly and macroglossia

Some 6% of cases of Wilms tumor are familial, have an early onset and are bilateral but are not associated with any other syndrome.

WAGR syndrome is due to a deletion in the short arm of chromosome 11 (11p13). Affected genes include the aniridia gene (PAX6) and ***WT1*, Wilms tumor gene 1.** WT1 is a DNA-binding transcription factor expressed in kidneys and gonads. Loss or mutation of one *WT1* allele leads to genitourinary anomalies. A defect in *PAX6* causes aniridia. One third of children with WAGR syndrome will develop Wilms tumors. The presence of a germline mutation in one *WT1* allele and loss of heterozygosity at this locus in the tumors of WAGR syndrome imply that acquired somatic mutation in the remaining *WT1* allele is needed for Wilms tumor to occur (similar to the pathogenesis of hereditary retinoblastoma; see Chapter 5). In contrast to deletions in WAGR syndrome, the mutations of the *WT1* gene in DDS are thought to be dominant negative mutations, possibly accounting for the fact that the DDS phenotype is far more severe than that of WAGR syndrome.

WT1 is a tumor-suppressor protein that regulates transcription of several other genes, including insulin-like growth factor-II (IGF-II) and platelet-derived growth factor (PDGF). WT1 protein also forms a complex with p53. Whereas Wilms tumors arising in the context of WAGR syndrome all have WT1 mutations, only 10% to 20% of sporadic Wilms tumors do. Thus, other genes probably are more critical than *WT1* in the genesis of sporadic Wilms tumors. Of sporadic Wilms tumors, 10% have a gain-of-function mutation in the β-catenin (*CTNNB1*) gene, a member of the developmentally important WNT signaling pathway.

Sporadic Wilms tumors often show loss of heterozygosity (LOH) at a second Wilms tumor susceptibility locus (*WT2*), on chromosome 11 (11p15.5). This site is distinct from, but close to, the *WT1* gene. *WT2* is also linked to BWS. Interestingly, in LOH at the *WT2* locus in sporadic Wilms tumors, the lost allele is invariably the maternal one, and some patients with BWS show germline duplication of the paternal *WT2* allele while others apparently inherited both of their normal copies of this gene from their father and none from the mother (*paternal uniparental isodisomy*). Normally, only the paternal allele of *WT2* may be expressed (*genomic imprinting*), so WT2 overexpression may lead to the overgrowth characteristic of BWS. Since the *IGF-II 2* gene also maps to chromosome 11p15 and is also paternally imprinted, increased dosage of *IGF-II 2* might also contribute to BWS and to tumorigenesis.

The *WTX* gene on the X chromosome is mutated in 20% to 30% of Wilms tumors. WTX may act as a tumor suppressor by downregulating WNT/β-catenin signalling. Mutations in WT1, CTNNB1, WT2 and WTX that are associated with Wilms tumor all activate the WNT signaling pathway, which thus appears to have a role in a final common pathway of tumorigenesis. Another possibility is that *WT2* is expressed only by the maternal allele acting as a tumor suppressor. Thus, loss of the maternal allele would contribute to tumorigenesis.

Nephrogenic rests (small foci of persistent primitive blastemal cells) are found in the kidneys of all children with syndromic Wilms tumors and in one third of sporadic cases. Given that such rests in the nontumorous kidney contain the same somatic mutations in *WT1* as are present in the tumors, these rests may represent clonal precursor lesions one or more steps along the pathway to tumor formation.

PATHOLOGY: Wilms tumors tend to be large when detected, with bulging, pale tan, cut surfaces enclosed by a thin rim of renal cortex and capsule (Fig. 16-86). Histologically, the tumor resembles normal fetal renal tissue (Fig. 16-87), including (1) metanephric blastema, (2) immature stroma (mesenchymal tissue) and (3) immature epithelial elements.

Although most Wilms tumors contain all three elements in varying proportions, occasionally only two elements or even only one is seen. The blastema-like component contains small ovoid cells with scanty cytoplasm, growing in nests and trabeculae. The epithelial component appears as small tubular structures. Structures resembling immature glomeruli may sometimes be seen. The tumor stroma contains spindle cells, which are mostly undifferentiated but may show smooth muscle or fibroblast differentiation. Skeletal muscle is the most common heterotopic stromal element, although bone, cartilage, fat or neural tissue may rarely be encountered.

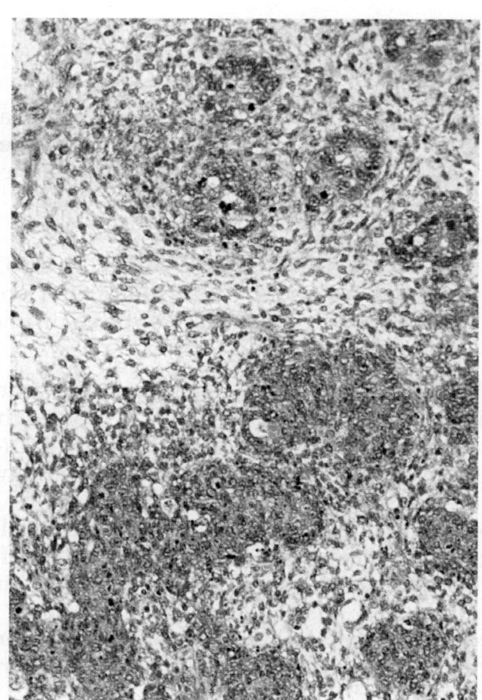

FIGURE 16-87. Wilms tumor (nephroblastoma). This photomicrograph of the tumor shows highly cellular areas composed of undifferentiated blastema, loose stroma containing undifferentiated mesenchymal cells and immature tubules.

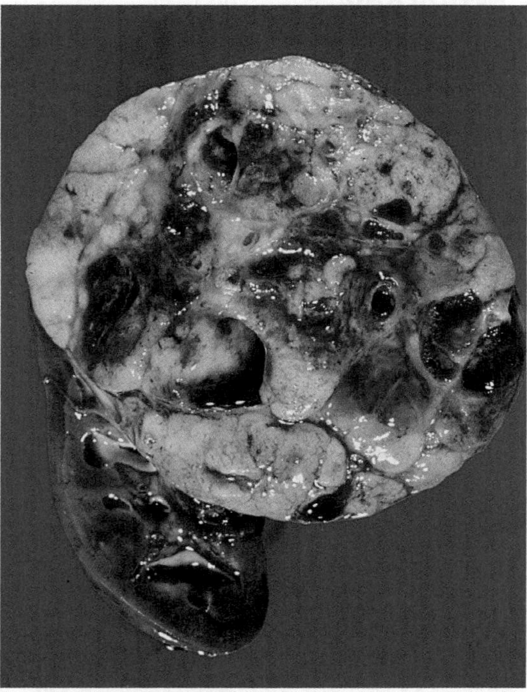

FIGURE 16-86. Wilms tumor. A cross-section of a pale tan neoplasm attached to a residual portion of the kidney.

CLINICAL FEATURES: Wilms tumors comprise 85% of pediatric renal neoplasms. They occur in 1 in 10,000 children, usually between 1 and 3 years of age, with 98% before age 10 years. The few familial cases usually exhibit autosomal dominant inheritance. Only 5% of sporadic cases are bilateral, contrasted with 20% of familial cases. Most often, the diagnosis is made after recognition of an abdominal mass. Additional manifestations include abdominal pain, intestinal obstruction, hypertension, hematuria and symptoms of traumatic tumor rupture.

Several histologic and clinical parameters have been used with varying success to predict the behavior of these tumors. Patients under 2 years of age tend to have a better prognosis. Presence of tumor outside the renal capsule at the time of surgery is a negative prognostic sign. Anaplasia (large, hyperchromatic nuclei and atypical mitoses) occurs more commonly in older patients, and contributes to their overall worse prognosis. Chemotherapy and radiation therapy, combined with surgical resection, have dramatically improved the outlook of patients with Wilms tumor, and many centers now report an overall long-term survival rate of 90%.

Renal Cell Carcinoma Is the Most Common Primary Cancer of the Kidney

RCC is a malignant neoplasm of renal tubular or ductal epithelial cells. It accounts for 80% to 90% of all primary renal cancers and over 30,000 cases occur each year in the United States.

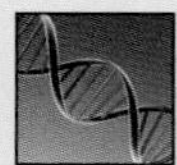

MOLECULAR PATHOGENESIS: Most RCCs are sporadic, but about 5% are inherited. Hereditary RCC occurs in the context of three distinct syndromes:

- **von Hippel-Lindau (VHL) syndrome,** an autosomal dominant cancer syndrome, with cerebellar hemangioblastomas, retinal angiomas, clear cell RCC (40% of all cases of VHL disease), pheochromocytoma and cysts in various organs
- **Autosomal dominant RCC,** in which a clear cell tumor is the primary manifestation and occurs in half of at-risk patients with genetic abnormalities like those in VHL syndrome
- **Hereditary papillary RCC,** an autosomal dominant inherited cancer characterized by multiple bilateral papillary tumors

Hereditary RCCs tend to be multifocal and bilateral, and appear at a younger age than do sporadic RCCs. A family history of RCC increases the risk for RCC by four- to fivefold.

A variety of translocations involving a breakpoint on chromosome 3 have been recognized in VHL syndrome and autosomal dominant RCC. Patients with sporadic RCC may have deletions and LOH in the short arm of chromosome 3 (3p) in the tumor tissue. Finally, the *VHL* gene is localized to 3p25-26. *VHL* is a tumor-suppressor gene. ***Loss of one VHL allele occurs in virtually all (98%) sporadic clear cell RCCs, and mutations in the gene are seen in more than half of these tumors.*** Thus, evidence strongly suggests that loss of *VHL* tumor-suppressive function is an important event in the pathogenesis of clear cell RCC. Abnormal VHL gene function causes the transcriptional regulatory molecule, hypoxia-inducible factor-α (HIF-α), to accumulate. In turn, genes that make proteins that activate kinase-dependent signalling pathways are transcriptionally upregulated. Components of these pathways are targets for kinase inhibitors and mTOR (mammalian target of rapamycin signalling) inhibitors that have proven useful for treating RCC.

Unlike clear cell RCC, hereditary papillary RCC is not associated with the *VHL* gene. Trisomies or tetrasomies of chromosomes 7, 16 and 17 and loss of the Y chromosome are seen in many cases. Mutations in c-*met* proto-oncogene (*MET*) at 7q31 are implicated in the development of hereditary papillary RCC.

Table 16-17

Categories of Renal Cell Carcinoma

Category	Frequency (%)
Clear cell type	70–80
Papillary type	10–15
Chromophobe type	5
Collecting duct type	1

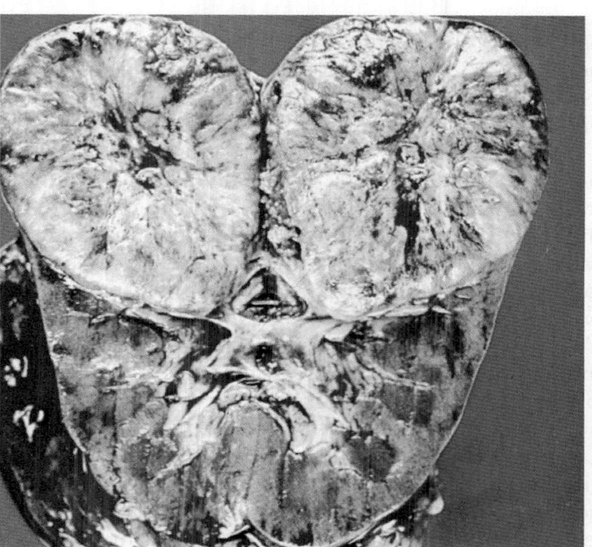

FIGURE 16-88. Clear cell renal cell carcinoma. The kidney contains a large irregular neoplasm with a variegated cut surface. Yellow areas correspond to lipid-containing cells.

Chromophobe RCCs derive from intercalated cells of the collecting ducts, and collecting duct RCCs originate in the ducts of Bellini of the medullary pyramids. Both of these tumors are associated with chromosome loss, including 1, 6 and 21.

Tobacco, whether smoked or chewed, increases risk of RCC: one third of these tumors are linked to tobacco use. Inherited and acquired renal cystic diseases may lead to RCC, especially papillary RCC. The cancer has also been tied to analgesic nephropathy.

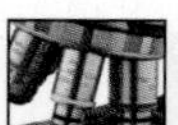

PATHOLOGY: The pathologic variants of RCC reflect differences in histogenesis and predict different outcomes. The histologic categories of RCC are shown in Table 16-17.

- **Clear cell RCC** is the most common type. It arises from proximal tubular epithelial cells. It is typically yellow-orange, solid or focally cystic, and focal hemorrhage and necrosis are common (Fig. 16-88). The removal of abundant cytoplasmic lipids and glycogen in tissue preparation accounts for the tumor cells' clear cytoplasm (Fig. 16-89).

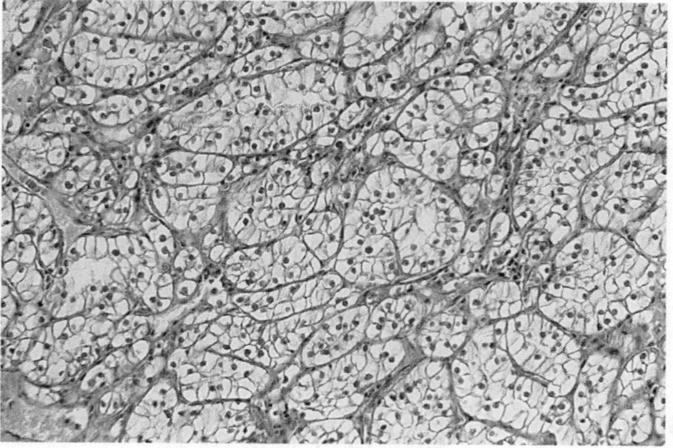

FIGURE 16-89. Clear cell renal cell carcinoma. Photomicrograph showing islands of neoplastic cells with abundant clear cytoplasm.

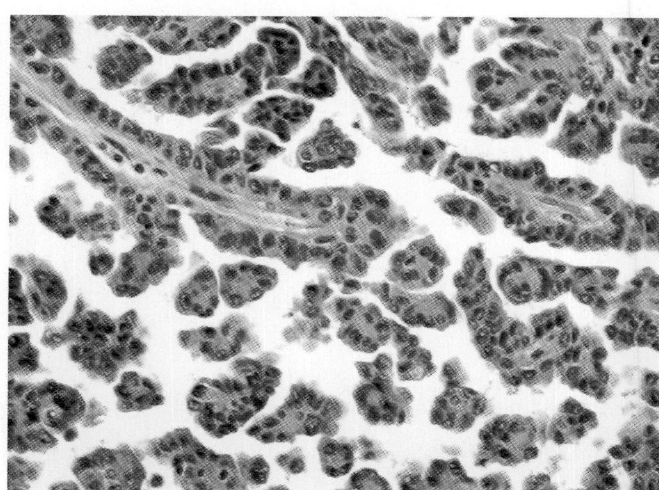

FIGURE 16-90. Papillary renal cell carcinoma. Photomicrograph showing papillary fronds covered by neoplastic cells.

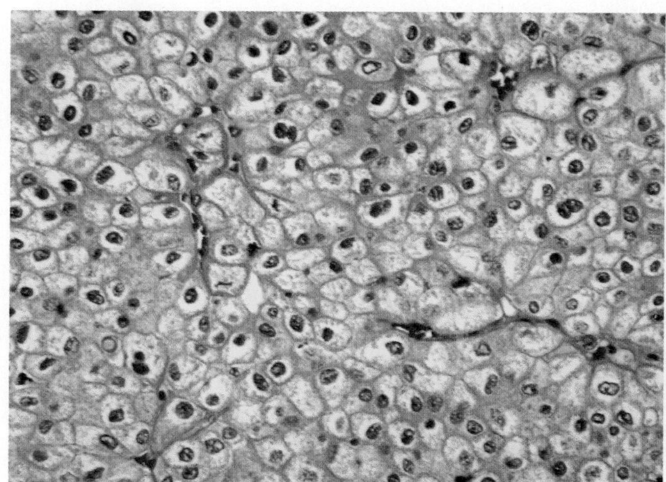

FIGURE 16-91. Chromophobe renal cell carcinoma. Photomicrograph showing pale acidophilic granular cells with prominent cell borders.

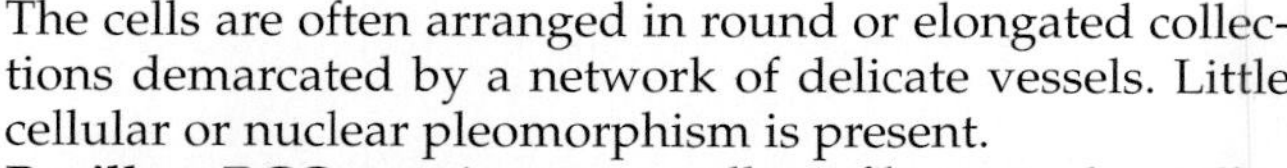

The cells are often arranged in round or elongated collections demarcated by a network of delicate vessels. Little cellular or nuclear pleomorphism is present.

- **Papillary RCC** contains tumor cells on fibrovascular stalks. Type 1 papillary RCC has small basophilic cells and type 2 has large acidophilic cells. The latter is more aggressive, with a worse prognosis. These tumors arise from proximal tubular epithelial cells (Fig. 16-90).
- **Chromophobe RCC** has a mixture of acidophilic granular cells and pale transparent cells with prominent cell borders, which impart a plant cell-like appearance (Fig. 16-91). Numerous cytoplasmic vesicles are filled with a distinctive mucopolysaccharide that stains with the Hale colloidal iron technique. These vesicles displace other organelles to the periphery, causing central cytoplasmic pallor. Chromophobe RCC appears to arise from intercalated cells of the renal collecting ducts.
- **Collecting duct RCC** is a rare variety that originates in medullary collecting ducts (ducts of Bellini) but may extend into the cortex. It is composed of tubular and papillary structures lined by a single layer of cuboidal cells with a hobnail appearance. Renal medullary carcinomas are variants of collecting duct carcinomas that develop almost exclusively in blacks with sickle cell trait or disease.
- **"Sarcomatoid" changes** may occur in any RCC and carry a worse prognosis.

The recommended histologic grading system for RCC is the Fuhrman system:

- **Grade I:** Nuclei round, uniform, 10 μm; nucleoli inconspicuous or absent
- **Grade II:** Nuclei irregular, 15 μm; nucleoli evident
- **Grade III:** Nuclei very irregular, 20 μm; nucleoli large and prominent
- **Grade IV:** Nuclei bizarre and multilobated, 20 μm or more; nucleoli prominent

CLINICAL FEATURES: Incidence of RCC peaks in the sixth decade. RCC occurs twice as often in men as in women. ***Hematuria is the single most common presenting sign, although many diagnoses are made incidentally during imaging studies of the abdomen performed for other reasons. The classic clinical triad of hematuria, flank pain and a palpable abdominal mass occurs in less than 10% of patients.*** RCC is known as a "great mimic," and the ectopic hormones it produces are frequently associated with fever and paraneoplastic syndromes. For example, secretion of a parathormone-like substance leads to symptoms of hyperparathyroidism; production of erythropoietin causes erythrocytosis; and RCC release of renin results in hypertension. Patients with RCC often come to medical attention because of symptoms from a metastasis. A sudden convulsion or a cough in a previously healthy person leads to discovery of an unsuspected tumor in the brain or lung, which on further examination proves to be RCC.

The prognosis for RCC is influenced by tumor size, extent of invasion and metastasis, histologic type and nuclear grade. Patients whose tumors show prominent sarcomatoid features rarely survive more than 1 year. By contrast, 1-year survival after nephrectomy for clear cell RCC is 50%. Papillary and chromophobe tumors have better prognoses than the clear cell type. Tumor stage (a measure of invasion and metastasis) is the most important prognostic factor. If the RCC is not beyond the renal capsule, 5-year survival is 90%; survival drops to 30% if there are distant metastases. The tumor spreads most frequently to the lungs and bones.

Transitional Cell Carcinoma

Between 5% and 10% of primary kidney cancers are transitional cell carcinomas of the pelvis or calyces (see Chapter 17). These are morphologically identical to the more common transitional cell carcinomas of the urinary bladder, and are associated with them in half of cases. Less than 5% of transitional cell carcinomas occur in the collecting system proximal to the bladder.

17 The Lower Urinary Tract and Male Reproductive System

Ivan Damjanov • Peter A. McCue

ANATOMY AND EMBRYOLOGY

Lower Urinary Tract

The ureters, urinary bladder and urethra—also known as the lower urinary tract—form the outflow part of the urinary system (Fig. 17-1). In males, the lower urinary tract is closely related to the reproductive system.

The Urinary Bladder Is in the Retroperitoneal Space of the Lower Abdomen

In males, the urinary bladder is anterior to the rectum and superior to the prostate. In females, it is anterior to the lower uterine corpus and anterior vaginal fornix.

The urinary bladder can be subdivided anatomically into several parts: apex (dome), midportion and base, the last composed of the trigone and bladder neck. The apex is

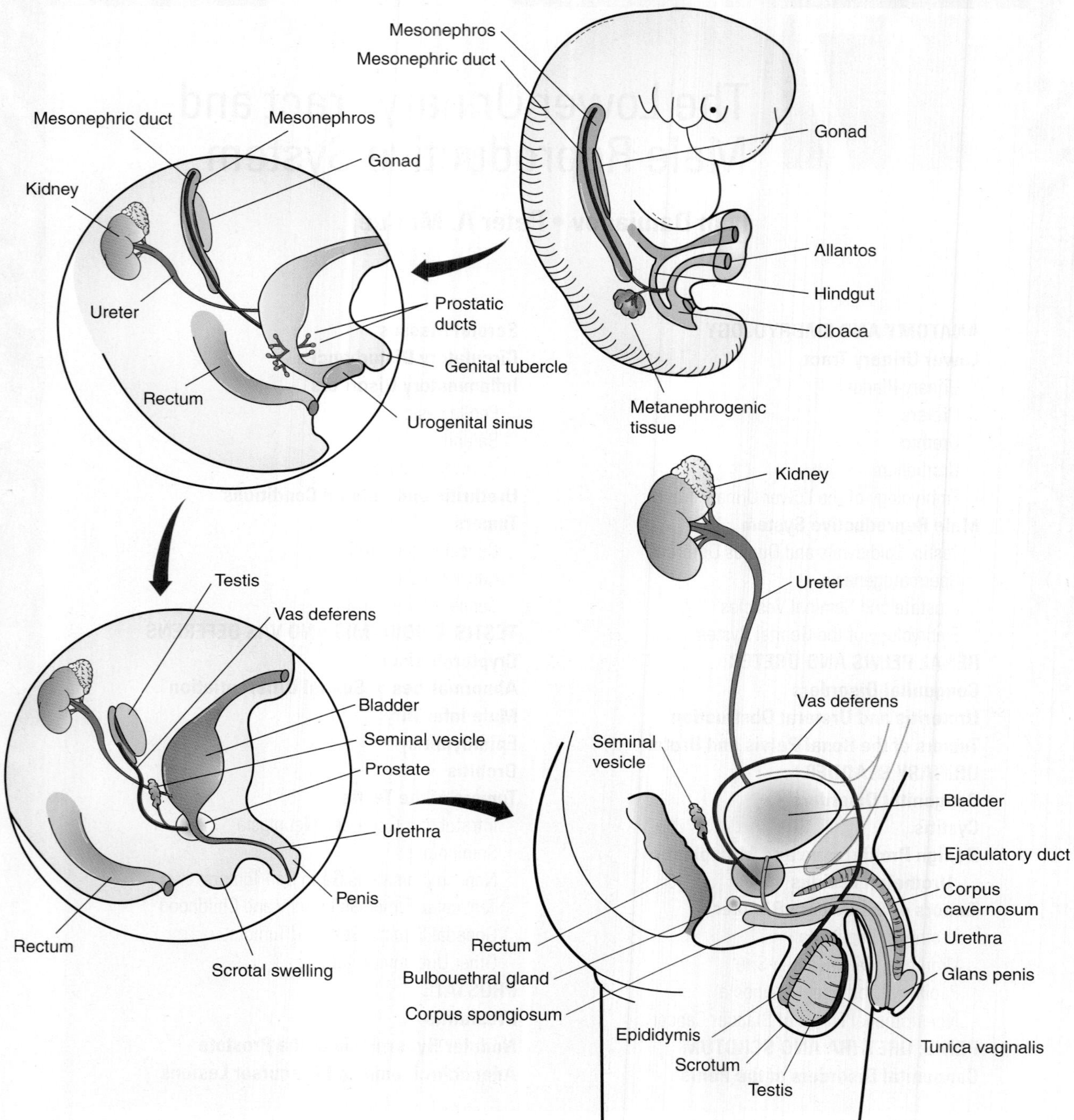

FIGURE 17-1. Embryologic development of the urinary tract and male reproductive system.

located behind the margin of the symphysis pubis and is linked in the midline to the umbilicus by the umbilical ligament, a fibrous strand representing the involuted fetal **urachus**. The bladder neck in males rests on the upper surface of the prostate, where the smooth muscle fibers of the two organs intertwine. Inside the bladder, the posterior aspect of the base of the bladder has a triangular shape and is called the **trigone,** a region that is devoid of mucosal folds and appears flattened. Superiorly, the trigone is bound by a muscular ridge joining the laterally placed orifices of the ureters. The inferior tip of the trigone is formed by the funnel-shaped internal orifice of the urethra.

The Ureters Are in the Posterior Retroperitoneal Space, Lateral to the Vertebrae

The ureters are paired organs linking each renal pelvis with the bladder. The lowermost part of the ureters is embedded in the wall of the urinary bladder, which forms the

ureterovesical valves. These valves allow urine to pass downward from the ureters into the urinary bladder but not in the opposite direction.

The Urethra Is the Terminal Conduit of the Urinary Outflow Tract

The male urethra, on average 20 cm long, is divided into the (1) **prostatic urethra**, extending through the prostate; (2) **membranous urethra**, penetrating through the pelvic floor; and (3) **spongy or penile urethra**, occupying the central portion of the penis. The prostatic urethra contains the ostia of ejaculatory and prostatic ducts. The posterior part of penile urethra, also termed the **bulbous urethra**, receives secretions from the mucous bulbourethral (Cowper) glands. The penile urethra terminates in the fossa navicularis, immediately proximal to the external orifice, or meatus, located on the tip of the penis.

The female urethra is shorter, measuring only 3 to 4 cm in length. It extends from its internal orifice at the urinary bladder to its external orifice in the vulva, immediately below the clitoris. The wall of the female urethra also contains mucous glands.

Transitional Epithelium (Urothelium) Lines the Ureters, Bladder and Posterior Urethra

The terminal urethra is lined by squamous epithelium. The urothelium consists of three epithelial zones. The **basal layer** lies on a basement membrane and contains cells that can divide and replace damaged superficial cells. Superficial to the basal layer are three to four layers of polygonal cells, the **intermediate zone.** Both the basal and the polygonal cells can flatten when the bladder dilates. The **superficial layer** of the urothelium consists of "umbrella cells," which are resistant to the urine that constantly bathes them.

Under the epithelium lies the lamina propria, composed principally of loose connective tissue and blood vessels. The muscularis mucosa is incomplete and poorly developed. The lamina propria is externally surrounded by a thick muscle layer that is covered by adventitia. Since the bladder, ureters and urethra are retroperitoneal, they do not have an external serosa. Only part of the bladder dome has a serosal covering.

The Lower Urinary Tract Develops Mostly From the Cloaca

The cloaca is a fetal structure that is partitioned early in ontogenesis into an anterior part, the urogenital sinus, and a posterior part, the primordium of the rectum (Fig. 17-1). The urogenital sinus is the anlage of the urinary bladder, the proximal urethra and the urachus, a temporary fetal structure connecting the urinary tract with the umbilicus. The caudal urogenital sinus makes contact with an invagination of the urogenital membrane, thereby forming the urethra. The urachus gradually involutes into the umbilical ligament. The fetal urinary bladder forms symmetric lateral outpouchings that grow cranially as ureteric buds. When these epithelial buds reach the nephrogenic zone, they induce formation of the metanephros, the kidney primordium.

Male Reproductive System

The male reproductive system includes the testis, epididymis, ductus (vas) deferens, seminal vesicles, prostate and penis (Fig. 17-1).

Testes Are Linked to the Epididymis and Located in the Scrotum

Testes are paired oval organs measuring $4 \times 3 \times 3$ cm and located in the scrotum. The epididymis lies along the lateral–posterior aspect of the testis and extends into the ductus deferens. The testis is invested with the **tunica vaginalis,** a layer of mesothelial cells that covers the outer fibrous capsule of the testis, which is called the **tunica albuginea.** This capsule has internal septal ramifications that divide the testis into about 250 **lobules**. Each lobule consists of coiled seminiferous tubules and loose interstitial tissue containing blood vessels and Leydig interstitial cells.

Arterial supply to the testis is via testicular arteries, which originate from the abdominal aorta. The right internal spermatic vein empties into the inferior vena cava, while the left drains into the left renal vein. This anatomic difference has several clinical implications, discussed below.

Spermatogenesis Occurs in the Seminiferous Tubules

Seminiferous tubules are the principal functional unit of the testes. They contain seminiferous epithelium and Sertoli cells, which provide support to **spermatogenesis**. **Sertoli cells** also secrete **inhibin**, which provides feedback information to the pituitary, thereby regulating secretion of **gonadotropins** (i.e., follicle-stimulating hormone [FSH] and luteinizing hormone [LH]). The interstitial spaces of the testis contain **Leydig cells,** the primary source of **testosterone.**

Seminiferous tubules in prepubertal testes contain two cell types: **germ cells** at the stage of spermatogonia and **Sertoli cells.** At puberty, LH stimulates Leydig cells to produce testosterone and initiate spermatogenesis, and FSH acts on both germ cells and Sertoli cells to support spermatogenesis.

Hormonal stimuli lead to increased numbers of germ cells, primarily **spermatogonia,** which also begin differentiating into primary **spermatocytes.** Meiotic division of primary spermatocytes produces **secondary spermatocytes,** which contain a haploid number (23) of chromosomes. Secondary spermatocytes mature to **spermatids,** and the latter to **spermatozoa,** which are discharged through the channels of rete testis into the epididymal ducts. In the **epididymis,** spermatozoa are admixed with fluid secreted by epididymal lining cells and are carried through the **vas deferens,** which empties its contents into the urethra. The final semen to be ejaculated through the penile urethra is a mixture of spermatozoa in the epididymal secretions and fluids produced by the **accessory glands,** namely, the seminal vesicles, prostate, Cowper bulbourethral glands and urethral glands.

The Prostate Is the Largest Accessory Gland

The prostate is an accessory gland located in the pelvis, in contact with the posterior and inferior external layers of the urinary bladder, close to the rectum. Posteriorly it is attached to **seminal vesicles.** Microscopically it is a tubuloalveolar gland with a rich fibromuscular stroma. It develops under the influence of testosterone, which is essential for maintaining its production of seminal fluid.

The traditional concept of prostate lobes has been supplanted by the functional organization of the prostate into three distinct zones. The **transition zone** is located around the prostatic urethra. The **central zone** sits slightly posterior and extends toward the seminal vesicles. The **peripheral zone** envelops the other zones and defines the boundaries of the prostate gland. In practice, it is difficult to recognize the precise demarcations of the zones by light microscopy. However, the biologic significance of the zones is readily apparent in that most carcinomas arise in the peripheral zone while hyperplasias generally arise in the transition zone.

The classic delineation of a true **prostatic capsule** is another concept that has been reinterpreted. In some areas of the prostate, the so-called capsule consists of a concentric band of fibromuscular tissue that melds into the adjacent glandular stroma. Thus, what constitutes capsule invasion by tumor is somewhat arbitrary. In the apex of the prostate, the capsular plane of dissection is essentially inseparable from the adjacent soft tissue. This lack of defined anatomic boundaries has important implications in the context of accurate cancer staging for the surgeon seeking to remove the organ, and for the pathologist looking to evaluate the extent of disease.

The Male Genital System Develops From Several Primordial Parts

The testes develop from the **genital ridges**, which form on the posterior surface of the celomic cavity. These ridges are populated by migratory **primordial germ cells** (initially formed in the yolk sac) that enter the fetal body through the midline and then migrate laterally into the right and left genital ridges. Complex interactions of germ cells and stromal cells in the genital ridges lead to formation of the fetal testes, which are on the posterior wall of the midabdomen. At the same time, the testes connect with the future epididymis and vas deferens, which develop from the **wolffian ducts.** At that point the testes begin their gradual descent into the inguinal canal, to the scrotum.

The scrotum and penis develop simultaneously with the testes but from another anlage that corresponds mostly to the genital tubercle and partly to the anterior urogenital sinus. These primordia of the external genital organs are initially identical in both sexes. In a male fetus, testosterone drives their development into penis, penile urethra and scrotum; in a female they become clitoris, labia minora and labia majora.

RENAL PELVIS AND URETER

Congenital Disorders

Developmental anomalies of the renal pelvis and ureters are found in 2% to 3% of all persons. They do not usually cause clinical problems, but on occasion may predispose to obstruction and urinary tract infections. The most important developmental anomalies include agenesis, ectopia, duplications, obstructions and dilations (Fig. 17-2).

AGENESIS OF THE RENAL PELVIS AND URETERS: This rare anomaly is always associated with agenesis of the corresponding kidney. Unilateral agenesis is usually asymptomatic. Bilateral agenesis of ureters and kidneys, a feature of **Potter syndrome,** is incompatible with extrauterine life (see Chapter 16).

ECTOPIC URETERS: Ureteric buds may develop at the wrong anatomic site during embryogenesis. The lower orifices of ectopic ureters can be found in many anomalous places, such as the midportion of the urinary bladder, seminal vesicles, urethra or vas deferens.

DUPLICATIONS: Single or multiple ureteric buds may be duplicated on the side of the fetal urinary bladder. These

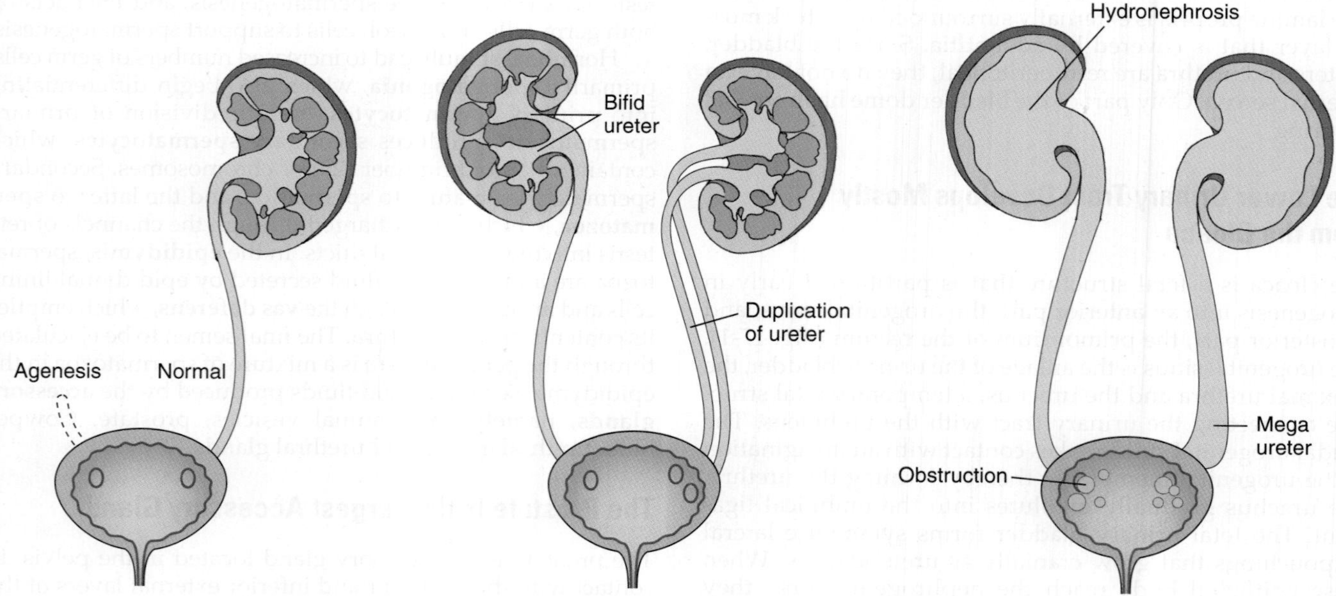

FIGURE 17-2. Anomalies of the renal pelvis and ureters.

duplications may be unilateral or bilateral, complete or partial. Usually there are two parallel ureters, each with its own renal pelvis and separate vesical orifice. **Bifid ureters** (subdivided by a septum), **bifurcate ureters** and many variations of this anomaly can be encountered, but most are not clinically significant.

URETERAL OBSTRUCTION: Obstructions can be traced to congenital **atresia** or abnormal **ureteral valves.** However, congenital **obstruction of the ureteropelvic junction,** the most common form of hydronephrosis in infants and children, cannot be explained in those terms. It is thought to be related to abnormal layering of smooth muscle cells and/or fibrous tissue replacing the smooth muscle cells at the ureteropelvic junction. Urinary obstruction in these children is usually unilateral, but is bilateral in 20% of cases. This form of hydronephrosis is often associated with other urinary tract anomalies and, in some cases, with agenesis of the contralateral kidney.

DILATIONS OF THE RENAL PELVIS OR URETERS: Dilations of the renal pelvis or ureters can be localized in the form of **diverticula.** Generalized dilation of the entire ureter, **congenital megaureter**, may be unilateral or bilateral. The pathogenesis of congenital megaureters is largely unknown. The ureters are tortuous and lack peristalsis. Resulting stagnation of urine (**hydroureter**) is typically associated with progressive hydronephrosis, ultimately leading to renal failure.

Ureteritis and Ureteral Obstruction

Ureteritis is inflammation of the ureters. It is a complication of descending infections from the kidneys or ascending infections if there is vesicoureteric reflux. Ureteritis is often associated with ureteral obstruction, which may be either intrinsic or extrinsic (Fig. 17-3).

Intrinsic causes of ureteral obstruction include calculi, intraluminal blood clots, fibroepithelial polyps, inflammatory strictures, amyloidosis and tumors of the ureter.

Extrinsic causes of ureteral obstruction include aberrant renal vessels to the lower pole of the kidney that cross the ureter, endometriosis and tumors in adjacent lymph nodes. In addition, a pregnant uterus may compress the ureters.

Ureteral obstruction can also result from diseases that involve urinary bladder, prostate and urethra (e.g., bladder cancer in the vicinity of the ureteral orifice or bladder neck, neurogenic bladder and prostatic hyperplasia). Proximal causes of ureteral obstruction tend to be unilateral, whereas more distal ones, such as prostatic hyperplasia, lead to bilateral hydronephrosis, with the possibility of renal failure in untreated cases.

Idiopathic retroperitoneal fibrosis is a rare cause of ureteral obstruction, characterized by dense fibrosis of retroperitoneal soft tissues and a modest, nonspecific, chronic inflammatory reaction. The etiology is unknown, although use of certain drugs (methysergide, β-adrenergic blockers) and autoimmunity have been proposed as causes. On occasion, idiopathic retroperitoneal fibrosis is accompanied by inflammatory fibrosis in other areas, including Riedel struma (thyroid), sclerosing cholangitis (liver) and mediastinal fibrosis. The disease may respond to treatment with corticosteroids and immunosuppressive agents.

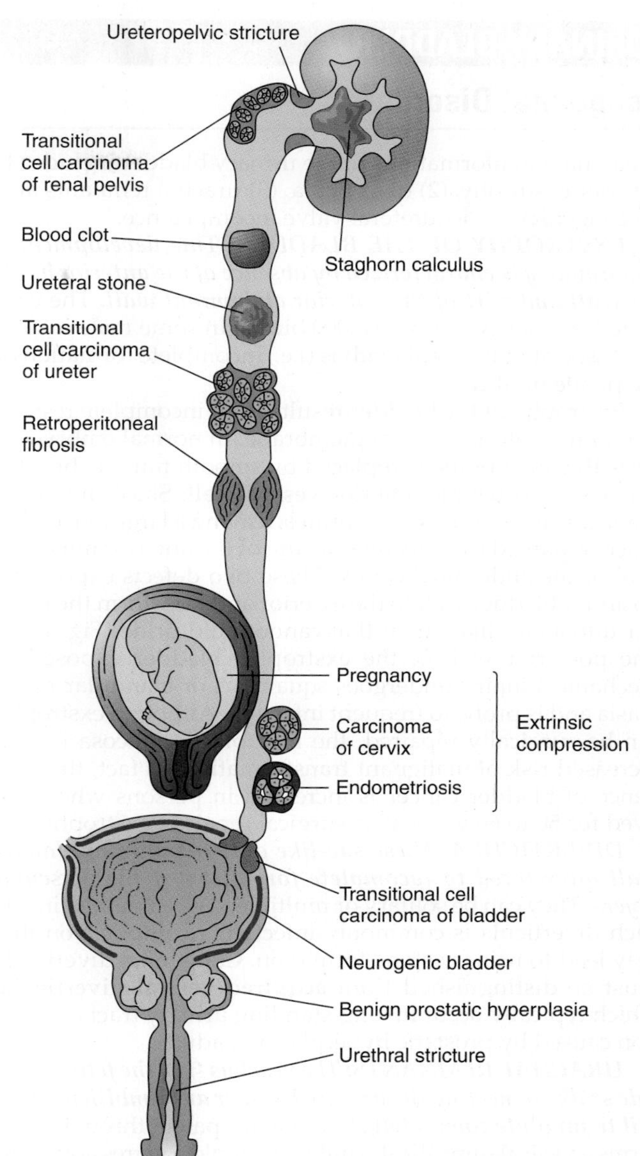

FIGURE 17-3. Most common causes of ureteral obstruction.

Tumors of the Renal Pelvis and Ureter

Tumors of the renal pelvis and ureter resemble those of the urinary bladder (see below) except that they are much less common. Histologically, most (>90%) are **urothelial cell carcinomas.** The etiologic factors associated with epithelial tumors of the renal pelvis and ureter are similar to those observed in bladder cancer, suggesting a "field effect" in which the entire urothelial mucosa represents a continuous "target organ." Five percent of urothelial tumors originate in the renal pelvis and ureters.

Patients most frequently present in their sixth and seventh decades with hematuria (80%) and flank pain (25%). Urothelial cell carcinoma of the ureter or renal pelvis requires radical nephroureterectomy. The entire ureter must be removed because of the high frequency of concurrent and subsequent urothelial cell carcinomas. The prognosis is related to tumor stage at the time of diagnosis.

URINARY BLADDER

Congenital Disorders

Congenital malformations of the urinary bladder include (1) bladder exstrophy, (2) diverticula, (3) urachal remnants and (4) congenital vesicoureteral valve incompetence.

EXSTROPHY OF THE BLADDER: ***This developmental abnormality is characterized by absence of the anterior bladder wall and part of the anterior abdominal wall.*** The estimated frequency is 1 per 50,000 births. In some male infants it is associated with **epispadias** (i.e., incomplete formation of the penile urethra).

Exstrophy of the bladder results from incomplete resorption of the anterior cloacal membrane. In normal embryogenesis this membrane is replaced by smooth muscle, but if it persists, it forms the anterior vesical wall. Since the membrane is thin, it ultimately ruptures, leaving a large defect that is accompanied by defective closure of the anterior muscular wall of the abdominal cavity. These two defects expose the posterior bladder wall to the exterior and transform the bladder into a cup-like organ that cannot hold urine (Fig. 17-4). The posterior wall of the exstrophic bladder exposed to mechanical injury undergoes squamous or glandular metaplasia and is prone to frequent infection. Although exstrophy can be surgically repaired, the metaplastic mucosa has an increased risk of malignant transformation. In fact, the incidence of bladder cancer is increased in persons who have lived for 50 to 60 years after surgical repair of exstrophy.

DIVERTICULA: ***These sac-like outpouchings of bladder wall are related to incomplete formation of the muscular layers.*** They can be solitary or multiple. Urine retained inside such diverticula is commonly infected, a complication that may lead to urinary stone formation. Congenital diverticula must be distinguished from **acquired vesical diverticula,** which typically occur in long-standing urinary tract obstruction caused by prostatic hyperplasia in adults.

URACHAL REMNANTS: ***The urachus (i.e., the fetal allantoic stalk connecting the urinary bladder and umbilicus) may fail to involute completely.*** If it remains patent throughout, it forms a **vesical–umbilical fistula.** Incomplete regression of the urinary end, midportion or umbilical end of the urachus results in an **urachal diverticulum, umbilical–urachal sinus** or **urachal cyst,** respectively. The columnar epithelium of urachal remnants may give rise to **adenocarcinoma.** Urachal remnants are the site of only 0.2% of bladder cancers, but represent one third of bladder adenocarcinomas.

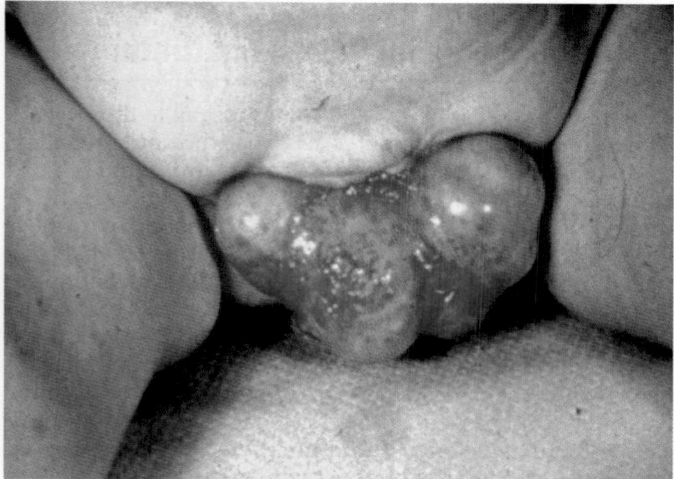

FIGURE 17-4. Exstrophy of the urinary bladder.

CONGENITAL INCOMPETENCE OF THE VESICOURETERAL VALVE: ***This anomaly results from an abnormal junction between the ureters and the urinary bladder.*** The ureters normally enter the wall of the bladder obliquely and have a long intravesical portion. The muscle layer of the urinary bladder serves as a sphincter that prevents backflow of urine into normal ureters during micturition. By contrast, ureters that enter the bladder perpendicularly have a short intravesical segment, which does not adequately prevent urine backflow during micturition. **Vesicoureteric reflux** (VUR) is more common in young girls than boys and is often familial. In 75% of cases, VUR is asymptomatic, but it may lead to reflux pyelonephritis. Congenital VUR is distinguished from the acquired form that occurs during pregnancy or in conditions associated with bladder hypertrophy.

Cystitis

Cystitis is inflammation of the bladder. It may be acute or chronic. It is the most common urinary tract infection and is often seen as a nosocomial infection in hospitalized patients.

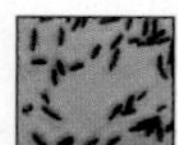

ETIOLOGIC FACTORS: ***In most cases cystitis is secondary to infection of the lower urinary tract.*** Factors related to bladder infection include the age and sex of the patient, presence of bladder calculi, bladder outlet obstruction, diabetes mellitus, immunodeficiency, prior instrumentation or catheterization, radiation therapy and chemotherapy. ***The risk of cystitis is increased in females because of a short urethra, especially during pregnancy.*** Bladder outlet obstruction due to prostatic hyperplasia predisposes men to cystitis. Introduction of pathogens into the bladder may also occur during instrumentation (cystoscopy) and is particularly common in patients in whom indwelling catheters remain for prolonged periods.

Coliform bacteria are the most common cause of cystitis, mostly *Escherichia coli, Proteus vulgaris, Pseudomonas aeruginosa* and *Enterobacter* sp. Tuberculosis of the bladder is almost always secondary to renal tuberculosis. Fungal cystitis may be seen in immunosuppressed patients. Gas-forming bacilli, usually in persons with diabetes, may produce characteristic interstitial bubbles in the lamina propria of the urinary bladder (**emphysematous cystitis**). Schistosomiasis as a cause of cystitis is common in North Africa and the Middle East, where *Schistosoma haematobium* is endemic. Cases in the Western world are restricted to immigrants from high-risk areas.

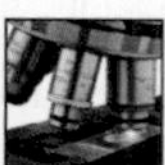

PATHOLOGY: Stromal edema, hemorrhage and a neutrophilic infiltrate of variable intensity are typical of acute cystitis (Fig. 17-5). Focal petechial mucosal hemorrhages (**hemorrhagic cystitis**) are often seen in acute bacterial cystitis. Bleeding diatheses (e.g., leukemia or treatment with cytotoxic drugs) and disseminated intravascular coagulation often cause extensive hemorrhagic cystitis. ***Lack of resolution of the inflammatory reaction of acute cystitis is***

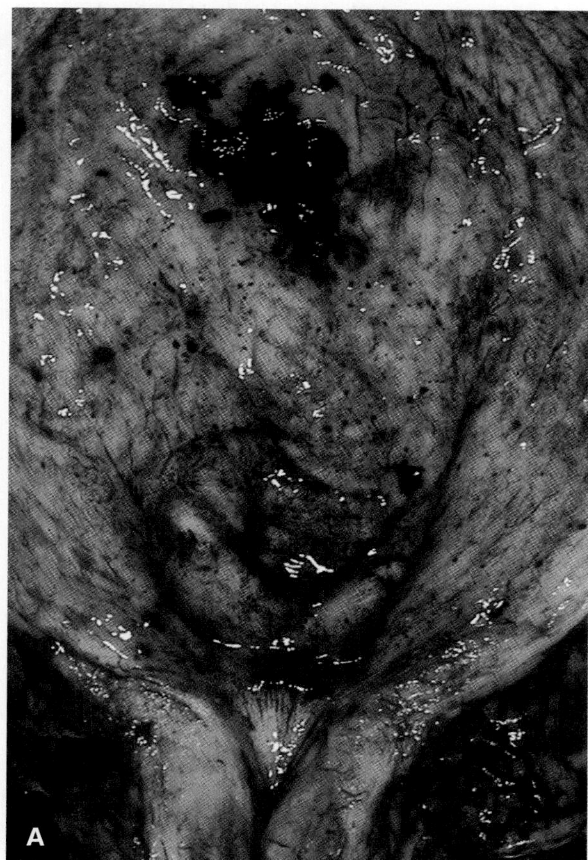

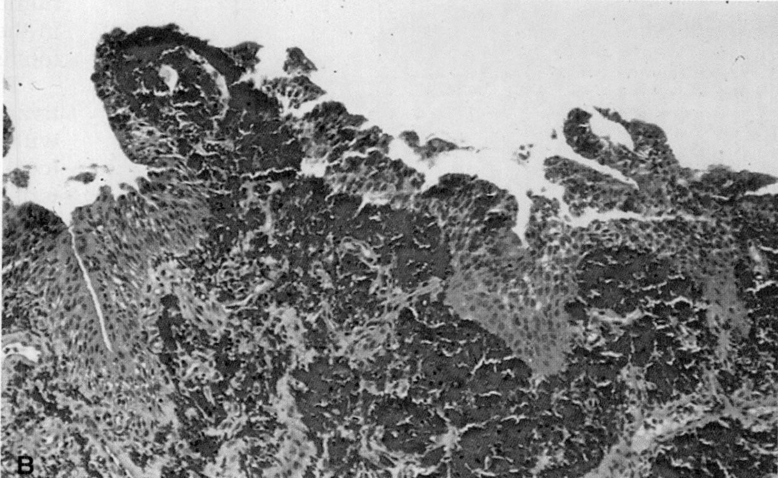

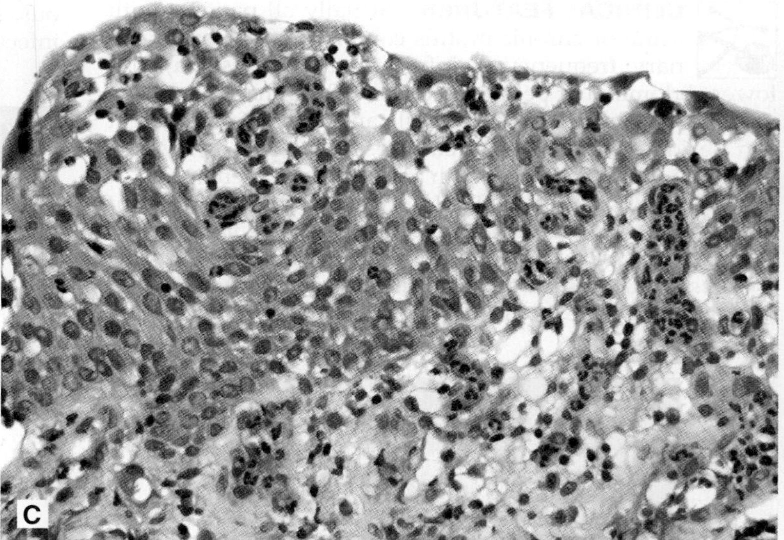

FIGURE 17-5. Acute cystitis. The patient died 2 days after surgery, and the cystitis was obviously caused by an indwelling catheter. **A.** Several foci of hemorrhage are seen on the hyperemic bladder mucosa. **B.** Foci of mucosal hemorrhage. **C.** Acute cystitis. Polymorphonuclear leukocytes infiltrate the mucosa.

associated with the hallmarks of chronic cystitis, including a predominance of lymphocytes, plasma cells (Fig. 17-6) and fibrosis of the lamina propria. Occasionally, the mucosa of an inflamed bladder may contain numerous lymphocytic follicles (**follicular cystitis**) or dense infiltrates of eosinophils (**eosinophilic cystitis**). **Granulomatous cystitis** is a feature of tuberculosis. Ova of *S. hematobium* can cause simultaneous granulomatous reactions and eosinophilic infiltrates. The specific pathologic forms of chronic cystitis include:

- **Ulcerative cystitis:** Chronic irritation caused, for example, by indwelling catheters or traumatic cystoscopy may lead to ulceration and focal mucosal hemorrhage. **Solitary mucosal ulcer** is also found in interstitial cystitis (see below).
- **Suppurative cystitis:** Pus may cover the bladder mucosa, fill the lumen or permeate the bladder wall. Suppurative cystitis may develop during local infection, but more often it is a complication of sepsis, pyelonephritis or purulent infections secondary to bladder surgery.
- **Pseudomembranous cystitis:** Pseudomembranes (i.e., shaggy layers of necrotic, gray or yellow material) sometimes cover the mucosa of the urinary bladder. They can be removed to expose the underlying hemorrhagic ulcerated mucosa. Pseudomembranous cystitis is typically a complication of infection that follows treatment with cytotoxic drugs, such as cyclophosphamide. Pseudomembranes consist of cell detritus, fibrin, inflammatory cells and blood.
- **Calcific cystitis:** This form of chronic inflammation is typically found in schistosomiasis. Calcification of ova produces encrustations of the bladder wall similar to grains of sand. These grains gradually coalesce and transform the entire urinary bladder into a calcified rigid vessel.

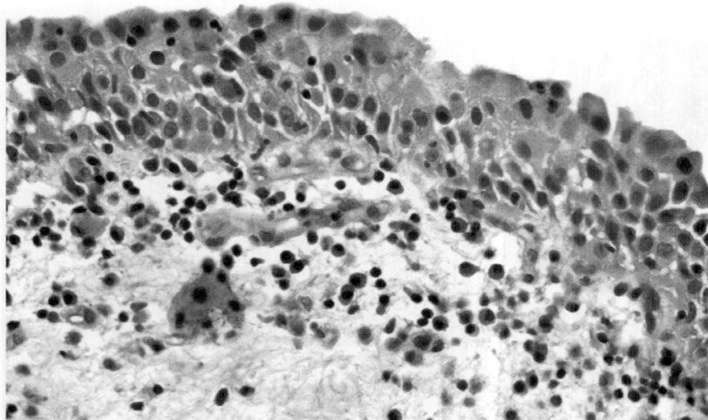

FIGURE 17-6. Chronic cystitis. A nonspecific inflammatory infiltrate composed of lymphocytes and plasma cells is present in the edematous lamina propria.

CLINICAL FEATURES: Virtually all patients with acute or chronic cystitis complain of excessive urinary frequency, painful urination (**dysuria**) and lower abdominal or pelvic discomfort. Examination of urine usually reveals inflammatory cells and the causative agent can be identified by urine culture. Most cases of cystitis respond well to treatment with antimicrobial agents.

CHRONIC INTERSTITIAL CYSTITIS: ***This disorder of unknown cause typically affects middle-aged women and features transmural inflammation of the bladder wall, which is occasionally associated with mucosal ulceration*** **(Hunner ulcer)** *(Fig. 17-7).* Chronic inflammation, including increased numbers of mast cells, and fibrosis are commonly observed in the mucosa and muscularis. A Hunner ulcer displays an intense acute inflammatory reaction.

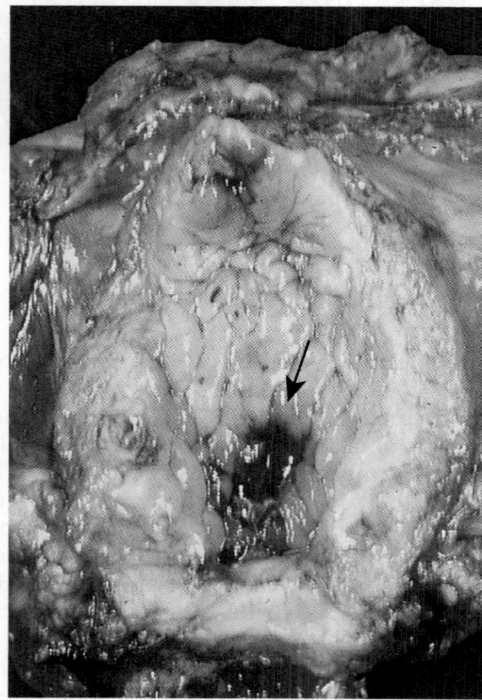

FIGURE 17-7. Interstitial cystitis. The hemorrhagic defect in the edematous mucosa of the posterior wall of the bladder is clinically known as Hunner ulcer.

The most common symptoms of chronic interstitial cystitis are long-standing suprapubic pain, frequency and urgency, with or without hematuria. At cystoscopy, mucosal edema, focal petechiae and irregular hemorrhagic areas are characteristic, most often in the dome and posterior wall. Urine cultures are usually negative. The disease is typically persistent and refractory to all forms of therapy.

MALAKOPLAKIA (from the Greek, **malakos,** *"soft"; plax, "plaque"):* ***An uncommon inflammatory disorder of unknown etiology, malakoplakia is identified by the accumulation of characteristic macrophages.*** The disorder, originally described in the bladder, has since been seen in numerous other sites, both within and outside the urinary tract. Malakoplakia is found in all age groups, the peak frequency being in the fifth to seventh decades. There is a marked female preponderance, regardless of the site.

Malakoplakia is often associated with urinary tract infection by *E. coli,* although a direct causal relationship is dubious. A clinical background of immunosuppression, chronic infections or cancer is common.

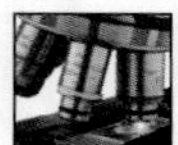

PATHOLOGY: Malakoplakia is characterized by soft, yellow plaques on the mucosal surface of the bladder. Histologically, the most striking feature is a chronic inflammatory cell infiltrate composed predominantly of large macrophages with abundant, eosinophilic cytoplasm containing periodic acid–Schiff (PAS)-positive granules (Fig. 17-8). Some of these macrophages exhibit laminated, basophilic calcospherites, termed **Michaelis-Gutmann bodies.** Ultrastructurally, these granules are engorged lysosomes that contain fragments of bacteria, suggesting that malakoplakia may reflect an acquired defect in lysosomal degrada-

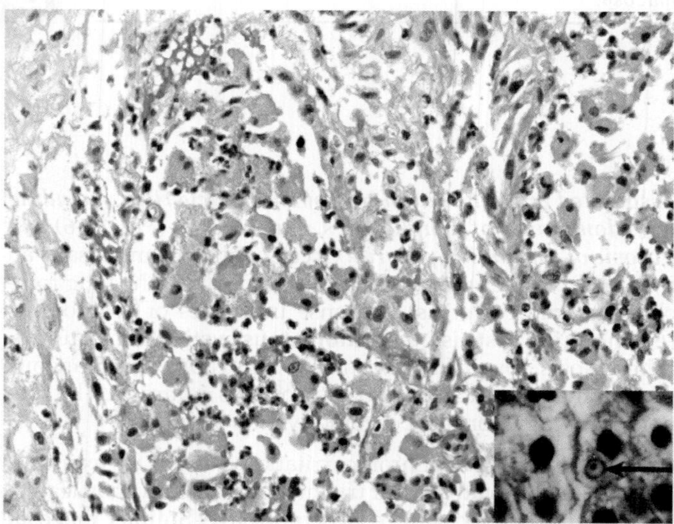

FIGURE 17-8. Malakoplakia. Inflammatory cells are composed principally of macrophages, with fewer lymphocytes. *Inset.* A Michaelis-Gutmann body (*arrow*) is seen at high magnification (periodic acid–Schiff stain).

tion. The Michaelis-Gutmann bodies result from calcium salt deposition in these enlarged lysosomes.

The urinary bladder is the most common site of malakoplakia: half of all cases occur in this organ. This enigmatic disorder has also been reported in other regions of the genitourinary system and many other organ systems. The clinical symptomatology of malakoplakia of the bladder is indistinguishable from that of other forms of chronic cystitis. Treatment is ineffective.

Benign Proliferative and Metaplastic Urothelial Lesions

Benign proliferative and metaplastic lesions of urothelium occur mostly in the urinary bladder but may be found in the entire urinary tract. These nonneoplastic lesions are characterized by hyperplasia (Fig. 17-9B) or by combined hyperplasia and metaplasia. They are mostly seen in association

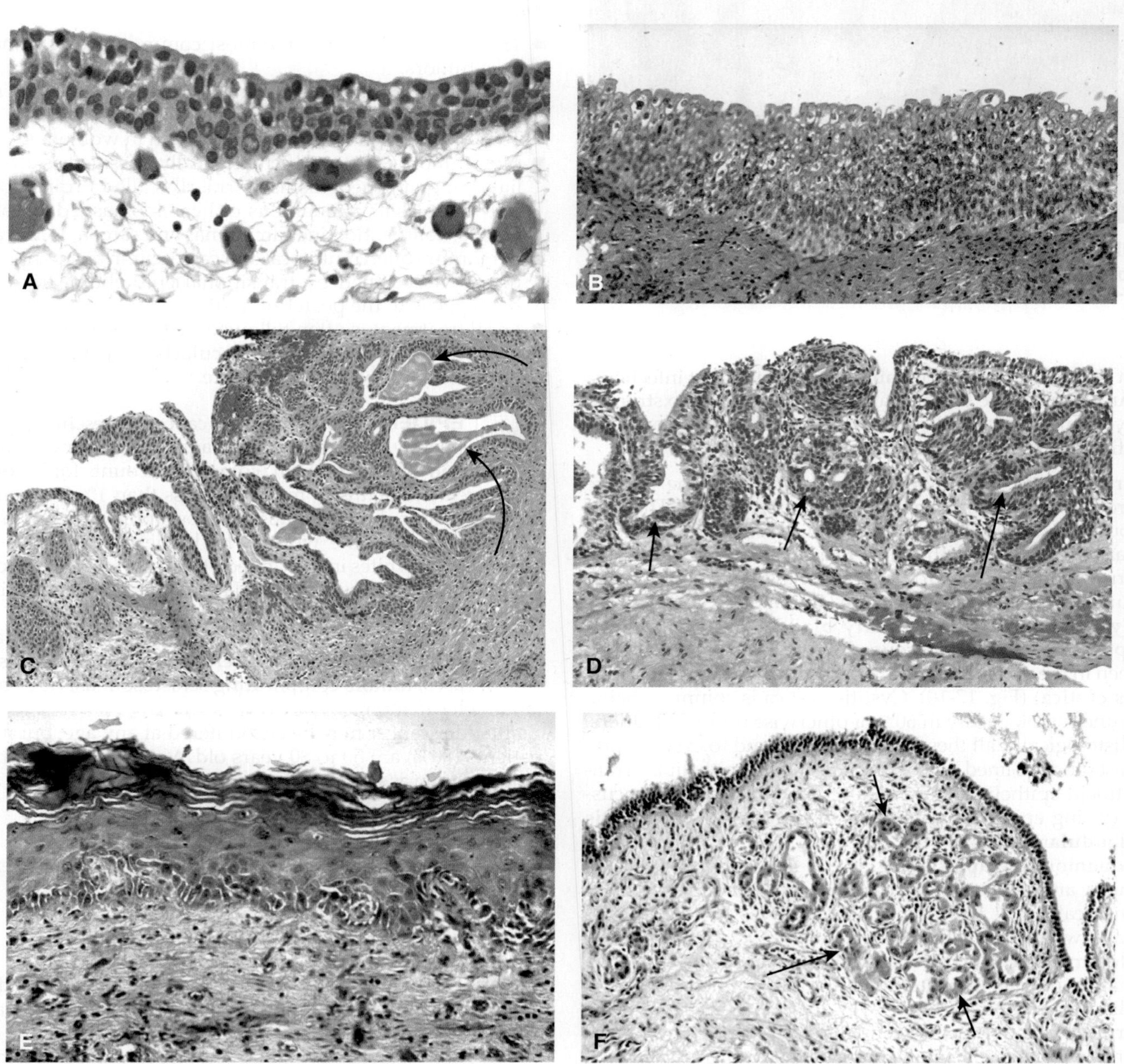

FIGURE 17-9. Proliferative and metaplastic changes of the urinary bladder. A. Normal bladder mucosa. B. Hyperplasia. Note the expansion of the normal six to seven layers of urothelial cells. **C. Cystitis cystica**. Brunn nests (*straight arrows*) and cysts (*curved arrow*) protrude into the lamina propria. **D. Cystitis glandularis.** Metaplastic glandular mucosa is highlighted by the arrows. **E. Squamous metaplasia**. Note the keratinizing layer on the superficial epithelium. **F. Nephrogenic metaplasia.** Proliferation of glandular structures resembling renal tubules (*arrows*).

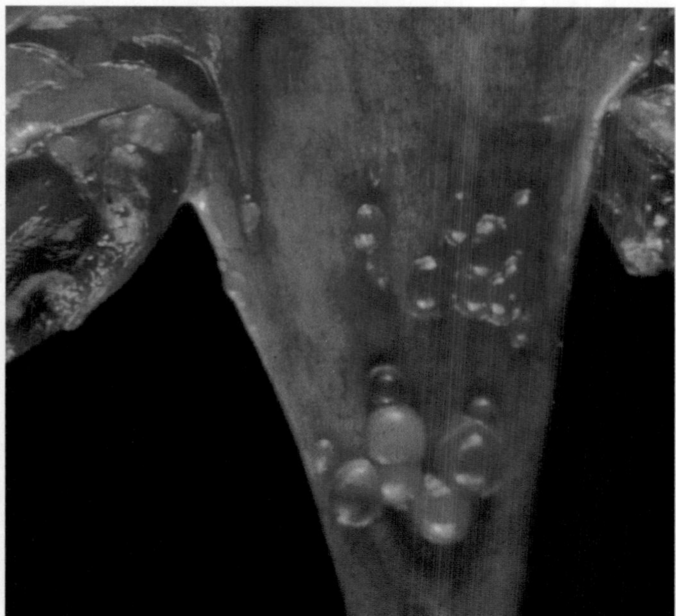

FIGURE 17-10. Ureteritis cystica. The mucosa of the proximal ureter exhibits small cystic structures.

with chronic inflammation caused by urinary tract infections, calculi, neurogenic bladder and (rarely) bladder exstrophy. They are also occasionally observed in the absence of any preexisting inflammatory condition.

- **Brunn buds** are bulbous invaginations of the surface urothelium into the lamina propria (Fig. 17-9C). They are found in over 85% of bladders and are considered normal variants of the urothelium. **Brunn nests** are similar to Brunn buds, but the urothelial cells have detached from the surface and are seen within the lamina propria.
- **Cystic lesions of the urinary bladder (cystitis cystica)** appear as fluid-filled grouped cysts. Similar cysts can be seen in the urethra or the ureter (**urethritis cystica, ureteritis cystica**) (Fig. 17-10). Cystitis cystica is common, being found histologically in 60% of otherwise normal bladders. Histologically, all these lesions correspond to cystic Brunn nests and are lined by normal transitional epithelium. Transitional epithelium may undergo metaplasia into mucus-secreting epithelium, which is then diagnosed as **cystitis glandularis** (Fig. 17-9D).
- **Squamous metaplasia** (Fig. 17-9E) is a reaction to chronic injury and inflammation, particularly when it is associated with calculi. It is present in as many as 50% of normal adult women and 10% of men.
- **Nephrogenic metaplasia** is a lesion caused by transformation of transitional epithelium into epithelium resembling renal tubules (Fig. 17-9F). It is most common in the urinary bladder but is seen less often in the urethra and ureter. Numerous small tubules clustered in the lamina propria produce a papillary exophytic nodule. The histogenesis is unsettled, but in some cases, the lesions seem to result from implants of detached renal tubular cells carried downstream by urine. The lesion may produce tumor-like protrusions in the urinary bladder. These may obstruct the ureters, in which case they require surgical treatment.

CLINICAL FEATURES: Proliferative and metaplastic urothelial lesions are of limited clinical significance, save that such lesions should not be confused with cancer. However, patients with these changes are at greater risk for urothelial bladder carcinoma and, in the case of cystitis glandularis, of **adenocarcinoma** as well. Yet there is no evidence to suggest that these lesions themselves are preneoplastic.

Tumors of the Urinary Bladder

The most important facts about bladder cancer are as follows:

- The urinary bladder is the most common site of urinary tract tumors.
- Most bladder tumors occur in older patients (median age 65 years) and are rare under the age of 50 years.
- Tumors are more common in men than in women.
- Most tumors (90%) are microscopically classified as urothelial malignant neoplasms (formerly called "transitional cell" neoplasms). Squamous cell carcinomas, adenocarcinomas, neuroendocrine carcinomas and sarcomas are rare.
- Tumors are often multifocal and can occur in any part of the urinary tract lined by transitional epithelium, from the renal pelvis to the posterior urethra.
- Local treatment is often followed by tumor recurrence.
- Tumor invasion into the muscularis propria markedly decreases the 5-year survival rate.

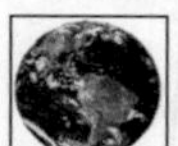

EPIDEMIOLOGY: Bladder cancer represents approximately 7% of all newly diagnosed cancers in males and 2% of cancers in women. It accounts for 3% of all cancer-related deaths in males and less than 1% in women. Bladder cancer shows significant geographic and sex differences throughout the world. The highest frequencies are among urban whites in the United States and western Europe, whereas it occurs less often in Japan and among American blacks.

A high incidence of bladder cancer in Egypt, Sudan and other African countries is due to endemic schistosomiasis. In 70% of cases, tumors complicating schistosomiasis are squamous cell carcinomas.

Bladder cancer may be encountered at any age, but most patients (80%) are 50 to 80 years old. Men are affected three times as often as women. The most important risk factors are:

- Cigarette smoking (fourfold increased risk)
- Industrial exposure to azo dyes
- Infection with *S. haematobium* (in Egypt and other endemic regions)
- Drugs, such as cyclophosphamide and analgesics
- Radiation therapy (cervical, prostate or rectal cancer)

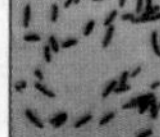

ETIOLOGIC FACTORS: The association of bladder cancer with occupational exposure to certain organic chemicals among workers in the German aniline dye industry was described in 1895 and was subsequently confirmed in similar workers in the United States. This was one of the first occupational cancers known. Later, increased risk of bladder cancer was noted in the leather, rubber, paint and organic chemical industries. Improved industrial hygiene has reduced this risk. ***Today, polycyclic hydrocarbons from cigarette smoke are the most important risk factor for urinary bladder carcinoma.***

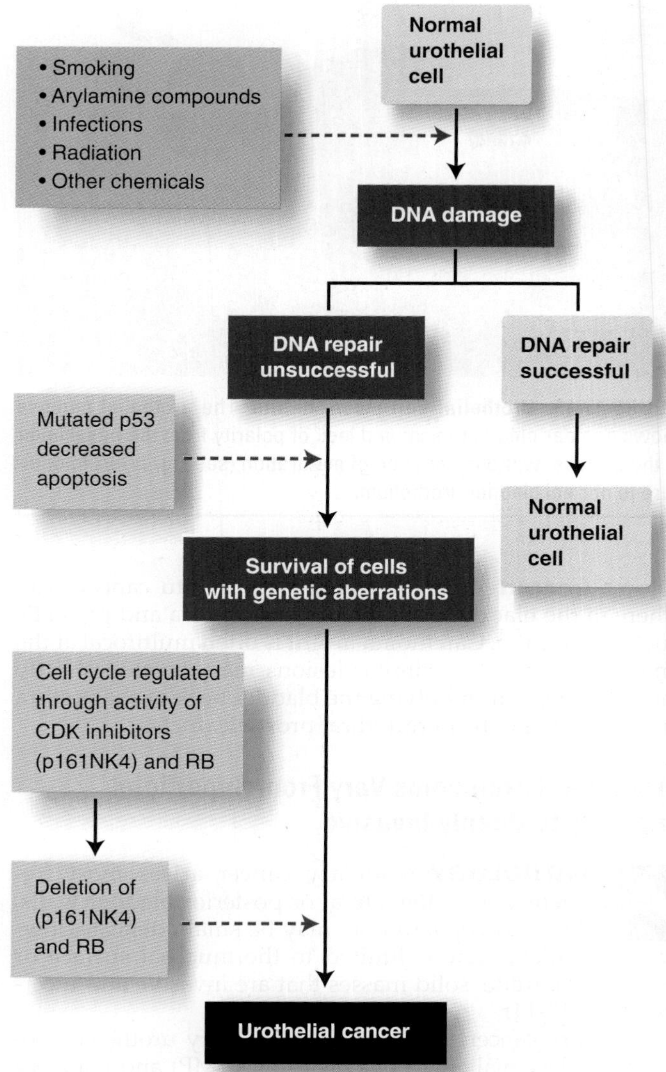

FIGURE 17-11. Hypothetical molecular model of urothelial neoplasms. The transition from normal urothelium to carcinoma occurs gradually in several steps.

A role for chemicals in bladder cancer has been strengthened by the demonstration that administration of β-naphthylamine, to which the dye industry workers were exposed, produces bladder cancer in dogs. The metabolism of naphthylamines explains their organ specificity. Arylamines are conjugated with glucuronic acid in the liver, after which the conjugates are excreted in the urine. In the bladder, β-glucuronidase hydrolyzes the glucuronic acid conjugate at the acidic pH of urine, producing reactive arylnitrenium ions, which bind guanines in DNA, and so act as mutagens.

MOLECULAR PATHOGENESIS: ***Specific cytogenetic abnormalities have been observed in 50% of bladder cancers.*** These include most often deletion of chromosome 9 or its short or long arm (9p- or 9q-) and deletions of 11p, 13p, 14q or 17p. Aneuploidy of chromosomes 3, 7 and 17 are well described. Chromosomal deletions in 9p, which contains the **tumor suppressor gene *p16***, are the only consistent finding in low-grade papillary tumors and flat carcinomas in situ. Deletions in 17p, the site of the ***p53* gene**, are often found in invasive bladder cancers.

A model for the development of urothelial carcinogenesis has evolved based on cytogenetic abnormalities observed in bladder tumors. Dysregulation of the cell cycle by a mutated *p53* allows propagation of genetically abnormal urothelial cells. Unregulated cell proliferation occurs secondary to accumulated mutations in cyclin-dependent kinase inhibitors (e.g., p16/INK4a) or deletion of the tumor suppressor gene *RB1* (Fig. 17-11).

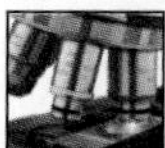

PATHOLOGY: Epithelial tumors, most of which are urothelial carcinomas, constitute more than 90% of all primary bladder tumors. Neoplastic urothelial lesions arising from the bladder mucosa comprise a spectrum that at one end includes benign papillomas and low-grade exophytic papillary carcinomas and at the other, invasive transitional cell carcinomas and highly malignant tumors (Fig. 17-12). Other tumors, listed in Table 17-1, are considerably less common.

Urothelial Papilloma Is a Rare Benign Tumor

Urothelial papillomas of the urinary bladder are uncommon, representing less than 1% of all bladder tumors. They are usually discovered incidentally in men above the age of 50 years during cystoscopy for an unrelated condition or for painless hematuria. There are two forms, classical exophytic papilloma and inverted papilloma.

Exophytic papilloma features papillary fronds lined by transitional epithelium that is virtually indistinguishable from normal urothelium. On cystoscopy, most patients show

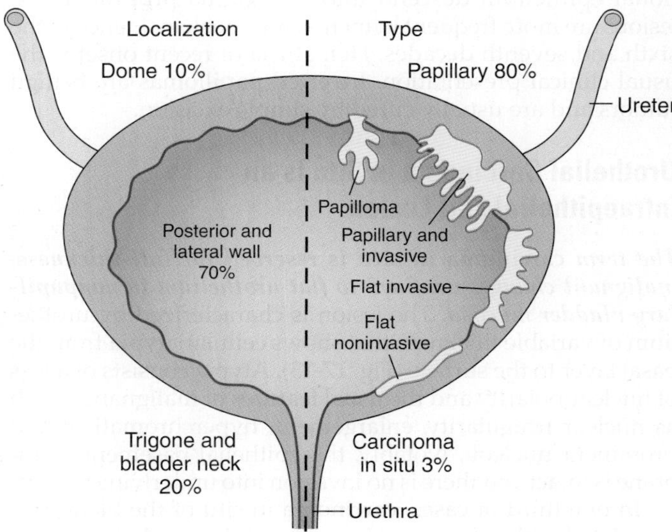

FIGURE 17-12. Urothelial neoplasms. Most tumors are localized on the posterior and lateral wall; trigone and bladder neck are involved less often and the dome least commonly. Malignant tumors may be papillary or flat. Both flat and papillary tumors may be invasive or noninvasive. Benign transitional cell papillomas are rare.

Table 17-1

Tumors of Urinary Bladder

Urothelial Tumors
Urothelial cell papilloma
Exophytic papilloma
Inverted papilloma
Urothelial carcinoma in situ
Papillary urothelial neoplasm of low malignant potential (PUNLMP)
Papillary urothelial carcinoma, low grade*
Papillary urothelial carcinoma, high grade*
Invasive urothelial carcinoma
Other Malignant Tumors
Squamous cell carcinoma
Adenocarcinoma
Neuroendocrine (small cell) carcinoma
Carcinosarcoma
Sarcomas

*Papillary carcinomas may be invasive or noninvasive.

single lesions 2 to 5 cm in diameter, but some tumors may be multiple. Although considered benign, some papillomas may recur or progress to carcinoma, mandating regular follow-up. In most instances, "recurrences" represent new tumors that develop elsewhere in the urinary bladder.

Inverted papillomas are rare and typically present as nodular mucosal lesions in the urinary bladder, usually in the trigone area. Less commonly they have also been observed in the renal pelvis, ureter and urethra. Inverted papillomas are covered by normal urothelium, from which cords of transitional epithelium descend into the lamina propria. These lesions are more frequent in men, with a peak incidence in the sixth and seventh decades. Hematuria of recent onset is the usual clinical presentation. Inverted papillomas are benign tumors and are usually cured by simple excision.

Urothelial Carcinoma in Situ Is an Intraepithelial Flat Lesion

The term* carcinoma in situ *is reserved for full-thickness, malignant changes confined to flat urothelium in nonpapillary bladder mucosa. The lesion is characterized by urothelium of variable thickness that shows cellular atypia from the basal layer to the surface (Fig. 17-13). Atypia consists of a loss of nuclear polarity and the usual features of malignancy, such as nuclear irregularity, enlargement, hyperchromatism and prominent nucleoli. Notably, the epithelial basement membrane is intact and there is no invasion into underlying stroma.

In one third of cases, carcinoma in situ of the bladder is associated with subsequent invasive carcinoma. In turn, most invasive transitional cell carcinomas arise from carcinoma in situ rather than from papillary transitional cell cancers. Confined to the mucosal surface, the in situ lesions most often appear as multiple, red, velvety, flat patches topographically close to exophytic papillary transitional cell carcinoma (see below). Concurrent involvement with in situ cancer elsewhere in the bladder or in the ureters, urethra and prostatic ducts is common. Carcinoma in situ is often multifocal at the time of discovery, or similar lesions may develop shortly thereafter. Lesions involving the bladder neck or the urethra may extend into the periurethral prostatic ducts.

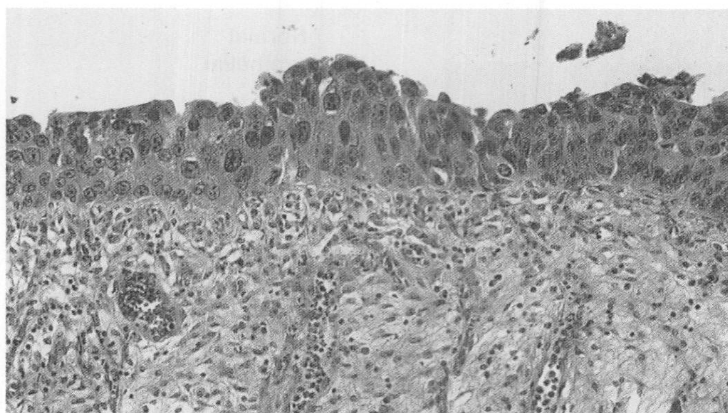

FIGURE 17-13. Urothelial carcinoma in situ. The urothelial mucosa shows nuclear pleomorphism and lack of polarity from the basal layer to the surface, without evidence of maturation (see Fig. 17-9A to compare to normal bladder urothelium).

Urothelial Carcinomas Vary From Superficial Papillary to Deeply Invasive

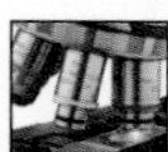

PATHOLOGY: Papillary cancer arises most frequently from the lateral or posterior bladder walls. At cystoscopy, tumors may be small, delicate, low-grade papillary lesions limited to the mucosal surface or larger, high-grade, solid masses that are invasive and ulcerated (Fig. 17-14).

Papillary cancers are graded as papillary urothelial neoplasms of low malignant potential (PUNLMP) and papillary urothelial carcinomas, low grade and high grade. Low-grade and high-grade urothelial papillary carcinomas may be invasive.

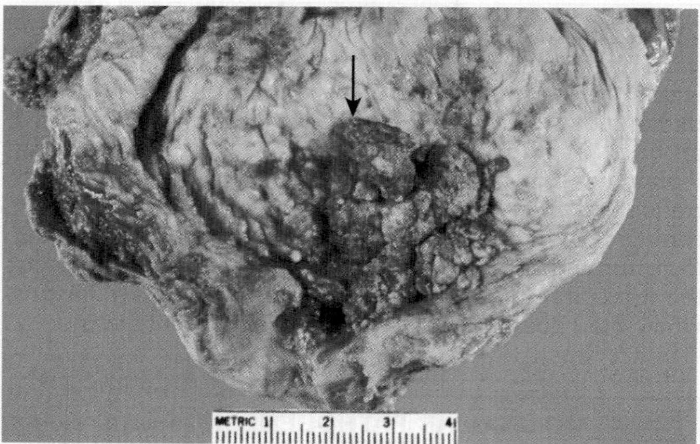

FIGURE 17-14. Urothelial carcinoma of the urinary bladder. A large exophytic tumor is situated above the bladder neck (*arrow*).

- **Papillary urothelial neoplasms of low malignant potential:** These are papillary tumors that resemble urothelial papillomas but exhibit increased cellularity. They are considered an intermediate between benign papilloma and low-grade papillary urothelial carcinoma. These lesions are usually larger than papillomas but do not show the architectural and cytologic atypia that are characteristic of low-grade carcinomas. PUNLMP may recur or occasionally progress to higher-grade tumors.
- **Low-grade papillary urothelial carcinoma:** Low-grade tumors have fronds lined by neoplastic urothelial epithelium with minimal architectural and cytologic atypia (Fig. 17-15A, B). The cells are moderately hyperchromatic with little nuclear pleomorphism and low mitotic activity. Papillae are long and delicate. Fusion of papillae is focal and limited. In about 10% of cases there is invasion of the lamina propria or into the deep muscle of the bladder (muscularis propria).
- **High-grade papillary urothelial carcinoma:** These tumors show significant nuclear hyperchromasia and pleomorphism. The epithelium is disorganized (Fig. 17-15C, D) and there are mitoses in all layers. Approximately 80% of all high-grade tumors show invasion into the lamina propria,

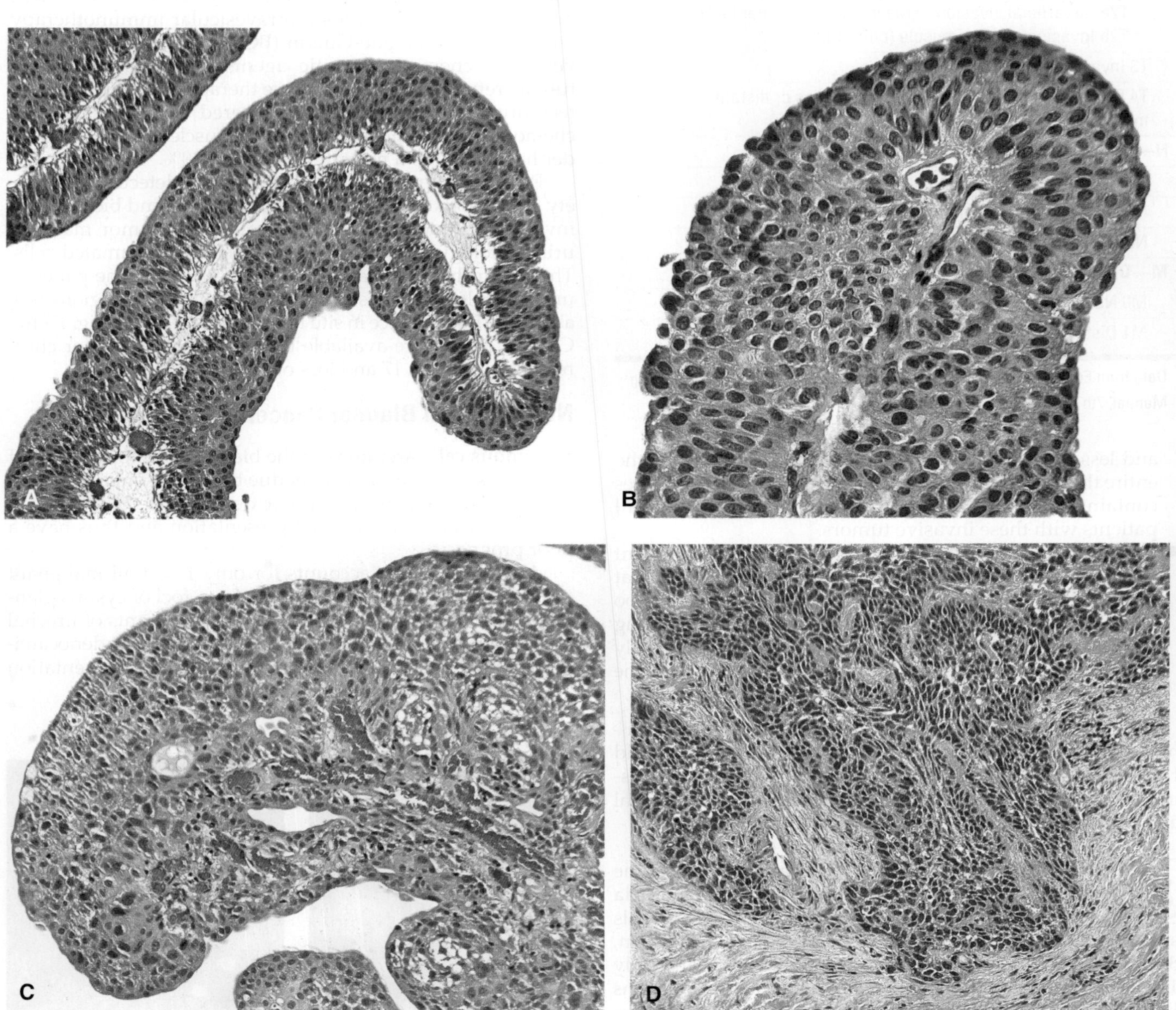

FIGURE 17-15. Urothelial tumors of the urinary bladder. A. Low-grade papillary urothelial carcinoma consists of exophytic papillae that have a central connective tissue core and are lined by slightly disorganized transitional epithelium. **B.** Low-grade papillary urothelial carcinoma at higher magnification shows mild architectural and cytologic atypia. **C.** High-grade papillary urothelial carcinoma shows prominent architectural disorganization of the epithelium, which contains cells with pleomorphic hyperchromatic nuclei. **D.** Invasive high-grade papillary urothelial carcinoma consists of irregular nests of hyperchromatic cells invading into the muscularis.

Table 17-2

TNM Staging of Urothelial Carcinoma of Urinary Bladder

T—Primary Tumor
T0 No grossly visible tumor
Ta Noninvasive papillary carcinoma
Tis Carcinoma in situ
T1 Invasion of the lamina propria
T2 Invasion of the muscularis propria T2a Superficial invasion of the muscularis (inner half) T2b Invasion of deep muscle (outer half)
T3 Invasion of the perivesical tissue
T4 Extravesical spread into adjacent organs or distant metastases
N—Regional Lymph Nodes
N0 No lymph node involvement
N1 Single lymph node metastasis
N2, N3 More lymph nodes involved
M—Distant metastases
M0 No metastases
M1 Distant metastases

Data from Edge SB, Byrd DR, Compton CC, et al., eds. AJCC Cancer Staging Manual, 7th ed. New York: Springer, 2009.

and less often into the muscularis propria or through the entire thickness of the bladder wall. Regional lymph nodes contain metastatic tumor in approximately half of all patients with these invasive tumors.

- **Invasive urothelial carcinoma:** These highly malignant tumors may evolve from preexisting papillary lesions or flat carcinoma in situ. In many cases the diagnosis is made too late to determine the nature of the initial or preexisting tumor. Most, if not all, invasive carcinomas are histologically high-grade tumors. The depth of invasion into the wall of the bladder, or beyond its confines, determines the prognosis.

Bladder cancers are staged according to the tumor–node–metastasis (TNM) classification system of the World Health Organization (WHO) (Table 17-2). In order of decreasing frequency, metastases of bladder cancer occur in regional and periaortic lymph nodes, liver, lung and bone.

CLINICAL FEATURES: Urothelial carcinoma of the bladder typically manifests as sudden **hematuria** and, less frequently, as **dysuria.** Cystoscopy reveals single or multiple tumors. At the time of initial presentation, 85% of tumors are confined to the urinary bladder and only 15% have regional or distant metastases. Papillary lesions limited to the mucosa or lamina propria (stage T1) are commonly treated conservatively by transurethral resection. Radical cystectomy is done for patients whose tumors show muscle invasion, and occasionally for advanced-stage tumors. In bladder cancer patients, the most common causes of death are uremia (from obstruction of the urinary outflow tract), extension into adjacent organs and effects of distant metastases.

The probability of tumor extension and subsequent recurrence correlates with a number of factors:

- Large size
- High stage
- High grade
- Presence of multiple tumors
- Vascular or lymphatic invasion
- Urothelial dysplasia (including carcinoma in situ) at other sites in the bladder

The overall 10-year survival rate with noninvasive or superficially invasive low-grade urothelial tumors is over 95% irrespective of the number of recurrences. Only 10% of low-grade tumors will progress to higher-grade tumors and, consequently, a worse prognosis. Conservative treatment involves tumor fulguration, intravesicular immunotherapy with bacillus Calmette-Guerin (BCG) or instillation of conventional chemotherapeutic agents. Invasive tumors or tumors refractory to conservative therapy are treated by cystectomy and patients may be offered adjuvant systemic chemotherapy. Tumors invading the muscle layer of the bladder have an overall mortality of 25% to 30%.

Recurrent or progressive disease can be detected by a variety of methods including repeat cystoscopy and biopsy. Less invasive techniques include urinalysis for tumor markers, urine cytology and cytogenic analysis of desquamated cells. This last technique analyzes cells isolated from the patient's urine for ploidy values of specific chromosomal regions (see above) by fluorescence in situ hybridization (FISH) (Fig. 17-16). Current probes are available to detect aneuploidy for chromosomes 3, 7 and 17 and loss of the 9p21 locus.

Nonurothelial Bladder Cancers Are Rare

Squamous cell carcinoma of the bladder develops in foci of squamous metaplasia, usually due to schistosomiasis. Virtually all patients with this tumor demonstrate bladder wall invasion at the time of initial presentation and thus have a poor prognosis.

Adenocarcinoma accounts for only 1% of all malignant tumors of the bladder. It originates from foci of cystitis glandularis or intestinal metaplasia or from remnants of urachal epithelium in the bladder dome. Most bladder adenocarcinomas are deeply invasive at the time of initial presentation and are not curable.

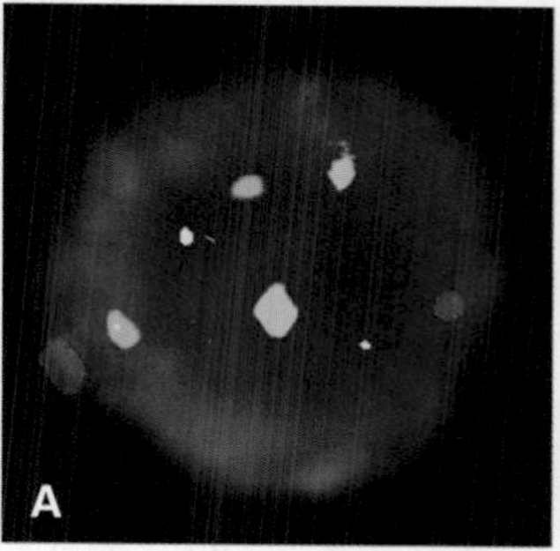

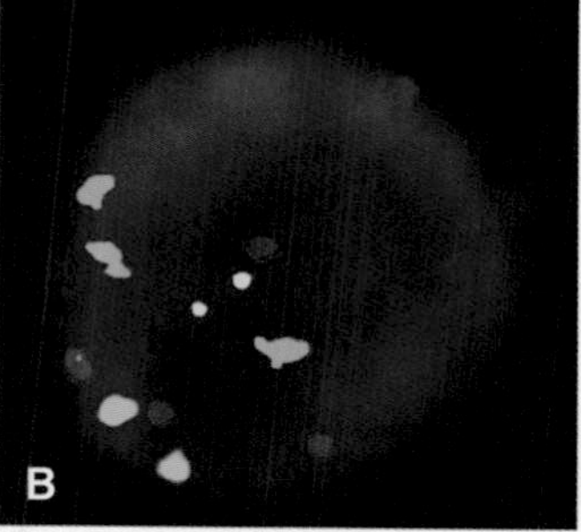

FIGURE 17-16. Fluorescence in situ hybridization of bladder cancer. A. Normal. Single urothelial cell collected from urine of normal person. Red fluorescence represents chromosome 3, green is chromosome 7, aqua is chromosome 17 and gold represents 9p21. The probe signals are present in two copies. **B. Urothelial carcinoma of the bladder.** There is aneuploidy of chromosome 3 (three copies) and chromosome 7 (four copies). Chromosome 17 and 9p21 locus are euploid.

Neuroendocrine carcinoma, resembling small cell lung carcinoma, is sometimes seen in the urinary bladder. The tumor is highly malignant and has a poor prognosis.

Sarcomas of the urinary bladder, resembling those of the soft tissues, are distinctly rare. These highly malignant tumors form bulky masses and are often inoperable. **Leiomyosarcoma** is the most common histologic form in adults.

Rhabdomyosarcoma, typically of the embryonal type, manifests most commonly in children as **sarcoma botryoides** (i.e., edematous, mucosal, polypoid masses that have been likened to a cluster of grapes). Combined treatment with radiation therapy and chemotherapy has greatly increased survival rates.

PENIS, URETHRA AND SCROTUM

Congenital Disorders of the Penis

Developmental anomalies of the penis include rare conditions such as agenesis and occasional abnormalities such as hypoplasia, as well as the more frequent anomalies that involve the penile urethra and prepuce.

HYPOSPADIAS: ***This term refers to a congenital anomaly in which the urethra opens on the underside (ventral) of the penis, so that the meatus is proximal to its normal glandular location on the tip of the penis.*** It results from incomplete closure of the urethral folds of the urogenital sinus.

Hypospadias occurs in 1 in 350 male neonates. Most cases are sporadic but familial occurrence has been reported. It also may be associated with other urogenital anomalies and complex, multisystemic, developmental syndromes. In 90% of cases, the meatus is located on the underside of the glans, or the corona (Fig. 17-17). Less often, it is found along the midshaft of the penis, in the scrotum and even in the perineum. Surgical repair is usually uncomplicated.

EPISPADIAS: ***In this rare congenital anomaly the urethra opens on the upper side (dorsal) of the penis.*** In the most common form of epispadias, the entire penile urethra is open along the entire shaft. Severe epispadias may be associated with bladder exstrophy (Fig. 17-4). In its mildest form, the defect is limited to the glandular urethra. Surgical treatment of epispadias is more complicated than that of hypospadias.

PHIMOSIS: ***The orifice of the prepuce may be too narrow to allow retraction over the glans penis.*** Phimosis predisposes the penis to infections. If a narrow prepuce is forcefully retracted, it may strangulate the glans and impede the outflow of venous blood, a condition termed **paraphimosis.** Congenital phimosis must be distinguished from acquired phimosis, which is usually a consequence of recurrent infections or trauma of the prepuce in uncircumcised men. Circumcision cures both phimosis and paraphimosis.

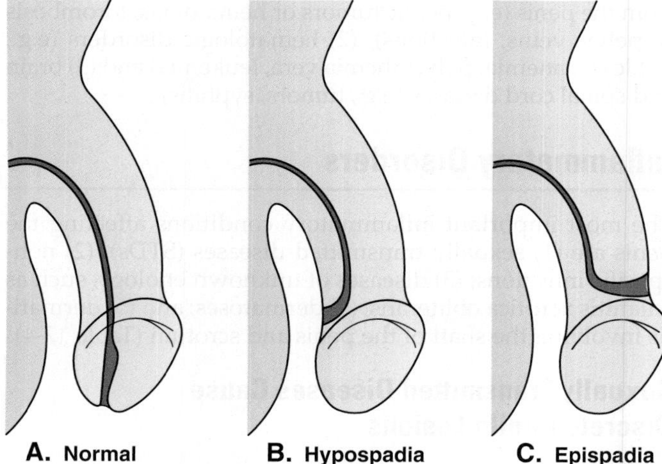

FIGURE 17-17. Congenital anomalies of the penis. A. Normal penis has the urethral opening on the tip of the glans. **B.** Hypospadia is characterized by a urethral opening on the ventral side of the penis. **C.** Epispadia is characterized by a urethral opening on the dorsal side of the penis.

Scrotal Masses

Scrotal masses and conditions that lead to scrotal swelling or enlargement often reflect abnormalities of testicular, epididymal and scrotal development. Clinical problems related to these pathologic conditions are most often encountered in children but may be found in adults (Fig. 17-18A–D).

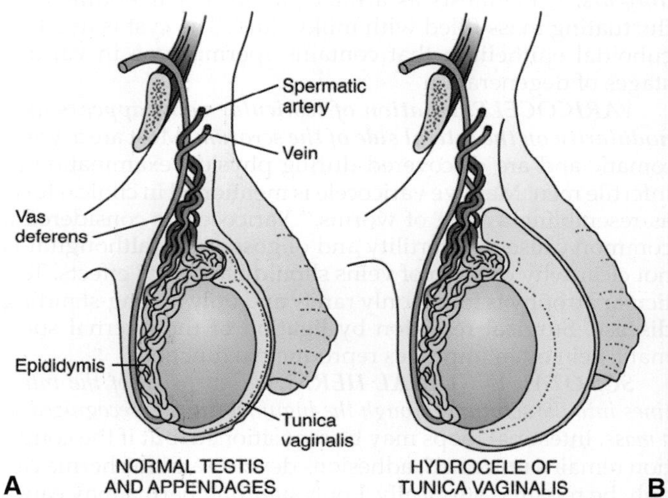

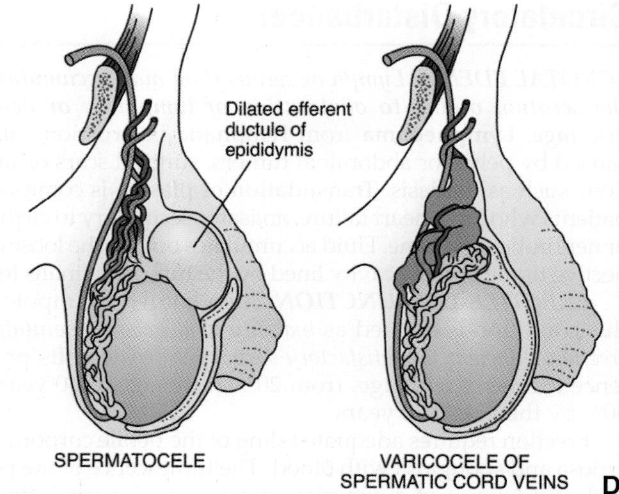

FIGURE 17-18. Scrotal masses. A. Normal testis. **B.** Hydrocele. **C.** Spermatocele. **D.** Varicocele.

HYDROCELE: This term refers to a collection of serous fluid in the scrotal sac between the two layers of the tunica vaginalis. The cavity is lined by mesothelium. Hydrocele may be congenital or acquired.

Congenital hydrocele reflects a patent processus vaginalis testis or its incomplete obliteration. It is the most common cause of scrotal swelling in infants and is often associated with inguinal hernia.

Acquired hydrocele in adults is secondary to some other disease affecting the scrotum, such as infection, tumor or trauma. The cause cannot be found. The diagnosis is made by ultrasound or by transluminating the fluid in the cavity. Hydrocele is a benign condition that disappears once the causal disease has been eliminated. However, long-standing hydrocele may cause testicular atrophy or compression of the epididymis, or the fluid may become infected and lead to **periorchitis.**

*HEMATOCELE: **Blood may accumulate between the layers of tunica vaginalis after trauma or hemorrhage into a hydrocele.*** Testicular tumors and infections may also lead to a hematocele.

*SPERMATOCELE: **This mass is a cyst formed from protrusions of widened efferent ducts of the rete testis or epididymis.*** It manifests as a hilar paratesticular nodule or a fluctuating mass filled with milky fluid. The cyst is lined by cuboidal epithelium that contains spermatozoa in various stages of degeneration.

*VARICOCELE: **Dilation of testicular veins appears as a nodularity on the lateral side of the scrotum.*** Most are asymptomatic and are discovered during physical examination of infertile men. Massive varicocele is mentioned in clinical texts as resembling a "bag of worms." Varicocele is considered a common cause of infertility and oligospermia, although it is not clear why dilation of veins should have such effects. Testicular atrophy is found only rarely and only in long-standing disease. Surgical resection by ligation of the internal spermatic vein often improves reproductive function.

SCROTAL INGUINAL HERNIA: Protrusion of the intestines into the scrotum through the inguinal canal is recognized as a mass. Intestinal loops may be repositioned, but if the condition remains untreated, adhesions develop and the hernia can only be repaired surgically. Long-standing hernia may cause testicular atrophy.

Circulatory Disturbances

*SCROTAL EDEMA: **Lymph or serous fluid may accumulate in the scrotum owing to obstruction of lymphatic or venous drainage.*** **Lymphedema** from lymphatic obstruction can be caused by pelvic or abdominal tumors, surgical scars or infections such as filariasis. **Transudation** of plasma is common in patients who have heart failure, anasarca secondary to cirrhosis or nephrotic syndrome. Fluid accumulates both in the loose connective tissue and the cavity lined by the tunica vaginalis testis.

ERECTILE DYSFUNCTION: Also known as impotence, this condition is defined as *inability to achieve or maintain an erection sufficient for satisfactory sexual performance.* Its prevalence increases with age, from 20% at the age of 40 years to 50% by the age of 70 years.

Erection requires adequate filling of the penile corpora cavernosa and spongiosa with blood. The tumescence of the penis is the end-result of a complex interaction of mental, neural, hormonal and vascular factors. Filling of these vascular spaces depends on nitric oxide (NO•)-mediated relaxation of vascular smooth muscle cells in the erectile cylinders. Since NO• release is related to cyclic guanosine 3′,5′-monophosphate (cGMP), drugs that inhibit the phosphodiesterase that degrades cGMP (e.g., sildenafil [Viagra], vardenafil hydrochloride [Levitra], tadalafil [Cialis]) are used to treat erectile dysfunction. Disorders associated with erectile dysfunction are listed in Table 17-3.

Table 17-3

Erectile Dysfunctions

Erectile Dysfunctions
Neuropsychiatric
Psychiatric disorders (e.g., depression)
Spinal cord injury
Nerve injury during surgery (e.g., pelvic or perineal surgery)
Endocrine
Hypogonadism
Pituitary diseases (e.g., hyperprolactinemia)
Hypothyroidism, Cushing syndrome, Addison disease
Vascular
Diabetic microangiopathy
Hypertension
Atherosclerosis
Drugs
Antihypertensives
Psychotropic drugs
Estrogens, anticancer drugs, etc.
Idiopathic
"Performance anxiety"
Age-related "impotence"

PRIAPISM: This term is used to describe ***continuous penile erection unrelated to sexual excitation.*** It may be primary or secondary. The cause of primary priapism is unknown and the treatment of this painful erection is usually ineffective. Secondary priapism may be a complication of several diseases, including (1) pelvic diseases that impede outflow of blood from the penis (e.g., pelvic tumors or hematomas, thrombosis of pelvic veins, infections), (2) hematologic disorders (e.g., sickle cell anemia, polycythemia vera, leukemia) and (3) brain and spinal cord diseases (e.g., tumors, syphilis).

Inflammatory Disorders

The most important inflammatory conditions affecting the penis are (1) sexually transmitted diseases (STDs); (2) nonspecific infections; (3) diseases of unknown etiology, such as balanitis xerotica obliterans; (4) dermatoses; and (5) dermatitis involving the shaft of the penis and scrotum (Table 17-4).

Sexually Transmitted Diseases Cause Discrete Penile Lesions

Sexually transmitted diseases (STDs) are reviewed here briefly in the context of other infections of the lower urinary tracts (Fig. 17-19) (for more detail, see Chapter 9).

- **Genital herpes** is most often caused by herpes simplex virus type 2 (HSV-2), but may be less commonly caused by HSV-1. It is the most common STD affecting the glans, and

Table 17-4

Inflammatory Lesions of the Penis

Sexually Transmitted Diseases
Herpes genitalis
Syphilis
Chancroid
Granuloma inguinale
Lymphogranuloma venereum
Human papillomavirus infections
Nonspecific Infectious Balanoposthitis
Bacterial, fungal, viral
Diseases of Unknown Etiology
Balanitis xerotica obliterans
Circinate balanitis
Plasma cell balanitis (Zoon balanitis)
Peyronie disease
Dermatitis Involving the Shaft of the Penis and Scrotum
Infectious (bacterial, viral, fungal)
Noninfectious (e.g., lichen planus, bullous skin diseases)

manifests typically as grouped vesicles that ulcerate and transform into crusts.

- **Syphilis** (*Treponema pallidum*) manifests as a solitary, soft ulcer (**chancre**).
- **Chancroid** is caused by *Haemophilus ducreyi* and manifests as a papule that transforms into a pustule and finally ulcerates. Shallow ulcers on the glans or the skin of the shaft are often associated with painful suppurative inguinal lymphadenitis.
- **Granuloma inguinale,** a tropical disease caused by *Calymmatobacterium granulomatis,* appears as a raised ulcer with a copious chronic inflammatory exudate and granulation tissue. Such ulcers tend to enlarge and heal very slowly.

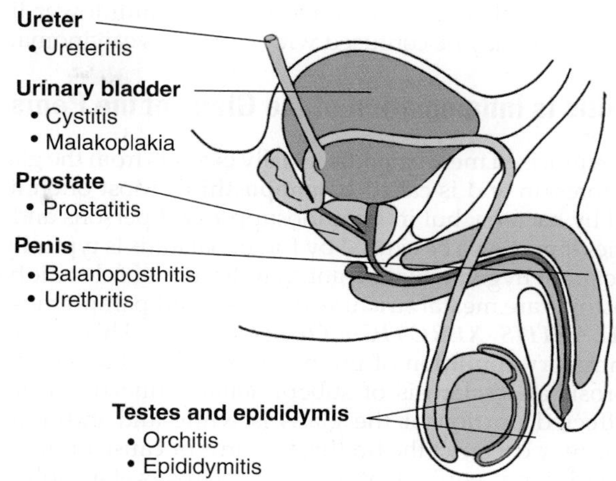

FIGURE 17-19. Infections of the lower urinary tract and male reproductive system.

- **Lymphogranuloma venereum** is caused by *Chlamydia trachomatis* and presents as a small, often innocuous, vesicle that ulcerates. It is typically accompanied by tender enlargement of inguinal lymph nodes, which adhere to the skin and form sinuses draining pus and serosanguineous fluid.
- **Condylomata acuminatum** is caused by human papillomavirus type 6 and, less often, type 11. It appears in the form of flat-topped warts on the shaft (Fig. 17-20), small polyps on

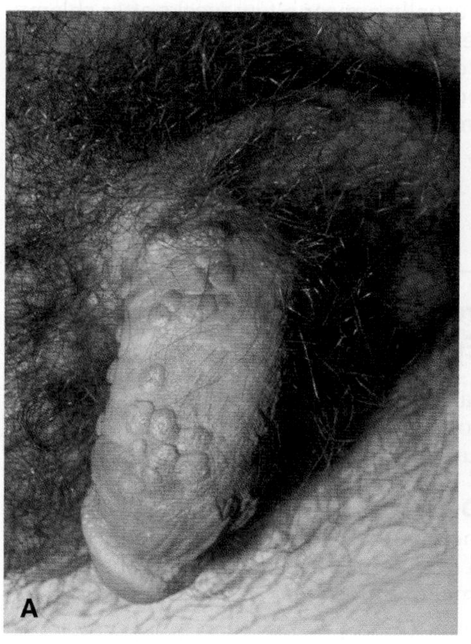

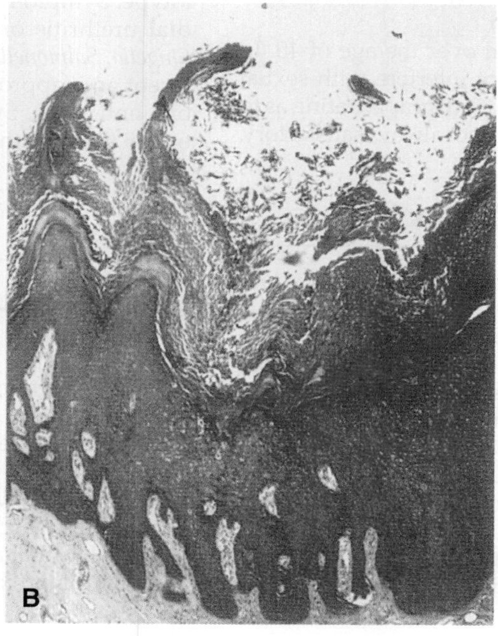

FIGURE 17-20. Condylomata acuminata of the penis. A. Raised, circumscribed lesions are seen on the shaft of the penis. **B.** Section of a lesion shows epidermal hyperkeratosis, parakeratosis, acanthosis and papillomatosis.

the glans and urethral meatus or larger cauliflower-like tumors that may be confused with verrucous carcinoma.

Balanitis Is Inflammation of the Glans of the Penis

In uncircumcised men, balanitis usually extends from the glans to the foreskin and is called **balanoposthitis.** Most often it is caused by bacteria, but in immunosuppressed persons and in diabetics it may also be caused by fungi. Balanitis is typically a result of poor hygiene. Significant complications of chronic balanoposthitis are meatal stricture, phimosis and paraphimosis.

BALANITIS XEROTICA OBLITERANS: This chronic inflammatory condition of unknown origin is characterized by fibrosis and sclerosis of subepithelial connective tissue. The affected portion of the glans is white and indurated. Fibrosis may constrict the urethral meatus or cause phimosis. This condition is equivalent to lichen sclerosus et atrophicus of the vulva (see Chapter 18).

CIRCINATE BALANITIS: In the course of **Reiter syndrome** (see below), the glans may show circular, linear or confluent plaque-like discolorations, occasionally associated with superficial ulcers.

PLASMA CELL BALANITIS: Also known as **Zoon balanitis,** this disease of unknown origin causes macular discoloration or painless papules on the glans. Histologically, the connective tissue shows infiltrates of plasma cells and lymphocytes and the overlying epithelium is thickened. The disease is chronic but innocuous.

DERMATOSES: Many inflammatory skin diseases may involve the penis. Such conditions are discussed in Chapter 24.

Peyronie Disease Is a Fibrous Induration of the Penis

Peyronie disease is a common malady of unknown etiology characterized by focal, asymmetric fibrosis of the penile shaft. Penile curvature is usually accompanied by pain during erection. The typical case is an ill-defined induration of the penile shaft in a young or middle-aged man, with no change in the overlying skin. On microscopic examination, dense fibrosis is associated with sparse, nonspecific, chronic inflammatory infiltration. Collagen focally replaces muscle in the septum of the corpus cavernosum.

Peyronie disease affects 1% of men over the age of 40. In most instances, it is mild and does not interfere with sexual function. Severe penile curvature may be so incapacitating as to require surgery, although the outcome is not always satisfactory.

Urethritis and Related Conditions

Urethritis is inflammation of the urethra. It may be either acute or chronic.

SEXUALLY TRANSMITTED URETHRITIS: ***Urethritis is the most common manifestation of STDs in men, in whom it typically presents with urethral discharge.*** Women rarely notice distinct urethral discharge and usually complain of vaginal discharge.

Gonococcal and nongonococcal urethritis have an acute onset and are related to recent sexual intercourse. The infection manifests with a typically purulent and greenish yellow urethral discharge. Symptoms include pain or tingling at the meatus of the urethra and pain on micturition (**dysuria**). Meatal redness and swelling are usually seen in both sexes. Acute gonococcal and nongonococcal urethritis can both become chronic.

The diagnosis is made by identifying the causative agent. In gonococcal urethritis the discharge contains *Neisseria gonorrhoeae,* which can be identified microscopically in smears of urethral exudates. Nongonococcal urethritis is mostly caused by *C. trachomatis* or *Ureaplasma urealyticum* but may be related to a variety of other pathogens.

NONSPECIFIC INFECTIOUS URETHRITIS: ***Uropathogens such as* E. coli *and* Pseudomonas *can cause urethritis.*** Typically infection is associated with cystitis but may be related to other diseases (e.g., prostatic hyperplasia or urinary stones). In men, infectious urethritis may be the only sign of prostatitis; in women, it may be a complication of vaginitis and vulvitis. In hospitalized patients it commonly follows cystoscopy and other urologic procedures and is almost inevitable in patients with indwelling urethral catheters.

Nonspecific infectious urethritis manifests clinically with urgency and a burning sensation during urination. Usually there is no discharge, although men can express some milky fluid by "stripping" or "milking" the urethra.

URETHRAL CARUNCLES: ***Polypoid inflammatory lesions near the female urethral meatus produce pain and bleeding.*** They occur exclusively in women, mostly after menopause. The etiology and pathogenesis are unclear; prolapse of the urethral mucosa and associated chronic inflammation have been suggested as the cause.

Urethral caruncle presents as an exophytic, often ulcerated, polypoid mass, 1 to 2 cm in diameter, at or near the urethral meatus. Microscopically, it exhibits acutely and chronically inflamed granulation tissue and ulceration and hyperplasia of transitional cell or squamous epithelium. Although complex patterns of papillomatosis and occasional dysplastic epithelium may give this inflammatory lesion a superficial resemblance to carcinoma, it does not lead to cancer. Treatment is surgical excision.

REITER SYNDROME: ***This condition is a triad of urethritis, conjunctivitis and arthritis of weight-bearing joints (e.g., knee, sacroiliac and vertebral joints).*** Other clinical findings encountered in variable proportions are circinate balanitis, cervicitis and skin eruptions. Reiter syndrome tends to affect young adults with human leukocyte antigen (HLA)-B27 haplotype. Symptoms usually appear a few weeks after chlamydial urethritis or enteric infection with such pathogens as *Shigella, Salmonella* or *Campylobacter*. It is thus thought to represent an inappropriate immune reaction to unknown microbial antigen(s). Symptoms usually disappear spontaneously over 3 to 6 months, but arthritis recurs in half of patients.

Tumors

Cancer of the Urethra May Arise From Squamous or Transitional Epithelium

Urethral carcinoma is an uncommon tumor usually found in elderly women. Some penile cancers arise in the terminal part of the penile urethra.

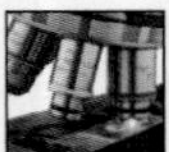

PATHOLOGY: Most urethral cancers are squamous cell carcinomas originating in the distal urethra. Urothelial carcinoma similar to that in the bladder arises in the proximal urethra.

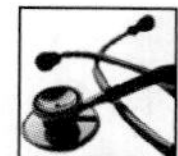

CLINICAL FEATURES: Urethral cancer develops most frequently in the sixth and seventh decades. Patients present with urethral bleeding and dysuria. Despite the accessible location and associated symptoms, most tumors have spread to adjacent tissues or regional lymph nodes at the time of presentation. Radical surgery is the main therapy.

Cancer of the Penis Occurs Mostly in Uncircumcised Men

Cancer of the penis originates from the squamous mucosa of the glans and contiguous urethral meatus or the prepuce and skin covering the penile shaft.

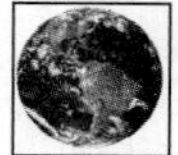

EPIDEMIOLOGY: In the United States, invasive squamous cell carcinoma of the penis is an uncommon tumor, accounting for less than 0.5% of all cancers in men. The average age of patients is 60 years. Penile cancer is much more common in less developed countries: in some parts of Africa, Asia and South America it constitutes 10% of cancers in men. Since it is virtually unknown in men who were circumcised at birth, these geographic variations have been attributed to differences in the frequency of circumcision.

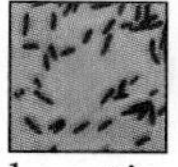

ETIOLOGIC FACTORS: No single agent has been identified as the cause of penile cancer. Current interest centers on the possible influence of accumulated keratin debris and inflammatory exudate (**smegma**) that accumulate beneath the prepuce. Most patients with cancer of the penis have had phimosis since an early age, suggesting that prolonged contact between smegma and the penile epithelium may play a role. Human papillomavirus (HPV) types 16 and 18 have also been suggested as factors in the pathogenesis of penile cancer.

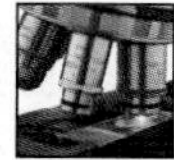

PATHOLOGY: Penile carcinoma occurs in a preinvasive form (carcinoma in situ) and an invasive variety.

SQUAMOUS CELL CARCINOMA IN SITU: Historically, carcinoma in situ of the penis was described in two forms: Bowen disease and erythroplasia of Queyrat. **Bowen disease** appears as a sharply demarcated, erythematous or grayish white plaque on the shaft. **Erythroplasia of Queyrat** manifests as solitary or multiple, shiny, soft, erythematous plaques on the glans and foreskin. Both of these conditions appear microscopically as **squamous cell carcinoma in situ** similar to that in other sites. The lesions show cytologic atypia of the keratinocytes of all layers of the epidermis, with parakeratosis or hyperkeratosis; papillomatosis with broad epidermal papillae; and thinning of the granular layer. By definition, the atypical keratinocytes do not invade the underlying dermis. The frequency of progression to invasive squamous cell carcinoma remains unsettled but is estimated to be less than 10% of cases.

Bowenoid papulosis of the penis is caused by HPV and affects young, sexually active men. In contrast to the solitary lesion of Bowen disease, bowenoid papulosis appears as multiple brownish or violaceous papules. Microscopically, it resembles other variants of carcinoma in situ, but occasionally there are some differences. In contrast to true carcinoma in situ, which slowly merges at the margins with normal epithelium, bowenoid papulosis is sharply demarcated from normal epidermis and thus resembles HPV-induced warts. The altered epidermis shows some superficial stratification and maturation and may contain giant keratinocytes with multinucleated atypical nuclei. HPV type 16 can be demonstrated in 80% of patients. Virtually all lesions of bowenoid papulosis regress spontaneously and do not progress to invasive carcinoma.

INVASIVE SQUAMOUS CELL CARCINOMA: The tumor presents as (1) an ulcer; (2) an indurated crater; (3) a friable hemorrhagic mass; or (4) an exophytic, fungating, papillary tumor. Squamous cell carcinoma usually involves the glans or prepuce and less commonly the penile shaft. Extensive destruction of penile tissue, including the urethral meatus, is observed in cases in which the tumor has been neglected. Microscopically, it is typically a well-differentiated, focally keratinizing, squamous cell carcinoma. Invasive tumors usually have a dense, chronic inflammatory cell infiltrate in the dermis. The adjacent epidermis often shows dysplastic changes. The tumor may invade deeply along the penile shaft and spread to inguinal lymph nodes, then to iliac nodes and ultimately to distant organs.

VERRUCOUS CARCINOMA: This tumor deserves to be separated from other penile cancers because it is a cytologically benign but clinically malignant exophytic squamous cell carcinoma (Fig. 17-21). It is grossly and cytologically similar to **condyloma acuminatum,** but unlike the latter, it shows local invasion. This low-grade squamous cell carcinoma usually does not metastasize and surgical removal is curative.

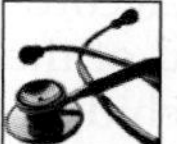

CLINICAL FEATURES: Most squamous cell cancers are confined to the penis at the time of initial presentation, but occult metastases to inguinal lymph nodes are not uncommon. Conversely, half of patients with enlarged regional lymph nodes do not have nodal metastases, but only reactive changes due to tumor-associated inflammation.

Survival of patients with penile cancer is related to the clinical stage and, to a lesser degree, the histologic grade of the tumor. Amputation of the penis is usually necessary. Patients with superficially invasive cancer have 90% 5-year survival; inguinal lymph node metastases reduce 5-year survival to 20% to 50%, depending on the extent of spread.

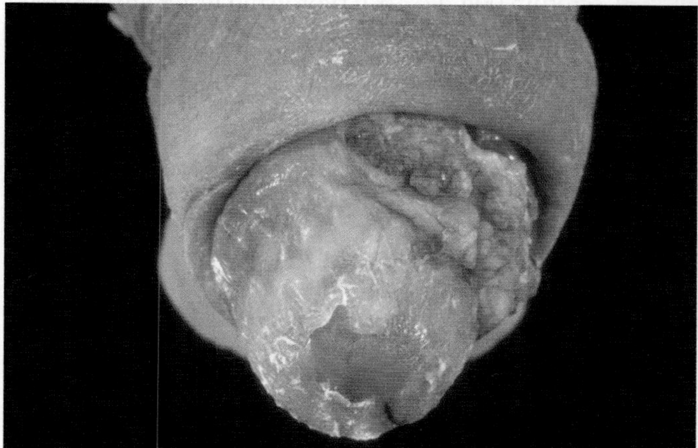

FIGURE 17-21. Carcinoma of the penis. This verrucous carcinoma arises on the glans and appears as an exophytic mass.

Cancer of the Scrotum Was First Identified in Chimney Sweeps

In 1775 Sir Percival Pott identified scrotal cancer as an occupational disease of chimney sweeps, thereby introducing the idea of chemical carcinogenesis (see Chapters 5 and 8). Pott implicated constant exposure to soot as the causative agent, but later investigators incriminated a large variety of industrial chemicals in the pathogenesis of this tumor. Industrial hygiene has improved so that scrotal cancer is today distinctly uncommon.

Squamous cell carcinoma of the scrotum typically affects older men and mostly in their sixth and seventh decades. At initial presentation, many patients show invasion of the scrotal contents and metastases to regional nodes. Therapy is surgical excision.

TESTIS, EPIDIDYMIS AND VAS DEFERENS

Cryptorchidism

Cryptorchidism, clinically known as **undescended testis,** *is a congenital abnormality in which one or both testes are not found in their normal position in the scrotum.* It is the most common urologic condition requiring surgical treatment in infants. In 5% of male infants born at term and 30% of those born prematurely, the testes are not in the scrotum or are easily retracted. In the large majority of these infants, testes descend into the scrotum during the first year of life. Accordingly, the prevalence of cryptorchidism from the end of the first year of life into adulthood is around 1%. Cryptorchidism is usually unilateral, but it is bilateral in 30% of affected men.

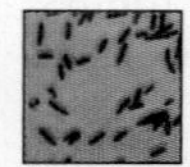

ETIOLOGIC FACTORS: The causes of testicular maldescent are usually unknown, but theoretically the condition could be related to (1) developmental disorders of the gonad, (2) endocrine factors or (3) mechanical factors that prevent passage of the fetal testis through the inguinal canal. It is usually an isolated developmental disorder, but may rarely be associated with other congenital anomalies.

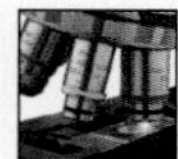

PATHOLOGY: Testicular descent may be arrested at any point from the abdominal cavity to the upper scrotum (Fig. 17-22). Cryptorchid testes are classified by their location as **abdominal, inguinal or upper scrotal.**

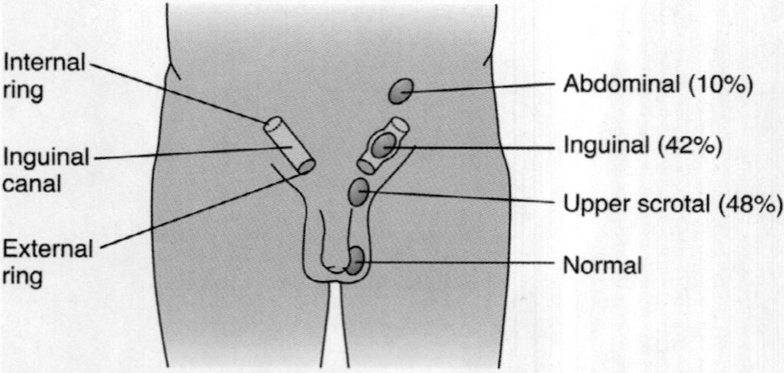

FIGURE 17-22. Cryptorchidism. In most instances, the testis has an upper scrotal location. It may be retained also in the inguinal canal and rarely in the abdominal cavity.

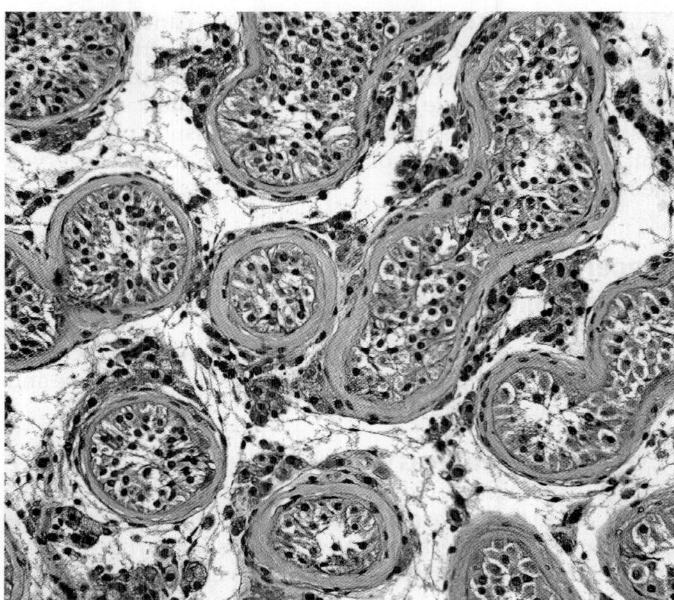

FIGURE 17-23. Cryptorchidism. This testis removed from a postpubertal man shows markedly thickened hyalinized basement membrane of seminiferous tubules, which show no signs of spermatogenesis.

Rarely, the testes are located in unusual locations, such as the perineum or calf.

Cryptorchid testes are smaller than normal even at an early age, and the difference between the affected and the normal testis becomes more prominent with age. Such testes appear firm, owing to parenchymal fibrosis.

The histology of cryptorchid testes varies with age. In infancy and early childhood the seminiferous tubules in affected testes are smaller and have fewer germ cells than normal. Postpubertal testes also contain fewer germ cells than normal and spermatogenesis is limited to a minority of tubules. Hyaline thickening of tubular basement membranes and prominent stromal fibrosis are observed (Fig. 17-23). Eventually, tubules become devoid of spermatogenic cells and are entirely hyalinized. **Orchiopexy** (surgical placement of a testis into the scrotum) performed either in childhood or after puberty does not prevent the loss of seminiferous epithelium and tubules; both the untreated and the repositioned testes show no signs of spermatogenesis in half of the cases. A few adult cryptorchid testes (2%) contain atypical germ cells corresponding to carcinoma in situ.

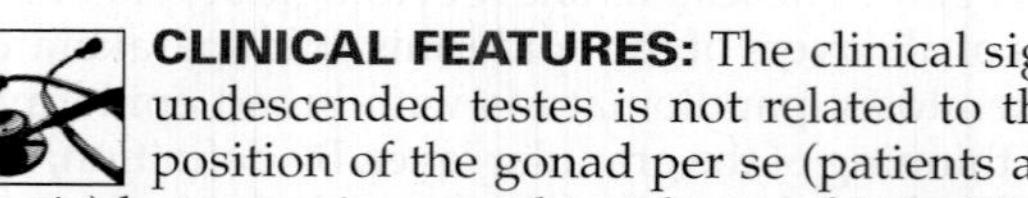

CLINICAL FEATURES: The clinical significance of undescended testes is not related to the abnormal position of the gonad per se (patients are asymptomatic) but to an increased incidence of **infertility** and **germ cell neoplasia.** All men with bilateral cryptorchid testes have **azoospermia** and are infertile. Unilateral cryptorchidism is associated with **oligospermia,** defined as a sperm count below 20 million/mL, in 40% of cases. Although oligospermia is a cause of reduced fertility, most men with one normal testis have a reasonable chance of fathering a child. Orchiopexy done in childhood or after puberty has no effect on the sperm count. Most urologists recommend orchiopexy between the ages of 6 months and 1 year, but it is not clear whether this treatment improves the eventual sperm count.

Cryptorchidism is associated with a 20- to 40-fold greater than normal risk for testicular cancer. Conversely, 10% of patients with germ cell neoplasia have cryptorchid testes. Intra-abdominal testes are at higher risk than those retained in the inguinal canal; in turn, inguinal testes are at higher risk than those high in the scrotum. The contralateral, normally descended testis is also at risk, but the incidence of cancer in there is only four times that in normal men. Unfortunately, orchiopexy does not reduce cancer risk.

Abnormalities of Sexual Differentiation

Disorders of gonadogenesis and formation of external genital organs, as well as development of secondary sex characteristics, can pertain to:

- Genetic sex; the presence or absence of X and Y chromosomes
- Gonadal sex; the presence or absence of testes or ovaries
- Genital sex; the appearance of external genital organs
- Psychosocial sexual orientation

Various conditions are listed in Table 17-5. Some of these, such as Klinefelter and Turner syndromes, are discussed in Chapter 6.

HERMAPHRODITISM: ***This rare developmental disorder is characterized by ambiguous genitalia in a person who has both male and female gonads.*** Gonads may become ovotestes (combination of ovary and testis) or one gonad may be testis and the other ovary. Half of these patients have a female karyotype (46,XX). The others are genetic males (46,XY) or mosaics or have a missing sex chromosome (45,X).

FEMALE PSEUDOHERMAPHRODITISM: ***Virilization of external genitalia may occur in genetic females (46,XX) who have normal ovaries and internal female genital organs.*** The vulva may show fusion into scrotal folds. Clitoromegaly is usually associated. This phenotype is most often seen in the adrenogenital syndrome caused by 21-hydroxylase deficiency (see Chapter 21). Lack of this enzyme leads to excess androgen production in the adrenal gland during fetal life, and the ambiguous genitalia are seen at birth. Excess androgens in a pregnant woman can have the same effects on the external genitalia of the baby.

A 46,XX karyotype is found in 1 of 25 patients with classical signs of Klinefelter syndrome. These 46,XX males carry the locus for the sex-determining region of chromosome Y (SRY) on one of their X chromosomes. It is not known how this translocation occurs, but it is probably related to a crossover during male meiosis.

MALE PSEUDOHERMAPHRODITISM: ***A spectrum of congenital disorders affects genetically male persons who have a normal 46,XY karyotype.*** The gonads are cryptorchid testes, but external genitalia appear feminine or ambiguously female with signs of virilization. Male pseudohermaphroditism occurs most often in **androgen insensitivity syndromes** due to a congenital deficiency of the androgen receptor, also known as **testicular feminization syndrome.**

Table 17-5

Disorders of Sexual Differentiation

Sex Chromosomal Abnormalities	
	Klinefelter syndrome and its variants
	Turner syndrome 46,XX males
Single Gene Defects	
	Adrenogenital syndromes
	Androgen insensitivity syndromes
	Müllerian inhibitory substance deficiency
Prenatal Hormonal Effects	
	Exogenous hormones during pregnancy
	Maternal hormone-producing tumors
Idiopathic Conditions	
	Hermaphroditism
	Gonadal dysgenesis

Male Infertility

Infertility is empirically defined as inability to conceive after 1 year of coital activity with the same sexual partner without contraception. Some 15% of couples are childless in the United States, but the true prevalence of infertility is difficult to assess because it is confounded by various cultural and social issues. The causes of infertility can be found in the male partner in 20% of cases, in the female in 40% and in both partners in 20%. In the remaining 20% of infertile couples, a cause cannot be identified. The causes of male infertility are listed in Table 17-6 and illustrated in Fig. 17-24.

Table 17-6

Causes of Male Infertility

Supratesticular Causes	
	Disorders of the hypothalamic–pituitary–gonadal axis
	Endocrine disease of the adrenal, thyroid; diabetes
	Metabolic disorders
	Major organ diseases (e.g., renal, hepatic, cardiopulmonary diseases)
	Chronic infectious and debilitating diseases (e.g., tuberculosis, acquired immunodeficiency syndrome)
	Drugs and substance abuse
Testicular Causes	
	Idiopathic: hypospermatogenesis or azoospermia
	Developmental (cryptorchidism, gonadal dysgenesis)
	Genetic disorders (e.g., Klinefelter syndrome)
	Orchitis (immune and infectious)
	Iatrogenic testicular injury (radiation, cytotoxic drugs)
	Trauma of the testis and surgical injury
	Environmental (? phytoestrogens)
Posttesticular Causes	
	Congenital anomalies of the excretory ducts
	Inflammation and scarring of excretory ducts
	Iatrogenic or posttraumatic lesions of excretory ducts

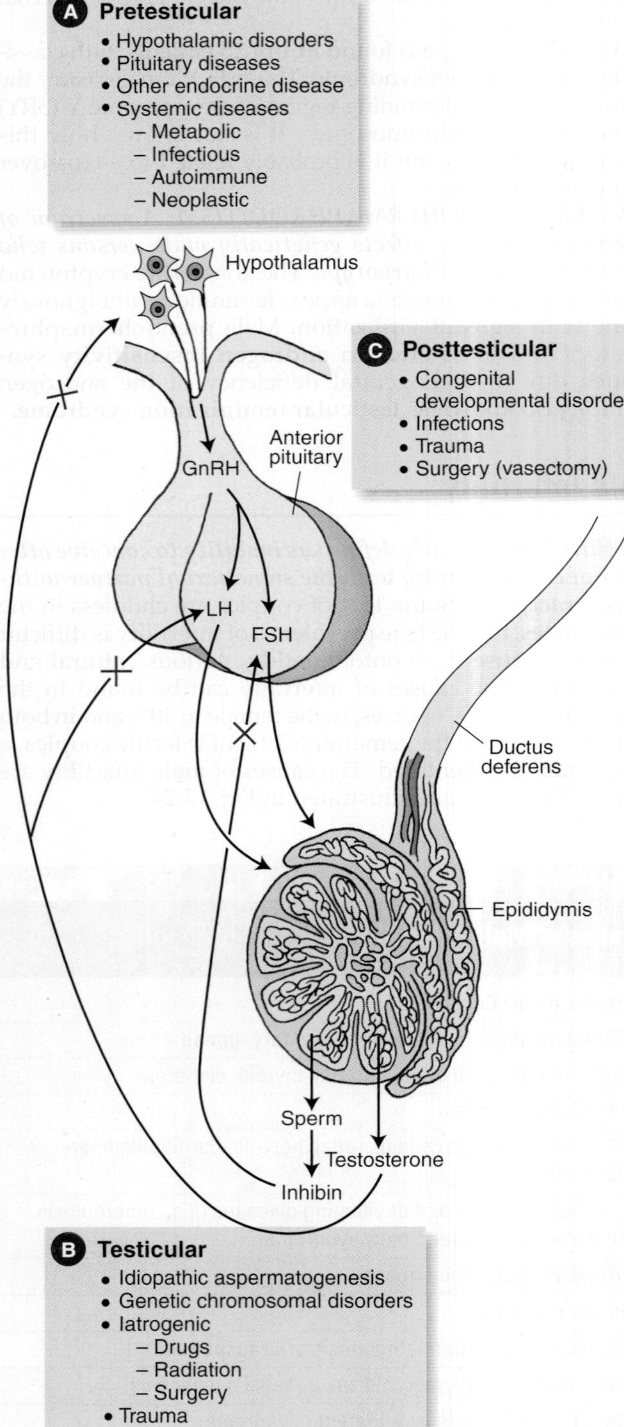

FIGURE 17-24. Causes of male infertility. A. Pretesticular infertility. FSH = follicle-stimulating hormone; LH = uteinizing hormone; GnRH = gonadotropin-releasing hormone. **B.** Testicular infertility. **C.** Posttesticular (obstructive) infertility.

Supratesticular causes of infertility are factors that influence or regulate hormonal and metabolic aspects of spermatogenesis. The best examples are injuries of the hypothalamic–pituitary area. Infertility can result from transection of the pituitary stalk, destruction of the hypothalamus by a brain tumor or pressure on the pituitary by a craniopharyngioma. A pituitary tumor secreting prolactin (prolactinoma) may act as a mass lesion that destroys gonadotropin-secreting pituitary cells or compresses the pituitary stalk. It also secretes prolactin, which suppresses spermatogenesis.

Testicular infertility, the most common variety of male infertility, is related to pathologic changes in the testis. A male infertility (andrologic) workup includes urologic examination, sonography, semen analysis, hormonal studies and, in some cases, testicular biopsy.

Posttesticular infertility refers to blockage of the excretory ducts through which sperm reach the urethra. Chronic infections of the epididymis or vas deferens are often responsible. Previous trauma or congenital atresia is the cause.

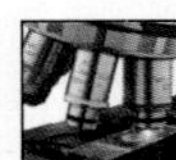

PATHOLOGY: Morphologic alterations detectable in testicular biopsies that may identify the cause of infertility include:

- **Immaturity of the seminiferous tubules** is typically found in hypogonadotropic hypogonadism caused by pituitary or hypothalamic diseases (Fig. 17-25). Seminiferous tubules show no signs of spermatogenic differentiation and resemble those of prepubertal testes.
- **Decreased spermatogenesis (hypospermatogenesis)** occurs in several systemic and endocrine diseases, including malnutrition and acquired immunodeficiency syndrome (AIDS). Hypospermatogenesis is also found in cryptorchid testes and following vasectomy.
- **Germ cell maturation arrest** is usually idiopathic. It can occur at the level of spermatogonia, spermatocytes or spermatids.
- **Germ cell aplasia** ("Sertoli cells only" syndrome) is mostly idiopathic (Fig. 17-26). An underlying genetic mutation has been identified in some patients. It can be seen in drug-induced and toxic injury of the seminiferous epithelium.
- **Orchitis** is caused by viruses (e.g., mumps) or autoimmune diseases.
- **Peritubular and tubular fibrosis** may be related to congenital disorders such as cryptorchidism or to previous infection, ischemia or radiation (Fig. 17-27).

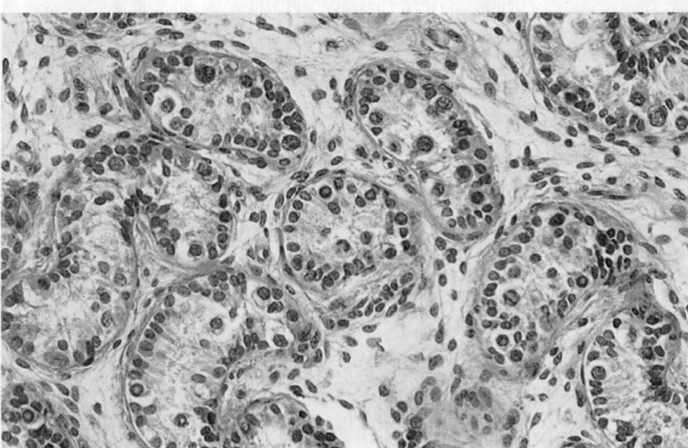

FIGURE 17-25. Hypogonadotropic hypogonadism. The testis of this 25-year-old man is composed of immature seminiferous tubules similar to those seen in prepubertal boys.

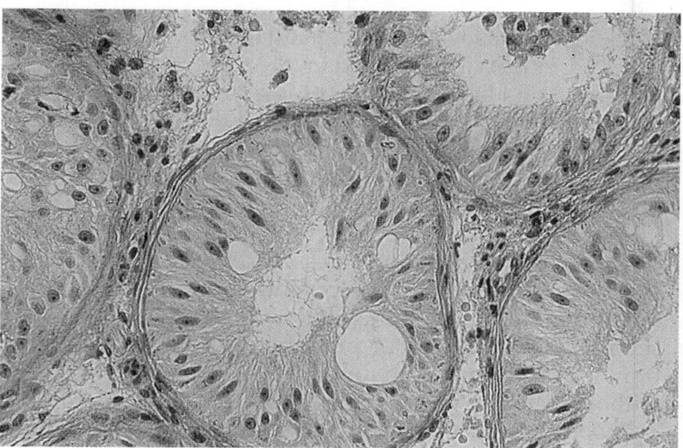

FIGURE 17-26. Germ cell aplasia–Sertoli cell only syndrome. The seminiferous tubules are lined by Sertoli cells and do not contain germ cells.

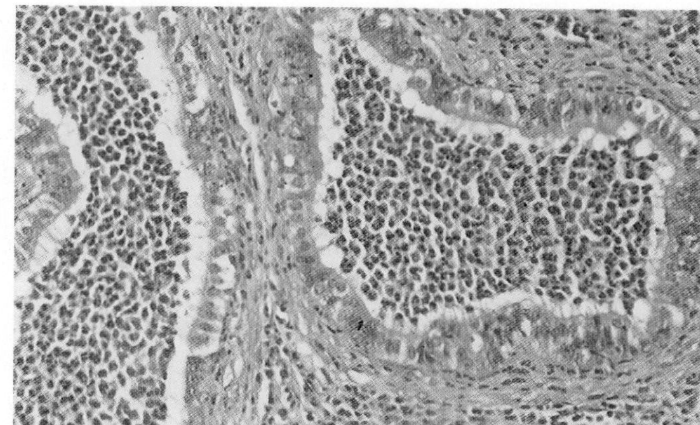

FIGURE 17-28. Bacterial epididymitis. The epididymal ducts contain numerous polymorphonuclear leukocytes.

Epididymitis

Epididymitis is acute or chronic inflammation of the epididymis, usually caused by bacteria.

Bacterial epididymitis in young men most often occurs in an acute form as a complication of gonorrhea or as a sexually acquired infection with *Chlamydia*. It is characterized by suppurative inflammation (Fig. 17-28). In older men, the most common causative agent is *E. coli* from associated urinary tract infections. Patients present with intrascrotal pain and tenderness, with or without associated fever. Epididymitis of recent origin shows the usual hallmarks of acute inflammation. Persistent chronic epididymitis is associated with accumulation of plasma cells, macrophages and lymphocytes and, ultimately, with fibrotic obstruction of infected ducts. Gonorrheal epididymitis is a common cause of male infertility.

Tuberculous epididymitis is now infrequent and is usually associated with previously established pulmonary and renal tuberculosis. The infection is manifested clinically by a palpable enlargement of the epididymis and beading of the vas deferens. Microscopically, the nodules consist of confluent caseating granulomas.

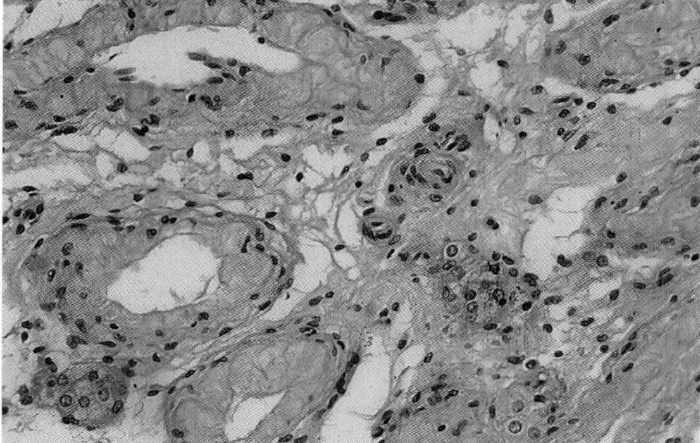

FIGURE 17-27. Postirradiation tubular atrophy of the testis. Seminiferous tubules are hyalinized, and there is no evidence of spermatogenesis.

Spermatic granulomas result from an intense inflammatory response to sperm that find their way into the interstitium of the epididymis. The reason for sperm extravasation is often obscure, but traumatic rupture of epididymal ducts may play a role. Patients present with scrotal pain and swelling, frequently lasting weeks or months. Microscopically, the epididymis displays a mixed inflammatory cell infiltrate with numerous extravasated sperm fragments and phagocytosis of sperm by macrophages. Ultimately, inflammation results in interstitial fibrosis, ductal obstruction and infertility.

Orchitis

Orchitis is acute or chronic inflammation of the testis. It may be part of epididymo-orchitis, usually caused by ascending infection, or it may occur as an isolated testicular inflammation. Orchitis is usually caused by hematogenous spread of pathogens, but some cases may be of autoimmune origin.

- **Gram-negative bacterial orchitis** is the most common form of the disease. It is often secondary to urinary tract infection and is typically associated with epididymitis. Infection may also manifest as intratesticular abscess or peritesticular suppuration and fibrosis.
- **Syphilitic orchitis** has two forms: (1) interstitial perivascular inflammation, characterized by infiltrates of lymphocytes, macrophages and plasma cells; or (2) granulomatous inflammation of testis in the form of gummas.
- **Mumps orchitis** occurs in 20% of adult males who develop mumps, but widespread immunization against mumps has reduced the incidence of the disorder. Viral infection is characterized by testicular pain and gonadal swelling, most commonly unilateral. Microscopically, it appears as an interstitial inflammation that also leads to destruction and loss of seminiferous epithelium (Fig. 17-29).
- **Granulomatous orchitis** of unknown cause is an infrequent disorder of middle-aged men that presents acutely as painful testicular enlargement or insidiously as testicular induration. It is characterized microscopically by noncaseating granulomas that fail to reveal either organisms or sperm remnants that might act as inciting agents. Variable numbers of seminiferous tubules are destroyed by the

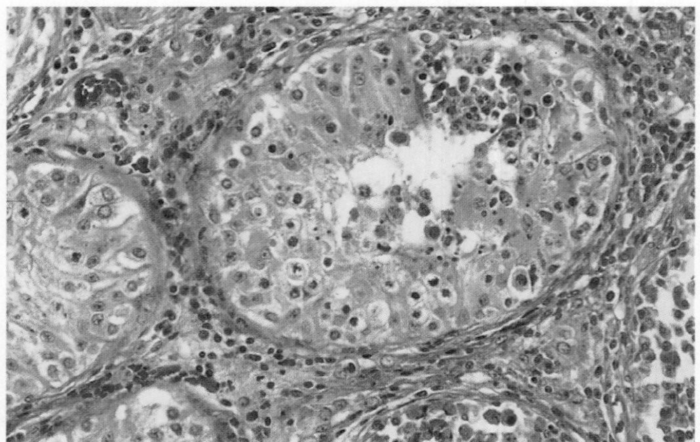

FIGURE 17-29. Viral orchitis. The interstitial spaces are infiltrated with mononuclear cells that spill focally into the lumen of seminiferous tubules (*arrow*). Note that the inflammation has interrupted normal spermatogenesis and that the seminiferous tubules do not contain sperm.

inflammatory process, which is considered to be a type IV (cell-mediated) hypersensitivity reaction.

- **Malakoplakia** of the testis has the same microscopic features and presumably the same histogenesis as malakoplakia elsewhere.

Tumors of the Testis

Tumors of the testis account for less than 1% of all malignancies in adult males. More than 90% of these tumors are characterized by:

- Diagnosis between 25 and 45 years of age
- Germ cell origin
- Malignancy
- Curable by a combination of surgery and chemotherapy
- Cytogenetic marker, namely, isochromosome p12
- Metastasis first to periaortic abdominal lymph nodes
- Most (65%) release markers that are detectable in the blood

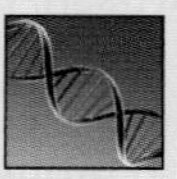

MOLECULAR PATHOGENESIS: The etiology of testicular tumors is unknown. There is a geographic variation in the incidence of testicular cancer. Incidence is highest in Denmark, Sweden and Norway, but is low in Finland and southern European countries. The tumors are five times more common among Americans of European descent than those of African heritage. Familial occurrence of testicular cancer in brothers or sons and fathers is on record but is rare and provides no support for a genetic theory of tumorigenesis. The only consistent cytogenetic abnormality is an additional fragment of chromosome 12 (isochromosome p12). As discussed previously, the only documented risk factors for testicular tumors are **cryptorchidism and gonadal dysgenesis.**

Malignant transformation of germ cells may occur during fetal development and involve (1) migrating primordial germ cells, (2) fetal germ cells interacting with stromal cells in the genital ridge or (3) early fetal spermatogonia. Since germ cell tumors rarely occur before puberty, some investigators believe that malignant transformation occurs in the peripubertal period and involves spermatogonia that are stimulated hormonally to proliferate and differentiate into spermatocytes. Although there is disagreement as to the initial events in testicular neoplasia, a consensus holds that germ cell tumors progress through two pathways (Fig. 17-30). Most commonly, a carcinoma in situ stage, also known as **intratubular testicular germ cell neoplasia** (ITGCN), precedes and progresses to invasive carcinoma (see below). This pathway accounts for most adult germ cell tumors, although ITGCN is not found in spermatocytic seminomas, teratomas of prepubertal testes or yolk sac tumors of infancy, which develop directly from germ cells without an in situ phase. It is possible that some migratory primordial germ cells may not find their way into the seminiferous tubules during fetal testicular organogenesis and that such "misplaced" cells become progenitors of yolk sac tumors and teratomas. Such germ cells can also give rise to extragonadal germ cell tumors in the retroperitoneum, sacral region, anterior mediastinum and area of the pineal.

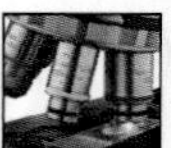

PATHOLOGY: Testicular tumors are classified histogenetically on the basis of their cell of origin into several groups (Table 17-7).

Tumor cells of ITGCN resemble spermatogonia or fetal germ cells but have much larger polyploid nuclei (Fig. 17-30). Like fetal germ cells, these cells express placental-like alkaline phosphatase on their surface. In infertile men with a history of cryptorchid testes, ITGCN can persist unchanged for 5 to 10 years, after which the neoplastic cells acquire invasive properties, penetrate the tubular basement membrane and give rise to infiltrating malignant tumors.

The malignant cells that retain the phenotypic features of spermatogonia give rise to **seminomas.** Alternatively, neoplastic germ cells can differentiate into malignant embryonic cells (**embryonal carcinoma**) by a process that resembles

Table 17-7

Testicular Tumors

Germ Cell Tumors—90%
Seminoma (40%)
Nonseminomatous germ cell tumors
Embryonal carcinoma (5%)
Teratocarcinoma (35%)
Choriocarcinoma (<1%)
Mixed germ cell tumors (15%)
Teratoma (1%)
Spermatocytic seminoma (1%)
Yolk sac tumor of infancy (2%)
Sex Cord Cell Tumors—5%
Leydig cell tumors (60%)
Sertoli cell tumors (40%)
Metastases—2%
Other Rare Tumors—3%

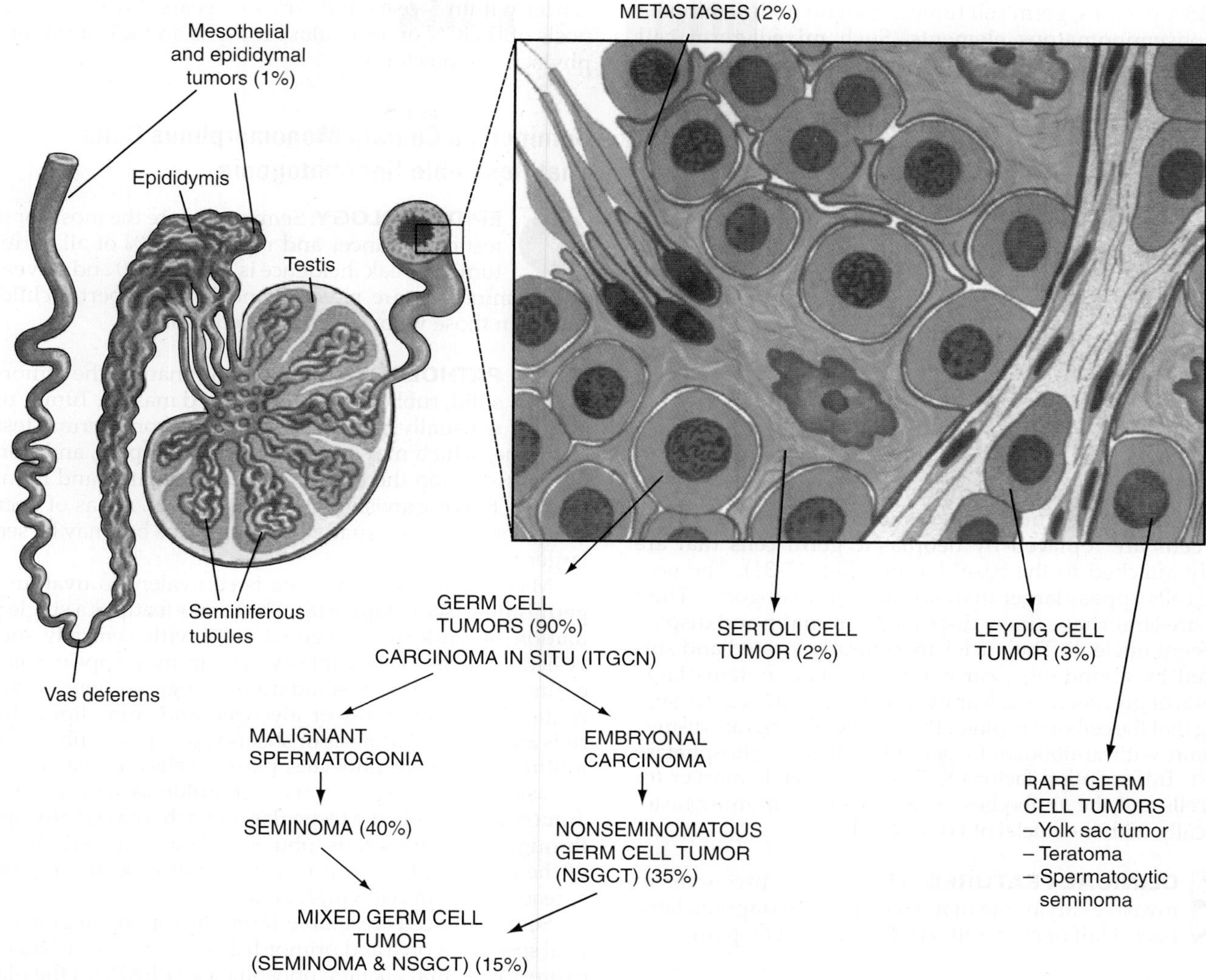

FIGURE 17-30. Tumors of the testis, epididymis and related structures. Most testicular tumors originate from germ cells and are preceded by a carcinoma in situ stage known as intratubular germ cell neoplasia (ITGCN). Germ cell tumors of adult testis can be classified as seminomas (40%) or nonseminomatous germ cell tumors (NSGCTs) (35%). In 15% of cases seminomatous elements are intermixed with NSGCT, forming mixed germ cell tumors. Some germ cell tumors (yolk sac tumor of childhood, childhood teratomas and spermatocytic seminomas) develop without passing through a preinvasive ITGCN stage. Tumors originating from sex cord stromal cells (Leydig and Sertoli cell tumors) account for 5% of testicular tumors. Epididymal tumors, tumors of the mesothelial lining of the tunica vaginalis (adenomatoid tumors) and metastases are rare.

parthenogenetic activation of oocytes in the female gonads of amphibians and reptiles.

In some cases, embryonal carcinoma cells proliferate in an undifferentiated form. In others, they differentiate into the three embryonic germ layers (ectoderm, mesoderm, endoderm) or extraembryonic tissues that form the fetal membranes and the placenta. Further differentiation of germ layer cells leads to formation of various somatic tissues. Ectoderm differentiates into skin, central nervous system, retinal pigment and other related tissues. Mesoderm gives rise to smooth and striated muscle, cartilage and bone. Endoderm forms intestinal tissue, bronchial epithelium, salivary glands and so forth. The extraembryonic derivatives of embryonal carcinoma cells give rise to chorionic epithelium (cytotrophoblast and syncytiotrophoblast) and yolk sac–like epithelium. These complex tumors composed of malignant undifferentiated embryonal carcinoma cells and their somatic and extraembryonic derivatives are called **teratocarcinomas** or **malignant teratomas.** When embryonal carcinoma cells proliferate without further differentiating and exhibit a single histologic pattern, the tumor is labeled **embryonal carcinoma.** In rare instances, extraembryonic components of teratocarcinomas overgrow and destroy all other components. Such tumors are composed of a single tumor type and are classified as **yolk sac carcinoma** or **choriocarcinoma.**

For clinical purposes, all germ cell tumors with embryonal carcinoma as their malignant stem cells are termed **nonseminomatous germ cell tumors (NSGCTs),** to distinguish them from seminomas. Pure yolk sac carcinomas of the adult testis and choriocarcinomas are also included in this group because it is assumed that these tumors must contain a few embryonal carcinoma cells that are not readily recognizable.

In 15% of cases, germ cell tumors contain both seminoma and nonseminomatous elements. Such **mixed germ cell tumors** are treated clinically as nonseminomatous neoplasms.

Intratubular Germ Cell Neoplasia Refers to Testicular Carcinoma in Situ

ITGCN represents a preinvasive form of germ cell tumors.

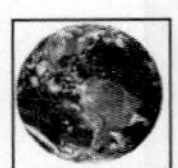

EPIDEMIOLOGY: ITGCN can be seen as (1) an isolated focal histologic change in 2% of cryptorchid testes or testicular biopsies performed for infertility, (2) widespread carcinoma in situ adjacent to almost all invasive germ cell tumors and (3) lesions in 5% of contralateral testes in patients who had an orchiectomy for a testicular germ cell tumor.

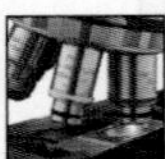

PATHOLOGY: ITGCN involves testes in a patchy manner, usually affecting less than 10% to 30% of the tubules. Seminiferous tubules harboring ITGCN have thick basement membranes and no sperm. The normal germ cells are replaced by neoplastic germ cells that are broadly attached to the basal lamina (Fig. 17-31). The neoplastic cells appear larger than normal spermatogonia. Their nuclei are large, have finely dispersed chromatin and display prominent nucleoli. The nuclei are centrally located and surrounded by abundant, clear cytoplasm that contains large amounts of glycogen. Nuclear DNA content is increased, suggesting that the cells are triploid. Plasma membranes are distinct and stain with antibodies to placental alkaline phosphatase (PLAP). Transcription factor OCT3/4 is a reliable marker for these cells and the antibodies to OCT3/4 react immunohistochemically with the nuclei of ITGCN cells.

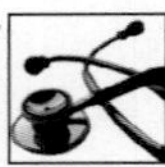

CLINICAL FEATURES: ITGCN is a precursor of invasive carcinoma that develops at an unpredictable pace. Half of men with ITGCN will develop invasive cancer within 5 years and 70% in 7 years. Microscopic diagnosis of ITGCN on testicular biopsy is an indication for prophylactic orchiectomy.

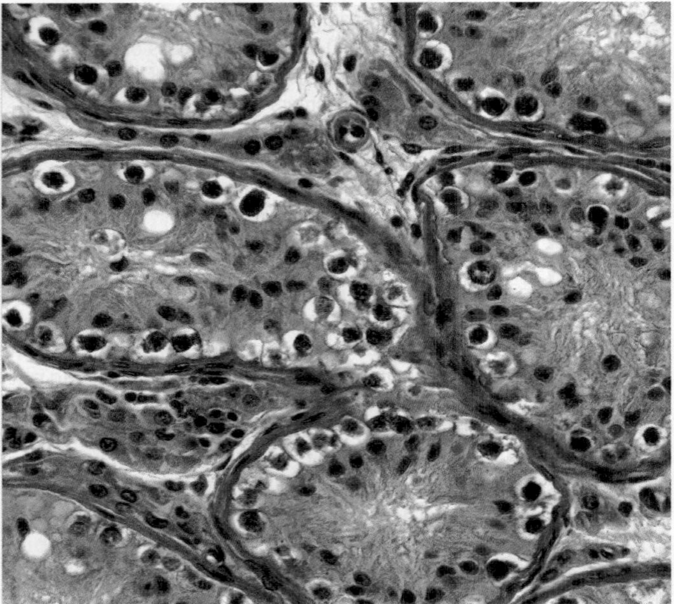

FIGURE 17-31. Intratubular germ cell neoplasia (ITGCN). The seminiferous tubules show no signs of spermatogenesis but instead contain large atypical cells corresponding to intratubular carcinoma in situ.

Seminomas Contain Monomorphous Cells That Resemble Spermatogonia

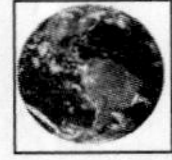

EPIDEMIOLOGY: Seminomas are the most common testicular cancer and represent 40% of all germ cell tumors. Peak incidence is between 30 and 40 years of age. Seminomas are never found in prepubertal children, except in those who have dysgenetic gonads.

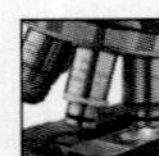

PATHOLOGY: On gross examination, the tumors are solid, rubbery-firm, bosselated masses. Tumor tissue is usually sharply demarcated from normal testicular tissue, which may be compressed, atrophic, and fibrotic. On cross-section the tumors appear lobulated and homogeneously tan or grayish yellow (Fig. 17-32). Areas of necrosis or hemorrhage are usually inconspicuous but may be seen in larger tumors.

Microscopically, seminoma is equivalent to **ovarian dysgerminoma** (see Chapter 18). The tumor features a single population of uniform polygonal cells with centrally located vesicular nuclei. The ample cytoplasm may appear pale and eosinophilic or clear in standard histologic sections because it contains large amounts of glycogen and some lipid. Tumor cells are arranged as nests or sheets separated by fibrous septa infiltrated with lymphocytes, plasma cells and macrophages. Occasionally, the septa contain granulomas with giant cells. Tumor cells invade the testicular parenchyma but also spread through the seminiferous tubules and into rete testis. Invasion of the epididymis is seen later in the disease, usually before spread to abdominal lymph nodes.

Seminoma cells resemble immature spermatogonia. Like fetal spermatogonia and primordial germ cells in the fetus, they express placental alkaline phosphatase (PLAP) on the plasma membrane. Immunohistochemically, seminoma cells also react with the antibodies to c-*KIT* (CD117) and the transcription factors OCT3/4, which are reliable markers for this tumor.

Pathologists recognize two subtypes of seminoma: (1) **seminoma with syncytiotrophoblastic giant cells** and (2) **anaplastic seminoma.** The first subgroup includes the 20% of tumors that contain syncytiotrophoblastic cells. These multinucleated giant cells are best demonstrated with antibodies to human chorionic gonadotropin (hCG). Although they secrete hCG, blood hCG levels are usually below detectable limits. Some 5% of seminomas show brisk mitotic activity and nuclear pleomorphism and are classified as anaplastic seminoma. There are no clinical differences between classical seminomas and these two microscopic tumor variants.

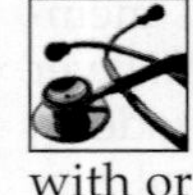

CLINICAL FEATURES: Seminoma manifests as a progressively growing scrotal mass and is usually diagnosed while it can still be cured by orchiectomy, with or without abdominal lymph node dissection. Seminomas are highly radiosensitive, and radiotherapy plays an important role in treating tumors that cannot be cured by surgery alone. Those in advanced stages of dissemination are treated with additional chemotherapy. ***The cure rate for all histologic subtypes of seminoma is over 90%.***

Spermatocytic seminoma is a rare tumor, which, despite its name, is unrelated to classical seminoma. These are benign

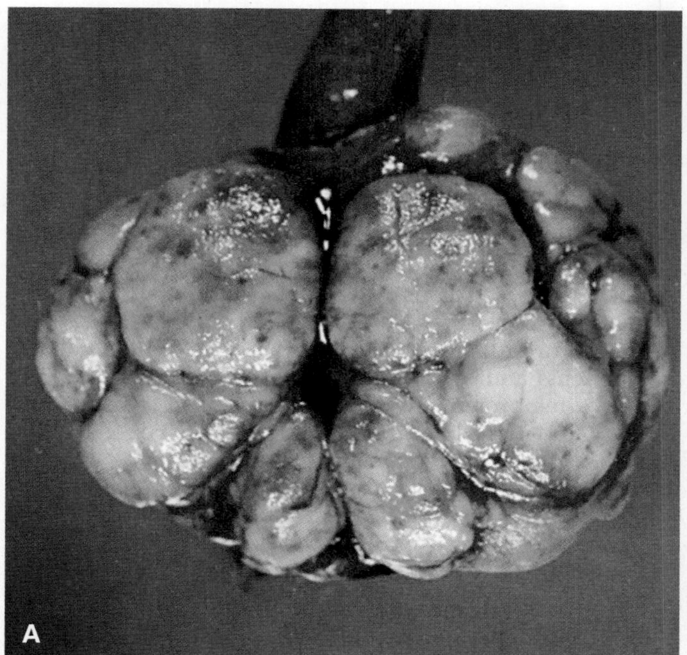

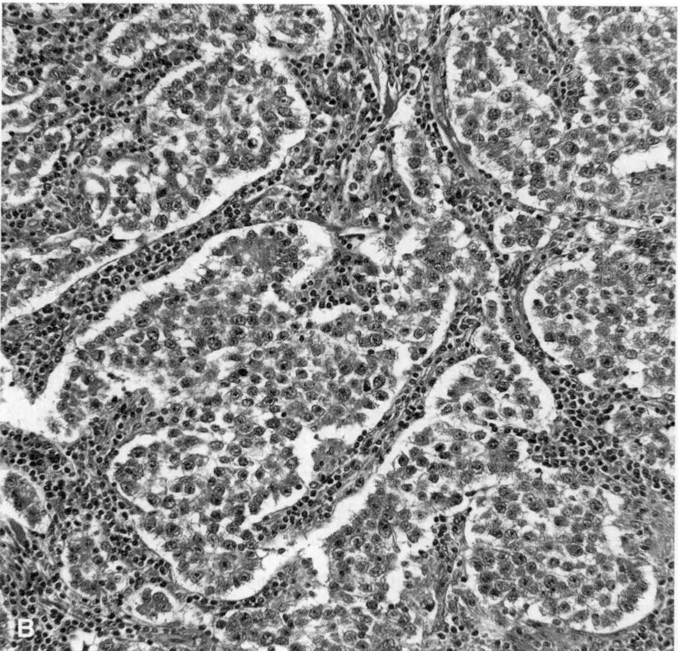

FIGURE 17-32. Seminoma. A. The cut surface of this nodular tumor is tan and bulging, suggesting that the tumor is firm and rubbery. **B.** Groups of tumor cells are surrounded by fibrous septa infiltrated with lymphocytes. Tumor cells have vesicular nuclei, which are much larger than the small round nuclei of the lymphocytes.

tumors in men over 40 years of age. They are not associated with ITGCN and do not elicit a lymphocytic reaction. Spermatocytic seminomas contain three cell types: large, small and intermediate cells. Immunohistochemically, the cells of these tumors do not express typical seminoma markers. Orchiectomy is curative.

Nonseminomatous Germ Cell Tumors Are Derived From Embryonal Cells

NSGCTs of the testis include several pathologic entities, two of which account for most of the cases: (1) pure embryonal carcinomas; and (2) teratocarcinomas, also known as **malignant teratomas** or **mixed germ cell tumors. Pure choriocarcinoma, pure yolk sac carcinoma of the adult testis** and the so-called **growing benign teratoma** are rare NSGCTs. Mixed germ cell tumors are NSGCTs combined with seminomas.

EPIDEMIOLOGY: NSGCTs constitute 55% of all testicular germ cell tumors. Teratocarcinomas account for two thirds of all NSGCTs, followed by mixed germ cell tumors and pure embryonal carcinomas. All other tumors of this group are extremely rare. Like seminomas, NSGCTs have peak incidence in the 25- to 40-year-old age group. At diagnosis, these patients are usually somewhat younger than those with seminomas.

PATHOLOGY: Nonseminomatous tumors vary in size and shape, and may be solid or partially cystic. Solid areas vary in color from white to yellow to red, indicating that they are composed of viable tumor cells, foci of necrosis and hemorrhage, respectively (Fig. 17-33).

The histology of NSGCTs is highly variable. Pure embryonal carcinomas are composed exclusively of undifferentiated embryonal carcinoma cells similar to cells from preimplantation-stage embryos (Fig. 17-34). Because the tumor cells have little cytoplasm, their hyperchromatic, disproportionately large nuclei seem to overlap. Embryonal carcinoma cells may be arranged as broad solid sheets, cords, gland-like tubules and acini, and sometimes even line papillary structures. Numerous mitoses and apoptotic cells are characteristic. Embryonal carcinoma invades the testis, epididymis and blood vessels and metastasizes to abdominal lymph nodes, lungs and other organs.

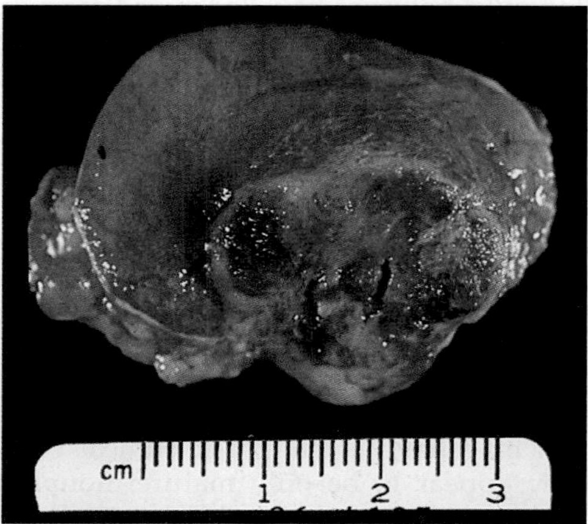

FIGURE 17-33. Nonseminomatous germ cell tumor of the testis. The cut surface of this small testicular tumor shows considerable heterogeneity, varying in color from white to dark red.

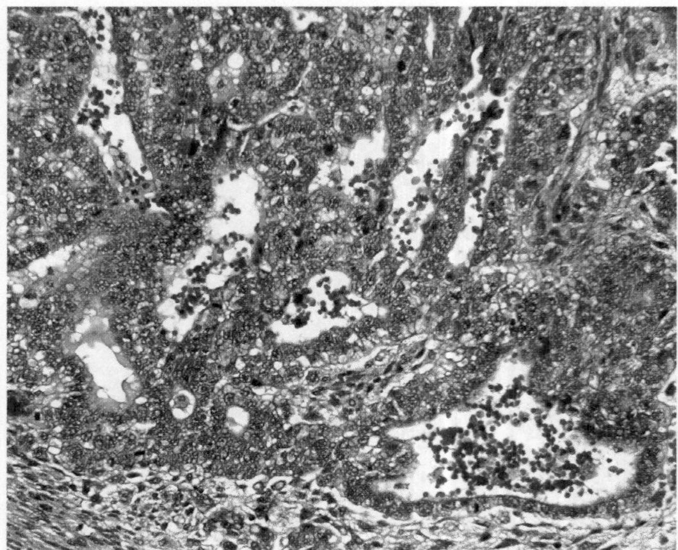

FIGURE 17-34. Embryonal carcinoma component of a nonseminomatous germ cell tumor. Because these undifferentiated cells have scant cytoplasm, their hyperchromatic nuclei impart a bluish color to the tumor. The nuclei appear crowded and seem to overlap each other. The cells form cords and sheets surrounding dilated vascular channels filled with red blood cells.

Embryonal carcinoma cells resemble seminoma cells in that they react with antibodies to PLAP and OCT3/4. However, embryonal carcinoma cells may be distinguished from seminoma and a host of other tumors by their expression of cytokeratins and CD30, but not c-KIT (CD117).

Embryonal carcinoma cells are the stem cells of **teratocarcinomas (malignant teratomas),** which feature differentiated somatic elements (i.e., tissues that are normally found in various organs, and extraembryonic elements, including yolk sac cells and trophoblastic cells). Microscopically, such nonseminomatous tumors thus reveal foci of embryonal carcinoma and a variety of other tissues (Fig. 17-35). For example, a tumor might be composed of embryonal carcinoma yolk sac components and trophoblastic components corresponding to choriocarcinoma. A similar tumor that also contains seminoma cells would, however, be called **mixed germ cell tumor.** In most tumors, the malignancy resides in the embryonal carcinoma cells. Interestingly, when these cells metastasize, they can differentiate into somatic or extraembryonic tissues, in which case the metastatic tumor can resemble the original one.

NSGCTs can give rise to clones of highly malignant cytotrophoblastic and syncytiotrophoblastic cells that overgrow other elements. Tumors composed exclusively of malignant chorionic epithelium are termed **choriocarcinomas.** Likewise, clones of malignant yolk sac epithelium produce **yolk sac carcinoma.**

Some histologically benign teratomas of postpubertal young men may have a malignant clinical course, even though they appear to be only mature, nonproliferating somatic tissues, without embryonal elements (Fig. 17-36). In some instances it is assumed that the tumor was actually a teratocarcinoma in which almost all embryonal cells have differentiated into mature somatic tissues but that a few remaining malignant cells were undetected by the pathologist or had metastasized before resection. These tumors are clinically known as the **growing teratoma syndrome.** In other cases, teratoma tissues remain undifferentiated and resemble embryonic organs or embryonic tumors such as neuroblastoma. These **immature teratomas** are also potentially malignant tumors.

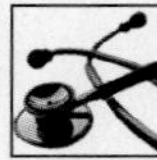

CLINICAL FEATURES: Most NSGCTs manifest as testicular masses. They tend to grow faster than seminomas and metastasize more readily and more widely. Hence, in some NSGCTs metastases may be the first sign of the neoplasm.

In contrast to seminomas, NSGCTs often contain yolk sac components and syncytiotrophoblastic cells. Yolk sac cells secrete α-fetoprotein (AFP), a fetal plasma protein not normally found in the blood. Syncytiotrophoblastic cells release hCG, a hormone of pregnancy, that is also not found in males. ***Elevated serum AFP or hCG is found in 70% of patients harboring NSGCTs and is thus a reliable tumor marker.*** These antigens are most useful in postoperative follow-up of patients who have been treated for NSGCT. Persistently elevated AFP and/or hCG indicate that a patient is not tumor free. Patients whose initially high levels of AFP and hCG normalize after treatment but subsequently rise again have metastases.

Treatment of NSGCT includes orchiectomy to remove the primary tumor, then platinum-based chemotherapy and, if indicated, surgical dissection of abdominal lymph nodes. Chemotherapy usually eliminates metastatic embryonal carcinoma cells, but differentiated tissues originating from them are resistant. Such tissues do not grow and are not likely to endanger the patient. Nevertheless, it is better to remove any residual tumor than to take a chance that a few malignant tumor cells might be hiding in the residuals tumors. Only three decades ago, patients with NSGCTs had only a 35% chance for 5-year survival. ***By contrast, complete cures are now recorded in over 90% of cases.***

Testicular Tumors Are Rare in Prepubertal Boys

In the first 4 years of life, most testicular neoplasms are yolk sac tumors. Benign teratomas are the most common testicular tumor in the age group between 4 and 12 years.

YOLK SAC TUMORS: These neoplasms are composed of cells arranged into structures reminiscent of parts of fetal yolk sac. The diagnosis is based on recognizing multiple microscopic tumor patterns and the so-called glomeruloid **Schiller-Duval bodies** (Fig. 17-37). The histology of neonatal tumors is similar to that of the yolk sac elements in NSGCTs. Yolk sac tumors of infancy and early childhood are considered malignant, but timely orchiectomy and removal of the tumor cure over 95% of patients.

TERATOMAS: These tumors of prepubertal testes are benign and are composed of mature somatic tissues. Orchiectomy, and even testis-sparing surgery, is curative.

Gonadal Stromal/Sex Cord Tumors Are Composed of Cells That Resemble Sertoli or Leydig Cells

Gonadal stroma/sex cord tumors constitute 5% of all testicular tumors.

LEYDIG CELL TUMORS: ***Rare neoplasms are composed of cells resembling interstitial (Leydig) cells of the testis.***

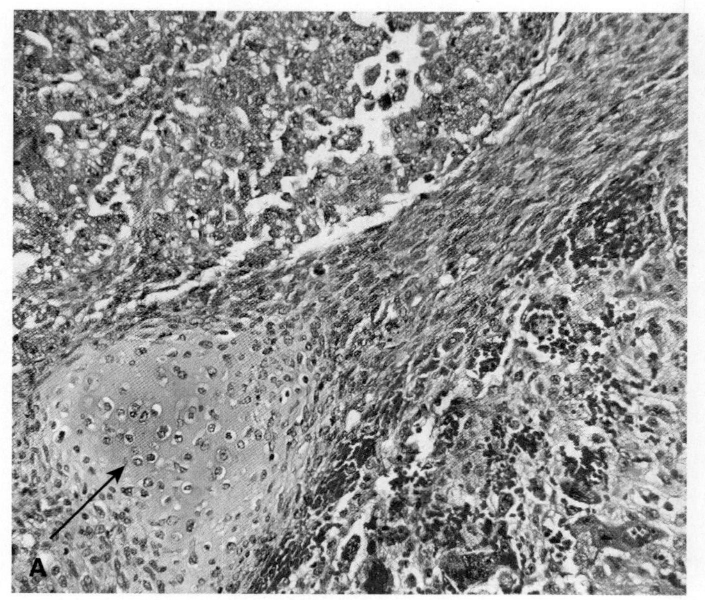

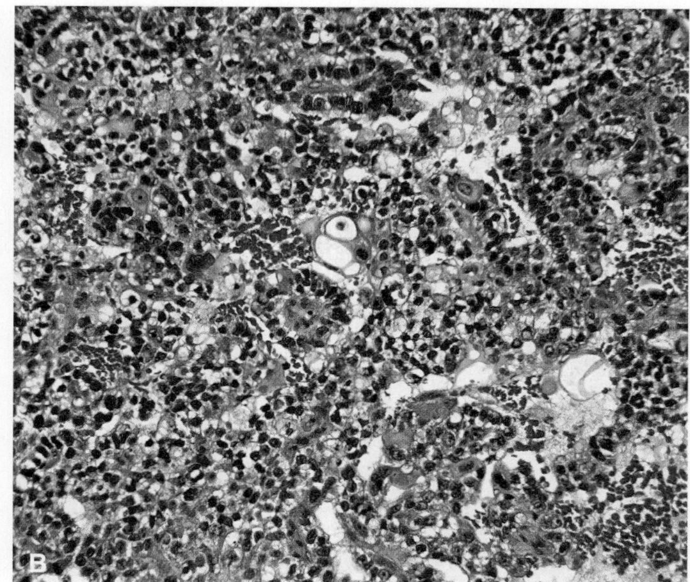

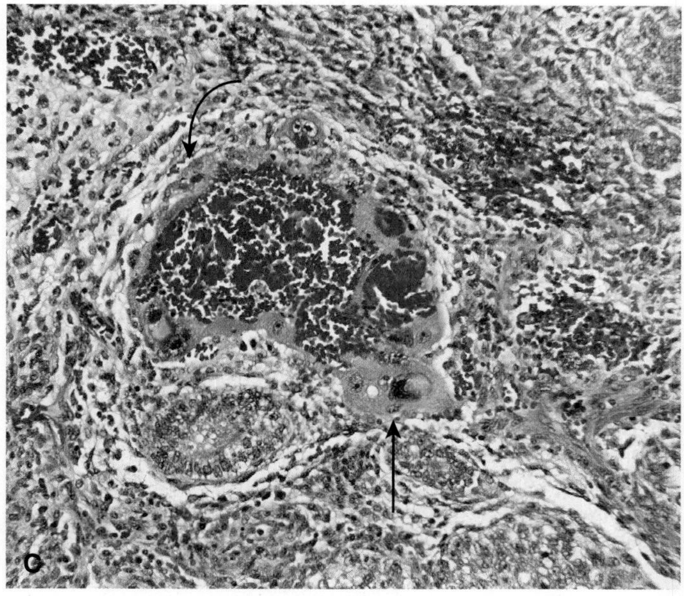

FIGURE 17-35. Nonseminomatous germ cell tumor (NSGCT). A. Somatic tissue of this tumor includes well-differentiated cartilage (*arrow*) and nondescript connective tissue separating the embryonal carcinoma (*upper left corner*) from the hemorrhagic choriocarcinoma (*right lower corner*). **B.** Yolk sac component consists of interlacing cord of epithelial cells surrounded by loose stroma resembling the early yolk sac. **C.** Choriocarcinoma component of the NSGCT consists of multinucleated syncytiotrophoblastic giant cells (*straight arrow*) and mononuclear cytotrophoblastic cells (*curved arrow*). Invasive growth of trophoblasts is usually associated with hemorrhage.

They can be hormonally active and secrete androgens, estrogens or both. Leydig cell tumors can occur at any age, with two distinct peaks, one in childhood and one in adults from the third to the sixth decade.

PATHOLOGY: Leydig cell tumors are well circumscribed, and some appear encapsulated. They vary from 1 to 10 cm in diameter. The cut surface is yellow to brown, and larger tumors have fibrous trabeculae, giving them a lobular appearance. Leydig cell tumors are composed of uniform cells with round nuclei and well-developed eosinophilic or vacuolated cytoplasm (Fig. 17-38). **Reinke crystals**—rectangular, eosinophilic, cytoplasmic inclusions—are typically found in normal Leydig cells and are present in 30% of tumors. Although most (90%) Leydig cell tumors are benign (only 10% are malignant), it is difficult to predict biological behavior on histologic grounds.

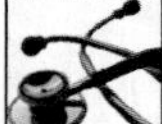

CLINICAL FEATURES: The androgenic effects of testicular Leydig cell tumors in prepubertal boys lead to precocious physical and sexual development. By contrast, feminization and gynecomastia are observed in some adults with this tumor. Either estrogen or testosterone levels may be elevated, but there is no characteristic pattern. All Leydig cell tumors in children and almost all tumors in adults are cured by orchiectomy.

SERTOLI CELL TUMORS: Some testicular sex cord stromal cell tumors are composed of neoplastic Sertoli cells. Most (90%) tumors are benign and produce few, if any, hormonal symptoms.

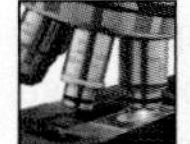

PATHOLOGY: Sertoli cell tumors tend to be small (1 to 3 cm), solid, well-circumscribed, yellow-gray nodules. Microscopically, they contain columnar tumor cells arranged into tubules or cords in a fibrous trabecular framework (Fig. 17-39). The rare malignant variant exhibits

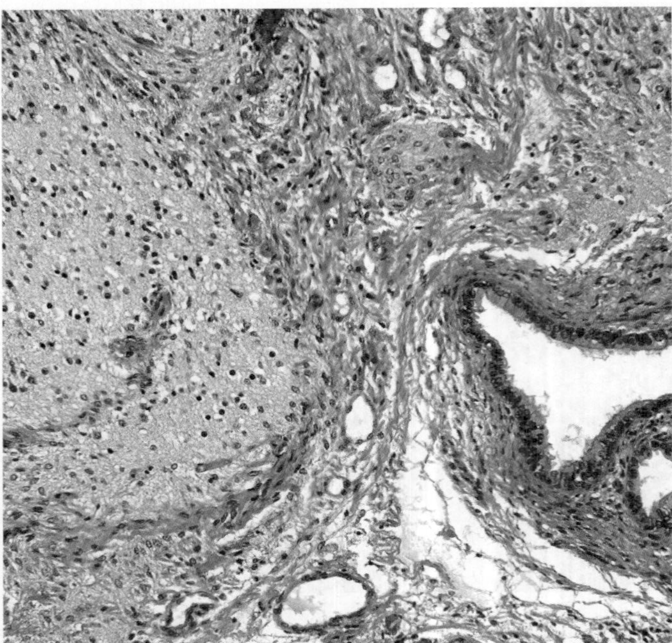

FIGURE 17-36. Teratoma. The tumor consists of neural tissue (*left*), connective tissue and smooth muscle cells (*midportion*) and glands lined by columnar epithelium (*right side of the picture*).

greater cellular pleomorphism, areas of necrosis and little tendency to form cords and tubules. Most patients with Sertoli cell tumors are under 40 years of age and come to medical attention because of a scrotal mass. Endocrine effects are uncommon and, if present, are vague. Orchiectomy is curative.

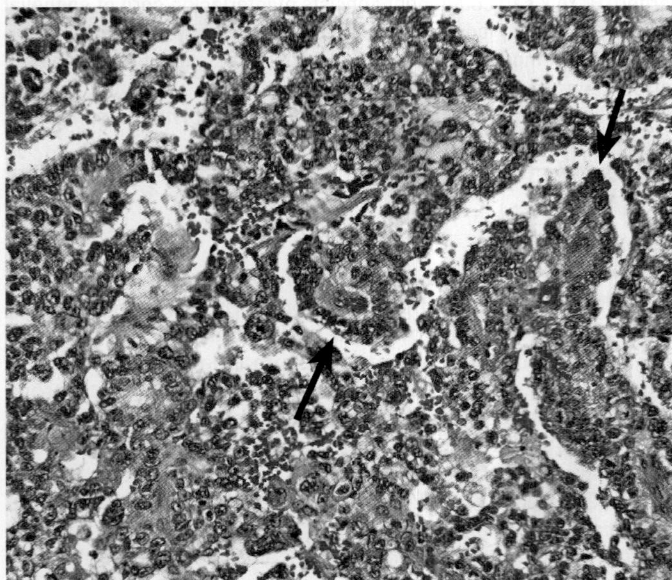

FIGURE 17-37. Yolk sac tumor. This childhood tumor is composed of interlacing strands of epithelial cells surrounded by loose connective stroma. The glomeruloid structures (Schiller-Duval bodies) are marked by arrows.

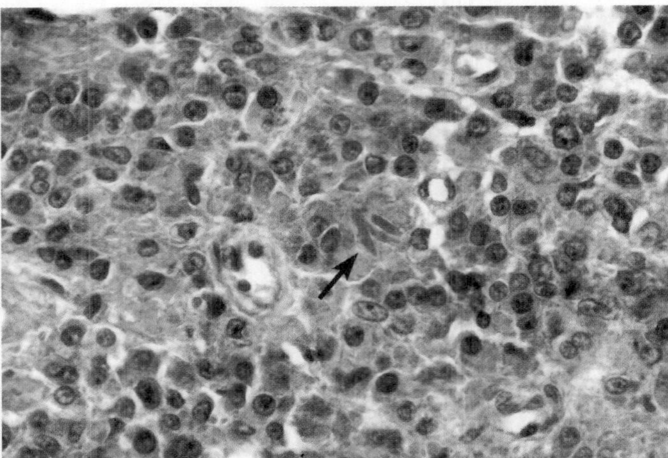

FIGURE 17-38. Leydig cell tumor. The tumor cells have uniform round nuclei and well-developed eosinophilic cytoplasm. Three cytoplasmic Reinke crystals are seen in the center of the field (*arrow*).

All Other Germ Cell Tumors Are Rare

Tumors may originate from the epithelium of the epididymis, from the connective tissue stroma and from the mesothelium and tunica vaginalis testis, but all these tumors are rare. Likewise, metastatic tumors, including lymphomas, are very uncommon. All these tumors account for less than 5% of all intrascrotal masses.

ADENOMATOID TUMOR: ***Adenomatoid tumor (benign mesothelioma) is a benign tumor that originates from the mesothelial layer of the testicular tunica vaginalis.*** These neoplasms are usually seen in the upper pole of the epididymis, with fewer cases involving the tunica vaginalis or spermatic cord. They are well-demarcated nodules discovered during palpation of the testis and epididymis. Microscopically, they are composed of mesothelial cells forming cords or small duct-like structures embedded in dense fibrous stroma.

METASTASES: Most of these result from a spread from primary cancers of the prostate, large intestine or bladder (i.e., organs that are located in the pelvis).

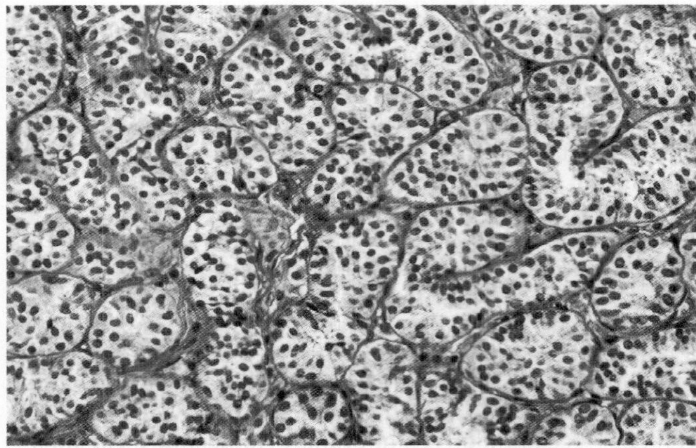

FIGURE 17-39. Sertoli cell tumor. The neoplastic cells are arranged in tubules surrounded by a basement membrane. These structures are reminiscent of seminiferous tubules devoid of germ cells.

MALIGNANT LYMPHOMA: This cancer is the most common neoplasm in the testes of men older than 60 years. It may be primary in the testis but more often represents secondary seeding of lymphoma from other sites, or in patients with leukemia. Most patients with lymphomatous involvement of the testis have a poor prognosis.

PROSTATE

The pathologic processes affecting the prostate can be simplified by considering just three processes: (1) inflammation, (2) hyperplasia and (3) neoplasia.

Prostatitis

Prostatitis is inflammation of the prostate. It occurs in acute and chronic forms. It is usually caused by coliform uropathogens, but often the cause cannot be determined.

ACUTE PROSTATITIS: Typically a complication of other urinary tract infections, acute prostatitis results from reflux of infected urine into the prostate. An acute inflammatory infiltrate is seen in prostatic acini and stroma. The disorder causes intense discomfort on urination and is often associated with fever, chills and perineal pain. Most patients respond well to standard antibiotic treatment.

CHRONIC BACTERIAL PROSTATITIS: This infection is of longer duration that may or may not be preceded by an episode of acute prostatitis. Most patients with chronic prostatitis complain of dysuria and burning at the urethral meatus. Suprapubic, perineal and low back pain or discomfort and nocturia may also be present. The urine usually contains bacteria. In addition to reflux of urine, factors such as prostatic calculi and local prostatic duct obstruction may contribute to development of chronic bacterial prostatitis. Microscopically, infiltrates of lymphocytes, plasma cells and macrophages are the rule. Prolonged antibiotic therapy is often, but not necessarily, curative.

NONBACTERIAL PROSTATITIS: There exists a form of chronic prostatitis in which no causative organism is identified. It is the most common form of inflammation in prostatic biopsy or prostatectomy specimens or at autopsy. Nonbacterial prostatitis typically affects men older than 50 years of age, but it is seen at virtually all ages. It has been hypothesized that some cases may be due to *C. trachomatis, Mycoplasma* or *U. urealyticum*. However, in practice this is a diagnosis of exclusion. The most common histologic pattern consists of dilated glands filled with neutrophils and foamy macrophages and surrounded by chronic inflammatory cells. The condition may be asymptomatic or it may cause symptoms similar to those in chronic bacterial prostatitis. Usually, no specific therapy is available.

GRANULOMATOUS PROSTATITIS: In most cases, the cause of granulomatous prostatitis cannot be established. Rarely, granulomatous prostatitis can be traced to specific causative agents, including *Mycobacterium tuberculosis*, BCG or fungal pathogens such as *Histoplasma capsulatum*. A granulomatous lesion resembling rheumatoid nodules has been recognized and related to previous transurethral resection of a portion of the prostate. The symptoms of chronic granulomatous prostatitis are vague and the diagnosis is made histologically. Caseating or noncaseating granulomas are associated with localized destruction of prostatic ducts and acini and, in later stages, with fibrosis.

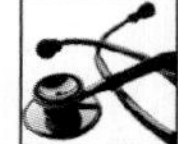

CLINICAL FEATURES: As indicated above, symptoms of chronic prostatitis are highly variable and treatment may be quite frustrating. Most importantly, chronic prostatitis may cause elevated serum prostate-specific antigen (PSA), raising the specter of prostatic malignancy. The diagnosis is thus often made by biopsy done to exclude carcinoma.

Nodular Hyperplasia of the Prostate

Nodular prostatic hyperplasia, also termed ***benign prostatic hyperplasia (BPH)****, is a common disorder characterized clinically by enlargement of the prostate and urinary outflow tract obstruction, and pathologically by proliferation of glands and stroma.*

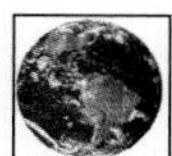

EPIDEMIOLOGY: BPH is most frequent in western Europe and the United States and least common in Asia. The prevalence of the disorder in the United States is higher among blacks than among whites. Clinical prostatism (i.e., BPH severe enough to interfere with urination) peaks in the seventh decade. However, the prevalence of BPH is far greater at autopsy than is suggested by clinically apparent prostatism. In fact, 75% of men 80 years of age or older have some degree of prostatic hyperplasia. The disorder is rare in men younger than 40 years of age.

MOLECULAR PATHOGENESIS: The earliest histogenetic events in BPH are still not understood owing to conflicting clinical evidence. Testosterone is necessary for prostatic development and for maintenance of secretory function. The active androgen form is dihydrotestosterone (DHT), a product of the enzyme 5 α-reductase. DHT binds to nuclear receptors in both glandular and stromal cells. In the adult male, exogenous testosterone does not induce hyperplastic change, and even does not stimulate atrophic glands. Advancing age is associated with a comparable reduction in circulating testosterone in men with and without BPH. Moreover, no change in serum DHT is observed in men with BPH, although the ratio of circulating testosterone to DHT may be abnormally low. Conversely, drugs that block 5α-reductase (e.g., finasteride or dutasteride) reduce the size of the prostate in men with BPH. Parenthetically, prepubertal castration prevents the development of age-related BPH and completely protects against prostate cancer.

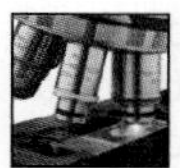

PATHOLOGY: Early nodular hyperplasia begins in the submucosa of the proximal urethra (**the transitional zone**). The enlarging nodules compress the centrally located urethral lumen and the more peripherally located normal prostate (Fig. 17-40). In well-developed BPH, the normal gland is actually limited to an attenuated rim of tissue beneath the capsule. On cut section, an individual nodule is demarcated by an enveloping fibrous pseudocapsule (Fig. 17-41B). Focal hemorrhage and infarction may be present, especially in larger nodules. On occasion, there are small stones within dilated hyperplastic acini.

Histologically, BPH features proliferation of epithelial cells of acini and ductules, smooth muscle cells and stromal

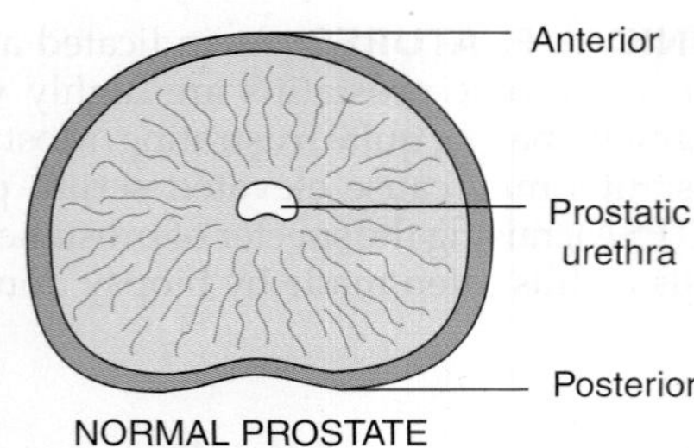

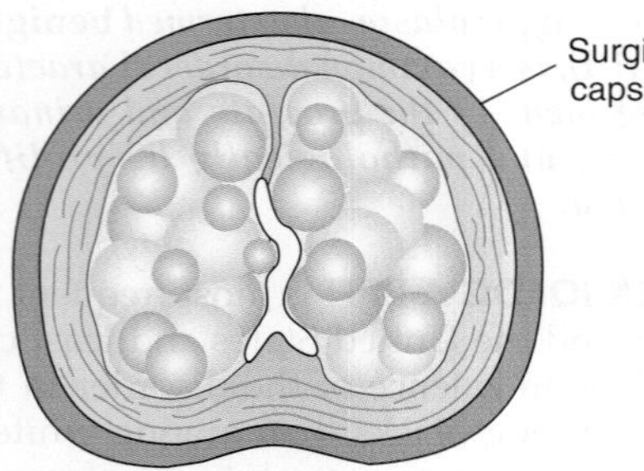

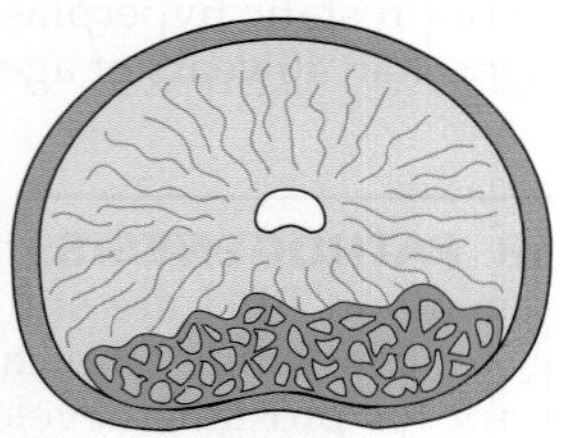

FIGURE 17-40. Normal prostate, nodular hyperplasia and adenocarcinoma. In prostatic hyperplasia, which involves predominantly the periurethral part of the gland, the nodules compress and distort the urethra. The expansion of the central prostatic glands leads to compression of the peripheral parts and fibrosis, resulting in the formation of so-called surgical capsule. Prostatic carcinoma usually arises from the peripheral glands, and compression of the urethra is a late clinical event.

fibroblasts, all in variable proportions. In these typical fibromyoadenomatous nodules, variably sized hyperplastic prostatic acini are randomly scattered throughout the stroma of the nodule. The epithelial (adenomatous) component is composed of a double layer of cells, with tall columnar cells overlying the basal layer (Fig. 17-41C). Papillary hyperplasia of glandular epithelium is characteristic. Hyperplastic nodules often contain chronic inflammatory cells and corpora amylacea (eosinophilic laminated concretions) are frequently seen within the acini. The glands of the uninvolved peripheral region of the prostate are frequently atrophic and compressed by the expanding nodules.

Nonspecific prostatitis is frequently seen in specimens with nodular hyperplasia. There is a dense intraglandular and periglandular infiltrate of lymphocytes, plasma cells and macrophages, often with acute inflammatory cells and focal gland destruction. Focal infarcts of varying age are observed in 20% of cases. Squamous metaplasia of ductal epithelium at the periphery of infarcts is typical.

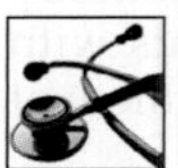

CLINICAL FEATURES: The clinical symptoms of nodular hyperplasia result from compression of the prostatic urethra and consequent bladder outlet obstruction (Fig. 17-42). A history of decreased vigor of the urinary stream and increasing urinary frequency is typical. Rectal examination reveals a firm, enlarged, nodular prostate. If the duration of severe obstruction is prolonged, backpressure results in hydroureter, hydronephrosis and ultimately renal failure and death.

Treatment of BPH is either surgical or pharmacologic with drugs that block the action of 5α-reductase. In addition, some patients receive an α_1-adrenergic blocker to enhance the flow of urine. In the surgical candidate, transurethral radiofrequency ablation and cryotherapy have supplanted traditional resection methods.

Adenocarcinoma and Precursor Lesions

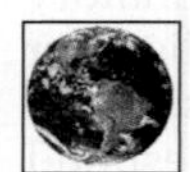

EPIDEMIOLOGY: ***In 1990, prostatic adenocarcinoma became the cancer most frequently diagnosed in American men, surpassing lung cancer for the first time.*** An estimated 220,000 new cases are diagnosed yearly in the United States. Approximately 30,000 American men die annually from it, a figure equivalent to that of colorectal carcinoma. Prostate cancer is largely a disease of elderly men: 75% of patients are 60 to 80 years of age. Autopsy studies confirm the correlation of increasing tumor frequency with increasing patient age. Prostate carcinoma is identified at autopsy in 20% of men in their 40s and in 70% after age 70. The cumulative lifetime probability of being diagnosed with either latent or symptomatic prostatic carcinoma is one in six for American men. There is considerable geographic variation in the age-related death rates for adenocarcinoma of the prostate throughout the world, the highest being in the United States and the Scandinavian countries, and the lowest in Mexico, Greece and Japan. Most western European countries have intermediate rates. American blacks, who exhibit a rate twice as high as white Americans, have proportionately the highest prostate carcinoma–related death rates in the world. Migrant studies have shown that in the United States, descendants of Polish and Japanese immigrants have a higher incidence of prostatic carcinoma than men in their original countries. Similarly, mortality from prostatic carcinoma among black American men exceeds that among blacks in Africa.

In addition to geography, racial and age differences, heredity and, possibly, diet influence the risk of prostate cancer. One tenth of cases have familial factors, with a significantly increased risk in persons whose first-degree relatives are afflicted with prostate cancer. There is some evidence that dietary fat content may increase the risk of prostate cancer, but neither environment nor dietary factors have been found to be causative.

Unfortunately, we cannot currently predict the clinical course of prostate cancer in many situations. Some tumors are amenable to therapy, while others are aggressive and lethal despite intervention. Most interestingly, there is a large subset of prostate cancers that are indolent (or latent) and may never become clinically significant during the lifetime of the patient.

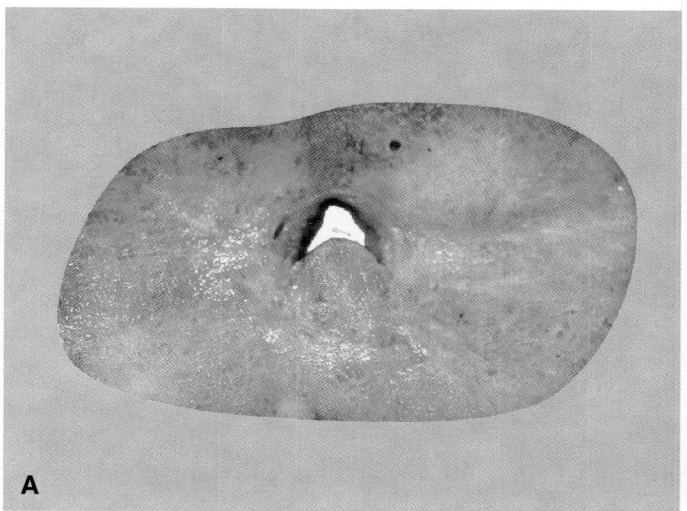

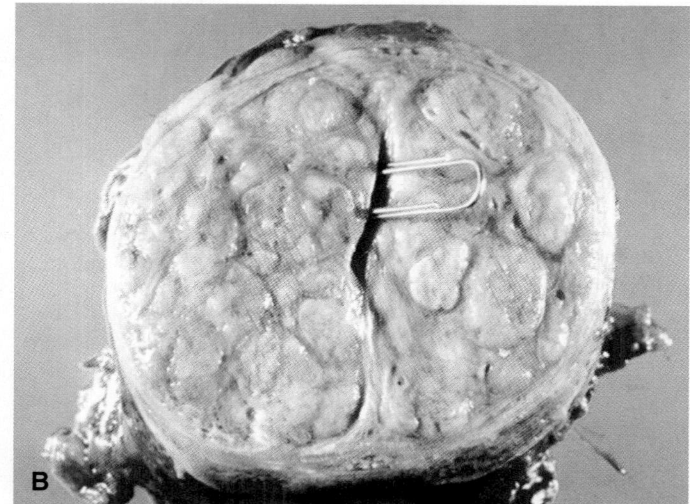

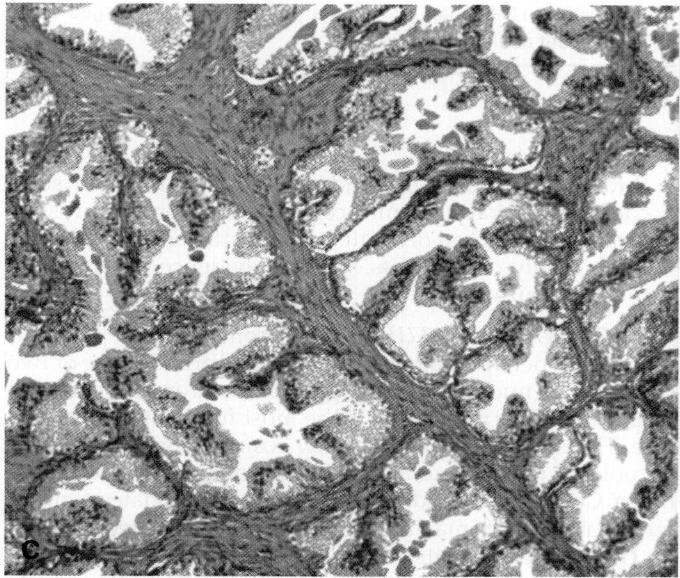

FIGURE 17-41. Nodular hyperplasia of the prostate. A. Normal prostate. **B.** The cut surface of a prostate enlarged by nodular hyperplasia shows numerous well-circumscribed nodules of prostatic tissue surrounded by pseudocapsules. The prostatic urethra (*paper clip*) has been compressed to a narrow slit. **C.** Hyperplastic prostate glands in nodular hyperplasia. The columnar epithelium lining the acini is composed of two cell layers: polarized clear cuboidal cells lining the acinar lumen and flattened basal cells interposed between the cuboidal acinar cells and the stroma. Hyperplastic cells line papillary projections protruding into the lumina of the acini.

MOLECULAR PATHOGENESIS: A principal focus of research interest is endocrine influences. Androgenic control of normal prostatic growth and the responsiveness of prostate cancer to castration and exogenous estrogens support a role for male hormones. Rats have developed the tumor after prolonged administration of testosterone. However, human patients with prostate cancer do not typically have higher levels of serum androgens. Elevated urinary estrone-to-testosterone ratios have been reported. The human androgen (AR) gene has shown considerable variation in CAG repeats in exon 1. Men with a lower number AR CAG repeats are at greater risk for developing prostate cancer. Some tumors show somatic mutations that place the transcription factor gene ETV1 under the control of the androgen-regulated TMPRSS2 promoter. Other cases show hypermethylation of the glutathione S-transferase gene. Altered regulation of the STAT family of transcription factors has been documented, as has dysregulation of the PTEN tumor suppressor gene.

There is consensus that intraductal dysplastic epithelial proliferation, termed **prostatic intraepithelial neoplasia (PIN),** is a precursor lesion of prostatic adenocarcinoma. ***PIN refers to prostatic ducts lined by cytologically atypical luminal cells and the concomitant decrease in basal cells.*** Nuclei of high-grade PIN are enlarged, contain nucleoli and show marked crowding (Fig. 17-43). Substantial evidence indicates that PIN lesions are premalignant and progress to adenocarcinoma. High-grade PIN is present in the vicinity of most invasive carcinomas. Such lesions may precede invasive cancer by as much as two decades, and their severity increases with increasing age.

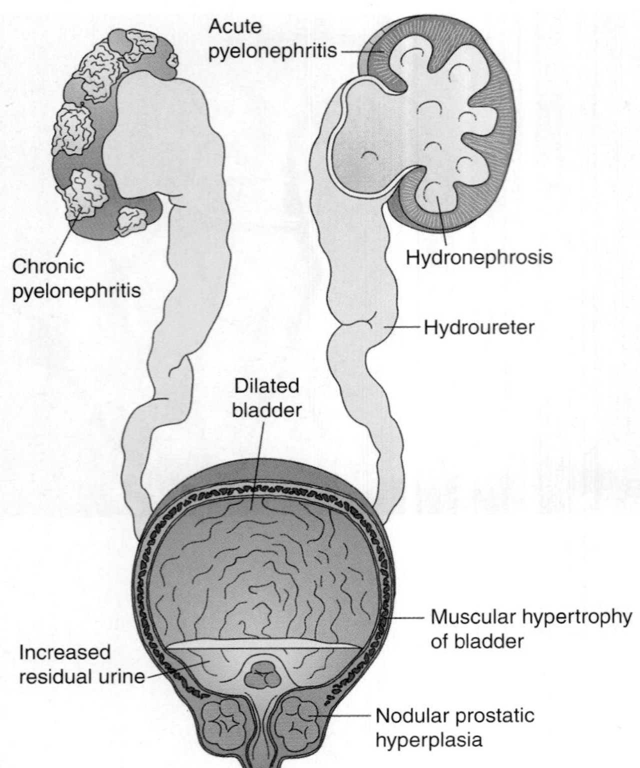

FIGURE 17-42. Complications of nodular prostatic hyperplasia.

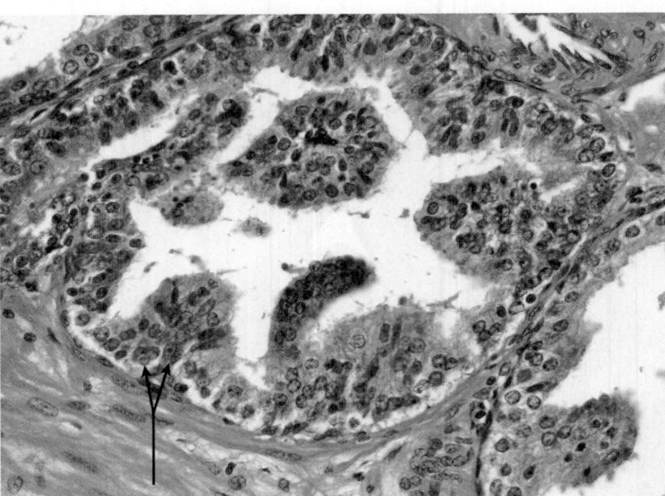

FIGURE 17-43. High-grade prostatic intraepithelial neoplasia (PIN). The large duct in the center is lined by atypical cells with enlarged nuclei and prominent nucleoli (*arrows*).

Morphologic evidence linking PIN to invasive prostate cancer includes (1) both lesions are mainly peripheral, (2) cytologic similarity of high-grade PIN to invasive cancer and (3) close topographic proximity of high-grade PIN to invasive cancer. Finally, PIN lesions are more frequent in prostates harboring cancer than in those without tumors. Certain markers are similar in high-grade PIN and invasive cancer (e.g., aneuploidy, transforming growth factor [TGF]-α, type IV collagenase and expression of *bcl*-2 and c-*erb*-2 oncogenes). High-grade PIN is important to recognize on needle biopsy because many patients with high-grade PIN on initial biopsy have invasive carcinoma on follow-up biopsy.

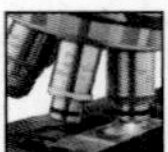

PATHOLOGY: Adenocarcinomas account for the vast majority of all primary prostatic tumors. They are commonly multicentric and located in the peripheral zones in over 70% of cases. The cut surface of the carcinomatous prostate shows irregular, yellow-white, indurated subcapsular nodules.

HISTOLOGIC FEATURES OF INVASIVE CARCINOMA: Most prostatic adenocarcinomas are of acinar origin and feature small to medium-sized glands that lack organization and infiltrate the stroma. Well-differentiated tumors show uniform medium-sized or small glands (Fig. 17-44) that are lined by a single layer of neoplastic epithelial cells. The malignant acini have lost their basal cells and no longer grow in a lobular fashion. Progressive loss of differentiation of prostatic adenocarcinomas is characterized by:

- Increasing variability of gland size and configuration
- Papillary and cribriform patterns
- Rudimentary (or no) gland formation, with only solid cords of infiltrating tumor cells. Uncommonly, a prostate cancer is composed of small undifferentiated cells growing individually or in sheets, without evidence of any structural organization.

CYTOLOGIC FEATURES: The prominence of pleomorphic and hyperchromatic nuclei is highly variable. One or two conspicuous nucleoli in a background of chromatin clumped near the nuclear membrane is the most frequent nuclear feature. The cytoplasm stains slightly eosinophilic or may be so vacuolated that it simulates the clear cells of renal cell carcinoma. Cell borders are distinct in better-differentiated tumors, but are not well demarcated in poorly differentiated ones.

GRADING: Prostatic adenocarcinoma is most commonly classified according to the **Gleason grading system** (Figs. 17-44 and 17-45), which is based on five histologic patterns of tumor gland formation and infiltration. Recognizing the high frequency of mixed tumor patterns, the Gleason score is the sum of the grades (1 through 5) attributed to the most prominent pattern and that of the minority pattern. The best-differentiated tumors have a Gleason score of 2 (1 + 1), while very poorly differentiated cancers have scores of 10 (5 + 5). Gleason patterns 1 and 2 are rare. The most common pattern is Gleason pattern 3. When combined with the tumor stage, the Gleason grading system has prognostic value: lower scores correlate with better prognoses.

INVASION AND METASTASIS: The high frequency of invasion of the prostatic capsule by adenocarcinoma relates to the subcapsular location of the tumor. Perineural tumor invasion within the prostate and adjacent tissues is usual. Since peripheral nerves are devoid of perineural lymphatic channels, this mode of invasion represents contiguous spread of the tumor along a tissue space that offers the plane of least resistance.

The seminal vesicles are almost always involved by direct extension of prostate cancer. Invasion of the urinary bladder is less common until late in the clinical course. The earliest metastases occur in the obturator lymph node, with subsequent dissemination to iliac and periaortic lymph nodes.

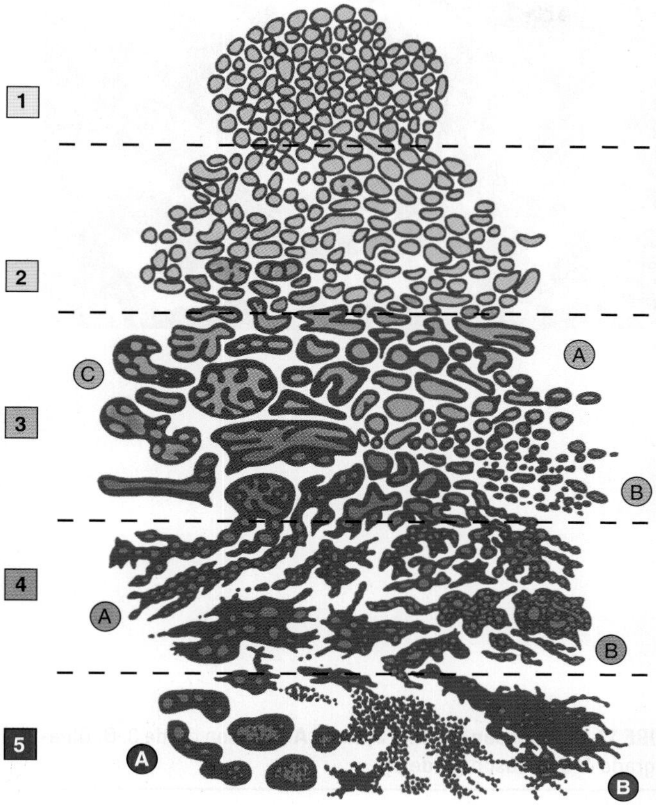

GLANDS

	Differentiation	Distribution
1	'Round,' lined by single layer of cuboidal cells	Close packed in rounded masses; definite edge
2	More variable in size and shape	Separated up to one gland diameter; 'loose' edge
3a	Irregular shape; medium to large size	Irregularly spaced apart; poorly defined 'edge'; surround normal strucutres
3b	Small to minute glands, not fused or 'chained'	Very irregular spacing and distribution; no 'edge'; surround normal structures
3c	Masses of cribriform or papillary epithelium with smooth outer surfaces	
4a	Ragged masses of fused glandular epithelium; bare tumor cells in stroma	Ragged infiltrating masses that overrun normal structures; No smooth surfaces against stroma
4b	Same as 4a; large clear cells	
5a	Smooth, cribriform to solid masses; often central necrosis 'comedocarcinoma'	Ragged infiltrating masses that infiltrate stromal fibers
5b	Anaplastic carcinoma with vacuoles and glands that suggest adenocarcinoma	

FIGURE 17-44. Prostate adenocarcinoma. Gleason grading system.

Metastases to the lung reflect further lymphatic spread through the thoracic duct and through dissemination from the prostatic venous plexus to the inferior vena cava. Bony metastases, particularly to the vertebral column (Fig. 17-46), ribs and pelvic bones, are painful and are difficult to manage.

CLINICAL FEATURES: Current screening programs for prostate cancer that use digital rectal examination in combination with serum PSA levels detect most malignancies. Patients with elevated serum PSA are further evaluated by needle biopsies. ***Preoperative PSA levels are correlated with cancer volume.*** Uncommonly, patients with prostate cancer present with bladder outlet obstruction or symptoms referable to metastatic tumor.

The principles of clinical staging of prostate cancer are shown in Fig. 17-47 and Table 17-8. At the time of initial presentation, 10% of prostate cancers are stage T1. In patients with tumors clinically judged to be localized to the prostate (stage T2), 60% show microscopic evidence of capsular penetration or seminal vesicle invasion (stage T3). Metastases are observed in lymph nodes, bones, lung and liver, in order of decreasing frequency. Widespread tumor dissemination (carcinomatosis), with pneumonia or sepsis, is the most common cause of death.

The immunohistochemical demonstration of **PSA** on biopsy specimens of metastatic sites has proved valuable in identifying the prostate as the primary site of the tumor. PSA is also detectable in the serum of patients with prostate cancer. Serum PSA is useful for tumor screening and as an indicator of recurrent disease after therapy. A new marker for prostate carcinoma, **α-methylacyl-CoA racemase** (AMCAR), is also useful for identifying prostatic adenocarcinoma inside the gland as well as in metastatic sites. PSA is also detectable in the serum of patients with prostate cancer. Serum PSA is used both for tumor screening and as an indicator of recurrent disease after therapy. **Serum alkaline phosphatase** levels are elevated in patients with osteoblastic bony metastases, because this enzyme is released from osteoblasts forming new bone at the site of metastasis.

Therapy for prostate cancer has become highly controversial, owing to recent studies that suggest that many tumors may best be left alone and considerable difficulty in distinguishing between tumors that are likely to benefit from treatment and those that are not. However, generally, treatments used depend on tumor stage. Patients with stage T1 and T2 cancers are treated by radical prostatectomy, radiofrequency ablation, cryogenic procedures or radiation therapy. Radiation therapy may be either external beam or implanted

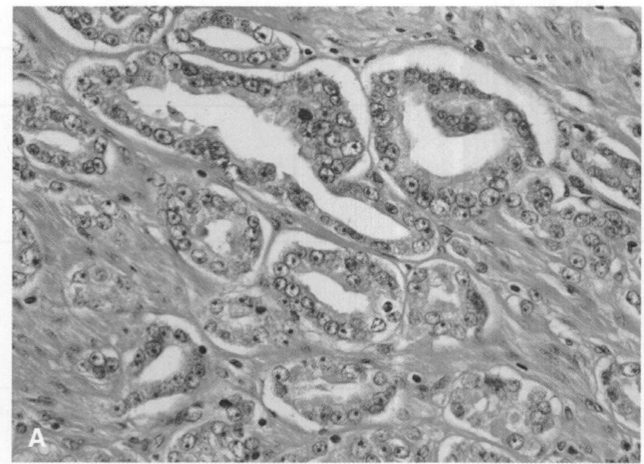

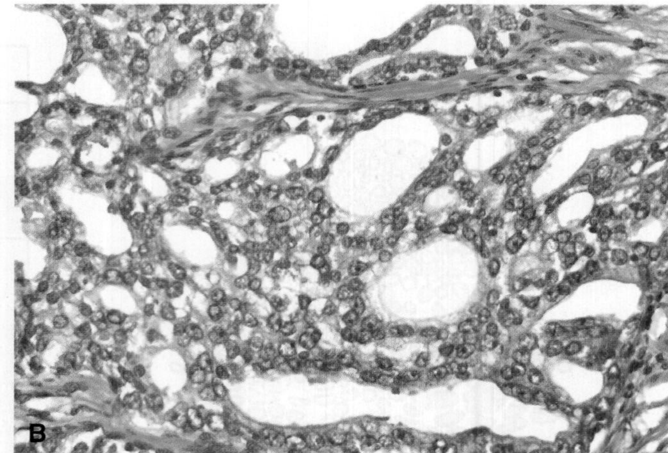

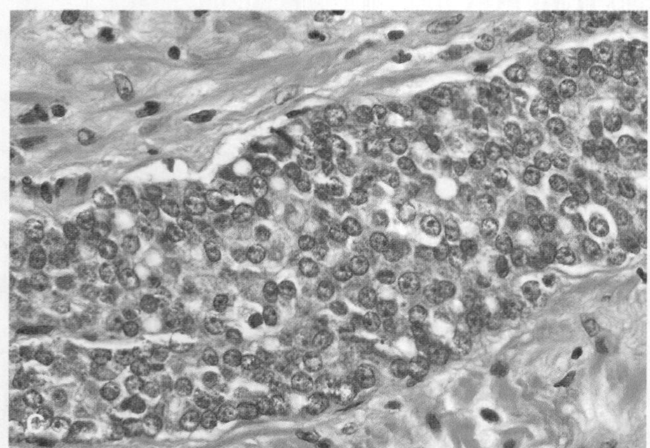

FIGURE 17-45. Gleason grading system. A. Gleason grade 3. **B**. Gleason grade 4. **C**. Gleason grade 5.

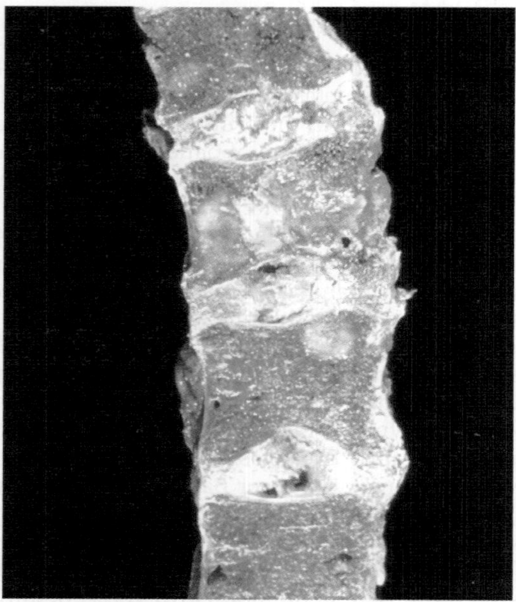

FIGURE 17-46. Prostatic adenocarcinoma metastatic to the spine. The vertebral bodies contain several nodular osteoblastic metastases.

Table 17-8

TNM Staging of Prostatic Carcinoma

T—Primary Tumor
T1 No clinically detectable tumor T1a Histologic tumor found in 5% or less of tissue examined T1b Histologic tumor found in more than 5% of tissue examined
T2 Tumor confined to the prostate T2a Tumor in one lobe only T2b Tumor in both lobes
T3 Tumor extends through the capsule T3a Extracapsular extension only T3b Tumor extends into seminal vesicles
T4 Tumor invades adjacent structures other than seminal vesicles
N—Regional Lymph Nodes
N0 No regional lymph node involvement
N1 Regional lymph node metastases present
M—Distant Metastases
M0 No distant metastases
M1 Distant metastases present

Data from Edge SB, Byrd DR, Compton CC, et al., eds. AJCC Cancer Staging Manual, 7th ed. New York: Springer, 2009.

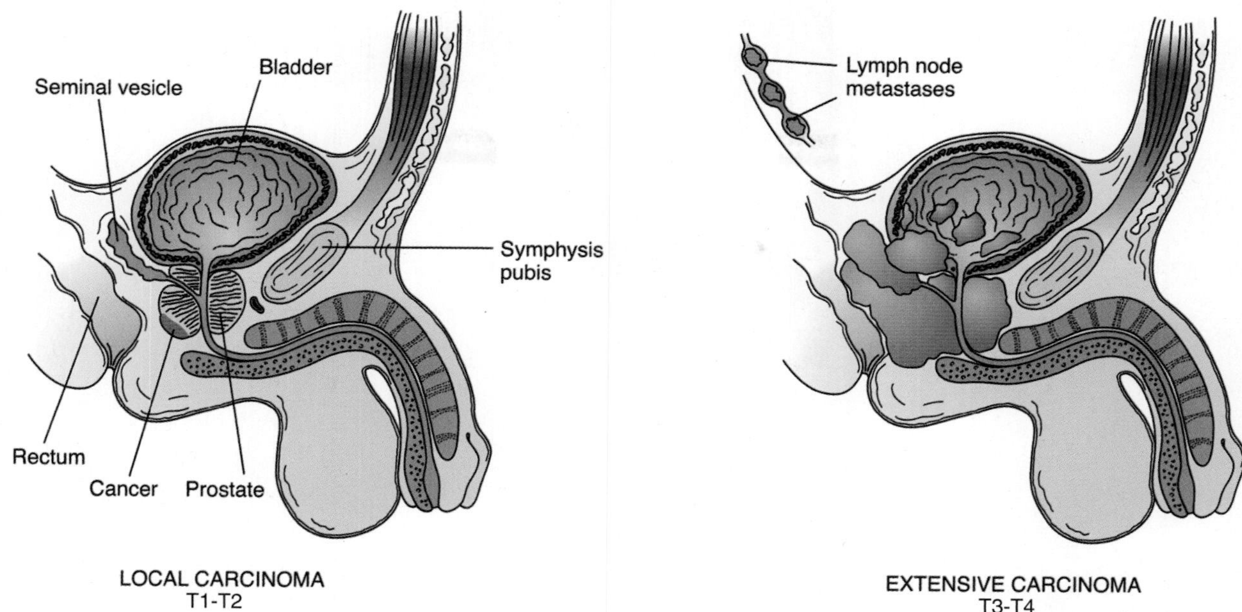

FIGURE 17-47. Staging of prostatic carcinoma. Tumor–node–metastasis (TNM) system is most widely used for staging of prostate carcinoma. Stage T1 and T2 tumors are localized to the prostate, whereas stage T3 and T4 tumors have spread outside the prostate.

radioactive seeds (brachytherapy). In stage T3 tumors, radiation therapy, combined with androgen deprivation therapy, is the treatment of choice, acknowledging that half of these patients have occult pelvic lymph node metastases (and possibly further systemic dissemination), which cannot be cured by surgical means. Patients with low-grade, low-volume tumors may opt to be managed by active surveillance only.

For patients with metastatic disease or whose tumors progress clinically, traditional chemotherapy combined with androgen deprivation is the principal strategy. Bone metastases can be treated with local radiation, bisphosphonates and supplements of calcium and vitamin D.

The 5-year survival rates depend on stage and Gleason grade (Fig. 17-44). Using staging data, survival is as follows: stages T1 and T2, 90%; stage T3, 40%; and stage T4, 10%.

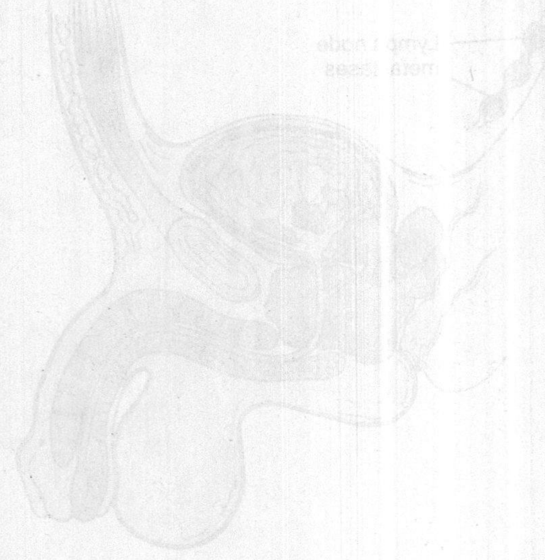

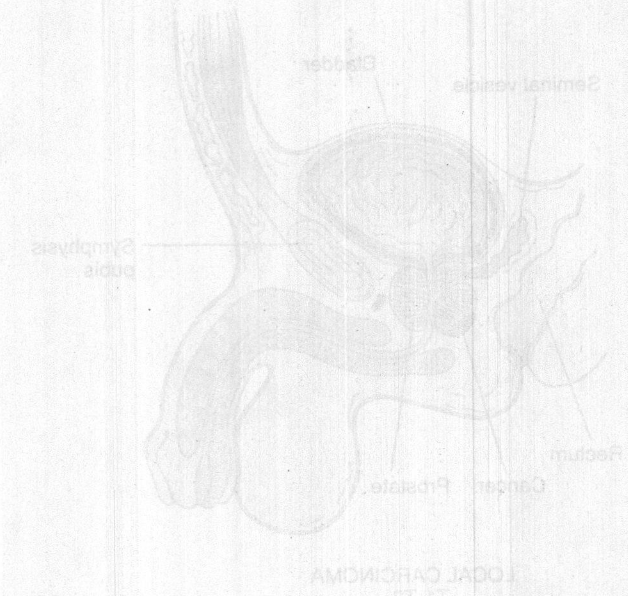

18 The Female Reproductive System, the Peritoneum and Pregnancy

George L. Mutter • Jaime Prat • David A. Schwartz

Embryology

The gonadal anlage, which forms as a swelling of the embryonic urogenital ridge, is initially in an indifferent state. Both sex chromosomes and autosomal chromosomes in gonadal stromal cells determine whether it will differentiate into testis or ovary. If the gonadal stroma is male, a gene on the Y chromosome (testis-determining gene) interacts with somatic components in the primitive gonad to initiate development of seminiferous tubules. An ovary develops if the gonadal stroma is female and there is no stimulus to form a testis. The ovary is derived from mesoderm, except for the germ cells, which are endodermal. By about the 40th day, the ovaries and testes are histologically distinct.

Wolffian (mesonephric) ducts begin to develop at about day 25, regardless of the embryo's sex. If stimulated by testosterone (secreted by Leydig cells starting about day 70), the ducts differentiate into vas deferens, epididymis and seminal vesicle. If not stimulated by day 84, the ducts regress and remain as vestigial rests in the female. They may form cysts in the cervix or vagina **(mesonephric cyst).**

Müllerian (paramesonephric) ducts, the anlage of the fallopian tubes, uterus and vaginal wall, appear at about day 37 as funnel-shaped openings of celomic epithelium. They develop into paired, undifferentiated tubes, using the wolffian ducts as "guide wires" to reach the area of the future hymen. If a wolffian duct is absent, as in renal agenesis, the vagina and cervix are almost always abnormal or absent. At day 54, müllerian ducts fuse into a straight uterovaginal canal.

A central tenet of genital tract development in both sexes is that müllerian tubes develop along female lines unless specifically impeded by embryonic testicular factors. In males, Sertoli cells in developing testes produce **antimüllerian hormone,** also called **müllerian-inhibiting substance,** which causes müllerian ducts to regress.

The external genitalia assume masculine form if testosterone is converted locally to dihydrotestosterone. Otherwise (i.e., relative estrogen excess), female external genitalia persist. The genital tubercle develops into the clitoris, genital folds into the labia minora and genital swellings into the labia majora. The basic layout of the female genital tract is done by day 120.

Genital Infections

Genital Infections Are Commonly Sexually Transmitted

Infectious diseases of the female genital tract are common and are caused by many organisms (Table 18-1; also see Chapter 9). Most of the important infectious diseases of the female genital tract are sexually transmitted.

Table 18-1

Infectious Diseases of the Female Genital Tract

Organism	Disease	Diagnostic Feature
Sexually Transmitted Diseases		
Gram-negative rods and cocci		
Calymmatobacterium granulomatis	Granuloma inguinale	Donovan body
Gardnerella vaginalis	*Gardnerella* infection	Clue cell
Haemophilus ducreyi	Chancroid (soft chancre)	
Neisseria gonorrhoeae	Gonorrhea	Gram-negative diplococcus
Spirochetes		
Treponema pallidum	Syphilis	Spirochete
Mycoplasmas		
Mycoplasma hominis	Nonspecific vaginitis	
Ureaplasma urealyticum	Nonspecific vaginitis	
Rickettsiae		
Chlamydia trachomatis type D-K	Various forms of pelvic inflammatory disease (PID)	
Chlamydia trachomatis type L_{1-3}	Lymphogranuloma venereum	
Viruses		
Human papillomavirus (HPV)	Condyloma acuminatum/planum Neoplastic potential	Koilocyte
Types 6, 11, 40, 42, 43, 44, 57	Low risk	Low-grade squamous intraepithelial lession (LSIL)
Types 16, 18, 31, 33, 35, 39, 45, 51, 52, 56, 58, 66	High risk	High-grade squamous intraepithelial lesion (HSIL)
Herpes simplex type 2	Herpes genitalis	Multinucleated giant cell with intranuclear homogenization and inclusion bodies
Cytomegalovirus (CMV)	Cytomegalic inclusion disease	Bulbous intranuclear inclusion body
Molluscum contagiosum	Molluscum infection	Molluscum body
Protozoa		
Trichomonas vaginalis	Trichomoniasis	Trichomonad
Selected Nonsexually Transmitted Diseases		
Actinomyces and related organisms		
Actinomyces israelii	PID (one of many organisms)	Sulphur granules
Mycobacterium tuberculosis	Tuberculosis	Necrotizing granulomas
Fungi		
Candida albicans	Candidiasis	*Candida* sp.

Bacterial Infections

Gonorrhea

Gonorrhea is caused by *Neisseria gonorrhoeae,* a fastidious, gram-negative diplococcus. A million cases of gonorrhea occur yearly in the United States. The infection is a frequent cause of acute salpingitis and pelvic inflammatory disease (PID) (Fig. 18-1).

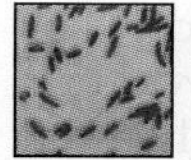

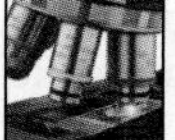

ETIOLOGIC FACTORS AND PATHOLOGY: The organisms ascend through the cervix and endometrial cavity, where they cause **acute endometritis.** They then attach to mucosal cells in the fallopian tube and elicit acute inflammation, which is confined to the mucosal surface **(acute salpingitis).** Infection may then spread to the ovary, sometimes causing a **tuboovarian abscess.** Pelvic and abdominal cavities may be affected, to cause subdiaphragmatic and pelvic abscesses.

Systemic complications of gonorrhea include septicemia and septic arthritis. At all sites of infection, the organisms induce purulent inflammatory reactions that rarely resolve completely. Dense fibrous adhesions often remain, distorting and destroying the plicae of the fallopian tube, and frequently leading to sterility.

Syphilis

Syphilis (see Chapter 9) is caused by *Treponema pallidum,* a thin, motile, spiral-shaped bacterium, called a spirochete. Spread is via sexual contact with an infected person, or transplacental spread (congenital syphilis). *T. pallidum* penetrates small cuts in the skin or normal mucosal surfaces.

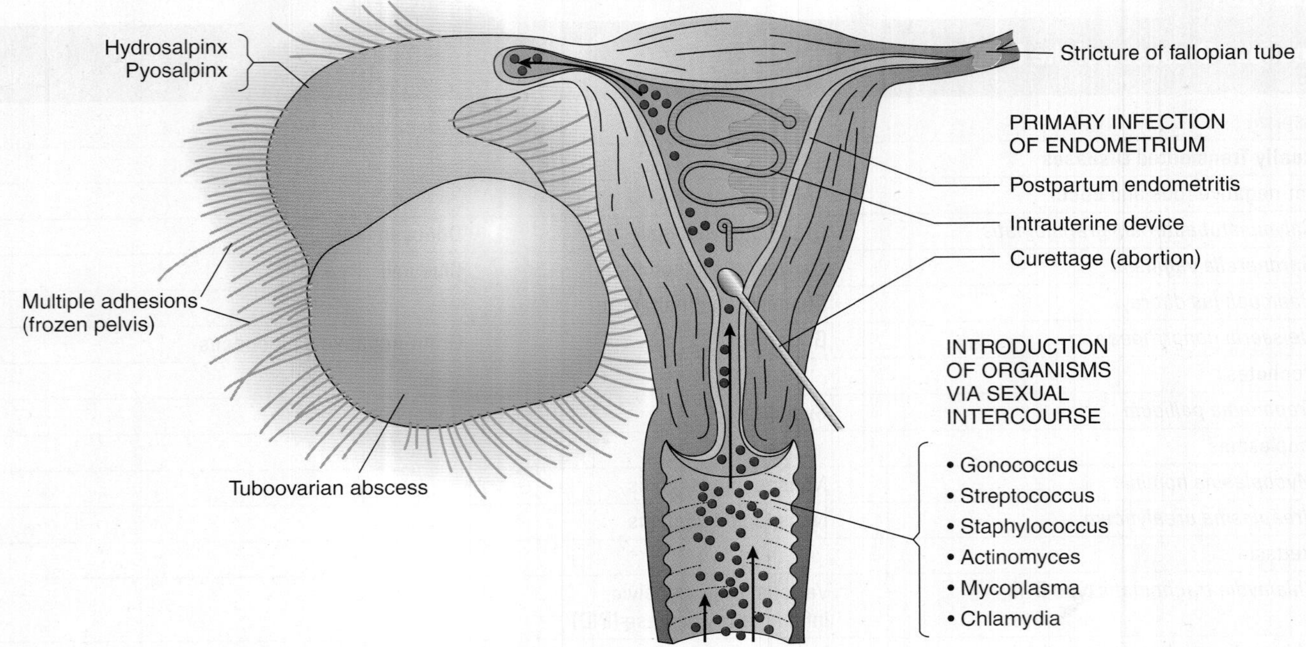

FIGURE 18-1. Pelvic inflammatory disease.

Untreated, syphilis persists, often waxing and waning, through three stages.

- In the **primary stage** a **chancre** usually appears after about 3 weeks at the portal of bacterial entry. It is a painless, indurated papule, 1 cm to several centimeters in diameter, surrounded by an inflammatory cuff that breaks down to form an ulcer. The lesion may persist for 2 to 6 weeks. It then heals spontaneously.
- **Secondary syphilis** appears after a latent period of several weeks to months, and features low-grade fever, headache, malaise, lymphadenopathy and highly very syphilitic lesions called **condylomata lata** (syphilitic warts). These secondary infectious lesions heal after 2 to 6 weeks and symptoms disappear spontaneously.
- The **tertiary stage** develops any time thereafter and may entail severe damage to the cardiovascular and nervous systems.

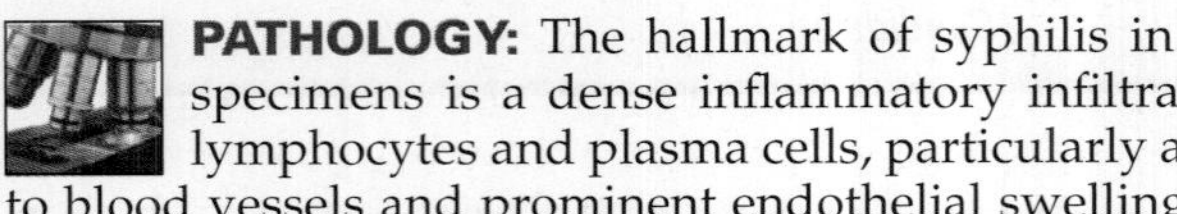

PATHOLOGY: The hallmark of syphilis in biopsy specimens is a dense inflammatory infiltrate with lymphocytes and plasma cells, particularly adjacent to blood vessels and prominent endothelial swelling. Silver impregnation techniques (Warthin-Starry stain or its modifications) help demonstrate the spirochetes. The more advanced stages of disease show greater obliterative endarteritis and subsequent tissue destruction.

Granuloma Inguinale

Granuloma inguinale is caused by *Calymmatobacterium granulomatis,* a sexually transmitted, gram-negative, encapsulated rod. The disease occurs with equal frequency in women and men.

PATHOLOGY: The primary lesion begins as a painless, ulcerated nodule involving genital, inguinal or perianal skin. The organisms invade through skin abrasions and spread locally by direct extension, destroying skin and underlying tissues. Extensive local spread and lymphatic permeation occur later. Vacuolated macrophages teem with characteristic intracellular bacteria **(Donovan bodies).** The organism, best seen with the Wright stain, resembles a closed safety pin. Hyperplasia of overlying squamous epithelium may be exuberant enough to be misinterpreted as a squamous cell carcinoma. Relapses after antibiotic therapy are common.

Chancroid

Chancroid, also called **soft chancre,** is caused by *Haemophilus ducreyi,* a gram-negative bacillus. This disease is rare in the United States but is common in underdeveloped countries.

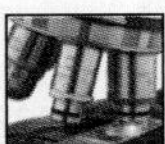

PATHOLOGY: Single or sometimes multiple small, vesiculopustular lesions appear on cervix, vagina, vulva or perianal region 3 to 5 days after sexual contact with an infected partner. At this stage examination shows granulomatous inflammation. The lesion may rupture to form a painful, purulent ulcer that bleeds easily. Inguinal lymphadenopathy, fever, chills and malaise may occur. A major complication is scarring during the healing phase, which may cause urethral stenosis.

Gardnerella

Sexual transmission of *Gardnerella vaginalis,* a gram-negative coccobacillus, causes many cases of "nonspecific vaginitis." Since the organism does not penetrate the mucosa, it causes no inflammation and biopsies appear normal. A wet mount specimen of a vaginal discharge or a Papanicolaou-stained smear (Pap smear) can identify the bacteria. **Clue cells,** squamous cells covered by coccobacilli, are pathognomonic. Other aids to diagnosis are a thin, homogeneous, milklike vaginal discharge, vaginal pH above 4.5 and a fishy odor when the discharge is alkalinized with 10% potassium hydroxide.

Mycoplasma

Mycoplasmas (see Chapter 9) are minute pleomorphic organisms that resemble the so-called L bacterial forms but differ by having no cell wall. They are common oropharyngeal and urogenital tract commensals, and colonize the lower genital tract through sexual contact. *Ureaplasma urealyticum* can be isolated from the lower genital tract in 40% of healthy women and may cause infertility, adverse effects on pregnancy and perinatal infections. *Mycoplasma hominis* is found in the lower genital tract of 5% of healthy women, and causes a small proportion of cases of symptomatic cervicitis and vaginitis. *M. hominis* is often isolated in association with *G. vaginalis* or *Trichomonas vaginalis* infection. Although the role of mycoplasma in genital tract infections is not completely understood, the organisms are encountered in PID, acute salpingitis, spontaneous abortion and puerperal fever. Affected tissue is usually unremarkable histologically.

Chlamydia Infections

Chlamydia trachomatis is a common, venereally transmitted gram-negative obligate intracellular rickettsia. Fifteen serotypes are known. *C. trachomatis* causes a variety of disorders in women, men and infants. It has been found in the genital tracts of about 8% of asymptomatic women and 20% of women with symptoms of lower genital tract infection. Chlamydia is easily confused with gonorrhea, as the symptoms of both diseases are similar.

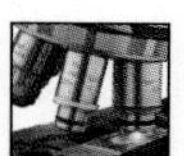

PATHOLOGY: Serotypes D through K cause the more common genital infections. The cervical mucosa is severely inflamed, and endocervical and metaplastic squamous cells contain small inclusion bodies. Cytologically, perinuclear intracytoplasmic inclusions with distinct borders and intracytoplasmic **coccoid bodies** are seen. Complications include ascending infection of the endometrium, fallopian tube and ovary, which may result in tubal occlusion and infertility. Chlamydia may also infect Bartholin glands and cause acute urethritis. Infants delivered vaginally to infected mothers may develop conjunctivitis, otitis media and pneumonia.

Lymphogranuloma Venereum

Lymphogranuloma venereum is a venereal infection of men and women that is endemic in tropical countries. It is caused by the L form of *C. trachomatis*, serotypes L1 through L3.

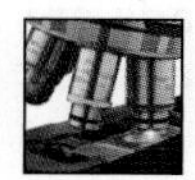

PATHOLOGY: After a few days to a month, a small painless vesicle forms at the site of inoculation. It heals rapidly and often is not even noticed. In the second stage, inguinal lymph nodes are enlarged and may rupture to form suppurative fistulas. Perirectal lymph nodes in women become matted and painful. In untreated patients, a third stage may appear after latency lasting several years. In this phase scarring causes lymphatic obstruction, resulting in genital elephantiasis and rectal strictures. Infected tissues in the second and third stages show necrotizing granulomas and neutrophil infiltrates. Inclusion bodies within macrophages may be seen.

Viral Infections

Human Papillomavirus

Human papillomavirus (HPV) is a DNA virus that infects several skin and mucosal surfaces, to produce wartlike lesions referred to as **verrucae** and **condylomata**. Over 100 HPV serotypes are known, one third of which cause genital tract lesions. The median time from infection to first detection of HPV is 3 months. In the United States, as many as two thirds of women graduating college have genital HPV infections, which result from sexual contact with an infected person. Even in women who have had only one sexual partner, the risk of acquiring cervical HPV by 3 years after first intercourse was 50% in one study. In another study, HPV prevalence among women aged 14 to 59 years exceeded 25%. About 20 million people are currently infected with HPV in this country, serotypes 6 and 11 accounting for over 80% of visible condylomata.

Several strains of HPV are the major etiologic factors for squamous cell cancer in the female lower genital tract, as well as anal and oropharyngeal cancers in both sexes. Types 16, 18, 31 and 45 are most often linked to intraepithelial neoplasia and invasive cancer (see below).

Most cases of HPV are diagnosed by cervical Pap smear. Recent tests directly assay for HPV DNA. Current treatment for HPV infections is inadequate, but most spontaneously disappear. The U.S. Food and Drug Administration (FDA) approved vaccines to prevent infection with HPV serotypes 6, 11, 16 and 18.

Condyloma Acuminatum

Condyloma acuminatum, caused by HPV infection, is a benign, exophytic, papillomatous lesion on the skin or mucous membranes of the lower female genital tract, which is often visible to the naked eye, but sometimes requires colposcopy to be seen. In the cervix and vagina these are known as low-grade squamous intraepithelial lesions (LSIL) (see below).

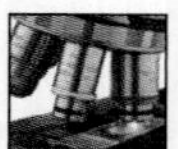

PATHOLOGY: Condylomata acuminata occur on the vulva, perianal region, perineum, vagina and cervix. They may also involve the urethra, bladder and rectum. Condylomata grow as papules, plaques or nodules and eventually as spiked or cauliflower-like excrescences (Fig. 18-2A). They show papillomatous squamous epithelial proliferation, with characteristic **koilocytes** (from the Greek *koilos*, "hollow"), epithelial cells with a perinuclear halo and wrinkled nucleus that contains HPV particles (Fig. 18-2B). Virus DNA typically remains episomal, and extensive virus replication causes extensive cytoplasmic injury, creating the koilocyte (Fig. 18-2C).

Herpesvirus

Herpes simplex type 2 is a very large double-stranded DNA virus that commonly causes sexually transmitted genital infections. After an incubation period of 1 to 3 weeks, small vesicles develop on the vulva and erode into painful ulcers. Similar lesions occur in the vagina and cervix. Epithelial cells adjacent to intraepithelial vesicles show ballooning degeneration and many contain large nuclei with eosinophilic inclusions.

Herpesvirus infections follow relapsing, remitting courses. While latent, the virus resides in the local (here, sacral) ganglia. If it reactivates in pregnancy, passage through the birth canal may transmit the virus to the newborn infant, often with fatal consequences. Active herpetic lesions in the vagina at the time of delivery are therefore an indication for Cesarean section.

Cytomegalovirus

Cytomegalovirus (CMV) is a ubiquitous double-stranded DNA virus of the *Herpesvirus* family. More than 80% of people over the age of 35 have antibodies to CMV. Several lines of evidence suggest that many cases are sexually transmitted: (1) seroprevalence of CMV has risen in young adults, (2) the virus is recovered more often from cervical secretions and semen than from any other body sites and (3) viral titers in semen are 100,000 times higher than in urine. Still, CMV only

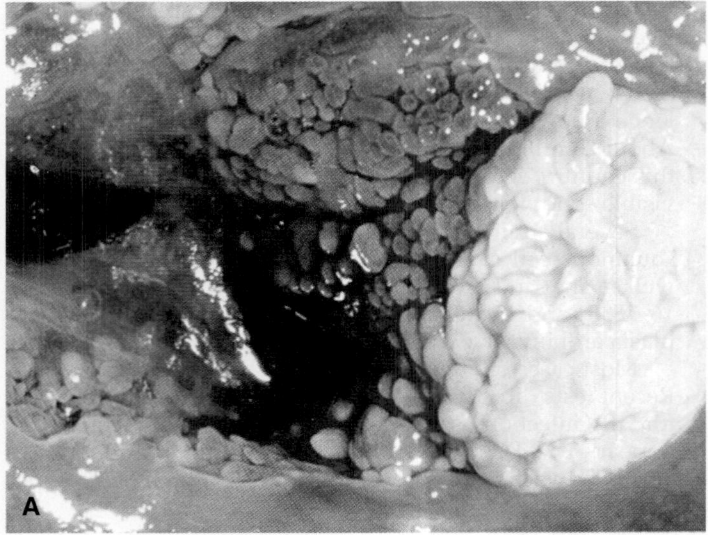

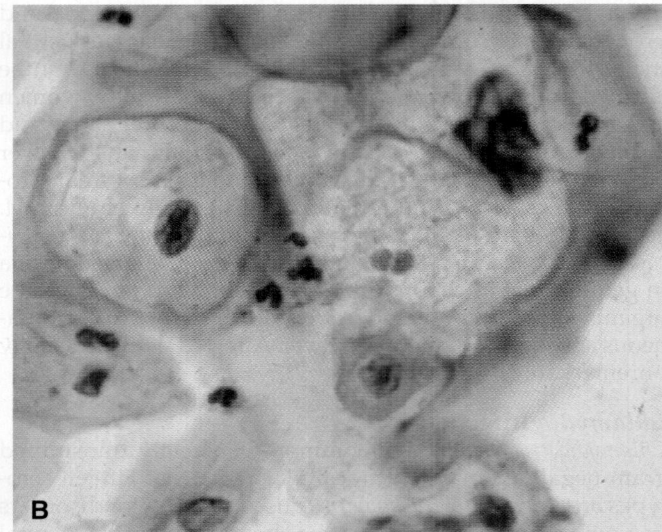

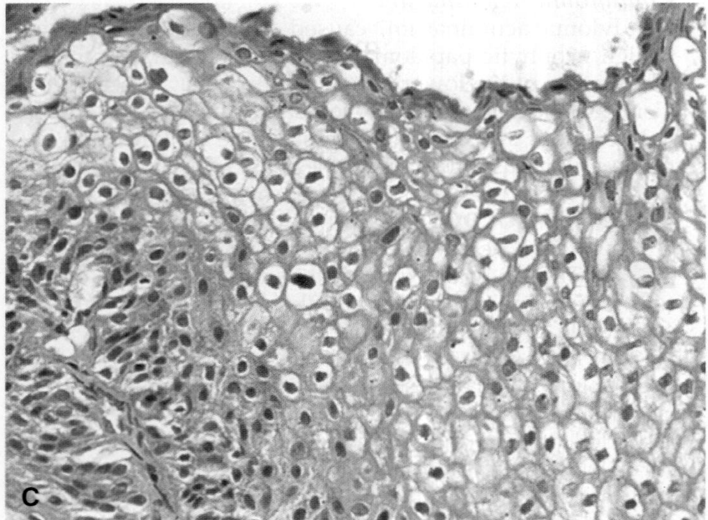

FIGURE 18-2. Human papillomavirus-induced condylomatous infections. A. Condyloma acuminatum on the cervix, visible with the naked eye as cauliflower-like excrescences. **B.** A cervical smear contains characteristic koilocytes, with a perinuclear halo and a wrinkled nucleus that contains viral particles. **C.** Biopsy of the condyloma shows koilocytes with perinuclear halos and significant nuclear pleomorphism and altered chromatin density.

rarely causes genital infections in women. Infection in the endometrium may result in spontaneous abortion or infection of the newborn. Infected cells exhibit characteristic large, eosinophilic, intranuclear inclusions and, occasionally, cytoplasmic inclusions.

Molluscum Contagiosum

Molluscum contagiosum (see Chapter 24) is a highly contagious double-stranded DNA poxvirus. Infection leads to multiple smooth, gray-white nodules that are centrally umbilicated and exude a cheesy material. Lesions occur predominantly in the genital region but may be found elsewhere as well. Large, cytoplasmic viral inclusions **(molluscum bodies)** are seen in infected epithelial cells. Most lesions regress spontaneously, but untreated ones may persist for years.

Trichomoniasis

T. vaginalis is a large, pear-shaped, flagellated protozoan that commonly causes vaginitis. It is transmitted sexually, and 25% of infected women are asymptomatic carriers. Infection manifests as a heavy, yellow-gray, thick, foamy discharge with severe itching, dyspareunia (painful intercourse) and dysuria (painful urination). The motile trichomonads are identified on wet mount preparations, and may also be demonstrated in Pap smears.

Pelvic Inflammatory Disease

PID refers to infection of pelvic organs due to extension of any of a variety of microorganisms beyond the uterine corpus (Fig. 18-1). Ascent of the infection results in bilateral acute salpingitis, pyosalpinx and tuboovarian abscesses. ***N. gonorrhoeae and* Chlamydia *are the main organisms responsible for PID, but most infections are polymicrobial.*** PID is far more common in sexually promiscuous women than in those who are monogamous. Occasionally, it occurs after postpartum endometritis or a complication of endometrial curettage.

Patients with PID typically present with lower abdominal pain. Examination reveals bilateral adnexal tenderness and marked discomfort when the cervix is manipulated (chandelier sign). Complications of PID include (1) rupture of a tuboovarian abscess, which may result in life-threatening peritonitis; (2) infertility from scarring of the healed tubal plicae; (3) increased rates of ectopic pregnancy; and (4) intestinal obstruction from fibrous bands and adhesions.

Some Genital Infections Are Not Transmitted Sexually

Tuberculosis

Mycobacterium tuberculosis may infect any part of the female genital tract. Genital tuberculosis is found in 1% of infertile women in the United States and in more than 10% of such women in less developed countries. Identification of acid-fast bacilli (AFB) confirms the diagnosis.

PATHOLOGY:

TUBERCULOUS SALPINGITIS: Salpingitis is usually the initial lesion of tuberculous genital infection, due to hematogenous dissemination from the respiratory tract. Tuberculous salpingitis results in fibrinous adhesions and scarring of the fallopian tube. These complications lead to multiple functional abnormalities (e.g., infertility, ectopic gestation, pelvic pain). The tubes may become nodular. **Pyosalpinx** (fallopian tube distended with pus) and **hydrosalpinx** (fluid-filled tube) are late sequelae, and the adjacent ovary may become infected.

TUBERCULOUS ENDOMETRITIS: Endometritis complicates half the cases of tuberculous salpingitis. Noncaseating, poorly formed granulomas with rare giant cells are typical. Although other afflicted areas may show well-formed granulomas with caseous necrosis and characteristic Langhans giant cells may be seen, menstrual shedding limits the time during which such mature granulomas may develop.

Candidiasis

Ten percent of women are asymptomatic carriers of fungi in the vulva and vagina, *Candida albicans* being the most common offender. However, only 2% of women present with clinically apparent candidal vulvovaginitis. However, diabetes mellitus, oral contraceptive use and pregnancy make women much more susceptible to vaginal candidiasis. Infection manifests as vulvar itching and a white discharge. Clinical examination reveals firmly adherent, small white plaques on mucous membranes ("thrush"). Biopsy shows submucosal edema and chronic inflammation. The fungi do not penetrate epithelium, and the white patches correspond to foci of desquamated, necrotic epithelial cells; cellular debris; bacterial flora; candidal spores; and pseudohyphae. Untreated infections wax and wane, and often disappear following delivery. Characteristic spores and pseudohyphae in a wet mount preparation or with a Pap stain are diagnostic.

Actinomycosis

Genital tract actinomycosis is uncommon but is increasingly reported in association with use of intrauterine devices (IUDs). *Actinomyces israelii,* the causative organism, is a gram-positive rod found in 4% of normal genital tracts. It enters the uterine cavity via the tail of the IUD; ascends to the fallopian tube, ovary and broad ligaments; and forms a tuboovarian abscess. Suppurating lesions display drainage tracts that contain dense microcolonies of organisms ("sulfur granules"). Actinomycosis results in extensive fibrosis and scarring of the female genital tract.

Toxic Shock Syndrome Is Associated With Vaginal Staphylococcal Infection

Toxic shock syndrome is an acute, sometimes fatal disorder characterized by fever, shock and a desquamative erythematous rash. In addition, vomiting, diarrhea, myalgias, neurologic signs and thrombocytopenia are common. Certain strains of *Staphylococcus aureus* release an exotoxin called **toxic shock syndrome toxin-1,** which alters the function of mononuclear phagocytes to impair clearance of other potentially toxic substances, such as endotoxin. Pathologic alterations are characteristic of shock, and lesions of disseminated intravascular coagulation are usually prominent. Toxic shock syndrome was first recognized when long-acting tampons were introduced, allowing sufficient time for the staphylococci to proliferate. Contraceptive "sponges" were also associated. The incidence of toxic shock syndrome has decreased markedly since recognition of the role of tampons in promoting colonization of the vagina by *S. aureus*.

VULVA

Anatomy

The vulva is composed of the mons pubis, labia majora and minora, clitoris and vestibule. At puberty, the mons pubis and lateral borders of the labia majora acquire increased subcutaneous fat and grow coarse hair. Sebaceous and apocrine glands in these regions develop concomitantly. The paired external openings of the paraurethral glands **(Skene glands)** flank the urethral meatus. **Bartholin glands**, immediately posterolateral to the introitus, are branching, mucus-secreting, tubuloalveolar glands drained by a short duct lined by transitional epithelium. In addition, microscopic mucous glands are scattered throughout the area bounded by the labia minora. The inguinal and femoral lymph nodes provide primary lymph drainage routes, except for the clitoris (the homolog of the penis), which shares the lymphatic drainage of the urethra.

Developmental Anomalies and Cysts

ECTOPIC BREAST TISSUE: Small, isolated nodules of ectopic breast tissue may extend in the "milk line" to the vulva and enlarge during pregnancy.

BARTHOLIN GLAND CYST: The paired Bartholin glands produce a clear mucoid secretion that continuously lubricates the vestibular surface. The ducts are prone to obstruction and consequent cyst formation (Fig. 18-3). Cyst infection may lead to **abscess formation.** Bartholin gland abscess was formerly associated with gonorrhea, but staphylococci, chlamydia and anaerobes are now more frequently the cause. Treatment consists of incision, drainage, marsupialization and appropriate antibiotics.

FOLLICULAR CYSTS: Follicular cysts recapitulate the most distal portion of the hair follicle. Also termed **epithelial inclusion cysts** or **keratinous cysts,** follicular cysts frequently appear on the vulva, especially the labia majora. They contain a white cheesy material and typically are lined by stratified squamous epithelium.

MUCINOUS CYSTS: Mucinous glands of the vulva, a normal but generally unrecognized finding, occasionally

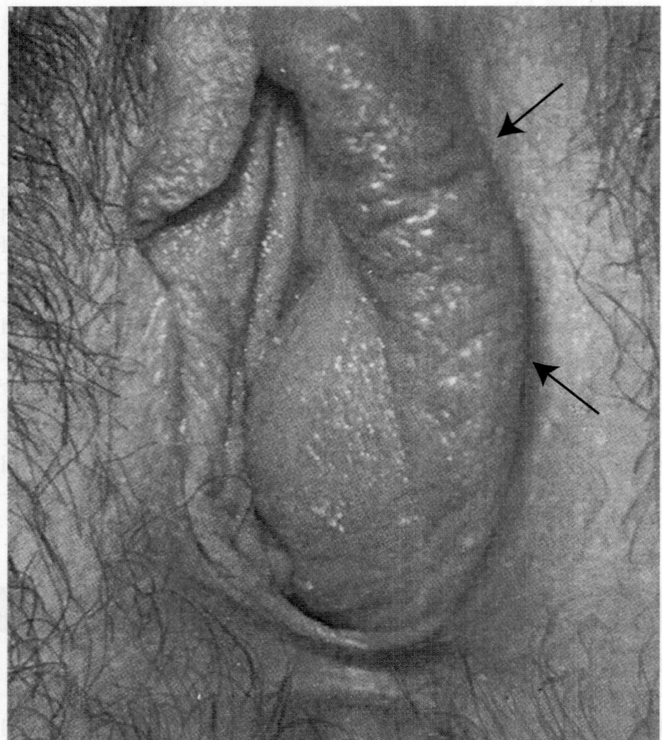

FIGURE 18-3. Bartholin gland cyst. The 4-cm lesion (*arrows*) is posterior to the vaginal introitus.

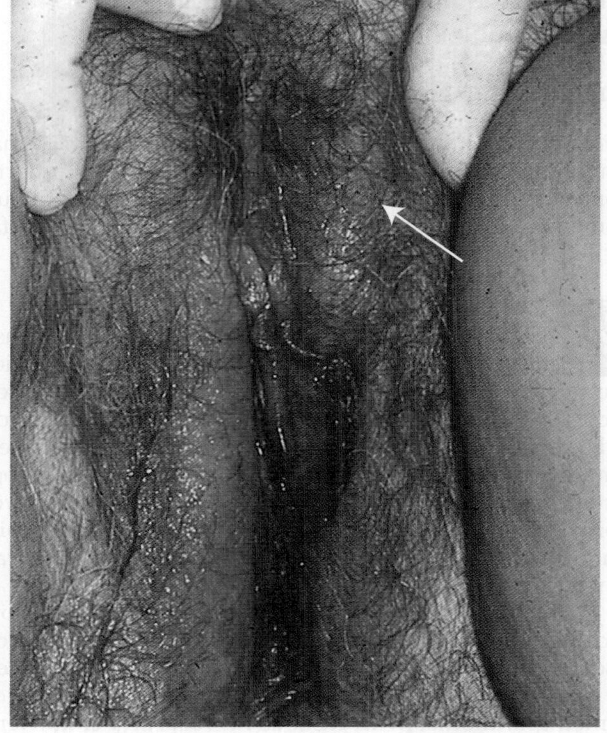

FIGURE 18-4. Vulvar acute dermatitis (eczema). Erythema, edema and weeping vesicles (*arrow*) are present.

become obstructed and subsequently cystic. Mucinous columnar cells line the cyst and may become infected.

Dermatoses

Acute Dermatitis of the Vulva Appears as Reddened Vesiculated Skin

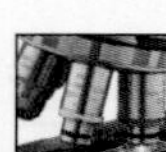

PATHOLOGY: As vesicles rupture (Fig. 18-4) onto the surface, the fluid forms a crust on the skin surface. The epidermis shows a range of inflammatory cells, and spongiotic areas form spongiotic vesicles that rupture to produce the exudative lesions. The dermis shows a perivascular lymphocytic infiltrate and edema, with separation of collagen fibers. Telangiectatic lymphatics and dilated capillaries are typical.

The most common endogenous types of acute dermatitis are **atopic (hypersensitivity) dermatitis** and **seborrheic dermatitis,** seen as a scaly macular eruption. Dermatitides with exogenous causes include irritant dermatitis (urine on the vulvar skin) and contact allergic dermatitis (type 4 delayed hypersensitivity reaction) and manifest as acute or chronic dermatitis.

Chronic Dermatitis, or Lichen Simplex Chronicus, Is the End Stage of Many Vulvar Inflammatory Diseases

Vulvar chronic dermatitis (Fig. 18-5) follows many diseases that are clinically pruritic and thus subject to repeated scratching in

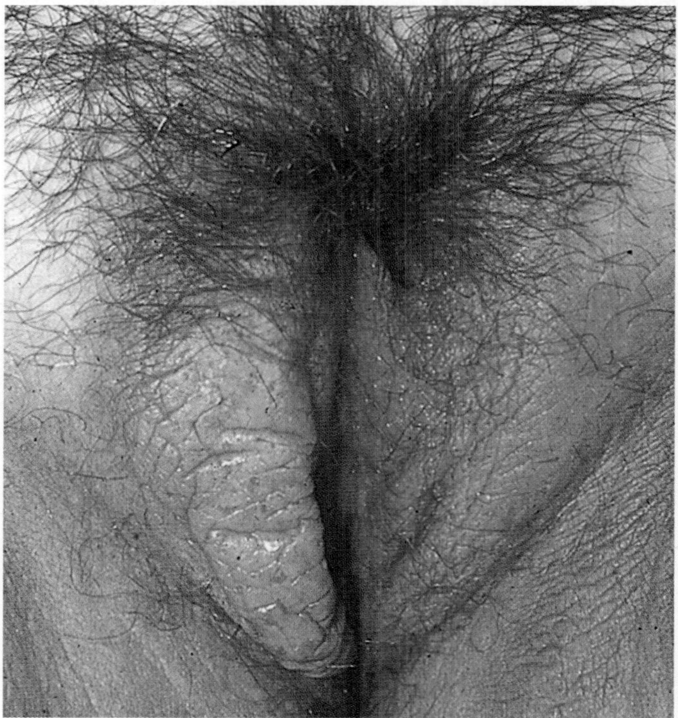

FIGURE 18-5. Lichen simplex chronicus of the right labium majus. There is thickening and accentuation of skin markings, with surface excoriation due to recent scratching.

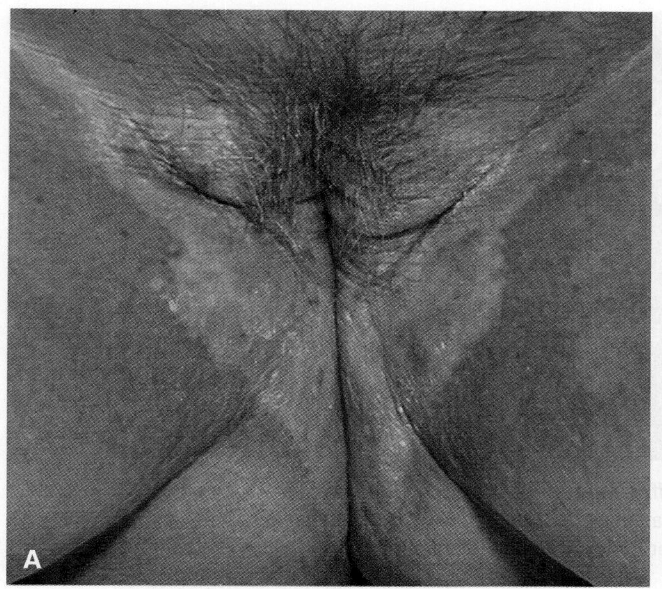

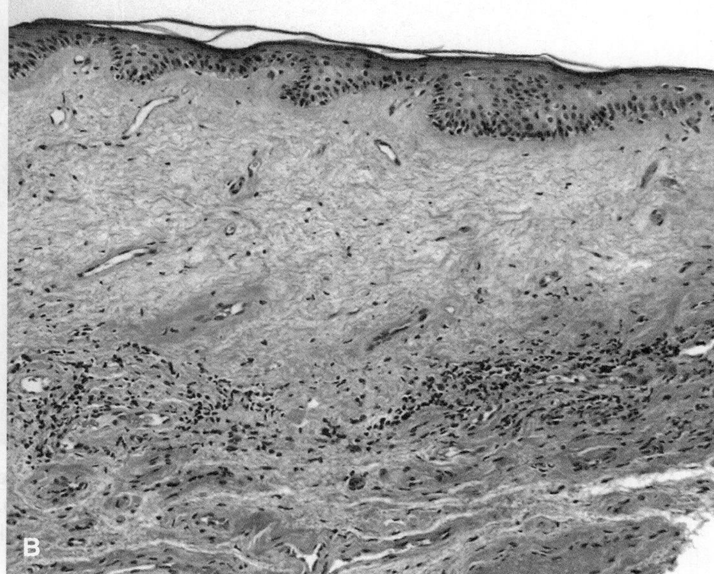

FIGURE 18-6. Lichen sclerosus of vulva. A. The sharply demarcated white lesion affects the vulva and perineum. **B.** The epidermis is thin and exhibits hyperkeratosis and a lack of the normal rete pattern. The dermis displays an acellular, homogeneous zone overlying a mild chronic inflammatory infiltrate.

their active phase. It may also occur in other disorders such as lichen planus, psoriasis and lichen sclerosus (see Chapter 24). The skin is thickened with exaggerated skin markings ("lichenification") and white, as a result of marked hyperkeratosis. Scaling is generally present, and excoriations due to recent scratching can often be seen.

LICHEN SCLEROSUS: Lichen sclerosus is an inflammatory disease associated with autoimmune disorders such as vitiligo, pernicious anemia and thyroiditis. Autoimmune etiology of lichen sclerosus is further suggested by the presence of activated T cells in the dermis.

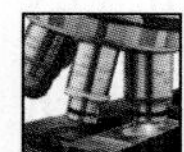
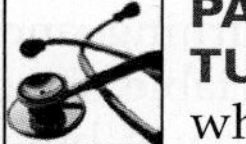

PATHOLOGY AND CLINICAL FEATURES: The condition is represented by white plaques, atrophic skin, a parchment-like or crinkled appearance and, occasionally, marked contracture of vulvar tissues (Fig. 18-6A). Hyperkeratosis, loss of rete ridges, epithelial thinning with flattening of rete pegs, cytoplasmic vacuolation of the basal layer and a homogeneous, acellular zone in the upper dermis are seen (Fig. 18-6B). A band of chronic inflammatory cells, lymphocytes with few plasma cells, typically lies beneath this layer. The most common symptoms are itching and dyspareunia. The disease develops insidiously and is progressive. Women with symptomatic lichen sclerosus have a 15% chance of developing squamous cell carcinoma.

Benign Tumors

HIDRADENOMA: This benign apocrine sweat gland tumor appears chiefly in the labia majora as a well-circumscribed nodule, rarely larger than 1 cm. Microscopically, it is composed of papillary tubules and acini lined by two layers of cells: an inner layer of apocrine columnar cells and an outer one of myoepithelial cells.

SYRINGOMA: An adenoma of eccrine glands, syringoma manifests as a flesh-colored papule within the dermis of labia majora. This asymptomatic tumor is composed of a proliferation of small ducts embedded in a dense fibrous and sclerotic stroma (see Chapter 24). The walls of the ducts have two layers of cells: an inner layer of serous cells and an outer one of myoepithelial cells. The lumen contains eosinophilic material or amorphous debris.

CONNECTIVE TISSUE TUMORS: **Senile hemangiomas** (cherry hemangiomas) are small, purple skin papules, which may bleed on surface trauma. **Lobular capillary hemangioma** (formerly termed pyogenic granuloma), previously thought to be a reaction to superficial wound infection, is a variant of hemangioma. Secondary infection occurs, as the surface of the lesion is fragile and easily traumatized. Soft tissue tumors found elsewhere in the body also occur in the vulva, including granular cell tumor, leiomyoma, fibroma, lipoma and histiocytoma.

PIGMENTED VULVAR LESIONS: **Lentigo** occurs in about 10% of women, and presents as small macules. **Nevi** and **seborrheic keratosis** also occur in this area (Chapter 24).

Malignant Tumors and Premalignant Conditions

Vulvar Intraepithelial Neoplasia Is a Precursor of Invasive Squamous Cell Carcinoma

Carcinoma of the vulva accounts for 3% of all female genital cancers and occurs mainly in women over 60 years. Squamous cell carcinoma is the most common type (86%). These tumors are divided into two groups: keratinizing squamous cell carcinomas unrelated to HPV (>70% of cases), and warty and basaloid carcinomas associated with high-risk HPV (<25% of cases).

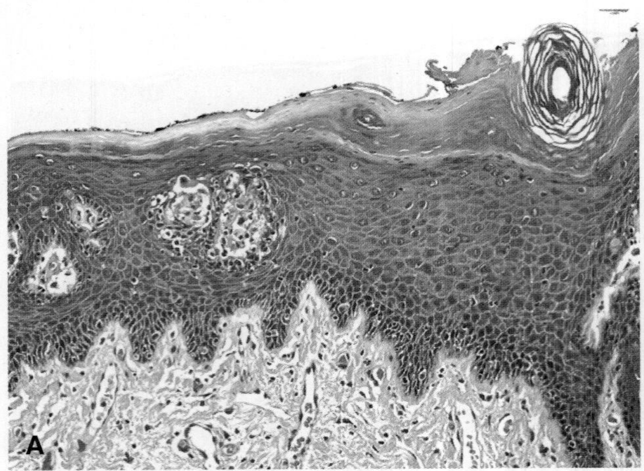

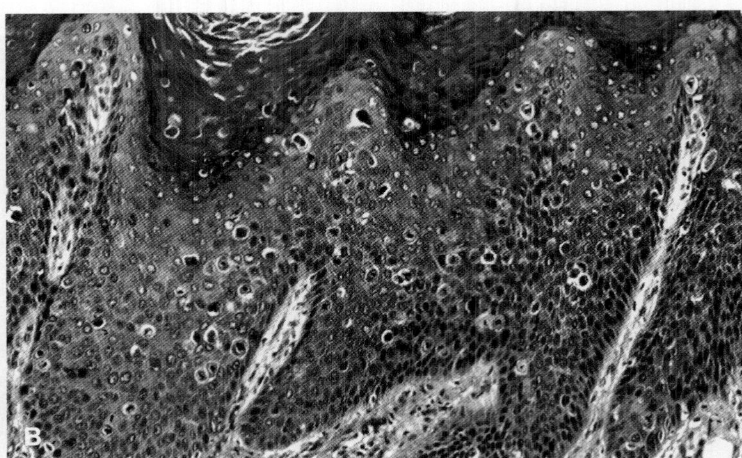

FIGURE 18-7. Vulvar intraepithelial neoplasia (VIN). A. Well-differentiated (*simplex*) type. The atypia is accentuated in the basal and parabasal layers. There is striking epithelial maturation in the superficial layers. **B. Human papilloma virus (HPV)-related undifferentiated (*classic*) VIN.** Beneath a hyperkeratotic surface the epithelial cells are dysplastic. There are numerous mitoses.

ETIOLOGIC FACTORS AND CLINICAL FEATURES: Keratinizing squamous carcinomas frequently develop in older women (mean age, 76 years), sometimes in the context of longstanding lichen sclerosus. The precursor lesion is referred to as **differentiated vulvar intraepithelial neoplasia (VIN)** or **VIN simplex** (Fig. 18-7A), which carries a high risk of cancer development. Carcinomas develop as nodules or masses in a background of "**leukoplakia**" (*white plaques*, a nonspecific, descriptive term). Cases of lichen sclerosus, differentiated VIN and invasive squamous cell carcinoma with identical p53 gene mutations have been reported. p53 gene mutation, however, is an uncommon and late event in vulvar carcinogenesis.

In contrast, the less common HPV-associated warty and basaloid carcinomas develop from a precursor lesion called **undifferentiated** or **classic VIN** (Fig. 18-7B). Since 1980 there has been a 5- to 10-fold increase in the frequency of classic VIN in women under age 40, typically related to **HPV 16.** HPV-associated VIN lesions have a low risk of progression to invasive carcinomas (approximately 6%), except in older or immunosuppressed women. Lesions associated with oncogenic HPV types generally demonstrate activated p16. Women with VIN may have squamous neoplasms similar to VIN elsewhere in the lower genital tract.

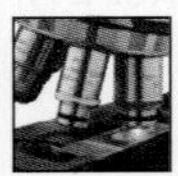

PATHOLOGY: VIN reflects a spectrum of neoplastic changes from minimal to severe cellular atypia. These lesions may be single or multiple, and macular, papular or plaquelike. Histologic grades are labeled VIN I, II and III, respectively, corresponding to mild, moderate and severe dysplasia. However, grade III (which includes squamous cell carcinoma in situ [CIS]) is by far the most common. Differentiated VIN shows severe nuclear atypia of the basal layer with striking epithelial maturation in the superficial layers (Fig. 18-7A). Keratinocytes of the latter contain rounded nuclei with enlarged nucleoli and ample eosinophilic cytoplasm with prominent intercellular bridges. Rete pegs often contain keratin pearls.

Like comparable lesions in the cervix (see below), criteria used in establishing the grade of classic VIN include (1) nuclear size and atypia, (2) number and degree of atypical mitoses and (3) loss of cytoplasmic differentiation toward the epithelial surface. In the undifferentiated form seen in younger women, the entire epithelium consists of cells with highly atypical nuclei and negligible cytoplasm. Mitoses, often atypical, are common (Fig. 18-7B). **Bowen disease,** a term still used in the dermatologic literature, is a synonym for VIN III.

Keratinizing squamous cell carcinomas usually follow differentiated VIN (VIN simplex). Two thirds of larger tumors are exophytic (Fig. 18-8A); the remainder are ulcerative and endophytic. Microscopically, the tumor is composed of invasive nests of malignant squamous epithelium with central keratin pearls (Fig. 18-8B). The tumors grow slowly, extending to contiguous skin, vagina and rectum. They metastasize initially to superficial inguinal lymph nodes, and then to deep inguinal, femoral and pelvic lymph nodes.

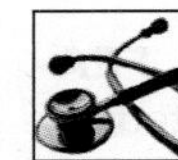

CLINICAL FEATURES: Most patients with VIN present with vulvar itching, burning and raised, well-defined skin lesions of variable sizes, which may be pink, red, brown or white. Carcinomas, but not VIN, may develop ulceration, bleeding and secondary infection. Spontaneous regression of VIN has been reported, frequently in younger women.

The 2009 International Federation of Gynecology and Obstetrics (FIGO) staging of vulvar cancer defines tumors of any size limited to the vulva as stage I carcinomas, tumors extending to perineal structures (lower third) as stage II, tumors with positive inguinofemoral lymph nodes as stage III and tumors invading perineal structures (upper third) or distant metastasis as stage IV (Table 18-2). Tumor grade and number, size and location of lymph node metastases determine survival. Better-differentiated tumors have a better mean survival, approaching 90% if nodes are negative. Two thirds of women with inguinal node metastases survive 5 years, but only one fourth of those with pelvic node metastases live that long.

Prognosis correlates with stage of disease and lymph node status. The number of inguinal lymph nodes with metastases is the most important single factor. The prognosis of patients with vulvar cancer is generally good, with an overall 5-year survival of 70%.

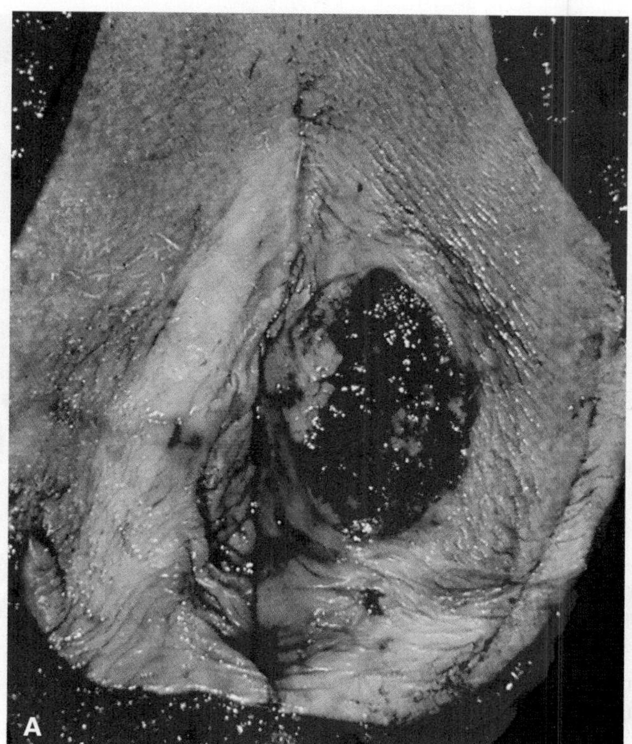

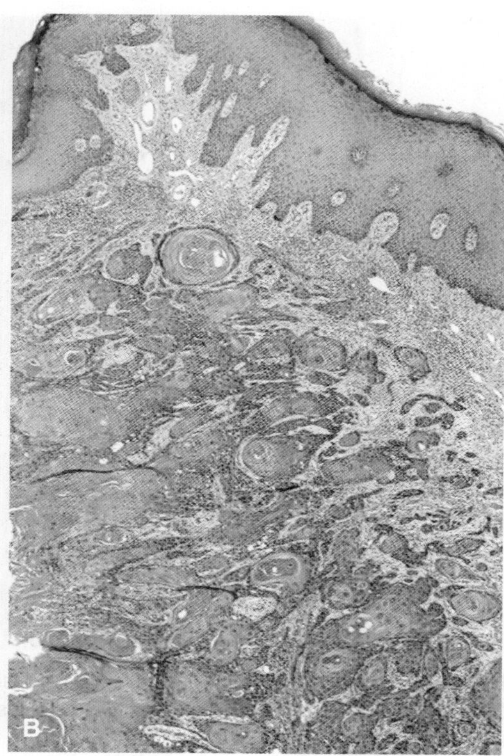

FIGURE 18-8. Squamous cell carcinoma of vulva. A. The tumor is situated in an extensive area of lichen sclerosus (*white*). **B.** Nests of neoplastic squamous cells, some with keratin pearls, are evident in this well-differentiated tumor.

Table 18-2

FIGO Staging of Carcinoma of the Vulva

Stage I	Tumor confined to the vulva
IA	Tumor ≤2 cm with stromal invasion ≤1.0 mm*
IB	Tumor >2 cm or with stromal invasion >1.0 mm*
Stage II	Tumor of any size with extension to adjacent perineal structures (one-third lower urethra, one-third lower vagina, anus)
Stage III	Tumor of any size with positive inguinofemoral nodes
IIIA	(i) With 1 lymph node metastasis (≥5 mm) or (ii) with 1–2 lymph node metastases (<5 mm)
IIIB	(i) With 2 or more lymph node metastases (≥5 mm) or (ii) with 3 or more lymph node metastases (<5 mm)
IIIC	With positive nodes with extracapsular spread
Stage IV	Tumor invades regional or distant structures
IVA	(i) Upper urethral and/or upper vaginal mucosa, bladder mucosa, rectal mucosa or pelvic bone, or
	(ii) Fixed or ulcerated inguinofemoral lymph nodes
IVB	Distant metastasis including pelvic lymph nodes

FIGO = International Federation of Gynecology and Obstetrics.
*The depth of invasion is defined as the measurement of the tumor from the epithelial–stromal junction of the adjacent most superficial dermal papilla to the deepest point of invasion.

Verrucous Carcinoma Is Well Differentiated

Vulvar verrucous carcinoma is a distinct variety of squamous cell carcinoma that manifests as a large fungating mass resembling a giant condyloma acuminatum. HPV, usually type 6 or 11, is commonly identified. The tumor is very well differentiated, with large nests of squamous cells with abundant cytoplasm and small, bland nuclei. Squamous pearls are common and mitoses are rare. The tumor invades with broad tongues, and the stromal interface frequently exhibits a heavy infiltrate of lymphocytes and plasma cells. Verrucous carcinomas rarely metastasize. Wide local surgical excision is the treatment of choice, but other forms of therapy (cryosurgery and retinoids) have been used successfully.

Basal Cell Carcinoma

Basal cell carcinomas of the vulva are identical to their counterparts in the skin. They are not associated with HPV, rarely metastasize and are usually cured by surgical excision.

Malignant Melanoma

Although uncommon, malignant melanoma is the second most frequent cancer of the vulva (5%). It occurs in the sixth and seventh decades but occasionally is found in younger women. The tumor has biological and microscopic characteristics of melanoma occurring elsewhere in the body. It is highly aggressive, and the prognosis is poor.

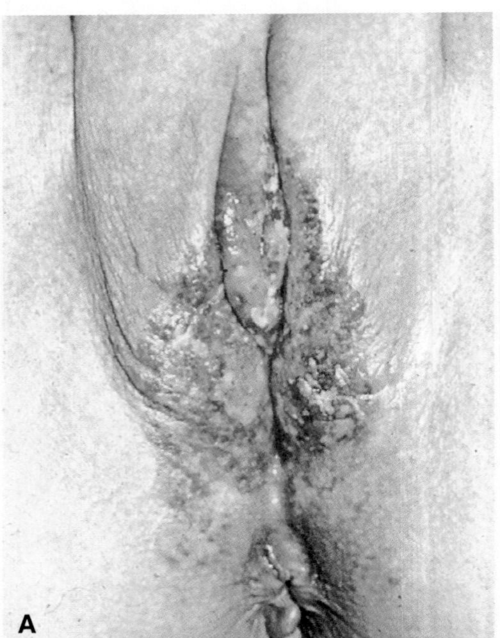

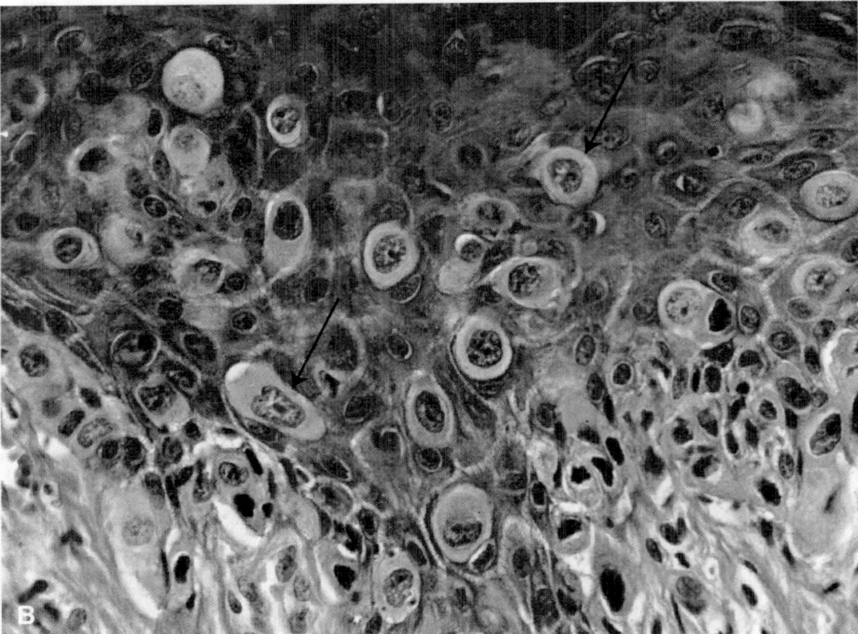

FIGURE 18-9. Paget disease of the vulva. A. The lesion is red, moist and sharply demarcated. **B.** Individual Paget cells (*arrows*), characterized by an abundant pale cytoplasm, infiltrate the epithelium and are interspersed among normal keratinocytes.

Extramammary Paget Disease Resembles Similar Tumors of the Breast and Elsewhere

The disorder usually occurs on the labia majora in older women. Women with Paget disease of the vulva complain of pruritus or a burning sensation for many years.

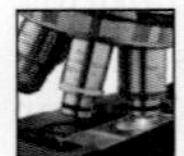

PATHOLOGY: The lesion of Paget disease is large, red, moist and sharply demarcated. The origin of the diagnostic cells (Paget cells) is controversial: they may arise in the epidermis or epidermally derived adnexal structures. Paget cells have pale, vacuolated cytoplasm (Fig. 18-9) with abundant glycosaminoglycans; they stain with periodic acid–Schiff (PAS) and mucicarmine and expresses carcinoembryonic antigen (CEA). They appear as large single cells or, less often, as clusters of cells that lack intercellular bridges and are usually confined to the epidermis.

Intraepidermal Paget disease may have been present for many years and is often far more extensive throughout the epidermis than preoperative biopsies indicate. Unlike Paget disease of the breast, which is almost always associated with underlying duct carcinoma, extramammary Paget disease is only rarely associated with carcinoma of the skin adnexa. Metastases rarely occur, so treatment requires only wide local excision or simple vulvectomy.

VAGINA

Anatomy

The vagina extends from the uterus to the vestibule of the vulva and is lined by hormone-responsive squamous epithelium. Estrogens stimulate—and progestogens inhibit—proliferation and maturation of vaginal epithelial cells. Thus, during the secretory phase of the menstrual cycle or during pregnancy—when progesterone levels are high—intermediate cells, rather than superficial ones, predominate in vaginal smears. Maturing epithelial cells accumulate glycogen, giving their cytoplasm a clear appearance.

Lymph drains through the lateral perivaginal plexus. Lymphatics from the vaginal vault and upper vagina communicate with branches from the cervix to drain into pelvic and then para-aortic nodes. The lower vagina also drains to inguinal and femoral nodes.

Nonneoplastic Conditions and Benign Tumors

Congenital Anomalies of the Vagina Are Rare

Congenital absence of the vagina is generally associated with anomalies of the uterus and urinary tract. If there is a functional uterus, absence of a vagina may lead to accumulation of menstrual blood in the uterus.

Septate vagina results from failure of embryonic müllerian ducts to fuse properly, and the resulting median wall does not resorb.

Vaginal atresia and imperforate hymen prevent transformation of the vaginal embryonic lining from a müllerian to a squamous epithelium, an effect that is a cause of vaginal adenosis.

Atrophic Vaginitis Results From Diminished Estrogenic Stimulation

Atrophic vaginitis is thinning and atrophy of the vaginal epithelium. The thinned epithelium is a poor barrier to infections or

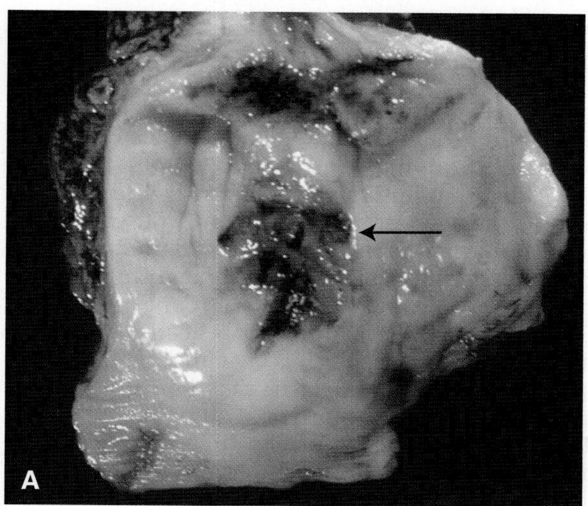

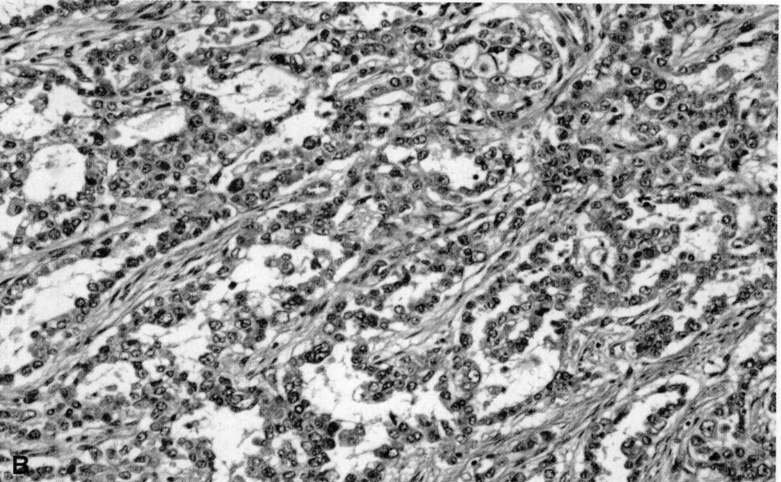

FIGURE 18-10. Clear cell adenocarcinoma of the vagina (in utero exposure to diethylstilbestrol [DES]). A. The tumor has arisen on the upper third of the anterior wall (*arrow*), corresponding to the most frequent site of adenosis. **B.** Microscopically, tubular glands are lined by hobnail cells.

abrasions. This occurs most commonly in postmenopausal women with low estrogen levels. Dyspareunia and vaginal spotting are common symptoms.

Vaginal Adenosis Occurs in Females Exposed to Diethylstilbestrol in Utero

In vaginal adenosis, the glandular epithelium that normally lines the embryonic vagina fails to be replaced during fetal life by squamous epithelium. Use of diethylstilbestrol (DES) to prevent miscarriages in women who were prone to repetitive abortions led, in the 1970s, to a substantial increase in this disorder in daughters of those women. Between the 10th and 18th weeks of gestation, the upgrowth of a squamous epithelium derived from the urogenital sinus replaces the glandular (müllerian) linings of the vagina and exocervix. DES exposure during this critical time arrests the transformation process and some glandular tissue (i.e., adenosis) remains.

Adenosis manifests as red, granular patches on the vaginal mucosa, which microscopically are composed of mucinous columnar cells (resembling those lining the endocervix) and ciliated cells (like those lining the endometrium and fallopian tubes). Clear cell adenocarcinomas typically arise in the upper one third of the vagina (Fig. 18-10). Many of these lesions have disappeared as the young women have grown older. Rare cases of **clear cell adenocarcinoma** of the vagina have also occurred in the daughters of women treated with DES. Clear cell adenocarcinomas are almost invariably curable when they are small and asymptomatic, but in more advanced stages, they may spread by hematogenous or lymphatic routes.

Fibroepithelial Polyp

Vaginal polyps are uncommon benign growths with a connective tissue core and an outer lining of vaginal squamous epithelium. They are usually single, gray-white, and smaller than 1 cm in diameter. Simple excision is usually curative.

Benign Mesenchymal Tumors

Most benign vaginal tumors resemble those elsewhere in the female genital tract (e.g., leiomyomas, rhabdomyomas and neurofibromas). These are solid submucosal tumors usually less than 2 cm in diameter.

Malignant Tumors of the Vagina

Primary malignant tumors of the vagina are uncommon, constituting about 2% of all genital tract tumors. **Most (80%) vaginal malignancies represent metastatic spread.** The most common symptoms are vaginal discharge and bleeding during coitus, but advanced tumors may cause pelvic or abdominal pain and edema of the legs. Tumors confined to the vagina are usually treated by radical hysterectomy and vaginectomy.

Squamous Cell Carcinoma Accounts for Over 90% of Primary Vaginal Malignancies

It is generally a disease of older women, with peak incidence between the ages of 60 and 70. It is most common in the anterior wall of the upper third of the vagina, where it usually manifests as an exophytic mass. **Vaginal intraepithelial neoplasia** (VAIN), a term replacing both "vaginal dysplasia" and "carcinoma in situ," frequently precedes invasive carcinoma. Vaginal squamous cell carcinoma may develop some years after cervical or vulvar carcinoma, suggesting that there may be a carcinogenic field effect in the lower genital tract, related to HPV infection.

Since most preinvasive and early invasive cancers are clinically silent, routine use of vaginal cytology is the most effective method to detect squamous carcinoma of the vagina. Prognosis is related to the extent of spread of the tumor at the time of its discovery (Table 18-3). The 5-year survival rate for tumors confined to the vagina (stage I) is 80%, whereas it is only 20% for those with extensive spread (stages III/IV).

Table 18-3

Clinical Staging of Carcinoma of Vagina

Stage	Description
0	Carcinoma in situ
I	Limited to vaginal wall
II	Involves subvaginal tissue, but does not extend to pelvic wall
III	Extends to pelvic wall
IV	Extends beyond true pelvis or involves mucosa of bladder or rectum
IVa	Spread to adjacent organs
IVb	Spread to distant organs

Embryonal Rhabdomyosarcoma Is a Rare Childhood Vaginal Tumor

This tumor often appears as confluent polypoid masses resembling a bunch of grapes, and hence may be called sarcoma botryoides (from the Greek *botrys*, "grapes") (Fig. 18-11). It occurs almost exclusively in girls under 4 years old. It arises in the lamina propria of the vagina and consists of primitive spindle rhabdomyoblasts (Fig. 18-11C), some of which show cross-striations. Myofibrils of myosin and actin are often demonstrable. A dense zone of round rhabdomyoblasts (the cambium layer) is present beneath the vaginal epithelium (Fig. 18-11B). Deep to this layer the stroma is myxomatous and shows fewer neoplastic rhabdomyoblasts. The tumor is usually detected because of spotting on the child's diaper. Tumors under 3 cm in greatest dimension tend to be localized and may be cured by wide excision and chemotherapy. Larger tumors have often spread to adjacent structures, regional lymph nodes or distant sites. Even in advanced cases, half of patients survive with radical surgery and chemotherapy.

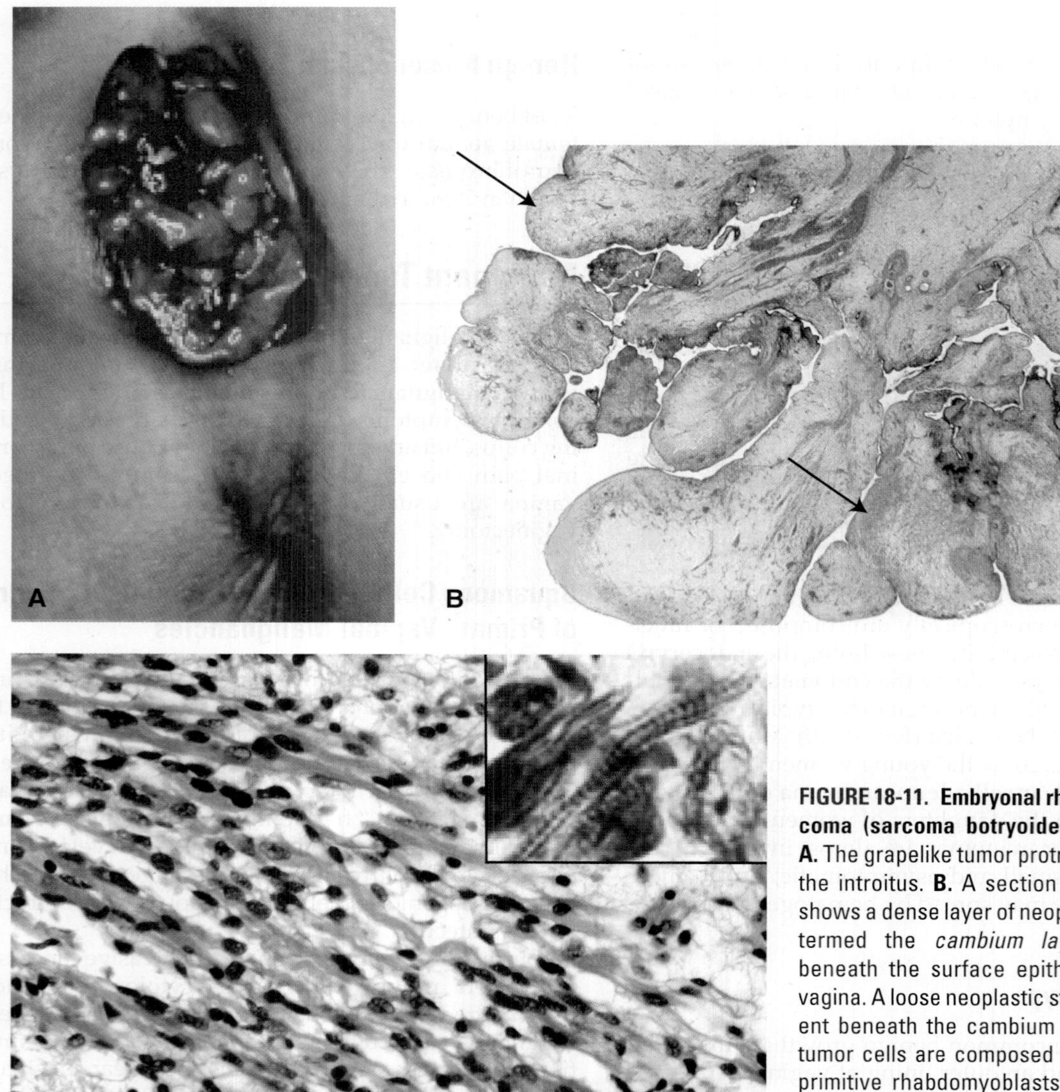

FIGURE 18-11. Embryonal rhabdomyosarcoma (sarcoma botryoides) of vagina. A. The grapelike tumor protrudes through the introitus. **B.** A section of the tumor shows a dense layer of neoplastic stroma termed the *cambium layer* (*arrows*) beneath the surface epithelium of the vagina. A loose neoplastic stroma is present beneath the cambium layer. **C.** The tumor cells are composed of elongated, primitive rhabdomyoblasts, with cross-striations. *Inset.* Electron micrograph.

CERVIX

Anatomy

The cervix (from the Latin *collare,* "neck") is the inferior portion of the uterus that connects the corpus to the vagina (Fig. 18-12). Its exposed portion (also termed the **exocervix, ectocervix** or **portio vaginalis**) protrudes into the upper vagina and is covered by glycogen-rich squamous epithelium. The **endocervix** is the canal that leads to the endometrial cavity. It is lined by longitudinal mucosal ridges made of fibrovascular cores lined by a single layer of mucinous columnar cells. Occasionally, the outlet of an endocervical gland becomes blocked and mucin is retained, which produces cystic dilations of these glands, termed **nabothian cysts.** The **external os** is the *macroscopic* junction between the exocervix and endocervix. The **squamocolumnar junction** is the *microscopic* junction of the squamous and mucinous columnar epithelia. The area between the endocervix and endometrial cavity is called the **isthmus** or **lower uterine segment.**

The exocervix remodels continuously throughout life. During embryonic development, the upward migration of squamous cells meets the columnar epithelium of the endocervix to form the initial squamocolumnar junction (Fig. 18-13). In some young women, this "original" squamocolumnar junction is located at the internal os. In most young women, however, the columnar epithelium extends onto the exocervix. In the latter case, the areas of the exocervix lined by columnar epithelium are termed **endocervical ectropion** and appear by colposcopic examination as reddish discolorations. With age, the columnar epithelium of the ectropion undergoes squamous metaplasia and a new squamocolumnar junction is found at the internal os.

The area between the most distal squamocolumnar junction and the external os is termed the **transformation zone.** The immature squamous epithelium of this zone displays progressive nuclear maturation and increasing amounts of glycogen-free cytoplasm toward the surface. Colposcopy reveals the development of a thin white membrane, which eventually becomes thicker and whiter as the squamous epithelium matures (Figs. 18-13 and 18-14). Subsequently, the cells accumulate glycogen and are indistinguishable from normal squamous epithelium lining the exocervix. The transformation zone is the site of cervical squamous carcinoma (see below).

Examination of the transformation zone by iodine staining is the basis of the **Schiller iodine test.** If squamous cells lining the exocervix are mature (glycogen rich), as is normal, they stain with iodine and the exocervix appears mahogany brown. If they are immature (glycogen poor), no iodine staining occurs and the exocervix is pale.

Cervicitis

Inflammation of the cervix is common and is related to constant exposure to bacterial flora in the vagina. Acute and chronic cervicitis are caused by many organisms, particularly endogenous vaginal aerobes and anaerobes, *Streptococcus, Staphylococcus* and *Enterococcus.* Other specific organisms include *Chlamydia trachomatis, Neisseria gonorrhoeae* and occasionally herpes simplex type 2. Some agents are sexually transmitted; others may be introduced by foreign bodies, such as residual fragments of tampons and pessaries.

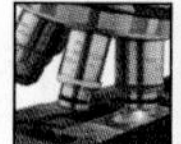

PATHOLOGY: In **acute cervicitis,** the cervix is grossly red, swollen and edematous, with copious pus "dripping" from the external os. Microscopically, the tissues exhibit an extensive infiltrate of polymorphonuclear leukocytes and stromal edema.

Chronic cervicitis is more common. The cervical mucosa is hyperemic (Fig. 18-15), and may show true epithelial

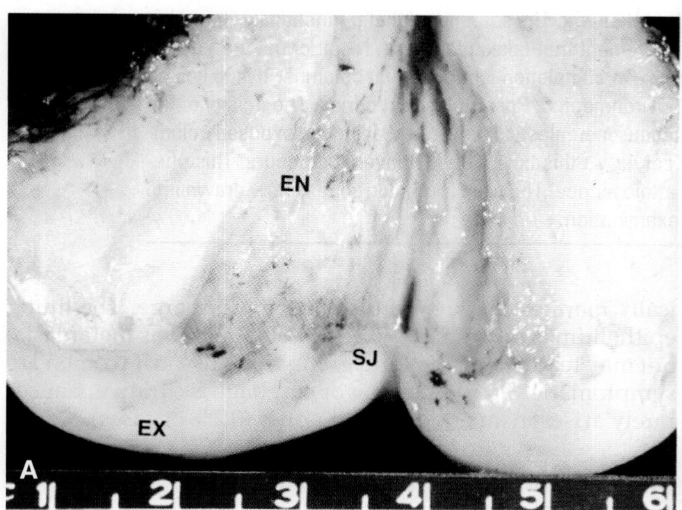

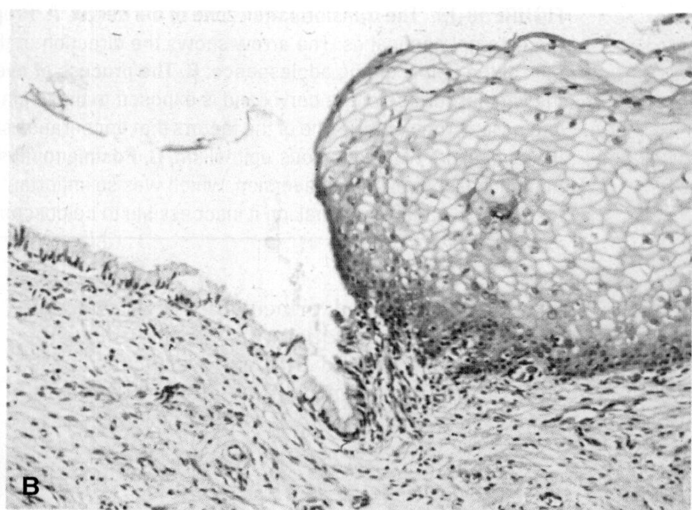

FIGURE 18-12. Anatomy of the cervix. A. The cervix has been opened to show the endocervix (EN), squamocolumnar junction (SJ) and exocervix (EX). The thick layer of squamous cells covering the exocervix accounts for its white color. **B.** A microscopic view of the squamocolumnar junction. The endocervix is lined by a single layer of columnar mucus-producing cells that abruptly meets the exocervix lined by mature squamous cells. *Note:* In specimens in which the squamocolumnar junction is on the ectocervix or in the endocervical canal, the region between it and the external os is called the *transformation zone* (see Fig. 18-13).

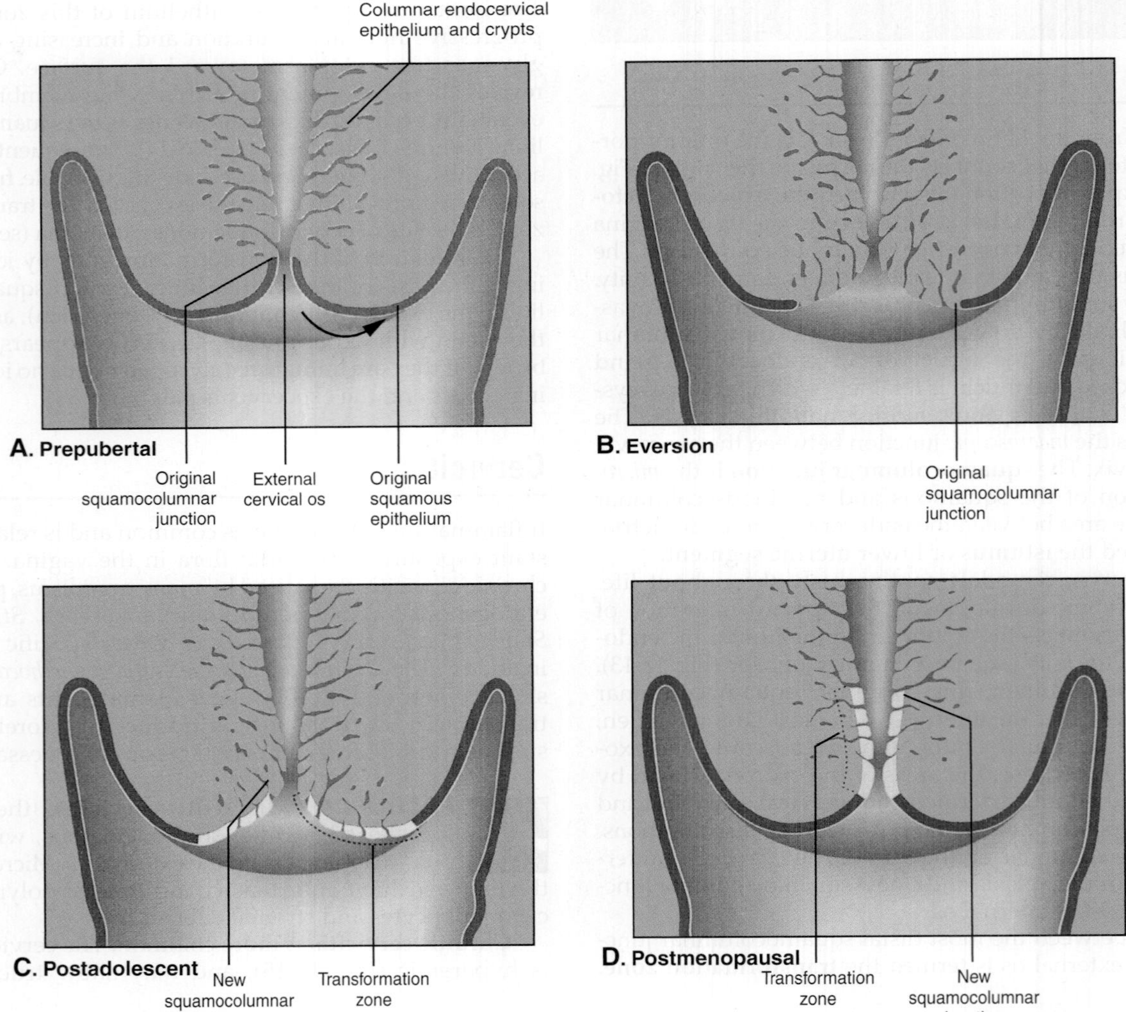

FIGURE 18-13. The transformation zone of the cervix. A. Prepubertal cervix. The squamocolumnar junction is situated at the external cervical os. The arrow shows the direction of the movement that takes place as a result of the increase in bulk of the cervix during adolescence. **B. The process of eversion.** On completion, endocervical columnar tissue lies on the vaginal surface of the cervix and is exposed to the vaginal environment. **C. Postadolescent cervix.** The acidity of the vaginal environmental is one of the factors that encourages squamous metaplastic change, replacing the exposed columnar epithelium with squamous epithelium. **D. Postmenopausal cervix.** At this time, cervical inversion occurs. This phenomenon is the reverse of eversion, which was so important in adolescence. The transformation zone is now drawn into the cervical canal, often making it inaccessible to colposcopic examination.

erosions. The stroma is infiltrated, principally by lymphocytes and plasma cells. Metaplastic squamous epithelium of the transformation zone may extend into endocervical glands, forming clusters of squamous epithelium, which must be differentiated from carcinoma.

Benign Tumors and Tumorlike Conditions of the Cervix

Endocervical Polyp Is Usually Benign

Endocervical polyps are the most common cervical growths (Fig. 18-16). They appear as single smooth or lobulated masses, usually under 3 cm in greatest dimension. They typically manifest as vaginal bleeding or discharge. The lining epithelium is mucinous, with variable squamous metaplasia, but may feature erosions and granulation tissue if women are symptomatic. Simple excision or curettage is curative. Cancer rarely arises in an endocervical polyp (0.2% of cases).

Microglandular Hyperplasia Reflects Progestational Stimulation

Cervical microglandular hyperplasia is a benign condition showing closely packed vacuolated glands lacking intervening stroma and mixed with a neutrophilic infiltrate. The glands vary in size and are lined by a flattened-to-cuboidal epithelium (Fig. 18-17). The nuclei are uniform, and mitoses are rare. Squamous metaplasia and reserve cell hyperplasia

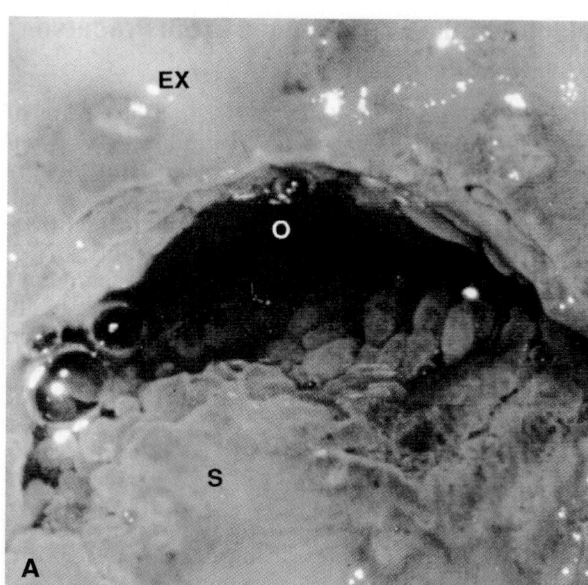

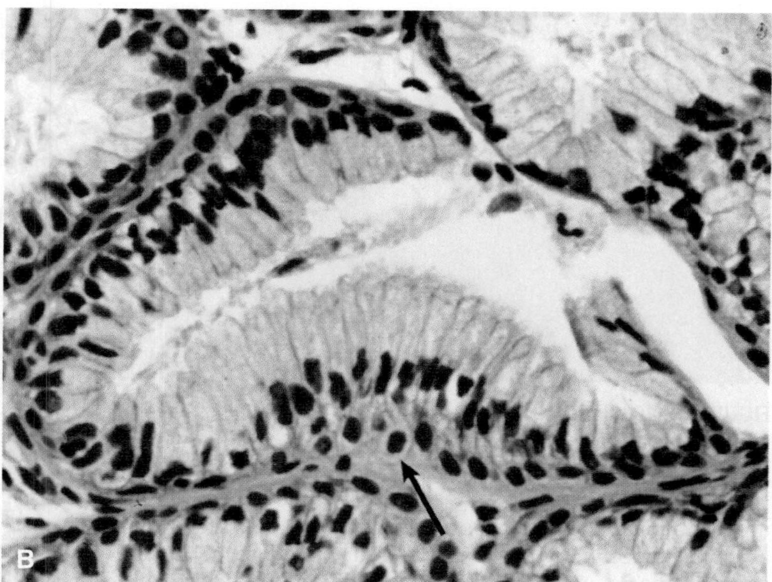

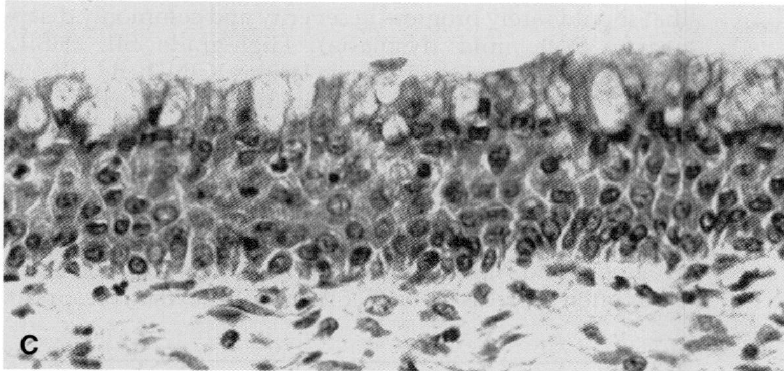

FIGURE 18-14. Squamous metaplasia in the transformation zone. A. In this colposcopic view of the cervix, a white area of metaplastic squamous epithelium (S) is situated between the exocervix (EX) and the mucinous endocervix (EN), which terminates at the internal os (O). **B.** In the early stages of squamous metaplasia of the transformation zone, the reserve cells, which normally constitute a single layer, begin to proliferate (*arrow*). **C.** At a later stage, the proliferating reserve cells displace the glandular epithelium. As a final step, the metaplastic cells mature into glycogen-rich squamous cells, resembling those in Figure 18-12B.

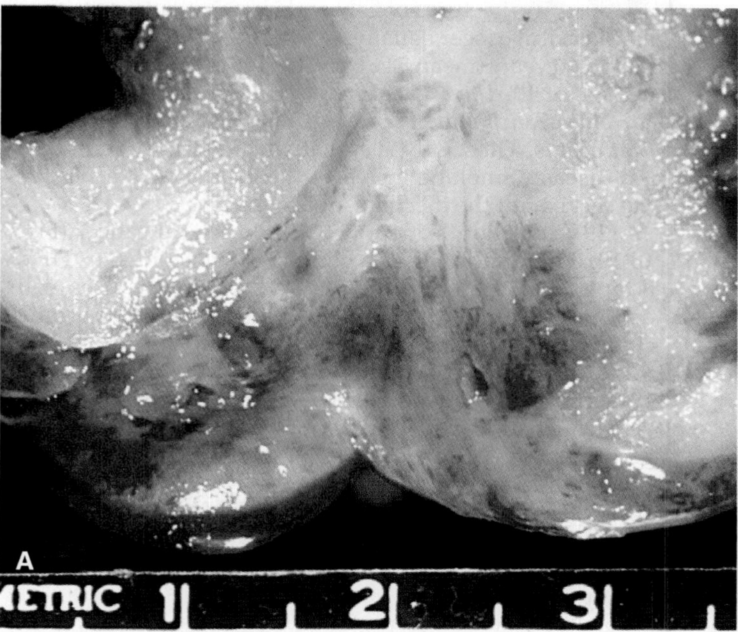

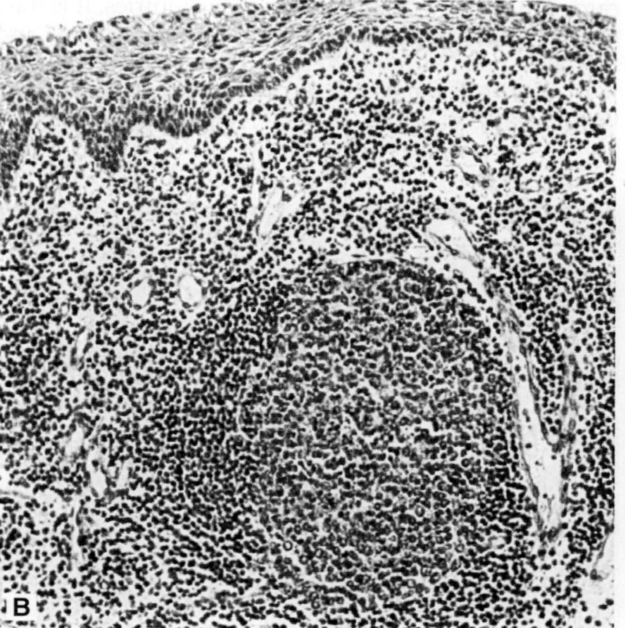

FIGURE 18-15. Chronic cervicitis. A. The cervix has been opened to reveal the reddened exocervix. **B.** Microscopic examination discloses chronic inflammation and the formation of a lymphoid follicle.

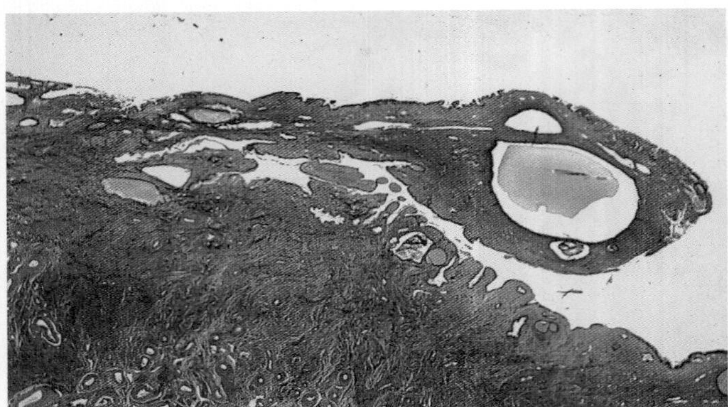

FIGURE 18-16. Endocervical polyp. An epithelial lining covers a fibrovascular core.

are common. It should not be confused with well-differentiated adenocarcinoma. Microglandular hyperplasia is usually asymptomatic and, as it is typically associated with progestin stimulation, it usually occurs during pregnancy, in the postpartum period and in women taking oral contraceptives.

Leiomyoma

Leiomyomas of the cervix can bleed or prolapse into the endocervical canal, leading to uterine contractions and pain resembling the early phases of labor. The appearance is similar to that of uterine leiomyomas (see below).

Squamous Cell Neoplasia

Fifty years ago, cervical cancer was the leading cause of cancer death in American women. The introduction and widespread use of cytologic screening decreased cervical carcinoma by 50% to 85% in Western countries. It is the sixth most common female cancer in the United States, and the mortality rate has fallen by 70%. However, worldwide, cervical cancer remains the second most common cancer in women.

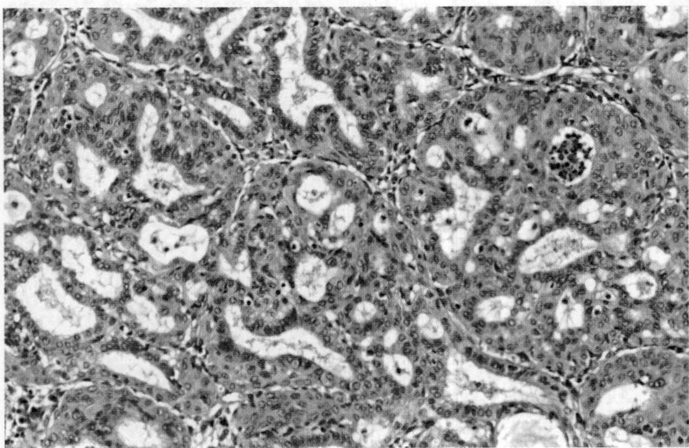

FIGURE 18-17. Microglandular hyperplasia. Small proliferated glands are admixed with a neutrophilic infiltrate.

Cervical Intraepithelial Neoplasia Is the Precursor of Invasive Cancer

Cervical intraepithelial neoplasia (CIN) is a spectrum of intraepithelial changes that begins with minimal atypia and progresses through stages of greater intraepithelial abnormalities to invasive squamous cell carcinoma (Fig. 18-18). The terms **CIN, dysplasia, CIS and squamous intraepithelial lesion (SIL)** are commonly used interchangeably.

Dysplasia in the cervical epithelium carries a risk for ***malignant transformation*** (Figs. 18-18 and 18-19). The concept of CIN emphasizes that dysplasia and carcinoma in situ are points on a disease spectrum, rather than separate entities. The grades of CIN are as follows:

- CIN-1: Mild dysplasia
- CIN-2: Moderate dysplasia
- CIN-3: Severe dysplasia and CIS

The Bethesda System for Reporting Cervical/Vaginal Cytologic Diagnoses groups these lesions slightly differently, calling them low- and high-grade squamous intraepithelial lesions (Fig. 18-18). Low-grade SIL (LSIL) reflects conditions that should rarely progress in severity and commonly disappear (CIN-1, mild dysplasia). High-grade SIL (HSIL) describes more severe histologic lesions (CIN-2 and CIN-3), which tend to progress and require treatment. Early phases of infection with all HPV types probably show episomal viral propagation throughout a polyclonal epithelial field, with an LSIL cytology. Oncogenic types of HPV are prone to monoclonal outgrowth of those cells, with genomic integration of virus, elaboration of transforming viral proteins (E6/E7) and progression to HSIL. Lesions associated with nononcogenic types often progress no further than LSIL and then disappear.

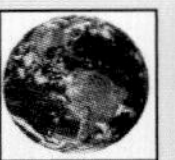 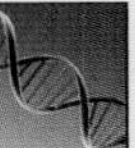

EPIDEMIOLOGY AND MOLECULAR PATHOGENESIS: Epidemiologic features of CIN and invasive cancer are similar. Cervical cancer usually manifests between the ages of 40 and 60 years (mean 54), but CIN generally occurs under the age of 40. ***The critical factor is HPV infection, which correlates with multiple sexual partners and early age at first coitus.*** Thus, CIN is essentially a **sexually transmitted disease.** Smoking increases the incidence of cancer of the cervix, but the mechanism is obscure.

HPV infection leads to CIN and cervical cancer (Fig. 18-19). Low-grade CIN is a permissive infection (i.e., HPV is episomal, freely replicates and thereby causes cell death). Huge numbers of virus must accumulate in the cytoplasm before being visible as a **koilocyte.**

In most cases of higher-grade CIN, viral DNA integrates into the cell genome. Proteins encoded by *E6* and *E7* genes of HPV 16 respectively bind and inactivate p53 and Rb proteins, thereby vitiating their tumor suppressor functions (see Chapter 5).

After HPV integrates into host DNA, copies of the whole virus do not accumulate and koilocytes are absent in many cases of high-grade dysplasia and all invasive cancers.

Some 85% of low-grade CIN lesions have low-risk HPV. Many genital warts (condylomata acuminata) on the cervix contain HPV 6 or 11, which are regarded as low-risk HPV types. By contrast, cells in high-grade CIN usually contain

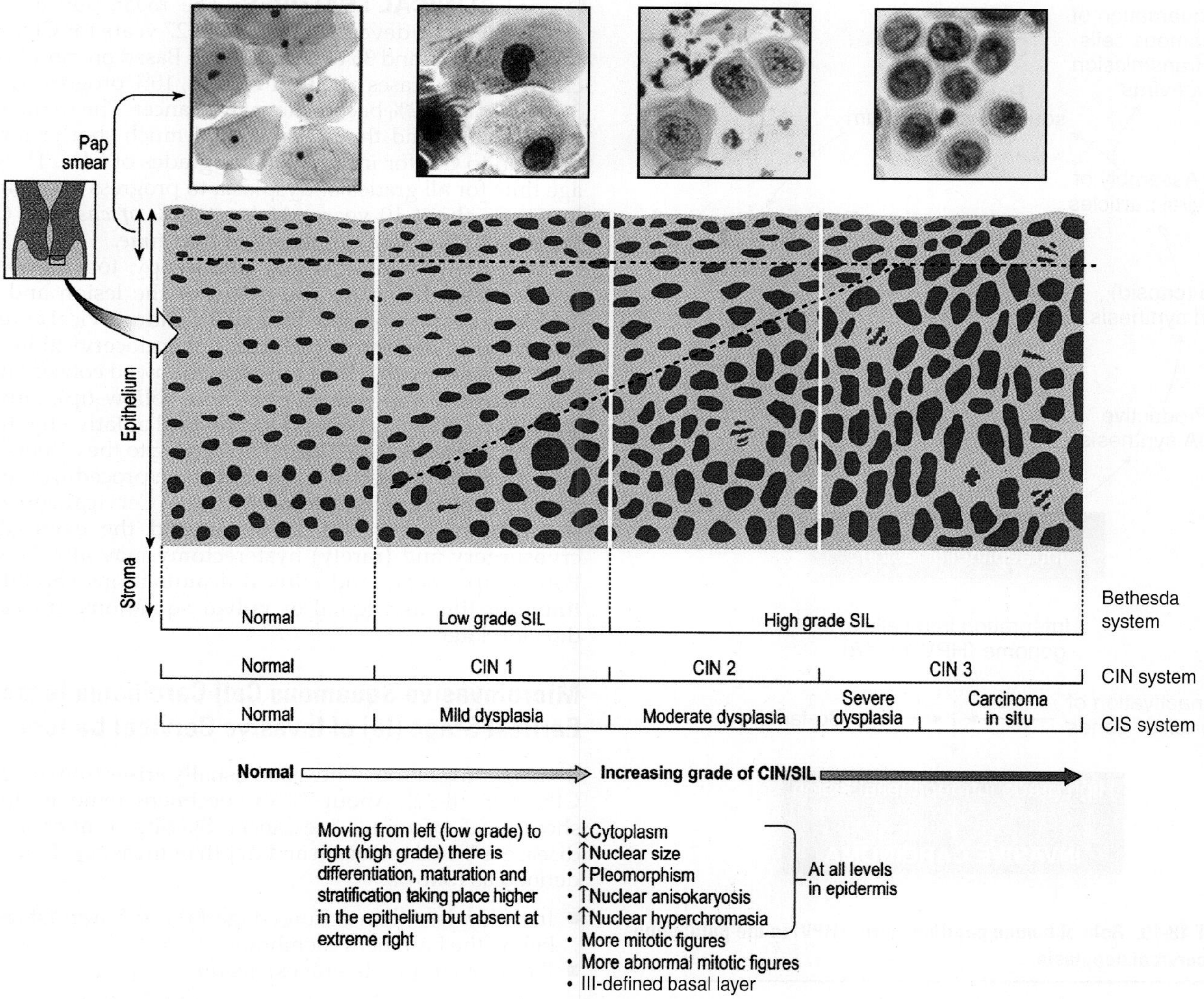

Pap smear

Epithelium

Stroma

Normal	Low grade SIL	High grade SIL			Bethesda system
Normal	CIN 1	CIN 2	CIN 3		CIN system
Normal	Mild dysplasia	Moderate dysplasia	Severe dysplasia	Carcinoma in situ	CIS system

Normal ⟹ Increasing grade of CIN/SIL ➡

Moving from left (low grade) to right (high grade) there is differentiation, maturation and stratification taking place higher in the epithelium but absent at extreme right

- ↓Cytoplasm
- ↑Nuclear size
- ↑Pleomorphism
- ↑Nuclear anisokaryosis
- ↑Nuclear hyperchromasia
- More mitotic figures
- More abnormal mitotic figures
- Ill-defined basal layer

At all levels in epidermis

FIGURE 18-18. Interrelations of naming systems in premalignant cervical disease. This chart integrates multiple aspects of the disease complex. It lists the qualitative and quantitative features that become increasingly abnormal as the premalignant disease advances in severity. It also illustrates the changes in progressively more abnormal disease states and provides translation nomenclature for the dysplasia/carcinoma in situ (CIS) system, cervical intraepithelial neoplasia (CIN) system and Bethesda system. Finally, the scheme illustrates the corresponding cytologic smear resulting from exfoliation of the most superficial cells, indicating that even in the mildest disease state, abnormal cells reach the surface and are shed. SIL = squamous intraepithelial lesion.

HPV types 16, 18, 31, 33, 35, 39, 45, 51, 52, 56, 58, 59 and 68. **HPV types 16 and 18** are found in 70% of invasive cancers; the other high-risk types account for another 25%.

Hormonally induced eversion of the cervix and an acidic vaginal environment encourage the development of the transformation zone. Under physiologic conditions, benign squamous metaplasia is the eventual outcome. In the presence of HPV or other carcinogenic agents, the benign metaplastic process is diverted into malignant transformation, resulting first in increasingly severe CIN, then progressing to invasive squamous cell carcinoma in an unknown proportion of women.

Cells at the early reserve cell hyperplasia stage are usually considered to be at greatest risk of transformation, and mature metaplastic squamous epithelium at no risk. Yet the potential for cells between these two extremes to undergo malignant transformation is unknown. Local and systemic immune defenses may be important in counteracting the changes generated by the carcinogenic agents.

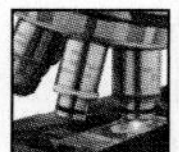

PATHOLOGY: CIN is nearly always a disease of metaplastic squamous epithelium in the transformation zone or endocervix. ***Practically, the location of the transformation zone on the exposed portion of the cervix determines the distribution of CIN, and hence cervical cancer.***

The normal process by which cervical squamous epithelium matures is disturbed in CIN, as evidenced morphologically by changes in cellularity, differentiation, polarity, nuclear features and mitotic activity. In **CIN-1 (mild dysplasia),** the most pronounced changes are in the basal third of the

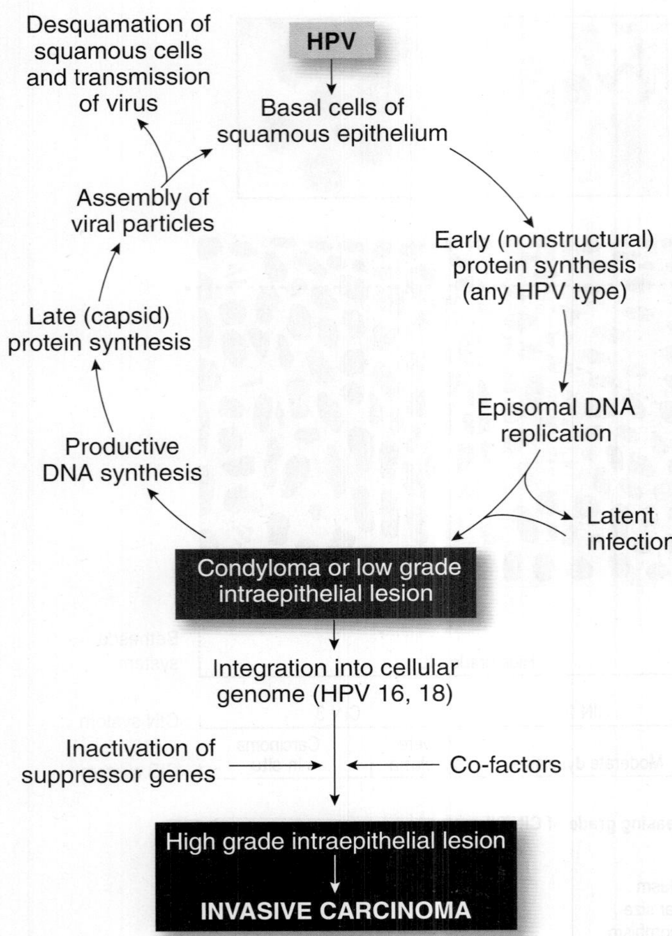

FIGURE 18-19. Role of human papillomavirus (HPV) in the pathogenesis of cervical neoplasia.

epithelium. However, abnormal cells are present throughout the thickness of the epithelium. Substantial cytoplasmic differentiation proceeds as abnormal cells migrate through the upper two thirds of the epithelium, but nuclei in the upper levels are still morphologically abnormal. Thus, the sloughed cells can be detected as abnormal in Pap smears. In **CIN-2 (moderate dysplasia),** most of the cellular abnormalities are in the lower and middle thirds of the epithelium. Cytodifferentiation occurs in cells in the upper third, but less than in CIN-1.

CIN-3 is synonymous with **severe dysplasia** and **CIS.** In severe dysplasia, cells in the superficial (upper) epithelium disclose some, albeit minimal, differentiation, but show none at all in CIS. The sequence of histologic changes from CIN-1 to CIN-3 is shown in Fig. 18-20. Dysplasia and CIS are often detected on colposcopic examination by signs associated with their altered vasculature and epithelial changes. Mosaicism (irregular surface resembling inlaid woodwork) (Fig. 18-21) and dots that differ from surrounding tissue surface by color and texture are the two patterns most often seen in high-grade CIN. The oncogenic process occurs more often on the anterior than the posterior cervical lip, and often involves the endocervical glands.

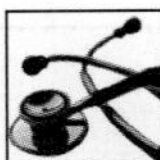

CLINICAL FEATURES: The mean age at which women develop CIN is 24 to 27 years for CIN-1 and CIN-2, and 35 to 42 for CIN-3. Based on morphologic criteria, half of cases of CIN-1 regress, 10% progress to CIN-3 and less than 2% become invasive cancer. The frequency is much greater and the time required much shorter for progression to CIS for initially higher grades of CIN. The average time for all grades of dysplasia to progress to carcinoma in situ is about 10 years. ***At least 20% of cases of CIN-3 progress to invasive carcinoma in that time.***

When CIN is discovered, colposcopy, together with a Schiller test, delineates the extent of the lesion and indicates areas to be biopsied. Diagnostic endocervical curettage also helps to determine the extent of endocervical involvement. Women with CIN-1 are often followed conservatively (i.e., repeated Pap smears plus close follow-up), although some gynecologists now advocate local ablative treatment. High-grade lesions are treated according to the extent of disease. LEEP (loop electrosurgical excision procedure), an outpatient procedure, is commonly used. Cervical conization (removal of a cone of tissue around the external os), cryosurgery and (rarely) hysterectomy may also be done. Follow-up smears and clinical examinations should continue for life, as vaginal or vulvar squamous cancer may develop later.

Microinvasive Squamous Cell Carcinoma Is the Earliest Stage (Ia) of Invasive Cervical Cancer

In this setting, stromal invasion usually arises from overlying CIN (Fig. 18-22). About 7% of specimens removed for CIS show focal microinvasive cancer. Staging of microinvasive disease is based on width and depth of invasion (Table 18-4), defined as follows:

- Invasion less than 3 mm (stage Ia1) or 5 mm (stage Ia2) below the basement membrane
- 7-mm maximum lateral extension

The earliest invasive changes ("early stromal invasion," or ESI) appear as tiny irregular epithelial buds emanating from the base of CIN-3 lesions (Fig. 18-23). These small (<1 mm) tongues of neoplastic epithelial cells do not affect the prognosis of CIN-3 lesions; hence, both can be treated similarly with conservative surgery. In the 2009 FIGO classification, ESI was excluded from stage Ia1. Most American gynecologic oncologists further limit microinvasive carcinoma to tumors lacking vascular invasion and lymph node metastases. Lymph node metastases are found in only 3% to 5% of stage Ia2 microinvasive tumors. Conization or simple hysterectomy generally cures microinvasive cancers less than 3 mm deep.

Invasive Squamous Cell Carcinoma Remains Common Worldwide

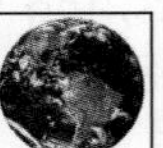

EPIDEMIOLOGY: Squamous cell carcinoma is by far the most common type of cervical cancer. Even in the United States (Table 18-5), 11,000 new cases occur annually, which is less than either endometrial or ovarian cancer. However, in underdeveloped areas, where cytologic screening is less available, cervical squamous cancer is still a major cause of cancer death. The HPV vaccine (often termed the **cervical cancer vaccine**) decreased risk of cervical cancer

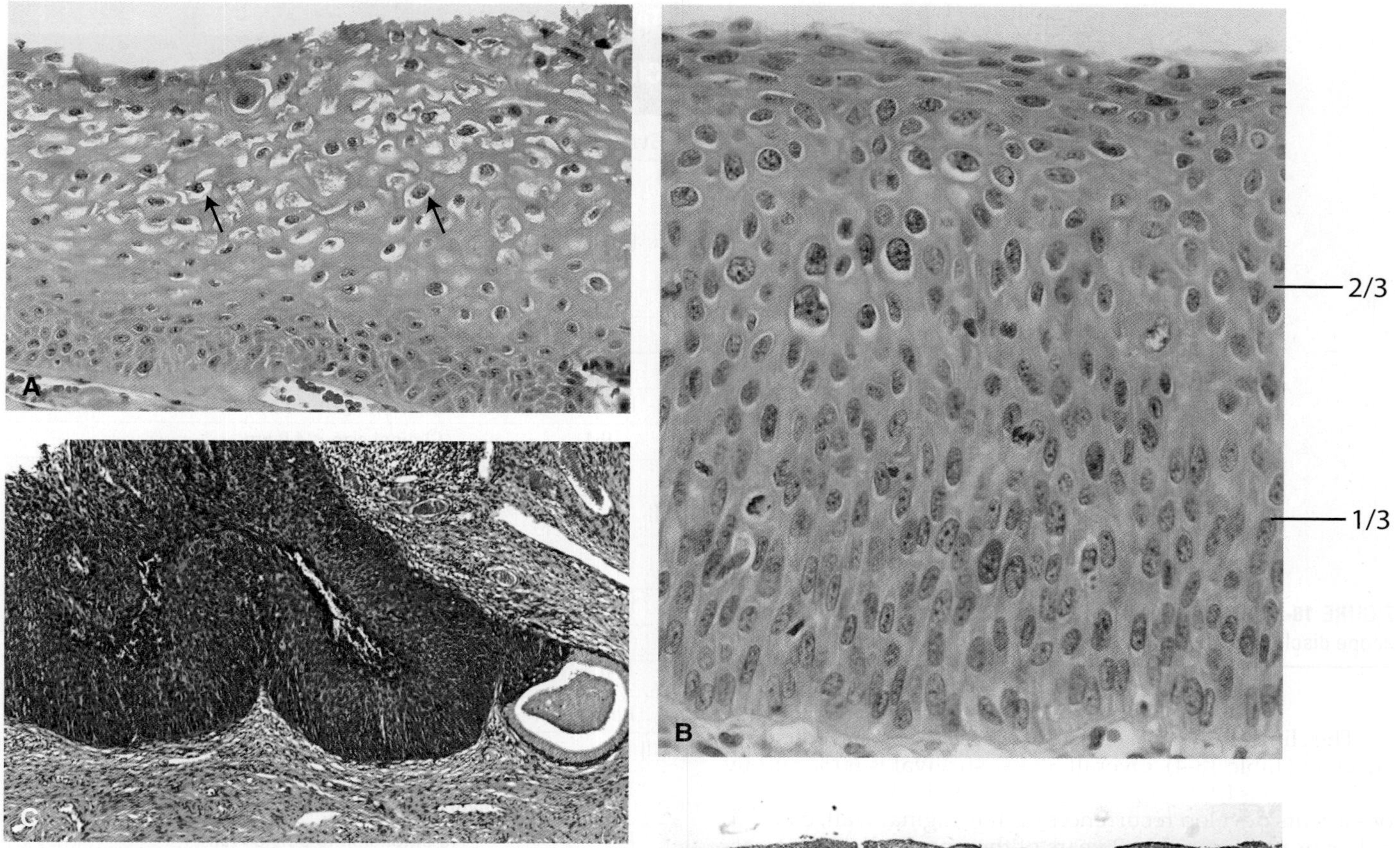

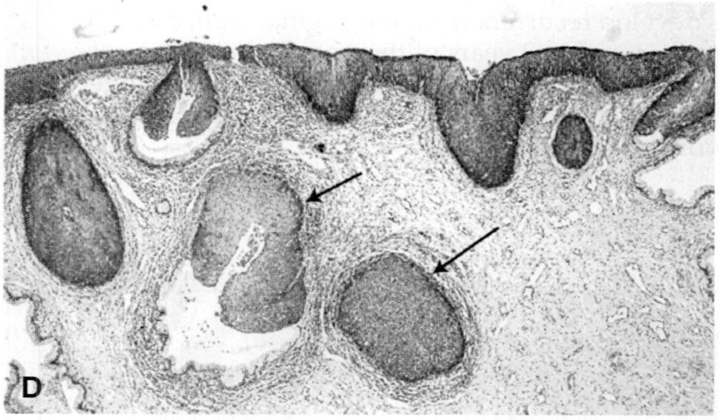

FIGURE 18-20. Cervical intraepithelial neoplasia (CIN). A. CIN-1: the cervical epithelium shows pronounced cellular atypia in the basal third. Some cells in the upper two thirds of the epithelium have abnormal nuclei indicative of HPV infection (*arrows*), but all show cytoplasmic differentiation. **B.** CIN-2 to CIN-3: the lower two thirds of the epithelium displays pronounced cell atypia. Although cytodifferentiation occurs in the upper third of the epithelium, it is less pronounced than in CIN-1. **C.** CIN-3 (carcinoma in situ, CIS): neoplastic cells are present throughout the entire epithelium. **D.** CIN-3: CIS partially or completely replaces the columnar epithelium of the endocervical glands (*arrows*).

by 97%. Vaccinated women developed neither HPV-associated precancer nor invasive cervical cancer.

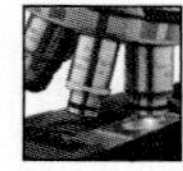

PATHOLOGY: Early stages of cervical cancer are often poorly defined, granular, eroded lesions or nodular and exophytic masses (Fig. 18-24A). If the tumor is predominantly within the endocervical canal, it can be an endophytic mass, infiltrate stroma and cause diffuse enlargement and hardening of the cervix. Most tumors are nonkeratinizing, with solid nests of large malignant squamous cells and no more than individual cell keratinization. Most remaining cancers show nests of keratinized cells in concentric whorls, so-called keratin pearls (Fig. 18-24B). The least common, and most aggressive, tumor is small cell carcinoma. It consists of infiltrating masses of small, cohesive, nonkeratinized, malignant cells, and has the worst prognosis.

Cervical cancer spreads by direct extension, through lymphatic vessels (Fig. 18-25) and only rarely by the hematogenous route. Local extension into surrounding tissues (parametrium) results in **ureteral compression** (stage IIIb; Table 18-4); the corresponding clinical complications are hydroureter, hydronephrosis and renal failure, the most common cause of death (50% of patients). Bladder and rectal involvement (stage IVa) may lead to fistula formation. Metastases to regional lymph nodes involve paracervical, hypogastric and external iliac nodes. Overall, tumor growth and spread are relatively slow, since the average age for patients with stage 0 tumor (CIN-3) is 35 to 40 years; for stage IA, 43 years; and for stage IV, 57 years.

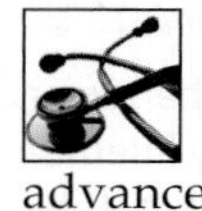

CLINICAL FEATURES: In the earliest stages of cervical cancer, patients complain most often of vaginal bleeding after intercourse or douching. With more advanced tumors, symptoms are referable to the route and degree of spread. The Pap smear remains the most reliable screening test for detecting cervical cancer.

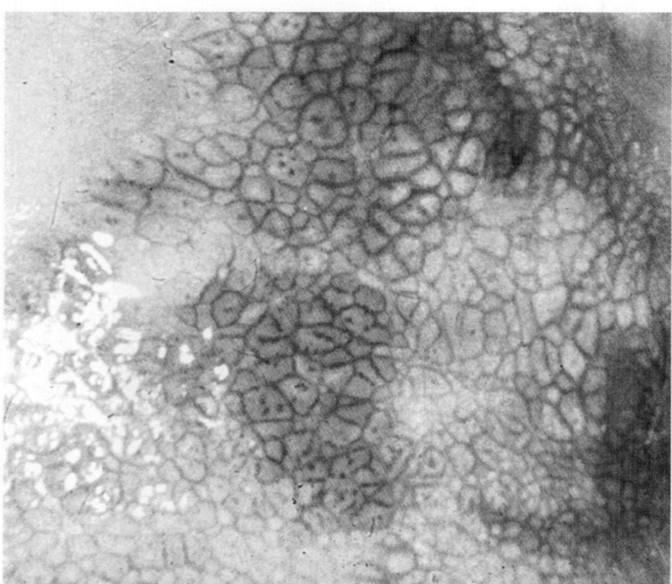

FIGURE 18-21. Dysplasia of the cervix. Examination with the colposcope discloses a mosaic pattern resembling inlaid woodwork.

The clinical stage of cervical cancer is the best predictor of survival (Table 18-4). Overall 5-year survival is 60%, and by each stage it is I, 90%; II, 75%; III, 35%; and IV, 10%. About 15% of patients develop recurrences on the vaginal wall, bladder, pelvis or rectum within 2 years of therapy. Radical hysterectomy is favored for localized tumor, especially in younger women; radiation therapy or combinations of the two are used for more advanced tumors.

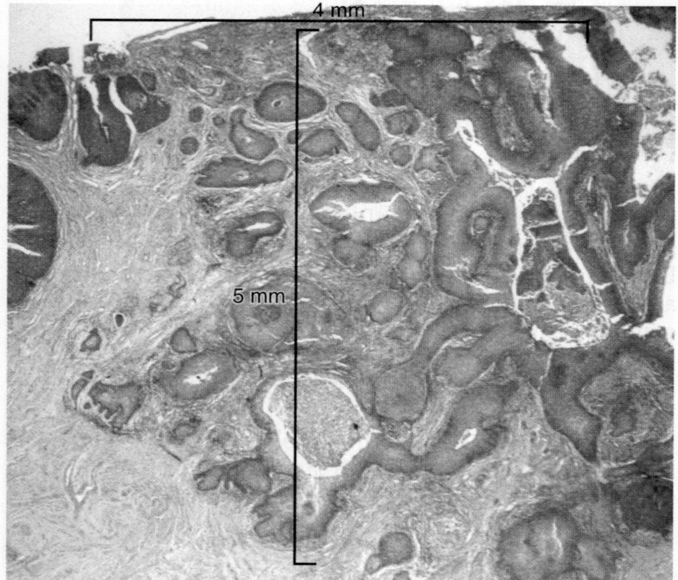

FIGURE 18-22. Microinvasive squamous cell carcinoma. The tumor invades 5 mm deep and 4 mm wide. This tumor is stage IA2 by International Federation of Gynecology and Obstetrics (FIGO) rules, but IB by Society of Gynecologic Oncology (SGO) rules.

Table 18-4

Clinical Staging of Cervical Cancer (FIGO)

Stage	Description
I	Carcinoma confined to cervix (extension to corpus disregarded)
Ia	Invasive cancer identified *only* microscopically. Maximum depth, 5.0 mm; maximum width, 7.0 mm*
Ia1	Depth ≤3.0 mm
Ia2	Depth 3.0–5.0 mm
Ib	Any cancer *grossly* visible
Ib1	Clinical size ≤4.0 cm
Ib2	Clinical size >4.0 cm
II	Carcinoma extending beyond cervix, but not to lateral pelvic wall; involvement of vagina limited to upper two thirds
IIa	Without parametrial invasion
IIa1	Clinical size ≤4.0 cm
IIa2	Clinical size >4.0 cm
IIb	With obvious parametrial invasion
III	Invasive carcinoma extending to lateral pelvic wall or lower one third of vagina or causing hydronephrosis or nonfunctioning kidney
IIIa	No extension to pelvic wall
IIIb	Extension to pelvic wall, hydronephrosis or nonfunctioning kidney
IV	Extended spread involving:
IVa	Mucosa of urinary bladder or rectum
IVb	Tissues beyond true pelvis

FIGO = International Federation of Gynecology and Obstetrics.
*Early stromal invasion: epithelial buds emanating from the base of cervical intraepithelial neoplasia (CIN)-3 lesions have no difference in outcome from CIN-3 lesions. Involvement of vascular (venous or lymphatic) spaces does not change the stage.

Endocervical Adenocarcinoma Makes up 20% of Malignant Cervical Tumors

The incidence of cervical adenocarcinoma has increased recently, with a mean age of 56 years at presentation. Most tumors are of the endocervical cell (mucinous) type, but the various subtypes have little importance for overall survival. Adenocarcinoma shares epidemiologic factors with squamous cell carcinoma of the cervix and spreads similarly. These tumors are often associated with adenocarcinoma in situ and are frequently infected with HPV types 16 and 18.

PATHOLOGY:
ADENOCARCINOMA IN SITU: Also called **cervical glandular intraepithelial neoplasia (CGIN),** this lesion generally arises by the squamocolumnar junction and extends into the endocervical canal. It displays tall columnar cells with eosinophilic or mucinous cytoplasm, sometimes resembling goblet cells. The pattern of spread and involvement

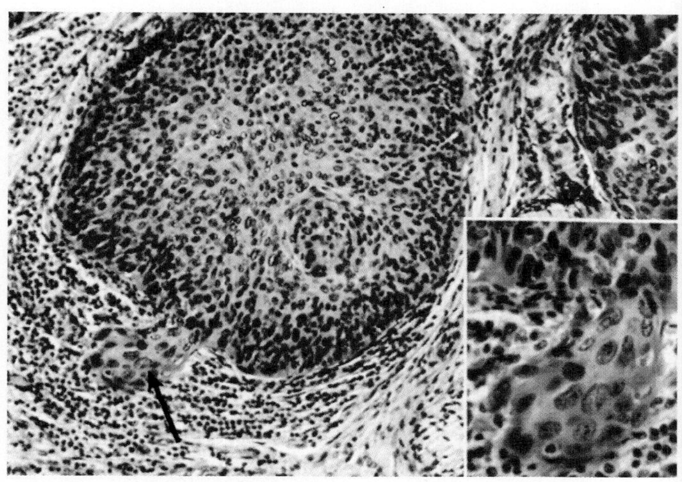

FIGURE 18-23. Early stromal invasion. Section of the cervix shows that carcinoma in situ in an endocervical gland has broken through the basement membrane (*arrow*) to invade the stroma. *Inset.* A higher-power view of the early invasive focus.

of endocervical glands resemble those of CIN. Adenocarcinoma in situ typically is intraepithelial, maintaining normal endocervical gland architecture. The cells show slight enlargement, atypical hyperchromatic nuclei, increased nuclear-to-cytoplasmic ratio and variable mitoses. Abrupt transitions help distinguish neoplastic from neighboring normal endocervical cells. Associated high-grade squamous cell CIN occurs in 40% of cases of adenocarcinoma in situ.

INVASIVE ADENOCARCINOMA: This tumor typically presents as a fungating polypoid (Fig. 18-26A) or papillary mass. Exophytic tumors often have a papillary pattern (Fig. 18-26B), whereas endophytic ones display tubular or glandular patterns. Poorly differentiated tumors are predominantly composed of solid sheets of cells.

Table 18-5

Incidence of Gynecologic Cancer in the United States (2004)

	New Cases		Death	
	Cases	%*	Cases	%*
Endometrium	40,320	6	7090	3
Ovary	25,580	4	16,090	6
Cervix, invasive	10,520	3	3900	2
Vulva, invasive	3970	<1	850	
Vagina, invasive	1000	<1		
Other	2000	<1		

*% = percentage of all cases of cancer in females.
Carcinoma in situ of cervix >50,000 new cases/year.

Adenocarcinoma of the endocervix spreads by local invasion and lymphatic metastases, but overall survival is somewhat worse than for squamous carcinoma. The tumor is treated similarly to squamous carcinoma.

UTERUS

Anatomy

The uterine corpus (body) is smaller than the cervix at birth and during childhood, but increases rapidly in size after puberty. The endometrium is composed of glands and stroma. It is thin at birth, when it consists of a continuous surface of cuboidal epithelium that dips to line a few sparse tubular glands. After puberty, it thickens. The superficial two thirds, the "zona functionalis," responds to hormones and is shed with each menstrual phase. The deepest third, the basal

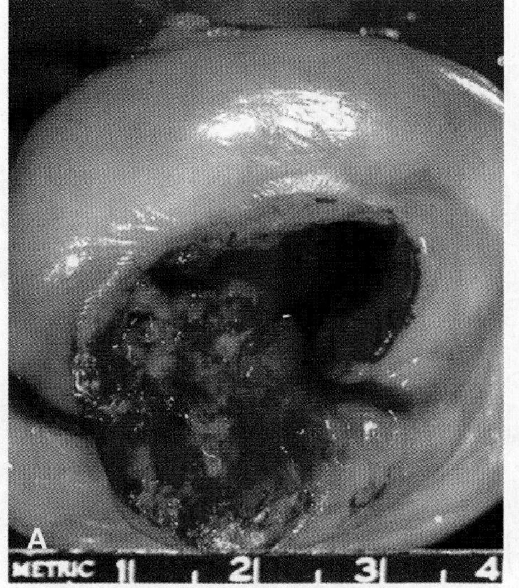

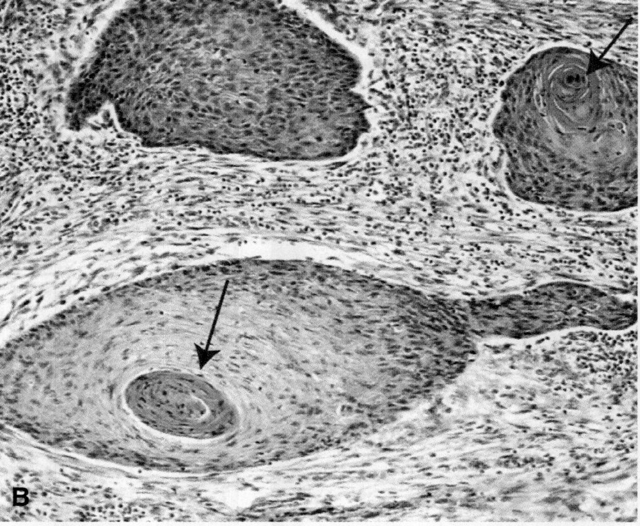

FIGURE 18-24. Squamous cell cancer. A. The cervix is distorted by the presence of an exophytic, ulcerated squamous cell carcinoma. **B.** The keratinizing pattern of the tumor is manifested as whorls of keratinized cells ("keratin pearls") (*arrows*).

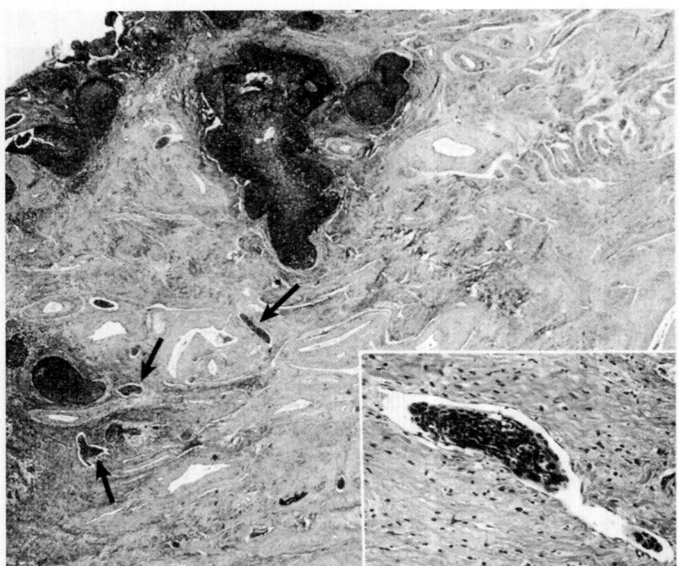

FIGURE 18-25. Squamous cell cancer of the cervix with lymphatic invasion. Low magnification shows a squamous cell carcinoma that has invaded the stroma and permeated the lymphatics (*arrows*). *Inset.* A high-power view of lymphatic invasion.

layer, is the germinative portion and with each cycle regenerates a new functional zone.

The endometrium is supplied by arcuate arteries that traverse the outer myometrium and give off two sets of vessels, one to the myometrium and the other, the radial arteries, to the endometrium. In turn, the radial arteries branch into two types of vessels. The basal arteries supply the basal endometrium and the spiral arteries nourish the superficial two thirds.

The Menstrual Cycle

The normal endometrium undergoes a series of sequential changes that support the growth of implanted fertilized ova (zygotes) (Fig. 18-27). If conception does not occur, the endometrium is shed, then regenerated to support a fertilized ovum in the next cycle.

MENSTRUAL PHASE: Without pregnancy (i.e., lacking a blastocyst to secrete human chorionic gonadotropin [hCG]), ovarian granulosa and thecal cells degenerate and progesterone levels fall. The endometrium becomes desiccated, spiral arteries collapse and the stroma disintegrates. Menses start on day 28, last 3 to 7 days and result in a flow of about 35 mL of blood. The denuded surface is reepithelialized by extension of the residual glandular epithelium.

PROLIFERATIVE PHASE: In days 3-15 of the menstrual cycle, the endometrium is under estrogenic stimulation. In the functional zone tubular to coiled glands are evenly distributed and supported by a cellular, monomorphic stroma (Fig. 18-27A). Early in the proliferative phase, glands are narrow, but they coil more and increase slightly in caliber over time. The columnar cells lining the tubules increase from one layer in thickness to a pseudostratified epithelium that is mitotically active. The glands produce a watery alkaline secretion that facilitates the passage of sperm through the endometrial cavity into the fallopian tubes. The stroma is also mitotically active. Spiral arteries are narrow and mostly inconspicuous.

SECRETORY PHASE: Ovulation occurs about 14 days after the last menstrual period. Then, the graafian follicle that discharged its ovum becomes a corpus luteum. The granulosa cells of the corpus luteum begin to secrete progesterone, which transforms the endometrium from a proliferative into a secretory state.

- **Days 17 to 19 (postovulatory days 3 to 5):** Endometrial glands enlarge, dilate and become more coiled. The lining cells develop abundant and prominent, glycogen-rich, subnuclear vacuoles (day 17). Over the next several days, these cells produce copious secretions that can support a zygote while it develops early chorionic villi capable of invading the endometrium.
- **Days 20 to 22 (postovulatory days 6 to 8):** The endometrium displays prominent stromal edema and glands have few discrete vacuoles but rather a homogenous cytoplasm. The glands dilate and are more tortuous.

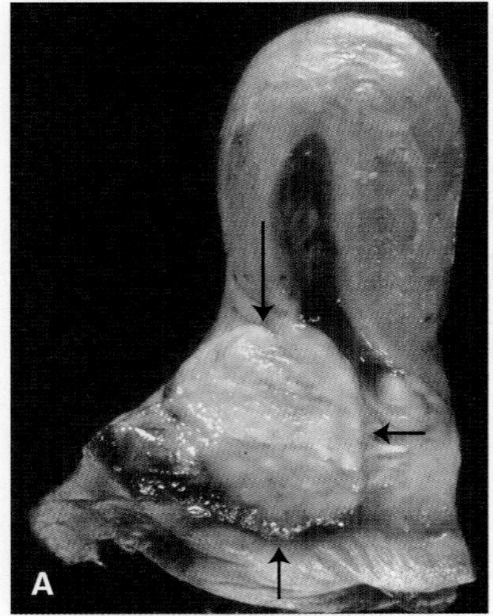

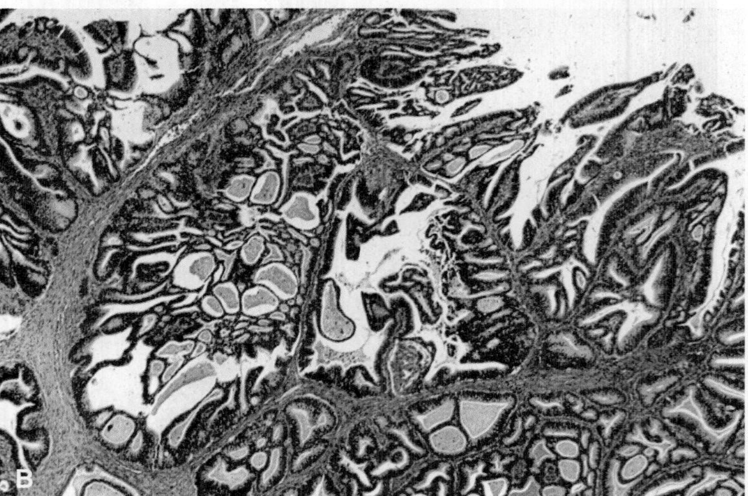

FIGURE 18-26. Endocervical adenocarcinoma. A. The endocervical tumor appears as a polypoid mass (*arrows*). **B.** Microscopic view of endocervical adenocarcinoma showing a papillary pattern of growth.

Day of Cycle		3—15	15–16	17	18	19–22	23	24–25	26–27	1—2
Post-ovulatory day			1–2	3	4	5–8	9	10–11	12–13	14+
Cycle phases		Proliferative	Interval	Early secretory		Mid-secretory			Late secretory	Menstrual
Key feature		Mitoses	Mitoses and subnuclear vacuoles	Maximum subnuclear vacuoles	Subnuclear vacuoles present	Stromal edema	Focal predecidua around spiral arteries	Patchy predecidua	Extensive predecidua	Stromal crumbling
Microscopic features of functional zone	Stroma	Loose stroma. Mitoses	Same as proliferative	Loose stroma. Scanty mitoses	Loose stroma	Stromal edema	Focal predecidua around spiral arteries. Edema prominent	Predecidua throughout stroma. Some edema	Extensive predecidua. Prominent granulated lymphocytes	Stromal crumbling. Hemorrhage
	Glands	Straight to tightly coiled tubules. Mitoses	Some subnuclear vacuoles, otherwise as proliferative	Extensive subnuclear vacuoles	Dilated glands. Some subnuclear vacuoles	Dilated glands with irregular outline. Luminal secretion		'Saw tooth' glands	Prominent 'saw tooth' glands	Disrupted glands. Secretory exhaustion. Regenerating epithelium
Appearances		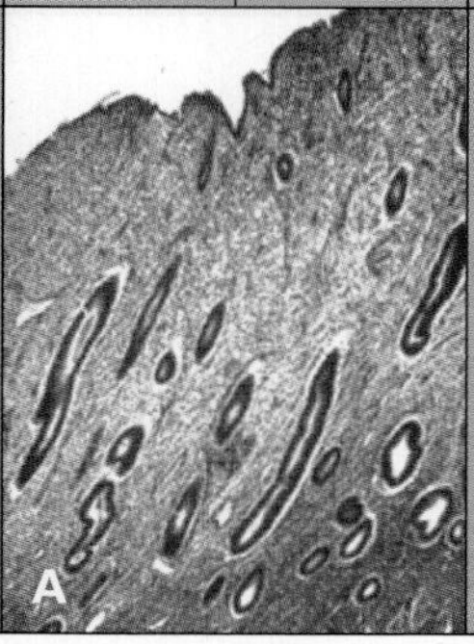 A				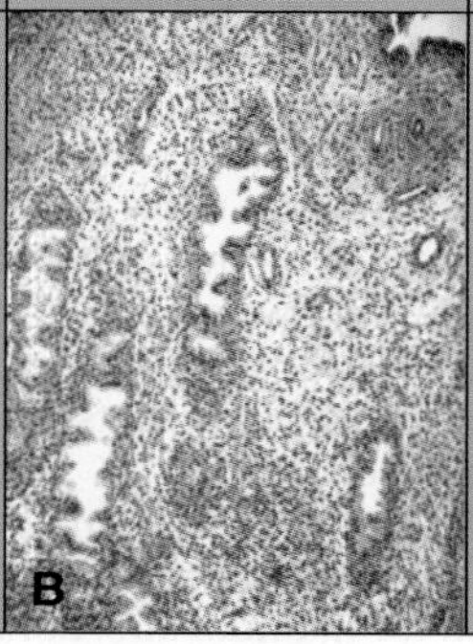 B			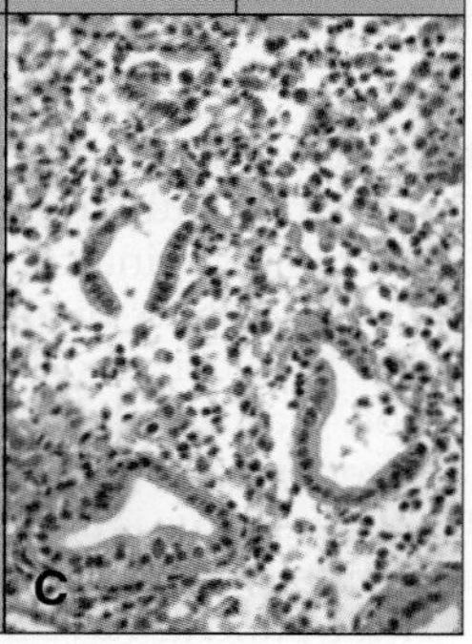 C	

FIGURE 18-27. Main histologic features of the endometrial phases of the normal menstrual cycle. A. Proliferative phase. Straight tubular glands are embedded in a cellular monomorphic stroma. **B.** Secretory phase, day 24. Dilated tortuous glands with serrated borders are situated in a predecidual stroma. **C.** Menstrual endometrium. Fragmented glands, dissolution of the stroma and numerous neutrophils are evident.

- **Day 23 (postovulatory day 9):** The stromal cells enlarge and exhibit large, round, vesicular nuclei and abundant eosinophilic cytoplasm in a specific distribution: surrounding spiral arterioles ("vascular cuffing"). With time, these cells become more extensively distributed until they fill the functionalis. These are the precursors of the decidual cells of pregnancy and are referred to as "predecidua."
- **Day 27 (postovulatory day 13):** The entire stroma is now predecidualized and prepared for menstruation. Tubular glands continue to dilate and develop serrated (saw-toothed) borders.

ATROPHIC ENDOMETRIUM: After menopause, the number of glands and quantity of stroma progressively decrease. Remaining glands often are oriented parallel to the surface and the stroma contains abundant collagen. The glands of the atrophic endometrium are often conspicuously dilated, an appearance termed **senile cystic atrophy of the endometrium.**

Endometrium of Pregnancy

The corpus luteum of pregnancy requires continuous stimulation by hCG secreted by placental trophoblast of the developing embryo. Trophoblast begins to develop about day 23. Under hCG stimulation, the corpus luteum increases its progesterone output, stimulating secretion of fluid by endometrial glands. In the hypersecretory endometrium of pregnancy, very dilated glands are lined by cells with abundant glycogen. These features can persist up to 8 weeks after delivery.

The hypersecretory response may become exaggerated with intrauterine pregnancy, ectopic pregnancy or trophoblastic disease. Nuclei of the glandular cells may enlarge and appear bulbous and polyploid, because their DNA has replicated, but the cells have not divided. Their nuclei protrude beyond the apparent cellular cytoplasmic limits into the gland lumen, an appearance referred to as the **Arias-Stella phenomenon** (Fig. 18-28). Enlarged nuclei are polyploid, not to be confused with aneuploidy, a condition sometimes seen in adenocarcinoma.

Congenital Anomalies of the Uterus

Congenital anomalies of the uterus are rare.

- **Congenital absence of the uterus (agenesis)** reflects failure of müllerian ducts to develop. Since elongation of these ducts during embryonic life requires the wolffian ducts as guides, uterine agenesis is almost always accompanied by other anomalies of the urogenital tract as well as an absent vagina and fallopian tubes.

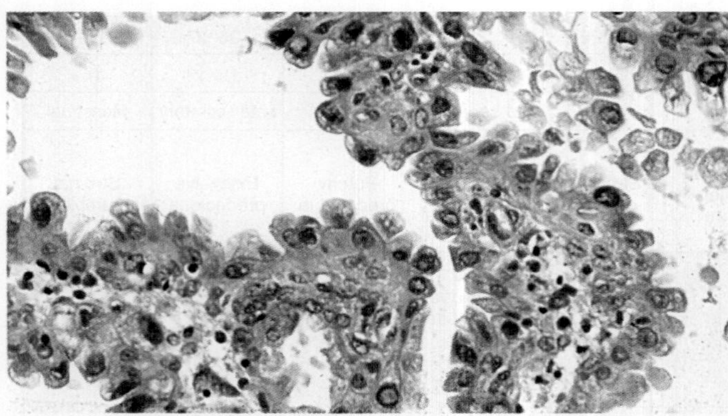

FIGURE 18-28. Arias-Stella reaction of pregnancy associated with human chorionic gonadotropin (hCG) stimulation. A section of endometrium shows enlarged, bulbous nuclei that protrude into the gland lumen.

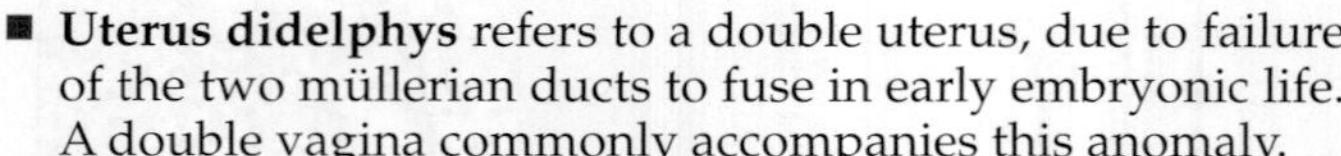

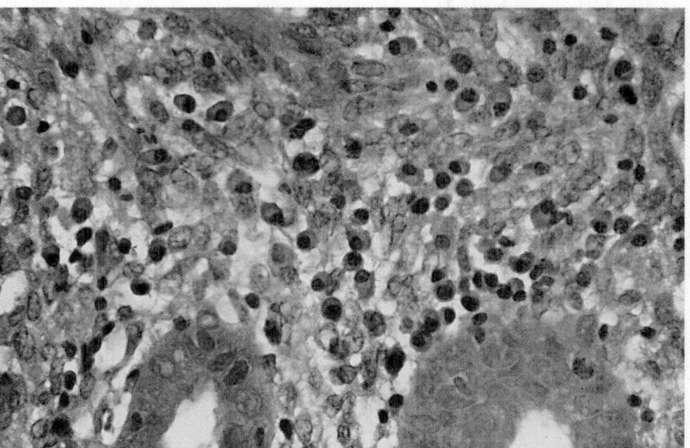

FIGURE 18-29. Chronic endometritis. The inflammatory infiltrate is composed largely of lymphocytes and plasma cells.

- **Uterus didelphys** refers to a double uterus, due to failure of the two müllerian ducts to fuse in early embryonic life. A double vagina commonly accompanies this anomaly.
- **Uterus duplex bicornis** is a uterus with a common fused wall between two distinct endometrial cavities. The common wall between the apposed müllerian ducts fails to degenerate to form a single uterine cavity.
- **Uterus septus** is a single uterus with a partial septum, due to incomplete resorption of the wall of the fused müllerian ducts. These patients have increased risk for habitual abortion.
- **Bicornuate uterus** refers to a uterus with two cornua (horns) and a common cervix. Didelphic and bicornuate uterine fusion defects slightly increase the risk of premature birth.

Endometritis

In endometritis, or an inflamed endometrium, there is an abnormal inflammatory infiltrate in the endometrium. It must be distinguished from the normal presence of polymorphonuclear leukocytes during menstruation and a mild lymphocytic infiltrate at other times. Findings in most cases of endometritis are nonspecific and rarely point to a specific cause.

ACUTE ENDOMETRITIS: This condition is defined as the abnormal presence of polymorphonuclear leukocytes in the endometrium. Most cases result from an ascending infection from the cervix (e.g., after the usually impervious cervical barrier is compromised by abortion, delivery or medical instrumentation). Curettage is diagnostic and often curative, because it removes necrotic tissue that has served as the nidus of the ongoing infection. Nowadays, the condition is of little significance, although it was quite dangerous before antibiotics.

CHRONIC ENDOMETRITIS: Although lymphocytes and lymphoid follicles are occasionally scattered in a normal endometrium, plasma cells in the endometrium are diagnostic of chronic endometritis (Fig. 18-29). The disorder is associated with IUDs, PID and retained products of conception after an abortion or delivery. Without a culture, the pathologic findings alone do not distinguish between infective and noninfective causes. Patients usually complain of bleeding, pelvic pain or both. The condition is generally self-limited.

PYOMETRA: Defined as pus in the endometrial cavity, pyometra is associated with gross anatomic defects such as fistulous tracts between bowel and uterine cavity, bulky or perforating malignancies or cervical stenosis. Long-standing pyometra may rarely be associated with development of endometrial squamous cell cancer.

Traumatic Lesions

INTRAUTERINE DEVICE: IUDs predispose bearers to (1) increased menstrual flow, (2) uterine perforation and (3) spontaneous abortion if conception occurs with the IUD in place. However, IUD use reduces endometrial cancer risk by half. Much of the adverse publicity about IUDs relates to early devices, and only 1% of women who desire contraception now use an IUD.

INTRAUTERINE ADHESIONS (ASHERMAN SYNDROME): Intrauterine fibrous adhesions sometimes develop after a uterus has been curetted, particularly for postpartum complications or therapeutic abortion. These bands traverse, but do not necessarily obliterate, the endometrial cavity. Additional complications include amenorrhea or, in the event of a subsequent pregnancy, increased abortion rates, preterm labor and placenta accreta.

Adenomyosis

Adenomyosis is the presence of endometrial glands and stroma within the myometrium. The most clinically significant correlation between symptoms of pain, dysmenorrhea or menorrhagia and pathologic finding of adenomyosis occurs if the glands are at least 1 mm or more beneath the endometrial myometrial junction. Adenomyosis is more likely to be symptomatic the more deeply it penetrates the myometrium. Pain occurs as foci of adenomyosis enlarge when blood is entrapped during menses. One fifth of all uteri removed at surgery show some adenomyosis.

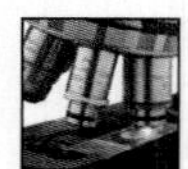

PATHOLOGY: The uterus may be enlarged. The myometrium discloses small, soft, tan areas, some of which are cystic (Fig. 18-30). Microscopic examination

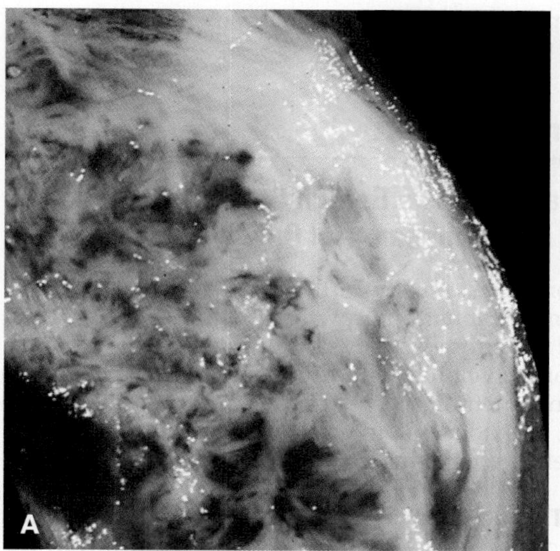

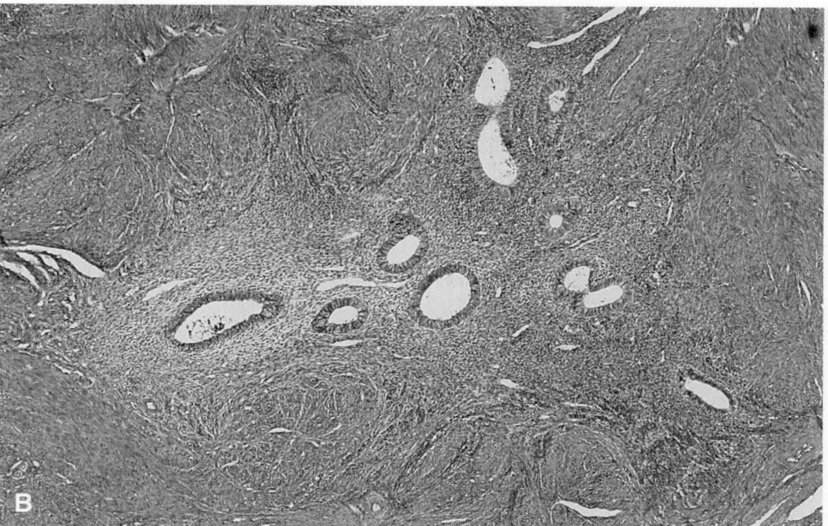

FIGURE 18-30. Adenomyosis. A. The cut surface of the uterus reveals small, red areas corresponding to endometrial glands in the myometrium. **B.** A microscopic view shows an endometrial gland and stroma in the myometrium.

reveals glands lined by proliferative to inactive endometrium and surrounded by endometrial stroma with varying degrees of fibrosis. Secretory changes are rare, except during pregnancy or in patients treated with progestins. Often myometrium nearby is locally hypertrophic and nodular. Over time, the uterus may also become enlarged from cyclic bleeding into these foci. Extension of hyperplastic or neoplastic endometrium from the endometrial functionalis into adenomyotic foci may occur.

CLINICAL FEATURES: Many patients with adenomyosis are asymptomatic, but varying degrees of pelvic pain, dysfunctional uterine bleeding, dysmenorrhea and dyspareunia are common. These symptoms appear in parous women of reproductive age and regress after menopause. The cause of adenomyosis remains unknown.

Hormonal Effects

Contraceptive Steroids Prevent Pregnancy and Many Gynecologic Cancers

Oral contraceptive agents induce endometrial changes that reflect the types, potencies and dosages of estrogens and progestins in individual formulations. Combined preparations generally contain potent progestins and weak estrogens. Pseudodecidual change thus appears early and overshadows the weak glandular growth. After several cycles, endometrial glands atrophy. Newer contraceptive combinations contain lower doses of hormones and correspondingly elicit less change. Women who use contraceptive steroids that include progestational agents have significantly lower rates of endometrial and ovarian cancer, reflecting the growth-inhibiting properties of progesterone, and in the ovary, a reduction in the number of ovulations (see below).

Dysfunctional Uterine Bleeding Occurs During or Between Menstrual Periods

The causes of dysfunctional bleeding lie outside the uterus. It is one of the most common gynecologic disorders of women of reproductive age but is still poorly understood. Most cases are related to a disturbance that involves an aspect of the hypothalamic–pituitary–ovarian axis (Table 18-6). Ovarian dysfunction is usual, especially in the presence of anovulation.

Some causes of menstrual irregularity are intrinsic to the uterus and are not considered dysfunctional. These include (1) growths (e.g., carcinoma, endometrial intraepithelial neoplasia [EIN], submucosal leiomyomata and polyps), (2) inflammation (e.g., endometritis), (3) pregnancy (e.g., complications of intrauterine or ectopic pregnancy) and (4) the effects of IUDs (Table 18-6).

Anovulatory Bleeding Is the Most Common Form of Dysfunctional Bleeding

Anovulatory bleeding is a complex syndrome of many causes that manifests as the absence of ovulation during the reproductive years. It is most often noted at either end of reproductive life (i.e., menarche and menopause).

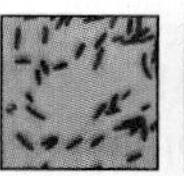 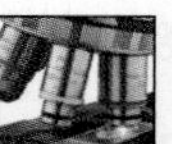

ETIOLOGIC FACTORS AND PATHOLOGY: In an anovulatory cycle, failure of ovulation leads to excessive and prolonged estrogen stimulation, without a postovulatory rise in progesterone. As a result, the endometrium remains in a proliferative state dominated by a disordered, cystic glandular appearance and excessive bulk. Lacking progesterone, the spiral arteries of the

Table 18-6

Causes of Abnormal Uterine Bleeding (Including Uterine and Extrauterine Causes)

Newborn	Maternal estrogen
Childhood	Iatrogenic (trauma, foreign body, infection of vagina)
	Vaginal neoplasms (sarcoma botryoides)
	Ovarian tumors (functional)
Adolescence	Hypothalamic immaturity
	Psychogenic and nutritional problems
	Inadequate luteal function
Reproductive age	Anovulatory
	Central: psychogenic, stress
	Systemic: nutritional and endocrine disease
	Gonadal: functional tumors
	End organ: benign endometrial hyperplasia
	Pregnancy: ectopic, retained placenta, abortion, mole
	Ovulatory
	Organic: neoplasia, infections (PID), leiomyomas
	Polymenorrhea: short follicular or luteal phases
	Iatrogenic: anticoagulants, IUD
Menopause	Irregular shedding
Postmenopause	Carcinoma, EIN, benign hyperplasias, polyps, leiomyomata
	Carcinoma, EIN, polyps, leiomyomata

EIN = endometrial intraepithelial neoplasia; IUD = intrauterine device; PID = pelvic inflammatory disease.

endometrium do not develop normally. "Breakthrough bleeding" can occur from damage to these fragile spiral arterioles. Resultant thrombosis causes local tissue breakdown resembling that of menstrual endometrium but with the addition of intravascular thrombi, which the patient experiences as symptomatic bleeding out of synchrony with other areas of the endometrium. Elevated estrogen levels usually decline eventually, either through delayed ovulation or involution of the stimulatory follicle. If estrogen decline is rapid, the endometrium undergoes a heavy synchronized menstrual flow.

Luteal Phase Defect Is Caused by Inadequate Progesterone

Luteal phase defect results in an abnormally short menstrual cycle: menses occur 6 to 9 days after the surge of luteinizing hormone (LH) associated with ovulation. A luteal phase defect occurs when a corpus luteum develops improperly or regresses prematurely. Luteal phase defects are responsible for 3% of cases of infertility, and so are mainly important in assessing infertility or in analysis of abnormal uterine bleeding. Diagnosis is confirmed by a biopsy showing an endometrium over 2 days out of synchrony with the chronologic day of the menstrual cycle.

Endometrial Tumors

Endometrial Polyp Is a Benign Stromal Neoplasm in the Endometrial Cavity

These tumors occur mostly in the perimenopausal period. Polyps are monoclonal outgrowths of endometrial stromal cells altered by chromosomal translocation, with secondary induction of polyclonal glandular elements. Stroma and glands of endometrial polyps respond poorly to hormonal stimulation, and do not slough upon menstruation. They do not occur before menarche.

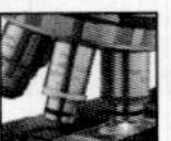

PATHOLOGY: Most endometrial polyps arise in the fundus (Fig. 18-31), but they are found anywhere within the endometrium. They vary from several millimeters to growths filling the entire endometrial cavity. Most are solitary but 20% are multiple. Polyp cores are composed of (1) endometrial glands, often cystically dilated and hyperplastic; (2) fibrous endometrial stroma; and (3) thick-walled, coiled, dilated blood vessels, derived from a straight artery that normally would have supplied the basal zone of the endometrium. They are covered by endometrial epithelium that usually is at a stage of the cycle different from adjacent normal endometrium.

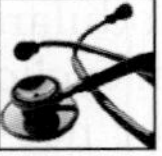

CLINICAL FEATURES: Endometrial polyps typically present with intermenstrual bleeding, owing to surface ulceration or hemorrhagic infarction. Since bleeding in an older woman may be due to endometrial cancer, this sign must be thoroughly evaluated. Endometrial polyps are not ordinarily precancerous, but up to 0.5% harbor adenocarcinoma.

Benign Endometrial Hyperplasia Is Caused by Abnormal Estrogenic Stimulation

It is characterized by diffuse, randomly distributed, architectural and cytologic changes **(Fig. 18-32).** Estrogenic stimulation of the endometrium beyond the normal 2-week proliferative phase causes progressive changes that are associated with a 2- to 10-fold increased risk of endometrial cancer. Aside from women with coexisting (see below), it is not possible to assign cancer risk within these patients by a single histologic examination. Endometrial histopathology does vary greatly, however, as a function of the sequence and tempo of hormonal stimulation among women with benign endometrial hyperplasia. The earliest changes are isolated cystic expansion of scattered proliferative glands without a substantial change in gland density, often designated **persistent proliferative** or **disordered proliferative** endometrium. Morphologic transition to **benign endometrial hyperplasia** is gradual and arbitrarily defined, but can be said to occur when gland density becomes irregular throughout, with some regions having more glands than stroma.

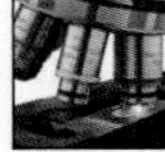

PATHOLOGY: Benign endometrial hyperplasia affects the entire endometrium, where remodeling of glands and stroma creates an irregular density of commingled cystic, slightly branching and tubular glands. In

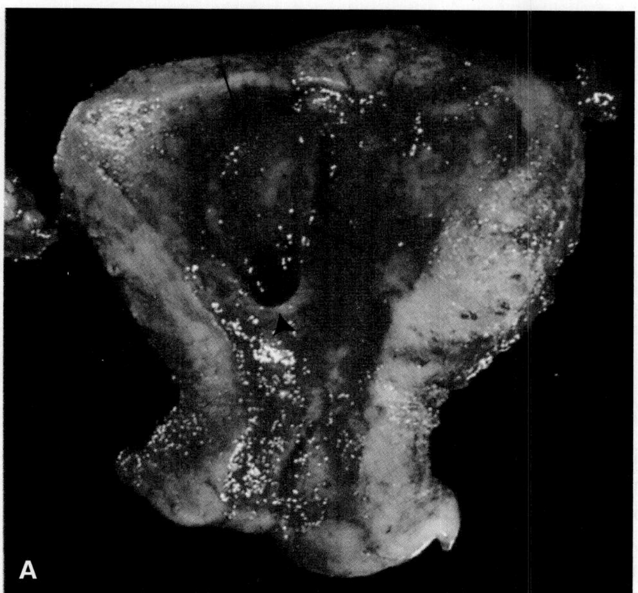

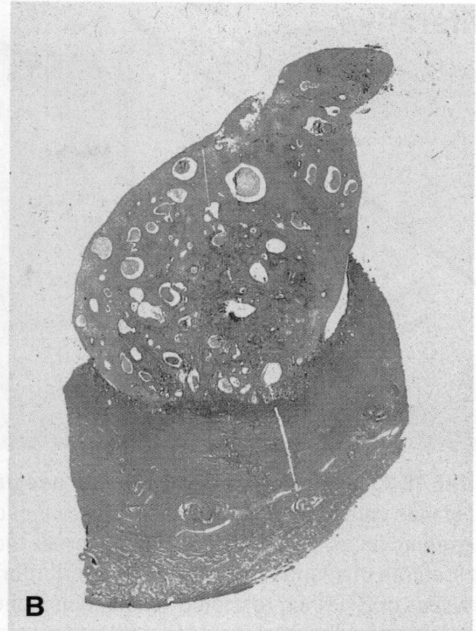

FIGURE 18-31. Endometrial polyp. A. A single polyp (*arrows*) extends into the endometrial cavity. The necrotic tip (*arrowhead*) is responsible for clinical bleeding. **B.** On microscopic section, a polyp exhibits slightly dilated endometrial glands embedded in a markedly fibrous stroma.

at least some areas the gland area should exceed the stromal area, but the cytology of the crowded foci is representative of that seen elsewhere. As long as circulating estrogens persist, glands are proliferative and, if ciliation occurs, this suggests tubal differentiation.

There are two classifications of endometrial hyperplasia: (1) the 1994 World Health Organization (WHO) scheme and (2) the benign hyperplasia–EIN schema compiled in the 1990s from new evidence. The former emphasized cytologic atypia and abnormal glandular architecture, had more subcategories and focused almost exclusively on cytologic atypia as the most important prognostic feature:

- **Simple hyperplasia:** This proliferative lesion shows minimal glandular complexity and crowding and no cytologic atypia. The epithelium is usually one cell layer thick and the stroma between the glands is abundant. Of these, 1% progress to adenocarcinoma.
- **Complex hyperplasia:** This variant exhibits marked glandular complexity and crowding but no cytologic atypia (Fig. 18-32). Glands are increased in number and may vary in size. The stroma between the glands is scanty. Adenocarcinoma develops in 3%.
- **Atypical hyperplasia:** This lesion shows cytologic atypia and marked glandular crowding, often as back-to-back glands. Gland architecture may be complex, with intraluminal papillary arrangements or glands appearing to bud in the stroma. Epithelial cells are large and hyperchromatic, with prominent nucleoli and increased nuclear-to-cytoplasm ratios. Of these, 25% progress to adenocarcinoma, which is almost always of the endometrioid type.

With increasing estrogen exposure, stromal breakdown and resultant gland collapse occur, often with fibrin vascular thrombi. Although prototypically an estrogenic lesion, architectural and metaplastic changes that persist after gradual weaning from a hyperestrogenic state can be construed as manifestations of benign endometrial hyperplasia in which proliferative activity is weak or absent. Stromal predecidualization caused by superimposed progestin therapy or delayed ovulation may develop between irregular glands of benign hyperplasia. Sudden loss of estrogen leads to massive shedding with attendant heavy menses.

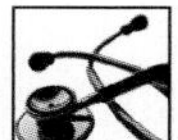

CLINICAL FEATURES: Benign endometrial hyperplasia may result from anovulatory cycles, polycystic ovary syndrome, an estrogen-producing tumor, estrogen administration or obesity. In such cases, therapy

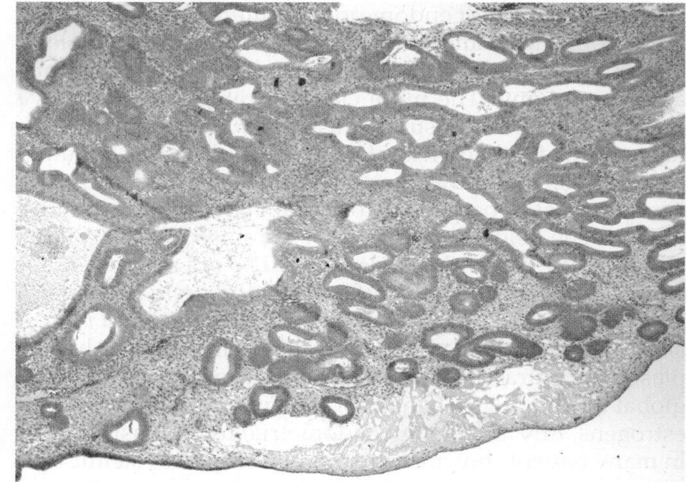

FIGURE 18-32. Benign endometrial hyperplasia. Proliferative endometrial glands are irregularly distributed and randomly dilated. Gland density varies locally, but crowded and uncrowded areas have a consistent cytology throughout. This is a benign endometrium altered by unopposed estrogen.

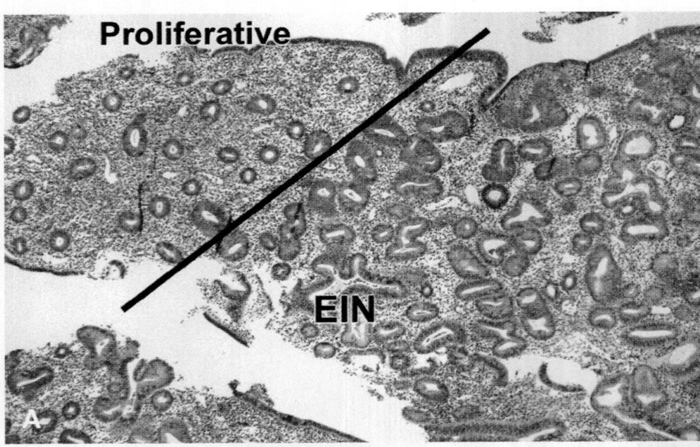

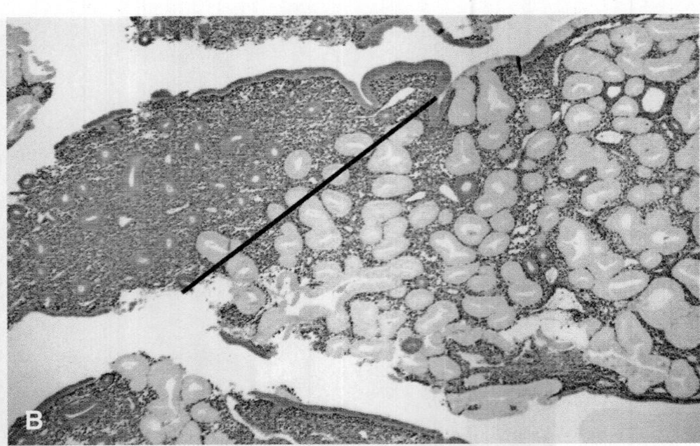

FIGURE 18-33. Endometrial intraepithelial neoplasia (EIN). A. Tight clusters of cytologically altered neoplastic endometrial glands with abundant cytoplasm and rounded nuclei (*right*) are offset from the background endometrium (*left*) in this geographic focus of EIN. Measurement across the perimeter of this aggregate of individual tubular glands exceeds 1 mm, and features of adenocarcinoma such as cribriform, mazelike, or solid architecture are lacking. **B.** Glands affected by EIN show loss of PTEN expression by immunohistochemistry (loss of brown staining).

aimed at the primary cause may alleviate estrogenic stimulation. Large doses of progestins can produce temporary symptomatic relief or objective remission, depending on persistence of the underlying hormonal condition. Short-term risk for endometrial cancer is low with benign endometrial hyperplasia, if extensive sampling of the endometrium shows no EIN. Long-term risks of refractory benign endometrial hyperplasia are best assessed by repeat biopsy.

Endometrial Intraepithelial Neoplasia and Adenocarcinoma Are Separate From Benign Endometrial Hyperplasia: Changing Terminology

Any classification of endometrial proliferations must incorporate our increasing understanding of molecular biology and biological behavior. Pathologic nomenclature is thus always evolving. The more classical categorization above may be supplanted or supplemented by groupings that better account for known molecular and biological parameters. Thus, we now understand the broad class of "endometrial hyperplasia" to contain two discrete entities: the estrogen field effects of benign endometrial hyperplasia, above, and EIN. ***In this paradigm, EINs are seen as monoclonal neoplastic growths of genetically altered cells with greatly increased risk of becoming the endometrioid type of endometrial adenocarcinoma.*** Benign endometrial hyperplasia, by contrast, is intrinsically normal endometrium with global morphologic changes of the influence of unopposed estrogens. EIN and benign endometrial hyperplasia coexist in many patients but are different histologies. Systemic hormonal factors are relevant to both, and can be positive or negative selection factors for mutated cells within an EIN lesion.

EIN is monoclonal neoplastic proliferation prone to malignant transformation. It shows a continuity of acquired genetic markers upon transformation into a malignant phase.

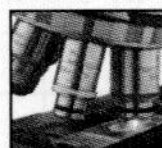

PATHOLOGY: EIN lesions have an epicenter that extends centripetally by interposing neoplastic glands between normal glands. The former are tight aggregates of discrete glands that differ cytologically from the background endometrium, have gland areas exceeding their stromal areas and measure more than 1 mm in dimension in a single fragment. Unlike the diffuse architectural and randomly dispersed cytologic changes of unopposed estrogen, EIN begins as a focus of cytologically altered glands, becoming diffuse only later (Fig. 18-33). Malignant transformation of EIN is evident when the glands develop solid, cribriform or mazelike patterns characteristic of adenocarcinoma.

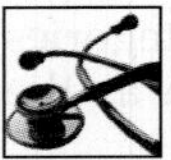

CLINICAL FEATURES: Women newly diagnosed with EIN have a 39% chance of having endometrial cancer diagnosed within 1 year. Thus, in most cases the cancer was already present at the time of the initial biopsy. This also explains the clinical adage, "not cancer but better out," as patients with a diagnosis of "atypical hyperplasia" in the older WHO classification system often had cancer if the uterus was removed immediately. Excluding women with concurrent cancer (i.e., only looking at those with a cancer-free interval of 1 year), EIN-positive patients have a 45-fold increased risk of developing of endometrial cancer.

Management aims to remove any coexisting cancer and prevent future cancer. Hysterectomy, which is usually the therapy of choice, meets both goals if a woman does not want more children. Women who want more children, or poor operative risks, may be treated with progestins.

Endometrial Adenocarcinoma

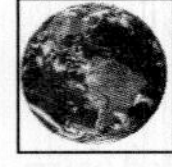

EPIDEMIOLOGY: Endometrial carcinoma is the fourth most frequent cancer in American women and the most common gynecologic cancer (Table 18-5). It caused 6000 deaths in the United States in 2002 (7% of all cancers in women). The incidence of this cancer was stable from 1950 to 1970, but then increased by 40% by 1975, possibly reflecting use of estrogens for easing the symptoms of menopause. By 1985, rates had returned nearly to 1950 levels,

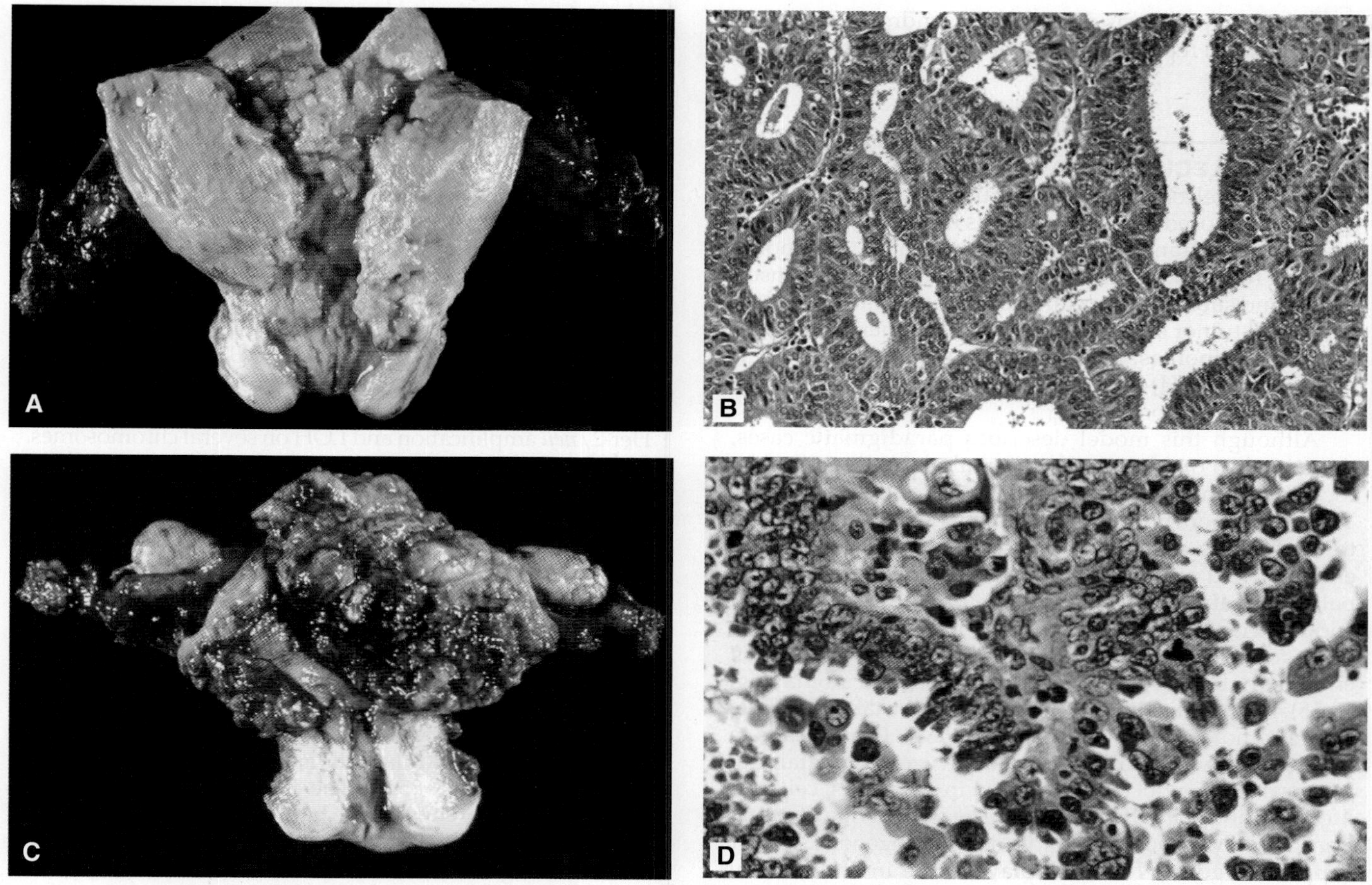

FIGURE 18-34. Adenocarcinoma of the endometrium. A, B. Endometrioid carcinoma. Polypoid tumor with only superficial myometrial invasion. Well-differentiated (grade 1) adenocarcinoma. The neoplastic glands resemble normal endometrial glands. **C, D. Nonendometrioid carcinoma.** Large hemorrhagic and necrotic tumor with deep myometrial invasion. Serous carcinoma (severe cytologic atypia) exhibiting stratification of anaplastic tumor cells and abnormal mitoses.

a trend that correlated with use of lower doses of estrogen, incorporation of progestins (estrogen antagonists) into estrogen replacement regimens and increased surveillance of women treated with estrogens.

The incidence of endometrial cancer varies with age, from 12 cases per 100,000 women at age 40, to 7-fold higher in 60-year-olds. Three quarters of women with endometrial cancer are postmenopausal. The median age at diagnosis is 63.

Endometrial carcinoma is classified into two different types (Fig. 18-34 and Table 18-7). Type I tumors (about 80%), endometrioid carcinomas, are often preceded by EIN precursors and are associated with estrogenic stimulation. They occur mainly in pre- or perimenopausal women and are associated with obesity, hyperlipidemia, anovulation, infertility and late menopause. Typically, most endometrioid carcinomas are confined to the uterus and follow a favorable course. In contrast, type II tumors (about 10%) are nonendometrioid, largely papillary serous carcinomas, arising occasionally in endometrial polyps or from precancerous lesions in atrophic endometria (endometrial "intraepithelial" carcinoma). Type II tumors are not associated with estrogen stimulation or hyperplasia, readily invade myometrium and vascular spaces and are highly lethal. The molecular alterations of endometrioid (type I) carcinomas are different from those of the nonendometrioid (type II) carcinomas.

Endometrial cancer also occurs in association with a higher incidence of both breast and ovarian cancer in closely related women, suggesting a genetic predisposition. It is also the most common extracolonic cancer in women with

Table 18-7

Clinicopathologic Features of Endometrial Carcinoma

	Type I: Endometrioid Carcinoma	Type II: Serous Carcinoma
Age	Pre- and perimenopausal	Postmenopausal
Unopposed estrogen	Present	Absent
Hyperplasia precursor	Present	Absent
Grade	Low	High
Myometrial invasion	Superficial	Deep
Growth behavior	Stable	Progressive
Genetic alterations	Microsatellite instability, PTEN, PIK3CA, β-catenin	p53 mutations, loss of heterozygosity (LOH)

hereditary nonpolyposis colon cancer syndrome, a defect in DNA mismatch repair that is also associated with breast and ovarian cancers.

MOLECULAR PATHOGENESIS: A dualistic model of endometrial carcinogenesis has been proposed. According to this model, normal endometrial cells transform into endometrioid carcinoma through replication errors, so-called "microsatellite instability," and subsequent accumulation of mutations in oncogenes and tumor suppressor genes. For nonendometrioid type of carcinomas, alterations of p53 and loss of heterozygosity (LOH) on several chromosomes drive malignant transformation.

Although this model describes paradigmatic cases, there is often overlap in clinical, pathologic, immunohistochemical and molecular characteristics of the tumors. Thus, some nonendometrioid (type II) carcinomas appear to develop as a result of progression from preexisting endometrioid carcinomas, and such tumors may share the pathologic and molecular features of both types I and II endometrial carcinomas.

Several genetic alterations occur in the transition from endometrial hyperplasia to endometrioid carcinoma (Fig. 18-35). In sporadic tumors, microsatellite instability results from promoter hypermethylation of *hMLH1* and leads to mutations in several critical target genes containing microsatellites, which are involved in apoptosis, cell proliferation and cell differentiation. The wide range of mutations is likely responsible for tumor heterogeneity. Tumor suppressor gene *PTEN* also plays a role in endometrial tumorigenesis (Figs. 18-33 and 18-35). *PTEN* is the most frequently inactivated tumor suppressor gene (2/3 of cases), resulting from deletion, mutation and/or promoter hypermethylation. *PIK3CA* is the most commonly mutated oncogene (up to 39% of cases) in endometrial carcinoma. *PTEN* inactivation frees the PI3K-AKT pathway, avoiding apoptosis and resulting in tumor growth advantage; *PIK3CA* mutations are rarely seen in such cases.

β-Catenin gene mutation occurs in 50% of atypical hyperplasias (with squamous differentiation) and 20% of endometrioid carcinomas. Mutations correlate with MMP-7 and cyclin D1 overexpression. Although they are found more frequently in early tumors associated with good prognosis, their clinical significance is not well established.

Thus, five main molecular alterations have been described in type I endometrioid carcinomas (Fig. 18-35): microsatellite instability (25% to 30% of the cases), *PTEN* mutations (30% to 60%), *PIK3CA* mutations (26% to 39%), *k-RAS* mutations (10% to 30%) and *β*-catenin (*CTNNB1*) mutations with nuclear protein accumulation (25% to 38%). In contrast, most type II nonendometrioid carcinomas have p53 mutations, Her-2/*neu* amplification and LOH on several chromosomes. Nonendometrioid carcinomas may also derive from endometrioid carcinoma with microsatellite instability through tumor progression and subsequent p53 mutations.

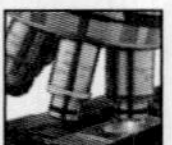

PATHOLOGY: Endometrial cancer grows in diffuse or exophytic patterns (Fig. 18-34). Regardless of its site of origin, the tumor often tends to involve multiple areas. Large tumors are usually hemorrhagic and necrotic.

ENDOMETRIOID ADENOCARCINOMA OF THE ENDOMETRIUM: This type of endometrial cancer is composed entirely of glandular cells and is the most common histologic variant (80%–85%). The FIGO system divides this tumor into three grades on the basis of the ratio of glandular to solid elements, the latter signifying poorer differentiation (Table 18-8; Fig. 18-36).

- **Grade 1:** Well differentiated; almost only neoplastic glands, with minimal (<5%) solid areas
- **Grade 2:** Moderately differentiated; mostly glands and less than half solid tumor
- **Grade 3:** Poorly differentiated; large (>50%) areas of solid tumor

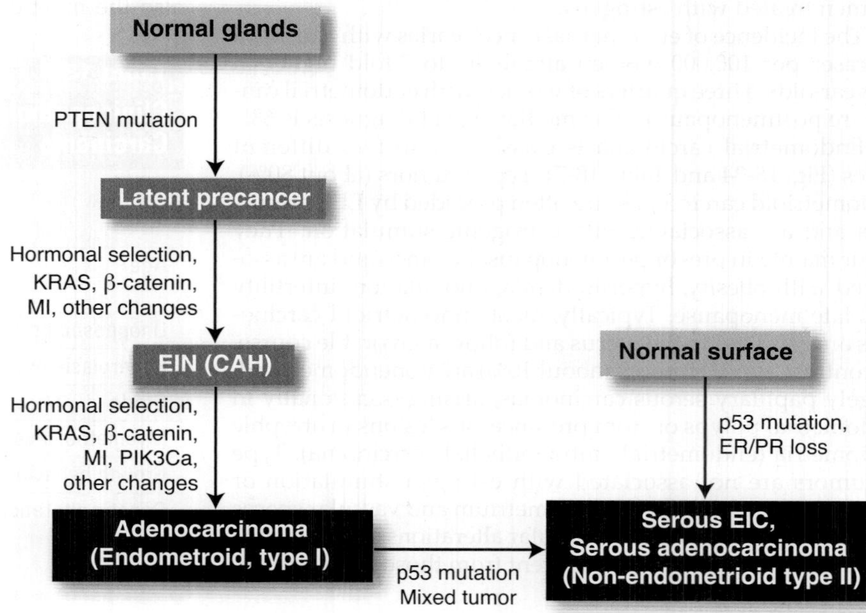

FIGURE 18-35. From endometrial hyperplasia to endometrioid carcinoma: molecular and genetic events. MI, microsattelite instability.

Table 18-8

Surgical Staging and Histopathologic Grading of Endometrial Cancer

Stage	Description
I	Confined to corpus
Ia	No or less than half myometrial invasion
Ib	Invades half or more of the myometrium
II	Invades cervical stroma*
III	Extends beyond uterus but not outside true pelvis
IIIa	Involves serosa or adnexa†
IIIb	Vaginal or parametrial involvement
IIIc	Metastases to pelvic and/or para-aortic lymph nodes
IIIc1	Positive pelvic lymph nodes
IIIc2	Positive para-aortic lymph nodes with or without positive pelvic lymph nodes
IV	Extends beyond true pelvis or involves the mucosa of bladder or rectum
IVa	Spread to adjacent organs
IVb	Spread to distant organs

*Endocervical glandular involvement only should be considered as stage I.
†Positive peritoneal cytology has to be reported separately without changing the stage.
Grading (International Federation of Gynecology and Obstetrics) of glandular tissue: G-1 = <5% solid (highly differentiated); G-2 = 5%–50% solid (differentiated with partly solid areas); G-3 = >50% solid (predominantly solid or entirely undifferentiated).

The nuclei of endometrial adenocarcinoma range from bland to markedly pleomorphic, usually with prominent nucleoli. Mitotic figures are abundant, and may be abnormal in less differentiated tumors. Tumor cells that grow in solid sheets generally are poorly differentiated.

ENDOMETRIOID ADENOCARCINOMA, WITH SQUAMOUS DIFFERENTIATION: One third of endometrial carcinomas contain squamous cells as well as glands. If the squamous element shows only minimal atypia, the tumor is a **well-differentiated adenocarcinoma with squamous differentiation** (previously, **adenoacanthoma**) (Fig. 18-37). If the squamous element appears malignant, the tumor is **poorly differentiated adenocarcinoma with squamous differentiation** (also known as **adenosquamous carcinoma**). These variants represent 22% and 7% of all endometrial cancers, respectively.

ENDOMETRIOID ADENOCARCINOMA, SECRETORY TYPE: This variant usually occurs in premenopausal women. It is an extremely well-differentiated but otherwise typical endometrial adenocarcinoma. Large subnuclear vacuoles of glycogen in some cases are due to progesterone stimulation and may be seen in only one of several serial specimens. Secretory carcinoma, perhaps because it is very well differentiated, has the most favorable prognosis.

OTHER TYPES (NONENDOMETRIOID) OF ENDOMETRIAL CARCINOMA: Nonendometrioid types of endometrial carcinoma are less common, and are not associated with estrogen exposure. They are aggressive as a group, and histologic grading is not clinically useful or separately diagnosed, all cases being considered high grade.

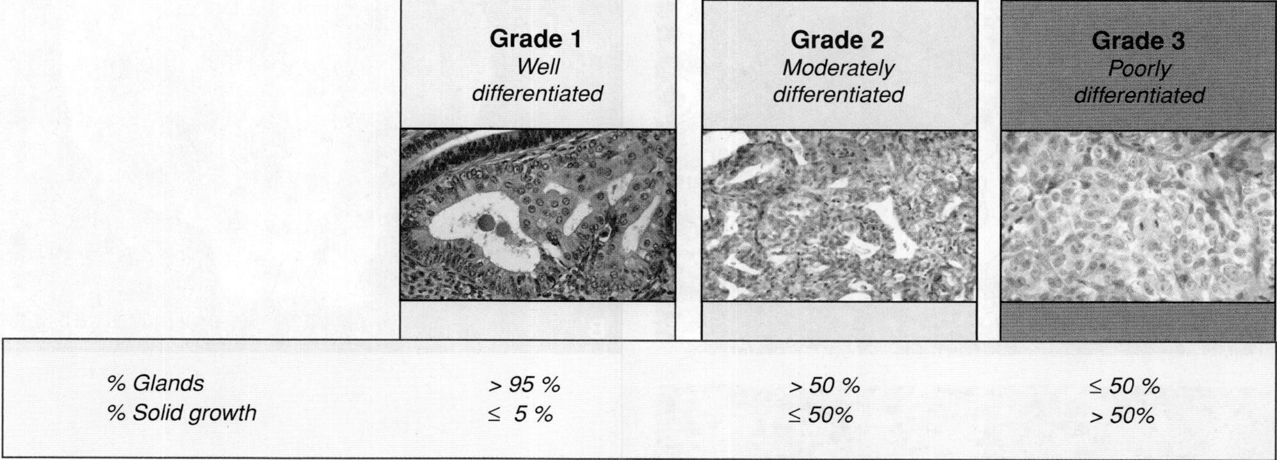

FIGURE 18-36. Grading of endometrial adenocarcinoma. The grade depends primarily on the architectural pattern, but significant nuclear atypia changes a grade 1 tumor to grade 2, and a grade 2 tumor to grade 3. Nuclear atypia is characterized by round nuclei; variation in shape, size and staining; hyperchromasia; coarsely clumped chromating; prominent nucleoli; and frequent and abnormal mitoses. Significant nuclear atypia if present increases the tumor grade.

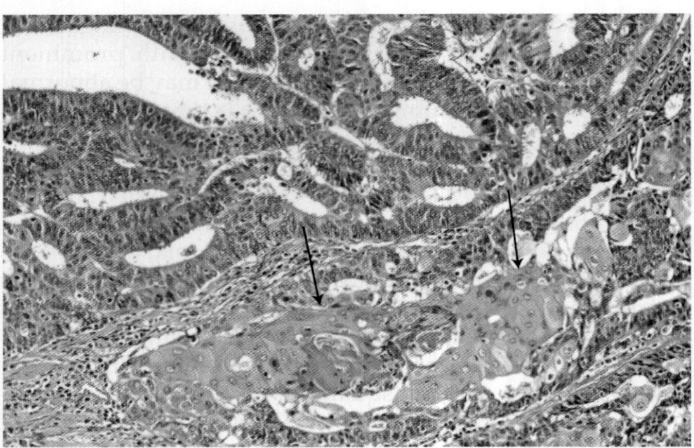

FIGURE 18-37. Squamous differentiation in endometrioid adenocarcinoma of the endometrium. The well-differentiated squamous cells (*arrows*) show minimal atypia. The pattern has been called adenoacanthoma when the squamous cells form squamous morules and nest among glands.

- **Serous adenocarcinoma** histologically resembles, and behaves like, serous adenocarcinoma of the ovary (Fig. 18-34D). It often shows transtubal spread to peritoneal surfaces. An in situ form has been termed "serous endometrial intraepithelial carcinoma" (serous EIC), not to be confused with EIN, described earlier. Patients with this type of tumor need to be staged and treated as if they had ovarian cancer.
- **Clear cell adenocarcinoma** is a tumor of older women. It contains large cells with abundant cytoplasmic glycogen ("clear cells") or cells with bulbous nuclei that line glandular lumina ("hobnail cells") (Fig. 18-38A). Serous and clear cell carcinomas have poor prognoses.
- **Carcinosarcoma (malignant mixed mesodermal tumor):** In this highly malignant tumor (Fig. 18-38B), pleomorphic **epithelial** cells intermingle with areas showing **mesenchymal** differentiation (Fig. 18-38C). These mixed neoplasms are derived from a common clone believed to be of epithelial origin. The prognosis is determined by the presence of a mesenchymal component admixed with the malignant epithelial component, rather than the specific type of mesenchymal histology displayed. Overall 5-year survival is 25%.

Although most endometrial carcinomas arise in the uterine corpus, a small proportion originate in the lower uterine segment (isthmus). These tumors often occur in women under the age of 50 and are often high grade and deeply invasive.

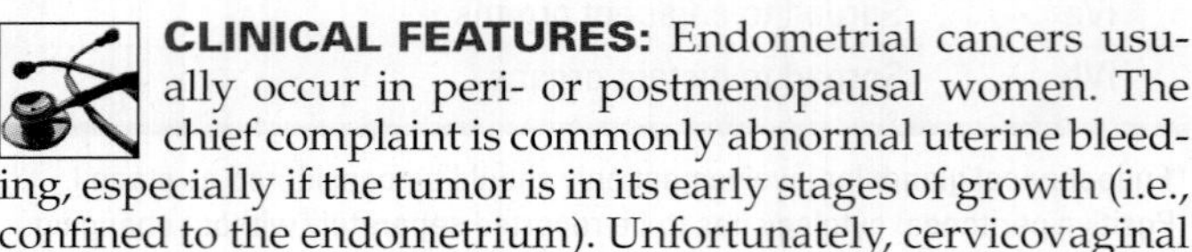

CLINICAL FEATURES: Endometrial cancers usually occur in peri- or postmenopausal women. The chief complaint is commonly abnormal uterine bleeding, especially if the tumor is in its early stages of growth (i.e., confined to the endometrium). Unfortunately, cervicovaginal

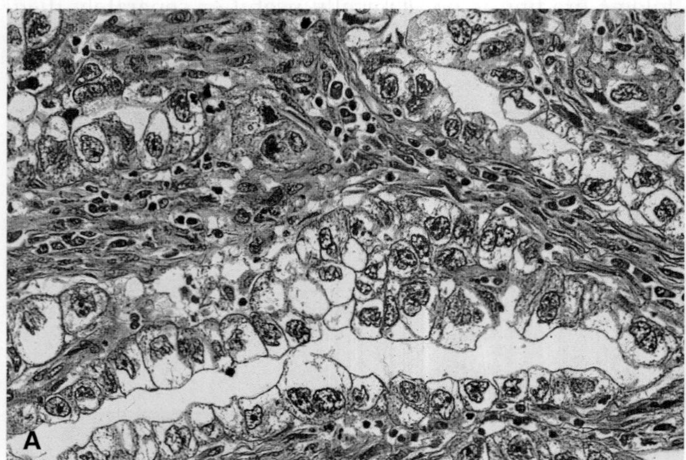

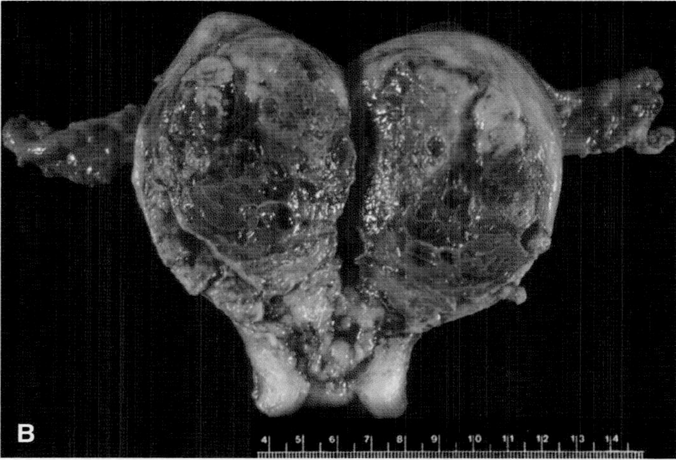

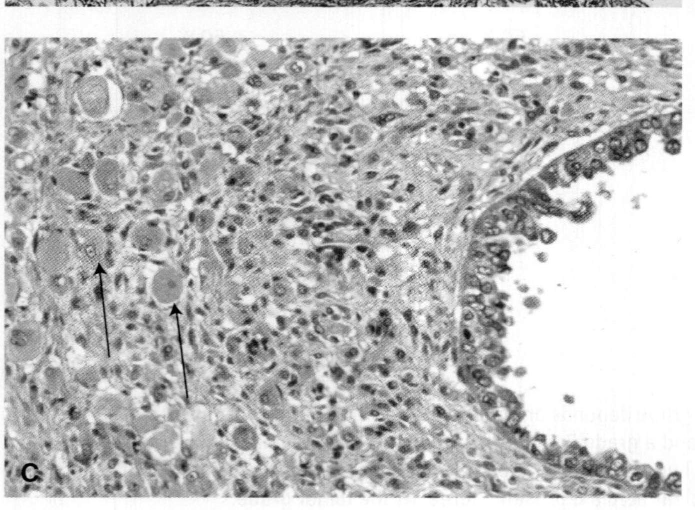

FIGURE 18-38. Nonendometrioid types of endometrial adenocarcinoma. A. Clear cell endometrial adenocarcinoma. The clear appearance of the cytoplasm is due to the dissolution of glycogen when the specimen was processed for microscopic examination. Hobnail cells with bulbous nuclei line glandular lumina. **B. Carcinosarcoma (malignant mixed mullerian tumor).** Solid, partially cystic and necrotic mass that expands the uterine cavity. **C.** Rhabdomyoblasts (*heterologous elements, arrows*) appear as pleomorphic, rounded cells with ample eosinophilic cytoplasm adjacent to malignant epithelium.

cytologic screening does not detect early endometrial cancer. Fractional curettage is needed to assess spread to the cervix, whereas peritoneal washing detects tubal reflux and abdominal contamination. Transvaginal ultrasonography is a valuable diagnostic modality; endometrium more than 5 mm thick is considered highly suspicious. Unlike cervical cancer, endometrial cancer may spread directly to para-aortic lymph nodes, thereby skipping pelvic nodes. Patients with advanced cancers may also develop pulmonary metastases (40% of cases with metastases).

Women with well-differentiated cancers confined to the endometrium are usually treated by simple hysterectomy. Postoperative radiation is considered if (1) the tumor is poorly differentiated or nonendometrioid in type, (2) myometrium is deeply invaded, (3) the cervix is involved or (4) lymph nodes contain metastases.

Survival in endometrial carcinoma is related to multiple factors: (1) stage, histotype and, for endometrioid tumors, grade (2) age; and (3) other risk factors, such as progesterone receptor activity, depth of myometrial invasion, extent of lymphovascular invasion and results of peritoneal washings. High tumor levels of estrogen and progesterone receptors and low mitotic rates correlate with a better prognosis. Actuarial survival of all patients with endometrial cancer following treatment is 80% after 2 years, decreasing to 65% after 10 years. Tumors that have penetrated the myometrium or invaded lymphatics are more likely to have spread beyond the uterus. Endometrial cancers involving the cervix have a poorer prognosis. Spread outside the uterus entails the worst outlook (Table 18-9).

Table 18-9

Stage, Grade and Survival for Endometrial Cancer

Stage	5-Year Survival (%)		
	G-1*	G-2	G-3
I	90	69	52
II	80	42	12
III, IV	25	33	17

*G = FIGO (International Federation of Gynecology and Obstetrics) grade.

Endometrial Stromal Tumors Account for Under 2% of All Uterine Cancers

Some endometrial stromal tumors are pure sarcomas; in others sarcomatous (stromal) and epithelial elements are intermingled. The nomenclature of these tumor types, the spectrum of their histologic components and the correlation of each tumor type with its potential for malignant behavior are presented in Table 18-10.

Endometrial Stromal Sarcoma

Pure stromal tumors are divided into two major categories, based on whether the tumor margin is expansile or infiltrating. Expansile lesions that do not invade are **benign stromal nodules**, which have little clinical significance. Tumors with infiltrating margins are termed **stromal sarcomas.**

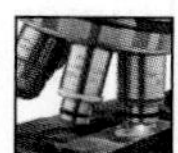

PATHOLOGY: Endometrial stromal sarcomas may be polypoid and fill the endometrial cavity, or they may diffusely invade the myometrium. Large masses of spindle cells with scant cytoplasm dissect the myometrium and invade vascular channels (Fig. 18-39). The tumor cells resemble endometrial stromal cells in the proliferative phase. Nuclear atypia may be minimal to severe and mitotic activity may be

Table 18-10

Nomenclature of Uterine Tumors

Tumor	Epithelium	Stroma	Clinical Behavior
Epithelium and Stroma			
Endometrial polyp	Polyclonal benign	Neoplastic	Benign
Benign endometrial hyperplasia	Polyclonal benign	Polyclonal benign	Benign
Endometrial intraepithelial neoplasia	Neoplastic	—	Premalignant
Endometrial adenocarcinoma	Neoplastic	—	Malignant
Endometrial stromal nodule	—	Neoplastic	Benign
Endometrial stromal sarcoma	—	Neoplastic	Low-grade malignant
Undifferentiated sarcoma	—	Neoplastic	Malignant
Adenosarcoma	Unknown	Neoplastic	Low-grade malignant
Carcinosarcoma	Neoplastic	Neoplastic, transformed epithelial cells	Malignant
Smooth Muscle			
Leiomyoma	—	Neoplastic	Benign
Cellular leiomyoma	—	Neoplastic	Benign
Intravenous leiomyomatosis	—	Neoplastic	Locally aggressive
Leiomyosarcoma	—	Neoplastic	Malignant

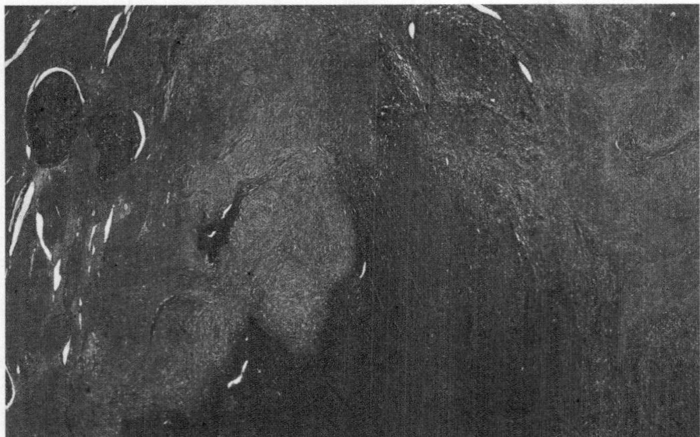

FIGURE 18-39. Endometrial stromal sarcoma, low grade. The myometrium is irregularly invaded by the tumor, which invades vascular spaces.

restrained. Expression of CD-10 and estrogen and progesterone receptors helps confirm the diagnosis. Higher-grade sarcomas originating in the endometrium lose all antigenic and morphologic resemblance to endometrial stroma and are thus designated as **undifferentiated endometrial sarcoma.**

CLINICAL FEATURES: Many years may elapse before endometrial stromal sarcomas recur clinically, and metastases may occur even if the original tumor was confined to the uterus at initial surgery. Recurrences usually involve the pelvis first, followed by lung metastases. Prolonged survival and even cure are feasible, despite metastases. By contrast, undifferentiated endometrial sarcomas recur early, generally with widespread metastases, even if there had been little myometrial invasion. Endometrial stromal sarcomas can be successfully treated with surgery and progestin therapy, with an expectation of 90% survival 10 years after diagnosis.

Uterine Adenosarcoma

Uterine (müllerian) adenosarcoma is a distinctive low-grade tumor with benign glandular epithelium and malignant stroma (Fig. 18-40). It should be distinguished from carcinosarcoma, in which both epithelial and stromal elements are malignant and which is highly aggressive.

Adenosarcoma typically presents as a polypoid mass within the endometrial cavity. The glandular epithelium resembles proliferative phase endometrial glands, but occasionally squamous epithelium and mucinous-type epithelium are seen. The stroma is cellular, may exhibit mitotic activity, is often densest about the glandular epithelium (periglandular cuffing) and resembles endometrial stromal cells in the proliferative phase of the cycle. One fourth of patients with adenosarcoma eventually succumb to local recurrence or metastatic spread.

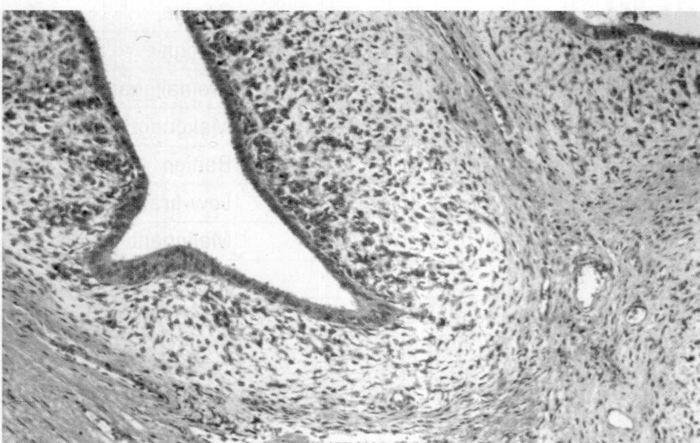

FIGURE 18-40. Adenosarcoma. There is periglandular cuffing by atypical stromal cells with mitotic activity.

Leiomyoma Is the Most Common Tumor of the Female Genital Tract

Leiomyomas, benign tumors of smooth muscle origin, are colloquially known as "myomas" or "fibroids." Including minute tumors, leiomyomas occur in 75% of women over age 30. They are rare before age 20, and most regress after menopause. Although often multiple, each tumor is monoclonal (see Chapter 5). Estrogen promotes their growth, but does not initiate them.

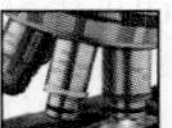

PATHOLOGY: Grossly, leiomyomas are firm, pale gray, whorled and without encapsulation (Figs. 18-41 and 18-42). They vary from 1 mm to over 30 cm in diameter. Their cut surface bulges and borders are smooth and distinct from neighboring myometrium. Most leiomyomas are intramural, but some are submucosal, subserosal or pedunculated. Many, especially larger ones, show areas of

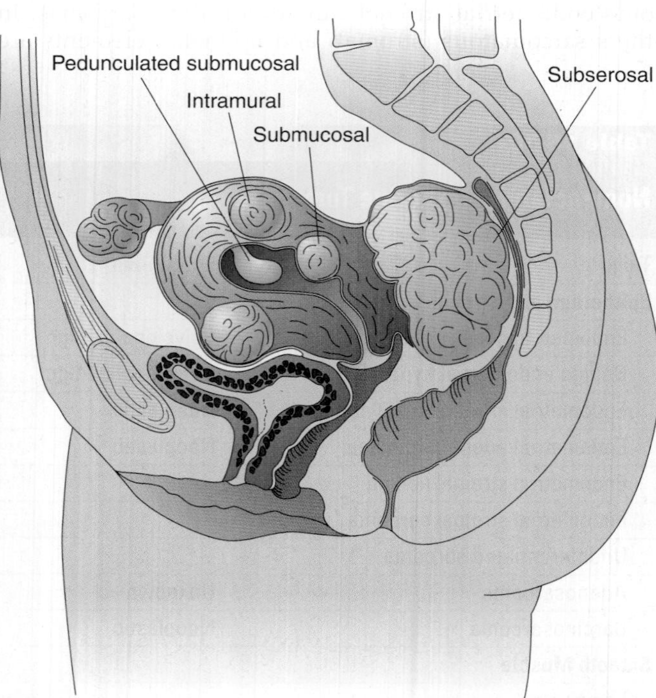

FIGURE 18-41. Leiomyomas of the uterus. The leiomyomas are intramural, submucosal (a pedunculated one appearing in the form of an endometrial polyp) and subserosal (one compressing the bladder and the other the rectum).

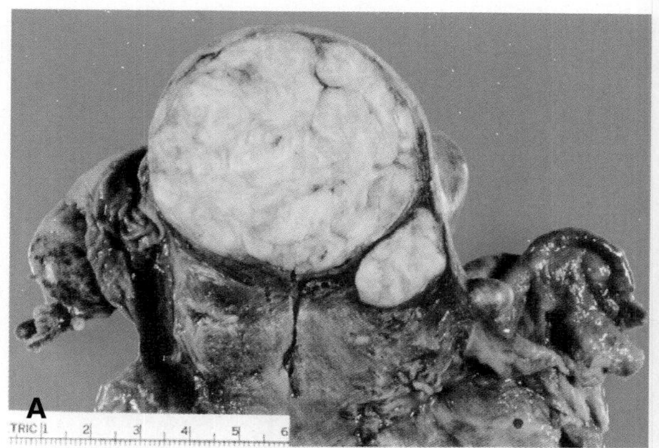

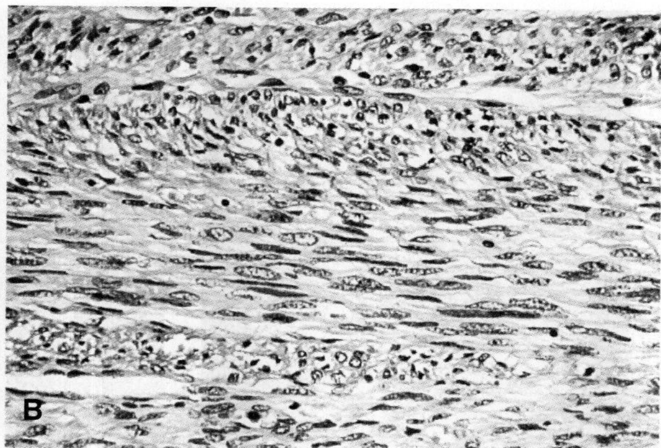

FIGURE 18-42. Leiomyoma of the uterus. A. A bisected uterus displays a prominent, sharply circumscribed, fleshy tumor. **B.** Microscopically, smooth muscle cells intertwine in bundles, some of which are cut longitudinally (elongated nuclei) and others transversely.

degenerative hyalinization that are sharply demarcated from adjacent normal myometrium. Leiomyomas show little mitotic activity (<4 mitoses per 10 high-power fields [HPFs]), lack nuclear atypia and geographical necrosis and have little or no malignant potential. "**Mitotically active leiomyoma,**" is one that shows brisk mitotic activity but is relatively small, is sharply demarcated from adjacent normal myometrium and lacks both geographical necrosis and significant cellular atypia. It is usually benign.

Microscopically, leiomyomas exhibit interlacing fascicles of uniform spindle cells, in which nuclei are elongated and have blunt ends (Fig. 18-42B). Cytoplasm is abundant, eosinophilic and fibrillar. The cells of leiomyomas and adjacent myometrium are cytologically identical, but leiomyomas are easily distinguished by their circumscription, nodularity and denser cellularity.

CLINICAL FEATURES: Submucosal leiomyomas may cause bleeding due to ulceration of thinned, overlying endometrium, or become pedunculated and protrude through the cervical os, eliciting cramping pains. Many intramural leiomyomas are symptomatic because of sheer bulk, and large ones may interfere with bowel or bladder function or cause dystocia in labor. Pedunculated leiomyomas on the uterine serosa may interfere with the function of neighboring viscera. Leiomyomas may also infarct and become painful if they undergo torsion.

Leiomyomas usually grow slowly, but occasionally enlarge rapidly during pregnancy. Large symptomatic leiomyomas are removed by myomectomy or hysterectomy. Ablation by arterial thrombosis has also been used recently.

Intravenous Leiomyomatosis Does Not Metastasize

Intravenous leiomyomatosis is a rare condition in which benign smooth muscle grows within uterine and pelvic veins. The condition may originate from vascular invasion by a preexisting uterine leiomyoma or growth of venous smooth muscle. It may be evident at surgery as wormlike extensions near the external uterine surface or as projections into uterine veins in the broad ligament. Although they may grow extensively inside blood vessels, these neoplasms do not metastasize. Rare fatalities have resulted from direct extension of leiomyomas from pelvic veins into the inferior vena cava and right atrium. Treatment consists of total abdominal hysterectomy.

Leiomyosarcoma Is Very Rare in Comparison to Leiomyoma

Leiomyosarcoma is a malignancy of smooth muscle origin whose incidence is only 1/1000 that of its benign counterpart. It accounts for 2% of uterine malignancies. Its pathogenesis is uncertain, but at least some appear to arise from within leiomyomas. Women with leiomyosarcomas are on average more than a decade older (age above 50) than those with leiomyomas, and the malignant tumors are larger (10 to 15 cm vs. 3 to 5 cm) (Fig. 18-43A).

PATHOLOGY: Leiomyosarcoma should be suspected if an apparent leiomyoma is soft, shows areas of necrosis on gross examination, has irregular borders (invasion of adjacent myometrium) or does not bulge above the surface when cut. Mitotic activity, cellular atypia and geographical necrosis are the best diagnostic criteria. There is usually a sharp transition from viable tumor to large zones of necrosis, with an intervening rim of partially viable tumor cells. Blood vessels, if present, may be surrounded by a thin rim of viable tumor cells. Evidence that a uterine smooth muscle tumor is a leiomyosarcoma includes (1) presence of geographical necrosis (Fig. 18-43B); (2) 10 or more mitoses per 10 HPFs (Fig. 18-43C), if the tumor is more than 5 cm in diameter; (3) 5 or more mitoses per 10 HPFs, with geographical necrosis and diffuse cytoplasmic/nuclear atypia; and (4) myxoid and epithelioid smooth muscle tumors with 5 or more mitoses per 10 HPFs. Size is important: tumors under 5 cm in diameter almost never recur.

Most leiomyosarcomas are large and are advanced when detected. They thus are usually fatal despite combinations of surgery, radiation therapy and chemotherapy. Nearly half of recurrences first present in the lung, and 5-year survival is about 20%.

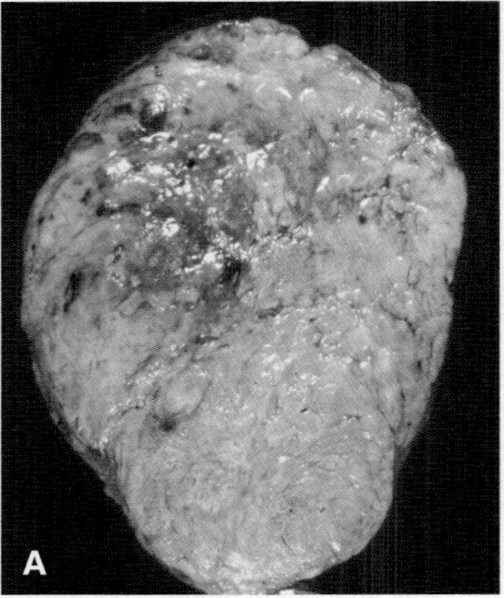

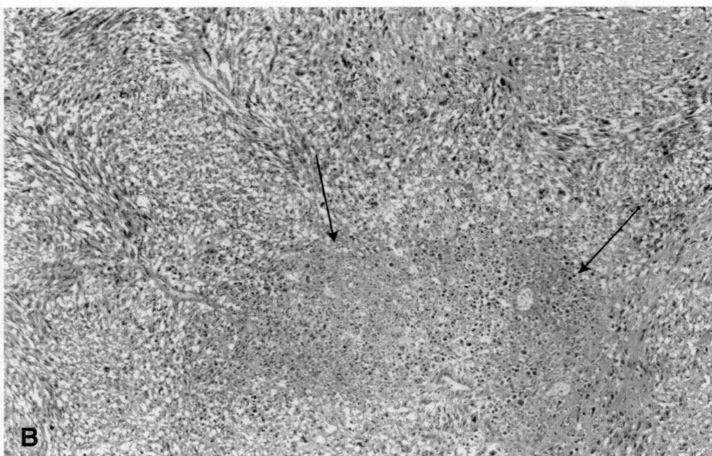

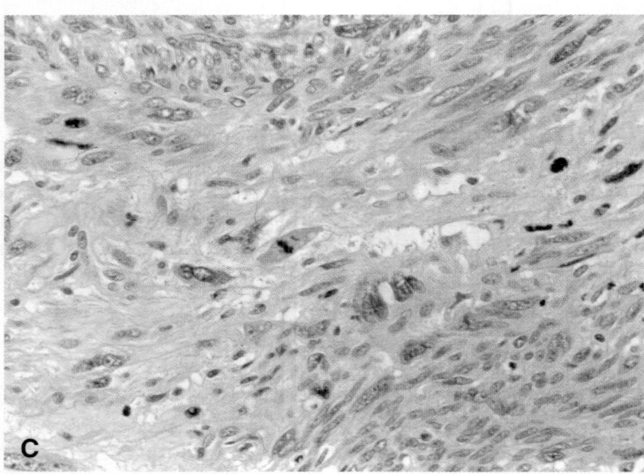

FIGURE 18-43. Leiomyosarcoma of the uterus. **A.** The uterus has been opened to reveal a large, soft leiomyosarcoma with extensive necrosis that replaces the entire myometrium. **B.** A zone of coagulative tumor necrosis (*arrows*) appears demarcated from the viable tumor. **C.** The tumor shows considerable nuclear atypia and abundant mitotic activity.

FALLOPIAN TUBE

Anatomy

The fallopian tubes extend from the uterine fundus to the ovaries. An interstitial portion, the **isthmus,** lies within the cornua of the uterus and connects the uterine cavity with the straight portion of the tube. As the tube extends to the ovary, it increases in diameter to form the **ampulla,** which merges with the **infundibulum.** The fimbriated end opens like the bell of a trumpet and has many fingerlike extensions that envelop the ovary. The lining cells are ciliated and are important in transport of ova.

Salpingitis

Salpingitis is inflammation of the fallopian tubes, typically due to infections ascending from the lower genital trac*t*. The most common causative organisms are *N. gonorrhoeae, Escherichia coli, Chlamydia* and *Mycoplasma,* and most infections are polymicrobial. Acute episodes of salpingitis (particularly if associated with chlamydia) may be asymptomatic. A fallopian tube damaged by prior infection is particularly susceptible to reinfection. In most cases, chronic salpingitis develops only after repeated episodes of acute salpingitis.

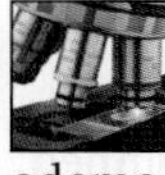
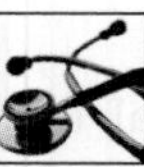

PATHOLOGY AND CLINICAL FEATURES: In acute salpingitis, there is marked polymorphonuclear infiltration, pronounced edema and congestion of mucosal folds (plicae). In chronic salpingitis the inflammatory infiltrate is mainly lymphocytes and plasma cells; edema and congestion are usually minimal. In late stages, the fallopian tube may seal and become distended with pus **(pyosalpinx)** or a transudate **(hydrosalpinx).**

The fallopian tube allows infections from the lower genital tract to ascend to the peritoneal cavity, leading to peritonitis and PID. Fibrinous adhesions between the fallopian tube serosa and surrounding peritoneal surfaces organize into thin fibrous adhesions ("violin string" adhesions). The adjacent ovary may also be involved, sometimes giving rise to a **tuboovarian abscess.**

Complications also ensue from damage to the fallopian tube itself. Destruction of the epithelium or deposition of fibrin on the mucosa leads to fibrin bridges, which cause the plicae to adhere to one another. In severe chronic salpingitis, adhesions are dense and form a blunted, clubbed end of the tube. The consequence of a blocked lumen may be hydrosalpinx or pyosalpinx. The damage wrought by chronic salpingitis may impair general tubal motility and passage of sperm, in which case **infertility** results. Chronic salpingitis is a common cause of **ectopic pregnancy,** since adherent mucosal plicae create pockets in which ova are entrapped.

Ectopic Pregnancy

Ectopic pregnancy implies implantation of a fertilized ovum outside the endometrium. The frequency of ectopic pregnancy in the United States has increased threefold, to 1.5% of live births, in the past two decades, although mortality has sharply declined. ***Over 95% of ectopic pregnancies occur in the fallopian tube, mostly in the distal and middle thirds.***

PATHOLOGY: Ectopic pregnancy results when passage of a conceptus along a fallopian tube is impeded, for example, by mucosal adhesions or abnormal tubal motility due to inflammatory disease or endometriosis. The trophoblast readily penetrates the tubal mucosa and musculature. Blood from the tubal implantation site enters the peritoneum, causing abdominal pain. Ectopic pregnancy is also associated with anomalous uterine bleeding after a period of amenorrhea, and Arias-Stella cells in the endometrium. The thin tubal wall usually ruptures by the 12th week of gestation. ***Tubal rupture is life-threatening as it can lead to rapid exsanguination.***

Rupture of the tube's interstitial portion produces greater intra-abdominal hemorrhage than rupture in other locations because vasculature there is richer and rupture occurs later in gestation. In the isthmus, the tube ruptures early (within the first 6 weeks), because its thick muscular wall does not allow much distention. Tubal pregnancies in the ampulla tend to be of longer duration, since the distensible tubal wall can accommodate a growing pregnancy for a longer time.

Ectopic pregnancy must be treated promptly with surgery or chemotherapy. Administration of methotrexate terminates ectopic pregnancy, and is used when the conceptus is smaller than 4 cm.

Fallopian Tube Tumors

Tumors of the fallopian tube are rare. The most common is the small, circumscribed **adenomatoid tumor,** which is of mesothelial origin. It arises in the mesosalpinx and shows benign mesothelial cells that line slitlike spaces.

Fallopian tube involvement by metastases or implants from adjacent ovarian and uterine neoplasms far exceeds the frequency of the rare primary cancer. Most primary malignancies are adenocarcinomas, with peak incidence among 50- to 60-year-olds. Recent observations suggest that many cases of high-grade serous carcinoma of the ovary (see below) may arise from the fimbriated end of the fallopian tube. The tumor is bilateral in 25% of cases. Prognosis is poor, as the disease is almost always detected at a late stage. Treatment is similar to ovarian cancer.

OVARY

Anatomy and Embryology

The ovaries are paired organs that flank the uterus. They are attached to the posterior surface of the broad ligament in a shallow peritoneal fossa between the external iliac vessels and the ureter. Each ovary consists of (1) an epithelial surface, (2) a mesenchymal stroma containing steroid-producing cells and (3) germ cells. It has an outer cortex and inner medulla.

Ovaries appear early in fetal life as swellings of the genital ridges. At the 19th gestational day germ cells migrate from the primitive yolk sac to the gonads and multiply by mitotic division. By the 40th day, ovaries and testes are histologically distinct. Toward the third trimester of fetal life, germ cells stop multiplying and instead continue to develop by meiosis. Of 1 million primordial follicles present at birth, only 70% remain by puberty and fewer than 15% persist to age 25 years. Only some 450 ova are actually shed during a woman's average 35-year reproductive lifetime.

The ovarian cortex mesenchyme consists of spindle-shaped, fibroblast-like cells. These give rise to granulosa and theca cells, which form a functional unit about each ovum (theca interna and theca externa). The complex of a germ cell and supporting granulosa cells is known first as a **primordial follicle**. During the reproductive period, a dominant follicle develops every month into a **graafian follicle,** which then ruptures during ovulation. Ovulation itself is often associated with mild cramping pain, which, if severe, is called **mittelschmerz** (i.e., midcycle pain). It is frequently confused with appendicitis. After ovulation the follicle granulosa cells luteinize, with hypertrophy and lipid accumulation. They then secrete progesterone in addition to estrogens. The collapsed follicle turns bright yellow and becomes the **corpus luteum** (yellow body).

The cells of ovarian stromal origin include hilus cells and those resembling luteinized cells of the theca interna, both of which respond to pituitary hormones. These specialized cells make and secrete both androgens and estrogens, which stimulate proliferation in end organs (e.g., uterus). They inhibit hypothalamic function by negative feedback loops.

Cystic Lesions of the Ovaries

Cysts are the most common cause of enlarged ovaries. Cysts arising from the invaginated surface epithelium (serous cysts) are quite common. Almost all of the rest derive from ovarian follicles.

Follicle Cysts Tend to Be Asymptomatic

Follicle cysts are thin-walled, fluid-filled structures lined internally by granulosa cells and externally by theca interna cells. They occur at any age up to menopause, are unilocular and may be single or multiple, unilateral or bilateral. These cysts arise from ovarian follicles and are probably related to abnormalities in pituitary gonadotropin release.

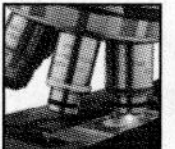

PATHOLOGY: Follicle cysts rarely exceed 5 cm in diameter. In an unstimulated state, the granulosa cells of the cyst have uniform, round nuclei and little cytoplasm. Thecal cells are small and spindle shaped. Occasionally, the layers may be luteinized, and the lumen wall contains fluid high in estrogen or progesterone. If the cyst persists, hormonal output can cause precocious puberty in a child and menstrual irregularities in an adult. The only significant complication is mild intraperitoneal bleeding (Fig. 18-44).

Corpus Luteum Cyst Can Bleed

A corpus luteum cyst results from delayed resolution of a corpus luteum's central cavity. Continued progesterone synthesis by the

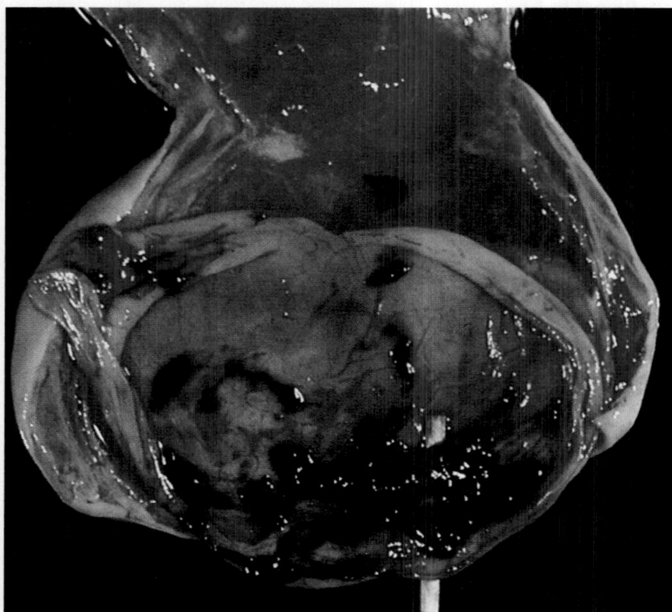

FIGURE 18-44. Follicle cyst of the ovary. The rupture of this thin-walled follicular cyst (dowel stick) led to intra-abdominal hemorrhage.

luteal cyst leads to menstrual irregularities. Rupture of a cyst can cause mild hemorrhage into the abdominal cavity. A corpus luteum cyst is typically unilocular, 3 to 5 cm in size and possessed of a yellow wall. Cyst contents vary from serosanguineous fluid to clotted blood. Microscopic examination shows numerous large, luteinized granulosa cells. The condition is self-limited.

Theca Lutein Cysts Relate to High Gonadotropin Levels

Theca lutein cysts are also known as *hyperreactio luteinalis* and are commonly multiple and bilateral. They are associated with high levels of circulating gonadotropin (as in pregnancy, hydatidiform mole, choriocarcinoma or exogenous gonadotropin therapy) or physical impediments (dense adhesions, cortical fibrosis) to ovulation. The excessive gonadotropin levels lead to exaggerated stimulation of the theca interna and extensive cyst formation.

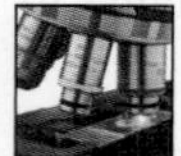

PATHOLOGY: Multiple thin-walled cysts filled with clear fluid and a markedly luteinized layer of theca interna replace both ovaries. Ovarian parenchyma shows edema and foci of luteinized stromal cells. Intra-abdominal hemorrhage due to torsion or rupture of the cyst may require surgical intervention.

Polycystic Ovary Syndrome

Presentation of polycystic ovary syndrome, or **Stein-Leventhal syndrome,** reflects (1) excess secretion of androgenic hormones, (2) persistent anovulation and (3) ovaries containing many small subcapsular cysts. It was described initially as a syndrome of **secondary amenorrhea, hirsutism and obesity.** However, clinical presentations are now known to be far more variable and include amenorrheic women who

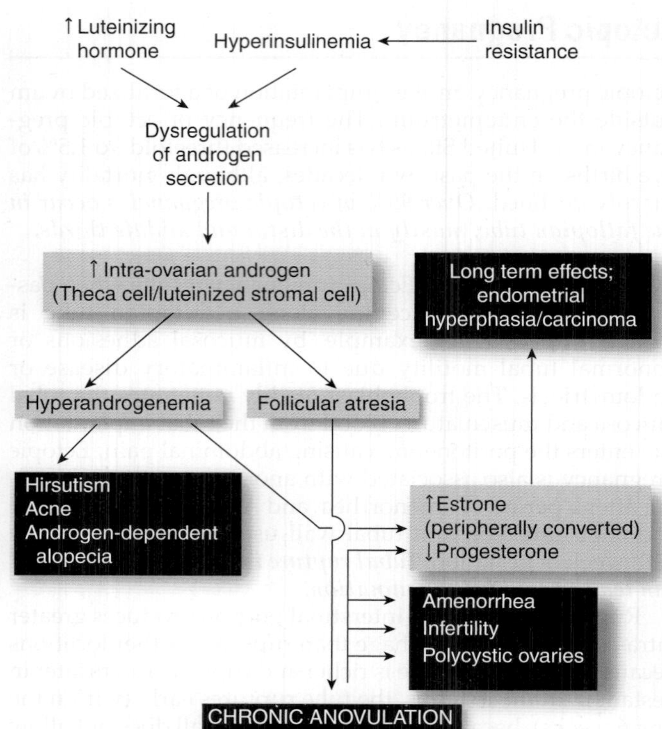

FIGURE 18-45. Pathogenesis of polycystic ovary syndrome.

appear otherwise normal and, even rarely, have ovaries lacking polycystic features. ***This condition is a common cause of infertility: up to 7% of women experience polycystic ovary syndrome.***

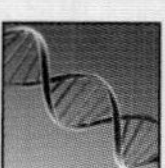

MOLECULAR PATHOGENESIS: Polycystic ovary syndrome is a state of functional ovarian hyperandrogenism with elevated levels of LH, although increased LH is probably a result, rather than a cause, of ovarian dysfunction (Fig. 18-45).

1. The central abnormality is thought to be increased ovarian production of androgens, although adrenal hypersecretion of androgens may also occur. The rate-limiting enzyme in androgen biosynthesis, cytochrome $P450_{c17\alpha}$ (17α-hydroxylase), which is expressed in both the ovary and the adrenal gland, is abnormally regulated.
2. Excess ovarian androgens act locally to cause (a) premature follicular atresia, (b) multiple follicular cysts and (c) a persistent anovulatory state. Impaired follicular maturation causes decreased secretion of progesterone. Peripherally, hyperandrogenism leads to hirsutism, acne and male-pattern (androgen-dependent) alopecia. These patients may have high levels of serum androgens, such as testosterone, androstenedione and dehydroepiandrosterone sulfate. But there are individual variations and some patients have normal androgen levels.
3. Excess androgens are converted to estrogens in peripheral adipose tissue, an effect that is exaggerated by obesity. Acyclic estrogen production and progesterone deficiency increase pituitary secretion of LH.

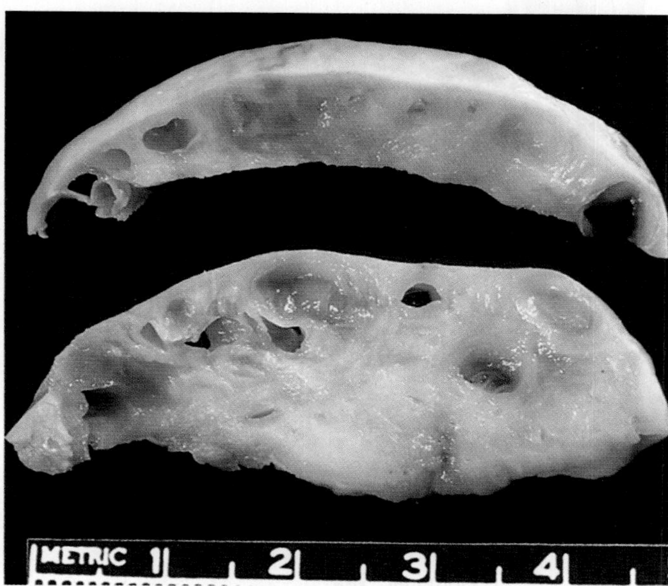

FIGURE 18-46. Polycystic disease of the ovary. Cut sections of an ovary show numerous cysts embedded in a sclerotic stroma.

> 4. Women with polycystic ovary syndrome exhibit marked peripheral insulin resistance, out of proportion to the degree of obesity. The mechanism appears to involve a post–insulin-receptor defect, possibly related to decreased expression of a glucose transporter. In any event, the resulting hyperinsulinemia seems to contribute to increased ovarian hypersecretion of androgens and direct stimulation of pituitary LH production.

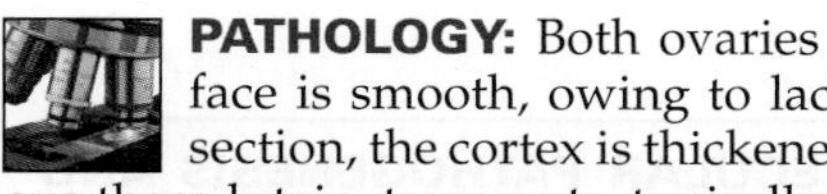

PATHOLOGY: Both ovaries are enlarged. The surface is smooth, owing to lack of ovulation. On cut section, the cortex is thickened and discloses numerous theca lutein–type cysts, typically 2 to 8 mm in diameter, arranged peripherally around a dense core of stroma or scattered throughout an increased amount of stroma (Fig. 18-46). Microscopic features include (1) numerous follicles in early stages of development; (2) follicular atresia; (3) increased stroma, occasionally with luteinized cells (hyperthecosis); and (4) signs of the absence of ovulation (thick, smooth capsule, and absence of corpora lutea and corpora albicantia). Many subcapsular cysts show thick zones of theca interna, in which some cells may be luteinized.

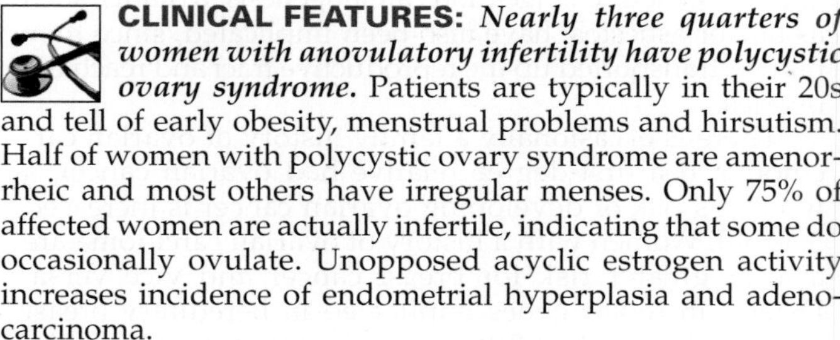

CLINICAL FEATURES: ***Nearly three quarters of women with anovulatory infertility have polycystic ovary syndrome.*** Patients are typically in their 20s and tell of early obesity, menstrual problems and hirsutism. Half of women with polycystic ovary syndrome are amenorrheic and most others have irregular menses. Only 75% of affected women are actually infertile, indicating that some do occasionally ovulate. Unopposed acyclic estrogen activity increases incidence of endometrial hyperplasia and adenocarcinoma.

Treatment of polycystic ovary syndrome encompasses two common problems in reproductive endocrinology—hirsutism and anovulation. Therapy is mostly hormonal and seeks to interrupt the constant excess of androgens. Wedge resection of the ovary provides temporary remission of the syndrome, but is rarely used today.

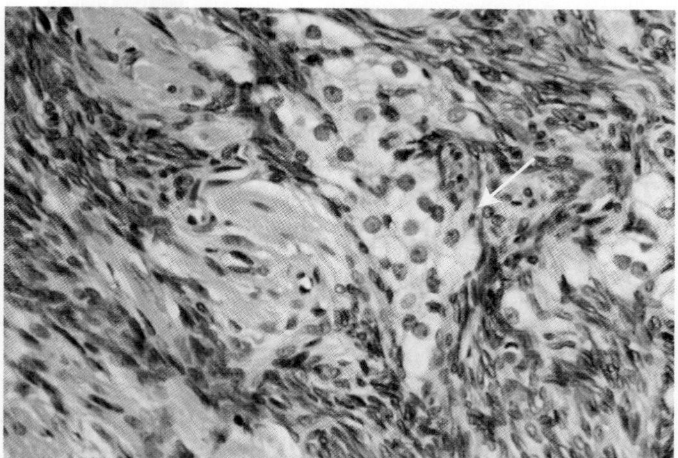

FIGURE 18-47. Hyperthecosis of the ovary. Nests of luteinized (lipid-rich) stromal cells are present (*arrow*).

Stromal Hyperthecosis

Stromal hyperthecosis is focal luteinization of ovarian stromal cells. These stromal cells are often functional and cause **virilization.** The condition is most common in postmenopausal women and, in a microscopic form, is found in one third of postmenopausal ovaries.

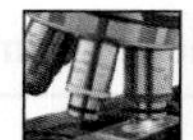

PATHOLOGY: If stromal hyperthecosis is detected clinically, usually due to masculinizing signs, both ovaries may be enlarged, sometimes up to 8 cm in greatest dimension. The serosa is smooth, and the cut surface is homogeneous, firm and brown to yellow. Single nests or nodules of luteinized stromal cells with deeply eosinophilic, often vacuolated cytoplasm are seen in the cortex or medulla (Fig. 18-47). The luteinized cells have a central large nucleus with a prominent nucleolus, a feature shared with all hormonally active stromal cells in the ovary.

Ovarian Tumors

There are many types of ovarian tumors including benign, borderline and malignant ones. About two thirds occur in women of reproductive age; less than 5% develop in children. Approximately 80% of ovarian tumors are benign. Almost 90% of malignant and borderline tumors are diagnosed after the age of 40 years.

Ovarian tumors are classified by the ovarian cell type of origin (Fig. 18-48). Most are **common epithelial tumors** (approximately 60%) and arise from serosal epithelium. Other important groups are germ cell tumors (30%), sex cord/stromal tumors (8%) and tumors metastatic to the ovary. In the Western world, common epithelial tumors account for about 90% of ovarian malignancies, serous adenocarcinoma being the most common among these.

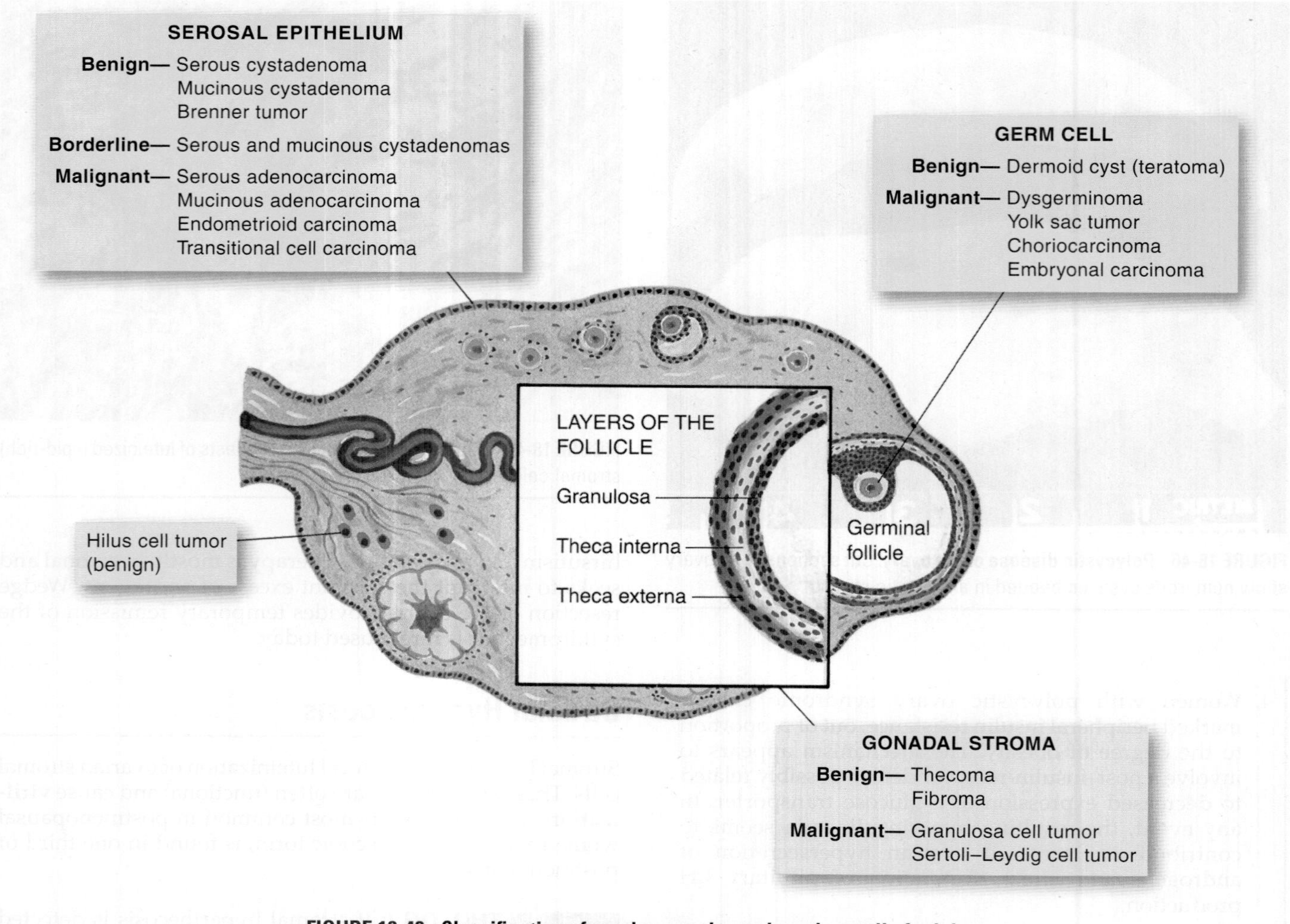

SEROSAL EPITHELIUM

Benign— Serous cystadenoma
Mucinous cystadenoma
Brenner tumor

Borderline— Serous and mucinous cystadenomas

Malignant— Serous adenocarcinoma
Mucinous adenocarcinoma
Endometrioid carcinoma
Transitional cell carcinoma

GERM CELL

Benign— Dermoid cyst (teratoma)

Malignant— Dysgerminoma
Yolk sac tumor
Choriocarcinoma
Embryonal carcinoma

LAYERS OF THE FOLLICLE
Granulosa
Theca interna
Theca externa
Germinal follicle

Hilus cell tumor (benign)

GONADAL STROMA

Benign— Thecoma
Fibroma

Malignant— Granulosa cell tumor
Sertoli–Leydig cell tumor

FIGURE 18-48. Classification of ovarian neoplasms based on cell of origin.

Ovarian cancer is the second most frequent gynecologic malignancy after endometrial cancer and carries a higher mortality rate than all other female genital cancers combined (Table 18-5). As it is difficult to detect early in its evolution when it is still curable, over three fourths of patients already have extraovarian tumor spread to the pelvis or abdomen at the time of diagnosis. There are 26,000 new cases of ovarian cancer diagnosed each year in the United States, and more than 16,000 women die from the disease (Table 18-5). The lifetime risk of developing ovarian cancer is 2%. These tumors predominate in women older than 60 years, but may occur in younger women with family history of the disease.

Epithelial Tumors Account for Over 90% of Ovarian Cancers

Tumors of common epithelial origin can be broadly classified, according to cell proliferation, degree of nuclear atypia and presence or absence of stromal invasion: (1) **benign**, (2) of **borderline malignancy** (also called **low malignant potential**) and (3) **malignant** (Fig. 18-49).

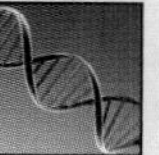
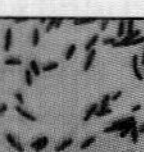

MOLECULAR PATHOGENESIS AND ETIOLOGIC FACTORS: Epidemiologic studies suggest that common epithelial neoplasms are related to repeated disruption and repair of the epithelial surface resulting from cyclic or "incessant" ovulation. Thus, tumors most commonly affect nulliparous women and, conversely, occur least often in women in whom ovulation has been suppressed (e.g., by pregnancy or oral contraceptives). Also, persistent, high concentrations of pituitary gonadotropins after menopause may stimulate surface epithelial cells, leading to accumulation of genetic changes and carcinogenesis. Irritants, such as talc or asbestos, have also been implicated, since they may be transported up the reproductive tract and reach the ovaries.

There is occasionally a family history of ovarian carcinoma. If a first-degree relative had ovarian cancer, a woman's risk of developing ovarian cancer is increased 3.5-fold. Women with a history of ovarian carcinoma are also at greater risk for breast cancer and vice versa. Defects in repair genes implicated in hereditary breast cancers, *BRCA-1* and *BRCA-2*, are incriminated in familial

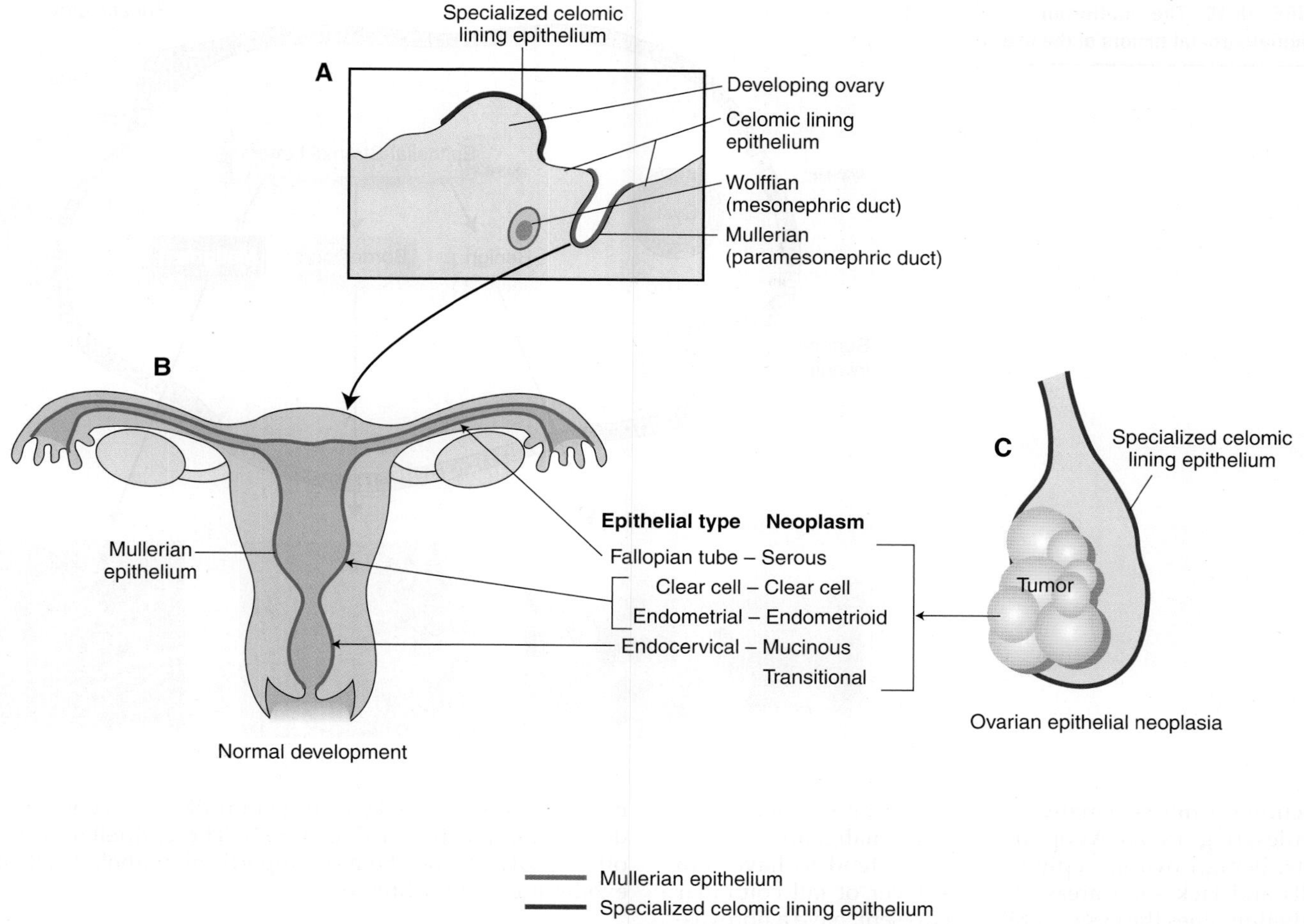

A
Specialized celomic lining epithelium
Developing ovary
Celomic lining epithelium
Wolffian (mesonephric duct)
Mullerian (paramesonephric duct)

B
Mullerian epithelium
Epithelial type Neoplasm
Fallopian tube – Serous
Clear cell – Clear cell
Endometrial – Endometrioid
Endocervical – Mucinous
Transitional
Normal development

C
Specialized celomic lining epithelium
Tumor
Ovarian epithelial neoplasia

Mullerian epithelium
Specialized celomic lining epithelium

FIGURE 18-49. Histogenesis of ovarian epithelial/stromal tumors.

ovarian cancers as well. Woman with BRCA-1 mutations tend to develop ovarian cancers at younger ages than those who develop sporadic ovarian tumors, but BRCA-1–related tumors have better prognoses. As for endometrial carcinoma, women with hereditary nonpolyposis colon cancer (HNPCC) are also at greater risk for ovarian cancer.

Most common epithelial tumors, especially serous carcinomas, arise from ovarian surface epithelium or serosa. A few, especially Brenner tumor, arise elsewhere in the ovary. During embryonic life, the celomic cavity is lined by mesothelium, parts of which specialize to form the serosal epithelium covering the gonadal ridge. The same mesothelial lining gives rise to müllerian ducts, from which the fallopian tubes, uterus and vagina arise (Fig. 18-50).

As the ovary develops, the surface epithelium may extend into the ovarian stroma to form glands and cysts. In some cases, these inclusion cysts become neoplastic and show a variety of müllerian-type differentiations (Fig. 18-49). Recent investigations suggest that epithelial ovarian tumors derive from epithelial precursor cells with differentiation pathways regulated by embryonic pathways involving *HOX* genes.

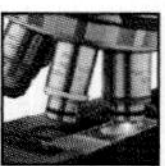

PATHOLOGY: In order of decreasing frequency, the **common epithelial tumors** are:

- **Serous tumors** that resemble fallopian tube epithelium
- **Mucinous tumors** that mimic the mucosa of the endocervix
- **Endometrioid tumors** that are similar to the glands of the endometrium
- **Clear cell tumors** with glycogen-rich cells like endometrial glands in pregnancy
- **Transitional cell tumors** that resemble the mucosa of the bladder
- **Mixed tumors**

Cystadenomas

Benign common epithelial tumors are almost always serous or mucinous adenomas and generally arise in women 20 to 60 years old. These tumors are frequently large, often 15 to 30 cm in diameter. Some, particularly mucinous ones, reach massive proportions, exceeding 50 cm in diameter, and may mimic the appearance of a term pregnancy. Benign epithelial tumors are typically cystic, hence the term **cystadenoma.** Serous cystadenomas are more often bilateral (15%) than mucinous cystadenomas and tend to be unilocular (Fig. 18-51). By contrast,

FIGURE 18-50. The müllerian relations of epithelial/stromal tumors of the ovaries.

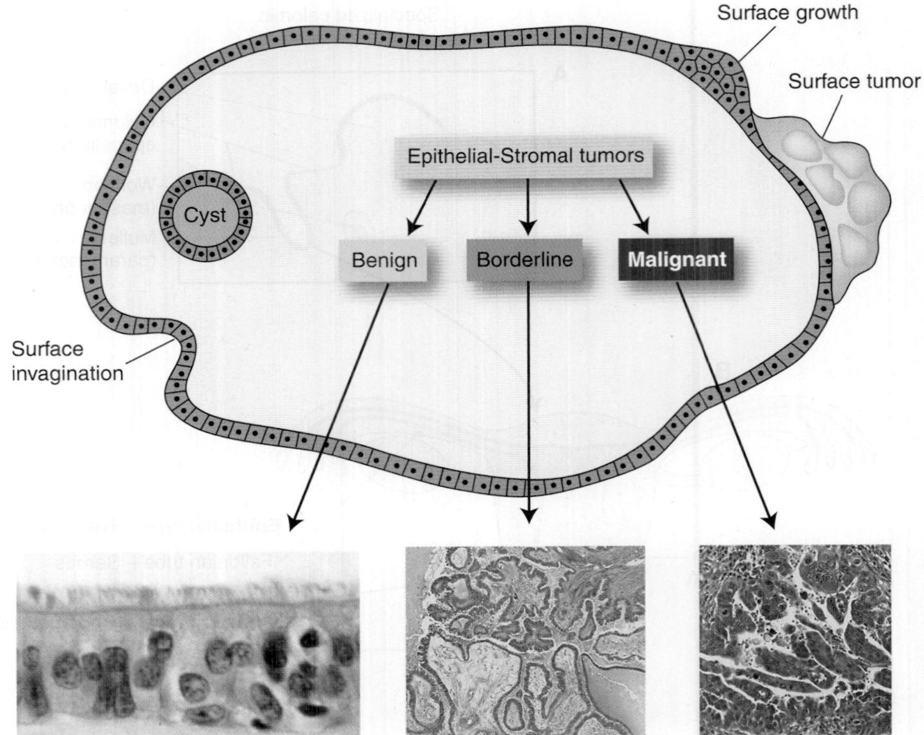

mucinous tumors usually show hundreds of small cysts (locules) (Fig. 18-52). As opposed to their malignant counterparts, benign ovarian epithelial tumors tend to have thin walls and lack solid areas. A single layer of tall columnar epithelium lines the cysts. Papillae, if present, have a fibrovascular core covered by a layer of tall columnar epithelium identical to the cyst lining.

Transitional Cell Tumor (Brenner Tumor)

The typical Brenner tumor is benign and occurs at all ages. Half of cases present in women over the age of 50. Size varies from microscopic foci to masses 8 cm or more in diameter. Brenner tumors are adenofibromas, typically showing solid nests of transitional-like (urothelium-like) cells encased in a dense, fibrous stroma (Fig. 18-53). The epithelial nests are often cavitated and the most superficial epithelial cells may exhibit mucinous differentiation.

Borderline Tumors (Tumors of Low Malignant Potential)

"Borderline tumors" are a well-defined group of ovarian tumors characterized by epithelial cell proliferation and nuclear atypia but not destructive stromal invasion. Despite histologic features suggesting aggressiveness, they share an excellent prognosis. Serous borderline tumors generally occur in women 20 to 50 years old (average, 46 years) but are also seen in older women. Surgical cure is almost always possible

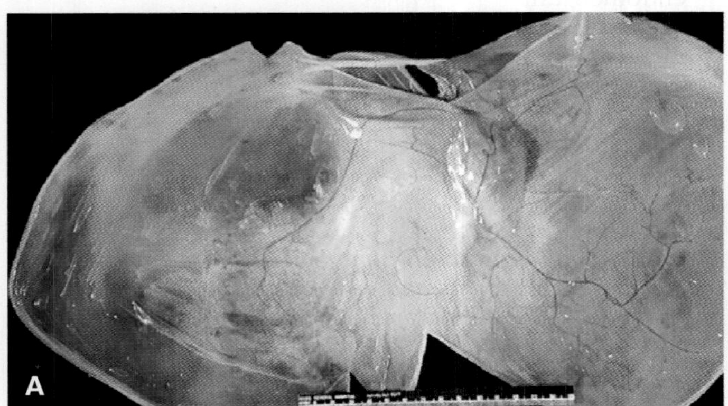

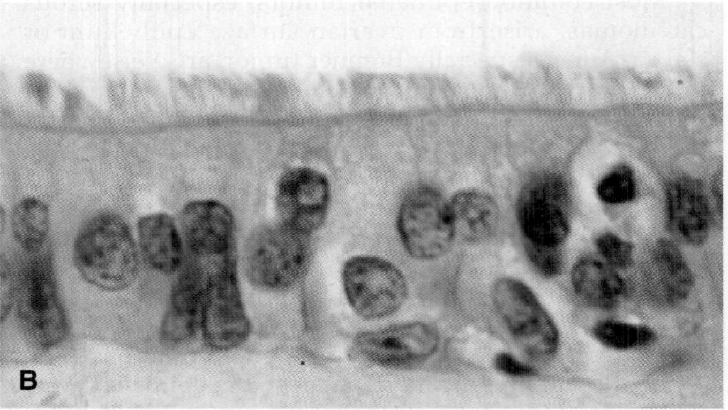

FIGURE 18-51. Serous cystadenoma of the ovary. A. Gross appearance of serous cystadenoma of the ovary. The fluid has been removed from this huge unilocular serous cystadenoma. The wall is thin and translucent. **B.** On microscopic examination, the cyst is lined by a single layer of ciliated tubal-type epithelium.

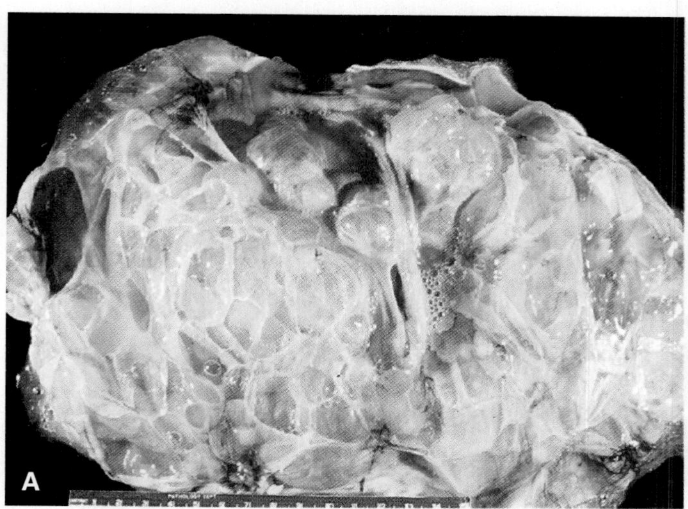
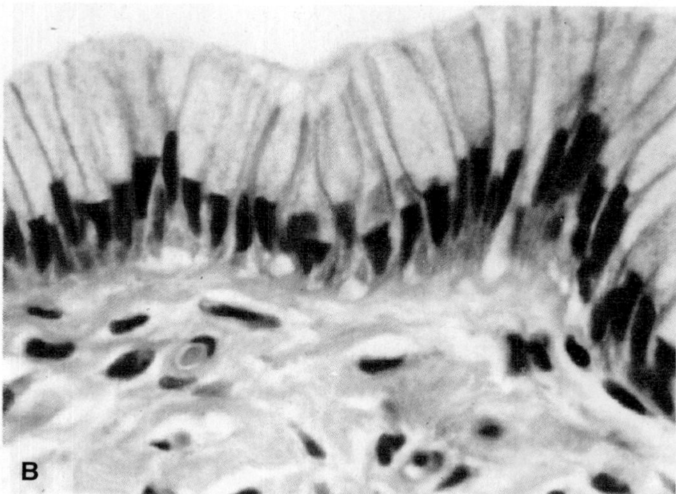

FIGURE 18-52. Mucinous cystadenoma of the ovary. A. The tumor is characterized by numerous cysts filled with thick, viscous fluid. **B.** A single layer of mucinous epithelial cells lines the cyst.

if the tumor is confined to the ovaries. Even if it has spread to the pelvis or abdomen, 80% of patients are alive after 5 years. Although there is a significant rate of late recurrence, the tumors rarely recur beyond 10 years. Late progression to low-grade serous carcinoma has been reported in approximately 7% of cases.

Serous tumors of borderline malignancy are more commonly bilateral (34%) than mucinous ones (6%) or other types. The tumors vary in size, although mucinous ones may be gigantic (100+ kg). In serous tumors of borderline malignancy, papillary projections, ranging from fine and exuberant to grapelike clusters arising from the cyst wall, are common (Fig. 18-54). These structures resemble papillary fronds in benign cystadenomas, but they show (1) epithelial stratification, (2) moderate nuclear atypia and (3) mitotic activity. The same criteria apply to borderline mucinous tumors, although papillary projections are less conspicuous. ***By definition, the presence of more than focal microinvasion (i.e., discrete nests of epithelial cells <3 mm into the ovarian stroma) identifies a tumor as low-grade invasive serous carcinoma, rather than a borderline tumor.*** However, borderline tumors with lymph node metastases or peritoneal implants (Fig. 18-55), whether noninvasive or invasive, are still "borderline," reflecting that this category is well defined and carries a prognosis far better than the usual adenocarcinoma. The presence of ovarian surface excrescences does not seem to predict progression of disease.

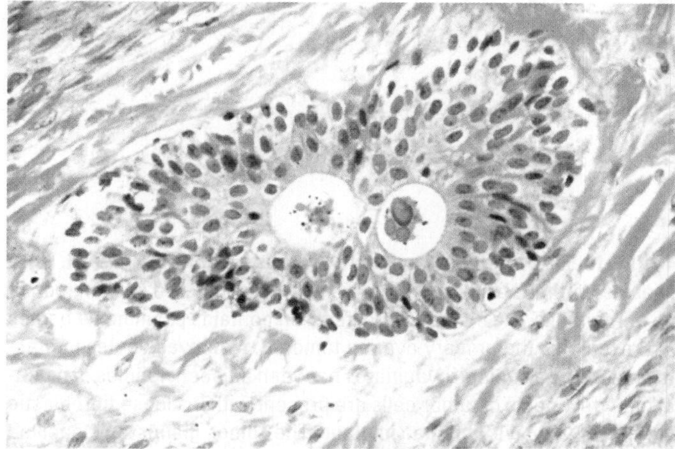

FIGURE 18-53. Brenner tumor. A nest of transitional-like cells is embedded in a dense, fibrous stroma.

Malignant Epithelial Tumors

Carcinomas of the ovary are most common in women 40 to 60 years old, and are rare under the age of 35. Based on light microscopy and molecular genetics, ovarian carcinomas are classified into five main subtypes (Table 18-11), which, in descending order of frequency, are high-grade serous carcinomas (>70%), endometrioid carcinomas (10%), clear cell carcinomas (10%), mucinous carcinomas (3% to 4%) and low-grade serous carcinomas (<5%). These subtypes, which account for 98% of ovarian carcinomas, can be reproducibly diagnosed and are inherently different diseases, as indicated by differences in epidemiologic and genetic risk factors, precursor lesions, patterns of spread, molecular events during oncogenesis, responses to chemotherapy and outcomes. With progress toward subtype-specific management of ovarian cancer, accurate subtype assignment is becoming increasingly important.

SEROUS ADENOCARCINOMAS:

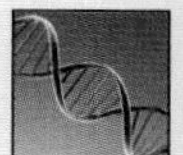

MOLECULAR PATHOGENESIS: Low-grade and high-grade serous carcinomas are fundamentally different tumors. Whereas low-grade tumors are frequently associated with serous borderline tumors and have mutations of *KRAS* or *BRAF* oncogenes, high-grade serous carcinomas appear to arise de novo without identifiable precursor lesions and have a high frequency of mutations in p53, but not in *KRAS* or *BRAF*. Interestingly, carcinomas arising in patients with germline *BRCA1* or *BRCA2* mutations (hereditary ovarian cancers)

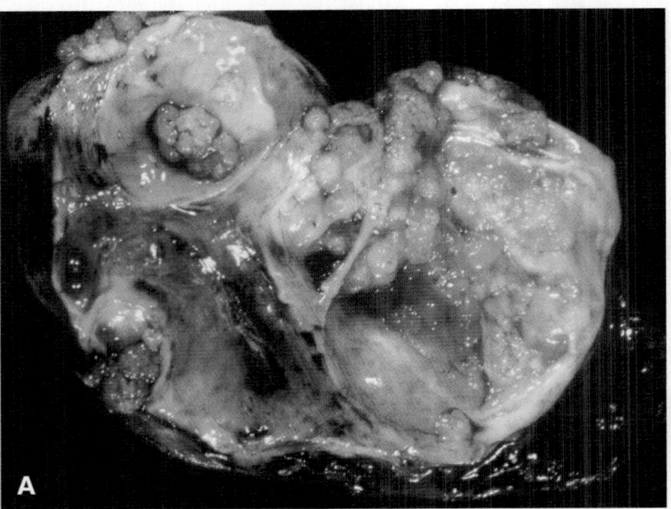

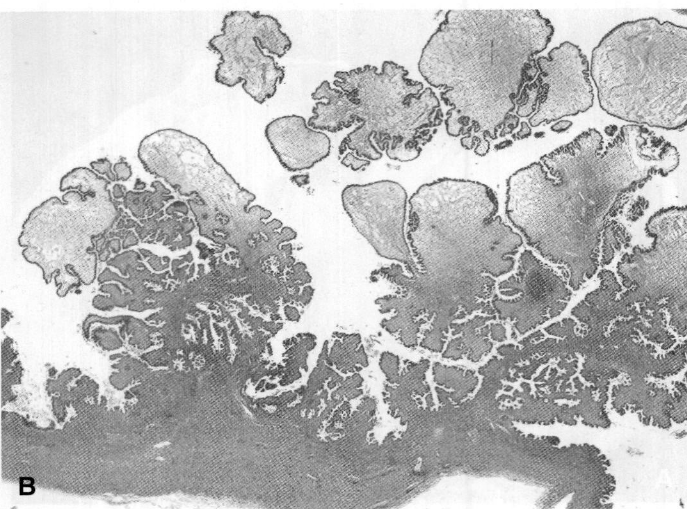

FIGURE 18-54. A. Serous cystic borderline tumor. A. The inner surface of the cysts is partly covered by closely packed papillae (endophytic growth). **B.** Microscopic view of the papillary tumor. The papillae show hierarchical and complex branching without stromal invasion. Some papillae have fibroedematous stalks.

are almost invariably the high-grade serous type and commonly have p53 mutations. A significant number of *BRCA1*- or *BRCA2*-related tumors arise from the epithelium of the fimbriated end of the fallopian tube, suggesting that at least some sporadic high-grade ovarian and "primary" peritoneal serous carcinomas may actually develop from the distal fallopian tube and "spill over" onto the adjacent tissues.

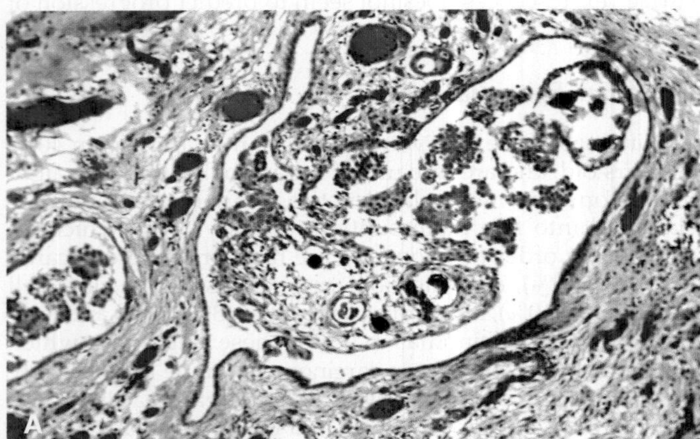

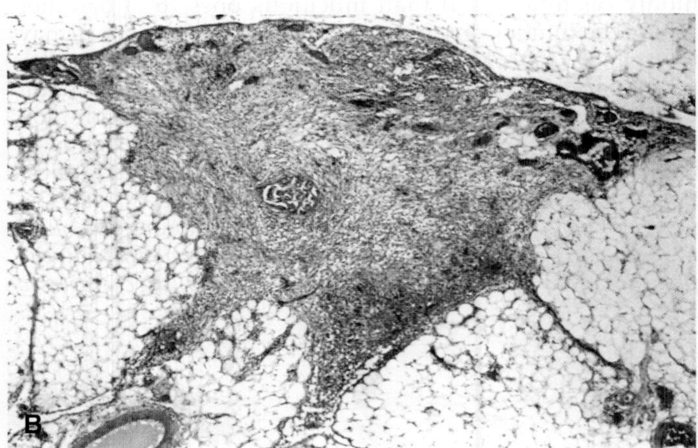

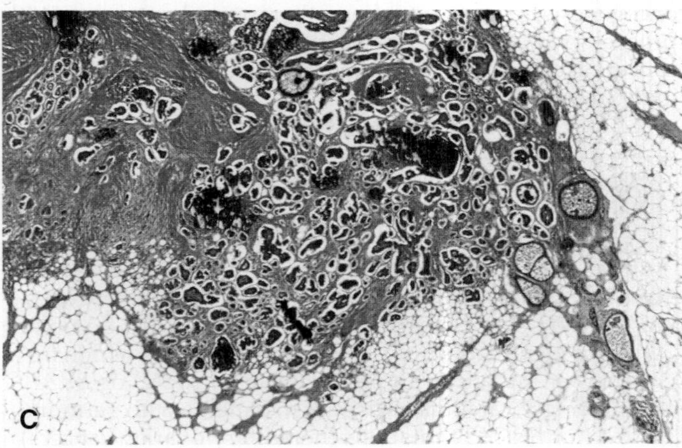

FIGURE 18-55. Peritoneal implants of serous borderline tumor. A. Noninvasive epithelial implant within a smoothly contoured invagination of the peritoneum. The epithelial proliferation contains psammoma bodies and resembles the primary ovarian tumor. **B. Noninvasive desmoplastic implant.** The implant invaginates between adjacent lobules of omental fat. A few nests of tumor cells are present within a loose fibroblastic stroma. **C. Invasive omental implant.** The tumor glands and papillae appear disorderly distributed within a dense fibrous stroma and resemble a low-grade serous carcinoma.

Table 18-11

Main Subtypes of Ovarian Carcinoma

	Low-Grade Serous	High-Grade Serous	Clear Cell	Endometrioid	Mucinous
Usual stage at diagnosis	Early or advanced	Advanced	Early	Early	Early
Presumed tissue of origin/ precursor lesion	Serous borderline tumor	Fallopian tube or tubal metaplasia in inclusions of ovarian surface epithelium	Endometriosis, adenofibroma	Endometriosis, adenofibroma	Adenoma–borderline–carcinoma sequence; teratoma
Genetic risk	?	BRCA1/2	?	HNPCC	?
Significant molecular abnormalities	BRAF or K-ras	p53 and pRb pathways	HNF-1β	PTEN, β-catenin, K-ras MI	K-ras
Proliferation	Low	High	Low	Low	Intermediate
Response to primary chemotherapy	26%–28%	80%	15%	?	15%
Prognosis	Favorable	Poor	Intermediate	Favorable	Favorable

PATHOLOGY: Low-grade serous carcinomas are characterized by irregular invasion of the ovary by small, tight nests of tumor cells within variable desmoplasia (Fig. 18-56). The uniformity of the nuclei is the principal criterion for distinguishing low- and high-grade serous carcinomas, with less than threefold variability. Low-grade serous carcinomas rarely progress to high-grade tumors.

High-grade serous carcinomas (commonly called "cystadenocarcinoma") are predominantly solid, multinodular masses, usually with necrosis and hemorrhage (Fig. 18-57A). By the time a tumor has reached 10 to 15 cm, it has often spread beyond the ovary and seeded the peritoneum. Two thirds of serous cancers with extraovarian spread are bilateral. High-grade serous cancers typically show obvious stromal invasion. Most tumors have a high nuclear grade with irregularly branching, highly cellular papillae with little or no stromal support and slitlike glandular lumens within more solid areas (Fig. 18-57B). The mitotic rate is very high. Psammoma bodies are often present.

MUCINOUS ADENOCARCINOMA:

MOLECULAR PATHOGENESIS: Mucinous ovarian tumors are often heterogeneous. Benign, borderline, noninvasive and invasive carcinoma components may coexist within the same tumor. Such a morphologic continuum suggests that tumor progression

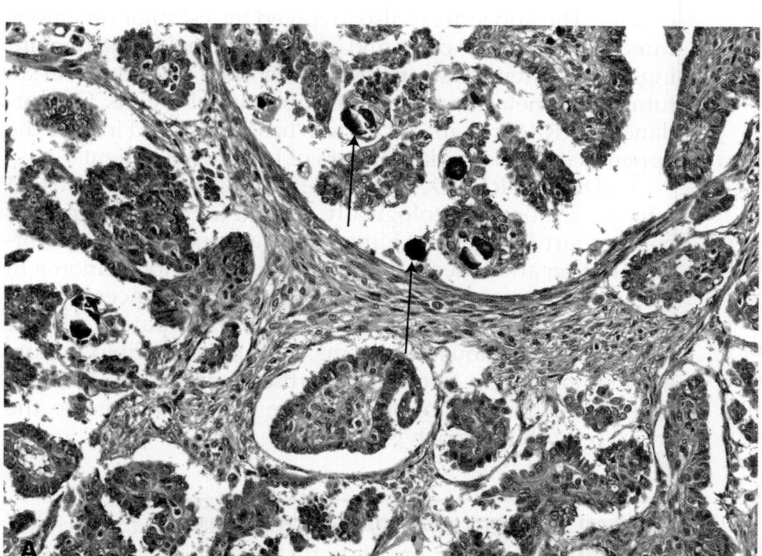

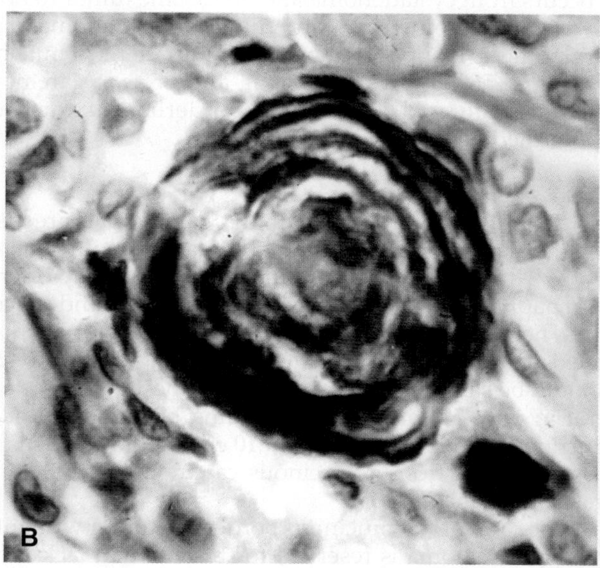

FIGURE 18-56. Low-grade serous carcinoma. A. The nests of tumor cells are disorderly distributed and appear surrounded by clefts. In contrast to high-grade serous carcinoma, the nuclei are low grade. Psammoma bodies (*arrows*) are seen. **B.** A higher-power view shows the laminated structure of a psammoma body.

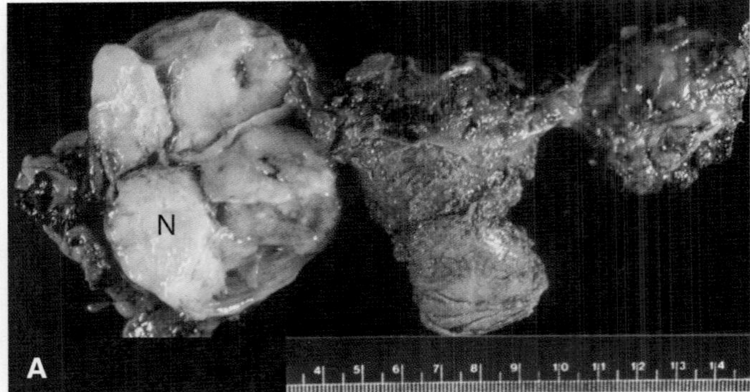

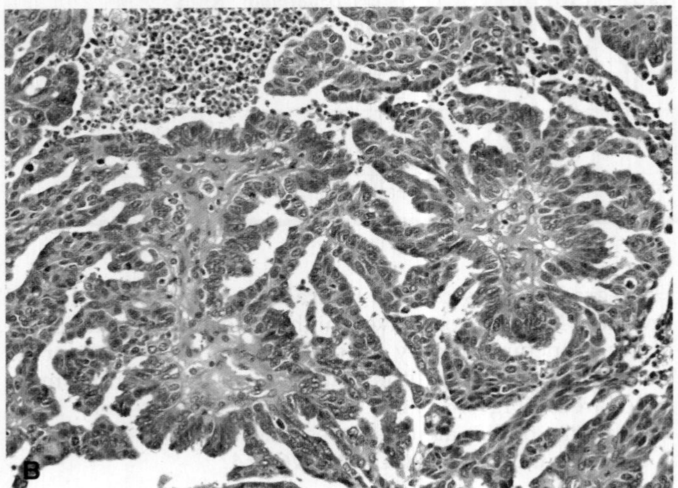

FIGURE 18-57. High-grade serous cystadenocarcinoma. A. In addition to cysts (*left*), the ovary is enlarged by a solid tumor that exhibits extensive necrosis (N). **B.** Microscopic examination shows complex papillae, lined by atypical nuclei, forming glomeruloid structures.

occurs from cystadenoma and borderline tumor to noninvasive, microinvasive and invasive carcinomas. This hypothesis is supported by KRAS mutations in mucinous tumors: 56% of cystadenomas and 85% of carcinomas express mutated *KRAS*, with borderline tumors being intermediate.

PATHOLOGY: Mucinous carcinomas are usually large, unilateral, multilocular or unilocular cystic masses containing mucinous fluid. They often contain papillary and solid areas that may be soft and mucoid or firm, hemorrhagic and necrotic. Malignant components may coexist within a single specimen, so mucinous ovarian tumors should be sampled extensively. Since these tumors are bilateral in only 5% of the cases, finding bilateral or unilateral mucinous tumors smaller than 10 cm should raise suspicion of metastases from a mucinous carcinoma elsewhere (e.g., gastrointestinal tract).

The category of mucinous borderline tumor with intraepithelial carcinoma is reserved for tumors that lack architectural features of invasive carcinoma but, focally, show unequivocally malignant cells lining glandular spaces. Mucinous borderline tumors with intraepithelial carcinoma have a very low likelihood of recurrence.

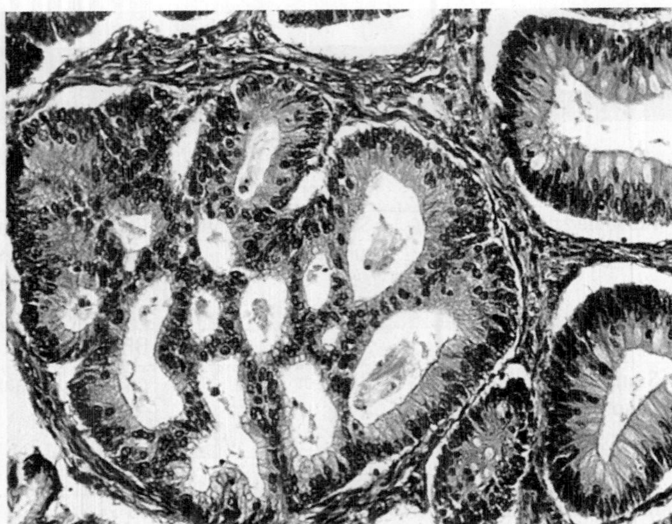

FIGURE 18-58. Mucinous cystadenocarcinoma. The malignant glands are arranged in a cribriform pattern and are composed of mucin-producing columnar cells.

Recent proposals further subdivide mucinous adenocarcinomas into (1) **expansile** or **confluent glandular pattern,** where destructive stromal invasion is absent (Fig. 18-58) but there are back-to-back or complex malignant glands with minimal or no intervening stroma, and (2) **infiltrative,** showing obvious glandular stromal invasion. The former appears to have a more favorable prognosis than the infiltrative type. The combination of extensive, infiltrative stromal invasion; high nuclear grade; and tumor rupture should be considered a strong predictor of recurrence for stage I mucinous adenocarcinomas.

Pseudomyxoma peritonei is a clinical condition of abundant gelatinous or mucinous ascites in the peritoneum, fibrous adhesions and frequently mucinous tumors involving the ovaries. The appendix is also involved by a similar mucinous tumor in 60% of the cases and appears normal in the remaining 40%. Current data suggest that in most cases the ovarian tumors are metastases from the appendiceal lesions. Concordance in *KRAS* mutational pattern has been found in both the appendiceal and ovarian tumors of individual patients.

ENDOMETRIOID ADENOCARCINOMA: Endometrioid adenocarcinoma histologically resembles its endometrial counterpart (Fig. 18-59A), may have areas of squamous differentiation and is second only to serous adenocarcinoma in frequency. It accounts for 10% of all ovarian cancers. These tumors occur most commonly after menopause. Unlike serous and mucinous neoplasms, most endometrioid tumors are malignant. Up to one half of these cancers are bilateral and, at diagnosis, most tumors are either confined to the ovary or within the pelvis.

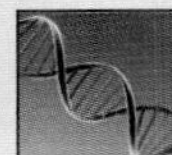

MOLECULAR PATHOGENESIS: Endometrioid carcinomas are thought to arise by malignant transformation of endometriosis, and not ovarian surface epithelium (Fig. 18-59B). The most common genetic abnormalities in sporadic endometrioid carcinoma of the ovary are somatic mutations of the β-catenin

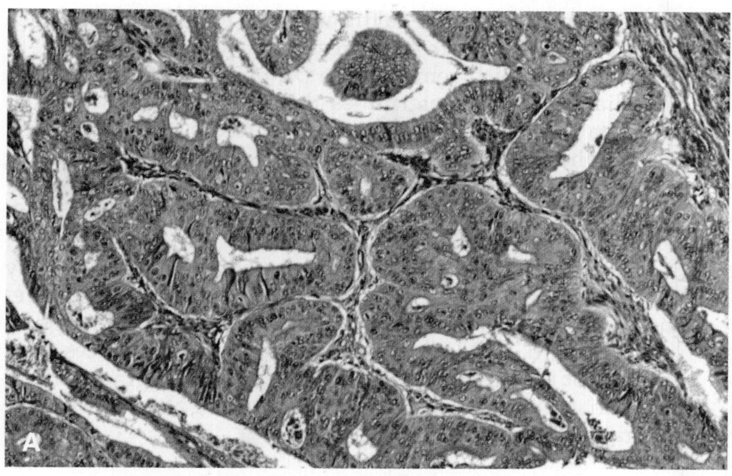

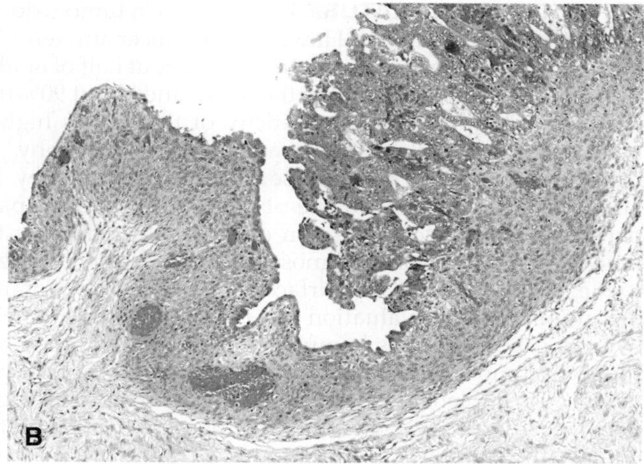

FIGURE 18-59. Endometrioid adenocarcinoma. A. The crowded neoplastic glands are lined by stratified non–mucin-containing epithelium. Nuclear atypia is moderate to severe. **B.** Endometrioid adenocarcinoma (*right*) arising in endometriosis. Note the stromal cells of endometriosis.

(*CTNNB1*) and *PTEN* genes and microsatellite instability. Endometrioid borderline tumors also have β-catenin gene mutations.

PATHOLOGY: Endometrioid carcinomas vary from 2 cm to more than 30 cm. Most are largely solid with areas of necrosis, although they may be cystic. Endometrioid tumors are graded like their endometrial counterparts. Between 15% and 20% of patients with endometrioid carcinoma of the ovary also harbor an endometrial cancer. Strong data suggest that if ovarian and endometrial cancers coexist, they generally arise independently, although some may be metastases from one or the other. This distinction has important prognostic implications. Clonality analysis using various molecular methods can be helpful including LOH, gene mutation and clonal X-inactivation analysis. The 5-year survival exceeds 85% in synchronous tumors. As with all malignant epithelial tumors of the ovary, prognosis depends on the stage at which it presents.

CLEAR CELL ADENOCARCINOMA: This enigmatic ovarian cancer is closely related to endometrioid adenocarcinoma, and often occurs in association with endometriosis (Fig. 18-60A). It constitutes 5% to 10% of all ovarian cancers usually occurring after menopause. Although patients typically present with stage I or II disease, clear cell carcinomas have a poor prognosis compared with other low-stage ovarian carcinomas. Sizes range from 2 to 30 cm, and 40% are bilateral. Most of these tumors are partially cystic and show necrosis and hemorrhage in the solid areas.

Clear cell ovarian adenocarcinomas resemble their counterparts in the vagina, and have sheets or tubules of malignant cells with clear cytoplasm (Fig. 18-60B). In its tubular form, malignant cells often display bulbous nuclei that protrude into the lumen of the tubule ("hobnail cell"), appearing like an Arias-Stella reaction in gestational endometrium (Fig. 18-28). The clinical course parallels that of endometrioid carcinoma.

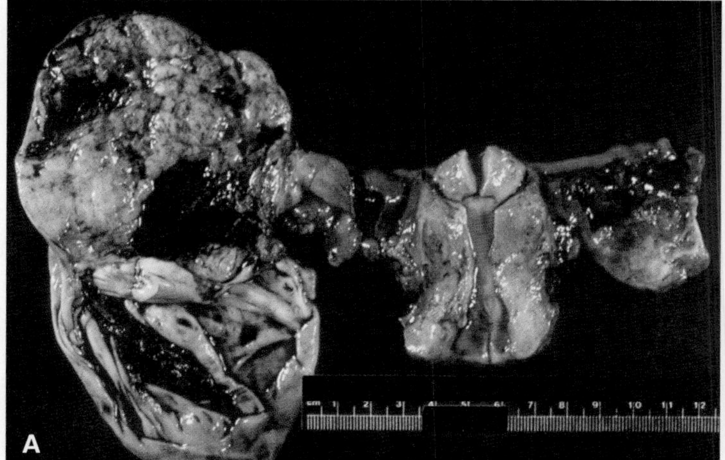

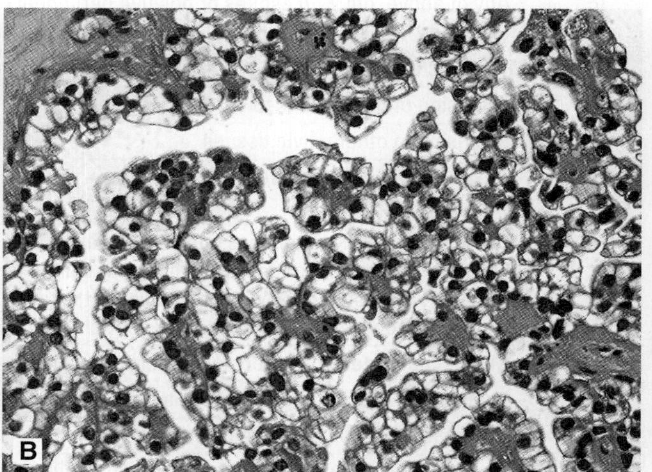

FIGURE 18-60. Clear cell adenocarcinoma. A. Clear cell adenocarcinoma arising as an ovarian mass in a large, hemorrhagic endometriotic cyst. **B.** The clear cells are polyhedral and have eccentric, hyperchromatic nuclei without prominent nucleoli.

CLINICAL FEATURES: Most ovarian tumors do not secrete hormones. However, the cancer antigen, CA-125, is detectable in the serum in about half of epithelial tumors that are confined to the ovary and about 90% that have already spread. The specificity of this test is highest when it is combined with transvaginal ultrasonography.

Ovarian masses rarely cause symptoms until they are large. When they distend the abdomen, they cause pain, pelvic pressure or compression of regional organs. By the time ovarian cancers are diagnosed, many have metastasized to (i.e., implanted on) the surfaces of the pelvis, abdominal organs or bladder. Evaluation of a patient with an epithelial ovarian cancer requires knowledge of staging, grading and routes of tumor spread. For example, ovarian tumors have a tendency to implant in the peritoneal cavity on the diaphragm, paracolic gutters and omentum. Lymphatic spread is preferentially to para-aortic lymph nodes near the origin of the renal arteries and to a lesser extent to external iliac (pelvic) or inguinal lymph nodes. In addition to specific symptoms, metastatic cancers may cause ascites, weakness, weight loss and cachexia.

Survival for patients with malignant ovarian tumors is generally poor. The most important prognostic index is the surgical stage of the tumor at the time it is detected (Table 18-12). Overall, 5-year survival is only 35%, because more than half of tumors have spread to the abdominal cavity (stage 3) or elsewhere by the time they are discovered. Prognostic indices for epithelial tumors also include grade, histologic type and the size of the residual neoplasm.

Surgery, which removes the primary tumor, establishes the diagnosis and determines the extent of spread, is the mainstay of therapy. The peritoneal surfaces, omentum, liver, subdiaphragmatic recesses and all abdominal regions must be visualized, and as much metastatic tumor removed as possible. Adjuvant chemotherapy is used to treat distant occult sites of tumor spread.

At some time after the initial operation, another exploratory (second-look) laparotomy may be used to assess the effectiveness of therapy. However, even if no residual disease is apparent, one third of older patients will develop recurrences. Risk factors for recurrence are (1) high stage, (2) high grade and (3) more than 2 cm of residual disease remaining after the primary operation.

Table 18-12

Clinical Staging of Ovarian Cancer

Stage	Description
I	Limited to ovaries; capsule intact; no tumor on the external surface
Ia	Limited to one ovary; ascitic fluid, if present, lacks malignant cells
Ib	Limited to both ovaries; capsule intact; no tumor on the external surface; ascitic fluid, if present, lacks malignant cells
Ic	Any of above, but with ascites or positive peritoneal washings
II	With pelvic extension
IIa	Extension or metastases to uterus or tubes
IIb	Extension to other pelvic tissues
IIc	Any of above, but with ascites or positive peritoneal washings
III	With intraperitoneal metastases outside the pelvis, or positive retroperitoneal nodes, or both. Tumor limited to true pelvis with histologically proven malignant extension to small bowel or omentum
IIIa	Microscopic seeding on abdominal-peritoneal surface
IIIb	Implants = 2 cm on abdominal peritoneal surface
IIIc	Implants >2 cm on abdominal peritoneal surface
IV	With distant metastases. If pleural effusion present, positive cytology required. Liver metastases must be parenchymal

Germ Cell Tumors Tend to Be Benign in Adults and Malignant in Children

Tumors derived from germ cells make up one fourth of ovarian tumors. In adult women, ovarian germ cell tumors are virtually all benign (mature cystic teratoma, dermoid cyst), but in children and young adults, they are largely cancerous. ***In children, germ cell tumors are the most common ovarian cancer (60%); they are rare after menopause.***

Neoplastic germ cells may differentiate along several lines (Fig. 18-61), producing:

- **Dysgerminomas** are composed of neoplastic germ cells, similar to oogonia of fetal ovaries.
- **Teratomas** differentiate toward somatic (embryonic or adult) tissues.
- **Yolk sac tumors** form extraembryonic tissue, like placental mesenchyme or its precursors.
- **Choriocarcinomas** feature cells similar to those covering the placental villi.

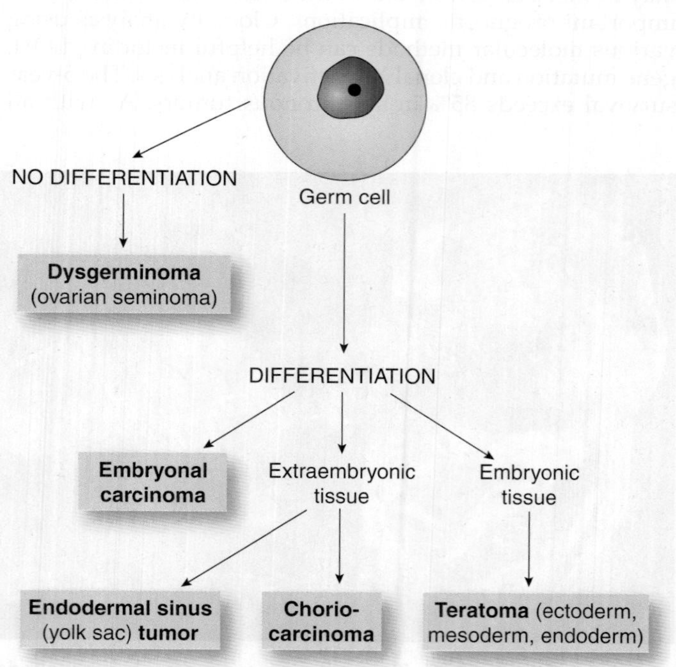

FIGURE 18-61. Classification of germ cell tumors of the ovary.

Germ cell tumors in infants tend to be solid and immature (e.g., yolk sac tumor and immature teratoma). Tumors in young adults show greater differentiation, as in mature cystic teratoma. Malignant germ cell tumors in women older than 40 years usually result from transformation of one of the components of a benign cystic teratoma.

Malignant germ cell tumors tend to be highly aggressive. While solid germ cell tumors of the ovary were once always fatal, with current chemotherapy survival rates for many exceed 80%.

Dysgerminoma

Dysgerminoma is the ovarian counterpart of testicular seminoma, and is composed of primordial germ cells. It accounts for less than 2% of ovarian cancers in all women, but constitutes 10% in women younger than 20 years. Most patients are between 10 and 30. The tumors are bilateral in about 15% of cases.

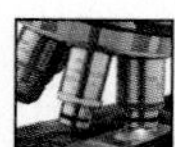

PATHOLOGY: Dysgerminomas are often large and firm and have a bosselated external surface. The cut surface is soft and fleshy. They contain large nests of monotonously uniform tumor cells that have clear glycogen-filled cytoplasm and irregularly flattened central nuclei (Fig. 18-62). Fibrous septa containing lymphocytes traverse the tumor.

Dysgerminomas are treated surgically; 5-year survival for patients with stage I tumor approaches 100%. Because the tumor is highly radiosensitive and also responsive to chemotherapy, even for higher-stage tumors 5-year survival rates still exceed 80%.

Teratoma

Teratoma is a tumor of germ cell origin that differentiates toward somatic structures. Most teratomas contain tissues from at least two, and usually all three, embryonic layers.

MATURE TERATOMA (MATURE CYSTIC TERATOMA, DERMOID CYST): This benign neoplasm accounts for one fourth of all ovarian tumors with a peak incidence in the third decade. Mature teratomas develop by **parthenogenesis.** Haploid (postmeiotic) germ cells endoreduplicate to give rise to diploid genetically female tumor cells (46,XX).

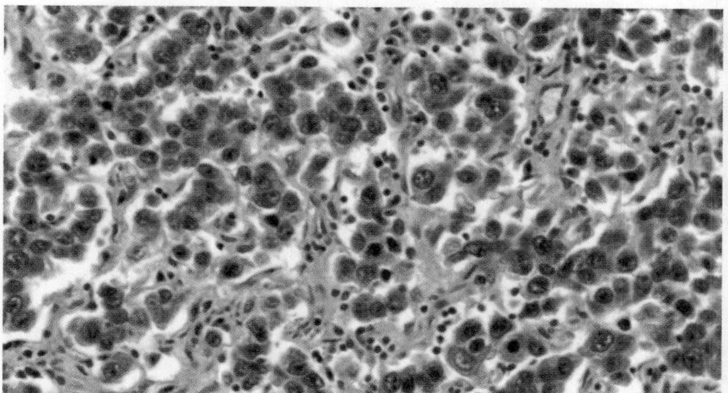

FIGURE 18-62. Dysgerminoma. The neoplastic germ cells are distributed in nests separated by delicate fibrous septa. The stroma contains lymphocytes.

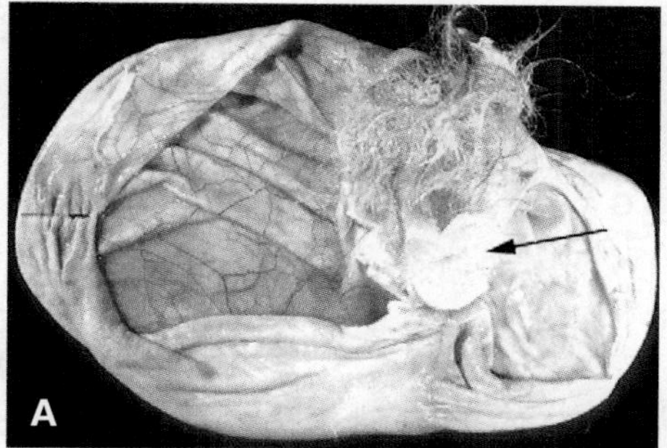

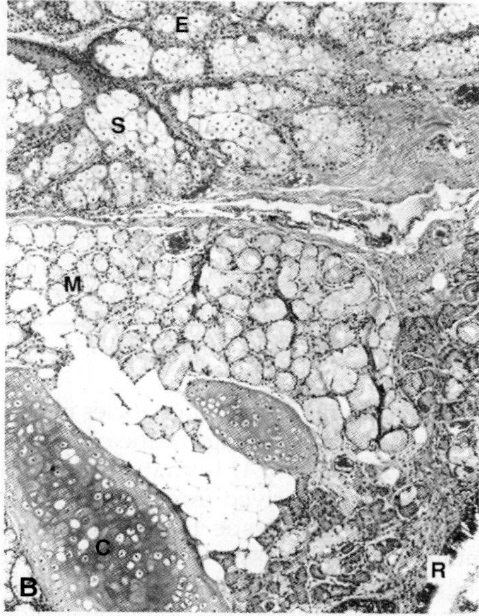

FIGURE 18-63. Mature cystic teratoma of the ovary. A. A mature cystic teratoma has been opened to reveal a solid knob (*arrow*) from which hair projects. **B.** A photomicrograph of the solid knob shows epidermal and respiratory components. Tissue resembling the skin exhibits an epidermis (E) with underlying sebaceous glands (S). The respiratory tissue consists of mucous glands (M), cartilage (C) and respiratory epithelium (R).

PATHOLOGY: Mature teratomas are cystic and almost all contain skin, sebaceous glands and hair follicles (Fig. 18-63). Half have smooth muscle, sweat glands, cartilage, bone, teeth and respiratory epithelium. Other tissues, like gut, thyroid and brain, are seen less often. If present, nodular foci in the cyst wall ("mammary tubercles" or "Rokitansky nodules") contain tissue elements of all three germ cell layers: (1) ectoderm (e.g., skin, glia), (2) mesoderm (e.g., smooth muscle, cartilage) and (3) endoderm (e.g., respiratory epithelium).

Struma ovarii is a cystic lesion composed predominantly of thyroid tissue (5% to 20% of mature cystic teratomas). Rare cases of hyperthyroidism may be associated with struma ovarii.

Very few (1%) dermoid cysts become malignant. These cancers usually occur in older women and correspond to the tumors that arise in other differentiated tissues of the body. Three fourths of cancers that arise in dermoid cysts are squamous cell carcinomas. The remainder are carcinoid tumors, basal cell carcinomas, thyroid cancers and others. Rarely, functional gut derivatives may cause carcinoid syndrome.

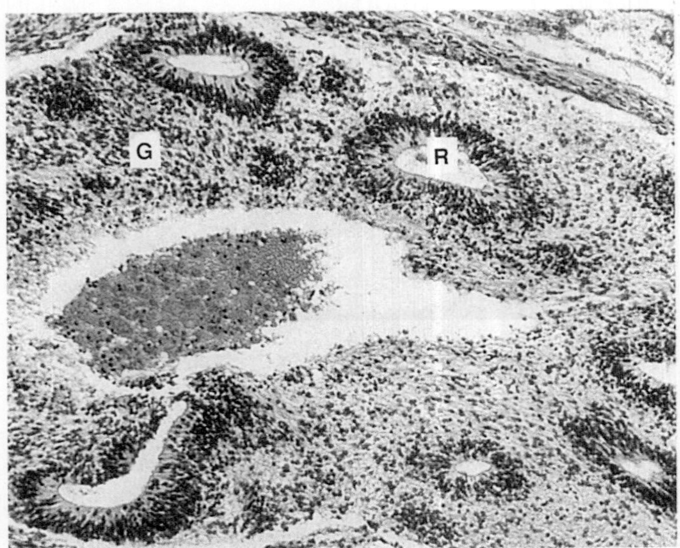

FIGURE 18-64. Immature teratoma of the ovary. Immature neural tissue exhibits rosettes (R) with multilayered nuclei. Embryonal glia (G) display densely packed, atypical nuclei.

The prognosis of patients with malignancies in mature cystic teratoma is related largely to stage of the cancer.

IMMATURE TERATOMA: Immature teratomas of the ovary contain elements derived from the three germ layers. However, unlike mature cystic teratomas, immature teratomas contain embryonal tissues. These tumors account for 20% of malignant tumors at all sites in women under the age of 20 but become progressively less common in older women.

PATHOLOGY: Immature teratomas are predominantly solid and lobulated, with numerous small cysts. Solid areas may contain grossly recognizable immature bone and cartilage. Multiple tumor components are usually seen, including those differentiating toward nerve (neuroepithelial rosettes and immature glia) (Fig. 18-64), glands and other structures found in mature cystic teratomas. Grading is based on the amount of immature tissue present. Metastases of immature teratomas are composed of embryonal, usually stromal, tissues. By contrast, rare metastases of mature cystic teratomas resemble epithelial adult-type malignancies.

Survival correlates with tumor grade. Well-differentiated immature teratomas generally have a good prognosis, but high-grade tumors (mainly embryonal tissue) are often lethal.

Yolk Sac Tumor

Yolk sac tumors are highly malignant tumors of women under the age of 30 that histologically resembles the mesenchyme of the primitive yolk sac. These are the second most common malignant germ cell tumors and are almost always unilateral.

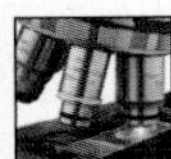

PATHOLOGY: Typically, yolk sac tumors are large, with extensive necrosis and hemorrhage. Multiple patterns are seen, the most common being a reticular, honeycombed structure of communicating spaces lined by primitive cells. **Schiller-Duval bodies** (Fig. 18-65A), which resemble the endodermal sinus of the rodent placenta, are found sparingly in a few tumors, but are characteristic. They consist of papillae that protrude into a space lined by tumor cells, resembling the glomerular Bowman space. The papillae are covered by a mantle of embryonal cells and contain a fibrovascular core and a central blood vessel.

Yolk sac tumor should not be confused with embryonal cell carcinoma, which is common in the testis. The former secretes α-fetoprotein, which can be demonstrated histochemically (Fig. 18-65B). Detection of α-fetoprotein in the blood is useful for diagnosis and for monitoring the effectiveness of therapy. Once uniformly fatal, 5-year survival with chemotherapy for stage I yolk sac tumors exceeds 80%.

Choriocarcinoma

Choriocarcinoma of the ovary is a rare tumor that mimics the epithelial covering of placental villi, namely, cytotrophoblast and syncytiotrophoblast. If it arises before puberty or together with another germ cell tumor, it most likely is of germ cell

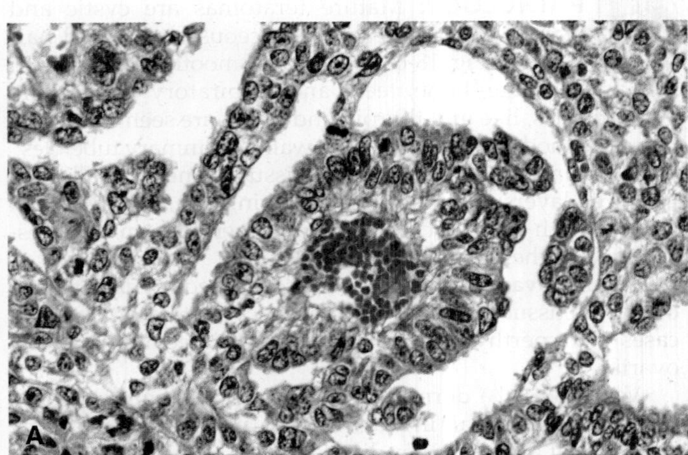

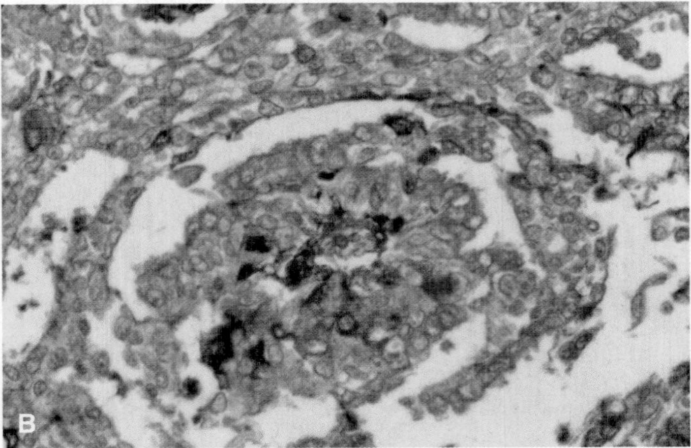

FIGURE 18-65. Yolk sac tumor of the ovary. A. Glomeruloid Schiller-Duval body that resembles the endodermal sinuses of the rodent placenta and consists of a papilla protruding into a space lined by tumor cells. **B.** Strong immunoreaction for α-fetoprotein.

origin. Young girls may show precocious sexual development, menstrual irregularities or rapid breast enlargement. In women of reproductive age, however, it may also be a metastasis from an intrauterine gestational tumor.

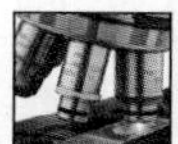

PATHOLOGY: Choriocarcinoma is unilateral, solid and widely hemorrhagic. Microscopically, it shows a mixture of malignant cytotrophoblast and syncytiotrophoblast (see placenta, choriocarcinoma, below). The syncytial cells secrete hCG, which accounts for the frequent finding of a positive pregnancy test result. Bilateral theca lutein cysts, a result of hCG stimulation, may also be found. Serial serum hCG determinations are useful both for diagnosis and follow-up. The tumor is highly aggressive but responds to chemotherapy.

Gonadoblastoma

Gonadoblastoma is a rare ovarian tumor that is distinctively associated with gonadal dysgenesis, especially in women who bear a Y chromosome. It occurs in phenotypic women under 30 years of age, although 20% are found in phenotypic men with cryptorchidism, hypospadias and female internal sex organs. Most affected women are virilized and suffer from primary amenorrhea and developmental abnormalities of the genitalia. Cellular nests show a mixture of germ cells and sex cord derivatives that resemble immature Sertoli and granulosa cells, and some consider the tumor to be an in situ form of germinoma. In half of cases, it is overgrown by dysgerminoma. Gonadoblastomas do not metastasize, but their overgrowths do.

Sex Cord/Stromal Tumors Are Clinically Functional

Tumors of sex cord and stroma originate from either primitive sex cords or from mesenchymal stroma of developing gonads. They represent 10% of ovarian tumors, vary from benign to low-grade malignant and may differentiate toward female (granulosa and theca cells) or male (Sertoli and Leydig cells) structures.

Fibroma

Fibromas account for 75% of all stromal tumors and 7% of all ovarian tumors. They occur at all ages, with a peak in the perimenopausal period, and are virtually always benign.

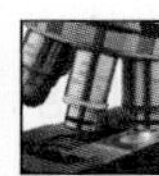

PATHOLOGY: Tumors are solid, firm and white (Fig. 18-66). Microscopically, the cells resemble the stroma of the normal ovarian cortex, being well-differentiated spindle cells, and variable amounts of collagen. Half of the larger tumors are associated with ascites and, rarely, with ascites and pleural effusions **(Meigs syndrome).**

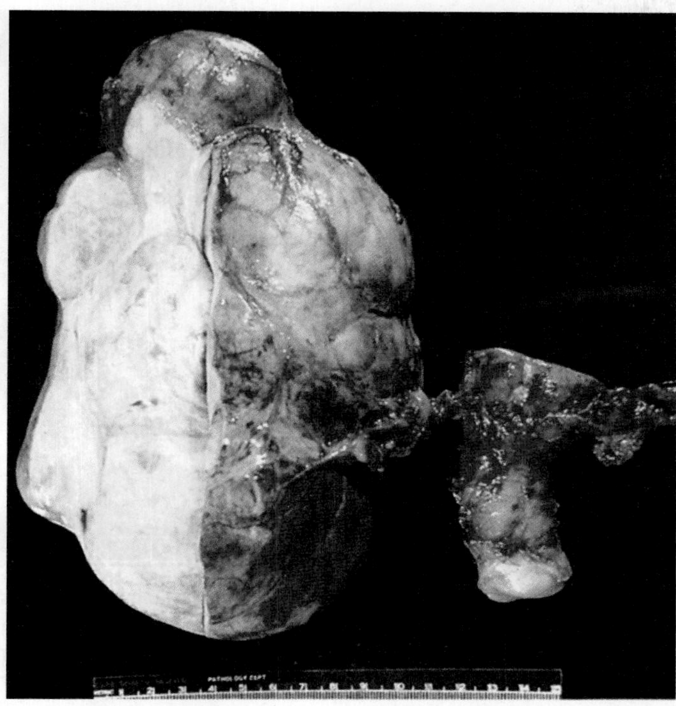

FIGURE 18-66. Fibroma of the ovary. The ovary is conspicuously enlarged by a firm, white, bosselated tumor.

Thecoma

Thecomas are functional ovarian tumors of postmenopausal women and are almost always benign. They are closely related to fibromas, but additionally contain varying amounts of steroidogenic cells that in many cases produce estrogens or androgen.

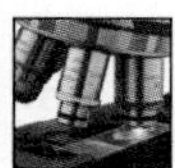

PATHOLOGY: Thecomas are solid, mostly 5 to 10 cm in diameter. Cut section is yellow, due to the many lipid-laden theca cells, which are large and oblong to round, with lipid-rich vacuolated cytoplasm (Fig. 18-67). Bands of hyalinized collagen separate nests of theca cells.

Because they produce estrogen, thecomas in premenopausal women may cause irregular menstrual cycles and breast enlargement. Endometrial hyperplasia and cancer are well-recognized complications.

Granulosa Cell Tumor

Granulosa cell tumors are the prototypical functional neoplasms of the ovary associated with estrogen secretion.

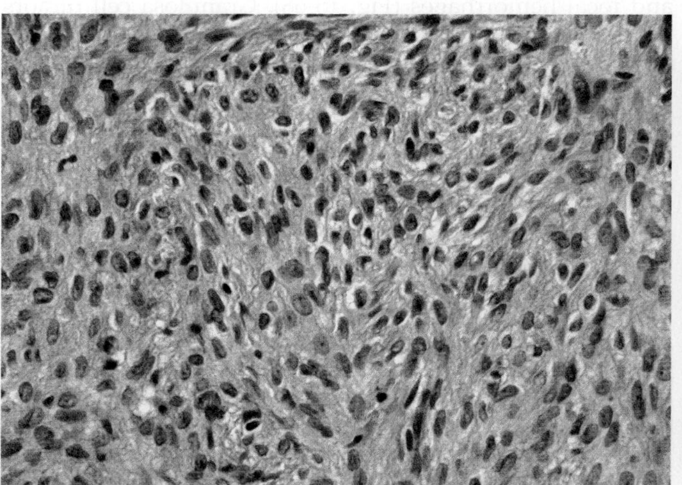

FIGURE 18-67. Thecoma of the ovary. Oblong cells are invested by collagen. The cytoplasm contains lipid.

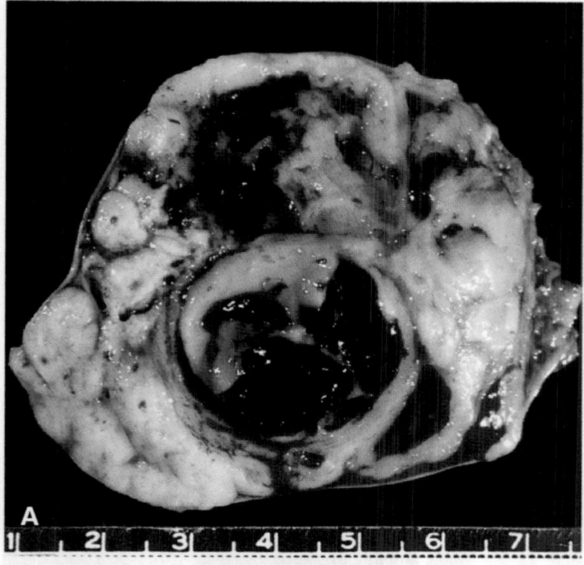

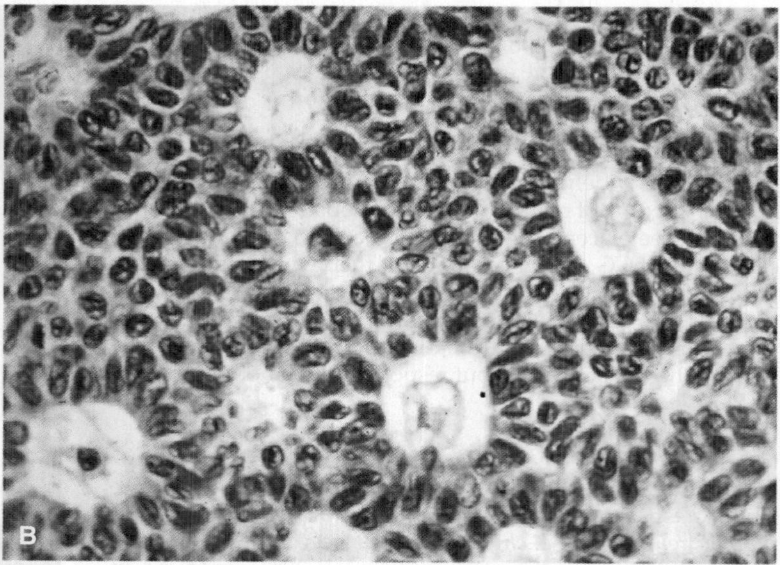

FIGURE 18-68. Granulosa cell tumor of the ovary. A. Cross-section of the enlarged ovary shows a variegated solid tumor with focal hemorrhages. The yellow areas represent collections of lipid-laden luteinized granulosa cells. **B.** The orientation of tumor cells about central spaces results in the characteristic follicular pattern (Call-Exner bodies).

They should be considered malignant because of their potential for local spread and the rare occurrence of distant metastases.

ETIOLOGIC FACTORS: Most granulosa cell tumors occur after menopause (adult form), and are unusual before puberty. A juvenile form occurs in children and young women and has distinct clinical and pathologic features (hyperestrinism and precocious puberty). Development of granulosa cell tumors is linked to loss of oocytes. Oocytes appear to regulate granulosa cells, and tumorigenesis occurs when follicles are disorganized or atretic.

PATHOLOGY: Adult-type granulosa cell tumors, like most ovarian tumors, are large and focally cystic to solid. The cut surface shows yellow areas, due to lipid-rich luteinized granulosa cells, white zones of stroma and focal hemorrhages (Fig. 18-68). Granulosa cell tumors show an array of growth patterns: (1) diffuse (sarcomatoid), (2) insular (islands of cells) or (3) trabecular (anastomotic bands of granulosa cells). Random nuclear arrangement about a central degenerative space **(Call-Exner bodies)** gives a characteristic follicular pattern (Fig. 18-68B). Tumor cells are typically spindle shaped and have a cleaved, elongated nucleus (coffee bean appearance). They secrete **inhibin,** a protein that suppresses pituitary release of follicle-stimulating hormone (FSH). These tumors can also express **calretinin,** a primarily neuronal protein, which suggests a possible neural differentiation or derivation for these neoplasms.

CLINICAL FEATURES: *Three fourths of granulosa cell tumors secrete estrogens.* Thus, endometrial hyperplasia is a common presenting sign. EIN or endometrial adenocarcinoma may develop if a functioning granulosa cell tumor remains undetected. At diagnosis, 90% of granulosa cell tumors are within the ovary (stage I). Over 90% of these patients survive 10 years. Tumors that have extended into the pelvis and lower abdomen have a poorer prognosis. Late recurrence after surgical removal is not uncommon after 5 to 10 years and is usually fatal.

Sertoli-Leydig Cell Tumors

Ovarian Sertoli-Leydig cell tumors **(arrhenoblastoma or androblastoma)** are rare androgen-secreting mesenchymal neoplasms of low malignant potential that resemble embryonic testis. Tumor cells typically secrete weak androgens (dehydroepiandrosterone), so tumors are usually quite large before patients complain of masculinization. Sertoli-Leydig cell tumors occur at all ages but are most common in young women of childbearing age.

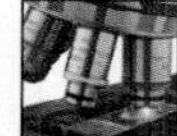

PATHOLOGY: Sertoli-Leydig cell tumors are unilateral, usually 5 to 15 cm, and tend to be lobulated, solid and brown to yellow. They vary from well to poorly differentiated and some have heterologous elements (e.g., mucinous glands and, rarely, even cartilage). Large Leydig cells have abundant eosinophilic cytoplasm and a central round to oval nucleus with a prominent nucleolus. The tumor cells are embedded in a sarcomatoid stroma (Fig. 18-69). The stroma in some areas often differentiates into immature solid tubules of embryonic Sertoli cells.

CLINICAL FEATURES: Nearly half of all patients with Sertoli-Leydig cell tumors exhibit signs of virilization: hirsutism, male escutcheon, enlarged clitoris and deepened voice. Initial signs are often defeminization, manifested as breast atrophy, amenorrhea and loss of hip fat. Once the tumor is removed, these signs disappear or at least lessen. Well-differentiated tumors are virtually always cured by surgical resection, but poorly differentiated ones may metastasize.

Steroid Cell Tumor

Steroid cell tumors of the ovary, also called **lipid cell** and **lipoid cell tumors,** are composed of cells that resemble lutein

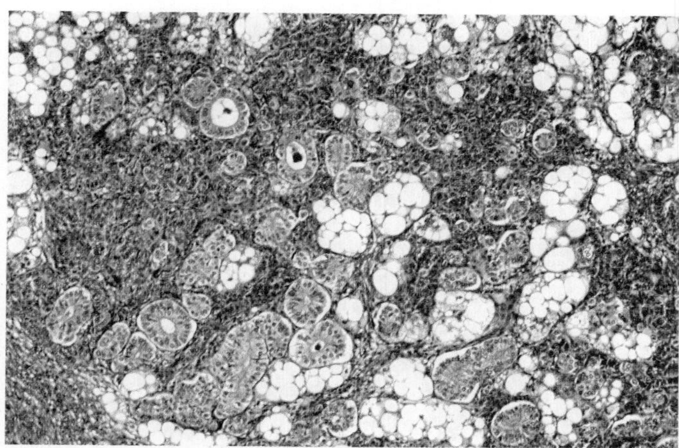

FIGURE 18-69. Sertoli-Leydig cell tumor, well differentiated. The hollow tubules are lined by mature Sertoli cells. The intervening stroma contains numerous Leydig cells with vacuolated cytoplasm.

cells, Leydig cells and adrenal cortical cells. Most steroid cell tumors are hormonally active, usually with androgenic manifestations. Some secrete testosterone; others synthesize weaker androgens. **Hilus cell tumor** is a specialized form of steroid cell tumor that is typically a benign neoplasm of Leydig cells. It arises in the hilus of the ovary, usually after menopause. As it secretes testosterone, the most potent of the common androgens, masculinizing signs are frequent (75%), even with small tumors. Most hilus cell tumors contain "crystalloids of Reinke" (rodlike cytoplasmic structures).

Tumors Metastatic to the Ovary May Mimic a Primary Tumor

About 3% of cancers found in the ovaries arise elsewhere, mostly in the breast, large intestine, endometrium and stomach, in descending order. These tumors vary from microscopic lesions to large masses. Those from the breast are usually tiny, and are seen in 10% of ovaries removed prophylactically in cases of advanced breast cancer. Metastatic tumors large enough to cause symptoms originate most often in the colon (Fig. 18-70). Commonly, the tumor cells stimulate ovarian stroma to differentiate into hormonally active cells (luteinized stromal cells), thereby inducing androgenic and sometimes estrogenic symptoms.

Krukenberg tumors are metastases to the ovary, composed of nests of mucin-filled "signet-ring" cells in a cellular stroma derived from the ovary (Fig. 18-71). The stomach is the primary site in 75% of cases and most of the rest are from the colon.

Bilateral ovarian involvement and multinodularity suggest a metastatic carcinoma, and both ovaries are grossly involved in 75% of cases. Even an ovary that grossly appears uninvolved may contain surface implants or minute foci of tumor within the parenchyma. Thus, when metastasis to one ovary is documented, the other should also be removed.

PERITONEUM

The peritoneum is a nearly continuous membrane that lines the peritoneal cavity and separates viscera from the abdominal wall. In men, the peritoneum is a closed system. In women, it is an "open system" interrupted in the pelvis by the fallopian tubes, which provide a final conduit for transmission of pathogens and chemicals from the genital tract to the peritoneal cavity.

The cells that line the peritoneal cavity and those that form the serosa of the ovary are both of celomic epithelial origin. ***Thus, it is not clear whether tumors and tumorlike lesions of peritoneum and ovary (i.e., müllerian epithelial lesions) are the same entity in both locations.***

Many inflammatory lesions involve the peritoneum, including granulomatous peritonitis as a response to suture materials, surgical glove powder and contrast media; intestinal contents following perforation (e.g., in Crohn disease or

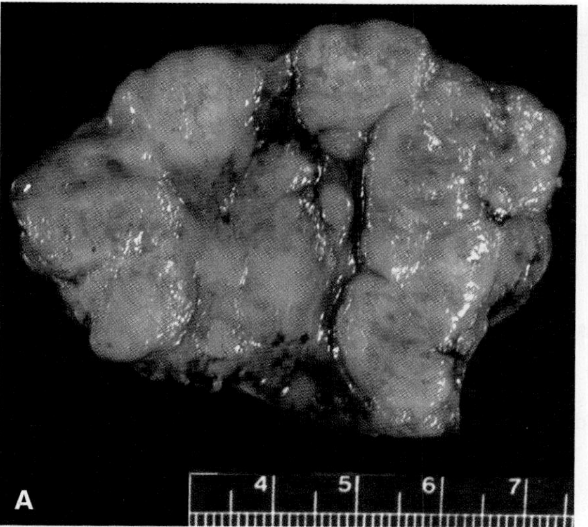

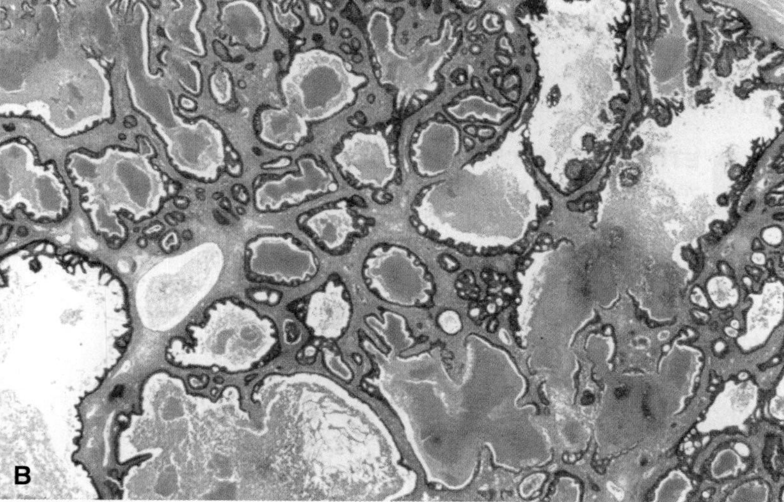

FIGURE 18-70. Metastatic adenocarcinoma from colon. A. The ovary is replaced by multinodular tumor. The sectioned surface appears solid. **B.** Microscopically, the tumor shows a garlandlike glandular pattern with focal segmental necrosis and abundant necrotic debris.

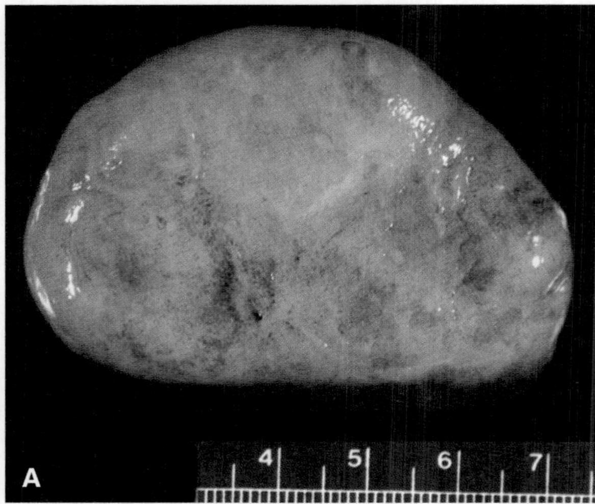

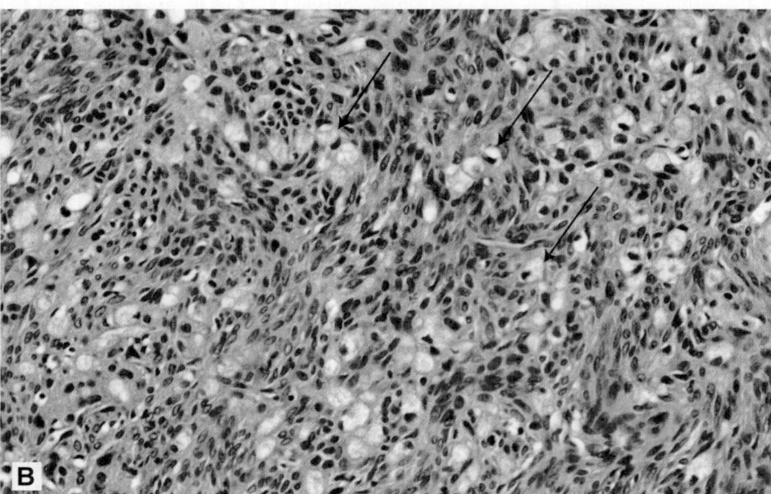

FIGURE 18-71. Krukenberg tumor. A. The ovary is enlarged and the cut surface appears solid, pale-yellow and partially hemorrhagic. **B.** A microscopic section of **A** reveals mucinous (signet-ring) cells (clear cells, *arrows*) infiltrating the ovarian stroma.

diverticulitis); rupture of a mature cystic teratoma (dermoid cyst) of the ovary; and, of course, tuberculosis. It is also the site of reactive mesothelial proliferation, which occurs with the slightest irritation. Peritonitis is discussed in Chapter 13.

Endometriosis

Endometriosis is the presence of benign endometrial glands and stroma outside the uterus. It afflicts 5% to 10% of women of reproductive age and regresses after natural or artificial menopause. The mean age at diagnosis is the late twenties to early thirties, although it may appear any time after menarche. Sites most frequently involved are the ovaries (>60%), other uterine adnexa (uterine ligaments, rectovaginal septum, pouch of Douglas) and the pelvic peritoneum covering the uterus, fallopian tubes, rectosigmoid colon and bladder (Fig. 18-72). Endometriosis can be even more widespread and occasionally affects the cervix, vagina, perineum, bladder and umbilicus. Even pelvic lymph nodes may contain foci of endometriosis. Rarely, distant areas such as lungs, pleura, small bowel, kidneys and bones contain lesions.

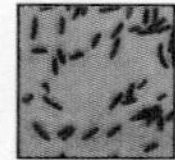

ETIOLOGIC FACTORS: Several theories, not necessarily mutually exclusive, are invoked to explain the histogenesis of endometriosis:

1. **Transplantation** of endometrial fragments to ectopic sites
2. **Metaplasia** of the multipotential celomic peritoneum
3. **Induction** of undifferentiated mesenchyme in ectopic sites to form lesions after exposure to substances released from shed endometrium

TRANSPLANTATION: The most widely accepted theory holds that menstrual endometrium refluxes through the fallopian tubes and implants at ectopic sites. It is known that retrograde menstruation through the fallopian tubes occurs in 90% of women. An extension of this theory is lymphatic and hematogenous dissemination, which would explain endometriosis in lymph nodes and at distant organ sites like the lungs and kidneys. The observation that pulmonary endometriosis occurs almost exclusively in women who have had uterine surgery supports this contention.

CELOMIC METAPLASIA: This theory proposes that endometriosis arises by endometrial metaplasia of peritoneal serosa or serosa-like structures. Thus, if appropriately stimulated, the pelvic peritoneum may differentiate into any type of müllerian epithelium.

INDUCTION THEORY: This concept suggests that a substance secreted by the endometrium induces development of endometrial epithelium and stroma in ectopic sites.

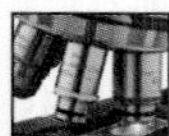

PATHOLOGY: The earliest lesions of endometriosis may be yellow-red stains, reflecting breakdown of blood products. Red lesions, which also occur early in the disease, are actively growing foci of endometriosis

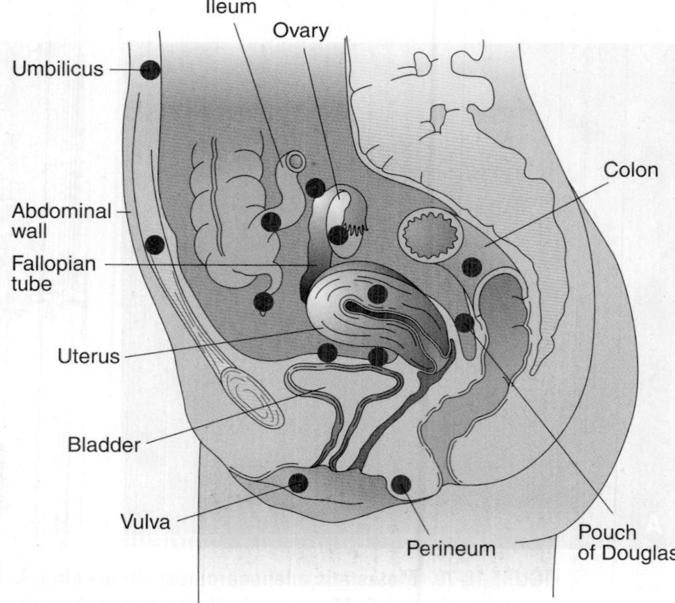

FIGURE 18-72. Sites of endometriosis.

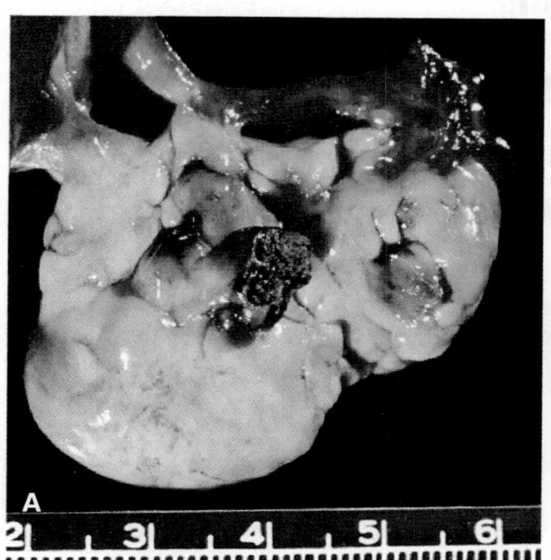

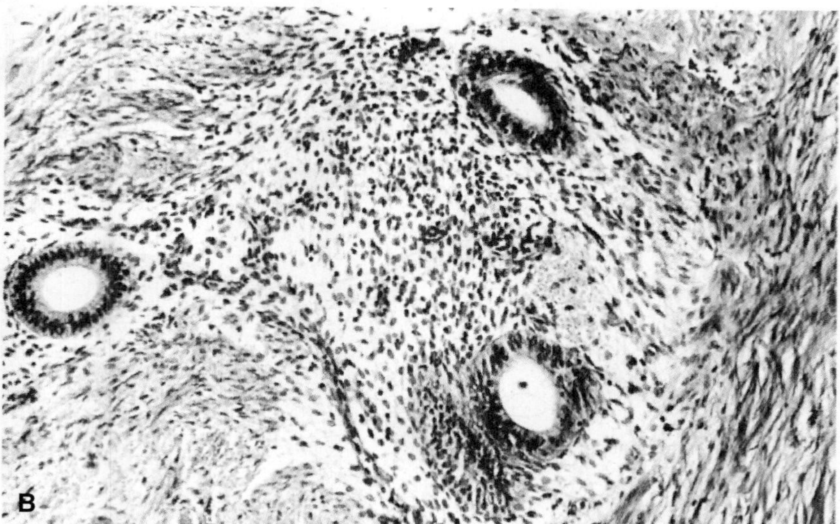

FIGURE 18-73. Endometriosis. A. Implants of endometriosis on the ovary appear as red-blue nodules. **B.** A microscopic section shows endometrial glands and stroma in the ovary.

(Fig. 18-73). Pathologists usually see black lesions in operative specimens, which show some degree of resolution. These 1- to 5-mm foci on the ovary and peritoneal surfaces are termed "mulberry" nodules. With repeated cycles, hemorrhage and the onset of fibrosis, affected surfaces may scar and become grossly brown ("powder burns"). Over time, fibrous adhesions may become more pronounced and may lead to complications, such as intestinal obstruction. In the ovaries, repeated hemorrhage may turn endometriotic foci into cysts up to 15 cm in diameter containing inspissated, chocolate-colored material ("chocolate cysts").

Endometriosis is characterized by ectopic normal endometrial glands and stroma (Fig. 18-73). Occasionally, healed foci may only contain fibrous tissue and hemosiderin-laden macrophages, features that by themselves are not diagnostic. Immunohistochemical demonstration of CD-10 can be diagnostic.

CLINICAL FEATURES: The symptoms of endometriosis depend on where the implants are located. Dysmenorrhea, caused by implants on uterosacral ligaments, is common. Lesions swell just before or during menstruation, producing pelvic pain. Half of all women with dysmenorrhea have endometriosis. Other symptoms include dyspareunia and cyclical abdominal pain.

Infertility is the primary complaint in a third of women with endometriosis (Fig. 18-74). The hormonal milieu in a woman who does not achieve pregnancy encourages development of endometriosis. In turn, once endometriosis develops, it contributes to the infertile state and a vicious circle is established. Conversely, pregnancy may alleviate the disease. Conservative surgery to restore pelvic anatomy helps many women with endometriosis to become pregnant.

Malignancy occurs in about 1% to 2% of cases of endometriosis (Fig. 18-60). Clear cell and endometrioid tumors are the most frequent forms. Adenosarcoma, although rare, is the most common sarcoma.

Mesothelial Tumors

Mesothelial tumors range from benign neoplasms to multicentric and aggressive malignancies.

Adenomatoid Tumor Is a Benign Mesothelial Tumor, Mainly of Fallopian Tubes

It is encountered in the fallopian tubes and in subserosal tissue of the uterine corpus near the fallopian tubes. It is rare elsewhere in the peritoneum.

Well-Differentiated Papillary Mesotheliomas Are Benign

Well-differentiated papillary mesotheliomas are rare tumors of women of reproductive age. They are typically asymptomatic and are usually found incidentally at operation. These tumors are typically solitary, small, broad-based, wartlike polypoid or nodular excrescences with a single layer of small bland cuboidal cells covering thick papillae (Fig. 18-75). These lesions often resemble serous epithelial tumors of the ovary, but the two are treated differently.

Diffuse Malignant Mesothelioma Is an Invariably Fatal Peritoneal Tumor

These tumors arise from peritoneal mesothelium. They are rare in women and constitute only a small proportion of all malignant mesotheliomas, most of which are pleural. These tumors should be distinguished from serous adenocarcinomas, including those arising from the peritoneal surface itself and those metastatic from the ovary, since the tumors are treated differently and have much different survival rates. Most patients are middle-aged or postmenopausal whose symptoms are nonspecific and include ascites, abdominal discomfort, digestive disturbances and weight loss. Asbestos exposure is uncommon in women with peritoneal mesothelioma, unlike pleural tumors, but up to 2 million fibers per gram of wet weight have been reported in some tumors.

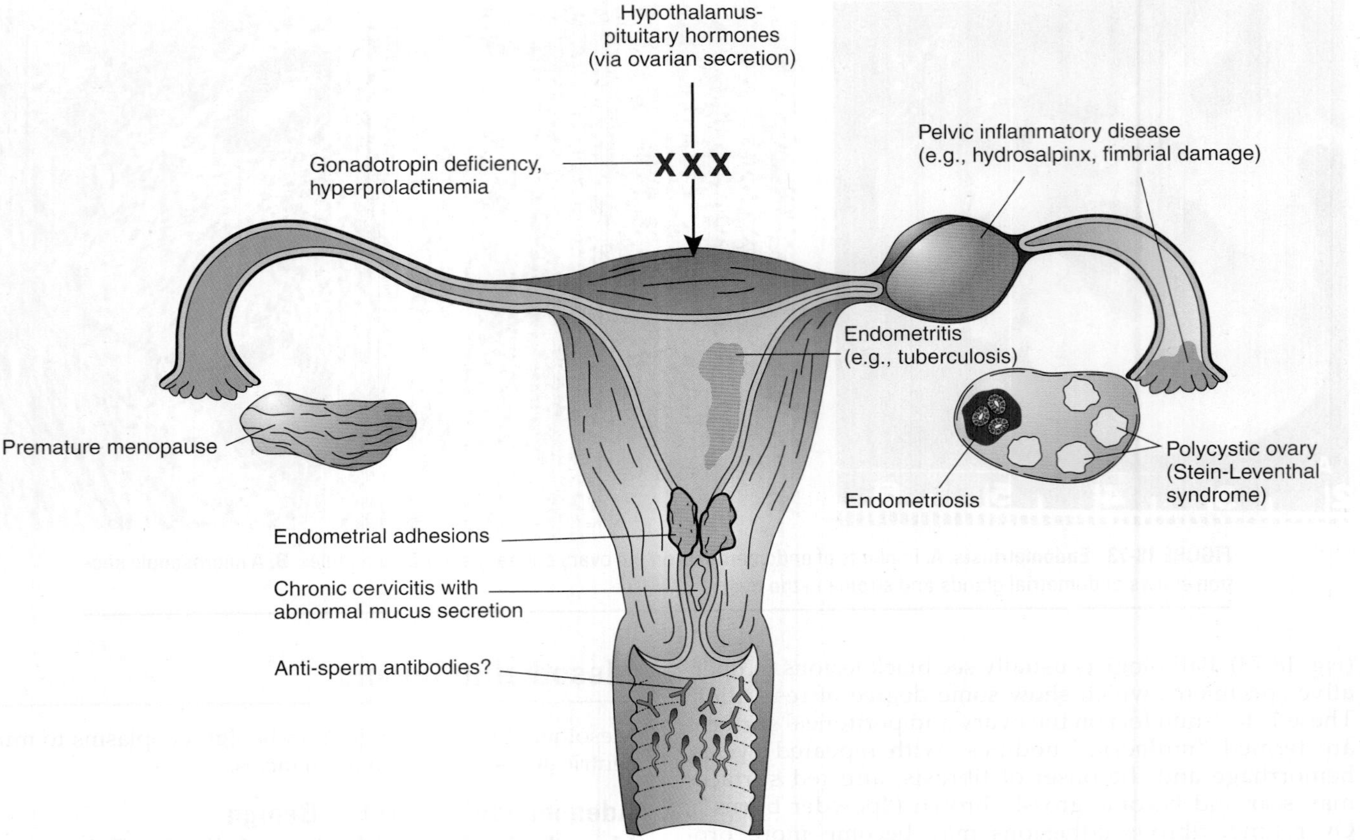

FIGURE 18-74. Causes of acquired infertility.

PATHOLOGY: Diffuse malignant mesothelioma extensively involves and thickens the peritoneum and serosa of the various abdominal and pelvic organs. It has a tubulopapillary to solid pattern. Unlike pleural mesothelioma, the sarcomatoid type is rare. The epithelial variant displays polygonal or cuboidal neoplastic cells with abundant cytoplasm. Thrombomodulin, calretinin, cytokeratin 5/6 and HBME-1 are markers of malignant mesothelioma, whereas CA-125, CEA and estrogen and progesterone receptors (ER and PR) are markers of ovarian epithelial tumors. No effective treatment is available.

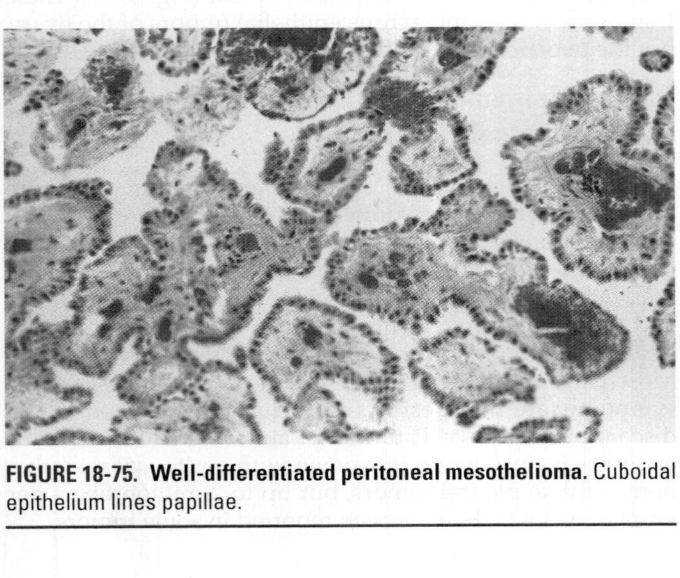

FIGURE 18-75. Well-differentiated peritoneal mesothelioma. Cuboidal epithelium lines papillae.

Serous Tumors (Primary and Metastatic)

Unlike the ovary, which features a wide range of tumors, serous tumors are virtually the only type found in the peritoneum. Mucinous tumors in the peritoneum are metastases from a primary cancer of the appendix or ovary.

Serous Tumors of Borderline Malignancy Resemble the Ovarian Neoplasm

Most serous borderline tumors in the peritoneum are metastases from the ovary, but some may be primary in the peritoneum. In the latter case, serous peritoneal tumors without evidence of invasion usually are benign; those that are invasive carry a worse prognosis.

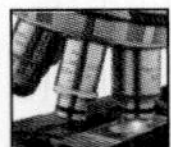

PATHOLOGY: Whether in the ovary or the peritoneum, borderline serous tumors are characterized by papillary processes, small clusters of cells, cell stratification, detached cellular clusters, nuclear atypia and mitotic activity in the absence of invasion. Implants appear as fine granularities or small nodules with clusters of blunt papillae or glandular structures, often having complex cellular tufts (Fig. 18-76). Psammoma bodies are common and may fill the core of the papillae. Mild to severe cytologic

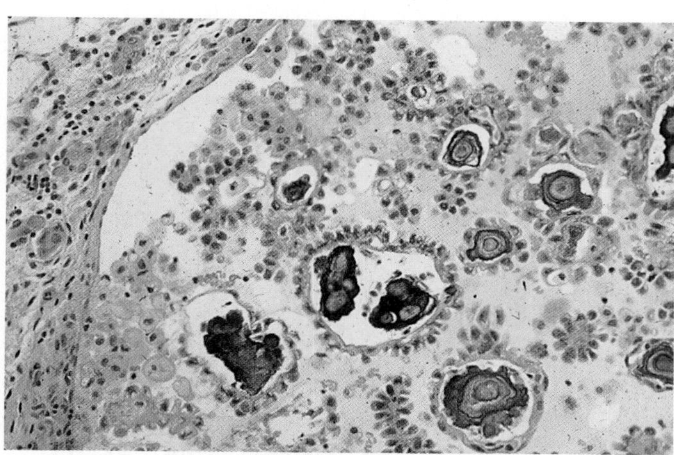

FIGURE 18-76. Noninvasive implants of borderline serous tumor on the peritoneum. The tumor exhibits epithelial tufts and psammoma bodies (compare to Fig. 18-56B).

atypia with some stratification is common but is substantially less than that seen in adenocarcinoma.

Serous Adenocarcinoma Occurs in Women With Normal Ovaries

The frequency of serous adenocarcinoma arising de novo in the peritoneum is estimated as 10% of its counterpart in the ovary. The mean age of women with this tumor is 50 to 65 years. The diagnosis of a primary peritoneal tumor requires demonstration of normal ovaries. Abdominal pain and ascites are frequent presentations. Like ovarian cancer, serous adenocarcinoma primarily in the peritoneum may have a familial basis and can metastasize to distant locations.

Pseudomyxoma Peritonei

Pseudomyxoma peritonei is the accumulation of jellylike mucus in the pelvis or peritoneum. Previously interpreted as spread from mucinous ovarian tumors, pseudomyxoma peritonei is now understood to derive largely from mucus-producing adenocarcinomas of the appendix.

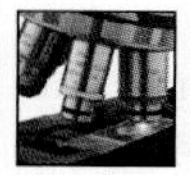

PATHOLOGY: The condition may be extensive and appear as semisolid gelatin covering all abdominal structures, or there may be little more than a slightly thickened gelatinous coat over a focal area of bowel or omentum. The appendix is commonly enlarged or adherent to an omentum covered with the gelatinous material. Within the gelatin are strips of very well-differentiated, intestinal-type, mucinous epithelium (Fig. 18-77). If only isolated foci are present, the epithelium may be so well differentiated that it resembles a simple mucinous adenoma. Cribriform patterns or other histologic features of malignancy, such as signet-ring cells or glands, are seen on occasion and warrant a diagnosis of adenocarcinoma.

Low-grade tumors are usually treated for cure, which entails aggressive surgical debulking and intraperitoneal chemotherapy. The 5-year survival is under 50%.

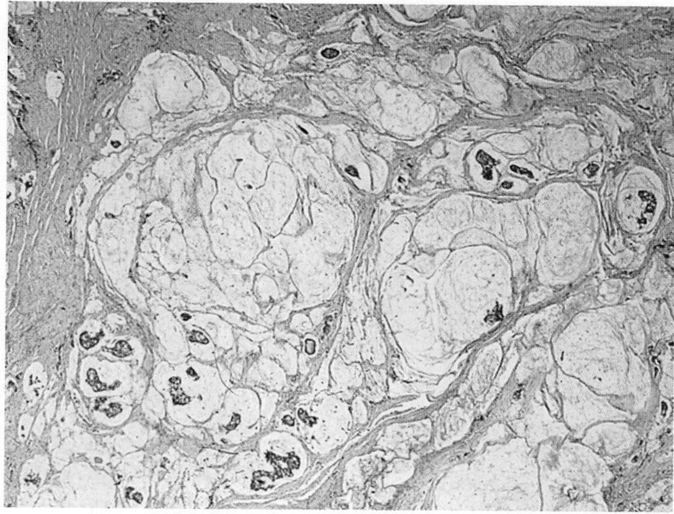

FIGURE 18-77. Pseudomyxoma peritonei. Multiple clusters of tumor cells are present in the mucinous material.

PATHOLOGY OF PREGNANCY

Placenta

Placental Anatomy

The placenta is a unique structure—it has two separate vascular supplies from two genetically distinct individuals (Fig. 18-78A). This complex organ has a fixed lifespan corresponding to the intrauterine gestation of the fetus. Although it is the largest organ of the developing fetus, it exists outside the fetal body, and includes the **placental disc, umbilical cord** and **extraplacental membranes.** The placenta is a flattened discoidal organ with two surfaces. One surface, facing the fetus **(fetal** or **chorionic surface)** is covered by membranes, the **amnion** and **chorion.** These are the "bag of water" with the **amniotic fluid** that surrounds the fetus. The opposite surface is the **maternal surface** (or the **decidual surface,** as the endometrium is termed the decidua during pregnancy).

Fetal blood enters the placenta through two umbilical arteries that spiral around an umbilical vein. Each artery supplies half of the placenta. The umbilical cord inserts into the chorionic surface on the placenta—the major branches of the umbilical arteries and vein (chorionic plate blood vessels) then branch along the surface of the disc and then penetrate into the placental disc to form the chorionic villous tree. Primary stem villi originate at the chorionic plate and contain the major branches of the umbilical arteries and veins. These villous trunks progressively subdivide into smaller branches, becoming the intermediate-sized secondary villi and, finally, the smaller terminal (tertiary) villi where oxygen transport occurs. At term, the terminal villi constitute almost 40% of the villous volume and nearly 60% of villous cross-sections.

The **decidua** forms the border between fetal tissue composing the villous trees, and the underlying uterus. The decidua contains approximately 80 to 100 small uterine arteries (**spiral arterioles,** branches of the myometrial arteries) that supply the placenta with oxygen- and nutrient-rich maternal blood. These arteries are normally remodeled to decrease vascular resistance to uterine blood flow. Each spiral

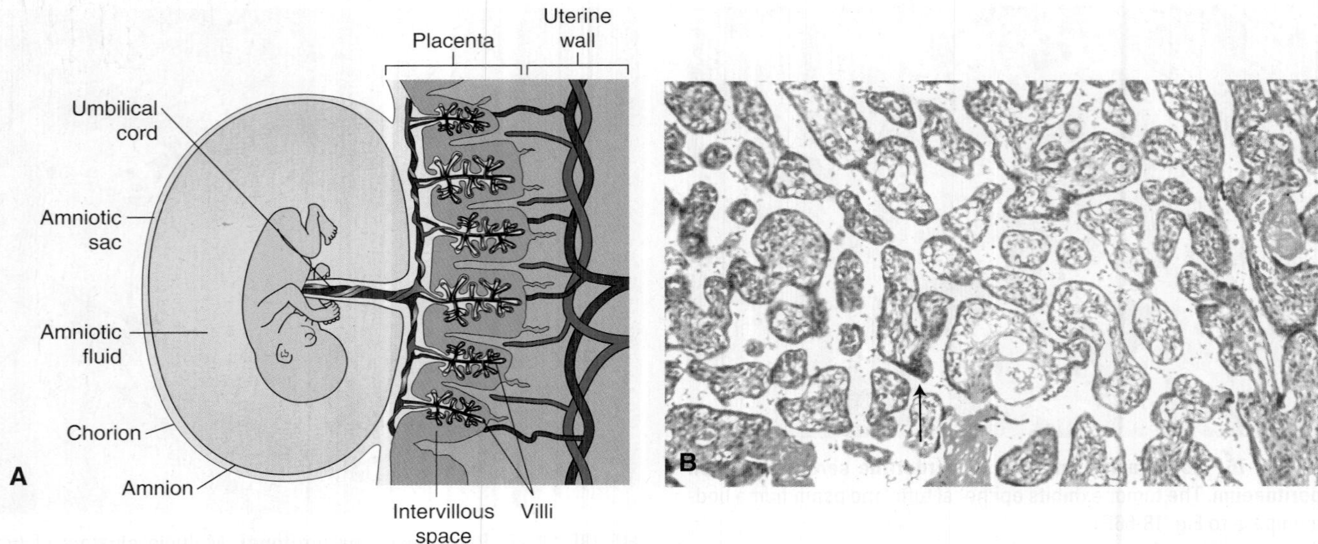

FIGURE 18-78. Normal placenta. A. Developing fetus within the uterus. B. Mature villi. *Arrow*: syncytial knot.

arteriole delivers its maternal blood to the center of an anatomic subunit of the placenta, the cotyledon. Maternal blood entering the placental disc is no longer confined to a vessel, but instead occupies a cavity, the **intervillous space.** The maternal blood flows around the villous tree, allowing exchange of oxygen and nutrients. Maternal blood is the sole source of oxygen and nutrients for the developing fetus.

The terminal villus is the placenta's functional unit of exchange. It consists of an inner layer of **cytotrophoblast (Langhans cells),** a middle layer of **intermediate trophoblast** and an outer layer of **syncytiotrophoblast.** The villous stroma is loose mesenchyme containing embryonal macrophages (Hofbauer cells). The tertiary villi decrease in size as gestation progresses. In the third trimester, syncytiotrophoblast nuclei aggregate to form multinuclear protrusions **(syncytial knots)** (Fig. 18-78B). In other areas along the villous surface, syncytium between the knots becomes markedly attenuated. At these points, the trophoblastic cytoplasm comes into direct contact with the endothelium of the fetal capillaries to form the vasculosyncytial membrane. These specialized zones facilitate gas and nutrient transfer across the placenta. In addition to releasing waste and absorbing oxygen and nutrients, the villi are hormonally active. ***Trophoblast secretes hCG and other biologically active compounds.***

Placental Size

To provide sufficient oxygen and nutrients to the developing fetus, the placenta increases in weight and size as gestation progresses. For example, its mean weight at 30 weeks' gestation is 316 grams, at 35 weeks it is 434 grams and at term (40 weeks) it averages 537 grams. The relationship between placental and fetal weights is also important. When the fetus is at term, 1 gram of optimally functioning placenta can oxygenate and nourish approximately 7 grams of fetal tissue. This relationship, called the **fetal–placental weight ratio,** is important to understand how chronic uteroplacental malperfusion, or placental insufficiency, arises. An abnormally small placenta, in which there is an increased fetal–placental weight ratio, may be too small to provide for the fetus, contributing to a poor obstetric outcome. Abnormally thin placentas (<2 cm thickness at term) can also be associated with poor obstetric outcomes.

Placental Shape

A typical placental disc is round or ovoid. In **bilobed placentas** (2% to 8% of placentas), two approximately equal-sized discs are separated by a segment of membranes through which fetal vessels (termed membranous vessels) run. A **succenturiate placenta** (5% to 6% of placentas) is a bilobed placenta in which one lobe is smaller than the other.

Placental Implantation

The placenta is normally implanted in the uterine wall, above the level of the internal cervical os. It may implant at the lower portion of the uterus and either partially or completely cover the internal os, a state called **placenta previa** (Fig. 18-79). Complete placenta previa is potentially hazardous, and must be recognized before delivery, to avoid the fetus being delivered through its own placenta, risking life-threatening hemorrhage. Placenta previa entails high risk of abruption, postpartum hemorrhage, fetal malpresentation and fetal and perinatal mortality.

Ectopic pregnancy occurs when a placenta implants outside the uterine cavity. It usually occurs in the fallopian tube, but about 2% of ectopic pregnancies occur in the ovary, cervix or abdomen. Abdominal pregnancy is associated with very high maternal morbidity and mortality.

Abnormalities of the Umbilical Cord

Some of the most common abnormalities of the umbilical cord involve the site at which it inserts into the fetal surface of the placenta. The point of insertion is usually at or near the center of the placental disc, but in about 7% of cases the cord inserts at the margin, termed **marginal insertion.** About 1% of umbilical cords insert into the membranes, termed a **velamentous** or **membranous insertion.** Velamentous and marginal

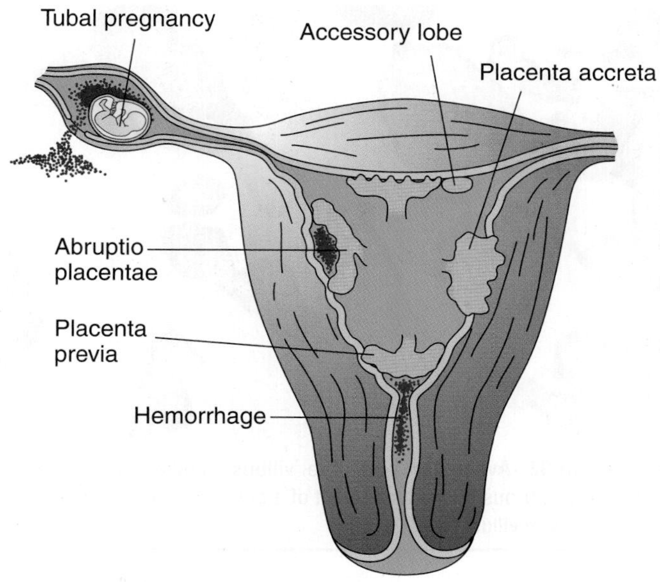

FIGURE 18-79. Uteroplacental abnormalities.

cord insertions are often seen in spontaneous abortions and fetuses with congenital anomalies. A serious potential complication of velamentous vessels is **vasa previa,** in which the membranous blood vessels of the cord cover the cervical os. Such vessels are easily ruptured during delivery, resulting in life-threatening hemorrhage.

Placental Infections

Chorioamnionitis Is the Histologic Hallmark of an Ascending Infection

Infectious organisms, almost exclusively bacteria, ascend from the maternal birth canal, pass through the cervical os and infect the decidua and placental tissues.

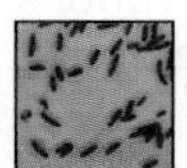

ETIOLOGIC FACTORS: Acute chorioamnionitis may be monomicrobial or polymicrobial, and is usually caused by bacteria that are normally present in the maternal cervicovaginal canal. The most common bacterial causes of chorioamnionitis are group B *Streptococcus* sp., *E. coli*, *Enterococcus*, other streptococcal species, *Staphylococcus* sp., gram-negative bacilli, *Bacteroides*, *Mycoplasma hominis* and *Ureaplasma*.

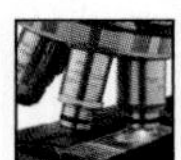

PATHOLOGY: Upon reaching the uterine cavity, the organisms elicit a maternal acute inflammatory response. Neutrophils from the mother migrate from the intervillous space of the placenta into the chorion and amnion of the placental disc and membranes, termed the maternal inflammatory response (MIR). The demonstration of neutrophils in the amnion and chorion identifies acute chorioamnionitis (Fig. 18-80). Amniotic fluid is usually cloudy, and membrane walls are slightly opaque, malodorous and edematous. If the infection is present for a while, the fetus may develop its own acute inflammatory response to the infection: fetal neutrophils migrate into the muscular walls of the umbilical vessels **(acute funisitis)** and large fetal vessels at the placental surface (acute **chorionic vasculitis**), called the **fetal inflammatory response.**

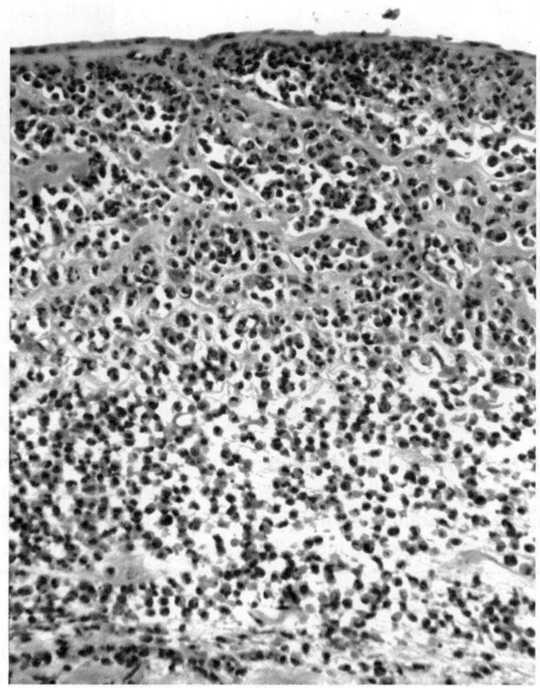

FIGURE 18-80. Acute chorioamnionitis. There is an intense infiltration of the amnion and chorion with neutrophils.

CLINICAL FEATURES: Acute chorioamnionitis is seen in about 10% of placentas, and can cause preterm labor, preterm and premature rupture of membranes, fetal and neonatal infections and intrauterine hypoxia. The mother may have fever, uterine tenderness, foul-smelling amniotic fluid and tachycardia. Major risks to the mother are postpartum endometritis and pelvic sepsis with venous thrombosis.

In preterm, low–birth-weight (<2500 grams) and especially very low–birth-weight (<1500 grams) infants, acute chorioamnionitis may lead to severe neurologic disease including cerebral palsy, as well as stillbirth, neonatal death and sepsis. However, it can also cause morbidity in full-term infants, particularly if (1) it is present for some time prior to delivery, (2) it is caused by highly pathogenic organisms or (3) there is a severe fetal inflammatory response. The risks of chorioamnionitis to the fetus include (1) pneumonia after inhalation of infected amniotic fluid; (2) skin or eye infections from direct contact with organisms in the fluid; and (3) neonatal gastritis, enteritis or peritonitis from ingestion of infected fluid.

Villitis Usually Reflects Hematogenous Infection

Villitis results from transplacental passage of organisms usually from the maternal circulation. The process is frequently focal. Although infection cannot be demonstrated in most cases, the microorganisms include (1) bacteria (*Listeria*, *T. pallidum*, *M. tuberculosis*, *Mycoplasma* sp., *Chlamydia* sp.), (2) viruses (rubella, CMV, herpes), (3) parasites and protozoa

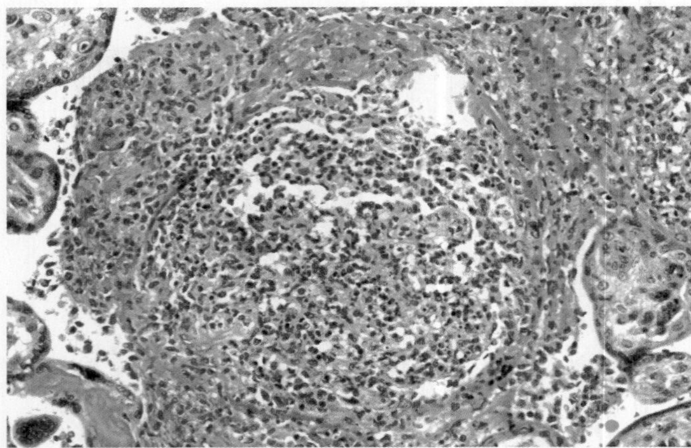

FIGURE 18-81. Acute villitis. Acute villitis caused by *Listeria monocytogenes*. The central villus has been destroyed by acute inflammation and has the appearance of a microabscess. The neutrophils extend from the inflamed villus into the intervillous space and adjacent villi.

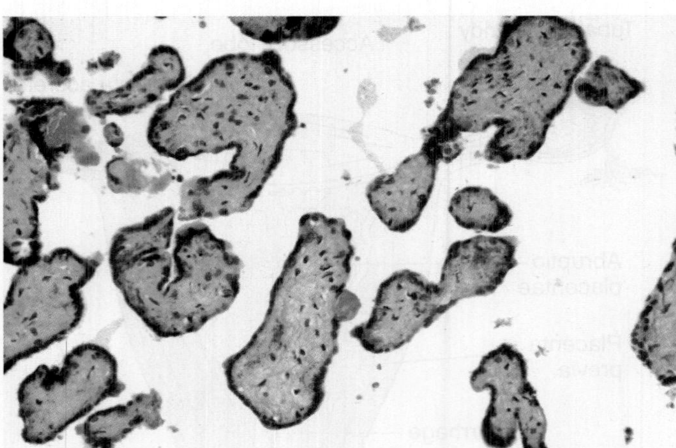

FIGURE 18-82. Avascular villi. The villous capillaries have been replaced by fibrous tissue as a result of a chronic thrombus in a larger upstream stem villus.

(*Toxoplasma* sp.) and (4) fungi (*Candida* sp.). The most important consequence of hematogenous placental infection is establishment of an inflammatory focus that infects the fetus secondarily. Perinatal morbidity and mortality can result from transplacental transmission of the microbial agent, inflammatory mediators, destruction of chorionic villi and placental insufficiency.

Recurrent Villitis of Unknown Etiology Is Associated With Reproductive Loss

Villitis of unknown etiology (VUE) is a significant cause of chronic placental insufficiency in which no infectious agent is found. VUE probably has multiple different etiologies, including as yet unidentified infectious agents and an immune reaction similar to a graft versus host reaction. VUE occurs in upwards of 5% to 10% of all pregnancies, and is associated with a significant rate of recurrence and with poor obstetric outcomes. Pregnancy failures occur in about 60% of pregnancies complicated by recurrent VUE. Infants who survive may have brain injury, including cerebral palsy.

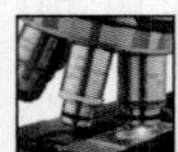

PATHOLOGY: Villitis may be focal or diffuse, and consist of acute and chronic inflammatory cells, or even granulomas. If it destroys chorionic villi, the prognosis for the fetus is ominous (Fig. 18-81). Not all infectious agents present in the maternal bloodstream cause villitis. For example, human immunodeficiency virus (HIV) does not. Villitis can cause microscopic abnormalities of chronic placental insufficiency, including fetal thrombotic vasculopathy with avascular villi and increased fibrin.

Vascular Disorders of the Placenta

Fetal Thrombotic Vasculopathy Results From Clotting in Placental Vessels

Risk factors for development of fetal thrombotic vasculopathy (FTV) include villitis and disorders of coagulation, particularly hypercoagulable syndromes (see Chapter 20). In some cases, there is no identifiable risk factor for thrombosis. Clots forming in the placental circulation can have fearsome complications for the fetus, as they cause placental insufficiency by obstructing blood flow and thus perfusion in part of the villous trees. A variety of poor outcomes are associated with FTV including stillbirth, neonatal death, intrauterine growth restriction and, in surviving infants, neurologic injury including cerebral palsy. Blood clots in the fetal placental circulation may occur together with blood clots in the fetal body, including lungs, brain and kidneys.

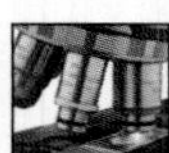

PATHOLOGY: Thrombi may be seen in chorionic villous blood vessels of all sizes. In chronic FTV, chorionic villi downstream from thrombosed vessels undergo progressive fibrosis, giving a distinctive appearance to clusters of scarred villi, termed **avascular villi** (Fig. 18-82). If larger chorionic vessels are thrombosed, the thrombus can attach to, and later be incorporated into, the vessel wall forming a mural thrombus, or **cushion defect.** Microcalcifications in avascular villi or mural thrombi are markers of the chronic-

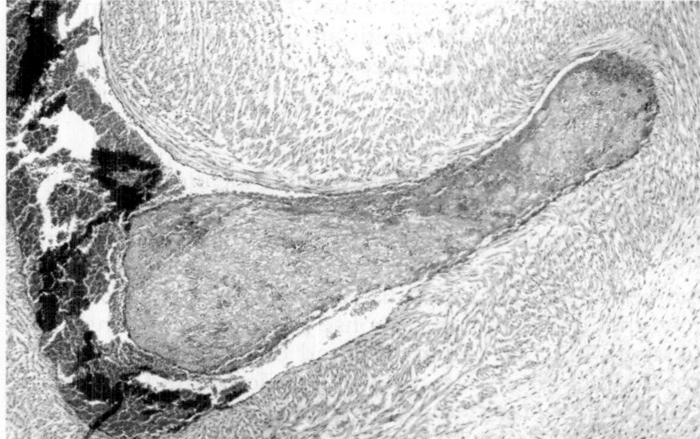

FIGURE 18-83. Thrombus within an umbilical cord blood vessel.

ity of the process. Thrombosis in the umbilical cord vessels (Fig. 18-83) can be catastrophic, as only three vessels (two umbilical arteries and one vein) transport all blood from the placenta to the fetus.

Abruptio Placentae May Cause Retroplacental Hematoma

Retroplacental hematoma occurs between the basal plate of the placenta and the uterine wall (Fig. 18-79). It is one of the most common causes of perinatal mortality, accounting for 8% of perinatal deaths. Hemorrhage usually comes from a ruptured maternal (spiral) artery or premature separation of the placenta. Retroplacental hemorrhage can be due to placental abruption **(abruptio placentae),** but in one third of cases it occurs without clinical abruption, and the reverse is also true. Abruptio placentae and retroplacental hematoma are often the final consequence of a chronic disorder, usually in the decidua and uterine blood vessels. Key risk factors for retroplacental hematoma include maternal smoking or hypertension, greater maternal age, acute chorioamnionitis and cocaine abuse. Trauma, as a motor vehicle accident or severe fall, can also precipitate retroplacental hemorrhage, but accounts for a small minority of cases.

PATHOLOGY: The hematomas may be small or may occupy the entire maternal surface of the placenta. Recent hematomas are soft, red and easily detached from the maternal surface. Older ones are firm and brown, and more adherent to the placental surface. Chronic retroplacental hematomas may indent the maternal surface of the placenta, indicating where they occupied space. When a retroplacental hematoma is present for some time, overlying villous tissue will begin to show ischemic degeneration, eventually causing an infarct. Adverse perinatal outcomes associated with retroplacental hematomas relate to size of the hematoma, coexistence of other placental abnormalities and severity of accompanying clinical conditions, such as preeclampsia. A large retroplacental hematoma can cause placental insufficiency and poor obstetric outcome.

Intervillous Thrombi Represent Fetomaternal Hemorrhage

Rupture of a chorionic villous blood vessel causes blood to accumulate in the placenta and to form an intervillous thrombus or hematoma. Since the pressure of the fetal circulation is higher than that of the maternal circulation in the placenta, fetal blood accumulates in the intervillous space, producing an intervillous thrombus. This represents a fetomaternal hemorrhage, and the entry of fetal blood into the maternal circulation can have clinical implications if there are blood group incompatibilities between the fetus and mother. Small intervillous thrombi occur in up to 20% of full-term-gestation placentas, and are usually clinically insignificant. A larger thrombus or multiple thrombi may have a deleterious effect on the fetus owing to fetal blood loss or hypoxia.

Placenta Accreta Is Abnormal Adherence of the Placenta to the Uterus

Placenta accreta is caused by failure to form decidua (Fig. 18-79). Normally, the decidual endometrium is present between the base of the placenta and the underlying uterine muscle. Placenta accreta occurs when the decidual layer is partially or totally deficient, and the villi are in direct contact with fibrin, extravillous trophoblast or uterine muscle. The placenta does not separate normally from the underlying uterine wall at the time of delivery, which may lead to life-threatening maternal hemorrhage. Risk factors for placenta accreta include placenta previa, prior cesarean sections, advanced maternal age, high parity and endometrial defects. Placenta accreta occurs in 10% of cases of placenta previa. A similar situation may arise when implantation occurs on scars from a previous cesarean section (termed Asherman syndrome). A woman who has had placenta previa and two previous cesarean sections has a 40% risk of placenta accreta.

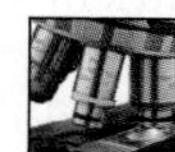

PATHOLOGY: Placenta accreta is classified by the depth of myometrial invasion by the villi:

- **Placenta accreta** refers to the attachment of villi to the surface of the uterine wall without further invasion (Fig. 18-84). It occurs in approximately 1 of 2500 pregnancies.
- **Placenta increta** defines villi invading the underlying myometrium.
- **Placenta percreta** describes villi penetrating the full thickness of the uterine wall.

CLINICAL FEATURES: Patients with placenta accreta can have a normal pregnancy and delivery. However, complications may occur during pregnancy, during delivery or especially in the immediate postpartum period. Third-trimester bleeding is the most common presenting sign: substantial fragments of placenta may

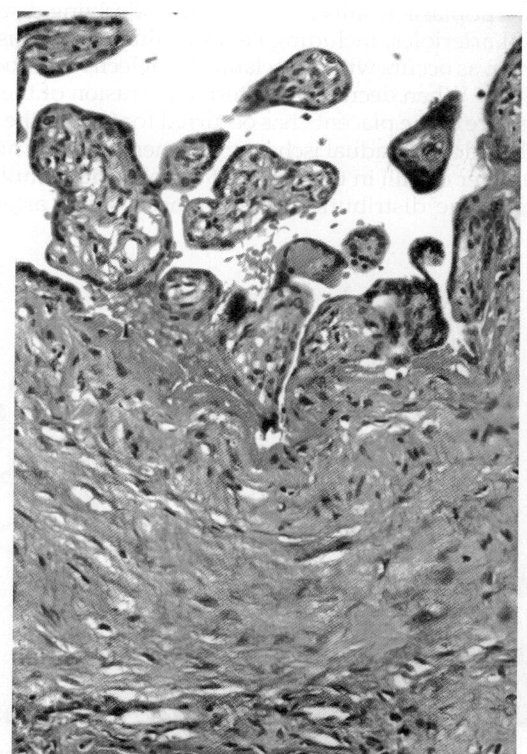

FIGURE 18-84. Placenta accreta. Some of the chorionic villi (top) are in contact with the underlying muscle.

remain adherent after delivery and cause postpartum hemorrhage. This bleeding can be difficult to control. It may threaten the lives of both mother and baby, and necessitate emergency hysterectomy. Attempts to remove attached placental fragments can cause hemorrhage and even uterine inversion. Placenta percreta can result in uterine rupture, and it can invade into the urinary bladder, resulting in hematuria. Placenta accreta is a serious complication of pregnancy, with a maternal death rate of 2% to 7%.

Chronic Uteroplacental Malperfusion Can Cause Poor Obstetric Outcomes

The placenta is perfused by 80 to 100 uterine spiral arterioles, which provide the placenta with oxygenated and nutrient-rich maternal blood. Inadequate delivery of maternal blood to the placenta can result from disorders affecting the spiral arterioles. When spiral arterial disease is chronic, it can lead to chronic uteroplacental malperfusion or chronic placental insufficiency. The latter is an important cause of perinatal morbidity and mortality. It can result in stillbirth, neonatal death, preterm birth, intrauterine growth restriction and, if the infant lives, neurologic injury. There are a variety of pathology abnormalities that can cause chronic placental insufficiency. In addition to fetal thrombotic vasculopathy and small placentas, the most prevalent histologic abnormalities causing chronic placental insufficiency include villous hyperplasia, increased fibrin, chronic villities, chronic cord abnormalities and multiple placental infarcts.

Villous Hypoplasia Occurs When Maternal Blood Flow to the Placenta Is Decreased

Villous hypoplasia results from chronic underlying disease of the spiral arterioles, including stenosis, fluctuating vasoconstriction or, as occurs with preeclampsia, defective remodeling (see below). When decreased maternal perfusion of the intervillous space of the placenta has occurred for weeks, the chorionic villi undergo gradual ischemic degeneration. The number and diameter of villi in the center of the placental lobule conforming to the distribution of a diseased spiral artery are decreased (Fig. 18-85A). Affected villi are shrunken from weeks of inadequate spiral arterial perfusion (Fig. 18-85B). In addition, their basement membranes are thickened, their stroma is fibrotic and trophoblast is often clumped and basophilic. The villi become much smaller, with smaller fetal vessels and more connective tissue than normal villi. The resulting fetal hypoxia can lead to such poor clinical outcomes as stillbirth, neonatal death, intrauterine growth restriction, preterm birth and neurologic injury in infants who survive.

Increased Fibrin Is an Abnormality of Decreased Maternal Perfusion of the Placenta

Increased perivillous fibrin can cause placental insufficiency. In some conditions, fibrin from maternal blood deposits in intervillous spaces and around chorionic villi. This fibrin can interfere with perfusion of the villi (and hence impair oxygen delivery to the fetus) by blocking oxygen-bearing maternal blood flow through the intervillous space. As intervillous fibrin deposits, fibrin in the maternal circulation accrues onto and around villi, blocks oxygen diffusion across villous surfaces and eventually causes ischemic necrosis of the villi (Fig. 18-86). In the its most severe forms, it may cause placental fibrin deposition and transmural villous necrosis from the maternal (decidual) to fetal (chorionic) surface, called **massive perivillous fibrin deposition** (MPFD). Fibrin can also deposit confluently throughout the lower half of the placenta including the decidua, termed **maternal floor infarction** (MFI). Increased villous fibrin, MPFD and MFI may lead to poor obstetric outcomes, including neurologic injury and cerebral palsy.

Infarcts Are Caused by Interruption of Maternal Blood Flow to the Placenta

The two most frequent causes of placental infarction are hemorrhage between the base of the placenta and the uterine wall (retroplacental hemorrhage and abruptio placentae), and occlusion or thrombosis of the uterine spiral artery. Like infarcts in other organs, placental infarcts change in gross and microscopic appearance over time. Small infarcts in placentas of full-term infants are common, and usually harmless.

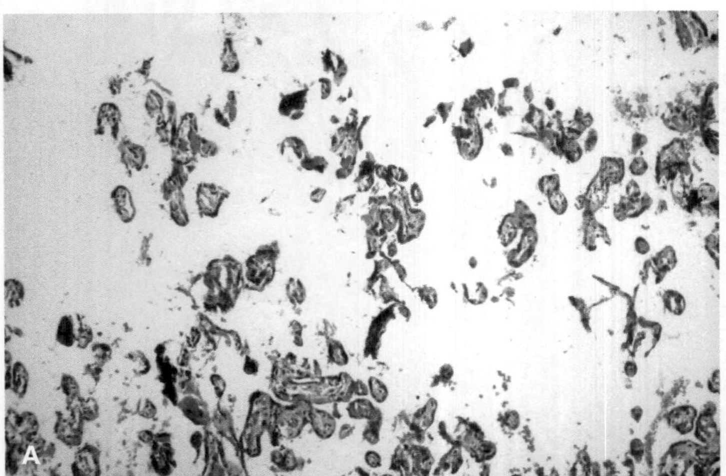

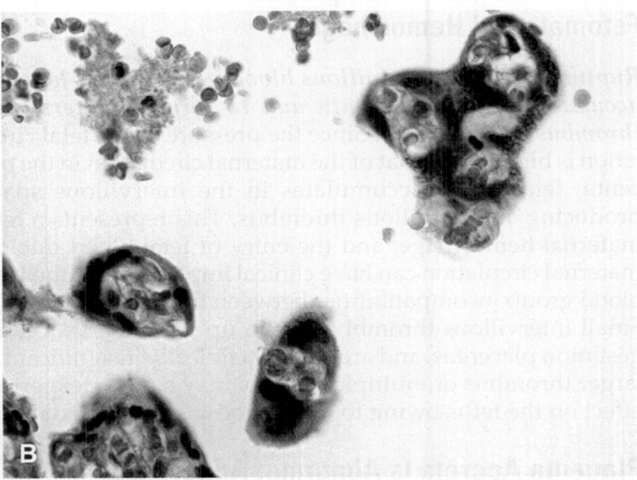

FIGURE 18-85. Villous hypoplasia. A. The diameter of the villi is decreased, resulting in an apparent increase in the intervillous space between villi **B. High magnification of villous hypoplasia.** The characteristic features of chronic ischemia are present, including small, shrunken villi with stromal fibrosis and clumped trophoblast.

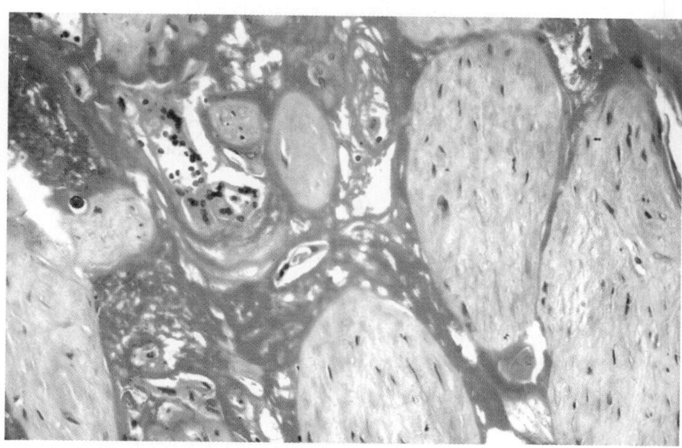

FIGURE 18-86. Increased villous fibrin. The fibrin has covered the chorionic villi, obstructed the intervillous space and resulted in villous necrosis.

However, multiple infarcts, especially if they are large or in the central part of the placenta, can compromise oxygenation of the fetus, result in placental insufficiency and lead to intrauterine growth restriction, neurologic injury and perinatal death. Placental infarcts often accompany preeclampsia, maternal thrombophilia and cigarette smoking.

Chorangiosis Is Abnormally Increased Chorionic Vessels Due to Chronic Fetal Hypoxia

Normal chorionic villi contain five to six or fewer fetal blood vessels. In chorangiosis, chorionic villi may contain 10 or more vessels in 10 or more villi in 10 or greater 10-power microscopic fields. The increased vascularity may be so prominent that some villi have 30 to 40 or more fetal vessels (Fig. 18-87). Chorangiosis can take many weeks to develop. Although it does not cause fetal damage, it is a marker of significant chronic placental insufficiency and fetal hypoxia due to other etiologies. Chorangiosis is correlated with perinatal circumstances that suggest long-standing hypoxia, and is seen more often in the placentas of infants with cerebral palsy.

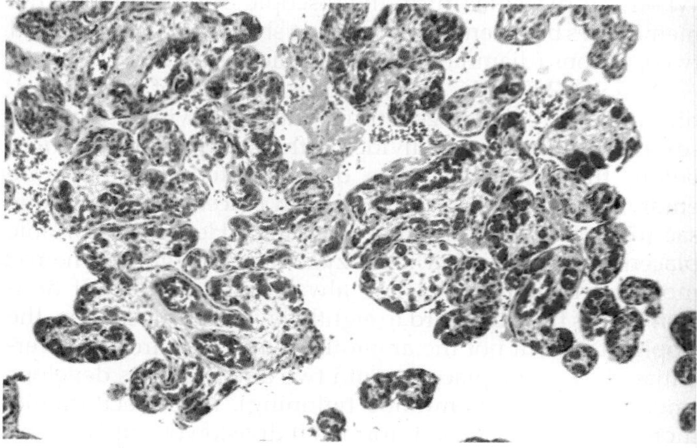

FIGURE 18-87. Chorangiosis. Chorangiosis results from chronic fetal hypoxia. Normal chorionic villi contain 5 or fewer capillaries (see Fig. 18-78B). The chorionic villi in these villi are hypervascular—most contain greater than 10 capillary cross-sections, and a few villi contain 20 or more vessels.

Increased Syncytial Knots Indicate Chronic Uteroplacental Malperfusion

Chorionic villi are covered by a layer of multinucleated cells termed the syncytiotrophoblast. If there has been chronic uteroplacental malperfusion, the syncytiotrophoblast forms prominent bulbous knots or folds, often bridging the intervillous space and touching the trophoblast of adjacent villi. This abnormality has also been called Tenney-Parker change and trophoblast hyperplasia. It is often present in placentas from all causes of chronic malperfusion, and may also be seen in placentas from pregnancies occurring at high altitudes.

Intrauterine Growth Restriction

Intrauterine growth restriction (IUGR) is a chronic abnormality of fetal growth and development that affects 3% to 10% of deliveries, depending on the diagnostic criteria. There are two major types: asymmetric (70% to 80% of all IUGR) and symmetric (20% to 30%). In the more common asymmetric form, the head size, length and weight are often normal, but there is loss of subcutaneous fat and muscle mass, and decreased abdominal circumference (see below). Symmetric IUGR results in an abnormally and proportionally small infant—low birth weight, small head and short stature. Symmetric IUGR begins early in pregnancy and is usually due to genetic disorders, early fetal infections and chromosomal and congenital anomalies. Mixed patterns make up 5% to 10% of IUGR cases, and combine features of both asymmetric and symmetric IUGR.

Asymmetric Intrauterine Growth Restriction Is Usually Due to Chronic Uteroplacental Insufficiency

Asymmetric IUGR, also termed "head-sparing IUGR," occurs when the placenta cannot provide adequate oxygen and nutrition to the fetus for a long period of time. Fetal soft tissues of its extremities (muscle mass) and body (subcutaneous fat, especially at the abdomen) are wasted. The resulting newborn with asymmetric IUGR has a 5 to 10 times increased risk for perinatal mortality and morbidity than for a neonate who is not growth restricted. Asymmetric IUGR is also associated with neonatal hypoglycemia, meconium aspiration, persistent fetal circulation and neurologic injury due to chronic fetal hypoxia. Asymmetric IUGR can become a mixed pattern of IUGR if the placental insufficiency lasts long enough or is sufficiently severe. A partial list of placental causes of asymmetric IUGR includes preeclampsia or chronic hypertension, thrombosis, villitis, maternal autoimmune disease, multiple placental infarcts, diabetes, chronic abruption, increased fibrin including maternal floor infarction and massive perivillous fibrin. ***Maternal cigarette smoking is the most important preventable cause of asymmetric IUGR.*** Prior to delivery, asymmetric IUGR may be suspected when obstetric ultrasonography shows abnormally small abdominal circumference (AC), or increased head circumference–to–abdominal circumference (HC/AC) ratio. The diagnosis can

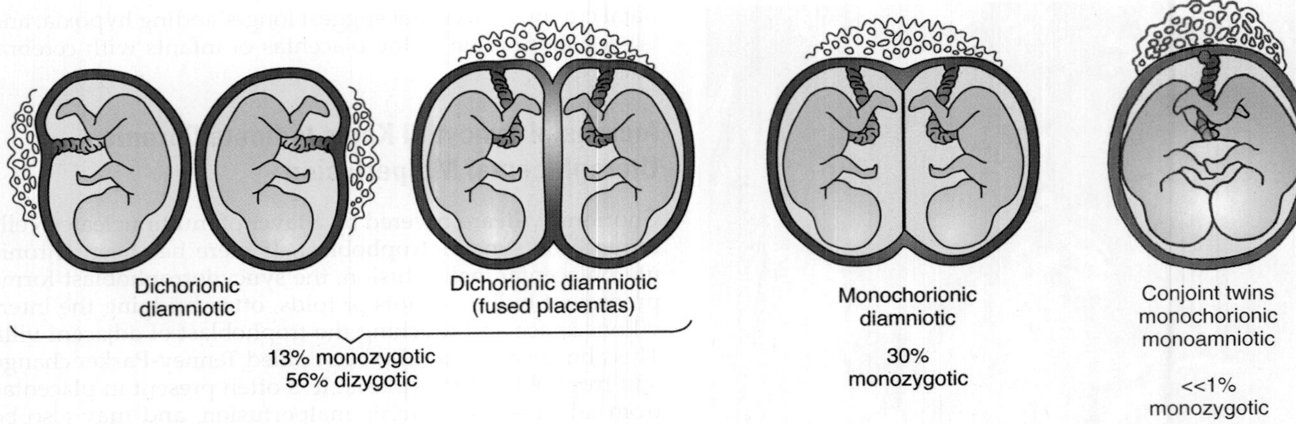

FIGURE 18-88. Placental structure in twin pregnancies. The percentages in the figure refer to the proportion of total twin pregnancies (100%) accounted for by each variant.

be made at the time of delivery by the Ponderal Index, a mathematical relationship between birth weight and length. A Ponderal Index below the 10th percentile is diagnostic of asymmetric IUGR.

Spontaneous Abortion

A pregnancy that ends with expulsion of a conceptus before the 20th week of gestation is called a spontaneous abortion, or miscarriage. Some 15% of recognized pregnancies abort spontaneously, and an additional 30% of women abort without being aware that pregnancy has occurred. Thus, almost 50% of pregnancies terminate in spontaneous abortion.

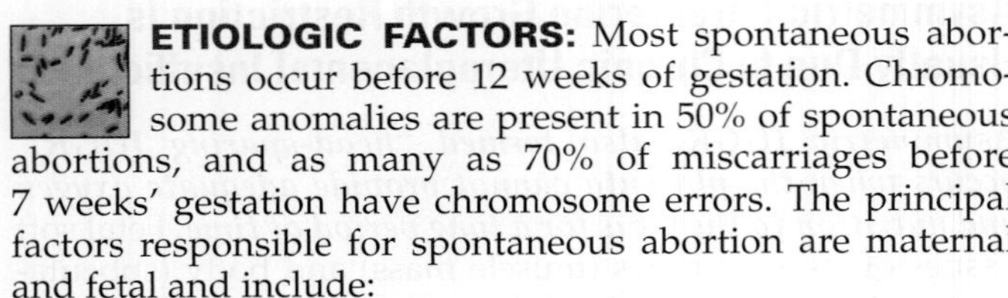

ETIOLOGIC FACTORS: Most spontaneous abortions occur before 12 weeks of gestation. Chromosome anomalies are present in 50% of spontaneous abortions, and as many as 70% of miscarriages before 7 weeks' gestation have chromosome errors. The principal factors responsible for spontaneous abortion are maternal and fetal and include:

- Infection early in pregnancy (e.g., *Listeria*, CMV, *Toxoplasma*, coxsackievirus)
- Mechanical factors (e.g., uterine leiomyoma, septate uteri, cervical incompetence)
- Endocrine factors (e.g., poorly controlled maternal diabetes, polycystic ovary, luteal phase defects)
- Immunologic factors
- Congenital fetal malformations (e.g., neural tube defects)
- Chromosomal abnormalities
- Multiple gestation (e.g., twins, triplets, quadruplets)

PATHOLOGY: An empty gestational sac with hydropic swelling of the chorionic villi (blighted ovum) suggests early fetal demise. The embryo may be grossly disorganized, or show defects such as spina bifida, anencephaly or cleft palate. Chorionic villi may be histologically normal for gestational age or show intravillous fibrosis or hydropic change. If infection preceded the miscarriage, there is often evidence of the infectious agent microscopically (see Chapter 9).

Multiple Gestations

Slightly fewer than 1% of pregnancies yield dizygotic or monozygotic twins (Fig. 18-88).

DIZYGOTIC TWINS: Fertilization of two separate ova results in genetically different twins, of the same or opposite sex. Dizygotic twinning has a strong hereditary component, which is confined to the maternal side. Dizygotic twinning and multiple gestations are more common in women who have used hormones to induce ovulation artificially or who have been impregnated after in vitro fertilization.

Separate placentas develop when two fertilized ova implant apart from one another. If they implant nearby each other, the two placentas show varying degrees of fusion, and may appear as one. When the ova implant apart, there are discrete conceptuses, each placenta having its own amniotic sac. When the placentas fuse, microscopic examination of the membranes between the two fetuses shows two amnions and two chorions (diamnionic, dichorionic gestation).

MONOZYGOTIC TWINS: Early division of a single fertilized ovum results in genetically identical twins of the same sex. If a fertilized ovum divides within 2 days of fertilization, before the trophoblast has differentiated, two separate embryos develop, each with its own placenta and amniotic sac (dichorionic, diamniotic twinning). Hence, dichorionic placentas may be either monozygotic or dizygotic, whereas monochorionic placentas are always monozygous. If division occurs from the third to eighth days after conception, the trophoblast (but not the amniotic cavity) has already differentiated. A single placenta with two amniotic sacs develops (monochorionic, diamniotic twinning). A monochorionic, monoamniotic placenta is formed if division occurs between the 8th and 13th day after conception, because the amniotic cavity has already developed. Incomplete separation of monozygous twins results in conjoint (formerly Siamese) fetuses within a monoamniotic, monochorionic placenta. The mechanisms by which triplet, etc., pregnancies arise may include one or more of the above.

Maternal Death

In spite of advances in the fields of obstetrics and maternal–fetal medicine, maternal death, defined as death of a woman while pregnant or up to 42 days after end of the pregnancy, is still an important public health problem in most parts of the world. The United States ranks 41st out of 171 nations in lifetime risk of maternal death; the risk has actually increased after remaining static for over 20 years. In 1987, the maternal mortality rate in the United States was 6.6 deaths per 100,000 births; by 2004, it had risen to 13 maternal deaths per 100,000 births.

Race is an important risk factor in maternal death in the United States; the death rate among black U.S. women is nearly four times higher than for white women (34.7 vs. 9.3 deaths per 100,000 births, respectively). Over 90% of maternal deaths occur in developing nations—in Sierra Leone, the maternal mortality rate is 2000 per 100,000 births (i.e., 1 in 50 births results in a maternal death); in Afghanistan, it is 1900 per 100,000 births. Causes of maternal death vary by region. Infectious diseases, including malaria, hemorrhagic fever, HIV/acquired immunodeficiency syndrome (AIDS) and bacterial disease, are most significant in tropical and developing nations. Septic abortion, or "back-alley abortion," is a common cause of maternal death in nations that prohibit elective pregnancy termination. In developed nations, the most common causes include hemorrhage, thrombosis, bacterial infection and puerperal sepsis, preeclampsia and HELLP syndrome and amniotic fluid embolism. A frequent complication arising from all of these conditions that contributes to maternal death is the onset of acute respiratory distress syndrome (ARDS) and disseminated intravascular coagulation (DIC). Less frequent causes of maternal death include ectopic pregnancy; uterine rupture; diseases of the heart, liver or kidney; and hyperemesis gravidarum.

Preeclampsia and Eclampsia

The hypertensive disorders of pregnancy—preeclampsia and eclampsia—define a syndrome of hypertension, proteinuria and edema, and, most severely, convulsions. Preeclampsia occurs in 6% of pregnant women in their last trimester, especially with the first child. If convulsive seizures appear, the syndrome is called eclampsia. (An archaic term, toxemia of pregnancy, is a misnomer and is rarely used anymore.) Preeclampsia causes approximately 50,000 maternal deaths worldwide each year.

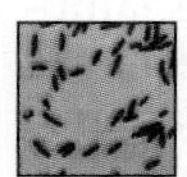

ETIOLOGIC FACTORS: The basis of preeclampsia is generally believed to be faulty remodeling of uterine spiral arteries that supply the placenta with oxygenated maternal blood (see Molecular Pathogenesis, below). Immunologic and genetic factors have been invoked as well as altered vascular reactivity, endothelial injury and coagulation abnormalities. Certain features of preeclampsia are characteristic (Fig. 18-89):

- Maternal blood flow to the placenta is markedly reduced because normal remodeling of the maternal spiral arteries of the decidua does not occur.
- Renal involvement contributes to hypertension and proteinuria.
- Disseminated intravascular coagulation may occur in preeclampsia, manifested as fibrin thrombi in the liver, brain and kidneys.
- The risk of preeclampsia in the first pregnancy is manyfold higher than in subsequent pregnancies.
- Rarely, preeclampsia may not occur clinically until the period of labor and delivery, or shortly thereafter. The latter is termed postpartum preeclampsia.
- Eclampsia is a cerebrovascular disorder characterized by seizures, worsening hypertension and cerebral edema. It is often the first sign of preeclampsia but does not necessarily evolve from it.

The pathologic changes in the placenta reflect reduced maternal blood flow to the uteroplacental unit, as the spiral arteries of the uteroplacental bed never fully dilate. Early in a normal pregnancy, fetal cytotrophoblast cells extend downward, into the decidua and uterus. They invade the uterine spiral arteries and progressively replace the maternal-derived endothelium, medial elastic tissue, smooth muscle and neural tissue. By the end of the second trimester, the normally narrow pre-pregnancy spiral arteries are dilated tubes lined by fetal-derived cytotrophoblast, forming a low-resistance arterial circuit that can supply the increasing oxygen and nutrient demand of the developing fetus.

In preeclampsia, many spiral arteries escape invasion by trophoblastic tissue and so never dilate. These spiral arteries commonly show fibrinoid necrosis, clusters of lipid-rich macrophages and a perivascular infiltrate of mononuclear cells, which together are termed **acute atherosis** (Fig. 18-90). Fibrin deposition is also seen. These vessels are often thrombosed, causing focal placental infarcts. The combination of vasoconstriction and structural changes in spiral arteries contributes to inadequate blood flow, placental ischemia, villous hypoplasia and fetal hypoxia.

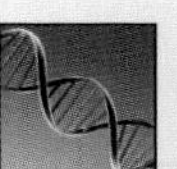

MOLECULAR PATHOGENESIS: The central pathogenetic abnormality in preeclampsia is placental ischemia, but many of the details of molecular pathogenesis are unclear. In normal pregnancy there are many hemodynamic and cardiovascular alterations—increased maternal cardiac output and plasma volume, reduction in total maternal vascular resistance and arterial pressure, increased renal plasma flow and decreased pressor response and vascular reactivity to vasoconstricting substances such as α-adrenergic agonists and angiotensin II. These changes are partially the result of physiologically enhanced endothelium-dependent vascular relaxation, as well as decreased vascular reactivity to vasoconstrictor agonists. In women developing preeclampsia, the latter beneficial vascular and hemodynamic modifications do not occur. The effectiveness of vasodilators in treating preeclampsia, including nitric oxide (NO•), prostacyclin (PGI_2) and endothelium-derived hyperpolarizing factor (EDHF), are further evidence for endothelial dysfunction in this condition.

Faulty cytotrophoblastic remodeling of the maternal uterine (spiral) arteries in early pregnancy (Fig. 18-80) is believed to result from abnormal expression of the adhesion molecule integrins by the fetal-derived cytotrophoblast, as well as generalized apoptosis of the cytotrophoblast. This leads to limited invasion of the decidua and spiral arteries. As a result, the spiral arteries cannot perfuse

FIGURE 18-89. Pathogenesis of preeclampsia. EDHF = endothelium-derived hyperpolarizing factor; IUGR = intrauterine growth retardation.

the growing fetus adequately. Resulting placental ischemia promotes release of cytokines such as tumor necrosis factor-α (TNF-α) and interleukin-6 (IL-6).

Upregulation and production of such placental antiangiogenic factors as fms-related tyrosine kinase 1 (vascular endothelial growth factor) and soluble endoglin may play a role in the onset of the clinical features of preeclampsia including hypertension and proteinuria. The roles, if any, of other factors are unclear, for example, oxidative stress, antibodies (antiendothelial cell, antiangiotensin type I receptor agonist), increased maternal plasma homocysteine and leptin concentrations, changes of contractile proteins in maternal smooth muscle and other mechanisms of vascular smooth muscle contraction and genetic factors.

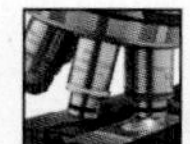

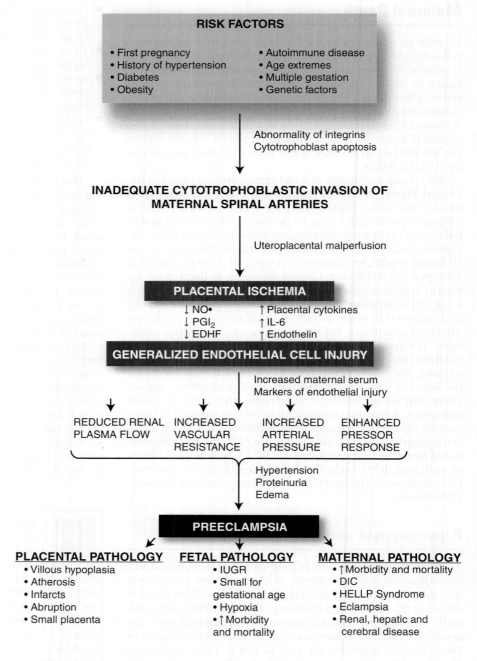

PATHOLOGY: Extensive placental infarction is seen in nearly one third of women with severe preeclampsia, although it is often negligible in mild preeclampsia. Retroplacental hemorrhage occurs in 15% of patients. Chorionic villi show signs of chronic maternal underperfusion (i.e., areas of ischemically shrunken and degenerated chorionic villi [villous hypoplasia]). Additional placental findings of maternal vascular underperfusion are often present, including villous agglutination, increased fibrin, increased placental site giant cells, syncytiotrophoblastic hyperplasia (Tenney-Parker change) and mural hypertrophy of membrane arterioles.

Maternal kidneys always show glomerular changes. Glomeruli are enlarged and endothelial cells are swollen, forming classic "bloodless" glomeruli of preeclampsia

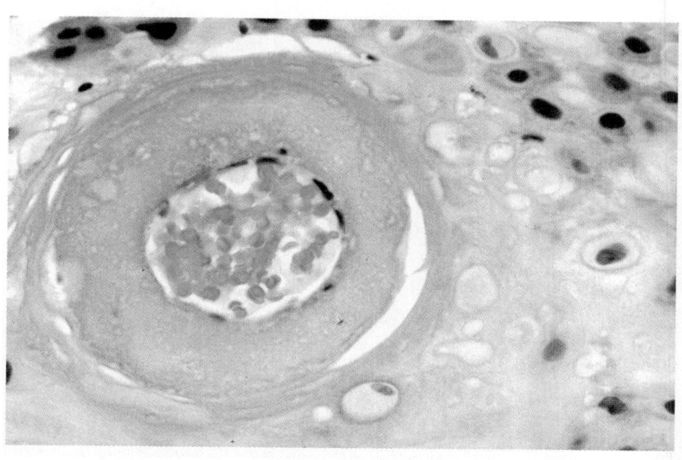

FIGURE 18-90. Decidual atherosis in preeclampsia. A small decidual artery shows fibrinoid thickening of the vessel wall.

(glomerular endotheliosis). Fibrin is seen between the endothelial cells and the glomerular capillary basement membrane. Mesangial cell hyperplasia is the rule. These maternal renal changes are reversible with therapy or after delivery. Fatal cases of eclampsia often show cerebral hemorrhages, ranging from petechiae to large hematomas.

Liver abnormalities are present in 60% of women dying from preeclampsia, including periportal fibrin deposits and necrosis (Fig. 18-91), periportal and hepatic plate hemorrhage and hepatic infarction. Rare hepatic complications include subcapsular hematoma and rupture.

CLINICAL FEATURES: Preeclampsia usually begins insidiously after the 20th week of pregnancy with (1) excessive weight gain occasioned by fluid retention, (2) increased maternal blood pressure and (3) proteinuria. As the preeclampsia progresses from mild to severe, diastolic pressure persistently exceeds 110 mm Hg, proteinuria is greater than 3 g/day and renal function declines. DIC often supervenes. Preeclampsia is treated with antihypertensive and antiplatelet drugs, but definitive therapy requires removing the placenta. Eclampsia is treated with magnesium sulfate, which reduces cerebrovascular tone.

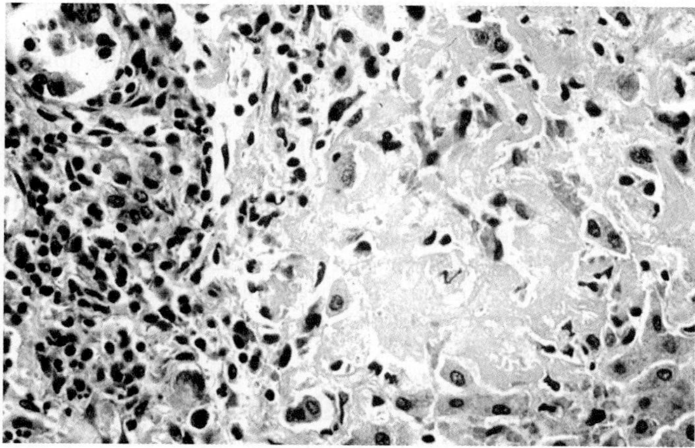

FIGURE 18-91. Liver of a woman with HELLP syndrome. The periportal area (zone 1) demonstrates fibrin deposition.

HELLP Syndrome

HELLP syndrome is a potentially fatal condition of pregnant women and their infants that most often follows the diagnosis of preeclampsia in the third trimester. Its name is an acronym for its major findings—**H**emolytic anemia, **El**evated **L**iver enzymes and **L**ow **P**latelet count. It occurs in 0.2% to 0.6% of all pregnancies, and in 4% to 12% of women with preeclampsia or eclampsia. When preeclampsia is not present, the diagnosis may be delayed. About 69% of cases occur antepartum and 31% develop in the postpartum period.

MOLECULAR PATHOGENESIS: Although the exact cause of HELLP syndrome remains unknown, generalized activation of the coagulation cascade is felt to be the major problem. The syndrome is the final manifestation of an event leading to microvascular endothelial damage and intravascular platelet activation. Platelet activation causes vasospasm, platelet agglutination and aggregation and further endothelial damage. Excessive platelet consumption results in DIC in about 20% of women with HELLP syndrome. Fibrin forms cross-linked networks in the small blood vessels, fragmenting red blood cells as they pass through the damaged vessels, leading to microangiopathic hemolytic anemia. Obstruction of hepatic blood flow by fibrin deposits in the sinusoids leads to liver cells becoming ischemic, resulting in periportal necrosis, increased liver enzymes and, in severe cases, intrahepatic hemorrhage, subcapsular hematoma formation or hepatic rupture. Additional complications of HELLP syndrome include hemorrhage from DIC, pulmonary edema, placental abruption, ARDS, acute hepatorenal failure and fetal demise. The mortality rate for women with HELLP syndrome is approximately 1%. Infant morbidity and mortality rates vary from 10% to 60% depending on the severity of maternal disease.

Amniotic Fluid Embolism

Amniotic fluid embolism (AFE) is a rare and incompletely understood life-threatening obstetric emergency. Its true frequency is debated, but may occur in 1 in 8000 to 1 in 30,000 pregnancies. AFE is believed to occur when amniotic fluid, fetal squamous cells, hair and other amniotic material enter the maternal circulation through the uterine veins in the decidual bed at the base of the placenta. Maternal mortality has historically been stated to be from 60% to 80%, but some other estimates are lower, at approximately 25%. AFE accounts for 5% to 10% of maternal deaths in the United States. Fetal mortality is lower than maternal mortality, but about 20% of infants die after their mothers develop AFE.

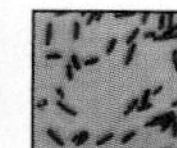

ETIOLOGIC FACTORS: The introduction of amniotic fluid elements into the maternal bloodstream is thought to be responsible for the acute onset of symptoms of AFE. However, amniotic fluid cellular elements are not always identified in women with AFE, and they may be present in women who do not develop AFE. In AFE, some amniotic fluid material(s) that enters the maternal

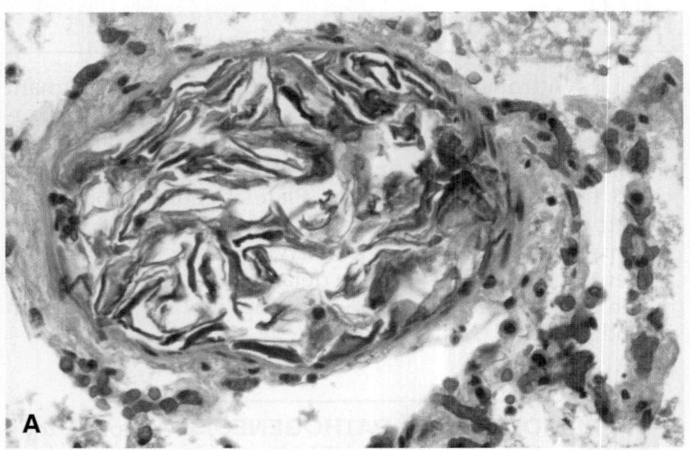

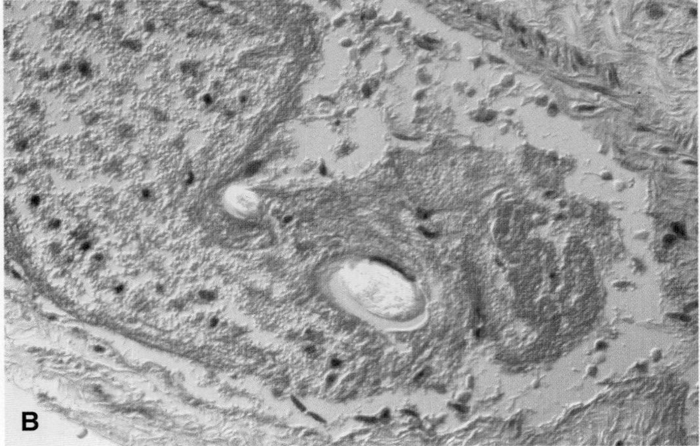

FIGURE 18-92. Amniotic fluid embolism. A. Lung from a woman who died from amniotic fluid embolism. Numerous tightly packed fetal squamous epithelial cells obstruct the lumen of this pulmonary blood vessel. **B.** Amniotic fluid embolism from another woman dying of this condition. Nomarski interference contrast highlights two golden brown cross-sections of a fetal hair in the maternal pulmonary circulation.

bloodstream around the time of labor and delivery triggers an anaphylactic reaction, complement activation or both.

PATHOLOGY: At the time of autopsy, the lungs usually show diffuse alveolar damage, the pathologic counterpart of ARDS. Microscopic platelet-fibrin aggregates are present in the pulmonary vessels and increased megakaryocytes are often present in the alveolar tissues, indicative of the onset of DIC. Careful search of pulmonary vessels will often reveal the distinctive fetal squamous epithelial cells in both alveolar capillaries or in larger blood vessels (Fig. 18-92A). In rare cases, other fetal elements are present, including fetal hair (Fig. 18-92B).

CLINICAL FEATURES: Initially, pulmonary arterial vasospasm, pulmonary hypertension and elevation of right ventricular pressure cause hypoxia. Myocardial and pulmonary capillary damage ensue, left heart failure occurs and ARDS develops, further endangering the patient. Women surviving the first phase of AFE may develop a second phase, including uterine atony, hemorrhage and DIC. A fatal consumptive coagulopathy may be the initial presentation.

Gestational Diabetes

In gestational diabetes a pregnant woman without previous diabetes develops abnormally high blood glucose levels. It occurs in 3% to 10% of pregnancies. Gestational diabetes usually reverses after delivery, but entails an increased risk (30% to 80%, depending on ethnicity) for developing gestational diabetes in a future pregnancy. There is also a higher risk for developing diabetes mellitus in the future. This risk is about 50% within 6 years postpartum, and is highest in women who need insulin treatment, had antibodies (e.g., anti-islet cell antibodies) associated with diabetes, had more than two previous pregnancies and who are obese.

MOLECULAR PATHOGENESIS: The hallmark of this condition is resistance to maternal insulin. Pregnancy hormones and other factors interfere with insulin binding to its receptor. This prevents glucose from entering the cells, so it remains in the blood, causing hyperglycemia. Pregnant women with gestational diabetes have insulin resistance for which increased insulin secretion by the pancreas cannot compensate. While maternal insulin does not pass the placenta, maternal glucose does, causing hypersecretion of insulin by the fetal pancreas. As insulin stimulates growth, its overproduction can lead to large fetal size **(macrosomia).** A similar effect may occur in the placenta; placentas from women with gestational diabetes may be abnormally thick and large (placentomegaly), and be more friable owing to decreased collagen and mucopolysaccharides. Villous structures may appear immature, and villous edema or chorangiosis may be present.

CLINICAL FEATURES: Mother and infant are both at risk for poor obstetric outcomes, largely owing to the effects of hyperglycemia. As mentioned above, infants of women with gestational diabetes may be abnormally large (macrosomia, birth weight >4000 grams), or they may be abnormally small or growth restricted. Macrosomia and increased fetal fat deposition (truncal obesity) may make for difficult vaginal delivery, with increased risk of shoulder dystocia. Congenital fetal malformations are increased with gestational diabetes, as are fetal and placental thrombosis. Neonates are at risk for a variety of metabolic abnormalities including hypoglycemia, jaundice, polycythemia, hypocalcemia and hypomagnesemia.

Acute Fatty Liver of Pregnancy

Acute fatty liver of pregnancy (AFLP) is a rare life-threatening condition of pregnancy caused by disordered metabolism of fatty acids by maternal mitochondria. It occurs in 1 of 7000 to

1 in 15,000 pregnancies, but is commonly associated with preeclampsia (50% to 100%). AFLP can recur in subsequent pregnancies. It usually occurs in the third trimester, and is characterized by the onset of nausea, vomiting, abdominal pain, jaundice and anorexia, with elevated liver enzymes and bilirubin. DIC may occur in severe cases; additional complications include pancreatitis and encephalopathy. AFLP is associated with significant mortality: maternal mortality is 18%, and there is a 23% fetal mortality rate.

MOLECULAR PATHOGENESIS: Acute fatty liver of pregnancy is caused by a mitochondrial dysfunction, generally thought to be a deficiency in long-chain 3-hydroxyacyl-coenzyme A dehydrogenase (LCHAD). Mitochondrial fatty acid β-oxidation includes a series of transport steps, as well as four enzyme-catalyzed reactions. Normally, carrier proteins transport fatty acids to the mitochondrial inner membrane, where they are broken down by four enzymes. LCHAD is the third enzyme in this process, and lack of LCHAD leads to accumulation of medium- and long-chain fatty acids. When this occurs in the fetus, unmetabolized fatty acids reenter the maternal bloodstream through the placenta, overwhelming maternal β-oxidation enzymes.

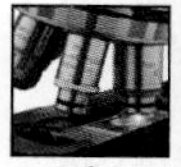

PATHOLOGY: Liver biopsy can be diagnostic of AFLP, showing characteristic microvesicular fat droplets in the cytoplasm of enlarged hepatocytes with central nuclei (see Chapter 14).

Effects of Cigarette Smoking During Pregnancy

Cigarette smoking is the leading avoidable cause of morbidity and mortality in pregnant women and their infants. (For more on smoking, consult Chapter 8.) About 13% of women report smoking during the last 3 weeks of pregnancy, even more among pregnant adolescents (27% to 37%). Cigarette smoking during pregnancy is associated with a variety of poor obstetric and infant outcomes (Table 18-13). However, cessation of maternal smoking when pregnancy is diagnosed in the first trimester virtually eliminates the majority of the excess morbidity and mortality. Second-hand smoke exposure has been linked to increased risk of attention-deficit hyperactivity disorder (ADHD), sudden infant death syndrome (SIDS) and low birth weight.

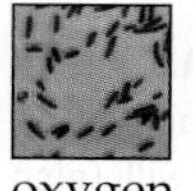

ETIOLOGIC FACTORS: Carbon monoxide in cigarette smoke binds hemoglobin better than does oxygen. Resulting carboxyhemoglobin cannot carry oxygen, and so decreases oxygen delivery to the fetus and causes fetal hypoxia. In heavy smokers, fetal oxygen-carrying capacity may be reduced by up to 25%.

Many of the obstetric complications of cigarette smoking result from vasoconstriction. In particular, nicotine in smoke is a potent vasoconstrictor. It reduces uterine and placental blood flow. It has both cardiac and central nervous system effects, can readily cross the placenta and reaches higher levels in the fetal tissues and amniotic fluid than in the mother. Vasoconstriction occurs in the blood vessels of all anatomic

Table 18-13

Effects of Cigarette Smoking in Pregnancy

Effects of Cigarette Smoking in Pregnancy
Umbilical Artery
Degeneration of arterial intima
Decreased production of vasodilators and antithrombotic compounds (nitric acid, prostacyclin)
Diminished blood flow to the fetus
Placental Villous Stem Vessels
Altered mechanical properties of villous arteries
Greater vasoconstrictive response to endothelin
Uterine Spiral Arteries
Increased fragility
Elevation of local platelet-activating factor (PAF) concentration
Vasoconstriction with decreased maternal blood flow to intervillous space of placenta
Persistence of diminished placental perfusion for 15 minutes after a cigarette is smoked
Fetal Physiology
Fetal acidosis
Fetal hypoxia
Higher serum and amniotic fluid nicotine concentration than in mother
Slower clearance of nicotine from blood than mother
Accumulation of nicotine in fetal tissues
Maternal Bloodstream
Increased levels of vasoconstrictors (e.g., endothelin-1)
Increased levels of cadmium (causes hemorrhagic necrosis of decidua)
Fetal Blood
Increased levels of toxic compounds (e.g., carbon monoxide, cyanide, thiocyanate, nicotine)
Placenta
Changes in placental enzymatic and synthetic functions
Villous hypoplasia
Trophoblast hyperplasia (Tenney-Parker change)
Infarcts
Chorangiosis
Additional microscopic findings of malperfusion
Abruptio placentae
Poor Obstetric Outcomes
Stillbirth
Neonatal death
Spontaneous abortion
Intrauterine growth restriction
Preterm delivery
Premature rupture of membranes
Low birth weight
Placenta previa
Abruptio placentae
Sudden infant death syndrome
Neurologic and behavioral disorders
Maternal and paternal infertility
Gestational diabetes

components of the uteroplacental unit, including the uterine spiral arteries perfusing the placenta with maternal blood, the placental villous vessels absorbing and transporting oxygen and nutrients and the umbilical vessels carrying placental blood to and from the fetus. Placentas of women who smoke can show a variety of findings of chronic uteroplacental malperfusion, including the small, atrophic and fibrotic chorionic villi of villous hypoplasia, Tenney-Parker change, placental infarcts, increased fibrin and chorangiosis.

Gestational Trophoblastic Disease

The term gestational trophoblastic disease is a spectrum of disorders with abnormal trophoblast proliferation and maturation, as well as neoplasms derived from trophoblast (Fig. 18-93).

Complete Hydatidiform Mole Does Not Contain an Embryo

Complete hydatidiform mole is a placenta with grossly swollen chorionic villi, resembling bunches of grapes, and showing varying degrees of trophoblastic proliferation. Villi are enlarged, often exceeding 5 mm in diameter (Fig. 18-94).

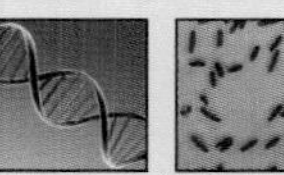
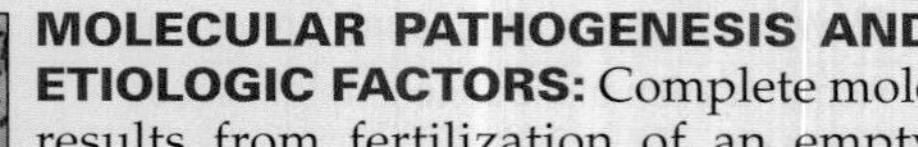

MOLECULAR PATHOGENESIS AND ETIOLOGIC FACTORS: Complete mole results from fertilization of an empty ovum that lacks functional maternal DNA. Most commonly, a haploid (23,X) set of paternal chromosomes introduced by monospermy duplicates to 46,XX, but dispermic 46,XX and 46,XY moles also occur. ***Moles characteristically lack maternal chromosomes.*** Paternally imprinted genes, such as *p57,* in which only the maternal allele is expressed, are not expressed in villous trophoblasts of androgenetic-derived complete moles. Since the embryo dies at a very early stage, before placental circulation has developed, few chorionic villi develop blood vessels and fetal parts are absent.

The risk of hydatidiform mole relates to maternal age and has two peaks. Girls under 15 years have a 20-fold higher risk than women 20 to 35 years old. Risk increases progressively for women over 40. In fact, women older than 50 years of age have 200 times the risk of those between 20 and 40. Ethnicity and obstetric history also affect the risk for hydatidiform mole. The incidence is manyfold higher in Asian women than white women. In Taiwan, the risk is 25 times that in the United States. Women with a prior hydatidiform mole have a 20-fold greater risk of a subsequent molar pregnancy than the general population.

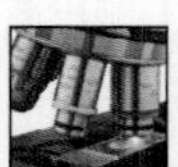

PATHOLOGY: Molar tissue is voluminous and consists of macroscopically visible villi that are obviously swollen (Fig. 18-94). Microscopically, many individual villi have cisternae, which are central, acellular, fluid-filled spaces devoid of mesenchymal cells. Trophoblast is hyperplastic and composed of syncytiotrophoblast, cytotrophoblast and intermediate trophoblast. Considerable cellular atypia is present.

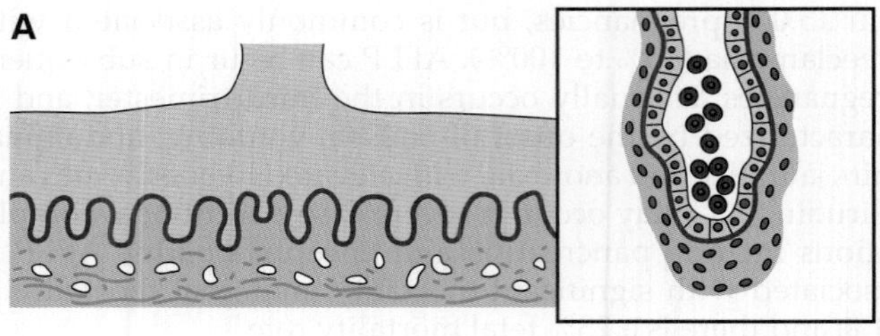

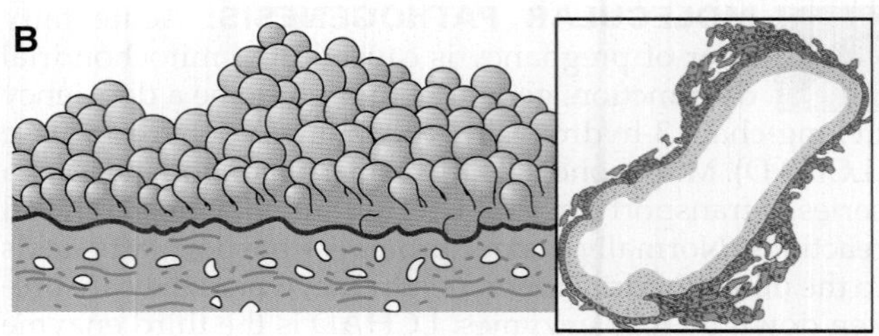

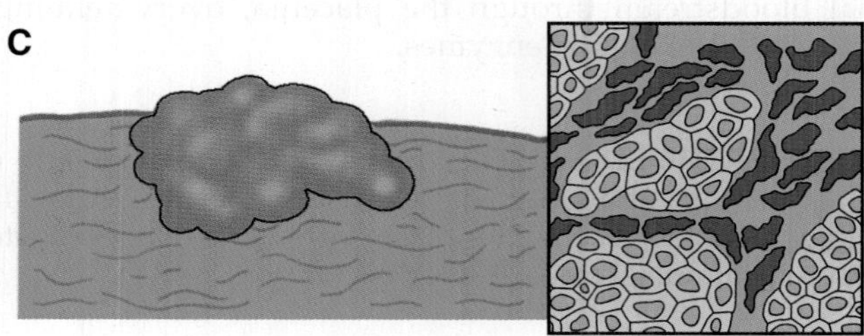

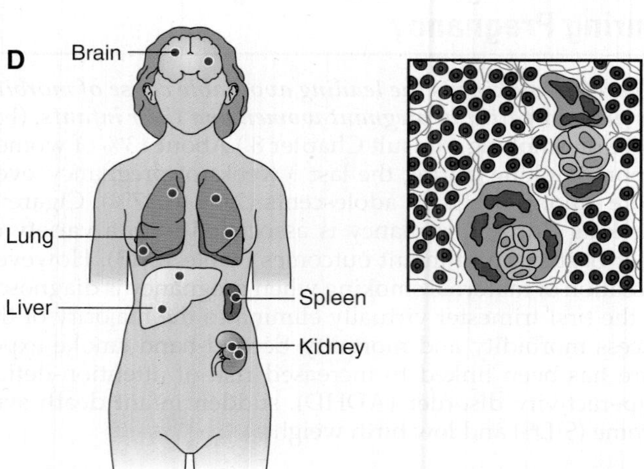

FIGURE 18-93. Proliferative disorders of the trophoblast. A. Normal chorionic villus of 8-week fetus, with blood vessel containing nucleated red blood cells. **B.** Complete hydatidiform mole with hydropic villi (also see Fig. 18-94). The villi are enlarged by an edematous stroma devoid of blood vessels. The trophoblastic epithelium is hyperplastic and exhibits variable atypia. **C.** Choriocarcinoma that has arisen in a molar pregnancy invades the myometrium and consists of admixed syncytiotrophoblastic and cytotrophoblastic elements. **D.** Common sites of metastasis from choriocarcinoma.

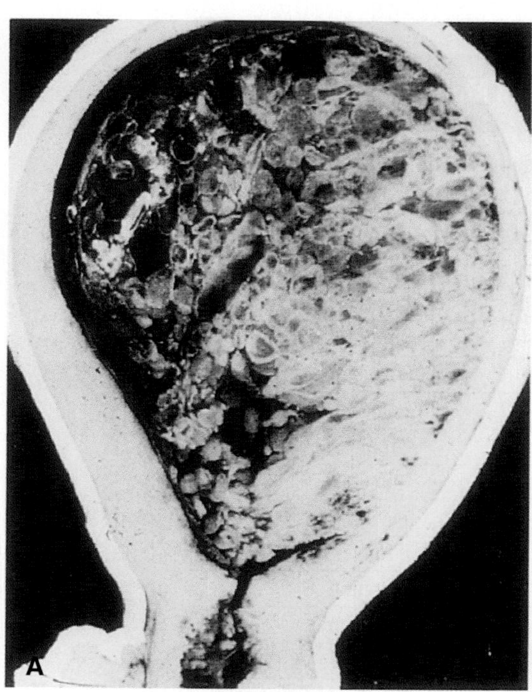

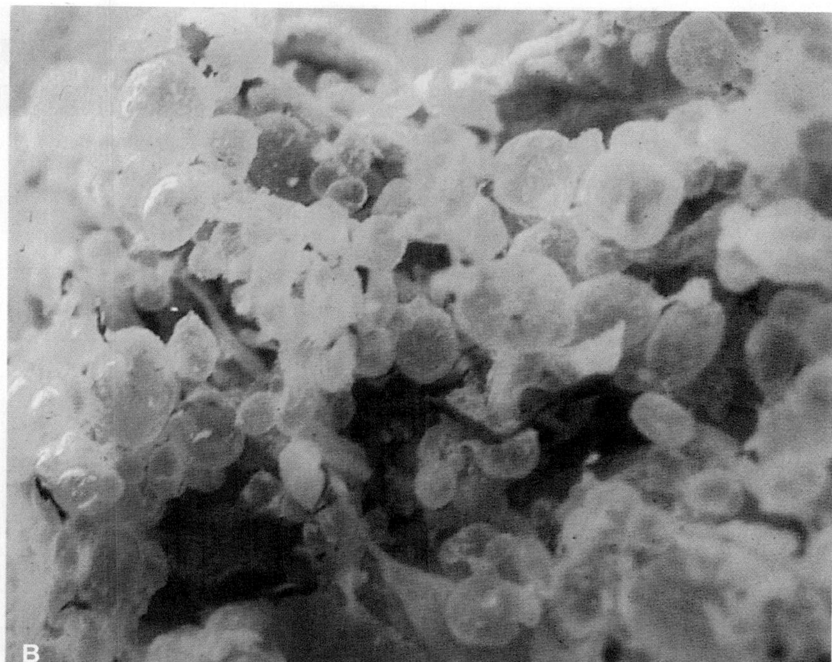

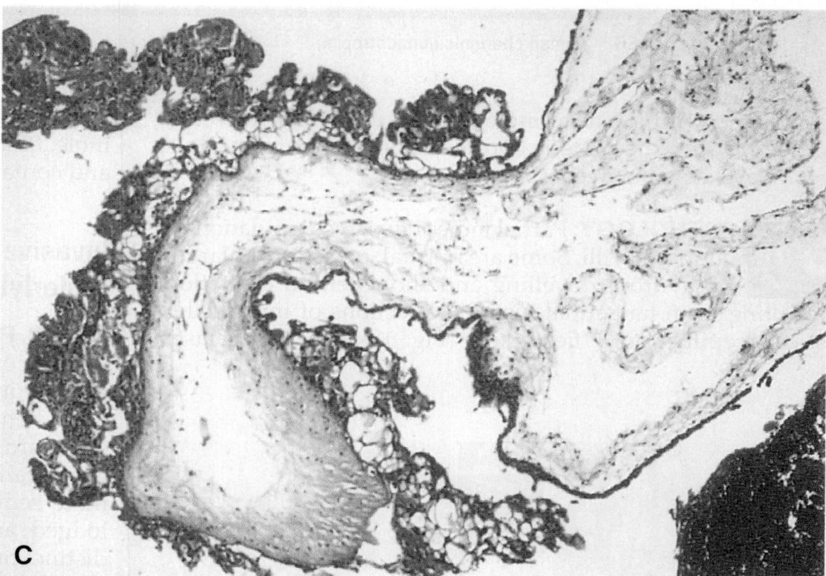

FIGURE 18-94. Complete hydatidiform mole. A. Complete mole in which the entire uterine cavity is filled with swollen villi. **B.** The villi are each 1 to 3 mm in diameter and appear grapelike. **C.** Individual molar villi, many of which have cavitated central cisterns, exhibit considerable trophoblastic hyperplasia and atypia. The blood vessels of the villi have atrophied and disappeared.

CLINICAL FEATURES: Patients with complete moles commonly present between the 11th and 25th weeks of pregnancy with excessive uterine enlargement and often abnormal uterine bleeding. Passage of tissue fragments, which appear as small grapelike masses, is common. Serum hCG levels are markedly elevated, and increase rapidly.

Complications of complete mole include uterine hemorrhage, DIC, uterine perforation, trophoblastic embolism and infection. The most important complication is development of choriocarcinoma, which occurs in about 2% of patients after the mole has been evacuated.

Treatment consists of suction curettage of the uterus and subsequent monitoring of serum hCG levels. Up to 20% of patients require adjuvant chemotherapy for persistent disease, judging by stable or rising hCG levels. Aneuploidy in the molar tissue may help to identify patients who will require adjuvant treatment. With such management, survival approaches 100%.

Partial Hydatidiform Mole Features Triploid Cells

Partial hydatidiform mole is a distinct form of mole that almost never evolves into choriocarcinoma (Table 18-14). Partial hydatidiform moles have 69 chromosomes (triploidy), of which one haploid set is maternal and two are paternal. This abnormal chromosomal complement results from fertilization of a normal ovum (23,X) by two normal spermatozoa, each with 23 chromosomes, or a single spermatozoon that failed meiotic reduction and has 46 chromosomes. The fetus

Table 18-14

Comparative Features of Complete and Partial Hydatidiform Mole

Features	Complete Mole	Partial Mole
Karyotype	46,XX	47,XXY or 47,XXX
Parental origin of haploid genome sets	Both paternal	1 maternal, 2 paternal
Preoperative diagnosis	Mole	Missed abortion
Marked vaginal bleeding	3+	1+
Uterus	Large	Small
Serum hCG	High	Less elevated
Hydropic villi	All	Some
Trophoblastic proliferation	Diffuse	Focal
Atypia	Diffuse	Minimal
hCG in tissue	3+	1+
Embryo present	No	Some
Blood vessels	No	Common
Nucleated erythrocytes	No	Sometimes
Persists after initial therapy	20%	7%
Choriocarcinoma	2% after mole	No choriocarcinoma

hCG = human chorionic gonadotropin.

associated with a partial mole usually dies after 10 weeks' gestation, and the mole is aborted shortly thereafter. Thus, fetal parts may be present.

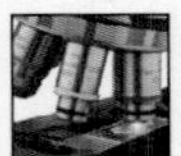

PATHOLOGY: Partial moles have two populations of chorionic villi. Some are normal; others are enlarged by hydropic swelling and show central cavitation, resulting from tangential histologic sections of invaginated surface epithelium ("fjordlike") (Fig. 18-95). Trophoblastic proliferation is focal and less pronounced than in complete mole. Blood vessels are typically found within chorionic villi and contain fetal (nucleated) erythrocytes.

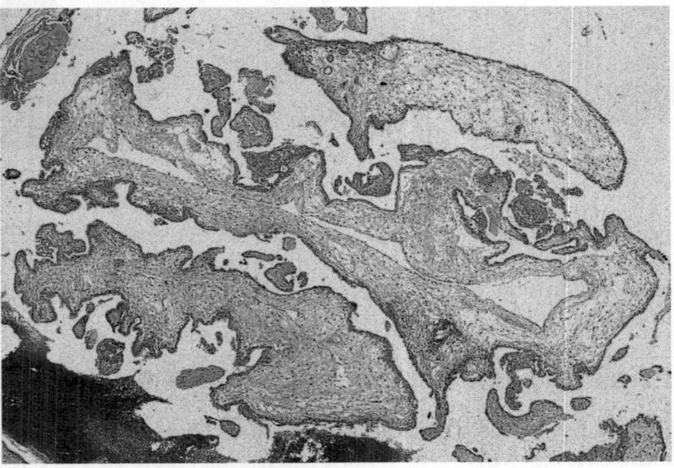

FIGURE 18-95. Partial hydatidiform mole. Two populations of chorionic villi are evident. Some are normal; others are conspicuously swollen. Trophoblastic proliferation is focal and less conspicuous than in a complete mole.

Invasive Hydatidiform Mole Penetrates the Underlying Myometrium

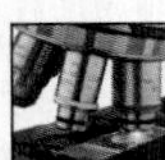

PATHOLOGY: The villi of a hydatidiform mole may only enter the superficial myometrium or they may invade the uterus, and even the broad ligament. They tend to enter dilated venous channels of the myometrium and one third spread to distant sites, mostly the lungs. Unlike choriocarcinoma (see below), distant deposits of an invasive mole remain within the blood vessels in which they are lodged, and death from such spread is unusual. The clinical distinction between invasive mole and choriocarcinoma is often difficult.

Histologically, invasive moles show less hydropic change than complete moles. Trophoblastic proliferation is usually prominent. Uterine perforation is a major complication, but occurs in only a minority of cases. Theca lutein cysts, which may occur with any form of trophoblastic disease as a result of hCG stimulation, are prominent with invasive moles.

Gestational Choriocarcinoma Is a Malignant Tumor Derived From Fetal Trophoblast

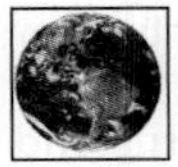

EPIDEMIOLOGY: Choriocarcinoma occurs in 1 in 30,000 pregnancies in the United States; in eastern Asia, the frequency is far greater. The incidence seems related to abnormalities of pregnancy. Thus, it occurs in 1 of 160,000 normal gestations, 1 of 15,000 spontaneous abortions, 1 of 5000 ectopic pregnancies and 1 of 40 complete molar pregnancies. In whites, 25% arise from term deliveries, 25% from spontaneous abortions and 50% from complete hydatidiform moles. Although the risk that a complete hydatidiform mole will transform into choriocarcinoma is only 2%, it is still several orders of magnitude higher than if the pregnancy were normal.

PATHOLOGY: The uterine lesions of choriocarcinoma range from microscopic foci to huge necrotic and hemorrhagic tumors. Viable tumor is usually confined to the rim of the neoplasm because, unlike most other cancers, choriocarcinomas lack intrinsic tumor vasculature. These tumors contain a dimorphic population of cytotrophoblast and syncytiotrophoblast, with varying degrees of intermediate trophoblast (Fig. 18-96). The tumor resembles the trophoblast of an early implanting blastocyst. Rims of syncytiotrophoblast surround central cytotrophoblastic cores, in addition to being arranged around maternal blood spaces, which resemble the intervillous space of normal placentation. hCG is localized to the syncytiotrophoblastic element. ***By definition, tumors containing any villous structures, even if metastatic, are considered hydatidiform mole and not choriocarcinoma.***

Choriocarcinoma invades mainly through venous sinuses in the myometrium. It metastasizes widely via the bloodstream, especially to lungs (over 90%), brain, gastrointestinal tract, liver and vagina (Table 18-15).

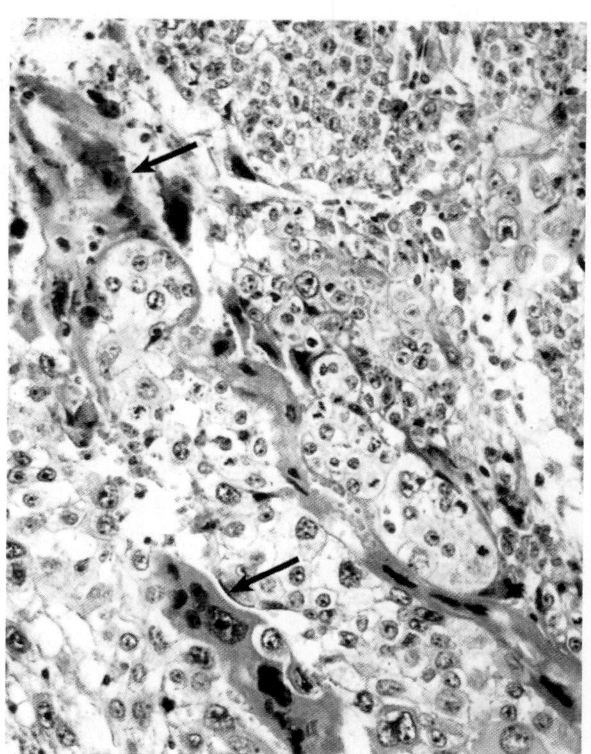

FIGURE 18-96. Choriocarcinoma. Malignant cytotrophoblast and syncytiotrophoblast (*arrows*) are present.

CLINICAL FEATURES: Abnormal uterine bleeding is the most common first symptom of choriocarcinoma. Occasionally, the tumor presents with metastases to lungs or brain. In some cases, it may only become evident 10 or more years after the last pregnancy.

With current chemotherapy, recognition of risk factors (high hCG levels and prolonged interval since antecedent pregnancy) and early treatment, most patients are cured. Survival rates exceed 70% for tumors that have metastasized, and virtually 100% remission is expected if a tumor is localized. Serial serum hCG levels are used to monitor the effectiveness of treatment.

Table 18-15

Clinical Staging of Gestational Trophoblastic Tumors

I	Confined to the uterus
Ia	0 risk factors
Ib	1 risk factor
Ic	2 risk factors
II	Extends outside of the uterus but limited to genital structures
III	Extends to lungs
IV	All other metastatic sites

Risk factors affecting stage include (1) human chorionic gonadotropin (hCG) >100,000 mIU/mL and (2) duration of disease >6 months from termination of antecedent pregnancy.

Placental Site Trophoblastic Tumor Outcomes Are Unpredictable

Placental site trophoblastic tumors are the least common trophoblastic tumors, and are mainly composed of intermediate trophoblastic cells.

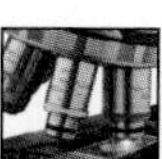

PATHOLOGY: The gross appearance of placental site trophoblastic tumor is more variable than that of choriocarcinoma. Often, the myometrium shows an ill-defined, yellowish tumor without conspicuous hemorrhage. The extent of myometrial invasion varies, and patterns of infiltration resemble that of normal trophoblast in the placental bed. Since intermediate trophoblast in a normal pregnancy functions to anchor the pregnancy into the superficial myometrium, the microscopic appearance of the tumor is typically that of an exaggerated placental site. Mononuclear and multinuclear trophoblast may be present as single cells or as cords, islands and sheets of cells interspersed among myometrial cells. Neither necrosis nor chorionic villi is present. Placental site trophoblastic tumor is also distinguished from choriocarcinoma by its monomorphic (intermediate) trophoblastic proliferation, unlike the dimorphic pattern of trophoblast in choriocarcinoma. Most trophoblastic cells express human placental lactogen (hPL), but a few express hCG.

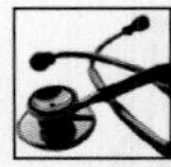

CLINICAL FEATURES: The age and parity of patients with placental site trophoblastic tumor resemble those of patients with choriocarcinoma. Half of patients report amenorrhea, whereas vaginal bleeding usually occurs with choriocarcinoma. Many fewer women with this tumor have had a preceding molar pregnancy than is seen in women with choriocarcinoma (5% vs. 50%).

Placental site trophoblastic tumor must be excised completely (hysterectomy) to prevent local recurrence. It sometimes metastasizes and may be fatal. Large tumors and mitotic indices of more than 5 mitoses/10 HPFs are associated with worse prognosis. Because of the short half-life of hPL, serum levels of hCG are more useful in monitoring response to treatment. Generally, conservative management suffices. If hCG persists, even at low levels, or mitotic count is elevated, aggressive treatment with hysterectomy or chemotherapy is indicated.

19 The Breast

Anna Marie Mulligan • Frances P. O'Malley

Development, Anatomy and Physiologic Change

During embryologic development, the human breast is first recognizable at about the fifth week, when ectodermal thickenings known as the mammary ridges, or "milk lines," extend from the axilla to the medial aspect of the thigh. Regression occurs except in the fourth intercostal space, where the breast will later develop. By the ninth week of gestation, solid epithelial cords grow from the epidermal layer into the underlying mesenchyme. From about the 20th to 32nd weeks of gestation, these solid cellular invaginations canalize and form a network of about 15 to 25 branching primary mammary ducts under the influence of maternal hormones. Toward the end of gestation, the breast is responsive to maternal and placental steroid hormones and to prolactin. These produce secretory activity, and breast development may be transiently prominent in male and female neonates before returning to the inactive state. Further breast development is accelerated at puberty, when ducts begin to elongate and branch (Fig. 19-1A). Estrogen and progesterone cause the terminal end buds and connective tissue stroma to proliferate, differentiate and remodel to form the terminal duct lobular unit (TDLU) of the adult breast (Fig. 19-1B).

The breasts are located on the upper chest wall between the second and the sixth ribs, extending medially to the sternum and laterally to the anterior axillary line, although the tail may extend farther into the axilla. Each breast is composed of skin, subcutaneous adipose tissue and the functional component composed of ducts, lobules and stroma. Collecting ducts, through which milk is secreted, open at the nipple. The nipple–areolar complex is centrally placed, and contains abundant sensory nerves and sebaceous and apocrine glands. The nipple consists predominantly of dense fibrous tissue mixed with fascicles of smooth muscle, which gives the nipple its erectile capability and contributes to expression of milk. Pigmentation increases in the nipple and areola at puberty and further increases during pregnancy. Stratified squamous epithelium that lines the nipple skin extends superficially into the collecting duct before an abrupt transition to glandular epithelium consisting of an inner luminal secretory epithelial cell layer and an outer myoepithelial cell layer.

Just beneath the nipple, collecting ducts dilate to form lactiferous sinuses, which subdivide into 15 to 25 lobes with segmental and subsegmental ducts, and terminate in the TDLU, where milk is made. The TDLU consists of (1) terminal ductules or acini, whose epithelium differentiates into secretory acini in pregnant or lactating glands; (2) the intralobular collecting duct; and (3) specialized intralobular stroma (Fig. 19-1B).

The TDLU is a dynamic structure that undergoes cellular alterations during the menstrual cycle. These cyclical changes include epithelial proliferation and apoptosis, as well as changes in the intralobular stromal components. During the follicular phase of the menstrual cycle, terminal ducts are few and are lined by a simple, two-cell layer of epithelium with surrounding myoepithelium. After ovulation, a conspicuous increase in mitoses in the luminal epithelium occurs with increased acini and edema of the intralobular stroma. Myoepithelial cells become more prominent due to cytoplasmic accumulation of glycogen. These changes may be perceived as progressive fullness of the breast and tenderness. The TDLUs return to their

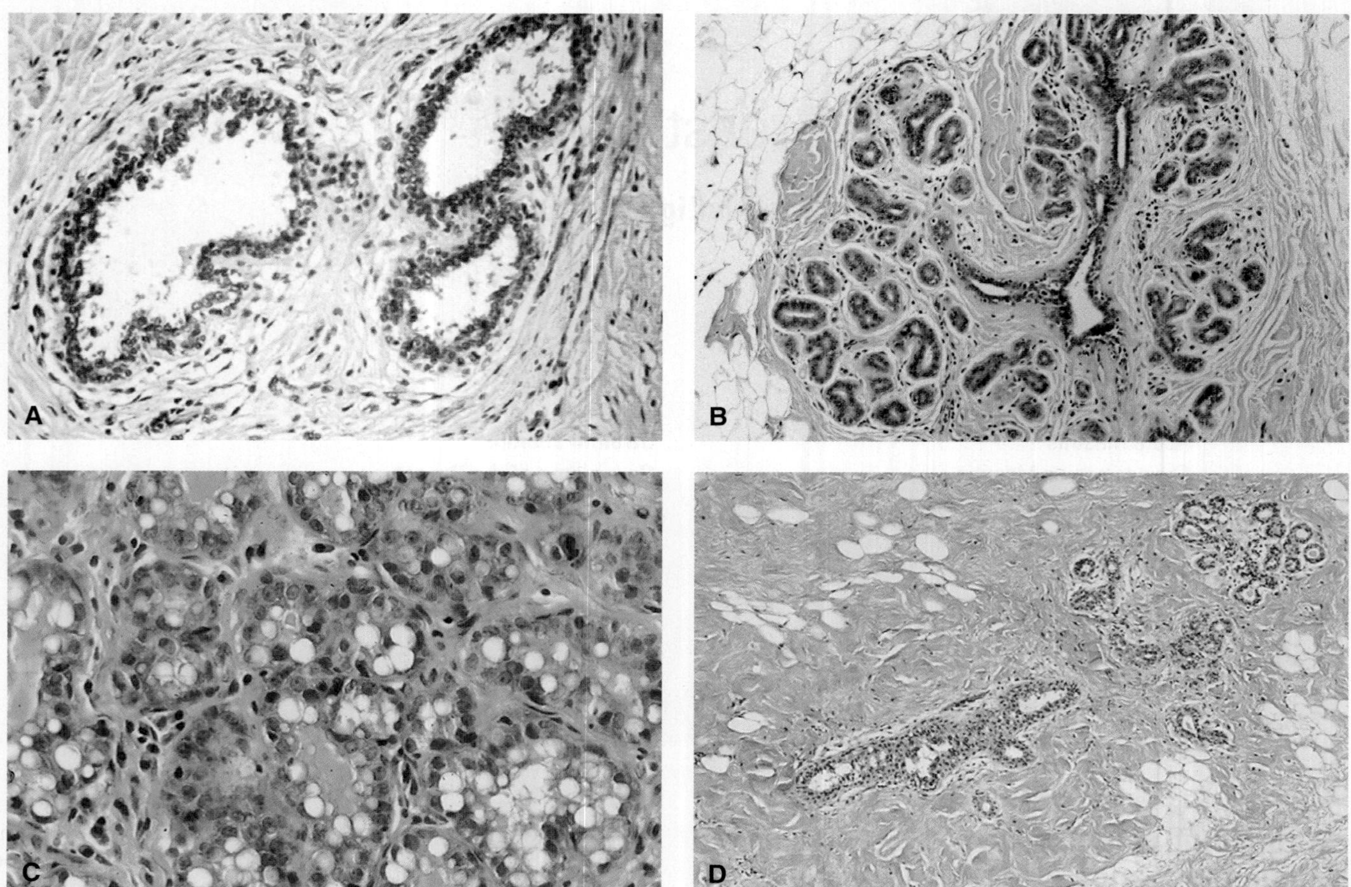

FIGURE 19-1. Normal breast architecture at various ages. A. Adolescent breast. Large and intermediate-size ducts are seen within a dense fibrous stroma. No lobular units are present. **B. Postpubertal breast.** The terminal duct lobular unit consists of small ductules arrayed around an intralobular duct. The two-cell-layered epithelium shows no secretory or mitotic activity. The intralobular stroma is dense and confluent with the interlobular stroma. **C. Lactating breast.** The terminal duct lobular units are conspicuously enlarged, with inapparent interlobular and intralobular stroma. The individual terminal ducts, now termed acini, show prominent epithelial secretory activity (cytoplasmic vacuolization). The acinar lumina contain secretory material. **D. Postmenopausal breast.** The terminal duct lobular units are absent. The remaining intermediate ducts and larger ducts are commonly dilated.

follicular phase state during menses when apoptosis occurs as estrogen and progesterone levels fall. At this time, a progressive increase in lymphocytic infiltration of the intralobular stroma occurs.

Full functional breast development is only realized with the hormonal changes of pregnancy and lactation. In pregnancy, glandular tissue increases markedly, compared to fibrous and fatty connective tissue. Early in pregnancy the TDLU grows rapidly. Stromal vascularity increases and chronic inflammatory cells increase. In later pregnancy, the lobular epithelial cells start to become vacuolated, with increased secretion into distended lobular units. This becomes more pronounced with lactation (Fig. 19-1C). At the end of lactation, a dramatic phase of glandular involution ensues with pronounced cell death and tissue remodeling and the breast returns eventually to its pre-pregnancy state.

In menopause, TDLUs atrophy, but large and intermediate-sized ducts persist (Fig. 19-1D). Fat predominates over fibrous tissue, although the latter typically cuffs the remaining ducts. With advancing age, fat increases as a percentage of total breast mass.

Outside of the TDLU, nonspecialized collagenous connective tissue and fat make up the bulk of the breast tissue. Intralobular stroma is more cellular than is interlobular stroma, and mucopolysaccharide ground substance is also more abundant, within which small numbers of lymphocytes, plasma cells, mast cells and macrophages are present.

The breast is very vascular and contains a complex lymphatic network, draining mainly into axillary lymph nodes, with a minority draining into internal mammary nodes. This rich lymphatic drainage may facilitate the metastatic spread of breast cancers.

Developmental Abnormalities

Very rarely, complete bilateral or unilateral absence of breast development occurs. More often, hypoplasia is seen. Minor asymmetry between breasts is common. Less frequently, marked differences in size may result from hypoplasia of one breast or unusual enlargement of the other breast **(juvenile hypertrophy).** However, juvenile hypertrophy is usually bilateral. Unless there is an underlying hormonal abnormality, juvenile breast hypertrophy regresses spontaneously.

The most common anomaly of breast development is **supernumerary nipples**, or **polythelia**, with or without associated breast tissue **(polymastia).** This results from persistent epidermal thickenings. These occur most frequently along the milk line, which extends from the axilla to the groin, but rarely other sites may be involved. Congenitally **inverted nipple** is due to failure of nipple eversion in development, usually unilaterally.

Inflammatory Diseases of the Breast

Acute Mastitis Is a Common Complication of Breast Feeding

Acute mastitis occurs mostly early in the postpartum period. It is caused by bacterial infection, usually with *Staphylococcus* or *Streptococcus*. Patients have pain, swelling or redness, often with fever and malaise. Cracks in the skin or lactational stasis predispose to infection. If minor, it usually resolves with antibiotics and continued lactation. If mastitis is severe or untreated, abscesses may form or systemic infection may occur.

Periductal mastitis is unrelated to lactation, age or history of pregnancy. It presents with a painful subareolar mass and overlying erythema. The vast majority of patients are cigarette smokers. Microscopically, nipple ducts show keratinizing squamous metaplasia and acute inflammation due to bacterial infection. The ducts often are dilated and may rupture or form fistulas. Surgical excision is curative.

Granulomatous Mastitis

Granulomatous inflammation of the breast can be caused by mycobacteria, parasites, fungi or foreign material. **Tuberculosis** (TB) of the breast is rare in Western countries but is more common in developing countries where TB is endemic. Patients typically present with a mass or sinus and it may be mistaken clinically for invasive carcinoma. Other infectious organisms that cause granulomas are discussed in Chapter 9. **Sarcoidosis** involves the breast rarely, presenting as single or multiple breast masses.

Leakage of **silicone gel** from breast implants leads to foreign body granulomatous inflammation, with a fibrous capsule. In severe cases, this may cause skin retraction, nipple inversion and formation of hard masses, which may simulate or obscure a malignancy. Draining lymph nodes may enlarge due to spread of vacuolated histiocytes with refractile particles. The use of saline, rather than silicone, in implants has greatly reduced implant-associated granulomatous mastitis.

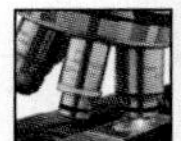

PATHOLOGY: Grossly, the breast tissue is firm, and may be gritty on sectioning if calcification is present. On microscopic evaluation, fat necrosis and foreign body giant cell reaction with varying degrees of inflammation and fibrosis are seen. During tissue processing, much of the silicone is lost from the tissue, leaving clear spaces behind. These spaces, and the histiocytes, may contain birefringent particles. The capsule is formed by a band of frequently calcified, collagenized fibrous tissue.

Idiopathic granulomatous mastitis is rare. It typically occurs in women 20 to 40 years of age with a history of recent pregnancy. It may be bilateral in up to 25% of women. Microscopically, granulomas are centered within lobules with frequent superimposed acute inflammation and microabscesses. Diagnosis is one of exclusion: absence of systemic causes of such inflammation, foreign material or identifiable organisms.

Sclerosing Lymphocytic Lobulitis Represents an Autoimmune Reaction

Sclerosing lymphocytic lobulitis, also called **lymphocytic** or **fibrous mastopathy**, is uncommon. It is frequently associated with other autoimmune diseases, in particular type 1 (insulin-dependent) diabetes mellitus and Hashimoto thyroiditis. Clinically, most patients have a hard mass that may be tender and sometimes bilateral. Circumscribed aggregates of small lymphocytes surround lobules, ducts and vessels, with lobular atrophy, basement membrane thickening and fibrosis. Germinal centers may be present. Interlobular stroma is fibrotic. As lesions progress, inflammation subsides, and diagnosis may be difficult. Recurrences can occur.

Duct Ectasia May Lead to Duct Rupture

Duct ectasia is common, characterized by dilatation, periductal inflammation and fibrosis of large and intermediate breast ducts, which contain inspissated material. Peri- or postmenopausal women are more likely to be symptomatic with a serous or bloody discharge, mass or pain. As disease progresses, duct wall fibrosis may cause the nipple to retract. Episodes of acute inflammation are occasionally complicated by abscess or sinus formation. Microscopically, dilated ducts contain amorphous debris and foamy macrophages (Fig. 19-2). The lining epithelium and periductal stroma contain inflammatory cells and foamy macrophages. Duct rupture may incite a chronic inflammatory response, often with foreign body granulomas. Over time, fibrosis increases, with or without obliteration of ducts.

Fat Necrosis May Mimic Carcinoma

Like carcinoma, fat necrosis commonly presents as a hard mass, often with associated skin tethering. Some patients may give a history of trauma. Necrotic fat cells, an acute inflammatory cell infiltrate, cholesterol clefts and hemorrhage

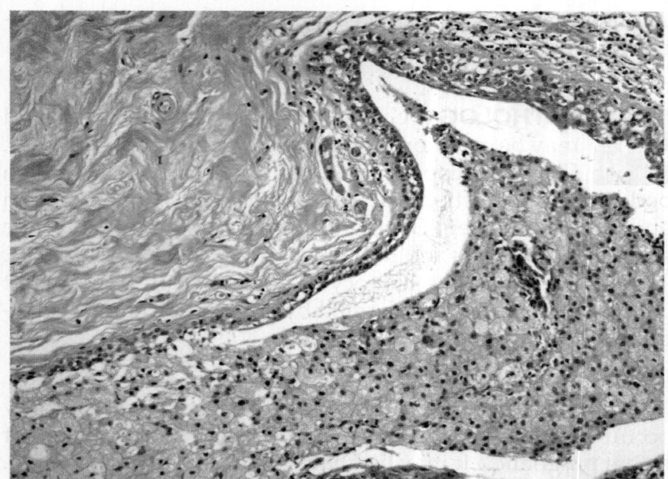

FIGURE 19-2. Duct ectasia. Dilated duct filled with foamy histiocytes. The duct epithelium is focally infiltrated by histiocytes and chronic inflammation of the periductal stroma is present.

are seen early in the course of fat necrosis. Foamy macrophages and multinucleated giant cells that engulf lipid droplets gradually accumulate (Fig. 19-3). With time, fibrosis and dystrophic calcification develop.

Benign Epithelial Lesions

Benign epithelial lesions can be classified based on their risk of developing into invasive carcinoma. Lesions not associated with an increased relative risk are referred to as **nonproliferative breast changes** (e.g., fibrocystic change). **Proliferative disease without atypia** is associated with a 1.5- to 2-fold relative risk of developing carcinoma over 5 to 15 years, and is classified simply as **proliferative breast disease. Proliferative lesions with atypia** entail an even greater relative risk (four- to fivefold risk). Such patients require close clinical follow-up. Patients at high risk may consider medical treatment options (e.g., estrogen antagonists).

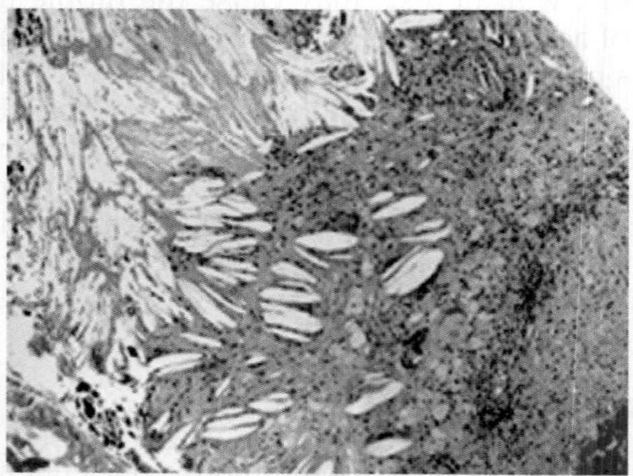

FIGURE 19-3. Fat necrosis. Abundant foamy histiocytes, multinucleated giant cells and cholesterol clefts are present. Calcification is seen on the left of the image.

Fibrocystic (Nonproliferative) Breast Change May Represent an Exaggerated Physiologic Response

Fibrocystic change (FCC) includes gross and microscopic cysts, apocrine metaplasia, mild epithelial hyperplasia and an increase in fibrous stroma. FCC affects over one third of women between 20 and 50 years of age, then declines after menopause. Most women are asymptomatic, but some present with nodularity occasionally associated with pain. FCC is typically multifocal and bilateral.

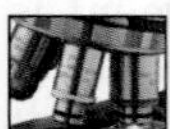

PATHOLOGY: The breast tissue consists grossly of firm fibrofatty tissue within which are multiple clear cysts or "blue dome" cysts (Fig. 19-4A), which contain dark, thin fluid that imparts a blue color to unopened cysts. Cysts vary from 1 to 2 mm to several centimeters in diameter, and may either lack an epithelial lining or be lined by attenuated epithelium and myoepithelium (Fig. 19-4C). Epithelium is often lined by apocrine type cells that are large with abundant granular eosinophilic cytoplasm and a basally located nucleus (Fig. 19-4D). Surrounding stroma is often sclerotic and with an inflammatory cell infiltrate caused by cyst rupture. Mild "usual" epithelial hyperplasia (see below) is frequent, with no more than three to four cell layers above the basement membrane (Fig. 19-4E). Acini are increased in number and size, are lined by columnar cells (columnar cell change) and frequently contain calcifications.

Proliferative Breast Disease Variably Increases Risk of Invasive Carcinoma

Usual Epithelial Hyperplasia

Usual epithelial hyperplasia within ducts or lobules is typified by increased numbers of cells relative to the basement membrane (Fig. 19-4E, F). There may be more than four cell layers, often bridging across duct lumens. Proliferating epithelial cells vary slightly in size, shape and location. Nuclei may be oriented so as to present a streaming pattern (Fig. 19-4F). Secondary spaces are slit-like, irregular and typically peripheral in location. Both luminal and basal epithelial cells proliferate, the latter expressing high–molecular-weight ("basal") cytokeratins.

Sclerosing Adenosis

In sclerosing adenosis (SA) the TDLU shows disordered epithelial, myoepithelial and stromal components. SA lesions vary from microscopic foci to mass lesions that may be palpable and that may be mistaken clinically and radiologically for carcinoma. SA often calcifies and may be targeted for core biopsies. It is not a precursor of invasive cancer but is grouped with proliferative lesions without atypia for risk assessment purposes.

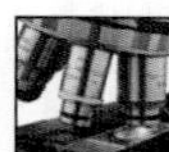

PATHOLOGY: SA lesions show disorderly proliferation of ducts, tubules and intralobular stromal cells resulting in distortion and expansion of lobules and obliterating duct spaces (Fig. 19-5). A lobulocentric architecture, best seen on low power, is maintained. In cases that are difficult to distinguish from invasive carcinoma, immunohistochemistry can highlight the preservation of myoepithelial cells around distorted ducts.

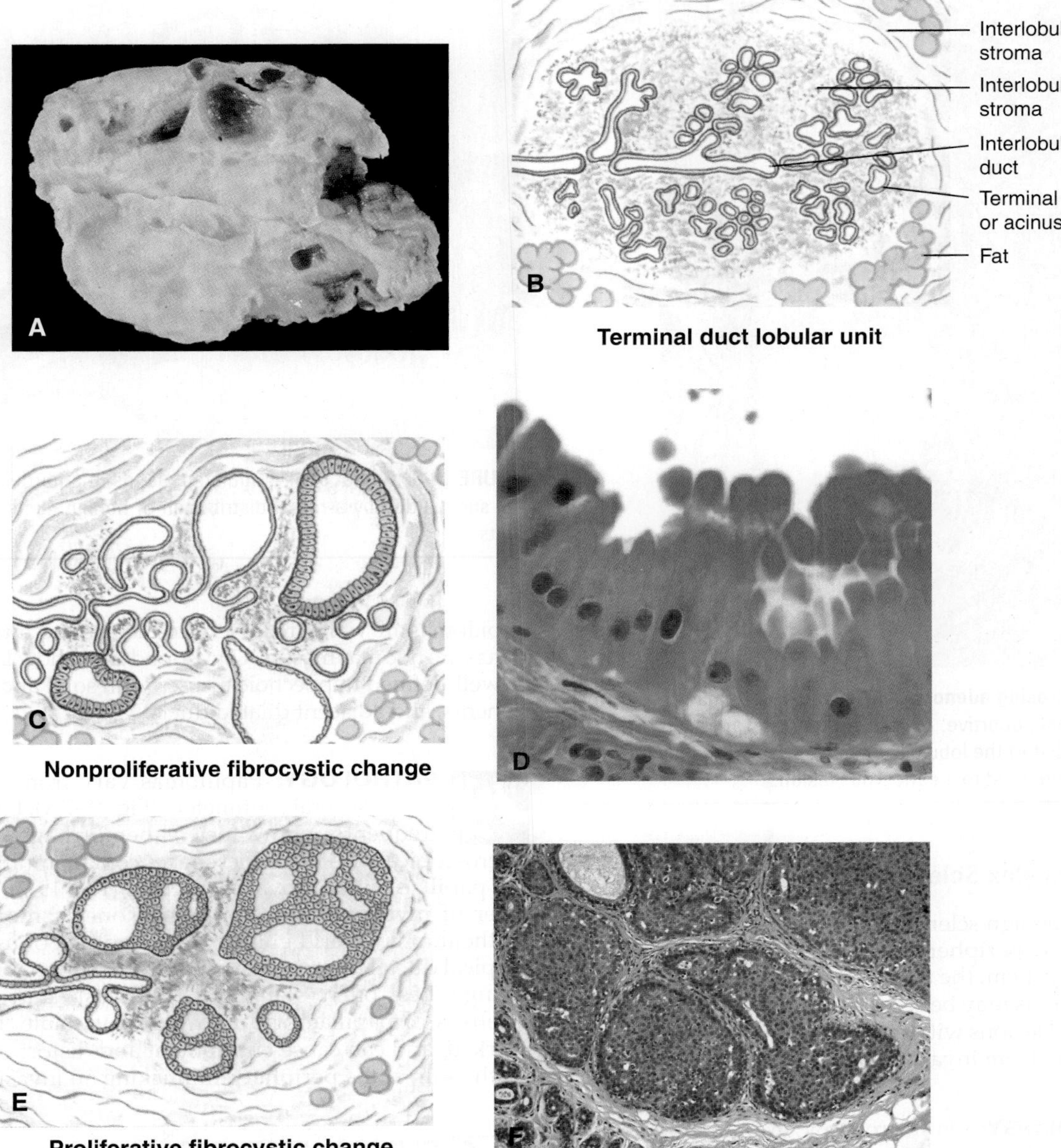

FIGURE 19-4. Fibrocystic change. A. Cysts of various sizes are dispersed in dense, fibrous connective tissue. Some of the cysts are large and contain old blood-tinged proteinaceous debris. **B. Normal terminal lobular unit. C. Nonproliferative fibrocystic change** combines cystic dilation of the terminal ducts with varying degrees of apocrine metaplasia of the epithelium and increased fibrous stroma. **D. Apocrine metaplasia.** Epithelial cells have apocrine features with eosinophilic cytoplasm. **E. Proliferative fibrocystic change**. Terminal duct dilation and intraductal epithelial hyperplasia are present. **F. Florid epithelial hyperplasia of usual type.** The epithelium within the ducts proliferates and almost fills the duct lumen, with residual "secondary" spaces remaining as peripheral slit-like spaces. Cytoplasmic borders are indistinct and the nuclei appear round to oval and frequently overlap, resulting in a streaming pattern.

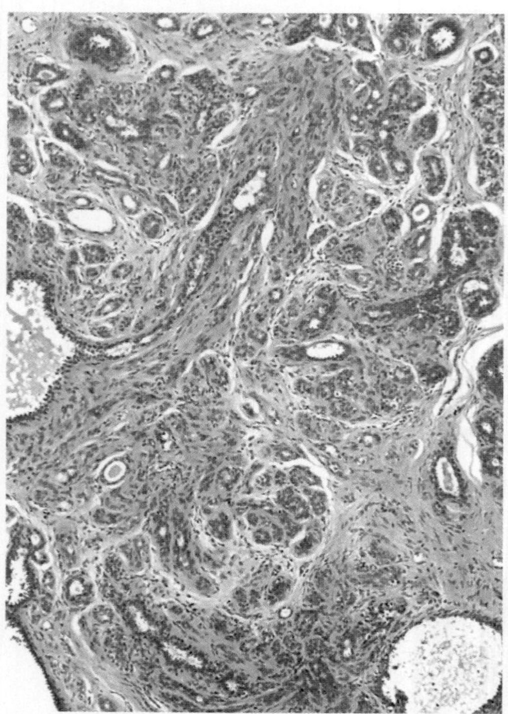

FIGURE 19-5. Sclerosing adenosis. This lesion is characterized by the proliferation of small, abortive, duct-like structures and myoepithelial cells expand and distort the lobule in which it arises. The lesion is well circumscribed, in contrast to a cancerous lesion.

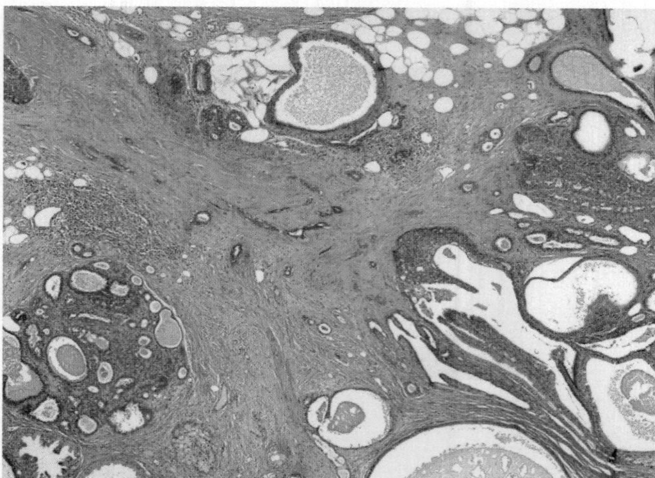

FIGURE 19-6. Radial scar. Angulated glands in a fibroelastotic center are surrounded by a radial distribution of benign ducts and apocrine cysts.

Radial Scar/Complex Sclerosing Lesion

Radial scar is a benign sclerosing lesion with a central fibroelastotic scar and peripheral radiating ducts and lobules. When larger than 1 cm, the term complex sclerosing lesion is used. Larger lesions may be seen mammographically as stellate or spiculated lesions with radiolucent central areas. Radiologic distinction from invasive cancer may be difficult.

PATHOLOGY: On microscopic examination, radial scars are characterized by central fibroelastotic cores, within which entrapped and distorted small ducts are found (Fig. 19-6). Around the periphery, radiating ducts and lobules exhibit a variety of benign alterations. Occasionally, atypical hyperplasia or carcinoma may be found.

CLINICAL FEATURES: Radial scars are associated with a twofold increase in breast cancer risk, and this risk is greater in women with coexisting proliferative disease with or without atypia. This increased risk pertains to both ipsilateral and contralateral breasts, indicating that radial scars are markers of generally increased risk. As carcinoma can occur in radial scars, surgical excision is recommended when these are diagnosed on core needle biopsy.

Intraductal Papilloma

Papillomas can be solitary or multiple and centrally or peripherally located. Patients may present with a nipple discharge, often bloody, or with a mass lesion. On mammography, solitary papillomas are well-circumscribed masses and multiple papillomas are nodular masses. Ultrasound may show larger lesions as well-defined hypoechoic masses with solid and cystic components, and adjacent dilated ducts.

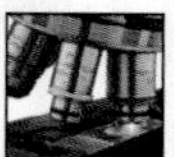

PATHOLOGY: Papillomas vary from microscopic foci to several centimeters (Fig. 19-7A). Larger lesions frequently show foci of hemorrhage or necrosis. Microscopically, dilated duct spaces contain multiple branching papillae with fibrovascular cores (Fig. 19-7B) lined by a layer of myoepithelium, on which one or more layers of epithelium lie. Florid epithelial hyperplasia of usual type or atypical ductal hyperplasia may be seen, often with apocrine change. Less often, squamous metaplasia may be present. Sclerosis of papillae or duct walls is variable, but may be marked, and can cause entrapment and distortion of benign epithelium at the periphery, mimicking an invasive process.

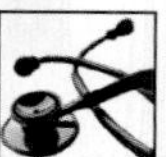

CLINICAL FEATURES: Multiple papillomas are more frequently associated with concurrent or subsequent development of breast carcinomas. The relative risk of breast cancer is twofold in patients with solitary papillomas and threefold if papillomas are multiple. If there is atypia within these lesions, relative risks are five- and sevenfold, respectively. Thus, patients with a diagnosis of papilloma require close follow-up, and if a papilloma is found on core biopsy, excision is generally recommended because of the possibility of coexisting atypia or carcinoma in areas not sampled in the biopsy.

Proliferative Disease With Atypia Are High-Risk Lesions and Precursors to Carcinoma

Atypical Ductal Hyperplasia

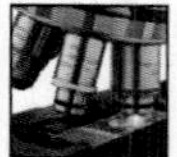

PATHOLOGY: Atypical ductal hyperplasia (ADH) is an intraductal epithelial proliferation composed of a dual population of low-grade neoplastic epithelial cells plus normal cells or epithelial cells of usual epithelial

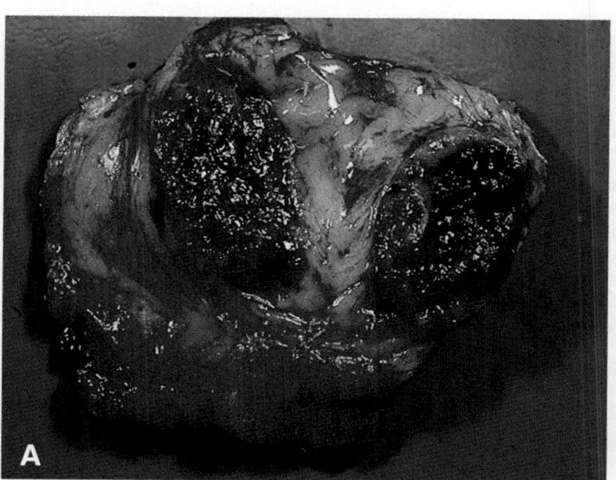

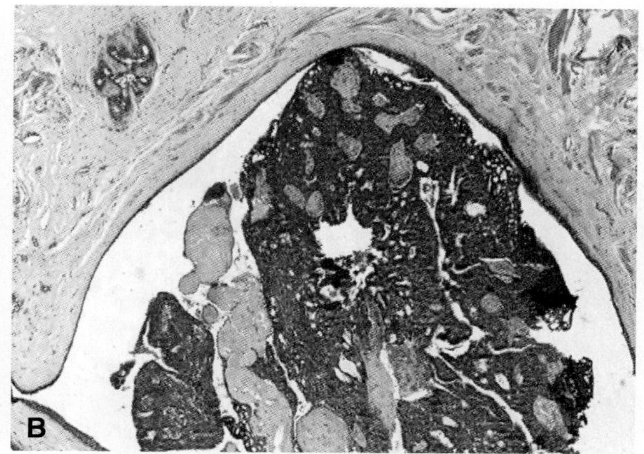

FIGURE 19-7. Intraductal papilloma. A. A large papillary mass is seen within dilated ducts. **B.** A photomicrograph shows a benign papillary growth in a subareolar duct.

hyperplasia (Fig. 19-8). The atypical population is monomorphic small cells that are evenly spaced, with well-defined cytoplasmic borders and round, hyperchromatic, uniform nuclei. The cells may form micropapillae, rigid bridges, bars, solid sheets or cribriform structures, where the atypical cells array around secondary spaces formed within the duct space. Residual normal epithelial cells, or proliferating cells with features of usual hyperplasia as described above, may be seen. If a duct is completely filled by neoplastic cells, and if two duct spaces extending at least 2 mm are involved, the lesion is considered low-grade ductal carcinoma in situ (DCIS). If these criteria are not met, most pathologists would designate the lesion ADH.

MOLECULAR PATHOGENESIS: One third to one half of ADHs show no genetic changes upon comparative genomic hybridization (CGH). The others, however, show alterations that overlap with low-grade DCIS, including loss of 16q and gain of 17p, corroborating studies in which similar changes at 16q and 17p were concurrently observed in paired ADH and DCIS.

In patients with ADH, the relative risk of subsequent breast cancer is increased four to five times over that of age-matched controls. Carcinoma may occur in ipsilateral and contralateral breasts equally frequently. Patients are followed closely. Hormonal therapy may be used to reduce the risk of developing breast cancer.

Atypical Lobular Hyperplasia

PATHOLOGY: Atypical lobular hyperplasia (ALH) is usually an incidental finding in a biopsy or excision done for another abnormality. In ALH, cells are indistinguishable from those seen in lobular carcinoma in situ (LCIS; see below), but the degree of involvement of the TDLU is less in ALH than LCIS: fewer acini are involved and those involved are less distended (Fig. 19-9A). Often, only a few atypical cells involve acini, without obliteration of the lumen. As in LCIS, cells of ALH can spread in a pagetoid fashion to involve ducts (Fig. 19-9B). The morphology of ALH and associated risk of subsequent breast cancer are detailed in the section on LCIS.

Flat Epithelial Atypia

Flat epithelial atypia (FEA) is a recently adopted term for a lesion of terminal duct lobular units in which acini are variably dilated and lined by one or several layers of epithelial cells with low-grade cytologic atypia. FEA most often presents as round, nonbranching mammographic microcalcifications.

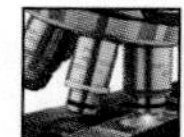

PATHOLOGY: On microscopy, the TDLU is enlarged with variably distended acini lined by cuboidal to columnar epithelial cells (Fig. 19-10). Cells appear uniform, with round to ovoid nuclei and a slight increase in the nuclear-to-cytoplasmic ratio. Cell polarity is lost, and nucleoli are variably prominent. Architectural complexity, in the form of micropapillae, bridges, bars or cribriform structures, is not a feature.

FEA may coexist with ADH, DCIS, ALH/LCIS and invasive carcinoma, particularly tubular carcinoma. The cells of

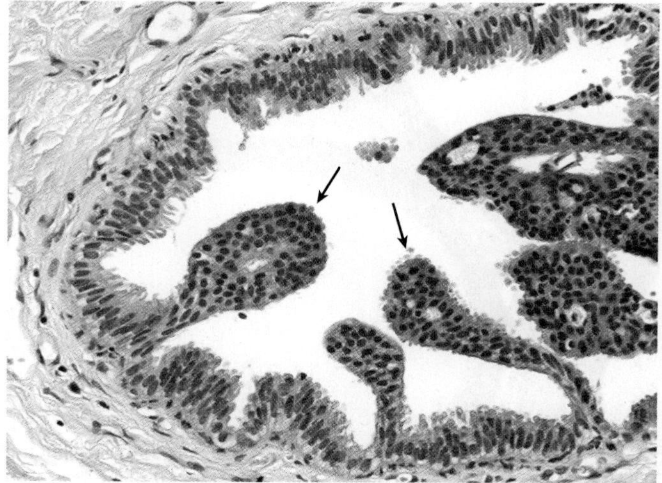

FIGURE 19-8. Atypical ductal hyperplasia (ADH). Micropapillae (*arrows*) project into the duct lumen and consist of cells with an increased nuclear:cytoplasmic ratio and nuclear hyperchromasia. Residual benign columnar cells are seen lining the duct.

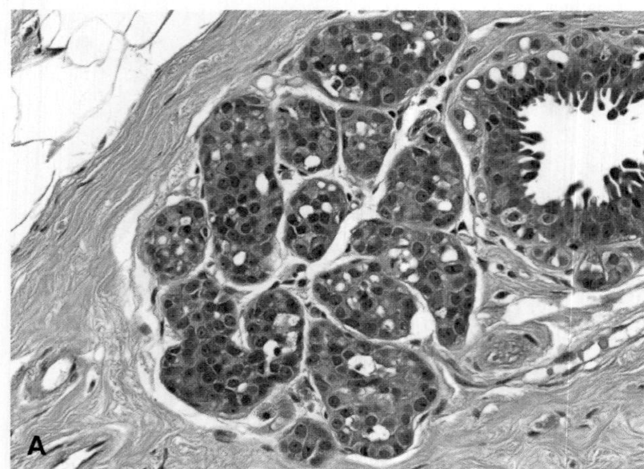

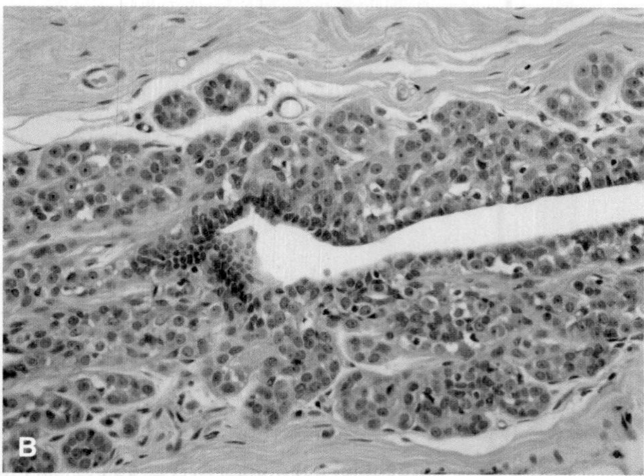

FIGURE 19-9. A. Atypical lobular hyperplasia (ALH). There is minimal distension of the lobular acini by a uniform population of cells with intracytoplasmic lumina and round nuclei containing small nucleoli. **B. Pagetoid spread** of lobular neoplastic cells into the terminal duct. Here the atypical cells lie beneath an attenuated surface layer of luminal epithelial cells.

FEA are similar in morphology to coexisting in situ and invasive carcinoma. Furthermore, loss of heterozygosity (LOH) is present in most cases, in patterns that are shared with coexistent DCIS or invasive carcinoma.

There are very few studies of clinical outcomes in patients with FEA on initial biopsy. Limited data suggest that local recurrence and progression to invasive carcinoma are low.

Fibroepithelial Lesions

These arise from intralobular stroma and contain both stromal and epithelial elements.

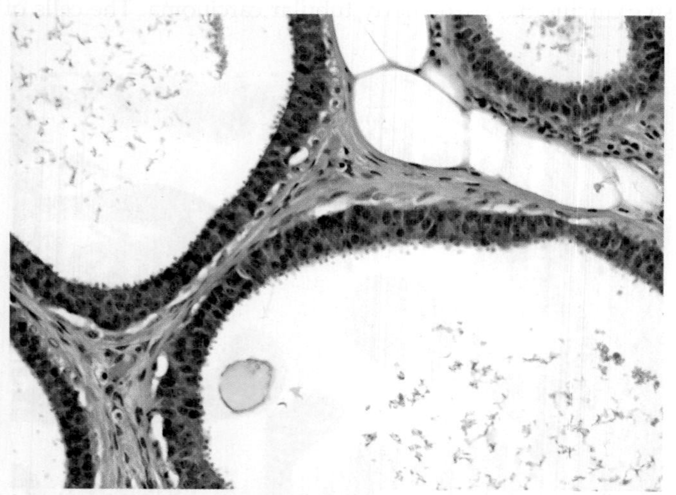

FIGURE 19-10. Flat epithelial atypia. The terminal duct lobular unit (TDLU) is enlarged as a result of dilatation of the lobular acini. These are lined by one to two layers of epithelial cells showing low-grade cytologic atypia. Nuclei appear round with variably conspicuous nucleoli and loss of their basal location (loss of polarity) is seen. Architectural complexity is not a feature.

Fibroadenoma Is a Benign Tumor With Epithelial and Stromal Components

Fibroadenomas are common, mobile, painless, well-defined breast lumps. They are most often diagnosed in women 20 to 35 years of age. Clinically silent lesions are particularly common, usually identified by mammography. These are well-defined masses, which may be calcified. They are most often solitary lesions, although they can be multiple and bilateral, most commonly in Afro-Caribbean women.

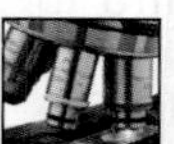

PATHOLOGY: Fibroadenomas are round or ovoid and rubbery (Fig. 19-11A), and are sharply demarcated from surrounding breast. Most are less than 3 cm in diameter, but they can rarely be much larger (up to 20 cm) in young women or adolescents.

Microscopically, there are two components: stroma and epithelium (Fig. 19-11B). The stroma is typically composed of spindle cells and shows variable, but usually low, cellularity. In younger women, the stroma is often myxoid. With age, stroma may be hyalinized and calcify. The epithelial component is formed from the normal TDLU constituents; the epithelial and myoepithelial layers are preserved. The relationship of the stroma to the epithelium is typically uniform throughout the lesion and two growth patterns may be seen. In the **intracanalicular** pattern, stromal growth compresses duct structures into curvilinear slits. In the **pericanalicular** pattern, ducts maintain a tubular configuration, surrounded by stromal proliferation. These patterns have no clinical or prognostic import.

The epithelial component often shows hyperplasia, particularly in young women. Rarely, atypical ductal hyperplasia, lobular neoplasia or DCIS can occur within fibroadenomas. Complex fibroadenomas show benign changes including epithelial calcifications, sclerosing adenosis, papillary apocrine change or cysts greater than 3 mm. Three-mm, non-complex fibroadenomas do not increase cancer risk.

Variants of fibroadenoma include **tubular adenoma**, in which small tubular structures are surrounded by a loosely

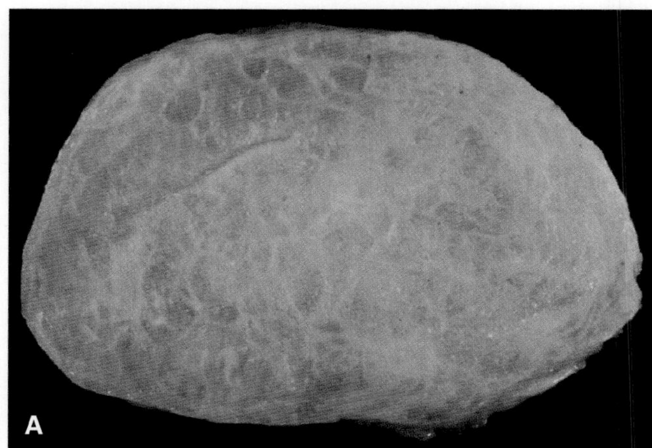

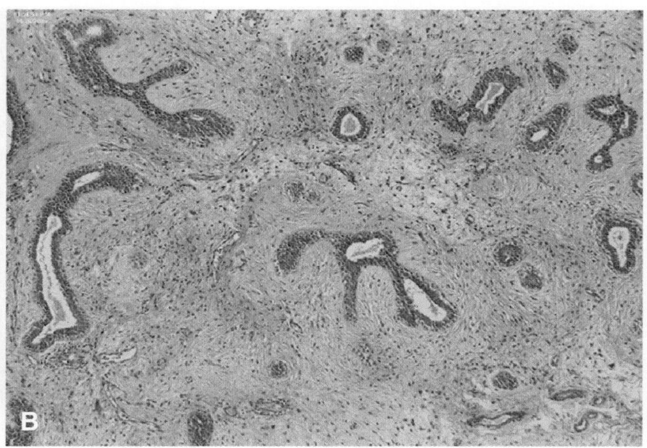

FIGURE 19-11. Fibroadenoma. A. Surgical specimen. This well-circumscribed tumor was easily enucleated from the surrounding tissue. The cut surface is characteristically glistening tannish-white and has a septate appearance. **B.** Microscopic section. Elongated epithelial duct structures are situated within a loose, myxoid stroma.

cellular vascularized stroma, and **juvenile fibroadenoma**, which are most common in adolescents (Fig. 19-12). These grow rapidly and may reach 20 cm in size, causing clinical concern. Juvenile fibroadenomas resemble fibroadenomas histologically, albeit with more cellular stroma.

Fibroadenomas are surgically excised if they are of clinical or radiologic concern, or if the patient prefers. They can recur. Ipsilateral or contralateral lesions may arise.

Phyllodes Tumor

Phyllodes tumors are rare. They have epithelial and stromal components, the latter being neoplastic. The name is derived from the Greek word *phyllos*, meaning "leaf," because they show a leaf-like growth pattern. Phyllodes tumors make up less than 1% of breast tumors. They can occur in any age group, but are most common in the sixth decade. They present as rapidly growing breast masses, and are well circumscribed or lobulated on mammography. Ultrasound may show internal hyperechoic areas in a hypoechoic mass.

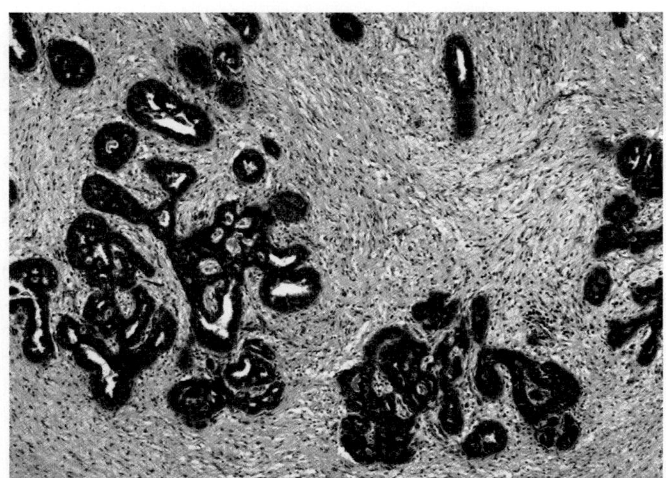

FIGURE 19-12. Juvenile fibroadenoma. The stroma shows hypercellularity, although mitoses and cellular atypia are not features. Epithelial hyperplasia of usual type is present in the glands.

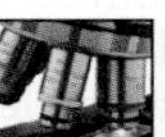

PATHOLOGY: Phyllodes tumors vary in size from a few centimeters to 20 cm. Grossly, **benign** phyllodes tumors are sharply circumscribed and their cut surfaces are firm, glistening and grayish white. Cleft spaces may be prominent. Malignant lesions may show infiltrative margins. On microscopy, fronds of hypercellular stroma lead to the formation of leaf-like structures, which project into cystic spaces (Fig. 19-13). These cystic spaces are lined by a dual layer of benign epithelium and myoepithelium. The stroma ranges from benign and hypercellular to frankly sarcomatous. Most phyllodes tumors are benign, with mild or moderately hypercellular stroma showing mild cytologic atypia and few mitoses (<5 per 10 high-powered fields [HPFs]). The stroma in **malignant** phyllodes tumors is markedly hypercellular, with considerable pleomorphism, abundant mitoses (>10 per 10 HPFs) and stromal overgrowth. Malignant heterologous elements, such as bone, cartilage or fat, may be seen. Phyllodes tumors that are not clearly benign or malignant are classified as **borderline**.

The risk of benign phyllodes tumors is local recurrence, which occurs 15% to 20% of the time, rather than metastasis. The best predictor of recurrence is completeness of excision; thus, a rim of normal tissue should be excised with these tumors. Recurrence is more common with malignant lesions. Metastases are rare overall, but with high-grade malignant phyllodes tumors, they may occur in 20% to 25% of patients. ***Only the stromal components are seen in metastases.*** Axillary lymph node metastases are very rare.

Stromal Lesions

Stromal lesions arise from nonspecialized interlobular stroma. Mesenchymal lesions that occur outside of the breast, such as lipomas or vascular tumors, can occur here. Stromal lesions specific to the breast, such as pseudoangiomatous stromal hyperplasia and myofibroblastoma, are also found.

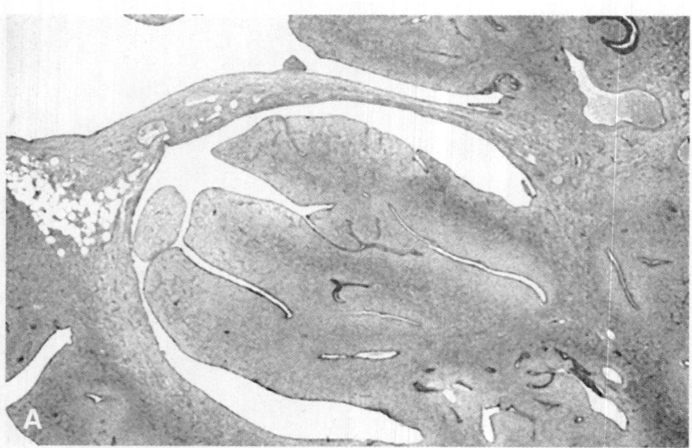

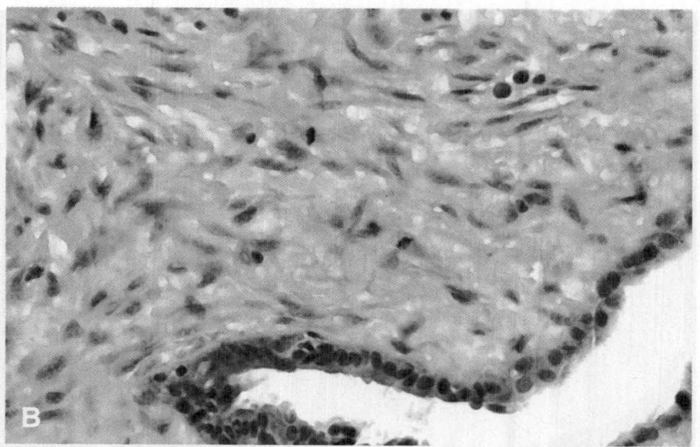

FIGURE 19-13. Phyllodes tumor. A. A polypoid tumor with a leaf-like pattern expands a duct. **B.** The stromal component adjacent to ductal epithelium is similar to a fibroadenoma, but is more cellular. The residual ductal structure is benign.

Pseudoangiomatous Stromal Hyperplasia

Pseudoangiomatous stromal hyperplasia (PASH) is a benign process that mimics a vascular lesion and is usually found incidentally in biopsies performed for other reasons. However, some PASH lesions can present as a discrete, painless, mobile mass, clinically indistinguishable from a fibroadenoma. It is frequently seen in gynecomastia and most female patients are premenopausal, suggesting that hormonal factors may play a role in their development and growth.

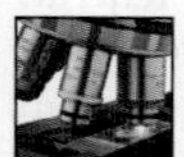

PATHOLOGY: On gross examination, PASH is a circumscribed mass with a homogeneous tan cut surface, approximately 1 to 7 cm in size. Microscopically, anastomosing spaces are seen in dense collagenous stroma (Fig. 19-14). Myofibroblasts close to these spaces mimic endothelial cells. Rarely, red blood cells are found within the spaces. True vascular channels can be seen within the stroma.

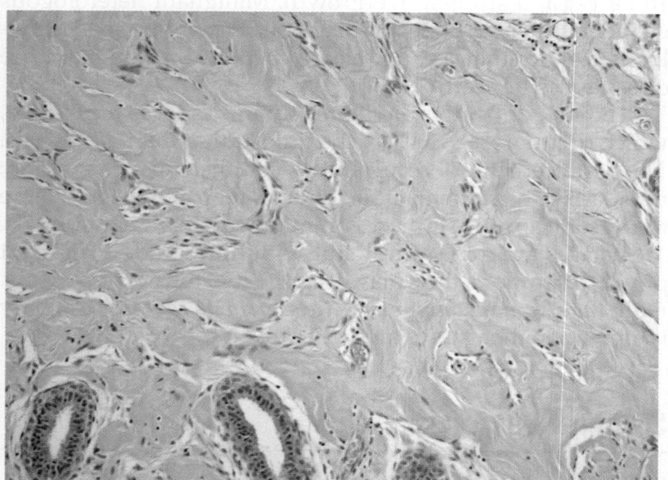

FIGURE 19-14. Pseudoangiomatous stromal hyperplasia. Slit-like spaces within a collagenized stroma are seen. Myofibroblasts are distributed singly at the margins of the spaces, resembling endothelial cells. True capillaries are also evident.

Fibromatosis

Fibromatosis is an infiltrative lesion of fibroblasts and myofibroblasts. These lesions can be locally aggressive but do not metastasize. They present predominantly as unilateral, painless, firm to hard masses.

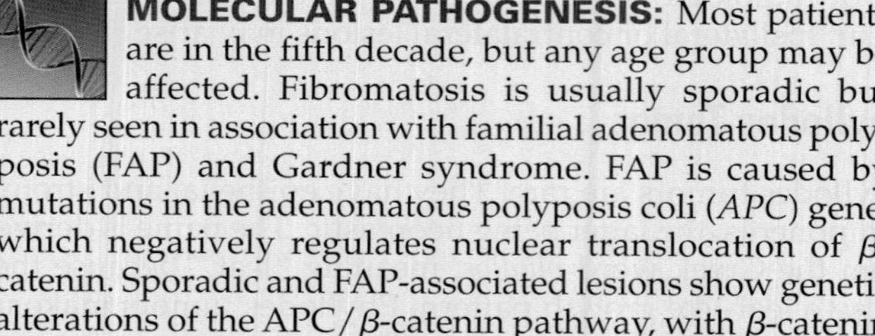

MOLECULAR PATHOGENESIS: Most patients are in the fifth decade, but any age group may be affected. Fibromatosis is usually sporadic but rarely seen in association with familial adenomatous polyposis (FAP) and Gardner syndrome. FAP is caused by mutations in the adenomatous polyposis coli (*APC*) gene, which negatively regulates nuclear translocation of β-catenin. Sporadic and FAP-associated lesions show genetic alterations of the APC/β-catenin pathway, with β-catenin mutation or mutation or allelic loss of 5q, the location of the APC gene. Breast fibromatosis may also occur during pregnancy, although hormonal factors are not thought to contribute to the pathogenesis.

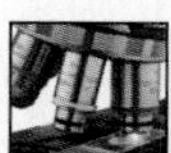

PATHOLOGY: On mammography, a stellate mass mimicking carcinoma is seen. Grossly, the lesion is poorly defined and firm, with infiltrative margins. Sizes vary from less than 1 cm to greater than 10 cm. Microscopically, broad sweeping fascicles and interlacing bundles of bland-appearing spindle or oval cells are seen (Fig. 19-15). Collagen may be prominent. Adjacent normal breast tissue is infiltrated by the proliferating spindled cells, and in many cases, lymphocytes may collect at the periphery. Cellular atypia is lacking and mitoses are rare (<3 per 10 HPFs). Immunochemical identification of the abnormal nuclear location of β-catenin may aid diagnosis, but is not entirely sensitive or specific.

Carcinoma of the Breast

Breast cancer is the most common malignancy of women in the United States, and the mortality from this disease among women is second only to that of lung cancer.

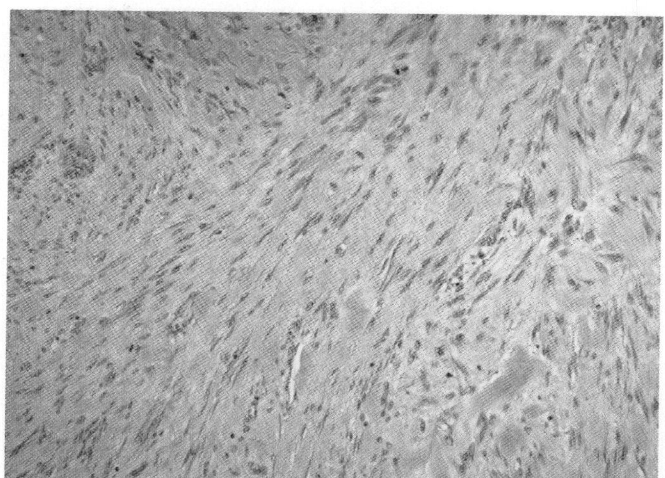

FIGURE 19-15. Fibromatosis. Interlacing bundles of spindle cells, without nuclear atypia, are present with focal bands of collagen.

EPIDEMIOLOGY: The incidence of breast cancer has increased slowly over the past 50 years. Women in the United States have a one in nine risk of developing breast cancer; however, as this represents lifetime risk, it overstates an individual's risk. One in five women with breast cancer will die of their disease. Age-specific incidence rates increase dramatically after 40 years of age. In industrialized countries with high rates of breast cancer, incidence increases with age, plateauing at 75 to 80 years. Among some groups, including Hispanic and black women, that plateau is reached at a younger age. Breast cancer is uncommon before the age of 35 in all populations. The incidence of estrogen receptor (ER)–negative cancers increases rapidly until age 50, after which it flattens or decreases. In contrast, ER-positive breast cancer continues to rise after that age. Thus, peak ages of onset for ER-negative and ER-positive breast cancers are 50 and 70 years, respectively.

Breast cancer occurs four to five times more frequently in Western industrialized countries. Risks in daughters and granddaughters of women who migrated from countries of low incidence to Western countries increase with successive generations. Dietary, environmental and lifestyle factors are implicated.

Widespread use of screening mammography in the 1980s led to a sharp increase in the proportion of breast cancers that are noninvasive (i.e., DCIS). The frequency of small invasive cancers has also increased. Overall mortality has declined from 30% to 20%, and stage-specific mortality has also improved.

However, the use of screening mammography has illustrated important gaps in our understanding of breast cancer. It is now apparent that routine screening mammography detects a significant percentage of tumors that will never cause clinical disease. Recent large-scale studies suggest that 20%, or possibly more, of invasive breast cancers that are found on screening mammography may actually regress without treatment. Among the important challenges in breast cancer, then, is to develop means of distinguishing tumors that need to be treated from those that may not.

Table 19-1

Risk Factors for Breast Cancer Development

Not Modifiable	Modifiable
Age	Body mass index
BRCA germline mutations	Diet
Family history	Alcohol
Chest radiation	Exogenous estrogen
Race/ethnicity	Exercise
Height	Smoking
Age at menarche	Reproductive history
Age at menopause	Age at first full-term delivery
Breast density	Lactation
Atypia on prior breast biopsy	

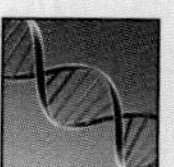
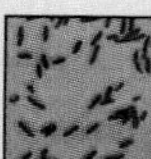

MOLECULAR PATHOGENESIS AND ETIOLOGIC FACTORS: Multiple risk factors for breast cancer have been identified, some of which cannot be modified and some of which are modifiable (Table 19-1). Women can be stratified by level of breast cancer risk. Women who carry a germline BRCA mutation (see below) or who have a history of chest radiation are considered high risk; women who have had multiple family members with breast cancer or who have multiple risk factors are at moderate risk. Risk assessment tools can be used to quantify risk for individual patients.

Nonmodifiable risk factors include age, race (greatest in non-Hispanic white population), family history, genetic factors (germline mutations in *BRCA1* or 2), breast density and early age at menarche. Modifiable risk factors include late age at first live birth, diet, high body mass index, alcohol consumption and use of exogenous hormones.

SPORADIC BREAST CANCER: Only about 25% of sporadic breast cancers have identifiable risk factors. Factors affecting the hormonal milieu modify breast cancer risk.

- ***The majority of breast cancers are stimulated by estrogens;*** cumulative lifetime exposure to estrogen determines the level of this risk. As such, early menarche (younger than 11 years), late menopause and older age at first term pregnancy increase risk. Pregnancy before age 20 is protective, and nulliparity and deferring childbearing until after 35 years of age are associated with a two- to threefold increased relative risk. Longer lactation reduces risk of breast cancer. Oophorectomy before age of 35, but not afterwards, dramatically lowers risk of breast cancer. Antiestrogens, including tamoxifen and aromatase inhibitors, decrease ER-positive breast cancer. Oral contraceptives do not increase breast cancer risk, although hormone replacement therapy (HRT) increases risk slightly, 1.2 to 1.7 times.
- **Radiation** increases risk of breast cancer, as documented in survivors of the atomic bomb and in women who received irradiation for Hodgkin lymphoma, etc. Irradiation earlier in life (i.e., in childhood or adolescence) poses the greatest risk; exposure after the age of 40 years has not been shown to increase incidence.

- The influence of **dietary fat** on breast cancer risk has been extensively studied, and there are limited data to suggest that total fat may increase risk of breast cancer after menopause but that the risk, if existent, is likely to be small. Prospective studies of the effects of carbohydrates have not shown consistent associations with breast cancer risk.
- **Alcohol consumption** consistently predicts higher breast cancer rates. A dose-response relationship without a threshold effect has been observed. Adequate folate intake, however, seems to reduce or eliminate excess risk due to alcohol.
- Postmenopausal women who are **overweight** or **obese** are at greater risk for breast cancer. Interestingly, heavier premenopausal women have a lower risk of breast cancer.
- Mammographic breast density reflects the proportions of stroma and epithelium rather than fat in breasts. Patients with **denser breasts** (i.e., >75% density) have a four- to fivefold greater risk of breast cancer. Density is influenced by age, parity, body mass index and menopausal status, but genetic factors may also play a role.
- Prior breast biopsies showing **atypical hyperplasia** or **nonatypical proliferative breast disease** increase relative risk of 4 to 5 times and 1.5 to 2 times, respectively (see above). Women with a previous breast carcinoma have a 10-fold greater chance of developing a second primary cancer in the ipsilateral or contralateral breast. Hormonal treatment with antiestrogens decreases this risk.

FAMILIAL BREAST CANCER: The strongest association with increased risk for breast cancer is a family history of breast cancer in first-degree relatives. The risk is greater if the relative was affected at a young age or had bilateral breast cancer. Familial disease accounts for approximately 10% of breast cancers. Two high-risk breast cancer susceptibility genes, *BRCA1* and *BRCA2*, account for 20% to 50% of these. A minority of familial breast cancers are attributable to mutations in highly penetrant genes, such as *p53* (Li-Fraumeni syndrome), *PTEN* (Cowden syndrome), *ATM* (ataxia telangiectasia), *CHEK2* (Li-Fraumeni variant syndrome) and *STK11* (Peutz-Jeghers syndrome).

BRCA1 and *BRCA2* are tumor-suppressor genes that display an autosomal dominant pattern of inheritance with variable penetrance. *BRCA1*, on chromosome 17q21, is involved in DNA repair, transcriptional regulation, chromatin remodeling and protein ubiquitination. Germline mutations in *BRCA1* confer a lifetime breast cancer risk of between 37% and 85% by age 70 years, with over half of the cancers occurring before age 50. In women older than 70 years, *BRCA1* germline mutations account for less than 2% of cancers; however, 30% of cancers in women under 45 years of age occur in mutation carriers. Carriers are also at significantly increased risk of other cancers, most notably ovarian cancer, with a lifetime risk of 15% to 40%, and cancers of the cervix, endometrium, fallopian tube, stomach, liver and prostate in male carriers. Approximately 0.1% of the population has *BRCA1* germline mutations, but rates are higher in Ashkenazi Jews and French Canadians. Breast cancers that develop in patients with germline mutations are typically high-grade ductal carcinomas of no special type; however, they show many of the features present in medullary-like cancers, with pushing margins, prominent inflammatory responses, absent tubule formation, high mitotic counts and significant nuclear pleomorphism (Fig. 19-16). The majority of cancers are ER, progesterone receptor (PR) and human epidermal growth factor receptor 2 (HER2) negative, and p53 mutations are more common. Young age of onset is typical.

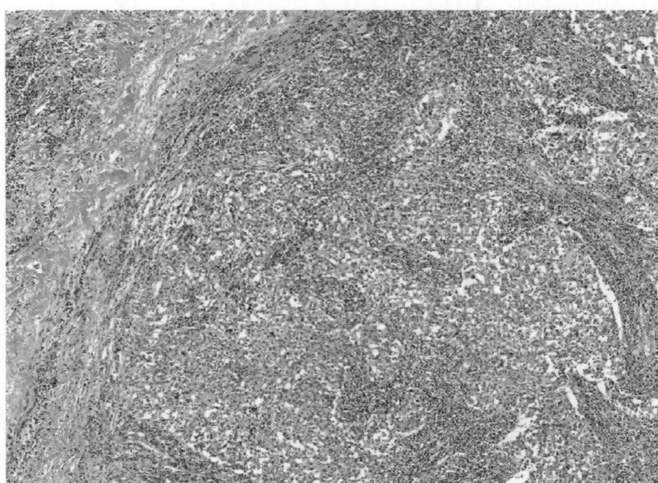

FIGURE 19-16. BRCA1-associated breast cancer. High-grade invasive ductal carcinoma, no special type, characterized by pushing margins and a prominent lymphocytic infiltrate.

Germline mutations in *BRCA2*, located on chromosome 13q12, are associated with a 30% to 40% lifetime risk of developing breast cancer and an increased risk of ovarian cancer, as well as uveal tract and skin melanoma and pancreatic, biliary tract and prostatic carcinomas. Male carriers of *BRCA2* mutations are also at risk for breast cancer. These patients mostly develop high-grade invasive ductal tumors of no special type. Unlike *BRCA1*-associated cancers, *BRCA2*-related cancers are mostly ER and PR positive. Similarly, p53 mutations are frequent. No significant difference in HER2 status is found.

MAMMARY STEM CELLS: Self-renewal of mammary stem cells involves a diverse network of regulatory pathways including Notch, Hedgehog, Wnt/β-catenin, epidermal growth factor receptor, TGF-β, integrins and ER/PR, among others. Current anticancer therapies mostly fail to eradicate stem cell clones and instead favor expansion of the stem cell pool and/or select for resistant clones. Eradicating these cells may greatly impact breast cancer survival. Pathways considered important in cancer stem cell biology, including Notch, Wnt/β-catenin and α6-integrin, are being investigated.

Carcinoma In Situ Is a Precursor of Invasive Carcinoma

Carcinoma of the breast may be **in situ** (confined by the gland's basement membrane) or **invasive**, where the malignant cells have infiltrated through the basement membrane into adjacent breast stroma. Further subclassification is based on morphology, immunohistochemistry and molecular profiling. Of women with biopsy-proven DCIS who received no further therapy, 20% to 30% subsequently developed invasive cancer.

Ductal Carcinoma In Situ

DCIS identifies a heterogeneous group of lesions that vary in their architectural and cytologic features, as well as in their natural history. These lesions are considered nonobligate precursors of invasive carcinoma, the chance of progressing to invasion varying with the histologic subtype, grade and extent. The incidence of DCIS has soared with the advent of screening mammography. It represented about 5% of breast cancers beforehand, and now represents 25% of breast cancers in screened populations.

MOLECULAR PATHOGENESIS: Several lines of evidence support that DCIS is a precursor of invasive breast carcinoma. DCIS is often seen together with invasive carcinomas. Noninvasive tumors and their invasive counterparts show similar cytologic appearance and nuclear grade. Also, DCIS and invasive carcinoma share distinct molecular and cytogenetic alterations as shown by CGH and LOH studies. The mechanisms involved in progression of DCIS to invasive carcinoma, however, are poorly understood. This progression may be determined less by intrinsic properties of tumor epithelial cells than by complex interactions between epithelial cells and all the cell types of the tumor microenvironment.

Molecular analyses have demonstrated differences in the numbers and type of chromosomal changes in low-, intermediate- and high-grade DCIS. More alterations are seen in the latter; however, these do not necessarily overlap with those seen in low-grade lesions. Loss of 16q and gain of chromosome 1q are the most frequent abnormalities in low-grade DCIS, but are rare in high-grade DCIS. In high-grade lesions, gains of 17q, 8q and 5p and losses of 11q, 14q, 8p and 13q are common, as is gene amplification involving loci on chromosomes 17, 6, 8 and 11. Intermediate-grade DCIS shares alterations of both groups. Invasive carcinomas occurring in association with DCIS share grade and molecular alterations. Thus, low-grade and high-grade DCIS, and also low-grade and high-grade invasive carcinomas, are fundamentally distinct entities and do not evolve into each other. ***Multiple pathways of carcinogenesis and progression are likely.***

PATHOLOGY: DCIS predominantly involves ducts but can extend into lobules and is characterized by a proliferation of malignant epithelial cells showing a range of histologic features (Fig. 19-17). Growth patterns may be cribriform, micropapillary, papillary, solid and comedo types, and multiple architectural patterns can coexist in one lesion. More important prognostically is the nuclear grade: low, intermediate and high.

- **High-grade DCIS** is composed of large, pleomorphic cells with marked variation in size and shape. The cells have abundant cytoplasm, irregular nuclei with prominent nucleoli and coarse chromatin. They proliferate rapidly. Intraductal necrosis is common (Fig. 19-18), and appears grossly as distended ducts with white necrotic material resembling comedos, hence the term **comedo necrosis**. The cellular necrotic debris often undergoes dystrophic calcification, which may be seen on mammography as linear, branching calcifications. Malignant cells are confined to duct spaces, but periductal chronic inflammation may be present with formation of new vessels. DCIS spreads through the duct system and often extends beyond clinically detected borders, making clear margins difficult to obtain. Cells with high nuclear grade can be seen with any of the above growth patterns.

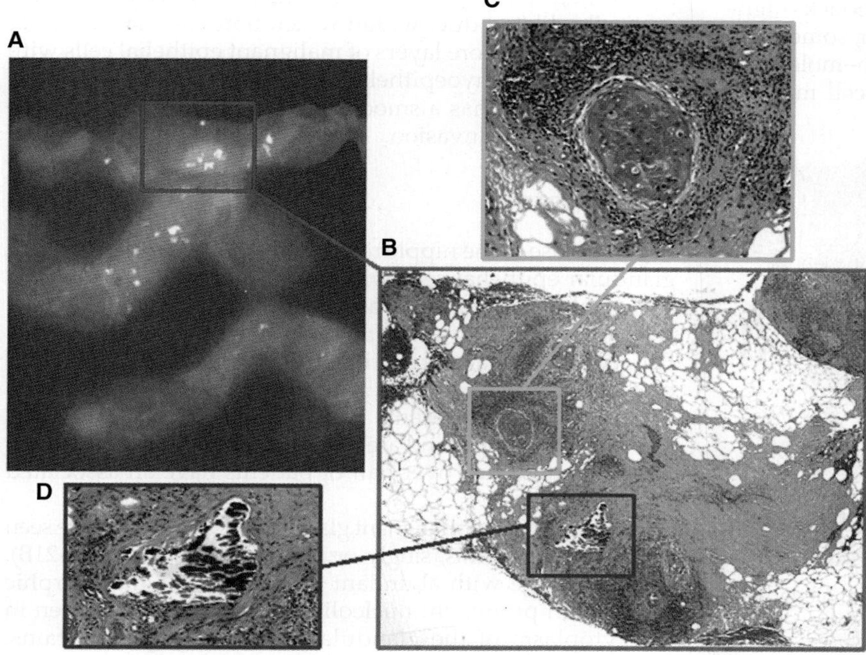

FIGURE 19-17. Ductal carcinoma in situ. A. Specimen radiograph of core biopsy shows linear and punctate atypical calcifications that are highly suspicious for cancer. **B.** Low-power photomicrograph showing high-grade in situ ductal carcinoma. **C.** High-power image of a duct expanded by in situ ductal carcinoma. **D.** High-power photomicrograph of tissue calcification.

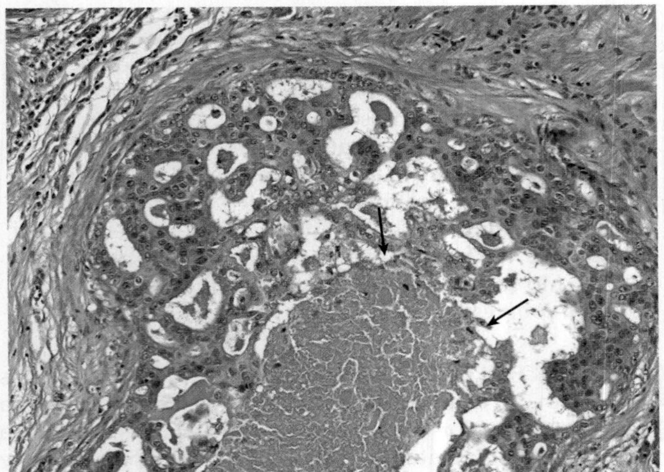

FIGURE 19-18. Ductal carcinoma in situ (DCIS) with comedo necrosis. Intraductal carcinoma with a cribriform architecture and central comedo necrosis (*arrows*).

- **Low-grade DCIS:** At the other end of the histologic spectrum, in low-grade DCIS cells are uniform, small and evenly spaced, with round, regular hyperchromatic nuclei (Fig. 19-19). Mitoses are infrequent. Micropapillary or cribriform growth is the rule, and solid growth patterns are less common.
- **Intermediate-grade DCIS:** Intermediate-grade DCIS falls between high- and low-grade DCIS. Cells show moderate pleomorphism, but maintain some degree of polarization. Solid or cribriform growth is typical.
- **Microinvasive carcinoma:** This pattern is defined as one or more foci of invasive carcinoma, none of which exceed 1 mm in diameter. ***This typically occurs in the setting of high-grade DCIS.***

Immunohistochemistry may occasionally be required to aid in the diagnosis of DCIS. DCIS is distinguished from epithelial hyperplasia of usual type because DCIS lacks high–molecular-weight cytokeratin staining. However, some high-grade DCIS may stain positively for "basal," high–molecular-weight cytokeratins. Stains for myoepithelial cell markers (smooth muscle myosin heavy chain, calponin, p63, etc.) will confirm that the lesion is in situ and help in cases with foci suspicious for microinvasion.

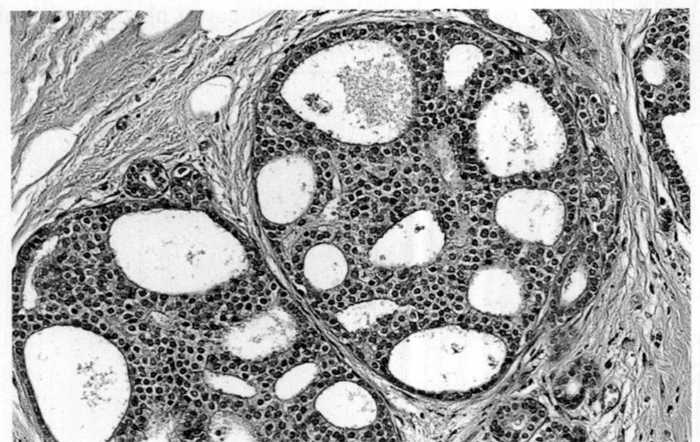

FIGURE 19-19. Ductal carcinoma in situ noncomedo type. A cribriform arrangement of tumor cells is evident.

Low- and intermediate-grade DCIS typically show strong diffuse staining with ER. High-grade lesions will show less frequent ER staining but often overexpress HER2 (50% to 60% of cases). This frequency is greater than what is seen in invasive carcinoma.

CLINICAL FEATURES: DCIS is most commonly detected on mammography as calcifications. A small proportion of women will, however, present symptomatically with a mass lesion or with Paget disease of the nipple (see below).

DCIS is treated by surgical excision. Breast-conserving surgery is possible in many cases and adjuvant radiation reduces the risk of recurrence. When tumors recur, they do so at the site of the previous surgery, and will be invasive carcinoma 50% of the time. Lymph node metastases occur in less than 1% of patients with DCIS. In those cases, foci of invasion were probably missed when examining the primary tumors.

Prospective clinical trials show that antihormone therapy reduces the risk of recurrence or progression for DCIS tumors that express estrogen or progesterone receptors. In all, the critical prognostic factors for patients with DCIS include lesion size, histopathologic subtype and grade, completeness of excision and hormone receptor status. Treatment for each patient is based on careful assessment of each of these factors.

Encapsulated Papillary Carcinoma

Encapsulated papillary carcinoma has been proposed to cover lesions previously called intracystic or encysted papillary carcinoma. Immunohistochemical studies have shown no myoepithelial cells at the periphery of these tumors. The true nature of these lesions (i.e., whether they are truly in situ or, perhaps, invasive) is unclear. These tumors behave indolently and metastases are rare.

Grossly, a well-circumscribed partially cystic, frequently hemorrhagic, solid mass is seen. Microscopically, there is a cystically dilated duct within which fibrovascular cores are lined by one or more layers of malignant epithelial cells with no intervening myoepithelial cell layer (Fig. 19-20). At its edge, the tumor has a smooth pushing border without evidence of stromal invasion.

Paget Disease

Paget disease of the nipple refers to the presence of malignant glandular epithelial cells within the epidermis of the nipple and areola. It is invariably associated with underlying DCIS, with or without an associated invasive ductal carcinoma. Paget disease is rare, occurring in approximately 1% to 4% of breast cancers.

Paget disease presents as erythema or an eczematous change to the nipple and areola (Fig. 19-21). Nipple retraction may be found. Just over half of patients have an associated palpable mass.

Microscopically, malignant glandular epithelial cells are seen within the epidermis, singly or in small groups (Fig. 19-21B). They are large with abundant cytoplasm and pleomorphic nuclei with prominent nucleoli. Mucin globules are seen in the cytoplasm of the glandular cells using special stains.

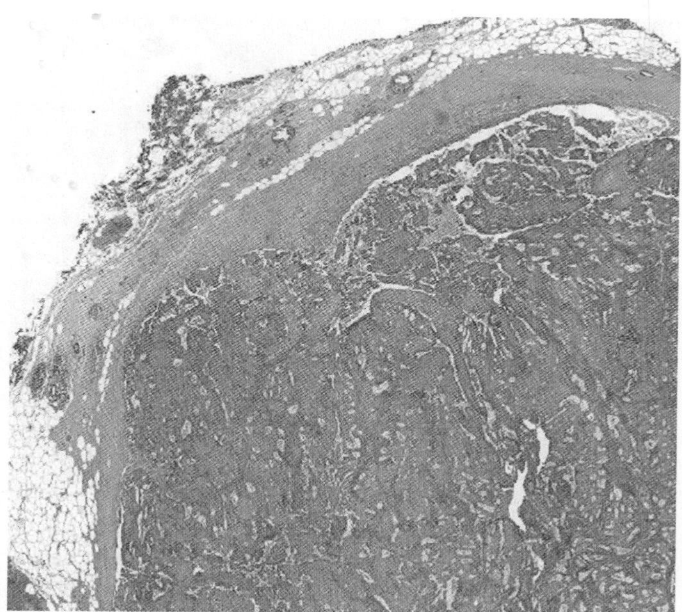

FIGURE 19-20. Encapsulated papillary carcinoma. Fibrovascular cores lined by malignant epithelial cells, without an intervening myoepithelial cell layer, fill the intraductal space. The edge of the tumor has a pushing front, without evidence of stromal invasion.

These cells express epithelial membrane antigen (EMA) and low–molecular-weight cytokeratins. These almost always show HER2 overexpression. The presence of Paget disease does not affect tumor stage: prognosis is a function of the stage of the underlying breast cancer.

Lobular Carcinoma In Situ

LCIS was first described by Foote and Stewart in 1941. The term lobular neoplasia (LN), introduced since then, encompasses ALH and LCIS. These entities are all atypical proliferations of loosely cohesive epithelial cells, but each of these entities entails significant differences in the relative risk of developing breast cancer.

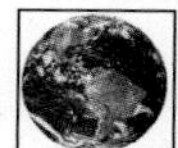

EPIDEMIOLOGY: LCIS is generally asymptomatic and so its true incidence is unknown. The estimated incidence is 1% to 3.8%. It is bilateral in up to 30% of patients and multicentric in up to 85% of patients. ALH and LCIS are more often felt to behave as risk factors than as direct precursors for breast cancer, since the cancers that develop are typically not at the same site as the LCIS, and may occur in the contralateral breast. The relative risk of subsequent cancer ranges from 3 to 5.5 times for ALH and 7 to 10 times for LCIS. For LCIS, this means an absolute risk of 1% to 2% per year, with a lifetime risk of 30% to 40%. A disproportionately high number of these will be invasive lobular carcinoma. Furthermore, coexistent LCIS and invasive lobular carcinomas often show the same genetic changes, suggesting that at least some LCIS are precursors to invasive carcinoma.

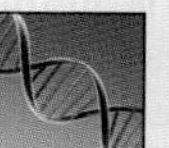

MOLECULAR PATHOGENESIS: CGH and LOH studies have shown loss of 16p, 16q, 17p and 22q and gains of 1q and 6q in both ALH and LCIS. These studies have identified recurrent 16q22.1 loss in LCIS, ALH and invasive lobular carcinoma, for which the target gene is *CDH1*. This gene encodes E-cadherin, a protein that plays an essential role in cell adhesion and in cell cycle regulation through the β-catenin/Wnt pathway. The *CDH1*

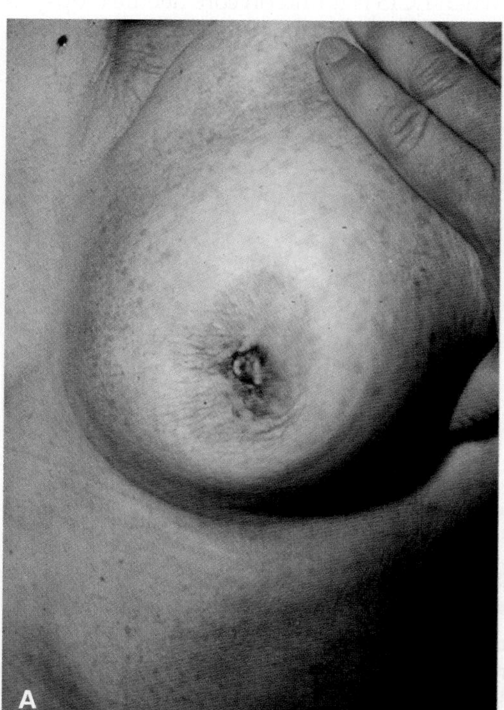

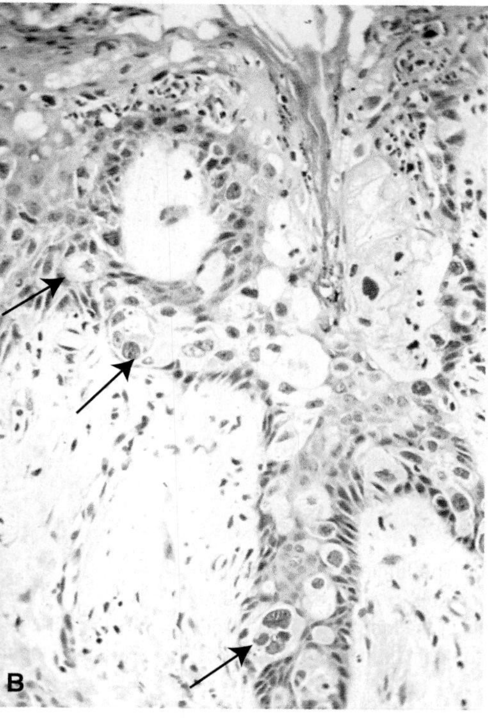

FIGURE 19-21. Paget disease of the nipple. A. An erythematous, scaly, and weeping "eczema" involves the nipple. **B**. The epidermis contains clusters of ductal-type carcinoma cells that are larger and have more abundant pale cytoplasm (*arrows*) than surrounding keratinocytes.

gene may be inactivated via various mechanisms including physical loss of chromosomal regions, missense mutations or gene promoter methylation. Patients with germline mutations in *CDH1* are at a high risk of developing lobular breast carcinoma and gastric signet ring cell carcinoma.

Array CGH has shown that paired LCIS and invasive lobular carcinomas share common genetic gains and losses, suggesting that LCIS is a precursor for invasive lobular carcinoma as well as being a risk factor. Additional other genetic events must precede tumor invasion.

LOH at 16q22.1 is also found in pleomorphic variants, supporting the view that it is biologically closely related to classic LCIS. Some cases of pleomorphic LCIS also show LOH at the p53, HER2 and *BRCA1* loci.

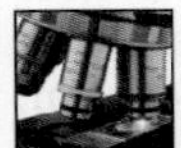

PATHOLOGY: LCIS is not detected mammographically, but associated calcifications may be due to residual nonneoplastic luminal epithelial cells. In the rare **pleomorphic variant,** dystrophic calcification with central necrosis is seen and is detectable on mammography.

A gross lesion is not seen. Microscopically, the cells are monotonous and small with round regular nuclei and minute nucleoli, although larger cells with conspicuous nucleoli may dominate (Fig. 19-22). Cytoplasmic mucin vacuoles may be surrounded by a distinct halo. Unlike DCIS, cells of LCIS do not form complex patterns, but rather solid clusters that pack and distend lobular acini. The growth pattern is loosely cohesive or dyshesive, with gaps between individual cells representing loss of cell–cell adhesion (see above). Pagetoid spread of lobular neoplastic cells is common in LCIS where the cells track along beneath the native luminal epithelial cells of the duct.

ALH and LCIS are differentiated by the degree of filling and distention of acini. In LCIS at least 50% of acini in a lobular unit are involved. Anything less is ALH.

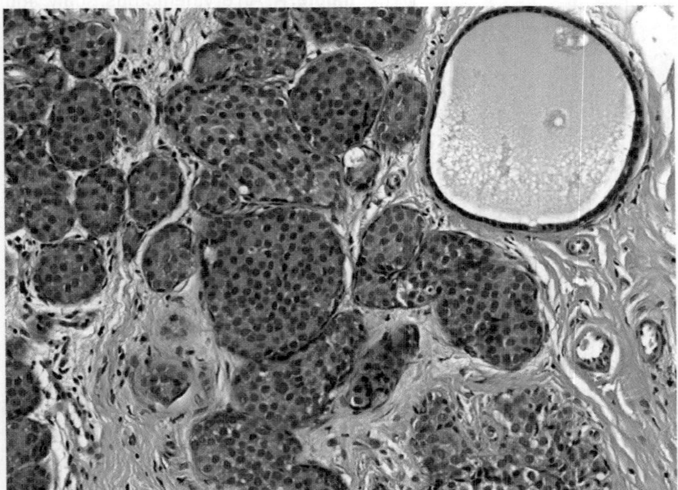

FIGURE 19-22. Lobular carcinoma in situ. The lumina of the terminal duct lobular units are distended by tumor cells, which exhibit round nuclei and small nucleoli. The cancer cells in the lobular form of carcinoma in situ are smaller and have less cytoplasm than those in the ductal type.

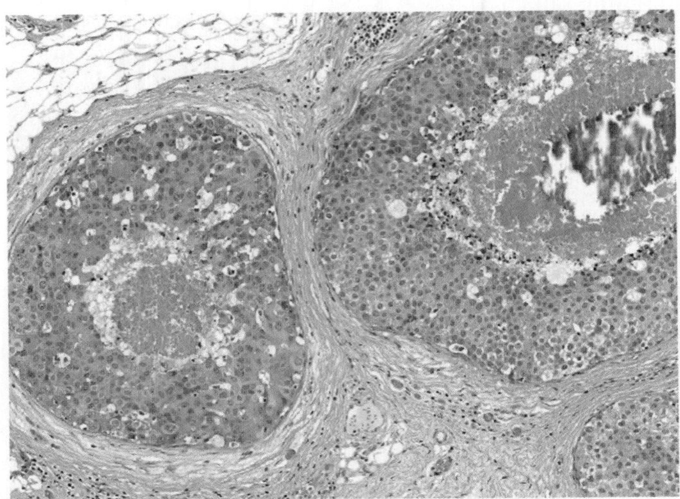

FIGURE 19-23. Pleomorphic lobular carcinoma in situ (PLCIS). A dyshesive population of markedly atypical epithelial cells with central comedo necrosis fill and distend the ducts. Dissociation of the neoplastic cells gives rise to spaces that may be misinterpreted as secondary spaces. E-cadherin expression was absent.

The pleomorphic variant shows moderate to marked variation in nuclear size and shape and nuclear hyperchromasia. Nucleoli and mitotic figures are variably prominent (Fig. 19-23). There is typically central comedo necrosis, often with microcalcifications, a feature rarely found in classic LCIS.

Distinguishing LCIS from low-grade solid DCIS is difficult. In such cases, immunohistochemistry can demonstrate the absence of staining for E-cadherin in LCIS and ALH (Fig. 19-24). Membranous staining is preserved in DCIS.

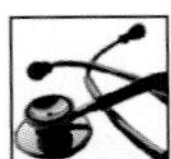

CLINICAL FEATURES: The management of a patient when LCIS is found on core needle biopsy is controversial. If classic LCIS is seen on excision

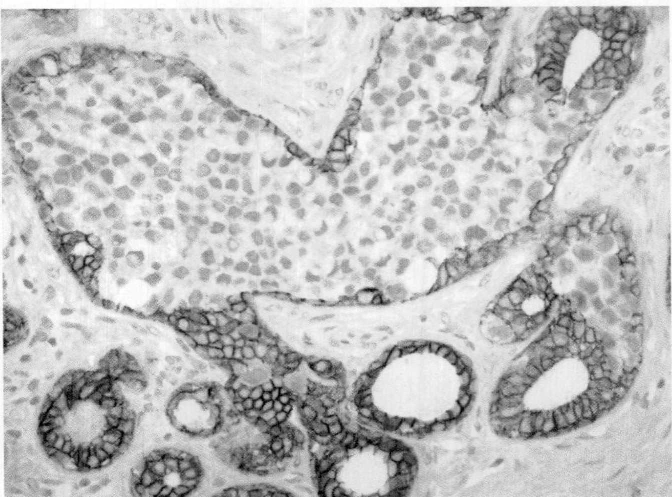

FIGURE 19-24. E-cadherin in lobular carcinoma in situ (LCIS). Membranous E-cadherin expression is seen in residual luminal epithelial cells, but the lobular neoplastic cells should show loss of staining.

biopsy, it is generally agreed that no further surgical management is required, but adjuvant hormonal therapy may be considered and lifelong follow-up is required. With the pleomorphic variant, surgically clear margins are required and adjuvant radiation therapy should be considered.

Invasive Breast Carcinoma

Invasive breast carcinoma is a malignant epithelial lesion derived from the TDLU. It can occur anywhere in the breast, but is most common in the upper outer quadrant. Patients most commonly present with an ill-defined breast mass that may be adherent to the skin or underlying muscle. Nonpalpable asymptomatic tumors are usually detected by mammography. These mostly appear radiologically as a spiculated mass or architectural distortion, with or without associated microcalcifications.

Current classification systems are based largely on pathologic appearances. Most breast cancers are classified as ductal, no special type (NST), and the remainder are special types or mixed morphologies.

Invasive Ductal Carcinoma, No Special Type

The proportion of invasive breast cancers in this category varies from 47% to 70%, with women younger than 35 years having this tumor type more than older patients. An irregular, dense mass is seen on mammography or ultrasound (Fig. 19-25A). Grossly, the tumor is moderately well defined or ill-defined, nodular or stellate, with a firm to hard cut surface (Fig. 19-25B). Microscopically, tumor cells form trabeculae, sheets, nests and glands (Fig. 19-25C). Nuclear pleomorphism and mitotic counts vary. The surrounding stroma ranges from desmoplastic to collagenous; higher-grade tumors may show tumor necrosis. Special histologic components may be present. If a special-type component represents greater than 50% of the tumor, the tumor is considered mixed (i.e., ductal with special-type features).

Most tumors (70% to 80%) are ER positive and 15% to 20% are HER2 positive. Overall, these tumors are associated with a 35% to 50% 10-year survival, depending on the status of traditional prognostic features including grade, tumor and lymph node stage and the presence of lymphovascular invasion.

Invasive Lobular Carcinoma

Invasive lobular carcinoma is the second most common form of invasive breast cancer, representing 5% to 15% of all invasive carcinomas. Stromal desmoplasia and fibrosis may be minimal, so patients often present with a poorly defined thickening of the breast or have clinically silent disease, often with subtle or absent mammographic features. Some studies report that multicentricity and bilaterality are more common, while others suggest that risk to be similar to that seen with ductal, NST cancers (i.e., 5% to 10%).

Tumors may be discrete firm masses or be poorly defined, making accurate gross measurement difficult. Lobular cancers characteristically show a dishesive population of malignant epithelial cells diffusely infiltrating the stroma, often without desmoplasia (Fig. 19-26). Cells frequently line up in single file, and may show a periductal "targetoid" arrangement. They do not form ducts, but may form solid sheets, trabeculae or nests. Cells typically contain intracytoplasmic lumina, with eccentrically placed nuclei, and are similar in appearance to those seen in LCIS.

Invasive lobular carcinomas are more often ER positive than ductal NST, although high-grade lobular cancers may lack ER or show HER2 positivity. E-cadherin is usually low or absent, reflecting biallelic loss of the CDH1 tumor-suppressor gene, which codes for E-cadherin. Lobular cancers often show increased copies of 1q and loss of 16q.

Lobular carcinoma shows a particular pattern of metastases with a tendency to spread to the peritoneum, retroperitoneum, ovary and uterus, leptomeninges and gastrointestinal tract. Matched for grade and stage, lobular carcinoma has a similar prognosis, in terms of disease-free and overall survival, to that of ductal, NST cancers.

Tubular Carcinoma

Tubular carcinoma is rare, representing 1% to 2% of invasive breast cancers. Mammography detects this tumor disproportionately frequently. Grossly, a well-defined stellate mass is

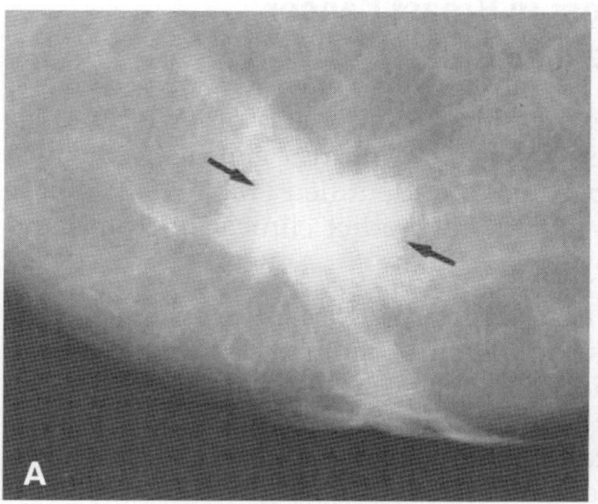

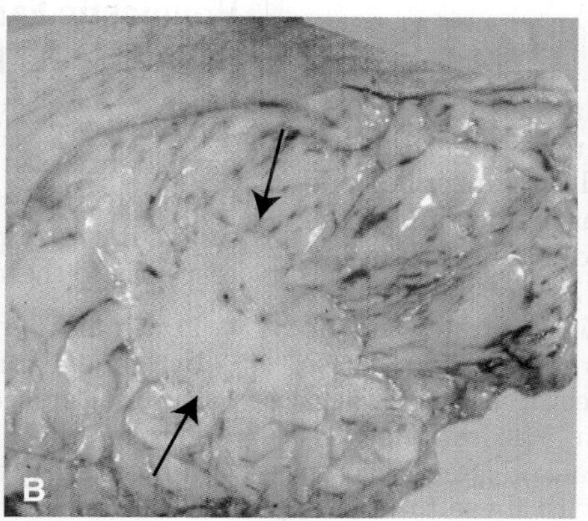

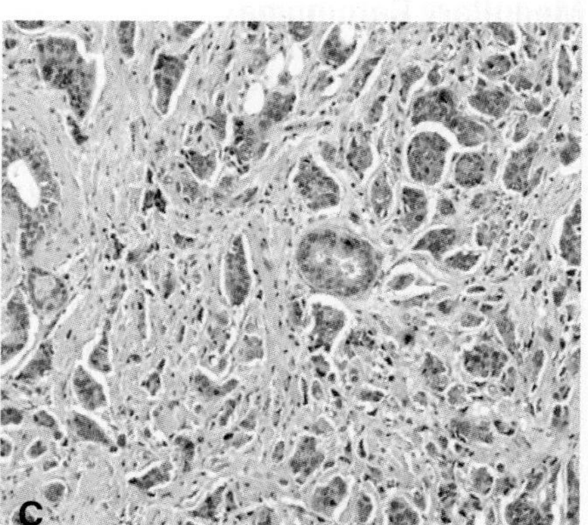

FIGURE 19-25. Carcinoma of the breast. A. Mammogram. An irregularly shaped, dense mass (*arrows*) is seen in this otherwise fatty breast. **B.** Mastectomy specimen. The irregular white, firm mass in the center is surrounded by fatty tissue. **C.** Photomicrograph showing irregular cords and nests of invasive ductal carcinoma cells invading stroma.

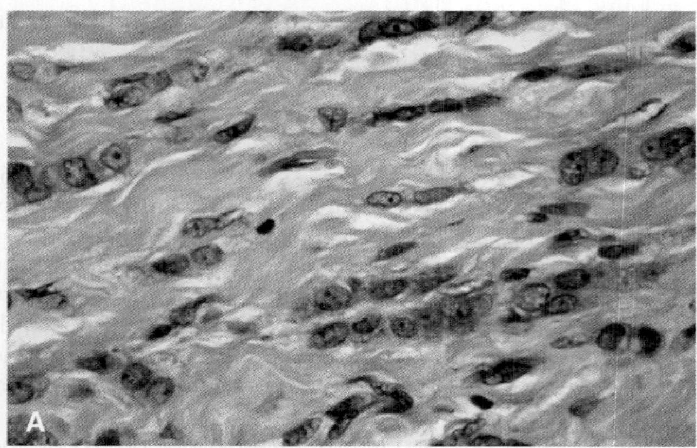

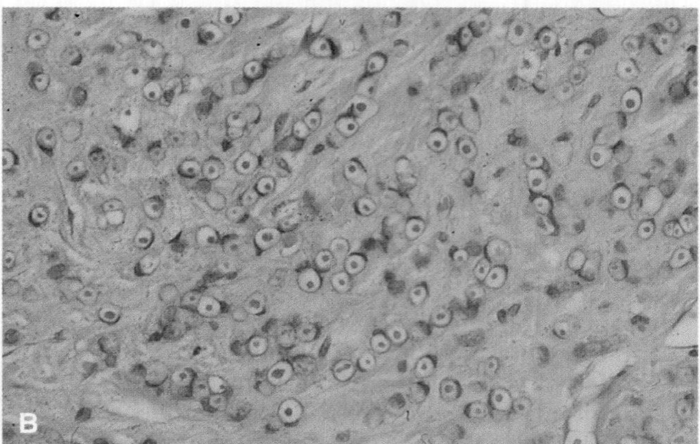

FIGURE 19-26. Lobular carcinoma. A. Invasive lobular carcinoma. In contrast to invasive ductal carcinoma, the cells of lobular carcinoma tend to form single strands that invade between collagen fibers in a single pattern. The tumor cells are similar to those seen in lobular carcinoma in situ. **B. Signet ring carcinoma.** The tumor cells contain large amounts of clear mucin.

seen. Microscopically, the tumor is composed almost entirely of open and angulated tubules lined by a single layer of mildly pleomorphic epithelial cells, often with prominent apical snouts (Fig. 19-27A). Over 95% of tubular carcinomas are ER positive and HER2 negative. Loss of 16q and gain of 1q are frequent. Lymph node metastases are rare, and patients with tubular carcinomas have an excellent prognosis.

Mucinous Carcinoma

Patients with mucinous carcinoma are typically older than those with other tumor types. This tumor makes up less than 1% to 6% of breast cancers, depending on criteria used for diagnosis. Grossly, they are well circumscribed, with a gelatinous texture. Low-grade malignant epithelial cells form acini, nests or trabeculae, which appear to float in pools of extracellular mucin (Fig. 19-27B). Direct stromal invasion by malignant epithelial cells is absent. Almost all mucinous carcinomas are ER positive and HER2 negative. Patients with pure mucinous carcinoma, strictly diagnosed, have an excellent prognosis.

Medullary Carcinoma

Medullary carcinomas are exceptionally rare, but are represented disproportionately in patients with germline *BRCA1* mutations. Almost half of all patients are younger than 50 years of age. These tumors are grossly well circumscribed and soft. Histologically, medullary carcinomas include all the following: grade 2 to 3 nuclei; circumscribed, pushing margins; syncytial growth pattern in greater than 75% of the tumor; a moderate or marked lymphoplasmacytic infiltrate; and no tubule formation (Fig. 19-27C). DCIS is uncommon. These tumors are typically ER, PR and HER2 negative ("triple negative"). p53 overexpression is common. The prognosis is uncertain as different diagnostic criteria are often used in making this diagnosis. The prognosis with these tumors is better than that for high-grade ductal, NST tumors. Lymph node metastases occur less frequently with medullary carcinoma. Most women who die from their disease do so within 5 years of diagnosis.

Micropapillary Carcinoma

Pure micropapillary carcinoma occurs rarely but is more frequently seen admixed with ductal, NST carcinoma. As these tumors show a high frequency of lymphovascular invasion and lymph node metastases, recognizing even a minor component of micropapillary carcinoma is important. Microscopically, malignant epithelial nests or acini are surrounded by a clear space (Fig. 19-27D). Lymph node metastases are very common with these tumors. However, overall prognosis of micropapillary carcinomas is similar to that of other tumor types.

Metaplastic Carcinoma

Metaplastic carcinomas are a heterogeneous group of tumors with malignant spindle cells, squamous cell carcinoma or heterologous elements such as bone or cartilage (Fig. 19-27E). Adenocarcinoma may not be present, but cytokeratin immunostains are at least focally present. These tumors typically cluster with the basal molecular subgroup on gene expression profiling (see below). Tumors are usually ER and HER2 negative.

Prognostic Factors in Breast Cancer Remain to Be Defined Clearly

Microarray gene expression profiling and other techniques have identified a set of genes, an "intrinsic gene list," of which five molecular subgroups are identified (Table 19-2). These molecular groups appear to predict clinical outcome and response to therapy.

- **Luminal A:** The luminal groups (A and B) are characterized by gene expression patterns similar to normal breast luminal epithelial cells, including low–molecular-weight cytokeratins 8/18, ER and ER-associated genes. Luminal A tumors are typically low grade with an excellent prognosis.
- **Luminal B** tumors are usually higher grade than luminal A tumors, exhibit higher proliferative indices and have a poorer prognosis.
- **HER2:** The HER2 group of tumors overexpress HER2 and genes associated with the HER2 pathway and with

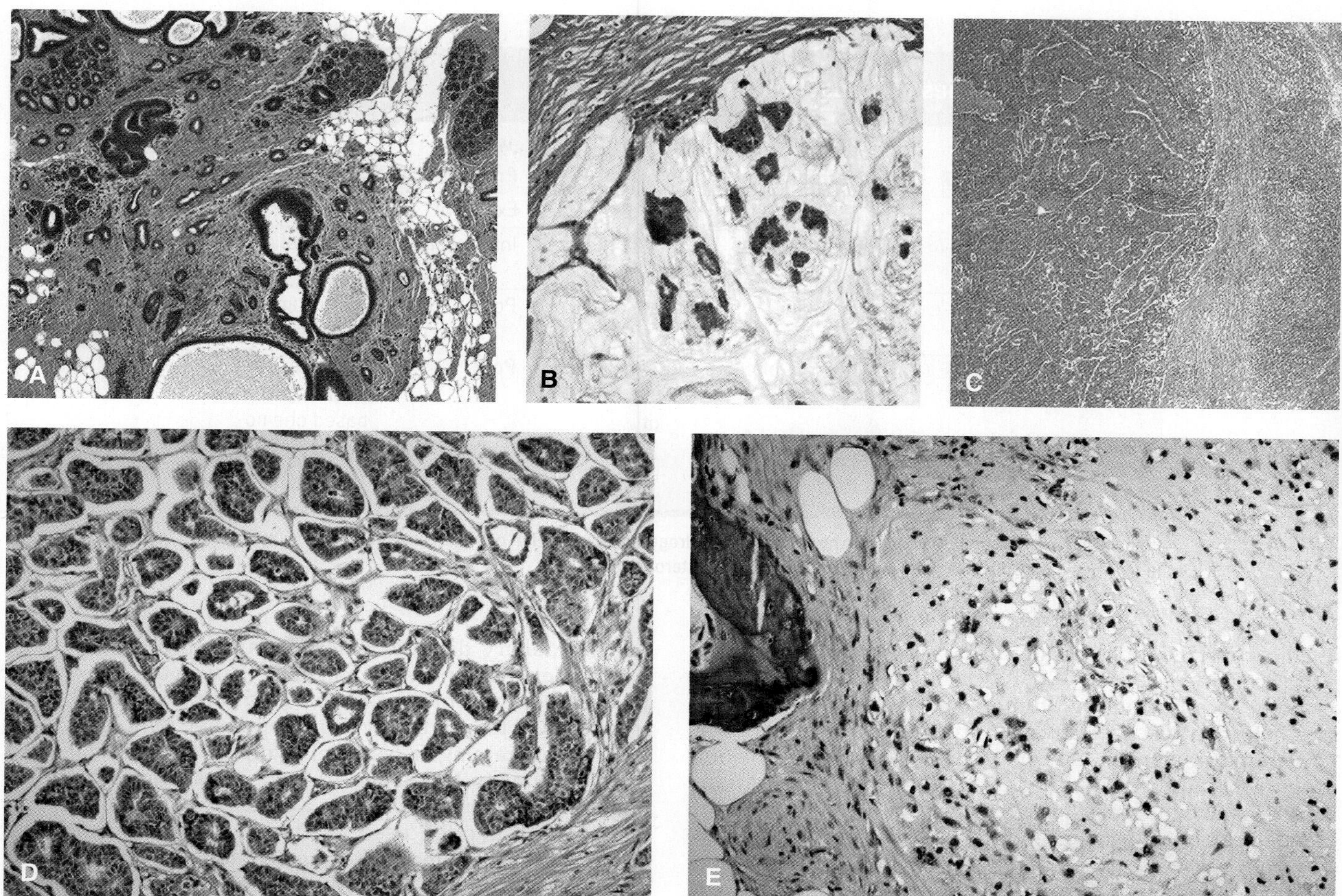

FIGURE 19-27. Patterns of breast carcinoma. A. Tubular carcinoma. Open and angulated malignant glands are dispersed between normal lobules and show extension into fat. A single layer of epithelium lines the tubules and myoepithelial cells are absent. **B. Colloid (mucinous) carcinoma.** Clusters of malignant cells float in large pools of extracellular mucin. **C. Medullary carcinoma.** The malignant cells are pleomorphic and grow in solid sheets, forming a blunt margin. There is no gland formation. Numerous mitoses are present. The tumor is surrounded by a dense lymphocytic infiltrate. **D. Micropapillary carcinoma.** Sponge-like pattern of empty spaces containing glands and small clusters of malignant epithelium. Focal serration of the outer borders of the glands is seen. **E. Metaplastic carcinoma.** Cartilaginous and osseus matrix in a metaplastic carcinoma with heterologous elements. Elsewhere, foci of poorly differentiated adenocarcinoma were seen.

ER negativity. These tumors behave aggressively, but targeting HER2 with the humanized monoclonal antibody trastuzumab has dramatically improved the course of these tumors.

- **Basal-like cancers:** These highly aggressive tumors constitute 10% to 20% of invasive breast carcinomas. They are mainly ER and HER2 negative. Their name derives from their consistent expression of genes in the basal or myoepithelial cells of the breast, including high–molecular-weight cytokeratins 5/6, 14 and 17; caveolins 1 and 2; nestin; p63; and epidermal growth factor receptor (EGFR). These tumors are distinctive, with high nuclear grade, many mitoses, pushing margins, central areas of necrosis or fibrosis and a lymphocytic infiltrate. Cancers with medullary features and metaplastic carcinomas are typically basal-like. Most cancers arising in patients with germline BRA1 mutations are basal-like.
- **Normal breast-like cancers:** These are poorly characterized and less reproducible than the other subgroups. Whether thy represent a truly distinctive molecular group or an artifact of gene expression profiling is not clear.

Breast Cancer Staging

Breast cancer survival is strongly influenced by tumor stage. The TNM (tumor [T], regional lymph nodes [N] and distant metastasis [M]) classification used for this purpose depends heavily on pathologic evaluation (Table 19-3). Breast cancer spreads by direct extension (e.g., to chest wall); via lymphatics to axillary, internal mammary and infra- and supraclavicular lymph nodes; and hematogenously to distant sites.

Tumor Size

Tumor size (T in staging protocol) is associated with prognosis: larger tumors correlate with poorer survival. Thus, breast screening programs aim to detect impalpable breast cancers

Table 19-2

Molecular Subtypes of Breast Cancer

Molecular Subgroup	ER	PR	HER2	Proliferation Index	Other	Prognosis	Treatment
Luminal A	+	+	−	Low	CK8/18	Excellent	Hormonal
Luminal B	+	+	−/+	Moderate	CK8/18	Intermediate	Hormonal and chemotherapy
HER2+	−	−	+	High	AR	Poor	Trastuzumab Anthracyclines
Basal	−	−	−	Very high	CK5/6, CK14, vimentin, EGFR, c-kit	Poor	Platinum- and anthracycline-based chemotherapy ?PARP inhibitors

+positive; −negative; −/+ sometimes positive; AR = androgen receptor; ER = estrogen receptor; PARP = poly (adenosine diphosphate-ribose) polymerase; PR = progesterone receptor.

at an early stage. In assessing tumor size, only the invasive part is considered.

Some locally advanced tumors are staged pT4, based on skin and/or chest wall invasion, regardless of tumor size. "Inflammatory breast cancer" carries a particularly poor prognosis, and features edema, erythema, induration, warmth and tenderness of overlying skin, resulting in an orange peel–like ("peau d'orange") appearance. Arm edema and pain may also occur, probably because of lymphatic obstruction by tumor. The corresponding histologic findings are dermal lymphatic invasion by tumor.

Lymph Node Status

The presence or absence of axillary lymph node metastases is a key prognostic indicator for patients with breast cancer, and requires pathologic evaluation of surgically resected lymph nodes. Axillary dissection risks significant morbidity (i.e., lymphedema and nerve damage). To reduce the risk of such postoperative morbidities, sentinel lymph node (SLN) biopsy is used. SLN biopsy involves intraoperative lymphatic mapping of the draining or "sentinel" lymph node, the node most likely to contain breast cancer metastases. If it is negative, axillary dissection can safely be avoided. Immunohistochemical staining is often used to identify cytokeratin-positive epithelial cells that may not be seen otherwise. Such detailed evaluation of the SLN has improved detection of micrometastases, although the prognostic significance of micrometastases in SLN biopsy is not known.

Table 19-3

Pathologic Tumor Staging

pTis:	Carcinoma in situ (ductal or lobar) or Paget disease without invasive carcinoma
pT1mic:	Microinvasion (≤1 mm)
pT1a:	Invasive tumor >1 mm but ≤5 mm
pT1b:	Invasive tumor >5 mm but ≤1 cm
pT1c:	Invasive tumor >1 cm but ≤2 cm
pT2:	Invasive tumor >2 cm but ≤5 cm
pT3:	Invasive tumor >5 cm
pT4:	Edema or tumor ulcerating through skin or satellite skin nodules and/or chest wall invasion* or inflammatory breast carcinoma

*Does not include invasion of the pectoralis muscle.

Data from Edge SB, Byrd DR, Compton CC, et al., eds. AJCC Cancer Staging Manual, 7th ed. New York: Springer, 2009.

Distant Metastases

Distant metastases portend a poor prognosis. Bone is the most frequently involved, being the site of presentation of metastatic disease in 25% of cases. Of women who die from their disease, 70% eventually develop bone involvement. Smaller percentages of patients develop metastases, usually to lung, liver, central nervous system, skin and adrenal glands.

Tumor Grade

Histopathologic grading of breast tumors is one of the critical components of treatment decision making. The Nottingham grading system, also called the modified Bloom and Richardson method, is most widely used. It combines scores for tubule formation, nuclear pleomorphism and mitotic count into a final grade of 1, 2 or 3, for low-, intermediate- and high-grade carcinomas, respectively (Fig. 19-28). Overall survival is significantly better in patients with grade 1 tumors than those with grade 2 or grade 3 tumors.

Other Prognostic Features

- **Lymphovascular invasion (LVI):** Finding tumor cells within lymphovascular spaces correlates well with lymph node metastases (Fig. 19-29) and is a poor prognostic sign.
- **Proliferative index and ploidy:** Tumors with a high proliferative index have poorer prognoses. Several parameters are used to evaluate proliferation in breast cancers, including

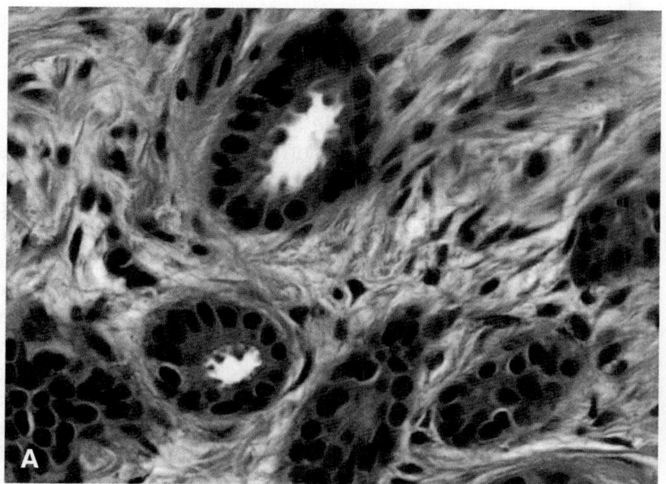

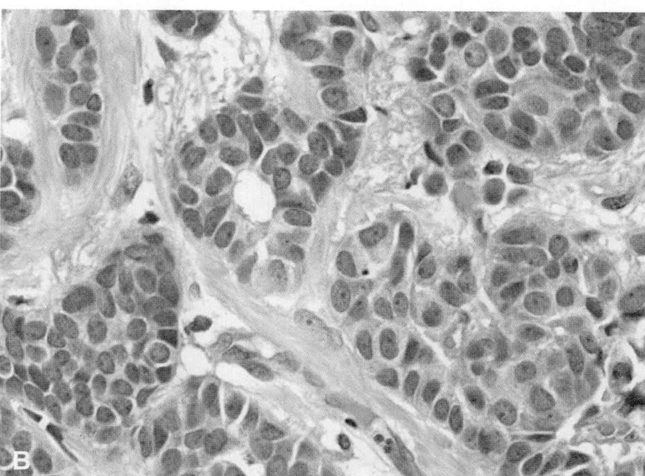

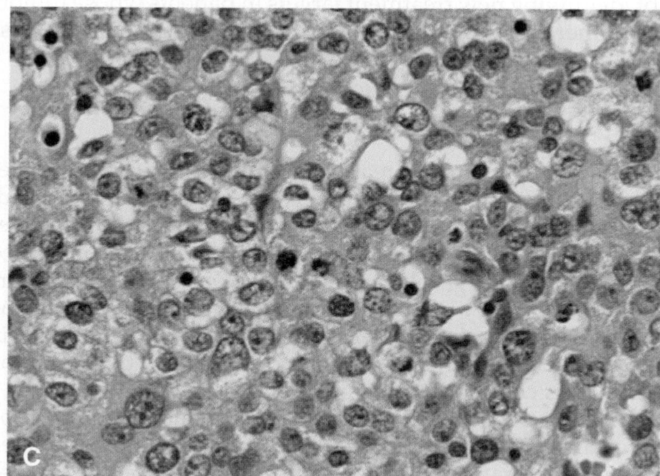

FIGURE 19-28. Tumor histologic grade. A. Low-grade invasive carcinoma showing good tubule formation, mild nuclear pleomorphism and inconspicuous mitoses. **B. Moderately differentiated** carcinoma with less tubule formation, moderate nuclear pleomorphism and variably prominent mitoses. **C. Poorly differentiated** carcinoma showing absent tubule formation, marked nuclear pleomorphism and frequent mitotic figures.

(1) mitotic index, assessed histologically; (2) the proportion of cells in S phase of the cell cycle by flow cytometry; (3) immunohistochemical staining for proteins (Ki67) expressed by actively proliferating cells; and (4) thymidine labeling index. Cell cycle analysis can also detect aneuploidy, which occurs in two thirds of breast cancers and is associated with a poorer prognosis.

- **Response to neoadjuvant therapy:** In patients receiving systemic treatment prior to surgery (neoadjuvant therapy), the degree of response to treatment is a strong prognostic factor: patients who show complete pathologic responses (i.e., who lack pathologic evidence of residual breast or nodal disease) show an excellent long-term survival. Poorly differentiated tumors with high proliferation indices are more likely to respond to neoadjuvant treatment than low-grade cancers.
- **Estrogen and progesterone receptors:** Steroid receptor proteins are expressed by benign breast epithelium and 70% to 80% of breast cancers. ER and PR status is determined by immunohistochemistry that detects nuclear staining by the respective commercially available antibodies (Fig. 19-30). The receptors bind their respective ligands (estrogen and progesterone) and stimulate cell growth. The greatest value of assessing hormone receptor status in breast cancer is for its predictive ability. Patients with ER/PR-negative tumors are unlikely to respond to hormonal therapies with antiestrogens. On the other hand, ER/PR-positive tumors show a greater probability of response.
- **HER2:** Overexpression and/or gene amplification of HER2 is seen in 15% to 20% of newly diagnosed breast cancers.

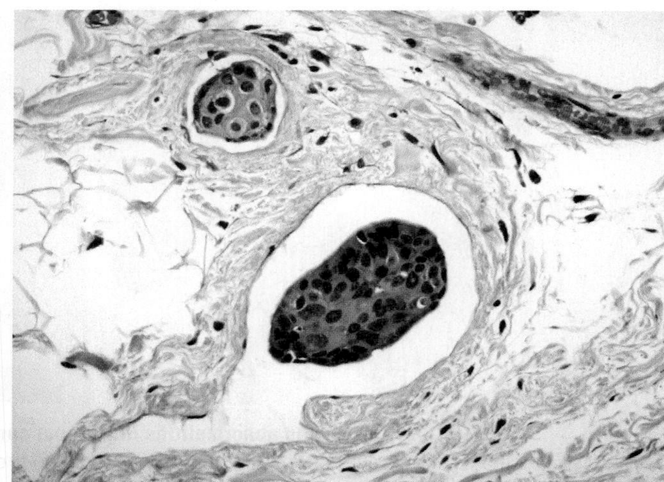

FIGURE 19-29. Lymphovascular invasion. Endothelial cell–lined lymphatic channels containing tumor emboli.

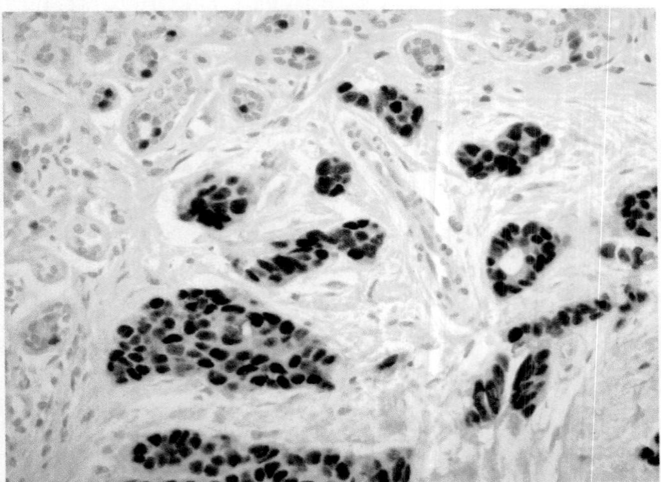

FIGURE 19-30. Estrogen receptor (ER). Strong nuclear positivity for estrogen receptor in this moderately differentiated invasive ductal carcinoma (immunohistochemical stain). Staining in normal breast lobules is seen in the upper left-hand corner.

HER2 positivity is an adverse prognostic factor irrespective of lymph node status. However, these patients may be treated with monoclonal antibodies or tyrosine kinase inhibitors that target HER2. As with hormone receptor status, many patients with HER2 positivity show de novo or eventual resistance to the targeting drugs. HER2 status can be determined either by immunohistochemistry to detect complete membranous expression of the protein or by in situ hybridization to identify gene amplification (Fig. 19-31). The latter is commonly detected using fluorescent probes (fluorescence in situ hybridization) and other newly available approaches.

- **Multigene analysis:** In recent years, gene expression profiling has facilitated decision-making processes and many of these tests are now commercially available. In guiding treatment decisions and evaluating prognosis, these tools complement, but do not replace, histopathology and clinical analyses.

Gene Expression

Newly commercially available approaches quantify mRNA levels for a panel of genes, whether by quantitative reverse transcriptase polymerase chain reaction (Q-RT-PCR) or by microarray analysis. For example, comparison of transcript levels for "cancer-related" genes and control genes provides an index that has been shown to be an independent predictor of risk of developing distant recurrence at 10 years after 5 years of tamoxifen therapy. Similarly, microarray-based multigene assays quantify expression of selected "cancer-related genes," with respect to 1800 reference genes, and helps stratify patients' risk for developing distant metastases at 10 years without adjuvant treatment. Both of these approaches may be useful in identifying patients who would, and would not, benefit from specific therapies. They also offer the hope of identifying new treatment targets in patients whose tumors are either unlikely to respond to treatment or in whom relapse has occurred following treatment.

Management of Breast Cancer

Primary treatment of breast cancer almost always involves surgery. Breast-conserving surgery (i.e., lumpectomy or quadrantectomy) is often used, while more extensive procedures may be needed in patients with bulky disease. As indicated above, sentinel lymph node sampling often replaces more extensive axillary lymph node chain removal, and dissection of axillary lymph nodes is often reserved for patients in whom the SLN is positive for tumor. Postoperative radiation therapy is commonly used as well.

Systemic therapies in the form of hormonal, chemotherapy and targeted molecular modalities are also often considered essential in managing patients with breast cancer. In general, patients with the greatest risk of mortality gain the most from such systemic therapies. Targeted therapies rely on the presence of a particular target in the tumor. Thus, for example, ER, PR and HER2 status is determined in all invasive breast cancers to see if hormonal or anti-HER2 therapy should be considered.

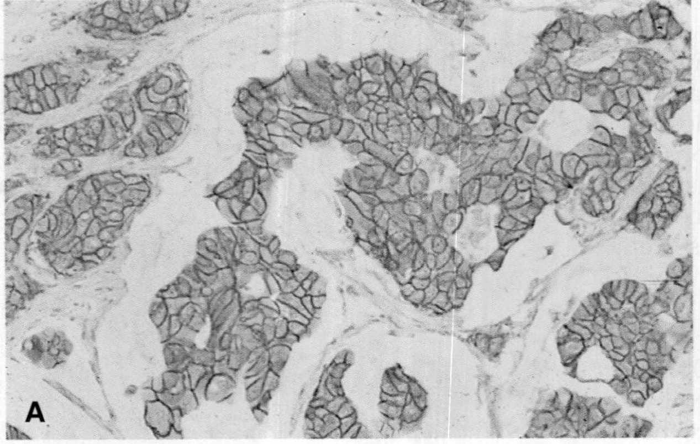

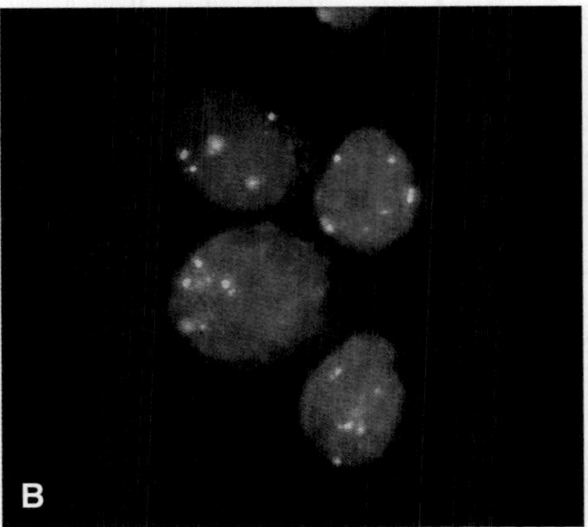

FIGURE 19-31. HER2/neu abnormalities in a breast cancer. A. Immunoperoxide staining of an invasive ductal carcinoma shows overexpression of the *HER2* (erbB-2) protein. **B.** Fluorescence in situ hybridization (FISH) methodology identifies the gene copies of *HER2* (erbB-2) in cancer cells. The *HER2* probe is red, and a normal cell should have two copies. More than two copies indicates *HER2* gene amplification. The green probe identifies the centromeric region of chromosome 17.

Emerging Therapeutic Targets

Other members of the HER tyrosine kinase family are implicated in tumor growth signaling and cross-talk and may mediate trastuzumab resistance mechanisms: HER1, 3 and 4 are activated by a variety of ligands to stimulate growth, migration and antiapoptotic pathways. Combination therapies or multitarget drugs that target multiple pathways simultaneously may reduce resistance to therapy.

Other potential therapeutic targets include TOP2A, which encodes topoisomerase IIα, the direct molecular target of anthracycline antitumor drugs. Its coamplification with HER2 is predictive of response to anthracycline-based chemotherapy. Agents that target vascular endothelial growth factor (VEGF) ligand or receptor have been developed and are currently in clinical trials. These drugs target tumor angiogenesis to inhibit new blood vessels and so limit tumor progression and metastases.

The Male Breast

Gynecomastia Is Enlargement of the Male Breast

Male breast tissue has receptors for androgens, estrogens and progesterone. Estrogen stimulates duct development and progesterone stimulates lobular development in the presence of luteinizing hormone, follicle-stimulating hormone and growth hormone. Androgens antagonize the effects of estrogen. Testosterone can be converted to estradiol by the enzyme aromatase, found especially in adipose tissue.

Physiologic gynecomastia occurs in most neonates, secondary to circulating maternal and placental estrogen and progesterone. Transient gynecomastia also affects over half of all boys during puberty because estrogen production peaks earlier than that of testosterone. With increasing age, a decline in free testosterone and increase in obesity leads to an increase in the prevalence of breast enlargement.

Gynecomastia is benign enlargement of the male breast due to a relative decrease in androgen effect or increase in estrogen effect. Breast enlargement due to adipose tissue is called **pseudogynecomastia.** Nonphysiologic gynecomastia results from drugs or disorders associated with low testosterone levels, high conversion of testosterone to estrogens, high estrogen levels and high sex hormone–binding globulin levels resulting in low free testosterone. It may occur in patients with hyperthyroidism, cirrhosis, renal failure, chronic lung disease and certain hormone-producing tumors including Leydig and Sertoli cell tumors, testicular germ cell tumors and tumors of the liver and lung. Drugs implicated in gynecomastia include digitalis, cimetidine, spironolactone, marijuana and tricyclic antidepressants.

Grossly, a rubbery discrete mass or ill-defined area of induration is seen, which may display either a florid or fibrous phase (Fig. 19-32). The florid phase typically occurs within 6 months of onset, and is characterized by epithelial hyperplasia with a flat or micropapillary architecture. Periductal stroma is hypercellular with edema, increased vascularity and chronic inflammation. The fibrous phase is seen after 1 year or more. Here, epithelial proliferation is usually absent and the stroma is more collagenous. Mixtures of both phases may be seen. Pseudoangiomatous stromal hyperplasia may be seen in either phase.

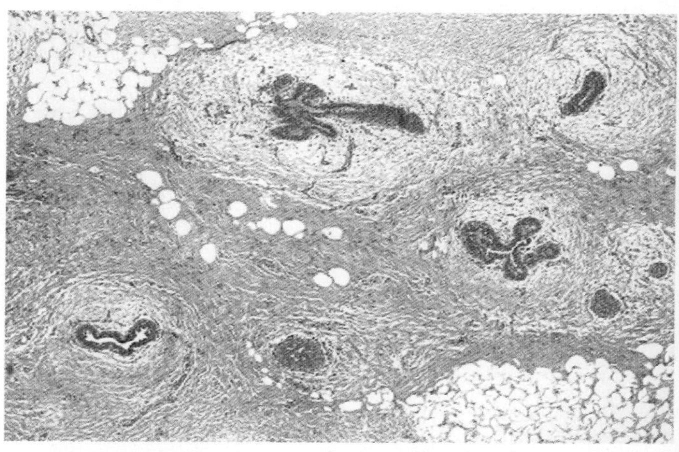

FIGURE 19-32. Gynecomastia. There is proliferation of branching, intermediate-sized ducts. The ductal epithelium is hyperplastic, and mitoses are present. A concomitant increase in the surrounding fibrous tissue causes a palpable mass.

Carcinoma of the Male Breast

Male breast cancers make up 1% of breast cancers in the United States, but 7% to 14% in sub-Saharan Africa. The higher rates may reflect endemic infectious diseases causing liver damage, leading to hyperestrogenism. In the United States, the rates are highest in black men, intermediate in non-Hispanic white men and Asian-Pacific Islanders and lowest in Hispanic men. The mean age at presentation is 65 years.

The risk of breast cancer is greater in high-estrogen states. Men with Klinefelter syndrome have an astonishing 58-fold higher risk than normal, with an absolute risk of up to 3%. Male–female transsexuals following castration and high-dose estrogen, and men treated with estrogen for prostate cancer, also are at greater risk. Men with inherited germline mutations in *BRCA2* show a cumulative risk of 7% of breast cancer by age 80 years. The risk in male *BRCA1* carriers is much less. Ionizing radiation is also implicated, being seen in Japanese men after the nuclear fallout and in patients treated with therapeutic chest irradiation at a young age.

Most patients present with a painless lump. Nipple involvement, including retraction, discharge or ulceration, is an early event. Paget disease is a presenting feature in just 1% of affected individuals. Delay in diagnosis may result in advanced disease at presentation.

Most male breast cancers are ductal, NST; however, papillary carcinoma is disproportionately represented in men, representing a higher proportion of cancers than that seen in women. Lobular carcinoma is rare. Ninety percent of cancers are ER and PR positive. Androgen receptor positivity is frequently seen.

Management of men with breast cancer largely reflects results of clinical studies done in women: simple mastectomy and sentinel lymph node biopsy and/or axillary dissection. Postoperative radiation may be given for large tumors or for close margins. Hormonal therapy with tamoxifen is frequently administered. Experience with the treatment of male breast cancer with aromatase inhibitors is limited. Adjuvant chemotherapy with or without trastuzumab may be indicated, depending on the aggressiveness of the disease and HER2 status, respectively.

20 Hematopathology

Riccardo Valdez • Mary Zutter • Alina Dulau Florea • Raphael Rubin

BONE AND NORMAL MYELOPOIETIC CELLS

Embryology

The origin of the hematopoietic stem cell is controversial, but it likely arises in the mesoderm of the intraembryonic aorta/gonad mesonephros region and/or the yolk sac itself. Blood cell formation shifts from the yolk sac to the fetal liver around the third month of embryogenesis. Hematopoietic stem cells and erythroid precursors comprise most of the hematopoietic tissue during the early stages of blood cell formation in the fetal liver, but production of megakaryocytes and mature neutrophils soon follows. A switch from the production of red blood cell embryonic hemoglobins to fetal hemoglobins also occurs during the hepatic phase of erythropoiesis.

Hematopoietic stem cells migrate from the liver to the bone marrow around the fourth month of embryogenesis, and by the 26th week of intrauterine life, the bone marrow becomes the primary site of hematopoiesis. At birth, blood cell formation in the liver virtually ceases, and bone marrow hematopoiesis becomes fully established.

From birth to puberty, all skeletal bone cavities are densely packed with hematopoietic tissue (red marrow), which is capable of producing all blood cell types—erythroid, myeloid and lymphoid. Red marrow is subsequently largely confined to the proximal epiphyseal regions of the humeri and femurs and the flat bones (skull, scapula, clavicles, sternum, ribs, vertebrae and pelvis). In the adult, adipose tissue occupies most of the available space within the medullary cavities of the skeleton, resulting in inactive "yellow marrow." The bone marrow in the axial skeleton continues to be active until old age, when resorption of cancellous bone enlarges the marrow cavities and leads to further fatty replacement. Remarkably, peripheral blood counts are maintained normally even with declining amounts of red marrow.

Local expansion of red (cellular) marrow and reactivation of peripheral yellow marrow allow the hematopoietic system to meet physiologic demands for increased blood cell formation. Reactivation of hepatic and splenic hematopoiesis rarely occurs during adult life. ***The finding of significant extramedullary hematopoiesis in adulthood usually suggests a clonal (malignant) disorder, rather than a reactive process.***

Bone Marrow

Hematopoietic Cells Derive From Multipotent Stem Cells

Bone marrow consists of a complex network of solid cords separated by sinusoids (Fig. 20-1). The cords are composed of stromal and hematopoietic cells, knitted together by extracellular matrix. The semipermeable barrier between sinusoids and cords consists of an endothelial cell layer, a thin basement membrane and an outer layer of interrupted

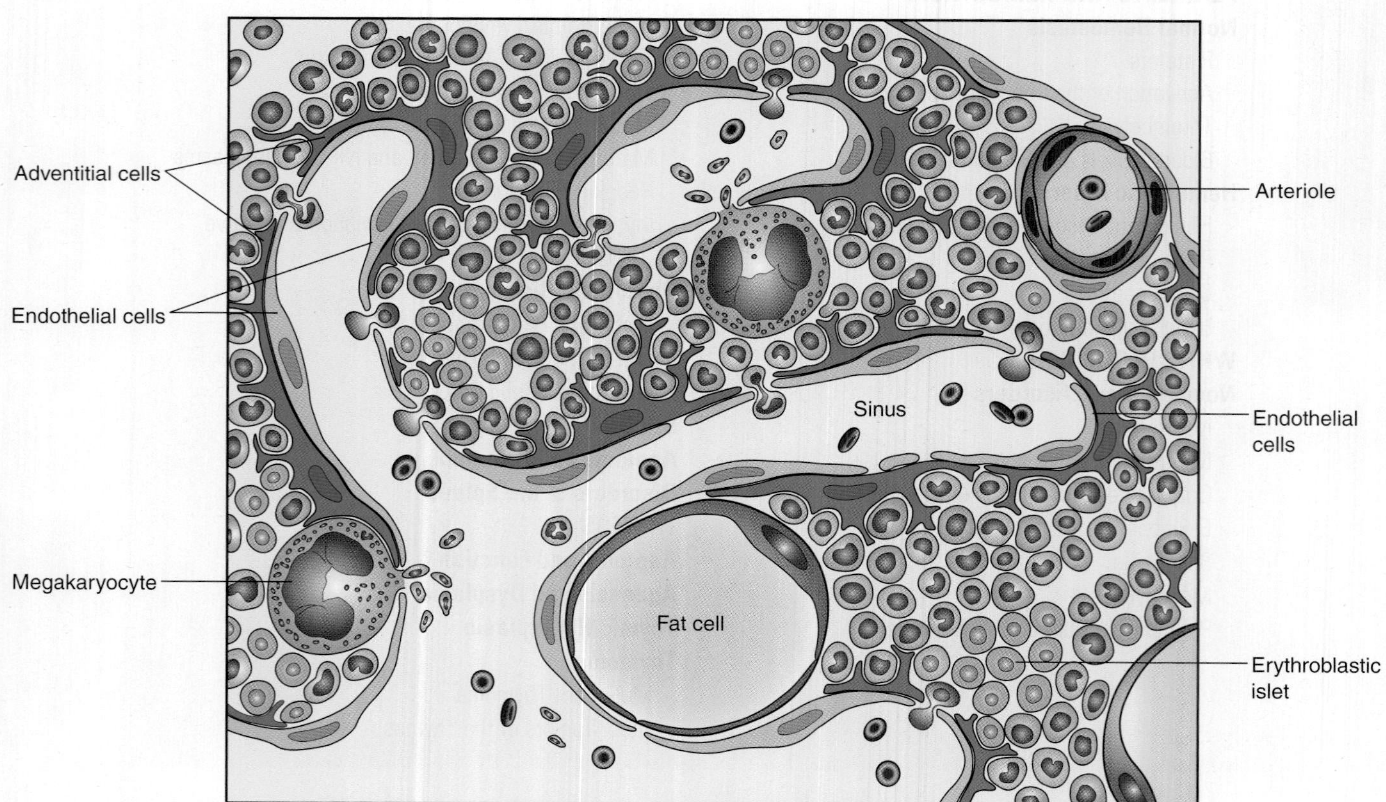

FIGURE 20-1. Structure of normal bone marrow. The sinusoids represent the major point of egress of hematopoietic cells from the bone marrow. Note that the bone marrow does not have lymphatic channels.

reticular adventitial cells. These reticular cells branch extensively throughout the cords and provide a scaffold for stromal and hematopoietic cells. Bone marrow stromal cells include macrophages, endothelial cells, lymphocytes and fibroblasts.

Islands of erythroblasts, usually located in concentric rings around a macrophage that stores excess iron (inappropriately termed a **"nurse cell"**), are present within the cords. The erythroid islands lie close to sinusoid walls, as do megakaryocytes. Granulocyte precursors are located deeper in the cords, adjacent to the bony trabeculae.

STEM CELLS: Pluripotent hematopoietic stems cells are a self-perpetuating pool, in which differentiation and exit are balanced by self-renewal (Fig. 20-2). The stem cells represent only a small proportion of the total hematopoietic cell mass, and they are admixed with progenitor and more mature hematopoietic cells. They are small, mononuclear, and difficult to identify by microscopic observation. Hematopoietic stem cells are semidormant (noncycling) cells that undergo differentiation to progenitor cells of a specific cell line as needed. When marrow elements are injected into irradiated mice, stem cells form visible colonies in the spleen **("colony-forming unit, spleen" [CFU-S])**. In bone marrow cultures, stem cells form colonies containing **multipotential cells** termed granulocyte, erythroid, macrophage and megakaryocyte elements **(CFU-GEMM)** and lymphoid precursor cells **(CFU-L)**.

PROGENITOR CELLS: Like stem cells, progenitor cells are small to medium-sized mononuclear cells that resemble mature lymphocytes. In culture, they give rise to colonies of differentiated progeny. The progenitor cell committed to production of **erythrocytes** forms luxuriant burst-shaped colonies **("burst-forming unit, erythroid" [BFU-E])**. Each subsequent generation of BFU-E makes smaller colonies, until a final progenitor cell, the "colony-forming unit, erythroid" **(CFU-E)**, produces only a small clone of mature erythroblasts.

Granulocytic and **monocytic** cell lines derive from a single progenitor cell. This cell, named "colony-forming unit, granulocyte-monocyte" **(CFU-GM),** makes a colony with both granulocytic and monocytic cells. As the cell matures, its progeny become increasingly committed to polymorphonuclear leukocytes **(CFU-G)** or monocyte/macrophages **(CFU-M). Eosinophils** and **basophils** also have specific progenitor cells (**CFU-Eo** and **CFU-Ba,** respectively). "Megakaryocytic progenitor cells" **(CFU-Meg)** produce colonies in vitro consisting of four to eight megakaryocytes.

GROWTH FACTORS: Hematopoietic cells in bone marrow help maintain the size of the circulating blood cell mass, adjusting to compensate for blood cell senescence or loss. Such regulation is mediated by growth factors that affect the rate of cellular proliferation, primarily in the progenitor cell compartment.

- **Stem cell factor** (SCF; also known as c-KIT ligand) and **Flt3 ligand** (Flt3L) support survival and proliferation of pluripotent stem cells, CFU-GEMM and various progenitor cells.
- **Interleukin (IL)-3** and **granulocyte-macrophage colony-stimulating factor (GM-CSF)** are important for proliferation of CFU-GEMM and multiple CFUs.
- **G-CSF and M-CSF** promote granulocytic and monocytic maturation from CFU-G and CFU-M, respectively.
- **Erythropoietin (EPO)** is released by interstitial peritubular cells of the kidney in response to hypoxia and activates erythroid progenitor cells.
- **Thrombopoietin** (**TPO**) facilitates production and maturation of megakaryocytes.

Several growth factors, notably GM-CSF, G-CSF and EPO, are widely used to treat conditions requiring stimulation of hematopoiesis (e.g., postchemotherapy pancytopenia, especially neutropenia, stem cell mobilization prior to bone marrow transplantation, renal failure).

PRECURSOR CELLS: The next step in hematopoiesis is maturation of progenitor cells to precursor cells called **blasts** (Fig. 20-2). ***It is only at the precursor stage and beyond that the cells are morphologically recognizable in terms of their lineage.*** The maturation of precursor cells to mature cells is characterized by progressive inactivation of the nuclear material and maturation of the cytoplasm, which contains the functional elements of the cells (e.g., hemoglobin in mature red blood cells, cytotoxic enzymes in neutrophils).

- **Erythroid precursor cells:** The **proerythroblast** represents the first stage in red blood cell maturation. Like other committed blast cells, these are relatively low in number compared to the subsequent mature forms in the cell series. Using standard light microscopy staining techniques, the proerythroblast is noted to have intensely basophilic (blue) cytoplasm with a large round nucleus with fine open chromatin and visible nucleoli. Maturation in the erythroid series is marked by a progressive decrease in the nuclear size and an increase in the density of the nuclear chromatin as well as progressive hemoglobinization of the cytoplasm, which is characterized by a gradual change of the cytoplasm from blue to pink. **Reticulocytes** are the final stage of erythroid cell maturation in the bone marrow. The nuclei are extruded from **orthochromatic erythroblasts**, leaving mitochondria and hemoglobin-producing polyribosomes in the reticulocyte. After release from the bone marrow, reticulocytes lose the capacity for aerobic metabolism and hemoglobin synthesis, and after 1 to 2 days become mature erythrocytes.
- **Granulocytic precursor cells: Myeloblasts** have round to oval nuclei with delicate chromatin, multiple visible nucleoli and a blue-gray cytoplasm. The next stage, **promyelocytes**, have similar nuclei, but their cytoplasm contains primary (azurophilic) granules. Maturation from **promyelocytes** to mature **neutrophils** involves (1) progressive condensation of nuclear chromatin, (2) increasing nuclear lobulation and (3) the appearance of secondary (specific) granules. **Basophils** and **eosinophils** derive from specific progenitor and precursor cells and, like neutrophils, are distinguished by their secondary granules.
- **Monocytic precursor cells:** The parallel formation of monocytes from monoblasts also involves a nuclear condensation process, but with less prominent nuclear lobation. Cytoplasm becomes gray, with only a few pink or purple granules. ***After a monocyte leaves the bloodstream, it becomes a member of the mononuclear phagocyte system.*** Depending on its tissue location and function as a **phagocyte** (fixed or wandering) or as an **immunoregulator** (dendritic reticulum cells, Langerhans cells), it may undergo further differentiation.
- **Megakaryocytic precursors:** Megakaryocytes in the bone marrow mature into multilobed giant cells by a number of endomitotic divisions. After reaching a certain ploidy, the cytoplasm becomes stippled and azurophilic and is eventually released into the sinusoids as long, platelet-containing ribbons. Some intact megakaryocytes are also released, and

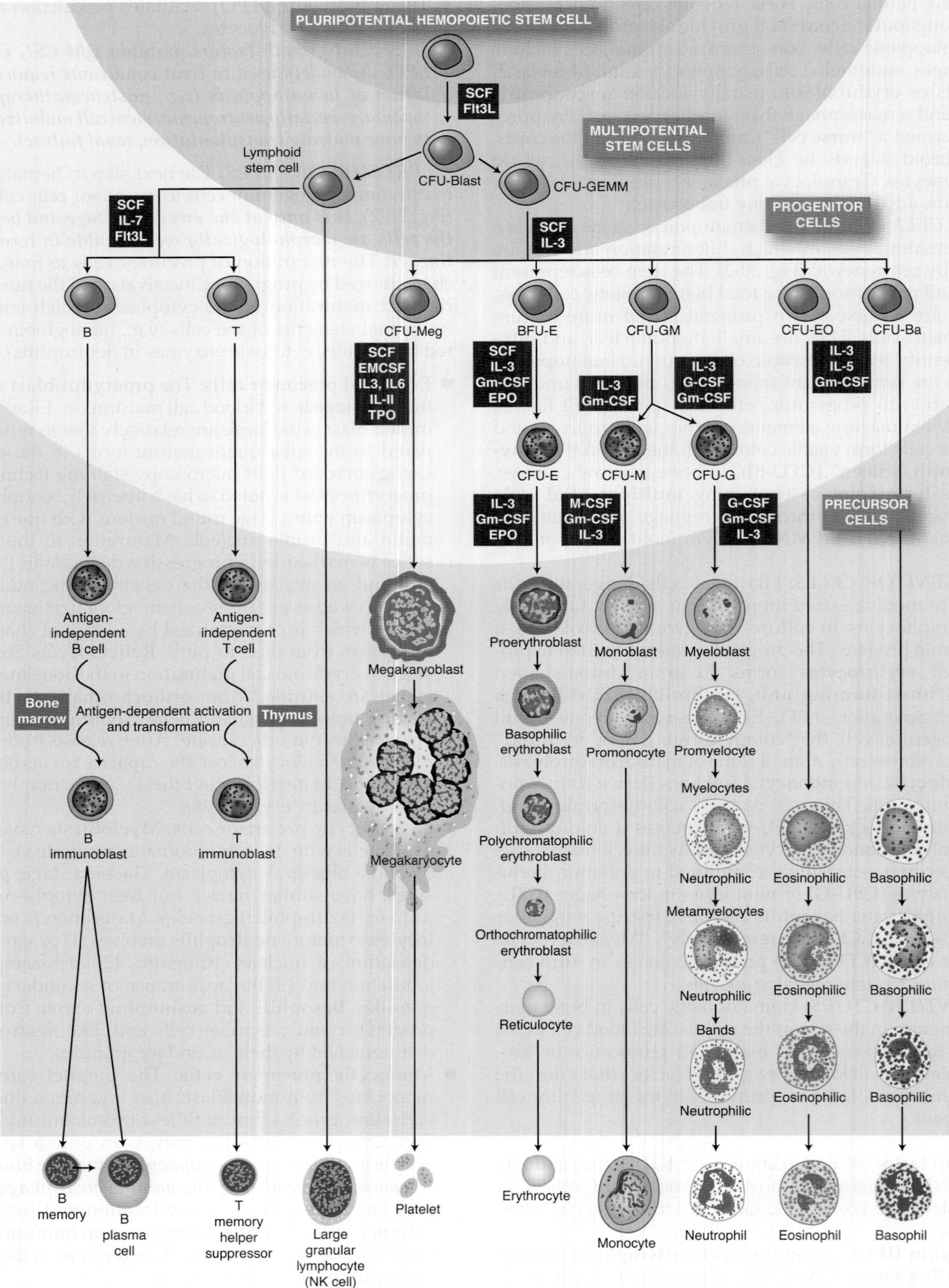

FIGURE 20-2. Cellular differentiation and maturation of the lymphoid and myeloid components of the hematopoietic system. Only the precursor cells (blasts and maturing cells) are identifiable by light microscopic evaluation of the bone marrow. BFU = burst-forming unit; CFU = colony-forming unit (Ba = basophils; E = erythroid; Eo = eosinophils; G = polymorphonuclear leukocytes; GM = granulocyte-monocyte; M = monocyte/macrophages; Meg = megakaryocytic); EPO = erythropoietin; Gm-CSF = granulocyte-macrophage colony-stimulating factor; IL = interleukin; NK = natural killer; SCF = stem cell factor; TPO = thrombopoietin.

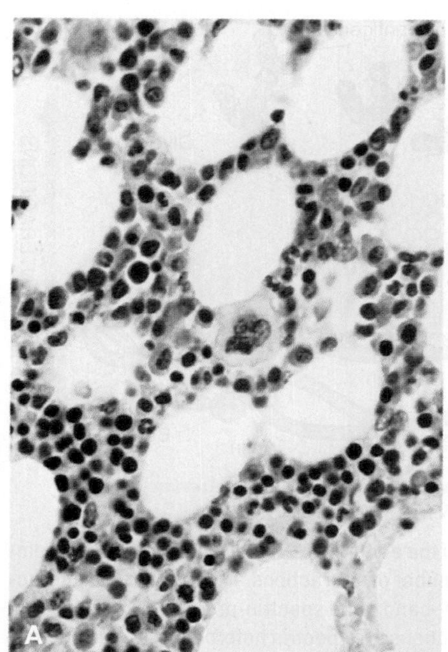

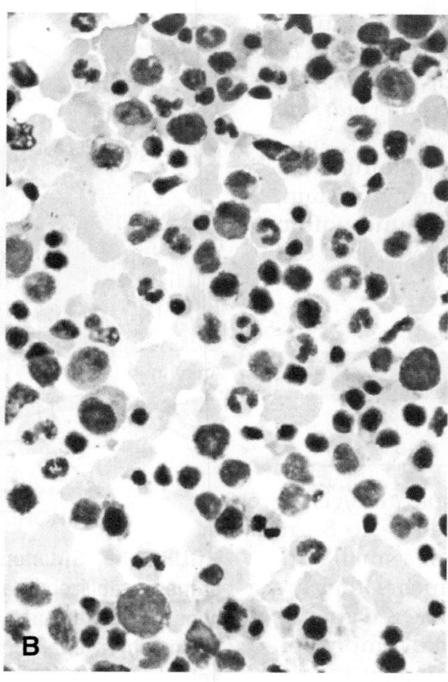

FIGURE 20-3. Normal bone marrow. A. Tissue section showing the normal relationship of cellular hematopoietic elements to fat cells, a normal myeloid-to-erythroid ratio (2:1) and a megakaryocyte in the center of the field (hematoxylin and eosin stain). **B.** Bone marrow aspirate smear from the same patient demonstrating normal hematopoietic elements in varying stages of differentiation (Wright-Giemsa stain).

platelet production occurs after they have been trapped in the pulmonary microcirculation.

RELEASE FROM THE MARROW: After maturation, the hematopoietic cells leave the bone marrow environment through the sinusoids and enter the blood circulation. ***Homeostasis of the hematopoietic system is highly regulated through cell-to-cell interactions in the bone marrow microenvironment and/or by various cytokines that may have a stimulatory or inhibitory effect.*** The cellular release mechanism in the bone marrow is responsive to the needs of the peripheral circulation and can quickly provide a boost of mature cells in an emergent situation (e.g., mature red blood cells and/or reticulocytes during acute hemorrhage or segmented neutrophils in the setting of acute infection).

Morphology

The cellular elements of the bone marrow are commonly evaluated by needle core biopsy and aspiration from the posterior iliac crest. Bone marrow can also be obtained in infants from the anterior tibia and from the sternum in adults (the latter performed rarely). Examination of bone marrow core biopsy sections allows for evaluation of the amount of hematopoietic elements and marrow architecture (Fig. 20-3A), whereas each of the specific bone marrow cell lineages are identified and evaluated in stained smears prepared from aspirated liquid bone marrow (Fig. 20-3B). In a normal middle-aged adult, about half of cells in the bone marrow core biopsy are fat cells and the other half are actively dividing and differentiating hematopoietic cells. The proportion of hematopoietic cells to fat is called the **cellularity,** and it varies with age. The bone marrow cellularity is high in children and lower in the elderly.

The cellular hematopoietic elements in the bone marrow consist of mostly maturing granulocytic precursors, erythroid precursors and megakaryocytes. This is often referred to as **trilineage hematopoiesis**. The proportion of myeloid to erythroid cells (i.e., the **M:E ratio**) typically ranges from 2:1 to 5:1 (Table 20-1). There are usually two to five megakaryocytes per high-power field. Monocytic cells, lymphocytes and plasma cells are found in low numbers under normal conditions. Normal bone marrow contains fewer than 3% plasma cells, up to 20% lymphocytes and only rare mast cells and macrophages. Importantly, blast cells are also few in number outside the setting of a myeloid disease (usually less than 3% in normal adults). A change in the normal number and distribution of mature cells compared to immature cells is often termed a **left shift** or a **shift to immaturity.** This can occur in reactive and neoplastic processes. ***The number of blast cells found in the bone marrow can be useful in distinguishing these two broad categories, since the number of blast cells in the bone marrow does not increase in truly reactive states.*** In addition to allowing for the determination of the cellularity and the proportion of the various cell types (done by differential cell counting), bone marrow examination also enables

Table 20-1

Normal Adult Bone Marrow (Age 18–70 Years)

Normal Adult Bone Marrow (Age 18–70 Years)
Fat-to-cell ratio: 50:50 ± 15%
Myeloid-to-erythroid ratio: 2:1 to 5:1
Cell distribution (% surface area)
Fat cells: 35%–65%
Erythroid series: 10%–20%
Granulocytic (myeloid) series: 40%–65%
Megakaryocytes: 2–5/high-power field
Plasma cells: <3% of nucleated cells
Lymphocytes: <20% of nucleated cells
No fibrosis

critical cytologic assessment for evidence of normal maturation of hematopoietic precursor cells. ***Dyssynchronization or aberration in the highly regulated process of nuclear and cytoplasmic maturation represents evidence of bone marrow disease.***

Finally, iron metabolism can be evaluated by staining the bone marrow aspirate with Prussian blue. Using this stain, storage and sideroblastic iron granules can be found within the cytoplasm of macrophages and nucleated red blood cell precursors, respectively.

RED BLOOD CELLS

Normal Structure and Function

Red blood cells (RBCs), or erythrocytes, transport oxygen to tissues. Mature erythrocytes are nonnucleated 7- to 8-μm biconcave disks, similar in size to the nucleus of a small lymphocyte (Fig. 20-4). On Wright-stained blood smears, they are round with reddish, eosinophilic cytoplasm. The red color is imparted by hemoglobin, their main cytoplasmic component. Because of their biconcave disk shape, RBCs display an area of central pallor approximately one-third the diameter of the cell. Erythrocytes are released from the marrow as reticulocytes, which are larger and have more diffusely basophilic gray cytoplasm than mature RBCs. Reticulocyte polychromatophilia results from their higher content of ribosomes, since these cells still synthesize hemoglobin.

RBC membranes are attached to an underlying cytoskeletal network (Fig. 20-5). Transmembrane proteins that act as receptors, channels and anchors for other membrane components, and the underlying cytoskeleton are inserted into the lipid bilayer. ***Addition of carbohydrate groups to some membrane proteins leads to formation of different red cell antigen groups.*** The erythrocyte cytoskeleton contains interconnected spectrin dimers and other stabilizing proteins (ankyrin, actin, band 4.1), which allows for the inherent deformability of RBCs. ***Changes in this membrane–cytoskeletal unit lead to increased cell rigidity and premature destruction of circulating erythrocytes.***

Hemoglobin accounts for the oxygen-carrying capacity of RBCs. Each hemoglobin molecule contains four heme groups and four globin chains and, when fully saturated, transports four molecules of oxygen. The heme portion of the molecule consists of a porphyrin ring (protoporphyrin IX), with one ferrous ion (Fe^{2+}). The globin portion of the molecule has pairs of two different protein chains. The most abundant normal hemoglobin, hemoglobin A, contains two alpha (α) and two beta (β) globin chains. Other hemoglobins are normally present in minor amounts in healthy adults and include hemoglobin F and hemoglobin A_2. These have, in addition to two α-chains each, two gamma (γ) and two delta (δ) globin chains, respectively, instead of β-globin chains.

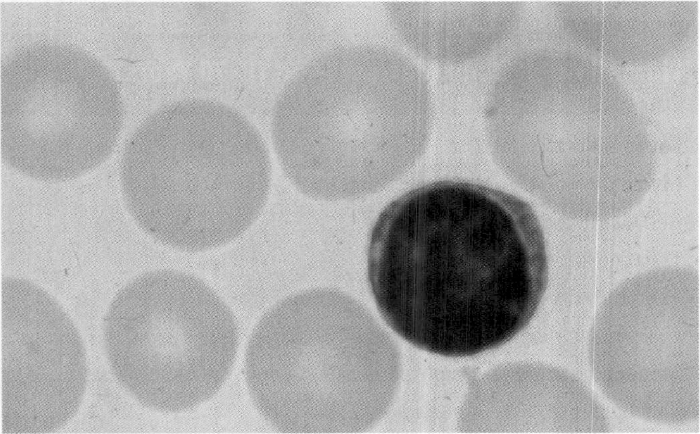

FIGURE 20-4. Normal red blood cells are approximately the same size as the nucleus of a small lymphocyte (approximately 7 μm).

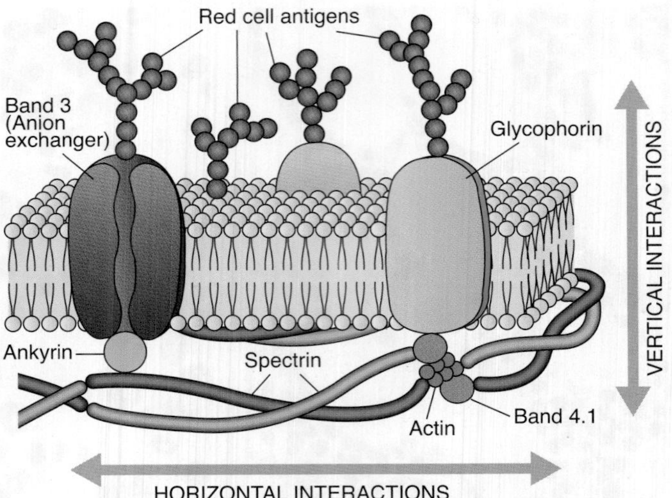

FIGURE 20-5. Structure of the erythrocyte plasma membrane. The membrane is stabilized by a number of interactions. The two vertical interactions are spectrin-ankyrin–band 3 and spectrin-protein 4.1–glycophorin. The two horizontal connections are spectrin heterodimers and spectrin-actin–protein 4.1.

Each heme group interacts with a hydrophobic pocket of one globin chain, and the entire molecule has a globular tertiary structure. Deoxygenated hemoglobin has low oxygen affinity and requires increased oxygen tension for heme–oxygen binding to occur. After this initial interaction, the hemoglobin molecule undergoes a conformational change that facilitates subsequent oxygen binding to the three remaining heme groups. The progressive increase in oxygen affinity is reflected in the sigmoid shape of the oxygen dissociation curve (Fig. 20-6). The slope of the oxygen dissociation curve can be shifted to the right by acidosis or increased 2,3-diphosphoglycerate (2,3-DPG) (a product of an alternate pathway of glycolysis), thus enhancing tissue oxygen delivery. Alkalosis shifts the curve to the left and results in increased oxygen binding.

The average life span of the erythrocyte in the blood is 120 days. Changes in membrane proteins and phospholipids appear in aged red cells and are likely signals for erythrocyte removal by mononuclear phagocytes.

The erythroid component of the blood is best analyzed by a complete blood count (CBC) plus microscopic examination of a blood smear (Table 20-2). The CBC measures hemoglobin (Hgb), red blood cell (RBC) count and mean corpuscular volume (MCV). From these values, additional parameters can be calculated including **hematocrit** (Hct = MCV × RBC), **mean corpuscular hemoglobin** (MCH = Hgb/RBC) and **mean**

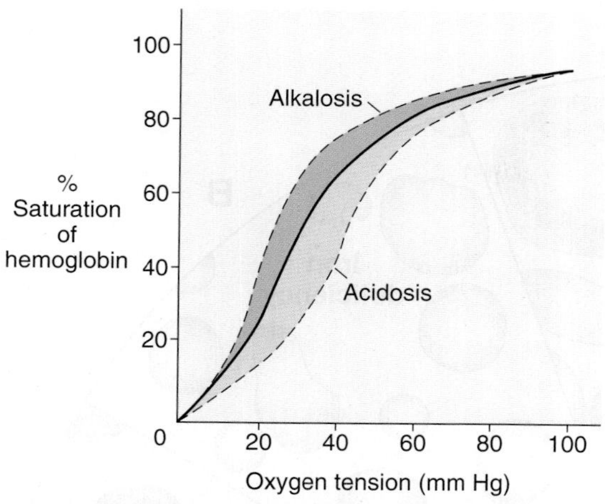

FIGURE 20-6. Oxygen dissociation curve of hemoglobin. With decreasing pH (acidosis) the oxygen affinity declines (shifts right); with increasing pH (alkalosis) the affinity increases (shifts left).

Table 20-2

Complete Blood Count (CBC): Normal Adult Values

Erythrocytes		
Hemoglobin	Male, 14–18 g/dL Female, 12–16 g/dL	
Hematocrit	Male, 40%–54% Female, 35%–47%	
Red blood cell (RBC) count	Male, 4.5–6 × $10^6/\mu$L Female, 4–5.5 × $10^6/\mu$L	
Reticulocytes	0.5%–2.5%	
Indices		
Mean corpuscular volume	82–100 μm^3	
Mean corpuscular hemoglobin	27–34 pg	
Mean corpuscular hemoglobin concentration	32%–36%	
Leukocytes		
	Absolute Count/μL	**Differential Count (%)**
White blood cells (WBCs)	4000–11,000	
Neutrophil granulocytes	1800–7000	50–60
Neutrophil bands	0–700	2–4
Lymphocytes	1500–4000	30–40
Monocytes	0–800	1–9
Basophils	0–200	0–1
Eosinophils	0–450	0–3
Platelets		
Quantitative normal value: 150,000–400,000/μL		
Qualitative estimation on smear: Number of platelets/oil immersion field × 10,000 = estimated platelet count		
Normal ratio of RBC to platelets = 15:1 to 20:1		

corpuscular hemoglobin concentration (MCHC = Hgb/Hct). The degree of variation in RBC size or red cell distribution width (RDW) is also derived. Reticulocytes can be accurately quantitated using supravital dyes that stain their cytoplasmic ribosome aggregates.

Anemia

Anemia is a reduction in circulating erythrocyte mass. A diagnosis of anemia is made by demonstrating a reduction in hemoglobin, hematocrit or RBC count. Anemia leads to decreased oxygen transport by the blood and ultimately tissue hypoxia.

Anemias Are Classified by Morphology or Pathophysiology

Anemias are classified by morphology or pathophysiology.

Morphologic classification of anemia is based on erythrocyte appearance, as determined by automated blood counters and microscopic evaluation of a blood smear. RBC size (generally measured by analyzers) is reflected in the MCV, which allows division of anemias into three groups: (1) **microcytic** (decreased MCV), (2) **normocytic** and (3) **macrocytic** (increased MCV) (Table 20-3). Blood smear analysis may show abnormally shaped RBCs **(poikilocytes),** which can be seen in a wide variety of anemias. The particular type of poikilocyte can aid in diagnosis (Fig. 20-7).

Pathophysiologic classification of anemia includes four major groups (Table 20-4):

1. **Acute blood loss**
2. **Decreased production** of red cells by the bone marrow, either by **stem cell or progenitor cell defects**
3. **Ineffective hematopoiesis** with reduced release of erythrocytes from marrow
4. **Increased destruction** of RBCs after release from the bone marrow, either **intracorpuscular** or **extracorpuscular**

Anemias associated with increased destruction of red cells are usually characterized by increased numbers of circulating

Table 20-3

Morphologic Classification of Anemia

Macrocytic	
Nutritional deficiency	Hypothyroidism
Alcohol use	Reticulocytosis
Liver disease	Primary bone marrow disease
Microcytic	
Iron deficiency	
Thalassemias	
Sideroblastic	
Normocytic	
Anemia of chronic disease/inflammation	
Anemia of renal disease	
Acute blood loss	

20 | Hematopathology

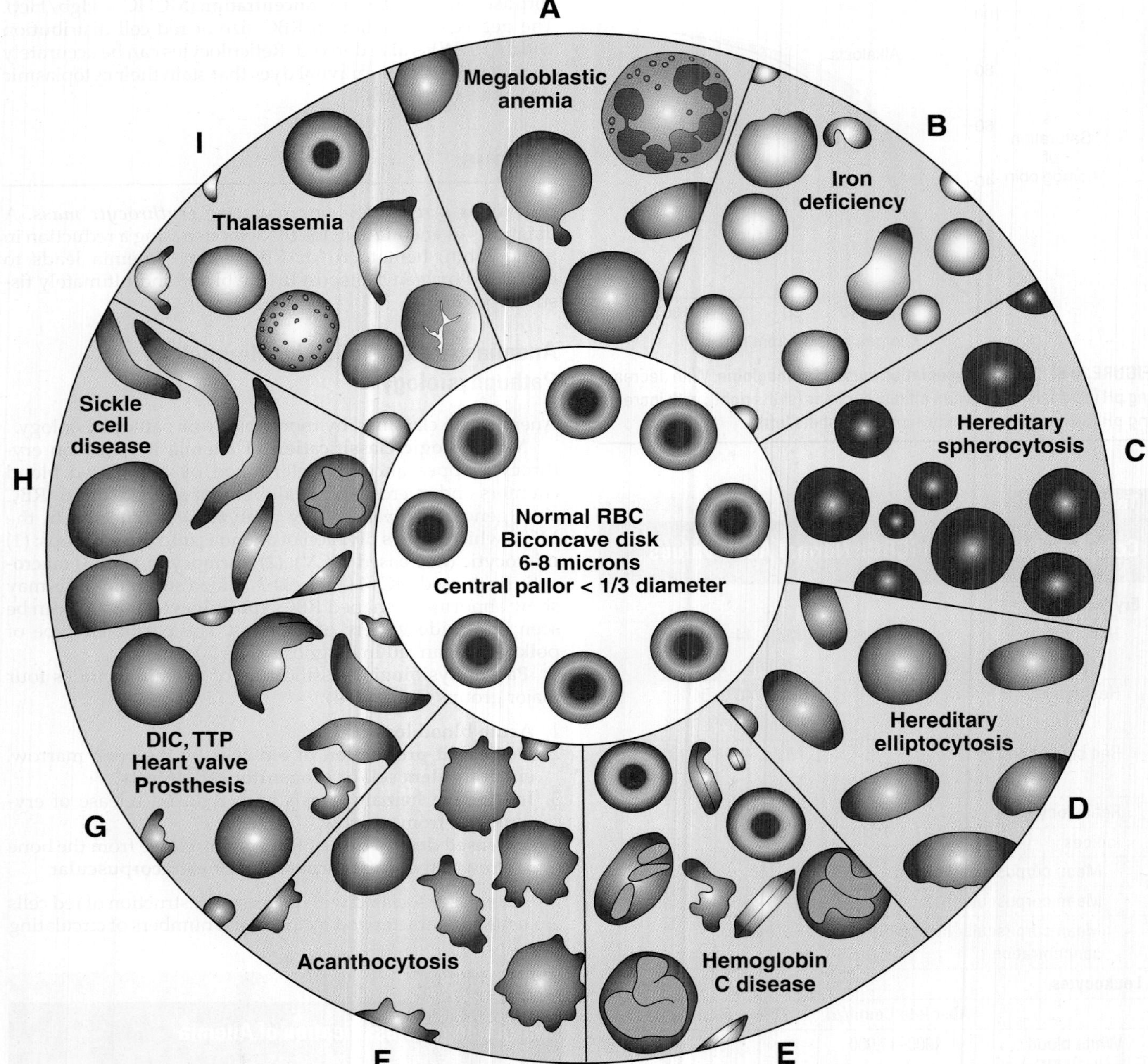

FIGURE 20-7. Abnormal red blood cell morphologies associated with various types of anemia. The morphology of normal erythrocytes is shown in the center. **A. Megaloblastic anemia (disturbance in DNA synthesis, most often caused by deficiency of vitamin B12 or folic acid):** Oval macrocytes, teardrop cells, and hypersegmented neutrophils. **B. Iron deficiency (disturbance in hemoglobin synthesis; lack of iron):** Hypochromic, microcytic erythrocytes. **C. Hereditary spherocytosis (membrane defect):** Spherocytes lacking central pallor. **D. Hereditary elliptocytosis (membrane defect):** Elliptocytes. **E. Hemoglobin C disease (abnormal globin chain):** Target cells, rhomboid crystals. **F. Acanthocytosis (membrane lipid defect, e.g., abetalipoproteinemia):** Irregular spiculation. **G. Microangiopathic hemolysis (mechanical damage to erythrocytes;** disseminated intravascular coagulation [DIC], thrombocytic thrombocytopenic purpura [TTP], heart valve prosthesis sequela): schistocytes/fragments. **H. Sickle cell disease (abnormal globin chain):** Sickle cells. **I. Thalassemia (disturbance in hemoglobin synthesis):** Hypochromic, microcytic erythrocytes; poikilocytosis; basophilic stippling; target cells.

Table 20-4

Pathophysiologic Classification of Anemia

Acute Blood Loss	
Decreased Production	
Stem Cell and Progenitor Cell Defects	
Iron deficiency	Leukemia
Anemia of chronic disease	Myelodysplastic syndromes
Aplastic anemia	Marrow infiltration
Pure red cell aplasia	Lead poisoning
Paroxysmal nocturnal hemoglobinuria	Anemia of renal disease
Ineffective Hematopoiesis	
Megaloblastic anemia	
Myelodysplastic syndromes	Thalassemia
Increased Destruction	
Intracorpuscular	
Membrane defect	Hemoglobinopathies
Enzyme defect	
Extracorpuscular	
Immunologic	
Autoimmune	Alloimmune
Nonimmunologic	
Mechanical	Infectious
Hypersplenism	Chemical

reticulocytes **(reticulocytosis),** which allows distinction from other groups.

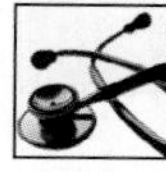

CLINICAL FEATURES: In the face of anemia, the body has several compensatory mechanisms, to enhance oxygen delivery to tissues.

- Increased cardiac output
- Increased respiratory rate
- Shunting of blood flow to provide increased tissue perfusion of vital organs
- Decreased hemoglobin–oxygen affinity
- Increased marrow erythrocyte production as a result of EPO stimulation

Clinical signs and symptoms (tachycardia, shortness of breath and systolic murmurs) may develop secondary to these compensatory processes. If anemia is sufficiently severe (i.e., hemoglobin levels below 7 g/dL), tissue hypoxia is uncompensated and additional clinical findings may include easy fatigability, faintness, angina and dyspnea on exertion.

Acute Blood Loss Leads to Normocytic Normochromic Anemia

Acute anemia reflects the loss of blood from the intravascular compartment.

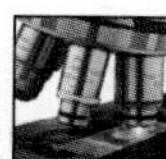
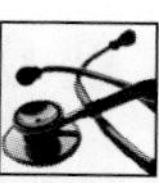

PATHOLOGY AND CLINICAL FEATURES: Initial manifestations of acute blood loss reflect volume depletion and decreased tissue perfusion. Since whole blood is lost, the severity of the anemia may not be appreciated initially. Within 24 to 48 hours after significant hemorrhage, however, fluid is mobilized from extravascular locations into the intravascular space to restore overall blood volume. This is when the extent of the anemia becomes apparent, since red cell replacement is not as rapid. If the underlying bleeding is stopped, EPO-driven bone marrow erythroid hyperplasia will gradually correct the anemia. Examination of the blood smear reveals no specific red cell abnormalities, but polychromasia is seen during the recovery phase.

Decreased Red Blood Cell Production Often Reflects Impaired Erythrocyte Precursor Development

Iron-Deficiency Anemia

Iron-deficiency interferes with normal heme (hemoglobin) synthesis and leads to impaired erythropoiesis and anemia. Iron deficiency is the most common cause of anemia worldwide.

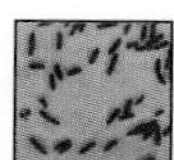

ETIOLOGIC FACTORS: The normal Western adult diet contains about 20 mg of iron, 1 to 2 mg of which is absorbed by the duodenum and proximal jejunum (see Chapter 14). The rate of iron absorption is regulated by normal losses, but with anemia (especially in cases of ineffective erythropoiesis), intestinal absorption is increased and may ultimately lead to iron overload. About 85% of absorbed iron is transported by a carrier protein, transferrin, to be incorporated into developing red cells through specific transferrin receptors on their surface. As senescent red cells are removed from circulation, hemoglobin is broken down into component parts and iron is recycled. Excess iron is stored as **hemosiderin** and as **ferritin.** Hemosiderin is large aggregates of iron with a disorganized structure, while ferritin is complexed with protein (apoferritin) and appears highly organized.

Many underlying conditions give rise to iron deficiency. In infants and children, dietary iron may be inadequate for growth and development. Iron need also increases during **pregnancy** and **lactation.** In adults, iron deficiency typically results from **chronic blood loss** or, less commonly, **intravascular hemolysis.** One milligram of iron is contained in 2 mL of whole blood lost from the body. In women of reproductive age, **gynecologic blood loss** (menstruation, parturition, vaginal bleeding) is most common. In postmenopausal women and men, unexplained iron deficiency should prompt study of the gastrointestinal tract for **tumors** or **vascular lesions,** as this is the most common site of chronic blood loss.

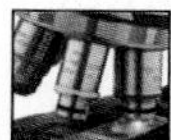

PATHOLOGY: Iron-deficiency anemia is characterized by a microcytic, hypochromic anemia (Fig. 20-8). Variation in erythrocyte size and shape **(anisopoikilocytosis)** is reflected in an increased RDW, which is a measure of **anisocytosis**. **Ovalocytes** may be found, some of which are very thin and are designated **pencil cells.** Because of the production defect in the marrow, there is no associated reticulocytosis. The bone marrow displays

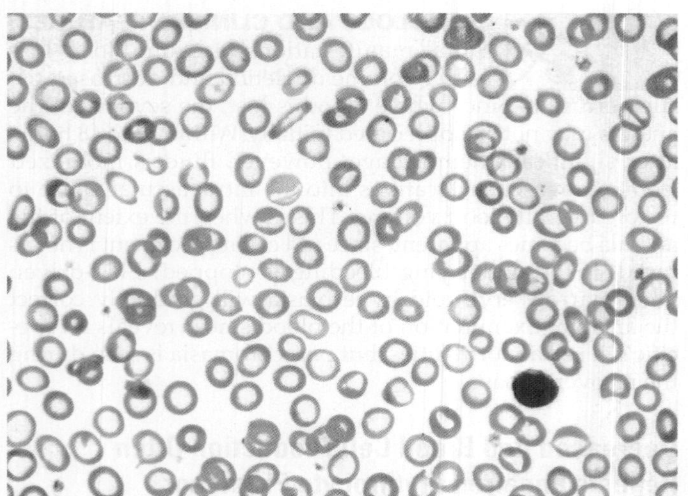

FIGURE 20-8. Microcytic hypochromic anemia caused by iron deficiency. Red blood cells (RBCs) are significantly smaller than the nucleus of a small lymphocyte, and they have increased central pallor (normal central pallor is about one third of the RBC diameter).

erythroid hyperplasia. Prussian blue staining shows absent storage or erythroid iron.

Serum iron and ferritin levels are decreased by iron deficiency, while total iron-binding capacity is increased (because of increased serum transferrin level). As a result, the percent saturation of transferrin is conspicuously lowered (often less than 5%).

CLINICAL FEATURES: The symptoms of iron deficiency are those of anemia in general. With advanced disease, a smooth and glistening tongue **(atrophic glossitis)** and inflammation at the corners of the mouth **(angular stomatitis)** may be encountered, as well as a spoon-shaped deformity of the fingernails **(koilonychia).** Treatment of iron deficiency involves correcting the source of chronic blood loss and oral iron supplementation. Parenteral iron is available for patients who are not compliant.

Anemia of Chronic Disease

Anemia of chronic disease arises in association with chronic inflammatory and malignant conditions.

MOLECULAR PATHOGENESIS: Chronic disease causes ineffective use of iron from macrophage stores in bone marrow, resulting in a functional iron deficiency, although iron stores are normal or even increased. Other factors that may contribute to anemia are decreased erythrocyte life span, blunted renal EPO responses to tissue hypoxia and impaired bone marrow response to erythropoietin. Inflammatory cytokines (lactoferrin, IL-1, tumor necrosis factor-α [TNF-α] and interferon) may interfere with iron mobilization.

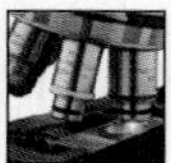

PATHOLOGY: The anemia of chronic disease is mild to moderate; red cells are often normocytic and normochromic, but can be microcytic. In bone marrow aspirates, Prussian blue staining shows normal or increased iron storage in macrophages, but reduced erythroid iron. Serum iron levels tend to be reduced. However, unlike iron-deficiency anemia, total iron-binding capacity also tends to be decreased (as is serum albumin). The reticulocyte count is not appropriately increased for the degree of anemia. Successful treatment of the underlying disease restores normal hemoglobin levels.

Aplastic Anemia

Aplastic anemia is a disorder of pluripotential stem cells that leads to bone marrow failure. The disorder features hypocellular bone marrow and pancytopenia (decreased circulating levels of all formed elements in the blood).

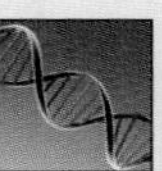
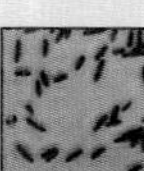

MOLECULAR PATHOGENESIS AND ETIOLOGIC FACTORS: Aplastic anemia results from injury to bone marrow stem cells. Most cases are idiopathic, and no specific initiating etiology can be identified (Table 20-5). There are two main mechanisms of stem cell injury. The first is a predictable, dose-dependent, toxic injury, typified by exposure to certain chemotherapeutic drugs, chemicals and ionizing radiation. The other is an idiosyncratic, dose-independent, immunologic injury, as seen in idiopathic cases or after certain drug exposures or viral infections. Rarely aplastic anemia (e.g., Fanconi anemia) may be inherited. Depending on its cause, stem cell injury may or may not be reversible.

The immune etiology of stem cell injury in some patients is supported by the clinical response to antithymocyte globulin or other immunosuppressive agents. An intrinsic abnormality of stem cells in other cases of aplastic

Table 20-5

Etiology of Aplastic Anemia

Idiopathic (two thirds of cases)
Ionizing radiation
Drugs
Chemotherapeutic agents
Chloramphenicol
Anticonvulsants
Nonsteroidal anti-inflammatory agents
Gold
Chemicals
Benzene
Viruses
Hepatitis C virus (HCV)
Epstein-Barr virus (EBV)
Human immunodeficiency virus (HIV)
Parvovirus B19
Hereditary
Fanconi anemia

anemia is suggested by the subsequent evolution of clonal stem cell disorders (paroxysmal nocturnal hemoglobinuria, myelodysplasia, acute leukemia). Aplastic anemia associated with **Fanconi anemia** (see below) is caused by germline mutations in *FANC* (Fanconi anemia complementation) genes, leading to chromosomal instability upon exposure to ionizing radiation or alkylating agents. Aplastic anemia in this syndrome usually manifests within the first decade of life.

PATHOLOGY: The bone marrow in aplastic anemia shows variably reduced cellularity, depending on the clinical stage of the disease. Myeloid, erythroid and megakaryocytic lineage cells are fewer, with a relative increase in marrow lymphocytes and plasma cells. As bone marrow cellularity decreases, there is a corresponding increase in fat (Fig. 20-9). Anemia, leukopenia (mainly granulocytopenia) and thrombocytopenia characterize aplastic anemia. Despite elevated EPO levels, reticulocytosis is not present, which underscores the underlying stem cell defect.

CLINICAL FEATURES: Patients with aplastic anemia present with signs and symptoms attributable to pancytopenia, namely, weakness, fatigue, infection and bleeding. For untreated aplastic anemia, the prognosis is grim, with a 3- to 6-month median survival. Only 20% survive over 1 year. Immunosuppressive therapy often leads to transient remissions and bone marrow or stem cell transplantation may be curative.

Pure Red Cell Aplasia

Pure red cell aplasia (PRCA) is selective suppression of committed erythroid precursors in the bone marrow. White blood cells and platelets are unaffected.

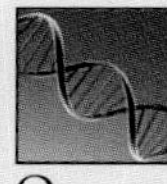

MOLECULAR PATHOGENESIS: PRCA most often results from immune suppression of red cell production, the stimulus for which is unknown. On occasion, it is secondary to viral infection (parvovirus B19) or thymic lesions (e.g., thymoma, thymic hyperplasia). The P antigen system on the red cell membrane is a receptor for parvovirus and explains the restricted infection of erythroid precursors by this agent.

Diamond-Blackfan syndrome is a PRCA caused by de novo or inherited mutations. It manifests within the first 2 years of life with anemia, with or without physical abnormalities including cleft lip or palate, micrognathia, limb abnormalities and short stature. Anemia is caused by defective erythroid precursors that show a diminished response to erythropoietin and decreased erythroid burst- and colony-forming capacities.

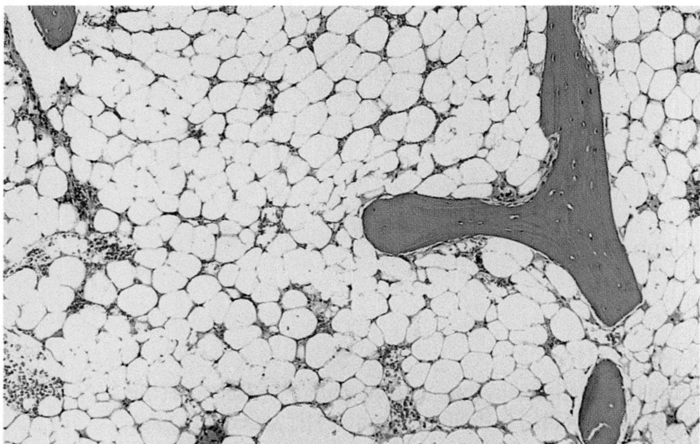

FIGURE 20-9. Aplastic anemia. The bone marrow consists largely of fat cells and lacks normal hematopoietic activity.

PATHOLOGY: In PRCA, overall marrow cellularity is normal, but there is a selective absence of erythroid precursors. Erythroid precursors are completely absent or are arrested at the erythroblast (pronormoblast) stage. In cases secondary to parvovirus B19, intranuclear viral inclusions in proerythroblasts can be observed. Myeloid and megakaryocytic precursors are adequate in number and show normal maturation.

Patients with PRCA develop moderate to severe anemia, often with macrocytic indices. Despite increased EPO, there is no accompanying reticulocytosis.

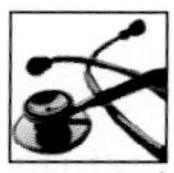

CLINICAL FEATURES: Acquired PRCA manifests as an acute self-limited illness or a chronic relapsing process. **Acute self-limited PRCA** is often caused by parvovirus B19. This condition may not be clinically apparent unless the patient suffers from an underlying chronic hemolytic anemia (e.g., hereditary spherocytosis, sickle cell anemia). Such cases may be complicated by a so-called aplastic crisis (i.e., sudden worsening of anemia).

Immunocompromised patients cannot clear parvovirus infection and anemia may be prolonged. **Chronic relapsing PRCA** may be idiopathic or associated with an underlying thymic lesion. In these cases, thymectomy may correct the anemia.

Anemia of Renal Disease

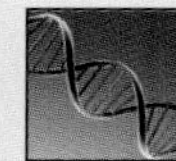

MOLECULAR PATHOGENESIS: Anemia associated with chronic renal disease of varying causes is associated with **decreased production of EPO** and subsequent development of anemia. The severity of anemia is proportional to the underlying degree of renal insufficiency. Administration of recombinant EPO is the treatment of choice. A "uremic toxin," which suppresses erythroid precursors, plus a minor hemolytic component have been suggested (but not proven) as contributing to the anemia of chronic renal disease.

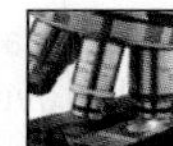

PATHOLOGY: The anemia of chronic renal disease is normocytic and normochromic. In some cases, erythrocytes with scalloped cell membranes can be seen (Burr cells). If renal insufficiency is secondary to malignant hypertension, red cell fragmentation with formation of schistocytes may be observed.

Anemia Associated With Marrow Infiltration (Myelophthisic Anemia)

Myelophthisic anemia is a hypoproliferative anemia associated with infiltration of bone marrow by a variety of processes.

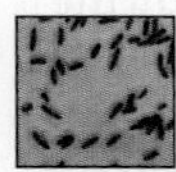

ETIOLOGIC FACTORS: Any infiltrative process (e.g., primary or secondary myelofibrosis, hematologic malignancies, metastatic carcinoma or granulomatous disease) may replace normal hematopoietic elements and cause anemia (and often leukopenia and thrombocytopenia). In an attempt to maintain blood cell production, extramedullary hematopoiesis may develop, mostly in the spleen and liver.

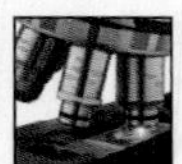

PATHOLOGY: Bone marrow infiltration causes moderate to severe normocytic anemia, with anisopoikilocytosis and teardrop cells. Circulating immature granulocytes and nucleated erythrocytes **(leukoerythroblastosis)** are frequently seen.

Anemia of Lead Poisoning

Lead poisoning results in anemia by interfering with several enzymes involved in heme synthesis (see Chapter 8).

In Ineffective Red Cell Production, There Are Fewer Circulating Erythrocytes

Various anemias reflect abnormal erythrocyte production caused by ineffective hematopoiesis. In contrast with stem cell or precursor cell disorders, the bone marrow erythrocyte precursor pool is expanded. Thus, sufficient erythrocyte precursors are formed in the bone marrow, but erythrocytes do not enter the circulation.

Megaloblastic Anemias

Megaloblastic anemias are caused by impaired DNA synthesis, usually because of either vitamin B_{12} or folic acid deficiency.

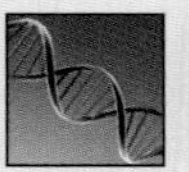
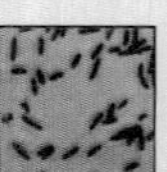

MOLECULAR PATHOGENESIS AND ETIOLOGIC FACTORS: Impaired DNA synthesis results in abnormal nuclear development, which in turn leads to ineffective erythrocyte maturation and anemia. In fact, all proliferating cell lines are affected. Certain chemotherapeutic agents (methotrexate, hydroxyurea) or antiretroviral drugs (5-azacytidine) may also cause megaloblastic anemia. Less commonly, inherited defects in purine or pyrimidine metabolism may be involved.

Folate and B_{12} are critical for normal DNA synthesis. Tetrahydrofolate is converted from methyl tetrahydrofolate by methyl transferase and vitamin B_{12}, which serves as a cofactor. Vitamin B_{12} is also required for converting homocysteine to methionine. Using tetrahydrofolate as a cofactor, thymidylate synthetase converts uridylate to thymidylate (Fig. 20-10). Dihydrofolate reductase restores tetrahydrofolate.

In the face of defective DNA synthesis, nuclear development is impaired, whereas cytoplasm matures normally. This situation, termed **nuclear-to-cytoplasmic asynchrony,** results in formation of large nucleated erythrocyte

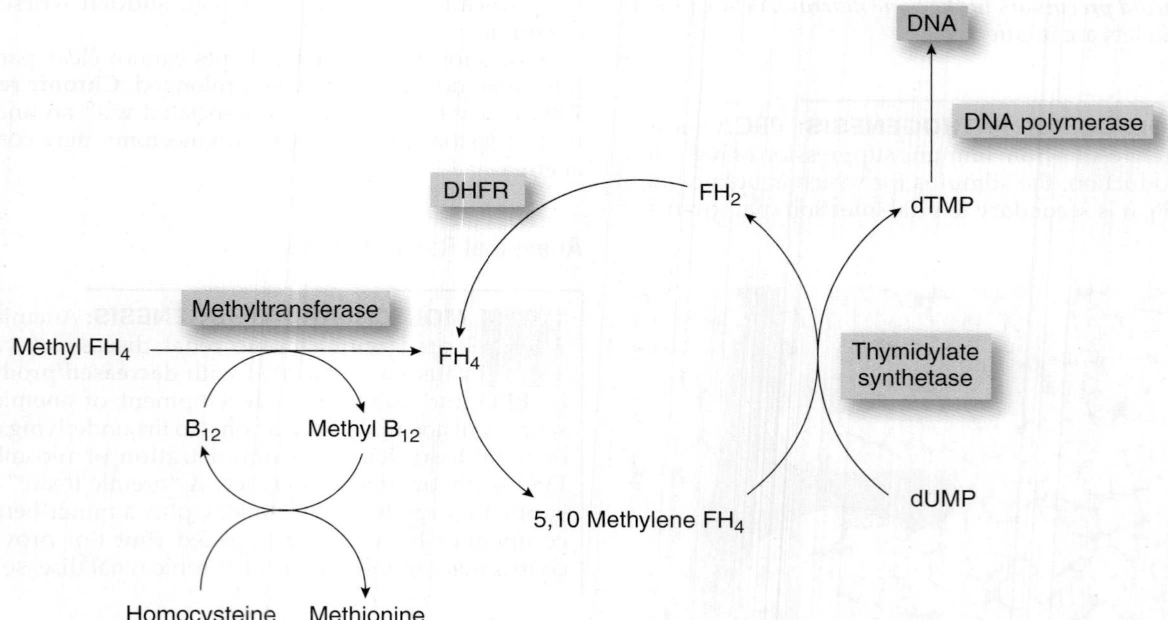

FIGURE 20-10. Relationship of folic acid to vitamin B_{12}. A 1-carbon transfer mediated by folic acid methylates dUMP to dTMP, which is then used for the synthesis of DNA. To enter this cycle, folate (methyl FH_4) is demethylated to FH_4, vitamin B_{12} acting as the cofactor. Thus, both vitamin B_{12} and folic acid deficiencies lead to impaired DNA synthesis and megaloblastic anemia. FH_4 = tetrahydrofolate; dUMP = deoxyuridine monophosphate; dTMP = deoxythymidine monophosphate; FH_2 = dihydrofolate; DHFR = dihydrofolate reductase.

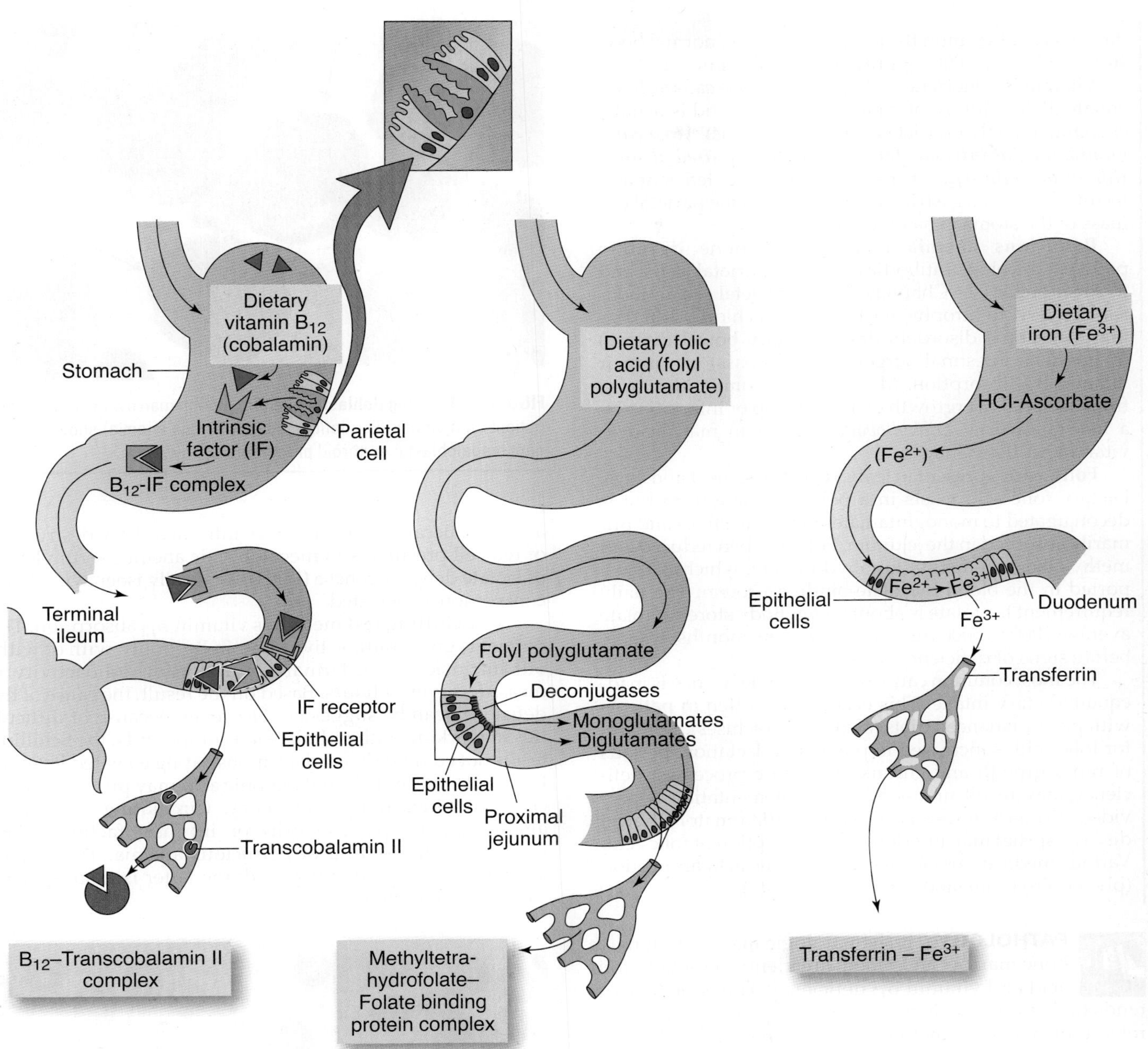

FIGURE 20-11. Absorption of vitamin B_{12}, folic acid and iron. Absorption of vitamin B_{12} requires initial complexing with intrinsic factor (IF), which is produced by the parietal cells of the gastric mucosa. Absorption then occurs in the terminal ileum, where there are receptors for the IF–B_{12} complex. Dietary folic acid is conjugated by conjugase enzymes to polyglutamate. Absorption occurs in the jejunum following deconjugation in the intestinal lumen. Reduction and methylation result in the generation of methyl tetrahydrofolate, which is then transported by folate-binding protein. Dietary ferric iron (Fe^{3+}) is reduced to ferrous iron (Fe^{2+}) in the stomach and absorbed principally in the duodenum. Iron is transported by transferrin in the circulation.

precursors **(megaloblasts).** Since megaloblast precursors do not mature enough to be released into the blood, they undergo intramedullary destruction. Released erythrocytes are macrocytic.

Vitamin B_{12} (cyanocobalamin) is found in a variety of animal food sources and is synthesized by intestinal microorganisms. Proper vitamin B_{12} absorption requires its binding to intrinsic factor, which protects vitamin B_{12} from degradation by intestinal enzymes (Fig. 20-11). Intrinsic factor is produced, along with hydrochloric acid, by gastric parietal cells. Vitamin B_{12} is absorbed in the distal ileum via specific receptors. In the blood, vitamin B_{12} is transported by a group of proteins called **transcobalamins,** of which transcobalamin II is the most important. The daily usage of vitamin B_{12} is 1 μg. Therefore, normal body stores of 1000 to 5000 μg provide several years of reserve.

Vitamin B_{12} deficiency arises from diverse causes. Inadequate dietary intake of vitamin B_{12} is rare and is usually encountered only in strict vegetarians (vegans). ***Most commonly, lack of intrinsic factor leads to impaired absorption of vitamin B_{12}.*** Intrinsic factor may be deficient as a result of previous gastric surgery in which the parietal cell mass of the stomach has been removed.

Pernicious anemia is an autoimmune disorder: patients develop antibodies against parietal cells and intrinsic factor (see Chapter 13). Antiparietal cell antibodies also lead to atrophic gastritis with achlorhydria. Primary intestinal disorders (inflammatory bowel disease) or previous intestinal surgery (ileal bypass) can impair vitamin B_{12} absorption. Microbiologic competition (e.g., from bacterial overgrowth of a blind loop or infestation by a fish tapeworm, *Diphyllobothrium latum*) may lead to vitamin B_{12} deficiency.

Folic acid is present in leafy vegetables, meat and eggs. Dietary folic acid exists in a polyglutamate form but is deconjugated to monoglutamates in the intestines and primarily absorbed in the jejunum. Folate is then reduced and methylated to 5-methyl tetrahydrofolate, which is transported in the blood by folate-binding protein. The daily requirement for folate is about 50 μg. Body stores of folate average 2000 to 5000 μg, providing a few months' reserve before signs of deficiency develop.

The most common cause of folic acid deficiency is inadequate dietary intake. This occurs most often in patients with poorly balanced diets (alcoholics, recluses). Demand for folic acid is increased in pregnancy, lactation, periods of rapid growth and chronic hemolytic processes; deficiency may result unless folate supplementation is provided. Primary intestinal diseases (inflammatory bowel disease, sprue) may interfere with absorption of folic acid. Various medications can also impair folic acid absorption (phenytoin) or metabolism (methotrexate).

PATHOLOGY: The hematologic manifestations, in bone marrow and blood, are identical for both folic acid and vitamin B_{12} deficiency. The bone marrow tends to demonstrate increased hematopoietic activity, but release of mature, functional cells is inadequate because of increased intramedullary cell death. This is termed **ineffective hematopoiesis.** Megaloblastic maturation, characterized by cellular enlargement with asynchronous maturation between the nucleus and cytoplasm (Fig. 20-12), is noted in bone marrow erythroid precursors. The changes within the myeloid series are characterized by giant bands and metamyelocytes, and hypersegmented nuclei of mature granulocytes. The megakaryocytes can also be large.

The degree of anemia varies but may be severe. Erythrocytes are macrocytic and may be oval (oval macrocytes). Anisopoikilocytosis is usually prominent and teardrop cells may be seen. Circulating neutrophils often show nuclear hypersegmentation (more than five lobes) (Fig. 20-13). No increase in reticulocytes occurs.

The distinction between folic acid and vitamin B_{12} deficiency can usually be established by measuring serum levels of these compounds. Occasionally, specific measurement of red cell folate provides more useful information than serum analyses. Because of the massive intramedullary destruction of red cell precursors in megaloblastic anemia, serum levels of lactate dehydrogenase (LDH), especially isoenzyme 1, are conspicuously elevated.

The **Schilling test** measures vitamin B_{12} absorption. The patient is given radioactive vitamin B_{12} orally, with or without intrinsic factor. Urinary excretion of radioactivity is measured over 24 hours. Based on the result, the cause of the deficiency can be suggested. However, because of difficulties in working with radiolabeled compounds, the Schilling test is not commonly used. Demonstrating elevated levels of homocysteine and methyl malonic acid may prove useful in cases of vitamin B_{12} deficiency. Circulating antibodies against gastric parietal cells or intrinsic factor can be detected in the setting of pernicious anemia. The former antibody is more often detected; the latter is more specific for pernicious anemia.

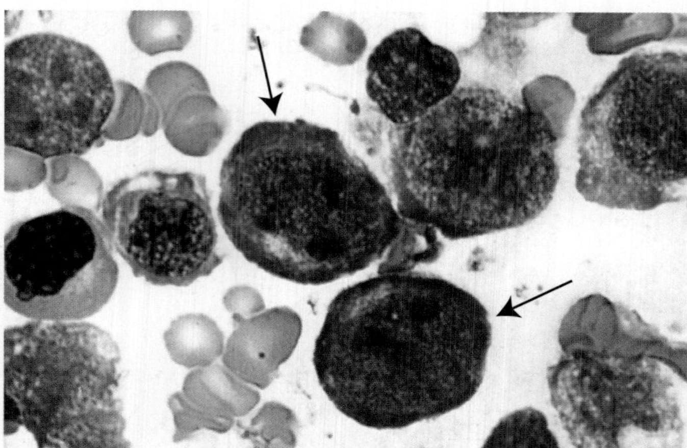

FIGURE 20-12. Megaloblastic anemia. A bone marrow aspirate from a patient with vitamin B_{12} deficiency (pernicious anemia) shows prominent megaloblastic erythroid precursors (*arrows*).

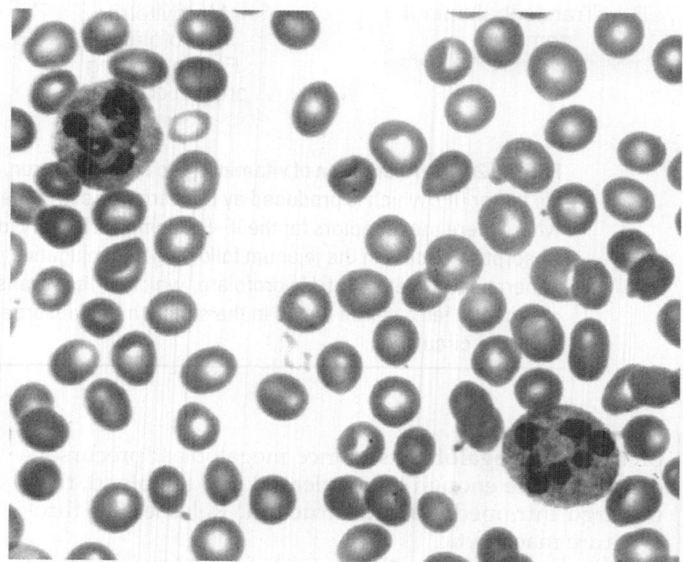

FIGURE 20-13. Hypersegmented granulocytes in a patient with vitamin B_{12} deficiency.

CLINICAL FEATURES: Whether a result of deficiency of vitamin B_{12} or folic acid, the clinical presentation of megaloblastic anemia is similar. In general, folate deficiency develops more rapidly (months) than does vitamin B_{12} deficiency (years). The most important difference clinically is the neurologic symptoms with vitamin B_{12} deficiency, secondary to demyelination of the posterior and lateral columns of the spinal cord, which may cause both sensory and motor deficiencies (see Chapter 28). Without appropriate and prompt therapy, neurologic symptoms may be irreversible. Such findings are not encountered with folate deficiency.

Thalassemia

Thalassemias are congenital anemias caused by deficient synthesis of globin chain subunits of the normal hemoglobins. Based on the affected globin chain, they are classified into β-thalassemia (defective β-chain production), α-thalassemia (defective α-chain production) and δ/β-thalassemia.

The basic defect is reduced or absent production of β-globin (in β-thalassemia) or α-globin (in α-thalassemia) chains. In a minority of thalassemia cases there are structural hemoglobin variants producing unstable globins. Since α- and β-chains normally pair to form hemoglobin tetramers, the lack of one type of chain leads to unpaired normal globin chains in thalassemic erythrocytes. In β-thalassemia, the resulting α-chains form an unstable structure that precipitates at the cell membrane, leading to excessive red blood fragility and erythrocyte destruction within the bone marrow. In α-thalassemia, there is an excess of β-chains (in extrauterine life), leading to hemoglobin composed only of β-chains. In intrauterine life, the excess of γ leads to hemoglobin composed only of γ-chains. In both cases, there is excessive red blood cell destruction caused by hemolysis.

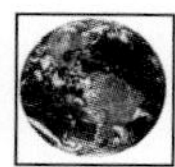

EPIDEMIOLOGY: Thalassemia is most common around the Mediterranean Sea, especially in Italy and Greece. It does, however, have a wide distribution, particularly in areas where malaria has been endemic (Middle East, India, Southeast Asia and China). A heterozygous state for thalassemia may provide a protective effect against malaria and increase the reproductive potential of heterozygotes, thereby explaining the persistence of thalassemic disorders. Many geographic areas with a higher incidence of thalassemia also exhibit an increased prevalence of structural hemoglobin defects (e.g., hemoglobin S). This situation leads double heterozygosity (e.g., sickle thalassemia), which demonstrates features of both disorders.

There are four α genes, paired on each chromosome 16. Non-α genes, two γ, one δ and one β gene per chromosome are on chromosome 11. Embryonic globin genes zeta (ζ) (α equivalent) and epsilon (ε) (non-α equivalent) are on chromosomes 16 and 11. The most important different types of hemoglobin and the globin chains that contribute to each are presented in Table 20-6.

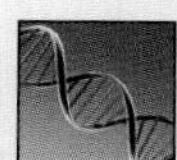

MOLECULAR PATHOGENESIS: Normal hemoglobin contains four globin chains: two α- and two non–α-chains. Three normal variants of hemoglobin are encountered, based on the nature of the non–α-chains (Fig. 20-14). ***Hemoglobin A ($\alpha_2\beta_2$) accounts for 95% to 98% of the total in adults; minor amounts of hemoglobin F ($\alpha_2\gamma_2$) and A2 ($\alpha_2\delta_2$) are present.***

Thalassemias are generally classified according to the affected globin chain. The two most clinically significant forms involve deficits of α- and β-chains. Thalassemias involving γ- and δ-globin chain synthesis have also been described but are not common.

β-Thalassemia

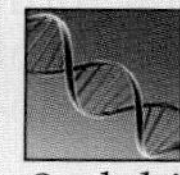

MOLECULAR PATHOGENESIS: β-Thalassemias are a heterogeneous group of disorders that are most often caused by point mutations in the β-globin gene. Mutations may be in the gene's promoter region, a splice site or other coding regions, or may lead to creation of an inappropriate stop codon. The result is that transcription of the gene is entirely (β^o) or partly (β^+) suppressed. Occasionally, a mutation may also affect the adjacent δ-globin gene, leading to a β–δ-thalassemia.

Table 20-6

Major Forms of Hemoglobin and Their Chain Composition

	Contribution of Globin Chains					
Type of Hemoglobin	α	β	γ	δ	ζ	**Explanation**
A	2	2				Principal normal hemoglobin (>95% of total) in postnatal life.
A_2	2			2		Usually <3% of total hemoglobin, but may be slightly increased in β-thalassemia.
F	2		2			Normal hemoglobin for most of intrauterine life. Production usually ends by early infancy; HbF is largely undetectable after 6 months of age. Persists in β-thalassemia.
H		4				Mainly seen in α-thalassemia, where deficiency of α-chains leads to hemoglobins composed of β-chain tetramers. Responsible for formation of Heinz bodies.
Bart's			4			Seen in babies with α-thalassemia. Heinz bodies seen.
Portland			2		2	Hemoglobin present very early in fetal life. May persist in very severe α-thalassemia.

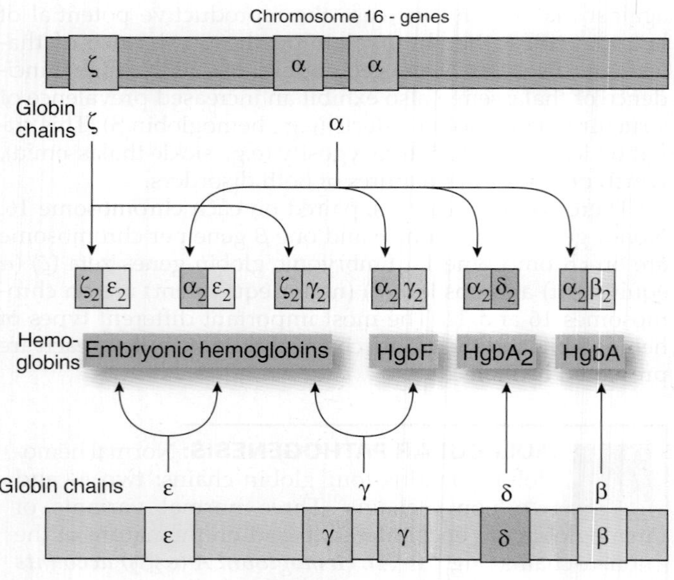

FIGURE 20-14. Hemoglobin assembly scheme using globin chains coded on chromosomes 11 and 16.

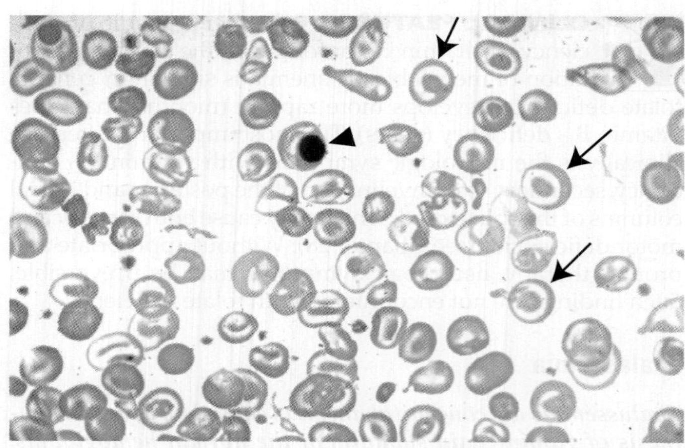

FIGURE 20-15. Thalassemia. The peripheral blood erythrocytes are hypochromic and microcytic and show anisopoikilocytosis with frequent target cells (*arrows*) and circulating nucleated red blood cells (*arrowhead*).

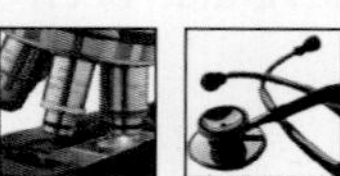

PATHOLOGY AND CLINICAL FEATURES: **Homozygous β-thalassemia (Cooley anemia)** is characterized by moderate to severe, microcytic and hypochromic anemia (Figs. 20-15 and 20-16). There is a marked excess of α-chains, which form unstable tetramers (α_4) that precipitate in the cytoplasm of developing erythroid precursors. In the β^o type, fetal hemoglobin accounts for most of the hemoglobin, although increased levels (5% to 8%) of hemoglobin A_2 are also present. In the case of β_1 type, some hemoglobin A may be detected (depending on the nature of the underlying defect) and hemoglobin A_2 is mildly increased. A modest increase in hemoglobin A_2 is characteristic of all forms of β-thalassemia, as δ-globin genes are upregulated.

In addition to microcytosis and hypochromia, blood smears demonstrate striking anisopoikilocytosis (uneven size and shape) with target cells, basophilic stippling and circulating normoblasts (especially after splenectomy). The

FIGURE 20-16. Pathogenesis of disease manifestations in β-thalassemia.

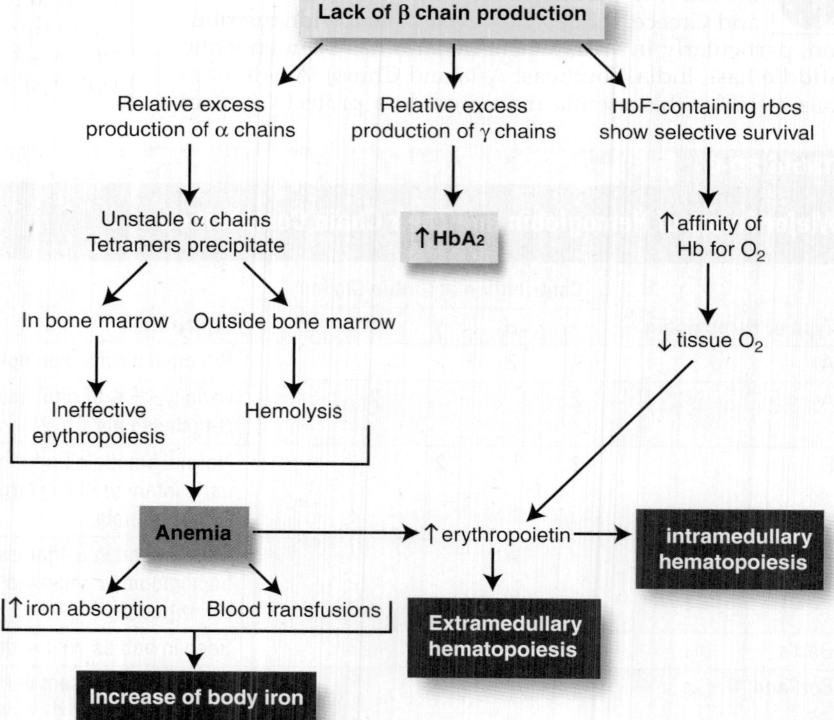

increased oxygen affinity of hemoglobin F plus the underlying anemia impair oxygen delivery and lead to increased EPO. The latter causes marked bone marrow erythroid hyperplasia. The marrow space is expanded, causing facial and cranial bone deformities. Extramedullary hematopoiesis contributes to hepatosplenomegaly and formation of soft tissue masses.

Excess erythropoiesis leads to increased iron absorption, which, together with repeated transfusions, creates iron overload. Excess iron deposition in tissues is a major cause of morbidity and mortality in thalassemic patients and often requires aggressive chelation therapy.

Heterozygous β-thalassemia (heterozygous carrier of β-thalassemia) is associated with microcytosis and hypochromia. The degree of microcytosis is disproportionate to the severity of the anemia, which is generally mild or absent. There is often an accompanying erythrocytosis (increased RBC count) but minimal anisocytosis (normal RDW). Target cells, basophilic stippling, increased reticulocytes and a mild increase in hemoglobin A_2 are present. Most patients are entirely asymptomatic. Iron absorption is increased.

α-Thalassemia

MOLECULAR PATHOGENESIS: Unlike β-thalassemias, α-thalassemias are most frequently caused by gene deletions. More syndromes are clinically observed because of the potential number (up to four) of α-globin genes that may be affected. The genetics of the several α-thalassemias are illustrated in Fig. 20-17. α-Thalassemia is associated with excess β- or γ-chains, which can then form the tetrameric hemoglobin H (β_4) and hemoglobin Bart (γ_4). Hemoglobins H and Bart are both unstable and precipitate in the cytoplasm, forming Heinz bodies, but to a lesser degree than α_4 tetramers. Further, they have high oxygen affinities and cause decreased tissue oxygen delivery. The relative amount of these tetrameric hemoglobins depends on the number of α genes involved and the patient's age. Because of the underlying impairment in hemoglobin synthesis, circulating red cells usually are microcytic and hypochromic.

PATHOLOGY AND CLINICAL FEATURES:

- **Silent carrier α-thalassemia** (one gene affected) is difficult to diagnose, because patients' only hematologic abnormality is small amounts of hemoglobin Bart, detectable only in infancy. There is no anemia, and patients are asymptomatic. **α-Thalassemia trait** (two genes affected) is associated with a mild microcytic anemia. Like heterozygous β-thalassemia, the degree of microcytosis is disproportionately low compared to the degree of anemia. Hemoglobin A_2 is not increased, allowing distinction between α- and β-thalassemia traits. Up to 5% hemoglobin Bart can be seen during infancy.

  Two different genotypes are possible in heterozygous α-thalassemia. There may be a single gene deleted from each chromosome 16 or, alternatively, both genes may be deleted from the same chromosome 16. The former scenario is more common in persons of Mediterranean and African descent; the latter is more frequent in Southeast Asia. Clinically, both genotypes present similarly, but homozygous α-thalassemia (see below) can only develop if both genes are deleted from the same chromosome.
- **Hemoglobin H disease** (three genes affected) is associated with moderate microcytic anemia. Increased hemoglobin Bart (up to 25% in infancy) and variable levels of hemoglobin H can be detected. Both hemoglobins H and Bart can be recognized by hemoglobin electrophoresis, since they migrate faster than hemoglobin A. Precipitated hemoglobin H (Heinz bodies) can also be demonstrated by supravital staining of a blood smear.

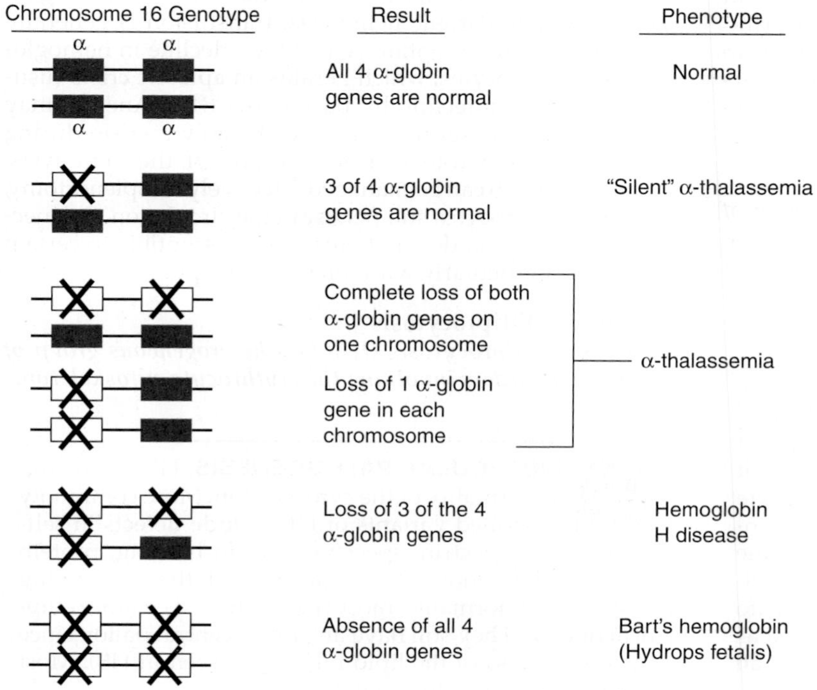

Chromosome 16 Genotype	Result	Phenotype
α α / α α	All 4 α-globin genes are normal	Normal
	3 of 4 α-globin genes are normal	"Silent" α-thalassemia
	Complete loss of both α-globin genes on one chromosome	α-thalassemia
	Loss of 1 α-globin gene in each chromosome	α-thalassemia
	Loss of 3 of the 4 α-globin genes	Hemoglobin H disease
	Absence of all 4 α-globin genes	Bart's hemoglobin (Hydrops fetalis)

FIGURE 20-17. Genetics of α-globin deficiencies and their manifestations.

- **Homozygous** (four genes affected) **α-thalassemia,** also termed α hydrops fetalis, is incompatible with life. Affected infants die in utero or shortly after birth with severe anemia, marked anisopoikilocytosis and large amounts of hemoglobin Bart. Severe impairment in tissue oxygen delivery is associated with heart failure and generalized edema. Massive hepatosplenomegaly is secondary to extramedullary hematopoiesis. It should be noted that a woman who carries a fetus with hemoglobin Bart is at increased risk for obstetric complications, including eclampsia and postpartum bleeding.

Hemolytic Anemias Feature Increased Red Cell Destruction

Hemolysis is the premature elimination of circulating erythrocytes. The resulting anemias are **hemolytic anemias.** These anemias are classified by the site of red cell destruction. In **extravascular hemolysis** the monocyte/macrophage system in the spleen and, to a lesser extent, the liver is involved. In **intravascular hemolysis**, erythrocytes are destroyed in the circulation.

Hemolytic anemias are characterized by a compensatory increase in red cell production and release. In the blood this manifests as polychromasia of red cells as a result of increased reticulocytes. Other laboratory findings commonly associated with hemolysis include increased LDH (particularly isoenzyme 1) and unconjugated (indirect) bilirubin, decreased haptoglobin, free (extracellular) hemoglobin in the blood and urine, increased urobilinogen and urine hemosiderin.

Erythrocyte Membrane Defects

Erythrocyte membranes are normally remarkably flexible and can deform to allow red cells to circulate unimpaired through the microcirculation and splenic vasculature. The red cell membrane consists of a lipid bilayer attached to an underlying cytoskeleton (Fig. 20-5). The main component of the cytoskeleton is spectrin, a dimer of α and β subunits. Ankyrin (band 2.1) anchors spectrin to transmembrane proteins (band 3, anion exchanger proteins), whereas spectrin is bound to actin and glycophorin by protein 4.1. ***Alterations in any portion of the red cell membrane can reduce the normal plasticity and render erythrocytes susceptible to hemolysis.***

Hereditary Spherocytosis

Hereditary spherocytosis (HS) is a heterogeneous group of inherited disorders of RBC cytoskeletons, characterized by a deficiency of spectrin or another cytoskeletal component (ankyrin, protein 4.2, band 3).

MOLECULAR PATHOGENESIS: The deficiency of a cytoskeletal protein in HS leads to a **"vertical"** defect in the red cell membrane, with uncoupling of the lipid bilayer from the underlying cytoskeleton. The result is progressive loss of membrane surface area and **spherocyte** formation. These abnormal red cells are more rigid and cannot easily traverse the spleen. While circulating through the spleen, spherocytes become "conditioned" and lose additional surface membrane before they ultimately succumb to extravascular hemolysis. Most forms of HS are inherited as autosomal dominant traits and the rare recessive cases all involve the α subunit of spectrin.

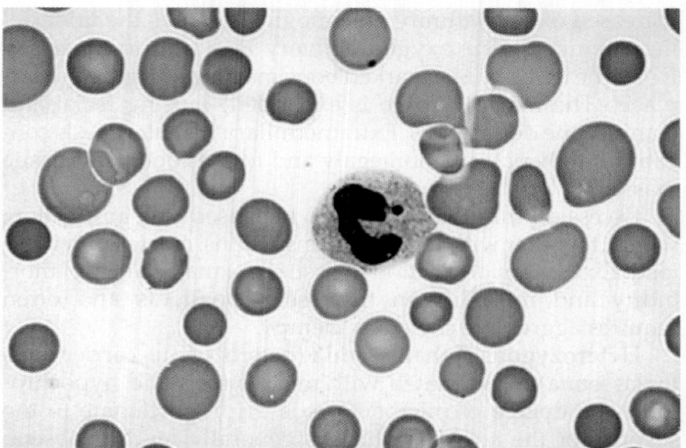

FIGURE 20-18. Hereditary spherocytosis. The peripheral blood smear shows frequent spherocytes with decreased diameter, intense staining and lack of central pallor (*arrows*).

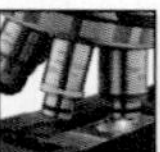

PATHOLOGY: Most patients with HS have a moderate normocytic anemia. Conspicuous spherocytes that appear hyperchromic (no central pallor) are typical, along with polychromasia and reticulocytosis (Fig. 20-18). The bone marrow shows erythroid hyperplasia. Although typical spherocytes have low MCV because of membrane loss and cell dehydration, these patients may have normal mean MCV because of increased reticulocytes (which are larger than average red blood cells).

Spherocytes show greater **osmotic fragility** than normal erythrocytes. Laboratory findings typical of hemolysis (decreased haptoglobin, increased indirect bilirubin, increased LDH) are often present.

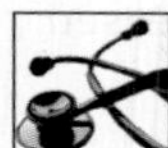

CLINICAL FEATURES: Most patients have splenomegaly caused by chronic extravascular hemolysis. They may appear jaundiced, and up to 50% develop cholelithiasis, with pigmented (bilirubin) gallstones. Despite chronic hemolysis, transfusion is generally not required. An exception is a sudden decline in hemoglobin and reticulocytes, which heralds an **aplastic crisis** (usually caused by infection by parvovirus B19). Anemia may also become more severe in so-called hemolytic crisis, during which there is a transient acceleration of the hemolysis. Patients with HS can be managed effectively by splenectomy, although spherocytes still persist in the circulation. Splenectomy, however, renders patients more susceptible to certain infections, particularly with *Streptococcus* spp.

Hereditary Elliptocytosis

Hereditary elliptocytosis (HE) is a heterogeneous group of inherited disorders involving the erythrocyte cytoskeleton.

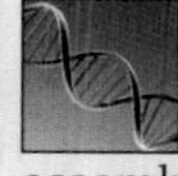

MOLECULAR PATHOGENESIS: HE features an abnormality of the cytoskeleton. More commonly described variants of HE include defects in self-assembly of spectrin, spectrin–ankyrin binding, protein 4.1 and glycophorin C. Regardless of the underlying molecular abnormality, most circulating red cells are elliptical or oval. They still have an area of central pallor, since there is no loss of the lipid bilayer (as seen in HS). Most forms of HE are autosomal dominant.

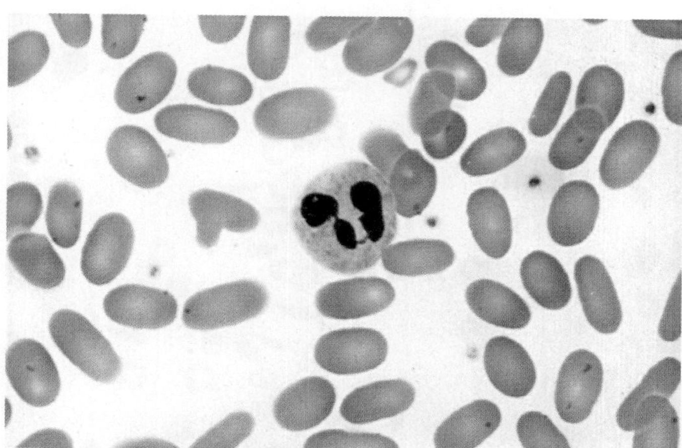

FIGURE 20-19. Hereditary elliptocytosis. A peripheral blood smear reveals that virtually all of the erythrocytes are elliptical with parallel sides.

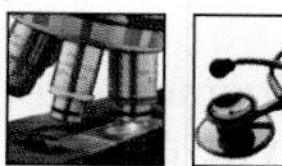

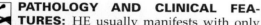

PATHOLOGY AND CLINICAL FEATURES: HE usually manifests with only mild normocytic anemia. Many patients are asymptomatic. Blood smears show numerous elliptocytes with only minimal reticulocytosis (Fig. 20-19). Generally, less hemolysis and subsequent anemia are seen than are seen with HS. Occasional patients with more severe hemolysis may require splenectomy.

Acanthocytosis

Acanthocytosis results from a defect within the lipid bilayer of the red cell membrane and features irregularly spaced spiny projections of the surface, which may be associated with hemolysis.

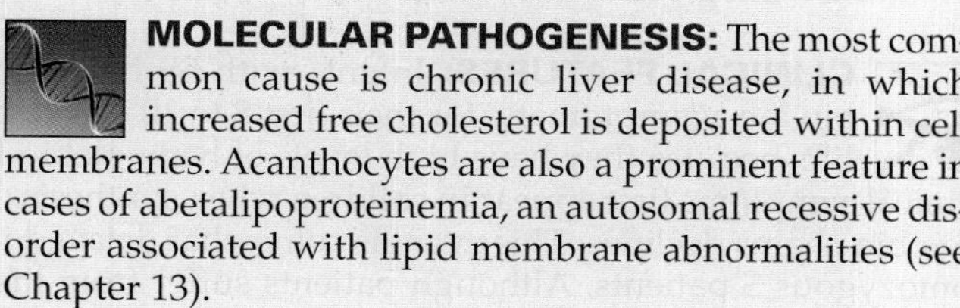

MOLECULAR PATHOGENESIS: The most common cause is chronic liver disease, in which increased free cholesterol is deposited within cell membranes. Acanthocytes are also a prominent feature in cases of abetalipoproteinemia, an autosomal recessive disorder associated with lipid membrane abnormalities (see Chapter 13).

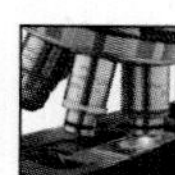
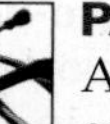

PATHOLOGY AND CLINICAL FEATURES: Abnormalities in the lipid membrane cause erythrocytes to become deformed and develop irregular spiny surface projections and centrally dense cytoplasm (no central pallor) (Fig. 20-20). These red cells are called **acanthocytes** (spur cells). They should be distinguished from burr cells (crenated cells, **echinocytes**), which have more uniform cell membrane scalloping and maintain an area of central pallor. Hemolysis and anemia in acanthocytosis are mild.

Enzyme Defects

Energy generation within erythrocytes occurs primarily by glycolysis. Inherited defects of enzymes in the glycolytic pathway can predispose circulating red cells to hemolysis. The most common enzyme defect involves glucose-6-phosphate dehydrogenase (G6PD), which catalyzes conversion of glucose-6-phosphate to 6-phosphogluconate. Deficiencies of other glycolytic enzymes are rare and autosomal recessive. Among these, pyruvate kinase deficiency is the most common. Clinically, these defects cause variable degrees of anemia and are designated **hereditary nonspherocytic anemias.**

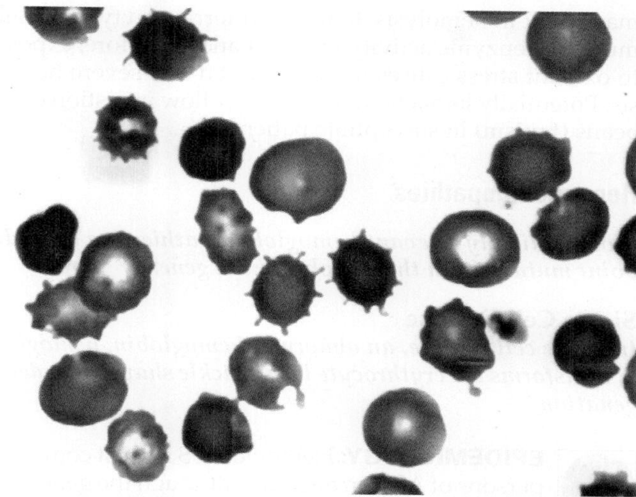

FIGURE 20-20. Acanthocytes. The red cells lack central pallor and display irregular spikes on the surface.

G6PD deficiency is an X-linked disorder in which abnormal red cell sensitivity to oxidative stress manifests as hemolytic anemia. G6PD deficiency has a variable worldwide distribution, with the highest prevalence in areas where malaria is historically endemic, notably Africa and the Mediterranean region. Various mutations have been identified. G6PD mutations appear to provide some protective effect against malaria.

MOLECULAR PATHOGENESIS: Because G6PD helps to recycle reduced glutathione, red cells deficient in this enzyme are susceptible to oxidative stress (e.g., infections, drugs or fava bean ingestion [favism]). Oxidation of hemoglobin leads to formation of methemoglobin, in which Fe^{2+} ions are converted to ferric (Fe^{3+}) ions. Methemoglobin cannot transport oxygen, is unstable and precipitates in the cytoplasm as Heinz bodies. Precipitated methemoglobin increases cell rigidity and leads to hemolysis.

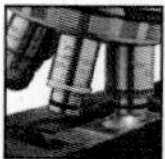

PATHOLOGY: In quiescent periods, erythrocytes in G6PD deficiency appear normal. However, in a hemolytic episode precipitated by oxidative stress, Heinz bodies can be demonstrated by supravital staining. After passage through the spleen, circulating red cells may have part of their membrane removed, forming so-called **bite cells**.

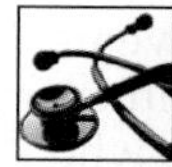

CLINICAL FEATURES: Full expression of G6PD deficiency is seen only in males, with females being asymptomatic carriers. The A variant of G6PD is seen in 10% to 15% of American blacks and is associated with reduced enzyme activity (10% of normal) because of instability of the molecule. In affected patients, exposure to oxidant drugs, such as the antimalarial agent primaquine, may result in hemolysis. In the Mediterranean type of G6PD mutation, enzyme activity is absent and, therefore, exposure to oxidant stress causes more sustained and severe hemolysis. Potentially lethal hemolysis may follow ingestion of fava beans **(favism)** in susceptible patients.

Hemoglobinopathies

Most clinically relevant hemoglobinopathies are caused by point mutations in the β-globin chain gene.

Sickle Cell Disease

In sickle cell disease, an abnormal hemoglobin, hemoglobin S, transforms the erythrocyte into a sickle shape upon deoxygenation.

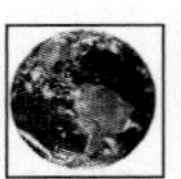

EPIDEMIOLOGY: Hemoglobin S is most common in persons of African ancestry, although the gene is also present in Mediterranean, Middle Eastern and Indian populations. In some regions of Africa, up to 40% of the population is heterozygous for hemoglobin S. Ten percent of American blacks are heterozygous and 1 in 650 is homozygous. Heterozygosity for hemoglobin S is thought to provide some protection against falciparum malaria. Infected erythrocytes selectively sickle and are removed from the circulation by splenic and hepatic macrophages, effectively destroying the parasite.

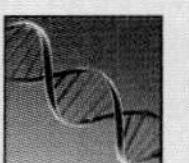

MOLECULAR PATHOGENESIS: In hemoglobin S a point mutation in the gene for the β-globin chain gene substitutes valine for glutamic acid at the sixth amino acid. This single change generates a structurally abnormal molecule that polymerizes under conditions of deoxygenation. Polymerization of hemoglobin S transforms the cytoplasm into a rigid filamentous gel and leads to the formation of less deformable sickled erythrocytes.

The rigidity of sickled erythrocytes results in obstruction of the microcirculation, with subsequent tissue hypoxia and ischemic injury in many organs. The inflexible nature of sickle cells also renders them susceptible to destruction (hemolysis) during circulation through the spleen. Thus, the two primary manifestations of sickle cell disease are recurrent ischemic events and chronic extravascular hemolytic anemia.

Erythrocyte sickling is initially reversible with reoxygenation, but after several cycles of sickling and unsickling, the process becomes irreversible. Sickled erythrocytes also have changes in the phospholipids of the membrane, and so adhere more strongly to endothelial cells, which further impairs capillary blood flow.

People who are homozygous for hemoglobin S show the full clinical presentation of sickle cell disease. A sickling disorder is also observed in patients who are doubly heterozygous for two β-chain mutations (e.g., hemoglobin SC disease, sickle/β-thalassemia). Heterozygotes for hemoglobin S (sickle cell trait), however, do not develop red cell sickling, because their hemoglobin A prevents hemoglobin S polymerization. Hemoglobin F also interferes with hemoglobin S polymerization, and patients who are homozygous for hemoglobin S and have increased levels of hemoglobin F have a milder form of disease.

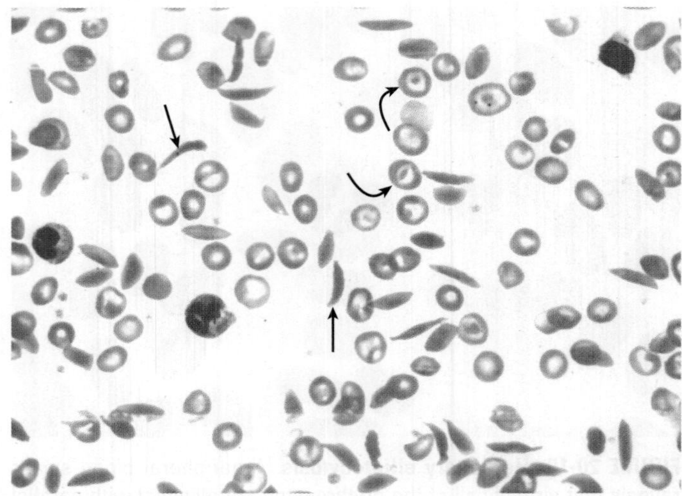

FIGURE 20-21. Sickle cell anemia. Sickled cells (*straight arrows*) and target cells (*curved arrows*) are evident in the blood smear.

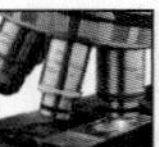

PATHOLOGY: Homozygous patients (hemoglobin SS) have severe normocytic or macrocytic anemia. The macrocytosis can be attributed to increased numbers of reticulocytes, secondary to chronic hemolysis. Blood smear examination reveals marked anisopoikilocytosis and polychromasia. Classic sickle cells and target cells, as well as a variety of other abnormally shaped erythrocytes, are observed (Fig. 20-21). Howell-Jolly bodies, representing nuclear remnants, are seen in most patients beyond childhood and reflect hyposplenism caused by ischemic loss of splenic tissue.

Electrophoretic analysis shows that hemoglobin S accounts for 80% to 95% of the total hemoglobin and hemoglobin A is absent. Hemoglobins F and A_2 account for the remaining hemoglobin.

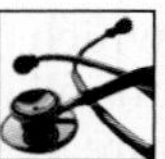

CLINICAL FEATURES: Infants with SS hemoglobin are asymptomatic for their first 8 to 10 weeks of life, because they have high levels of hemoglobin F. Clinical symptoms first appear in children when synthesis of γ-globin chains declines. This event is somewhat delayed in homozygous S patients. Although patients suffer from lifelong hemolysis, adaptation occurs over time and most may not require regular transfusions. Instead, the clinical picture is dominated by sequelae of repeated **vaso-occlusive disease.** In an attempt to minimize these complications by decreasing the amount of hemoglobin S in circulation, a chronic exchange transfusion program may become necessary. Sickle cell anemia is a systemic disorder and is eventually responsible for impaired function in most organ systems and tissues (Fig. 20-22).

Patients with sickle cell disease develop episodic painful crises, the number of which varies. Capillary occlusion leads to ischemia and hypoxic cell injury, which cause severe pain, especially in the chest, abdomen and bones. Painful crises can be triggered by various stimuli (e.g., underlying infection, acidosis or dehydration).

APLASTIC CRISIS: In aplastic crisis, the bone marrow fails to compensate for the high level of red cell loss. Hemoglobin levels drop rapidly and there is no reticulocyte response. Parvovirus B19 is the most frequent cause of an

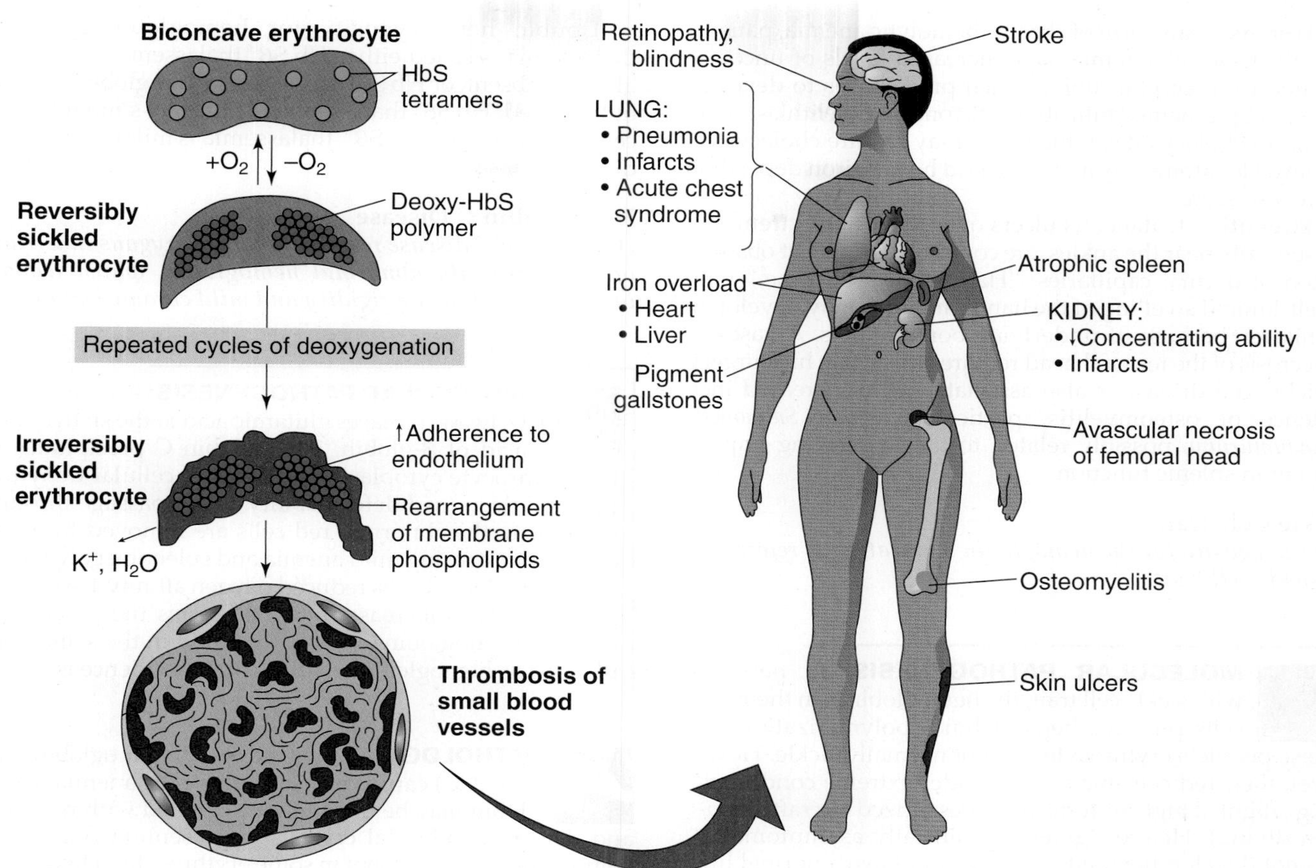

FIGURE 20-22. Pathogenesis of the vascular complications of sickle cell anemia. Substitution of valine for glutamic acid leads to an alteration in the surface charge of the hemoglobin molecule. Upon deoxygenation ($-O_2$), sickle hemoglobin (HbS) tetramers aggregate to form poorly soluble polymers. The erythrocytes change shape from a biconcave disk to a sickle form with the polymerization of HbS. This process is initially reversible upon reoxygenation ($+O_2$), but with repeated cycles of deoxygenation and reoxygenation, the erythrocytes become irreversibly sickled. Irreversibly sickled cells display a rearrangement of phospholipids between the outer and inner monolayers of the cell membrane, in particular an increase in aminophospholipids in the outer leaflet. Potassium (K^+) and water (H_2O) are lost from the cells. The erythrocytes are no longer deformable and are more adherent to endothelial cells, properties that predispose to thrombosis in small blood vessels. The resulting vascular occlusions lead to widespread ischemic complications.

aplastic crisis, although other viral and bacterial infections may also cause transient bone marrow suppression.

SEQUESTRATION CRISIS: In this case, sudden pooling of erythrocytes, especially in the spleen, results in a decreased circulating blood volume and low hemoglobin levels. The etiology is not well understood, but it most frequently develops in young children, who still have a functioning spleen. This complication is followed by hypovolemic shock and is the most frequent cause of death early in life.

- **Heart:** Chronic demand for increased cardiac output may lead to cardiomegaly and congestive heart failure. In addition, obstruction of coronary microcirculation may cause myocardial ischemia. Myocyte function may also be impaired by excess iron deposition, as a result of the chronic hemolysis and repeated transfusions.
- **Lungs:** Up to one third of patients with sickle cell anemia show a rapid decrease in respiratory function, associated with pulmonary infiltrates on chest radiography. This **acute chest syndrome** may be fatal. Pulmonary infarction may occur, and sickle cell patients are more susceptible to a variety of pulmonary infections.
- **Spleen:** Although splenomegaly is often found in childhood, repeated splenic infarction leads to a functional autosplenectomy. In most adults, only a small fibrous remnant of the spleen remains. The asplenic state renders the patient prone to infections with encapsulated bacteria, especially pneumococcus.
- **Brain:** Patients with sickle cell anemia develop neurologic complications related to vascular obstruction, including transient ischemic attacks, overt strokes and cerebral hemorrhages. Occlusion of retinal microvasculature may lead to retinal hemorrhage and detachment, proliferative retinopathy and blindness.
- **Kidney:** Sickling commonly occurs in the renal medulla because of the hypoxic, acidotic and hypertonic environment that normally exists there. Complications include inability to form concentrated urine, renal infarcts and papillary necrosis. Male patients may develop priapism, which, if not treated promptly, may lead to permanent erectile dysfunction.

- **Liver:** As in any form of chronic hemolytic anemia, patients with sickle cell anemia have increased levels of unconjugated (indirect) bilirubin, which predisposes to development of pigmented bilirubin gallstones. Cholelithiasis may lead to cholecystitis, which then may require cholecystectomy. Hepatomegaly and increased hepatic iron deposition are also seen.
- **Extremities:** Cutaneous ulcers over the lower extremities, especially near the ankles, are common and reflect obstruction of dermal capillaries. "Hand–foot syndrome," with self-limited swelling of the hands and feet, may develop in children because of underlying bone infarcts. A vascular necrosis of the femoral head requires corrective hip surgery. Sickle cell disease is also associated with increased incidence of osteomyelitis, particularly with *Salmonella typhimurium*, possibly related to the underlying impairment in splenic function.

Sickle Cell Trait

Heterozygosity for the hemoglobin S mutation is referred to as sickle cell trait.

MOLECULAR PATHOGENESIS: In persons with sickle cell trait, the hemoglobin A in their red cells prevents hemoglobin S polymerization, so these people's erythrocytes do not normally sickle. However, their red cells may sickle under extreme conditions (e.g., flight at high altitude in unpressurized aircraft, deep-sea diving). Heterozygotes are clinically asymptomatic, do not develop hemolytic anemia and have a normal life span.

Double Heterozygosity for Hemoglobin S and Other Hemoglobinopathies

Some patients with a sickling disorder are actually heterozygous for both hemoglobin S and other abnormal hemoglobins (e.g., hemoglobin C or D) or for thalassemia.

MOLECULAR PATHOGENESIS: The presence of an additional abnormal hemoglobin or thalassemic gene does not prevent polymerization of hemoglobin S, and the clinical expression and severity of disease may be affected. Doubly heterozygous individuals may have less frequent crises, higher baseline hemoglobin values, microcytic red cell indices or persistent splenomegaly into adult life.

CLINICAL FEATURES: Double heterozygosity for hemoglobins S and C produces a less severe sickle phenotype than does homozygosity for hemoglobin S. These patients have episodic skeletal or abdominal pain. However, they develop a retinopathy that is relatively common and severe. As well, they are prone to undergo necrosis of the heads of their femurs. These features are thought to reflect the high blood viscosity conferred by hemoglobin SC.

Blood smears from hemoglobin SC patients reveal mild reticulocytosis, target cells and relatively few sickled erythrocytes. However, red blood cells with hemoglobin crystals caused by hemoglobin C are seen.

Double heterozygosity for hemoglobin S and β-thalassemia is called either Hb Sβ^0 thalassemia, in which β-globin is absent, or Hb Sβ^+ thalassemia, if β-globin is present but reduced. Hb Sβ^0 thalassemia is clinically similar to sickle cell disease in severity. Sβ^+ thalassemia is milder than Hb SC disease.

Hemoglobin C Disease

Hemoglobin C disease results from homozygous inheritance of a structurally abnormal hemoglobin, which leads to increased erythrocyte rigidity and mild chronic hemolysis.

MOLECULAR PATHOGENESIS: In hemoglobin C, lysine replaces glutamic acid at the sixth amino acid of β-globin. Hemoglobin C precipitates in the erythrocyte cytoplasm and leads to cellular dehydration and decreased deformability. Upon passage through the spleen, the abnormal red cells are removed from the circulation, causing mild anemia and splenomegaly. Given that hemoglobin C has reduced oxygen affinity, tissue oxygen delivery is increased, which lessens the severity of disease. Hemoglobin C is mostly found in the same populations as hemoglobin S, although its incidence is less.

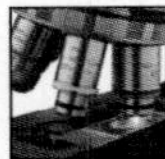

PATHOLOGY: Homozygosity for hemoglobin C disease (CC) causes a mild normocytic anemia. Hemoglobin may be unevenly distributed within red cells and dense, rhomboidal crystals (representing precipitated hemoglobin C) are present in some erythrocytes. Hemoglobin electrophoresis reveals no hemoglobin A and more than 90% hemoglobin C.

Two to 3% of American blacks are heterozygous for hemoglobin C and are asymptomatic (hemoglobin C trait). In such people, about 40% of hemoglobin is hemoglobin C. Red cell morphology is normal, except for some target cells.

Hemoglobin E Disease

Hemoglobin E disease is a result of homozygosity for a structurally abnormal hemoglobin, leading to a thalassemia-like defect that is associated with mild chronic hemolysis.

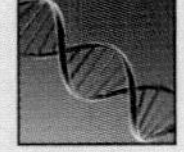

MOLECULAR PATHOGENESIS: In hemoglobin E, lysine substitutes for glutamic acid at position 26 of the β-globin chain. This position is at a splice site in the gene, so the mutation results in a structurally abnormal molecule, decreased transcription of the gene and unstable β-globin messenger RNA (mRNA). The latter defects diminish synthesis of hemoglobin E, creating a situation akin to that seen with thalassemia. Hemoglobin E is relatively unstable and may precipitate within the cell, leading to hemolysis. Hemoglobin E is most prevalent in Southeast Asia and globally is second in incidence only to hemoglobin S. Hemoglobin E is believed to exert a protective effect against malaria.

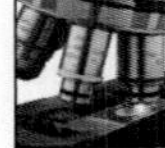

PATHOLOGY: Patients homozygous for hemoglobin E (EE) have a mild microcytic anemia. MCV is decreased, and there is often erythrocytosis because of the thalassemia-like component. Blood smear examination reveals microcytic, hypochromic red cells, and target cells. More than 90% of hemoglobin is hemoglobin E.

Other Hemoglobinopathies

Several hundred additional hemoglobin variants have been described that result from mutations in α- or β-globin genes. These mutations may lead to structural abnormalities or to a functional derangement of the hemoglobin molecule.

MOLECULAR PATHOGENESIS: Some mutations alter the tertiary structure of hemoglobin, leading to its destabilization and precipitation in the cytoplasm. As a group, these hemoglobins are referred to as **unstable hemoglobins** and are often named after the geographic location in which they were first discovered (e.g., hemoglobin Köln). Unstable hemoglobins precipitate and form Heinz bodies within the erythrocytes that can be shown with supravital staining. Heinz bodies bind to cell membranes, increasing their rigidity and leading to mild chronic hemolysis. Patients may suffer jaundice and splenomegaly.

Other hemoglobin mutations cause **abnormal oxygen affinity. Increased oxygen affinity** leads to decreased tissue oxygen delivery. Resulting hypoxia leads to increased EPO production and erythroid hyperplasia in the bone marrow. This in turn causes erythrocytosis. Patients are mostly asymptomatic, but in some cases they may have symptoms related to hyperviscosity. Abnormal hemoglobins with **decreased oxygen affinity** readily release oxygen at the tissue level. EPO levels are low, and most patients have mild anemia. Because of increased of deoxyhemoglobin, patients appear cyanotic.

Immune and Autoimmune Hemolytic Anemias

In immune hemolytic anemias, red cell destruction (hemolysis) is caused by antibodies against antigens at the erythrocyte surface. The red cells themselves are intrinsically normal but are targets for an immune-mediated attack. Immune hemolytic anemia can develop secondary to either auto- or alloantibodies, and the site of hemolysis may be **extravascular** or **intravascular**.

Autoimmune hemolytic anemia (AIHA) features autoantibodies against red cells. Autoantibodies can be classified as either **warm** or **cold antibodies.**

Warm Antibody Autoimmune Hemolytic Anemia

MOLECULAR PATHOGENESIS: Warm autoantibodies have optimal reactivity at 37°C (98.6° F) and account for 80% of all cases of AIHA. They are usually immunoglobulin G (IgG) and directed against erythrocyte membrane antigens such as **Rh group proteins.** They do not bind complement, but "coat" red blood cells, followed by removal of these RBCs by macrophages of the reticuloendothelial system (extravascular hemolysis), primarily in the spleen. Splenic macrophages have Fc receptors that recognize erythrocyte-bound warm antibodies and remove segments of the membrane with attached antibody. Progressive loss of membrane leads to formation of spherocytes, which ultimately undergo hemolysis.

Warm antibody AIHA affects women more often than men, and half of cases are idiopathic. In the remaining cases, warm antibody reflects an underlying condition, such as infection, collagen vascular disease, lymphoproliferative disorders and drug reactions.

Drug-induced warm antibodies may arise by several different mechanisms (see Chapter 4). In the **hapten** mechanism, a drug such as penicillin binds to erythrocyte surfaces. With this modification, the red cell–drug complex elicits antibodies, some of which react with the erythrocyte itself. In the **immune complex** mechanism, a drug (such as quinidine) reacts with specific circulating antibody to form immune complexes, which are then bound to red cell membranes. In the **autoantibody** mechanism, a drug (e.g., α-methyldopa) leads to the formation of antibodies that cross-react with red cell membrane components. In both hapten and immune-complex models, the drug is required for hemolysis, whereas in the autoantibody model, hemolysis occurs in the absence of the initiating drug.

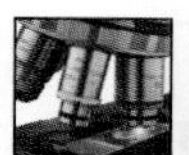
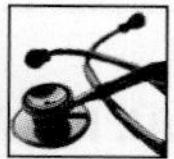

PATHOLOGY AND CLINICAL FEATURES: Warm antibody AIHA is associated with normocytic or occasionally macrocytic anemia, with spherocytes and polychromasia. Extravascular hemolysis results in increased serum bilirubin, mostly unconjugated bilirubin, but hemoglobinemia (excess of hemoglobin in the blood) and hemoglobinuria (hemoglobin in the urine) are usually absent. The direct antiglobulin (Coombs) test is usually positive and is useful in distinguishing immune from nonimmune spherocytosis. In the direct Coombs test, the patient's red cells are incubated with antihuman globulin serum. Agglutination indicates antibody is present on the cell surface. Warm antibody AIHA is treated with corticosteroids or other immunosuppressive agents. Refractory cases may require splenectomy or transfusions.

Cold Antibody Autoimmune Hemolytic Anemia

Cold antibodies have maximal reactivity at 4°C (39.2°F). Some 20% of cases of AIHA are caused by cold IgM or IgG antibodies, which occur as cold agglutinins or hemolysins.

MOLECULAR PATHOGENESIS: Cold agglutinins are mostly IgM directed against the I/i antigen system on red cells. At cooler temperatures in the peripheral circulation, these antibodies bind and agglutinate red cells (Fig. 20-23) and fix complement, followed by complement activation through the C3 stage. These complement-coated red cells may undergo extravascular hemolysis in the liver, because Kupffer cells have more complement receptors than do splenic macrophages. Occasionally, IgM autoantibodies are reactive at greater than 30°C (high thermal amplitude) and activate the classic complement pathway on the RBC membrane, starting with C1q binding and going all the way to the membrane attack complex. This process leads to intravascular hemolysis, resulting in hemoglobinemia, hemoglobinuria and decreased haptoglobin levels (free hemoglobin released into the circulation binds haptoglobin, which causes a decline in haptoglobin). Cold agglutinins may be idiopathic or develop secondary to an underlying condition, mostly infections (Epstein-Barr virus [EBV], *Mycoplasma*) or lymphoproliferative disorders.

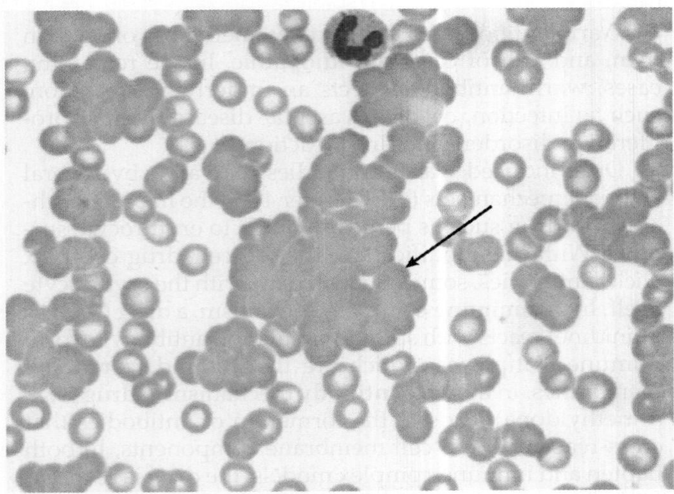

FIGURE 20-23. Red blood cell clumping (agglutination) caused by cold agglutinins (*arrow*). Note that this is not the same phenomenon as rouleaux formation.

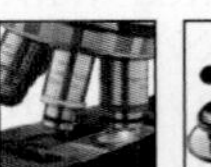
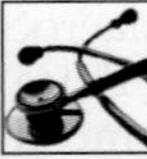

PATHOLOGY AND CLINICAL FEATURES: Cold agglutinins often are activated upon cooling of blood to room temperature, and erythrocyte agglutination in vitro can be noted on blood smears (Fig. 20-23). Agglutination leads to falsely low RBCs and hematocrit (Hct) and falsely elevated MCV and MCHC. Warming a blood sample to 37°C (98.6°F) prior to analysis corrects the spurious results. The direct Coombs test is positive but usually only for the presence of complement on red cells. Significant hemolysis is uncommon with cold agglutinins and patients are more likely to develop peripheral vascular symptoms (Raynaud phenomenon) upon cold exposure, because of red cell agglutination.

Cold Hemolysin Disease

MOLECULAR PATHOGENESIS: Cold hemolysins (Donath-Landsteiner antibodies) are usually biphasic IgGs and directed against the P antigen system on red cells. Cold hemolysins have biphasic activity and rarely cause AIHA. The antibody binds to erythrocytes at low temperatures and fixes complement, but intravascular hemolysis does not occur at these temperatures. Because the antibody is IgG, red cells do not agglutinate. Upon warming to 37°C, the cold hemolysin remains attached, complement is activated and intravascular hemolysis occurs.

The clinical syndrome related to cold hemolysins is designated **paroxysmal cold hemoglobinuria (PCH).** PCH most often follows a viral illness. Immunosuppressive therapy and splenectomy are usually ineffective. Cold avoidance and supportive therapy such as RBC transfusions are required.

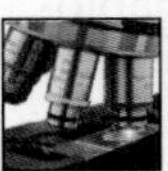

PATHOLOGY: Patients with PCH may develop severe anemia, decreased haptoglobin levels and hemoglobinuria secondary to intravascular hemolysis. The direct Coombs test is positive for complement but may be negative for IgG, since cold hemolysins may readily dissociate from red cells in vitro.

Hemolytic Transfusion Reactions

An **immediate hemolytic transfusion** reaction occurs when grossly incompatible blood is administered to a patient with preformed alloantibodies, usually because of a clerical error. Massive hemolysis of the transfused blood may be associated with severe complications, including hypotension, renal failure and even death. Hemolytic transfusion reaction and hemolytic disease in the newborn (see below) are examples of **alloimmune hemolytic anemia,** which refers to the destruction of fetal red cells by alloantibodies.

Delayed hemolytic transfusion reactions usually involve antibodies to minor red cell antigens. Following initial exposure to such antigens, antibody levels rise, but then may decline to the point where they are undetectable in routine pretransfusion screening tests. Subsequent reexposure to the offending antigen elicits an anamnestic antibody response, with hemolysis occurring several days later. Delayed hemolytic transfusion reactions are usually less severe than immediate reactions and may be clinically undetectable. In both types of hemolytic transfusion reactions, the direct antiglobulin test is positive.

Hemolytic Disease of the Newborn

Hemolytic disease of the newborn (HDN) reflects incompatibility of blood types between a mother and her developing fetus; the mother lacks an antigen that is expressed by the fetus. Maternal IgG alloantibodies can then cross the placenta and cause hemolysis of fetal erythrocytes and erythroblastosis detectable in peripheral blood smears (Fig. 20-24). Erythroblasts (immature red blood cells) are released from the fetal bone marrow in an effort to compensate for the RBC loss. Most commonly, HDN antibodies react to ABO or Rh antigens.

With ABO-type HDN, the mother is type O and the fetus is usually type A. Naturally occurring maternal anti-A antibodies cause hemolysis in the fetus. No prior exposure through pregnancy or transfusion is required for hemolysis to develop. The anemia associated with ABO incompatibility is usually mild. Affected babies develop hyperbilirubinemia, spherocytosis and a positive direct antiglobulin test.

With Rh-type HDN, the mother is Rh negative and the fetus is Rh positive. The D antigen is most frequently involved,

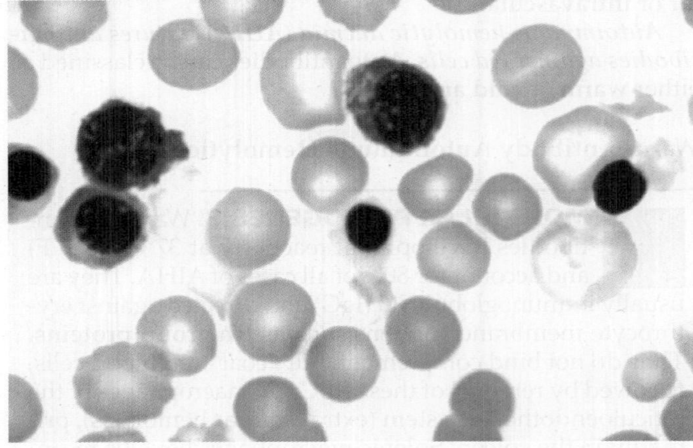

FIGURE 20-24. Hemolytic disease of the newborn (HDN). The presence of nucleated red blood cells in the peripheral blood is abnormal. They are often present in various types of hemolytic disorders, but are particularly numerous in HDN.

although minor Rh antigens can also cause disease. Prior maternal exposure reflects previous pregnancy or transfusion. The severity of the disease varies, but hemolysis in Rh incompatibility is generally more significant than in ABO-type HDN. Severely affected fetuses may develop **hydrops fetalis,** characterized by heart failure, generalized edema, ascites and intrauterine death (see Chapter 6). Fortunately, today most cases of D-related HDN are preventable by passive immunization of Rh-negative mothers during pregnancy with injections of Rh immune globulin. Laboratory findings are similar to those described above for ABO HDN.

Nonimmune Hemolytic Anemias

In nonimmune hemolytic anemias, red cell destruction is caused by factors other than antibodies against red cell antigens. Examples include red cell fragmentation syndromes and march hemoglobinuria.

Mechanical Red Cell Fragmentation Syndromes (Microangiopathic Hemolytic Anemia)

In red cell fragmentation syndromes, intrinsically normal erythrocytes are subjected to mechanical disruption as they circulate in the blood (intravascular hemolysis).

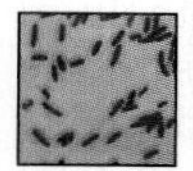

ETIOLOGIC FACTORS: In **microangiopathic** hemolytic anemia, mechanical fragmentation of red cells is caused either by their contact with an abnormal surface (e.g., prosthetic heart valve, synthetic vascular graft) or alteration of the endothelial surface of small blood vessels with resulting fibrin deposition (with capillary thrombosis) and platelet aggregation. As erythrocytes travel through these damaged vessels, they are fragmented by these fibrin meshworks (Fig. 20-7). Classic examples of microangiopathic hemolysis include **disseminated intravascular coagulation** (DIC), **thrombotic thrombocytopenic purpura** (TTP) and hemolytic uremic syndrome. Alterations in blood flow, as are encountered in malignant hypertension or vasculitis syndromes, may also lead to mechanical fragmentation of erythrocytes.

Long-distance running or walking ("march hemoglobinuria") or prolonged vigorous exercise can cause repetitive trauma to red cells and lead to hemolysis.

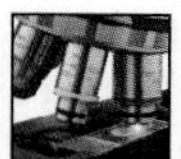

PATHOLOGY: Laboratory findings seen in microangiopathic hemolytic anemias are similar regardless of the underlying etiology. Anemia is mild to moderate and an appropriate reticulocyte response is seen. Blood smears show fragmented erythrocytes (schistocytes) and polychromasia (Fig. 20-25). Abnormalities in coagulation and thrombocytopenia characterize DIC, whereas thrombocytopenia alone is seen in cases of TTP (see below).

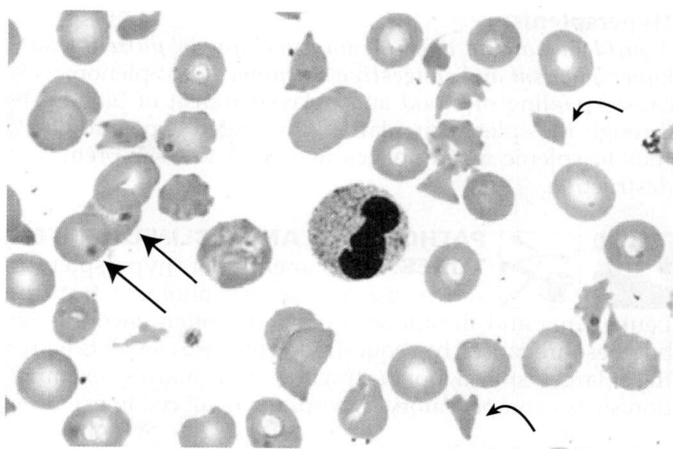

FIGURE 20-25. Microangiopathic hemolytic anemia (MAHA). Irregular, fragmented erythrocytes (schistocytes, *curved arrows*) are seen in the blood smear of a patient with disseminated intravascular coagulation. Howell-Jolly bodies are also present (*straight arrows*).

Paroxysmal Nocturnal Hemoglobinuria

Paroxysmal nocturnal hemoglobinuria (PNH) is an acquired clonal stem cell disorder characterized by episodic intravascular hemolytic anemia resulting from increased sensitivity of erythrocytes to complement-mediated lysis.

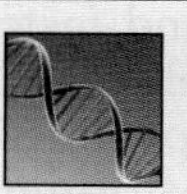

MOLECULAR PATHOGENESIS: The underlying defect in cases of PNH involves somatic mutation of the *phosphatidylinositol glycan-class A (PIG-A)* gene, on the short arm of the X chromosome (Xp22.1) in hematopoietic stem cells. Mutation of the *PIG-A* gene leads to disrupted synthesis of glycosyl phosphatidylinositol (GPI), which normally anchors many proteins (e.g., cluster designation [CD]14, CD16, CD55, CD59) to red cell membranes. Consequent loss of **decay acceleration factor** (CD55) and more importantly **membrane inhibitor of reactive lysis** (CD59) from erythrocyte surfaces renders the cells susceptible to complement-mediated hemolysis. Leukocytes and platelets derived from the abnormal stem cells also show loss of GPI-linked membrane proteins.

PNH may develop as a primary disorder or evolve from preexisting aplastic anemia. Because the defect is clonal, it may progress to **myelodysplasia** or overt **acute leukemia.** Some patients exhibit several abnormal clonal erythrocyte populations, with varying susceptibility to complement.

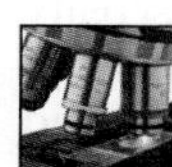

PATHOLOGY: During hemolytic episodes, patients develop varyingly severe normocytic or macrocytic anemia, with an appropriate reticulocyte response. Because the hemolysis is intravascular, hemoglobinuria is present, and iron deficiency may develop over time from recurrent iron loss in the urine. Traditionally, increased lysis of patient red cells when incubated with sugar (sucrose hemolysis test) or acidified serum (Ham test) suggest PNH. Both manipulations enhance complement binding to red cells. ***Today, PNH is diagnosed by demonstrating loss of GPI-anchored proteins on blood cells by flow cytometry.*** Leukopenia and thrombocytopenia are frequently detected, and sensitivity to complement may lead to inappropriate platelet activation.

CLINICAL FEATURES: Patients develop intermittent intravascular hemolysis, although it is nocturnal in only a minority of cases. Venous and arterial thrombosis, notably Budd-Chiari syndrome (hepatic vein thrombosis), are increased in PNH as a result of complement-mediated platelet activation. Thrombocytopenia may lead to bleeding. Treatment is supportive; bone marrow transplantation is curative.

Hyperspenism

A mild hemolytic anemia may develop in patients with hypersplenism and congestive splenomegaly. Splenomegaly causes pooling of blood and delayed transit of blood cells through the splenic circulation. Prolonged exposure of red cells to splenic macrophages may lead to their premature destruction.

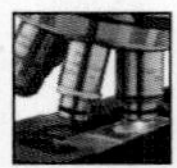
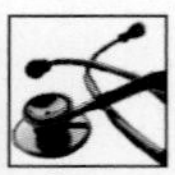

PATHOLOGY AND CLINICAL FEATURES: The anemia of hypersplenism shows no specific morphologic features. Leukopenia and thrombocytopenia are often encountered, but these are caused by sequestration of these elements within the enlarged spleen, not destruction. Bone marrow examination shows compensatory hyperplasia of all cell lines.

Other Hemolytic Anemias

Severe thermal burns lead to intravascular hemolysis of erythrocytes. Normal red cells undergo membrane disruption and fragmentation when exposed to temperatures over 49°C (120.2°F). Blood smears reveal numerous schistocytes and microspherocytes, as well as polychromasia. The direct Coombs test is negative.

Several **infectious microorganisms** specifically parasitize erythrocytes and can cause significant hemolysis. All species of *Plasmodium* have an intraerythrocytic life cycle, which upon completion results in lysis of the red cell (see Chapter 9). Infected red cells are also removed from circulation by splenic macrophages. *Babesiosis,* found in more temperate climates (northeastern United States), is also associated with hemolysis after the intraerythrocytic life cycle is over. In both cases, blood smears reveal the parasites within red cells.

Polycythemia

Polycythemia (erythrocytosis) refers to an increase in the RBC mass.

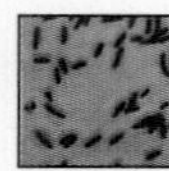

ETIOLOGIC FACTORS: Polycythemia can be arbitrarily defined as an Hct greater than 54% in men and 47% in women. At Hcts above 50%, blood viscosity increases exponentially, and cardiac function and peripheral blood flow may be impaired. With an Hct above 60%, blood flow may be so compromised as to lead to tissue hypoxia.

Polycythemia can be further divided on the basis of overall red cell mass into relative and absolute categories.

- **Relative polycythemia,** seen in dehydration, is characterized by decreased plasma volume with a normal red cell mass. This syndrome, sometimes called Gaisböck syndrome or spurious polycythemia, is not a true increase in red cell mass, but rather a reflection of altered total blood volume.
- **Absolute polycythemia** is a true increase in red cell mass and can be subclassified as primary and secondary.
  - **Primary polycythemia,** or **polycythemia vera (PV),** is an autonomous, EPO-independent proliferation of erythroid cells caused by an acquired, clonal, hematopoietic stem cell disorder. PV is considered to be a chronic myeloproliferative disorder, and is discussed below.
  - **Secondary polycythemia** arises from EPO-dependent stimulation of erythropoiesis, usually as a compensatory response to general tissue hypoxia. Causes of tissue hypoxia include chronic lung disease, cigarette smoking, residence at high altitudes, a right-to-left shunt in the heart and the presence of an abnormal hemoglobin with high oxygen affinity.

    Secondary polycythemia can also occur under certain circumstances unrelated to generalized tissue hypoxia. Neoplasms may produce ectopic EPO as a paraneoplastic syndrome, particularly renal cell carcinoma, hepatocellular carcinoma, cerebellar hemangioblastoma and uterine leiomyoma. Some nonneoplastic conditions of the kidney may cause secondary polycythemia. Renal cysts or hydronephrosis may exert direct pressure on the kidney, thereby leading to localized hypoxia and increased EPO production.

PLATELETS AND HEMOSTASIS

Normal Hemostasis

Normal hemostasis requires an exquisite balance of platelets, endothelial cells and coagulation factors to maintain a resting nonthrombotic state but maintain the ability to respond instantly to vascular damage and form a clot. Following vascular injury, platelets adhere to the vascular endothelium to form a hemostatic plug. Platelet activation leads to the recruitment and activation of additional platelets and subsequent **platelet aggregation** and **thrombin generation.** Platelet aggregates are stabilized by fibrin after the coagulation cascade is activated.

Platelets Develop From Hematopoietic Stem Cells by Thrombopoiesis

Under homeostatic conditions, the platelet count ranges from 150 to 350 × $10^9/\mu l$. To maintain platelets at this level requires continues proliferation, differentiation and release into the peripheral blood. Platelets are derived from megakaryocytes via the process of proplatelet formation and fragmentation. Thrombopoiesis requires the marrow microenvironment and stimulation from thrombopoietin (TPO). TPO, which is produced by the liver, binds the TPO receptor, c-Mpl, a member of the type I hematopoietic cytokine receptor family, to stimulate megakaryocyte proliferation and differentiation. Mature megakaryocytes undergo proplatelet formation and fragmentation to release 1000 to 4000 anucleate platelets.

Morphology and Function

Platelets are small discoid cells, 2 to 3 μm in diameter (Fig. 20-26), with a lifespan of about 10 days. On Wright-stained smears they are pale blue with faint pink granules. By electron microscopy, they contain mitochondria, glycogen particles, dense granules and α granules. Dense granules contain various nucleotides, including the potent aggregating molecule adenosine diphosphate (ADP) and adenosine triphosphate (ATP), calcium, histamine, serotonin and epinephrine. α Granules express the adhesive proteins P-selectin on their membranes and contain fibrinogen, von Willebrand factor (vWF), fibronectin and thrombospondin, as well as the chemokines platelet factor 4, neutrophil-activating peptide 2, platelet-derived growth factor (PDGF) and transforming growth factor-α (TGF-α).

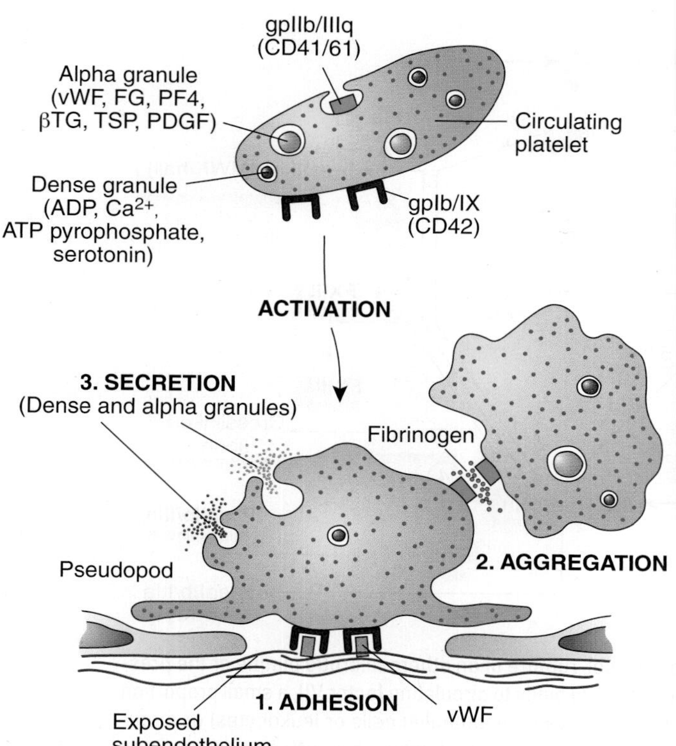

FIGURE 20-26. Platelet activation involves three overlapping mechanisms. (1) Adhesion to the exposed subendothelium is mediated by the binding of von Willebrand factor (vWF) to Gp Ib/IX (CD42) and is the initiation signal for activation. **(2)** Exposure of Gp IIb/IIIa (CD41/61) to the fibrinogen (FG) receptor on the platelet surface allows for platelet aggregation. **(3)** At the same time, platelets secrete their granule contents, which facilitates further activation. α-Granules contain vWF, fibrinogen, platelet factor 4 (PF4), thromboglobulin (TG), thrombospondin (TSP) and platelet-derived growth factor (PDGF).

Platelet Activation

When the vascular endothelium is disrupted, platelets respond by creating a platelet plug to minimize bleeding. After contact with the extracellular matrix, particularly type I collagen, platelets undergo a sequence of steps of platelet activation (Fig. 20-26):

1. **Platelets adhere** to subendothelial matrix proteins with specific platelet surface glycoproteins (Gps). Major adhesive ligands include collagen (via the Gp Ia/IIa [$\alpha_2\beta_1$ integrin] and Gp VI receptors) and vWF (via Gp Ib/IX).
2. **Shape change,** from discoid to spherical to stellate, follows initial adhesion.
3. **Secretion of platelet granule contents from both the dense granules and α granules** results in the release of ADP, epinephrine, calcium, vWF and PDGF.
4. **Thromboxane A_2** is generated by cyclooxygenase 1.
5. **Membrane changes** expose P-selectin and procoagulant anionic phospholipids such as phosphatidylserine.
6. **Aggregation of platelets** occurs through fibrinogen receptor Gp IIb/IIIa cross-linking.

Each of these functional steps has specific consequences. Initial adhesion signals platelet activation. Secreted granule contents and thromboxane A_2 provide positive feedback to activate additional platelets via their surface receptors. The stellate shape projects the procoagulant membrane surface and activated Gp IIb/IIIa/fibrinogen to the site of interaction with coagulation factors and other platelets, respectively. ***Thus, the surface of activated platelets is an optimal environment for propagating assembly of the coagulation–factor complex, including the prothrombinase complex. The resulting thrombin has many consequences, particularly further platelet activation.*** Finally, P-selectin participates in binding leukocytes and localizing them to participate in healing, together with substances secreted by platelets such as PDGF. ***As a result of these concerted steps, activated platelets form a strong primary plug and then an aggregate within a platelet–fibrin meshwork, which stops bleeding and initiates healing.***

Activation of the Coagulation Cascade Completes Blood Clot Formation

Platelets and leukocytes circulate in an inactive state. Similarly, coagulation factors are present as inactive zymogen forms. Activation of platelets and coagulation factors is concerted and highly constrained in space and time, to limit dissemination of clots through the circulation. The localization of coagulation–factor complexes to activated surfaces of blood cells, especially platelets, accelerates activation of coagulation factors and avoids the many anticoagulant factors in plasma.

Activation of the coagulation cascade by damaged tissue results in the exposure of tissue factor and culminates in conversion of prothrombin (factor II) to thrombin (factor IIa), and generation of fibrin from fibrinogen (Fig. 20-27). Thrombin has additional roles, namely, (1) activation of platelets and (2) feedback activation of factors that sustain the coagulation response (see Chapter 10).

There are three essential procoagulant complexes and one anticoagulant complex (Figs. 20-27 and 20-28). ***As a general rule, each active enzyme in the cascade is assisted by a cofactor and localized to a phospholipid surface (PL).***

PROCOAGULANT PATHWAYS: Factor Xa, together with its cofactor Va (Xa/Va complex), cleaves factor II (prothrombin) to IIa (thrombin). There are two complexes that activate factor X, the so-called Xase complexes.

1. The complex of **tissue factor (TF) and factor VIIa** initiates coagulation. Its activation is controlled by exposure to subendothelial cells or activated monocytes and endothelial cells. Microparticles derived from activated leukocytes and endothelial cells contribute to a pool of circulating TF that participates in hemostasis and thrombosis. TF/VIIa/PL initiates factor X activation but is then rapidly shut off by **TF pathway inhibitor (TFPI)** (Fig. 20-28). The TF/VIIa/PL complex also cleaves and thus activates a small amount of factor IX.
2. The **IXa/VIIIa/PL complex** also initiates factor X activation, with ongoing activation of factor IX by XIa.

The coagulation pathways are presented in detail in Chapter 10.

Note that thrombin activates the Xase complexes by activating factors XI, VIII and V. ***In summary, the three procoagulant complexes are the prothrombinase complex, Xa/Va/PL, and the two Xase complexes, TF/VIIa/PL and IXa/VIIIa/PL.***

ANTICOAGULANT PATHWAYS: ***An anticoagulant complex (α-thrombin-thrombomodulin) activates protein C***

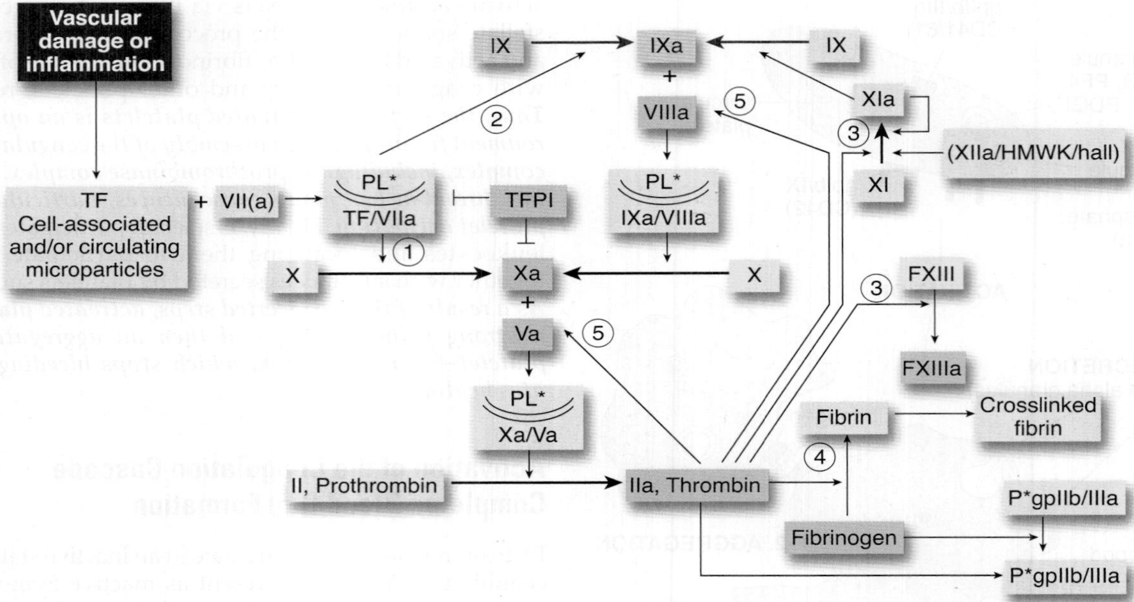

FIGURE 20-27. Hemostasis and thrombosis. Following injury to a vessel, rupture of an atherosclerotic plaque or the presence of major inflammation, coagulation is initiated when tissue factor (TF) binds to circulating factor VII, a small proportion of which is activated (VIIa). TF is located on cells (subendothelial or activated endothelial cells or leukocytes) or circulating microparticles. The TF/VIIa complex is activated by localizing to an activated phospholipid surface (PL*) such as that provided by activated platelets. TF/VIIa activates factor X to form Xa (*1*) and IX to form IXa (*2*). However, TF pathway inhibitor (TFPI) inhibits both (*1*) and (*2*). Sustained amplification is achieved through the actions of factors XI, IX and VIII. Factor XI is activated through the small amount of initial thrombin formed and, to a limited extent, by autoactivation or factor XIIa. Cofactors V and VIII, when activated by thrombin, form complexes with X (Xa/Va) and IX (IXa/VIIIa), respectively, on activated PL surfaces. Note the central and multiple roles for thrombin (*4*), which converts fibrinogen to fibrin, activates cofactors V and VIII (*5*), activates factors XI and XIII (*3*) and activates platelets. Fibrinogen binds to the Gp IIb/IIIa integrin receptor on activated platelets (P*). Note the extensive control in time and space of these concerted surface reactions. The combined result is the platelet–fibrin thrombus.

(Fig. 20-28). The **protein $\mathbf{C_{ase}}$ complex** is composed of thrombin and thrombomodulin in the endothelial cell plasma membrane. Endothelial protein C receptor also participates in forming this cell surface complex. Activated protein C, with its cofactor protein S, inactivates the key cofactors VIIIa and Va, thus limiting further generation of Xa and IIa (see Chapter 10).

Antithrombin III inhibits thrombin activity. Antithrombin III also cleaves activated factors IXa, Xa, XIa and XIIa. In vivo this effect is accentuated by heparan sulfate proteoglycans and, most dramatically, by therapeutic administration of heparin.

Thrombolysis Is Mediated by Plasminogen Activation

After a thrombus is firmly established, its growth is curtailed further by removal of platelet-activating factors and coagulation proteins. Endothelial cells near the thrombus produce plasminogen activators, which activate circulating plasminogen to plasmin and initiate thrombolysis (also known as **fibrinolysis**). There are two major plasminogen activators, **tissue plasminogen activator** (t-PA) and **urokinase-type plasminogen activator** (u-PA). Plasminogen cleavage to plasmin and plasmin action are tightly regulated by several naturally occurring inhibitors, including plasminogen activator inhibitor-I (PAI-I), antiplasmin and thrombin-activatable fibrinolysis inhibitor (TAFI). Together, the protease plasmin and the activity of macrophages dissolve the thrombus. Plasmin targets specific sites in the fibrin meshwork for degradation, helping to localize its activity to sites where it is needed (see Chapter 10).

Thrombolysis is also coincident with the start of wound repair (see Chapter 7). The latter involves migration and proliferation of fibroblasts and endothelial cells, secretion of new extracellular matrix and restoration of blood vessel patency. Angiogenesis (i.e., new blood vessels budding from existing ones) occurs in the setting of tissue ischemia or damage. Many products of coagulation and fibrinolysis pathways are potent angiogenic agents.

Blood Vessels and Endothelial Cells Interact With Platelets

The above discussion highlights the many roles of endothelial cells in regulating platelets and coagulation (Fig. 20-28). Endothelial cells rest on a basement membrane that contains collagens, elastin, laminin, fibronectin, vWF and other structural

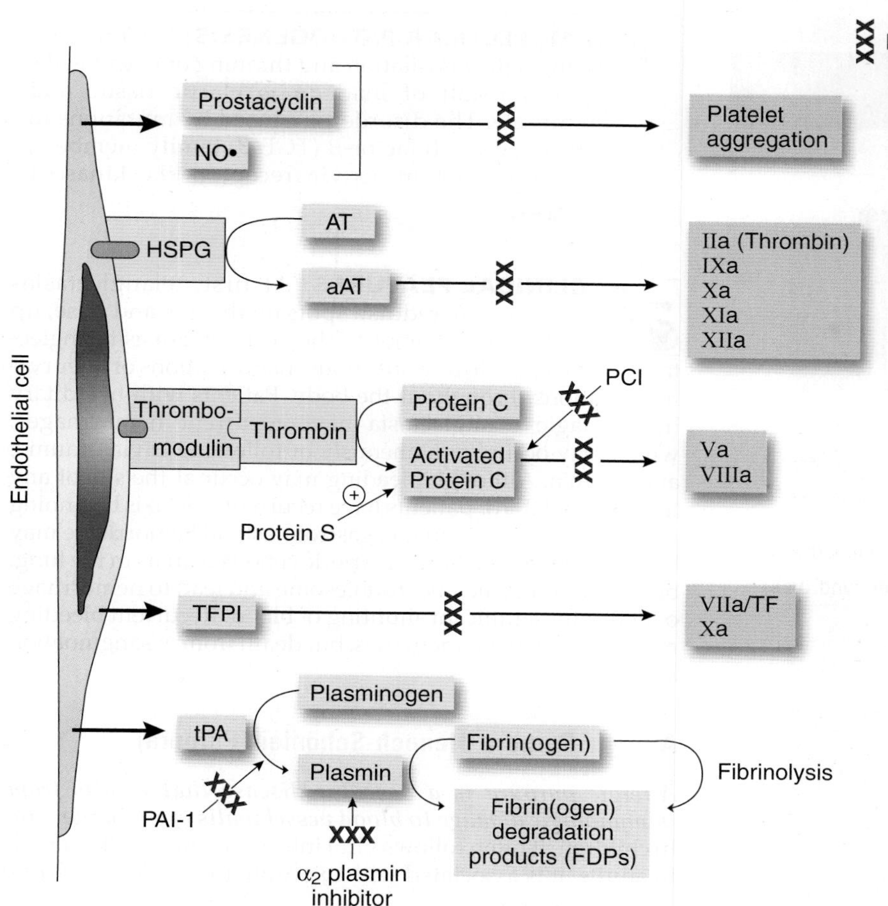

FIGURE 20-28. The role of endothelium in anticoagulation, platelet inhibition and thrombolysis. The endothelial cell plays a central role in the inhibition of various components of the clotting mechanism. Heparan sulfate proteoglycan potentiates the activation of antithrombin (AT) 15-fold. Thrombomodulin stimulates the activation of protein C by thrombin 30-fold. NO• = nitric oxide; HSPG = heparan sulfate proteoglycan; PCI = protein C inhibitor; tPA = tissue plasminogen activator; PAI-I = plasminogen activator inhibitor-I.

and adhesive proteins. The subendothelial cells are a potent source of TF. When exposed, the matrix of the intima is intensely thrombogenic. Its adhesive proteins bind corresponding platelet membrane glycoprotein receptors and cause them to adhere to the exposed matrix. TF binds circulating activated factor VIIa to activate factors X and IX (Fig. 20-27).

The endothelium provides a smooth, nonthrombogenic surface. The synthesis of anticoagulant molecules on the endothelium prevents unstimulated platelets from adhering to, or penetrating, the endothelial barrier. Endothelial cells also synthesize the potent vasodilator prostacyclin, which inhibits platelet activation. Nitric oxide exerts similar effects. These actions prevent the development of a clot until injury to the endothelium exposes subendothelial tissue (see Chapters 2 and 10).

Hemostatic Disorders

Defects in the hemostatic system result when the balance of procoagulant or anticoagulant activity results in either bleeding or clotting and fall into two categories: **hemostatic** disorders and **thrombotic** disorders. Failure of the hemostatic system to restore the integrity of an injured vessel causes **bleeding.** Inability to maintain the fluidity of blood results in **thrombosis.**

The clinical manifestations of hemorrhage associated with disorders of each component of the hemostatic system tend to be distinctive (Table 20-7). Platelet abnormalities result in both petechiae and purpuric hemorrhages in the skin and mucous membranes. Deficiencies of coagulation factors lead to hemorrhage into muscles, viscera and joint spaces. Disorders of the blood vessels usually cause purpura.

Hemostatic Disorders of Blood Vessels Reflect Dysfunction of Vascular or Extravascular Tissues

Dysfunction of the extravascular or vascular tissues may cause hemorrhages ranging from cosmetic blemishes to life-threatening blood loss.

Extravascular Dysfunction

SENILE PURPURA: The most common disorder in extravascular dysfunction, senile purpura, is age-related atrophy of supporting connective tissues. Senile purpura is associated with superficial, sharply demarcated, persistent purpuric spots on the forearms and other sun-exposed areas.

PURPURA SIMPLEX: A similar type of purpura occurs principally in women during menses. Purpura simplex occurs in the deep dermis and resolves quickly.

SCURVY: Collagen synthesis is disturbed in vitamin C deficiency, and purpura is a common manifestation (see Chapter 8). Perifollicular hemorrhages are characteristic.

Table 20-7

Principal Causes of Bleeding

Vascular Disorders
Senile purpura
Purpura simplex
Glucocorticoid excess
Dysproteinemias
Allergic (Henoch-Schönlein) purpura
Hereditary hemorrhagic telangiectasia
Platelet Abnormalities
Thrombocytopenia (see Table 20-7)
Qualitative disorders
Inherited
Glycoprotein IIb/IIIa deficiency (Glanzmann thrombasthenia)
Glycoprotein Ib/IX/V deficiency (Bernard-Soulier syndrome)
Storage pool diseases (α and δ)
Abnormal arachidonic acid metabolism
Acquired
Uremia
Drugs
Cardiopulmonary bypass
Myeloproliferative disorders
Liver disease
Coagulation Factor Deficiencies
Inherited
von Willebrand disease
Hemophilia A
Hemophilia B
Acquired
Vitamin K deficiency/antagonism
Liver disease
Disseminated intravascular coagulation

Vascular Dysfunction

Deposition of immunoglobulin fragments in vessel walls may occur in **amyloidosis** (see Chapter 23), **cryoglobulinemia and other paraproteinemias** and can cause vessel wall weakness and purpura. Certain types of **arteritis** also injure the vessel wall and may lead to hemorrhage (see Chapter 10).

Hereditary Hemorrhagic Telangiectasia (Rendu-Osler-Weber Syndrome)

Hereditary hemorrhagic telangiectasia is an autosomal dominant disorder of blood vessel walls (venules and capillaries) characterized by arteriovenous malformations (AVMs) of multiple solid organs and telangiectases of the mucous membranes and dermis that results in tortuous, dilated vessels (telangiectasias). The incidence is approximately 1 to 2 individuals per 10,000.

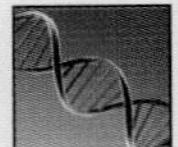

MOLECULAR PATHOGENESIS: The underlying defect is dilation and thinning of vessel walls as a result of inadequate elastic tissue and smooth muscle. The disorder is caused by mutations in transforming growth factor-β (TGF-β) family members, endoglin (ENG) or an activin receptor–like kinase 1 (ALK1).

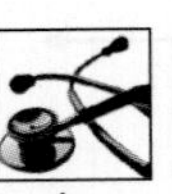

CLINICAL FEATURES: At first, telangiectasias are punctate reddish spots on the lips and nose, up to 0.5 cm in diameter. They can remain as telangiectasias or progress to arteriovenous malformations or aneurysmal dilations throughout the body. Patients with hereditary hemorrhagic telangiectasia have recurrent hemorrhages, which may occur spontaneously or following trivial trauma, and anemia. Although bleeding may occur at the site of any lesion, over 80% of patients have recurrent epistaxis beginning at an early age. Later in life, gastrointestinal hemorrhage may be the dominant symptom. Arteriovenous fistulas in the lung, brain and retina may be troublesome and lead to hemorrhage or clinically significant shunting of blood. Recurrent bleeding may limit a patient's activities, but death from exsanguination is rare.

Allergic Purpura (Henoch-Schönlein Purpura)

Allergic purpura is a vascular disease that results from immunologic damage to blood vessel walls (see Chapter 16). In children, it often follows viral infections and is self-limited. In adults, it is associated with exposure to a variety of drugs and may be chronic.

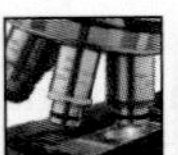

PATHOLOGY: Histologically, Henoch-Schönlein purpura is characterized by **leukocytoclastic vasculitis,** with perivascular infiltration of neutrophils and eosinophils, fibrinoid necrosis of vessel walls and platelet plugs in vascular lumens. IgA and complement complexes circulate in the blood and are often seen in vessel walls. Purpuric spots are often accompanied by raised urticarial lesions. Intestinal cramps and bleeding indicate gastrointestinal involvement. If kidneys are affected, renal failure may ensue.

Platelet Disorders Impair Hemostasis

Platelet disorders can result from an insufficient number of platelets, because of decreased production, increased destruction or abnormal function of existing platelets. Patients may have a history of easy bruising; mucocutaneous bleeding, including gingival bleeding, epistaxis and menorrhagia; or life-threatening bleeds into the gastrointestinal tract, genitourinary tract and brain. Petechiae, which are characteristic of platelet disorders, are nonblanching red lesions less than 2 mm in size. They usually occur in lower extremities, in dependent regions of the body, on the buccal mucosal and soft palate and at pressure points (waistband, wristwatch band). Petechiae may also occur in vascular disorders. Platelet disorders reflect:

1. Decreased production
2. Increased destruction
3. Impaired function

Thrombocytopenia

Thrombocytopenia, defined as platelet counts under 150,000/μL, results from either decreased production or increased destruction. Manifestations of thrombocytopenia include spontaneous bleeding, prolonged bleeding time and a normal prothrombin time (PT) and partial thromboplastin time (PTT). The lower the platelet count, the greater the risk of bleeding. Patients with fewer than 10,000 platelets/μL are at greatest risk of spontaneous hemorrhage (Table 20-8).

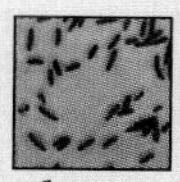
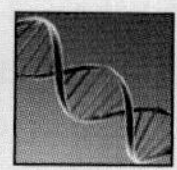

ETIOLOGIC FACTORS AND MOLECULAR PATHOGENESIS: Decreased platelet production can result from multiple congenital or acquired defects in megakaryocytopoiesis, including diseases that affect the marrow generally, abnormalities that selectively impair platelet production and defects that lead to ineffective megakaryocytopoiesis. Marrow infiltration with leukemic cells or metastatic cancer and bone marrow failure in patients with aplastic anemia or who received radiotherapy or chemotherapy produce pancytopenia, including thrombocytopenia. Certain viral infections such as cytomegalovirus and human immunodeficiency virus (HIV) and certain drugs impair platelet production. (HIV may also elicit increased platelet destruction; see below.) Megaloblastic anemia and myelodysplasia may cause severe thrombocytopenia as a result of ineffective megakaryopoiesis.

May-Hegglin anomaly, a congenital form of thrombocytopenia, characterized by decreased platelet production, is the most common entity of a group of inherited thrombocytopenias now called the myosin heavy chain 9 (MYH9)-related platelet disorders. These result from mutation in the *MYH9* gene, whic nonmuscle myosin heavy chain IIA (NM cytoskeletal contractile protein. The three other overlapping disorders include Epstein syndrome, Fechtner syndrome and Sebastian platelet syndrome. Large platelets (macrothrombocytopenia) result from these mutations that lead to abnormal megakaryocyte maturation. In addition, neutrophils are slightly abnormal morphologically with blue cytoplasmic inclusions (**Döhle-like bodies;** true Döhle bodies are seen in acute infections).

Increased platelet destruction can result from immune-mediated damage and removal of circulating platelets, as in idiopathic thrombocytopenic purpura and drug-induced thrombocytopenia. Alternatively, excessive platelet destruction occurs by nonimmunologic conditions such as intravascular platelet aggregation (e.g., in TTP).

Abnormal platelet distribution, or pooling, is seen in disorders of the spleen and hypothermia.

Table 20-8

Principal Causes of Thrombocytopenia

Decreased Production
Aplastic anemia
Bone marrow infiltration (neoplastic, fibrosis)
Bone marrow suppression by drugs or radiation
Ineffective Production
Megaloblastic anemia
Myelodysplasias
Increased Destruction
Immunologic (idiopathic, HIV, drugs, alloimmune, posttransfusion purpura, neonatal)
Nonimmunologic (DIC, TTP, HUS, vascular malformations, drugs)
Increased Sequestration
Splenomegaly
Dilutional
Blood and plasma transfusions

DIC = disseminated intravascular coagulation; HIV = human immunodeficiency virus; HUS = hemolytic–uremic syndrome; TTP = thrombocytic thrombocytopenic purpura.

Idiopathic (Autoimmune) Thrombocytopenic Purpura

Idiopathic thrombocytopenic purpura (ITP) is a syndrome characterized by decreased blood platelets and caused by antibodies against platelet or megakaryocytic antigens. It is, thus, more appropriately called **immune thrombocytopenic purpura.** ITP occurs in two forms: an acute, self-limited, hemorrhagic syndrome in children and a chronic bleeding disorder in adolescents and adults. The antibodies are often directed against the platelet membrane glycoproteins, Gp IIb/IIIa or Ib/IX, the proteins involved in platelet adhesion and clot formation.

MOLECULAR PATHOGENESIS: Like autoimmune hemolytic anemia, ITP reflects antibody-mediated destruction of platelets or their precursors. In most patients, these autoantibodies are of the IgG class, but IgM antiplatelet antibodies also occur.

Acute ITP typically appears in children of either sex after a viral illness and is likely caused by virus-induced changes in platelet antigens that elicit autoantibodies. Complement bound at the surface causes platelets to be lysed in the blood or phagocytosed and destroyed by splenic and hepatic macrophages.

Chronic ITP occurs mainly in adults (male-to-female ratio of 1:2.6) and may be associated with collagen vascular diseases (e.g., systemic lupus erythematosus) or a malignant lymphoproliferative disease, especially chronic lymphocytic leukemia. It is also common in people infected with HIV. The extent of thrombocytopenia in ITP is determined by the balance between (1) levels of antiplatelet antibodies; (2) the degree of inhibition of platelet production in the bone marrow, as some antibodies may bind to megakaryocytes; and (3) expression of Fc and complement receptors on the surface of macrophages. This expression is upregulated in infection and pregnancy but is ameliorated by certain drugs, for example, corticosteroids, danazol and intravenous γ-globulin, all of which are used to treat ITP.

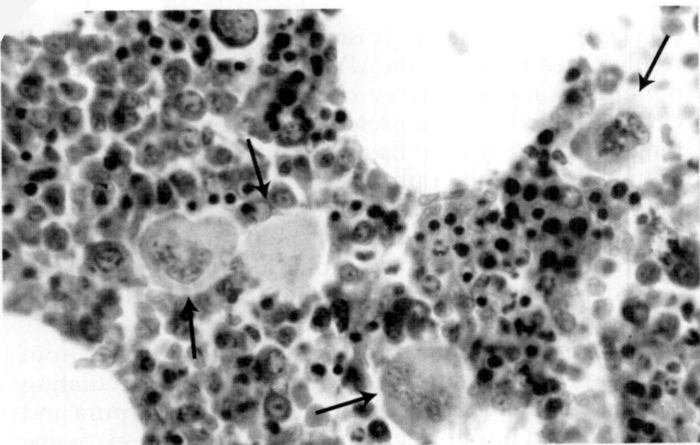

FIGURE 20-29. Idiopathic thrombocytopenic purpura. A section of the bone marrow reveals increased megakaryocytes (*arrows*).

PATHOLOGY: In acute ITP, the platelet count is typically less than 20,000/μL. In chronic adult ITP, platelet counts vary from a few thousand to 100,000/μL. Peripheral blood smears show numerous large platelets, which reflect accelerated release of young platelets by bone marrow actively engaged in platelet production. Accordingly, bone marrow examination reveals compensatory increases in megakaryocytes (Fig. 20-29). IgG is detected on the platelets in more than 80% of patients with chronic ITP, and in half of these, increased platelet-associated C3 can be demonstrated.

CLINICAL FEATURES: Children with **acute ITP** experience sudden onset of petechiae and purpura but are otherwise asymptomatic. Spontaneous recovery occurs within 6 months in over 80% of cases. The major threat (<1% of cases) is intracranial hemorrhage. Treatment is rarely necessary, but with serious disease, corticosteroids and intravenous immunoglobulin may be needed. Glucocorticoids decrease production of antiplatelet antibodies and downregulate macrophage Fc receptors. γ-Globulin interferes with clearance of IgG-coated platelets from the circulation via multiple mechanisms.

Chronic ITP in adults manifests as bleeding episodes, such as epistaxis, menorrhagia or ecchymoses, and excessive bleeding after trauma and minor procedures (e.g., tooth extraction). Life-threatening hemorrhages are uncommon. Occasionally, asymptomatic people are discovered to have thrombocytopenia on a routine blood cell count. Most adults with chronic ITP improve when given corticosteroids and intravenous γ-globulin. Danazol (a synthetic anabolic steroid) acts similarly to glucocorticoids. In 70% of patients who do not respond adequately to drug therapy within 2 to 3 months, splenectomy produces complete or partial remission. In patients with severe ITP, studies are ongoing to evaluate the efficacy of thrombopoietic agents that activate the TPO receptor.

Drug-Induced Autoimmune Thrombocytopenia

Many drugs are known to cause immune-mediated platelet destruction: quinine, quinidine, heparin, sulfonamides, gold salts, antibiotics, sedatives, tranquilizers and anticonvulsants. The drug often forms a complex with a platelet-related protein to make a neoepitope that elicits antibody production. By contrast, chemotherapeutic agents, ethanol and thiazides cause thrombocytopenia by suppression of platelet production.

Heparin-induced thrombocytopenia (HIT) is a distinct type of drug-induced thrombocytopenia. There are two types of HIT. About 25% of patients experience a mild, transient thrombocytopenia within the first 2 to 5 days of treatment. This mild form of HIT is self-limited, entails aggregation of platelets by nonimmune mechanisms and follows a relatively benign course.

Type II HIT is immunologically mediated, caused by acquired IgG antibodies against platelet factor 4–heparin complexes. It occurs in 1% to 3% of patients treated with heparin, after 7 to 10 days of therapy, and these individuals develop profound consumptive thrombocytopenia, platelet activation and consequently a hypercoagulable state. Because this form of HIT entails hypercoagulability, platelet aggregation predisposes patients to arterial and venous thromboembolic events that may be lethal.

Pregnancy-Associated Thrombocytopenia

Minimal thrombocytopenia occurs frequently during the third trimester of pregnancy, as a result of dilution of platelets. Since platelet counts are usually above 100,000/μL, no special management is needed. Conversely, preeclampsia/eclampsia syndromes can result in maternal thrombocytopenia. A condition related to preeclampsia is called **HELLP** (hemolysis, elevated liver enzyme tests and low platelets; see Chapter 18). The latter two syndromes can be life-threatening.

Neonatal Thrombocytopenia

Neonatal thrombocytopenias are either **inherited** or **acquired.**

Inherited causes associated with increased platelet destruction include **Wiskott-Aldrich syndrome** (WAS), an X-linked recessive disorder, which is caused by a defect in the Wiskott-Aldrich syndrome protein (*WASP*) gene. Affected boys have small platelets, eczema and immunodeficiency. A variant of WAS is **X-linked thrombocytopenia,** which displays defects in the same gene but features only thrombocytopenia. Other inherited defects associated with poor platelet production include amegakaryocytic thrombocytopenia, thrombocytopenia-absent radius syndrome and Fanconi anemia. Thrombocytopenia can also be seen in infants with trisomy 13, 18 or 21.

Fanconi anemia is an inherited, autosomal recessive, bone marrow failure disorder manifesting often with thrombocytopenia and RBC macrocytosis. A family of genes that are mutated and defective in Fanconi anemia have been identified. These genes are involved in DNA repair and genetic stability. There is a high incidence of associated congenital anomalies, such as skin hypopigmentation and hyperpigmentation, short stature, microcephaly, microphthalmia and radial/thumb abnormalities (see Chapters 5 and 6).

Neonatal alloimmune thrombocytopenia (NAIT) is caused by increased destruction of platelets, resulting from the alloimmunization to HPA-1a and other platelet-specific antigens that occurs during pregnancy. Alloimmunization in this condition results from antibodies produced by the mother recognizing the paternal HPA-1a–positive antigen present on the fetus' platelets, whereas the mother is HPA-1a negative. In NAIT, the fetus or neonate but not the mother is thrombocytopenic. NAIT predisposes to fetal and neonatal intracranial hemorrhage.

Nonimmune causes of thrombocytopenia in the neonate are similar to those in adults, with additional considerations such as birth asphyxia, hypoxic injury, sepsis and DIC, necrotizing enterocolitis, hemangiomas and thrombosis.

Posttransfusion Purpura

This complication of blood transfusion typically develops in women who are HPA-1 negative, and who were sensitized to HPA-1 as a result of previous pregnancies. It may also be seen in men who have had previous blood transfusions. Thus, whether following pregnancy or transfusion involving HPA-1–positive platelets, HPA-1–negative persons may develop antibodies to HPA-1–positive platelets. Subsequently, infused HPA-1–positive platelets are then destroyed by those antibodies. Curiously, the patient's own HPA-1–negative platelets are also destroyed, perhaps related to the passive acquisition of the antigen by these platelets or the development of immune complexes. In any event, a self-limited thrombocytopenia occurs about a week after the transfusion.

Thrombotic Thrombocytopenic Purpura

The thrombotic microangiopathies (TMAs) represent a heterogeneous group of syndromes with common features including thrombocytopenia, microangiopathic hemolytic anemia, neurologic symptoms, fever and renal impairment. These disorders include TTP and hemolytic–uremic syndrome. The pathology of these disorders results from widespread platelet aggregation and the deposition of hyaline thrombi in the microcirculation.

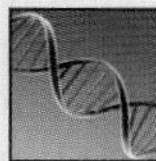

MOLECULAR PATHOGENESIS: The pathogenesis of TTP is obscure, but the most tenable hypothesis holds that it results from the introduction of one or more platelet-aggregating substances into the circulation. The theory that has received the most attention is the cross-linking of platelets by inappropriate vWF multimers from injured endothelial cells. vWF monomers are normally assembled into multimeric molecules of varying size (up to millions of daltons) within endothelial cells and released locally in response to endothelial stimulation. ADAMTS13 is a metalloprotease that normally cleaves large vWF multimers. *In TTP, ADAMTS13 is deficient, resulting in the accumulation of ultralarge vWF multimers, which bind platelets, leading to thrombocytopenia and formation of thrombi in the microvasculature.* ADAMTS13 is genetically absent or defective in familial TTP as a result of mutations of the ADAMTS13 gene, and is inactivated by autoantibodies in idiopathic TTP. Prophylactic plasma infusion, which replaces the missing ADAMTS13, is most effective in familial forms of TTP, and plasma exchange is preferred in acquired types.

Although most cases arise in otherwise normal persons, TTP may also complicate autoimmune collagen vascular disorders (systemic lupus erythematosus, rheumatoid arthritis, Sjögren syndrome) and drug-induced hypersensitivity reactions. It has also been triggered by infections, cancer chemotherapy, bone marrow transplantation and pregnancy. Occurrence of TTP in siblings suggests a hereditary predisposition.

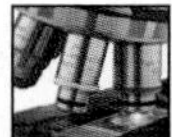

PATHOLOGY: The morphologic hallmark of TTP is the deposition of periodic acid–Schiff (PAS)-positive hyaline microthrombi in arterioles and capillaries throughout the body, mainly in the heart, brain and kidneys (Fig. 20-30). These microthrombi contain platelet aggregates, fibrin and a few erythrocytes and leukocytes. Unlike immune-mediated vasculitis, there is no inflammation in TTP. Fragmented erythrocytes (schistocytes) are always evident in peripheral blood smears (Fig. 20-31) and are caused by RBC shearing that occurs in the vessels narrowed by thrombi. RBC polychromasia is also a feature and reflects an increase in reticulocytes in response to anemia. Serum LDH and unconjugated bilirubin are increased.

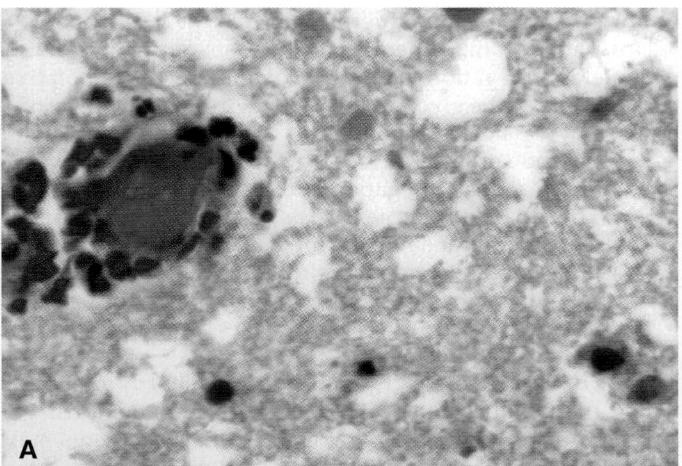

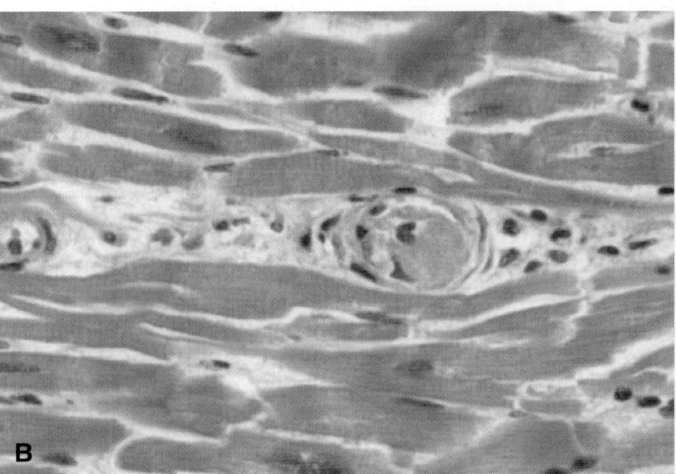

FIGURE 20-30. Thrombotic thrombocytopenic purpura. Microthrombi are present in the brain **(A)** and heart **(B)** of a patient who died of thrombotic thrombocytopenic purpura.

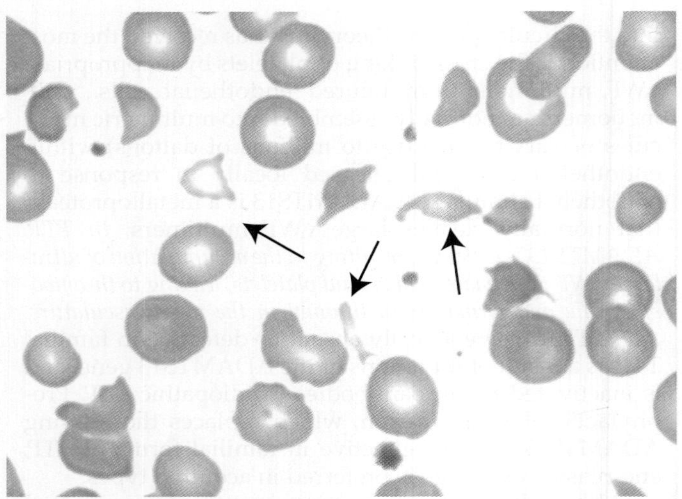

FIGURE 20-31. Microangiopathic hemolytic anemia. Numerous schistocytes (*arrows*) are present in a patient with thrombotic thrombocytopenic purpura.

CLINICAL FEATURES: TTP occurs at virtually any age, but is most common in women in the fourth and fifth decades. It may be chronic and recurrent for years or, more frequently, occur as an acute, fulminant disease that is often fatal. Most patients present with neurologic symptoms, including seizures, focal weakness, aphasia and alterations in the state of consciousness. Widespread purpura is often present and vaginal bleeding may occur in women. Hemolytic anemia is a constant feature; hemoglobin levels are often below 6 g/dL. Jaundice caused by hemolysis may be severe. Renal dysfunction includes proteinuria, hematuria and mild renal insufficiency.

More than half of patients with TTP have platelet counts below 20,000/μL. Despite the presence of aggregated platelets, activation of the coagulation cascade does not occur. Consequently, the PT, PTT, and fibrinogen concentration remain normal, distinguishing this syndrome from DIC (see below). Acute TTP was formerly fatal, but the cure rate is approximately 80% with plasma infusion and plasmapheresis.

Hemolytic–Uremic Syndrome

Hemolytic–uremic syndrome (HUS) is a thrombotic microangiopathy that resembles TTP, but the pathogenesis of the two syndromes is different. HUS is characterized by thrombocytopenia, microangiopathic hemolysis and acute renal failure.

Classic HUS occurs in children, usually after an acute infectious hemorrhagic gastroenteritis caused by *Escherichia coli* strain O157:H7 or *Shigella dysenteriae* (see Chapter 16). The production of a Shiga-like toxin damages the endothelium and initiates platelet activations, followed by binding of fibrinogen to activated platelet Gp IIb/IIIa complex and platelet aggregation. In HUS, aggregated platelet thrombi are found primarily in the renal microvasculature. Kidney failure, rather than neurologic abnormalities, is the main clinical feature.

Splenic Sequestration of Platelets

Many patients with splenomegaly, irrespective of the cause, show **hypersplenism,** a syndrome that includes sequestration of platelets in the spleen. One third of platelets are normally stored temporarily in the spleen, but in massive splenomegaly, up to 90% of the total platelet pool may be captured in that organ. Interestingly, the platelet life span is normal or only slightly reduced. Thrombocytopenia associated with hypersplenism is rarely severe and by itself does not produce a hemorrhagic diathesis.

Other Causes of Thrombocytopenia

Vascular malformations, including hemangiomas and arteriovenous malformations, can cause thrombocytopenia. In hemangiomas, consumption of platelets has been called the **Kasabach-Merritt syndrome.** Platelet loss occurs in patients who have massive hemorrhage, such as in bleeding from a peptic ulcer or during surgery with heavy blood loss. Transfused blood does not contain viable platelets because it is stored at 4°C (39.2°F) before administration. Thus, thrombocytopenia in transfused patients is a result of platelet loss and dilution. Platelet transfusion may be used to prevent development of thrombocytopenia.

Hereditary Disorders of Platelets

Bernard-Soulier Syndrome (Giant Platelet Syndrome)

Bernard-Soulier syndrome is an autosomal recessive platelet disorder in which platelets have a quantitative or qualitative defect in the membrane glycoprotein complex (Gp Ib/IX [CD42] and sometimes Gp V) that serves as a receptor for vWF. The complex plays a prominent role in the adhesion of normal platelets to vWF in injured subendothelial tissues. The platelets in Bernard-Soulier syndrome vary widely in size and shape, and the diagnosis is suggested by the presence of *thrombocytopenia and giant platelets* on the blood smear. Bernard-Soulier syndrome manifests in infancy or childhood with a bleeding pattern characteristic of *abnormal platelet function:* ecchymoses, epistaxis and gingival bleeding. At a later age, traumatic hemorrhage, gastrointestinal bleeding and menorrhagia occur. Many patients have only a mild bleeding disorder, but others suffer more severe hemorrhage that requires frequent platelet transfusions and that may even be fatal.

Glanzmann Thrombasthenia

Glanzmann thrombasthenia is an autosomal recessive defect in platelet aggregation caused by a quantitative or qualitative abnormality in the glycoprotein complex IIb/IIIa (CD41/61). In normal platelets, this complex is activated during platelet adhesion and serves as a receptor for fibrinogen and vWF, mediating platelet aggregation and the generation of a solid plug. The IIb/IIIa complex is also linked to the platelet cytoskeleton and transmits the force of contraction to adherent fibrin, a mechanism that promotes clot retraction. In Glanzmann thrombasthenia the lack of aggregation and clot retraction impairs hemostasis and causes bleeding, despite a normal platelet count.

The disease becomes clinically apparent shortly after birth when an infant has mucocutaneous or gingival hemorrhage, epistaxis or bleeding after circumcision. Later, patients may suffer unexpected hemorrhage after trauma or surgery. Disease severity varies, and only a few patients experience life-threatening hemorrhage. Platelet transfusions correct the condition temporarily.

α Storage Pool Disease (Grey Platelet Syndrome)

A rare inherited disease, α storage pool disease, is characterized by the absence of morphologically recognizable α granules in platelets. The defect resides in abnormal granule membranes. Thrombocytopenia is common; platelets are large and pale. The bleeding diathesis tends to be mild.

δ Storage Pool Disease

This heterogeneous illness affects the dense granules of platelets. It is sometimes associated with other multisystem hereditary disorders, including Chédiak-Higashi syndrome or Hermansky-Pudlak syndrome (both of which are characterized by oculocutaneous albinism). Bleeding manifestations are mild to moderate.

Acquired Qualitative Disorders of Platelets

A variety of acquired disorders may adversely affect platelet function (Table 20-8).

- **Drugs:** Various drugs can impair platelet function. Aspirin irreversibly acetylates cyclooxygenase (COX), primarily COX-1, and thus blocks production of platelet thromboxane A_2, which is important in platelet aggregation. Platelets cannot synthesize cyclooxygenase, so the aspirin effect lasts for the life span of platelets (7 to 10 days). Nonsteroidal analgesics, such as indomethacin or ibuprofen, impair platelet function, but as their inhibition of cyclooxygenase is reversible, their effect on platelets is short. Antibiotics, particularly β-lactams (penicillin and cephalosporins), can cause platelet dysfunction. Ticlopidine, which is used to suppress platelet function in patients with thromboembolic disease, causes marked impairment of platelet function and even TTP.
- **Renal failure:** End-stage kidney disease is often accompanied by a qualitative platelet defect that results in a prolonged bleeding time and a tendency toward hemorrhage. The platelet abnormality is heterogeneous and is aggravated by uremic anemia. Restoring a normal hematocrit by administering EPO may restore bleeding time to normal without affecting the azotemia.
- **Cardiopulmonary bypass:** Platelet dysfunction caused by platelet activation and fragmentation occurs in the extracorporeal circuit during bypass surgery.
- **Hematologic malignancies:** In chronic myeloproliferative disorders and myelodysplastic syndromes, platelet dysfunction is caused by intrinsic platelet defects. In dysproteinemias, platelets are impaired because they are coated with plasma paraprotein.

Thrombocytosis

Reactive Thrombocytosis

An increase in platelet counts occurs in association with (1) iron-deficiency anemia, especially in children; (2) splenectomy; (3) cancer; and (4) chronic inflammatory disorders. Reactive thrombocytosis is rarely symptomatic, but it has been associated with thrombotic episodes, especially in patients bedridden after splenectomy.

Clonal Thrombocytosis

Patients with myeloproliferative neoplasms such as polycythemia vera and essential thrombocythemia have a malignant proliferation of megakaryocytes (see below). Resulting increases in circulating platelets may lead to episodes of thrombosis or bleeding (see below).

Coagulopathies Are Caused by Deficient or Abnormal Coagulation Factors

Quantitative and qualitative disorders of all of the coagulation factors have been identified. These conditions may be **hereditary** or **acquired.** Only the hereditary deficiencies of factor VIII (hemophilia A), factor IX (hemophilia B) and vWF are common. Most of these disorders result from deficiency of the protein factor, leading to inadequate hemostasis and concomitant bleeding. Occasionally the protein factor is present but dysfunctional.

Hemophilia is an X-linked recessive disorder of blood clotting that results in delayed bleeding along with joint and muscle bleeding. Classic hemophilia is actually two distinct diseases resulting from mutations in the genes for **factor VIII (hemophilia A)** and **factor IX (hemophilia B).**

Hemophilia is one of the oldest genetic diseases recorded, having been described in the Talmud almost 2000 years ago: male infants of Jewish families with a history of fatal bleeding after circumcision were excused from this ritual. Transmission of a bleeding tendency to boys from unaffected mothers has been known for 200 years. Subsequently, the dissemination of hemophilia throughout Europe's royal families by Queen Victoria's daughters highlighted this disease. The gene for factor VIII was cloned in 1984, allowing investigation of the molecular basis of hemophilia A.

Hemophilia A (Factor VIII Deficiency)

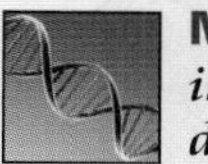

MOLECULAR PATHOGENESIS: *Hemophilia A is the most common X-linked inherited bleeding disorder (1 per 5000 to 10,000 males).* Causative mutations in the very large factor VIII gene at the tip of the long arm of the X chromosome (Xq28) include deletions, inversions, point mutations and insertions. Each family with a history of hemophilia actually harbors a different mutation (private mutant allele). In half of cases, hemophilia A can be traced through many generations, but in the other half, de novo mutations arise within two generations of the index case. In most of these de novo mutations, an origin in the mother, maternal grandfather or maternal grandmother has been identified.

CLINICAL FEATURES: Patients with hemophilia A have mild, moderate or severe bleeding tendencies. In most, the severity of the illness parallels the activity of factor VIII in the blood. Half of patients have virtually no factor VIII activity and often suffer spontaneous bleeding. A third of patients, in whom the factor VIII activity level is 1% to 5%, bleed spontaneously only occasionally, but often do so after minor trauma. One fifth have factor VIII activity levels greater than 5% to 40% and bleed only after significant trauma or surgery.

The most frequent complication of hemophilia A is a degenerative joint disease caused by repeated bleeding into many joints. Although uncommon, bleeding into the brain was formerly the most common cause of death. Hematuria, intestinal obstruction and respiratory obstruction may all occur with bleeding into the respective organs.

Management consists of factor VIII replacement, either prophylactically to prevent bleeding or therapeutically in response to bleeding episodes. The aim is to correct factor VIII levels to control the bleeding diathesis and prevent long-term sequelae. Unfortunately, in the 1980s many of these patients developed acquired immunodeficiency syndrome (AIDS) and viral hepatitis from contamination of pooled factor VIII preparations (from plasma-derived concentrates). These complications have been virtually eliminated by screening blood donors and heat treatment of purified factor VIII to inactivate HIV. The availability of human recombinant factor VIII now avoids these infectious complications. Screening to detect female carriers and prenatal diagnosis using DNA markers are highly accurate.

Hemophilia B

MOLECULAR PATHOGENESIS: ***Hemophilia B is an X-linked inherited disorder of factor IX deficiency.*** At 1 in 20,000 male births, hemophilia B is four times less common than hemophilia A and accounts for 15% of all cases of hemophilia. Factor IX is a vitamin K–dependent protein that is made in the liver. Many different mutations, from single base substitutions to gross deletions, have been linked to hemophilia B.

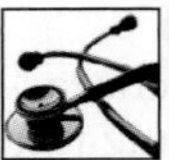

CLINICAL FEATURES: The bleeding manifestations in hemophilia B are like those of hemophilia A. Treatment relies on infusion of purified or recombinant factor IX concentrates.

von Willebrand Disease

von Willebrand disease (vWD) is a heterogeneous complex of hereditary bleeding disorders related to deficiency or abnormality of vWF. Over 20 distinct subtypes are known. A simplified classification (see below) recognizes three major categories. Variable expression of vWF (especially type I) confounds estimates of prevalence, although some hold that vWD is the most common inherited coagulopathy (1% to 2% of the population).

MOLECULAR PATHOGENESIS: vWF is an adhesive molecule produced by endothelial cells and megakaryocytes as a 250-kd monomer that polymerizes to multimers with molecular weights in the millions. It is stored in cytoplasmic Weibel-Palade bodies of endothelial cells, from which it is released into subendothelial tissues and plasma. After endothelial injury, subendothelial vWF binds to platelet glycoprotein receptors (Gp Ib/IX or CD42), promoting platelet adherence and sealing the endothelial injury (Fig. 20-32). vWF can also bind to Gp IIb/IIIa (CD41/61) to promote platelet

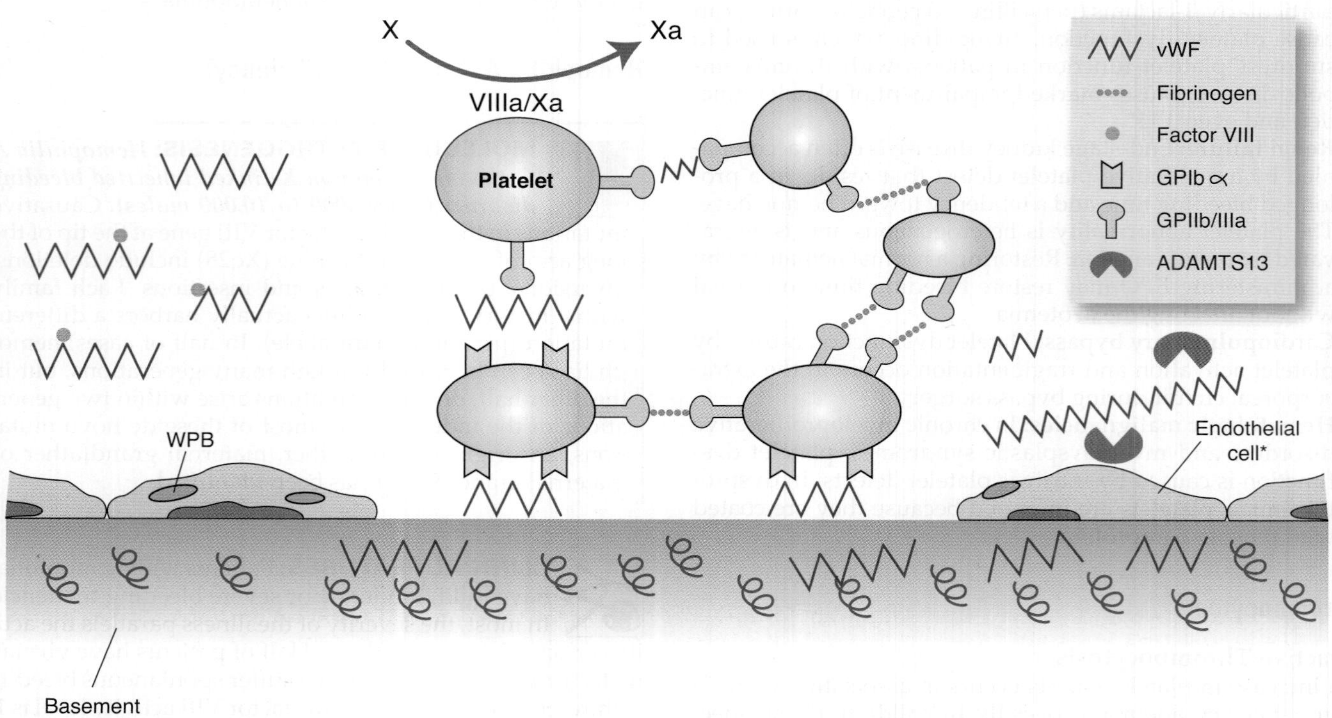

FIGURE 20-32. von Willebrand factor. vWF is stored in Weibel-Palade bodies (WPBs) of endothelial cells and is secreted from activated endothelial cells (*) into the subendothelial space. vWF is also secreted from platelet α granules. After endothelial injury, vWF binds to platelet glycoprotein receptors Gp Ibα and promotes platelet adherence and protects factor VIII. Released vWF stabilizes platelet adhesion to the damaged vessel wall and promotes platelet–fibrin interactions. vWF also binds Gp IIB/IIA on the activated platelet surface to promote platelet aggregation. ADAMTS13 is the protease that cleaves ultralarge multimers of vWF.

aggregation. In plasma, it binds to and protects factor VIII; its absence is always associated with impaired factor VIII activity.

vWD is an autosomal disease, affecting men and women. The *vWF* gene on chromosome 12 is large and complex (180 kb with 52 exons). Three types of the disease are recognized, each of which is heterogeneous:

- **Type I vWD:** These variants constitute 75% of all cases of vWD and are inherited as autosomal dominant traits with variable penetrance. Type I vWD is a **quantitative deficiency in vWF,** in which levels of **all** multimers are reduced, though their relative concentrations remain unchanged.
- **Type II vWD: Qualitative defects in vWF** characterize type II variants, which account for 20% of vWD. In type II disease, interactions of vWF and the blood vessel wall are defective. The plasma activities of both vWF and factor VIII are low. In type IIa, higher-molecular-weight multimers are **absent** from platelets and plasma. Type IIb is caused by synthesis of an **abnormal** vWF with increased affinity for platelets, and may be associated with thrombocytopenia.
- **Type III vWD:** This severe form of vWD is least common and is inherited as an autosomal recessive trait. Some patients are compound heterozygotes (different mutations in the two vWF alleles). vWF activity is absent and plasma levels of factor VIII are less than 10% of normal.

CLINICAL FEATURES: Most cases of vWD are associated with only a mild bleeding diathesis, with the exception of type III.

In contrast to hemophilia-related bleeding, patients with vWD manifest immediate, mucocutaneous bleeding such as easy bruising, epistaxis, gastrointestinal bleeding and (in women) menorrhagia. The presenting symptom is often excessive hemorrhage after trauma or surgery. Patients with type III vWD may have life-threatening hemorrhage from the gut; hemarthroses like those in hemophilia are not infrequent.

The bleeding tendency in all forms of vWD is treated successfully with vWF concentrates or cryoprecipitate. The vasopressin analog desmopressin (DDAVP) is the treatment of choice in types I and IIa vWD because it increases release of preformed vWF from endothelial storage pools. Intranasal sprays of DDAVP are now available.

Other Coagulation Factor Deficiencies

Deficiencies of all coagulation factor proteins, including factors VII, X, V, XI and II (prothrombin) and fibrinogen, have been noted in humans. As expected, the severity of bleeding usually correlates with the level of functional protein activity. Prolonged PT or PTT in patients with bleeding manifestations helps to identify a problem with coagulation factors. Factor-specific assays confirm the diagnosis. The thrombin time helps to screen for deficiency or dysfunction of fibrinogen. Deficiency of fibrinogen causes bleeding. By contrast, dysfibrinogenemia may cause bleeding but more often leads to thrombosis.

Liver Disease

Many coagulation factors are produced in the liver (e.g., II, V, VII, IX, X). In addition, the liver has an essential role in vitamin K absorption. Severe liver disease may cause impaired secretion of coagulation factors as a manifestation of the general protein synthetic defect. In this case, levels of all liver-synthesized coagulation factors are low, affecting both the intrinsic and extrinsic pathways. Both PT and PTT are prolonged.

In comparison to DIC (see below), in liver disease the PT is much more prolonged compared to the PTT, because vitamin K–dependent factors are disproportionately affected.

Vitamin K Deficiency

Liver-derived coagulation factors depend on vitamin K as an essential cofactor in γ-carboxylation of glutamic acid residues to Gla residues. Only if Gla residues are present are the secreted proteins functional. By contrast, factor V is made in the liver but does not require vitamin K. Thus, in vitamin K deficiency (see Chapter 8), activities of factors II, VII, IX and X are low but factor V activity is normal. However, in severe liver disease, all of these factors have low activity.

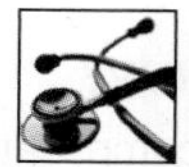

CLINICAL FEATURES: Levels of vitamin K are physiologically low in neonates, and it is standard practice to administer vitamin K to newborns to prevent hemorrhagic disease. In adults, vitamin K deficiency may reflect inadequate dietary intake. Since bacteria in the colon produce the form of vitamin K that is best absorbed, prolonged antibiotic intake, or large colonic resections, may lead to vitamin K deficiency.

Inhibitors of Coagulation Factors

Acquired inhibitors of coagulation factors, **circulating anticoagulants,** are usually IgG autoantibodies. Most are directed against factor VIII and vWF, although rarely antibodies against most of the other coagulation factors are seen. In hereditary coagulation disorders, especially hemophilia, circulating anticoagulants arise in response to administration of plasma concentrates containing the deficient factor. Anticoagulants also develop in some patients with autoimmune disorders (e.g., systemic lupus erythematosus, rheumatoid arthritis), presumably as a result of abnormal immune regulation. Finally, acquired anticoagulants often appear in apparently normal persons.

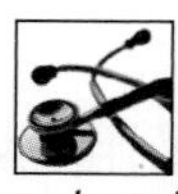

CLINICAL FEATURES: Acquired anticoagulants may be asymptomatic laboratory findings, or they may cause life-threatening hemorrhage. These autoantibodies are difficult to eliminate, but one third of patients have spontaneous remissions. Treatment includes plasma concentrates, corticosteroids and immunosuppressive agents.

Disseminated Intravascular Coagulation

DIC refers to widespread intravascular activation of coagulation with generation of thrombin and microvascular fibrin thrombi and subsequent fibrinolysis, which are accompanied by consumption of platelets and coagulation factors and a hemorrhagic diathesis. DIC is a serious, often fatal disorder that typically occurs as a complication of massive trauma, burns, sepsis from numerous organisms and obstetric emergencies. It is also associated with metastatic cancer, hematopoietic malignancies, cardiovascular and liver disease and many other conditions.

MOLECULAR PATHOGENESIS: DIC begins with activation of the clotting cascades within the vascular compartment by tissue injury, endothelial damage or both. ***Subsequent generation of substantial amounts of thrombin (Fig. 20-33), combined with the initial failure of the natural inhibitory mechanisms to neutralize thrombin, triggers DIC.*** With the consequent uncontrolled intravascular coagulation, the delicate balance between coagulation and fibrinolysis is disrupted. This leads to consumption of clotting factors, platelets and fibrinogen and a consequent hemorrhagic diathesis.

Procoagulant TF is released into the circulation after injury in a variety of circumstances, including direct trauma, brain injury and obstetric accidents (e.g., premature separation of the placenta) (see Chapter 18). **Bacterial endotoxin** also stimulates macrophages to release TF. **Certain tumor cells** cause DIC by releasing TF. With activation of the clotting cascade, intravascular fibrin microthrombi are deposited in the smallest blood vessels. Stimulation of the fibrinolytic system by fibrin generates fibrin split products, which possess anticoagulant properties and contribute to the bleeding diathesis.

Endothelial injury often plays an important role in the pathogenesis of DIC. The anticoagulant properties of the endothelium (Fig. 20-28) are impaired by widely varying injuries, including (1) TNF in gram-negative sepsis; (2) other inflammatory mediators, such as activated complement, IL-1 or neutrophil proteases; (3) viral or rickettsial infections; and (4) trauma (e.g., burns). Thus, platelet aggregates form in the microvasculature.

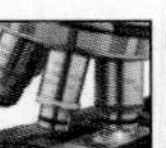

PATHOLOGY: Arterioles, capillaries and venules throughout the body are occluded by **microthrombi** composed of fibrin and platelets (Fig. 20-34). However, because of the enhancement of fibrinolysis, these thrombi may no longer be visualized at the time of autopsy.

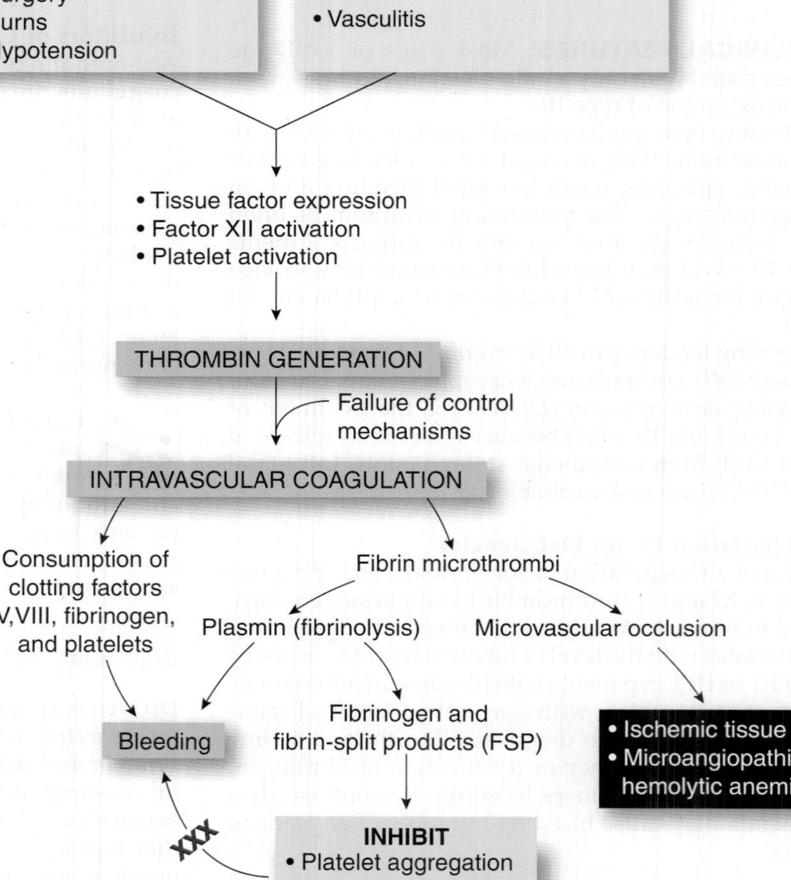

FIGURE 20-33. The pathophysiology of disseminated intravascular coagulation (DIC). The DIC syndrome is precipitated by tissue injury, endothelial cell injury or a combination of the two. These injuries trigger increased expression of tissue factor on cell surfaces and activation of clotting factors (including XII and V) and platelets. With the failure of normal control mechanisms, generation of thrombin leads to intravascular coagulation.

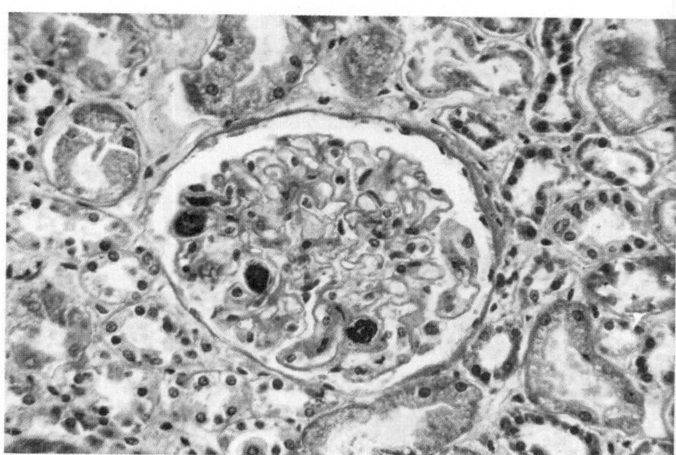

FIGURE 20-34. Disseminated intravascular coagulation. A section of a glomerulus stained with phosphotungstic acid hematoxylin (PTAH), which colors fibrin deep purple, demonstrates several microthrombi.

Microvascular obstruction is associated with widespread **ischemic changes,** particularly in the brain, kidneys, skin, lungs and gastrointestinal tract. These organs are also sites of bleeding, which, in the case of the brain and gut, may be fatal.

Erythrocytes become fragmented **(schistocytes)** by passage through webs of intravascular fibrin, resulting in **microangiopathic hemolytic anemia.** Consumption of activated platelets leads to **thrombocytopenia,** while **depletion of clotting factors** is reflected in prolonged PT and PTT and decreased plasma fibrinogen. Plasma fibrin split products prolong the thrombin time. Fibrinopeptide A and D-dimers are elevated (as markers of coagulation and fibrinolytic activation, respectively).

CLINICAL FEATURES: The symptoms of DIC reflect both microvascular thrombosis and a bleeding tendency. Ischemic changes in the brain lead to seizures and coma. Depending on the severity of DIC, renal symptoms range from mild azotemia to fulminant acute renal failure. Acute respiratory distress syndrome may supervene, and acute gastrointestinal ulcers may bleed. The bleeding diathesis is evidenced by cerebral hemorrhage, ecchymoses and hematuria. Patients with DIC are treated with (1) heparin anticoagulation to interrupt the cycle of intravascular coagulation and (2) replacement of platelets and clotting factors to control the bleeding.

Hypercoagulability Causes Widespread Thrombosis

Hypercoagulability is defined as an increased risk of thrombosis in circumstances that would not cause thrombosis in a normal person. Laboratory evaluation of an underlying hypercoagulable state is warranted in persons who have unexplained thrombotic episodes that show one or more of the following:

- Recurrence
- Development at a young age
- Family history of thrombotic episodes
- Thrombosis in unusual anatomic locations
- Difficulty in controlling with anticoagulants

Disorders that enhance thrombosis have been considered elsewhere (Chapters 7, 10 and 11).

Table 20-9

Principal Causes of Hypercoagulability

Inherited
Activated protein C resistance (factor V Leiden)
Antithrombin deficiency
Protein C deficiency
Protein S deficiency
Dysfibrinogenemias
Acquired
Lupus inhibitor
Malignancy
Nephrotic syndrome
Therapy
Factor concentrates
Heparin
Oral contraceptives
Hyperlipidemia
Thrombotic thrombocytopenic purpura

Hypercoagulable states are divided into inherited and acquired forms (Table 20-9).

Inherited Hypercoagulability

Inherited hypercoagulable states are caused by genetic mutations that affect one of the natural anticoagulant mechanisms. The hereditary tendency to develop thrombosis, irrespective of its origin, is referred to as **thrombophilia.**

- **Activated protein C (APC) resistance—factor V Leiden:** A point mutation in the *factor V* gene (factor V Leiden) renders it resistant to the inhibitory effect of APC. ***Resistance APC action is the most common genetic disorder associated with hypercoagulability, and its prevalence in patients with venous thrombosis has been reported to be as high as 65%.*** The factor V Leiden mutation is found worldwide, but more so in whites (up to 5% of the general population) and much less so in Africans (near 0%). Compared with normal persons, the risk for deep venous thrombosis is increased sevenfold in heterozygotes and 80-fold in homozygotes.
- **Antithrombin deficiency:** This autosomal dominant disorder, which has incomplete penetrance, occurs in 0.2% to 0.4% of the general population and can result in either a quantitative or a qualitative effect on antithrombin. The risk of a thrombotic event (usually venous) ranges between 20% and 80% in different families.
- **Protein C and protein S deficiencies:** Homozygous protein C deficiency causes life-threatening neonatal thrombosis with **purpura fulminans.** Up to 0.5% of the general population has heterozygous protein C deficiency, but many of these persons are symptom free. The clinical presentations for deficiencies of protein C and protein S are similar to that for ATIII deficiency.
- **Other causes of hypercoagulability:** Prothrombin also has a known genetic variant (G20210A) in the 3′ untranslated

region of the mRNA that is associated with thrombosis. The mechanism is not defined but may involve excessively high prothrombin levels in persons with the variant. Unusually high levels of fibrinogen, factor VII and factor VIII are associated with thrombosis, although the molecular basis for the elevated levels remains to be elucidated. Some dysfibrinogenemias are also associated with thrombosis.

Acquired Hypercoagulability

Venous stasis contributes to the hypercoagulability associated with prolonged immobilization and congestive cardiac failure. Increased platelet activation probably accounts for the clotting tendency in patients with myeloproliferative disorders, heparin-associated thrombocytopenia and TTP.

Antiphospholipid Antibody Syndrome

Antibodies directed against several negatively charged protein/phospholipid complexes are associated with the development of antiphospholipid antibody syndrome. This is an autoimmune disorder, which features (1) arterial and venous thrombosis, (2) spontaneous abortions and (3) immune-mediated thrombocytopenia or anemia. Combinations of laboratory tests help to confirm the diagnosis of antiphospholipid syndrome. Antibodies (IgG primarily but not exclusively) react with proteins that bind anionic phospholipids such as phosphatidylserine (PS) or cardiolipin. These membrane lipids are only exposed when cells such as platelets are activated. Many plasma proteins and Gla domain–containing procoagulant proteins (e.g., prothrombin) bind to PS and related anionic phospholipids. The laboratory tests are (1) detection of lupus-type anticoagulant activity, (2) anticardiolipin antibodies and (3) antibodies to plasma protein β_2-GPI. Anticardiolipin antibodies bind to β_2-GPI in the presence of cardiolipin.

Lupus anticoagulants (which are not restricted to patients with systemic lupus erythematosus) are antiphospholipid antibodies in patients with systemic lupus erythematosus and other autoimmune conditions or in otherwise asymptomatic persons. Although they prolong PTT in vitro (because of phospholipid inhibition), these patients, instead of bleeding manifestations, have a hypercoagulable (thrombotic) tendency.

The antiphospholipid antibody syndrome is the leading acquired hematologic cause of thrombosis. The thrombosis in this syndrome has several proposed mechanisms, including platelet activation, endothelial cell activation and alterations in the coagulation factor assembly on membranes. Thrombosis in the uteroplacental vasculature is the likely mechanism in recurrent fetal loss.

Table 20-10

Principal Causes of Neutropenia

Decreased Production
Irradiation
Drug induced (long and short term)
Viral infections
Congenital
Cyclic
Ineffective Production
Megaloblastic anemia
Myelodysplastic syndromes
Increased Destruction
Isoimmune neonatal
Autoimmune
Idiopathic
Drug induced
Felty syndrome
Systemic lupus erythematosus
Dialysis (induced by complement activation)
Splenic sequestration
Increased margination

WHITE BLOOD CELLS

The reader is referred to Chapters 2 through 4 for discussions of white blood cell structure and function.

Nonmalignant Disorders

Neutropenia Is an Absolute Neutrophil Count Below 1500/μL

The clinical consequences of neutropenia are entirely dependent on the severity of neutropenia, ranging from mild with an absolute neutrophil count (ANC) ranging from 1000 to 1500/μL, to moderate (ANC 500 to 1000/μL), to severe (<500/μL). In patients with mild neutropenia **(granulocytopenia),** the number of neutrophils is adequate to defend against microorganisms. With moderate neutropenia, patients become vulnerable to microbial infections; with severe neutropenia, the risk of serious infection is high. The term **agranulocytosis** denotes virtual absence of neutrophils, caused by depletion of both the marginated pool and the bone marrow reserve.

Neutropenia reflects either decreased production or increased destruction of neutrophils (Table 20-10). Most cases of neutropenia are asymptomatic and unexplained, and the term **chronic benign neutropenia** is used. In some cases, the total granulocyte pool is normal, but excessive neutrophils are stored in the marrow or marginated in blood vessels.

DECREASED PRODUCTION OF NEUTROPHILS: Radiation or chemotherapeutic drugs interfere with generation of neutrophils by suppressing normal marrow hematopoiesis. Certain drugs, such as phenothiazines, phenylbutazone, antithyroid drugs and indomethacin, can cause **idiosyncratic** marrow suppression. Viral infection and alcohol intake may also suppress myelopoiesis.

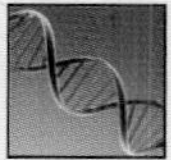

MOLECULAR PATHOGENESIS: Decreased production of granulocytes can also result from constitutional genetic alterations that lead to a number of rare hereditary disorders, including **Kostmann syndrome** and **infantile genetic agranulocytosis.** The genetic basis of several of these disorders has been identified. Mutations in the neutrophil elastase gene cause the most common form of congenital agranulocytosis.

Mutations in *HAX*, a gene regulating apoptosis, have been identified in Kostmann syndrome. Ineffective myelopoiesis is involved in the neutropenia of megaloblastic anemias and myelodysplastic syndromes. In **cyclic neutropenia,** episodes recur regularly about every 21 days.

INCREASED PERIPHERAL DESTRUCTION OF GRANULOCYTES: Accelerated elimination of granulocytes is caused by:

- Increased consumption of neutrophils in overwhelming infections
- Increased sequestration in hypersplenism
- Increased destruction by antibodies

Many **drugs** can lead to immunologically mediated neutrophil destruction, especially sulfonamides, phenylbutazone and indomethacin. The toxic effect results from attachment of circulating antigen–antibody complexes to granulocyte surfaces, with subsequent complement-mediated injury.

Neutropenia is a common feature in AIDS and is multifactorial. Virus-induced depression of neutrophil production is aggravated by infectious consumption of neutrophils and often by antiretroviral drugs (e.g., zidovudine).

Neutrophilia Is an Absolute Neutrophil Count Above 7000/μL

Neutrophilia has many causes (Table 20-11) and reflects (1) **increased mobilization** of neutrophils from bone marrow storage, (2) **enhanced release** from the peripheral blood marginal pool or (3) **stimulation of granulopoiesis** in the bone marrow. Increased mobilization of neutrophils from the bone marrow pool or from the peripheral marginal pool occurs in acute traumatic or infectious disorders. A mild neutrophilia occurs in 20% of women during the third trimester of pregnancy, but the mechanism is poorly defined.

LEUKEMOID REACTION: In acute infections and occasionally in settings of severe hemorrhage or acute hemolysis, the elevation in white blood cells (and, implicitly, neutrophils) may be so pronounced that it may be mistaken for leukemia, especially chronic myeloid leukemia (CML). Such nonneoplastic increase in leukocyte counts is called a **leukemoid reaction.** Clues to the benign (or reactive) nature of a leukemoid reaction include the following: (1) the cells in the peripheral blood are usually segmented neutrophils and fewer neutrophilic myeloid precursors, (2) leukocyte alkaline phosphatase activity is high in a leukemoid reaction but low in CML, (3) the WBC count is usually less than 50,000/μl in reactive conditions and (4) reactive neutrophils often contain large blue cytoplasmic inclusions **(Döhle bodies)** or prominent blue-black granulation of the cytoplasm **(toxic granulation).** If uncertain, the absence of the Philadelphia chromosome (see below) or other cytogenetic abnormality supports the reactive, nonneoplastic nature of the disorder.

Qualitative Disorders of Neutrophils Are Associated With Impaired Function

If granulocyte functionality is impaired, resistance to infection may decrease despite a normal granulocyte count. A number of rare hereditary disorders of granulocytes have been described earlier (see Chapter 2), including chronic granulomatous disease, myeloperoxidase deficiency and Chédiak-Higashi syndrome.

Table 20-11

Principal Causes of Neutrophilia

Infections
Primarily bacterial
Immunologic/Inflammatory
Rheumatoid arthritis
Rheumatic fever
Vasculitis
Neoplasia
Hemorrhage
Drugs
Glucocorticoids
Colony-stimulating factors (CSFs)
Lithium
Hereditary
CD18 deficiency
Metabolic
Acidosis
Uremia
Gout
Thyroid storm
Tissue Necrosis
Infarction
Trauma
Burns

Eosinophilia Occurs With Allergic Reactions and Malignancies

Eosinophils differentiate in the bone marrow under the influence of eosinophil growth factors (e.g., IL-5). They circulate briefly in the blood, then migrate preferentially to the gastrointestinal and respiratory tracts and the skin. Eosinophils respond to chemotactic substances produced by mast cells or are induced by the presence of persistent antigen–antibody complexes, such as occur in chronic parasitic, dermatologic and allergic conditions. The principal causes of eosinophilia are listed in Table 20-12.

Idiopathic hypereosinophilic syndrome refers to an increase in circulating eosinophils above 1500/μL for more than 6 months without evident underlying disease. Eosinophil counts in this condition may reach 50,000 to 100,000/μL.

Hypereosinophilia may accompany mast cell disease (see below), neoplasms such as Hodgkin or non-Hodgkin lymphoma or myeloproliferative disorders (see below). Some of these neoplasms are associated with platelet-derived growth factor receptor (PDGFR) or fibroblast growth factor receptor-1 (FGFR-1) gene rearrangements.

Table 20-12

Principal Causes of Eosinophilia

Principal Causes of Eosinophilia
Allergic Disorders
Skin Diseases
Parasitic (helminth) Infestations
Malignant Neoplasms
Hematopoietic
Solid tumors
Collagen Vascular Disorders
Miscellaneous
Hypereosinophilic syndromes
Eosinophilia–myalgia syndrome
Interleukin-2 therapy

Regardless of the basis for eosinophilia, accumulation of eosinophils in tissues often leads to necrosis, particularly in the myocardium, where it produces endomyocardial disease (see Chapter 11). Neurologic dysfunction may also develop. Eosinophil-mediated cell injury is related to constituents of the eosinophil granules, particularly major basic protein and cationic protein (see Chapter 2).

The prognosis of untreated idiopathic hypereosinophilic syndrome is serious: only 10% of untreated patients survive 3 years. With aggressive corticosteroid therapy, 70% survive more than 5 years, even with cardiac involvement. The prognosis of hypereosinophilia associated with malignancies is mainly a function of the effectiveness of antineoplastic therapy (see below).

Basophilia Is Associated With Allergic Reactions and Myeloproliferative Diseases

The basophil, the least abundant of all leukocytes, differentiates in the bone marrow, circulates briefly in the blood and then passes to the tissues. Its relationship to mast cells is controversial. Basophil granules contain a number of preformed mediators of the inflammatory response, including histamine and chondroitin sulfate. Upon stimulation, these cells also synthesize leukotrienes and other mediators. The principal causes of basophilia are listed in Table 20-13. Basophilia is most commonly observed in immediate-type hypersensitivity reactions and in association with chronic myeloproliferative neoplasms.

Monocytosis Is Seen in Malignant and Inflammatory Conditions

Monocytosis is defined as a peripheral blood monocyte count above 800/μL. The main causes include hematologic malignancies, immunologic and inflammatory conditions, infectious diseases and solid cancers. The former account for at least half of peripheral blood monocytoses. For example, monocytes may constitute a component of myeloproliferative neoplasms, or myelodysplastic/myeloproliferative neoplasms such as chronic myelomonocytic leukemia. In such cases, they may be either morphologically normal or immature and dysplastic cytologically. Monocytosis often occurs in neutropenic states, probably as a compensatory mechanism. Peripheral blood monocytosis may also accompany malignant lymphomas, either Hodgkin or non-Hodgkin.

Table 20-13

Principal Causes of Basophilia

Principal Causes of Basophilia
Allergic (drug, food)
Inflammation
Juvenile rheumatoid arthritis
Ulcerative colitis
Infection
Viral (chickenpox, influenza)
Tuberculosis
Neoplasia
Myeloproliferative syndromes
Basophilic leukemia
Carcinoma
Endocrine
Diabetes mellitus
Myxedema
Estrogen administration

Proliferative Disorders of Mast Cells Release Inflammatory Mediators

Mast cell disorders are heterogeneous and include a wide spectrum of both benign and malignant disorders. The benign, nonneoplastic, reactive conditions of mast cells are important to recognize and differentiate from the malignant syndromes. Mast cells derive from precursor cells in the bone marrow and are found in the connective tissues, usually in close proximity to blood vessels (see Chapter 2). Mast cell granules contain inflammatory mediators, such as histamine, heparin, eosinophil and neutrophil chemotactic factors and certain proteases. The symptoms of mast cell proliferative diseases are caused by the release of these substances and include flushing, pruritus and hives. The secretion of heparin also causes bleeding from the nasopharynx or gastrointestinal tract.

Reactive mast cell hyperplasia is a nonmalignant process that occurs in immediate- and delayed-type hypersensitivity reactions and in lymph nodes that drain the sites of malignant tumors. It is also observed in Waldenström macroglobulinemia, in the bone marrow of women with postmenopausal osteoporosis, in myelodysplastic syndromes and after chemotherapy for leukemia.

Leukemias and Myelodysplastic Syndromes

Malignant leukocytes originate from either myeloid cells or lymphoid cells. Malignant proliferations of myeloid cells are derived from bone marrow cells and manifest as **myelodysplastic syndromes,** or **myeloproliferative neoplasms.** By contrast, **malignant lymphocytes** can arise anywhere there are lymphoid cells. The World Health Organization (WHO) classification is based on conventional morphologic criteria, immunophenotype, cytogenetics and molecular abnormalities. In 2008, the WHO made significant changes to the classification of hematopoietic malignancies.

Myeloproliferative Neoplasms Are Clonal Stem Cell Disorders

Myeloproliferative neoplasms (MPNs) are clonal hematopoietic, stem cell disorders with unregulated, increased proliferation of one or more myeloid lineages (granulocytes, erythrocytes or megakaryocytes). Based on the new WHO classification, four additional and four well-established types are distinguished: **chronic myelogenous leukemia, *BCR-ABL1* positive; polycythemia vera; primary myelofibrosis; essential thrombocythemia; chronic neutrophilic leukemia; chronic eosinophilic leukemia; mastocytosis; and myeloproliferative neoplasm, unclassifiable** (Table 20-14).

Myeloproliferative neoplasms typically affect adults between 40 and 80 years old. They are relatively uncommon, with a yearly incidence of 6 to 10 cases per 100,000. The cause is usually unknown, although radiation or benzene exposure has been implicated in only limited cases. There is also evidence of an inherited susceptibility to MPNs. Characteristic features of all subtypes include hypercellularity of the bone marrow with effective hematopoietic maturation and increased numbers of red cells, granulocytes and/or platelets. Bone marrow fibrosis of different degrees often accompanies MPNs. Specific oncogene mutations and/or translocations are diagnostic of certain myeloproliferative neoplasms (see below).

Chronic Myelogenous Leukemia

CML is derived from an abnormal pluripotent bone marrow stem cell and results in prominent neutrophilic leukocytosis over the full range of myeloid maturation. A **Philadelphia chromosome,** or molecular demonstration of the ***BCR/ABL* fusion gene,** is

Table 20-14

Myeloproliferative Neoplasms*

	Chronic Myelogenous Leukemia, BCR-ABL1 Positive	Polycythemia Vera	Primary Myelofibrosis	Essential Thrombocythemia
Clinical Features				
Peak age range (years)	25–60	40–60	50–70	50–70
Splenomegaly	90%	75%	100%	30% (slight)
Hepatomegaly	50%	40%	80%	40% (slight)
Acute leukemic conversion	80%	5%–10%	5%–10%	2%–5%
Median survival (years)	3–4	13	5	>10
Bone Marrow				
Histopathology	Panhyperplasia (predominantly granulocytic)	Panhyperplasia (predominantly erythroid)	Panhyperplasia with fibrosis	Large megakaryocytes in clusters
M:E ratio	10:1 to 50:1	≤2:1	2:1 to 5:1	2:1 to 5:1
Fibrosis	<10%	15%–20%	90%–100%	<5%
Laboratory Findings				
Hemoglobin	Mild anemia	>20 g/dL	Mild anemia	Mild anemia
RBC morphology	Slight aniso- and poikilocytosis	Slight aniso- and poikilocytosis	Immature erythrocytes and marked aniso- and poikilocytosis	Hypochromic microcytes
Granulocytes	Moderate to markedly increased with spectrum of maturation	Normal to mildly increased; may show a few immature forms	Normal to moderately increased; some immature WBCs	Normal to slightly increased
Platelets	Normal to moderately increased	Normal to moderately increased	Increased to decreased	Markedly increased with abnormal forms
Genetics	Philadelphia chromosome: *BCR/ABL* gene rearrangement	JAK2 activating mutation	JAK2 activating mutation	JAK2 activating mutation

M:E ratio = ratio of myeloid to erythroid; RBC = red blood cell; WBC = white blood cell.

*Other myeloproliferative neoplasms include chronic neutrophilic leukemia, chronic eosinophilic leukemia, mastocytosis and myeloproliferative neoplasm, unclassifiable.

required to establish the diagnosis. CML is the most common myeloproliferative disease and accounts for 15% to 20% of all cases of leukemia.

MOLECULAR PATHOGENESIS: The cause of CML is unknown in most cases. Radiation exposure and myelotoxic agents, such as benzene, have been implicated in a small number of cases. The leukemic cells in CML represent clonal pluripotent stem cells with the ability to differentiate along myeloid or lymphoid pathways; however, most cases show predominantly granulocytic differentiation. A reciprocal balanced translocation involving exchange of genetic material between chromosomes 9 and 22, resulting in a Philadelphia chromosome [t(9;22)(q34;q11)], can be found in 95% of cases using conventional cytogenetic and/or fluorescence in situ hybridization (FISH) techniques (Fig. 20-35A). The Philadelphia chromosome itself is a derivative (shortened) chromosome 22 [der(22q)]. The *BCR* (breakpoint cluster region) gene on chromosome 22 is fused to the *ABL* gene on chromosome 9 to form the *BCR/ABL* fusion gene. A small number of cases have cryptic translocations involving 9q34 and 22q11 that cannot be identified by conventional cytogenetics. In these cases, the *BCR/ABL* fusion gene can be detected by FISH (Fig. 20-35B) or molecular techniques, such as reverse transcriptase polymerase chain reaction (RT-PCR).

In the vast majority of cases, the abnormal BCR/ABL fusion gene encodes for a 210-kd fusion protein (p210), with constitutively active tyrosine kinase activity, central to the pathogenesis of this neoplasm. This activated tyrosine kinase leads to autophosphorylation of the oncoprotein and subsequent activation of downstream signaling pathways implicated in cell proliferation, differentiation, survival and adhesion. Much less commonly, the *BCR/ABL* fusion gene results from a breakage in the minor breakpoint cluster regions yielding alternative fusion proteins such as p190 and p230. While small amounts of the p190 fusion product can be found in CML, this form of BCR/ABL is more commonly seen in **Philadelphia chromosome–positive acute lymphoblastic leukemia occurring outside the setting of CML.** RT-PCR can be used to determine the specific BCR/ABL product fusion present in the leukemic cells as well as to quantitate the amount of fusion product, which is useful for monitoring patient response to therapy. Acquisition of additional chromosomal abnormalities (e.g., second Philadelphia chromosome or trisomy 8) indicates disease progression to a clinically aggressive form.

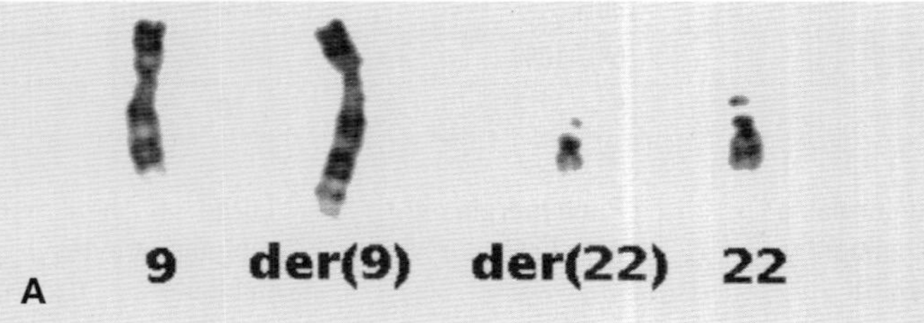

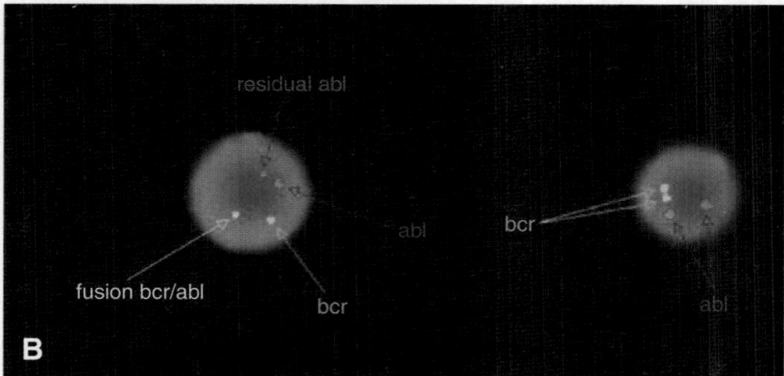

FIGURE 20-35. Chronic myelogenous leukemia. A. The Philadelphia chromosome der(22) is shown. **B.** Fluorescence in situ hybridization (FISH) in a patient with t(9;22) (Philadelphia chromosome)-positive chronic myeloid leukemia. *Right image.* A normal cell contains two separate bcr (chromosome 22) and abl (chromosome 9) genes. *Left image.* A leukemic cell with a fusion bcr/abl signal; residual abl signal; and two normal abl and bcr signals derived from normal chromosomes 9 and 22, respectively.

PATHOLOGY: CML may present in **chronic, accelerated** or **blast phase**.

- **CML, chronic phase (CP),** presents with leukocytosis, consisting of neutrophils in all stages of maturation with a peak of myelocytes and mature neutrophils. By definition, blasts represent less than 10% of circulating or bone marrow leukocytes. Basophilia and eosinophilia are frequent. The platelet count is normal or increased and may exceed $10^6/\mu L$. Bone marrow biopsy shows hypercellularity, usually with total effacement of the marrow space by predominantly myeloid cells and their precursors (Fig. 20-36). Megakaryocytes often form clusters and show abnormal morphologic features, including micromegakaryocytes and hypolobation of nuclei. Reticulin fibers are normal or moderately increased.
- **CML, accelerated phase (AP),** represents disease progression of CML-CP. CML-AP is defined by one of the following criteria: (1) increasing WBC count, (2) increasing splenomegaly unresponsive to therapy, (3) persistent thrombocytopenia or thrombocytosis unresponsive to therapy, (4) additional chromosomal abnormalities, (5) more than 20% blood basophils and (6) 10% to 20% blasts in the blood or bone marrow.
- **CML, blast phase (BP),** is the evolution to acute leukemia and features (1) at least 20% blasts in the peripheral blood or bone marrow, (2) extramedullary proliferation of blasts (skin, lymph nodes, spleen, bone, brain) and (3) clusters of blasts in the bone marrow biopsy. Blast phase heralds a poor prognosis. In 70% of blast crises, the leukemic blasts exhibit morphology and immunophenotype of myeloid lineage; in 30%, they are lymphoblasts, usually with a B-cell precursor immunophenotype (expressing CD10, CD19, CD34 and terminal deoxynucleotidyl transferase [TdT]). In 80% of cases, transformation to accelerated phase or blast crisis is associated with additional cytogenetic alterations such as additional Philadelphia chromosome, trisomy of chromosome 8 or 19 or isochromosome 17q.

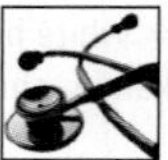

CLINICAL FEATURES: Peak incidence is in the fifth and sixth decades, with a slight male predominance. Patients with CML report fatigue, anorexia,

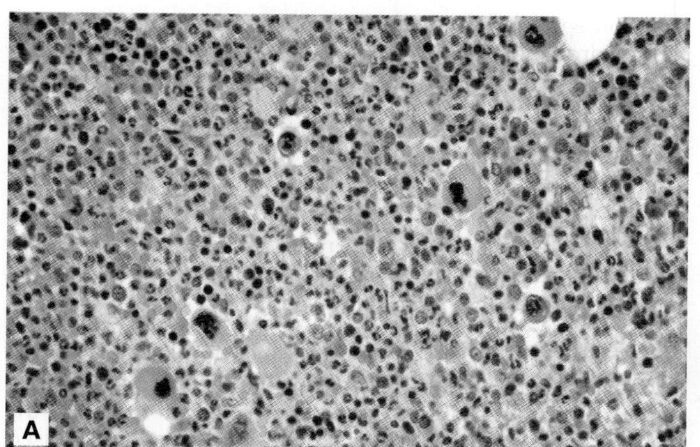

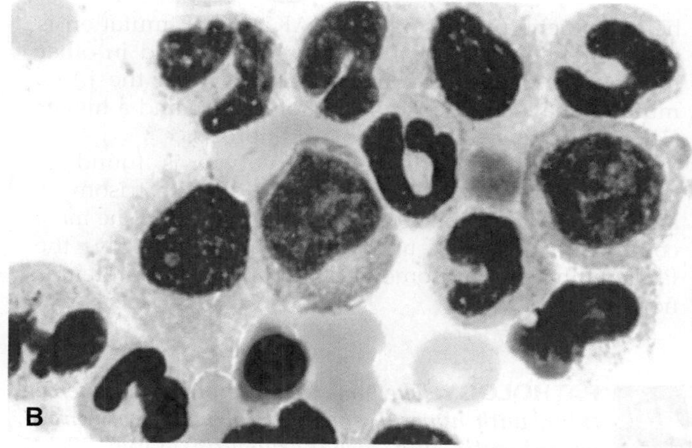

FIGURE 20-36. Chronic myelogenous leukemia. A. The bone marrow is conspicuously hypercellular because of an increase in granulocyte precursors, mature granulocytes and megakaryocytes. **B.** A smear of the bone marrow aspirate from the same patient reveals numerous granulocytes at various stages of development.

weight loss and vague abdominal discomfort caused by hepatosplenomegaly. Acute left upper quadrant pain is often a symptom of splenic infarction. Blood findings include mild to moderate anemia, leukocytosis and absolute basophilia. Peripheral granulocytes are markedly increased with a full maturation range with peaks in myelocytes and segmented neutrophils. Clinical deterioration often heralds blast phase.

CML is a paradigm for a malignancy with a well-defined cytogenetic abnormality that can be targeted by specific drug therapy. The drug imatinib successfully competes for the ATP-binding site on the *BCR/ABL* tyrosine kinase, thereby inactivating it. Improved survival of 70% to 90% overall has been achieved with imatinib. However, resistance to imatinib as a result of development of subclones with point mutations within the ATP-binding pocket has been increasingly reported. Allogeneic bone marrow transplantation is also used with curative intent in some patients with CML.

Polycythemia Vera

PV is a myeloproliferative neoplasm arising from a clonal hematopoietic stem cell characterized by autonomous production of RBCs, not regulated by EPO. *It is a clonal proliferation not only of erythroid elements but also of megakaryocytes and granulocytes in the bone marrow.* As secondary polycythemia and other myeloproliferative neoplasms resemble PV both clinically and pathologically, the WHO established diagnostic criteria for polycythemia. A diagnosis of PV requires that both major criteria and one minor criterion, or the first major criterion and two minor criteria be present. Major criteria include (1) increased RBC mass or hemoglobin greater than 18.5 g/dL in men and greater than 16.5 g/dL in women and (2) presence of Janus kinase 2 (JAK2) V617F mutation or a similar mutation of JAK2. Minor criteria include (1) no elevation of erythropoietin (EPO); (2) hypercellular marrow with panmyelosis involving erythroid, granulocytic and megakaryocytic hyperplasia; and (3) erythroid colony formation in vitro in the absence of growth factor stimulation (endogenous production).

MOLECULAR PATHOGENESIS: PV derives from malignant transformation of a single hematopoietic stem cell with primary commitment to the erythroid lineage. Proliferation of the neoplastic clone occurs mainly in the bone marrow but may involve such extramedullary sites as the spleen, lymph nodes and liver **(myeloid metaplasia).**

As mentioned at the beginning of this chapter, EPO is the primary regulator of erythropoiesis, and its synthesis by the kidney is controlled by transcription factors produced in response to tissue hypoxia.

The neoplastic erythroid progenitor cells of PV are sensitive to EPO, like their normal counterparts. In semisolid culture media, they form luxuriant clusters of erythroid cells (BFU-E) when exposed to EPO. However, at the more mature colony-forming stage (CFU-E), the neoplastic cells form erythroid colonies in semisolid culture media even without erythropoietin stimulation. These autonomous erythroid colonies, "endogenous CFU-E," are characteristic of PV throughout the disease. By contrast, CFU-E formation in normal erythroid progenitor cells requires added EPO ("exogenous CFU-E"). Autonomous proliferation of the more mature cells confers a proliferative advantage to neoplastic clones, since the increased erythrocyte mass suppresses normal EPO secretion and the function of the remaining normal progenitors. Serum EPO levels are thus either normal or low in PV, unlike secondary (functional) erythrocytosis, in which EPO levels are increased.

A somatic mutation in Janus kinase 2 (JAK2; V617F) is found in greater than 95% of patients with PV. This gain-of-function mutation, which occurs in the hematopoietic stem cell and is found in all myeloid lineages, causes the hematopoietic cells to be hypersensitive to growth factors and cytokines, including EPO. The JAK2 family of transcription factors plays a critical role in cytokine signaling in normal hematopoietic cells primarily by activating signal transducers and activators of transcription (STAT) proteins. In vitro studies indicate that the activating JAK2 mutation confers a proliferative and survival advantage to hematopoietic precursors. The JAK2 V617F mutation is not entirely specific for PV, as it can be found in other myeloproliferative neoplasms. Patients with the JAK2 mutation have a longer duration of disease and a higher risk for bleeding complications and fibrosis.

An abnormal cytogenetic karyotype is found in approximately 20% of patients with PV, with trisomy 8 and/or 9 and deletion 20q, 13q and/or 9p being the most commonly observed abnormalities. Importantly, the Philadelphia chromosome or BCR/ABL fusion protein is not found in PV.

PATHOLOGY: *The bone marrow in PV is hypercellular, with hyperplasia of all elements: erythroid, granulocytic and megakaryocytic* (Table 20-14). Although panmyelosis is characteristic, the morphologic findings and clinical course vary depending on the stage of disease. The three stages include the prepolycythemic, the overt polycythemic and the postpolycythemic myelofibrosis phases. In the pre- and polycythemic stages, erythroid precursors predominate, and the myeloid-to-erythroid ratio is less than 2:1. Erythroid maturation is normal. The granulocyte series also shows normal maturation. Megakaryocytes are typically increased in number, are of variable size and tend to cluster. In 90% of cases, marrow-stainable iron is decreased or absent. A mild to moderate increase in reticulin is common in the early stages. In the later stage of postpolycythemic myelofibrosis, or the "spent phase," erythropoiesis decreases and the marrow becomes replaced by reticulin and collagen fibrosis.

The spleen is typically enlarged, with prominent accumulation of erythrocytes in the red pulp cords and sinuses. In the polycythemic phase, there is minimal if any evidence of extramedullary hematopoiesis (EMH). This phenomenon increases in the postpolycythemic myelofibrotic phase and is characterized by formation of blood cell precursors outside the marrow. Although the principal site of extramedullary hematopoiesis is the spleen, liver and lymph nodes are other possible sites and contain foci of erythroid precursor cells, immature granulocytes and megakaryocytes.

Blood hemoglobin concentration may exceed 20 g/dL, and the Hct surpasses 60% (Table 20-14). A mild to moderate leukocytosis of 10,000 to 25,000/μL occurs initially in two thirds of cases. A mild to moderate thrombocytosis (400,000 to 800,000 platelets/μL) occurs initially in half of cases, often with abnormal morphologic features. Anemia is one criterion of the later, spent phase of PV. Hyperuricemia and secondary gout may be present and are related to rapid cell turnover.

The peripheral blood smear in the polycythemic phase reveals crowding of RBCs, which are usually normochromic normocytic. Hypochromia and microcytosis are seen if there is iron deficiency. Iron-deficiency anemia is common in PV, largely because storage iron is diverted to the increased red cell mass or caused by phlebotomy or gastrointestinal bleeding. In the later stages of PV, anemia develops and the peripheral blood smear shows a leukoerythroblastic picture, poikilocytosis with teardrop-shaped RBCs.

CLINICAL FEATURES: In North America, 8 to 10 cases of PV per million are seen annually. The mean age at diagnosis is 60 years. Onset tends to be insidious, and symptoms are generally nonspecific, typically relating to the increased erythrocyte mass. Plethora and splenomegaly are early findings. Headache, dizziness and visual problems result from hypertension and/or vascular disturbances in the brain and retina. Angina pectoris, secondary to slowing of coronary artery blood flow, and intermittent claudication caused by sluggish peripheral blood flow in the lower extremities may be observed. Gastric or duodenal ulcers may result from circulatory problems in the gastrointestinal tract and possibly (in part) from histamine release by basophils. Major thrombotic complications occur in approximately 20% of cases, including stroke and myocardial infarction.

The clinical course of PV tends to proceed in the three phases described above. The **prepolycythemic phase** is the prodromal phase characterized by borderline or mild erythrocytosis with mild erythroid hyperplasia, but not to the degree diagnostic of PV. The diagnosis can be rendered based on a low EPO level, the identification of JAK2 or similar mutation or endogenous erythroid colony (EEC) formation. Later, when red cell mass is definitively increased, the polycythemic stage has been reached. In 10% of cases, the disease evolves to the postpolycythemic (spent) phase when excessive proliferation of erythroid cells ceases, resulting in decreased erythrocyte mass and anemia. Another 10% of cases progress to myelofibrosis with extramedullary hematopoiesis, like that in other myeloproliferative neoplasms **(postpolycythemic myelofibrosis). Acute myelogenous leukemia or myelodysplasia** occurs in up to 15% of cases of PV and may be caused in part by treatment with ^{32}P or alkylating agents. The disease progression is often the result of karyotypic evolution with the acquisition of complex chromosomal abnormalities.

Median survival with PV is 13 years. Specific causes of death related to the disease itself include thrombosis, hemorrhage, acute myeloid leukemia (AML) and the spent phase. Therapeutic reduction of erythrocyte mass, by repeated phlebotomy or chemotherapy, is effective management in most cases.

Primary Myelofibrosis

Primary myelofibrosis (PMF) is a clonal myeloproliferative neoplasm in which marrow fibrosis is accompanied by prominent megakaryopoiesis and granulopoiesis. Extramedullary hematopoiesis is present in fully developed disease.

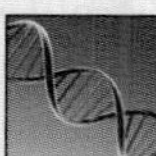

MOLECULAR PATHOGENESIS: As in other types of myeloproliferative neoplasia, exposure to benzene or radiation has occasionally been implicated in primary myelofibrosis (chronic idiopathic myelofibrosis). The neoplastic megakaryocytes produce PDGF and TGF-β, both of which are powerful fibroblast mitogens. Ultimately, the entire marrow space is displaced by connective tissue, although fibroblasts are not part of the clonal stem cell disorder. In the fibrotic phase, clonal stem cells enter the circulation and give rise to extramedullary hematopoiesis at multiple anatomic sites, especially the spleen. Approximately 50% of patients with PMF have JAK2 V617F mutation, which is important in the pathogenesis of the disease. A minority of cases have mutations of MPL, a gene encoding the thrombopoietin (TPO) receptor.

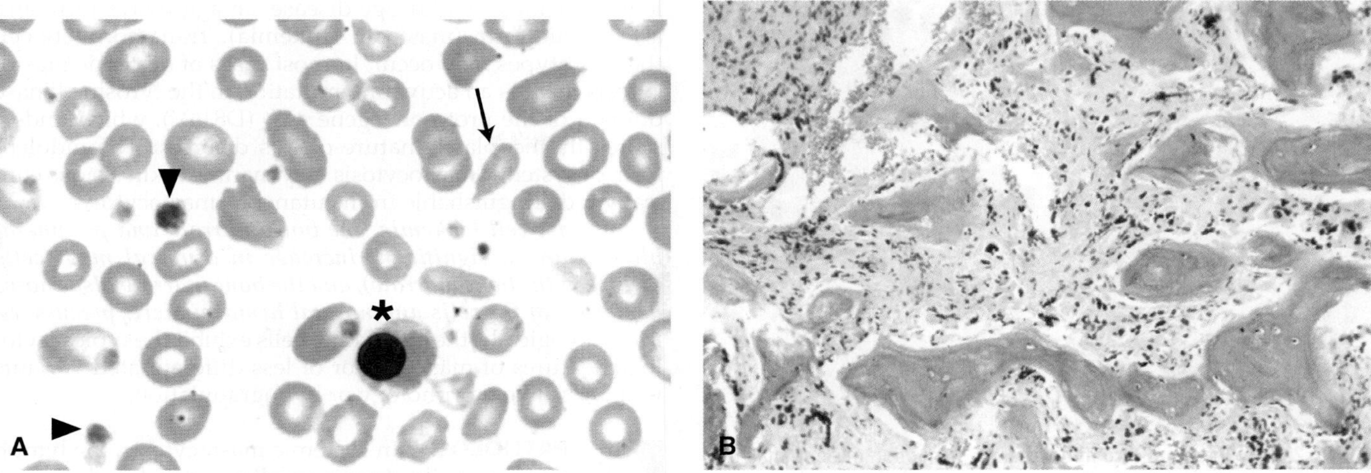

FIGURE 20-37. Chronic idiopathic myelofibrosis. A. Peripheral smear shows anisocytosis (red blood cells of different sizes), poikilocytosis with teardrop forms (*arrow*) and nucleated erythrocytes (*). Giant platelets are also seen (*arrowheads*). **B.** A section of bone marrow shows collagenous fibrosis, osteosclerosis and numerous abnormal megakaryocytes.

PATHOLOGY: PMF evolves through two stages, the prefibrotic and early stage and the fibrotic stage. The majority of patients are diagnosed at the fibrotic stage, but 30% to 40% are first detected in a prefibrotic stage. The **prefibrotic stage** usually presents with unexplained thrombocytosis and features a hypercellular bone marrow, with predominant neutrophilic and megakaryocytic proliferation and minimal fibrosis. The megakaryocytes are densely clustered and atypically lobated with "cloud-like" nuclei. In the **fibrotic stage,** the blood shows either leukopenia or marked leukocytosis, and myeloid precursors and nucleated RBCs (leukoerythroblastosis) are usually present. The red cells exhibit poikilocytosis and teardrop forms (Fig. 20-37A). The bone marrow cellularity gradually decreases, and foci of hematopoiesis containing mostly atypical megakaryocytes alternate with hypo- or acellular regions. Conspicuous reticulin or collagen fibrosis in the marrow defines this stage (Fig. 20-37B). Extramedullary hematopoiesis leads to splenomegaly, hepatomegaly and lymphadenopathy, and may be seen in other organs.

The WHO requires the presence of three major criteria and two minor criteria for a diagnosis of PMF. The major criteria include the presence of megakaryocyte proliferation with or without fibrosis, the absence of features of other well-defined MPNs and demonstration of a clonal genetic marker, such as JAK2 mutation. Minor criteria include leukoerythroblastosis, anemia and splenomegaly.

CLINICAL FEATURES: The annual incidence of idiopathic myelofibrosis is estimated at 0.5 to 1.5 per 100,000. It is a disease of the elderly, with a peak incidence in the seventh decade. A quarter of patients with idiopathic myelofibrosis are asymptomatic at diagnosis, the disease being detected by splenomegaly on physical examination or by demonstration of teardrop red cells or thrombocytosis. Early clinical symptoms are nonspecific and include fatigue, low-grade fever, night sweats and weight loss. Platelet function may be impaired and associated with either increased platelet aggregation and thrombosis or decreased platelet aggregation with a bleeding diathesis. Transformation to AML occurs in 5% to 30% of cases (Table 20-14).

Essential Thrombocythemia

Essential thrombocythemia (ET) is an uncommon neoplastic disorder of hematopoietic stem cells, characterized by uncontrolled proliferation of megakaryocytes. A marked and sustained increase in circulating platelets (>450,000/μL) is accompanied by recurrent episodes of thrombosis and hemorrhage. The disease affects middle-aged persons, with a slight male predominance (Table 20-14).

MOLECULAR PATHOGENESIS: ET is a clonal disorder believed to derive from neoplastic transformation of a single hematopoietic stem cell with principal, but not exclusive, commitment to megakaryocytic lineage. The disease features a marked proliferation of megakaryocytes, with up to a 15-fold or greater increase in platelet production and consequent marked thrombocytosis (sometimes exceeding 1 million/μL). Approximately 40% to 50% have a JAK2 V617F mutation or other functionally similar abnormality. One to 2% of cases have an MPL gene mutation. Chromosomal abnormalities include deletion 20q and trisomy 8 and are identified in approximately 5% to 10% of cases.

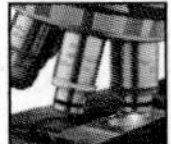
PATHOLOGY: The diagnosis of ET requires exclusion of other chronic myeloproliferative neoplasms. Abnormalities of platelet function are common in primary thrombocythemia. Recurrent episodes of thrombosis in arteries or veins are attributed to severe thrombocytosis, and hemorrhage reflects defects in platelet function. Thromboses in the spleen, with subsequent infarctions, may result in splenic atrophy. Iron-deficiency anemia follows hemorrhage from gastrointestinal or urogenital tracts. The bone marrow is normocellular or markedly hypercellular, with decreased fat cells (Fig. 20-38). Increased numbers of large, hyperlobulated, "stag-horn–shaped" megakaryocytes form cohesive clusters or sheets in the marrow. Reticulin fibers in the marrow are increased in one third of cases, but post-ET myelofibrosis is rare. Iron stores are normal or low.

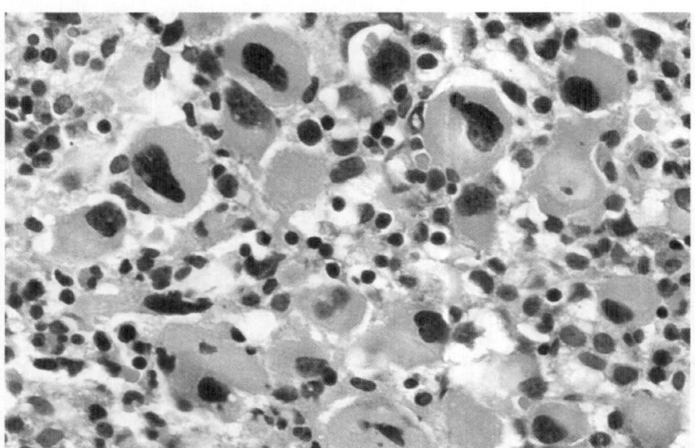

FIGURE 20-38. Essential thrombocythemia. A section of bone marrow exhibits a conspicuous increase in the number of megakaryocytes, which display atypical features and hypolobated forms.

The spleen is mildly enlarged in half the cases of primary thrombocythemia. Microscopically, extramedullary hematopoiesis is common, but extensive myeloid metaplasia only occurs when myelofibrosis develops. The peripheral blood shows thrombocytosis.

CLINICAL FEATURES: The clinical course of primary thrombocythemia is protracted, with a median survival of over 10 to 15 years. In untreated cases, thrombosis of large arteries and veins is common, especially in the legs, heart, intestine and kidneys. Hemorrhage is less common, usually from mucosal surfaces, and is mild, not life-threatening. AML supervenes in up to 5% of cases. The disease is treated with platelet pheresis and myelosuppressive chemotherapy.

Mastocytosis

Mastocytosis is a clonal hematopoietic disorder characterized by an abnormal accumulation of mast cells in certain tissues, mainly skin and bone marrow. The recent WHO classification has placed the systemic neoplastic mast cell disorders in the category of MPN. The distinct subtypes are characterized by tissue involvement and clinical manifestations.

CUTANEOUS MASTOCYTOSIS: This lesion can present as either as a single, tan-brown, cutaneous nodule in newborns or as several groups of skin nodules in young children. The most common subtype is called **urticaria pigmentosa.** This entity presents as multiple, symmetrically distributed, tan-brown, cutaneous macules or papules, most commonly in infants and young children. The skin of the trunk is predominantly affected, but any cutaneous site may be involved. ***Microscopically, a disseminated perivascular and periadnexal dermal infiltrate of mast cells is observed.*** Spontaneous resolution usually occurs at puberty and systemic involvement is not present.

SYSTEMIC MASTOCYTOSIS: This is a rare myelogenous neoplasm, characterized by infiltration of many organs with mast cells, including the skin, lymph nodes, spleen, liver, bones, bone marrow and gastrointestinal tract. Systemic mastocytosis has a number of possible manifestations, including an indolent form, a subtype associated with clonal hematologic non–mast cell lineage disease, an aggressive form and a leukemic form (mast cell leukemia). Transition between these subtypes may occur. In most cases of systemic mastocytosis there is an activating mutation in the tyrosine kinase domain of the proto-oncogene *c-kit* (D816V), which underscores the neoplastic nature of this disorder. The indolent form of systemic mastocytosis may manifest skin lesions clinically indistinguishable from cutaneous mastocytosis.

In mast cell leukemia, the bone marrow and peripheral blood show a significant increase in atypical mast cells (>20% in the bone marrow), and the bone marrow also shows depletion of fat cells and normal hematopoietic precursors. Morphologically, the circulating cells exhibit the typical cytologic features of mast cells or of less differentiated variants with blast-like morphology or hypogranulation.

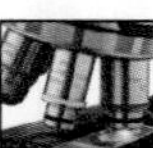

PATHOLOGY: In systemic mastocytosis, the lymph nodes initially show perifollicular and perivascular infiltration by mast cells (Fig. 20-39). Compact aggregates of mast cells within the paracortical areas can also be seen. The spleen exhibits nodular aggregates of mast cells with accompanying dense fibrosis in the red and white pulp. In the liver, the portal triads are first involved. Involvement of the bone marrow may be peritrabecular, perivascular or diffuse, and there is often accompanying fibrosis and eosinophilia.

CLINICAL FEATURES: Systemic mastocytosis occurs at any age, but adults in the sixth and seventh decades of life are most commonly affected. Patients with systemic mastocytosis suffer symptoms related to the overproduction of a number of mediators normally produced by mast cells and basophils, including histamine, prostaglandin D_2 and thromboxane B_2. Most experience gastrointestinal pain and diarrhea. The serum tryptase levels are usually elevated. Anaphylactic episodes—with pruritus, flushing and asthmatic symptoms—are common. Extensive mast cell infiltration of the bone marrow leads to secondary anemia, leukopenia and thrombocytopenia. The indolent form of systemic mastocytosis follows a chronic course, with about half of patients surviving for 5 years. Symptomatic

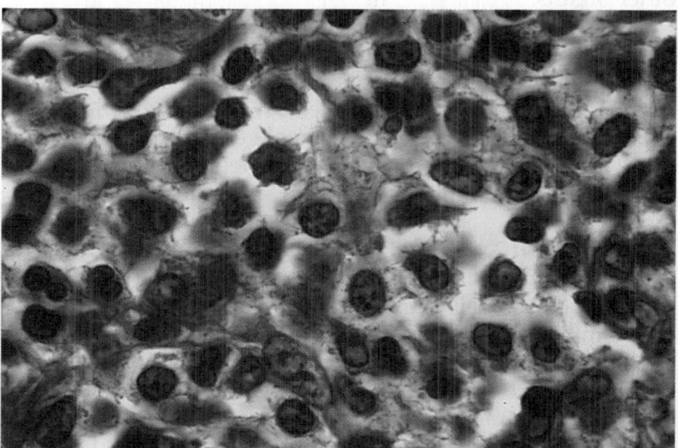

FIGURE 20-39. Mastocytosis. A section of lymph node shows effacement of the normal architecture by sheets of mast cells. The centrally situated nuclei are round to elongated, and occasionally indented. The cytoplasm is pale pink and finely granular.

relief is obtained, at least partially, with H_1- and H_2-receptor antagonists. There is no effective therapy for the underlying disease process.

Myelodysplastic Syndromes Are Clonal Disorders That Cause Ineffective Hematopoiesis

Myelodysplastic syndromes (MDSs) are characterized by peripheral blood cytopenia, marrow failure and dysplastic morphology in one or more hematopoietic lineages. There is discrepancy between the paucity of peripheral blood elements and the hypercellularity in the bone marrow because of ineffective hematopoiesis and increased apoptosis in the marrow. The WHO classifies several subtypes of MDS depending on whether dysplasia involves one or more cell lineages and the percentage of blasts in the peripheral blood or bone marrow. ***All subtypes manifest refractory anemia and/or other cytopenia. MDS does not display erythrocytosis, leukocytosis or thrombocytosis, in contrast to the MPNs discussed above.*** MDS exhibits less than 20% blasts in the peripheral blood or bone marrow, in contrast to acute leukemia, which manifests greater than 20% blasts in the peripheral blood or bone marrow. Progression of MDS to AML (i.e., progression from marrow failure to a proliferative state) occurs in 30% to 40% of cases that usually have genetic instability. This subset of MDS is referred to as **preleukemic syndrome.** Some low-grade subsets of MDS have a more stable clinical course and no progression or a very low rate of progression to AML.

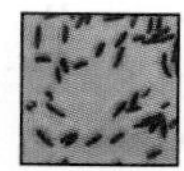

ETIOLOGIC FACTORS: MDSs may be either primary (de novo) or secondary (therapy related). Patients with secondary myelodysplasia usually have a history of treatment with chemotherapy (particularly alkylating agents or topoisomerase II inhibitors) or radiation therapy. Other risk factors for MDS include benzene exposure, cigarette smoking, and congenital disorders such as Fanconi anemia or Kostmann syndrome.

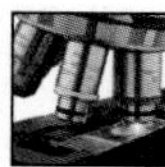

PATHOLOGY: The subclassification of MDS is based on the presence of **dysplasia** in one or more of the hematopoietic lineages and the proportion of myeloblasts. Dysplasia is most frequently observed in erythroid precursors, which show megaloblastoid changes, multinucleation, nuclear budding, bridging between nuclei and karyorrhexis (Fig. 20-40). Erythroid precursors with iron-laden mitochondria around the nuclei **(ringed sideroblasts)** are found in several subtypes of MDS (Fig. 20-41A). Dysgranulopoietic features include nuclear hyposegmentation (pseudo-Pelger-Huët cells) and cytoplasmic hypogranulation. Dysplastic megakaryocytes may be mononuclear or hypolobated, or show nuclear separation (Fig. 20-41B). Careful elucidation of the blast percentage is critical to the subcategory of MDS and clinical course of the disease.

Cytogenetic and molecular studies are essential for the diagnosis and prognosis of myelodysplastic syndromes. Clonal abnormalities are identified in approximately 50% of cases. Isolated deletion of chromosome 5 (5q−), when accompanied by macrocytic anemia, megaloblastoid erythropoiesis with or without ringed sideroblasts and normal or increased platelet counts with monolobated megakaryocytes, defines a clinicopathologic entity that occurs primarily in elderly women and indicates a more favorable prognosis. Other favorable chromosomal abnormalities are −y and 20q−. By contrast, deletion of chromosome 7 (7q−) has an unfavorable prognosis. ***The more chromosomal abnormalities there are, the less favorable is the outcome.***

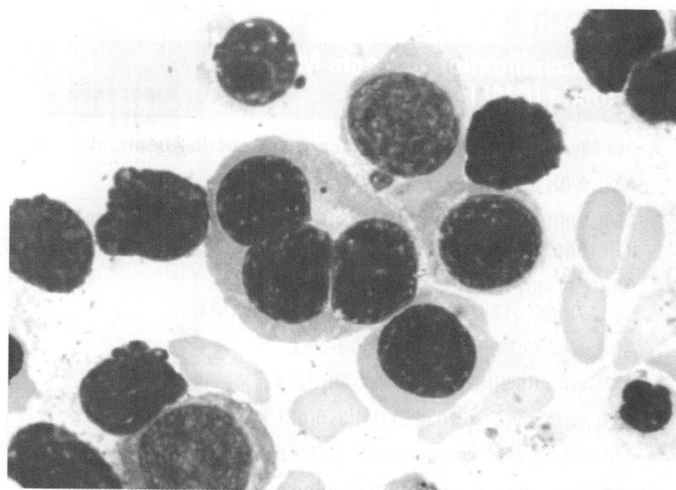

FIGURE 20-40. Myelodysplastic syndrome. Dysplastic, multinucleated, megaloblastoid erythroid precursors are shown.

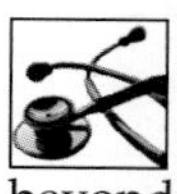

CLINICAL FEATURES: MDS usually occurs in older patients with a median age of 70 years. The various subtypes of MDS classified by the WHO are beyond the scope of the current discussion. ***However, as a general common feature, MDS presents with symptoms related to peripheral blood cytopenias: weakness in anemia, recurrent infections in neutropenia and bleeding in thrombocytopenia. Up to 40% of patients with MDS progress to AML.*** Progression to AML and overall prognosis are dependent of the morphologic subtype of MDS. Increased numbers of blasts, complex cytogenetic abnormalities and increased cytopenia confer a worse prognosis.

Acute Myeloid Leukemia Is a Clonal Proliferation of Myeloblasts in the Marrow With Their Subsequent Appearance in Blood and Possibly in Extramedullary Tissues

A diagnosis of AML requires greater than 20% myeloblasts in the peripheral blood or bone marrow. These criteria are relaxed in the cases of several AML types with specific

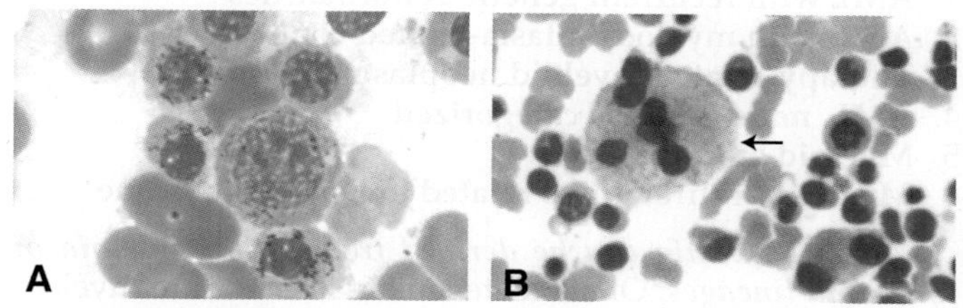

FIGURE 20-41. Myelodysplastic syndrome. A. Smear of a bone marrow aspirate stained with Prussian blue shows an erythroid precursor cell containing iron-laden mitochondria that encircle the nuclei (ringed sideroblast). **B.** Dysplastic megakaryocyte with nuclear separation (*arrow*).

20 | Hematopathology

Table 20-15

WHO Classification of Acute Myeloid Leukemia (AML)

Acute Myeloid Leukemia with Recurrent Genetic Abnormalities
AML with t(8;21)(q22;q22); RUNX1-RUNX1T1
AML with abnormal bone marrow eosinophils inv(16)(p13q22) or t(16;16)(p13;q22); CBFβ/MYH11
Acute promyelocytic leukemia [AML with t(15;17)(q22;q12)(PML/RARα] and variants (**M3**)
AML with (9;11)(p22;q23) MLLT3-MLL
AML with t(6;9)(p23:q34); DEK-NUP214
AML with inv(3)(q21q24.2) or t(3;3)(q21;126.2); RPN1-EVI1
AML (megakaryoblastic) with t(1;22)(p13;q13); RBM15-MKL1
Acute Myeloid Leukemia with Myelodysplasia-Related Changes
Following a myelodysplastic syndrome or myelodysplastic syndrome/myeloproliferative disorder
Without antecedent myelodysplastic syndrome
Therapy-Related Myeloid Neoplasms
Alkylating agent related
Topoisomerase type II inhibitor related (some may be lymphoid)
Other types
Acute Myeloid Leukemia Not Otherwise Categorized
AML minimally differentiated (**M0**)
AML without maturation (**M1**)
AML with maturation (**M2**)
AML (**M4**)
Acute monoblastic and monocytic leukemia (**M5**)
Acute erythroid leukemia (**M6**)
Acute megakaryoblastic leukemia (**M7**)
Myeloid sarcoma
Myeloid proliferations related to Down syndrome

PML = promyelocytic leukemia; RAR = retinoic acid receptor; WHO = World Health Organization.

cytogenetic abnormalities. Such types are defined as AML regardless of blast cell count. When less than 20% blasts are present in AMLs without recurrent cytogenetic abnormalities, the disease should be considered in the MDS or MPN categories. AML is classified into six distinct types (Table 20-15):

1. **AML with recurrent genetic abnormalities**
2. **AML with myelodysplasia-related changes**
3. **Therapy-related myeloid neoplasms**
4. **AML, not otherwise categorized**
5. **Myeloid sarcoma**
6. **Myeloid proliferations related to Down syndrome**

Acute leukemia can be derived from either myeloid or lymphoid lineages. Of all acute leukemias, 70% are myeloid leukemias. The remainder are lymphoblastic leukemias (discussed below under lymphoid malignancies).

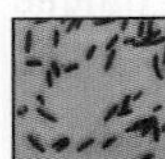

ETIOLOGIC FACTORS: Most cases of AML are of unknown etiology, but in a few instances, a causal relationship between radiation, cytotoxic chemotherapy or benzene exposure has been documented. An increased incidence in AML was noted after the detonation of atomic bombs in Hiroshima and Nagasaki (see Chapter 8). Cigarette smoking doubles the risk for AML.

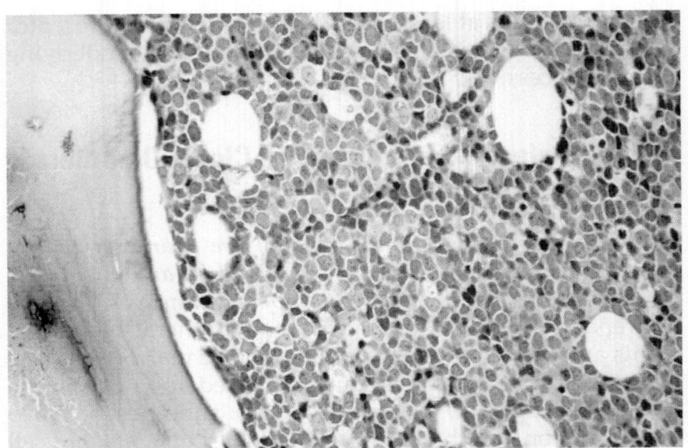

FIGURE 20-42. Acute myelogenous leukemia. A bone marrow section is hypercellular, resulting from effacement of the normal architecture by myeloblasts.

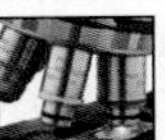

PATHOLOGY: Malignant myeloblasts of AML are detectable in the bone marrow and, in most instances, in the blood. Typically, the malignant cells pack the bone marrow and displace normal hematopoietic cells (Fig. 20-42). Myeloblasts are medium-sized to large cells with round or slightly irregular nuclei and immature nuclear chromatin. Depending on the AML subtype, eosinophilic, slender cytoplasmic inclusions, *Auer rods,* may be present in the cytoplasm (Fig. 20-43). These inclusions, which are coalesced primary granules, are specific for the myeloid lineage and preclude a diagnosis of lymphoblastic leukemia.

Immunophenotyping by flow cytometry and cytogenetic studies is essential for correct classification of AML. Myeloid antigens frequently expressed include CD13, CD15, CD33

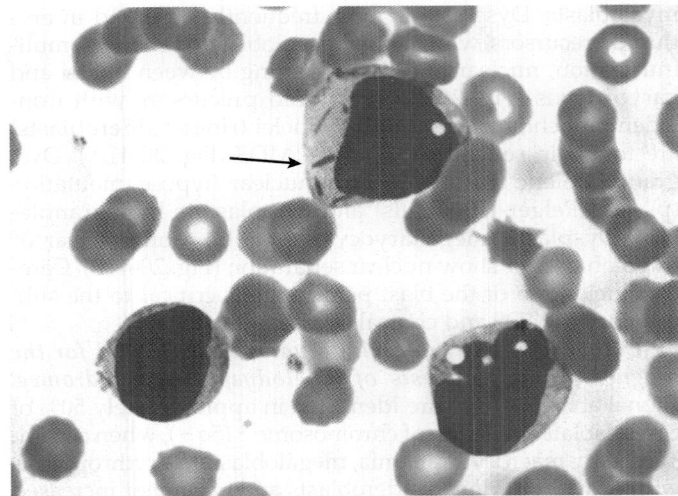

FIGURE 20-43. Acute promyelocytic leukemia. Auer rods are prominent (*arrow*).

and CD117 (c-kit), in addition to the progenitor cell marker CD34. AML with megakaryoblastic differentiation may show the platelet/megakaryocyte markers CD41 and CD61 (platelet Gp IIb/IIIa complex).

Although cytochemical markers, including myeloperoxidase, Sudan black and nonspecific esterase (NSE), were critical to the diagnosis of AML in the past, flow cytometric characterization is now preferred for diagnosis and subtyping.

CLINICAL FEATURES: ***Most cases of AML occur in adults, with a median age of 67 years at onset. The major problems associated with AML reflect the progressive accumulation in the marrow of immature myeloid cells that lack the potential for further differentiation and maturation.*** Whereas leukemic myeloblasts replicate at a slower rate than do normal hematopoietic precursor cells, the frequency of spontaneous cell death is also less than normal. The expanded pool of abnormal leukemic blasts encroaches on the marrow and suppresses normal hematopoiesis. ***Thus, the major clinical problems in AML are granulocytopenia, thrombocytopenia and anemia.*** Infections, particularly with opportunistic organisms (e.g., fungi), are common, as are cutaneous bleeding (petechiae and ecchymoses) and serosal hemorrhages over viscera. Untreated AML carries a dismal prognosis. Chemotherapy leads to remission in over 50% of patients, but overall 5-year survival is less than 30%. Bone marrow transplantation is a common mode of treatment for high-risk forms of AML, and for AML in relapse.

Selected Acute Myeloid Leukemia Subtypes

ACUTE MYELOID LEUKEMIA WITH RECURRENT GENETIC ABNORMALITIES: There are multiple cytogenetic abnormalities associated with this category of AML. These include t(8;21)(q22;q22), inv(16)(p13,1q22) or t(16;16)(p13.1;q22); t(15;17)(q22;q12), t(9;11)(p22;q23). t(6;9)(p23;q34); inv(3)(q21q26.2) or t(3;3)(q21;q26.2), t(1;22)(p13;q13) and AML with mutated *NPM1* or *CEBPA*. AML with t(15;17)(q22;q12) is also named **acute promyelocytic leukemia (APL).** ***APL is defined by the chromosomal translocation involving the*** **promyelocytic leukemia 1 (PML1)** ***gene on chromosome 15q22 and the retinoic acid receptor (RAR) gene on chromosome 17q12.*** APL mainly affects middle-aged patients and accounts for 5% to 10% of all cases of AML.

APL is a paradigm for a molecularly defined disease in which the underlying genetic defect determines the type of treatment. The translocation results in the *PML/RARα* fusion gene that encodes a functional retinoic acid receptor. The receptor can be targeted by all-*trans*-retinoic acid (ATRA), which mediates maturation of the tumor cells. The bone marrow is packed with tumor cells that have promyelocytic morphologic features. Auer rods may be abundant. Leukemic cells are strongly reactive for myeloperoxidase or Sudan black. ***Patients with APL frequently present with DIC.*** Senescent leukemic cells degranulate and activate the coagulation cascade. Treatment with ATRA induces maturation of the tumor cells and prevents both degranulation and DIC. The prognosis for APL is more favorable than for all other AMLs.

THERAPY-RELATED MYELOID NEOPLASMS: Cytotoxic chemotherapy or radiation therapy for a prior malignancy can induce mutational changes that lead to hematopoietic neoplasms several years after treatment. Included in this category are therapy-related AML, myelodysplastic syndrome and myelodysplastic/myeloproliferative neoplasms. Alkylating agents and radiation most often give rise to myelodysplasia and subsequent AML after 5 to 10 years. In contrast, topoisomerase II inhibitors (epipodophyllotoxins) lead to overt AML with a latency of 1 to 5 years.

ACUTE MYELOID LEUKEMIA, NOT OTHERWISE CATEGORIZED: This set of leukemias does not meet the characteristics of any of the other subtypes of AML. They are therefore groups based on the older French-American-British (FAB) classification. The WHO classification incorporates the FAB scheme (Fig. 20-44):

- **AML, minimally differentiated:** The leukemic cells are immature myeloblasts with no defining morphologic criteria of the myeloid lineage. Immunophenotyping by flow cytometry establishes the myeloid nature of the tumor cells. The prognosis is unfavorable.
- **AML without maturation:** Less than 10% of the myeloid cells are promyelocytes or more mature myeloid cells. The disease occurs most often in middle-aged persons.
- **AML with maturation:** More than 10% maturing myeloid cells (promyelocytes and later) are present.
- **Acute myelomonocytic leukemia (AMML):** Some 20% to 80% of tumor cells show monocytoid features. AMML accounts for 20% of all AMLs.

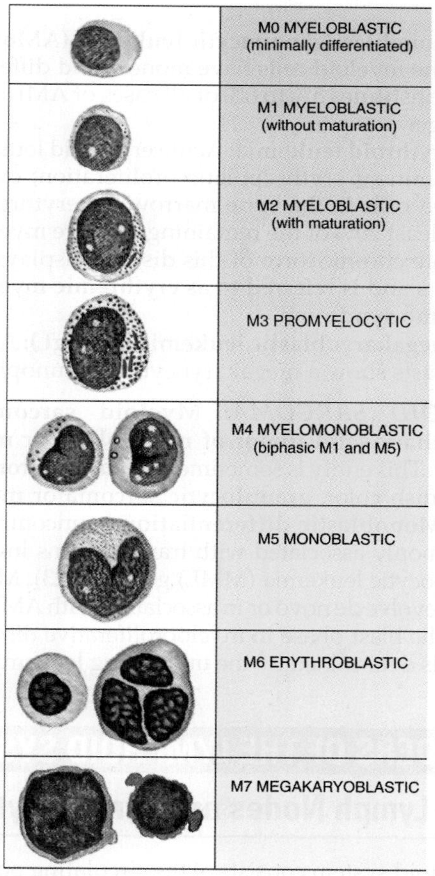

M0 MYELOBLASTIC (minimally differentiated)
M1 MYELOBLASTIC (without maturation)
M2 MYELOBLASTIC (with maturation)
M3 PROMYELOCYTIC
M4 MYELOMONOBLASTIC (biphasic M1 and M5)
M5 MONOBLASTIC
M6 ERYTHROBLASTIC
M7 MEGAKARYOBLASTIC

FIGURE 20-44. Morphology of acute myeloid leukemia (AML) in the traditional French-American-British (FAB) classification, now within the framework of the World Health Organization (WHO) classification "AML-not otherwise categorized."

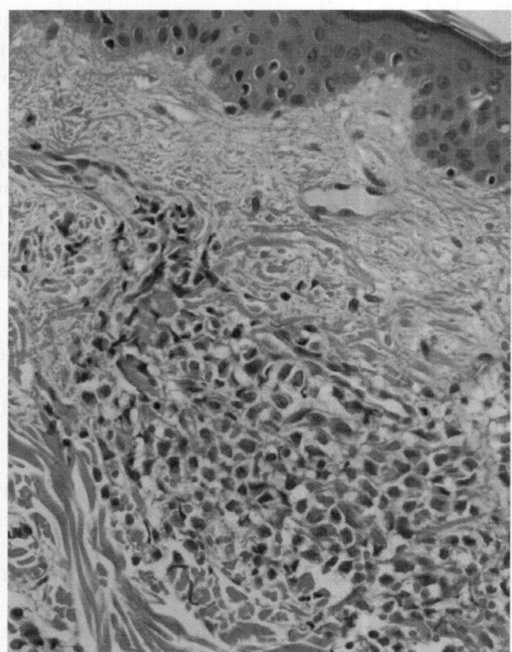

FIGURE 20-45. Myeloid sarcoma. The skin from a patient with acute monoblastic leukemia (leukemia cutis) shows neoplastic myeloid cells.

- **Acute monoblastic/monocytic leukemia (AMoL):** At least 80% of the myeloid cells have monocytoid differentiation. AMoL constitutes 5% to 8% of all cases of AML and is seen in younger patients.
- **Acute erythroid leukemia:** Acute erythroid leukemias feature prominent erythropoietic proliferation; over 50% of nucleated cells in the bone marrow are erythroid precursors. At least 20% of the remaining cells are myeloblasts. A rare, more chronic form of this disease displays pure erythroblasts and is referred to as **erythremic myelosis** or **di Guglielmo syndrome.**
- **Acute megakaryoblastic leukemia (AMegL):** At least 50% of the blasts show a megakaryocytic immunophenotype.

MYELOID SARCOMA: **Myeloid sarcoma is an extramedullary solid tumor of myeloblasts or monoblasts** (Fig. 20-45). This entity is sometimes called a **chloroma** because of its greenish color, **granulocytic sarcoma** or **monoblastic sarcoma. Monoblastic differentiation** is uncommon and is most commonly associated with translocations involving the myelomonocytic leukemia (MML) gene (11q23). Myeloid sarcoma may evolve de novo or in association with AML, or it may represent the blast phase in myeloproliferative disorders. The prognosis is determined by the underlying leukemic process.

DISORDERS OF THE LYMPHOID SYSTEM

Normal Lymph Nodes and Lymphocytes

The lymphoid system consists of the circulating pool of T and B lymphocytes, natural killer cells and the secondary lymphoid organs, which mainly includes the lymph nodes, spleen and thymus. In addition to the tonsils in the oro- and nasopharynx (Waldeyer ring), aggregates of organized lymphoid tissue known as mucosa-associated lymphoid tissue (MALT) are also present in extranodal sites, such as the gastrointestinal tract, lungs and skin. The Peyer patches in the terminal ileum represent a prototypic example of MALT.

The lymphocytes in tonsils and Peyer patches arrive in those sites by migration through the tall endothelial cells of vessels, which are comparable to the postcapillary venules found in lymph nodes. ***Mucosa-associated lymphoid tissue plays an important role in immunologic protection of the host in areas vulnerable to potential invaders.*** IgA secretion is a prominent component of this protective function.

All three major types of lymphocytes (T cells, B cells and natural killer cells) are derived from lymphoid stem cells in the bone marrow (Fig. 20-2). The T cells mature and differentiate in the thymus, whereas the B cells undergo activation, transformation and selection in lymph nodes and spleen. The natural killer cells do not go through a thymic or lymph node education phase, but rather they are released into the peripheral circulation where they are recognized as large granular lymphocytes. Regardless of type, lymphocyte development is associated with a tightly controlled sequence of gene expression and silencing, which results in a sequential gain and loss of nuclear, cytoplasmic and/or surface antigen expression in these cells. ***The pattern of antigenic expression identifies the lineage and maturation stage of both benign and neoplastic lymphoid cells*** (discussed below). The reader is referred to Chapter 4 for a detailed discussion of T- and B-lymphocyte development and function.

LYMPH NODES: Lymph nodes are located along lymphatic vessels throughout the body. By palpation and gross examination, normal lymph nodes are typically round to bean shaped and measure less than 1 cm in diameter. Lymph nodes that are larger than 1 cm are considered clinically enlarged, and they may be abnormal microscopically. Regional collections of lymph nodes are known as chains or groups (e.g., cervical lymph node chain, inguinal lymph node chain), and sometimes many nodes within a chain or group may be enlarged and/or matted together, often a feature of malignancy. The identification of abnormal chains is important for malignancy staging.

Individual lymph nodes are surrounded by a thin fibrous capsule with internally radiating trabeculae, which provides structural support (Fig. 20-46). Subjacent to the fibrous capsule sits the subcapsular sinus, which receives the lymph fluid (potentially containing antigen) from the **afferent lymphatic vessels** that penetrate the lymph node at several points along the capsule. The **subcapsular sinus** extends along the fibrous trabeculae, forming the trabecular sinuses, which ultimately connect to the efferent limb of the lymphatic vessels. The sinuses are lined by mononuclear phagocytes, which are involved in antigen presentation. The arrangement of the sinuses maximizes exposure of foreign antigens present in the lymph fluid to the macrophages and immunoreactive lymphocytes.

Lymph nodes are composed of an **outer cortex** and an **inner medulla** (Fig. 20-46). The cortex can be subdivided into the follicular area (which contains mostly B cells) and the paracortical area (which consists of predominantly T cells and contains many postcapillary venules). Lymphocytes from the circulation enter the lymph node cortex by migrating through the tall endothelial cells of the postcapillary venules in the **paracortex.** The T lymphocytes tend to remain in the paracortex, while the B lymphocytes home to the **follicle germinal centers.**

The B-cell–rich cortex contains two types of follicles: (1) immunologically inactive follicles, termed **primary follicles,**

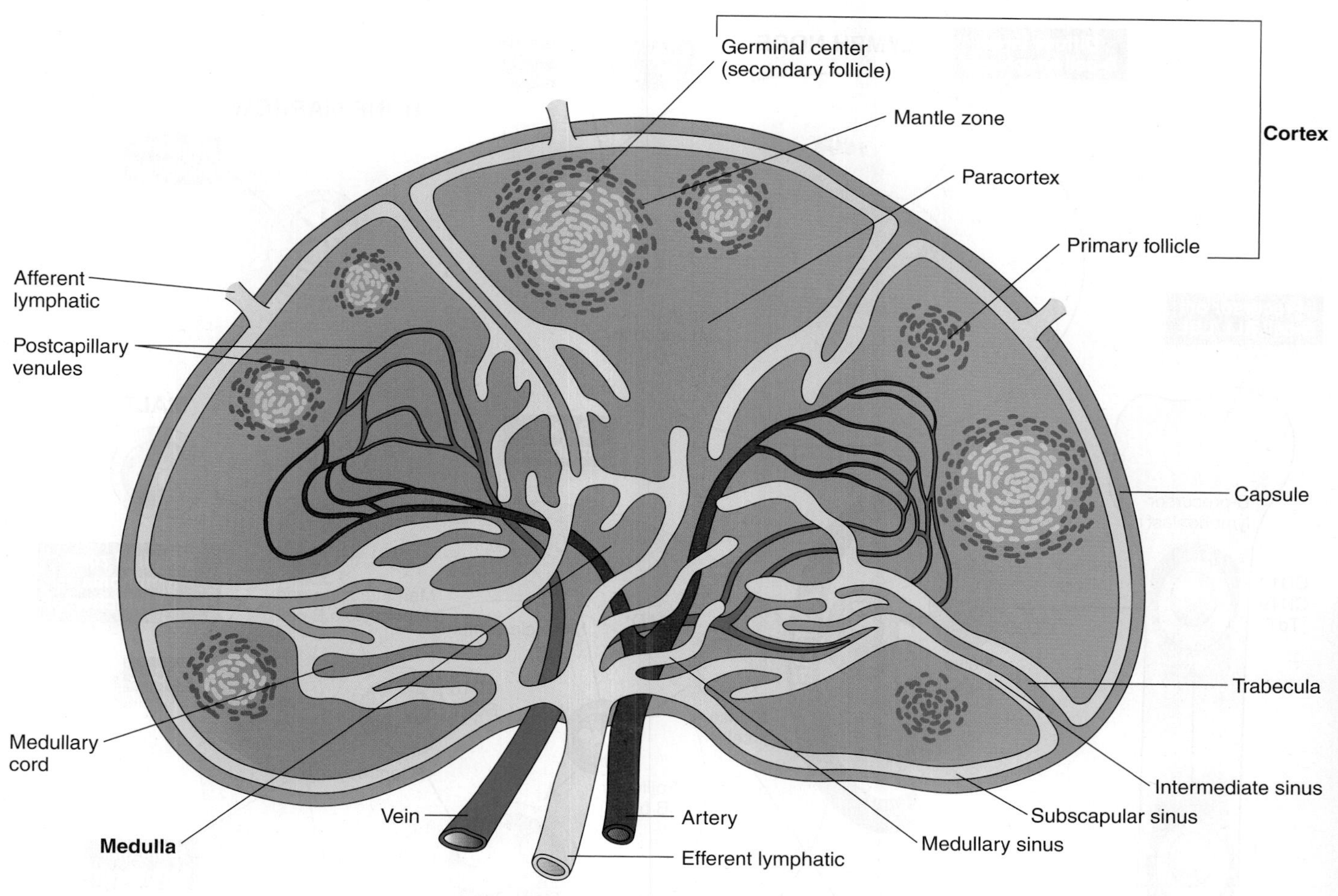

FIGURE 20-46. Structure of normal lymph node.

that consist of cohesive aggregates of small lymphocytes without well-defined germinal centers or mantle zones and (2) immunologically active follicles, termed **secondary follicles,** that contain germinal centers. The germinal centers contain large noncleaved lymphocytes **(centroblasts)** admixed with small and larger lymphocytes with cleaved nuclei **(centrocytes).**

The germinal centers also contain scattered macrophages that contain phagocytized nuclear and cytoplasmic debris ("tingible body" macrophages) and follicular dendritic cells important for antigen presentation. **Follicular dendritic cells (FDCs)** are stellate cells with long cytoplasmic processes. They present antigens to follicular lymphocytes. Macrophages, and to a lesser extent dendritic cells, provide growth factors for activated B cells.

The T-cell–rich paracortex, also known as the deep cortex, lies between the B-cell follicles and deep to them. In addition to T lymphocytes, scattered macrophages and interdigitating dendritic cells (IDCs) are found in the paracortex. The IDCs process and present antigens to the T lymphocytes.

B-LYMPHOCYTE DEVELOPMENT: Normal **B-cell progenitor cells** arise in the bone marrow (Fig. 20-47) (termed hematogones). These normal B-lymphoid cells have a similar phenotype to the cells of **precursor B-cell acute lymphoblastic leukemia,** and they are present in relatively low numbers in the bone marrow. Similar to their leukemic counterparts, the normal B-cell progenitors express the early B-cell surface antigens **CD10** (common acute leukemia/lymphoma antigen [CALLA]) and **CD19,** as well as the nuclear antigen **terminal deoxynucleotidyl transferase.** These cells lack or have minimal expression of CD20, a marker found at high levels on the more mature B-cell populations, and they also lack surface immunoglobulin light-chain expression. Increased numbers of hematogones can be seen during viral infections and in bone marrow recovery after chemotherapy or stem cell transplantation.

A fraction of the bone marrow–derived B cells subsequently home to the lymph node germinal centers where further development and selection occurs. Specifically, B cells with sufficient affinity for antigen survive the germinal center reaction and eventually leave the follicle compartment. As the B lymphocytes mature, the genes for immunoglobulin heavy chains are rearranged in preparation for the synthesis of IgM molecules. In precursor (progenitor) B cells, IgM is expressed in the cytoplasm. Mature B cells express the pan B-cell antigens CD19, CD20 and CD22 and surface immunoglobulin light and heavy chains. After activation and clonal expansion in germinal centers, B lymphocytes migrate to the B-cell–dependent medullary cords of the lymph nodes and become immunoglobulin-secreting **plasma cells** or exit lymph nodes as **memory B lymphocytes.** Plasma cells have eccentric nuclei with clumped chromatin marginated at the nuclear membrane, traditionally described as "clock-face

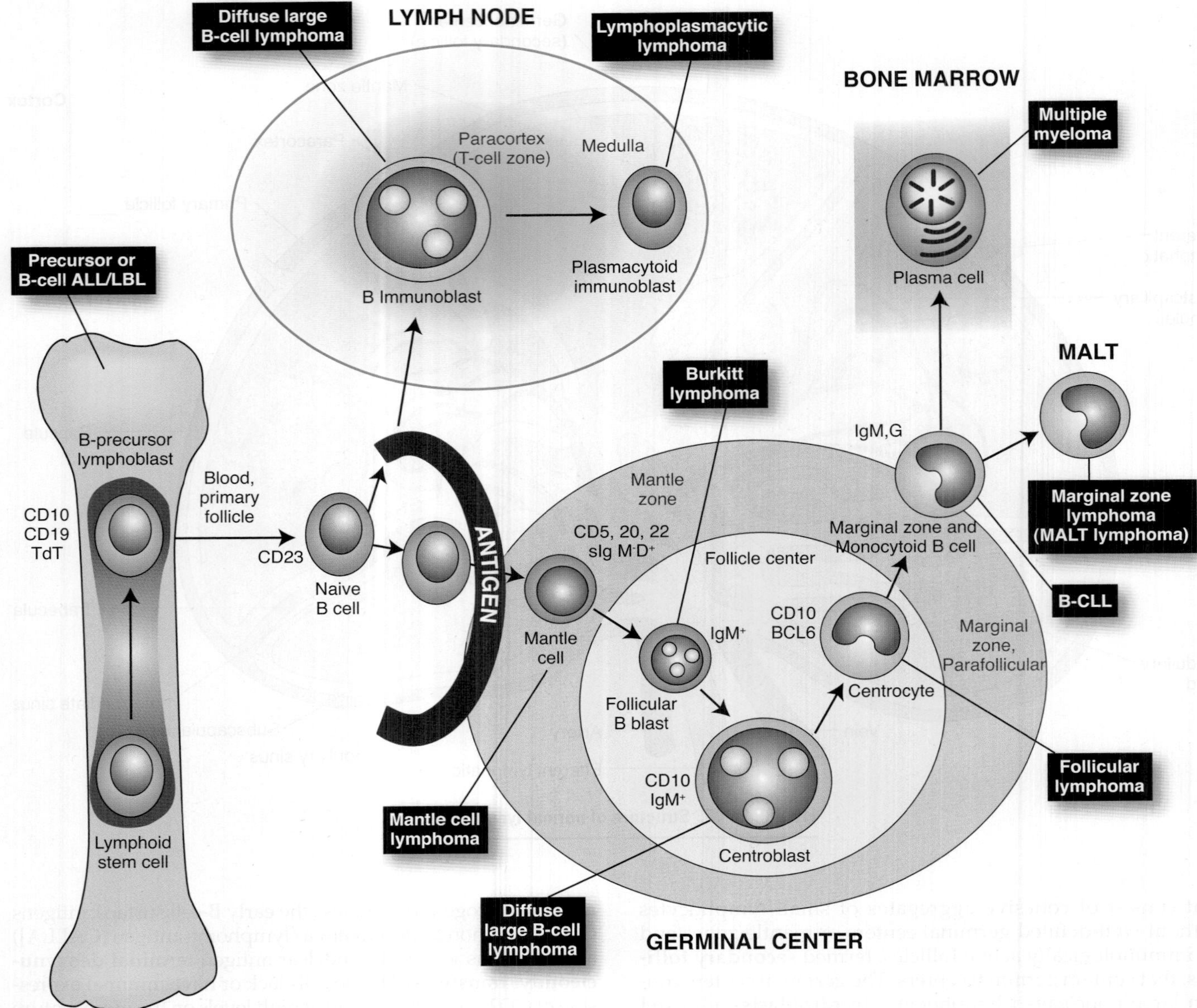

FIGURE 20-47. Pathway of normal B-cell differentiation and corresponding B-cell neoplasms. Following the lymphoid stem cell and precursor stage in the bone marrow, B cells mature into naive B lymphocytes and home to the secondary lymphoid organs (primarily lymph nodes). The germinal-center reaction represents an important turntable for immunoglobulin variable-region gene mutations, Ig heavy-chain switch and differentiation into plasma cells and memory B cells. Cluster designation (CD) markers are shown. B-cell immunoblasts and plasmacytoid immunoblasts reside in the T-cell–rich paracortex and medulla, respectively. Marginal zone B cells home to mucosa-associated lymphoid tissue (MALT) sites and bone marrow. Neoplastic transformation occurs at all phases of B-cell differentiation. ALL/LBL = acute lymphoblastic leukemia/lymphoma; B-CLL = B-cell chronic lymphocytic leukemia; Ig = immunoglobulin.

chromatin." The abundant blue-purple cytoplasm of plasma cells often displays a clear paranuclear clear zone representing the Golgi complex. At the plasma cell stage, the lymphoid cells no longer normally express CD20 or surface immunoglobulin.

T LYMPHOCYTES: The lymphoid stem cells that migrate from the bone marrow to the thymus are exposed to a number of thymic hormones that induce sequential expression of pan T-cell surface antigens such as CD2, CD3, CD5 and CD7, and CD4 or CD8 (Fig. 20-48). ***Recombination of the T-cell receptor genes leads to generation of a diverse population of T cells, each of which has the ability to recognize a single antigen.*** T cells without the ability to recognize foreign antigen with high affinity and T cells that recognize self-antigens are negatively selected and undergo apoptosis. Once mature and educated, the T cells migrate from the thymus to lymph

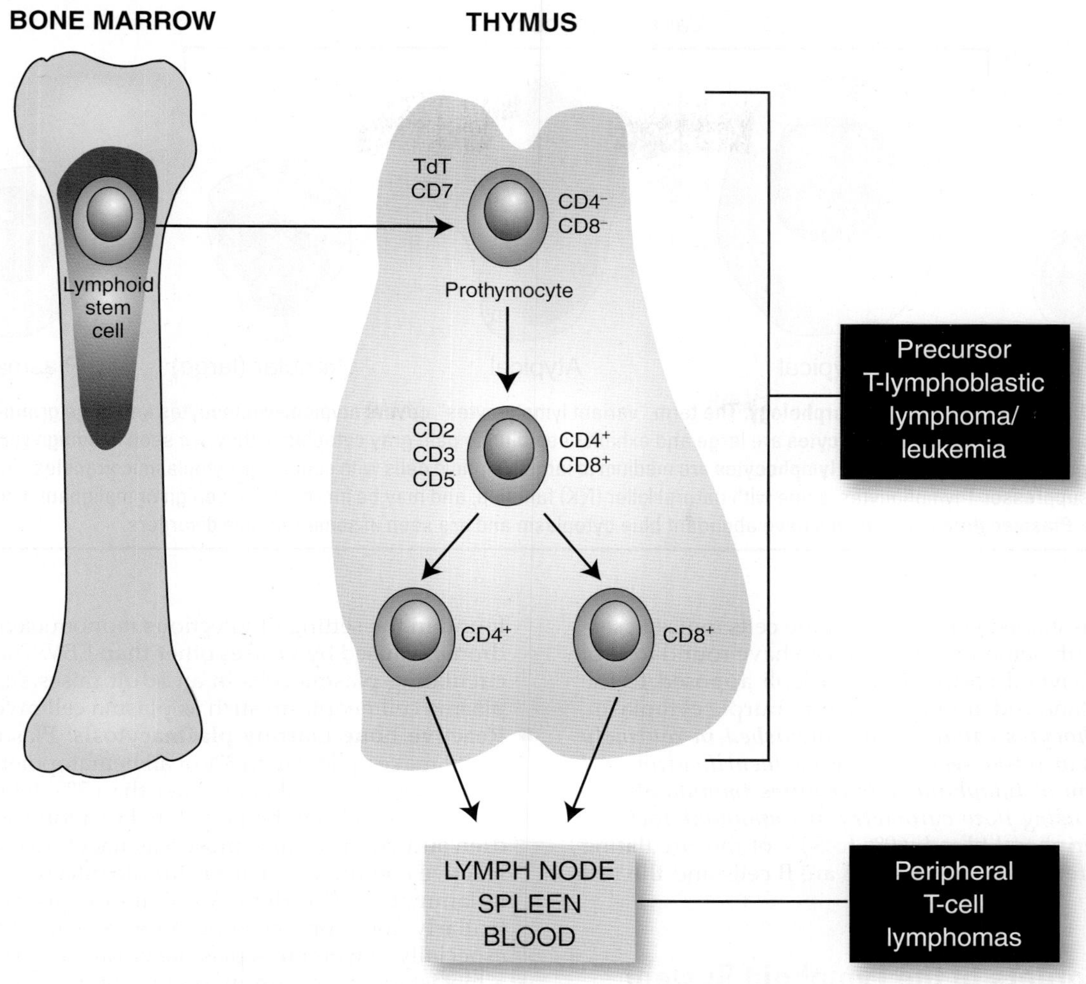

FIGURE 20-48. Pathways of normal T-cell development and corresponding T-cell neoplasms. CD = cluster designation; TdT = terminal deoxynucleotidyl transferase.

nodes, spleen and peripheral blood to become **postthymic T cells.**

When exposed to foreign (nonself) receptor-specific antigen in the context of major histocompatibility complex (MHC) class II molecules, the $CD4^+$ T cells become activated via the release of mitogenic growth factors, such as IL-1 and IL-2. The antigens presented to the T-helper cells are peptide fragments derived from the partial digestion of foreign proteins by macrophages and/or other antigen-presenting cells. The T-helper cells in turn interact with B lymphocytes that express the same antigenic specificity, prompting the latter to proliferate and inducing them to differentiate to plasma cells, which will produce antigen-specific antibody.

$CD8^+$ cells are activated when their receptors recognize peptide antigens presented in association with MHC class I HLA molecules, after which they become suppressor/cytotoxic cells. $CD8^+$ cells limit expansion of activated B cells and stop their immune response in a negative feedback response loop.

NATURAL KILLER AND CYTOTOXIC LYMPHOCYTES: A small subset of the total lymphocyte pool lacks expression of the usual T- or B-cell antigens, known as **natural killer (NK) cells.** These cytotoxic cells do not require antigenic recognition to initiate their killing function. Natural killer cells are large lymphocytes with granular cytoplasm, also known as **large granular lymphocytes** (Fig. 20-49). These cells are distinguished from mature T cells by their lack of surface CD3 expression and by their positivity for other surface antigens, such as CD16 and CD56.

Lymphocytes exhibit a heterogeneous morphologic appearance in stained peripheral blood and bone marrow smears, as well as in tissue sections. Similar to other blast cells, immature lymphoid cells have high nuclear-to-cytoplasmic ratios, fine nuclear chromatin and visible nucleoli. During the process of maturation and differentiation, the lymphoid cells can range from large to small, but they generally exhibit more clumped nuclear chromatin and variable amounts of cytoplasm (with or without granules) compared to the immature (blast) cells. While a variety of cell sizes (including frequent large transformed or activated cells) are normally found in the secondary lymphoid organs, the lymphocytes that circulate in the peripheral blood and those found in the bone marrow are predominantly small and heterogeneous (Fig. 20-49). In peripheral blood smears, transformed cytotoxic T cells are recognized as **variant lymphocytes** (and sometimes called "**atypical lymphocytes**"). The variant lymphocytes tend to have abundant blue-gray cytoplasm and multiple nucleoli in

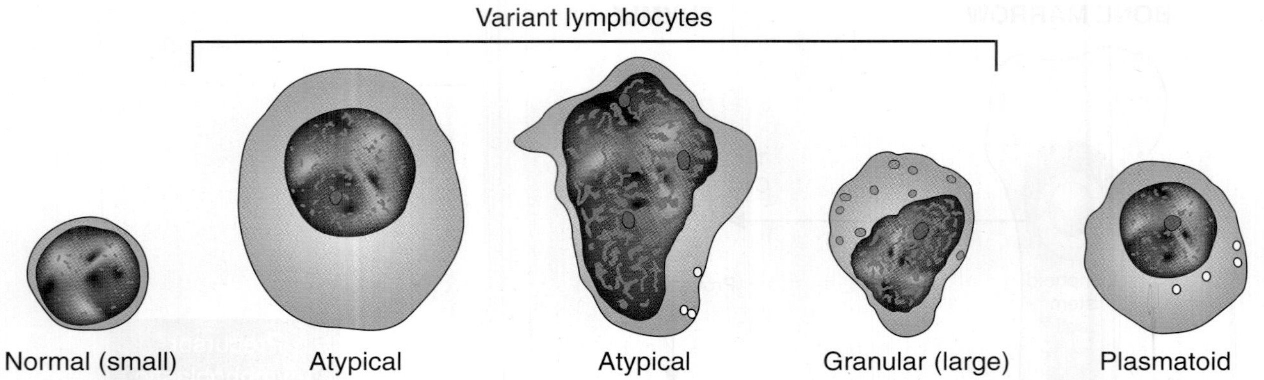

Variant lymphocytes

Normal (small) Atypical Atypical Granular (large) Plasmatoid

FIGURE 20-49. Lymphocyte morphology. The term "variant lymphocytes" covers atypical lymphocytes and large granular lymphocytes. **Atypical lymphocytes** are large and exhibit deep blue to pale gray cytoplasm; they are seen in benign reactive processes. **Large granular lymphocytes** are medium to large lymphoid cells with some pink cytoplasmic granules. They are suppressor T lymphocytes, some with natural killer (NK) function, and may be increased in benign or malignant disorders. **Plasmacytoid lymphocytes** have abundant blue cytoplasm and are seen in some reactive disorders.

Wright-Giemsa–stained smears. The same cells in tissue sections stained with hematoxylin and eosin have round to oval nuclei, one to several eosinophilic nucleoli apposed to the nuclear membrane and abundant clear to purple cytoplasm. ***T and B lymphocytes cannot be distinguished in routinely stained smears or tissue sections. Precise identification and characterization of lymphoid cells requires immunophenotypic analysis using flow cytometry or immunohistochemistry.*** In the peripheral blood, 60% to 80% of the circulating lymphocytes are T cells, 10% to 15% are B cells and the rest are NK cells.

Benign Disorders of the Lymphoid System

Lymphocytosis Denotes Elevated Peripheral Blood Lymphocyte Counts

Benign lymphocytosis is characterized by a transient increase in the absolute number of circulating lymphocytes. The upper limits of normal are 4000/μL in adults, 7000/μL in children and 9000/μL in infants. The lymphocytes in benign lymphocytoses are usually reactive appearing and morphologically heterogeneous, but atypical lymphocytes may also be seen (Figs. 20-49 and 20-50). Infectious mononucleosis as a result of EBV infection is the most common cause of reactive lymphocytosis; however, other viral infections can produce similar syndromes (e.g., cytomegalovirus [CMV]). Other less common causes of reactive lymphocytosis include whooping cough, chronic bacterial infections such as tuberculosis and brucellosis, stress and cigarette smoking. Persistent absolute lymphocytosis over 4000/μL, particularly in adults, raises suspicion for a lymphoproliferative disorder and deserves further evaluation.

Bone Marrow Plasmacytosis Most Often Signifies a Plasma Cell Disorder

- **Plasma cells in peripheral blood:** It is uncommon to find plasma cells circulating in the peripheral blood. When seen, they are usually part of the spectrum of lymphoid cells found in the setting of infectious mononucleosis–like syndromes caused by viruses other than EBV. The presence of circulating plasma cells in an adult raises suspicion for a plasma cell neoplasm such as plasma cell myeloma.
- **Reactive bone marrow plasmacytosis:** Plasma cells normally make up less than 3% of all hematopoietic cells in the bone marrow. Numbers greater than 3% define a plasmacytosis, which may be polyclonal or monoclonal. In children and young adults, most plasmacytoses are caused by reactive conditions such as chronic infections or systemic inflammatory disorders. Autoimmune diseases are a particularly common cause of bone marrow plasmacytosis, especially in women. A plasmacytosis can also accompany a metastatic neoplasm involving the bone marrow. ***Bone marrow plasmacytosis greater than 10% is typically associated with a plasma cell disorder.*** In both reactive and neoplastic plasma cell proliferations, immunoglobulin may accumulate in the cytoplasm to form prominent eosinophilic globules, which are known as Russell bodies. Similarly,

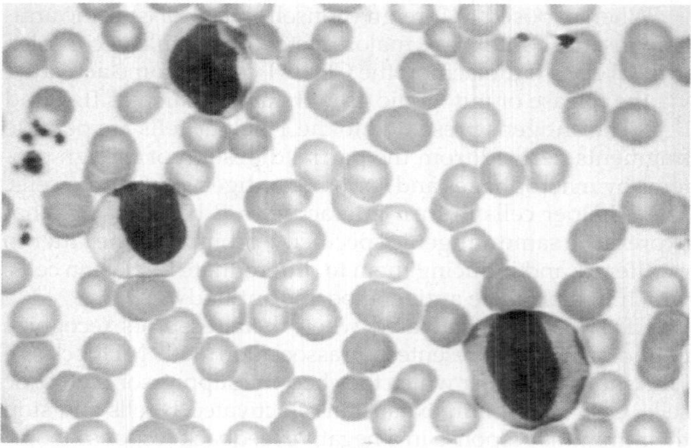

FIGURE 20-50. Infectious mononucleosis. An absolute lymphocytosis caused by a heterogeneous population of small and larger lymphoid cells, including atypical lymphocytes, is characteristic of this Epstein-Barr virus–driven disorder.

benign and neoplastic plasma cells may contain nuclear pseudoinclusions known as Dutcher bodies. These pseudoinclusions represent immunoglobulin invaginated into the nucleus and seen in cross-section.

Lymphocytopenia Usually Reflects a Decrease in T-Helper Lymphocytes

Peripheral blood lymphocytopenia is defined as a decrease in blood lymphocytes to less than 1500/μL in adults or less than 3000/μL in children. Since the predominant lymphocytes in the blood are T-helper ($CD4^+$) cells, lymphocytopenia generally indicates that this population of lymphocytes is decreased. There are several mechanisms by which lymphocytopenia occurs:

- **Decreased production of lymphocytes:** A variety of congenital and acquired immunodeficiency syndromes are characterized by reduced production of lymphocytes. Decreased production of T cells also occurs with some lymphomas, such as Hodgkin lymphoma, particularly in advanced stages.
- **Increased destruction of lymphocytes:** Lymphocytes are destroyed by medical treatments, such as irradiation, chemotherapy, administration of antilymphocyte globulin, adrenocorticotropic hormone (ACTH) and corticosteroids. Some viral infections, particularly HIV, are associated with T-cell destruction and lymphopenia.
- **Loss of lymphocytes:** Intestinal disorders associated with damage to lymphatics can result in the loss of lymph and lymphocytes into the intestinal lumen. These disorders include protein-losing enteropathies, Whipple disease and disorders associated with increased central venous pressure (e.g., right-sided heart failure and chronic constrictive pericarditis). Immunologic damage to lymphocytes may occur in collagen vascular diseases, such as systemic lupus erythematosus.

Reactive Lymph Node Hyperplasia Is a Response to Infections, Inflammation or Tumors

Lymph nodes may exhibit hyperplasia of all cellular compartments or any combination of B lymphocytes, T lymphocytes and mononuclear phagocytic cells in response to a variety of infectious, inflammatory and neoplastic disorders (Fig. 20-51).

The histopathology and degree of lymph node enlargement in reactive hyperplasia is related to (1) the age of the patient (children tend to exhibit more pronounced immunoreactivity than adults), (2) the immunologic competence of the host and (3) the type of infectious agent or inflammatory disorder.

Acute suppurative and necrotizing lymphadenitis occurs in lymph nodes that drain sites of acute bacterial or fungal infections. Suppurative lymph nodes enlarge rapidly because of edema and hyperemia, and they are usually tender to palpation because of distention of the capsule. Microscopically, the lymph node sinuses and stroma are infiltrated by polymorphonuclear leukocytes (neutrophils) and variable numbers of bland macrophages. Well-formed or ill-defined granulomas are usually present, and necrosis can be focal and geographic or extensive. The anatomic site of the reactive lymphadenopathy often provides a clue to its cause. For example, posterior auricular lymph nodes are commonly enlarged in rubella infection; occipital lymph nodes in scalp infections; posterior cervical lymph nodes in toxoplasmosis; axillary lymph nodes in infections of the arms or chest wall; and inguinal lymph nodes in venereal infections and infections of the legs. Generalized lymphadenopathy may occur in systemic infections, hyperthyroidism, drug hypersensitivity reactions and collagen vascular diseases.

Follicular Hyperplasia

Hyperplasia of secondary follicles (germinal centers) and plasmacytosis of medullary cords indicate B-cell immunoreactivity. In **nonspecific reactive follicular hyperplasia,** prominent hyperplastic follicles occur principally in the cortex of the lymph node (Figs. 20-51 and 20-52). Follicles are round or irregularly shaped and may be confluent or fused. The activated B cells in the follicles range from small cells with irregular, cleaved nuclei to large immunoblasts. Numerous mitotic figures reflect the rapid proliferation of activated B lymphocytes. Scattered benign macrophages, with abundant pale cytoplasm containing pyknotic nuclear and cytoplasmic debris, impart the characteristic "starry sky" pattern in the benign follicle centers. A well-defined mantle of normal small B lymphocytes surrounds the follicles, sharply separating them from the interfollicular regions.

The cause of nonspecific reactive follicular hyperplasia is frequently unknown, although a viral, drug or inflammatory etiology is often suspected. The clinical course features rapid and complete resolution of the lymphadenopathy following removal of the stimulus.

Reactive lymphadenopathy (either localized or generalized) caused by follicular hyperplasia and interfollicular plasmacytosis is common in rheumatoid arthritis. Follicular hyperplasia is also encountered in the early stages of HIV infection. It is worth noting here that the lymph nodes in persons with HIV/AIDS show a high incidence of superimposed malignant neoplasms (such as diffuse B-cell lymphomas, Burkitt lymphoma, Hodgkin lymphoma and Kaposi sarcoma) or opportunistic infection (such as atypical mycobacteria and CMV).

Interfollicular Hyperplasia

Hyperplasia of the deep cortex or paracortex (interfollicular or diffuse hyperplasia) is characteristic of T-lymphocyte immunoreactivity.

Nonspecific reactive interfollicular hyperplasia (Fig. 20-51) is most commonly caused by viral infections or immunologic reactions. Although the precise cause is often undetermined, the condition usually resolves promptly. Interfollicular lymph node hyperplasia is a common finding in viral diseases, including infectious mononucleosis, varicella-herpes zoster infection, measles and CMV lymphadenitis.

Systemic lupus erythematosus (SLE) is often associated with lymphadenopathy characterized by interfollicular hyperplasia with prominent immunoblasts and plasma cells and focal to massive necrosis. Arteriolitis, with fibrinoid necrosis of vessel walls, is frequently observed. Unlike acute suppurative and necrotizing lymphadenitis, neutrophils are not present in the lymphadenitis associated with SLE.

Mixed Patterns of Reactive Hyperplasia of Lymph Nodes

Some infectious diseases are associated with mixed patterns of lymph node hyperplasia, in which several different

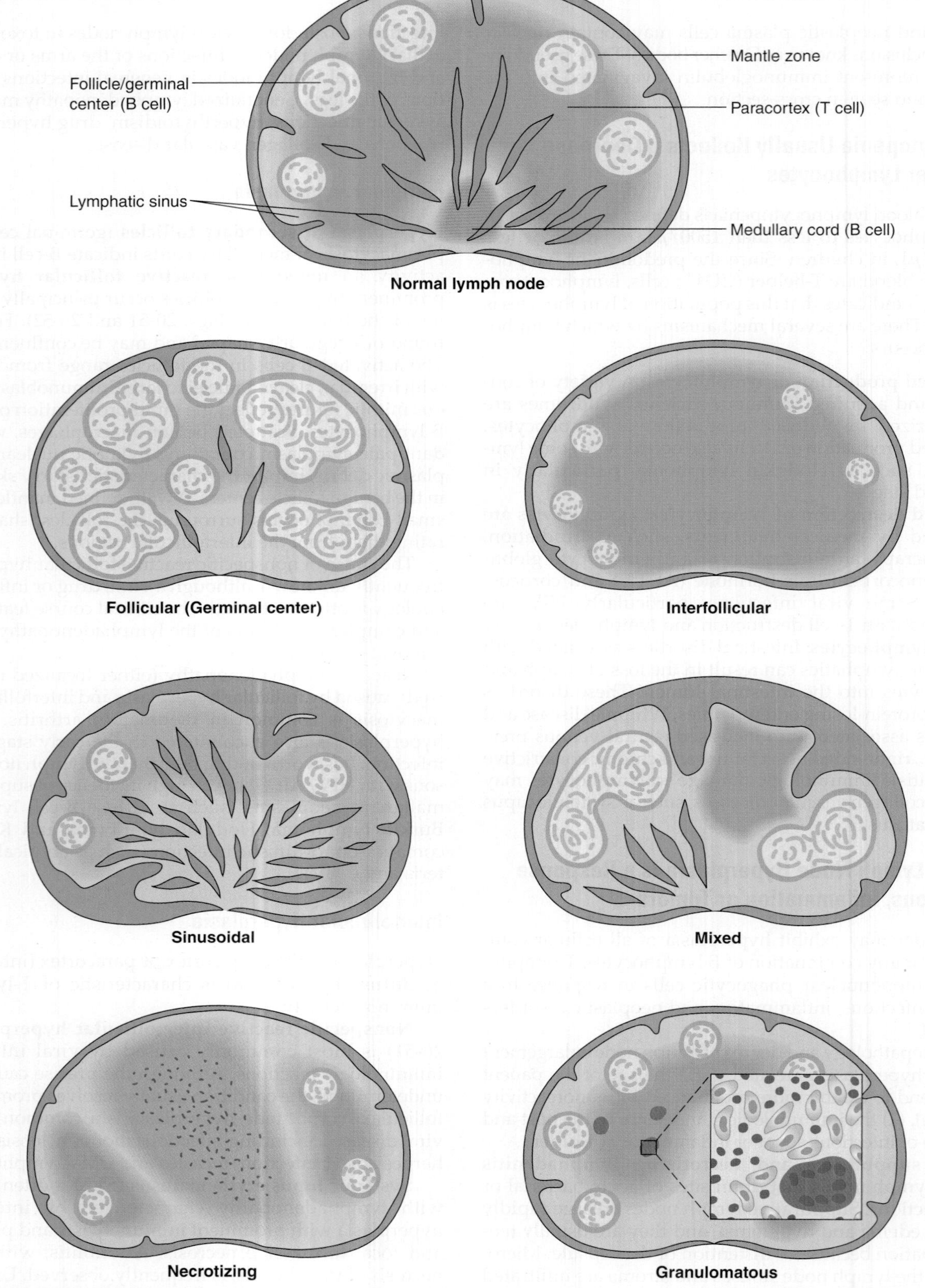

FIGURE 20-51. Patterns of reactive lymphadenopathy. The major patterns of reactive hyperplasia are contrasted with the architecture of a normal lymph node. **Follicular hyperplasia,** with an increased number of enlarged and irregularly shaped follicles, is characteristic of B-cell immunoreactivity. **Interfollicular hyperplasia** with expansion of the paracortex is typical of T-cell immunoreactivity. The **sinusoidal pattern** is typified by expansion of sinuses by bland macrophages. This pattern is seen in reactive proliferations of the mononuclear–phagocyte system. A **mixed pattern** of follicular, interfollicular and sinusoidal hyperplasia is common in a variety of complex immune reactions. In **necrotizing lymphadenitis,** variable zones of necrosis are found within the lymph nodes, with or without the presence of neutrophils. Cohesive clusters of macrophages and occasional multinucleated giant cells are characteristic of the **granulomatous inflammation pattern.**

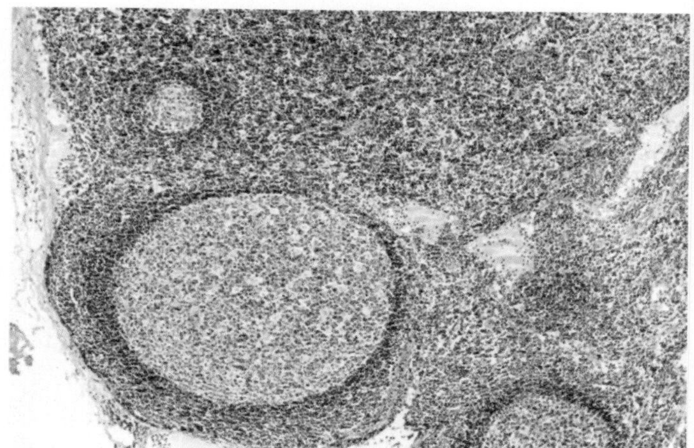

FIGURE 20-52. Lymph node with reactive follicular hyperplasia. A section of a hyperplastic lymph node shows prominent follicles (germinal centers) containing numerous macrophages with pale cytoplasm.

features are prominent. For example, in **toxoplasmosis** one sees prominent follicular hyperplasia and small collections of epithelioid macrophages in the interfollicular regions and surrounding the hyperplastic follicles (Figs. 20-51 and 20-53). **Cat-scratch disease** elicits follicular hyperplasia and suppurative granulomas with a stellate appearance. Lymphadenitis caused by **lymphogranuloma venereum** and **tularemia** (see Chapter 9) is indistinguishable from cat-scratch disease.

Sinus Histiocytosis Represents an Increase in Macrophages

Sinus histiocytosis is an increase in tissue macrophages (histiocytes) within the subcapsular and trabecular sinuses of the lymph nodes (Fig. 20-51). Sinus histiocytes are derived from blood monocytes. Sinus histiocytosis is common in lymph nodes draining sites of carcinoma and, less often, inflammatory and infectious foci. The nature of the phagocytic debris in the cytoplasm of the macrophages helps identify the origin of the sinus histiocytosis. For example, anthracotic pigment is frequently seen in the macrophages of mediastinal lymph nodes that exhibit sinus histocytosis. Macrophages containing erythrocytes and hemosiderin pigment occur with autoimmune hemolytic anemia.

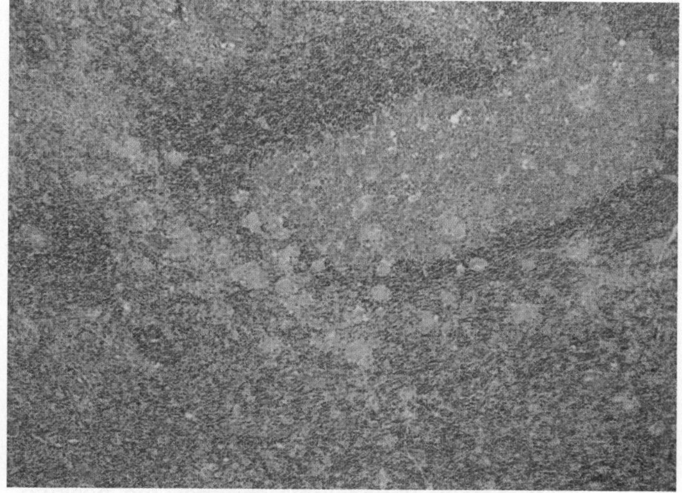

FIGURE 20-53. Toxoplasmosis. A section of a lymph node displays clusters of pink epithelioid macrophages and follicular hyperplasia.

Lymph nodes with sinus histiocytosis may or may not be pathologically enlarged. Common sinus histiocytosis should not be confused with **sinus histiocytosis with massive lymphadenopathy (Rosai-Dorfman disease),** which is characterized by prominent bilateral lymphadenopathy (usually cervical) caused by a marked expansion of the lymph node sinuses by histocytes containing intact lymphocytes (emperipolesis). The majority of cases of Rosai-Dorfman disease occur in the second decade of life, and the disease is often associated with systemic findings including fever, leukocytosis and hypergammaglobulinemia.

Dermatopathic Lymphadenopathy Features Paracortical T-Cell Proliferation

Dermatopathic lymphadenopathy refers to specific reactive changes in lymph nodes that are caused by a variety of chronic dermatoses. This reaction is a result of drainage of lipid, melanin and hemosiderin from the affected skin to the regional lymph nodes. The lymph nodes demonstrate an immunologic reaction to antigenic material draining from the skin, which accumulates principally in paracortical macrophages. The paracortex is expanded by a heterogeneous cell population that consists of Langerhans cells, interdigitating reticulum cells and macrophages whose cytoplasm contains lipid or granular, brown, melanin pigment.

Malignant Lymphomas

Lymphomas are malignant proliferations of lymphocytes. B-cell, T-cell and NK-cell lymphomas are categorized as **immature** (derived from precursor cells; lymphoblasts) or **mature** (derived from mature effector cells). The latter are more common. While all lymphomas are malignant neoplasms, there is a wide spectrum of clinical behavior, with some following an indolent clinical course (sometimes not even requiring treatment) and others behaving in an aggressive manner (causing death in a short time frame if left untreated). Lymphomas mostly affect the lymph nodes, but any tissue or organ may be involved (e.g., gastrointestinal tract, thyroid, liver, skin, lungs, brain, gonads). When lymphoma involves the peripheral blood and/or bone marrow, it is said to be leukemic or peripheralized.

Beyond the broad categories of B-cell, T-cell and NK-cell types, lymphomas are further classified according to their postulated cell of origin, normal cellular counterpart, immunophenotype, molecular/genetic alterations, clinical features and morphology. In addition, a distinction between non-Hodgkin lymphoma (NHL) and Hodgkin lymphoma (HL) continues to exist. The WHO classification of lymphoid tumors, which takes all of these parameters into account, is the classification scheme currently used by physicians and pathologists alike. The major types of recognized B-, T- and NK-cell lymphomas are shown in Tables 20-16 and 20-17. Selected examples are discussed in the following sections.

Table 20-16

WHO Histologic Classification of B-Cell Neoplasms

Precursor B-Cell Neoplasm
Precursor B-cell lymphoblastic leukemia/lymphoma
Mature B-Cell Neoplasms
Chronic lymphocytic leukemia/small lymphocytic lymphoma
B-cell prolymphocytic leukemia
Lymphoplasmacytic lymphoma
Splenic marginal zone lymphoma
Hairy cell leukemia
Plasma cell myeloma
Monoclonal gammopathy of undetermined significance (MGUS)
Solitary plasmacytoma of bone
Extraosseous plasmacytoma
Primary amyloidosis
Heavy-chain diseases
Extranodal marginal zone B-cell lymphoma of mucosa-associated lymphoid tissue (MALT lymphoma)
Nodal marginal zone B-cell lymphoma
Follicular lymphoma
Mantle cell lymphoma
Mediastinal (thymic) large B-cell lymphoma
Intravascular large B-cell lymphoma
Primary effusion lymphoma
Burkitt lymphoma/leukemia

WHO = World Health Organization.

Table 20-17

WHO Histologic Classification of T-Cell and NK-Cell Neoplasms

Precursor T-Cell Neoplasm
Precursor T-cell lymphoblastic leukemia/lymphoma
Mature T-Cell Neoplasms
Leukemic/Disseminated
T-cell prolymphocytic leukemia
T-cell large granular lymphocytic leukemia
Aggressive NK-cell leukemia
Adult T-cell leukemia/lymphoma
Cutaneous
Mycosis fungoides
Sézary syndrome
Primary cutaneous anaplastic lymphoma
Large cell lymphoma
Lymphomatoid papulosis
Other Extranodal
Extranodal NK-/T-cell lymphoma, nasal type
Enteropathy-type T-cell lymphoma
Hepatosplenic T-cell lymphoma
Subcutaneous panniculitis-like T-cell lymphoma
Nodal
Angioimmunoblastic T-cell lymphoma
Peripheral T-cell lymphoma, unspecified
Anaplastic large cell lymphoma
Neoplasm of Uncertain Lineage and Stage of Differentiation
Blastic NK-cell lymphoma

NK = natural killer; WHO = World Health Organization.

Precursor B-Cell Acute Lymphoblastic Leukemia/Lymphoma Is a Malignancy of B Lymphoblasts

The malignant lymphocytes in precursor B-cell acute lymphoblastic leukemia (B-ALL) and B-cell lymphoblastic lymphoma (B-LBL) are immature (precursor) cells known as **lymphoblasts.** When the B-lymphoblast proliferation involves the bone marrow and/or peripheral blood, the term **acute lymphoblastic leukemia** is used, whereas when the proliferation of lymphoblasts predominantly involves extramedullary tissues (e.g., lymph nodes), the term **acute lymphoblastic lymphoma** is preferred.

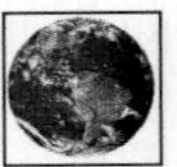

EPIDEMIOLOGY: ***Precursor B-cell acute lymphoblastic leukemia is the most common form of childhood leukemia.*** Approximately 75% of cases occur in children younger than 6 years of age, although the disease can present at all ages. The worldwide incidence is estimated to be 1 to 4.75 per 100,000 people and at the turn of the century, there were approximately 3200 new cases diagnosed in the United States alone. Several environmental and genetic factors have been incriminated in the etiology of ALL, such as Down syndrome, Bloom syndrome, ataxia-telangiectasia, neurofibromatosis type I, exposure in utero to ionizing radiations and solvents. Unlike precursor T-cell ALL, most cases of precursor B-cell ALL are leukemic rather than lymphomatous in presentation.

MOLECULAR PATHOGENESIS: Chromosomal abnormalities are present in the majority of cases of precursor B-cell ALL. Numerical and structural abnormalities are typical of the chromosomal lesions found in precursor B-cell ALL. Translocations are frequent, including those involving chromosomes 9 and 22 (*BCR/ABL* fusion; Philadelphia chromosome) and chromosome 11 at the *mixed lineage leukemia* (*MLL*) gene locus (11q23). In most cases of precursor B-cell ALL with a t(9;22) translocation occurring in children, the BCR/ABL fusion protein is a 190-kd product (p190). This is in contrast to most cases of Philadelphia chromosome–positive ALL occurring in adults, which usually show the 210-kd product (p210). The latter is the fusion protein form seen in CML, a chronic leukemia that affects mostly adults. As such, many cases of Philadelphia chromosome–positive ALL in adults with p210 represent a lymphoid blast crisis of CML, and this has implications for prognosis and treatment. Cases with an increased number of chromosomes (hyperdiploidy) tend to have a better prognosis compared to cases with less than the normal human chromosome number (hypodiploidy).

PATHOLOGY: Lymphoblasts are small to medium-sized cells with high nuclear-to-cytoplasmic ratios, fine nuclear chromatin, inconspicuous nucleoli and agranular cytoplasm (Fig. 20-54). The lymphoblasts typically make up at least 20% of the bone marrow cellularity, and variable numbers of blast cells can be found circulating in the peripheral blood. Flow cytometric immunophenotyping is needed to confirm the diagnosis. While all cases have evidence of B-lymphoblast differentiation, the immunophenotypic patterns seen in precursor B-cell ALLs are variable and reflect the different stages of early B-cell maturation (Fig. 20-47). The earliest antigens that indicate B-cell differentiation are CD10, CD19 and TdT. B-cell neoplasms that express surface Ig are not considered precursor neoplasms since surface Ig expression is a feature of mature B cells.

CLINICAL FEATURES: The leukemic cells of precursor B-cell ALL proliferate in the bone marrow and displace the normal marrow elements, resulting in anemia, thrombocytopenia and neutropenia. Organomegaly and central nervous system involvement are common as the disease disseminates from the bone marrow. The rapidly growing tumor cells in the bone marrow cause bone pain and arthralgias, and these may be the earliest presenting symptoms in children.

The prognosis for childhood precursor B-cell ALL is generally excellent with complete remission rates of greater than 90% using modern treatment protocols. Among other variables, age younger than 1 year or older than 12 years, older adult onset and/or the presence of certain cytogenetic abnormalities [e.g., t(9;22), t(1;19), t(4;11), hypodiploidy] are poor prognostic indicators. All translocations involving the *MLL* gene at 11q23 are associated with a poor prognosis regardless of age.

The treatment includes chemotherapeutic agents or stem cell transplantation for patients with high-risk features or who are unresponsive to chemotherapy.

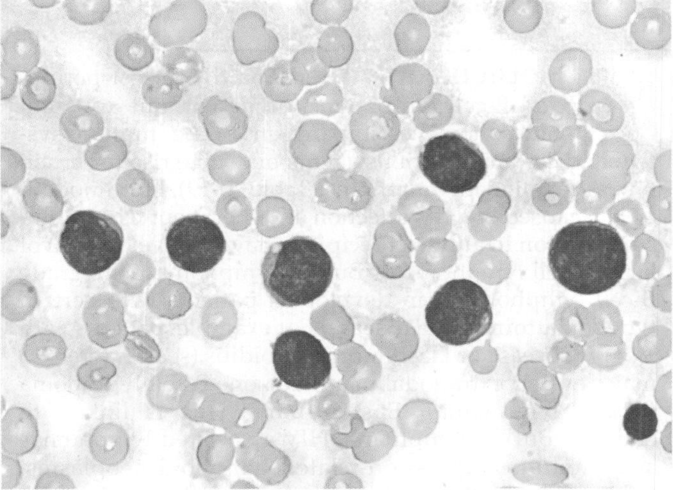

FIGURE 20-54. Acute lymphoblastic leukemia. The lymphoblasts in peripheral blood have irregular and indented nuclei with fine nuclear chromatin, visible nucleoli and variable amounts of agranular cytoplasm.

Precursor T-Cell Acute Lymphoblastic Leukemia/Lymphoma Is a Neoplasm of T Lymphoblasts

Precursor T-cell acute lymphoblastic leukemia (T-ALL) and T-cell lymphoblastic lymphoma (T-LBL) are immature T-cell neoplasms. Whether the term **leukemia** or **lymphoma** applies is often arbitrary, and the considerations are similar to those described for precursor B-ALL.

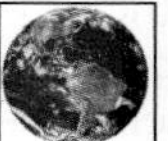

EPIDEMIOLOGY: Precursor T-cell ALL can be seen in any age group. It accounts for approximately 15% of all cases of childhood ALL. Adolescents are more commonly affected than younger children, and the neoplasm is more common in males than females. Approximately 25% of all acute lymphoblastic leukemias in adults are classified as precursor T-cell ALL. Compared to its B-cell counterpart, precursor T-cell ALL is more likely to have a lymphomatous presentation, with **mediastinal adenopathy** being common particularly in adolescent males.

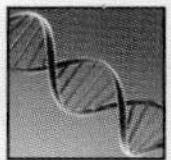

MOLECULAR PATHOGENESIS: The genes encoding the four T-cell receptor chains (α-, β-, γ-, δ-chains) often participate in chromosomal translocations with transcription factor genes such as *MYC, TAL1, RBTN1, RBTN2* and *HOX11*. Juxtaposition of the T-cell receptor loci to one of the transcription partner genes often results in disturbed transcriptional regulation.

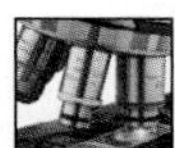

PATHOLOGY: The morphologic appearance of T lymphoblasts is similar to that of B lymphoblasts (Fig. 20-54). Antigenic expression in T-ALL reflects normal T-cell differentiation and maturation in the bone marrow and thymus (Fig. 20-48). The earliest T-cell antigen is CD7, followed by CD2 and CD5. During thymic differentiation, T cells become positive for CD1a and cytoplasmic CD3 (cCD3; CD3*e*), CD4 and CD8. The immunophenotypes observed in precursor T-cell ALL reflect the sequence of antigen expression seen in the normal counterparts. Like precursor B-cell ALL, the lymphoblasts in most cases of T-cell ALL are positive for TdT.

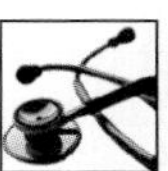

CLINICAL FEATURES: The blood and bone marrow are almost always involved in precursor T-cell ALL. The presenting white blood cell count is usually high, and a mediastinal mass or other tissue mass (lymphoma) is often present. Lymphadenopathy and organomegaly are common, and pleural effusions are frequently found. The neoplasm usually shows rapid growth, and patients with mediastinal involvement may present with a respiratory emergency because of compression of the central airways or the superior vena cava syndrome. In general, precursor T-cell ALL has a poorer prognosis compared to precursor B-cell ALL in children, but it has a slightly better outcome than B-ALL in adults for unclear reasons.

Mature (Peripheral) B-Cell Lymphomas Are the Most Common Type of Lymphoma in the Western World

Mature B-cell malignancies are derived from clonal proliferation of peripheral B cells. As B cells progress through the multiple steps of differentiation and maturation from naïve B lymphocytes to mature plasma cells, lymphomas may arise at any point along the way (Fig. 20-47).

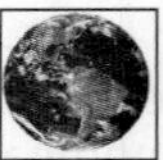

EPIDEMIOLOGY: Mature B-cell lymphomas make up over 90% of all lymphoid neoplasms worldwide. They are more common in developed countries, particularly the United States, Australia, New Zealand and western Europe, and their incidence is increasing. In the United States, the incidence of all lymphoid neoplasms is approximately 34 cases per year per 100,000 persons, whereas the incidence of B-cell lymphomas alone is approximately 26 per year per 100,000. The frequency of the specific types of B-cell lymphoma varies in different parts of the world. For example, Burkitt lymphoma is endemic in equatorial Africa (where it is the most common childhood malignancy), but it accounts for only 1% to 2% of all lymphomas in the United States and western Europe. Similarly, the frequency of follicular lymphoma is higher in the United States and western Europe relative to the frequency in South America, eastern Europe and Asia. ***Worldwide, the most common lymphomas are follicular lymphoma and diffuse large cell lymphoma, exclusive of Hodgkin lymphoma and plasma cell myeloma (Table 20-18).***

The majority of mature B-cell lymphomas occur in the sixth and seventh decades of life. A variant of diffuse large B-cell lymphoma known as mediastinal large B-cell lymphoma represents an exception, as it occurs at a median age of 35 years. With the exclusion of Burkitt lymphoma and diffuse large B-cell lymphoma, mature B-cell lymphomas are distinctly uncommon in children.

Risk factors for development of B-cell lymphoma include abnormalities of the immune system (such as immunodeficiency [e.g., AIDS, iatrogenic immunosuppression] and autoimmune diseases [e.g., Hashimoto's thyroiditis, Sjögren disease]), certain infectious agents (e.g., EBV, hepatitis C, *Helicobacter pylori*, and *Chlamydia*), environmental exposures (e.g., herbicides and pesticides), and even genetic polymorphisms in a number of immunoregulatory genes.

Table 20-18

Frequency of B- and T-/NK-Cell Lymphomas

Diagnosis	% of Total Cases
Diffuse large B-cell lymphoma	30.6
Follicular lymphoma	22.1
MALT lymphoma	7.6
Mature T-cell lymphomas (except ALCL)	7.6
Chronic lymphocytic leukemia/small lymphocytic lymphoma	6.7
Mantle cell lymphoma	6.0
Mediastinal large B-cell lymphoma	2.4
Anaplastic large cell lymphoma	2.4
Burkitt lymphoma	2.5
Nodal marginal zone lymphoma	1.8
Precursor T-cell lymphoblastic lymphoma	1.7
Lymphoplasmacytic lymphoma	1.2
Other types	7.4

ALCL = anaplastic large cell lymphoma; MALT = mucosa-associated lymphoid tissue; NK = natural killer.

Table 20-19

Disorders With Increased Risk of Secondary Malignant Lymphoma

Sjögren syndrome
Hashimoto thyroiditis
Renal and cardiac transplant recipients
AIDS
EBV infection
HHV-8 infection
Helicobacter pylori–positive gastritis
Hepatitis C
Congenital immune deficiency syndromes
Chediak-Higashi
Wiskott-Aldrich
Ataxia telangiectasia
IgA deficiency
Severe combined immune deficiency
α Heavy-chain disease
Celiac disease
Hodgkin lymphoma (posttreatment)

AIDS = acquired immunodeficiency syndrome; EBV = Epstein-Barr virus; HHV = human herpesvirus; Ig = immunoglobulin.

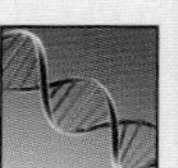

MOLECULAR PATHOGENESIS: Most peripheral B-cell lymphomas occur without apparent cause; however, impairment of the immune system and certain infectious agents may give rise to certain types of malignant lymphoma (Table 20-19). Immunodeficiency caused by HIV infection and therapeutic **immunosuppression in allograft recipients** favors development of large B-cell lymphoma or Burkitt lymphoma. Low-grade B-cell lymphomas can develop in patients with certain types of **autoimmune disease.** For example, patients with Sjögren disease or Hashimoto thyroiditis (see Chapter 21) may develop extranodal marginal zone B-cell lymphoma (MALT lymphoma). **Epstein-Barr virus** is linked to endemic Burkitt lymphoma, HIV-associated lymphomas and immunosuppression-related lymphoid neoplasms. Other **viruses** that predispose to B-cell malignancies include human herpesvirus 8 (HHV-8) in primary effusion lymphoma and hepatitis C virus in lymphoplasmacytic lymphoma associated with type 2 cryoglobulinemia. MALT lymphoma is frequently associated with *H. pylori*

infection of the stomach (see Chapter 13) and often regresses following antibiotic treatment.

As discussed earlier, lymphomas are currently classified according to their respective normal lymphocyte counterparts (Fig. 20-47). After the precursor stage, B cells undergo immunoglobulin *VDJ* gene rearrangements and mature to surface IgM- and IgD-positive naïve B cells that often express CD5. These cells give rise to **mantle cell lymphoma.** Large activated B cells **(centroblasts)** home to germinal centers where they mature into smaller cells with cleaved nuclei **(centrocytes).** Centroblasts and centrocytes lack expression of the apoptosis inhibitor BCL-2, and they express the germinal center cell markers BCL-6 and CD10. **Follicular lymphomas** are derived from germinal center B cells and consist of a mixture of centroblasts and centrocytes. **Burkitt lymphoma** and some diffuse large **B-cell lymphomas** are also derived from germinal center lymphocytes.

Late-stage memory B cells reside in the marginal zone, which is the outermost compartment of the lymphoid follicle. Variants of **marginal zone lymphomas** include **splenic marginal zone lymphoma** and **MALT lymphomas** of the stomach and other mucosal surfaces. In addition, late-stage memory B cells can give rise to chronic lymphocytic leukemia/small lymphocytic lymphoma **(CLL/SLL).** Ultimately, some B cells differentiate into plasma cells. These cells are the only B cells that secrete immunoglobulins, although they lack immunoglobulin expression on the cell surface. Plasma cells home to the bone marrow, where they may give rise to **multiple myeloma.**

CLINICAL FEATURES: The various types of mature B-cell lymphoma can behave in a clinically indolent or aggressive manner. The behavior can be predicted by the morphology, immunophenotype, genetic lesions and clinical presentation (including stage) associated with the lymphoma. ***In general terms, and with a few exceptions, mature B-cell lymphomas composed of small lymphocytes usually follow an indolent clinical course, whereas those composed of mostly large cells follow an aggressive course that is rapidly fatal if left untreated.*** Examples of indolent mature B-cell lymphomas include (but are not limited to) B-cell chronic lymphocytic leukemia/small lymphocytic lymphoma, follicular lymphoma, extranodal marginal zone B-cell lymphoma (MALT lymphoma) and lymphoplasmacytic lymphoma; examples of aggressive mature B-cell lymphoma are diffuse large B-cell lymphoma, Burkitt lymphoma and mantle cell lymphoma (MCL). The latter represents an important exception to the general rule of small cell morphology predicting indolent behavior (see MCL discussion below). Ironically, although indolent lymphomas follow a prolonged clinical course, they are usually incurable using standard therapy. By contrast, aggressive lymphomas progress rapidly, but many of them are curable with conventional therapies. Unfortunately, from a clinical standpoint, not all lymphomas fall unequivocally into either category.

Our subsequent discussion of B-cell lymphomas follows the B-cell development paradigms outlined in Fig. 20-47.

Mantle Cell Lymphoma

Mantle cell lymphoma is a $CD5^+$ mature B-cell neoplasm composed of a monotonous population of small to medium-sized lymphocytes with irregular nuclear contours, resembling the normal lymphocytes found in the mantle zone surrounding germinal centers.

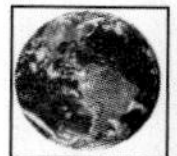

EPIDEMIOLOGY: Mantle cell lymphoma accounts for less than 10% of all types of B-cell lymphoma. It is a disease of adults with a median age of 60 years, and it affects men about twice as often as it affects women; it does not occur in children.

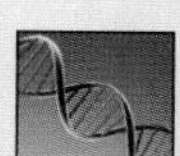

MOLECULAR PATHOGENESIS: The reciprocal chromosomal translocation t(11;14)(q13;q32) is present in nearly all cases of MCL and is considered the primary genetic event. The translocation results in overexpression of the Bcl-1 (PRAD1) gene, which codes for cyclin D1. Cyclin D1 exerts cell cycle control at the transition from the G_1 to S phase by complexing with Cdk4/6. This event results in phosphorylation of retinoblastoma (Rb) and subsequent activation of transcription factors promoting G_1- to S-phase progression of the cell cycle (see Chapter 5). Several other oncogenic alterations have been identified in MCL, including inactivating mutation of the ataxia-telangiectasia mutated (ATM) gene at 11q22–23. Immunoglobulin variable-region genes are unmutated, indicating derivation from a pregerminal center B cell.

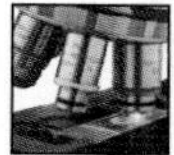

PATHOLOGY: Lymph nodes involved by MCL show a diffuse to vaguely nodular lymphoid infiltrate composed of small to medium-sized B cells with irregular nuclear contours. In some cases, the MCL lymphocytes are round and resemble the lymphocytes of B-cell CLL/SLL, which is often in the differential diagnosis (see below). One of the characteristic features in typical cases of MCL is the striking monotony of lymphoma cells with respect to size and shape. Unlike many other small B-cell lymphomas, large transformed cells and/or centroblasts are absent or rare in MCL. The presence of scattered epithelioid histiocytes and hyalinized small blood vessels completes the picture of typical cases.

Two major variants are recognized: one with a more nodular-appearing pattern where the lymphoma cells surround the germinal centers **(mantle zone pattern)** and another where the cells are larger and resemble lymphoblasts **(blastic/blastoid variant).** The mantle zone pattern is thought to behave less aggressively compared to the typical type, while the blastic/blastoid variant is known to be more aggressive. While primarily a nodal-based disease, MCL involves many different tissues and organs, with the spleen, bone marrow and gastrointestinal tract being common sites of disease. Multifocal mucosal involvement of the gastrointestinal tract (mostly small intestine and colon) results in a pattern known as **lymphomatous polyposis.**

Mantle cell lymphomas express the B-cell markers CD19 and CD20, and they show surface light-chain restriction. The lymphoma cells are also positive for CD5, but they are negative for CD10 and CD23. ***Importantly, MCL cells are positive for cyclin D1*** (Fig. 20-55). This immunophenotype, combined with the morphologic features, helps distinguish MCL from other small B-cell lymphomas with a more indolent course.

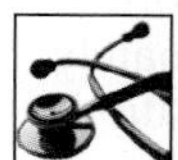

CLINICAL FEATURES: Most patients with MCL present with high-stage disease (III or IV). Approximately one third of patients have peripheral blood

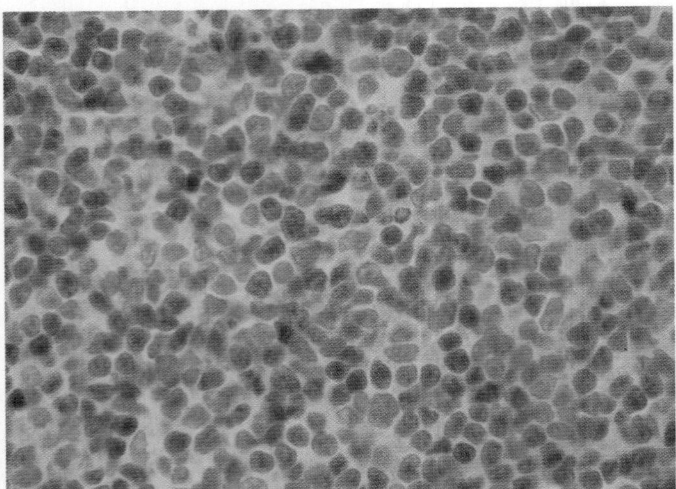

FIGURE 20-55. Mantle cell lymphoma (MCL). A nuclear stain for Bcl-1 (cyclin D1) is positive. This finding correlates with the presence of t(11;14), the typical translocation in MCL.

involvement at diagnosis. Despite its small cell morphology, MCL is clinically aggressive and is considered incurable by standard chemotherapy. The median survival is approximately 5 years for the typical type of MCL and about 3 years with the blastic/blastoid variant.

Diffuse Large B-Cell Lymphoma

Diffuse large B-cell lymphomas (DLBCLs) are a heterogeneous group of aggressive but potentially curable B-cell neoplasms. The heterogeneity of DLBCL is evident at the morphologic, immunophenotypic, genetic and clinical levels. While some cases of DLBCL arise de novo, others represent transformation or progression from an indolent lymphoma.

EPIDEMIOLOGY: Diffuse large B-cell lymphoma is the most common B-cell lymphoma worldwide. The disease has been the single largest contributor to the increasing incidence of non-Hodgkin lymphoma over the past few decades. Diffuse large B-cell lymphoma occurs in all age groups, but it is most prevalent between the ages of 60 and 70 years. It is slightly more common in males than females.

MOLECULAR PATHOGENESIS: The cause of DLBCL is unknown, but alterations of immune function are known to be important since a number of cases are associated with viral infections, such as EBV, HIV and rarely HHV-8. The frequency of EBV-positive cases is highest in immunosuppressed patients and in those older than the age of 50 years. Similar to the morphologic heterogeneity discussed below, the pathogenetic mechanisms involved in DLBCL are also variable. The *BCL6* gene locus at 3q27, which codes for a DNA-binding zinc-finger transcriptional regulator required for normal germinal center formation, is rearranged in approximately 30% of all cases. Other cases have acquired point mutations in the *BCL6* promoter sequences leading to transcriptional dysregulation and translocation. Approximately 20% to 30% of DLBCL cases show rearrangement of the *BCL2* gene, with approximately 20% to 30% harboring the t(14;18) translocation, which is the characteristic abnormality of follicular lymphoma (see below). Rearrangement of the *MYC* gene occurs in about 10% of cases and is usually associated with other complex genetic abnormalities and a poor outcome.

PATHOLOGY: DLBCL is characterized by a diffuse proliferation of large neoplastic B cells (Fig. 20-56). The large lymphoma cells are comparable in size to the nucleus of a histiocyte (macrophage) or roughly twice the size of a normal lymphocyte. Variants (e.g., centroblastic, immunoblastic) are described. The malignant cells of DLBCL are sometimes pleomorphic and/or anaplastic appearing, or they may resemble the cells seen in other malignant neoplasms such as carcinoma, melanoma or seminoma. Immunohistochemical stains on fixed tissue sections are therefore usually necessary to establish a correct diagnosis of DLBCL. ***While DLBCL most often involves lymph nodes, it frequently presents in extranodal tissues with the gastrointestinal tract being a common site of disease.***

The malignant cells of DLBCL express pan B-cell antigens, including CD19 and CD20. These common markers are sometimes lost, and analysis using additional markers of B-cell differentiation such as CD22, CD79a and PAX-5 may be investigated. DLBCL cells are variably positive CD10 and BCL-6, which indicates germinal center cell differentiation, and they sometimes express CD5. Surface immunoglobulin light-chain restriction can be identified in most cases, and all cases are negative for TdT and cyclin D1, helping to distinguish DLBCL from B-cell lymphoblastic lymphoma (TdT positive) and MCL, respectively.

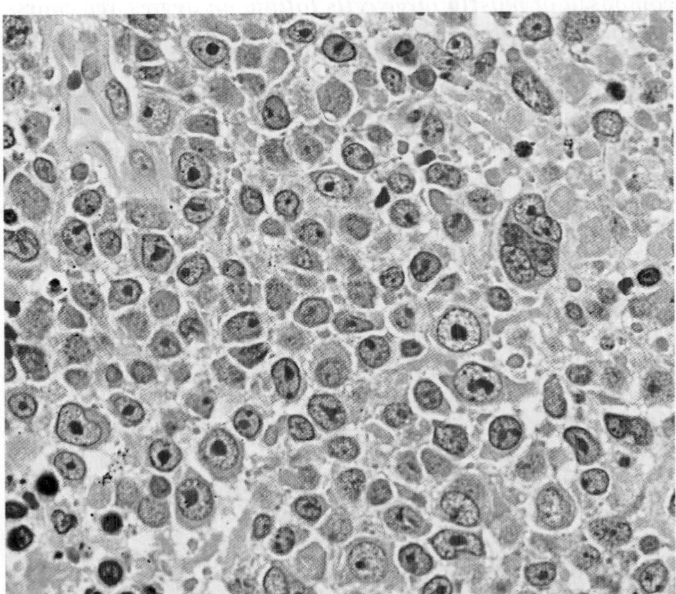

FIGURE 20-56. Diffuse large B-cell lymphoma. Sheets of large lymphoma cells with prominent nucleoli are present.

CLINICAL FEATURES: Patients with DLBCL most often present with a rapidly growing tumor in nodal and/or extranodal sites. Single or multiple sites may be involved, but approximately 50% of patients have low-stage disease (stage I or II) at presentation. Bone marrow involvement can occur, but it is usually late in the course of disease. Peripheral blood involvement is rare. Symptoms tend to be related to the site(s) of involvement. For example, a large mass in the colon can produce obstruction or bowel perforation, whereas a rapidly growing mass in the mediastinum can result in obstruction of the superior vena cava (SVC) leading to the SVC syndrome. Systemic manifestations such as fever, fatigue and night sweats ("B symptoms") are not uncommon in patients with DLBCL.

In general terms, diffuse large B-cell lymphomas are aggressive neoplasms that are rapidly fatal if left untreated. Because these tumors are generally rapidly proliferating neoplasms, however, they are susceptible to chemotherapeutic agents, and complete remissions can be achieved in 60% to 80% of patients. Patient outcome is dependent on tumor stage, and those with limited disease do better compared to those with widespread (high-stage) disease at diagnosis.

Burkitt Lymphoma

Burkitt lymphoma (BL), one of the most rapidly growing malignancies, is defined by a chromosomal translocation involving 8q24, which harbors the *MYC* oncogene (see Chapter 5). It is composed of a monomorphic population of medium-sized cells, often presents at extranodal sites and has a propensity toward leukemia. While MYC translocation is highly characteristic, it is not specific and a combination of diagnostic features is required to confirm the diagnosis.

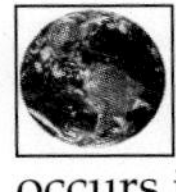

EPIDEMIOLOGY: BL occurs in three distinct variants, each with different clinical presentations, morphologic features and pathobiology. **Endemic BL** occurs in equatorial Africa and Papua, New Guinea. It is the most common childhood malignancy in these areas with a peak incidence in 4- to 7-year-olds. The jaw, other facial bones and the abdominal viscera are commonly involved in endemic cases. **Sporadic BL** is seen worldwide and mainly affects children and young adults. While it has a low incidence among all lymphomas in the Western world (1% to 2%), it accounts for approximately 30% to 50% of all childhood lymphomas. The median age for adult patients is 30 years. Like most other B-cell lymphomas, males are affected more than females. In contrast to endemic BL, sporadic BL often presents as an abdominal mass involving the ileocecum. **Immunodeficiency-associated BL** mainly occurs in HIV-infected persons and may be the initial manifestation of AIDS.

MOLECULAR PATHOGENESIS: All cases are associated with a translocation involving the *c-MYC* gene on chromosome 8. The *immunoglobulin heavy-chain* gene locus on chromosome 14 is the usual partner for c-MYC, resulting in the classic t(8;14) abnormality; however, the immunoglobulin light-chain loci can also be involved, resulting in the alternate translocations t(2;8) (κ light chain) and t(8;22) (λ light chain). In endemic cases, the breakpoint on chromosome 14 occurs in the heavy-chain–joining region, as seen in early B cells. In sporadic BL, the translocation occurs in the Ig switch region, which is more characteristic of mature B lymphocytes. In these cases, expression of *MYC* gene driven by the Ig heavy-chain promoter leads to uncontrolled tumor cell growth (see Chapter 5).

EBV is present in virtually all cases of endemic BL, but it is found in less than 30% of sporadic and immunodeficiency-related cases. EBV-positive sporadic BL is associated with low socioeconomic status. Many patients experience a prodromal stage of polyclonal B-cell activation caused by bacterial, viral or parasitic infections (e.g., malaria).

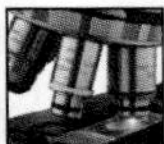

PATHOLOGY: BL typically produces extranodal tumors rather than lymphadenopathy. All variants of this lymphoma have a high risk for central nervous system involvement. The classic presentation for endemic BL is a destructive tumor in the jaws or other facial bones (Fig. 20-57A). Patients with sporadic BL typically present with abdominal masses. All types may involve ovaries, kidneys and breast. Patients with sizable bulky tumors sometimes present with Burkitt leukemia and extensive bone marrow involvement.

Microscopically, BL cells are medium sized and lack significant cytologic atypia. Tissue sections reveal a high number of mitotic figures, which attests to the extremely high proliferation rate in this tumor. The cellular debris of apoptotic tumor cells is cleared by macrophages, whose scattered appearance imparts a "starry sky" pattern under low microscopic magnification (Fig. 20-57B). Aspirate smears stained with Wright-Giemsa demonstrate numerous lipid vacuoles in the deeply basophilic cytoplasm of the tumor cells (Fig. 20-57C).

Burkitt lymphoma cells express surface IgM and immunoglobulin light chain, and they are positive for common B-cell antigens (CD19, CD20, CD22). They also mark for CD10 and BCL-6, supporting their postulated origin from the germinal center. BL cells do not express TdT, helping to distinguish these tumors from precursor B-cell acute lymphoblastic leukemia/lymphoma.

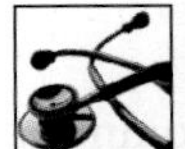

CLINICAL FEATURES: All variants of BL are highly aggressive, and most patients present with bulky extranodal tumors and a high tumor burden. Most patients present after a short symptomatic period with high-stage disease (III or IV). Because of its marked proliferative rate, BL is responsive to intensive chemotherapy, and cure rates of up to 90% can be achieved in patients with low-stage disease and of 60% to 80% in patients with high-stage disease. Children and young adults tend to fare better than adults with BL. Tumor lysis syndrome can occur upon initiation of therapy as a result of rapid tumor cell death, and this can lead to early patient mortality.

Follicular Lymphoma

Follicular lymphoma (FL) is a mature B-cell neoplasm composed of follicle center B cells (germinal center cells). In contrast to diffuse B-cell lymphomas, follicular lymphomas must have at least a partially follicular architecture to meet diagnostic criteria. The neoplastic cells of FL are heterogeneous and consist of small and large cleaved cells and centroblasts.

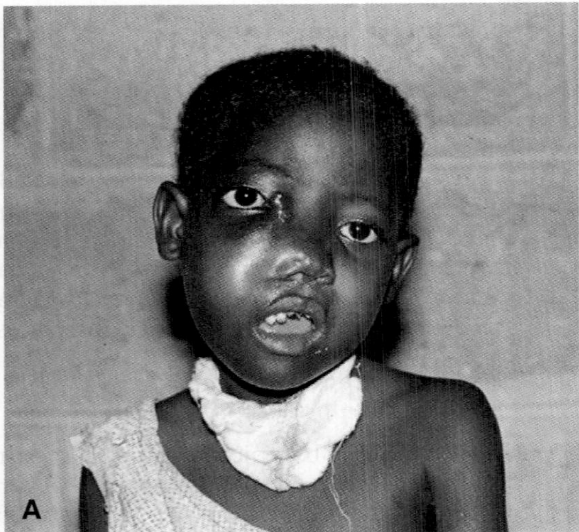

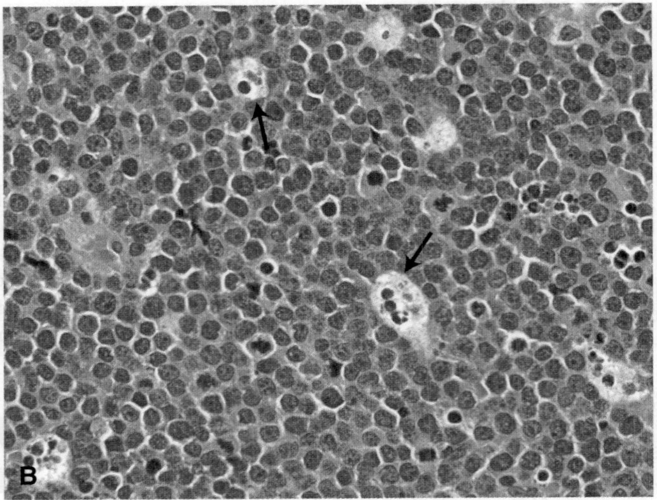

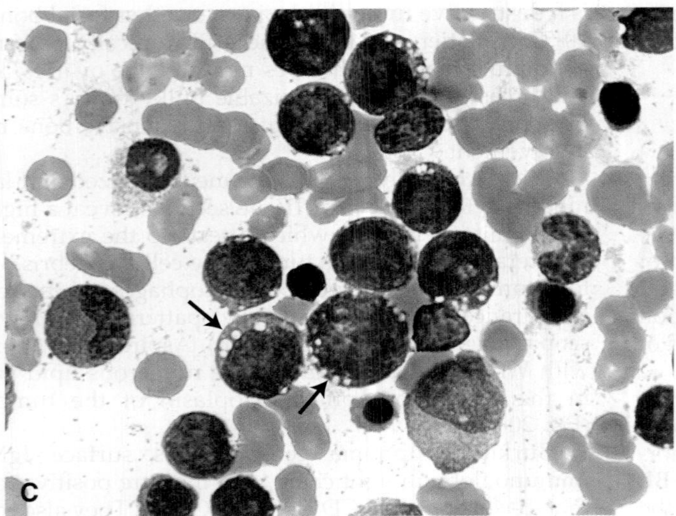

FIGURE 20-57. Burkitt lymphoma. A. A tumor of the jaw distorts the child's face. **B.** Lymph node is effaced by neoplastic lymphocytes with several starry-sky macrophages (*arrows*). **C.** Bone marrow aspirate smear showing typical cytologic features of Burkitt lymphoma. Note the deeply basophilic cytoplasm and lipid vacuoles (*arrows*).

FL exhibits variable clinical behavior ranging from indolent to aggressive, and the behavior is somewhat predictable by histologic grade, which is predicated upon the number of centroblasts present in the neoplastic follicles.

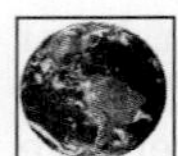

EPIDEMIOLOGY: FL is the second most common lymphoma worldwide, but it is the most common form of non-Hodgkin lymphoma in the United States, where it constitutes 20% of all adult lymphomas. It is predominantly a disease of adults with a peak incidence in the sixth decade of life. FL only rarely occurs in individuals younger than age 20. In contrast to most other B-cell lymphomas, FL occurs more commonly in women than men.

MOLECULAR PATHOGENESIS: The t(14:18)(q32;q21) is the characteristic chromosomal translocation associated with FL, and it is found in up to 90% of grade I and II FLs. This translocation, which juxtaposes the *BCL2* gene on chromosome 18 and the immunoglobulin heavy-chain (IgH) gene on chromosome 14, results in overexpression of the Bcl-2 protein. ***The Bcl-2 protein is an inhibitor of apoptosis and is thought to give the lymphoma cells a survival advantage.*** In addition to the *Bcl-2/IgH* rearrangement, several other genetic alterations have been found in FL, and some of them are associated with progression/transformation from the low-grade indolent forms to the more aggressive higher-grade form or DLBCL (e.g., inactivation of p53 and activation of MYC).

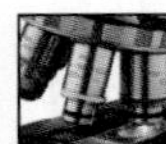

PATHOLOGY: At low magnification, lymph nodes (or other tissues) involved by follicular lymphoma will have a distinctly nodular (follicular) pattern or a combination of nodular and diffuse architectural patterns (Fig. 20-58). The neoplastic follicles are present in high density, and they are often found in a back-to-back arrangement with very little intervening paracortex. The neoplastic follicle centers (germinal centers) are composed of a mixture of small and large cells with irregular nuclear contours (centrocytes/cleaved cells) and scattered centroblasts, which have round nuclear contours and multiple nucleoli attached to the nuclear membrane.

Histologic grade is one of the features that determines prognosis in FL. There are three histologic grades of FL, distinguished by the number of centroblasts found per high-power

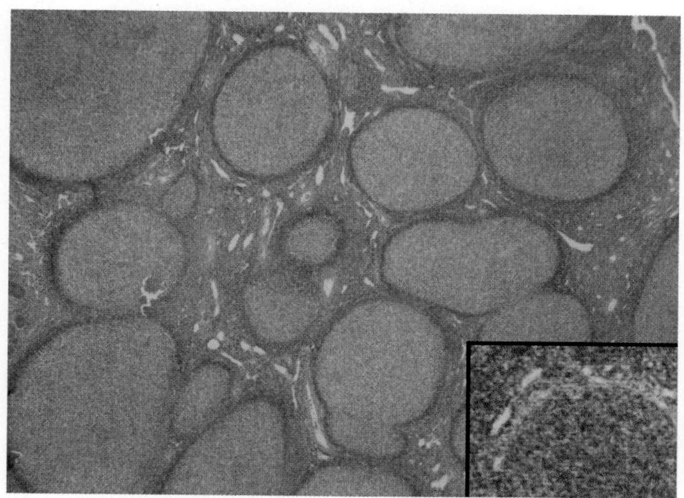

FIGURE 20-58. Follicular lymphoma. The normal lymph node architecture is replaced by malignant lymphoid follicles in a back-to-back pattern. *Inset.* Malignant lymphoid follicle germinal centers can be distinguished from normal/reactive germinal centers using immunohistochemistry for Bcl-2.

field (Fig. 20-59). Diffuse areas are not uncommon in FL, but they generally do not impact prognosis unless they are composed of large B cells, in which case a diagnosis of concurrent DLBCL is made. The bone marrow is involved in approximately 40% to 60% of cases; a characteristic paratrabecular pattern of involvement is found. Circulating follicular lymphoma cells are found in the peripheral blood in about 10% of cases.

Follicular lymphomas express pan B-cell antigens including CD19, CD20, CD22 and CD79a, and surface immunoglobulin expression and light-chain restriction are found in most cases. In addition, FLs also express the germinal center cell markers CD10 and Bcl-6, as would be expected given their origin from the follicle center. Unlike MCL and B-cell CLL/SLL, FLs do not express CD5. The follicular lymphoma cells express Bcl-2 protein in greater than 90% of cases (Fig. 20-58, *inset*). This latter finding is often useful in distinguishing FL from follicular hyperplasia, which has Bcl-2–negative follicles.

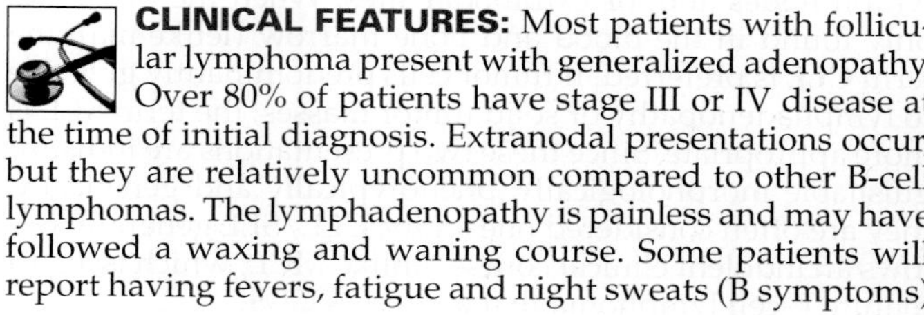

CLINICAL FEATURES: Most patients with follicular lymphoma present with generalized adenopathy. Over 80% of patients have stage III or IV disease at the time of initial diagnosis. Extranodal presentations occur, but they are relatively uncommon compared to other B-cell lymphomas. The lymphadenopathy is painless and may have followed a waxing and waning course. Some patients will report having fevers, fatigue and night sweats (B symptoms)

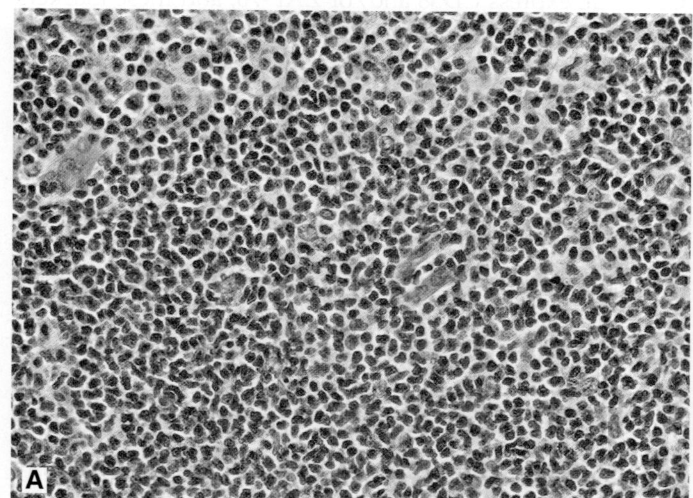

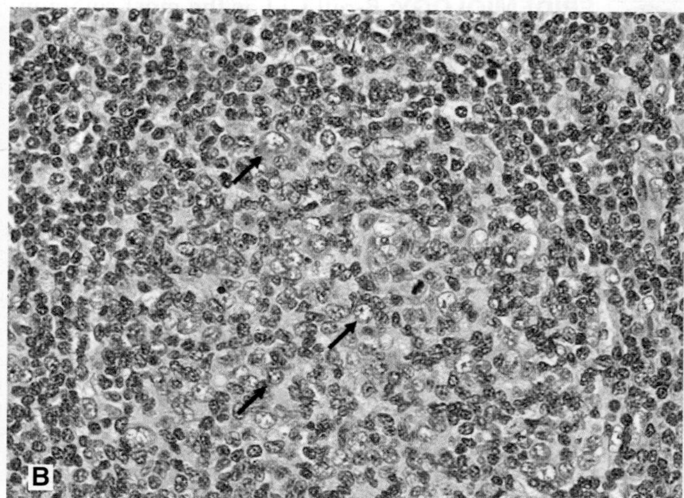

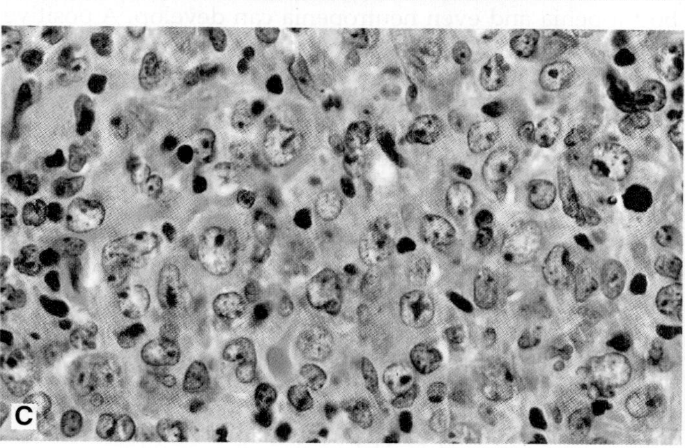

FIGURE 20-59. Follicular lymphoma grading. A. Follicular lymphoma, grade 1. The neoplastic follicles are composed of predominantly small cleaved cells (centrocytes) and only a few scattered centroblasts are present. **B. Follicular lymphoma, grade 2.** The neoplastic follicle shows a mixture of small and large cleaved cells and centroblasts characterized by multiple nucleoli (*arrows*). **C. Follicular lymphoma, grade 3.** The neoplastic follicle shows a predominance of centroblasts with only rare admixed centrocytes. The persistence of a follicular pattern helps distinguish this entity from diffuse large B-cell lymphoma.

during the course of disease. Most cases of FL follow an indolent clinical course, and because the disease is usually incurable, treatment is not always indicated at diagnosis. The overall median survival is approximately 7 to 9 years, and this is not dramatically improved with high-dose chemotherapy. As discussed above, the clinical course is linked to histologic grade, and progression/transformation to more aggressive disease occurs in up to 50% of cases over time.

B-Cell Chronic Lymphocytic Leukemia/Small Lymphocytic Lymphoma

B-cell CLL/SLL is a common, mature $CD5^+$ B-cell neoplasm composed of a monomorphic population of predominantly small lymphocytes with round to slightly irregular nuclear contours admixed with a lesser population of larger cells with round nuclei and single basophilic nucleoli known as prolymphoyctes (in blood) or paraimmunoblasts (in tissue). B-cell CLL/SLL involves peripheral blood, bone marrow, lymph nodes and/or extranodal sites. When the disease is only found in the blood and bone marrow (leukemia), the term **CLL** is preferred. If tumor cells predominantly give rise to lymphadenopathy or solid tumor masses, the term **SLL** is more appropriate. Since these two presentations are indistinguishable morphologically, phenotypically and genetically, they are often considered one entity. CLL/SLL generally follows an indolent clinical course, unlike MCL, which is also a mature B-cell lymphoma that expresses CD5.

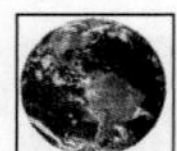

EPIDEMIOLOGY: B-cell CLL is the most common form of leukemia in adults in the Western world. The annual incidence is approximately 2 to 6 cases per 100,000 persons, but the incidence increases with age to approximately 12.8 per 100,000 at age 65, which is the average age at diagnosis. The diagnosis of CLL/SLL is made more frequently in males compared to females. SLL accounts for approximately 7% of all non-Hodgkin lymphomas diagnosed in tissue biopsies.

MOLECULAR PATHOGENESIS: The vast majority of CLL/SLL cases have cytogenetic abnormalities that can be detected by FISH testing. The most common abnormalities are deletion of 13q12–14, deletion of 11q, trisomy 12 and deletion of 17p (p53). Approximately half of B-CLL cases have not undergone somatic mutations in variable-region genes (i.e., unmutated), and thus they have the genotype of naïve B cells. The other half have undergone *VH* gene mutations (i.e., mutated) and resemble postgerminal center B cells. Cases with unmutated immunoglobulin segments tend to follow a more aggressive clinical course for unknown reasons.

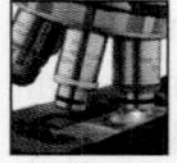

PATHOLOGY: Lymph nodes involved by CLL/SLL are effaced by a proliferation of predominantly small lymphocytes in a diffuse to vaguely nodular or pseudofollicular pattern (Fig. 20-60). The peripheral blood in CLL/SLL shows an absolute lymphocytosis composed of mostly small monotonous lymphocytes with round to slightly irregular nuclear contours and scant blue-gray cytoplasm (Fig. 20-60B). Peripheral smear also contains a high number of disrupted cells (smudge cells; Fig. 20-60B). The nuclear chromatin is clumped and often has a blotchy appearance resembling cracked mud; nucleoli are absent in the small cells. In addition to the small cells, all cases also show a population of larger cells with round nuclear contours, less condensed chromatin and a single prominent central nucleolus; these cells are known as prolymphocytes in the blood, and they usually account for less than 10% of total lymphocytes. In order to establish a diagnosis of CLL in the absence of tissue-based disease, the total number of circulating monoclonal B cells must exceed 5000/μL.

The vaguely nodular gross pattern is most apparent at low-power magnification, and further examination of lighter-staining areas reveal the so-called proliferation centers, which contain a small number of large cells known as paraimmunoblasts (Fig. 20-60C). Large confluent sheets of paraimmunoblasts or other large lymphoid cells may represent transformation to diffuse large B-cell lymphoma **(Richter transformation).** CLL/SLL infiltrates the splenic white and red pulp and the portal areas of the liver. Bone marrow involvement ranges from complete effacement of the marrow space to a patchy interstitial or nonparatrabecular distribution.

The immunophenotype of B-cell CLL/SLL is distinct. The neoplastic cells express pan B-cell antigens, including CD19, CD20, CD22 and CD79, as well as CD5, CD23 and surface immunoglobulin light chain. It is important to note that CLL/SLL cells show weaker CD20 and immunoglobulin light-chain expression compared to other mature B-cell neoplasms, and these findings are diagnostically useful. CLL/SLL is negative for cyclin D1 and CD10. Some cases of CLL/SLL express CD38 and/or ZAP-70, and these markers serve as prognostic indicators often used in conjunction with other molecular and FISH tests to help predict individual patient outcome.

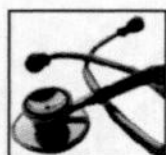

CLINICAL FEATURES: Most patients with CLL/SLL are asymptomatic, and many cases are diagnosed incidentally. Often the first hint of the disease comes from the finding of an abnormal complete blood count showing an absolute lymphocytosis. The total lymphocyte count is variable, but currently, an absolute monoclonal B-cell count of at least 5000 cells/μL is needed to establish a diagnosis of CLL outside the setting of tissue-based disease. Flow cytometric analysis of the peripheral blood is sufficient to establish the diagnosis in most cases. The other peripheral counts may be normal or abnormal, and findings such as platelet count and hemoglobin level are used to stage CLL/SLL. The erythrocyte and platelet counts are initially normal, but as the disease advances, severe anemia, thrombocytopenia and even neutropenia can develop. A positive Coombs test is observed during the course of disease in up to 20% of cases, and this may be associated with immune-mediated hemolytic anemia. A small monoclonal paraprotein is present in some patients.

Immunologic deficiencies, mainly of B cells but also of T cells, are common. The cause of B-cell dysfunction is unknown. Hypogammaglobulinemia occurs in 50% to 75% of cases at some point in the course of disease, and the degree of hypogammaglobulinemia generally correlates with disease stage and is responsible for infectious complications. Patients with B-CLL also have increased peripheral blood T cells (>3000/μL). There is an increase in $CD8^+$ T cells and a corresponding decrease in $CD4^+$ cells, with a resulting decrease in the $CD4^+/CD8^+$ ratio. The T cells often show impaired delayed-type hypersensitivity in vitro, which also contributes to the increased risk of infection. The most common infectious complications are bacterial infections, followed by viral and fungal infections.

The median survival of patients with CLL/SLL is approximately 4 to 6 years, but the disease course and prognosis are highly variable. For instance, patients with low disease burden can survive for greater than 10 years, whereas others with extensive disease or poor prognostic features experience rapid progression and succumb within 2 to 3 years. The presence of certain molecular lesions such as trisomy 12 and deletions of 11q and 17q portends a worse prognosis.

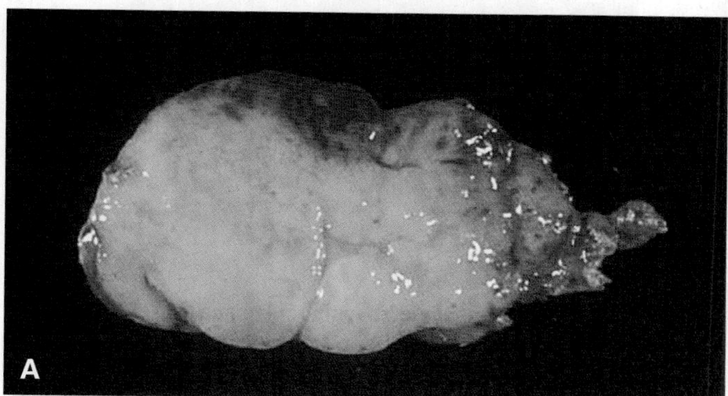

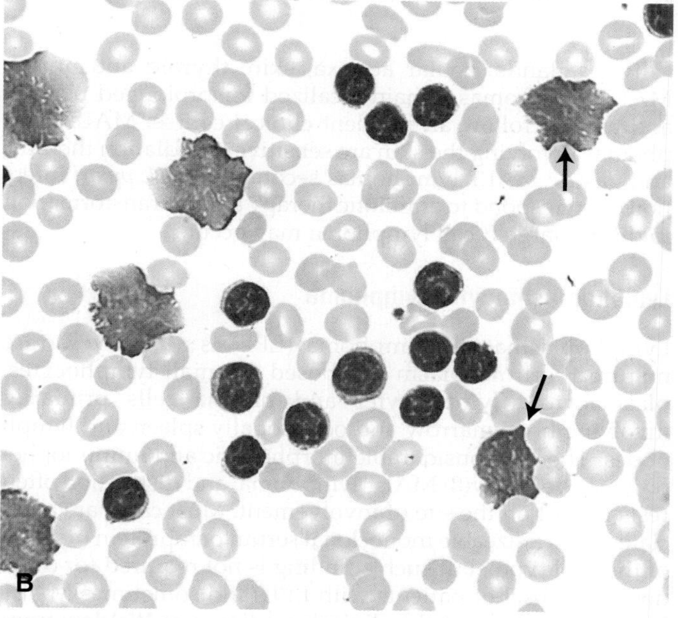

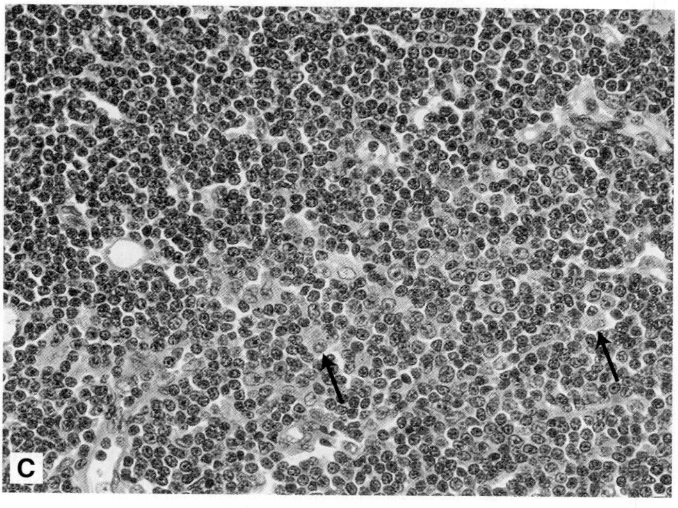

The survival of patients with CLL/SLL is also impacted by the risk of transformation or progression to a more aggressive B-cell neoplasm. ***Transformation to prolymphocytic leukemia is the most common form of progression, occurring in approximately 15% to 30% of cases.*** This form of transformation is characterized by worsening cytopenias, increasing splenomegaly and a progressive increase in the number of prolymphocytes in the peripheral blood or paraimmunoblasts in lymph nodes or other tissues. Transformation of diffuse large B-cell lymphoma, known as **Richter syndrome,** occurs in about 10% of cases. This form of progression is marked by the appearance of a rapidly enlarging mass, worsening of systemic symptoms and a high lactate dehydrogenase level in the serum. Other rare forms of transformation also occur, including a Hodgkin lymphoma or Hodgkin-like transformation. Most patients experiencing prolymphocytic or Richter transformation survive less than 1 year.

Asymptomatic patients with CLL/SLL who have stable lymphocyte counts may not require treatment. Multiagent chemotherapy and/or treatment with humanized monoclonal antibodies (e.g., Rituxan) is used in patients with high-stage or aggressive disease, but the disease generally remains incurable.

Marginal Zone Lymphomas

The marginal zone lymphomas consist of a heterogeneous group of mature B-cell neoplasms that arise in lymph nodes, spleen and extranodal tissues. The lymphoma cells are postulated to arise from the marginal zone of the lymphoid follicle, which contains memory B cells that have gone through the germinal center reaction (postgerminal center). Regardless of the primary site of involvement, all marginal zone lymphomas share similar morphologic and immunophenotypic features. Because they represent the prototype for marginal zone lymphoma, further discussion will be limited to the extranodal marginal zone B-cell lymphomas, which are also known as the MALT lymphomas.

MALT lymphomas are indolent B-cell lymphomas composed of a heterogeneous population of small B cells including centrocyte-like cells (marginal zone cells), monocytoid lymphocytes, small lymphocytes and scattered larger lymphoid cells resembling centroblasts and immunoblasts occurring at extranodal sites, such as the gastrointestinal tract, salivary glands, ocular adnexa, lungs and skin. Plasma cell differentiation is present in a variable proportion of cases.

FIGURE 20-60. B-cell small lymphocytic lymphoma/chronic lymphocytic leukemia. A. Gross image of a bisected, enlarged lymph node shows the characteristic uniform, glistening, fish-flesh appearance seen in tissues involved by lymphoma. **B.** A smear of peripheral blood exhibits numerous small to medium-sized lymphocytes with clumped nuclear chromatin. Scattered smudge cells (osmotically fragile cells) are present (*arrows*). **C.** On microscopic examination, the nodal architecture is replaced by a diffuse proliferation of small lymphocytes admixed with a low number of larger cells known as paraimmunoblasts (*arrows*) found in scattered proliferation centers.

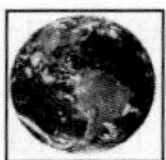

EPIDEMIOLOGY: MALT lymphomas account for approximately 5% to 10% of all B-cell lymphomas, and they represent the most common type of gastric lymphoma. Most cases occur in adults with a median age of 60; they only rarely occur in children and young adults. There is a slight female predominance in part because of their association with autoimmune diseases (e.g., Sjögren syndrome, Hashimoto thyroiditis). Immunoproliferative small intestinal disease (IPSID), also termed α-chain disease or **Mediterranean lymphoma,** is a subtype of MALT lymphoma that produces α heavy chains.

MOLECULAR PATHOGENESIS: MALT lymphomas arise in the setting of chronic inflammation, most often caused by autoimmunity or infection. The monoclonal B-cell neoplasm develops in the background of what begins as a benign polyclonal reaction following the acquisition of genetic mutations and/or chromosomal lesions in B cells. T lymphocytes are necessary to maintain growth and survival of the neoplastic B-cell population. ***The prototypical infection-driven MALT lymphoma is gastric lymphoma associated with* H. pylori *gastritis*** (see Chapter 13). Gastric MALT lymphomas found at the earliest phases of development may regress with antibiotic therapy aimed to eradicate *H. pylori*. MALT lymphomas that have progressed to acquire chromosomal translocations, such as t(11;18) or t(1;14), no longer respond to antibiotic therapy alone. Dissemination to distant sites and/or transformation to diffuse large B-cell lymphoma occurs as additional genetic lesions are acquired. A similar progression from a polyclonal to monoclonal lymphoid infiltrate is observed in EBV-related lymphomas.

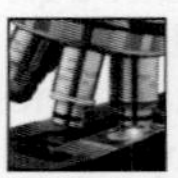

PATHOLOGY: Early-stage MALT lymphomas present microscopically with expanded marginal zone lymphocytes surrounding and infiltrating reactive B-cell follicles. The malignant B lymphocytes are heterogeneous and include varying proportions of small angulated lymphocytes, medium-sized monocytoid lymphocytes with abundant cytoplasm, plasmacytoid lymphocytes and even admixed clonal plasma cells. The tumor cells invade glandular epithelium or epithelia of mucosal surfaces, resulting in **lymphoepithelial lesions** (Fig. 20-61). Occasionally, transformation of (indolent) MALT lymphoma into large cell B-cell lymphoma occurs.

There is no specific immunophenotype that characterizes the MALT lymphomas. Most tumor cells express IgM and show light-chain restriction. MALT lymphomas express B-cell–associated antigens, and they are negative for CD5, CD23 and cyclin D1, which distinguishes them from B-CLL/SLL and mantle cell lymphoma. They are also negative for CD10, which differentiates them from follicular lymphoma.

MALT lymphomas typically show somatic mutation of variable-region genes. The most common cytogenetic abnormalities are trisomy 3 and t(11;18), the latter involving the apoptosis inhibitor gene *API2* and the *MALT1* gene. In cases with subtle lymphocytic infiltrates in the gastric mucosa, demonstration of clonal *IgH* gene rearrangement helps to establish the diagnosis.

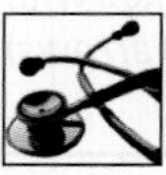

CLINICAL FEATURES: Most MALT lymphomas involve the stomach or other mucosal sites, including the respiratory tract. They may also be seen in the salivary glands, ocular adnexa, skin, thyroid and breast. MALT lymphomas remain localized for prolonged periods and tend to follow an indolent clinical course. MALT lymphomas involving the skin are sensitive to radiation therapy, and gastric MALT lymphomas secondary to *H. pylori* infection often respond to antibiotic therapy alone. Transformation to diffuse large B-cell lymphoma may occur.

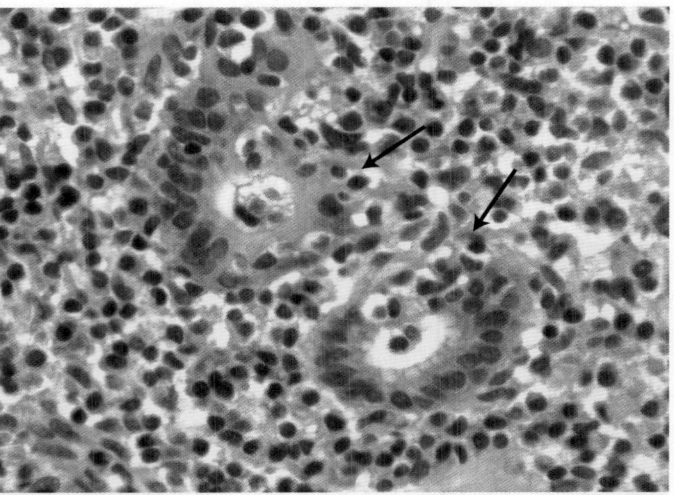

FIGURE 20-61. Mucosa-associated lymphoid tissue (MALT) lymphoma. A stomach biopsy showing the characteristic lymphoepithelial lesions seen in MALT lymphomas (*arrows*). The infiltrating lymphocytes are B cells.

Lymphoplasmacytic Lymphoma

Lymphoplasmacytic lymphoma (LPL) is a relatively rare mature B-cell neoplasm composed of small lymphocytes, plasmacytoid lymphocytes and plasma cells primarily involving bone marrow and occasionally spleen and lymph nodes. There is considerable morphologic and immunophenotypic overlap with MALT lymphoma, and distinction often rests in part on the site of involvement. Most cases are associated with a sizeable monoclonal serum paraprotein (usually of the IgM type), but such a finding is not required for diagnosis. A subset of patients with LPL (and sometimes MALT lymphoma) develop the clinical syndrome of **Waldenstrom macroglobulinemia,** which can be associated with a **hyperviscosity syndrome.** The disease usually occurs in adults in their fifth to sixth decades of life, and there is a slight male predominance.

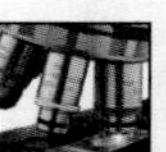

PATHOLOGY: Bone marrow involved by LPL shows a variably dense lymphoid infiltrate composed of a heterogeneous population of small lymphocytes, plasmacytoid lymphocytes and mature plasma cells in a diffuse and nonparatrabecular pattern. A low number of large transformed lymphoid cells can be found in some cases. Lymphoplasmacytic cells with nuclear pseudoinclusions known as Dutcher bodies (immunoglobulin) are commonly found in tissue sections. Stained bone marrow aspirate smears show the cytologic features to advantage and also reveal an increased number of normal mast cells in most cases. Lymphoplasmacytic lymphoma may involve the peripheral blood, but it only rarely produces an absolute lymphocytosis like CLL/SLL. An interfollicular pattern of involvement is most commonly seen in lymph nodes affected by LPL, and in many cases the nodal architecture is generally preserved.

Lymphoplasmacytic lymphomas express pan B-cell antigens, and they are negative for CD5, CD10, CD23 and cyclin D1. The plasma cell component can be highlighted with the plasma cell marker CD138, and in addition, clonality of the plasma cells can be documented in tissue sections using immunohistochemical stains for k and λ immunoglobulin light chains. No specific chromosomal or oncogenic abnormalities have been found in LPL.

CLINICAL FEATURES: Fatigue, weakness and weight loss are the most frequent presenting complaints of persons with LPL. These nonspecific findings are usually related to anemia caused by marrow infiltration or immune-mediated hemolysis. About one half of patients will have lymphadenopathy and/or organomegaly at diagnosis. The majority of patients will have an IgM paraprotein in the serum; some may have a different paraprotein (IgG, IgA) or no paraprotein at all. Increased blood viscosity caused by the presence of macroglobulinemia occurs in approximately 30% of patients, and the serum hyperviscosity may be associated with visual impairment, neurologic problems, bleeding and cryoglobulinemia. Therapeutic plasma exchange (plasmapheresis) is often necessary to control the complications of the hyperviscosity syndrome until definitive therapy is initiated.

Lymphoplasmacytic lymphoma is an indolent disease that follows a progressive course. The median survival is approximately 5 to 10 years. Like other small B-cell lymphomas, it is generally incurable, and transformation to diffuse large B-cell lymphoma can occur during the course of disease in a small proportion of cases. The latter is associated with poor survival.

Hairy Cell Leukemia

Hairy cell leukemia (HCL) is a clonal B-cell neoplasm composed of small to medium-sized lymphocytes with abundant pale cytoplasm and hair-like cell cytoplasmic protrusions involving bone marrow and peripheral blood (Fig. 20-62A). The malignant cell is postulated to arise from a postgerminal center–stage peripheral B cell (late activated memory B cell). Hairy cell leukemia is rare and affects mainly middle-aged to elderly men, with a male-to-female ratio of 5:1. Marked splenomegaly is a common presentation.

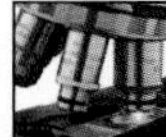

PATHOLOGY: Hairy cell leukemia exhibits subtle interstitial infiltrates that do not disturb normal marrow architecture. Hairy cells have abundant clear cytoplasm compared to normal small lymphocytes, which gives

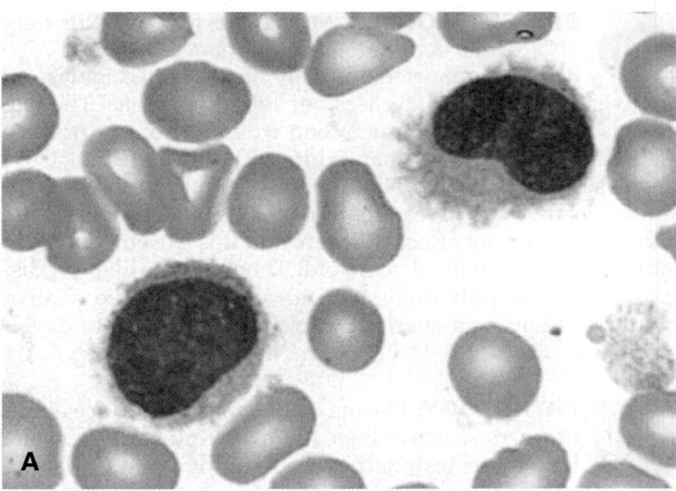

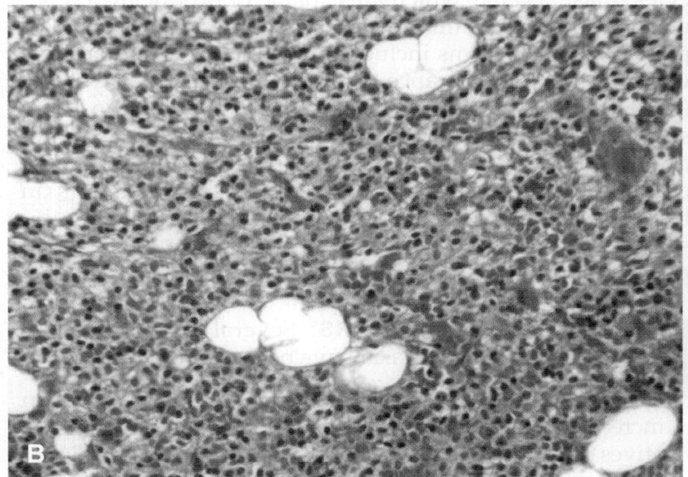

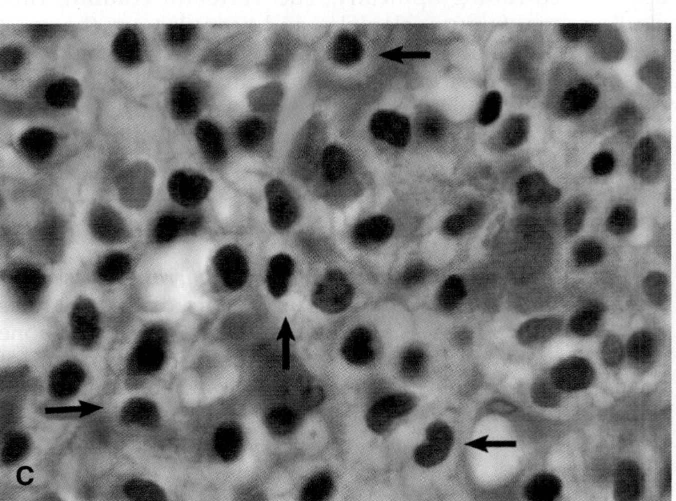

FIGURE 20-62. Hairy cell leukemia. A. Peripheral smear demonstrating "hairy" appearance of the leukemic cells in hairy cell leukemia. **B.** Bone marrow biopsy, showing infiltration of bone marrow by small to medium-sized lymphocytes with oval to reniform nuclei and pale cytoplasm with circumferential hair projections seen in peripheral blood and bone marrow aspirate smears. **C.** Higher-power photomicrograph of the lymphocytes infiltrating the bone marrow in hairy cell leukemia. Typical "fried egg" cells, with round-oval to kidney-shaped nuclei, are shown (*arrows*).

them a "fried egg" appearance (Fig. 20-62B,C). Both liver and spleen are prominently involved, but lymph nodes are generally spared. The immunophenotypic features of HCL are characteristic, allowing distinction from other small B-cell neoplasms. The hairy cells express the pan B-cell antigens CD19 and CD20 as well as CD11c, CD22, CD25 and CD103. Occasional cases will show variable expression of CD5, CD10 and even cyclin D1. The neoplastic cells are positive for tartrate-resistant acid phosphatase (TRAP), but the use of this cytochemical stain has been largely supplanted by more robust immunophenotyping techniques in clinical practice. No specific cytogenetic abnormalities have been found in HCL.

CLINICAL FEATURES: Most patients with HCL present with splenomegaly, leukopenia and monocytopenia, or sometimes pancytopenia. Hepatosplenomegaly is less common, and peripheral lymphadenopathy is rare. Infections are frequent, occurring in about one third of patients during the course of disease. The disorder is otherwise indolent, and complete and durable remissions can be achieved with purine analogs such as deoxycoformycin or 2-chlorodeoxyadenosine (2-CDA).

Plasma Cell Neoplasia

Plasma cell neoplasms are a group of disorders resulting from the clonal expansion of terminally differentiated B lymphocytes (plasma cells), which are capable of producing a monoclonal paraprotein **(monoclonal gammopathy).** The major plasma cell neoplasms include monoclonal gammopathy of undetermined significance (MGUS), plasma cell myeloma (multiple myeloma), plasmacytoma, immunoglobulin deposition disease (amyloidosis and light-chain disease) and osteosclerotic myeloma (POEMS disease: polyneuropathy, organomegaly, endocrine disorders, myeloma and skin lesions). These are diseases that affect adults almost exclusively. Further discussion will be limited to MGUS and plasma cell myeloma.

ETIOLOGIC FACTORS: Several risk factors for plasma cell neoplasia have been identified.

- A **genetic predisposition** is suggested by an increased incidence of multiple myeloma in first-degree relatives of patients with plasma cell neoplasia and the higher frequency of multiple myeloma in blacks.
- **Ionizing radiation** has been incriminated in the etiology of plasma cell neoplasia. Long-term survivors of the bombing of Hiroshima and Nagasaki had a fivefold increased incidence of multiple myeloma.
- **Chronic antigenic stimulation** may constitute a risk factor. Some cases of multiple myeloma have been associated with chronic infections, such as HIV and chronic osteomyelitis, and with chronic inflammatory disorders (e.g., rheumatoid arthritis). A two-hit hypothesis been proposed by which (1) antigenic stimulation leads to reactive, polyclonal proliferation of B lymphocytes and (2) a subsequent mutagenic event establishes a single malignant clone.

Monoclonal Gammopathy of Undetermined Significance

MGUS is found in about 3% of persons older than age 50 and in more than 5% older than age 70. It is defined by the presence of a monoclonal paraproteinemia of less than 3.0 g/dL, fewer than 10% plasma cells in the bone marrow, lack of end-organ damage (CRAB: hypercalcemia, renal insufficiency, anemia, bone lesions) and exclusion of other B-cell neoplasms or diseases known to produce a monoclonal paraprotein (M-protein). IgM MGUS is most often associated with a clone of immunoglobulin-secreting B cells and can progress to a small B-cell lymphoma with plasma cell differentiation such as lymphoplasmacytic lymphoma. Non-IgM MGUS is most often associated with the presence of clonal plasma cells and may progress to a bona fide malignant plasma cell neoplasm. Although non-IgM MGUS is associated with an expanded clone of immunoglobulin-secreting plasma cells that have been shown to have similar genetic lesions to multiple myeloma, it is considered a preneoplastic condition with a rate of progression to overt plasma cell neoplasia (e.g., multiple myeloma, amyloidosis) of about 1% per year for the life of affected individuals.

Plasma Cell Myeloma

Plasma cell myeloma (PCM) is a malignant neoplasm of plasma cells that is associated with an M-protein in the serum and/or urine. The disease is primarily bone marrow based and tends to be multifocal. There is a broad clinical spectrum of disease ranging from asymptomatic and indolent to highly aggressive with leukemic involvement. The diagnosis is based on a combination of clinicopathologic findings, which routinely includes radiographic and laboratory studies.

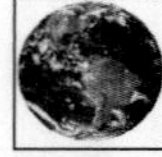

EPIDEMIOLOGY: PCM accounts for approximately 10% of all hematologic malignancies. About 7500 cases are reported annually in the United States, for an overall incidence of 3 cases per 100,000 persons. The disease is more common in men than women and occurs twice as frequently in blacks than whites. The incidence of PCM increases with age, and the median age at diagnosis is 70 years. Over 90% of cases occur in persons older than 50 years old. PCM does not affect children, and it is extremely rare in adults younger than 30 years old. There is a familial predisposition, with individuals who have a first-degree relative with PCM having a nearly fourfold increased risk of developing the disease.

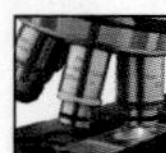

PATHOLOGY: Plasma cell myeloma produces multifocal destructive bone lesions throughout the skeleton; these lesions have a lytic or "punched out" appearance radiographically. The vertebral column, ribs, skull, pelvis, femurs, clavicles and scapulae are the most common bones affected. Pathologic fractures occur as the plasma cell tumors focally fill the medullary cavity, erode cancellous bone and eventually destroy the bony cortex. Grossly, the affected bone contains gelatinous red soft tissue masses that are sharply demarcated from the surrounding normal tissue (Fig. 20-63). Extension beyond the medullary cavity into the surrounding soft tissue may be evident if the bony cortex has been breached.

Pathologic examination of the bone marrow is essential in the diagnosis of PCM. Interstitial clusters, distinct nodules and/or confluent sheets of plasma cells may be seen in bone marrow core biopsy sections. Because of the patchy nature of the malignant plasma infiltrates in PCM, variable amounts of normal bone marrow are present in many cases. These marrow reserves, however, are not seen in all cases and are less likely in advanced disease. Plasma cell infiltrates involving over 30% of the bone marrow volume and large confluent

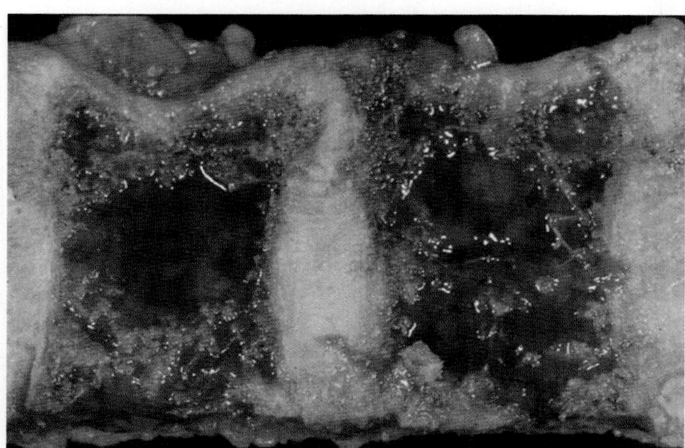

FIGURE 20-63. Plasma cell myeloma. Multiple lytic bone lesions are present in the vertebra. Bones such as this are prone to pathologic fracture.

masses of plasma cells without admixed background normal hematopoietic cells strongly favor a diagnosis of PCM even in the absence of the other typical clinicopathologic findings. Immunohistochemical stains for plasma cells (e.g., CD138) are extremely useful for assessing the degree and pattern of bone marrow infiltration in tissue sections. Bone marrow aspirate smears stained with Wright-Giemsa show a variable plasmacytosis in PCM, again in part because of the patchy distribution of the disease. The myeloma plasma cells may resemble their normal counterparts (with an eccentric nucleus showing clock-face chromatin, lack of visible nucleoli and abundant basophilic cytoplasm with a prominent perinuclear hof) (Fig. 20-64A), or they may display an immature, plasmablastic or pleomorphic appearance (Fig. 20-64B). Plasma cells with cytoplasmic and nuclear inclusions, representing accumulated or partially degraded immunoglobulin, may be observed in some cases.

Erythrocyte rouleaux formation is the key finding in peripheral blood smears and is associated with the type and quantity of circulating paraprotein. High levels of M-protein cause the red blood cells to stick together end on end, resembling a stack of coins. Circulating plasma cells are found in low percentages in a minority of cases of PCM, but marked peripheral blood plasmacytosis can occur in the setting of plasma cell leukemia. Renal abnormalities are seen in over half of cases (see Chapter 16).

The plasma cells in PCM usually express the B-lymphoid marker CD79a, the plasma cell markers CD38 and CD138 and monotypic cytoplasmic immunoglobulin. Unlike normal plasma cells, myeloma cells generally lack CD19, and in contrast to mature B cells, they are negative for CD20. Aberrant expression of various markers such as CD56, CD117, CD52, CD10 and CD20 can be seen in a variable number of cases. Some cases are cyclin D1 positive and possess a t(11;14) translocation, and those cases must be distinguished from MCL. In most cases, the heavy chain in the monoclonal paraprotein is IgG or IgA. Rarely, IgD or IgE is secreted. Complete immunoglobulin is produced in 85% of cases; only light chains are produced in the remaining 15% **(light-chain disease).** Some cases are nonsecretory.

Clonal rearrangement of the immunoglobulin light and heavy chains is present in all cases. The pattern of somatic hypermutation in the variable region of the immunoglobulin heavy chain is consistent with the postgerminal center origin of the neoplastic cells in PCM. Approximately 30% of plasma cell myelomas have chromosomal abnormalities detectable by conventional cytogenetic analysis; this is known to be a poor prognostic sign. Greater than 90% of cases have chromosomal lesions detectable only by FISH. Both numerical and structural abnormalities are found, with trisomies, deletions and translocations being common findings. The immunoglobulin heavy chain (IgH) gene is a frequent partner in translocations. The following oncogenes are most commonly involved in IgH translocations: *cyclin D1, C-MAF, FGFR3/MMSET, cyclin D3* and *MAFB*. Together these lesions

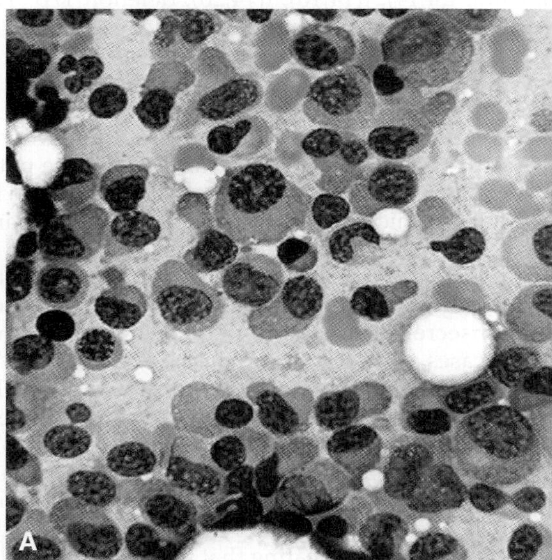

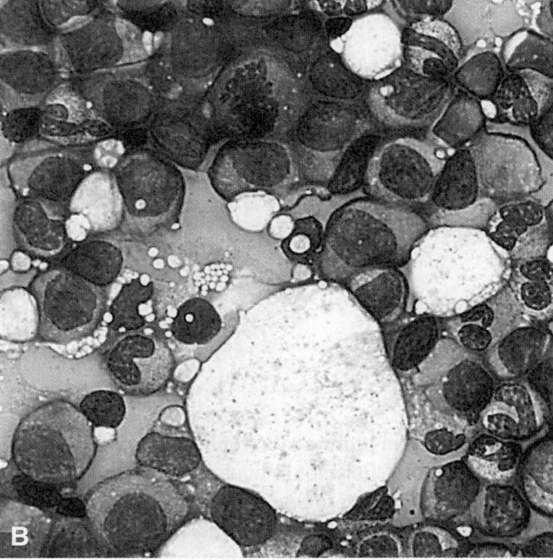

FIGURE 20-64. Plasma cell myeloma (PCM). Neoplastic plasma cells can show variable cytologic features ranging from normal-appearing cells **(A)** to cells resembling blasts **(B)**. Total number, clonality and clinicopathologic findings help distinguish PCM from other plasma cell proliferations.

are found in approximately 40% of cases. Monosomy or partial deletion of chromosome 13 is found in nearly 50% of cases by FISH and is thought to be an early genetic event in plasma cell neoplasia.

CLINICAL FEATURES: As stated above, the diagnosis of PCM rests on a constellation of clinicopathologic findings. The most important disorder to consider in the differential diagnosis of PCM is MGUS, which is a more common entity.

Symptomatic myeloma is characterized by the presence of end-organ damage (CRAB) in a patient with an M-protein in the serum or urine and a clonal population of plasma cells in the bone marrow. Radiographic studies reveal lytic bone lesions in approximately 70% of cases; these lesions are often associated with bone pain and hypercalcemia. A pathologic bone fracture can be the presenting manifestation of PCM. Bone destruction in multiple myeloma is a result of both progressive tumor growth and secretion of osteoclast-activating factor by malignant plasma cells. Osteoclasts may also be activated by IL-6, whose activity is increased in patients with PCM. The calcium released from the injured bone may precipitate in the kidneys and cause renal damage (nephrocalcinosis).

Monoclonal light-chain proteinuria can cause damage to the renal tubular epithelium, resulting in renal failure. Suppression of normal immunoglobulin production by the M-protein can lead to infectious complications. Approximately 70% of patients develop anemia as a result of normal bone marrow displacement or loss of erythropoietin production because of kidney damage. An M-protein is found in the serum or urine in 97% of patients. Laboratory assessment for monoclonal gammopathy is performed by serum (or urine) protein electrophoresis followed by immunofixation if a restricted protein (spike) is found (Fig. 20-65). The immunofixation test confirms the spike to be monoclonal κ or λ and also identifies the heavy-chain type. IgG is the most common M-protein in PCM, accounting for 50% of cases, followed by IgA (20%), light chain (20%), and IgD, IgE and biclonal (<10% combined). Approximately 3% of cases are nonsecretory.

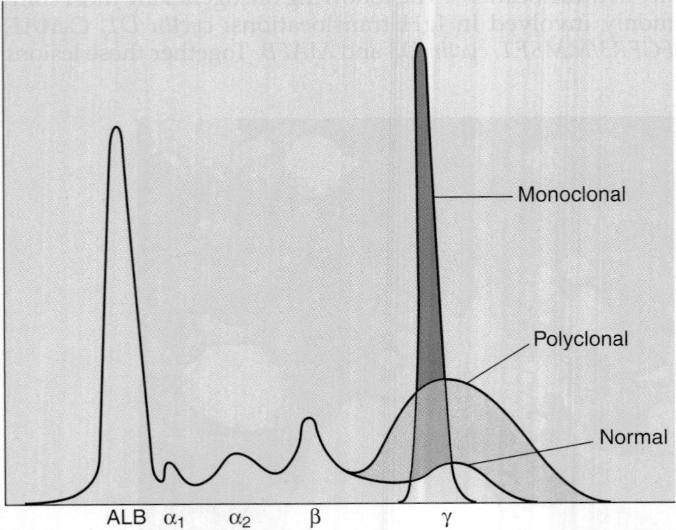

FIGURE 20-65. Abnormal serum protein electrophoretic patterns contrasted with a normal pattern. Polyclonal hypergammaglobulinemia, characteristic of benign reactive processes, shows a broad-based increase in immunoglobulins as a result of immunoglobulin secretion by myriad reactive plasma cells. Monoclonal gammopathy of unknown significance (MGUS) or plasma cell neoplasia shows a narrow peak, or spike, as a result of the homogeneity of the immunoglobulin molecules secreted by a single clone of aberrant plasma cells. ALB = albumin.

The type of M-component determines the course of the disease and its prognosis.

- **IgG myeloma** is "typical" myeloma. Mean survival is 3 to 4 years. Infectious complications are common.
- **IgA myeloma** causes serum hyperviscosity because IgA tends to form dimers.
- **IgD myeloma** is an aggressive clinical disorder that tends to occur in middle-aged men. Mean survival is 1 year.
- **IgE myeloma** is an uncommon and aggressive clinical disorder that also tends to occur in young adult men.
- **Light-chain disease** is an aggressive variant in which only κ or λ light chains are made. κ-chain disease is twice as common as λ-chain disease, reflecting the normal ratio of κ and λ light chains in plasma cells. The serum protein pattern is normal until secondary renal disease prevents glomerular filtration of light chains.

While nonspecific, the finding of rouleaux formation in the peripheral blood smear sometimes leads to the initial screening of serum protein analysis and the subsequent diagnosis of a plasma cell disorder. ***Additional findings and complications associated with PCM include amyloidosis, hyperviscosity syndrome, coagulation abnormalities, humoral immune deficiency and treatment-related myeloid malignancies such as myelodysplasia and acute myeloid leukemia.***

Plasma cell myeloma remains an incurable disease; however, recent advances in the understanding of its pathogenesis and novel treatments are showing a trend toward improved outcomes. The median survival is approximately 3 years but is highly variable, ranging from less than 6 months to greater than 10 years. Total disease burden (as assessed by serum β_2-microglobulin and albumin levels) and genetic abnormalities are the most important factors influencing prognosis. The most important negative prognostic indicators include t(4;14), t(14;16), t(14;20), deletion 17p/TP53 and an increased serum β_2-microglobulin level.

Clinical Variants of Plasma Cell Myeloma

- **Asymptomatic myeloma** is a condition where the diagnostic criteria for PCM are fulfilled but the patient has no evidence of end-organ damage. This condition is similar to MGUS, which also shows a lack of clinical manifestations (i.e., CRAB), but it is more likely to progress to symptomatic PCM. Approximately 8% of patients with PCM are initially asymptomatic and fall into this disease category.
- **Nonsecretory myeloma** accounts for approximately 3% of all cases of PCM. In this variant, there is an absence of detectable M-protein on immunofixation. This lack of serum or urine M-protein is a result of either impaired immunoglobulin secretion from malignant plasma cells (85% of cases) or lack of immunoglobulin synthesis from nonproducer malignant plasma cells (15% of cases). Free immunoglobulin light chains are produced in the majority of these cases, indicating that they are minimally secretory. The clinical features of nonsecretory PCM are otherwise similar to secretory PCM.
- **Plasma cell leukemia (PCL)** is an aggressive variant of PCM that features greater than 20% circulating malignant

plasma cells in the peripheral blood. Unlike in typical PCM, patients with PCL often have widespread extramedullary involvement at presentation with the lymph nodes, spleen, liver, body cavities and cerebrospinal fluid being common sites of disease. Plasma cell leukemia may be the initial presentation of a plasma cell neoplasm (primary) or it may evolve as a late complication of PCM (secondary). Many cases of PCL are IgD, IgE or light chain only rather than IgG or IgA. An abnormal cytogenetic karyotype is common in PCL, and the incidence of unfavorable genetic lesions is higher compared to typical PCM. As such, plasma cell leukemia is usually an aggressive disease with a short survival.

- **Solitary plasmacytoma of bone (osseous plasmacytoma)** presents as a single lytic skeletal lesion (most commonly involving the ribs, vertebrae or pelvic bones) and accounts for approximately 3% to 5% of all plasma cell neoplasms. Patients most frequently present with pain at the site of the tumor or with a pathologic fracture. An M-protein can be found in a variable number of patients (25% to 75%), but importantly, patients do not have the clinical features of PCM and their bone marrow shows no evidence of a plasmacytosis. ***Microscopically, plasmacytomas consists of diffuse sheets of plasma cells without admixed normal hematopoiesis.*** The natural history of solitary osseous myeloma is progression to multiple myeloma (70%), local extension or recurrence (15%) or extension to a distant skeletal site (15%). Local control with radiation therapy is often the first line of treatment. The median survival is approximately 10 years.
- **Extramedullary (extraosseous) plasmacytomas** are localized plasma cell tumors that occur in tissues other than bone. Approximately 80% arise in the upper respiratory tract, including nasal sinuses, nasopharynx and tonsils. The rest occur in other soft tissue sites, such as lungs, breast and lymph nodes. Given their anatomic distribution, they must be distinguished from B-cell lymphoma with plasma cell differentiation such as MALT lymphomas. Extramedullary plasmacytoma can be definitively treated by surgery or local irradiation in most cases. Local recurrences occur in up to 25% of cases, and progression to PCM is seen in about 15%.
- **Primary amyloidosis** is a disorder caused by a plasma cell neoplasm (or B-cell lymphoma with plasma cell differentiation) that secretes light-chain–type amyloid protein (AL amyloid) (see Chapter 23). It is a disease of older adults with a median age of 65 years. Approximately 20% of patients with amyloidosis have PCM, but most only meet criteria for MGUS. The clinical presentation is typically related to deposition of amyloid in organs, resulting in organomegaly or organ dysfunction (e.g., congestive heart failure, nephrotic syndrome, malabsorption). Purpura, bone pain, peripheral neuropathy and carpal tunnel syndrome are early signs of disease. Similar to the plasma cell disorders, an M-protein can be found in greater than 90% of cases, and the vast majority of cases are of the λ light-chain type. Grossly, tissues infiltrated by amyloid deposits have a dense lardaceous appearance. The median survival of patients with primary amyloidosis is approximately 2 years from diagnosis. Patients with PCM and amyloidosis have a poorer outcome compared to those with PCM or amyloidosis alone. Amyloid-related cardiac disease is the most common cause of death.

Peripheral T-Cell and NK-Cell Lymphomas

Peripheral T-cell and NK-cell neoplasms share a heterogeneous group of mature lymphoid malignancies that originate from postthymic T cells and arise in lymphoid tissues outside of the thymus, such as lymph nodes, spleen, gastrointestinal tract and skin (Fig. 20-48). They are relatively rare compared to their B-cell counterparts, and they generally have a poorer prognosis.

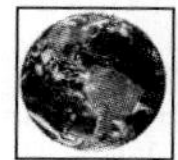

EPIDEMIOLOGY: Mature T-cell neoplasms account for approximately 12% of all non-Hodgkin lymphomas worldwide. The incidence of T-cell and NK-cell lymphomas is higher in Asia compared to the Western world. Major risk factors for T-cell neoplasia include the prevalence of human T-cell leukemia virus type 1 (HTLV-1) and EBV in the environment combined with the racial genetic predisposition to those viruses (see Chapter 5). In southwestern Japan where HTLV-1 is endemic and approximately 8% to 10% of the population is seropositive, the lifetime risk of developing adult T-cell leukemia/lymphoma (ATLL) is about 5%. EBV-associated T-cell lymphomas are more common in Asians compared to other racial groups.

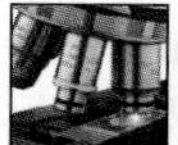

PATHOLOGY: Peripheral T-cell and NK-cell neoplasms show variable morphologic features. Involved lymph nodes and other tissues are usually diffusely effaced by a heterogeneous population of malignant lymphoid cells ranging from small to large size and either relatively bland or overtly anaplastic in appearance. Eosinophils and benign macrophages are often found in association with the neoplastic T-cell infiltrate, most likely recruited to the site of involvement by cytokines elaborated by the lymphoma cells. Prominent vascularity is seen in certain types of T-cell lymphoma.

Immunophenotypically, mature T-cell lymphomas are characterized by the expression of surface CD3; a variable number of other pan T-cell antigens such as CD2, CD5 and CD7; CD4 or CD8; and either α-β or γ-δ T-cell receptor subunits. ***Because α-β T cells are more common, most peripheral T-cell lymphomas are of the α-β type.*** γ-δ T cells constitute less than 5% of the T-cell repertoire, and they are found in association with epithelial surfaces and within the splenic red pulp. γ-δ T cells do not express CD4, CD5 or CD8.

Some mature T-cell lymphomas have a **cytotoxic** phenotype and are positive for the granule-associated proteins perforin, granzyme B and T-cell intracellular antigen (TIA-1). In contrast to immature T-cell neoplasms (such as T-cell lymphoblastic lymphoma), mature T-cell neoplasms are negative for TdT.

Natural killer cells lack surface CD3 expression, but they do express the CD3 *e* subunit, which is intracellular. NK cells also express other T-cell–associated markers including CD2, CD7 and CD8, as well as CD16 and CD56.

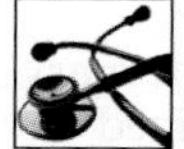

CLINICAL FEATURES: Peripheral T-cell and NK-cell neoplasms are clinically grouped into **leukemic, nodal, extranodal** and **cutaneous** forms. *They are usually widely disseminated at presentation (high stage), and hence, they are generally more aggressive compared to B-cell neoplasms.* Systemic manifestations such as fever, pruritus, eosinophilia, fever and weight loss are common. T- and NK-cell lymphomas are treated with multiagent chemotherapy similar to that used for other aggressive lymphomas;

20 | Hematopathology

however, most T-cell neoplasms respond poorly to treatment, and the overall 5-year survival is approximately 20% to 30%.

Adult T-Cell Leukemia/Lymphoma

ATLL is caused by the human retrovirus **HTLV-1.** The normal counterpart of ATLL is a mature, activated, CD4$^+$ T cell.

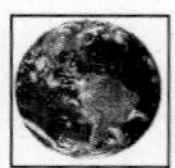

EPIDEMIOLOGY: In addition to southwestern Japan, ATLL is also endemic in the Caribbean basin and parts of Central Africa. Worldwide, it accounts for approximately 10% of all mature T-cell neoplasms. Most cases occur in persons from endemic regions of the world, but sporadic cases are also seen. The disease has a long latency period, and individuals from geographic areas with a high prevalence of the causative virus are exposed early in life. ATLL occurs only in adults, with a mean age of 58 years old. HTLV-1 may be transmitted in breast milk and through exposure to blood and blood products.

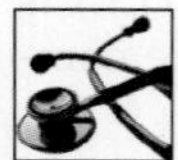

CLINICAL FEATURES: ATLL is a systemic disease with multiorgan manifestations and peripheral leukocytosis. Acute, smoldering and chronic variants are recognized. Hypercalcemia, with or without lytic bone lesions, is typical. The skin is the most important extranodal site of involvement. Acute ATLL has a poor prognosis, with most patients surviving less than 1 year despite aggressive systemic chemotherapy. Death frequently occurs from infectious complications, like those seen in HIV-infected patients. Chronic and smoldering forms have a somewhat better prognosis.

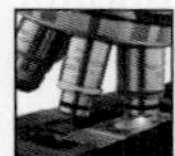

PATHOLOGY: ATLL is most often disseminated at presentation. Usual sites of involvement include lymph nodes, spleen, bone marrow, peripheral blood and skin. The latter is the most common extralymphatic site of disease, occurring in greater than 50% of cases. The neoplastic lymphoid cells vary widely in appearance, but most often, they display prominent nuclear convolutions and lobations and are described as having a flower-like appearance (flower cells). The neoplastic cells in ATLL express T-cell–associated antigens including CD2, CD3 and CD5, but they usually lack CD7. Most cases express CD4, and CD25 is strongly expressed in nearly all cases. ***The tumor cells show a clonal T-cell receptor gene rearrangement pattern, and they are positive for clonally integrated HTLV-1.*** A viral protein known as p40 tax leads to transcriptional activation of several genes in infected lymphocytes. While HTLV-1 is causally linked to ATLL, infection alone is insufficient to result in neoplastic transformation in infected cells, and other genetic lesions are required for progression from lymphocyte infection to malignancy.

Mycosis Fungoides and Sézary Syndrome

Mycosis fungoides (MF) is the most common form of primary cutaneous T-cell lymphoma (CTCL). It is characterized by infiltration of the epidermis by malignant CD4$^+$ (helper-type) T cells with marked nuclear folding. Sézary syndrome is an overlapping variant of MF defined by the triad of erythroderma, generalized lymphadenopathy and the presence of circulating lymphoma cells in the peripheral blood (Sézary cells).

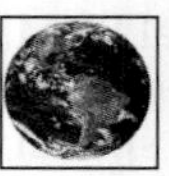

EPIDEMIOLOGY: Mycosis fungoides occurs mainly in adults and the elderly. The disease affects men twice as often as women.

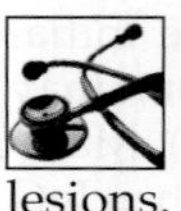

CLINICAL FEATURES: MF is an indolent lymphoma that progresses slowly over years (and sometimes decades) from patches to plaques to mass lesions.

- The **premycotic or eczematous stage** lasts some years and is difficult to distinguish from many benign chronic dermatoses. A skin biopsy specimen is not diagnostic of lymphoma and shows a nonspecific perivascular and periadnexal lymphocytic infiltration with accompanying eosinophils and plasma cells.
- The **plaque stage** follows the premycotic stage. It is characterized by well-demarcated, raised cutaneous plaques. A definitive diagnosis of MF can usually be made in this stage. There is a dense subepidermal band-like infiltrate of variably sized lymphoid cells with irregular nuclear contours. Distinctive medium to large lymphoid cells with hyperchromatic nuclei and cerebriform nuclear contours, **mycosis cells,** are typical. Pautrier microabscesses in intraepidermal clear spaces are highly characteristic, but not often observed.
- The **tumor stage** features raised cutaneous tumors, mostly on the face and in body folds, which frequently ulcerate and become secondarily infected. The name **mycosis fungoides** derives from the raised, fungating, mushroom-like appearance of these tumors. Extracutaneous involvement is common, particularly of lymph nodes, spleen, liver, bone marrow and lungs.

The clinical stage (i.e., extent of disease) is the single most important factor impacting prognosis. Patients with limited disease generally have an excellent prognosis with survival rates similar to the general population. Extracutaneous involvement heralds a poor prognosis. The 5-year survival of patients with Sézary syndrome is approximately 10% to 20%.

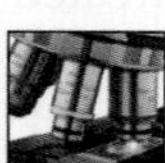

PATHOLOGY: The histologic features of MF vary with the stage of the disease (see Chapter 24). A superficial band-like infiltrate or lichenoid lymphoid infiltrate with early epidermotropism is seen in the initial patch stage. The diagnostic plaque stage is marked by pronounced infiltration of the epidermis (epidermotropism) by an atypical lymphoid infiltrate composed of mostly small to medium-sized lymphoid cells with irregular nuclear contours (cerebriform nuclei). Pautrier microabscesses, which are focal nests of intraepidermal lymphoma cells, are found in some cases. Diffuse dermal infiltrates composed of small, medium, and/or large lymphoma cells and loss of epidermotropism characterize the tumor stage. Identification of MF cells in extracutaneous sites such as lymph nodes may be difficult, and T-cell receptor gene rearrangement studies are necessary as an adjunct to the histologic evaluation.

The characteristic cerebriform nuclei of Sézary cells aid in their identification in peripheral blood smears of patients with MF (Fig. 20-66).

The MF cells have a T-helper cell immunophenotype and generally express CD2, CD3, CD5, CD4 and T-cell receptor (TCR)-α,β. Similar to other mature T-cell lymphomas, the pan T-cell antigen CD7 is aberrantly absent. Clonal T-cell receptor gene rearrangements are common, which helps to distinguish subtle cases of MF from inflammatory dermatoses.

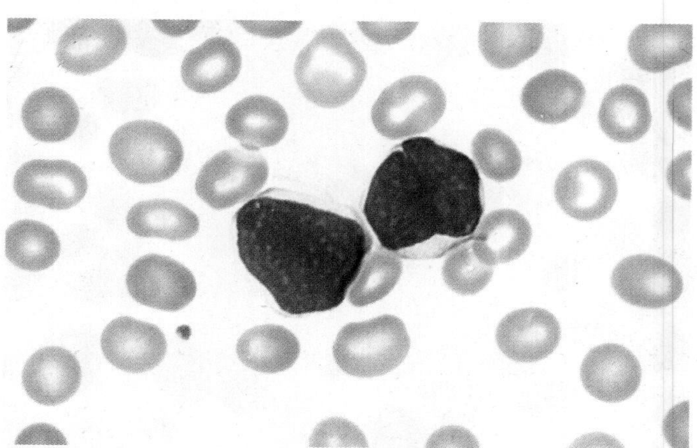

FIGURE 20-66. Sézary cells. Typical cells are medium to large with prominent nuclear convolutions resulting in a cerebriform appearance. This represents the leukemic phase of the cutaneous T-cell lymphoma, mycosis fungoides.

Anaplastic Large Cell Lymphoma

Anaplastic large cell lymphomas (ALCLs) are mature T-cell neoplasms composed of large pleomorphic lymphoid cells that express the lymphoid activation marker CD30 and involve nodal and extranodal sites (frequently skin). The disease has a bimodal age distribution; one peak occurs in the young and a second peak in older persons.

MOLECULAR PATHOGENESIS: A translocation involving the *anaplastic lymphoma kinase* (*ALK*) gene on chromosome 2 and the *nucleophosmin* (*NPM*) gene on chromosome 5 is found in some cases, especially those that occur in children and young adults. The lymphoma cells in cases with t(2;5) express ALK protein, and these cases are associated with a relatively good prognosis. ALK-negative ALCL cases tend to behave more aggressively and have a prognosis similar to unspecified types of peripheral T-cell lymphoma.

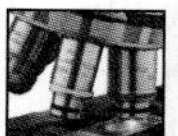

PATHOLOGY: The histologic features of ALCL are variable, but all cases contain a population of cells with irregularly shaped nuclei (often horseshoe or kidney shaped) and abundant cytoplasm that often has a distinct eosinophilic area near the nucleus (Fig. 20-67). These diagnostic cells, which are usually large, are called hallmark cells, and they are positive for CD30. ALCL cells express a variety of pan T-cell antigens and cytotoxic T-cell antigens (TIA-1, granzyme B); however, most cases are negative for CD3. Greater than 90% of cases will show a T-cell receptor rearrangement by molecular testing even if the lymphoma cells do not express T-cell antigens. ALK expression can be assessed by immunohistochemistry, or cytogenetic analysis can be performed to identify a translocation involving the ALK gene on chromosome 2.

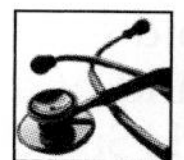

CLINICAL FEATURES: The majority of patients present with advanced stage disease (i.e., stage III or IV). Peripheral and central adenopathy are common, and extranodal and bone marrow involvement occurs in many cases as well. Patients often have B symptoms, particularly fever. The overall 5-year survival of patients with ALK-positive ALCL is about 80%, and this drops to 48% in those with ALK-negative tumors.

Angioimmunoblastic T-Cell Lymphoma

Angioimmunoblastic T-cell lymphoma (AILT) is an aggressive peripheral (mature) T-cell lymphoma. Patients present with generalized adenopathy and symptoms consistent with a systemic disease process. The neoplastic T-cell infiltrate

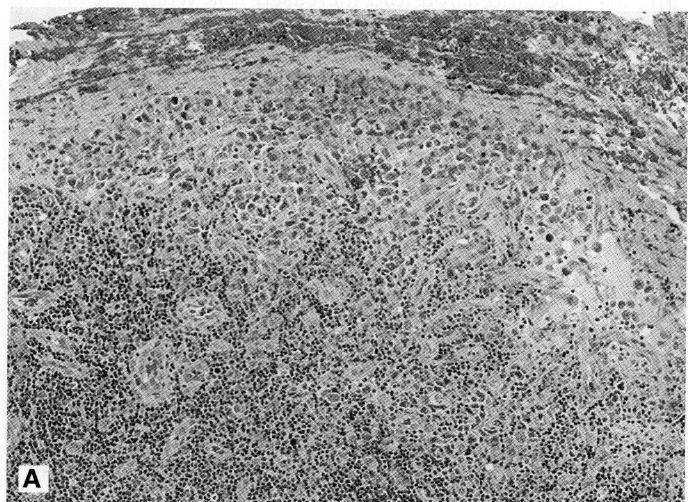

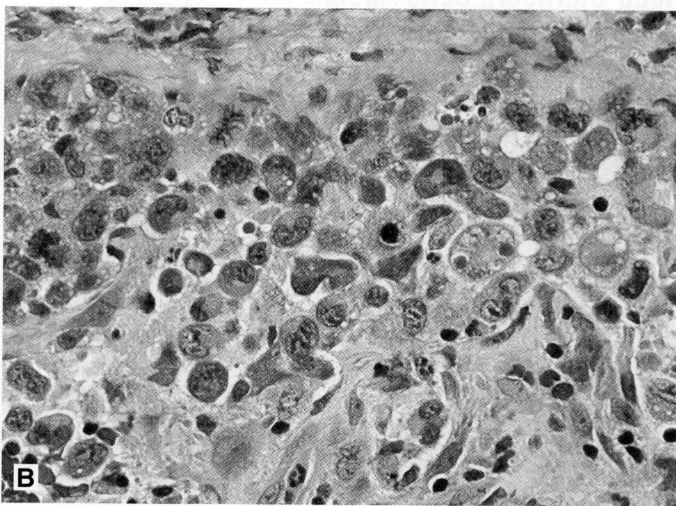

FIGURE 20-67. Anaplastic large cell lymphoma (ALCL). A. Partially effaced lymph node with accumulation of malignant cells in the subcapsular sinus. This common ALCL pattern may be confused with metastatic carcinoma. **B.** The intrasinusoidal lymphoma cells are large and pleomorphic. Cells with kidney-shaped nuclei and an eosinophilic zone near the nucleus are known as hallmark cells and are seen in all variants of ALCL.

expands the paracortical regions of lymph nodes and is associated with a striking proliferation of high endothelial venules. Evidence of EBV is found in nearly all cases; however, the EBV is found in B cells and not the neoplastic T cells.

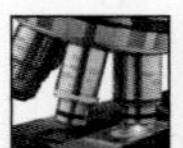

CLINICAL FEATURES: AILT occurs in adults and elderly persons. Most patients present with high-stage disease and usually exhibit generalized lymphadenopathy, hepatosplenomegaly, bone marrow involvement, hypergammaglobulinemia and body cavity effusions. A pruritic skin rash is also a common finding. Other laboratory findings include cold agglutinins, hemolytic anemia, circulating immune complexes and positive rheumatoid factor. Persons with AILT are immunodeficient as a result of the neoplastic process, and the high incidence of EBV-positive B cells in these patients is a consequence of altered immune function. AILT is an aggressive lymphoma with a median survival of less than 3 years. Patients often die from infectious complications. Some patients develop a concomitant large B-cell lymphoma.

PATHOLOGY: Lymph nodes involved by AILT show partial or complete architectural effacement by a heterogeneous population of atypical lymphoid cells ranging from small to medium size in the background of a prominent arborizing high endothelial venule network. Some cases contain lymphoma cells with abundant clear cytoplasm and minimal atypia and others show a population of atypical large lymphoid cells. The neoplastic T cells express most pan T-cell antigens (CD2, CD3, CD5 and CD7) and CD4 in most cases. Importantly, the lymphoma cells show a phenotype of follicular T-helper cells with expression of CD10, CXCL13 and PD-1. Clonal rearrangement of the T-cell receptor is found in most cases, and in addition, a minority of cases also demonstrate a clonal immunoglobulin gene rearrangement (because of the expanded EBV-positive B-cell population).

Hodgkin Lymphoma Features Hodgkin Cells and Reed-Sternberg Cells Against an Inflammatory Background

These lymphomas were first recognized and described by Thomas Hodgkin of Guy's Hospital, London, in 1832, and the first descriptions of the distinctive malignant cell were by Sternberg in 1898 and Reed in 1902 (hence termed Reed-Sternberg cells, Fig. 20-68). Two types of HL are recognized: **classical Hodgkin lymphoma** and **nodular lymphocyte-predominant Hodgkin lymphoma.** In contrast to the non-Hodgkin lymphomas discussed above, the HLs usually arise in a single lymph node or chain of lymph nodes, frequently spread in a contiguous fashion, occur in mostly younger persons and contain a low number of neoplastic cells in a prominent mixed inflammatory cell background. ***In the vast majority of cases, the neoplastic cells in both types of HL are derived from lymphoid cells at the germinal center stage of B-cell differentiation.***

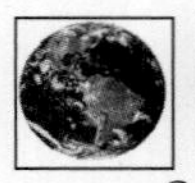 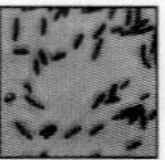

EPIDEMIOLOGY AND ETIOLOGIC FACTORS: *HL is the most common malignancy of Americans between the ages of 10 and 30 years.* Some 8000 cases are reported annually in the United States, for an incidence of 3 per 100,000 persons. It is somewhat more common in men than in women (4:2.5) and in whites than in blacks (3.5:2).

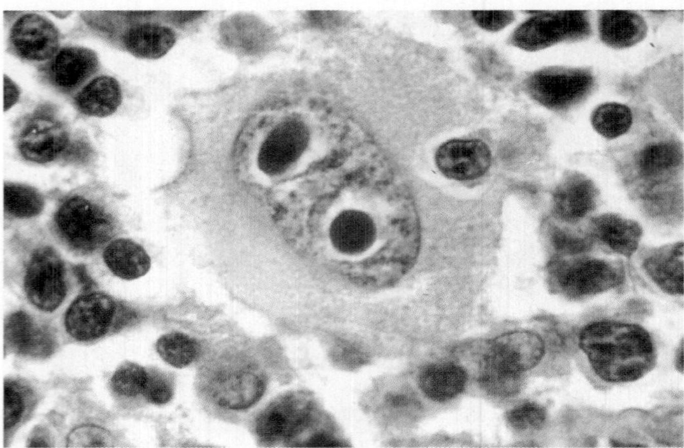

FIGURE 20-68. Classic Reed-Sternberg cell. Mirror-image nuclei contain large eosinophilic nucleoli.

The geographic variation in HL incidence and some clinicopathologic features that simulate an infectious process suggest a viral etiology, but proof is still lacking. The possibility of horizontal transmission (i.e., by interpersonal contact) of an infectious agent has been suggested by several self-limited "mini-epidemics" of HL in children. However, such apparent case clustering is predictable on statistical grounds and has not been confirmed by broader epidemiologic studies. A possible relationship between HL and infection with EBV has been suggested. Young adults who have had EBV infection (infectious mononucleosis) have a threefold increased risk of developing HL, and the EBV genome is frequently identified in the Reed-Sternberg cell.

Genetic factors may play a role in the pathogenesis of HL. The frequency of certain HLA subtypes, particularly HLA-B18, is higher in patients diagnosed with HL. Moreover, there is a sevenfold increased risk of HL in siblings of patients with this disorder and a 100-fold increased risk when the sibling is a monozygotic twin.

Immune status also seems to be a factor in at least some cases of HL. HL is more frequent in patients with compromised immunity or with autoimmune diseases, such as rheumatoid arthritis, and HL accounts for approximately 7% of the malignancies seen in individuals with ataxia-telangiectasia, who have a 100-fold increased incidence of cancer overall.

Historically, the pathogenesis of HL has been difficult to study, in part because of the inability to define the lineage and clonality of Hodgkin/Reed-Sternberg (HRS) cells, which frequently constitute less than 1% of the total cell population. Recent studies have indicated that in most patients with HL, EBV is present in HRS cells. EBV antigens can be demonstrated in situ in the tumor cells by immunohistochemistry or in situ hybridization (Fig. 20-69). Mixed-cellularity HL is associated with EBV in 70% to 80% of cases but in less than 40% of those of the nodular sclerosis type.

Classical Hodgkin Lymphoma

This lymphoma, formerly known as Hodgkin disease, is a B-cell neoplasm (in most cases) composed of mononuclear

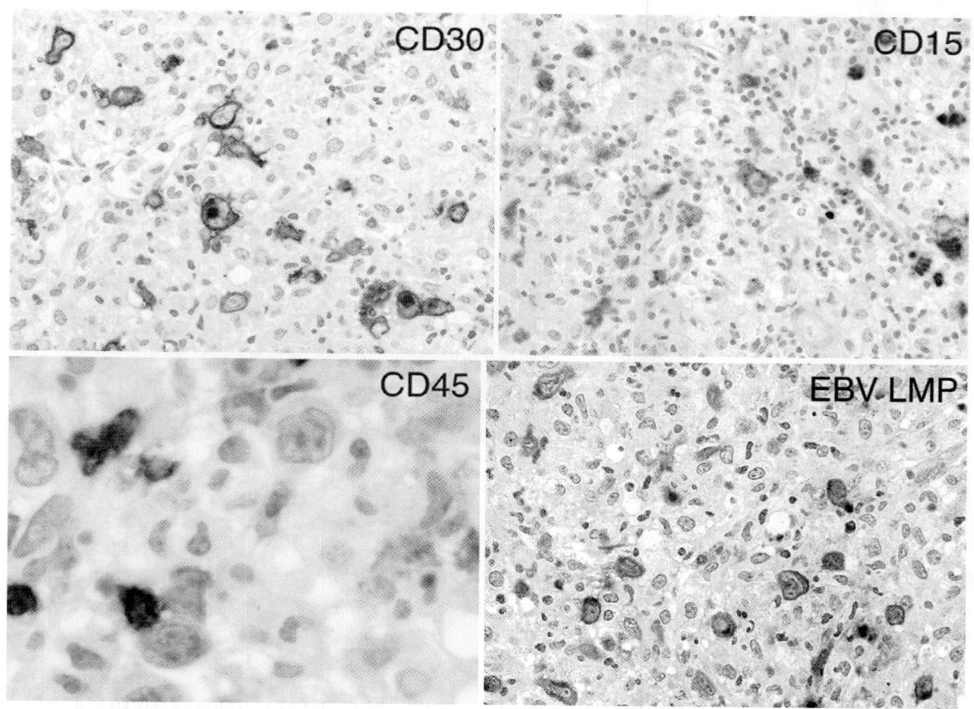

FIGURE 20-69. Immunophenotype of Reed-Sternberg and Hodgkin cells. Hodgkin/Reed-Sternberg (HRS) cells show uniform expression of the activation marker, CD30. HRS cells are variably positive for CD15, and they do not express the common leukocyte antigen, CD45. Epstein-Barr virus latent membrane protein (EBV LMP) can be detected by immunohistochemistry in a subset of cases.

Hodgkin cells and multinucleate Reed-Sternberg (Fig. 20-68) cells in a reactive inflammatory cell milieu consisting of small lymphocytes (mostly T cells), plasma cells, bland histiocytes and eosinophils. It is associated with a variable increase in fibroblasts and/or with distinct bands of collagen fibrosis (Fig. 20-70). In the vast majority of cases, the HRS cells are singly scattered and account for only a small fraction of all the cells in the involved lymph node. Classical Hodgkin lymphoma can be divided into four histologic subtypes, which are largely based on the nature of the associated inflammatory and fibroblast cell background and the appearance of the HRS cells: (1) **nodular sclerosis**, (2) **mixed cellularity,** (3) **lymphocyte rich** and (4) **lymphocyte depleted.** All four subtypes share similar immunophenotypes and genetic alterations, and the outcomes are essentially the same with current radiation and chemotherapy protocols.

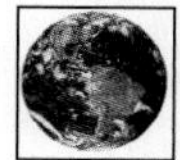

EPIDEMIOLOGY: Approximately 95% of all HLs are classical Hodgkin lymphomas. The disease has a bimodal age distribution, with one peak at 15 to 35 years and a second in older adults. Individuals with a history of infectious mononucleosis caused by EBV have a higher incidence of classical HL.

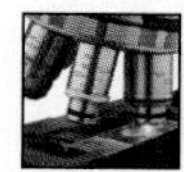

PATHOLOGY: Lymph nodes involved by classical HL show architectural effacement by a variable number of HRS cells in a mixed inflammatory cell background and variable amounts of fibrosis (sclerosis) (Fig. 20-70). Prototypical Reed-Sternberg cells are large with at least two nuclear lobes or nuclei and abundant light blue cytoplasm (Fig. 20-68). Moreover, the classical HRS cell nuclei have irregular nuclear contours, prominent eosinophilic nucleoli and a perinuclear halo giving the cells the appearance of "owl's eyes" or a viral inclusion. Occasionally, HRS cells undergo apoptosis, resulting in mummified-appearing cells with condensed cytoplasm and pyknotic nuclei. ***Despite their unique appearance, the HRS cells can be hard to find in the dense reactive background as they typically account for 1% to 3% of total cells in the involved tissue.***

The HRS cells express the lymphoid activation marker CD30 in nearly all cases (Fig. 20-69). In addition, they also express the macrophage/monocyte marker CD15 in 85% of cases. Unlike B-cell non-Hodgkin lymphomas, the neoplastic HRS cells do not typically express the usual B-cell antigens such as CD20 and CD79a, and they are also negative for CD45 (leukocyte common antigen).

The peculiar HRS immunophenotype, including the lack of markers indicative of B-cell differentiation, resulted in decades of confusion regarding the origin of the HRS cells, and it was not until the advent of advanced molecular diagnostic techniques in the late 1990s that the cells were found to be clonally related B cells of germinal center cell origin. ***A clonal immunoglobulin gene rearrangement can be found in over 98% of HRS cells isolated from whole tissue sections using laser microdissection techniques.***

HRS cells produce several cytokines that elicit characteristic tissue effects. Eosinophils are attracted by the combined effects of IL-5 and eotaxin, and IL-6 can attract plasma cells. TGF-β activates fibroblasts and may account for nodular fibrosis. Other growth factors and cytokines made by HRS cells include IL-2, -7, -9, -10 and -13.

Nodular Sclerosis Hodgkin Lymphoma

Nodular sclerosis Hodgkin lymphoma (NSHL) is characterized by a fibrous thickening of the lymph node capsule, with bands of sclerosis extending from the capsule into the nodal cortex resulting in the formation of nodules (Fig. 20-70A). **Lacunar cells** result from a retraction artifact in formaldehyde-fixed tissue (Fig. 20-70C). The nodules are composed of the mixed inflammatory cell population described above and a variable number of classical HRS cells and lacunar cells. This subtype accounts for about 70% of cases of classical HL,

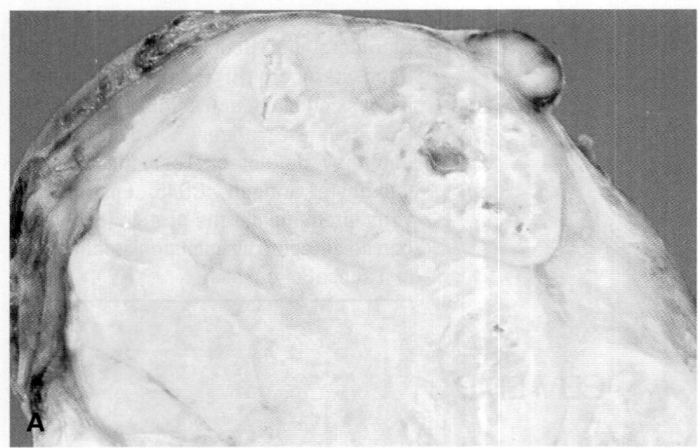

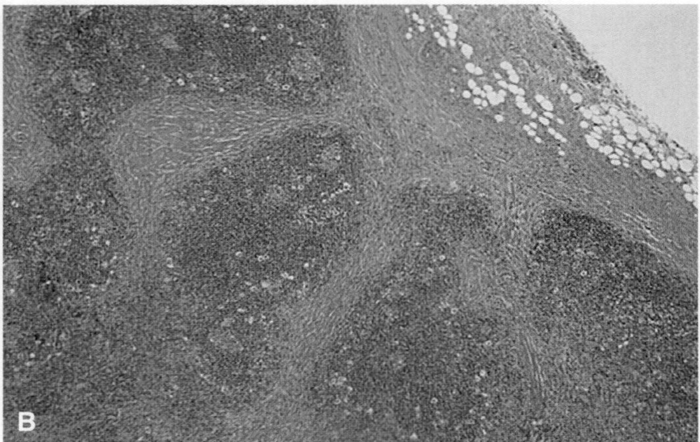

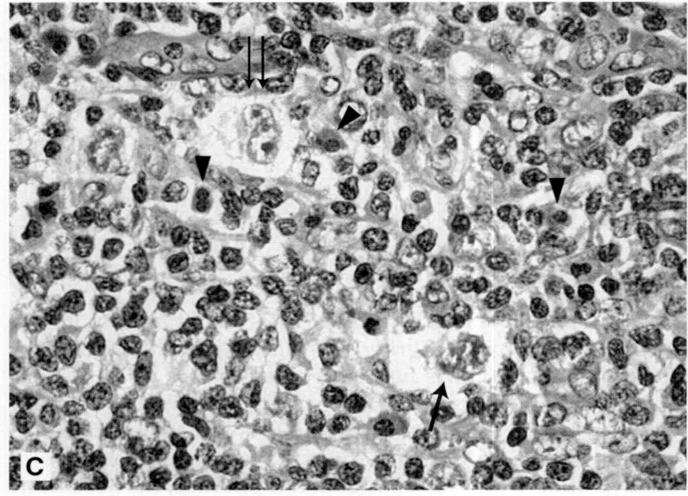

FIGURE 20-70. Nodular sclerosis Hodgkin lymphoma (NSHL). A. Gross photograph showing an enlarged lymph node with a thickened capsule and broad bands of fibrosis dividing the parenchyma into distinct nodules. Several foci of necrosis are evident (red-brown discolorations). **B.** A low-power photomicrograph demonstrates broad bands of fibrosis. There is a dense inflammatory background. Reed-Sternberg cells are rare. **C.** A photomicrograph of NSHL shows a mixed inflammatory background with eosinophils (*arrowheads*), Reed-Sternberg cells (*double arrow*) and lacunar cells (*arrow*).

with most cases occurring in the 15- to 30-year-old age group. Mediastinal involvement is found in over 80% of patients, and the disease is bulky in over half of these patients. B symptoms (see Table 20-20) occur in up to 40% of patients. Bone marrow involvement and association with EBV are low relative to other types. As such, this subtype has a better prognosis compared to the other subtypes.

Mixed Cellularity Hodgkin Lymphoma

Mixed cellularity Hodgkin lymphoma (MCHL) contains HRS cells in a mixed inflammatory background of eosinophils, neutrophils, macrophages and plasma cells (Fig. 20-71) but lacks the nodular fibrosis seen in NSHL. MCHL accounts for approximately 25% of classical HLs, is the most frequent subtype in HIV-1–infected patients and shows the highest association with EBV. MCHL is most common in the fourth and fifth decades of life. Cervical neck lymph nodes are the most common site of initial involvement, and unlike in NSHL, mediastinal involvement is uncommon in MCHL. The overall outcome for patients is similar to that of NSHL with modern treatment regimens.

Lymphocyte-Rich Hodgkin Lymphoma

Cases of lymphocyte-rich Hodgkin lymphoma (LRHL) are marked by presence of classical HRS cells in the background of a nodular (or rarely diffuse) lymphoid infiltrate composed of small B cells and absence of eosinophils, neutrophils and

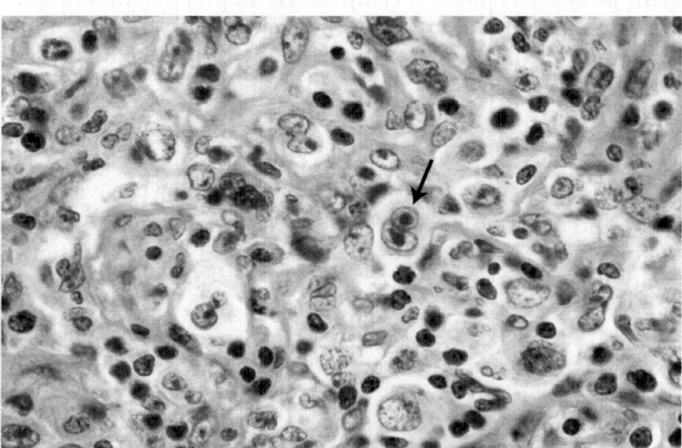

FIGURE 20-71. Mixed cellularity Hodgkin lymphoma. A photomicrograph of a lymph node shows classic, binucleated and mononuclear Reed-Sternberg cells (*arrow*) in a mixed inflammatory background that includes many small lymphocytes (T cells). Note the absence of fibrotic bands, which helps distinguish this subtype from nodular sclerosis Hodgkin lymphoma.

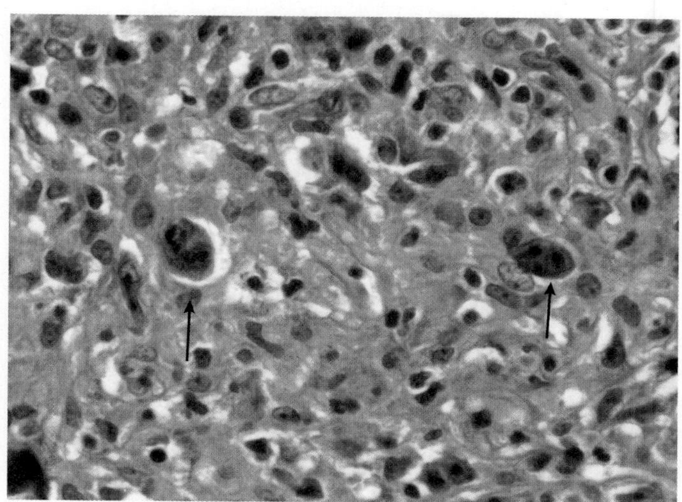

FIGURE 20-72. Lymphocyte-depleted Hodgkin lymphoma. Two Hodgkin/Reed-Sternberg cells are seen (*arrows*). The number of reactive lymphocytes in the fibrotic background is markedly reduced. The differential diagnosis in cases like this includes large cell lymphoma.

sclerosis. This subtype is rare, accounting for only 5% of cases of classical HL, and it tends to occur in older persons. Patients generally present with low-stage disease and do not usually manifest B symptoms. The overall survival is better than that of all other subtypes of classical HL and similar to that seen in nodular lymphocyte predominant HL (see below).

Lymphocyte-Depleted Hodgkin Lymphoma

Lymphocyte-depleted Hodgkin lymphoma (LDHL) is the least common type of classical HL, accounting for less than 1% of cases. Histologically, it shows a predominance of HRS cells and/or a marked absence (depletion) of background lymphocytes (Fig. 20-72). Most patients diagnosed with LDHL are male with a median age range of 30 to 40 years. This subtype is frequently associated with HIV infection. There is a predilection for involvement of retroperitoneal lymph nodes (rare in other subtypes), abdominal organs and bone marrow. While a poor prognosis is seen in cases associated with HIV infection, the disease course and outcome are otherwise similar to the other subtypes. Distinction from non-Hodgkin lymphoma is often more difficult with this subtype of classical HL.

CLINICAL FEATURES: HL usually manifests as nontender peripheral adenopathy involving a single lymph node or group of lymph nodes. The cervical and mediastinal nodes are involved in over half of cases, and the anterior mediastinum is frequently involved, especially in the nodular sclerosis type. Less commonly, axillary, inguinal and retroperitoneal lymph nodes are initially enlarged. Peripheral lymph node groups, such as antecubital, popliteal and mesenteric lymph nodes, tend to be spared. Initially, HL spreads predictably between contiguous lymph node groups via efferent lymphatics. As the disease progresses, spread is less predictable because of vascular invasion and hematogenous dissemination (Fig. 20-73). Constitutional ("B") symptoms are found in 40% of HL patients. These include low-grade fever, which is occasionally cyclical (Pel-Ebstein fever); night sweats; and weight loss exceeding 10% of body

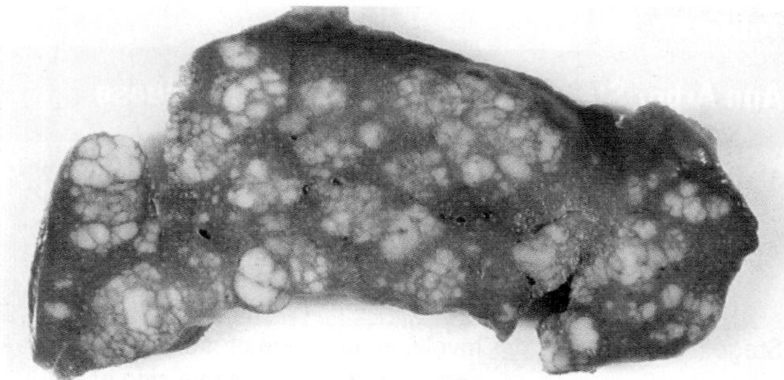

FIGURE 20-73. Hodgkin lymphoma involving the spleen. Multiple masses replace the normal splenic parenchyma. Laparotomy and splenectomy are no longer routinely performed for diagnostic and staging purposes.

weight. Pruritus may occur as the disease progresses. For unknown reasons, drinking alcoholic beverages induces pain at involved sites in 10% of patients.

Deficient T-lymphocyte function is characteristic of HL. Subtle defects of delayed-type hypersensitivity, which can be detected in most patients even at the time of initial diagnosis, tend to become more pronounced as the disease progresses. Anergy to skin test antigens is often noted early in HL. Such immune dysfunction is by the immunosuppressive effects of therapy. An absolute lymphocytopenia ($<$1500 cells/μL) is seen in half of cases, most often in advanced HL. Humoral immunity is usually intact until late in the course of the disease.

The prognosis in HL depends mainly on the patient's age and the anatomic extent of the disease (i.e., the stage). A better prognosis is associated with (1) younger age, (2) lower clinical stage (localized disease) and (3) absence of "B" signs and symptoms. The comprehensive Ann Arbor Staging System (Table 20-20), which is based on clinical evaluation and radiographic and pathologic findings, is used to assign stage. In the past, abdominal exploratory surgery (staging laparotomy) was performed to search for abdominal involvement, but this is currently an uncommon practice. The bone marrow is also examined as part of the staging process.

Complications of HL include compromise of vital organs by progressive tumor growth and secondary infections as a result of both the primary defect in delayed-type hypersensitivity and the immunosuppressive effects of therapy. Development of second malignancies after therapy is of special concern, since more than 15% of treated patients may eventually suffer this complication. AML develops in 5% of patients and aggressive large cell lymphomas occur somewhat less frequently.

Nodular Lymphocyte-Predominant Hodgkin Lymphoma

This type of Hodgkin lymphoma is distinct from classical HL discussed above. While classified as an HL, it has immunomorphologic and clinicopathologic features more akin to indolent B-cell non-Hodgkin lymphomas than classical HL. The characteristic cells in nodular lymphocyte-predominant Hodgkin lymphoma (NLPHL) are Hodgkin variant

Table 20-20

Ann Arbor Staging System for Hodgkin Disease

Stage		
Stage I A or B*	I	Involvement of a single lymph node region
		or
	I_E	A single extralymphatic organ or site
Stage II A or B	II	Involvement of two or more lymph node regions on the same side of the diaphragm
		or
	II_E	With localized contiguous involvement of an extralymphatic organ site
Stage III A or B	III	Involvement of lymph node regions on both sides of the diaphragm
		or
	III_E	With localized contiguous involvement of an extralymphatic organ or site
		or
	III_S	With involvement of spleen
		or
	III_{ES}	Both extralymphatic organ or site and spleen involvement
Stage IV A or B	IV	Diffuse or disseminated involvement of one or more extralymphatic organs with or without associated lymph node involvement

*A = asymptomatic; B = presence of constitutional symptoms (fever, night sweats and weight loss exceeding 10% of baseline body weight in preceding 6 months).

cells known as L&H (lymphocyte and histiocytic) cells, or "popcorn" cells, because of their histologic appearance. As in classical HL, the neoplastic cells in NLPHL are found in low numbers in involved tissues.

NLPHL is also a neoplasm of germinal center B-cell origin. In contrast to classical HL, the lymphoma cells in NLPHL express specific B-cell lineage antigens (including CD20, CD79a and surface Ig), and they are negative for CD15 and CD30 expression. Clonal immunoglobulin gene rearrangement is found in almost all cases. The rearranged immunoglobulin heavy-chain genes show a high degree of somatic hypermutation in the variable region, indicating that they are most likely of germinal center B-cell origin.

NLPHL represents about 5% of all HLs. It affects predominantly males in the 30- to 50-year-old age group; it also occurs in younger persons, including children. The disease is typically localized at the time of diagnosis (i.e., stage I). Cervical, axillary or inguinal lymph nodes are common sites of disease. In contrast to classical HL, mediastinal, splenic and bone marrow involvement is rare. Visceral involvement is also uncommon. Unlike classical HL, NLPHL tends to skip anatomic lymph node regions (i.e., noncontiguous spread). B signs and symptoms are present in only 20% of cases. NLPHL follows an indolent clinical course and is rarely fatal. The 10-year survival for patients with low-stage disease (stage I or II) is greater than 80%. The outcome is less favorable for patients with advanced stage disease. Complications include recurrences, which are common, and progression to diffuse large B-cell lymphoma, which occurs in 3% to 5% of cases.

Lymphoproliferative Disorders Are Associated With Immune Deficiency

While several of the non-Hodgkin and Hodgkin lymphomas discussed above are associated with immune dysfunction, a specific group of lymphoproliferative disorders associated with immunodeficiency is also recognized. These disorders include lymphoproliferative diseases associated with primary immune disorders (such as CD40 ligand and CD40 deficiencies, common variable immunodeficiency, Wiskott-Aldrich syndrome, ataxia-telangiectasia, Nijmegen breakage syndrome and X-linked lymphoproliferative disorder), lesions associated with HIV infection, posttransplant lymphoproliferative disorders and immune deficiency–associated lymphoproliferative disorders resulting from other iatrogenic causes of immunosuppression.

Posttransplant Lymphoproliferative Disorders

Posttransplant lymphoproliferative disorders (PTLDs) occur in individuals who are immunosuppressed as a result of being a recipient of a solid organ, bone marrow or stem cell allograft. These disorders are either lymphoid or plasmacytic and range from proliferations resembling infectious mononucleosis to overt large cell lymphomas, which are mostly B-cell type. Occasional PTLDs have a T-cell phenotype, and some resemble Hodgkin lymphoma or plasma cell neoplasms such as multiple myeloma and plasmacytoma. ***The majority of these disorders have a pathogenesis rooted in Epstein-Barr virus infection.*** The most important risk factor for EBV-driven PTLD is EBV seronegativity at the time of transplantation.

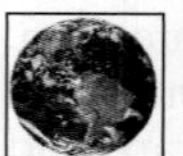

EPIDEMIOLOGY: Several factors are linked to the risk of developing PTLD, including patient characteristics, allograft types and immunosuppressive regimens, which may vary from institution to institution. The incidence of PTLD most closely parallels the extent of immunosuppression. Patients with renal allografts have the lowest frequency of PTLD (<1%), whereas those who receive heart/lung or intestinal allografts have the highest frequency of PTLD (>5%). Patients receiving stem cell or bone marrow allografts have a low risk of PTLD (approximately 1%). The risk in these individuals is associated with the degree of HLA matching, with unrelated or HLA-mismatched transplants resulting in higher rates of PTLD. The incidence of PTLD is higher in children, and this is most likely a result of primary EBV infection in this patient population.

MOLECULAR PATHOGENESIS: Most cases are caused by EBV, with an average latency period of less than 1 year. However, EBV-negative cases may evolve more than 5 years after transplantation. In solid organ recipients, ***host*** lymphocytes become infected with EBV, but in bone marrow allograft recipients, PTLD is caused by infected ***donor*** lymphocytes.

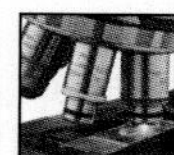

PATHOLOGY: The histologic features of PTLD are variable and form the basis for categorizing these lesions.

- **Early lesions:** These lesions are characterized by plasmacytic hyperplasia or infectious mononucleosis–like changes. They tend to occur in younger patients, particularly those who have not had prior EBV infection. Early lesions involve lymph nodes, or tonsils and adenoids, more often than true extranodal sites. Spontaneous regression or regression with a reduction in immunosuppression is the usual course; however, some infectious mononucleosis–like lesions can occasionally be fatal. Early lesions can be followed by other PTLD categories over time.
- **Polymorphic PTLD:** These lesions are composed of a heterogeneous population of cells, including immunoblasts, plasma cells and small to medium-sized lymphocytes. The atypical lymphoplasmacytic and immunoblastic proliferation tends to efface the lymph node architecture and/or form destructive extranodal masses. This is the most common type of PTLD seen in children and frequently follows primary EBV infection. The clinical presentation is indistinguishable from other types of PTLD. A variable number of cases regress with reduction in immunosuppression, but others progress and require cytotoxic treatment for lymphoma. The atypical cells in polymorphic PTLD show clonally rearranged immunoglobulin genes, although detectable clones are less prominent compared to the level seen in monomorphic PTLD (see below).
- **Monomorphic PTLD:** These are proliferations composed of transformed monoclonal B lymphocytes or plasma cells that fulfill a diagnosis of diffuse large B-cell lymphoma, or less commonly Burkitt lymphoma or plasma cell myeloma/plasmacytoma (Fig. 20-74). The presentation of monomorphic PTLD is similar to the presentation of other lymphomas or plasma cell neoplasms. Virtually all cases show clonal immunoglobulin gene rearrangements; the majority of cases contain clonal EBV genomes. Cytogenetic abnormalities are common. Treatment for lymphoma is required in the majority of cases; this type of PTLD does not typically respond to a reduction in immunosuppression like the other PTLD types discussed above.
- **Classical Hodgkin lymphoma-type PTLD:** This rare type of PTLD occurs more often in renal transplant patients, is almost always EBV positive and has features identical to those described for classical Hodgkin lymphoma.

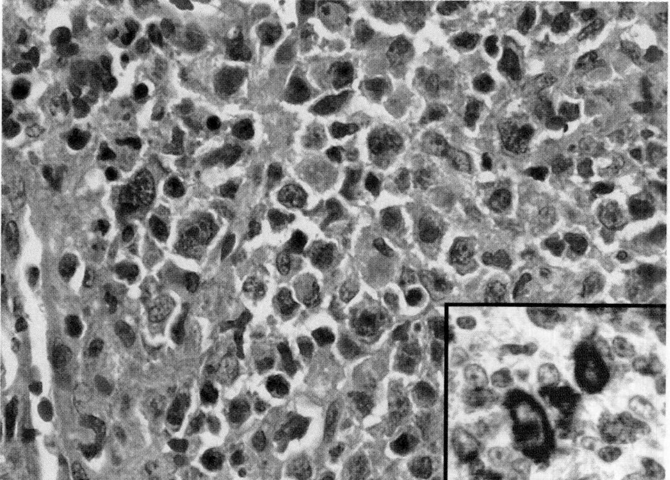

FIGURE 20-74. Posttransplant lymphoproliferative disorder (PTLD). Monomorphic-type PTLD is characterized by a diffuse proliferation of large lymphoid cells with clonal immunoglobulin gene rearrangements. The histologic features are most often similar to diffuse large B-cell lymphomas occurring in immunocompetent patients. Neoplastic lymphocytes in many cases are positive for Epstein-Barr virus, which can be readily assessed by immunohistochemistry (inset).

CLINICAL FEATURES: Patients with PTLD present with nonspecific symptoms, such as lethargy, malaise, weight loss and fever. Lymphadenopathy and allograft dysfunction are also common. Some patients, primarily children, may present with obstructive airway symptoms because of enlarged tonsils. In addition to lymph nodes and tonsils, PTLDs frequently involve extranodal sites, and the gastrointestinal tract, lungs and liver are common sites of disease. Moreover, PTLDs frequently involve the allograft itself, and this may cause diagnostic confusion because allograft rejection can present with similar clinical and histologic features. The prognosis of PTLD is variable and largely dependent on the type of lesion encountered. The so-called "early" lesions tend to regress with reduction in immunosuppression without graft loss. Other forms that resemble outright lymphomas may also regress with a reduction in immunosuppression; however, many of these cases require additional cytotoxic therapy, such as anti-CD20 therapy or chemotherapy or a combination of both. Bone marrow/stem cell allograft recipients tend to show a higher mortality as a result of PTLPD compared to solid organ allograft recipients, and mortality may be lower in children than in adults. EBV viral load monitoring of seronegative patients is a common practice in many transplant centers, and this has led to a decreased incidence in the number of patients presenting with disseminated PTLD.

Iatrogenic Immunodeficiency-Associated Lymphoproliferative Disorders

These disorders primarily occur in patients being treated with immunosuppressive drugs for autoimmune diseases or other conditions (excluding transplantation). The lymphoid proliferations seen in this group of patients are similar to those seen in patients with PTLD and range from polymorphic disorders to outright diffuse large B-cell lymphoma, peripheral T-cell lymphoma or classical Hodgkin-type lymphomas. Methotrexate, which has long been used to treat rheumatoid arthritis (RA), was the first immunosuppressive agent reported to be associated with lymphoproliferative disorders. Newer agents used to treat RA, such as the tumor necrosis factor-α antagonists, have also been associated with a higher prevalence of lymphoma compared to a healthy age-matched population. Like most PTLDs, the iatrogenic lymphoproliferative disorders are often associated with EBV, but EBV alone is not the only important risk factor, as the chronic antigenic stimulation caused by the patient's inflammatory disease as well as his or her genetic background are also important determinants in the development of lymphoma. Close to 50% of all cases have an extranodal presentation, with the gastrointestinal tract, skin, liver, spleen, lung, kidney, thyroid gland, bone marrow and soft tissue being frequent sites of involvement. The remaining clinical features are similar to those associated with lymphomas occurring in immunocompetent patients. Histologically, many of these tumors resemble diffuse large B-cell lymphoma or classical Hodgkin lymphoma. Like the PTLDs, many of the iatrogenic lymphoproliferative disorders show at least a partial response following withdrawal of the immunosuppressive medication. The majority of the responses occur in cases with EBV-positive cells. The overall survival of patients with DLBCL is approximately 50% in this setting.

Histiocytic Disorders

Histiocytic Proliferations May Occur in Both Neoplastic and Non-Neoplastic Settings

Among the non-neoplastic disorders are Rosai-Dorfman disease (sinus histiocytosis with massive lymphadenopathy (see above), storage disorders such as Niemann-Pick disease, Gaucher disease and Tangier disease (see Chapter 6) and hemophagocytic syndromes.

Hemophagocytic Disorders

All hematophagocytic disorders share the common features of an immunologic defect that results in dysregulation of the immune system and consequent increases in certain cytokines, resulting in inadequately regulated T cell and macrophage activation. Natural killer (NK) cells are normal in number but show inadequate ability to regulate antigen-presentinig cells, leading to uncontrolled activation of CD8+ T cells. Consequently, levels of proinflammatory cytokines (see Chapter 4), such as TNF-α, IL-6 and IFNγ, are elevated. Hemophagocytic syndromes may be genetic or acquired. The diagnosis is made by a combination of clinical and pathologic criteria that include: (1) fever above 38.5°C, (2) splenomegaly, (3) anemia, (4) thrombocytopenia, (5) hypertriglyceridemia, (6) hypofibrinogenemia, accompanied by hemophagocytosis in bone marrow, spleen or lymph nodes. In these organs, one may find macrophages engulfing normal hematopoietic cells (Fig. 20-75).

Inherited hemophagocytic syndromes commonly involve mutations of the *PFR1* gene. These disorders typically present in children, are associated with activation and proliferation of benign macrophages and are characterized by hemophagocytosis, systemic symptoms (fever, etc.) and decreased hemaotpoietic elements of one or more series in the blood. Cellular immune defects may also accompany these clinical manifestations.

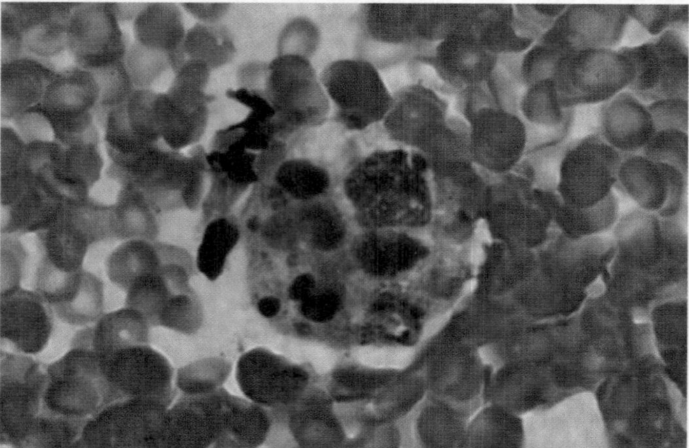

FIGURE 20-75. Hemophagocytic syndrome. This disorder is characterized morphologically by phagocytosis of hematopoietic cells by tissue macrophages. Shown here is a macrophage engulfing bone marrow cells.

Acquired hemophagocytic syndrome may occur in several settings. These include viral infections (primary infections with EBV, CMV, HIV, parvovirus), malaria, *E. coli*, histoplasmosis and hematologic malignancies such as T cell and NK cell lymphomas. Autoimmune diseases (juvenile rheumatoid arthritis, systemic lupus erythematosus) are also occasionally implicated in this syndrome.

Histiocytic Neoplasms are Rare Disorders Derived from Macrophages, Dendritic Cells or Histiocytes

The true incidence of these tumors is unknown since many have been poorly recognized and characterized until only recently. The clinicopathologic features of this group of neoplasms is broad and ranges from indolent to aggressive. Recognized entities in this group of neoplasms includes: **Langerhans cell histiocytosis, histocytic sarcoma** and **follicular and interdigitating dendritic cell sarcomas.** Only the former will be discussed.

Langerhans Cell Histiocytosis is Neoplastic Proliferation of Langerhans cells Occuring Mainly in Children

Langerhans cell histiocytosis (LCH) represents a spectrum of uncommon proliferations of Langerhans cells. The diseases arising from these cells range from asymptomatic involvement at a single site, such as bone or lymph nodes, to an aggressive systemic multiorgan disorder. Langerhans cells are mononuclear phagocytes derived from precursor cells in the bone marrow. They are found in the epidermis, lymph nodes, spleen, thymus and mucosal tissues. Langerhans cells ingest, process and present antigens to T lymphocytes. In lymph nodes, Langerhans cells are termed **interdigitating reticulum cells** (IDCs).

The etiology and pathogenesis of LCH are unknown. The recent demonstration of the frequent, but not invariable, clonality of Langerhans cells in all forms of LCH strongly suggests that it is a neoplastic disorder. Infants, children and young adults are most affected. The extent of disease and rate of progression correlate inversely with the age at presentation. Certain eponyms were traditionally attached to the various presentations of LCH, but these terms are used infrequently.

The least aggressive form, is called an **eosinophilic granuloma.** It is a localized, usually self-limited, disorder, usually of the bone. Lymph nodes, skin and lungs may less often be involved. Eosinophilic granuloma affects older children (5- to 10-years-old) and young adults (under 30 years), mostly males, and accounts for almost 75% of LCH.

In some cases, these lesions present as a multifocal and typically indolent disorder, affecting one organ system, largely bone. Children 2 to 5 years of age will generally present with multiple bone lesions sometimes associated with soft tissue masses. This manifestation was once termed **Hand-Schüller-Christian disease.**

The rarest of all forms of these diseases (less than 10% of cases) is an acute, disseminated variant of LCH that usually presents in infants and children under 2 years of age. There is no sex predominance. Skin lesions and hepatosplenomegaly and lymphadenopathy, and bone lesions, along with pancytopenia are characteristic. In the older literature, this is referred to as **Letterer-Siwe disease.**

PATHOLOGY: Despite their clinical heterogeneity, LCHs share common histopathological findings (Fig. 20-76). The cells accumulate in an environment containing eosinophils, histiocytes and small lymphocytes. The Langerhans cells are large (15–25 μm in diameter), with grooved nuclei, delicate vesicular chromatin and small nucleoli. By electron microscopy, a distinctive rod-shaped or tubular cytoplasmic inclusion with a dense core and a double outer sheath, the **Birbeck granule,** is commonly observed. Frequently, one end of the granule is bulbous, in which case it resembles a tennis racket. Characteristic immunologic cell markers identical to those of epidermal Langerhans cells include S-100 protein and CD1a.

CLINICAL FEATURES: The clinical manifestations of LCH reflect the sites involved. Skin involvement, principally in the Letterer-Siwe variant, takes the form of seborrheic or eczematoid dermatitis, most prominent on the scalp, face and trunk. Otitis media is common. Painless localized or generalized lymphadenopathy and hepatosplenomegaly are frequent. Lytic lesions of bone cause pain or tenderness to palpation. Bone manifestations of LCH are discussed in Chapter 26. Proptosis (protrusion of the eyeball) may be a complication of infiltration of the orbit. Diabetes insipidus occurs when the hypothalamic–pituitary axis is affected. ***The classic triad of diabetes insipidus, proptosis, and defects in membranous bones occurs in only 15% of cases of Hand-Schüller-Christian disease.*** The prognosis in LCH depends mainly on age at presentation, extent of disease and rate of progression. In general, the disorder is self-limited and benign in older persons (eosinophilic granuloma), whereas children younger than 2 years (Letterer-Siwe disease) tend to do poorly. Rarely, the clinical course is aggressive and indistinguishable from that of a malignant neoplasm.

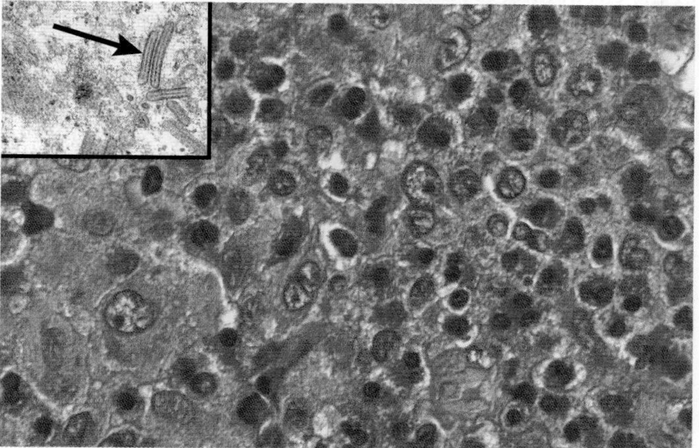

FIGURE 20-76. Eosinophilic granuloma. A section of an affected rib shows proliferated Langerhans cells and numerous eosinophils. *Inset.* Electron micrograph showing a Birbeck granule (*arrow*) in Langerhans histiocytosis.

SPLEEN

Anatomy and Function

The spleen is a lymphoid organ that plays a major role in blood filtration for removal of abnormal or senescent cells, immune complexes and opsonized bacteria. The normal spleen weighs between 100 and 170 g and is not palpable on clinical examination. The spleen's supporting structure consists of a fibrous capsule, radiating fibrous trabeculae and a delicate stromal framework of reticulum fibers (Fig. 20-77). The splenic artery enters at the hilum and branches into trabecular arteries, following the course of the fibrous trabeculae. The spleen is subdivided into the areas of red and white pulp. This division is useful, since most diseases affect one compartment or the other.

THE WHITE PULP: The lymphoid tissue of the spleen, called the white pulp, is composed of masses of T and B lymphocytes ensheathing a central artery. The T-cell domain is located in the periarteriolar lymphoid sheath; the B-cell domain consists of the follicles and perifollicular marginal zone. Arising from the central artery, follicular arteries enter the B-cell follicles and terminate in the marginal sinus at the junction between the white and red pulp. Circulating lymphocytes exit the vascular system from the marginal sinus and travel to their respective B-cell and T-cell domains. Lymphocytes leave the white pulp and enter the red pulp by way of the same marginal sinuses.

As part of the peripheral lymphoid system, effector B and T lymphocytes of the white pulp perform an immunologic function for the circulatory system comparable to the immunologic function of the lymph nodes. The white pulp is (1) the source of protection from blood-borne infection, (2) a major locale for the synthesis of opsonizing IgM antibody and (3) a site of production of lymphocytes and plasma cells.

THE RED PULP: The red pulp is composed of a network of stromal cords and vascular sinuses. Blood from the penicilliary arteries empties directly into the sinuses (closed circulation), with subsequent drainage to the trabecular veins and ultimately to the splenic vein. A small fraction (5% to 10%) is diverted into the splenic cords (open circulation) and slowly percolates through a meshwork studded with phagocytic macrophages. The blood then reenters the sinusoids through narrow slits composed of longitudinally oriented, slender endothelial cells and radially oriented ring fibers.

The red pulp is primarily a filter designed to screen and eliminate defective or foreign cells. In the splenic cords, erythrocytes are subjected to the sustained scrutiny of mononuclear phagocytes and must be deformable to traverse the narrow interstices between the lining endothelial cells. The erythrocytes must also be able to withstand the hypoxia, hypoglycemia and acidosis that are characteristic of the stromal cord microenvironment. Senescent and damaged erythrocytes are recognized and phagocytosed by splenic macrophages. The spleen ordinarily accounts for the removal of about half of aged erythrocytes, the remainder being destroyed in the liver, bone marrow and other components of the mononuclear phagocyte system. Following phagocytosis and breakdown of erythrocytes, the iron is first stored as hemosiderin in macrophages. It is then released, bound to transferrin, and transported to the bone marrow for reuse in

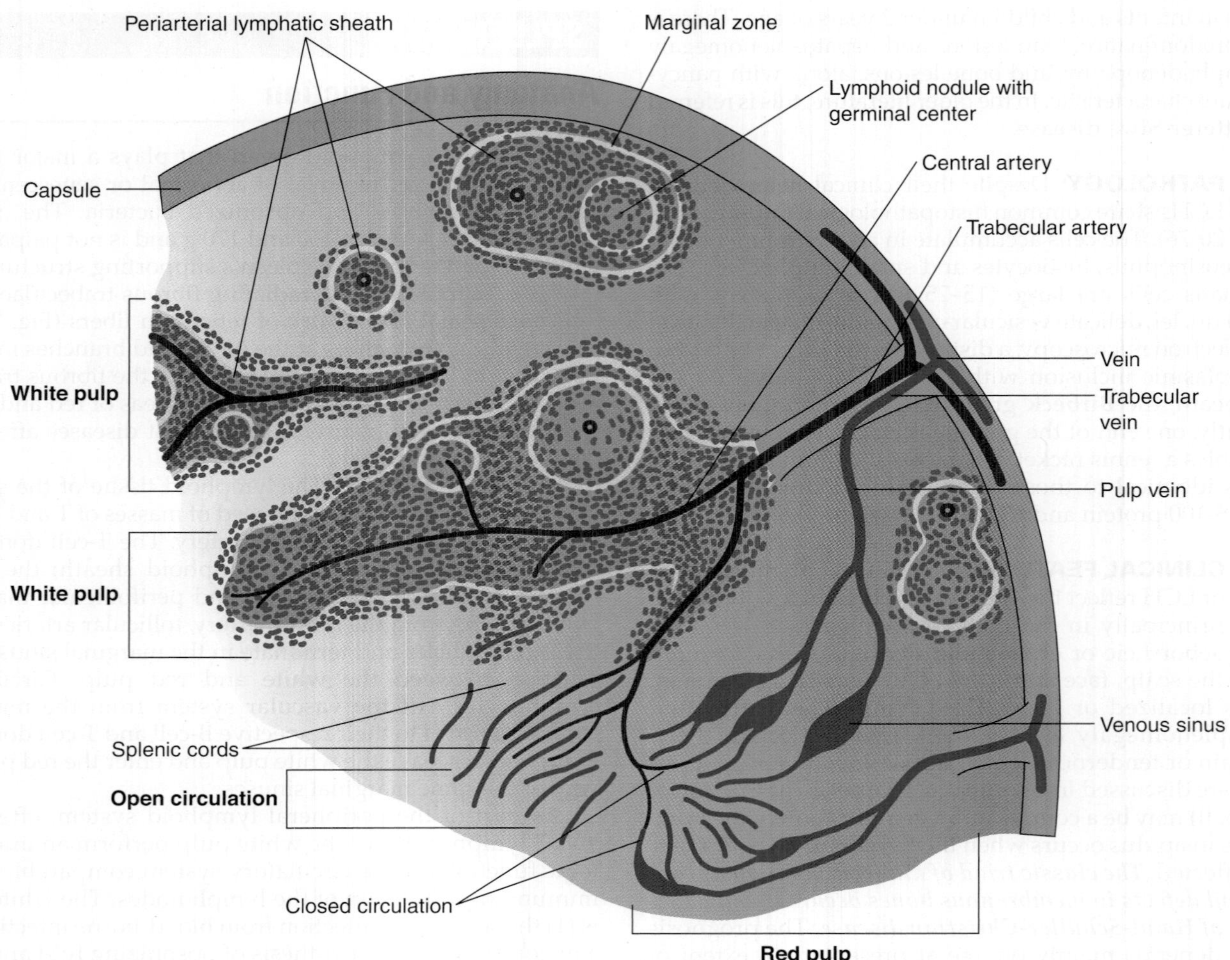

FIGURE 20-77. Structure of the normal spleen.

erythropoiesis. Abnormal erythrocyte inclusions, such as Howell-Jolly bodies (remnants of nuclear DNA), Heinz bodies (denatured hemoglobin) and siderotic granules (iron), are recognized and removed (pitted) by macrophages, without destroying the erythrocyte.

Some membrane lipids of maturing erythrocytes are removed in the red pulp. In the absence of this function, such as after splenectomy, there may be excess erythrocyte membrane in relation to hemoglobin content, which leads to central pooling of hemoglobin and a "target cell" appearance.

Most normal erythroid cells survive, as do granulocytes and platelets. They ultimately enter the trabecular veins and leave the hilum by way of the splenic vein. One third of the blood platelet pool and a small fraction of granulocytes are normally sequestered in the spleen without causing any damage to the cells. By contrast, there is no significant splenic sequestration of erythrocytes and splenectomy is followed only by an increase in platelet and granulocyte counts.

Disorders of the Spleen

Hypersplenism is a functional disorder, which, as noted above (see hemolytic anemia), is characterized by anemia, leukopenia, thrombocytopenia and compensatory bone marrow hyperplasia. Hyposplenism is a situation in which normal splenic functions are reduced by disease or are absent after splenectomy. Impaired filtering leads to increased risk of severe bacteremia and mild leukocytosis and thrombocytosis. Nuclear remnants and Howell-Jolly bodies are found in many of the circulating erythrocytes.

Asplenia, congenital absence of the spleen, is rare, being seen in 1 in 40,000 births, and is often seen with other congenital anomalies. **Acquired asplenia,** following a period of hypersplenism, is common in young adults with sickle cell anemia. In these patients, multiple infarctions eventually result in atrophy and hyposplenism. The infarctions are often painful because of the complication of fibrinous perisplenitis. In the absence of splenic sequestration of erythrocytes, with consequent lack of removal of excess membrane and intracellular debris, many erythrocytes become target cells and contain nuclear remnants, Howell-Jolly bodies or even intact nuclei.

Accessory spleen is the most common congenital anomaly, encountered in about 16% of pediatric splenectomies. Accessory spleens are usually solitary and located in the splenic hilum, in the tail of the pancreas or in the gastrosplenic ligament. After splenectomy, accessory spleens may increase considerably in size, but they rarely become large enough to restore the functions of the lost spleen. Other congenital anomalies of the spleen include polysplenia with multiple small splenic masses, fusion, hamartomas and cysts.

Reactive Splenomegaly

The spleen is a prominent member of the lymphopoietic and mononuclear phagocyte systems and **splenomegaly** is common in a variety of unrelated benign and malignant diseases (Table 20-21). Acute splenitis arises as a result of many blood-borne infections. The spleen typically becomes congested, with infiltration of the red and white pulp by neutrophils and plasma cells. In most cases the spleen in moderately enlarged (400 g).

In **acute and chronic parasitemias,** the red pulp may be engorged with parasites and their breakdown products. The spleen is often massively enlarged in chronic malaria (up to 10 kg). It shows fibrous thickening of the capsule and trabeculae, with a slate gray to black coloration of the pulp as a result of phagocytosed malarial pigment (hematin).

Splenomegaly is seen in about half of patients with infectious mononucleosis and is occasionally complicated by fatal splenic rupture. Infiltration of the capsular and trabecular systems and of blood vessels by lymphoid elements weakens the supporting structure of the spleen and accounts for **traumatic splenic rupture** in infectious mononucleosis. Microscopically, the red pulp cords and sinuses are infiltrated by a polymorphic population of T and B immunoblasts that may include large multinucleated forms.

In **chronic inflammatory disorders,** splenomegaly is caused by hyperplasia of the white pulp. Germinal centers are prominent, as in rheumatoid arthritis, and the red pulp displays an associated increase in mononuclear phagocytes, immunoblasts, plasma cells and eosinophils. In systemic lupus erythematosus, fibrinoid necrosis of the capsule and concentric, or "onion skin," thickening of the penicilliary arteries and central arterioles of the white pulp are seen.

Table 20-21

Principal Causes of Splenomegaly

Infections
Acute
Subacute
Chronic
Immunologic Inflammatory Disorders
Felty syndrome
Lupus erythematosus
Sarcoidosis
Amyloidosis
Thyroiditis
Hemolytic Anemias
Immune Thrombocytopenia
Splenic Vein Hypertension
Cirrhosis
Splenic or portal vein thrombosis or stenosis
Right-sided cardiac failure
Primary or Metastatic Neoplasm
Leukemia
Lymphoma
Hodgkin disease
Myeloproliferative syndromes
Sarcoma
Carcinoma
Storage Diseases
Gaucher
Niemann-Pick
Mucopolysaccharidoses

Congestive Splenomegaly

Chronic passive congestion of the spleen causes splenomegaly and hypersplenism. This is most common in patients with portal hypertension caused by cirrhosis, thrombosis of the portal or splenic veins or right-sided heart failure. Splenic congestion is also seen in hereditary hemolytic anemias and hemoglobinopathies. Common inherited causes of hemolytic anemia include hereditary spherocytosis and elliptocytosis and the hemoglobinopathies such as thalassemia and sickle cells anemia. The erythrocytes in the conditions are inflexible and become trapped as they attempt to pass through the splenic cords.

The Spleen in Sickle Cell Anemia

The spleen is modestly enlarged (300 to 700 g) and has a thickened, fibrotic capsule. Focal accentuation of the capsular fibrosis leads to a "sugar-coated" appearance. The cut surface is firm, and the color varies from pink to deep red, depending on the extent of fibrosis. Microscopically, the venous sinuses are distended with red cells and are surrounded by hemosiderin-laden macrophages. Later, as a consequence of hypoxia and infarcts, the parenchyma becomes fibrotic, and the red pulp is hypocellular. Foci of old hemorrhages persist as **Gamna-Gandy bodies,** which are fibrotic nodules containing iron and calcium salts encrusted on collagenous and elastic fibers. The white pulp tends to be atrophic.

Infiltrative Splenomegaly

The spleen may be enlarged by an increase in cellularity or by deposition of extracellular material, as in amyloidosis. Splenic macrophages accumulate in chronic infections, hemolytic anemias and a variety of storage diseases, Gaucher disease being the prototype (see Chapter 6). A variety of neoplastic and reactive bone marrow disorders are accompanied by extramedullary hematopoiesis and a corresponding increase in the size of the spleen. Splenomegaly is also caused by infiltration of malignant cells in hematologic proliferative disorders, such as leukemias and lymphomas, and virus-associated hemophagocytic syndrome.

Splenomegaly Caused by Cysts and Tumors

Splenic cysts are rare, and the most common are actually pseudocysts. The latter are lined by a fibrous wall and are the residue of previous hemorrhage or infarction. **Hydatid or echinococcal cysts** are the most common cysts worldwide, in areas endemic for *Echinococcus granulosus* (see Chapter 9), but are very rare in the United States.

Primary splenic tumors are also distinctly uncommon. Vascular neoplasms are the most common nonhematopoietic neoplasm to involve the spleen. These tumors include benign tumors (i.e., hemangiomas and lymphangiomas). Usually of the cavernous type, they contain large endothelial-lined spaces and vary from minute foci to lesions that occupy most of the spleen. The spaces in hemangiomas are occupied by erythrocytes, and in lymphangiomas by lymph. Other benign tumors include littoral cell angiomas and hemangioendotheliomas.

The most common primary malignant tumor of the spleen is the hemangiosarcoma. Splenic hemangiosarcoma is a rare, highly malignant neoplasm of vascular endothelial cells that tends to metastasize to the liver by way of the portal drainage. Other malignancies, such as malignant lymphomas or HL, are usually part of a generalized disease. Despite its large blood supply and filtering function, the spleen is only rarely involved by metastatic tumors. The microenvironment, with its abundance of macrophages and lymphocytes, is apparently not favorable for tumor growth. Metastatic tumors are usually observed only late in the course of a widely metastasizing neoplasm.

THYMUS

Theories underlying the historical categorization of the thymus as an endocrine organ have long been discredited. Nevertheless, we know that the thymus elaborates a number of factors (thymic hormones) that play a key role in the maturation of the immune system and the development of immune tolerance. On this basis, we discuss certain entities associated with thymus abnormalities in this chapter.

Anatomy and Function

The thymus derives embryologically from the third pair of pharyngeal pouches, with an inconstant contribution from the fourth pair. The organ is irregularly pyramidal, with its base located inferiorly and its two lobes fused in the midline. Its fibrous capsule extends into the parenchyma, forming septa that delimit lobules. The thymus is largest in relation to total body size and weight at birth, when it averages about 15 g. It continues to grow until puberty, and then may weigh 30 to 40 g.

Microscopically, the lobules display an **outer cortex** and an **inner medulla.** The cortex consists of densely packed lymphocytes, which in this location are termed **thymocytes.** Thymocytes are admixed with a few epithelial and mesenchymal cells. The medulla contains many more epithelial cells and fewer thymocytes. **Hassall corpuscles** are medullary structures that are focally keratinized, concentric aggregates of epithelial cells characteristic of the thymus.

The thymus is the key site for T-lymphocyte differentiation (see Chapter 4). It also has a small population of neuroendocrine cells, which may explain the occurrence of neuroendocrine tumors in this organ. The thymus also exhibits a complement of myoid cells, which resemble striated muscle cells but are nevertheless regarded as epithelial cells. Myoid cells may play a role in the autoimmune pathogenesis of myasthenia gravis.

Beginning at puberty, the thymus starts to involute and continues to diminish in size into adulthood. Initially, cortical thymocytes are decreased relative to epithelial cells. Eventually, the thymus consists of islands of epithelial cells depleted of lymphocytes and aggregates of Hassall corpuscles separated by adipose tissue.

Agenesis and Dysplasia

Alterations in the thymus vary from complete absence **(agenesis)** or severe **hypoplasia** to a situation in which the thymus is small but exhibits a normal architecture. Some small glands exhibit **thymic dysplasia,** characterized by an absence of thymocytes, few if any Hassall corpuscles and only epithelial components. Various developmental abnormalities are associated with immune deficiencies (see Chapter 4) and hematologic disorders.

- **Severe combined immunodeficiency (SCID)** represents a group of genetically distinct syndromes all characterized by defects of both T and B lymphocytes and associated with severe thymic dysplasia. Both X-linked and autosomal recessive modes of inheritance have been observed. SCID can be caused by mutations in at least 10 different genes. The most common form is the X-linked type, caused by mutations in *IL-2RG*, a cytokine-receptor gene. Common autosomal recessive inherited forms include the adenosine deaminase deficiency and IL-7Ra.
- **Chromosome 22q11.2 deletion syndrome (DiGeorge, velocardiofacial, Shprintzen, conotruncal anomaly face and Cayler syndromes)** is a spectrum of overlapping conditions caused by 22q11.2 deletions. It is one of the most common genetic syndromes associated with variable clinical manifestations (180 at least). Patients with DiGeorge syndrome have a failure in development of the third and fourth branchial pouches, resulting in agenesis or hypoplasia of the thymus and parathyroid glands, congenital heart defects, dysmorphic facies and a variety of other congenital anomalies. As a result, patients have hypocalcemia and a deficiency of cellular immunity, with a particular susceptibility to *Candida* infection. Recent reports indicate that patients with 22q11.2 deletion syndrome are also at increased risk for psychotic illnesses. Endocrine abnormalities include hypocalcemia, thyroid dysfunction and short stature. The diagnosis, suspected on clinical grounds, can be readily established by FISH analysis.
- **Nezelof syndrome** is characterized by lymphopenia, hypoplastic lymphoid tissue, abnormal thymus architecture and abnormal T-cell function. It is like DiGeorge syndrome save for the lack of parathyroid and cardiac involvement.
- **Wiskott-Aldrich syndrome** is an X-linked, recessive immunodeficiency caused by mutations in the gene encoding WAS protein and characterized by a hypoplastic thymus, recurrent infections, eczema and thrombocytopenia (see Chapter 4). Patients have increased susceptibility to lymphoid malignancies and autoimmune disorders.
- **Reticular dysgenesis (RD)** is a very rare, severe form of immune deficiency characterized by a vestigial thymus and developmental failure of bone marrow stem cells, resulting in lymphopenia, granulocytopenia and death in utero or in the neonatal period. The primary defect that disturbs the differentiation of the myeloid and lymphoid cell precursors is currently unknown.
- **Swiss-type hypogammaglobulinemia** is an autosomal recessive disorder featuring severe thymic hypoplasia or

dysplasia. Infants with this condition have no lymphocytes or Hassall corpuscles in the thymus and die within a few years from a variety of infections. The anomaly represents a failure of the thymic anlage in the neck to descend into the mediastinum.

- **Ataxia telangiectasia (A-T)** is an autosomal recessive cerebellar ataxia associated with immunodeficiency, telangiectasia, increased sensitivity to ionizing radiation and frequent occurrence of lymphoma. The involuted thymus lacks epithelial differentiation and Hassall corpuscles. Classic A-T results from two truncating ATM mutations that cause complete loss of ATM protein kinase.

Thymic Hyperplasia

Thymic hyperplasia denotes the presence of lymphoid follicles in the thymus irrespective of the size of the gland (Fig. 20-78). The total weight of the thymus is usually within the normal range, although it may be increased. The follicles contain germinal centers and are composed largely of B lymphocytes that contain IgM and IgD. The follicles tend to occupy and distort the medullary zones.

The best-known association of thymic hyperplasia is with **myasthenia gravis** (see Chapter 27), in which two thirds of patients exhibit this thymic abnormality. Interestingly, thymic epithelial and myoid cells contain nicotinic acetylcholine receptor protein, suggesting a potential source for the development of antibodies directed against this receptor. Thymic follicular hyperplasia may also be found in other diseases in which autoimmunity is believed to play a role, including Graves disease, Addison disease, systemic lupus erythematosus, scleroderma and rheumatoid arthritis.

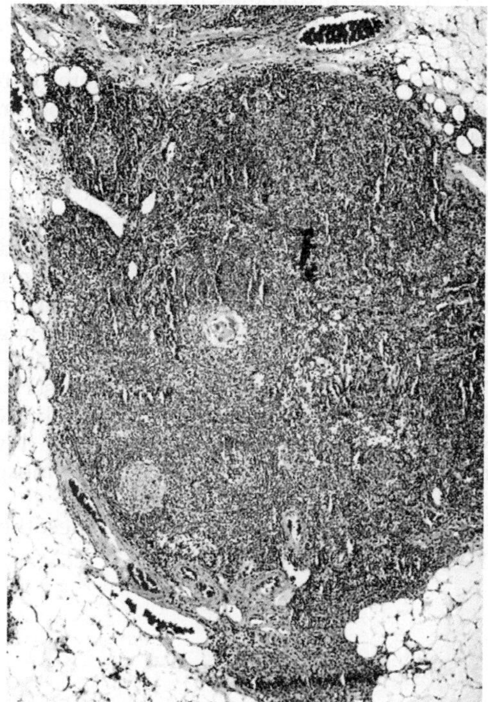

FIGURE 20-78. Thymic hyperplasia. This thymus removed from a patient with myasthenia gravis shows lymphoid follicles with germinal centers.

Thymoma

Thymoma is a neoplasm of thymic epithelial cells. This tumor almost always occurs in adult life and most (80%) are benign.

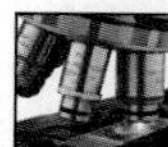

PATHOLOGY: Most thymomas are in the anterosuperior mediastinum, although a few have been described in other locations where thymic tissue is found, including the neck, middle and posterior mediastinum and pulmonary hilus. Benign thymomas are irregularly shaped masses that range from a few centimeters to 15 cm or more in greatest dimension. They are encapsulated, firm and gray to yellow tumors that are divided into lobules by fibrous septa (Fig. 20-79). Large tumors show foci of hemorrhage, necrosis and cystic degeneration. In some instances, the entire thymoma becomes cystic and multiple sections are required to identify the true nature of the lesion.

On microscopic examination (Fig. 20-80), thymomas consist of a mixture of neoplastic epithelial cells and nontumorous lymphocytes. The proportions of these elements vary in individual cases and even among different lobules. The epithelial cells are plump or spindle shaped and have vesicular nuclei. In cases in which epithelial cells predominate, they may exhibit an organoid differentiation, including perivascular spaces containing lymphocytes and macrophages, tumor cell rosettes and whorls suggesting abortive Hassall corpuscle formation.

MYASTHENIA GRAVIS: Fifteen percent of patients with myasthenia gravis have thymoma. Conversely, one third to one half of patients with thymoma develop myasthenia gravis. The occurrence of thymoma in persons with myasthenia gravis is more common in men older than age 50.

When thymoma is associated with myasthenic symptoms, the epithelial cells are of the plump, rather than spindle cell, variety. Antigens related to the nicotinic acetylcholine receptor have also been detected in thymomas. Thymic hyperplasia is almost always present in the nontumorous thymic tissue and lymphoid follicles may even be present in the thymoma itself.

OTHER ASSOCIATED DISEASES: Thymoma is also associated with many other immune disorders. More than 10% of

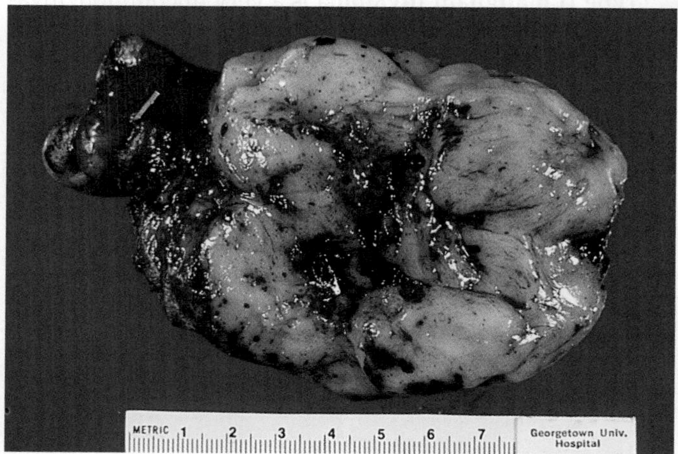

FIGURE 20-79. Thymoma. The tumor in cross-section is whitish and has a bulging surface with areas of hemorrhage. Note the attached portion of normal thymus.

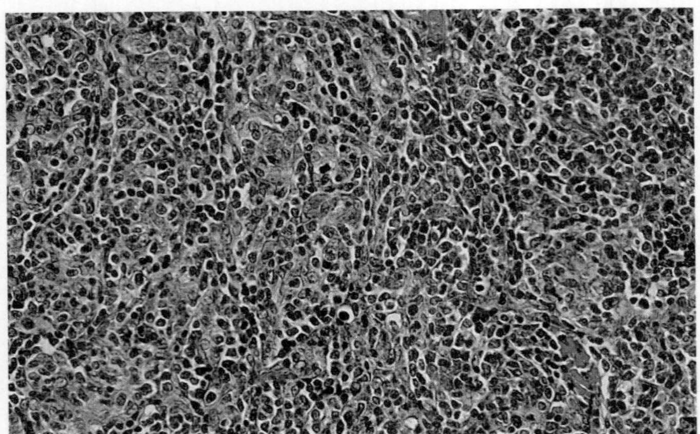

FIGURE 20-80. Microscopic features of thymomas. The tumor consists of a mixture of neoplastic epithelial cells and nontumorous lymphocytes.

patients have hypogammaglobulinemia and 5% have erythroid hypoplasia. In contrast to the situation with myasthenia gravis, the epithelial component of the thymoma is spindle shaped in these cases. Other associated diseases include myocarditis, dermatomyositis, rheumatoid arthritis, lupus erythematosus, scleroderma and Sjögren syndrome. Certain malignant tumors have also been associated with thymoma, including T-cell leukemia/lymphoma and multiple myeloma.

Malignant Thymoma Invades Locally and May Metastasize

One fourth of thymomas are not encapsulated and exhibit malignant features.

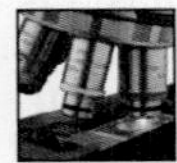

PATHOLOGY: **Type I malignant thymoma** is the most common cancer of the thymus and is virtually indistinguishable histologically from encapsulated, benign thymoma. However, it penetrates the capsule, implants on pleural or pericardial surfaces and metastasizes to lymph nodes, lung, liver and bone.

Type II malignant thymoma is a very uncommon, invasive tumor that is also termed **thymic carcinoma.** Its morphology is highly variable and takes the form of squamous cell carcinoma, lymphoepithelioma-like carcinoma (identical to that found in the oropharynx; see Chapter 25), a sarcomatoid variant (carcinosarcoma) and a number of other rare patterns. These variants share a distinct epithelial appearance and a mediastinal tumor that lacks this feature is probably not a thymic carcinoma.

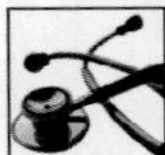

CLINICAL FEATURES: Malignant thymoma is treated by surgical excision and radiation therapy. Chemotherapy is added in cases with distant metastases. The prognosis for benign thymoma is excellent. The presence or absence of myasthenic symptoms has little prognostic value. For type I malignant thymomas, prognosis correlates with the extent of disease. Most patients with type II thymomas die within 5 years of diagnosis.

Other Tumors of the Thymus Are Uncommon

NEUROENDOCRINE TUMORS: Several neuroendocrine tumors, which are similar in appearance and natural history to comparable tumors elsewhere, arise in the thymus. These include carcinoids (typical and atypical) and carcinomas (small and large cell). Neuroendocrine tumors are immunoreactive for cytokeratins (AE1/AE3, CAM5.2) and endocrine markers (synaptophysin, chromogranin, NSE). ACTH may be produced in such tumors that cause Cushing syndrome. Interestingly, nuclear expression of thyroid transcription factor 1 (TTF-1) is reportedly negative in many thymic neuroendocrine tumors.

CARCINOID: Thymic carcinoid tumors are malignant and tend to invade locally and metastasize widely, although if well circumscribed they may be cured by local excision. Interestingly, one third of these patients show Cushing syndrome, but carcinoid syndrome is exceedingly rare. Thymic carcinoid tumors occur both sporadically, in familial forms, and in the context of multiple endocrine neoplasia (MEN)-1 and -2A. Association with neurofibromatosis type I is also described. Most thymic carcinoids are atypical (intermediate category) with frequent mitoses and/or necrosis.

SMALL CELL CARCINOMA: Small cell carcinomas (SCCs), indistinguishable from those in the lung, may also arise in the thymus. Thymic SCCs may be admixed with squamous cell carcinomas.

GERM CELL TUMORS: Thymic germ cell tumors account for 20% of all mediastinal tumors. It is felt that these arise from cells left behind when germ cells migrate during embryogenesis. The histologies of mediastinal germ cell tumors are like those in the gonads (see Chapters 17 and 18). Mature cystic teratoma is most common. Seminoma, embryonal carcinoma, endodermal sinus tumor, teratocarcinoma, immature teratoma and choriocarcinoma all occur. Mixed germ cell tumors are common. Mediastinal germ cell tumors may on occasion contain a somatic-type malignant component of sarcoma, carcinoma or hematologic malignancies. Save for mature cystic teratoma, which affects both sexes equally, the other tumors occur mostly in males and thymic seminoma arises only in men. Prognosis is similar to that of comparable gonadal tumors, except for mediastinal nonseminomatous germ cell tumors, which are more aggressive.

Other lesions include benign and malignant stromal tumors. **Thymolipoma** is a benign, well-circumscribed mass composed of mature adipose tissue and unremarkable thymic parenchyma. **Thymic stromal sarcomas** are low-grade malignant mesenchymal tumors with variable morphology, but frequently of a liposarcomatous nature.

Nonneoplastic masses include thymic, mesothelial and enteric-type cysts.

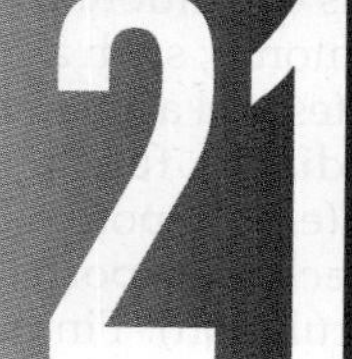

21 The Endocrine System

Maria J. Merino • Martha Quezado

The main function of the endocrine system is communication. The nervous and endocrine systems overlap in the soluble mediators they use and the functions they serve, but the defining characteristic of the endocrine system is its ability to communicate at a distance using soluble mediators, hormones.

The term **hormone** (from the Greek *horman,* "set in motion") applies to chemicals secreted by "ductless" (i.e., endocrine) glands into the circulation, which carries it to the target organ. Many hormones, such as thyroid hormone, corticosteroids and pituitary hormones, fit this definition. By contrast, some traditionally recognized hormones, such as catecholamines, are produced in a variety of sites and act either locally or through the circulation. Other mediators function only in restricted circulation compartments (e.g., hypothalamic hormones only act on the pituitary and reach it via portal tributaries without entering the systemic circulation). Finally, many hormones exert their effects in the same tissues in which they are formed, such as müllerian-inhibiting substance. These diverse forms of chemically mediated cell-to-cell communication are summarized in Figure 21-1.

To qualify as a hormone, a chemical messenger must bind to a receptor, either on the surface of the cell or within it. Hormones act either on the final effector target or on other glands that in turn produce another hormone. For instance, thyroid hormone acts directly on many types of peripheral cells, whereas thyroid-stimulating hormone (TSH) is released by the pituitary and induces the thyroid gland to secrete thyroid hormone. Diseases of the endocrine system may lead to excessive or insufficient production of hormones. In addition, insensitivity of target tissues leads to effects similar to those associated with underproduction of hormones.

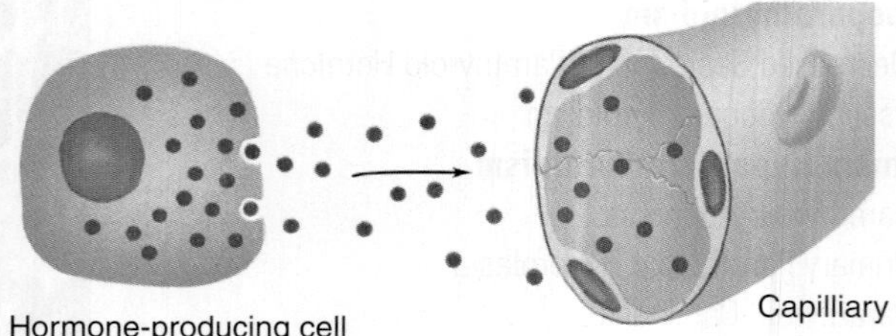

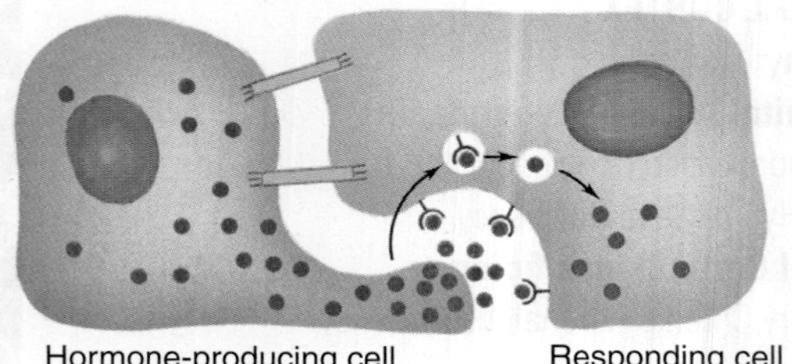

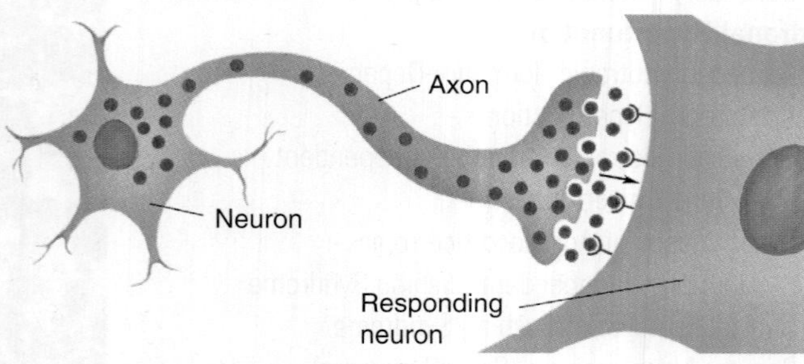

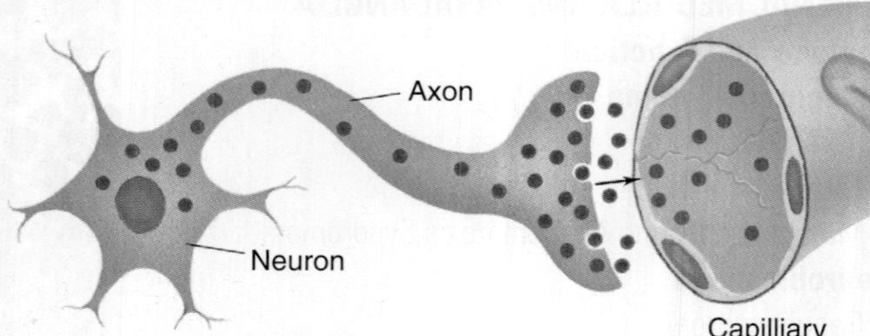

FIGURE 21-1. Mechanisms of chemically mediated cell-to-cell communication. Biological messages may be transmitted by mechanisms other than the classic endocrine pathway via the circulation. These include paracrine, synaptic and neuroendocrine modes of communication.

PITUITARY GLAND

Anatomy

The pituitary gland, also termed the **hypophysis,** resides within the sella turcica, located within the sphenoid bone at the base of the brain. The gland is composed of two lobes: the **adenohypophysis** or anterior lobe, which makes up 80% of the gland and is populated by epithelial cells, and the posterior lobe or **neurohypophysis,** which is a neural structure (Fig. 21-2). The adult gland measures about $1.3 \times 0.9 \times 0.6$ cm

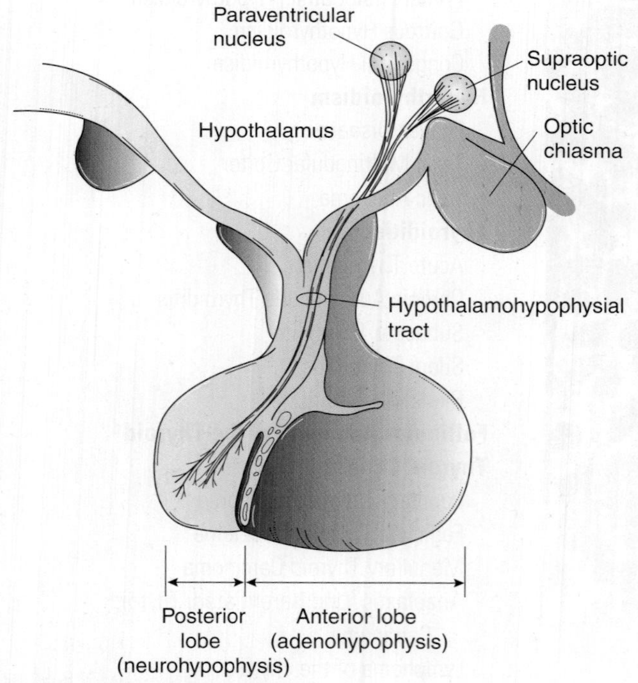

FIGURE 21-2. The pituitary gland.

and weighs 0.6 g. The pituitary is near the optic chiasm and cranial nerves III, IV, V and VI; so tumors of the gland may produce partial blindness or various cranial nerve palsies.

The two lobes of the pituitary are anatomically distinct and derive from different embryologic anlagen. The anterior lobe develops from the Rathke pouch, an endodermal evagination of the developing oral cavity. Along its migration tract, this craniopharyngeal duct may leave intrasphenoidal squamous epithelial rests that later serve as the origin of a tumor known as craniopharyngioma. The neurohypophysis originates as a downward projection of the brain and remains connected to the hypothalamus by the hypophyseal stalk. Flanked on either side by the anterior and posterior lobes is the vestigial intermediate lobe, composed of a few cystic cavities lined by cuboidal or columnar epithelium.

The pituitary has a dual circulation, composed of a complex portal system that originates in the hypothalamus, and by a separate arterial and venous blood supply. The hypophysial portal system transports hypothalamic stimulatory and inhibitory releasing hormones to the anterior pituitary. The venous drainage of the pituitary follows the cavernous sinus to both inferior petrosal sinuses.

Axons and unmyelinated nerve fibers originate in the hypothalamus and proceed along the pituitary stalk to enervate the neurohypophysis. These nerves regulate secretion of arginine vasopressin (antidiuretic hormone [ADH]) and oxytocin, which are made in the hypothalamus, stored in the posterior lobe, then released into the systemic circulation.

The cells of the anterior pituitary are arranged in cords or nests in a highly vascular stroma. On the basis of staining with hematoxylin and eosin, these cells were classically divided into two groups of equal number (i.e., stainable and *chromophobe*, or unstainable, cells). The cytoplasmic granules of stainable cells either stained *acidophilic* (eosinophilic) (40%) or *basophilic* (10%). ***However, as the tinctorial properties of the granules proved to be unrelated to their function, these cells are now categorized according to the hormone secreted,*** as determined by immunohistochemical staining (Fig. 21-3):

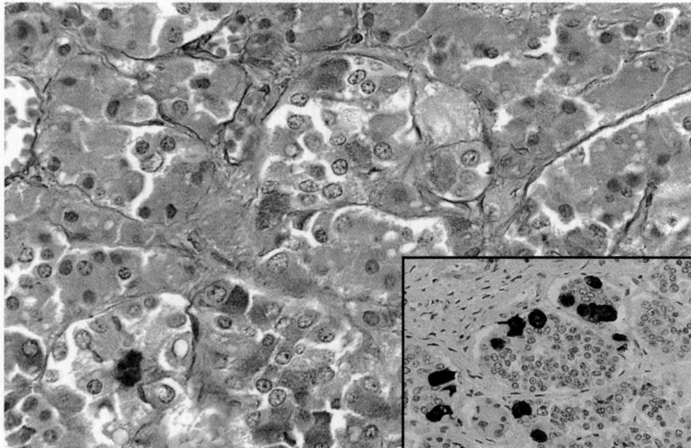

FIGURE 21-3. Normal anterior lobe of pituitary. In a periodic acid–Schiff (PAS)–orange G stain, the cytoplasm of somatotropic and prolactin-secreting cells take up the orange G stain. Most of the cells with a lavender cytoplasm produce adrenocorticotropic hormone (ACTH) (corticotropes). An immunohistochemical stain (*inset*) demonstrates cells that synthesize growth hormone (somatotropes).

- **Corticotrophs:** These basophilic cells secrete **proopiomelanocortin** (POMC) and its derivatives including **adrenocorticotropic hormone** (ACTH, corticotropin), which controls adrenal secretion of corticosteroids; **melanocyte-stimulating hormone** (MSH); **lipotropic hormone** (LPH); and **endorphins.** Basophilic corticotrophs of the *pars intermedia* may cluster and spread deep into the posterior lobe, a phenomenon called "basophil invasion." Corticotrophs are mainly located in the median wedge of the gland.
- **Lactotrophs:** These acidophilic cells secrete **prolactin,** which is essential for lactation and many other metabolic activities. They are mainly seen in the posterolateral wings of the gland.
- **Somatotrophs:** These acidophilic cells, located mainly in the lateral wings, elaborate **growth hormone** and constitute half of all hormone-producing cells of the adenohypophysis.
- **Thyrotrophs: Thyroid-stimulating hormone** (TSH) is produced by pale basophilic or amphophilic cells, which constitute only 5% of the cells of the anterior lobe; these cells are scattered in the parenchyma concentrating in the anterior median/wedge of the gland.
- **Gonadotrophs: Follicle-stimulating hormone** (FSH) and **luteinizing hormone** (LH) are secreted by the same basophilic cells that are distributed throughout the gland. In the ovary, FSH stimulates formation of Graafian follicles and LH induces ovulation and formation of corpora lutea.

The posterior lobe of the pituitary is composed of **pituicytes**, modified glial cells without secretory function; **axon terminals;** and **unmyelinated nerve fibers** containing **ADH** and **oxytocin.** These hormones are made in the nerve cell bodies in the hypothalamus and transported along axons to the neurohypophysis. ADH promotes water resorption from the distal renal tubules; oxytocin stimulates the pregnant uterus to contract at term and cells around the lactiferous ducts of the mammary gland.

Hypopituitarism

In hypopituitarism secretion of one or more pituitary hormones is lacking. This entity has many causes and various clinical presentations, but its incidence and prevalence are still unknown. Most often, only one or a few of pituitary hormones are deficient. Occasionally, total failure of pituitary function, or **panhypopituitarism,** occurs. The effects of hypopituitarism depend on (1) the extent of the loss, (2) the specific hormones involved and (3) the age of the patient. Symptoms usually relate to deficient function of the thyroid and adrenal glands and the reproductive system. Growth retardation and delayed puberty may occur in children.

PITUITARY TUMORS: More than half of all cases of hypopituitarism in adults are caused by pituitary tumors, usually adenomas. The tumor itself may be functional, but symptoms of hypopituitarism often result from compression of adjacent tissue by the mass.

SHEEHAN SYNDROME: Panhypopituitarism may be caused by ischemic necrosis of the gland, commonly due to severe hypotension caused by postpartum hemorrhage. It may rarely occur without massive bleeding or after normal delivery. Enlargement of the pituitary reduces its blood flow, rendering it particularly vulnerable. Agalactia, amenorrhea, hypothyroidism and adrenocortical insufficiency are

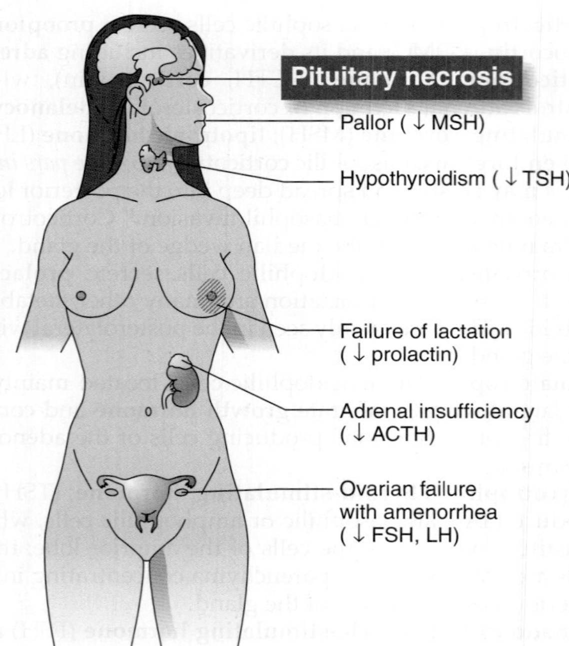

FIGURE 21-4. Major clinical manifestations of panhypopituitarism. ACTH = adrenocorticotropic hormone; FSH = follicle-stimulating hormone; LH = luteinizing hormone; MSH = melanocyte-stimulating hormone; TSH = thyroid-stimulating hormone.

important consequences (Fig. 21-4). With modern obstetric care, Sheehan syndrome is rare.

PITUITARY APOPLEXY: Hemorrhage/infarction can occur in the normal pituitary, but at least half of the cases occur in association with endocrinologically inactive adenomas. On occasion, pituitary apoplexy leads to hypopituitarism.

IATROGENIC HYPOPITUITARISM: Radiation damage to the hypothalamic–pituitary axis during therapy or prophylactic irradiation may cause neuroendocrine abnormalities, including hypopituitarism. Similarly, neurosurgical procedures may damage the pituitary.

TRAUMA: Traumatic brain injury is associated with significant risk to the pituitary gland, with potential development of diabetes, hypopituitarism and other endocrinopathies.

INFILTRATIVE DISEASES: Bacterial and viral infections may lead to inflammation, which can damage the gland. Hypothalamic–pituitary axis involvement in Langerhans cell histiocytosis (formerly Hand-Schüller-Christian syndrome; see Chapters 20, 26) results in endocrine abnormalities including diabetes insipidus in 5% to 50% of patients and panhypopituitarism in 5% to 20%. Hemochromatosis may cause panhypopituitarism (see Chapter 14).

GENETIC ABNORMALITIES OF PITUITARY DEVELOPMENT:

MOLECULAR PATHOGENESIS: Congenital growth hormone deficiency may occur in isolation, in the so-called **isolated growth hormone deficiency** (IGHD) or in association with other anterior and posterior pituitary hormone deficiencies. Four types of IGHD are described. They may be familial or sporadic. In familial forms, inheritance can be autosomal recessive (AR), autosomal dominant (AD) or X-linked recessive. The autosomal forms are linked to the human growth hormone (GH) gene or in the gene encoding the growth hormone–releasing hormone (GHRH) receptor. DNA deletions, amino acid substitutions and splice site mutations are known. The availability of recombinant human GH has permitted the safe and effective treatment of children with this disorder.

Several mutations targeting transcription factors during embryogenesis have been identified:

- **Pit-1:** Pit-1 is a POU homeodomain transcription factor important for development of somatotrophs, lactotrophs and thyrotrophs. It is encoded by the *POU1F1* gene on human chromosome 3p11. Mutations in this gene, most commonly arginine to tryptophan at codon 271 (R271W), cause combined pituitary hormone deficiency (CPHD) with low or zero levels of GH, prolactin (PRL) and TSH.
- **PROP1 (5q):** Prop 1 is a pituitary-specific pairedlike homeodomain transcription factor. Mutations in this transcription factor inactivate LH, FSH, GH, PRL and TSH. Phenotypes associated with such mutations are variable. Mutations seem to be rare in sporadic cases, but in familial cases a prevalence of more than 25% is seen.
- **HESX1 (3p21):** This gene is a member of the pairedlike class of the homeobox genes, important for optic nerve and pituitary development. Its expression begins before that of other developmental genes. About 14 *HESX1* mutations, with both recessive and dominant inheritance, are associated with septo-optic dysplasia and/or hypopituitarism patients. Septo-optic dysplasia is a rare congenital anomaly with midline forebrain abnormalities, optic nerve hypoplasia and hypopituitarism. Also described is an ectopic/undescended posterior pituitary. Endocrinopathies are characterized by GHD followed by TSH and ACTH deficiency.
- **PITX2:** This gene is expressed in fetal pituitary and in most cells of the adult gland. Mutations are associated with **Rieger syndrome** in humans, an autosomal dominant condition with variable phenotype including pituitary abnormalities.
- **LX3/LX4:** These genes of the LIM family of homeobox genes are expressed early in the Rathke pouch. *LHX3* is at chromosome 9q, and mutations are associated with GH, TSH, LH, FSH and PRL deficiencies. In a single report of a mutation within the *LX4* gene, the patient presented with GH, TSH and ACTH deficiency.
- **GLI2:** Patients with *GLI2* mutations have abnormal pituitary function.

GROWTH HORMONE INSENSITIVITY (LARON SYNDROME): Laron dwarfism is a rare, autosomal recessive form of short stature due to extreme resistance to GH secondary to abnormalities in the growth hormone receptor (GHR). Clinically, patients tend to be obese, with high levels of serum GH and low concentrations of insulin-like growth factor-I (IGF-I). This condition is seen predominantly in people of Mediterranean origin, especially Sephardic Jews. Interestingly, the same lesion is responsible for the dwarfism of African pygmies.

Laron syndrome is caused by more than 30 *GHR* mutations, all involving the extracellular domain of the receptor.

Clinical presentations are heterogeneous, and most cases are unique to particular families or geographical areas. As GH acts by promoting secretion of IGF-I, the latter hormone provides effective replacement therapy for Laron syndrome, recapitulating most effects ascribed to GH itself.

ISOLATED GONADOTROPIN DEFICIENCY (KALLMANN SYNDROME): Kallmann syndrome is characterized by **hypogonadotropic hypogonadism** (due to gonadotropin-releasing hormone [GnRH] deficiency) and **anosmia** (absent sense of smell). Cleft lip/palate and other anomalies may also be present. Kallmann syndrome is usually diagnosed at puberty due to delayed appearance of secondary sex characteristics. It is three to five times more common in males than in females (1:8000). Most cases are sporadic, although X-linked and autosomal recessive and dominant familial forms of the disease have been described. X-linked Kallmann syndrome (KAL1) is associated with mutations of the *KAL1* gene (Xp23.3), which codes for an extracellular matrix component with putative antiprotease activity and cell adhesion function. As a result of this mutation, neurons destined to secrete GnRH fail to migrate from their origin in the olfactory anlage to their normal location in the hypothalamus. The autosomal dominant form of the disease (KAL2) is associated with mutations of the gene encoding the fibroblast growth factor receptor 1 (8p11). A third form of Kallmann syndrome (KAL3) appears to show autosomal recessive inheritance, but no affected gene is yet known.

EMPTY SELLA SYNDROME: This is primarily a radiologic term that describes an enlarged sella containing a thin, flattened pituitary at the base (Fig. 21-5). It is secondary to a congenitally defective or absent diaphragma sella, which permits transmission of cerebrospinal fluid pressure into the sella. Empty sella syndrome can cause various degrees of pituitary dysfunction and endocrine abnormalities. Although its pathogenesis is still controversial, it has been linked to both pituitary and nonpituitary causes. Hormonal abnormalities previously felt to be uncommon are now recognized as not so rare, including hyperprolactinemia, oligomenorrhea or amenorrhea, frank hypopituitarism, acromegaly, diabetes insipidus and Cushing syndrome.

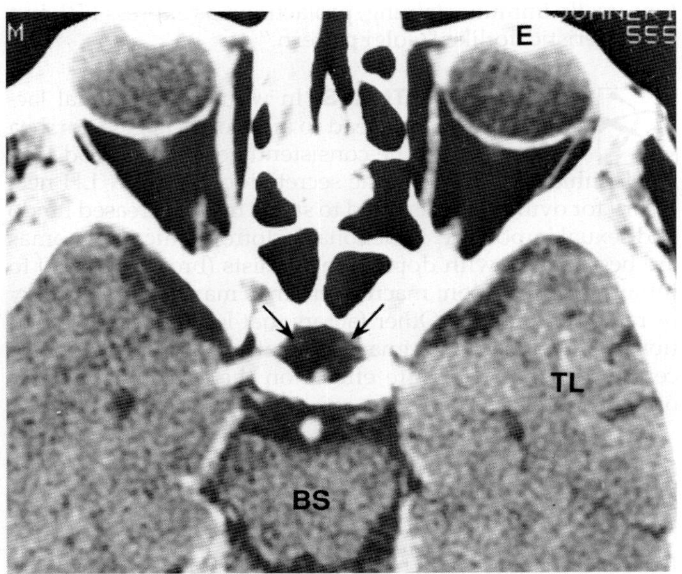

FIGURE 21-5. Empty sella syndrome. A computed tomography (CT) scan of the cranium in an axial section demonstrates an empty sella turcica (*arrows*). BS = brainstem; E = eye; TL = temporal lobe.

Pituitary Adenomas

Pituitary adenomas are benign neoplasms of the anterior lobe of the pituitary and are often associated with excess secretion of pituitary hormones and evidence of corresponding endocrine hyperfunction (Table 21-1). Most of these tumors are sporadic but about 5% occur in a familial setting and in association with multiple endocrine neoplasia type 1 (MEN1), Carney complex and familial isolated pituitary adenomas (FIPAs). They occur in both sexes, but are more common in adults, making up only 2% of all adenomas in children. PRL-producing adenomas are the most common hormone-secreting tumors in both adults and children. Gonadotroph adenomas are more common in the elderly. Small, apparently nonfunctioning pituitary adenomas are found incidentally in as many as 27% of adult autopsies.

MOLECULAR PATHOGENESIS: The etiology of pituitary adenomas is still obscure, but the pathogenesis involves hormonal and genetic factors. In rare instances and in familial settings, they occur in the context of MEN1, a hereditary disposition to pituitary adenomas, parathyroid hyperplasia or adenoma and pancreatic islet cell adenomas (see Chapter 15). Nevertheless, the MEN1 gene is not downregulated in pituitary tumors and there is no evidence for mutations in MEN1 in sporadic pituitary adenomas.

A syndrome of myxomas, pigmentation and endocrine overactivity including development of pituitary adenomas comprises the Carney complex. Mutations in the gene for protein kinase A regulatory subunit Iα (*PRKAR1A*) are seen in more than 50% of these patients, who can

Table 21-1

Frequency of Adenomas of the Anterior Pituitary

Cell Type	Hormone	Frequency (%)
Lactotrope	Prolactin	26
Null cell	None	17
Corticotrope	ACTH (corticotropin)	15
Somatotrope	Growth hormone	14
Plurihormonal	Multiple	13
Gonadotrope	FSH, LH	8
Oncocytoma	None	6
Thyrotrope	TSH	1

ACTH = adrenocorticotropic hormone; FSH = follicle-stimulating hormone; LH = luteinizing hormone; TSH = thyroid-stimulating hormone.

develop acromegaly due to GH/prolactin-secreting pituitary adenomas.

Patients with FIPAs are younger and about 15% have mutations in the *aryl hydrocarbon receptor-interacting protein gene (AIP).* Pituitary adenomas from patients with *AIP* mutations appear to have a more aggressive clinical course.

The most important oncogene involved in sporadic pituitary tumorigenesis is *gsp.* Acquired activating point mutations in the stimulatory subunit of the G_s protein that activates adenylyl cyclase are seen in 40% of growth hormone–secreting pituitary adenomas. Elevated intracellular cyclic adenosine 3′,5′-monophosphate (cAMP) levels may stimulate hypersecretion of GH and cell proliferation. Some human pituitary tumors express a kinase-containing variant of fibroblast growth factor/receptor (FGFR4), which is linked to pituitary tumor formation in transgenic mice. Mutations or overexpression of several regulatory genes are described in pituitary adenomas, including *cyclin* D_1, *CREB, ras* and *pituitary tumor transforming gene (PTTG).* Recent data suggest that *GADD45γ* and bone morphogenic protein (BMP)4 may participate in pituitary tumorigenesis. Epigenetic regulation may also be related to pituitary tumor formation.

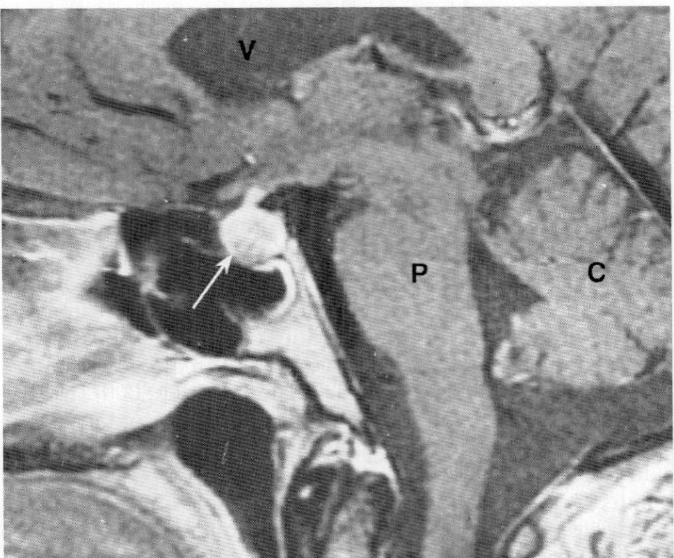

FIGURE 21-6. Pituitary adenoma. A magnetic resonance sagittal view of the brain shows a distinct pituitary tumor (*arrow*). C = cerebellum; P = pons; V = lateral ventricle.

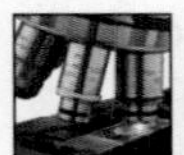

PATHOLOGY: Pituitary adenomas were once classified by the tinctorial properties of the constituent cells as either acidophil, basophil or chromophobe adenomas. These were respectively associated with overproduction of GH or ACTH, or with no endocrine hyperfunction. Since hematoxylin and eosin (H&E) staining properties of the tumor cells correlated poorly with hormonal function, pituitary adenomas are currently classified according to the hormone(s) elaborated. The current classification takes into account the histologic, histochemical, immunohistochemical and electron microscopic features.

Pituitary adenomas range from small lesions that do not enlarge the gland to expansive tumors that erode the sella turcica and impinge on adjacent cranial structures (Fig. 21-6). In general, adenomas less than 10 mm in diameter are referred to as **microadenomas,** whereas larger tumors are termed **macroadenomas.** Microadenomas are not symptomatic until they secrete hormones. Alternatively, macroadenomas tend to cause local compressive symptoms, by virtue of their size, and systemic manifestations, as a result of the overproduction of hormones.

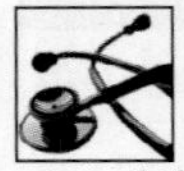

CLINICAL FEATURES: Pituitary macroadenomas may impinge on the optic chiasm, causing severe headaches, bitemporal hemianopsia (loss of lateral visual fields in both eyes) and loss of central vision. Oculomotor palsies occur if a tumor invades the cavernous sinus. Extension into the hypothalamus may interfere with hypothalamic input to the pituitary, causing loss of temperature regulation, hyperphagia and hormonal syndromes.

Lactotroph Adenomas (Prolactinomas) Cause the Most Common Pituitary Endocrinopathy

Hyperprolactinemia is the most common endocrinopathy associated with pituitary adenomas. Almost half of all pituitary microadenomas contain PRL, but many fewer appear to secrete this hormone. PRL-producing microadenomas are most often symptomatic in young women, but over half of all prolactinomas are found in men. This difference in sex distribution is related to the greater frequency of endocrinologic symptoms in women. The true incidence in unselected autopsies is similar in both sexes. In general, larger adenomas secrete more PRL.

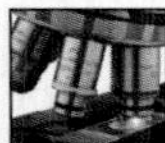

PATHOLOGY: Lactotroph adenomas tend to be chromophobic and contain spheroid nuclei with prominent nucleoli. Deposition of endocrine amyloid (see Chapter 23) and presence of psammoma bodies (calcospherites) are characteristic, but not pathognomonic, of these tumors. By immunostaining, prolactinomas express PRL in a characteristic dotlike "Golgi pattern."

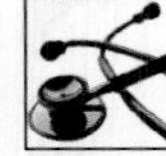

CLINICAL FEATURES: In women, functional lactotroph adenomas lead to amenorrhea, galactorrhea and infertility. The consistently elevated blood PRL levels inhibit the surge in the secretion of pituitary LH necessary for ovulation. Men tend to suffer from decreased libido and sexual impotence. Functional lactotroph microadenomas are best treated with dopamine agonists (bromocriptine) to inhibit PRL secretion; macroadenomas may require surgery or radiation therapy. Other factors that lead to excess secretion of PRL include pregnancy, lactation, administration of certain drugs or pressure effects on the hypothalamus by other tumors.

Somatotrope Adenomas Secrete Growth Hormone

Dramatic changes result from excess secretion of GH. A somatotroph adenoma that arises in a child or adolescent before the epiphyses close results in **gigantism.** By contrast, after long bone epiphyses have fused and adult height is achieved, the same tumor produces **acromegaly.** Most tumors are

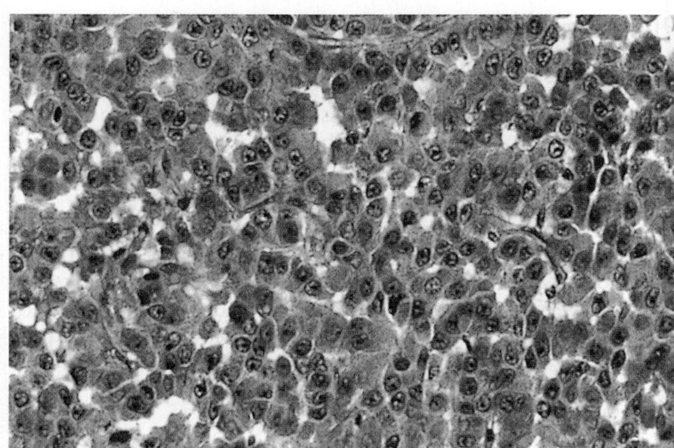

FIGURE 21-7. Pituitary somatotrope adenoma from a man with acromegaly. The tumor cells are arranged in thin cords and ribbons.

macroadenomas and cause mass effects and tumor-induced adenohypophyseal hypofunction.

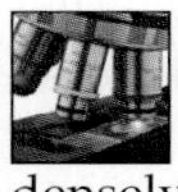

PATHOLOGY: Of patients with acromegaly, 75% have a somatotroph macroadenoma. Most of the rest have microadenomas. Two variants include the densely granulated and sparsely granulated somatotroph adenomas. Densely granulated somatotroph adenomas contain acidophilic cells (Fig. 21-7) with strong, diffuse immunopositivity for GH. Sparsely granulated adenomas are composed of chromophobe cells with characteristic spheroid cytoplasmic inclusions known as "fibrous bodies," containing keratin intermediate filaments, especially keratin 8. By electron microscopy, acidophilic tumors tend to have abundant secretory granules, while chromophobic tumor cells are sparsely granular. Acidophilic somatotroph adenomas usually grow slowly and remain within the sella. The chromophobic variant usually grows faster, is invasive and shows cellular and nuclear pleomorphism.

Mixed somatotroph–lactotroph adenomas contain two cell types, one elaborating GH and the other PRL. In **mammosomatotroph adenomas** a single cell type expresses both GH and PRL. **Acidophil stem cell adenomas** are monomorphous, slightly acidophilic tumors with nuclear pleomorphism and large cytoplasmic vacuoles. Key diagnostic features of these tumors include giant mitochondria, keratin 8–positive fibrous bodies and misplaced exocytosis. This subtype is more clinically aggressive.

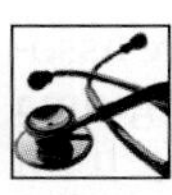

CLINICAL FEATURES: Acromegaly is an uncommon disorder, with an annual incidence of only three per million. Over many years, patients with acromegaly gradually develop coarse facial features (Fig. 21-8). They exhibit overgrowth of the mandible (prognathism) and maxilla, with increased space between the upper incisor teeth and a thickened nose. Hands and feet are often enlarged and the hat size increases.

Acromegaly has significant impact on health beyond simple cosmetic disfigurement. Incidence of cardiovascular, cerebrovascular and respiratory deaths is increased. Most patients suffer from neurologic and musculoskeletal symptoms, including headaches, paresthesias, arthralgias and muscle weakness. One third have hypertension, and half of nor-

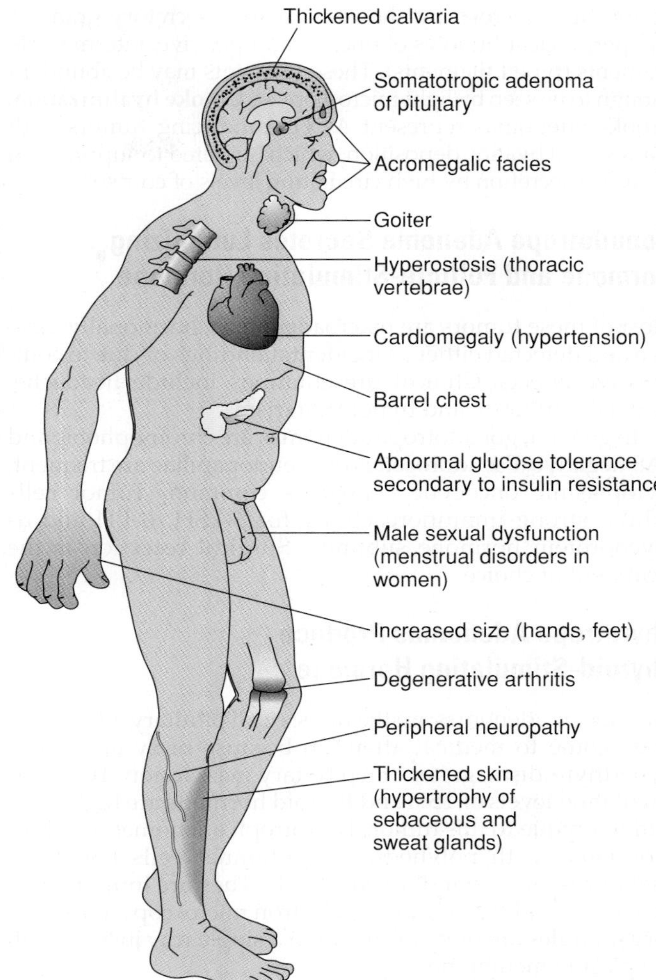

FIGURE 21-8. Clinical manifestations of acromegaly.

motensive acromegalics have increased left ventricular mass and are at risk to develop congestive heart failure. Visceral hypertrophy is common. Diabetes occurs in as many as 20%, and hypercalciuria and renal stones occur in another fifth of patients. Half of patients with acromegaly have symptomatic hyperprolactinemia (see above).

The treatment of choice for somatotroph adenomas is transsphenoidal removal of the pituitary, after which circulating GH levels may decline to normal levels within hours. Radiation therapy is an alternative if surgery is contraindicated. A long-acting analog of somatostatin, an antagonist of GH, is a useful therapeutic adjunct.

Corticotrope Adenomas Produce Adrenocorticotropic Hormone

ACTH excess induces adrenal cortical hypersecretion to produce **Cushing disease** (see below). The tumors are usually microadenomas that are intensely basophilic and periodic acid–Schiff (PAS) positive. Immunohistochemistry documents production of ACTH and also related peptides, such as endorphins and lipotropin. A few functional corticotroph adenomas are chromophobic and tend to be more aggressive than their basophilic counterparts.

Electron microscopy shows numerous secretory granules and perinuclear bundles of fine, keratin-positive, intermediate filaments (type I filaments). These filaments may be abundant enough to be seen by light microscopy as **Crooke hyalinization.** Crooke adenomas represent ACTH-producing tumors with massive cell hyaline deposition, which is related to suppression of ACTH secretion by high circulating levels of cortisol.

Gonadotrope Adenoma Secretes Luteinizing Hormone and Follicle-Stimulating Hormone

Most of these tumors are macroadenomas, hormonally inactive and detected either as incidental findings or due to compressive effects. Clinical presentations include headache, visual disturbance and hypopituitarism.

In general, gonadotrope adenomas are chromophobic and PAS negative. Pseudorosettes or pseudopapillae are frequent. Cytoplasmic oncocytic change is common. Tumor cells exhibit strong immunoreactivity for β-FSH, β-LH and α-glycoprotein hormone subunits. Surgical resection is the treatment of choice.

Thyrotrope Adenomas Produce Thyroid-Stimulating Hormone

Thyrotrope adenomas are the rarest of all pituitary adenomas. They come to medical attention because of symptoms of hyperthyroidism, goiter or a pituitary mass lesion. Typically, circulating levels of TSH and thyroid hormone are high, a situation unique to this tumor. Thyrotroph adenomas are chromophobic, with polyhedral or columnar cells that form pseudorosettes around blood vessels. They are immunopositive for α- and β-TSH, and by electron microscopy, the secretory granules are often arranged in a single row just beneath the plasma membrane.

Patients with long-standing hypothyroidism may show hyperplasia of pituitary thyrotrophs (thyroid deficiency cells) presumably due to inadequate feedback inhibition by thyroid hormone.

Nonfunctional Pituitary Adenomas Are Not Associated With Endocrinopathies

One fourth of all pituitary tumors removed surgically do not secrete hormones. The tumors are slowly growing macroadenomas that are diagnosed in older people because of mass effect.

Null cell adenomas are usually chromophobic, are PAS negative and show pseudopapillary growth. By immunohistochemistry, tumor cells are either negative for all anterior pituitary hormones or contain a few cells immunoreactive for chromogranin A and synaptophysin.

Oncocytomas are variants of nonfunctional null cell adenomas characterized by enlarged, eosinophilic and often granular tumor cells. The neoplastic cells are packed with mitochondria but are otherwise similar to other null cell adenomas.

Silent adenomas are distinguished from other nonfunctional pituitary adenomas by their well-differentiated ultrastructural appearance and, in many cases, immunoreactivity for ACTH and other hormones. Silent GH-producing, ACTH-producing tumors may have higher mitotic rates and more aggressive biological behavior.

Plurihormonal Adenomas Show Immunoreactivity for Multiple Hormones

The most common combinations include GH, PRL and one or more glycoprotein hormone subunits.

Pituitary Carcinomas Are Exceedingly Rare

The diagnosis of pituitary carcinoma implies the existence of cerebrospinal and/or systemic metastases. Histologic distinction between pituitary adenoma and carcinoma is not possible. Adults are usually affected, without age or sex preponderance. When functional, they primarily produce PRL or ACTH.

Nonadenomatous Lesions Involving the Pituitary Gland

Nonneoplastic conditions that can involve the pituitary include cysts (Rathke cleft, arachnoid and dermoid), inflammatory lesions and hyperplasia. Various neoplasms, benign and malignant, are described including craniopharyngiomas, gliomas, meningiomas, schwannomas, hematologic malignancies and metastatic lesions (most commonly from breast, lung and prostate).

Posterior Pituitary

MOLECULAR PATHOGENESIS: Central diabetes insipidus (Fig. 21-9) is the only significant condition associated with disease of the posterior pituitary. This disorder is characterized by an inability to concentrate the urine and consequent chronic water diuresis (polyuria), thirst and polydipsia. The biochemical basis of the disease is a deficiency of ADH (vasopressin), which is secreted by the posterior pituitary under the influence of the hypothalamus. One third of cases of central diabetes insipidus are of unknown etiology or can be attributed to sporadic or familial mutations in the vasopressin–neurophysin II gene. Currently, more than 50 mutations have been linked with familial neurohypophysial diabetes insipidus. Mutations or deletions in the vasopressin V2 receptor (Xq28) and the vasopressin-sensitive aquaporin-2 water channel genes have also been described in the context of **nephrogenic diabetes insipidus.**

One fourth of cases of central diabetes insipidus are associated with brain tumors, particularly **craniopharyngioma** (Fig. 21-10). This tumor arises above the sella turcica from remnants of Rathke pouch and invades and compresses adjacent tissues (see Chapter 28). Two variants of this tumor are well characterized: adamantinomatous (predominant in children, and associated with mutations of the β-catenin gene) and papillary. Trauma and hypophysectomy for anterior pituitary tumors account for most of the remaining cases of diabetes insipidus. Uncommonly, localized hemorrhage or infarction, Langerhans cell histiocytosis or granulomatous infiltrates involve the posterior pituitary stalk or body. Polyuria may be controlled by powdered posterior pituitary or vasopressin administered as snuff. Ectopic secretion of

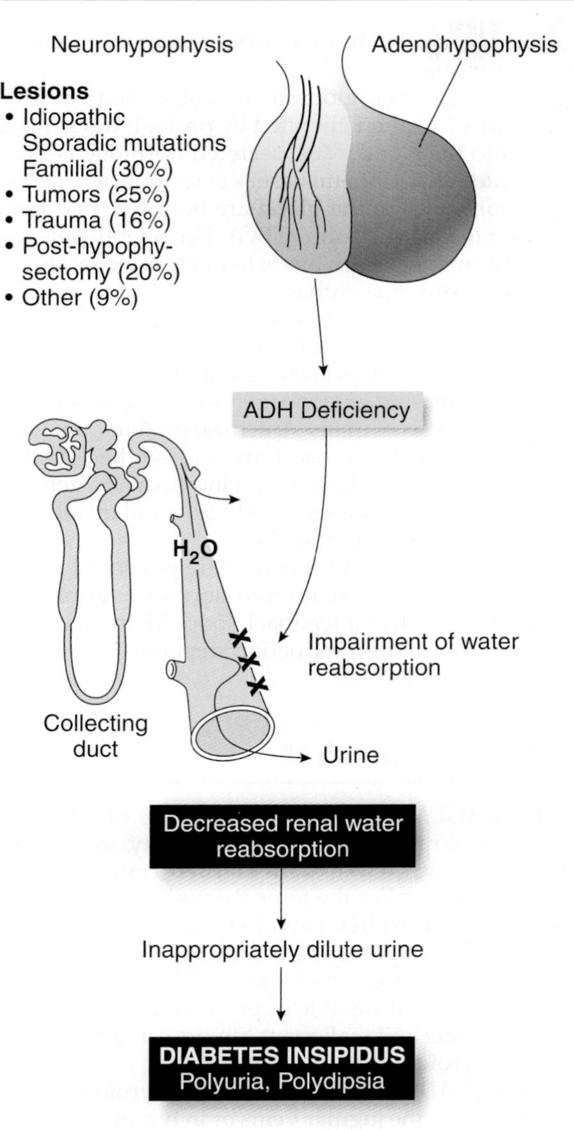

FIGURE 21-9. Mechanism of diabetes insipidus.

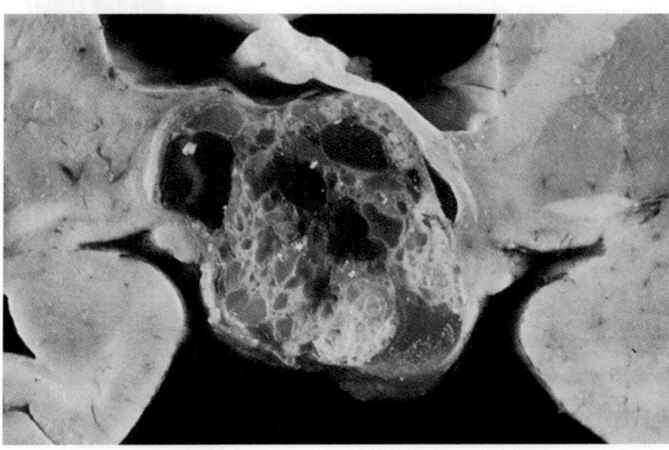

FIGURE 21-10. Craniopharyngioma. Coronal section of the brain shows a large, cystic tumor mass replacing the midline structures in the region of the hypothalamus.

ADH and a syndrome of inappropriate ADH secretion (SIADH) may be caused by paraneoplastic secretion of ADH by tumor cells.

Hypothalamic–Pituitary Axis

The hypothalamus, pituitary stalk and pituitary gland constitute an anatomically and functionally integrated "neuroendocrine system." Neuron groups in the hypothalamus secrete a number of factors that stimulate the anterior pituitary lobe (Table 21-2). Secretion of these hypothalamic factors is, in turn, antagonized by hormones secreted by the peripheral target organs, thereby completing the feedback loop. In addition, specific hypothalamic inhibitory hormones have been identified. For example, dopamine inhibits the pituitary secretion of prolactin.

The hypothalamus may be damaged by a variety of primary and metastatic tumors, viral infections and granulomatous inflammations and several types of degenerative and

Table 21-2

Hormones of the Hypothalamic–Pituitary–Target Gland Axis

Hypothalamus	Pituitary	Target Gland	Peripheral Inhibitory Hormone
CRH	ACTH	Adrenal	Corticosteroids
TRH	TSH	Thyroid	T_3, T_4
GHRH	Growth hormone	Varied	IGF-I
Somatostatin	Growth hormone	Varied	IGF-I
LHRH	LH	Gonads	Estradiol, testosterone
	FSH	Gonads	Inhibin, estradiol, testosterone
Dopamine	Prolactin	Breast	Unknown

ACTH = adrenocorticotropic hormone; CRH = corticotropin (ACTH)-releasing hormone; FSH = follicle-stimulating hormone; GHRH = growth hormone–releasing hormone; IGF-I = insulin-like growth factor-I; LH = luteinizing hormone; LHRH = luteinizing hormone–releasing hormone; T_3 = triiodothyronine; T_4 = tetraiodothyronine (thyroxine); TRH = thyrotropin-releasing hormone; TSH = thyroid-stimulating hormone.

hereditary disorders. In many instances, hypothalamic dysfunction occurs in the absence of an identifiable anatomic abnormality. Diverse conditions result from disturbances of hypothalamic function and include, among others, hypogonadism, precocious puberty, amenorrhea and eating disorders (obesity or anorexia). Some pituitary disorders characterized by increased or decreased hormone secretion have their origin in hypothalamic dysfunction. A detailed description of the hypothalamic syndromes is beyond the scope of this chapter.

THYROID GLAND

Anatomy

The thyroid is one of the largest endocrine organs. It forms early in fetal life and can be recognized as early as 24 days of development. The primitive thyroid descends to its eventual location in the lower anterior neck by elongation of its tubular attachment to the tongue, the thyroglossal duct, which then atrophies around the seventh week of life. The adult thyroid has two lobes connected by an isthmus, and is situated below the thyroid cartilage anterior to the trachea. Each lobe is about 4 cm in greatest dimension. The entire gland weighs 25 to 35 g. The cut surface has a glistening, light brown, lobulated appearance. In its early development, the gland contains cords of cells that will give origin to the follicles or acini, which constitute the functional unit of the thyroid gland. Follicles average about 200 μm in diameter and are formed by a single row of cuboidal cells surrounded by a delicate basement membrane. Approximately 20 to 40 follicles comprise a thyroid lobule, supplied by a lobular artery and sustained by a diffuse mesh of fibrous stroma, lymphatics and connective tissue. The follicles eventually become filled by an eosinophilic, proteinaceous material called **colloid.** This substance represents secreted thyroglobulin, from which active thyroid hormones are released. Immunohistochemical staining for thyroglobulin has become a powerful marker to identify follicular cells. Nuclear staining with thyroid transcription factor (TTF1) also identifies follicular epithelium.

In addition to follicular epithelial cells, the thyroid also contains **parafollicular** or **C cells,** located in the lateral aspects of the upper portion of both thyroid lobes and in close proximity with the follicles. These cells may derive from the neural crest, and they are more prominent in children. C cells produce calcitonin, a calcium-lowering hormone. C cells are difficult to identify using routine stains, but they are readily seen by immunostaining for **calcitonin.** They also express neuroendocrine markers such as chromogranin and synaptophysin.

Function

The main function of the thyroid gland is to make the thyroid hormones triiodothyronine (T_3) and tetraiodothyronine (thyroxine, T_4). T_4 is principally a prohormone; the major effector of thyroid function is T_3. These molecules are formed by iodination of tyrosines in thyroglobulin by the follicular cells. Thyroid hormone synthesis requires H_2O_2 produced by dual oxidases and thyroperoxidase. Iodinated thyroglobulin is then secreted into the lumen of the follicle. Alone among endocrine glands, the thyroid can store a large amount of preformed hormone.

On demand, thyroglobulin is reabsorbed by follicular cells. T_4 and T_3 are then liberated by proteolytic cleavage and released into the blood. Most secreted hormone is T_4, which is deiodinated in peripheral tissues to its more active form, T_3. Thyroid hormones in the blood are both free and bound to thyronine-binding globulin (TBG). Peripheral cells take up only free hormone, which binds to nuclear receptors and initiates specific protein synthesis.

Thyroid hormone affects almost all organs. It stimulates basal metabolic rate and metabolism of carbohydrates, lipids and proteins. It increases body heat and hepatic glucose production by increasing gluconeogenesis and glycogenolysis. It promotes synthesis of many structural proteins, enzymes and other hormones. Glucose use, fatty acid synthesis in the liver, and adipose tissue lipolysis are all increased. In general, thyroid hormone upregulates the body's overall metabolic activities, both anabolic and catabolic.

Thyroid structure and function are governed principally by pituitary TSH. In turn, thyroid hormone suppresses TSH secretion, to complete a feedback loop. Maintenance of normal thyroid hormone production depends on an adequate dietary supply of iodine.

Congenital Anomalies

THYROID AGENESIS: Complete absence of thyroid tissue (athyrosis) is a rare congenital abnormality, usually not discovered until several weeks after birth because maternal thyroid hormone supplies the fetus through the placenta.

ECTOPIC THYROID: Thyroid tissue can be found outside the thyroid gland in a variety of locations as a result of abnormal migration during development. These tissues are functionally normal and capable of producing thyroid hormone. Hyperplastic foci and malignant tumors can develop from the displaced thyroid tissue.

LATERAL ABERRANT THYROID: Thyroid tissue may be located lateral to the jugular veins or in lymph nodes and soft tissue adjacent to the normal gland. A lateral aberrant thyroid may sometimes actually represent well-differentiated metastases from an occult thyroid cancer, while they may be embryonal rests lateral to the thyroid. If the aberrant thyroid tissue is histologically malignant (see below), the lesion should be considered a metastasis.

LINGUAL THYROID: If the thyroid fails to descend during embryogenesis, it remains at its origin as a nodule at the base of the tongue. This happens more in females and usually is found because of difficulty in swallowing, speaking or breathing. Removal may result in total hypothyroidism. These tissues resemble normal thyroid histologically.

HETEROTOPIC THYROID TISSUE: Nests of thyroid tissue may be found anywhere along the path of its descent into the lower neck. Thyroid tissue is also occasionally encountered in the pericardium or mediastinum.

THYROGLOSSAL DUCT CYST: If a thyroglossal duct fails to involute completely, a cystic, fluid-filled remnant may be seen anywhere along the route of the duct. Thyroglossal duct cysts may present at any age as cystic masses of variable size (1 to 4 cm), often in the middle of the neck and attached to the hyoid bone or soft tissues. The cysts can be lined by squamous or respiratory-type epithelium, and contain variable amounts of thyroid tissue. Malignant tumors can develop in the cysts, usually papillary carcinoma. Surgical excision is curative, and portions of the hyoid bone should be removed to avoid recurrences.

Nontoxic Goiter

Goiter, or thyroid enlargement, may be nodular or diffuse. It is classified by its functionality.

Nontoxic goiter (from the Latin, guttur, "throat"), also called simple, colloid, multinodular goiter or nodular hyperplasia, is thyroid enlargement without functional, inflammatory or neoplastic alterations. These patients are euthyroid and without any thyroiditis (see below). They are far more likely to be women than men (8:1). Diffuse goiter is common in adolescence and during pregnancy, whereas the multinodular type usually occurs in people older than 50 years.

ETIOLOGIC FACTORS: In nontoxic goiter, the capacity of the gland to make thyroid hormone leads to thyroid enlargement, which maintains the euthyroid state. The etiology of the decrease in thyroid hormone production is unknown. Goiters can develop in patients taking certain medications (e.g., sulfonamides) or consuming excess iodine. However, in some endemic cases, decreased hormone production is due to low content of iodine in the water.

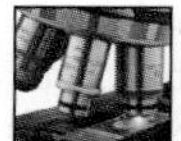

MOLECULAR PATHOGENESIS: Simple nodular thyroid enlargement tends to be familial, suggesting a genetic factor in the disorder. Mutations in the thyroglobulin gene have been detected in some families affected by simple goiter. Linkage analyses in some families identified two chromosomal regions (MNG-1 in chromosome 14q, and Xp22) as possible loci for multinodular goiter. The cells of the nodules may be monoclonal or polyclonal.

PATHOLOGY: Nontoxic goiters range from double the size of a normal gland (40 g) to massive thyroid weighing hundreds of grams (Fig. 21-11).

Diffuse nontoxic goiter occurs early in the disease. The gland is diffusely enlarged and shows hypertrophy and hyperplasia of follicular epithelial cells. On occasion, the epithelium is papillary. At this stage, the amount of colloid in the follicles is decreased.

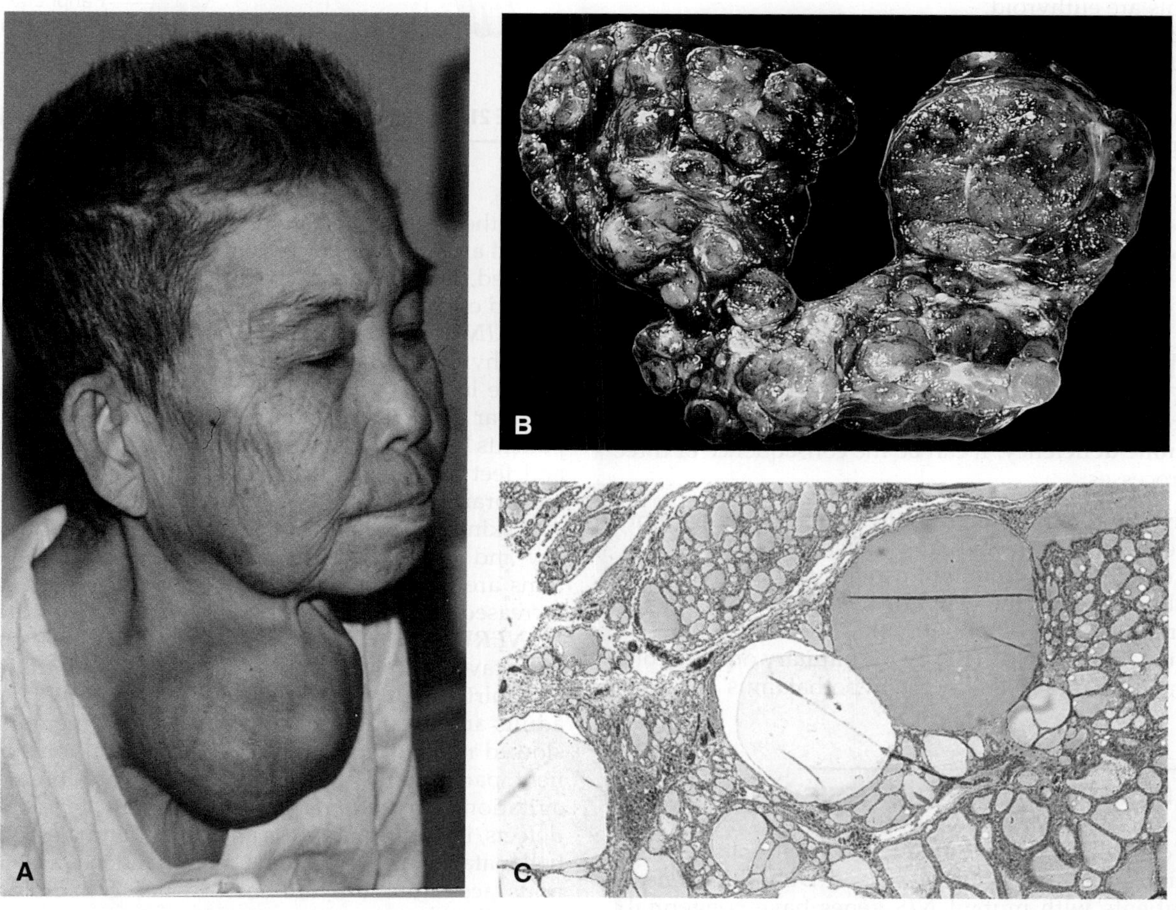

FIGURE 21-11. Nontoxic goiter. A. In a middle-aged woman with nontoxic goiter, the thyroid has enlarged to produce a conspicuous neck mass. **B.** Coronal section of the enlarged thyroid gland shows numerous irregular nodules, some with cystic degeneration and old hemorrhage. **C.** Microscopic view of one of the macroscopic nodules shows marked variation in the size of the follicles.

Multinodular nontoxic goiter reflects more chronic disease. The enlarged gland becomes increasingly nodular, and the cut surface is typically studded with numerous irregular nodules. If these nodules contain large amounts of colloid, the thyroid tends to be soft, glistening and reddish. Microscopically, nodules vary considerably in size and shape. Some are distended with colloid; others are collapsed. Large colloid-containing follicles may fuse to form even larger "colloid cysts." Lining epithelial cells are flat to cuboidal and may be arrayed as papillae that project into the follicular lumen. Hemosiderin deposition and cholesterol granulomas are evidence of old hemorrhage. Individual follicles or groups of follicles are separated by dense fibrosis and dystrophic calcifications. Hemorrhage and chronic inflammation are common.

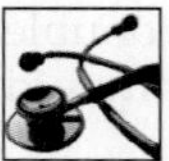

CLINICAL FEATURES: Patients with nontoxic goiter are typically asymptomatic and come to medical attention because of a mass in the neck. Large goiters may cause dysphagia or inspiratory stridor by compressing the esophagus or trachea. Pressure on neck veins may cause venous congestion of the head and face. Hoarseness may result from recurrent laryngeal nerve compression. Occasionally, a single nodule may be the initial manifestation. Hemorrhage into a nodule or cyst may lead to local pain. Blood concentrations of T_4, T_3 and (usually) TSH are normal and patients are euthyroid.

Nontoxic goiter is most commonly treated with thyroid hormone to reduce TSH levels and, thus, the stimulation of thyroid growth. In older patients with low TSH levels, further suppression by exogenous thyroid hormone may be ineffective, and radioactive iodine therapy is indicated. Surgery is ordinarily contraindicated, but may be necessary if local obstructive symptoms become troublesome. Many patients with nontoxic goiter eventually develop hyperthyroidism, in which case the term **toxic multinodular goiter** is applied (see below).

Hypothyroidism

Hypothyroidism refers to the clinical manifestations of thyroid hormone deficiency. It can be the consequence of three general processes:

- **Defective thyroid hormone synthesis,** with compensatory goitrogenesis (goitrous hypothyroidism)
- **Inadequate thyroid function,** usually due to thyroiditis, surgical resection of the gland or therapeutic administration of radioiodine
- **Inadequate secretion of TSH** by the pituitary or of thyroid-releasing hormone (TRH) by the hypothalamus

MOLECULAR PATHOGENESIS: Defects in thyroid H_2O_2 generation in some patients may cause congenital hypothyroidism. These include loss-of-function mutations in *DUOX2* and *DUOXA2* genes. Some patients with mutant *NIS* genes have congenital hypothyroidism due to an iodide transport defect.

Symptoms of hypothyroidism develop insidiously and reflect decreased circulating thyroid hormone (Fig. 21-12).

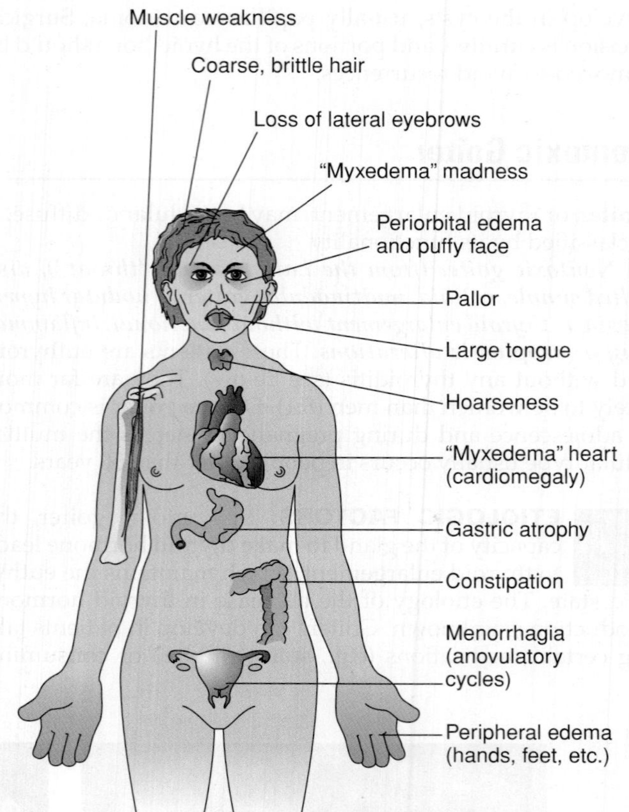

FIGURE 21-12. Dominant clinical manifestations of hypothyroidism.

Often the first manifestations are fatigue, lethargy, sensitivity to cold and inability to concentrate. Many organ systems are affected, but all are hypofunctional. Hypothyroidism is treated effectively with thyroid hormone replacement.

SKIN: Almost all patients with clinically apparent hypothyroidism have cutaneous signs. Proteoglycans accumulate in the extracellular matrix, bind water and cause a peculiar form of edema termed **myxedema.** Myxedematous patients have boggy facies, puffy eyelids, edema of the hands and feet and enlarged tongues. Thickening of the mucous membranes of the larynx causes patients to be hoarse. A pale, cool skin reflects cutaneous vasoconstriction. The skin is also dry and coarse, because sebaceous and sweat gland secretions are inadequate. Ecchymoses are common because of increased capillary fragility. Skin wounds heal slowly.

NERVOUS SYSTEM: Hypothyroidism during pregnancy has grave neurologic consequences for the fetus, expressed after birth as cretinism (see below, Chapter 6). Hypothyroid adults are lethargic and somnolent, show memory loss and slowed mental processes. Psychiatric symptoms are prominent: paranoid ideation and depression are common. Severe agitation, "**myxedema madness,**" may develop. Sensory defects, including deafness and night blindness, occur. Cerebellar ataxia may appear and tendon reflexes are slow. Mucinous accumulations are seen in nerve fibers and in the cerebellum.

HEART: In early hypothyroidism heart rate and stroke volume are reduced, resulting in decreased cardiac output. Left untreated, **myxedema heart** develops, with a dilated heart and pericardial effusion. These hearts are flabby, with interstitial edema and swelling of myocytes. Coronary atherosclerosis is common.

GASTROINTESTINAL TRACT: Decreased peristalsis leads to constipation, which may be severe enough to lead to fecal impaction **(myxedema megacolon).**

REPRODUCTIVE SYSTEM: Women with hypothyroidism suffer ovulatory failure, progesterone deficiency and irregular and excessive menstrual bleeding. In men, erectile dysfunction and oligospermia are common.

Primary (Idiopathic) Hypothyroidism Is Often Autoimmune

Primary hypothyroidism occurs most often in the fifth and sixth decades and, like most thyroid disorders, is more common in women than in men. Three fourths of patients have circulating antibodies to thyroid antigens, suggesting that these cases represent the end stage of autoimmune thyroiditis (see below). Nongoitrous hypothyroidism may also result from antibodies that block TSH or TSH receptor without activating the thyroid. Some cases of primary hypothyroidism are part of multiglandular autoimmune syndrome, including insulin-dependent diabetes, pernicious anemia, hypoparathyroidism, adrenal atrophy and hypogonadism (see below).

Goitrous Hypothyroidism Reflects Inadequate Secretion of Thyroid Hormone

Thyroid enlargement (goiter) may occur in hypothyroidism. The etiology includes iodine deficiency, antithyroid agents (drugs or dietary goitrogens), long-term iodide intake and a number of hereditary defects in thyroid hormone synthesis. ***The evolution of the pathology of goitrous hypothyroidism is similar to that described earlier for nontoxic goiter.***

Endemic Goiter

Endemic goiter is goitrous hypothyroidism due to dietary iodine deficiency in locales with a high prevalence of the disease. Since salt water and seafood are rich sources of iodides, goiters are (or were) common far inland. The Great Lakes area of the United States, alpine Europe, central Africa, parts of China and the Himalayas are such places. The availability of iodized salt has eliminated endemic goiter in many areas. Nevertheless, more than 200 million persons worldwide still have the disease.

The pathologic evolution of endemic goiter is like that of nontoxic goiter (see above), but, unlike the latter, endemic goiter rarely causes hyperthyroidism. Iodine supplements may reverse the early, diffuse stage of endemic goiter, but have little effect on fully developed multinodular goiter. Thyroid hormone replacement therapy is indicated, and local symptoms may necessitate surgical resection.

Goiter Induced by Antithyroid Agents

Several drugs and naturally occurring chemicals in foods suppress thyroid hormone synthesis and so are goitrogenic. Such goiters may or may not be associated with hypothyroidism. Goitrogenic drugs include **lithium,** which is used to treat bipolar disorders; phenylbutazone; and *p*-aminosalicylic acid. Certain cruciferous vegetables (turnips, rutabaga, cassava) contain goitrogens, and can potentiate an iodine-deficient diet to produce goitrous hypothyroidism.

Iodide-Induced Goiter

Goiter and/or hypothyroidism may occur in persons who consume large amounts of iodide, either as a medicinal component (potassium iodide-containing expectorants) or in foods particularly rich in this halide (e.g., seaweed in Japan). In most cases, iodide-induced goiter develops in the context of preexisting thyroid disease, such as thyroiditis. Women given large doses of iodine during pregnancy may deliver goitrous infants.

Congenital Hypothyroidism Is Also Termed Cretinism

Cretinism may be endemic, sporadic or familial, and is twice as frequent in girls as boys. In nonendemic regions, 90% of cases result from developmental defects of the thyroid **(thyroid dysgenesis).** The remainder principally have a variety of inherited metabolic defects, including mutations in genes for TRH and its receptor, TSH and its receptor, sodium-iodide symporter, thyroglobulin and thyroid oxidase.

CLINICAL FEATURES: Symptoms of congenital hypothyroidism appear in the early weeks of life. Infants are apathetic and sluggish. Their abdomens are large and often show umbilical hernias. Body temperatures are often below 35°C (95°F) and the skin is pale and cold. Refractory anemia and a dilated heart are frequent. By the age of 6 months, the clinical syndrome of congenital hypothyroidism is well developed. Mental retardation, stunted growth (owing to defective osseous maturation) and characteristic facies are evident. Serum T_4 and T_3 are low, and TSH levels are high (unless the problem relates to a lack of TSH secretion itself).

Prompt thyroid hormone replacement therapy is needed to prevent mental retardation and stunted growth. Although treatment may prevent dwarfism, its effects on mental development are more variable. Children in whom hypothyroidism is detected early with neonatal screening respond well to thyroid hormone treatment and are apparently normal mentally. Delayed treatment leads to irreversible brain damage.

Endemic cretinism refers to congenital hypothyroidism in areas of endemic goiter. Both parents are usually goitrous. The disease encompasses two overlapping clinical presentations, a neurologic syndrome and a predominantly hypothyroid one.

- **Neurologic cretinism** features mental retardation, ataxia, spasticity and deaf-mutism. In the pure form of neurologic cretinism, children may be of normal stature and virtually euthyroid. It is postulated that iodine deficiency in the first trimester of pregnancy damages the developing nervous system independently of its effect on thyroid hormone production.
- **Hypothyroid cretinism** is thought to arise from iodine deficiency in late fetal life and in the neonatal period. The clinical course in these children is similar to that of other forms of congenital hypothyroidism.

Hyperthyroidism

Hyperthyroidism refers to the clinical consequences of excessive circulating thyroid hormone. Signs and symptoms of hyperthyroidism reflect a hypermetabolic state of target tissues. Prolonged hypersecretion of thyroid hormone can result from (1) an abnormal thyroid stimulator (Graves disease), (2) intrinsic disease of the thyroid gland (toxic multinodular goiter or functional adenoma) and (3) excess TSH production by a pituitary adenoma (rare).

Graves Disease Is the Most Common Cause of Hyperthyroidism in Young Adults

Also known as **diffuse toxic goiter** and **Basedow disease** in continental Europe, Graves disease is an autoimmune disorder characterized by diffuse goiter, hyperthyroidism, exophthalmos (Fig. 21-13), tachycardia weight loss and dermopathy. It is the most prevalent autoimmune disease in the United States, affecting 0.5% to 1% of the population under 40 years of age. The disease can also affect children.

MOLECULAR PATHOGENESIS: The etiology of Graves disease is not fully understood and seems to involve an interplay between immune mechanisms, heredity, gender and possibly emotional factors.

IMMUNE MECHANISMS: Graves patients have immunoglobulin G (IgG) antibodies that bind specific domains of the plasma membrane TSH receptor on thyrocytes (Fig. 21-14). ***These antibodies act as agonists;*** that is, they stimulate the TSH receptor, thereby activating adenylyl cyclase and increasing thyroid hormone secretion. With this continued stimulation, the thyroid becomes diffusely hyperplastic and excessively vascular.

Production of such antibodies requires helper ($CD4^+$) T cells that recognize multiple epitopes of the TSH receptor and stimulate autoreactive B cells, which then produce thyroid-stimulating immunoglobulins. Graves autoantibodies are heterogeneous, and those that stimulate thyroid hormone secretion represent only one component. Other antibodies seem to be cytotoxic and may cause the thyroid failure that often follows long-standing Graves disease. These include antibodies against thyroglobulin, thyroid peroxidase and the sodium–iodide symporter, all of which may also play roles in the pathogenesis of chronic lymphocytic thyroiditis (Hashimoto disease; see below). Patients with Graves disease have low levels of suppressor $CD8^+$ cells, which may play a role in the lack of immune tolerance.

GENETIC FACTORS: The biggest risk factor for Graves disease is positive family history. No one gene is responsible or necessary for Graves disease, and concordance in monozygotic twins is only 30% to 50%, while in dizygotic twins it is merely 5%. Thus, both genetic and environmental factors are probably involved. Human leukocyte antigen (HLA) class II molecules on thyrocytes (e.g., HLA-DR3, HLA-DQA1) are considered to be susceptibility loci, with several of these increasing the relative risk of Graves disease up to fourfold. Graves disease is also associated with polymorphism of cytotoxic T-lymphocyte antigen-4 (CTLA-4), on chromosome 2q33, which indicates the importance of autoreactive T cells. Patients with Graves disease and their relatives have a considerably higher incidence of other autoimmune diseases, including pernicious anemia and Hashimoto thyroiditis. Some asymptomatic, first-degree relatives of these patients also have increased ^{131}I uptake. White patients with Graves disease more often express HLA-B8 and HLA-DR3, while Chinese patients are more likely to be positive for HLA-Bw46, and Japanese ones for HLA-Bw35.

A new polymorphic gene family called the *major histocompatibility complex class I chain-related gene A* (MICA) has been linked to regulation of Graves disease. Genotype *MICA A5* is a risk factor for development of Graves disease, whereas genotype *MICA A6/A9* may be preventive.

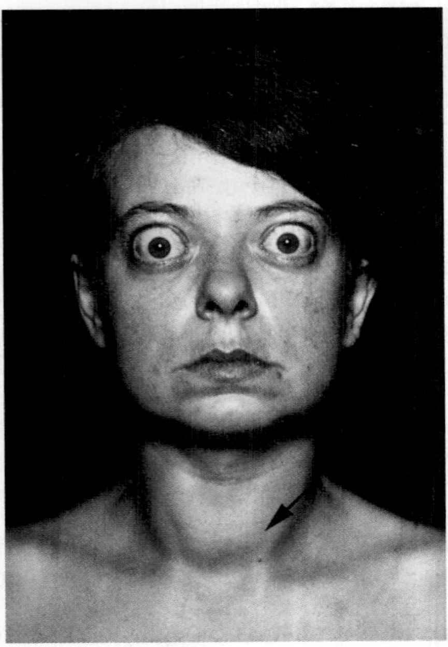

FIGURE 21-13. Graves disease. A young woman with hyperthyroidism displays a mass in the neck and exophthalmos.

ETIOLOGIC FACTORS:

SEX: Like other autoimmune diseases, Graves disease is far more common (7 to 10 times) in females. Interestingly, it tends to arise at times of hormonal imbalance, including puberty, pregnancy and menopause. Men with Graves disease are usually older, and while they may show greater thyroid hyperfunction, their symptoms tend to be less severe.

EMOTIONAL INFLUENCES: Endocrinologists have long observed that onset of Graves disease often follows a period of emotional stress, such as separation anxiety, death of a loved one or near injury in an accident. Quantitative data are lacking.

SMOKING: Smoking is associated with increased risk of Graves disease, and it increases the severity of the eye disease in patients who develop ophthalmopathy.

OPHTHALMOPATHY: Although exophthalmos (protrusion of eyeballs) is common in Graves disease (Fig. 21-13), its occurrence and severity correlate poorly with thyroid hormone levels. A combination of humoral and cell-mediated

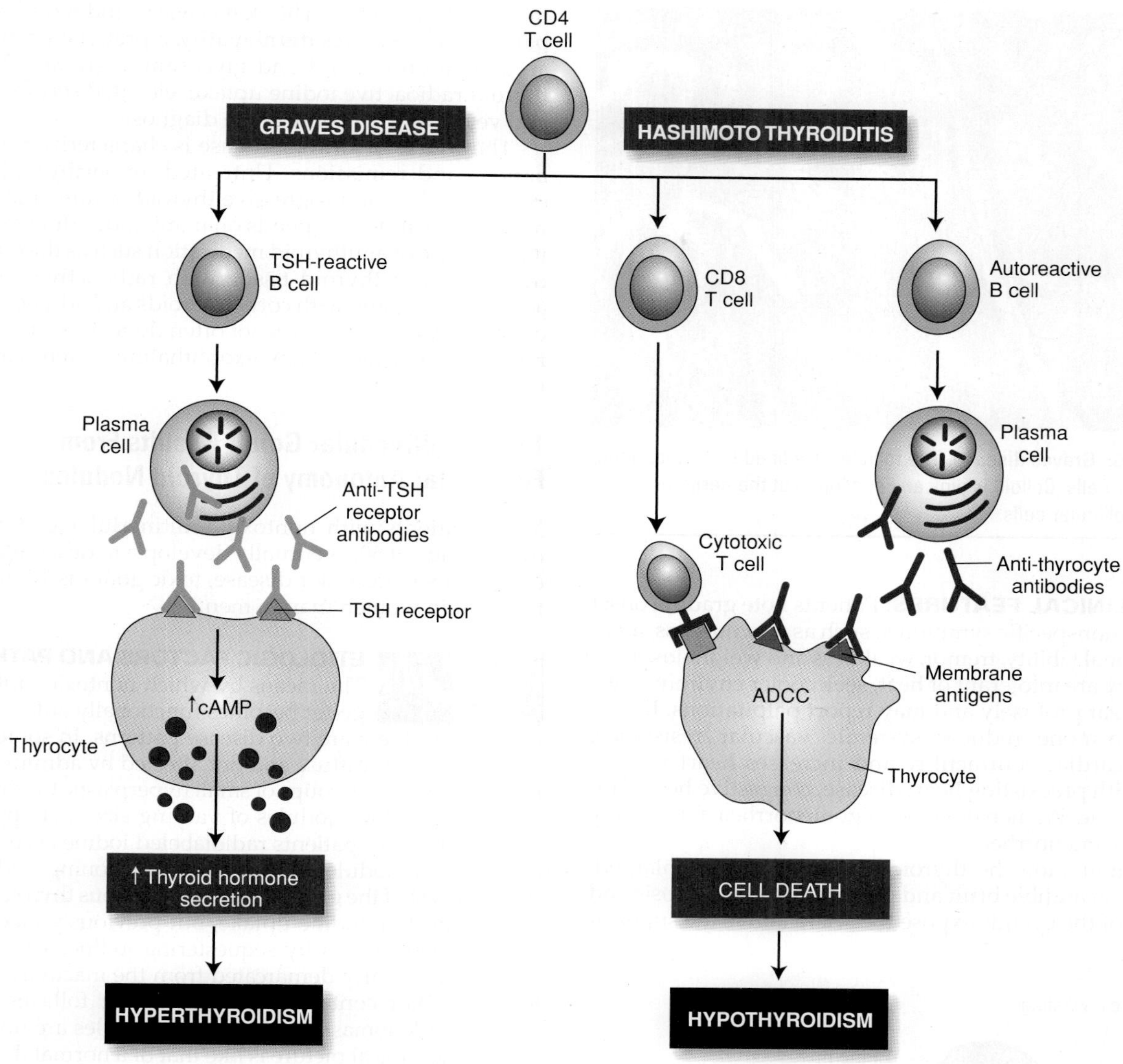

FIGURE 21-14. Immune mechanisms of Graves disease and Hashimoto thyroiditis. $CD4^+$ T cells stimulate antibody production by autoreactive B cells. Anti–thyroid-stimulating hormone (TSH) receptor antibodies stimulate thyroid hormone synthesis in Graves disease. Antibodies induce thyrocyte cell death in Hashimoto thyroiditis by complement-dependent cytotoxicity and antibody-dependent cell-mediated cytotoxicity (ADDC). Thyrocyte death also results from attack by $CD8^+$ (cytotoxic) T cells. cAMP = cyclic adenosine 3′,5′-monophosphate.

immune mechanisms is likely involved. T lymphocytes sensitized to antigens shared by thyroid follicular cells and orbital fibroblasts (possibly TSH receptor) accumulate around the eye and secrete cytokines that activate fibroblasts. Systemic or local production of antibodies may stimulate orbital fibroblasts to proliferate and produce collagen and glycosaminoglycans.

PATHOLOGY: The thyroid in Graves disease is symmetrically enlarged, usually 35 to 100 g. Cut surfaces are firm and dark red. The tan translucence of normal thyroid, due to stored colloid, is notably absent. The gland is diffusely hyperplastic and highly vascular. The epithelial cells are tall and columnar and are often arranged as papillae that project into the lumen of the follicles. This papillary proliferation can be misdiagnosed as papillary carcinoma. However, the nucleus is hyperchromatic, not clear as it is in cancer. Colloid appears depleted and is pale, scalloped or "moth-eaten" where it abuts epithelial cells (Fig. 21-15). Scattered B and T lymphocytes and plasma cells infiltrate the interstitial tissue, and germinal centers may be seen. Hyperplastic follicles are occasionally found outside the gland's capsule and even in adjacent muscle.

Therapy with antithyroid medication (e.g., methimazole or propylthiouracil) commonly results in increased thyroid hyperplasia and complete lack of colloid.

Exophthalmos is caused by enlargement of orbital extraocular muscles. These muscles themselves are normal, but are swollen by mucinous edema, accumulation of fibroblasts and lymphocyte infiltration. The increased orbital contents displace the eye forward **(proptosis).**

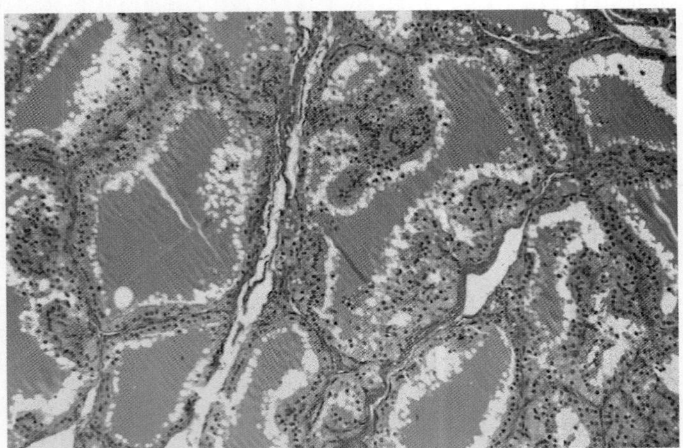

FIGURE 21-15. Graves disease. The follicles are lined by hyperplastic, tall columnar cells. Colloid is pink and scalloped at the periphery adjacent to the follicular cells.

CLINICAL FEATURES: Patients note gradual onset of nonspecific symptoms, such as nervousness, emotional lability, tremor, weakness and weight loss (Fig. 21-16). They are intolerant of heat, seek cooler environments, tend to sweat profusely and may report palpitations. Excess thyroid hormone reduces systemic vascular resistance, enhances cardiac contractility and increases heart rate. In patients with preexisting heart disease, congestive heart failure may ensue. Women develop oligomenorrhea, which may progress to amenorrhea.

On examination the thyroid is symmetrically enlarged, often with an audible bruit and palpable thrill. Proptosis and retraction of the eyelids expose the sclera above the superior margin of the limbus. The skin is warm and moist, and some patients have **Graves dermopathy,** a pretibial edema due to accumulation of fluid and glycosaminoglycans. Increased thyroid radioactive iodine uptake, elevated serum T_4 and T_3 and very low TSH confirm the diagnosis.

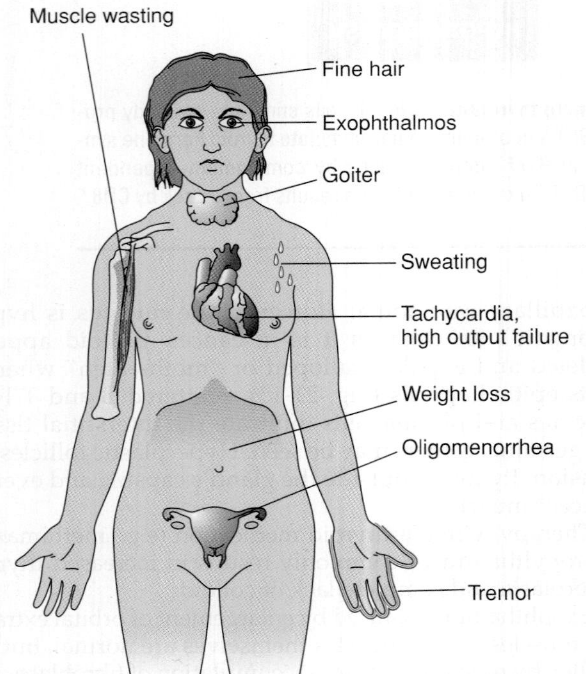

FIGURE 21-16. Major clinical manifestations of Graves disease.

The course of Graves disease is characterized by exacerbations and remissions. Untreated, hyperthyroidism may eventually lead to progressive thyroid failure and hypothyroidism. Treatment depends on many individual factors and includes use of antithyroid medication such as thioisocyanate, destruction of thyroid tissue with radioactive iodine and adjunctive therapy with corticosteroids and adrenergic antagonists. Surgical ablation is not often done. Despite successful relief of hyperthyroidism, exophthalmos often persists and may even worsen.

Toxic Multinodular Goiter Results From Functional Autonomy of Thyroid Nodules

Many patients with nontoxic multinodular goiter, usually over the age of 50, eventually develop a toxic form of the disease. Like its precursor disease, toxic goiter is 10 times more frequent in women than in men.

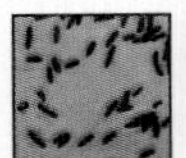
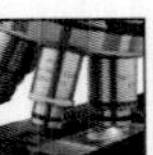

ETIOLOGIC FACTORS AND PATHOLOGY: The means by which nontoxic multinodular goiter becomes functionally autonomous are unclear, but there are two disease patterns. In some patients, iodine uptake is diffuse and not affected by administration of thyroid hormone. Groups of small hyperplastic thyroid follicles mingle with other nodules of varying size that appear to be inactive. In other patients radiolabeled iodine accumulates in one or more nodules. These hyperfunctioning nodules suppress the rest of the gland. Further exogenous thyroid hormone has no effect on iodine uptake, but previously inactive areas will respond to TSH by sequestering iodine. The functional nodules are clearly demarcated from the inactive areas histologically. They contain large hyperplastic follicles, and thus resemble adenomas. The functional nodules are not neoplastic, but the clinical picture is like that of a normal thyroid with a single hyperfunctioning adenoma.

CLINICAL FEATURES: Patients with toxic multinodular goiter usually have less severe symptoms of hyperthyroidism than those with Graves disease and never develop exophthalmos. Since patients with toxic goiter tend to be older, cardiac complications, including atrial fibrillation and congestive heart failure, may dominate the clinical presentation. Serum T_4 and T_3 levels are often minimally elevated, and radiolabeled iodine uptake may be normal or only slightly elevated. Antithyroid medication followed by radioiodine is the most common therapy.

Toxic Adenoma Is a Benign, Solitary, Hyperfunctioning Thyroid Neoplasm

These follicular tumors develop in an otherwise normal thyroid and are infrequent causes of hyperthyroidism. They (1) display autonomous function, (2) are independent of TSH and (3) are not suppressed if thyroid hormone is given. A hyperfunctioning toxic adenoma will eventually suppress the rest of the thyroid, which then atrophies. At that point, a ^{131}I scintiscan shows a lone focus of iodine uptake ("hot nodule") in a gland with minimal uptake. Many, but not all, toxic adenomas carry somatic mutations of the TSH receptor gene, causing constitutive activation of the cAMP cascade and less commonly the inositol phosphate-diacylglycerol system.

CLINICAL FEATURES: Toxic thyroid adenomas occur most often in the fourth and fifth decades of life. Symptoms of hyperthyroidism usually begin when the adenoma is about 3 cm in diameter. Spontaneous necrosis and hemorrhage may occur within an adenoma and relieve the hyperthyroidism. In this case the rest of the gland resumes its normal function, and the adenoma appears as a "cold" nodule in a scintigram, simulating thyroid cancer.

Since normal thyroid tissue is suppressed, toxic adenomas are treated effectively with radiolabeled iodine. Large nodules may be excised surgically, especially in young patients to minimize risk of thyroid cancer that may occur years after radiolabeled iodine administration.

Thyroiditis

Thyroiditides are a heterogeneous group of inflammatory disorders of the thyroid gland, including those caused by autoimmune mechanisms and infectious agents.

Acute Thyroiditis Usually Reflects Thyroid Involvement in Acute Systemic Infections

The responsible infectious agent reaches the thyroid by hematogenous spread. The most common causative organisms are *Streptococcus*, *Staphylococcus* and *Pneumococcus*. Other causes include fungi, *Pneumocystis* and cytomegalovirus. Patients of all ages can be affected, but children, elderly or immunocompromised patients are most commonly affected.

Patients present with fever, chills, malaise and a painful, swollen neck. Infection may involve one lobe or the entire gland, with diffuse acute and chronic inflammation and focal microabscess formation. Rarely, acute thyroiditis is complicated by extension of the infection into the trachea, mediastinum and esophagus. The prognosis is excellent with prompt antibiotic therapy.

Chronic Autoimmune Thyroiditis (Hashimoto Thyroiditis) Is the Most Common Cause of Goitrous Hypothyroidism in the United States

Hashimoto thyroiditis (HT) occurs predominantly in women 30 to 50 years of age, although both sexes and all ages can be affected. Patients present with diffuse thyroid enlargement and mild hyperthyroidism or hypothyroidism. HT can affect several family members who often also suffer other autoimmune conditions such as lupus, Graves disease, arteritis and scleroderma.

MOLECULAR PATHOGENESIS: The autoimmune process in HT arises from activation of CD4 (helper) T lymphocytes sensitized to thyroid antigens (Fig. 21-14). Helper T-cell activation may be initiated by viral or bacterial infection.

In turn, these $CD4^+$ cells stimulate proliferation of autoreactive cytotoxic ($CD8^+$) T cells, which attack thyrocytes. The activated lymphocytes secrete interferon-γ, causing thyrocytes to express major histocompatability complex (MHC) class II molecules (HLA-DR, DP, DQ), thereby expanding the autoreactive T-cell population. These effects account for the striking accumulation of lymphocytes in the glands of patients with autoimmune thyroiditis.

Activated CD4 cells also recruit autoreactive B cells to produce antibodies against thyroid antigens, including thyroid microsomal peroxidase (95%), thyroglobulin (60%) and TSH receptor. Cytotoxic antibodies that fix complement are described in some patients. Antibody-dependent cell-mediated cytotoxicity (ADCC) may further magnify thyroid injury. Unlike the stimulatory anti-TSH receptor antibodies in Graves disease, autoantibodies in HT block TSH action. Similar blocking antibodies are detectable in 10% of patients with goitrous autoimmune thyroiditis and in 20% of those with end-stage atrophy of the gland. Half of all first-degree relatives of patients with HT have antithyroid antibodies, suggesting autosomal dominant transmission. Moreover, both Graves disease and chronic autoimmune thyroiditis are described in these family members. A familial tendency for HT is further suggested by the higher prevalence of other autoimmune diseases in patients and their relatives, including MEN syndrome type 2, insulin-dependent diabetes, pernicious anemia, Addison disease and myasthenia gravis. Autoimmunity and thyroiditis occur disproportionately in people with Down syndrome and familial Alzheimer disease, which has focused attention on chromosome 21, but no genetic causes of these disorders are known. Interestingly, half of adults with Turner syndrome, especially those with an X isochromosome, have antithyroid antibodies, and a third develop hypothyroidism. Only association with HLA and CTLA-4 genes has been seen consistently, but how these contribute to autoimmune thyroiditis remains obscure.

HT is highest in regions with the greatest **intake of iodine,** for example, Japan and the United States. In iodine-deficient areas, iodine supplementation increases the prevalence of chronic inflammation of the thyroid and the presence of thyroid autoantibodies.

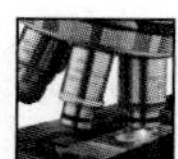

PATHOLOGY: Thyroids of patients with HT are diffusely enlarged and firm, weighing 60 to 200 g. The cut surfaces are pale tan and fleshy with a vaguely nodular pattern (Fig. 21-17). The capsule is intact; perithyroid tissues are not involved. Microscopically, the gland shows (1) a conspicuous infiltrate of lymphocytes and plasma cells, (2) destruction and atrophy of follicles and (3) oxyphilic metaplasia of follicular epithelial cells **(Hürthle or Askanazy cells).** Lymphoid follicles, often with germinal centers, are present. The Askanazy cells are filled with mitochondria and frequently show nuclear atypia, which may be mistaken for cancer. Interstitial fibrosis is present to a varying extent and in 10% of cases is particularly conspicuous (fibrous variant). The thyroid eventually atrophies in some patients, leaving a small, fibrotic gland infiltrated by lymphocytes. Thyroid lymphoma is a rare complication of HT.

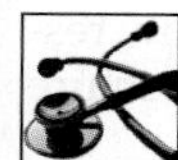

CLINICAL FEATURES: HT mainly affects women 30 to 50 years old, but no age group is spared. Patients present with diffuse thyroid enlargement

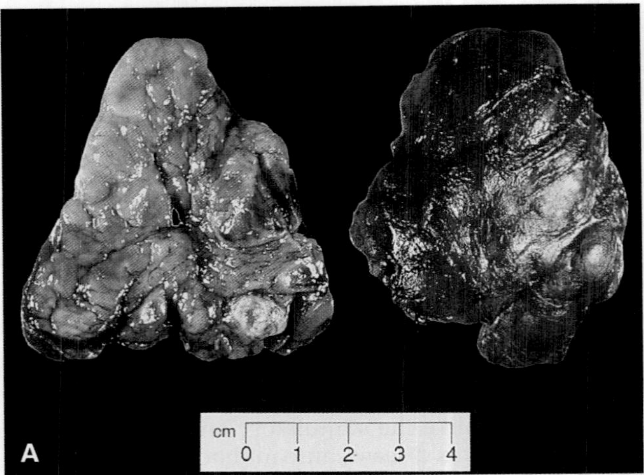

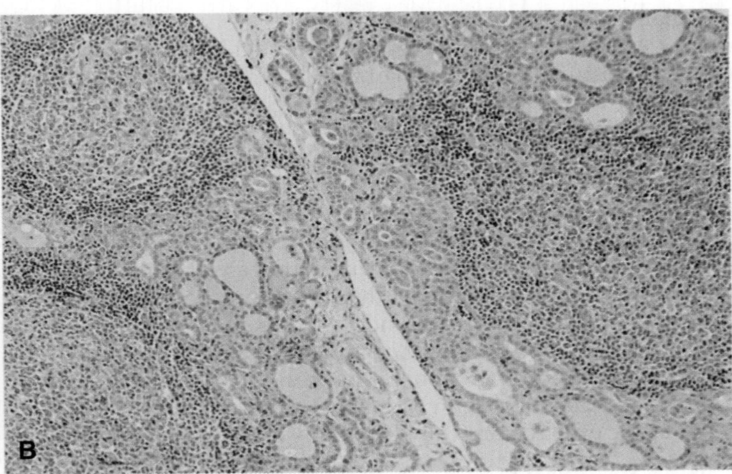

FIGURE 21-17. Chronic autoimmune (Hashimoto) thyroiditis. The thyroid gland is symmetrically enlarged and coarsely nodular. **A.** A coronal section of the right lobe shows irregular nodules and an intact capsule. **B.** A microscopic section of the thyroid reveals a conspicuous chronic inflammatory infiltrate and many atrophic thyroid follicles. The inflammatory cells form prominent lymphoid follicles with germinal centers.

and either mild hyperthyroidism or hypothyroidism. Goiter usually begins insidiously, although sometimes the gland enlarges rapidly. In time, one third to one half of patients—men disproportionately more than women—develop overt hypothyroidism. Rarely, hyperthyroidism may occur **(hashitoxicosis).** HT is now diagnosed by detecting circulating antithyroid antibodies (seen in 95% of patients), antithyroglobulin and cell membrane antibodies. Patients show low T_4 levels, elevated serum thyrotropin and thyroxine index and elevated TSH. HT may often coexist with papillary cancer.

Many patients require no treatment. Thyroid hormone is given to alleviate hypothyroidism and decrease the size of the gland. Surgery is reserved for patients who do not respond to suppressive hormone therapy or with troublesome pressure symptoms.

Subacute Thyroiditis (de Quervain, Granulomatous or Giant Cell Thyroiditis) Is Caused by a Viral Infection

This nonsuppurative thyroiditis is an infrequent, self-limited disorder characterized by granulomatous inflammation. It typically occurs after upper respiratory viral infections, such as with influenza virus, adenovirus, echovirus and coxsackievirus. Mumps virus has occasionally been incriminated as well. De Quervain thyroiditis principally affects women 30 to 50 years old. Its true incidence is unknown as many infectious thyroiditides are reported under this name.

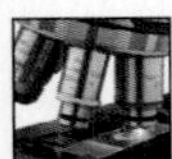

PATHOLOGY: The thyroid is enlarged to 40 to 60 g, and its cut surface is firm and pale. Acute inflammation, often with microabscesses, is followed by a patchy infiltrate of lymphocytes, plasma cells and macrophages throughout the gland. Colloid released as follicles are destroyed elicits a florid granulomatous reaction (Fig. 21-18). Numerous foreign body–type multinucleated giant cells, often containing colloid, are present. Fibrosis may follow resolution of the inflammation, but normal thyroid architecture is usually restored.

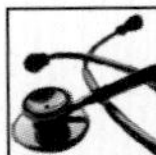

CLINICAL FEATURES: Patients with subacute thyroiditis typically notice pain in the anterior neck or radiating to the jaw, sometimes accompanied by fever, malaise and fatigue. Other patients follow a mild course with only minimal symptoms. The disorder is often mistaken for pharyngitis, because of a preceding respiratory tract infection and the presence of hoarseness and dysphagia. On physical examination, the thyroid is moderately enlarged and exquisitely tender. Subacute thyroiditis generally resolves within a few months without any clinical sequelae. Iodine uptake is usually suppressed in the early stages of the disease.

Destruction of follicles releases preformed thyroid hormone. Serum T_4 and T_3 may be high, sometimes high enough to cause transient clinical hyperthyroidism. The consequent suppression of TSH leads to decreased uptake of radiolabeled iodine. This phase is followed by decreased serum T_4 and T_3 levels, but as subacute thyroiditis resolves, a euthyroid state is restored.

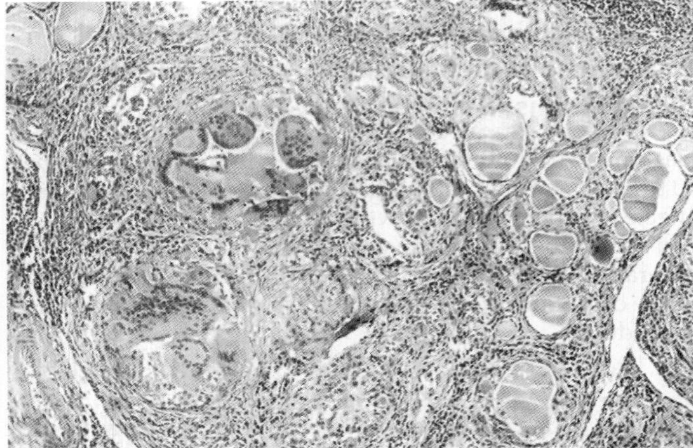

FIGURE 21-18. Subacute thyroiditis. The release of colloid into the interstitial tissue has elicited a prominent granulomatous reaction, with numerous foreign body giant cells.

Silent Thyroiditis Causes Transient Hyperthyroidism

Silent thyroiditis, also termed **painless subacute thyroiditis** or **lymphocytic thyroiditis,** is characterized by painless thyroid enlargement, self-limited hyperthyroidism, destruction of gland parenchyma and lymphocytic infiltration. Thus, it clinically resembles subacute thyroiditis but pathologically is more similar to HT. Importantly, silent thyroiditis differs from the latter by the lack of antithyroid antibodies or other evidence of autoimmune thyroiditis. However, association with HLA-DR3 has been reported. As in subacute thyroiditis, the hyperthyroid state reflects release of preformed thyroid hormone from injured glands.

Silent thyroiditis mainly affects women, often in the postpartum period. Hyperthyroidism usually lasts 2 to 4 months. Treatment is symptomatic, and most patients become euthyroid.

Riedel Thyroiditis Causes Fibrosis of the Thyroid

The "thyroiditis" in Riedel thyroiditis is something of a misnomer, as this rare disease also involves the soft tissues of the neck and may accompany progressive fibrosis in other locations, including the retroperitoneum, mediastinum and orbit. Riedel thyroiditis is mainly a disease of middle age. The female-to-male ratio is 3:1. The etiology is unknown, but it does not appear to be related to other forms of thyroiditis.

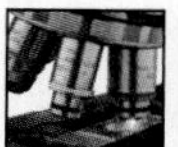

PATHOLOGY: Grossly, part or all of the thyroid is stony hard and "woody." The process is usually asymmetric and often affects only one lobe. The fibrous infiltrate extends into the thyroid gland and other tissues of the neck, including skeletal muscle and nerves, and may also surround and infiltrate lymph nodes and parathyroid glands. The surgeon may have extreme difficulty identifying a tissue plane. Dense, hyalinized fibrous tissue and a chronic inflammatory infiltrate are seen throughout involved portions of the thyroid (Fig. 21-19). Eosinophils may be also present. Follicles are normal in the unaffected parts of the gland. Fibrosis may surround and infiltrate skeletal muscle, nerves, fat, blood vessels and, sometimes, the parathyroids.

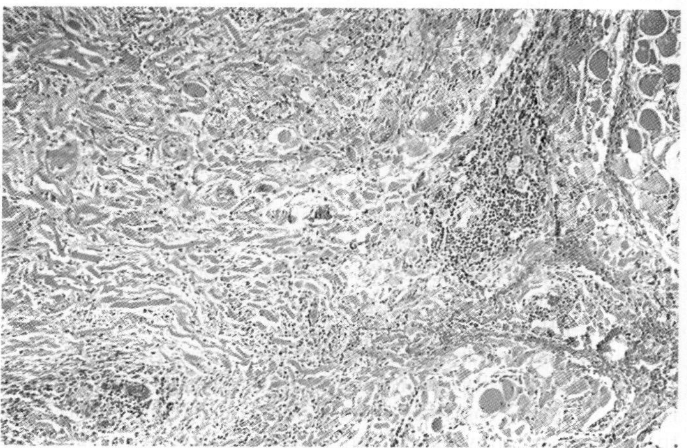

FIGURE 21-19. Riedel thyroiditis. The thyroid parenchyma is largely replaced by dense, hyalinized fibrous tissue and a chronic inflammatory infiltrate.

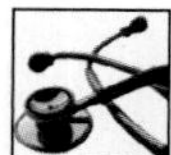

CLINICAL FEATURES: Patients notice gradual onset of painless goiter and present with a hard thyroid mass. Fibrosing lesions in other sites, such as the retroperitoneum, mediastinum and retro-orbital tissues, may be present. Immunophenotyping shows a predominance of T cells with few B cells. Compression of neck organs may lead to stridor (trachea), dysphagia (esophagus) or hoarseness (recurrent laryngeal nerve). Involvement of the entire thyroid is rare, and may cause hypothyroidism. Surgery is needed to relieve the compression of the local organs.

Follicular Adenoma of the Thyroid

Follicular adenoma is a benign neoplasm showing follicular differentiation. It is the most common thyroid tumor, and typically presents in euthyroid persons as a "cold" nodule (i.e., a tumor that does not take up radiolabeled iodine). It is a solitary encapsulated neoplasm in which the cells are arranged in follicles resembling normal thyroid gland or mimicking stages in the gland's embryonic development. Multiple adenomas may occur. In up to 90% of cases, palpable, solitary follicular lesions are actually the dominant nodule in a multinodular goiter, and follicular adenomas are correspondingly infrequent. Follicular adenoma is most common in the fourth and fifth decades, with a female-to-male ratio of 7:1. The clonal origin of follicular adenomas has been established. Follicular adenomas occur frequently in iodine-deficient areas. They can also occur in irradiated glands and as part of Cowden syndrome.

MOLECULAR PATHOGENESIS: Adenomas are clonal in over 60% of cases. Molecular changes include trisomy 7, translocations in 19q13 and deletions in chromosomes 3p, 10 and 13. The oncocytic variants of adenomas have been known to have alterations in mitochondrial DNA.

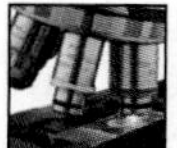

PATHOLOGY: Follicular adenomas are solitary, circumscribed, 1- to 3-cm nodules that protrude from the surface of the thyroid and are completely surrounded by a thin fibrous capsule. The tumor cut surface is soft and paler than the surrounding gland. Hemorrhage, fibrosis and cystic change are common. There are several distinctive histologic patterns (Fig. 21-20), the main significance of which is to aid in distinguishing such adenomas from thyroid cancers.

- **Embryonal adenoma** is distinguished by a trabecular pattern with poorly formed follicles containing little or no colloid (Fig. 21-20B).
- **Fetal adenoma** displays cells that are similar to those of embryonal adenoma but tend to be arranged in microfollicles containing little colloid (Fig. 21-20C).
- **Simple adenoma** exhibits mature follicles with a normal amount of colloid.
- **Colloid adenoma** resembles simple adenoma but follicles are larger, with more colloid (Fig. 21-20A).
- **Hürthle (oncocytic) cell adenoma** is a solid tumor with oxyphil cells, small follicles and scant colloid (Fig. 21-20D). These often become infarcted after needle aspiration biopsy.

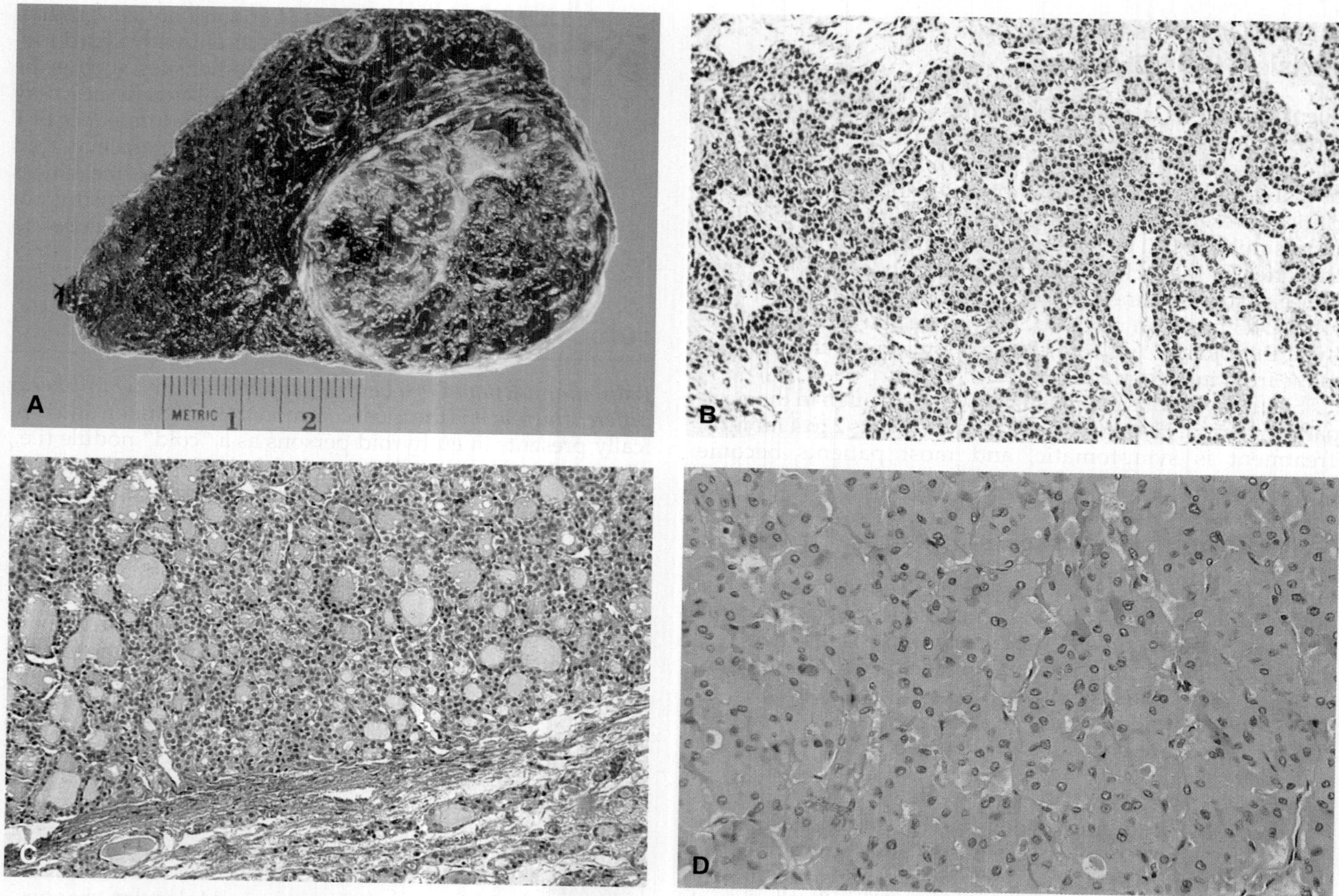

FIGURE 21-20. Follicular adenoma. A. Colloid adenoma. The cut surface of an encapsulated mass reveals hemorrhage, fibrosis and cystic change. **B.** Embryonal adenoma. The tumor features a trabecular pattern with poorly formed follicles that contain little if any colloid. **C.** Fetal adenoma. A regular pattern of small follicles is noted. **D.** Hürthle cell adenoma. The tumor is composed of cells with small, regular nuclei and abundant eosinophilic cytoplasm.

- **Atypical adenoma** shows mitoses, excessive cellularity, nuclear atypism or equivocal capsular invasion, but a diagnosis of carcinoma cannot be established with certainty.

These benign lesions should be differentiated from follicular carcinomas (see below), which usually have thicker capsules. Careful evaluation of the capsule for capsular or vascular invasion is mandatory to make this distinction. ***Malignancies can develop in association with, or within, benign nodules.*** Surgical lobectomy to remove the lesion is curative.

Papillary Hyperplastic Nodules

Papillary hyperplastic nodules occur mainly in children and young women. These solitary lesions are well circumscribed and well encapsulated. They are made of variably sized papillae in which the stalks may contain small follicles. Papillae are lined by cuboidal cells with characteristic follicular nuclei (i.e., dense and dispersed chromatin). The centers of nodules are often cystic and can contain colloidlike material. These lesions are commonly misdiagnosed as papillary cancer.

Thyroid Cancer

Malignant thyroid tumors cause 0.4% of all cancer deaths in the United States. Approximately 10,000 new cases are diagnosed each year. Mortality from thyroid cancer exceeds that from malignant tumors of all other endocrine organs.

The difficulty of distinguishing clinically between nonneoplastic lesions, benign tumors and thyroid cancer is a major clinical and pathologic concern. Thyroid nodules are found in 1% to 10% of the population, but malignant thyroid tumors make up only about 1% of all cancers. A single nodule has up to a 12% chance of being malignant; these odds decrease significantly (to about 3%) if a nodule is palpable.

Most cases of thyroid carcinoma occur between the third and seventh decades, but children can also be affected. Tumors occur in women 2.5 times more often than in men.

Fine-needle biopsy of thyroid nodules makes a diagnosis in most cases. Prognosis is a function of the morphology of the tumor, and may range from a very indolent clinical course to a rapidly fatal disease. The latter outcome is fortunately uncommon.

Radioscintigraphy of the gland may help in assessing thyroid tumors, since hyperfunctioning nodules are usually benign. "Cold" or nonfunctioning nodules, on the other hand, although more frequently malignant, may also be benign.

Papillary Thyroid Carcinoma Is the Most Common Thyroid Cancer

Up to 90% of sporadic cases of thyroid cancer in the United States are papillary thyroid carcinoma (PTC). It can affect any age, even children, but is most frequent between 20 and 50 years of age, with a female-to-male ratio of 3:1. PTC is the most common thyroid tumor in children and young adolescents. Elderly men have a worse prognosis with this type of thyroid cancer.

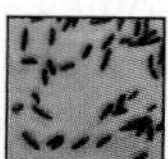

ETIOLOGIC FACTORS: The etiology of PTC is unknown, but several associations have been identified.

- **Iodine excess:** PTC can be produced in animals by administering excess iodine. In areas with endemic goiter, adding iodine to the diet increased the proportion of thyroid cancers showing papillary, as compared with follicular, morphology.
- **Radiation:** External radiation to the neck of children and adults increases the incidence of later PTC, as exemplified by a greater than expected incidence in survivors of atomic bomb explosions in Japan and an almost 100-fold increase of PTC in children living in contaminated areas around Chernobyl, the site in Ukraine of a nuclear reactor catastrophe in 1986. The younger the children, the higher the risk, since younger children take up more radioactive iodine. With regard to PTC, radiation produces double-strand breaks in DNA that can affect *RET* rearrangements (see below). On the other hand, treatment with radiolabeled iodine does not increase the risk of this tumor.

MOLECULAR PATHOGENESIS: Epidemiologic studies show that first-degree relatives of patients with PTC have a 4- to 10-fold higher risk for PTC. Concordance for PTC has been described in monozygotic twins. A familial form of PTC accounts for some 5% of all cases, but the genes responsible have not been identified. PTC also occurs in association with familial adenomatous polyposis syndrome.

- **Somatic mutations:** Somatic rearrangements of the *RET* proto-oncogene on chromosome 10 (10q11.2) are common in PTC, and 60% of such tumors in children exposed to radiation from the Chernobyl accident showed this mutation. The same mutation occurs after external radiation to the thyroid. These rearrangements link the tyrosine kinase domain of *RET* to various other genes, creating *RET/PTC* fusion oncogenes. The frequency of *RET/PTC* rearrangements in PTC varies geographically from none in Korea to 2% in Saudi Arabia and 60% in the United States and Great Britain. RET/PTC rearrangements also vary with age, being higher in children and young adults. Many types of RET/PTC are described. RET/PTC1 and RET/PTC3 are the most common. RET/PTC2 is less frequent, accounting for fewer than 5% of all the rearrangements. Illegitimate recombination of the *NTRK1* gene on chromosome 1, which encodes the high-affinity nerve growth factor receptor (*NGFR*), with another gene on the same chromosome (*TPM3*) has also been described in some PTCs.
- **BRAF mutations:** Gene expression profiling has shown that point mutations of the T1799A B-type Raf kinase (*BRAF*) gene are detected in up to 70% of PTCs. This mutation appears to be associated with specific clinicopathologic characteristics that predict tumor behavior and progression. *BRAF* mutation occurs only in PTC and PTC-derived anaplastic thyroid cancer.
- **RAS mutations:** *RAS* proto-oncogenes are mutated in less than 10% of PTC.

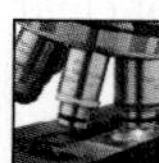

PATHOLOGY: PTCs vary in size from microscopic to larger than a normal gland. Serial sections of ostensibly normal glands at autopsy revealed many papillary cancers under 1 mm across, but lymph node metastases in such cases are distinctly rare. Papillary cancers may arise anywhere in the gland including the isthmus. They are firm, solid and white-yellowish, with irregular and infiltrative borders. Lesions may be multiple, and occasionally encapsulated (Fig. 21-21A).

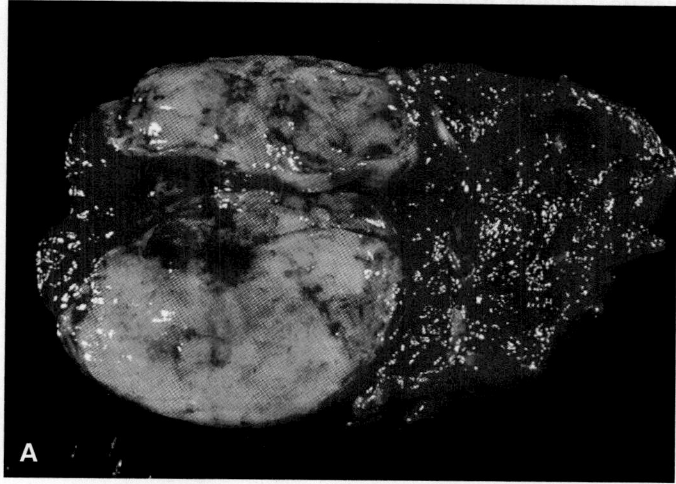

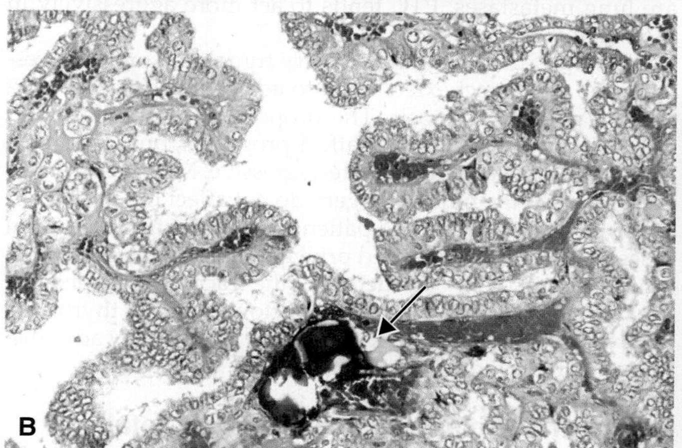

FIGURE 21-21. Papillary carcinoma of the thyroid. A. The cut surface of a surgically resected thyroid displays a circumscribed pale tan mass with foci of cystic change. **B.** Branching papillae are lined by neoplastic columnar epithelium with clear nuclei. A calcospherite, or psammoma body, is evident (arrow).

Branching papillae have central fibrovascular cores and a single or stratified lining of cuboidal to columnar cells (Fig. 21-21B). Irregularly shaped or tubular neoplastic follicles are usually seen in the tumor, but the proportions of the papillary and follicular elements are highly variable. Nuclear atypia is an important diagnostic feature and includes clear **(ground-glass or "Orphan Annie")** nuclei, eosinophilic pseudoinclusions (which are invaginations of the cytoplasm into the nucleus) and nuclear grooves. Many papillary cancers show dense fibrosis. Calcospherites **(*psammoma bodies*)** are seen in half the cases and are virtually diagnostic of PTC. The stroma may be infiltrated by lymphocytes and Langerhans cells. In over 75% of cases, careful sectioning of resected thyroids reveals multiple microscopic foci of tumor, but it is not clear if these reflect multifocal origin of the tumor or spread from a solitary primary. Vascular invasion is rare.

Several morphologic types of papillary carcinoma have been described, some with good prognoses such as **micro-carcinoma** (1 cm in size), **follicular variant of papillary cancer, encapsulated tumors** and **papillary tumors of the usual type. Diffuse sclerosis type** and the **tall cell** and **columnar variants** generally have worse outcomes.

PTC typically invades lymphatics and spreads to regional cervical lymph nodes. Lymph node metastases vary from microscopic foci in otherwise normal lymph nodes to large masses that dwarf the primary lesion. Direct extension of PTC into soft tissues of the neck occurs in one quarter of cases. Hematogenous metastases occur less often than in other varieties of thyroid cancer, but occur occasionally, mostly to the lungs.

CLINICAL FEATURES: PTC presents as (1) a painless, palpable nodule in an otherwise normal gland; (2) a nodule with enlarged cervical lymph nodes; or (3) cervical lymphadenopathy with no palpable thyroid nodule. Tumors over 0.5 cm appear as cold areas in thyroid scintiscans.

In general, the prognosis of PTC is excellent, and life expectancy for these patients differs little from that of the general population. The prognosis is more serious in men over 50 years, whereas in children, the outlook is good even if there are lung metastases. PTC tends to act more aggressively in men than in women.

As a rule, the larger the primary tumor, the more aggressive it is, and direct extension into adjacent soft tissues portends a poorer prognosis. The proportion of papillary and follicular elements does not affect prognosis, but less differentiated tumors tend to be more aggressive. Metastases to cervical nodes at the time of surgery do not affect the prognosis, as fewer than 10% of these patients die of the tumor. In fatal cases of PTC, death is caused principally by metastases to the lungs or brain or by obstruction of the trachea or esophagus.

Therapies include surgery (lobectomy or total thyroidectomy) with or without neck dissection, followed by administration of radioiodine.

Follicular Thyroid Carcinoma Is Rarely Fatal

Follicular thyroid carcinoma (FTC) is a purely follicular malignant tumor with no papillary or other elements. It makes up 15% to 20% of thyroid tumors. Most patients are older than 40 years of age, and the female-to-male ratio is 3:1. However, in areas where iodine is added to salt, such as the United States, FTC is uncommon, accounting for as few as 5% of all thyroid cancers. It is extremely rare in children. The incidence of follicular carcinoma is higher in endemic goiter areas among people who do not receive iodine supplements. Irradiation to the gland increases the frequency of these tumors.

MOLECULAR PATHOGENESIS: Between 20% and 45% of FTCs have point mutations in *RAS* oncogene and rearrangement of the *PAX8/PPARG* (paired box 8/peroxisome proliferator-activated receptor-γ). *PPARG* gene rearrangements are more frequent in low-grade tumors with vascular invasion and aggressive follicular carcinomas. Mutations of *p53* and *PTEN* tumor suppressor genes may occur. FTC has been reported in Cowden syndrome. Imbalances in several chromosomes including 3p, 7q, 11 and 10q are reported, among others.

PATHOLOGY: FTCs vary in size, are yellow-tan and have thick white fibrous capsules. Hemorrhage and necrosis are common as are foci of cystic degeneration. FTCs are subdivided into minimally invasive and widely invasive variants.

Minimally invasive FTC is grossly a well-defined, encapsulated tumor. On cut section it is soft and pale tan to pink and bulges from its capsule. Most lesions resemble follicular adenoma histologically, but tend more to microfollicular or trabecular patterns. Occasionally, hemorrhagic necrosis is seen in the center of a tumor. Mitoses, uncommon in adenomas, are common in FTCs. The key distinction from adenoma is spread into or through the tumor capsule.

Minimally invasive cancer is diagnosed when tumor extends into, but not entirely through, the capsule. **Invasive FTC** usually presents few diagnostic problems, since it extends through its capsule or shows vascular invasion (Fig. 21-22), often within or adjacent to the capsule. The tumor may also extend into the surrounding soft tissues. Proliferative markers such as Ki67 may assist in the diagnosis of carcinoma.

Oncocytic (Hürthle cell) carcinomas are tumors of follicular derivation composed mainly (>75%) of oncocytic cells. Criteria for malignancy are the same as for follicular cancer: capsular and vascular invasion. These tumors account for

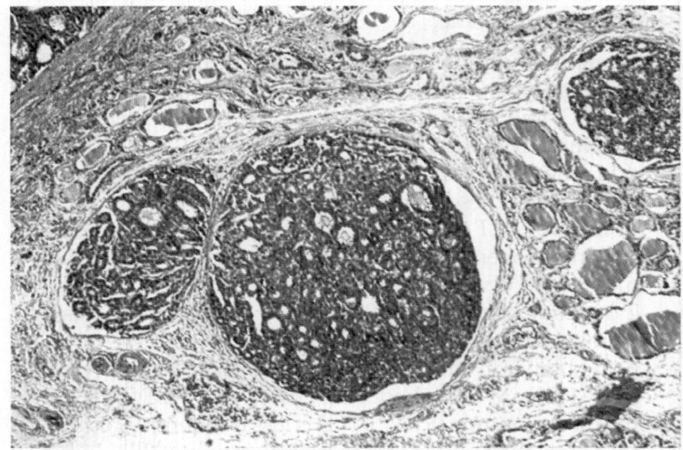

FIGURE 21-22. Follicular carcinoma of the thyroid. A microfollicular tumor has invaded veins in the thyroid parenchyma.

4% to 5% of all thyroid malignancies, and are thought to behave more aggressively than regular follicular cancer.

Unlike PTC, FTC metastases are blood-borne, not lymphatic, and go mainly to the bones of the shoulder and pelvic girdles, sternum and skull.

CLINICAL FEATURES: Most follicular cancers are detected clinically as solitary palpable nodules or enlarged thyroids. However, in some cases, they present as pathologic fractures through bony metastases or pulmonary lesions. Both primary tumors and metastases take up radiolabeled iodine, although a thyroid scintiscan may suggest a cold nodule as the normal gland accumulates iodine more efficiently. However, the affinity for ^{131}I may be used therapeutically. ***Minimally invasive follicular tumors have a cure rate of at least 95%, compared with survival of about 50% for the widely invasive form.*** FTC is treated with unilateral lobectomy. Metastases can be treated with radioiodine.

Medullary Thyroid Carcinoma Is Derived From C Cells of the Thyroid

These cells originate from the branchial pouches and secrete calcitonin and other peptides such as serotonin, ACTH and somatostatin. Medullary thyroid carcinoma (MTC) represents no more than 5% of all thyroid cancers.

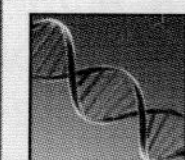

MOLECULAR PATHOGENESIS: The disease occurs in sporadic and familial forms, the latter accounting for 20% of cases. Patients with the familial form of medullary carcinoma often have MEN type 2B and 2A. In patients with MEN2B, tumors occur in infancy, and the tumors of MEN2A occur in adolescents. Sporadic cases present later in life. There is a slight female predominance (1.5:1). In familial cases, inheritance is autosomal dominant, and sex distribution is equal.

Somatic mutations in the *RET* proto-oncogene occur in 25% to 70% of sporadic MTC, mostly at codon 918 (ATG to ACG) in the protein's tyrosine kinase domain. This mutation signifies a poorer prognosis. *RET* is discussed more fully in the section on MEN syndromes (below). Other studies show loss of heterozygosity in chromosomes 1p, 3p, 3q, 11p, 13q, 22q and others.

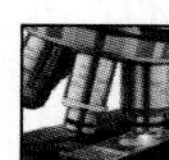

PATHOLOGY: MTC tends to arise in the superior portion of the thyroid, the area richest in C cells. MEN2 tumors are often multicentric and bilateral. MTCs are not encapsulated, but are usually circumscribed. Cut surfaces are firm and grayish white. MTC histology is highly variable. Tumors are usually solid, with polygonal, granular cells separated by a distinctly vascular stroma (Fig. 21-23). However, architectural patterns and cellular

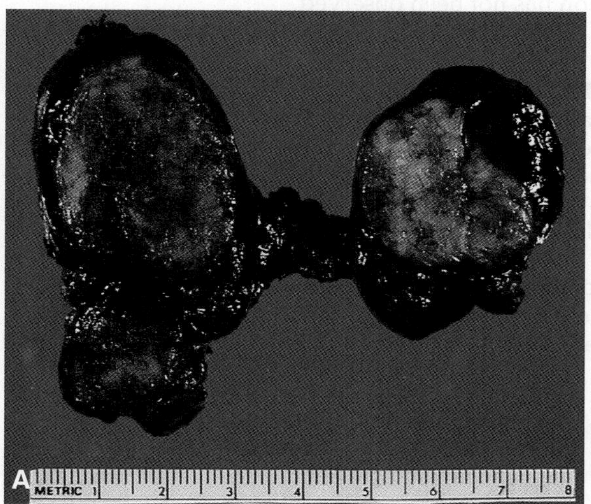

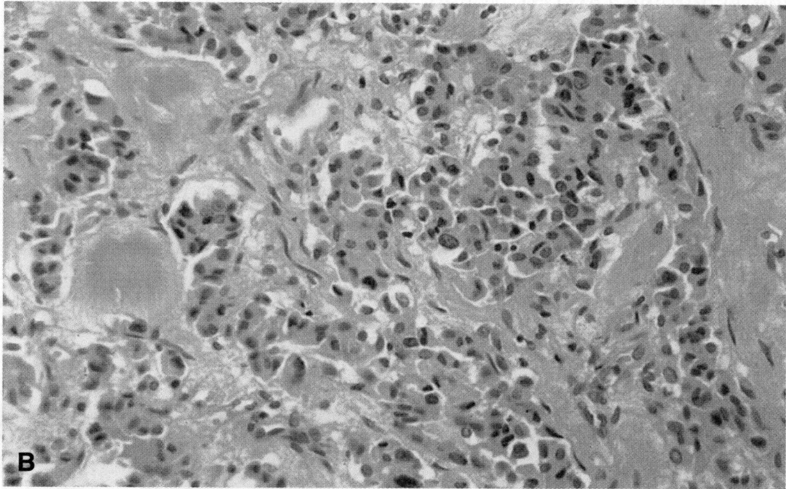

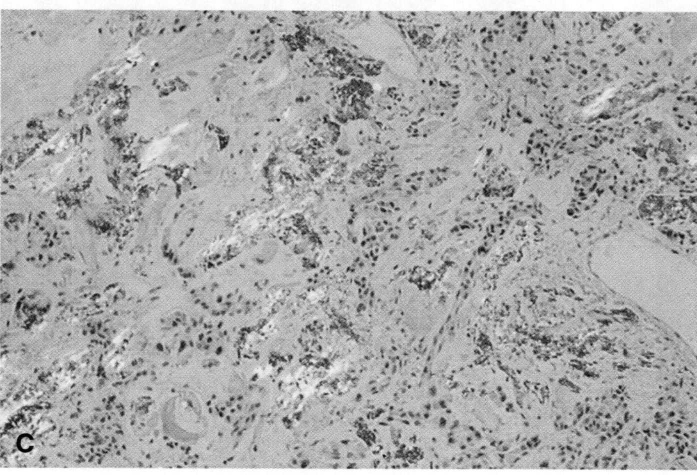

FIGURE 21-23. Medullary thyroid carcinoma. A. Coronal section of a total thyroid resection shows bilateral involvement by a firm, pale tumor. **B.** The tumor features nests of polygonal cells embedded in a collagenous framework. The connective tissue septa contain eosinophilic amyloid. **C.** A section stained with Congo red and viewed under polarized light demonstrates the pale green birefringence of amyloid.

appearances are highly variable. ***Stromal amyloid, representing deposition of procalcitonin, is conspicuous.*** Nests of tumor cells are embedded in a hyalinized collagenous framework. Focal calcification is common, and may be extensive enough to be detected radiologically. Besides amyloid, these tumors may contain mucin, melanin and many polypeptide hormones, detected by immunohistochemistry.

By electron microscopy, the neoplastic C cells have dense-core secretory granules that are positive for several endocrine markers, including calcitonin, synaptophysin and chromogranin. Almost all MTCs express carcinoembryonic antigen (CEA), and many also produce ACTH, serotonin, substance P, glucagon, insulin and human chorionic gonadotropin (hCG).

MTCs extend by direct invasion into soft tissues and metastasize to regional lymph nodes, lung, liver and bone. Sometimes, the initial presentation may be as metastatic disease. Metastases resemble primary tumors and tend to contain amyloid.

The precursor lesion of the familial variety of MTC is C-cell hyperplasia. Thus, patients with MEN types 2A and 2B (see section on adrenal medulla) who are at risk for MTC are monitored by periodic measurement of serum calcitonin, CEA and sometimes chromogranin. When these are elevated, the patient is treated by total thyroidectomy.

CLINICAL FEATURES: Patients with MTC often suffer symptoms related to endocrine secretion, including carcinoid syndrome (serotonin) and Cushing syndrome (ACTH). Watery diarrhea in one third of patients is caused by secretion of vasoactive intestinal peptide (VIP), prostaglandins and several kinins. In familial MTC, patients may exhibit hyperparathyroidism, or symptoms (e.g., episodic hypertension) due to catecholamine secretion by pheochromocytomas.

The tumor usually presents as a firm thyroid nodule or cervical lymphadenopathy. By scintiscan, a cold nodule is characteristic. Treatment is total thyroidectomy, but tumors recur locally in one third of patients. Prognosis depends on age (women have better prognosis) and tumor size and stage. Patients with MEN2A younger than 5 years of age should undergo thyroidectomy to improve survival. Other prognostic parameters include histologic type, mitotic count, necrosis and amount of calcitonin present. The 5-year survival rate is 60% to 75%.

Anaplastic (Undifferentiated) Thyroid Carcinoma Is Usually Fatal

Anaplastic thyroid cancer principally afflicts women (female-to-male ratio of 4:1) over the age of 60. This tumor constitutes 10% of thyroid cancers and is more common in areas of endemic goiter, and at least half of patients have long-standing goiter. In addition, there is often a history of a lower-grade thyroid cancer. Thus, anaplastic thyroid cancer may develop by transformation from a benign or lower-grade thyroid neoplasm. There is evidence that the risk of such an event is enhanced by external radiation.

MOLECULAR PATHOGENESIS: Anaplastic carcinomas have more chromosomal imbalances than do other thyroid tumors. Comparative genomic hybridization (CGH) studies show gains and losses at chromosomes 1q, 1p, 11, 17p, 22q, 9p, 16p and others. Tumors originating from preexisting well-differentiated tumors show similar genetic alterations, but the anaplastic component may have higher mutation rates. Anaplastic tumors often show mutations in *p53*, but *RET* activation has not been observed.

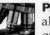

PATHOLOGY: Anaplastic thyroid carcinoma is usually a large poorly circumscribed mass that frequently extends into the soft tissues of the neck. The cut surface is hard and grayish white. The most common histology is a sarcoma-like proliferation of bizarre spindle and giant cells, with polyploid nuclei, many mitoses, necrosis and stromal fibrosis (Fig. 21-24). Other microscopic patterns include distinct epithelial differentiation. These tumors tend to invade blood vessels, often occluding them and causing focal infarcts in the tumor. Immunohistochemistry is positive

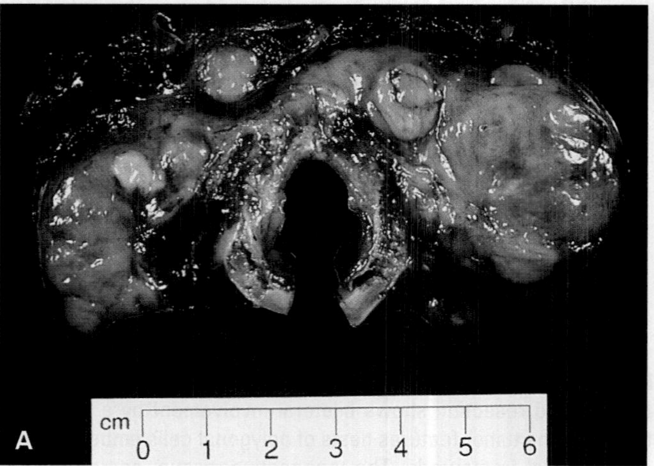

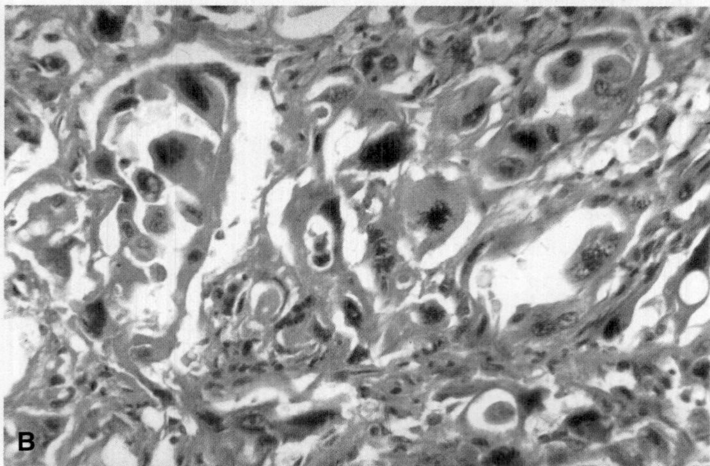

FIGURE 21-24. Anaplastic carcinoma of the thyroid. A. The tumor in transverse section partially surrounds the trachea and extends into the adjacent soft tissue. **B.** The tumor is composed of bizarre spindle and giant cells with polyploid nuclei and numerous mitoses.

for cytokeratins and epithelial membrane antigen (EMA) in many cases. However, TTF1 is negative.

CLINICAL FEATURES: Local structures are compressed or disrupted. Accordingly, these tumors present as rapidly enlarging neck masses and cause dysphagia, hoarseness, dyspnea and enlargement of cervical nodes. Dysphagia and dyspnea are caused by tracheal compression or invasion. The prognosis is dismal, and widespread metastases are frequent. Fewer than 10% of patients survive for 5 years. Treatment with radiation and chemotherapy has had little success.

Lymphomas of the Thyroid Are Largely B-Cell Tumors

Primary thyroid lymphomas are quite uncommon, and account for 2% of thyroid malignancies. Most are B-cell lymphomas arising in the setting of chronic thyroiditis; in regions where this disorder is frequent, up to 10% of malignant thyroid tumors are lymphomas. Patients present with dyspnea, hoarseness and a mass in the neck. Like chronic thyroiditis, thyroid lymphoma is more common in women than men (4:1). The mean age at presentation is in the seventh decade. Histologically, they resemble lymphomas at other sites; the most common subtype is the diffuse large cell pattern. These patients should be staged and treated as primary nodal lymphomas.

PARATHYROID GLANDS

Anatomy and Physiology

The parathyroid glands are derivatives of branchial clefts III and IV. Most people have 4 glands, but numbers vary from 1 to 12. Normally, they are on the posterior thyroid surface, but they may occur elsewhere, such as in the mediastinum or pericardium or by the recurrent laryngeal nerve.

They measure between 4 to 6 mm in length and are the color of saffron-cooked rice. All glands combined weigh about 130 mg. Individual gland weights vary considerably, but a gland over 50 mg is probably enlarged. Microscopically, about three fourths of the parathyroids are composed of chief cells and oxyphil cells, the remainder being adipose tissue scattered throughout the parenchyma. Fat cells appear after puberty, and then vary throughout life.

Chief cells secrete parathyroid hormone (PTH) and PTH-related protein. They are polyhedral cells with pale, eosinophilic-to-amphophilic cytoplasm containing glycogen and fat droplets. Electron microscopy reveals cytoplasmic membrane-bound secretory granules. Chief cells produce cytokeratins, chromogranin A and synaptophysin, and are very sensitive to calcium concentrations. **Clear cells** are chief cells whose cytoplasm is packed with glycogen. **Oxyphil cells** appear after puberty, are larger than chief cells and have deeply eosinophilic cytoplasm, owing to numerous mitochondria. They have no secretory granules and do not secrete PTH.

The parathyroids respond to blood levels of ionized calcium and magnesium. In turn, PTH controls plasma calcium. Magnesium, a cation closely related to calcium, acts as a brake on PTH secretion. PTH is degraded in the liver and kidney. Other PTH functions include renal excretion of phosphates, increased tubular and intestinal reabsorption of calcium and bone resorption.

Hypoparathyroidism

Hypoparathyroidism results from **decreased secretion of PTH** or **end-organ insensitivity to it (pseudohypoparathyroidism)** owing to congenital or acquired conditions. It is clinically characterized by hypocalcemia and hyperphosphatemia.

Hypoparathyroidism Is Most Often Due to Surgical Removal of the Parathyroids at the Time of Thyroidectomy

Symptoms of hypoparathyroidism relate to hypocalcemia. Increased neuromuscular excitability may cause mild tingling in the hands and feet, severe muscle cramps, tetany, laryngeal stridor and convulsions. Neuropsychiatric manifestations include depression, paranoia and psychoses. High cerebrospinal fluid pressure and papilledema may mimic a brain tumor. Patients with all forms of hypoparathyroidism can be treated with vitamin D and calcium supplementation. Of patients undergoing surgery for primary hyperparathyroidism, 1% develop irreversible hypoparathyroidism. Radioactive iodine therapy can also cause hypoparathyroidism.

Familial hypoparathyroidism may be part of a polyglandular syndrome that includes adrenal insufficiency and mucocutaneous candidiasis (see below). **Familial isolated hypoparathyroidism** has variable inheritance patterns, is rare and reflects deficient PTH secretion. **Idiopathic hypoparathyroidism** is a heterogeneous group of rare disorders, sporadic and familial, that share deficient secretion of PTH. **Agenesis of the parathyroid glands** is part of the DiGeorge syndrome (see Chapter 4).

Pseudohypoparathyroidism Is Caused by Target Organ Insensitivity to Parathyroid Hormone

MOLECULAR PATHOGENESIS: Hypocalcemia in this group of hereditary conditions reflects mutation of the *GNAS1* gene on the long arm of chromosome 20, resulting in decreased activity of G_s, the G protein that couples hormone receptors to stimulation of adenyl cyclase. Consequently, renal tubular cell production of cAMP in response to PTH is impaired, leading to inadequate resorption of calcium from glomerular filtrate. Patients with pseudohypoparathyroidism are also often resistant to other cAMP-coupled hormones, including TSH, glucagon, FSH and LH. These patients have a characteristic phenotype **(Albright hereditary osteodystrophy)**, including short stature, obesity, mental retardation, subcutaneous calcification and congenital anomalies of bone, particularly abnormally short metacarpals and metatarsals (Fig. 21-25).

Some patients with pseudohypoparathyroidism have normal G_s activity and a normal phenotype. The basis for their resistance to PTH is unclear.

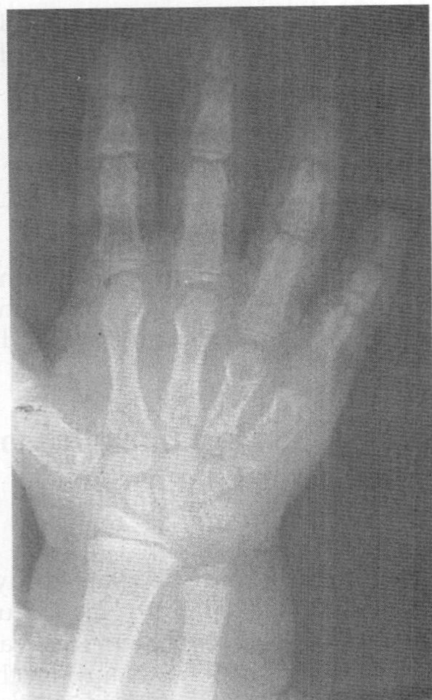

FIGURE 21-25. Pseudohypoparathyroidism. A radiograph of the hand reveals the characteristic shortness of the fourth and fifth metacarpal bones.

Pseudopseudohypoparathyroidism refers to rare cases in which Albright hereditary osteodystrophy is associated with normal cAMP responses to PTH. These patients also have reduced G_s activity similar to cases of pseudohypoparathyroidism. They lack *GNAS1* mutations, although a candidate gene maps to a nearby region on chromosome 20.

Primary Hyperparathyroidism

Primary hyperparathyroidism defines a persistent production of PTH in the absence of intestinal or renal stimulation of the parathyroid glands. The incidence of this condition is about 1:1000. It is most common in women in the fifth decade. Patients have hypercalcemia, hypophosphatemia, nephrolithiasis and bone disease. Some are asymptomatic, with the only clinical finding being elevated serum calcium. Hyperparathyroidism may be caused by a parathyroid adenoma (80% to 90%), hyperplasia of all parathyroids (10% to 15%) or (rarely) parathyroid carcinoma (1% to 5%). It can be sporadic, or part of familial syndromes such as MEN1 and MEN2A.

Parathyroid Adenoma Accounts for Most Cases of Hyperparathyroidism

MOLECULAR PATHOGENESIS: Parathyroid adenomas arise sporadically or (in 20%) in the context of MEN1 (see below), and cause 85% of primary hyperparathyroidism. In a small minority of sporadic adenomas, genetic analysis identified rearrangement and overexpression of the cyclin D_1 (*PRAD1*) proto-oncogene on chromosome 11. *HRPT2*, on chromosome 1q, is the cause of the familial *hyperparathyroidism–jaw tumor syndrome*. CGH studies of parathyroid adenomas may show gains or losses in chromosomes 11q13, 11q23, 13q, 15q and others.

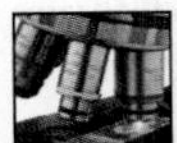

PATHOLOGY: Parathyroid adenomas are circumscribed, reddish brown, solitary masses, 1 to 3 cm in diameter, weighing 0.05 to 200 g. Hemorrhagic areas are common, and cystic changes are occasionally noted. They show sheets of neoplastic chief cells in a rich capillary network. A rim of normal parathyroid tissue is usually seen outside the capsule, and distinguishes adenomas from parathyroid hyperplasia (Fig. 21-26). Most cells resemble normal chief cells and are positive for PTH by immunostaining. The other three glands tend to be atrophic. Surgical resection of the tumor relieves symptoms of hyperparathyroidism. Although most parathyroid adenomas only involve one gland, rare patients may have two. Parathyroid adenomas can also occur within the thyroid gland or in ectopic parathyroid tissue. Mitoses are infrequent, and a proliferative index over 5% should raise the possibility of an atypical gland or a cancer.

Primary Parathyroid Hyperplasia Causes 15% of Hyperparathyroidism

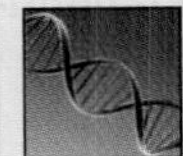

MOLECULAR PATHOGENESIS: About 75% of cases occur in women. Of these, about 20% are associated with familial hyperparathyroidism or MEN types 1 or 2A. One third of sporadic primary parathyroid hyperplasias are monoclonal, suggesting neoplastic proliferation. In such instances, both chief cell hyperplasia and multiple small adenomas occur in the same gland. Sporadic primary hyperparathyroidism may be due to external radiation and lithium ingestion.

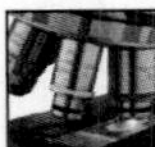

PATHOLOGY: All four parathyroid glands are enlarged, with combined weights ranging from under 1 g to 10 g. In half of patients, one gland is noticeably larger than the others, which may make the distinction from adenoma difficult. Microscopically, the normal glandular adipose tissue is replaced by hyperplastic chief cells arranged in sheets or trabecular or follicular patterns (Fig. 21-27). Scattered oxyphil cells are common, and small foci of adipose tissue may remain.

Parathyroid Carcinoma Accounts for 1% of Hyperparathyroidism

Parathyroid carcinoma is rare. It occurs in both sexes, mainly between the ages of 30 and 60. These are usually functioning tumors: most patients have symptoms of hyperparathyroidism. Hypercalcemia may be severe, with serum calciums in excess of 14 mg/dL.

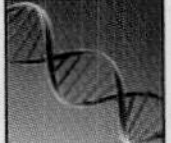

MOLECULAR PATHOGENESIS: The etiology of these tumors is not known, but neck radiation and hereditary syndromes with history of parathyroid adenoma are risk factors. As in functioning parathyroid adenomas, overexpression of cyclin D_1 has

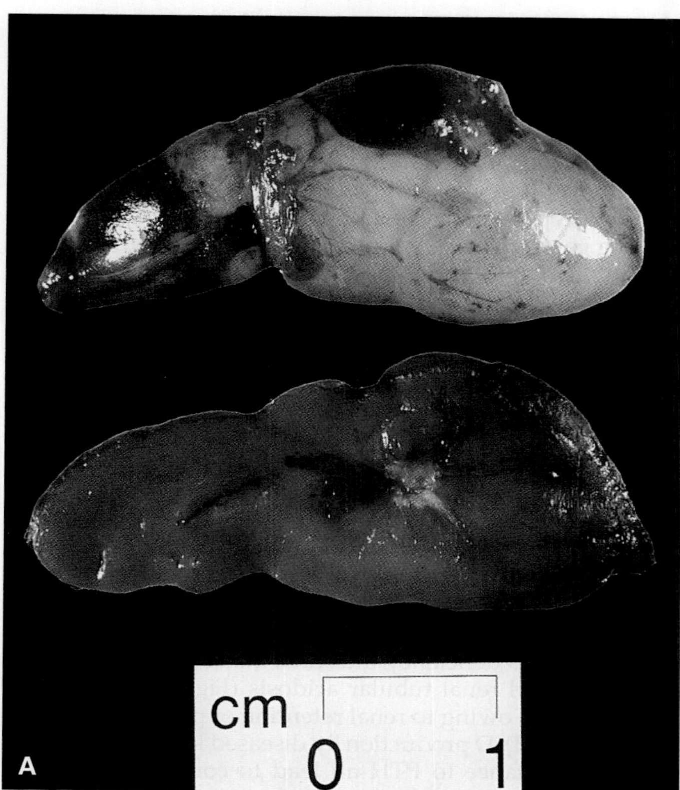

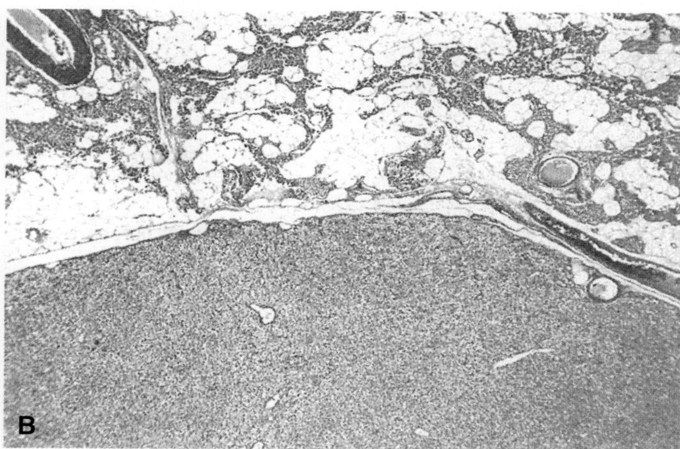

FIGURE 21-26. Parathyroid adenoma. A. External (*top*) and cross-section views (*bottom*) show a tan fleshy tumor. **B.** The tumor consists of sheets of neoplastic chief cells and is separated from normal parenchyma by a thin capsule.

also been described in some parathyroid carcinomas, suggesting that deregulation of this proto-oncogene is an important feature of parathyroid neoplasia in general. Most parathyroid carcinomas are negative for retinoblastoma protein (another cell cycle regulator); adenomas usually display normal staining. Molecular studies have shown losses in chromosome 13q and mutations of the *HRPT2* gene. This tumor suppressor gene is located in chromosome 1q25-31 and is responsible for the hyperparathyroidism–jaw tumor syndrome. This gene encodes for parafibromin, whose expression is reduced or negative in hyperparathyroid–jaw tumor syndrome and carcinomas.

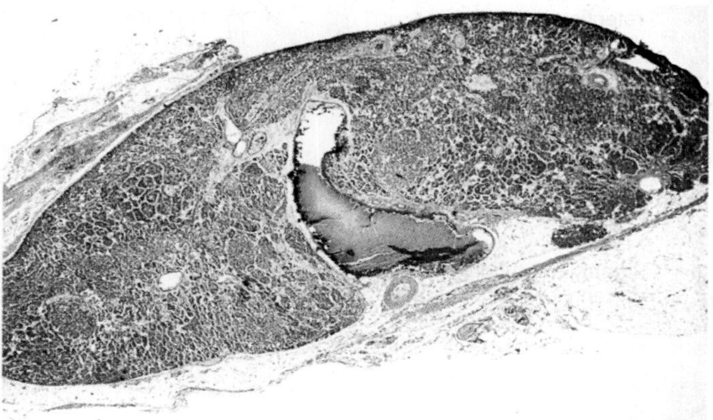

FIGURE 21-27. Primary parathyroid hyperplasia. The normal adipose tissue of the gland has been replaced by sheets and trabeculae of hyperplastic chief cells.

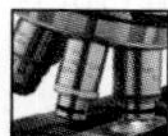

PATHOLOGY: Parathyroid carcinomas tend to be larger than adenomas, and appear as lobulated, firm, tannish, unencapsulated masses, often adherent to surrounding soft tissues. Most show a trabecular histology, with significant mitotic activity and thick fibrous bands. Capsular or vascular invasion may be seen. Importantly, cell atypism often seen in parathyroid adenomas is rare in carcinomas. Proliferative markers such as MIB1 show a high proliferative index.

After surgical removal, local recurrence is common: about a third of patients develop metastases to regional lymph nodes, lungs, liver and bone. Tumor-related death is most often due to hyperparathyroidism rather than carcinomatosis. Ten-year survival is approximately 50%.

Clinical Features of Hyperparathyroidism Are Highly Variable

Hypercalcemia and hypophosphatemia are characteristic. Some patients are asymptomatic, with the ion imbalance picked up on routine blood analysis, while others show florid systemic, renal and skeletal disease (Fig. 21-28). Excessive PTH leads to calcium loss from bones and enhanced calcium resorption by renal tubules. Production of the activated form of vitamin D (1,25[OH]$_2$D) by renal tubules is also stimulated by PTH, increasing intestinal calcium absorption. The action of PTH on the kidney, together with hypercalcemia, leads to hypophosphatemia. Common symptoms include nausea, vomiting, fatigue, weight loss, anorexia, polyuria and polydipsia. A neck mass is palpable in many patients. Other systems affected are:

SKELETAL SYSTEM: The classic bone lesions of hyperparathyroidism, known as **osteitis fibrosa cystica** (see

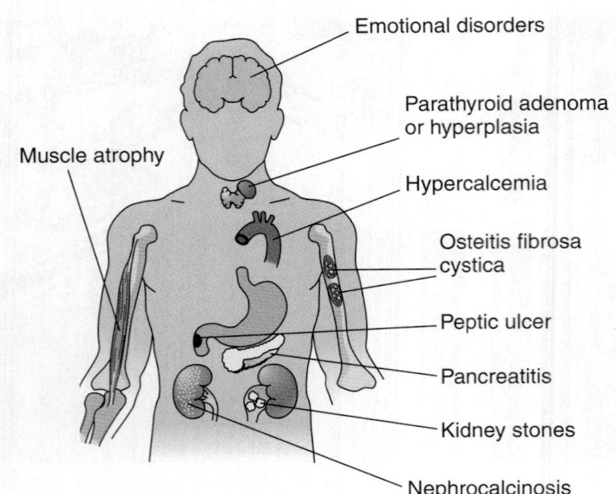

FIGURE 21-28. Major clinical features of hyperparathyroidism.

Chapter 26), are seen in a minority of patients who follow an accelerated course and have a serious form of the disease. These patients present with bone pain, bone cysts, pathologic fractures and localized bone swellings (brown tumors and epulis of the jaw). Chondrocalcinosis may be a complication of hyperparathyroidism.

KIDNEY: Ten percent of patients with primary hyperparathyroidism present with renal colic due to kidney stones. Nephrocalcinosis, noted radiologically as diffuse renal calcification, may also occur (see Chapter 16). Polyuria is caused by hypercalciuria, and leads to polydipsia.

NERVOUS SYSTEM: Psychiatric changes are common, including depression, emotional lability, poor mentation and memory defects. Hyperactive reflexes are seen. Peripheral neuropathy with type 2 fiber atrophy of skeletal muscles leads to muscle weakness.

GASTROINTESTINAL TRACT: Patients with hyperparathyroidism tend to develop gastric ulcers, possibly because hypercalcemia increases serum gastrin, thus stimulating gastric acid secretion. Peptic ulcers in patients with MEN1, which includes parathyroid hyperplasia or adenoma, may be secondary to Zollinger-Ellison syndrome (see Chapter 15). Hypercalcemia may also cause constipation and chronic pancreatitis, but the pathogenesis is not understood.

OTHER SYSTEMS: Half of patients with hyperparathyroidism are hypertensive, although the mechanism is not clear. Anemia of unknown cause is also frequent.

Secondary Hyperparathyroidism

Secondary parathyroid hyperplasia is seen mainly in patients with chronic renal failure, but it also occurs in association with vitamin D deficiency, intestinal malabsorption, Fanconi syndrome and renal tubular acidosis (Fig. 21-29). Chronic hypocalcemia owing to renal retention of phosphate, inadequate 1,25(OH)$_2$D production by diseased kidneys and some skeletal resistance to PTH all lead to compensatory PTH hypersecretion. Secondary hyperplasia causes all glands to produce excess levels of PTH, which cause skeletal pain and deformities, osteomalacia and osteitis fibrosis cystica and bony manifestations of hyperparathyroidism, termed **renal osteodystrophy** (see Chapter 26). Joint pain, swelling and

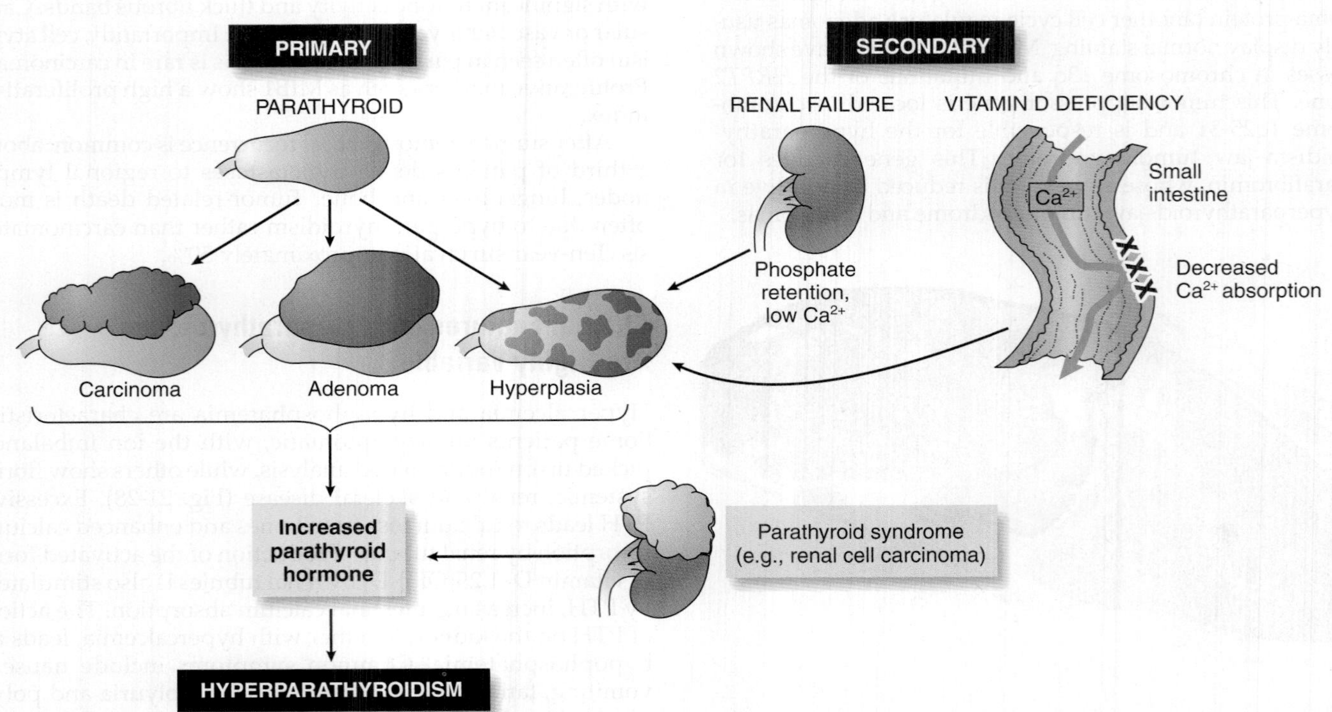

FIGURE 21-29. Major pathogenetic pathways leading to clinical primary and secondary hyperparathyroidism.

stiffness may be due to deposits of calcium around the joints. The parathyroids in secondary hyperplasia resemble those in primary chief cell hyperplasia. Treatment is surgical removal of the enlarged glands with or without reimplantation.

Tertiary hyperparathyroidism is the development of autonomous parathyroid hyperplasia after long-standing hyperplasia secondary to renal failure. In these cases parathyroid hyperplasia may not regress after renal transplantation, and surgery to remove parathyroids is required. Two thirds of patients with long-standing uremia have monoclonal hyperplastic parathyroid proliferations.

ADRENAL CORTEX

Anatomy

Each adrenal gland contains two independent endocrine organs: the cortex and the medulla. Each is distinct anatomically, functionally and embryologically. The cortex arises from celomic mesenchymal cells near the urogenital ridge. The medulla is formed by neuroectodermal cells invading fetal adrenal glands.

Adult adrenal glands are pyramidal organs found anteriorly in the retroperitoneum, above each kidney. Each gland is 4 to 6 cm in greatest dimension and weighs about 4 g. The cortex secretes steroid hormones and corticosteroids. Grossly, and on cut section, the cortex is yellow and the medulla is paler gray-tan. Microscopically, the cortex shows three layers or zones.

- The **zona glomerulosa** is the outermost layer where aldosterone production is stimulated by angiotensin and potassium, and inhibited by atrial natriuretic peptide and somatostatin. The zona glomerulosa makes up 15% of the cortex and is composed of indistinct spherical nests of cells with dark-staining nuclei and a moderate number of fat droplets in the cytoplasm.
- The **zona fasciculata** makes up 75% of the cortex and is not distinctly separated from the zona glomerulosa. Radial cords of larger cells, each with a small nucleus and a large, foamy, clear cytoplasm, representing stored lipid, are readily appreciated.
- The **zona reticularis** is the innermost layer, adjacent to the medulla. Irregular anastomosing cords are composed of compact smaller cells with a lipid-poor, slightly granular eosinophilic cytoplasm and bland nuclei.

The cells of the fasciculata and reticularis secrete glucocorticoids and sex hormones under the control of ACTH. In addition, ACTH stimulates adrenal growth. These zones also produce dehydroepiandrosterone, a weak adrenal androgen. Electron microscopy shows that the cells have abundant smooth endoplasmic reticulum and numerous mitochondria with lamellar cristae, findings that are common to steroid-producing cells.

Ectopic adrenal tissue can be present in many locations outside the gland, commonly including the retroperitoneum, the broad ligament near the ovary, near the epididymis, the kidney and the liver. Ectopic adrenal tissue does not contain medullary cells. Small nodules of adrenocortical cells are frequently found in the fibroadipose tissue that surrounds the adrenal gland.

Congenital Adrenal Hyperplasia

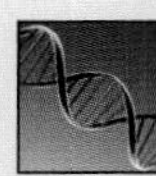

MOLECULAR PATHOGENESIS: Congenital adrenal hyperplasia (CAH) results from several autosomal recessive enzyme defects in the biosynthesis of cortisol from cholesterol (Fig. 21-30). The extent of the defects varies from mild to complete deficiencies. In general, a deficiency in corticosteroid synthesis results in unopposed action of ACTH and hence adrenal hyperplasia. CAH occurs equally in males and females and is the most common cause of ambiguous genitalia in newborn girls (Fig. 21-31A).

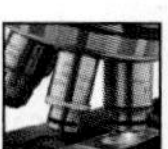

PATHOLOGY: Adrenal glands are enlarged, weighing as much as 30 g (Fig. 21-31B). The cut surface is soft, tan to brown and either diffusely enlarged or nodular. The cortex is widened between the medulla and the zona glomerulosa. The hyperplastic zone is filled by compact, granular, eosinophilic cells. In most cases, the zona glomerulosa is also hyperplastic, although not to the extent of the other zones, especially the zona fasciculata. Ectopic adrenal tissue or nodules may also be hyperplastic, and if the stimulation persists, adenomas can develop.

21-Hydroxylase, or $P450_{C21}$, Deficiency Is the Major Cause of Congenital Adrenal Hyperplasia

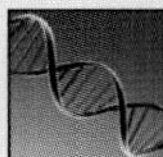

MOLECULAR PATHOGENESIS: The gene for the microsomal enzyme, $P450_{C21}$ (*CYP21*), is linked to the *MHC* locus on the short arm of chromosome 6 (6p21.3) and is closely associated with *HLA-B* and the *C4A* and *C4B* complement genes. The incidence of CAH varies from about 1 in 10,000 in whites to 1 in 500 in Alaskan Eskimos. $P450_{C21}$ converts 17-hydroxyprogesterone to 11-deoxycortisol. A deficiency in this enzymatic activity impairs cortisol biosynthesis, and accumulated precursors are instead converted to androgens.

Clinical manifestations result from cortisol stimulation or accumulation of steroids that may need to be synthesized in different pathways. There are different forms of CAH: (1) "classic"; (2) "nonclassic," which is a common disorder in the white population; and (3) "cryptic," in which the biochemical abnormalities are present, but patients have no symptoms.

Classic CAH caused by $P450_{C21}$ deficiency manifests as several genetically distinct syndromes. Two variants affect newborns. One is simple virilizing CAH; the other is a salt-wasting form that is linked to HLA-Bw47. There is also a less severe late-onset (nonclassic) variant. Mutations that completely inactivate 21-hydroxylase lead to salt-wasting CAH, while those that reduce activity to 2% cause simple virilizing CAH. Late-onset CAH features intermediate values.

SIMPLE VIRILIZING CONGENITAL ADRENAL HYPERPLASIA: Female infants exhibit pseudohermaphroditism; males exhibit no abnormalities of the sexual organs. Conversion of cortisol precursors into adrenal androgens is amplified by the ACTH-dependent increase in the size of the gland. Female newborns exposed to a large excess of adrenal

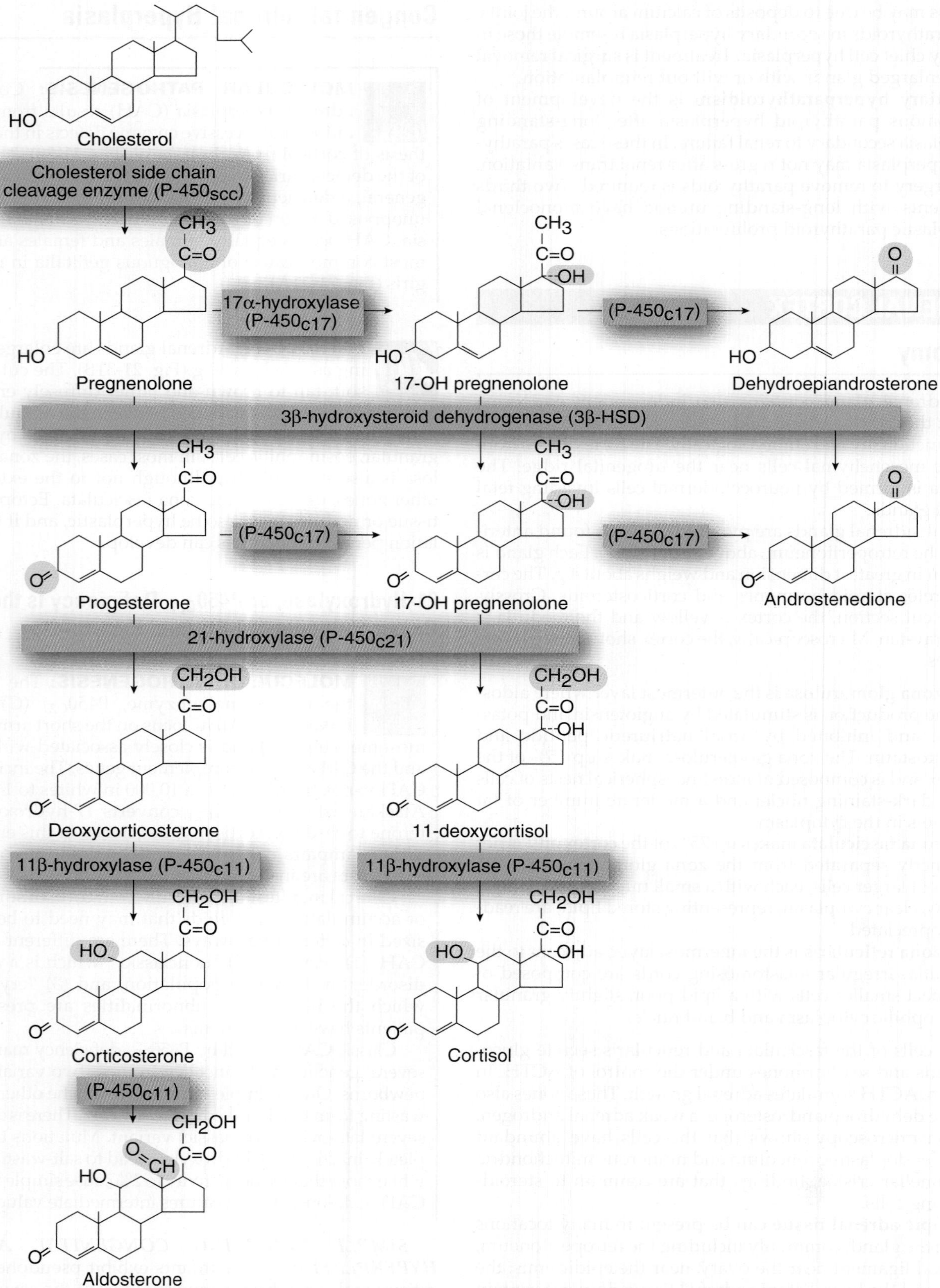

FIGURE 21-30. Biosynthetic pathways in the synthesis of adrenal corticosteroids.

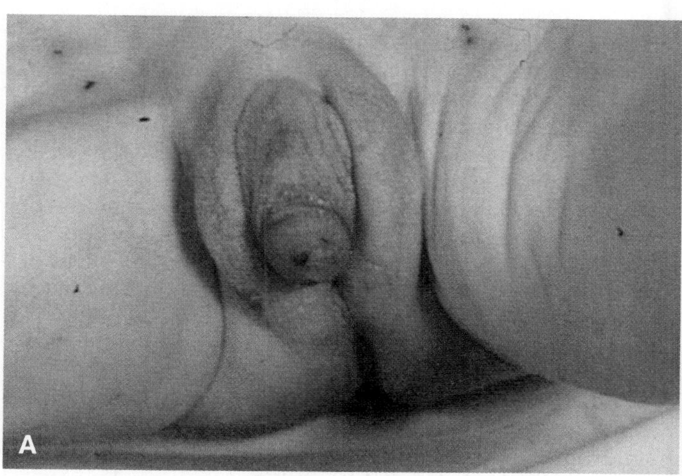

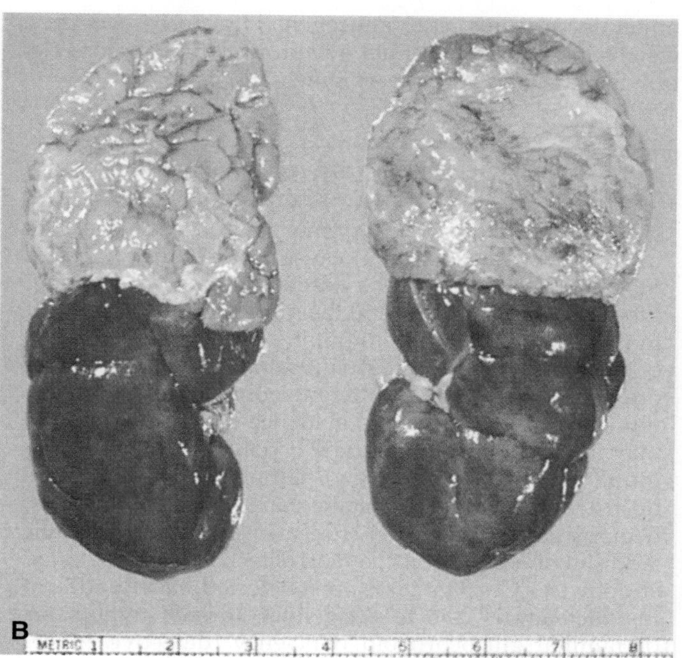

FIGURE 21-31. Congenital adrenal hyperplasia. A. A female infant is markedly virilized with hypertrophy of the clitoris and partial fusion of labioscrotal folds. **B.** A 7-week-old male died of severe salt-wasting congenital adrenal hyperplasia. At autopsy, both adrenal glands were markedly enlarged.

androgens in utero are born with fused labia, an enlarged clitoris and a urogenital sinus that may be mistaken for a penile urethra (Fig. 21-31A). The sexual ambiguity may cause the infant to be mislabeled as male.

Female external genitalia are not necessarily abnormal at birth, but infant girls may develop a syndrome of androgen excess, with clitoral enlargement and pubic hair. Infant boys exhibit sexual precocity. High levels of adrenal androgens lead to premature closure of epiphyses and short stature. Women with CAH tend to be infertile, since high androgen and progestogen levels interfere with the hypothalamic–pituitary–gonadal axis, disturb the menstrual cycle and inhibit ovulation. Men with CAH may be fertile, but some exhibit azoospermia.

SALT-WASTING CONGENITAL ADRENAL HYPERPLASIA: Owing to 21-hydroxylase deficiency, aldosterone synthesis may be impaired. Hypoaldosteronism develops in the first few weeks of life in two thirds of babies with CAH, manifested as hyponatremia, hyperkalemia, dehydration, hypotension and increased renin secretion. These effects may be rapidly fatal if the disease is untreated (Fig. 21-31B).

Both infantile variants of CAH caused by $P450_{C21}$ deficiency are treated with glucocorticoids and mineralocorticoids to suppress ACTH and replace steroids. Reconstructive surgery may be necessary for virilized girls with ambiguous genitalia.

LATE-ONSET CONGENITAL ADRENAL HYPERPLASIA: Patients with nonclassic variants of 21-hydroxylase deficiency show no abnormalities at birth but show virilization at puberty. In young women, late-onset CAH may be difficult to distinguish from polycystic ovary syndrome. Most young men with the disorder are asymptomatic. This form of CAH is probably more common than is classic CAH, particularly among Ashkenazi Jews, Italians and people from the former Yugoslavia.

11β-Hydroxylase Deficiency Causes 5% of Congenital Adrenal Hyperplasia

MOLECULAR PATHOGENESIS: This disorder is uncommon in the general population, but it is the most common cause of CAH among Jews of Iranian or Moroccan ancestry in Israel. The gene for 11β-hydroxylase is located on chromosome 8. There is thus no linkage to the *HLA* locus. 11β-Hydroxylase catalyzes terminal hydroxylation in cortisol biosynthesis. Its absence leads to high levels of 11-deoxycortisol, a weak mineralocorticoid. Thus, in addition to androgenic complications of CAH, excess mineralocorticoid activity often causes sodium retention and accompanying hypertension.

Rare forms of CAH have been described, including deficiencies of several enzymes involved in the biosynthesis of adrenocorticosteroids. These result in variable combinations of electrolyte abnormalities and anomalies of the sex organs.

Adrenal Cortical Insufficiency

Deficient production of adrenal cortical hormones can result from (1) adrenal gland destruction, (2) pituitary or hypothalamic dysfunction with decreased ACTH production or (3) chronic corticosteroid therapy.

Primary Chronic Adrenal Insufficiency (Addison Disease) Often Reflects an Autoimmune Destruction of the Adrenal

Addison disease is a fatal wasting disorder caused by failure of the adrenal glands to produce glucocorticoids, mineralocorticoids and androgens. It causes weakness, weight loss, gastrointestinal symptoms, hypotension, electrolyte imbalance and hyperpigmentation.

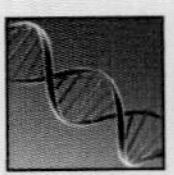
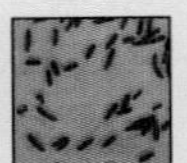

MOLECULAR PATHOGENESIS AND ETIOLOGIC FACTORS: When Addison described primary adrenal insufficiency in 1855, the most common cause of the syndrome was tuberculosis involving the adrenal glands. Worldwide, tuberculosis probably is still the most common cause, but in Western societies, autoimmunity is responsible for 75% of cases. Autoimmune adrenalitis may be an isolated disorder or a part of two different polyglandular autoimmune syndromes. There is evidence that sporadic cases may in fact be variants of type II polyglandular autoimmune syndrome (see below). Other causes of adrenal destruction include metastatic carcinoma, amyloidosis, hemorrhage, sarcoidosis and fungal infections. In idiopathic Addison disease, the biochemical defect of adrenoleukodystrophy (see Chapter 28) is often detected. Rarely, adrenal insufficiency is due to congenital adrenal hypoplasia or familial glucocorticoid deficiency (defective ACTH receptor).

The autoimmune pathogenesis of most cases of Addison disease is supported by:

- Lymphoid infiltrates in the adrenal gland
- The presence of circulating antibodies to adrenal antigens
- Abnormalities of cellular immunity
- Associations with other autoimmune endocrinopathies
- Genetic linkage with *HLA* loci

IMMUNE MECHANISMS: Cell-mediated immunity is probably responsible for the destruction of the adrenal gland in Addison disease. Increased numbers of Ia^+ T lymphocytes and decreased suppressor T-cell function have been detected in blood from patients with the disorder. As well, antibodies against all three zones of the adrenal cortex are reported in two thirds of patients with chronic adrenal insufficiency, the major autoantigens being adrenal steroidogenic enzymes, particularly $P450_{C21}$.

POLYGLANDULAR ENDOCRINOPATHIES: Half of patients with autoimmune adrenal insufficiency suffer from other autoimmune endocrine diseases. These are grouped into two polyglandular endocrine syndromes.

Type I polyglandular autoimmune syndrome is a rare autosomal recessive condition with a slight female predominance. It is seen in older children and adolescents. In addition to adrenal insufficiency, most (60%) patients also have hypoparathyroidism and chronic mucocutaneous candidiasis. Insulin-dependent diabetes (type I, see Chapter 22) is common. Premature ovarian failure, hypothyroidism, malabsorption syndromes, pernicious anemia, chronic hepatitis, alopecia totalis and vitiligo are also encountered.

Type I polyglandular disease is prevalent among Finns and Iranian Jews. The *AIRE* gene (autoimmune regulator) on chromosome 21q22 is associated with type I disease. It is expressed in thymus, lymph nodes and fetal liver, all tissues involved in the maturation of the immune system and in immune tolerance. Similar to the common form of autoimmune Addison disease, sera from patients with type I polyglandular disease recognize steroidogenic autoantigens and other targets.

Type II polyglandular autoimmune syndrome (Schmidt syndrome) is more common than type I and always includes adrenal insufficiency. Women are affected twice as often as are men. It usually manifests between 20 and 40 years of age. Half of cases are familial, but several modes of inheritance are known. Hashimoto thyroiditis and occasionally Graves disease occur in more than two thirds of cases. Insulin-dependent diabetes mellitus and premature ovarian failure are common. Only rarely are other autoimmune diseases present. This condition is considered to be a polygenic disorder with linkage to HLA-DR3.

GENETIC FACTORS: Half of patients with autoimmune adrenal insufficiency as part of a polyglandular syndrome have familial histories of autoimmune endocrinopathy. When Addison disease occurs alone, one third have an affected relative. There is a strong linkage between autoimmune adrenalitis and HLA-B8, HLA-DR3 and HLA-DR4, except for cases that are part of polyglandular syndrome type I, which is not linked to any *HLA* alleles.

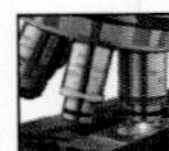

PATHOLOGY: Over 90% of the adrenal gland must be destroyed before chronic adrenal insufficiency is symptomatic. If specific infectious, neoplastic or metabolic disorders are involved, there is corresponding evidence of the underlying disorder in the adrenals. Autoimmune adrenalitis leads to pale, irregular, shrunken glands, weighing 2 to 3 g or less. The medulla is intact but surrounded by fibrous tissue containing small islands of atrophic cortical cells (Fig. 21-32). Depending on the stage of the disease, lymphoid infiltrates, predominantly T cells, of varying density are encountered.

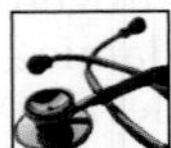

CLINICAL FEATURES: Addison's original description of the clinical features of chronic adrenal insufficiency still applies to untreated cases. Patients had "general languor and debility, remarkable feebleness of the

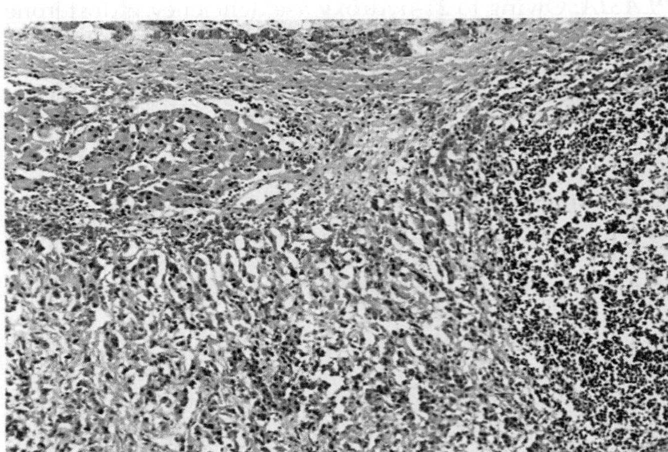

FIGURE 21-32. Autoimmune adrenalitis. A section of the adrenal gland from a patient with Addison disease shows chronic inflammation and fibrosis in the cortex, an island of residual atrophic cortical cells and an intact medulla.

heart's action, irritability of the stomach and a peculiar change of the colour of the skin." Typically, the first symptom is insidious onset of weakness, which may lead to a patient being bedridden. Anorexia and weight loss are invariably present. Diffuse, tan skin pigmentation usually develops, and dark patches may appear on mucous membranes. This hyperpigmentation is related to pituitary proopiomelanocortin (POMC) stimulation of skin melanocytes. Hypotension, with blood pressures in the range of 80/50 mm Hg, is the rule. Most patients have gastrointestinal complaints, including vomiting, diarrhea and abdominal pain. Addison disease often causes marked personality changes and even organic brain syndromes.

Impaired mineralocorticoid secretion, plus the other metabolic derangements, lowers serum sodium and raises serum potassium. Lack of glucocorticoids leads to lymphocytosis and mild eosinophilia. The diagnosis is made by testing corticosteroid blood levels after ACTH injection. Glucocorticoid and mineralocorticoid replacement allows patients to live normal lives.

Acute Adrenal Insufficiency Is a Life-Threatening Emergency

Acute adrenal insufficiency, or adrenal crisis, reflects a sudden loss of adrenal cortical function. Symptoms are related more to mineralocorticoid deficiency than to inadequate glucocorticoids. Adrenal crisis occurs in three settings:

- Abrupt withdrawal of corticosteroid therapy in patients with adrenal atrophy that is due to long-term use of these steroids. This is the most common cause of acute adrenal insufficiency.
- Sudden, devastating deterioration of chronic adrenal insufficiency may be precipitated by the stress of infection or surgery.
- **Waterhouse-Friderichsen syndrome** is acute, bilateral, hemorrhagic infarction of the adrenal cortex, most often due to meningococcus or *Pseudomonas* septicemia (see Chapter 7). Adrenal hemorrhage in these circumstances is thought to be a local manifestation of a generalized Shwartzman reaction with disseminated intravascular coagulation. Acute adrenal insufficiency due to adrenal hemorrhage is also seen in newborns subjected to birth trauma.

CLINICAL FEATURES: The initial manifestations of adrenal crisis are usually hypotension and shock. Nonspecific symptoms commonly include weakness, vomiting, abdominal pain and lethargy, which may progress to coma. Typically in Waterhouse-Friderichsen syndrome, a young person suddenly develops hypotension and shock, together with abdominal or back pain, fever and purpura. Adrenal crisis is almost invariably fatal unless the patient is treated promptly and aggressively with corticosteroids and supportive measures.

Secondary Adrenal Insufficiency Reflects a Lack of Adrenocorticotropic Hormone

Destruction of the pituitary and consequent panhypopituitarism result in secondary adrenal insufficiency. Causes include pituitary tumors, craniopharyngioma, empty sella syndrome and pituitary infarction. Trauma, surgery and radiation therapy also may result in loss of pituitary function. Isolated ACTH deficiency is often associated with autoimmune endocrinopathies.

Any disorder that interferes with secretion of corticotropin (ACTH)-releasing hormone (CRH) by the hypothalamus (e.g., tumors, sarcoidosis) can cause inadequate production of ACTH. Glucocorticoid response to ACTH distinguishes secondary from primary adrenal insufficiency. Pigmentary and electrolyte abnormalities are unusual in secondary adrenal insufficiency since these processes are not regulated by ACTH.

Adrenal Hyperfunction

Excess corticosteroid secretion occurs in adrenal hyperplasia or neoplasia (Fig. 21-33), and may entail either **hypercortisolism** (Cushing syndrome) or **hyperaldosteronism** (Conn syndrome), which reflect the two major classes of adrenal steroid hormones.

Early in the 20th century, the neurosurgeon Harvey Cushing associated "painful obesity, hypertrichosis and amenorrhea" with the presence of a pituitary tumor. The combination of pituitary hyperfunction and the signs and symptoms produced by chronic glucocorticoid excess was termed Cushing disease. These clinical features are caused by high glucocorticoid levels of any origin (i.e., from an adrenal adenoma or carcinoma, ectopic production of ACTH or CRH by a tumor or exogenous administration of corticosteroids). Thus, hypercortisolism from any cause is now called **Cushing syndrome;** the term **Cushing disease** is reserved for excessive secretion of ACTH by pituitary corticotrope tumors.

The most common cause of Cushing syndrome in the United States is chronic corticosteroid administration to treat immune and inflammatory disorders. The next most common cause is a paraneoplastic syndrome in which nonpituitary cancers inappropriately produce ACTH. Cushing disease is five times more frequent than is Cushing syndrome caused by adrenal tumors.

Adrenocorticotropic Hormone–Dependent Adrenal Hyperfunction Is of Pituitary or Ectopic Origin

ETIOLOGIC FACTORS: Women, usually 25 to 45 years old, are five times more likely than men to develop Cushing disease. Excessive secretion of ACTH leads to adrenal cortical hyperplasia. ACTH-dependent adrenal hyperfunction results from:

- Ectopic ACTH production by a nonpituitary tumor
- Primary hypersecretion of ACTH by the pituitary (Cushing disease)
- Inappropriate secretion of CRH by tumors arising outside the hypothalamus, with secondary pituitary hypersecretion of ACTH

ECTOPIC PRODUCTION OF ADRENOCORTICOTROPIC HORMONE: Inappropriate secretion of ACTH by a malignant tumor accounts for most cases of ACTH-dependent hyperadrenalism. Cancer of the lung, particularly small cell carcinoma, is responsible for more than half of the cases of ectopic ACTH syndrome. The remainder are attributable principally to carcinoids and neural crest tumors (pheochromocytoma, neuroblastoma, medullary carcinoma of the thyroid), thymoma and islet cell adenoma of the pancreas.

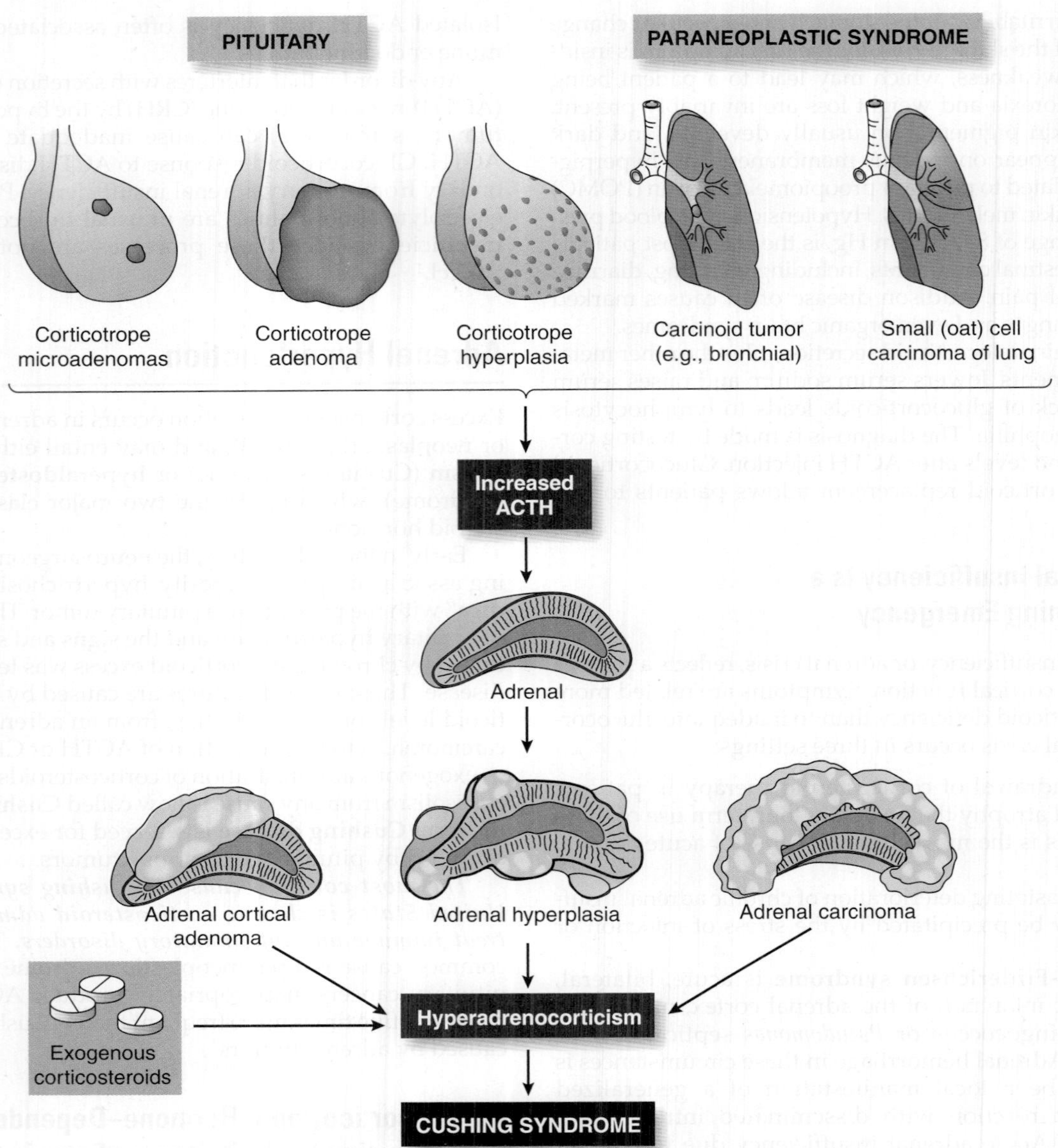

FIGURE 21-33. The pathogenetic pathways of Cushing syndrome. The ACTH-dependent pathway is referred to as Cushing disease. ACTH = adrenocorticotropic hormone (corticotropin).

PRIMARY HYPERSECRETION OF ADRENOCORTICOTROPIC HORMONE: Pituitary-derived Cushing disease usually results from corticotrope microadenomas of the pituitary, but is occasionally due to a macroadenoma or, in a few patients, diffuse corticotrope hyperplasia. Adenomas are monoclonal, arising from a single progenitor cell, but corticotrope hyperplasia is caused by chronic CRH hypersecretion.

ECTOPIC CORTICOTROPIN-RELEASING HORMONE PRODUCTION: Ectopic CRH syndrome is similar to ectopic ACTH syndrome, except that a malignant tumor secretes CRH. In turn, CRH stimulates pituitary ACTH secretion, leading to adrenal hyperplasia.

PATHOLOGY: Cushing disease is characterized by bilateral, diffuse (75%) or nodular (25%) hyperplasia of adrenal glands. Each gland usually weighs 8 to 10 g but may be as much as 20 g.

In **diffuse adrenal hyperplasia** the cortex is grossly visible and broadened, with an inner brown layer and a yellow, lipid-rich cap. The inner third of the cortex is composed of a compact cell layer, and the outer zone, corresponding to the zona fasciculata, has large clear cells packed with lipid. The appearance of the zona glomerulosa varies, sometimes being prominent and at other times difficult to identify.

Nodular adrenal hyperplasia describes grossly visible nodules up to 2.5 cm in diameter, since microscopic nodules are common in diffuse hyperplasia. Bilateral, multiple nodules compress the overlying cortex, and the intervening parenchyma exhibits diffuse hyperplasia. However, nodular hyperplasia may be asymmetric, and the two glands may differ significantly in weight. Microscopically, the nodules are composed of large, lipid-laden, clear cells.

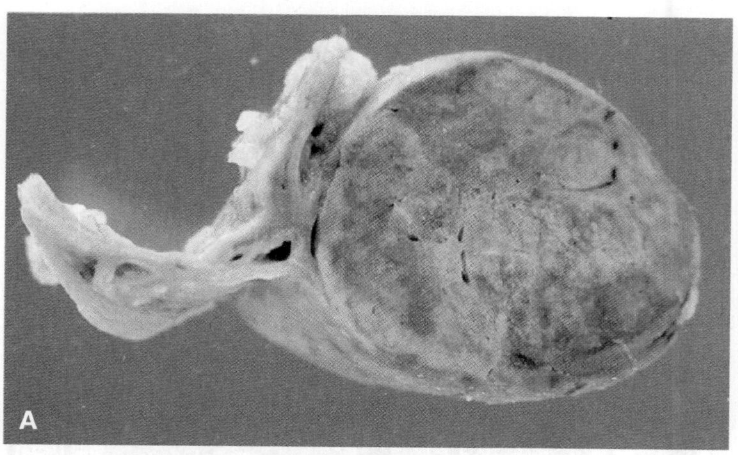

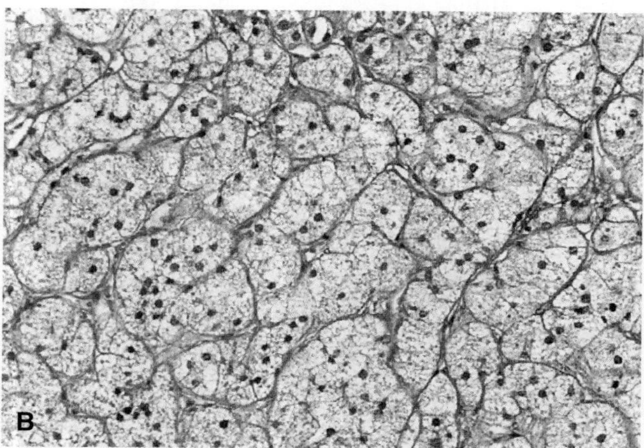

FIGURE 21-34. Adrenal adenoma. A. The cut surface of an adrenal tumor removed from a patient with Cushing syndrome is a mottled yellow with a rim of compressed normal adrenal tissue. **B.** A microscopic view reveals nests of clear, lipid-laden cells.

Adrenocorticotropic Hormone–Independent Adrenal Hyperfunction Is Caused by Adrenal Tumors

In adults, incidence of adrenal carcinoma peaks at 40 years of age and that of adenoma a decade later. In children, adrenal carcinoma accounts for one half of cases of Cushing syndrome; 15% are caused by adenoma. At all ages, the female-to-male ratio is 4:1.

Adrenal Adenoma

Adrenocortical adenomas can produce hormones, the most common being cortisol and aldosterone. They can also produce SF-1Ad4BP, a binding protein secreted by adrenocortical cells. The incidence of these lesions is unknown, as they are often asymptomatic. Adenomas are commonly seen in syndromes such as MEN1, Carney complex and McCune-Albright syndrome.

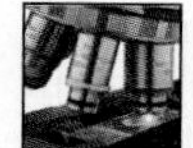

PATHOLOGY: Typical adrenal adenomas are from 1 to 4 cm in diameter (Fig. 21-34), firm, yellow, encapsulated and slightly lobulated. They usually weigh 10 to 50 g, but may rarely reach 100 g. The cut surface is mottled yellow and brown and occasionally black, from deposition of lipofuscin pigment. A thin rim of normal adrenal cortex surrounds the tumor. Necrosis and calcifications are rare. Clear, lipid-laden (fasciculata-type) cells are arranged in sheets or nests, often with interspersed clusters of compact, lipid-depleted, eosinophilic cells (reticularis type). The nontumorous cortex of the involved and contralateral gland is generally atrophic.

Nonfunctional adrenal cortical adenomas are seen in up to 5% of adult autopsies, but less than 10% of surgically removed benign tumors of the adrenal are hormonally silent. Morphology alone cannot distinguish nonfunctional adenomas from their functional counterparts.

Adrenocortical Carcinoma

Adrenal cortical carcinoma is a rare and aggressive tumor that has an incidence of one case per million per year. Eighty percent of adrenal cortical carcinomas are functional with glucocorticoid and androgen secretion. They occur more frequently in women and have poor prognosis. Computed tomography (CT) scans show a mass, usually larger than 5 cm. Median survival is 30 months. The tumor metastasizes to lung, liver and lymph nodes. Local recurrences are common.

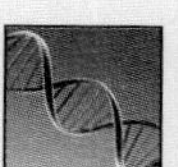

MOLECULAR PATHOGENESIS: Most cases of adrenocortical carcinoma are sporadic, but adrenal cancer has been reported in association with Li-Fraumeni and Beckwith-Wiedemann syndromes. No specific genetic alterations are associated with adrenocortical carcinomas, but there have been reports of overexpression of IGF-2 in sporadic tumors, duplication of the paternal allele and loss of heterozygosity (LOH) at chromosomes 11p15 and 17p13 (p53 locus).

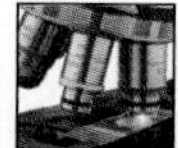

PATHOLOGY: Tumors vary in weight, with the largest ranging up to 5 kg. They are soft, circumscribed, lobulated and bulky (Fig. 21-35). The cut surface has a variegated pink, brown or yellow appearance, often with necrosis, hemorrhage and cystic change. Local invasion is common, and remnants of normal adrenal are difficult to identify. Tumors are composed of both clear and compact cells, showing variable nuclear pleomorphism. Mitotic figures (>5 per high-powered field), necrosis or vascular invasion may or may not be apparent. Other criteria of malignancy include atypical mitoses, diffuse architecture and capsular and vascular invasion. In functional carcinomas, the contralateral adrenal cortex is atrophic.

Most adrenal cortical carcinomas cannot be resected completely. Even when a surgeon believes he or she has removed the entire tumor, micrometastases in other organs, especially lung, liver and bone, are already likely to be present. Most patients survive only 1 to 3 years.

Nonfunctional adrenal cortical carcinomas tend to be highly malignant, and may exceed 1 kg. They are morphologically indistinguishable from functional cancers.

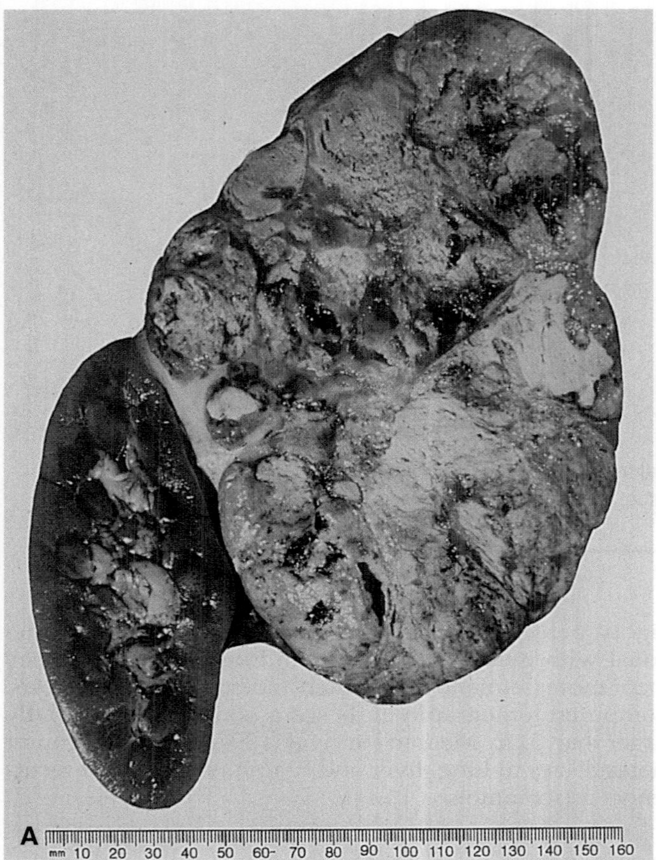

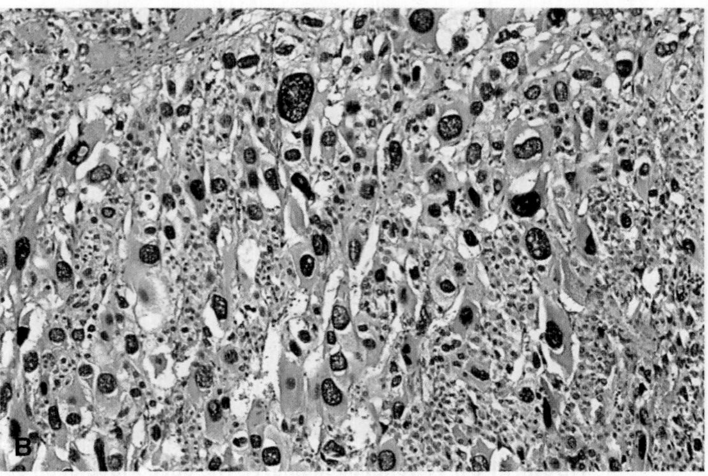

FIGURE 21-35. Adrenal cortical carcinoma. A. The bulky tumor on section is yellow to tan with areas of necrosis and cystic degeneration. **B.** A microscopic section demonstrates marked anisocytosis and nuclear pleomorphism.

Other Causes of Adrenocorticotropic Hormone–Independent Cushing Syndrome Include Chronic Corticosteroid Administration and Bilateral Micronodular Hyperplasia

Many immunologic and inflammatory diseases are treated with glucocorticoids, constituting by far the most common cause of Cushing syndrome. The synthetic hormones ordinarily used (e.g., dexamethasone, prednisone) have only glucocorticoid activity, with few or no mineralocorticoid or androgen effects. Thus, hypertension and hirsutism, which are common in Cushing syndrome due to adrenal hyperplasia or neoplasia, are usually absent in this iatrogenic disorder.

Bilateral adrenal cortical micronodular hyperplasia (Carney complex or **primary pigmented nodular adrenocortical disease)** is a rare cause of ACTH-independent Cushing syndrome, usually in children or young adults. Half have an adrenocortical disease characterized by pigmented skin lesions over much of the body, a variety of myxomas, testicular tumors and pituitary somatotrope adenomas. The adrenals contain small, brown or black nodules, up to 0.5 cm in diameter, with large eosinophilic cells laden with lipofuscin granules. These lesions are termed primary pigmented nodular adrenocortical disease. Half of patients with Carney complex have a mutation in a tumor suppressor gene (17q22-24), *PRKAR1A*, that codes for a regulatory subunit of protein kinase A. Another gene in 2p16 has also been mapped to the disease.

Clinical Features of Cushing Syndrome Affect Many Organ Systems

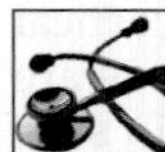

CLINICAL FEATURES: The manifestations of Cushing syndrome (Fig. 21-36) depend on the degree and duration of excessive corticosteroid levels, as well as on the levels of adrenal androgens and mineralocorticoids. Approximately 70% of the patients are females, with fewer than 20% of the cases occurring before puberty.

OBESITY: Typically, patients note gradual enlargement of the face (moon face) (Fig. 21-37), neck (buffalo hump), trunk and abdomen. Arms and legs are unaffected, or even thinner.

SKIN: The skin is atrophic. Subcutaneous fat is decreased. Enlargement of the abdomen and other areas of fat deposition stretches the thin skin and produces purplish striae, which represent venous channels that are visible through the attenuated dermis. Hyperpigmentation, similar to, but less severe than, that in Addison disease, may occur because of pituitary hypersecretion of POMC. Acanthosis nigricans is increased in frequency in Cushing syndrome.

MUSCULOSKELETAL SYSTEM: Increased bone resorption causes osteoporosis. Back pain is common, and up to a fifth of patients have radiologic evidence of vertebral compression fractures. Fractures of ribs and occasionally long bones may occur. Proximal muscle wasting **(steroid myopathy)** causes weakness, which may be so severe that the patient cannot rise from sitting or climb a flight of stairs.

CARDIOVASCULAR SYSTEM: Hypertension is common, often reflecting excessive mineralocorticoid activity. In older patients, congestive heart failure is a frequent sequel.

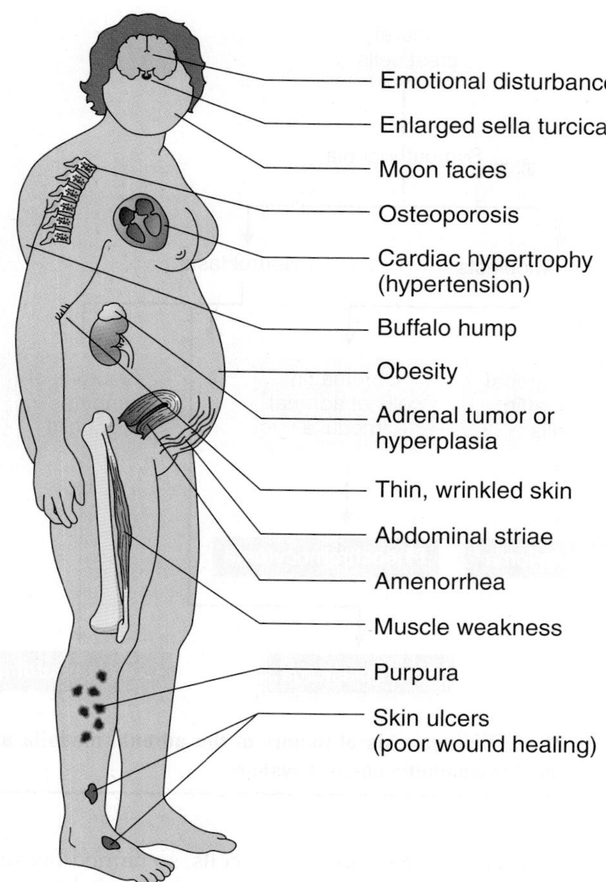

FIGURE 21-36. Major clinical manifestations of Cushing syndrome.

SECONDARY SEX CHARACTERISTICS: Women with Cushing syndrome tend to be virilized, with increased facial hair, thinning of scalp hair, acne and oligomenorrhea. Men may complain of erectile dysfunction, and both sexes experience decreased libido.

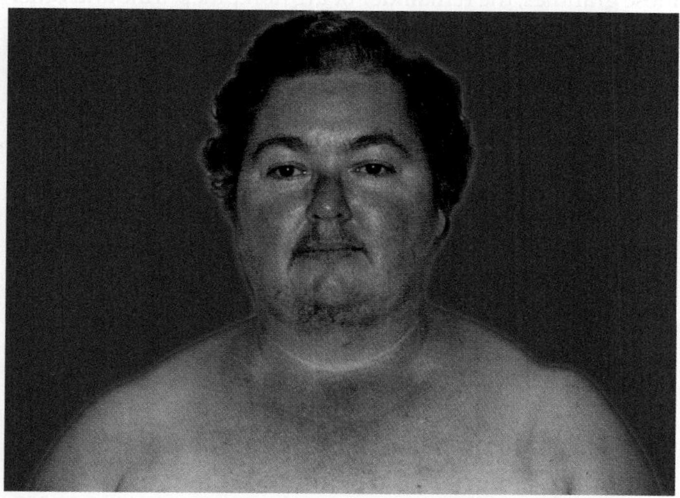

FIGURE 21-37. Cushing syndrome. A woman who had a pituitary adenoma that produced adrenocorticotropic hormone (ACTH) exhibits a moon face, buffalo hump, increased facial hair and thinning of the scalp hair.

EYES: One fourth of patients have increased intraocular pressure, which may be a problem in the event of preexisting glaucoma.

GLUCOSE INTOLERANCE: Glucocorticoid-stimulated gluconeogenesis leads to glucose intolerance and hyperinsulinemia. Diabetes mellitus develops in 15% of patients, usually those with a family history of diabetes.

PSYCHOLOGICAL CHANGES: Cushing syndrome, whether endogenous or iatrogenic, usually causes distinct personality changes. These include irritability, emotional lability, depression and paranoia. These may be so severe that patients become suicidal.

LABORATORY FINDINGS: Half of patients show lymphopenia, and one third have abnormally low eosinophil counts. Hypercalciuria is common, although serum calcium levels remain unchanged. Blood cholesterol and triglyceride levels are frequently elevated.

All forms of Cushing syndrome show increased glucocorticoids. The dexamethasone suppression test distinguishes ACTH-dependent and ACTH-independent forms of Cushing syndrome. Dexamethasone suppresses pituitary ACTH secretion, and hence hypercortisolism, if the latter is dependent on ACTH. However, this test has no effect on adrenal tumors.

Cushing syndrome is treated by (1) extirpation (surgery or irradiation) of pituitary, adrenal or ectopic ACTH-producing tumors; (2) discontinuation of corticosteroid therapy; or (3) administration of adrenal enzyme inhibitors (e.g., aminoglutethimide, ketoconazole, metapyrone). Except for ectopic ACTH syndrome and adrenal carcinoma, in which patients die of cancer rather than of hypercortisolism, Cushing syndrome is highly curable.

Primary Aldosteronism (Conn Syndrome) Leads to Hypertension and Hypokalemia

Inappropriate secretion of aldosterone is caused by adrenal adenomas or hyperplasia. Overproduction of aldosterone causes loss of potassium in the urine and retention of sodium.

Aldosterone-secreting adenomas are more common in women than in men (3:1) and usually occur between the ages of 30 and 50 years.

MOLECULAR PATHOGENESIS: About 75% of causes of primary aldosteronism are caused by solitary adrenal adenomas (aldosteronoma). In a quarter of cases, adrenal hyperplasia is involved. The remainder reflect bilateral hyperplasia of the adrenal zona glomerulosa. Rarely, primary aldosteronism is caused by adrenal carcinomas.

Three types of familial hyperaldosteronism (FH) are known. Type I (glucocorticoid suppressible) is an autosomal dominant disease in which fusion of ACTH-responsive regulatory elements of the 11β-hydroxylase gene to the aldosterone synthase gene results in a hybrid gene that is ectopically and constitutively activated in the zona fasciculata. Bilateral hyperplasia of this zone results. Exogenous glucocorticoids suppress ACTH and ameliorate type I disease. Type II FH is associated with adrenal cortical adenomas and so cannot be suppressed by glucocorticoids. It is suggested that the locus responsible for type II FH is at 7p22. Type III FH has only recently been described, and entails early onset of severe hypertension. The genetic defect in type III FH is unknown.

Aldosterone hypersecretion enhances renal tubular sodium reabsorption, thus increasing body sodium. Hypertension is caused not only by retention of sodium and consequent volume expansion, but also by increased peripheral vascular resistance. Hypokalemia reflects aldosterone-induced loss of potassium in the distal renal tubule.

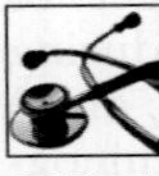

PATHOLOGY: Most aldosterone-secreting adenomas are yellow, less than 3 cm in diameter and under 6 g. However, the size varies, and tumors up to 50 g are reported. Histologically, the dominant cells are clear and lipid rich, resembling the zona fasciculata, and arranged in cords or alveoli. Little nuclear pleomorphism is noted. In hyperaldosteronism, the uninvolved cortex is not atrophic, because aldosterone does not inhibit ACTH secretion by the pituitary.

Bilateral nodular adrenal hyperplasia in Conn syndrome is characterized by yellow cortical nodules less than 2 cm in diameter and composed of clear cells with no nuclear pleomorphism.

CLINICAL FEATURES: Most patients with primary aldosteronism are diagnosed after detection of asymptomatic diastolic hypertension. Muscle weakness and fatigue are caused by the effects of potassium depletion on skeletal muscle. Polyuria and polydipsia result from a disturbance in the concentrating ability of the kidney, probably secondary to hypokalemia. Metabolic alkalosis and an alkaline urine are common.

Primary aldosteronism due to an adenoma is cured when the tumor is removed. Dietary sodium restriction and treatment with the aldosterone antagonist spironolactone are also often effective. Bilateral adrenal hyperplasia is treated medically with aldosterone antagonists and sometimes with dexamethasone in the case of glucocorticoid-suppressible hyperaldosteronism.

Miscellaneous Adrenal Tumors

Adrenal myelolipoma is a mixture of mature adipose tissue and hematopoietic marrow and is notable for its occasional large size.

Adrenal cysts are rare. Most are actually pseudocysts that occur as a result of degenerative changes in benign adrenal tumors or resolution of hemorrhage. In some cases, they represent remnants of an underlying vascular lesion.

Metastatic cancers to adrenal glands usually are from primary lung or breast carcinomas, or malignant melanomas. The glands may be unilaterally or bilaterally hugely enlarged, up to 20 to 45 g. They are largely replaced by carcinoma, often with necrosis and hemorrhage. Sufficient functional adrenal cortex usually remains so that Addison disease does not develop.

ADRENAL MEDULLA AND PARAGANGLIA

Anatomy and Function

The adrenal medulla is entirely surrounded by the cortex and accounts for 10% of the weight of the gland. It consists of neuroendocrine cells, **chromaffin cells,** derived from primitive pheochromoblasts of the developing sympathetic nervous system (Fig. 21-38). Chromaffin cells, so named because catecholamines in their cytoplasmic granules bind chromium salts and darken on oxidation by potassium dichromate, are also present at such extra-adrenal sympathetic nervous system sites as the preaortic sympathetic plexuses and paravertebral sympathetic chain.

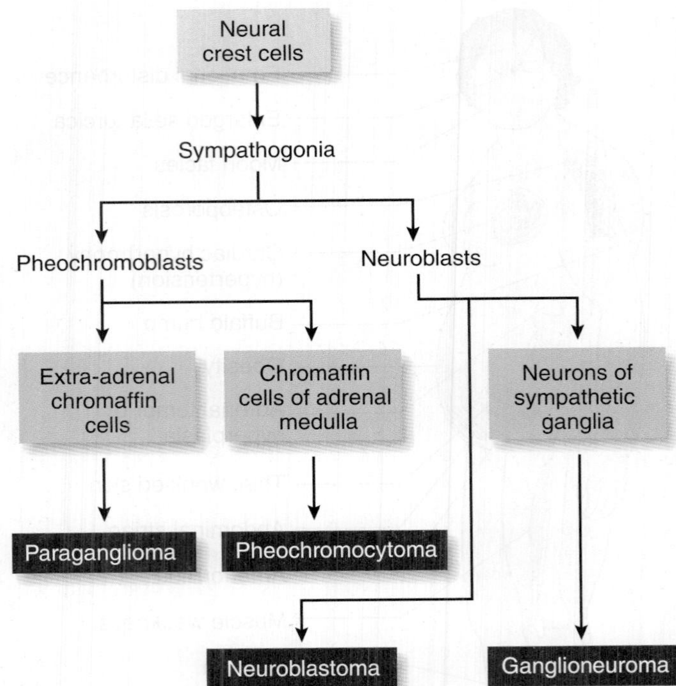

FIGURE 21-38. Histogenesis of tumors of the adrenal medulla and extra-adrenal sympathetic nervous system.

Chromaffin cells appear as nests of small polyhedral cells with pale amphophilic cytoplasm and vesicular nuclei. These cells have many electron-dense 100- to 300-nm chromaffin (catecholamine-containing) granules, like those of sympathetic nerve endings. Epinephrine accounts for 85% of the content of these granules, the remainder being norepinephrine and other noncatecholamine hormones. Interspersed among the chromaffin cells are postganglionic neurons and small autonomic nerve fibers. Stored catecholamines are secreted upon sympathetic stimulation in response to stress (exercise, cold, fasting, trauma) or excitement (e.g., fear, anger).

The adrenal medulla is supplied by arterial and portal venous circulations that originate in the zona reticularis of the cortex. Most of the blood to the hormonally active cells of the medulla is from the portal system. The medulla is innervated from the splanchnic nerves by cholinergic preganglionic sympathetic neurons.

Pheochromocytoma

Pheochromocytomas Are Rare Catecholamine-Secreting Tumors of Chromaffin Cells of the Adrenal Medulla

If pheochromocytomas arise in extra-adrenal sites, they are called **paragangliomas.** Other catecholamine-producing tumors (e.g., chemodectoma, ganglioneuroma) may also cause a syndrome similar to that associated with pheochromocytoma.

Pheochromocytomas are rare tumors, somewhat more frequent in women than in men. They occur at any age, including infancy, but are uncommon after 60 years of age. ***Hypertension, sustained or episodic, is the key symptom.*** Other symptoms include pallor, anxiety and cardiac arrhythmias. Pheochromocytomas account for fewer than 0.1% of cases of hypertension, but should be considered in evaluating any hypertensive patient. If detected early, they are amenable to surgical resection, but untreated patients can die of the complications of prolonged hypertension. Most pheochromocytomas are unexpected findings at autopsy, indicating that some curable cases of hypertension escaped clinical detection. Imaging using iodine-metaiodobenzylguanidine (I-MIBG), an analog of guanethidine, may help to localize these and other neuroendocrine tumors.

Pheochromocytomas are mostly sporadic. A minority are inherited, either alone or as part of hereditary syndromes, such as MEN types 2A and 2B (see below), von Hippel-Lindau disease, neurofibromatosis type 1 and McCune-Albright syndrome.

PATHOLOGY: Of sporadic pheochromocytomas, 80% are unilateral, 10% are bilateral and 10% occur in extra-adrenal locations; 10% are malignant and 10% occur in children. By contrast, two thirds of tumors occurring in the context of MEN (see below) are bilateral. Tumors range from 1 cm to masses of more than 2 kg. Most are 5 to 6 cm in diameter and weigh 80 to 100 g.

Pheochromocytomas tend to be encapsulated, spongy, reddish masses, with prominent central scars, hemorrhage and foci of cystic degeneration (Fig. 21-39A). Histology is highly variable. Typically, circumscribed nests **(zellballen)** of neoplastic cells are present. Tumor cells range from polyhedral to fusiform, with granular, amphophilic or basophilic cytoplasm and vesicular nuclei. Eosinophilic cytoplasmic globules are seen. Cellular pleomorphism is often prominent and may include multinucleated tumor giant cells (Fig. 21-39B). These tumors are very vascular. Less commonly, trabecular or solid patterns are seen, with only indistinct **zellballen.**

By electron microscopy, membrane-bound, dense core granules are seen, corresponding to stored catecholamines. Immunohistochemical stains attest to the neuroendocrine nature of the tumor and show neuron-specific enolase, chromogranin (Fig. 21-39C) and synaptophysin.

In 5% to 10% of cases, pheochromocytomas are malignant, but this figure may be higher for extra-adrenal tumors. Malignancy can only identified by biological behavior (i.e., metastases), and not from histologic appearance. Benign and malignant pheochromocytomas show mitoses, cellular pleomorphism, capsular or vascular invasion and necrosis. Metastases are most common in the regional lymph nodes, bone, lung and liver.

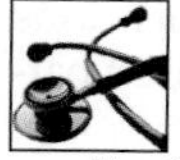

CLINICAL FEATURES: With few exceptions, the clinical features of pheochromocytomas reflect catecholamine release by the tumor. Patients may come to medical attention because of (1) asymptomatic hypertension

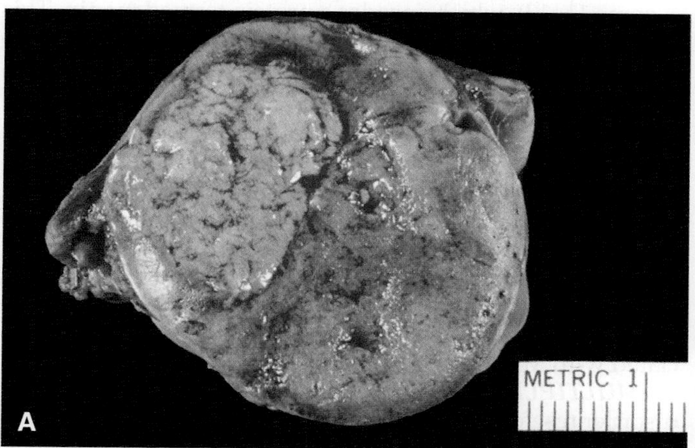

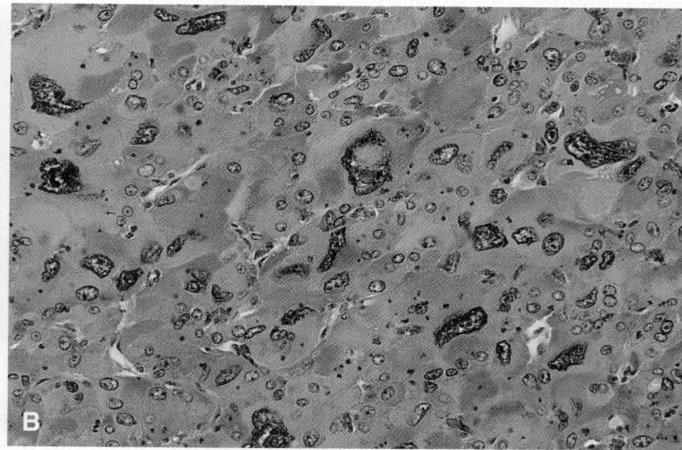

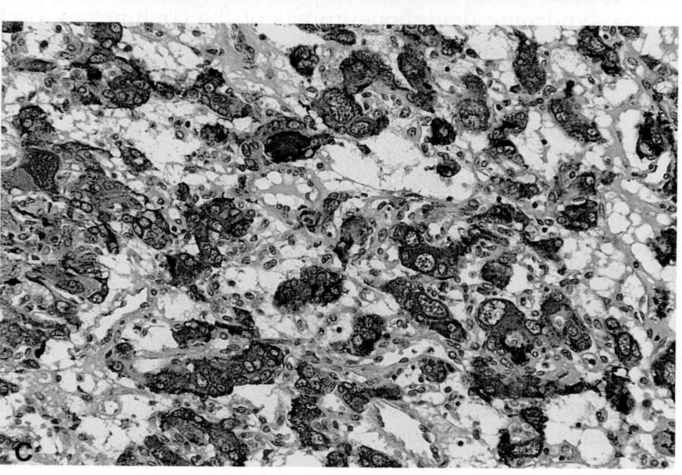

FIGURE 21-39. Pheochromocytoma. A. The cut surface of an adrenal tumor from a patient with episodic hypertension is reddish brown with a prominent area of fibrosis. Foci of hemorrhage and cystic degeneration are evident. **B.** A photomicrograph of the tumor shows polyhedral tumor cells with ample finely granular cytoplasm. Note the enlarged hyperchromatic nuclei. **C.** Many of the tumor cells show positive immunohistochemical staining for chromogranin A, a marker of neuroendocrine differentiation.

found on routine examination, (2) symptomatic hypertension resistant to antihypertensive therapy, (3) malignant hypertension (e.g., encephalopathy, papilledema, proteinuria), (4) myocardial infarction or aortic dissection or (5) paroxysms of convulsions, anxiety or hyperventilation.

Typically, episodic catecholamine release leads to a paroxysm or crisis, of up to several hours, with severe throbbing headache, sweating, palpitations, tachycardia, abdominal pain and vomiting. Blood pressure may be elevated, often extremely so. Paroxysms can be precipitated by activities that place pressure on the abdominal contents (including the tumor), such as exercise, lifting, bending or vigorous abdominal palpation. Anxiety may occur during a paroxysm, but it is not an initiating factor.

More than 90% of patients with pheochromocytoma show hypertension, which is sustained in two thirds of patients and resembles essential hypertension. In these patients, blood pressure rises even higher during a paroxysm. One third of patients have episodic hypertension, which becomes sustained. In many untreated patients, it evolves into malignant hypertension.

There are other consequences of excess catecholamine levels. Orthostatic hypotension results from decreased plasma volume and poor postural tone. Increased basal metabolism, sweating, heat intolerance and weight loss may mimic hyperthyroidism. Angina and myocardial infarction occur in the absence of coronary artery disease. The cardiac complications are attributed to myocardial necrosis caused by elevated catecholamine levels **(catecholamine cardiomyopathy).**

Increased urinary levels of catecholamine metabolites, particularly vanillylmandelic acid (VMA), metanephrine and unconjugated catecholamines, are diagnostic for these tumors. Treatment for pheochromocytoma is surgical. β-Adrenergic blocking agents may be used to control hypertensive crises, and β-adrenergic receptor antagonists are helpful adjuncts.

Paragangliomas Are Pheochromocytomas Arising at Extra-Adrenal Sites

Paragangliomas arise in paraganglia in any location, including the retroperitoneum, neck, posterior mediastinum and urinary bladder. They may also arise in the base of the skull, neck or vagal or aortic bodies, or in any organ that contains paraganglionic tissue, such as the larynx and small intestine. Bladder paragangliomas may present with a syndrome of headaches and paroxysmal hypertension on urination. Paragangliomas originate in such paraganglia as the glomus jugulare, carotid body and other vasoreceptor bodies. Most (90%) paragangliomas of the head and neck are benign; those in the retroperitoneum are more often malignant.

Carotid body tumors are prototypical paragangliomas, arising at the carotid bifurcation. They form palpable masses in the neck. Interestingly, carotid body tumors are 10 times more frequent in people living at high altitude than in those at sea level, suggesting that these tumors may represent a hyperplastic response to prolonged carotid body sensing of hypoxia.

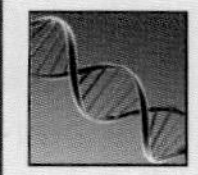

MOLECULAR PATHOGENESIS: Autosomal dominant transmission of paragangliomas is seen in some families, and hereditary paraganglioma was the first hereditary tumor syndrome reported to be caused by a germline mutation in a gene encoding a mitochondrial protein. Genetic linkage is traced to the *SDHD* gene (11q23), which encodes a subunit of cytochrome B that has been proposed to participate in oxygen sensing. Curiously, all affected persons, whether male or female, inherited the disease from their fathers. About 10% of these tumors can be malignant and metastasize to distant organs such as lung and bone.

Multiple Endocrine Adenomatosis Syndromes Are Inherited Disorders in Which Multiple Endocrine Organs Are Affected by Diverse Cellular Proliferations

The features of the autosomal dominant MEN syndromes are (Fig. 21-40):

- **MEN type 1 (Wermer syndrome)** includes (1) pituitary adenoma, (2) parathyroid hyperplasia or adenoma and (3) islet cell tumors of the pancreas (insulinoma, gastrinoma). The pancreatic neoplasms tend to be multicentric and more aggressive than in sporadic cases. Two thirds of patients have adenomas of two or more endocrine organs, and one fifth develop tumors of three or more. Carcinoid, adrenocortical and lipoid tumors may also occur in MEN1. Almost all people with MEN type 1 (>95%) have primary hyperparathyroidism. The disease is caused by mutation of the MEN1 tumor suppressor gene (chromosome 11q13), which encodes a protein termed **menin.** This nuclear protein is thought to interact with the transcription factor junD.
- **MEN type 2 syndromes** feature MTC in virtually all patients and pheochromocytoma in about half.

MULTIPLE ENDOCRINE NEOPLASIA TYPE 2A (SIPPLE SYNDROME): Most (95%) MEN2 patients are classified as 2A. In addition to MTC and pheochromocytoma, a third of patients show hyperparathyroidism due to parathyroid hyperplasia or adenoma. A variety of neural crest tumors may be seen with MEN type 2A, including gliomas, glioblastomas and meningiomas. Hirschsprung disease is also associated with MEN type 2A.

MULTIPLE ENDOCRINE NEOPLASIA TYPE 2B: This disorder resembles MEN2A, but develops some 10 years earlier. Parathyroid disease is uncommon. The **mucosal neuroma syndrome** (ganglioneuromas of the conjunctiva, oral cavity, larynx and gastrointestinal tract) is a feature of MEN2B. Mucosal neuromas are always encountered, but only half of patients express the full phenotype. Many patients have a habitus similar to that in Marfan syndrome.

FAMILIAL MEDULLARY THYROID CARCINOMA: There are families who have at least four members with this tumor and no evidence of other features of MEN2.

Adrenal medullary hyperplasia has been reported in some patients with both MEN2A and MEN2B. Just as C-cell hyperplasia precedes thyroid medullary carcinomas, adrenal medullary hyperplasia is thought to antedate pheochromocytoma in these cases. Lesions are usually less than 1 cm. Grossly, an enlarged adrenal shows an expanded medulla. The chromaffin cells are larger than normal and are arranged in distinct nests or cords.

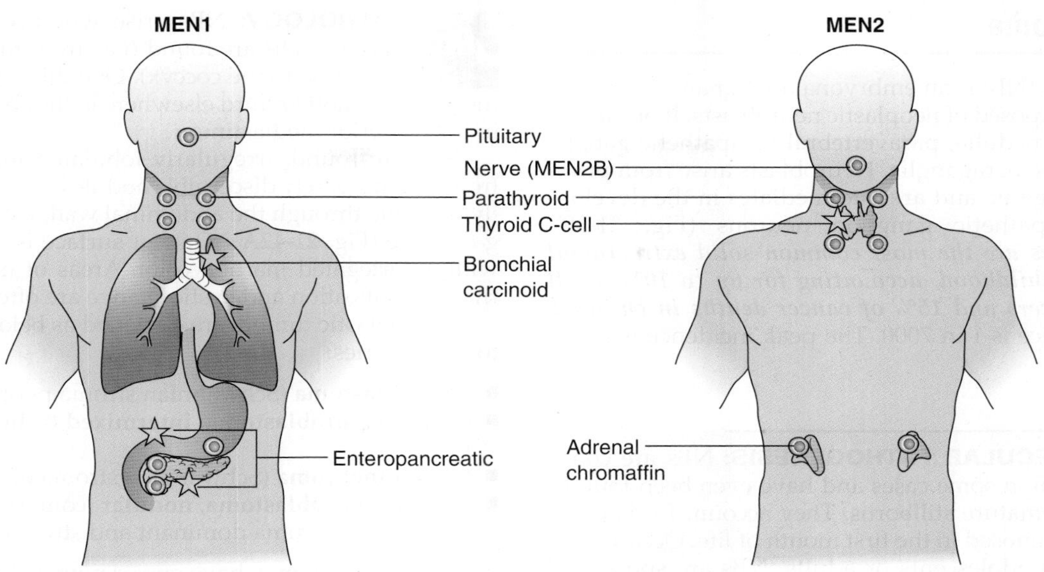

FIGURE 21-40. Multiple endocrine neoplasia (MEN) syndromes. The locations of the most common endocrine tumors in hereditary MEN syndromes types 1 and 2 are shown.

MOLECULAR PATHOGENESIS: The *RET* **proto-oncogene** on chromosome 10q11.2 is responsible for MEN2 syndromes. *RET* encodes a transmembrane tyrosine kinase receptor that binds glia-derived growth factor and neurturin. Several germline, missense and activating mutations in the cysteine-rich extracellular domain of RET have been identified in 95% of families with MEN2A and 85% of those with familial thyroid carcinoma (Fig. 21-41). The most common mutation (codon 634) constitutively activates the receptor by promoting its dimerization, recapitulating the result of ligand binding.

A point mutation at codon 918 of the tyrosine kinase domain of *RET* is seen in 95% of patients with MEN2B. This mutation constitutively activates the tyrosine kinase function of the receptor, and also causes it to phosphorylate substrates ordinarily preferred by other kinases (e.g., c-*src* and c-*abl*).

Identification of* RET *mutations is used to confirm the diagnosis of MEN2 and identify asymptomatic family members. People who carry *RET* mutations are screened for thyroid cancer, pheochromocytoma and hyperparathyroidism between 6 and 35 years of age, and are offered prophylactic thyroidectomy.

Somatic mutations in *RET* have been found in 10% to 20% of patients with sporadic pheochromocytomas. In addition, some sporadic pheochromocytomas exhibit mutations in the von Hippel-Lindau (*VHL*) and neurofibromatosis type 1 (*NF1*) genes.

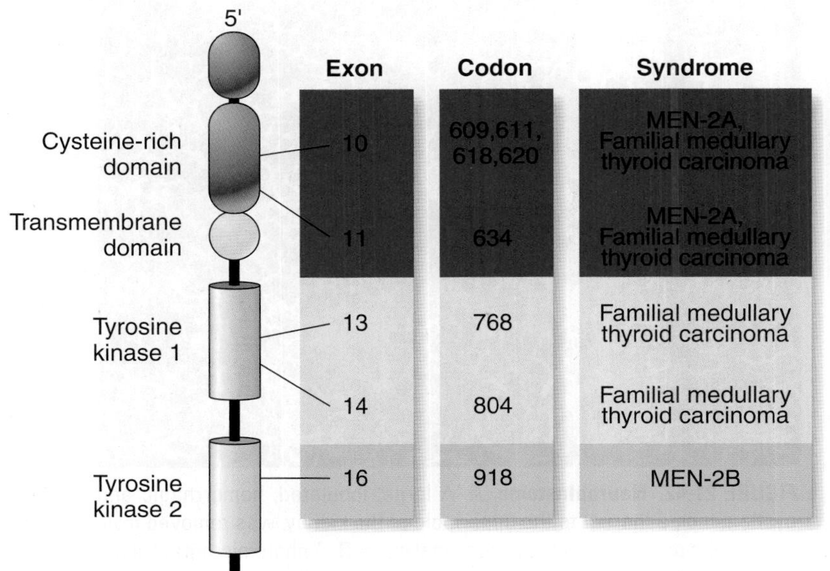

5'
3'
Cysteine-rich domain
Transmembrane domain
Tyrosine kinase 1
Tyrosine kinase 2
Exon
Codon
Syndrome
10
609,611, 618,620
MEN-2A, Familial medullary thyroid carcinoma
11
634
MEN-2A, Familial medullary thyroid carcinoma
13
768
Familial medullary thyroid carcinoma
14
804
Familial medullary thyroid carcinoma
16
918
MEN-2B

FIGURE 21-41. Representative *RET* proto-oncogene mutations in multiple endocrine neoplasia type 2 (MEN2).

Neuroblastoma

Neuroblastoma (NB) is an embryonal malignancy of neural crest origin composed of neoplastic neuroblasts. It originates in the adrenal medulla, paravertebral sympathetic ganglia and sympathetic paraganglia. Neuroblasts arise from primitive sympathogonia and are intermediates in the development of sympathetic ganglion neurons (Fig. 21-38). ***Neuroblastomas are the most common solid extracranial neoplasms of childhood, accounting for up to 10% of all childhood cancers and 15% of cancer deaths in children.*** Overall incidence is 1 in 7000. The peak incidence is in the first 3 years.

MOLECULAR PATHOGENESIS: NBs are congenital in some cases and have even been found in premature stillborns. They account for half of all cancers diagnosed in the first month of life. Occasional cases occur in adolescents or adults. NBs are sporadic. However, rare autosomal dominant familial NBs are reported, which tend to be multifocal tumors and to occur at an early age. The short arm of chromosome 16 appears to be the affected locus. NBs may occur with neurofibromatosis type 1, Beckwith-Wiedemann syndrome and Hirschsprung disease.

The embryologic adrenal medulla, and presumably other parts of the sympathetic nervous system, continue to develop during the first year of life. ***Persistence and transformation of these embryonal structures may be related to the pathogenesis of NB.*** Deletions on chromosome 1 (1p35-36) are frequent, with unbalanced translocation with 17q. Extrachromosomal double minutes and homogeneously staining regions (HSRs) are found on chromosome 2. The HSRs represent amplification of N-*myc;* this abnormality is key in determining the aggressiveness of neuroblastoma. The locus on chromosome 1 may encode a gene that suppresses N-*myc* amplification.

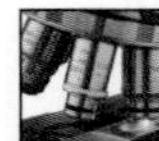

PATHOLOGY: NBs arise wherever neural crest–derived cells are found (i.e., from the posterior cranial fossa to the coccyx). One third of tumors are in the adrenal, another third elsewhere in the abdomen and 20% in the posterior mediastinum.

NBs are round, irregularly lobulated masses that vary from minute, barely discernible nodules to large masses readily palpable through the abdominal wall, weighing 50 to 150 g or more (Fig. 21-42A). The cut surface is soft and friable, with a variegated maroon color. Areas of necrosis, hemorrhage, calcification and cystic change are often present.

Neuroblastic tumors are classified as belonging to one of four categories:

- **Neuroblastoma** (Schwannian stroma poor)
- **Ganglioneuroblastoma, intermixed** (Schwannian stroma rich)
- **Ganglioneuroma** (Schwannian stroma dominant)
- **Ganglioneuroblastoma, nodular** (composite Schwannian stroma rich/stroma dominant and stroma poor)

Each category may have one or more subtypes.

Dense sheets of small, round to fusiform cells with dark nuclei and scant cytoplasm, which are often compared with lymphocytes, make up the tumor. Limited or no Schwannian proliferation is seen and mitoses are frequent. Characteristic Homer Wright rosettes are defined by a rim of dark tumor cells in a circumferential arrangement around a central pale fibrillar core (Fig. 21-42B). By electron microscopy, malignant neuroblasts show peripheral dendritic processes with longitudinally oriented microtubules and neurosecretory granules and filament.

NBs readily infiltrate surrounding structures and metastasize to regional lymph nodes, liver, lungs, bones and other sites. The tumor may differentiate into a ganglioneuroma (see below).

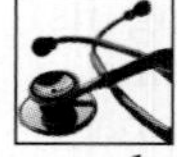

CLINICAL FEATURES: The presentation of NB is highly variable, a consequence of the many sites of the primary tumors and metastases. The first sign is often an enlarging abdomen in a young child. Physical examination

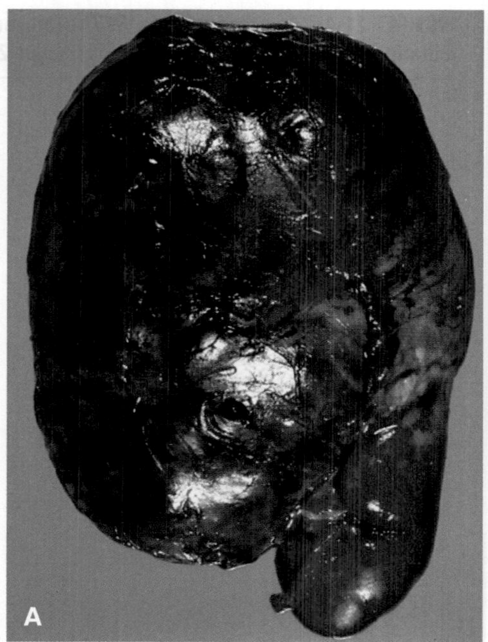

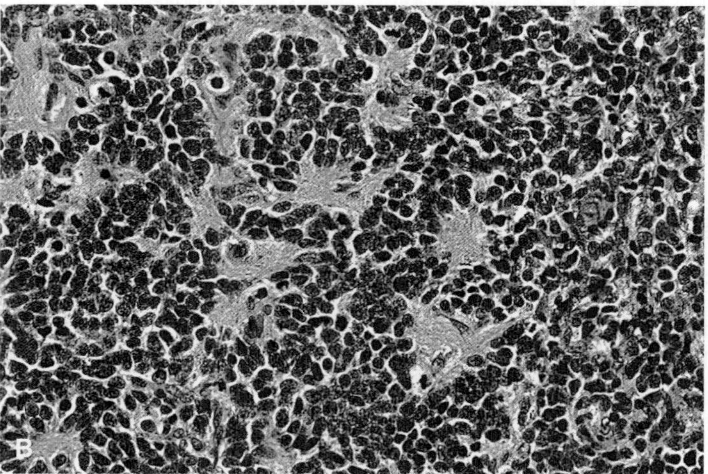

FIGURE 21-42. Neuroblastoma. A. A large, lobulated, hemorrhagic and cystic tumor, adherent to the upper pole of the kidney, was removed from a child who presented with an abdominal mass. **B.** A photomicrograph illustrates the characteristic rosettes, formed by small, regular, dark tumor cells arranged around a central, pale fibrillar core.

discloses a firm, irregular, nontender mass. Hepatic metastases enlarge the liver and may cause ascites. Marked irritability may reflect pain from bony metastases. Respiratory distress accompanies large masses in the thorax, and tumors in the pelvis obstruct the bowel or ureters. Spinal cord compression may lead to gait disturbance and sphincter dysfunction. Severe diarrhea may be caused in tumors secreting vasoactive intestinal peptide. Some patients show paraneoplastic opsoclonus-myoclonus syndrome, which usually indicates an excellent prognosis, although some may develop permanent neurologic deficits.

Urinary excretion of catecholamines and their metabolites is almost invariably elevated in patients with NB. The urine contains increased amounts of **norepinephrine, VMA, homovanillic acid** (HVA) and **dopamine.**

Several factors are useful in predicting the outcome of NB:

- **Age:** Age at diagnosis is one of the most important indicators of survival. Children under 1 year old do better than older patients with the same stage of disease. Spontaneous tumor regression is common at this age.
- **Site:** Extra-adrenal tumors tend to be better differentiated and so less aggressive.
- **Stage:** Survival is 90% in stage I (tumor confined to the organ of origin), and decreases to less than 3% in stage IV (widespread metastases). An exception is stage IVS (special), in which tumors lack the chromosomal abnormalities characteristic of neuroblastoma. Even with liver and bone marrow metastases, patients with stage IVS may have spontaneous remissions; survival is 60% to 90%.
- **Tumor histology:** Low-grade (better-differentiated) tumors have better prognoses than high-grade (undifferentiated) tumors. If the **VMA/HVA ratio** is less than 1, the tumor is deficient in dopamine β-hydroxylase and likely to be more aggressive.
- **DNA ploidy:** DNA indices near diploid/tetraploid range are unfavorable, while hyperdiploid or near-triploid neuroblastomas have a good prognosis. DNA ploidy has less prognostic value in patients older than 2 years of age.
- **Genomic alterations:** N-*myc* amplification occurs in 20% to 25% of cases, and is associated with poor outcome. Tumors with N-*myc* amplification often have deletion of chromosome 1p (especially deletion of 1p36.3). Allelic gain of 17q is associated with more aggressive tumors.

NBs can express three tyrosine kinase neurotrophin receptors: TrkA, TrkB and TrkC. High levels of TrkA correlate with younger age, lower stage, absence of MYCN amplification and a better prognosis. Conversely, TrkB expression correlates with an invasive phenotype, high-risk disease and chemoresistance. Expression of TrkC is found in lower-stage tumors. High-level expression of *EPHB6, CD44, EFNB2* and *EFNB3* genes is associated with good clinical outcome.

Localized NBs are treated by surgery alone. Disseminated tumors require chemotherapy and sometimes irradiation.

Ganglioneuromas Are Mature Variants of Neuroblastic Tumors

Ganglioneuroma, like NB, is a neural crest tumor. It is seen in older children and young adults. ***Ganglioneuromas are benign and arise in sympathetic ganglia, typically in the posterior mediastinum.*** Up to 30% occur in the adrenal medulla. Ganglioneuromas do not show the chromosomal abnormalities characteristic of NB.

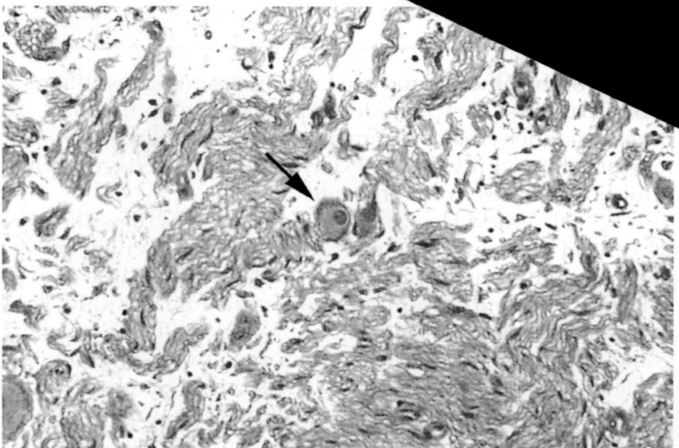

FIGURE 21-43. Ganglioneuroma. A photomicrograph shows mature ganglion cells (*arrow*) interspersed among wavy spindle cells embedded in a myxoid matrix.

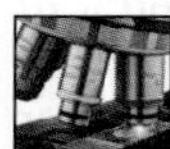

PATHOLOGY: Ganglioneuromas are well encapsulated with myxoid, glistening, cut surfaces. They contain well-differentiated, mature ganglion cells, associated with spindle cells in a loose, abundant fibrillar stroma (Fig. 21-43). The fibrils represent neurites extending from tumor cell bodies. Cytoplasmic processes of ganglion cells contain neurosecretory granules and may form synaptic junctions. Neuroendocrine substances, such as neuron-specific enolase and certain peptide hormones, are detectable. As mentioned above, a NB may differentiate into a ganglioneuroma.

PINEAL GLAND

Anatomy and Function

The pineal gland, shaped like a minute pine cone, is located below the posterior edge of the corpus callosum and is suspended from the roof of the third ventricle over the superior colliculi.

The gland shows a lobulated architecture, compartmentalized by fibrovascular septa. It is composed of cords and clusters of large epithelial-like cells, **pinealocytes,** which have modified photosensory and neuroendocrine functions. Astrocytes make up about 10% of pineal cells.

The gland produces a number of neurotransmitter substances, among the most important of which is **melatonin.** Although in lower animal species melatonin has a significant depigmenting effect, this is not evident in mammals. Since melatonin levels are higher at night than during waking hours, it has been suggested that it may function to induce sleep.

Serotonin and several other peptides are produced by the pineal. The most significant peptide is arginine vasotocin, a hormone that has important antigonadotropic activity. It is postulated that melatonin acts as a releasing factor for arginine vasotocin.

Beginning at about the time of puberty, calcifications (corpora arenacea or "brain sand") can be identified in autopsy specimens in the pineal gland or by various radiologic techniques. Accumulation of these mineralized concretions increases with age and is accompanied by cystic degeneration and gliosis.

...e, representing less than 1% ...eoplasms originating from the ...ably from the pineocyte, and ...ot derived from pineocytes, plus, ...ther sites.

...lth Organization (WHO) classification of ... system (CNS) tumors divides pineal paren... ...ors (PPTs) into **well-differentiated pineocytomas, ... differentiated pineoblastomas** and **PPTs of intermedia... differentiation.** Tumors located in the pineal gland region include germ cell tumors; astrocytomas, in particular pilocytic astrocytomas; glioblastomas; gangliogliomas; ependymomas; meningiomas; and curiosities such as lipoma, hemangioma, paraganglioma, primary melanoma, fibrosarcoma and extraskeletal osteosarcoma. Metastatic neoplasms include primaries originating from lung, breast, stomach, esophagus, rectum, gallbladder and kidney.

PATHOLOGY:

- **Germ cell tumors:** ***These make up about 60% of pineal neoplasms, and are apparently derived from germ cells misplaced during embryogenesis.*** They occur primarily in young people. In morphology and biological behavior they resemble their gonadal/extragonadal counterparts. Components of this group include germinomas, the most common pineal gland tumor, as well as embryonal carcinomas, choriocarcinomas, teratomas and mixed germ cell tumors. CNS germ cell tumors are described in association with Klinefelter syndrome, Down syndrome, neurofibromatosis type 1 and neurocutaneous melanosis. Cytogenetic abnormalities in the pineal region germ cell tumors include numerical and structural abnormalities involving chromosome 12. Mutations of the *p53* tumor suppressor gene have been reported, but it is still unclear if this gene plays a pathogenetic role in germ cell neoplasms of the CNS. Histology is the most important factor predictive of outcome for this tumor group. Of note, intracranial germinomas are extremely radiosensitive and potentially curable.
- **Pineocytoma:** About 45% of pineal parenchymal tumors are pineocytomas. They appear primarily at 25 to 35 years of age. Grade I tumors are usually solid, well-circumscribed masses that replace the pineal body and may compress surrounding structures including the aqueduct, brainstem and cerebellum, with occasional extension into the third ventricle. Clinical features are variable with signs and symptoms related to their impact on surrounding structures, and include headaches and visual and behavioral disturbances. Microscopically, these tumors often have small, uniform tumor cells with round nuclei and eosinophilic cytoplasm that aggregate in poorly defined nests separated by thin strands of connective tissue. Alternatively, the neoplastic cells show a sheetlike growth, occasionally interrupted by irregular nuclear free zones known as pineocytomatous rosettes (Fig. 21-44). Mitoses are inconspicuous and necrosis, if identified, usually occurs in large tumors with compromised vasculature. A rare, poorly characterized papillary variant has been described and is noted for its aggressive behavior. Tumor cells typically show strong immunoreactivity for synaptophysin and neuron-specific enolase (NSE). Cytogenetic studies have been done in few cases, and reveal numerical and structural abnormalities of various chromosomes, including monosomy/loss of chromosomes 22, 11 and 1. ***Pineocytomas do not metastasize, and 5-year event-free survival is 100%.***
- **Pineoblastoma:** This highly malignant tumor predominantly affects children. It constitutes about 45% of all pineal parenchymal tumors. These are soft masses, often with hemorrhagic and necrotic areas, that invade and infiltrate surrounding structures with frequent craniospinal dissemination. Clinical signs and symptoms are similar to those of other tumors in the region. Pineoblastomas consist of small oval cells, with dark nuclei and scanty cytoplasm, resembling medulloblastoma or PNET (see Chapter 28). Homer Wright and Flexner Wintersteiner rosettes may be seen. Mitoses are usually numerous. Like pineocytomas, pineoblastomas show variable immunoreactivity to NSE and synaptophysin. Pineoblastomas may occur in patients with bilateral/familial retinoblastoma, the so-called "trilateral retinoblastoma syndrome." Association with familial adenomatous polyposis is also reported.

  Pineoblastomas have shown normal karyotype and complex chromosomal abnormalities; monosomy of chromosomes 20 and 22 and trisomy of chromosome 14 have been reported. The extent of disease at presentation determines prognosis. About 58% of patients with pineoblastoma survive 5 years.
- **Pineal parenchymal tumor of intermediate differentiation:** These tumors contain areas of well-differentiated pineocytoma and poorly differentiated pineoblastoma, and regions of intermediate histologic differentiation between these tumors. They represent about 10% of all pineal parenchymal tumors and occur at all ages, with highest incidence in adults. Clinical behavior is variable, with reports of survival longer than 4 years. These are moderately cellular tumors, with mild nuclear atypia, occasional mitosis and Homer Wright rosettes.

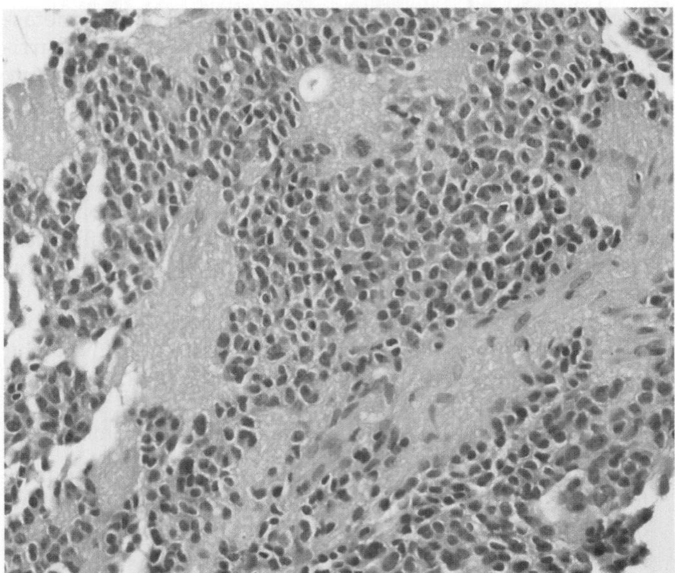

FIGURE 21-44. Pineocytoma. A photomicrograph shows nests of tumor cells with round nuclei and eosinophilic cytoplasm separated by connective tissue.

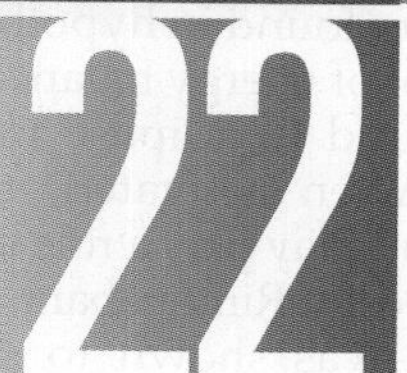

22 Obesity, Diabetes Mellitus and the Metabolic Syndrome

Kevin Jon Williams • Elias S. Siraj

OBESITY

Only three decades ago, obesity was relatively uncommon, but its prevalence has been increasing rapidly. Astonishingly, on a global scale, 1 billion adults might be classified as overweight, and at least 400 million meet established criteria for obesity. Approximately one third of the adults in the United States are obese, but there is some indication that this prevalence might be leveling off. In the developed world, obesity is more common among women and the poor, whereas in developing countries, it affects primarily the well-to-do. The explosion in obesity rates indicates that the fundamental problem is a recent change in environment, not genetics. It is especially worrisome that at least one in seven children in the United States is obese; a recent longitudinal study showed that obesity in children more than doubles the risk of death before the age of 55 years from endogenous causes.

Energy Intake and Expenditure

Weight gain other than water occurs when energy intake exceeds expenditure: you are what you eat, minus what you burn. Energy intake is conceptually straightforward: many populations consume an overabundance of calories, and the normal human gastrointestinal tract absorbs essentially all simple fuels presented to it. As little as 300 extra calories per day—two cans of regular soda or three 8-ounce servings of fruit juice—can result in 120 kg of weight gain from age 15 to age 25. Thus, a child who ingests a high-caloric snack on the way to and from school assumes a substantial risk for obesity. Some of these behaviors have a significant inherited component: offspring of mothers with high prepregnancy body weights exhibit eating in the absence of hunger (EAH) and seek out foods of high energy density (kcal/g). Total daily energy expenditure (TDEE) consists of several regulated components:

1. **Basal metabolic rate (BMR):** The BMR is the energy expended at complete rest, lying down, in the postabsorptive state. It includes maintenance levels of breathing, circulation of blood and essential metabolic functions. For individuals with sedentary occupations, BMR accounts for ~60% of TDEE. Over three quarters of the variance in BMR reflects differences in lean body mass.
2. **Calories spent to digest, absorb and store ingested calories** (6% to 12% of TDEE).
3. **Energetic costs of emotion, medication and adaptive thermogenesis in response to the environment** (e.g., changes in temperature, exposure to infectious agents).
4. **Activity thermogenesis** generated by physical movement during purposeful exercise and nonexercise activity thermogenesis (NEAT). Importantly, levels of NEAT vary substantially among apparently normal individuals, by as much as 2000 calories per day, and lower NEAT correlates strongly with obesity. Obese individuals sit approximately 2.5 more hours each day than their sedentary lean counterparts. The cumulative effect on energy balance over the years can be substantial, and public health strategies have been proposed to increase NEAT during work and leisure time.

The Brain Is the Central Homeostatic Controller of Body Weight

The brain receives hormonal and neuronal signals from the periphery about food deficits or surpluses and the rate of fuel utilization. To maintain homeostasis, it then coordinates responses, modulating behavior and the endocrine and autonomic nervous systems to adjust energy balance.

The **hypothalamus** is the main processor of signals from the periphery and is crucial to management of energy balance. Many hypothalamic nuclei regulate metabolism, but the arcuate nucleus plays a central role in integrating peripheral signals via two distinct populations of neurons with opposing actions on food intake. One population produces **anorexigenic** (appetite-suppressing) neuropeptides including proopiomelanocortin (POMC) and cocaine- and amphetamine-regulated transcript (CART). POMC is cleaved into α-melanocyte stimulating hormone (α-MSH), which binds melanocortin receptors MC3R and MC4R to decrease appetite.

The other group of neurons produces two **orexigenic** (appetite-stimulating) neuropeptides: neuropeptide Y (NPY) and agouti-related protein (AgRP). NPY is among the most abundant neuropeptides in the mammalian brain and is a potent stimulator of feeding. It may bind any of six G-protein–coupled NPY receptor subtypes (Y1 through Y6), but Y1 and Y2 NPY receptors seem to be most involved with feeding. AgRP antagonizes the melanocortin receptors, thereby blocking the anorexigenic effects of α-MSH, leading to increased food intake.

- **Leptin:** The discovery of **leptin** revealed a key link between neural and nonneural systems in the control of appetite and energy expenditure. Leptin (from the Greek λεπτός, meaning "thin") is the protein product of the *LEP* gene, known historically as the *Ob* gene, and is produced mainly by adipocytes. Its serum concentration is proportional to body fat mass (i.e., it is lower in lean individuals and rises with obesity). Its chief physiologic role appears to be signaling the brain that body adipose stores are sufficient. Low serum leptin levels increase appetite and decrease energy expenditure, in part by dampening the thyroidal axis; normal leptin levels decrease food intake.

  Leptin enters the brain and interacts with leptin receptors on both POMC/CART and NPY/AgRP neurons, regulating them in opposite ways. Leptin directly activates (anorexigenic) POMC/CART neurons while blocking the activity of (orexigenic) NPY/AgRP neurons. The result is decreased food intake. As noted before, blood levels of leptin are above normal in most obese individuals, but unfortunately, this increased leptin fails to halt excessive fat accumulation. There is evidence to support several explanations, including an inability of leptin to reach its neuronal targets, a failure of intracellular signaling by the leptin receptor despite occupancy with leptin (desensitization) and increased responsiveness to hedonic cues to overeat that overwhelm physiologic restraints. Leptin injections to treat obesity have not been successful to date.
- **Circadian rhythms** affect, and are affected by, caloric flux. Mice with genetic disruption of the circadian system develop obesity, hyperleptinemia, hyperlipidemia and hyperglycemia. In humans, shift workers, who must alter their sleep rhythms, exhibit increased prevalence of high body mass indexes (BMIs), the metabolic syndrome (see below) and cardiovascular events. Forced sleep restriction in humans disturbs appetite control and glucose tolerance, which is a particular concern given the disturbances in sleep caused by obstructive apnea in individuals who are already obese.
- **Endocannabinoids** are recently discovered endogenous lipids that bind to cannabinoid receptors 1 and 2 (CB1, CB2). CB1 receptors are found in hypothalamic nuclei that are involved in control of energy balance and weight. CB1 receptors are also found in adipose tissue and the gastrointestinal tract. When activated, the CB1 receptor induces food intake and may play a role in the development and maintenance of obesity. Rimonabant, a synthetic blocker of the CB1 receptor, was shown to suppress appetite, decrease weight and improve metabolic parameters in obese subjects, but its side effects have prevented its being used to treat obesity.
- The **gastrointestinal tract** is another major participant in energy homeostasis. It contains a diverse group of mechanoreceptors and chemosensitive receptors that relay information via vagal afferent fibers that terminate on the nucleus tractus solitarii in the brainstem. For example, activation of the vagus from gastric distension causes satiety and meal termination. Additionally, several hormones produced by the gastrointestinal tract signal to the central nervous system (CNS) to regulate energy intake. Notably, **glucagon-like peptide 1** (GLP-1) is produced by posttranslational processing of proglucagon by L cells located primarily in the mucosa of the distal ileum and colon. GLP-1 decreases food intake, slows gastric emptying, generates a feeling of satiety, augments postprandial glucose-stimulated insulin secretion and decreases secretion of glucagon, a hormone that opposes insulin action (see Chapter 21). These combined effects reduce the rate of caloric delivery into the intestines, and hence to the rest of the body, while enhancing insulin secretion and action. Long-acting GLP-1 analogs (exenatide and liraglutide) are used to treat type 2 diabetes mellitus and also cause weight reduction.
- **Ghrelin** is a hormone that stimulates hunger. It is produced primarily by gastric endocrine cells but also to a lesser extent in the duodenum, ileum and colon. Ghrelin stimulates orexigenic NPY neurons in the arcuate nucleus of the hypothalamus. Circulating ghrelin levels increase during fasting, and its administration to normal subjects increases caloric intake. Patients with anorexia nervosa have high plasma concentrations of ghrelin; however, administration of exogenous ghrelin to treat this condition has not been successful. A fall in plasma ghrelin is seen after gastric bypass, and may contribute to the continued weight loss after the procedure. Conversely, patients with Prader-Willi syndrome exhibit hyperphagia and very high plasma ghrelin levels. Moreover, serum ghrelin concentrations increase after diet-induced weight loss, which may contribute to the long-term failure of clinical weight loss programs.
- **Cholecystokinin (CCK)** is produced by gastrointestinal mucosa and is mainly concentrated in the duodenum and jejunum. It is released in response to fat and protein intake and acts on two distinct receptors. CCK stimulates release of enzymes from the pancreas and gallbladder to aid digestion, slows gastric emptying and reduces food intake. Regulation of food intake is mediated via vagal afferent signals to the brain.
- **Peptide YY** (PYY) is secreted along the entire gastrointestinal tract, but is concentrated in the ileum and colon. Of its two forms, PYY(3-36) is the major circulating form. It is released in response to food intake, and its numerous actions include delaying pancreatic and gastric secretions, gallbladder emptying and gastric emptying. PYY(3-36) decreases appetite, duration of food intake and total caloric intake.

- **Pancreatic polypeptide** (PP) is in the same peptide family as PYY. It is primarily produced in the pancreas, but is also found in the colon and rectum. The main stimulus to its release is food intake: it acts to reduce appetite and decrease food intake.
- **Amylin** is a peptide mainly produced by pancreatic beta cells, but also found in gut endocrine cells, visceral sensory neurons and the hypothalamus. It is a potent inhibitor of gastric emptying and decreases food intake. An analogue of amylin known as pramlintide is currently available for treatment of diabetes mellitus. It is associated with weight reduction in these patients and is in clinical trials for obesity.
- **Insulin** is well known for its role in peripheral glucose uptake, but it also affects appetite. Injection of insulin into the third ventricle of rats decreases food intake via insulin receptors in the arcuate nucleus of the hypothalamus, where it increases messenger RNA (mRNA) for POMC (anorexigenic) and suppresses mRNA for NYP (orexigenic). Clinically, however, administration of insulin often increases appetite, which can cause already overweight patients to eat more. Part of the explanation may be hypoglycemia.
- **Other substances** have been found to regulate hunger, satiety, fat deposition and so forth, in rodents, including galanin, adipocyte complement-related protein (ACRP), peroxisome proliferator-associated receptors (PPARs) and others.
- **Gut flora** affect body weight. Germ-free mice are protected from diet-induced obesity, and colonization of these mice with intestinal flora from conventionally raised mice enhances caloric uptake from complex dietary plant polysaccharides and modulates the expression of specific host genes to increase caloric storage in adipose tissue. In humans, distal gut flora from obese individuals have a different microbial composition from flora in lean individuals and a greater ability to extract calories from the diet than do microbiota from lean individuals.

Known orexigenic and anorexigenic factors are illustrated in Fig. 22-1.

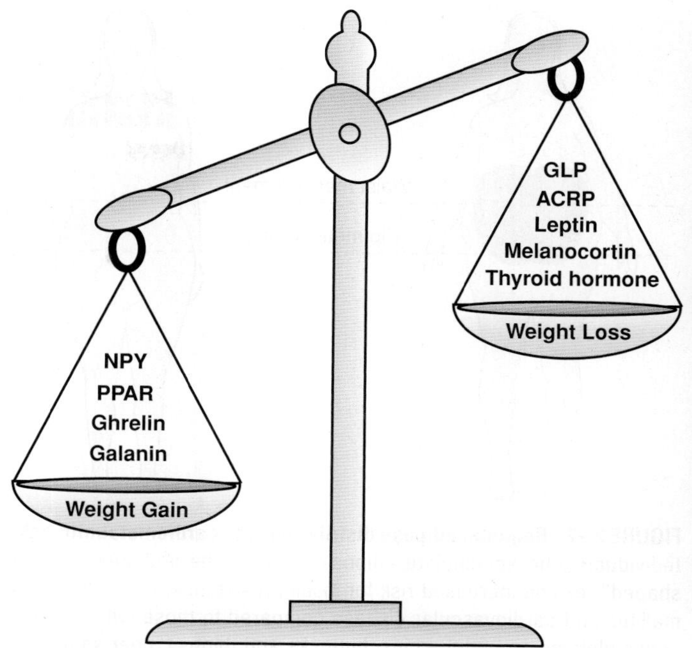

FIGURE 22-1. The balance of chemical mediators that promote fat accumulation (weight gain) and those that promote fat loss (weight loss). ACRP = adipocyte complement-related protein; GLP = glucagon-like peptide; NPY = neuropeptide Y; PPAR = peroxisome proliferator-activated receptor.

Body Mass Index and Obesity

The standard most often used to define obesity is the BMI:

$$\text{BMI} = [\text{weight (kg)}] \div [\text{height (m)}]^2$$

Although BMI is an excellent indicator of obesity, it does not formally distinguish between fat mass and lean mass. For example, a muscular person with little body fat could be misclassified as obese, and a person with excess adipose tissue and reduced muscle mass, such as an elderly or chronically ill individual, could have a normal BMI. There may also be ethnic variations in the amounts of adipose tissue at a given BMI.

Most health organizations define overweight to mean a BMI between 25 and 29.9 kg/m^2. Someone whose BMI is 30 kg/m^2 or greater is considered obese, and a BMI greater than 40 kg/m^2 denotes morbid obesity. These classifications are based on epidemiologic studies that show that high BMI correlates with excess morbidity and mortality, as well as metabolic abnormalities, particularly hyperglycemia, dyslipoproteinemia, hypertension and risk of developing overt type 2 diabetes. There is substantial variation in susceptibilities of various populations worldwide to metabolic abnormalities at similar BMIs, possibly related to differences in body composition, lifestyle (e.g., diet, physical activity, tobacco) and genetics. Most importantly, the appropriate BMI values to define obesity—and hence a need for intervention—may substantially differ among populations.

Regional body fat distribution is an important determinant of health risk associated with obesity. Fat depots in different parts of the body play various roles including energy metabolism, secretion of circulating proteins and metabolites into the bloodstream and the physical cushioning and protection of internal organs. Abdominal obesity (also known as central adiposity, visceral–abdominal obesity, or "apple shaped") carries a greater risk of diabetes, hypertension, heart disease and some forms of cancer compared to gluteal–femoral obesity (termed lower body obesity or "pear shaped"; Fig. 22-2).

The BMI does not account for fat distribution, so abdominal obesity is better assessed by measuring waist circumference or the waist:hip ratio. An increased risk for adverse health outcomes is associated with waist circumferences greater than 102 cm (40 inches) or waist:hip ratios greater than 0.9 in men, and waist circumferences greater than 88 cm (35 inches) or waist:hip ratios greater than 0.85 in women.

The Causes of Obesity Are Complex

Obesity is a multifactorial condition that involves complex interaction of genetic, metabolic, physiologic, social and behavioral factors. Rarely, severe clinical obesity has monogenic causes, but most cases are due to combined effects of multiple genes, lifestyle and environmental factors.

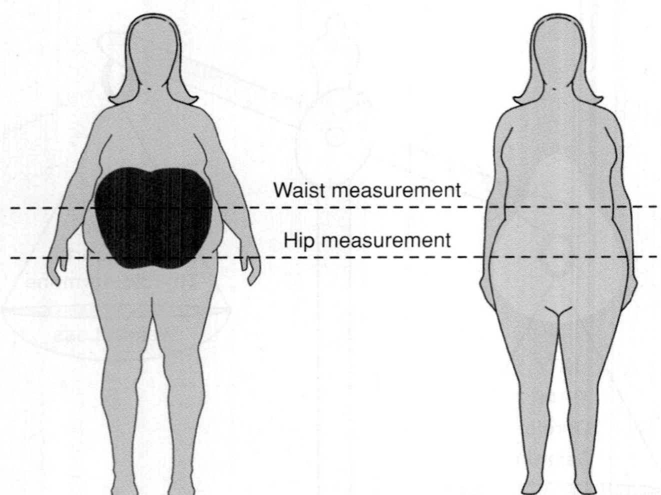

FIGURE 22-2. Regional adipose distribution and cardiometabolic risk. Individuals who accumulate adipose tissue in the abdomen ("apple shaped") exhibit increased risk for insulin resistance, type 2 diabetes mellitus and cardiovascular disease compared to those with adipose accumulations around the hips, buttocks and thighs ("pear shaped"). Standard methods to assess abdominal obesity include waist circumference and the waist:hip ratio.

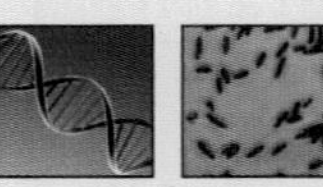

MOLECULAR PATHOGENESIS AND ETIOLOGIC FACTORS: Essentially everyone living in developed countries is exposed to a calorie-rich environment, yet BMIs vary considerably, from extremely thin to morbidly obese. An inherited propensity toward obesity is clear: comparisons of BMI values between monozygotic and dizygotic twins, between genetically full or half-siblings raised apart after adoption in infancy and in multigenerational kindreds have given estimates of heritability ranging from 20% to 80%. Most of these studies were done on people born before the recent increase in obesity. A recent study of twin children growing up during the obesity epidemic found that BMI and waist circumference each showed 77% heritability. Behaviors linked to obesity (e.g., eating in the absence of hunger, impaired responses to internal signals of satiety but exaggerated responses to external food cues, rapid eating [increased bites/min] and low levels of physical activity) all exhibit substantial inherited components.

To date, the wealth of genetic studies has identified specific gene variants that seem to play only minor roles in the development of obesity:

- **Leptin gene mutations** have been linked to rare monogenic syndromes of severe obesity in humans. Homozygotes present with hyperphagia and severe, early-onset obesity. They die more readily after childhood infections and develop hypothalamic hypogonadism, insulin resistance and diabetes as adults. Heterozygotes have reduced blood levels of leptin and increased body weight compared with unaffected siblings. Replacement therapy with recombinant leptin by injection is very effective in these individuals.
- **Leptin receptor gene mutations** have been found in rare families with severe early-onset obesity. The phenotype is similar to that in patients with mutations in the leptin gene, except that patients with the receptor mutation have markedly elevated serum leptin levels. They also have hypogonadotropic hypogonadism, failure of pubertal development, growth delay and secondary hypothyroidism. As expected, leptin supplementation is ineffective in these individuals.
- **Melanocortin-4 receptor gene (*MC4R*) mutations** are the leading cause of severe, monogenic childhood-onset obesity. Mutations in *MC4R* are estimated to occur in approximately 5% of cases of severe childhood-onset obesity. As this syndrome is rare, *MC4R* mutations have a minor effect on population-wide prevalence of obesity. Patients tend to have no phenotype other than obesity. Both dominant and recessive inheritance are described.
- Isolated cases of obesity have been linked to mutations or deficiencies in POMC/α-MSH, α-MSH, prohormone convertase 1 and hypothalamic transcription factor SIM1.
- **The Human Genome Initiative** has led to genome-wide association (GWA) studies to discover links between obesity and polymorphisms throughout the entire genome. Several genes have been identified that encode brain/hypothalamic proteins and are associated with variations in BMI. However, all of the specific gene polymorphisms identified to date can account for less than 1% of the genetic basis for obesity.
- **Epigenetic programming** during fetal or immediate postnatal life may influence adult physiology. Remarkably, large maternal weight loss from obesity surgery before pregnancy seems to prevent transmission of obesity to subsequent children. In contrast, children born to the same mothers before weight loss surgery show high rates of obesity.

The impact of sociologic and psychological factors on development of obesity cannot be underestimated. Insights gained by GWA studies and investigations into monogenic causes of obesity notwithstanding, the vast majority of obesity is probably caused by complex interactions of multiple genes and an individual's environment. The marked increase in obesity in the past 20 years underscores the role of environmental influences in the genesis of obesity. Body weight control mechanisms are believed to have evolved to protect from weight loss in times of scarcity, not obesity in times of plenty.

Striking examples of environmental influence on genetic predisposition include the Pima Native Americans in Arizona and the Aboriginal population of northern Australia. Pimas are now largely sedentary and eat a diet in which 50% of energy derives from fat, unlike their traditional low-fat diets. They have experienced dramatic increases in obesity and diabetes. In contrast, the genetically related Pimas in the Sierra Madre Mountains of Northern Mexico are more physically active, have maintained more traditional low-fat diets and have much lower rates of obesity and type 2 diabetes mellitus (T2DM). Similarly, urbanized Aboriginal people in Australia have a high prevalence of diabetes and hypertriglyceridemia, compared with their nonurbanized counterparts. As little as a 7-week reexposure of urbanized Aboriginals with T2DM and hypertriglyceridemia to the traditional lifestyle led to weight loss, improved glucose tolerance and fasting glucose, insulin and triglyceride concentrations.

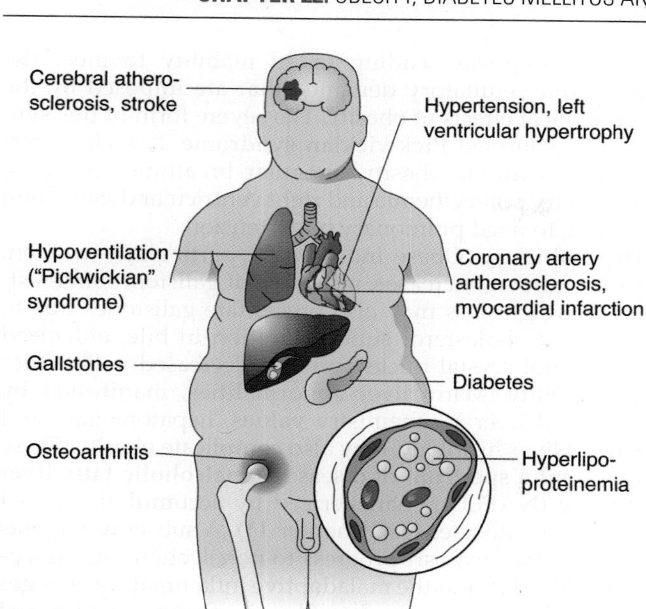

FIGURE 22-3. Medical complications of obesity.

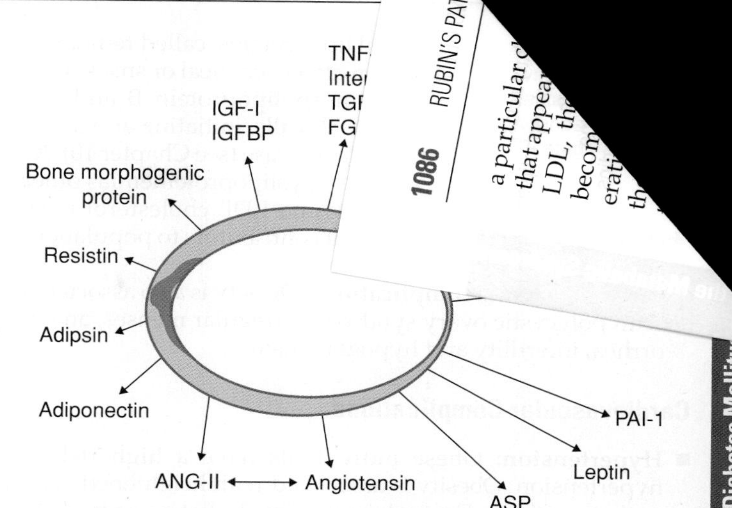

FIGURE 22-4. Many proteins and metabolites are secreted from adipose tissue and act locally or at a distance in other organs. They have been shown to have a strong influence on food intake, energy expenditure, insulin signaling, vascular function and other homeostatic processes in the body. ANG-II = angiotensin II; ASP = acetylation-stimulating protein; EGF = epidermal growth factor; FGF = fibroblast growth factor; IGF = insulin-like growth factor; IGFBP = insulin-like growth factor–binding protein; PAI-1 = plasminogen activator inhibitor-1; TGF = transforming growth factor; TNF = tumor necrosis factor.

The Complications of Obesity Affect Most Organ Systems

Many epidemiologic studies have shown that obesity and central adiposity are associated with increased mortality (Fig. 22-3). Fat cells undergo both hyperplasia and hypertrophy. The excess from the imbalance between energy intake and energy expenditure is stored in adipocytes that enlarge and/or increase in number: an extremely obese adult can have four times as many adipocytes as a lean adult, each one containing twice as much lipid.

The nature of the connection of excess adiposity with dysregulation of glucose and lipid metabolism and cardiovascular risk is an area of active research. Current theories include the portal/visceral hypothesis, the idea of adipose tissue as an endocrine organ, and the metabolic consequences of ectopic fat storage in metabolically active tissues like liver and skeletal muscle. The portal/visceral hypothesis proposes that increased central adiposity increases delivery of nonesterified fatty acids to the liver, where they directly block insulin action. Hepatic insulin resistance has been implicated in the development of hyperglycemia in diabetes (see below).

The endocrine paradigm derives from recent research showing that adipose tissue is an active secretory organ that releases many different types of factors into the blood. These substances include hormones and cytokines such as leptin, interleukin (IL)-6, angiotensin II, adiponectin, and resistin, among others. Importantly, obesity changes the profile of molecules secreted by adipose tissue, thereby promoting insulin resistance in liver and skeletal muscle (Fig. 22-4). Interestingly, many of these factors are also believed to contribute to endothelial dysfunction and maladaptive inflammatory changes in the vasculature during the development of atherosclerosis, potentially linking adiposity with cardiovascular disease.

The ectopic fat storage hypothesis proposes that obesity promotes the storage of excess lipid in liver, skeletal muscle and pancreatic insulin-secreting beta cells, where it influences insulin signaling and secretion, contributing to development of T2DM. Inherited defects in mitochondrial metabolism in skeletal muscle can lead to lipid accumulation there, eventuating in insulin resistance and type 2 diabetes.

Endocrine Complications

- **T2DM:** This disorder is strongly associated with obesity: more than 80% of cases of T2DM are attributed to obesity. Risk of diabetes increases linearly with BMI and with increments in abdominal fat mass, waist circumference, or waist:hip ratio at any given BMI. Conversely, weight loss and exercise decrease risk of type 2 diabetes and can prevent progression of insulin resistance to diabetes. In a large American population with impaired glucose tolerance, simply engaging in brisk walking for 150 minutes per week and loss of 7% of body weight reduced the rate of progression of blood glucose levels to overt T2DM in 58% of subjects. Using more drastic measures for morbid obesity, weight loss occurring after gastric bypass surgery resulted in complete resolution of diabetes in 77% of patients. Thus, these harmful effects appear reversible.
- **Dyslipidemia and dyslipoproteinemia:** By far, the major killer in obesity and diabetes is atherosclerotic cardiovascular disease. Several deleterious plasma lipid and lipoprotein abnormalities often occur in obesity, including elevated fasting triglycerides and nonesterified fatty acids, reduced high-density lipoprotein (HDL) and increased circulating low-density lipoprotein (LDL) particles. These abnormalities are strongly associated with increased risk of cardiovascular disease, particularly in individuals with central adiposity. In addition, recent studies have shown that nonfasting plasma triglyceride concentrations independently predict subsequent heart attacks and strokes. Nonfasting plasma triglyceride concentrations reflect the persistence of

lass of harmful lipoproteins, called remnants, in the circulation after each meal or snack. Like se particles contain apolipoprotein B and can e trapped within arterial walls, initiating and accel- ng atherosclerotic vascular disease (see Chapter 10). As e prevalence of obesity rises, dyslipoproteinemias other than simple elevations in plasma LDL cholesterol have become increasingly important contributors to population-wide cardiovascular risk.

- **Other endocrine complications:** Obesity is also associated with polycystic ovary syndrome, irregular menses, amenorrhea, infertility and hypogonadism.

Cardiovascular Complications

- **Hypertension:** Obese individuals have a high risk of hypertension. Obesity is associated with heightened sympathetic activity. The high insulin levels that occur in obese patients with insulin resistance act on pathways unrelated to glucose importation, such as enhancing renal reabsorption of sodium, which contributes to hypertension, and stimulating endothelial production of endothelin-1, a vasoconstrictor. As noted above, obese adipose tissue also secretes substances that directly cause vasoconstriction and increase blood pressure, including angiotensin II and its precursors. By interfering with the action of antihypertensive agents, obesity makes hypertension more difficult to control. Even a small reduction in weight may decrease blood pressure in this population.
- **Coronary heart disease:** BMI has a modest and graded association with myocardial infarction, but body fat distribution, especially the waist:hip ratio, is a stronger indicator of risk. Dyslipoproteinemia and hypertension are the best predictors of cardiovascular disease linked to obesity.
- **Congestive heart failure:** Obesity is associated with increased risk of heart failure owing to eccentric cardiac dilatation. Additionally, the combination of obesity and hypertension leads to ventricular wall thickening and larger heart volume. Obese patients are also at increased risk of atrial fibrillation and atrial flutter.
- **Thromboembolic disease:** Deep venous thromboses and pulmonary embolism are more common in obese patients. Lower extremity venous thromboembolic disease may be related to increased abdominal pressure, impaired fibrinolysis and increased circulating mediators of inflammation, particularly with abdominal obesity.

Additional Complications of Obesity

- **Neurologic:** Obesity increases risk of fatal and nonfatal ischemic strokes progressively as BMI increases. It is also associated with a higher prevalence of idiopathic intracranial hypertension. Marked weight loss in severely obese individuals can lead to a decline in intracranial pressure and resolution of symptoms.
- **Pulmonary:** Obesity may interfere mechanically with lung function. Increased weight, particularly excess abdominal obesity, decreases ventilatory drive, respiratory compliance and ventilation, particularly ventilation of lung bases. It thus contributes to ventilation–perfusion mismatching. Obesity is a major risk factor for development of **obstructive sleep apnea,** in which patients are prone to apnea and hypopnea during sleep. Obesity-hypoventilation syndrome is decreased ventilatory responsiveness to hypercapnia and/or hypoxia, leading to an inability to meet the increased ventilatory demands that are imposed by the mechanical effects of obesity. The severe form of this syndrome is termed **Pickwickian syndrome**. It is characterized by extreme obesity, irregular breathing, cyanosis, secondary polycythemia and right ventricular dysfunction leading to fixed pulmonary hypertension.
- **Hepatobiliary:** Obese individuals, particularly women, suffer from an increased incidence of gallstones. Interestingly, weight loss may also precipitate gallstones due to increased cholesterol supersaturation in bile, enhanced cholesterol crystal nucleation and decreased gallbladder contractility. Many liver abnormalities, manifested by increased liver biochemistry values, hepatomegaly and altered liver histology, may also complicate obesity. These represent a spectrum of disease, **nonalcoholic fatty liver disease** (NAFLD), characterized by accumulation of fat within hepatocytes (see Chapter 14). A subset of patients with simple steatosis progress to nonalcoholic steatohepatitis (NASH), and the maladaptive inflammatory changes within the liver can lead to fibrosis, cirrhosis and portal hypertension. NASH is considered the leading cause of so-called "idiopathic" cirrhosis.
- **Gastrointestinal:** Most large epidemiologic studies have found that gastroesophageal reflux is more common in obese individuals.
- **Cancer:** Certain cancers occur with greater frequency in people who are obese. Specifically, risk of esophageal, gallbladder, pancreatic, breast, renal, uterine, cervical and prostate cancers is increased. Once cancer is diagnosed, obesity is associated with a worse prognosis.
- **Musculoskeletal:** Hyperuricemia and gout are more common in obese people. Obesity increases the risk of osteoarthritis, particularly of weight-bearing joints such as the knees. However, non–weight-bearing joints can also be affected, suggesting mechanisms other than increased mechanical load. Weight loss decreases the risk of osteoarthritis.
- **Skin:** Obesity causes **striae**, stretching and thinning of the epidermis in a ribbonlike pattern. **Acanthosis nigricans** is a velvety, hypertrophic, hyperpigmented alteration especially at skinfold areas (axillae, nape of the neck) in the epidermis. It is believed to be a response to high circulating insulin levels in obese individuals with insulin resistance. Excessive hair growth, **hirsutism**, can result from increases in circulating androgens in susceptible women.
- **Psychological and social:** Obesity has also been associated with impaired quality of life, increased sick leave absences and disability claims and depression.

INSULIN RESISTANCE AND THE METABOLIC SYNDROME

Insulin resistance is a common consequence of obesity, and leads to type 2 diabetes mellitus. To understand the relationship of obesity, insulin resistance and diabetes, an understanding of the insulin receptor and its function is needed.

The insulin receptor is a tetrameric glycoprotein composed of two extracellular α-subunits that bind insulin and two transmembrane β-subunits that contain an insulin-stimulated tyrosine kinase activity. Activation of the receptor kinase leads to tyrosine phosphorylation of several insulin receptor substrate (IRS) proteins, causing transmission of the insulin signal into the cell. Adaptor proteins then bind to the newly phosphorylated sites on IRS molecules, which activates their downstream signaling. Thus, signaling kinases activated by phosphorylation of IRS proteins phosphorylate lipid and protein substrates, leading to translocation of glucose transport proteins from the interior of the cell to the plasma membrane and regulation of glucose and lipid metabolism, depending on the specific target cell type (i.e., liver, skeletal muscle or adipocyte). As noted above, insulin has several functions unrelated to glucose importation, including activation of mitogen-activated protein (MAP) kinases that then increase endothelin-1 production.

Several processes contribute to insulin resistance. In obese people, adipose tissue releases inhibitory mediators (including nonesterified fatty acids and cytokines such as tumor necrosis factor-α [TNF-α]) that interfere with insulin signaling by disrupting propagation of protein–tyrosine phosphorylation. An overabundance of nonesterified fatty acids can lead to intracellular accumulations of triglyceride and acyl coenzyme A (CoA) derivatives, particularly diacylglycerol. These molecules can activate intracellular serine kinase pathways that induce insulin resistance by blocking the insulin receptor tyrosine kinase signal cascade. Plasma levels of nonesterified fatty acids and TNF-α are strongly influenced by body fat distribution, in particular, visceral–abdominal (upper body) versus subcutaneous (hips/buttocks; lower body) adiposity (Fig. 22-2). Insulin resistance and T2DM are more prevalent in people with upper body–visceral obesity. Levels of nonesterified fatty acids and TNF-α are preferentially increased in visceral adiposity. Adiponectin, which promotes insulin action on its target tissues, is reduced in visceral adiposity. Hyperinsulinemia, caused by insulin resistance, can downregulate the number of insulin receptors on the plasma membrane, which may further contribute to cellular resistance to insulin action. Resistance to insulin is usually selective, meaning that it impairs signaling pathways leading to translocation of glucose transport proteins but leaves MAP kinase signaling intact.

Mitochondrial abnormalities have recently been shown to contribute to the development of T2DM (see below). In diabetics who are obese, abnormal intracellular triglyceride accumulation in liver and skeletal muscle suggests a defect in mitochondrial lipid oxidation. A genetic component for defective mitochondrial oxidative phosphorylation has been suggested.

Resistance to the action of insulin in target tissues and compensatory hyperinsulinemia are closely tied to a diverse set of cardiovascular risk factors that are prevalent in obese, sedentary people and patients with type 2 ("adult onset") diabetes mellitus. These risk factors, together termed the **metabolic syndrome,** include abdominal adiposity with increased waist circumference; mild hypertension (perhaps related to failure of endothelium-dependent vascular relaxation); impaired fasting plasma glucose levels; and a dyslipoproteinemia characterized by reduced HDL cholesterol and elevated fasting and nonfasting plasma triglyceride concentrations (Table 22-1). These features should be evaluated in the context of other important contributors to cardiovascular risk, such as plasma LDL levels, age, sex and smoking.

Table 22-1

Frequently Observed Concomitants of the Insulin Resistance/Metabolic Syndrome

Clinical Signs
Central (upper body) obesity with increased waist circumference
Acanthosis nigricans (hypertrophic, hyperpigmented skin changes)
Laboratory Abnormalities
Elevated fasting and/or postprandial glucose
Insulin resistance with hyperinsulinemia
Dyslipidemia characterized by increased triglycerides and low high-density lipoprotein cholesterol
Abnormal thrombolysis
Hyperuricemia
Endothelial and vascular smooth muscle dysfunction
Albuminuria
Comorbid Illnesses
Hypertension
Atherosclerosis
Hyperandrogenism with polycystic ovary syndrome

DIABETES MELLITUS

Almost a century ago, the noted physician Sir William Osler defined diabetes mellitus as "a syndrome due to a disturbance in carbohydrate metabolism from various causes, in which sugar appears in the urine, associated with thirst, polyuria, wasting and imperfect oxidation of fats." With the advent of insulin and other therapeutic agents, however, these extreme features are unusual in properly managed patients with diabetes. Long-term consequences persist, however. Hence, diabetes mellitus in the modern setting has been redefined as "a state of premature cardiovascular death that is associated with chronic hyperglycemia and may also be associated with blindness and renal failure." This emphasis reflects the fact that cardiovascular disease continues to kill ~70% of individuals with diabetes, compared to 50% of the general population in industrialized countries, and it affects them earlier in life, with greater morbidity.

Today, diabetes is a major health problem that affects increasing numbers of people throughout the world. Two major forms of diabetes mellitus are recognized, distinguished by their underlying pathophysiology. **Type 1 diabetes mellitus (T1DM)**, formerly known as **insulin-dependent (IDDM)** or **juvenile-onset diabetes**, is caused by autoimmune destruction of the insulin-producing beta cells in the pancreatic islets of Langerhans. It affects fewer than 10% of all patients with diabetes. By contrast, **T2DM**, formerly known as **non–insulin-dependent (NIDDM)** or **maturity-onset diabetes,** is usually associated with obesity, and results from a complex interrelationship between resistance to the metabolic action of insulin in its target tissues and inadequate secretion of insulin by the pancreas (Table 22-2).

Gestational diabetes develops in a percentage of pregnant women, owing to the insulin resistance of pregnancy combined with a beta cell defect, but almost always abates after parturition. Diabetes can also occur secondary to other endocrine conditions or drug therapy, especially in Cushing

Table 22-2

Comparison of Type 1 and Type 2 Diabetes Mellitus

	Type 1 Diabetes	Type 2 Diabetes
Age at onset	Usually before 20	Usually after 30
Type of onset	Abrupt; symptomatic (polyuria, polydipsia, dehydration); often severe with ketoacidosis	Gradual; usually subtle; often asymptomatic
Usual body weight	Normal; recent weight loss is common	Overweight
Family history	<20%	>60%
Monozygotic twins	50% concordant	90% concordant
HLA associations	+	No
Antibodies to islet cell antigens (insulin, glutamic acid decarboxylase [GAD-65], IA-2)	+	No
Islet lesions	Early—inflammation Late—atrophy and fibrosis	Late—fibrosis, amyloid
Beta cell mass	Markedly reduced	Normal or slightly reduced
Circulating insulin level	Markedly reduced	Elevated or normal
Clinical management	Insulin absolutely required	Insulin usually not needed initially; insulin supplementation may be needed at later stages; weight loss typically improves the condition

HLA = human leukocyte antigen; IA-2 = islet cell antigen-512.

syndrome or during treatment with glucocorticoids. Other rare clinical syndromes are associated with abnormal glucose metabolism or overt **hyperglycemia**. Because these conditions are uncommon and have well-defined genetic etiologies that differ from the more common forms of diabetes, they will not be considered in detail. The classification of diabetes as recommended by the American Diabetes Association (ADA) is shown in Table 22-3.

Current criteria for the diagnosis of diabetes mellitus are based on abnormal glucose threshold levels that have been shown to be closely associated with the chronic complications of this disorder. In particular, hyperglycemia causes the microvascular changes of diabetic retinopathy and renal glomerular damage. In a younger patient with abrupt onset of hyperglycemia and elevated plasma ketones or frank ketoacidosis, the diagnosis of T1DM due to absolute insulin deficiency is obvious. In contrast, T2DM typically develops gradually over many years before it is recognized, most often in an overweight, middle-aged person with a genetic predisposition.

The ADA suggests any of four criteria to diagnose diabetes (Table 22-4). One of the four criteria has to be present for the diagnosis, but some criteria need repeat testing to confirm. In addition, the ADA recognizes three categories of increased risk for diabetes (Table 22-5). Some of those categories have been commonly referred to as "prediabetes," even though this term has recently fallen out of favor because only half of those patients will ultimately develop diabetes.

Table 22-3

Etiologic Classification of Diabetes Mellitus

I. Type 1 diabetes (beta cell destruction, absolute insulin deficiency)
   - A. Immune mediated
   - B. Idiopathic

II. Type 2 diabetes (insulin resistance with relative insulin deficiency)

III. Other specific types
   - Genetic defects of beta cell function (e.g., maturity-onset diabetes of the young)
   - Genetic defects in insulin action (e.g., type A insulin resistance)
   - Diseases of the exocrine pancreas
   - Endocrinopathies (e.g., Cushing disease, acromegaly, etc.)
   - Drug or chemical induced (e.g., glucocorticoids)
   - Infections (e.g., cytomegalovirus, rubella)
   - Uncommon forms of immune-mediated diabetes (e.g., "stiff-man syndrome")
   - Other genetic syndromes (e.g., Turner syndrome, Down syndrome)

IV. Gestational diabetes mellitus

Table 22-4

Criteria for the Diagnosis of Diabetes

1. HbA_{1C}* ≥6.5%
OR
2. FPG ≥126 mg/dL (7.0 mmol/L). Fasting is defined as no caloric intake for at least 8 h
OR
3. 2-h plasma glucose ≥200 mg/dL (11.1 mmol/L) during an OGTT
OR
4. In a patient with classic symptoms of hyperglycemia or hyperglycemic crisis, a random plasma glucose ≥200 mg/dL (11.1 mmol/L)

FPG = fasting plasma glucose; HbA_{1C} = hemoglobin A_{1C}; OGTT = oral glucose tolerance test.

*In the absence of unequivocal hyperglycemia, criteria 1–3 should be confirmed by repeat testing.

Type 2 Diabetes Mellitus

T2DM is a heterogeneous disorder characterized by a combination of reduced tissue sensitivity to insulin and inadequate secretion of insulin from the pancreas. The disease usually develops in adults, with an increased prevalence in obese persons and in the elderly. Recently, T2DM has been appearing in increasing numbers in younger adults and adolescents, owing to worsening obesity and lack of exercise in this age group. ***Hyperglycemia in T2DM is a result of the failure of the beta cells to meet the body's increased demand for insulin.*** As of 2007, T2DM is estimated to affect more than 23 million Americans (7.8% of the population, or 10.7% of those older than 20 years of age), almost a quarter of whom are undiagnosed. About 23% of people older than 60 years of age have diabetes. An additional 57 million Americans (25% of adults older than 20 years of age) are believed to be at increased risk for diabetes as indicated by impaired fasting glucose (IFG). T2DM is most prevalent in all nonwhite ethnic groups in the United States, including blacks, Hispanics, Asians and Native Americans.

Table 22-5

Categories of Increased Risk for Diabetes*

FPG 100 mg/dL (5.6 mmol/L) to 125 mg/dL (6.9 mmol/L) (IFG)
2-h PG in the 75-g OGTT 140 mg/dL (7.8 mmol/L) to 199 mg/dL (11.0 mmol/L) (IGT)
HbA_{1C} 5.7%–6.4%

FPG = fasting plasma glucose; HbA_{1C} = hemoglobin A_{1C}; IFG = impaired fasting glucose; IGT = impaired glucose tolerance; OGTT = oral glucose tolerance test; PG = plasma glucose.

*For all three tests, risk is continuous, extending below the lower limit of the range and becoming disproportionately greater at the higher ends of the range.

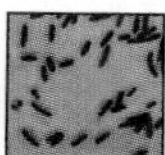

ETIOLOGIC FACTORS:

Type 2 Diabetes Mellitus Is the Result of Insulin Insensitivity

T2DM results from a complex interplay between underlying resistance to the action of insulin in its metabolic target tissues (liver, skeletal muscle, adipose tissue) and lower glucose-stimulated insulin secretion, which fails to compensate for the increased demand for insulin. Progression to overt diabetes occurs most commonly in patients with both of these defects (Fig. 22-5).

Several risk factors have been clearly associated with T2DM. The three most important ones are **obesity, diet and lack of physical activity.** As noted above, the risk of T2DM increases linearly with BMI. More than 80% of cases of T2DM can be attributed to obesity. Upper body/central or male-type obesity ("apple shaped") is more associated with insulin resistance and T2DM than is lower body or female-type

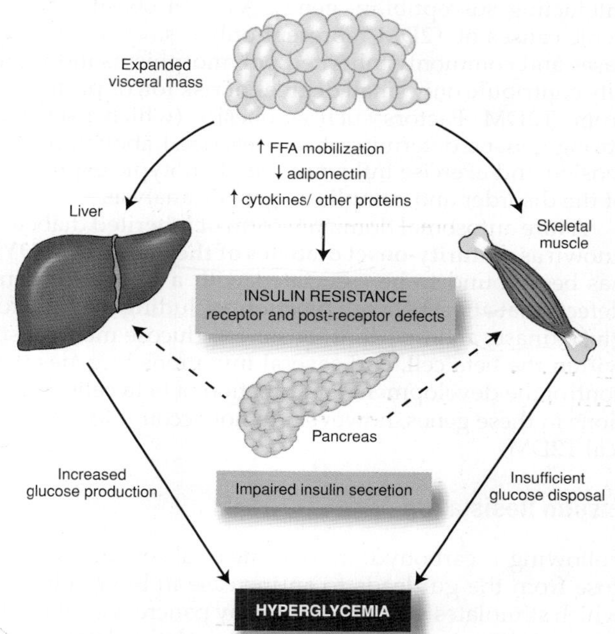

FIGURE 22-5. Pathogenesis of obesity-related type 2 diabetes mellitus (T2DM). The expanded visceral fat mass in upper body obesity elaborates several factors that contribute to tissue insulin resistance. These include an increase in circulating free (nonesterified) fatty acids (FFAs) and other cytokines and proteins that inhibit insulin action, as well as a decrease in factors that enhance insulin signaling, such as adiponectin. These changes result in a block to insulin action in liver and skeletal muscle at the level of the insulin receptor and at postreceptor signaling sites, resulting in a failure of insulin to suppress hepatic glucose production and to promote glucose uptake into muscle. The resulting hyperglycemia is normally countered by increased insulin secretion by pancreatic beta cells. In persons with T2DM, the combination of resistance to insulin action and a genetically determined impairment of the beta cell response to hyperglycemia results in hyperglycemia, and T2DM ensues.

obesity ("pear shaped"). Conversely, weight loss lowers the risk of T2DM and can prevent progression of insulin resistance to diabetes.

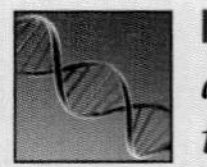

MOLECULAR PATHOGENESIS: ***Multifactorial and multigenic inheritance is a key contributor to the development of T2DM.*** Several observations demonstrate genetic influences in the development of T2DM:

- More than a third of patients with T2DM have at least one parent with T2DM.
- Among monozygotic twins, concordance for T2DM approaches 100%.
- The prevalence of T2DM among different ethnic groups who are living in similar environments varies tremendously.
- First-degree relatives of patients with T2DM have significantly higher lifetime risk of T2DM compared with matched subjects without family history.

Despite the high familial prevalence of the disease, inheritance is complex and thought to involve multiple interacting susceptibility genes. As with obesity, monogenic causes of T2DM represent only a small fraction of cases and commonly inherited polymorphisms individually contribute only small degrees of risk for, or protection from, T2DM. Factors such as obesity (which itself has strong genetic determinants as described above), hypertension and exercise influence the phenotypic expression of the disorder and complicate genetic analysis.

A rare autosomal dominant form of inherited diabetes, known as **maturity-onset diabetes of the young (MODY),** has been found to be associated with a variety of gene defects that affect beta cell function, including the gene for glucokinase, an important sensor for glucose metabolism within the beta cell, and several mutations in genes that control the development and function of beta cells. Mutations in these genes, however, do not account for the typical T2DM.

Insulin Resistance

Following a carbohydrate-rich meal, absorption of glucose from the gut leads to an increase in blood glucose, which stimulates insulin secretion by pancreatic beta cells. Insulin in turn increases glucose uptake by skeletal muscle and adipose tissue. At the same time, insulin suppresses hepatic glucose production by (1) inhibiting gluconeogenesis, (2) enhancing glycogen synthesis, (3) blocking the effects of glucagon on the liver and (4) antagonizing glucagon release from the pancreas.

All of these effects of insulin are diminished in insulin resistance. Initially, insulin resistance is subclinical. As the condition progresses, there is evidence of impaired fasting glucose and/or impaired glucose tolerance. Eventually, frank hyperglycemia sets in and T2DM can be diagnosed (Fig. 22-6). Insulin resistance leads to increased hepatic glucose production and reduced glucose uptake by peripheral tissues, primarily muscles and adipose tissue.

Insulin resistance alone rarely causes T2DM, since increased insulin secretion (hyperinsulinism) by beta cells will compensate for insulin resistance and thereby prevent blood glucose levels from rising. It is only when the beta cells start showing evidence of dysfunction that blood glucose levels start to increase (Fig. 22-6).

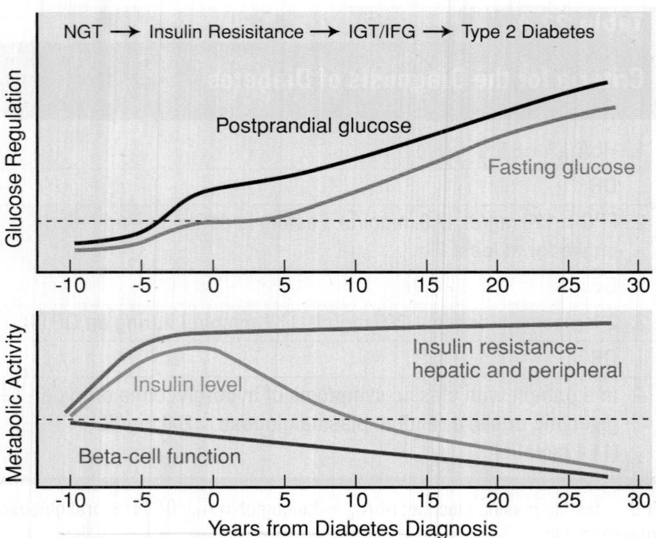

FIGURE 22-6. Glucose regulation and metabolic activity during the development of Type 2 diabetes mellitus. NGT, normal glucose tolerance; IGT, impaired glucose tolerance; IFG, impaired fasting glucose.

The molecular basis for insulin resistance is a subject of intense research. In animals, desensitization of the insulin receptor by posttranslational modification has been demonstrated in models of diabetes. Whether derangement of insulin receptor signaling occurs in human T2DM has not been resolved.

Beta Cell Dysfunction

At first, this is characterized by impairment in the first phase of insulin secretion following glucose stimulation, and may precede the onset of glucose intolerance in T2DM. Later in the disease, the second phase, release of newly synthesized insulin, is impaired (Fig. 22-7). This effect can be reversed, at least in part in some patients, by restoring good control of glycemia. This partially reversible reduction in insulin secretion is the result of a paradoxical inhibitory effect of glucose upon insulin release that is sometimes seen with high blood glucose levels ("glucose toxicity").

Impaired first-phase insulin secretion can serve as a marker of risk for T2DM in family members of subjects with T2DM and may be seen in patients with prior gestational diabetes. Over a long period of time, insulin secretion in T2DM gradually declines. There is also an associated decline in beta cell mass.

The Role of Incretins

In the 1960s, it was discovered that the ability of an oral glucose load to stimulate insulin secretion was significantly greater than that evoked from an intravenous infusion of glucose when plasma glucose concentrations were matched. This discrepancy was named the incretin effect (Fig. 22-8). Incretins are peptides secreted by the gut in

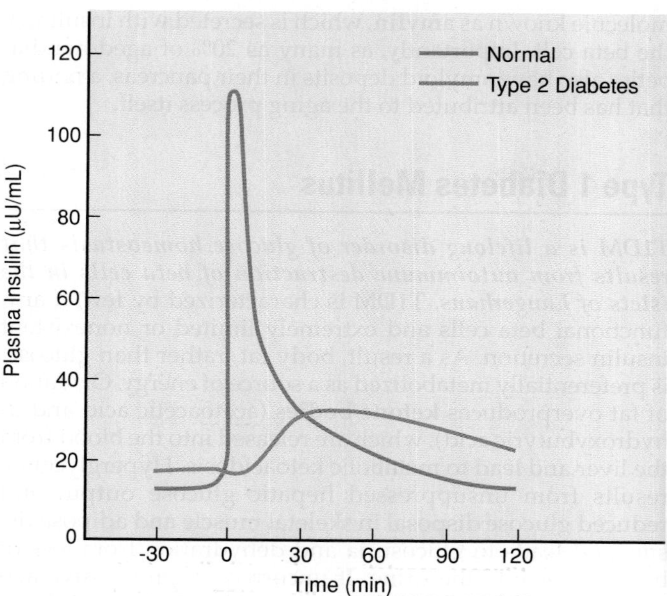

FIGURE 22-7. Insulin response in diabetes. Typical patterns of insulin production in response to glucose challenge in normal (*blue*) and type 2 diabetic (*red*) patients.

response to meals that increase insulin secretion and decrease glucagon secretion. Most of this effect is now thought to be due to glucose-dependent insulinotropic peptide (GIP) and glucagon-like peptide-1 (GLP-1). Incretins are rapidly inactivated in the circulation by the enzyme dipeptidyl peptidase 4 (DPP-4). Effects of incretins include (1) glucose-dependent stimulation of insulin secretion by beta cells, (2) inhibition of glucagon secretion by alpha cells, and (3) inhibition of appetite.

In patients with T2DM, the incretin effect is markedly reduced (Fig. 22-8B), which has been attributed to defects in secretion of GLP-1 and GIP. The role, if any, of these changes in incretins in the pathogenesis of T2DM has not yet been clarified.

Therapeutic Implications

Early in T2DM, insulin resistance and hyperinsulinemia are the predominant presentations. Insulin-sensitizing drugs are most often used to manage those patients. Over the years, with the development of beta cell dysfunction, hyperglycemia is managed by insulin secretagogues, incretin mimetics and, ultimately, exogenous insulin.

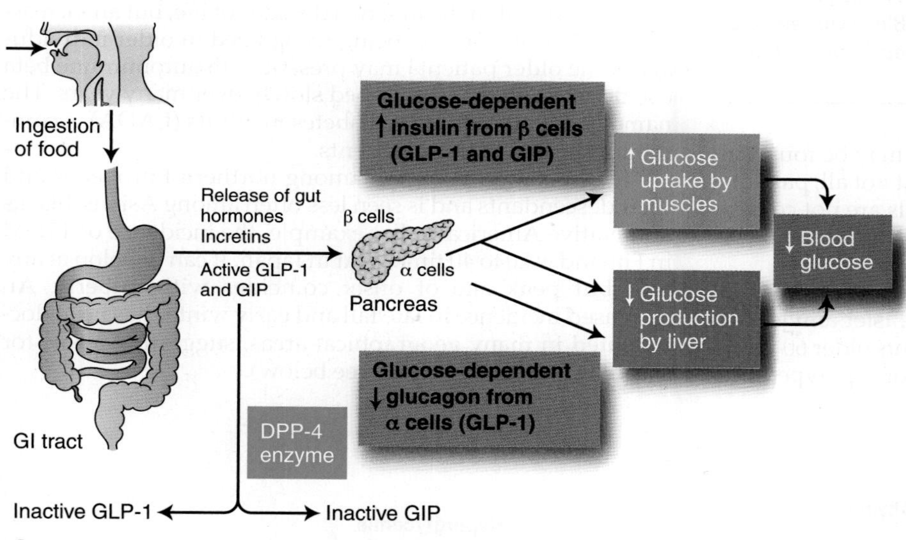

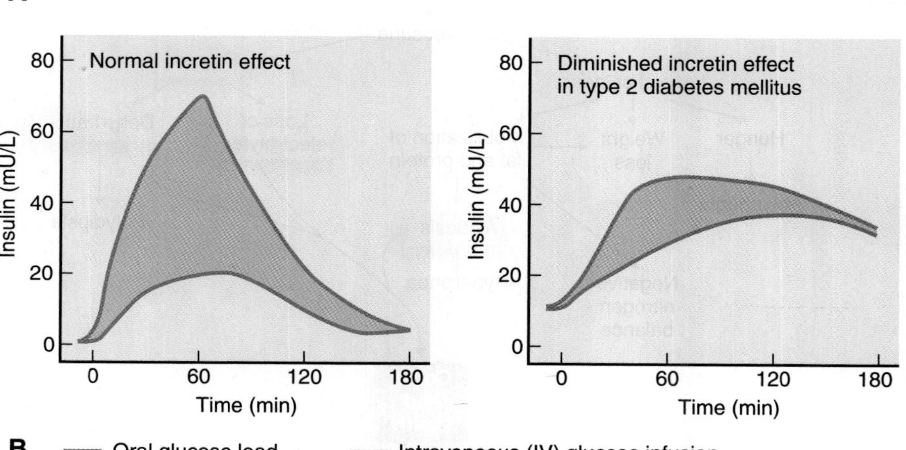

FIGURE 22-8. Incretins. A. Physiologic roles of incretins in glucose metabolism. Involvement of incretins in regulating the responses of the body to a caloric load. GIP = glucose-dependent insulinotropic peptide; GLP-1 = glucagon-like peptide-1. **B. Diminished incretin responsiveness in type 2 diabetes mellitus.**

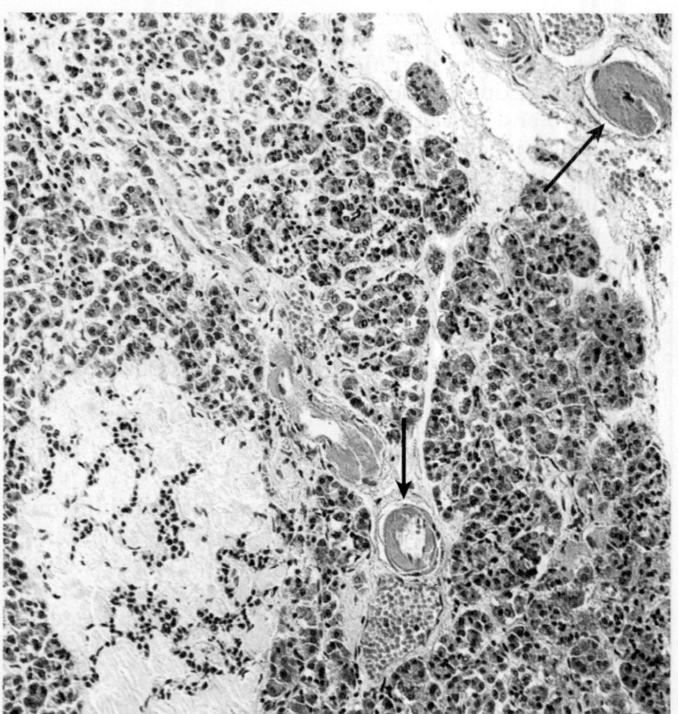

FIGURE 22-9. Amyloidosis (hyalinization) of an islet in the pancreas of a patient with type 2 diabetes mellitus (*lower left*). Blood vessels adjacent to the islet show the advanced hyaline arteriolosclerosis (*arrows*) characteristic of diabetes.

PATHOLOGY: Microscopic lesions may be found in the islets of Langerhans of many, but not all, patients with T2DM. Unlike T1DM, beta cells are not consistently reduced in T2DM, and no morphologic lesions of these cells have been found by light or electron microscopy.

In some islets, fibrous tissue accumulates, sometimes to such a degree that the islets are obliterated. Islet amyloid is often present (Fig. 22-9), particularly in patients older 60 years of age. This type of amyloid is composed of a polypeptide molecule known as **amylin**, which is secreted with insulin by the beta cell. Importantly, as many as 20% of aged nondiabetics also have amyloid deposits in their pancreas, a finding that has been attributed to the aging process itself.

Type 1 Diabetes Mellitus

T1DM is a lifelong disorder of glucose homeostasis that results from autoimmune destruction of beta cells in the islets of Langerhans. T1DM is characterized by few, if any, functional beta cells and extremely limited or nonexistent insulin secretion. As a result, body fat, rather than glucose, is preferentially metabolized as a source of energy. Oxidation of fat overproduces **ketone bodies** (acetoacetic acid and β-hydroxybutyric acid), which are released into the blood from the liver and lead to metabolic ketoacidosis. Hyperglycemia results from unsuppressed hepatic glucose output and reduced glucose disposal in skeletal muscle and adipose tissue, and leads to glucosuria and dehydration from loss of body water into the urine. If uncorrected, progressive acidosis and dehydration ultimately lead to coma and death (Fig. 22-10).

EPIDEMIOLOGY: It is estimated that nearly 1 million people in the United States are afflicted with T1DM. Most patients are diagnosed and classified with T1DM within the first two decades of life, but an increasing number of cases are being recognized in older individuals. Some older patients may present with autoimmune beta cell destruction that developed slowly over many years. The name latent autoimmune diabetes in adults (LADA) is commonly applied to those patients.

T1DM is most common among northern Europeans and their descendants and is seen less often among Asians, blacks and Native Americans. For example, the incidence of T1DM in Finland is 20 to 40 times that in Japan. It can develop at any age, but peak age of onset coincides with puberty. An increased incidence in late fall and early winter has been documented in many geographical areas, suggesting a role for seasonal infectious agents (see below).

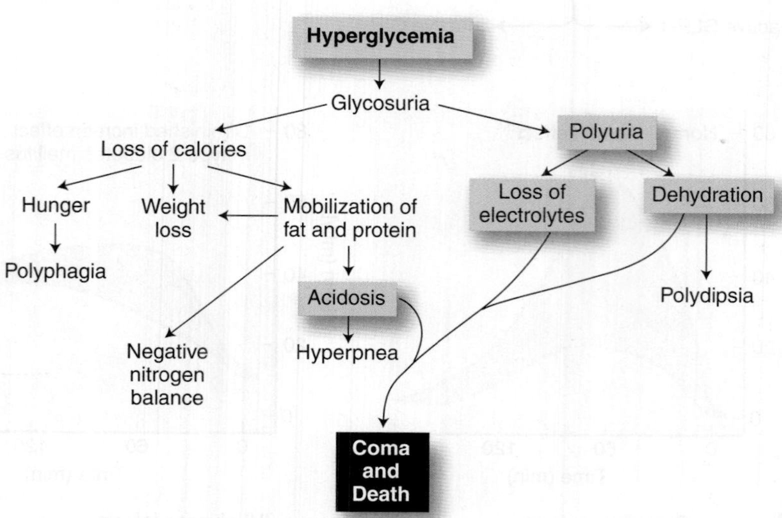

FIGURE 22-10. Symptoms and signs of uncontrolled hyperglycemia in diabetes mellitus.

MOLECULAR PATHOGENESIS:
GENETIC FACTORS: Evidence for the role of genetic factors in the pathogenesis of T1DM include:

1. Relatives of people with T1DM have increased risk for development of T1DM. The lifetime risk of T1DM in the U.S. general population is 0.4%, but is 3% to 8% for first-degree relatives of people with T1DM. An identical twin has a 30% to 50% risk of developing T1DM once the other twin develops it. Interestingly, children of fathers with T1DM are three times more likely to develop the disease than are children of mothers with T1DM, suggesting genetic imprinting involving paternal susceptibility genes.
2. There are differences in risk among different ethnic groups who live in similar environments.
3. There are many susceptibility genes (major histocompatibility complex [MHC] and non-MHC genes) linked to T1DM. There is a strong linkage of T1DM to the highly polymorphic human leukocyte antigen (HLA) class II immune recognition molecules—DR and, later, DQ—on chromosome 6. Over the years, extensive studies have revealed a large number of high- and low-risk HLA alleles. For example, whereas only 45% of the population in the United States expresses DR3 or DR4, 95% of those who develop T1DM express these haplotypes. Because of the known role of HLA molecules in antigen presentation, the HLA linkage and association supports the hypothesis that T1DM has an autoimmune component.
4. Many other, independent chromosomal regions (several of them non-HLA) have thus far been associated with susceptibility to T1DM.

AUTOIMMUNITY: The concept of an autoimmune pathogenesis for T1DM is supported by the observation that pancreatic islets from patients who die shortly after the onset of the disease often exhibit an infiltrate of mononuclear cells, termed **insulitis** (Fig. 22-11). Among the inflammatory cells, $CD8^+$ T lymphocytes predominate, although some $CD4^+$ cells are also present. The infiltrating inflammatory cells also elaborate cytokines, for example, IL-1, IL-6, interferon-α and nitric oxide, which may further contribute to beta cell injury.

An autoimmune origin for T1DM was initially suggested by the finding of circulating antibodies against components of the beta cells (including insulin itself) in most newly diagnosed children with this disease. Major target antigens include (1) insulin; (2) glutamic acid decarboxylase (GAD); and (3) insulinoma-associated protein 2 (IA-2), also known as islet cell antigen 512 (ICA-512). Many patients develop anti-islet cell antibodies months or years before insulin production decreases and clinical symptoms appear, a clinical state known as "pre-type 1 diabetes" (Fig. 22-12). However, these antibodies are regarded as a response to beta cell antigens released during destruction of beta cells by cell-mediated immune mechanisms, rather than the cause of beta cell depletion. Nevertheless, detection of serum antibodies to islet cells and target islet antigens is a useful clinical tool for differentiating T1DM, which has an autoimmune basis, from T2DM, which does not.

Cell-mediated immune mechanisms are fundamental to the pathogenesis of T1DM. Cytotoxic T lymphocytes sensitized to beta cells in T1DM persist indefinitely, possibly for a lifetime. Patients transplanted with a donor pancreas or a preparation of purified islets must be treated with immunosuppressive drugs. Ten percent of patients with T1DM manifest at least one other organ-specific autoimmune disease, including Hashimoto thyroiditis, Graves disease, myasthenia gravis, Addison disease or pernicious anemia. Interestingly, most patients with polyendocrine immune syndromes (see Chapter 21) also possess HLA-DR3 and -DR4 histocompatibility antigens.

Beta cell destruction in T1DM generally develops slowly over years, and specific stages of the disease have been described (Fig. 22-12). Studies in first-degree relatives of subjects with T1DM have shown that antibodies against islet cells are present several years before the onset of the disease. T1DM with hyperglycemia or ketoacidosis is clinically evident only when 90% or more of insulin-secreting cells are eliminated and insulin deprivation is severe.

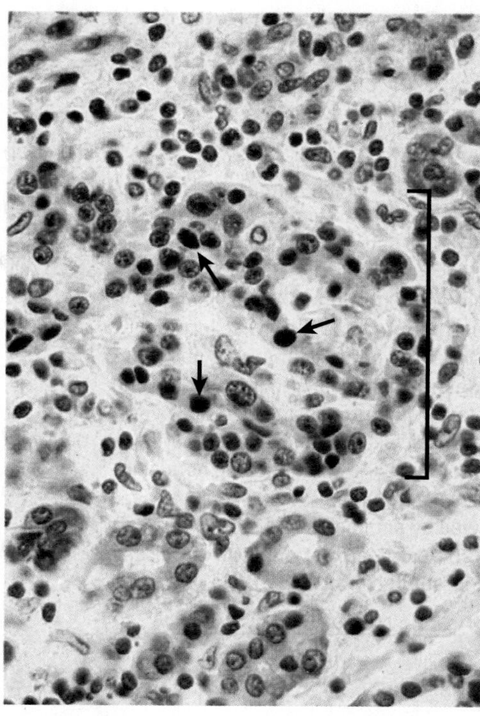

FIGURE 22-11. Insulitis in type 1 diabetes mellitus. A lymphocytic inflammatory infiltrate (*arrows*) is seen in and around the islet (*left of bracket*).

ETIOLOGIC FACTORS:
ENVIRONMENTAL FACTORS: Evidence for the role of environmental factors in the pathogenesis of T1DM include the following:

- Only 33% to 50% of monozygotic twins of T1DM patients develop T1DM.
- Recent increases in T1DM incidence in some populations suggests a possible etiologic role of environment.
- About 80% to 90% of subjects with T1DM have no family history of the disease.
- There are seasonal differences in the incidence of T1DM.

Viruses have been implicated as causative factors in at least some cases of T1DM. Thus, the disease occasionally develops after infection with coxsackie B viruses and, less often,

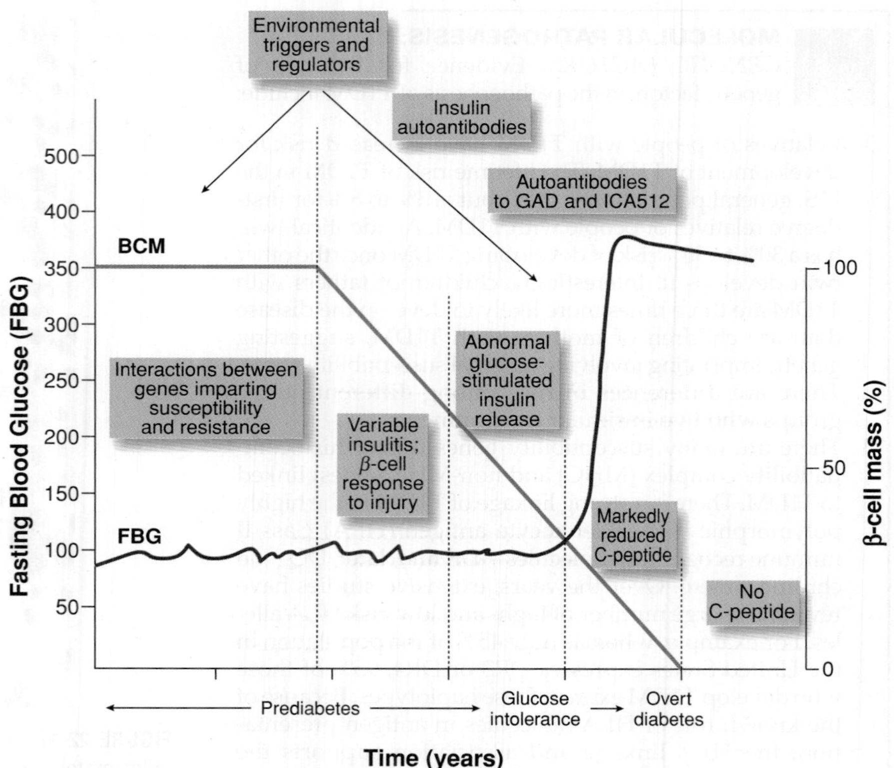

FIGURE 22-12. Pathogenetic stages in the development of type 1 diabetes (T1DM). The disease develops from an initial genetic susceptibility to defective recognition of beta cell epitopes and ends with essentially complete beta cell destruction in most patients. An environmental event is believed to trigger the immune attack, and persons with certain genetic markers (human leukocyte antigen [HLA]-DR3 and -DR4) are particularly susceptible to the autoimmune disease. Patients with islet cell antibodies and normal blood glucose levels are considered to have a state of "pre-type 1 diabetes." The rate of decline in beta cell mass (*blue line*) determines the length of time between onset of beta cell destruction and eventual hyperglycemia (*red line*, fasting blood glucose) owing to loss of greater than 90% of functioning beta cells. In the serum, autoantibodies to insulin appear early, followed by antibodies to the beta cell antigen glutamic acid decarboxylase (GAD-65) and the islet cell antigen (ICA-512). BCM, beta cell mass.

mumps viruses. Certain proteins may share antigenic epitopes with human cell surface proteins and trigger the autoreactive disease process by "molecular mimicry." For example, a coxsackie B virus protein has close homology to the human GAD-65 islet protein.

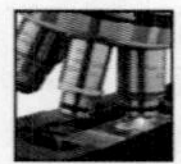

PATHOLOGY: As noted above, the most characteristic early lesion in the pancreas of T1DM is a mononuclear infiltrate in the islets (insulitis), composed chiefly of lymphocytes, sometimes accompanied by a few macrophages and neutrophils (Fig. 22-11). As the disease becomes chronic, islet beta cells become progressively depleted; eventually insulin-producing cells are no longer discernible. Loss of beta cells results in variably sized islets, many of which appear as ribbonlike cords that may be difficult to distinguish from surrounding acinar tissue. Fibrosis of the islets is uncommon. Unlike T2DM, amyloid deposition in pancreatic islets is not seen in T1DM. The exocrine pancreas in chronic T1DM often exhibits diffuse interlobular and interacinar fibrosis, accompanied by atrophy of the acinar cells.

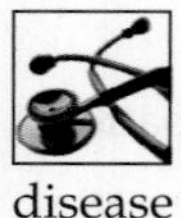

CLINICAL FEATURES: The clinical presentation of T1DM results from lack of insulin, which has a unique role in energy metabolism in the body. The disease classically presents with acute metabolic decompensation characterized by hyperglycemia and ketoacidosis. Depending on the degree of absolute insulin deficiency, severe ketoacidosis may be preceded by weeks to months of increased urine output **(polyuria)** and increased thirst **(polydipsia).** Excessive diuresis results from glucosuria. Weight loss in spite of increased appetite (polyphagia) results from unregulated catabolism of body stores of fat, protein and carbohydrate with inefficient energy use. Often the clinical onset of T1DM coincides with another acute illness, such as a febrile viral or bacterial infection (Fig. 22-10).

Complications of Diabetes

The discovery of insulin in the early 20th century promised to cure diabetes, but as patients with diabetes lived longer, they became subject to numerous complications. ***It is now clearly established that the severity and chronicity of hyperglycemia in both T2DM and T1DM are the major pathogenetic factors leading to the "microvascular" complications of diabetes including retinopathy, nephropathy and neuropathy. Thus, control of blood glucose remains the major means by which the development of microvascular diabetic complications can be minimized.*** It has been more difficult to demonstrate that glucose control can prevent "macrovascular" (large-vessel) complications, meaning atherosclerosis and its sequelae (coronary artery disease, peripheral vascular disease and cerebrovascular disease). These macrovascular complications are especially common in insulin-resistant patients with T2DM, because the patients tend to be older and frequently harbor additional cardiovascular risk factors.

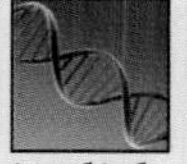

MOLECULAR PATHOGENESIS: Several biochemical mechanisms have been proposed to account for the development of pathologic changes in diabetes.

EXCESSIVE REACTIVE OXYGEN SPECIES: In various cell types in culture, hyperglycemia increases production of reactive oxygen species (ROS) as byproducts of mitochondrial oxidative phosphorylation. ROS are implicated

Diabetic Nephropathy

leading cause of renal failure in U.S.

of pts w/ T1DM 30–40% develop renal failure

T2DM (20%)

T1DM can die of uremia.

hyperglycemia leads to glomerular hypertension + renal hyperperfusion (8) leads to glomerulosclerosis + renal failure

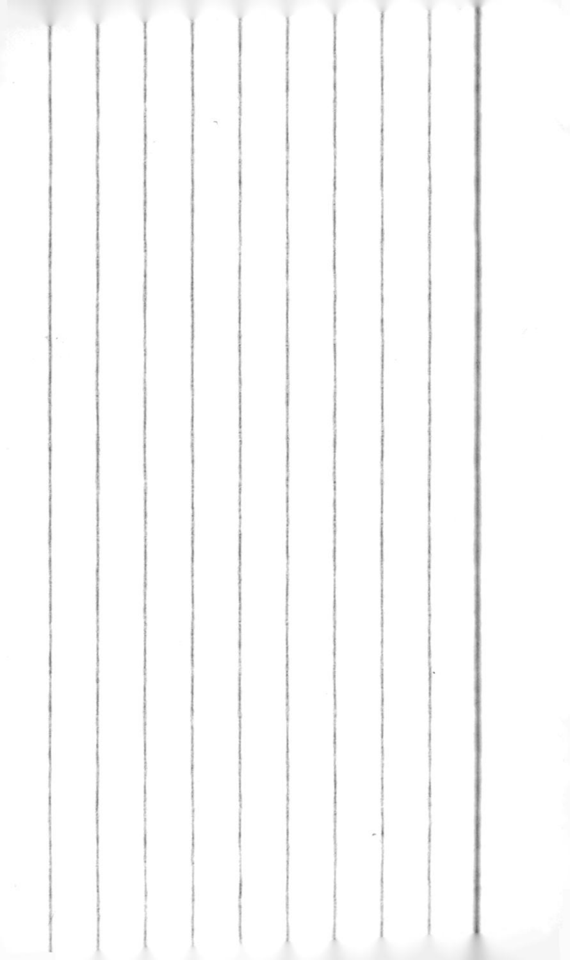

type1 diabetes mellitus (T1DM) aka. insulin dependent, or juvenile onset T1DM

- caused by autoimmune destruction of insulin producing β cells in pancreatic islets of Langerhans. few if any functional β cells & extremely limited or non existent insulin secretion
- body fat rather than glucose is preferentially metabolized as source of energy

early characteristic pancreas lesion
(mononuclear infiltrate in islets
composed chiefly of lymphocytes)

β cell dysfunction

...ulin secretion ↑ blood glucose
inc. glucose uptake by skeletal
adipose tissue
suppresses hepatic glucose production by:
gluconeogenesis
glycogenolysis
effects of glucagon on liver
• antagonize glucagon release from pancreas
all diminished w/ T2DM

type 2 diabetes mellitus T2DM

aka non-insulin dependent/maturity onset diabetes

- associated w/ obesity
- results from complex interrelationship bet resistance to metabolic action of insulin in target tissues + inadequate secretion of insulin by pancreas
- failure of β cells to meet body's inc demand for insulin!
- insulin insensitivity

risk factors:

obesity / diet / lack of physical activity

Expanded visceral fat mass in upper
are stored freely circulating:

$\uparrow$ Fatty acids
$\uparrow$ cytokines/other proteins that inhibit
$\downarrow$ in factors that enhance insulin signa
(i.e. adiponectin)

leads to insulin resistance (receptor + post receptor defects).
Block to insulin action in liver & skeletal muscle
at level of receptors. So results in failure of insulin to suppress
hepatic glucose prdn & to promote glucose uptake into
muscle. Resulting hyperglycemia (in normal ppl this is
counteracted by sufficient insulin secretion by pancreatic
β cells. in T2DM not the case).

in many types of cellular injury (see Chapter 1). Proposed mediators of glucose-induced oxidative damage include nitric oxide, superoxide anions and aldose reductase. Nevertheless, numerous therapeutic trials of aldose reductase inhibition and antioxidant supplementation in diabetes (and other conditions) have failed to show clinical benefit. Thus, there is no direct causal evidence in humans that excessive ROS contribute to diabetes or its complications.

PROTEIN GLYCATION: Glucose covalently attaches to an assortment of proteins nonenzymatically, a process termed **glycation** (also termed **nonenzymatic glycosylation**). Glycation occurs roughly in proportion to the severity of hyperglycemia. Numerous cellular proteins are modified in this manner, including hemoglobin, components of the crystalline lens and cellular basement membrane proteins. A specific fraction of glycated hemoglobin in circulating red blood cells (hemoglobin A_{1c}) is used routinely to monitor the overall degree of hyperglycemia during the preceding 6 to 8 weeks. Nonenzymatic glycation of hemoglobin is irreversible, so hemoglobin A_{1c} levels serve as a marker for glycemic control.

The initial glycation products (known chemically as Schiff bases) are labile and can dissociate rapidly. With time, these labile products undergo complex chemical rearrangements to form stable **advanced glycosylation end-products (AGEs),** consisting of a glucose derivative covalently bound to the protein amino group. As a result, the structure of the protein is permanently altered and its function may be affected. For example, albumin and immunoglobulin G (IgG) do not normally bind to collagen, but they adhere to glycated collagen. Unstable chemical bonds in proteins containing AGEs can lead to physical cross-linking of nearby proteins, which may contribute to the characteristic thickening of vascular basement membranes in diabetes. Importantly, unlike the initial labile glycation products, AGEs can continue to cross-link proteins even if blood glucose returns to normal. Patients with diabetic retinopathy have higher levels of AGEs than do diabetics without this complication. The role of AGEs in diabetic microvascular disease is uncertain. Although compounds that inhibit formation of AGEs (e.g., aminoguanidine) provide some protection against diabetic complications in experimental animals, human studies so far have been disappointing.

AGE peptides are normally excreted in the urine, and so as patients with diabetes develop renal failure, plasma and tissue levels of AGEs markedly increase. Increased AGEs in diabetic renal failure are believed to contribute to the acceleration of microvascular and macrovascular complications.

THE ALDOSE REDUCTASE PATHWAY: By mass action, hyperglycemia also increases uptake of glucose into tissues that do not depend on insulin. Some of the increased flux of glucose is metabolized by aldose reductase, which catalyzes the reaction:

$$\text{Glucose} + \text{NADPH} \rightarrow \text{Sorbitol} + \text{NADP}$$

This reaction depletes cellular reducing equivalents, thereby altering redox status, and leads to sorbitol accumulation. There is speculation that sorbitol may be involved in tissue complications of diabetes, by mechanisms that are not understood. Although aldose reductase has a low affinity for glucose, it generates appreciable amounts of sorbitol in these tissues when blood glucose levels are elevated. In the lens of the eye, excess sorbitol may simply create an osmotic gradient that causes influx of fluid and consequent swelling. Increased intracellular sorbitol has been linked to decreased myoinositol (a precursor of phosphoinositides), lower protein kinase C activity and inhibition of the plasma membrane sodium pump. However, the role of aldose reductase and sorbitol in the complications of diabetes is unclear: inhibition of aldose reductase has shown occasional benefit in animal models, but not in human clinical trials.

PROTEIN KINASE C ACTIVATION: In patients with hyperglycemia, specific protein kinase C (PKC) isoforms, mainly PKC-β and PKC-δ, are activated by diacylglycerol (DAG) synthesized from glycolytic intermediates and from high plasma concentrations of nonesterified fatty acids. PKC activation may lead to (1) increased production of extracellular matrix and cytokines, (2) enhanced microvascular contractility, (3) increased microvascular permeability, (4) proliferation of endothelial and smooth muscle cells and (5) insulin resistance. PKC also activates phospholipase A_2 and inhibits the activity of Na^+/K^+-ATPase. Selective inhibition of PKC-β prevents or reverses a number of vascular abnormalities in vitro and in vivo.

Atherosclerosis Is a Frequent and Deadly Complication of Diabetes

Cardiovascular disease, including atherosclerotic heart disease and ischemic stroke, accounts for more than half of all deaths among adults with diabetes. The extent and severity of atherosclerotic lesions in medium-sized and large arteries are increased in patients with long-standing diabetes. Diabetes eliminates the usual protective effect of being female, and coronary artery disease develops at a younger age than in nondiabetic persons. Moreover, mortality from myocardial infarction is higher in patients with diabetes than in those without. As indicated above, patients with T2DM frequently exhibit multiple risk factors of the metabolic syndrome that contribute to development of atherosclerosis.

Atherosclerotic peripheral vascular disease, particularly of the lower extremities, is a common complication of diabetes. Vascular insufficiency leads to ulcers and gangrene of the toes and feet, complications that ultimately necessitate amputation. ***Indeed, diabetes accounts for more than 60% of nontraumatic limb amputations in the United States.***

Even though epidemiologic analyses suggest a correlation between chronic hyperglycemia and higher rates of cardiovascular disease, the extent to which glucose levels per se are involved is far from clear. In most randomized clinical trials, improvements in HbA_{1c} levels do not lead to improved macrovascular outcomes in T2DM.

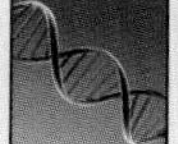

MOLECULAR PATHOGENESIS: The mechanism whereby diabetes promotes atherosclerosis has been the subject of considerable study. There are at least three general schools of thought to account for this pathogenetic relationship:

1. **Direct effects of diabetes or hyperglycemia on the arterial wall.** As noted above, however, none of the clinical therapies based on this idea (e.g., aldose reductase

inhibitors, antioxidants, intensive glycemic control) has reduced this type of complication of T2DM.
2. **Side effects of diabetic therapy,** such as high insulin concentrations associated with certain forms of treatment.
3. **Exacerbation of general risk factors for atherosclerosis** (e.g., dyslipoproteinemia, hypertension and hypercoagulability). The dyslipoproteinemia of T2DM arises in part from a defect in lipoprotein lipase that impairs clearance of chylomicrons and leads to postprandial hypertriglyceridemia, and a defect in hepatic uptake of atherogenic postprandial remnant lipoprotein particles. At this point, the most successful strategies to reduce cardiovascular events in T2DM involve management of these risk factors (e.g., administration of statins, antihypertensive agents and aspirin). Gastric bypass surgery for weight loss has been associated with substantial decreases in cardiovascular deaths.

Diabetic Microvascular Disease Is Responsible for Many of the Complications of Diabetes, Including Renal Failure and Blindness

***Arteriolosclerosis and capillary basement membrane thickening are characteristic vascular changes in diabetes* (see Chapter 10).** The frequent occurrence of hypertension contributes to the development of the arteriolar lesions. Deposition of basement membrane proteins, which may also become glycated, increases in diabetes. Aggregation of platelets in smaller blood vessels and impaired fibrinolytic mechanisms may also play a role in the pathogenesis of diabetic microvascular disease.

Whatever the pathogenetic processes, the effects of microvascular disease on tissue perfusion and wound healing are profound. Blood flow to the heart, already compromised by large-vessel disease (coronary atherosclerosis), is reduced. Healing of chronic ulcers that develop from trauma and infection of the feet in diabetic patients is commonly defective, in part because of microvascular disease. The major complications of diabetic microvascular disease involve the kidney and the retina (Fig. 22-13).

Diabetic Nephropathy

Diabetes is the leading cause of renal failure in the United States, accounting for about 44% of new cases. Of patients with T1DM, 30% to 40% ultimately develop renal failure. A somewhat smaller proportion (up to 20%) of patients with T2DM are similarly affected. Although some patients with T1DM die from uremia, most who develop nephropathy succumb to cardiovascular disease, the risk of which is 40 times greater in patients with T1DM who have end-stage renal disease. The prevalence of diabetic nephropathy increases with the severity and duration of hyperglycemia. ***Kidney disease due to diabetes is the most common reason for renal transplantation in adults.***

Initially, hyperglycemia leads to glomerular hypertension and renal hyperperfusion (Fig. 22-14). Increased glomerular pressure favors deposition of protein in the mesangium, resulting in glomerulosclerosis and, eventually, renal failure. Advanced glycosylation products and lipoprotein abnormalities may contribute to changes in the chemical composition of the glomerular basement membrane. In addition, growth factors, particularly transforming growth factor-β (TGF-β), that are induced in the diabetic kidney have been implicated in some of the cellular abnormalities in diabetic nephropathy. Inhibition of TGF-β in animal models of diabetes attenuates renal disease. Regardless of the underlying mechanism, strict control of blood glucose levels and blood pressure retards development of diabetic nephropathy. Treatment with angiotensin-converting enzyme (ACE) inhibitors or angiotensin receptor blockers—which reduce systemic blood pressure, glomerular hypertension and renal perfusion—retard progression of diabetic nephropathy.

Eventually, glomeruli in diabetic kidneys exhibit a unique lesion termed **Kimmelstiel-Wilson disease** or **nodular glomerulosclerosis** (see Chapter 16), which assumes two microscopic patterns. In the more common one, spherical masses of basement membrane–like material accumulate in glomerular lobules (Fig. 22-15). The other form is characterized by more diffuse, somewhat irregular, deposition of this material throughout the glomerulus. This must be differentiated from membranous nephropathy. Onset of glomerular disease is heralded clinically by the appearance in the urine of small amounts of serum albumin, termed **microalbuminuria**. Proteinuria increases with time and with progressive decline in renal function.

Diabetic Retinopathy

Diabetic retinopathy is the leading cause of blindness in the Unites States in adults younger than the age of 74 years. The risk is higher in T1DM than in T2DM. In fact, 10% of patients with T1DM of 30 years' duration become legally blind. Nevertheless, there are many more patients with T2DM, so they are the most numerous patients with diabetic retinopathy. Retinopathy is the most devastating ophthalmic complication of diabetes, although glaucoma, cataracts and corneal disease are also increased. Like nephropathy, the prevalence of diabetic retinopathy reflects the duration and degree of glycemic control (also see Chapter 29).

Diabetic Neuropathy Affects Sensory and Autonomic Innervation

Peripheral sensory impairment and autonomic nerve dysfunction are among the most common and distressing complications of diabetes. Changes in the nerves are complex, and abnormalities in axons, the myelin sheath and Schwann cells have all been found. Microvasculopathy involving the small blood vessels of nerves contributes to the disorder. Evidence suggests that hyperglycemia increases the perception of pain, independent of any structural lesions in the nerves.

Peripheral neuropathy is initially characterized by pain and abnormal sensations in the extremities. However, fine touch, pain detection and proprioception are ultimately lost. As a result, diabetics tend to ignore irritation and minor trauma to feet, joints and legs. Peripheral neuropathy can thus lead to foot ulcers, which often plague patients with severe diabetes. It also plays a role in the painless destructive joint disease that occasionally occurs.

Although autonomic nerve dysfunction is subtle, abnormalities in neurogenic regulation of cardiovascular and gastrointestinal functions frequently lead to postural hypotension

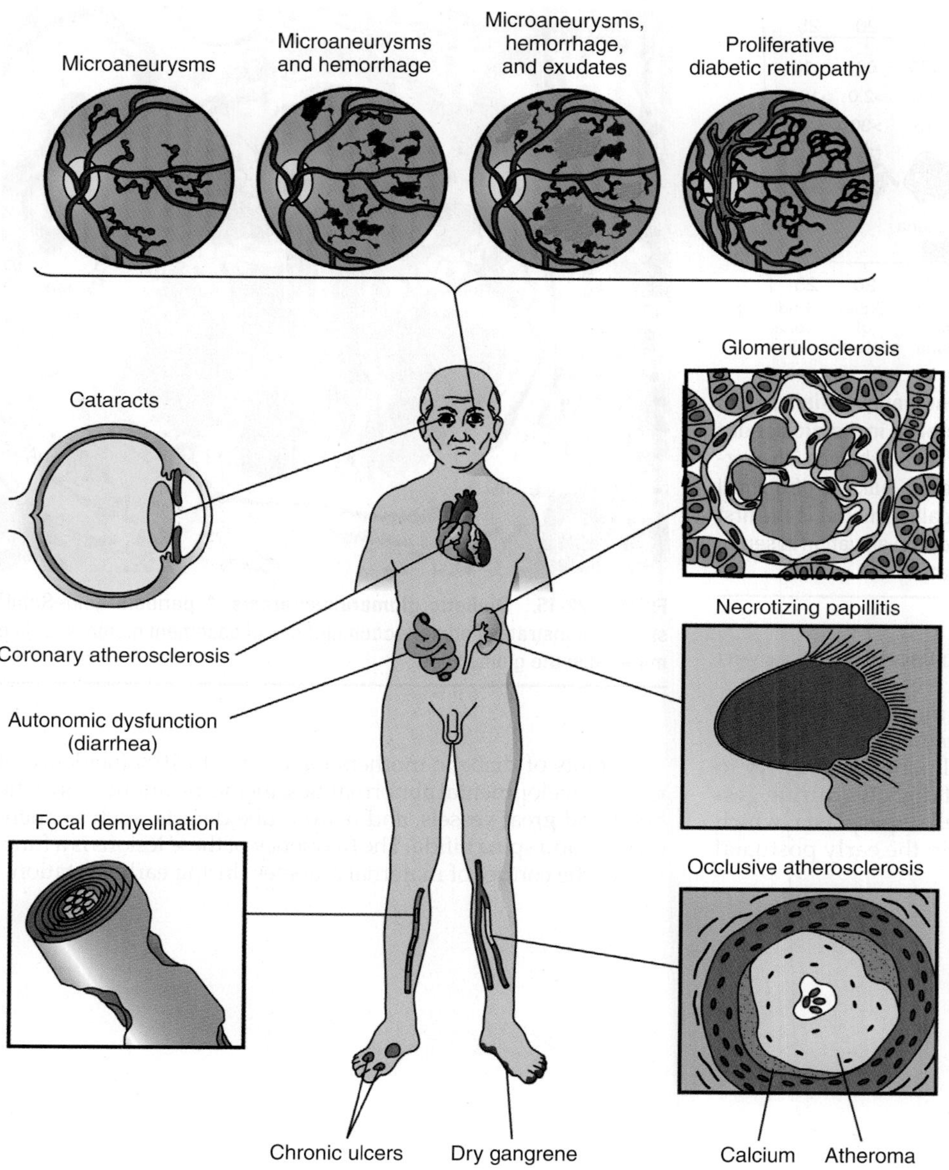

FIGURE 22-13. Secondary complications of diabetes. The effects of diabetes on a number of vital organs result in complications that may be incapacitating (cerebral and peripheral vascular disease), painful (neuropathy) or life-threatening (coronary artery disease, pyelonephritis with necrotizing papillitis).

and problems of gut motility, such as gastroparesis and diarrhea. Erectile dysfunction and retrograde ejaculation are common complications of autonomic dysfunction, although vascular disease is often a contributing factor. Hypotonic urinary bladder develops occasionally, results in urinary retention and predisposes to infection.

Bacterial and Fungal Infections Occur in Diabetic Patients Whose Hyperglycemia Is Poorly Controlled

Multiple abnormalities in host responses to microbial pathogens are described in patients with poorly controlled diabetes. Leukocyte function is compromised and immune responses are blunted. Before the use of insulin, tuberculosis and purulent infections were often life-threatening. Now, patients with well-controlled diabetes are much less susceptible to infections. However, **urinary tract infections** continue to be problematic because glucose in the urine provides an enriched culture medium. This is further complicated if patients have developed autonomic neuropathy leading to urinary retention from poor bladder emptying. Infection ascending from the bladder to the kidney (i.e., **pyelonephritis**), is thus a constant concern. **Renal papillary necrosis** may be a devastating complication of bladder infection.

A dreaded infectious complication of poorly controlled diabetes is **mucormycosis**. This often fatal fungal infection tends to originate in the nasopharynx or paranasal sinuses and spreads rapidly to the orbit and brain (see Chapter 9).

Diabetes Occurring During Pregnancy May Put Both Mother and Fetus at Risk

Gestational diabetes develops in only a few percent of seemingly healthy women during pregnancy. It may continue after parturition in a small proportion of these patients. Pregnancy is a state of insulin resistance, but only pregnant women with impaired beta cell secretion of insulin become diabetic. Abnormalities in the amount and timing of pancreatic insulin

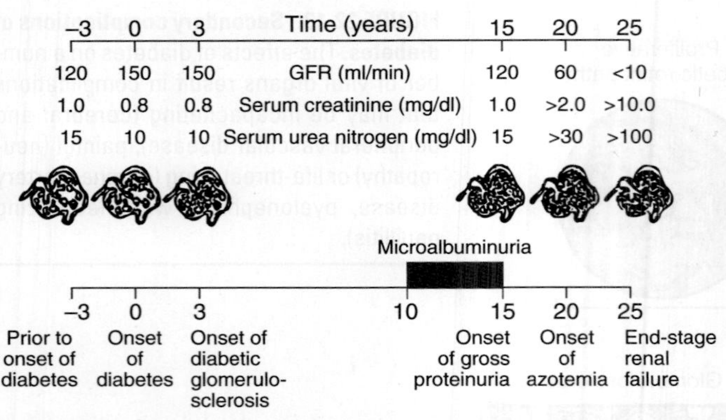

FIGURE 22-14. Natural history of diabetic nephropathy. Initially, renal hypertrophy and hyperfiltration lead to an increase in the glomerular filtration rate (GFR). Once the decline in renal function begins, on average at least 10 years after the onset of diabetes, leakage of a small amount of serum albumin into the urine (microalbuminuria) is the first abnormality that is easily and reliably measured. The elevation in serum creatinine and gross proteinuria occur much later.

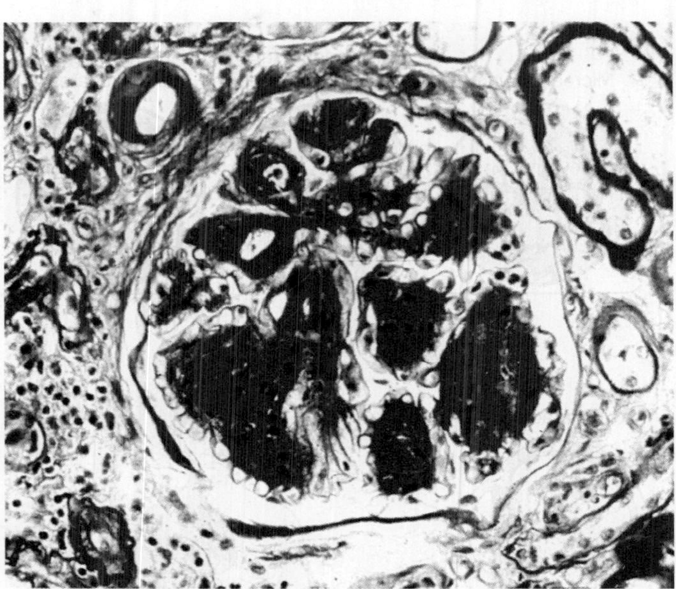

FIGURE 22-15. Diabetic glomerulosclerosis. A periodic acid–Schiff stain demonstrates nodular accumulations of basement membrane–like material in the glomerulus.

secretion make these women highly susceptible to overt T2DM later in life.

Poor control of gestational diabetes may lead to the birth of large infants, make labor and delivery more difficult and necessitate a cesarean section. The fetal pancreas may try to compensate for poor maternal control of diabetes during gestation. Such fetuses may develop beta cell hyperplasia, which may lead to hypoglycemia at birth and in the early postnatal period.

Infants of diabetic mothers have a 5% to 10% incidence of major developmental abnormalities, including anomalies of the heart and great vessels, and neural tube defects, such as anencephaly and spina bifida. The frequency of these lesions is a function of the control of maternal diabetes during early gestation.

23 The Amyloidoses

Philip Hawkins • Robert Kisilevsky

Constituents of Amyloid

Amyloid refers to a group of diverse extracellular protein deposits that have (1) common morphologic properties, (2) affinities for specific dyes and (3) a characteristic appearance under polarized light. All proteins that form amyloid are folded so they share common ultrastructural and physical properties, despite different amino acid sequences. **Amyloidosis** encompasses the clinical disorders caused directly by localized or systemic amyloid deposition.

Diseases associated with amyloid deposition have been recognized for more than 300 years, but only in the mid-19th century were attempts made to define these tissue deposits by their staining properties. Amyloid stained blue with acidified iodine, a method that demonstrates cellulose or starch. Hence, the term **amyloid** (Greek for "starchlike") was coined, and has been retained, although the protein nature of these deposits has been recognized for over 100 years. Protein misfolding and aggregation are increasingly being recognized in various other diseases, but amyloidosis—the disease directly caused by extracellular amyloid deposition—is a precise term with critical implications for patients with a specific group of life-threatening disorders.

More than 25 different unrelated proteins can form amyloid in vivo, and clinical amyloidosis is classified by the identity of the fibril protein. Amyloid deposition is remarkably diverse: it can be systemic or localized, acquired or hereditary, life-threatening or merely incidental. Clinical consequences occur when amyloid accumulates sufficiently to disrupt the structure of tissues or organs, and to impair function. Patterns of organ involvement vary among the amyloidoses, but clinical phenotypes overlap greatly. In **systemic amyloidosis,** virtually any tissue may be involved. This form of the disease is often fatal, although prognosis has improved due to better treatments for many of the underlying conditions. **Localized amyloid deposits** are confined to a particular organ or tissue, and range from being clinically silent to life-threatening (e.g., cardiac amyloidosis). In addition to clinical disorders classified as amyloidoses, local amyloid deposits are seen in other important disorders including Alzheimer disease (see Chapter 28), prion disorders and pancreatic islets in type II diabetes mellitus (see Chapter 22).

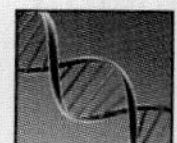

MOLECULAR PATHOGENESIS: Amyloidosis defies the dogma that tertiary structure of proteins is determined solely by primary amino acid sequence. Amyloid-forming proteins can exist in two completely different stable structures: (1) **a native form** and (2) transformation by massive refolding of the native form into predominantly **β-sheets** that can autoaggregate in a highly ordered manner to produce characteristic fibrils. Such amyloid fibrils are rigid, nonbranching, 10 to 15 nm in diameter and indeterminate in length. Acquired biophysical properties that are common to all amyloid fibrils include insolubility in physiologic solutions, relative resistance to proteolysis and the ability to bind **Congo red dye** in a spatially ordered manner to produce the diagnostic green birefringence under cross-polarized light (Fig. 23-1).

There are several circumstances in which amyloid deposition occurs (Fig. 23-2):

- *Sustained, abnormally high abundance of certain proteins that are normally present at low levels,* such as serum amyloid A protein (SAA) in chronic inflammation and β_2-microglobulin in renal failure, which underlie susceptibility to AA and Aβ_2M amyloidosis, respectively (see below)
- *Normal concentrations of a normal, but to some extent inherently amyloidogenic, protein over a very prolonged period,* such as transthyretin in senile amyloidosis (ATTR) and β-protein in Alzheimer disease
- *Presence of an acquired or inherited variant protein with an abnormal, markedly amyloidogenic structure,* such as certain monoclonal immunoglobulin light chains in AL amyloidosis and the genetic amyloidogenic variants of transthyretin, lysozyme, apolipoprotein AI and fibrinogen Aα chain in hereditary amyloidosis

Although it is not clear why only the 20 or so known amyloidogenic proteins adopt the amyloid fold and persist as fibrils in vivo, a unifying theme is that amyloid precursors are relatively unstable. Even under normal physiologic conditions, these proteins can exist in partly

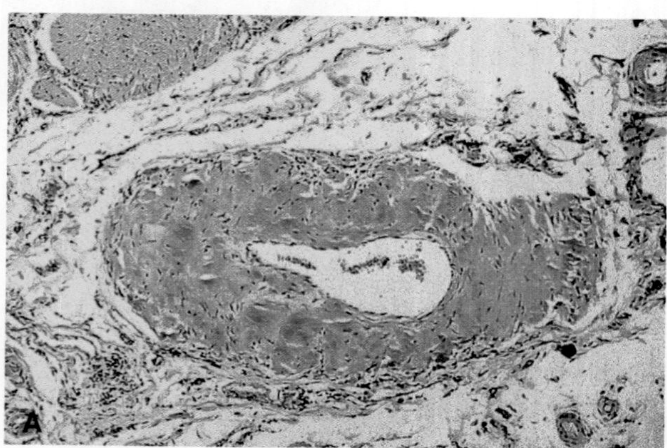

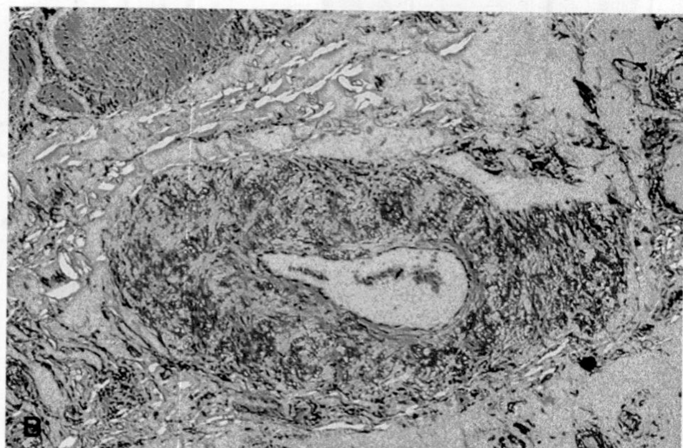

FIGURE 23-1. AL amyloid involving the wall of an artery stained with Congo red is shown under (**A**) ordinary light and (**B**) polarized light. Note the red-green birefringence of the amyloid. Collagen has a silvery appearance.

unfolded states involving loss of tertiary structure but retention of β-sheet secondary structure, and which can autoaggregate into protofilaments and thence mature amyloid fibrils.

Amyloid deposits consist mainly of these protein fibrils, but also contain some common minor constituents, including certain **glycosaminoglycans** (GAGs), the normal plasma protein **serum amyloid P component** (SAP) and various other trace proteins such as **apolipoprotein E** (apoE), **laminin** and **collagen IV** (Fig. 23-3).

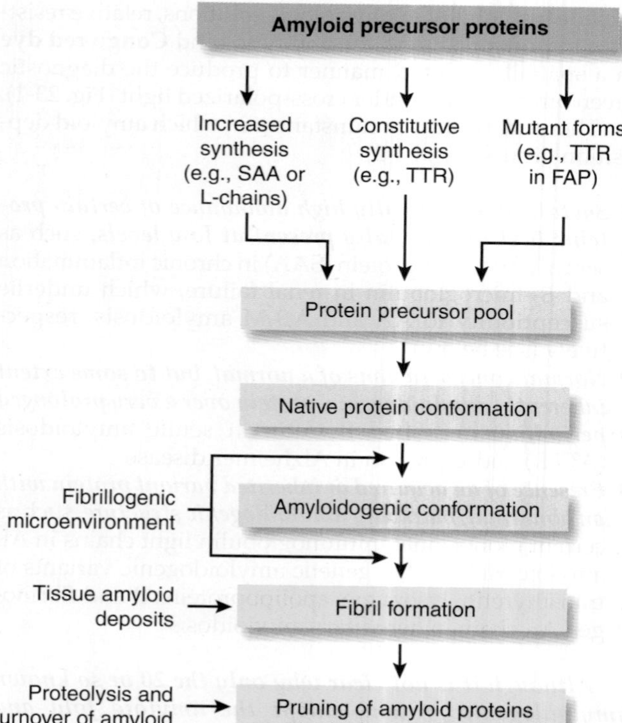

FIGURE 23-2. General scheme for amyloidogenesis. FAP = familial amyloidotic polyneuropathy; SAA = serum amyloid A protein; TTR = transthyretin.

- SAP binds in a specific calcium-dependent manner to a domain that is present on all amyloid fibrils but not on their respective precursor proteins. This phenomenon is the basis for the use of SAP scintigraphy for diagnostic imaging and quantitative monitoring of amyloid deposits. Animal studies indicate that SAP contributes to amyloidogenesis. SAP is also a minor, structural component of normal basement membranes.
- Amyloid fibril-associated GAGs are mainly heparan and dermatan sulphates. Their universal presence, restricted heterogeneity and intimate relationship with the fibrils are consistent with their contribution to the development or stability of amyloid deposits. This hypothesis has been supported by the inhibitory effect of low–molecular-weight GAG analogs on the experimental induction of AA amyloidosis in mice and people.

The genetic and/or environmental factors that determine the individual susceptibility and timing of amyloid deposition are unclear, although several factors may be at play:

- Once the process has begun, further accumulation of amyloid is unremitting so long as there is a continuous supply of the respective precursor protein. Initiation of amyloid accumulation may involve a "seeding" process, consistent with observations that amyloid deposition can be remarkably rapid following its initiation. Seeding may be a stochastic event. The notion of seeding is supported by observations in experimental murine AA amyloidosis, in which nanogram quantities of parenterally administered amyloid material result in massive amyloid deposition within 24 hours of developing an acute phase SAA response. The existence of an "amyloid-enhancing factor" (AEF) has been proposed.
- Both increasing age and male sex appear to be potent susceptibility factors in wild-type TTR amyloid deposition. Clinical sequelae of this kind of amyloid are almost unheard before age 60 years, and more than 90% of patients are male.
- The factors that influence the anatomic distribution of amyloid deposits are also unclear, but there is reasonable consistency among the organ involvement associated

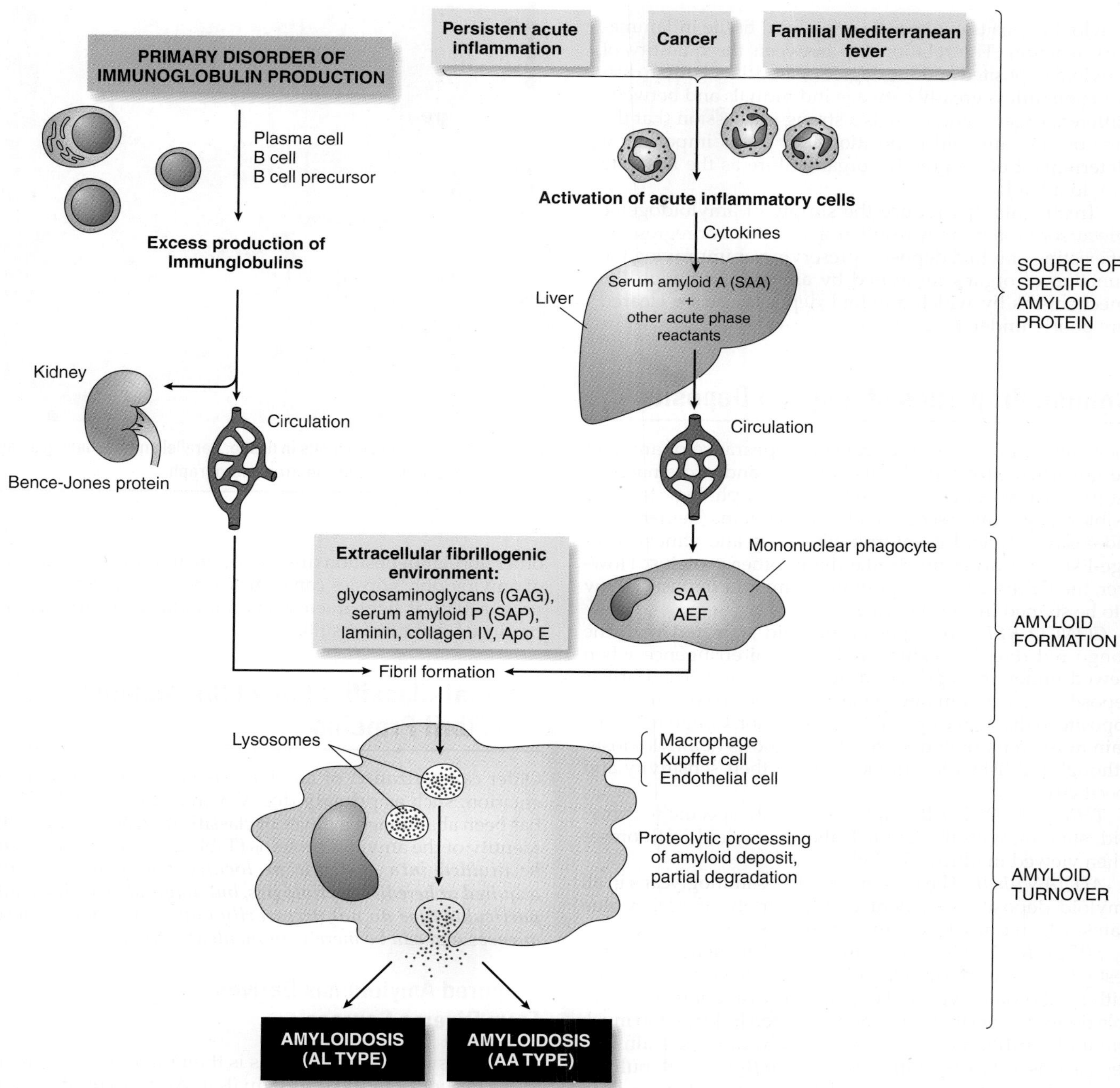

FIGURE 23-3. The mechanisms of amyloid deposition. For **AL amyloid**: Certain lymphocyte- and plasma cell–derived immunoglobulin light chains are amyloidogenic within a fibrillogenic environment. For **AA amyloid** deposition: A variety of diseases are associated with the activation of polymorphonuclear leukocytes and macrophages, which in turn leads to the synthesis and release of acute phase reactants by the liver, including serum amyloid A protein (SAA). SAA may undergo cleavage by macrophages, and its conversion into AA fibrils is promoted by amyloid-enhancing factor (AEF). In a fibrillogenic environment the released products complex with glycosaminoglycans and serum amyloid P component (SAP). Macrophages are also involved in turnover of amyloid.

with AA and most hereditary types of amyloidosis in which the fibril protein has the same structure in all individuals. By contrast, the organ distribution in AL amyloidosis is extremely heterogeneous, probably reflecting the unique sequence of the respective monoclonal immunoglobulin light chain in each patient.

The pathologic effects of amyloid are due to its physical presence. Extensive deposits may total kilograms, are structurally disruptive and impair normal function, as do strategically located smaller deposits (e.g., in glomeruli or nerves). It is possible that amyloid fibrils or prefibrillar aggregates may sometimes be directly cytotoxic, but amyloid deposits evoke little or no local tissue inflammatory reaction. The relationship between the quantity of amyloid deposited and the degree of associated organ dysfunction differs greatly between individuals and between different organs, and there is a strong impression that the rate of new amyloid deposition may be as important a determinant of progressive organ failure as the absolute amyloid load.

Treatments that reduce the supply of amyloidogenic precursor proteins may result in stabilization or regression of existing amyloid deposits, preserving or improving the function of organs infiltrated by amyloid, although the mechanisms by which amyloid deposits can be cleared are poorly understood.

Staining Properties of Amyloid Deposits

The staining properties and general appearance of amyloid are governed primarily by its compact and proteinaceous nature. Because of this, amyloid has few morphologic features visible on light microscopy. With routine stains (hematoxylin and eosin), amyloid is amorphous, glassy and almost cartilage-like, appearing much like many other proteins. However, the nature and organization of amyloid deposits allow it to be stained in specific ways.

CONGO RED: All types of amyloid stain red with the Congo red dye, but exhibit red-green birefringence when viewed under cross-polarized light (Fig. 23-1). The fibrillar deposits organized in one plane exhibit one color, and those opposite to that plane appear the other color. Congo red is the stain most commonly used for the diagnosis of amyloidosis, although published techniques vary in their sensitivity and specificity.

THIOFLAVIN T: Although not entirely specific for amyloid, staining with thioflavin T allows amyloid to fluoresce when viewed in ultraviolet light.

ALCIAN BLUE: The presence of glycosaminoglycans in all amyloid deposits is evident with a variety of Alcian blue stains, which cause GAGs to appear blue.

SPECIFIC ANTIBODIES: Immunohistochemistry is the best way to characterize amyloid, although its success varies with fibril protein type and depends on availability of a suitable tissue sample that contains neither too little nor too much amyloid. Antibodies to SAA virtually always stain AA deposits, as is the case with antibodies to β_2-microglobulin in hemodialysis-associated amyloid. In AL amyloid, deposits in fixed specimens are stained convincingly with antibodies to κ or λ immunoglobulin light chains in only about two thirds of cases, in part because AL fibrils are chiefly variable light chain domains with unique sequences in each case. Immunohistochemical staining of TTR and other hereditary amyloid fibril proteins may require pretreatment of sections with formic acid, alkaline guanidine or deglycosylation, and even then, does not always yield definitive results. Demonstration of SAP, the most abundant nonfibrillar protein present in all types of amyloid, helps to corroborate that deposits are indeed amyloid, and can be particularly useful in excluding light chain deposition disease.

ELECTRON MICROSCOPY: By electron microscopy, amyloid is straight, rigid nonbranching fibrils of indeterminate length, 10 to 15 nm in diameter (Fig. 23-4). Electron microscopy should be used to supplement other diagnostic tools, since other fibrillar deposition diseases occur. Immunogold staining of amyloidotic biopsies can sometimes be diagnostic of fibril protein type if light microscopic immunochemistry has not produced definitive results.

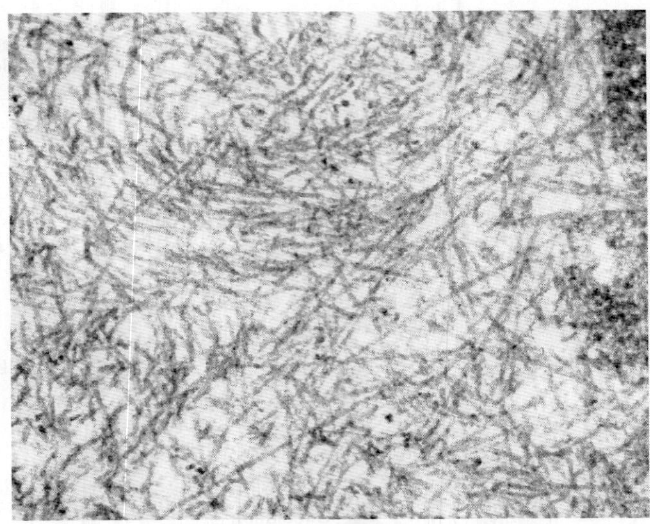

FIGURE 23-4. Amyloid deposits in tissue. Parallel and interlacing arrays of fibrils are evident in this electron micrograph.

Clinical Classification of the Amyloidoses and Fibril Proteins

Older categorization of amyloidosis based on clinical presentation, such as primary (for AL) and secondary (for AA), has been abandoned in favor of classification according to the identity of the amyloid proteins (Table 23-1). ***The disease can be divided into systemic or localized distributions and acquired or hereditary etiologies, but amyloid deposits of any particular type do not necessarily have any clinical consequences and can be merely an incidental finding.***

Acquired Amyloidosis Derives From Diverse Sources

Acquired systemic amyloidosis is thought to be the cause of death in about 1 in 1000 individuals in Western countries, and is probably underdiagnosed among the elderly, who are likely to be at greatest risk of developing it. Systemic AL amyloidosis is the most common and serious type, accounting for over 60% of cases. Although less serious, dialysis-related β_2-microglobulin amyloidosis affects about 1 million patients on long-term renal replacement therapy worldwide. Senile transthyretin amyloidosis, which predominantly involves the heart, occurs in about one quarter of individuals older than 80 years, a sector of the population that is ever rising.

Reactive Systemic Amyloidosis, AA Amyloidosis

AA amyloidosis is a complication of chronic infections and inflammatory diseases, or any condition that leads to long-term overproduction of the acute phase reactant SAA. The amyloid fibrils are composed of an N-terminal cleavage fragment of

Table 23-1

Classification of Human Amyloids

Amyloid Protein	Protein Precursor	Clinical Setting
AL	κ or λ immunoglobulin light chain	Multiple myeloma, plasma cell dyscrasias and primary amyloid
AH	γ Immunoglobulin chain	Waldenström macroglobulinemia
Aβ_2M	β_2-Microglobulin	Hemodialysis related
ATTR	Transthyretin	Familial amyloidotic polyneuropathy (FAP), normal TTR in senile systemic amyloid
AA	Apo serum AA	Persistent acute inflammation; familial Mediterranean fever; certain malignancies
AApoAI	Apolipoprotein AI	Hereditary systemic amyloidosis
AApoAII	Apolipoprotein AII	Familial
AApoAIV	Apolipoprotein AIV	Sporadic, age associated
Aβ	β-Protein precursor	Alzheimer disease, Down syndrome, hereditary cerebral hemorrhage with amyloid (HCHWA), Dutch
ABri	ABriPP	Familial dementia, British
ADan	ADanPP	Familial dementia, Danish
APrP	Prion protein	CJD, scrapie, BSE, GSS, Kuru
ACys	Cystatin C	HCHWA, Icelandic
ALys	Lysozyme	Hereditary systemic amyloidosis
AFib	Fibrinogen	Hereditary renal amyloidosis
AGel	Gelsolin	Familial amyloidosis, Finnish
ACal	(Pro)calcitonin	Medullary carcinoma of the thyroid
AANF	Atrial natriuretic factor	Isolated atrial amyloid
AIAPP	Islet amyloid polypeptide	Type 2 diabetes, insulinomas
AIns	Insulin	Iatrogenic
APro	Prolactin	Pituitary, age associated
AMed	Lactadherin	Senile aortic, media
AKer	Keratoepithelin	Cornea, familial
ALac	Lactoferrin	Cornea

Apo = apolipoprotein; BSE = bovine spongiform encephalopathy; CJD = Creutzfeldt-Jakob disease; GSS = Gerstmann-Straussler-Sheinker syndrome; TTR = transthyretin.

SAA (i.e., AA protein). AA amyloidosis occurs in 1% to 5% of patients with rheumatoid arthritis, juvenile idiopathic arthritis and Crohn disease, and is more common in those with untreated lifelong autoinflammatory diseases such as familial Mediterranean fever. Most patients present with proteinuria, and although liver and gastrointestinal involvement may occur later, clinically significant cardiac or neuropathic involvement is very rare.

MOLECULAR PATHOGENESIS: ***AA protein is a single nonglycosylated polypeptide chain usually of mass ~8 kd making up the 76-residue N-terminal portion of the 104-residue SAA.*** Smaller and larger AA fragments occur. SAA is an apolipoprotein of high-density lipoprotein particles and is the polymorphic product of a set of genes located on chromosome 11. It is highly conserved in evolution and is a major acute phase reactant. Most SAA in plasma is produced by hepatocytes under transcriptional regulation by cytokines, especially interleukin 1 (IL-1), IL-6 and tumor necrosis factor-α (TNF-α). After secretion, SAA rapidly associates with high-density lipoproteins, from which it displaces apolipoprotein AI. Circulating SAA can rise from normal levels ($\leq$3 mg/L) to over 2000 mg/L within 24 to 48 hours of an acute stimulus, and remains elevated indefinitely in the presence of chronic inflammation.

Cleavage of circulating SAA to AA can be done by macrophages and several proteinases, but it is not known whether cleavage of SAA occurs before and/or after aggregation of monomers during AA fibrillogenesis. Long-term overproduction of SAA is a prerequisite for deposition of

AA amyloid, but it is not known why the latter occurs in only some individuals. SAA isoforms are complex, but homozygosity for particular types seems to favor amyloidogenesis, as may ethnic differences in susceptibility.

SAA function is not known, but it may modulate effects on reverse cholesterol transport and on lipid functions in the microenvironment of inflammatory foci. Regardless of its physiologic role, SAA as an exquisitely sensitive acute phase protein with enormous dynamic range, making it a very valuable empirical clinical marker. It can be used to monitor the extent and activity of many infective, inflammatory, necrotic and neoplastic diseases. Frequent long-term monitoring of SAA is vital in managing all patients with AA amyloidosis, as the primary inflammatory process must be controlled sufficiently to reduce SAA production if amyloid deposition is to be halted or enabled to regress. Automated immunoassays for SAA are available standardized on a World Health Organization International Reference Standard.

AA amyloidosis occurs in association with chronic inflammatory disorders, chronic local or systemic microbial infections and, occasionally, neoplasms. In the Western world the most common predisposing conditions are chronic inflammatory diseases, particularly rheumatoid arthritis. Amyloidosis is exceptionally rare in ulcerative colitis or systemic lupus erythematosus and related connective tissue diseases, since these conditions provoke only modest acute phase responses. Tuberculosis and leprosy are important causes of AA amyloidosis in some parts of the world. Chronic osteomyelitis, bronchiectasis, chronically infected burns and decubitus ulcers and the chronic pyelonephritis of paraplegia are other well-recognized associations. Hodgkin disease and renal carcinoma often cause a major acute phase response and are the malignancies most commonly associated with systemic AA amyloid. The associated chronic inflammatory disease in about 7% of patients with AA amyloidosis may not be clinically evident, and these patients may be erroneously assumed to have AL amyloidosis.

AA amyloid deposits are widely distributed, and so random rectal and other biopsies are often used to make the diagnosis. However, clinically AA amyloidosis is dominated by progressive proteinuria. Treatment entails measures to suppress the underlying inflammatory disorder. Prognosis is now often excellent among patients in whom the causative acute phase response can be substantially suppressed, but about 50% of patients with persistent uncontrolled inflammation die within 10 years of diagnosis.

Amyloidosis Associated With Monoclonal B-Cell Dyscrasias, AL Amyloidosis

Systemic AL, once known as "primary," amyloidosis occurs in about 2% of people with monoclonal B-cell dyscrasias. AL fibrils are derived from monoclonal immunoglobulin light chains. These are unique in each patient, so that AL amyloidosis is highly heterogeneous in terms of organ involvement and overall clinical course. Virtually any organ other than the brain may be directly affected, but the kidneys, heart, liver and peripheral nerves bear the brunt of the clinical consequences. As the underlying monoclonal gammopathy is often missed by routine screening techniques, very sensitive methods, such as serum free light chain analysis, may be needed to identify the causative subtle B-cell dyscrasias.

MOLECULAR PATHOGENESIS: ***AL amyloid fibrils are usually derived from the N-terminal region of monoclonal immunoglobulin light chains and consist of the whole or part of the variable (V_L) domain.*** The molecular weight of the fibril subunit protein thus varies between 8 and 30 kd. Monoclonal light chains are unique to each individual, and only a small percentage are amyloidogenic, but it is not possible to predict which light chains will form AL amyloid.

The property of "amyloidogenicity" is inherent in certain monoclonal light chains. Thus, when purified human Bence Jones proteins (urinary light chain proteins) were injected into mice, animals receiving light chains from patients with AL amyloid developed typical amyloid deposits, whereas mice given light chains from myeloma patients without amyloid did not. AL fibrils develop more commonly from λ than κ light chains, despite the fact that κ-chains are more common among normal immunoglobulins and monoclonal gammopathies. Compared to light chains that do not form amyloid, some amyloidogenic light chains have distinctive amino acid replacements or insertions that can promote aggregation and insolubility, including replacement of hydrophilic framework residues by hydrophobic ones. Certain light chain types, notably $V\lambda_{VI}$, are especially amyloidogenic, and some tend to be deposited as amyloid in particular organs. For example, $V\lambda_{VI}$ light chains often deposit in the kidney, whereas $V\lambda_{II}$ chains prefer the heart.

B-cell dyscrasias underlying systemic AL amyloidosis are also heterogeneous, and include almost any clonal proliferation of differentiated B cells: multiple myeloma, Waldenström macroglobulinemia and occasionally other malignant lymphomas or leukemias. However, over 80% of cases are associated with low-grade and otherwise "benign" monoclonal gammopathies that may be difficult to detect. Histologically, minor and clinically insignificant amyloid deposits are seen in up to 10% of patients with myeloma, and similarly in a smaller proportion of patients with monoclonal gammopathy of undetermined significance (MGUS). Cytogenetic abnormalities common in multiple myeloma and MGUS, such as 14q translocations and 13q deletion, are also observed in AL amyloidosis, but their prognostic significance is not yet understood.

Localized AL Amyloidosis

A localized monoclonal B-cell dyscrasia may lead to AL deposits at the site of that B-cell lesion, almost anywhere in the body. Characteristic sites include the skin, airways, lungs, conjunctiva and urogenital tract. Deposits may be nodular or confluent, but the clonal B-cell infiltrate that is the culprit, producing the amyloidogenic L chains, may be inconspicuous. Lichenoid and macular forms of cutaneous amyloid are distinct and are thought to be derived from keratin or related proteins. Nodular cutaneous amyloid deposits are usually localized AL type, but can also be part of systemic AL amyloidosis. Localized AL amyloid deposits can exert serious space-occupying effects or cause serious hemorrhage, but otherwise are benign and enlarge slowly.

Dialysis-Related Amyloidosis, β_2-Microglobulin Amyloidosis

β_2-Microglobulin amyloid deposition occurs in patients with dialysis-dependent chronic renal failure, mainly affecting articular and periarticular structures, and typically causing arthralgia of the shoulders, knees, wrists and small joints of the hand, joint swelling and carpal tunnel syndrome. The amyloid fibril precursor protein is β_2-microglobulin, which is the invariant chain of the major histocompatibility complex (MHC) class I molecule, and is expressed by all nucleated cells. It is synthesized at an average rate of 150 to 200 mg/day and is normally filtered freely at the glomerulus, reabsorbed and catabolized by proximal tubular cells. Decreasing renal function causes a proportionate rise in concentration. β_2-Microglobulin amyloidosis was first described in 1980 and occurs in patients who have been on hemodialysis for several years and peritoneal dialysis for 5 to 10 years. Infrequently, it occurs in patients with long-term severe chronic renal impairment. DRA is present in 20% to 30% of patients within 3 years of starting dialysis for end-stage renal failure. Although it is a systemic disease, manifestations outside of the musculoskeletal system are unusual: there have been notable reports of DRA causing congestive cardiac failure and gastrointestinal bleeding, perforation and pseudo-obstruction.

Senile Transthyretin Amyloidosis, ATTR Amyloidosis

In the elderly, clinically silent systemic deposits of wild-type "senile" TTR amyloid are common, involving the heart and blood vessel walls, smooth and striated muscle, fat tissue, renal papillae and alveolar walls. Unlike most other forms of systemic amyloidosis, including hereditary transthyretin amyloid caused by point mutations in the transthyretin gene, the spleen and renal glomeruli are rarely affected. Neither is the brain involved, although symptomatic leptomeningeal deposits can occasionally occur in familial TTR amyloidosis. Senile transthyretin amyloidosis almost always presents with restrictive cardiomyopathy, and other than carpal tunnel syndrome, deposits elsewhere rarely ever attain clinical significance. About one quarter of patients can be demonstrated to have gastrointestinal amyloid deposits on rectal biopsy. Most patients are at least 70 years of age, and there is a very strong male preponderance. Cardiac failure progresses and death usually occurs within about 5 years.

Endocrine Amyloidosis

Many hormone-producing tumors of APUD cells have amyloid deposits in their stroma (see Chapter 21). These are probably composed of the hormone peptides, and in the case of medullary carcinoma of the thyroid, fibril subunits are derived from procalcitonin.

In insulinomas, the amyloid fibril protein is called islet amyloid polypeptide (or **amylin**) and shows appreciable homology with calcitonin gene–related peptide. It has subsequently been shown to be the same protein as in the amyloid of the islets of Langerhans in type 2 diabetes. Islet polypeptide amyloid is almost always seen in the pancreatic islets in type 2 diabetes, and becomes more extensive with increasing duration and severity of the disease. The amyloid itself probably does not initiate the metabolic defect in type 2 diabetes, but progressive amyloid deposition may facilitate islet destruction.

Amyloid and the Brain

The brain is a common and important site of amyloid deposition, although there are never any deposits in the cerebral parenchyma itself in any form of acquired systemic visceral amyloidosis. However, cerebrovascular and oculoleptomeningeal amyloid deposits that can be clinically significant do occasionally occur in hereditary TTR amyloidosis.

The common and major forms of brain amyloid are associated with Alzheimer disease, the most common type of dementia (see Chapter 28). In brief, intracerebral and cerebrovascular amyloid deposits derived from β-protein (Aβ), a 39- to 43-residue cleavage product of the large amyloid precursor protein, are neuropathologic hallmarks of Alzheimer disease. It is unclear whether or how Aβ per se, small prefibrillar aggregates or the amyloid fibrils that it forms contribute to the neuronal loss that underlies the dementia.

Intracerebral amyloid plaques derived from the normal physiologic cellular prion protein PrP^C are sometimes seen in acquired and hereditary spongiform encephalopathies. The pathogenetic significance of amyloid in these disorders is not clear. However, the amyloid-like proteinase-resistant conformational isoform of PrP^C, called PrP^{Sc}, is the transmissible agent of these spongiform encephalopathies. Neuron damage may be caused by cytotoxic interaction between prefibrillar PrP^{Sc} aggregates and normal PrP^C, or by other mechanisms entirely.

In Hereditary Amyloidosis Genetically Variant Proteins Accumulate as Amyloid

In hereditary systemic amyloidosis mutations in the genes for transthyretin, cystatin C, gelsolin, lysozyme, fibrinogen A α-chain, apolipoprotein AI and, extremely rarely, apolipoprotein AII lead to deposition of these mutant proteins as amyloid. These diseases are all inherited dominantly with variable penetrance, and present clinically from teenage to old age, though usually in midadult life. Hereditary transthyretin amyloidosis is by far the commonest, most often presenting as a syndrome of familial amyloid polyneuropathy with peripheral and autonomic neuropathy and/or cardiomyopathy. Cystatin C amyloidosis presents as cerebral amyloid angiopathy with recurrent cerebral hemorrhage and clinically silent systemic deposits, and has been reported only in Icelandic families. Gelsolin amyloidosis presents with cranial neuropathy but is also extremely rare. Apolipoprotein AI, lysozyme and fibrinogen A α-chain amyloidosis usually present as nonneuropathic systemic amyloidosis that can affect any or all major viscera, with renal involvement usually being prominent. Since a family history is often absent, these latter conditions are readily misdiagnosed as acquired "primary" AL amyloidosis, and are much less rare than previously thought. ***Of patients presenting with non-AA systemic amyloidosis, 5% to 10% have hereditary*** *forms of the disease.* It is imperative that hereditary amyloidosis is identified correctly, since prognosis, treatment and implications for family members differ substantially, compared to acquired amyloidosis.

Familial Amyloidotic Polyneuropathy, Variant Transthyretin (ATTR) Amyloidosis

Familial amyloidotic polyneuropathy (FAP) is associated with heterozygous point mutations in the TTR gene. It is an autosomal dominant syndrome with onset between the third and seventh decades. Over 100 TTR variants are associated with FAP, and amyloid fibrils are a mixture of variant and wild-type TTR protein. There are probably several thousand patients with FAP in the world. The disease is characterized by progressive and disabling peripheral and autonomic neuropathy and varying degrees of visceral amyloid involvement, prominently including cardiac amyloidosis, which can be the sole clinical feature in some cases. Deposits within the vitreous of the eye are well recognized and are pathognomonic, whereas deposits in the kidneys, thyroid, spleen and adrenals are usually asymptomatic. There is considerable phenotypic variation in age of onset, rate of progression, involvement of different systems and disease penetrance, even within one family. Typically the disease progresses inexorably, causing death within 5 to 15 years.

Familial Amyloid Polyneuropathy With Predominant Cranial Neuropathy

This is a very rare dominant form of hereditary amyloidosis that presents in mid- to late adult life with cranial neuropathy, lattice corneal dystrophy and mild distal peripheral neuropathy. It was first described in Finland but has since been reported in other ethnic groups. There may be skin, renal and cardiac manifestations, but these are usually covert and life expectancy approaches normal. There is no specific treatment and the disorder is progressively disfiguring and very distressing in its late stages. The responsible mutant gene encodes a variant form of gelsolin, which is an actin-modulating protein. The functional role of circulating gelsolin is unknown but may be related to clearance of actin filaments released by apoptotic cells.

Nonneuropathic Variants of Hereditary Systemic Amyloidosis

Hereditary lysozyme systemic amyloidosis has been ascribed to six lysozyme variants, all of which are very rare. Most patients present in middle age with proteinuria, sicca syndrome or upper gastrointestinal and liver involvement. Acute gastrointestinal hemorrhage or perforation and spontaneous liver rupture are well recognized and potentially fatal complications.

Apolipoprotein AI is a major constituent of high-density lipoprotein. Known amyloidogenic variants include single amino acid substitutions, deletions and a deletion/insertion. Associated clinical syndromes vary but often entail substantial amyloid deposits in the liver, spleen and kidneys; some mutations cause cardiomyopathy, and patients with the arginine 26 variant may develop polyneuropathy. In several C-terminal variants, laryngeal amyloid deposits lead to hoarseness. Other manifestations seen with particular mutations include male infertility and skin lesions. Many patients eventually develop renal failure, but liver function usually remains normal despite extensive hepatic amyloid deposits. Normal wild-type apolipoprotein AI amyloid is itself weakly amyloidogenic, and is the precursor of small amyloid deposits that occur quite frequently in aortic atherosclerotic plaques.

Hereditary fibrinogen A α-chain amyloid is the commonest type of hereditary renal amyloidosis, caused by some 10 different mutations, the commonest being substitution of valine for glutamic acid at position 526. Penetrance in most families is low and a family history is often lacking. Most patients present in late middle age with proteinuria or hypertension and progress to end-stage renal failure during the next 5 years or so. Amyloid deposition occurs in the kidneys, spleen and sometimes the liver, but it is usually asymptomatic in the latter two sites.

Morphologic Features of Amyloidosis

Amyloid fibrils are usually first deposited near subendothelial basement membranes (Fig. 23-5). Because amyloid accumulates along stromal networks, deposits take on the configurations of the organs involved. Morphologic differences in amyloid deposition among organs simply reflect organ-to-organ differences in stromal organization. For example, in the renal medulla, amyloid is laid down longitudinally, parallel to tubules and vasa recta, while in glomeruli amyloid (Fig. 23-6) it follows lobular glomerular architecture. In the

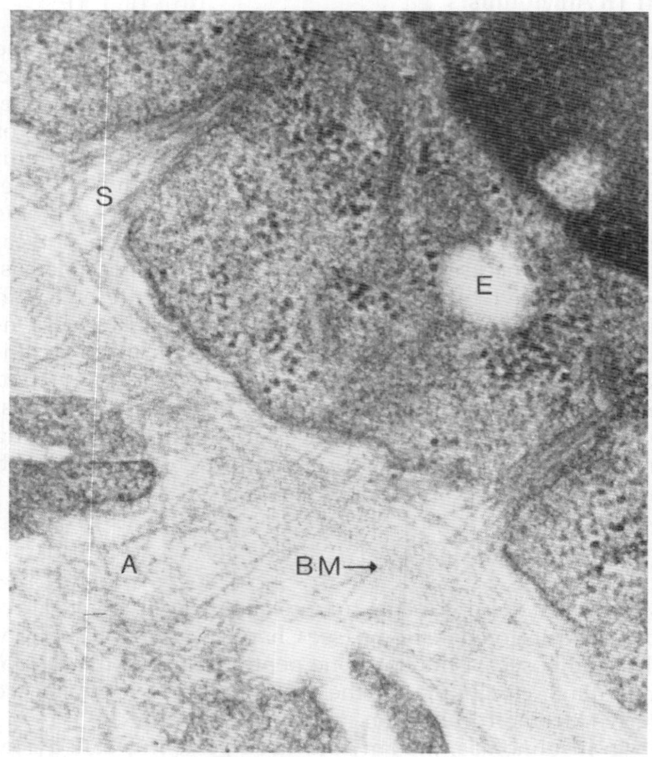

FIGURE 23-5. Electron micrograph of glomerular amyloid (*A*) illustrating its location relative to the basement membrane (*BM*). Amyloid spicules (*S*) extend into the cytoplasm of the glomerular epithelial cells (*E*).

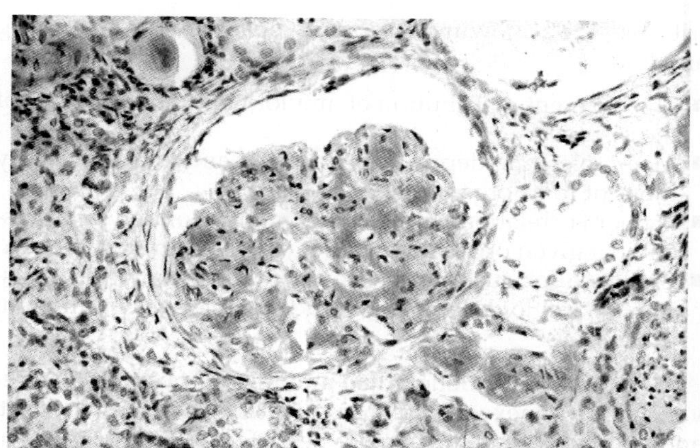

FIGURE 23-6. Microscopic appearance of AA amyloid in a glomerulus. Note the lobular pattern of the amyloid deposit and the involvement of the afferent arteriole.

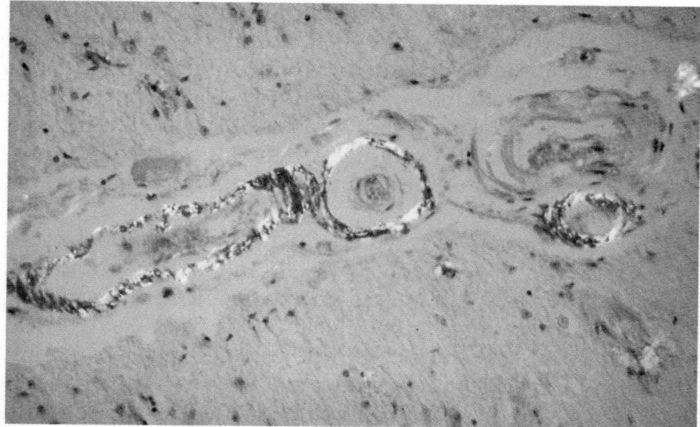

FIGURE 23-8. Cerebrovascular amyloid in a case of Alzheimer disease. The section was stained with Congo red and examined under polarized light.

spleen, amyloid may be mostly in the stroma of the red pulp or that of the white pulp. Grossly, amyloid in the red pulp imparts a diffusely pale and waxy appearance, the so-called lardaceous spleen. A spleen containing white pulp amyloid shows multiple pale foci scattered throughout the organ, which is called sago spleen. Deposits in the liver follow the arteries of the portal triads or are laid down along central veins and radiate into the parenchyma along liver cell plates (Fig. 23-7).

Amyloid adds interstitial material at sites of deposition, thereby increasing the size of affected organs. This increase may be counterbalanced by the deposition of amyloid in blood vessels (Fig. 23-8), which might impair circulation and lead to organ atrophy. Affected organs may thus increase or decrease in size. Amyloid deposits are essentially avascular, so the involved organs are commonly pale and firm.

Regardless of whether amyloid is laid down in a systemic or local fashion, deposits tend to occur between parenchymal cells and their blood supply, interfering with normal nutrition and gas exchange. Amyloid may eventually entrap parenchymal cells. Alternatively, it may have an additional toxic effect on these cells through the interaction of protofibrils and cell membranes. In each case, amyloid deposits may lead to cell strangulation, atrophy and death (Fig. 23-9).

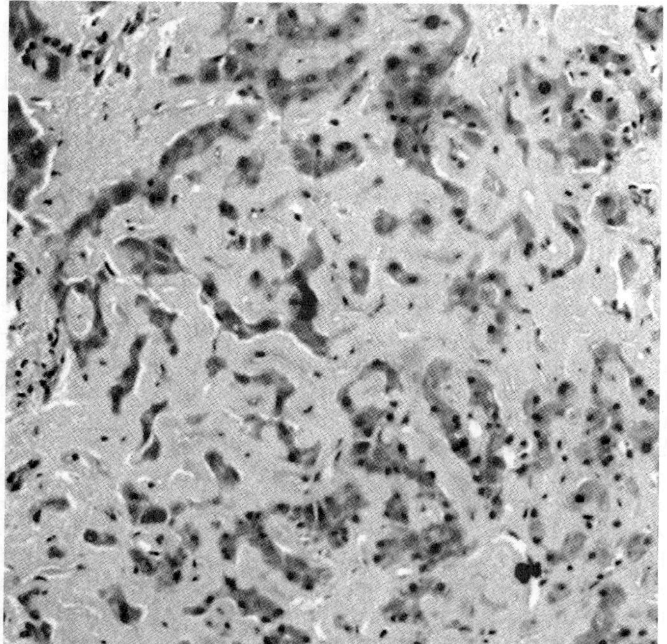

FIGURE 23-7. Hepatic amyloidosis. Amyloid is deposited along the sinusoids. Note the atrophic hepatocytes.

Clinical Features and Organ Involvement in Amyloidosis

No single set of symptoms points unequivocally to amyloidosis as a diagnosis. The symptoms of amyloidosis depend on the underlying disease and the type and organ locations of the amyloid deposits. Amyloidosis may also be diagnosed unexpectedly in the course of evaluation for something unrelated, with no clinical manifestations referable to the amyloidosis itself. In other cases, for example, unexplained renal and cardiac dysfunction may be the presenting conditions.

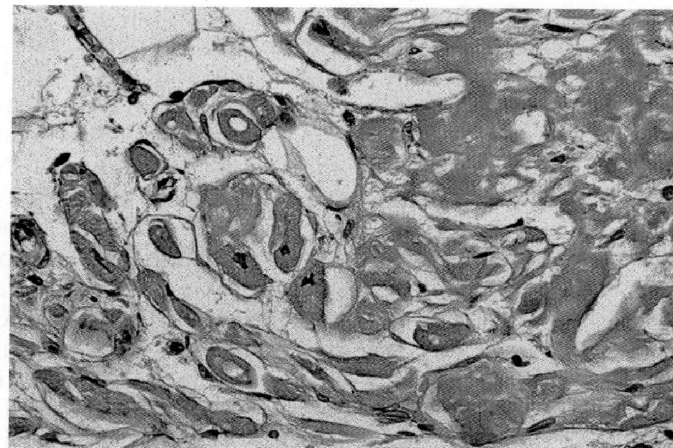

FIGURE 23-9. Myocardial amyloid (AL type), showing the encroachment upon, and strangulation of, individual myocardial fibers.

KIDNEY: Patients with multiple myeloma and other clonal B-cell dyscrasias or long-standing inflammatory disorders who develop **nephrotic syndrome** should be suspected of having amyloidosis. Proteinuria, particularly in patients with plasma cell dyscrasias, may be overlooked if the patient is already excreting a Bence Jones protein. Progressive glomerular obliteration may ultimately lead to renal failure and uremia.

HEART: Amyloid involvement of the myocardium should be suspected in all patients with AL and TTR amyloidosis, and in any patient with unexplained concentric thickening of the myocardium, especially if the latter is not associated with abnormally large voltage complexes on electrocardiography. Myocardial amyloid deposits cause **restrictive cardiomyopathy** in which diastolic dysfunction is often associated with well-preserved systolic function. Short of biopsy, two-dimensional echocardiography and Doppler studies are helpful in suggesting the diagnosis. Cardiac magnetic resonance imaging with late gadolinium enhancement has been reported to be useful as well. Serum cardiac troponin and NT-pro BNP concentrations appear to be powerful predictors of cardiac involvement, as well as prognosis and survival after chemotherapy in AL amyloidosis. Cardiac amyloidosis is also associated with conduction abnormalities that cause arrhythmias and sudden death.

GASTROINTESTINAL TRACT: The ganglia, smooth muscle, vasculature and submucosa of the gastrointestinal tract may all be affected by amyloid. Deposits in these locations can alter gastrointestinal motility and absorption, but are often clinically silent. Patients complain of either constipation or diarrhea, and insidious malnutrition is common. Enlargement of the tongue is virtually pathognomonic of AL amyloidosis, and interference with its motor function may be severe enough to affect speech and swallowing.

LIVER: AL, AA and familial forms of amyloidosis often cause amyloid deposits in the liver, but rarely lead to clinically significant hepatic dysfunction. Substantial hepatomegaly may occur before any abnormalities in serum liver function tests are seen. Liver amyloidosis is typically associated with progressive elevation of serum alkaline phosphatase and γ-glutamyl transferase in these patients, but jaundice generally occurs late and is associated with frank liver failure and a very poor prognosis, particularly the AL type.

PERIPHERAL NERVES: The familial polyneuropathic forms of amyloid usually manifest as paresthesias, with loss in temperature and pain sensation of the extremities.

The diagnosis of amyloidosis generally requires histologic confirmation, although the mere demonstration of amyloid deposition does not by itself establish that it is clinically significant. While amyloidosis does not occur in the absence of amyloid deposits, the latter may be an incidental histologic finding, especially in older subjects. Immunohistochemical staining is the most accessible method for characterizing amyloid fibril protein type, but it does not always produce definitive results, especially in AL type. Amyloid deposits can be quite patchy and histology can never provide information about the overall whole body load or distribution of amyloid deposits, nor does it permit monitoring of the natural history of amyloidosis or its response to treatment. Radiolabeled human SAP is a specific, noninvasive, quantitative in vivo tracer for amyloid deposits, and has been used in scintigraphy and metabolic turnover studies. This approach facilitates the diagnosis, monitoring and response of amyloidosis to treatment, and has contributed the following important observations regarding amyloid:

- The different distribution of amyloid in different forms of the disease
- Major systemic deposits in forms of amyloid previously thought to be organ limited
- A poor correlation between the quantity of amyloid present in a given organ and the degree of organ dysfunction
- Evidence for surprisingly rapid progression and regression of amyloid deposits with different rates in different organs

The long-held belief that amyloid deposition is irreversible and inexorably progressive is evidently incorrect, and simply reflects the usually persistent nature of the conditions that underlie it. Many case reports have described improvement in amyloidotic organ function when the underlying conditions have been controlled, suggesting that amyloid deposits may regress.

Treatment of Amyloidosis

Systemic amyloidosis is a progressive disease that, without effective treatment, is ultimately fatal in most cases. Although no treatments yet exist that specifically promote the mobilization of amyloid, there have been substantial recent advances in the management of systemic amyloidosis, in particular active measures to support failing organ function while attempts are made to reduce the supply of the amyloid fibril precursor protein. Serial SAP scintigraphy has shown that control of the primary disease process, or removal of the source of the amyloidogenic precursor, often allows gradual regression of existing deposits and recovery or preservation of organ function. Thus, aggressive intervention, and relatively toxic drug regimens or other radical approaches, can be justified by the poor prognosis. However, clinical improvement is often delayed long after the underlying disorder has remitted, reflecting the very gradual regression of the deposits that is now recognized to occur in most patients. Continuing production of amyloid precursor protein should be monitored closely over time, to determine the requirement for, and intensity of, treatment for the underlying primary condition. In AA amyloidosis this means frequent estimation of plasma SAA levels; in AL amyloidosis it requires monitoring of serum free light chains or other markers of the underlying monoclonal plasma cell proliferation.

The treatment of AA amyloidosis ranges from potent anti-inflammatory, cytokine-inhibiting and immunosuppressive drugs in patients with rheumatoid arthritis, to lifelong prophylactic colchicine in familial Mediterranean fever, and surgery in conditions such as refractory osteomyelitis and the tumors of Castleman disease. Treatment of AL amyloidosis is based on that for myeloma, including oral administration of melphalan and dexamethasone, thalidomide-based regimens and the new agents such as the proteasome inhibitor bortezomib and the immunomodulatory agent lenalidomide. High-dose chemotherapy with autologous peripheral blood stem cell transplantation has high response rates but much toxicity and is restricted to selected patients. The disabling arthralgia of β_2-microglobulin amyloidosis usually responds dramatically to renal transplantation. The basis for this remarkable clinical response is unclear since although transplantation rapidly restores normal β_2-microglobulin metabolism, regression of β_2-microglobulin amyloid may not be evident for many years.

Liver transplantation is effective in familial amyloid polyneuropathy associated with transthyretin gene mutations since the variant amyloidogenic protein is produced mainly in the liver. Outcomes are best among younger patients with the methionine 30 variant, though even in this group the peripheral neuropathy usually only stabilizes. Unfortunately, paradoxical progression of established cardiac amyloidosis with wild-type transthyretin has been noted in many older patients. On a similar basis, hepatic transplantation has proven promising in some patients with hereditary fibrinogen A α-chain and apolipoprotein AI amyloidosis.

Supportive therapy remains critical in systemic amyloidosis, notably including attention to nutrition, rigorous control of hypertension in renal amyloidosis and diuretic and fluid balance management in cardiac amyloidosis. Dysrhythmias may respond to conventional pharmacologic therapy or to pacing. Replacement of vital organ function, notably dialysis, may be necessary, and cardiac and renal transplantation has been very successful in selected cases.

24 The Skin

Craig A. Storm • David E. Elder

The skin is an optimal organ for studying fundamental principles of pathology because lesions on its surface are readily apparent and easily biopsied. Except for diseases of highly specialized tissues—for instance, those of the alveolus or glomerulus or the demyelinating diseases of the central nervous system—all classes of disease are seen in the skin. Some diseases, such as the blistering ones, are manifested only in the skin (except for some involvement of the mucous membranes).

Considering the imperatives of appearance in human interactions, a changed appearance of the skin may at times be the most important feature of cutaneous disease. Many cutaneous diseases have only minor symptoms and some have no symptoms at all. Few are life-threatening, and many are self-limited. However, even self-limited, asymptomatic cutaneous diseases are often of great concern to the patient. For example, the symptoms of acne are systemically minor, but the disease can change a life. Although scalp hair is unneeded, baldness may cause considerable distress. Vitiligo, a completely asymptomatic, progressive, depigmentation disorder, may create emotional havoc for an otherwise normal black person.

Anatomy and Physiology of the Skin

The skin is a protective barrier; microorganisms find it almost impossible to penetrate the epidermis from the outside, and water loss is limited from the inside. The skin is vital in regulating temperature and protecting against ultraviolet light. A variety of sensory receptors communicate details related to the immediate environment. The skin plays a prominent role in immune regulation through skin-associated lymphoid tissues, which consist of lymphocytes and antigen-presenting cells that travel between the skin and regional lymph nodes via the lymphatics and bloodstream. Keratinocytes, Langerhans cells, mast cells, lymphocytes and macrophages all serve functions related to immunity. Epidermal keratinocytes produce a variety of cytokines, notably interleukin (IL)-1α and IL-1β, as well as eicosanoids. This ability of keratinocytes to produce products that mediate immunity and inflammation is necessary in an organ relentlessly exposed to the external environment. Langerhans cells, the dendritic antigen-presenting cells of the skin, are bone marrow–derived, epidermal, immigrant cells. They play an important role in the development and regulation of contact hypersensitivity, allograft rejection and graft-versus-host disease.

KERATINOCYTES: The epidermis is a multilayered sheet of keratin-producing cells. A progressive change in morphology occurs from the replicating columnar cells of the basal layer **(stratum basalis)** through the spinous layer **(stratum spinosum)** and the granular layer **(stratum granulosum)** to the nonviable flattened cells of the cornified layer **(stratum corneum)** (Figs. 24-1 and 24-2). The basal cells harbor most of the mitotic activity of the epidermis. As keratinocytes approach the surface, they lose their nuclei and form flattened plates of dead cells on the outer boundary of the skin (the cornified layer). Keratinocytes synthesize a sulfur-poor, filamentous protein, the **tonofibril,** which is related to the keratin molecules of the stratum corneum. Tonofibrils are composed of varying blends of acidic and basic intermediate keratin filaments, resulting in over 30 different keratins that are responsible for structures such as the stratum corneum, hair and nails. Bundles of tonofibrils converge on, and terminate at, the plasma membrane in attachment plates called **desmosomes** (Fig. 24-3).

Keratinocytes are also distinguished by two other structural products: "keratohyaline granules" and **"Odland bodies."** Keratohyaline granules are the defining feature of the granular layer and are composed of a histidine-rich, electron-dense, basophilic protein—profilaggrin—which is associated with intermediate filaments. Odland bodies, also known as keratinosomes or membrane-coating granules, are the only structurally distinctive, secretory product of the epidermis (Fig. 24-3). They form in the outer spinous and granular layers and discharge their contents into the intercellular spaces,

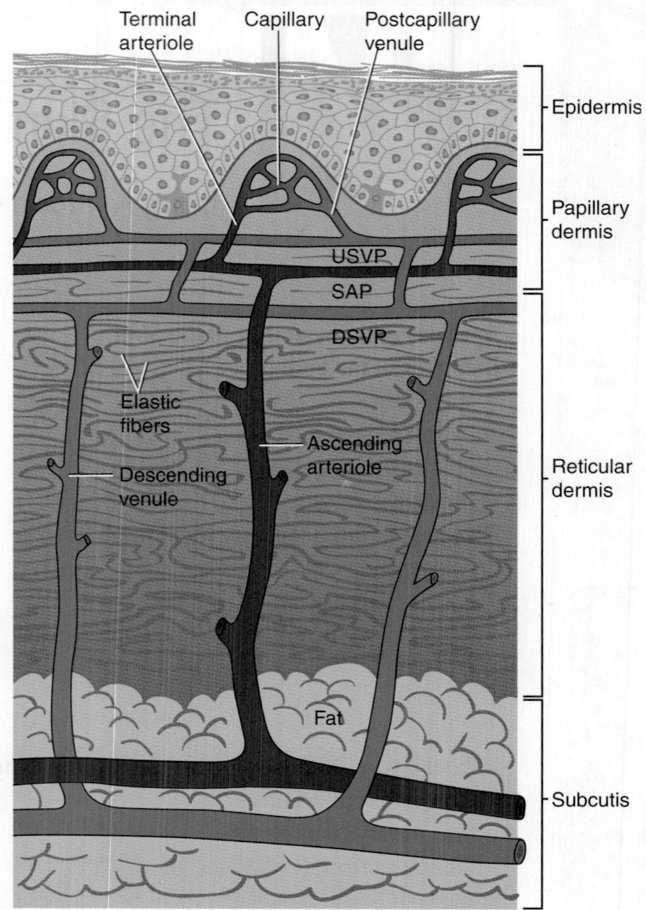

FIGURE 24-1. The dermis and its vasculature. The dermis is divided into two distinct anatomic regions. The papillary dermis with its vascular plexus and the epidermis usually react together in diseases that are primarily limited to the skin. The reticular dermis and the subcutis are altered in association with systemic diseases that manifest in the skin. DSVP = deep superficial venular plexus; SAP = superficial arterial plexus; USVP = upper superficial venular plexus.

FIGURE 24-2. Normal epidermis and the epidermal immigrant cells. Keratinocytes form the multilayered epidermis, protecting against water loss and bacterial invasion. Melanocytes provide color as well as protection against ultraviolet radiation. Langerhans cells are among the cells responsible for the skin's function as an immunologic organ. Merkel cells may represent one of the enablers of tactile function of the skin.

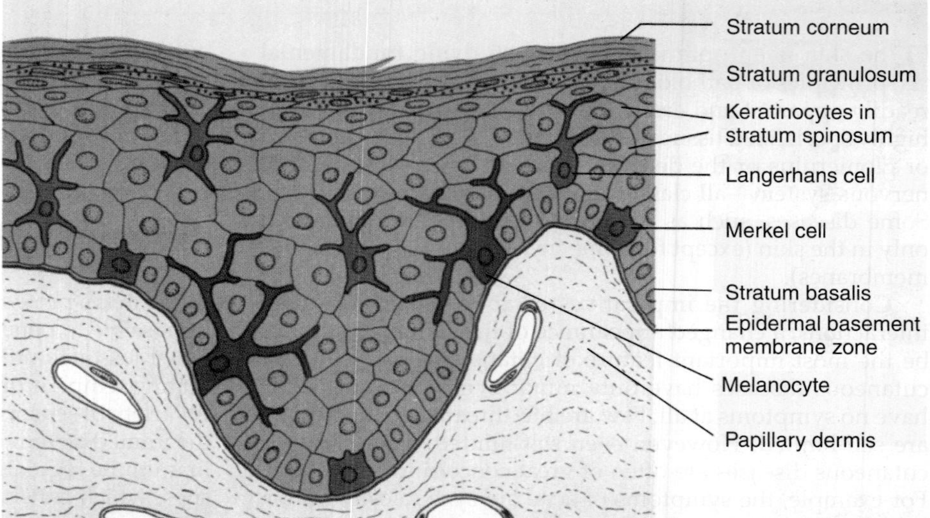

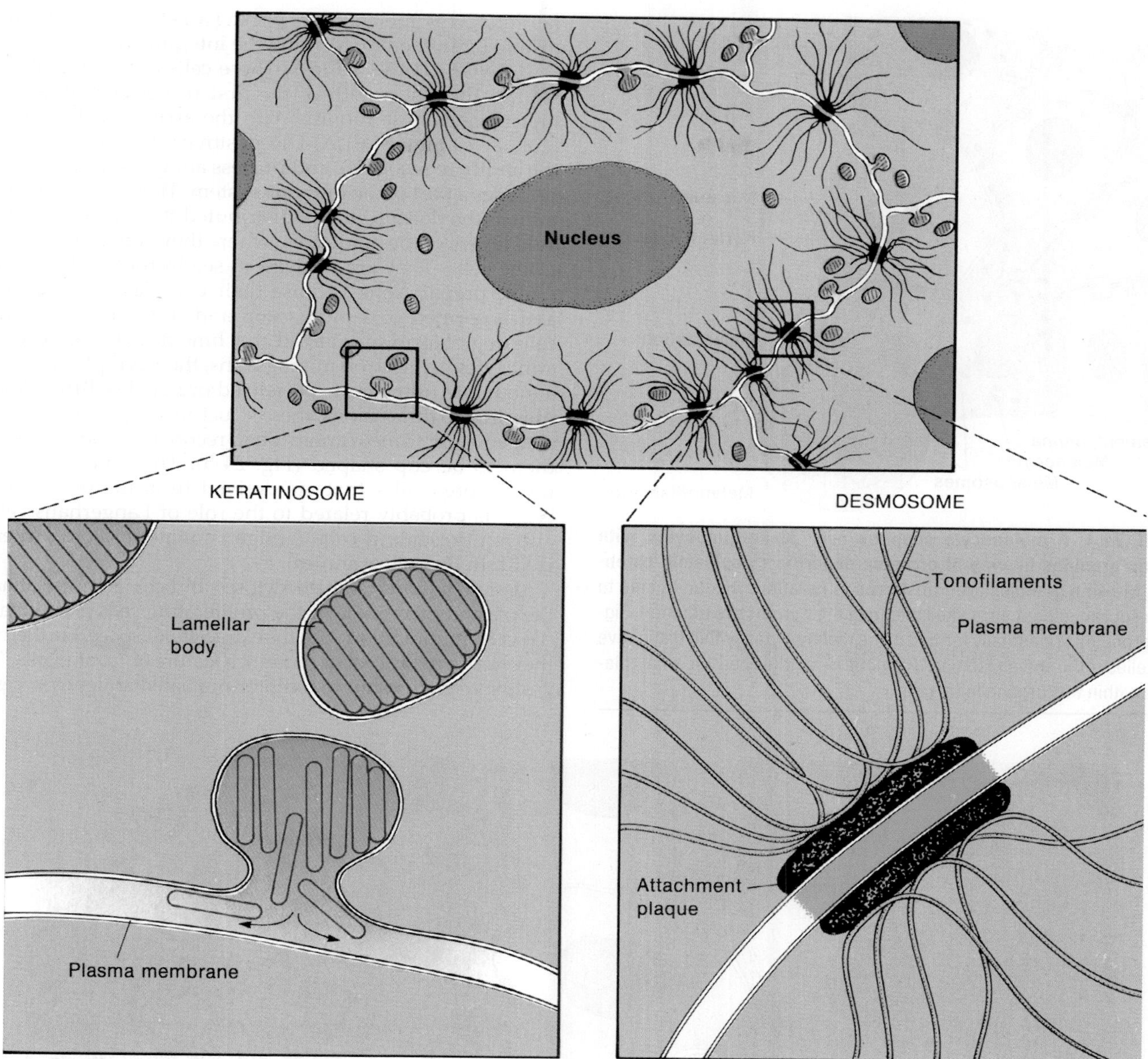

FIGURE 24-3. The keratinocyte, keratinosome and desmosome. The keratinocyte cytoplasm is dominated by delicate keratin fibrils, the tonofilaments. These are part of the cytoskeleton of the cell and loop within the attachment plaque of the desmosome. The lamellar body of the keratinocyte extrudes its contents into the intercellular space. This material probably has a role in cellular cohesion.

appearing there as lamellar masses parallel to the surface of the skin. Odland bodies and the discharged lamellated products are most obvious in the outer granular layer and are related to epidermal barrier function.

The epidermis harbors immigrant cells of neuroectodermal and mesenchymal origin that do not synthesize keratin but which have their own highly distinctive organelles. Their numbers vary among the several different levels of the epidermis. Two of these cells, **melanocytes** and **Langerhans cells,** are dendritic. The third, the **Merkel cell,** is associated with a terminal neuronal axon (Fig. 24-2).

MELANOCYTES: Melanocytes are dendritic cells of neural crest origin that are largely responsible for skin color. They lie in the basal layer of the epidermis and are separated from the dermis by the epidermal basement membrane zone. A single melanocyte may supply dendrites to over 30 keratinocytes (Fig. 24-4).

The **melanosome** is a cytoplasmic membrane–bound complex in which melanin is synthesized. When melanin synthesis is active, melanosomes contain filaments arranged in a parallel array along the long axis of the organelle (Fig. 24-4). As it matures, the melanosome's orderly internal structure is progressively obliterated, whereupon it appears as an electron-opaque granule. Such granules are transferred to keratinocytes, where they form a supranuclear cap, protecting the nuclear material from ultraviolet light.

Skin color is largely based on the number, size and packaging of melanosomes in keratinocytes. In hair and epidermal

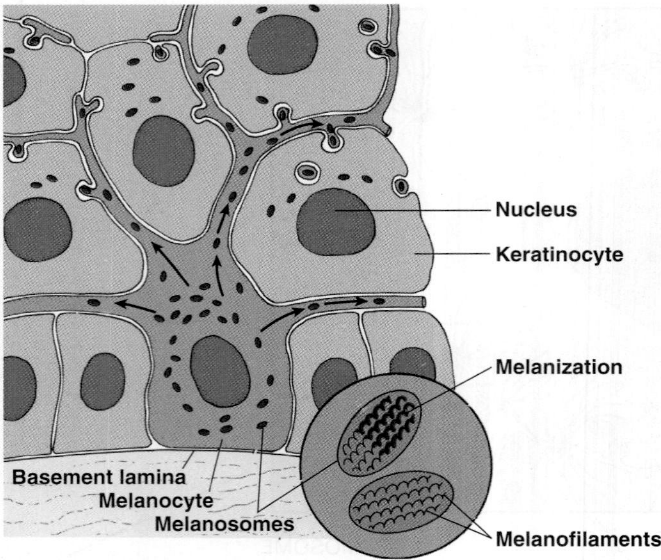

FIGURE 24-4. A melanocyte supplies over 30 keratinocytes with melanin granules by way of complex dendritic cytoplasmic extensions. Melanin granules are transferred to keratinocytes and come to lie in a supranuclear cap, a site indicating their protective function. Pigment granules are actually formed in the melanocytes within distinctive organelles—the melanosomes. Pigment is synthesized on small filaments within this organelle (*inset*).

keratinocytes, melanins are packaged, and absorb and reflect visible light, thereby forming the integumentary colors.

LANGERHANS CELLS: These cells arrive in embryonic skin in the last month of the first trimester, following the melanocytes by a month. With the arrival of these human leukocyte antigen (HLA)-DR–positive cells, the skin acquires the ability to recognize and process antigens, at which time it becomes a part of the immune system. These cells are uncommon in the dermis but are distributed throughout the nucleated layers of the epidermis, where they constitute about 4% of the cells. They are difficult to see in routine light microscopic preparations because their cytoplasm is translucent and is formed of a perikaryon and dendrites. Langerhans cells do not form specialized attachments to the apposed keratinocytes. In electron micrographs, their cytoplasm contains a moderate number of specialized organelles, **Birbeck granules.** In two dimensions, these structures appear to be racquet shaped, but three-dimensional reconstruction has shown them to be cup shaped (Fig. 24-5). The function of these unique organelles that are derived from the plasma membrane is probably related to the role of Langerhans cells as antigen-presenting cells (antigenic material being internalized into Birbeck granules).

In Langerhans cell histiocytoses, Birbeck granules attach to the plasma membrane of the proliferating cells and remain in direct communication with the extracellular space. Furthermore, they have a fuzzy coat of clathrin, a feature of "coated pits," suggesting a relationship to receptor-mediated antigen processing

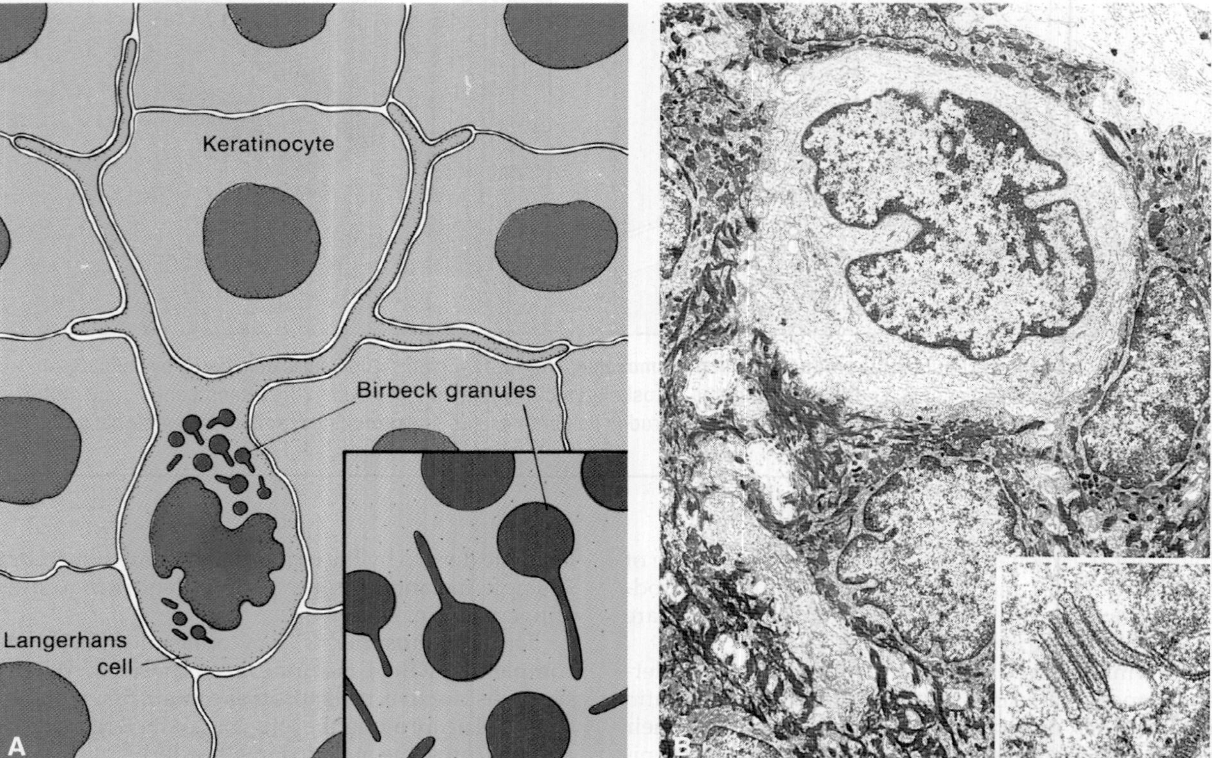

FIGURE 24-5. The dendritic Langerhans cell can recognize and process antigens. A. The unique racket-shaped organelles, called *Birbeck granules,* may be important in antigen presentation. **B.** An electron micrograph of a Langerhans cell shows a high-power view of the racket-shaped organelles (*inset*). The Langerhans cell body (*mid-upper portion*) is pale compared to the surrounding keratinocytes, whose cytoplasm contains electron-dense packets of tonofilaments. A dendrite is present (*arrow*).

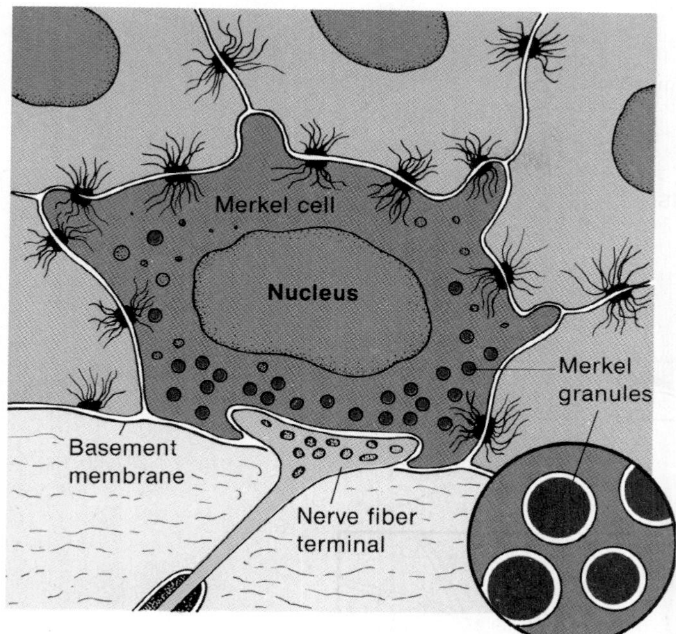

FIGURE 24-6. The Merkel cell, which differs from other immigrant cells, forms desmosomes with keratinocytes and is attached to a small nerve plate (nerve fiber terminal). The membrane-delimited, dense core granule is distinctive (*inset*).

and recognition. Langerhans cells express major histocompatibility complex (MHC)-I, MHC-II and receptors for Fc immunoglobulin (Ig) G and Fc IgE. They are identified immunohistochemically by CD1a or, less specifically, by S-100 protein.

MERKEL CELLS: Although sometimes classified as "immigrant" cells, Merkel cells may be specialized basal keratinocytes. They form desmosomes with keratinocytes and express keratins in a fashion similar to that of keratinocytes. They project short, blunt cytoplasmic fingers into adjacent keratinocytes. Merkel cells do not appear in all areas of the epidermis, but are seen in special regions such as the lips, oral cavity, external root sheath of the hair follicles and palmar skin of the digits. They have a distinctive organelle, a membrane-bound, dense-core granule, 100 nm or wider (Fig. 24-6). Immunohistochemical and ultrastructural studies suggest that Merkel cells have a neurosecretory function. The basal aspect of the cell is apposed to a small nerve plate, which is connected to a myelinated axon by a short, nonmyelinated axon. This complex structure may function as a tactile mechanoreceptor.

BASEMENT MEMBRANE: The basement membrane zone (BMZ) is an interface between the dermis and epidermis and is as diverse in function as it is complex in structure (Fig. 24-7). It is responsible for dermal–epidermal adherence and probably functions as a selective macromolecular filter. It is also a site of immunoglobulin and complement deposition in certain cutaneous diseases. Most of the structures of the BMZ are elaborated by cells of the epidermis. The basal lamina is the primary organizational feature of the BMZ and is responsible for epithelial cell polarity as well as some keratin gene expression. Ultrastructurally, the basal lamina includes:

- **Deep aspects of basal keratinocytes** including plasma membrane and tonofilaments that attach to the deep face of the hemidesmosome
- **Hemidesmosome,** with its subdesmosomal dense plate
- **Anchoring filaments** that extend from subdesmosomal dense plates across the lamina lucida and insert into the lamina densa
- **Lamina lucida,** an electron-lucent layer containing adherence proteins
- **Lamina densa,** composed principally of type IV collagen
- **Anchoring fibrils,** which are arrays of type VII collagen extending from the inner face of the lamina densa for a short distance into the papillary dermis
- **Microfibrils,** which feature delicate, long, elastic fibrils that blend with the underlying elastic fibrillary system of the skin

Certain antigenic components have been identified in the BMZ, some of which play identified roles in cutaneous disease, particularly blistering disorders. **Laminin** is a glycoprotein present in the lamina lucida and lamina densa of all BMZs. It assists in organizing BMZ macromolecules and promotes cell attachment to extracellular matrix. Laminin binds to **type IV collagen.** Bullous pemphigoid (BP) antigens were identified with antibodies from patients with the blistering disorder bullous pemphigoid (discussed below). The antigens BPAG1 and BPAG2 **(type XVII collagen)** are normal constituents of the dermal–epidermal junction, but are absent in BMZs around adnexal structures and blood vessels. These BP antigens are located in the hemidesmosomes and cytoplasm of basal keratinocytes. Type IV collagen is present in the lamina densa of all BMZs. It is the most superficial component of the complex collagen fiber network of the dermis and is important in dermal–epidermal attachment. **Type VII collagen** is present on the deep aspect of the basal lamina in anchoring fibrils. Anchoring fibril antigens (AF-1 and AF-2) reside within anchoring fibrils and possibly within the lower lamina densa.

The **dermis** is a complex organization of connective tissue deep to the BMZ and is composed predominantly of collagen, which is embedded in a ground substance rich in hyaluronic acid. The dermis consists of two zones:

PAPILLARY DERMIS: The papillary dermis is a narrow zone immediately deep to the BMZ of the epidermis. This region is pale pink with hematoxylin and eosin stain and has little organization when viewed with the light microscope (Figs. 24-1 and 24-2). Delicate collagen fibrils are the most apparent structures. This delicate connective tissue extends as a sheath about blood vessels, nerves and adnexal structures. This entire network of collagen is known as the **adventitial dermis.**

The papillary dermis is generally altered in conjunction with epidermal disease and disorders affecting the superficial vascular bed. The epidermis, papillary dermis and superficial vascular bed react jointly and influence each other in complex ways. Some primary skin diseases with few, if any, systemic manifestations, such as psoriasis and lichen planus, involve these superficial structures.

RETICULAR DERMIS: The reticular dermis is deep to the papillary dermis and contains most of the dermal collagen, which is organized into coarse bundles and associated with elastic fibers (Fig. 24-1). The reticular dermis and subcutis (also recognized as a cutaneous structure) are less common sites of pathologic change. If they are diseased, it is often as a manifestation of systemic disease (e.g., scleroderma [progressive systemic sclerosis] and erythema nodosum).

CUTANEOUS VASCULATURE: Cutaneous circulating blood has a number of functions. The skin, via its vascular

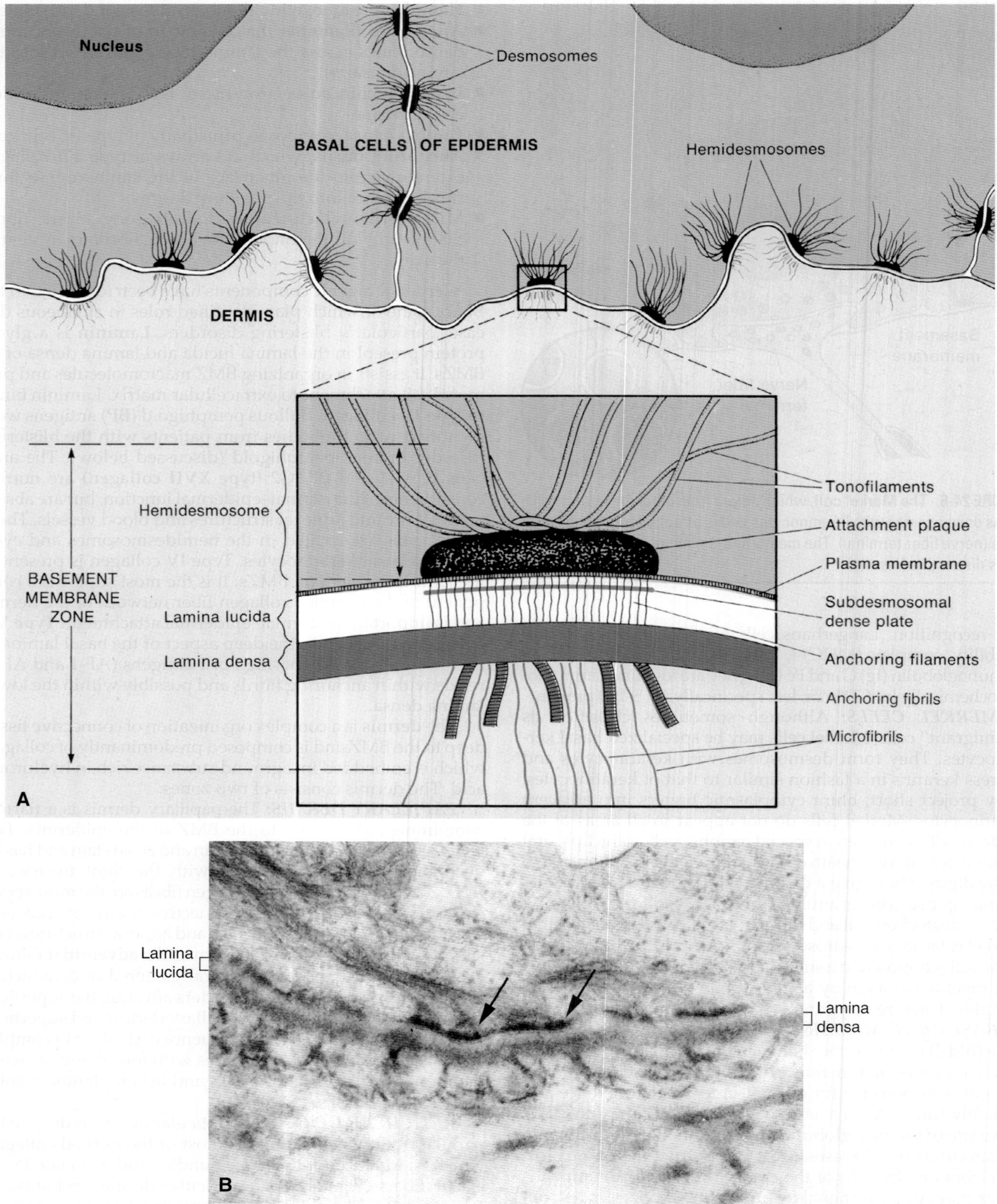

FIGURE 24-7. The dermal–epidermal interface and the basement membrane zone. A. This epithelial–mesenchymal interface is the site of the basement membrane zone, a complex structure that is mostly synthesized by the basal cells of the epidermis. Each of its complex structures is a site of change in specific disease, from tonofilaments and attachment plaques of basal cells to anchoring fibrils and microfibrils. **B.** An electron micrograph shows the hemidesmosomal attachment plaques with their inserting tonofilaments (*arrow*). The subdesmosomal dense plates, the lamina lucida, the lamina densa and the subjacent anchoring fibrils are well demonstrated.

network, is important in temperature regulation. Many aspects of cutaneous inflammation involve the superficial cutaneous vasculature.

An ascending arteriole arises from arteries in the subcutis and directly crosses much of the reticular dermis (Fig. 24-1). In the outer part of the reticular dermis, in conjunction with other similar ascending arterioles, a superficial arteriolar plexus is formed. A terminal arteriole extends from this plexus into each dermal papilla, where an arterial capillary is formed. The arterial capillary makes a U-turn and on its descent becomes a venous capillary and then a postcapillary venule. These venules join to form a complex venular plexus in the reticular dermis, immediately deep to the papillary dermis. The venular end of this vascular structure is important in cutaneous inflammatory responses.

Cutaneous lymphatic vessels form a random network, beginning as lymphatic capillaries near the epidermis. A superficial lymphatic plexus is then formed, from which lymphatic channels drain to regional lymph nodes. Lymphatic channels are involved in drainage of tissue fluids and metastasis of cutaneous cancers, especially malignant melanoma. Cutaneous lymphatics have, at best, an incomplete basal lamina.

Mast cells are derived from the bone marrow and are normally present around dermal venules. Mast cells release vasoactive and chemotactic substances, mediate all types of inflammation and proliferate in a spectrum of diseases termed **urticaria pigmentosa** (Fig. 24-8).

HAIR FOLLICLES: Hair follicles originate in the primitive epidermis and grow downward through the dermis as well as upward through the epidermis. Growing hairs of the scalp and beard have bulbs of epithelial and mesenchymal tissue firmly embedded within the subcutis. A vertical cross-section of a bulb reveals a cap of actively dividing, keratin-synthesizing cells that become arrayed in layers that join at the top of the bulb to form the cylindrical hair shaft. The differentiating hairs form the roof of the epithelial bulb and interact with an island of melanocytes that contribute melanin to the passing keratinocytes. This process results in hair color. The colored keratinocytes lose their nuclei as they form the final product, the cylindrical hair shaft. Curly hair is formed from angulated bulbs; straight hair develops from round bulbs.

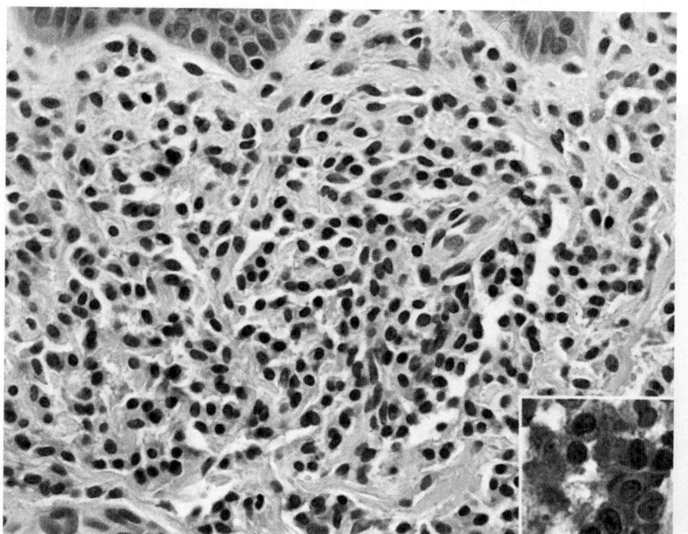

FIGURE 24-8. Urticaria pigmentosa. Mast cells fill and expand the papillary dermis. The cytoplasm of mast cells contains chloracetate esterase-rich granules, giving them a red hue in this Leder stain (*inset*), a useful distinguishing feature.

THE HAIR CYCLE: Hair grows in a cyclical fashion. At any given time, 90% of hairs are normally in the **anagen,** or actively growing, phase. These have a mosaic distribution and are interspersed with hairs that show no evidence of active growth, **telogen** hairs. Hairs in the process of ceasing growth, **catagen** hairs, still have hair shafts. Catagen hairs end in the lower reticular dermis as slightly widened club-like structures, each surrounded by a rim of nucleated keratinocytes. The hair bulbs are no longer evident, and the lamina densa surrounding the catagen hair is strikingly thickened.

As the telogen phase (resting follicle) is reached, the end of the hair retreats to the level of the arrector pili muscle. The hair shaft may be missing, since it is no longer tethered at the base, leaving only a remnant of the original follicle. However, a delicate vascularized mesenchymal tract, the telogen tract, extends from the attenuated tip. At the top of this tract, the early anagen hair forms again from the follicular stem cells. With growth, it follows the delicate pathway through the reticular dermis into the panniculus, there forming a mature anagen follicle and a new hair.

ALOPECIA: Alopecia, commonly known as baldness, refers to the loss of hair. **Common alopecia,** which affects both men and women, results from a complex and poorly understood interaction of heritable and hormonal factors. Men castrated before puberty retain scalp hair and fail to grow a beard. On the other hand, administering testosterone to such castrated men results in growth of a beard and may lead to male-pattern baldness. Loss of scalp hair results in replacement of a large terminal hair follicle by a diminutive "vellus" hair follicle, the source of the delicate "fuzz" on the cheeks of women and the upper cheeks of men.

Growing hair is a site of active mitosis, and many systemic diseases cause cessation of mitosis in this location and subsequent alopecia. If the malady passes, mitotic activity is renewed and regrowth occurs. If a patient is subjected to a potent antimitotic regimen (e.g., chemotherapy), hair follicles stop growth, hair is lost and a telogen follicle follows. When therapy stops, hair cycling resumes. Almost any kind of follicular inflammation can induce the telogen phase. If fibrosis distorts the telogen tract (the regrowth pathway), scarring alopecia with permanent loss of that follicle is the result.

Alopecia areata is a circumscribed area of hair loss, usually on the scalp, although other body areas may be involved. A brisk lymphocytic infiltrate is found around the hair bulb and results in formation of telogen hairs and hair loss. Alopecia areata may actually result from several diseases. This histologic pattern and the association of this phenomenon with the inheritance of HLA class II alleles (especially HLA-DQ3) have been interpreted as evidence for an autoimmune etiology. Generally, scarring does not occur and hair may regrow normally after varying time periods.

VELLUS HAIRS: These fine hairs may play a role in touch perception in many mammals, but in humans they have no function. Microscopically, vellus hairs are diminutive anagen hairs, with a small active bulb high in the reticular dermis, together with small sebaceous glands.

SEBACEOUS FOLLICLES: These structures develop with puberty and are clinically important because they are the sites of **acne.** Sebaceous follicles have a minute vellus hair at the base. The central face has large sebaceous glands that dwarf the vellus hairs and fill the follicular canal with sebum.

Diseases of the Epidermis

Ichthyoses Feature Epidermal Thickening and Scales

Ichthyosiform dermatoses, many of which are heritable, are a heterogeneous group of diseases characterized by striking thickening of the stratum corneum. The term **ichthyosis** reflects the similarity of the diseased skin to coarse, fish-like scales (Fig. 24-9). Several rare ichthyoses are associated with other abnormalities such as abnormal lipid metabolism, neurologic disorders, bone diseases and cancer.

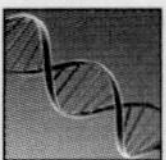

MOLECULAR PATHOGENESIS: Three general defects are involved in the excessive epidermal cornification of the ichthyoses:

- **Increased cohesiveness** of the cells of the stratum corneum, possibly related to altered lipid metabolism
- **Abnormal keratinization,** manifested as impaired tonofilament formation and keratohyaline synthesis and as excessive cornification
- **Increased basal cell proliferation,** associated with a decrease in transit time of keratinocytes across the epidermis

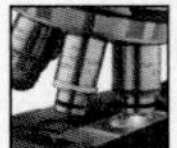

PATHOLOGY: All ichthyoses (with the possible exception of lamellar ichthyosis) have a stratum corneum that is disproportionately thick in comparison with the nucleated epidermal layers. Virtually all diseases characterized by thickening of the nucleated epidermal layers also exhibit hyperkeratosis. For example, chronic scratching or rubbing of normal skin causes a thickened epidermis, hyperkeratosis and dermal fibrosis, a condition known as **lichen simplex chronicus.** In this entity, the nucleated epidermis and stratum corneum may each be three times normal thickness. By contrast, in ichthyosis, the stratum corneum may be five times thicker than normal, but it overlies a disproportionately thin nucleated epidermis.

Ichthyosis Vulgaris

Ichthyosis vulgaris is an autosomal dominant disorder of keratinization characterized by hyperkeratosis and reduced or absent epidermal keratohyaline granules (Fig. 24-10). Scaly skin results from increased cohesiveness of the stratum corneum. The attenuated stratum granulosum is a single layer with small, defective keratohyaline granules. *Decreased or absent synthesis of* **profilaggrin,** *a keratin filament "glue," is responsible for these defects.*

Ichthyosis vulgaris is the prototype of disproportionate corneal thickening. The stratum corneum is loose and has a basket-weave appearance, which differs from normal only in amount. The granular layer is greatly diminished and often appears absent (Fig. 24-9B). Ultrastructurally, the keratohyaline granules are small and sponge-like, a feature indicating defective synthesis. Basal and spinous layers appear normal. Thus, the primary defect in ichthyosis vulgaris is in the granular and cornified layers, the epidermal zones responsible for the final stage of keratinization and cornification.

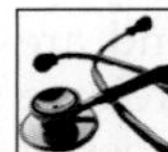

CLINICAL FEATURES: Ichthyosis vulgaris is the most common of the ichthyoses and begins in early childhood. A family history of this condition is often obtained. Small white scales occur on the extensor surfaces of extremities and on the trunk and face. The disease is lifelong, but most patients can be maintained free of scales with topical treatment.

A clinical and histologic state similar to ichthyosis vulgaris is occasionally associated with other diseases or may follow the use of drugs. Lymphomas, especially Hodgkin disease and other neoplasms; systemic granulomatous disorders; and connective tissue disease may be associated with ichthyosis. Drugs may produce ichthyosis by interfering with similar pathways of lipid metabolism.

X-Linked Ichthyosis

This condition is a heritable epidermal disorder that, in the recessive form, is characterized by delayed dissolution of desmosomal disks in the stratum corneum, owing to a

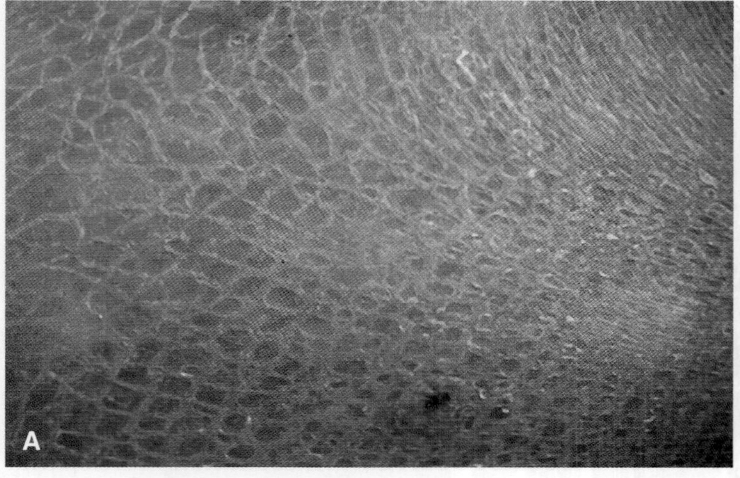

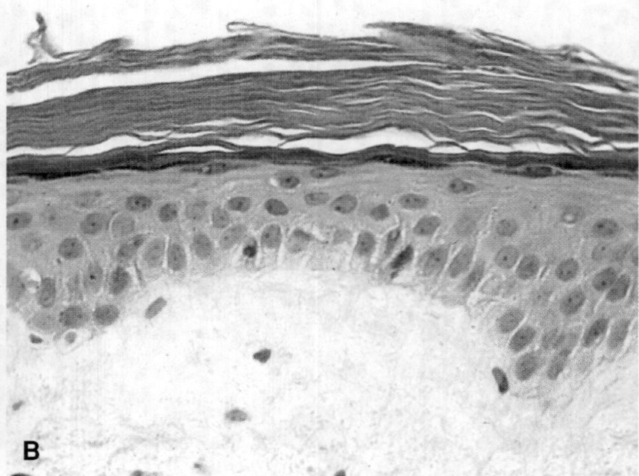

FIGURE 24-9. Ichthyosis vulgaris. A. Noninflammatory fish-like scales are evident on the thigh of a patient with a strong family history of ichthyosis vulgaris. **B.** There is disproportionate thickening of the stratum corneum relative to the normal thickness of the nucleated epidermal layer. The stratum granulosum is thin and focally absent.

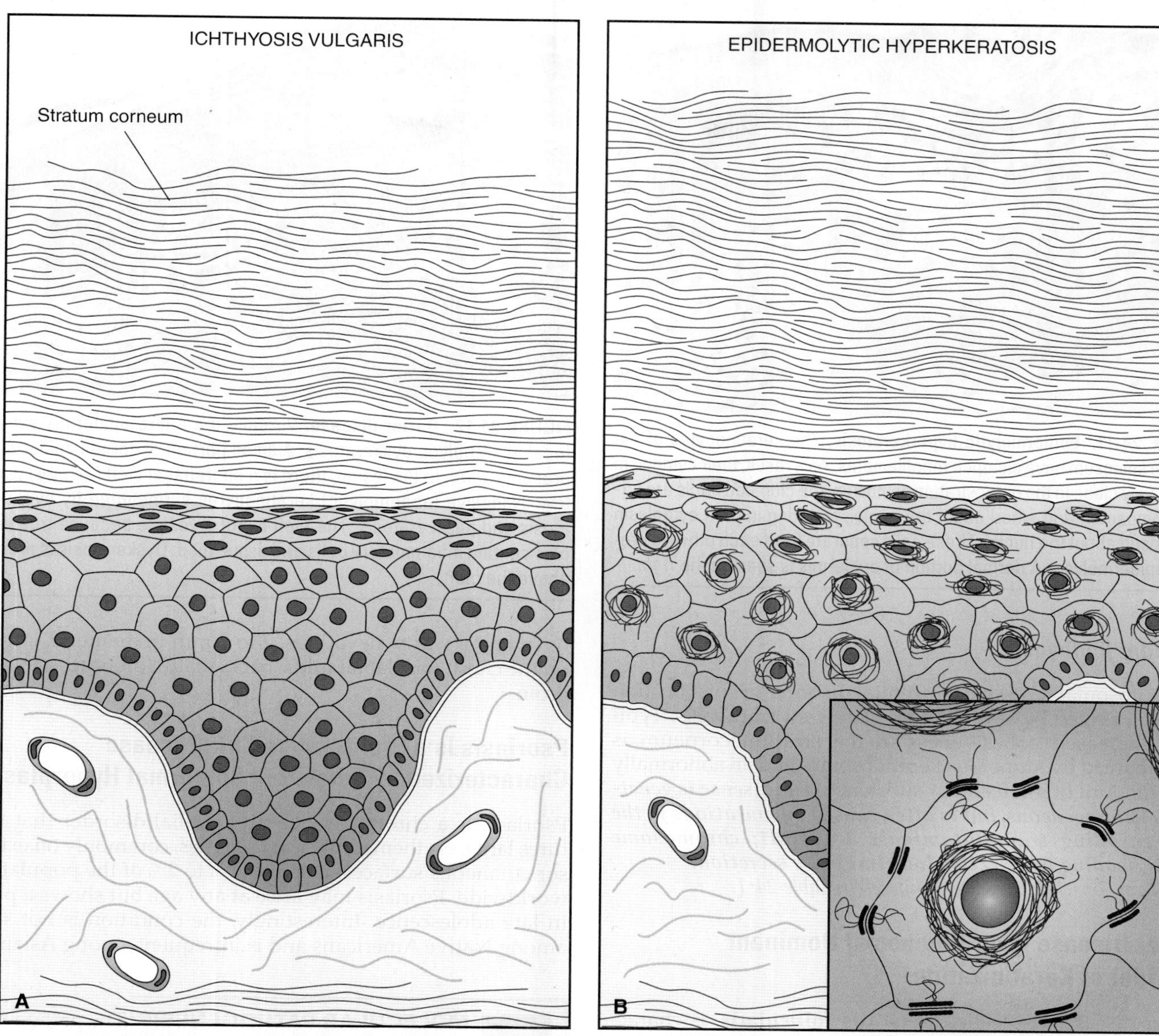

FIGURE 24-10. A. Ichthyosis vulgaris. B. Epidermolytic hyperkeratosis. Both diseases are characterized by thickening of the stratum corneum relative to the nucleated layers. Epidermolytic hyperkeratosis is characterized by abnormal keratin synthesis, manifested by whorled keratin filaments about the nucleus (*inset*).

deficiency of steroid sulfatase. Steroid sulfatase normally degrades the Odland body product, cholesterol sulfate, which provides cellular adhesion in the lower stratum corneum. Failure of steroid sulfatase action on cholesterol sulfate leads to persistent cohesion of the stratum corneum, but in this disease the granular layer is preserved.

Epidermolytic Hyperkeratosis

This congenital, autosomal dominant ichthyosis features generalized erythroderma, ichthyosiform skin and blistering. ***The disease results from mutations in the K1 or K10 keratin genes (chromosomes 12 and 17, respectively), which encode the keratins in the suprabasal epidermis.*** These mutations cause faulty assembly of keratin tonofilaments and impair their insertion into desmosomes. Normal development of the cytoskeleton is impaired, resulting in epidermal "lysis" and a tendency to form vesicles.

In epidermolytic hyperkeratosis, suprabasal keratinocytes contain thick, eosinophilic tonofilaments that whorl around the nucleus in a concentric fashion (Fig. 24-11). The cytoplasm has a clear zone (vacuolization) peripheral to the perinuclear tonofilaments, but at the periphery of the cell these filaments again become condensed. Enlarged keratohyaline granules are present. The stratum corneum is disproportionately thickened (Fig. 24-10).

CLINICAL FEATURES: Epidermolytic hyperkeratosis manifests with blistering at or shortly after birth. It may be generalized or localized to only several areas of the body. Lesions tend to appear dark and even verrucous. Other than cosmetic disfigurement, the major problem is secondary bacterial infection.

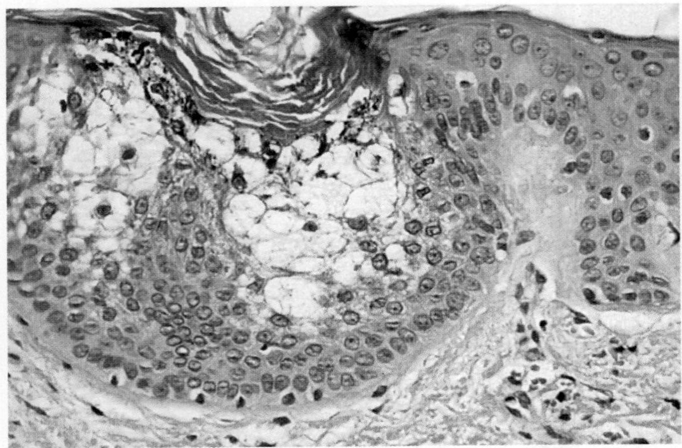

FIGURE 24-11. Epidermolytic hyperkeratosis. The keratinocytes of the stratum spinosum have clumped tonofilaments. As a result, their cytoplasm is relatively clear. In the outer stratum spinosum, the clumped fibrils are further compacted and whorl about the nuclei, resulting in dark cytoplasm condensed about the nuclei. These cells separate from each other to produce epidermolysis. A normal portion of epidermis is seen on the *right*.

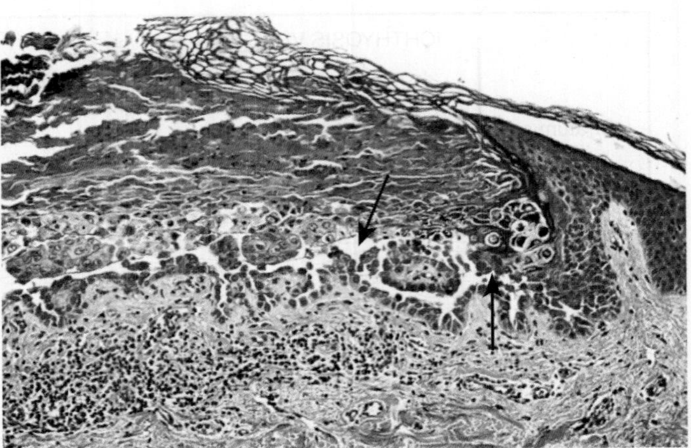

FIGURE 24-12. Darier disease. Virtually the entire epidermis exhibits focal acantholytic dyskeratosis. A small portion of normal epidermis is present (*right*). In the lesion, there is a suprabasal cleft (*arrows*) with a few dyshesive (acantholytic) keratinocytes surmounted by hyperkeratosis and parakeratosis. The cleft is not a vesicle because true vesicles contain inflammatory cells and tissue fluid. Dyskeratosis is present above the cleft.

Lamellar Ichthyosis

This autosomal recessive congenital disorder of cornification is characterized by severe and generalized ichthyosis. Typically, increased cohesiveness of the stratum corneum is accompanied by numerous keratinosomes and an abnormally large amount of intercellular substance. ***The disease is genetically heterogeneous, but is often caused by mutations in the gene encoding transglutaminase 1 (TGM1; chromosome 14q11), leading to defective lamellar body secretion.***

The major ichthyoses are compared in Table 24-1.

Darier Disease Is an Autosomal Dominant Disorder of Keratinization

Darier disease, also called **keratosis follicularis,** is characterized by multifocal keratoses.

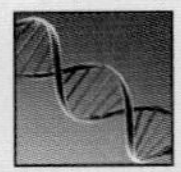

MOLECULAR PATHOGENESIS: Darier disease is linked to a defect in the intercellular matrix. The specific gene, *ATP2A2* on chromosome 12q23–24, encodes a calcium pump of the endoplasmic reticulum, and its mutation may exert a direct effect on calcium-dependent assembly of desmosomes. The many neuropsychiatric problems among these patients may also be related to *ATP2A2* mutations.

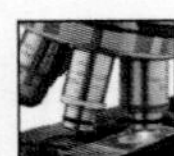

PATHOLOGY: Microscopically, the warty papule of Darier disease has a suprabasal cleft. Above and to the side of the cleft, dyskeratotic keratinocytes with eosinophilic cytoplasm contain keratin fibrils that whorl about the nucleus (Fig. 24-12). The roof of the cleft is formed by a column of compact keratotic material.

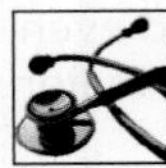

CLINICAL FEATURES: Darier disease first appears late in childhood or in adolescence as skin-colored papules that later become crusted. Affected areas have many warty elevations, 2 to 4 mm in diameter, largely on the chest, nasolabial folds, back, scalp, forehead, ears and groin.

Psoriasis Is a Proliferative Skin Disease Characterized by Persistent Epidermal Hyperplasia

Psoriasis is a chronic, frequently familial disorder that features large, erythematous, scaly plaques, commonly on extensor cutaneous surfaces. It affects 1% to 2% of the population worldwide. Psoriasis may arise at any age but shows a peak in late adolescence. Interestingly, the condition is not seen among Native Americans and is infrequent among Asians.

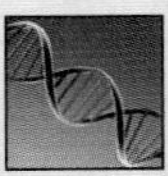

MOLECULAR PATHOGENESIS: The pathogenesis of psoriasis is poorly understood and is likely multifactorial.

GENETIC FACTORS: Psoriasis unquestionably has a genetic component, although only one third of patients with psoriasis have a family history of the disease. The more severe the illness, the greater the likelihood is of a familial background. The genetic basis for psoriasis rests on a number of observations: (1) increased incidence among relatives and offspring of patients with psoriasis; (2) 65% concordance for psoriasis in monozygotic twins; and (3) increased prevalence in individuals with certain HLA haplotypes, especially HLA-B13, HLA-B17, HLA-Bw57 and particularly HLA-Cw6. In fact, persons with HLA-Cw6 are 10 to 15 times more likely to develop psoriasis than the general population. A 300-kb segment in the MHC-I region of chromosome 6p21, known as PSORS1, is thought to be the major genetic determinant of susceptibility.

IMMUNOLOGIC FACTORS: T lymphocytes are now considered key to the pathogenesis of psoriatic lesions. Eruption of psoriatic lesions coincides with T-cell infiltration into the epidermis. By contrast, resolution of psoriatic plaques, whether spontaneous or induced by treatment,

Table 24-1

A Comparison of the Major Ichthyoses

Type of Ichthyosis	Mode of Inheritance	Present at Birth	Pathogenetic Mechanism	Histology
Ichthyosis vulgaris	Autosomal dominant	No; onset in childhood	Normal epidermal turnover Retention keratosis due to defective dissolution of adhesive mechanisms in the stratum corneum	Hyperkeratosis, loosely woven, disproportionately thick in relationship to a relatively thin stratum spinosum Thin granular layer with abnormal keratohyaline granules
Sex-linked ichthyosis	X-linked recessive	Yes; onset may be in infancy	Normal epidermal turnover Constitutional absence of steroid sulfatase and arylsulfatase-C Retention keratosis due to a failure to break down cholesterol sulfate, an important substance in stratum corneum adhesion	Compact, disproportionately thick stratum corneum Normal granular layer Stratum spinosum only slightly thick
Epidermolytic hyperkeratosis	Autosomal dominant	Yes	Increased germinative cell replication and decreased cellular transit time through the epidermis Defect in keratin genes *K1* and *K10*, the differentiation-specific keratins of the suprabasal epidermis	Tonofilaments aggregate at the cell periphery and have a distorted association with desmosomes, which may lead to dyshesion (acantholysis) of epidermal keratinocytes and vesicle formation; entire skin is rarely involved
Lamellar ichthyosis	Autosomal recessive	Yes	Increased number of keratinosomes and increased intercellular substance; defects in transglutaminase acylation and in lamellar body secretion	Moderate hyperkeratosis; normal or thickened granular layer

follows disappearance, or reduction in, epidermal T cells. Streptococcal superantigens reportedly induce expression of cutaneous lymphocyte antigens, which enable T cells to migrate to the skin. Finally, T lymphocytes from psoriatic patients can produce psoriasis-like plaques when transferred to nude mice.

ENVIRONMENTAL FACTORS: Clinical lesions may occur anywhere on the skin. In this context, a variety of stimuli, such as physical injury ("Köbner's phenomenon"), infection, certain drugs and photosensitivity, may produce psoriatic lesions in apparently normal skin. The pathogenesis of psoriatic plaques may be appreciated by contrasting the effect of chronic cutaneous trauma in persons with and without psoriasis. Chronic irritation of a normal person's skin, as in repeated rubbing, produces a tough, scaly, cutaneous plaque that is both clinically and histologically psoriasiform. However, the lesion disappears when the trauma ceases. In psoriatic patients, even less trauma leads to psoriatic plaques that may persist for years after the initial injury.

ABNORMAL CELLULAR PROLIFERATION: There is evidence to suggest that deregulation of epidermal proliferation and an abnormality in dermal microcirculation produce psoriatic lesions (Fig. 24-13). Abnormal proliferation of keratinocytes is possibly related to defective epidermal cell surface receptors. Decreased adenylyl cyclase activity in the lower proliferative compartment of the epidermis has been attributed to faulty β-adrenergic receptors. The decrease in cyclic adenosine 3′,5′-monophosphate (cAMP) alters cutaneous responses to trauma in complex ways that are not fully understood.

Increased cAMP-regulated proteinases and augmented polyamines of low molecular weight are postulated to be associated with a growth factor–like effect. Acute inflammation follows an increase in phospholipase A_2, which enhances production of arachidonic acid. In turn, lipooxygenase metabolites of arachidonic acid, notably leukotriene B_4, exert potent neutrophilic chemotactic effects.

MICROCIRCULATORY CHANGES: In psoriatic skin, the capillary loops of the dermal papillae become venular, showing multiple layers of basal lamina material, wide lumina and "bridged" fenestrations between endothelial cells. The vascular change, which occurs in concert with a striking increase in neutrophilic chemotactic factors, leads to diapedesis of many neutrophils at the tips of dermal papillae and subsequent migration into the epidermis (the "squirting papillae") (Fig. 24-13). This unusual pattern of neutrophilic inflammation is responsible for the dense collections of neutrophils in the stratum corneum **(Munro microabscesses)** as well as for the scattering of neutrophils throughout the epidermis **(spongiform pustules of Kogoj).**

In summary, keratinocytes of persons afflicted with psoriasis possess a genetic predisposition to hyperproliferation and altered differentiation (Fig. 24-13). Environmental stimuli may trigger release of cytokines and growth factors by keratinocytes and other epidermal cells, and ensuing immune and inflammatory responses lead to the full development of psoriatic lesions.

PATHOLOGY: The most distinctive pathologic changes are seen at the periphery of a chronic psoriatic plaque. The epidermis is thickened and shows **hyperkeratosis** and **parakeratosis** (persistence of nuclei in cells of the stratum corneum). Parakeratosis may be circumscribed and focal, or it may be diffuse, in which case the granular layer is diminished or absent. The nucleated layers of the epidermis are thickened severalfold in the rete pegs and are frequently thinner over the dermal papillae (Fig. 24-14). In turn, the papillae are elongated and appear as sections of cones, with their apices toward the dermis. In chronic lesions, dermal papillae tend to appear as bulbous "clubs" with short handles (Figs. 24-14 and 24-15). The rete ridges of the epidermis have a profile reciprocal to that of the dermal papillae, resulting in interlocked dermal and epidermal "clubs," with alternately reversed polarity. The capillaries of dermal papillae are dilated and tortuous (Fig. 24-15). In a very early lesion, changes may be limited to capillary dilation with a few neutrophils "squirting" into the epidermis. Epidermal hyperplasia and hyperkeratosis are hallmarks of chronic lesions.

Ultrastructurally, the capillaries are venule-like; neutrophils may emerge at their tips and migrate into the epidermis above the apices of the papillae. Neutrophils may become localized in the epidermal spinous layer or in small microabscesses in the stratum corneum and may be associated with circumscribed areas of parakeratosis (Fig. 24-16).

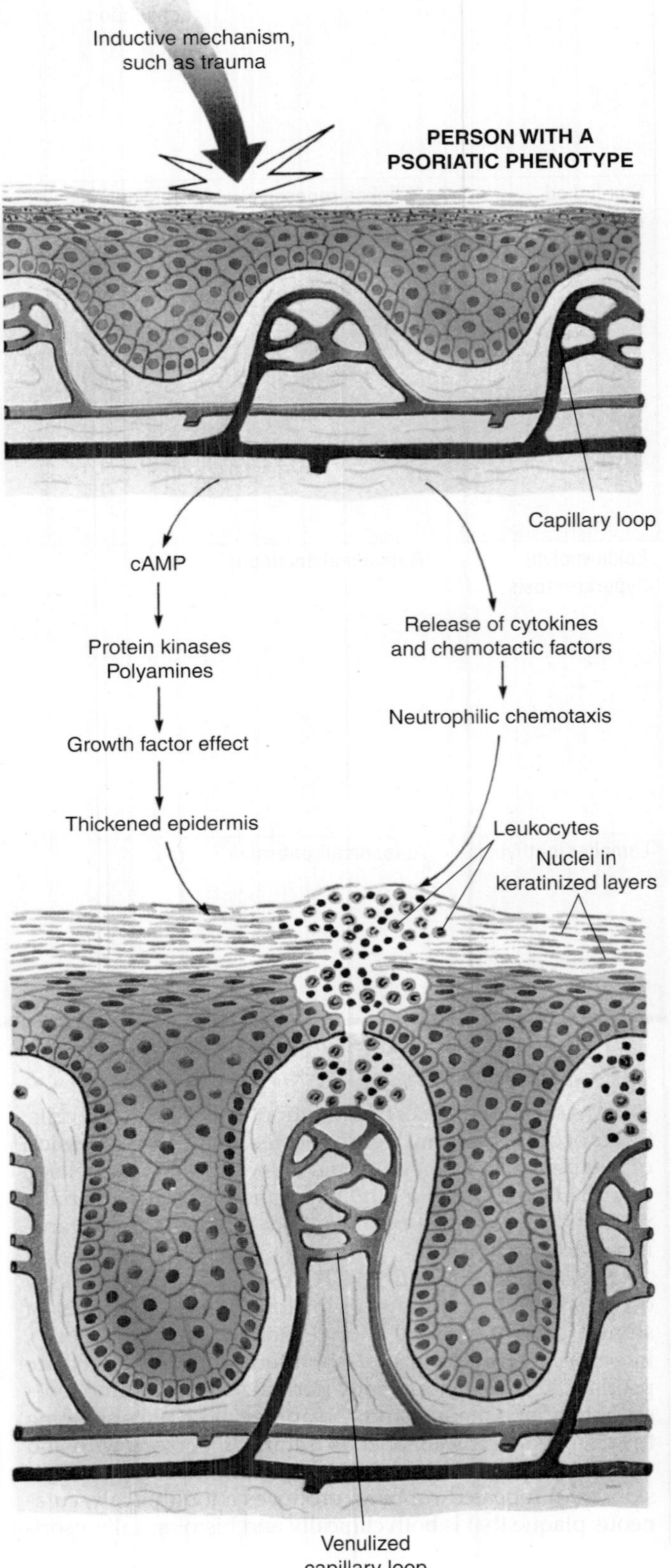

FIGURE 24-13. Pathogenetic mechanisms in psoriasis. The drawing depicts the deregulation of epidermal growth, venulization of the capillary loop and a unique form of neutrophilic inflammation. The altered epidermal growth is thought to be caused by defective epidermal cell surface receptors. This results in a decrease in cyclic adenosine 3′,5′-monophosphate (cAMP), together with the effects indicated. The decrease in cAMP is also likely to be related to the increased production of arachidonic acid, which in turn leads to activation of leukotriene B_4 (LTB-4). This potent neutrophilic chemotactic agent acts on a venulized capillary loop. Neutrophils then emerge from the tips of the capillary loop at the apex of the dermal papilla rather than from the post-capillary venule, as is the rule in most inflammatory skin diseases.

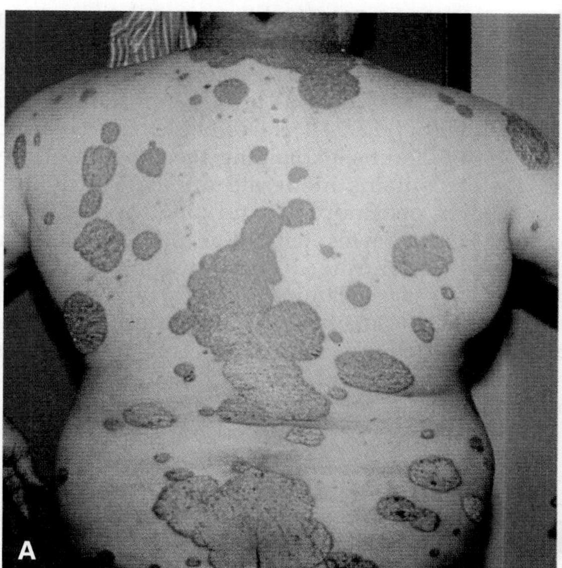

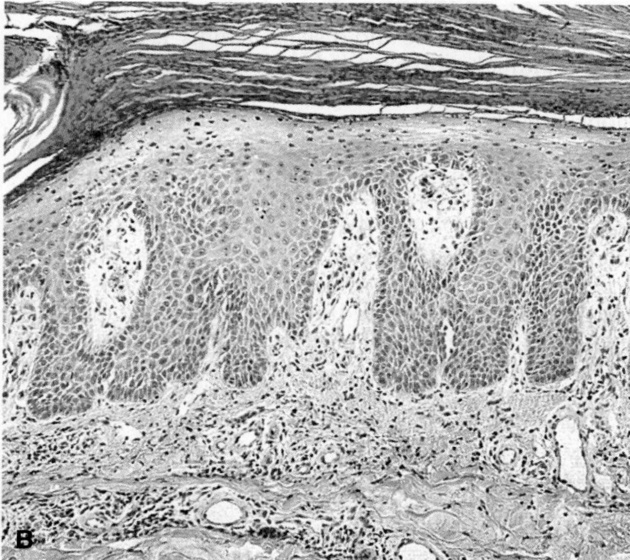

FIGURE 24-14. Psoriasis. This disorder is the prototype of psoriasiform epidermal hyperplasia. **A.** A patient with psoriasis shows large, confluent, sharply demarcated, erythematous plaques on the trunk. **B.** Microscopic examination of a lesion demonstrates that the rete ridges are uniformly elongated, as are the dermal papillae, giving an interlocking pattern of alternately reversed "clubs." The dermal papillae are edematous and reside beneath a thinned epidermis (suprapapillary thinning). There is striking parakeratosis, which is the scale observed clinically.

The dermis below the papillae contains a variable mononuclear inflammatory infiltrate, mostly lymphocytes, around the superficial vascular plexus. The inflammatory process does not extend into the subjacent reticular dermis.

The psoriasiform histologic pattern is common in cutaneous pathology. Seborrheic dermatitis, reaction to chronic trauma (lichen simplex chronicus) and cutaneous T-cell lymphoma (mycosis fungoides) all exhibit psoriasiform epidermal change.

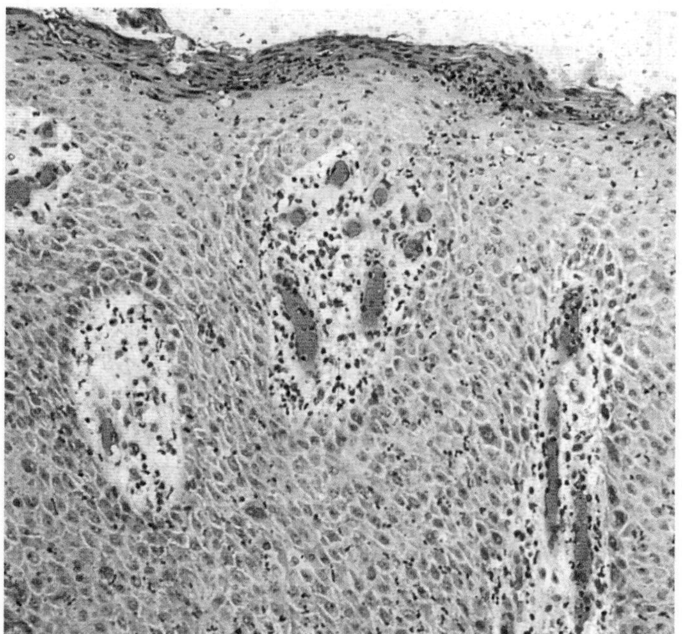

FIGURE 24-15. Psoriasis. The clubbed papillae contain tortuous dilated venules. The prominent venules are part of the venulization of capillaries, which may be of histogenetic importance in psoriasis. The papilla to the *right* has one cross-section of its superficial capillary venule loop, which is normal. The papilla in the *center* shows numerous cross-sections of its venule, indicating striking tortuosity.

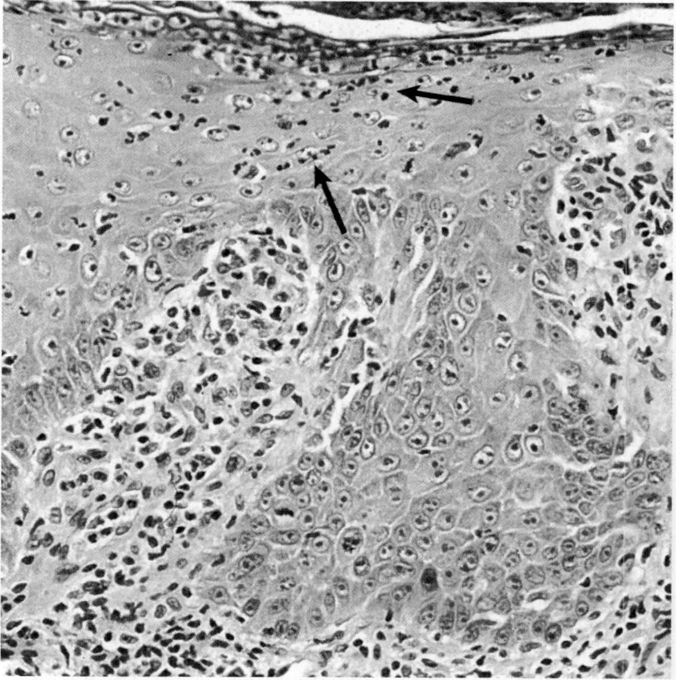

FIGURE 24-16. Psoriasis. Neutrophils migrate into the epidermis, emerging from the venulized capillaries at the tips of the dermal papillae. They migrate to the upper stratum spinosum and stratum corneum (*arrows*). In some forms of psoriasis, pustules are common clinical lesions.

CLINICAL FEATURES: The initial presentation of psoriasis is variable and disease activity is intermittent. Familial psoriasis tends to be more severe than sporadic types, but disease severity varies from annoying scaly lesions over the elbows to a serious debilitating disorder involving most of the skin and often associated with arthritis. A single lesion of psoriasis may be a small focus of scaly erythema or an enormous confluent plaque covering much of the trunk (Fig. 24-14A). A typical plaque is 4 to 5 cm in diameter, is sharply demarcated at its margin and is covered by a surface of silvery scales. When the scales are detached, pinpoint foci of bleeding, originating from the dilated capillaries in the dermal papillae, dot the underlying glossy erythematous surface ("Auspitz sign").

Seronegative arthritis develops in 7% of patients with psoriasis. The tendency to arthropathy is linked to several HLA haplotypes, particularly HLA-B27. Psoriatic arthritis closely resembles its rheumatoid counterpart, but it is usually milder and causes little disability.

In some variations of the disease, neutrophilic pustules dominate **(pustular psoriasis).** Severe intractable psoriasis has been observed in some patients with acquired immunodeficiency syndrome (AIDS).

Psoriasis has long been treated with coal tar or wood tar derivatives and anthralin, a strong reducing agent. Topical and systemic corticosteroids have also been used. Severe, generalized psoriasis justifies systemic treatment with methotrexate. Phototherapy ("PUVA") after administration of psoralens, an ultraviolet-absorbing compound that binds to DNA, is often effective. Synthetic vitamin A and vitamin D derivatives have also been used. More recently, treatment modalities that target immunologic aspects of psoriasis have been used, such as those targeting surface markers of T cells or interfering with intracellular signaling of T cells.

Pemphigus Vulgaris Is a Blistering Skin Disorder Caused by Antibodies to Keratinocytes

Dyshesive disorders are cutaneous diseases in which blister formation is secondary to diminished cohesiveness between epidermal keratinocytes. Pemphigus vulgaris (PV) (Greek, *pemphix*, "bubble"), the prototype of dyshesive diseases, is a chronic, blistering skin disorder that is most common in people between 40 and 60 years of age, but is seen in all age groups, including children. All races are susceptible, but persons of Jewish or Mediterranean heritage are at greater risk.

MOLECULAR PATHOGENESIS: PV is an autoimmune disease: circulating IgG antibodies in patients with PV react with an epidermal surface antigen called **desmoglein 3,** a desmosomal protein. Antigen–antibody union results in dyshesion, which is augmented by release of plasminogen activator and, hence, activation of plasmin. This proteolytic enzyme acts on the intercellular substance and may be the dominant factor in dyshesion. Internalization of the pemphigus antigen–antibody complex, disappearance of attachment plaques and retraction of perinuclear tonofilaments may all act in concert with proteinases to cause dyshesion and vesiculation (Fig. 24-17). The blisters that form in PV are intraepidermal. In other blistering disorders that affect the basement membrane zone, discussed in the next sections, subepidermal blisters are formed.

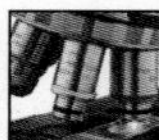

PATHOLOGY: The blister in PV forms because the outer epidermal layers separate from the basal layer. This suprabasal dyshesion results in a blister that has an intact basal layer as a floor and the remaining epidermis as a roof (Fig. 24-18). Desmoglein 3 is concentrated in the lower epidermis, explaining the location of the blister. The blister contains moderate numbers of lymphocytes, macrophages, eosinophils and neutrophils. Distinctive, rounded keratinocytes, termed acantholytic cells, are shed into the vesicle during dyshesion. The basal cells remain adherent to the basal lamina and form a layer of "tombstone cells." Dyshesion may extend along dermal adnexa and is not always strictly suprabasal. The subjacent dermis shows a moderate infiltrate of lymphocytes, macrophages, eosinophils and neutrophils, predominantly around the capillary venular bed.

CLINICAL FEATURES: The characteristic lesion of PV is a large, easily ruptured blister that leaves extensive denuded or crusted areas. Lesions are most common on the scalp and mucous membranes and in periumbilical and intertriginous areas. Without corticosteroid treatment, PV is progressive and usually fatal, and much of the skin surface may become denuded. Immunosuppressive agents are also useful for maintenance therapy. With appropriate treatment, the 10-year mortality rate for PV is less than 10%.

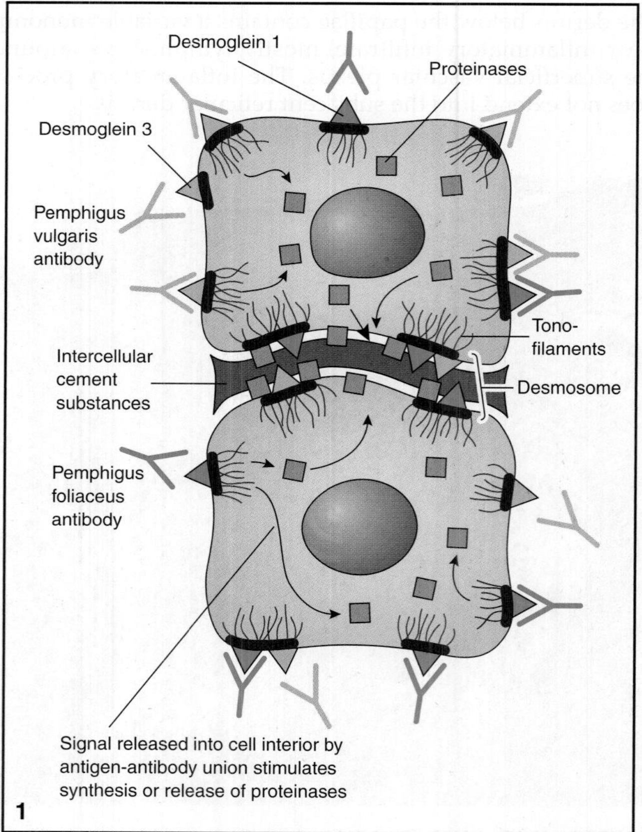

FIGURE 24-17. Pemphigus vulgaris. A pathogenetic mechanism of suprabasal dyshesion is shown. **(1)** A circulating autoantibody binds to an antigen on the outer leaflet of the plasma membrane (desmosome) of the keratinocyte, especially in the basal regions.

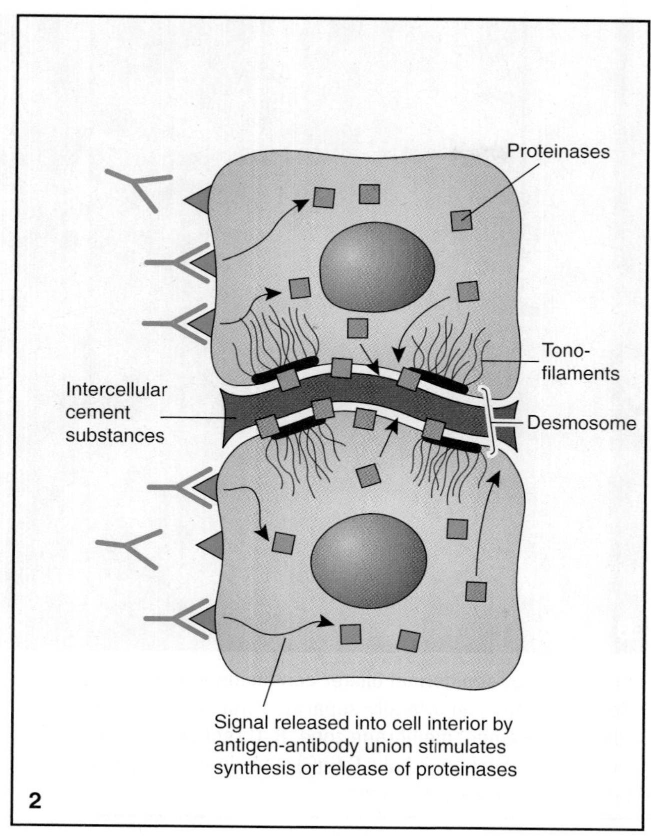

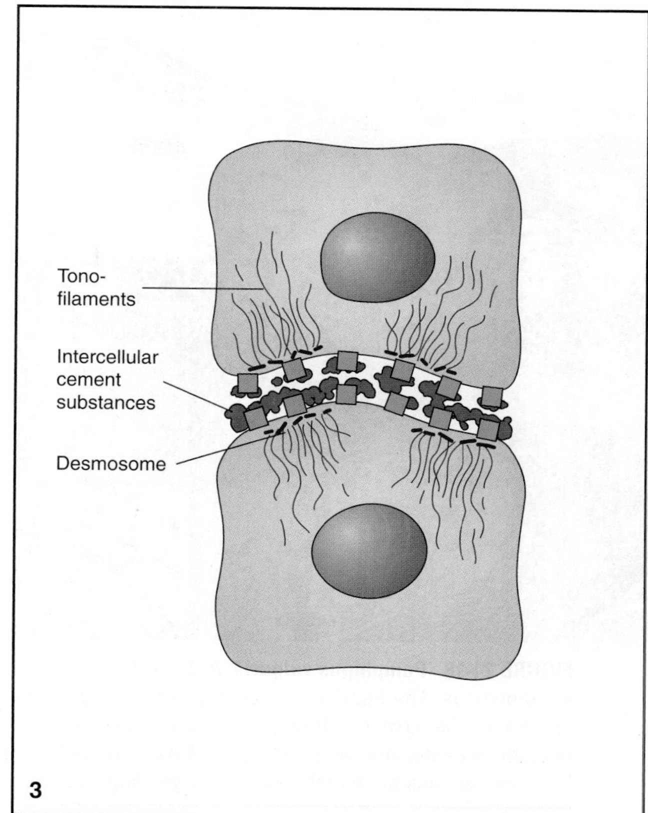

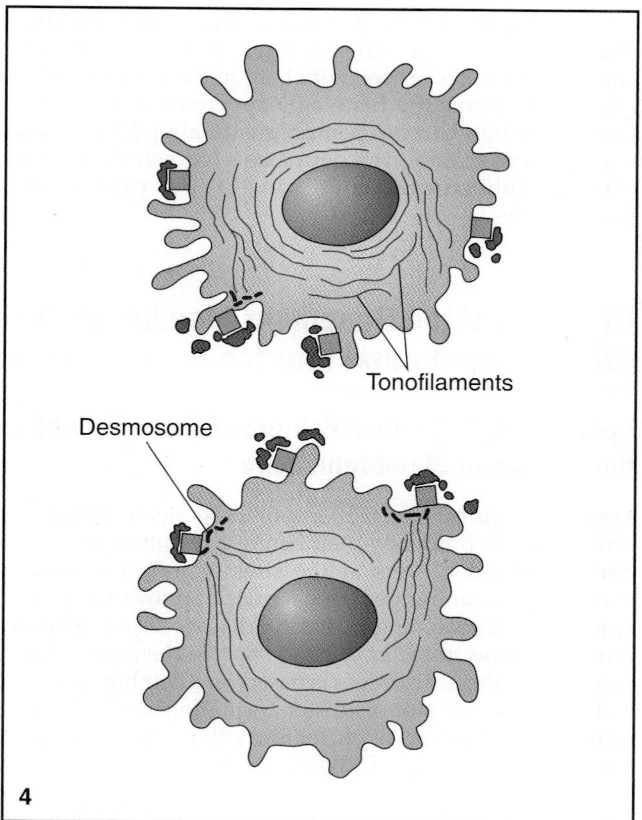

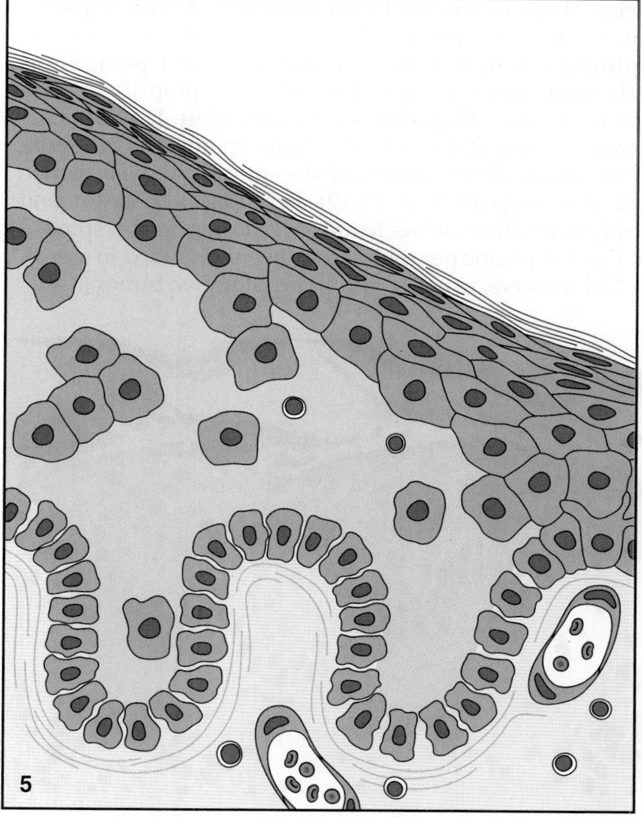

FIGURE 24-17. (*continued*) **(2)** Antigen–antibody union results in release of a proteinase (plasmin). **(3)** The proteinase interacts with intercellular cement, initiating dyshesion. **(4)** Desmosomes deteriorate, tonofilaments clump about the nucleus, the cells round up and separation is complete. **(5)** A vesicle, which is usually suprabasal, forms. Alternatively, acantholysis may occur by direct interference with desmosomal and adherence junction attachments.

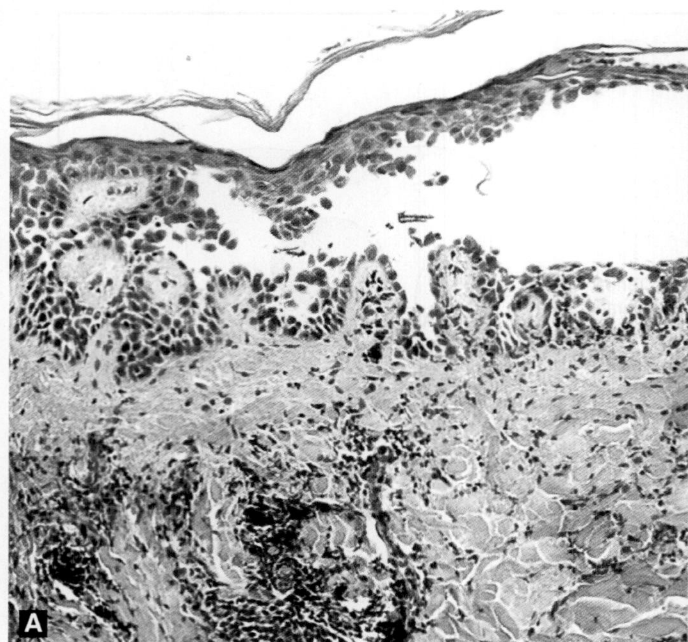

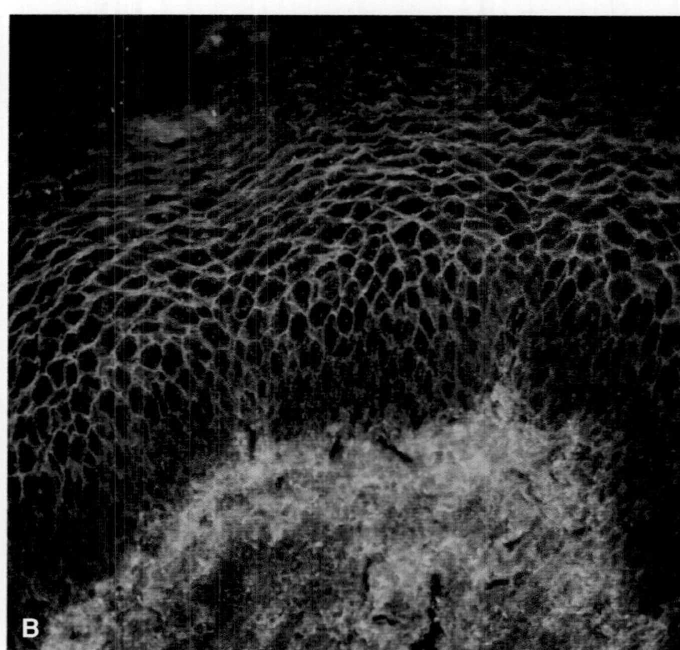

FIGURE 24-18. Pemphigus vulgaris. A. Suprabasal dyshesion leads to an intraepidermal blister containing acantholytic keratinocytes. The basal keratinocytes are slightly separated from each other and totally separated from the stratum spinosum. The basal keratinocytes are firmly attached to the epidermal basement membrane zone. **B.** Direct immunofluorescence examination of perilesional skin reveals antibodies, usually of the immunoglobulin G (IgG) type, deposited in the intercellular substance of the epidermis, yielding a lace-like pattern outlining the keratinocytes.

Other diseases caused by dyshesion that have a pathogenetic mechanism similar to PV include **pemphigus foliaceus, pemphigus erythematosus** and **drug-induced pemphigus** (mostly associated with penicillamine and captopril). In pemphigus foliaceus, IgG antibodies to **desmoglein 1,** a desmosomal protein, cause dyshesion in the outer spinous and granular epidermal layers (in contrast with the suprabasal dyshesion in pemphigus vulgaris) (Fig. 24-19). Pemphigus foliaceus and pemphigus erythematosus feature dyshesion in the spinous layer. Paraneoplastic pemphigus has been described in association with cancers, usually lymphoproliferative tumors.

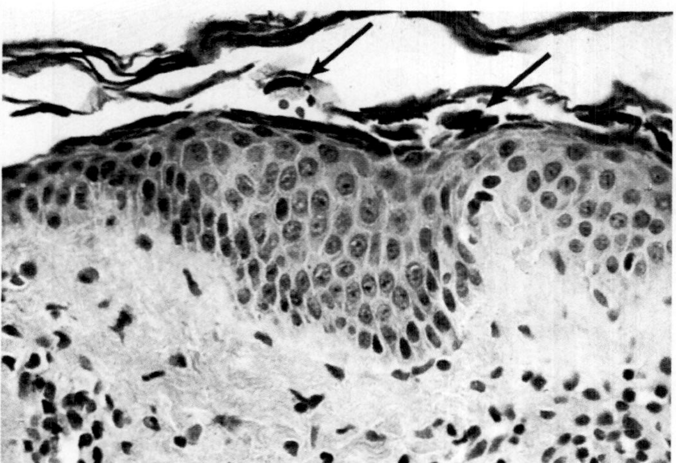

FIGURE 24-19. Pemphigus foliaceus. The dyshesion develops in the outer stratum spinosum and stratum granulosum. (Compare with that of pemphigus vulgaris; Fig. 24-18.) Dyshesive and dyskeratotic keratinocytes of the stratum granulosum (*arrows*) are important hallmarks.

Pemphigus may be associated with other autoimmune diseases, such as myasthenia gravis and lupus erythematosus, and may also be seen with benign thymomas. Other diseases may mimic the histologic appearance of PV, namely, familial benign chronic pemphigus (Hailey-Hailey disease) and transient acantholytic dermatosis (Grover disease). However, IgG antibodies do not react with epidermal antigens in these entities.

Diseases of the Basement Membrane Zone (Dermal–Epidermal Interface)

Epidermolysis Bullosa Features Blister Formation in the Basement Membrane Zone

Epidermolysis bullosa (EB) is a heterogeneous group of disorders loosely bound by their hereditary nature and by a tendency to form blisters at the sites of minor trauma. The clinical spectrum ranges from a minor annoyance to a widespread, life-threatening blistering disease. ***These blisters are almost always noted at birth or shortly thereafter.*** The classification of these disorders is based on a combination of clinical features and site of blister formation in the BMZ. The different mechanisms of blister formation underlie each of the four major categories of EB (Fig. 24-20).

Epidermolytic Epidermolysis Bullosa

This disorder, also known as **EB simplex,** is a group of autosomal dominant and autosomal recessive skin diseases in which blisters form as a result of disruption of basal keratinocytes. The

EPIDERMOLYTIC EB

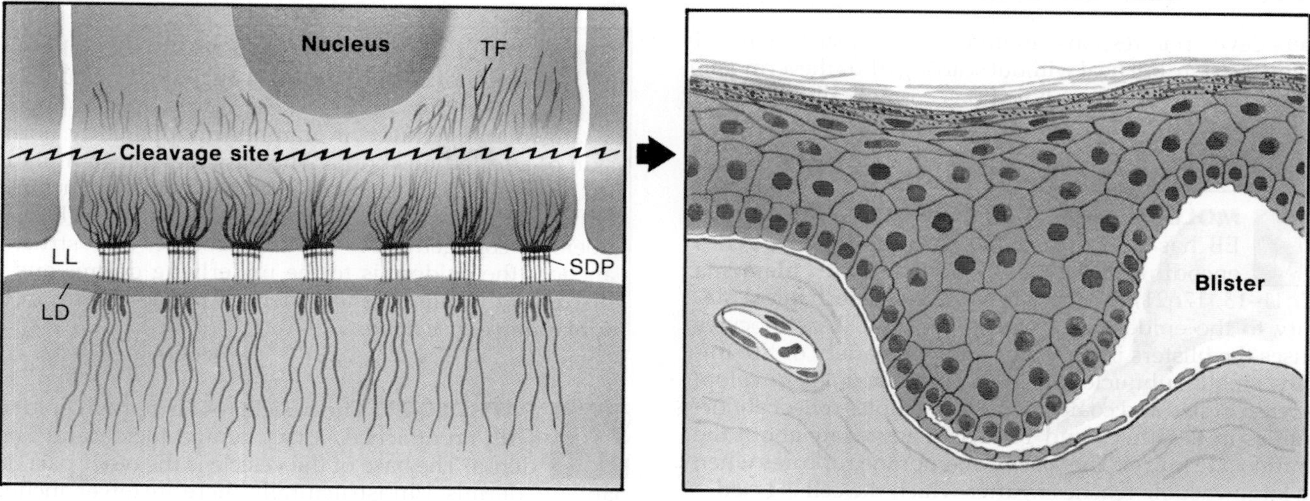

JUNCTIONAL EB

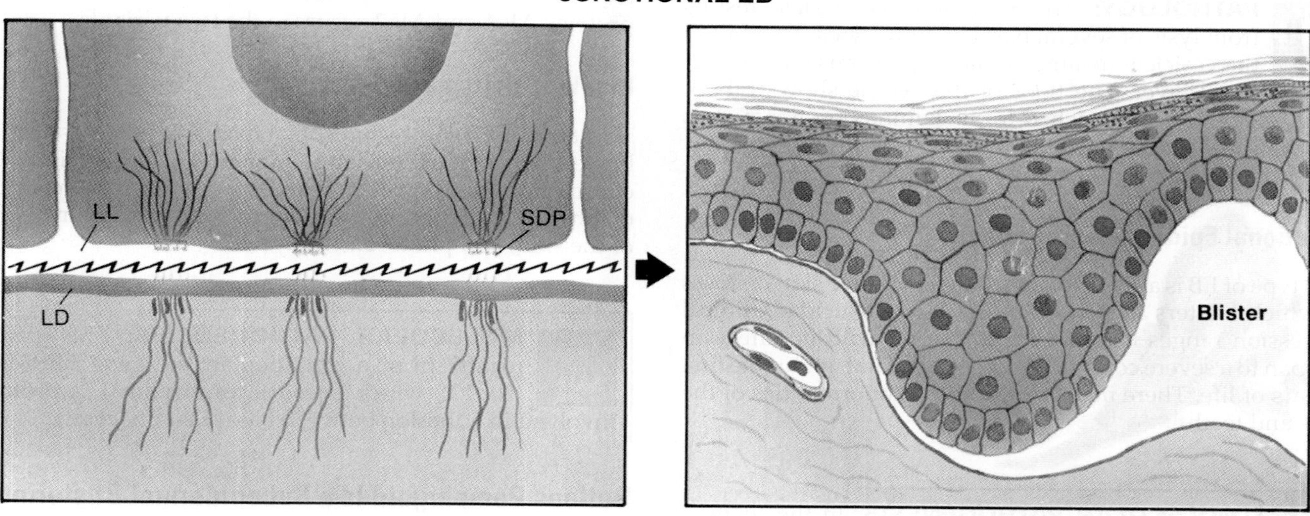

DERMOLYTIC EB

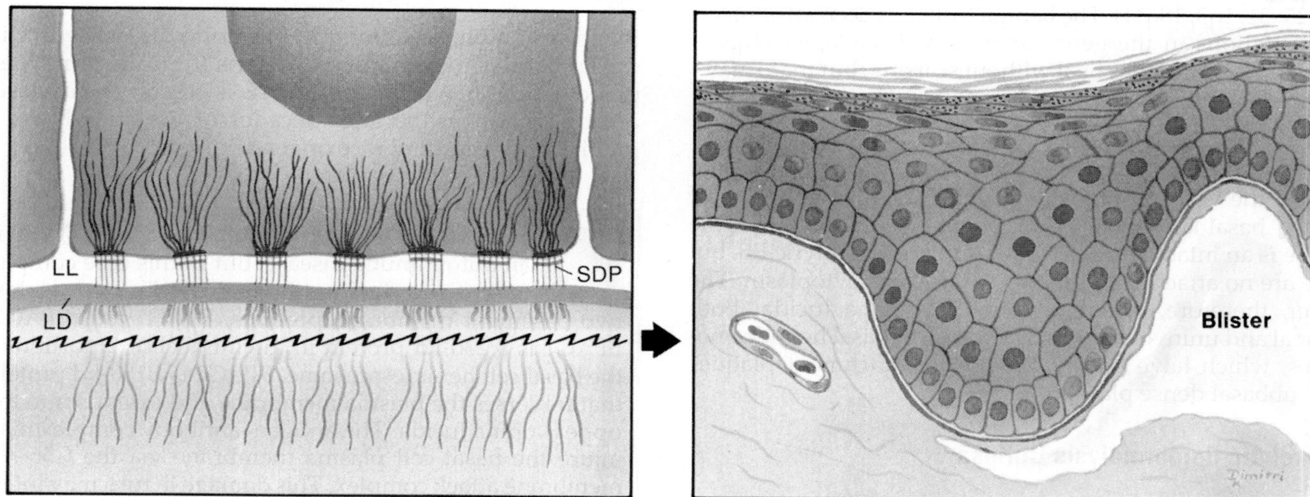

FIGURE 24-20. Epidermolysis bullosa (EB). Three distinct mechanisms of blister formation are shown. Electron microscopic images are diagrammed on the *left*; light microscopic images are on the *right*. **Epidermolytic EB** is caused by disintegration of the lowermost regions of the epidermal basal cells. The bottom portions of the basal cells cleave, and the remainder of the epidermis lifts away. Small fragments of basal cells remain attached to the basement membrane zone. **Junctional EB** is characterized by cleavage in the lamina lucida. **Dermolytic EB** is associated with rudimentary and fragmented anchoring fibrils. The entire basement membrane zone and epidermis split away from the dermis in relationship to these flawed anchoring fibrils. LL = lamina lucida; LD = lamina densa; SDP = subdesmosomal dense plate.

blisters develop in response to minor trauma, such as merely rubbing the skin, but heal without scarring (thus the term "simplex"). Although epidermolytic EB is cosmetically disturbing and sometimes debilitating, it is not life-threatening.

MOLECULAR PATHOGENESIS: Epidermolytic EB has been attributed to mutations of genes encoding cytokeratin intermediate filaments (12q11–13, 17q21), which likely provide mechanical stability to the epidermis. Cytolysis of basal keratinocytes causes the blisters in the epidermolytic variety of EB. Initially, small, subnuclear, cytoplasmic vacuoles develop, increase in size and coalesce. These vacuoles reflect abnormalities in keratins 5 and 14, which aggregate about the keratinocyte nuclei. The plasma membrane ruptures when the large vacuole reaches it, after which the cell is lysed.

PATHOLOGY: An intraepidermal vesicle results from lysis of several basal keratinocytes. The roof of the vesicle is an almost intact epidermis with a fragmented basal layer. The floor of the vesicle shows bits of basal cell cytoplasm attached to the lamina densa, which is seen as a well-preserved pink line at the base of the vesicle. Inflammatory cells are sparse.

Junctional Epidermolysis Bullosa

This type of EB is a group of autosomal recessive skin diseases in which blisters form within the lamina lucida. Clinical expression ranges from a benign disease with no effect on lifespan to a severe condition that may be fatal within the first 2 years of life. There may be associated abnormalities of the nails and teeth.

MOLECULAR PATHOGENESIS: In the severe form, mutations in the genes for certain isoforms of laminin and the integrins have been reported (1q25–31, 1q3, 18q11). The benign form has been attributed to mutations in the gene for type XVII collagen (1q32, 10q23). Both varieties heal without scarring, but there may be residual atrophy of the skin.

PATHOLOGY: An intact epidermis forms the roof of the vesicle in junctional EB. Plasma membranes of basal keratinocytes are unchanged. The floor of the vesicle is an intact lamina densa, as in epidermolytic EB, but there are no attached fragments of basal cell cytoplasm. The blister, therefore, occurs within the lamina lucida. Both lesional and uninvolved skin shows fewer basal hemidesmosomes, which have poorly developed attachment plaques and subbasal dense plates.

Dermolytic Epidermolysis Bullosa

Also known as **dystrophic EB,** dermolytic EB is a group of autosomal dominant and autosomal recessive diseases in which blisters are located immediately deep to the lamina densa. The recessive variant is more severe. In both variants, healed blisters are characterized by atrophic ("dystrophic") scarring. Nails and teeth may be involved.

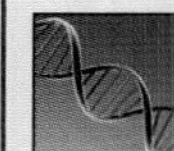

MOLECULAR PATHOGENESIS: The development of dermolytic EB is attributed to a defect in anchoring fibrils. These fibrils are abnormally arranged and reduced in number in apparently normal skin of affected newborns. The basic defect is a mutation in the gene encoding collagen type VII (3p21). Anchoring fibrils comprise a net in the upper dermis through which fibers of collagen types I and III course. This structure anchors the epidermis to the underlying dermis and its disruption results in subepidermal bullae arising in the sublamina densa zone.

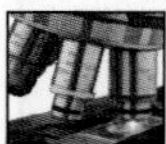

PATHOLOGY: The vesicle roof is normal epidermis with an attached, intact lamina lucida and lamina densa. The base of the vesicle is the outer part of the papillary dermis. Ultrastructurally, there are fewer anchoring fibrils in the dominant variant and virtually no fibrils in the recessive form. A corresponding decrease in anchoring fibril proteins AF-1 and AF-2 occurs in the two variants.

Kindler Syndrome

This type of EB shows autosomal recessive transmission and blisters with mixed cleavage planes. There are distinctive clinical findings, however, that set it apart from other forms of inherited EB, namely, poikiloderma (mottled pigmentation of the skin) and photosensitivity.

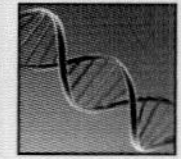

MOLECULAR PATHOGENESIS: This entity results from a mutation in the gene FERMT1 (20p12), which encodes for kindlin-1, a protein involved in adhesion between basal keratinocytes.

Bullous Pemphigoid Is a Subepidermal Blistering Disease Caused by Autoantibodies Against Basement Membrane Proteins

BP is a common, autoimmune, blistering disease with clinical similarities to pemphigus vulgaris (thus the term "pemphigoid") but in which acantholysis is absent. The disease is most common in the later decades of life and shows no predilection regarding race or gender.

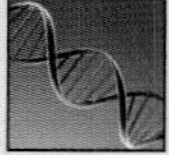

MOLECULAR PATHOGENESIS: Like PV, BP is an autoimmune disease, but in this case complement-fixing IgG antibodies are directed against two basement membrane proteins, BPAG1 and BPAG2. BPAG1 is a 230-kd protein in the intracellular portion of the basal cell hemidesmosome. BPAG2 is a 180-kd protein that traverses the plasma membrane and extends into the upper lamina lucida. The antigen–antibody complex may injure the basal cell plasma membrane via the C5b–C9 membrane attack complex. This damage in turn may interfere with elaboration of adherence factors by basal keratinocytes. Of greater importance is production of the anaphylatoxins C3a and C5a following complement activation. These molecules cause degranulation of mast cells and release of factors chemotactic for eosinophils, neutrophils and lymphocytes. Levels of IL-5 and eotaxin, known to play significant roles in recruitment and function of eosinophils, are increased in the blister fluid of patients with BP. Eosinophil granules contain tissue-damaging substances, including eosinophil peroxidase and major basic protein. These molecules, together with proteases of neutrophilic and mast cell origin, cause dermal–epidermal separation within the lamina lucida (Fig. 24-21).

PATHOLOGY: The blisters of BP are subepidermal: the roof is intact epidermis and the base is the lamina densa of the BMZ (Fig. 24-22). The blisters contain numerous eosinophils, together with fibrin, lymphocytes and neutrophils. In BP, apparently normal skin shows migration of mast cells from the venule toward the epidermis. With the onset of erythema, eosinophils appear in the upper dermis and are occasionally arranged along the epidermal BMZ. Ultrastructurally, dermal–epidermal separation begins with disruption of anchoring filaments of the lamina lucida. Immunofluorescence studies demonstrate linear deposition of C3 and IgG along the epidermal BMZ and serum antibodies against BPAG1 and BPAG2 (Fig. 24-23).

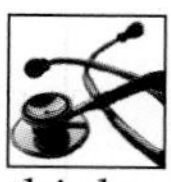

CLINICAL FEATURES: The blisters of BP are large and tense and may appear on normal-appearing skin or on an erythematous base (Fig. 24-22). The medial thighs and flexor aspects of the forearms are commonly affected, but the groin, axillae and other cutaneous sites may also develop blisters. The disease is self-limited but chronic. The patient's general health is usually unaffected. The course of the disease is greatly shortened by systemic administration of corticosteroids.

Dermatitis Herpetiformis Reflects Gluten Sensitivity and Immune Complex Deposition

Dermatitis herpetiformis (DH) is an intensely pruritic cutaneous eruption characterized by urticaria-like plaques and small subepidermal vesicles over the extensor surfaces of the body.

MOLECULAR PATHOGENESIS: DH is associated with gluten sensitivity in patients with HLA-B8, HLA-DR3 and HLA-DQw2 haplotypes. The gluten-sensitive enteropathy may be subclinical but most patients will show features of celiac sprue on small intestinal biopsy. Gluten is a protein in wheat, barley, rye and oats. The cutaneous lesions are related to granular deposits of IgA mainly at the tips of dermal papillae (Fig. 24-24). IgA immune complexes at the tips of dermal papillae are more prominent in perilesional skin than in normal-appearing skin. A gluten-free diet controls the disease; reintroduction of gluten provokes new lesions.

Genetically predisposed patients may develop IgA antibodies to components of gluten in the intestines. Resulting IgA complexes then gain access to the circulation and are deposited, possibly through binding to an as yet unknown ligand, in the dermal papillae (Fig. 24-24). Patients with DH have increased levels of IgA autoantibodies to tissue transglutaminase, suggesting that there is a dermal autoantigen related to tissue transglutaminase. Antibodies to smooth muscle endomysium are also increased in many patients with DH.

IgA immune complexes are inefficient in complement activation (alternate pathway), and few neutrophils are attracted to the site. However, those neutrophils that do accumulate elaborate leukotrienes, which attract more neutrophils. The neutrophils release lysosomal enzymes that degrade laminin and type IV collagen, cleaving the epidermis from the dermis and eventually causing blisters (Fig. 24-24).

CLINICAL FEATURES: The lesions of DH are especially prominent over the elbows, knees and buttocks (Fig. 24-25A). These intensely pruritic vesicles may become grouped similarly to herpes simplex infections (therefore the term "herpetiformis") and are almost invariably rubbed until broken. Thus, patients may present with only crusted lesions and no intact vesicles. Although DH is of varying severity and characterized by remissions, it is disturbingly chronic. The healing lesions often leave scars. Other than a gluten-free diet, treatment with dapsone or sulfapyridine controls the signs and symptoms of DH by an unknown mechanism. Increased risk of lymphoproliferative disorders and systemic lupus erythematosus has been reported.

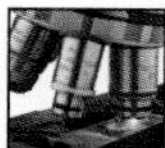

PATHOLOGY: A delicate perivenular lymphocytic infiltrate appears first, together with a row of neutrophils just deep to the lamina densa in the dermal papillae. During the next 12 hours, the neutrophils aggregate in clusters of 10 to 25 at the tips of the dermal papillae to create a diagnostic histologic appearance.

There are two related mechanisms of dermal–epidermal separation. One is associated with the sheet-like spread of a layer or two of neutrophils at the dermal–epidermal interface. In this situation, the entire epidermis detaches from the papillary dermis (Fig. 24-25B). The roof of such a vesicle contains the epidermis; the floor is composed of the lamina densa and the papillary dermis. In contrast to BP, eosinophils are uncommon early in the course of DH. The IgA deposits at the dermoepidermal junction are detected on direct immunofluorescence analysis (Fig. 24-25C).

In the second mechanism of vesicle formation, many neutrophils accumulate rapidly in the tips of the dermal papillae. Release of neutrophilic lysosomal enzymes in the superficial portion of the dermal papillae results in (1) uncoupling of the epidermis from the dermis at the tips of dermal papillae, (2) disruption of the BMZ in the lamina lucida and superficial part of the papillae and (3) tearing of the epidermis across the adjacent rete ridges. The roof of the resulting vesicle has alternating tears across its epidermal covering and the floor shows residual epidermal pegs alternating with the basal half of dermal papillae.

Erythema Multiforme Is Often a Reaction to a Drug or Infection

Erythema multiforme (EM) is an acute, self-limited disorder that varies from a few annular or ring-like and targetoid erythematous macules and blisters (EM minor) to a life-threatening, widespread ulceration of the skin and mucous membranes (EM major; Stevens-Johnson syndrome). ***This phenomenon is usually a reaction to a drug or an infectious agent, in particular, herpes simplex infection.***

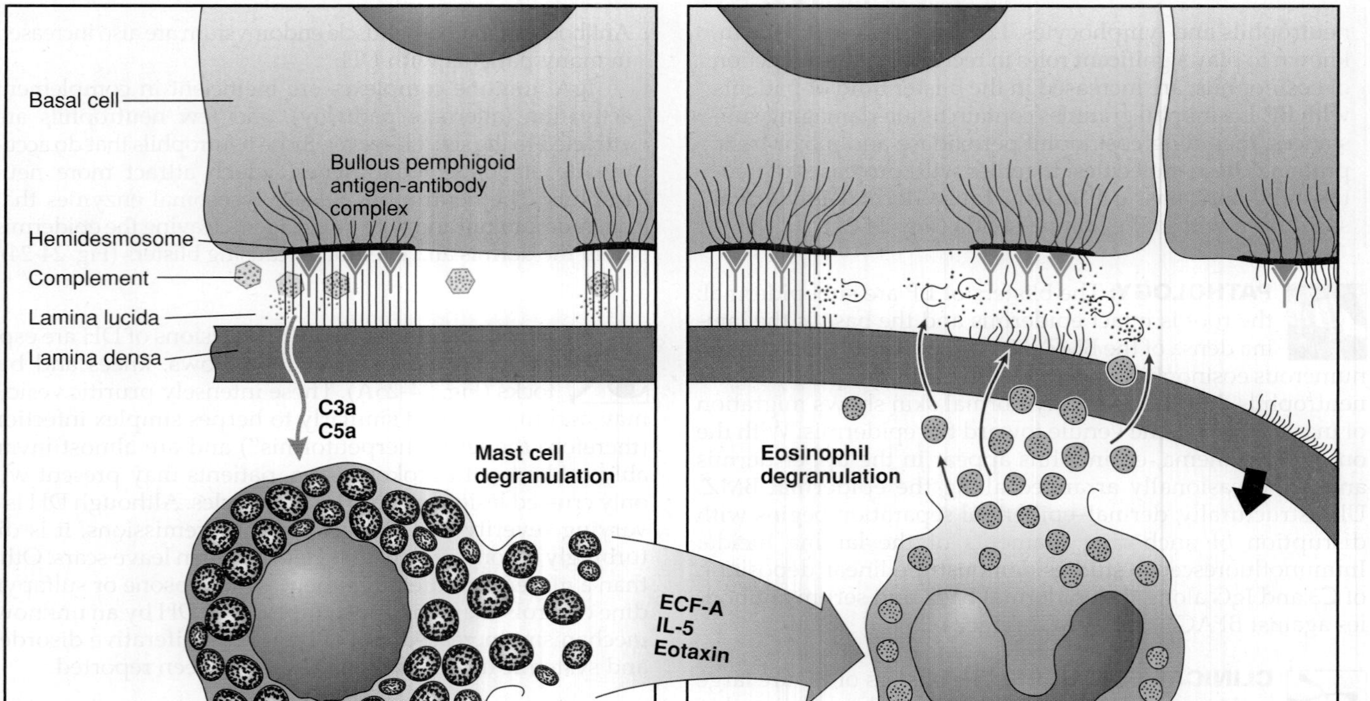

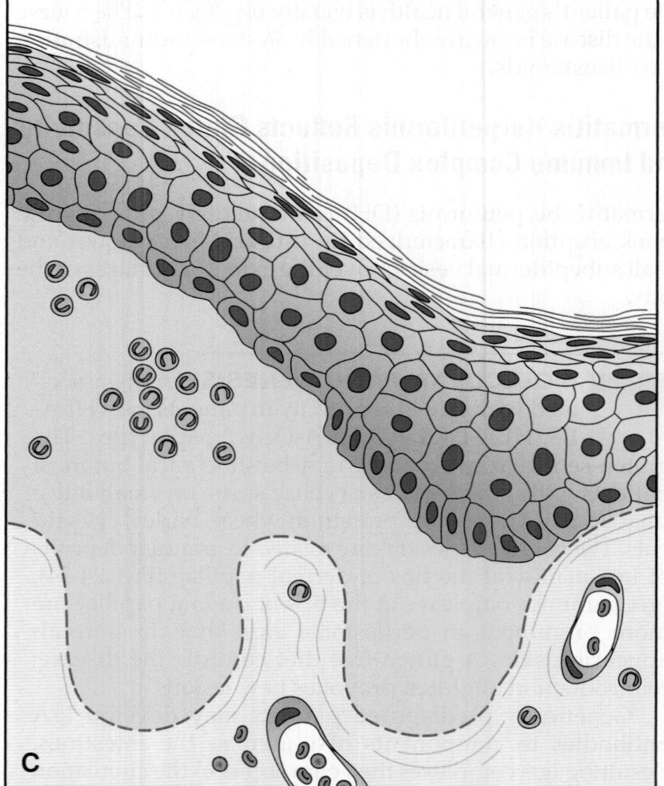

FIGURE 24-21. Bullous pemphigoid (BP). Pathogenetic mechanisms of blister formation are outlined. A circulating antibody to an apparently normal glycoprotein—BP antigen—in the lamina lucida precipitates the pathogenetic events in bullous pemphigoid. **A**. Antigen–antibody union activates complement, and the anaphylatoxins C3a and C5a are produced. These degranulate mast cells, resulting in the release of eosinophilic chemotactic factors. **B, C**. The tissue-damaging substances of eosinophilic granules cause vesicle formation at the lamina lucida, with some breakdown of the lamina densa. ECF-A = eosinophil chemotactic factor-A.

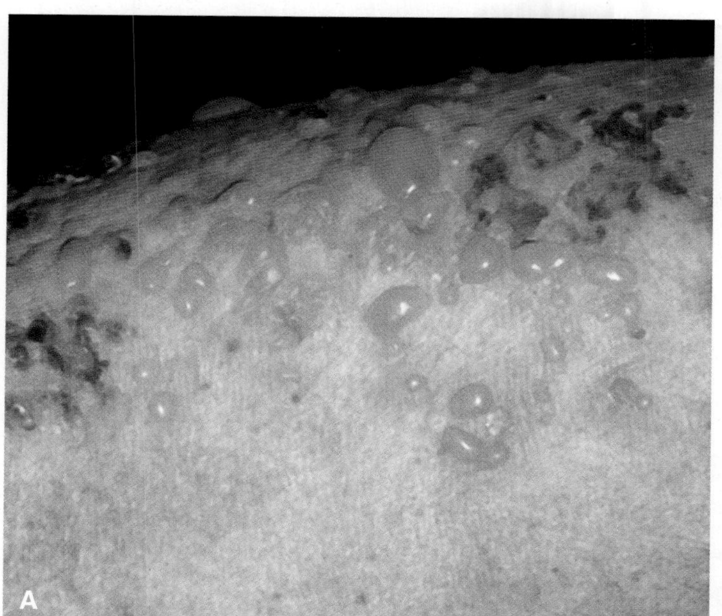

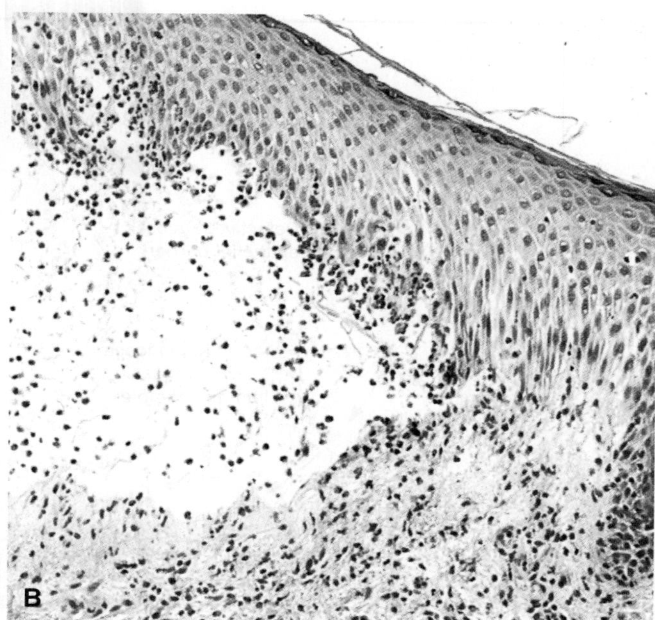

FIGURE 24-22. Bullous pemphigoid. A. The skin shows multiple tense bullae on an erythematous base and erosions, distributed primarily on the medial thighs and trunk. **B.** A subepidermal blister has an edematous papillary dermis as its base. The roof of the blister consists of the intact, entire epidermis, including the stratum basalis. Inflammatory cells, fibrin and fluid fill the blister.

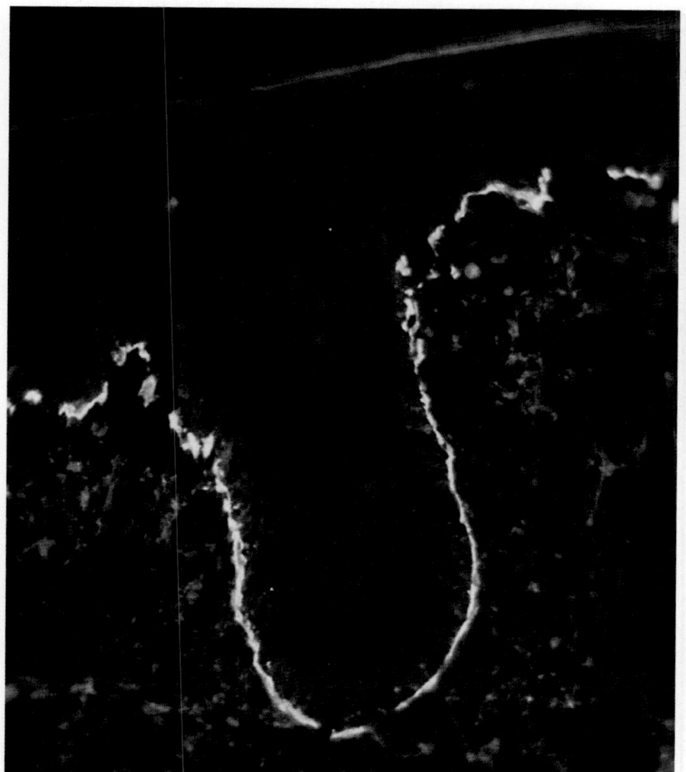

FIGURE 24-23. Bullous pemphigoid. Direct immunofluorescence study discloses linear deposition of immunoglobulin G (IgG) (and C3) along the dermal–epidermal junction. Ultrastructurally, these antibodies and complement are present in the lamina lucida.

ETIOLOGIC FACTORS: The list of agents that may provoke EM is long and includes Herpesvirus, *Mycoplasma* and sulfonamides. However, precipitating factors are identified in only half of cases. In postherpetic EM, viral antigens, IgM and C3 are deposited in a perivascular location and at the epidermal BMZ. The combination of infiltrating lymphocytes and antigen–antibody complexes within the lesions suggests that both humoral and cellular hypersensitivity are involved.

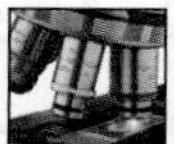

PATHOLOGY: The dermis in EM shows a sparse lymphocyte infiltrate about the superficial vascular bed and at the dermal–epidermal interface. The characteristic morphologic feature in the epidermis is the presence of apoptotic keratinocytes, which have a pyknotic nucleus and eosinophilic cytoplasm. Apoptosis may be extensive and associated with a subepidermal vesicle, whose roof is an almost completely necrotic epidermis. Because of the acute onset of the disease, in most cases there is little or no change in the stratum corneum.

CLINICAL FEATURES: The characteristic "target" or "iris" lesions of EM have a central, dark red zone, occasionally with a blister, surrounded by a paler area (Fig. 24-26). In turn, the latter is encompassed by a peripheral red rim. Urticarial plaques are common. The presence of vesicles and bullae usually predicts a more severe course. EM is a common condition, with a peak incidence in the second and third decades of life. It is occasionally encountered in association with other presumably immunologic cutaneous disorders, including erythema nodosum, toxic epidermal necrolysis and necrotizing vasculitis. **Stevens-Johnson syndrome** refers to an unusually severe form of EM that

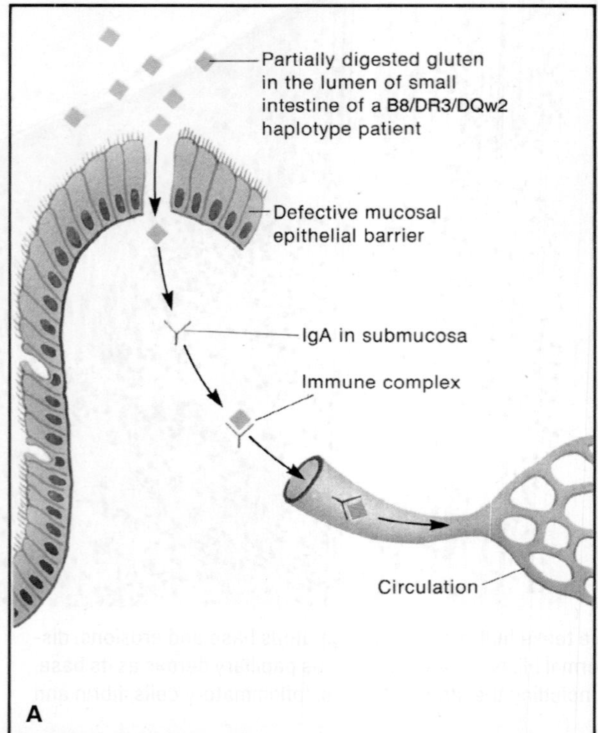

1. Formation of immune complexes in submucosa of small intestine. Passage of immune complexes into **the circulation.**

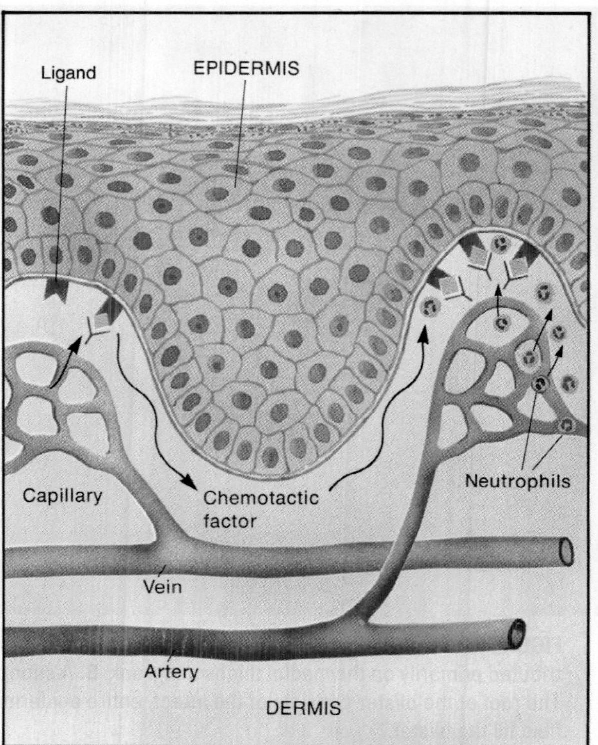

2. Ligand–immune complex union releases neutrophil chemotactic factor. Neutrophils migrate to the tips of the papillae.

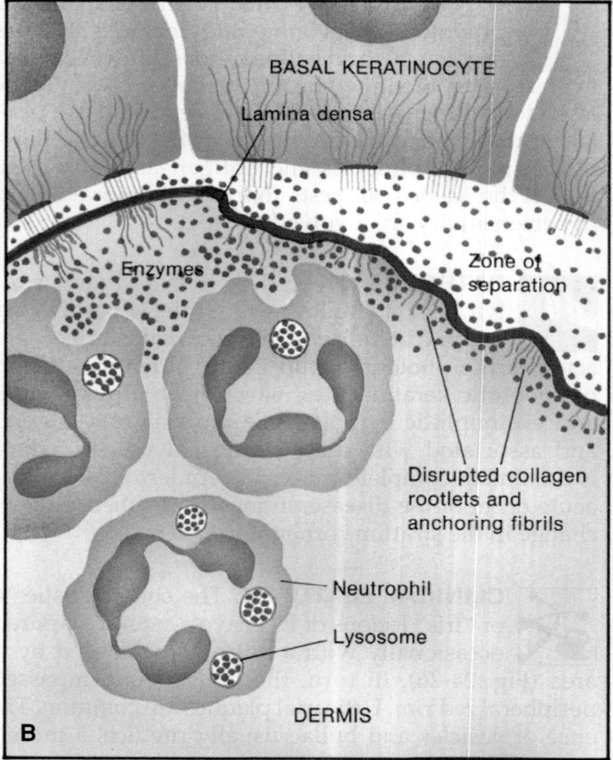

3. Dissolution of basal rootlets and anchoring fibrils by enzymes released by neutrophils. Early dermo-epidermal separation.

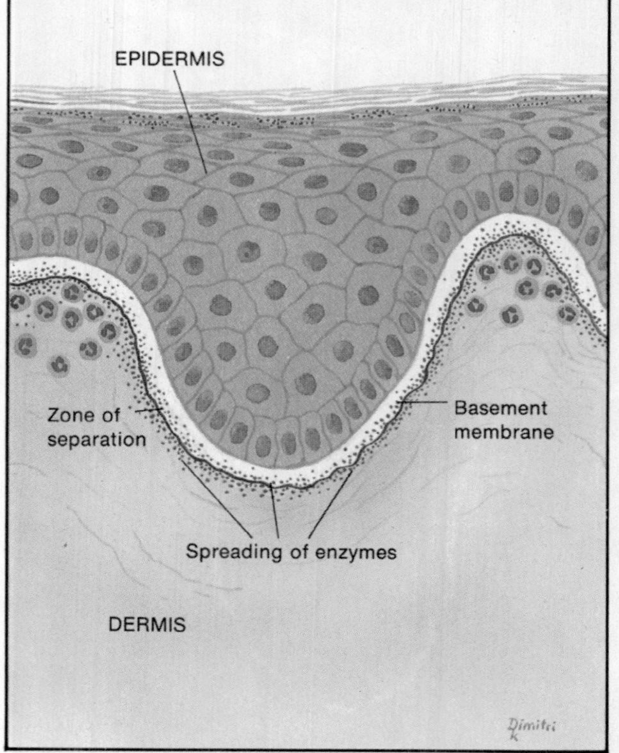

4. Concentration of neutrophils at the tips of the papillae. Spreading of enzymes along basement membrane. Lifting away of lamina densa.

FIGURE 24-24. Dermatitis herpetiformis. Proposed pathogenesis for cutaneous lesions. The disease is initiated in the small intestine and is likely expressed in the skin because of the presence of a ligand immediately deep to the lamina densa. IgA = immunoglobulin A.

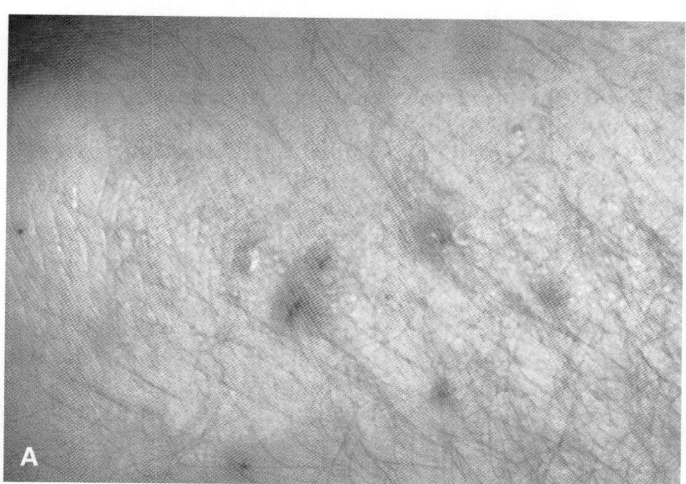

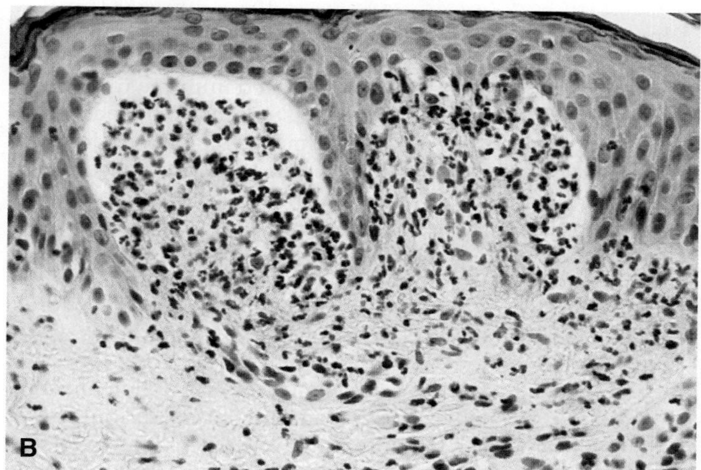

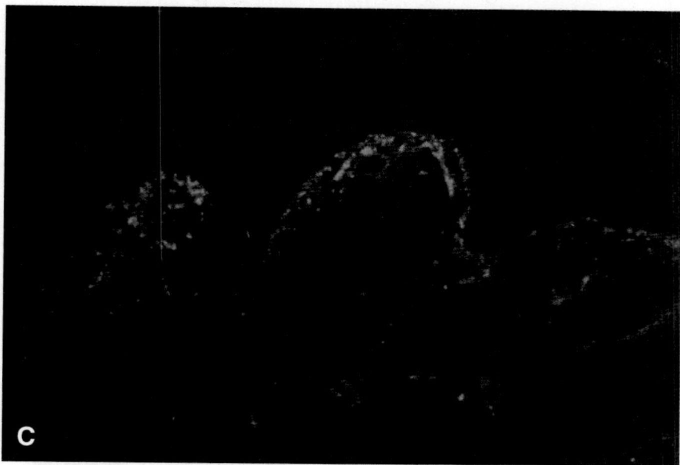

FIGURE 24-25. Dermatitis herpetiformis. A. Pruritic, symmetric, grouped vesicles on an erythematous base are seen on the elbows and knees. **B.** Dermal papillary abscesses of neutrophils with vesicle formation at the dermal–epidermal junction are characteristic. **C.** Direct immunofluorescence reveals immunoglobulin A (IgA) deposited in dermal papillae in association with (but not necessarily directly upon) anchoring fibrils and elastic tissue fibers. This is the site of neutrophil infiltration and subepidermal vesicle formation.

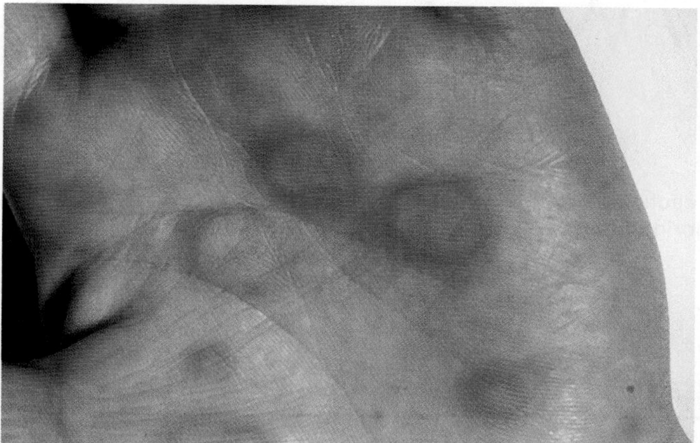

FIGURE 24-26. Erythema multiforme. Steroid-responsive "target" papules, characterized by central bullae with surrounding erythema, appeared after antibiotic therapy.

involves mucosal surfaces and internal organs and is frequently fatal. Toxic epidermal necrolysis (TEN or Lyell disease) is a related condition that may be generalized and may be life-threatening.

Systemic Lupus Erythematosus Is an Immune Complex Disease Characterized by Autoantibodies and Other Immune Abnormalities

Cutaneous involvement may be severe and cosmetically devastating, but is not life-threatening. However, the nature and pattern of immune reactants in the skin are an excellent guide to the likelihood of systemic disease.

MOLECULAR PATHOGENESIS: Immune complexes are present in both lesional and normal-appearing skin in systemic lupus erythematosus (SLE), and are not likely to be solely responsible for the cutaneous lesions of SLE. Deposition of immune reactants along the epidermal BMZ of normal-appearing skin is important in the diagnosis of SLE. Epidermal injury seems to be initiated by exogenous agents such as ultraviolet light and perpetuated by cell-mediated immune reactions similar to those in graft-versus-host disease. The manifestations of epidermal injury include (1) vacuolization of basal keratinocytes, hyperkeratosis and diminished epidermal thickness; (2) release of DNA and other nuclear and cytoplasmic antigens to the circulation; and (3) deposition of DNA and other antigens in the epidermal BMZ (lamina densa and immediately subjacent dermis) (Fig. 24-27). Thus, epidermal injury, local immune complex formation, deposition of circulating immune complexes and lymphocyte-induced cellular injury all seem to act in concert.

The various forms of cutaneous lupus erythematosus have been classified according to their chronicity, but considerable overlap in features is possible. There is an inverse relationship between the prominence of skin lesions and the extent of systemic disease.

CHRONIC CUTANEOUS (DISCOID) LUPUS ERYTHEMATOSUS: This form of lupus is usually limited to the skin. Disease generally manifests above the neck, on the face (especially the malar area), scalp and ears. Lesions begin as slightly elevated violaceous papules with a rough scale of keratin. As they enlarge, they assume a disc shape, with a hyperkeratotic margin and a depigmented center. The cutaneous lesions may culminate in disfiguring scars. Elevated circulating antinuclear antibodies (ANAs) are seen in fewer than 10% of patients.

PATHOLOGY: In discoid lupus, nucleated epidermal layers are modestly thickened or somewhat thin. Hyperkeratosis and plugging of hair follicles are prominent. The rete–papillae pattern of the dermal–epidermal interface is partially effaced. Basal keratinocytes are vacuolated, and eosinophilic apoptotic bodies are noted. The lamina densa is greatly thickened and reduplicated. On periodic acid–Schiff (PAS) staining, multiple layers of lamina densa extend into the subjacent dermis. The excessive quantity of lamina densa, a product of the basal keratinocytes,

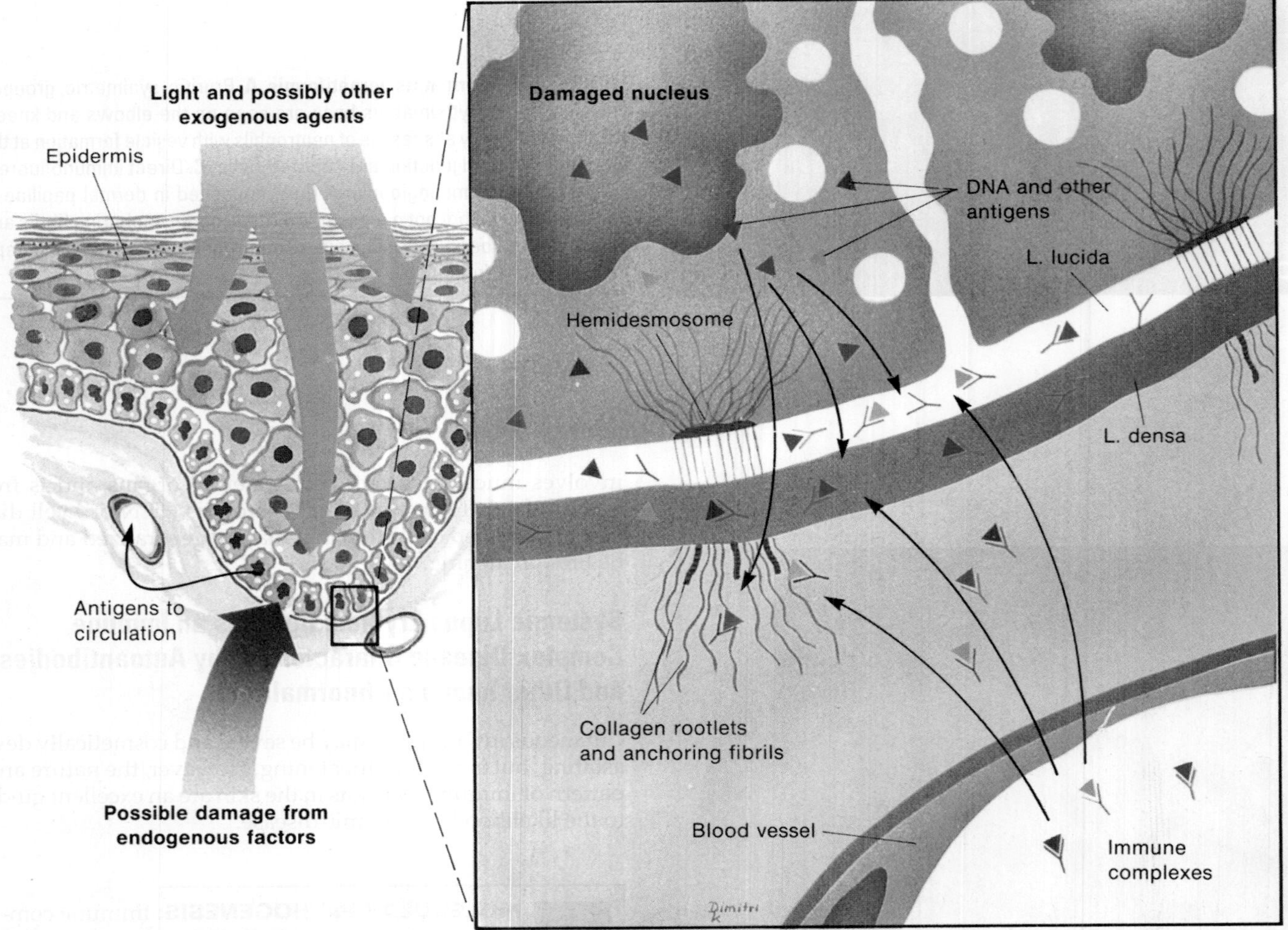

FIGURE 24-27. Lupus erythematosus. A cell-mediated immune reaction leads to epidermal cellular damage when initiated by light or other exogenous agents as well as endogenous ones. Such injury releases a large number of antigens, some of which may return to the skin in the form of immune complexes. Immune complexes are also formed in the skin by a reaction of local DNA with antibody that may also be deposited beneath the epidermal basement membrane zone. L = lamina.

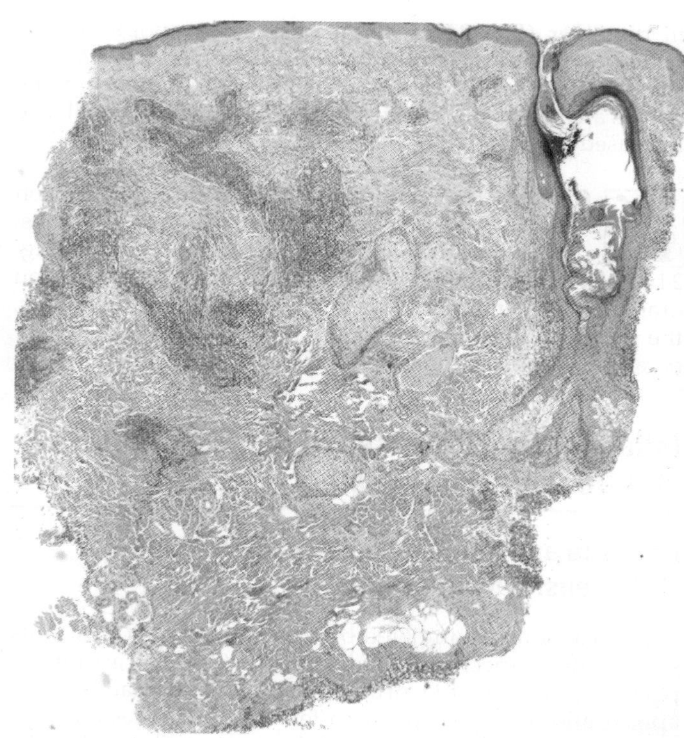

FIGURE 24-28. Lupus erythematosus. Perivascular and periappendageal lymphocytic inflammation is present in the superficial and deep dermis. A hair follicle plugged with keratin is present near the right edge.

reflects a response of basal cells to damage. These changes all suggest that injury to basal keratinocytes is an essential pathogenetic characteristic of skin disease associated with lupus (Figs. 24-28 through 24-30).

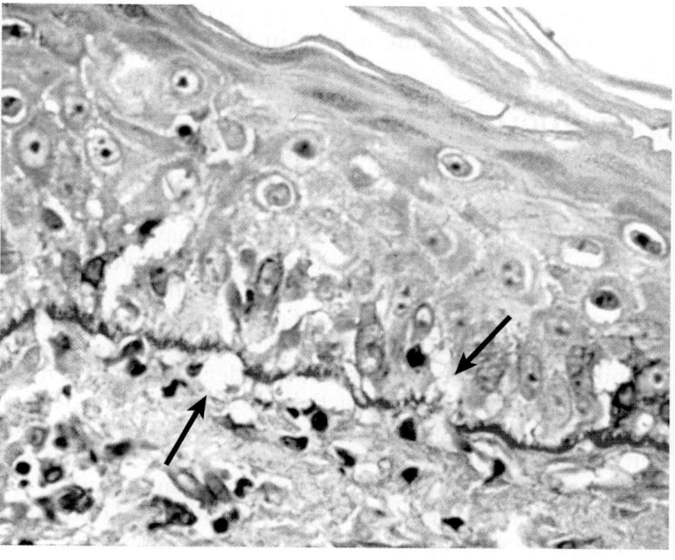

FIGURE 24-29. Lupus erythematosus. Basal cell necrosis with resultant basal keratinocytic migration and synthesis of new basement membrane zone leads to thickening of the epidermal basement membrane zone (BMZ), as evident in this periodic acid–Schiff (PAS) stain. Notice the vacuoles (*arrows*) on either side of the BMZ, an indicator of cellular injury.

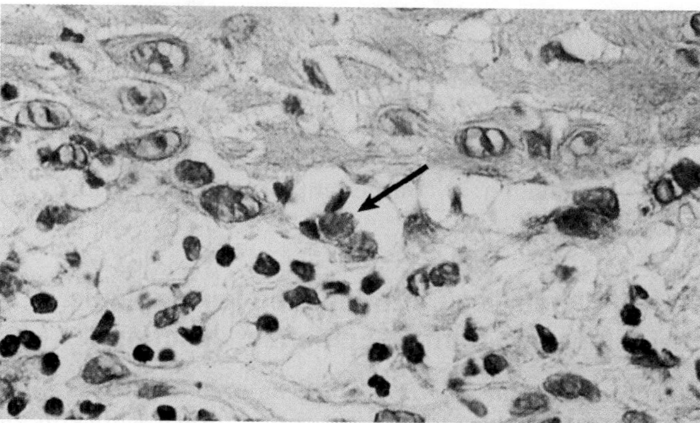

FIGURE 24-30. Lupus erythematosus. An active lesion shows striking basal vacuolization, with keratinocyte necrosis (*arrow*) forming a dense eosinophilic body (apoptotic/fibrillary/colloid body) that is surrounded by lymphocytes (satellitosis).

The basal keratinocytes and BMZ contain a diffuse lymphocytic infiltrate that penetrates the basal layer focally. Deeper in the dermis, dense patches of helper and cytotoxic/suppressor T lymphocytes, often with plasma cells, are commonly found around skin appendages. Immune complexes are predominantly located deep to the lamina densa, but are also seen by immunofluorescence as granular deposits on the lamina densa and within the lamina lucida. This pattern contrasts with that of BP in which there are only two antigens, both precisely localized to the lamina lucida, resulting in a linear staining pattern.

SUBACUTE CUTANEOUS LUPUS ERYTHEMATOSUS: This disorder primarily afflicts young and middle-aged white women. Unlike discoid lupus, subacute cutaneous lupus may also involve the musculoskeletal system and kidneys. Initially, scaly erythematous papules develop and then enlarge into psoriasiform or annular lesions, which may fuse. Skin changes are seen in the upper chest, upper back and extensor surfaces of the arms, a distribution indicating that light exposure plays a role in the pathogenesis of the disorder. Significant scarring does not occur. About 70% of patients have circulating anti-Ro (SS-A) antibodies. ANA levels are elevated in 70%.

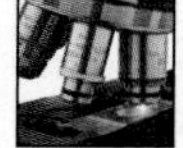

PATHOLOGY: Subacute cutaneous lupus features edema of the papillary dermis, thickening of the lamina densa and prominent vacuolar degeneration of basilar keratinocytes. There is some lymphocytic infiltration of the BMZ but deeper patches of lymphocytes are not observed.

ACUTE SYSTEMIC LUPUS ERYTHEMATOSUS: Over 80% of patients with SLE have acute cutaneous manifestations during their illness, in association with disease of the kidneys and joints. The rash is often the first manifestation of the disease and may precede the onset of systemic symptoms by a few months. The typical "butterfly" rash of SLE is a delicate erythema of the malar area of the face, which may pass in a few hours or a few days. Many patients exhibit a maculopapular eruption of the chest and extremities, often developing after sun exposure. Both rashes heal without scarring. Lesions indistinguishable from discoid lupus may occur. ANA levels are elevated in more than 90% of patients.

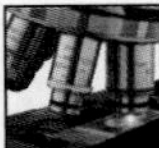

PATHOLOGY: Histologically, the earliest malar blush of acute cutaneous lupus may show only edema of the papillary dermis. More often, the changes are similar to those in the subacute form of lupus. In **bullous SLE,** blisters may occur subepidermally and beneath the lamina densa, where an autoantibody against type VII collagen, a component of anchoring fibrils, is deposited.

Lichen Planus Is a Cell-Mediated Immunologic Reaction at the Dermal–Epidermal Junction

"Lichenoid" tissue reactions are so named because the clinical lesions resemble certain lichens that form a scaly growth on rocks or tree trunks. Histologically, lichenoid infiltrates are characterized by a band-like congregation of lymphocytes that obscures the dermal–epidermal junction. Epidermal turnover is decreased, leading to hyperkeratosis without parakeratosis. Lichen planus (LP) is the prototypic disorder of this group, which includes entities such as lichen nitidus and lichenoid drug eruptions.

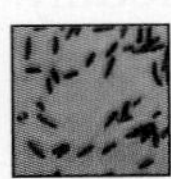

ETIOLOGIC FACTORS: The etiology of LP is unknown. It is occasionally familial and may also accompany a variety of autoimmune disorders, such as SLE and myasthenia gravis. LP is more frequent in patients with ulcerative colitis. Drugs such as gold, chlorothiazide and chloroquine may induce lichenoid reactions. External agents such as photographic chemicals may evoke a lichenoid response (presumably reduced in incidence with the advent of digital cameras). LP-like lesions are also often observed in the later stages of chronic graft-versus-host disease. Thus, it seems that immunologic mechanisms play a role in the pathogenesis of LP (Fig. 24-31). The presence of apoptotic bodies and reduced epidermal cell turnover suggest that the lesions of LP result from basal layer cell destruction leading to reduced and subsequent reactive epidermal proliferation. Evidence supports the notion that LP is a delayed type of hypersensitivity reaction, initiated and amplified by cytokines such as interferon-γ (IFN-γ) and IL-6, produced both by infiltrating lymphocytes and by stimulated keratinocytes. Association of LP with hepatitis C infection has been observed.

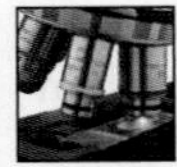

PATHOLOGY: The epidermis in LP features compact hyperkeratosis with little or no parakeratosis. The stratum granulosum is thickened, frequently in a distinctive, focal, wedge-shaped pattern, with the base of the wedge abutting the stratum corneum. The stratum spinosum is variably thickened.

The distinctive pathologic changes of LP are at the dermal–epidermal interface. The basal row of cuboidal cells is replaced by flattened or polygonal keratinocytes. The undulating interface between the dermal papillae and the rounded profiles of the rete ridges is obscured by a dense infiltrate of lymphocytes and macrophages, many of the latter containing melanin pigment **(melanophages)** (Fig. 24-32). The lymphocytes are principally of the helper/inducer phenotype. Sharply pointed ("saw-toothed") rete ridges of keratinocytes project into the inflammatory infiltrate.

Commonly admixed with the infiltrate (in the epidermis or dermis) are globular, fibrillary, eosinophilic bodies, 15 to 20 μm in diameter (Fig. 24-32), which represent apoptotic keratinocytes. These structures are variably termed *apoptotic, colloid, Civatte* or *fibrillary bodies*. The fibrils within the apoptotic bodies are keratin filaments. Epidermal Langerhans cells are increased early in LP.

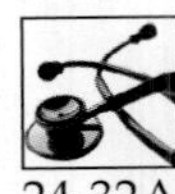

CLINICAL FEATURES: LP is a chronic eruption characterized by violaceous, flat-topped papules, usually on the flexor surfaces of the wrists (Fig. 24-32A). White patches or streaks may also be present on oral mucous membranes (Wickham striae). In most patients, the pruritic lesions resolve in less than a year, but they may occasionally persist longer.

Inflammatory Diseases of the Superficial and Deep Vascular Bed

Urticaria and Angioedema Are IgE-Dependent Hypersensitivity Reactions

These reactions are initiated by degranulation of mast cells sensitized to a specific antigen. **Urticaria** ("hives") are raised, pale, well-demarcated pruritic papules and plaques that appear and disappear within a few hours. The lesions represent edema of the superficial portion of the dermis. **Angioedema** refers to a condition in which the edema involves the deeper dermis or subcutis, resulting in an egg-like swelling. Both entities have a rapid onset and range in severity from simply annoying lesions to life-threatening anaphylactic reactions. The mainstays of treatment are avoiding the offending agent and prompt administration of antihistamines.

Dermatographism is a linear hive with a rich pink flare produced by briskly stroking the skin, present in approximately 4% of the population. It represents an exaggerated IgE-dependent response. One may write on the skin of such persons and create a hive in the form of a legible word.

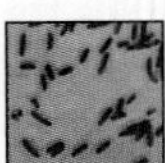

ETIOLOGIC FACTORS: Most cases of urticaria are IgE dependent and reflect exaggerated venule permeability owing to mast cell degranulation. An almost endless list of materials may react with IgE antibodies on the surface of the mast cell. Urticaria may occur in both atopic and nonatopic persons. Atopic persons have intensely pruritic skin eruptions, a family history of similar eruptions and a personal or family history of allergies. They commonly have elevated circulating IgE.

Initially, cutaneous venules react to degranulation of mast cells and release of their vasoactive mediators with increased permeability, resulting in rapidly forming edema. If the reaction persists, inflammatory cells are attracted to the area, causing an urticarial plaque (lasting more than a day).

Hereditary angioedema is a serious autosomal dominant disorder caused by mutation of C1-esterase inhibitor.

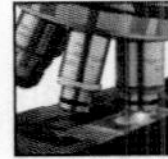

PATHOLOGY: In urticaria, collagen fibers and fibrils are splayed apart by excess fluid. Lymphatic vessels are dilated; venules show margination of neutrophils and eosinophils. Vessels are cuffed by a few lymphocytes. In persistent urticaria, lymphocytes and eosinophils are increased, but neutrophils are sparse.

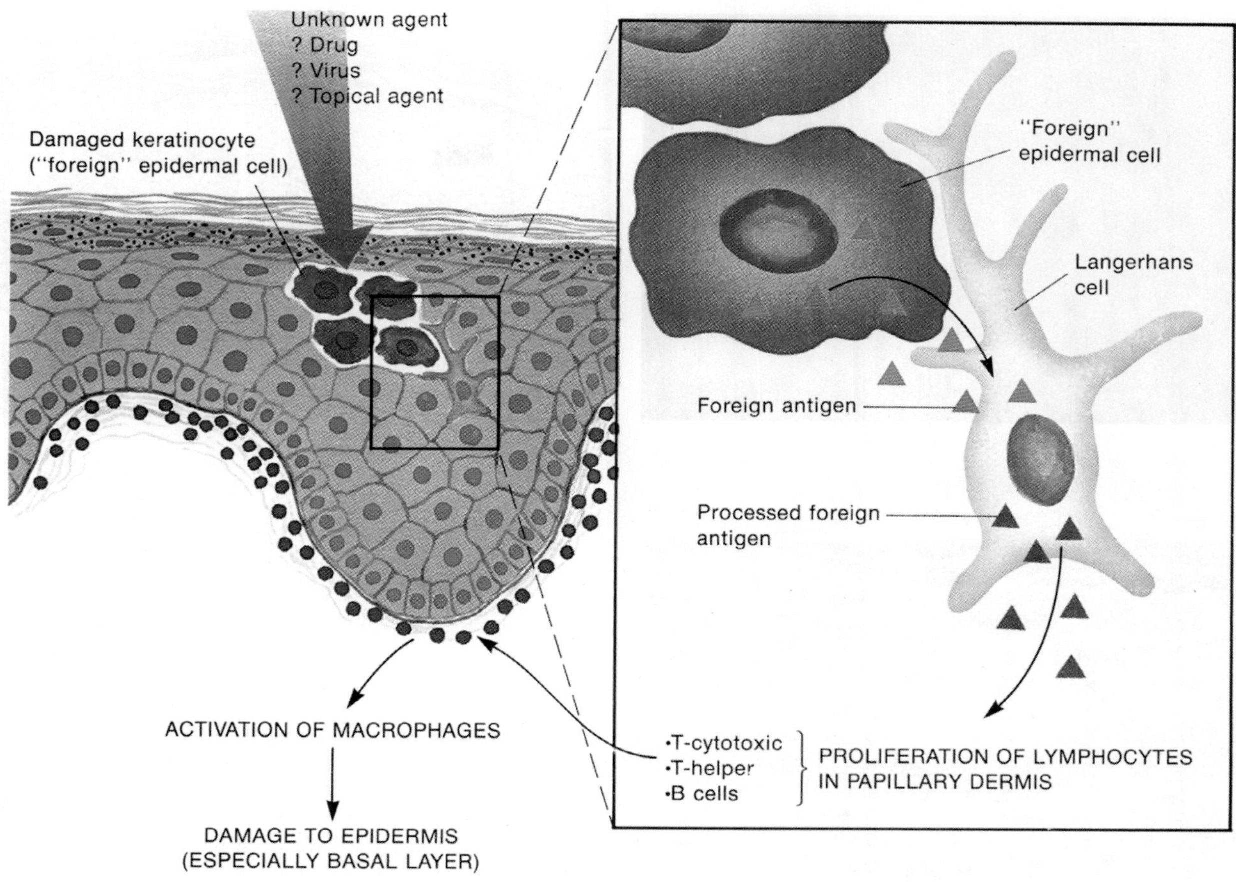

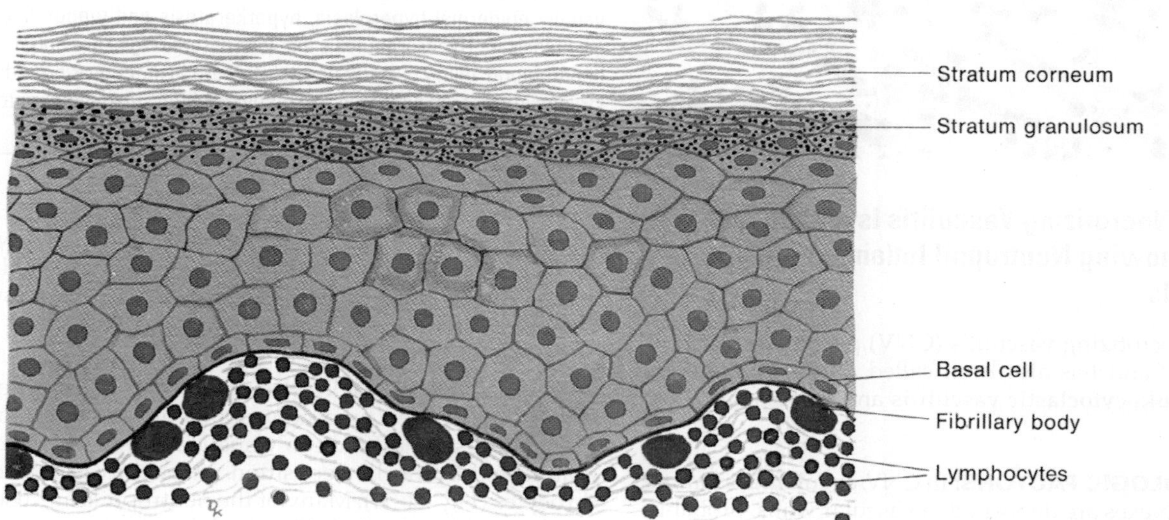

FIGURE 24-31. Lichen planus. Pathogenetic mechanisms are outlined. The disease is apparently initiated by epidermal injury. This injury causes some epidermal cells to be treated as "foreign." The antigens of such cells are processed by Langerhans cells. The processed antigen induces lymphocytic proliferation and macrophage activation. Macrophages, along with T lymphocytes, kill the epidermal basal cells, resulting in a reactive epidermal proliferation and the formation of fibrillary bodies.

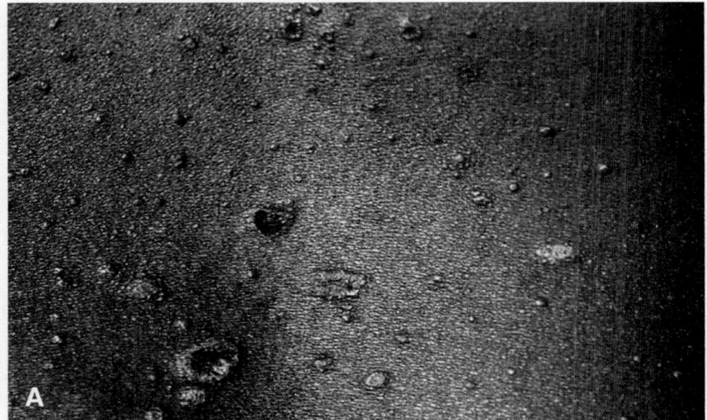

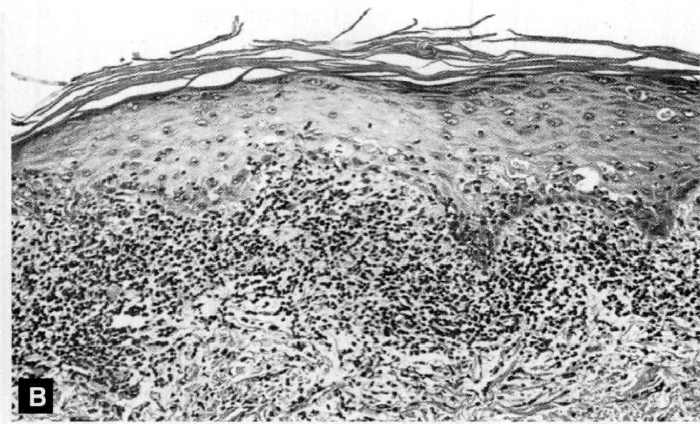

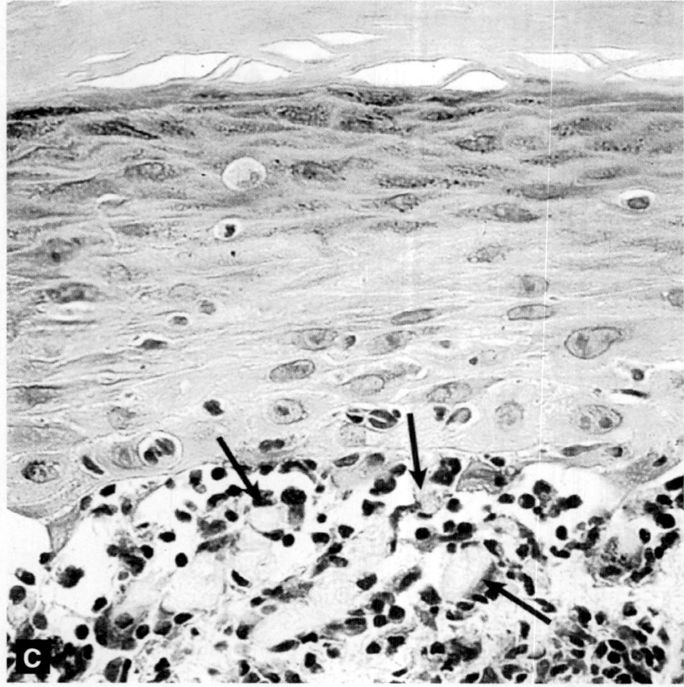

FIGURE 24-32. Lichen planus. A. The skin displays multiple flat-topped violaceous polygonal papules. **B.** A cell-rich, band-like, lymphocytic infiltrate disrupts the stratum basalis. Unlike lupus erythematosus, there is usually epidermal hyperplasia, hyperkeratosis and wedge-like hypergranulosis. **C.** Hypergranulosis and loss of rete ridges are noted. The site of pathologic injury is at the dermal-epidermal junction where there is a striking infiltrate of lymphocytes, many of which surround apoptotic keratinocytes (*arrows*).

Cutaneous Necrotizing Vasculitis Is an Immune Reaction Showing Neutrophil Inflammation of Vessel Walls

Cutaneous necrotizing vasculitis (CNV) presents as "palpable purpura," and has also been called **allergic cutaneous vasculitis, leukocytoclastic vasculitis** and **hypersensitivity angiitis.**

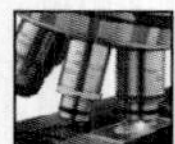

ETIOLOGIC FACTORS: In CNV, circulating immune complexes are deposited in vascular walls, probably at sites of injuries, at branch points where turbulence is increased or where venous circulation is slowed, as in the lower extremities. The elaborated C5a complement component attracts neutrophils, which degranulate and release lysosomal enzymes, causing endothelial damage and fibrin deposition (Fig. 24-33).

CNV may be either primary, without a known precipitating event in about half of the cases, or associated with a specific infectious agent (e.g., hepatitis B virus [HBV] or hepatitis C virus [HCV]). It may also be a secondary process in a variety of chronic diseases, such as rheumatoid arthritis, SLE and ulcerative colitis. CNV may also be associated with (1) underlying malignancies such as lymphoma, (2) a drug or some other allergy or (3) a postinfectious process such as Henoch-Schönlein purpura.

PATHOLOGY: The lesions of CNV show vessel walls obliterated by a neutrophilic infiltrate. Endothelial cells are difficult to visualize and vessel damage is manifested by fibrin deposition and extravasation of erythrocytes (Fig. 24-34). Many of the neutrophils are also damaged, resulting in dust-like nuclear remnants, a process known as "leukocytoclasia." The collagen fibers between affected vessels are separated by neutrophils, eosinophils and leukocytoclastic cellular remnants, as well as the extravasated erythrocytes that account for the characteristic palpable purpura.

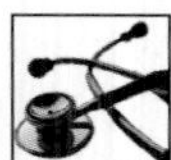

CLINICAL FEATURES: CNV is distinguished by 2- to 4-mm purpuric papules that are red, palpable lesions that do not blanch under pressure ("palpable

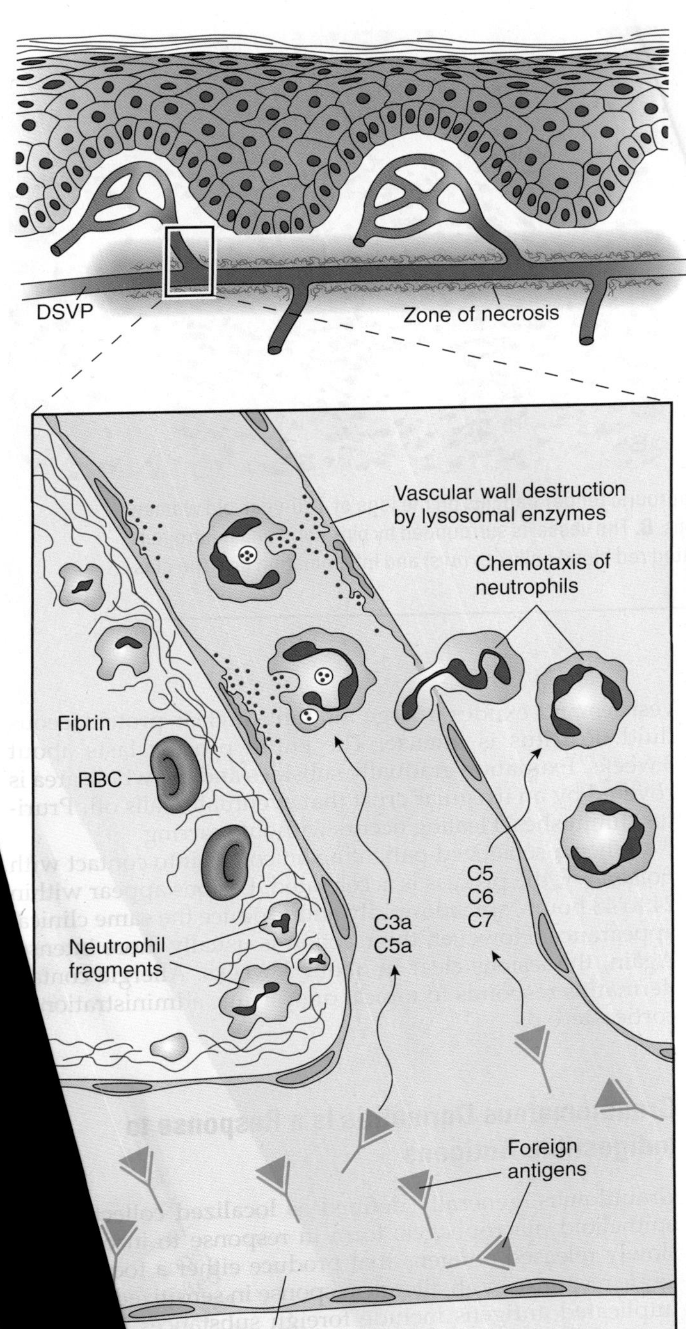

Cutaneous necrotizing vasculitis. The pathogenesis of … is depicted. The site of the vascular pathology is indi… …pper diagram. Circulating immune complexes activate … …ere is neutrophilic chemotaxis (*C5a*) and neutrophilic … …cular damage occurs, with extravasation of erythro… …sition and leukocytoclasia. DSVP = deep superficial … …C = red blood cell.

…4-34). Multiple lesions characteristically … the lower extremities or at sites of pres… …be confined to the skin in an otherwise … may involve small blood vessels in the …l (GI) tract or kidney. Individual lesions … …onth and then resolve, leaving hyperpigmentation or atrophic scars. Despite removal of the offending agent, episodes of CNV may recur.

Allergic Contact Dermatitis Is Cell-Mediated Hypersensitivity to Exogenous Sensitizing Agents

Some of the most common sensitizing agents are members of the *Rhus* genus of plants. Some 90% of the population of the United States is sensitive to the common offenders: *Rhus radicans* (poison ivy), *Rhus diversiloba* (poison oak) and *Rhus vernix* (poison sumac). These plant dermatitides are so well known that the resultant disease is commonly labeled according to the offending plant. Patients definitively state "I have poison ivy" and go to the physician for relief rather than for diagnosis.

ETIOLOGIC FACTORS: The offending plant contains low–molecular-weight compounds called **haptens,** in particular, oleoresins. These are not active in sensitization unless they combine with a carrier protein. This likely happens at the cell membrane of the Langerhans cell in the **sensitization phase,** a process that has been studied as a prototype of antigenic sensitization in delayed-type hypersensitivity. Formation of a hapten–carrier complex requires about 1 hour, after which it is processed as an antigen by the Langerhans cells. These cells carry the antigen through the lymphatics to regional lymph nodes and present the antigen to $CD4^+$ T lymphocytes (Fig. 24-35). After 5 to 7 days, some clones of these T lymphocytes become sensitized to the antigen, become activated, multiply and circulate in the blood as memory cells. Some migrate to the skin, ready to react with the antigen if they encounter it. IL-1, produced by Langerhans cells, supports proliferation of $CD4^+$ Th1 lymphocytes, the effector cells of delayed hypersensitivity.

In the **elicitation phase,** specifically sensitized T lymphocytes in the circulation enter the skin. At the site of antigen challenge, Langerhans cells, endothelial cells, perivascular dendritic cells and monocytes process the antigen and present it to the specifically sensitized T cells, which then migrate into the epidermis. Cytokine production leads to the accumulation of more T cells and macrophages. This inflammatory infiltrate is responsible for epidermal cell injury.

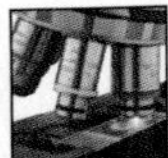

PATHOLOGY: Allergic contact dermatitis is a model of **spongiotic dermatitis.** In the 24 hours after reexposure to the offending plant (elicitation phase), numerous lymphocytes and macrophages accumulate about the superficial venular bed and extend into the epidermis. The epidermal keratinocytes are partially separated by the edema fluid, creating a sponge-like appearance **(spongiosis)** (Fig. 24-36). The stratum corneum contains coagulated eosinophilic fluid and plasma proteins. Later, numerous mononuclear inflammatory cells and eosinophils accumulate. Vesicles containing lymphocytes and macrophages are present, and large amounts of eosinophilic coagulated fluid accumulate in the stratum corneum.

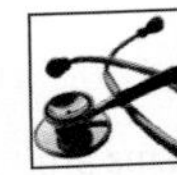

CLINICAL FEATURES: When a person first comes into contact with poison ivy, no immediate reaction occurs. Five to 7 days after reexposure, the site of contact becomes intensely pruritic, after which erythema and small vesicles rapidly develop (Fig. 24-36). Over the next few days, the area enlarges, becomes fiery red, develops numerous

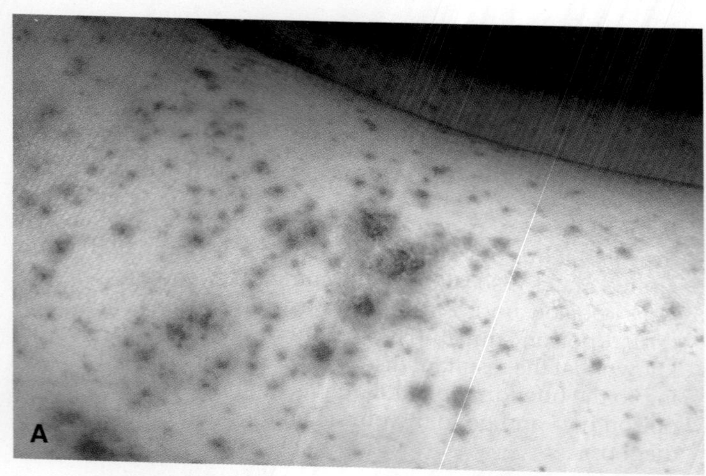
A

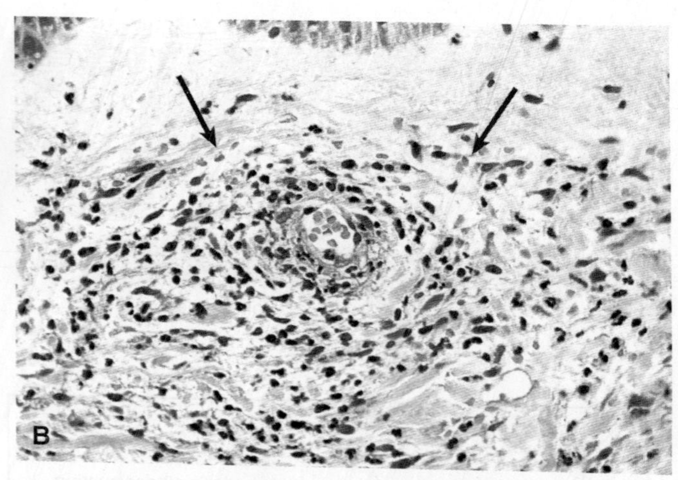
B

FIGURE 24-34. Cutaneous necrotizing vasculitis. A. Palpable purpuric tender papules on the legs of a 25-year-old woman. The condition resolved after therapy for streptococcal pharyngitis. **B.** The vessel is surrounded by pink fibrin and neutrophils, many of which have disintegrated (leukocytoclasis). Extravasated red blood cells (*arrows*) and inflammation give the classic clinical appearance of "palpable purpura."

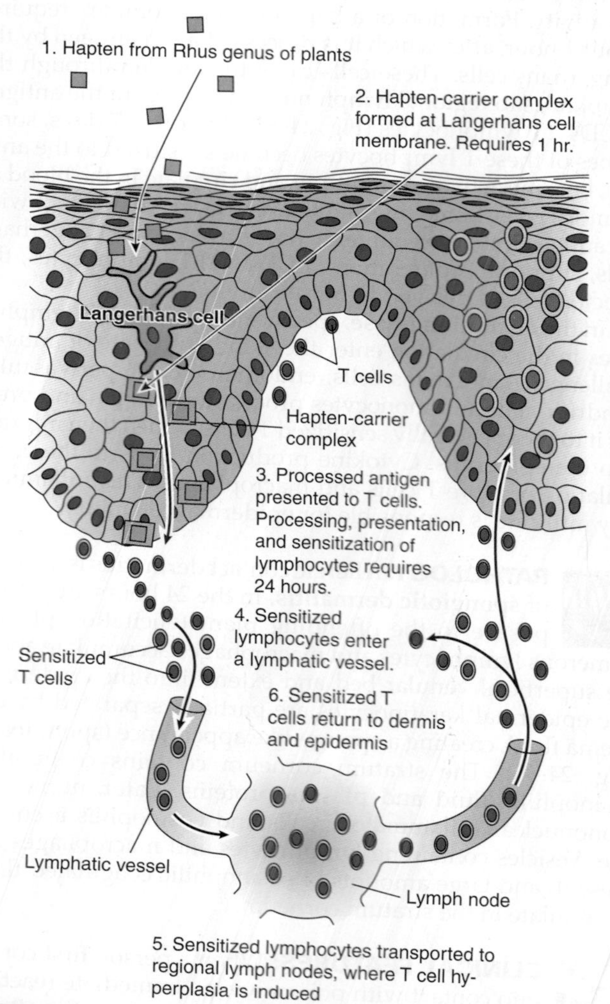
1. Hapten from Rhus genus of plants
2. Hapten-carrier complex formed at Langerhans cell membrane. Requires 1 hr.
Langerhans cell
T cells
Hapten-carrier complex
3. Processed antigen presented to T cells. Processing, presentation, and sensitization of lymphocytes requires 24 hours.
4. Sensitized lymphocytes enter a lymphatic vessel.
Sensitized T cells
6. Sensitized T cells return to dermis and epidermis
Lymphatic vessel
Lymph node
5. Sensitized lymphocytes transported to regional lymph nodes, where T cell hyperplasia is induced

FIGURE 24-35. Allergic contact dermatitis. Pathogenetic mechanisms are shown.

vesicles and exudes a large amount of clear proteinaceo fluid. Pruritus is intense. The entire process lasts ab 3 weeks. Exudation gradually subsides and the whole ar covered by an irregular crust that eventually falls off. tus diminishes. Healing occurs without scarring.

When a sensitized patient again comes into con poison ivy, the process is accelerated. Lesions app 24 to 48 hours, spread rapidly and produce the sa appearance. However, the reaction is usually m Again, the lesions clear in about 3 weeks. Al dermatitis responds to topical or systemic ad corticosteroids.

Granulomatous Dermatitis Is a Re Indigestible Antigens

Granulomas, generally defined as epithelioid macrophages, form in slowly released antigens that p lergic response or an allergic re Implicated antigens include accidentally into the skin (e. endogenous antigens such include mycobacterial an annulare. In many cases ing sarcoidosis, an incit cytosis of the forei of protein antigens macrophages as th tous epithelioid c

Sarcoidosi

Sarcoidosi ogy that skin, lymp

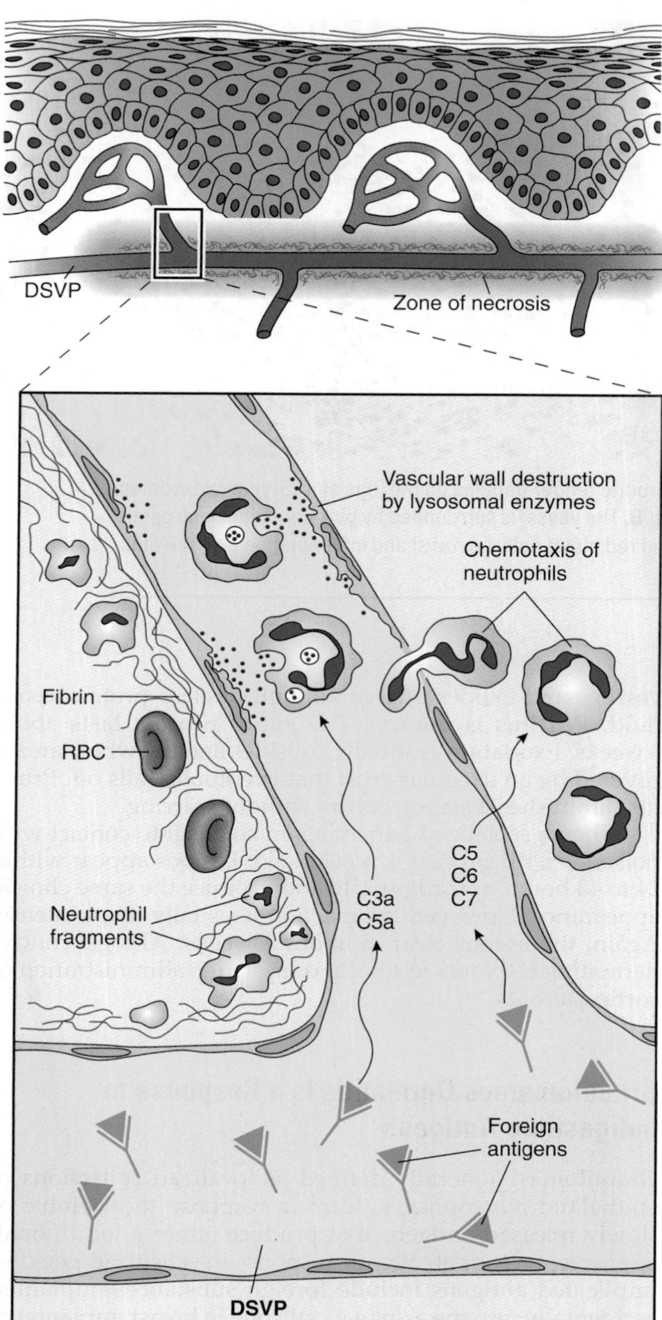

FIGURE 24-33. Cutaneous necrotizing vasculitis. The pathogenesis of vessel damage is depicted. The site of the vascular pathology is indicated in the *upper diagram.* Circulating immune complexes activate complement. There is neutrophilic chemotaxis (*C5a*) and neutrophilic destruction. Vascular damage occurs, with extravasation of erythrocytes, fibrin deposition and leukocytoclasia. DSVP = deep superficial venular plexus; RBC = red blood cell.

purpura") (Fig. 24-34). Multiple lesions characteristically appear in crops on the lower extremities or at sites of pressure. Lesions may be confined to the skin in an otherwise healthy person, or may involve small blood vessels in the joints, gastrointestinal (GI) tract or kidney. Individual lesions persist for up to a month and then resolve, leaving hyperpigmentation or atrophic scars. Despite removal of the offending agent, episodes of CNV may recur.

Allergic Contact Dermatitis Is Cell-Mediated Hypersensitivity to Exogenous Sensitizing Agents

Some of the most common sensitizing agents are members of the *Rhus* genus of plants. Some 90% of the population of the United States is sensitive to the common offenders: *Rhus radicans* (poison ivy), *Rhus diversiloba* (poison oak) and *Rhus vernix* (poison sumac). These plant dermatitides are so well known that the resultant disease is commonly labeled according to the offending plant. Patients definitively state "I have poison ivy" and go to the physician for relief rather than for diagnosis.

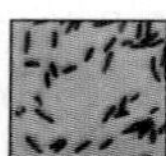

ETIOLOGIC FACTORS: The offending plant contains low–molecular-weight compounds called **haptens,** in particular, oleoresins. These are not active in sensitization unless they combine with a carrier protein. This likely happens at the cell membrane of the Langerhans cell in the **sensitization phase,** a process that has been studied as a prototype of antigenic sensitization in delayed-type hypersensitivity. Formation of a hapten–carrier complex requires about 1 hour, after which it is processed as an antigen by the Langerhans cells. These cells carry the antigen through the lymphatics to regional lymph nodes and present the antigen to CD4$^+$ T lymphocytes (Fig. 24-35). After 5 to 7 days, some clones of these T lymphocytes become sensitized to the antigen, become activated, multiply and circulate in the blood as memory cells. Some migrate to the skin, ready to react with the antigen if they encounter it. IL-1, produced by Langerhans cells, supports proliferation of CD4$^+$ Th1 lymphocytes, the effector cells of delayed hypersensitivity.

In the **elicitation phase,** specifically sensitized T lymphocytes in the circulation enter the skin. At the site of antigen challenge, Langerhans cells, endothelial cells, perivascular dendritic cells and monocytes process the antigen and present it to the specifically sensitized T cells, which then migrate into the epidermis. Cytokine production leads to the accumulation of more T cells and macrophages. This inflammatory infiltrate is responsible for epidermal cell injury.

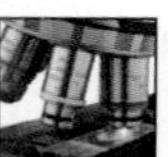

PATHOLOGY: Allergic contact dermatitis is a model of **spongiotic dermatitis.** In the 24 hours after reexposure to the offending plant (elicitation phase), numerous lymphocytes and macrophages accumulate about the superficial venular bed and extend into the epidermis. The epidermal keratinocytes are partially separated by the edema fluid, creating a sponge-like appearance **(spongiosis)** (Fig. 24-36). The stratum corneum contains coagulated eosinophilic fluid and plasma proteins. Later, numerous mononuclear inflammatory cells and eosinophils accumulate. Vesicles containing lymphocytes and macrophages are present, and large amounts of eosinophilic coagulated fluid accumulate in the stratum corneum.

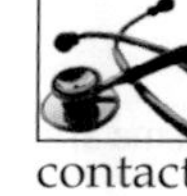

CLINICAL FEATURES: When a person first comes into contact with poison ivy, no immediate reaction occurs. Five to 7 days after reexposure, the site of contact becomes intensely pruritic, after which erythema and small vesicles rapidly develop (Fig. 24-36). Over the next few days, the area enlarges, becomes fiery red, develops numerous

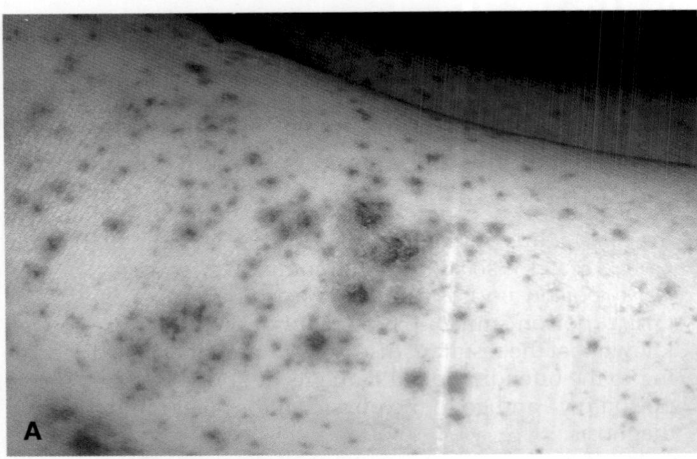
A

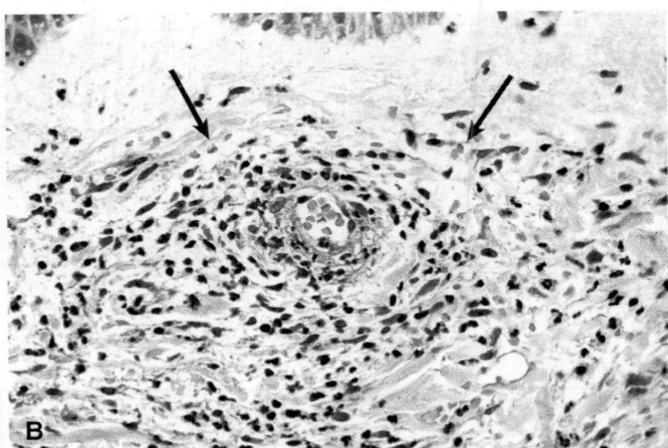
B

FIGURE 24-34. Cutaneous necrotizing vasculitis. A. Palpable purpuric tender papules on the legs of a 25-year-old woman. The condition resolved after therapy for streptococcal pharyngitis. **B.** The vessel is surrounded by pink fibrin and neutrophils, many of which have disintegrated (leukocytoclasis). Extravasated red blood cells (*arrows*) and inflammation give the classic clinical appearance of "palpable purpura."

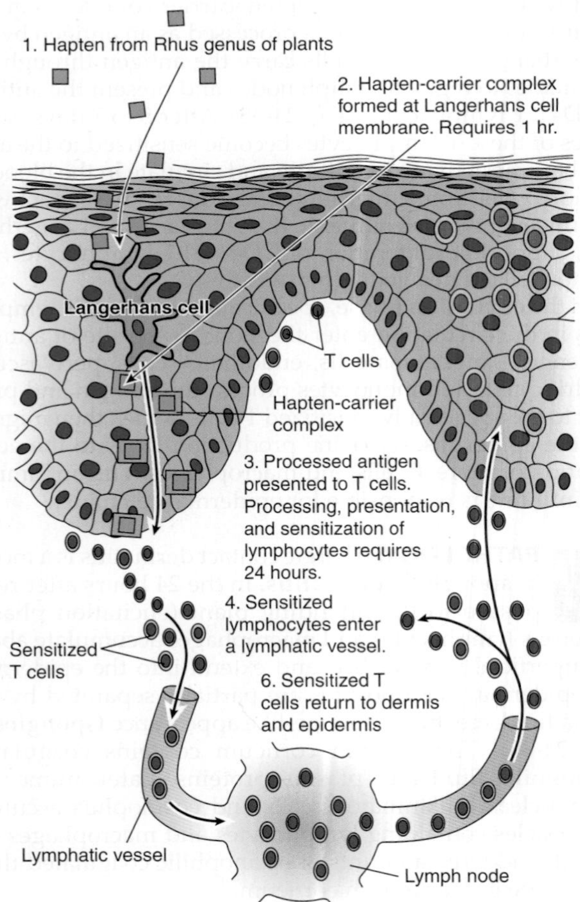
1. Hapten from Rhus genus of plants
2. Hapten-carrier complex formed at Langerhans cell membrane. Requires 1 hr.
Langerhans cell
T cells
Hapten-carrier complex
3. Processed antigen presented to T cells. Processing, presentation, and sensitization of lymphocytes requires 24 hours.
4. Sensitized lymphocytes enter a lymphatic vessel.
Sensitized T cells
6. Sensitized T cells return to dermis and epidermis
Lymphatic vessel
Lymph node
5. Sensitized lymphocytes transported to regional lymph nodes, where T cell hyperplasia is induced

FIGURE 24-35. Allergic contact dermatitis. Pathogenetic mechanisms are shown.

vesicles and exudes a large amount of clear proteinaceous fluid. Pruritus is intense. The entire process lasts about 3 weeks. Exudation gradually subsides and the whole area is covered by an irregular crust that eventually falls off. Pruritus diminishes. Healing occurs without scarring.

When a sensitized patient again comes into contact with poison ivy, the process is accelerated. Lesions appear within 24 to 48 hours, spread rapidly and produce the same clinical appearance. However, the reaction is usually more intense. Again, the lesions clear in about 3 weeks. Allergic contact dermatitis responds to topical or systemic administration of corticosteroids.

Granulomatous Dermatitis Is a Response to Indigestible Antigens

Granulomas, generally defined as localized collections of epithelioid macrophages, form in response to insoluble or slowly released antigens that produce either a focal nonallergic response or an allergic response in sensitized persons. Implicated antigens include foreign substances implanted accidentally into the skin (e.g., silicone in breast implants) or endogenous antigens such as keratin. Other common causes include mycobacterial and other infections and granuloma annulare. In many cases of granulomatous dermatitis, including sarcoidosis, an inciting antigen may not be known. Phagocytosis of the foreign particulate matter, or processing of protein antigens, is central to the activation of tissue macrophages as they become the characteristic granulomatous epithelioid cells.

Sarcoidosis May Lead to Skin Lesions

Sarcoidosis is a granulomatous disorder of unknown etiology that primarily affects the lungs but may also involve the skin, lymph nodes, spleen, eyes and other organs. Sarcoidal

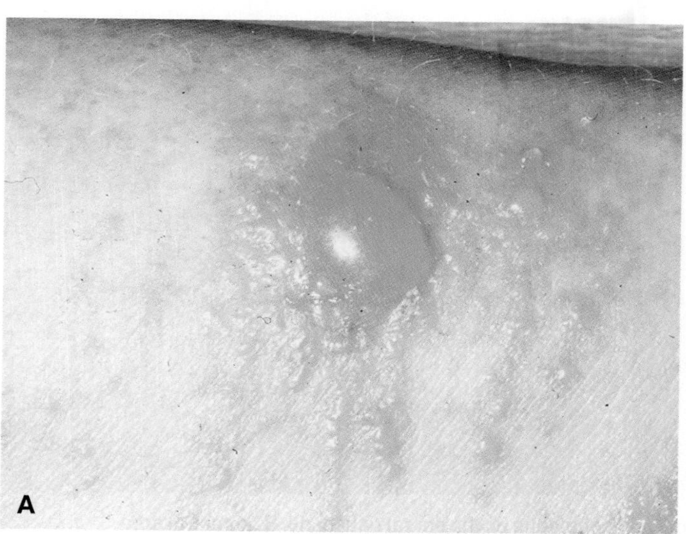
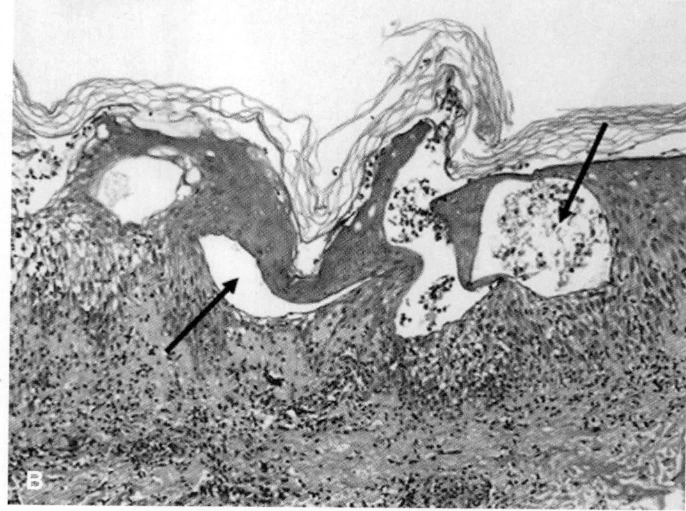

FIGURE 24-36. Allergic contact dermatitis. A. Vesicles and bullae developed on the volar forearm after application of perfume. **B.** Epidermal spongiosis and spongiotic vesicles (*arrows*) are present in this biopsy of "poison ivy." Infiltrating lymphocytes are apparent in the epidermis, where they effect the cell-mediated delayed hypersensitivity reaction.

granulomas are the classic epithelioid cell type, without caseation necrosis (Fig. 24-37). Cutaneous manifestations of sarcoidosis are asymptomatic papules, plaques and nodules in the dermis and subcutis. Some dermal plaques may be annular, and those that involve the subcutis appear as irregular nodules. In severe cases, cutaneous lesions may be so prominent that they simulate a diffuse infiltrative neoplasm.

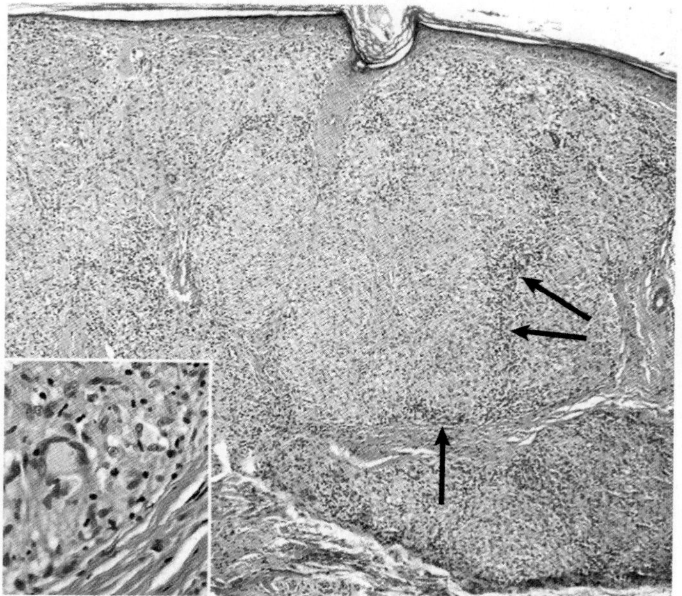

FIGURE 24-37. Sarcoidosis. Numerous large granulomas fill the reticular dermis. Around some of the granulomas are small cuffs of lymphocytes (*arrows*). The granulomas are composed of epithelioid macrophages, some of which are multinucleated (*inset*).

Granuloma Annulare Is a Reaction to an Unknown Antigen

Granuloma annulare is a benign, self-limited disorder of unknown etiology, characterized by palisading "necrobiotic" granulomas in the skin.

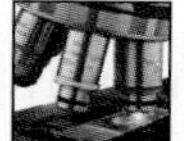

ETIOLOGIC FACTORS: Granuloma annulare may be an immunologically mediated reaction to an unknown antigen. It can occur following insect bites, sun exposure and viral infections. Antigenic stimuli are thought to include viral antigens, altered dermal collagen or elastic fibers or proteins in the saliva of biting arthropods. The precise type of immune reaction is unclear, but both circulating immune complexes and cell-mediated immunity may be involved. The activated macrophages may themselves contribute to the disease process by releasing lysosomal enzymes and cytokines that in turn cause the focal collagen degeneration ("necrobiosis") characteristic of granuloma annulare.

PATHOLOGY: Well-developed lesions contain a central area of acellular degenerated collagen and mucin in the superficial to midreticular dermis (Fig. 24-38). This central area is surrounded by palisaded macrophages, each with the long axis of the nucleus radiating outward.

CLINICAL FEATURES: The most common type of granuloma annulare occurs on the dorsum of the hands and feet, primarily in children and young adults (Fig. 24-38A). The disease features asymptomatic, skin-colored or erythematous annular plaques. About 15% of patients have disseminated granuloma annulare, with 10 or more lesions involving the trunk and neck. Granuloma annulare rarely requires treatment and usually has no medical consequences. In patients with significant cosmetic disfigurement, lesional injection of steroids is usually effective.

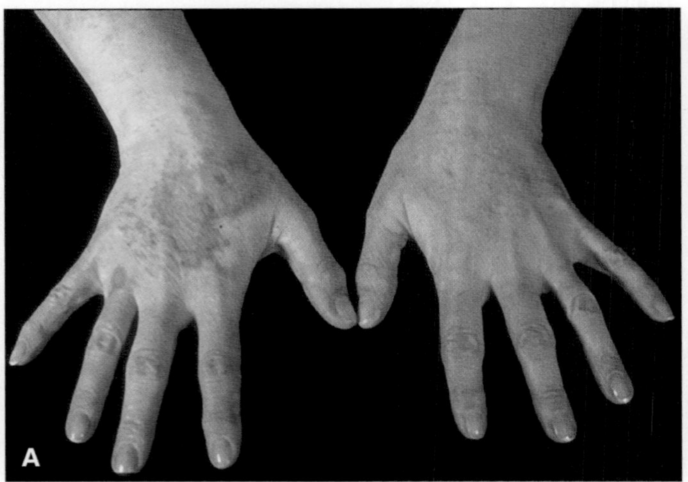

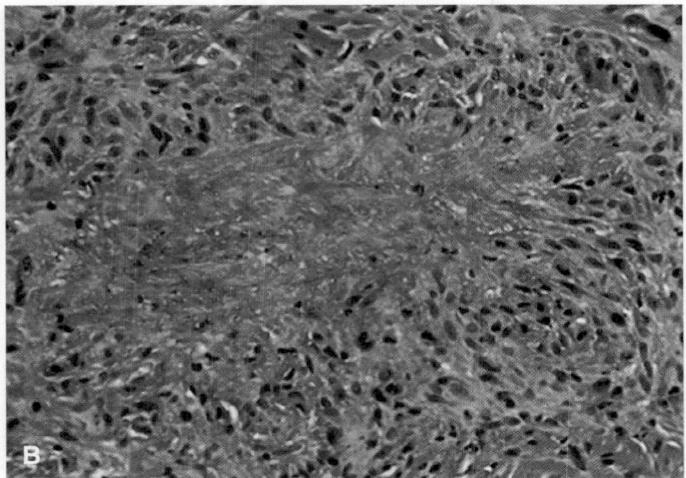

FIGURE 24-38. Granuloma annulare. A. The skin exhibits a typical annular plaque on the dorsal right hand. **B.** A central area of acellular degenerated collagen is surrounded by palisaded macrophages with the long axes of their nuclei radiating outward.

Scleroderma: A Disorder of the Dermal Connective Tissue

Scleroderma (Greek, *skleros*, "hard") also displays variable structural and functional involvement of internal organs, including the kidneys, lungs, heart, esophagus and small intestine. **Morphea** is similar to scleroderma, but involves only patchy, circumscribed areas of the skin. The pathogenesis and systemic manifestations of scleroderma are discussed elsewhere (see Chapters 4 and 16).

PATHOLOGY: The initial cutaneous lesions of scleroderma are in the lower reticular dermis, but eventually the entire reticular dermis and even the papillary dermis are involved. There is diminished space among collagen bundles in the reticular dermis and a tendency for the collagen bundles to be enlarged, hypocellular and parallel to each other. A patchy lymphocytic infiltrate containing a few plasma cells is common and may also be present in the underlying subcutaneous tissue. Sweat ducts are entrapped in the thickened fibrous tissue and the fat that is usually around them is lost. Hair follicles are completely obliterated (Fig. 24-39). In late stages of the disease, large areas of subcutaneous fat are replaced by newly formed collagen.

CLINICAL FEATURES: Scleroderma shows a peak incidence in persons between 30 and 50 years of age. Women are afflicted four times as often as men. Patients with early scleroderma usually present with Raynaud phenomenon or nonpitting edema of the hands or fingers. Affected areas become hard and tense. The skin of the face becomes mask-like and expressionless, and the skin around the mouth exhibits radial furrows. In late stages of the disease, the skin over large parts of the body is thickened, densely fibrotic and fixed to the underlying tissue. Prognosis is related to the extent of disease in visceral organs, particularly the lung and kidney.

Inflammatory Disorders of the Panniculus

Panniculitis denotes a heterogeneous group of diseases characterized by inflammation, mainly in the subcutis (panniculus). The various disorders gathered under the umbrella of

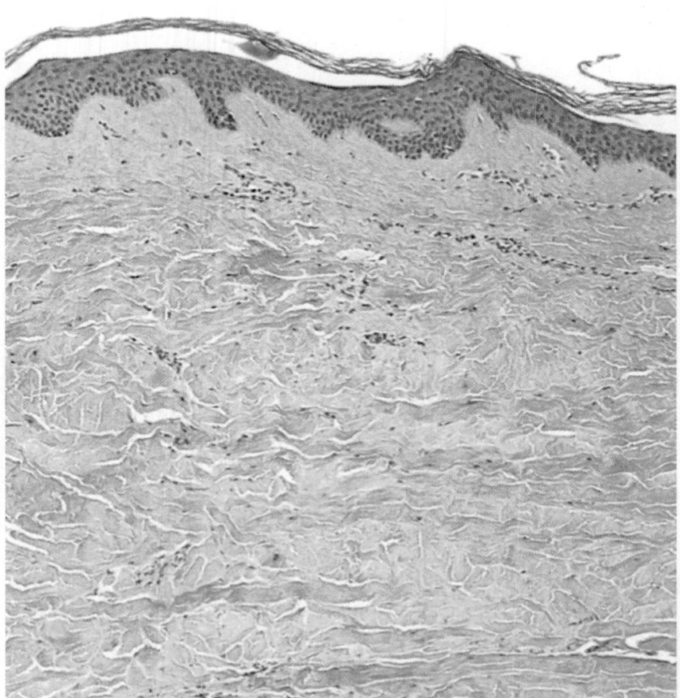

FIGURE 24-39. Scleroderma. The dermis is characterized by large, reticular collagen bundles that are oriented parallel to the epidermis. The large size and loss of basket-weave pattern of these collagen bundles are abnormal. No appendages are apparent because these structures have been destroyed.

panniculitis are classified according to their location. **Septal panniculitis** is inflammation in connective tissue septa, whereas **lobular panniculitis** denotes involvement of fat lobules. These two entities may occur with or without accompanying vasculitis.

Erythema Nodosum Is Related to Toxic and Infectious Agents

Erythema nodosum (EN) is a cutaneous disorder that manifests as self-limited, nonsuppurative, tender nodules over the extensor surfaces of the lower extremities. The disease has a peak incidence in the third decade of life and is three times more common in women than in men.

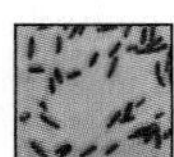

ETIOLOGIC FACTORS: EN is triggered by exposure to a variety of agents, including drugs and microorganisms, and occurs in association with a number of benign and malignant systemic diseases. Common infections complicated by EN include streptococcal diseases (especially in children), tuberculosis and *Yersinia* infection. In endemic areas deep fungal infections (blastomycosis, histoplasmosis, coccidioidomycosis) are common causes. EN also frequently occurs after acute respiratory tract infections of unknown etiology, but which are likely viral. The agents most commonly implicated in drug-induced EN are sulfonamides and oral contraceptives. Finally, Crohn disease and ulcerative colitis may be complicated by EN.

It is thought that EN represents an immunologic response to foreign antigens, although the evidence is indirect. For example, patients with tuberculosis or coccidioidomycosis do not develop EN until skin tests for reactions to antigens of those infectious agents become positive, and testing with Frei antigen for lymphogranuloma venereum may itself induce EN. The early neutrophilic inflammation suggests that EN may be a response to complement activation, with resulting neutrophilic chemotaxis. Subsequent chronic inflammation, foreign body giant cells and fibrosis are secondary to adipose tissue necrosis at the interface of septa and lobules.

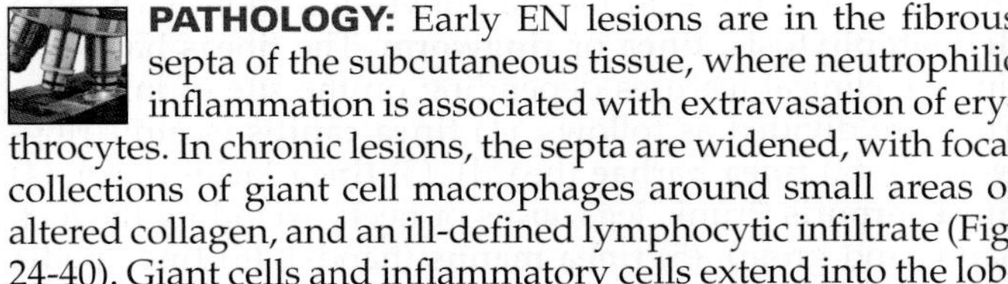

PATHOLOGY: Early EN lesions are in the fibrous septa of the subcutaneous tissue, where neutrophilic inflammation is associated with extravasation of erythrocytes. In chronic lesions, the septa are widened, with focal collections of giant cell macrophages around small areas of altered collagen, and an ill-defined lymphocytic infiltrate (Fig. 24-40). Giant cells and inflammatory cells extend into the lobule from the interface between the septum and the fat lobule.

CLINICAL FEATURES: EN typically manifests acutely on the anterior aspects of the lower limbs as dome-shaped, exquisitely tender, erythematous nodules. These nodules eventually become firm and less tender, and disappear in 3 to 6 weeks. As some nodules heal, others may arise, but all lesions resolve without residual scarring within 6 weeks.

Erythema Induratum Is Frequently Associated With *Mycobacterium tuberculosis*

Erythema induratum (EI) refers to chronic, recurrent subcutaneous nodules or plaques on the legs, predominantly in women. EI was traditionally considered a "tuberculid" (i.e., a hypersensitivity reaction to mycobacteria or associated antigens at a distant site). Although lesional tissue does not yield mycobacteria in culture or in laboratory animals, a specific *Mycobacterium tuberculosis* DNA sequence is detectable in over 75% of skin biopsy specimens with EI.

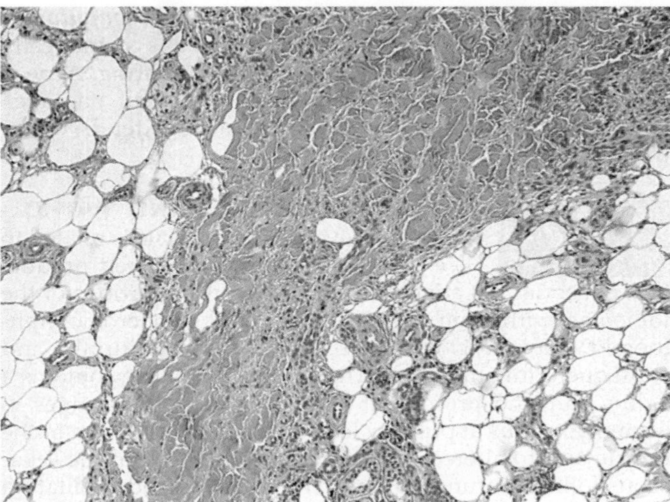

FIGURE 24-40. Erythema nodosum. The reticular dermis is present in the *upper right*. Within the panniculus is a widened septum (*extending through the middle of the field*). Lymphocytes and macrophages are present at its interface with the adipose tissue lobules. The vessels palisading along the interface of the septum are infiltrated by lymphocytes.

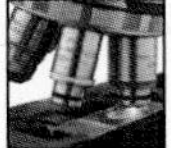

PATHOLOGY: In contrast to EN, which is a septal panniculitis, EI manifests initially as a lobular panniculitis, secondary to a vasculitis that produces ischemic necrosis of the fat lobule. The panniculus exhibits a dense, chronic inflammatory infiltrate within the lobules, which can form prominent tuberculoid granulomas or result in areas of coagulative necrosis. The septa around the lobules are relatively spared. Vascular changes are usually extensive and include (1) prominent infiltration of small and medium-sized arteries and veins by a dense lymphoid or granulomatous infiltrate; (2) endothelial swelling, which may progress to thrombosis; and (3) fibrous thickening of the intima. These changes give rise to the alternative nomenclature of this condition as "nodular vasculitis." Extensive ischemic necrosis leads to subsequent ulceration of the overlying epidermis. Eventually, lesions heal by fibrosis.

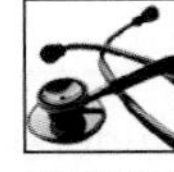

CLINICAL FEATURES: Patients with EI present with recurrent, tender, erythematous, subcutaneous nodules on the legs, particularly the calves (as opposed to the shins, which are the usual location of EN). Lesions tend to ulcerate and heal with an atrophic scar. The course may last many years, and systemic steroids are usually necessary to control the disease.

Acne Vulgaris: A Disorder of the Pilosebaceous Unit

Acne vulgaris is a self-limited, inflammatory disorder of sebaceous follicles that typically afflicts adolescents,

results in intermittent formation of discrete papular or pustular lesions and may lead to scarring. It is cosmetically disfiguring and often psychologically debilitating. Acne is so common that many regard it as a "rite of passage" through adolescence. In some cases, acne extends to the third decade.

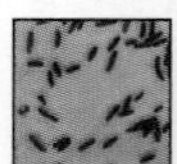
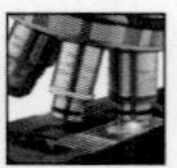

ETIOLOGIC FACTORS AND PATHOLOGY: The development of acne is related to (1) excessive hormonally induced production of sebum, (2) abnormal cornification of portions of the follicular epithelium, (3) a response to the anaerobic diphtheroid *Propionibacterium acnes* and (4) follicle rupture and subsequent inflammation. The sebaceous follicle contains a vellus hair and prominent sebaceous glands. Changes in hormonal status at puberty lead to sebum production in the follicle and to altered cornification in the neck of the sebaceous follicle (infundibulum). These effects lead to dilation of the follicular canal. Another round of excessive sebum production is associated with desquamation of squamous cells and accretion of keratinous debris, providing a rich environment for *P. acnes* proliferation. These combined changes produce a distended, plugged follicle: a **comedone.** Neutrophils attracted to the area by chemotactic factors released by *P. acnes* release hydrolytic enzymes to form a follicular abscess **(pustule).** They also attack the follicle wall, thereby permitting escape of sebum, keratin and bacteria into perifollicular tissue, where they stimulate further acute inflammation and a perifollicular abscess (Fig. 24-41). The development of allergy to *P. acnes* intensifies the inflammatory response. Fully evolved lesions show intense neutrophilic inflammation surrounding a ruptured sebaceous follicle. In addition, numerous macrophages, lymphocytes and foreign body giant cells accumulate in response to sebaceous follicle rupture.

CLINICAL FEATURES: Acne vulgaris features a variety of skin lesions in different stages of development, including comedones, papules, pustules, nodules, cysts and pitted scars. Comedones, the primary noninflammatory lesions of acne, are either open **(blackheads)** or closed **(whiteheads).** More advanced inflammatory lesions vary from small, erythematous papules to large, tender, purulent nodules and cysts.

Acne vulgaris is treated with topical cleansing and keratolytic and antibacterial agents. Severe cases are managed with topical vitamin A, systemic antibiotics or synthetic oral retinoids (isotretinoin).

Infections and Infestations

The skin is under constant assault from countless marauders and is an effective but imperfect barrier against them: bacteria, fungi, viruses, parasites and insects sometimes penetrate this first line of defense.

Impetigo Is a Cutaneous Infection by Staphylococci or Streptococci

Superficial bacterial infections of the skin, known as **impetigo,** occur mostly in children, who are often infected through minor breaks in the skin. Adults tend to contract impetigo after an underlying disease process that somehow compromises the barrier function of the skin. Honey-colored crusted erosions or ulcers, often with central healing, are present most commonly on exposed areas such as the face, hands and extremities (Fig. 24-42). A combination of topical and systemic antimicrobial agents against staphylococci or streptococci is the mainstay of therapy. **Ecthyma** occurs when the organisms invade the superficial aspects of the skin to form a necrotizing ulcerated lesion with neutrophils present in the floor of the ulcer and in the dermis.

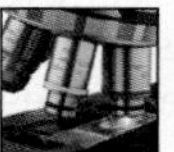

PATHOLOGY: Microscopically, neutrophils accumulate beneath the stratum corneum. Bacteria may be identified with special stains. Vesicles or bullae form and eventually rupture, allowing a thin, seropurulent discharge to appear. This discharge dries and forms the characteristic layers of exudate containing neutrophils and cellular debris. Reactive epidermal changes (spongiosis and elongation of rete ridges) and superficial dermal inflammation are usually present.

Superficial Fungal Infections Are Caused by Dermatophytes

Dermatophytes are fungi that can infect nonviable keratinized epithelium, including stratum corneum, nails and hair. They synthesize keratinases that digest keratin and provide sustenance for the organisms. Superficial fungal infections are often caused by a change in the microenvironment of the skin, which allows overgrowth of transient or resident flora. For example, use of immunosuppressive agents such as topical or systemic glucocorticoids may impair cell-mediated immune responses that normally eliminate dermatophytes. Excessive sweating or occlusion of a body part may provide an environment that "tips the balance" between fungal proliferation and elimination in favor of proliferation.

Of the 10 or so dermatophyte species that often cause human cutaneous infection, *Trichophyton rubrum* is the most common. A superficial dermatophyte infection is called a **dermatophytosis, tinea** or **ringworm.** The tineas have distinctive clinical features depending on the site of infection. They are divided as follows: (1) **tinea capitis** (scalp; "ringworm"), (2) **tinea barbae** (beard), (3) **tinea faciei** (face), (4) **tinea corporis** (trunk, legs, arms or neck, excluding the feet, hands and groin), (5) **tinea manus** (hands), (6) **tinea pedis** (feet; "athlete's foot"; Fig. 24-43A), (7) **tinea cruris** (groin, pubic area and thigh; "jock itch") and (8) **tinea unguium** (nails; "onychomycosis").

Other causes of superficial fungal infections are *Candida* sp. and *Malassezia furfur. Candida* sp. require a warm, moist environment in which to flourish, such as that found when a baby's bottom is encased in a wet diaper. *M. furfur* requires a moist, lipid-rich environment. **Tinea versicolor,** caused by *M. furfur,* is more common in young adults when sebum production is greatest. Variably sized, pigmented, sharply demarcated, round or oval macules with fine scales are present, predominantly on the upper trunk.

Special stains such as PAS show budding yeast and hyphal forms in the most superficial layers of the stratum corneum. Hyperkeratosis, epidermal hyperplasia and chronic perivascular inflammation are noted in the dermis (Fig. 24-43B, C).

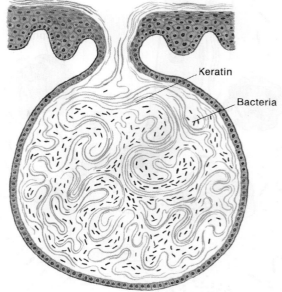

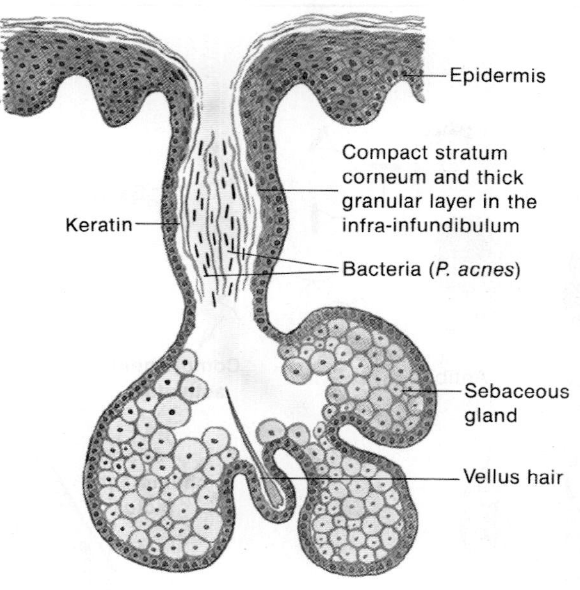

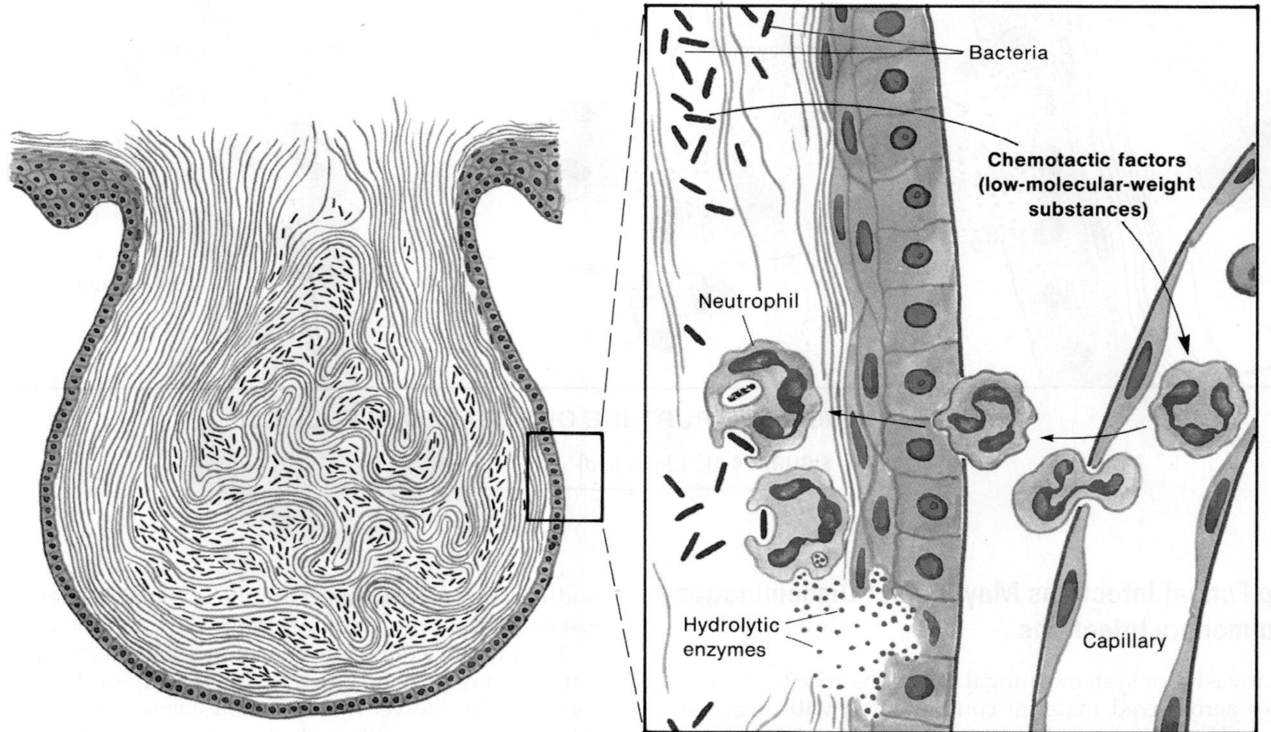

FIGURE 24-41. Acne vulgaris. The pathogenesis of follicular distention, rupture and inflammation is depicted. Acne is a disease of the follicular canal of a sebaceous follicle. A compact stratum corneum and a thickened granular layer in the infrainfundibulum are the beginning of the formation of a comedone. Microcomedones **(A)** and closed **(B)** and open **(C)** comedones form. Excessive sebum secretion occurs, and the bacterium *Propionibacterium acnes* proliferates. The organism produces chemotactic factors, leading to neutrophil migration into the intact comedone. Neutrophilic enzymes are released, and the comedone ruptures, inducing a cycle of chemotaxis and intense neutrophilic inflammation **(D, E)**. (*continued*)

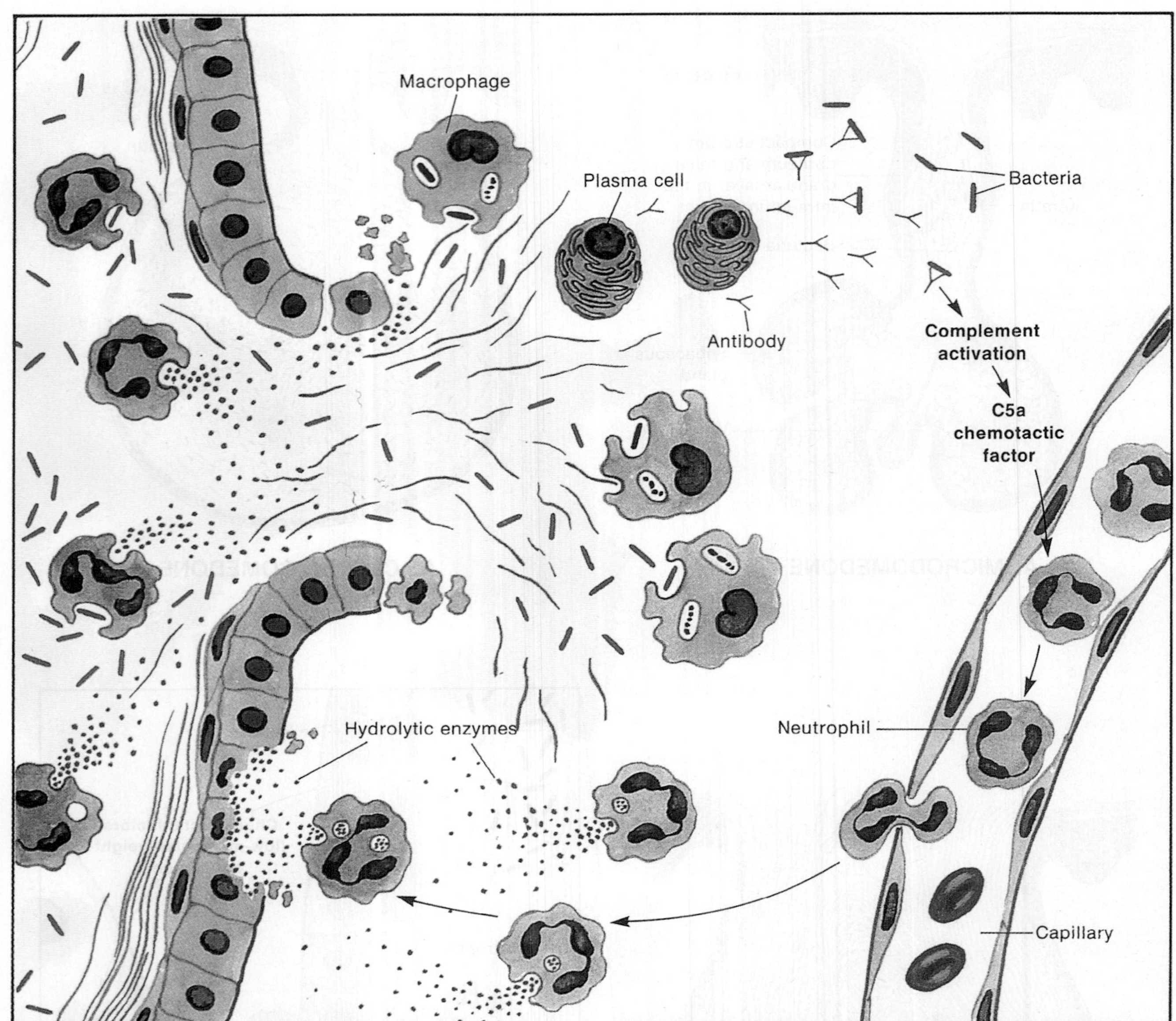

FIGURE 24-41. (*continued*)

Deep Fungal Infections May Reflect Dissemination of Pulmonary Infections

Most invasive or systemic fungal infections arise from inhalation of aerosolized material contaminated with organisms such as *Histoplasma* or *Blastomyces*. A primary pulmonary infection may then spread to the skin or mucosa. Locally invasive fungal infections of the skin are rare and usually arise from traumatic implantation of organisms such as *Sporothrix* or *Fonsecaea*. An underlying immunocompromised state increases the likelihood of dissemination of fungal organisms.

Deep extension of a local cutaneous infection often results in a chancre-like lesion at the site of implantation. Intervening lymphatic vessels may become indurated and thickened. Nodules and ulcers, especially those found bilaterally, suggest an internal source of infection.

The presence of certain morphologic features or staining patterns may provide clues to the identity of the organism. For example, the yeast form of *Blastomyces dermatitidis* has notably refractile walls and a broad-based budding pattern, whereas the yeast form of *Histoplasma capsulatum* is much smaller, is often found within macrophages and shows a narrow-based budding pattern. Staining a smear with India ink, or a tissue biopsy with mucicarmine, may show the thick capsule characteristic of the yeast *Cryptococcus neoformans*. Marked epidermal hyperplasia, intraepidermal microabscesses and suppurative granulomatous inflammation in the dermis may be associated with these deep-seated fungal infections (Fig. 24-44).

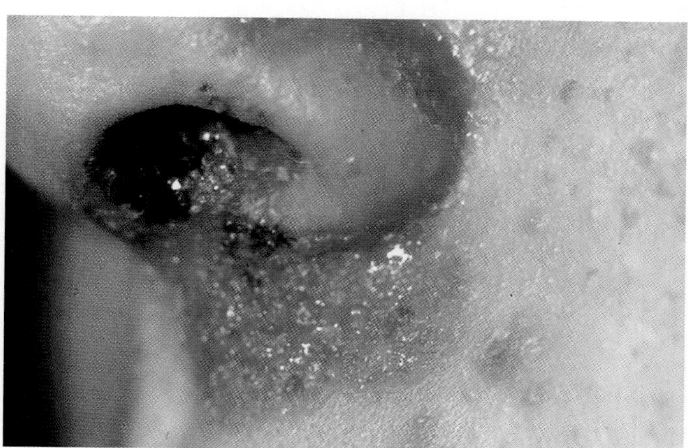

FIGURE 24-42. Impetigo contagiosa. Honey-colored crusts secondary to rupture of vesicopustules are seen in the nasal area of a child, an area commonly colonized by *Staphylococcus aureus.*

Viral Skin Infections Are Common and Cause a Variety of Clinical Manifestations

Some viruses, such as the poxvirus **molluscum contagiosum** or **human papillomaviruses** (HPVs), cause transient benign epithelial proliferations that resolve spontaneously. Others (e.g., measles or *parvovirus* [**erythema infectiosum**]) cause febrile illnesses with self-limited cutaneous eruptions **(exanthems).** Primary infection by most **human herpesviruses** is often asymptomatic but results in a state of latent infection. Upon reactivation, the virus causes a painful, vesicular eruption.

Molluscum contagiosum is a common infection among children and sexually active adults. It is a self-limited infection that is easily spread by direct contact. Firm, dome-shaped, smooth-surfaced papules with a characteristic central umbilication are usually found on the face, trunk and anogenital area. Microscopic examination shows epidermal cells containing large intracytoplasmic inclusion bodies ("molluscum bodies"), which are found within cup-shaped areas that also exhibit verrucous (papillomatous) epidermal hyperplasia. Numerous viral particles are present within these inclusion bodies (Fig. 24-45).

Arthropod Infestations Produce Pruritic Skin Lesions

Mites and lice, other insects and spiders produce local lesions that may be intensely pruritic.

- *Scabies* is a severely pruritic, eczematous dermatitis caused by the mite *Sarcoptes scabei*. The female mite burrows beneath the stratum corneum on the fingers, wrists, trunk and genital skin (Fig. 24-46). Intense lymphocytic and

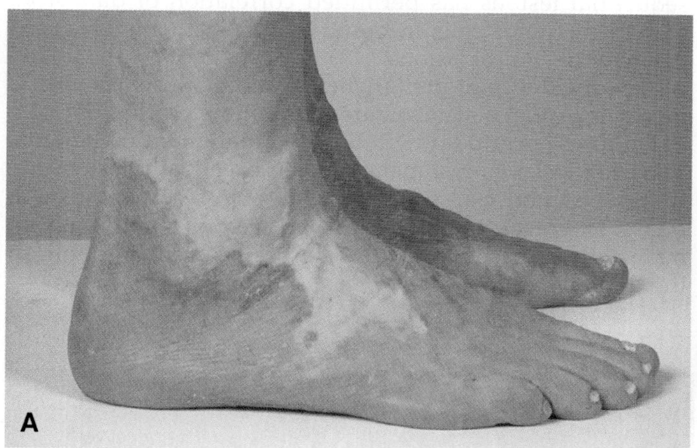

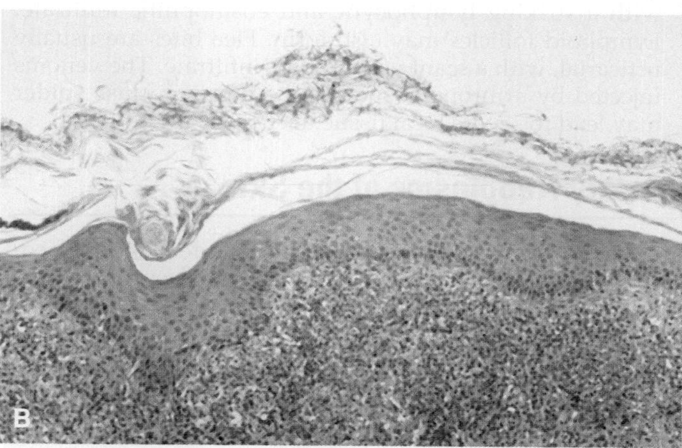

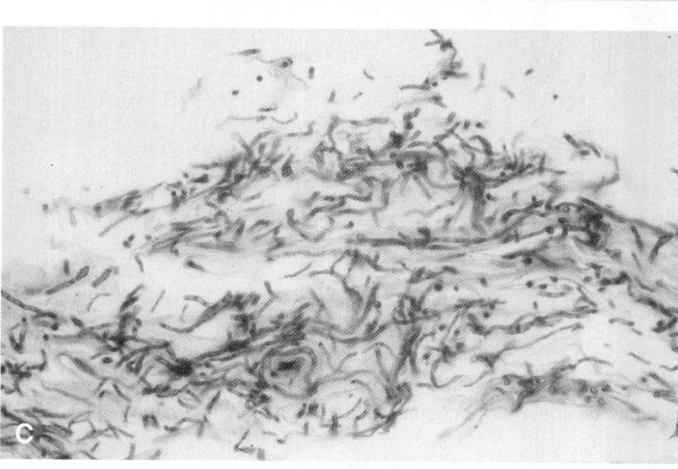

FIGURE 24-43. Dermatophytosis. A. Tinea pedis. A leading edge of scale and erythema in a moccasin distribution characterizes this infection, most commonly caused by *Trichophyton rubrum.* **B.** A dense inflammatory infiltrate is present in the epidermis and dermis and is associated with the presence of fungal hyphae in the stratum corneum. **C.** A higher power view of the fungal hyphae in the stratum corneum.

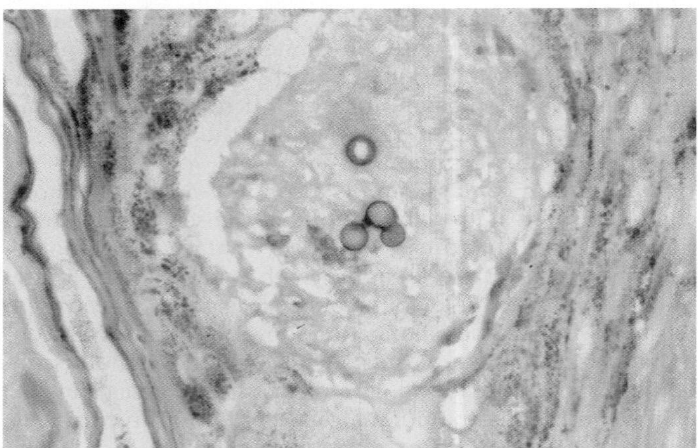

FIGURE 24-44. Blastomycosis. A Gomori methenamine silver stain highlights the organisms, which are thick-walled spores 8 to 15 microns in diameter. One of the organisms demonstrates broad-based budding.

eosinophilic dermatitis is induced as a hypersensitivity reaction to the mite and its eggs and feces.

- *Pediculosis,* another pruritic dermatosis, may be caused by a variety of human lice. Eggs ("nits") of the lice may be found attached to hair shafts.
- **Biting insects** produce lesions that vary from small, pruritic papules to large, weeping nodules. The reaction depends on the particular arthropod species and the host immune response. For example, tick bites tend to be large, with a striking lymphocytic and eosinophilic infiltrate. Lymphoid follicles may also form. Flea bites are usually urticarial, with a scant neutrophilic infiltrate. The venoms injected by arthropods such as the brown recluse spider may lead to severe local tissue necrosis.

Primary Neoplasms of the Skin

Cutaneous tumors are a paradigm for understanding neoplasia in general. These lesions are on the body surface where their development and evolution may be readily observed. The availability of tumor tissue from the developmentally sequential lesions has permitted correlation of data from studies of tumor cells in tissue culture with the observed behavior of clinical lesions.

The incidence of malignant melanoma, in particular, is increasing at an alarming rate. It is estimated that over 1% of children born today will develop malignant melanoma. The prognosis of most melanomas is excellent if lesions are recognized and excised before entering a vertical growth phase. However, a patient is at increased risk of dying from metastatic disease if the tumor exceeds a critical depth in the dermis.

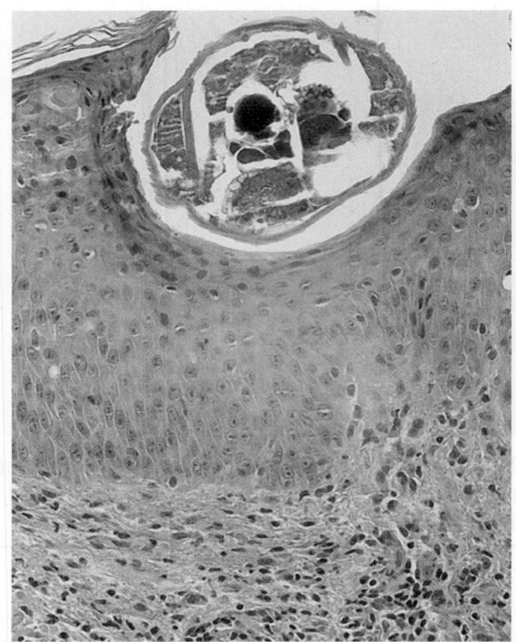

FIGURE 24-46. Scabetic nodule. A scabies mite is present in the stratum corneum.

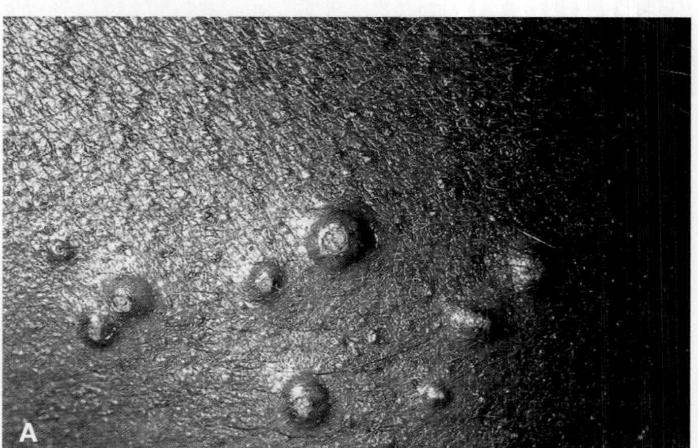

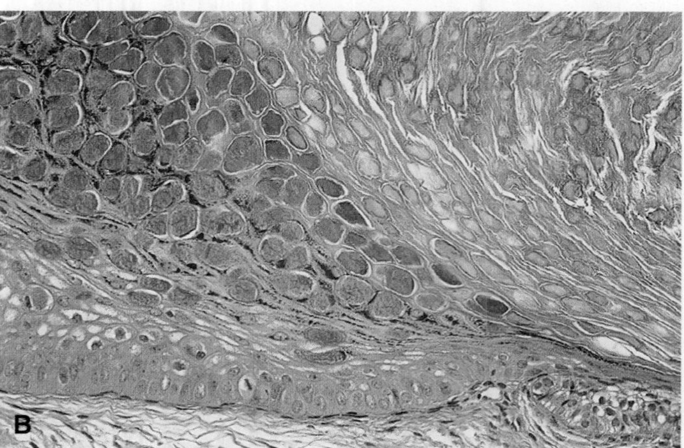

FIGURE 24-45. Molluscum contagiosum. A. Multiple umbilicated papules in a human immunodeficiency virus (HIV)-positive patient. **B.** The keratinocytes that are infected with this poxvirus show large eosinophilic cytoplasmic inclusions called "molluscum bodies."

Common Acquired Melanocytic Nevi (Moles) Are Localized Benign Neoplastic Proliferations of Melanocytes Within the Epidermis and/or Dermis

ETIOLOGIC FACTORS: Most people, regardless of skin color, develop 10 to 50 nevi on their skin. The total number of nevi depends on light exposure and innate susceptibility. Except for occasional cosmetic significance, nevi are important mainly in relation to melanoma, as markers of individuals at increased risk of developing melanoma and as potential precursors of melanoma. Even though about 30% of melanomas may arise in relation to a nevus, nevi are vastly more common than melanomas and most of them are stable or undergo senescent changes over time. Thus, wholesale excision of nevi is not recommended as a means to prevent melanoma.

Black skin can develop nevi, but less commonly, and those nevi that develop in the skin of darkly pigmented people are usually not associated with increased risk of melanoma or progression to melanoma. However, the risk of melanoma on the palms of the hands, the soles of the feet or the genital skin is the same in all races. Nevi, like melanomas, do not ordinarily develop in areas protected from light by at least two layers of clothing, such as the breasts of women. There is an unequivocal causal relationship between ultraviolet light and melanocytic nevi (and malignant melanoma), but the relationship is complex: some people with fair skin form relatively few nevi, whereas some with dark skin develop numerous nevi. The ability to form nevi is partly under genetic control and has been correlated with polymorphic variants of the melanocortin receptor and with subsequent variation in the ratio of pheomelanin to eumelanin, which are the pigments associated with red and brown hair respectively, and also with susceptibility to burning and tanning. There are at least two distinguishable profiles of individuals at risk for melanoma. One group prototypically has skin that may burn but can tan, and has an increased number of nevi. The other group consists of red-haired, blue-eyed persons with milk-white skin, who are exquisitely sensitive to light, do not tan well but form freckles and do not develop a significant number of nevi.

MOLECULAR PATHOGENESIS: A majority of nevi have recently been found to have an activating mutation of the gene encoding the oncogene *BRAF*, which can lead to growth stimulation through the mitogen-activated protein kinase (MAPK) pathway. However, after an initial period of growth, nevi are stable lesions that may regress or senesce. Such senescence is mediated by increased activity of p16, which is encoded by the gene CDKN2A on chromosome 9p21 and is an inhibitor of cyclin-dependent kinase 4 (CDK4). p16 suppresses cell proliferation and promotes end-stage differentiation of the nevus cells.

Epidemiologic studies have shown melanocytic nevi to be strong risk markers for development of melanomas. A person with 100 or more nevi that are 2 to 5 mm in greatest dimension has a threefold greater risk of developing melanoma than does a person with fewer than 25 similar nevi. Patients with clinically atypical-appearing nevi or histologically proven dysplastic nevi are at even greater risk for melanoma. Only 10 or more such clinically atypical or dysplastic nevi may be associated with a 12-fold increased risk for melanoma. As nevi are very common and melanomas are rare, the risk of progression of any one nevus is small.

Melanocytic nevi begin to appear between the first and second years of life and continue to emerge for the first two decades of life. A nevus first appears as a small tan dot no bigger than 1 to 2 mm in diameter. During the next 3 to 4 years, the dot enlarges to become a uniform tan to brown circular or oval area. The peripheral outline usually remains regular. When it reaches 4 to 5 mm in diameter, it is flat or slightly elevated, stops enlarging peripherally and is sharply demarcated from surrounding normal skin. Over the next 10 years, the lesion elevates and its color pales to the point of becoming a tan tag-like protrusion. For the next decade or two, it gradually flattens and the skin may approximate a normal appearance. In most people, the number of nevi gradually decreases over time. Notably, many melanoma patients tend to retain increased numbers of nevi, including atypical ones, in the later decades of life.

PATHOLOGY: At the inception of a melanocytic nevus, melanocytes are increased in the basal epidermis, with subsequent hyperpigmentation. The melanocytes eventually form nests, frequently at tips of rete ridges, and then migrate into the dermis where they form small clusters. As the lesion becomes elevated, the dermal nevus cells begin to differentiate in a manner reminiscent of Schwann cells (melanocytes like Schwann cells are derived from embryonic neural crest), an evolution that gradually encompasses the entire dermal component, leaving a core of delicate neuromesenchyme. The nevus may eventually flatten and possibly even disappear. The histologic classification of melanocytic nevi reflects their evolution:

- **Junctional nevus:** Melanocytes form nests at the tips of epidermal rete ridges. They are then by definition known as "nevus cells," and they also tend to lose their dendritic morphology and retain pigment in their cytoplasm
- **Compound nevus:** Nests of melanocytes are seen in the epidermis and some of the cells have migrated into the dermis (Fig. 24-47).
- **Dermal nevus:** Intraepidermal melanocytic growth has ceased and melanocytes are present only in the dermis (Fig. 24-48). Pigment tends to be lost at this stage, but the presence of a residual nested architecture is an important clue to the diagnosis of a nevus versus another tumor.

Dysplastic (Atypical) Nevus Is a Risk Marker for Melanoma

An increased number of total nevi is a significant risk factor for melanoma, as is the presence of large nevi. Some common acquired nevi do not follow the pattern of growth, differentiation and disappearance described above, and are termed "dysplastic nevi." These are especially strong risk factors. Such lesions persist and are often more than 5 mm in greatest dimension. These nevi may show foci of aberrant melanocytic growth and become larger and somewhat irregular peripherally (although less so than melanomas). The

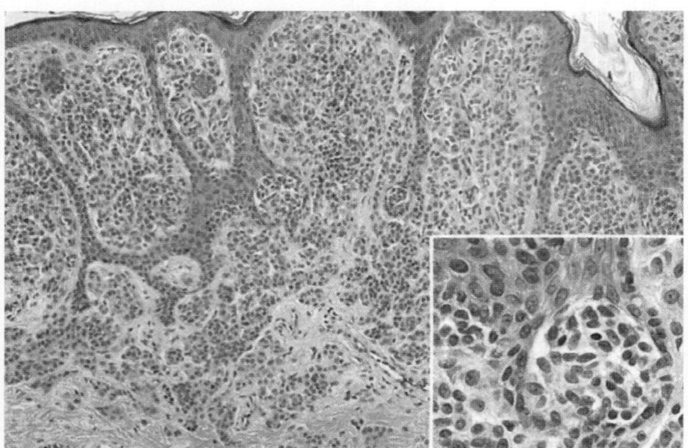

FIGURE 24-47. Compound melanocytic nevus. Melanocytes are present as nests within the epidermis and dermis. An intraepidermal nest of melanocytes is surrounded by keratinocytes (*inset*).

peripheral area is flat (macular) and extends symmetrically from the parent nevus. Some clinically dysplastic nevi are entirely macular.

Dysplastic nevi were first described in melanoma kindreds, families in which there is a greatly increased incidence of melanoma. In these families and in general population members, patients with dysplastic nevi are at increased risk of developing melanoma (although not all patients with dysplastic nevi will develop melanomas, and not all melanomas occur in patients with dysplastic nevi). The magnitude of this risk varies with the number of nevi, and is especially high in patients with a prior melanoma and/or family history of melanoma. The genetics of dysplastic nevi are not completely understood, and contributions from multiple genes are likely.

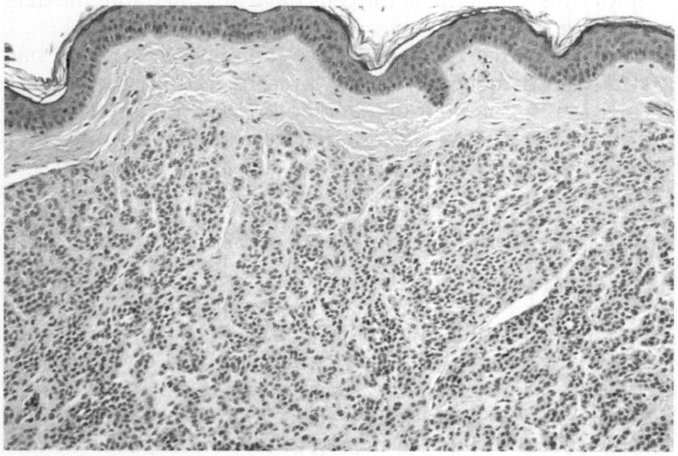

FIGURE 24-48. Dermal melanocytic nevus. The melanocytes are entirely confined to the dermis.

Melanocytic Dysplasia Features Architectural Disorder and Cytologic Atypia

Initially, growth of melanocytes in the basal epidermis of a dysplastic nevus appears similar to that seen in the early stages of a common nevus. This area is abnormal in architectural pattern, not in cytologic features. A band of eosinophilic connective tissue ("lamellar fibroplasia") is seen around the rete ridges, which contain aberrantly growing melanocytes. These aberrant melanocytes may grow to become continuous horizontal streams of melanocytes extending from rete to rete ("bridging"). As these architectural features become more prominent, melanocytes with large atypical nuclei that are reminiscent of malignant cells may also appear in the areas of architectural disorder. This combination of architectural disorder and cytologic atypia constitutes a dysplastic nevus (Figs. 24-49 and 24-50). Areas of dysplasia may also be associated with a subjacent lymphocytic infiltrate. More than one third of malignant melanomas have precursor nevi, most of which show melanocytic dysplasia. However, most dysplastic nevi are stable and never progress to melanoma. That is, dysplastic nevi are much more common in the population than melanomas. Between 7% and 20% of the population has at least one dysplastic nevus, depending on the diagnostic criteria applied. In this regard, controversy about the significance of dysplastic nevi largely reflects diagnostic variation.

The Prognosis of Malignant Melanoma Is a Function of the Depth of Invasion

Malignant melanoma is a neoplasm of melanocytes. The term "melanoma" in current practice is synonymous with "malignant melanoma." Malignant melanoma, although not one of the most common cancers overall, is a leading cause of cancer mortality in young adults. It is rare in adolescence, and exceedingly rare in childhood. Melanomas may evolve

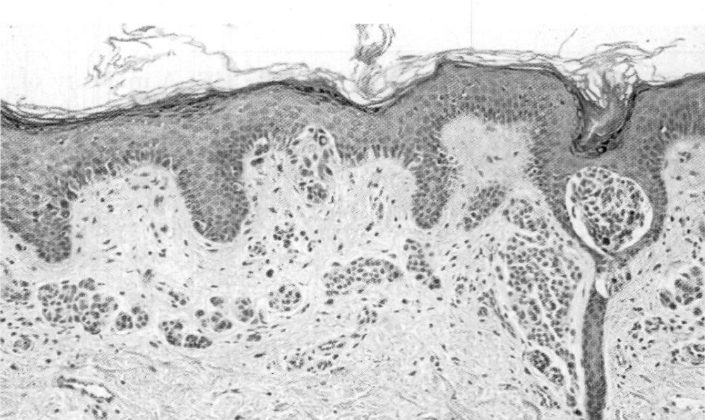

FIGURE 24-49. Compound nevus with melanocytic dysplasia. On the *right*, a compound nevus is apparent with both intraepidermal and dermal components. To the *left*, within the epidermis, are single, atypical melanocytes within the basal layer, as well as incipient lamellar fibroplasia. Dermal melanocytes are present *below*.

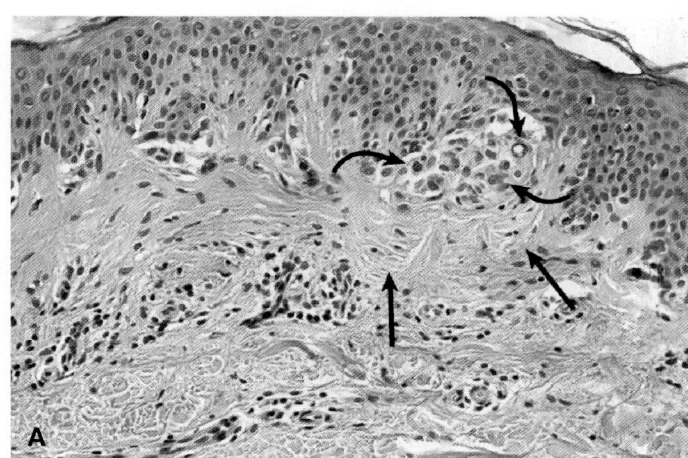

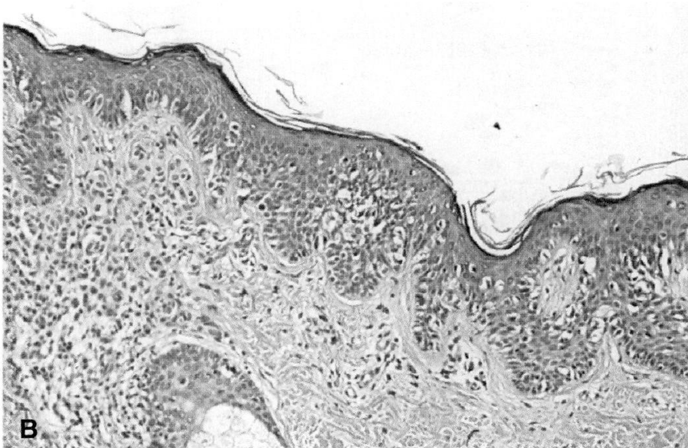

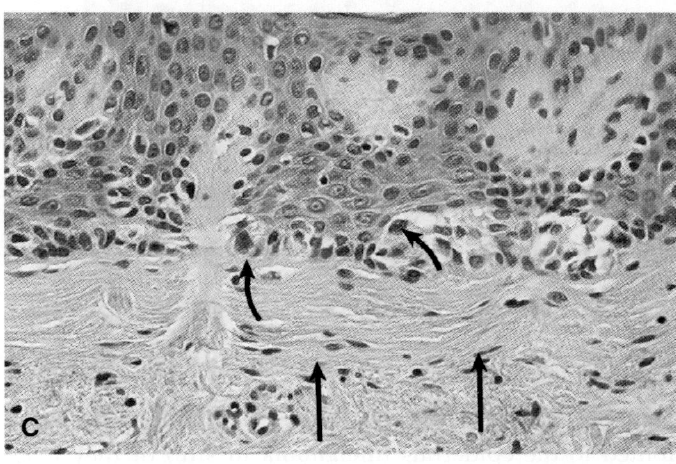

FIGURE 24-50. Dysplastic nevus. A. There is bridging of rete ridges by nests of melanocytes, melanocytes with cytologic atypia (*curved arrows*), lamellar fibroplasia (*straight arrows*) and a scant perivascular lymphocytic infiltrate. **B.** To the *left* is a zone containing typical dermal nevus cells of a compound melanocytic nevus. In the epidermis on the *right* is a proliferation of atypical melanocytes with lamellar fibroplasia. This photomicrograph is taken from the junction of the papular and macular components of this dysplastic nevus. Dysplasia usually develops in the macular portion, which takes up most of the field. **C.** Irregular melanocytic nests resting above lamellar fibroplasia (*straight arrows*) exhibit large epithelioid melanocytes with atypia (*curved arrows*).

through two major stages of progression. In the "radial growth phase" (RGP), the lesion spreads along the radii of an imperfect circle in the skin but remains superficial and thin as measured by micrometer in the method originally described by Breslow. In the "vertical growth phase" (VGP), there is a focal area in which the lesion expands in a more or less spherical manner to form a tumor mass, with increasing Breslow thickness. In recent years, it has become clear that melanomas are dependent, to a greater or lesser extent, on an activated oncogene, *B-RAF*, which is also mutated in benign nevi. The histopathologic subtypes of melanoma, discussed below, are related to the particular oncogenes involved in their pathogenesis. Loss of p16 (and/or in some cases other tumor suppressors) is a common event in melanomas, leading to relatively unrestrained proliferation and the potential for future progression "from bad to worse."

Radial Growth Phase Melanoma

The most frequently encountered type of melanoma is **superficial spreading melanoma,** which can present in the radial growth phase or the vertical growth phase (Fig. 24-51). Excision for histologic examination is the gold standard for diagnosis of melanoma of any sort.

PATHOLOGY: In a superficial spreading melanoma, large epithelioid melanocytes are dispersed in nests and as individual cells through the entire thickness of the epidermis ("pagetoid spread"), not just along the basal layer as in nevi and in the lentiginous forms of melanoma

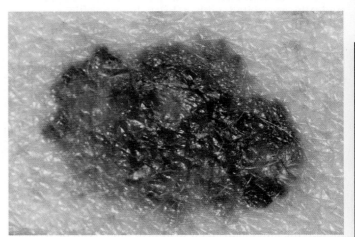

FIGURE 24-51. The clinical appearance of the radial growth phase in malignant melanoma of the superficial spreading type. The larger diameter is 1.8 cm.

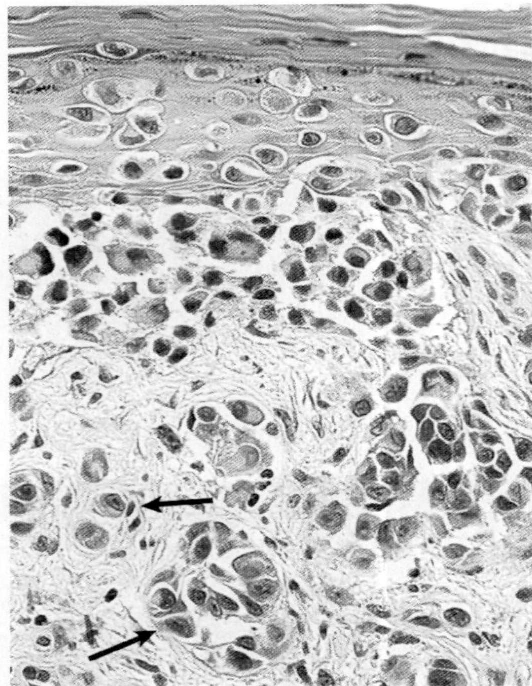

FIGURE 24-52. Malignant melanoma, superficial spreading type, radial growth phase. Melanocytes grow singly within the epidermis at all levels and as large, irregularly sized nests at the dermal–epidermal junction. Tumor cells are present in the papillary dermis (*arrows*), but no nest shows preferential growth over the others.

described in the next sections. These melanocytes may be limited to the epidermis **(melanoma in situ)** or they may invade into the papillary dermis. In the radial growth phase, no nest has growth preference (larger size) over the other nests (Fig. 24-52), so cells grow evenly in all directions: upward in the epidermis, peripherally in the epidermis and downward into the dermis **(invasion).** Mitoses are not seen in dermal melanocytes but may be present in the epidermal component. These lesions enlarge at the periphery, hence the term **radial.** Melanocytes of the radial growth phase are typically associated with a brisk lymphocytic response. Melanomas in the radial growth phase rarely metastasize.

CLINICAL FEATURES: Superficial spreading melanoma (SSM) has been associated with a history of intermittent sun exposure and sunburn and with activating mutations of the *B-RAF* oncogene. Early melanomas in the radial growth phase have slightly elevated and palpable borders. The neoplasm is usually variably and haphazardly pigmented. Some parts are black or dark brown, whereas other areas may be lighter brown, possibly mixed with pink or light blue tints. The entire lesion may be purely dark brown (Fig. 24-51). With regard to lesions that are eventually documented to be melanoma, patients frequently state that a change occurred in a nevus. Such changes can include itching, increase in size, darkening or bleeding and oozing, though the latter signs tend to appear later. With or without such observations on the part of the patient, any lesion that prompts clinical suspicion of melanoma warrants an excisional biopsy. The "ABCDE rule" is a convenient mnemonic that is commonly taught to patients to help them recognize changes in nevi that should prompt them to seek medical

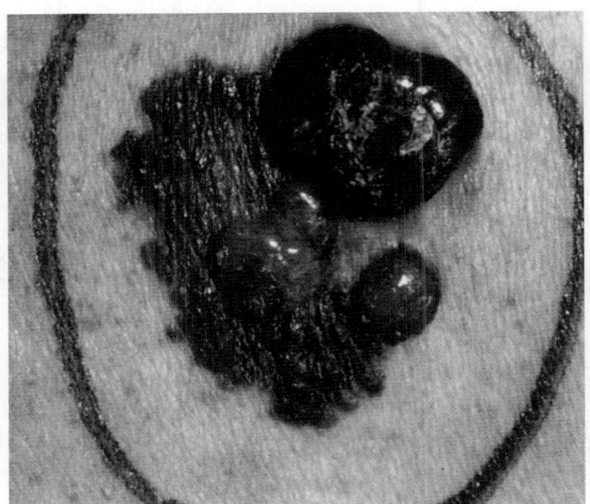

FIGURE 24-53. Malignant melanoma. The superficial spreading type is represented by the relatively flat, dark, brown–black portion of the tumor. Three areas in this lesion are characteristic of the vertical growth phase. All are nodular in configuration; two have a pink coloration, and the largest is a rich, ebony black.

attention: **A**symmetry of shape, **B**order irregularity, **C**olor variation and a **D**iameter more than 6 mm. The letter "E" can stand for "**E**levation" or more importantly "**E**volution." However, not all early melanomas exhibit these attributes, and any changing lesion should be evaluated for excisional biopsy.

Vertical Growth Phase Melanoma

After a variable time (usually 1 to 2 years), the character of growth begins to change. Melanocytes exhibit mitotic activity in both the epidermal and dermal components and grow as expanding spheroid nodules in the dermis (Fig. 24-53). The net direction of growth tends to be perpendicular to that of the radial growth phase, hence the term **vertical** (Figs. 24-53 through 24-56).

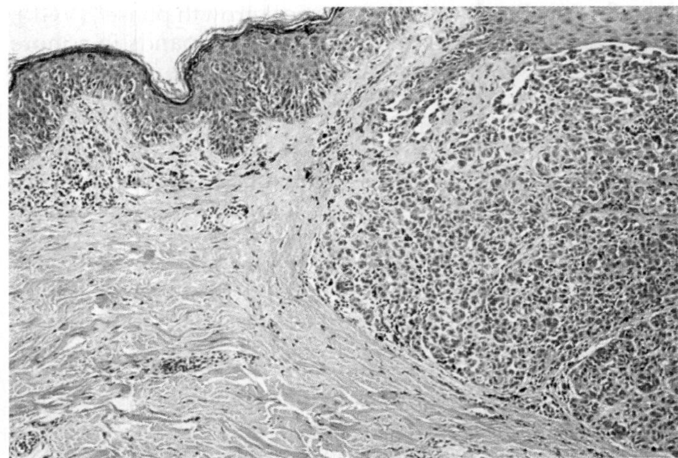

FIGURE 24-54. Malignant melanoma, superficial spreading type, vertical growth phase. Vertical growth is manifested by the distinct spheroid tumor nodule to the *right*. This focus of melanocytes clearly has a growth advantage (larger size of the aggregate) over nests in the adjacent radial growth phase (*left*).

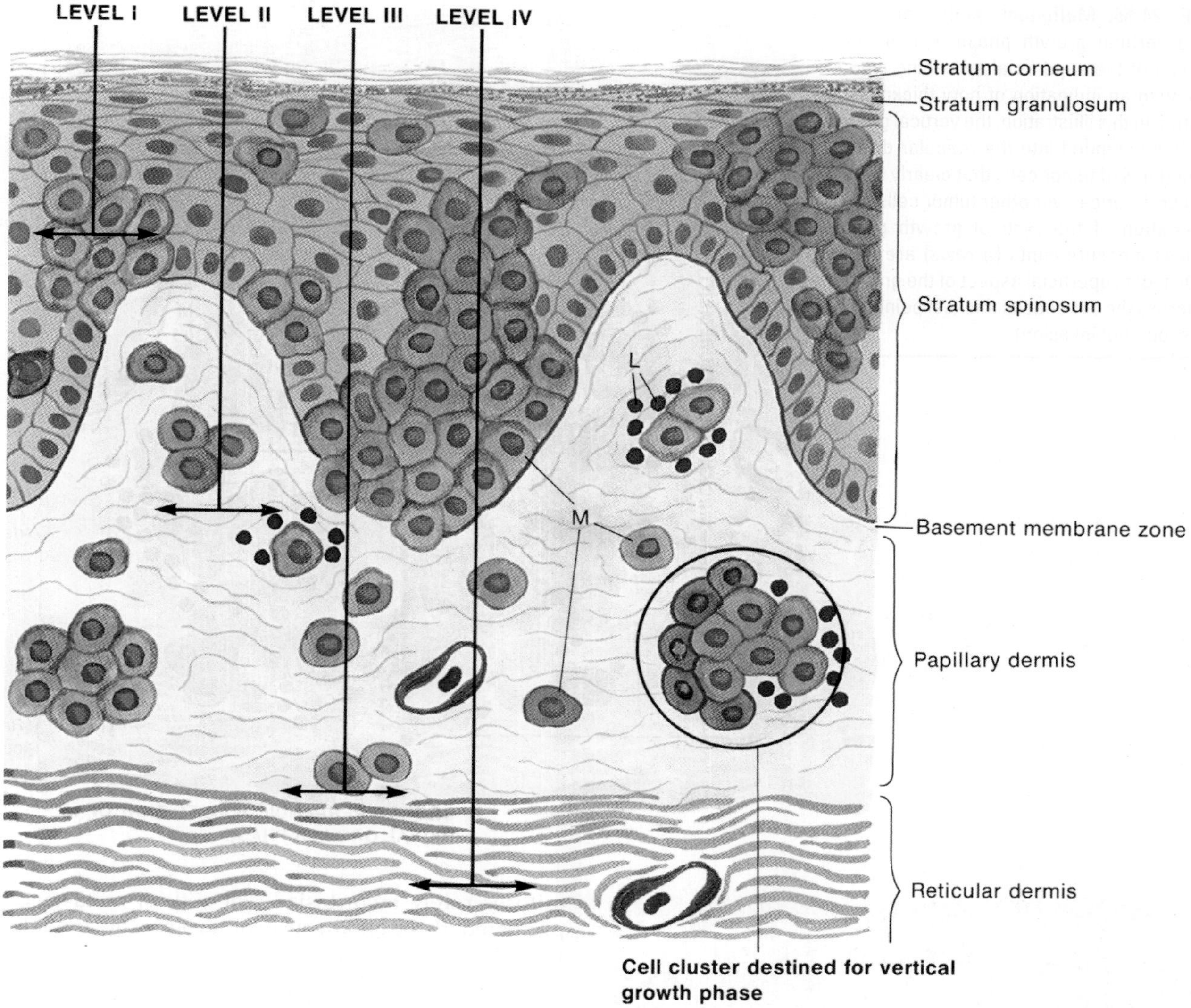

FIGURE 24-55. Malignant melanoma. In the radial growth phase, cells grow in the epidermis and are present in the dermis. They grow in all directions: outward, peripherally and downward. The net direction of growth is peripheral—along the radii of an imperfect circle. Growth is predominantly in the epidermis. No cells in the dermis seem to have a growth preference over others. A nest depicted here is shown as it evolves into the vertical growth phase. The anatomic landmarks of the levels of invasion are shown. Level III is not simply the occasional impingement of a tumor cell against the reticular dermis but indicates a collection of cells that fills and widens the papillary dermis and broadly abuts the reticular dermis. Level III invasion is usually a manifestation of the vertical growth phase. Level IV invasion should be designated only when tumor cells clearly permeate between otherwise unaltered collagen bundles of the reticular dermis. L = lymphocyte; M = melanocyte.

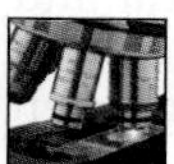

PATHOLOGY: The more specific characteristics of the vertical growth phase are:

- The melanocytes tend to differ in appearance from those of the radial growth phase. For example, they may contain little or no pigment, whereas the cells of the radial growth phase are melanotic.
- The cellular aggregate that characterizes the vertical growth phase is larger than the clusters of melanocytes that form the epidermal and dermal (invasive) components of the radial growth phase. It is important to note that invasion can occur in both the radial growth phase and the vertical growth phase, but the dominant direction of tumor growth shifts from the epidermis to the dermis in the vertical growth phase.
- Tumors that extend into the reticular dermis are usually considered to be in the vertical growth phase.
- The host immune response (manifested by lymphocytic inflammation; Fig. 24-57) may be absent or reduced at the base of the vertical growth phase, compared to the radial growth phase.
- Markers of cell cycle progression, such as Ki-67, increase in cells of the vertical growth phase.

Even when tumors enter the vertical growth phase, they may still lack the propensity to metastasize. Thus, vertical growth phase melanomas less than 1 mm thick that lack

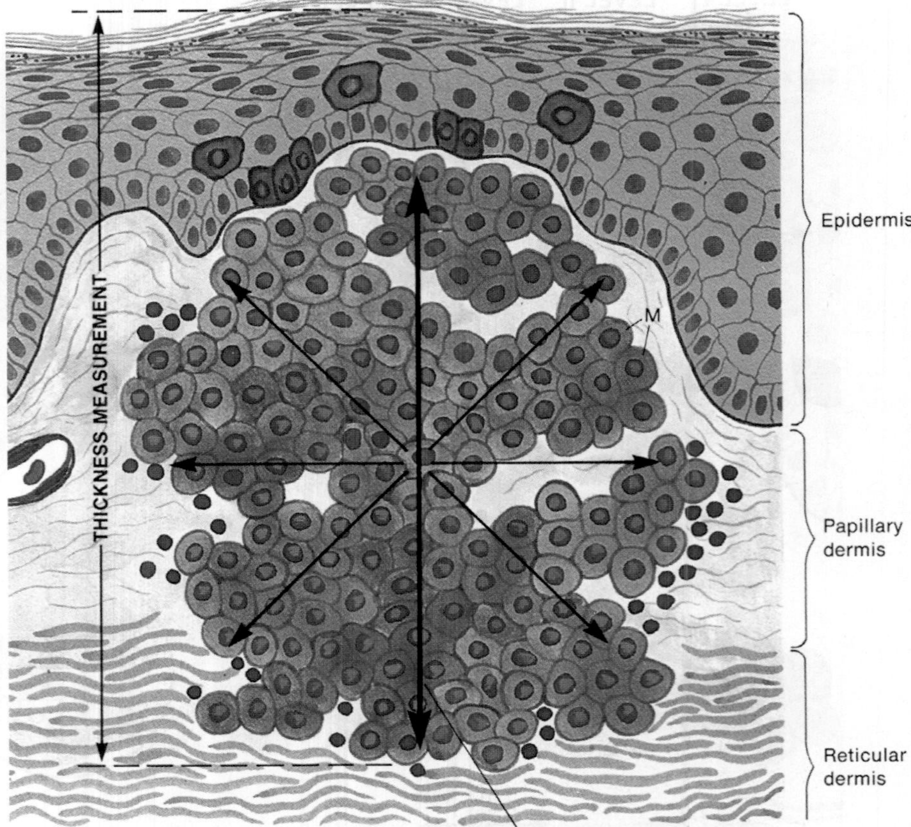

FIGURE 24-56. Malignant melanoma. The evolved vertical growth phase in malignant melanoma of the superficial spreading type is shown, with an indication of how thickness is measured. In this illustration, the vertical growth phase has extended into the reticular dermis. Small nodules of tumor cells that clearly have a growth preference over other tumor cells are a manifestation of the vertical growth phase. Thickness measurements (*arrows*) are taken from the most superficial aspect of the granular layer across the tumor at its thickest point (to its deepest point of invasion).

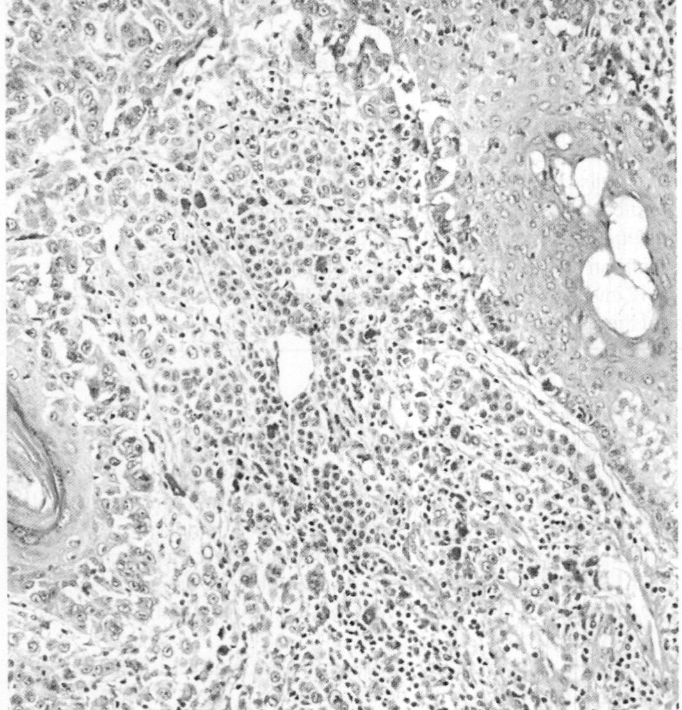

FIGURE 24-57. Malignant melanoma, vertical growth phase. The host response consists of lymphocytes infiltrating amid the melanocytes ("tumor-infiltrating lymphocytes").

mitoses rarely metastasize. The risk of metastasis can be predicted through the use of prognostic models, albeit imperfectly.

Nodular Melanoma

Occasionally, a melanoma "bypasses" the stepwise tumor progression described above and manifests all of its malignant characteristics in the initial lesion. Nodular melanoma is an uncommon form of the tumor (10%). It appears as a circumscribed, elevated, spheroidal nodule. It does not develop through a radial growth phase but is in the vertical growth phase when initially observed (Fig. 24-58). Nodular melanoma is composed of one or more nodules of cells that grow in an expansile fashion in the dermis (Fig. 24-59). These lesions lack most of the ABCD criteria and may be advanced in thickness, and thus at high risk of metastasis at the time of diagnosis, despite being often quite small in diameter, symmetric and homogeneous in color.

Lentigo Maligna Melanoma

Lentigo maligna melanoma, also known as **Hutchinson melanotic freckle,** is a large, pigmented macule that occurs on sun-damaged skin. It develops almost exclusively in fair-skinned, usually elderly, whites, often with history of being outdoor workers. Because it occurs on exposed body surfaces, often without history of acute sunburn injury, it is probably related to chronic ultraviolet light exposure. Lentigo maligna

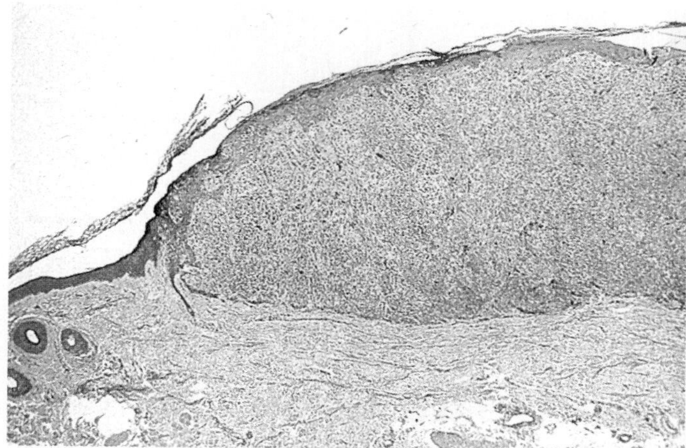

FIGURE 24-58. Malignant melanoma, nodular type. Intraepidermal growth is essentially absent. There is no radial growth lateral to the nodule. This tumor expands the papillary dermis and distorts the reticular dermal junction; it is therefore level III.

melanoma, like acral and mucosal melanomas (see below), is less likely than superficial spreading melanoma to be associated with mutation of *B-RAF*. Some of these have activating mutations of the receptor tyrosine kinase c-Kit and may be responsive, at least for a time, to c-kit inhibitors such as Gleevec.

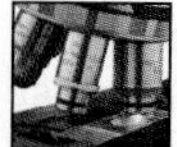

PATHOLOGY: In the radial growth phase, lentigo maligna melanoma (LMM) is a flat, irregular, brown-to-black patch that may cover a large part of the face or dorsal hands (Fig. 24-60). The cells of the radial growth phase are predominantly in the basal layer, often forming contiguous or nearly contiguous rows of atypical single melanocytes but occasionally forming small nests that hang down into the papillary dermis (Fig. 24-61). Cells of the radial growth phase of LMM vary in size and are usually associated with effacement of rete ridges and thinning of the epidermis. The subjacent dermis often shows a modest lymphocytic infiltrate and, with only rare exceptions, solar degeneration of the connective tissue.

The clinical appearance of LMM in the vertical growth phase is shown in Fig. 24-62. Histologically, the cells in this phase tend to be spindle shaped. They will occasionally provoke a connective tissue response to form a firm plaque

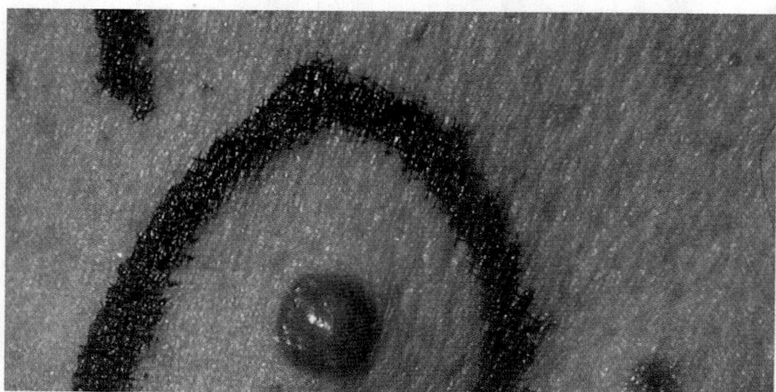

FIGURE 24-59. Malignant melanoma of the nodular type. The primary focus of growth of this 0.5-cm lesion is in the dermis.

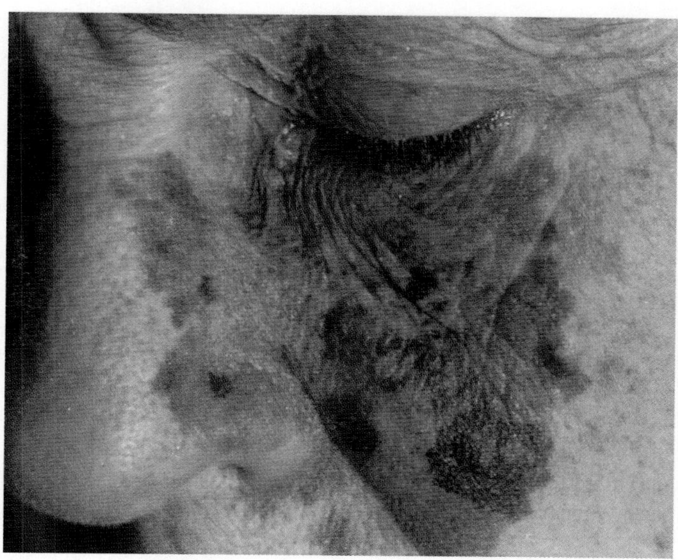

FIGURE 24-60. Malignant melanoma of the lentigo maligna type, radial growth phase.

(**desmoplastic melanoma** that may mimic a scar or a neuroma and be difficult to diagnose histologically). Cells of the vertical growth phase may also grow along small nerves ("neurotropism").

Acral Lentiginous Melanoma

Acral lentiginous melanoma is the most common form of melanoma in dark-skinned people and, as the name implies, is generally limited to palms, soles and subungual regions.

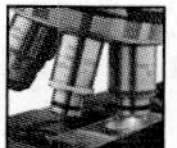

PATHOLOGY: In the radial growth phase, acral lentiginous melanoma forms an irregular, brown-to-black patch that covers a part of the palm or sole or arises under a nail, usually on a thumb or great toe

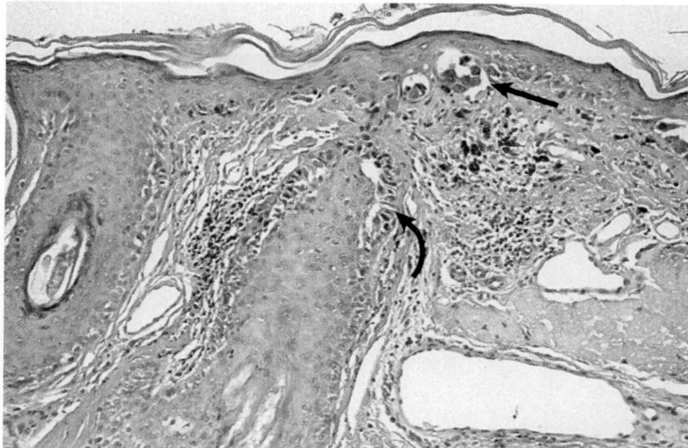

FIGURE 24-61. Lentigo maligna. Atypical melanocytes grow mostly at the dermal–epidermal interface (*straight arrow*), with extension down the external root sheath of follicles (*curved arrow*). Upward growth of melanocytes is much less prominent than in malignant melanoma of the superficial spreading type.

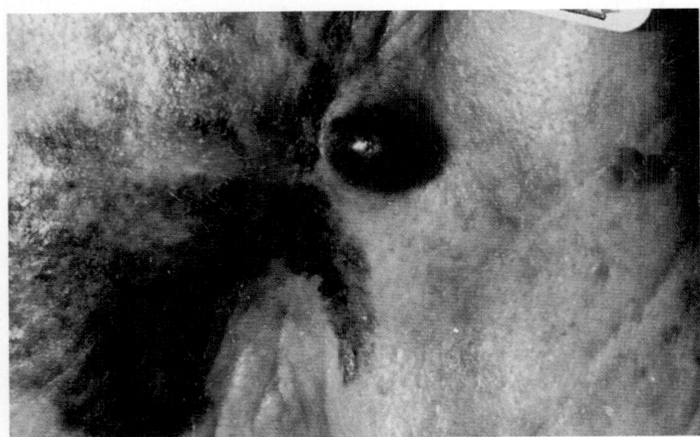

FIGURE 24-62. Lentigo maligna. The clinical appearance of the radial and vertical growth phase in malignant melanoma of the lentigo maligna type is shown. The lesion is 1 cm in diameter.

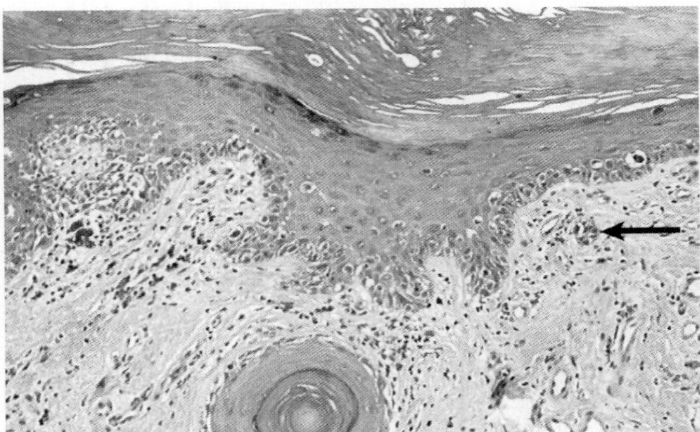

FIGURE 24-64. Malignant melanoma, acral lentiginous type, principally intraepidermal radial growth. Atypical melanocytes are present along the dermal–epidermal junction. A small dermal nest of atypical melanocytes is present (*arrow*).

(Fig. 24-63). Microscopically, cells are mostly confined to the basal layer of the epidermis and tend to maintain long dendrites (Figs. 24-64 and 24-65). A brisk lichenoid lymphocytic infiltrate is often seen.

The vertical growth phase (Figs. 24-66 and 24-67) is similar to that of lentigo maligna melanoma in that it commonly consists of spindle cells and occasionally includes desmoplasia and neurotropism.

Metastatic Melanoma

Metastatic melanoma arises from the melanocytes of the vertical growth phase of any of the various forms of melanoma. Initial metastases usually involve regional lymph nodes, although hematogenous spread to organs is also possible. When the latter occurs, metastases are unusually widespread in comparison with other neoplasms; virtually any organ may be involved. Metastatic melanomas may remain dormant and clinically undetectable for long periods after the apparently successful excision of a primary melanoma, only to reappear years later.

Staging and Prognosis of Melanoma

The prognosis of a patient with a melanoma is based on a number of attributes:

TUMOR THICKNESS: Tumor thickness, originally described by Breslow, is the strongest prognostic variable for melanomas that are apparently confined to their primary sites (stages 1 and 2 in the current staging system of the American Joint Committee on Cancer [AJCC]). The "Breslow thickness" of a melanoma is measured from the most superficial aspect of the stratum granulosum to the point of deepest penetration of the tumor into the dermis (Fig. 24-56). Outcome may be predicted with some accuracy by dividing tumors into groups based on thickness. Cutoffs at 1-mm intervals have been established in the current AJCC staging system. Prognosis up to 10 years after removal of the primary lesion may then be estimated from Table 24-2.

ULCERATION: Ulceration in a primary melanoma is associated with decreased survival. In one study, survival rates were 66% and 92% for patients with and without ulceration,

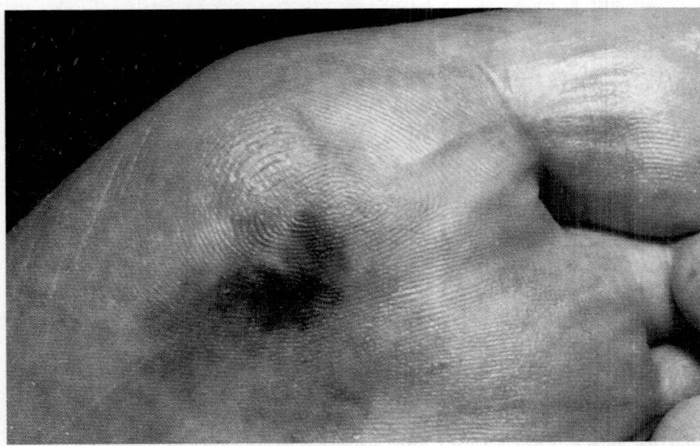

FIGURE 24-63. Malignant melanoma, acral lentiginous type (radial growth phase). The clinical appearance of the sole of the foot is depicted.

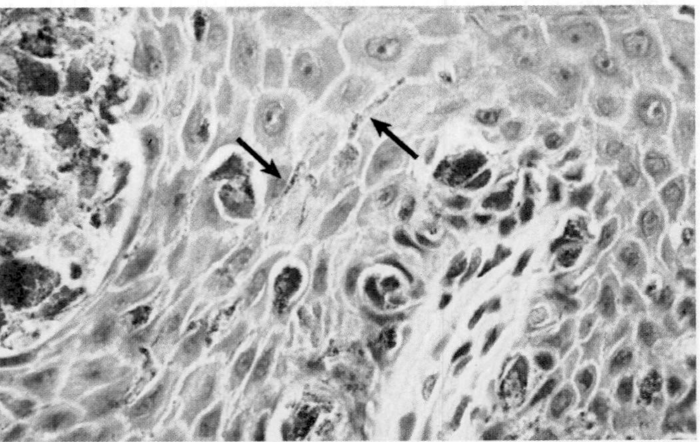

FIGURE 24-65. Malignant melanoma, acral lentiginous type. Large melanocytes with prominent dendrites (*arrows*) are present in the basilar region of the epidermis. The tumor cells contain numerous melanosomes, making the perinuclear and dendritic cytoplasms brown.

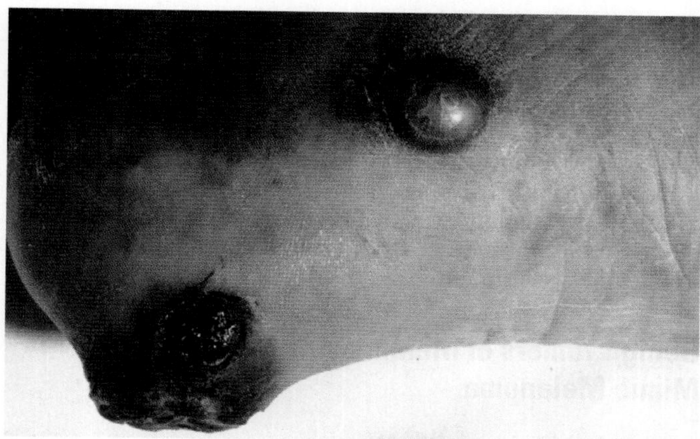

FIGURE 24-66. Malignant melanoma, acral lentiginous type. The lesion on the heel is the primary tumor. The flat portion represents the radial growth phase, whereas the elevated portion indicates the vertical growth phase. The dark nodule on the instep is a metastasis.

respectively. Ulceration is used as a stage modifier in the AJCC system; its presence raises a lesion to the next stage in each thickness group.

DERMAL MITOTIC RATE: For tumor cells in the vertical growth phase, the mitotic rate is highly predictive of survival. Survival becomes progressively worse as the mitotic rate increases. The 5-year survival is 99% for patients whose tumors show no mitoses, 85% with a mitotic rate of 0.1 to 6.0/mm^2 and 68% with over 6 mitoses/mm^2. Mitogenicity, or the presence of any mitoses in the dermis, has been identified as a risk factor for recurrence in otherwise early-stage ("thin") melanomas, and will be included in the forthcoming (2010) AJCC staging system as a modifier of stage 1 (melanomas of thickness <1 mm).

LYMPHOCYTIC RESPONSE: Interaction of lymphocytes with tumor cells in the vertical growth phase is an important prognostic indicator. A cellular response is reported to be "infiltrative" when the lymphocytes actually infiltrate and disrupt the tumor, frequently forming rosettes around tumor cells (Figs. 24-57 and 24-68). If tumor-infiltrating lymphocytes (TILs) are present throughout the vertical growth phase or are seen across the entire base of the vertical growth phase, the infiltrate is said to be "brisk." The more prevalent the TILs, the better the prognosis is. Although widely accepted as having potential relevance, this and the other attributes listed below are not included in the AJCC staging system, which is the current standard of care.

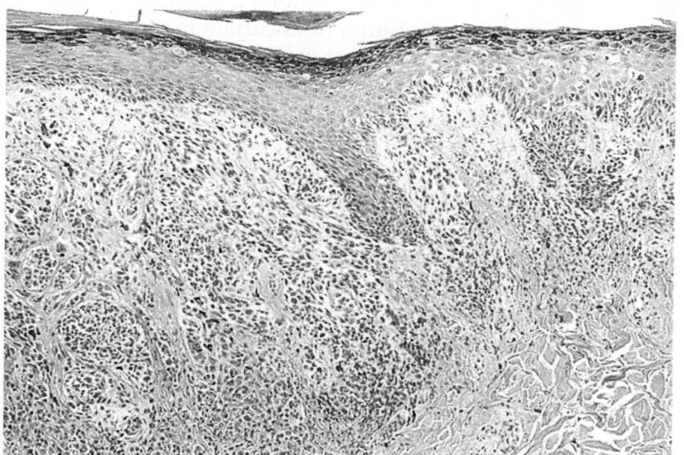

FIGURE 24-67. Malignant melanoma, acral lentiginous type, vertical growth phase. On the *left* is confluent growth of atypical dermal melanocytes filling and expanding the papillary dermis.

Table 24-2

Tumor Thickness as Sole Predictor of Outcome 10 Years After Definitive Therapy of Primary Melanoma

Thickness (mm)	Survival (%)
≤1	83–88
1.01–2	64–79
2.01–4	51–64
>4	32–54

LOCATION: Melanomas on the extremities have a better prognosis than those on the head, neck or trunk (axial). However, melanomas on the sole of the foot or the subungual region have a prognosis similar to, or worse than, axial lesions.

SEX: For every site and thickness, women have better prognoses than men. For example, women with axial melanomas 0.8 to 1.7 mm thick have almost 90% 10-year survival after excision of the lesion, whereas the comparable figure in men is only 60%.

REGRESSION: Many primary melanomas show some spontaneous regression in the radial growth phase component, indicated clinically by a color change to blue-white or

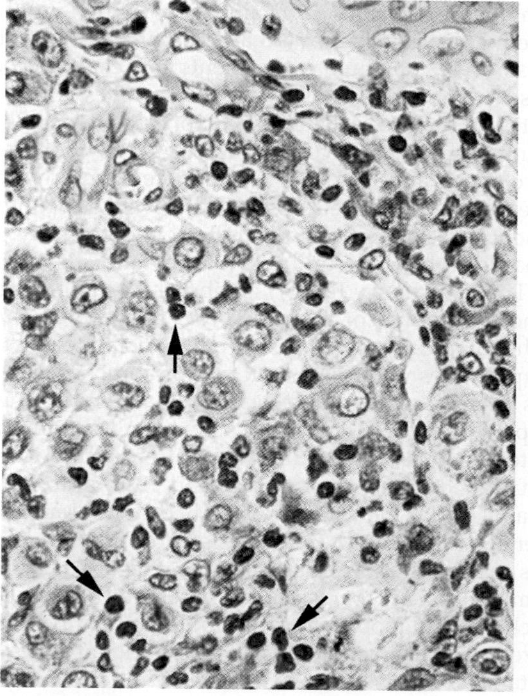

FIGURE 24-68. Malignant melanoma, vertical growth phase. Numerous tumor-infiltrating lymphocytes (*arrows*) are arranged among individual tumor cells.

white. Microscopically, such regression is characterized by a widened papillary dermis, containing melanophages and a lymphocytic infiltrate, with an absence of melanoma cells in the epidermis overlying these dermal changes. Patients whose tumors show such changes have a somewhat worse prognosis than those in whom regression is absent.

LEVELS OF INVASION: The Clark level system describes the degree of tumor penetration within the anatomic layers of the skin (Fig. 24-55). The Clark levels are not as accurate as tumor thickness in predicting the risk of metastasis, and are no longer included in the AJCC system. However, the levels have descriptive value and are of prognostic significance in some subsets of cases.

- **Level I:** Tumor cells are entirely above the basement membrane (in situ).
- **Level II:** Invasive cells are present only in the papillary dermis without filling or expanding it (radial growth phase).
- **Level III:** The tumor has usually entered the vertical growth phase and impinges on the reticular dermis, forming small expansile nodules that expand and fill the papillary dermis.
- **Level IV:** Tumor cells invade between the collagen bundles of the reticular dermis.
- **Level V:** The tumor extends into the subcutaneous fat.

LYMPHATIC INVASION: Although intuitively important, this property has not been included in prognostic models because it is rarely observed in routine sections. There is recent evidence that lymphatic invasion may be more common than previously thought when enhanced detection techniques are used, and that it is prognostically significant.

STAGE: The stage of the disease is the most important single factor influencing a patient's survival. Metastasis to regional lymph nodes is now determined routinely by sentinel lymph node staging, which involves biopsy of a single node that lies first in the regional node drainage pattern. Lymph node involvement is associated with an estimated 40% decrease in 5-year survival, compared with patients with clinically localized tumors. The number of involved lymph nodes is also highly predictive of prognosis. Patients with one positive node have a 10-year survival of 40%, compared with 25% with two to four positive nodes, and 15% with five or more nodes involved.

The tumor–node–metastasis (TNM) system of tumor staging incorporates features related to the primary tumor, regional lymph nodes and soft tissues and distant metastases. The **T** (primary tumor) attributes of tumor thickness, presence or absence of ulceration and mitogenicity are classified histologically after excision of the melanoma. Numbers of lymph nodes with metastatic tumor and characterization of this tumor as micrometastasis or macrometastasis are a large part of the **N** (node) classification. **Micrometastasis** refers to nodal metastases diagnosed after sentinel or elective lymphadenectomy; **macrometastasis** refers to clinically detectable nodal metastases confirmed by therapeutic lymphadenectomy. The **M** (metastasis) properties incorporate results of evaluation for distant metastases at various anatomic sites. A TNM classification scheme based primarily on thickness and modified by ulceration and mitogenicity, for localized primary melanomas and for regional and systemic metastatic disease, is used to determine the pathologic stage of disease, which in turn reflects the probability of survival.

The current recommendations regarding excisional removal of confirmed melanomas state that a 5-mm margin of uninvolved tissue should be obtained with in situ melanoma, a 1-cm margin should be obtained with a tumor thickness of 1 mm or less, and a 2-cm margin may be considered with a tumor thickness greater than 1 mm or with Clark level IV or greater with any thickness. However, many clinicians would use a 1-cm margin, at least for tumors in the lower end of these ranges, and margins are typically adjusted so as to spare important structures, such as the eyes. Sentinel lymph node sampling is generally considered with tumor thickness greater than 1 mm or with other risk factors, including ulceration or mitogenicity (dermal mitotic activity).

Benign Tumors of Melanocytes May Mimic Melanoma

Congenital Melanocytic Nevus

About 1% of white children are born with some form of pigmented lesion on their skin, sometimes as inconspicuous as a small patch of pale tan hyperpigmentation. Much more rarely, the trunk or an extremity is covered by a large pigmented patch or plaque that is cosmetically deforming ("giant hairy" or "garment" nevus). Such areas display a striking increase in intraepidermal and dermal melanocytes, which may extend deep into the subcutaneous tissue. Malignant melanoma may develop in these large congenital melanocytic nevi. Attempts are sometimes made to remove these large lesions, but in many instances their size makes surgical removal problematic.

Spitz Tumor

Spitz tumors (also known as spindle and epithelioid cell nevi) occur in children or adolescents and, less often, in adults. The Spitz tumor is an elevated, spheroid, pink, smooth nodule, usually on the head or neck. It grows rapidly, increasing to a diameter of 3 to 5 mm within 6 months. The lesion is composed of large spindle or epithelioid melanocytes that are present in the epidermis and the dermis (Fig. 24-69). The cells are so atypical that an incorrect diagnosis of melanoma may be made even though melanoma is rare in childhood. Although most Spitz tumors are benign, a few may metastasize. Therefore, the prognosis is to some extent uncertain, especially in adults. Sometimes in these lesions, as in other rare categories of melanocytic tumors, a descriptive diagnosis, such as "melanocytic tumor of uncertain malignant potential," or "MELTUMP," is all that can be rendered.

Blue Nevus

Blue nevi appear in childhood or late adolescence as dark blue, gray or black, firm, well-demarcated papules or nodules on the dorsal hands or feet or on the buttocks, scalp or face. The clinical appearance may prompt an excisional biopsy to rule out nodular melanoma. Melanin-containing melanocytes with long, thin dendrites are present in the superficial to middermis, where they are often admixed with numerous melanin-containing macrophages (Fig. 24-70). There are also rare examples of "cellular blue nevi" and "malignant blue nevi."

Freckle and Lentigo

Freckles, or **ephelides,** are small, brown macules that occur on sun-exposed skin, especially in people with fair skin (Fig. 24-71). They usually appear at about age 5. The pigmentation

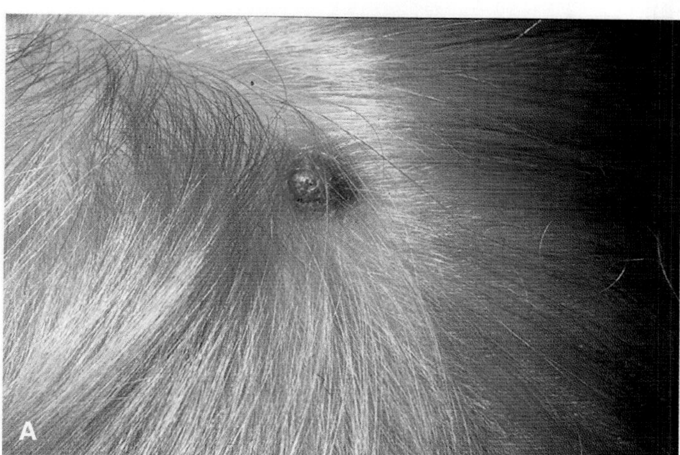

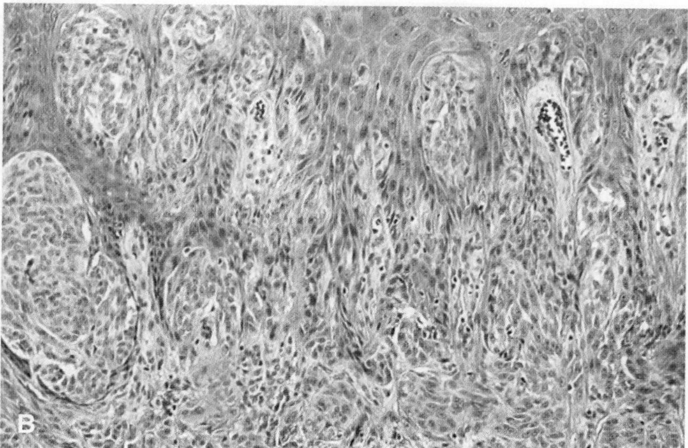

FIGURE 24-69. Spindle and epithelioid cell (Spitz) nevus. A. A symmetric pink nodule appeared suddenly in a child but then remained stable for several weeks until it was excised. **B.** Spitz tumors are composed of large melanocytes with prominent nuclei. Within a hyperplastic epidermis, the melanocytes are present in large nests. Even though the cells are large and, at first glance, suggest melanoma, they are much more uniform than the cells of most malignant melanomas.

of a freckle deepens with exposure to sunlight and fades when light exposure ceases. A **lentigo** is a discrete, brown macule that appears at any age and on any part of the body (though a **solar lentigo,** or "liver spot," appears at an older age after long-term sun exposure) (Fig. 24-72). Unlike a freckle, the pigmentation of a lentigo does not depend on sun exposure. Freckles show hyperpigmentation of basal keratinocytes without concomitant increases in the number of melanocytes. Lentigines, on the other hand, display elongated rete ridges, increased melanin pigment in both basal keratinocytes and melanocytes and increased melanocytes. Larger lesions may need to be biopsied to rule out lentigo maligna melanoma.

Verrucae Are Warts Caused by Human Papillomavirus

Verrucae are cutaneous tumors. They are elevated, circumscribed, symmetric, epidermal proliferations that often appear papillary. ***HPV is the cause of verrucae.***

PATHOLOGY:

- **Verruca vulgaris,** also known as the **common wart,** is an elevated papule with a verrucous (papillomatous) surface. Such lesions may be single or multiple and are most frequent on the dorsal surfaces of the hands or on the face. Histologically, verruca vulgaris displays hyperkeratosis and papillary epidermal hyperplasia (Fig. 24-73). **Koilocytes** (i.e., enlarged keratinocytes with a pyknotic nucleus surrounded by a halo-like cleared area) are observed within the upper epidermis. Viral inclusions are difficult to identify (Fig. 24-74). HPV, especially serotypes 2 and 4, are commonly found in verruca vulgaris. There is no malignant potential.
- **Plantar warts** are benign, frequently painful, hyperkeratotic nodules on the soles of the feet. Occasionally, similar lesions appear on the palms of the hands **(palmar warts).** Histologically, plantar warts are endophytic or exophytic, papillary, squamous epithelial proliferations. The cells contain abundant cytoplasmic inclusions that are similar in appearance to

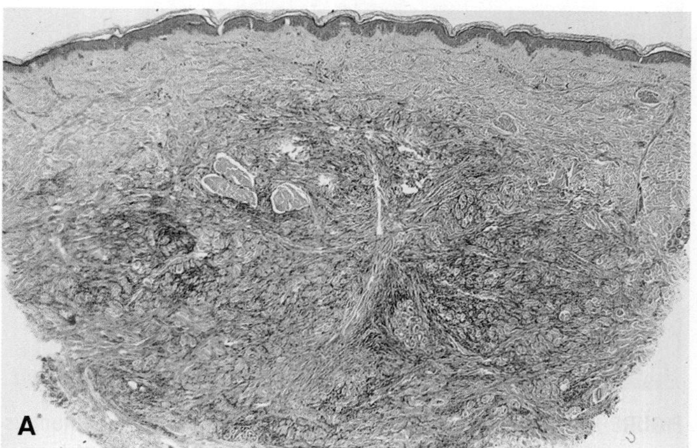

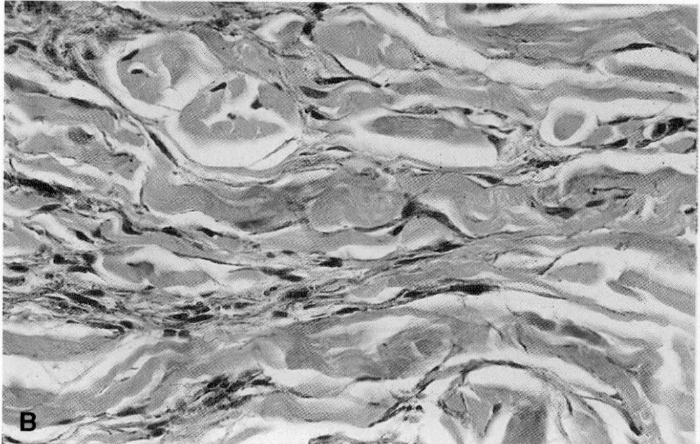

FIGURE 24-70. Blue nevus. A. Within the dermis there is a poorly defined but symmetric spindle cell proliferation that is dark brown. **B.** The lesion is composed of elongated cells with heavily pigmented dendrites and small bland nuclei.

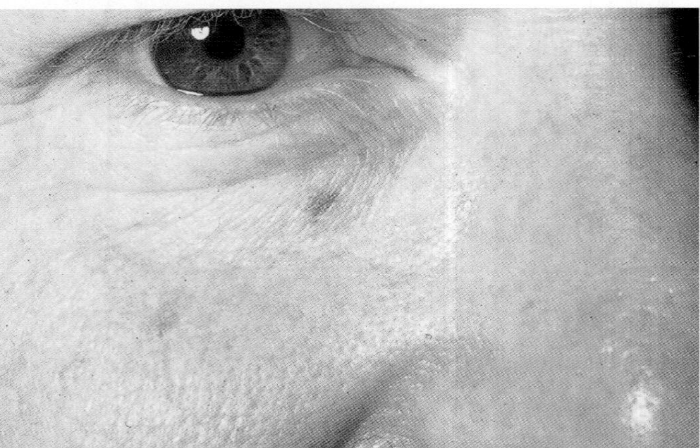

FIGURE 24-71. Freckle. A fair-complexioned man has a prominent brown macule that darkens in sunlight.

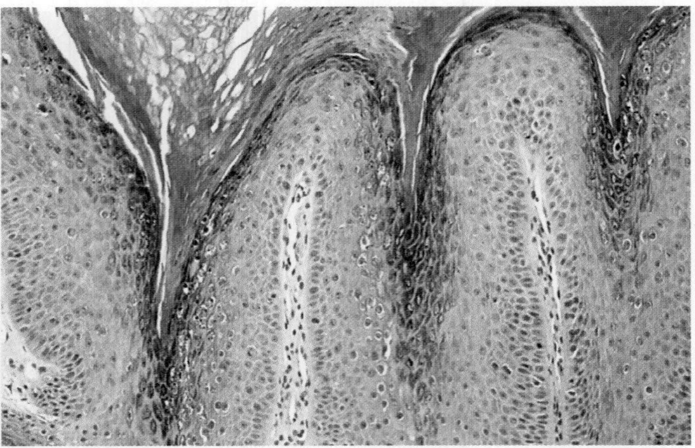

FIGURE 24-73. Verruca vulgaris. Verruca vulgaris is the prototype of papillary epidermal hyperplasia. Squamous epithelial-lined fronds have fibrovascular cores. The blood vessels within the cores extend close to the surface of verrucae, which makes them susceptible to traumatic hemorrhage and the resultant black "seeds" that patients observe.

the darker-staining keratohyaline granules. The nuclei of keratinocytes near the base of these warts also contain pink nuclear inclusions. HPV type 1 is the etiologic agent.

- **Verruca plana,** or "flat warts," are small flat papules that appear on the face. Microscopically, they display slight elongation of rete ridges (acanthosis), striking hypergranulosis and superficial koilocyte formation. HPV types 3 and 10 often elicit these lesions. The lesions do not progress to cancer.
- **Condyloma acuminatum** is a venereally transmitted wart usually caused by HPV serotypes 6 and 11, and occurring primarily around the genitalia. Histologically, lesions are papillary squamous proliferations. Koilocytosis and an almost continuous cap of parakeratosis are usually present. Squamous carcinomas may develop, especially when HPV types 16 and 18 are involved.
- **Bowenoid papulosis,** also caused by HPV types 16 and 18, is characterized by multiple hyperpigmented papules on the genitalia. Lesions may be histologically identical to squamous cell carcinoma (SCC) in situ in that they display disordered epithelial maturation and scattered keratinocyte atypia. The lesions also exhibit parakeratosis and irregular acanthosis. Bowenoid papulosis often regresses but may progress to dysplasia or malignancy.
- **Epidermodysplasia verruciformis** is a rare autosomal recessive disease characterized by impaired cell-mediated immunity and subsequently enhanced susceptibility to HPV infection. Warts similar to those of verruca plana, with confluence into patches, are widespread. It first appears in childhood, and SCC develops in 30% to 60% of patients. HPV types 5, 8, 9 and 47 are most commonly encountered.

Keratosis Is a Benign Horny Growth Composed of Keratinocytes

Seborrheic Keratosis

Seborrheic keratoses are scaly, frequently pigmented, elevated papules or plaques with scales that are easily rubbed

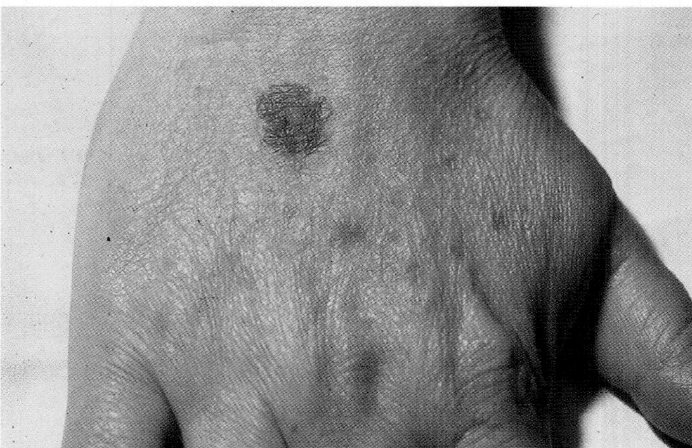

FIGURE 24-72. Lentigo. A 1-cm irregular patch of slightly variegated hyperpigmentation is present with a background of chronic solar damage.

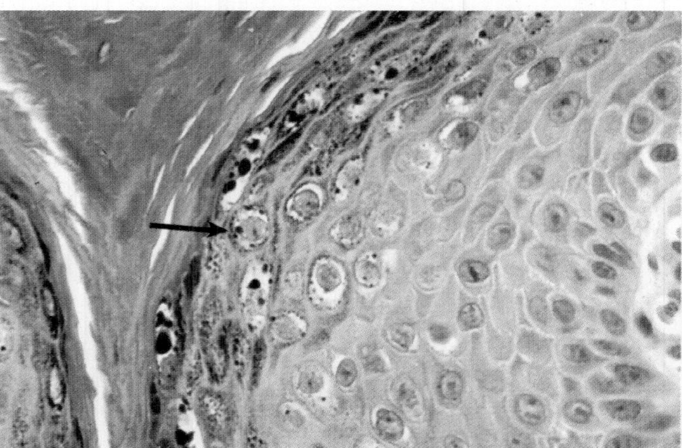

FIGURE 24-74. Verruca vulgaris. Characteristic cytopathic changes occur in the outer portion of the stratum spinosum and stratum granulosum, in which there is perinuclear vacuolization and prominent keratohyaline granules, with homogeneous blue inclusions (*arrow*).

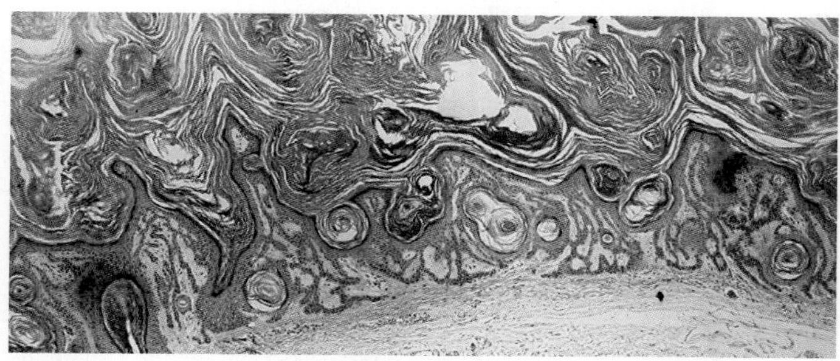

FIGURE 24-75. Seborrheic keratosis. Broad anastomosing cords of mature stratified squamous epithelium are associated with small keratin cysts.

off. Although they are among the most common keratoses, the etiology is unknown. The lesions generally occur in later life and tend to be familial. Clinically and microscopically, they appear "pasted on" and are composed of broad anastomosing cords of mature stratified squamous epithelium associated with small cysts of keratin (horn cysts) (Fig. 24-75). Seborrheic keratoses are innocuous but are a cosmetic nuisance. The sudden appearance of numerous seborrheic keratoses has been associated with internal malignancies ("sign of Leser-Trélat"), especially gastric adenocarcinoma.

Actinic Keratosis

Actinic keratoses ("from the sun's rays") are keratinocytic neoplasms that develop in sun-damaged skin as circumscribed keratotic patches or plaques, commonly on the backs of the hands or the face. Microscopically, the stratum corneum is no longer loose and basket-weaved but is replaced by a dense parakeratotic scale. The basal keratinocytes display significant atypia (Fig. 24-76). With time, actinic keratoses may evolve into squamous cell carcinoma in situ and finally into invasive squamous cell carcinoma. However, most are stable, and many regress.

Keratoacanthoma

Keratoacanthomas are rapidly growing keratotic papules on sun-exposed skin that develop over 3 to 6 weeks into crater-like nodules. They reach a maximum diameter of 2 to 3 cm.

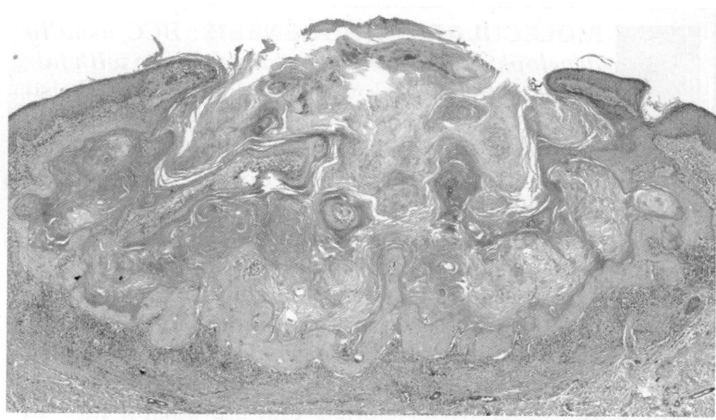

FIGURE 24-77. Keratoacanthoma. A keratin-filled crater (*center*) is lined by glassy proliferating keratinocytes.

Spontaneous regression usually follows within 6 to 12 months, leaving an atrophic scar. Some lesions may cause considerable damage before they regress, and some fail to regress. Keratoacanthomas are considered by some to be variants of SCC.

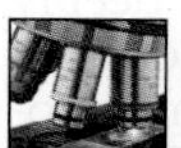

PATHOLOGY: Histologically, keratoacanthomas are endophytic papillary proliferations of keratinocytes. The lesion is cup shaped, with a central, keratin-filled umbilication and overhanging ("buttressing") epidermal edges (Fig. 24-77). At the base of the keratin, keratinocytes are large and have abundant homogeneous, eosinophilic ("glassy") cytoplasm. At the lower aspect of the lesion, irregular tongues of squamous epithelium infiltrate the collagen of the reticular dermis. Older lesions show active fibroplasia in the dermis around these tongues. There may be focal lichenoid inflammation and the dermis may be markedly infiltrated with neutrophils, lymphocytes and eosinophils. Microabscesses of neutrophils and entrapped dermal elastic fibers may be present within the lesion.

Basal Cell Carcinoma Is a Locally Invasive Epidermal Neoplasm

Basal cell carcinoma (BCC) is the most common malignant tumor in persons with pale skin. Although it may be locally aggressive, metastases are exceedingly rare.

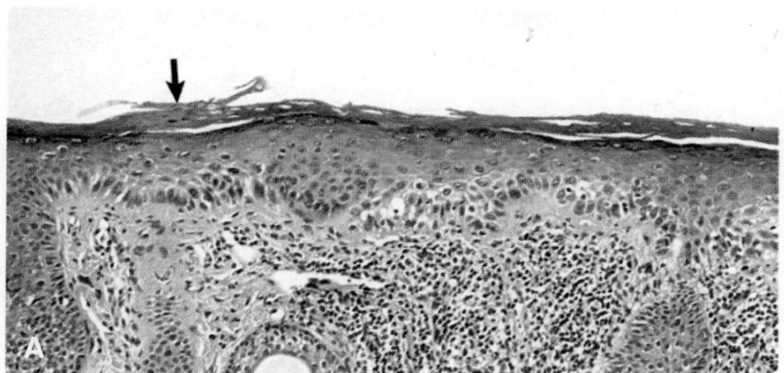

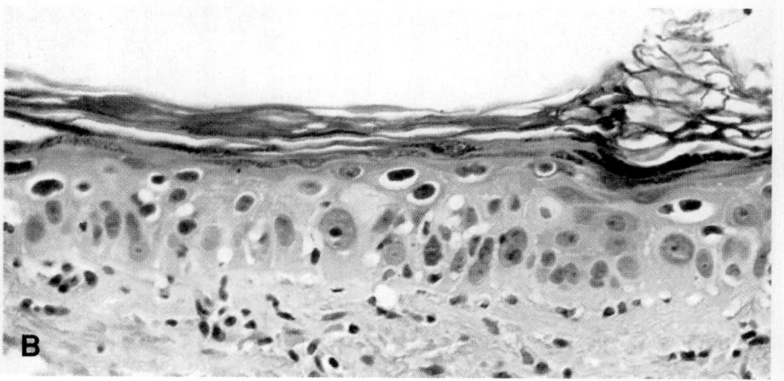

FIGURE 24-76. Actinic keratosis. A. A low-power view reveals cytologic atypia within the stratum basalis and lower stratum spinosum with loss of polarity. A lichenoid, band-like, lymphocytic infiltrate is frequently present. Parakeratosis is present here only in a small focus (*arrow*). **B.** High-power examination of an actinic keratosis reveals striking cytologic atypia of the basal keratinocytes, the hallmark of actinic keratoses.

MOLECULAR PATHOGENESIS: ***BCC usually develops on sun-damaged skin of people with fair skin and freckles.*** However, unlike SCC, BCC also arises on areas not exposed to intense sunlight. It is unusual to find BCC on the fingers and dorsal surfaces of the hands. The tumor is thought to derive from pluripotential cells in the basal layer of the epidermis, more specifically, in the bulge region of the hair follicle.

In several heritable syndromes, BCC originates on skin that has had little light exposure. **Nevoid BCC syndrome** refers to the occurrence of multiple tumors in the context of a complex multisystem disease. The syndrome also includes pits (dyskeratoses) on the palms and soles, mandibular cysts, hypertelorism and a predisposition to other neoplasms, including medulloblastoma. The BCCs of this syndrome appear at a young age and may number in the hundreds.

Germline mutations in the *PTCH* tumor suppressor gene on chromosome 9q22 cause nevoid BCC syndrome. Somatic mutations in *PTCH* have been implicated in up to 67% of sporadic BCCs.

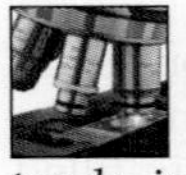

PATHOLOGY: BCC is composed of nests of deeply basophilic epithelial cells with narrow rims of cytoplasm that are attached to the epidermis and protrude into the subjacent papillary dermis (Fig. 24-78). The central part of each nest contains closely packed keratinocytes that are slightly smaller than the normal epidermal basal keratinocytes and show occasional apoptosis. The periphery of each nest shows an organized layer of polarized, columnar keratinocytes, with the long axis of each cell perpendicular to the surrounding BMZ ("peripheral palisading"). **Superficial, multicentric BCC** is composed of apparently isolated, but actually interconnected, nests that usually remain confined to the papillary dermis and manifest clinically as a spreading plaque. **Nodulocystic BCC** is also attached to the epidermis and exhibits the same cytologic and architectural features as the superficial type of BCC, but grows more deeply into the dermis. Usually, tumor cells of the dermal islands are associated with a mucinous ground substance and are surrounded by an array of fibroblasts and lymphocytes. Tumor nests are often separated from adjacent stroma by thin clefts ("retraction artifact"), a feature that may sometimes help distinguish BCC from other adnexal neoplasms displaying basaloid cell proliferation. BCCs with particularly dense sclerotic stroma are called **morpheaform BCCs** because of a clinical resemblance to lesions of localized scleroderma (also known as "morphea").

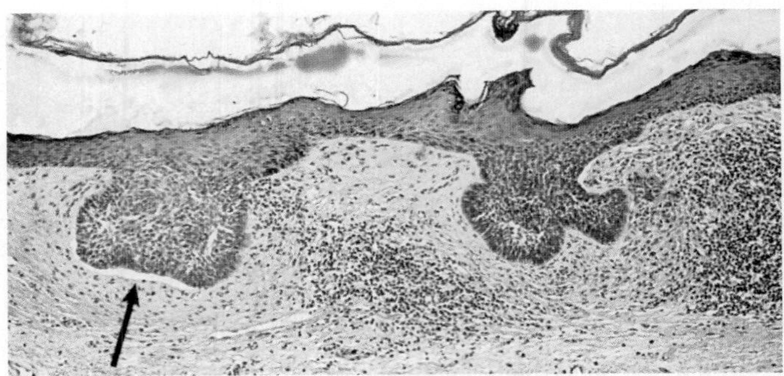

FIGURE 24-78. Basal cell carcinoma, superficial type. Buds of atypical basaloid keratinocytes extend from the overlying epidermis into the papillary dermis. The peripheral keratinocytes mimic the stratum basalis by palisading. The separation artifact (*arrow*) is present because of poorly formed basement membrane components and the hyaluronic acid-rich stroma that contains collagenase.

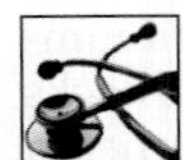

CLINICAL FEATURES: Some common forms of BCC are recognized:

- **Pearly papule** is the prototypic nodulocystic type of lesion, so named because it resembles a 2- to 3-mm pearl (Fig. 24-79). It is covered by tightly stretched epidermis and is laced with small, delicate, branching vessels (telangiectasia).
- **Rodent ulcer** is a small crater in the center of the pearl.
- **Superficial BCC** appears as a scaly, red, sharply demarcated plaque.

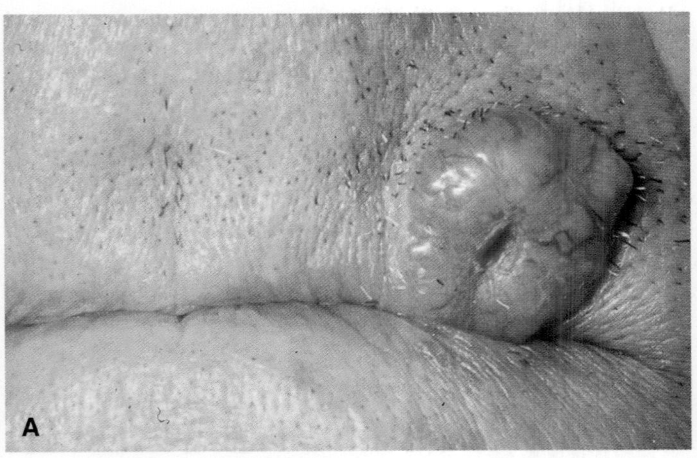

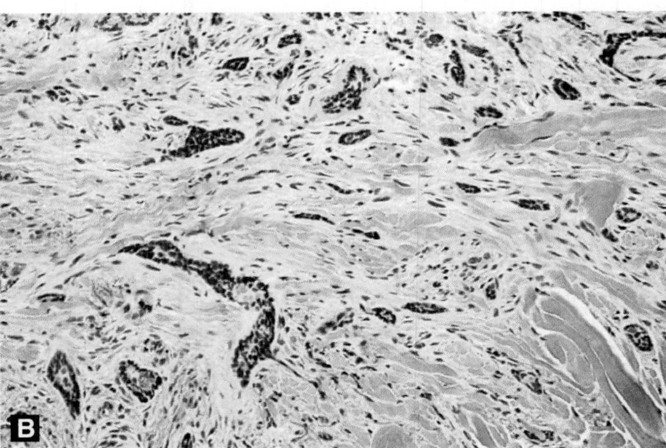

FIGURE 24-79. Basal cell carcinoma (BCC). A. Pearly papule: the tumor exhibits typical rolled pearly borders with telangiectases and central ulceration. **B.** Microscopic examination of morpheaform BCC shows a sclerosing and infiltrative lesion. Irregularly branching strands of tumor cells permeate the dermis, with induction of a cellular, fibroblastic, hyaluronic acid-rich stroma.

- **Morpheaform BCC** is a pale, firm, scar-like tumor that is ill-defined on and especially beneath the skin surface, making it particularly difficult to eradicate.
- **Pigmented BCC** may grossly resemble malignant melanoma. The pigment comes from reactive melanocytes that populate the tumor.

Treatment usually involves various excision or eradication procedures.

Cells of Squamous Cell Carcinomas Typically Resemble Differentiated Keratinocytes

SCC is second only to BCC in skin cancer incidence and may be caused by ultraviolet light, ionizing radiation, chemical carcinogens and HPV. SCC is most common on sun-damaged skin of fair persons with light hair and freckles, and often originates in actinic keratoses. It is exceedingly rare on normal black skin.

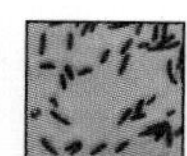

ETIOLOGIC FACTORS: SCC has multiple causes, ultraviolet light being the most common. SCC arising in sun-damaged skin metastasizes rarely (<2%). It may also arise in chronic scarring processes such as osteomyelitis sinus tracts, burn scars ("Marjolin ulcers") and areas of radiation dermatitis. In these settings, SCC metastasizes more often. Over 90% of SCCs, and many actinic keratoses, have mutated *p53* genes.

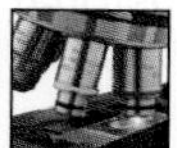

PATHOLOGY: SCC is composed of tumor cells that mimic epidermal stratum spinosum in varying degrees and extend into the subjacent dermis (Fig. 24-80). The edges of many tumors show changes typical of actinic keratosis, namely, a variably thickened epidermis with parakeratosis and significant atypia of basal keratinocytes.

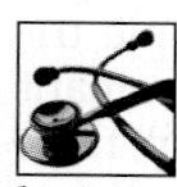

CLINICAL FEATURES: SCC characteristically arises in chronically sun-exposed areas such as the backs of the hands, face, lips and ears (Fig. 24-80A). Early lesions are small, scaly or ulcerated, erythematous papules, which may be pruritic. SCCs are usually treated by electrosurgery, topical chemotherapy, excision or radiation therapy.

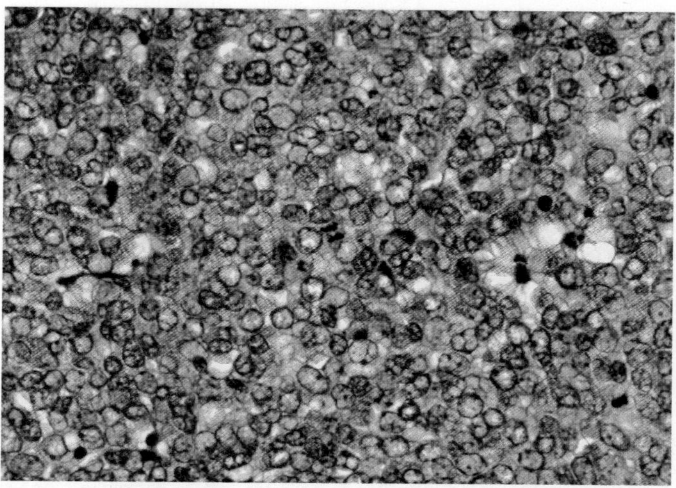

FIGURE 24-81. Merkel cell carcinoma. The tumor is composed of solid nests of undifferentiated cells that resemble small cell carcinoma of the lung.

Merkel Cell Carcinoma Is an Aggressive Tumor of Neurosecretory Cells That Shows Epithelial Differentiation

Merkel cell carcinoma (MCC) is typically a solitary, dome-shaped, red to violaceous nodule or indurated plaque that arises on the skin of the head and neck in elderly white patients. These are aggressive tumors that cause death in 25% to 70% of patients within 5 years.

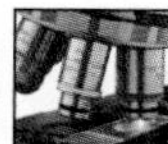

PATHOLOGY: Most MCCs consist of large solid nests of undifferentiated cells that resemble small cell carcinoma of the lung (Fig. 24-81). At its periphery, the tumor may show a trabecular pattern. Nuclear chromatin is dense and evenly distributed, cytoplasm is scant and mitotic figures and nuclear fragments are frequently present. Immunostaining shows cytokeratin 20 distributed in a "perinuclear dot" cytoplasmic pattern. Tumor cells also

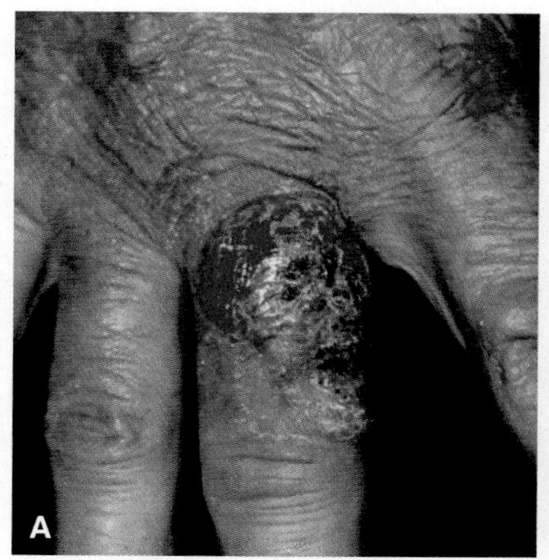

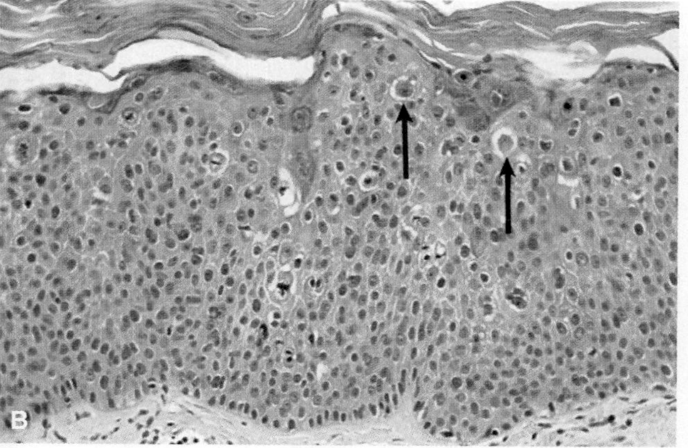

FIGURE 24-80. Squamous cell carcinoma. A. An ulcerated, encrusted and infiltrating lesion is seen on the sun-exposed dorsal aspect of a finger. **B.** A microscopic view of the periphery of the lesion shows squamous cell carcinoma in situ. The entire epidermis is replaced by atypical keratinocytes. Mitoses are apparent, as is apoptosis (*arrows*).

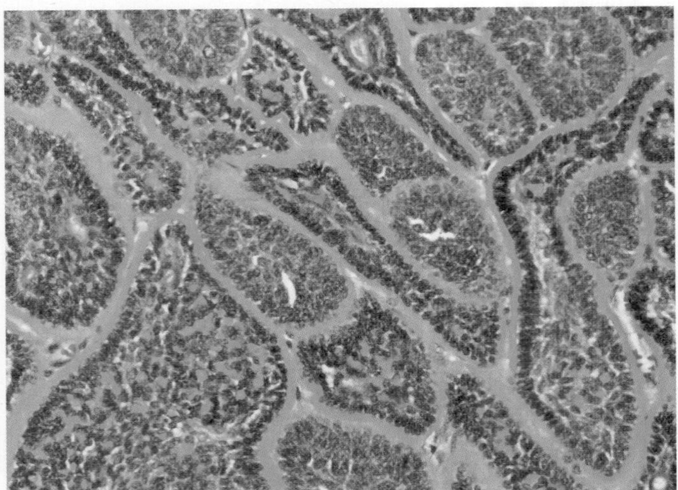

FIGURE 24-82. Cylindroma. Sharply circumscribed islands of basophilic epithelial cells reside in a jigsaw puzzle–like array. Dense eosinophilic hyaline sheaths surround each island.

stain positively for neuroendocrine markers such as chromogranin and synaptophysin.

MOLECULAR PATHOGENESIS: Recent evidence suggests that an infection with a relatively common polyomavirus, called Merkel cell polyoma virus (MCV), may play a role in the etiology of about 80% of cases of this rare and dangerous tumor. Tumorigenicity is associated with a mutation truncating the *TAg* gene of MCV.

Adnexal Tumors Differentiate Toward Skin Appendages

Adnexal tumors generally appear as elevated small skin nodules that often occur in people with a familial history of similar tumors. Frequently, the lesions appear at puberty. Although most are benign, malignant behavior is sometimes observed.

Cylindroma

Cylindromas are adnexal neoplasms with features of sweat gland differentiation. They may be solitary or multiple elevated nodules around the scalp. An autosomal dominant, heritable variant features multiple tumors. Occasionally, cylindromas become large and cluster about the head ("turban tumors"). Microscopic examination shows sharply circumscribed nests of deeply basophilic cells surrounded by a hyalinized, thickened BMZ (Fig. 24-82).

Syringoma

Syringomas typically occur about the eyelid and upper cheek as small, elevated, flesh-colored papules. Microscopically, small ducts resembling intraepidermal portions of eccrine sweat ducts are seen (Fig. 24-83).

Poroma

Poroma is a common, solitary neoplasm histologically similar to seborrheic keratosis but with narrow ductal lumina and occasional cystic spaces (Fig. 24-84). The pattern has been interpreted as eccrine sweat gland differentiation. The tumor is a firm, raised lesion, usually less than 2 cm in diameter, that develops on the sole or sides of the foot or on the hands or fingers. Microscopically, poromas extend from the lower portion of the epidermis into the dermis as broad, anastomosing bands of uniform, cuboidal cells. Occasional malignant lesions with similar differentiation are termed **porocarcinomas.**

Trichoepithelioma

Trichoepithelioma is a neoplasm that differentiates toward hair structures. It is usually a solitary lesion but in "multiple trichoepithelioma syndrome" it occurs as an autosomal dominant trait. Lesions begin to appear at puberty, on the face, scalp, neck and upper trunk. Microscopically, they resemble basal cell carcinomas but contain many "horn cysts" (keratinized centers surrounded by basophilic epithelial cells) (Fig. 24-85).

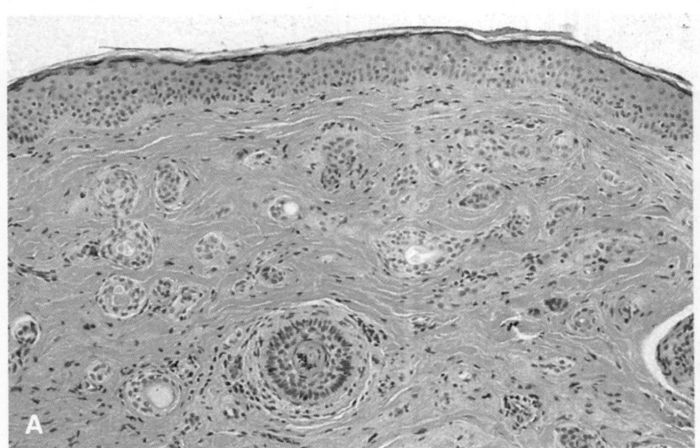

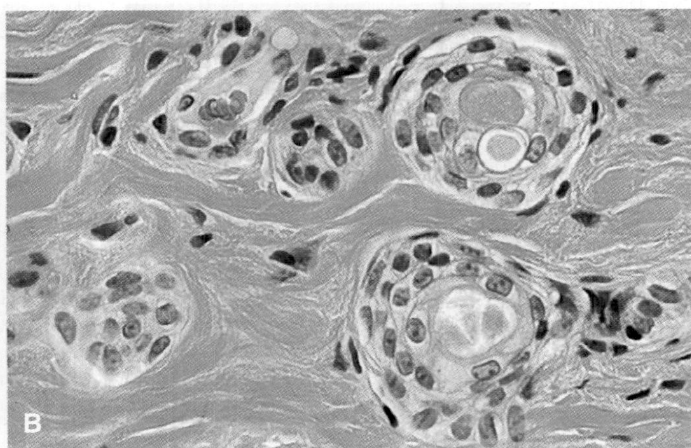

FIGURE 24-83. Syringoma. A. Within the upper dermis is an epithelial proliferation forming ducts, tubules and solid islands amid a dense fibrous stroma. **B.** The ductal differentiation closely mimics that of the straight dermal eccrine duct, with a central lumen and cuticle formation.

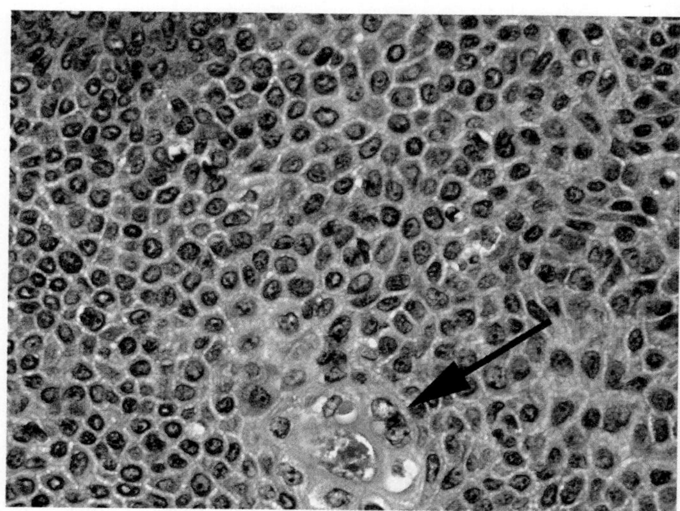

FIGURE 24-84. Poroma. Poroma displays uniform cells with narrow ductal lumina (*arrow*).

Fibrohistiocytic Tumors of the Skin Show a Varied Spectrum of Differentiation

Dermatofibroma

Dermatofibroma is a common, benign tumor of fibroblasts and macrophages. The former are the neoplastic cells. It occurs on the extremities as a dome-shaped, firm, rubbery nodule with ill-defined borders and pigmentation ranging from pink to dark brown. They are rarely more than 3 to 5 mm in diameter. Microscopically, the papillary and reticular dermis are replaced by fibrous tissue that forms ill-defined small cartwheels with small central vascular spaces (Fig. 24-86). The tumors are not well demarcated and blend with the surrounding dermis. The overlying epidermis is hyperplastic and often hyperpigmented.

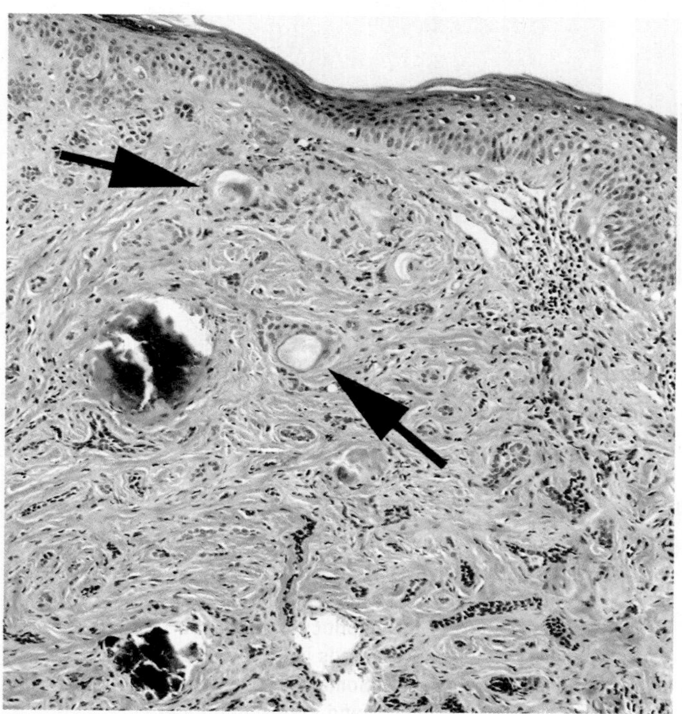

FIGURE 24-85. Trichoepithelioma. The tumor is composed of keratinized centers surrounded by basophilic epithelial cells ("horn cysts"; *arrows*).

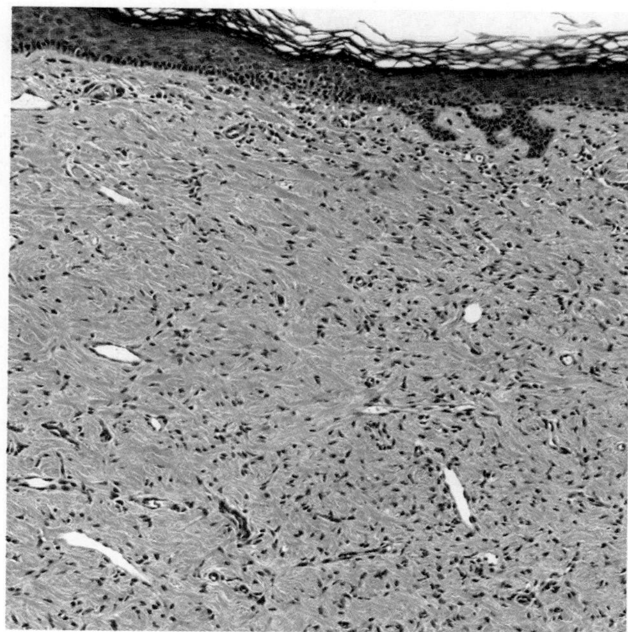

FIGURE 24-86. Dermatofibroma. Fibrous tissue replaces the dermis and forms poorly defined cartwheels.

Dermatofibrosarcoma Protuberans

Dermatofibrosarcoma protuberans, a tumor with intermediate malignant potential, is a slowly growing nodule or indurated plaque that appears mostly on the trunk of young adults. Local recurrence after attempted complete excision is common, but metastases are rare. The most common histologic pattern is a poorly circumscribed, monotonous population of spindle cells arranged in a dense "storiform" (pinwheel-like) array (Fig. 24-87). The tumor extends into the subcutis along fat septa and interstices, creating an infiltrative, honeycomb-like pattern. Tumor cells display CD34, a marker of endothelial cells and some neural tumor cells, as well as dermal fibroblast-like dendritic cells, the probable cell of origin. Positivity for CD34 may help distinguish this tumor from a dermatofibroma, which does not express this antigen.

Atypical Fibroxanthoma

Atypical fibroxanthoma is a low-grade malignant neoplasm that appears as a dome-shaped nodule on the sun-damaged skin of elderly persons. Microscopically, atypical spindle cells and epithelioid cells infiltrate and disrupt the dermis. Multinucleated cells, some with a finely vacuolated cytoplasm, may be prominent. Mitoses are numerous. It is negative for cytokeratins and S-100 protein, thereby differentiating it from spindle cell squamous cell carcinoma and spindle cell

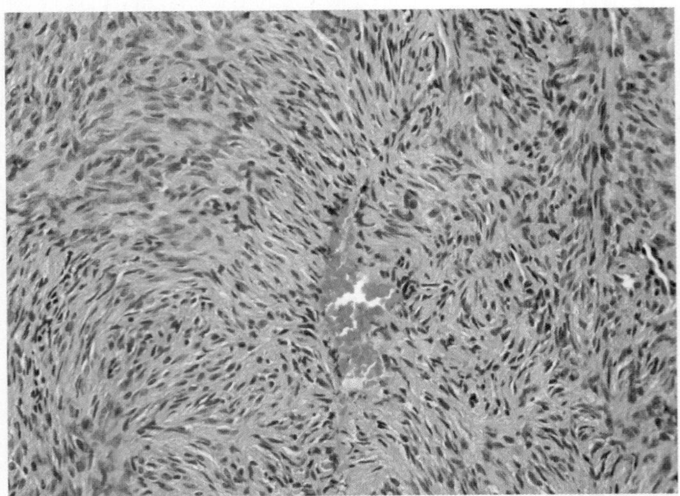

FIGURE 24-87. Dermatofibrosarcoma protuberans. Tumor cells form small cartwheels with central vascular spaces.

melanoma, respectively. Treatment is by excision, but local recurrence is common.

Mycosis Fungoides Is a Variant of Cutaneous T-Cell Lymphoma

The etiology of mycosis fungoides (MF) is unknown, but it is thought that malignancy of helper T cells ($CD4^+$) may be a pathologic response to chronic exposure to an antigen.

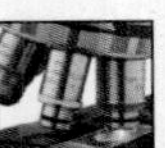

PATHOLOGY: In the early stages of the disease, delicate, erythematous plaques appear, often by the buttocks. Microscopically, these plaques show psoriasiform changes in the epidermis. The early inflammatory cell infiltrates in the dermis are polymorphic and are often not diagnostic of MF.

Skin involvement becomes progressively more prominent and infiltrative (Fig. 24-88). The most important histologic feature of MF is the presence of lymphocytes in the epidermis ("epidermotropism"). In late stages, the dermal infiltrate becomes dense to the point of forming tumor nodules. Increasing numbers of atypical lymphocytes that display hyperchromatic, convoluted ("cerebriform") nuclei are seen in the papillary dermis and epidermis. Circumscribed nests of these atypical lymphocytes ("Pautrier microabscesses")

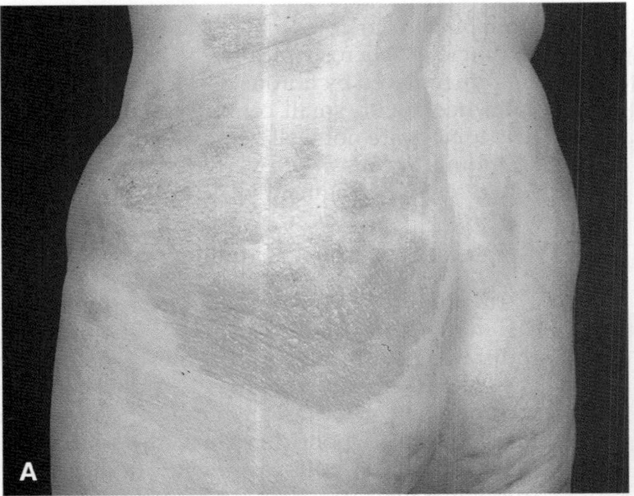

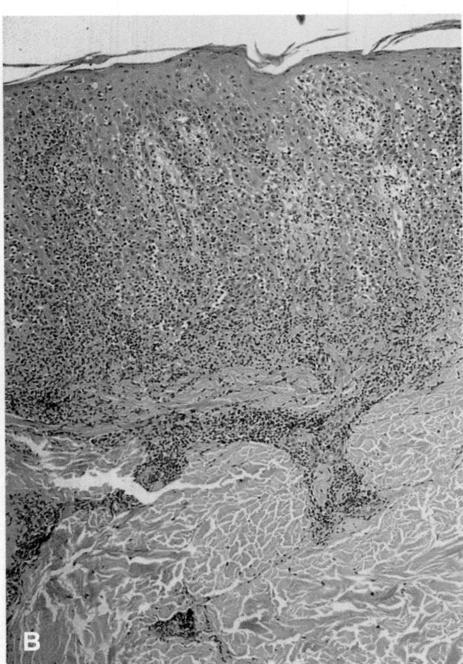

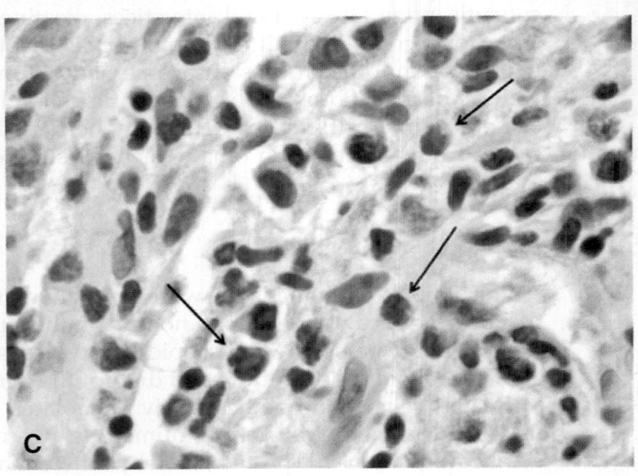

FIGURE 24-88. Mycosis fungoides. A. A 66-year-old woman presented with a 30-year history of erythematous scaly patches and plaques with telangiectases, atrophy and pigmentation. **B.** An atypical infiltrate of lymphocytes expands the papillary dermis and extends into the epidermis ("epidermotropism"). **C.** Some of the lymphocytes display hyperchromatic and convoluted ("cerebriform") nuclei (*arrows*).

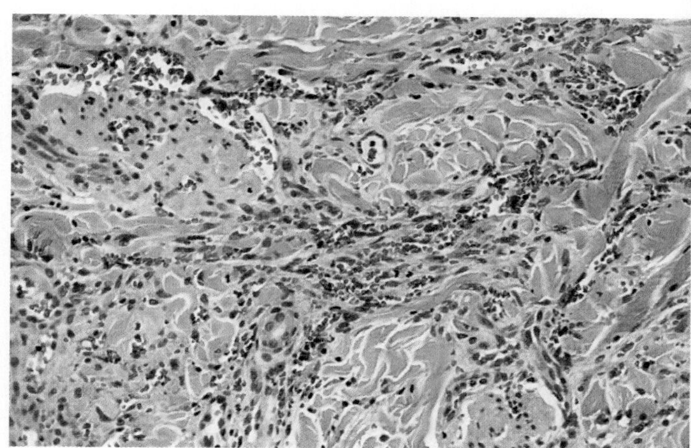

FIGURE 24-89. Kaposi sarcoma, plaque stage. Extending along the vascular arcades and amid reticular dermal collagen is a proliferation of endothelial cells. They form delicate vascular channels filled with red blood cells. Some endothelial cells are not canalized (have not formed lumina.)

eventually appear in the epidermis. Polymerase chain reaction and Southern blotting techniques may reveal a T-cell receptor gene rearrangement, indicative of a clonal cell population.

Sézary syndrome refers to the systemic dissemination of MF. The characteristic feature is the presence of cerebriform lymphocytes in the peripheral circulation.

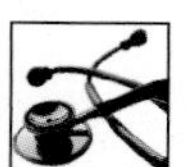

CLINICAL FEATURES: MF affects older age groups, has a slight male predominance and preferentially affects blacks over whites. It is classically divided into three stages: patch, plaque and tumor. In the patch stage, which may persist for months, eruptions consist of scaly, erythematous macules that may be slightly indurated. They are usually found on the lower abdomen, buttocks and upper thighs as well as the breasts of women, and can mimic other dermatitides such as psoriasis or eczema (Fig. 24-88A). Plaque-stage lesions are more infiltrated and circumscribed. As these coalesce, involvement becomes more widespread. Large, variably shaped tumor nodules can form on existing indurated plaques or on apparently normal skin. Spread to lymph nodes or visceral involvement portends reduced survival. Therapy includes ultraviolet light, topical nitrogen mustard and electron beam therapy.

Human Immunodeficiency Virus Infection Is Associated With Various Skin Diseases

Kaposi Sarcoma

Kaposi sarcoma (KS) is a malignant tumor of endothelial cells of blood vessels. This neoplasm was once seen only in older people of Mediterranean descent or in Africans. Since the advent of human immunodeficiency virus (HIV) infection, KS is most commonly seen in patients with AIDS. ***Human herpesvirus 8 (HHV-8) is the etiologic agent of KS.***

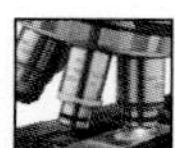

PATHOLOGY: All cases of Kaposi sarcoma, whether associated with HIV or not, evolve through three stages: patch, plaque and nodule. In the patch stage, a subtle proliferation of irregular vascular channels, lined by a single layer of mildly atypical endothelial cells, radiates from preexisting blood vessels and extends almost imperceptibly into the surrounding reticular dermis. Extravasated red blood cells, hemosiderin deposition and a sparse inflammatory infiltrate of lymphocytes and plasma cells are commonly observed.

In the plaque stage (Fig. 24-89), the entire reticular dermis is involved, with frequent extension into the subcutis and formation of bundles of spindle cells. In the nodule stage (Fig. 24-90), well-circumscribed dermal nodules are composed of anastomosing fascicles of spindle cells surrounding numerous slit-like spaces.

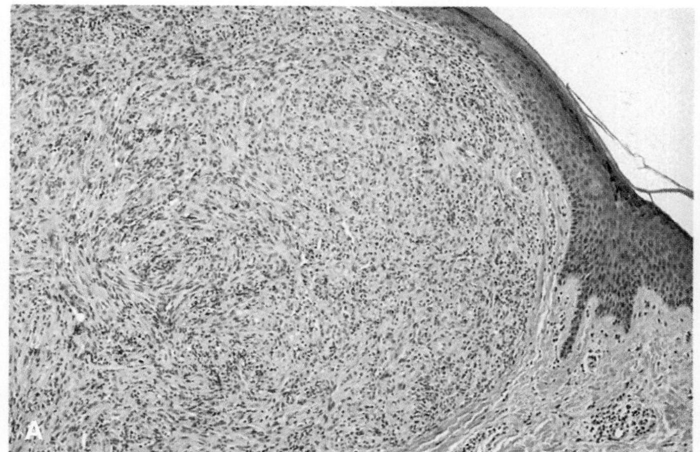

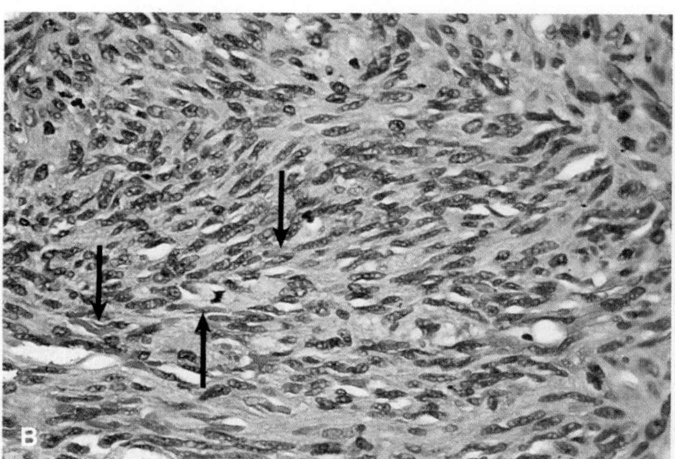

FIGURE 24-90. Kaposi sarcoma, nodule stage. A. A large nodule is composed of proliferating endothelial cells forming fascicles and vascular spaces. **B.** A higher-power view shows cytologic atypia of the spindle cells. Red blood cells appear agglutinated (*arrows*). The endothelial cells, in which the agglutinated red blood cells are present, form slit-like spaces.

Bacillary Angiomatosis

Bacillary angiomatosis is a pseudoneoplastic proliferation of capillaries that arises in response to infection with *Bartonella* species. Patients with late-stage AIDS are at risk for infection with these organisms. The proliferative lesions appear as red-to-brown papules, often in large numbers, and may be confused with Kaposi sarcoma. Silver impregnation stains show dense masses of bacilli within the basophilic deposits. The lesions clear with antibiotic treatment.

Eosinophilic Folliculitis

Eosinophilic folliculitis (EF) is a chronic pruritic eruption of papules that are centered on hair follicles. Patients infected with HIV are a distinct population that displays EF, although variants that are not related to HIV infection occur in other populations. The lesions are most often found on the trunk and proximal extremities. An infiltrate composed of lymphocytes, macrophages and numerous eosinophils is present in the intrafollicular and perifollicular areas and around dermal blood vessels.

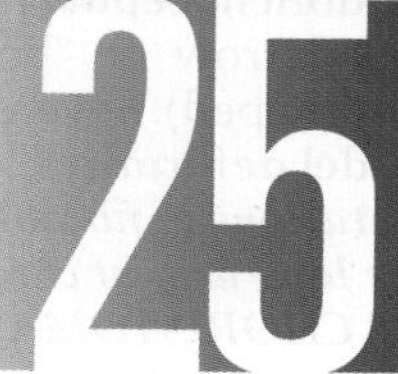

The Head and Neck

Diane L. Carlson • Bruce M. Wenig

ORAL CAVITY

The oral cavity extends from the lips to the pharynx. Its anatomic borders include:

- The vermilion border of the lips (anterior)
- A line from the junction of the hard and soft palate to the circumvallate papillae of the tongue (posterior)
- The hard palate until its junction with the soft palate (superior)
- The anterior two thirds of the tongue to the line of the circumvallate papillae (inferior)
- The buccal mucosa of the cheeks (lateral)

The oral mucosa consists of keratinized tissues of the attached gingiva, hard palate mucosa and specialized keratinized gustatory mucosa of the dorsum of the tongue. It also includes nonkeratinized mucosal surfaces of the inner lip and inner cheek, the nonattached, movable gingiva that continues into the maxillary and mandibular sulci, ventral tongue, floor of the mouth, soft palate and tonsillar pillars. The epithelium is three to four times the thickness of skin epidermis. Beneath the epithelium is the lamina propria of fibrous tissue and blood vessels, underneath which is the densely fibrous periosteum of the hard palate or the alveolus of the maxilla and mandible. The term **submucosa** is sometimes loosely applied to the deep connective tissue just above the muscle layer, in which the minor salivary glands are often embedded.

Minor salivary glands are scattered, unencapsulated small lobules within the mucosa and submucosa throughout the oral cavity. There are mucous glands in the lamina propria, particularly in the posterior hard palatal mucosa. Minor salivary glands of pure mucous type exist in the anterior ventral portion of the tongue (called Blandin, or Nunn, glands). Serous salivary glands are found near circumvallate papillae on the posterior and lateral tongue (von Ebner glands). Mixed mucoserous and mainly mucous glands predominate within the remainder of the oral cavity. Minor salivary glands are present in the retromolar mandibular ridge but the anterior hard palate and gingiva typically lack minor salivary glands.

The anterior two thirds of the dorsum of the tongue is covered by keratinized stratified squamous epithelium that is specialized to form **filiform papillae** (pointed projections of keratin). Between these are **fungiform papillae**, mushroom-shaped mucosal elevations containing taste buds. **Circumvallate papillae** separate the anterior two thirds from the posterior one third, and contain taste buds at their base. The last group of papillae is the **foliate papillae** located in the posterior lateral tongue in a series of ridges. Each taste bud is a barrel-shaped collection of modified epithelial cells that extend vertically from the basal lamina to the epithelial surface, opening via a taste pore.

Developmental Anomalies

FACIAL CLEFTS: If facial structures fail to fuse in the seventh week of embryonic life, facial clefts form. The most common of these is cleft upper lip **(harelip).** It may be unilateral or bilateral and frequently occurs in association with cleft palate (see Chapter 6).

Crouzon syndrome (craniofacial dysostosis) and **Apert syndrome** (acrocephalosyndactyly) are autosomal dominant disorders associated with craniosynostosis (premature fusion of the cranial sutures). This can lead to **brachycephaly** (flat head), **scaphocephaly** or **dolichocephaly** (the head is disproportionately long and narrow or "boat" shaped) and **trigonocephaly** (triangular shaped). Severe craniosynostosis may lead to **Kleeblattschadel deformity** ("cloverleaf" skull). ***Both syndromes reflect mutations in fibroblast growth factor receptor 2 (FGFR2), on the long arm of chromosome 10.***

HAMARTOMAS AND CHORISTOMAS: These are common in the oral cavity. **Fordyce granules** are aggregates of sebaceous glands in the oral cavity (choristoma). They occur on the buccal mucosa, lingual surface and lip, in 70% to 95% of the adult population; they may rarely coalesce to form mass lesions.

Abnormal descent of the thyroid during development may lead to submucosal foci of **ectopic thyroid** between the tongue and suprasternal notch. The base of the tongue between the foramen cecum and epiglottis is the most common site for ectopic thyroid **(lingual thyroid).** Normally located cervical thyroid is absent in over 75% of patients with lingual thyroid ("total migration failure"). Thus, surgical removal of a lingual thyroid may lead to hypothyroidism. The absence of a normally descended thyroid may also affect parathyroid gland development and localization. Seventy percent of patients with symptomatic lingual thyroid are hypothyroid and 10% suffer from cretinism. Malignancies are rare but will generally be papillary thyroid carcinomas.

Thyroglossal duct cysts result from persistence and cystic dilatation of the thyroglossal duct midline in the neck. The anomaly usually occurs above the thyroid isthmus but below the hyoid bone. Patients are usually symptomatic before age 40. Surgery is the treatment of choice.

*BRANCHIAL CLEFT CYST: **Branchial cleft cysts originate from branchial arch remnants*** (Fig. 25-1). They occur in

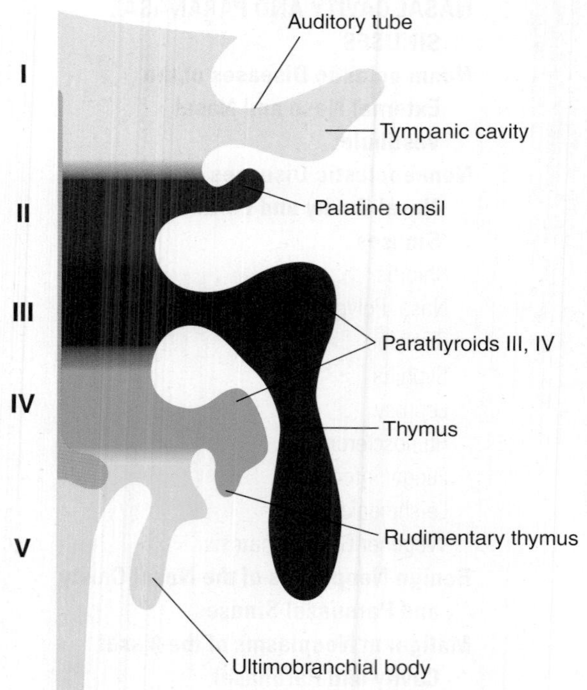

FIGURE 25-1. Branchial apparatus in humans. Schematic diagram of the pharyngeal pouches (*left half, ventral view*) in a human embryo of 6 weeks. Five pairs of pouches give rise to many important structures of the head, neck and chest. A wide spectrum of congenital malformations results from abnormalities of the branchial apparatus.

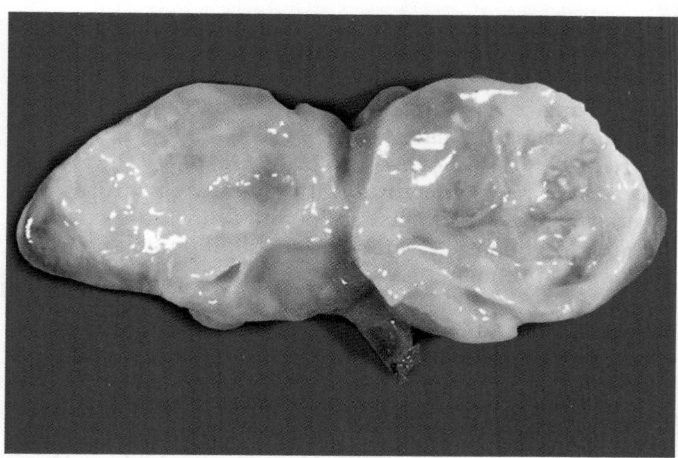

FIGURE 25-2. Branchial cleft cyst. Most of these cysts arise from the second branchial cleft and occur laterally in the neck. The cysts have a thin wall, contain turbid fluid and are lined by stratified squamous or respiratory-type epithelium.

the lateral anterior neck or parotid gland, mostly in young adults, and contain thin, watery fluid, and mucoid or gelatinous material (Fig. 25-2). These cysts are usually lined by squamous epithelium, with occasional foci of ciliated respiratory or pseudostratified columnar epithelium.

Infections of the Oral Cavity

Bacteria, spirochetes, viruses and fungi are normally present in the oral cavity, and are usually harmless. If the mucosa is injured or immunity is impaired, these otherwise normal oral flora can become pathogenic (see Chapter 9 for further discussion).

These terms are used to describe localized inflammation of the oral cavity:

- **Cheilitis** (lips)
- **Gingivitis** (gum)
- **Glossitis** (tongue)
- **Stomatitis** (oral mucosa)

Bacterial and Fungal Infections Commonly Affect the Oral Cavity

SCARLET FEVER: Predominantly a disease of children, scarlet fever is caused by several strains of β-hemolytic streptococci (*Streptococcus pyogenes*). Damage to vascular endothelium by the erythrogenic toxin results in a rash on the skin and oral mucosa. The tongue acquires a white coating, through which the hyperemic fungiform papillae project as small red knobs ("strawberry tongue"). Untreated, it can lead to glomerulonephritis and heart disease (**acute rheumatic fever**; see Chapters 11 and 16).

APHTHOUS STOMATITIS (CANKER SORES): Aphthous stomatitis is a common disease characterized by painful, recurrent, solitary or multiple, small ulcers of oral mucosa. The cause is unknown. Bacteria, mycoplasma, viruses and autoimmune and hypersensitivity reactions have been implicated but are unproved. The lesion consists of a shallow ulcer covered by a fibrinopurulent exudate. The underlying inflammatory infiltrate is composed of mononuclear and polymorphonuclear leukocytes. The lesions heal without scar formation.

ACUTE NECROTIZING ULCERATIVE GINGIVITIS (VINCENT ANGINA): Vincent angina is an acute necrotizing ulcerative gingivitis caused by infection by two symbiotic organisms, a fusiform bacillus and a spirochete (*Borrelia vincentii*). The term **fusospirochetosis** is used for this infection. These organisms are found in the mouths of many healthy people, suggesting that other factors are involved, particularly decreased resistance to infection due to inadequate nutrition, immunodeficiency or poor oral hygiene. Vincent angina is characterized by punched-out erosions of the interdental papillae. The process tends to spread and eventually involve all gingival margins, which become covered by a necrotic pseudomembrane.

Noma (cancrum oris) is a severe fusospirochetal infection in people who are malnourished, debilitated from infections or weakened by blood dyscrasias. It features rapidly spreading gangrene of oral and facial tissues. Large masses of tissue slough and leave the bones exposed, especially in children (see Chapter 9).

LUDWIG ANGINA: Ludwig angina is a rapidly spreading cellulitis, which originates in the submaxillary or sublingual space but extends locally to involve both. The responsible bacteria originate from oral flora; a variety of aerobic or anaerobic bacteria have been implicated. This potentially life-threatening inflammatory process is uncommon in developed countries save in patients with chronic illnesses associated with immunosuppression.

Ludwig angina is most often related to dental extraction or trauma to the floor of the mouth. After extraction of a tooth, hairline fractures may occur in the lingual cortex of the mandible, providing microorganisms ready access to the submaxillary space. Infection may dissect into the parapharyngeal space along fascial planes and from there into the carotid sheath. An infected (mycotic) aneurysm of the internal carotid artery may result, erosion of which may cause massive hemorrhage. The inflammation may also dissect into the superior mediastinum, to involve the pleural space and pericardium.

DIPHTHERIA: Infection with *Corynebacterium diphtheriae* is characterized by a patchy pseudomembrane, which often begins on the tonsils and pharynx but may also involve the soft palate, gingiva or buccal mucosa (see Chapter 9).

TUBERCULOSIS: Primary tuberculosis of the oral mucosa is rare. Most lesions are the result of pulmonary disease. The bacilli are carried in sputum and enter through small breaks in the mucosa, where they produce irregular, painful ulcers, mostly on the tongue. Biopsy reveals caseating granulomatous inflammation typical of tuberculous granulomas.

SYPHILIS: A chancre of primary syphilis may form on lips, tongue or oropharyngeal mucosa after contact with a lesion of primary or secondary syphilis (see Chapter 9). Regional lymphadenitis follows, and heals spontaneously in a few weeks. Without therapy, a diffuse mucocutaneous eruption of the secondary stage develops. Syphilitic lesions in the oral mucosa appear as multiple gray-white patches overlying ulcerated surfaces. They may spontaneously remit but may also recur. **Gummas** on the palate and tongue may appear years after initial infection. They are firm nodular masses that eventually ulcerate and may lead to palatal perforation.

ACTINOMYCOSIS: Actinomycetes are common inhabitants of the oral cavity in healthy people, so that culture of these anaerobic bacteria does not necessarily denote infection. Invasive actinomycosis is most often due to *Actinomyces bovis*, but *Actinomyces israelii* is sometimes seen. The organisms produce chronic granulomatous inflammation and abscesses that drain by fistula formation, with suppurative infection evidenced by characteristic yellow "sulfur granules." It is customary to distinguish cervicofacial (the most common form), pulmonary and abdominal forms of actinomycosis according to the site of the infection. In the cervicofacial form, soft tissue infection may extend to adjacent bones, most commonly to the mandible.

CANDIDIASIS: Also termed **thrush** or **moniliasis**, oral candidiasis is caused by *Candida albicans* (see Chapter 9), which is common on the surfaces of the oral cavity, gastrointestinal tract and vagina. To cause disease, it must penetrate tissues, albeit superficially. Oral candidiasis is mostly seen in people with compromised immune systems and in diabetics. The incidence in patients with acquired immunodeficiency syndrome (AIDS) is 40% to 90%. The lesions are white, slightly elevated, soft patches that consist mainly of fungal hyphae.

Viral Infections Present as Vesicular or Ulcerative Lesions

HERPES SIMPLEX VIRUS TYPE 1: Herpes labialis (cold sores, fever blisters) and herpetic stomatitis are caused by herpes simplex virus (HSV) type 1 and are among the most common viral infections of the lips and oral mucosa in both children and young adults. Transmission occurs by droplet infection, and the virus can be recovered from saliva of infected people. Disease starts with painful inflammation of the affected mucosa, followed shortly by formation of vesicles. The vesicles rupture and form shallow, painful ulcers, ranging from punctate size to a centimeter in diameter. Herpetic vesicles form as a result of "ballooning degeneration" of epithelial cells, some of which show intranuclear inclusions (Fig. 25-3). Ulcers heal spontaneously without scarring.

Once HSV enters the body, it survives in a dormant state in the trigeminal ganglion. Stresses such as trauma, allergy, menstruation, pregnancy, exposure to ultraviolet light and other viral infections may reactivate it to cause recurrent lesions. Recurrent oral cavity vesicles almost invariably develop on a mucosa that is tightly bound to periosteum, for example, the hard palate.

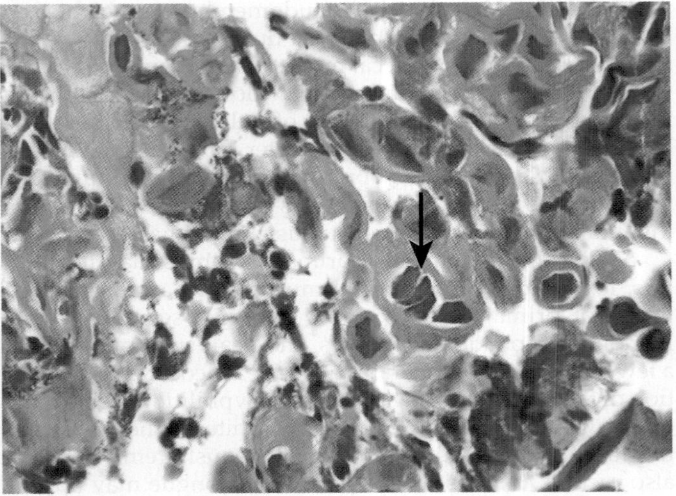

FIGURE 25-3. Herpes simplex virus type 1. A biopsy from a nonhealing ulcer on the tongue demonstrates intranuclear viral inclusions (*arrow*) within squamous cells infected by the virus.

HUMAN PAPILLOMAVIRUS–RELATED DISEASES: The human papillomavirus (HPV) family of viruses (see Chapter 9) causes epithelial proliferations including papillomas (e.g., sinonasal, Schneiderian papillomas and other mucosal papillomas of various upper aerodigestive tract sites). "High-risk" HPV, predominantly types 16 and 18, as well as 31, 33 and 35, is strongly associated with the development of oropharyngeal squamous cell carcinoma (see below).

EPSTEIN BARR VIRUS–RELATED DISEASES: Epstein-Barr virus (EBV; a human herpes virus, HHV 4) is the cause of infectious mononucleosis, oral hairy leukoplakia and lymphoid malignancies (e.g., nasal-type natural killer [NK]/T-cell lymphoma, Hodgkin lymphoma; see Chapter 20) and epithelial malignancies (e.g., nasopharyngeal-type differentiated and undifferentiated carcinomas, salivary gland undifferentiated carcinoma).

HUMAN HERPES VIRUS 8: HHV8 (also known as KS-associated herpes virus) is associated with **Kaposi sarcoma.** This malignancy occurs most commonly in the skin (see Chapter 24), but can also involve lymph nodes and viscera and, less commonly, sites such as the tongue and oral cavity. These tumors show proliferation of vascular endothelial cells that form slitlike vascular channels with extravasation (or "spilling out") of red blood cells. Patients with human immunodeficiency virus (HIV) are at very high risk for this disease. It is also seen in elderly men of Mediterranean/East European descent and in non–HIV-infected middle-aged adults and children in Equatorial Africa. KS is also seen in transplant patients on high doses of immunosuppressive agents.

HHV8 is a causative agent in **multicentric Castleman disease** (MCD) and **primary effusion lymphomas** (PELs) (see Chapter 20).

OTHER VIRAL INFECTIONS: Coxsackievirus causes **herpangina**, an acute vesicular oropharyngitis. A brief course of infection confers lasting immunity. **Cytomegalovirus** (CMV) infection typically presents with surface ulceration. Other virus infections that involve the oral mucosa include measles, rubella, chickenpox and herpes zoster.

Benign Tumors

Benign tumors found elsewhere in the body are seen also in the oral cavity. These include pigmented nevi, fibromas, hemangiomas, lymphangiomas and squamous papillomas. Trauma may lead to ulceration of these lesions, in which case they may bleed or become infected.

PAPILLOMA: Squamous papilloma is a benign, exophytic epithelial tumor made of branching fronds of squamous epithelium with fibrovascular cores. These are the most common benign oral cavity neoplasms, and have been associated with HPV types 6 and 11, which are low-risk serotypes not associated with malignancy. They occur mainly in the third to fifth decades. The tongue, palate, buccal mucosa, tonsil and uvula are most often involved.

BENIGN MINOR SALIVARY GLAND TUMORS: **Pleomorphic adenoma** (benign mixed tumor) is the most common

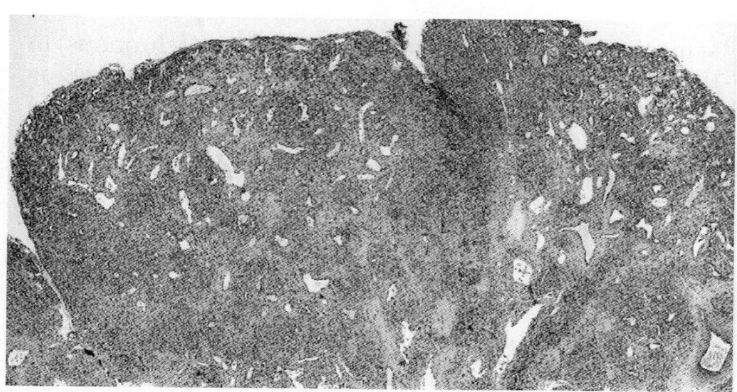

FIGURE 25-4. Lobular capillary hemangioma (pyogenic granuloma). Submucosal lesion characterized by the presence of cellular lobules consisting of dilated, irregularly shaped vascular spaces and surrounded by granulation tissue with a chronic inflammatory cell infiltrate.

oral salivary gland tumor (see below). Monomorphic adenomas such as myoepithelioma and oncocytoma occur less frequently. Benign mesenchymal tumors may occur in the oral cavity, including hemangiomas, leiomyomas and lipomas.

LOBULAR CAPILLARY HEMANGIOMA (PYOGENIC GRANULOMA; PREGNANCY TUMOR): Lobular capillary hemangiomas are benign polypoid capillary hemangiomas that occur mainly on the skin and mucous membranes and, most often, gingiva. The term pyogenic granuloma is a misnomer: it is neither infectious nor granulomatous. In the oral cavity, they range from a few millimeters to a centimeter and are elevated, soft, red or purple, with smooth, lobulated, ulcerated surfaces. They show submucosal vascular proliferation arranged in lobules or clusters with central capillaries and smaller ramifying tributaries (Fig. 25-4). In time, the lesions may become less vascular and may resemble a fibroma.

In pregnant women, particularly near the end of the first trimester, a gingival lesion may develop that grossly and microscopically is identical to lobular capillary hemangioma. Termed **pregnancy tumor,** it may or may not regress after delivery.

Preneoplastic or Epithelial Precursor Lesions

Premalignant lesions of the upper aerodigestive tract include leukoplakia, erythroplakia or speckled leukoplakia, the terms reflecting the presence of a white, red or mixed white/red lesion, respectively. ***Leukoplakia** (from the Greek,* leukos, *"white," and* plax, *"plaque")* ***is an asymptomatic white lesion on the surface of a mucous membrane*** that affects both sexes equally, mostly after the third decade of life. Some of these lesions may become squamous cell carcinomas (SCCs). A variety of diseases appear clinically as leukoplakia, including various keratoses, hyperkeratosis and squamous carcinoma in situ. ***Thus, leukoplakia is not a histologic diagnosis but rather a descriptive clinical term.*** Other clinical entities may also have white plaques on the oral mucosa (e.g., candidiasis, lichen planus, psoriasis, syphilis).

The causes of leukoplakia are diverse, and include use of tobacco products, alcoholism and local irritation. The same factors also appear to be important in the etiology of oral carcinoma.

Erythroplakia is the red equivalent of leukoplakia. It occurs less often than leukoplakia. Red areas associated with leukoplakic lesions are termed **speckled leukoplakia (erythroleukoplakia; speckled mucosa).** Erythroplakia may represent moderate to severe dysplasia or carcinoma. Not all red erythroplakic lesions herald dysplasia/carcinoma, as many red oral mucosal lesions may be inflammatory in nature.

PATHOLOGY: Leukoplakia (Fig. 25-5) occurs mostly on the buccal mucosa, tongue and floor of mouth. Plaques may be solitary or multiple and vary from small lesions to large patches. Erythroplakia is commonly associated with ominous histopathologic alterations, including severe dysplasia, carcinoma in situ or invasive carcinoma. In contrast, leukoplakic lesions are not necessarily premalignant; they may show a spectrum of histopathologic changes, from increased surface keratinization without dysplasia to invasive keratinizing squamous carcinoma. Leukoplakic lesions, unlike erythroplakic ones, tend to be well defined with demarcated margins. The risk of malignant transformation in leukoplakia is 10% to 12%. Speckled leukoplakia has an intermediate risk between "pure" leukoplakic and "pure" erythroplakic lesions for development of a malignancy, but speckled leukoplakia should be viewed as a variant of erythroplakia.

Oral hairy leukoplakia exhibits shaggy parakeratosis and edema, and may or may not have an associated inflammatory infiltrate. It is mainly seen in HIV-positive individuals, and over half of the lesions have associated candidiasis. The EBV-infected epithelial cells have vacuolated cytoplasm and are superficially located just beneath the keratin. Nuclei show dense central eosinophilic inclusions. Oral hairy leukoplakia and candidiasis are important markers in HIV immune status; together they are indicative of low $CD4^+$ counts and high viral load.

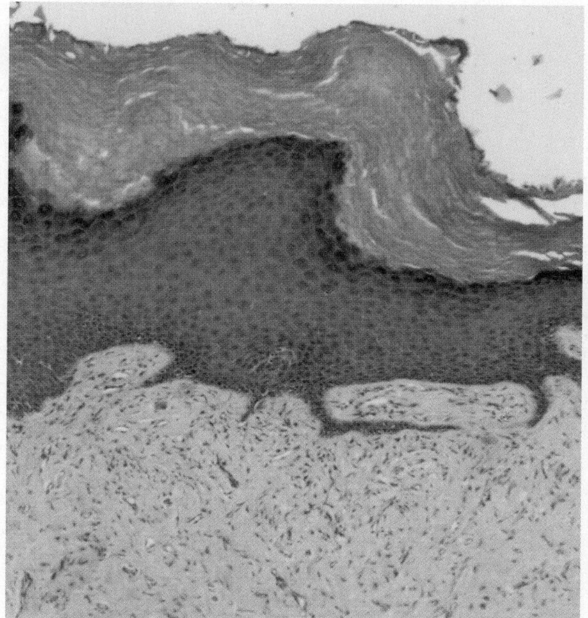

FIGURE 25-5. Leukoplakia. The lesion was seen as a white patch on the buccal mucosa of a heavy smoker. Histologically, epithelial hyperplasia and hyperkeratosis are evident.

Squamous Cell Carcinoma

SCC is the most common malignant tumor of the oral mucosa and may occur at any site. In the United States, there are over 35,000 cases yearly, most often involving the tongue, then, in descending order the floor of the mouth, alveolar mucosa, palate and buccal mucosa. The male:female ratio is 2:1 for the gums but 10:1 for the lip. There are substantial variations in geographic distribution for oral cancer; for example, it is the single most common cancer of men in India, where it is associated with betel nut quid chewing, also known as *pan*.

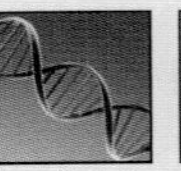
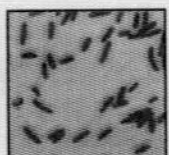

MOLECULAR PATHOGENESIS AND ETIOLOGIC FACTORS: Predisposing factors in the pathogenesis of oral cancer include use of tobacco products, alcoholism, iron deficiency (Plummer-Vinson syndrome), Fanconi anemia, physical and chemical irritants, chewing of betel nuts, ultraviolet light on the lips and poor oral hygiene (craggy teeth and ill-fitting dentures). Not surprisingly, several of these factors are also connected with leukoplakia. Multiple separate squamous cell carcinomas may be found at the same time (synchronous) or at intervals (metachronous) in the oral mucosa ("field cancerization"). Worldwide, as many as 25% of head and neck squamous cell carcinomas are associated with high-risk HPV, mostly HPV 16.

Midline carcinomas of the upper aerodigestive tract with rearrangement of the *nuclear protein of the testis (NUT)* gene (NUT midline carcinoma) generally occur in children, but are also seen in adults. These tumors have a balanced translocation (t15;19), resulting in the BRD4-NUT oncogene. They tend to occur in midline structures of the upper aerodigestive tract (e.g., sinonasal tract) and non-head and neck (e.g., mediastinum) but may occur away from the midline (e.g., parotid gland). NUT midline carcinomas are undifferentiated or poorly differentiated malignancies, but squamous cell differentiation can be seen.

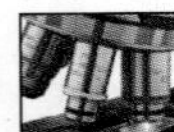

PATHOLOGY: ***Invasive SCC of the oral cavity is similar to the same tumor in other sites and is generally preceded by carcinoma in situ.*** SCC ranges from well to poorly differentiated, including undifferentiated and sarcomatoid variants. Well-differentiated, or grade I, tumors are frequently keratinizing (Fig. 25-6). At the other

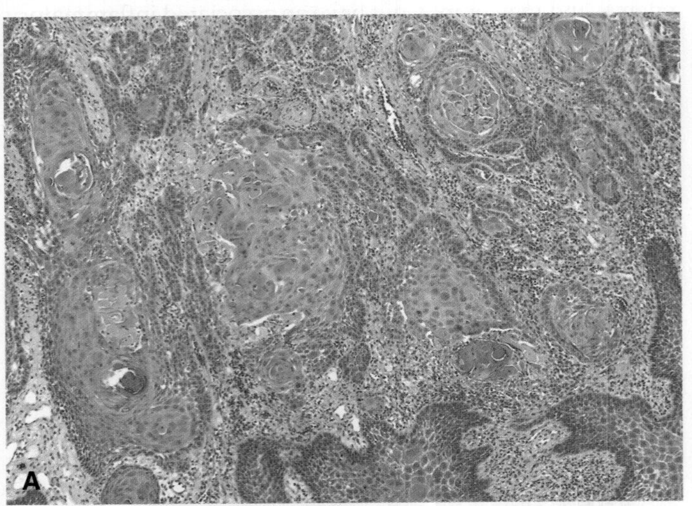

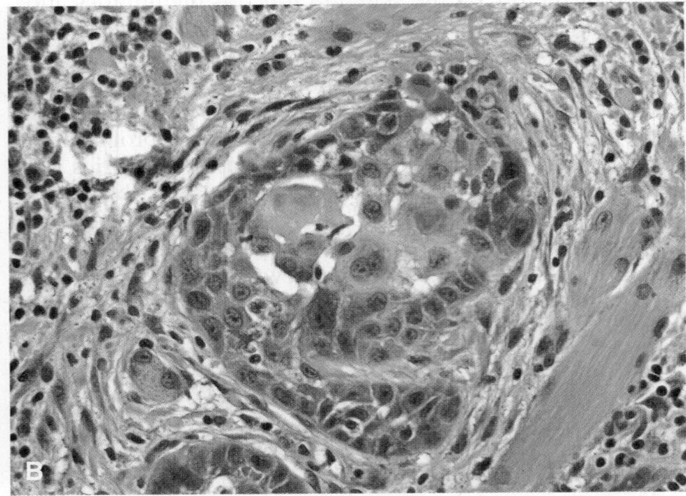

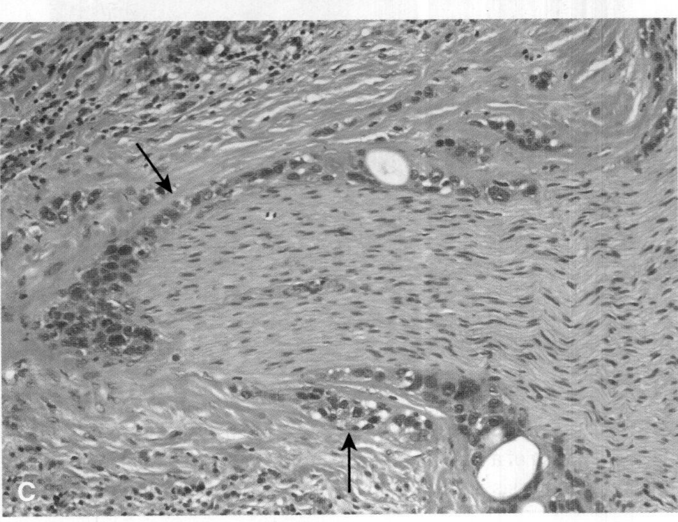

FIGURE 25-6. Squamous cell carcinoma. A. An infiltrative neoplasm is composed of cohesive nests of tumor. **B.** A less differentiated tumor displays cells with pleomorphic nuclei, prominent nucleoli, brightly eosinophilic cytoplasm indicating keratinization and intercellular bridges connecting adjacent cells. **C.** Perineural invasion by squamous cell carcinoma. Tumor surrounds a nerve (*arrows*).

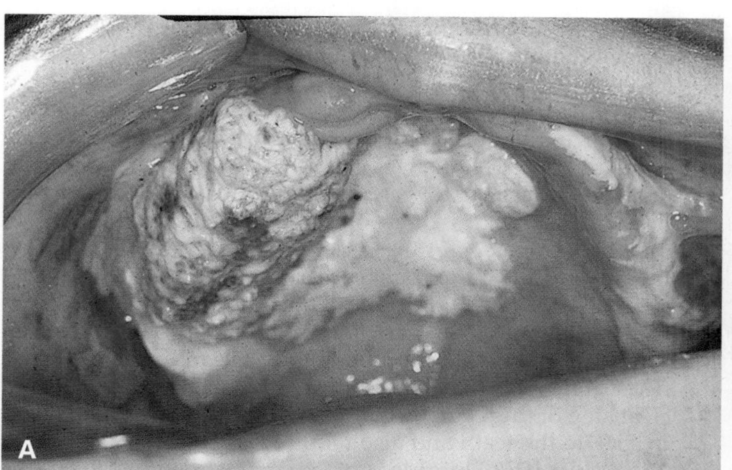

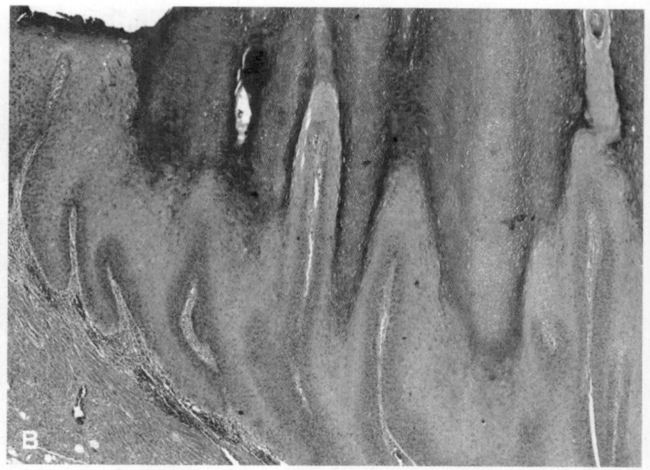

FIGURE 25-7. Verrucous carcinoma. A. The tumor is white with an exophytic appearance involving the alveolar ridge. Note the confluent flat white (leukoplakic) appearance of the palate. **B.** Microscopically, there is prominent surface keratinization ("church-spire" keratosis) composed of bland-appearing uniform squamous cells without dysplasia, and broad or bulbous rete pegs with a pushing margin into the submucosa.

end of the spectrum, tumors may be so poorly differentiated that their origin is difficult to determine.

Oral SCC mainly metastasizes to submandibular, superficial and deep cervical lymph nodes. More than half of patients who die of SCC of the head and neck have distant, blood-borne metastases, most commonly in lungs, liver and bones. Autopsy studies have shown that nearly 20% of these patients have axillary metastases.

Local recurrence is affected by the pattern of tumor infiltration; single cell infiltration is more unfavorable than a broad, "pushing" border. Other prognostic factors include depth of tumor invasion, perineural invasion and lymphovascular tumor emboli. As one would expect, negative margins are another key factor in maintaining local and regional control of the tumor.

Verrucous carcinoma (VC) is a highly differentiated variant of squamous cell carcinoma, which is locally destructive but does not metastasize. It generally occurs in the sixth and seventh decades of life. VCs may arise anywhere in this region but are most common on buccal mucosa, gingiva and larynx. VCs are usually white, warty to fungating, or exophytic and are generally attached by a broad base (Fig. 25-7A). They exhibit a benign-appearing squamous epithelium (without dysplasia or atypia), marked surface keratinization and a pushing border of bulbous rete pegs (Fig. 25-7B). The tumor carries a good prognosis if it is completely removed.

Malignant Minor Salivary Gland Neoplasms

About 50% of intraoral minor salivary gland tumors are malignant. These include mucoepidermoid carcinoma, adenoid cystic carcinoma and polymorphous low-grade adenocarcinoma (see below). Some of the more common malignant tumors of major salivary glands are uncommon in minor salivary glands (e.g., acinic cell adenocarcinoma), whereas polymorphous low-grade adenocarcinoma and clear cell carcinoma are more common in the palate rather than in major salivary glands.

Benign Diseases of the Lips

The lips are affected by a variety of degenerative, inflammatory and proliferative processes. Some of these, particularly those expressed in the skin and mucous membranes, are systemic; others reflect localized disease. **Mucocele** is a mucus-filled cystic lesion associated with minor salivary glands that is probably caused by trauma (Fig. 25-8).

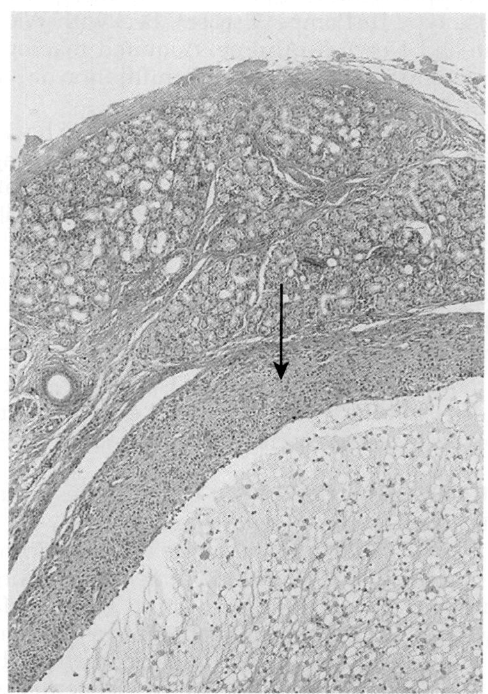

FIGURE 25-8. Mucocele of lower lip. This cystic lesion is associated with the minor salivary glands and is probably caused by trauma that permits escape of mucus. The cyst has a fibrous wall and is lined by granulation tissue (*arrow*). The lumen is filled with mucus that contains numerous macrophages.

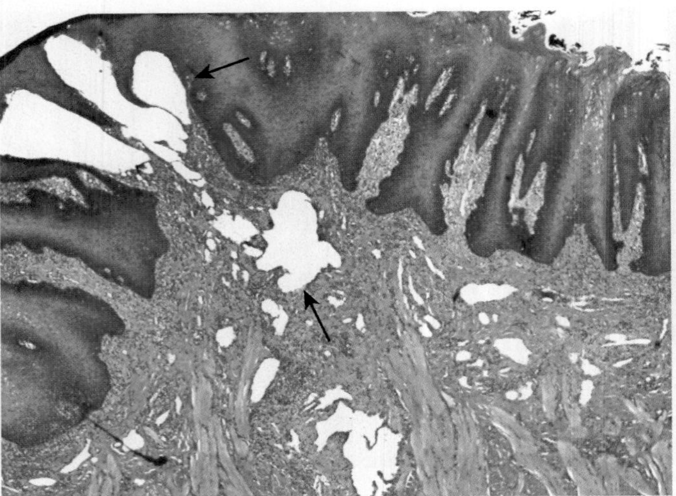

FIGURE 25-9. Lymphangioma of the tongue. Submucosal dilated lymphatics (*arrows*) splay skeletal muscle fibers.

Benign Diseases of the Tongue

MACROGLOSSIA: ***All components of the tongue may be involved by various localized or systemic diseases, some of which can lead to tongue enlargement.*** If present at birth, macroglossia is usually due to diffuse lymphangioma (Fig. 25-9) or hemangioma, although it may rarely be caused by congenital neurofibromatosis or true muscle hypertrophy. An enlarged tongue that protrudes from the mouth occurs in congenital hypothyroidism, Hurler syndrome, glycogen storage disease type II (Pompe disease), Beckwith-Wiedemann syndrome and Down syndrome. Acquired macroglossia is due to amyloidosis, acromegaly and infiltration or lymphatic obstruction by tumors.

GLOSSITIS: Inflammation of the tongue can be caused by various microorganisms, physical effects, chemical agents or systemic diseases. Some forms of glossitis are associated with vitamin deficiencies, including pernicious anemia, riboflavin deficiency, pellagra and pyridoxine deficiency.

Dental Caries (Tooth Decay)

Caries is the most prevalent chronic disease of the calcified tissues of teeth, affecting both sexes and every age group. Its incidence has markedly increased with modern civilization.

ETIOLOGIC FACTORS: Dental caries results from the interactions of several factors:

BACTERIA: Dental caries is a chronic infectious disease of tooth enamel, dentin and cementum, the organisms being part of the indigenous oral flora. Tooth surfaces are normally colonized by many microorganisms, and unless the surface is cleaned thoroughly and frequently, bacterial colonies coalesce into a soft mass known as **dental plaque**.

Carious lesions result primarily from leaching of mineral in dental tissues by acids produced from food residues by microorganisms on tooth surfaces. Numerous streptococci, lactobacilli and actinomycetes in the oral flora have these characteristics. Indirect evidence points strongly to *Streptococcus mutans* as the primary etiologic agent that initiates caries. Organisms other than *S. mutans* may be more capable of maintaining the destructive process deeper in the enamel and dentin.

SALIVA: Saliva has a high buffering capacity that helps neutralize microbially produced acids in the mouth. It also contains bacteriostatic factors such as lysozyme, lactoferrin, lactoperoxidases and secretory immunoglobulins. **Xerostomia** (chronic dryness of the mouth from lack of saliva), which may be iatrogenic, for example, due to surgery or radiation therapy, results in rampant caries.

DIETARY FACTORS: One of the most important factors in the pathogenesis of caries is a high-carbohydrate diet. Roughage in raw and unrefined foods cleanses the teeth and necessitates more mastication, which further contributes to cleansing of the teeth. By contrast, soft and refined foods tend to stick to the teeth and also require less chewing.

FLUORIDE: Fluoride protects against dental caries. It is incorporated into the crystal lattice structure of enamel, where it forms fluoroapatite, which is less acid soluble than is the apatite of enamel. Fluoridation of drinking water in many communities led to dramatic reductions in dental caries in children whose teeth were formed while they drank fluoride-containing water.

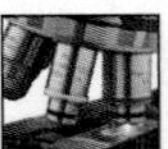

PATHOLOGY: Caries begins with disintegration of enamel prisms after decalcification of the interprismatic substance, events that lead to accumulation of debris and microorganisms (Fig. 25-10). These changes produce a small pit or fissure in the enamel. When the process reaches the dentinoenamel junction, it spreads laterally and also penetrates the dentin along the dentinal tubules. A substantial cavity then forms in the dentin, producing a flask-shaped lesion with a narrow orifice. Decalcification of dentin leads to focal coalescence of the destroyed dentinal tubules. Only when the vascular pulp of the tooth is invaded does an inflammatory reaction **(pulpitis)** appear, accompanied for the first time by pain.

Diseases of the Pulp and Periapical Tissues

The dental pulp is delicate connective tissue enclosed within the calcified walls of dentin. The pulp chamber is lined by odontoblasts and has a minute apical foramen through which blood vessels, lymphatics and small nerves penetrate.

- **Pulpitis** results from invasion by oral bacteria involved in dental caries. Pain in acute pulpitis reflects increased pressure caused by edema and exudate in the pulp chamber.
- **Apical (or periapical) granuloma,** the most common sequel of pulpitis, is chronically inflamed periapical granulation tissue. The inflammation gradually becomes surrounded by a fibrous capsule, which, on extraction, may be seen attached to the root of the tooth.
- **Radicular cyst (apical periodontal cyst)** occurs when the squamous epithelium of an apical granuloma proliferates, forming a cavity or cyst.
- **Periapical abscess** may follow pulpitis.
- **Osteomyelitis** may complicate a periapical abscess, and is usually caused by *Staphylococcus aureus, Staphylococcus epidermidis,* various streptococci or mixed organisms. Infection may traverse the cortical bone and spread to tissue spaces of the head and neck or, rarely, mediastinum.

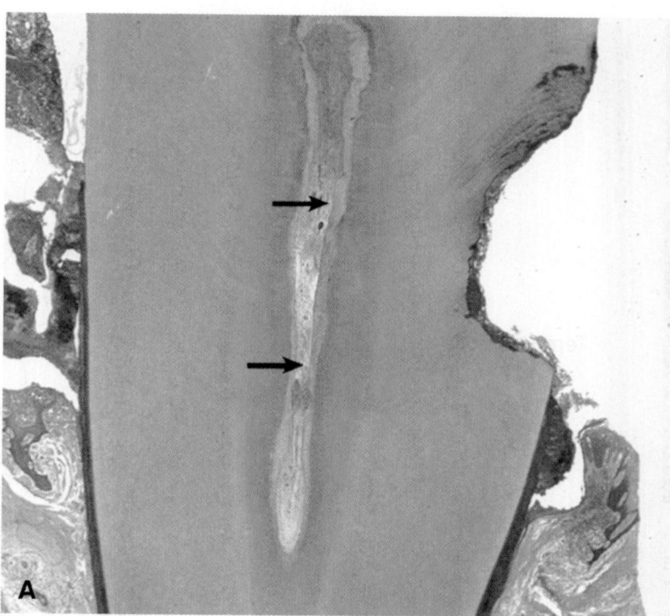

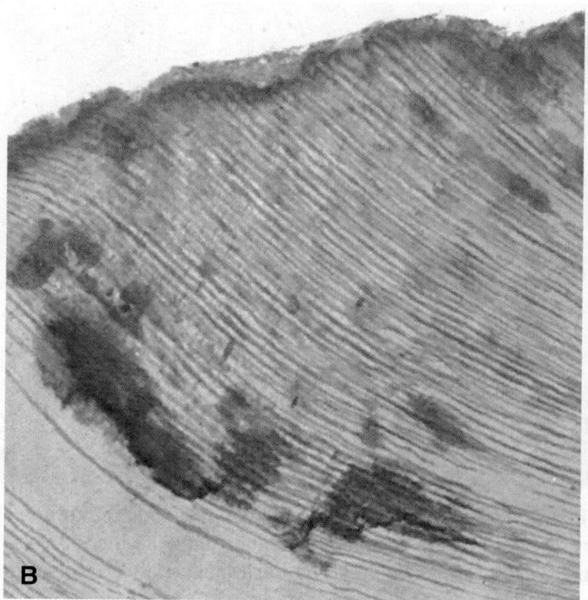

FIGURE 25-10. Dental caries. A. A large cavity close to the gingival margin is illustrated. *Arrows* indicate band of secondary dentin that lines the pulp chamber. This newly formed dentin is opposite the area of tooth destruction and was produced by the stimulated odontoblasts. **B.** Deposits of debris cover the surface. Bacterial colonies (*dark purple*) have extended into dentinal canals.

Periodontal Disease

The gingiva (gum) is that part of the oral mucosa that surrounds the teeth. It ends in a thin edge (free gingiva) that adheres closely to the teeth. A periodontal ligament of collagen fibers holds teeth in position in the socket (alveolus) of the jawbone. These structures form the periodontium.

Periodontal disease denotes acute and chronic disorders of the soft tissues around the teeth, which eventually lead to loss of supporting bone. Chronic periodontal disease typically occurs in adults with poor oral hygiene, but may develop even in people with apparently impeccable habits who have a strong family history of periodontal disease. Chronic periodontitis causes loss of more teeth in adults than does any other disease, including caries.

Periodontal disease is caused by bacterial accumulation under the gingiva in the periodontal pocket. The mass of bacteria adhering to the surface of tooth **(dental plaque)** ages and mineralizes and forms **calculus (tartar).** Adult periodontitis is mostly associated with *Bacteroides gingivalis. Bacteroides intermedius*, *Actinomyces* sp., *Haemophilus* sp. and other microorganisms may also participate.

The inflammation often starts as a marginal gingivitis. If untreated, it progresses to chronic periodontitis, which continues to progress in the absence of treatment. Chronic inflammation weakens and destroys the periodontium, causing loosening and eventual loss of teeth.

Hematologic disorders may affect oral tissues. Agranulocytosis causes necrotizing ulcers anywhere in the oral and pharyngeal mucosa, but especially in the gingiva. Infectious mononucleosis often results in gingivitis and stomatitis, with exudation and ulceration. Acute and chronic leukemias of all types cause oral lesions. In **acute monocytic leukemia,** 80% of patients show gingivitis, gingival hyperplasia, petechiae and hemorrhage. Necrosis and ulceration of the gingiva lead to severe superimposed infection, which may cause loss of teeth and alveolar bone. A hemorrhagic diathesis may be reflected in gingival hemorrhage.

Mild scurvy (vitamin C deficiency; see Chapter 8) is still encountered, particularly in those of lower socioeconomic status or neglected individuals. It affects the marginal and interdental gingiva, which become swollen and bright red, and bleed and ulcerate readily. Hemorrhage into the periodontal membrane causes loosening and loss of teeth.

Odontogenic Cysts and Tumors

Odontogenic cysts may be inflammatory and developmental. The most common are **radicular**, or **apical, periodontal cysts**, which involve the apex of an erupted tooth, usually after infection of the dental pulp. **Dentigerous cysts** are associated with the crowns of impacted, embedded or unerupted teeth, most often involving the mandibular and maxillary third molars. They form after the crown has completely developed: fluid accumulates between the crown and the overlying enamel epithelium. Dentigerous cysts may be complicated by ameloblastoma or SCC.

Ameloblastomas are tumors of odontogenic epithelia and are the most common clinically significant odontogenic tumor. They are slow-growing, locally invasive tumors that generally follow a benign clinical course, but can be locally destructive. Most arise in the mandibular ramus or molar area, maxilla or floor of the nasal cavity. The tumor tends to grow slowly as a central lesion of bone. They often show a characteristic "soap bubble" radiographic appearance. These tumors resemble the enamel organ in its various stages of differentiation, and a single tumor may show

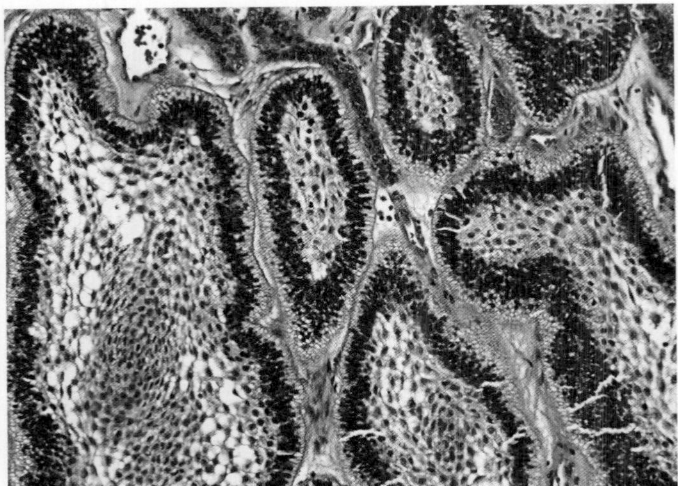

FIGURE 25-11. Ameloblastoma. A common histologic pattern is characterized by islands of odontogenic epithelium with a central stellate reticulum-like area, surrounded by basal cells with a "picket fence" appearance, due to subnuclear vacuoles.

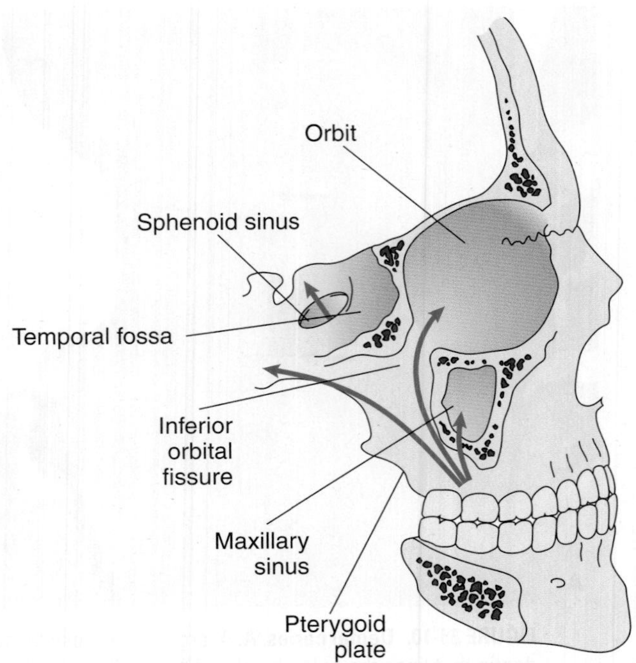

FIGURE 25-12. Pathways of infection to the intracranial cavity. Osseous pathways of infection from the jaws. *Arrows* indicate the direction of spread from the teeth to the maxillary sinus and through the inferior orbital fissure to the orbit. A deeper route is along the lateral pterygoid lamina up to the base of the skull, where, medial to the foramen ovale, a small aperture admits the vein of Vesalius. Through this small vein, the pterygoid plexus communicates with the cavernous sinus.

several histologic patterns. Thus, tumor cells resemble ameloblasts at the edges of epithelial nests or cords, where columnar cells are oriented perpendicularly to the basement membrane (Fig. 25-11). The prognosis is favorable. Incompletely excised tumors recur. Some may metastasize and yet remain histologically benign **(metastasizing ameloblastoma). Ameloblastic carcinomas** are frankly malignant, with atypia, necrosis, nuclear pleomorphism and abundant mitoses. Nuclei of ameloblastomas may show aberrant β-catenin expression, and the APC (adenomatous polyposis coli) missense mutation, which plays a role in colon cancer, may play a role in the pathogenesis of odontogenic tumors.

NASAL CAVITY AND PARANASAL SINUSES

The **nostril apertures** (anterior nares) lead into the **nasal vestibule**, a space lined by skin that contains hairs and sebaceous glands. Beyond the nares, the median septum divides the nasal cavity into two symmetric chambers, the **nasal fossae**. Each nasal fossa has an **olfactory region**, consisting of the superior nasal concha and the opposed part of the septum, and a **respiratory region**, which constitutes the rest of the cavity. Laterally, the inferior, middle and superior nasal conchae **(turbinates)** overhang the corresponding nasal passages or meatus.

The paranasal sinuses are paired air spaces that communicate with the nasal cavity. The mucous membrane covering the respiratory portion of the nasal cavity has a ciliated, columnar epithelium with interspersed goblet cells.

These anatomic interrelations determine routes of disease spread (Fig. 25-12). Infections can spread to maxillary, ethmoid, frontal and sphenoid sinuses, causing intraorbital and intracranial disease. The vein of Vesalius, medial to the foramen ovale, puts the cavernous sinus at risk.

Nonneoplastic Diseases of the External Nose and Nasal Vestibule

Virtually all diseases of the skin can occur on the external nose, including lesions due to solar damage (e.g., actinic keratosis, basal cell carcinoma, SCC, malignant melanoma). The numerous sebaceous glands of the nose are commonly involved by acne vulgaris.

Rosacea is a chronic cutaneous disorder of the cheeks, nose, chin and central forehead, characterized by telangiectasias, flushing, erythema, papules, pustules, rhinophyma and ocular manifestations. The etiology of rosacea is unknown. **Rhinophyma** is a protuberant bulbous mass on the nose caused by marked hyperplasia of sebaceous glands and chronic inflammation of the skin in acne rosacea.

Nosebleed (epistaxis) is most often due to trauma, but may be caused by hypertension, diverse hematologic abnormalities, inflammatory conditions and nasal mucosal tumors. Epistaxis frequently originates in a triangular area of the anterior nasal septum called "Little area," where the epidermis is thin and the anterior ethmoid, greater palatine, sphenopalatine and superior labial arteries anastomose to form the **Kiesselbach plexus**. Many dilated blood vessels, or telangiectasias, are often apparent. Little area is also the location of ulcers and perforations, which may be caused by various diseases or by trauma to the nasal septum (Table 25-1).

Table 25-1

Causes of Nasal Septum Perforation

Causes of Nasal Septum Perforation
Trauma
Specific infections (tuberculosis, syphilis, leprosy)
Wegener granulomatosis
Lupus erythematosus
Chronic exposure to dust (containing arsenic, chromium, copper, etc.)
Cocaine abuse
Malignant tumors

Nonneoplastic Diseases of the Nasal Cavity and Paranasal Sinuses

Rhinitis Is Usually Viral or Allergic

Rhinitis is inflammation of the mucous membranes of the nasal cavity and sinuses. Causes range from the common cold to unusual infections such as diphtheria, anthrax and glanders. The latter may be transmitted from animals to humans, and is caused by a bacterium, *Burkholderia mallei*.

VIRAL RHINITIS: The most common cause of acute rhinitis is viral infection, especially the common cold **(acute coryza).** The virus replicates in epithelial cells, causing the degenerating epithelial cells to be shed. The mucosa is edematous and engorged, and infiltrated by neutrophils and mononuclear cells. Clinically, mucosal swelling is manifested as nasal stuffiness. Abundant mucus secretion and increased vascular permeability lead to **rhinorrhea** (free discharge of a thin nasal mucus).

Secondary infection caused by normal nasal and pharyngeal flora may follow viral rhinitis by a few days. The abundant serous discharge then becomes mucopurulent, after which the surface epithelium is shed. The epithelial cells regenerate rapidly after the inflammation subsides.

ALLERGIC RHINITIS: Numerous allergens are constantly present in our environment, and sensitivity to any one of them can cause allergic rhinitis. Often called **hay fever,** allergic rhinitis may be acute and seasonal or chronic and perennial.

MOLECULAR PATHOGENESIS: In this condition, air-borne allergens (e.g., pollens, molds, animal dander) deposit on the nasal mucosa. The few plasma cells present in the nasal mucosa normally produce IgE. Mast cells in the nasal mucosa or free in nasal secretions also bear specific IgE directed against allergens. On contact with an allergen, mast cells release cytoplasmic granules ("degranulate") with a variety of chemical mediators and enzymes. Some mediators are preformed and thus act rapidly (e.g., histamine); others elute slowly from the granule matrix (e.g., heparin or trypsin); still others (e.g., leukotrienes) are newly synthesized. Thus, an immediate, rapidly apparent reaction may give way to a prolonged inflammatory reaction as the various mediators exert their specific effects. The released mediators cause the signs and symptoms of allergic rhinitis, and many of the responses are attributable to histamine, acting through its H_1 receptor.

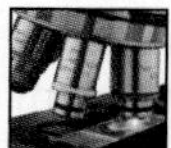

PATHOLOGY: Increased capillary permeability mediated by vasodilator substances results in edema of the nasal mucosa, especially of the inferior turbinates. Numerous eosinophils may be seen in the nasal secretions or mucosa. The late phase of mast cell–mediated reactions is associated with persistent mucosal edema, and is seen clinically as nasal obstruction.

CHRONIC RHINITIS: Repeated bouts of acute rhinitis may lead to chronic rhinitis. A deviated nasal septum is often a contributory factor. In chronic rhinitis the nasal mucosa is thickened by persistent hyperemia, mucous gland hyperplasia and lymphocyte and plasma cell infiltration.

Nasal Polyps Are Focal Inflammatory Swellings

Inflammatory polyps are nonneoplastic mucosal lesions of the nose and sinuses (Fig. 25-13). Most arise from the lateral nasal wall or ethmoid recess. They may be unilateral or bilateral, single or multiple. Symptoms include nasal obstruction, rhinorrhea and headaches. The etiology involves multiple factors, including allergy, cystic fibrosis, infections, diabetes mellitus and aspirin intolerance. These polyps are lined by respiratory epithelium and have mucous glands within a loose mucoid stroma, infiltrated by plasma cells, lymphocytes and many eosinophils.

Sinusitis Is a Bacterial Infection

Sinusitis is inflammation of the mucous membranes of paranasal sinuses.

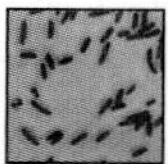

ETIOLOGIC FACTORS: Any condition (inflammation, neoplasm, foreign body) that interferes with sinus drainage or aeration renders it liable to infection. If a sinus ostium is blocked, secretions or exudate accumulate behind the obstruction.

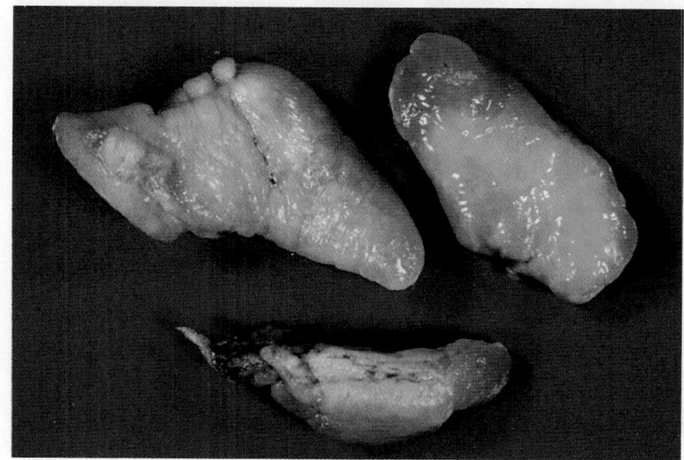

FIGURE 25-13. Nasal polyps. These smooth, pale, polypoid masses were removed from a patient with chronic rhinitis.

Acute sinusitis is a disorder of less than 3 weeks' duration, largely caused by extension of infection from the nasal mucosa. *Haemophilus influenzae* and *Branhamella catarrhalis* are the most common organisms. Maxillary sinusitis may also be caused by odontogenic infections, in which case bacteria from the roots of the first and second molars penetrate the thin bony plate that separates them from the floor of the maxillary sinus. Incomplete resolution of infection or recurrent acute sinusitis may lead to chronic sinusitis, in which the purulent exudate almost always includes anaerobic bacteria.

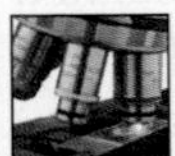

PATHOLOGY: Acute or chronic sinusitis may be followed by a number of complications:

- **Mucocele:** Mucocele is an accumulation of mucous secretions in a nasal sinus. If infected, a mucocele may lead to a sinus being filled with mucopurulent exudate, called a **pyocele**. Purulent exudation in a sinus is **empyema** (Fig. 25-14). Mucoceles occur most often in the anterior compartments ("cells") of frontal and ethmoid sinuses. They develop slowly and cause bone resorption by the pressure they exert. Mucoceles of anterior ethmoid or frontal sinuses may be large enough to displace the contents of the orbit and occasionally erode into the central nervous system.
- **Osteomyelitis:** Bone infection occurs when suppurative infection in the frontal sinus reaches a bone. Infection of nasal sinus walls may spread through Volkmann canals to the periosteum, producing periostitis and subperiosteal abscess. If these occur on the orbital side of the bone, orbital cellulitis or an orbital abscess forms. Skin overlying the infection is often markedly edematous, and subcutaneous cellulitis or a subcutaneous abscess also may develop. Osteomyelitis also may spread rapidly between the outer and inner tables of the skull.
- **Septic thrombophlebitis:** Infection in the sinuses may penetrate the bone and spread to the frontal and diploe venous systems. Spread of septic thrombophlebitis to the cavernous venous sinus through the superior ophthalmic veins is a life-threatening complication.
- **Intracranial infections:** Sinusitis may also lead to spread of infection to the cranial cavity. Lesions include epidural, subdural and cerebral abscesses and purulent leptomeningitis. Spread may be via lymphatics and veins, and need not involve extensive destruction of bone.

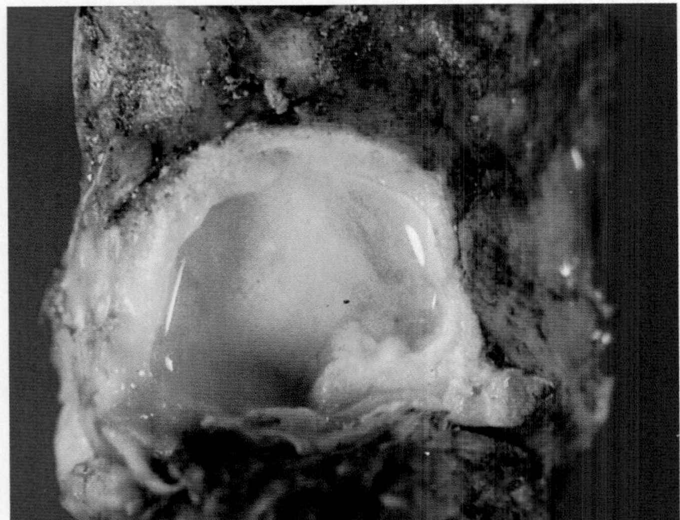

FIGURE 25-14. Empyema of the maxillary sinus (sagittal section). Infection followed chronic obstruction of the orifice caused by adenocarcinoma of the nasal mucosa.

Syphilis May Destroy the Nasal Bridge

Primary chancres in the nose are rare, but mucosal lesions of secondary syphilis are common in the nose and nasopharynx. In tertiary syphilis, inflammation may involve large portions of the nasal mucosa, underlying cartilage and bone. Perichondrial or periosteal gummas may destroy nasal cartilage and bone, causing the nasal bridge to collapse, and producing "saddle nose." Destruction of nasal bony walls may also lead to perforation of the nasal septum, hard palate, wall of the orbit or maxillary sinus.

Leprosy Is Spread Through Nasal Secretions

Mycobacterium leprae multiplies best at lower temperatures, and so prefers cooler body sites, such as the nares and anterior nasal mucosa. Nasal involvement is often the first manifestation of leprosy. Tuberculoid and intermediate forms of leprosy account for most cases (see Chapter 9). The skin around the nares and anterior nasal mucosa shows nodules, ulceration or perforations. Nasal involvement is important as leprosy is spread via nasal secretions teeming with bacilli.

Rhinoscleroma Is a Chronic Bacterial Infection of the Nose

Rhinoscleroma (scleroma) is a chronic inflammatory process caused by a gram-negative diplobacillus, *Klebsiella rhinoscleromatis*. It usually begins in the nose and remains localized to that site, but may extend slowly into the nasopharynx, larynx and trachea. Rarely, rhinoscleroma is seen elsewhere, including paranasal sinuses, orbital tissues, skin, lips, oral mucosa, cervical lymph nodes and gastrointestinal tract. It is endemic in some Mediterranean countries and parts of Asia, Africa and Latin America. Indigenous cases also occur in the United States. It affects both sexes and any age. Most patients have poor domestic and personal hygiene.

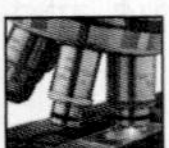

PATHOLOGY: Infected tissues appear firm, greatly thickened, irregularly nodular and often ulcerated. The granulation tissue is strikingly rich in plasma cells, lymphocytes and foamy macrophages (Fig. 25-15). The characteristic large macrophages, or Mikulicz cells, contain masses of phagocytosed bacilli. Immunohistochemistry can now identify the organisms, which may be intracellular or extracellular. Serologic tests, including indirect immunofluorescence done on serum, are valuable in establishing the diagnosis of rhinoscleroma, because specific antibodies are present in many patients. The disease is successfully treated with antibiotics.

Fungal Infections of the Nose and Paranasal Sinuses Are Usually Opportunistic

Pathogenic fungi may involve the nose and paranasal sinuses as part of cutaneous or mucocutaneous infection, particularly in a setting of immunodeficiency (see Chapter 9).

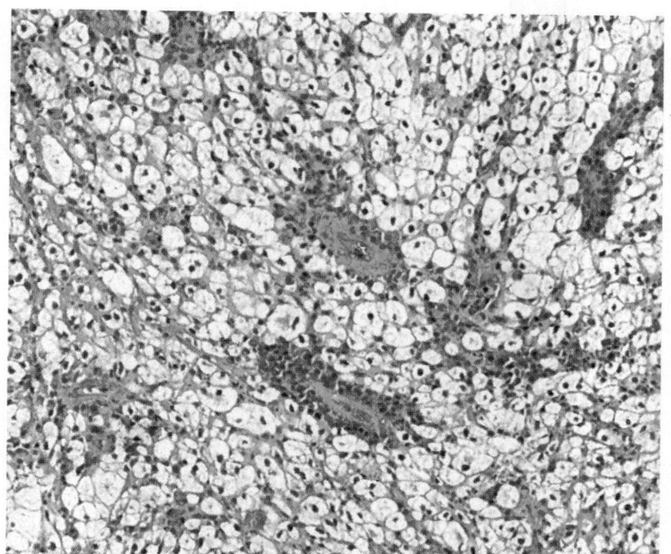

FIGURE 25-15. Rhinoscleroma. Granulation tissue contains numerous foamy macrophages (Mikulicz cells).

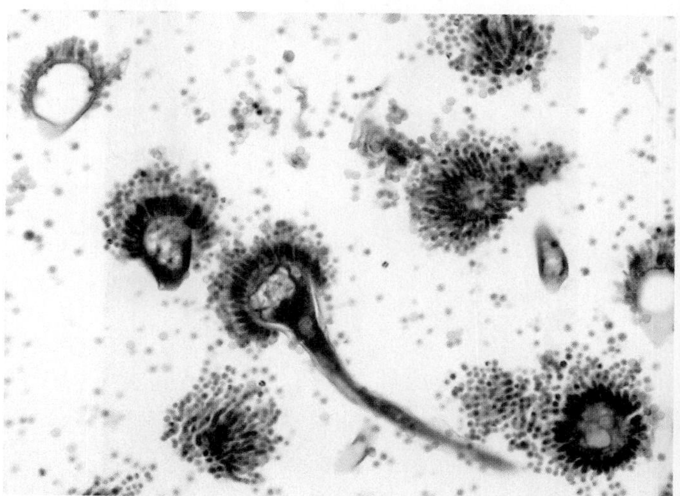

FIGURE 25-16. Aspergillus. A nasal, green mass in a patient with lymphoma demonstrated abundant fruiting bodies.

Candidiasis is the most common fungus infection of the nasal mucosa, usually accompanying oral and pharyngeal candidiasis **(thrush)**. **Aspergillosis** is uncommon, and when it occurs it generally involves a paranasal sinus. Fungi may disseminate to venous sinuses, meninges and the brain. Aspergillosis of the sinonasal tract may be noninvasive or invasive, including angioinvasive. Noninvasive types of aspergillus sinusitis include **allergic fungal sinusitis** (AFS) and **sinus mycetoma** (so-called fungus balls).

AFS is a hypersensitivity reaction to fungal antigens, like allergic bronchopulmonary aspergillosis (see Chapter 12), and affects patients who are atopic or immunologically "hypercompetent." The disease occurs at all ages but is most common in children or young adults. Any sinus may be affected but the maxillary and ethmoid sinuses are most often involved.

Fungus balls or **aspergillomas** occur in immunologically competent patients, usually with chronic sinus disease associated with poor drainage. In this setting, fungi proliferate and form a dense mass of hyphae that causes nasal obstruction. Evidence of bone destruction and ocular symptoms may be present.

Invasive fungal sinusitis usually affects immunocompromised or immunosuppressed patients (Fig. 25-16). In the rare **rhinocerebral aspergillosis**, the organisms spread to venous sinuses, meninges and brain, and few patients survive.

Mucormycosis is a potentially life-threatening fungus infection, particularly in diabetic patients. It typically involves the nasopharynx, but can invade the skin, bone, orbit and brain.

Nasal **rhinosporidiosis** is caused by *Rhinosporidium seeberi*, an organism that is classified as a fungus, but that has not been grown in culture nor transmitted experimentally. The disease is endemic in Sri Lanka and in parts of India, and Central and South America. Affected nasal mucosa contains vascular polyploid masses. Microscopically, the polyps show marked chronic inflammation and characteristic spherical 50- to 350-μm-diameter sporangia.

Leishmaniasis (Also Known as Kala-Azar)

The nose is a frequent site of mucocutaneous leishmaniasis, caused by *Leishmania braziliensis* (see Chapter 9). The nasal disease, known as **espundia,** occurs in Central and South America. Initial lesions are skin sores that heal within a few months. In some patients, mucocutaneous lesions develop in the nose or upper lip after an interval of months or years. The infection probably spreads by nasal contact with contaminated fingers. The infected mucosa has polypoid inflammatory lesions and superficial ulcers. Early in infection, many macrophages contain parasites. Later, a tuberculoid type of granulomatous response develops. Such lesions contain few recognizable parasites. Bacterial infection may supervene and lead to soft tissue destruction and collapse of the anterior cartilaginous nasal septum.

Wegener Granulomatosis May Present in the Nose

Wegener granulomatosis affects the lower airways (see Chapter 12).

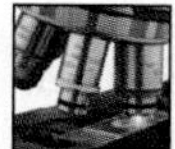

PATHOLOGY: If fully developed, this Wegener granulomatosis involves the lungs, kidneys and small arteries throughout the body. The sinonasal tract may be affected as part of systemic disease or the process may be localized to this region. Septal perforation and mucosal ulceration may be followed by slowly progressive destruction of the nose and paranasal sinuses, leading to a saddle nose deformity (Fig. 25-17). Constitutional symptoms, such as fever, malaise and weight loss, may accompany resulting "runny nose," sinusitis and nosebleeds. Nasal lesions show ischemic-type necrosis, vasculitis, mixed chronic inflammation, scattered multinucleated giant cells and microabscesses. Well-formed granulomas are not seen. Elevated serum antineutrophil cytoplasmic antibodies (ANCAs) and proteinase 3 (PR3) are associated with active disease.

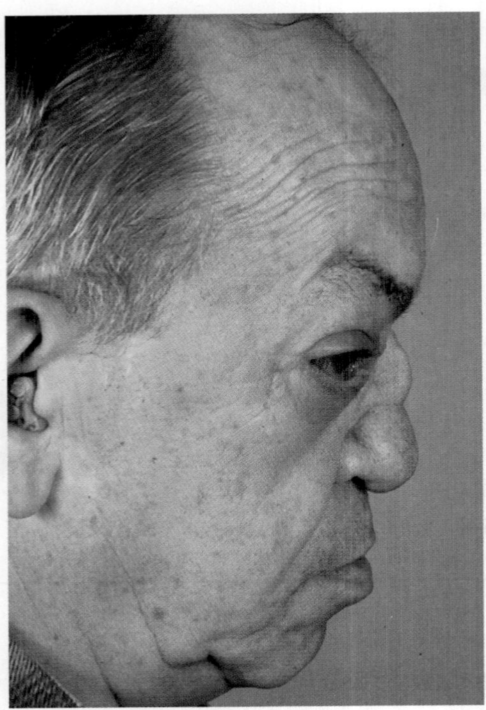

FIGURE 25-17. Saddle nose deformity of Wegener granulomatosis.

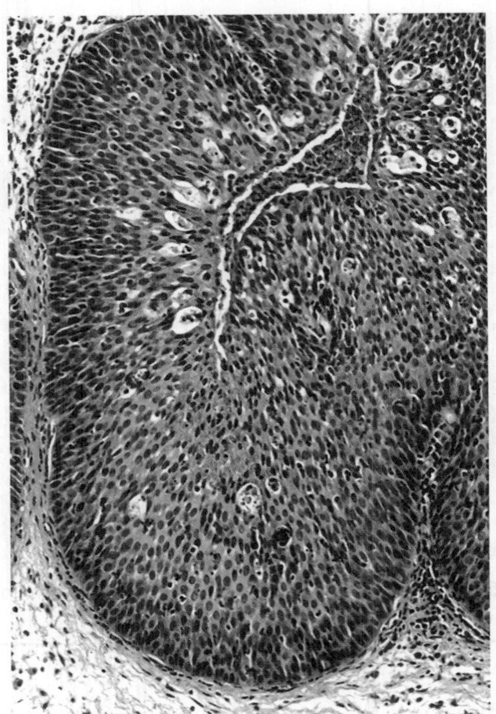

FIGURE 25-18. Sinonasal inverted papilloma. Epithelial nests are growing downward (inverted) into the submucosa. They are composed of a uniform cellular proliferation, which displays an inflammatory cell infiltrate and scattered microcysts.

Benign Neoplasms of the Nasal Cavity and Paranasal Sinuses

SQUAMOUS PAPILLOMA: The most common benign tumor of the nasal cavity is squamous papilloma, which almost always occurs in the nasal vestibule. The lesion is often indistinguishable from a wart (verruca vulgaris).

SCHNEIDERIAN PAPILLOMAS: Schneiderian papillomas are a group of benign neoplasms composed of a squamous or columnar epithelial proliferation with associated mucous cells, and arising from the sinonasal (Schneiderian) mucosa. The ectodermally derived lining of the sinonasal tract, the Schneiderian membrane, may give rise to three morphologically distinct benign papillomas collectively called Schneiderian or sinonasal-type papillomas: **inverted**, **oncocytic** (cylindrical or columnar cell) and **fungiform** (exophytic, septal) papillomas. In all, Schneiderian papillomas represent less than 5% of all sinonasal tract tumors.

INVERTED PAPILLOMA: This tumor involves the lateral nasal wall and may spread to the paranasal sinuses. Inverted papillomas occur mainly in middle-aged persons. As the name implies, they show inversions of surface epithelium into underlying stroma (Fig. 25-18). HPV types 6 and 11 and rarely other types (16, 18, 33, 40, 57) have been identified in inverted papillomas, but a cause-and-effect relationship is unproven. Although benign, these tumors may erode bone by pressure. Surgical resection must extend beyond the boundaries of grossly visible lesions, or they may recur. In 5% of cases, inverted papillomas give rise to SCC.

Malignant Neoplasms of the Nasal Cavity and Paranasal Sinuses

Squamous Cell Carcinoma Is Often Associated With Occupational Risk Factors

Over half of carcinomas of the nasal cavity and paranasal sinuses originate in the maxillary sinus antrum, one third in the nasal cavity, 10% in the ethmoid sinus and 1% in sphenoid and frontal sinuses (Fig. 25-19). Most of these cancers are squamous cell tumors (either keratinizing or

Table 25-2

Variants of Squamous Cell Carcinoma
Acantholytic squamous cell carcinoma
Adenosquamous carcinoma
Basaloid squamous cell carcinoma
Carcinoma cuniculatum
Papillary squamous cell carcinoma
Spindle cell squamous carcinoma
Verrucous carcinoma
Lymphoepithelial carcinoma (nonnasopharyngeal)

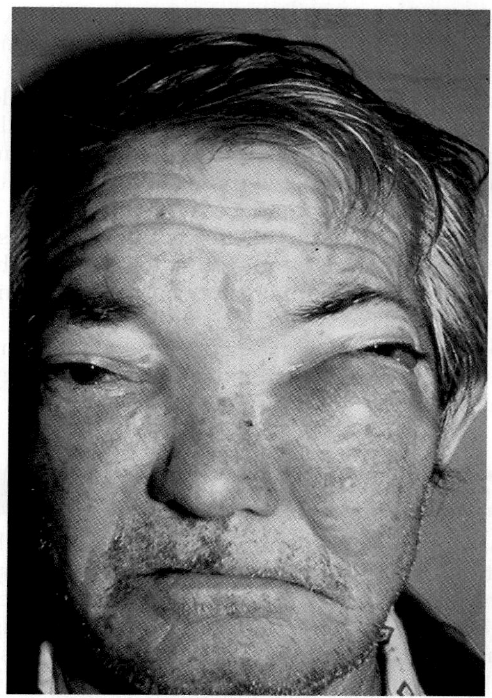

FIGURE 25-19. Squamous cell carcinoma of the maxillary sinus caused an obvious facial deformity, owing to invasion outside the confines of the sinus. Involvement of the orbit and facial nerve is evident. The latter is defined by drooping of the mouth to the side of the facial nerve paralysis.

nonkeratinizing; Table 25-2). Some 15% are adenocarcinomas, or undifferentiated carcinomas.

MOLECULAR PATHOGENESIS: Several industrial chemicals may cause cancer of the nose and sinuses, including nickel, chromium and aromatic hydrocarbons. Occupational settings reportedly with increased risk for cancer of the nose and sinuses (but for which a specific chemical agent is not identified) are woodworking in the furniture industry, use of cutting oils and leather textile industries.

Nickel workers are prone to SCCs, mostly from the middle turbinate, with latencies from 2 to 32 years. Most other occupational exposures mainly lead to adenocarcinomas and occur mostly in the maxillary and ethmoid sinuses. Because of the occupational risk factors, cancers of the nose and sinuses are far more common in men and occur after age 50 years.

Cancers of the nasal cavity and sinuses grow relentlessly and invade adjacent structures but typically do not give rise to distant metastases. Survival is usually only a few years.

Olfactory Neuroblastoma, or Esthesioneuroblastoma, Is of Neural Crest Origin

This tumor is an unusual malignancy of the nose. It has a slight male predominance and occurs over a wide age range from 3 years to the ninth decade.

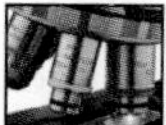

PATHOLOGY: This cancer arises from the olfactory mucosa covering the superior third of the nasal septum, cribriform plate (Fig. 25-20A) and superior turbinate. The tumor is usually polypoid and highly vascular and displays diverse histologic patterns, depending on the amount of intercellular neurofibrillary material. Tumor cells are slightly larger than lymphocytes, with round nuclei with an even distribution of chromatin and inconspicuous cytoplasm (Fig. 25-20B). Tumor cells may form pseudorosettes (Homer Wright rosettes) or true neural rosettes (Flexner-Wintersteiner rosettes). The World Health Organization (2005) adopted a four-tiered grading system, based on lobular architecture, mitosis, necrosis, nuclear pleomorphism, fibrillary matrix and rosettes. Immunohistochemistry is useful in

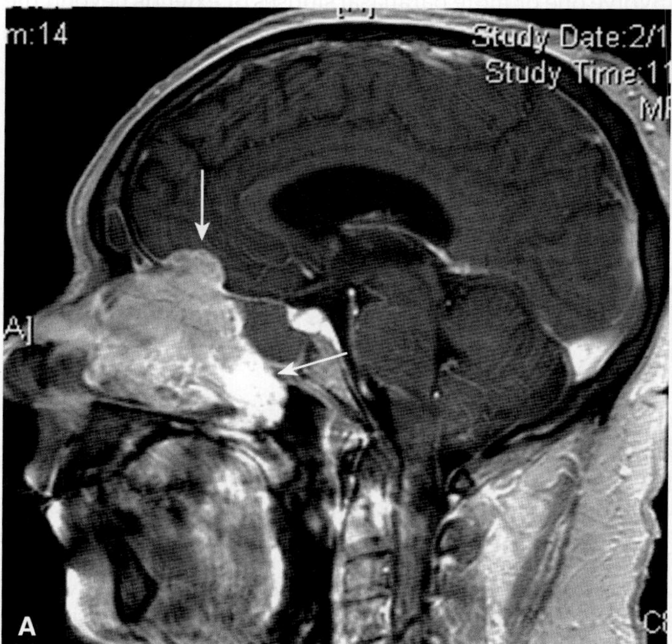

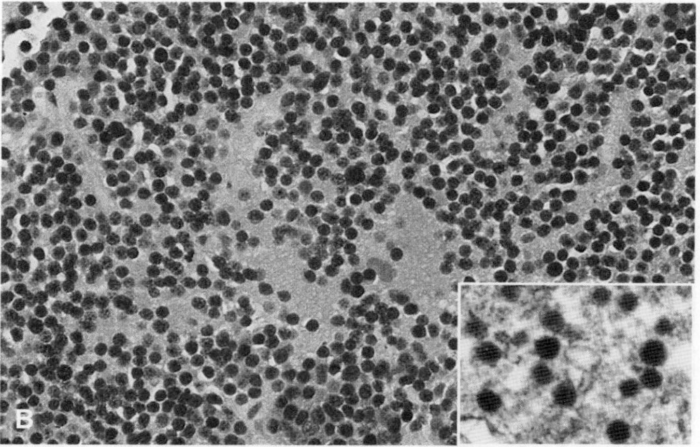

FIGURE 25-20. Olfactory neuroblastoma. A. Sagittal T1 postcontrast magnetic resonance image (MRI) demonstrates a hyperintense mass (*arrows*) arising from the cribriform plate and filling the nasal cavity. **B.** The tumor is composed of small round cells with hyperchromatic nuclei and a background eosinophilic stroma representing neurofibrillary matrix. *Inset.* An electron micrograph shows intracytoplasmic, secretory-type, membrane-bound granules with dense cores.

diagnosing olfactory neuroblastomas, which stain strongly for synaptophysin and neuron-specific enolase (NSE) but not cytokeratin and epithelial membrane antigen (EMA). S-100 protein often surrounds the nests or lobules **(sustentacular cells),** mostly in lower-grade tumors. By electron microscopy, olfactory neuroblastoma cells have intracytoplasmic secretory granules similar to those of neuroblastomas at other sites.

CLINICAL FEATURES: Olfactory neuroblastomas invade and destroy bony structures slowly, and spread readily via lymphatics to regional and distant lymph nodes. Hematogenous spread is less frequent. Differences in survival, including disease-free survival, usually correspond to tumor grade. In the past, clinical staging based on whether tumor is confined to the nasal cavity, extends to involve one or more paranasal sinuses or extends beyond the sinonasal cavities had been predictive of prognosis. However, complete removal is critical. Overall, craniofacial resection with chemotherapy and/or radiation therapy may provide 85% 5-year survival.

Nasal-Type Angiocentric Natural Killer/T-Cell Lymphoma Is an Aggressive, Highly Lethal Disease

Nasal-type angiocentric NK/T-cell lymphoma was once called **lethal midline granuloma**, midline malignant reticulosis and polymorphic reticulosis. This aggressive lymphoma presents as necrotizing, ulcerating mucosal lesions of the upper respiratory tract.

PATHOLOGY: The polymorphism of the atypical lymphocytic infiltrate is a characteristic feature that distinguishes the nasal-type NK/T-cell lymphoma from many other lymphomas. Similar necrotizing infiltrates may occur in the upper airways, lungs and alimentary tract, but any organ can be involved. The malignant infiltrate characteristically surrounds small to medium-sized blood vessels (angiocentric), infiltrates through vascular walls (angioinvasion), often occludes vessel lumens like a thrombus and causes necrosis in adjacent tissues (ischemic type) (Fig. 25-21). ***EBV infection is associated with this type of lymphoma.***

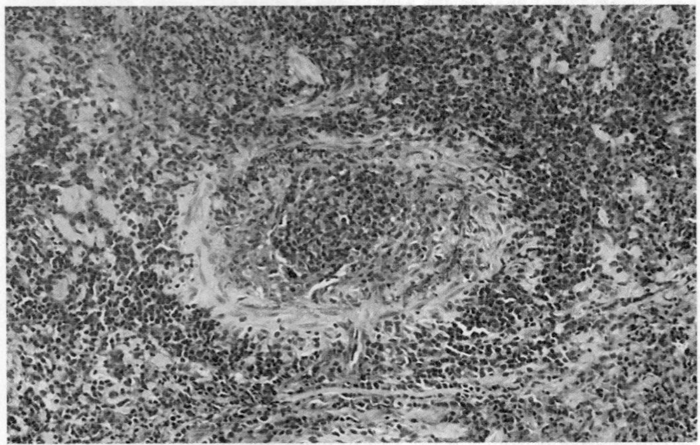

FIGURE 25-21. Angiocentric natural killer (NK)/T-cell lymphoma. A malignant cellular infiltrate growing around and into a medium-sized blood vessel with disruption of the external elastic membrane and occlusion of the vessel lumen.

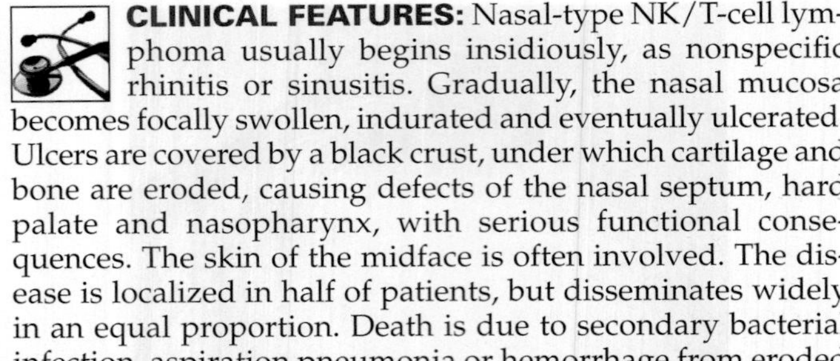

CLINICAL FEATURES: Nasal-type NK/T-cell lymphoma usually begins insidiously, as nonspecific rhinitis or sinusitis. Gradually, the nasal mucosa becomes focally swollen, indurated and eventually ulcerated. Ulcers are covered by a black crust, under which cartilage and bone are eroded, causing defects of the nasal septum, hard palate and nasopharynx, with serious functional consequences. The skin of the midface is often involved. The disease is localized in half of patients, but disseminates widely in an equal proportion. Death is due to secondary bacterial infection, aspiration pneumonia or hemorrhage from eroded large blood vessels.

The infiltrates of nasal-type NK/T-cell lymphoma are, at least initially, radiosensitive and remission with cytotoxic agents has also been reported.

NASOPHARYNX AND OROPHARYNX

The nasopharynx is continuous anteriorly with the nasal cavities; its roof is formed by the body of the sphenoid bone and its posterior wall by the cervical vertebrae. Eustachian tube openings are on the lateral walls of the nasopharynx. In newborns it is covered by pseudostratified ciliated columnar epithelium. With advancing age, it is replaced by a stratified squamous epithelium over large areas (80%). The mucosa contains numerous mucous glands and abundant lymphoid tissue.

Waldeyer ring *is a circular band of lymphoid tissue at the opening of the oropharynx into the respiratory and digestive tracts.* Lymphoid tissue on the superior posterior wall forms the nasopharyngeal tonsils, which, when hyperplastic, are called **adenoids**. The palatine tonsils are lateral, where the pharynx connects with the oral cavity, and are covered by stratified squamous epithelium, which lines the infoldings **(tonsillar crypts)** into the lymphoid tissue. Crypts normally contain desquamated epithelium, lymphocytes, some neutrophils and saprophytic organisms, such as bacteria, *Candida* and actinomycetes. Pathogens (e.g., *Corynebacterium diphtheriae,* meningococcus) may also be seen in the pharynx of healthy people.

Waldeyer ring is well developed in children and contains follicles with germinal centers. In fact, the tonsils contain the largest collection of B lymphocytes in a normal child. Pharyngeal lymphoid tissue diminishes considerably by adulthood. It gradually involutes with age, but does not totally disappear. Tonsillectomy and adenoidectomy are less common now than previously, and lead to decreased secretory IgA in the nasopharynx, but do not decrease serum antibody levels or alter antibody responses to several human respiratory viruses.

Hypoplasia and Hyperplasia of Pharyngeal Lymphoid Tissue

Bruton sex-linked agammaglobulinemia (see Chapter 4) affects only males, who have minimal or no lymphoid tissue in their tonsils, pharynx and intestines (Peyer patches and appendix). They have a normally developed thymus.

Atrophy of pharyngeal lymphoid tissue is common in chronically immunosuppressed patients. Local radiation therapy also causes marked loss of lymphoid tissue in the Waldeyer ring.

Hyperplasia of nasopharyngeal lymphoid tissue follows infections or chronic irritation due to dust, smoke and fumes. In some primary immunodeficiencies (dysgammaglobulinemia type I or nodular lymphoid hyperplasia), the tonsils may be enlarged, presumably reflecting an adaptive response by the immune system.

Infections

Pharyngitis and tonsillitis are among the most common diseases of the head and neck. Nasopharyngeal inflammation occurs mainly in children, but is also common in adolescents and young adults. Viral or bacterial infections may be limited to the palatine tonsils, but may also involve nasopharyngeal tonsils or adjacent pharyngeal mucosa, often as part of a general upper respiratory tract infection. In the latter case, initial infecting agents are mostly viruses spread by droplet or by direct contact: usually influenza, parainfluenza, adenovirus, respiratory syncytial virus and rhinovirus.

S. pyogenes is the most important cause of pharyngitis and tonsillitis, because of the possibility of serious suppurative and nonsuppurative sequelae. **Diphtheria** is still an important cause of pharyngitis in some countries. These infections are characterized by an exudate or, in the case of diphtheria, a pseudomembrane, on the tonsils and pharynx.

Acute tonsillitis is a bacterial infection, usually with *S. pyogenes* (group A β-hemolytic streptococci). In follicular tonsillitis pinpoint exudates may be extruded from the crypts.

In **pseudomembranous tonsillitis** a necrotic mucosa is covered by a coat of exudate, as in diphtheria or in **Vincent angina.** The latter is caused by fusiform bacilli and spirochetes that are present in the normal bacterial flora of the mouth. These organisms become pathogenic when local or systemic resistance is low (e.g., after mucosal injury or in malnutrition).

Recurrent or chronic tonsillitis is not as common as once believed, and enlarged tonsils in children do not necessarily signify chronic tonsillitis. However, repeated infections can cause tonsils and adenoids to enlarge and obstruct air passages. Repeated streptococcal tonsillitis may lead to rheumatic fever or glomerulonephritis in children, who may benefit from tonsillectomy.

Peritonsillar abscess (quinsy) is a collection of purulent material behind the posterior capsule of the tonsil, usually due to α- and β-hemolytic streptococci. About one third of patients have a prior history of tonsillitis. Untreated, such abscesses may lead to life-threatening situations: (1) aided by gravity, they may dissect inferiorly to the pyriform sinus and obstruct, or rupture into, the airway; (2) they may extend laterally into the parapharyngeal space (parapharyngeal abscess) and weaken the carotid artery wall; or (3) they may penetrate along the carotid sheath inferiorly into the mediastinum or, superiorly, to the base of the skull or cranial cavity, with disastrous consequences.

Infectious mononucleosis (associated with EBV infection) often presents with exudative tonsillitis and pharyngitis, commonly with posterior cervical lymphadenopathy. **Adenoids** represent chronic inflammatory hyperplasia of the pharyngeal lymphoid tissue. This condition is often accompanied by chronic tonsillitis or rhinitis, almost always in children. Enlarged adenoids may cause partial or complete obstruction of the eustachian tube, leading to otitis media.

Neoplasms

Nasopharyngeal Angiofibroma Is a Tumor of Adolescent Boys

This tumor is an uncommon, highly vascular neoplasm of the nasopharynx. It is histologically benign but locally aggressive. Also referred to as "juvenile nasopharyngeal angiofibroma," these tumors most commonly arise in adolescent males. However, as they are not restricted to this age group, the designation of "juvenile" is no longer encouraged.

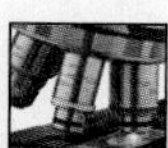

PATHOLOGY: These tumors are multinodular, lobulated or smooth pink-white masses, which may show surface ulceration and obvious blood vessels (Fig. 25-22A). They typically arise submucosally in the **posterolateral nasal wall** posterior to the sphenopalatine foramen, and tend to expand into adjacent structures, causing local mass effects. Angiofibromas may grow into fissures and foramina of the skull or destroy bone and spread into adjacent structures, such as the nasal cavity, paranasal sinuses, orbit, middle cranial fossa or pterygomaxillary fossa. Diagnosis is usually made on clinical examination and imaging studies.

Angiofibromas have vascular and stromal components (Fig. 25-22B). Blood vessels vary in size and shape; their walls lack a smooth muscle layer and show irregularly arranged smooth muscle. Aberrant nuclear β-catenin is expressed in stromal fibroblasts (Fig. 25-22C).

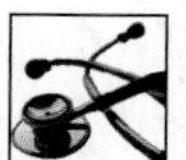

CLINICAL FEATURES: Many angiofibromas regress spontaneously after puberty. They respond to estrogen therapy, and so are thought to be hormonally regulated and androgen-dependent. Vessel wall defects preclude vasoconstriction, leading to brisk bleeding after trauma. Biopsies may thus be dangerous, and are contraindicated. Radiation therapy is also effective. Preoperative embolization may be used to reduce vascularity prior to surgery. There is a familial tendency for the development of these tumors; they occur 25 times more often in patients with familial adenomatous polyposis (FAP) syndrome.

Oropharyngeal Squamous Cell Carcinomas Are Usually Associated with Human Papillomavirus Infection

In the United States, approximately 80% of oropharyngeal squamous cell carcinomas are associated with high-risk HPV. These carcinomas, termed HPV-associated head and neck squamous cell carcinoma (HPV-HNSCC), arise mainly from the palatine and lingual tonsils, and are nonkeratinizing carcinomas of the basaloid cell type. Such carcinomas may be small and difficult to detect, and often present as metastatic cancer to a cervical lymph node. The primary lymphatics drain into the superior deep jugular and submandibular lymph nodes and, to a lesser degree, into retropharyngeal lymph nodes.

In contrast with non–HPV-associated head and neck squamous cell carcinomas, HPV-HNSCC often occur in patients with no known risk factors for HNSCC (i.e., nonsmokers, nondrinkers), present in younger patients, are radiosensitive and have better outcomes.

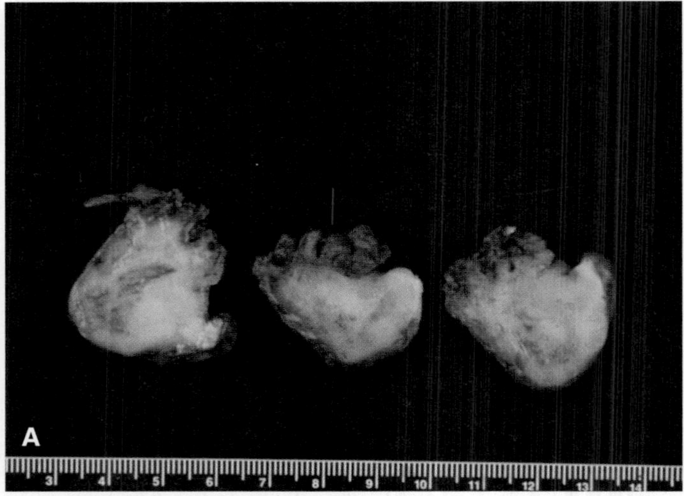
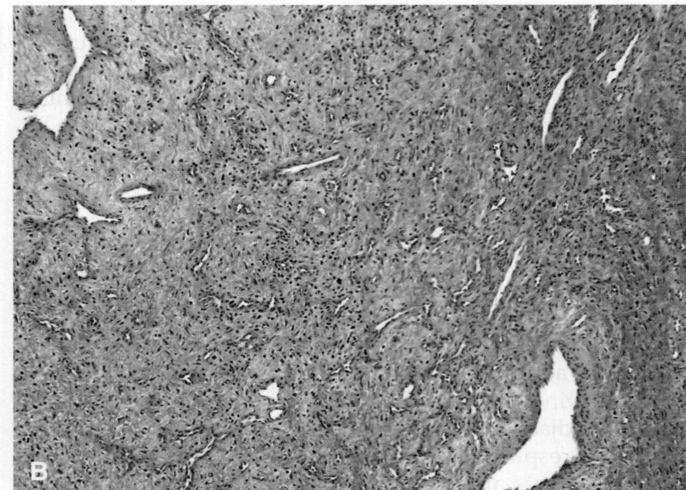
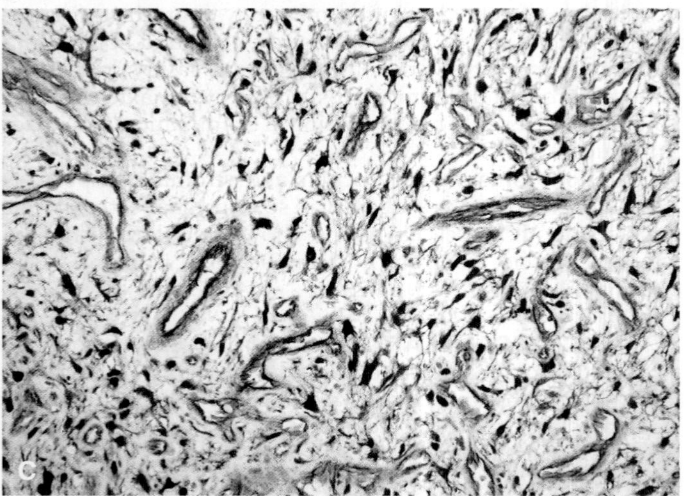

FIGURE 25-22. Nasopharyngeal angiofibroma. A. The cut surface of the tumor appears dense and spongy. **B.** Microscopically, it is composed of slitlike vascular structures in a collagenous stroma. **C.** Immunohistochemistry for β-catenin demonstrates aberrant nuclear labeling.

MOLECULAR PATHOGENESIS: As in the uterine cervix, high-risk HPV viral oncoproteins E6 and E7 transform oral squamous epithelial cells. These proteins bind with p53 and Rb, respectively, and interfere with their tumor suppressor functions, leading to cell cycle dysregulation and genetic instability. Diagnostically, immunohistochemical detection of p16 (a surrogate marker for HPV 16) and/or polymerase chain reaction (PCR) or in situ hybridization for HPV facilitate diagnosis of these carcinomas. Further, the presence of p16 (in fine needle aspiration material or tissue sampling) in a carcinoma metastatic to a cervical neck lymph node from an unknown primary tumor is presumptive evidence of a primary carcinoma originating in the oropharynx (i.e., base of tongue or tonsil). The advent of the HPV vaccine is expected to reduce the incidence of HPV-HNSCC.

Nasopharyngeal Carcinoma Is Related to Epstein-Barr Virus

Nasopharyngeal carcinoma (NPC) is a malignancy of the nasopharynx that is subclassified into keratinizing and nonkeratinizing types. The latter are associated with EBV infection, and may be differentiated or undifferentiated.

EPIDEMIOLOGY: ***Undifferentiated nonkeratinizing carcinomas are particularly common in southeast Asia and parts of Africa.*** By far the most common cancer of the nasopharynx, NPC is the most frequent of all malignant tumors in China. In Hong Kong, it represents 18% of all cancers, compared with 0.25% worldwide. Chinese born in the United States have about a 20-fold greater mortality from nasopharynx carcinoma than people of other races.

MOLECULAR PATHOGENESIS: Despite considerable effort, environmental risk factors for NPC have not been positively identified, although recent studies suggest possible combined roles for environmental and genetic factors. There is an association with the A2/sin HLA profile in the Chinese, suggesting a genetic susceptibility. Loss of heterozygosity (LOH) studies have demonstrated deletions on several chromosomes, in particular 3p, 9p and 14q, in high frequency in nasopharyngeal carcinoma, possibly reflecting an association with tumor suppressor genes located on these loci.

Antibodies to EBV are detected in 85% of patients with NPC. EBV genomes are found in 75% to 100% of nonkeratinizing and undifferentiated types of NPC. In the keratinizing NPC, EBV is more variable. See Chapters 5 and 9 for a more detailed discussion.

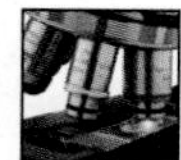

PATHOLOGY: NPC may be keratinizing or nonkeratinizing, differentiated or undifferentiated (squamous) tumors. The former tend to occur in older people and do not bear the same relation to EBV as nonkeratinizing types. Differentiated nonkeratinizing NPCs have a stratified appearance and distinct cell margins. By contrast, in undifferentiated tumors, clusters of poorly delimited or syncytial cells have large oval nuclei and scant eosinophilic cytoplasm (Fig. 25-23A). A lymphoid infiltrate may be prominent in the undifferentiated variety, accounting for the obsolete (and misleading) term "lymphoepithelioma." Both subtypes are immunoreactive with cytokeratin (Fig. 25-23B). The tumor cells express cytokeratin but not hematologic or lymphoid markers. In situ hybridization usually demonstrates Epstein-Barr virus DNA (Fig. 25-23C).

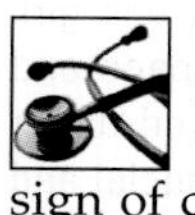

CLINICAL FEATURES: Owing to their location, most NPCs are asymptomatic for a long time. Palpable cervical lymph node metastases are the first sign of disease in about half of cases, and even then, many patients have no complaints referable to the nasopharynx. Tumors invade nearby regions, such as the parapharyngeal space, orbit and cranial cavity, causing neurologic symptoms and hearing disturbances. Invasion of the base of the skull leads to cranial nerve involvement. Tumors in the fossa of Rosenmüller and the lateral wall of the nasopharynx lead to symptoms referable to the middle ear. Eustachian tube obstruction is common. The abundant local lymphatic network leads to frequent and early metastases to cervical lymph nodes.

Nasopharyngeal undifferentiated carcinoma is radiosensitive, and most patients with tumors restricted to the nasopharynx survive 5 or more years. Cervical lymph node metastases cloud the prognosis greatly, and survival with cranial nerve involvement or distant metastasis is dismal.

Lymphomas of the Waldeyer Ring Are Mostly Diffuse B-Cell Tumors

Lymphomas make up 5% of head and neck cancers. The Waldeyer ring is by far the most common site of origin of lymphoma in this region: the palatine tonsils first, followed by the nasopharynx and the base of the tongue. Enlargement of a single tonsil in any age group, or bilateral painless tonsillar enlargement in adults, should suggest the possibility of lymphoma. In these cases, cervical lymph nodes are most often

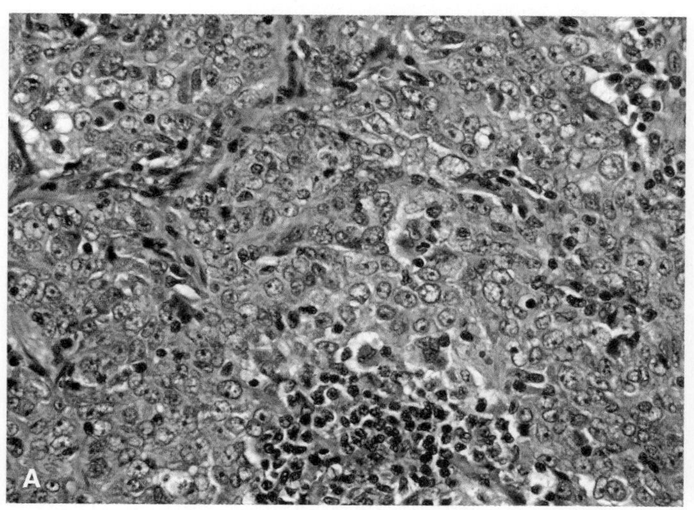

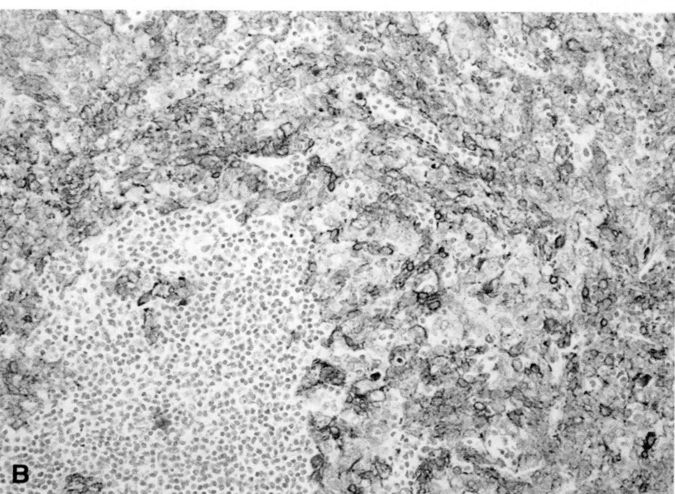

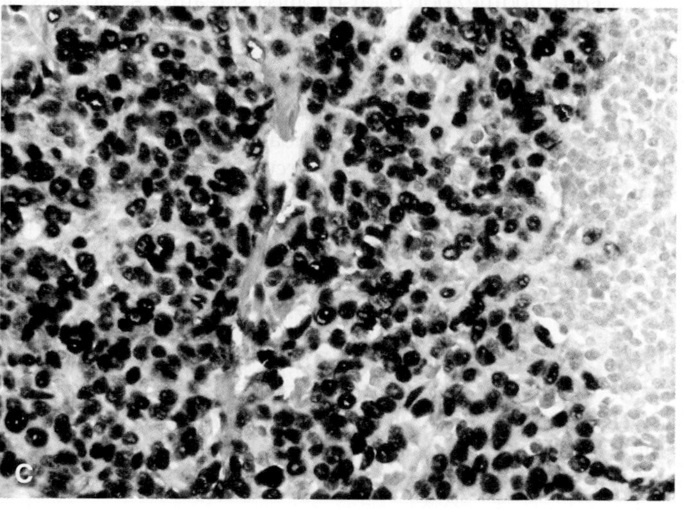

FIGURE 25-23. Nasopharyngeal nonkeratinizing carcinoma, undifferentiated type. **A.** The cells have large nuclei and prominent eosinophilic nucleoli. **B.** The cells are cytokeratin positive (by immunohistochemistry), indicating an epithelial cell proliferation. **C.** In situ hybridization for Epstein-Barr virus (EBER-ISH).

involved. Nasopharyngeal lymphomas are histologically diffuse (90%), and more than half are large cell lymphomas. In the United States and Asia, the vast majority of lymphomas of the Waldeyer ring are of B-cell origin.

Three Quarters of Extramedullary Plasmacytomas Occur in the Head and Neck

These tumors show a strong predilection for the nasopharynx, nasal cavity and paranasal sinuses. They behave like other extramedullary plasmacytomas, and may remain localized or may evolve into systemic plasma cell myeloma (see Chapter 20).

Chordomas Are Malignancies Derived From Remnants of Embryonic Notochord

These tumors are uncommon in people under 40. In one third of cases, chordomas extend into the nasopharynx. In the cranial region, they originate from the area of the sphenooccipital synchondrosis or **clivus**. They are characterized by large vacuolated (physaliferous) cells surrounded by abundant intercellular matrix (Fig. 25-24). Chordomas usually grow slowly, but they infiltrate bone and are ordinarily impossible to remove completely by surgery. Few patients with chordomas of the cranial region survive longer than 5 years.

Other Malignant Tumors of the Nasopharynx Are Rare

They may derive from various components of mucosa or adjacent supportive soft tissues and skeleton. **Embryonal rhabdomyosarcoma** (Fig. 25-25) arises in the pharyngeal tissues of young children. This highly malignant tumor invades contiguous structures and metastasizes by both the bloodstream and lymphatics. **Kaposi sarcoma** has been reported in the nasopharyngeal mucosa of patients with AIDS, in association with HHV8.

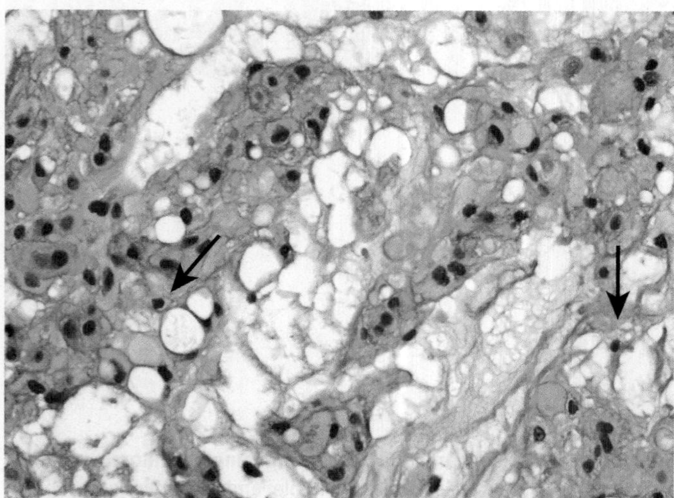

FIGURE 25-24. Chordoma. Large vacuolated (physaliferous) tumor cells (*arrows*) are evident.

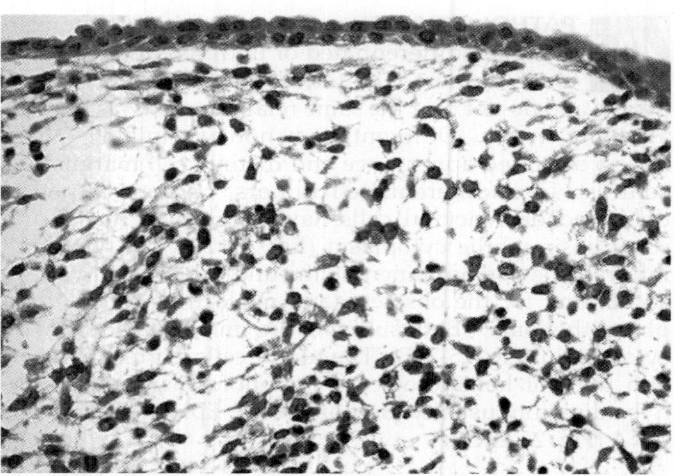

FIGURE 25-25. Embryonal rhabdomyosarcoma from a 3-year-old girl. This highly malignant tumor arose in the parapharyngeal space and invaded the adjacent structures. The oval or tadpole-shaped tumor cells under the epithelium have hyperchromatic, eccentric nuclei and immunohistochemical and ultrastructural features of rhabdomyoblasts.

LARYNX AND HYPOPHARYNX

Infections

EPIGLOTTITIS: Inflammation of the epiglottis is most commonly caused by *H. influenzae* type B. Occurring in infants and young children, this may be a life-threatening emergency. Swelling of the acutely inflamed epiglottis may obstruct airflow. Inspiratory stridor (a loud wheezing sound on inspiration) occurs and the onset of cyanosis may indicate airway obstruction so severe as to require tracheostomy.

CROUP: Croup is a laryngotracheobronchitis of young children who have symptoms of inspiratory stridor, cough and hoarseness, due to varying degrees of laryngeal obstruction. It is a complication of an upper respiratory infection, and is marked by edema of the larynx.

Vocal Cord Nodule and Polyp

Vocal cord nodule/polyp (also called screamer's, singer's or preacher's nodule) is a stromal reactive process related to inflammation and/or trauma. They may be seen in all age groups but are most common between the third and sixth decades (Fig. 25-26). Symptoms related to vocal cord polyps and nodules are similar and include hoarseness or voice changes ("cracking" of the voice). Lesions occur after voice abuse, infection (laryngitis), alcohol, smoking or endocrine dysfunction (e.g., hypothyroidism). Histologic appearances vary from a myxoid, edematous, fibroblastic stroma in the early stages to a hyalinized, densely fibrotic stroma in the later stages.

Neoplasms of the Larynx

SQUAMOUS PAPILLOMA AND PAPILLOMATOSIS: Squamous papillomas of the larynx are solitary or multiple papillary growths of mature squamous cells that line the surface

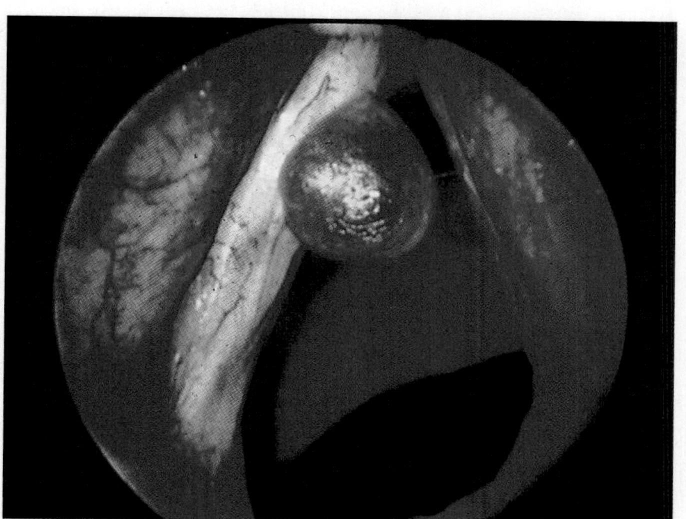

FIGURE 25-26. Vocal cord polyp. A solitary polypoid lesion with a glistening appearance is seen arising from the true vocal cord.

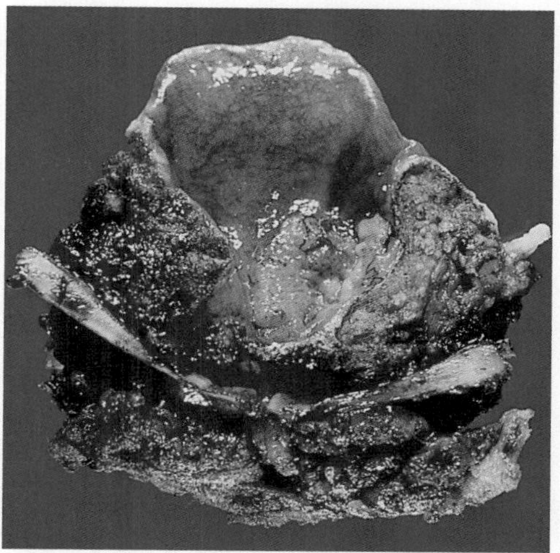

FIGURE 25-27. Supraglottic laryngectomy specimen for squamous cell carcinoma. The carcinoma appears as an irregular raised granular-appearing area in the right supraglottic larynx.

of fibrovascular cores. They may be multiple in children or adolescents (juvenile laryngeal papillomatosis), and may extend into the trachea and bronchi. HPV, especially types HPV-6 and HPV-11, are the principal causes. The condition may cause life-threatening respiratory obstruction and, rarely, evolve into an overt SCC, particularly in smokers or after radiation therapy. Surgical excision may not be curative, as viral infection of the mucosa is often widespread, and the tumors tend to recur over many years. Solitary laryngeal squamous papilloma occurs in adults, predominantly in men, and is usually cured surgically.

SQUAMOUS CELL CARCINOMA: Almost all laryngeal cancers are SCCs. Virtually all of these patients are men, most of whom are cigarette smokers.

- **Glottic carcinoma** is limited to one or both true vocal cords and accounts for almost two thirds of laryngeal cancers. It is slow to metastasize to lymph nodes and has a good prognosis.
- **Supraglottic carcinomas** arise in the ventricle, false cords or epiglottis and, by definition, do not involve the true cords. Up to one third of laryngeal carcinomas arise in this location. Nodal metastases are more common than in glottic tumors.
- **Transglottic carcinoma**, by definition, involves the true and false cords (Fig. 25-27). This uncommon tumor metastasizes to lymph nodes and often requires total laryngectomy.
- **Infraglottic carcinoma** is an uncommon tumor located below the true cords or involving the true cords, with considerable infraglottic extension and frequent extension into the trachea. Nodal metastases are common, and total laryngectomy is generally required.

CHONDROSARCOMA: Chondrosarcoma, a rare malignant tumor of cartilage, accounts for 75% of nonepithelial laryngeal malignancies. In the larynx, it usually grows as an exophytic, polypoid mass, which may lead to airway obstruction. Most patients are men in their seventies. It also occurs in mandible, maxilla, nasal, and paranasal sinuses and nasopharynx. Patients present with hoarseness, airway obstruction and dyspnea.

SALIVARY GLANDS

The salivary glands develop as buds of oral ectoderm. They are tubuloalveolar structures that secrete saliva. All major salivary glands are paired organs. Parotid glands secrete serous saliva, and submandibular and sublingual glands produce mixed serous and mucous saliva. Minor salivary glands are widespread under the mucosa of the lips, cheeks, palate and tongue. Lymph nodes, which are normally embedded in the parotid gland, may be involved in a variety of inflammatory, reactive or proliferative processes, including malignant lymphoma.

XEROSTOMIA: Xerostomia, which is chronic mouth dryness due to lack of saliva, has many causes. Diseases that involve the major salivary glands and produce xerostomia include mumps, Sjögren syndrome, sarcoidosis, radiation-induced atrophy (Fig. 25-28) and drug sensitivity (antihistamines, tricyclic antidepressants, hypotensive drugs, phenothiazines).

SIALORRHEA: Increased salivary flow is associated with many conditions, including acute inflammation of the oral cavity, as in aphthous stomatitis, Parkinson disease, rabies, mental retardation, nausea and pregnancy.

ENLARGEMENT: Unilateral enlargement of major salivary glands is usually caused by cysts, inflammation or neoplasms. Bilateral enlargement is due to inflammation (mumps, Sjögren syndrome; see below), granulomatous disease (sarcoidosis) or diffuse neoplastic involvement (leukemia or malignant lymphoma).

SIALOLITHIASIS: Calcific stones occur in salivary gland ducts, mostly in the submandibular gland. The most important consequence of stone formation is duct obstruction, which is often followed by inflammation distal to the occlusion.

PAROTITIS: Bacteria (usually *S. aureus*) ascending from the oral cavity when salivary flow is reduced cause acute suppurative parotitis. It is most often seen in debilitated or postoperative patients. Salivary duct stricture or obstruction by stones may cause acute or chronic parotitis. Stagnant secretions serve as a medium for retrograde bacterial invasion.

Epidemic parotitis (mumps) is an acute viral disease of the parotid glands that spreads with infected saliva. The submandibular and sublingual salivary glands also may be

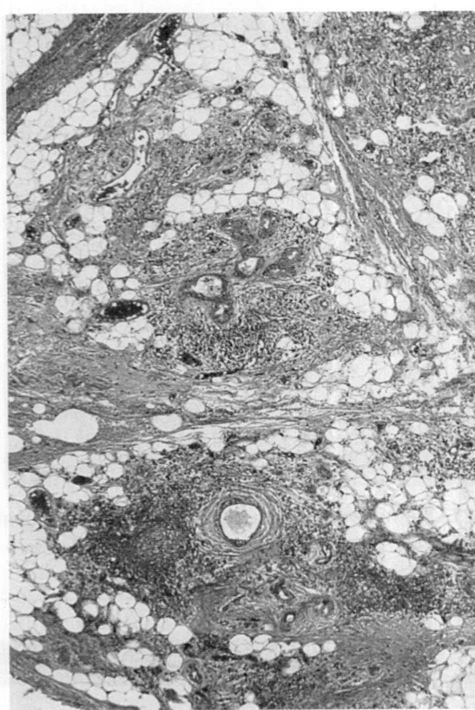

FIGURE 25-28. Chronic sialadenitis. Severe chronic inflammation and marked atrophy of the submandibular gland are present after irradiation of an adjacent oral cancer. The atrophic acini have been replaced by fat.

involved. Mumps infection may also cause pancreatitis and orchitis. Microscopically, salivary glands contain dense lymphocytic and macrophage infiltrates, and show epithelial degeneration and necrosis.

Sjögren Syndrome

Sjögren syndrome is an autoimmune chronic inflammatory disorder of salivary and lacrimal glands; it may be limited to these sites, or be associated with a systemic autoimmune disease. Involvement of the salivary glands leads to xerostomia, and involvement of the lacrimal glands results in dry eyes **(keratoconjunctivitis sicca)**. The pathogenesis and clinical features of Sjögren syndrome are discussed in Chapter 4.

PATHOLOGY: In Sjögren syndrome, parotid glands, and sometimes submandibular glands, are unilaterally or bilaterally enlarged, but their lobulation is preserved. Initial periductal chronic inflammation gradually extends into the acini, until the glands are completely replaced by a sea of polyclonal lymphocytes, immunoblasts, germinal centers and plasma cells. Proliferating myoepithelial cells surround remnants of damaged ducts and form so-called epimyoepithelial islands (lymphoepithelial sialadenitis; Fig. 25-29). Similar changes can be seen in the lacrimal glands and minor salivary glands. Focal lymphocytic sialadenitis is also seen in minor salivary glands sampled by labial biopsy in most patients with Sjögren syndrome. Late in the course of the disease, affected glands become atrophic, with fibrosis and fatty infiltration of the parenchyma. The lymphoid infiltrates in Sjögren syndrome may contain monotypic cells that have restricted immunoglobulin patterns, which may not be invasive and may remain localized.

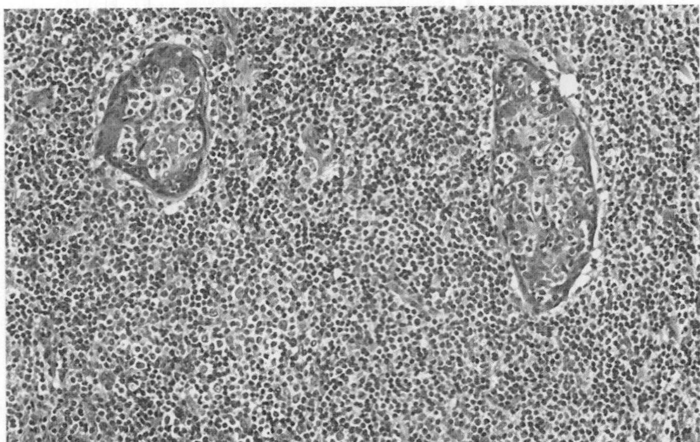

FIGURE 25-29. Sjögren syndrome. There is infiltration of the involved salivary gland by a mixed chronic inflammatory cell infiltrate. Extension of the infiltrate into epithelial (ductal) structures results in metaplasia and characteristic epimyoepithelial islands.

Benign Salivary Gland Neoplasms

Pleomorphic Adenoma Is the Most Common Tumor of Salivary Glands

These neoplasms, also called mixed tumors, are benign proliferations characterized by admixed epithelial and stromal elements. Two-thirds of major salivary gland tumors, and about half of those in the minor glands, are pleomorphic adenomas. The tumors occur nine times more often in the parotid than in the submandibular gland, and usually arise in the superficial lobe of the parotid. Middle-aged people and women are most affected.

MOLECULAR PATHOGENESIS: Loss of heterozygosity of chromosome 8q17p and rearrangements in 3p21 and 12q13-15 have been found in pleomorphic adenomas. PLAG1 (pleomorphic adenoma gene 1), which encodes a zinc finger protein, is developmentally regulated and is rearranged in most of these tumors. It is activated by reciprocal chromosomal translocations involving 8q12 in a subset of these tumors. Development of carcinomas from pleomorphic adenomas involves rearrangements of 8q12, alterations in 12q13-15 and mutations in *HMGIC* and *MDM2* genes.

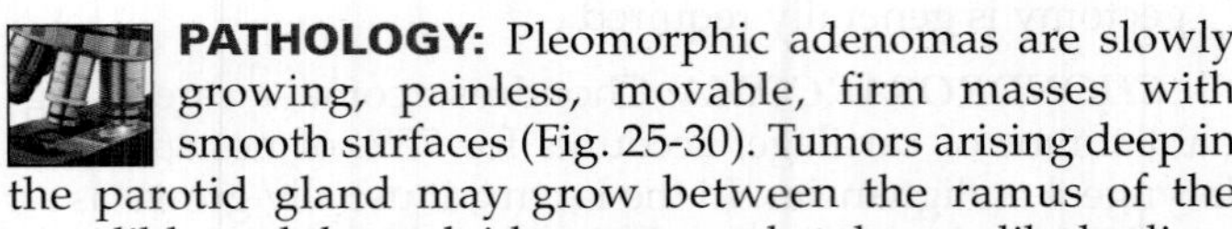

PATHOLOGY: Pleomorphic adenomas are slowly growing, painless, movable, firm masses with smooth surfaces (Fig. 25-30). Tumors arising deep in the parotid gland may grow between the ramus of the mandible and the styloid process and stylomandibular ligament into the parapharyngeal space, where they are swellings of the lateral pharyngeal or tonsillar regions. Pleomorphic adenomas show epithelial tissue intermingled with myxoid, mucoid or chondroid areas (Fig. 25-31B), hence the older term

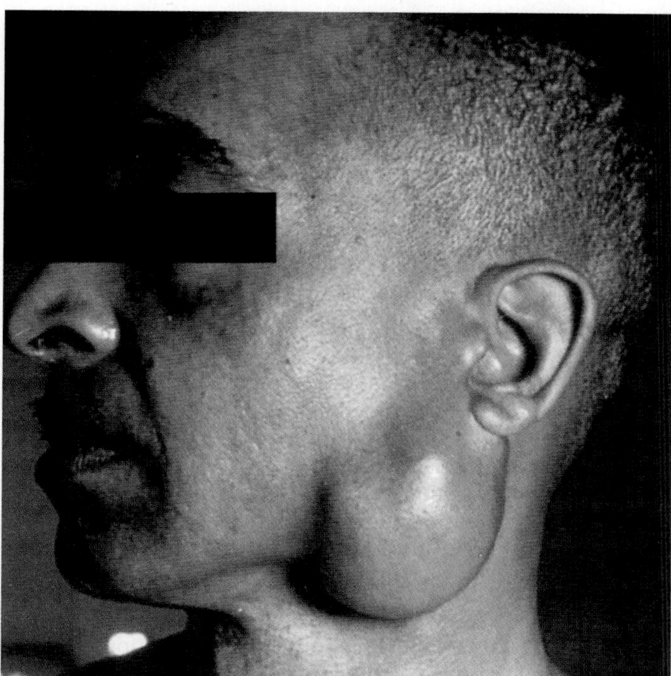

FIGURE 25-30. Pleomorphic adenoma of the parotid. A conspicuous tumor mass is seen at the angle of the jaw.

mixed tumor. However, the neoplasm is now considered to be of epithelial origin.

The epithelial component of pleomorphic adenomas consists of ductal and myoepithelial cells. The cells lining the ducts form tubules or small cystic structures and contain clear fluid or eosinophilic, periodic acid–Schiff (PAS)-positive material. Around ductal epithelial cells are smaller myoepithelial cells, which are the main cellular component. These cells form well-defined sheaths, cords or nests and are often separated by a cellular ground substance that resembles cartilaginous, myxoid or mucoid material.

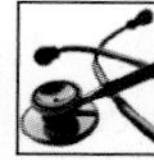

CLINICAL FEATURES: Pleomorphic adenomas have fibrous capsules. As they grow, the surrounding fibrous tissue condenses around them. The tumors expand and tend to protrude focally into adjacent tissues, becoming nodular (Fig. 25-31A). These tumor projections can be missed if a tumor is not carefully removed with an intact capsule and an adequate margin of surrounding glandular parenchyma. Tumor implanted during surgery or tumor nodules left behind continue to grow as recurrences in scars from previous operations. Recurrence represents local regrowth, not malignancy, and further surgery may necessitate sacrificing the facial nerve.

Carcinomas may rarely arise in pleomorphic adenomas, **carcinoma ex pleomorphic adenoma.** Usually, the tumor has been present for many years, then begins to grow rapidly or becomes painful. Histologically, carcinoma, usually a high-grade malignancy such as poorly differentiated or undifferentiated adenocarcinoma, is seen in an otherwise benign pleomorphic adenoma. However, virtually any type of salivary gland malignancy may occur in this setting, including mucoepidermoid or adenoid cystic carcinomas. If the carcinoma is fully confined to the tumor capsule and does not invade the adjacent salivary gland parenchyma, it is considered **in situ** or **noninvasive carcinoma ex pleomorphic adenoma.** If there is invasion beyond the tumor capsule less than or equal to 1.5 mm, it is considered **minimally invasive.** Both of these entities have an excellent prognosis, but invasion beyond 1.5 mm (i.e., ***widely invasive tumor***) behaves aggressively, recurs frequently, metastasizes and has a poor prognosis.

Monomorphic Adenomas Are 5% to 10% of Benign Salivary Gland Tumors

In these tumors, the epithelium is arranged in a regular, usually glandular, pattern with no mesenchyme-like component. Monomorphic adenomas include (1) Warthin tumor (papillary cystadenoma lymphomatosum), (2) basal cell adenoma, (3) oxyphilic adenoma or oncocytoma, (4) canalicular adenoma, (5) myoepithelioma and (6) clear cell adenoma.

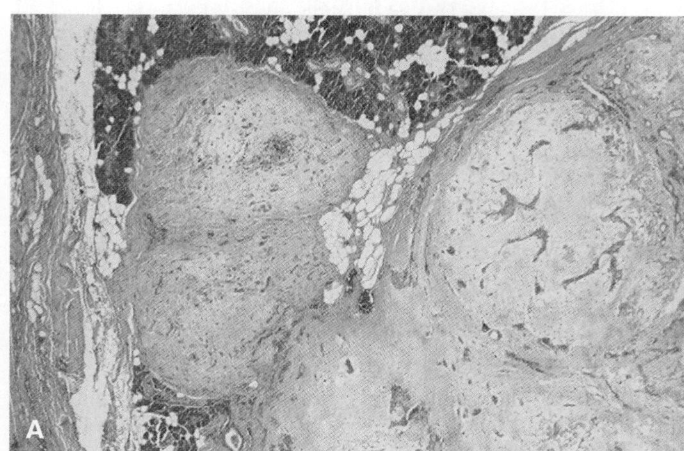

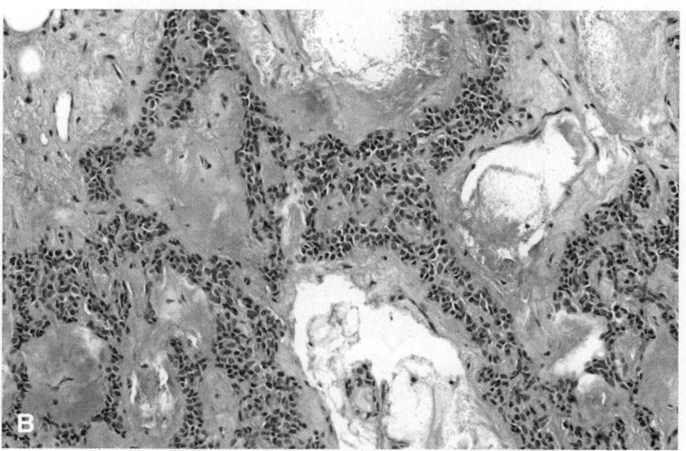

FIGURE 25-31. Pleomorphic adenoma of the parotid gland. A. The tumor contains characteristic myxoid and chondroid portions. The tumor is partly encapsulated, but a nodule protruding into the parotid gland lacks a capsule. If such nodules are not included in the resection, the tumor will recur. **B.** Cellular components of pleomorphic adenomas include an admixture of glands and myoepithelial cells within a chondromyxoid stroma.

Warthin Tumor

Warthin tumors are benign parotid gland neoplasms composed of cystic glandular spaces within dense lymphoid tissue. This is the most common monomorphic adenoma. Although it is clearly benign, it may be bilateral (15% of cases) or multifocal within one gland. These are the only salivary gland tumors that are more common in men than in women. They generally occur after age 30, with most arising after age 50.

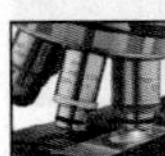

PATHOLOGY: Warthin tumors are composed of glandular spaces that tend to become cystic and show papillary projections. The cysts are lined by characteristic eosinophilic epithelial cells (oncocytes) and are embedded in dense lymphoid tissue with germinal centers (Fig. 25-32).

The histogenesis of this tumor is uncertain. Lymph nodes are normally found in the parotid gland and in its immediate vicinity, and usually contain a few ducts or small islands of salivary gland tissue. Warthin tumors may arise from proliferation of these salivary gland inclusions.

Oncocytoma (Oxyphil Adenoma)

Oncocytes are benign epithelial cells swollen with mitochondria, which impart a granular appearance to the cytoplasm. Normally, they are scattered or in small clusters among epithelial cells of various organs (e.g., thyroid, parathyroid glands). They first appear in early adulthood, and increase in number with age. Their function is unknown. Rare benign tumors composed of nests or cords of these cells occur in the parotid glands of elderly persons.

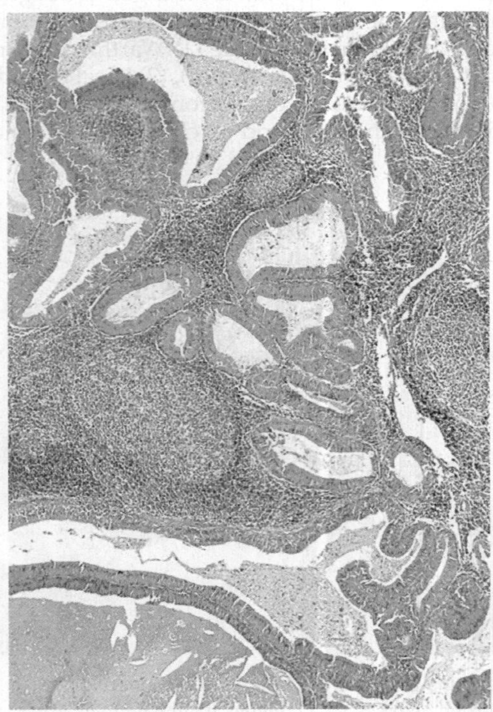

FIGURE 25-32. Warthin tumor. Cystic spaces and ductlike structures are lined by oncocytes. Follicular lymphoid tissue is present.

Malignant Salivary Gland Tumors

Salivary gland tumors make up about 5% of all head and neck malignancies. Most (75%) arise in the parotid glands, 10% in submandibular glands and 15% in minor salivary glands (mucoserous glands) of the upper aerodigestive tract. Malignancies of the sublingual glands are rare.

Mucoepidermoid Carcinomas Show Neoplastic Epidermoid, Mucus-Secreting and Intermediate Cells

These tumors derive from ductal epithelium, which has a considerable potential for metaplasia. They account for 5% to 10% of major salivary gland tumors and 10% of those in the minor salivary glands. More than half of mucoepidermoid carcinomas in the major glands arise in the parotid gland. In minor salivary glands, they develop mostly in the palate. The tumor may occur in adolescents, but most arise in adults. They are more common in women.

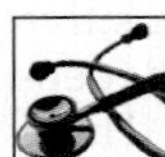

PATHOLOGY: Mucoepidermoid carcinomas grow slowly and present as firm, painless masses. Microscopically, low-grade (well-differentiated) tumors form irregular solid, ductlike and cystic spaces that include squamous cells, mucus-secreting cells and intermediate cells (Fig. 25-33). Intermediate-grade tumors tend to (1) be more solid in growth, (2) contain a greater percentage of epidermoid and intermediate cells and (3) possess fewer mucus-secreting cells. High-grade (poorly differentiated) carcinomas are markedly pleomorphic, without evidence of differentiation save, perhaps, for scattered mucus-secreting cells.

CLINICAL FEATURES: Even low-grade (well-differentiated) mucoepidermoid carcinomas can metastasize, but over 90% of patients survive 5 years,

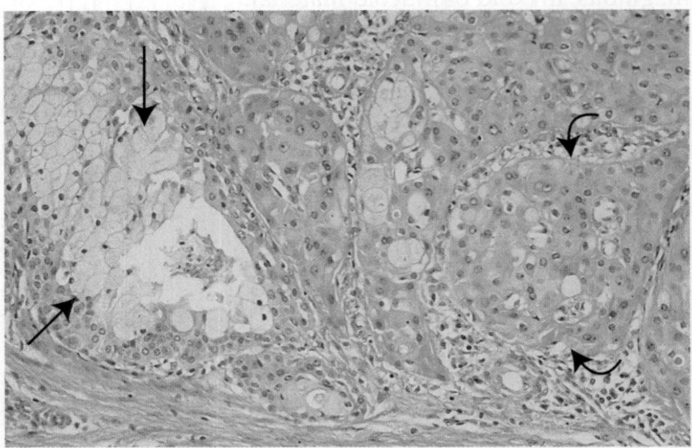

FIGURE 25-33. Mucoepidermoid carcinoma is characterized by an admixture of mucocytes (*straight arrows*), epidermoid cells (*curved arrows*) and intermediate cells. The mucocytes are clustered and have a clear cytoplasm with eccentrically situated nuclei. Epidermoid cells are squamouslike cells but lack keratinization and intercellular bridges. Intermediate cells (best seen at *lower left*) are smaller than epidermoid cells.

regardless of the primary site. Survival with high-grade (poorly differentiated) tumors is much worse (20% to 40%).

Adenoid Cystic Carcinomas Invade Locally and Often Recur After Resection

Adenoid cystic carcinomas are slowly growing salivary gland malignancies. They represent 5% of major salivary gland tumors and 20% of those of the minor salivary glands. One third arise in the major salivary glands and two thirds in the minor ones. They occur not only in the oral cavity but also in lacrimal glands, nasopharynx, nasal cavity, paranasal sinuses and lower respiratory tract. They are most common in people 40 to 60 years of age.

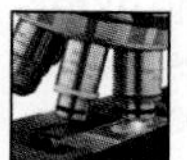

PATHOLOGY: Adenoid cystic carcinomas show variable histologies. The tumor cells are small, have scant cytoplasm and grow in solid sheets or as small groups, strands or columns. Within these structures, the tumor cells interconnect to enclose cystic spaces, resulting in a solid, tubular or cribriform (sievelike) arrangement (Fig. 25-34). Grading these tumors on the basis of the proportions of tubular and cribriform patterns may be done, with over 30% solid growth defining "high grade." Tumor cells make a homogeneous basement membrane material that gives them the characteristic "cylindromatous" appearance.

The tumors probably arise from cells that are differentiating toward intercalated ducts and myoepithelium. ***Adenoid cystic carcinomas tend to infiltrate perineural spaces and are often painful.*** Although most do not metastasize for many years, they are often diagnosed late, are difficult to eradicate completely and have poor long-term prognosis.

Acinic Cell Adenocarcinomas Arise From Epithelial Secretory Cells

These are uncommon parotid tumors (10% of all salivary gland tumors). They arise occasionally in other salivary glands and occur principally in young men between the ages of 20 and 30. They are encapsulated, round masses, usually less than 3 cm and may be cystic. Acinic cell carcinomas are composed of uniform cells with a small central nucleus and abundant basophilic cytoplasm, similar to the secretory (acinic) cells of normal salivary glands (Fig. 25-35). They may spread to the regional lymph nodes. After surgery, most (90%) patients survive for 5 years, but local recurrence may be expected in one third of patients. Only half survive for 20 years.

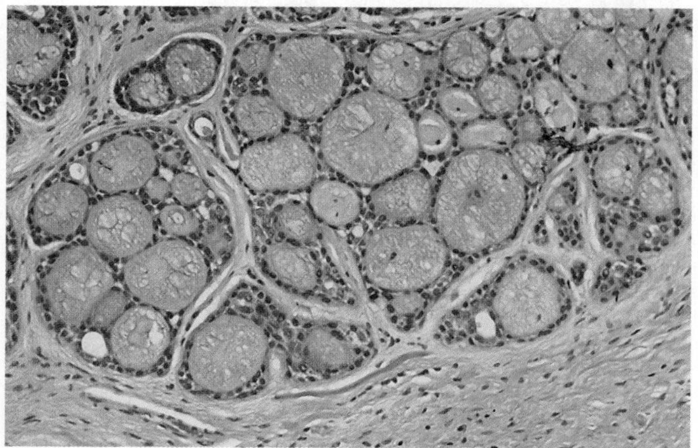

FIGURE 25-34. Adenoid cystic carcinoma showing cribriform growth in which cystlike spaces are filled with basophilic material. The cyst spaces are really pseudocysts surrounded by myoepithelial cells.

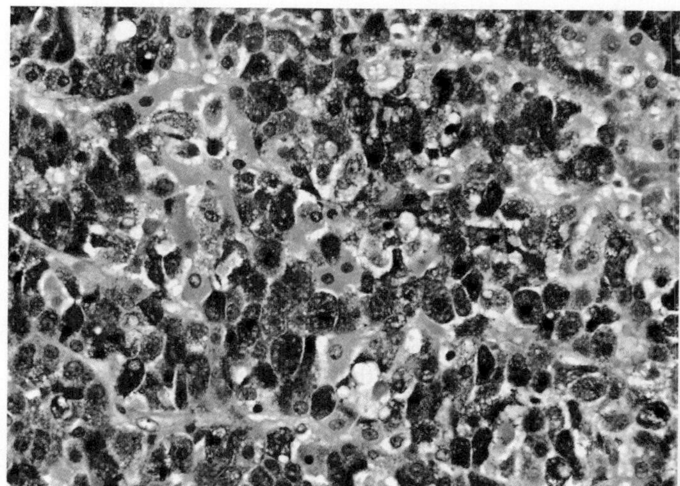

FIGURE 25-35. Acinic cell adenocarcinoma. This tumor demonstrates a solid growth pattern and is composed of basophilic cells with abundant cytoplasm filled with zymogen granules.

THE EAR

External Ear

The outer portion of the external ear includes the auricle or pinna leading into the external auditory canal. The external auditory canal or meatus extends from the concha to its medial limit, which is the outer aspect of the tympanic membrane. The lateral portion of its wall consists of cartilage and connective tissue, and the medial part is bone. The tympanic membrane (eardrum) is situated obliquely at the end of the external auditory canal, sloping medially both from above downward and from behind forward. It separates the external ear from the middle ear.

The auricle is composed of keratinizing, stratified squamous epithelium with associated adnexa that include hair follicles, sebaceous glands and eccrine sweat glands. The outer third of the external auditory canal also contains ceruminal glands, modified apocrine glands that replace the eccrine glands of the auricular dermis. These glands produce cerumen and contain clusters of cuboidal cells with eosinophilic cytoplasm often containing granular, golden yellow pigment and secretory droplets along their luminal border. Peripheral to the secretory cells are flattened myoepithelial cells. Ceruminal gland ducts terminate in hair follicles or on the skin. The inner portion of the external auditory canal has no adnexal structures. The outer surface of this airtight membrane is covered by squamous epithelium that is continuous with the skin of the external ear canal. Its inner surface is lined by the cuboidal epithelium of the middle ear. Between these two epithelial covers of the tympanic membrane is a middle layer of dense fibrous tissue.

KELOIDS: Keloids are particularly common on the ear lobes after piercing for earrings or other trauma (see Chapter 3). They occur much more frequently in blacks and Asians than in whites. Keloids can attain considerable size and tend to recur. They are composed of thick, hyalinized bundles of collagen in the deep dermis (see Chapter 3).

CAULIFLOWER EARS: These deformities are particularly common in wrestlers and boxers and result from repeated mechanical trauma to the external ear. Blows to the ears cause subperichondrial hematomas, which organize and deform the ears.

RELAPSING POLYCHONDRITIS: This rare, chronic disorder of unknown origin is characterized by intermittent inflammation that destroys the cartilage of the ears, nose, larynx, tracheobronchial tree, ribs and joints. It may involve hyaline, elastic or fibro-cartilage.

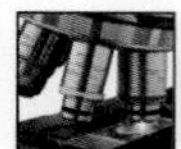

MOLECULAR PATHOGENESIS: The etiology of relapsing polychondritis is obscure, but immune mechanisms are suspected. Serum antibodies to cartilage, type II collagen and chondroitin sulfate have been found in patients during acute attacks. Immune complexes can be detected in involved cartilage. Relapsing polychondritis occurs alone or together with one of the connective tissue diseases. Noncartilaginous tissues, such as the sclera and cardiac valves, also may be affected. Aortic involvement may lead to fatal rupture of the aorta.

PATHOLOGY: The perichondrium is infiltrated by lymphocytes, plasma cells and neutrophils, which also extend into the adjacent cartilage (Fig. 25-36). Chondrocytes die, the cartilaginous matrix degenerates and it fragments. Ultimately, the cartilage is destroyed and replaced by granulation tissue and fibrosis.

"MALIGNANT" OTITIS EXTERNA: This infection of the external auditory canal is caused by *Pseudomonas aeruginosa*. Infection may spread through the skin and cartilage to cause mastoiditis or osteomyelitis of the skull, venous sinus thrombosis, meningitis and death. Malignant otitis externa occurs mainly in elderly diabetics but has also been reported in patients with blood dyscrasias (e.g., leukemia, granulocytopenia).

AURAL POLYPS: These benign inflammatory lesions arise from within the external ear canal or extrude into the canal from the middle ear. Aural polyps are composed of ulcerated and inflamed granulation tissue, which bleeds readily. Those arising in the middle ear result from chronic otitis media.

NEOPLASMS: Benign and malignant tumors of the external ear include the gamut of skin-related neoplasms: squamous papillomas, seborrheic keratosis, basal cell carcinoma, SCC and benign and malignant adnexal tumors.

Ceruminal gland tumors are unique to this area. Benign tumors arising from ceruminal glands include ceruminoma (ceruminal gland adenoma) and salivary gland–type tumors (e.g., pleomorphic and monomorphic adenomas). Malignant tumors include adenocarcinoma and malignant salivary gland–type tumors (e.g., adenoid cystic and mucoepidermoid carcinomas).

Middle Ear

The middle ear, or tympanic cavity, is an oblong space in the temporal bone lined by a mucous membrane. Together with the mastoid, it forms a closed mucosal compartment, also

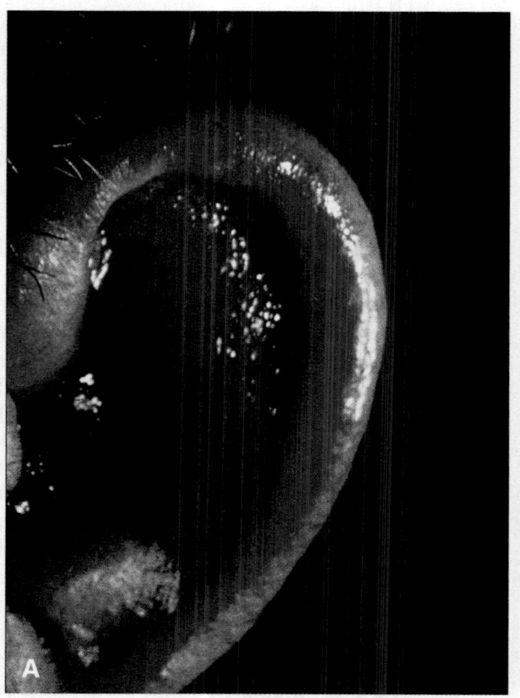

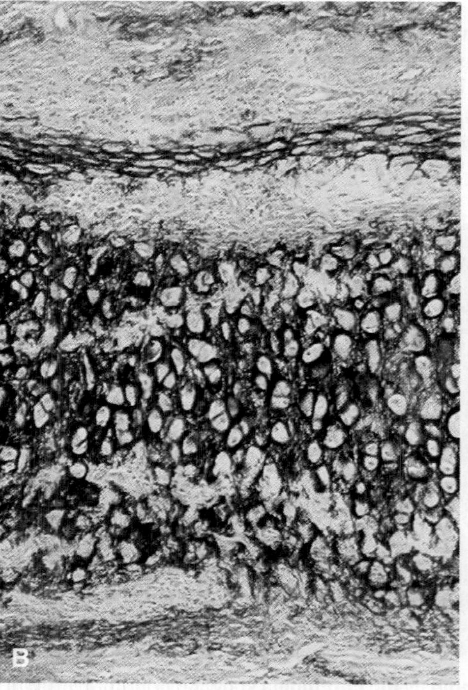

FIGURE 25-36. Relapsing polychondritis. A. The ear is beefy red. **B.** The perichondrium and elastic cartilage are infiltrated and partially destroyed by inflammatory cells and replaced by fibrosis.

called the **middle ear cleft**. Most of the lateral wall consists of the tympanic membrane. Anteriorly, the eustachian tube connects the middle ear with the nasopharynx. It is an air passage that allows air pressure on both sides of the tympanic membrane to equalize. The three auditory ossicles—the malleus, incus and stapes—are a chain that connects the tympanic membrane with the oval window (on the medial wall of the tympanic cavity). They conduct sound across the middle ear. Freedom of motion of the ossicles, mainly the stapes in the oval window, is more important for hearing than is an intact tympanic membrane. The middle ear opens posteriorly into the mastoid antrum, a honeycomb of small, aerated, bony compartments (air cells) lined by a thin mucous membrane continuous with that of the middle ear.

Otitis Media Often Results From Obstruction of the Eustachian Tube

Otitis media is inflammation of the middle ear. It usually results from an upper respiratory tract infection that extends from the nasopharynx.

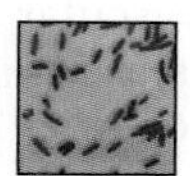

ETIOLOGIC FACTORS: The infection almost invariably penetrates through the mastoid antrum into the mastoid cells. During an infection in the nasopharynx, microorganisms ascend through the eustachian tube to reach the middle ear. Acute otitis media may be due to viral or bacterial infection, or sterile obstruction of the eustachian tube. Viral otitis media may resolve without suppuration or lead to secondary invasion by pus-forming bacteria.

Obstruction of the eustachian tube is important in production of middle ear effusions. When the pharyngeal end of the eustachian tube is swollen, air cannot enter the tube. Air in the middle ear is absorbed through the mucosa, and negative pressure causes transudation of plasma and occasionally bleeding. Antibiotics usually cure or suppress the condition.

ACUTE SEROUS OTITIS MEDIA: Obstruction of the eustachian tube may result from sudden changes in atmospheric pressure (e.g., during flying in an aircraft or deep-sea diving). This effect is particularly severe if there is an upper respiratory tract infection, acute allergic reaction or viral or bacterial infection at the eustachian tube orifice. Inflammation may also occur without bacterial invasion of the middle ear. More than half of children in the United States have had at least one episode of serous otitis media before their third birthday. Repeated bouts of otitis media in early childhood often contribute to unsuspected hearing loss, which is due to residual (usually sterile) fluid in the middle ear.

CHRONIC SEROUS OTITIS MEDIA: Recurrent or chronic serous effusion of the middle ear is due to the same conditions that cause acute obstruction of the eustachian tube. Carcinoma of the nasopharynx may cause chronic serous otitis media in adults and should always be suspected when a unilateral effusion occurs in the middle ear of an adult.

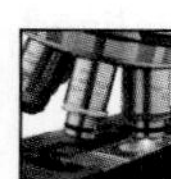

PATHOLOGY: In chronic serous otitis media, mucus-producing (goblet) cell metaplasia may be seen in the mucosal lining of the middle ear. If the obstruction is acute, there may be accompanying hemorrhage, for example, in the mastoid cells. Extravasation of blood and degradation of erythrocytes liberate cholesterol. Cholesterol crystals stimulate a foreign body response and granulation tissue, called a **cholesterol granuloma.** Large cholesterol granulomas may destroy tissue in the mastoid or antrum. If cholesterol granulomas are allowed to persist for many months, the granulation tissue may become fibrotic, which may eventually lead to complete obliteration of the middle ear and mastoid by fibrous tissue.

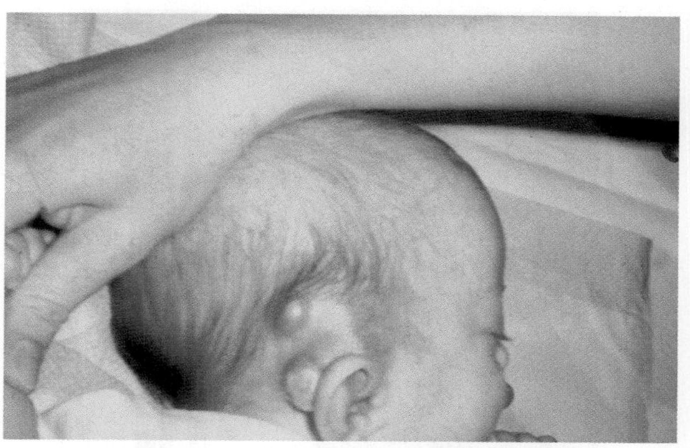

FIGURE 25-37. Acute mastoiditis. An unusual complication of otitis media, acute mastoiditis, appears as large bulging lesions above the child's ear.

ACUTE SUPPURATIVE OTITIS MEDIA: One of the most common infections of childhood, acute suppurative otitis media, is caused by pyogenic bacteria that invade the middle ear, usually via the eustachian tube. *Streptococcus pneumoniae* (pneumococcus) is the most common causative agent in all age groups (30% to 40%). *H. influenzae* causes about 20% of cases, but is less frequent with increasing age. If a purulent exudate accumulates in the middle ear, the eardrum ruptures and the pus is discharged. In most cases, infection is self-limited, and may heal even without therapy.

ACUTE MASTOIDITIS: Infection of the mastoid bone was a common complication of acute otitis media before the advent of antibiotics. It is still seen, rarely, when otitis media is not treated adequately. Mastoid air cells are filled with pus, and their thin osseous intercellular walls are destroyed. Extension of infection to contiguous structures causes complications (Fig. 25-37).

CHRONIC SUPPURATIVE OTITIS MEDIA AND MASTOIDITIS: Neglected or recurrent infection of the middle ear and mastoid process may eventually produce chronic inflammation of the mucosa or destruction of the periosteum covering the ossicles (Fig. 25-38). Chronic otitis media is much more common in people who had ear disease in early childhood, which may have arrested normal development of the air cells in the mastoid.

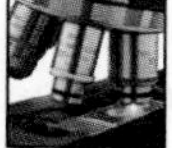

PATHOLOGY: Inflammation tends to be insidious, persistent and destructive. By definition, the eardrum is always perforated in chronic otitis media. Painless discharge **(otorrhea)** and varying degrees of hearing loss are constant symptoms. Exuberant granulation tissue may form polyps, which can extend through the perforated eardrum into the external ear canal.

A **cholesteatoma** is a mass of accumulated keratin and squamous mucosa due to growth of squamous epithelium from the external ear canal thorough a perforated eardrum into the middle ear. There, it continues to produce keratin. Microscopically, cholesteatomas are identical to epidermal inclusion cysts, and are surrounded by granulation tissue

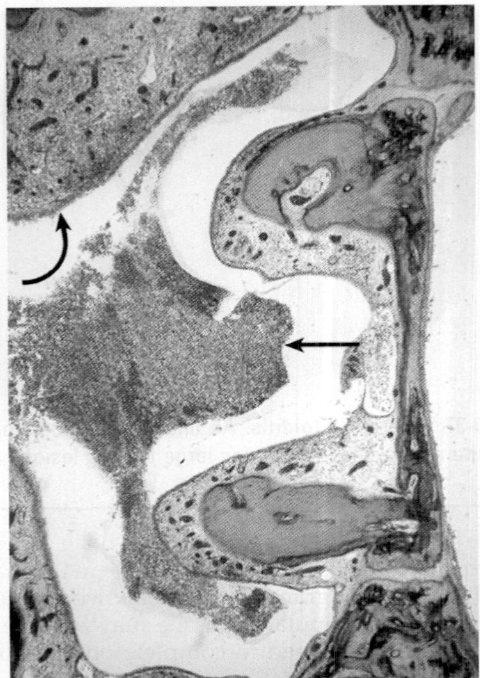

FIGURE 25-38. Chronic suppurative otitis media. A purulent exudate (*straight arrow*) is present in the middle ear cavity. The entire mucosa (*curved arrow*) is thickened by chronic inflammation and granulation tissue. The footplate and the crura of the stapes are at right.

and fibrosis. The keratin mass frequently becomes infected and shields the bacteria from antibiotics. The principal dangers of cholesteatoma arise from erosion of bone, a process that may lead to destruction of important contiguous structures (e.g., auditory ossicles, facial nerve, labyrinth).

COMPLICATIONS OF ACUTE AND CHRONIC OTITIS MEDIA: With antibiotic therapy, complications of otitis media are now rare. However, the following serious or even fatal consequences may still follow suppurative infections of the middle ear:

- Destruction of the facial nerve
- Deep cervical or subperiosteal abscess, if the cortical bone of the mastoid process is eroded
- Petrositis, when infection spreads to the petrous temporal bone through the chain of air cells
- Suppurative labyrinthitis, due to infection of the internal ear
- Epidural, subdural or cerebral abscess, when infection extends through the inner table of the mastoid bone
- Meningitis, when infection reaches the meninges
- Sigmoid sinus thrombophlebitis, if infection traverses the dura to the posterior cranial fossa

Jugulotympanic Paragangliomas Arise From Middle Ear Paraganglia

Jugulotympanic paragangliomas are the most common benign tumors of the middle ear. They grow slowly but, over years, may destroy the middle ear and extend into the internal ear and cranial cavity. Metastases are rare.

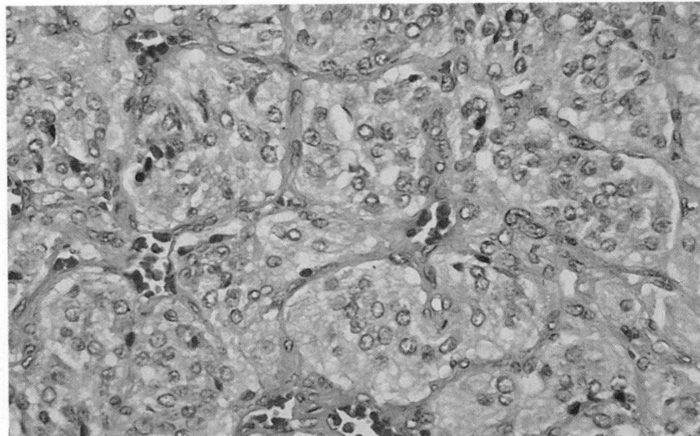

FIGURE 25-39. Jugulotympanic paraganglioma. Tumor cell nests are composed of cells with ill-defined cell borders and prominent eosinophilic cytoplasm (chief cells).

Middle ear paragangliomas resemble those arising elsewhere, with characteristic lobules of cells in richly vascular connective tissue (Fig. 25-39). The paraganglial cells are of neural crest origin and contain varying amounts of catecholamines, mostly epinephrine and norepinephrine.

Internal Ear

The petrous portion of the temporal bone contains the labyrinth, which shelters the end organs for hearing (cochlea) and equilibrium **(vestibular labyrinth).** The complex cavities of the osseous labyrinth contain the membranous labyrinth, a series of communicating membranous sacs and ducts. The osseous labyrinth is filled with a clear fluid, the perilymph, which connects to the subarachnoid space and mingles with the cerebrospinal fluid via the cochlear aqueduct, which provides direct exchange with the cerebrospinal fluid. The membranous labyrinth contains a different fluid, the endolymph, which circulates in a closed system. Because of the lack of barriers between the cochlear and vestibular labyrinths, injury or disease of the inner ear frequently affects both hearing and equilibrium.

The **cochlea** is coiled upon itself like a snail shell and makes two and one-half turns. It has three compartments: two that contain perilymph and a third (the cochlear duct) with endolymph. The cochlear duct encompasses the end organ for hearing, **the organ of Corti,** which rests on the basement membrane, and is arranged as a spiral, with three rows of outer hair cells and a row of inner hair cells. When the hairs of these neuroepithelial cells are bent or distorted by vibration, the mechanical force is converted into electrochemical impulses and interpreted in the temporal cortex as sound. The vestibular part of the membranous labyrinth consists of the utricle, saccule and semicircular canals, each with specialized neuroepithelium that determines equilibrium.

Otosclerosis Is Formation of New Spongy Bone About the Stapes and Oval Window

Otosclerosis causes progressive deafness. ***It is an autosomal dominant hereditary defect, and is the most common cause of***

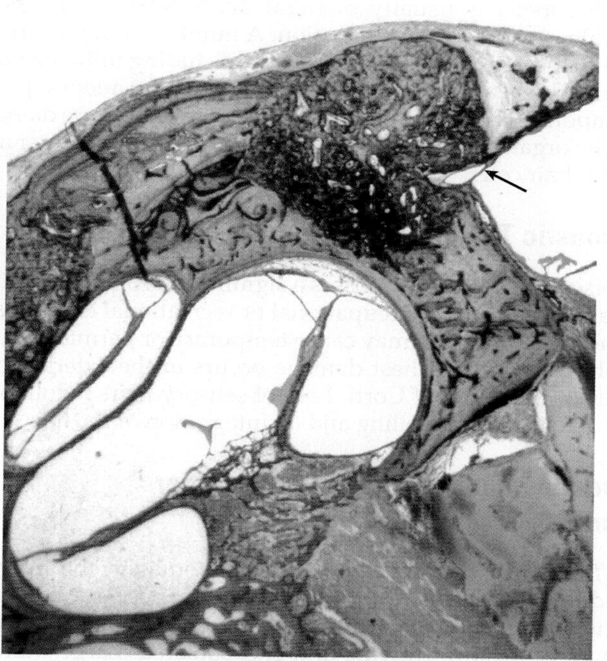

FIGURE 25-40. Otosclerosis. Otosclerotic foci appear as dark purple areas in the bony labyrinth. At the anterior margin of the oval window (*arrow*), otosclerosis has immobilized the footplate of the stapes by bony ankylosis.

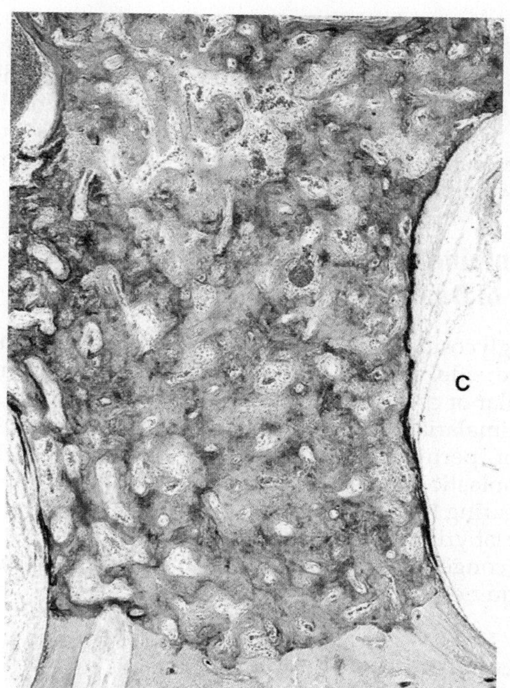

FIGURE 25-41. Otosclerosis. In the lateral wall of the cochlea, the basophilic and more vascular bone is well demarcated. C = organ of Corti.

conductive hearing loss in young and middle-aged adults in the United States, affecting 10% of white and 1% of black adult Americans, although 90% of cases are asymptomatic. The female-to-male ratio is 2:1. Both ears are usually affected. The pathogenesis of otosclerosis is obscure.

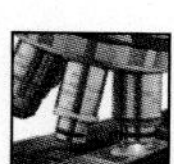

PATHOLOGY: Although any part of the petrous bone may be affected, otosclerotic bone tends to form at particular points. The most frequent (80% to 90%) site is immediately anterior to the oval window. The focus of sclerotic bone extends posteriorly and may infiltrate and replace the stapes, progressively immobilizing the footplate of the stapes. The developing bony ankylosis (Fig. 25-40) is functionally manifested as a slowly progressive conductive hearing loss.

The initial lesion of otosclerosis is resorption of bone and formation of highly cellular fibrous tissue, with wide vascular spaces and osteoclasts. The focus of resorbed bone is later replaced by immature bone, which, with repeated remodeling, becomes mature bone (Fig. 25-41).

Otosclerosis is successfully treated by surgical mobilization of the auditory ossicles.

Ménière Disease Is the Triad of Vertigo, Sensorineural Hearing Loss and Tinnitus

Several etiologic factors have been suggested, but the cause of **Ménière disease** is uncertain. Its pathologic correlate is hydropic distention of the endolymphatic system of the cochlea. Ménière disease is most common in the fourth and fifth decades and is bilateral in 15% of patients.

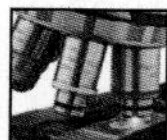

PATHOLOGY: The earliest change is dilatation of the cochlear duct and saccule. As the disease **(hydrops)** progresses, the entire endolymphatic system dilates and the membranous wall may tear (Fig. 25-42). Ruptures can be followed by collapse of the membranous labyrinth, but atrophy of sensory and neural structures is rare. The symptoms of Ménière disease are felt to occur when endolymphatic hydrops causes rupture and endolymph escapes into the perilymph.

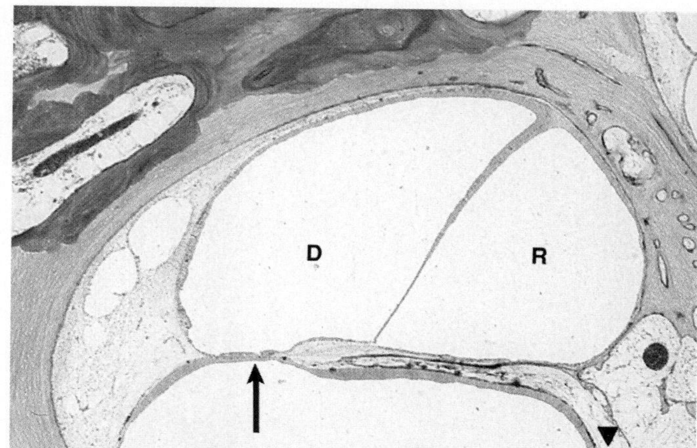

FIGURE 25-42. Ménière disease. The cochlear duct (D) is markedly distended, and the Reissner membrane (R) is pushed back by endolymphatic hydrops. Neither the organ of Corti (*arrow*) nor the spiral ganglion (*arrowhead*) is in its usual location.

CLINICAL FEATURES: Attacks of vertigo, accompanied by often incapacitating nausea and vomiting, last less than 24 hours. Weeks or months go by before another episode, and in time, remissions become longer. Hearing loss recovers between attacks but later becomes permanent. Ménière disease seems to be improved by a low-salt diet and use of diuretics.

Labyrinthine Toxicity Is a Drug-Induced Cause of Deafness

Aminoglycoside antibiotics are the most common drugs with ototoxic side effects. They cause irreversible damage to vestibular or cochlear sensory cells. Other antibiotics, diuretics, antimalarial drugs and salicylates may also cause transient or permanent sensorineural hearing loss. Among antineoplastic agents, cisplatin causes temporary or permanent hearing loss.

The labyrinth of the embryo is especially sensitive to some drugs (congenital deafness due to thalidomide, quinine and chloroquine).

Viral Labyrinthitis Can Result in Congenital Deafness

Viral infections are increasingly recognized as causes of inner ear disorders, particularly deafness, mostly due to viral invasion of the labyrinth. CMV and rubella are the best-known prenatal viral infections that lead to congenital deafness through maternal-to-fetal transmission. CMV antigen has been shown in the cells of the organ of Corti and neurons of the spiral ganglia.

Mumps is the most common postnatal viral cause of deafness. It can cause rapid hearing loss, which is unilateral in 80% of cases. By contrast, prenatal infection of the labyrinth with rubella is usually bilateral, with permanent loss of cochlear and vestibular function. A number of other viruses are suspected to cause labyrinthitis, including influenza and parainfluenza viruses, EBV, herpesviruses and adenoviruses. Temporal bone specimens of such cases reveal severe damage to the organ of Corti, with almost total loss of both inner and outer hair cells.

Acoustic Trauma

Noise-induced hearing loss is a significant problem in industrialized countries. Occupational or recreational exposure to loud tones or noises may cause temporary or permanent loss of hearing. The earliest damage occurs in the external hair cells of the organ of Corti. Loss of sensory hairs is followed by deformation, swelling and disintegration of the hair cells.

The Most Common Tumor of the Inner Ear Is Schwannoma

SCHWANNOMA: Nearly all schwannomas in the internal auditory canal arise from the vestibular nerves. Vestibular schwannomas, which account for about 10% of all intracranial tumors, are slow growing and encapsulated. Larger tumors protrude from the internal auditory meatus into the cerebellopontine angle and may deform the brainstem and adjacent cerebellum (see Chapter 28). Schwannomas cause slowly progressive vestibular and auditory symptoms. In neurofibromatosis type 2, bilateral vestibular schwannomas occur frequently. These tumors are indistinguishable from other vestibular schwannomas (see Chapter 28 for more detail).

MENINGIOMA: Meningiomas of the cerebellopontine angle originate from the meningothelial cells in the arachnoid villi. The favored sites for these tumors are the sphenoid ridge and petrous pyramid. Meningiomas may extend into the adjacent temporal bone or dural sinuses (see Chapter 28).

26 Bones and Joints

Roberto A. Garcia • Michael J. Klein • Alan L. Schiller

BONES

The functions of bone are mechanical, mineral storage and hematopoietic. Mechanical functions of bone include protection for the brain, spinal cord and chest organs; rigid internal support for limbs; and deployment as lever arms in the skeletal muscle. Bone is the principal reservoir for calcium and stores other ions such as phosphate, sodium and magnesium. The bones also serve as hosts for hematopoietic bone marrow.

The mechanical properties of bone are related to its construction and internal architecture. Although extremely light, it has high tensile strength. This combination of strength and light weight results from its hollow tubular shape, layering of bone tissue and internal buttressing of the matrix.

The term **bone** can refer to both an organ and a tissue. The "organ" is composed of bone tissue, cartilage, fat, marrow elements, vessels, nerves and fibrous tissue. Bone "tissue" is described in microscopic terms and is defined by the relation of its collagen and mineral structure to the bone cells.

Anatomy

Macroscopically, two types of bone are recognized:

- **Cortical bone** is dense, compact bone, whose outer shell defines the shape of the bone. It comprises 80% of the skeleton. Because of its density, its functions are mainly biomechanical.
- **Coarse cancellous bone** (also termed **spongy, trabecular** or **medullary bone**) is found at the ends of long bones within the medullary canal. Cancellous bone has a high surface-to-volume ratio and contains many more bone cells per unit volume than does cortical bone. Changes in the rate of bone turnover are manifested principally in cancellous bone.

All bones contain both cancellous and cortical elements (Fig. 26-1), but their proportions differ. The body or shaft of a long tubular bone, such as the femur, is composed of cortical bone and its marrow is mainly fat. Toward the ends of the femur, the cortex becomes thin and coarse cancellous bone becomes the predominant structure. By contrast, the skull is formed by outer and inner tables of compact bone, with only a small amount of cancellous bone within the marrow space, called the **diploë.**

The anatomy of bone is defined in relation to a transverse cartilage plate, which is present in the growing child. This structure is termed the **growth plate**, the **epiphyseal cartilage plate** or **the physis** (Fig. 26-2). The terms **epiphysis, metaphysis** and **diaphysis** are defined in relation to the growth plate.

- The **epiphysis** is the area of the bone that extends from the subarticular bone plate to the base of the growth plate.
- The **metaphysis** contains coarse cancellous bone and is the region from the side of the growth plate facing away from the joint to the area where the bone develops its fluted or funnel shape. The **diaphysis** corresponds to the body or shaft of the bone and is the zone between the two metaphyses in a long tubular bone.

The metaphysis blends into the diaphysis and is the area where coarse cancellous bone dissipates. This area of bone is particularly important in hematogenous infections, tumors and skeletal malformations.

Two additional terms are essential to an understanding of bone organization:

- **Endochondral ossification** is the process by which bone tissue replaces cartilage.
- **Intramembranous ossification** refers to the mechanism by which bone tissue supplants membranous or fibrous tissue laid down by the periosteum.

All bones are formed by at least some intramembranous ossification. Some bones (e.g., the calvaria of the skull) are forged purely by intramembranous ossification. Microscopically, it cannot be determined whether a bone resulted from replacement of cartilage or of fibrous tissue. Because bone tumors tend to recapitulate their embryologic origins, it is not surprising that cartilaginous tumors of the frontal bone have not been seen, because the calvaria of the skull do not originate from cartilage.

The Bone Marrow Resides in the Marrow Space, or Medullary Canal

The marrow space is enclosed by cortical bone. It is supported by a delicate connective tissue framework that enmeshes marrow cells and blood vessels. Three types of marrow are evident to the naked eye:

- **Red marrow** corresponds to hematopoietic tissue and is found in virtually all bones at birth. At adolescence, it is

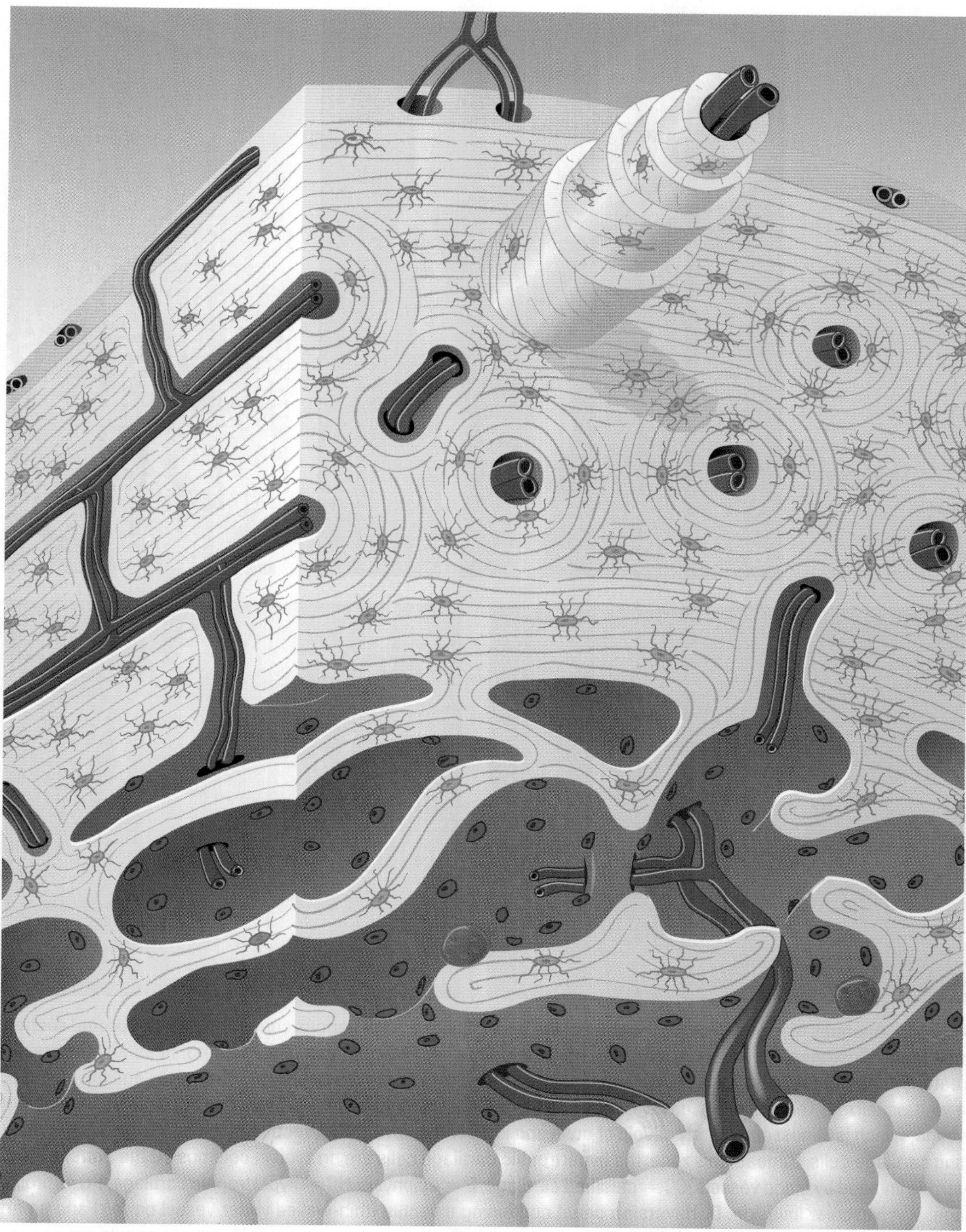

FIGURE 26-1. Anatomy of bone. A schematic representation of cortical and trabecular bone. The longitudinal section (*left*) shows the vasculature entering the periosteum via the periosteal perforating arteries and coursing through the bone perpendicular to the long axis in Volkmann canals. The vessels that proceed longitudinally, or parallel to the long axis, are located in haversian canals. Each artery is accompanied by a vein. Within the cortex, osteocytes reside in lacunae, and their cell processes extend into the canaliculi. The cross-sectional view (*right*) illustrates the various types of lamellar bone in the cortex. Circumferential lamellar bone is located adjacent to the periosteum and borders the marrow space. Concentric lamellar bone surrounds the central haversian canals to form an **osteon.** Each layer of the concentric lamellar bone displays a change in the pitch of the collagen fibers, such that each layer has a different arrangement of collagen. The interstitial lamellar bone occupies the space between osteons. The marrow space is filled with fat, and its trabecular bone is contiguous with the cortex. Multinucleated osteoclasts are present, and palisaded osteoblasts surround the bone surfaces. The perforating arteries from the periosteum and the nutrient artery from the marrow space communicate within the cortex via haversian and Volkmann canals.

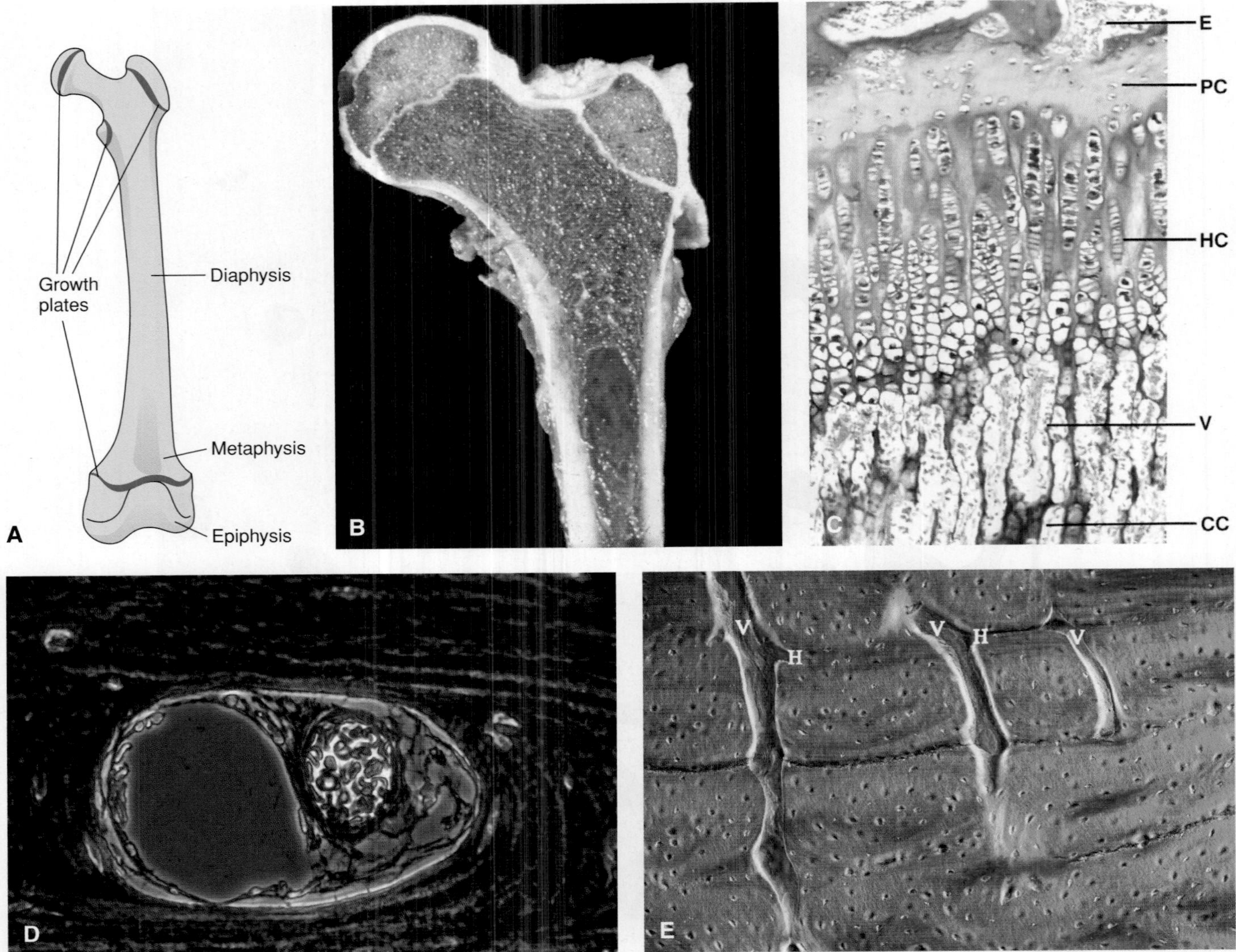

FIGURE 26-2. Anatomy of a long bone. A. Diagram of the femur illustrates the various compartments. **B. Coronal section of the proximal femur** illustrates the various anatomic parts of a long bone. The epiphysis of the femoral head and the apophysis of the greater trochanter are separated from the metaphysis by their respective growth plates. The cortex and the medullary cavity are well visualized. The medullary cavity contains cancellous bone until the metaphysis narrows into the diaphysis (shaft) of the bone, which is almost completely devoid of bone and filled with marrow. **C. A section of the epiphysis** with a zone of proliferating cartilage cells. Beneath this zone, the hypertrophic cartilage cells are arrayed in columns. At the *bottom,* the calcifying matrix is invaded by blood vessels. CC = calcified cartilage; E = epiphysis; HC = hypertrophic cartilage; PC = proliferative cartilage; V = vascular invasion. **D. Haversian canal** containing a venule (thin-walled wider vessel on *left*) and an arteriole (thicker-walled narrow vessel on the *right*). **E. Volkmann canals.** In this photograph, three Volkmann canals are seen running parallel to each other (*V*) and perpendicular to the cortex. The openings of two Haversian canals (*H*) are visible.

confined to the axial skeleton, which includes skull, vertebrae, sternum, ribs, scapulae, clavicles, pelvis and proximal humerus and femur. Its presence may also be pathologic, depending on the patient's age and the site of the marrow. For example, red marrow in the femoral diaphysis of a 55-year-old man is abnormal and may reflect underlying disease, such as leukemia.

- **Yellow marrow** is fat tissue and is found in the limb bones. In a normally hematopoietic area, such as a vertebral body, yellow marrow is abnormal at any age.
- **Gray or white marrow** is deficient in hematopoietic elements and is often fibrotic. ***It is always a pathologic tissue in a nongrowing adult bone or in areas distant from the growth plate in a child.***

Blood Supply Enters Bone Through Specialized Canals

The long tubular bones are provided with blood from two sources and contain canals to supply the tissues.

- **Nutrient arteries** enter bone through a nutrient foramen and supply the marrow space and the internal one third to one half of the cortex.

- **Perforating arteries** are small straight vessels that extend inward from periosteal arteries on the external surface of the periosteum (the fibrous capsule of the bone). Perforating arteries anastomose in the cortex with branches from nutrient arteries coming from the marrow space.
- **Haversian canals** are spaces in cortical bone that course parallel to the long axis of the bone for a short distance and then branch and communicate with other similar canals. Each canal contains one or two blood vessels, lymphatics and some nerve fibers.
- **Volkmann canals** are spaces within the cortex that run perpendicular to the long axis of the cortex to connect adjacent haversian canals. Volkmann canals also contain blood vessels.

Each artery has its paired vein and, perhaps, free nerve endings. Venous drainage proceeds from the cortex outward to the periosteal veins, or inward into the marrow space and out the nutrient veins.

Periosteum Covers All Bones and Can Form Bone

The internal layer of the periosteum, the **cambium layer**, is applied to the surface of the bone and consists of loosely arranged collagenous bundles, with spindle-shaped connective tissue cells and a network of thin elastic fibers. The outer **fibrous layer** is contiguous with soft tissue planes and fascia. It is composed of dense connective tissue containing blood vessels.

Bone Matrix Is Organic and Heavily Mineralized

Bone tissue is composed of cells (10% by weight), a mineralized phase (hydroxyapatite crystals, representing 60% of the total tissue) and an organic matrix (30%). ***Thus, except for its cells, bone is a biphasic structure composed of an organic and an inorganic matrix.***

The **mineralized matrix** consists of poorly crystalline hydroxyapatite, $Ca_{10}(PO_4)_6(OH)_2$. Because of its net negative charge, it can neutralize substantial amounts of acid. Other important ions in bone are carbonate, citrate, fluoride, chloride, sodium, magnesium, potassium and strontium.

The **organic matrix** consists of 88% type I collagen, 10% other proteins and 1% to 2% lipids and glycosaminoglycans. ***Thus, type I collagen basically defines the organic matrix.*** Other proteins include:

- **Osteocalcin** is produced by osteoblasts. Blood levels of this protein are a useful marker of bone formation.
- **Osteopontin** and **sialoprotein** are bone matrix proteins containing the amino acid sequence *Arg-Gly-Asp*, which is recognized by **integrins**. Thus, osteopontin and bone sialoprotein probably help anchor cells to the bone matrix.

The Cells of the Bone Are Responsible for Maintaining Its Structure

There are four types of cells in bone tissue, each of which has specific functions related to the formation, resorption and remodeling of bone:

OSTEOPROGENITOR CELL: The osteoprogenitor cell, which differentiates ultimately into osteoblasts and osteocytes, is itself derived from a primitive stem cell. The stem cell can develop into adipocytes, myoblasts, fibroblasts or osteoblasts. Osteoprogenitor cells are found in marrow, periosteum and all supporting structures within the marrow cavity. They are not readily recognized by light microscopy as they are small, nonspecific, stellate or spindle-shaped cells. In response to an appropriate signal, the osteoprogenitor gives rise to an osteoblast.

OSTEOBLAST: Osteoblasts are the protein-synthesizing cells that produce and mineralize bone tissue. They are derived from mesenchymal progenitors that also give rise to chondrocytes, myocytes, adipocytes and fibroblasts. These large mononuclear and polygonal cells are arrayed in a line along the bone surface (Fig. 26-3A). Underlying the layer of osteoblasts is a thin, eosinophilic zone of organic bone matrix that has not yet been mineralized, termed **osteoid**. The time from the deposition of osteoid to its mineralization is known as the **mineralization lag time** (approximately 12 days). Its protein synthetic capacity is reflected in its abundant endoplasmic reticulum, prominent Golgi apparatus and mitochondria with calcium-containing granules. Cytoplasmic processes that extend into the osteoid contact cells embedded in the matrix called **osteocytes**. The syncytium of osteocytes and osteoblasts probably prevents bone calcium (99% of the body's calcium) from equilibrating with the general extracellular space. When an osteoblast is inactive, it flattens on the surface of bone tissue. It contains alkaline phosphatase, manufactures osteocalcin and has parathyroid hormone (PTH) receptors. Collagenase secreted by osteoblasts may also facilitate osteoclastic activity. Finally, a number of growth factors, including transforming growth factor-β (TGF-β), insulin-like growth factor-I (IGF-I), IGF-2, platelet-derived growth factor (PDGF), interleukin-1 (IL-1), fibroblast growth factor (FGF) and tumor necrosis factor-α (TNF-α), are produced by osteoblasts and are important in regulating bone growth and differentiation. Furthermore, the osteoblast possesses surface receptors for various hormones (e.g., PTH, vitamin D, estrogen, glucocorticoids, etc.) as well as for cytokines and growth factors. ***The osteoblast ultimately controls the activation, maturation and differentiation of the osteoclast.***

OSTEOCYTE: The osteocyte is an osteoblast that is completely embedded in bone matrix and is isolated in a lacuna (Fig. 26-3B). Osteocytes deposit small quantities of bone around lacunae, but with time they lose the capacity for protein synthesis. They have small hyperchromatic nuclei and numerous processes that extend through bony canals called **canaliculi** that communicate with those from other osteocytes and osteoblasts (Fig. 26-3C). ***The osteocytes may be the bone cells that recognize and respond to mechanical forces, and are also important regulators of bone remodeling.***

OSTEOCLAST: ***Osteoclasts are the exclusive bone-resorptive cells.*** They are of hematopoietic origin, being members of the monocyte/macrophage family. Three major factors are required for osteoclastogenesis: (1) TNF-related receptor RANK (receptor activator for nuclear factor-κB [NF-κB]), (2) RANK ligand (RANKL) and (3) macrophage colony-stimulating factor (M-CSF). RANK is expressed by osteoclast precursors. RANKL and M-CSF are produced by osteoblasts and stromal cells. Binding of RANKL to RANK activates NF-κB signaling, which leads to increased osteoclastogenesis. M-CSF is required for the survival of cells of macrophage/osteoclast lineage. **Osteoprotegerin**, another protein produced by osteoblasts and also a member of the TNF family, blocks the interaction between RANK and RANKL and consequently inhibits osteoclastogenesis.

Osteoclasts are multinucleated cells that contain many lysosomes and are rich in hydrolytic enzymes. They are found

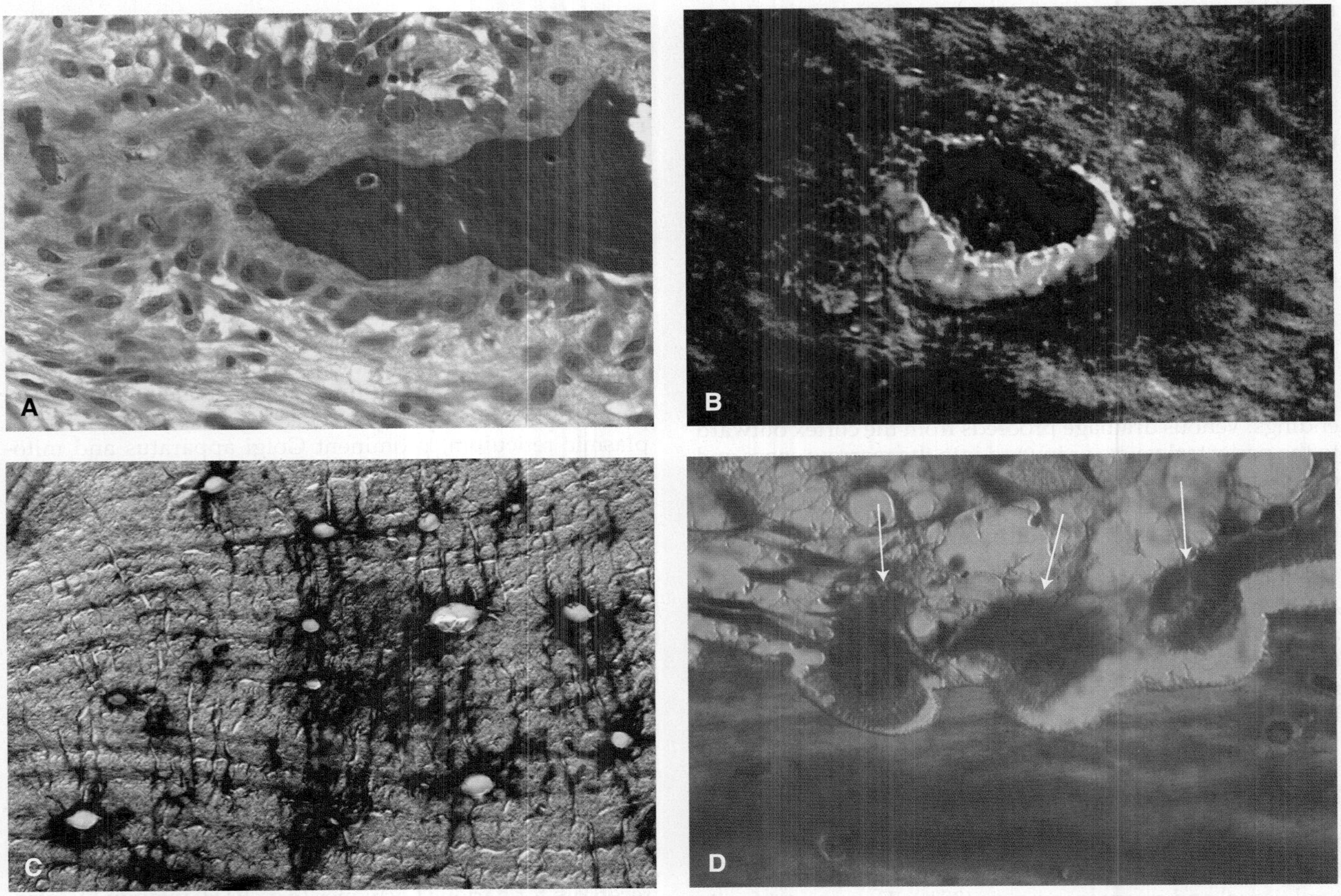

FIGURE 26-3. The cells of bones. A. A **developing bone spicule** demonstrates a prominent layer of plump osteoblasts lining the pink osteoid seam. The dark purple layer beneath the osteoid seam is mineralized bone. **B. Osteocytes.** Osteocytes represent trapped osteoblasts surrounded by bone matrix. The space surrounding the cell is called a **lacuna.** At this power, a few cytoplasmic extensions of the cell can be seen extending into narrow channels in the bone, called **canaliculi. C.** The extensive **intercommunication of osteocyte processes** via their canalicular network in cortical bone is visible in this section. **D. Osteoclasts.** These are multinucleated giant cells (*arrows*) found on bone surfaces within small scalloped reabsorption pits, called **Howship lacunae.**

in small depressions, termed **Howship lacunae,** on bone surfaces (Fig. 26-3D). By electron microscopy, they form a polarized ruffled plasmalemmal membrane (Fig. 26-4) when the cell is in contact with and is actively degrading bone. Osteoclastic resorption is a multistep process that involves attachment of the cell to bone by integrins. A tight gasket-like seal isolates an extracellular compartment that forms between bone and the osteoclast ruffled membrane. A proton pump then acidifies this compartment to a pH of 4.5, in effect creating a giant extracellular lysosome. This proton-rich environment mobilizes bone mineral, thereby exposing the organic bone matrix to degradation by lysosomal enzymes. Degraded fragments of bone are transported to the opposite side of the osteoclasts and then released to the extracellular space.

Although the machinery of an osteoclast is superbly suited for bone resorption, it functions only if the matrix is mineralized. ***In fact, any bone that is lined by osteoid or unmineralized cartilage is protected from osteoclastic activity.*** In rickets (see below), the growth plate does not calcify normally; it thus grows without osteoclastic resorption and becomes very thick.

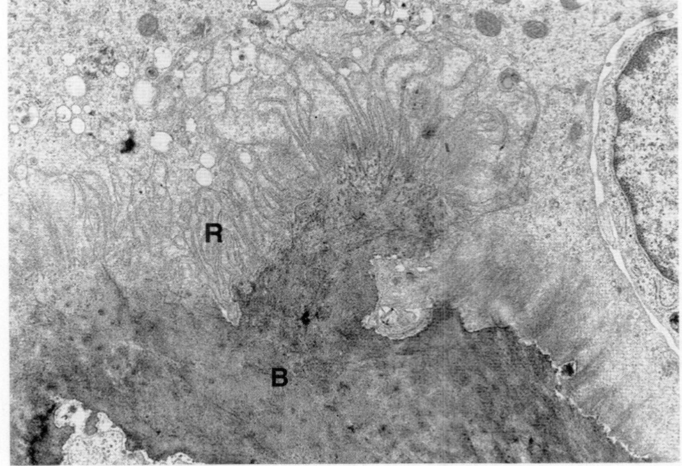

FIGURE 26-4. Osteoclast. An electron micrograph shows the ruffled membrane (*R*), which consists of a complex infolding of the plasma membrane juxtaposed to bone (*B*).

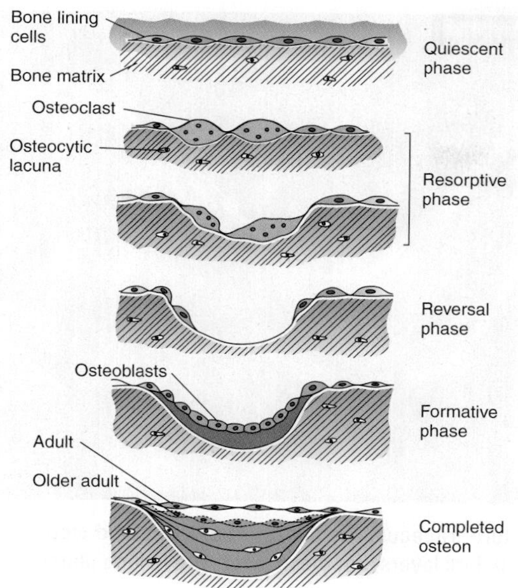

FIGURE 26-5. Bone-remodeling sequence. Bone remodeling is initiated by the appearance of osteoclasts on a bone surface previously lined by fusiform cells. After development of a resorption bay, osteoclasts are replaced by osteoblasts, which deposit new bone. The bone loss that attends aging (senile osteoporosis) is due to incomplete filling of resorption bays.

Constant bone remodeling is a normal part of skeletal maintenance (Fig. 26-5). It is initiated by activation of the cytokine receptor RANK on osteoclasts. Soluble factors released during resorption and PTH aid in recruitment of osteoblasts to the site and their activation to form new bone. Osteoclasts possess receptors for **calcitonin**, which inhibits osteoclast activity. ***Thus, bone remodeling involves replacing old bone with newly formed bone via the functional coupling of osteoclasts and osteoblasts, termed the* bone-remodeling unit.** Bone remodeling enables bone to adapt to mechanical stress, maintain its strength and regulate calcium homeostasis.

There Are Two Types of Bone Tissue: Lamellar Bone and Woven Bone

Both may be mineralized or unmineralized. Unmineralized bone is called **osteoid**.

Lamellar Bone

Lamellar bone is made slowly and is highly organized. As the stronger bone tissue, it forms the adult skeleton. ***Anything other than lamellar bone in the adult skeleton is abnormal.*** Lamellar bone is defined by (1) a parallel arrangement of type I collagen fibers, (2) few osteocytes in the matrix and (3) uniform osteocytes in lacunae parallel to the long axis of the collagen fibers. There are four types of lamellar bone (Fig. 26-6):

- **Circumferential bone** forms the outer periosteal and inner endosteal lamellar envelopes of the cortex.
- **Concentric lamellar bone** is arranged around the haversian canals. In two dimensions, concentric lamellar bone and its haversian artery and vein constitute the **osteon** (Fig. 26-1). In three dimensions, osteons comprise the **haversian system**. These cylinders of bone around haversian canals run parallel to the long axis of the cortex and are the strongest bone made. The osteons form only if there is appropriate stress. Thus, a paralyzed limb has a cortex composed exclusively of poorly formed haversian systems and circumferential lamellar bone.
- **Interstitial lamellar bone** represents remnants of either circumferential or concentric lamellar bone that have been remodeled and are wedged between the osteons.
- **Trabecular lamellar bone** forms the coarse cancellous bone of the medullary cavity. It exhibits plates of lamellar bone perforated by marrow spaces.

Woven Bone

Woven bone is identified by (1) an irregular arrangement of type I collagen fibers, hence the term *woven*; (2) numerous osteocytes in the matrix; and (3) variation in osteocyte size and shape (Fig. 26-7A,B).

26 | Bones and Joints

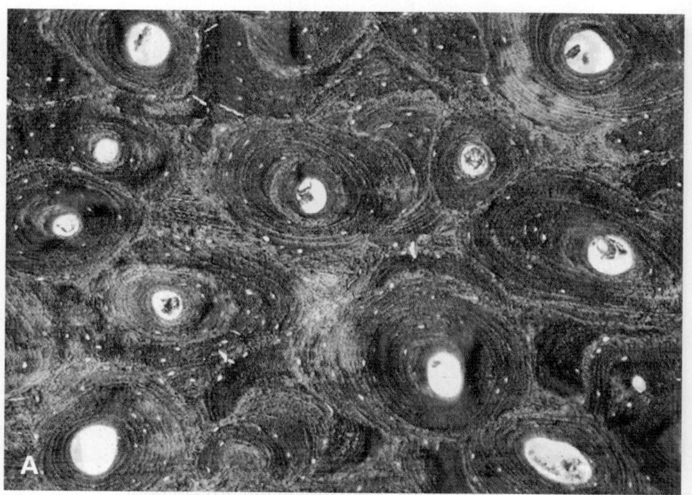

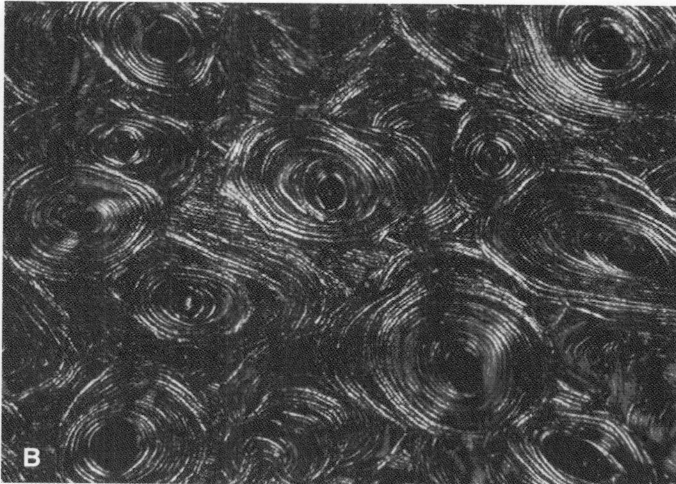

FIGURE 26-6. Cortical lamellar bone. A. Lamellae of the compacta (cortex) are arranged concentrically about haversian canals. **B.** The same field in polarized light shows the alternating light and dark layered arrangement of the collagen fibers (*continued*).

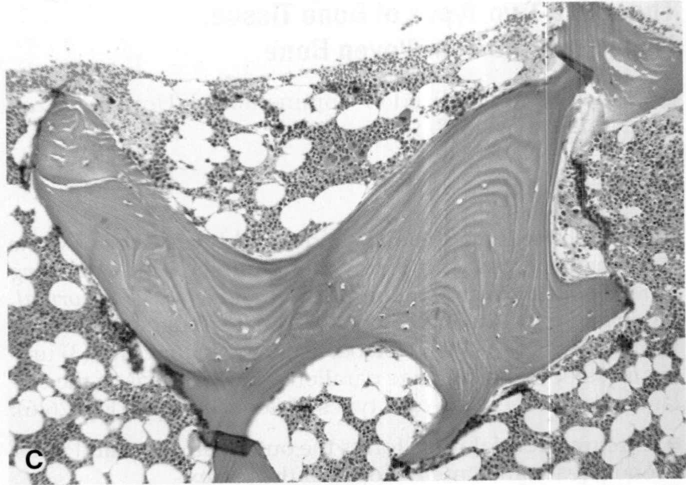

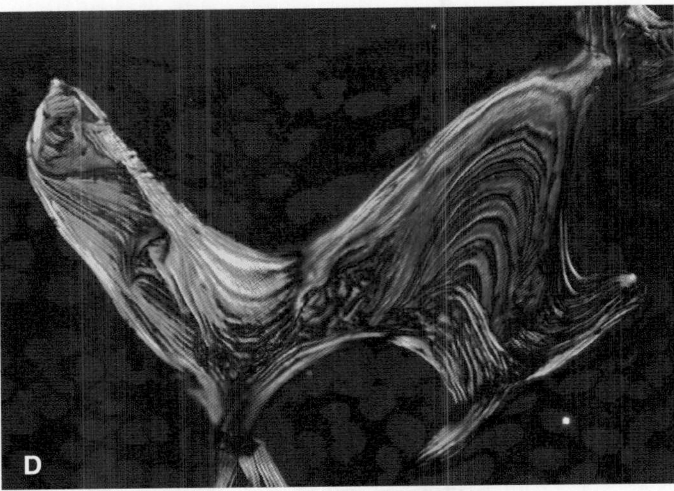

FIGURE 26-6. (*Continued*) **C. Lamellae of the spongiosa** in a single mature trabecula are shown in a bright field view. **D.** Polarized light demonstrates that the lamellae are arranged in light and dark layers, but these layers are in long plates rather than in a concentric arrangement.

Woven bone is deposited more rapidly than lamellar bone. It is haphazardly arranged and of low tensile strength, serving as a temporary scaffolding for support. It is not surprising that woven bone is found in the developing fetus, in areas surrounding tumors and infections and as part of a healing fracture. ***Its presence in the adult skeleton is always abnormal, and indicates that reactive tissue has been produced in response to some stress in the bone.***

Cartilage, Unlike Bone, Contains No Blood Vessels, Nerves or Lymphatics

Cartilage may be focally calcified to provide some internal strength in the appropriate areas.

Cartilage Matrix

Like bone, cartilage may be viewed as an organic and inorganic biphasic material. The inorganic phase is composed of calcium hydroxyapatite crystals, equivalent to those found in bone matrix. However, the organic matrix is quite different from that of bone. Essentially, cartilage is a hyperhydrated structure, with water forming some 80% of its weight. The remaining 20% is composed principally of two types of macromolecules, type II collagen and proteoglycans. The water content is extremely important in the function of articular cartilage as it enhances the resilience and lubrication of the joint. Proteoglycans are complex macromolecules composed of a central linear protein core, to which long side arms of polysaccharides called **glycosaminoglycans** are attached.

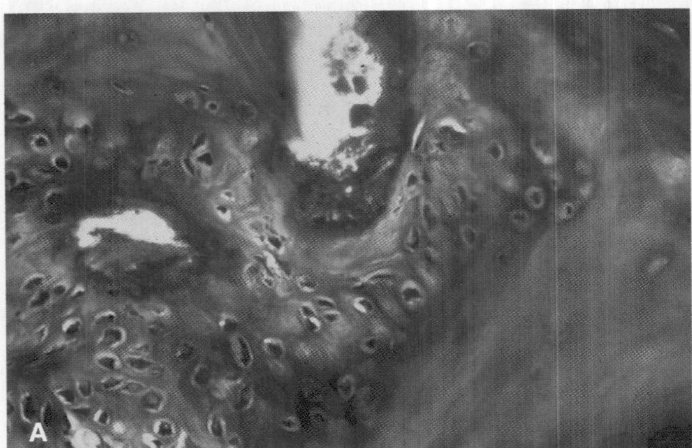

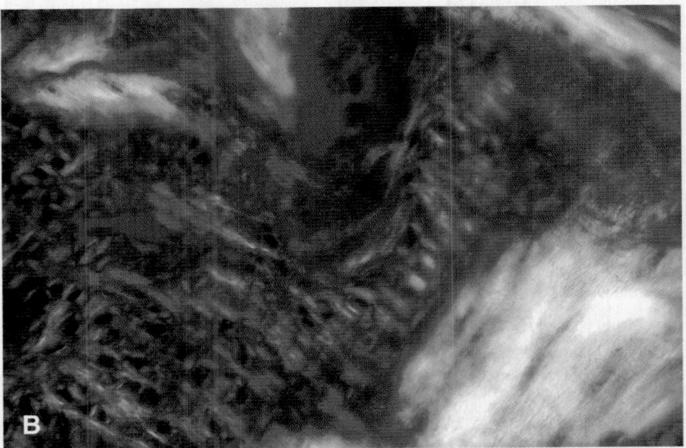

FIGURE 26-7. Woven bone. A. In this section, the woven bone constitutes early fracture repair. Note that in the area of new bone there are many osteocytes that vary in size but are mainly large with prominent lacunae (compare with area of mature bone at *lower right*). **B.** This is the same section viewed in polarized light. Note that the collagen fibers are disposed in a pattern resembling the loose fiber pattern of coarsely woven burlap.

These molecules are polyanionic because of the regular presence of carboxyl groups and sulfates along the molecules. Cartilage glycosaminoglycans comprise three long-chain, unbranched, repeating, polydimeric saccharides: chondroitin-4-sulfate, chondroitin-6-sulfate and keratan sulfate. The chondroitin sulfates are the most abundant, accounting for 55% to 90% of the cartilage matrix, depending on the age of the tissue.

Types of Cartilage

There are three types of cartilage:

- **Hyaline cartilage:** This is the prototypic cartilage, constituting the articular cartilage of joints; cartilaginous anlage of developing bones; growth plates; costochondral cartilages; cartilages of the trachea, bronchi and larynx; and nasal cartilages. Hyaline cartilage is the most common cartilage in tumors, in fracture callus and in areas of relative avascularity.
- **Fibrocartilage:** This tissue is essentially hyaline cartilage that contains numerous type I collagen fibers for tensile and structural strength. It is found in the annulus fibrosus of the intervertebral disk, tendinous and ligamentous insertions, menisci, the symphysis pubis and insertions of joint capsules. Fibrocartilage may also occur in a fracture callus.
- **Elastic cartilage** is found in the epiglottis, in the arytenoid cartilages of the larynx and in the external ear.

Chondrocytes

Chondrocytes are derived from primitive mesenchymal cells that are similar to the precursors of bone cells. The chondroblast gives rise to the chondrocyte. Activation of SOX9 transcription factor is essential for chondrocyte formation and SOX9 is expressed in cartilaginous neoplasms. As in bone, the cell that destroys calcified cartilage is the osteoclast.

Bone Formation and Growth

Bone tissue grows only by appositional growth, defined as deposition of new matrix on a preexisting surface by adjacent surface osteoblasts. By contrast, virtually all other tissues, especially cartilage, increase by interstitial cell proliferation within the matrix as well as by appositional growth.

Bone development in the fetus follows a stereotyped sequence. Most of the skeleton (except the calvaria and clavicles) develops from cartilage anlagen present during fetal development. This cartilage is eventually resorbed and replaced by bone, a process termed **endochondral ossification.** Development of bone can be illustrated by using a limb as an example.

The Process of Primary Ossification Follows a Defined Temporal Sequence

1. **Cartilage anlage:** By 5 weeks of gestation, a thin layer of mesenchymal cells forms between the ectoderm and endoderm of the limb bud and condenses into a core of hyaline cartilage. This cartilaginous anlage is the precursor of the future long bone of that limb. The fibrous capsule of the cartilage anlage is called a **perichondrium.** The width of the cartilaginous anlage is increased by appositional growth of chondroblasts, which deposit cartilage matrix on the internal surface of the perichondrium. At the same time, the anlage increases in length by both appositional and interstitial growth of the chondrocytes. At this stage, the long "bone" is actually composed of cartilage.
2. **The primary center of ossification:** The vascular bed increases, and the perichondrium deposits woven bone on the surface of the cartilage core. This circumferential sleeve of woven bone is the primary center of ossification, because it is the first bone tissue to be formed. The perichondrium is thereafter termed **periosteum** (Fig. 26-8A).
3. **Cylinderization:** Within the cartilaginous anlage, chondrocytes form proliferating columns, which eventually

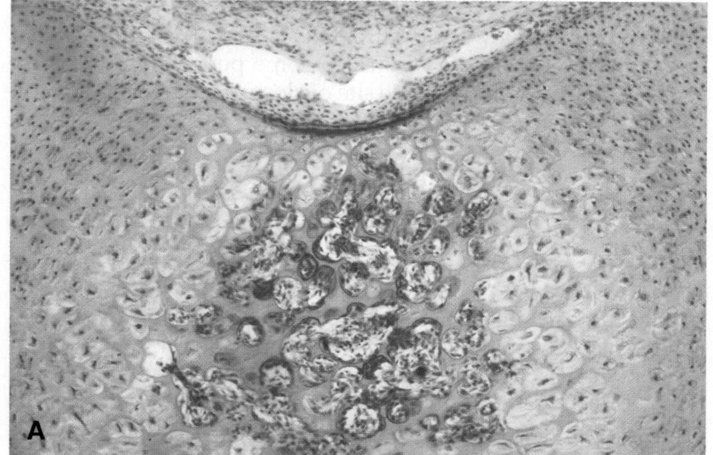

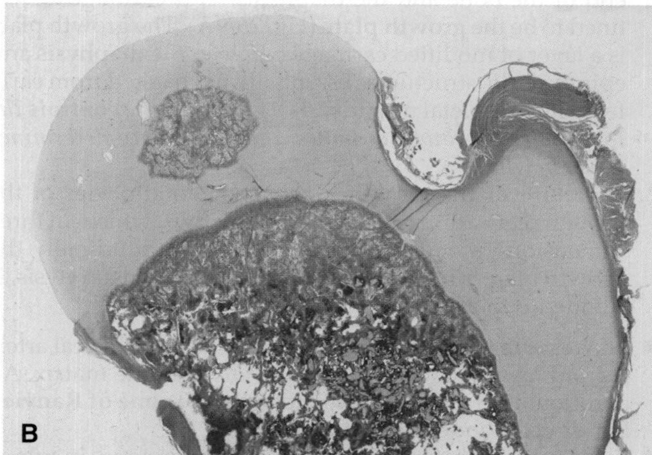

FIGURE 26-8. Primary ossification. A. This section of a short tubular bone demonstrates the first true bone tissue deposited on the outside of the midshaft of the cartilage model along with very early hollowing of the center of the cartilage model to form mixed spicules of cartilage and bone (primary spongiosa). **B.** The **secondary ossification center** is demonstrated in this femoral head.

undergo focal calcification. Calcification is the signal for osteoclastic resorption and invasion of vessels into the cartilaginous mass. Thus, the earliest endochondral ossification occurs after the cartilage is hollowed out from the center of the anlage. This "cavitation" of the cartilaginous core forms the future marrow space. The progressive hollowing of the diaphysis is termed **cylinderization.**

4. **Primary spongiosum:** The swollen, hypertrophied chondrocytes within the central cartilage begin to die. Capillary invasion increases. The surfaces of the calcified cartilage cores become enveloped by woven bone laid down by osteoblasts, which arrive through the pluripotential mesenchymal tissue that enters with the capillaries. This cartilaginous core, surrounded by woven bone, is called **primary spongiosum,** or **primary trabecula.** It is the first bone formed after the replacement of cartilage.

Cavitation continues along the future diaphysis toward each end of the bone. Meanwhile, the bone enlarges in width by appositional bone growth from the ever-increasing periosteal sleeve, which makes additional woven bone for the future cortex.

In Secondary Ossification, Cartilage Is Stimulated and Transformed Into Bone

Programmed events similar to those in the primary spongiosum take place in the cartilaginous ends of the future bone. Resting (reserve) cartilage is stimulated to become columns of proliferating cartilage, which then progress to hypertrophied chondrocytes and, eventually, calcified cartilage.

1. **The secondary center of ossification** (Fig. 26-8B): Also termed the **epiphyseal center of ossification,** this structure is formed at the ends of the bone when cartilage is resorbed. The centrifugal enlargement of the secondary ossification is called **hemispherization** and occurs simultaneously with the longitudinal development of the marrow cavity of the diaphysis.
2. **Formation of the growth plate:** As the bony ends expand during hemispherization and cylinderization occurs in the future diaphysis, a zone of cartilage is trapped between the end of the bone and the diaphysis. This cartilage is destined to be the **growth plate** (Fig. 26-9A). The growth plate is a layer of modified cartilage between the diaphysis and epiphysis. Its structure is essentially unchanged from early fetal life to skeletal maturity. ***The growth plate controls the longitudinal growth of bones and ultimately determines adult height.***
3. **Structure of the growth plate:** The chondrocytes of the growth plate are arranged in vertical rows, which, in three dimensions, are really helices. Viewed longitudinally, the growth plate, proceeding from epiphysis to metaphysis, is divided into zones (Figs. 26-2B and 26-9).

- The **reserve (resting) zone** is supplied by epiphyseal arteries and has small chondrocytes and very little matrix. An additional peripheral zone, known as the **zone of Ranvier,** lies directly under the perichondrium.
- The **proliferative zone** is the next deeper zone, in which active proliferation of chondrocytes occurs both longitudinally and transversely, although the main growth thrust is longitudinal. In a very active growth plate, proliferative zones comprise over half the thickness of the growth plate.
- The **hypertrophic zone** is next, and demonstrates a substantial increase in chondrocyte size. The intercellular matrix is prominent, and a dense zone, the **territorial matrix,** surrounds chondrocytes.
- The **zone of calcification** is the cartilaginous zone closest to the metaphysis, where the matrix becomes mineralized.
- The **zone of ossification** is the area where a coating of bone is laid down on the surface of the calcified cartilage. Capillaries grow into the calcified cartilage and give access to osteoclasts, which resorb much of the calcified matrix. Residual vertical walls of calcified cartilage act as scaffolding for the deposition of bone.

The molecular mechanisms governing endochondral growth are beginning to be understood. Parathyroid hormone–related protein (PTHrP) is secreted from perichondrial cells and chondrocytes and maintains chondrocyte proliferation. PTHrP deficiency leads to severe growth retardation and distorted growth plates. The developmental regulator Indian hedgehog (Ihh) is also involved in growth plate maturation by acting in conjunction with PTHrP. A third major factor involved in growth plate regulation is fibroblast growth factor (FGF). FGF receptor-3 (FGFR3) is expressed on proliferating chondrocytes, and its activation leads to inhibition of growth plate proliferation. Mutations of FGFR3 lead to growth arrest (e.g., achondroplasia or other forms of dwarfism) or growth acceleration.

Formation of the Metaphysis Is Called Funnelization

It occurs at the ring of Delacroix, a periosteal cuff of bone surrounding the epiphyseal cartilage. A wave of periosteal osteoclasts resorbs the cortex, so that a fluted or funnel shape begins to appear. At the same time, endosteal osteoblastic bone is deposited to keep pace with, and offset, some of the osteoclastic resorption. The net result is the funnel or fluted shape of the bone.

The Growth Plate Is Normally Obliterated at a Specific Age for Each Bone

Closure of the growth plate (Fig. 26-9B) is induced by sex hormones and occurs earlier in girls than in boys. Renewal of chondrocytes slows and ultimately ceases. The entire plate is eventually replaced by bone. In some persons, a transverse bony plate representing the site of closure can be seen on radiography.

Disorders of the Growth Plate

Cretinism Leads to Defective Cartilage Maturation

Cretinism results from **maternal iodine deficiency** (see Chapter 21) and has profound effects on the skeleton. Thyroid hormone plays a role in regulating chondrocytes, osteoblasts and osteoclasts through production of cytokines and other factors involved in bone development and growth. Linear growth is severely impaired, resulting in dwarfism, with limbs disproportionately short in relation to the trunk. Delayed closure of the fontanelles of the skull causes an unusually large head. There is a delay in closure of the epiphyses, as well as radiologic stippling of these zones. Shedding of deciduous teeth and eruption of permanent teeth are retarded.

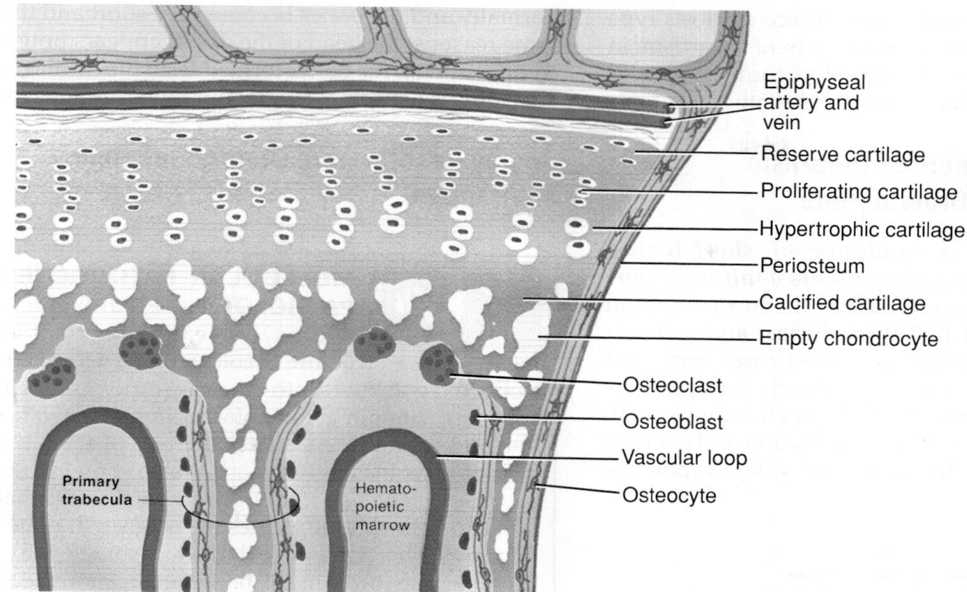

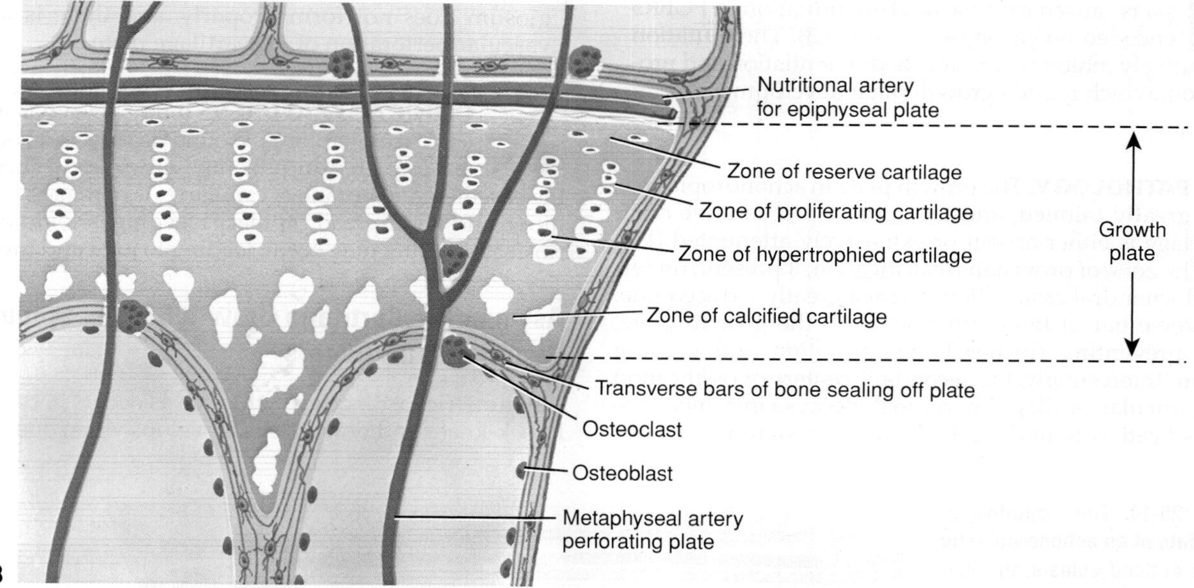

FIGURE 26-9. Anatomy of the epiphyseal growth plate. A. Normal growing epiphyseal plate. The epiphysis is separated from the epiphyseal plate by transverse plates of bone that seal the plate so that it grows only toward the metaphysis. The various zones of cartilage are illustrated. As the calcified cartilage migrates toward the metaphysis, the chondrocytes die, and the lacunae are empty. At the interface of the epiphyseal plate and the metaphysis, osteoclasts bore into the calcified cartilage, accompanied by a capillary loop from the metaphyseal vessels. Osteoblasts follow the osteoclasts and lay down osteoid on the cartilage core, thereby forming the primary spongiosum or primary trabeculae. **B. Normal closure.** The epiphyseal cartilage has ceased to grow, and metaphyseal vessels penetrate the cartilage plate. Transverse bars of bone separate the plate from the metaphysis.

PATHOLOGY: In cretinism, chondrocytes do not follow the orderly endochondral sequence. Instead, maturation of the hypertrophied zone is retarded, and the zone of proliferative cartilage is narrow. Endochondral ossification, therefore, does not proceed appropriately, and transverse bars of bone in the metaphysis seal off the growth plate. Although growth plates may remain open, the failure of endochondral ossification produces severe dwarfism. The misshapen epiphyses seen on radiography reflect incomplete penetration of the secondary centers of ossification of the epiphysis.

Morquio Syndrome Features Mucopolysaccharide Deposition in Chondrocytes

Many of the mucopolysaccharidoses (see Chapter 6) involve skeletal deformities, attributable to deposition of mucopolysaccharides (glycosaminoglycans) in developing bones. An

26 | Bones and Joints

example is Morquio syndrome (mucopolysaccharidosis type IV), which leads to a particularly severe form of dwarfism, in addition to dental defects, mental retardation, corneal opacities and increased urinary excretion of keratan sulfate.

Achondroplasia Is an Inherited Dwarfism Caused by Arrest of the Growth Plate

Achondroplasia refers to a syndrome of short-limbed dwarfism and macrocephaly and represents a failure of normal epiphyseal cartilage formation. It is the most common genetic form of dwarfism (1:15,000 live births) and is inherited as an autosomal dominant trait. Most cases represent new mutations. The mean adult height in achondroplasia is 131 cm (51 inches) in men and 125 cm (49 inches) in women. Achondroplastic dwarfs have normal mentation and average life spans. However, some patients develop severe kyphoscoliosis and its complications.

MOLECULAR PATHOGENESIS: Achondroplasia is caused by an **activating** mutation in FGFR3 encoded on chromosome 4(p16.3). The mutation constitutively inhibits chondrocyte differentiation and proliferation, which retards growth plate development.

PATHOLOGY: The growth plate in achondroplasia is greatly thinned, and the zone of proliferative cartilage is either absent or extensively attenuated (Fig. 26-10). The zone of provisional calcification, if present, undergoes endochondral ossification, but at a greatly reduced rate. A transverse bar of bone often seals off the growth plate, thereby preventing further bone formation and causing dwarfism. Interestingly, the secondary centers of ossification and the articular cartilage are normal. Because intramembranous ossification is undisturbed, the periosteum functions normally and the bones become very short and thick. For the same reasons, the head of the dwarf appears unusually large, compared with the bones formed from the cartilage of the face. The spine is of normal length, but limbs are abnormally short.

Scurvy Results From Dietary Deficiency of Vitamin C

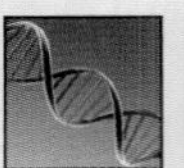
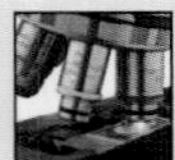

MOLECULAR PATHOGENESIS AND PATHOLOGY: Hydroxyproline and hydroxylysine are important in stabilizing the helical structure of collagen and in cross-linking the tropocollagen fibers into the proper molecular structure of collagen. Vitamin C is a cofactor in hydroxylation of proline and lysine. The skeletal changes of scurvy reflect the lack of osteoblastic function. Woven bone is not formed because osteoblasts cannot produce and normally cross-link collagen. Chondrocytes at the growth plate continue to grow. The zone of calcified cartilage may actually become more prominent, because it is more heavily calcified. Osteoclasts resorb this zone, but the primary spongiosum does not form properly, and there is irregular vascular perforation of the cartilage plate.

CLINICAL FEATURES: Today, scurvy is a rare disease (see Chapter 8). Wound healing and bone growth are impaired in patients with scurvy. Furthermore, the basement membrane of capillaries is damaged by this condition and widespread capillary bleeding is common. Subperiosteal bleeding may occur, leading to joint and muscle pain.

Asymmetric Cartilage Growth Causes Spinal Disorders and Tumors

Asymmetric cartilage growth, such as occurs in patients with knock-knees and bowed legs, develops when one part of the

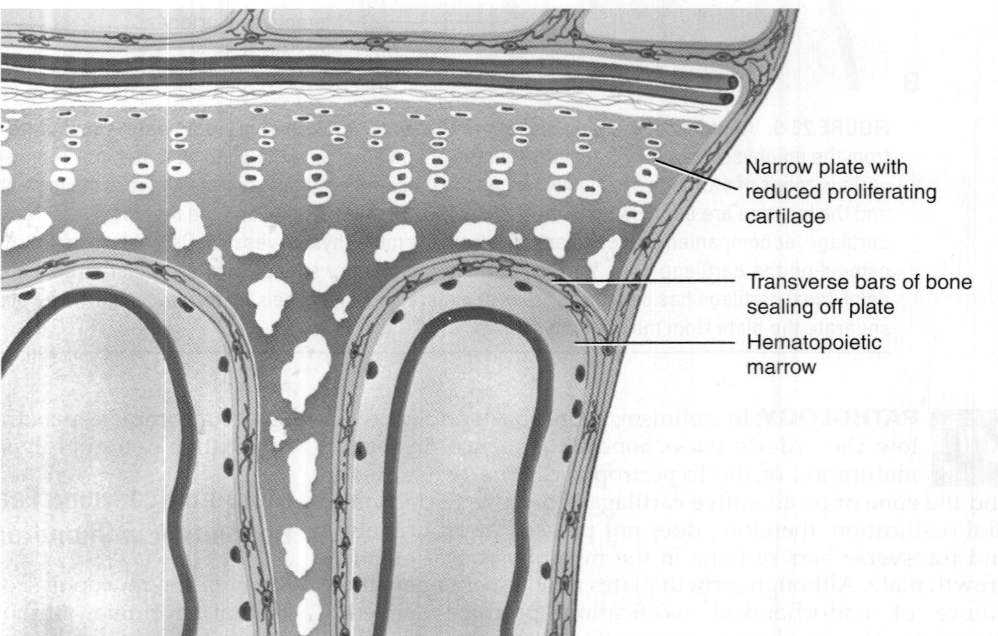

FIGURE 26-10. The epiphyseal growth plate of an achondroplastic dwarf. In achondroplasia, the epiphyseal plate is reduced in thickness, and the zones of proliferating cartilage are attenuated. Osteoclastic activity is inconspicuous, and the interface between the plate and the metaphysis is often sealed by transverse bars of bone that prevent further endochondral ossification. As a result, the bones are shortened.

growth plate, either medial or lateral, grows faster than the other. Most cases are hereditary, but mechanical forces, such as trauma near the growth plate, may stimulate one side to grow faster or in an asymmetric fashion. Aside from the cosmetic appearance, these conditions may require correction to prevent future incongruity, eventual loss of articular cartilage and joint destruction.

Scoliosis and Kyphosis

Scoliosis ***is an abnormal lateral curvature of the spine, usually affecting adolescent girls.*** **Kyphosis** ***refers to an abnormal anteroposterior curvature.*** When both conditions are present, the term **kyphoscoliosis** is used.

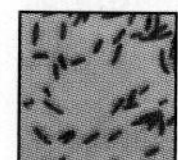

ETIOLOGIC FACTORS: A vertebral body grows in length (height) from the endplates of the vertebrae, which correspond to the growth plates of long tubular bones. As in tubular bones, vertebral bodies increase in width by appositional bone growth from the periosteum. In scoliosis, for unknown reasons, one portion of the endplate grows faster than the other, producing lateral curvature of the spine.

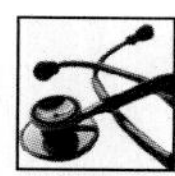

CLINICAL FEATURES: The treatment is appropriate stress on the vertebral body through use of braces or internal fixation to straighten the spine. If kyphoscoliosis is severe, the patient may eventually develop chronic pulmonary disease, cor pulmonale and joint problems, particularly involving the hip.

Osteochondroma

Osteochondroma is a developmental defect of the skeleton, which arises from a defect at the ring of Ranvier of the growth plate. Solitary osteochondroma is the most common form of the lesion. The tumor may have to be removed if it is cosmetically displeasing or presses upon an artery or nerve. A number of cases where the tumor increased in size have been related to pregnancy and lactation.

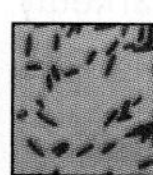

ETIOLOGIC FACTORS: The ring of Ranvier guides the growth of the growth plate cartilage toward the metaphysis. If the ring of Ranvier is absent or defective, the growth plate cartilage grows laterally into the soft tissue. Vessels originating in the marrow cavity of the bone extend into this cartilage mass. Continuation of this process results in a cartilage-capped, bony, stalked osteochondroma (Fig. 26-11), which is in direct continuity with the marrow cavity of the parent bone.

MOLECULAR PATHOGENESIS: Cytogenetic aberrations have been characterized in sporadic and hereditary osteochondromas, including chromosomes 8q24, 11p11–p13 and 19p, where the tumor suppressor genes *EXT1*, *EXT2* and *EXT3* are located, respectively. The *EXT* genes may be involved in chondrocyte proliferation and differentiation by affecting the Indian hedgehog–PTH-related protein (Ihh–PTHrp) pathway, which is vital for the proper development of endochondral bones. *EXT* mutations induce increased chondrocyte proliferation and disrupt the differentiation process, which may alter the direction of chondrocyte growth and lead to the development of osteochondromas.

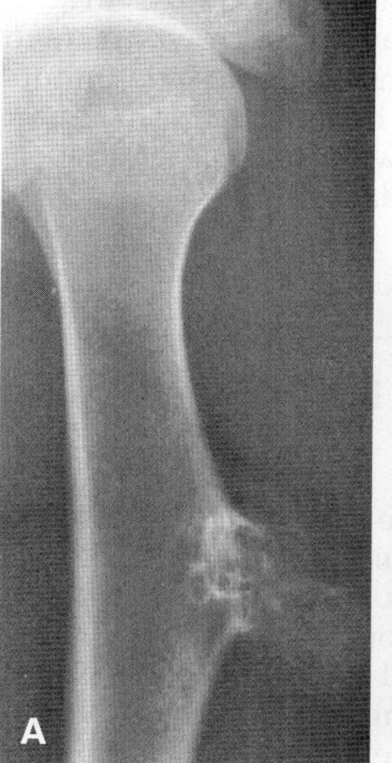

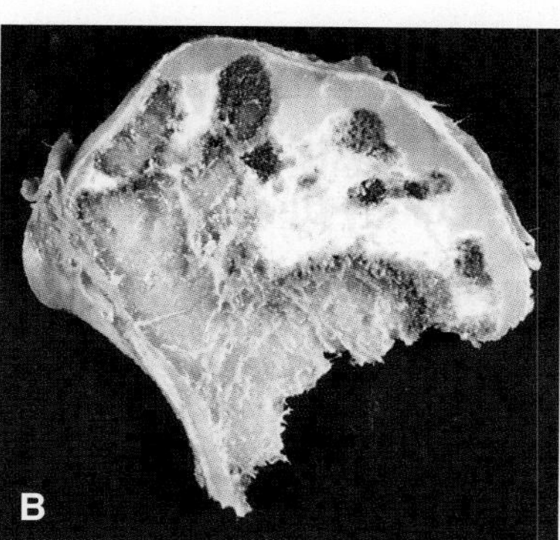

FIGURE 26-11. Osteochondroma. A. A radiograph of an osteochondroma of the humerus shows a lesion that is directly contiguous with the marrow space. **B.** The cross-section of an osteochondroma shows the cap of calcified cartilage overlying poorly organized cancellous bone.

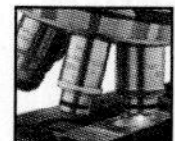

PATHOLOGY: Osteochondromas tend to grow away from the joint. In radiographs, the cartilaginous mass is in direct continuity with the parent bone and lacks an underlying cortex. Histologically, a cartilage-capped, bony mass is surrounded by a surface fibrous membrane, which is the perichondrium. Active endochondral ossification deep to the cartilage cap allows the bony protuberance to lengthen.

HEREDITARY MULTIPLE OSTEOCHONDROMATOSIS: This inherited autosomal dominant disorder is characterized by numerous osteochondromas. Hereditary multiple osteochondromatosis (HMO) is one of the most common inherited musculoskeletal disorders, and is caused by loss of *EXT1* or *EXT2* gene function. Although not as common as solitary osteochondroma, the heritable variety is not rare, with an incidence of about 1 in 50,000. It occurs predominantly in men, but because of its variable expression, a seemingly unaffected woman from an afflicted family may transmit the disorder.

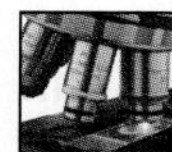

PATHOLOGY: Each individual lesion in multiple osteochondromatosis is identical to a solitary osteochondroma. In severe cases of hereditary osteochondromatosis, dwarfism may result because of lateral displacement of the longitudinal growth plate by the osteochondroma. Metacarpals may be shortened and fixed pronation or supination may develop if the lesions occur in the forearm and interfere with wrist function. Further difficulties may be caused by unequal leg length and disturbed joint function because of encroaching osteochondromas. Chondrosarcoma is a rare complication.

Hemihypertrophy

Hemihypertrophy describes several conditions in which one limb's growth plate is stimulated to undergo rapid and prolonged endochondral ossification. That limb becomes much longer than the contralateral one. Infection in the metaphyseal area may stimulate the growth plate to grow rapidly. An arteriovenous malformation may also cause one growth plate to grow faster than its counterpart, as may fractures and tumors near the growth plate. In some cases, hemihypertrophy is part of an inherited syndrome. Children with isolated hemihypertrophy are at increased risk for neoplasms.

Modeling Abnormalities

Osteopetrosis Is Characterized by Abnormally Dense Bone

Osteopetrosis, *also known as* **marble bone disease** *or* **Albers-Schönberg disease,** *is a heterogeneous group of rare inherited disorders in which skeletal mass is increased as a result of abnormally dense bone.* The most common autosomal recessive form is a severe, sometimes fatal disease affecting infants and children. Death of infants with this severe variant is attributable to marked anemia, cranial nerve entrapment, hydrocephalus and infection. A more benign form, transmitted as an autosomal dominant trait and seen in adulthood or adolescence, is associated with mild anemia or no symptoms at all.

MOLECULAR PATHOGENESIS: *The sclerotic skeleton of osteopetrosis is the result of failed osteoclastic bone resorption.* The disease is caused by mutations in genes that govern osteoclast formation or function. The most common mutations cause defects in bone acidification, which is necessary for osteoclastic bone resorption. These include mutations in the *TCIRG1* gene (osteoclast proton pump; autosomal dominant), the *CLCN7* gene (osteoclast chloride channel; autosomal recessive) and the **carbonic anhydrase II** gene (autosomal recessive). Other mutations that cause osteopetrosis involve transcription factors or cytokines necessary for the osteoclast differentiation.

PATHOLOGY: Because osteoclast function is arrested, osteopetrosis is characterized by (1) retention of the primary spongiosum with its cartilage cores, (2) lack of funnelization of the metaphysis and (3) a thickened cortex. The result is short, block-like, radiodense bones, hence the term **marble bone disease** (Fig. 26-12). These bones are extremely radiopaque and weigh two to three times more than normal bone. However, they are basically weak because their structure is intrinsically disorganized and cannot remodel along lines of stress. The mineralized cartilage is also weak and friable so that the bones in osteopetrosis fracture easily. Grossly, bones in osteopetrosis are widened in the metaphysis and diaphysis, causing the characteristic "Erlenmeyer flask" deformity. Histologically, the bone tissue is extremely irregular, and almost all areas contain a cartilage core. Depending on the mutation, osteoclasts may be absent, present in normal numbers or even abundant. In the case of osteopetrosis characterized by normal or increased numbers of osteoclasts, the molecular defect lies in a gene involved in the function of osteoclasts, rather than their formation.

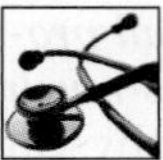

CLINICAL FEATURES: Suppression of hematopoiesis in osteopetrosis is due to replacement of the marrow by sheets of abnormal osteoclasts or extensive fibrosis. Marrow suppression in patients with the malignant form of osteopetrosis may be severe enough to lead to severe anemia or pancytopenia. To compensate for loss of marrow hematopoiesis, extramedullary hematopoiesis occurs in the liver, spleen and lymph nodes, and these structures are enlarged. Narrowing of neural foramina causes cranial nerve involvement, and subsequent strangulation of nerves leads to blindness and deafness. Osteopetrosis can be treated by bone marrow transplantation, which gives rise to a new clone of functional osteoclasts.

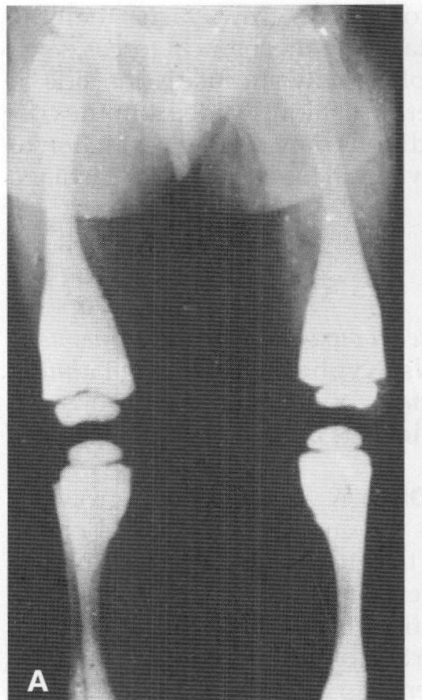

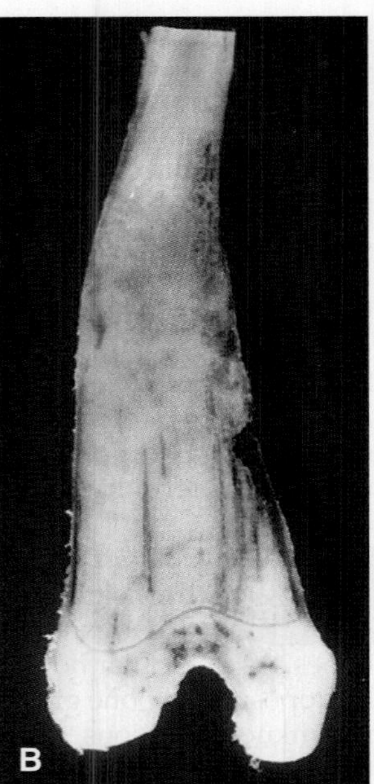

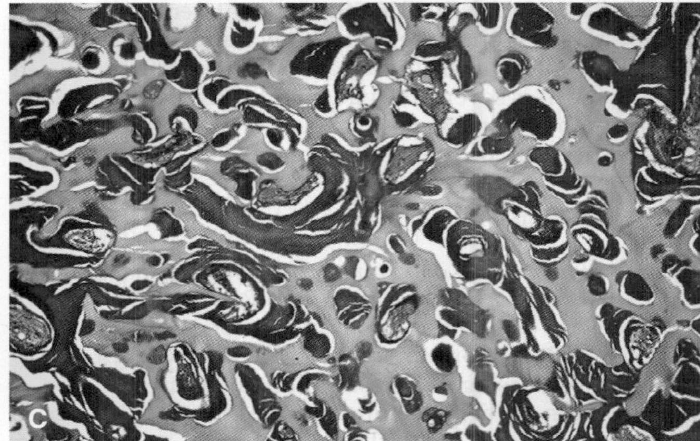

FIGURE 26-12. Osteopetrosis. A. A radiograph of a child shows markedly misshapen and dense bones of the lower extremities, characteristic of "marble bone disease." **B.** A gross specimen of the femur shows obliteration of the marrow space by dense bone. **C.** A photomicrograph of the bone of a child with autosomal recessive osteopetrosis demonstrates disorganization of bony trabeculae by retention of primary spongiosa (mixed spicules) and further obliteration of the marrow space by secondary spongiosa. The result is complete disorganization of the trabeculae and absence of marrow.

Progressive Diaphyseal Dysplasia Features Thickened Long Bones

Progressive diaphyseal dysplasia (Camurati-Engelmann disease) is an autosomal dominant disorder of children in which cylinderization does not proceed appropriately, resulting in symmetric thickening and increased diameter of the diaphyses of long bones. It is due to increased bone formation linked to a mutation in the propeptide of TGF-β. The disease particularly affects the femur, tibia, fibula, radius and ulna. Patients have pain over the affected areas, fatigue, muscle wasting, atrophy and gait abnormalities.

Delayed Maturation of Bone

Osteogenesis Imperfecta Is Characterized by Abnormal Type I Collagen

Osteogenesis imperfecta (OI) refers to a group of mainly autosomal dominant, heritable disorders of connective tissue, caused by mutations in the gene for type I collagen, affecting the skeleton, joints, ears, ligaments, teeth, sclerae and skin (see Chapter 6). There are four well-characterized types of OI, each different genetic structurally and clinically.

MOLECULAR PATHOGENESIS: The pathogenesis of OI involves mutations of *COL1A1* and *COL1A2* genes, which encode the α_1- and α_2-chains of type I procollagen, the major structural protein of bone. These genes are in chromosomes 17 (17q21.3–q22) and 7 (7q21.3–q22), respectively. A point mutation that affects a glycine residue in either *COL1A1* or *COL1A2* is the most typical abnormality found in OI. While *COL1A1* mutations are seen in all types of OI, mutations of *COL1A2* are found in types II, III and IV OI. Mutations of *COL1A1* affect three fourths of the type I collagen molecules, with half of the molecules containing one abnormal pro–α_1-chain and one quarter containing two abnormal pro–α_1-chains. By contrast, mutations in *COL1A2* affect only half of the synthesized collagen molecules. The resulting phenotype will range from mild to lethal depending on which gene is affected, the location in the collagen triple helix at which the substitution occurs and which amino acid is substituted for glycine.

Osteogenesis Imperfecta Type I

OI type I is the mildest phenotype. It is inherited as an autosomal dominant trait, characterized by multiple fractures after birth, blue sclera and hearing abnormalities. In some patients abnormalities of the teeth are also conspicuous (dentinogenesis imperfecta).

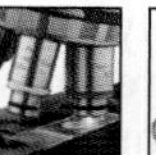
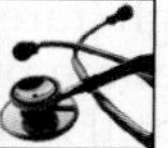

PATHOLOGY AND CLINICAL FEATURES: Initial fractures usually occur after the infant begins to sit and walk. There may be hundreds of fractures a year with minor movement or trauma. On radiologic examination, bones are extremely thin, delicate and abnormally curved (Fig. 26-13A). The collagen has reduced tensile strength and bone mineralization is abnormal. The combination of these abnormalities accounts for the brittleness of OI bone. In OI, insufficient bone is formed, leading to decreased cortical thickness and reduced trabecular bone. When a fracture occurs, the fracture callus may be extensive enough to resemble a tumor (Fig. 26-13B). As the child grows, fractures tend to decrease in severity and frequency, and stature is generally unaffected.

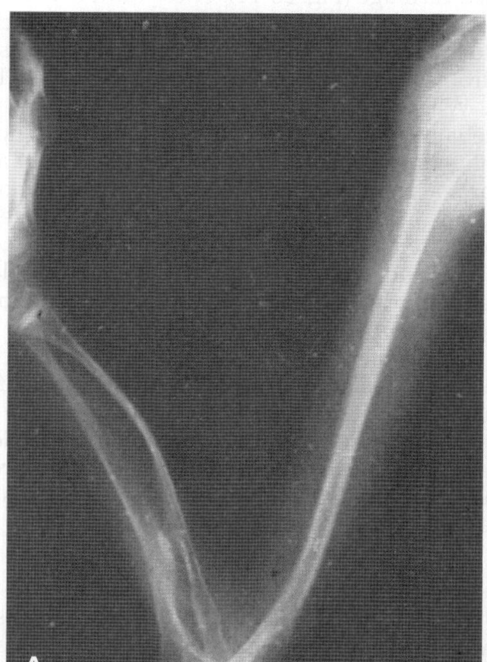

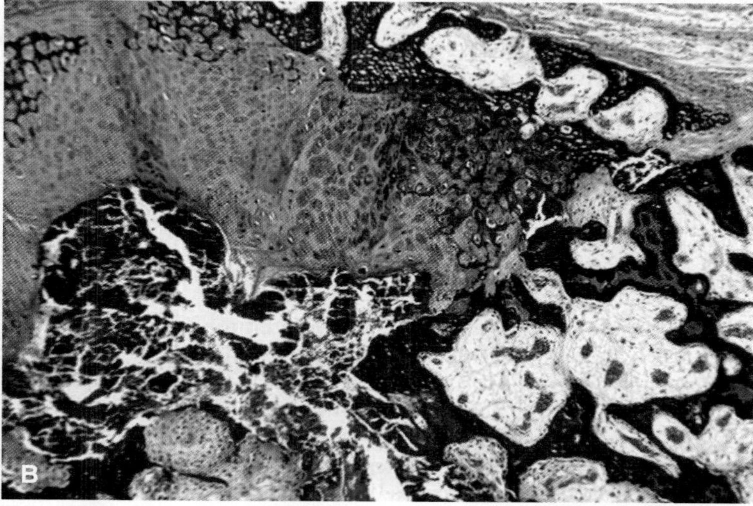

FIGURE 26-13. Osteogenesis imperfecta. A. A radiograph illustrates the markedly thin and attenuated humerus and bones of the forearm. There is a fracture callus in the proximal ulna. **B.** A photomicrograph of the fracture callus with prominent cartilage (*upper left*). The cortex is thin and composed of hypercellular woven bone.

The sclerae are very thin, with a blue color attributable to the underlying choroid. Progressive hearing loss, which develops to total deafness in adulthood, results from fusion of the auditory ossicles. The joint laxity associated with the condition eventually leads to kyphoscoliosis and flat feet. Because of hypoplasia of the dentine and pulp, the teeth are misshapen and bluish yellow.

Osteogenesis Imperfecta Type II

OI type II is a lethal, perinatal disease with an autosomal dominant inheritance pattern. Affected infants are stillborn or die within a few days after birth, in a sense being crushed to death. They are markedly short in stature, with severe limb deformities. Almost all bones sustain fractures during delivery or during uterine contractions in labor. As in OI type I, sclerae are blue.

Osteogenesis Imperfecta Type III

OI type III is the progressive, most severely deforming type of disease and is characterized by many bone fractures, growth retardation and severe skeletal deformities. Inheritance is usually autosomal dominant, although (rarely) autosomal recessive forms are reported. Fractures are present at birth, but bones are less fragile than in the type II form. These patients eventually develop severe shortening of their stature because of progressive bone fractures and severe kyphoscoliosis. Although sclerae may be blue at birth, they become white shortly thereafter. Dental abnormalities are common.

Osteogenesis Imperfecta Type IV

OI type IV is similar to type I except that sclerae are normal. The condition is heterogeneous in presentation, and there may or may not be dental disease. In this disorder, abnormal cross-linkages of collagen result in thin, delicate and weak collagen fibrils. This inappropriate collagen does not allow the bone cortex to mature, so that at birth the cortex of the bone resembles that of a fetus. The cortex is composed of woven bone and small areas of lamellar bone. Over a period of years, the cortex matures, but this may not occur until adolescence or even later. In any event, the frequency of fractures tends to decrease over a long period. These patients are vigorously treated with orthopedic devices, including rods inserted into the medullary cavities to prevent the dwarfing effect of multiple fractures.

Additional types of OI (types V, VI, VII and VIII) have recently been identified from within the heterogeneous type IV group based on distinct clinical, genetic and bone histologic features.

There is no single treatment for OI. Osteoprogenitor cells for bone marrow transplantation, growth factors, bisphosphonates and gene therapy to improve collagen synthesis have been undergoing clinical trials in an attempt to modify the course and severity of the disease. Because exuberant fracture callus occurs, it is not surprising that rare cases of OI have been interpreted as osteosarcoma.

Enchondromatosis Is Marked by Multiple Cartilaginous Tumors

Enchondromatosis, *also termed* **Ollier disease,** *is characterized by development of numerous cartilaginous masses that lead to bony deformities.* The condition is not strictly a disease of delayed maturation of bone, but one in which residual hyaline cartilage, anlage cartilage or cartilage from the growth plate does not undergo endochondral ossification and remains in the bones. As a consequence, bones show multiple, tumor-like masses of abnormally arranged hyaline cartilage (enchondromas), with zones of proliferative and hypertrophied cartilage (Fig. 26-14). These tumors tend to be located in the metaphyses. As growth continues, the enchondromas settle in the diaphysis of adolescents and adults.

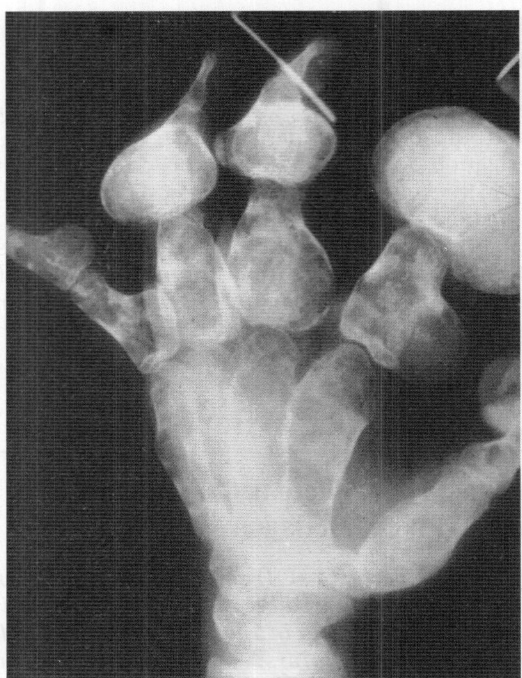

FIGURE 26-14. Multiple enchondromatosis (Ollier disease). A radiograph of the hand shows bulbous swellings that represent nodular masses composed of hyaline cartilage, which is sometimes admixed with more primitive myxoid cartilage.

Enchondromatosis is asymmetric and may cause bone deformities. Whether enchondromas represent true neoplasms is debated, but they exhibit a strong tendency to undergo malignant change into chondrosarcomas in adult life. Therefore, a patient with enchondromatosis who has increasing pain or an increasing abnormality at one site should be evaluated to rule out an underlying sarcoma.

Solitary enchondroma has histologic features similar to Ollier disease and principally affects the tubular bones of the hands and feet. It rarely undergoes malignant change.

Maffucci syndrome is characterized by multiple enchondromas and cavernous or spindle cell hemangiomas of soft tissue. It usually manifests in early childhood and may lead to significant skeletal deformities. Chondrosarcoma develops in as many as half of all patients with Maffucci syndrome. The incidence of malignant tumors in other organs is also greatly increased in patients with Maffucci syndrome.

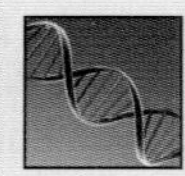

MOLECULAR PATHOGENESIS: Most cases of enchondromatosis are sporadic, but a familial form possibly with autosomal dominant inheritance has been reported. Recent studies have disclosed mutations in the *PTHR1* gene, encoding a receptor for PTH and PTH-related protein, in some cases of enchondromatosis. The mutation results in a substitution in the receptor's extracellular domain, increasing cyclic adenosine 3′,5′-monophosphate (cAMP) signaling. The mutant receptor may delay chondrocyte differentiation by activating Hedgehog signaling, which results in the formation of the multiple cartilaginous masses characteristic of the disease.

Fracture

The most common bone lesion is a fracture, which is defined as a discontinuity of the bone. A force perpendicular to the long axis of the bone results in a **transverse fracture**. A force along the long axis of the bone yields a **compression fracture**. Torsional force results in **spiral fractures,** and combined tension and compression shear forces cause angulation and displacement of the fractured ends.

A force powerful enough to fracture a bone also injures adjacent soft tissues. In this situation, there is often (1) extensive muscle necrosis; (2) hemorrhage because of shearing of capillary beds and larger vessels of soft tissues; (3) tearing of tendinous insertions and ligamentous attachments; and (4) even nerve damage, caused by stretching or direct tearing of the nerve.

Fracture Healing Is Divided Into Inflammatory, Reparative and Remodeling Phases

The duration of each phase (Fig. 26-15) depends on the patient's age, the site of fracture, the patient's overall health and nutritional status and the extent of soft tissue injury. Local factors, such as vascular supply and mechanical forces at the site, also play a role in healing. ***In repairing a bone fracture, anything other than formation of bone tissue at the fracture site represents incomplete healing.***

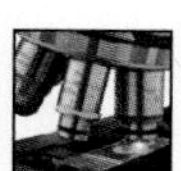

PATHOLOGY:

The Inflammatory Phase

In the first 1 to 2 days after a fracture, rupture of blood vessels in the periosteum and adjacent muscle and soft tissue leads to extensive hemorrhage. Extensive bone necrosis at the fracture site also occurs because of disruption of large vessels in the bone and interruption of cortical vessels (i.e., Volkmann and haversian canals). ***Dead bone is characterized by the absence of osteocytes and empty osteocyte lacunae.***

In 2 to 5 days, the hemorrhage forms a large clot, which must be resorbed so that the fracture can heal. Neovascularization begins to occur peripheral to this blood clot. By the end of the first week, most of the clot is organized by invasion of blood vessels and early fibrosis.

The earliest bone, which is invariably woven bone, is formed after 7 days. ***This corresponds to the "scar" of bone.*** Since bone formation requires a good blood supply, woven bone spicules begin to appear at the periphery of the clot. Pluripotential mesenchymal cells from the soft tissue and within the bone marrow give rise to the osteoblasts that synthesize woven bone. In most fractures, cartilage also is formed and is eventually resorbed by endochondral ossification. Granulation tissue containing bone or cartilage is termed a **callus**. Woven bone also forms inside the marrow cavity at the edge of the blood clot because vascular tissue is also present there.

The Reparative Phase

The reparative phase follows the first week after a fracture and may last for months, depending on the degree of movement and the fixation of the fracture. By this time, acute inflammation has dissipated. Pluripotential cells differentiate into fibroblasts and osteoblasts. Repair proceeds from the periphery toward the center of the fracture site and accomplishes two objectives: (1) to organize and resorb the blood clot and, more importantly, (2) to neovascularize construction of the callus, which will eventually bridge the fracture site. Events leading to repair are as follows:

1. Armies of osteoclasts within the haversian canals form **cutting cones** that bore into the cortex toward the fracture site. A new vessel accompanies the cutting cone, supplying nutrients to these cells and providing more pluripotential cells for cell renewal.
2. At the same time, the external callus, which is found on the surface of the bone and is formed from the periosteum and the soft tissue mesenchymal cells, continues to grow toward the fracture site.
3. Simultaneously, an endosteal or internal callus forms within the medullary cavity and grows outward toward the fracture site.
4. The cortical cutting cones reach the fracture site and the ends of the fractured bone begin to appear beveled and smooth, as the site is remodeled by osteoclasts.
5. The same is true of the endosteal surface of the cortex, as the internal callus works its way to the fracture site.
6. Where there are large areas of cartilage, new blood vessels invade the calcified cartilage, after which the endochondral sequence duplicates the normal formation of bone at the growth plate.

The Remodeling Phase

Several weeks after a fracture, the ingrowth of callus has sealed the bone ends and remodeling begins. In this phase, the bone is reorganized so that the original cortex is restored. Occasionally, the bone is strong enough to qualify as a clinically healed fracture, but biologically, the fracture may not be truly healed and may continue to undergo remodeling for years. For instance, the callus of rib fractures may remain throughout life because the continual respiratory movement of the ribs shears blood vessels and preserves extensive cartilage callus. In a child, in whom the growth plates are still open, normal modeling of growing bone overtakes the callus, so that a fracture may not be recognizable in later life. Similarly, normal modeling in a child may correct the angulation of a bone at a fracture site. If a fracture is near the growth plate, differential growth rates of the growth plate also correct the angulation. In an adult, however, because the plates are closed, angulation often requires correction with external or internal devices.

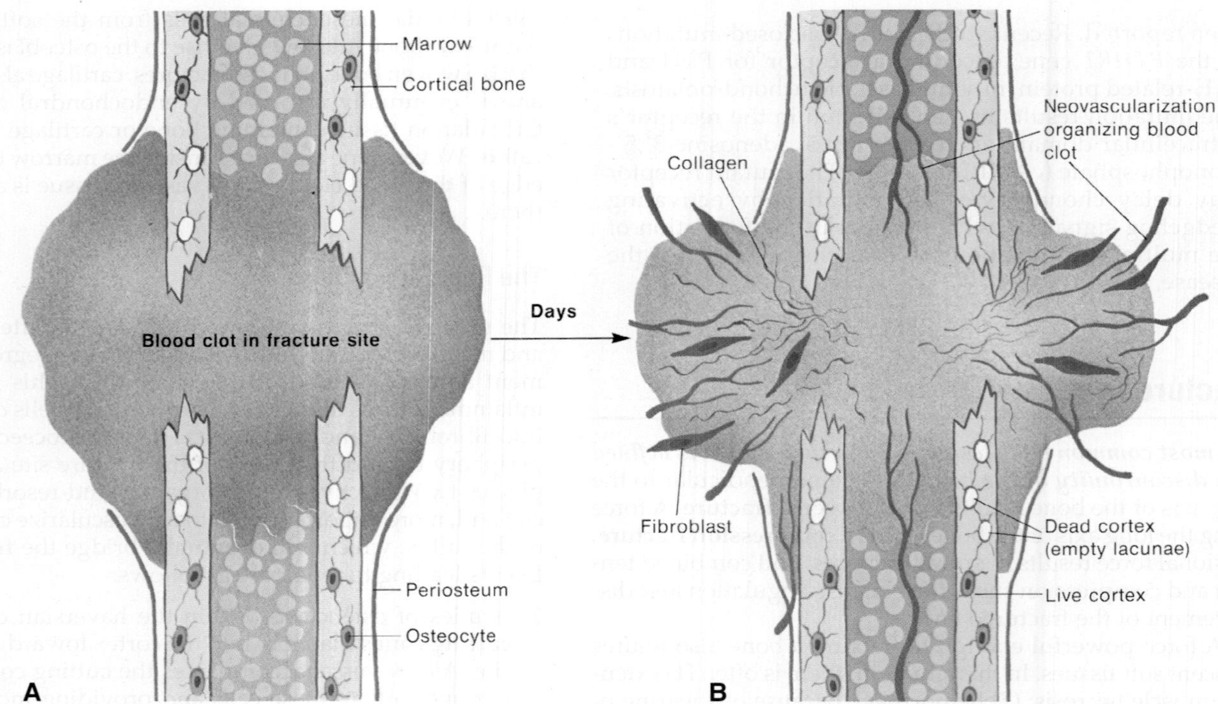

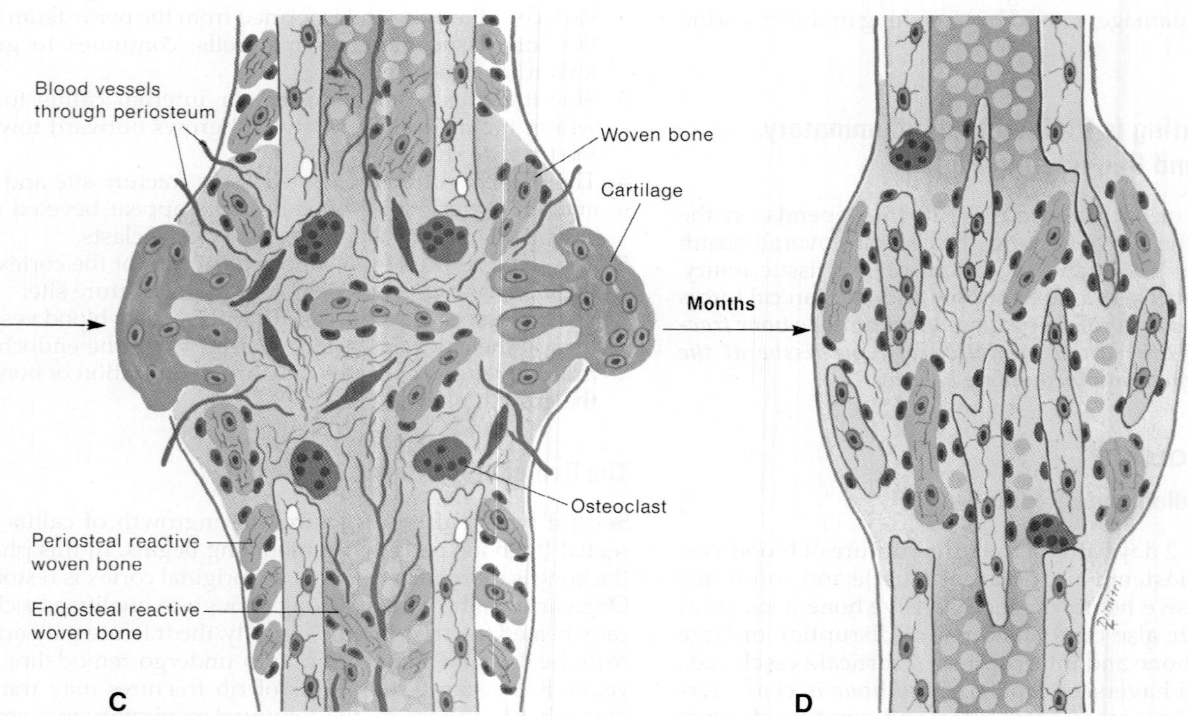

FIGURE 26-15. Healing of a fracture. A. Soon after a fracture is sustained, an extensive blood clot forms in the subperiosteum and soft tissue, as well as in the marrow cavity. The bone at the fracture site is jagged. **B.** The **inflammatory phase** of fracture healing is characterized by neovascularization and beginning organization of the blood clot. Because the osteocytes in the fracture site are dead, the lacunae are empty. The osteocytes of the cortex are necrotic well beyond the fracture site, owing to the traumatic interruption of the perforating arteries from the periosteum. **C.** The **reparative phase** of fracture healing is characterized by the formation of a callus of cartilage and woven bone near the fracture site. The jagged edges of the original cortex have been remodeled and eroded by osteoclasts. The marrow space has been revascularized and contains reactive woven bone, as does the periosteal area. **D.** In the **remodeling phase**, during which the cortex is revitalized, the reactive bone may be lamellar or woven. The new bone is organized along stress lines and mechanical forces. Extensive osteoclastic and osteoblastic cellular activity is maintained.

Special Considerations

There are unusual nuances to fracture healing that deserve mention.

PRIMARY HEALING: A fracture does not necessarily result in bone displacement and soft tissue injury. For example, a drill hole in the bone cortex or a controlled fracture, such as an osteotomy created with a fine saw during orthopedic surgery, does not displace bone. In this situation, there is almost no soft tissue reaction and callus formation because the bone is rigidly fixed. The fracture callus grows directly into the fracture site by a process called **primary healing.** This results in rapid reconstitution of the cortex, including restoration of the haversian systems. Similarly, if a fracture site is held in rigid alignment by metal screws and plates, there is also little external callus. The cortical cutting cones will then be prominent and will heal the fracture site quickly.

NONUNION: If a fracture site does not heal, the condition is termed **nonunion**. Causes of nonunion include interposition of soft tissues at the fracture site, excessive motion, infection, poor blood supply and other factors mentioned above. Continued movement at the unhealed fracture site may also lead to **pseudoarthrosis**, a condition in which joint-like tissue is formed. Pluripotential cells become histologically indistinguishable from synovial cells, secrete synovial fluid and form a joint-like structure. In such cases, the fracture never heals and the abnormal tissue must be removed surgically for the fracture to heal properly.

Stress Fractures Result From Accumulation of Stress-Induced Microfractures

In these fractures, also known as* fatigue or march fractures, *repeated microfractures eventually result in a true fracture through the bone cortex.

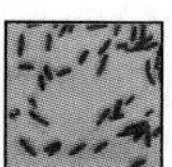

ETIOLOGIC FACTORS: A stress fracture occurs in bones in which the cortex has few osteons and forms only when stress is applied to the cortex. If the ill-prepared cortex (e.g., in the fifth metatarsal) undergoes repeated mechanical stress (e.g., from jogging, skiing or ballet dancing), the bone produces cutting cones in an attempt to implant osteons. If the stress continues and microfractures accumulate, periosteal and endosteal calluses develop to strengthen the bone while active remodeling takes place. An actual fracture occurs as the last event if the stresses are continually applied during remodeling.

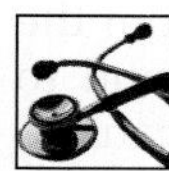

CLINICAL FEATURES: Stress fractures produce pain and swelling over the affected bone. ***At the site of a future stress fracture, a callus forms before a fracture occurs.*** When the actual fracture takes place, the pain becomes more severe. In the early stages of this condition, before the actual fracture, the radiologic appearance may resemble that of a tumor. A biopsy will show that the cortex is riddled with cutting cones for remodeling, which is also seen in the reactive bone at the edge of an invasive tumor.

Osteonecrosis (Avascular Necrosis, Aseptic Necrosis)

Osteonecrosis refers to the death of bone and marrow in the absence of infection (Fig. 26-16). Causes of osteonecrosis are listed in Table 26-1. Necrotic bone heals differently in the cortex and in the underlying coarse cancellous bone.

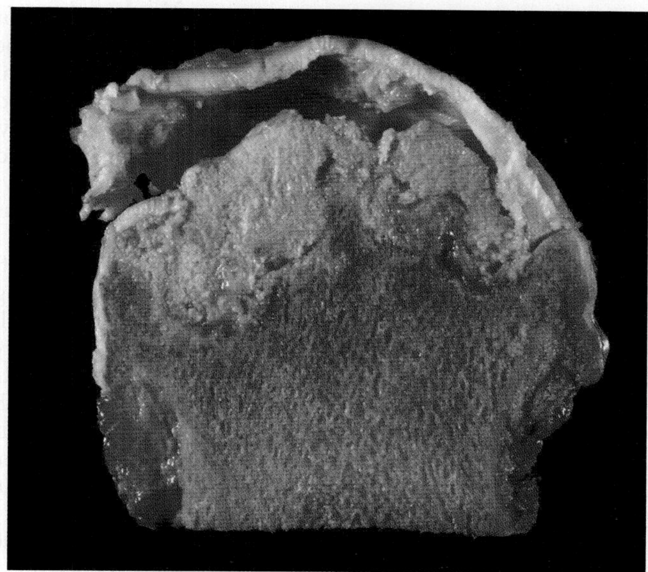

FIGURE 26-16. Osteonecrosis of the head of the femur. A coronal section shows a circumscribed area of subchondral infarction with partial detachment of the overlying articular cartilage and subarticular bone.

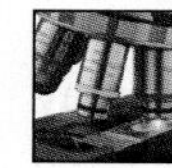

PATHOLOGY: Necrotic coarse cancellous bone heals by **creeping substitution,** in which the necrotic marrow is replaced by invading or creeping neovascular

Table 26-1

Causes of Osteonecrosis

Causes of Osteonecrosis
Trauma, including fracture and surgery
Emboli, producing focal bone infarction
Systemic diseases, such as polycythemia, lupus erythematosus, Gaucher disease, sickle cell disease and gout
Radiation, either internal or external
Corticosteroid administration
Specific focal bone necrosis at various sites—for instance, in the head of the femur (Legg-Calvé-Perthes disease) or in the navicular bone (Köhler disease)
Organ transplantation, particularly renal, in patients with persistent hyperparathyroidism
Osteochondritis dissecans, a condition of unknown etiology in which a piece of articular cartilage and subchondral bone breaks off into a joint. It is thought that a focal area of bone necrosis occurs and eventually detaches.
Autografts and allografts
Thrombosis of local vessels secondary to the pressure of adjacent tumors or other space-occupying lesions
Idiopathic factors, as in the high incidence of osteonecrosis of the head and the femur in alcoholics. Necrotic bone heals differently in the cortex and in the underlying coarse cancellous bone.

tissue, which provides the pluripotential cells needed for bone remodeling. Although necrotic bony trabeculae may be resorbed directly by osteoclastic activity, they are more commonly surrounded by new woven or lamellar bone generated by the osteoblastic activity of granulation tissue. Eventually, the sandwich composed of necrotic bone in the center and surrounding viable bone is remodeled by osteoclastic activity, and new bone is laid down through intramembranous bone formation.

Necrotic cortical bone is healed by a cutting cone. The cutting cone, as discussed above, forms by way of preexisting vascular channels in the cortex. The appropriate signals reach this vascular channel and stimulate neovascularization by surrounding pluripotential mesenchymal tissue. Osteoclasts make their way into the necrotic compact cortical bone, with osteoblasts trailing behind. As a result, tunnels bore their way into the necrotic cortex, leading to new bone formation. This is a slow process, and the bone is often laid down de novo as lamellar bone.

Legg-Calvé-Perthes disease is osteonecrosis in the femoral head in children; **idiopathic osteonecrosis** occurs in a similar location in adults. In both conditions, collapse of the femoral head may lead to joint incongruity and eventual severe osteoarthritis. Collapse of the subchondral bone results from several mechanisms:

- Necrotic bone may sustain stress fractures and compaction over a long period.
- The portion peripheral to the necrotic bone may undergo neovascularization. On radiologic examination, there is a lucent area surrounding the necrotic zone.
- The rigid articular cartilage and subchondral bone may actually crack as the subchondral necrotic zone collapses, producing a fracture.

A radiograph in avascular necrosis often shows the necrotic zone to be radiodense because of (1) relative osteoporosis in the surrounding viable bone compared with the unchanged necrotic bone; (2) addition of new bone through creeping substitution; (3) formation of calcium soaps, which arise as a result of the necrosis of marrow fat; and (4) actual compaction of the preexisting dead bone. Focal end-arterial vascular insufficiency may precede these events, as the necrotic zone tends to be wedge shaped.

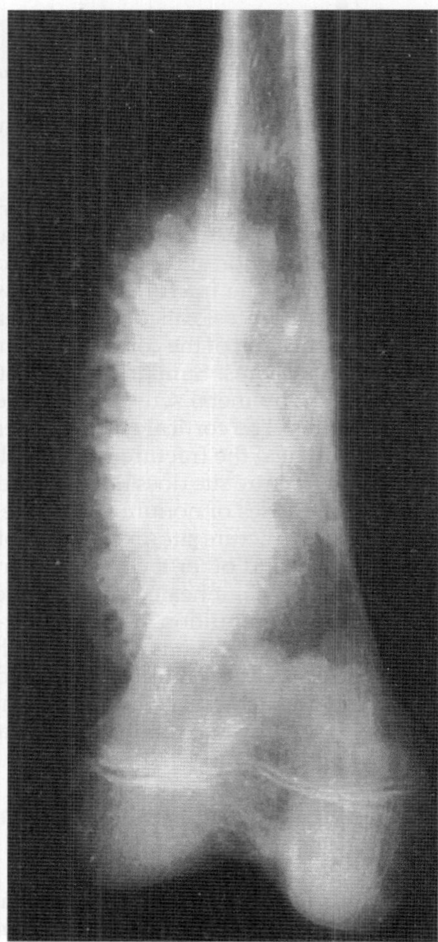

FIGURE 26-17. Reactive bone formation. A radiograph of a resected femur bearing an osteosarcoma shows a sunburst pattern of hyperdense new bone in the distal diaphysis and metaphysis. This radiodensity is due to woven bone produced by the sarcoma and the periosteal reaction of the host bone. The epiphyseal plate is represented as a transverse lucent line that separates the metaphysis from the epiphysis. The radiating radiodense bone extends beyond the periosteum into the soft tissues, obscuring the underlying bone architecture.

Reactive Bone Formation

Reactive bone is intramembranous bone formed in response to stress on bone or soft tissue. Conditions such as tumors, infections, trauma or generalized or focal disease can stimulate bone formation.

PATHOLOGY: The periosteum may respond with a so-called **sunburst** pattern (Fig. 26-17), as seen with certain tumors, or progressive layering of the periosteum, which yields an **onionskin pattern** of the cortex. The endosteal or the marrow surface may produce new bone, so that on radiologic studies, the cortex appears to be thickened, and the coarse cancellous bone appears to be denser.

Reactive bone may be either woven or lamellar, depending on the rates of deposition of the reactive bone. Around an indolent infection, as in chronic osteomyelitis, reactive bone may be laid down de novo as lamellar bone from the periosteum. In this case, the bone has time to respond to the persistent stress. Similarly, a benign tumor may cause a lamellar bone reaction. By contrast, a rapidly enlarging tumor is more likely to promote woven bone. Invariably, reactive bone is of the intramembranous type, because it is derived from the periosteum or the endosteal tissue of the marrow.

Heterotopic Ossification Is Bone Formation Outside the Skeletal System

Heterotopic ossification (HO) is formation of reactive bone (woven and/or lamellar) in extraskeletal sites such as the skin, subcutaneous tissue, skeletal muscle and fibroconnective tissue around joints. HO is not associated with any metabolic disease reflected in the fact that patients have normal serum calcium and phosphorous levels. HO occurs in five major clinical settings: genetic, posttraumatic, neurogenic, postsurgical and as distinctive reactive lesions such as myositis ossificans. A genetic disorder known as **fibrodysplasia ossificans progressiva** is characterized by massive deposits of bone around multiple joints. HO may form in hematomas or skeletal muscle after trauma. Neurogenic HO occurs in muscle and periarticular fibrous tissue at multiple sites in patients with head trauma, spinal cord injury or prolonged coma. HO can form in periarticular soft tissue following joint surgery.

Heterotopic Calcification Is Deposition of Calcium Salts in Soft Tissues

Radiologically, heterotopic ossification and heterotopic calcification are usually distinctive. Bone formation is characterized by a spicular or trabeculated pattern, whereas heterotopic calcification has an irregular, splotchy, amorphous appearance. Heterotopic calcification tends to occur in necrotic soft tissue or in cartilage and is usually denser than bone on radiography. Heterotopic calcification appears in two forms:

- **Metastatic calcification** occurs when there is an increase in the calcium–phosphorus product. Thus, hypercalcemic states or hyperphosphatemic conditions predispose normal soft tissues to calcification.
- **Dystrophic calcification** is seen in abnormal or damaged soft tissues such as tumors, degenerative diseases such as arteriosclerosis and areas subjected to trauma. In addition, loss of neurologic function as seen in quadriplegia and hemiplegia predisposes the affected parts to soft tissue calcification.

Myositis Ossificans Is Formation of Reactive Bone in Muscle After Injury

Myositis ossificans is a distinctive form of heterotopic ossification that affects young persons and, although it is entirely benign, often mimics a malignant neoplasm. It is a self-limited process and carries an excellent prognosis. Spontaneous regression has been observed. No treatment is required once the diagnosis is established.

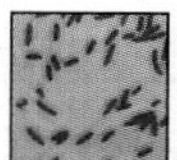

ETIOLOGIC FACTORS: The lesion typically results from blunt trauma to the muscle and soft tissues, usually of the lower limb. However, some cases occur spontaneously. Peripheral neovascularization and fibrosis at the site of damaged tissue with associated hemorrhage leads in a short time to bone spicule formation. These changes are similar to those that occur at the initial hematoma in a healing fracture. Because myositis ossificans often occurs near a bone such as the femur or tibia, it may be misdiagnosed on radiography as a malignant bone-forming tumor.

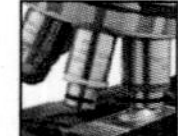

PATHOLOGY: Histologically, woven bone is formed within granulation tissue and reactive fibrous tissue (Fig. 26-18B). The center of an early lesion of myositis ossificans is characterized by proliferating fibroblasts and more peripheral osteoblastic cells beginning to form woven bone. The fibroblasts are often cytologically atypical and show abundant mitoses, a histologic appearance that also resembles a malignant tumor. ***The key feature that distinguishes myositis ossificans from a neoplasm is that the bone matures peripherally, whereas it is immature or not formed at all in the center of the lesion.*** The phenomenon of peripheral maturity with central immaturity, the **zonation effect,**

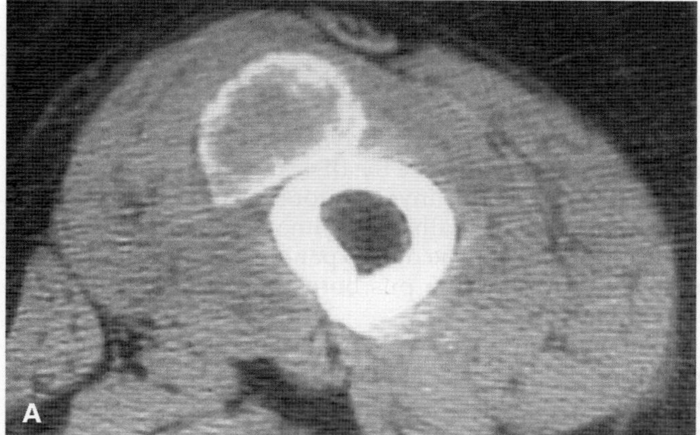

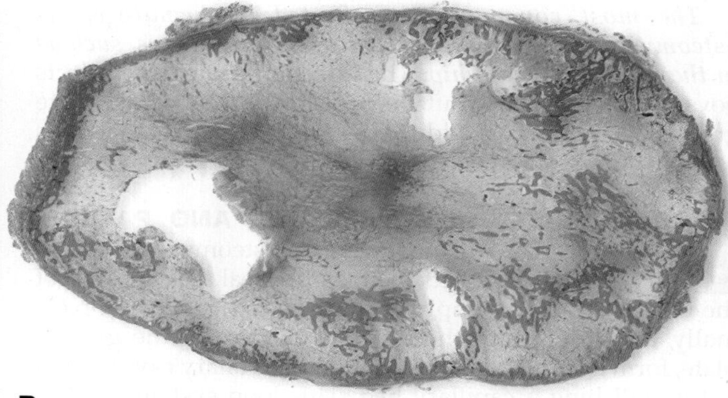

FIGURE 26-18. Myositis ossificans circumscripta. A. Computed tomography scan of the thigh shows an axial view of an ovoid, intramuscular mass adjacent to the femoral cortex with a radiolucent center and ossification that becomes denser at the periphery. **B.** The mass at low-power magnification with woven bone at the periphery and fibrous tissue in the center.

clearly indicates a reactive process. In a well-developed lesion, this phenomenon may be seen radiographically (Fig. 26-18A). A neoplasm has an opposite zonation effect: the most mature tissue of the tumor is located centrally.

The growth pattern of myositis ossificans reflects the ingrowth of neovascular tissue from the periphery into the center of the damaged area. In the late stages, the lesion may contain cartilage and even lamellar bone. Thus, in a well-developed lesion, it may mimic a sesamoid bone in the soft tissue.

Infections

Osteomyelitis Is Inflammation, Usually Caused by a Bacterial Infection of Bone and Bone Marrow

Any infectious agent may be responsible, but the most common pathogens are *Staphylococcus* sp. Other organisms, such as *Escherichia coli, Neisseria gonorrhoeae, Haemophilus influenzae* and *Salmonella* sp., are also seen. The organisms gain entry either via the bloodstream or by direct introduction into the bone.

Direct Penetration

Infection by direct penetration or extension of bacteria is now the most common cause of osteomyelitis in the United States. Bacterial organisms are introduced directly into bone by penetrating wounds, open fractures or surgery. Staphylococci and streptococci are still commonly incriminated, but in 25% of postoperative infections, anaerobic organisms are detected. Rarely, a gram-negative organism may seed a hip after a urologic or gastrointestinal surgical procedure.

Hematogenous Osteomyelitis

Infectious organisms may reach the bone from a focus elsewhere in the body through the bloodstream. Often the focus itself (e.g., a skin pustule or infected teeth and gums) poses little threat. Even the mere brushing of teeth may create a temporary bacteremia, which may allow organisms to reach the bone.

The most common sites affected by hematogenous osteomyelitis are the metaphyses of the long bones, such as in the knee, ankle and hip. The infection principally affects boys aged 5 to 15 years, but it is occasionally seen in older age groups as well. Drug addicts may develop hematogenous osteomyelitis from infected needles.

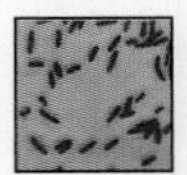
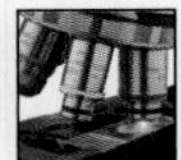

ETIOLOGIC FACTORS AND PATHOLOGY: Hematogenous osteomyelitis primarily affects the metaphyseal area because of the unique vascular supply in this region (Fig. 26-19). Normally, arterioles enter the calcified portion of the growth plate, form a loop, then drain into the medullary cavity without establishing a capillary bed. This loop system permits slowing and sludging of blood flow, thereby allowing bacteria enough time to penetrate blood vessel walls and establish infective foci within the marrow. If the organism is virulent and continues to proliferate, it creates increased pressure on the adjacent thin-walled vessels because they lie in a closed space, the marrow cavity. Such pressure further compromises the vascular supply in this region and produces bone necrosis. The necrotic areas coalesce into an avascular zone, thereby allowing further bacterial proliferation.

If infection is not contained, pus and bacteria extend into the endosteal vascular channels that supply the cortex and spread throughout the Volkmann and haversian canals of the cortex. Eventually, pus forms underneath the periosteum, shearing off the perforating arteries of the periosteum and further devitalizing the cortex. The pus flows between the periosteum and the cortex, isolating more bone from its blood supply, and may even invade the joint. Eventually, the pus penetrates the periosteum and the skin to form a draining sinus (Fig. 26-20). A sinus tract that extends from the cloaca (see below) to the skin may become epithelialized by epidermis that grows into the sinus tract. When this occurs, the sinus tract invariably remains open, continually draining pus, necrotic bone and bacteria.

Periosteal new bone formation and reactive bone formation in the marrow tend to wall off the infection. At the same time, osteoclastic activity resorbs bone. If the infection is virulent, this attempt to contain it is overwhelmed and it races through the bone, with virtually no bone formation but extensive bone necrosis. More commonly, pluripotential cells modulate into osteoblasts in an attempt to wall off the infection. Several lesions may develop:

- **Cloaca** is the hole formed in the bone during the formation of a draining sinus.
- **Sequestrum** is a fragment of necrotic bone that is embedded in the pus.
- **Brodie abscess** consists of reactive bone from the periosteum and the endosteum, which surrounds and contains the infection.
- **Involucrum** refers to a lesion in which periosteal new bone formation forms a sheath around the necrotic sequestrum. An involucrum that involves an entire bone may exist for several years before a patient seeks medical attention.

In very young children (1 year old or younger) afflicted with osteomyelitis, the adjacent joint is often involved because the periosteum is loosely attached to the cortex. From the age of 1 year to puberty, subperiosteal abscesses are common. Spread to adjacent joints may also occur in adults.

Vertebral Osteomyelitis

In adults, osteomyelitis frequently involves vertebral bodies (Fig. 26-21). The intervertebral disk is not a barrier to bacterial osteomyelitis, particularly staphylococcal infection. Infections directly traverse the disk and travel from one vertebra to the next. Some investigators consider that the intervertebral disk is actually the primary source of infection, so-called "diskitis." The disk expands with pus and is eventually destroyed as the pus bores into adjacent vertebral bodies.

Half or more of cases of vertebral osteomyelitis are caused by *Staphylococcus aureus*. Twenty percent involve *E. coli* and other enteric organisms, often originating from the urinary tract. *Salmonella* sp. are also seen in the vertebral bodies, as are *Brucella* sp. Predisposing factors are intravenous drug abuse, upper urinary tract infections, urologic procedures and hematogenous spread of organisms from other sites. Back pain, with point tenderness over the area of infection, is associated with low-grade fever and an increased sedimentation rate.

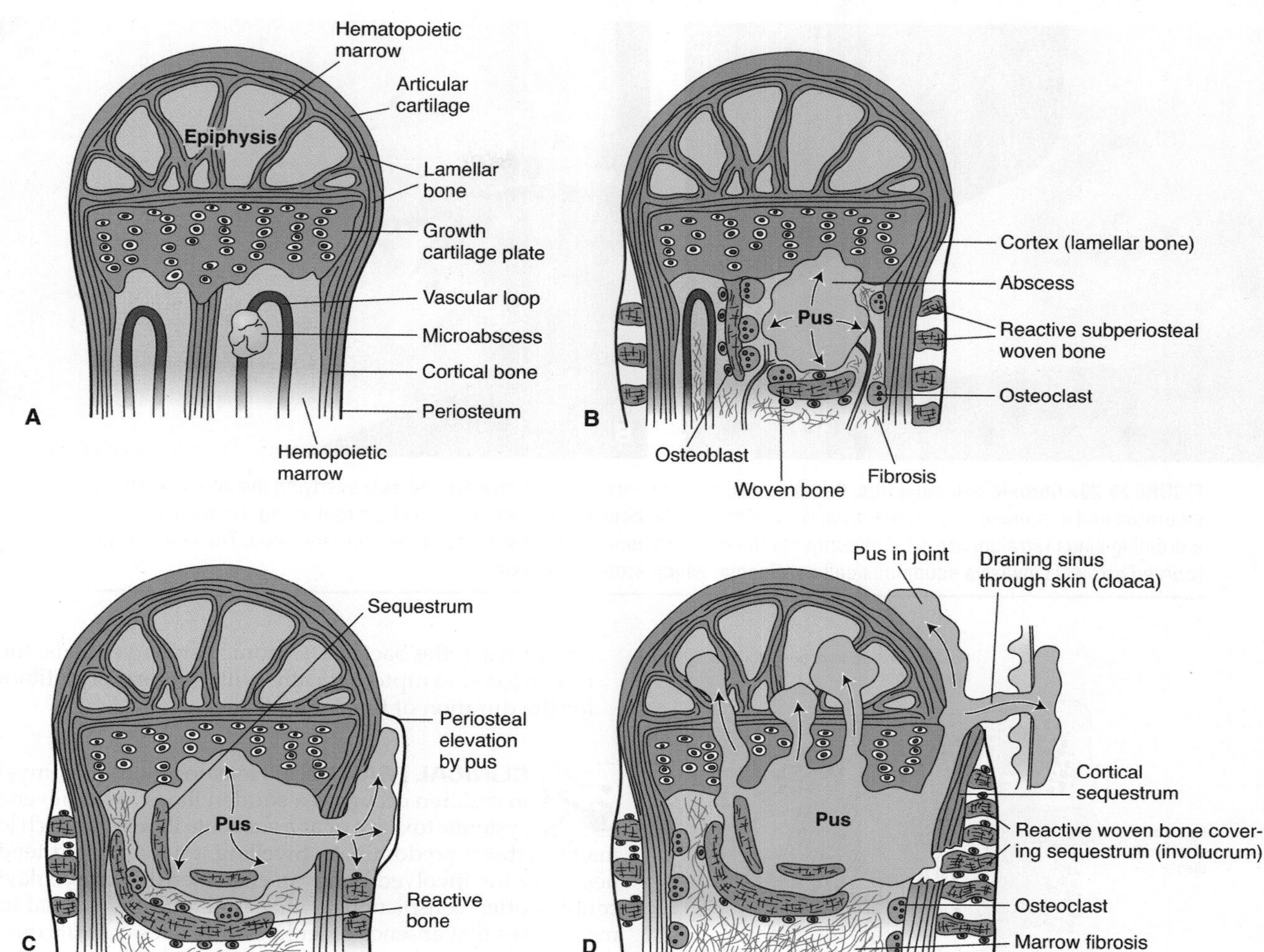

FIGURE 26-19. Pathogenesis of hematogenous osteomyelitis. A. The epiphysis, metaphysis and growth plate are normal. A small, septic microabscess is forming at the capillary loop. **B.** Expansion of the septic focus stimulates resorption of adjacent bony trabeculae. **Woven bone** begins to surround this focus. The abscess expands into the cartilage and stimulates reactive bone formation by the periosteum. **C.** The **abscess,** which continues to expand through the cortex into the subperiosteal tissue, shears off the perforating arteries that supply the cortex with blood, thereby leading to necrosis of the cortex. **D.** The extension of this process into the joint space, the epiphysis and the skin produces a **draining sinus.** The necrotic bone is called a **sequestrum.** The viable bone surrounding a sequestrum is termed the **involucrum.**

Occasionally, a paravertebral abscess draining the bone may "point" and emerge in the groin or elsewhere. Vertebral osteomyelitis may lead to (1) vertebral collapse with paravertebral abscesses; (2) spinal epidural abscesses, with cord compression from the abscess or from displaced fragments of the infected bone; and (3) compression fractures of the vertebral body, leading to neurologic deficits.

Complications

The complications of osteomyelitis include:

- **Septicemia:** Dissemination of organisms through the bloodstream may occur as a result of bone infection. It is unusual for osteomyelitis to result from septicemia.
- **Acute bacterial arthritis:** Joint infection is secondary to osteomyelitis at all ages, and represents a medical emergency. Direct digestion of cartilage by inflammatory cells destroys the articular cartilage and produces osteoarthritis. Rapid intervention to prevent this complication is mandatory.
- **Pathologic fractures:** Osteomyelitis may lead to fractures, which heal poorly and may require surgical drainage.
- **Squamous cell carcinoma:** This cancer develops in the bone or the sinus tract of long-standing chronic osteomyelitis, often years after the initial infection. In such cases, squamous tissue arises from the epithelialization of the sinus tract and eventually undergoes malignant transformation (Fig. 26-20).
- **Amyloidosis:** Amyloidosis used to be a common consequence of chronic osteomyelitis, but is now only rarely seen in industrialized countries.
- **Chronic osteomyelitis:** Chronic osteomyelitis may follow acute osteomyelitis. It is difficult to treat, especially if it involves the entire bone, because necrotic bone or sequestra function as foreign bodies in avascular areas, and antibiotics

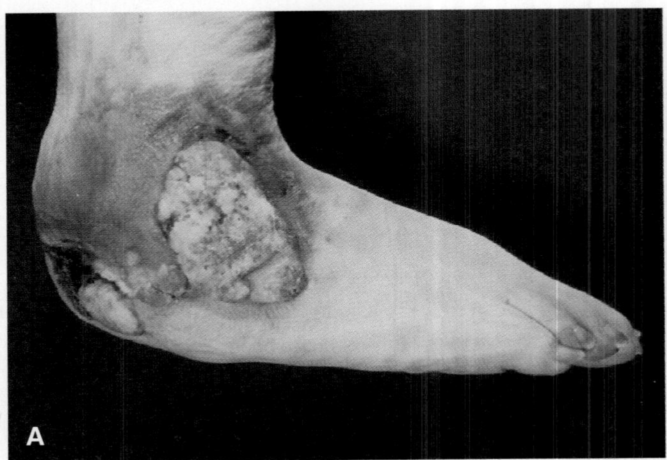

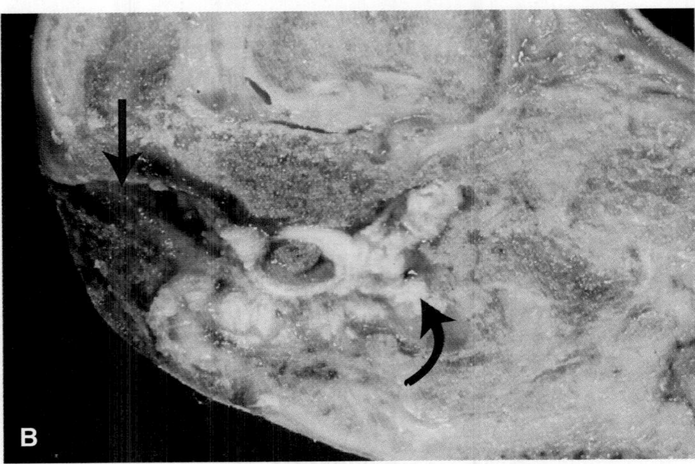

FIGURE 26-20. Chronic osteomyelitis. A. In this patient with chronic osteomyelitis, the skin overlying the infected bone is ulcerated and a draining sinus (*dark area*) is evident over the heel. **B.** After amputation of the foot, a sagittal section shows a draining sinus (*straight arrow*) that connects the infected bone with the surface of the ulcerated skin. The white tissue (*curved arrow*) is invasive squamous cell carcinoma, which arose in the skin.

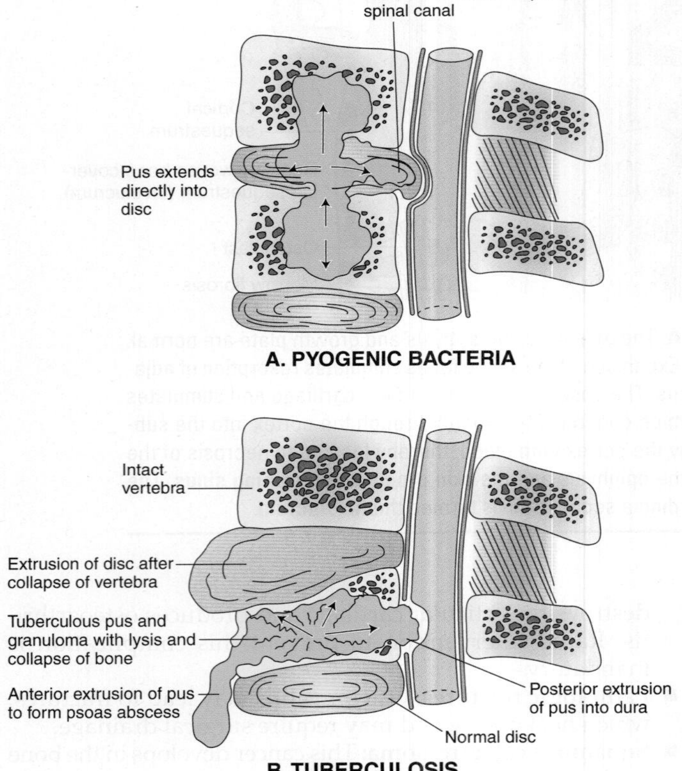

FIGURE 26-21. Osteomyelitis of the vertebral body. A. Bacterial osteomyelitis expands from one vertebral body to the next by direct invasion of the intervertebral disk and may actually push posteriorly into the spinal canal. The sequence of events in the marrow cavity is similar to that in a long bone. **B.** In **tuberculous osteomyelitis**, the bone is destroyed by resorption of bony trabeculae, which results in mechanical collapse of the vertebrae and extrusion of the intervertebral disk. Tuberculous organisms cannot penetrate the intervertebral disk directly; rather, they extend from one vertebra to the next after mechanical forces destroy and extrude the intervertebral disk.

do not reach the bacteria. Chronic osteomyelitis is, therefore, treated symptomatically with surgery or antibiotics for the duration of the patient's life.

CLINICAL FEATURES: Hematogenous osteomyelitis in children occurs as a sudden illness, with fever and systemic toxicity, or as a subacute illness in which local manifestations predominate. Swelling, erythema and tenderness over the involved bone are characteristic. The leukocyte count is often conspicuously increased, but it is normal in so many cases that absence of leukocytosis does not rule out the disease. Erythrocyte sedimentation rate and C-reactive protein are usually elevated but are not specific. Radiologic workup including radiography, computed tomography (CT), magnetic resonance imaging (MRI) and bone scan are very helpful. Bone biopsy is necessary for a definitive diagnosis since it provides material for histologic examination, microbiological culture and antibiotic sensitivity.

The treatment depends on the stage of the infection. Early osteomyelitis is treated with intravenous antibiotics for 6 or more weeks. Surgery is used to drain and decompress the infection within the bone or to drain abscesses that do not respond to antibiotic therapy. In long-standing, chronic osteomyelitis, antibiotics alone are not curative and extensive surgical débridement of necrotic bone is often required.

Tuberculosis of Bone Represents Spread From a Primary Focus Elsewhere

Tuberculosis of bone usually originates in the lungs or lymph nodes (see Chapter 9). When the bone infection is caused by the rare bovine type of tubercle bacillus, the initial focus is often in the gut or tonsils. The mycobacteria spread to the bone hematogenously, and only rarely is there direct spread from the lungs or lymph nodes.

Tuberculous Spondylitis (Pott Disease)

Tuberculous spondylitis (i.e., infection of the spine) is a feared complication of childhood tuberculosis. The disease affects

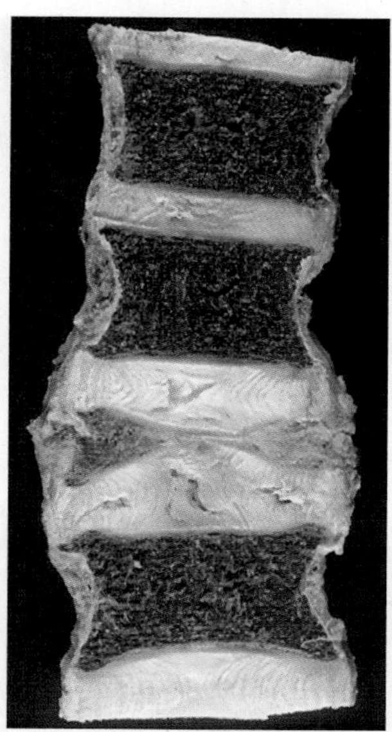

FIGURE 26-22. **Tuberculous spondylitis (Pott disease).** A vertebral body is almost completely replaced by tuberculous tissue. Note the preservation of the intervertebral disks.

vertebral bodies, sparing the lamina and spines and adjacent vertebrae (Figs. 26-21 and 26-22). Thoracic vertebrae are usually affected, especially the 11th thoracic vertebra. The lumbar and cervical vertebrae are less often involved. As a result of currently available effective antibiotic treatment, Pott disease is now rare.

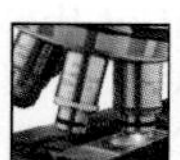

PATHOLOGY: The pathology in tuberculous spondylitis is similar to tuberculosis at other sites. The granulomas first produce caseous necrosis of the bone marrow, which leads to slow resorption of bony trabeculae and, occasionally, to cystic spaces in the bone. Since there is little or no reactive bone formation, affected vertebrae usually collapse, leading to kyphosis and scoliosis. The intervertebral disk is crushed and destroyed by the compression fracture, rather than by invasion of organisms. The typical hunchback of bygone days was often the victim of Pott disease.

If the infection ruptures into the soft tissue anteriorly, pus and necrotic debris drain along the spinal ligaments and form a **cold abscess** (i.e., an abscess lacking acute inflammation). A **psoas abscess**—which forms near the lower lumbar vertebrae and dissects along the pelvis, to emerge through the skin of the inguinal region as a draining sinus—may be the first manifestation of tuberculous spondylitis. Paraplegia results from vascular insufficiency of the spinal nerves, rather than from direct pressure.

Tuberculous Arthritis

Hematogenous spread of tuberculosis may bring organisms to the joint capsule, synovium or intracapsular portion of the bone. Tuberculosis induces granulomas in synovial tissue, which then becomes edematous and papillary and may fill the entire joint space. Massive destruction of the articular cartilage results from undermining granulation tissue in the bone. The destroyed joint is replaced by bone, an effect that leads to an immovable joint (**bony ankylosis**).

Tuberculous Osteomyelitis of the Long Bones

Infection of long bones is the least common bone manifestation of tuberculosis. Tuberculosis of a long bone occurs near the joint, where it also produces arthritis. For unknown reasons, the greater trochanter of the femur is a common site for this disease.

Syphilis of Bone Is Today Rare

Syphilis causes a slowly progressive, chronic, inflammatory disease of bone, characterized by granulomas, necrosis and marked reactive bone formation. It may be acquired through sexual contact or transmitted transplacentally from mother to fetus (see Chapter 9). The bone changes in syphilis depend on the patient's age, endosteal and periosteal changes and the presence or absence of gummas.

Congenital Syphilis

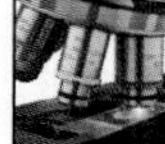

PATHOLOGY: Bone involvement in congenital syphilis may appear as early as the fifth month of gestation and is fully developed at birth. Spirochetes are ubiquitous in the epiphysis and periosteum, where they produce osteochondritis (epiphysitis) and periostitis, respectively (Fig. 26-23). In severe disease, an epiphysis may become dislocated, leaving the child with a functionless limb (**pseudoparalysis of Parrot**).

The knee is most often affected by congenital syphilis. The growth plate is irregularly widened and displays a yellow discoloration. The zone of calcified cartilage is destroyed and a sea of lymphocytes, plasma cells and spirochetes fills the marrow spaces. Because the periosteum is stimulated to produce reactive new bone, the thickness of the cortex may actually be doubled. The inflammatory infiltrate permeates the cortex through the Volkmann and haversian canals and settles in the elevated periosteum. Ultimately, as the affected bones grow, they become short and deformed.

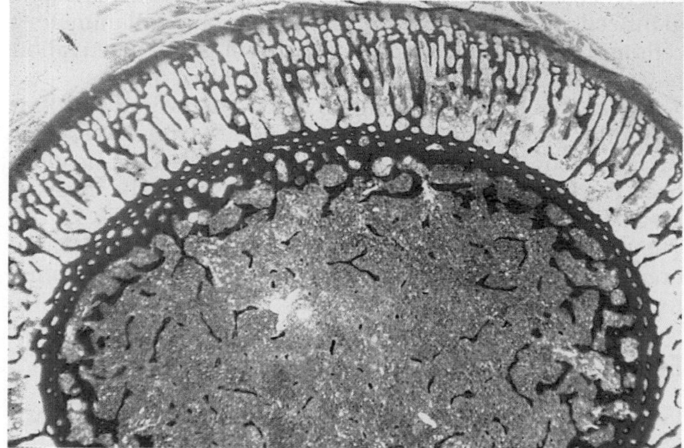

FIGURE 26-23. **Congenital syphilis of bone.** A cross-section of a tubular bone infected by syphilis shows marked periosteal new bone formation. The medullary cavity is filled with a lymphoplasmacytic infiltrate that replaces the normal marrow fat. The cortex is irregularly destroyed by osteoclastic resorption, a process that stimulates periosteal new bone formation.

Acquired Syphilis

Acquired syphilis in adults produces lesions of the bone early in the tertiary stage, 2 to 5 years after inoculation of the organisms. Periostitis is predominant because the growth plates have already closed. The bones most commonly affected are the tibia, nose, palate and skull. Tibial lesions are marked by periostitis, with deposition of new bone on the medial and anterior aspects of the shaft, which leads to the **saber shin** deformity. The skull thickness also increases because of periosteal stimulation.

Gumma formation is seen most often in tertiary syphilis. Bone adjacent to gummas is slowly replaced by fibrous marrow. Ultimately, perforations occur through the cortex. The markedly irregular, thickened periosteal surfaces, which are perforated by pits and serpiginous ulcerations, are characteristic of syphilis. Lysis and collapse of nasal and palatal bones produce the classic **saddle nose**—perforation, destruction and collapse of the nasal septum (see Chapter 25).

Langerhans Cell Histiocytosis

Langerhans cell histiocytosis (LCH) is a generic term (previously referred to as **histiocytosis X**) for three entities characterized by proliferation of Langerhans cells in various tissues: (1) **eosinophilic granuloma**, a localized form; (2) **Hand-Schüller-Christian disease,** a disseminated variant; and (3) **Letterer-Siwe disease**, a fulminant and often fatal generalized disease (see Chapter 20).

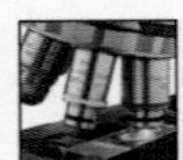

PATHOLOGY: The histologic appearance of the bones in all three variants of LCH is identical and is characterized by collections of large, phagocytic cells with pale, eosinophilic cytoplasm and convoluted or grooved nuclei (see Figs. 12-68 and 20-33). By electron microscopy these cells have the typical racquet-shaped, tubular structures, **"Birbeck granules,"** seen in normal Langerhans cells of the skin (see Fig. 20-34). There are many eosinophils throughout these lesions, occasionally forming collections called "eosinophilic abscesses." Multinucleated **osteoclastic** giant cells are often observed, as are chronic inflammatory cells and neutrophils. Studies of X-chromosome inactivation have shown that LCH is a clonal proliferative disease.

Lesions of LCH may occur anywhere in the body, including bones, skin, brain, lungs, lymph nodes, liver and spleen. Radiologic findings in the bones in all three diseases are identical. The lesions may occur in the metaphysis or diaphysis of long bones, or in a flat bone, especially in the skull (Fig. 26-24). They are punched-out lytic defects, with virtually no reactive bone. Such lesions may lead to fractures and periosteal callus formation.

Eosinophilic Granuloma Is a Self-Limited Disease

Eosinophilic granuloma, in either its solitary or multiple varieties, accounts for 70% of all cases of LCH. It is usually seen in the first two decades of life, but occasionally occurs in older persons. There are typically one or two lytic areas in bones of the axial or appendicular skeleton (Fig. 26-24) or the vertebrae. These lesions may cause mild pain or may be incidental findings on routine chest radiographs. Foci of disease in the lower thoracic or upper lumbar vertebrae may lead to collapse and pathologic fractures. Eventual recovery is the rule.

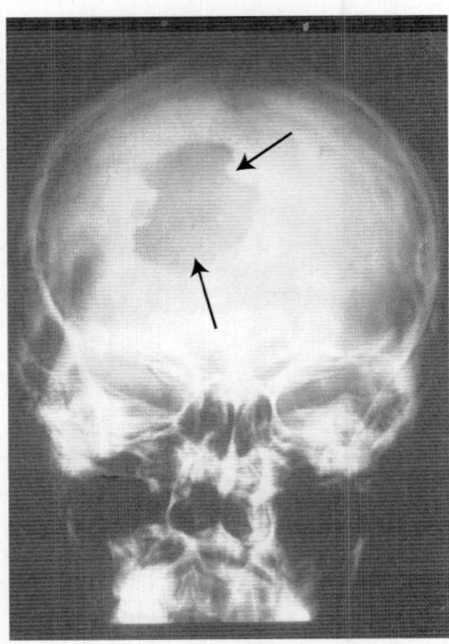

FIGURE 26-24. Eosinophilic granuloma. A radiograph of the skull shows a large, lytic lesion (*arrows*).

Hand-Schüller-Christian Disease Is a Multiorgan Disease of Childhood

Hand-Schüller-Christian disease occurs in children 2 to 5 years old. The lesions are more widespread than eosinophilic granuloma. It represents some 20% of all cases of LCH. Radiolucent bony lesions characterize the disorder, most frequently in the calvaria, ribs, pelvis and scapulae. Involvement of the jaw bone results in loss of teeth, evident radiologically as "floating teeth." Infiltration of the retro-orbital space causes exophthalmos; infiltration of the hypothalamic stalk by Langerhans cells leads to diabetes insipidus. One fifth of patients have lymphadenopathy and lung infiltrates.

Crusty, red, weepy skin lesions occur at the hairline and on the extensor surfaces of the extremities, the abdomen and occasionally the soles of the feet. Deafness results from involvement of the external auditory canal and mastoid air cells. One third of affected patients have disease in the liver and spleen, and 40% have bone lesions, half of which involve the skull. Thus, the classic triad of Hand-Schüller-Christian disease, **(1) radiolucent lesions of the skull, (2) diabetes insipidus and (3) exophthalmos,** occurs in only one third of patients.

Letterer-Siwe Disease Is an Aggressive, Potentially Fatal Disease of Infants

It accounts for 10% of cases of LCH. Affected children fail to thrive and become cachectic. Multiple organ involvement culminates in massive hepatosplenomegaly, lymphadenopathy, anemia, leukopenia and thrombocytopenia. Widely scattered, seborrheic skin lesions, which are often hemorrhagic, are usual. Bone lesions are not prominent initially, but progressive marrow replacement and pulmonary infiltration occasionally cause death.

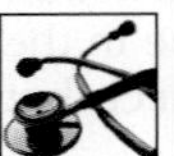

CLINICAL FEATURES: Eosinophilic granuloma is a self-limited disease, and most lesions disappear if left alone. A bone lesion may have to be curetted and packed with bone chips. Sometimes biopsy itself is enough to stimulate repair of the lytic lesion. A collapsed vertebra may actually reconstitute itself over time. Hand-Schüller-Christian disease may require radiation therapy for some bone and retro-orbital lesions. Diabetes insipidus seems to be irreversible, despite irradiation of the pituitary region. Drugs such as corticosteroids, cyclophosphamide and tumoricidal agents may also be used to treat Hand-Schüller-Christian disease. Aggressive chemotherapy for Letterer-Siwe disease may improve the prognosis.

METABOLIC BONE DISEASES

Metabolic bone diseases are defined as disorders of metabolism that result in secondary structural effects on the skeleton, including diminished bone mass due to decreased synthesis or increased destruction, reduced bone mineralization or both. Because metabolic bone diseases are systemic, a biopsy of any bone should reveal the abnormality, even though severity may differ in various parts of the skeleton (Fig. 26-25).

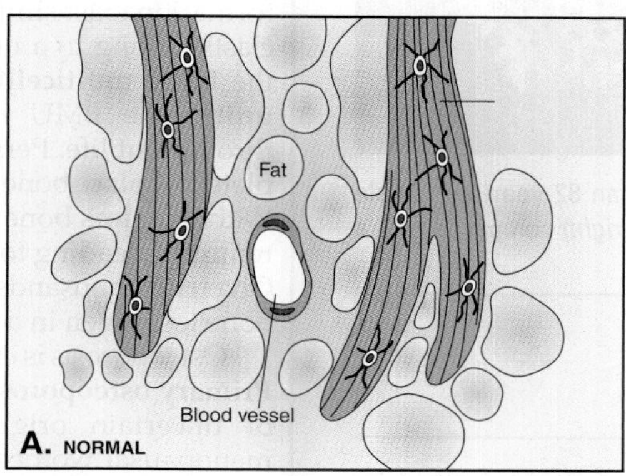

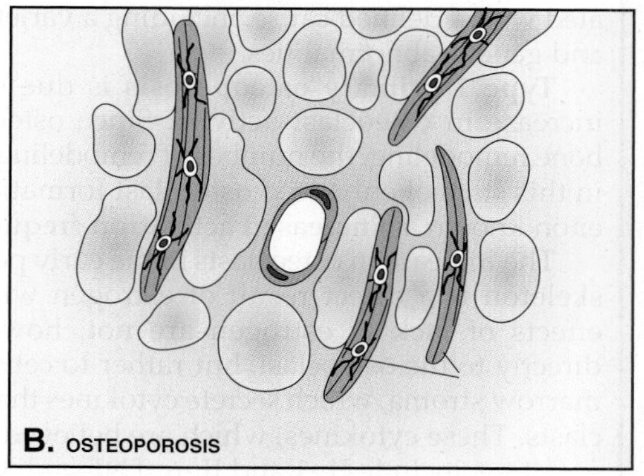

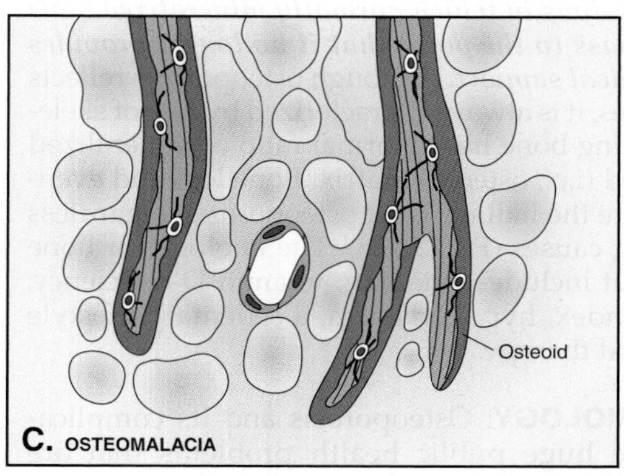

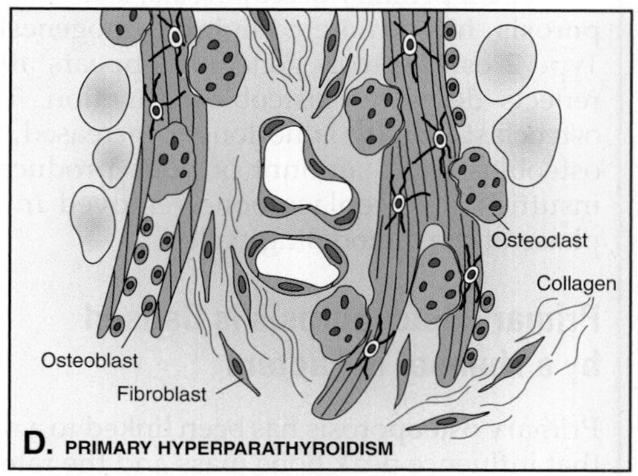

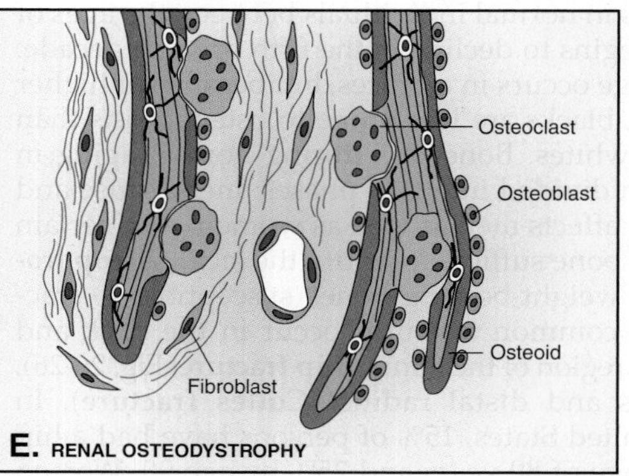

FIGURE 26-25. Metabolic bone diseases. A. Normal trabecular bone and fatty marrow. The trabecular bone is lamellar and contains evenly distributed osteocytes. **B. Osteoporosis.** The lamellar bone exhibits discontinuous, thin trabeculae. **C. Osteomalacia.** The trabeculae of the lamellar bone have abnormal amounts of nonmineralized bone (osteoid). These osteoid seams are thickened and cover a larger than normal area of the trabecular bone surface. **D. Primary hyperparathyroidism.** The lamellar bone trabeculae are actively resorbed by numerous osteoclasts that bore into each trabecula. The appearance of osteoclasts dissecting into the trabeculae, a process termed **dissecting osteitis,** is diagnostic of hyperparathyroidism. Osteoblastic activity also is pronounced. The marrow is replaced by fibrous tissue adjacent to the trabeculae. **E. Renal osteodystrophy.** The morphologic appearance is similar to that of primary hyperparathyroidism, except that prominent osteoid covers the trabeculae. Osteoclasts do not resorb osteoid, and wherever an osteoid seam is lacking, osteoclasts bore into the trabeculae. Osteoblastic activity, in association with osteoclasts, is again prominent.

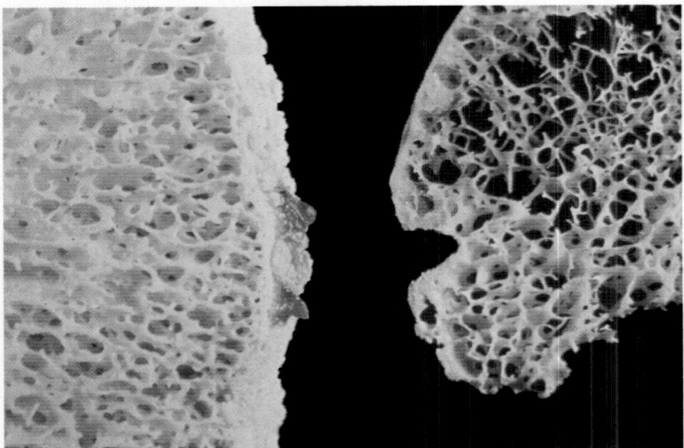

FIGURE 26-26. Osteoporosis. Femoral head of an 82-year-old female with osteoporosis and a femoral neck fracture (*right*) compared with a normal control cut to the same thickness (*left*).

Osteoporosis

Osteoporosis is a metabolic bone disease characterized by diffuse skeletal lesions in which normally mineralized bone is decreased in mass to the point that it no longer provides adequate mechanical support. Although osteoporosis reflects a number of causes, it is always characterized by loss of skeletal mass. Remaining bone has a normal ratio of mineralized to nonmineralized (i.e., osteoid) matrix. Bone loss and eventually fractures are the hallmarks of osteoporosis, regardless of the underlying causes (Fig. 26-26). The etiology for bone loss is diverse but includes smoking, vitamin D deficiency, low body mass index, hypogonadism, a sedentary lifestyle and glucocorticoid therapy.

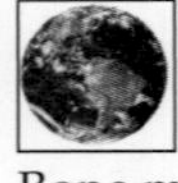

EPIDEMIOLOGY: Osteoporosis and its complications are huge public health problems that are expected to expand as life expectancy increases. Bone mass peaks in normal individuals between the ages of 25 and 35 and begins to decline in the fifth or sixth decade. Bone loss with age occurs in all races, but because of higher peak bone mass, blacks are less prone to osteoporosis than are Asians and whites. Bone loss during normal aging in women has been divided into two phases: menopause and aging. The latter affects men as well as women. At a certain point, the loss of bone suffices to justify the label **osteoporosis** and renders weight-bearing bones susceptible to fractures. The most common fractures occur in the neck and intertrochanteric region of the femur (**hip fracture**; Fig. 26-26), vertebral bodies and distal radius (**Colles fracture**). In whites in the United States, 15% of persons have had a hip fracture by the age of 80 years and 25% by age 90. Women have twice the risk of hip fracture as men, although among blacks and some Asian populations, the incidence is equal among the sexes. Compared with other osteoporotic fractures, hip fractures incur the greatest morbidity, mortality (up to 20% within a year) and direct medical costs. The female predominance of 8:1 is particularly striking for vertebral fractures. A subset of women in the early postmenopausal years is at particular risk of vertebral fractures, which are rare in middle-aged men. The propensity of men to sustain hip fractures as opposed to vertebral ones also reflects factors other than bone mass, such as loss of proprioception.

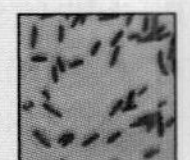 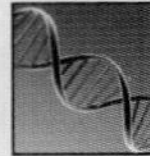

ETIOLOGIC FACTORS AND MOLECULAR PATHOGENESIS: *Regardless of the cause of osteoporosis, it always reflects enhanced bone resorption relative to formation.* Thus, this family of diseases should be viewed in the context of the remodeling cycle. Bone resorption and bone formation exist simultaneously. All osteoblasts and osteoclasts belong to a unique temporary structure, known as the **basic multicellular unit** (BMU or **bone remodeling unit**). The BMU is responsible for bone remodeling throughout life. Persons younger than 35 or 40 years completely replace bone resorbed during the remodeling cycle. With age, less bone is replaced in resorption bays than is removed, leading to a small deficit at each remodeling site. Given the thousands of remodeling sites in the skeleton, net bone loss, even in a short time, can be substantial.

Osteoporosis is classified as either primary or secondary. **Primary osteoporosis,** by far the more common variety, is of uncertain origin and occurs principally in postmenopausal women (type 1) and elderly persons of both sexes (type 2). **Secondary osteoporosis** is a disorder associated with a defined cause, including a variety of endocrine and genetic abnormalities.

Type 1 primary osteoporosis is due to an absolute increase in osteoclast activity. Since osteoclasts initiate bone remodeling, the number of remodeling sites increases in this state of enhanced osteoclast formation, a phenomenon known as **increased activation frequency.**

The increase in osteoclasts in the early postmenopausal skeleton is a direct result of estrogen withdrawal. The effects of lack of estrogen are not, however, targeted directly to the osteoclast, but rather to cells derived from marrow stroma, which secrete cytokines that recruit osteoclasts. These cytokines, which are believed to be estrogen sensitive, include IL-1 and IL-6, TNF and M-CSF.

Type 2 primary osteoporosis, also called **senile osteoporosis**, has a more complex pathogenesis than type 1. Type 2 osteoporosis generally appears after age 70 and reflects decreased osteoblast function. Thus, although osteoclast activity is no longer increased, the number of osteoblasts and amount of bone produced per cell are insufficient to replace bone removed in the resorptive phase of the remodeling cycle.

Primary Osteoporosis Is Caused by a Number of Factors

Primary osteoporosis has been linked to a number of factors that influence peak bone mass and the rate of bone loss:

- **Genetic factors:** Environmental factors and an individual's genotype both play a role in determining peak bone mass and risk of osteoporosis. The development of clinically significant osteoporosis is related, in largest part, to the maximal amount of bone in a given person, referred to as the **peak bone mass.** In general, peak bone mass is greater in men than in women and in blacks than in whites or Asians. There is a higher concordance of

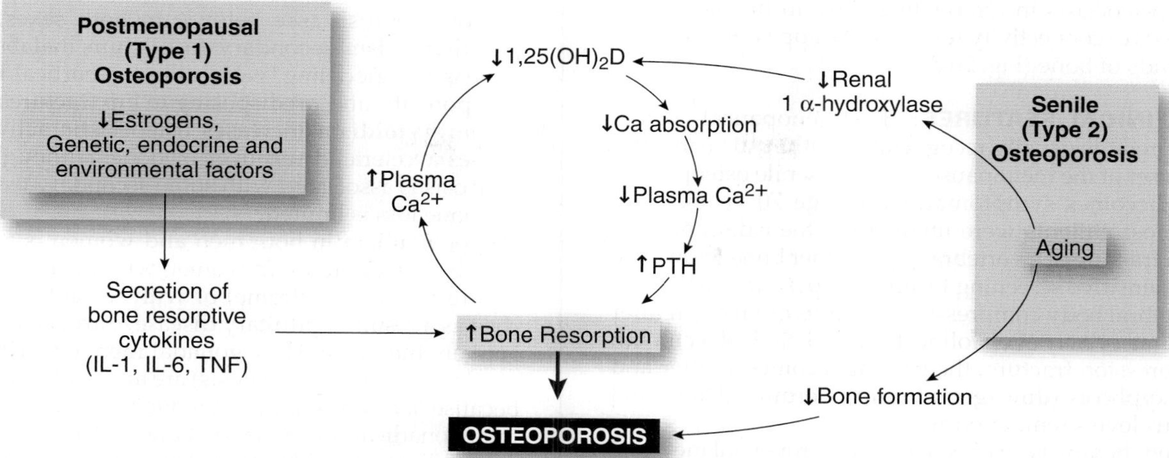

FIGURE 26-27. Pathogenesis of primary osteoporosis. Ca^{2+} = calcium; IL = interleukin; PTH = parathyroid hormone; TNF = tumor necrosis factor.

peak bone mass in monozygotic than in dizygotic twins. Women of reproductive age whose mothers have postmenopausal osteoporosis exhibit a lower bone mineral density (BMD) than do women in the general population. BMD is the most commonly used index for defining and studying osteoporosis. Genetic factors are thought to play an important role in regulating BMD. In fact, genetic variations explain as much as 70% of the variance in BMD. Sequence variance in the vitamin D receptor (VDR), *Col1A1* collagen gene, estrogen receptor-*a* (ESR1), IL-6 and low-density lipoprotein (LDL) receptor–related protein-5 (LRP5) are significantly associated with differences in BMD. Furthermore, VDR and IL-6 interact with environmental and hormonal factors (e.g., calcium intake, estrogen) to modulate BMD.

- **Calcium intake:** The average calcium intake of postmenopausal women in the United States is below the recommended value of 800 mg/d. However, whether this apparent shortfall contributes to development of osteoporosis is controversial, in view of a number of studies to the contrary. Nevertheless, it has been recommended that both premenopausal and postmenopausal women increase the intake of calcium and vitamin D.
- **Calcium absorption and vitamin D:** Calcium absorption by the intestine decreases with age. Because calcium absorption is largely under the control of vitamin D, attention has been directed to the role of this steroid hormone in osteoporosis. Compared with controls, persons with osteoporosis have lower circulating levels of 1,25-dihydroxyvitamin D, [$1,25(OH)_2D$], the active form of vitamin D that promotes calcium absorption in the intestine. This decrease has been attributed to age-related decreases in 1α-hydroxylase activity in the kidney. This enzyme catalyzes formation of $1,25(OH)_2D$. The lower 1α-hydroxylase activity has been attributed to diminished stimulation of the enzyme by parathyroid hormone (PTH), as well as an age-related decrease in responses of renal tubules to PTH. Interestingly, giving estrogens to postmenopausal women with osteoporosis increases both circulating $1,25(OH)_2D$ and calcium absorption. It has been suggested that decreased 1α-hydroxylase activity in the kidney may stimulate PTH secretion, thereby contributing to bone resorption.
- **Exercise:** Physical activity is necessary to maintain bone mass, and athletes often have increased bone mass. By contrast, immobilization of a bone (e.g., prolonged bed rest, application of a cast) leads to accelerated bone loss. The weightlessness of space flight results in severe bone loss (33% of trabecular bone mass in 25 weeks), and vigorous exercise in this setting does not seem to increase bone mass substantially or help prevent osteoporosis.
- **Environmental factors:** Cigarette smoking in women has been correlated with an increased incidence of osteoporosis. It is possible that the decreased level of active estrogens produced by smoking (see Chapter 8) is responsible for this effect.

In summary, the two major determinants of primary osteoporosis are estrogen deficiency in postmenopausal women and the aging process in both sexes. The possible mechanisms for these effects are summarized in Fig. 26-27.

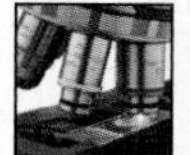

PATHOLOGY: ***The ratio of osteoid to mineralized bone is normal in persons with osteoporosis.*** Because of the abundance of cancellous bone in the spine, osteoporotic changes are generally most conspicuous there. In vertebral body fractures caused by osteoporosis, the vertebra is deformed, with anterior wedging and collapse. If the vertebral body is not fractured, there is a general outline of both endplates, with a virtual absence of cancellous bone.

Osteoporosis is characterized histologically by decreased thickness of the cortex and reduction in the number and size of trabeculae of the coarse cancellous bone. Whereas senile osteoporosis tends to feature reduced trabecular thickness, postmenopausal osteoporosis exhibits disrupted connections between trabeculae. The loss of trabecular connectivity, which is attended by diminished biomechanical strength and ultimately leads to fracture, is due to perforation of trabeculae by resorbing osteoclasts in remodeling sites. In histologic sections, the loss of connectivity results in the appearance of "isolated" islands of bone (Fig. 26-25).

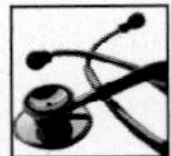

CLINICAL FEATURES: Postmenopausal osteoporosis is usually recognizable within 10 years after onset of the menopause, whereas senile osteoporosis generally becomes symptomatic after age 70 years. Until recently, most patients were unaware of their disease until they had a fracture of a vertebra, hip or other bone. However, the use of sensitive screening techniques permits early diagnosis. Vertebral body compression fractures often occur after trivial trauma or may even follow lifting a heavy object. With each compression fracture, the patient becomes shorter and develops kyphosis (**dowager's hump**). Serum calcium and phosphorus levels remain normal.

Estrogen therapy is an effective yet controversial means of preventing postmenopausal osteoporosis. Because hormone treatment carries with it increased risks of breast and endometrial cancers, other bone-specific antiosteoporotic drugs have been developed. **Bisphosphonates** are currently the most popular therapeutic agents used. All successful antiosteoporotic agents thus far developed block or slow the rate of bone resorption but do not stimulate bone formation. Thus, the drugs may prevent disease progression but cannot cure a patient who already has osteoporosis. Dietary calcium supplementation in elderly patients reduces the risk of osteoporotic fractures by half.

Secondary Osteoporosis Reflects Extraosseous Metabolic Disorders

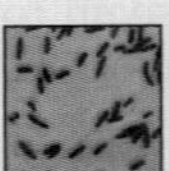
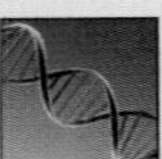

ETIOLOGIC FACTORS AND MOLECULAR PATHOGENESIS: Causes of secondary osteoporosis include adverse effects of drug therapy, endocrine disorders, eating disorders, immobilization, marrow-related disorders, disorders of the gastrointestinal or biliary tracts, renal disease and cancer.

- **Endocrine conditions:** The most common form of secondary osteoporosis is iatrogenic and results from corticosteroid administration. Bone loss may also result from an excess of endogenous glucocorticoids, as in Cushing disease (see Chapter 21). Corticosteroids inhibit osteoblastic activity, thereby reducing bone formation. They also impair vitamin D–dependent intestinal calcium absorption, an effect that leads to increased secretion of PTH and increased bone resorption.

  Estrogen is a key hormone for maintaining bone mass. Estrogen deficiency is the major cause of age-related bone loss in both sexes; estrogen deficiency or a low level of bioavailable estrogen decreases bone mass in elderly males. Its role in bone metabolism is focused on the role of proinflammatory cytokines: IL-1, IL-6, TNF-α, RANK-L, granulocyte-macrophage colony-stimulating factor (GM-CSF), M-CSF and prostaglandin E_2 (PGE_2). It is thought that these cytokines act upon both osteoclasts and osteoblasts via mediation by estrogen receptors.
- **Hyperparathyroidism** causes osteoclast recruitment and increased osteoclastic activity, resulting in secondary osteoporosis (see below). In both sexes, hyperparathyroidism secondary to calcium malabsorption increases remodeling, worsening the cortical thinning and porosity, and predisposing to hip fractures.
- **Hyperthyroidism** increases osteoclastic activity and causes accelerated turnover of bone. Although thyrotoxicosis is associated with some secondary osteoporosis, bone loss is limited.
- **Hypogonadism** in both men and women is accompanied by osteoporosis. In women with primary gonadal failure (Turner syndrome) or with secondary amenorrhea as a result of pituitary disease, estrogen deficiency is likely the cause. Hypogonadal men (e.g., Klinefelter syndrome, hemochromatosis) are at risk of osteoporosis because of a deficiency of anabolic androgens. Similarly, hypogonadism contributes to bone loss in 25% of elderly males. There is evidence of decreased bone density in androgen deprivation therapy for prostatic carcinoma.
- **Hematologic malignancies:** A variety of hematologic cancers, particularly multiple myeloma, are accompanied by significant bone loss. The malignant plasma cells of multiple myeloma secrete osteoclast-activating factor, which is presumably responsible for secondary osteoporosis. Some leukemias and lymphomas are also associated with osteoporosis. Even in the absence of skeletal metastases, some neoplasms (e.g., squamous cell carcinoma of lung) are associated with severe hypercalcemia due to bone resorption. Osteoclastic activity is enhanced in these patients, owing to secretion of PTH-related protein by the tumor (paraneoplastic syndrome).
- **Malabsorption:** Gastrointestinal and hepatic diseases that cause malabsorption often contribute to osteoporosis, probably because of impaired absorption of calcium, phosphate and vitamin D.
- **Alcoholism:** Chronic alcohol abuse also has been linked to development of osteoporosis. Alcohol is a direct inhibitor of osteoblasts and may also inhibit calcium absorption.

Osteomalacia and Rickets

Osteomalacia (soft bones) *is a disorder of adults characterized by inadequate mineralization of newly formed bone matrix.* **Rickets** *refers to a similar disorder in children, in whom the growth plates (physes) are open.* Thus, children with rickets manifest defective mineralization not only of bone (osteomalacia) but also of the cartilaginous matrix of the growth plate. Diverse conditions associated with osteomalacia and rickets include abnormalities in vitamin D metabolism, phosphate deficiency states and defects in the mineralization process itself.

Vitamin D Metabolism Influences Bone Mineralization

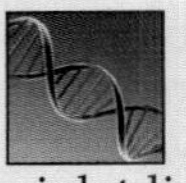

MOLECULAR PATHOGENESIS: Vitamin D is ingested in food or synthesized in the skin from 7-dehydrocholesterol under the influence of ultraviolet light (Fig. 26-28). The vitamin is first hydroxylated

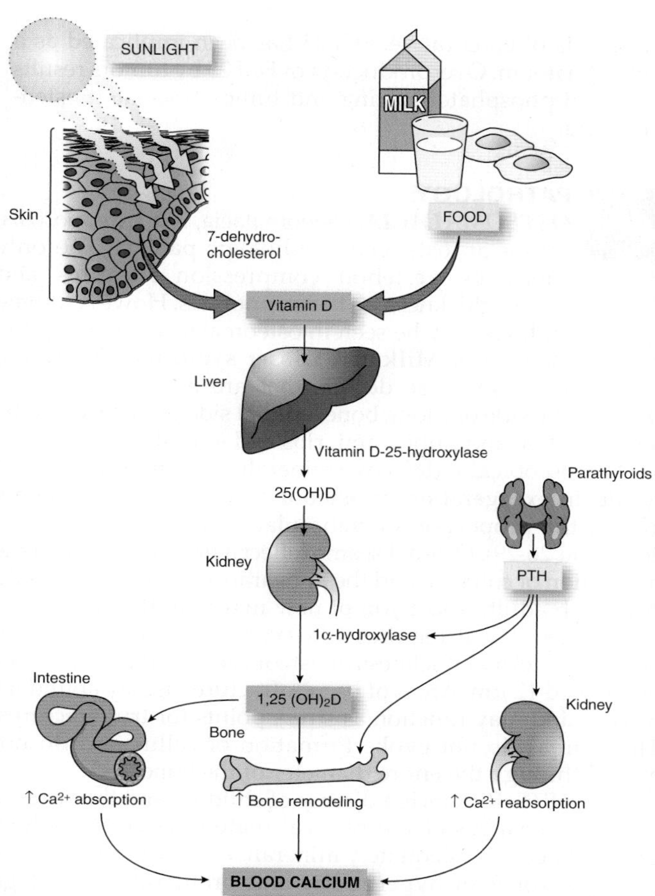

FIGURE 26-28. Metabolism of vitamin D and the regulation of blood calcium.

in the liver to form its major circulating metabolite, 25-hydroxyvitamin D, then hydroxylated again in proximal renal tubules to produce the active hormone $1,25(OH)_2D$. Exposure to sunlight provides sufficient vitamin D for bone growth and mineralization, even if there is an inadequate dietary source.

Receptors for $1,25(OH)_2D$ are present not only in classic targets, such as intestine, bone and kidney, but also in many other cell types. This hormone is a general inducer of differentiation, for example, influencing maturation of hematopoietic and dermal cells, as well as many cancers. In the intestine, $1,25(OH)_2D$ stimulates calcium and phosphate absorption. It is also essential for osteoclast maturation. Regardless of mechanism, $1,25(OH)_2D$, in concert with PTH, maintains blood calcium and phosphate at levels that are required for proper mineralization of bone. ***The key determinant of the formation of $1,25(OH)_2D$ is blood calcium concentration.*** Decreases in blood calcium stimulate release of PTH, which augments renal synthesis of $1,25(OH)_2D$.

Hypovitaminosis D can result from (1) inadequate exposure to sunlight, (2) deficient dietary intake or (3) defective intestinal absorption. There are also hereditary and acquired disorders of vitamin D metabolism.

Dietary Deficiency of Vitamin D and Inadequate Exposure to Sunlight Cause Rickets

Rickets plagued children of the industrial cities of the United States and Europe from the 17th century through the 19th century. Of urban children in these regions, about 85% had rickets. These children had insufficient sun exposure, and their dietary intake of vitamin D was inadequate to avert hypovitaminosis D. Use of vitamin D–rich cod liver oil and later fortification of milk and other foods with vitamin D effectively ended widespread rickets in Western countries. However, nutritional vitamin D deficiency remains a problem elsewhere in the world, in neglected elderly persons and food faddists.

Intestinal Malabsorption Decreases the Availability of Vitamin D

In industrialized countries, diseases associated with intestinal malabsorption cause osteomalacia more often than does poor nutrition. ***Intrinsic diseases of the small intestine, cholestatic disorders of the liver, biliary obstruction and chronic pancreatic insufficiency are the most frequent causes of osteomalacia in the United States.***

Malabsorption of vitamin D and calcium complicates a number of small-intestinal diseases, including celiac disease, Crohn disease, scleroderma and the postsurgical blind-loop syndrome. In obstructive jaundice, the lack of bile salts in the intestine impairs absorption of lipids and lipid-soluble substances, among which is fat-soluble vitamin D. Furthermore, hydroxylation of vitamin D is reduced with severe liver damage. Oddly, biliary cirrhosis, a disease characterized by intestinal malabsorption and vitamin D deficiency, leads to osteoporosis rather than osteomalacia. Thus, vitamin D is essential not only for mineralization but also for the synthesis of bone collagen.

Disorders of Vitamin D Metabolism Are Inherited or Acquired

Vitamin D metabolism can be disturbed either by defective 1α-hydroxylation of vitamin D in the kidney or by insensitivity of the target organ to $1,25(OH)_2D$. Two autosomal recessive diseases associated with rickets are together known as **vitamin D–dependent rickets.**

- **Vitamin D–dependent rickets type I** results from an inherited deficiency of renal 1α-hydroxylase activity. The clinical and biochemical changes of rickets appear during the first year of life, and these children exhibit hypocalcemia, hypophosphatemia and high levels of serum PTH and alkaline phosphatase. The disease is controlled by the administration of $1,25(OH)_2D$.
- **Vitamin D–dependent rickets type II** involves inherited mutations of the vitamin D receptor, so that end organs are insensitive to $1,25(OH)_2D$. The disease usually manifests early in life but may appear at any time up to adolescence. Serum concentrations of $1,25(OH)_2D$ are very high. Patients do not respond to $1,25(OH)_2D$ but are helped by repeated intravenous administration of calcium.
- **Acquired alterations in vitamin D metabolism** include defective renal 1α-hydroxylation and end-organ

insensitivity. Some of the causes of impaired α-hydroxylation are hypoparathyroidism, tumor-induced osteomalacia, chronic renal diseases and osteomalacia of old age. Osteomalacia occasionally complicates the treatment of epilepsy with anticonvulsant drugs, particularly phenobarbital and phenytoin. It is believed that these drugs block the action of 1,25(OH)$_2$D on target organs.

Renal Disorders of Phosphate Metabolism Interfere With Vitamin D Metabolism

Both rickets and osteomalacia may result from impaired reabsorption of phosphate by the proximal renal tubules, with resulting hypophosphatemia.

MOLECULAR PATHOGENESIS:
X-LINKED HYPOPHOSPHATEMIA: This condition, also termed **vitamin D–resistant rickets** or **phosphate diabetes,** is the most common type of hereditary rickets and is inherited as a dominant trait. Mutations in the *PHEX* (phosphate-regulating) gene on the X chromosome (Xp22) impair transport of phosphate across the luminal membrane of proximal renal tubular cells. The gene product of *PHEX* is a protease that inactivates fibroblast growth factor-23 (FGF23). Increased levels of FGF23 produced renal phosphate wasting. Renal phosphate wasting is central to the disease, but osteoblast function is also impaired. In boys, florid rickets appears during childhood, but girls often suffer only hypophosphatemia. Treatment is with lifelong administration of phosphate and 1,25(OH)$_2$D. Microscopically, the bones of patients with X-linked hypophosphatemia show severe osteomalacia and wide osteoid seams. They also exhibit characteristic hypomineralized areas surrounding osteocytes, known as **halos.** The presence of these structures indicates that osteocytes are responsible for the terminal mineralization of bone.

FANCONI SYNDROMES: These inborn errors of metabolism are characterized by renal wastage of phosphate, glucose, bicarbonate and amino acids. They are all characterized by renal tubular acidosis and lead to rickets and osteomalacia. Fanconi syndromes include Wilson disease, tyrosinemia, galactosemia, glycogen storage disease and cystinosis. Renal tubular damage that leads to phosphate wastage may also be acquired, as in lead or mercury intoxication, amyloidosis and Bence-Jones proteinuria.

TUMOR-ASSOCIATED OSTEOMALACIA: This disorder is a phosphate-wasting syndrome that is associated with predominantly benign and occasionally malignant tumors of soft tissue and bone. The typical laboratory features are hypophosphatemia, hyperphosphaturia, low serum concentrations of 1,25-(OH)$_2$D and elevated serum alkaline phosphatase. Oncogenic osteomalacia mimics the clinical phenotype of X-linked hypophosphatemia and autosomal dominant hypophosphatemia. The paraneoplastic phosphaturic factors secreted by the tumor, known as **phosphatonins,** cause renal tubular phosphate wasting and prevent tubular conversion of 25-hydroxyvitamin D into 1,25(OH)$_2$D. Phosphatonins thus appear to have the same effect as inherited mutations of the *PHEX* gene seen in X-linked hypophosphatemia. Removal of the primary tumor is often curative. FGF23 has been implicated as a phosphatonin. Overproduction of FGF23 by tumors results in renal phosphate wasting and tumor-associated osteomalacia.

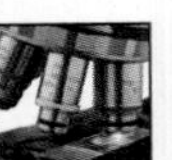

PATHOLOGY:
OSTEOMALACIA: Osteomalacia, like osteoporosis, causes an osteopenic radiologic pattern. The only findings may be vertebral compression fractures and decreased bone thickness, as in osteoporosis. However, some specific findings may be seen in osteomalacia, including the pseudofractures of **Milkman-Looser syndrome.** These are radiolucent transverse defects that are most common on the concave side of a long bone, medial side of the neck of the femur, ischial and pubic rami, ribs and scapula.

Microscopically, defective mineralization in osteomalacia results in **exaggeration of osteoid seams,** both in thickness and in the proportion of trabecular surface covered (Figs. 26-25 and 26-29). Osteoid seams reflect a time lag between the deposition of collagen and the appearance of the calcium salt. Although adults add 1 μm of new matrix to the surfaces of bone every day, it requires 10 days to mineralize this new bone. The normal thickness of osteoid seams, therefore, does not exceed 12 μm. Areas of pseudofracture display abundant osteoid and may function as stress points for true fractures. These areas do not evoke formation of callus and do not extend through the entire diameter of the bone.

RICKETS: Rickets is a disease of children and thus causes extensive changes at the physeal plate (Fig. 26-30), which does not become adequately mineralized. The calcified cartilage and zones of hypertrophy and proliferative cartilage continue to grow because osteoclastic activity does not resorb the cartilage growth plate. As a consequence, the growth plate is conspicuously thickened, irregular and lobulated. Endochondral ossification proceeds very slowly and preferentially at the peripheral portions of the metaphysis. The result is a flared, cup-shaped epiphysis. The largest part of the primary spongiosum is composed of lamellar or woven bone that, importantly, remains unmineralized.

Microscopically, the growth plate exhibits striking changes. The resting zone is normal, but the zones of proliferating

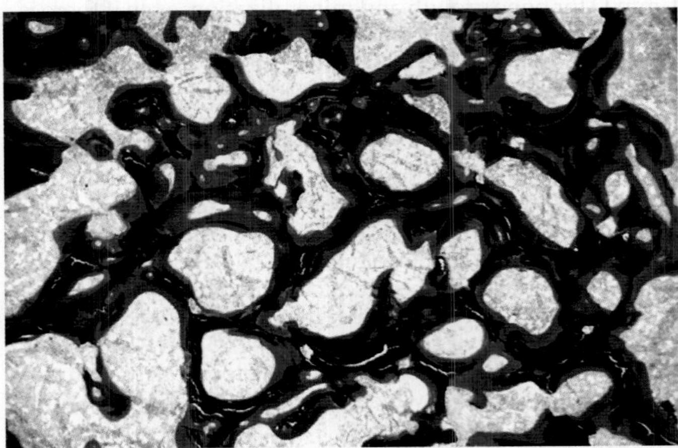

FIGURE 26-29. Osteomalacia. The surfaces of the bony trabeculae (*black*) are covered by a thicker than normal layer of osteoid (*red*) with the von Kossa stain, which colors calcified tissue black.

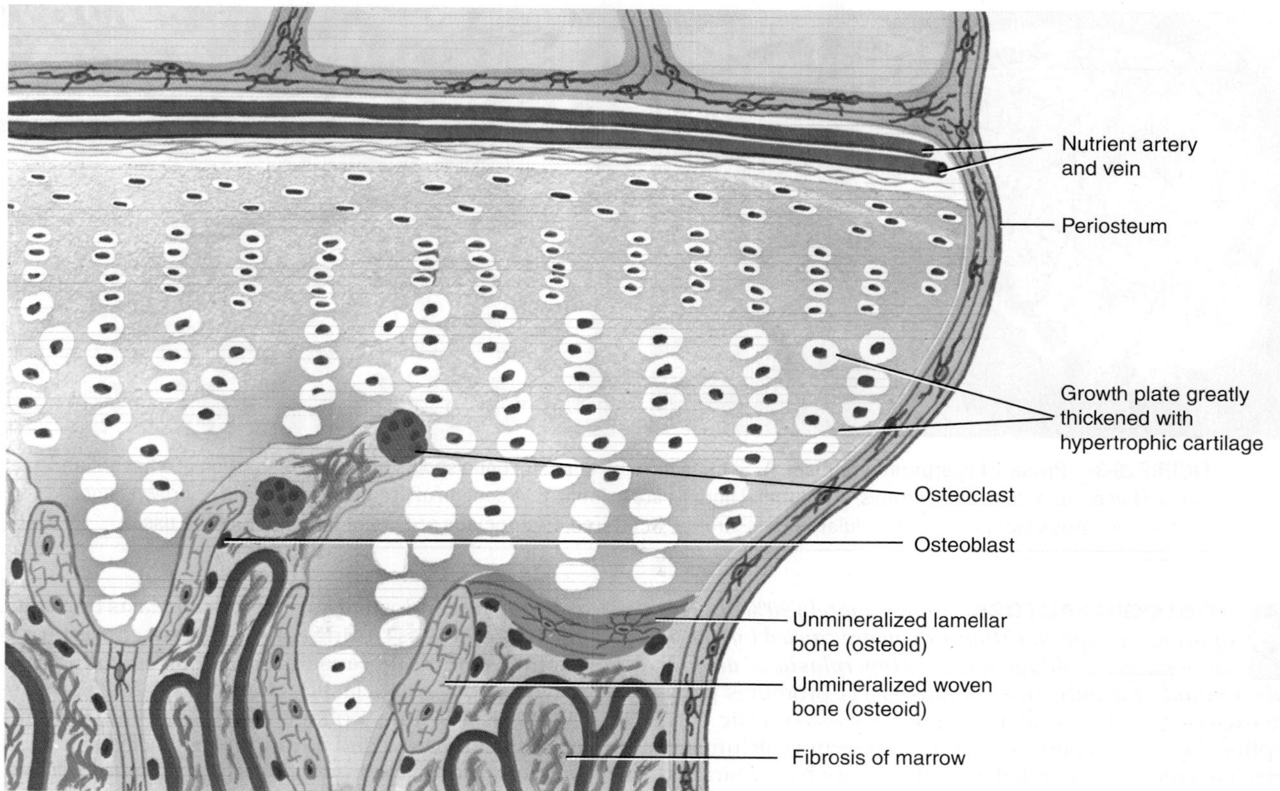

FIGURE 26-30. The growth plate in rickets. The growth plate is thickened and disorganized, with a large zone of hypertrophic cartilage cells. Irregular perforation of the cartilage plate by osteoclasts occurs because there is little calcified cartilage. The woven bone on the surface of some of the primary trabeculae is unmineralized and therefore easily fractured. Such microfractures often lead to hemorrhage at the interface between the plate and the metaphysis.

cartilage are greatly distorted. The ordered progression of helix-forming chondrocytes is lost and is replaced by a disorderly profusion of cells separated by small amounts of matrix. Resulting lobulated masses of proliferating and hypertrophied cartilage are associated with increasing width of the growth plate, which may be 5 to 15 times the normal width. The zone of provisional calcification is poorly defined, and only a minimal amount of primary spongiosum is formed. Masses of proliferating cartilage extend into the metaphyseal region, without any apparent vascular invasion and with little osteoclastic activity.

CLINICAL FEATURES:

OSTEOMALACIA: Clinical diagnosis of osteomalacia is often difficult. Patients have nonspecific complaints, such as muscle weakness or diffuse aches and pains. In mild forms of the disease, only slowly progressive changes in bone are seen, and many patients are totally asymptomatic for years. In advanced cases, poorly localized bone pain and tenderness are common, especially in the spine, pelvis and proximal parts of the extremities. In such cases, the diagnosis may be made only after an acute fracture, the most common sites being the femoral neck, pubic ramus, spine or ribs. Muscular weakness and hypotonia lead to a waddling gait in severe cases, and some patients are unable to walk.

RICKETS: Children with rickets are apathetic and irritable and have short attention spans. They are content to be sedentary, assuming a "Buddha-like" posture. They are short, with characteristic changes of bones and teeth. Flattening of the skull, prominent frontal bones (**frontal bossing**) and conspicuous suture lines are typical. There is delayed dentition, with severe dental caries and enamel defects. The chest has the classic **rachitic rosary** (a grossly beaded appearance of the costochondral junctions due to enlargement of the costal cartilages) and indentations of the lower ribs at the insertion of the diaphragm. **Pectus carinatum** ("pigeon breast") reflects an outward curvature of the sternum.

The overall musculature is weak, and abdominal weakness leads to a "potbelly." The limbs are shortened and deformed, with severe bowing of the arms and forearms, and frequent fractures. The femoral head may dislocate from the growth plate (slipped capital femoral epiphysis).

Primary Hyperparathyroidism

Primary hyperparathyroidism is a metabolic bone disease characterized by generalized bone resorption due to inappropriate secretion of PTH. Early in the 20th century, bone disease in patients diagnosed with primary hyperparathyroidism was often advanced and crippling. Owing to screening of hospitalized patients for abnormalities of serum calcium, severe primary hyperparathyroidism is rarely encountered and clinically significant bone disease is unusual.

The histologic changes of primary hyperparathyroidism are known as **osteitis fibrosa.** This term applies to all circumstances of markedly accelerated bone remodeling and may be seen in Paget disease, in hyperthyroidism and even in some patients with postmenopausal osteoporosis.

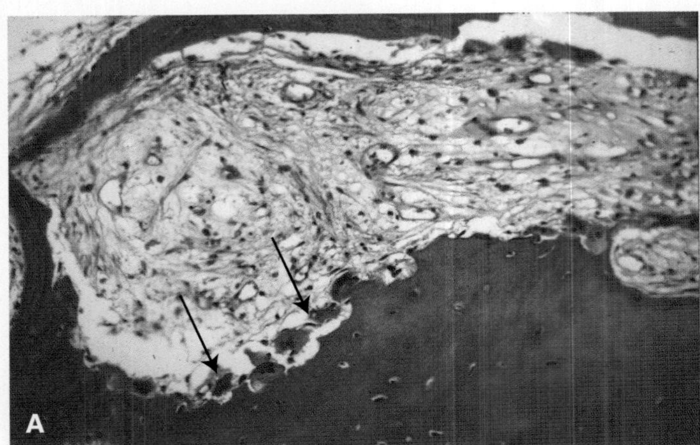

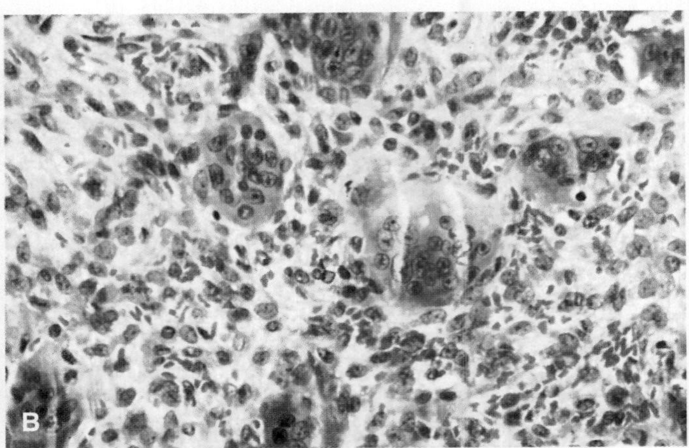

FIGURE 26-31. Primary hyperparathyroidism. A. Section through compact bone shows tunneling resorption of a haversian canal. Numerous osteoclasts (*arrows*) and stromal fibrosis are evident. **B.** A section of tissue obtained from a "brown tumor" reveals numerous giant cells in a cellular fibrous stroma. Scattered erythrocytes are present throughout the tissue.

ETIOLOGIC FACTORS: *Approximately 90% of cases of primary hyperparathyroidism are caused by one or more parathyroid adenomas. Hyperplasia of all four glands accounts for only 10%.* Because PTH promotes phosphate excretion in the urine and stimulates osteoclastic bone resorption, low serum phosphate and high serum calcium levels are characteristic. A familial type of primary hyperparathyroidism is associated with mutations in the calcium-sensing receptor (*CASR*) gene, located on chromosome 3 (3q13.3).

The effects of PTH are mediated by its effects on bone, kidney and (indirectly) intestine.

BONE: PTH mobilizes calcium from bone (the major reservoir of calcium in the body) by causing increased osteoclasis by extant osteoclasts and by recruitment of new osteoclasts from pre-osteoclastic histiocytic cells. This action is indirect and is mediated by direct stimulation of osteoblasts by PTH, causing them to synthesize and secrete RANK-L, which then binds to RANK in osteoclasts and osteoclast precursors and results in bone resorption. Under physiologic circumstances, PTH secretion is shut down by increases in ionic calcium and the osteoblast stimulation by PTH tends to cause balanced remodeling and does not cause a net loss of bone mass. Under pathologic conditions, the release of large amounts of PTH and continued RANK-L secretion prevents osteoclast apoptosis, prolongs osteoclast life and activation and results in a net loss of bone mass.

KIDNEY: PTH stimulates reabsorption of calcium by the thick ascending and granular portions of the distal renal tubules. It also enhances phosphate excretion in the proximal and distal convoluted tubules by directly inhibiting sodium-dependent phosphate transport. PTH also augments the activity of 1α-hydroxylase in the proximal tubules, thereby stimulating production of 1,25$(OH)_2$D.

INTESTINE: PTH does not act directly on the intestine, but rather enhances intestinal calcium absorption indirectly by increasing renal synthesis of 1,25$(OH)_2$D.

PATHOLOGY: The histogenesis of osteitis fibrosa may be classified into three stages:

- **Early stage:** Initially, osteoclasts are stimulated by the increased PTH levels to resorb bone. From the subperiosteal and endosteal surfaces, osteoclasts bore their way into the cortex as cutting cones. This process is termed **dissecting osteitis** because each osteon is continually hollowed out by osteoclastic activity (Figs. 26-25 and 26-31A). At the same time, collagen fibers are laid down in the endosteal marrow and additional osteoclasts penetrate the bone. In contrast to myelofibrosis of hematologic origin, in which fibrous tissue is randomly distributed in the marrow space, the collagen of osteitis fibrosa is deposited adjacent to trabeculae. This observation suggests that the stromal cells depositing matrix material are osteoblast precursors.
- **Osteitis fibrosa:** In the second stage, the trabecular bone is resorbed and marrow is replaced by loose fibrosis, hemosiderin-laden macrophages, areas of hemorrhage from microfractures and reactive woven bone. These features constitute the "osteitis fibrosa" portion of the complex.
- **Osteitis fibrosa cystica:** As primary hyperparathyroidism progresses and hemorrhage continues, cystic degeneration ultimately occurs, leading to the final stage of the disease. The areas of fibrosis that contain reactive woven bone and hemosiderin-laden macrophages often display many osteoclast giant cells. Because of its macroscopic appearance, this lesion has been termed a **brown tumor** (Fig. 26-31B). This is not a neoplasm, but rather a repair reaction as an end stage of hyperparathyroidism.

The skeletal radiographs of most persons with primary hyperparathyroidism are normal. Some patients exhibit mottled bone cortices, with an irregular frayed surface in the outer table of the skull, tufts of the terminal digits and shafts of the metacarpals (Fig. 26-32). A distinctive radiologic peculiarity, referred to as **subperiosteal bone resorption,** is evident in the subperiosteal outer surface of the cortex and reflects dissecting osteitis. Resorption around tooth sockets causes the lamina dura of the teeth to disappear, a well-known finding on radiography.

A classic feature of osteitis fibrosa cystica is the presence of multiple, localized, lytic lesions, which represent hemorrhagic cysts or masses of fibrous tissue. These eccentric and well-demarcated lesions are separated from the soft tissue by a periosteal shell of bone. The focal, tumor-like, lytic lesions always occur in the context of an abnormal skeleton produced

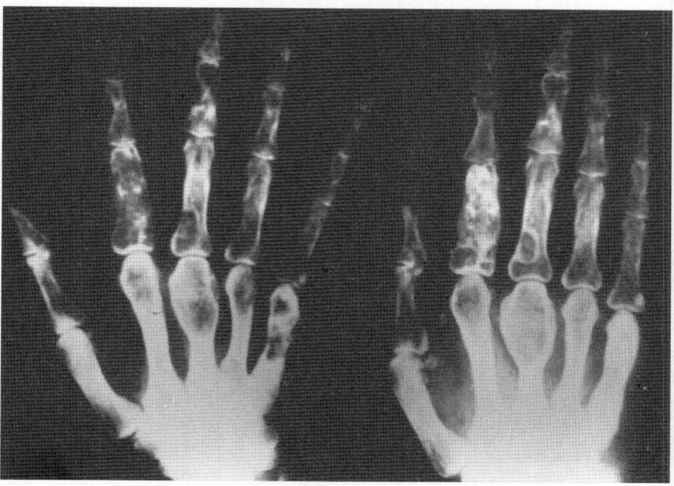

FIGURE 26-32. Primary hyperparathyroidism. A radiograph of the hands reveals bulbous swellings ("brown tumors") and numerous cavities, both representing bone resorption.

by hyperparathyroidism. If a single lesion is examined in isolation, it may be mistaken for a primary giant cell neoplasm of bone.

CLINICAL FEATURES: The symptoms of primary hyperparathyroidism are related to the abnormality of calcium homeostasis and have been summarized as "stones, bones, moans and groans." The "stones" refer to kidney stones and the "bones" to the skeletal changes. The "moans" describe psychiatric depression and other abnormalities associated with hypercalcemia and the "groans" characterize the gastrointestinal irregularities associated with a high serum calcium level.

Primary hyperparathyroidism is treated by surgical removal of the parathyroid adenomas. If parathyroid hyperplasia is the cause of the disease, three and a half glands are usually removed. The remaining fragment suffices to ensure that the patient does not develop hypocalcemia. After surgery, the histologic appearance of the affected skeleton gradually normalizes.

Renal Osteodystrophy

Renal osteodystrophy is a complex metabolic bone disease that occurs in the context of chronic renal failure. Severe renal osteodystrophy is most common in patients maintained on long-term dialysis, because they live long enough to develop conspicuous bone disease.

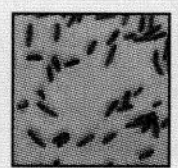
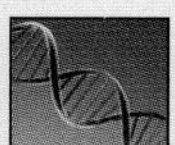

ETIOLOGIC FACTORS AND MOLECULAR PATHOGENESIS: The pathogenesis of renal osteodystrophy is similar to that of osteomalacia, with secondary hyperparathyroidism exerting its influence by way of osteoclastic bone resorption (Fig. 26-25). The development of renal osteodystrophy may be summarized as follows:

1. In chronic renal disease, a reduced glomerular filtration rate leads to retention of phosphate, thereby producing **hyperphosphatemia.** High serum phosphate levels drive down the serum calcium levels.
2. Tubular injury reduces 1α-hydroxylase activity, with a resulting deficiency of $1{,}25(OH)_2D$.
3. Intestinal calcium absorption is, in turn, decreased, worsening the **hypocalcemia.**
4. Hypocalcemia stimulates **PTH production.** In fact, most patients with end-stage renal disease have substantial hyperparathyroidism. However, PTH does not effectively promote intestinal calcium absorption or renal tubular resorption of calcium because of failure to produce adequate $1{,}25(OH)_2D$.
5. Perhaps because of hyperparathyroidism and hyperphosphatemia, a substantial proportion of patients with end-stage renal disease have increased bone mass. Renal osteosclerosis is particularly prominent in vertebrae where, owing to alternating bands of radiopaque and normally dense bone, the lesion is named "rugger jersey spine."
6. Osteomalacia may result from the disturbances of vitamin D pathway or from aluminum deposition at the mineralization front of bones. Aluminum negatively affects bone formation through inhibition of osteoblastic activity, as well as hydroxyapatite crystal formation (bone mineralization). Aluminum is present in dialysate solutions or aluminum-containing phosphate-binding agents used to combat the hyperphosphatemia of renal failure.

The **adynamic variant of renal osteodystrophy (ARO)** is characterized by arrested bone remodeling. More than 40% of adults who are treated with hemodialysis and more than 50% of those who are treated with peritoneal dialysis have bone biopsy evidence of ARO. Adynamic bone is characterized microscopically by an overall reduction in cellular activity in bone, with fewer or absent osteoblasts and osteoclasts. These changes can be due to either direct inhibitory effects of systemic factors on osteoblast function or indirect changes in osteoblast activity mediated through PTH-dependent mechanisms. Old bone accumulates because it is not remodeled, thereby leading to structural compromise of the skeleton and increased tendency to fractures.

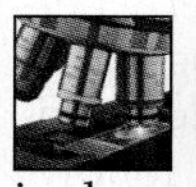
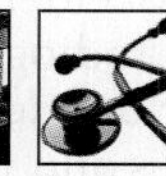

PATHOLOGY AND CLINICAL FEATURES: As a result of these effects of chronic renal failure, renal osteodystrophy is characterized by varying degrees of osteitis fibrosa, osteomalacia, osteosclerosis and adynamic bone disease (Fig. 26-33). Combinations of osteitis fibrosa and osteomalacia are particularly common. Hyperphosphatemic patients with terminal chronic renal disease may display metastatic calcification at various sites, including the eyes, skin, muscular coats of arteries and arterioles and periarticular soft tissues.

Management of renal osteodystrophy involves not only treatment of renal failure but also control of phosphate levels by appropriate drug therapy and infusions. Occasionally, parathyroidectomy is required to control hyperparathyroidism and the administration of vitamin D may also be necessary.

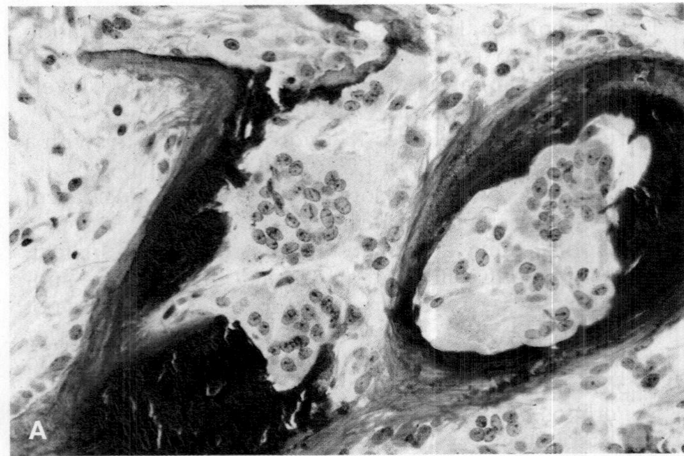

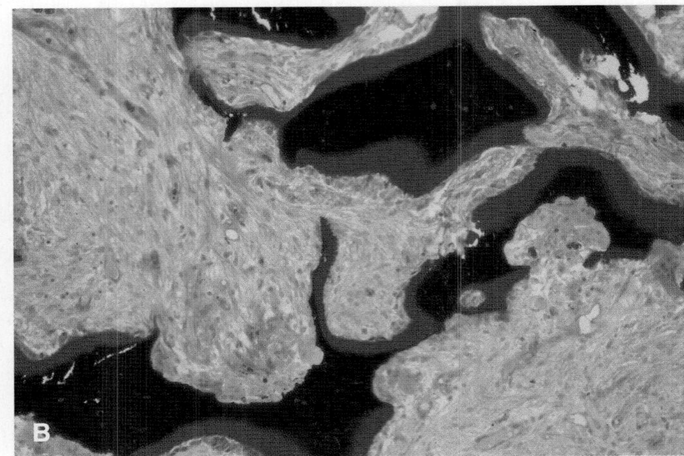

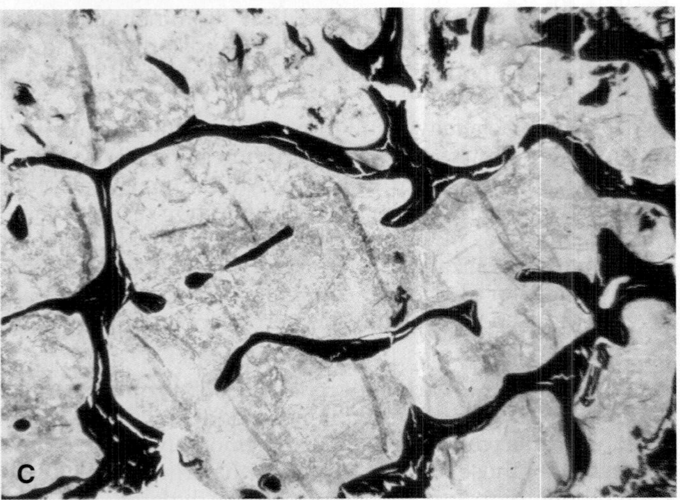

FIGURE 26-33. Renal osteodystrophy. A. Osteitis fibrosa. Several large multinucleated osteoclasts are resorbing these bone spicules, and the paraosseous tissue is fibrotic. Note that the osteoclastic resorption takes place only on the mineralized (*blue*) portions of the trabeculae. In this undecalcified section, the unmineralized bone (osteoid) appears *red*. **B. Osteomalacia.** This is a von Kossa stain prepared on an undecalcified section. The mineralized bone is *black* and the abundant osteoid appears *magenta*. Osteoid is thick and lines a large proportion of the bone surfaces. Surfaces not covered by the osteoid demonstrate scalloped Howship lacunae and contain abundant osteoclasts. **C. Adynamic bone disease** in which remodeling is attenuated, with a paucity of osteoblasts, osteoclasts and osteoid (von Kossa stain).

Paget Disease of Bone

Paget disease is a chronic condition characterized by lesions of bone resulting from disordered remodeling, in which excessive bone resorption initially results in lytic lesions, to be followed by disorganized and excessive bone formation.

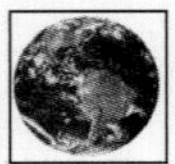

EPIDEMIOLOGY: Paget disease is common and generally affects men and women older than 50 years. In predisposed populations, 3% of elderly persons manifest the disease at autopsy or on radiographic examination. The disorder has an unusual worldwide distribution, afflicting populations of the British Isles and following their migrations throughout the world. Persons of English descent living in the United States, Australia, New Zealand and Canada have a high incidence of the disease. Northern Europeans have more Paget disease than southern Europeans. The disorder is almost nonexistent in Asia and in the indigenous populations of Africa and South America. For unknown reasons the incidence of Paget disease appears to have decreased worldwide over the last several decades.

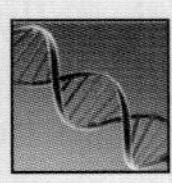

MOLECULAR PATHOGENESIS: Sir James Paget coined the term **osteitis deformans** for this disease over a century ago, but until recently its etiology has been obscure. Paget disease resembles a metabolic disease histologically and there is a slight increase in bone turnover in affected patients, but its clinical tendency to involve one bone or only a few bones does not fulfill the definition of a metabolic disorder.

A hereditary predisposition has been suggested by reports of almost 100 families in which Paget disease is generally transmitted as an autosomal dominant trait with incomplete penetrance that increases with age. There is evolving evidence that Paget disease and some related diseases are caused by mutations in genes encoding proteins in the RANK signaling pathway. Specifically, mutations in *Sequestosome 1* (*SQSTM1*) have been found in familial and sporadic forms of Paget disease. The *SQSTM1* gene encodes a protein also known as p62, which may act as a scaffold protein in the RANK signaling pathway. It is currently unknown how this mutated protein leads to accelerated osteoclast activity. Inactivation of *SQSTM1* causes defects in RANKL-induced osteoclastogenesis, indicating a significant role of p62 in osteoclast function.

Some evidence indicates that Paget disease is of viral origin. Virtually all patients exhibit nuclear inclusions consistent with the structure of a virus in osteoclasts and osteoclast precursors, which are not found in any other skeletal disease other than giant cell tumors of bone. They consist of microfilaments in a paracrystalline array and have been compared with the inclusions in the brains of patients with subacute sclerosing encephalitis (see Chapter 28). This similarity has suggested that a slow virus may be involved (Fig. 26-34). Support for this hypothesis has come from the finding that the marrow of Paget disease patients contains paramyxovirus nucleocapsid transcripts. Infection of osteoclast precursor cells with paramyxovirus can increase expression of RANK and thereby increase osteoclastic activity. In addition, paramyxoviruses stimulate osteoblasts to produce IL-6, which contributes to osteoclastogenesis. Although a viral etiology seems plausible, actual live viruses have not been isolated from pagetic bone, and it is difficult to explain monostotic bone involvement by a systemic viral infection.

Overall, Paget disease is characterized by localized increases in osteoclast formation that lead to bone resorption and associated osteoblastic activity. The increased osteoclastogenic nature of the bone microenvironment is mediated by increases in IL-6 and the RANK signaling pathway. These are perturbed in Paget disease as a result of genetic factors such as *SQSTM1* mutations and possibly a slow virus infection that may serve as a catalyst for developing the pagetic phenotype in genetically predisposed individuals. The result is uncoupling of the normal osteoclast/osteoblast remodeling unit.

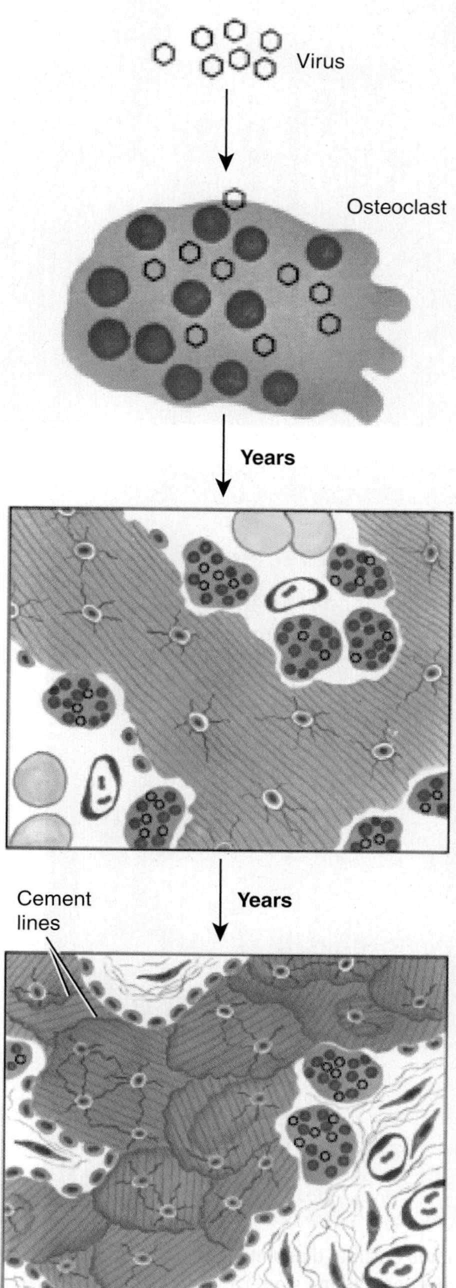

FIGURE 26-34. Hypothetical viral etiology of Paget disease of bone. A virus infects osteoclastic progenitors or osteoclasts in a genetically predisposed individual and stimulates osteoclastic activity, thereby leading to excessive resorption of bone. Over a period of years, the bone develops a characteristic mosaic pattern, produced by chaotically juxtaposed units of lamellar bone that form irregular cement lines. The adjacent marrow is often fibrotic, and there is a mixture of osteoclasts and osteoblasts on the surface of the bone.

PATHOLOGY: The lesions of Paget disease may be solitary or may occur at multiple sites. They tend to localize to the bones of the axial skeleton, including the spine, skull and pelvis. The proximal femur and tibia may also be involved in the polyostotic form of the disease. Solitary Paget disease rarely involves the humerus, but in polyostotic disease, lesions involving this bone are common.

Paget disease is an example of bone remodeling gone awry. The disease is triphasic:

1. **"Hot" or osteoclastic resorptive stage:** Radiologically, there is a characteristic, sharply defined, flame-shaped or wedge-shaped lysis of the cortex, which may mimic a tumor (Fig. 26-35A). Histologically, there is widespread **osteolysis** with marked osteoclastic resorption, marrow fibrosis and dilation of marrow sinusoids.
2. **Mixed stage of osteoblastic and osteoclastic activity:** By radiography, the bones are larger than normal. In fact, Paget disease is one of only two diseases that produce **larger than normal bones** (the other is fibrous dysplasia, discussed below). The cortex in the mixed phase is thickened, and the accentuation of the coarse cancellous bone makes the bone look heavy and enlarged (Fig. 26-35B,C). Involvement of vertebral bodies leads to a "picture frame" appearance (Fig. 26-35D), as cortices and endplates become greatly exaggerated compared with the coarse cancellous bone of the vertebral body. Although the bone is abnormal, the distorted, coarse cancellous bone and cortex still tend to align along stress lines. The pelvis is often thickened in the area of the acetabulum. Histologically, there is evidence of both increased osteoclastic and osteoblastic activity (Fig. 26-36).
3. **"Cold" or burnt-out stage:** This period is characterized histologically by little cellular activity and radiologically by thickened and disordered bones.

The disease need not progress through all three stages, and in polyostotic disease, various foci may appear in different stages.

The osteoclast is the pathologic cell of Paget disease, and its appearance is characteristic. Whereas normal osteoclasts contain fewer than a dozen nuclei, those of Paget disease are

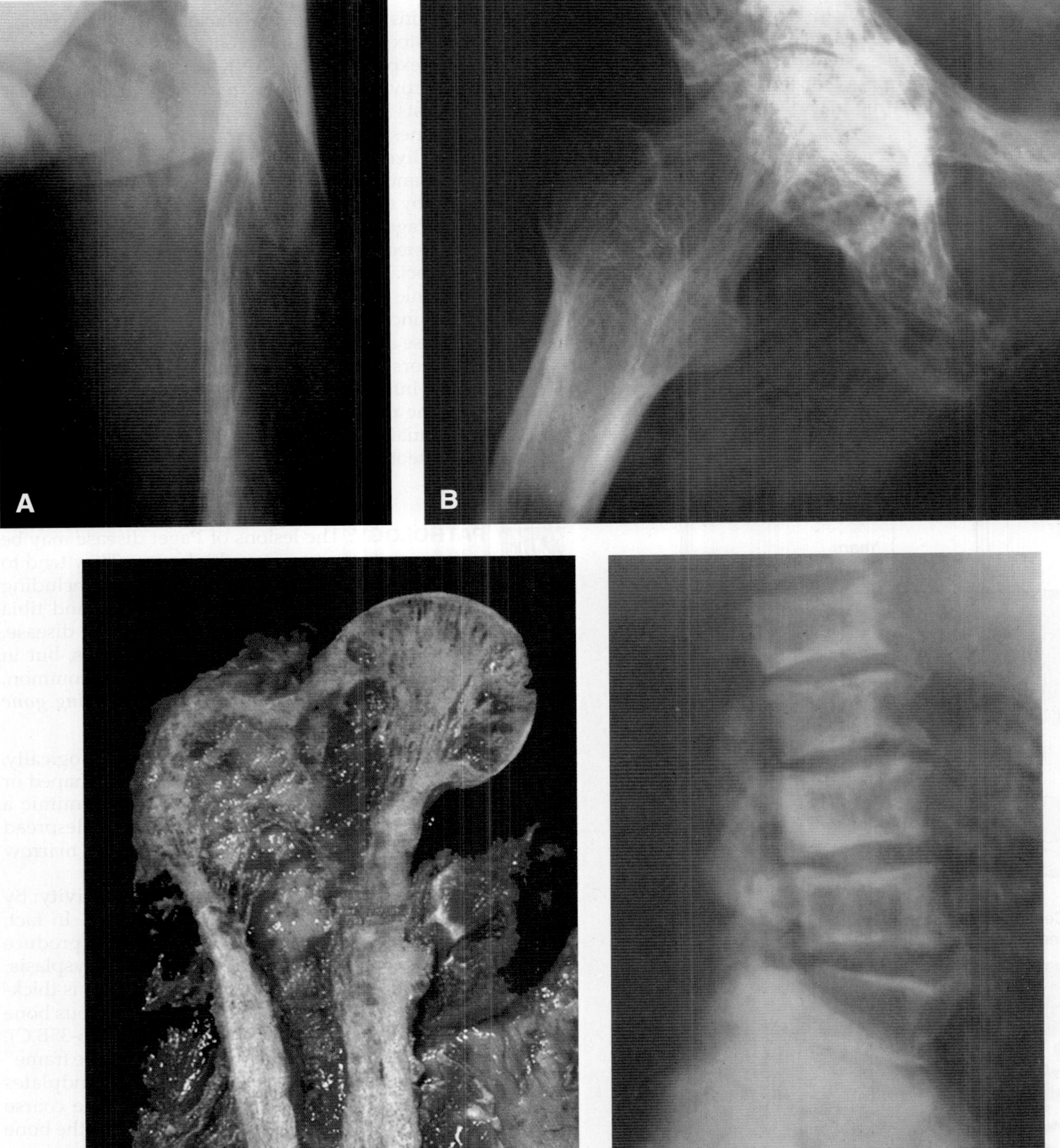

FIGURE 26-35. Paget disease. A. A radiograph of early Paget disease shows cortical dissolution, increased diameter of the diaphysis and an advancing, wedge-shaped area of cortical resorption ("flame sign"). Proximal to the edge of this wedge, the femur appears entirely normal. **B.** Later, Paget disease of the proximal femur and pelvis shows cortical disorganization and irregular coarse trabeculations. **C.** Gross specimen of proximal femur showing cortical thickening and coarse trabeculations of the femoral head and neck. **D.** Paget disease of the spine shows shortening and widening of the lumbar vertebral bodies. Their cortices and endplates are thickened and have a "picture-frame" appearance.

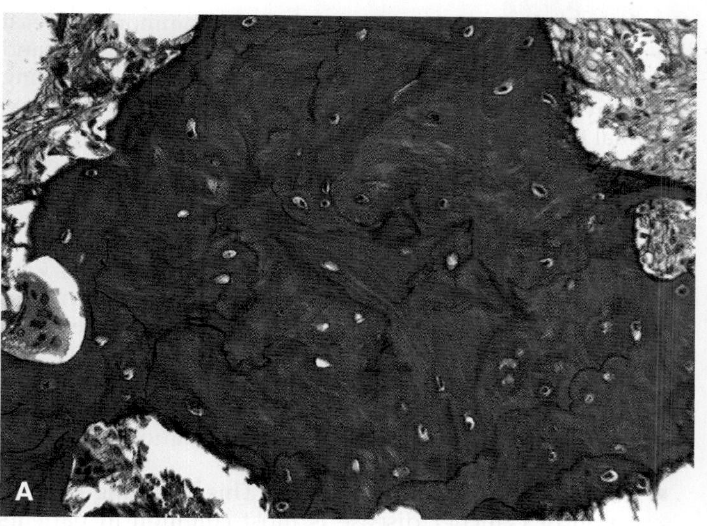

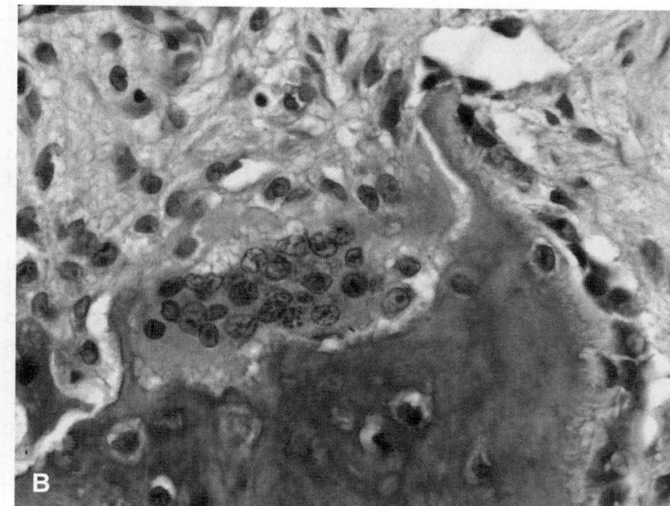

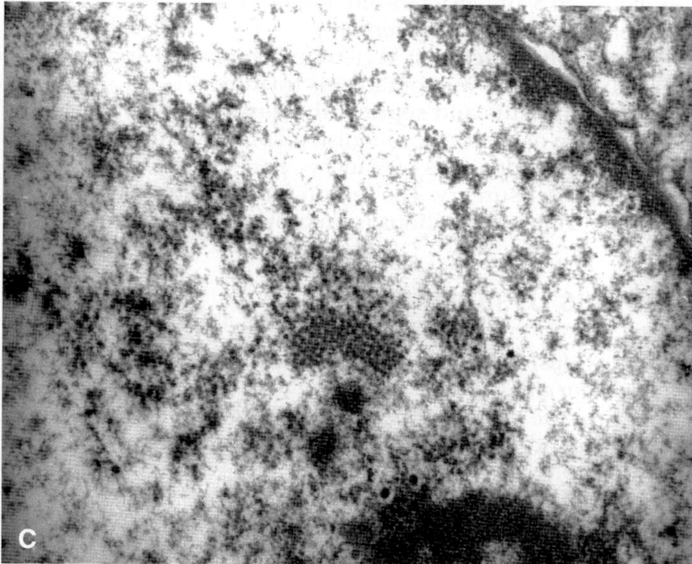

FIGURE 26-36. Paget disease. A. A section of bone shows prominent and irregular basophilic cement lines and numerous lining osteoclasts and osteoblasts. **B.** An osteoclast in pagetic bone contains many more nuclei than a usual osteoclast. A few of the nuclei contain eosinophilic intranuclear inclusion-like particles. **C.** On electron microscopy, the nuclei of the osteoclasts contain particles that resemble paramyxovirus in their shape and orientation.

huge and may have over 100 (Fig. 26-36B). Nuclei may contain intranuclear inclusions that contain virus-like particles (Fig. 26-36C).

Because active Paget disease is a disorder of accelerated remodeling, its histologic features are those of severe osteitis fibrosa. Numerous osteoclasts, large active osteoblasts and peritrabecular marrow fibrosis are encountered. The rapid remodeling leads to disruption of the trabecular architecture. Trabeculae are characteristically distorted and irregular, with a high surface-to-volume ratio. Bone collagen is often arranged in a woven rather than lamellar pattern.

With time, the lesions of Paget disease burn out and become inactive. The diagnostic hallmark of this stage is the abnormal arrangement of lamellar bone, in which islands of irregular bone formation resembling pieces of a jigsaw puzzle are separated by prominent **cement lines.** The result is a **mosaic pattern** in the bone, which can be seen particularly well under polarized light. In the cortex of an affected bone, the osteons tend to be destroyed, and concentric lamellae are incomplete. Although the changes in lamellar bone are diagnostic, it is common to see woven bone as part of the pathologic process. In this situation, the woven bone is a reactive phenomenon, as in a microcallus, and represents a temporary bridge between islands of the mosaic bone of Paget disease.

CLINICAL FEATURES: The most common focal symptom of Paget disease is pain in the affected bone, although its cause is not clear. The pain may be related to microfractures, stimulation of free nerve endings by dilated blood vessels adjacent to the bones or weight bearing in weaker bones. The diagnosis is primarily made by radiologic findings.

SKULL: Involvement of the skull is particularly common. The skull exhibits localized lysis, generally in the frontal and parietal bones, which is termed **osteoporosis circumscripta.** Alternatively, there may be thickening of the outer and inner tables, which is most pronounced in the frontal and occipital bones. The skull becomes very heavy and may collapse over the C1 vertebra, compressing the brain and spinal cord. Hearing loss follows involvement of the ossicles and bony impingement on the eighth cranial nerve at the foramen. **Platybasia** (flattening of the base of the skull) impinges on the foramen magnum, thereby compressing the medulla and upper spinal cord.

The jaws may be grossly misshapen and the teeth may fall out. Often, facial bones increase in size, especially the maxillary bones, producing the so-called **leontiasis ossea** (lion-like face).

PAGETIC STEAL: Occasionally, patients feel lightheaded, due to so-called pagetic steal, in which blood is shunted from the internal carotid system to the bones rather than directed to the brain.

FRACTURES AND ARTHRITIS: Bone fractures are common in Paget disease, the bones snapping transversely like a piece of chalk. Incomplete fractures without displacement are called **infractions.** Involvement of the pelvis leads to hip problems. The loss of subchondral bone compliance causes secondary osteoarthritis and destruction of the articular cartilage.

HIGH-OUTPUT CARDIAC FAILURE: With extensive Paget disease, blood flow to the bones and subcutaneous tissue increases remarkably, requiring increased cardiac output. In the presence of underlying cardiac disease, it may be severe enough to result in cardiac failure.

SARCOMATOUS CHANGE: Neoplastic transformation may occur in a focus of Paget disease, usually in the femur, humerus or pelvis. This complication occurs in less than 1% of all cases and usually arises in patients with severe Paget disease. However, the incidence of bone sarcoma is 1000 times higher than that in the general population. Interestingly, the skull and vertebrae, the bones most commonly involved by Paget disease, rarely undergo sarcomatous change. Sarcomas are usually osteogenic but may be fibrosarcoma or chondrosarcoma.

Serum calcium and phosphorus levels in Paget disease are normal, even though bone turnover increases more than 20-fold. Hypercalcemia is rare, but does occur if a patient is immobilized. The collagen structure of bone in Paget disease is entirely normal, but because of the accelerated bone turnover, levels of collagen breakdown products (hydroxyproline and hydroxylysine) increase in the serum and urine. Hydroxyproline excretion may reach 1000 mg/d (normal, <40 mg). The serum alkaline phosphatase level is the most useful laboratory test in diagnosing Paget disease. It increases enormously and correlates with osteoblastic activity. The alkaline phosphatase levels are disproportionately high with skull involvement, but tend to be lower when only the pelvis is affected. A sudden increase in the activity of serum alkaline phosphatase may reflect sarcomatous change within a lesion.

Fortunately, most patients with Paget disease are asymptomatic and require no treatment. Fractures, osteoarthritis and other orthopedic complications are treated symptomatically. Drugs directed at abnormal osteoclast function, including calcitonin, bisphosphonates and mithramycin, may be useful.

GIANT CELL TUMOR: This is not a neoplasm but rather a reactive phenomenon, similar to the "brown tumor" of hyperparathyroidism. Giant cell tumor is an overshoot of osteoclastic activity and an associated fibroblastic response. Radiation therapy to the giant cell tumor is curative in many cases.

Gaucher Disease

This autosomal recessive hereditary storage disease is discussed in Chapter 6. We consider here only its skeletal manifestations. These include:

- **Failure of remodeling:** This is the most common, and least problematic, skeletal abnormality. Flaring is absent and funnelization and cylinderization are abnormal, leading to an Erlenmeyer flask shape of the distal femur and proximal tibia.
- **Crisis:** This rare but very painful event results from acute infarction of a large segment of one or more bones, often after an acute viral illness. It last about 2 weeks, then gradually improves.
- **Localized and diffuse bone loss:** Radiolucent lesions with overlying cortical thinning are usually asymptomatic unless a fracture occurs at the site. These lesions are packed with Gaucher cells.
- **Osteosclerotic lesions:** These reflect increased bone formation, usually in the medullary cavity of the long bones and pelvis. Reactive new bone formation following osteonecrosis may be involved.
- **Corticomedullary osteonecrosis:** This disabling complication of Gaucher disease is most common in patients between 8 and 35 years old. It mostly involves the femoral head or proximal humerus.
- **Pathologic fractures:** Vertebrae, long bones and even the pelvis may show spontaneous fractures.
- **Osteomyelitis and septic arthritis:** Commonly caused by coliform or anaerobic organisms, spread via bloodstream to the bones and joints of Gaucher patients is common, especially after surgery. The reason for the increased susceptibility to these infections is unknown.

Fibrous Dysplasia

Fibrous dysplasia is a developmental abnormality characterized by a disorganized mixture of fibrous and osseous elements in the medullary region of affected bones. It occurs in children and young adults and may affect one (monostotic) or multiple bones (polyostotic) or other systems (McCune-Albright Syndrome).

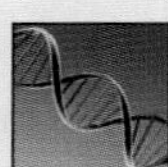

MOLECULAR PATHOGENESIS: Activating mutations in the *GNAS1* gene encoding the α subunit of the stimulatory guanine nucleotide-binding protein (Gsα), which is linked to adenyl cyclase, have been described in bone cells from patients with fibrous dysplasia and McCune-Albright syndrome. The result would be constitutive activation of adenyl cyclase and increased levels of cAMP, thereby enhancing certain functions of the affected cells (e.g., c-*fos* and c-*jun* proto-oncogenes, IL-6 and IL-11).

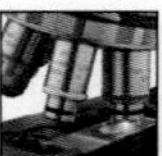
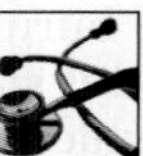

PATHOLOGY AND CLINICAL FEATURES: *MONOSTOTIC FIBROUS DYSPLASIA:* Monostotic fibrous dysplasia is the most common form of the disease and is most often seen in the second and third decades, with no predilection for either sex. The bones commonly involved are the proximal femur, tibia, ribs and facial bones, although any bone may be affected. The disease may be asymptomatic or it may lead to a pathologic fracture.

POLYOSTOTIC FIBROUS DYSPLASIA: One fourth of patients with polyostotic fibrous dysplasia exhibit disease in more than half of the skeleton, including the facial bones.

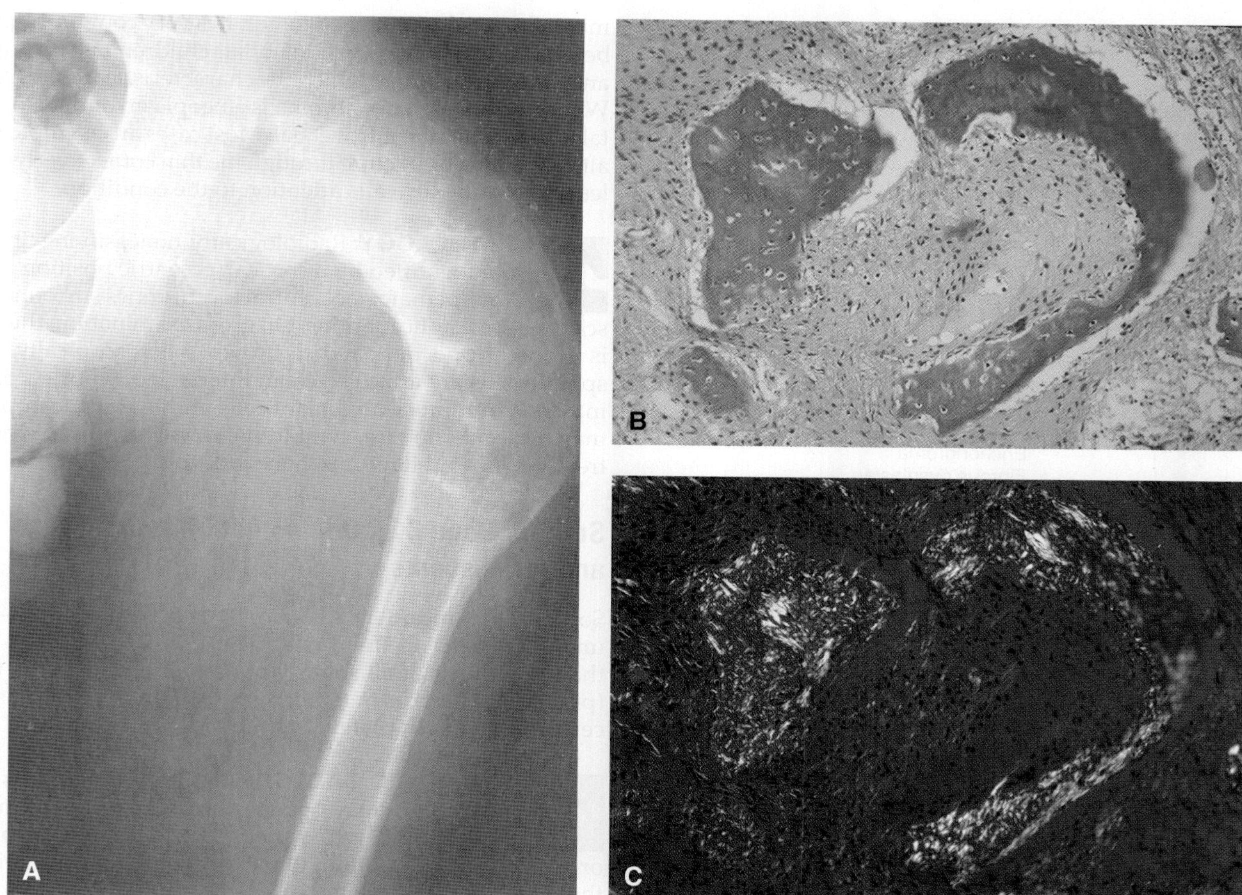

FIGURE 26-37. Fibrous dysplasia. A. A radiograph of the proximal femur shows the "shepherd's crook" deformity caused by fractures sustained over the years. Irregular, marginated, ground-glass lucencies are surrounded by reactive bone. The shaft has an appearance that has been likened to a soap bubble. **B.** Histologically, fibrous dysplasia consists of moderately cellular fibrous tissue in which irregular, curved spicules of woven bone develop without discernible appositional osteoblast activity. **C.** The same section in polarized light demonstrates not only that the spicules are woven, but also that their fiber pattern extends imperceptibly into the fiber pattern of the surrounding stroma.

Symptoms usually are seen in childhood, and almost all patients have pathologic fractures, limb deformities or limb-length discrepancies. Polyostotic fibrous dysplasia is more common in females. Sometimes the disease becomes quiescent at puberty, whereas pregnancy may stimulate the growth of lesions.

MCCUNE-ALBRIGHT SYNDROME: This condition is characterized by endocrine dysfunction, including acromegaly, Cushing syndrome, hyperthyroidism and vitamin D–resistant rickets. The most common endocrine abnormality is precocious puberty in girls (boys rarely have McCune-Albright syndrome). As a result, premature closure of the growth plates may lead to abnormally short stature. The most common extraskeletal manifestations of McCune-Albright syndrome are characteristic skin lesions: pigmented macules ("café-au-lait" spots) with irregular ("coast of Maine") borders that do not cross the midline of the body and are usually located over the buttocks, back and sacrum. These often overlie the skeletal lesions.

The radiographic features of fibrous dysplasia are distinctive. The bone lesion has a lucent ground-glass appearance with well-marginated borders and a thin cortex. The bone may be ballooned, deformed or enlarged and involvement may be focal or may encompass the entire bone (Fig. 26-37A).

All forms of fibrous dysplasia have an identical histologic pattern (Fig. 26-37B,C). Benign fibroblastic tissue is arranged in a loose, whorled pattern. Irregularly arranged, purposeless spicules of woven bone that lack osteoblastic rimming are embedded in the fibrous tissue. In 10% of cases, irregular islands of hyaline cartilage are also present. Occasionally, cystic degeneration occurs, with hemosiderin-laden macrophages, hemorrhage and osteoclasts congregated about the cyst. Rarely (1<% of cases), malignant degeneration (osteosarcoma, chondrosarcoma or fibrosarcoma) has been reported, but most of these cases involved prior radiation therapy. Treatment of fibrous dysplasia consists of curettage, repair of fractures and prevention of deformities.

Benign Tumors of Bone

Bone tumors of all kinds are uncommon but are nevertheless important neoplasms because many occur in children and young persons and are potentially lethal. A primary bone tumor may arise from any of the cellular elements of bone.

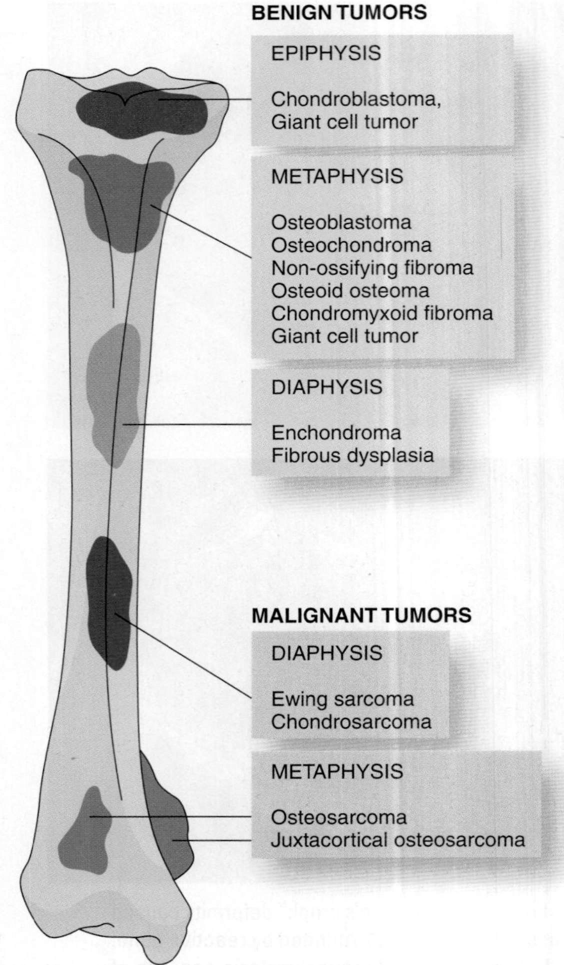

FIGURE 26-38. Location of primary bone tumors in long tubular bones.

Most neoplasms of bone occur near the metaphyseal area, and more than 80% of primary tumors occur in the distal femur or proximal tibia (Fig. 26-38). In a growing child, these areas show conspicuous growth activity.

Osteoma Is a Benign Tumor Composed of Compact Cortical Bone

Osteoma is a benign, slow-growing tumor composed of cortical-type dense bone. These lesions can be divided into four major clinicopathologic subtypes: (1) calvarial and mandibular osteomas, (2) osteomas of the sinonasal and orbital bones, (3) bone islands occurring in medullary bone and (4) surface osteomas of long bones. Some osteomas are likely developmental or hamartomatous in nature. However, sinonasal osteomas may be benign osteoblastic neoplasms. Interestingly, multiple osteomas are associated with colonic familial adenomatous polyposis in Gardner syndrome (see Chapter 13).

Nonossifying Fibroma Is a Solitary Lesion of Childhood

Nonossifying fibroma, also termed **fibrous cortical defect**, is a benign tumor that occurs in the metaphysis of a long bone, most commonly the tibia or femur. It is very common and may be present in as many as 25% of all children between ages 4 and 10 years, after which it characteristically regresses. Whether nonossifying fibroma is a neoplasm or developmental lesion remains controversial. Most cases are asymptomatic, although pain or fracture through the thin cortex overlying the lesion occasionally calls attention to the condition.

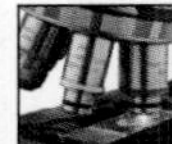

PATHOLOGY: Radiologically, nonossifying fibromas are identified by a cortical, eccentric position and by well-demarcated, central lucent zones surrounded by scalloped, sclerotic margins. On gross examination, the lesion is granular and dark red to brown. Microscopically, bland spindle cells are arranged in an interlacing, whorled pattern in which multinucleated giant cells and foamy macrophages may be seen. The rare, symptomatic or expanded lesions are treated with curettage and bone grafting.

Solitary Bone Cyst Occurs in Children and Adolescents

Solitary, or unicameral, bone cyst is a benign, fluid-filled, unilocular lesion. There is a male predilection (3:1). More than two thirds of all solitary bone cysts occur in the upper (proximal) humerus or femur, usually in the metaphysis adjacent to the growth plate.

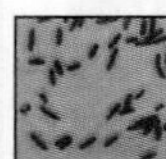

ETIOLOGIC FACTORS: Solitary bone cysts seem not to be true neoplasms but rather disturbances of bone growth with superimposed trauma. Secondary organization of a hematoma or some abnormality of the metaphyseal vessels causes accumulation of fluid. The "tumor" then grows by expansion of the fluid cavity. The resulting pressure causes bone resorption, mediated by neighboring osteoclasts. The process is slow, so that as the endosteal surface of the cortex is resorbed, a thin periosteal shell of new bone is laid down. This sequence results in a thin, well-marginated, radiolucent bone lesion (Fig. 26-39), which is never greater in diameter than the growth plate and is particularly susceptible to pathologic fracture.

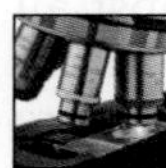

PATHOLOGY: Solitary bone cyst is not a true cyst since there is no epithelial lining, but is rather lined by fibrous tissue, a few osteoclastic giant cells, hemosiderin-laden macrophages, chronic inflammatory cells and reactive bone. Osteoclasts are present in the advancing front of the cyst and allow expansion of the lesion. The cyst wall may contain characteristic masses of amorphous, calcified, proteinaceous material.

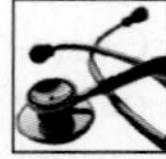

CLINICAL FEATURES: Most solitary bone cysts are entirely asymptomatic until a pathologic fracture calls attention to it. Once the diagnosis is confirmed by other imaging studies and by finding clear fluid by needle aspiration, intralesional corticosteroids may be given. Curettage and deposition of bone chips are performed only when the cyst is not controlled by injection.

Aneurysmal Bone Cyst May Be Primary or Secondary

Aneurysmal bone cyst (ABC) is an uncommon, expansive lesion arising within a bone or on its surface. It occurs in

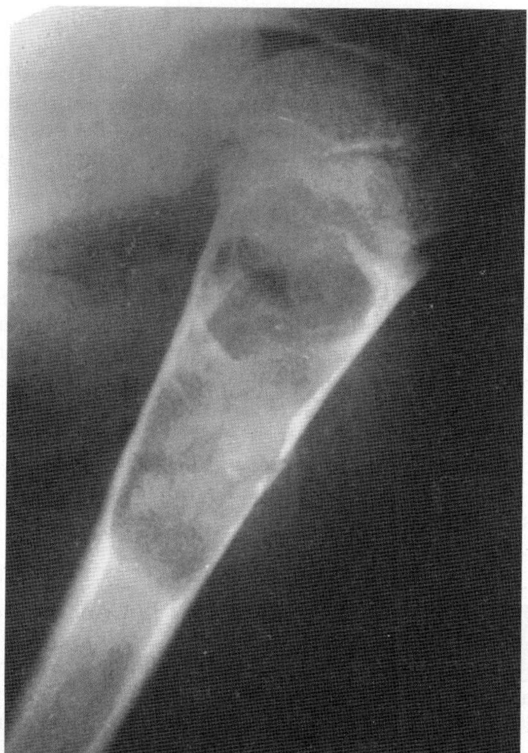

FIGURE 26-39. **Solitary bone cyst.** A radiograph of the proximal humerus of a child (note the epiphyseal plate) shows a large, well-demarcated, lytic epiphyseal and diaphyseal lesion. The cortex is thinned, but there is no cortical distortion or malformation of the shape of the bone.

children and young adults, with a peak incidence in the second decade. The lesion has been observed at every skeletal site but is most frequent in the long bones and the vertebral column.

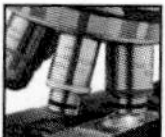

MOLECULAR PATHOGENESIS: The pathogenesis of ABC is controversial. Some cases represent cystic and hemorrhagic transformation of an underlying lesion, most commonly chondroblastoma, osteoblastoma, fibrous dysplasia, giant cell tumor and osteosarcoma (termed "secondary ABC"). Other cases of ABC have no detectable associated lesion (termed "primary ABC"). Primary ABC may be a true neoplasm since it is associated with a recurring chromosomal translocation t(16;17)(q22;p13). This translocation fuses the promoter region of the osteoblast cadherin 11 gene (*CDH11*) on chromosome 16q22 to the coding sequence of the ubiquitin protease (*USP6*) gene on chromosome 17p13. USP6 is thought to have a role in regulating actin remodeling. However, the possible mechanism of neoplastic transformation by upregulation of USP6 has not been elucidated.

PATHOLOGY: The periosteum around an aneurysmal bone cyst is ballooned but intact. In the spine, aneurysmal bone cyst may actually extend across more than one bone. By magnetic resonance imaging (MRI), fluid-fluid levels may be seen as blood cells separate from plasma. The cut surface of the lesion resembles a sponge permeated with blood and blood clots (Fig. 26-40A). The walls and septa are composed of fibrous tissue with

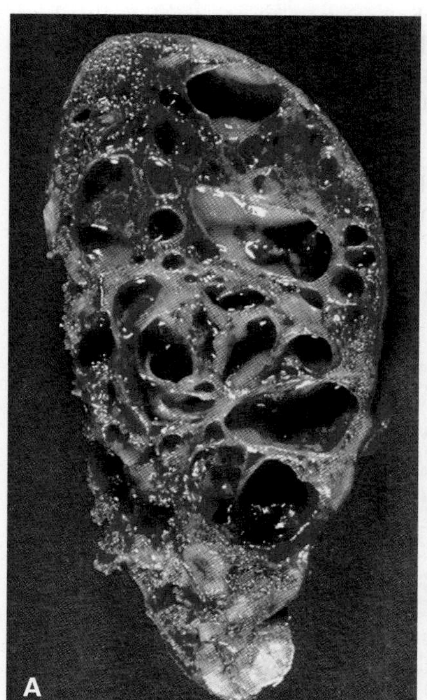

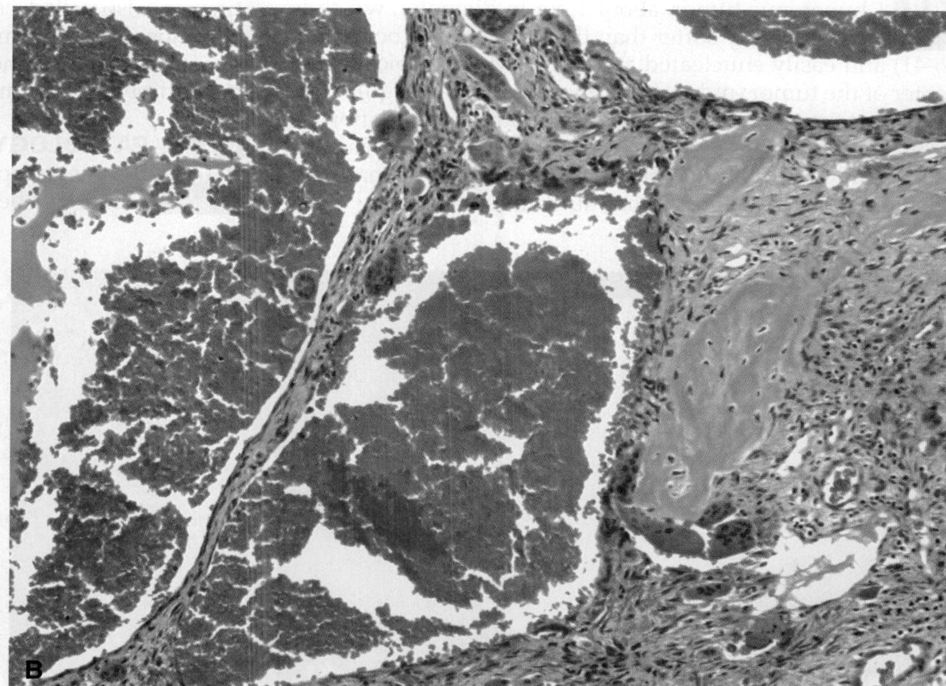

FIGURE 26-40. **Aneurysmal bone cyst. A.** In cross-section, the lesion consists of a spongy mass containing multiple blood-filled cysts. Some of the septa between the cysts contain bony tissue. **B.** Microscopically, the blood-filled spaces are separated by cellular fibrous septa with scattered osteoclast-like giant cells and reactive bone.

multinucleated giant cells and occasional osteoid trabeculae (Fig. 26-40B).

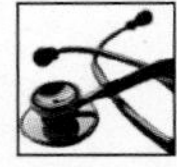

CLINICAL FEATURES: Although some aneurysmal bone cysts tend to grow slowly, most expand rapidly and may be enormous. They usually manifest with pain and swelling, sometimes in relation to trauma, and often develop in a short period of time. A bone cyst may "blow out," that is, rupture and produce local hemorrhage. Treatment is usually extraperiosteal excision and curettage. At surgery, incising the cyst decreases its internal pressure, causing brisk bleeding that may be difficult to control. In sites such as the vertebral column or the pelvis, selective arterial embolization has been successful.

Osteoid Osteoma Is a Benign, Painful Lesion

It is composed of osseous tissue (the nidus) and surrounded by a halo of reactive bone formation. The typical patient is between 5 and 25 years old. Boys are affected more often than girls (3:1). Osteoid osteomas frequently arise in the diaphyseal cortex of the tubular bones of the leg but may occur elsewhere. Osteoid osteomas have limited growth potential and do not metastasize.

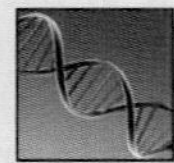

MOLECULAR PATHOGENESIS: Chromosomal analysis of a few osteoid osteomas has disclosed abnormalities of chromosome 22q13 and loss of part of 17q, which suggests that osteoid osteomas are neoplasms.

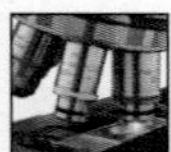

PATHOLOGY: Osteoid osteoma is a spherical, hyperemic tumor, about 1 cm in diameter, which is considerably softer than the surrounding bone (Fig. 26-41) and easily enucleated at surgery. Microscopically, the center of the tumor (nidus) is composed of thin, irregular trabeculae of woven bone within a cellular and vascular fibrous stroma containing many osteoblasts and osteoclasts. The trabeculae are more mature in the center, which is often partially calcified. Reactive sclerotic bone surrounds the nidus.

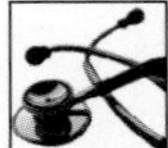

CLINICAL FEATURES: Pain is typically nocturnal and out of proportion to the size of the lesion. Interestingly, the pain is often exacerbated by drinking alcohol and promptly relieved by aspirin, possibly because of the high prostaglandin content and abundant nerve fibers within the tumor. Surgical excision or radioablation (electric probe inserted into the tumor) is curative.

Osteoblastoma Is Not Painful

Osteoblastoma is an uncommon, benign neoplasm histologically similar to osteoid osteoma but larger and not accompanied by nocturnal pain relieved by aspirin. It stimulates less bone reaction and appears as a purely radiolucent lesion, with only a thin shell of surrounding bone. Osteoblastoma occurs in persons between the ages of 10 and 35 years, with no sex predilection, and mainly affects the spine and long bones. Curettage cures small osteoblastomas, but larger lesions may require wide resection.

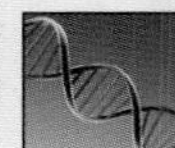

MOLECULAR PATHOGENESIS: Several chromosomal and molecular abnormalities have been described in osteoblastoma. However, no consistent abnormality has emerged. Aneuploid to hyperdiploid karyotypes have been demonstrated. *MDM2* gene amplification and *TP53* gene deletion implicate cell cycle abnormalities in the pathogenesis of osteoblastoma.

Solitary Chondroma Is a Benign Intraosseus Tumor of Mature Hyaline Cartilage

Although their neoplastic nature has been questioned, these tumors, also called enchondromas, may occasionally show chromosomal abnormalities, suggesting that they are in fact neoplasms. The diagnosis is made at any age, and many cases are entirely asymptomatic.

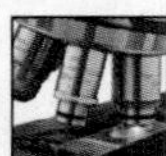

PATHOLOGY: Most solitary chondromas occur in the metacarpals and phalanges of the hands, the remainder being in almost any other tubular bone.

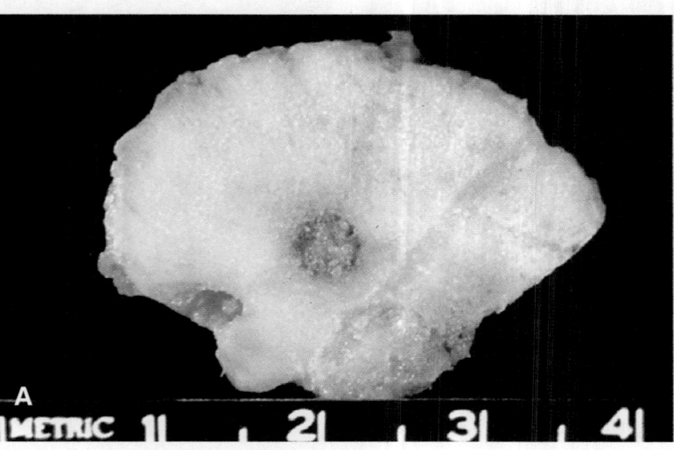

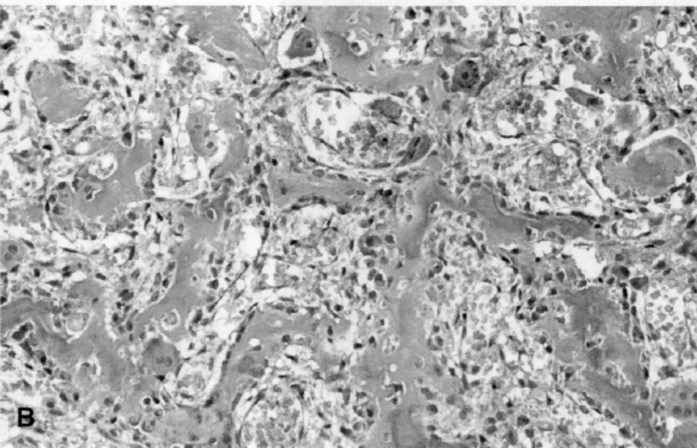

FIGURE 26-41. Osteoid osteoma. A. A gross specimen of an osteoid osteoma shows the central nidus, which is embedded in dense bone. **B.** A photomicrograph of the nidus reveals irregular trabeculae of woven bone surrounded by osteoblasts, osteoclasts and fibrovascular marrow.

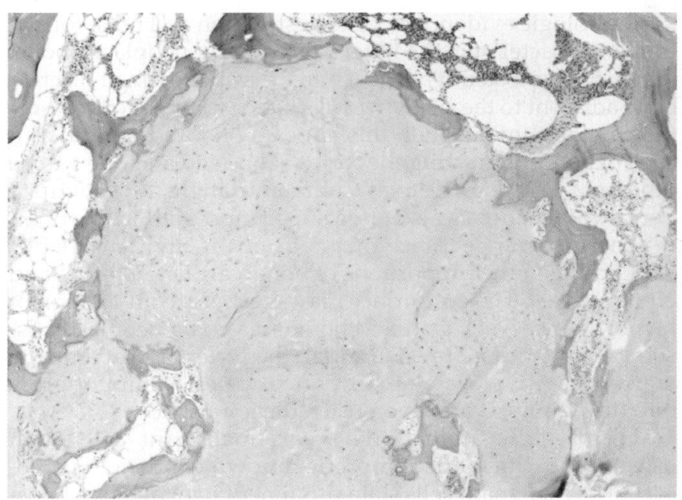

FIGURE 26-42. Enchondroma. The tumor is composed of lobules of hypocellular hyaline cartilage without atypia.

The tumor is small and grows slowly. Radiologically, it appears as a well-delimited radiolucent area, sometimes containing stippled calcifications. On gross examination, solitary chondromas have the semitranslucent appearance of hyaline cartilage, often with a few calcified areas. Microscopically, the cartilaginous tissue is well differentiated, with sparse chondrocytes (Fig. 26-42). Asymptomatic chondromas are best left untreated. When pain intervenes, curettage and bone grafting are the treatment of choice.

Chondroblastoma Is a Benign Tumor of the Epiphyses of Long Bones

Chondroblastoma is an uncommon, chondrogenic tumor with predilection for the proximal femur, tibia and humerus. It is more common in males than in females (2:1) and 90% of cases occur in young persons between the ages of 5 and 25.

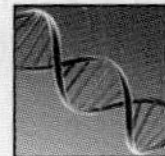

MOLECULAR PATHOGENESIS: Genetic abnormalities suggest a neoplastic origin of chondroblastoma including aneuploidy, abnormalities involving chromosomes 5 and 8 and mutations in the *p53* gene.

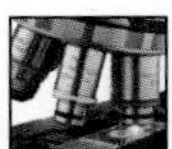

PATHOLOGY: Chondroblastoma grows slowly, and on radiologic examination, displays an eccentric, radiolucent appearance with sharply defined borders (Fig. 26-43). On gross examination, the tumor is soft and compact with scattered gray or hemorrhagic areas. Microscopically, primitive chondroblasts are arranged as sheets of round to polyhedral cells that have well-defined cytoplasmic borders and large, ovoid nuclei, often with prominent nuclear grooves. The cartilage matrix is variably calcified and appears primitive. This accounts for the mottled pattern often seen in CT scans. Well-developed hyaline cartilage as seen in enchondroma is not found in chondroblastoma. Chondroblastoma causes bone destruction by stimulating osteoclastic resorption. In fact, these tumors may perforate the cortex, although they remain confined by the periosteum.

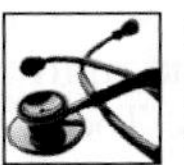

CLINICAL FEATURES: Because of its para-articular location, chondroblastoma tends to cause joint pain, with mild swelling and functional limitation of joint movement. If neglected, it may rarely attain a large size, destroy the epiphyseal area and invade the joint. Curettage is the treatment of choice, although in over 10% of cases, the tumor recurs.

Malignant Tumors of Bone

Osteosarcoma Is the Most Common Primary Malignant Bone Tumor

Osteosarcoma, also termed **osteogenic sarcoma,** *is a highly malignant bone tumor characterized by formation of bone*

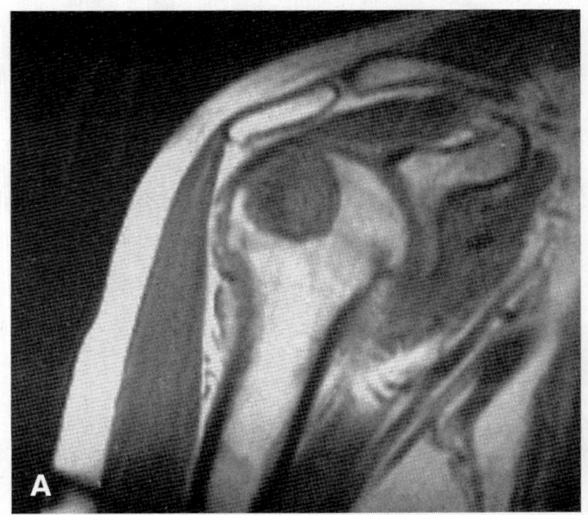

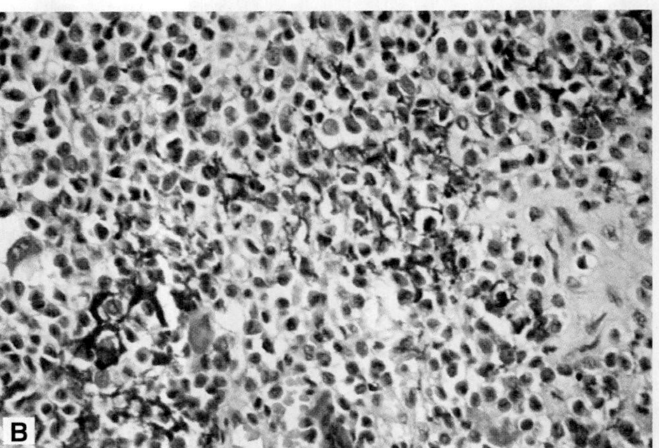

FIGURE 26-43. Chondroblastoma. A. A magnetic resonance image of the shoulder of a child shows a prominent lytic lesion of the head of the humerus that involves the epiphysis and extends across the epiphyseal plate. **B.** The histologic appearance of a chondroblastoma is defined by plump, round cells (chondroblasts) surrounded by a mineralized primitive chondroid matrix.

tissue by tumor cells. It represents one fifth of all bone cancers and is most frequent in adolescents between 10 and 20 years old, affecting boys more often than girls (2:1).

MOLECULAR PATHOGENESIS: Osteosarcomas are associated with mutations in tumor suppressor genes: almost two thirds show mutations in the retinoblastoma (*Rb*) gene (see Chapter 5) and many also have mutations in the *p53* gene. There are also many other chromosomal and molecular abnormalities pertaining to apoptosis, replicative potential, insensitivity to growth inhibitory signals and cell cycle regulation that contribute in some part to the development of osteosarcoma. For example, amplification of *MDM2*, *CDK4* and *PRIM1* as well as overexpression of *MET* and *FOS* have been detected in a significant proportion of cases.

ETIOLOGIC FACTORS: These tumors are more common in tall persons. Interestingly, they occur more frequently in taller breeds of dogs. In older people, they usually occur in the context of Paget disease or radiation exposure. For example, radium watch dial painters who wetted their brushes by licking them developed osteosarcoma many years later due to radium depositing in their bones. Today, osteosarcoma can develop in adults and children previously subjected to external therapeutic radiation for some other tumor such as lymphoma. Several preexisting benign bone lesions are associated with an increased risk of developing osteosarcoma, including fibrous dysplasia, osteomyelitis and bone infarcts. Although trauma may call attention to an existing osteosarcoma, there is no evidence that it ever causes the tumor.

PATHOLOGY: Osteosarcomas often arise near the knee, in the lower femur (Fig. 26-44A), upper tibia or fibula, although any metaphyseal area of a long bone may be affected. The proximal humerus is the second most common site: 75% arise adjacent to the knee or shoulder.

Radiologic evidence of bone destruction and bone formation is characteristic, the latter representing neoplastic bone. Often, the periosteum produces an incomplete rim of reactive bone adjacent to the site where it is lifted from the cortical surface by the tumor. When this appears on a radiograph as a shell of bone intersecting the cortex at one end and open at the other end, it is referred to as **Codman triangle.** A "sunburst" periosteal reaction is also often superimposed (Fig. 26-17).

The gross appearance of the tumor is highly variable, depending on the proportions of bone, cartilage, stroma and blood vessels. The cut surface may show any combination of hemorrhagic, cystic, soft and bony areas. The neoplastic tissue may invade and break through the cortex, spread into the marrow cavity, elevate or perforate the periosteum or grow into the epiphysis and even reach the joint space.

Histologic examination reveals malignant cells with osteoblastic differentiation producing woven bone (Fig. 26-44B). The malignant cells stain prominently for alkaline phosphatase and osteonectin. The tumorous bone is laid down haphazardly and not aligned along stress lines. Often, foci of malignant cartilage cells or pleomorphic giant cells are intermixed. In areas of osteolysis, nonneoplastic osteoclasts are found at the advancing front of the tumor.

Osteosarcoma spreads through the bloodstream to the lungs. In fact, almost all patients (98%) who die of this disease have lung metastases. Less commonly, the tumor metastasizes to other bones (35%), the pleura (33%) and the heart (20%).

CLINICAL FEATURES: Osteosarcoma presents with mild or intermittent pain around the knee or other involved areas. As pain intensifies, the area becomes swollen and tender. The adjacent joint becomes functionally limited. Serum alkaline phosphatase is increased in half of patients and may decrease after amputation, only to increase again with recurrence or metastasis. Metastatic disease heralds rapid clinical deterioration and death.

Historically, osteosarcoma was treated exclusively by amputation or disarticulation of the involved limb, but the prognosis for 5-year survival did not exceed 20%. Today, standard therapy

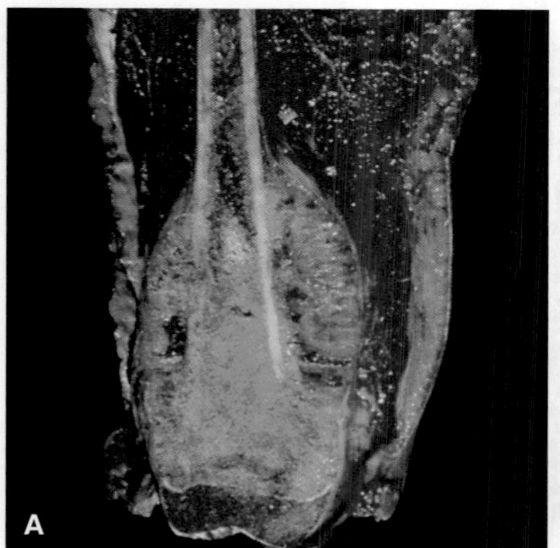

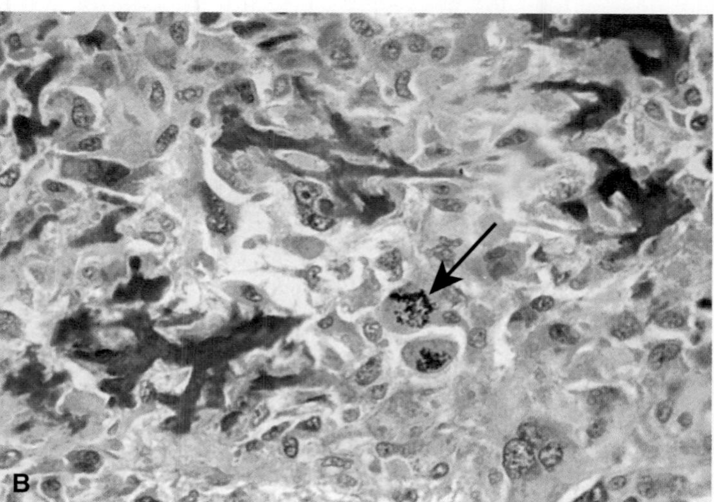

FIGURE 26-44. Osteosarcoma. A. The distal femur contains a dense osteoblastic malignant tumor that extends through the cortex into the soft tissue and the epiphysis. **B.** A photomicrograph reveals pleomorphic malignant cells, tumor giant cells and mitoses (*arrow*). The tumor produces woven bone that is focally calcified.

of chemotherapy and limb-sparing surgery gives 5-year disease-free rates from 60% to 80%. Resection of isolated pulmonary metastases may prolong survival.

Juxtacortical osteosarcoma is a rare variant of osteosarcoma that occurs on the periosteal surface of the bone, especially the lower posterior metaphysis of the femur (72% of cases). Unlike classic osteosarcoma, most patients are older than 25 years, and the tumor is more common in women. Juxtacortical osteosarcoma spares the deep cortex and medulla of the bone and grows external to the shaft. Usually, Codman triangle is not evident radiologically, because the periosteum is not elevated. Most juxtacortical osteosarcomas are low-grade lesions and do not require adjunctive chemotherapy. Surgical excision is the treatment of choice. The prognosis is good, with a 5-year survival of more than 80%.

Chondrosarcoma Is a Cartilaginous Malignancy Whose Grade Determines Prognosis

Chondrosarcoma is a malignant tumor of cartilage that arises from a preexisting cartilage rest or enchondroma. Some patients have a history of enchondromas, solitary osteochondroma or hereditary multiple osteochondromas. Most have no known preexisting lesion. ***Chondrosarcoma is the second most common primary malignant bone tumor and is more common in men than in women (2:1).*** It is most frequently seen in the fourth to sixth decades (average age, 45 years).

MOLECULAR PATHOGENESIS: Numerous nonrandom chromosomal abnormalities have been discovered in chondrosarcoma. There probably is a different molecular mechanism resulting in tumor development between central chondrosarcoma and secondary peripheral chondrosarcoma (tumors arising in the cartilaginous cap of an osteochondroma) (see below). The latter may develop by upregulation of PTHrP and Bcl-2 expression in an osteochondroma, along with mutations in other genes such as *p53* and nonspecific chromosomal abnormalities. Development of central chondrosarcoma is related at least in part to abnormalities of chromosome 9p12-22, which may involve the *CDKN2A* tumor suppressor gene. The transcription factor *SOX9*, which plays a critical role in normal chondrocyte development, is expressed in chondrosarcomas.

PATHOLOGY: Chondrosarcoma occurs in three anatomic variants:

CENTRAL CHONDROSARCOMA: This form arises in the medullary cavity of pelvic bones, ribs and long bones, although any site may be affected. Radiologically, poorly defined borders, a thickened shaft and perforation of the cortex characterize these tumors. There are usually stippled radiopacities or ring-like ossifications representing calcification or endochondral ossification in the tumor (Fig. 26-45A). Although central chondrosarcoma may penetrate the cortex, extension beyond the periosteum is uncommon. On gross examination, the neoplastic cartilaginous tissue is compressed inside the bone and exhibits areas of necrosis, cystic change and hemorrhage (Fig. 26-45B). The cortex of the bone and the intertrabecular spaces of the marrow are infiltrated by the tumor.

Central chondrosarcoma begins with deep pain, which becomes more intense with time. The tumor is only rarely palpable, but in untreated cases, large masses may eventually form.

PERIPHERAL CHONDROSARCOMA: This variant is less common than the central variety of chondrosarcoma and arises outside the bone, almost always in the cartilaginous cap of an osteochondroma. It occurs after the age of 20 years and never before puberty. The most frequent location of peripheral chondrosarcoma is the pelvis, followed by the femur, vertebrae, sacrum, humerus and other long bones. It arises only rarely distal to the knee or elbow. Radiologically, characteristic radiopacities representing calcification or ossification of the neoplastic cartilage are virtually pathognomonic for the lesion. Macroscopically, peripheral chondrosarcoma tends to be a large bosselated mass that surrounds the base of an osteochondroma and invades the bone.

Peripheral chondrosarcoma is usually seen as a slowly growing mass. Expansion of the mass causes pain and local symptoms. In the pelvis, the lumbosacral plexus may be compressed and tumors in the vertebrae may cause paraplegia.

JUXTACORTICAL CHONDROSARCOMA: This is the least common variety of chondrosarcoma and is similar to central chondrosarcoma in its predilection for middle-aged men. It tends to be situated in the metaphysis of long bones, lying on the outer surface of the cortex. Thus, it is probably periosteal or parosteal in origin. Radiologically, it may be entirely translucent or focally calcified. The symptoms of juxtacortical chondrosarcoma are dominated by swelling, with little accompanying pain.

Histologically, chondrosarcomas are composed of malignant cartilage cells in various stages of maturity (Fig. 26-45C). Occasionally, a well-differentiated chondrosarcoma is difficult to distinguish from a benign tumor on cytologic grounds alone. Zones of calcification are often conspicuous and are seen radiographically as splotches or bulky masses. Chondrosarcoma expands by stimulating osteoclastic resorption of bone and often breaks through the cortex. Most chondrosarcomas grow slowly, but hematogenous metastases to the lungs are common in poorly differentiated variants.

There is a positive correlation between histologic grade, histomorphology and the degree of karyotypic complexity. Trisomy 7 is associated with chondrosarcoma. Rearrangement of the short arm of chromosome 17 is associated with high-grade chondrosarcoma. Alterations of 12q13 are associated with tumors exhibiting myxoid features. Extraskeletal myxoid chondrosarcomas have a classical translocation (9;22)(q31;q12).

OTHER VARIANTS OF CHONDROSARCOMA: The above forms of chondrosarcoma are conventional forms in that they are characterized by a hyaline cartilage matrix. Uncommon histopathologic variants of chondrosarcoma include **clear cell chondrosarcoma,** which occurs almost exclusively in the proximal epiphysis of the femur or humerus and is composed of chondrocytes with abundant clear cytoplasm, areas of woven trabecular bone and areas with a hyaline cartilage matrix. The prognosis for this tumor following complete excision is close to that of conventional low-grade chondrosarcoma. **Dedifferentiated chondrosarcoma** is defined as a high-grade nonchondrogenic pleomorphic sarcoma (e.g., osteosarcoma or fibrosarcoma) arising in association with a low-grade conventional chondrosarcoma

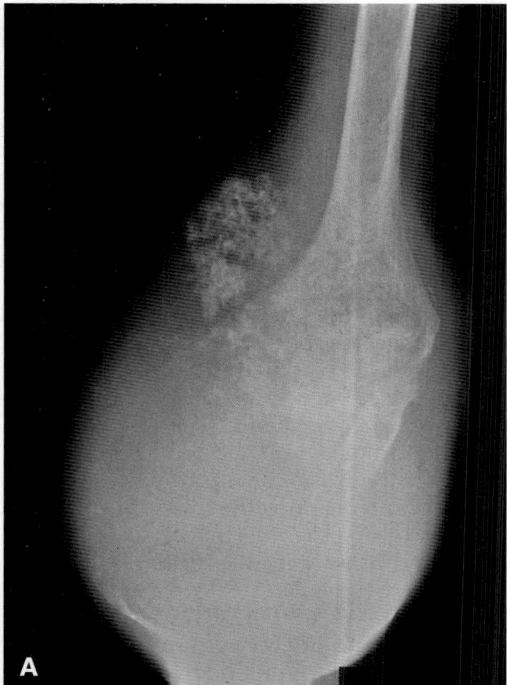

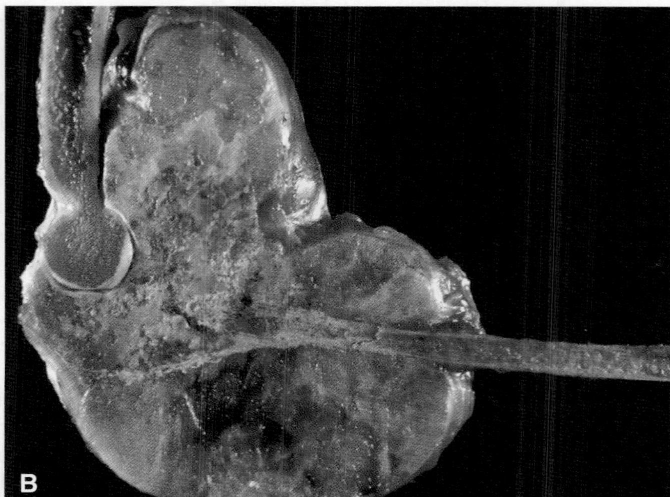

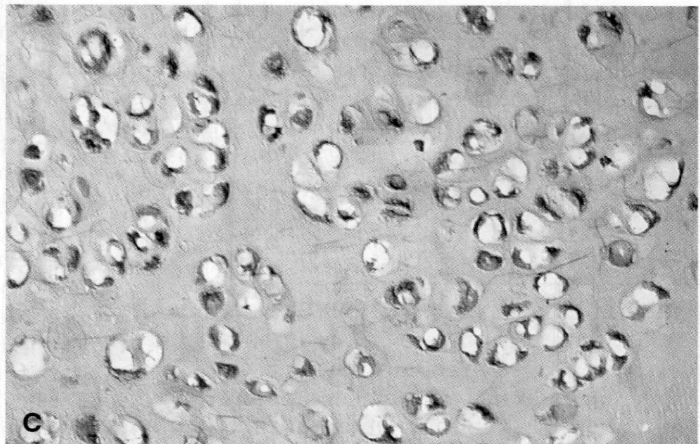

FIGURE 26-45. Chondrosarcoma. A. Radiograph demonstrates a large, destructive mass replacing the proximal ulna. There is a huge soft tissue mass containing aggregates of ring-shaped and popcorn-like calcifications. **B.** Resected gross specimen demonstrates lobulated hyaline cartilage with calcifications, ossification and focal liquefaction. **C.** A photomicrograph of a chondrosarcoma shows malignant chondrocytes with pronounced atypia.

or enchondroma. This tumor usually arises in flat bones of the pelvis or long bones of the extremities and has a dismal prognosis, with less than 10% of patients surviving 5 years despite surgery and chemotherapy. One other variant is known as **mesenchymal chondrosarcoma** and is histologically characterized by two distinct components. The first is a high-grade malignant, small, round, blue cell tumor that resembles Ewing sarcoma. Sheets of these cells are interrupted by discrete islands of malignant hyaline cartilage tumor histologically similar to conventional chondrosarcoma. The bones of the jaw and the chest wall are the most commonly affected sites. The prognosis for these tumors is poor.

CLINICAL FEATURES: Patients generally present with pain at the affected site. Chondrosarcoma is one of the few tumors in which microscopic grading has a significant prognostic value. The 5-year survival rate for low-grade conventional chondrosarcomas is 80%, for moderate-grade tumors about 50%, and for high-grade tumors only 20%. Wide excision is the usual treatment since response to radiation and chemotherapy is usually poor.

Giant Cell Tumors of Bone Rarely Metastasize

Giant cell tumor (GCT) of bone is a benign, locally aggressive neoplasm characterized by the presence of osteoclastic, multinucleated giant cells, randomly and uniformly distributed in a background of proliferating mononuclear cells. It usually occurs in the third and fourth decades, has a slight predilection for women and seems to be more common in Asia than in Western countries. GCTs in the elderly may be secondary to irradiation. Paget disease may produce a giant cell reactive lesion that closely resembles a true GCT.

MOLECULAR PATHOGENESIS: GCT is composed of osteoclastic giant cells and two lineages of mononuclear cells. One population of mononuclear cells is believed to be of macrophage-monocyte origin and is likely nonneoplastic. The other mononuclear cell population has chromosomal abnormalities and molecular alterations in oncogenes such as *p53* and c-*myc*.

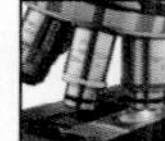

PATHOLOGY: In most cases (90%), GCT of bone originates at the junction between the metaphysis and the epiphysis of a long bone, with more than half being situated in the knee area (distal femur and proximal tibia; Fig. 26-46A). The lower end of the radius, humerus and fibula are also occasionally involved. The neoplasm is often a lytic lesion that grows slowly enough to allow a periosteal reaction. Thus, radiologically, the tumor tends to be

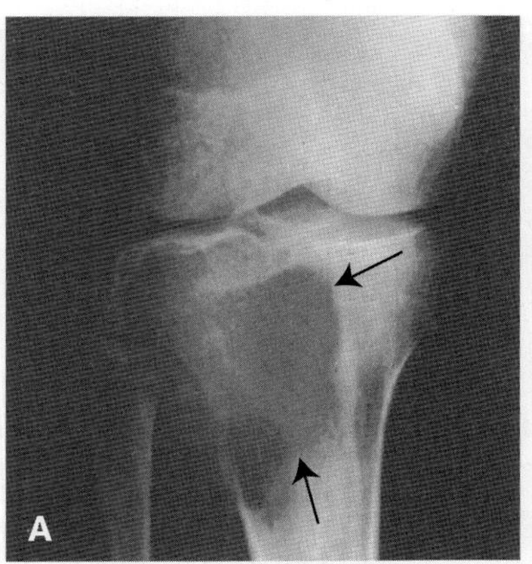

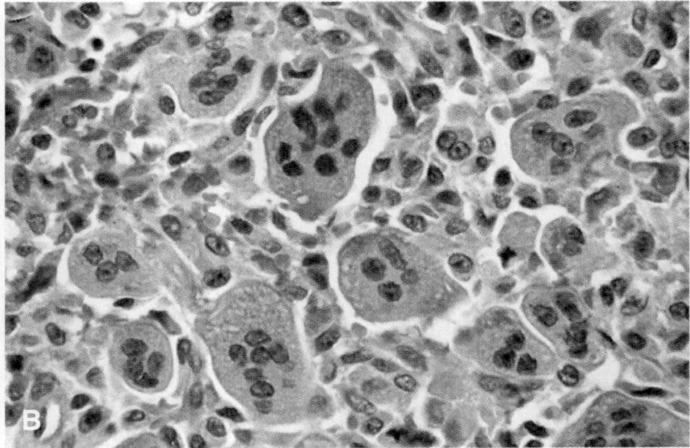

FIGURE 26-46. Giant cell tumor of bone. A. Radiograph of the proximal tibia shows an eccentric lytic lesion with virtually no new bone formation (*arrows*). The tumor extends to the subchondral bone plate and breaks through cortex into the soft tissue. **B.** Photomicrograph shows osteoclast-type giant cells and plump, oval, mononuclear cells. The nuclei of both types of cells are identical.

surrounded by a thin, bony shell and expands the bone. Often, it has a multiloculated or "soap bubble" appearance, representing endosteal resorption of the bone.

On gross examination, GCT is clearly circumscribed, and its cut surface is soft and light brown, without bone or calcification. Numerous hemorrhagic areas result in the appearance of a sponge full of blood. In some cases, cystic cavities and necrotic areas are present. GCT is often limited by the periosteum, although aggressive forms penetrate the cortex and the periosteum, even reaching the joint capsule and the synovial membrane.

Microscopically, GCT exhibits two types of cells (Fig. 26-46B). The mononuclear ("stromal") cells are plump and oval, with large nuclei and scanty cytoplasm. Large osteoclastic giant cells, some with more than 100 nuclei, are scattered throughout the richly vascularized stroma. Diffuse interstitial hemorrhage is common. On low-power examination, the tumor often appears as a syncytium of nuclei with poor demarcation of cytoplasmic borders and random distribution of the giant cells. It is evident that the mononuclear cells are the neoplastic and proliferative components of GCT (mitotic activity is common in the mononuclear cells but is not observed in the giant cells). Indeed, the diagnosis of malignancy in a GCT depends on the morphology of the mononuclear cells rather than that of the multinucleated cells.

CLINICAL FEATURES: The vast majority of GCTs are considered benign, but locally aggressive tumors have the potential to recur locally after simple curettage and to rarely metastasize to distant sites, particularly the lungs. Virtually all metastases have occurred after an initial surgical intervention and have the benign histology of the primary tumor. In contrast to patients with lung metastases from other malignant bone tumors, most of these patients may enjoy an essentially normal life span, especially if the metastatic deposits are few and can be surgically removed. Thus, historical belief has been that local recurrence of the tumor reflects inadequate resection rather than biological aggressiveness and that distant metastases may result from dislodgment of tumor fragments during surgery.

True malignancy in GCT may be occasionally observed as either a sarcomatous lesion arising in a typical GCT or as a pure sarcoma after a GCT has been curetted. Recurrence as pure sarcoma may occur spontaneously or after local radiation therapy. About 1% of GCTs demonstrate sarcomatous transformation.

GCTs manifest with pain, usually in the joint adjacent to the tumor. Microfractures and pathologic fractures are frequent, owing to thinning of the cortex. The tumor is usually treated with thorough curettage and bone grafting, although more aggressive management, including en bloc resection or even amputation, may be necessary. Local recurrence after simple curettage has been reported in one third to one half of cases, and 2% to 5% metastasize.

Ewing Sarcoma Is a Primitive Neuroectodermal Tumor of Childhood

Ewing sarcoma (EWS) is an uncommon malignant bone tumor composed of small, uniform, round cells. It represents only 5% of all bone tumors and is found in children and adolescents, with two thirds of cases occurring in patients younger than 20 years. Boys are affected more often than girls (2:1). EWS is very rare in blacks.

MOLECULAR PATHOGENESIS: EWS is thought to arise from primitive marrow elements or immature mesenchymal cells. Approximately 90% of these tumors have a reciprocal translocation between chromosomes 11 and 22 [t(11;22)(q24;q12)], which results in the fusion of the amino terminus of the *EWS1* gene to the carboxy terminus of the *FLI-1* gene, which encodes a transcription factor. The resulting fusion protein, EWS/FLI-1, is an aberrant transcription factor whose target genes are not yet fully identified. A less common translocation, t(21;22)(q22;q12), leads to *EWS/ERG* gene fusion and gives rise to a variant of EWS with a significantly worse prognosis.

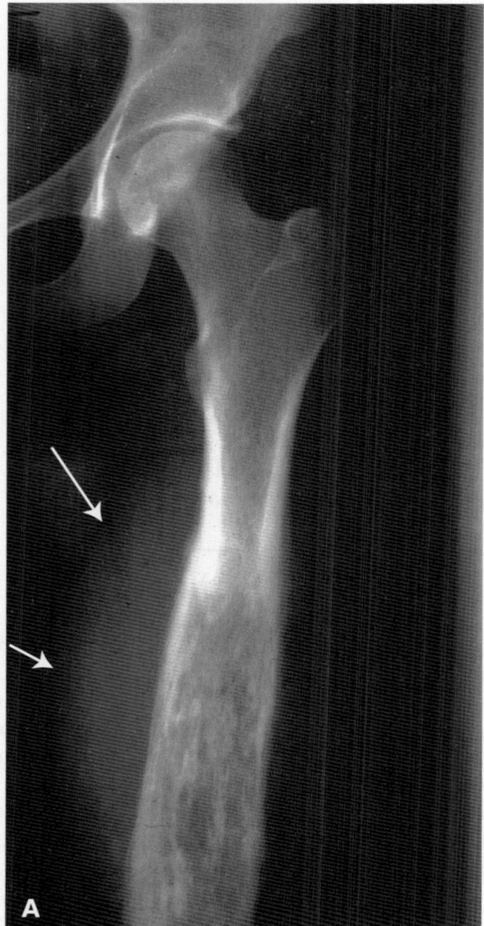

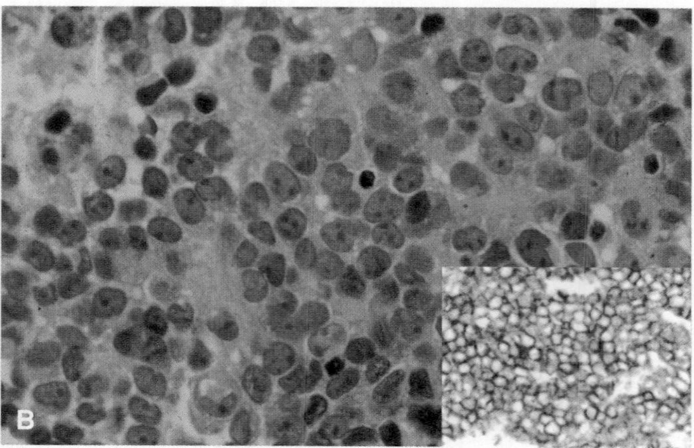

FIGURE 26-47. Ewing sarcoma. A. A clinical radiograph demonstrates expansile cortical destruction with poor circumscription and a delicate interrupted periosteal reaction (*arrows*). **B.** A biopsy specimen shows fairly uniform small cells with round, dark blue nuclei and poorly defined cytoplasm. Immunohistochemical stain for CD99 shows a membranous pattern (*inset*).

PATHOLOGY: EWS is primarily a tumor of the long bones in childhood, especially the humerus, tibia and femur, where it occurs as a midshaft or metaphyseal lesion. It tends to parallel the distribution of red marrow, so when it arises in the third decade or later, it affects the pelvis and spine. However, no bone is immune from involvement.

The radiographic findings are variable and depend on the interaction of the tumor with the host bone. There is often a destructive process in which the border between normal bone and the lesion is indistinct (Fig. 26-47A). The onion-skin pattern of periosteal bone that is sometimes seen on radiologic examination represents circumferential discontinuous layers of periosteal new bone associated with a lytic lesion involving the medulla and endosteal surface of the cortex. Some patients present with fever and weakness as well as bone pain, so it is not surprising that their condition may be mistaken for osteomyelitis.

On gross examination, EWS is typically soft and grayish white, often studded by hemorrhagic foci and necrotic areas. The tumor may infiltrate the medullary spaces without destroying the bony trabeculae. It may also diffusely infiltrate the cortical bone or form nodules in which the bone is completely resorbed. In many cases, the tumor mass penetrates the periosteum and extends into the soft tissues.

Microscopically, EWS cells appear as sheets of closely packed, small, round cells with little cytoplasm, which are up to twice the size of a lymphocyte (Fig. 26-47B). Fibrous strands separate the sheets of cells into irregular nests. There is little or no interstitial stroma, and mitoses are frequent. In some areas, the neoplastic cells tend to form rosettes. An important diagnostic feature is the presence of substantial amounts of glycogen in the cytoplasm of the tumor cells, which is well visualized with the periodic acid–Schiff (PAS) stain. EWS cells also express characteristic antigens that can be detected by immunohistochemistry (Fig. 26-47B, *inset*), some of which are part of the translocation product (e.g., FLI-1 and CD99).

EWS metastasizes to many organs, including the lungs and brain. Other bones, especially the skull, are common sites for metastases (50% to 75% of cases).

CLINICAL FEATURES: EWS initially presents with mild pain, which becomes more intense and is followed by swelling of the affected area. Nonspecific symptoms, including fever and leukocytosis, commonly follow. In some cases, a soft tissue mass is encountered.

Although EWS prognosis used to be dismal, with current use of chemotherapy plus radiation and/or surgery, 5-year disease-free survival is between 60% and 75%.

Multiple Myeloma Produces Lytic Lesions in Bone

Malignant plasma cell tumors may be either localized (plasmacytoma) or diffuse (see Chapter 20). Multiple myeloma occurs mostly in older persons (average age, 65 years) and affects men twice as often as women. Because myeloma cells secrete cytokines that recruit osteoclasts, the lesions are unique in that they are almost exclusively lytic. The bones most

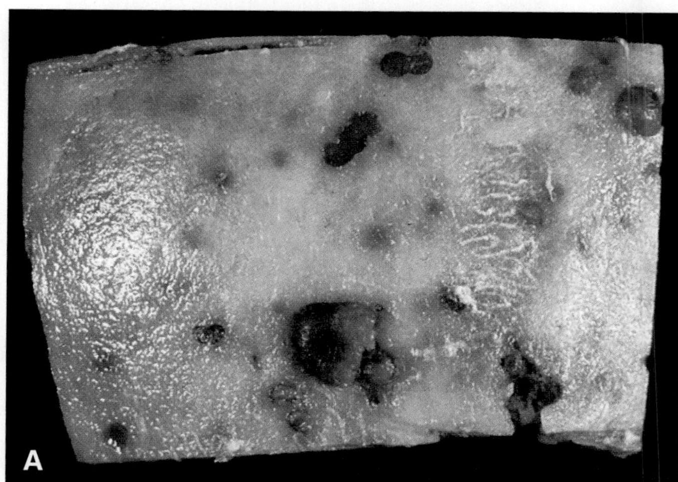

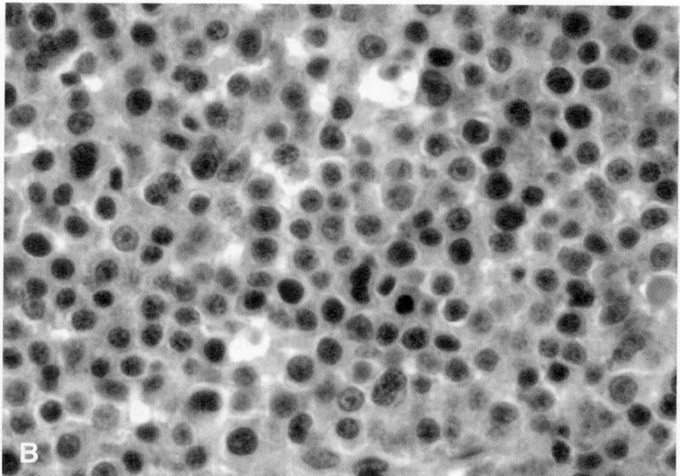

FIGURE 26-48. Multiple myeloma. A. A segment of the skull from a patient with multiple myeloma reveals numerous punched-out, lytic lesions. **B.** Microscopically, the lesions are composed of sheets of plasma cells with atypia, binucleation and discernible nucleoli.

frequently involved are the skull (Fig. 26-48A), spine, ribs, pelvis and femur. Pathologic fractures are common. On microscopic examination, sheets of plasma cells show varying degrees of maturity (Fig. 26-48B). Amyloid deposits, in both skeletal and extraskeletal sites, are seen in 10% of patients.

Despite irradiation and chemotherapy, the prognosis is poor (median survival is 32 months). Death is usually due to infection or renal failure. Solitary plasmacytoma has a better prognosis, with a 60% 5-year survival.

Metastatic Tumors Are the Most Common Malignant Tumors in Bone

In adults, most metastatic lesions to bone are carcinomas, particularly of the breast, prostate, lung, thyroid and kidney. ***In children, the most common bone metastases are from rhabdomyosarcoma, neuroblastoma, Wilms tumor and clear cell sarcoma of the kidney.*** It is estimated that skeletal metastases are found in at least 85% of cancer cases that have run their full clinical course. The vertebral column is the most common site in adults, and the appendicular skeleton is the most common site in children. Tumor cells usually arrive in the bone via the bloodstream; in the case of spinal metastases, the vertebral veins often transport them.

Some tumors (e.g., thyroid, gastrointestinal tract, kidney, neuroblastoma) produce mostly lytic lesions by stimulating osteoclasts. A few neoplasms (e.g., prostate, breast, lung, stomach) stimulate osteoblastic components to make bone (Fig. 26-49A), creating dense foci on radiographs (blastic or sclerotic lesions). However, most deposits of metastatic

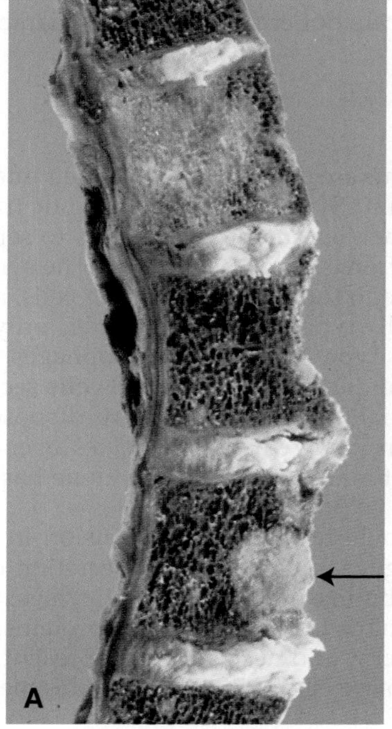

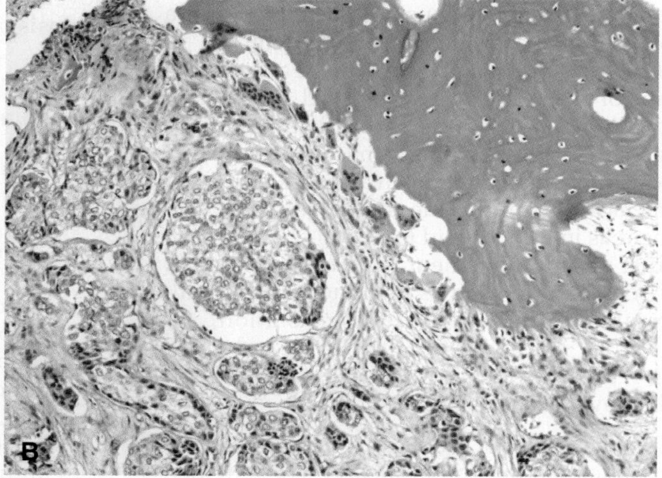

FIGURE 26-49. Metastatic carcinoma to bone. A. A section through the vertebral column reveals conspicuous tan nodules of metastatic tumor (*arrow*). **B.** Tumor-induced osteolysis. Breast cancer metastatic to bone recruits numerous osteoclasts, which resorb bone and lead to osteolytic lesions.

cancer in the bones have mixtures of both lytic and blastic elements (Fig. 26-49B).

JOINTS

A joint (or articulation) is a union between two or more bones, whose construction varies with the function of that joint. There are two types of joints: (1) a **synovial** or **diarthrodial joint,** which is a movable joint, such as the knee or elbow, that is lined by a synovial membrane; and (2) a **synarthrosis,** which is a joint that has little movement.

Synarthroses are further divided into four subclassifications:

- A **symphysis** is an articulation joined by fibrocartilaginous tissue and firm ligaments that allows little movement. Examples are the symphysis pubis and the ends of vertebral joints.
- **A synchondrosis** is found at the ends of bones and has articular cartilage but is not associated with synovium or a significant joint cavity (e.g., the sternal manubrial joint).
- **A syndesmosis** connects bones by fibrous tissue without any cartilaginous elements. The distal tibiofibular articulation and the cranial sutures are syndesmoses.
- **A synostosis** is a pathologic bony bridge between bones as, for example, in ankylosis of the spine.

Diseases of diarthrodial joints are among the oldest pathologic conditions known, having been found in the fossil bones of dinosaurs. One third of the population of the United States older than 50 years develop some form of clinically significant joint disease.

Classification of Synovial Joints

The synovial, or diarthrodial, joints are classified according to the type of movement they permit.

- A **uniaxial joint** allows movement around only one axis. Examples include a hinge joint such as the elbow and a pivot (rotational) joint such as the radioulnar joint.
- A **biaxial joint** allows movement around two axes, as the condyloid joint of the wrist axis is oriented in the long diameter and the other along the short diameter of the articular surfaces. This allows four-way movement: flexion, extension, abduction and adduction. In a saddle joint, such as the carpometacarpal joint of the thumb, joint surfaces allow movement as in a condyloid joint.
- **Polyaxial joints** permit movement in virtually any axis. In a ball-and-socket joint, such as is found in the shoulder and hip, all movements, including rotation, are possible.
- A **plane joint,** represented by the patella, allows articular surfaces to glide over one another.

UNIT LOAD: The concept of unit load is the most important principle in understanding joint function. The unit load is the compressive force, expressed as kilograms per cubic centimeter of articular cartilage. It is fairly constant over the hip, knee and ankle (20 to 26 kg/cm^3 along the articular surfaces). Because the articular cartilage is injured if a load exceeds these values, several mechanisms protect a joint from exceeding the unit load.

Adjacent muscles are the major shock-absorbing structures that protect the joint. Deformation, even to the extent of microscopic fractures of the coarse cancellous bone, also helps protect the joint. Joint deformation allows the contact area to increase with increasing load. Diarthrodial joints may have intra-articular structures such as ligaments and menisci. Menisci hold distributed force along the articular surface and allow two planes of motion, such as flexion and rotation. However, 90% or more of energy absorption across the knee joint is by active muscle contraction and only 10% or less is by secondary mechanisms, such as by the coarse cancellous bone of the knee joint. A properly functioning joint also requires support from ligaments and tendons, periarticular connective tissues such as the joint capsule and nerves that provide proprioception. Thus, to protect the articular cartilage from forces that exceed the critical unit load, virtually any structure is sacrificed, even to the point of a bone fracture.

Once there is an insult to one component of the joint, the resulting dysfunction can lead to degeneration of other components of the joint. For example, knee ligament injuries sustained by athletes, such as a torn anterior cruciate ligament, can result in joint instability, which, over time, contributes to degeneration of articular cartilage due to changes in movement and load on the joint (secondary osteoarthritis).

ARTHRITIS: Arthritis is joint inflammation, usually accompanied by pain, swelling and sometimes change in structure. Arthritis can generally be divided into two major forms: (1) **inflammatory arthritis** usually involves the synovium and is mediated by inflammatory cells (e.g., rheumatoid arthritis) and (2) **noninflammatory arthritis,** as featured in primary osteoarthritis, may involve cytokines in its pathogenesis (see below).

Structures of the Synovial Joint

Movement plays a major role in joint formation. Lack of movement retards joint development and may cause **arthrogryposis,** a rare but crippling disease characterized by joint fusion.

Synovium

Synovial joints are partially lined on their internal aspects by the synovium. Synovial linings are not true membranes since they lack basement membranes to separate synovial lining cells from subsynovial tissue. The synovium is composed of one to three layers of lining cells, and is made up of two cell types distinguishable only by electron microscopy. **Type A cells** are macrophages with lysosomal enzymes and dense bodies. **Type B cells** secrete hyaluronic acid. Synovial cell membranes are disposed in villi and microvilli, an arrangement that creates an enormous surface area. It is estimated that the knee alone has 100 m^2 of synovial lining.

The synovium controls (1) diffusion in and out of the joint; (2) ingestion of debris; (3) secretion of hyaluronate, immunoglobulins and lysosomal enzymes; and (4) lubrication of the joints by secreting glycoproteins. Synovial fluid is clear, sticky and viscous. It is present only in small amounts, not exceeding 1 to 4 mL, and is the main source of

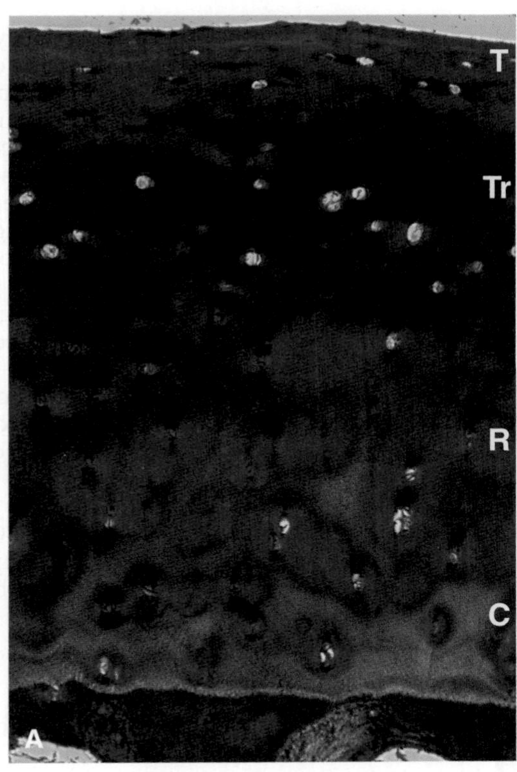

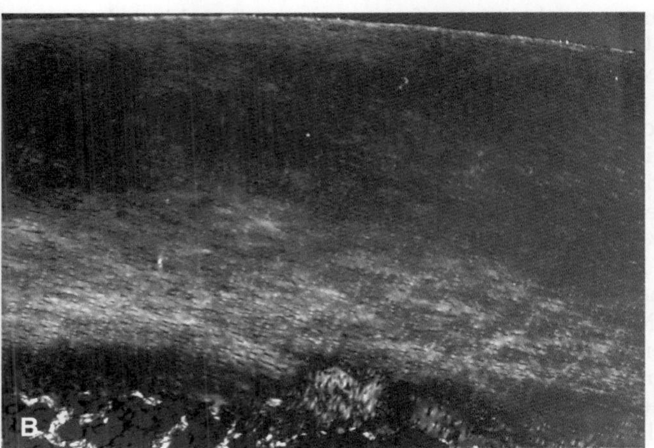

FIGURE 26-50. Articular hyaline cartilage. A. Demonstrating tangential zone (T), transitional zone (Tr), radial zone (R) and calcified zone (C). The chondrocyte lacunae change shape in conformation with the direction of the collagen arcades in the cartilage. **B.** Articular cartilage, polarized light. The tangential and radial zones have the highest concentration of collagen fibers and appear bright yellow.

nourishment for chondrocytes of the articular cartilage, which lacks a blood supply. Synovial fluid is an ultrafiltrate that acts as a molecular sieve. It does not contain tissue thromboplastin and so cannot clot. Hyaluronate is a very large molecule. Because it is highly charged, it has a high affinity for water.

Articular Cartilage

The hyaline cartilage that covers the articular ends of bones does not participate in endochondral ossification and is well suited for its dual role of absorbing shocks and lubricating the surfaces of movable joints. On gross examination, the articular cartilage is glistening, smooth, white and semirigid, and is generally not thicker than 6 mm.

Joint Histology

The articular surface appears smooth to the eye, but scanning electron microscopy reveals gentle waves and pits that correspond to the underlying lacunae of the surface chondrocytes. There are four zones in articular cartilage (Fig. 26-50).

- **Tangential** or **gliding zone:** This is the region closest to the articular surface, where chondrocytes are elongated, flattened and parallel to the long axis of the surface. Within this zone, a condensation of type II collagen fibers forms the so-called skin of the articular cartilage.
- **Transitional zone:** Chondrocytes in this slightly deeper zone are larger, ovoid and more randomly distributed than those in the tangential zone. The standard hyaline cartilage matrix is present and by electron microscopy, the collagen fibers are arranged transverse to the articular surface.
- **Radial zone:** The next deeper zone is the radial zone, where chondrocytes are small and are arranged in short columns like those seen in the epiphyseal plate. In this area, collagen fibers are large and oriented perpendicular to the long axis of the articular surface.
- **Calcified zone:** Small chondrocytes and a heavily calcified matrix characterize the deepest region.

The calcified zone is separated from the radial zone by a transverse, undulating, heavily calcified "blue line" (evident on hematoxylin–eosin staining) called the **tidemark.** The tidemark is the interface between mineralized and unmineralized cartilage. Above the tidemark on the joint side, all of the cartilage is nourished by diffusion from the synovial fluid. Deep to the tidemark, the calcified cartilage is nourished by epiphyseal blood vessels.

The tidemark is the area where the cartilage cells are renewed. As a result of cell division, true articular chondrocytes migrate upward toward the joint surface. Cell division below the tidemark occurs in the calcified cartilage, if there is appropriate stimulation. For example, in acromegaly, when the epiphyseal plates have already closed, the bones may grow in minute increments, because growth hormone stimulates the calcified cartilage remnant of the epiphyseal cartilage anlage. Because the joints in acromegaly do not keep pace, joint incongruity leads to severe osteoarthritis. Deep to the calcified cartilage, the transverse bony plate, termed the **subchondral bone plate,** supports the articular cartilage. It is directly contiguous with the coarse cancellous bone of the epiphysis.

Osteoarthritis

Osteoarthritis is slowly progressive destruction of articular cartilage that affects weight-bearing joints and fingers of

older persons or the joints of younger persons subjected to trauma. Osteoarthritis is the single most common form of joint disease and the major form of noninflammatory arthritis. It is a group of conditions that have in common the mechanical destruction of a joint.

In **primary osteoarthritis,** destruction of joints results from intrinsic defects in the articular cartilage. The prevalence and severity of primary osteoarthritis increase with age. About 4% of individuals ages 18 to 24 are affected, versus 85% of those 75 to 79 years. Before age 45, the disease mainly affects men. After age 55, osteoarthritis is more common in women. Many cases of primary osteoarthritis exhibit a familial clustering, suggesting a hereditary predisposition.

In primary osteoarthritis, also called **wear-and-tear arthritis** and **degenerative joint disease,** progressive degradation of articular cartilage leads to joint narrowing, subchondral bone thickening and eventually a nonfunctioning, painful joint. Although osteoarthritis is not primarily an inflammatory process, a mild inflammatory reaction may occur within the synovium.

Secondary osteoarthritis has a known underlying cause, including congenital or acquired incongruity of joints, trauma, crystal deposits, infection, metabolic diseases, endocrinopathies, inflammatory diseases, osteonecrosis and hemarthrosis.

Chondromalacia is a term applied to a subcategory of osteoarthritis that affects the patellar surface of the femoral condyles of young persons and produces pain and stiffness of the knee.

ETIOLOGIC FACTORS: *INCREASED UNIT LOAD:* Abnormal force on the cartilage may have many causes, but is often attributable to incongruities of the joint. Thus, in congenital hip dysplasia, a fairly common abnormality, the socket of the acetabulum is shallow, covering only 30% to 40% of the femoral head (normal, 50%). Less surface area is covered by articular cartilage, which thus bears an increased load. When the critical unit load is exceeded, chondrocyte death causes degradation of articular cartilage.

RESILIENCE OF THE ARTICULAR CARTILAGE: Because articular cartilage binds extensive amounts of water, it normally has a swelling pressure of at least 3 atm. Disruption in water bonding leads to decreased resilience.

STIFFNESS OF SUBCHONDRAL COARSE CANCELLOUS BONE: The structure of bone adjacent to a joint is important in maintaining articular cartilage. Mechanical forces are not transferred to articular cartilage by normal stress, but rather are dissipated by microfractures of coarse cancellous bone. Damage to coarse cancellous bone results in an increased unit load on the cartilage because of an increase in the stiffness of subchondral bone (e.g., in Paget disease).

MOLECULAR PATHOGENESIS: *BIOCHEMICAL ABNORMALITIES:* The biochemical changes of osteoarthritis mainly involve proteoglycans. Proteoglycan content and aggregation decrease, and glycosaminoglycan chain length is reduced. Collagen fibers are thicker than normal and the water content of osteoarthritic cartilage increases. The reduction in proteoglycans allows more water to be bound to the collagen. Thus, osteoarthritic cartilage, or any cartilage that is fibrillated, swells more than normal cartilage.

Although matrix synthesis by chondrocytes is increased early in osteoarthritis, protein synthesis eventually declines, suggesting that the cells reach a point at which they fail to respond to reparative stimuli. Similarly, chondrocytes in early osteoarthritic cartilage replicate, but cell replication diminishes with advanced disease. Acid cathepsin, which attacks the protein cores of the matrix macromolecules, increases in osteoarthritic cartilage. Collagenase is absent in normal cartilage, but is found in osteoarthritic cartilage.

Chondrocyte apoptosis, decreased type II collagen synthesis and extracellular matrix breakdown also occur and have been correlated with local increases in IL-1β and TNF-a, which, in turn, induce increased production of matrix metalloproteinases (MMP), nitric oxide and PGE_2. Mechanical stress appears to be the triggering factor for these signaling cascades.

Studies of identical twins have demonstrated genetic contributions to the prevalence of osteoarthritis. Genetic analysis of patients with a type of familial, early-onset osteoarthritis revealed a variety of mutations in the gene for type II collagen (*COL2A1*), the major collagen species of articular cartilage.

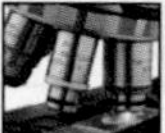

PATHOLOGY: Joints commonly affected by osteoarthritis are the proximal and distal interphalangeal joints, as well as the joints of the arms, knees, hips and cervical and lumbar spine. Radiologically, osteoarthritis is characterized by (1) narrowing of the joint space, which represents the loss of articular cartilage; (2) increased thickness of the subchondral bone; (3) subchondral bone cysts; and (4) large peripheral growths of bone and cartilage, called **osteophytes**. Histologic changes follow a well-described sequence.

1. First, loss of proteoglycans from the surface of the articular cartilage is seen histologically as decreased metachromatic staining. At the same time, empty lacunae in articular cartilage indicate that chondrocytes have died (Fig. 26-51). Viable chondrocytes enlarge, aggregate into groups or clones and become surrounded by basophilic staining matrix called the **territorial matrix.**
2. Osteoarthritis may arrest at this stage for many years before progressing to the next stage, which is characterized by fibrillation (i.e., development of surface cracks parallel to the long axis of the articular surface). These fibrillations may persist for many years before further progression occurs.
3. As fibrillations propagate, synovial fluid begins to flow into the defects. The cracks are progressively oriented more vertically, parallel to the long axis of the collagen fibrils. Synovial fluid penetrates deeper into the articular cartilage along these cracks. Eventually, pieces of articular cartilage break off and lodge in the synovium, inducing inflammation and a foreign-body giant cell reaction. The result is a hyperemic and hypertrophied synovium.
4. As the crack extends down toward the tidemark and eventually crosses it, neovascularization from the epiphysis and subchondral bone extends into the area of the crack, inducing subchondral osteoclastic bone resorption. Adjacent osteoblastic activity also occurs and results in a thickening of the subchondral bone plate in the area of the crack. As neovascularization progressively extends into

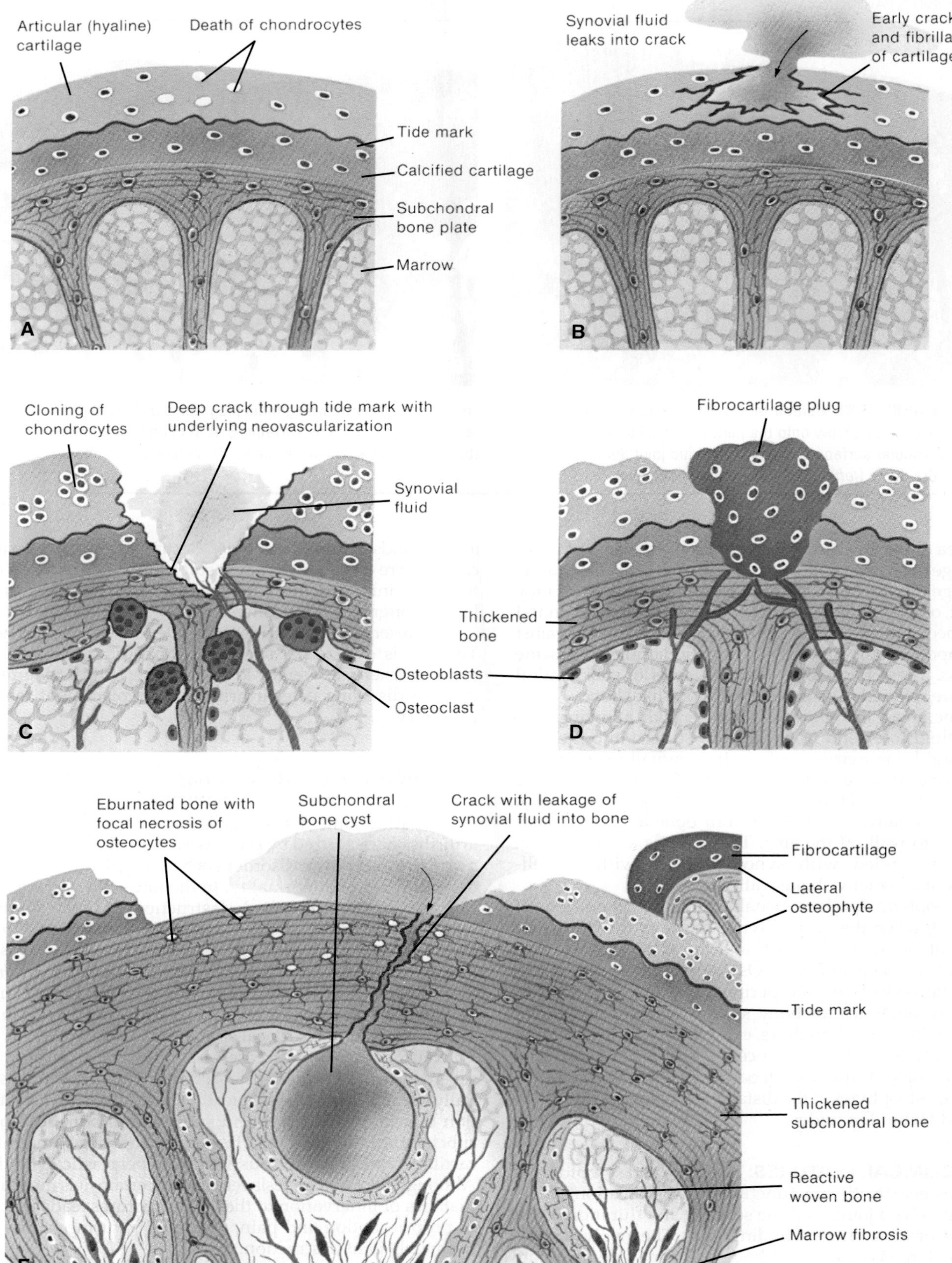

FIGURE 26-51. Histogenesis of osteoarthritis. A, B. The death of chondrocytes leads to a crack in the articular cartilage that is followed by an influx of synovial fluid and further loss and degeneration of cartilage. **C.** As a result of this process, cartilage is gradually worn away. Below the tidemark, new vessels grow in from the epiphysis, and fibrocartilage (**D**) is deposited. **E.** The fibrocartilage plug is not mechanically sufficient and may be worn away, thus exposing the subchondral bone plate, which becomes thickened and eburnated. If there is a crack in this region, synovial fluid leaks into the marrow space and produces a subchondral bone cyst. Focal regrowth of the articular surface leads to the formation of osteophytes.

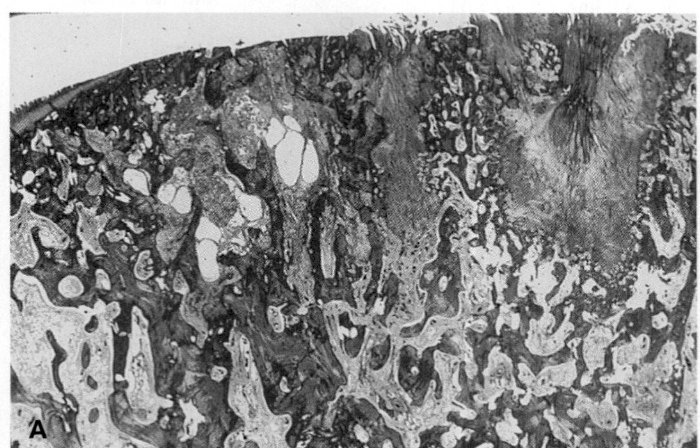
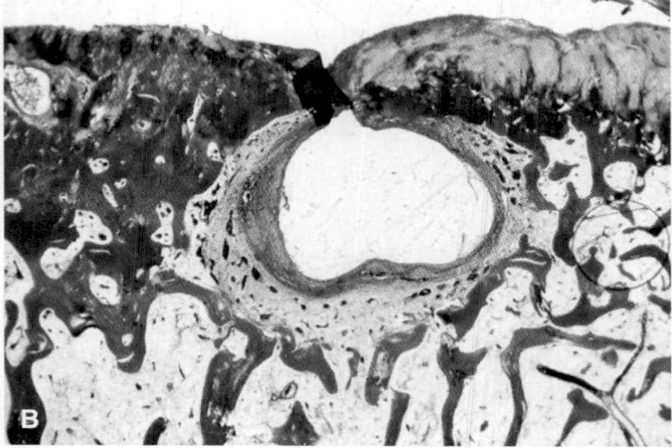

FIGURE 26-52. Osteoarthritis. A. A femoral head with osteoarthritis shows a fibrocartilaginous plug (*far right*) extending from the marrow onto the joint surface. Eburnated bone is present over the remaining surface. **B.** A section through the articular surface of an osteoarthritic joint demonstrates focal absence of the articular cartilage, thickening of subchondral bone (*left*) and a subchondral bone cyst.

the area of the crack, mesenchymal cells invade and fibrocartilage forms as a poor substitute for the articular hyaline cartilage (Fig. 26-52A). These fibrocartilaginous plugs may persist, or they may be swept into the joint. The subchondral bone becomes exposed and burnished as it grinds against the opposite joint surface, which is undergoing the same process. These thick, shiny, smooth areas of subchondral bone are referred to as **eburnated** (ivory-like) bone.

5. In some areas, the eburnated bone cracks, allowing synovial fluid to extend from the joint surface into the subchondral bone marrow, where it eventually produces a **subchondral bone cyst** (Fig. 26-52B). These cysts increase in size as synovial fluid is forced into the space but cannot exit. Eventually, osteoclasts resorb bone and osteoblasts attempt to wall off the area. The result is a subchondral bone cyst filled with synovial fluid, with a well-marginated, reactive bone wall.
6. An osteophyte develops, usually in the lateral portions of the joint, when the mesenchymal tissue of the synovium differentiates into osteoblasts and chondroblasts to form a mass of cartilage and bone. Osteophytes are pearly grayish bone nodules on the periphery of the joint surface. These osteophytes, or bony spurs, also occur at lateral edges of intervertebral disks, extending from the adjacent vertebral bodies. They produce the "lipping" pattern seen on radiologic studies as osteoarthritis of the spine. In the fingers, osteophytes at the distal interphalangeal joints are termed **Heberden nodes.**

CLINICAL FEATURES: The signs and symptoms of osteoarthritis are functions of the location of the involved joints and the severity and duration of the joint deterioration. Physical findings vary. The involved joints may be enlarged, tender and boggy and may demonstrate crepitus. Deep, achy joint pain that follows activity and is relieved by rest is the clinical hallmark of osteoarthritis. Pain is usually a sign of significant joint destruction and arises in the periarticular structures, since articular cartilage lacks a nerve supply. Discomfort also is caused by short periods of stiffness, which is frequently experienced in the morning or after periods of minimal activity. Restricted joint motion indicates severe disease and may result from joint or muscle contractures, intra-articular loose bodies, large osteophytes and loss of congruity of the joint surfaces.

At present, osteoarthritis cannot be prevented or arrested. Therapy is directed at specific orthopedic conditions and includes exercise, weight loss and other supportive measures. In disabling osteoarthritis, joint replacement may be necessary.

Neuropathic Joint Disease (Charcot Joint)

Neuropathic joint disease is a form of noninflammatory arthritis characterized by progressive joint destruction due to a primary neurologic disorder such as peripheral neuropathy or central motor abnormality. In the mid-19th century, Jean-Martin Charcot described destruction of knee joints in patients with syphilitic tabes dorsalis (Charcot joint). ***Today, the most common form of neuropathic joint disease is destruction of foot joints in people with diabetic peripheral neuropathy.*** Destruction of shoulder or other upper extremity joints can occur in patients with syringomyelia, an abnormality affecting the cervical spinal cord.

Neuropathic joint disease can be viewed as a rapid and severe form of secondary osteoarthritis in which a joint essentially fragments. Microscopically, there is marked destruction of articular cartilage and subchondral bone leading to subchondral sclerosis, cyst formation and large amounts of cartilage and bone detritus within hyperplastic synovium. Although the pathogenesis remains uncertain, it is most likely that loss of innervation to the joint structures leads to a lack of proprioception and pain, abnormal joint mechanics and ultimately joint destruction.

Rheumatoid Arthritis

Rheumatoid arthritis (RA) is a systemic, chronic inflammatory disease in which chronic polyarthritis involves diarthrodial

joints symmetrically and bilaterally. The proximal interphalangeal and metacarpophalangeal joints, elbows, knees, ankles and spine are most commonly affected. RA may occur at any age, but usually begins in the third or fourth decade, and prevalence increases until age 70. The disease afflicts 1% to 2% of the adult population and its incidence is greater in women than in men (3:1). The excess incidence of RA in women is firmly established before menopause, after which the frequency for men and women increases uniformly. Commonly, extremity joints are simultaneously affected, often in a symmetric fashion. The course of the disease varies and is often punctuated by remissions and exacerbations. The broad spectrum of clinical manifestations ranges from barely discernible to severe, destructive, mutilating disease.

It is now thought that classic RA comprises a heterogeneous group of disorders. Patients who are persistently seronegative for rheumatoid factor probably have disease of a different etiology than those who are seropositive. There are also rheumatoid-like diseases associated with underlying conditions, such as inflammatory bowel disease and cirrhosis.

MOLECULAR PATHOGENESIS:

GENETIC FACTORS: A contribution of hereditary factors to RA susceptibility is suggested by the increased frequency of the disease in first-degree relatives of affected persons and by the concordance for the illness in monozygotic twins (30%). In addition, it is generally agreed that certain major histocompatibility genes are expressed in a nonrandom manner in patients with RA. An important genetic locus that predisposes to RA is present in human leukocyte antigen (HLA) II genes, and a specific set of HLA-DR alleles (DR4, DR1, DR10, DR14) is consistently increased in these patients. These alleles share a pentapeptide sequence motif (shared epitope) in a hypervariable segment of the *HLA-DRB1* gene, which forms the rheumatoid pocket on the HLA molecule. It is likely that the binding properties of this pocket influence the type of peptides that can be bound by RA-associated HLA-DR molecules, thereby affecting the immune response to these peptides. Interestingly, seropositive RA (poor prognosis) is associated with a high frequency of an arginine in the shared epitope, whereas seronegative disease (good prognosis) commonly exhibits a lysine in the same position, further suggesting that the physical characteristics of the rheumatoid pocket influence the immune response in RA. Several non-HLA loci have been linked to RA, including a region of chromosome 18q21 that encodes RANK.

HUMORAL IMMUNITY: Immunologic mechanisms are important in the pathogenesis of RA. Lymphocytes and plasma cells accumulate in the synovium, where they produce immunoglobulins, mainly of the immunoglobulin (Ig) G class. In addition, immune complex deposits are present in the articular cartilage and the synovium. Increased serum levels of IgM, IgA and IgG are also seen.

Some 80% of patients with classic RA are positive for rheumatoid factor (RF). RF represents multiple antibodies, mostly IgM, but sometimes IgG or IgA, directed against the Fc fragment of IgG. Significant titers of RF are also found in patients with related collagen vascular diseases, such as systemic lupus erythematosus, progressive systemic sclerosis and dermatomyositis. RF also occurs in many nonrheumatic disorders, including pulmonary fibrosis, cirrhosis, sarcoidosis, Waldenström macroglobulinemia, tuberculosis, kala-azar, lepromatous leprosy and viral hepatitis. Even healthy elderly persons, particularly women, occasionally test positive for RF.

Although patients with classic RA may be seronegative, the presence of RF in high titer is frequently associated with severe and unremitting disease, many systemic complications and a serious prognosis. The presence of IgG type RF is sometimes associated with the development of systemic complications, such as necrotizing vasculitis.

Immune complexes (IgG RF + IgG) and complement components are found in the synovium, synovial fluid and extra-articular lesions of patients with RA. Furthermore, patients with seropositive RA have lower levels of complement in their synovial fluid than do those who are seronegative.

Anticitrullinated protein antibody (ACPA) is a recently developed serologic test that, like RF, is positive in approximately 67% of cases of RA. It is rarely positive if RA is not present, giving a specificity of approximately 95%. The test may be positive even before the onset of clinical disease. Currently, the most common test for ACPAs is the anticyclic citrullinated peptide test.

CELLULAR IMMUNITY: It has also been postulated that cell-mediated immunity contributes to RA. Abundant T lymphocytes in rheumatoid synovium are frequently Ia positive ("activated") and of the helper type. They are often in close contact with HLA-DR–positive cells, which are either macrophages or dendritic Ia-positive cells.

T cells may directly or indirectly interact with macrophages through production of cytokines that inhibit migration and proliferation of the latter. Such substances have been found in rheumatoid synovial fluid and in supernatants from rheumatoid tissue explants. These studies provide strong evidence that joint destruction in RA reflects local production of cytokines, especially TNF and IL-1.

INFECTIOUS AGENTS: Infectious bacteria and viruses are not detected in joints of patients with RA, although structures resembling viruses have been reported early in the disease. Most patients with RA develop antibodies against a nuclear antigen in B cells infected with Epstein-Barr virus (EBV). This antigen, RA-associated nuclear antigen (RANA), is closely related to the nuclear antigen encoded by EBV (EBNA). Moreover, EBV is a polyclonal B-cell activator that stimulates production of RF. Interestingly, the blood of many patients with RA has increased numbers of EBV-infected B cells.

LOCAL FACTORS: Synovial cells cultured from rheumatic joints exhibit a decreased response to glucocorticoids and increased production of hyaluronate. These cells release a peptide (connective tissue–activating peptide) that may influence the function of other cells, producing increased amounts of prostaglandins, particularly PGE_2.

A hypothetical scenario consistent with the evidence presented earlier might be constructed as follows:

1. In a genetically susceptible person, an unknown agent (possibly a virus, such as EBV) infects a joint or some other tissue and stimulates antibody formation.
2. These immunoglobulins act as new antigens, triggering production of anti-idiotype antibodies (RF).
3. Immune complexes containing RF are deposited in the synovium and activate complement. This increases

vascular permeability and uptake of immune complexes by leukocytes, which in turn release lysosomal enzymes, activated oxygen species and other injurious products.
4. Activated macrophages in the synovium present unknown antigens to T cells, thus stimulating production of cytokines, which amplify inflammation, tissue injury and synovial cell proliferation.

PATHOLOGY: The early synovial changes of RA are edema and accumulation of plasma cells, lymphocytes and macrophages (Fig. 26-53). Vascularity increases, with exudation of fibrin into the joint space, which may result in small fibrin nodules that float in the joint (**rice bodies**).

PANNUS FORMATION: Synovial lining cells, normally only one to three layers thick, undergo hyperplasia and form layers 8 to 10 cells deep. Multinucleated giant cells are often found among the synovial cells. The synovial lining is thus thrown into numerous villi and frond-like folds that fill the peripheral recesses of the joint (Fig. 26-54A). This inflammatory synovium now contains mast cells, creeps over the surface of the articular cartilage and adjacent structures and is termed **pannus** (cloak). Pannus covers the articular cartilage and isolates it from the synovial fluid. Lymphocytes aggregate and eventually develop follicular centers (Fig. 26-54B). The pannus erodes the articular cartilage and adjacent bone, probably through the action of collagenase produced by the pannus. Since PGE_2 and IL-1 stimulate osteoclasts and are actively produced in the rheumatoid synovium, they may mediate bone erosion.

The characteristic bone loss of RA is juxta-articular; that is, it is immediately adjacent to both sides of the joint. The pannus penetrates the subchondral bone; it may involve tendons and ligaments, leading to deformities and instabilities. Eventually, the joint is destroyed and undergoes fibrous fusion, termed **ankylosis** (Fig. 26-55). Long-standing cases may lead to bony bridging of the joint (**bony ankylosis**). The pannus may destroy cartilage by depriving it of nourishment; alternately, it may stimulate T lymphocytes to secrete a factor causing release of lysosomal enzymes. In turn, this process may lead to secondary osteoarthritis.

Changes in synovial fluid include a massive increase in volume, increased turbidity and decreased viscosity. The protein content and the number of inflammatory cells in the fluid increase, correlating with the activity of the rheumatoid process. In some cases, the leukocyte count exceeds 50,000/μL, with 95% polymorphonuclear leukocytes.

RHEUMATOID NODULES: RA is a systemic disease that also involves tissues other than joints and tendons. A characteristic lesion, termed the "rheumatoid nodule," is found in extra-articular locations. It has a central core of fibrinoid necrosis, which is a mixture of fibrin and other proteins, such as degraded collagen (Fig. 26-56). A surrounding rim of macrophages is arranged in a radial or palisading fashion. Beyond the macrophages is a circle of lymphocytes, plasma cells and other mononuclear cells. The overall appearance resembles a peculiar granuloma surrounding a core of fibrinoid necrosis. Rheumatoid nodules, which are usually found in areas of pressure (e.g., the skin of elbows and legs), are movable, firm, rubbery and occasionally tender. A large nodule may ulcerate. They often recur after surgical removal.

Rheumatoid nodules may also be seen in lupus erythematous and rheumatic fever. They are sometimes found in visceral organs, such as the heart, lungs and intestinal tract and even the dura. Nodules in the bundle of His may cause cardiac arrhythmias; in the lungs, they produce fibrosis and even respiratory failure (see Chapter 12). RA also may be accompanied by **acute necrotizing vasculitis**, which can affect any organ.

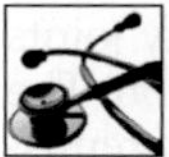

CLINICAL FEATURES: The clinical diagnosis of RA is imprecise and is based on a number of criteria, such as the number and types of joints involved, the presence of rheumatoid nodules and RF and radiographic features characteristic of the disease.

The onset of RA may be acute, slowly progressing or insidious. Most patients describe slowly developing fatigue, weight loss, weakness and vague musculoskeletal discomfort, which eventually localizes to the involved joints. Diseased joints tend to be warm, swollen and painful. The pain is heightened by motion and is most severe after periods of disuse. Unabated disease causes progressive destruction of the joint surfaces and periarticular structures. Eventually, patients manifest severe flexion and extension deformities, associated with joint subluxation, which may terminate in joint ankylosis.

The natural history of RA is variable. In most patients, disease activity waxes and wanes. One fourth of patients seem to recover completely. Another quarter have only slight functional impairment for many years. However, half develop serious progressive and disabling joint disease. There is increased mortality from infection, gastrointestinal hemorrhage and perforation, vasculitis, heart and lung involvement, amyloidosis and subluxation of the cervical spine. In fact, survival of patients with active RA is comparable to that in Hodgkin disease and diabetes.

Three types of drugs are used to suppress synovial inflammation and to induce a remission:

- **Nonsteroidal anti-inflammatory drugs (NSAIDs).**
- **Corticosteroids,** which have both anti-inflammatory and immunoregulatory activity.
- **Disease modifying antirheumatic drugs (DMARDs),** which have been shown to alter the course of the disease and improve outcome. These include cytotoxic drugs such as methotrexate, leflunomide, cyclosporin, cyclophosphamide, azathioprine, sulfasalazine, gold salts, penicillamine, antimalarial drugs (hydroxychloroquine), TNF inhibitors, T-cell costimulatory blockers, B-cell–depleting agents and IL-1 receptor antagonists. They are now recommended early in the course of the disease to prevent progression, induce remission and prevent joint deformities and functional disabilities.

Spondyloarthropathy Is a Seronegative Arthritis Mostly Linked to HLA-B27

A number of clinical entities were formerly classified as variants of RA but are now recognized to be distinct disorders. These forms of arthritis are now termed **spondyloarthropathies** and include ankylosing spondylitis, Reiter syndrome, psoriatic arthritis and arthritis associated with inflammatory bowel disease. They share several features:

- Seronegativity for RF and other serologic markers of RA
- Association with class I histocompatibility antigens, particularly HLA-B27
- Sacroiliac and vertebral involvement

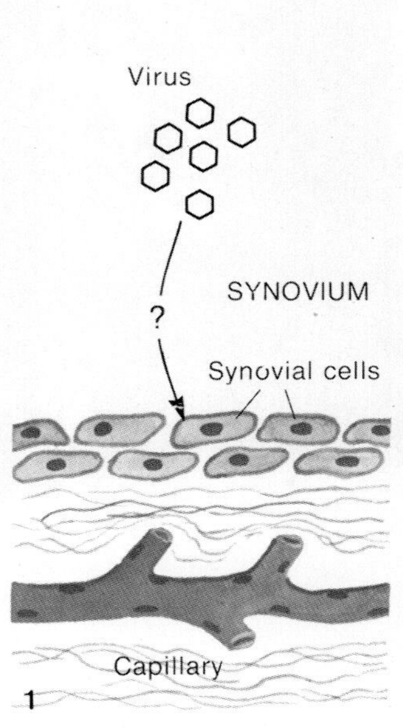

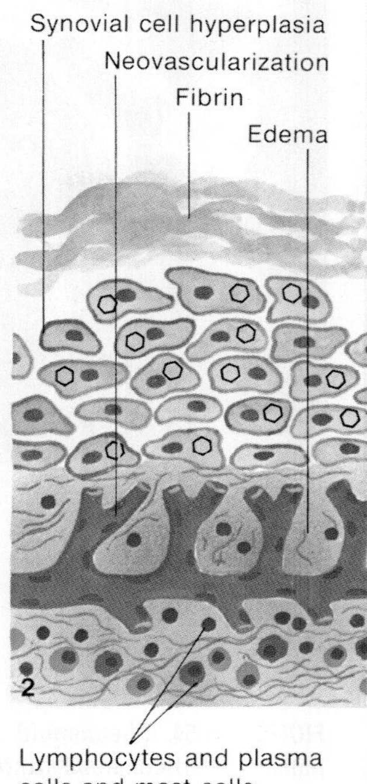

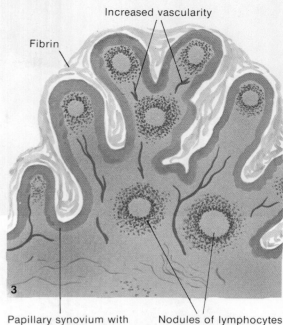

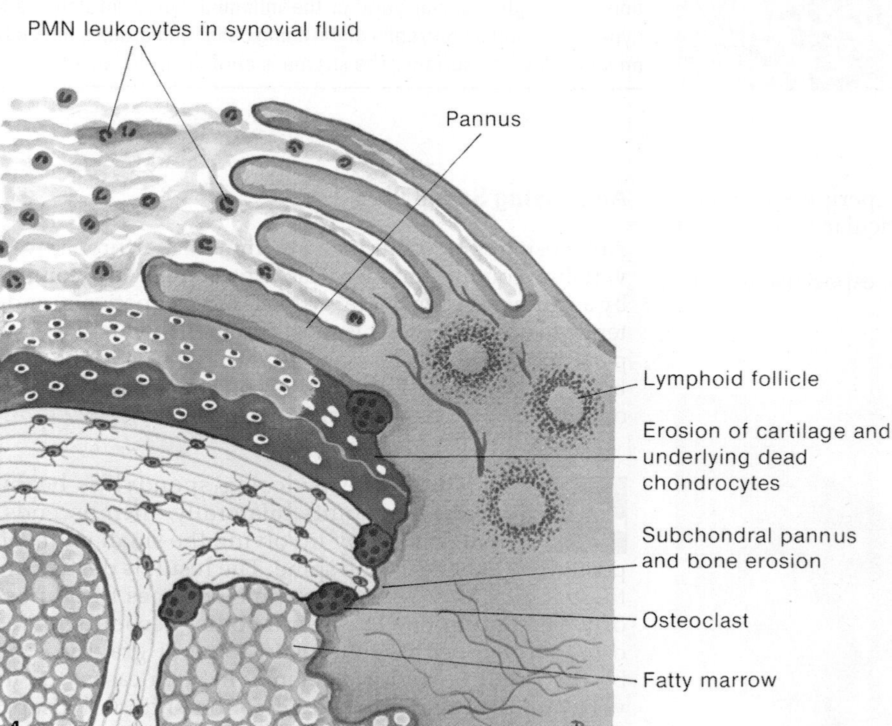

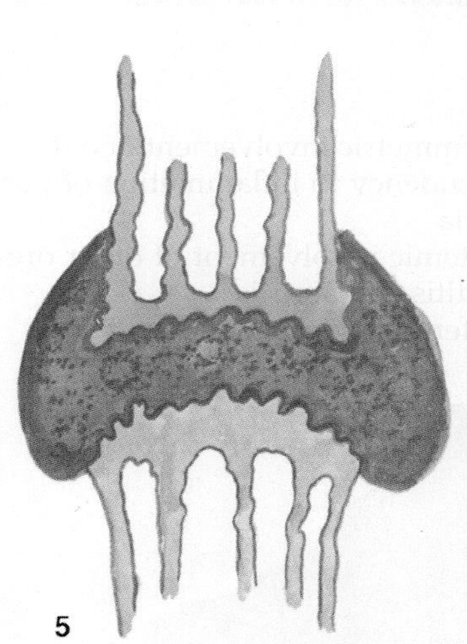

FIGURE 26-53. Histogenesis of rheumatoid arthritis. 1. A virus or an unknown stress may stimulate the synovial cells to proliferate. **2.** The influx of lymphocytes, plasma cells and mast cells, together with neovascularization and edema, leads to hypertrophy and hyperplasia of the synovium. **3.** Lymphoid nodules are prominent. **4.** Proliferating synovium extends into the joint space, burrows into the bone beneath the articular cartilage and covers the cartilage as a pannus. The articular cartilage is eventually destroyed by direct resorption or deprivation of its nutrient synovial fluid. The synovial tissue continues to proliferate in the subchondral region, as well as in the joint. **5.** Eventually, the joint is destroyed and becomes fused, a condition termed **ankylosis.**

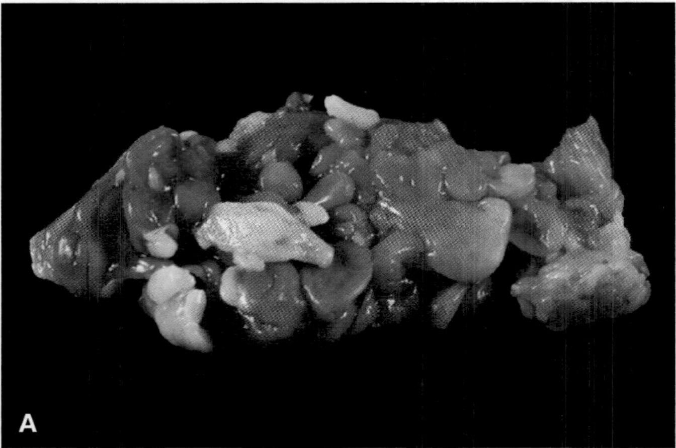

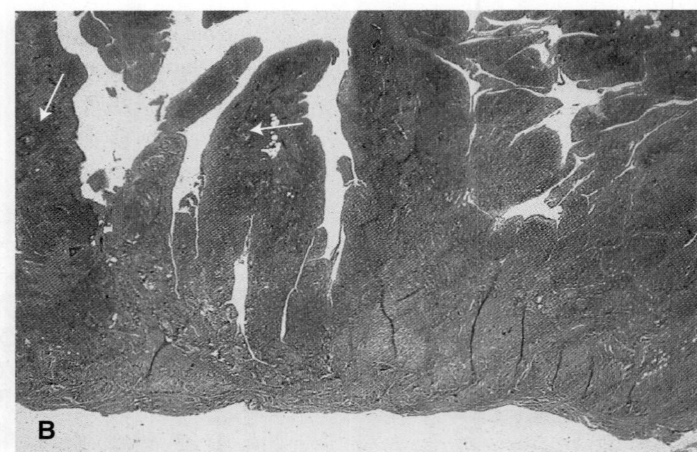

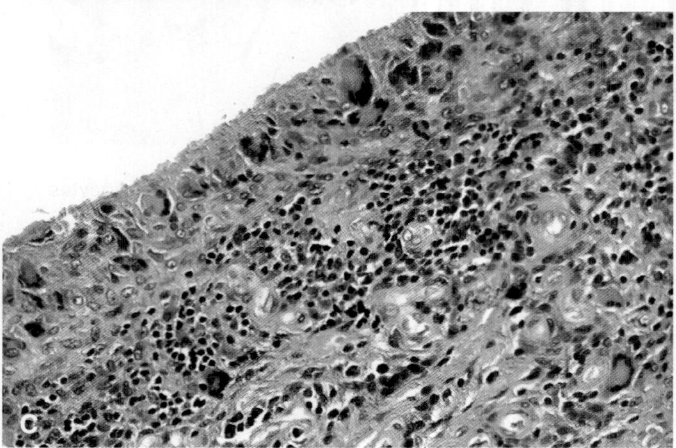

FIGURE 26-54. Rheumatoid arthritis. A. Hyperplastic synovium from a patient with rheumatoid arthritis shows numerous finger-like projections, with focal pale areas of fibrin deposition. The brownish color of the synovium reflects hemosiderin accumulation derived from old hemorrhage. **B.** A microscopic view reveals prominent lymphoid follicles (Allison-Ghormley bodies; *arrows*), synovial hyperplasia and hypertrophy, villous folds and thickening of the synovial membrane by fibrosis and inflammation. **C.** A higher-power view of the inflamed synovium demonstrates hyperplasia and hypertrophy of the lining cells. Numerous giant cells are on and below the surface. The stroma is chronically inflamed.

- Asymmetric involvement of only a few peripheral joints
- A tendency to inflammation of periarticular tendons and fascia
- Systemic involvement of other organs, especially uveitis, carditis and aortitis
- Preferential onset in young men

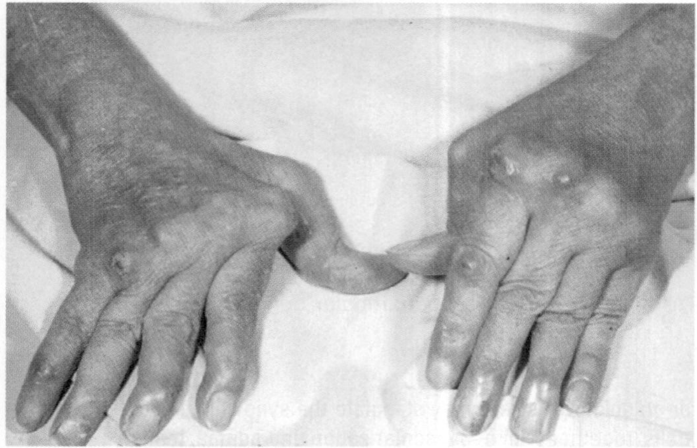

FIGURE 26-55. Rheumatoid arthritis. The hands of a patient with advanced arthritis show swelling of the metacarpophalangeal joints and the classic ulnar deviation of the fingers.

Ankylosing Spondylitis

Ankylosing spondylitis is an inflammatory arthropathy of the vertebral column and sacroiliac joints. It may be accompanied by asymmetric, peripheral arthritis (30% of patients) and systemic manifestations. It is most common in young men, with peak incidence at about age 20. Over 90% of patients have HLA-B27 (normal, 4% to 8%), although the disorder affects only 1% of persons with this haplotype.

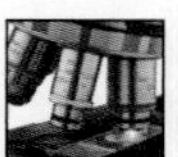

PATHOLOGY: Ankylosing spondylitis begins at the sacroiliac joints bilaterally, then ascends the spinal column by involving the small joints of the posterior elements of the spine. The result is destruction of these joints, after which the spine becomes fused posteriorly. The unburdened vertebral bodies become square and osteoporotic, because the main force of gravity is borne by the fused posterior elements. In such cases, the intervertebral disk undergoes ossification and may disappear. Eventually, bony fusion of the vertebral bodies ensues (Fig. 26-57).

Although a few patients with ankylosing spondylitis rapidly develop crippling spinal disease, most are able to maintain their employment and live a normal life span. However, up to 5% of patients develop AA amyloidosis and uremia and a few manifest severe cardiac involvement.

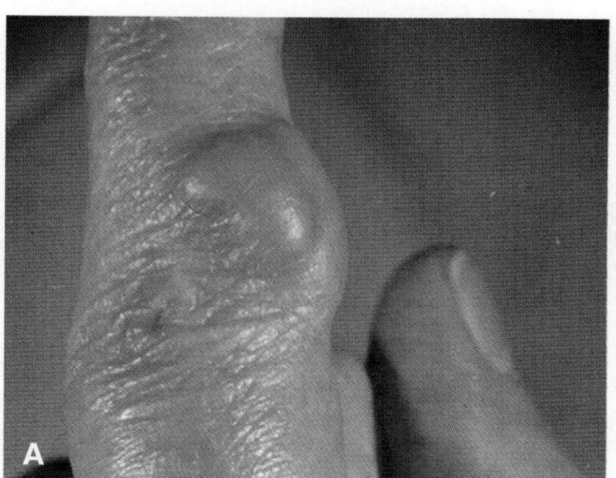

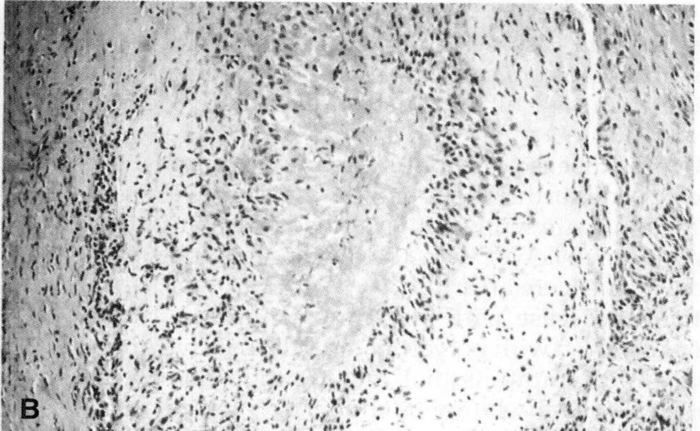

FIGURE 26-56. Rheumatoid nodule. A. A patient with rheumatoid arthritis has a subcutaneous mass on a digit. **B.** Microscopic view of a rheumatoid nodule shows a central area of necrosis surrounded by palisaded macrophages and a chronic inflammatory infiltrate.

Reiter Syndrome

Reiter syndrome (a.k.a. reactive arthritis) is a triad that includes (1) seronegative polyarthritis, (2) conjunctivitis/uveitis and (3) nonspecific urethritis. It occurs almost exclusively in men and usually follows venereal exposure or an episode of bacillary dysentery. As in ankylosing spondylitis, Reiter syndrome is associated with HLA-B27 antigen in up to 90% of patients. In fact, after an attack of dysentery, 20% of HLA-B27–positive men develop Reiter syndrome.

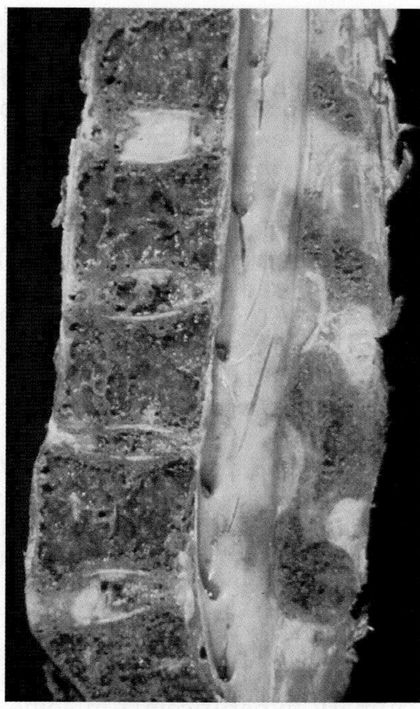

FIGURE 26-57. Ankylosing spondylitis. The vertebrae have been cut longitudinally. The vertebral bodies are square and have lost most of their trabecular bone, owing to osteoporosis from disuse. Bone bridges fuse one vertebral body to the next across the intervertebral disks. Portions of the intervertebral disk are replaced by bone marrow. Bony bridges also fuse the posterior elements (**ankylosis**).

The pathologic features of Reiter arthritis are comparable to those of RA. More than half of patients develop mucocutaneous lesions similar to those of pustular psoriasis (**keratoderma blennorrhagica**) over the palms, soles and trunk. In most patients, the disease remits within a year, but in 20%, progressive arthritis develops, including ankylosing spondylitis.

Psoriatic Arthritis

Of all patients with psoriasis, particularly in those with severe disease, 7% develop an inflammatory seronegative arthritis. HLA-B27 has been linked to psoriatic spondylitis and inflammation of distal interphalangeal joints, and HLA-DR4 has been associated with a rheumatoid pattern of involvement. Joint disease is usually mild and slowly progressive, although a mutilating form is occasionally encountered.

Enteropathic Arthritis

Ulcerative colitis and Crohn disease are accompanied by seronegative peripheral arthritis in 20% of cases and spondylitis in 10%. This form of arthritis also is seen in patients with Whipple disease and after certain bacterial infections of the gut. No particular tissue type is associated with peripheral arthritis, but most patients with ankylosing spondylitis are HLA-B27 positive. It has been proposed that HLA-B27 and proteins from enteric bacteria are structurally related in a manner that potentially affects antigen presentation to the T-cell receptor. Resection of the affected bowel in ulcerative colitis relieves the arthritis, but in Crohn disease, this complication often does not resolve.

Juvenile Arthritis Includes Any Inflammatory Arthritis in Children

Several different chronic arthritic conditions in children are included in this designation, also called Still disease. In addition to RA, many children with juvenile arthritis eventually develop ankylosing spondylitis, psoriatic arthritis and other connective tissue diseases.

- **Seropositive arthritis:** Fewer than 10% of children with arthritis are positive for RF and have a polyarticular presentation.

26 | Bones and Joints

Females predominate (80%) among children with seropositive Still disease and in most cases (75%), antinuclear antibodies are present. HLA-D4 is often present, and more than half of the children eventually develop severe arthritis.

- **Polyarticular disease without systemic symptoms:** One fourth of juvenile arthritis patients (90% girls) have disease of several joints, are seronegative and do not manifest systemic symptoms. Fewer than 15% of these patients eventually develop severe arthritis.
- **Polyarticular disease with systemic symptoms:** Twenty percent of children with polyarticular arthritis have prominent systemic symptoms that include high fever, rash, hepatosplenomegaly, lymphadenopathy, pleuritis, pericarditis, anemia and leukocytosis. Most (60%) are boys who are negative for RF and one fourth of all of these children are left with severe arthritis.
- **Pauciarticular arthritis:** Children with involvement of only a few large joints, such as the knee, ankle, elbow or hip girdle, account for half of all cases of juvenile arthritis and fall into two general groups. The larger group (80%) is mainly girls who are negative for RF but exhibit antinuclear antibodies and are positive for HLA-DR5, HLA-DRw6 or HLA-DRw8. Of these patients, one third have ocular disease characterized by chronic iridocyclitis (inflammation of the iris and ciliary body). Only a small minority of these children have residual polyarthritis or ocular damage. The smaller group of children with a pauciarticular presentation is composed almost exclusively of boys, is negative for both RF and antinuclear bodies and is positive for HLA-B27 (75%). A few have acute iridocyclitis, which resolves spontaneously. Some of these boys subsequently develop ankylosing spondylitis.

Lyme Disease

Lyme disease usually involves the knee or other large joints and is caused by the spirochete* Borrelia burgdorferi *transmitted by the Ixodes tick (see Chapter 9). Patients generally present with joint effusion and other manifestations of Lyme disease. Although there may be a transient arthritis with acute infection, patients can develop chronic Lyme arthritis, which is microscopically identical to rheumatoid arthritis. Sequelae do not occur.

Gout

Primary Gout Is a Disorder of Uric Acid Metabolism

Gout is a heterogeneous group of diseases collectively characterized by increased serum uric acid, and urate crystal deposition in joints and kidneys. All such patients have hyperuricemia, but fewer than 15% of people with hyperuricemia have gout. Gout is characterized by acute and chronic arthritis. Gout is classified as primary or secondary, depending on the etiology of the hyperuricemia. In **primary gout** hyperuricemia occurs without any other disease, while **secondary gout** occurs in association with another illness that results in hyperuricemia. Of all cases of hyperuricemia, one third are primary and the remainder secondary.

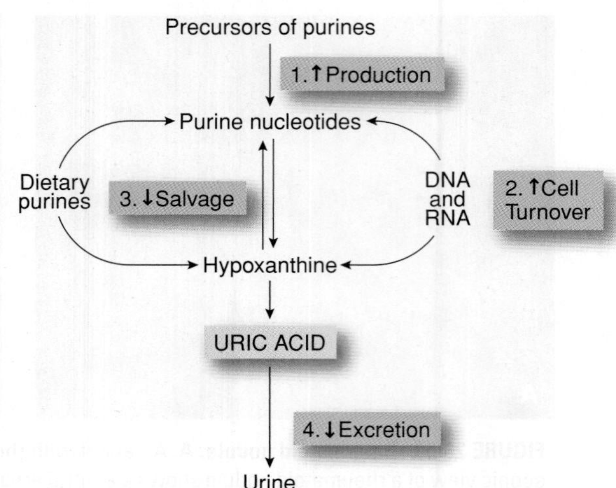

FIGURE 26-58. Pathogenesis of hyperuricemia and gout. Purine nucleotides are synthesized de novo from nonpurine precursors or derived from preformed purines in the diet. Purine nucleotides are catabolized to hypoxanthine or incorporated into nucleic acids. The degradation of nucleic acids and dietary purines also produces hypoxanthine. Hypoxanthine is converted to uric acid, which in turn is excreted into the urine. Hyperuricemia and gout result from (1) increased de novo purine synthesis, (2) increased cell turnover, (3) decreased salvage of dietary purines and hypoxanthine and (4) decreased uric acid excretion by the kidneys.

MOLECULAR PATHOGENESIS: Uric acid results from purine catabolism, due either to a high-purine diet or increased de novo synthesis. In humans, there is a tight balance between uric acid production and tissue deposition of urates. Uric acid is only eliminated in the urine. Thus, the blood uric acid level (normal, >7.0 mg/dL in men, <6.0 mg/dL in women) reflects the difference between the amount of purines ingested and synthesized and renal excretion. Gout can result from (1) overproduction of purines, (2) increased catabolism of nucleic acids due to greater cell turnover, (3) decreased salvage of free purine bases or (4) decreased urinary uric acid excretion (Fig. 26-58). A high dietary intake of purine-rich foods, particularly meat, by an otherwise normal person does not lead to hyperuricemia and gout.

Most cases (85%) of idiopathic gout result from an as-yet-unexplained impairment of renal uric acid excretion. In the remainder, there is a primary overproduction of uric acid, but only in a minority of cases has the underlying abnormality been identified.

A *familial tendency* to gout has been recognized since the time of Galen. Hyperuricemia is common among relatives of persons with gout. It has been proposed that primary hyperuricemia in some persons is inherited as an autosomal dominant trait with variable expression, in some as an X-linked abnormality and in others as instances of multifactorial inheritance. Precocious gout exhibits a strong familial tendency. The consensus today is that multiple genes control the level of serum uric acid.

Gout Can Be Due to Inborn Errors of Metabolism

The rate-limiting step in purine synthesis is condensation of glutamine with phosphoribosyl pyrophosphate (PP-ribose-P) to form phosphoribosylamine. Increased intracellular PP-ribose-P accelerates purine biosynthesis. PP-ribose-P, through the activity of hypoxanthine phosphoribosyl transferase (HPRT), also condenses with, and thereby salvages, purine bases (hypoxanthine and guanine) derived from the catabolism of nucleic acids. Although the specific cause of an abnormally high rate of urate production is not known in most cases of primary gout, two inborn errors of metabolism are known to lead to elevated PP-ribose-P.

Lesch-Nylan syndrome is an inherited, X-linked (Xq26–q27) deficiency of HPRT, a defect that leads to accumulation of PP-ribose-P, and in turn to enhanced purine synthesis. Children with this syndrome are clinically normal at birth but exhibit delays in development and neurologic dysfunction within the first year. Most are mentally retarded and exhibit self-mutilation. They are hyperuricemic and eventually develop gouty arthritis. In addition, obstructive nephropathy and hematologic abnormalities are often present.

Secondary Gout Often Results From DNA Turnover

A number of conditions result in hyperuricemia and secondary gout. As in primary gout, secondary hyperuricemia may reflect overproduction or decreased urinary excretion of uric acid. Increased production is most often associated with increased nucleic acid turnover, as seen in leukemias and lymphomas and after chemotherapy. Accelerated adenosine triphosphate (ATP) degradation may also lead to overproduction of uric acid and occurs in glycogen storage diseases and tissue hypoxia. Ethanol intake leads to secondary hyperuricemia, in part owing to accelerated ATP catabolism and (to a lesser degree) decreased renal excretion of uric acid. Reduced urate excretion may result from primary renal disease. Dehydration and diuretics increase tubular reabsorption of uric acid and lead to hyperuricemia. In fact, various drugs are implicated in 20% of patients with hyperuricemia.

Saturnine gout was described in 18th-century England, where this disease was prevalent among the upper classes with lead plumbing in their houses (Saturn is the symbol for lead). It is now recognized that these patients were afflicted with lead nephropathy. The Romans had a similar problem, because they drank from vessels containing lead.

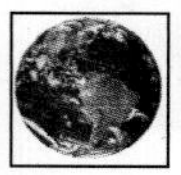

EPIDEMIOLOGY: Primary gout usually afflicts adult men; only 5% of cases occur in women. It is rare in children before puberty and in women during the reproductive years. Peak incidence is in the fifth decade. This sex distribution can be traced to the fact that at all ages, mean serum urate concentrations in women are lower than in men, although they increase after menopause. Many patients have a family history of gout, but environmental factors are also important. Positive correlations exist between the prevalence of hyperuricemia in a population and mean weight, protein intake, alcohol consumption, social class and intelligence. Thus, gout is a disease that exemplifies the interplay between genetic predisposition and environmental influences.

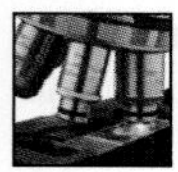

PATHOLOGY: When sodium urate crystals precipitate from supersaturated body fluids, they absorb fibronectin, complement and a number of other proteins on their surfaces. Neutrophils that have ingested urate crystals release activated oxygen species and lysosomal enzymes, which mediate tissue injury and promote an inflammatory response.

The presence of long, needle-shaped crystals that are negatively birefringent under polarized light is diagnostic of gout (Fig. 26-59). Monosodium urate monohydrate crystals may be found intracellularly in leukocytes of the synovial fluid. A **tophus** is an extracellular soft tissue deposit of urate crystals surrounded by foreign body giant cells and an associated inflammatory response of mononuclear cells. These granuloma-like areas are found in cartilage, in any of the soft tissues around joints and even in the subchondral bone marrow adjacent to joints.

Macroscopically, any chalky white deposit on intraarticular surfaces, including articular cartilage, suggests gout. Radiologically, gouty arthritis exhibits characteristic, punched-out, juxta-articular, lytic ("rat bite") lesions that are associated with only minimal reactive new bone (Fig. 26-60). In contrast to RA, there is no juxta-articular osteopenia in gout.

Renal urate deposits are between the tubules, especially at the apices of the medulla. These deposits are grossly visible as small, shiny, golden-yellow, linear streaks in the medulla.

CLINICAL FEATURES: The clinical course of gout is divided into four stages: (1) asymptomatic hyperuricemia, (2) acute gouty arthritis, (3) intercritical gout and (4) chronic tophaceous gout. Renal stones may occur in any stage except the first. In most cases, symptomatic gout appears before renal stones, which usually require 20 to 30 years of sustained hyperuricemia.

- **Asymptomatic hyperuricemia** often precedes clinically evident gout by many years.
- **Acute gouty arthritis** was well characterized by Thomas Sydenham, who described his own disease in the 1600s. It is a painful condition that usually involves one joint, without constitutional symptoms. Later in the course of the disease, polyarticular involvement with fever is common. At least half of patients are first seen with a painful and red first metatarsophalangeal joint (great toe), designated **podagra.** Eventually, 90% of all patients have such an attack. Commonly, a gouty attack begins at night and is exquisitely painful, simulating an acute bacterial infection of the affected joint. A large meal or drinking alcoholic beverages may trigger an attack, but other specific events such as trauma, certain drugs and surgery may also be responsible. Even when untreated, acute attacks of gout are self-limited.
- The **intercritical period** is the asymptomatic interval between the initial acute attack and subsequent episodes. These periods may last up to 10 years, but later attacks tend to be increasingly severe, prolonged and polyarticular.
- **Tophaceous gout** eventually appears in the untreated patient in the form of tophi in the cartilage, synovial membranes, tendons and soft tissues.

Renal failure is responsible for 10% of deaths in persons with gout. One third of patients have mild albuminuria, reduced glomerular filtration and decreased renal concentrating ability. However, the contribution of urate nephropathy to chronic renal dysfunction is unclear, and hypertension, preexisting kidney disease and the intake of analgesic drugs may be more important. In patients with severe gout caused by inherited enzyme deficiencies and in those with a

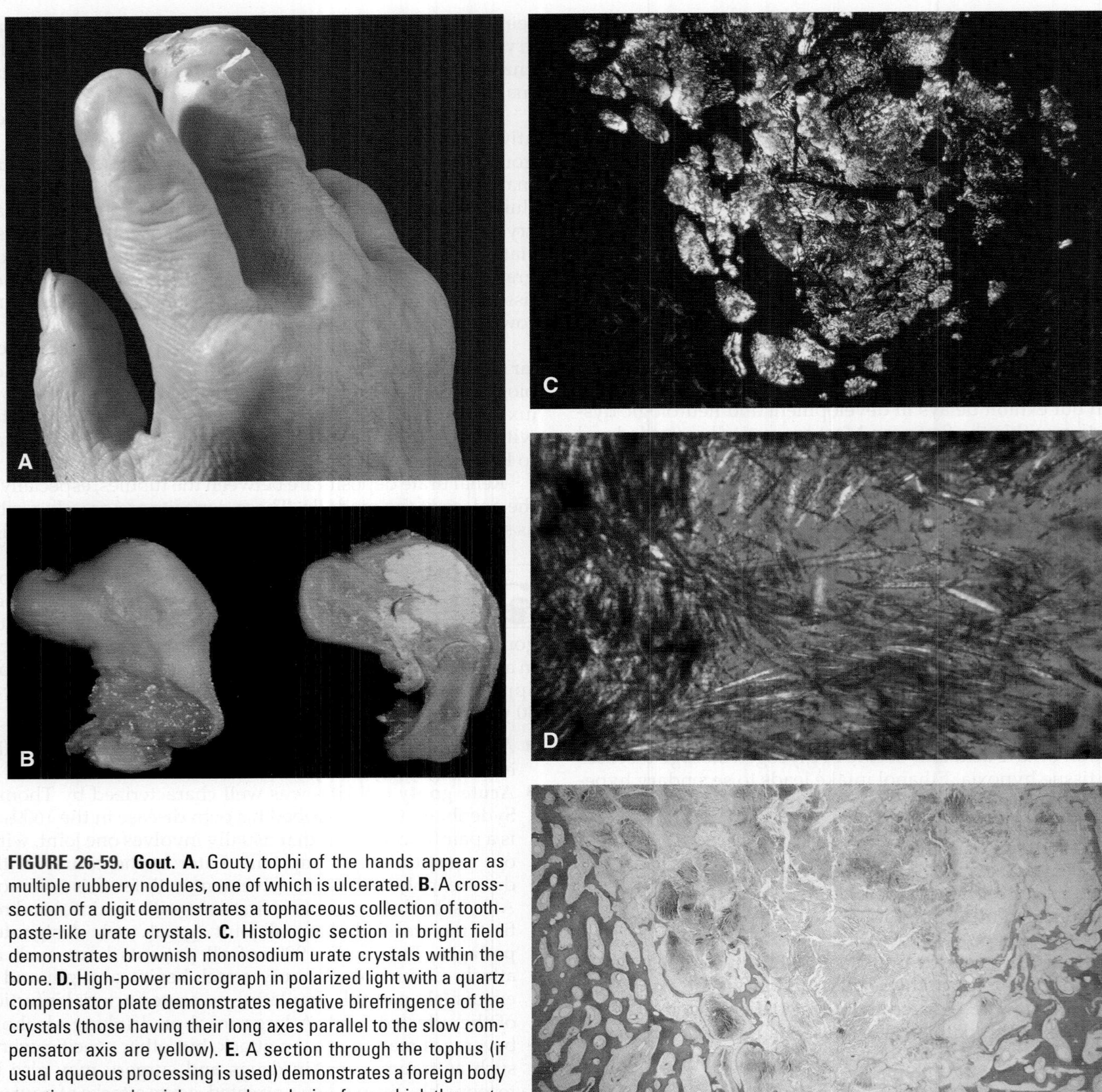

FIGURE 26-59. Gout. A. Gouty tophi of the hands appear as multiple rubbery nodules, one of which is ulcerated. **B.** A cross-section of a digit demonstrates a tophaceous collection of toothpaste-like urate crystals. **C.** Histologic section in bright field demonstrates brownish monosodium urate crystals within the bone. **D.** High-power micrograph in polarized light with a quartz compensator plate demonstrates negative birefringence of the crystals (those having their long axes parallel to the slow compensator axis are yellow). **E.** A section through the tophus (if usual aqueous processing is used) demonstrates a foreign body reaction around a pink, amorphous lesion from which the urate crystals have been dissolved during processing.

precocious presentation, urate nephropathy is a prominent feature of the clinical course. **Urate stones** are 10% of all renal calculi in the United States and up to 40% in Israel and Australia. The prevalence of urate stones correlates with the serum concentration of uric acid and affects up to 25% of gout patients. They also have an increased frequency of calcium-containing stones, in which case the uric acid may serve as a nidus for a calcium stone.

Treatment of gout is designed to (1) decrease the severity of acute attacks, (2) reduce serum urate, (3) prevent future attacks, (4) promote dissolution of urate deposits and (5) alkalinize the urine to prevent stone formation. The main drugs used to interrupt the inflammatory process, thus preventing or controlling the acute attack, are nonsteroidal anti-inflammatory agents. Colchicine has been used for hundreds of years and has been administered prophylactically during the intervals between gouty attacks to prevent recurrent episodes. Uricosuric drugs that interfere with urate reabsorption by the renal tubule are often useful.

Allopurinol is a competitive inhibitor of xanthine oxidase, the enzyme that converts xanthine and hypoxanthine to uric acid. This drug causes a prompt decrease in uricosemia and uricosuria and is used in people with renal insufficiency and those who are resistant to other uricosuric drugs. It also may

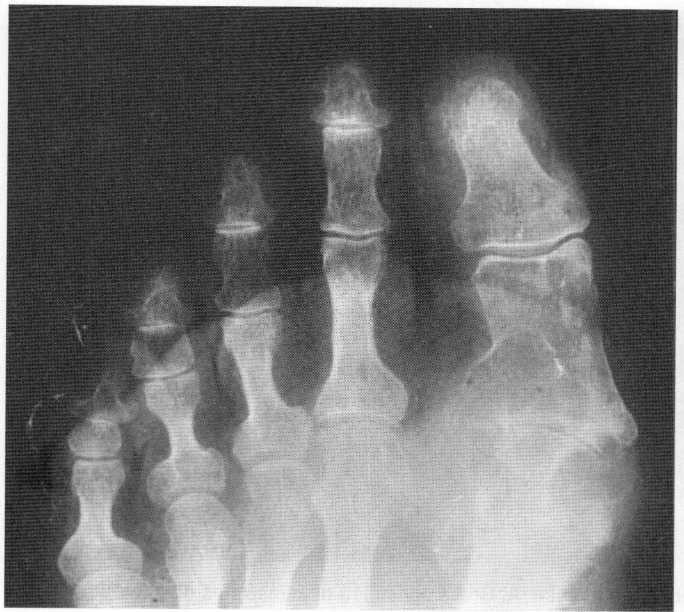

FIGURE 26-60. Gout. A radiograph of the first metatarsophalangeal joint shows a lytic lesion that destroys the joint space. There is an adjacent soft tissue tophus, as well as surrounding edema.

be administered to patients undergoing chemotherapy for hematopoietic proliferative disorders, which increases the rate of urate production.

Calcium Pyrophosphate Dihydrate Deposition Disease (Chondrocalcinosis and Pseudogout)

Calcium pyrophosphate dihydrate (CPPD) deposition disease refers to the accumulation of this compound in synovial membranes (pseudogout), joint cartilage (chondrocalcinosis), ligaments and tendons. The disease can be idiopathic, associated with trauma, linked to a number of metabolic disorders or, in rare cases, hereditary.

CPPD deposition disease is principally a condition of old age: half of those over 85 years are afflicted. Most cases in the elderly are asymptomatic. Because fully two thirds of these patients manifest preexisting joint damage, it is believed that trauma and the aging process in cartilage promote nucleation of CPPD crystals. In asymptomatic cases, punctate or linear calcifications may be present in any fibrocartilage or hyaline cartilage surface. For example, radiography of the knee may disclose linear streaks that outline the menisci.

MOLECULAR PATHOGENESIS: The major predisposing abnormality in patients with CPPD deposition disease is an excessive level of inorganic pyrophosphate in the synovial fluid. This material derives from hydrolysis of nucleoside triphosphates in joint chondrocytes. Increased pyrophosphate levels in synovial fluid can result from either increased production or decreased catabolism.

CPPD deposition is commonly found in the knees after trauma and after surgical removal of the meniscus. Nucleotides released after injury to articular cartilage may act as substrates for nucleotide triphosphate pyrophosphohydrolase (NTP), thereby increasing production of pyrophosphate. A number of other disorders are associated with deposition of CPPD crystals, including hyperparathyroidism, hypothyroidism, hemochromatosis, Wilson disease and ochronosis. Iron and copper are presumed to inhibit pyrophosphatase, accounting for decreased degradation of pyrophosphate.

Mutations in the *ANKH* gene cause familial autosomal dominant CPPD chondrocalcinosis. The *ANKH* gene is thought to encode a membrane pyrophosphate transporter that inhibits mineralization of several tissues including joints, articular cartilage and tendons. Mutated ANKH elevates intracellular pyrophosphate and reduces extracellular pyrophosphate.

Hypophosphatasia is a heritable condition in which activity of alkaline phosphatase (the enzyme that hydrolyzes pyrophosphate) in serum and tissue is deficient. As a result, pyrophosphate is not adequately metabolized and accumulates in synovial fluid.

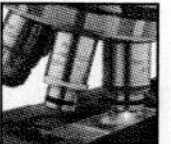 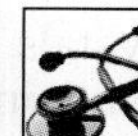

PATHOLOGY AND CLINICAL FEATURES: A minority of patients symptomatic with CPPD deposition disease are classified according to the nature of joint involvement.

- **Pseudogout** refers to self-limited attacks of acute arthritis lasting from 1 day to 4 weeks and involving one or two joints. Some 25% of patients with CPPD deposition disease have an acute onset of gout-like symptoms manifesting as inflammation and swelling of the knees, ankles, wrists, elbows, hips or shoulders. Metatarsophalangeal joints, which are frequently affected in gout, are usually spared. The synovial fluid exhibits abundant leukocytes containing CPPD crystals.
- **Pseudorheumatoid arthritis** is a variant of CPPD deposition disease in which multiple joints are chronically involved. The symptoms are mild and resemble those of RA.
- **Pseudo-osteoarthritis** has symptoms similar to those of osteoarthritis.
- **Pseudoneurotrophic disease** is characterized by joint destruction severe enough to resemble a neurotrophic joint.

On gross examination, CPPD deposits appear as chalky white areas on cartilaginous surfaces (Fig. 26-61A). Unlike needle-shaped urate crystals, they are stubby, short and rhomboid ("coffin shaped") and have weak positive birefringence under polarized light. In contrast to urate crystals, CPPD crystals do not dissolve in water and are easily found in tissue sections (Fig. 26-61B). Only a few mononuclear cells and macrophages surround foci of crystal deposition.

Calcium Hydroxyapatite Deposition Disease

Calcium hydroxyapatite deposition disease is an acute or chronic arthritis characterized by hydroxyapatite crystals within leukocytes and mononuclear cells in joint tissue and synovial fluid. Calcium hydroxyapatite (HA) is the major mineral of bone and teeth and is the compound deposited in

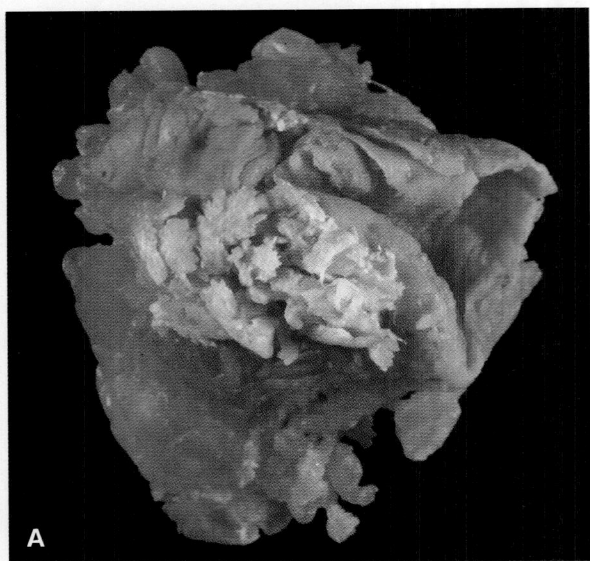

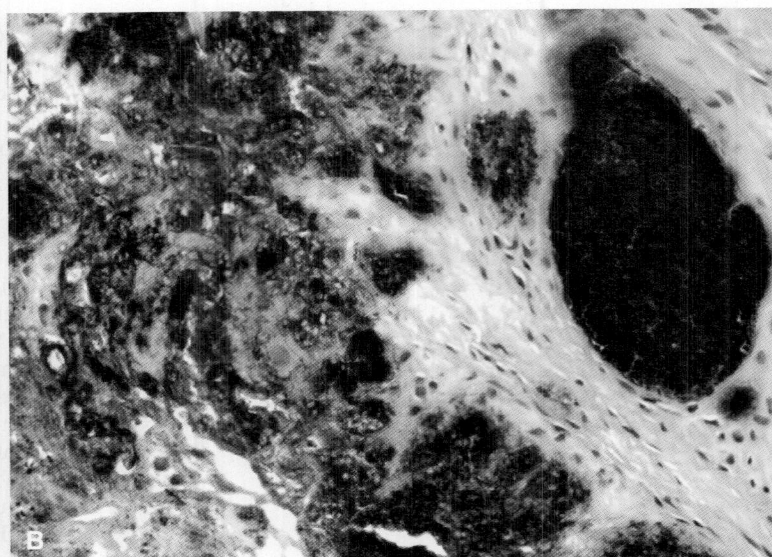

FIGURE 26-61. Calcium pyrophosphate dihydrate (CPPD) deposition disease. A. Gross specimen demonstrates chalky-white calcific material. **B.** Microscopically, the deposits are deep purple with discernible rhomboid-shaped crystals.

dystrophic and metastatic calcification. HA crystals are frequently encountered in the synovial fluid of joints involved by osteoarthritis, but there is reason to believe that severe HA deposition is a distinct entity. The joints most frequently involved are the knee, shoulder, hip and fingers. Attacks may last several days.

Hemophilia, Hemochromatosis and Ochronosis

Hemophilia, hemochromatosis and ochronosis (see Chapter 6) all produce joint disease with degradation of the matrix and destruction of the articular cartilage.

- **Hemophilia** gives rise to severe forms of arthritis because of extensive bleeding into joints (hemarthrosis), particularly the knees, elbows, ankles, shoulders and hips. In addition to the effects within the articular cartilage matrix, synovial proliferation also simulates RA.
- **Hemochromatosis** is complicated by arthritis in half of affected patients. The hands, hips and knees may be involved in recurrent attacks.
- **Ochronosis** is a rare, autosomal recessive disease caused by a defect in homogentisic acid oxidase. The deposition of ochronotic pigment in the cartilage of the joints, including the intravertebral disks, eventually causes them to become brittle and degenerate.

Tumors and Tumor-Like Lesions of Joints

True neoplasms of the joints are rare. The most common malignant lesions of the synovium are metastatic carcinomas, particularly adenocarcinoma of the colon, breast and lung. Lymphoproliferative diseases (e.g., leukemia) may also involve the synovium, mimicking other conditions, such as RA. It is unusual for primary malignant bone tumors to extend into the joint, although they may invade the joint capsule from the soft tissues.

A Ganglion Is a Small Fluid-Filled Cyst

A ganglion is a thin-walled, simple cyst containing clear mucinous fluid, which occurs most commonly on the extensor surfaces of the hands and feet, especially the wrist. It is more common in females between 25 and 45 years. The cyst arises either from the synovium or from areas of myxoid change in the connective tissue, possibly after trauma. The wall is composed of fibrous tissue and there is no cell lining. The lesion may be painful and can be readily removed surgically, although a blow with the family Bible was the traditional treatment for a ganglion on the dorsum of the wrist.

A **Baker cyst** is a herniation of the synovium of the knee joint into the popliteal space. It is most often seen in association with various forms of arthritis, in which the intra-articular pressure is increased.

Synovial Chondromatosis Features Cartilage Nodules in a Joint

Synovial chondromatosis is a benign, self-limited disease in which hyaline cartilage nodules form in the synovium, detach from that structure and float in the synovial fluid, like grains of sand between gears. The chronic irritation produced by these foreign bodies stimulates the synovium to secrete large amounts of synovial fluid and also causes bleeding in the synovial membrane. Synovial chondromatosis involves the large diarthrodial joints of young and middle-aged men, affecting the knee in most cases, but also the hip, elbow, shoulder and ankle. Patients have pain, stiffness and locking of the joint, with associated bloody effusions.

Unlike cartilage that detaches from articular surfaces in osteoarthritis, in synovial chondromatosis fragments of hyaline cartilage are formed de novo in the synovium (Fig. 26-62).

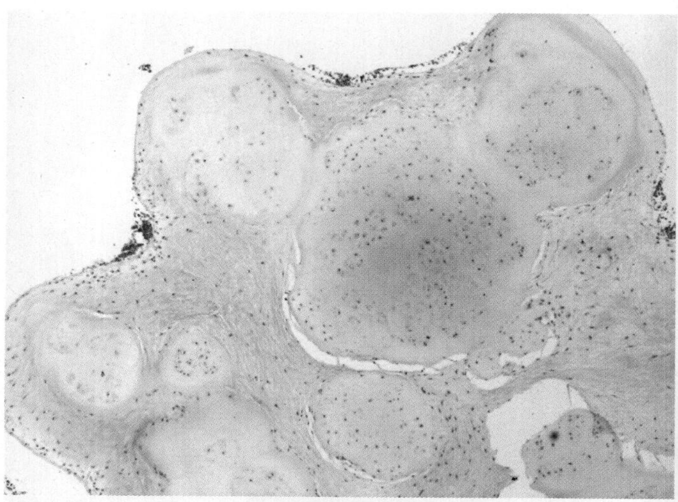

FIGURE 26-62. Synovial chondromatosis. Nodules of benign hyaline cartilage form in the synovium.

They do not have a tidemark and thus differ from true articular cartilage. Occasionally, the cartilage nodules, while still in the synovium, undergo endochondral ossification, in which case the disease is called **synovial osteochondromatosis**. If these nodules detach, the bony portions die, but the cartilage fragments remain viable and enlarge because they are nourished by synovial fluid. Evacuating the joint and performing a partial synovectomy treat the condition.

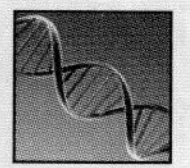

MOLECULAR PATHOGENESIS: Dysregulation of Hedgehog signaling is a factor in the development of synovial chondromatosis in animal models and suggests that this disorder is a neoplasm.

Tenosynovial Giant Cell Tumor Is a Benign Neoplasm of Synovial Lining

This is the most common neoplasm of synovium and tendon sheath and occurs in a localized and a diffuse form. The lesions may be intra- or extra-articular.

- **Localized tenosynovial giant cell tumor or giant cell tumor of the tendon sheath** involves tendon sheaths of the hands and feet. It is the most common soft tissue tumor of the hand. It occurs mostly in young and middle-aged women (30 to 50 years) and involves flexor surfaces of the middle or index fingers. The tumor is usually well circumscribed and grows slowly.
- **Diffuse tenosynovial giant cell tumor or pigmented villonodular synovitis (PVNS)** is characterized by an ill-defined, exuberant proliferation of synovial lining cells arising from periarticular soft tissues, with extension into the subsynovial tissue. It involves a single joint, usually in young adults, and is seen equally in males and females. The most common site is the knee (80%), but it also occurs in the hip, ankle, calcaneocuboid joint, elbow and, less frequently, the tendon sheaths of the fingers and toes.

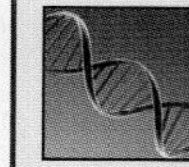

MOLECULAR PATHOGENESIS: In the past, these lesions were regarded as reactive/inflammatory but recurrent chromosomal aberrations have been described in both forms, supporting a neoplastic nature. Translocations involving the short arm of chromosome 1 have been detected, most commonly t(1;2)(p11;q35-36) or (p13;q37), with evidence of a fusion of colony-stimulating factor-1 (CSF-1) with COL6a3. Trisomies for chromosomes 5 and 7 have been found only in the diffuse form. The association of these anomalies with tumor pathogenesis is unclear.

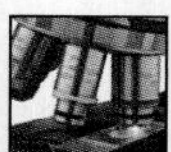

PATHOLOGY: The localized tenosynovial giant cell tumor is characterized by a small (<4 cm), multinodular, smooth contoured, partially encapsulated, exophytic mass attached to a tendon sheath. The diffuse form is usually larger than 5 cm and poorly circumscribed. It invades the joint and erodes the bone (Fig. 26-63A). It may insinuate through joint capsules into soft tissue and encompass nerves and arteries, sometimes necessitating radical surgical excision. The synovium develops enlarged folds and nodular excrescences that are brown colored owing to their iron pigment content (Fig. 26-63B). Microscopically, both tumors have very similar histology. They are composed of bland mononuclear cells resembling histiocytes, admixed with scattered multinucleated giant cells, fibroblasts and foam cells. Hemosiderin-laden macrophages reflect previous hemorrhage (Fig. 26-63C,D). The diffuse form extensively infiltrates the surrounding tissue and frequently displays a villous configuration.

Treatment for these lesions is surgical excision. Radiation therapy has been used for unresectable cases. Amputation is occasionally necessary for local control. Tumors recur in 10% to 20% of cases of localized tenosynovial giant cell tumor in contrast to 40% to 50% in the diffuse form. Metastases do not occur. A malignant counterpart has been described but it is very rare.

SOFT TISSUE TUMORS

Soft tissue tumors are neoplasms that arise in certain extraskeletal mesodermal tissues of the body, including skeletal muscle, fat, fibrous tissue, blood vessels and lymphatics. Tumors of peripheral nerves may be included in the category of soft tissue tumors, despite their derivation from the neuroectoderm (see Chapter 28). Malignant soft tissue tumors are rare, accounting for less than 1% of all malignancies in the United States. Benign soft tissue neoplasms are 100 times more common than malignant ones.

Soft tissue tumors are believed to arise from multipotential mesenchymal stem cells that reside in soft tissues and are generally classified according to the phenotype they exhibit (e.g., fibroblastic, adipocytic, vascular, myoid, etc.). Many have characteristic and unique chromosomal abnormalities that are diagnostically useful.

In the context of soft tissue tumors, the term **benign** is somewhat relative because so-called benign tumors may invade and may recur locally (e.g., fibromatosis). Malignant soft tissue tumors (sarcomas) can metastasize via the bloodstream, usually to the lungs. ***Patients generally die of metastatic disease rather than local invasion at the primary tumor site.***

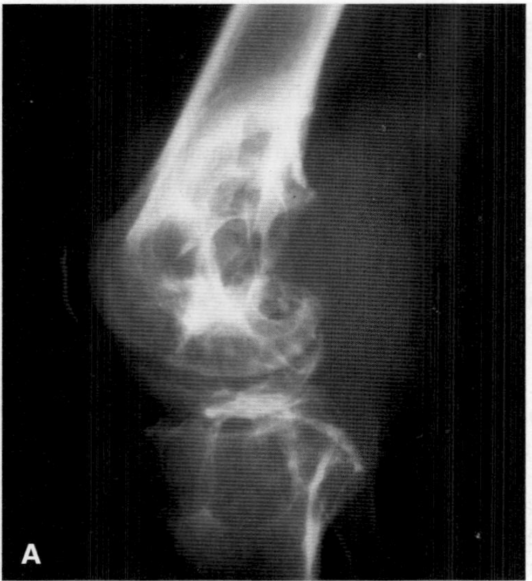

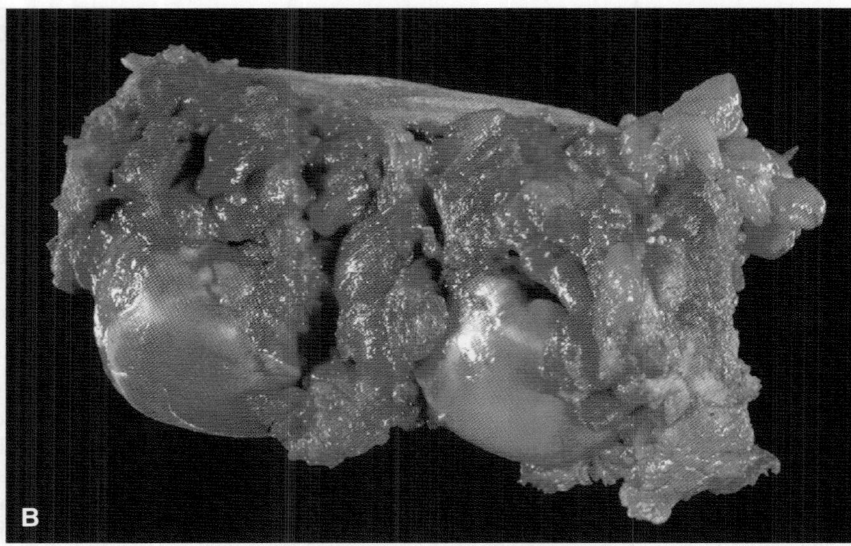

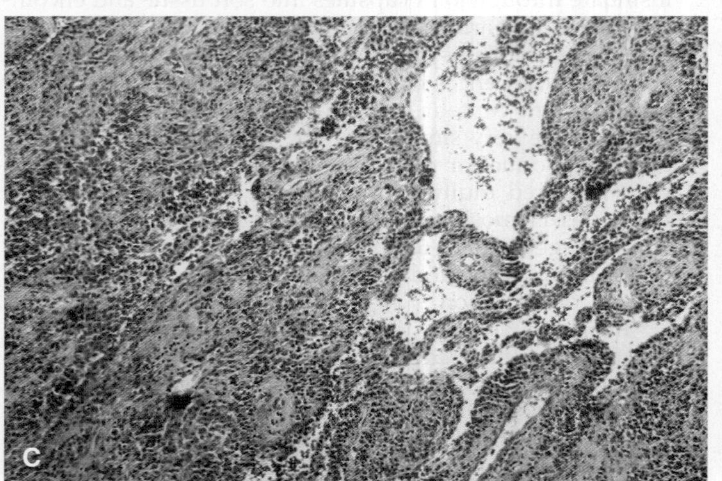

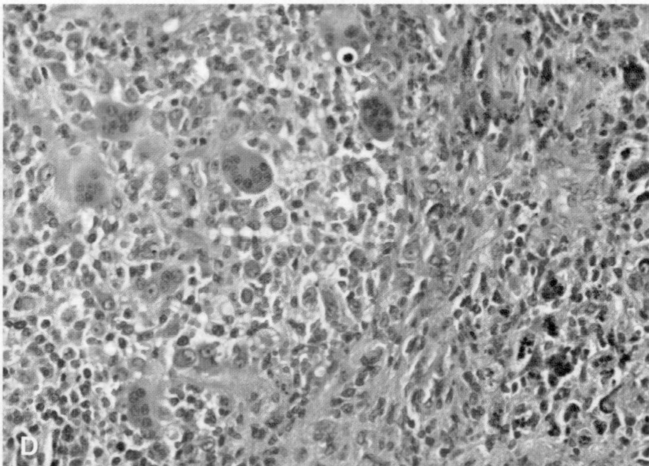

FIGURE 26-63. Pigmented villonodular synovitis. A. Radiograph of the knee demonstrates confluent erosions of the distal femur and proximal tibia and a soft tissue mass within the joint. **B.** Gross specimen shows massive destruction of the femoral condyles. Note brown color and nodular thickenings. **C.** Low-power microscopy demonstrates thickened villous synovium. **D.** At higher power, the cellular infiltrate mainly consists of mononuclear histiocytic synoviocytes, many of which contain brown hemosiderin pigment, and multinucleated giant cells.

A group of genetic disorders associated with soft tissue tumors includes neurofibromatosis type 1, tuberous sclerosis, Osler-Weber-Rendu disease and mesenteric fibromatosis in Gardner syndrome. Burns in childhood produce scars, which in rare instances lead to soft tissue fibroblastic tumors many years later. Radiation injury has been reported to be associated with the development of sarcomas years after exposure. There is no scientific evidence to support the association of trauma with the development of soft tissue tumors, and injury merely draws attention to a preexisting tumor.

A few important general principles relate to soft tissue tumors:

- Superficial tumors tend to be benign.
- Deep lesions are often malignant.
- Large tumors are more often malignant than small ones.
- Rapidly growing tumors are more likely to be malignant than tumors that develop slowly.
- Calcification may exist in both benign and malignant tumors.
- Benign tumors are relatively avascular, whereas most malignant ones are hypervascular.
- Some soft tissue tumors are classified on the basis of genetic or molecular findings.

Tumors and Tumor-Like Conditions of Fibrous Origin

Nodular Fasciitis Is a Benign Lesion That May Mimic a Sarcoma

Nodular fasciitis is a rapidly growing reactive lesion that probably results from trauma and commonly affects superficial tissues of the forearm, trunk and back. Most cases occur in young adults and the lesion's rapid growth usually prompts a patient to seek medical attention. Histologically, it may be mistaken for a sarcoma, because it is hypercellular and has abundant mitoses and numerous polymorphic, spindle-shaped fibroblasts and myofibroblasts in a myxoid stroma (Fig. 26-64). Its true nature is revealed when it is recognized that the entire "mass" is the counterpart of granulation tissue or an exuberant scar in response to trauma. Cytogenetic abnormalities involving chromosome 15 have been reported in some cases. The affected region on chromosome 15 codes for proteins involved in tissue repair (e.g., FGF-7) and oncogenic proteins. Nodular fasciitis is self-limited and is cured by surgical excision.

Fibromatosis Is a Locally Aggressive Proliferation of Fibroblasts

Also known as desmoid tumor, fibromatosis is a locally invasive, slowly growing mass that may occur virtually anywhere in the body. They do not metastasize, but surgical resection is often followed by local recurrence. Diabetics, alcoholics and epileptics have an increased incidence of fibromatosis, as do patients with familial adenomatous polyposis.

MOLECULAR PATHOGENESIS: Inactivating mutations in the *APC* gene are found mostly in cases of fibromatosis that are associated with familial adenomatous polyposis. The APC protein binds to β-catenin and enhances its degradation. Thus, loss of APC indirectly stabilizes β-catenin. β-catenin in turn promotes Wnt pathway signaling, which modulates developmental genes and presumably plays a role in the development of fibromatosis. Many sporadic cases of fibromatosis have activating mutations in the gene for β-catenin, which make it resistant to the inhibitory effect of APC. In short, mutations in both the *APC* and β-catenin genes result in persistent stabilization of β-catenin.

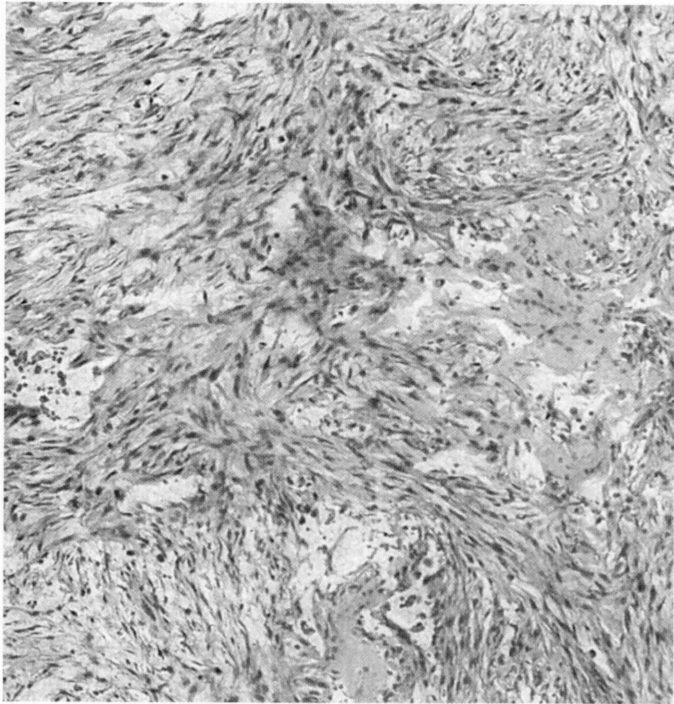

FIGURE 26-64. Nodular fasciitis. Swirls of tightly woven uniform spindle cells and collagen are admixed with a few lymphoid cells and vascular channels.

PATHOLOGY: On gross examination, the lesions of fibromatosis tend to be large, firm and whitish, with poorly demarcated borders and a whorled cut surface. They frequently originate in a muscular fascia. Microscopic examination reveals sheets and interdigitating fascicles of benign-appearing spindle cells (fibroblasts) with little mitotic activity (Fig. 26-65). Because microscopic tongues of tumor extend between preexisting structures, surgical "shelling out" of the lesion is followed by recurrences in half of cases. Complete surgical excision is curative.

Specific forms of fibromatosis are identified by their characteristic locations:

- **Palmar fibromatosis** (Dupuytren contracture) is the most common form of fibromatosis. It affects 1% to 2% of the general population but as many as 20% of persons older than 65 years. In half of cases, the lesion is bilateral, and in 10% of cases it is associated with fibromatosis in other locations. Fibrous nodules and cord-like bands in the palmar fascia eventually lead to flexion contractures of the fingers, particularly the fourth and fifth digits.
- **Plantar fibromatosis** is similar to palmar fibromatosis, except that it is less frequent and involves the plantar aponeurosis.
- **Penile fibromatosis** (Peyronie disease) is the least common of the localized fibromatoses. It is characterized by

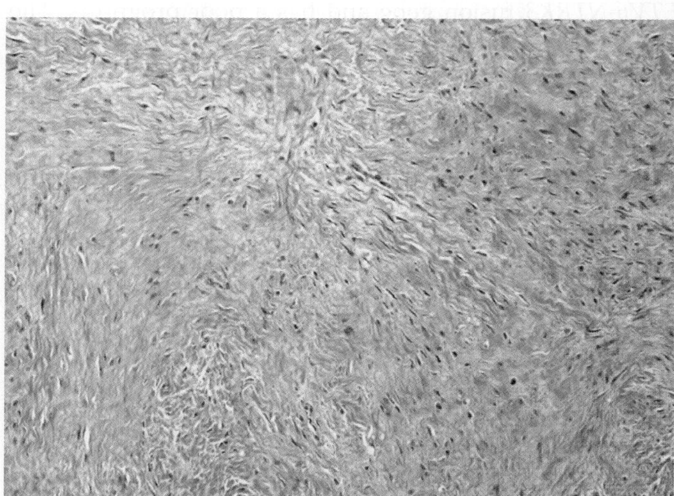

FIGURE 26-65. Fibromatosis. Microscopically, the lesion is composed of fascicles of bland spindle cells in a collagenous stroma.

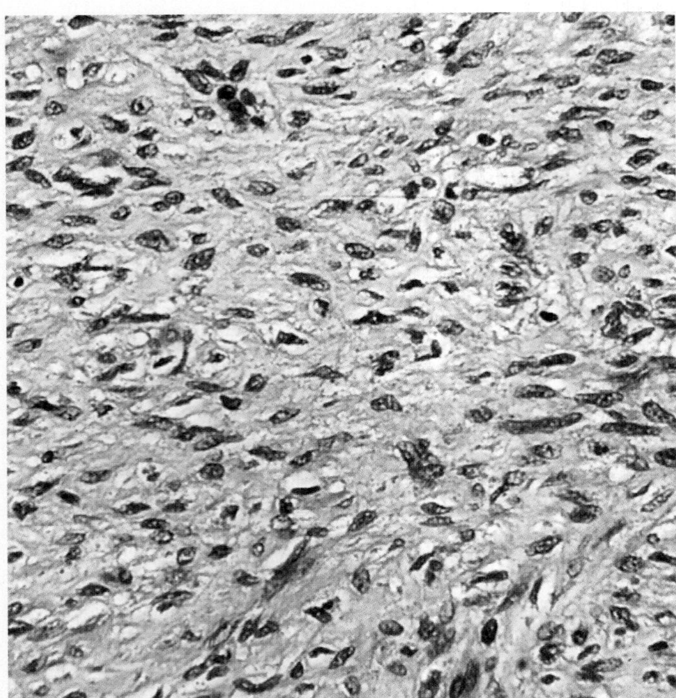

FIGURE 26-66. Fibrosarcoma. A photomicrograph demonstrates irregularly arranged malignant fibroblasts characterized by dark, irregular and elongated nuclei of varying sizes.

induration of, or a mass in, the penile shaft, causing it to curve toward the affected side (**penile strabismus**). The lesion leads to urethral obstruction and pain on erection.

Fibrosarcoma Is a Malignant Tumor of Fibroblasts

Fibrosarcoma is most common in the thigh, particularly around the knee. This tumor typically occurs in adults, although it may be seen in any age group and may even be congenital. Congenital (infantile) fibrosarcoma has a chromosomal translocation, t(12;15)(p13;q26), that contains an *ETV6-NTRK3* fusion gene and has a poor prognosis. The adult form shows no characteristic cytogenetic abnormality. Fibrosarcomas arise from deep connective tissue, such as fascia, scar tissue, periosteum and tendons. Macroscopically, the tumors are sharply demarcated and frequently exhibit necrosis and hemorrhage. They are characterized histologically by malignant-appearing fibroblasts (Fig. 26-66), which often form densely interlacing bundles and fascicles, producing a "herringbone" pattern. There are also several morphologic variants including low-grade (less aggressive) tumors. The prognosis for high-grade conventional adult fibrosarcoma is guarded; the survival at 5 years is only 40% and that at 10 years, 30%.

Undifferentiated Pleomorphic Sarcoma (Malignant Fibrous Histiocytoma) Is the Most Common Soft Tissue Sarcoma

Malignant fibrous histiocytoma (MFH) was historically considered to be a malignant soft tissue tumor with fibroblastic and histiocytic (macrophage) differentiation. However, the term "MFH" now refers to a microscopic appearance that actually represents a phenotypically heterogeneous group of sarcomas generically termed "undifferentiated pleomorphic sarcomas." More recent immunohistochemical and ultrastructural studies have shown that the histologic pattern of MFH/undifferentiated pleomorphic sarcoma can be seen in pleomorphic variants of liposarcoma, leiomyosarcoma, rhabdomyosarcoma, myofibroblastic sarcoma and fibrosarcoma. Collectively, the MFH/undifferentiated pleomorphic sarcoma group of tumors is the most common sarcoma in patients over the age of 40, but cases have been recorded at all ages. In half of cases, these tumors arise in the deep fascia or within skeletal muscle of the lower limbs and have been reported in association with surgical scars and foreign bodies or after radiation treatment. In general, these tumors have complex, nonspecific cytogenetic abnormalities. Several oncogenes may play a role in the pathogenesis of MFH-like tumors including *SAS, TP53, RB1* and *CDKN2A,* among others.

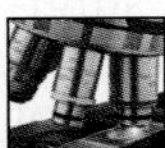

PATHOLOGY: Adult undifferentiated pleomorphic sarcomas are usually unencapsulated, gray-white or tan tumors that may have areas of hemorrhage and necrosis. Microscopically, MFH-like tumors display a highly variable morphologic pattern, with areas of spindle-shaped tumor cells arrayed in an irregularly whorled (storiform) pattern adjacent to fields with bizarre pleomorphic cells (Fig. 26-67). The spindle cells tend to be better differentiated and may resemble fibroblasts. There are occasional plump cells (resembling histiocytes), abundant mitoses, a few xanthomatous cells and a moderate chronic inflammatory reaction. Some tumors contain numerous tumor giant cells, which exhibit intense cytoplasmic eosinophilia. The extent of collagen deposition varies and sometimes dominates the microscopic pattern. Necrosis is often present and may be extensive. A few tumors reveal a conspicuous myxoid stroma. Immunohistochemical and ultrastructural studies are generally performed to establish a specific line of differentiation (smooth muscle, skeletal muscle, adipose tissue, etc.). If no such line of differentiation can be demonstrated, then the

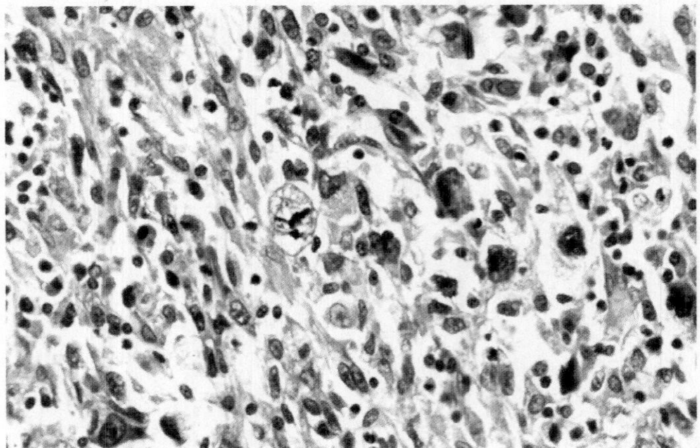

FIGURE 26-67. Undifferentiated pleomorphic sarcoma ("malignant fibrous histiocytoma"). An anaplastic tumor exhibits spindle cells, plump polygonal cells, bizarre tumor giant cells, an abnormal mitosis (*center*) and scattered chronic inflammatory cells. This appearance can be seen in pleomorphic sarcomas with other lines of differentiation (e.g., pleomorphic liposarcoma).

tumor can be considered to be an **undifferentiated pleomorphic sarcoma**.

The prognosis of adult undifferentiated pleomorphic sarcomas depends on the degree of cytologic atypia, the extent of mitotic activity and the degree of necrosis. Almost half of the patients develop a local recurrence after surgery and a comparable proportion later manifest metastatic disease, particularly in the lungs. The overall 5-year survival ranges from 50% to 60%.

Radiation-induced sarcomas are a form of adult undifferentiated pleomorphic sarcoma that arise in bone or soft tissue, usually 10 to 20 years after radiotherapy for a malignancy in that field. A typical story is development of osteosarcoma of a rib or vertebral body (uncommon sites for de novo osteosarcomas) after radiation to the thorax as treatment for mediastinal lymphoma or breast cancer. The incidence of postradiation sarcoma is low (<1% of irradiated patients).

Tumors of Adipose Tissue

Lipomas Are the Most Common Soft Tissue Mass and Closely Resemble Normal Fat

Composed of well-differentiated adipocytes, these benign, circumscribed tumors can originate at any site in the body that contains adipose tissue. Most occur in the subcutaneous tissues of the upper half of the body, especially the trunk and neck. Lipomas are seen mainly in adults, and patients with multiple tumors often have relatives with a similar history.

MOLECULAR PATHOGENESIS: Numerous cytogenetic abnormalities have been documented in lipomas. In general, lipomas can be subclassified into three major groups: (1) tumors with aberrations involving 12q13–15, (2) tumors with abnormalities involving 6p21–23 and (3) tumors with loss of portions of 13q. Some tumors have the translocation t(3;12)(q27–28;q13–15), which results in the generation of a fusion gene involving the *HMGIC* gene (a member of the high-mobility group of proteins) and the *LPP* gene (a member of the LIM protein family). However, the molecular pathways that are responsible for the development of lipomas are unknown. Some lipomas have no cytogenetic abnormalities and may represent localized adipocyte hyperplasia.

PATHOLOGY: On gross examination, lipomas are encapsulated, soft, yellow lesions that vary in size and may become very large. Deeper tumors are often poorly circumscribed. Histologically, a lipoma is often indistinguishable from normal adipose tissue (Fig. 26-68). Lipomas are adequately treated by simple local excision.

An **angiolipoma** is a small, well-circumscribed, subcutaneous lipoma with extensive vascular proliferation that usually occurs in the upper extremities and trunk of young adults. They are often multiple and painful.

Liposarcomas Are the Second Most Common Sarcoma in Adults

Liposarcomas comprise 20% of all malignant soft tissue tumors. The neoplasm arises after age 50 years and is most common in the deep thigh and retroperitoneum. Liposarcomas tend to grow slowly but may become extremely large. There are several subtypes of liposarcoma including myxoid/round cell liposarcoma, well-differentiated liposarcoma and pleomorphic liposarcoma.

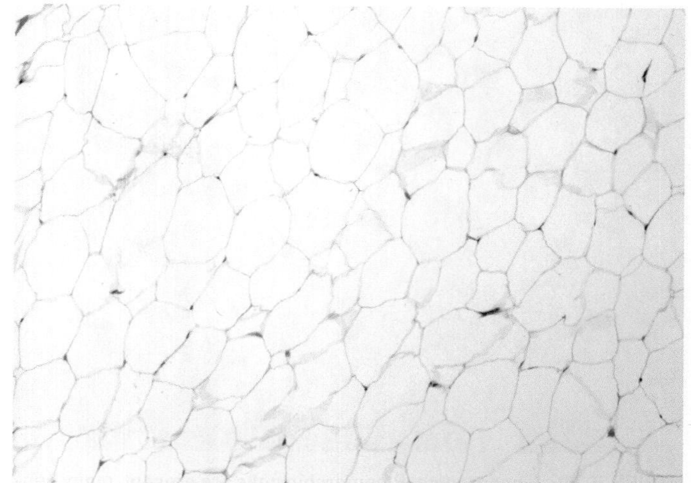

FIGURE 26-68. Lipoma. The tumor is composed of mature adipocytes with small eccentric nuclei.

MOLECULAR PATHOGENESIS: Myxoid/round cell liposarcomas exhibit a translocation between chromosomes 12 and 16, [t(12;16)(q13;p11)], in which the *TLS/FUS* gene on chromosome 16 is fused with the *CHOP* gene on chromosome 12. The *TLS/FUS* gene product is a novel RNA-binding protein with substantial homology to the EWS protein of Ewing sarcoma, whereas CHOP protein is a transcriptional repressor. Atypical lipomas/well-differentiated liposarcomas are defined by a giant marker chromosome or a supernumerary ring chromosome with amplification of the 12q14–15 region, which includes the *MDM2* gene. MDM2 is involved in regulating growth and signaling survival, in part by inhibition of p53 (see Chapter 5).

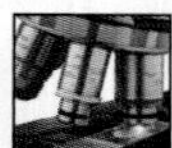

PATHOLOGY: Liposarcomas typically measure 5 to 10 cm in diameter, although some measure 40 cm in diameter and weigh in excess of 20 kg. Gross appearances vary depending on the proportions of adipose, mucinous and fibrous tissue. Poorly differentiated liposarcomas grossly appear similar to brain tissue and display necrosis, hemorrhage and cysts. Microscopically, myxoid/round cell liposarcoma consists of variably differentiated "signet ring" lipoblasts and variable amounts of primitive round cells embedded in a vascularized myxoid stroma. Well-differentiated liposarcomas are often composed of large amounts of mature fat, and therefore can be confused with lipomas. Pleomorphic liposarcomas have an MFH-like histologic appearance with numerous large, bizarre tumor cells but also contain **lipoblasts** ***(Fig. 26-69). It is the lipoblast, a malignant-appearing cell with univacuolated or multivacuolated cytoplasmic fat vesicles indenting the nucleus, that essentially defines a tumor as a liposarcoma.***

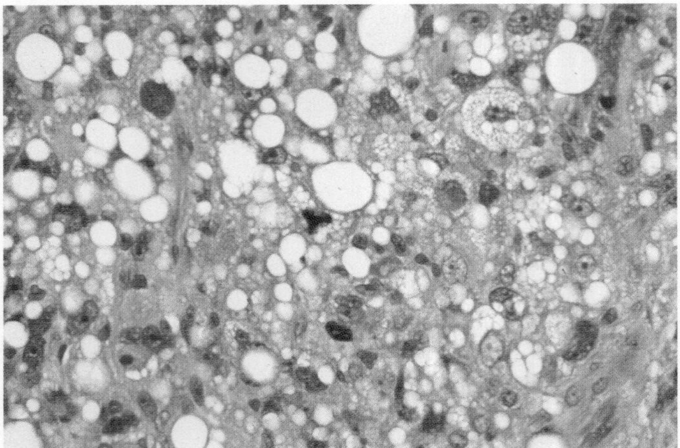

FIGURE 26-69. Liposarcoma. Pleomorphic cells are present, many containing lipid vacuoles that indent the nuclei or completely displace them to one side (lipoblasts).

Local recurrence rates and metastases after surgery are high for round cell and pleomorphic liposarcomas, and the 5-year survival for these tumors is less than 20%. By contrast, 5-year survival for patients with well-differentiated and pure myxoid variants exceeds 70%.

Rhabdomyosarcoma

Rhabdomyosarcoma is a malignant tumor that displays features of striated muscle differentiation. It is uncommon in mature adults but is the most frequent soft tissue sarcoma of children and young adults. Its pathogenesis is controversial, but probably most of these tumors derive from primitive mesenchyme that has retained the capacity for skeletal muscle differentiation. Alternatively, rhabdomyosarcoma may arise from embryonal muscle tissue that is displaced into the soft tissues during embryogenesis.

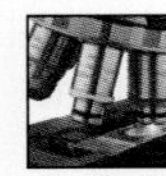

PATHOLOGY: Most cases of rhabdomyosarcoma can be classified in one of four subtypes. In addition to their light microscopic features, all subtypes of rhabdomyosarcoma show immunohistochemical evidence of skeletal muscle differentiation. Tumors may express nonspecific myoid markers such as actin and desmin, or more specific markers such as the skeletal muscle–specific transcription factors myogenin and MyoD1.

EMBRYONAL RHABDOMYOSARCOMA: This form is most common in children between 3 and 12 years old and frequently involves the head and neck, genitourinary tract and retroperitoneum. Its appearance varies from that of a highly differentiated tumor containing rhabdomyoblasts, with large eosinophilic cytoplasm and cross-striations (Fig. 26-70A), to that of a poorly differentiated neoplasm.

BOTRYOID EMBRYONAL RHABDOMYOSARCOMA: This tumor, also known as **sarcoma botryoides**, is distinguished by the formation of polypoid, grape-like tumor masses. Microscopically, the malignant cells are scattered in an abundant myxoid stroma. Botryoid foci may occur in any type of embryonal rhabdomyosarcoma, but they are most common in tumors of hollow visceral organs, including the vagina (see Chapter 18) and urinary bladder.

ALVEOLAR RHABDOMYOSARCOMA: This neoplasm occurs less frequently than the embryonal type and principally affects persons between ages 10 and 25; rarely, it may be seen in elderly patients. It is most common in the upper and lower extremities, but it can also be distributed in the same sites as the embryonal type. Typically, club-shaped tumor cells are arranged in clumps that are outlined by fibrous septa. The loose arrangement of the cells in the center of the clusters leads to the "alveolar" pattern (Fig. 26-70B). The tumor cells exhibit intense eosinophilia and occasional multinucleated giant cells are identified. Malignant rhabdomyoblasts, recognizable by their cross-striations, occur less commonly in the alveolar variant than in embryonal rhabdomyosarcoma, being present in only 25% of cases.

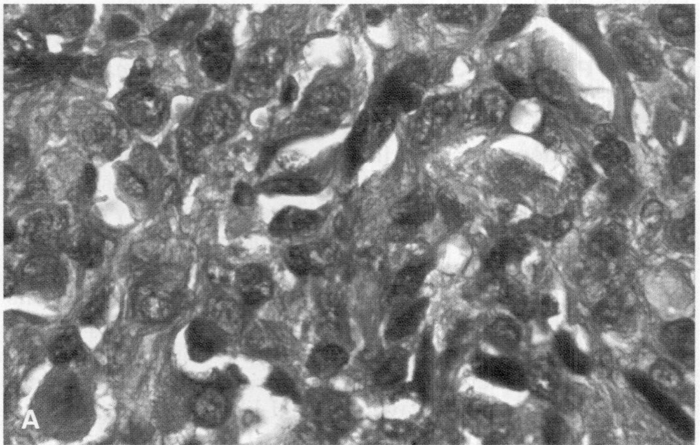

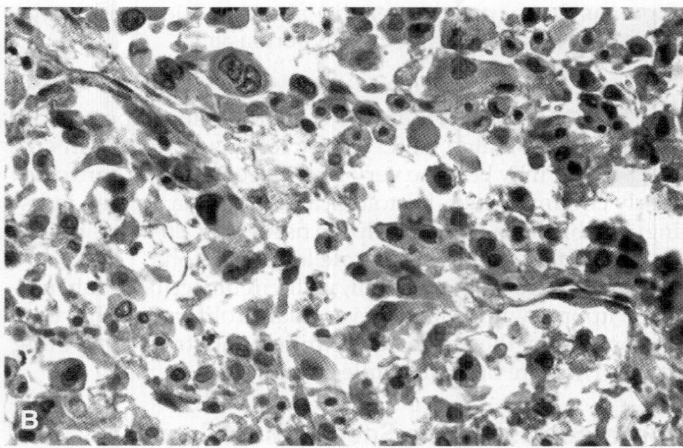

FIGURE 26-70. Rhabdomyosarcoma. A. The tumor contains polyhedral and spindle-shaped tumor cells with enlarged, hyperchromatic nuclei and deeply eosinophilic cytoplasm. A few cells have clearly visible cross-striations. **B.** Alveolar rhabdomyosarcoma. The neoplastic cells are arranged in clusters that display an alveolar pattern.

MOLECULAR PATHOGENESIS: Most alveolar rhabdomyosarcomas express *PAX3-FKHR* or *PAX7-FKHR* gene fusions, resulting from t(2;13)(q35;q14) or t(1;13)(p36;q14) translocations, respectively. In patients with localized tumors, the type of fusion does not correlate with the clinical outcome. However, in the presence of metastatic disease, *PAX3-FKHR*–positive tumors have a worse prognosis than do *PAX7-FKHR*–positive ones.

PLEOMORPHIC RHABDOMYOSARCOMA: The least common form of rhabdomyosarcoma is found in the skeletal muscles of older persons, often in the thigh. This tumor differs from the other types of rhabdomyosarcoma in the pleomorphism of its irregularly arranged cells and can be categorized as one type of adult undifferentiated pleomorphic sarcoma. Large, granular, eosinophilic rhabdomyoblasts, together with multinucleated giant cells, are common. Cross-striations are virtually nonexistent.

The historically dismal prognosis associated with most rhabdomyosarcomas has improved in the past two decades as a result of the introduction of combined therapeutic modalities, including surgery, radiation therapy and chemotherapy. Today, more than 80% of patients with localized or regional disease are cured. Factors indicating a worse prognosis include age older than 10, tumor size greater than 5 cm, alveolar and pleomorphic histologic subtypes and advanced stage of disease.

Smooth Muscle Tumors

These tumors are characterized histologically by fascicles of spindled cells with light, eosinophilic cytoplasm; cylindrical nuclei; and immunohistochemical expression of smooth muscle actin, muscle-specific actin and desmin.

LEIOMYOMA: This benign soft tissue tumor usually arises in subcutaneous tissues, or from blood vessel walls in deep somatic tissues. Leiomyomas are painful lesions that appear as firm, gray-white, well-circumscribed nodules. Microscopically, they are composed of intersecting fascicles of relatively uniform spindled cells with cigar-shaped nuclei and very low mitotic activity. Some display prominent blood vessels (angiomyoma). Simple excision is curative.

LEIOMYOSARCOMA: This malignant soft tissue neoplasm is an uncommon tumor of adults that typically arises from the wall of blood vessels in the soft tissue of the extremities or in retroperitoneum. Macroscopically, leiomyosarcomas tend to be well circumscribed but are larger and softer than leiomyomas and often exhibit necrosis, hemorrhage and cystic degeneration. Histologically, the tumor cells are arranged in fascicles, often with palisaded nuclei. Well-differentiated tumor cells have elongated nuclei and eosinophilic cytoplasm; poorly differentiated ones show marked increased cellularity and severe cytologic atypia (Fig. 26-71). Leiomyosarcoma is differentiated from leiomyoma mainly by a high mitotic activity, which also indicates the prognosis. Most leiomyosarcomas eventually metastasize, although dissemination may occur as late as 15 or more years after resection of the primary tumor. Chromosomal abnormalities occur in leiomyosarcoma, but no specific alterations have been documented. Retroperitoneal tumors have poor prognosis.

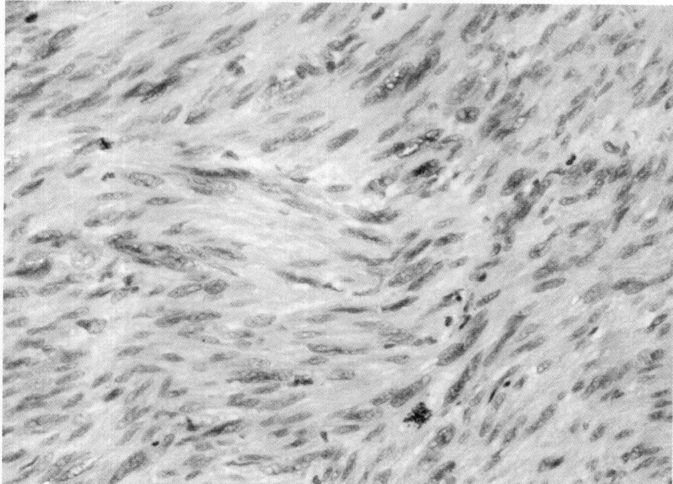

FIGURE 26-71. Leiomyosarcoma. The tumor is composed of spindle cells with elongated, hyperchromatic nuclei; a variable degree of pleomorphism; and frequent mitoses.

EBV-associated smooth muscle tumors comprise a distinctive subgroup of smooth muscle tumors that occur in immunocompromised patients, mostly children and young adults who are human immunodeficiency virus (HIV) positive or are status post–organ transplant. The tumors may be multifocal or multicentric. Their histology is quite variable and all display a certain degree of mitotic activity and numerous intralesional T lymphocytes. Death from these tumors is rare but most patients have persistent disease.

Vascular Tumors

Benign vascular tumors (hemangiomas) are among the most common soft tissue tumors and are the most frequent neoplasms of infancy and childhood. By contrast, angiosarcomas are among the rarest of soft tissue tumors, accounting for less than 1% of all sarcomas, and are more common in older adults. Vascular tumors are discussed in detail in Chapter 10.

Synovial Sarcoma

Synovial sarcoma is a highly malignant soft tissue tumor that arises in the region of a joint, usually in association with tendon sheaths, bursae and joint capsules. Fewer than 10% of synovial sarcomas are intra-articular. This tumor may also arise in other soft tissue sites away from joints as well as within organs. Although the tumor bears a microscopic resemblance to synovium, its origin from this tissue has not been established. Thus, it is currently considered to be a malignant soft tissue tumor with both epithelial and mesenchymal differentiation. Synovial sarcoma occurs principally in adolescents and young adults as a painful or tender mass, usually in the vicinity of a large joint, particularly the knee.

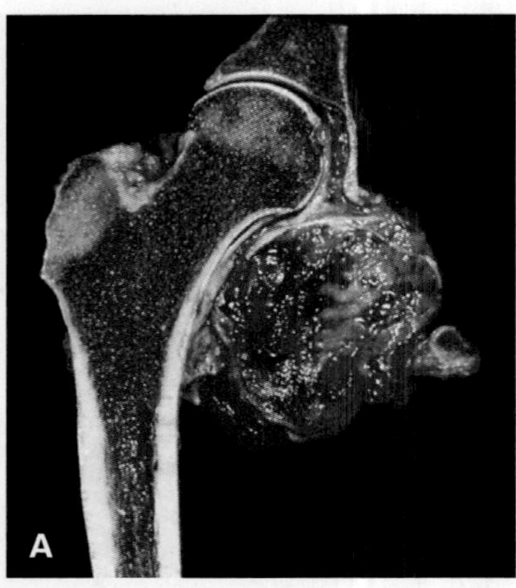

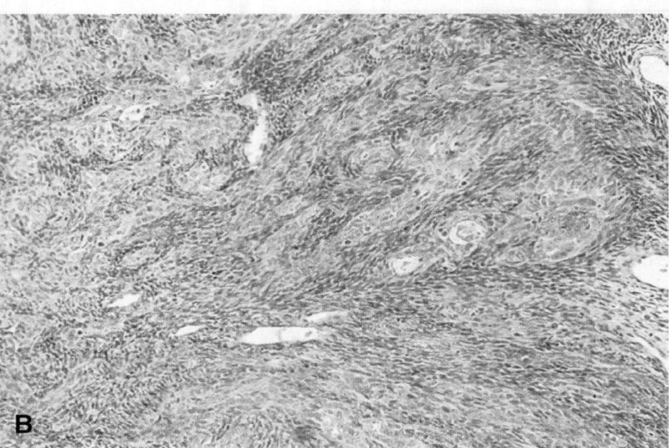

FIGURE 26-72. Synovial sarcoma. A. Section of the upper femur and acetabulum reveals a tumor adjacent to the hip joint and the neck of the femur. **B.** A microscopic view demonstrates the biphasic appearance of a synovial sarcoma. Irregular glandular spaces are lined by plump, epithelial-like neoplastic cells. The intervening tissue contains smaller and darker-staining spindle cells.

MOLECULAR PATHOGENESIS: Synovial sarcomas display a specific, balanced chromosomal translocation involving chromosomes X and 18 [t(x;18)(p11.2;q11.2)]. This translocation results in fusion of the *SYT* (synteny) gene on chromosome 18 to the *SSX* gene (a transcriptional repressor) on the X chromosome, leading to production of a hybrid protein, SYT-SSX1 or SYT-SSX2. The SYT-SSX2 protein is associated with a better prognosis if the disease is localized.

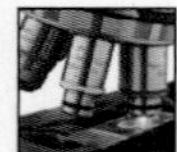

PATHOLOGY: On gross examination, synovial sarcomas are usually circumscribed, round or multilobular masses attached to tendons, tendon sheaths or the exterior wall of the joint capsule (Fig. 26-72A). The tumors tend to be surrounded by a glistening pseudocapsule and in many instances are cystic. Areas of hemorrhage, necrosis and calcification may be seen. They range from small nodules to masses of 15 cm or more in diameter, the average being 3 to 5 cm.

Microscopically, synovial sarcoma is classically described as having a **biphasic pattern** (Fig. 26-72B). Fluid-filled glandular spaces lined by epithelium-like tumor cells are embedded in a sarcomatous, spindle cell background. These elements vary in proportion, distribution and cellular differentiation, with the spindle cells usually considerably more numerous than the glandular elements. If the "epithelial" component is lacking, the tumor is referred to as **monophasic synovial sarcoma**. Although monophasic synovial sarcoma resembles fibrosarcoma, its atypical spindle cells are plumper and swirled rather than being arranged in a herringbone pattern. Calcifications may be conspicuous within the tumor. Poorly differentiated morphology imparts a poorer prognosis. Synovial sarcoma usually expresses cytokeratin or epithelial membrane antigen, further evidence of epithelial differentiation.

The recurrence rate of synovial sarcoma is high, and metastases occur in over 60% of cases. The 5-year survival rate is about 50%, and those who die usually have extensive lung metastases.

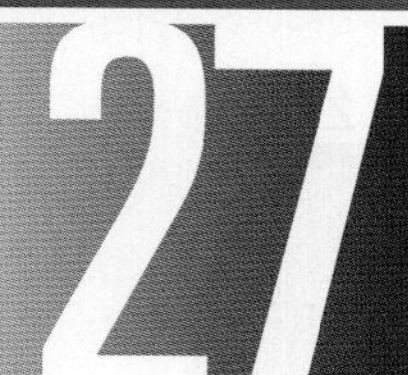

27 Skeletal Muscle

Lawrence C. Kenyon

Embryology and Anatomy

The myoblast is a primitive cell that fuses with other myoblasts to form a cylindrical multinucleated myotube. The periphery of the myotube rapidly accumulates myofibrils, containing myosin and actin, which become arrayed in the cross-banded pattern characteristic of striated muscle (Fig. 27-1). The myofiber has a distinctive architecture when visualized by electron microscopy (Fig. 27-2).

The myotube matures completely when it is innervated by the terminal axon of a lower motor neuron. Before innervation, the sarcolemma of the myotube contains diffusely distributed nicotinic receptors for acetylcholine on its surface membrane. Upon innervation, these receptors become highly concentrated at the motor endplate. Although an individual muscle fiber is innervated by only a single nerve ending, each motor neuron innervates numerous muscle fibers. After innervation, the nuclei of each fiber move from the center to arrange themselves in a regular pattern beneath the sarcolemma (Fig. 27-3A). Mature skeletal muscle cells are syncytia (multiple nuclei within a single cytoplasm) and can be several centimeters in length.

The muscle fibers responsible for movement are **extrafusal fibers**, whereas those contained within stretch receptors (muscle spindle organs) are known as **intrafusal fibers.** ***Most primary myopathies feature damage to extrafusal fibers but not intrafusal fibers.*** Thus, muscle spindle organs, which are usually inconspicuous in routine histologic preparations, become relatively more prominent as extrafusal fibers disappear.

Myofiber Structure

The myofiber consists of distinct functional units (Figs. 27-1 and 27-2):

- **Sarcomere:** Functional unit of the myofibril that extends from one Z band to the next
- **Z band:** A distinct electron-dense band that anchors the thin actin filaments
- **I band:** Zone of the actin filaments as they extend from the Z band into the A band
- **A band:** Structure composed of the thick myosin filaments. Actin filaments overlap myosin filaments to a variable extent, depending on the degree of muscle contraction. The thin filaments form a hexagonal array around each thick filament (best seen in cross-section).
- **H zone:** Pale region in the midportion of the A band where actin filaments end
- **M line:** Zone of intermolecular bridging and thickening of myosin filaments at the midline of the A band, which forms a thin, slightly darker electron-dense band

During contraction, actin filaments slide past myosin filaments. The sliding actin filaments advance farther into the A band, decreasing sarcomere length. As a result, the I band

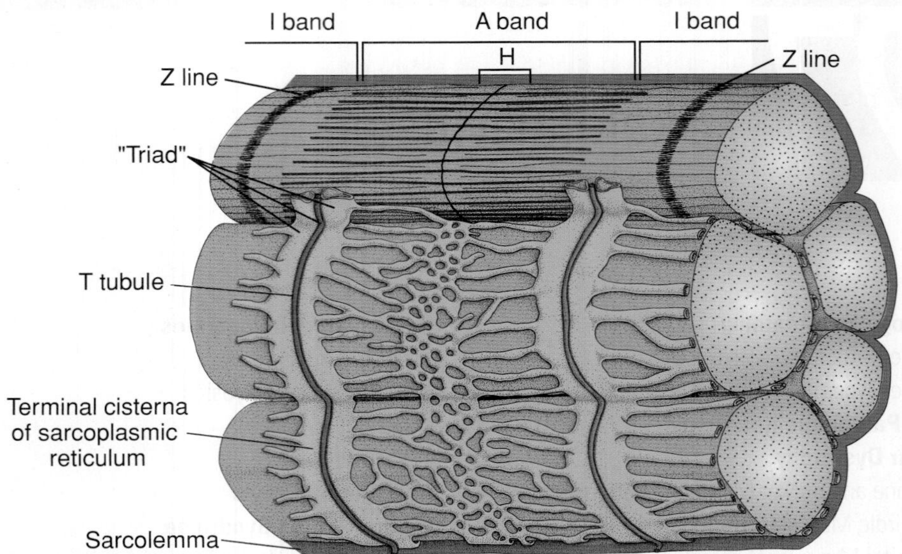

FIGURE 27-1. Normal striated muscle. Cross-striations of striated muscle are created by the arrangement of the myofilaments of the myofibril (compare to Fig. 27-2). The dark A band results from the thick myosin filaments and the thinner, partially overlapping actin filaments. In the middle portion of the myosin filaments where the actin does not overlap, there is a lighter band called the H zone or H band. In the middle of the H band, the center of each myosin filament thickens, forming intermolecular bridging with the adjacent myosin filament and giving rise to the M line (see Fig. 27-2). The finer actin filaments are anchored on the dark Z disk of the lighter I band. With contraction, the myosin filaments pull the actin filaments, causing the H zone to disappear, the I band to shrink and the A band to remain the same. The mitochondria are scattered throughout the sarcoplasm among the myofibrils. The endoplasmic reticulum (sarcoplasmic reticulum) forms an extensive, complex tubular network with periodic dilations (cisternae) around each myofibril. The cisternae are closely apposed to the transverse tubules, which are derived from the cell membrane (sarcolemma) and form a transverse network, which resembles chicken wire, around each myofibril, giving extensive communication between the internal and external environments. A triad consists of a T tubule and adjacent terminal cisternae of the sarcoplasmic reticulum.

and H zone shorten, whereas the A band remains nearly constant. There are numerous filamentous proteins that comprise the sarcomeres, and multiple proteins that anchor sarcomeres to the sarcolemma. These proteins may be mutated or abnormally regulated in muscular dystrophies (see below).

The **sarcoplasmic reticulum** surrounds each myofibril and forms an elaborate membranous network that has irregular dilations (cisternae) juxtaposed to a transverse tubular network derived from the sarcolemma (Fig. 27-1). The **transverse tubular system** (T-tubule system) is arranged across the fiber like chicken wire, each ring wrapping around an individual myofibril. This arrangement allows an electrical stimulus to proceed along the muscle fiber surface and become diffusely and rapidly internalized via the transverse tubular system. The electrical signal is translated into a chemical signal between the transverse tubule and the cisternae of the sarcoplasmic reticulum. This process releases calcium from the sarcoplasmic reticulum into the vicinity of myofibrils, where the chemical signal triggers muscle contraction.

The lower motor neurons and the fibers they innervate are the **motor units**, which vary in size. In limb muscles, one motor unit can include as many as several hundred myofibers. By contrast, each motor unit of extraocular muscles may have as few as 20 myofibers. The muscles of the eye are also exceptional in that a single fiber may have more than one motor endplate.

Myofibers Are Classified as Slow Twitch or Fast Twitch

After innervation, a characteristic metabolic profile develops for different muscle fibers. Muscle fiber types can be broadly classified according to the rate of contraction and fatigueability, as type I or type II, or slow-twitch fibers and fast-twitch fibers, respectively. These can be further subdivided into slow twitch, fatigue resistant (type I); fast twitch, fatigue resistant (type IIA); and fast twitch, fatigue sensitive (type IIB). There are also type IIC fibers, which are an immature fiber type. In lower mammals, some muscles are deep red (type I), whereas others are pale (type II).

TYPE I FIBERS (RED, SLOW TWITCH): If a nerve stimulates a dark (red) muscle, the resulting contraction is slower and more prolonged than when a nerve excites a pale (white) muscle. For this reason, red muscles have been classified as "slow twitch." Type I fibers tend to have more mitochondria and more myoglobin, the red, oxygen-storing pigment. Krebs cycle enzymes and the carrier proteins of the electron-transport chain–mitochondrial constituents are all present in greater amounts in slow-twitch muscle than in fast-twitch muscle. The alkaline histochemical reaction for myosin ATPase gives a crisp distinction between the two fiber types. Type I fibers stain poorly at high (alkaline) pH, but type II fibers stain darkly (Fig. 27-3B).

Functionally, type I muscles have a greater capacity for long, sustained contractions and resist fatigue. A training

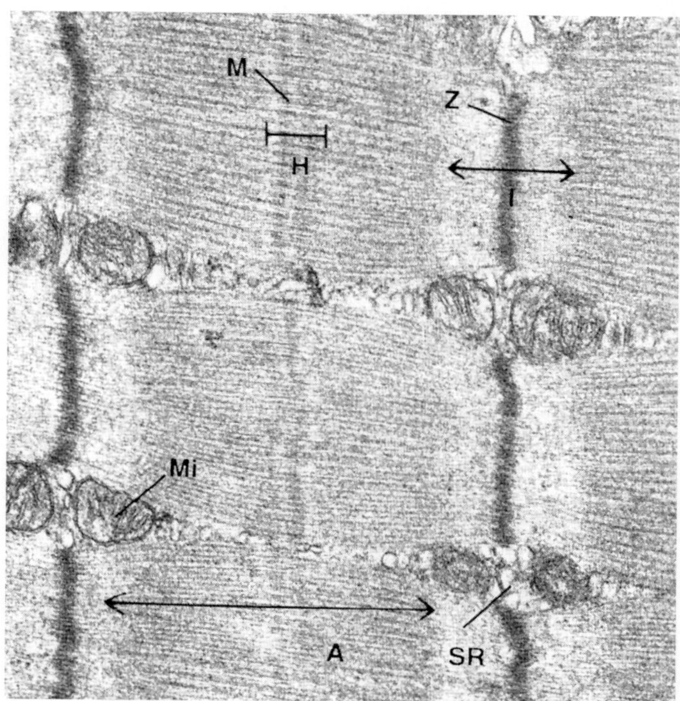

FIGURE 27-2. Normal muscle. This electron micrograph of the biceps muscle demonstrates the ultrastructure of the sarcomere. The thin dark band, the Z disk (*Z*), bisects the broad, pale I band (*I*), a zone composed of the thin actin filaments. The broad, dark band, made up of the thick myosin filaments and overlapping actin filaments, is the A band (*A*). The middle of the A band consists of the pale H zone (*H*), which in turn is bisected by a slightly darker M line (*M*), representing a zone of intermolecular bridging of myosin. Small membrane-bound vesicles compose the sarcoplasmic reticulum (*SR*) and the transverse tubules. Pairs of mitochondria (*Mi*) tend to be located between myofibrils at the level of the I bands.

program that increases endurance produces little change in size of type I fibers, but conditioning of these fibers results in a proliferation of mitochondria and an expanded capacity for generating energy.

TYPE II FIBERS (WHITE, FAST TWITCH): Stimulation of type II fibers elicits faster, shorter and stronger contractions than occur in type I fibers. Glycogen, phosphorylase and other enzymes that produce energy by anaerobic glycolysis in the Embden-Meyerhof pathway are present in higher concentrations in white muscle. Type II muscle fibers are used for rapid, brief contractions, and react to strength training with hypertrophy. Androgenic steroids induce type II fiber hypertrophy, and disuse of muscle results in their selective atrophy.

The lower motor neuron influences fiber type. During embryonic development, early muscle cells begin to express type-specific contractile proteins before muscle is innervated. Thus, the phenotype of a myofiber seems to be a programmed characteristic of the cell, rather than one induced by the nerve supply. However, the kind of innervation can alter the types of myofibers. For example, after denervation injury, reinnervation of a slow-twitch muscle (type I) by a nerve from a fast-twitch muscle (type II) causes the newly innervated type I fibers to resemble type II fibers. It is thought that the pattern or rate of discharge of the lower motor neuron plays an important role in this process. Because lower motor neurons can determine fiber type, it follows that all muscle fibers in a given motor unit are of the same type. A cross-section of muscle stained with the alkaline ATPase reaction shows a random mixture of fiber types (Fig. 27-3B), because motor units interdigitate extensively with each other.

In humans, no muscles are composed exclusively of one fiber type. However, proportions of fiber types do vary from muscle to muscle. For example, the soleus muscle is composed of predominantly (≥80%) type I fibers. The pattern of fiber types in a given muscle is apparently genetically determined, and varies between people. Some evidence indicates

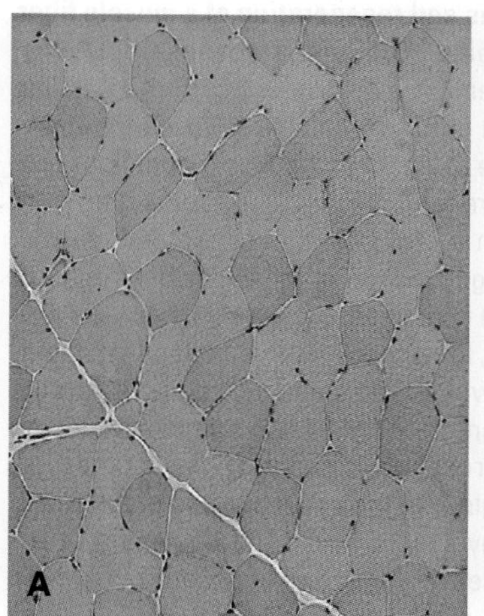

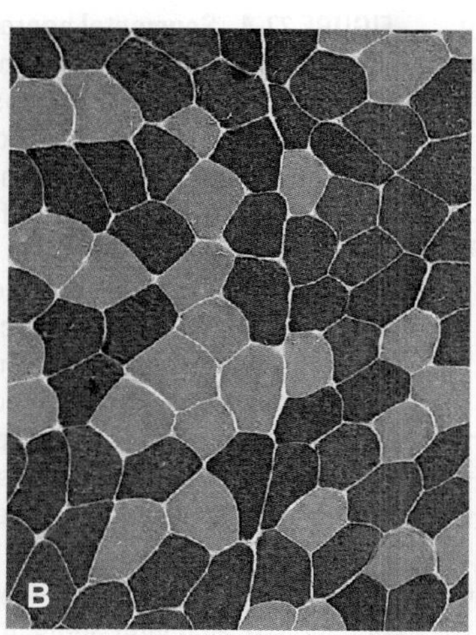

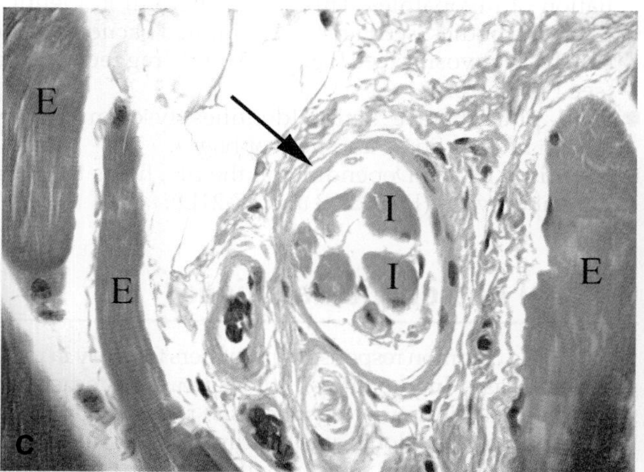

FIGURE 27-3. Normal muscle. A. Hematoxylin and eosin stain. In this transverse frozen section of the vastus lateralis, the polygonal myofibers are separated from each other by an indistinct, thin layer of connective tissue, the endomysium. The thicker band of connective tissue, the perimysium, demarcates a bundle or fascicle of fibers. All of the nuclei in this field are located at the periphery of the cells. Satellite cell nuclei are contained within the basement membrane of the muscle cell and cannot be distinguished from those of the myofibers by light microscopy. **B. Myofibrillar (myosin) ATPase.** Type I fibers are pale, at high (alkaline) pH; type II fibers are dark. Note the intermixture of fiber types. **C. Muscle spindle organ (stretch receptor).** The *arrow* marks the capsule of the muscle spindle organ. I = intrafusal fibers; E = extrafusal fibers.

that changing the use of a muscle through lengthy, intensive training may alter the pattern of muscle fiber types.

MUSCLE BIOPSY: Since normal muscle patterns are more constant within a specific muscle, the same muscles are biopsied from case to case. Samples from the quadriceps femoris or biceps brachii are suitable for biopsy diagnosis in most primary muscle diseases (myopathies). Biopsies of the sural nerve and gastrocnemius muscle are often done if a peripheral neuropathy is suspected. However, as some neuromuscular conditions are more focal, locations for muscle biopsies are not invariable.

Biopsy sampling from a moderately involved muscle is the most informative. Unaffected muscles may show few or no pathologic changes, whereas a severely weak muscle may be largely replaced by adipose and fibrous connective tissue (see end-stage muscle, Fig. 27-5).

Cryostat (i.e., fresh frozen) sections of muscle are stained by several histochemical reactions:

- **Nonspecific esterase:** Important for identifying denervation atrophy (see Fig. 27-22).
- **NADH-tetrazolium reductase (NADH-TR):** Type I fibers appear dark owing to abundant mitochondria. This stain is useful in identifying central cores (see Fig. 27-11) and signs of denervation (see Fig. 27-23).
- **Succinate dehydrogenase (SDH):** Sensitive histochemical index of mitochondrial proliferation caused by mutations of mitochondrial DNA (mtDNA) (see Fig. 27-20C).
- **Cytochrome C oxidase:** Fibers containing abnormal mitochondria lacking the terminal component of the electron transport chain will fail to stain (see Fig. 27-20B).
- **Alkaline phosphatase:** Regenerating fibers are selectively stained.
- **Periodic acid–Schiff (PAS):** Helpful in identification of glycogen and the diagnosis of glycogen storage diseases.
- **Oil red orcein (Oil red O):** Marks neutral lipid and is particularly useful in evaluating lipid storage myopathies such as carnitine deficiency (see Fig. 27-19).
- **Modified Gomori trichrome stain:** Versatile stain in evaluation of myopathies. This stain is helpful in identifying nemaline bodies (see Fig. 27-12), rimmed vacuoles of inclusion body myositis (see Fig. 27-15) and "ragged red fibers" (see Fig. 27-20A).
- **Acid phosphatase stain:** Identifies lysosomal activity within muscle fibers and macrophages.
- **Myosin ATPase**: Depending on the pH, helps to differentiate fiber types (Figs. 27-3 and 27-21D).

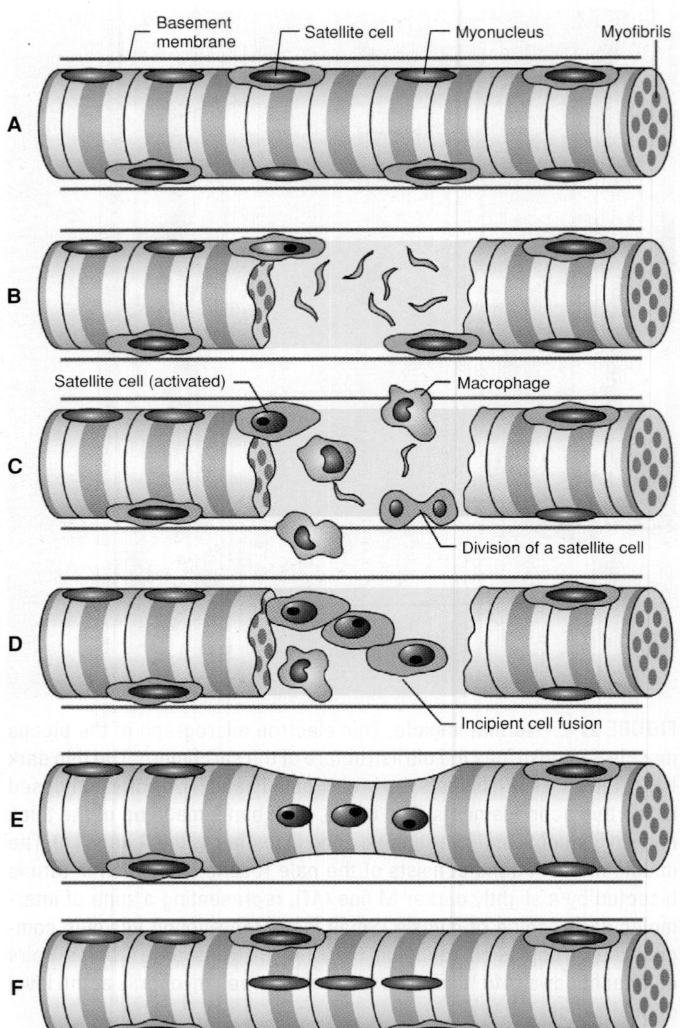

FIGURE 27-4. Segmental necrosis and regeneration of a muscle fiber. **A.** A normal muscle fiber contains myofibrils and subsarcolemmal nuclei and is covered by a basement membrane. Scattered satellite cells are situated on the surface of the sarcolemma, inside the basement membrane. These cells are dormant myoblasts, capable of proliferating and fusing to form differentiated fibers. They constitute 3% to 5% of the nuclei, as observed in a cross-section of skeletal muscle. **B.** In many muscle diseases (e.g., Duchenne muscular dystrophy or polymyositis), injury to the muscle fiber causes segmental necrosis with disintegration of the sarcoplasm, leaving a preserved basement membrane and nerve supply (not shown). **C.** The damaged segment attracts circulating macrophages that penetrate the basement membrane and begin to digest and engulf the sarcoplasmic contents (myophagocytosis). Regenerative processes begin with the activation and proliferation of the satellite cells, forming myoblasts within the basement membrane. Macrophages gradually leave the site of injury with their load of debris. **D.** At a later stage, the myoblasts are aligned in close proximity to each other in the center of the fiber and begin to fuse. **E.** Regeneration of the fiber segment is prominent, as indicated by the large, pale, vesicular, centrally located nuclei. **F.** The fiber is nearly normal except for a few persistent central nuclei. Eventually, the normal state (A) is restored.

General Pathologic Reactions

Necrosis is a common response of myofibers to injury in primary muscle diseases **(myopathies)**. Widespread acute necrosis of skeletal muscle fibers **(*rhabdomyolysis*)** releases cytosolic proteins, including myoglobin, into the circulation, which may lead to myoglobinuria and acute renal failure. In many human myopathies, segmental necrosis occurs along the length of a fiber, with intact muscle flanking the site of damage (Fig. 27-4). The injury quickly elicits two responses: an influx of blood-borne macrophages into the necrotic cytoplasm and activation of the satellite cells, a population of dormant myoblasts located close to each fiber. As monocytes gradually phagocytose necrotic debris and remove it, satellite cells proliferate and become active myoblasts. Within 2 days, they begin to fuse to each other and to the ends of the intact fiber remnants, to form a joining multinucleated segment. This regenerating fiber is smaller in diameter than the parent fiber, and has basophilic cytoplasm (due to increased ribosomes) and large, vesicular nuclei with prominent nucleoli arranged in long chains (see Fig. 27-14B).

Regeneration can restore normal structure and function of muscle fibers within a few weeks after a single episode of injury, as in the inherited disorder myophosphorylase deficiency (see below). With subacute or chronic disorders, fiber necrosis proceeds concurrently with fiber regeneration, gradually leading to atrophy of muscle fibers and fibrosis.

Muscular Dystrophy

In the middle of the 19th century, physicians discovered that progressive weakness of the voluntary muscles could be caused by either a disorder of the nervous system or primary degeneration of muscles. **Muscular dystrophy** was the name applied to primary muscular degeneration. It was found to be frequently hereditary (or at least familial) and relentlessly progressive. Muscle from these patients showed fiber necrosis, with regeneration, progressive fibrosis and infiltration by fatty tissue (Fig. 27-5). Little or no inflammation was seen. In ensuing years, numerous variants of this type of muscle disease were described, and a classification of hereditary, progressive, noninflammatory degenerative conditions of muscle has evolved.

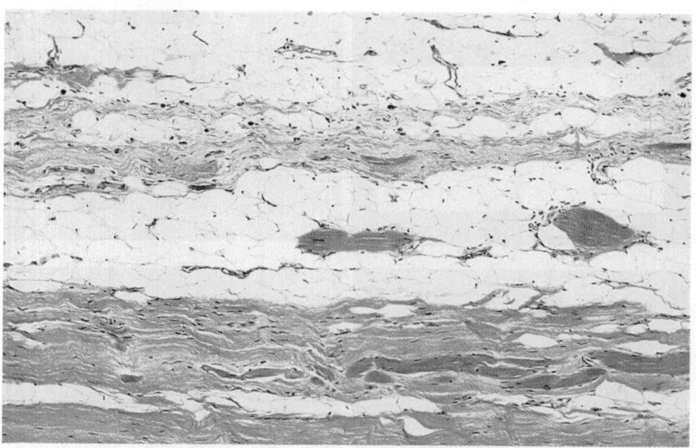

FIGURE 27-5. End-stage neuromuscular disease. In this section of the deltoid muscle stained by hematoxylin and eosin, skeletal muscle has been largely replaced by fibrofatty connective tissue. The few surviving muscle fibers have a deeper eosinophilia than does the abundant collagenous component.

Duchenne Muscular Dystrophy Is a Severe, Progressive, X-Linked Disease

Duchenne muscular dystrophy is characterized by progressive degeneration of muscles, particularly those of the pelvic and shoulder girdles. It is the most common noninflammatory myopathy in children. A milder form of the disease is known as **Becker muscular dystrophy** (see Chapter 6 for the molecular genetics of both diseases). Serum creatine kinase is usually greatly increased in both conditions.

MOLECULAR PATHOGENESIS: Duchenne and Becker muscular dystrophies are caused by various mutations of a large gene on the short arm of the X chromosome (Xp21). This gene codes for **dystrophin**, a 427-kd protein located on the inner sarcolemma surface. Dystrophin links the subsarcolemmal cytoskeleton to the exterior of the cell through a transmembrane complex of proteins and glycoproteins that binds to laminin (Fig. 27-6).

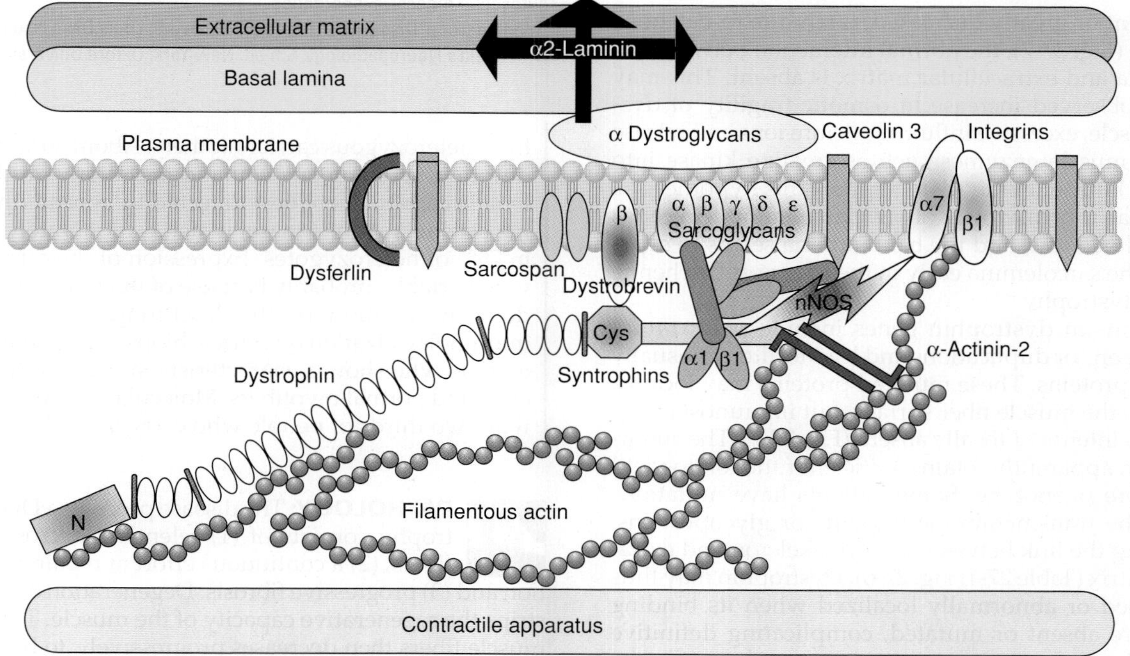

FIGURE 27-6. Diagrammatic representation of proteins linking dystrophin to the plasma membrane and the contractile apparatus. Several of these linking proteins are associated with known myopathies (see Table 27-1).

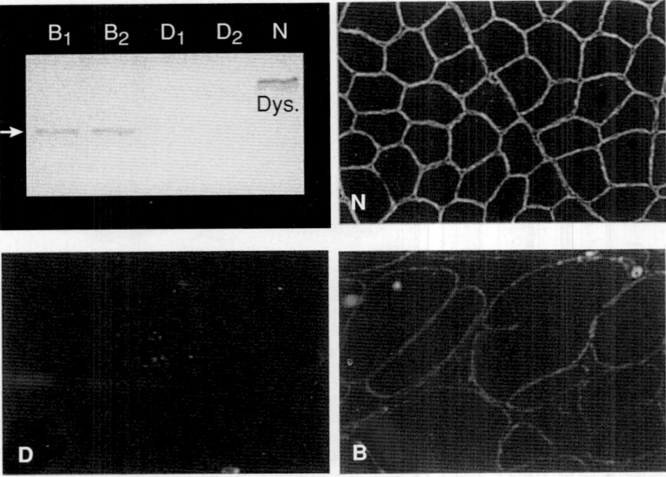

FIGURE 27-7. Dystrophin analysis in Duchenne and Becker muscular dystrophies. Immunofluorescence stain for dystrophin. The sections illustrate a normal subject (*N*), a patient with Duchenne dystrophy (*D*) and one with Becker dystrophy (*B*). Dystrophin is normally concentrated at the surface membrane of every muscle fiber, but in Duchenne dystrophy, the protein is absent or is only barely detected in a small proportion of muscle fibers. Becker dystrophy exhibits hypertrophic muscle fibers with reduced expression of dystrophin. The immunoblot (*upper left*) of normal muscle shows a band near the top of the gel corresponding to the 427-kd protein dystrophin. Dystrophin is undetectable in Duchenne dystrophy (two patients, D_1, D_2). In Becker dystrophy, a weaker band has migrated farther down the gel relative to the normal protein, and it corresponds to a smaller, truncated protein (two patients, B_1, B_2). The combined analysis (immunolocalization and immunoblot) of the dystrophin protein is diagnostic of this group of dystrophies (*dystrophinopathies*).

If it is absent or greatly decreased, often due to deletions of the gene (Fig. 27-7), the normal interaction between the sarcolemma and extracellular matrix is absent. This may cause the observed increase in osmotic fragility of dystrophic muscle, excessive influx of calcium ions and release of soluble muscle enzymes such as creatine kinase into the serum. Further evidence to support this hypothesis is the fact that a breakdown of the sarcolemma precedes muscle cell necrosis, and the basal lamina seems to separate from the sarcolemma early in the course of Duchenne muscular dystrophy.

Mutations in dystrophin genes include point mutations, deletions or duplications and lead to altered, usually truncated, proteins. These mutated proteins may localize correctly to the muscle fiber surface, but immunostaining is often less intense or focally absent (Fig. 27-7). The abnormal protein apparently retains sufficient function to yield a less severe phenotype. Some patients have mutations affecting the transmembrane proteins or glycoproteins, interrupting the link between the cytoskeleton and extracellular matrix (Table 27-1; Fig. 27-6). Dystrophin may thus be decreased or abnormally localized when its binding partners are absent or mutated, complicating definitive diagnosis (see below).

Because Duchenne muscular dystrophy is inherited as an X-linked recessive disease, the abnormal gene is passed from heterozygous carrier mothers. About 30% of cases are due to a spontaneous somatic mutation. Until recently, female carriers were best detected by repeatedly measuring serum creatine kinase, which is moderately increased in 75% of heterozygotes. Expression of the carrier state is very variable, probably because of fluctuations in the random inactivation of the X chromosome. Dystrophin immunolocalization on muscle biopsy also identifies some carriers who show a characteristic mosaic pattern of deficient and normal myofibers. Molecular probes detect more than two thirds of people who carry large deletions.

Table 27-1

Limb-Girdle Muscular Dystrophies

Limb-Girdle Muscular Dystrophies*	Defective Protein	Subcellular Location
LGMD1A	Myotilin	Sarcomere
LGMDIB	Lamin	Nuclear envelope
LGMD1C	Caveolin 3	Sarcolemma
LGMD1D	?	
LGMD1E	?	
LGMD1F	?	
LGMD1G	?	
LGMD2A	Calpain 3	Sarcoplasm
LGMD2B/Miyoshi	Dysferlin	Sarcolemma
LGMD2C	γ-Sarcoglycan	Sarcolemma
LGMD2D	α-Sarcoglycan	Sarcolemma
LGMD2E	β-Sarcoglycan	Sarcolemma
LGMD2F	δ-Sarcoglycan	Sarcolemma
LGMD2G	Telethion	Sarcomere
LGMD2H	Trim32	Sarcoplasm
LGMD2I	Fukutin-related protein	Golgi
LGMD2J	Titin	Sarcomere
LGMD2K	POMT1	Endoplasmic reticulum
LGMD2L	Eukutin	Golgi
LGMD2M	DOMGnT1	Golgi

*LMGD1s show autosomal dominant inheritance, whereas LMGD2s show autosomal recessive inheritance.

Adapted from "Diseases of Muscle." In Love S, Louis DN, Ellison DW, eds. Greenfield's Neuropathology, 8th ed. New York: Oxford University Press, 2008.

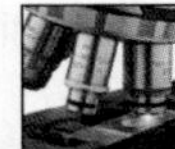

PATHOLOGY: The disease process in Duchenne dystrophy consists of (1) relentless necrosis of muscle fibers, (2) a continuous effort at repair and regeneration and (3) progressive fibrosis. Degeneration eventually outstrips the regenerative capacity of the muscle. The number of muscle fibers then decreases progressively, to be replaced by fibrofatty connective tissue. In the end stage, skeletal muscle fibers disappear almost completely (Fig. 27-5), but muscle spindle fibers (intrafusal fibers) are relatively spared.

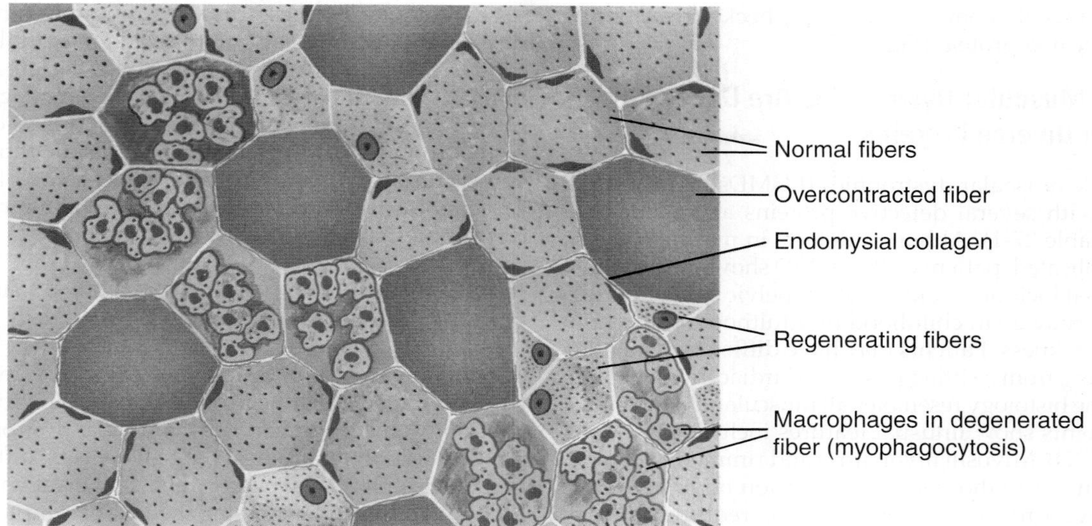

FIGURE 27-8. Duchenne muscular dystrophy. The pathologic changes in skeletal muscle (illustration of modified Gomori trichrome stain). Some fibers are slightly larger and darker than normal. These represent overcontracted segments of sarcoplasm situated between degenerated segments. Other fibers are packed with macrophages (myophagocytosis), which remove degenerated sarcoplasm. Other fibers are smaller than normal and have granular sarcoplasm. These fibers have enlarged, vesicular nuclei with prominent nucleoli and represent regenerating fibers. Developing endomysial fibrosis is represented by the deposition of collagen around individual muscle fibers. The changes are those of a chronic, active noninflammatory myopathy.

In the early stage of the disease, necrotic fibers and regenerating fibers tend to occur in small groups, together with scattered, large, hyalinized dark fibers. The latter are overly contracted and are thought to precede fiber necrosis (Figs. 27-8 and 27-9). Breakdown of the sarcolemma is one of the earliest ultrastructural changes. Macrophages invade necrotic fibers and reflect a scavenging function rather than an inflammatory process.

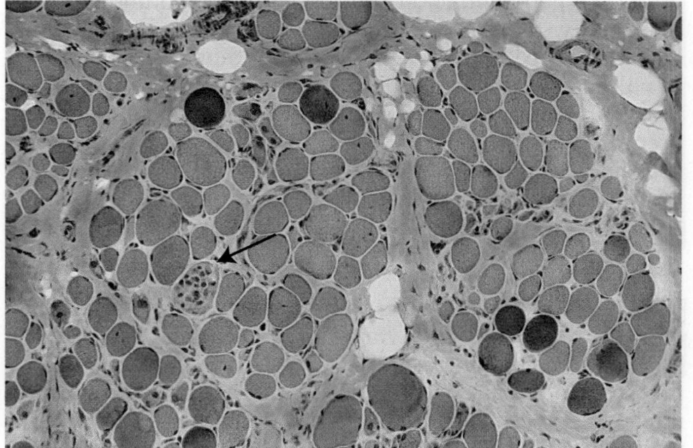

FIGURE 27-9. Duchenne muscular dystrophy. Modified Gomori trichrome stain. A section of vastus lateralis muscle shows necrotic muscle fibers, some of them invaded by macrophages (*arrow*). Dark-staining, enlarged fibers represent overly contracted fibers. Calcium influx across the defective surface membrane overwhelms mechanisms that maintain a low resting Ca^{2+} concentration and triggers excessive contraction. There is conspicuous perimysial and endomysial fibrosis.

CLINICAL FEATURES: The diagnosis of Duchenne dystrophy can be established by polymerase chain reaction (PCR) analysis of genomic DNA from leukocytes. In practice, diagnosis using this method is limited to large deletions of the gene. About 30% of patients have small rearrangements or point mutations and can be evaluated by muscle biopsy, which shows little or no detectable dystrophin by immunoblot or immunocytochemistry. Prenatal diagnosis of chorionic villus samples is useful, especially when the mutation of an affected family member is known.

Boys with Duchenne muscular dystrophy have markedly increased serum creatine kinase levels from birth and morphologically abnormal muscle, even in utero. Clinical weakness is not detectable during the first year, but is usually evident by age 3 or 4 years, mainly around pelvic and shoulder girdles (proximal muscle weakness). It progresses relentlessly. "Pseudohypertrophy" (enlargement of a muscle when muscle fibers are replaced by fibroadipose tissue) of calf muscles eventually develops. Patients are usually wheelchair bound by the age of 10 and bedridden by 15. Death is usually from complications of respiratory insufficiency caused by muscular weakness or cardiac arrhythmia owing to myocardial involvement. Other extraskeletal manifestations include gastrointestinal dysfunction (from degeneration of smooth muscle) and intellectual impairment. Many boys with Duchenne dystrophy exhibit variable degrees of mental retardation, apparently due to lack of dystrophin in the central nervous system (CNS).

While the clinical presentation of patients with Becker muscular dystrophy is typically milder and of later onset, affected individuals often have exercise intolerance with muscle cramping, occasional rhabdomyolysis and myoglobinuria. In contrast with Duchenne dystrophy, where dystrophin is usually completely absent, Becker dystrophy features a truncated protein (Fig. 27-7).

Limb-Girdle Muscular Dystrophies Are Caused by Mutations in Diverse Proteins

The limb-girdle muscular dystrophies (LGMDs) are a group of disorders with several defective proteins and modes of inheritance (Table 27-1). Although defects in many proteins have been implicated, patients with LGMD show similar clinical features that include weakness of the pelvic and shoulder girdles. Onset may be in childhood or adulthood with variable muscle weakness. Patients may have difficulty walking, running or rising from a sitting position. Cardiac involvement is common. The histology resembles all muscular dystrophies, but some variants show unusual features including inflammation (LGMD2B, Miyoshi myopathy) and rimmed vacuoles (LGMD1A) similar to those seen in inclusion body myositis (see below). As a result, proper diagnosis requires both a detailed clinical history and a battery of immunohistochemical, immunoblotting and genetic tests. LGMD (2C through 2F) are also known as the sarcoglycanopathies.

Congenital Muscular Dystrophies Present at Birth or Shortly Thereafter

These diseases are characterized by hypotonia, weakness and contractures (Table 27-2). Depending on the variant, patients may also present with a leukoencephalopathy (white matter disease), brain malformations and eye involvement.

Table 27-2

Congenital Myopathies Caused by Abnormalities in the Sarcolemma or Extracellular Matrix

Congenital Muscular Dystrophy (CMD)	Protein	Location and/or Function of Protein
Merosin-deficient CMD	Laminin $\alpha 2$	Extracellular matrix
Ullrich syndrome	Collagen VI	Extracellular matrix
Integrin $\alpha 7$ deficiency	Integrin $\alpha 7$	Plasma membrane
Fukuyama CMD	Fukutin	Possible substrate for glycosyltransferase
Muscle-eye-brain	POMGnT1 (*O*-mannose β-1,2-*N*-acetyl-glucosaminyl-tranferase	Glycosyltransferase
Walker-Warburg syndrome	POMT1 (protein-*O*-mannosyl-transferase)	Glycosyltransferase
	Fukutin-related protein	Possible phosphor-sugar transferase
Rigid spine syndrome	Selenoprotein N1	Glycoprotein of the endoplasmic reticulum

Adapted from "Diseases of Muscle." In Love S, Louis DN, Ellison DW, eds. Greenfield's Neuropathology, 8th ed. New York: Oxford University Press, 2008.

Pathologically, these diseases resemble other muscular dystrophies, with variable fibrosis and fatty infiltration of the muscle. Many of these disorders are associated with mutations in extracellular matrix proteins (e.g., collagens, laminin, integrins) or abnormal glycosylation of α-dystroglycan (α-dystroglycanopathies) and sarcoplasmic reticulum (rigid spine muscular dystrophy). Note that some of the affected proteins are also responsible for certain limb-girdle muscular dystrophies, albeit with different mutations.

Nucleotide Repeat Syndromes May Be Associated With Muscular Dystrophies

Several human genetic diseases are caused by abnormal numbers of intragenic oligonucleotide repeats. While both myotonic dystrophy and oculopharyngeal muscular dystrophy are trinucleotide repeat syndromes, they show very different muscle pathologies. Both, however, exhibit "anticipation" (i.e., an earlier age at onset and increasing severity of symptoms in successive generations associated with increased numbers of repeats).

Myotonic Dystrophy Is the Most Common Form of Adult Muscular Dystrophy

Myotonic dystrophy is an autosomal dominant disorder characterized by slowing muscle relaxation (myotonia), progressive muscle weakness and wasting. The prevalence has been estimated to be as high as 14 per 100,000, although it may be higher because of the difficulty in detecting minimally affected persons. The age at onset and severity of symptoms are very variable. Myotonic dystrophy is classified as either adult onset or congenital.

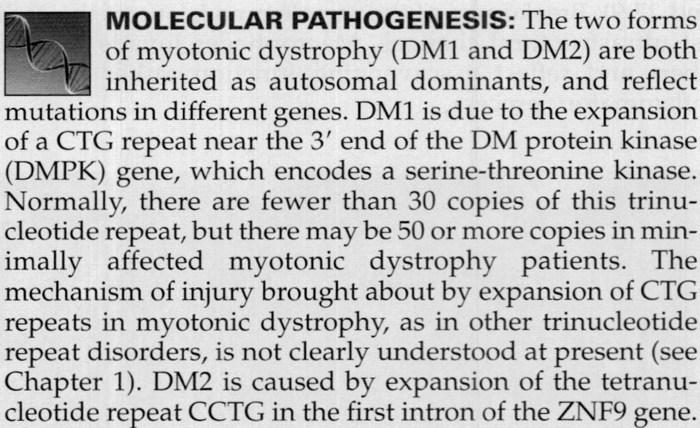

MOLECULAR PATHOGENESIS: The two forms of myotonic dystrophy (DM1 and DM2) are both inherited as autosomal dominants, and reflect mutations in different genes. DM1 is due to the expansion of a CTG repeat near the 3′ end of the DM protein kinase (DMPK) gene, which encodes a serine-threonine kinase. Normally, there are fewer than 30 copies of this trinucleotide repeat, but there may be 50 or more copies in minimally affected myotonic dystrophy patients. The mechanism of injury brought about by expansion of CTG repeats in myotonic dystrophy, as in other trinucleotide repeat disorders, is not clearly understood at present (see Chapter 1). DM2 is caused by expansion of the tetranucleotide repeat CCTG in the first intron of the ZNF9 gene.

PATHOLOGY: The pathology of adult myotonic dystrophy is highly variable, even in muscles from the same patient. Most patients display type I fiber atrophy and hypertrophy of type II fibers. Internally situated nuclei are a constant feature. The ATPase reaction shows many ring fibers, with circumferential concentration of heavily stained sarcoplasm. In these fibers, the outer sarcomeres are oriented circumferentially, instead of the usual longitudinal arrangement along the fiber axis (Fig. 27-10). Necrosis and regeneration, although occasionally present, are not prominent (as they are in Duchenne muscular dystrophy).

Muscles in congenital myotonic dystrophy show myofiber atrophy, frequent central nuclei and failure of fiber differentiation. These features closely resemble those of the

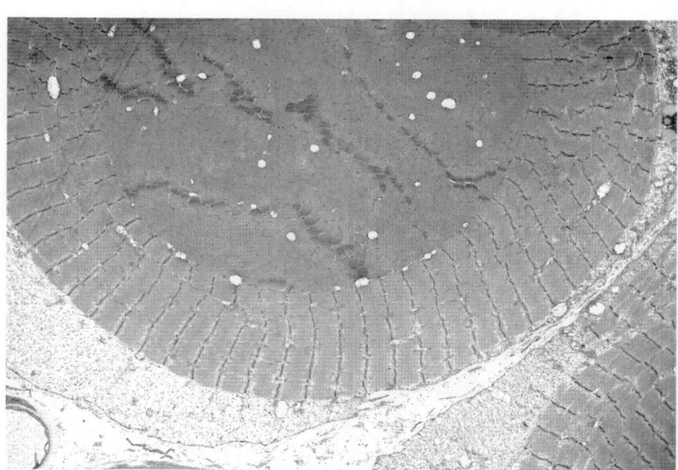

FIGURE 27-10. Ring fiber. Electron micrograph (magnification ×1900). The outer sarcomeres are oriented perpendicular to the axis of the myofiber.

X-linked recessive type of myotubular myopathy (see below).

CLINICAL FEATURES: In DM1, slowly progressive muscle weakness and stiffness are seen, principally in the distal limbs (proximal weakness is more common in DM2). Facial and neck weakness as well as ptosis are typical of DM1, but less common in DM2. Extramuscular features sometimes present in myotonic dystrophy include cataracts, testicular atrophy with diminished fertility and variable degrees of personality deterioration. A few patients exhibit involvement of smooth muscle, with disorders of the gastrointestinal tract, gallbladder and uterus. Other features include frontal balding, gonadal atrophy, cataracts and endocrine abnormalities. Cardiac arrhythmias and, less commonly, cardiomyopathy have been reported.

The diagnosis is based on clinical features, family history and characteristic electromyography, which exhibits myotonic discharges. The demonstration of an expanded CTG repeat (DM1) or CCTG (DM2) is predictive in utero and can be diagnostic in patients.

Congenital myotonic dystrophy is seen only in the offspring of women with DM1 who themselves show symptoms of myotonic dystrophy. Affected infants are born with severe muscle weakness. Myotonia is inconspicuous or absent, but appears in later childhood. A significant number of these patients suffer mental retardation. Congenital DM2 has not been identified.

Oculopharyngeal Muscular Dystrophy Usually Presents in Adults

Oculopharyngeal muscular dystrophy (OPMD) is typically diagnosed in middle age (older than 45 years) and most often shows autosomal dominant inheritance. An autosomal recessive form exists. Patients develop slowly progressive eyelid ptosis and dysphagia, and weakness of other muscle groups including the face and limbs. The autosomal dominant form is prevalent among French-Canadians in Quebec and Bukhara Jews living in Israel. Both autosomal dominant and recessive forms are due to abnormally increased numbers of GCG repeats in the poly(A) binding protein nuclear 1 gene (PABPN1), but differ in where these increased repeats are within the gene. Muscle biopsy shows intranuclear inclusions, rimmed vacuoles and filamentous inclusions similar to those observed in inclusion body myositis (see below and Fig. 27-15). Unlike inclusion body myositis, the intranuclear inclusions contain 8.5-nm filamentous inclusions.

Facioscapulohumeral Muscular Dystrophy Usually Begins in Childhood

Facioscapulohumeral muscular dystrophy (FSHD) is an autosomal dominantly inherited relatively common muscular dystrophy with onset in childhood or young adulthood. Patients suffer from facial and shoulder girdle weakness. Scapular winging is prominent. Other muscles may also be affected. Life expectancy is usually normal and extraskeletal involvement includes bundle branch block, hearing loss and retinal vasculopathy. FSHD is caused by deletion of part of a repetitive DNA fragment in the subtelomeric region of chromosome 4q. Thus, affected patients have fewer repeats than normal. Mononuclear inflammation is prominent, to the point of resembling an inflammatory myopathy such as polymyositis (see below), but does not correlate with the disease course. A detailed clinical history is essential to making the proper diagnosis.

Congenital Myopathies

A newborn occasionally manifests generalized hypotonia, with decreased deep tendon reflexes and muscle bulk. Many of these children have a difficult perinatal period because of weak respiration and consequent pulmonary complications. Some have "malignant" hypotonia, which is progressive and results in death within the first 12 months of life. **Werdnig-Hoffman disease** and **infantile acid maltase deficiency (Pompe disease)** are examples.

In other hypotonic patients, hypotonia may persist with little or no progression. These people become ambulatory and live a normal life span, although sometimes with secondary skeletal complications of hypotonia. This group of patients is subsumed in the category of "congenital myopathies." Muscle from these patients rarely reveals distinctive structural abnormalities of myofibers. Three of the most common forms of congenital myopathies are **central core disease** (Fig. 27-11), **nemaline (rod) myopathy** (Fig. 27-12) and **central nuclear myopathy** (Fig. 27-13). All show congenital hypotonia, decreased deep tendon reflexes, decreased muscle bulk and delayed motor milestones. In all three conditions abnormal muscle morphology is usually limited to type I fibers, with type I fiber predominance in some disorders and type I hypotrophy in others. Often, type I fibers are unusually predominant, or possibly, type II fibers fail to develop. There is no active myofiber necrosis or fibrosis, and patients have normal serum creatine kinase.

Central Core Disease Is an Autosomal Dominant Condition Characterized by Congenital Hypotonia and Proximal Muscle Weakness

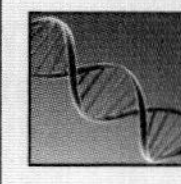

MOLECULAR PATHOGENESIS: Afflicted patients have decreased deep tendon reflexes and delayed motor development. The disease has been traced

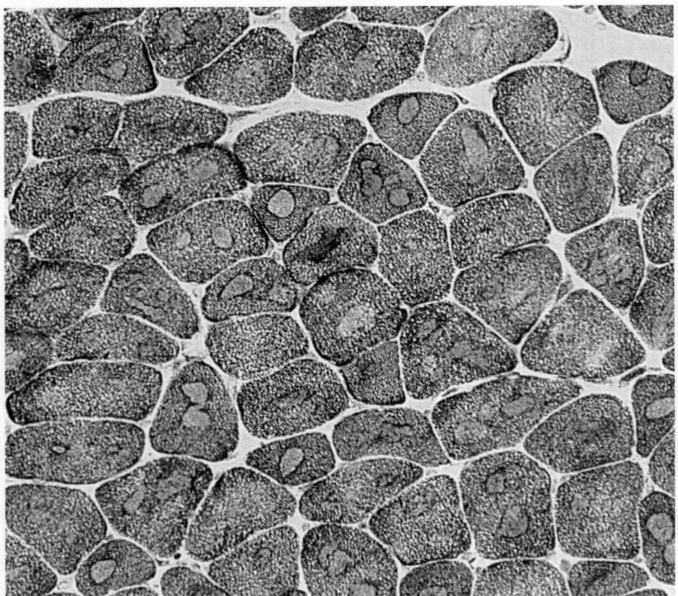

FIGURE 27-11. Central core disease. A section of vastus lateralis muscle stained for NADH-tetrazolium reductase shows a distinct circular zone of pallor in the center of most muscle fibers. A thin zone of excessive staining surrounds the core lesion. All of the myofibers in this case were type I, as demonstrated by the myofibrillar ATPase stain (not shown). Note the close resemblance of the core lesions to the target formations found in the muscle fibers of neurogenic disorders (see Fig. 27-23).

to a mutation on the long arm of chromosome 19 (19q13.1) that codes for the ryanodine receptor, the calcium-release channel of the sarcoplasmic reticulum. Occasional cases are sporadic or show autosomal recessive inheritance. Typical patients become ambulatory, but muscle strength remains less than normal.

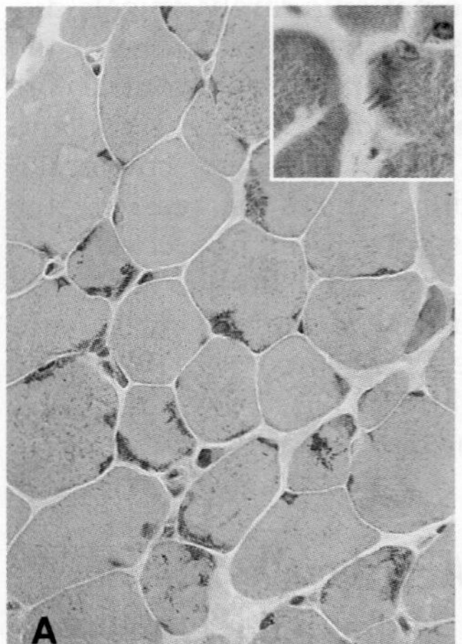

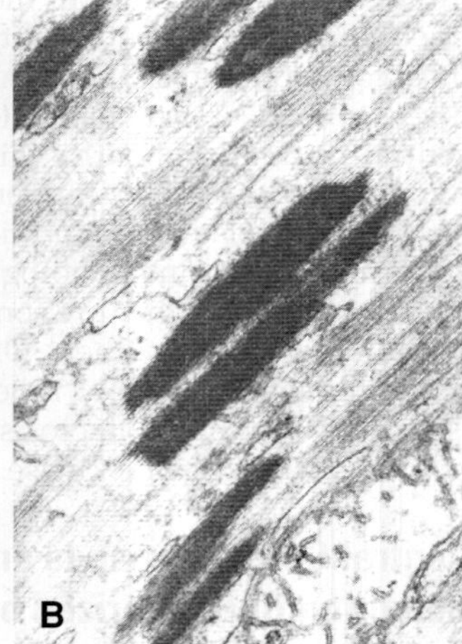

FIGURE 27-12. Rod (nemaline) myopathy. A. Muscle fibers contain dark aggregates of rods and granules (modified Gomori trichrome stain). As shown in the *inset*, these rods tend to be located at the fiber periphery near nuclei. **B.** An electron micrograph of the same biopsy shows that the structures are rod shaped and are derived from the Z disk.

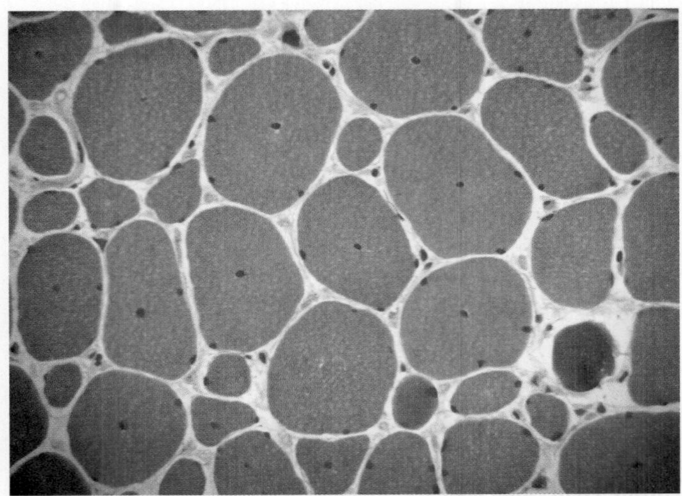

FIGURE 27-13. Central nuclear myopathy. Hematoxylin and eosin stain. Many muscle fibers contain a single central nucleus, and most of the affected muscle fibers are abnormally small. In addition, there are radiating spokes emanating from the central nuclei. These fibers resemble the late myotube stage of fetal development of skeletal muscle.

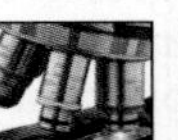

PATHOLOGY: There is a striking predominance of type I fibers, often showing a central zone of degeneration with loss of NADH-TR reaction staining (Fig. 27-11) and extending the entire length of the fiber. By electron microscopy, mitochondria and other membranous organelles are lost in the central cores, with or without myofibril disorganization. Membranous organelles tend to condense around the margin of the central core. The periphery of the fiber is unremarkable.

The central core anomaly may resemble the target fibers seen in active denervating conditions (see Fig. 27-23), although target fibers typically have dark rims around the areas of pallor and there is no evidence of denervation in central core disease.

Mutations of the ryanodine receptor 1 gene also cause **malignant hyperthermia**, a potentially fatal disorder triggered by succinylcholine and some anaesthetic agents, particularly halothane, characterized by rhabdomyolysis (see Chapter 8). As central core disease and malignant hyperthermia may coexist in some patients, patients with central core disease are possibly at risk for malignant hyperthermia. However, patients with malignant hyperthermia often have no abnormal histologic changes. Malignant hyperthermia is suspected by family history and confirmed by an in vitro muscle contraction test.

In Rod (Nemaline) Myopathy Sarcoplasmic Inclusions Derive From the Z Band

Rod myopathy includes a group of diseases in which rodlike inclusions accumulate within skeletal muscle sarcoplasm. The disease was initially named "nemaline" myopathy because the inclusions within the muscle fiber were interpreted as a tangled, threadlike mass. In reality, they are clusters of rod-shaped structures.

In the classic congenital form of rod myopathy patients show congenital hypotonia, delayed motor milestones of variable clinical severity and secondary skeletal changes such as kyphoscoliosis. Some exhibit severe involvement of muscles of the face, pharynx and neck. Later-onset (childhood and adult) forms tend to be associated with some muscle degeneration, increased serum creatine kinase levels and a slowly or nonprogressive course.

MOLECULAR PATHOGENESIS: Autosomal dominant and recessive patterns of inheritance are described. Genes responsible for rod myopathy so far identified include nebulin (most common), skeletal muscle α-actin, α- and β-tropomyosin and slow troponin T. Mutations in the ryanodine receptor gene have also been associated with nemaline rod formation.

PATHOLOGY: There is variable predominance of type I fibers and accumulation of rod-shaped structures within their sarcoplasm. Aggregates of these inclusions often occur in subsarcolemmal regions, near nuclei. They are brilliant red to dark red using modified Gomori trichrome stain (Fig. 27-12A), but are often not visible with hematoxylin and eosin. The inclusions are rod shaped and arise from the Z band, which they resemble ultrastructurally (Fig. 27-12B).

Rods have been described in a variety of neuromuscular diseases, including denervation atrophy, muscular dystrophy and inflammatory myopathies. Experimental tenotomy (cutting a tendon) induces formation of rods in the muscle when the nerve supply remains intact. In rod myopathy, however, the inclusions are the predominant pathologic change.

Central Nuclear Myopathy and Myotubular Myopathy Resemble the Myotubular Stage of Embryogenesis

MOLECULAR PATHOGENESIS: Central nuclear myopathy and myotubular myopathy were previously considered synonymous. Central nuclear myopathy is a group of clinically and genetically heterogeneous inherited conditions that have in common the presence of a centrally located nucleus in skeletal muscle cells. Autosomal recessive and autosomal dominant varieties are known. The latter tends to manifest in adolescence, and shows modestly increased serum creatine kinase. It progresses slowly and, like rod myopathy, resembles the so-called limb-girdle muscular dystrophy syndrome. Some patients exhibit a striking involvement of facial and extraocular musculature. Bilateral ptosis is almost always present. The gene responsible, dynamin 2, is involved in endocytosis, membrane trafficking and centrosome and actin assembly.

Myotubular myopathy is an X-linked disorder caused by myotubularin gene mutations. Myotubularin is a phosphatase expressed in most tissues and involved in phosphatidylinositol signaling cascades, but its precise function is unknown. Clinically, myotubular myopathy is characterized by marked neonatal hypotonia and respiratory failure at birth. Pathologically, like central nuclear myopathy, there are centrally placed nuclei within both fiber types.

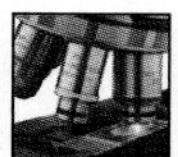

PATHOLOGY: Biopsies show predominance of type I fibers (Fig. 27-13), many of which are small and round, with a single central nucleus (hence the name of the disease). They resemble the myotubular stage in skeletal muscle embryogenesis. This apparent immature state suggests a possible defect in the nerve supply to the muscle fiber because the lower motor neuron requires subsequent maturation of the fiber. However, lower motor neurons in these patients, including motor endplates, are not demonstrably abnormal.

Later-onset forms of myotubular myopathy are characterized morphologically by more-mature muscle fibers, in which fibers are larger, have more numerous myofibrils and display single central nuclei that appear more mature.

Inflammatory Myopathies

Inflammatory myopathies are a heterogeneous group of acquired disorders, all of which feature symmetric proximal muscle weakness, increased serum levels of muscle-derived enzymes and nonsuppurative inflammation of skeletal muscle.

These are uncommon diseases, the annual incidence being 1 in 100,000. ***Dermatomyositis afflicts children and adults, but polymyositis almost always begins after 20 years of age.*** Both disorders are more frequent in females than males. By contrast, inclusion body myositis usually occurs after age 50 years and is three times more common in men than women.

These myopathies are thought to have an autoimmune origin because (1) they are seen with other autoimmune and connective tissues diseases, (2) pathology suggests autoimmune muscle cell injury, (3) serum autoantibodies are detected and (4) polymyositis and dermatomyositis (but not inclusion body myositis) respond to immunosuppressive treatment. No specific target autoantigens in muscle or blood vessels have been identified but antinuclear and anticytoplasmic antibodies exist in all of these diseases, with specificity to several different antigens.

The most common morphologic characteristics in the inflammatory myopathies are (1) the presence of inflammatory cells, (2) necrosis and phagocytosis of muscle fibers, (3) a mixture of regenerating and atrophic fibers and (4) fibrosis.

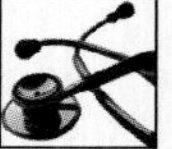

CLINICAL FEATURES: All inflammatory myopathies manifest as insidious proximal and symmetric muscle weakness, gradually increasing over weeks to months. Patients have problems with simple activities that require use of proximal muscles, including lifting objects, climbing steps or combing hair. Dysphagia and difficulty in holding up the head reflect involvement of pharyngeal and neck-flexor muscles. Some patients with inclusion body myositis have distal muscle weakness of the limbs that equals or exceeds that of proximal muscles. In advanced cases, respiratory muscles may be affected. Weakness progresses over weeks or months and leads to severe muscular wasting.

Dermatomyositis is distinguished from the other myopathies by a characteristic rash on the upper eyelids, face, trunk and occasionally elsewhere. It may occur alone or in association with scleroderma, mixed connective tissue disease or other autoimmune conditions. Its occurrence in a middle-aged man is associated with increased risk of epithelial cancer, mostly lung carcinoma. Polymyositis and inclusion body myositis are not associated with malignancy.

In Polymyositis Direct Muscle Damage Is Mediated by Cytotoxic T Cells

MOLECULAR PATHOGENESIS: In polymyositis there is no detectable microangiopathy as is seen in dermatomyositis (see below). In these disorders, healthy muscle fibers are initially surrounded by $CD8^+$ T lymphocytes (Fig. 27-14) and macrophages, after which the fibers degenerate. Unlike normal muscle, muscles affected in polymyositis express major histocompatibility complex (MHC) I antigens. Since cytotoxic T cells attack antigenic targets associated with MHC I molecules, an autoimmune etiology is likely.

The pathogenetic role of autoantibodies against nuclear antigens and cytoplasmic ribonucleoproteins in muscle injury is unknown. Polymyositis often has detectable anti-Jo-1, an antibody against histidyl-transfer RNA (tRNA) synthetase, with concomitant interstitial lung disease, Raynaud phenomenon and nonerosive arthritis.

Viral infections may precede polymyositis, but virus cultures of muscle are negative. An inflammatory myopathy indistinguishable from polymyositis occurs in many cases of human immunodeficiency virus (HIV-1) infection, but the role of the virus is unclear.

PATHOLOGY: Inflammatory cells infiltrate connective tissue mostly within fascicles (i.e., endomysial inflammation) and invade apparently healthy muscle fibers (Fig. 27-14). Angiopathy is absent. Isolated degenerating or regenerating fibers are scattered throughout fascicles. Perifascicular atrophy is not present in polymyositis (see below).

Inclusion Body Myositis Is Characterized by β-Amyloid Deposits

Inclusion body myositis resembles polymyositis pathologically, showing single-fiber necrosis and regeneration, with predominantly endomysial cytotoxic T cells. Basophilic granular material is seen at the edge of slitlike vacuoles (rimmed vacuoles) within muscle fibers. The fibers also have small eosinophilic cytoplasmic inclusions, often near the rimmed vacuoles (Fig. 27-15A, B). These inclusions are stained by Congo red and are a form of intracellular amyloid (Fig. 27-15C) that is immunoreactive for β-amyloid protein, the same type of amyloid as in the senile plaques of Alzheimer disease. Additional proteins associated with Alzheimer disease are also present including phosphorylated tau, α-synuclein, ubiquitin and presenilins (see Chapter 28). Parkin, a protein associated with hereditary Parkinson disease as well as the prion precursor protein, has also been localized to the inclusions. The pathogenic significance of these inclusions is unclear. Small groups of angulated fibers are present. By electron microscopy, the granules of rimmed vacuoles contain membranous whorls. Distinctive filaments are found nearby the rimmed vacuoles (Fig. 27-15D). The pathognomonic features of inclusion body myositis include the Congo red–positive inclusions and the characteristic filaments in the cytoplasm (or rarely in nuclei) of muscle fibers. An autosomal recessive hereditary form of the disease shows similar features but may be manifest in late adolescence or adulthood.

Dermatomyositis Is Caused by an Immune-Mediated Microangiopathy

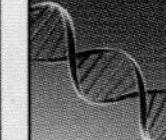

MOLECULAR PATHOGENESIS: This myopathy is characterized by (1) deposition of immune complexes of IgG, IgM and complement components, including membrane attack complex C5b-9 in the

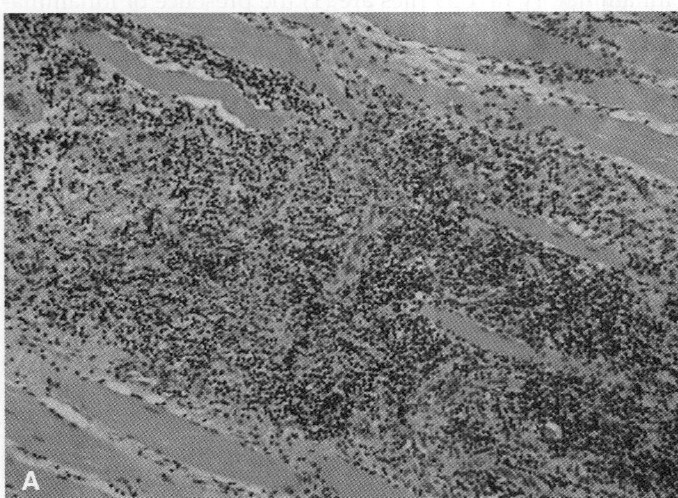

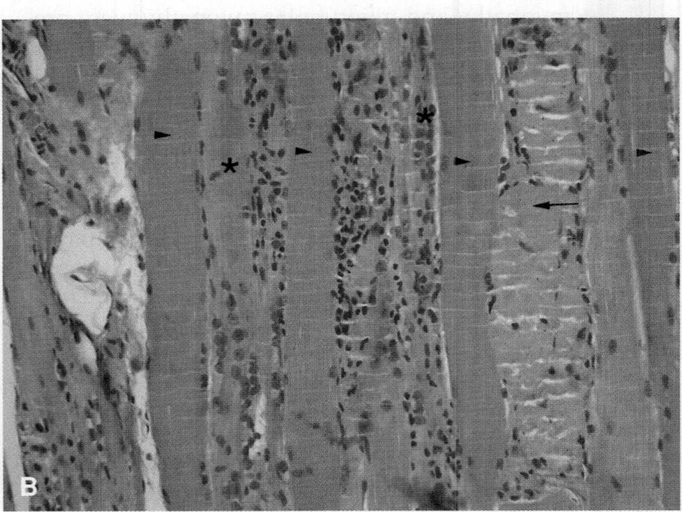

FIGURE 27-14. Polymyositis. A. Hematoxylin and eosin stain. A section of affected muscle shows an inflammatory myopathy. Mononuclear inflammatory cells infiltrate chiefly the endomysium. The field includes single-fiber necrosis. **B.** Region of healing inflammatory myopathy demonstrates intact fibers (*arrowheads*), necrotic fibers (*arrow*) and regenerating fibers characterized by enlarged nuclei and basophilic cytoplasm (*asterisk*).

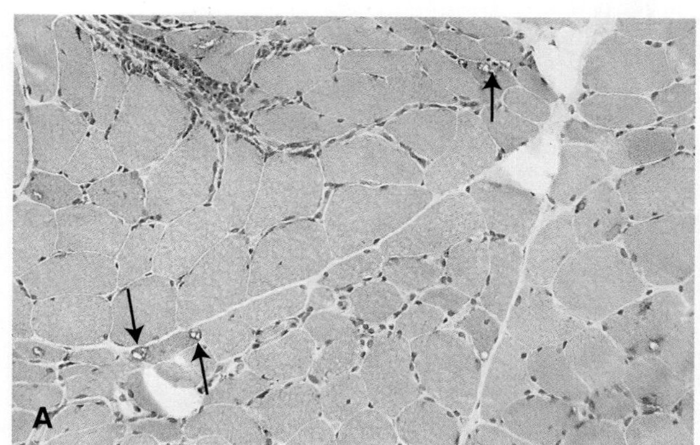

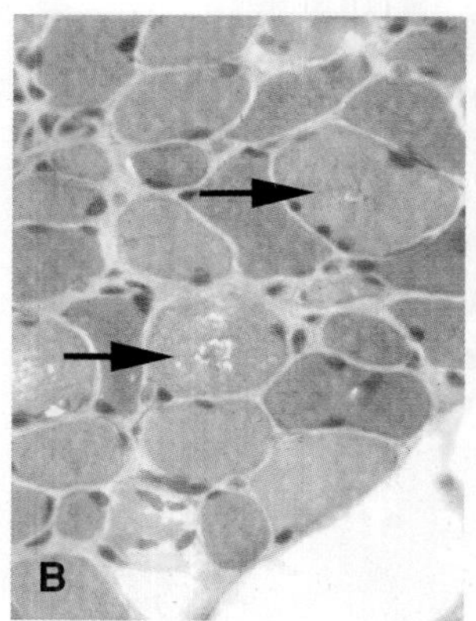

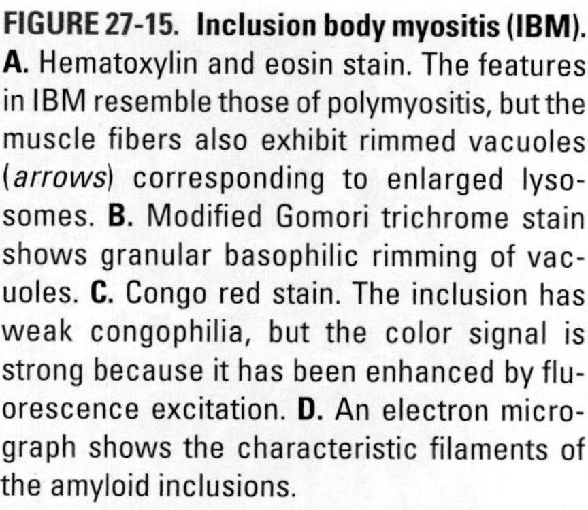

FIGURE 27-15. Inclusion body myositis (IBM). **A.** Hematoxylin and eosin stain. The features in IBM resemble those of polymyositis, but the muscle fibers also exhibit rimmed vacuoles (*arrows*) corresponding to enlarged lysosomes. **B.** Modified Gomori trichrome stain shows granular basophilic rimming of vacuoles. **C.** Congo red stain. The inclusion has weak congophilia, but the color signal is strong because it has been enhanced by fluorescence excitation. **D.** An electron micrograph shows the characteristic filaments of the amyloid inclusions.

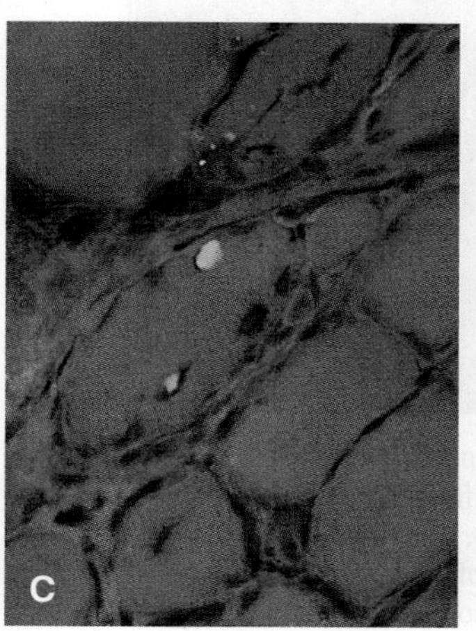

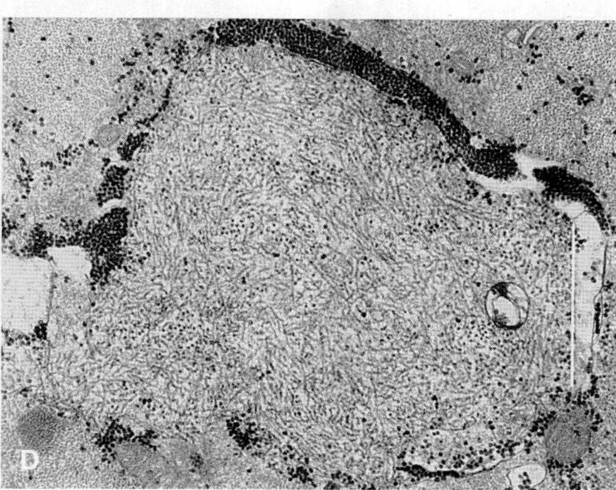

walls of capillaries and other blood vessels; (2) microangiopathy with loss of capillaries; (3) signs of injury and atrophy of myofibers; and (4) perivascular infiltrates of B cells and CD4$^+$ helper T cells (Fig. 27-16). These features suggest that muscle injury in dermatomyositis is mainly mediated by complement-fixing cytotoxic antibodies against skeletal muscle microvasculature. Complement detected in the capillaries before inflammation or damage to muscle fibers is the most specific finding of dermatomyositis. This microangiopathy is thought to lead to ischemic injury of individual muscle fibers and eventually to fiber atrophy. True infarcts may result from involvement of larger intramuscular arteries. The rash, which clinically distinguishes dermatomyositis from the other inflammatory myopathies, is presumably related to the same microangiopathy.

PATHOLOGY: Lymphocytes infiltrate around blood vessels and in perimysial connective tissue. B cells and T cells are involved, with a high CD4$^+$ (helper):CD8$^+$ (cytotoxic/suppressor) T-cell ratio. Immune complexes in the walls of blood vessels (Fig. 27-16, inset) are associated with microangiopathy. Intramuscular blood vessels exhibit endothelial hyperplasia, fibrin thrombi and obliteration of capillaries. One or more layers of atrophic fibers are seen at the periphery of the fascicles (perifascicular atrophy; Fig. 27-16). The combination of perifascicular atrophy and immune complexes in capillary walls is virtually diagnostic of dermatomyositis, even without inflammation. The abnormal staining of the endomysial connective tissue with the alkaline phosphatase reaction reflects damage to the blood vessels.

Vasculitis May Occur in Skeletal Muscle as Part of Systemic Vasculitides

Vasculitis can be present in skeletal muscle in polyarteritis nodosa (PAN), Wegener granulomatosis, collagen vascular disease and immune-mediated hypersensitivity states. In such instances, skeletal muscle may show neurogenic changes secondary to nerve damage.

Myasthenia Gravis

Myasthenia gravis is an acquired autoimmune disease characterized by abnormal muscular fatigability and caused by antibodies to the acetylcholine (Ach) receptor at the myoneural junction. It occurs in all races and is twice as common in women as in men. The disease typically begins in young adults, but cases in children and the very old have also been described.

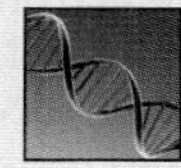

MOLECULAR PATHOGENESIS: In myasthenia gravis, antibodies bind the Ach receptor of the motor endplate. Complement activation leads to

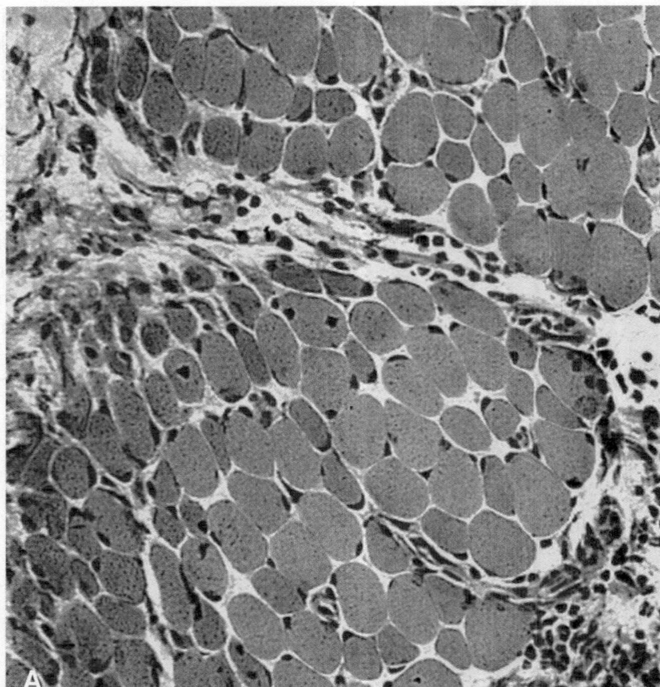

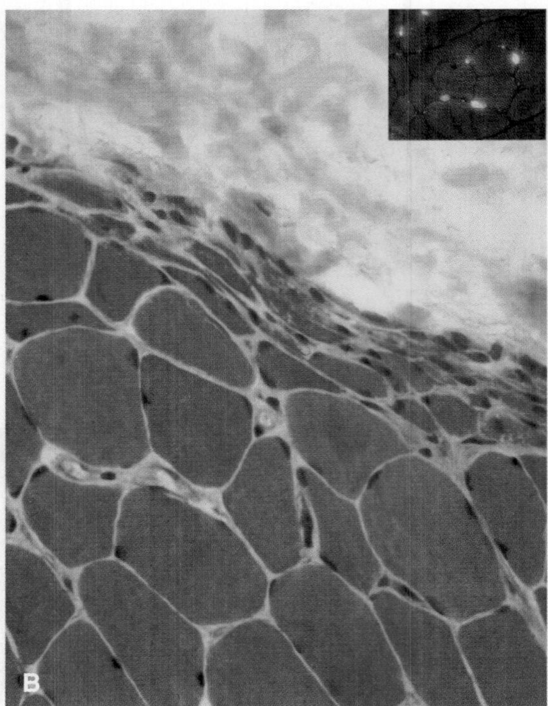

FIGURE 27-16. Dermatomyositis. A. Hematoxylin and eosin stain. The inflammatory cells infiltrate predominantly the perimysium rather than the endomysium. The periphery of muscle fascicles shows most of the muscle fiber atrophy and damage, resulting in a pattern of injury characteristic of dermatomyositis, termed *perifascicular atrophy*. **B.** High-magnification image of perifascicular atrophy demonstrating the flattening and shrinkage of fibers at the periphery of the fascicle. Immunofluorescence (*inset*) reveals that the walls of many capillaries display C5b-9 (membrane attack complex), reflecting the altered microvasculature typical of dermatomyositis. A few small regenerating fibers are also stained by this method.

shedding of the Ach receptor–rich terminal portions of the folds of the neuromuscular junction. The bivalent IgG antibodies also cross-link receptor proteins that remain in the postsynaptic membrane. This leads to Ach receptor endocytosis faster than the muscle fiber can replace them. The combination of reduced postsynaptic membrane area, decreased numbers of Ach receptors per unit area and widened synaptic space impairs signal transmission and causes muscle weakness and abnormal fatigability. The antireceptor antibodies do not directly block binding of Ach to prevent neuromuscular transmission.

Most patients with myasthenia gravis have thymic hyperplasia and about 15% have an associated thymoma. Surgical removal of the hyperplastic thymic tissue or the thymoma is often an effective treatment for myasthenia gravis. Ach receptors have been demonstrated on the surface of some thymic cells in both thymoma and thymic hyperplasia. Thus, thymic T lymphocytes may activate B lymphocytes to produce antireceptor antibodies.

PATHOLOGY: Light microscopy may reveal atrophy of type II muscle fibers and focal collections of lymphocytes within the fascicles. However, electron microscopy shows that most muscle endplates are abnormal, even in muscles that are not weakened. Sarcolemmal secondary folds are simplified with breakdown, loss of the crests of the folds and widening of the clefts.

CLINICAL FEATURES: The clinical severity of the condition is quite variable, and symptoms tend to wax and wane as in other autoimmune diseases. Weakness of extraocular muscles is typically severe and causes ptosis and diplopia. Sometimes, the disease may be confined to these muscles. More commonly, it progresses to other muscles (e.g., those associated with swallowing, the trunk and extremities). Patients with myasthenia gravis often have other autoimmune diseases.

The overall mortality from myasthenia gravis is about 10%, often because muscle weakness leads to respiratory insufficiency. In addition to thymectomy, corticosteroids, methotrexate and anticholinesterase drugs are used, alone or in combination. Plasmapheresis reduces anti–Ach receptor antibody titers, but any consequent clinical improvements are short-lived.

Lambert-Eaton Syndrome

Lambert-Eaton syndrome is a paraneoplastic disorder that manifests as muscle weakness, wasting and fatigability of proximal limbs and trunk. Also termed **myasthenic–myopathic syndrome,** it is usually associated with small cell lung carcinoma, but may also occur with other malignancies, and rarely in the absence of underlying cancer. Neurophysiologic evidence suggests a defect in Ach release at nerve terminals. IgG from patients can transfer the disease to mice. The pathogenic

IgG autoantibodies target voltage-sensitive calcium channels expressed in motor nerve terminals and in the cells of the lung cancer. These calcium channels are necessary for Ach release and are greatly reduced in presynaptic membranes in these patients, thus reducing neuromuscular transmission. Lambert-Eaton syndrome responds to corticosteroid treatment.

Inherited Metabolic Diseases

Skeletal muscle is dramatically affected by a variety of endocrine and metabolic diseases, such as Cushing syndrome, Addison disease, hypothyroidism, hyperthyroidism (see Chapter 21) and conditions associated with hepatic or renal failure. Only primary hereditary abnormalities in metabolism of skeletal muscle resulting in abnormal muscular function will be discussed here.

Glycogen Storage Diseases Are Genetic Disorders With Variable Effects on Muscle

Glycogen storage diseases (glycogenoses) are autosomal recessive, inherited, metabolic disorders characterized by an inability to degrade glycogen (see Chapter 6). There are many glycogenoses, but only some of them affect skeletal muscle. Only the most important glycogenoses affecting skeletal muscle will be described.

Type II Glycogenosis (Acid Maltase [α-1,4-Glucosidase] Deficiency, Pompe Disease)

MOLECULAR PATHOGENESIS: Various mutations affect muscle acid maltase activity and lead to distinctly different clinical syndromes. Acid maltase is a lysosomal enzyme that is expressed in all cells and participates in glycogen degradation. When the enzyme is deficient, glycogen is not broken down, accumulates within lysosomes and remains membrane bound (Fig. 27-17B).

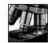

PATHOLOGY: In all forms of glycogenosis due to acid maltase deficiency, the morphologic changes are distinctive and almost pathognomonic (Fig. 27-17A). In the severe form, Pompe disease, muscle shows massive accumulation of membrane-bound glycogen. The myofilaments and other sarcoplasmic organelles disappear. Surprisingly, there is very little regeneration, and apparently inactive satellite cells are present at the surfaces of muscle fibers that have been almost completely destroyed by the disease process.

Late infantile, juvenile and adult-onset forms of type II glycogenosis are milder. Changes range from overt vacuolar myopathy seen on routine histology to very subtle accumulation of membrane-bound glycogen particles only detectable by electron microscopy. Vacuoles observed by light microscopy are empty or contain glycogen.

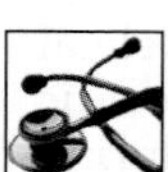

CLINICAL FEATURES: Pompe disease occurs in neonates or young infants and is the most severe form of acid maltase deficiency. Patients have severe hypotonia and areflexia, and clinically resemble patients with Werdnig-Hoffmann disease (see below under Denervation). Some have enlarged tongues and cardiomegaly, and die of cardiac failure, usually within their first 2 years. Many tissues are affected, but the most significant involvement is in skeletal and cardiac muscle, the CNS and liver. The serum creatine kinase level is slightly to moderately increased. Later-onset forms of the disease entail milder, but relentlessly progressive, myopathy. Glycogen accumulates in other organs, but clinical expression of the disorder is usually limited to muscle.

Type III Glycogenosis (Debranching Enzyme Deficiency, Cori Disease, Limit Dextrinosis, Amylo-1,6-Glucosidase Deficiency)

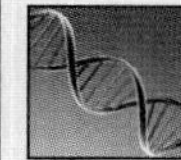

MOLECULAR PATHOGENESIS: Type III glycogenosis is a rare, autosomal recessive disease that affects children or adults. Because the debranching enzyme is absent, phosphorylase hydrolyzes the

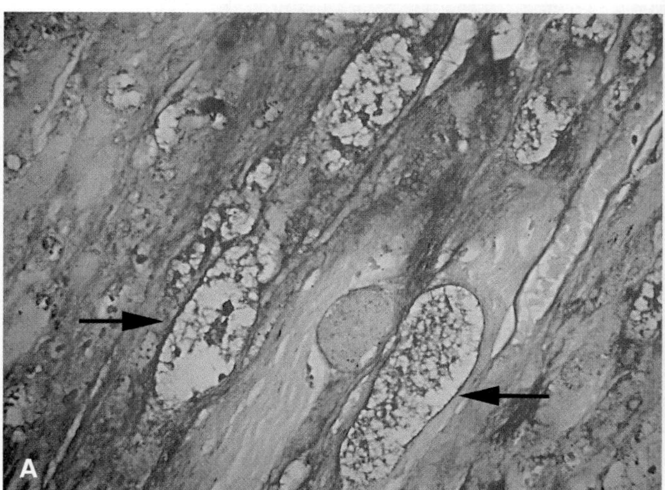

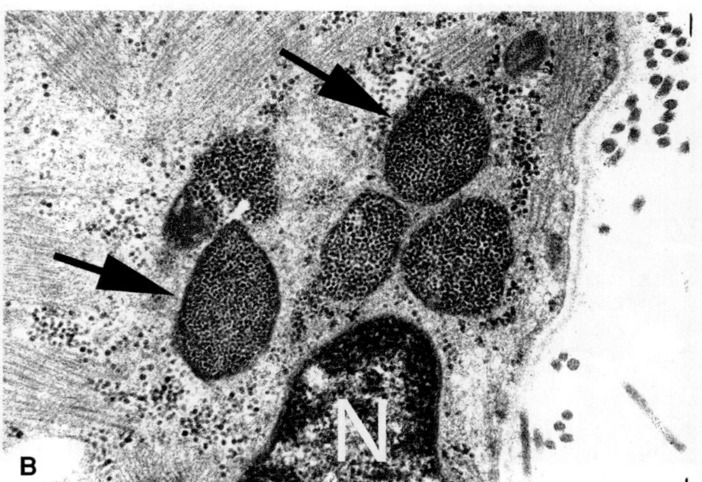

FIGURE 27-17. Acid maltase deficiency—adult onset. A. Periodic acid–Schiff (PAS) stain demonstrating large vacuoles filled with PAS-positive glycogen granules (*arrows*). **B.** Electron micrograph demonstrating membrane-bound glycogen granules (*arrows*). The structure marked *N* is a nucleus.

1,4-glycosidic linkages of the terminal glucose chains of glycogen, but not beyond branch points. Hepatomegaly and growth retardation are usual. Muscle symptoms vary, and the most severe and consistent involvement is related to liver dysfunction in children.

Type V Glycogenosis (McArdle Disease, Myophosphorylase Deficiency)

MOLECULAR PATHOGENESIS: Type V glycogenosis is a more common metabolic myopathy that is usually not progressive or severely debilitating. The deficient enzyme, myophosphorylase, is specific for skeletal muscle. Lacking this enzyme, skeletal muscle glycogen cannot be cleaved at 1,4-glycosidic chains to produce glucose for energy production during physical exertion. Thus, muscles cramp with exercise. Patients also cannot produce lactate during ischemic exercise. This defect is the basis for a metabolic test for the condition.

PATHOLOGY: Tissue may appear completely normal, except for the absence of phosphorylase activity. However, there is usually subtle evidence of abnormal accumulation of glycogen granules within the sarcoplasm, mainly in the subsarcolemmal area (Fig. 27-18). The specific diagnosis can be made by a histochemical reaction for myophosphorylase, but must be confirmed by biochemical assay of the muscle enzyme activity or by analysis of genomic DNA.

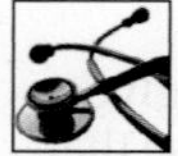

CLINICAL FEATURES: If patients avoid strenuous exercise, myophosphorylase deficiency does not seriously interfere with their lives. However, prolonged, vigorous exercise can lead to widespread necrosis of myofibers and release of soluble muscle proteins like creatine kinase and myoglobin into the circulation. This event, in turn, can produce myoglobinuria and renal failure.

Muscle biopsy should be performed several weeks after an episode of symptoms to allow regeneration of the muscle.

Type VII Glycogenosis (Phosphofructokinase Deficiency, Tarui Disease)

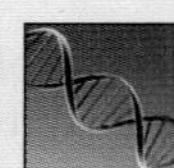

MOLECULAR PATHOGENESIS: Phosphofructokinase (PFK) deficiency is less common than McArdle disease but causes an identical syndrome. PFK catalyzes conversion of fructose-6-phosphate to fructose-1,6-diphosphate and is a key enzyme in the Embden-Meyerhof pathway. In muscle, this enzyme has four identical subunits (M_4), while in erythrocytes, it contains two different (M and L) subunits, each under separate genetic control. Genetic lack of the muscle subunit thus leads to complete absence of muscle PFK activity, but reduces erythrocyte PFK by 50%. In the latter cells, the remaining active enzyme is made up of four normal L subunits.

Patients with type VII glycogenosis often have slight anemia or low-grade hemolysis, but muscle histology resembles that in McArdle disease, save that phosphorylase activity is present. By contrast, a histochemical reaction for PFK shows little or no staining for the enzyme. The diagnosis is substantiated by biochemical analysis of the enzyme activity in muscle.

Lipid Myopathies Are Caused by Defective Fat Metabolism

Occasionally, a muscle biopsy from a patient with exercise intolerance or muscle weakness shows excess neutral lipids. This occurs in several metabolic disorders that affect lipid metabolism, more than a dozen of which have been identified. In brief, lipid myopathies may involve deficiencies in (1) fatty acid transport into mitochondria (carnitine-deficiency

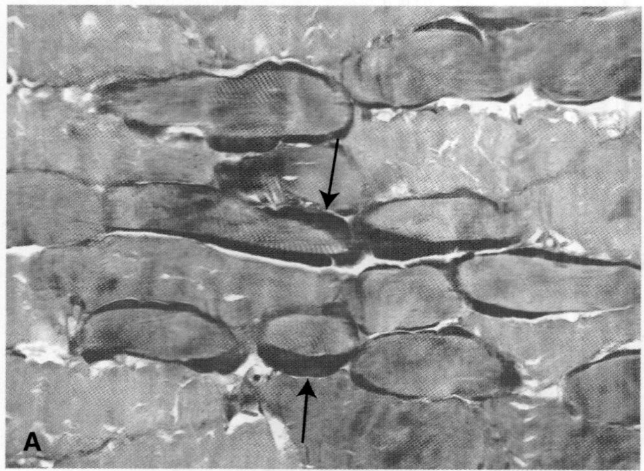

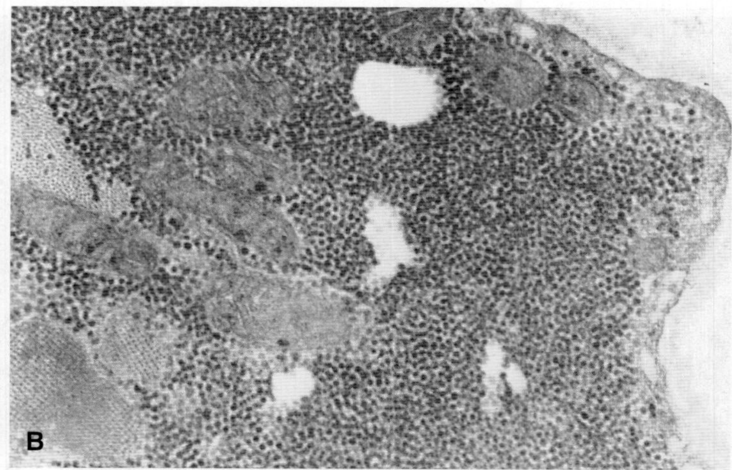

FIGURE 27-18. McArdle disease (myophosphorylase deficiency). A. Prominent periodic acid–Schiff (PAS)-positive glycogen accumulation in a subsarcolemmal distribution (*arrows*). **B.** An electron micrograph demonstrates an abnormal mass of glycogen particles just beneath the sarcolemma. The glycogen is not surrounded by a membrane, in contrast to the lysosomal glycogen storage of acid maltase deficiency.

syndromes, carnitine palmityl transferase deficiency), (2) a variety of enzymes that mediate β-oxidation of fatty acids, (3) respiratory chain enzymes and (4) triglyceride use. Only disorders involving carnitine metabolism are discussed here.

Carnitine Deficiency

Carnitine, which is synthesized in the liver and is present in large quantities in skeletal muscle, is necessary for transport of long-chain fatty acids into mitochondria. Muscle carnitine deficiency is an autosomal recessive condition, characterized by progressive proximal muscle weakness and atrophy, often with signs of denervation and peripheral neuropathy. The absence of carnitine leads to massive accumulation of lipid droplets in the sarcoplasm outside mitochondria, which is readily evident in muscle biopsies (Fig. 27-19). Sometimes oral carnitine therapy alleviates the symptoms. Carnitine deficiency in skeletal muscle also occurs as part of a systemic disorder that can affect the CNS, heart and liver. Structural abnormalities of mitochondria may be present.

Carnitine Palmitoyltransferase Deficiency

As in carnitine deficiency, patients with carnitine palmitoyltransferase deficiency cannot metabolize long-chain fatty acids owing to an inability to transport these lipids into mitochondria, where they undergo β-oxidation. After heavy exercise, these patients have muscular pain, which may progress to myoglobinuria. Prolonged fasting can produce the same symptoms. After such an episode, fibers regenerate and restore muscle structure. Biopsies are microscopically normal; the diagnosis depends on a biochemical assay for carnitine palmitoyltransferase activity.

Mitochondrial Diseases Reflect Mutant Nuclear DNA or Mitochondrial DNA

Inherited defects of mitochondrial metabolism are an uncommon but conceptually important group of disorders. Historically, diseases of muscle were recognized first and designated mitochondrial myopathies, but others affect both CNS and muscle and are known as **mitochondrial encephalomyopathies.** The nervous system, skeletal muscle, heart, kidney and other organs can be affected in different combinations as part of a multisystem disease.

Inherited diseases of mitochondria are classified genetically into two broad groups, defects of either **nuclear DNA** (nDNA) or **mitochondrial DNA** (mtDNA). Point mutations, deletions and duplications of mtDNA have been identified and linked to several mitochondrial encephalomyopathies. This group of syndromes is discussed here.

MOLECULAR PATHOGENESIS: Genes for most mitochondrial proteins are in nDNA, but mtDNA encodes 13 of the approximately 80 polypeptide subunits of the respiratory chain complexes. Defects in these proteins lead to mitochondrial encephalomyopathies.

Unlike Mendelian inheritance of nDNA mutations, mtDNA diseases are transmitted in the maternal mtDNA, because mtDNA derives only from the oocyte. The zygote and its daughter cells have many mitochondria, each of which contains maternally derived mitochondrial DNA. Mutations in mtDNA are passed on randomly to subsequent generations of cells. During fetal or later growth, some cells may thus contain only mutant genomes (mutant homoplasmy), others will have only normal genomes (wild-type homoplasmy) and still others receive a mixed population of mutant and normal mtDNA (heteroplasmy). Clinical expression of a disease produced by a given mutation of mtDNA depends on the proportion of the total content of mitochondrial genomes that is mutant. ***The fraction of mutant mtDNA must exceed a critical value for a mitochondrial disease to be symptomatic.*** This threshold varies in different organs and is presumably related to cellular energy requirements.

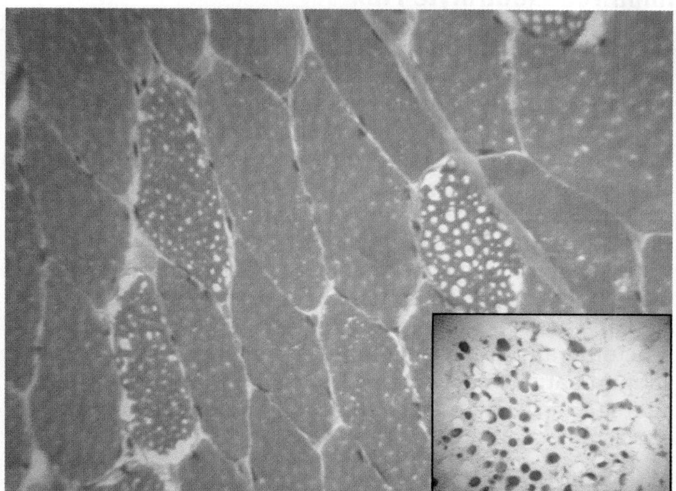

FIGURE 27-19. Lipid storage myopathy. Hematoxylin and eosin–stained frozen section. Numerous cytoplasmic vacuoles are present in the muscle fibers. Oil red-orcein stain (*inset*) demonstrates that the cytoplasmic vacuoles contain neutral lipid.

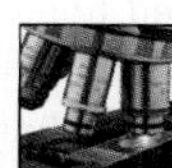

PATHOLOGY: In skeletal muscle, defects of mtDNA lead to accumulation of mitochondria, excessive numbers of which may, with modified Gomori trichrome stain, appear as aggregates of reddish granular material in the sarcoplasm (Fig. 27-20A). This has been termed a **ragged red fiber** because of the irregular contours of these deposits at the fiber periphery. Three subunits of complex IV (cytochrome oxidase) are encoded by mtDNA and are required for the assembled electron transport carrier to be functional. Pathogenic mutations of mtDNA may impair complex IV activity, so that ragged red fibers are often deficient in cytochrome oxidase activity (Fig. 27-20B). By contrast, they stain intensely for SDH (complex II); this complex is exclusively encoded by nDNA (Fig. 27-20C). This increased SDH presumably reflects the proliferation of mitochondria. The mitochondrial defects cause atrophy of myofibers and accumulation of sarcoplasmic lipid and glycogen. Ultrastructurally, mitochondria may display striking paracrystalline inclusions (Fig. 27-20D).

Death of nerve cells and reactive astrocytosis occur in the CNS. Increased ragged red fibers and cytochrome oxidase–negative fibers have also been seen in elderly patients with unexplained muscle weakness ("mitochondrial cytopathy

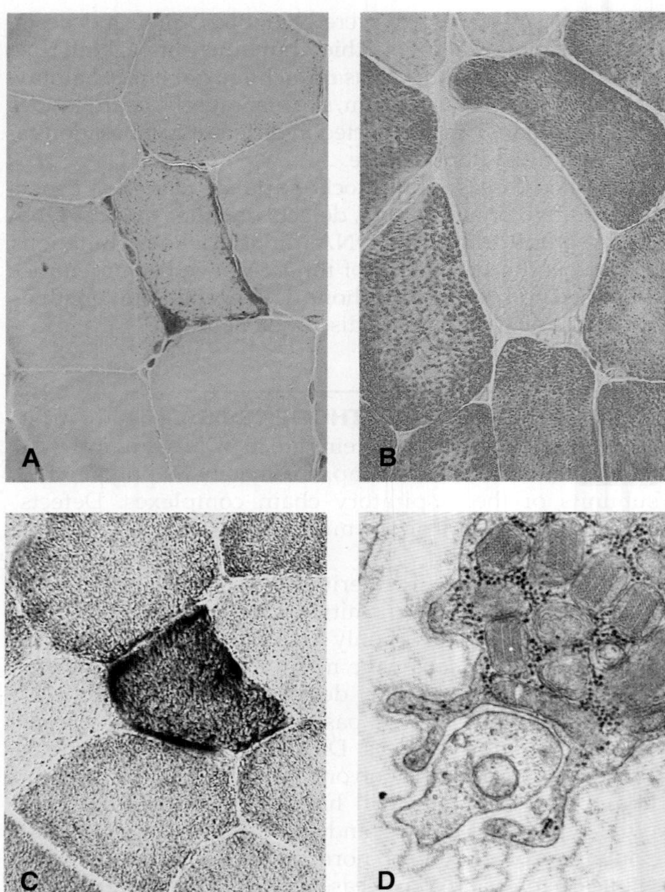

FIGURE 27-20. Mitochondrial myopathy caused by deletions of mitochondrial DNA (mtDNA). A. Modified Gomori trichrome. A ragged red fiber shows prominent proliferation of reddish, granular mitochondria, located chiefly in a subsarcolemmal region. **B.** A ragged red fiber displays lack of **histochemical staining for cytochrome oxidase** (central pale fiber). Three subunits of this electron-transport carrier are coded by mtDNA, and the mutations have interfered with function in this fiber. **C. Succinate dehydrogenase (SDH) stain**. A ragged red fiber shows overexpression of SDH, an enzyme that is entirely encoded by nuclear DNA (nDNA). **D.** An electron micrograph reveals mitochondria with ultrastructural abnormalities, including paracrystalline inclusions.

of old age"), presumably owing to increased numbers of mutant mitochondria that occurs with aging. Ragged red fibers, cytochrome oxidase–negative fibers and intra-mitochondrial paracrystalline inclusions are characteristic of a mitochondrial disorder, but are not specific, as similar changes may be seen in some muscular dystrophies, in inclusion body myositis and after AZT therapy. Conversely, the absence of such changes does not exclude a mitochondrial disorder.

CLINICAL FEATURES: Clinical manifestations of the encephalomyopathies vary, but usually begin in childhood. Some patients start with muscle weakness and then develop a brain disorder. Others present with CNS disease with or without overt muscle weakness, even though muscle biopsy indicates a mitochondrial disorder. Other organs, such as the heart, are often affected as part of a multisystem disorder.

Three neurologic syndromes have been delineated: (1) **Kearns-Sayre syndrome** (progressive ophthalmoplegia, retinal pigmentary degeneration, cardiac arrhythmias and other features), (2) **MELAS** (mitochondrial myopathy, encephalopathy, lactic acidosis and strokelike episodes) and (3) **MERRF** (myoclonic epilepsy and ragged red fibers). Most patients with Kearns-Sayre syndrome have large deletions of mtDNA that are not familial. MELAS and MERRF usually involve point mutations in mitochondrial genes for transfer RNAs, mostly—but not exclusively—leucine tRNA (MELAS) and lysine tRNA (MERRF). Mitochondrial genetic disorders are inherited from maternal mtDNA. Other syndromes affecting mitochondrial proteins encoded by nuclear genes show autosomal or X-linked patterns of inheritance.

Myoadenylate Deaminase Deficiency Is a Frequent Cause of Mild Weakness

MOLECULAR PATHOGENESIS: Large amounts of adenosine monophosphate deaminase (AMP-DA) are present in skeletal muscle, particularly in type II fibers. AMP-DA is important in regulating purine nucleotide cycles and in maintaining the adenosine triphosphate/adenosine diphosphate (ATP/ADP) ratio during exercise. A group of patients with mild proximal muscle weakness and exercise intolerance completely lack AMP-DA activity. It is a common, autosomal recessive condition, seen in 1% to 2% of all muscle biopsies. AMP-DA deficiency may thus not actually be a separate disease, but one that is unmasked by other neuromuscular diseases.

Familial Periodic Paralysis Reflects Impaired Electrolyte Flux

Familial periodic paralysis encompasses several autosomal dominant disorders characterized by episodic muscular weakness or even complete paralysis, followed by a rapid recovery. These disorders reflect abnormalities in sodium and potassium fluxes into and out of muscle cells. During an attack, the muscle fiber surface does not propagate action potentials, although delivery of calcium into the muscle fiber causes contraction. Muscle biopsies taken during an attack show no detectable abnormalities of recent onset. Later, permanent mild myopathic changes and sarcoplasmic vacuoles appear. These vacuoles are dilated or remodeled sarcoplasmic reticulum and transverse tubules. In some cases, a distinct subpopulation of fibers (type IIB) contains numerous tubular aggregates derived from the tubular network of the sarcoplasmic reticulum.

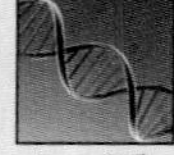

MOLECULAR PATHOGENESIS: Three clinically and genetically distinct syndromes are hypokalemic, hyperkalemic and normokalemic periodic paralysis. The hypokalemic type is linked to mutations of the gene that encodes a voltage-gated calcium channel of skeletal muscle; the hyperkalemic and normokalemic forms involve mutations in the *SCN4A* gene on chromosome 17q, which codes for the sodium channel.

Rhabdomyolysis

Rhabdomyolysis is dissolution of skeletal muscle fibers and release of myoglobin into the blood, which may cause myoglobinuria and acute renal failure. The disorder may be acute, subacute or chronic. During acute rhabdomyolysis, muscles are swollen, tender and profoundly weak.

Episodes of rhabdomyolysis may be precipitated by diverse stimuli. They may complicate or follow bouts of influenza. Some patients develop rhabdomyolysis with apparently mild exercise and probably have some form of metabolic myopathy. A spectrum of muscle dysfunction, from pain (myalgia) to rhabdomyolysis, is also well known during treatment with statin cholesterol-lowering agents. Biopsies after recovery may show morphologically normal muscle. Rhabdomyolysis also may complicate heat stroke or malignant hyperthermia. Alcoholism is occasionally associated with either acute or chronic rhabdomyolysis.

Pathologic changes in rhabdomyolysis are those of an active, noninflammatory myopathy, with scattered necrosis of muscle fibers and varying degrees of degeneration and regeneration. Clusters of macrophages without other inflammatory cells are seen in and around muscle fibers.

Denervation

The pathology of denervation reflects lesions of the lower motor neuron. Lower motor neuron lesions can be detected by muscle biopsy, but patterns of denervation do not identify the cause of the lesion. The morphology may indicate whether denervation is recent or chronic but does not distinguish between, for example, amyotrophic lateral sclerosis, a disorder of motor neurons, and neuropathy due to diabetes mellitus. Lesions of upper motor neurons, as in multiple sclerosis or stroke, lead to paralysis and atrophy, but lower motor neurons in these conditions remain intact. Pathologic changes thus reflect nonspecific diffuse atrophy rather than denervation atrophy.

When a skeletal muscle fiber becomes separated from contact with its lower motor neuron, it invariably atrophies, owing to progressive loss of myofibrils. On cross-section, atrophic fibers have characteristic angular configurations, seemingly compressed by surrounding normal muscle fibers (Fig. 27-21). If a fiber is not reinnervated, atrophy progresses to complete loss of myofibrils, with nuclei condensing into aggregates. In the end stage, muscle fibers disappear and are replaced chiefly by adipose tissue.

Early in denervation, fibers are irregularly scattered, angular and atrophic. As the disease progresses, these fibers are first seen in small clusters of several fibers, and then in progressively larger groups (Fig. 27-21B). They stain excessively darkly for nonspecific esterase (Fig. 27-22) and NADH-TR, in contrast to atrophy caused by disuse or wasting. By ATPase staining, groups of denervated fibers are a mixture of type I and type II fibers: **denervating conditions are not selective for only one type of motor neuron.**

"Target fibers" (Fig. 27-23) are seen in 20% of cases of denervation. This apparently transient change occurs during or shortly after denervation or reinnervation, and indicates that the process is active. The lesion consists of central pallor of the muscle fiber, which is surrounded by a condensed zone that in turn is surrounded by a normal zone of sarcoplasm. Target fibers are difficult to see with hematoxylin and eosin stain, but the NADH-TR stain shows greatly reduced staining in the central zone, reflecting reduced or absent mitochondria.

Every episode of denervation is followed by an effort at reinnervation. If denervation proceeds slowly, reinnervation may keep pace. New sprouting nerve endings make synaptic contact with the muscle fiber at the site of the previous motor endplate. As in the myotubular phase of embryogenesis, nicotinic Ach receptors (extrajunctional receptor) cover muscle fibers soon after denervation. This denervated state induces sprouting of new nerve endings from adjacent surviving nerves. With reinnervation, extrajunctional receptors again disappear from the sarcolemma, except at the point of synaptic contact.

In a chronic denervating condition, reinnervation of each surviving motor unit gradually enlarges. As a specific type of lower motor neuron takes over innervation of a given field of fibers, fiber groups of one type are seen adjacent to groups of another type. This pattern, called **type grouping,** is pathognomonic of denervation followed by reinnervation (Fig. 27-21C).

Patients with striking fiber–type grouping often have symptoms of muscle cramping in addition to progressive muscular weakness. After a single episode of denervation, such as in poliomyelitis, reinnervation often leads to remarkable recovery of strength. Years later, a biopsy shows a conspicuous pattern of type grouping, with scattered pyknotic nuclear clumps. In such cases, there are neither angular atrophic fibers nor target fibers.

Occasionally, a biopsy reveals abnormal prominence of one fiber type (either type I or type II) over the other, **type predominance**. There is frequently evidence of denervation. It is possible that in this case, reinnervation may favor one type of lower motor neuron over another.

Occasional muscle fibers may undergo necrosis or regeneration in neuropathic conditions. In such patients, a modest increase in serum creatine kinase levels reflects muscle degeneration. This is common in slowly progressive forms of spinal muscular atrophy (e.g., Kugelberg-Welander disease and Kennedy disease [X-linked spinobulbar muscular atrophy]).

Spinal Muscular Atrophy Reflects Progressive Degeneration of Anterior Horn Cells

Spinal muscular atrophy (SMA) is the second most common lethal autosomal recessive disorder after cystic fibrosis. Childhood SMA is classified into type I **(Werdnig-Hoffmann disease)**, type II (intermediate) and type III **(Kugelberg-Welander disease)**. The survival motor neuron gene (5q11.2-13.3) is absent in virtually all (99%) cases of SMA.

WERDNIG-HOFFMANN DISEASE (INFANTILE SPINAL MUSCULAR ATROPHY): In ***Werdnig-Hoffmann disease infants show progressive and severe weakness,*** and seldom survive beyond 1 year of life. Denervation seems to begin in utero after motor units are established. The histology is virtually pathognomonic (Fig. 27-24). Groups of minute,

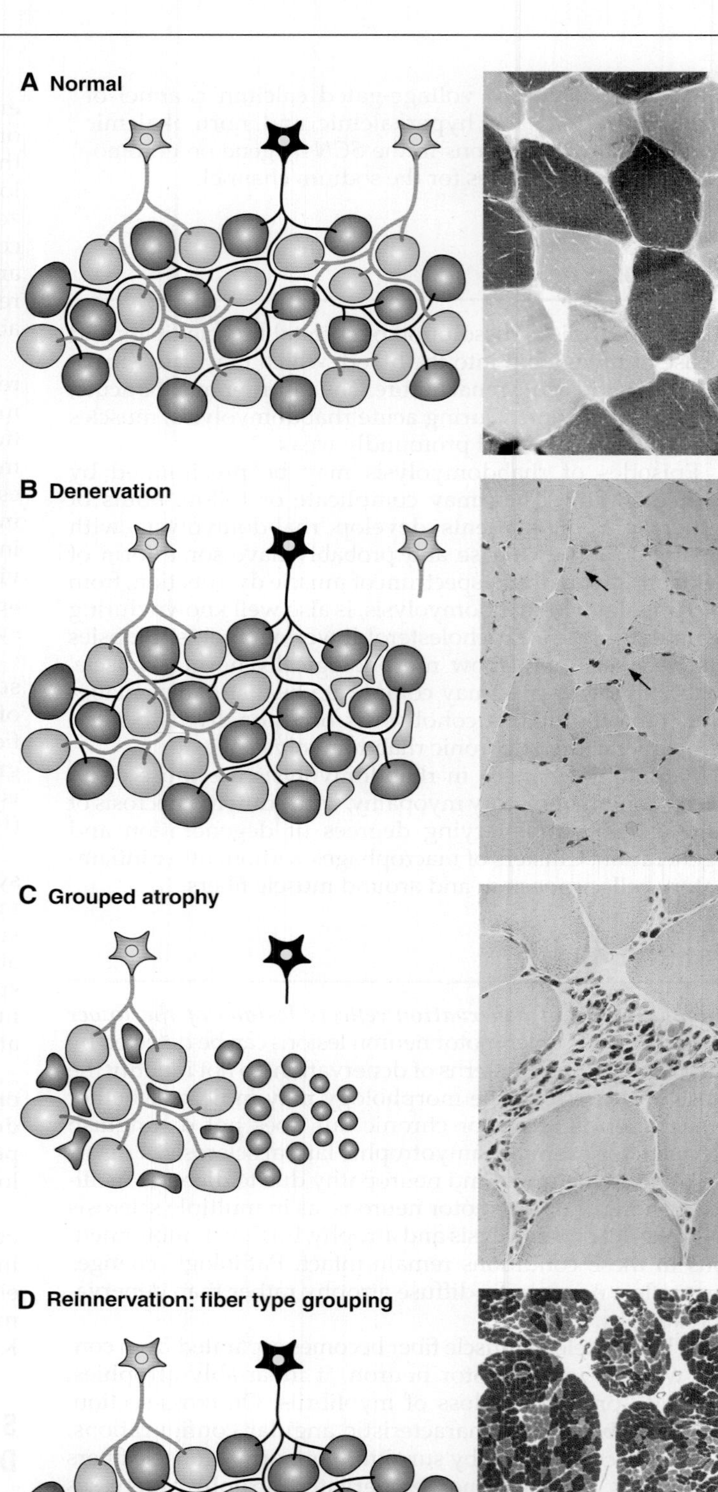

FIGURE 27-21. Denervation/reinnervation. A. As shown in the photomicrograph, the normal intermixed distribution of type I (*pale*) and type II (*dark*) muscle fibers is shown by staining for ATPase. In the drawing, two neurons (*blue*) innervate type I muscle fibers, and two neurons (*brown*) supply type II fibers. **B.** Denervation; hematoxylin and eosin stain. With early (mild) denervation, portions of the axonal tree degenerate, resulting in angular atrophy of scattered type I and II muscle fibers (*arrows*). **C.** With more advanced (severe) denervation, entire lower motor neurons or numerous axonal processes degenerate, causing small groups of angular atrophic fibers (grouped atrophy) to appear as illustrated in the photomicrograph. **D.** Reinnervation; myofibrillar ATPase. As neurons degenerate, surviving neurons sprout more nerve endings and reinnervate some of the denervated fibers. These reinnervated fibers become either type I or type II, according to the type of neuron that reinnervates them. This process results in fewer, but larger, motor units and the appearance of clusters of fibers of one type adjacent to clusters of the other type, a pattern called "type grouping." The photomicrograph demonstrates type grouping. This field would appear normal except for a few atrophic fibers if it were stained with hematoxylin and eosin.

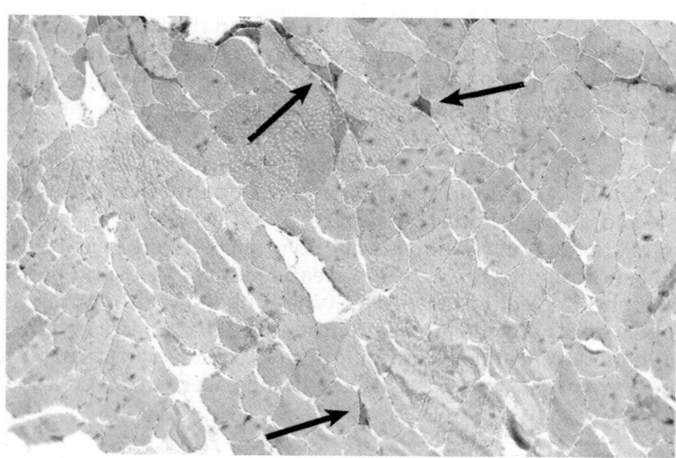

FIGURE 27-22. Denervation. In this frozen section of the biceps muscle subjected to the nonspecific esterase reaction, a few irregularly scattered, angular, atrophic fibers (*arrows*) are excessively dark stained. This pattern is highly characteristic of atrophy due to denervation.

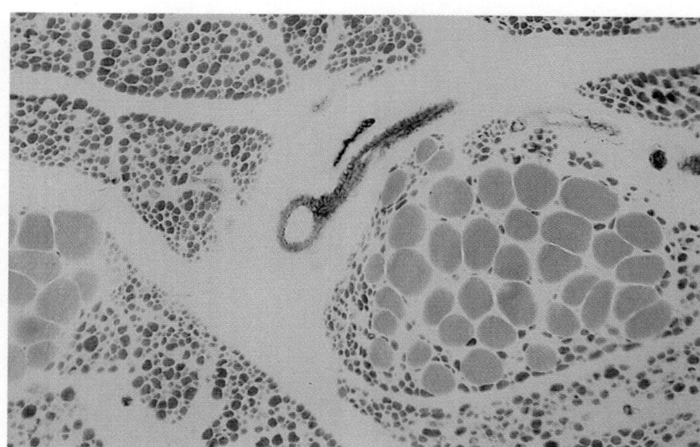

FIGURE 27-24. Werdnig-Hoffman disease (infantile spinal muscular atrophy). This cross-section of skeletal muscle stained for myofibrillar ATPase is derived from an infant with severe hypotonia. It shows groups of extremely atrophic, rounded type I and type II fibers and clusters of markedly hypertrophied pale type I fibers.

rounded, atrophic fibers are still identifiable with the ATPase reaction as being either type I or type II. There are also fascicles of normal muscle fibers and almost invariably clusters of hypertrophied type I fibers. In addition to the absent survival motor neuron gene, a second gene (neuronal apoptosis inhibitory protein gene) has also been implicated in the pathogenesis of Werdnig-Hoffmann disease.

KUGELBERG–WELANDER DISEASE (JUVENILE SPINAL MUSCULAR ATROPHY): ***This variant is a later-onset form of SMA and is not necessarily progressive.*** These patients had often been designated as having limb-girdle muscular dystrophy, but the electromyographic pattern of denervation helps to make the diagnosis. Muscle biopsies show type grouping and other evidence of a neurogenic disorder but can resemble a myopathy in a small sample because of coexisting necrotic fibers and regenerating fibers.

Type II Fiber Atrophy Resembles Denervation Myopathy

A commonly misinterpreted pathologic pattern in muscle biopsy specimens is atrophy from disuse, wasting, upper motor neuron disease and corticosteroid toxicity. This diffuse, nonspecific atrophy is a selective angular atrophy of type II fibers, and may resemble denervation atrophy on hematoxylin and eosin stain. However, the ATPase reaction shows that all angular atrophic fibers are type II (Fig. 27-25),

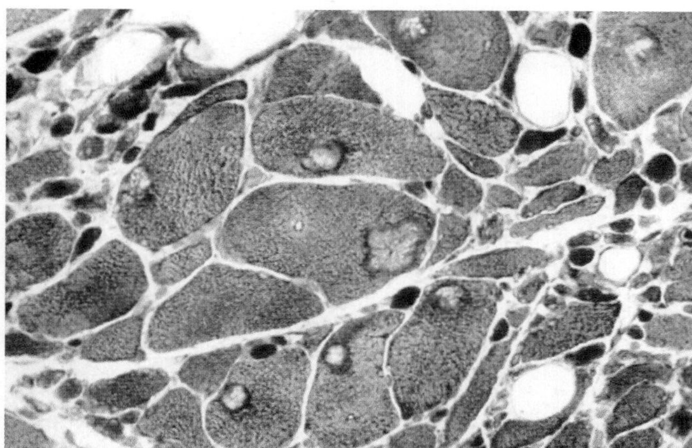

FIGURE 27-23. Target fiber. A cross-section of striated muscle treated with the NADH-tetrazolium reductase (NADH-TR) stain demonstrates several "target fibers," a characteristic feature of some cases of denervation. Because the enzyme reaction creates a product (formazan) that selectively fixes to membranous organelles, the centers of the target areas appear devoid of mitochondria and sarcoplasmic reticulum. The myofibrils may or may not be intact.

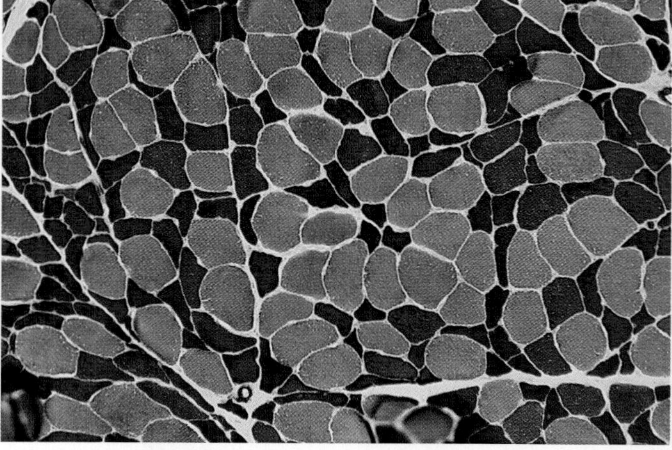

FIGURE 27-25. Type II fiber atrophy. This biopsy of the vastus lateralis muscle was taken from a 48-year-old man with proximal muscle weakness because of endogenous corticosteroid toxicity (Cushing syndrome). Virtually all of the angular atrophic fibers are type II. This form of atrophy closely mimics denervation atrophy when visualized with the hematoxylin and eosin stain.

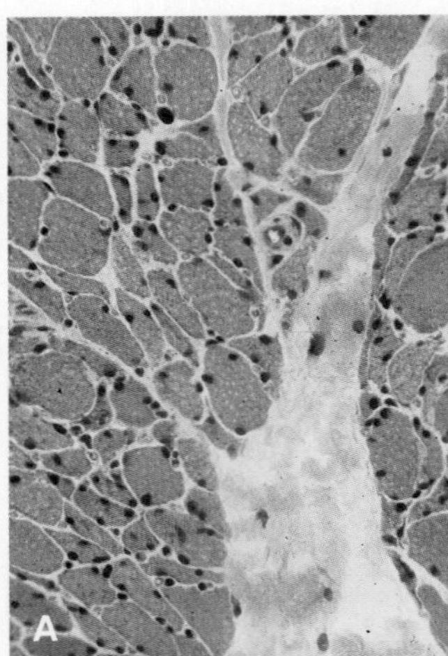

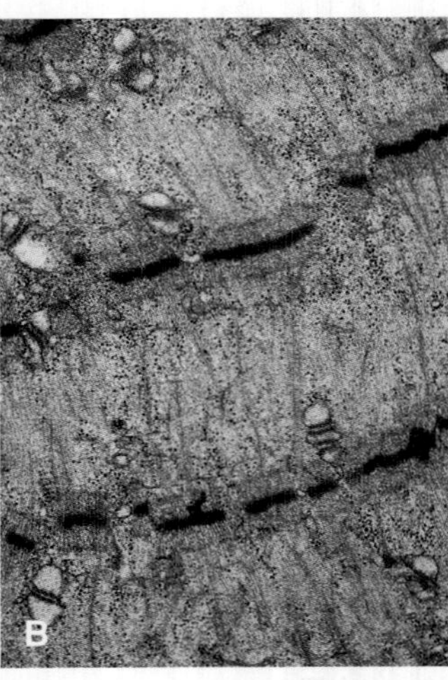

FIGURE 27-26. Critical illness myopathy. A. The condition frequently shows atrophic muscle with angular fibers (hematoxylin and eosin). **B**. By electron microscopy, there is marked loss of thick myosin filaments, whereas α-actin (thin) filaments are intact (compare to Fig. 27-2).

and do not stain heavily by nonspecific esterase or NADH-TR reactions. Type II fiber atrophy is common and is often related to a more chronic problem.

STEROID MYOPATHY: Corticosteroid therapy can cause muscle weakness with type II atrophy. This feature raises an important point clinically, as patients with polymyositis often receive large doses of corticosteroids. If a patient's weakness worsens, the physician must decide if this development represents a relapse of polymyositis, requiring increased corticosteroids, or if it represents steroid myopathy, in which case steroid dosage should be decreased.

Patients with weakness due to corticosteroid toxicity do not show an increased serum creatine kinase level and biopsies show selective atrophy of type II fibers, without muscle fiber degeneration and inflammation. By contrast, fiber degeneration and inflammation are expected in recurrent polymyositis, a process reflected in increased serum creatine kinase activity.

Critical Illness Myopathy Is Associated With Corticosteroid Therapy

If patients on high-dose steroids and neuromuscular blocking agents experience severe weakness in spite of removal of paralyzing agents, they may have **critical illness myopathy,** also known as **myosin heavy chain depletion syndrome.** These patients show loss of thick myosin filaments from muscle fibers (Fig. 27-26). The underlying mechanism of the myosin depletion is unclear, though myosin thick filaments reappear with discontinuation of corticosteroids, and muscle strength returns.

28 The Nervous System

Gregory N. Fuller (Central Nervous System) •
J. Clay Goodman (Central Nervous System) •
Thomas W. Bouldin (Peripheral Nervous System)

THE CENTRAL NERVOUS SYSTEM

The nervous system is the most complex organ system in the body. It is responsible for sensory processing and synthesis and motor control, and is the organ of thought, emotion and personality—in short, the basis of humanity itself. The vast majority of its operations occur without conscious supervision. Disorders of the central nervous system (CNS) strike at the core of our being as sentient organisms, and so inspire fear and dread. Diseases of the nervous system are common throughout the human life span and are major contributors to mortality and morbidity. Examples include stroke, Alzheimer disease, mental retardation, traumatic brain and spinal cord injury, epilepsy, migraine, meningitis and tumors.

TOPOGRAPHY: The functions of the nervous system have fine topographic localization, so that focal disease processes can produce myriad signs and symptoms that permit a skilled clinician to locate the affected site precisely. In addition, most neurons are organized in functional arrays, which, if damaged, eventuate in some of the most vexing neurodegenerative and neuropsychiatric disorders. Selective vulnerability of different nervous system cells and CNS regions to specific disease processes is one of the most profound unresolved enigmas of neurologic illnesses. For example, Huntington disease is primarily characterized by selective degeneration of neurons in the caudate nuclei; Parkinson disease targets the nigrostriatal system; amyotrophic lateral sclerosis (ALS) selectively singles out upper and lower motor neurons of cerebrum, brainstem and spinal cord. Some infectious diseases also have topographic predilections: poliomyelitis involves anterior horn cells of the spinal cord and motor nuclei of the brainstem, while herpes simplex preferentially affects the temporal lobes. Vascular diseases and demyelinating conditions display regional preferences within the nervous system, and a degree of topographic predictability characterizes some brain tumors. The basis for the topographic vulnerability to most nervous system diseases is obscure.

AGE: The nervous system is affected by neurologic disorders throughout the life span, but individual diseases commonly have a predilection for selected age groups. For example, inborn errors of metabolism, such as Tay-Sachs disease, the leukodystrophies and several posterior fossa tumors, are encountered largely in childhood. The reckless exuberance of youth leads to a spike in traumatic brain and spinal cord injury during adolescence and emerging adulthood that subsides with maturity, only to return with the infirmities of age. Multiple sclerosis shows a strong preference for young adults, rarely having its onset before puberty or after the age of 40 years. Neuropsychiatric disorders such as schizophrenia often make their appearance in late adolescence and young adulthood when the brain is undergoing striking neurodevelopmental transformations. Huntington disease typically strikes youthful and middle-aged adults, while Parkinson disease and stroke are rarely evidenced before the later decades of life, and Alzheimer disease tends to be a malady of the aged brain.

Cells of the Nervous System

The diversity and complexity of the central nervous system is reflected at all levels in its organization, from the morphologic and functional subspecialization of the many unique cellular constituents, to the regional localization of sensory, motor and cognitive functions.

GRAY MATTER AND THE NEUROPIL: Gray matter includes all regions of the CNS rich in neurons, including the cerebral cortex, cerebellar cortex, basal ganglia and central gray matter of the spinal cord. Gray matter consists of the cell bodies (perikarya) of neurons and supporting glial cell nuclei, plus the intervening delicate interwoven meshwork of neuronal and glial cell processes that is referred to as the **neuropil** (Fig. 28-1). Focal circumscribed collections of neuronal cell

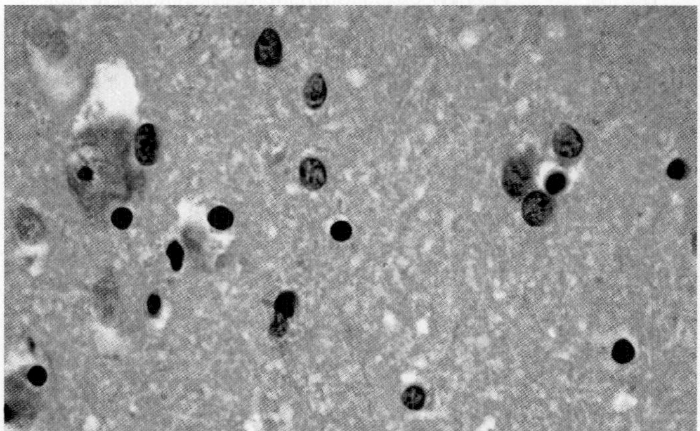

FIGURE 28-1. Gray matter and the neuropil. Gray matter by definition contains neuronal cell bodies. In addition, the nuclei of supporting glial cells, astrocytes and satellite oligodendroglia, are also present. The remaining finely fibrillar background meshwork is called the neuropil and consists of intimately intermingled axons, dendrites and astrocytic cytoplasmic processes.

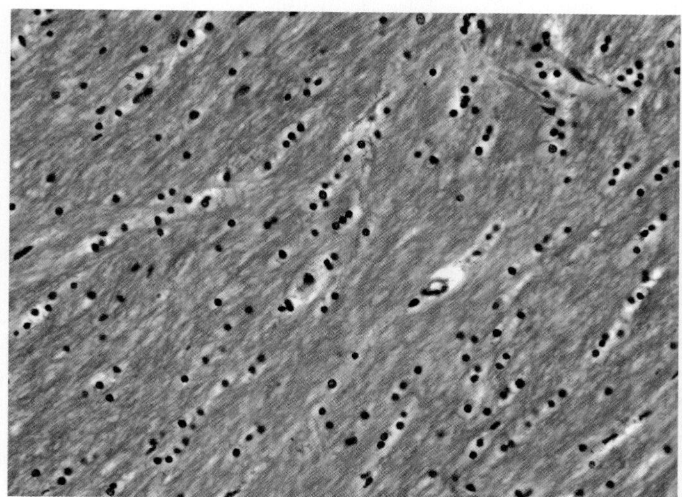

FIGURE 28-2. White matter. In contrast to gray matter, white matter is composed almost entirely of myelinated axons and the cells that produce and maintain their myelin sheaths, the oligodendroglia, whose small round nuclei are seen in between the fiber bundles.

bodies that share a common functional task are referred to as "nuclei."

WHITE MATTER: White matter consists of compact bundles **(tracts, fascicles)** of myelinated axons with abundant oligodendrocytes and interspersed astrocytes (Fig. 28-2).

NEURONS: The morphology of neuronal subtypes in the gray matter varies as a result of functional subspecialization, ranging from large motor and primary sensory neurons to diminutive "granular cell" neurons (Fig. 28-3A). For example, pigmented neurons, found only in specific nuclei of the brainstem, are an important subclass of neurons that are distinguished by cytoplasmic brown neuromelanin pigment, a byproduct of catecholaminergic neurotransmitter synthesis (Fig. 28-3B). These clusters of pigmented catecholaminergic neurons are dense enough to be visible to the naked eye in the midbrain (substantia nigra) and pons (locus ceruleus).

ASTROCYTES: Astrocytes outnumber neurons by at least 10-fold and play a critical supportive role in regulating the CNS microenvironment. They also constitute one of two primary CNS cell types that respond to a wide variety of pathologic insults to the CNS (the other being microglia). A major hallmark of the acute response of "reactive astrocytes" is upregulated synthesis of glial fibrillary acidic protein (GFAP) and its assembly into intracytoplasmic intermediate filaments, resulting in prominent cell bodies and cytoplasmic processes (Fig. 28-4A). With advancing age, astrocyte peripheral processes tend to accumulate spherical inclusion bodies, corpora amylacea, which are glucose polymers that are especially numerous in subpial, subependymal and perivascular sites and in the olfactory tracts (Fig. 28-4B). Cytoplasmic straplike densities, Rosenthal fibers (Fig. 28-4C), are densely compacted glial intermediate filaments with entrapped cytosolic proteins and form in long-standing astrogliosis.

OLIGODENDROGLIA: Oligodendroglia produce and maintain myelin sheaths of axons in the CNS and are thus the CNS counterparts of the Schwann cells of the peripheral nervous system. Oligodendroglia cell bodies are dominated by uniform round nuclei that, in formalin-fixed paraffin-embedded tissue sections, are characteristically surrounded by only a small clear rim of vacuolated cytoplasm ("perinuclear halo") (Fig. 28-5).

MICROGLIA: Microglia are the bone marrow–derived mononuclear phagocytes of the CNS. In the healthy state, they are inconspicuously distributed throughout the brain and spinal cord but respond quickly to CNS insults such as ischemia, trauma or viral infection. They adopt an infiltrative phenotype, characterized by thin, elongated nuclei, which

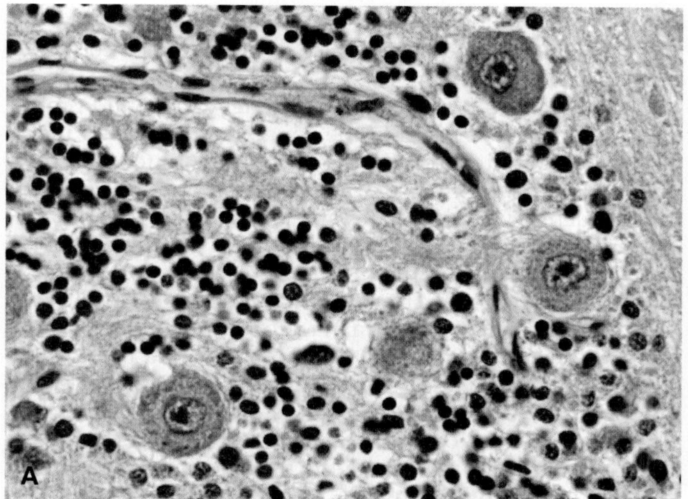

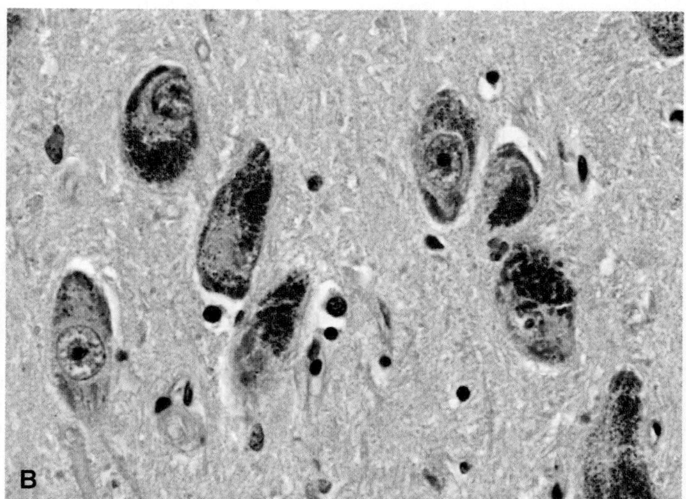

FIGURE 28-3. Neurons. A. The different neuronal populations of the central nervous system (CNS) subserve different functions, and this diversity is reflected in their morphology. Illustrative of the extremes are the large cell bodies of Purkinje cell neurons juxtaposed next to the diminutive granular cell neurons of the cerebellar cortex; the entire granular neuron cell body is not much bigger than the nucleolus of a Purkinje cell neuron! **B.** The pigmented catecholaminergic neurons with their prominent neuromelanin content serve as an additional, striking example of diversity in form and function among CNS neuronal populations.

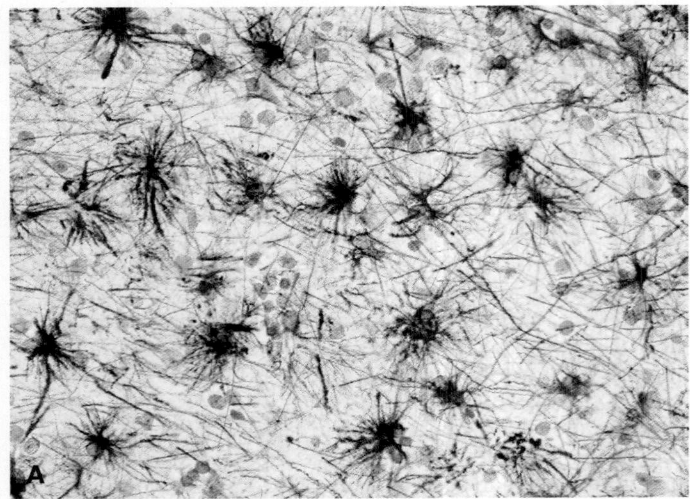

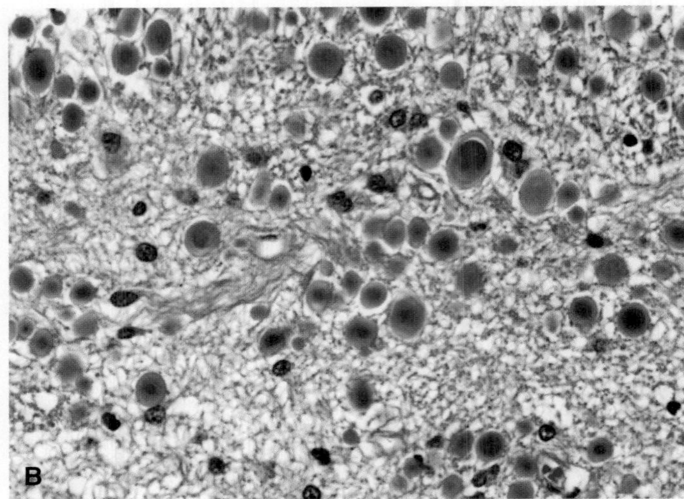

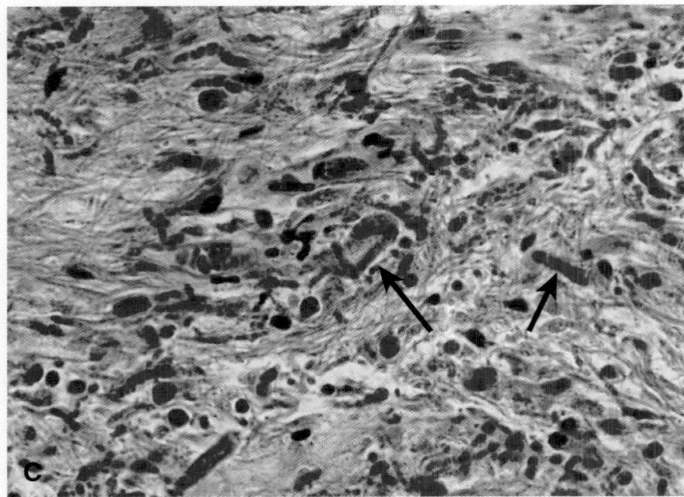

FIGURE 28-4. Astrocytes. A. Astrocytes have been called "the fibroblast of the central nervous system," referring to their role as the ubiquitous supporting cell of the brain and spinal cord that reacts to any pathologic insult. As seen in this immunostain directed against glial fibrillary acidic protein, astrocytes occupy adjacent domains and send cytoplasmic process radiating out in all directions to fill their individual fiefdoms. **B.** With advancing age, astrocytes are prone to develop glucose polymer inclusion bodies, termed **corpora amylacea,** in the distal distribution of their cell processes, particularly around blood vessels and subjacent to the pia and ependyma. **C. Rosenthal fibers** are another astrocytic inclusion body formed as a response to long-standing astrogliosis; they are composed of densely compacted glial intermediate filaments together with entrapped cytosolic proteins (*arrows*).

facilitates their ability to migrate through the CNS parenchyma and localize to the site of injury (Fig. 28-6A,B).

EPENDYMA: The ependymal lining of the ventricular system forms a barrier between the cerebrospinal fluid and brain parenchyma and regulates fluid transfer between these two compartments. The normal ependyma is lined by ciliated cuboidal-to-columnar simple epithelium (Fig. 28-7).

Specialized Regions of the Central Nervous System

CHOROID PLEXUS: The choroid plexus produces the cerebrospinal fluid (CSF). It is found in the cerebral ventricles including the temporal horns bilaterally, the interventricular foramen of Monro, the roof of the third ventricle and the roof and lateral recesses of the fourth ventricle. The choroid plexus is composed of cuboidal epithelium (derived embryologically from ependyma) that covers a fibrovascular core (Fig. 28-8A). The highly vascular core is critical to CSF formation, develops from the leptomeninges (pia and arachnoid) and contains scattered nests of arachnoid (meningothelial) cells (Fig. 28-8B). This explains the occasional occurrence of "intraventricular" meningiomas (which are in fact choroid plexus meningiomas).

MENINGES: Three layers of meninges cover and protect the CNS. The **dura** forms the tough outer fibrous membrane composed primarily of collagen. Its outer surface is the inner periosteum of the cranial bones, and its inner surface attaches weakly to the subjacent arachnoid via cell junctions. The two dural layers separate in several sites to form the dural venous sinuses, the largest of which is the superior sagittal sinus. The underlying arachnoid is bound to the overlying dura via a loosely cohesive layer of cells, the **dural border cell (DBC) layer.** This layer is the path of least resistance to pathogenic fluids, which easily dissect the weak intercellular junctions to form so-called "subdural" hematomas, hygromas and empyemas. The meningeal layer just beneath the DBC layer, the **arachnoid barrier cell (ABC) layer,** in contrast, forms a cohesive outer limiting membrane of the subarachnoid space via profuse intercellular junctions (desmosomes) that weld together elongated, interlacing arachnoid (meningothelial) cell processes. Whorls of arachnoid cells are common in thicker areas of the arachnoid (Fig. 28-9); this feature is often recapitulated in tumors derived from the arachnoid (meningiomas).

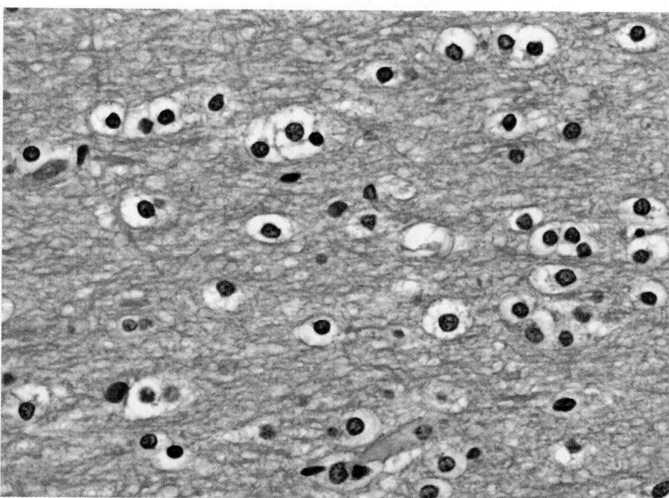

FIGURE 28-5. Oligodendroglia. Oligodendroglia are the myelin-forming glia of the central nervous system (CNS; including the optic "nerves," which are actually CNS tracts). On routine histologic imaging, oligodendroglia are easily recognized by their monotonous small dark round nuclei surrounded by a halo of vacuolated cytoplasm ("fried egg" appearance). This characteristic appearance is recapitulated in neoplastic oligodendrogliomas.

PINEAL GLAND: The pineal gland contains pineal parenchymal cells (pineocytes), plus supporting glial cells (pineal astrocytes), arranged in cell clusters separated by collagenous septa (Fig. 28-10). Inconspicuous autonomic peripheral nerve fibers coming from cell bodies in the superior cervical ganglia provide sympathetic nervous system (noradrenergic) innervation.

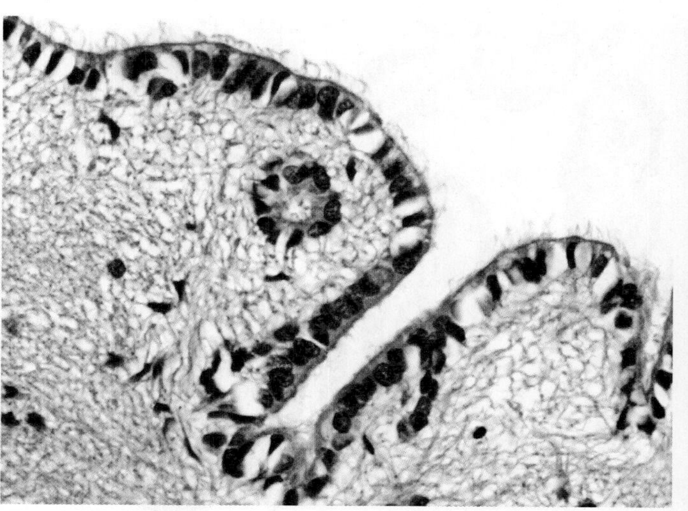

FIGURE 28-7. Ependyma. Ependymal cells form a ciliated cuboidal-to-columnar epithelium that lines the cerebral ventricles and spinal cord central canal. Ependymal cell clusters and true rosettes, as seen here, commonly are scattered beneath the ependymal lining.

Increased Intracranial Pressure and Herniation Occur With Space-Occupying Lesions

ETIOLOGIC FACTORS: From a pathophysiologic viewpoint, the single most important aspect of the brain's existence is that it ***lives in a closed box***! The brain, the CSF and the blood going to and from the brain occupy the intracranial volume, which in the adult is fixed.

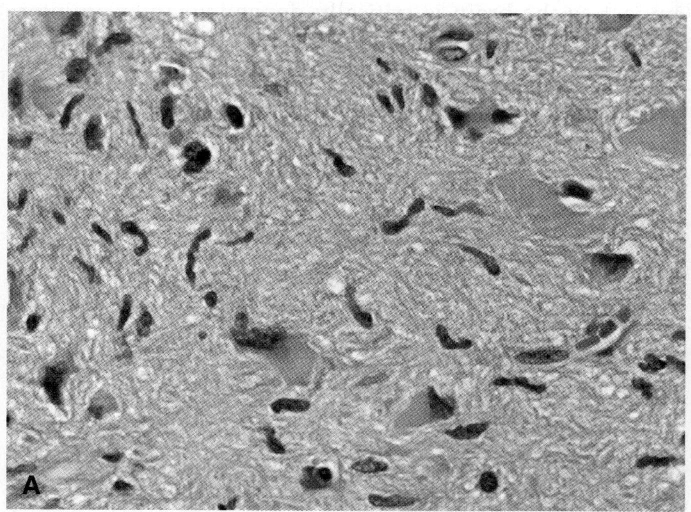

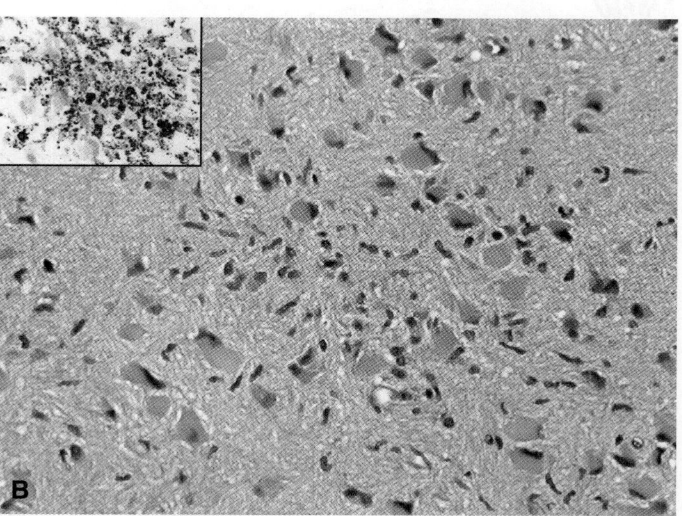

FIGURE 28-6. Microglia. A. Microglia are the resident representatives of the monocyte–macrophage system in the brain and spinal cord. While inconspicuous in normal healthy brain ("resting microglial"), they become very prominent when responding to central nervous system (CNS) injury and are easily recognized by their elongated nuclei ("rod cells"), which reflect their infiltrative phenotype. **B.** Actively migrating through CNS parenchyma, they commonly cluster around foci of disease; such collections are known as "microglial nodules." Microglia demonstrate strong immunohistochemical reactivity for the macrophage marker CD68 (*inset*).

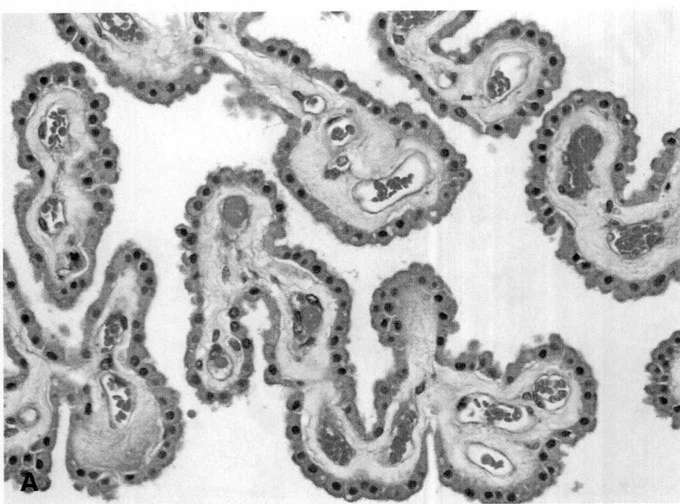

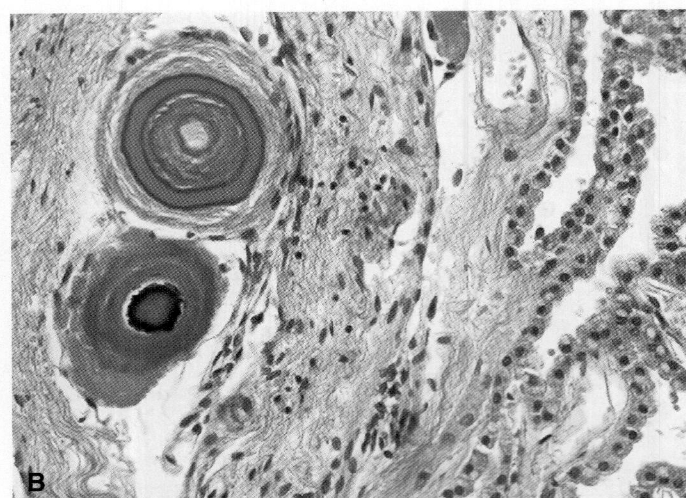

FIGURE 28-8. Choroid plexus. A. Choroid plexus is the central nervous system (CNS) organ responsible for producing cerebrospinal fluid and consists of innumerable papillae with a highly vascular core covered by cuboidal epithelium that is derived embryologically from the ependyma. **B.** The core also contains arachnoid (meningothelial) cell nests (by virtue of its embryologic derivation from the pia-arachnoid) that tend to mineralize with age, forming psammoma bodies (B).

Any disease process that takes up space does so at the expense of brain, CSF or blood. This is a verbal expression of the Monro-Kellie hypothesis that states:

$$\text{Intracranial volume} = \text{Volume}_{\text{CNS}} + \text{Volume}_{\text{CSF}} + \text{Volume}_{\text{blood}} + \text{Volume}_{\text{lesion}}$$

Space-occupying lesions may occur in diseases from every major category of disease with the exception of degenerative disorders. Examples include brain tumors, abscesses, swollen brain contusions following trauma and stroke with brain swelling.

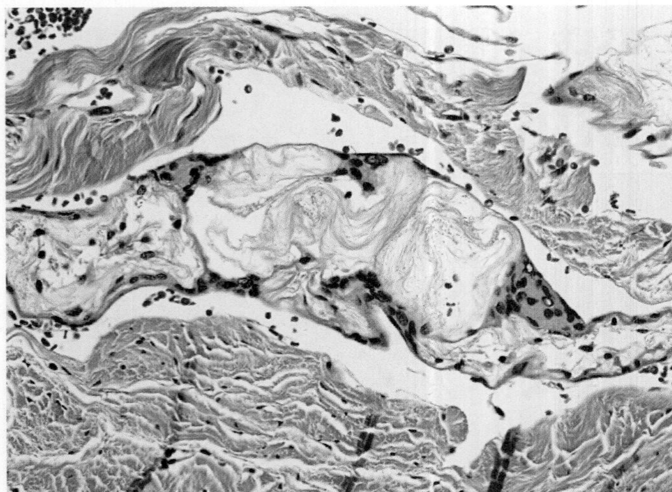

FIGURE 28-9. Arachnoid villi. The arachnoid membrane forms the outer boundary of the subarachnoid space and also protrudes into the dural venous sinuses, as seen here, to form arachnoid villi whose function is to return cerebrospinal fluid (CSF) into the venous circulatory system. The villi are covered by a layer of meningothelial cells, termed arachnoid cap cells, that varies in thickness from a single cell to multilayered whorls.

The immediate result of trying to fit more volume into the fixed space of the intracranial vault is increased intracranial pressure (ICP). The normal mean ICP is less than 200 mm H_2O or 15 mm Hg for a patient in the lateral decubitus position. The pressure can be measured by lumbar puncture or by placement of an intracranial pressure transducer. As ICP increases, the patient has headaches, confusion and drowsiness and may develop papilledema. To compensate, CSF volume is reduced; hence, the ventricles are compressed to small slits and sulci are effaced.

If the lesion takes up more space than a reduction in CSF volume can accommodate, blood volume is then reduced. Such lower cerebral blood flow may have immediate adverse impact as the brain is critically dependent upon uninterrupted supply of oxygen and nutrients. If the lesion expands

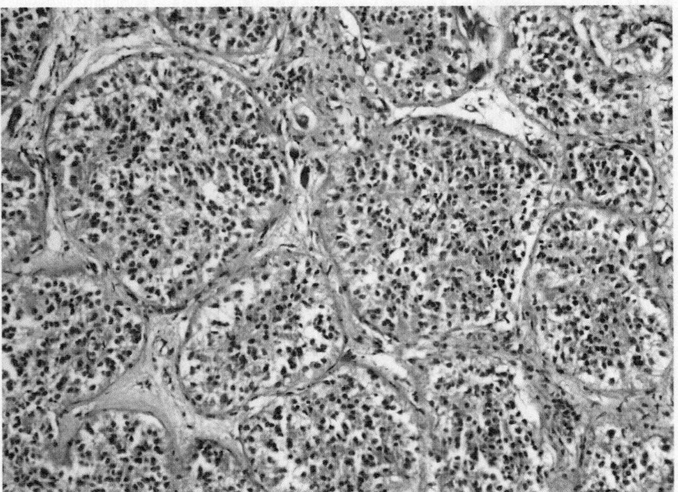

FIGURE 28-10. Pineal gland. The pineal is composed of pineal parenchymal cells (pineocytes) organized into lobules by fibrovascular septa.

further, the only structure remaining to "give" is the brain itself. The intracranial compartment is subdivided by the dura—the tentorium cerebelli divides the vault into the supra- and infratentorial compartments, and the falx divides the supratentorial compartment into the right and left compartments. Depending on the location of the space-occupying lesion, the brain may be forced out of one compartment into another; such shifts are called brain herniations.

CLINICAL FEATURES:

CINGULATE HERNIATION: If one hemisphere is forced under the falx, the cingulate lobe is the first part of that hemisphere to be displaced. Such herniations are called **subfalcine** or **cingulate herniations.** Someone experiencing such a herniation becomes confused and drowsy. The anterior cerebral artery is also displaced beneath the falx, and infarction within this vessel's territory may occur, leading to contralateral lower extremity weakness and urinary incontinence.

UNCAL HERNIATION: If one hemisphere is forced from the supratentorial compartment toward the infratentorial compartment, the medial temporal lobe (the uncus) is the first portion of the hemisphere displaced; thus, this is an **uncal,** or **transtentorial, herniation** (Fig. 28-11). The ipsilateral oculomotor nerve (cranial nerve III) is crushed by the displaced temporal lobe, leading to ipsilateral pupillary dilatation and paresis of all extraocular muscles except the lateral rectus (cranial nerve VI) and superior oblique (cranial nerve IV). The unopposed action of the lateral rectus leads to the eye "looking" laterally. A dilated unresponsive or minimally responsive pupil indicates extreme danger and necessitates immediate measures to arrest the herniation.

As medial displacement continues, the midbrain shifts away from the displaced hemisphere, with the contralateral cerebral pedicle driven into the unyielding tentorium. This crushing injury of the cerebral pedicle **(Kernohan notch)** results in hemiparesis on the same side of the body as the offending mass. A hemispheric mass will normally cause hemiparesis on the opposite side of the body; ipsilateral hemiparesis, which may be clinically confusing, is called a "false localizing" sign.

The downward and medial displacement of the hemisphere through the tentorial opening may also result in compression of one or both posterior cerebral arteries as they travel from the infratentorial compartment to the now crowded supratentorial compartment. Such compression may impair blood flow to the occipital lobes, resulting in infarction with attendant visual field disturbances bearing no obvious relationship to the inciting mass. This occipital lobe infarction and its attendant signs are also "false localizing."

The uncal herniation syndrome is very ominous but is reversible with removal of the offending mass. Temporary measures to reduce intracranial pressure include intravenous mannitol to shrink the brain osmotically and hyperventilation to reduce PCO_2-inducing cerebral vasospasm and so decrease cerebral blood volume and therefore pressure. These actions may gain the patient sufficient time for definitive neurosurgical treatment.

CENTRAL HERNIATION: If both hemispheres herniate transtentorially, the central herniation syndrome is said to be present. Both pupils dilate; flaccidity and coma ensues. The downward displacement of the brainstem may wrench vessels from their parenchymal beds within the midbrain and pons and cause multiple linear hemorrhages known as **Duret hemorrhages** or secondary hemorrhages of herniation (Fig. 28-12).

CEREBELLAR TONSILLAR HERNIATION: If the infratentorial compartment becomes crowded either from migrating supratentorial contents or from a mass arising in the infratentorial compartment, the brainstem and cerebellum may be forced through the foramen magnum. The compressed cerebellar tonsils and medulla may lead to lethal compression of vital medullary centers. This bleak situation is called tonsillar herniation.

FUNGUS CEREBRI: If a traumatic or surgical defect is present in the skull, brain under increased pressure may ooze from the opening. This process is known as fungus cerebri.

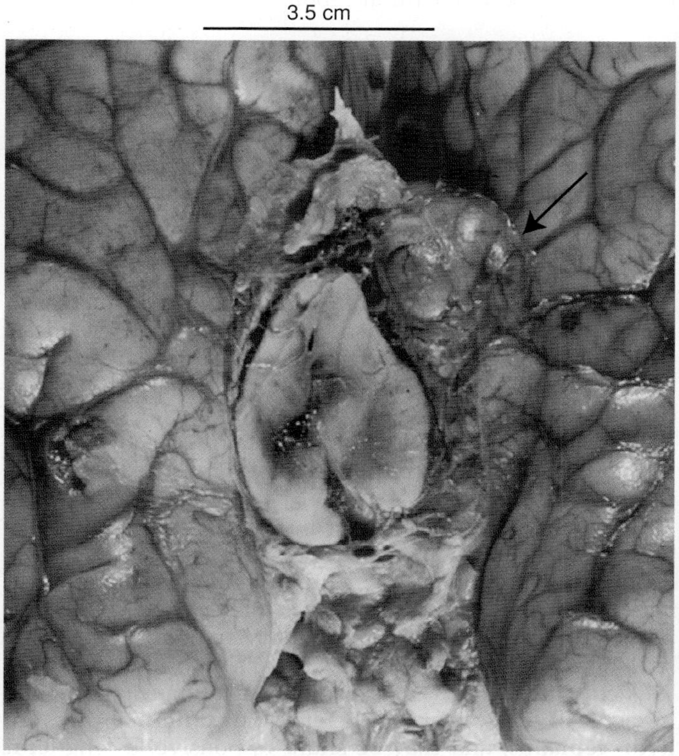

3.5 cm

FIGURE 28-11. Transtentorial herniation. The uncus (*arrow*) of the parahippocampal gyrus is herniated downward to displace the midbrain, resulting in distortion of the midbrain with increased anterior to posterior and diminished left to right dimensions. The oculomotor nerve may be compromised, leading to an ipsilateral third nerve palsy.

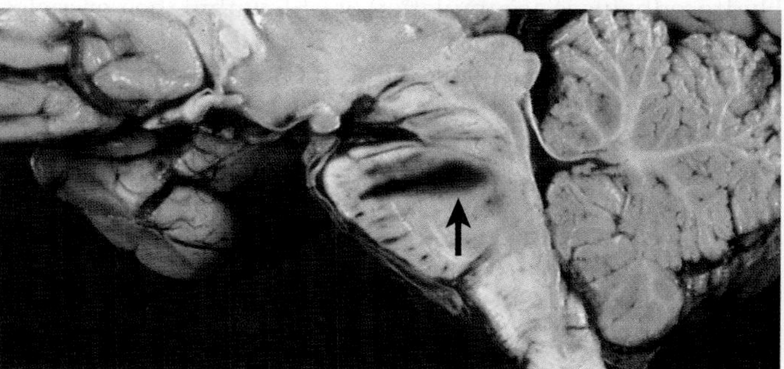

FIGURE 28-12. Duret hemorrhages (*arrow*) in a case of transtentorial herniation tend to be midline and to occupy the brainstem from the upper midbrain to midpons. (Courtesy of Dr. F. Stephen Vogel, Duke University.)

Cerebral Edema

Cerebral edema may complicate any process that gives rise to increased intracranial pressure and can set up a self-perpetuating cycle in which increasing edema begets increasing pressure, which in turn begets more edema.

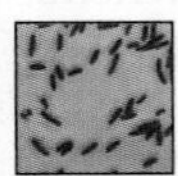

ETIOLOGIC FACTORS: Cerebral edema is an absolute increase in brain water content. The amount of water in brain tissue is tightly controlled by the production of CSF, rate of egress of CSF from the cranial vault and flux of water across the blood-brain barrier. The blood-brain barrier separates the brain from the blood so that only lipid-soluble molecules, or molecules that can access specialized transport systems, enter the brain. The structural basis of the blood-brain barrier is endothelial cell tight junctions lining the cerebral vessels. Water can enter the brain uncontrollably if the barrier is disrupted or if osmotic forces across the barrier are sufficient to drive water into the cerebral tissues. Three major forms of cerebral edema may occur:

- **Cytotoxic edema:** Water is driven across an intact blood brain barrier by osmotic forces arising either because of failure of cells within the brain to maintain osmotic homeostasis or because of systemic water overload. In either case, water is driven down its concentration gradient into the cerebral tissues until osmotic equilibrium is reestablished.
- **Vasogenic edema:** The blood-brain barrier loosens, permitting uncontrolled entry of water into the tissues. ***This is the most common cause of edema*** and is seen with neoplasms, abscesses, meningitis, hemorrhage, contusions and lead poisoning. A combination of cytotoxic and vasogenic edema is common in infarcts. The above processes may disrupt the barrier properties of the endothelium, or the vessels formed in neoplasms may be defective from their inception. Vasogenic edema often responds dramatically to the administration of corticosteroids that restore barrier integrity even in tumors.
- **Interstitial edema:** While cytotoxic and vasogenic edema involve water fluxes across the endothelium, interstitial edema involves overproduction or failure of egress of CSF so that the fluid seeps across the ependymal lining of the ventricles to accumulate within the white matter.

Hydrocephalus Can Be Noncommunicating or Communicating

Hydrocephalus is accumulation of CSF within the ventricles resulting in dilatation of these structures (Fig. 28-13). When the ventricular distension is sufficiently advanced, fluid will leak trans-ependymally into the white matter, causing interstitial edema. Accumulation of CSF can arise from one of two processes: (1) ***overproduction of CSF, which is very rare,*** occurring only in the context of tumors of the choroid plexus; and (2) ***failure of CSF egress from the cranial vault, which is the most common mechanism.*** If the blockage occurs within the ventricular system itself, ventricles proximal to the block will dilate, whereas those situated downstream from the block will be spared. This form of hydrocephalus is **obstructive**, or **noncommunicating, hydrocephalus.** The most frequent site of block is at the ventricular system's narrowest strait—the aqueduct of Sylvius connecting the third and fourth ventricles.

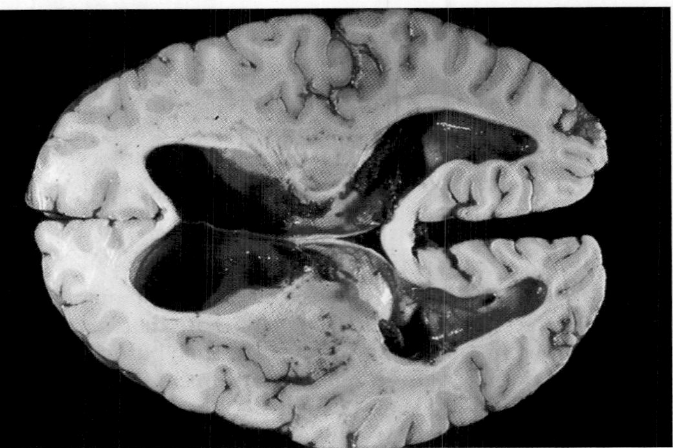

FIGURE 28-13. Hydrocephalus. Horizontal section of the brain from a patient who died of a brain tumor that obstructed the aqueduct of Sylvius shows marked dilation of the lateral ventricles.

If the block exists after the CSF has left the ventricular system and is traveling over the cerebral convexities to the arachnoid granulations that usher the fluid into the venous sinuses, then all of the ventricles dilate and the process is referred to as **communicating hydrocephalus,** meaning that the ventricles are in unobstructed fluidic communication. Communicating hydrocephalus may complicate subarachnoid hemorrhage or inflammation, resulting in arachnoid scarring, or may result from thrombosis of the dural venous sinuses themselves.

CLINICAL FEATURES: The clinical features of hydrocephalus depend on the age of the patient. In infancy and childhood, before the cranial sutures have fused, the head enlarges sometimes to grotesque proportions as the ventricles dilate. Since hydrocephalus is common in infants and treatable by shunting, measurement of the head circumference is a fundamental part of the pediatric physical examination.

After suture fusion has occurred, hydrocephalus finds its expression not in head enlargement, but in increased intracranial pressure with headache, confusion, drowsiness, papilledema and vomiting. Ventricular enlargement proceeds at the expense of cerebral tissue volume so that in advanced cases only a mantle of several millimeters thickness remains. Remarkably, such individuals may retain substantial cognitive abilities, although spasticity may cloak the expression of this intelligence.

In older persons, hydrocephalus may develop insidiously with gradual enlargement of the ventricles being clinically expressed as progressive dementia, gait impairment and urinary incontinence as the long white matter fibers connecting portions of cortex to one another and lower motility centers are stretched apart by the relentless expansion of the ventricles. This condition is usually accompanied by normal baseline intracranial pressure and is therefore called **normal-pressure hydrocephalus,** and may be shunt responsive. If long-term CSF pressure monitoring is conducted, periodic waves of elevated intracranial pressure are seen.

All of the above forms of hydrocephalus result from disturbance of CSF dynamics and should be distinguished from **hydrocephalus ex vacuo,** which is compensatory enlargement of the ventricles in response to loss of CNS tissue from

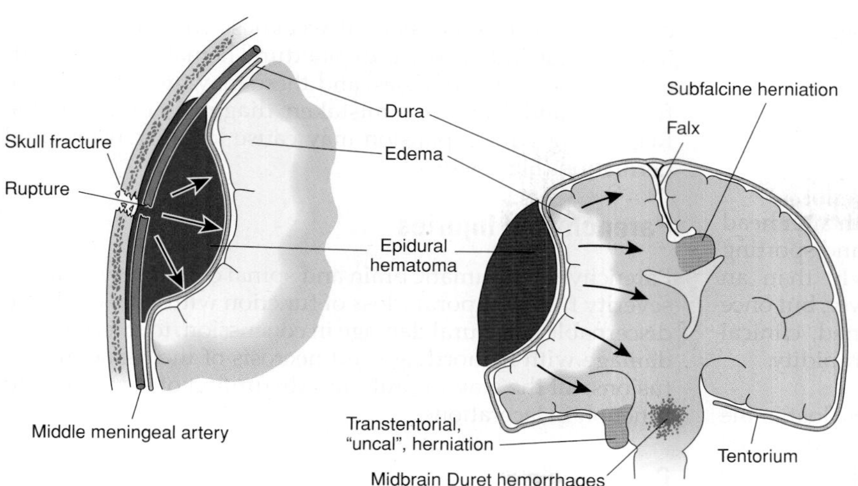

FIGURE 28-14. Development of an epidural hematoma. Laceration of a branch of the middle meningeal artery by the sharp bony edges of a skull fracture initiates bleeding under arterial pressure that dissects the dura from the calvaria and produces an expanding hematoma. After an asymptomatic interval of several hours, subfalcine and transtentorial herniation occur, and if the hematoma is not evacuated, lethal Duret hemorrhages will occur.

other diseases. This is most commonly seen in diffuse cortical atrophy, although focal destruction such as occurs at the site of an old infarct may lead to focal compensatory ventricular enlargement.

Trauma

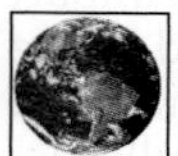

EPIDEMIOLOGY: Physical injury of the brain, spinal cord and peripheral nervous system constitutes a major cause of loss of life and productivity. Populations at highest risk for such injuries include children, men in late adolescence and early adult life, and the elderly.

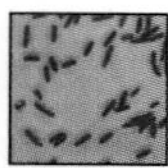

ETIOLOGIC FACTORS: The brain and spinal cord are enclosed in protective bony cases that serve to dissipate forces delivered to these delicate nervous system structures; however, evolutionary selection has not yet adequately responded to the need to survive motor vehicle crashes, personal assaults or dives into shallow pools. Injury to the nervous system results from the transfer of kinetic energy to the neural tissues—the degree of injury correlates with the quantity of energy delivered and the time over which it was delivered. This energy transfer may directly disrupt tissues in penetrating injuries, or the energy may be translated into movement and compression of neural structures within the confines of the skull or spinal canal in a closed injury. Importantly, extreme injury of the brain and cord is possible with minimal disruption of the overlying tissues. Conversely, very dramatic injury of the superficial tissues can occur with no damage to the underlying nervous system.

Epidural Hematoma Is Often Fatal

Epidural hematoma usually results from a blow to the head with skull fracture, and unless treated promptly, can be fatal. The intracranial dura is securely bound to the inner aspect of the calvaria and is thus analogous to the intracranial periosteum. The middle meningeal arteries reside in grooves in the inner table of the bone between the dura and the calvaria, and their branches splay across the temporal–parietal area. The temporal bone is one of the thinnest bones of the skull and is particularly vulnerable to fracture, so seemingly minor trauma may fracture the bone, which may in turn lacerate branches of the middle meningeal artery, resulting in a life-threatening epidural hemorrhage (Fig. 28-14).

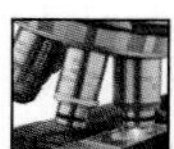

PATHOLOGY: Transection of the middle meningeal artery permits the escape of blood under arterial pressure into the epidural space, thereby separating the dura from the calvaria. The dura is tightly bound to the calvarium at the coronal suture lines; therefore, the epidural blood accumulation will not extend beyond the suture lines. This leads to a lens-shaped accumulation of fresh blood that stops at the coronal suture lines (Fig. 28-15).

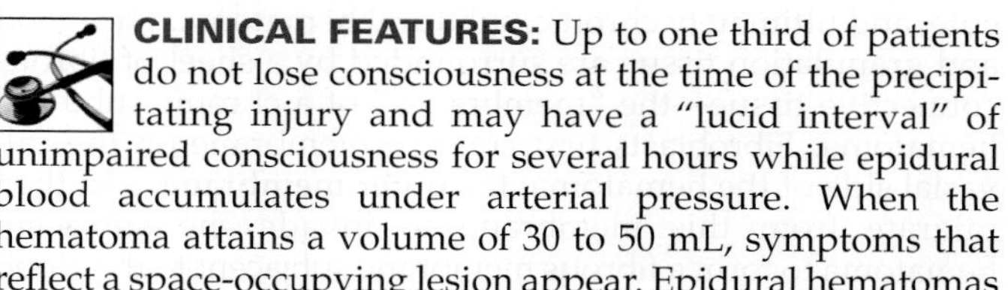

CLINICAL FEATURES: Up to one third of patients do not lose consciousness at the time of the precipitating injury and may have a "lucid interval" of unimpaired consciousness for several hours while epidural blood accumulates under arterial pressure. When the hematoma attains a volume of 30 to 50 mL, symptoms that reflect a space-occupying lesion appear. Epidural hematomas

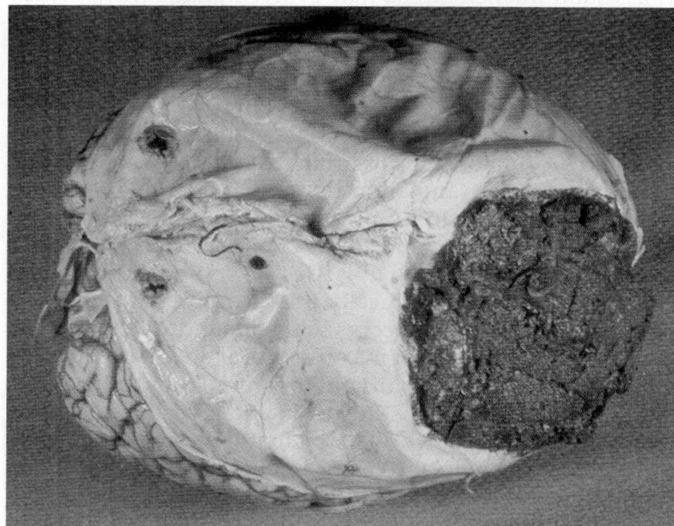

FIGURE 28-15. Epidural hematoma. A discoid mass of fresh hemorrhage overlies the dura covering frontal–parietal cortex but does not transgress the coronal sutures.

are invariably progressive and, when not recognized and evacuated, may be fatal in 24 to 48 hours.

Subdural Hematoma Develops Slower Than Epidural Hematoma

Subdural hematoma is a significant cause of death after head injuries from falls, assaults, vehicular accidents and sporting mishaps. The hematomas expand more slowly than an epidural hematoma, so the clinical tempo is slower, but once critical increased intracranial pressure is attained, clinical deterioration and death can occur with horrific rapidity.

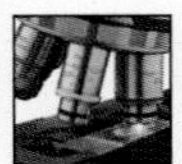

PATHOLOGY: The cerebral hemispheres float in the CSF, tethered loosely by blood vessels and cranial nerves. Blood draining from the cerebral hemispheres flows through veins that cross the subarachnoid space and arachnoid to breach the dura and enter the dural sinus. There is no true subdural space per se, but the inner layer of meningothelial cells of the dura has fewer tight junctions than those in the outer layers of the dura. Shearing forces will separate these cells, allowing blood to seep between the cells. Since bleeding in this situation is under low venous pressure, it is slow and may stop spontaneously after an accumulation from a local tamponade effect. The bleeding is within the dura itself and readily extends beyond the coronal sutures, causing a hematoma that can extend along the entire anterior to posterior dimensions of the calvarium (Fig. 28-16). Granulation tissue forms in reaction to the blood, and the delicate capillaries of this tissue may themselves leak, leading to gradual accumulation of an ever enlarging subacute, and ultimately chronic, subdural hematoma. The blood and granulation tissue are surrounded by a sheet of fibrous connective tissue—the "membranes" of a chronic subdural hematoma. Fibroblasts first create a membrane on the calvarial side of the hematoma, the **outer membrane,** and then migrate from this membrane to invade the subjacent hematoma to form a fibrous membrane subjacent to the blood clot. This **inner membrane** is visible in about 2 weeks (Fig. 28-17). A subdural hematoma may evolve in three ways. It may (1) be reabsorbed and leave only a small amount of telltale hemosiderin; (2) remain static, and perhaps calcify; or (3) enlarge as a result of recurrent microhemorrhages in the granulation tissue.

Expansion of the hematoma, together with the onset of symptoms, commonly results from rebleeding, usually within 6 months. Since granulation tissue is vulnerable to minor trauma, even that caused by shaking the head, a subdural hematoma can rebleed and create a new hematoma subjacent to the outer membrane. Episodes of sporadic rebleeding expand the lesion periodically and at unpredictable intervals. Since the bleeding occurs in the inner dural border cell zone rather than an imaginary subdural space, no blood is seen in the CSF. In addition to granulation tissue and blood, other cellular constituents include plasma cells, lymphocytes and extramedullary hematopoiesis, which may contribute to the cellular dynamics of the subdural hematoma by releasing cytokines, resulting in cerebral edema in the underlying brain.

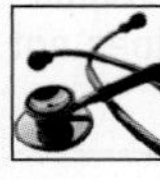

CLINICAL FEATURES: Symptoms and signs of subdural hematomas are diverse. Stretching of meninges induces headaches, pressure on the motor cortex produces contralateral weakness, and focal cortical irritation can initiate seizures. Subdural hematomas are bilateral in 15% to 20% of cases, and these may impair cognitive function and lead to a mistaken diagnosis of dementia. Rebleeding with expansion may cause lethal transtentorial herniation (Fig. 28-16A).

Parenchymal Injuries

Parenchymal traumatic brain and spinal cord injury range in severity from temporary loss of function with little or absent discernable structural damage in concussion, to intermediate damage with hemorrhage and necrosis of the tissue in contusions, all the way to profound disruption of structure and function in lacerations.

Concussion

Concussion is a transient loss of consciousness caused by biomechanical forces acting on the central nervous system. A blow that causes an epidural hematoma does not necessarily produce a concussion. Consciousness depends on a functional brainstem reticular formation interacting with the two cerebral hemispheres and is lost if either the reticular formation or both cerebral hemispheres are damaged. The classic example of concussion occurs in the boxing ring as the consequence of a blow that deflects the head upward and posteriorly, often with a rotatory component. These motions impart a quick rotational acceleration to the brainstem and cause dysfunction of reticular formation neurons. By contrast, a blow to the temporal–parietal area may lead to a skull fracture and lethal epidural hematoma but may not cause loss of consciousness because lateral movement of the cerebral hemispheres does not occur.

Classically, concussion is not associated with gross neuropathologic findings, and since the condition is not lethal, microscopic examination is not possible. Recent advances in diffusion tensor imaging suggest that axonal injury leads to functional disconnection of the reticular activating system from the cerebral hemispheres. Axonal injury and disconnection may also account for cognitive and memory difficulties, vertigo and feelings that "things are just not quite right" that bedevil individuals with "mild" traumatic brain injury.

Cerebral Contusion

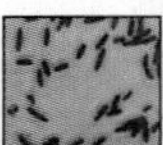

ETIOLOGIC FACTORS: A cerebral contusion is basically a brain bruise—an area of tissue disruption and seepage of blood—usually when the brain strikes the irregular bony contours of the skull as a result of abrupt acceleration or deceleration. If a moving object strikes the head, acceleration will be imparted to skull and its delicate cargo, the brain. In contrast, a fall results in an abrupt deceleration. When a contusion occurs at a point of impact, the lesion is referred to as a **coup** (from the French, "blow") injury (Fig. 28-18). If the side of the brain opposite the impact site strikes the skull, resulting contusions are contralateral to the point of initial contact and are a **contrecoup** injury. Coup injuries are maximal when the head is stationary and struck by an object, while contrecoup contusions are more severe when the head is in motion and abruptly stops. If an individual is struck by an assailant with a baseball bat, a large coup contusion will be present. In contrast, if a person falls off of a ladder, a large contrecoup contusion will result.

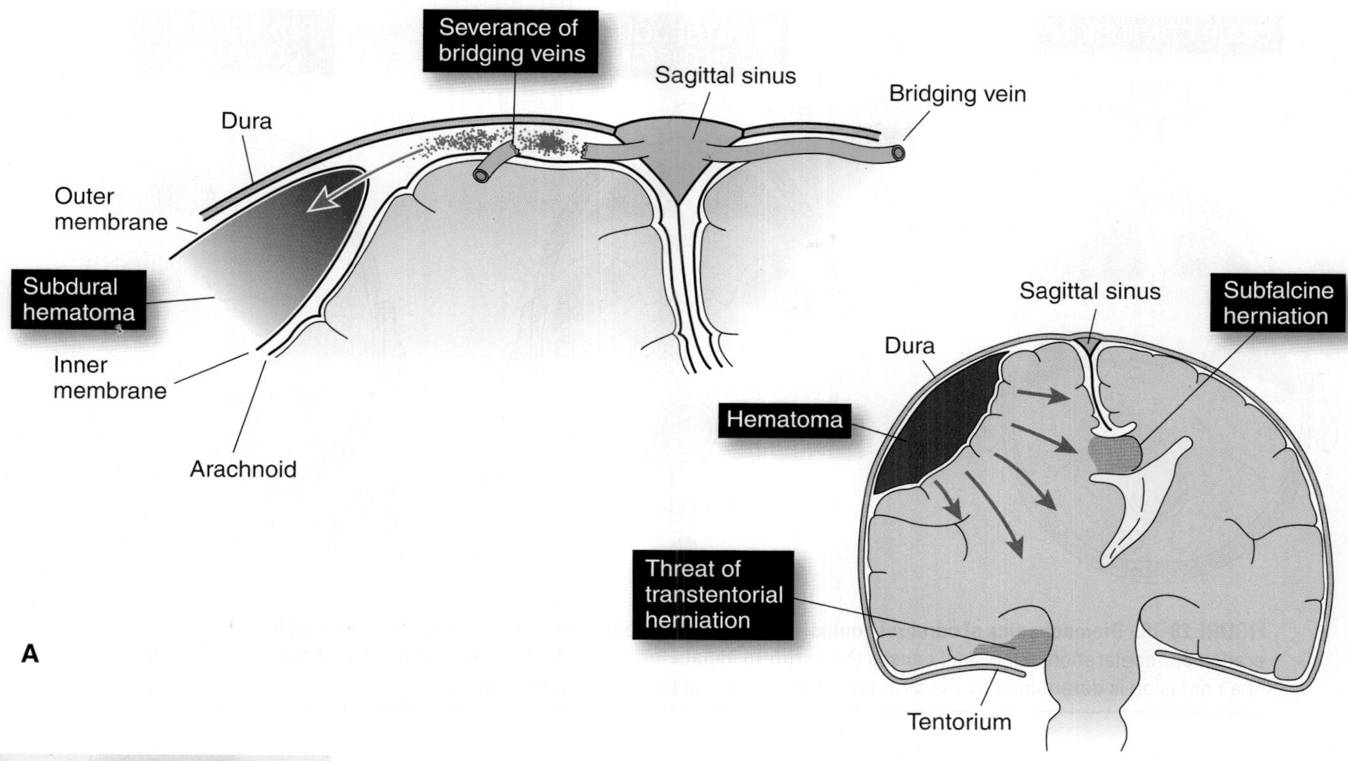

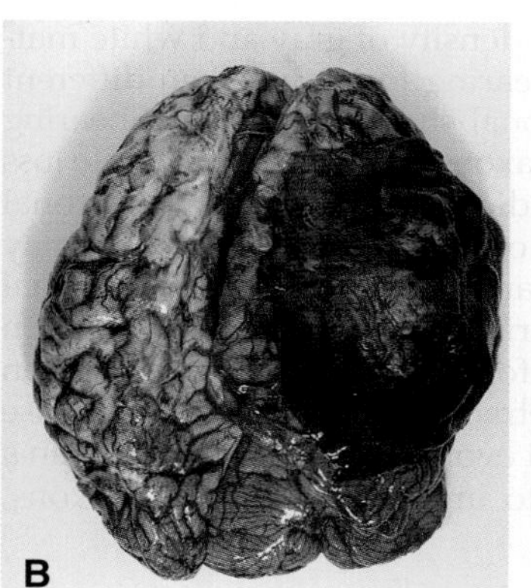

FIGURE 28-16. Development of a subdural hematoma. A. With head trauma, the dura moves with the skull, and the arachnoid moves with the cerebrum. As a result, the bridging veins are sheared as they cross between the dura and the arachnoid. Venous bleeding creates a hematoma in the expansile subdural space. Subsequent transtentorial herniation is life-threatening. **B.** The right hemisphere exhibits a large collection of blood in the "subdural space", owing to rupture of the bridging veins.

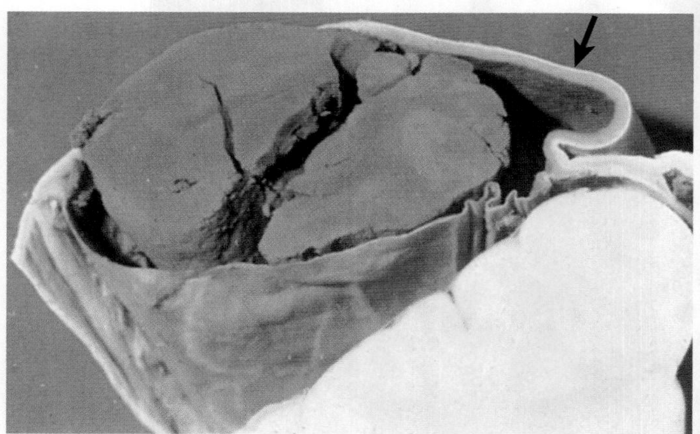

FIGURE 28-17. Chronic subdural hematoma with well-developed surrounding membranes. The thicker membrane (*arrow*) is the exterior membrane and the thinner membrane is adjacent to the brain. (Courtesy of Dr. F. Stephen Vogel, Duke University.)

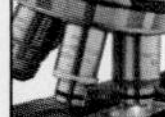

PATHOLOGY: If the force of impact is mild, cerebral contusion is limited to the cortex and the crowns of gyri (Fig. 28-19A). Greater force destroys larger expanses of cortex, creating cavitary lesions that may extend into the white matter or may lacerate the cortex, causing intraparenchymal hemorrhage (Fig. 28-19B). Together, edema and hemorrhage in a contusion may result in expansion of the contusion over several days that can become life-threatening as a result of increased intracranial pressure.

Contusions leave permanent marks on the brain. Bruised, necrotic tissue is phagocytosed by macrophages and eliminated in large part via the bloodstream. Astrocytosis then leads to local scar formation, which persists as telltale evidence of a prior contusion. Usually some residual hemosiderin imparts an orange brown hue to the old contusion (Fig. 28-20).

Diffuse Axonal Injury

Diffuse axonal injury (DAI) is a very common result of traumatic brain injury and may result in severe neurologic deficits

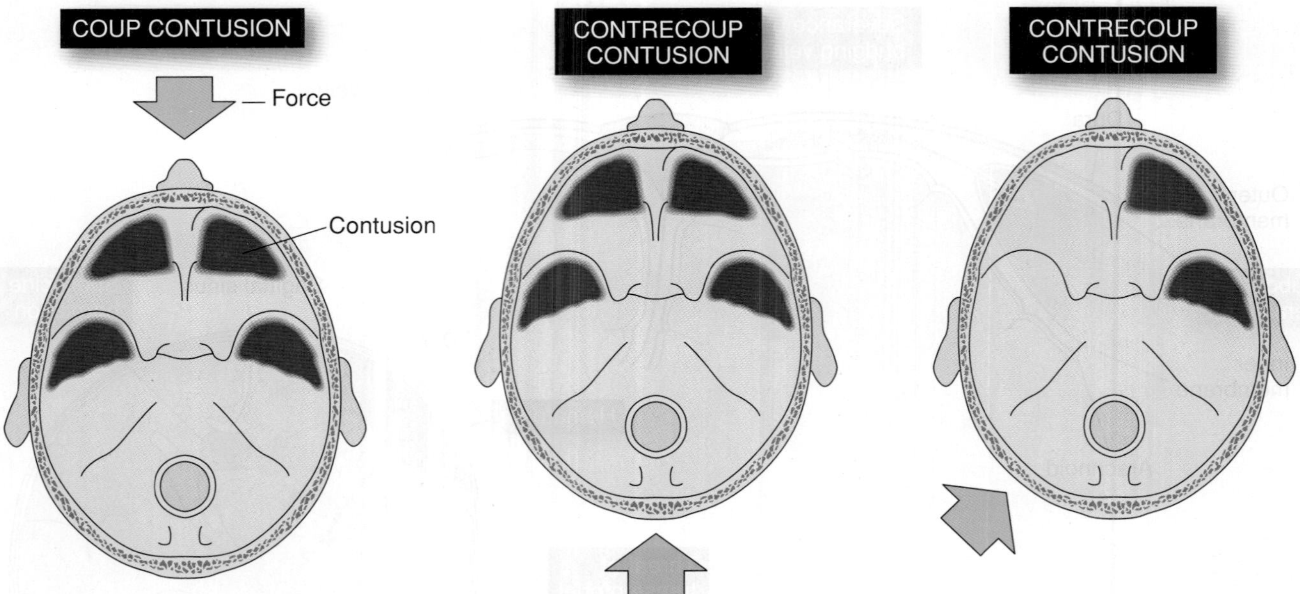

FIGURE 28-18. Biomechanics of cerebral contusion. The cerebral hemispheres float in the cerebrospinal fluid. Rapid deceleration or acceleration of the skull causes the cortex to impact forcefully into the anterior and middle fossae. The position of a contusion is determined by the direction of the force and the intracranial anatomy.

and coma in patients without gross hematomas, contusions or lacerations. Advances in imaging techniques allow better detection and quantification of this type of injury, and it appears to be a major contributor to morbidity and mortality. There is also increased interest in DAI as a component of blast injury from improvised explosive devices (IEDs) used in war and against civilian populations.

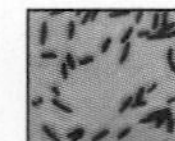

ETIOLOGIC FACTORS: The parasagittal cerebral hemispheres are anchored to arachnoid villi **(pacchionian granulations),** whereas the lateral aspects of the cerebrum move more freely. This anatomic feature, together with the differential density of gray and white matter, permits generation of shearing forces between different brain regions, leading to axonal shearing injuries. Shearing injuries can distort or disrupt axons, leading to immediate loss of function. Experimental studies indicate that diffuse axonal injury evolves over a period of hours to days, so axons may be injured at the time of primary injury, with impaired axonal transport and cytoskeletal disruption leading to accumulation of axoplasm at sites of injury, followed by physical separation of the axons to form axonal retraction spheroids. Since diffuse axonal injury is a process that evolves over time rather than a catastrophic event leading to immediately severed axons,

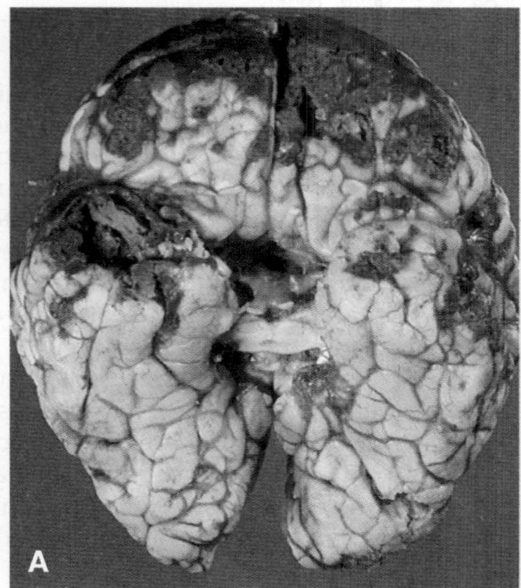

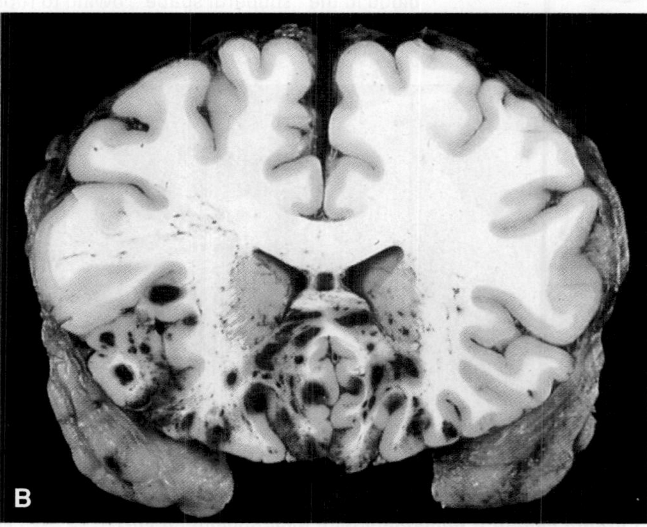

FIGURE 28-19. Acute contusions of the brain. A. After an automobile accident, the brain exhibits necrosis and hemorrhage involving the frontal and temporal lobes. **B.** In addition, there are some underlying white matter hemorrhages. (A and B Courtesy of Dr. F. Stephen Vogel, Duke University.)

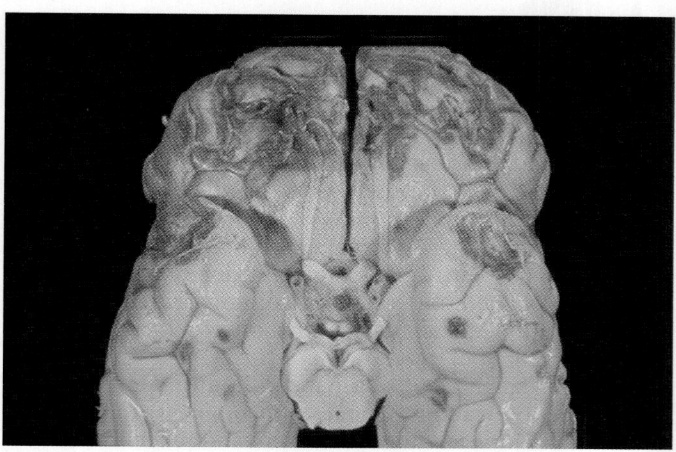

FIGURE 28-20. Remote contusions of the brain. Bilateral large frontal and smaller temporal tip contusions were cleared out by macrophages, leaving residual hemosiderin-stained divots. Also, note the involvement of the olfactory bulbs—anosmia (loss of sense of smell) is the most common cranial neuropathy following traumatic brain injury.

there may be opportunities to arrest its progression and preserve axonal structural integrity. If an injury is severe, the functional loss of axonal activity may immediately render the patient comatose, but imaging may show only small hemorrhages and focal edema, particularly in the corpus callosum and midbrain. However, more widely distributed axonal swelling and retraction spheroids may be seen in the cerebral white matter, corpus callosum and brainstem. These can be highlighted by immunostaining for amyloid precursor protein (APP), which is normally transported along axons and accumulates at sites of injury where transport is impaired. Diffusion tensor imaging (DTI), a specialized magnetic resonance imaging (MRI) technique, detects and quantifies DAI.

Penetrating Traumatic Brain Injury

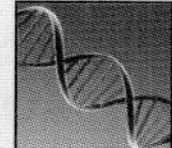

MOLECULAR PATHOGENESIS: Penetrating objects such as bullets and knives enter the cranium and traverse the brain with variable velocities. In the absence of direct damage to the vital brain centers, the immediate threat to life is hemorrhage (Fig. 28-21).

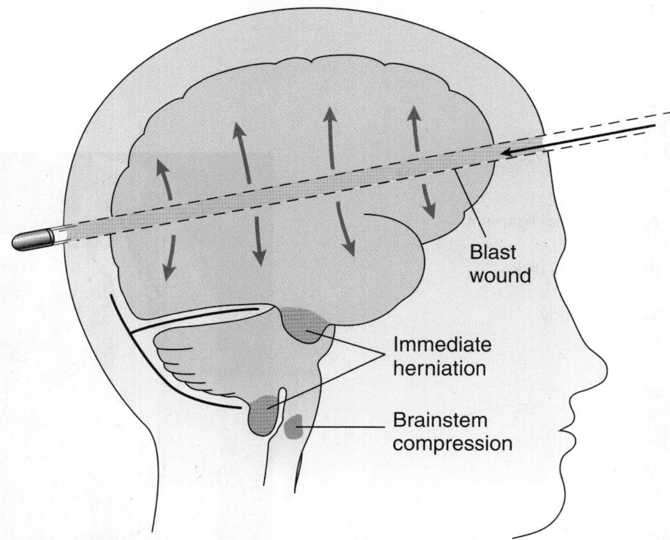

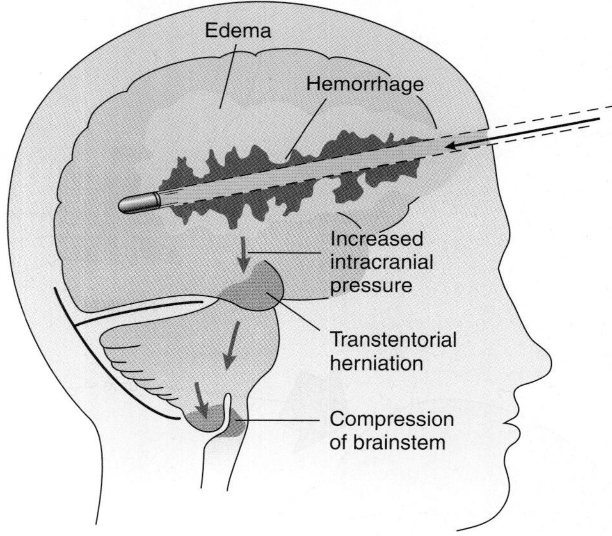

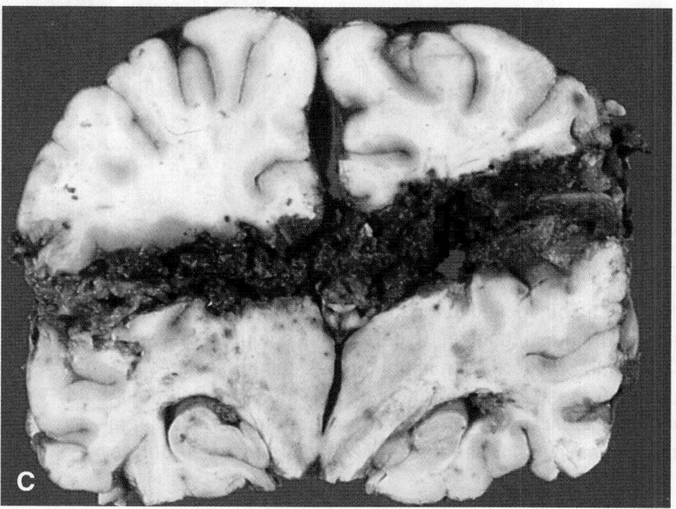

FIGURE 28-21. Consequences of high- and low-velocity bullet wounds. A. The "blast effect" of a high-velocity projectile causes an immediate increase in supratentorial pressure and results in death because of impaction of the cerebellum and medulla into the foramen magnum. **B.** A low-velocity projectile increases the pressure at a more gradual rate through hemorrhage and edema. **C. Bullet track in a through-and-through penetrating injury.** The "blast effect" of a high-velocity projectile causes an immediate increase in supratentorial pressure and may result in death because of impaction of the cerebellum and medulla into the foramen magnum. A lower-velocity projectile increases the pressure at a more gradual rate through hemorrhage and edema. (Courtesy of Dr. F. Stephen Vogel, Duke University.)

The amount of damage that a projectile does depends on how much kinetic energy is involved. Kinetic energy equals mass multiplied by velocity squared; thus, projectile velocity is the key determinant of injury. The kinetic energy of a high-velocity bullet directly disrupts tissues by its own mass as well as by a centrifugal blast zone whose diameter is determined by the original kinetic energy of the projectile. Thus, a high-velocity bullet can cause an explosive increase in intracranial pressure, which forcefully herniates the cerebellar tonsils into the foramen magnum, causing immediate death.

Spinal Cord Injury

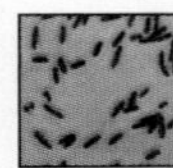

ETIOLOGIC FACTORS: Traumatic lesions of the spinal cord may result from direct injury by penetrating wounds (e.g., stab wounds, bullets) or indirect injury from vertebral fractures or displacement. The spinal cord may be contused not only at the site of injury but also above and below the point of trauma. Traumatic injury may be complicated by compromise of the arterial supply to the cord, with resulting infarction.

Vertebral bodies are separated by intravertebral disks and are stabilized in normal alignment by two longitudinal ligaments and the posterior bony processes. The anterior spinal ligament adheres to the ventral surface of the vertebral bodies, whereas the posterior spinal ligament is affixed to the dorsal vertebral column. After extreme flexion or extension, the angulation of the bony vertebral column brings the spinal cord forcefully into contact with bone or interferes with regional circulation.

The consequences of a spinal cord injury depend on the severity of the trauma. **Concussion of the spinal cord** is the mildest injury, leading to transient and reversible disturbance of spinal cord function. **Contusion of the spinal cord** is the result of more severe trauma, from a minor transient bruise to hemorrhagic spinal cord necrosis (Fig. 28-22). The

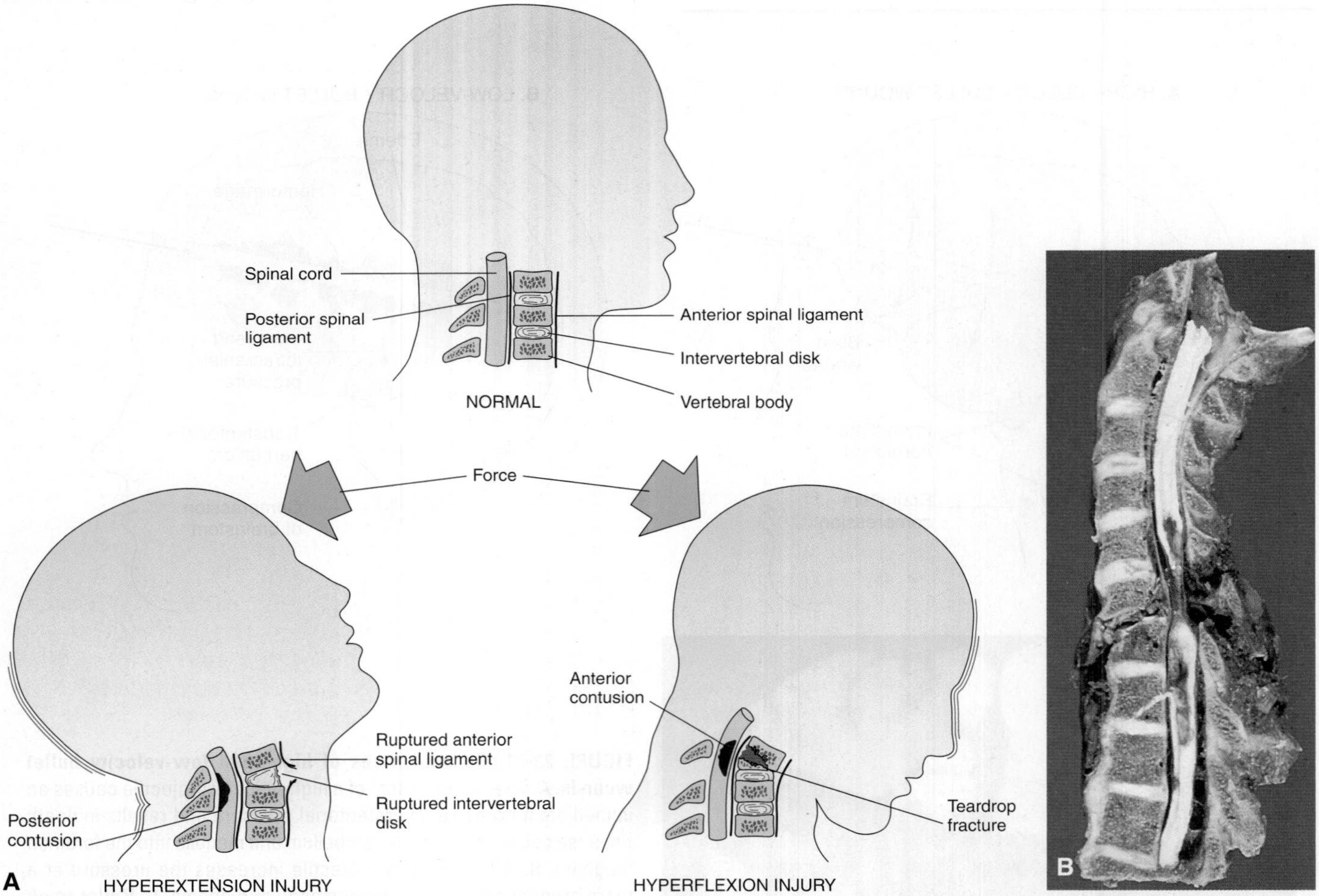

FIGURE 28-22. Spinal injury. A. Numerous different angles of force can be applied to the highly vulnerable cervical spine. Posterior (hyperextension) and anterior (hyperflexion) injuries are the most common. Hyperextension injury causes rupture of the anterior spinal ligament and excessive posterior angulation. Hyperflexion injury causes compression associated with a "teardrop" fracture of a vertebral body and produces excessive forward angulation of the cord. **B.** Fracture dislocation of the spinal column may result in spinal cord contusion, laceration, necrosis or frank transection. Preservation of a relatively small cross-sectional area of the spinal cord can have major beneficial effects on recovery. (Courtesy of Dr. F. Stephen Vogel, Duke University.)

spinal cord necrosis and edema caused by a severe contusion are referred to as **myelomalacia,** and a hematoma within the spinal cord is termed **hematomyelia. Lacerations and transections of the spinal cord** are usually produced by penetrating wounds or severely displaced spinal fractures. They are irreversible and result in complete loss of function below the spinal level of the injury. Paralysis of the legs **(paraplegia)** or all four extremities **(quadriplegia)** ensues, depending on the spinal level and extent of the injury. Preservation of as little as 10% to 15% of the cross-sectional diameter of the spinal cord can allow much better functional recovery than complete transection.

Cerebrovascular Disorders

Stroke is the third leading cause of death after myocardial infarction and cancer. As elsewhere, vascular disease can result from either vessel blockage, causing ischemia, or leaking of the vessels, resulting in hemorrhage. Vascular disorders of the nervous system lead to either (1) globally or focally inadequate blood flow (ischemia), which, if sufficiently protracted, leads to tissue necrosis (infarction) or (2) rupture of vascular structures leading to hemorrhage that is either intraparenchymal or in the subarachnoid space.

Ischemic Stroke Often Follows Shock

ETIOLOGIC FACTORS: The brain receives about 20% of basal cardiac output. Aerobic glycolysis is virtually the sole source of energy of the mature brain. CNS glycogen reserves are meager and oxygen reserves are nil; hence, an uninterrupted supply of oxygenated blood is essential for brain integrity. The blood supply of the brain comes via paired internal carotid and vertebral arteries. The carotids are the "anterior circulation," supplying most superficial and deep structures of the cerebral hemispheres; the vertebral arteries supply the "posterior circulation," which feeds the brainstem, cerebellum and the territory of the posterior cerebral arteries. The posterior and anterior circuits anastomose via the circle of Willis. This anastomotic network at the base of the brain is quite variable, but in some fortunate individuals, the blood supply of the brain is sufficiently redundant that complete blockage of two carotids and one vertebral can be asymptomatic. Despite these elaborate hemodynamic precautions, many people experience global or focal ischemia leading to cerebral infarction. Global ischemia leads to widespread tissue injury, resulting in **ischemic encephalopathy.** ***Global ischemia usually results from cardiopulmonary arrest or extreme hypotension in severe shock.*** If perfusion failure is brief (minutes), neurologic functions may quickly be restored with only transient postischemic confusion. Some patients may come back more slowly and suffer subtle impairments of higher intellectual function, which may preclude complete resumption of societal activities. More severe injury may lead to dementia and spasticity. If the ischemic period is protracted, the patient may not regain consciousness, exhibit decorticate posturing and seizures and remain in a vegetative state indefinitely.

Although the entire brain is inadequately perfused, there is surprising focality to the pathologic alterations seen.

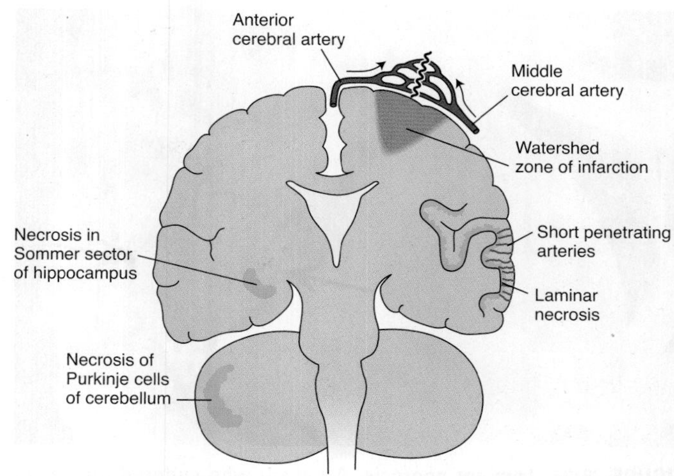

FIGURE 28-23. Mechanisms of injury in global ischemia. A global insult induces lesions that reflect the vascular architecture (watershed infarcts, laminar necrosis) and the selective vulnerability of individual neuronal systems (pyramidal cells of the Sommer sector, Purkinje cells, laminar necrosis). Both rheologic (blood flow) and neurochemical (excitotoxicity) factors may be operational in laminar necrosis.

Certain cell populations are selectively vulnerable to ischemic injury, including large neurons in the Sommer sector of the hippocampus, Purkinje cells of the cerebellum and neurons of layers 3 and 5 of the cerebral cortex (Fig. 28-23).

The basis of this selective vulnerability is not clear, but it may be related to local energy metabolism requirements, hemodynamic factors and local neurotransmitters. In particular, when ischemia leads to brain energy failure, membranes depolarize, permitting uncontrolled release of the amino acid neurotransmitters glutamate and aspartate. These neurotransmitters bind ligand-gated cation channels on the postsynaptic cell, opening the floodgates for entry of calcium and sodium. The sodium depolarizes the cell membrane, and calcium may activate intracellular proteases and quench mitochondrial energy production, propagating the energy failure and magnifying cellular injury. Injury done by abnormally released neurotransmitters is termed **"excitotoxicity."** This mechanism may play a role in neurodegenerative disorders and epilepsy, as well as stroke. In excitotoxicity, the areas of brain injury depend on the local use of toxic neurotransmitters. For example, high levels of amino acid neurotransmitters make the midcortex more vulnerable to ischemic injury, resulting in a midcortical band of necrosis with relatively preserved cortex in deep and superficial layers on either side of this band. As infarcted tissue is infiltrated by macrophages, it becomes grossly conspicuous and is called **"laminar necrosis"** (Fig. 28-24).

Hemodynamic factors cause **watershed** or **borderzone infarcts,** which occur at junctions of major arterial supply zones (Fig. 28-25). The zones are at the precarious distal regions of arterial supply, and if perfusion pressure drops, these are the first areas to experience perfusion insufficiency. The classic border zone lies between the anterior and middle cerebral arteries' distal territories (Fig. 28-25). With global ischemia, this area in both hemispheres may undergo infarction, leading to symmetric wedge-shaped parasagittal high-convexity infarcts.

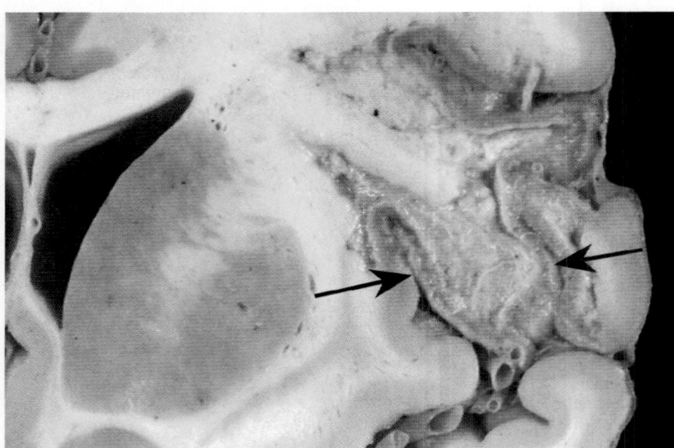

FIGURE 28-24. Laminar necrosis. A patient who suffered prolonged anoxia during a cardiac arrhythmia developed selective necrosis of layers in the cerebral cortex (*arrows*). (Courtesy of Dr. F. Stephen Vogel, Duke University.)

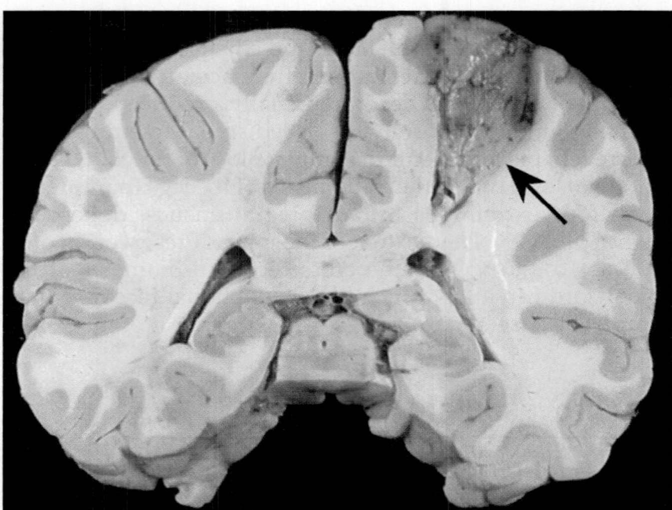

FIGURE 28-25. Watershed infarct. In global hypoperfusion, the most precarious perfusion zones are at the distal overlapping portions of the major cerebral vessels. Here an acute infarct is seen at the watershed of the anterior and middle cerebral arteries (*arrow*). (Courtesy of Dr. F. Stephen Vogel, Duke University.)

Regional Ischemia Causes Localized Cerebral Infarction

The high prevalence and progressive nature of atherosclerosis is reflected in the fact that cerebrovascular occlusive disease remains a major cause of morbidity and death. ***Atherosclerosis predisposes to vascular thrombosis and embolic events, both of which result in localized ischemia and subsequent cerebral infarction.***

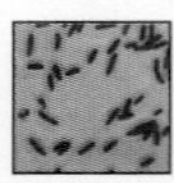

ETIOLOGIC FACTORS: Cerebral infarcts are usually designated either **"hemorrhagic"** or **"bland."** ***In general, infarcts caused by embolization are hemorrhagic, whereas those initiated by local thrombosis are ischemic (or bland).*** Emboli occlude vascular flow abruptly, after which the distal segments of affected blood vessels become necrotic and leak blood into the region during reperfusion (Fig. 28-26A). Atherosclerotic plaques in the common and internal carotid arteries may lead to emboli, but the heart is also a rich source of emboli, whether from infected or defective valves, hypokinetic thrombogenic endocardial wall after myocardial infarction or atrial thrombi in atrial fibrillation, particularly when associated with mitral insufficiency. Fat emboli and deep vein thrombi from the systemic venous circulation may find their way to the brain via a patent foramen ovale through paradoxic embolization. Tumor emboli, usually from atrial myxoma, or amniotic emboli are well recognized, although rarely seen.

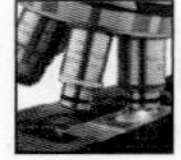

PATHOLOGY: Most infarcts caused by thrombosis are anemic or bland and are difficult to see grossly for several hours, after which softening and discoloration are increasingly prominent (Fig. 28-26B). Swelling and liquefaction follow within 3 to 5 days, during which time the patient is in peril from the mass effect of the infarct. The infarct then matures over weeks to months into a cystic space (Fig. 28-27), sometimes accompanied by compensatory ventricular enlargement. If blood flow is restored to a bland infarct, as often occurs in embolic or compressive vascular disease, blood may seep into the softened tissues, resulting in a hemorrhagic infarct, which is readily discernible grossly and radiologically (Fig. 28-28).

As in other tissues, an orderly procession of gross and histopathologic alterations permits estimation of an infarct's age. If a patient survives for minutes to several hours, no changes are seen. If the patient survives for 6 to 24 hours, shrunken eosinophilic neurons ("red neurons") with nuclear pyknosis are present in the infarct (Fig. 28-29), while grossly, the infarct is slightly discolored and softened with blurring of the border between gray and white matter. These changes become more pronounced as the infarct ages. By 24 to 72 hours, the tissue is infiltrated by neutrophils and blood vessels are prominent. The tissue is soft and edematous and may be sufficiently swollen to cause lethal mass effect.

By 72 to 96 hours, neutrophils are replaced by macrophages that clear debris in the infarct at a rate of about 1 mL per month. The infarct is now frankly mushy. In the second week, proliferating astrocytes join the macrophages and, for the ensuing weeks to months, form a dense fibrillary glial meshwork around the dead tissue so that as the macrophages dispose of debris in the infarct over weeks to months, the infarct evolves into a glial lined cyst, crossed at points by delicate glial sheets and small vessels and invested with residual lipid and hemosiderin-laden macrophages.

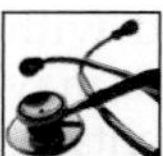

CLINICAL FEATURES: The diversity of the neurologic deficits caused by stroke directly reflects the functional eloquence of the brain. For example, the lengthy and slender striate arteries, which take origin from the proximal middle cerebral artery, are commonly occluded by atherosclerosis and thrombosis. Resultant infarcts often impact the internal capsule to produce hemiplegia (Fig. 28-26A). Similarly, the middle cerebral artery trifurcation is a favored site for lodgment of emboli and for thrombosis secondary to atherosclerotic damage. Middle cerebral artery occlusion at this site deprives much of the lateral

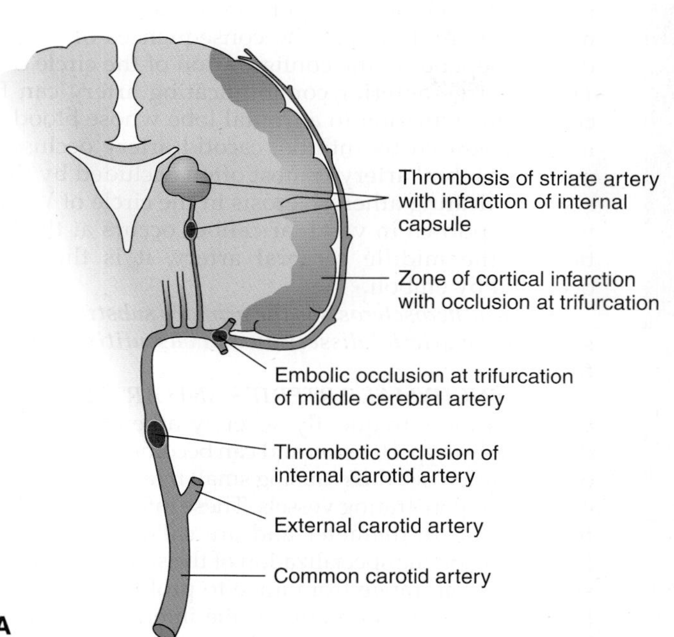

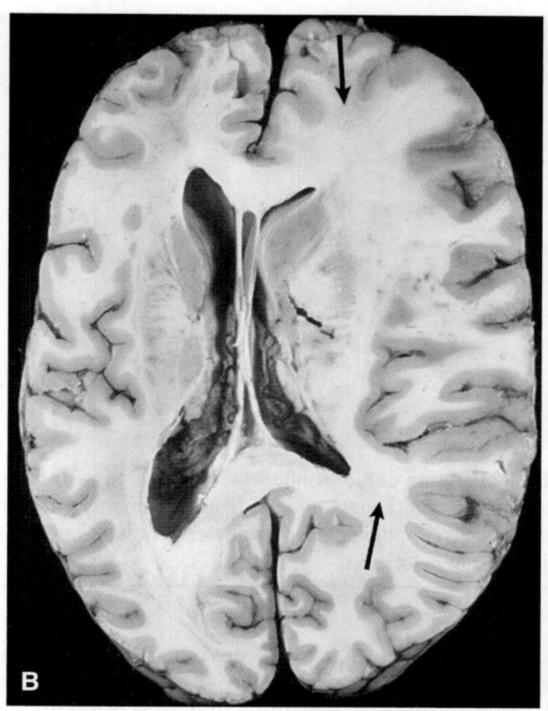

FIGURE 28-26. A. Distribution of cerebral infarcts. The normal distribution of the cerebral vasculature defines the pattern and size of infarcts and, consequently, their symptoms. Occlusion at the trifurcation causes cortical infarcts with motor and sensory loss and often aphasia. Occlusion of a striate branch transects the internal capsule and causes a motor deficit. **B. Acute middle cerebral artery distribution infarct.** An axial section of the brain of a patient who suffered thrombosis of the middle cerebral artery reveals a large infarct of the right hemisphere (*between arrows*) with swelling and focal dusky discoloration. (Courtesy of Dr. F. Stephen Vogel, Duke University.)

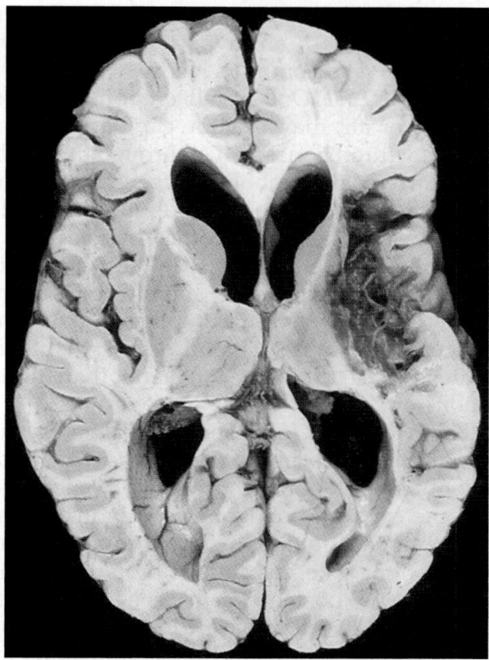

FIGURE 28-27. Remote middle cerebral artery distribution infarct. An axial section of the brain shows a remote middle cerebral artery distribution cystic infarct. The brain in Fig. 28-26B would transform to this state as a result of clearing out of the large infarct by macrophages. (Courtesy of Dr. F. Stephen Vogel, Duke University.)

hemispheric cortex of blood, producing motor and sensory deficits. If the dominant hemisphere is involved, aphasia may develop.

Localized ischemia may be associated with three distinct clinical syndromes:

- **Transient ischemic attack (TIA)** refers to focal cerebral dysfunction of less than 24 hours, and often lasting only a

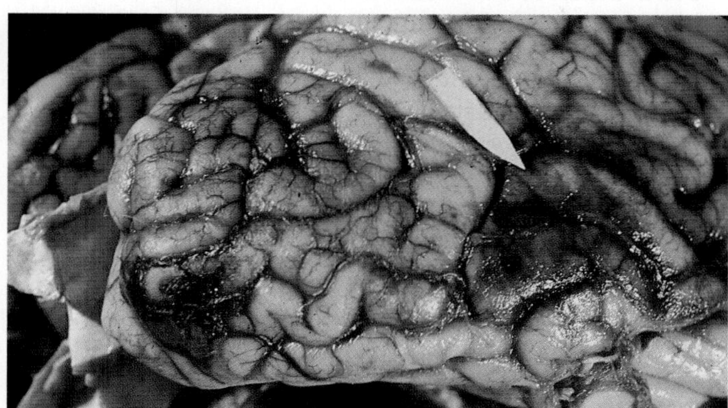

FIGURE 28-28. Hemorrhagic embolic infarct. Emboli from a carotid endarterectomy resulted in hemorrhagic infarcts in the territory of the middle cerebral artery (*arrow*). Such hemorrhagic infarcts may expand because of seepage of blood or frank hemorrhage and become life-threatening.

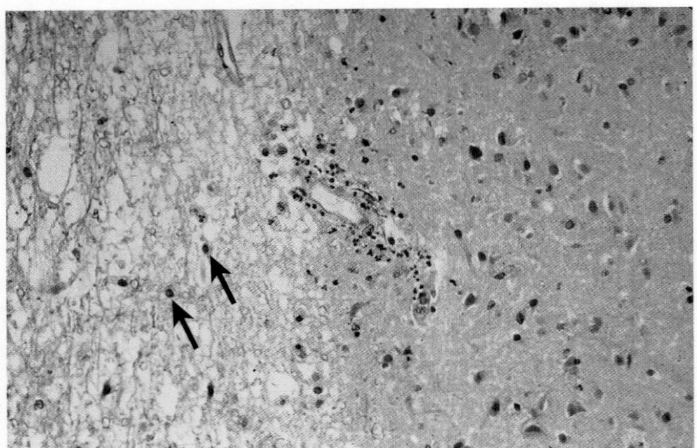

FIGURE 28-29. Acute cerebral infarct histopathology. An 18-hour-old cerebral infarct (*left*) shows edema, hypereosinophilic neurons and perivascular polymorphonuclear leukocytes. Pyknotic nuclei of dying neurons are shown (*arrows*).

few minutes. Although complete neurologic recovery follows, a TIA heralds increased risk of cerebral infarction. TIAs, like angina, are warnings that all is not well with the blood supply of a critical organ, and their occurrence often triggers diagnostic and therapeutic activity. A patient having TIAs is at risk for later cerebral infarction; about one third of patients with TIAs will experience a stroke within 5 years of the onset of TIAs, the period of highest risk being the first 30 days after TIAs begin; in one third of patients the TIAs will simply continue; and about one third of patients with TIAs will have no more TIAs, nor will they suffer a stroke. ***Although TIAs often are harbingers of a stroke, it must be emphasized that many people (50% to 85%) who have a cerebral infarct never have a TIA.*** If a TIA lasts more than a few minutes, some tissue damage does occur as evidenced by MRI abnormalities on diffusion water inversion (DWI) sequences.

- **Stroke in evolution** describes the often stuttering progression of neurologic symptoms as a patient is being observed. This syndrome reflects propagation of a thrombus in the carotid or basilar arteries and is a clinically unstable situation requiring urgent treatment.
- **Completed stroke** is the term for a stable or fixed neurologic deficit caused by a cerebral infarct. Two to three days after a completed stroke, there can be sufficient cerebral cytotoxic and vasogenic edema in the infarct that increased intracranial pressure and herniation become issues.

Regional Occlusive Cerebrovascular Disease

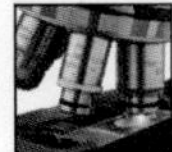

PATHOLOGY: The various occlusive cerebrovascular diseases that lead to cerebral infarcts may be classified by the caliber and nature of the involved vessel.

LARGE EXTRACRANIAL AND INTRACRANIAL ARTERIES: These arteries are frequent sites of atherosclerosis. Most notably, atherosclerotic plaques occur quite often in the common carotid artery at its bifurcation into external and internal branches. Occlusion or stenosis of an internal carotid artery affects the ipsilateral hemisphere, but this can be offset by the variable collateral circulation through the anterior and posterior communicating arteries. Most often, occlusion of a carotid artery produces infarcts restricted to all or some portion of the distribution of the middle cerebral artery. The consequences of large vessel disease depend on the configuration of the circle of Willis. Thus, a large anterior communicating artery can furnish collateral circulation to a frontal lobe whose blood supply is compromised by internal carotid artery occlusion. The middle cerebral artery is most often occluded by thrombosis complicating atherosclerosis in the circle of Willis. As a major stepdown in vascular caliber occurs at the trifurcation of the middle cerebral artery, it is the main site occluded by emboli.

While atherosclerosis is the primary substrate of ischemic stroke, both arterial dissection and vasculitis may also lead to stroke.

PARENCHYMAL ARTERIES AND ARTERIOLES: These vessels are less frequently severely atherosclerotic but are damaged by hypertension and can become narrowed because of atherosclerosis, thus causing small infarcts in the territories of the deep penetrating vessels. These infarcts are usually less than 15 mm in diameter and are called **lacunar infarcts.** Depending on the specialization of the small region supplied, symptoms can range from none to profound—contralateral hemiparesis from an infarct in the internal capsule or pure hemisensory loss caused by a thalamic lacunar infarct. When multiple, these minute infarcts can lead to impaired cognition called **multiple infarct dementia.**

Hypertensive encephalopathy refers to the acute neurologic complications of malignant hypertension. As in other affected organs, hypertension can cause fibrinoid necrosis of small arteries and arterioles, as well as minute hemorrhages **(petechiae).** Cerebral edema may complicate the vascular pathology. Hypertensive encephalopathy usually manifests clinically as headache and vomiting that progress to coma and death. With modern antihypertensive therapy, malignant hypertension is uncommon.

MICROCIRCULATION: Small emboli, composed, for example, of fat or air, may occlude capillaries. **Fat emboli,** usually from fractured bones, travel through the cerebral vessels until the size of the embolus exceeds that of the blood vessel, at which point they lodge and block blood flow. The distal capillary endothelium becomes hypoxic and permeable, and petechiae develop, mostly in the white matter (Fig. 28-30). **Air emboli** liberate many bubbles that further fragment as they encounter vascular bifurcations, until they impede vascular flow in small blood vessels. In this situation, petechiae are less restricted to white matter than those caused by fat emboli.

VENOUS CIRCULATION: The cerebral veins empty into large venous sinuses, the largest of which is the sagittal sinus, which accommodates venous drainage from the superior portions of the cerebral hemispheres. Venous sinus thrombosis in the brain is a potentially lethal complication of systemic dehydration, phlebitis caused by adjacent infections such as mastoiditis, obstruction by a neoplasm such as a meningioma or sickle cell disease. Since venous obstruction causes stagnation upstream, abrupt sagittal sinus thrombosis results in bilateral hemorrhagic infarction of the frontal lobe regions (Fig. 28-31). A more indolent occlusion of the sinus (e.g., caused by invasion by a meningioma) permits recruitment of collateral circulation through the inferior sagittal sinus, which lies at the lower edge of the falx and empties into the straight sinus.

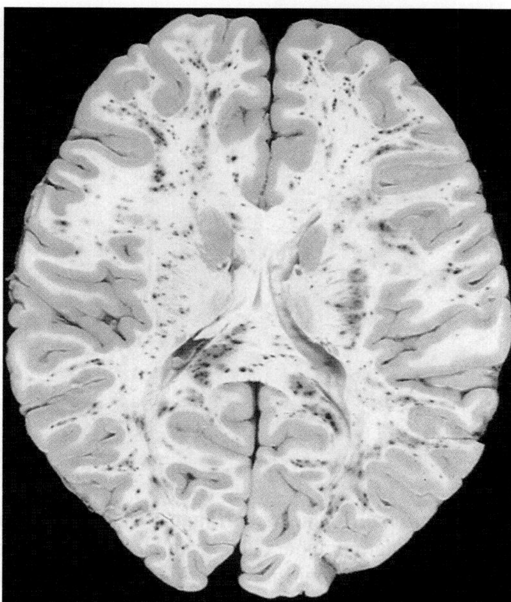

FIGURE 28-30. Fat emboli. An axial section of the brain in a patient with polytrauma with multiple bone fractures leading to cerebral fat emboli manifested by numerous small petechiae throughout the white matter where the small emboli lodge in the microcirculation. (Courtesy of Dr. F. Stephen Vogel, Duke University.)

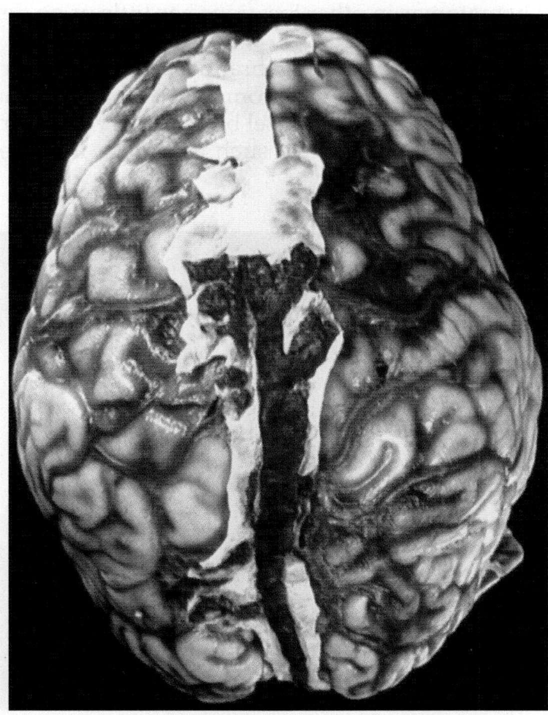

FIGURE 28-31. Superior sagittal sinus thrombosis. Upon opening of the superior sagittal sinus, a thrombus filling the sinus is seen. The thrombus impeded venous drainage of the cerebral hemisphere, leading to bilateral hemorrhagic infarcts of the cerebral hemispheres. Venous thrombosis is seen in hypercoagulable states such as dehydration, pregnancy, hereditary defects of thrombolysis, sickle cell disease or extension of an infection or neoplasm into the sinus. (Courtesy of Dr. F. Stephen Vogel, Duke University.)

Intracranial Hemorrhage Can Be Intraparenchymal or in the Subarachnoid Space

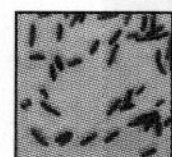

ETIOLOGIC FACTORS: Intraparenchymal hemorrhage is called intracerebral hemorrhage (ICH) and usually results from rupture of small fragile vessels or vascular malformations. Subarachnoid hemorrhage (SAH) is mostly caused by rupture of aneurysms or vascular malformations.

Intracerebral Hemorrhage

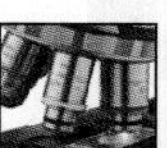

PATHOLOGY: Cerebral hemorrhages that occur without trauma are usually caused by vascular malformations or are consequences of long-standing hypertension. **Hypertensive intracerebral hemorrhage (ICH)** occurs at preferential sites, which in order of frequency are (1) basal ganglia–thalamus (65%), (2) pons (15%) and (3) cerebellum (8%). Hypertensive ICH can also occur in the white matter of the cerebral hemispheres, where it is called **lobar ICH.** Lobar ICH should suggest possible amyloid angiopathy, vascular malformation, coagulopathy or bleeding into a tumor, in addition to simple hypertensive hemorrhage.

Hypertension compromises the integrity of cerebral arterioles by causing lipid and hyaline material to deposit in their walls, an alteration referred to as **lipohyalinosis.** Weakening of the wall leads to formation of **Charcot-Bouchard aneurysms,** which are located mainly along the trunk of an arteriole rather than sites where it bifurcates (Fig. 28-32).

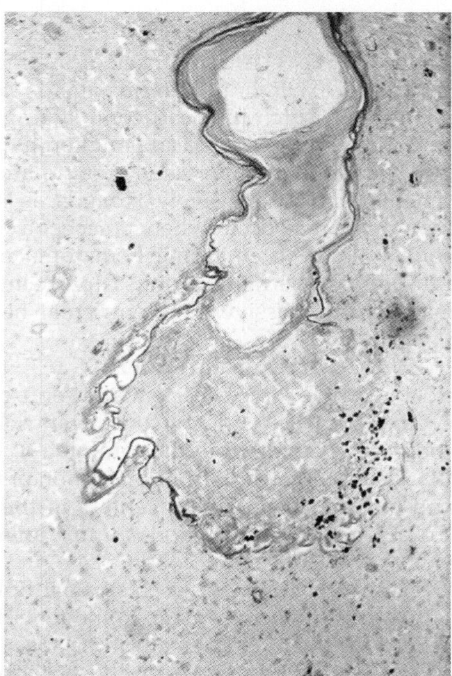

FIGURE 28-32. Charcot-Bouchard aneurysm. The combination of small penetrating cerebral vessels and high perfusion pressure leads to small microaneurysms that may rupture, leading to intracerebral hemorrhage. Effective treatment of hypertension reduces the formation of microaneurysms and the frequency of intracerebral hemorrhage. (Courtesy of Dr. F. Stephen Vogel, Duke University.)

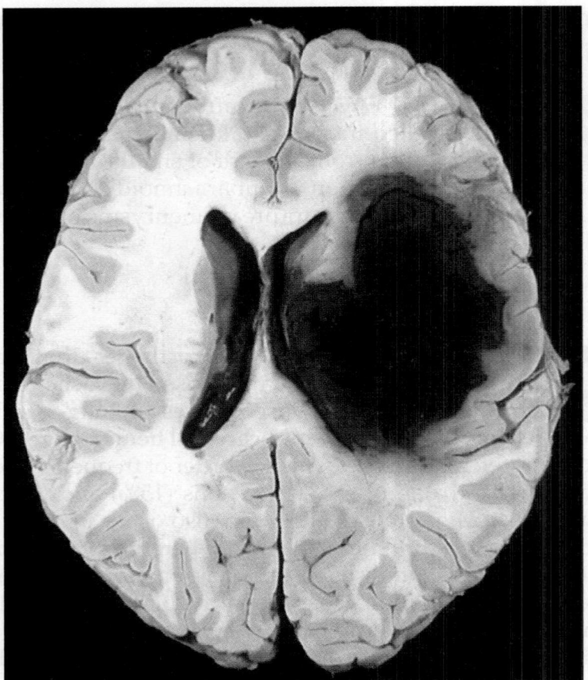

FIGURE 28-33. Intracerebral hemorrhage in the basal ganglia. A hypertensive patient bled into the basal ganglia, resulting in acute severe headache, contralateral hemiparesis and rapid decline in level of consciousness. The deep cerebral nuclei (basal ganglia) and thalamus are the most common locations of intracerebral hemorrhages. (Courtesy of Dr. F. Stephen Vogel, Duke University.)

CLINICAL FEATURES: Onset of symptoms of a hypertensive cerebral hemorrhage is abrupt. A patient may clutch his head complaining of severe headache and lapse into coma. Basal ganglion hypertensive intracerebral hemorrhages may cause contralateral hemiparesis. If a hematoma progressively expands, as is common in the first day, death may occur when it reaches a critical volume of about 30 mL. An enlarging hematoma may cause death by transtentorial herniation, or its rupture into a lateral ventricle may lead to massive intraventricular hemorrhage (Fig. 28-33).

INTRAVENTRICULAR HEMORRHAGE: Extension of the ICH into a ventricle rapidly distends the entire ventricular system with blood, including the fourth ventricle (Fig. 28-34). The blood may emerge from the foramina of Magendie and Luschka. Death may result from distention of the fourth ventricle and compression of vital centers in the medulla. Ventricular drainage allows reduction of intracranial pressure and removal of intraventricular blood.

PONTINE HEMORRHAGE: In this catastrophic event, loss of consciousness reflects damage to the reticular formation, an injury that overshadows all other specific cranial nerve deficits. The hemorrhage generally starts in the midpons (Fig. 28-35). It encroaches upon vital medullary centers with minimal enlargement, commonly resulting in death or severe disability.

CEREBELLAR HEMORRHAGE: Bleeding into the cerebellum causes abrupt ataxia with a severe occipital headache and vomiting (Fig. 28-36). The expanding hematoma threatens life acutely by compressing the medulla or via cerebellar

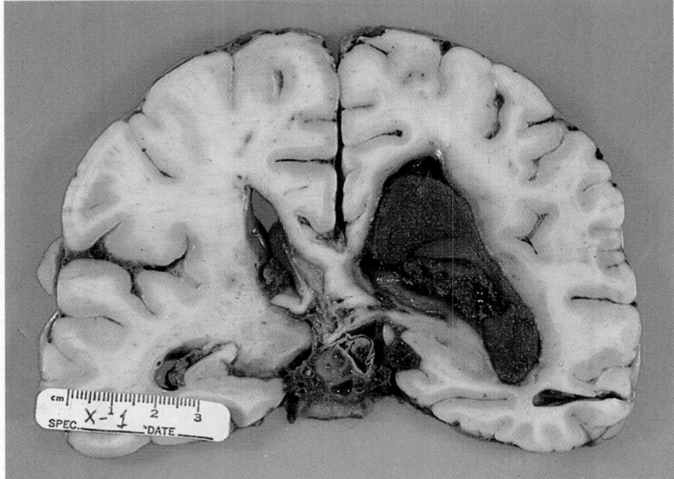

FIGURE 28-34. Intraventricular hemorrhage. A sagittal section of the brain shows ventricular chambers filled with blood that extended from a more anterior basal ganglionic intracerebral hemorrhage. The patient died rapidly from compression of the brainstem by blood in the fourth ventricle.

herniation through the foramen magnum. Surgical evacuation of the hematoma is life saving and may leave few serious neurologic deficits, whereas surgical intervention for intracerebral hematomas in other locations has little or no demonstrated benefit.

Causes of spontaneous cerebral hemorrhages other than hypertension include leakage from an arteriovenous malformation, erosion of a blood vessel by a primary or secondary neoplasm, endothelial injury such as occurs in rickettsial

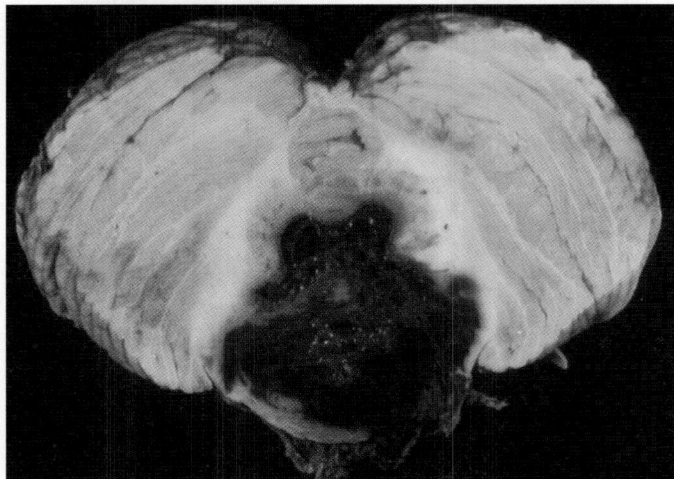

FIGURE 28-35. Pontine hemorrhage. Rupture of microaneurysms in the pons leads to rapid decline in level of consciousness as a result of disruption of the reticular activating system. Multiple cranial neuropathies, dysconjugate gaze, pupillary abnormalities, paralysis and dysregulation of respiration and cardiovascular systems are common. This is the second most common location of intracranial hemorrhage, and hemorrhage in the pons is often lethal. (Courtesy of Dr. F. Stephen Vogel, Duke University.)

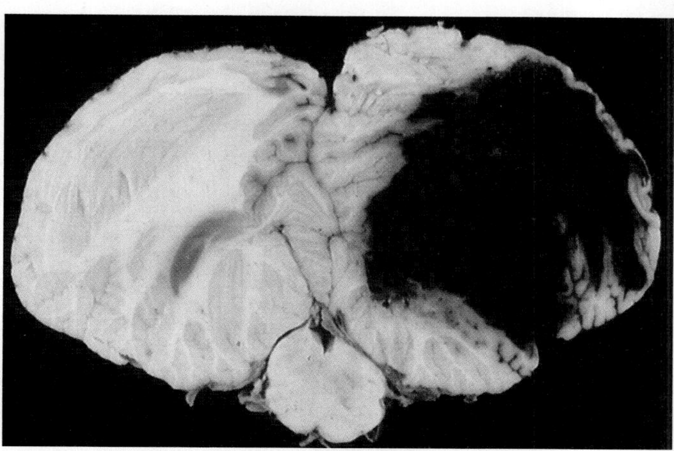

FIGURE 28-36. Cerebellar hemorrhage. Intracerebral hemorrhage in the cerebellum leads to acute-onset occipital headache, nausea, vomiting, vertigo and ataxia. If the hematoma expands rapidly, fatal compression of the medulla may ensue. Surgical evacuation of the cerebellar intracranial hemorrhage can be life-saving and is a neurosurgical emergency. (Courtesy of Dr. F. Stephen Vogel, Duke University.)

infections, a bleeding diathesis or embolic infarction with consequent hemorrhage into the area of necrosis (hemorrhagic conversion).

AMYLOID ANGIOPATHY: This vascular change results from deposition of β-amyloid protein in vascular walls, rendering them weak and friable (Fig. 28-37). Small intraparenchymal vessels in the lobar white matter are most affected, and their rupture may lead to lobar ICH. Amyloid angiopathy increases in frequency with increasing age and is an important cause of ICH in the elderly, where the angiopathy may coexist with Alzheimer disease, a neurodegenerative disease in which β-amyloid protein processing is abnormal (see below).

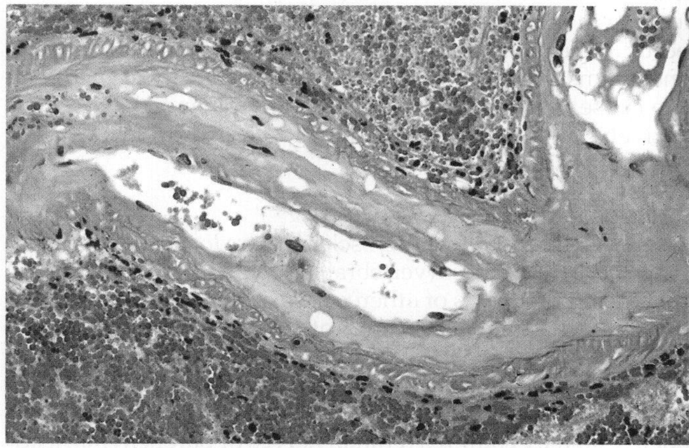

FIGURE 28-37. Amyloid angiopathy. While hypertension is the most common cause of intracerebral hemorrhage in the classic locations—basal ganglia and thalamus, pons and cerebellum—hemorrhage in the white matter of the cerebral hemispheres has a broader range of possible etiologies. These hemorrhages, called lobar hemorrhages, may be caused by amyloid angiopathy in which β-amyloid protein is deposited in the walls of vessels, rendering them weak and friable. This is the same protein as is involved in plaque formation in Alzheimer disease; amyloid angiopathy and Alzheimer disease frequently coexist.

Subarachnoid Hemorrhage

Intravascular pressure and weakness in arterial walls lead to formation of cerebral aneurysms that may rupture, leading to subarachnoid hemorrhage. Ruptured aneurysms cause about 85% of subarachnoid hemorrhage (SAH), while vascular malformations account for approximately 15%.

Saccular (Berry) Aneurysms

Saccular aneurysms are balloonlike outpouchings of cerebral arteries that may rupture to cause catastrophic subarachnoid hemorrhage. They tend to occur at branch points of the cerebral vasculature in or near the circle of Willis (Fig. 28-38).

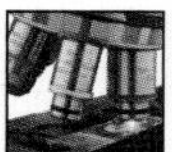

PATHOLOGY: When a developing blood vessel bifurcates into two branches, the muscularis layer may not adequately span the branch point, creating an area of congenital muscularis thinning covered only by endothelium, the internal elastic membrane and a thin adventitia. Over time, pressure from the pulsatile blood flow from the parent vessel expands the congenital defect. The internal elastic membrane may degenerate or fragment, after which a saccular aneurysm evolves that is precariously covered only by a layer of adventitia. There is active vascular wall remodeling that may contribute to the evolution of the aneurysm.

More than 90% of saccular aneurysms occur at proximal branch points in the anterior circulation fed by the carotid system; however, some may arise on branches of the posterior circulation, particularly on the posterior communicating and posterior cerebral arteries (Fig. 28-39). They are equally distributed at the junctions of the (1) anterior cerebral and anterior communicating arteries, (2) internal carotid–posterior communicating–anterior cerebral–anterior choroidal arteries and (3) trifurcation of the middle cerebral artery. In 15% to 20% of cases, multiple aneurysms are present. The incidence of cerebral aneurysms is increased in polycystic kidney disease, coarctation of the aorta and Ehlers-Danlos syndrome.

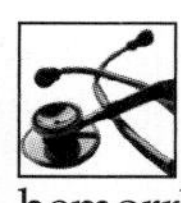

CLINICAL FEATURES: Rupture of a saccular aneurysm leads to life-threatening subarachnoid hemorrhage, with a 35% mortality during the initial hemorrhage. Blood may jet under arterial pressure to produce intracerebral or intraventricular hemorrhage in up to one third of patients. The subarachnoid blood irritates pain-sensitive vessels and dura, leading to a sudden severe headache that the patient may describe as "the worst headache in my life." The patient may lapse rapidly into coma. Those who survive 3 to 4 days may develop vasospasm, leading to fluctuating levels of consciousness and focal neurologic deficits. Survivors of the initial episode often rebleed within 21 days, and 50% of patients who rebleed will perish. Therapy is directed at preventing rebleeding by isolating the aneurysm from the circulation by surgical occlusion of the vascular stalk or neck that connects the sac of the aneurysm to the parent vessel. A metallic clip, positioned across the neck of the aneurysm, renders the aneurysm bloodless. Alternatively, an endovascular approach can be taken using a catheter inserted through the femoral artery and guided to the cerebral circulation, whereupon thin thrombogenic metallic coils are threaded into the aneurysm sac, causing the blood

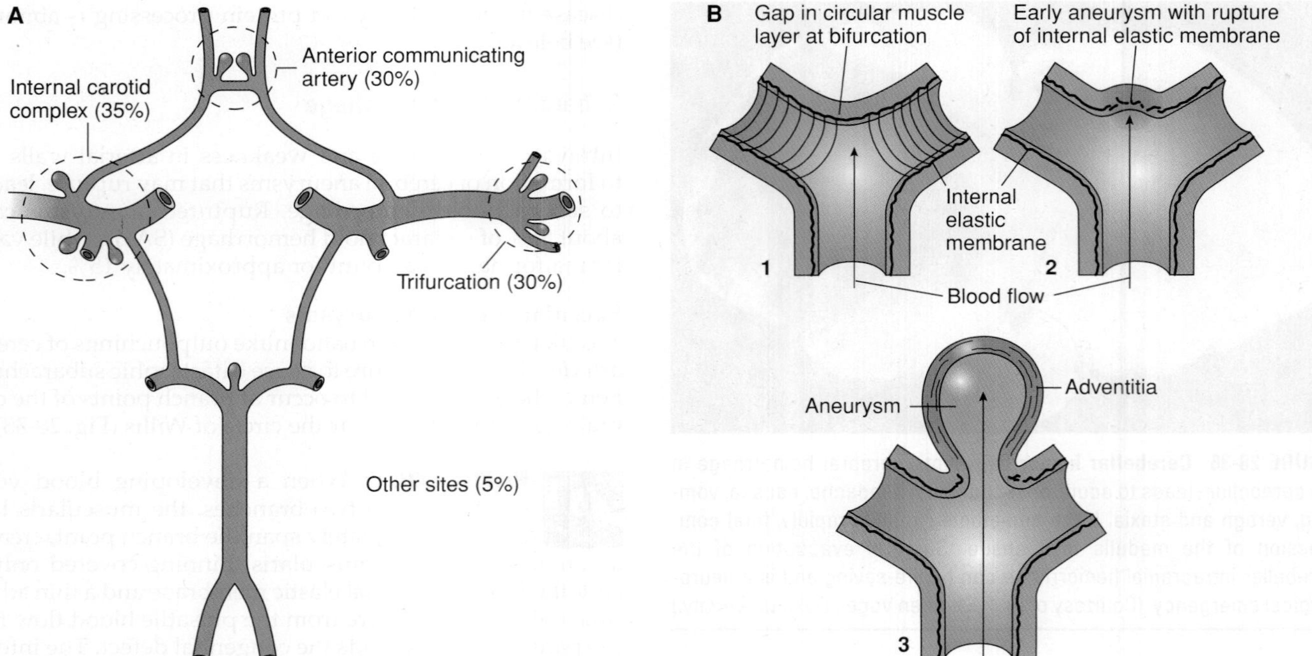

FIGURE 28-38. Pathophysiology of saccular aneurysm. A. The incidence of saccular aneurysms (berry aneurysms), which preferentially involve the proximal carotid tributaries, is shown. **B.** The lesion evolves as a result of blood under pressure acting on an early embryonic defect of the vascular wall at bifurcations.

in the aneurysm to clot. Aneurysmal coiling is less invasive than clipping and appears to be equally effective and durable.

At times, rather than rupturing, a saccular aneurysm enlarges to form a mass that may compress cranial nerves and produce palsies or impinge on parenchymal structures and induce neurologic symptoms. Classically, for example, a posterior communicating artery aneurysm may compress the third cranial nerve, leading to an isolated oculomotor nerve palsy with dilated pupil.

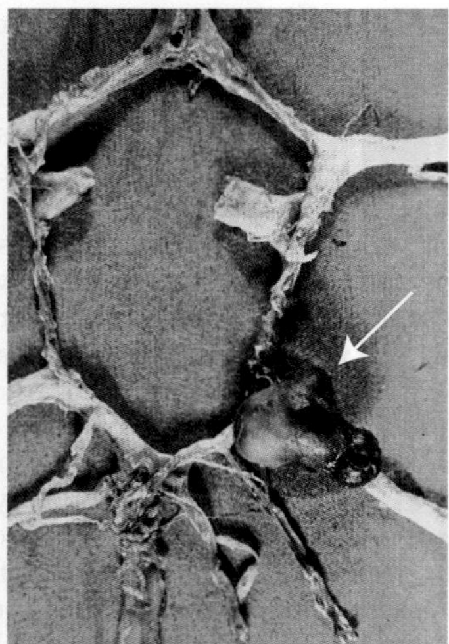

FIGURE 28-39. Berry aneurysm. A saccular aneurysm (*arrow*) arises from the posterior cerebral artery. The dark color is a result of subarachnoid blood from this aneurysm that ruptured.

Mycotic (Infectious) Aneurysms

Infections, either bacterial or fungal, of an arterial wall may result in a focal dilatation called a mycotic aneurysm. These usually result from septic emboli originating in an infected cardiac valve. The embolus usually flows through the carotid circulation and lodges in the vasa vasorum of a distal branch of the middle cerebral artery, where microbes proliferate, induce inflammation and destroy the affected arterial wall, leading to the formation of an aneurysm. Mycotic aneurysms occur in the distal cerebral circulation, in contrast to saccular aneurysms, which occur proximally. Rupture of the aneurysm can cause intracerebral or subarachnoid hemorrhage. Alternatively, microorganisms may be released and produce a cerebral abscess or meningitis.

Atherosclerotic Aneurysms

Aneurysms caused by atherosclerosis are localized mainly in major cerebral arteries (vertebral, basilar and internal carotid) that are favored sites of atherosclerosis. Fibrous replacement of the media and destruction of the internal elastic membrane weaken the arterial wall and cause aneurysmal dilation. As they enlarge, atherosclerotic aneurysms tend to be fusiform and elongate. An enlarging atherosclerotic aneurysm may compress cranial nerves or parenchyma, leading to focal neurologic deficits. For example, an atherosclerotic aneurysm of the basilar artery may encroach upon the cerebellopontine angle, leading to compression of the eighth cranial nerve, causing deafness and vertigo. Basilar aneurysms may compress cranial nerve V, leading to trigeminal neuralgia, or cranial nerve VII, and lead to hemifacial spasm. Atherosclerotic aneurysms rarely rupture leading to subarachnoid hemorrhage, but intraplaque hemorrhage may lead to vascular occlusion or a complicated plaque may lead to arterial thrombosis and ischemic stroke.

Vascular Malformations

Vascular malformations arise during embryogenesis but evolve as a result of angiogenesis, vascular remodeling and recruitment of vessels from normal parenchyma. They are named according to the nature of vascular channels in the malformation and the intervening neuroglial parenchyma that may be normal, gliotic or absent. Vascular malformations may bleed to cause subarachnoid or intraparenchymal hemorrhage or both. They may also irritate normal cerebral cortex, resulting in seizures, or they may divert blood flow from adjacent structures, leading to focal neurologic deficits.

ARTERIOVENOUS MALFORMATION: An arteriovenous malformation (AVM) is a tangle of arteries and veins of varying caliber and wall thickness separated by abnormal gliotic parenchyma (Fig. 28-40). The abnormal blood vessels form in embryogenesis as a result of a focal communication between cerebral arteries and veins without intervening capillaries. Resulting congeries of abnormal vessels are typically located in the cerebral cortex and the contiguous underlying white matter. The malformation enlarges with time and recruits vessels from adjacent tissue.

CLINICAL FEATURES: Seizure disorders result from irritation of neural tissue; focal neurologic deficits caused by vascular steal; and intracranial hemorrhages, usually subarachnoid or intracerebral, which commonly arise in the second or third decades. The hemorrhage is not usually catastrophic but may be recurring.

CAVERNOUS ANGIOMA: This congenital anomaly is less common than AVMs and consists of capacious, irregular, thin-walled vascular channels with no intervening neural parenchyma. Although most cavernous angiomas are asymptomatic, they may cause intracranial bleeding, seizures or focal neurologic disturbances. Cavernous angiomata may be multiple in 15% to 20% of cases. Many patients have autosomal dominant cerebral cavernous malformations (CCMs), the most common form of which, CCM1, results from *krit* mutations.

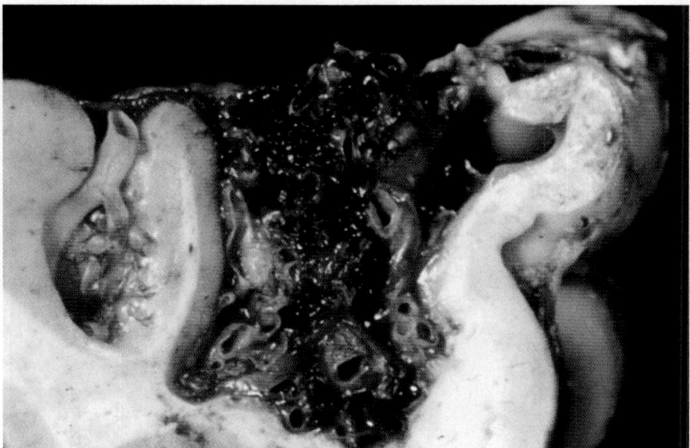

FIGURE 28-40. Arteriovenous malformation (AVM). A disorganized collection of arteries and veins is seen within the substance of the brain extending to the surface. AVMs may result in subarachnoid hemorrhage if they bleed on the surface or intraparenchymal hemorrhage if deeper vascular channels rupture. The hemorrhage is usually not as catastrophic as that seen in aneurysm subarachnoid hemorrhage or hypertensive intracerebral hemorrhage.

TELANGIECTASIA: This focal aggregate of uniformly dilated, thin-walled small capillary-sized vessels with normal intervening neural parenchyma may very rarely initiate seizures but infrequently ruptures. These are usually incidentally discovered during imaging for other conditions or at autopsy.

VENOUS ANGIOMA: This malformation consists of a solitary or a few enlarged veins residing in normal parenchyma. They are distributed randomly in the spinal cord or brain and are generally asymptomatic.

Infectious Disorders

Many of the infections of the nervous system are devastating or lethal if untreated. The clinical course may be swift and ferocious or indolent and progressive and can mimic many other disorders. Clinical vigilance, thorough diagnostic evaluation and emphatic therapeutic response are essential for effective management. The clinical context of nervous system infections is crucial. Patients' age, socioeconomic situation, risky behaviors, immune status and travel history are very important in assessing CNS infections. Acquired immunodeficiency syndrome (AIDS), iatrogenic immunocompromise, economic stagnation, environmental change, bioterrorism and transglobal travel and immigration continue to change the face of infectious diseases.

Assessment of CNS infections should take into account three issues: the location and extent of the infection, the nature of the host response to the infection and the inciting organism.

Empyema in the epidural or subdural space is usually related to trauma or spread from contiguous infection in the sinuses or ear. These infections are usually bacterial.

In leptomeningitis **(meningitis)** the inflammatory response and the majority of inciting organisms reside in the subarachnoid space floating in the CSF. The vigor of the inflammatory response may lead to parenchymal involvement including cerebral edema and vasculitis with thrombosis, hemorrhage or infarction. The war between host and organisms may involve the parenchyma, resulting in **cerebritis**. Long-term complications of meningitis include effusions, obstruction of CSF flow with hydrocephalus, and cranial neuropathies, particularly deafness from involvement of the eighth cranial nerve.

Cerebritis is a purulent parenchymal infection that is usually bacterial or fungal. Brain tissue is soft and soupy and the borders of the infection cannot be easily discerned. If a host can mount a containment response, a brain abscess is formed when the cerebritis is walled off. Abscesses have many polymorphonuclear leukocytes within a necrotic core surrounded by granulation tissue, a dense fibrovascular capsule and a gliotic rind.

Encephalitis, like cerebritis, is a parenchymal infection, but the term usually refers to viral infections with necrosis, perivascular lymphocytic cuffing and microglial nodules. Intranuclear or cytoplasmic viral inclusions may be seen, as may gliosis, demyelination and status spongiosus.

Different classes of infectious organisms produce distinctive host inflammatory responses, and while not absolute, the inflammatory reaction provides clues about the inciting organism. Bacterial infections tend to produce vigorous polymorphonuclear (purulent) responses. Fungi and mycobacterial infections elicit more indolent granulomatous reactions. In viral infections, a lymphocytic response predominates, while protozoa tend to incite a lymphoplasmacytic infiltrate. Metazoan parasites generate eosinophilic and lymphocytic inflammation. Host responses to prions entail no inflammation but rather vigorous gliosis.

Bacterial Infections Produce Inflammation in the Subarachnoid Space

This response, called **leptomeningitis,** is located between the pia and arachnoid layers of the meninges. The CSF filling this compartment is an excellent culture medium for most bacteria. The inflammatory response in the CSF to infections varies with the virulence of the organism and the tempo of the infection. Changes are detectable in CSF cellular constituents as well as glucose and protein concentrations. Organisms can sometimes be identified microscopically in the CSF and they can be definitively characterized by culture, antigenicity and in some cases polymerase chain reaction (PCR).

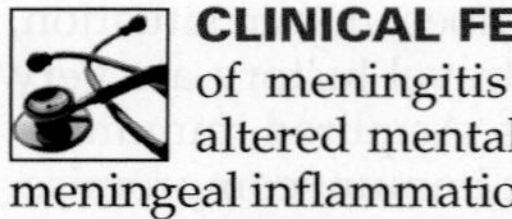

CLINICAL FEATURES: The signs and symptoms of meningitis include headache, vomiting, fever, altered mental status and seizures. Classic signs of meningeal inflammation include neck rigidity, knee pain with hip flexion (Kernig sign) and knee/hip flexion when the neck is flexed (Brudzinski sign). At the extremes of age—newborn and senescence—clinical manifestations can be more variable. A newborn may have autonomic instability and fragmentary seizures, while the elderly may have altered mental status without fever or headache.

Bacterial Meningitis

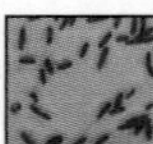

ETIOLOGIC FACTORS: Because most bacteria initiate purulent responses, the presence of neutrophils in the CSF is strong evidence of meningitis. In many instances CSF glucose will be decreased and the protein elevated. The causes of bacterial meningitis depend on the age of the patient. Gram-negative *Escherichia coli* and β-hemolytic *Streptococcus* sp. predominate in the neonate, *Haemophilus influenza* in early childhood in unvaccinated populations and *Neisseria meningitidis* in adolescence and early adult life. *Streptococcus pneumoniae* is the most common cause thereafter. Routes of entry to the intracranial vault are shown in Fig. 28-41A.

ESCHERICHIA COLI: In newborns, whose resistance to gram-negative bacteria has not yet fully developed, *E. coli* is a major cause of meningitis. Transplacental transfer of maternal immunoglobulin (Ig) G protects the newborn against many bacteria, but *E. coli* and similar gram-negative organisms require IgM for neutralization, and IgM does not cross the placenta. Thus, in infancy gram-negative organisms quickly produce purulent meningitis with a high mortality.

HAEMOPHILUS INFLUENZAE: Environmental exposure to *H. influenzae,* a gram-negative organism, is somewhat delayed, and the incidence of meningitis peaks between 3 months and 3 years. The incidence of *H. influenza* meningitis has decreased in recent years owing to widespread vaccination against the organism.

STREPTOCOCCUS PNEUMONIAE: *Pneumococcus* is the main cause of meningitis later in life. Patients with a history of basilar skull fracture with CSF leak have an unusually

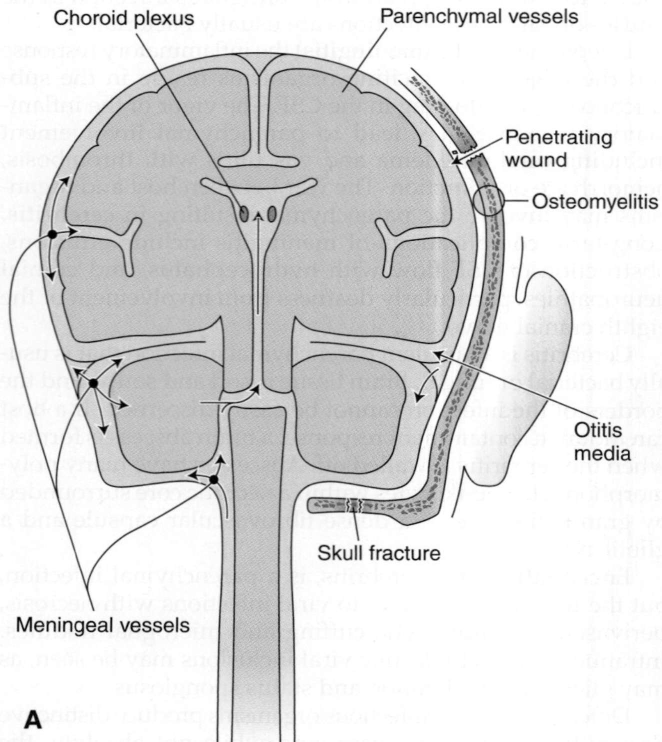

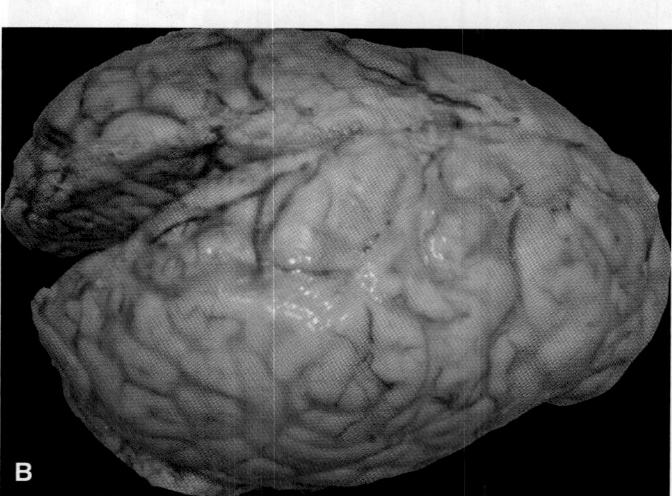

FIGURE 28-41. Purulent meningitis. A. Routes of entry of infectious organisms into the cranial cavity. B. A creamy exudate opacifies the leptomeninges in bacterial meningitis. The superficial veins are engorged and may develop thrombosis and the arteries on the surface of the brain may also develop thrombosis, leading to infarcts.

high incidence of pneumococcal meningitis, which often recurs after treatment. Alcoholics and patients who are asplenic have increased susceptibility to this form of meningitis.

NEISSERIA MENINGITIDIS: The meningococcus resides in the nasopharynx, and airborne transmission in crowded places (e.g., schools or barracks) causes "epidemic meningitis." Initially, bacteremia causes fever, malaise and petechial rash, but intravascular coagulopathy may cause lethal adrenal hemorrhage **(Waterhouse-Friderichsen syndrome).** Untreated meningococcal bacteremia is prone to initiate an acute fulminant meningitis. A polyvalent vaccine is available and is recommended for all young people; this vaccine is extremely effective but there are strains of *N. meningitidis* that are not covered by the vaccine. It is also important to recognize that vaccines are not widely available in many parts of the world. In 1996, the sub-Saharan "meningitis belt" of Africa experienced the largest epidemic of meningococcal meningitis in history, with over 250,000 cases and 25,000 deaths.

LISTERIA MONOCYTOGENES: Listerial meningitis is increasing in all ages and may account for up to 10% of cases of bacterial meningitis. The course is less fulminant than the other bacterial meningitides and CSF cellular responses may be lymphocyte predominant.

BACILLUS ANTHRACIS: Anthrax produces a fulminant hemorrhagic meningitis in up to 50% of cases. During the bioterrorism attacks in 2001, the index case was diagnosed as a result of the presence of large gram-positive rods in the CSF.

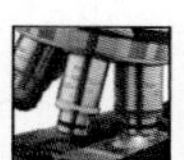

PATHOLOGY: In bacterial meningitis, an exudate of leukocytes and fibrin opacifies the arachnoid. The exudate may be mild and equivocal to the naked eye or prominent enough to obscure blood vessels. Purulent exudates are most conspicuous over the cerebral hemispheres (Fig. 28-41B) but may extend to the base of the brain and from intracranial to intraspinal and subarachnoid spaces. Although the pia is an effective barrier against the intraparenchymal spread of infection, cerebral abscesses rarely complicate meningitis. The pia forms sleeves around blood vessels that penetrate the brain **(Virchow-Robin spaces)** in continuity with the subarachnoid space. The subarachnoid space including the Virchow-Robin domain is usually packed with neutrophils and organisms (Fig. 28-42). A vigorous host response is essential to clear the infection, but significant vascular and neuropil damage results from cytotoxic substances such as free radicals and cytokines released by inflammatory cells. Also, those cells may compete with the brain for glucose; low CSF glucose in bacterial meningitis is caused more by consumption by inflammatory cells than by bacteria. In contemporary practice, corticosteroids are given with antibiotics to mitigate this host response–induced damage.

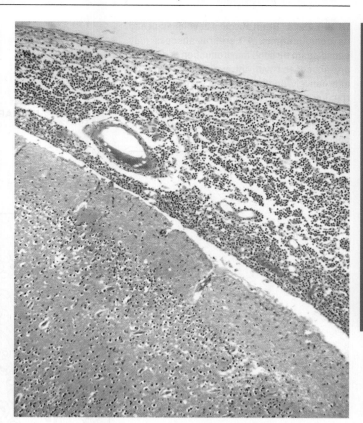

FIGURE 28-42. Bacterial meningitis. A microscopic section shows the accumulation of numerous neutrophils in the subarachnoid space.

Cerebral Abscess

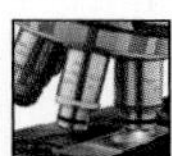

PATHOLOGY: A localized intraparenchymal abscess begins when bacteria or fungi lodge in the neuropil and incite an acute inflammatory and edematous reaction termed **cerebritis.** The tissue is soft and soupy, and within days, liquefactive necrosis causes an expanding mass that may threaten life by herniation or rupture into a ventricle (Fig. 28-43). Vigorous reactive astrogliosis is triggered, and fibroblasts make a rare appearance in the brain by invading from the cerebral microvasculature to encapsulate the nascent abscess. As the abscess matures over days to weeks, three layers surround a central core of purulent debris—an inner layer of vigorous granulation tissue where host and microbes engage in open warfare, a second layer of a dense meshwork of fibroblasts and collagen that forms a tough rind around the core and granulation tissue and finally a zone of intense astrogliosis, microglial activation and edema (Fig. 28-44). The granulation tissue layer lacks a blood-brain barrier and will leak contrast, causing a smooth ring of enhancement. If the abscess is not drained or treated with antibiotics, pressure builds within it that may extrude microbes into adjacent parenchyma to spawn "daughter" abscesses. Or, the abscess may rupture catastrophically into the ventricles. The bacteria that cause brain abscesses are often anaerobic or microaerophilic, and so may be difficult to culture. They often spread to the brain hematogenously from the heart or lungs; as showers of organisms repeatedly enter the circulation, abscesses are multiple in 15% to 20% of cases. Brain invasion may also be a result of contiguous spread from infected frontal or mastoid sinuses or neurosurgical wound infections.

Neurosyphilis

Syphilis is caused by a spirochete, *Treponema pallidum,* which by aligning its transmission with the carnal impulses of the host has assured its status as a centuries old scourge of mankind. The organism enters the bloodstream from the primary lesion, the chancre (see Chapter 9). Secondary syphilis is heralded by a maculopapular rash on the skin and mucous membranes. A few lymphocytes and plasma cells and increased protein in the CSF reflect entry

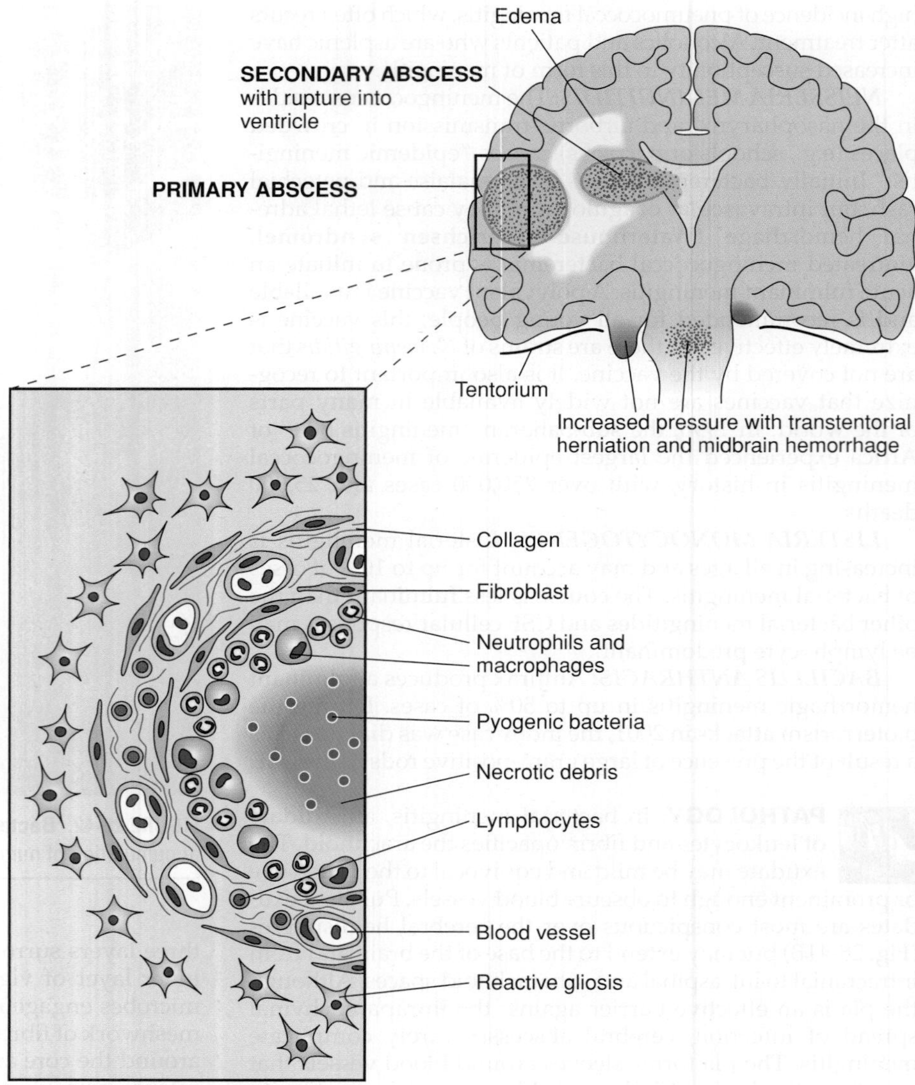

FIGURE 28-43. Brain abscess development and its complications. A cerebral abscess may cause death through the production of secondary abscesses with intraventricular rupture; alternatively, death may result from transtentorial herniation. The abscess consists of a necrotic purulent core, a layer of granulation tissue, a layer of fibrosis and, finally, the abscess is surrounded by gliosis.

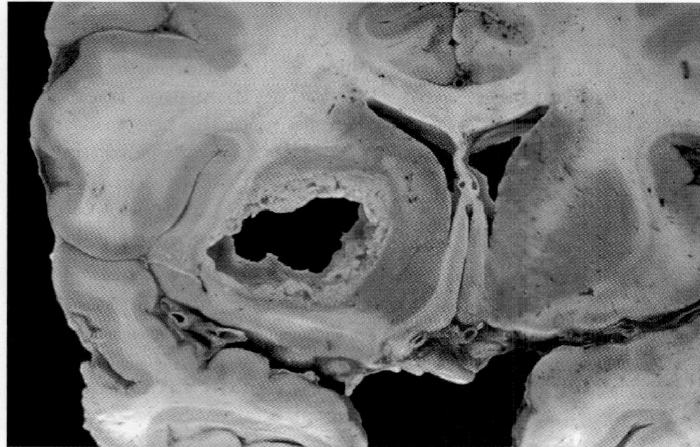

FIGURE 28-44. Cerebral abscess. A young man with bacterial endocarditis developed an abscess in the left basal ganglia.

of bloodborne spirochetes into the meninges, leading to a transient and often asymptomatic meningitis. The organisms usually do not survive for long and the CSF reverts to normal. On occasion, however, the transient spirochete initiates a meningeal fibroblastic response, accompanied by obliterative endarteritis that induces multiple small cerebral cortex or brainstem infarcts. The classical eponymic brainstem strokes described in the 18th and 19th centuries were largely the product of syphilitic obliterative endarteritis. Plasma cells, the inflammatory hallmark of syphilis, surround arterioles of the cerebral cortex in meningovascular syphilis (Fig. 28-45).

Tabes Dorsalis

Tabes dorsalis is impairment of spinal dorsal column function, as manifested by loss of joint position sense and fine touch (Fig. 28-46). The dorsal nerve roots proximal to dorsal root ganglia are met by a conical sleeve of arachnoid filled with CSF, which can be the site of syphilitic inflammation.

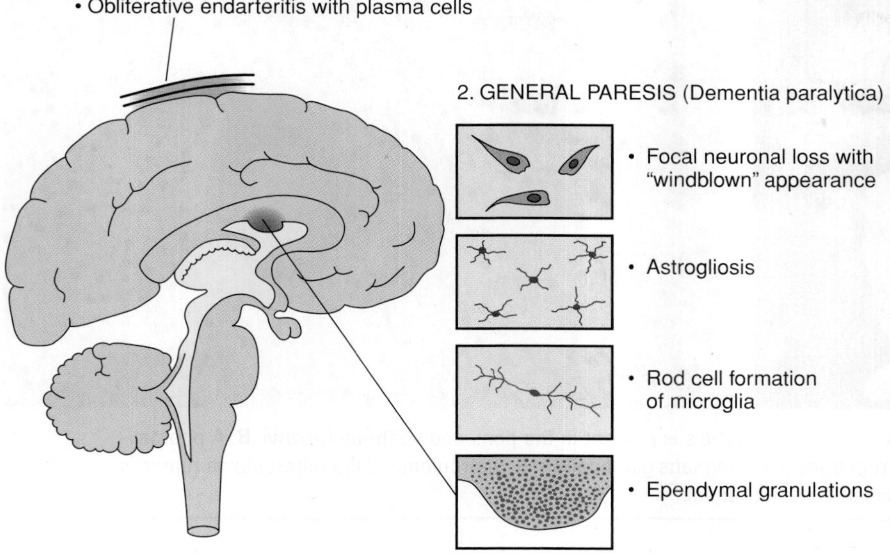

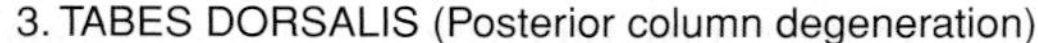

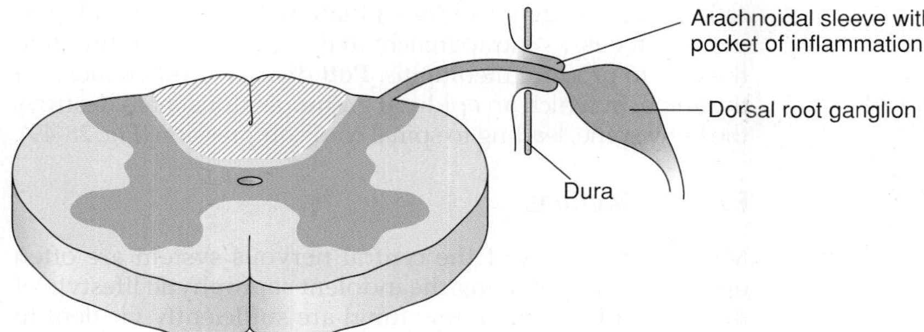

FIGURE 28-45. Involvement of the central nervous system in syphilis. Hallmarks of neurosyphilis are meningovascular inflammation leading to pachymeningitis and strokes caused by obliterative endarteritis tabes dorsalis caused by inflammation of posterior roots and meninges, and intraparenchymal involvement leading to dementia.

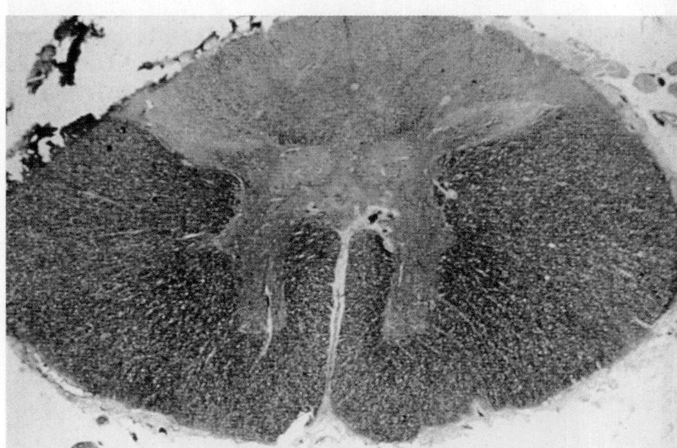

FIGURE 28-46. Tabes dorsalis. The spinal cord of a patient with tertiary syphilis displays posterior column degeneration (sliver impregnation stain). The patient would be unable to walk without visual cues because he has lost proprioception.

Fibrous tissue triggered by the inflammation constricts nerve roots, causing axonal (wallerian) degeneration. Since axons that course cephalad in the posterior columns do not synapse with intramedullary neurons, unlike spinothalamic afferents, wallerian degeneration initiated in the dorsal spinal nerves extends the length of the posterior fasciculi. The patient loses position sense in the legs and comes to rely on visual cues for the position of his or her feet and legs in space. In darkness or with his or her eyes closed, the patient becomes unsteady and may even fall. This inability to remain standing with eyes closed is called a positive Romberg sign and reflects severe posterior column dysfunction.

Luetic Dementia

T. pallidum may reside in a latent state in the brain for decades. The spirochetes replicate sluggishly and escape eradication, resulting in dementia and psychosis years after the initial infection. The morphologic features include focal loss of cortical neurons, disfigurement of the residual nerve cells ("wind-blown appearance"), marked gliosis and conversion of microglia into elongated forms encrusted with iron ("rod cells") associated with nodular ependymitis.

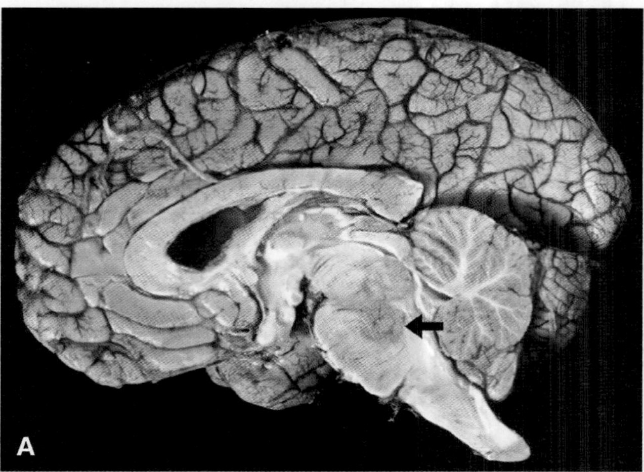

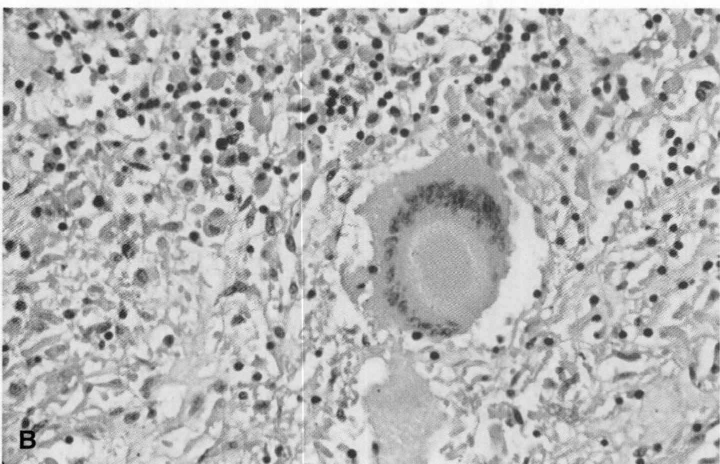

FIGURE 28-47. Tuberculoma. A. A focus of caseous necrosis is present in the pons and midbrain (*arrow*). **B.** A photomicrograph shows caseous necrosis, macrophages and Langhans giant cells in a tuberculoma. If the tuberculoma ruptures into the cerebrospinal fluid, tuberculous meningitis will ensue.

Mycobacterial and Fungal Nervous System Infections Elicit Granulomatous Responses

PATHOLOGY: Mycobacterial and fungal infections progress more slowly than bacterial infections. Multinucleate giant cells are admixed with lymphocytes and plasma cells. The exudate tends to accumulate at the base of the brain, surrounding the brainstem, rather than over the convexities as in bacterial meningitis.

CLINICAL FEATURES: This chronic basilar meningitis may block CSF flow through the foramina of Magendie and Luschka, leading to hydrocephalus, headache, nausea and vomiting. Multiple cranial nerve palsies can occur as cranial nerves emerging from the brainstem traverse the exudate.

Tuberculous Meningitis and Tuberculomas

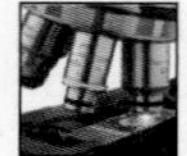

PATHOLOGY: Tuberculous meningitis is a chronic infection inciting a granulomatous host response with multinucleated giant cells and lymphocytes surrounding areas of caseous necrosis (Fig. 28-47). Like neurosyphilis, mycobacterial meningitis may lead to meningeal fibrosis, communicating hydrocephalus and arteritis that may result in infarcts. As tuberculous meningitis has a predilection for the base of the brain, these infarcts are usually in the distribution of the penetrating striate and brainstem arteries. Untreated tuberculous meningitis is usually fatal in 4 to 6 weeks, but may progress faster in immunocompromised individuals. Parenchymal tuberculosis produces **tuberculomas,** individual masses with central caseous necrosis surrounded by granulomatous inflammation (Fig. 28-48). In parts of the world where tuberculosis is endemic, mycobacterial granulomas are the most common cause of brain masses. In childhood, these granulomas tend to be located in the posterior fossa, which is also the most common site of childhood brain tumors. Confluent tuberculomas are seen in miliary tuberculous infections. Tuberculous meningitis usually reflects hematogenous dissemination from an initial pulmonary focus, as intraparenchymal granulomas rupture into the CSF to produce meningitis. **Pott disease** is tuberculosis of the spine, in which an epidural granulomatous mass destroys the bony spine, leading to spinal cord compression (Fig. 28-49).

Fungal Infections

Mycotic infections of the central nervous system are often opportunistic, reflecting the indolent saprophytic lifestyle of these organisms, but a few fungi are sufficiently virulent to produce disease in immunocompetent individuals. Fungi invading tissue may be round to oval, often budding, yeast

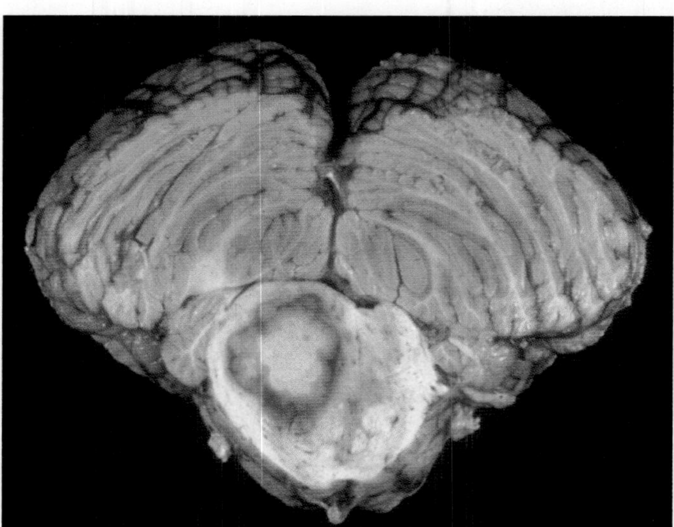

FIGURE 28-48. Tuberculoma. A focus of caseous necrosis is present in the pons and midbrain. In parts of the world where tuberculosis is endemic, tuberculomas are among the most common brain masses seen. (Courtesy of Dr. F. Stephen Vogel, Duke University.)

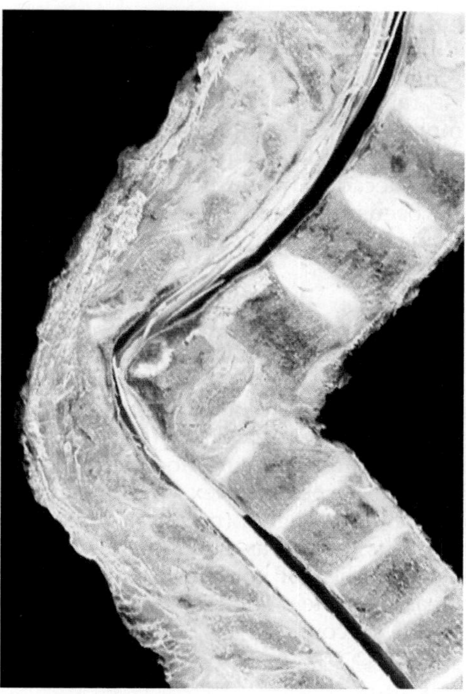

FIGURE 28-49. Pott disease. Tuberculosis involving the spinal column leads to slow vertebral collapse and acute angulation of the spine ("gibbus" deformity). Spinal cord compression may result, with myelopathic findings. (Courtesy of Dr. F. Stephen Vogel, Duke University.)

forms or branching hyphae. In some infections yeast and hyphae are both seen in infected tissues. This morphologic dichotomy allows tentative identification of fungi in tissue sections, but ultimate identification requires antigenic, PCR or culture confirmation.

Cryptococcus

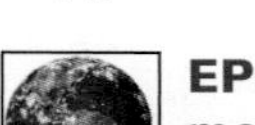

EPIDEMIOLOGY: Cryptococcal meningitis is the most common fungal meningitis. In most instances, *Cryptococcus* acts opportunistically in immunocompromised patients, but it can rarely establish meningitis in an immunologically competent host. *Cryptococcus neoformans* enters the host by inhalation, with birds being the major reservoir. Their inhaled fungus-laden excreta initiate a lung infection that may remain confined to the lungs, but may disseminate to involve other organs including the brain.

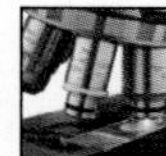

PATHOLOGY: Meningeal responses to *C. neoformans* are typically granulomatous, with infectious foci appearing as discrete white nodules, a millimeter or so in diameter. *C. neoformans* may remain confined to the subarachnoid space, but in some cases infection spreads to the brain parenchyma. The gelatinous fungal capsule appears clear and glistening, so that microabscesses resemble soap bubbles and are sometimes called "soap bubble" abscesses (Fig. 28-50).

The organisms are abundant particularly in the Virchow-Robin spaces. An occasional multinucleated giant cell, sometimes with phagocytosed organisms, is accompanied by scant epithelioid cells and a few lymphocytes. The organisms are encapsulated, budding yeast forms that are large by fungal standards (5 to 15 μ). They have an external gelatinous capsule, seen as a clear halo around the organism, which can be highlighted by mixing a drop of contaminated CSF with India ink (Fig. 28-51). This capsule shields the organism from the host's immune response, accounting for the usually feeble inflammatory reaction. The capsule sheds specific antigens that can be detected in the CSF by the latex cryptococcal antigen test.

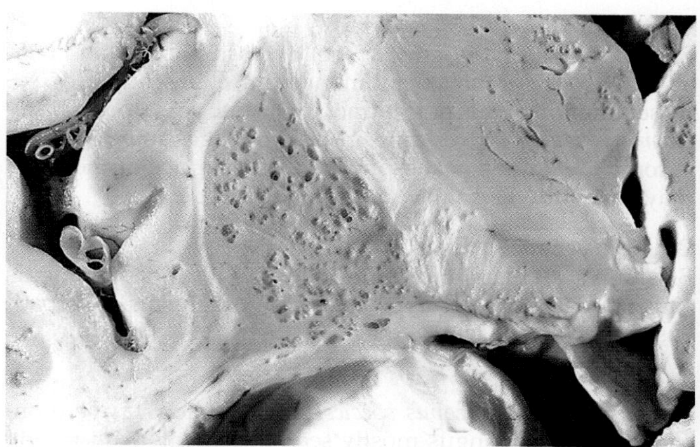

FIGURE 28-50. Cryptococcal "soap bubble" abscesses. The encapsulated organisms occur in great abundance in the Virchow-Robin space and in microabscesses within the parenchyma. The microbial capsule imparts a glistening clear appearance to these collections that has been likened to soap bubbles. (Courtesy of Dr. F. Stephen Vogel, Duke University.)

Coccidioidomycosis

Coccidioidomycosis results from a tissue yeast form of *Coccidioides immitis* that is endemic in arid regions of the Southwest and San Joaquin Valley in California. Initial pulmonary infection is usually asymptomatic and rarely spreads. A combination of suppurative and granulomatous inflammation is seen sometimes, with an arteritis that may be complicated by infarction. The organism appears in tissue as an eye-catching refractile endosporulating spherule.

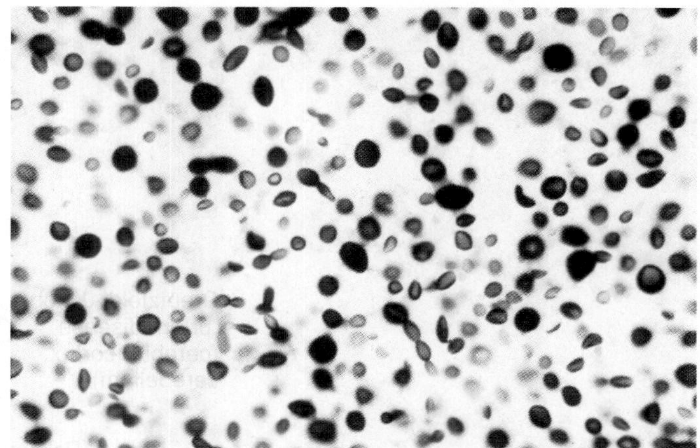

FIGURE 28-51. Cryptococcal meningitis. The cryptococcal organisms vary in size (5 to 15 microns in diameter), placing them among the largest of the yeast-form fungi (GMS stain). They reproduce by budding. (Courtesy of Dr. F. Stephen Vogel, Duke University.)

Histoplasmosis

Histoplasmosis is endemic in the Mississippi basin and usually causes asymptomatic pulmonary infections, but rare CNS dissemination of this tiny, intracytoplasmic yeast form (*Histoplasma capsulatum*) residing in macrophages may occur. A chronic meningitis ensues in which the surface of the brain may be studded by small granulomata.

Blastomycosis

Blastomycosis is an uncommon cause of mycotic meningitis caused by *Blastomyces dermatitidis*. The organisms are broad-based budding yeasts.

Mucormycosis

Mucormycosis (*Rhizopus species*) is an angioinvasive, non-septate, hyphal fungus mostly seen in patients with poorly controlled diabetes or immunocompromised patients. The large vessels at the skull base, orbit and neck are subject to invasion with occlusion and distal infarction. Black nasal mucosa indicating mucosal infarction is sometimes seen and can be used for diagnosis.

Aspergillosis

Aspergillus is an angiocentric septated hyphal fungus (*Aspergillus fumigatus*) seen mainly in immunocompromised hosts. Vascular involvement produces multiple gray necrotic abscesses within the parenchyma. The lung is the primary site of infection, but the brain is the second most commonly involved organ.

Candidiasis

Candidiasis results from infection by a ubiquitous opportunistic fungus (*Candida albicans*) that shows both yeast and pseudohyphae morphology in infected tissues. This infection is common in immunocompromised patients, producing numerous microabscesses. Systemic involvement is the rule, and in large hospital-based autopsy series this is the most common systemic fungal infection.

Viral Infections

The manifestations of viral infections of the CNS are remarkably diverse, ranging from non–life-threatening viral meningitis to more ominous viral encephalitis affecting the parenchyma. These diseases may unfold over a period of hours or span decades. In addition to producing infections, viruses have been implicated in some autoimmune and neurodegenerative diseases.

Viral Meningitis

Infection of the meninges may be the most common viral disease of the CNS, but, unlike bacterial meningitis, it is usually benign and resolves without sequelae. The most common causative agents are enteroviruses (e.g., coxsackievirus B, echovirus), but mumps, lymphocytic choriomeningitis, Epstein-Barr and herpes simplex viruses cause many sporadic cases. Viral meningitis (mainly a disease of children and young adults) begins as a sudden febrile illness with a severe headache. The CSF contains excess lymphocytes and a slight increase in protein but, unlike bacterial meningitis, no decrease in CSF glucose.

Viral Encephalitis

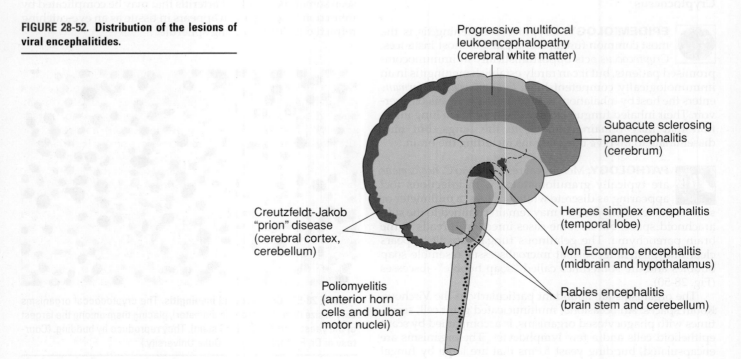

The manifestations of viral infections of CNS parenchyma are clinically and pathologically heterogeneous (Fig. 28-52). For example, poliomyelitis affects spinal and brainstem motor neurons, while herpes simplex targets the temporal lobes. Subacute sclerosing panencephalitis afflicts the gray matter, while progressive multifocal leukoencephalopathy (PML) is a white matter disorder. The mechanisms of viral tropism may reflect specific binding of viruses to sites on the plasma membranes of CNS cells, the ability of viruses to remain latent, or selective replication in specific intracellular microenvironments. Viruses may exploit axonal transport to travel to

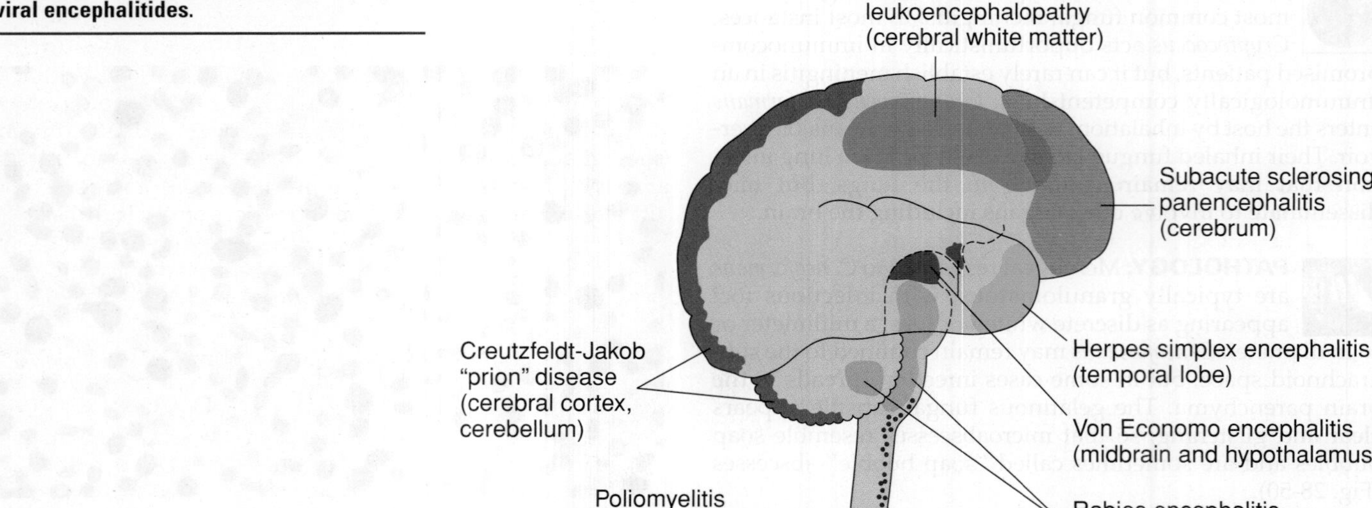

FIGURE 28-52. Distribution of the lesions of viral encephalitides.

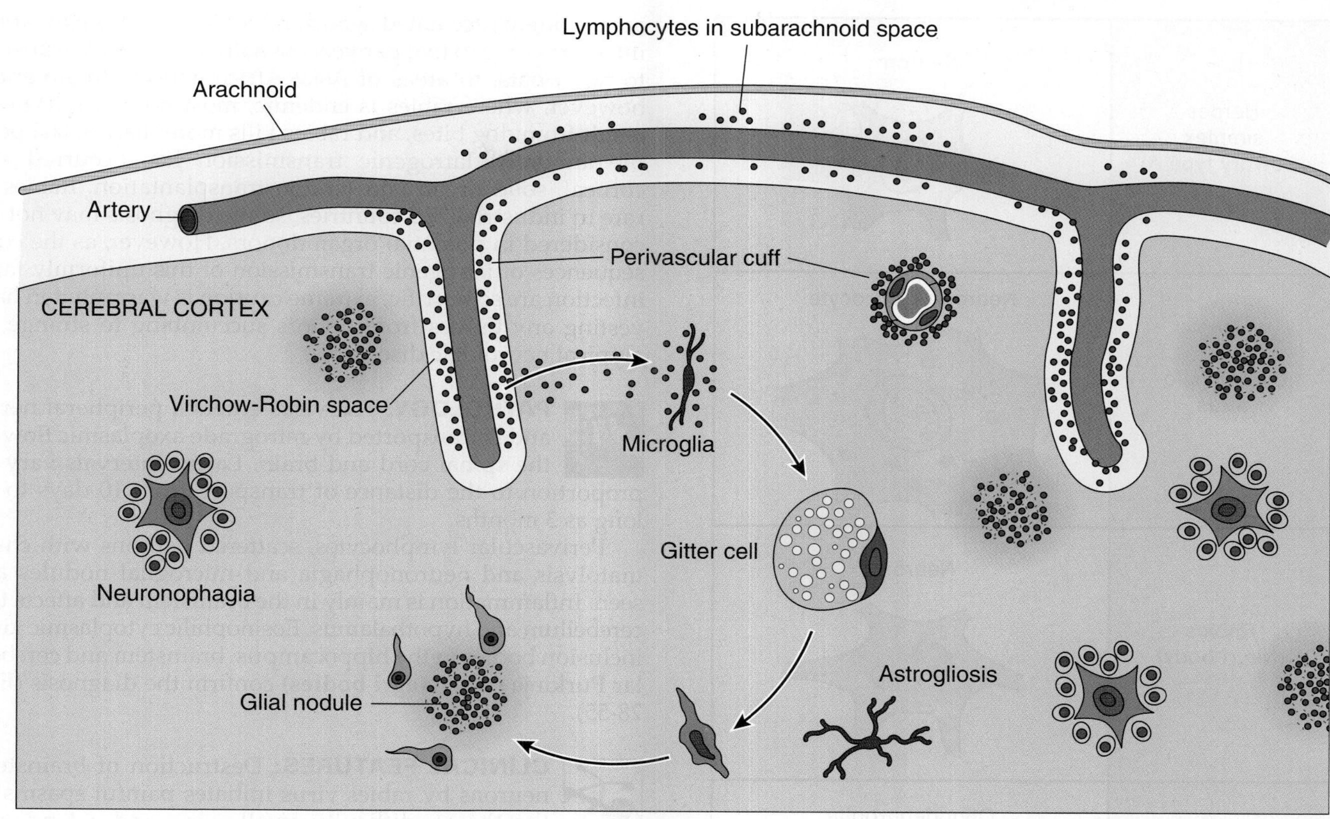

FIGURE 28-53. The lesions of viral encephalitis.

sites far distant from their point of entry, as exemplified by rabies and herpesviruses.

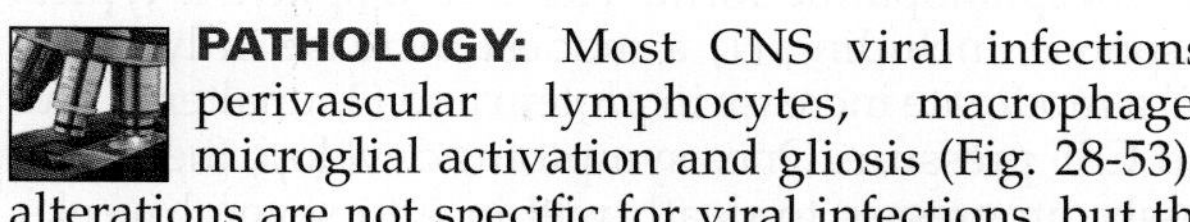

PATHOLOGY: Most CNS viral infections elicit perivascular lymphocytes, macrophage and microglial activation and gliosis (Fig. 28-53). These alterations are not specific for viral infections, but the presence of viral inclusions provides compelling evidence of viral infection (Fig. 28-54). Unfortunately, inclusion bodies are not seen in all viral infections. Viral particles also may be seen by electron microscopy, but in situ hybridization, PCR and immunochemistry are now more often used to establish a diagnosis.

CLINICAL FEATURES: The onset of most viral encephalitides is usually abrupt. The more specific neurologic deficits (e.g., paralysis of poliomyelitis or difficulty in swallowing in rabies) reflect the localization of the infection. Although most encephalitides run a rapid course, the tempo can vary. For example, the clinical course of subacute sclerosing panencephalitis may last years. Herpes simplex and varicella-zoster viruses may reside latently in sensory ganglia for years, only to be reactivated decades after initial infection.

Poliomyelitis

The term **poliomyelitis** describes any inflammation of the gray matter of the spinal cord, but in common usage it implies an infection by poliovirus. The organism is one of the enteroviruses, which are small, nonenveloped, single-stranded RNA viruses.

Historical evidence suggests that poliomyelitis has occurred in epidemics since antiquity. Affected people shed large amounts of virus in their stools, and spread is by the fecal–oral route.

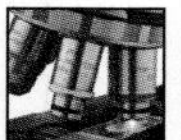

PATHOLOGY: Binding sites on motor neurons permit the virus to enter these cells and replicate. Infected cells may undergo chromatolysis, after which they are phagocytosed by macrophages (neuronophagia). Initial inflammatory responses transiently include neutrophils, which are followed by lymphocytes that surround blood vessels in the spinal cord and brainstem. The motor cortex usually shows no inflammation but may contain microglial nodules, which are focal collections of microglia and lymphocytes. Host immune responses to the virus, although limited, may halt progression of clinical disease. Sections of spinal cord in cases of healed poliomyelitis show a paucity of neurons, with secondary degeneration of corresponding ventral roots and peripheral nerves.

CLINICAL FEATURES: After infection with poliovirus, nonspecific symptoms such as fever, malaise and headache are followed in several days by signs of meningitis and then by paralysis. In severe cases, the muscles of the neck, trunk and all four limbs may be rendered powerless, and paralysis of the respiratory muscles may become life-threatening. Patients with milder cases exhibit an asymmetric and patchy paralysis, most prominently in the lower limbs.

Improvement begins in about a week, and only some of the muscles affected at the outset may remain permanently

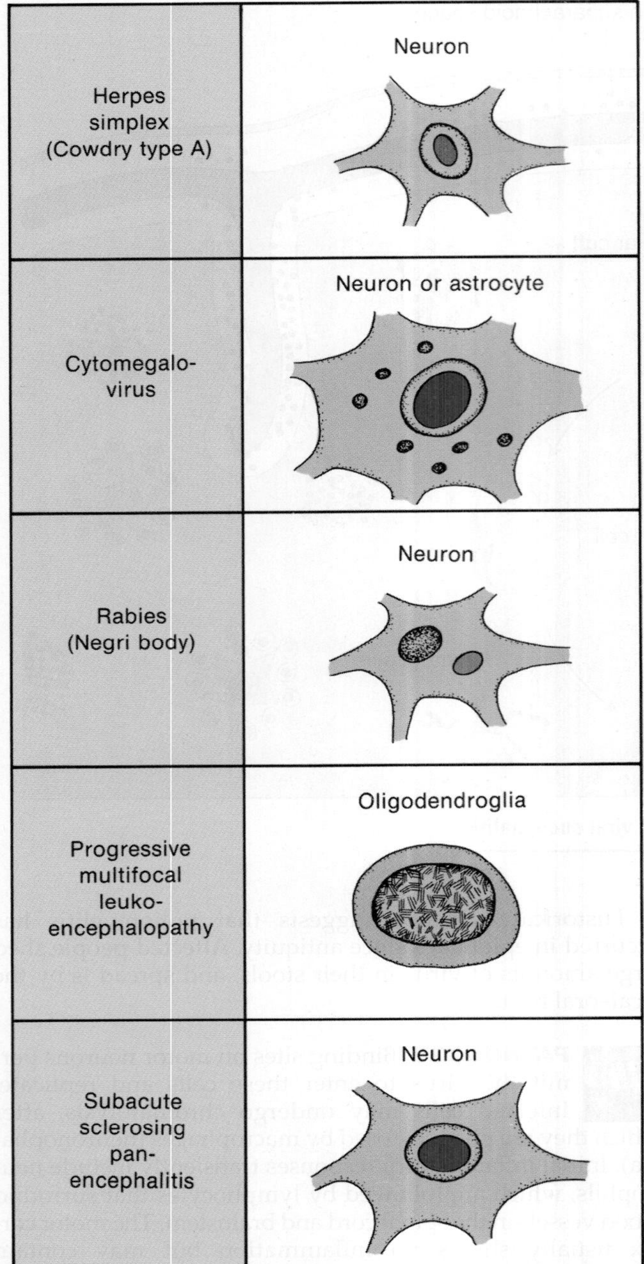

FIGURE 28-54. Inclusion bodies in viral encephalitides.

paralyzed. Mortality varies from 5% to 25%, with death usually resulting from respiratory failure. The development in the 1950s of effective vaccines against poliovirus has largely eliminated the disease in most of the world.

Rabies

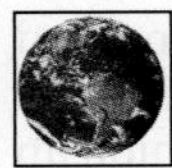

EPIDEMIOLOGY: Rabies is an encephalitis caused by an enveloped, single-stranded RNA virus of the rhabdovirus group. Dogs, wolves, foxes and skunks are the main reservoirs, but bats and domestic animals, including cattle, goats and swine, may also carry the disease. Rabies virus is transmitted to humans via contaminated saliva, introduced by a bite. In the United States, where dogs are routinely vaccinated against rabies, the few human rabies infections (one to five per year) usually result from exposure to rabid bats. In areas of Asia, Africa and South America, however, where rabies is endemic, most human infections result from dog bites, and rabies kills more than 50,000 people annually. Iatrogenic transmission has occurred via corneal, solid organ and tendon transplantation. Rabies is rare in industrialized countries, so the diagnosis may not be considered in potential organ donors. However, as the consequences of iatrogenic transmission of this uniformly fatal infection are so horrific, extreme caution is warranted in harvesting any tissues from donors succumbing to strange or atypical neurologic disorders.

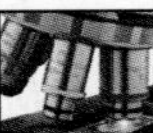

PATHOLOGY: The virus enters a peripheral nerve and is transported by retrograde axoplasmic flow to the spinal cord and brain. Latent intervals vary in proportion to the distance of transport, from 10 days to as long as 3 months.

Perivascular lymphocytes, scattered neurons with chromatolysis and neuronophagia and microglial nodules are seen. Inflammation is mainly in the brainstem and affects the cerebellum and hypothalamus. Eosinophilic cytoplasmic viral inclusion bodies in the hippocampus, brainstem and cerebellar Purkinje cells **(Negri bodies)** confirm the diagnosis (Fig. 28-55).

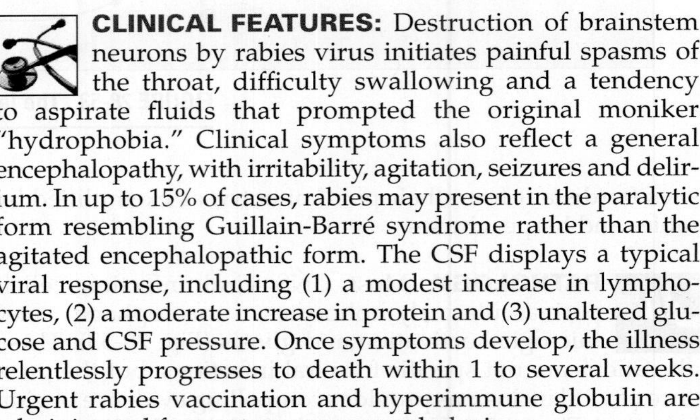

CLINICAL FEATURES: Destruction of brainstem neurons by rabies virus initiates painful spasms of the throat, difficulty swallowing and a tendency to aspirate fluids that prompted the original moniker "hydrophobia." Clinical symptoms also reflect a general encephalopathy, with irritability, agitation, seizures and delirium. In up to 15% of cases, rabies may present in the paralytic form resembling Guillain-Barré syndrome rather than the agitated encephalopathic form. The CSF displays a typical viral response, including (1) a modest increase in lymphocytes, (2) a moderate increase in protein and (3) unaltered glucose and CSF pressure. Once symptoms develop, the illness relentlessly progresses to death within 1 to several weeks. Urgent rabies vaccination and hyperimmune globulin are administered for postexposure prophylaxis.

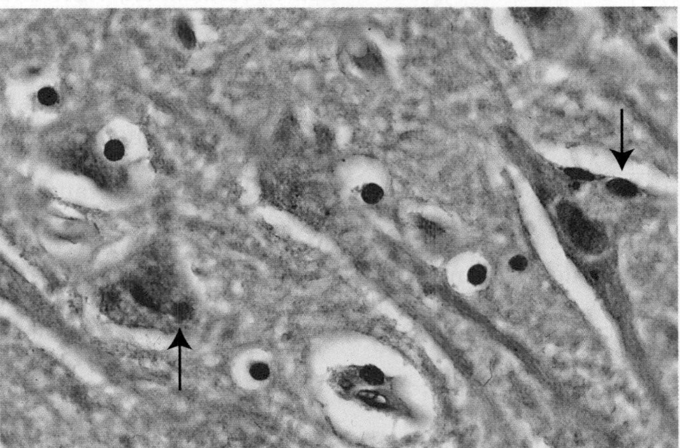

FIGURE 28-55. Negri body. Rabies encephalitis is characterized by round, eosinophilic cytoplasmic inclusions that resemble an erythrocyte (*arrows*).

Herpes Viruses

Herpes viruses include herpes simplex (types 1 and 2), varicella-zoster virus, cytomegalovirus, Epstein-Barr virus and simian B virus.

HERPES SIMPLEX TYPE 1: Herpes simplex virus type 1 (HSV-1) is largely responsible for "cold sores." The region of the vesicular lesion on the lip is innervated by sensory axons from the trigeminal ganglion. HSV-1 may reside latently in the trigeminal ganglion, where it proliferates during periods of stress and is transmitted centrifugally through the nerve trunk to the lip. Reactivation and spread of HSV-1 to the CNS results in herpes encephalitis, which is the most common sporadic (i.e., nonepidemic) viral encephalitis.

PATHOLOGY: This encephalitis localizes mainly in one or both temporal lobes. Herpes encephalitis is a fulminant infection. The temporal lobes become swollen, hemorrhagic and necrotic (Fig. 28-56). Inflammation is predominantly lymphocytic, with perivascular cuffing (Fig. 28-57). The small arteries and arterioles become hemorrhagic and edematous. Intranuclear eosinophilic inclusions, usually surrounded by a halo (Cowdry A), occur in both neurons and glial cells (Fig. 28-58). Detection of viral proteins by immunohistochemistry is diagnostically reliable. The diagnosis is often made by PCR of CSF and viral culture.

HERPES SIMPLEX TYPE 2: In women, herpes simplex virus type 2 (HSV-2) initiates a vesicular lesion on the vulva **(genital herpes),** coupled with a latent infection in the pelvic ganglia. Newborns acquire HSV-2 during passage through the birth canal and thereafter may develop a fulminant encephalitis causing extensive liquefactive necrosis in the cerebrum and cerebellum.

VARICELLA-ZOSTER: Herpes zoster virus (HZV) causes childhood exanthem "chicken pox" whereupon HZV may become latent in dorsal root ganglia. In later life, particularly after age 60 years, the virus may reactivate and be transported down the sensory axon to the skin, leading to an exquisitely painful cutaneous vesicular eruption called "shingles" in the dermatomal distribution of the dorsal root ganglion harboring the virus. The infection elicits only mild inflammation and rarely spreads to the CNS. Intranuclear Cowdry A inclusions like those of herpes simplex are present. Rarely, HZV may also cause a fatal encephalitis, and the virus has been implicated in isolated giant cell arteritis of the CNS leading to stroke. "Shingles" reflects reemergence of latent infection by the HZV and may be the initial manifestation of

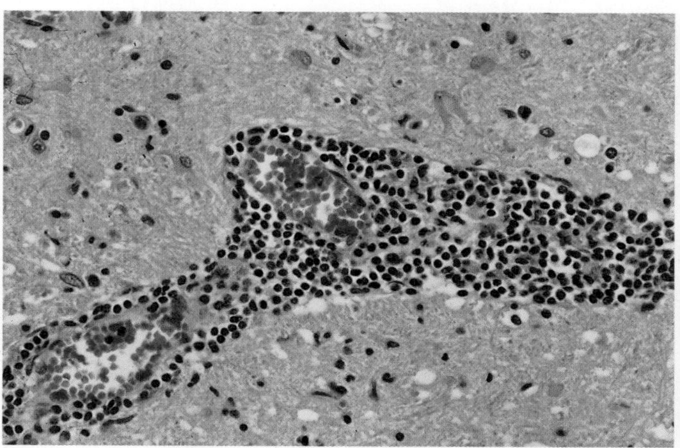

FIGURE 28-57. Herpes simplex encephalitis. Microscopically, the specimen exhibits pronounced perivascular lymphocytic inflammation. This finding indicates that active inflammation is present, but is not etiologically specific.

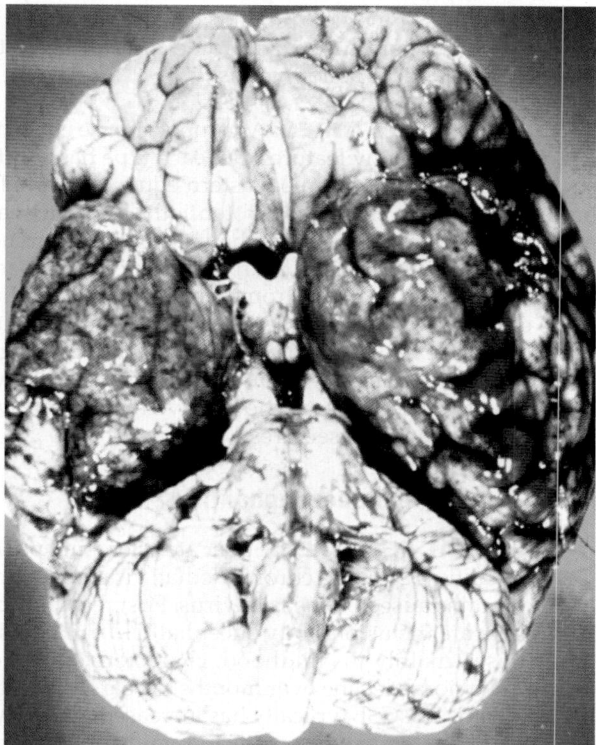

FIGURE 28-56. Herpes simplex encephalitis. Grossly, there are swollen hemorrhagic necrotic temporal lobes. The patient may experience memory disturbances and complex partial seizures as a result of this selective involvement of the temporal lobes. (Courtesy of Dr. F. Stephen Vogel, Duke University.)

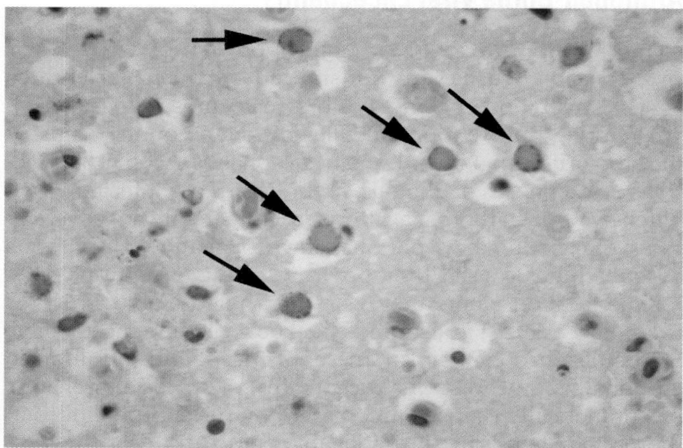

FIGURE 28-58. Herpes simplex encephalitis. The infected neurons display intranuclear, eosinophilic viral inclusions (Cowdry A inclusions) that fill the nuclei (*arrows*). The presence of these findings is extremely valuable in guiding diagnostic evaluation as a limited number of viruses produce Cowdry A inclusions.

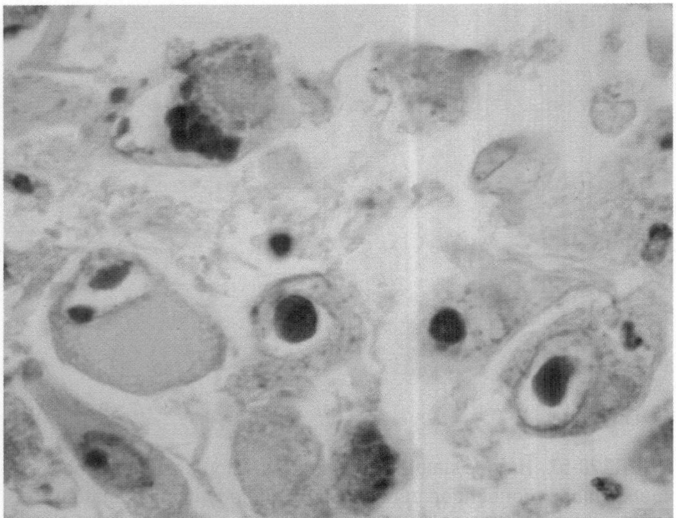

FIGURE 28-59. Cytomegalovirus ependymitis. Ependymal cells display large intranuclear inclusions in grotesquely enlarged infected cells.

immune dysfunction. The pain and vesicular eruption can be severe and disabling, but an HZV vaccine is now available and is recommended for individuals over 60 years of age.

CYTOMEGALOVIRUS: Cytomegalovirus (CMV) crosses the placenta to induce encephalitis in utero. Lesions in the embryonic CNS are characterized by periventricular necrosis and calcification. Because of the proximity of these lesions to the third ventricle and the aqueduct, they may induce obstructive hydrocephalus. CMV is a "TORCH" complex agent (**t**oxoplasmosis, **o**ther [congenital syphilis and viruses], **r**ubella, **c**ytomegalovirus and **h**erpes simplex virus) of newborns. In adults, CMV initiates encephalitis in immunocompromised hosts. Eosinophilic viral inclusions are seen in the nuclei and cytoplasm of astrocytes and neurons, most conspicuously in enlarged nuclei, where they are sharply defined and surrounded by a halo (Fig. 28-59).

Arthropod-Borne Viral Encephalitis

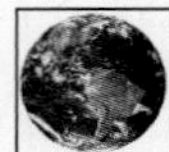

EPIDEMIOLOGY: Arthropod-borne viruses, or **arboviruses,** are transmitted between vertebrates by blood-sucking vectors (e.g., mosquitoes, ticks). Togaviridae, Bunyaviridae and Flaviviridae account for most of the arboviruses that cause human encephalitis. Arbovirus infections are zoonoses of animals, and humans are infected when bitten by virus-harboring arthropods. Humans are not generally reservoirs, nor do they continue viral propagation. The various encephalitides caused by arboviruses are named principally for the location where they were first noted (Table 28-1); for example, Eastern, Western and Venezuelan equine encephalitis; St. Louis encephalitis; Japanese B encephalitis; California encephalitis; and West Nile encephalitis. West Nile encephalitis has numerically eclipsed all other arbovirus encephalitides in the United States since its initial appearance in 1999.

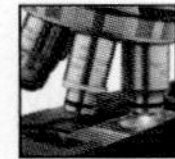

PATHOLOGY: The lesions of the several arbovirus encephalitides resemble each other, and vary from mild meningitis with scattered lymphocytes to severe inflammation of gray matter, thrombosis of small blood vessels and prominent necrosis. There are no inclusions in infected neurons. In necrotic foci, neuronophagia is evident, and if the patient survives, demyelination and gliosis may develop. West Nile encephalitis has a propensity for spinal cord and may produce a syndrome clinically indistinguishable from classical poliomyelitis.

Table 28-1

Insect-Borne Viral Encephalitis

Virus	Insect Vector	Distribution
St. Louis encephalitis	Mosquito	North and South America
Western equine encephalitis	Mosquito	North and South America
Venezuelan equine encephalitis	Mosquito	North and South America
Eastern equine encephalitis	Mosquito	North America
California encephalitis	Mosquito	North America
Murray Valley encephalitis	Mosquito	Australia, New Papua
Japanese B encephalitis	Mosquito	Eastern and southeastern Asia
Tick-borne encephalitis	Tick	Eastern Europe, Scandinavia
West Nile encephalitis	Mosquito	Global

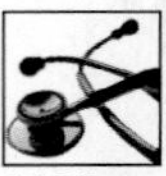

CLINICAL FEATURES: Arthropod-borne encephalitides share many features, but each type has a different course. For example, Eastern equine encephalitis is commonly a more fulminant potentially lethal disease, whereas Venezuelan equine encephalitis tends to pursue a more benign course. Mild cases of arbovirus encephalitis may entail only a mild flulike syndrome and may not be diagnosed as encephalitis. In more severe cases, onset is abrupt, often with high fever, headache, vomiting and meningeal signs, followed by lethargy and coma. Death is more likely at the extremes of age, and those who survive may be left with cognitive impairment and seizures.

Subacute Sclerosing Panencephalitis

CLINICAL FEATURES: Subacute sclerosing panencephalitis (SSPE) is a chronic, lethal, viral infection of the brain caused by measles virus. First recognized in 1933 as "subacute inclusion-body encephalitis," SSPE has an insidious onset, mainly in childhood, characterized by cognitive and behavioral decline over months to years, ultimately leading to death. The CSF typically has increased antibody to measles virus. The course is protracted, and inflammation occurs primarily in cerebral gray matter. In adults, SSPE may follow a more rapid course.

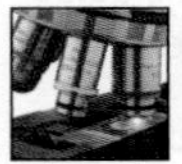

PATHOLOGY: SSPE is a consequence of infection with the measles virus, and most patients have a history of measles. SSPE develops 6 to 8 years after the

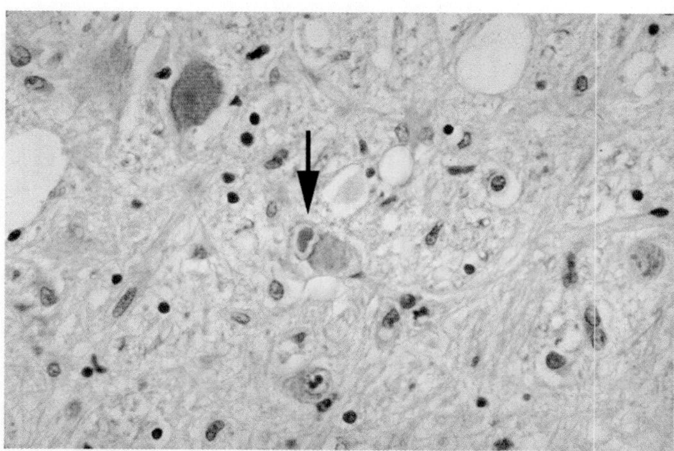

FIGURE 28-60. Subacute sclerosing panencephalitis. The brain shows loss of myelin and reactive gliosis. An intranuclear inclusion is present (*arrow*).

initial infection and is caused by a measles virus with defective expression of the viral M (Matrix) protein. Intranuclear inclusions are prominent in neurons and oligodendroglia, as are marked gliosis in affected gray and white matter, patchy loss of myelin and ubiquitous perivascular lymphocytes and macrophages (Fig. 28-60). The intranuclear inclusions are basophilic, rimmed by a prominent halo. Affected neurons may contain neurofibrillary tangles.

Progressive Multifocal Leukoencephalopathy

Progressive multifocal leukoencephalopathy (PML) is an increasingly common infectious demyelinating disease caused by a ubiquitous polyoma virus that infects oligodendrocytes, leading to cytolysis and patchy multifocal demyelination. Astrocytes are also infected, but instead of dying, they show extreme pleomorphism.

ETIOLOGIC FACTORS: The JC virus is a polyoma virus, closely related to simian virus 40 (SV40). The "JC" derives from the initials of the first patient in whom the disease was described. This virus is present in over 50% of people where it resides in a latent state in the bone marrow after asymptomatic acquisition earlier in life. If the host becomes immunocompromised, viremia ensues with specific viral strains having a propensity for neurovirulence.

CLINICAL FEATURES: The disease occurs mostly in immunocompromised patients and manifests as dementia, weakness, visual loss and ataxia, usually leading to death within 6 months. PML is a terminal complication in immunosuppressed patients, such as those treated for cancer or lupus erythematosus, organ transplant recipients and people with AIDS. PML may complicate the use of drugs that inhibit T-cell adherence to endothelial cells as a treatment of immunologic disorders. Natalizumab is such a drug and was temporarily withdrawn from the market after the appearance of PML in patients treated for multiple sclerosis or Crohn disease. The drug has been reintroduced to clinical use with stringent guidelines.

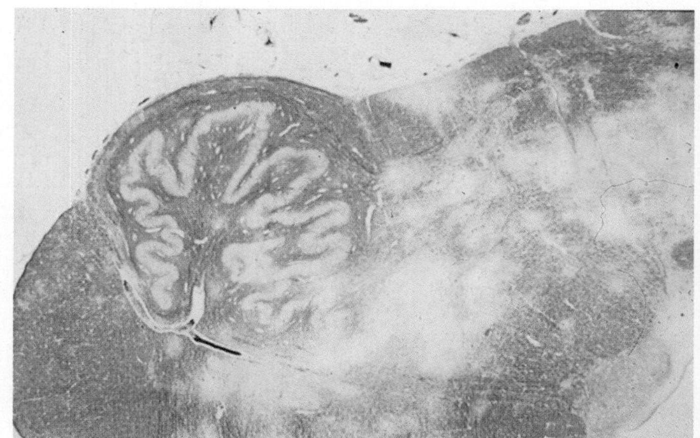

FIGURE 28-61. Progressive multifocal leukoencephalopathy. A Luxol fast blue stain of the medulla reveals severe patchy loss of myelin.

PATHOLOGY: The typical lesions of PML appear as widely scattered discrete foci of demyelination near the gray–white junction in the cerebral hemispheres and brainstem (Fig. 28-61). They are characteristically spherical and several millimeters in diameter with a central area largely devoid of myelin. Axons are retained, a few oligodendrocytes are seen and the lesion is infiltrated by macrophages. At the edge of the demyelinated area, there are oligodendrocytes with enlarged nuclei occupied by homogeneously dense, hyperchromatic, "ground-glass" intranuclear inclusions lacking a halo. Electron microscopy discloses intranuclear, crystalline arrays of spherical virions, 35 to 40 nm in diameter (Fig. 28-62). Infected astrocytes are highly pleomorphic and may contain multiple irregular nuclei with dense chromatin (Fig. 28-63). These astrocytes can be so pleomorphic that a diagnosis of astrocytoma may be entertained.

Human Immunodeficiency Virus

Neurologic disorders are common in AIDS. Some patients have opportunistic CNS infections, such as toxoplasmosis,

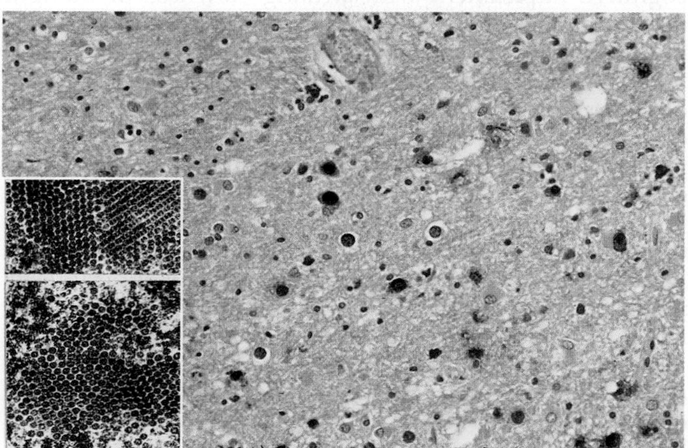

FIGURE 28-62. Progressive multifocal leukoencephalopathy. An immunohistochemical stain for JC virus demonstrates numerous infected oligodendroglia in the white matter. By electron microscopy, there are intranuclear paracrystalline arrays of viral particles (*insets*).

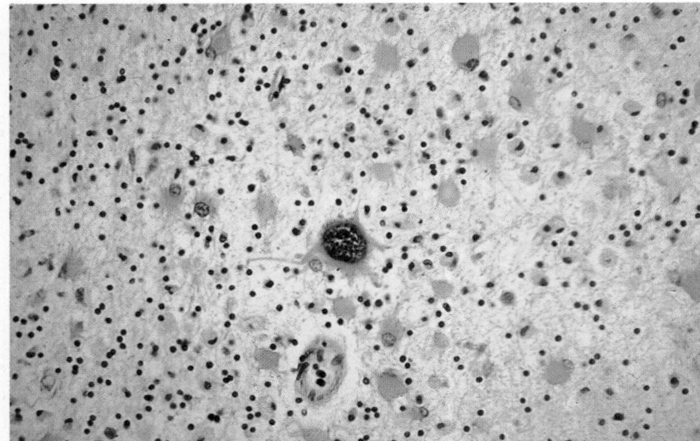

FIGURE 28-63. Progressive multifocal leukoencephalopathy (PML). A bizarre astrocyte is present (*center*) and may mimic neoplasia. The presence of macrophages and ground-glass inclusions should direct diagnostic consideration away from neoplasia and toward PML.

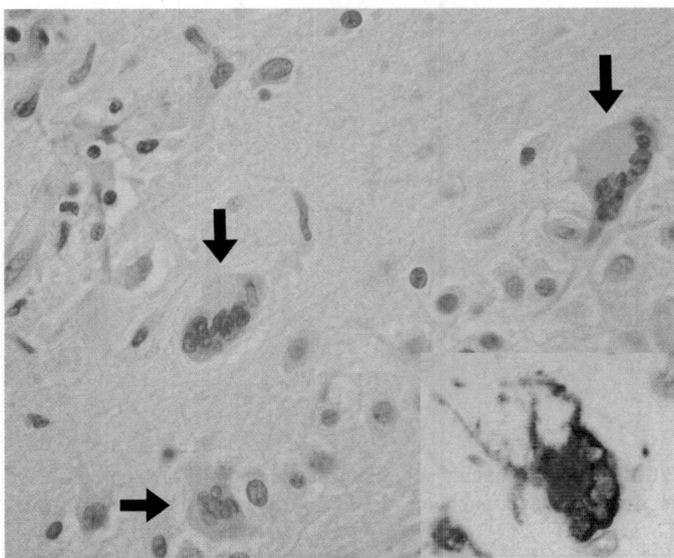

FIGURE 28-64. Human immunodeficiency virus (HIV) encephalitis or encephalopathy (HIVE). Multinucleated giant cells (*arrows*) often in a perivascular location are characteristic of HIV encephalitis. *Inset.* Immunohistochemical stain for HIV anti-p24.

cytomegalovirus, herpes simplex or PML, or have EBV-driven primary CNS lymphoma (PCNSL). In AIDS, cryptococcal meningitis is the most common fungal meningitis, toxoplasmosis is the most common intracranial mass and PCNSL is the most common neoplasm. These are indicator diseases of AIDS; that is, the occurrence of any of these in any patient should trigger diagnostic consideration of underlying AIDS. There are many other opportunistic nervous system infections that may complicate AIDS, and it is important to remember that the clinical presentation may be more fulminant or atypical than in immunocompetent individuals.

HIV Encephalopathy

Many AIDS patients have diffuse encephalopathy that is attributable to active CNS infection by the human immunodeficiency virus type 1 (HIV-1) retrovirus itself, variously called HIV encephalopathy (HIVE) or HIV-associated neurologic disease (HAND). Dementia, once the most common clinical manifestation of HIVE, may range from mild to severe cognitive impairment with striking slowness of thought (bradyphrenia) often accompanied by marked bradykinesis mimicking Parkinson disease. CNS macrophages and microglial cells are productively infected by HIV-1. Infection of neurons and astrocytes is probably not clinically significant. Rather, these cells are injured indirectly by cytokines or neurotoxic viral proteins, which elicit oxidant-mediated cell injury.

The advent of highly active antiretroviral therapy (HAART) has dramatically extended the life span and quality of life of AIDS patients, including reducing opportunistic infections and primary CNS lymphoma. HAART drugs largely do not cross the blood-brain barrier and, since the virus enters the CNS via infected blood monocytes very soon after it enters the body, HAART has not altered the incidence of HIVE. Rather, frank dementia has become less common, but a combination of sensory, motor and other defects causing minor cognitive motor disease (MCMD) affects as many as 30% of HIV-1–positive patients. As HIV-1–positive people age, this prevalence is augmented by an additional approximately 5% of the HIV-1–positive population yearly. Initiation of HAART may also be complicated by immune reconstitution inflammatory syndrome (IRIS). In the brain, IRIS may lead to potentially lethal cerebral edema and exacerbation of focal symptoms and may contribute to fulminant HIVE.

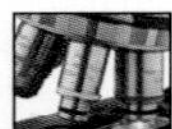

PATHOLOGY: HIVE is characterized by mild cerebral atrophy, dilation of the lateral ventricles and slight prominence of gyri and sulci. Histologic changes are usually in the subcortical gray and white matter. Multinucleated giant cells of the monocyte/macrophage lineage are associated with microglial nodules (Fig. 28-64). In addition, myelin pallor, reflecting diffuse demyelination, intense astrogliosis and loss of neurons, is common (Fig. 28-65).

Vacuolar myelopathy is another disorder attributed to HIV infection, although it is less frequent than encephalopathy. It is characterized by marked vacuolation of the posterior and lateral columns, principally at the thoracic level of the spinal cord. Ataxia and spastic paraparesis dominate the clinical presentation.

Parasitic Central Nervous System Infections Include Both Protozoan and Metazoan Pathogens

Protozoan Infections

- **Toxoplasmosis** is a ubiquitous protozoan to which most of us have protective immunity. Immunocompromised patients lose the ability to limit proliferation of these organisms. Small commalike tachyzoites and large polyorganismal cysts (bradyzoites) are seen in association with chronic inflammation, tissue necrosis and vasculitis. Toxoplasmosis is the most frequent cause of multiple intracranial masses in AIDS patients (Fig. 28-66).
- ***Naegleria* spp.** cause primary amoebic meningoencephalitis, a fulminant and rapidly fatal meningitis with diffuse brain swelling. Brain inoculation occurs via the nasal route through the cribriform plate in people who swim in stagnant

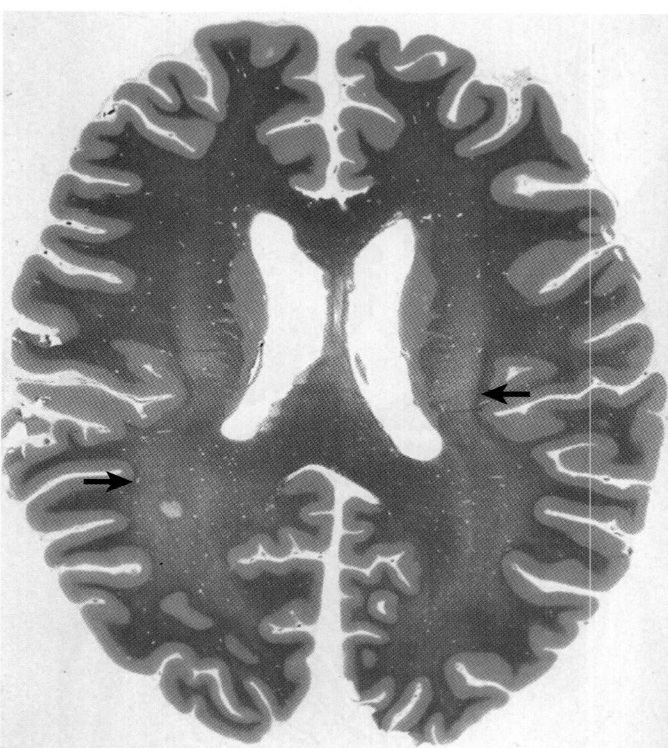

FIGURE 28-65. Human immunodeficiency virus (HIV) encephalitis or encephalopathy (HIVE). An axial whole brain section in HIVE shows symmetric myelin pallor (*arrows*) caused by HIVE. Demyelination caused by progressive multifocal leukoencephalopathy would be less symmetric and patchy. (Courtesy of Dr. F. Stephen Vogel, Duke University.)

warm freshwater ponds. *Naegleria* trophozoites resemble macrophages (Fig. 28-67).

- *Acanthamoeba* produces granulomatous amoebic encephalitis, a subacute, usually fatal illness characterized by multiple granulomatous abscesses. This condition is usually seen in immunocompromised hosts.
- ***Entamoeba histolytica*** leads to amebic brain abscess from spread from a gastrointestinal or hepatic locus. Amebae in tissue sections can be difficult to distinguish from foamy macrophages.
- **CNS malaria** is most commonly caused by *Plasmodium falciparum*. During attacks of cerebral malaria, the CSF shows elevated protein and pressure but pleocytosis is uncommon. In fatal cases, the brain is diffusely swollen and may be otherwise unremarkable, but one may see microinfarcts with gliosis (Dürck granulomata) in white matter or numerous small hemorrhages. Both the infarcts and microhemorrhages may be caused by obstruction of blood flow in small vessels as a result of parasitemia. Severity of cerebral malaria is also related to tumor necrosis factor release from the host immune system.

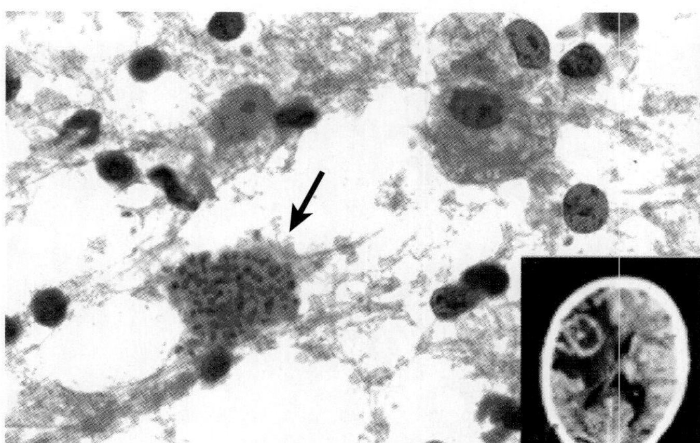

FIGURE 28-66. Toxoplasmosis in a human immunodeficiency virus (HIV) patient. This previously asymptomatic patient presented with an irregularly enhancing mass with surrounding edema that was initially thought to be a high-grade neoplasm. *Toxoplasma gondii* bradyzoites (*arrow*) are present in a necrotic inflammatory background. Toxoplasmosis is the most common mass lesion in patients with AIDS and is an indicator disease of HIV infection.

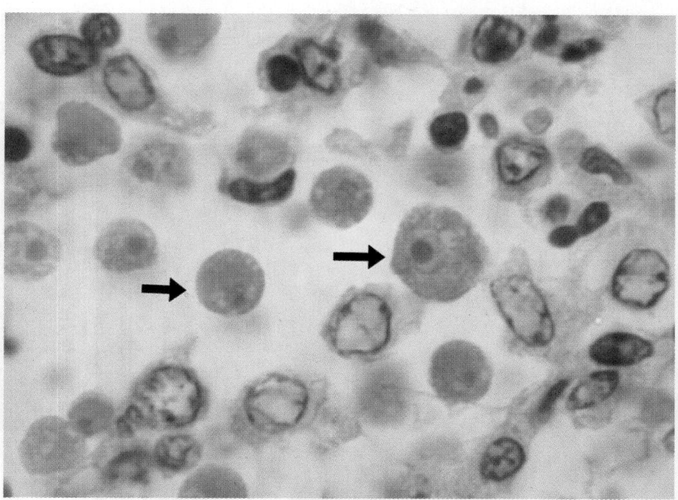

FIGURE 28-67. *Naegleria* meningoencephalitis. Amebic organisms (*arrows*) resemble macrophages but have much more prominent nucleoli.

Metazoan Infections of the Nervous System

- **Cysticercosis** caused by infection by *Taenia solium*, the pig tapeworm, may lead to multiple parasitic cysts up to 1 cm in the parenchyma, intraventricularly or in the basal cisterns. The intraparenchymal disease usually becomes symptomatic when the organism dies and is recognized immunologically by the host (Fig. 28-68). A peculiar form of this infection is racemose neurocysticercosis, in which grapelike clusters and sheets of worm tissues are made, without a fully formed worm. Racemose cysticercosis can be regarded as invertebrate tissue culture in the CSF and is resistant to therapy that is effective against intact parasites. Treatment of neurocysticercosis may lead to massive cerebral edema caused by massive host immune responses to the suddenly necrotic metazoan tissue. From a global health perspective, neurocysticercosis is one of the most common causes of epilepsy and intracranial mass lesions.
- **Echinococcosis** is caused by *Taenia echinococcus* or *Echinococcus granulosus*, the dog tapeworm, and produces cerebral cysts that are usually solitary and may be huge, in contrast to the smaller multiple cysts of cysticercosis.

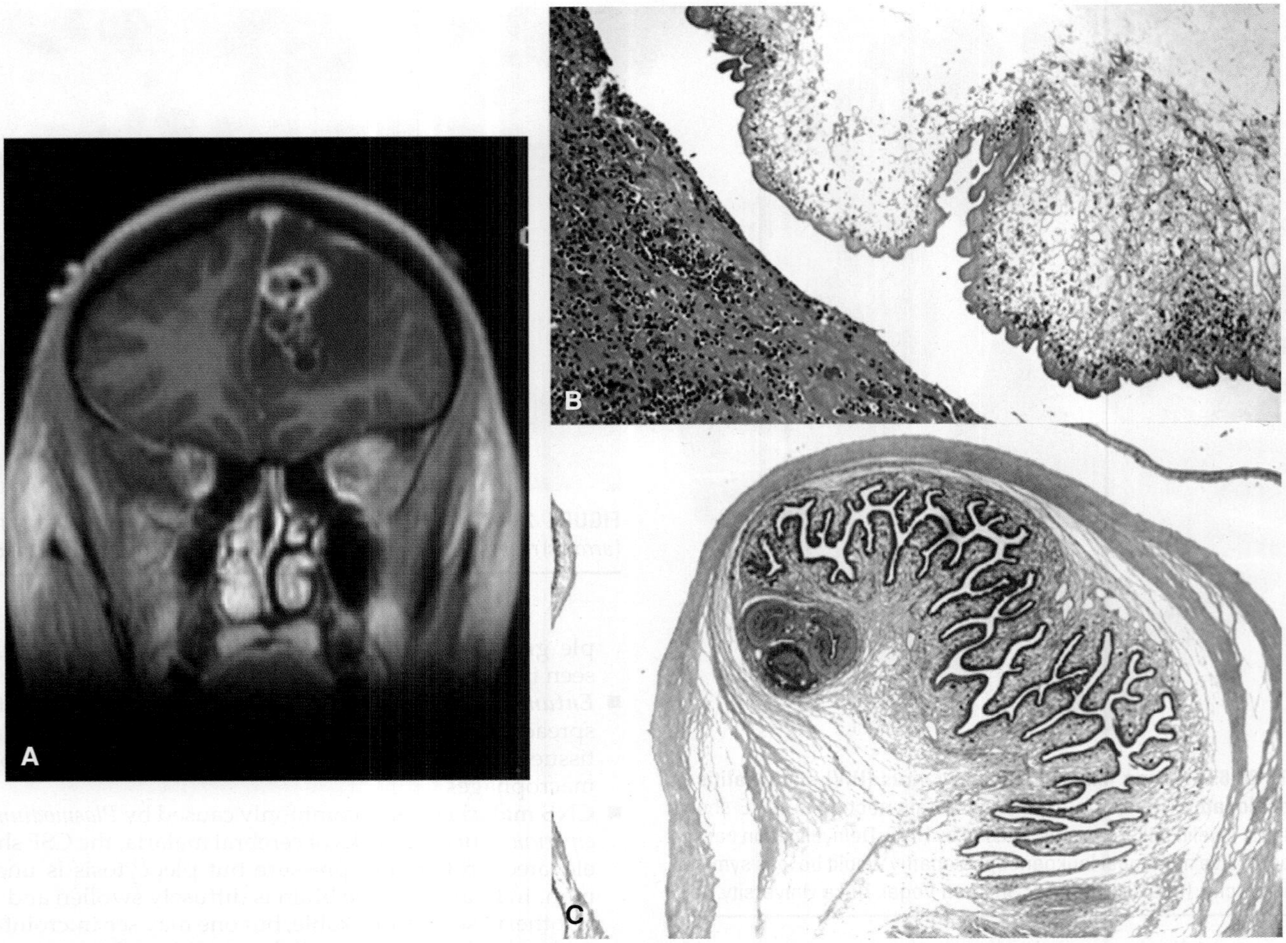

FIGURE 28-68. Neurocysticercosis. A. Radiographic appearance. Brain involvement by *Taenia solium* may result in solitary or multiple contrast-enhancing masses with surrounding edema. **B.** As the parasite begins to die and is detected by the host immune response, the lesions may become symptomatic. The corrugated cuticular surface forms an eosinophilic interface with inflamed adjacent brain. **C.** At low magnification the worm scolex and gastrointestinal tract can sometimes be seen.

The brain lesion is frequently accompanied by hepatic cysts.

- **Trichinosis** results from *Trichinella spiralis* infection of skeletal and cardiac muscle, producing an acute eosinophilic myositis during the invasive phase. Larvae may then die and calcify, producing fibrosis and low-grade inflammation. The infection may rarely encroach on the CNS, producing lymphocytic-eosinophilic aseptic meningitis.

Prion Diseases (Spongiform Encephalopathies) Are Transmissible Neurodegenerative Diseases Caused by Particles Containing Modified Proteins

Prion diseases are characterized clinically by rapidly progressive ataxia and dementia and pathologically by accumulations of fibrillar or insoluble prion proteins, degeneration of neurons and vacuolization termed **spongiform encephalopathy** (Fig. 28-69). The spongiform encephalopathies are biologically remarkable because the causative infectious entity is

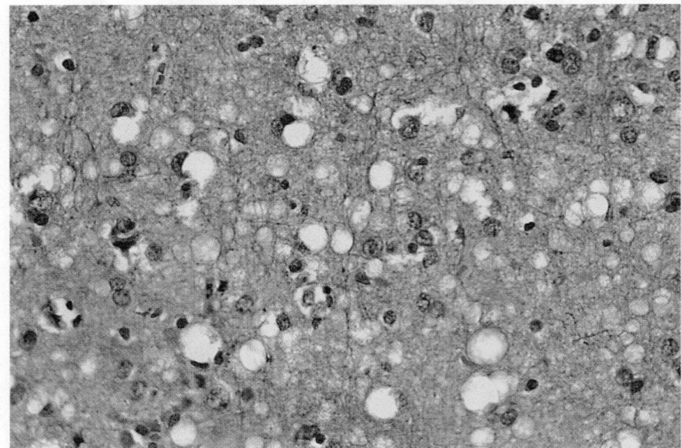

FIGURE 28-69. Creutzfeldt-Jakob disease. Spongiform degeneration of the gray matter is characterized by individual and clustered vacuoles, with no evidence of inflammation. (Courtesy of Dr. F. Stephen Vogel, Duke University.)

devoid of nucleic acids. These infectious agents are called **prions** (proteinaceous infectious particles).

EPIDEMIOLOGY: The classic spongiform encephalopathies in humans include several diseases: kuru, Creutzfeldt-Jakob disease (CJD), Gerstmann-Sträussler-Scheinker syndrome (GSS) and fatal familial insomnia (Table 28-2). Similar diseases occur in animals, including scrapie in sheep and goats, bovine spongiform encephalopathy (BSE; mad cow disease), transmissible mink encephalopathy and chronic wasting disease in mule deer and elk. BSE is of particular interest because it resulted from inadvertent introduction of prion-contaminated feed to cattle, thus establishing that prions can be transmitted by the oral route. BSE is also more easily transmitted and does not exhibit the species selectivity of other prions. It decimated the cattle industry in the United Kingdom and has spread to other regions of the world and to other species including zoo animals, pets and humans.

Table 28-2

Prion Diseases

I. Human
A. Creutzfeldt-Jakob disease (CJD)
1. Sporadic (85% of all CJD cases; incidence 1 per million worldwide)
2. Inherited mutation of the prion gene, autosomal dominant transmission (15% of all CJD cases)
3. Iatrogenic
a. Hormone injection: human growth hormone, human pituitary gonadotropin
b. Tissue grafts: dura mater, cornea, pericardium
c. Medical devices: depth electrodes, surgical instruments (none definitely proven)
4. New variant CJD (vCJD)
B. Gerstmann-Sträussler-Scheinker disease (GSS; inherited prion gene mutation, autosomal dominant transmission)
C. Fatal familial insomnia (FFI; inherited prion gene mutation, autosomal dominant transmission)
D. Kuru (confined to the Fore people of Papua New Guinea, formerly transmitted by cannibalistic funeral ritual)
II. Animal
A. Scrapie (sheep and goats)
B. Bovine spongiform encephalopathy (BSE; "mad cow disease")
C. Transmissible mink encephalopathy
D. Feline spongiform encephalopathy
E. Captive exotic ungulate spongiform encephalopathy (nyala, gemsbok, eland, Arabian oryx, greater kudu)
F. Chronic wasting disease of deer and elk
G. Experimental transmission to many species, including primates and transgenic mice

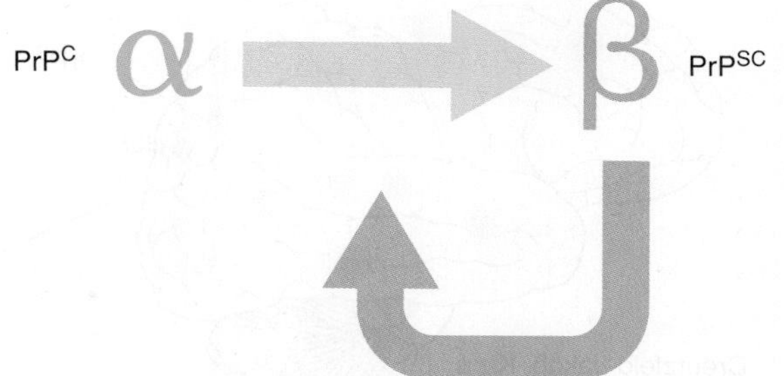

FIGURE 28-70. Creutzfeldt-Jakob disease. The unique mode of "reproduction" of the prion is the autocatalytic conversion of native α-helix–rich cellular prion protein into a β-sheet–rich pathogenic form that has a strong tendency toward aggregation.

MOLECULAR PATHOGENESIS: The signal molecular event in prion disorders is conversion of a native α-helix–rich protein into a pathogenic β-sheet–rich isoform that tends to polymerize with subsequent fibril formation (Figs. 28-70 and 28-71). Uniquely, conversion of the native protein to the pathogenic form is autocatalyzed by the pathogenic form itself. The pathogenic protein begets more pathogenic protein from the limitless supply of native protein! The native protein is coded by a human prion gene (*PRNP*) on the short arm of chromosome 20, which contains a single exon encoding 254 amino acid residues. The normal prion gene product, prion protein (PrP), is a constitutively expressed cell-surface glycoprotein that is bound to the neuronal plasmalemma by a glycolipid anchor. PrP is made widely throughout the body, but the highest levels of PrP mRNA are in CNS neurons. Its function is unknown. The normal cellular prion protein, termed cellular PrP or PrP^{C}, and the pathogenic (infectious) prion protein, known as scrapie PrP or PrP^{SC}, have the same primary amino acid sequence but different three-dimensional conformations and patterns of glycosylation. Specifically, PrP^{C} is rich in α-helix configuration, whereas the β-pleated sheet configuration predominates in PrP^{SC}. The pathogenic conformation is extremely stable so that PrP^{SC} is extremely resistant to conventional microbial decontamination methods. If PrP^{SC} gains access to the brain either through infectious transmission or by spontaneous misfolding of native protein, it will change other PrP^{C} proteins into pathogenic PrP^{SC}, leading to autocatalytic, exponentially expanding accretion of abnormal PrP^{SC}. The masses of PrP^{SC} compromise cell function and result in neurodegeneration by mechanisms that remain to be elucidated but may be similar to those of other neurodegenerative diseases characterized by fibrillogenesis.

All spongiform encephalopathies are transmissible, and inadvertent human transmission of CJD has followed administration of contaminated human pituitary growth hormone, corneal transplantation from a diseased donor, insufficiently sterilized neurosurgical instruments and surgical implantation of contaminated dura (Table 28-2).

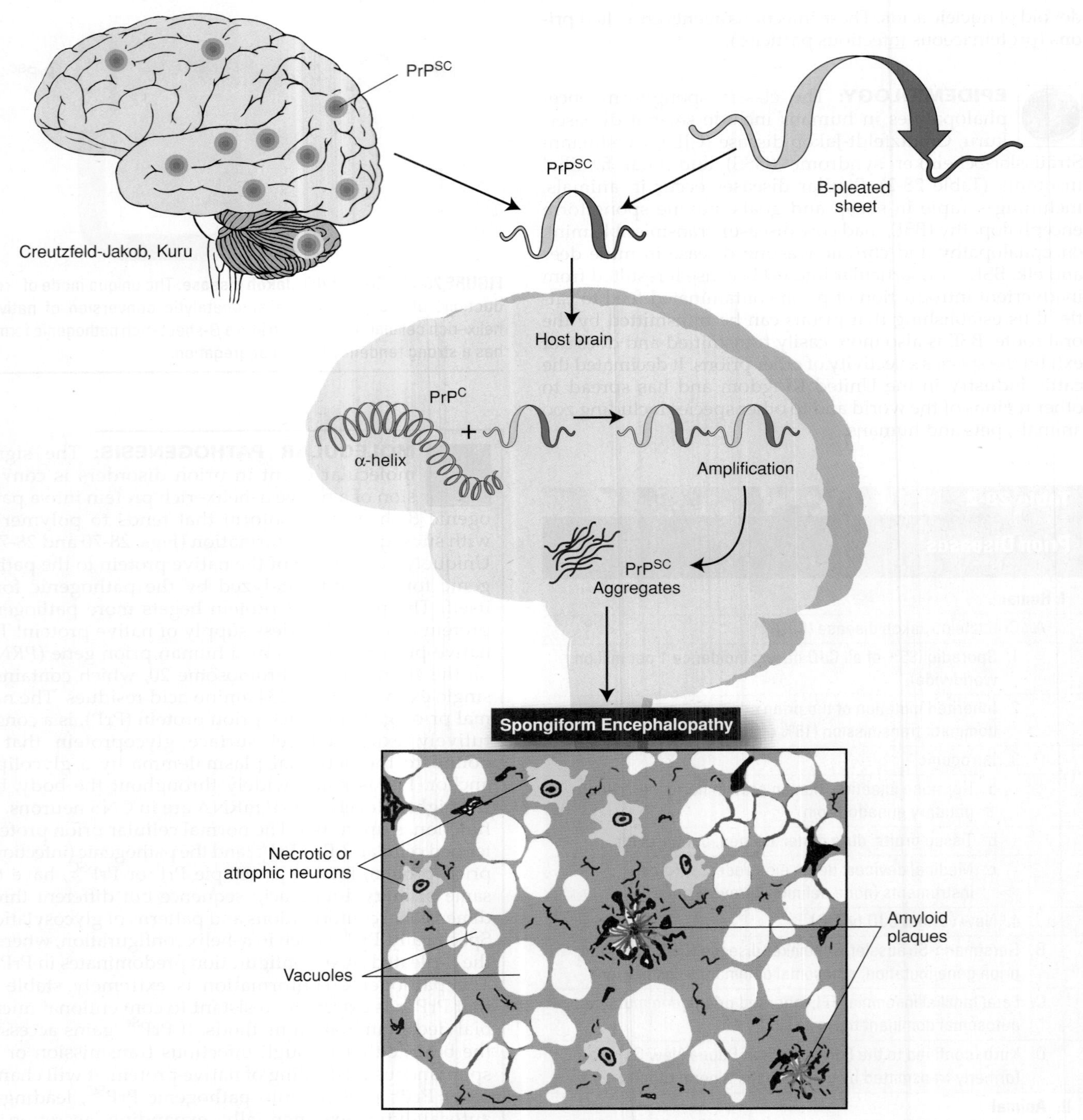

FIGURE 28-71. Molecular pathogenesis of prion disorders.

PATHOLOGY: Prion diseases feature neuron degeneration; gliosis; spongiform degeneration; many small, clear, often confluent microcysts in the neuropil; and accumulations of insoluble prions forming extracellular plaques (Fig. 28-71). These occur most in cortical gray matter but also involve deeper nuclei of the basal ganglia, thalamus, hypothalamus and cerebellum.

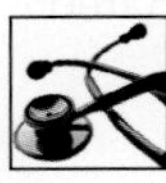

CLINICAL FEATURES: The various human prion diseases have distinctive features.

KURU: In 1956, a medical officer in New Guinea provided an account of kuru, a progressive, fatal neurologic disorder, in members of the isolated Fore tribe. The disease takes its name from the word "trembling" in their language. Transmission of kuru was linked to ritualistic funereal cannibalism in which women and children ate brains of deceased relatives.

Kuru was the first human prion disease shown to be transmissible. It attained epidemic proportions in the Fore people but was eliminated when cannibalism ceased. The initial and most prominent clinical feature of kuru is ataxia of the limbs and trunk, owing to severe involvement of the cerebellum. In

70% of cases, insoluble, fibrillar prion proteins accumulate extracellularly in plaques. Spongiform change is present in both the cerebral hemispheres and cerebellum.

CREUTZFELDT-JAKOB DISEASE: CJD is the most common form of spongiform encephalopathy. Symptoms begin insidiously, but usually within 6 months to 3 years, patients exhibit severe dementia leading to death. Cerebellar involvement produces ataxia, which helps to distinguish CJD from Alzheimer disease. Myoclonus often occurs for some weeks to months during the afflicted person's decline. CJD can be classified into four types based on etiology: sporadic, familial, iatrogenic and new variant:

- **Sporadic CJD:** The sporadic form occurs worldwide, with an incidence of 1 per million, and accounts for 75% of all cases of CJD. The mode of acquisition is unknown; patients do not exhibit the mutations associated with the inherited forms of CJD or other prion diseases, and there is no history of iatrogenic exposure. A polymorphism in PRNP codon 129 confers differential susceptibility to CJD: homozygosity for either methionine (M) or valine (V) at this codon confers disproportionate susceptibility to prion disorders, while heterozygotes (M/V) are resistant. Codon frequencies for the white population are 51% M/V, 37% M/M and 12% V/V.
- **Inherited CJD: Familial CJD** constitutes 15% of prion diseases, with an incidence of 1 per 10 million. Several different PRNP mutations are documented in various kindreds. In those cases, the PrP^{C} has a greater propensity to misfold into the pathogenic isoform. The mutated PRNP causes familial CJD, fatal familial insomnia and Gerstmann-Sträussler-Scheinker disease.
- **Iatrogenic CJD:** As listed in Table 28-2, several iatrogenic causes of CJD are known, but most of the causes for iatrogenic CJD now have been eliminated. Thus, recombinant human growth hormone has supplanted human pituitary-derived preparations for therapy. When brain biopsies or autopsies are performed in prion disease cases, special protocols are used to limit exposure of staff and patients to prions. Disposable instruments are used if possible, and surfaces and instruments are treated with 2 N NaOH. Conventional autoclaving and most standard disinfectants do not eradicate this hardy infectious agent.
- **New variant CJD (vCJD or nvCJD):** This form was identified by a surveillance program in the United Kingdom after the BSE epidemic (see above) between 1980 and 1996. A group of patients was identified that differed from other patients with sporadic CJD in several key characteristics, most importantly, age. The mean age at onset of symptoms for sporadic CJD is 65 years; it is 26 years for vCJD patients. Also, vCJD patients had a longer duration of illness (median, 12 months vs. 4 months) and an atypical clinical presentation, including various behavioral changes or sensory disturbances (dysesthesias) and none of the usual electroencephalographic (EEG) findings of sporadic CJD. At autopsy, vCJD is characterized by prominent spongiform change in the basal ganglia and thalamus and extensive PrP plaques in the cerebrum and cerebellum. The plaques are distinctive in that they resemble those of kuru. Finally, brains from vCJD patients contain much more PrP than brains of sporadic CJD patients. Physicochemical analysis showed different characteristics for vCJD PrP^{SC} from CJD PrP^{SC}, but similar to prions in BSE that were transmitted to mice and primates. Thus, BSE is considered to be the source of nvCJD. Current evidence suggests that vCJD cases have peaked and are declining. Of concern, essentially all vCJD cases were in codon 129 homozygotes (who are more susceptible), and a recent case in a heterozygote raises the unsettling specter of a longer incubation type of vCJD in this population.

Demyelinating Diseases

In demyelinating diseases the primary problem is disruption of the myelin economy including flawed manufacture **(dysmyelination),** destruction of myelin **(demyelination)** or disruption of myelin metabolism **(leukodystrophies).** Central myelin is made by oligodendrocytes, while peripheral myelin is made by Schwann cells. These two types of myelin differ biochemically. Operationally, the border between the CNS and the peripheral nervous system can be considered to be the point of transition between myelin made by oligodendrocytes and that made by Schwann cells. This transition usually occurs about 2 to 3 mm after a cranial nerve or spinal root exits the brainstem or spinal cord. Myelin disorders affect central or peripheral myelin, or both.

Multiple Sclerosis Is the Most Common Demyelinating Disease

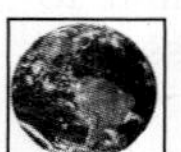

EPIDEMIOLOGY: Multiple sclerosis (MS) is a chronic demyelinating disease that is the most common chronic CNS disease of young adults in the United States. Its prevalence is 1 per 1000. MS is characterized by exacerbations and remissions over many years. It becomes symptomatic at a mean age of 30 years, and women are afflicted almost twice as often as men.

MOLECULAR PATHOGENESIS: The etiology of MS remains obscure, but experimental and clinical studies suggest a genetic predisposition and an immune pathogenesis. MS is principally a disease of temperate climates. People who emigrate before the age of 15 years from areas with a low prevalence of MS to more temperate endemic areas assume an increased risk for the disease, suggesting that environmental factors are important.

A genetic predisposition to MS may be inferred from the fact that there are familial aggregates of the disease, increased risk in second- and third-degree relatives of MS patients and 25% concordance for MS in monozygotic twins. Susceptibility is also linked to a number of major histocompatibility complex (MHC) alleles (e.g., HLA-DR2), thereby implying that immune mechanisms are involved in the pathogenesis.

Evidence supporting a role for immune mechanisms in MS also comes from the lesions' microscopic appearance. For example, chronic MS lesions show perivascular lymphocytes, macrophages and many $CD4^{+}$ (helper-inducer subset) as well as $CD8^{+}$ T cells. Moreover, $CD4^{+}$ T cells from the CSF of MS patients appear to be oligoclonal. Although a target antigen has not been identified, data suggest an immune response to a specific CNS protein. Further support for immune mechanisms comes from experimental production of an antigen-specific, T-cell–mediated, autoimmune disease,

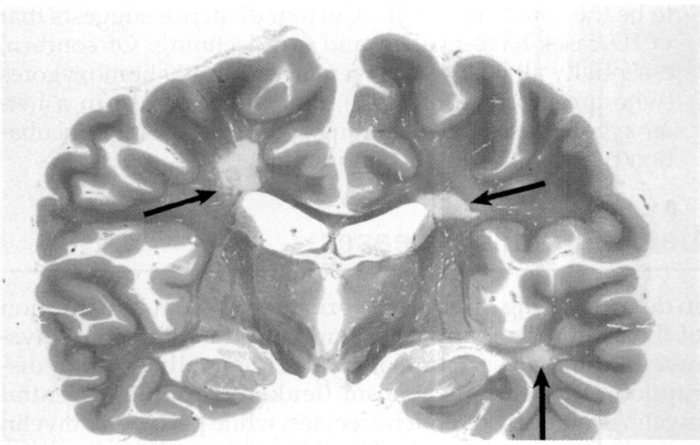

FIGURE 28-72. Multiple sclerosis. This myelin-stained coronal whole brain section of the brain of a patient with long-standing multiple sclerosis shows many areas of myelin loss—plaques (*arrows*)—with characteristic periventricular demyelination especially prominent at the superior angles of the lateral ventricles. (Courtesy of Dr. F. Stephen Vogel, Duke University.)

termed **experimental allergic encephalitis (EAE).** Injecting myelin basic protein experimentally, including into nonhuman primates, elicits a demyelinating disorder similar to MS. However, unlike MS, EAE is a monophasic illness.

Although an assortment of viruses have been implicated in the etiology of MS, to date there is no compelling evidence for the involvement of any infectious agent.

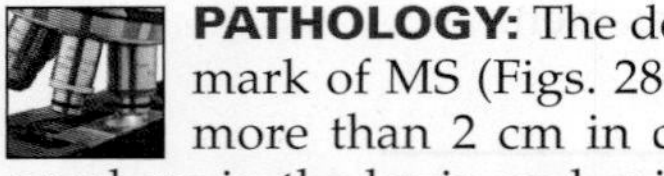

PATHOLOGY: The demyelinated plaque is the hallmark of MS (Figs. 28-72 and 28-73). Plaques, rarely more than 2 cm in diameter, accumulate in great numbers in the brain and spinal cord (Fig. 28-74). They are discrete, with smoothly rounded contours, and are usually in white matter, although they may breach the gray matter. The lesions exhibit a preference for the optic nerves, chiasm, paraventricular white matter and spinal cord, but any part of the CNS may be affected.

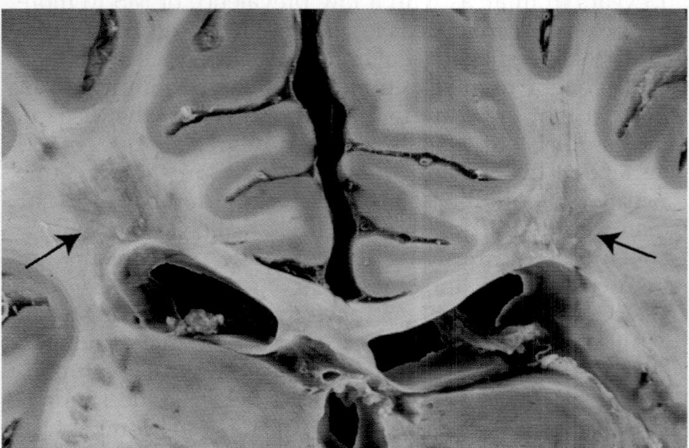

FIGURE 28-73. Multiple sclerosis. This fresh coronal section shows darker hues of the somewhat irregular periventricular plaques (*arrows*) reflecting the loss of myelin, which imparts the normal glistening white appearance of white matter.

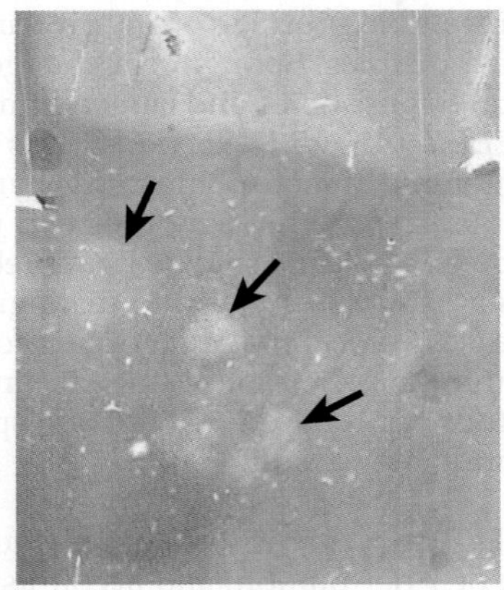

FIGURE 28-74. Multiple sclerosis. The subcortical white matter of a patient with multiple sclerosis showing multiple small irregular, partially confluent areas of demyelination (*arrows*). Normal intact myelin stains blue in this Luxol fast blue–stained section.

The evolving plaque is marked by selective loss of myelin in a region of relative axonal preservation, lymphocytes that cluster about small veins and arteries, an influx of macrophages and considerable edema.

Neuronal bodies within the boundaries of a plaque are remarkably spared, but the axons may degenerate. The number of oligodendrocytes is moderately diminished. As plaques age, they become more discrete and less edematous. This sequence emphasizes the focal nature of the injury, its selectivity and its severity, since demyelination is total within a plaque. Usually, axons within plaques lose their myelin abruptly. Old MS plaques are dense and gliotic.

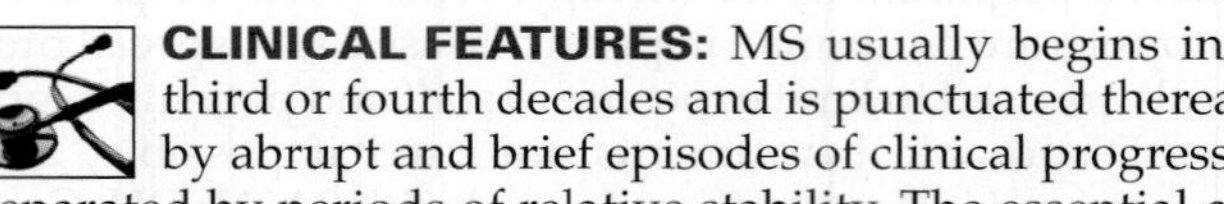

CLINICAL FEATURES: MS usually begins in the third or fourth decades and is punctuated thereafter by abrupt and brief episodes of clinical progression, separated by periods of relative stability. The essential clinical criterion for MS is dissemination of lesions in space and time; that is, multiple separate areas of the CNS must be affected at differing times. Our understanding of disease activity in MS has been revolutionized by use of serial MRI studies, which show ongoing disease activity despite apparent clinical quiescence. New plaques emerge and regress, only occasionally causing clinical manifestations. Contemporary diagnostic criteria for MS strongly incorporate imaging to provide evidence of plaques disseminated in space on the initial scan and disseminated in time with serial imaging. Thus, MS is an ongoing active process even between clinical exacerbations. The therapeutic focus is now suppression of this ongoing disease activity using a variety of immune system modulators such as β-interferon, and MRI efficacy is an endpoint in drug trials and clinical management. Neuropathologic studies have confirmed increased inflammatory activity in brains of MS patients between exacerbations.

Many patients with MS pursue relapsing remitting clinical courses, but some suffer a relentless course without remissions. Each exacerbation reflects the formation of additional demyelinated MS plaques. MS typically begins with symptoms relating to lesions in the optic nerves, brainstem or spinal cord. Blurred vision or the loss of vision in one eye as a result of optic neuritis is often the presenting complaint. When the initial lesion is in the brainstem, double vision and vertigo occur. In particular, internuclear ophthalmoplegia, caused by disruption of the medial longitudinal fasciculus, strongly suggests demyelinating disease when it occurs in a young person. Acute demyelination within the spinal cord is called **transverse myelitis** and produces weakness of one or both legs and sensory symptoms in the form of numbness in the lower extremities. Many of the initial symptoms are partially reversible within a few months.

Despite the fact that most patients have a chronic relapsing and remitting course, neurologic deficits accumulate gradually and relentlessly. Even in relatively quiescent plaques there may be axonal attrition leading to irreversible lesions. In established cases, the degree of functional impairment is highly variable, ranging from minor disability to severe incapacity, with widespread paralysis, dysarthria, ataxia, severe visual defects, incontinence and dementia. Patients with severe disability usually die of respiratory paralysis or urinary tract infections. Most patients with MS survive 20 to 30 years after the onset of symptoms.

Neuromyelitis Optica Is a Demyelinating Disease Common in Japan

Neuromyelitis optica (NMO) is a demyelinating disorder showing a striking predilection for the optic nerves and spinal cord. Once regarded as simply a variant of MS, NMO is now recognized as resulting from autoantibodies against a water channel, aquaporin 4, and is thus pathophysiologically fundamentally distinct from MS. This disorder responds poorly to conventional MS therapy.

Postinfectious and Postvaccinal Encephalomyelitis Are Immune Responses to Viral Antigens

Some viral infections (e.g., measles, varicella, rubella) may rarely be followed in 3 to 21 days by an encephalomyelitis. The disease is characterized by focal perivascular demyelination and conspicuous mononuclear cell infiltrates around small to medium-sized venules in the white matter of the brain and spinal cord. This disorder is suspected to be immune mediated, but its precise pathogenesis remains unclear. Onset of postinfectious encephalomyelitis is heralded by headache, vomiting, fever and meningismus that may be followed by paraplegia, incontinence and stupor. Up to 15% to 20% of patients die. A similar syndrome, **postvaccinal encephalomyelitis,** may follow immunization against infectious agents (e.g., smallpox, rabies) (Fig. 28-75). The use of more-purified vaccines that are free of cross-reacting antigenic contaminants has dramatically reduced the frequency of this complication.

Leukodystrophies Are Inherited Disturbances in Myelin Formation and Preservation

These disorders often impact both central and peripheral myelin and usually manifest in infancy or childhood, although milder adult phenotypes may occur. Disruption of central myelin leads to blindness, spasticity and loss of developmental milestones, while loss of peripheral myelin leads to weakness and loss of reflexes.

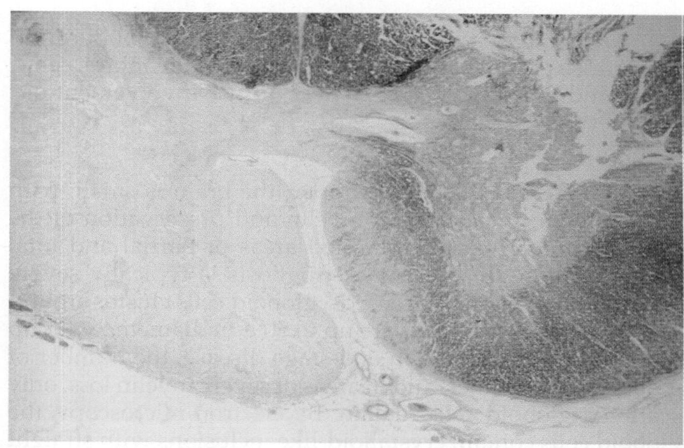

FIGURE 28-75. Postvaccinal encephalomyelitis involving the spinal cord with marked myelin loss in the lateral and anterior regions of the spinal cord on the left.

Metachromatic Leukodystrophy

Metachromatic leukodystrophy (MLD), the most common leukodystrophy, is an autosomal recessive disorder characterized by accumulation of a cerebroside (galactosyl sulfatide) in the white matter of the brain and peripheral nerves. MLD predominates in infancy, but rare juvenile or adult cases are described. It is lethal within several years.

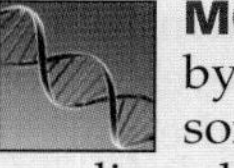

MOLECULAR PATHOGENESIS: MLD is caused by deficiency in arylsulfatase A activity. This lysosomal enzyme is involved in the degradation of myelin sulfatides. Accordingly, there is progressive accumulation of sulfatides within the lysosomes of myelin-forming Schwann cells and oligodendrocytes.

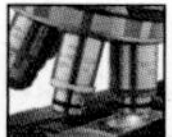

PATHOLOGY: In MLD, the accumulated sulfatides form cytoplasmic spherical granules, 15 to 20 microns in diameter, which stain metachromatically with cresyl violet and toluidine blue. Normal staining is orthochromatic; that is, cresyl violet or toluidine blue stains tissue violet or blue. In metachromasia the color of dyes shifts: tissue stained with cresyl violet or toluidine blue looks rusty brown to red. The brain shows diffuse myelin loss, accumulation of metachromatic material in white matter and astrogliosis. Demyelination of peripheral nerves is less severe.

Krabbe Disease

MOLECULAR PATHOGENESIS: Krabbe disease is a rapidly progressive, fatal, autosomal recessive neurologic disorder caused by a deficiency of galactocerebroside β-galactosidase. The condition appears in infancy and is characterized by the presence of perivascular aggregates of mononuclear and multinucleated "globoid cells" in the white matter, leading to the alternative name **globoid cell leukodystrophy.** The globoid cells are simply multinucleated macrophages containing undigested galactocerebroside (galactosylceramide).

Krabbe disease appears in the early months of life and progresses to death within 1 to 2 years. Severe motor, sensory and cognitive defects reflect diffuse involvement of the nervous system.

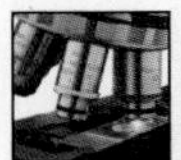

PATHOLOGY: At autopsy, the brain is small, with widespread loss of myelin and preservation of the cerebral cortex. Marbled areas of partial and total demyelination are present. Astrogliosis is typically severe and, as demyelination proceeds, globoid cells cluster around blood vessels. These cells are up to 50 μ in diameter, with up to 20 peripheral nuclei. In end-stage disease, the number of globoid cells declines, and in areas of severe myelin loss, only scattered globoid cells remain. By electron microscopy, the globoid cells contain crystalloid-like inclusions with straight or tubular profiles.

Adrenoleukodystrophy

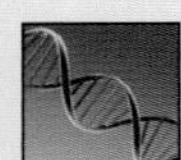

MOLECULAR PATHOGENESIS: Adrenoleukodystrophy (ALD) is an X-linked (Xq28) inherited disorder in which dysfunction of the adrenal cortex and nervous system demyelination are associated with high levels of saturated very-long-chain fatty acids (VLCFAs) in tissue and body fluids. The enzyme mutation in ALD impairs degradation of VLCFAs by preventing normal activation of free VLCFAs by the addition of coenzyme A (CoA). Pathology in the brain and adrenal are a result of accumulation of abnormal cholesterol esters and VLCFA toxicity.

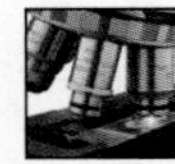

PATHOLOGY: In the brain there is confluent, bilaterally symmetric demyelination. The most severe lesions are in the subcortical white matter of the parieto-occipital region, which then extend rostrally (while sparing cortex) to result in severe loss of myelinated axons and oligodendrocytes. Gliosis and perivascular infiltrates of mononuclear cells (mostly lymphocytes) are prominent in affected areas. Scattered macrophages contain periodic acid–Schiff (PAS)-positive and sudanophilic material. Peripheral nerves are affected, but to a lesser degree than the brain. The adrenal glands are atrophic, and electron microscopy of cortical cells reveals pathognomonic cytoplasmic, membrane-bound, curvilinear inclusions or clefts (lamellae) containing VLCFAs. Similar inclusions occur in Schwann cells and CNS macrophages.

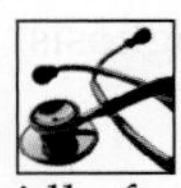

CLINICAL FEATURES: ALD occurs in children 3 to 10 years old, and neurologic symptoms precede signs of adrenal insufficiency. The disease progresses rapidly for 2 to 4 years, and the patient is quickly reduced to a vegetative state, which may persist for several years before death. Manipulation of dietary lipid composition and quantity using a 4:1 mixture of glycerol trioleate and glycerol trierucate ("Lorenzo's oil") reduces serum VLCFAs and slows progression of the disease in some cases. If the patient survives through childhood, the diet can be liberalized.

Toxic and Metabolic Disorders

Given the enormous appetite of the brain for oxygen and amino acids and other metabolic morsels, it is not surprising that the brain is subject to malfunction as a result of lack or malutilization of essential substances, intoxication and hereditary metabolic disorders. These disorders are particularly important since correction of the underlying metabolic derangement restores function. In most instances, these disturbances, while functionally profound, have no morphologic correlate; however, in some cases, pathologic alterations are seen.

Metabolic Storage Diseases Reflect Lack of Key Enzymes

Neuronal storage diseases are inherited enzyme defects that lead to accumulation of normal metabolic products within lysosomes. Unlike leukodystrophies, which produce blindness and spasticity, neuronal storage diseases impact neurons, leading to seizures and cognitive decline.

Tay-Sachs Disease

Tay-Sachs disease is a lethal, autosomal recessive disorder caused by an inborn deficiency of hexosaminidase A. Thus, ganglioside accumulates in CNS neurons. The disease is fatal in infancy and early childhood. Retinal involvement increases macular transparency and causes a **cherry-red spot** in the macula.

The brain is the major site of ganglioside storage, and it progressively enlarges in infancy. Lipid droplets are seen in the cytoplasm of distended CNS nerve cells and peripheral nervous system (Fig. 28-76A). Electron microscopy reveals the lipid within lysosomes in the form of whorled "myelin figures" (Fig. 28-76B). The neural tissues develop diffuse astrogliosis. An affected infant appears normal at birth but, by age 6 months, shows delayed motor development. Thereafter, progressive deterioration leads to flaccid weakness, blindness and severe mental impairment. Death usually supervenes before the end of the second year.

Hurler Syndrome

Hurler syndrome is an autosomal recessive disturbance in glycosaminoglycan metabolism that results in intraneuronal accumulation of mucopolysaccharides. Clinical variants of this syndrome are distinguished by variable involvement of visceral organs and the nervous system. The disease is typically expressed in infancy or early childhood as reduced stature, corneal opacities, skeletal deformities and hepatosplenomegaly. The intraneuronal storage distends the cytoplasmic compartment and is accompanied by astrogliosis and progressive mental deterioration.

Gaucher Disease

Gaucher disease is an autosomal recessive genetic deficiency of glucocerebrosidase, leading to the accumulation of glucocerebroside, principally in macrophages. The CNS is most severely involved in the infantile type (type II) of Gaucher disease. Although intraneuronal accumulation of glucocerebroside is not conspicuous, neuronal loss is severe and is accompanied by diffuse astrogliosis. These infants fail to thrive and die at an early age.

Niemann-Pick Disease

Niemann-Pick disease is an autosomal recessive disorder in which intraneuronal storage of sphingomyelin results from a

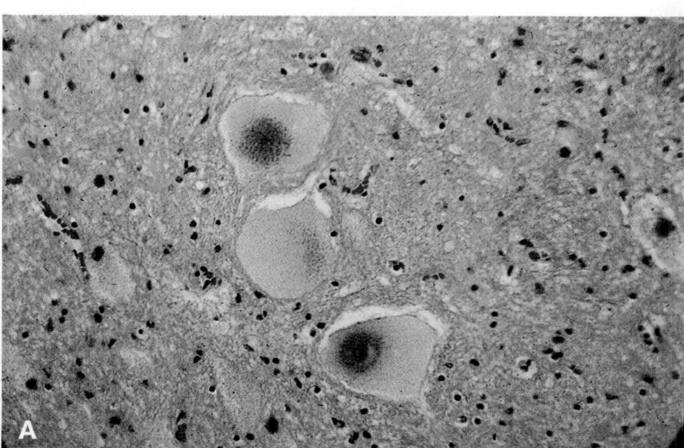

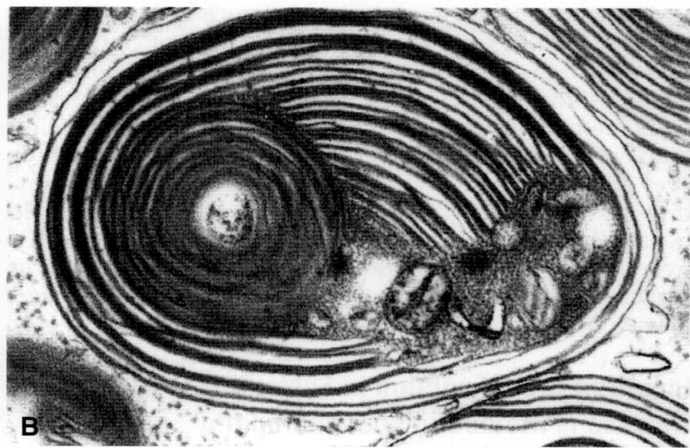

FIGURE 28-76. Tay-Sachs Disease A. The cytoplasm of the neurons is distended by the accumulation of eosinophilic storage material. **B.** Ultrastructurally, whorled "myelin bodies" composed of accumulated gangliosides are present within the cytoplasm.

deficiency of sphingomyelinase. The clinical symptoms occur early, and the disease is marked by failure of the infant to develop and thrive. The mononuclear phagocyte system is targeted for storage, but the nervous system may predominate symptomatically during infancy. The brain becomes atrophic and shows marked astrogliosis. Retinal degeneration may produce a cherry-red spot, similar to that in Tay-Sachs disease.

Alexander Disease

Alexander disease is an astrocytic storage disease. It is an uncommon neurologic disorder of infants, children and rarely adults that is characterized by a loss of myelin in the brain and striking accumulation of eosinophilic collections of GFAP in astrocytic processes (Rosenthal fibers; Fig. 28-77). The Rosenthal fibers are extremely abundant, particularly in a perivascular and subpial distribution. Clinically, children have psychomotor retardation, progressive dementia and paralysis, and eventually die. The disease is caused by mutations in the gene encoding GFAP. It is not yet clear how this process impairs myelin formation and induces degeneration of oligodendrocytes and myelin.

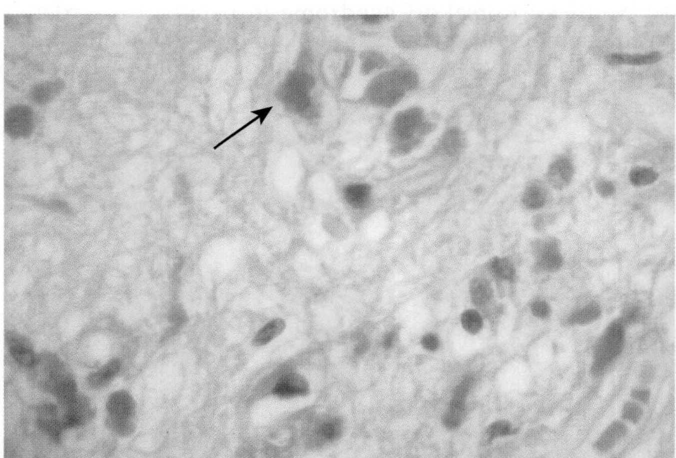

FIGURE 28-77. Alexander disease. This disease reflecting a mutation in the glial fibrillary acidic protein (GFAP) gene is characterized by accumulation of aggregated GFAP into eosinophilic bodies called Rosenthal fibers (*arrows*). Rosenthal fibers are seen in Alexander disease, in pilocytic astrocytoma and as a reaction adjacent to chronic compressive lesions.

Phenylketonuria Is a Deficiency in Phenylalanine Hydroxylase

Phenylketonuria (PKU) is an autosomal recessive disease (see Chapter 6) in which phenylalanine accumulates in the blood and tissues because its conversion to tyrosine is blocked. The condition becomes apparent in the early months of life and leads to mental retardation, seizures and impaired physical development. Treatment consists of restricting dietary phenylalanine. Untreated patients rarely obtain an intelligence quotient (IQ) above 50, but those on the diet do well. Since the morbidity of this condition is preventable by a simple dietary restriction, all newborns are now screened for the condition. Although there are no consistent morphologic alterations, the brain may be underweight and deficient in myelination.

Wilson Disease Is an Autosomal Recessive Disorder of Copper Metabolism

Wilson disease, also called "hepatolenticular degeneration," affects brain and the liver and is caused by mutations of the *WD* gene (see Chapter 14). Defective excretion of copper in the bile leads to copper deposition in the brain.

CLINICAL FEATURES: Symptoms of cerebral involvement appear clinically as a movement disorder with a propensity to choreoathetosis, usually in the second decade, but symptoms may start as late as the eighth decade. The movement disorder may be associated with psychosis. Before, during or after the appearance of neurologic symptoms, an insidiously developing cirrhosis may result in hepatic failure. Copper deposition in the limbus of the cornea produces a visible golden-brown band, the **Kayser-Fleischer ring,** seen on slit lamp examination.

The lenticular nuclei of the brain show a light golden discoloration, and 25% of cases have small cysts or clefts in the putamen or in deep layers of the neocortex. Mild neuron loss and gliosis are characteristic.

Some patients are "presymptomatic," never developing high enough levels of copper to accumulate in the brain or eyes or developing cirrhosis. Diagnosis is critical as this condition is treatable and failure to treat can lead to irreversible hepatic and CNS damage. Any individual presenting with a hyperkinetic movement disorder, particularly with onset in early adult life in association with psychiatric or hepatic manifestations, must be evaluated for Wilson disease.

Impaired Brain Function in Systemic Metabolic Disease Is Metabolic Encephalopathy

Brain malfunctions in systemic metabolic derangements caused by cardiopulmonary, renal, hepatic or endocrine diseases occurring singly or in combination are called **metabolic encephalopathy.** Clinically, patients show declining level of consciousness starting with inattentiveness sometimes with rowdiness, progressing to lethargy and finally lack of arousal, regardless of level of stimulation. The change in consciousness may be accompanied by tremor, asterixis and changing multifocal neurologic signs. Computed tomography (CT) and MRI scans show no structural abnormality, and EEG demonstrates a progressive slowing of the rhythmic cortical activity sometimes accompanied by periodic high-amplitude discharges known as triphasic waves (triphasic waves are seen most commonly in hepatic encephalopathy, but they are not specific for this condition). Biochemically, metabolic encephalopathy is characterized by diminished cerebral glucose and oxygen utilization regardless of the inciting derangement. No specific morphologic features are seen in metabolic encephalopathy, although the presence of Alzheimer type II astrocytes is suggestive but not diagnostic of hepatic encephalopathy.

Hepatic Encephalopathy

Hepatic encephalopathy is a common clinical expression of liver failure, manifested as delirium, seizures and coma. In general, clinical symptoms greatly exceed their morphologic correlates, which are restricted to the appearance of altered astroglia (termed **Alzheimer type II astrocytes**) with enlarged nuclei and marginated chromatin, especially in the thalamus.

Osmotic Demyelination Syndrome (Central Pontine Myelinolysis)

Central pontine myelinolysis is a rare demyelinating disorder of the pons, where discrete areas of selective demyelination occur (Fig. 28-78). Lesions often are too small to manifest clinically and are discovered only at autopsy. In a few patients, quadriparesis, pseudobulbar palsy or locked-in syndrome may occur. Central pontine myelinolysis arises from overly rapid correction of hyponatremia in alcoholics, malnourished persons or patients with marked electrolyte instability, including those with renal failure and liver transplant recipients.

Vitamin Deficiencies

Vitamin deficiencies and their systemic consequences are discussed in depth in Chapter 8.

Wernicke Syndrome

Wernicke syndrome results from thiamine (vitamin B_1) deficiency and is characterized clinically by rapid onset of altered consciousness with dramatically impaired short-term memory, ophthalmoplegia and nystagmus. Lesions are seen in the hypothalamus and mamillary bodies, the periaqueductal regions of the midbrain and the tegmentum of the pons (Fig. 28-79). The syndrome is most common in chronic alcoholics, although it may appear in others whose diets lack thiamine. It may progress rapidly to death, but it is reversed by administration of thiamine. In fatal cases, petechiae form around capillaries in the mamillary bodies, hypothalamus, periaqueductal region and floor of the fourth ventricle (Fig. 28-80). Over time, hemosiderin deposition identifies regions where petechiae occurred. Neurons and myelin are generally spared, but the mamillary bodies atrophy and capillary proliferation may be prominent.

Wernicke-Korsakoff syndrome is a state of disordered recent memory often compensated for by confabulation. The histologic changes are similar to those of Wernicke syndrome,

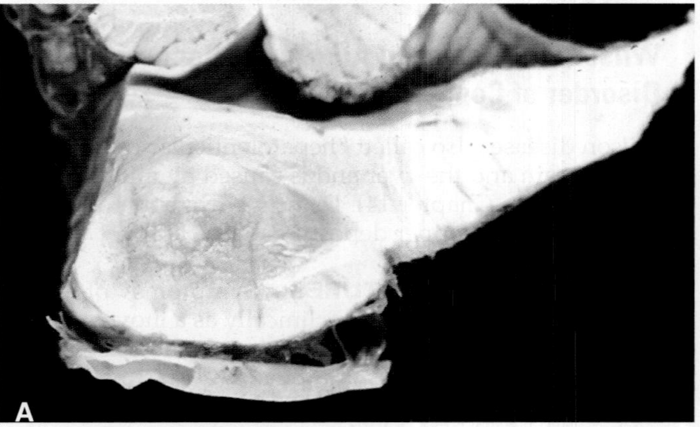

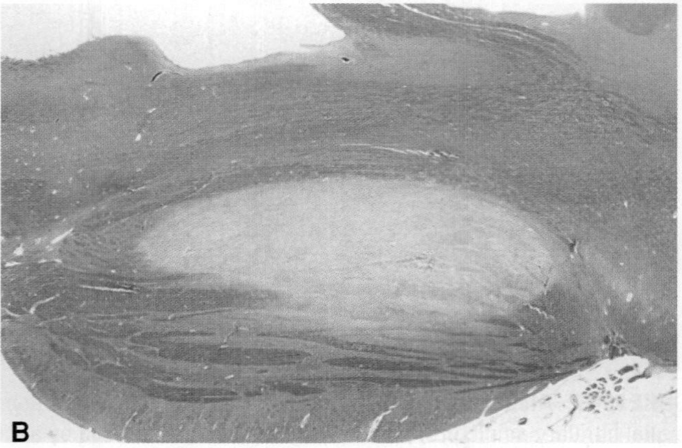

FIGURE 28-78. Osmotic demyelination syndrome with central pontine myelinolysis. A. This sagittal section of the brainstem shows a soft, discolored, midpontine lesion. **B.** A myelin-stained section reveals a sharply demarcated loss of myelin appearing as a pink ovoid zone. (A and B Courtesy of Dr. F. Stephen Vogel, Duke University.)

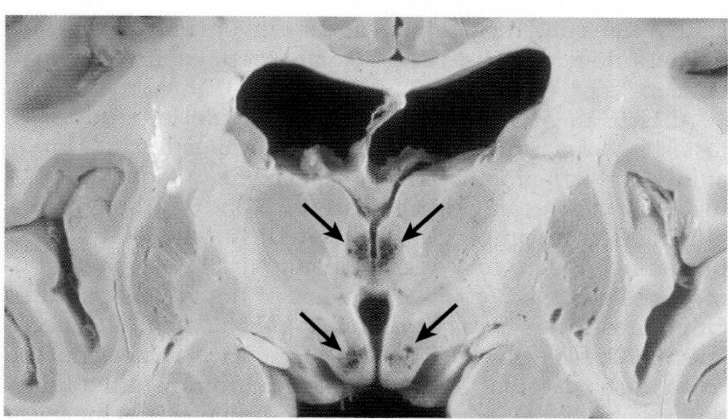

FIGURE 28-79. Wernicke encephalopathy. This coronal section shows hemorrhagic petechiae in the mamillary bodies and periventricular anterior thalamus (*arrows*). (Courtesy of Dr. F. Stephen Vogel, Duke University.)

but there may be prominent degeneration of neurons in the medial–dorsal nucleus of the thalamus.

Many chronic alcoholics have cerebral atrophy of uncertain cause and for which the relative roles of alcohol toxicity, malnutrition and other factors are not defined. Similar uncertainties prevail with regard to atrophy of the Purkinje and granular cells of the cerebellum. These alterations are common in chronic alcoholism and are the cause of truncal ataxia, which persists during periods of sobriety.

Subacute Combined Degeneration

Subacute combined degeneration of the spinal cord results from a lack of vitamin B_{12} (pernicious anemia) and leads to lesions in the posterolateral portions of the spinal cord. Initially, there is symmetric myelin and axonal loss at the thoracic level of the spinal cord. Astrogliosis is mild in the acute lesions, but with time, an affected spinal cord exhibits gliosis and atrophy, especially in the posterolateral areas of the cord. A burning sensation in the soles of the feet and other paresthesias herald the onset of this rapidly progressive and poorly reversible neurologic disorder. Weakness emerges in all four limbs, then defective postural sensibility, incoordination and ataxia. In addition to pernicious anemia, subacute combined degeneration may complicate a rare case of extensive gastric resection and other malabsorption syndromes. As vitamin B_{12} is not found in plants, some extreme vegetarians who eschew all animal products, even milk and eggs, develop subacute combined degeneration after many years on the restricted diet.

Iatrogenic, occupational or recreational exposure to the anesthetic gas nitrous oxide may lead to a condition clinically and morphologically indistinguishable from combined system degeneration. This anesthetic interferes with vitamin B_{12}–dependent enzymes. Hypocupric (low serum copper) myelopathy following bariatric surgery or zinc overdosage is also similar.

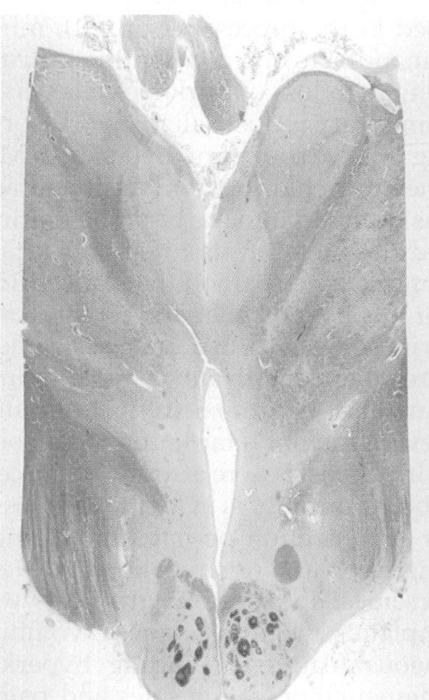

FIGURE 28-80. Wernicke encephalopathy with petechial hemorrhage in mammillary bodies. (Courtesy of Dr. F. Stephen Vogel, Duke University.)

Intoxication

Neurotoxicology is a major aspect of contemporary neuropathology. The breadth of this area far exceeds the scope of this chapter, so we concentrate on the more common and better-understood toxic injuries to the brain.

ETHANOL: Acute and chronic alcohol intake has widespread harmful effects and more widespread societal repercussions as a result of its behavioral effects. Acute alcohol intoxication signs and symptoms correspond to dose-related blood level, such that 0.05 to 0.1 mg/dL is associated with disinhibition and motor impairment; 0.1 to 0.3 mg/dL with frank inebriation and ataxia; and 0.3 to 0.35 mg/dL with extreme intoxication and sleepiness, nausea and vomiting. Greater than 0.35 mg/dL is potentially lethal because of respiratory depression and inability to protect the airway from aspiration. Lethal intoxication tragically occurs when drinking takes on a competitive quality as in "chugging" contests, fraternity initiations and other rituals of youth.

Chronic alcohol use is associated with neurologic complications caused by nutritional deficiencies, including Wernicke-Korsakoff syndrome and possibly peripheral neuropathy; liver failure with hepatic encephalopathy and non-Wilsonian hepatocerebral degeneration; and metabolic derangements including central pontine myelinolysis from rapid correction of hyponatremia (Fig. 28-81). Also seen in alcoholics is central necrosis of the corpus callosum, called Marchiafava-Bignami disease, which was initially thought to occur only in Italian drinkers of red wine but is now known to have a more cosmopolitan distribution. Marchiafava-Bignami disease is now known to be part of the osmotic demyelination syndrome caused by overly rapid correction of hyponatremia. Less well understood is anterior superior vermal cerebellar degeneration, which occurs mainly in alcoholic men, presents with truncal ataxia and is grossly evident as atrophy of the vermis (Fig. 28-82).

METHANOL: In their quest for ethanol, alcoholics may from time to time drink methanol, which is oxidized to formaldehyde and formic acid. Patients dying of methanol intoxication have severe cerebral edema with hemorrhagic necrosis of the lateral putamen. Retinal edema and ganglion cell degeneration are observed and account for the blindness that afflicts these patients. Blindness may result from ingestion of as little as 4 mL, whereas a lethal dose is in the range of 8 to 10 mL of pure methanol, although usually 70 to 100 mL is consumed in fatal cases.

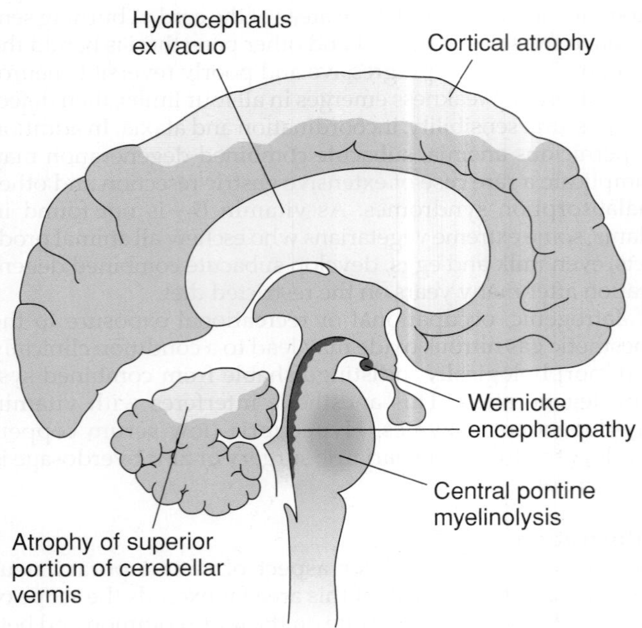

FIGURE 28-81. Regions of the brain with lesions associated with chronic ethanol abuse.

ETHYLENE GLYCOL: Similarly, ethylene glycol (automotive antifreeze) is sometimes consumed as an alternative to ethanol or by children or animals because of its sweet taste. Oxalate is its metabolic product. Severe organic acidosis may lead to coma and renal failure, and survivors may have residual neurologic deficits. Tissue oxalate crystal deposition may be seen.

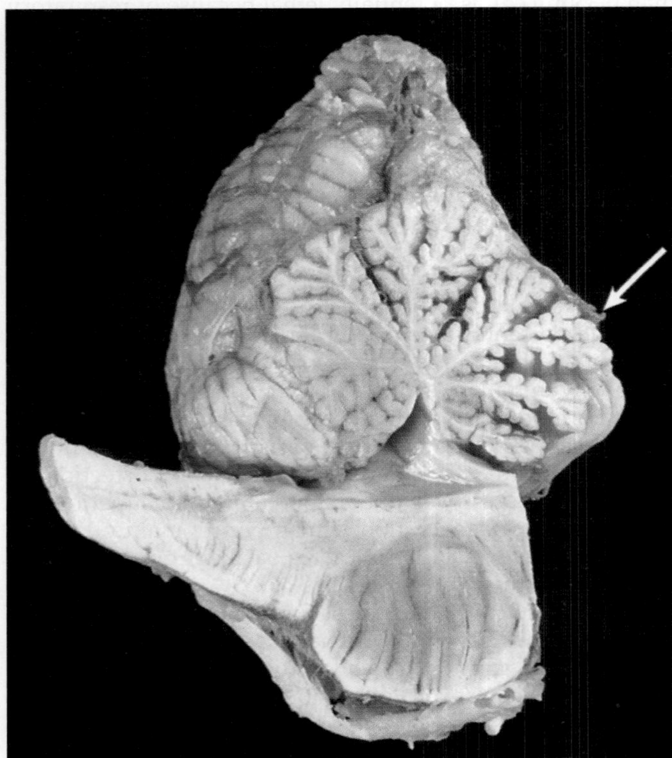

FIGURE 28-82. Chronic alcoholism. The superior and anterior portions of the cerebellar vermis are atrophic (*arrow*), leading to truncal ataxia. (Courtesy of Dr. F. Stephen Vogel, Duke University.)

CARBON MONOXIDE (CO): This colorless, odorless, tasteless gas is formed by incomplete combustion. CO binds avidly to hemoglobin forming carboxyhemoglobin, reducing the oxygen-carrying capacity of blood. Carboxyhemoglobin is red and imparts a "cherry-red" hue to victims of CO poisoning. Severe intoxication results in almost pathognomonic bilateral liquefactive necrosis of the globus pallidus. Other areas of CNS ischemic injury may be seen. The mechanism of the selective globus pallidus injury is unclear, but the recent discovery that CO may act as a neurotransmitter raises the possibility that areas rich in heme-iron (such as the basal ganglia) may use CO under physiologic conditions for cell-to-cell signaling. Analogous to the amino acid excitotoxicity story, an excess of a neurotransmitter such as CO might inflict injury in the areas where it normally plays a physiologic role.

METAL INTOXICATION: A number of metals employed in industry and medicine can result in neurologic disease; additionally, the biocidal properties of some of these substances such as arsenic and thallium have made them favorite tools of murderers, suicidal individuals and pesticide users.

- **Lead:** Lead intoxication produces an edema-based encephalopathy in acute poisoning, especially in childhood. An amorphous exudate is present around microvessels, and some vascular proliferation may be seen. Children may acquire lead intoxication by ingesting lead-based paint, fishing sinkers and other lead weights. In adults, poisoning more commonly presents as a neuropathy rather than as an encephalopathy.
- **Mercury:** Chronic inorganic mercury intoxication may present with dementia, delirium, tremor, irritability and insomnia. Intoxication of this type is now rare, but in the 19th century, it decimated workers in cinnabar mines, hat manufacturing ("mad as a hatter" possibly derives from the psychic state of felt hat factory workers exposed to mercury used in the processing of felt), mirror silvering plants and manufacturing of scientific instruments. Cerebellar atrophy with loss of Purkinje cells was seen.
- In the contemporary industrialized world, organomercurial poisoning is more prevalent. In Japan, in Minamata Bay, industrial mercuric chloride from the manufacture of vinyl chloride was dumped into the bay. The marine food chain concentrated the metal. Fishermen and local inhabitants then ate contaminated seafood that caused 1500 people to be injured or to die. Cerebellar and cerebrocortical atrophy were seen with some cortical damage elsewhere, and these patients were afflicted with ataxia and blindness. Congenital methylmercury neurotoxicity from in utero exposure results in severe mental retardation, athetosis, ataxia and spastic quadriparesis. Severe atrophy of the cerebrum with milder cerebellar atrophy is evident, with loss of the cortical lamellar organization perhaps indicating a defect in neuronal migration and organization in development.
- **Arsenic:** Arsenical intoxication manifests with gastrointestinal complaints including nausea, vomiting and diarrhea; cutaneous features including hyperkeratosis and increased pigmentation of the soles and palms and Mees lines on the nails; and a severe axonal neuropathy. In the brain, swelling and petechiae may be present. Long-term exposure is strongly associated with increased risk of cancer.

- **Thallium:** Like arsenic, gastrointestinal disturbances are evident, with major cutaneous manifestations consisting of late alopecia and Mees lines occasionally, and a severe axonal neuropathy.
- **Manganese:** Basal ganglionic damage producing parkinsonism is seen in manganese miners. This may be associated with a psychosis known as "manganese madness."

Neurodegenerative Disorders

Neurodegenerative disorders involve death of functionally related neurons; hence, these disorders can be classified by the primary functional system involved. **Cortical** degeneration leads to dementia, **basal ganglia** degeneration to movement disorders, **spinocerebellar** degeneration to ataxia and **motor neuron** degeneration to upper and lower motor neuron weakness. ***Neuropathologically, there is loss of neurons in these systems. There are often characteristic microscopic cellular inclusions and extracellular protein accumulations in these disorders and variable degrees of glial and microglial activation.***

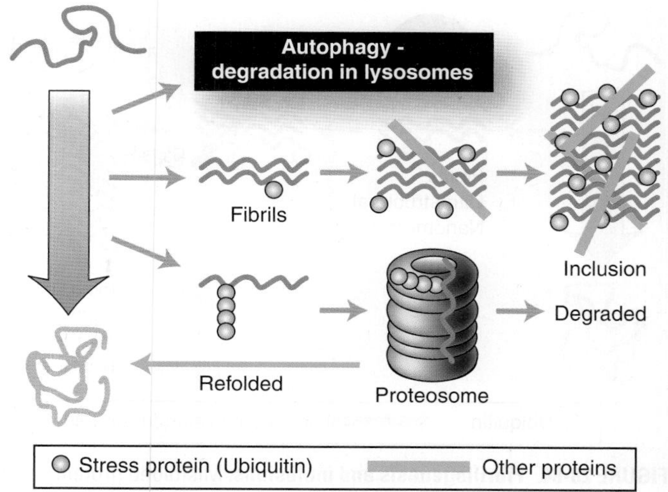

FIGURE 28-83. Possible fates of misfolded proteins. Many of the neurodegenerative diseases appear to be, at least in part, disorders of proteostasis, which consist of the cellular pathways that control protein synthesis, folding, trafficking, aggregation, disaggregation and degradation.

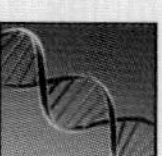

MOLECULAR PATHOGENESIS: Biochemical study of the composition of intracellular and extracellular protein accumulations has recently led to major insights into these disorders. Currently neurodegenerative disorders are classified according to which neuronal systems are most involved and the biochemistry of the proteins that accumulate in those cells.

Intracellular, and particularly intracytoplasmic, inclusions have a history that is inextricably linked to neurodegenerative disorders, as these engaging features of diseased cells were among the first histologic abnormalities of the nervous system recognized. Modern techniques have shown them to be markers of cellular stress. They are cytoplasmic landfills made of deranged cellular proteins and heat shock proteins. Evidence is mounting that abnormal protein homeostasis is key to the molecular pathogenesis of these disorders (Fig. 28-83; see Chapter 1).

When a cell is stressed, the intermediate filament network collapses into perinuclear bundles or clumps. This may reflect increased phosphorylation or proteolysis of these proteins as a result of the influx of calcium into the stressed cell. If the stress is not lethal, the cell deploys an adaptive **heat shock response,** first recognized in cells exposed to thermal stress: the cell produces several proteins that may restore functional activity of partially denatured proteins or, if the denaturing is too severe to permit restoration, the proteins are polyubiquitinated for subsequent proteolysis, but their highly stable β-pleated sheet structure leads to aggregation, preventing effective removal by proteasomal or other means. Other stress proteins may include crystallin and a family of heat shock proteins. If the proteins conjugated to these stress proteins are not successfully degraded, the conjugated complexes aggregate as intracellular inclusions.

The inclusions in neurodegenerative disorders ***reflect damaged native cellular proteins and their stress response conjugates.*** A stress response is evoked any time a cell is damaged; thus, the presence of stress response inclusions does not identify an inciting insult. Neuropathologic inclusions are made from relatively few permutations of cytoskeletal and stress proteins—fewer, in fact, than the number of apparently discrete types of inclusions described. Ubiquitin is present in many intracellular inclusions. While itself not "diagnostic" of any particular disease, ubiquitin immunostaining is the most sensitive technique for detecting such aggregated proteins. Combined with the morphology, cellular distribution and clinical context, it may be helpful diagnostically. Available antibodies allow identification of the ubiquitinated proteins as tau, neurofilament, α-synuclein and others. In summary, inclusions give limited data about the precise stress damaging the cell, their biochemical composition overlaps in many cases, and final diagnostic categorization often is dependent on clinical data, immunohistochemical characterization of inclusions and analysis of the population of cells affected.

These protein aggregates may cause disease (Fig. 28-84; Table 28-3) by several routes. Sequestering a protein or other macromolecules makes them unavailable for their normal functions. As aggregates enlarge, they may physically obstruct axons, dendrites or movement of material within the cytoplasm. They may also act as ubiquitin sinks, sequestering ubiquitin that cannot be recycled, since the polyubiquitinated proteins are not available for proteasomal processing. Thus, cellular protein recycling and homeostasis are impaired. As these proteins aggregate, they initially form ultrastructural fibrils that may be extremely cytotoxic. Thus, it appears that cellular stress from a variety of causes may disrupt proteostasis and result in formation of toxic fibrils that themselves can perpetuate and amplify the cellular stress. In view of parallels between the brain amyloidoses in many of these neurodegenerative disorders, clarification of pathogenesis in one disease could have a significant impact on understanding mechanisms underlying all of these disorders.

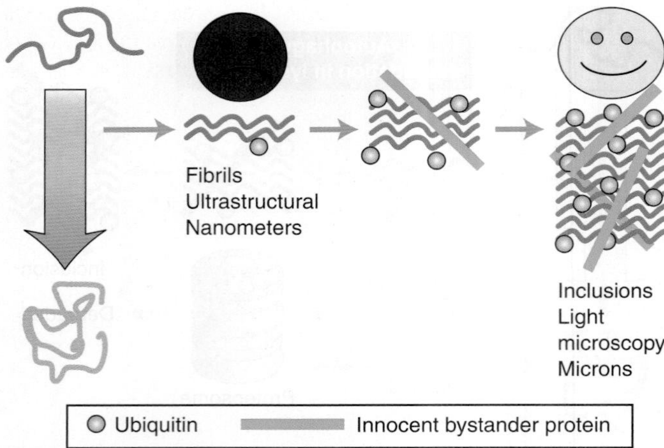

FIGURE 28-84. Fibrillogenesis and inclusions. Misfolded proteins with a tendency toward polymerization may form extremely cytoxic fibrils that are only visible by electron microscopy. The cellular stress response may facilitate hyperaggregation to inclusions that are visible by light microscopy. Such inclusions may be considered "toxic landfills" and may be protective.

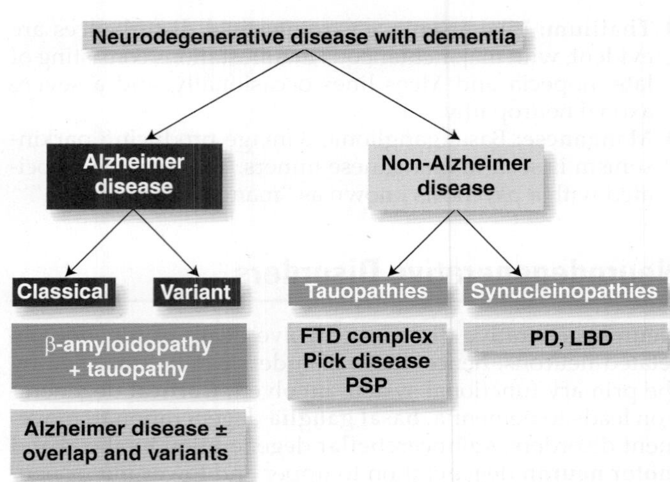

FIGURE 28-85. Protein fibrillogenesis. Molecular classification of the dementias and other neurodegenerative diseases now recognizes disorders based on the proteins that undergo fibrillogenesis. Alzheimer disease (AD) is a combination of a β-amyloidopathy and a tauopathy. Most of the frontotemporal lobar degenerations (FTDs) such as Pick disease and progressive supranuclear palsy (PSP) are pure tauopathies. Lewy body dementia (LBD) and Parkinson disease (PD) complex are α-synucleinopathies.

There Are Three Major Distinctive Cerebral Cortical Neurodegenerative Diseases

The clinical, gross and microscopic features are distinctive, with accumulation of different polymerized proteins (Fig. 28-85). These cortical degenerations ultimately lead to dementia.

- **Alzheimer disease (AD)** accounts for the majority of neurodegenerative dementia and is characterized by abnormal accumulation of two proteins: β-amyloid and tau.
- **Pick disease,** which is the prototypical frontotemporal lobar dementia, is characterized by accumulation of abnormal tau without β-amyloid.
- **Lewy body dementia** features accumulation of α-synuclein.

Alzheimer Disease

EPIDEMIOLOGY: Alzheimer disease is an insidious progressive neurologic disorder characterized clinically by loss of memory, cognitive impairment and, eventually, dementia. Although Alzheimer's original patients

Table 28-3

Representative Neurodegenerative Diseases With Fibrillogenesis

Disease	Lesion	Components	Location
Alzheimer disease	Senile plaques	β-Amyloid	Extracellular
	Neurofibrillary tangles	Tau	Intracytoplasmic
Amyotrophic lateral sclerosis	Spheroids	Neurofilament Superoxide dismutase (SOD-1) TDP43 FUS	Intracytoplasmic
Dementia with Lewy bodies	Lewy bodies	α-Synuclein	Intracytoplasmic
Frontotemporal dementias	Neurofibrillary tangles	Tau	Intracytoplasmic
		TDP43, progranulin and other proteins	
Multiple system atrophy	Glial inclusions	α-Synuclein	Intracytoplasmic
Parkinson disease	Lewy bodies	α-Synuclein	Intracytoplasmic
Prion diseases	Prion deposits	Prions	Extracellular
Trinucleotide repeat diseases	Inclusions	Polyglutamine tracts	Intranuclear and cytoplasmic

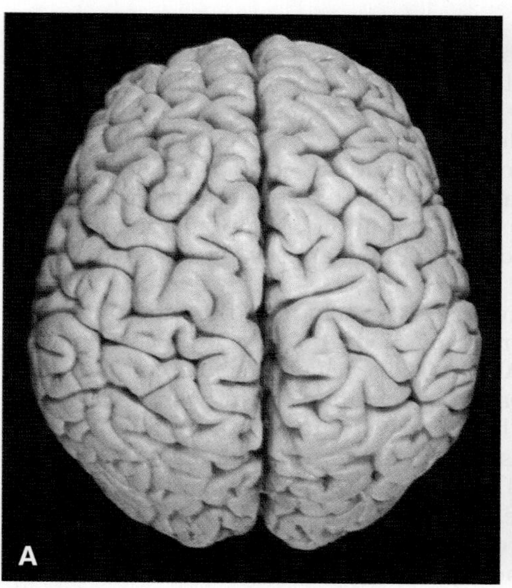

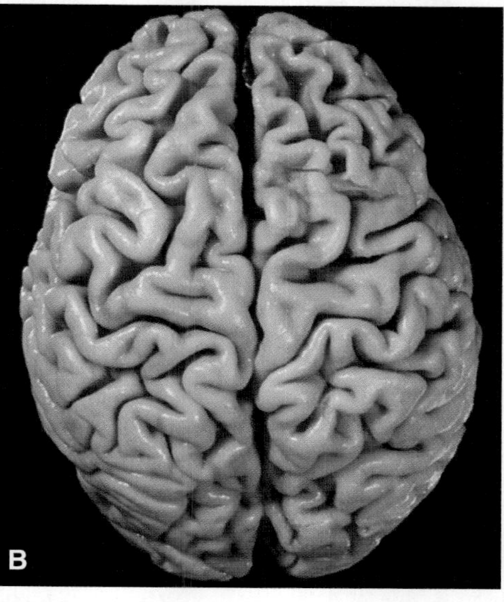

FIGURE 28-86. Cortical atrophy. A normal brain is shown on the left **(A)** and a brain with cortical atrophy caused by Alzheimer disease is shown on the right **(B)** with thinning of the gyri and prominent sulci. (Courtesy of Dr. F. Stephen Vogel, Duke University.)

were younger than 65 years and were said to suffer "presenile dementia," the term is now used for dementia at any age that displays characteristic pathologic changes. ***It is the most common dementia in the elderly, accounting for more than half of all cases.*** The prevalence of the condition is closely related to age. In patients younger than 65 years, the prevalence of Alzheimer disease is at most 1% to 2%, but it is 40% or more in patients older than 85 years. Women are affected twice as often as men. Most cases are sporadic, but familial variants are reported.

PATHOLOGY: AD brains show cortical atrophy with hydrocephalus ex vacuo (Figs. 28-86 and 28-87). Gyri narrow, sulci widen and cortical atrophy is especially apparent in the parahippocampal regions. However, as the disease progresses, atrophy of temporal, frontal and parietal cortex becomes more severe.

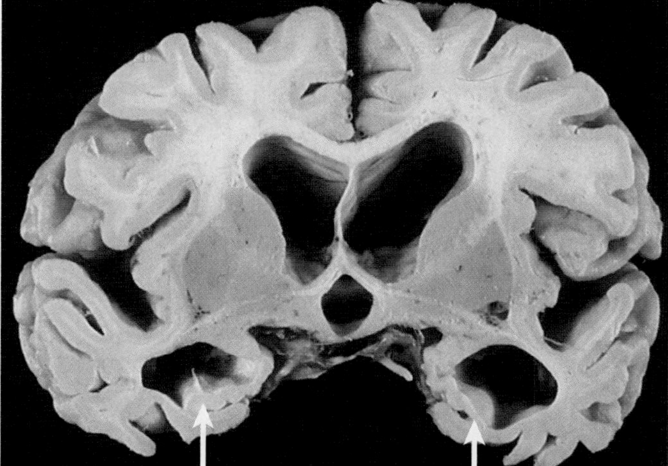

FIGURE 28-87. Cerebral atrophy with hydrocephalus ex vacuo in Alzheimer disease. Note also the severe atrophy of the hippocampus (*arrows*) leading to early memory disturbances in this disease. (Courtesy of Dr. F. Stephen Vogel, Duke University.)

Senile plaques and neurofibrillary tangles (NFTs) dominate AD histology. Small numbers of plaques and tangles are common in elderly patients with mild forgetfulness and mild cognitive impairment, which in about 50% of cases is a prodrome of AD.

NEURITIC PLAQUES: The most conspicuous histologic lesions, senile or neuritic plaques, are ***extracellular*** spherical deposits of β-amyloid several hundred microns in diameter. In end-stage disease, senile plaques occupy large volumes of affected cerebral gray matter (Fig. 28-88). They stain positively using planar amyloid binding dyes such as Congo red and thioflavin S, bind silver containing dyes (argentophilic) and are immunoreactive for β-amyloid protein (Aβ) at the core and periphery. They are surrounded by reactive astrocytes and microglia and display swollen distorted neuronal processes (dystrophic neurites). While detection of plaques is necessary for pathologic diagnosis of AD, their number and distribution do not correlate well with clinical disease severity.

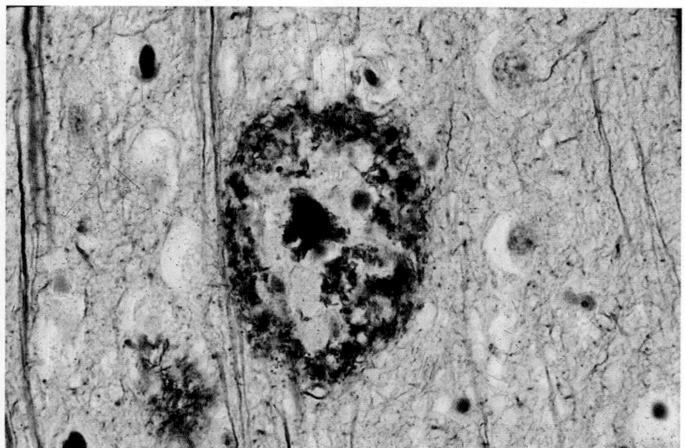

FIGURE 28-88. Neuritic plaques are extracellular accumulations of polymerized β-amyloid centrally with a rim of dystrophic neuritic processes. The number of plaques in the cerebral cortex does not correlate well with the severity of dementia in Alzheimer disease.

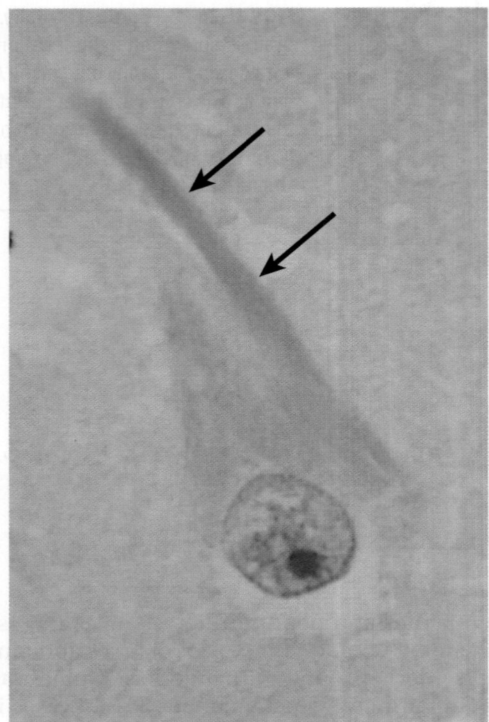

FIGURE 28-89. Neurofibrillary tangles are intracytoplasmic intraneuronal accumulations of polymerized hyperphosphorylated tau protein (*arrows*). The sites and degree of distribution of neurofibrillary tangles correlate with clinical symptoms.

NEUROFIBRILLARY TANGLES: NFTs are ***intracytoplasmic*** collections of polymerized tau filaments (Fig. 28-89). NFTs contain irregular bundles of fibrils that are positive for Congo red and thioflavin S and immunoreactive for tau. The tangles are composed of paired, 10-nm-thick, helical filaments. Western blots demonstrate abundant insoluble tau proteins. Distribution of these tangles correlates with the clinical severity of AD. Tangles in the entorhinal cortex and parahippocampal gyrus can be seen in asymptomatic individuals decades before the usual age of onset of AD, and may represent the earliest phases of the disorder. As more temporal neocortex comes to possess tangles, mild cognitive impairment may develop. Finally, with large swaths of neocortex, deep nuclei and brainstem involved, full-blown AD is present. As this concept of gradual accretion of neurofibrillary tangles is increasingly validated, efforts are increasingly directed at early diagnosis in the asymptomatic phase and development of drugs that will arrest progression.

NFTs are not unique to AD, as they also occur in other neurodegenerative diseases including dementia pugilistica (punch drunk syndrome in boxers), postencephalitic parkinsonism, Guam ALS/parkinsonism dementia complex, Pick disease, corticobasal degeneration, sporadic frontotemporal dementias and hereditary frontotemporal lobe dementia with parkinsonism associated with mutations on chromosome 17 (FTDP-17). These hereditary and sporadic neurodegenerative diseases characterized by aggregation of abnormal forms of tau are called **tauopathies** and they may share common mechanisms of brain degeneration. ***Alzheimer disease is both a tauopathy and a β-amyloidopathy leading to intracellular and extracellular tangles and plaques, respectively, seen in this disorder.***

There are minor histologic changes—granulovacuolar degeneration and Hirano bodies—in AD and normal aging that can be visually arresting but lack diagnostic significance. **Granulovacuolar degeneration** is largely restricted to the cytoplasm of hippocampal pyramidal cells, where it is evident as circular clear zones containing basophilic and argentophilic granules (Fig. 28-90A). **Hirano bodies,** like granulovacuolar degeneration, are seen almost exclusively in hippocampal pyramidal neurons, especially in their processes (Fig. 28-90B). Hirano bodies are 10- to 15-micron-thick eosinophilic rods composed of polymerized action.

MOLECULAR PATHOGENESIS: The cause of Alzheimer disease has not been fully elucidated, but there have been significant advances in our understanding of the origin of both Alzheimer disease–associated amyloid and NFTs.

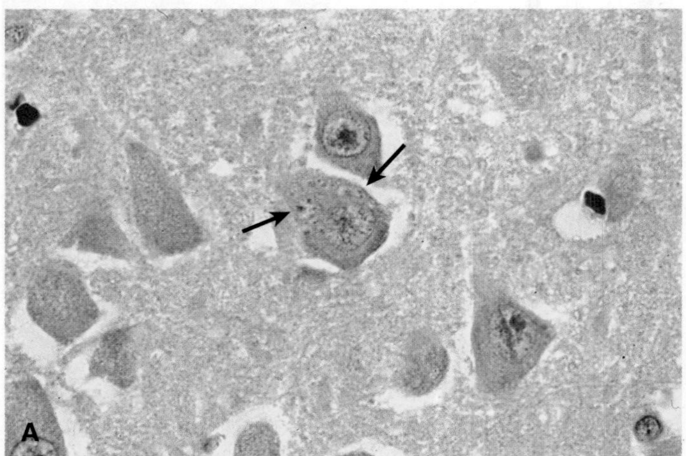

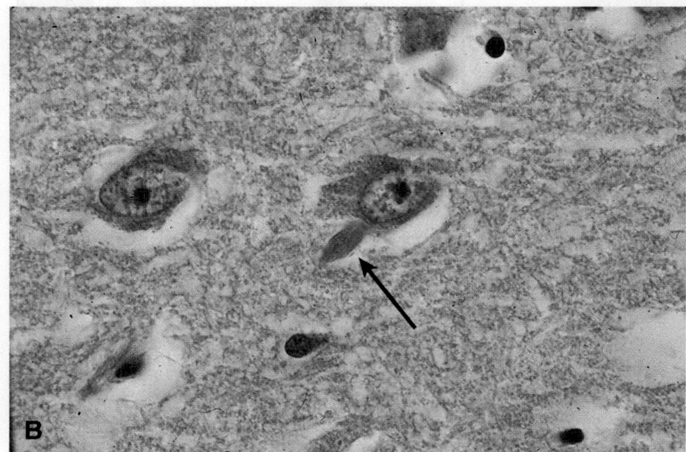

FIGURE 28-90. A. Granulovacuolar degeneration (*arrows*) is seen in hippocampal pyramidal neurons in both normal aging and Alzheimer disease. **B. Hirano bodies** are eosinophilic cytoplasmic accumulations of actin (*arrow*) seen in the cytoplasm of hippocampal pyramidal neurons in normal aging and Alzheimer disease.

- **β-Amyloid protein (Aβ):** Increasing evidence points to the importance of deposition of Aβ protein in **neuritic plaques** of Alzheimer disease. The core of these plaques contains a distinct form of Aβ peptide, which is mainly 42 amino acids long. Aβ is derived by proteolysis from a much larger (695 amino acids) membrane-spanning APP. Full-length APP has an extracellular region, a transmembrane sequence and a cytoplasmic domain. The region comprising Aβ anchors the amino-terminal portion of APP to the membrane. The physiologic functions of APP and Aβ remain obscure.

  The normal degradation of APP involves proteolytic cleavage in the middle of the Aβ domain, to release a nonamyloidogenic fragment extending from the middle of the Aβ domain to the amino terminus of APP. Proteolysis at either end of the Aβ domain then releases intact and highly amyloidogenic Aβ that accumulates in senile plaques as amyloid fibrils.

  Deposition of Aβ appears to be necessary for Alzheimer disease to develop because of the following:

  1. Patients with **Down syndrome** (trisomy 21) develop clinical and pathologic features of Alzheimer disease, including deposition of Aβ in neuritic plaques, generally by age 40. The gene for APP is on chromosome 21, and the additional dose of the gene product in trisomy 21 may predispose to precocious accumulation of Aβ.
  2. Some patients with familial Alzheimer disease carry mutant *APP* genes or mutant presenilin genes. These mutations lead to increased production of Aβ, the amyloidogenic part of APP.
  3. Transgenic mice expressing mutant human *APP* genes develop senile plaques in the brain very similar to those of Alzheimer disease. However, these mice lack other critical features of Alzheimer disease such as NFTs and evidence of neurodegeneration, such as significant loss of neurons.

  Neurons and glial cells are sites of APP synthesis in the brain, but Aβ also accumulates in the walls of cerebral blood vessels.

- **Neurofibrillary tangles:** NFTs are composed of paired helical filaments that contain tau abnormally phosphorylated at aberrant sites, resulting in a protein that does not associate with microtubules but instead aggregates to form paired helical filaments. Release of tau from microtubules may deprive cells of tau's microtubule-stabilizing effects, thereby impairing axonal transport and compromising neuronal function. Alternatively, fibril formation occurring as the hyperphosphorylated tau aggregates may itself be cytotoxic.

There are several genetic risk factors for AD. Mutations in the *APP* gene have been associated with early-onset familial variants of Alzheimer disease. Additional genetic associations (Table 28-4) involve the apolipoprotein E (apoE) genotype and the genes for presenilin 1 (*PS1*) and 2 (*PS2*).

APOLIPOPROTEIN E: ApoE has long been known for its role in cholesterol metabolism. Its relevance to dementia was uncovered in 1993, when it was reported that specific apoE isoforms confer differential susceptibility to sporadic and late-onset familial subtypes of AD. The human apoE gene is found on chromosome 19 (19q13.2). The three common alleles—ε2, ε3 and ε4—all occur in North American apoE genotypes. An increased risk of late-onset familial and sporadic AD is associated with inheritance of the ε4 allele, particularly the homozygous ε4/ε4 genotype, which occurs in 2% of the population. Conversely, the ε2 allele may confer some protection. The age at which symptoms appear in late-onset AD also correlates with the ε4 allele, with ε4/ε4 homozygotes exhibiting the earliest age at onset (younger than 70 years), whereas patients with the ε2 allele experience the latest onset (older than 90 years). The ε4 allele also correlates with increased numbers of senile plaques in patients with Alzheimer disease, but the apoE genotype is not an absolute determinant of the disease and does not predict who will develop it. How these different apoE alleles influence the risk of Alzheimer disease remains poorly understood.

PRESENILIN: Two genes with significant homology are associated with different kindreds of familial AD. Mutations of the *PS1* gene, on chromosome 14, are associated with the most common form of autosomal dominant early-onset Alzheimer disease. The *PS2* gene is on chromosome 1 and is associated with Alzheimer disease in Volga German pedigrees (Table 28-4). Presenilin mutations occur in half of cases of inherited Alzheimer disease, compared with only a few percent for mutant *APP* genes. There is some evidence that mutant PS1 and PS2 proteins alter processing of β-APP to favor increased production and deposition of Aβ. Cell processing of APP releases Aβ fragments of varying lengths, but the Aβ42 variant seems to be especially amyloidogenic. It is the Aβ molecule whose production is enhanced by mutant *PS1*.

Proposed mechanisms leading to development of Alzheimer disease are shown in Fig. 28-91.

Table 28-4

Genetic Factors in Alzheimer Disease

Gene	Chromosome	Disease Association
Amyloid precursor protein (*APP*)	21	Mutations of the *APP* gene are associated with early-onset familial Alzheimer disease
Presenilin 1 (*PS1*)	14	Mutations of the *PS1* gene are associated with early-onset familial Alzheimer disease
Presenilin 2 (*PS2*)	1	Mutations of the *PS2* gene are associated with Volga German familial Alzheimer disease
Apolipoprotein E (*apoE*)	19	Presence of the ε4 allele is associated with increased risk and younger age of onset of both inherited and sporadic forms of late-onset Alzheimer disease

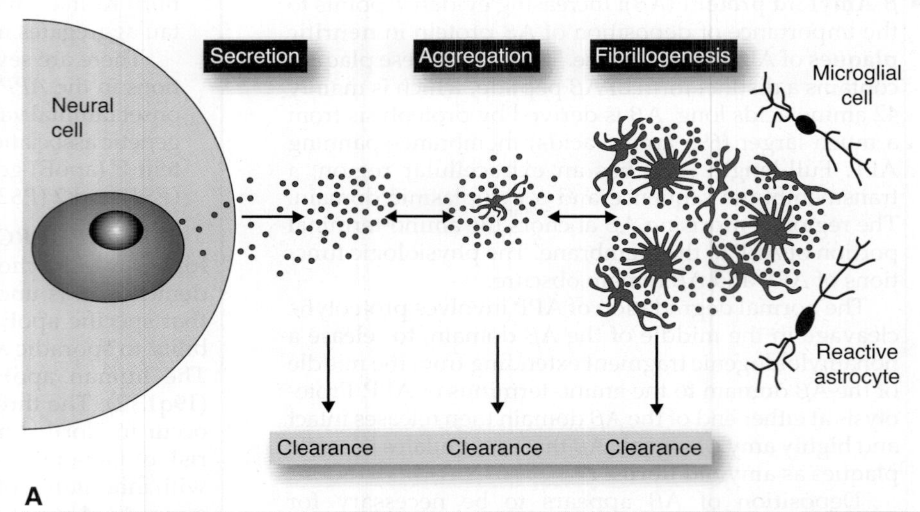

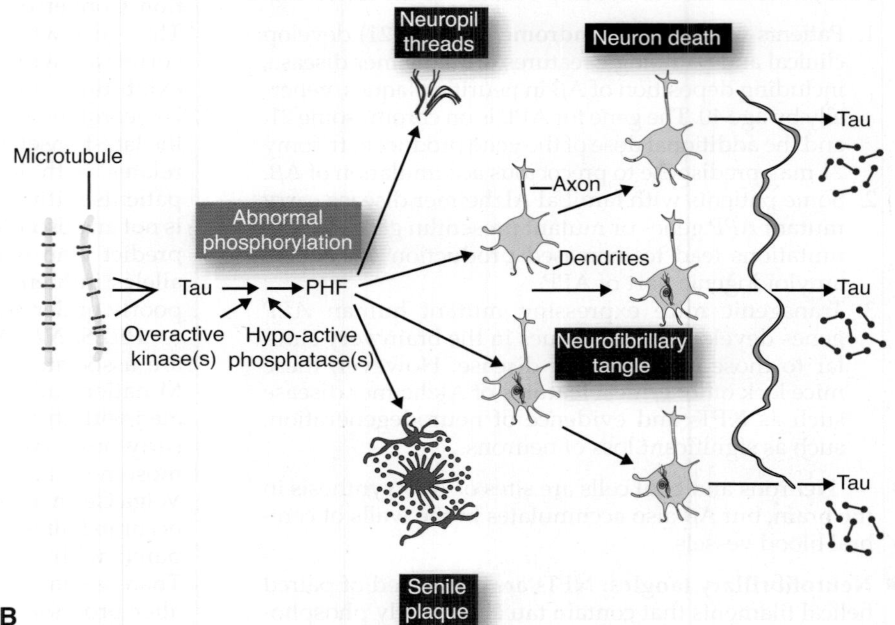

FIGURE 28-91. Mechanisms of amyloidosis and brain degeneration in Alzheimer disease. A. This schematic illustrates a hypothetical mechanism for the formation of senile plaques (SPs) from soluble Aβ peptides produced inside cells and secreted into the extracellular space. Amyloidogenic Aβ may encounter fibril-inducing cofactors and go on to form A fibrils to deposit in SPs (*far right*). SPs are surrounded by reactive astrocytes and microglial cells, which secrete cytokines that may contribute to the toxicity of the SPs. These steps may be reversible. Increasing Aβ clearance or reducing its production, as well as modulating the inflammatory response, may be effective therapeutic interventions for Alzheimer disease, in combination with therapies that target brain degeneration caused by neurofibrillary tangles (NFTs). **B.** This schematic illustrates a hypothetical mechanism leading to the conversion of normal human central nervous system (CNS) tau overlying two microtubules into paired helical filaments (PHFs). PHFs are generated in neuronal perikarya and their processes. Overactive kinase(s) or hypoactive phosphatase(s) may contribute to this effect. Abnormally phosphorylated tau forms PHFs in neuronal processes (neuropil threads) and neuronal perikarya (NFTs). Tau in PHFs loses the ability to bind microtubules, thus causing their depolymerization, disruption of axonal transport and degeneration of neurons. Accumulation of PHFs in neurons could exacerbate this process by physically blocking transport in neurons. The death of affected neurons would release tau and increase the levels of tau in the cerebrospinal fluid (CSF) of patients with Alzheimer disease. NFT formation may be reversible, and drugs that block NFT formation, reverse it or stabilize microtubules may be effective therapeutic interventions for Alzheimer disease.

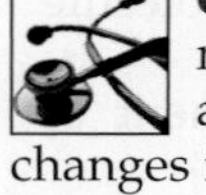

CLINICAL FEATURES: Patients with AD come to medical attention because of gradual loss of memory and cognitive function, difficulty with language and changes in behavior. Those with mild cognitive impairment are increasingly being recognized, since they move on to full-blown dementia at a rate of about 15% per year. Alzheimer disease progresses inexorably, so that previously intelligent and productive people become demented, mute, incontinent and bedridden. Bronchopneumonia, urinary tract infections and pressure decubiti are common medical complications that lead to death in Alzheimer disease.

Frontotemporal Lobar Degeneration: Pick Disease Complex

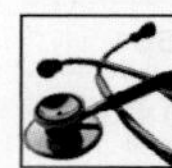

CLINICAL FEATURES: The frontotemporal lobar degenerations (FTLDs) are predominantly tauopathies in which the frontal and temporal lobes bear the early brunt of the disease. The prototype eponymic disorder of the FTLDs is **Pick disease,** which is manifested clinically as loss of frontal executive function causing disinhibition, loss of judgment about social propriety and inability to plan or foresee the consequences of one's actions. Most cases are sporadic, although Pick disease kindreds have been described. Sporadic Pick disease becomes symptomatic in midadult life and progresses relentlessly to death over a period of 3 to 10 years. A respected pillar of the community may be reduced to a vulgar, disheveled derelict as this tragic disease progresses. Unlike AD, which generally begins with memory difficulties, FTLD begins with very disruptive inappropriate behavior. These dementias converge clinically at the end.

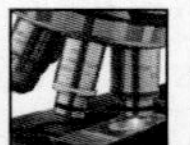

PATHOLOGY: Cortical atrophy in Pick disease predominantly involves the frontotemporal regions (Fig. 28-92) and the atrophy may attain extreme proportions, so that affected gyri are reduced to thin slivers

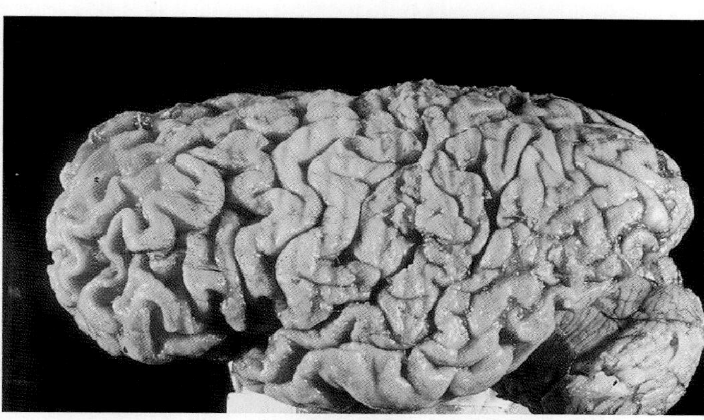

FIGURE 28-92. Severe cortical atrophy with marked frontotemporal atrophy is characteristic of the frontotemporal lobar degenerations, such as Pick disease, but may be seen in Alzheimer disease. Frontal atrophy correlates with loss of executive function, impaired judgement and disinhibition.

(knife-edge atrophy). The involved cortex is severely depleted of neurons and displays intense astrogliosis. Residual neurons contain intensely argentophilic and tau immunoreactive round cytoplasmic inclusions termed **Pick bodies** (Fig. 28-93A, B)**.** These structures are formed by densely aggregated straight tau filaments.

Pick disease is the prototypical FTLD, but there are others that only recently have begun to reveal their molecular secrets. In any cohort of patients with clinical FTLD, many at autopsy have Pick disease, but a significant number do not. Often, their neurons are immunoreactive for ubiquitin, implying an as yet unidentified protein triggering an unfulfilled degradative response. These are classified at FTLD-U, the U for ubiquitin immunoreactivity. Several of these proteins have recently been identified. The protein TDP43 bears brief consideration, since abnormal accumulation of this protein is seen in both FTLD and motor neuron disease. This molecular commonality is reflected by the increasingly recognized clinical coexistence of frontotemporal dementia and motor neuron disease.

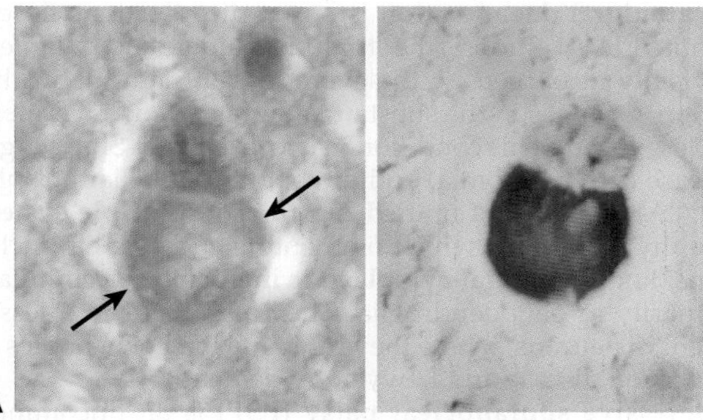

FIGURE 28-93. Pick bodies. A. In hematoxylin and eosin–stained sections, Pick bodies are basophilic, spherical, intracytoplasmic, intraneuronal aggregates of tau protein (*arrows*). They tend to be round rather than angular like the neurofibrillary tangles (NFTs) in Alzheimer disease, but like NFTs, they are argentophilic (silver impregnation) (**B**).

Lewy Body Dementia

Lewy body dementia (LBD), also known as Lewy body disease or diffuse Lewy body disease, is characterized by intracytoplasmic α-synuclein immunoreactive inclusions in a relatively small number of cortical neurons, predominantly in the cingulate cortex. AD pathology often coexists with Lewy body inclusions at the end stage of the disease.

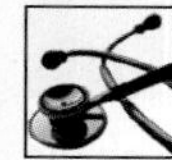

CLINICAL FEATURES: LBD is distinctive in that cognitive function fluctuates greatly from day to day, subtle extrapyramidal manifestations may be present and the patient may experience fascinating well-formed visual hallucinations. LBD exists on a continuum with the other α-synucleinopathies that include Parkinson disease and multiple system atrophy.

Neurodegeneration of the Basal Ganglia

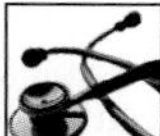

CLINICAL FEATURES: Movement disorders may result in too little **(bradykinetic)** or too much involuntary **(hyperkinetic)** movement. Parkinson disease is the prototypical bradykinetic movement disorder, characterized by difficulty initiating and sustaining voluntary movement, resting tremor and postural instability. This clinical triad is "parkinsonism," and while the most common cause is Parkinson disease, there are other disorders such as progressive supranuclear palsy, multiple system atrophy and even neuro-AIDS that may result in parkinsonism.

The prototypical hyperkinetic movement disorder is Huntington disease, in which there is progressive development of involuntary rapid twitching movements (chorea) and writhing dancelike movements (athetosis) that may conflate as choreoathetosis.

Parkinson Disease

First described in 1817, Parkinson disease (PD) is characterized clinically by tremors at rest, cogwheel rigidity, expressionless countenance, postural instability and, less commonly, cognitive impairment. Pathologically, PD shows loss of neurons, primarily in the substantia nigra, and accumulation of Lewy bodies, made of filamentous aggregates of α-synuclein. Neurochemically there is loss of dopaminergic neurons that project from the substantia nigra to the striatum.

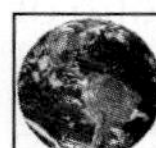

EPIDEMIOLOGY: Parkinson disease typically appears in the sixth to eighth decades of life. The disease is common, and 1% to 2% of the population in North America eventually develops it. The prevalence has remained unchanged for at least the past 40 years. No racial differences are apparent, but men are more affected than women.

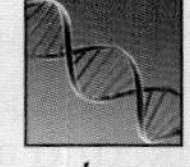

MOLECULAR PATHOGENESIS: Most cases are sporadic, but missense mutations in the α-synuclein gene are responsible for rare cases of autosomal dominant, early-onset, familial PD. The finding that wild-type α-synuclein is the major polymerized protein in Lewy bodies led to consideration of fibrillogenesis as a major contributor to the pathogenesis of neurodegenerative diseases. Accumulating evidence suggests that

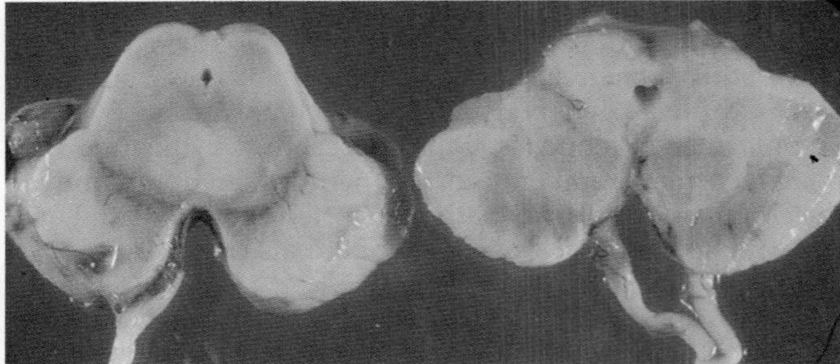

FIGURE 28-94. Parkinson disease. The normal substantia nigra on the left in an adult is heavily pigmented, while the substantia nigra in a patient with Parkinson disease has lost pigmented neurons and the nucleus now blends inconspicuously with the rest of the midbrain. The locus ceruleus in the pons is also depigmented (not shown). (Courtesy of Dr. F. Stephen Vogel, Duke University.)

oxidative stress produced by the autooxidation of catecholamines during melanin formation injures neurons in the substantia nigra by promoting misfolding of α-synuclein and formation of filamentous inclusions.

In addition to PD, accumulation of filamentous α-synuclein inclusions is seen in a number of other diseases, including multiple system atrophy, dementia with Lewy bodies, progressive autonomic failure and rapid eye movement (REM) sleep behavior disorder. These disorders are now called **α-synucleinopathies** and, like the tauopathies, are considered brain-specific amyloidoses.

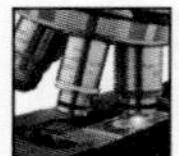

PATHOLOGY: Brains of Parkinson disease patients reveal loss of pigmentation in the substantia nigra and locus ceruleus (Fig. 28-94). Other brain regions are affected to a lesser extent. Pigmented neurons are scarce, and small extracellular deposits of melanin are derived from dying neurons. Some residual neurons are atrophic, and a few contain Lewy bodies, which are visualized as spherical, eosinophilic cytoplasmic inclusions (Fig. 28-95). By electron microscopy, Lewy bodies exhibit amyloid-like filaments formed by insoluble α-synuclein.

Other Disorders Causing Parkinsonism

PD is not the sole cause of parkinsonism. There is a group of disorders where the common theme is loss of pigmented dopaminergic neurons in the substantia nigra. Normal aging is associated with some neuron loss in the substantia nigra and reduced levels of dopamine, but these features are exaggerated in PD and these other causes of parkinsonism. At times, mechanistic insights have been gleaned in these other less common causes of parkinsonism that have led directly to greater understanding of PD and other neurodegenerative conditions.

- **MPTP-induced parkinsonism** was discovered the late 1970s when there was an epidemic of parkinsonism among intravenous drug abusers that was ultimately linked to a toxic byproduct of the illicit synthesis of a meperidine. That contaminant, 1-methyl-4-phenyl-1,2,3,6-tetrahydropyridine (MPTP), is transformed by the brain's own monoamine oxidase into a highly reactive free radical. The MPTP saga led to consideration that there may be environmental and endogenous free radicals that led to initiation and progression of neurodegenerative disorders, and therapeutic interventions directed against these targets are being developed and tested.

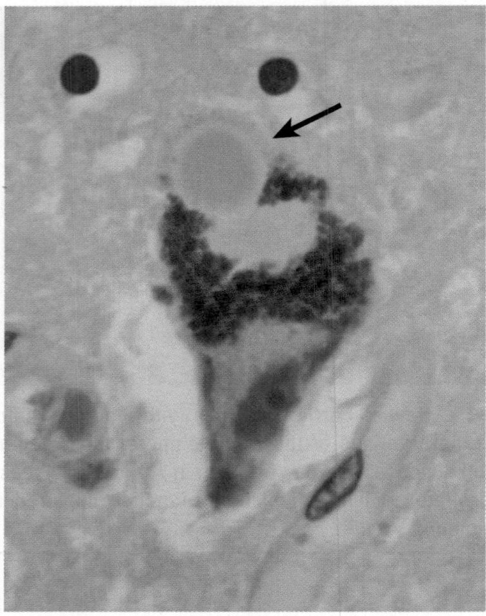

FIGURE 28-95. Lewy body in Parkinson disease. Examination of residual neurons in the substantia nigra show intracytoplasmic, intraneuronal, spherical eosinophilic inclusions composed of polymerized α-synuclein called Lewy bodies (*arrow*). These inclusions often have a thin clear halo.

- **Postinfectious parkinsonism** was seen after viral encephalitis (von Economo encephalitis) associated with the influenza pandemic during World War I and has not recurred to a major degree since that time. This condition was characterized by loss of substantia nigra neurons but no Lewy bodies being present. How this disorder develops is unknown, but there is concern that a similar combination of influenza antigens may lead to a recurrence of this epidemic. The 2009 H1N1 influenza virus, for example, was very similar antigenically to the influenza seen in the earlier pandemic.
- **Striatonigral degeneration** is a rare disorder that closely mimics PD. At autopsy, the striatum (caudate and putamen) is visibly atrophied, with severe loss of neurons in this region. Changes in the substantia nigra and locus ceruleus are less severe. This condition may coexist with Shy-Drager disease (dysautonomia) and olivopontocerebellar atrophy (OPCA) as part of a unified disorder of **multiple system atrophy (MSA),** in which filamentous α-synuclein inclusions, known as **glial cytoplasmic inclusions,** accumulate primarily in oligodendroglia. They also occur to a lesser extent in neurons, where they resemble the Lewy bodies of Parkinson disease and Lewy body dementia.
- **Progressive supranuclear palsy (PSP)** is an uncommon disorder characterized by parkinsonism, severe postural instability with falls and progressive paralysis of vertical eye movements. Pathologic changes in the brain are more widespread than in Parkinson disease, but the hallmark is atrophy of the midbrain tegmentum, leading to an exaggerated contribution of the cerebral peduncles to the profile

of the midbrain in axial sections—a profile that is referred to by some as "Mickey Mouse" midbrain. Since the midbrain, as well as the substantia nigra, is the locus of integration of vertical eye movement, the combination of parkinsonism and vertical gaze dysfunction makes anatomic sense. PSP is a **tauopathy:** the sole inclusions are tau-rich NFTs. PSP spreads throughout the nervous system, and cognitive impairment complicates the disease course.

Huntington Disease

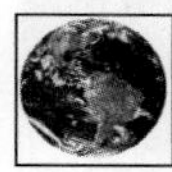

EPIDEMIOLOGY: First described in 1872, Huntington disease (HD) is an autosomal dominant genetic disorder characterized by involuntary movements, deterioration of cognitive function and often severe emotional disturbances. It principally affects whites of northwestern European ancestry, with an incidence of 1 in 20,000. Genealogic studies indicate that all cases derive from an original founder in northern Europe; the disease is very rare in Asia and Africa.

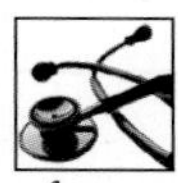

CLINICAL FEATURES: The symptoms of HD are usually first seen by age 40, but 5% of patients with the disorder develop neurologic signs before 20 years of age, and a comparable proportion develop manifestations after age 60. Cognitive and emotional disturbances precede the onset of abnormal movements by several years in over half of patients. Once it develops, choreoathetosis may be incapacitating. Cortical involvement leads to a severe loss of cognitive function and intellectual deterioration, often accompanied by paranoia and delusions. The interval from the onset of symptoms to death averages 15 years.

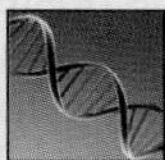

MOLECULAR PATHOGENESIS: The *HD* gene, on chromosome 4 (4p16.3), codes for the protein **huntingtin.** In 1993, it was discovered that the aberration at this locus is expansion of a trinucleotide (CAG) repeat. The repeat is within a coding region of the gene and results in production of an altered protein, with a polyglutamine tract near the N-terminus. In agreement with the dominant mode of inheritance, the triplet expansion causes a toxic gain of function.

Huntingtin is widely expressed in tissues throughout the body and in all regions of the CNS by neurons and glia, but its function is unknown. As with other CAG repeat expansion diseases (see Chapter 6), the longer the CAG repeat, the more severe the disease phenotype and the earlier the age of clinical onset. In HD, CAG length is more unstable and tends to be longer when inherited from the father than in maternal transmission. As a result, transmission of the *HD* mutation from the father results in clinical disease some 3 years earlier than when it is passed on from the mother. Of children with juvenile-onset HD, the ratio of those who inherit the expanded CAG allele from their father to those who inherit it from their mother is 10:1.

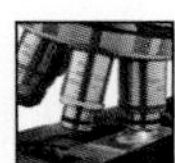

PATHOLOGY: The frontal cortex is symmetrically and moderately atrophic, whereas the lateral ventricles appear disproportionately enlarged as a result of the loss of the normal convex curvature of the caudate nuclei (Fig. 28-96). There is symmetric atrophy of the caudate nuclei, with lesser involvement of the putamen. Neuronal populations of the caudate and putamen, particularly the small neurons, are severely depleted, with accompanying astrogliosis. The cerebral cortical neurons are similarly, but less severely, lost. Aggregates of huntingtin are seen in neurons, especially in nuclei, but also in neuronal processes, potentially impairing axodendritic transport. γ-Aminobutyric acid (GABA) and glutamic acid decarboxylase are markedly decreased.

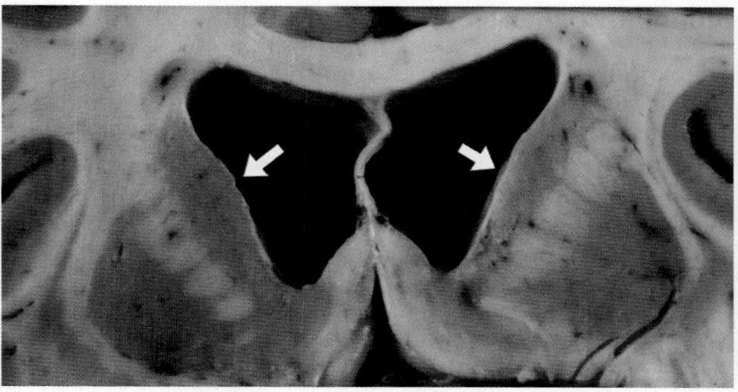

FIGURE 28-96. Huntington disease. The caudate nuclei (*arrows*) bilaterally are atrophic, leading to enlarged lateral ventricles. Some cortical atrophy is also seen, but it is usually not as severe as that seen in the primary cortical dementias such as Alzheimer and Pick disease.

Nucleotide Repeat Expansion Disorders

Huntington disease is one of an ever-increasing group of neurologic diseases that are now classified as nucleotide repeat expansion syndromes (see Chapter 6). These disorders are not rare, but rather include the most common cause of mental retardation in boys (fragile X syndrome), the most common adult-onset muscular dystrophy (myotonic dystrophy) and the most common hereditary spinocerebellar ataxia (Friedreich ataxia).

MOLECULAR PATHOGENESIS: Trinucleotide repeats are a normal feature of many genes, and expansion of the number of triplet repeats confers pathogenicity. Some triplet repeat diseases show only a small expansion compared with their normal counterparts (e.g., Huntington disease), but in others, the expansion is quite large (e.g., fragile X syndrome and Friedreich ataxia). This class of diseases includes examples of all forms of inheritance: X-linked, autosomal dominant and autosomal recessive. In most of the autosomal dominant CAG expansion disorders, the abnormal expansion is in the coding region of a gene and results in production of an abnormal ("toxic") protein. In other disorders, the expansion occurs in a noncoding region of the gene and probably interferes with transcription or message processing. The resulting decrease in protein levels constitutes a loss-of-function mutation (as appears to be the case with GAA expansion in Friedreich ataxia). In myotonic dystrophy, a noncoding region expansion produces a transcript that interferes with correct mRNA splicing for multiple gene products, leading to the multiorgan multiprotein manifestations of this condition. The discovery of these mutations allows for better understanding of the functions of these normal proteins, elucidating the pathogenesis of these diseases and, hopefully, better therapies.

Spinocerebellar Neurodegeneration

The spinocerebellar ataxias are a heterogeneous group of genetic disorders that impact cerebellar inflow and outflow pathways, or the cerebellar parenchyma itself. The cerebellum plays a key role in assisting the motor cerebral cortex and basal ganglia program with motor actions, and in ensuring the smooth performance of repetitive motor tasks such as playing the piano, riding a bicycle or speaking. Once the cerebellum is exposed to motor tasks, it serves as a repository of motor programs sometimes called "motor memory." Dysfunction of the cerebellum leads to ataxia—the inability to execute motor tasks smoothly, particularly those requiring rapid alternating movement or precise motor control. Ataxia may result from defects in the major cerebellar input pathways including the middle cerebellar peduncle, which conveys motor execution commands from the cerebral motor and premotor cortex, and the inferior cerebellar peduncle, which receives proprioceptive data from the spinal cord via the spinocerebellar tracts. If the cerebellar parenchyma itself degenerates, ataxia will result in a distribution congruent with the functional portion of the cerebellum involved—vermal degeneration leads to truncal ataxia, while cerebellar hemispheric degeneration leads to appendicular ataxia. Finally, the cerebral outflow—the dentatorubrothalamic pathway—may degenerate, leading to a peculiarly high-amplitude ataxia called "wing-beating ataxia."

Friedreich Ataxia

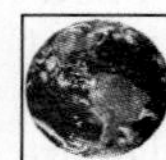

EPIDEMIOLOGY: Friedreich ataxia is the most common inherited ataxia. Its prevalence in European populations is 1 in 50,000. Although the inheritance pattern is autosomal recessive, many cases arise sporadically as new mutations without a family history.

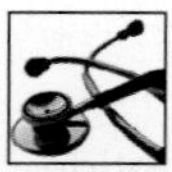

CLINICAL FEATURES: Symptoms usually begin before age 25 years, followed by an unremittingly progressive course of about 30 years to death. Friedreich ataxia is a cerebellar inflow disorder characterized by ataxia of both the upper and lower limbs, dysarthria, lower limb areflexia, extensor plantar reflexes and sensory loss reflecting concurrent degeneration of spinal long tracts. Common concomitants include deformities of the skeletal system (e.g., scoliosis, pes cavus), hypertrophic cardiomyopathy (which commonly causes death) and diabetes mellitus.

MOLECULAR PATHOGENESIS: The genetic defect in Friedreich ataxia is autosomal recessive loss of function of the genes encoding a mitochondrial protein **(frataxin),** which is involved in iron transport into mitochondria. In most cases the mutation is an unstable expansion of a trinucleotide (GAA) repeat in the first intron of this gene (9q13.3–21.1). The recessive pattern of inheritance means that both frataxin alleles must be lost—both may bear the trinucleotide repeat expansion, or one may have the repeat expansion while the other allele may be compromised by a different mutation. The expansion mutation probably interferes with transcription or RNA processing. In unaffected people, levels of frataxin protein are highest in the heart and spinal cord. Lack of frataxin is thus probably responsible for the neuropathologic manifestations of Friedreich ataxia and the cardiomyopathy. The longer the trinucleotide repeat, the earlier the age of disease onset, the faster the rate of clinical progression and the higher the frequency of hypertrophic cardiomyopathy.

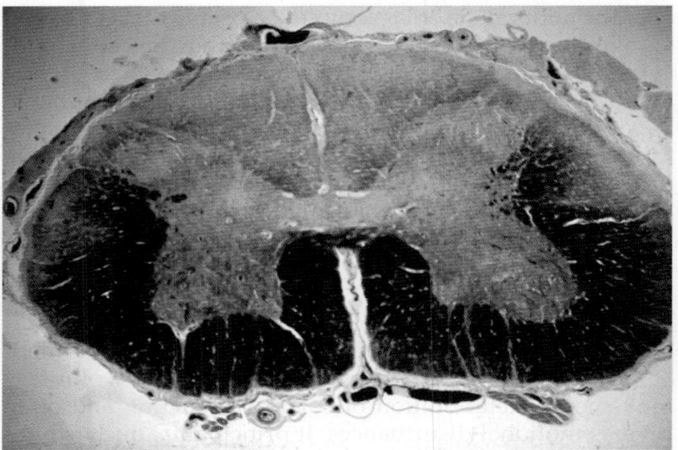

FIGURE 28-97. Friedreich ataxia. This is the most common hereditary ataxia. Myelin-stained sections show secondary degeneration of the dorsal columns, lateral corticospinal tracts and spinocerebellar tracts. This is predominantly an inflow ataxia and the cerebellum is usually not atrophic.

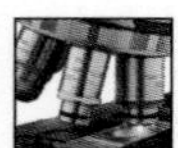

PATHOLOGY: The most prominent postmortem findings in Friedreich ataxia are in the spinal cord, where classic features are degeneration of the posterior columns, corticospinal pathways and spinocerebellar tracts (Fig. 28-97). Posterior column degeneration accounts for the sensory loss experienced by patients with Friedreich ataxia and results from loss of the parent neuronal cell bodies in the dorsal root ganglia. In advanced cases, this degeneration can be appreciated grossly as shrinkage of the dorsal spinal roots and posterior funiculi. Similarly, atrophy of the spinocerebellar tracts, with attendant ataxia, follows neuronal degeneration in the dorsal nucleus of Clarke. The corticospinal tracts show the most pronounced degeneration more distally in the cord leading to weakness and release of the plantar extensor reflex.

The Most Common Motor Neuron Disease Is Amyotrophic Lateral Sclerosis

Amyotrophic Lateral Sclerosis

ALS is a degenerative disease of upper and lower motor neurons of the brain and spinal cord, with progressive weakness and wasting of the extremities and tongue, a sometimes confusing combination of hyperreflexia and hyporeflexia and eventual impairment of respiratory muscles.

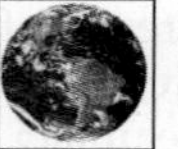

EPIDEMIOLOGY: ALS is a worldwide disease with an incidence of 1 in 100,000. It peaks in the fifth decade, and it is rare in persons younger than 35 years. There is a 1.5- to 2-fold excess of ALS in men.

Restricted geographic areas with a particularly high incidence of ALS exist in Guam and parts of Japan and Papua New Guinea, but these cases differ from ALS in the rest of the world. Cases in the Chamorro people indigenous to Guam are characterized by abundant accumulations of tau-rich NFTs and are now classified as **tauopathies.** Moreover, ALS in Guam is part of a spectrum of disorders that includes dementia and parkinsonism.

MOLECULAR PATHOGENESIS: Familial ALS cases, with an autosomal dominant pattern, account for 5% of ALS, and the most common form has been associated with missense mutations in the gene that codes for the cytosolic form of the antioxidant enzyme superoxide dismutase (Cu/Zn SOD, or SOD1). Since SOD1 is a key free radical detoxifying enzyme, SOD1 mutations might lead to increased free radical damage. However, the extent to which enzyme activity is lost is unclear, but mutant SOD1 is more prone to aggregation than wild-type SOD1, so familial ALS may be a member of the pantheon of **protein conformational disorders.**

PATHOLOGY: ALS affects lower motor neurons, including anterior horn cells of the spinal cord and the motor nuclei of the brainstem, particularly the hypoglossal nuclei; and the upper motor neurons of the cerebral cortex. Loss of the upper motor neurons leads to degeneration of their axons, with secondary demyelination visualized in myelin-stained axial sections of the spinal cord as loss of the lateral and anterior corticospinal pathways (Fig. 28-98).

The defining histologic change in ALS is a loss of large motor neurons accompanied by mild gliosis (Fig. 28-99). This change is most apparent in the anterior horns of the lumbar and cervical enlargements of the spinal cord, and the hypoglossal nuclei. There is also a loss of the giant pyramidal Betz cells in the motor cortex of the cerebrum. The anterior nerve roots bearing the few remaining axons of the dying lower motor neurons become atrophic, and the affected muscles are pale and shrunken, reflecting severe neurogenic atrophy.

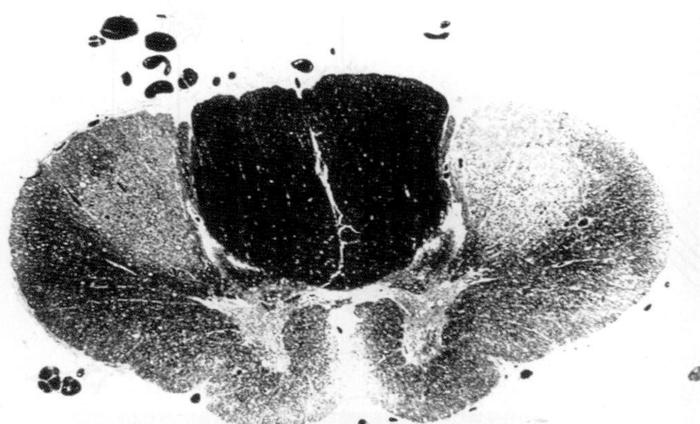

FIGURE 28-98. Amyotrophic lateral sclerosis (ALS) spinal cord showing upper motor neuron loss. Myelin-stained sections show degeneration of the lateral corticospinal tracts reflecting degeneration of the axons of the upper motor neurons originating in the motor strip of the cerebral cortex. Note the preservation of the dorsal columns, spinothalamic tracts and spinocerebellar pathways.

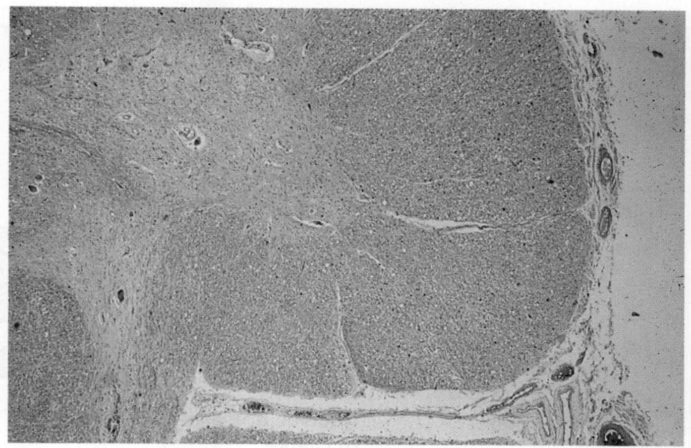

FIGURE 28-99. Amyotrophic lateral sclerosis (ALS) spinal cord showing lower motor neuron loss. The anterior horn of the spinal cord normally contains numerous very large lower motor neurons. In ALS there is anterior horn cell loss and gliosis.

CLINICAL FEATURES: ALS often begins asymmetrically as weakness and wasting of the muscles of a hand. Irregular rapid involuntary contractions of small muscle groups (fasciculations) are characteristic and are believed to arise from hyperirritability of the terminal arborizations of dying lower motor neurons. The disease is inexorably progressive, with increasing weakness of the limbs leading to total disability. Speech may become unintelligible, and respiratory weakness supervenes. Despite the dramatic wasting of the body, intellectual capacity tends to be preserved to the end, although some patients with ALS also suffer dementia of the frontotemporal lobar type. The clinical course does not usually extend beyond a decade.

Spinal muscular atrophy (Werdnig-Hoffman disease) is the second most common lethal autosomal recessive condition in Caucasian populations. It usually presents in infancy with extreme muscle weakness and atrophy caused by severe loss of anterior horn cells. Death from respiratory failure or aspiration pneumonia is usually within a few months of diagnosis. Accurate diagnosis is critical for genetic risk management. This disorder results from a loss-of-function mutation of a neuronal apoptosis inhibitor protein resulting in neurons having an extremely low threshold for initiating programmed cell death.

Several neurodegenerative, infectious and vitamin deficiency disorders impact the spinal long tracts and are summarized in Fig. 28-100.

Paraneoplastic Neurologic Disorders

Systemic benign or malignant tumors may occasionally elicit autoimmune attack on the brain or peripheral nervous system. Paraneoplastic neurologic disorders (PNDs) occur when an antitumor immune response is directed against an antigen, usually a protein, present on both the cancer cells and a nervous system cell **(onconeural antigens).** Antionconeural antibodies can often be identified in a patient's serum or CSF.

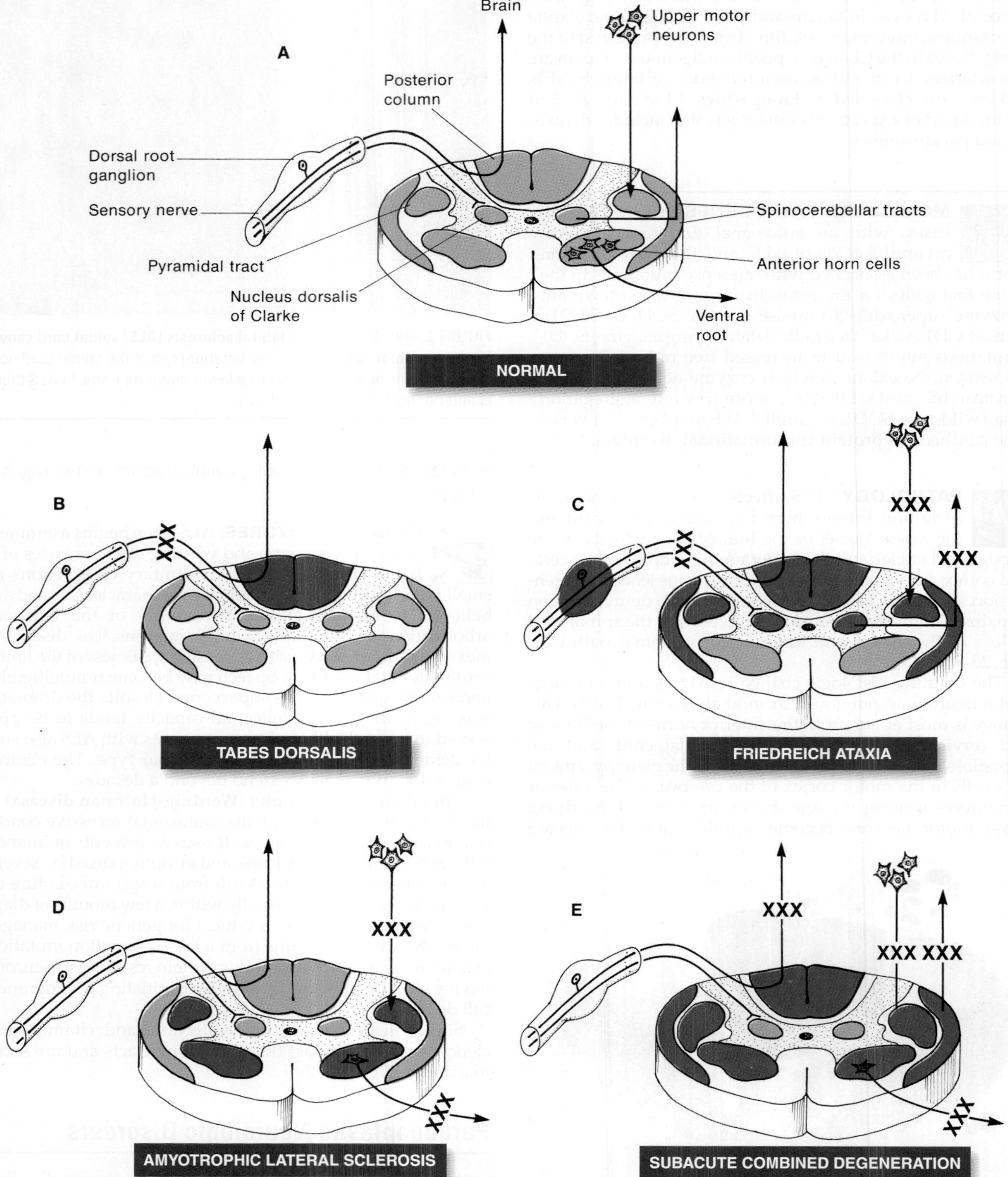

FIGURE 28-100. Tract degeneration in diseases of the spinal cord. Ascending (*blue*) sensory and descending (*green*) pathways travel through the spinal cord. These tracts may be differentially affected (*red*) depending on the nature of the underlying disease, as shown in this example of four diseases that we have considered.

PND may precede the clinical presentation of the primary tumor, sometimes by several years, and successful treatment of the cancer often results in resolution of the PND.

The clinical signs and symptoms of a given PND depend on the anatomic distribution of the neurons that express the particular onconeural antigen under attack. In some PNDs the antigen is broadly expressed in neuron populations throughout the brain and spinal cord, and so results in a **diffuse encephalomyelitis.** A prominent example is the Hu antigen, for which the most commonly associated cancer is small cell lung carcinoma (SCLC). In other PNDs, the antigen is more restricted, as in **cerebellar degeneration** resulting from immune attack against cerebellar Yo or Ri antigens, typically associated with breast or ovarian cancer, or **limbic encephalitis** targeting the Ma or Ma2 antigen, which is often associated with SCLC or testicular cancer.

Two major classes of neuron proteins serve as targets of PND-associated autoimmune attack: (1) **intracellular antigens,** such as the Hu, Yo, Ri and Ma antigens mentioned above, and (2) **neuronal cell surface antigens,** such as potassium channel proteins, and AMPA, GABA(B), glycine, glutamate and NMDA receptor proteins. The latter exemplifies the importance of clinical recognition and accurate diagnosis of PNDs. The paraneoplastic limbic encephalitis resulting from anti-NMDA receptor autoantibodies is potentially a lethal disease that can be completely cured by simple surgical resection of the triggering benign ovarian teratoma!

Developmental Malformations

CNS development unfolds according to a precise schedule, with each morphologic event being the foundation for those that follow. Thus, congenital anomalies reflect interruptions in the completion of critical developmental processes. ***The characteristics of a congenital malformation are defined more by the timing of an insult than the nature of the injury itself.***

ETIOLOGIC FACTORS: There are three critical stages of CNS development: (1) neurulation, (2) segmentation and cleavage and (3) proliferation and migration. Neurulation is complete by 4 weeks of gestation, often before a mother is aware that she is pregnant, and consists of formation and closure of the neural tube. This step establishes cranial to caudal, dorsal to ventral and left to right axes of the embryo. Between weeks 4 and 8, the neural tube segments into neighborhoods that will ultimately become the spinal cord, medulla, pons and cerebellum, midbrain, diencephalon and telencephalon. The diencephalon and telencephalon then cleave to form the paired basal ganglia, thalami and cerebral hemispheres. By the end of 8 weeks of gestation, basic CNS architecture is established. For the rest of gestation and beyond into postnatal life, cell proliferation creates the *trillions* of neuroglia that ultimately populate the mature CNS. These cells are predominantly born in the periventricular germinal matrix and must successfully migrate to their ultimate destinations. In humans, defects of proliferation and migration mainly impact the formation of cerebral cortex and lead to mental retardation and seizures. Once neurons and glia reach their destinations, they must correctly wire the brain using axonal pathfinding and oligodendroglial myelination.

Defects of Neurulation Are the Neural Tube Defects

Anencephaly

Anencephaly is the congenital absence of all or part of the brain as a result of unsuccessful closure of the cephalad (anterior neuropore) portion of the neural tube.

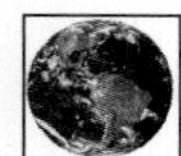

EPIDEMIOLOGY: Anencephaly is the second most common CNS malformation after spina bifida (0.5 to 2.0 per 1000 births, with a modest female predominance) and is the most common lethal CNS malformation. Anencephalic fetuses are stillborn or die in the first few days of life.

Anencephaly is a multifactorial birth defect exhibiting geographic variation in incidence. In the United States, it occurs in 0.3 per 1000 live births and stillbirths. In Ireland, the frequency is 20-fold greater (5 to 6 per 1000). Incidence declines to 2 to 3 per 1000 among Irish immigrants to North America. The incidence of this disorder is low in blacks.

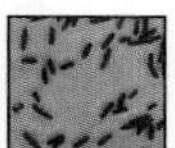

ETIOLOGIC FACTORS: Anencephaly is a dysraphic defect of neural tube closure (Fig. 28-101). Its concurrence with other neural tube defects (NTDs), such as spina bifida, suggests shared pathogenic mechanisms. During development, the neural plate invaginates and is transformed into the neural tube by fusion of the posterior surfaces. Mesenchymal tissue overlying the primitive neural tube then forms the skull and vertebral arches posterior to the spinal cord, while ectoderm forms the skin of the head and back. Failure of the neural tube to close results in the lack of closure of the overlying bony structures of the cranium and an absence of the calvarium, skin and subcutaneous tissues of this region. The exposed brain is incompletely formed or even entirely absent. In most cases, the base of the skull contains only fragments of neural and ependymal tissue and residues of the meninges.

Genetic factors play a role in the pathogenesis of anencephaly. The anomaly is twice as common in female as in male fetuses, and it occurs with higher frequency in certain families. The risk of a second anencephalic fetus is 2% to 5%, and after two anencephalic fetuses the risk rises to 25% for each subsequent pregnancy.

Folic acid supplied in the periconceptional period lowers the incidence of NTDs. In 1998, the U.S. Food and Drug Administration began requiring manufacturers of enriched flour, bread and some other products to supplement these foods with folate. This led to a significant decrease in the incidence of NTDs of all types.

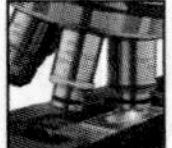

PATHOLOGY: The cranial vault is absent, and in place of the cerebral hemispheres is a mass of highly vascularized, disorganized neuroglial tissue, the **cerebrovasculosa** (Fig. 28-102), on the flattened base of the skull, behind two well-formed eyes, which mark the anterior margin of disturbed organogenesis. A well-differentiated retina attests to the preservation of the eyes, and short segments of the optic nerve extend posteriorly. The posterior aspect of the malformation forms a variable transitional zone with a recognizable midbrain, but most often the entire brainstem and cerebellum are rudimentary. The upper spinal cord is hypoplastic, and a dysraphic bony defect of the posterior spinal column **(rachischisis)** may involve the cervical area. Vertebral and basilar arteries usually are identifiable in a tangle of meningeal vessels.

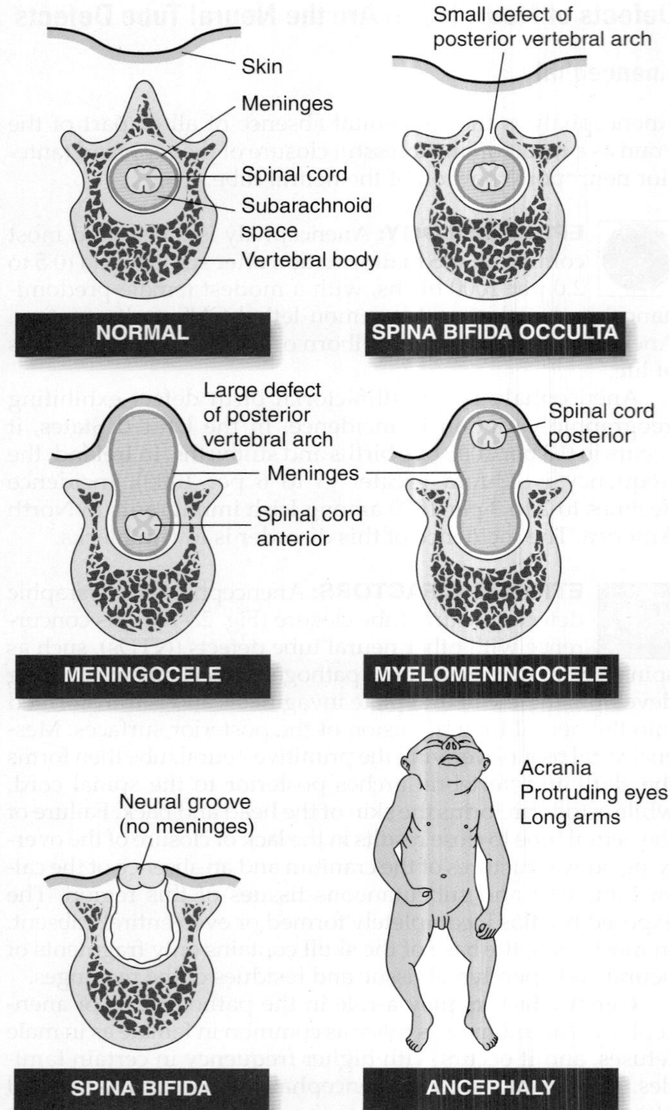

FIGURE 28-101. Defects of the neural tube. The first critical step in neural development is neurulation—formation and closure of the neural tube. Incomplete fusion of the neural tube and overlying bone, soft tissues or skin leads to several defects, varying from mild anomalies (e.g., spina bifida occulta) to severe anomalies (e.g., anencephaly).

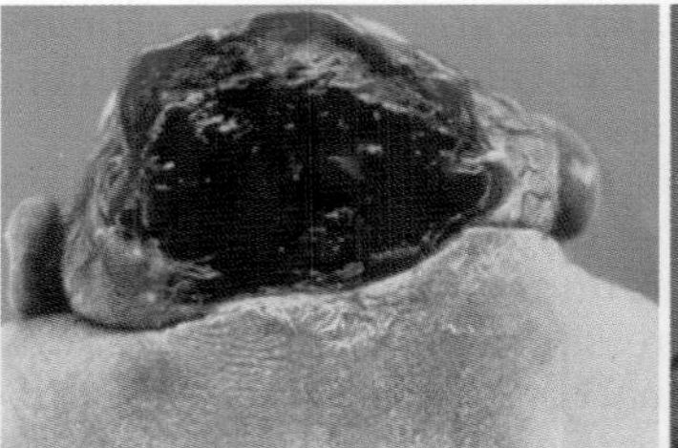
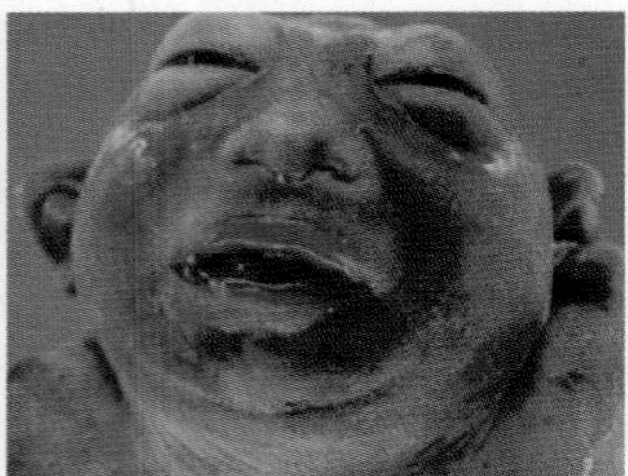

FIGURE 28-102. Anencephaly is the most severe defect of neurulation. The cerebral vault is absent (*right panel*), and the absence of a calvarium exposes a mass of vascularized tissue (cerebrovasculosa, *left panel*), in which there are rudimentary neuroectodermal structures. The lesion is bounded anteriorly by normally formed eyes and posteriorly by the brainstem.

The cerebrovasculosa typically contains islands of immature neural tissue. It also encloses cavities partially lined by ependyma with or without choroid plexus. However, the mass is composed predominantly of abnormal vascular channels that vary considerably in size.

Two thirds of anencephalic fetuses die in utero, and those that are alive at birth rarely survive for more than a week. Screening of pregnant women for serum α-fetoprotein and ultrasonography detect virtually all anencephalic fetuses.

Spina Bifida

Spina bifida is a set of NTDs resulting from failure of neural tube closure in the more caudal regions. This anomaly is usually localized to the lumbar region and varies in clinical severity from asymptomatic to disabling, but is not usually lethal. Spina bifida results from an insult between the 25th and 30th days of gestation, reflecting the sequential closure of the neural tube. It is subclassified according to the severity of the defect:

- **Spina bifida occulta:** This defect is restricted to the vertebral arches and is usually asymptomatic. It is frequently manifested externally only by a dimple or small tuft of hair on the lower back.
- **Meningocele:** This condition features a more extensive bony and soft tissue defect that permits protrusion of the meninges as a fluid-filled sac visible on the external surface of the back, in the midline. The lateral aspects of the sac are characteristically covered by a thin layer of skin, whereas the apex may become ulcerated, allowing entry of microorganisms into the CSF.
- **Meningomyelocele:** This term refers to a still more extensive defect that exposes the spinal canal and causes nerve roots (particularly those of the cauda equina) and spinal cord to be entrapped in an externally visible protruding CSF-filled sac (Fig. 28-103). Usually, the spinal cord is a flattened, ribbonlike structure. Severe neurologic consequences include lower extremity motor and sensory defects and compromise of bowel and bladder neurogenic control.
- **Rachischisis:** In this extreme defect, the spinal column is a gaping canal, often without a recognizable spinal cord (Fig. 28-104). This defect is usually lethal and seen in abortuses.

Spina bifida is induced readily in rats and chicks at the eighth to ninth gestational day by chemicals such as trypan blue or by hypervitaminosis A. It probably results from failure of the neural tube to close, but the validity of this concept is uncertain. As mentioned above, maternal folic acid deficiency has been implicated in NTDs, and folic acid supplementation in food has reduced NTDs. Some drugs, notably retinoids used for acne and valproic acid used to manage seizures, must be avoided by women of child-bearing age because of their association with NTDs.

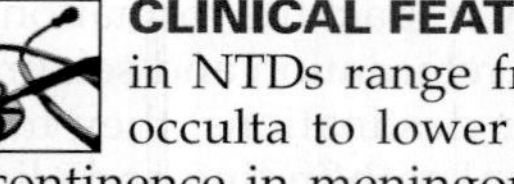

CLINICAL FEATURES: Clinical neurologic deficits in NTDs range from no symptoms in spina bifida occulta to lower limb paralysis, sensory loss and incontinence in meningomyelocele. One must be aware of potential associated malformations such as Arnold-Chiari

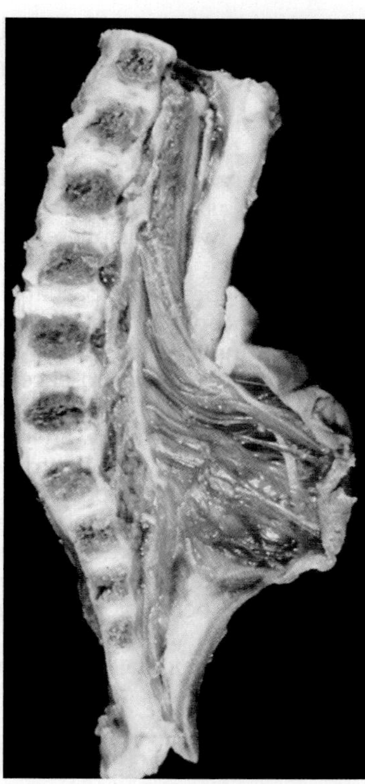

FIGURE 28-103. Meningomyelocele. This dysraphic defect, which is caused by lack of fusion of the spinal canal usually in the lumbar region, reveals disorganized spinal cord tissue with entrapment of nerve roots in a cerebrospinal fluid–filled sac. (Courtesy of Dr. F. Stephen Vogel, Duke University.)

malformation, hydrocephalus, polymicrogyria and hydromyelia of the spinal central canal (see below).

Malformations of the Spinal Cord

Other congenital spinal cord malformations that are less apparent at birth than NTDs include rare duplications, from complete **(dimyelia)** to partial duplication of spinal cord into two separate structures **(diastematomyelia). Hydromyelia** is dilation of the central spinal cord canal.

Syringomyelia is a congenital malformation, a tubular cavitation (syrinx), which may or may not communicate with the central canal that extends for variable distances within the spinal cord. Many cases represent congenital malformations, but the condition progresses slowly and is usually clinically manifested in adults. Some cases of syringomyelia are not malformational but are caused by trauma, ischemia or tumors. The syrinx is filled with a clear fluid similar to CSF. **Syringobulbia** is a variant of syringomyelia in which the syrinx is located in the medulla.

CLINICAL FEATURES: The symptoms of syringomyelia are present at the spinal level of the syrinx where, because of the central location of the syrinx, the segmentally crossing secondary axons of the spinothalamic pathway are disrupted. This leads to loss of pain and thermal sensation bilaterally at the spinal level of the syrinx with relative sparing of fine touch and proprioception as well as motor pathways.

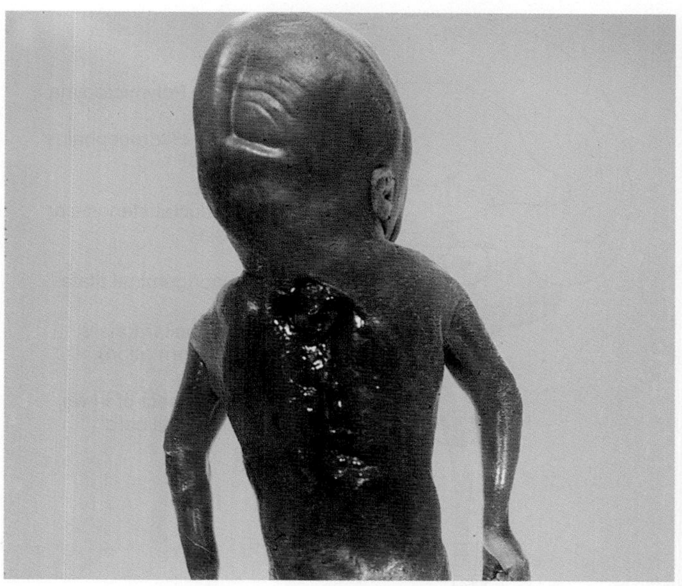

FIGURE 28-104. Rachischisis. A view of the vertebral column shows a bony, cutaneous defect with segmental thoracic absence of the spinal cord and overlying vertebral arches and soft tissues.

Arnold-Chiari Malformation

Arnold-Chiari malformation is a complex condition in which the brainstem and cerebellum are compacted into a shallow, bowl-shaped posterior fossa with a low-positioned tentorium. It is often associated with syringomyelia or a lumbosacral meningomyelocele. Symptoms depend on the severity of the defect (Fig. 28-105). ***Since this malformation involves segmentation of the medulla and cerebellum as well as neural tube closure, it may be considered a defect of both neurulation and segmentation.***

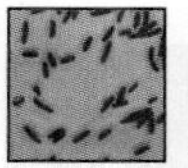

ETIOLOGIC FACTORS: The pathogenesis of the Arnold-Chiari malformation is obscure and has spawned much speculation, but no one theory explains all features of the condition. One theory posits that a meningomyelocele anchors the lower end of the spinal cord, causing downward growth of the vertebral column, thereby creating traction on the medulla. However, other features of this malformation (curvature of the medulla, beaking of the quadrigeminal plate) are not explained by this mechanism. Other proposed mechanisms include increased intracranial pressure associated with hydrocephalus or limited size of the posterior fossa.

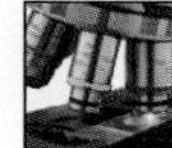

PATHOLOGY: In Arnold-Chiari malformation, the caudal aspect of the cerebellar vermis is herniated through an enlarged foramen magnum and protrudes onto the dorsal cervical cord, often reaching C3 to C5 (Fig. 28-106). The herniated tissue is bound in position by thickened meninges and shows pressure atrophy (i.e., depletion of Purkinje and granular cells). The brainstem also is displaced caudally. Typically, the displacement is more exaggerated dorsally than ventrally, and landmarks such as the obex of the fourth ventricle are more caudal than ventral structures such as the inferior olive. From a lateral perspective, the lower medulla is angulated in its midsegment, thereby creating a dorsal

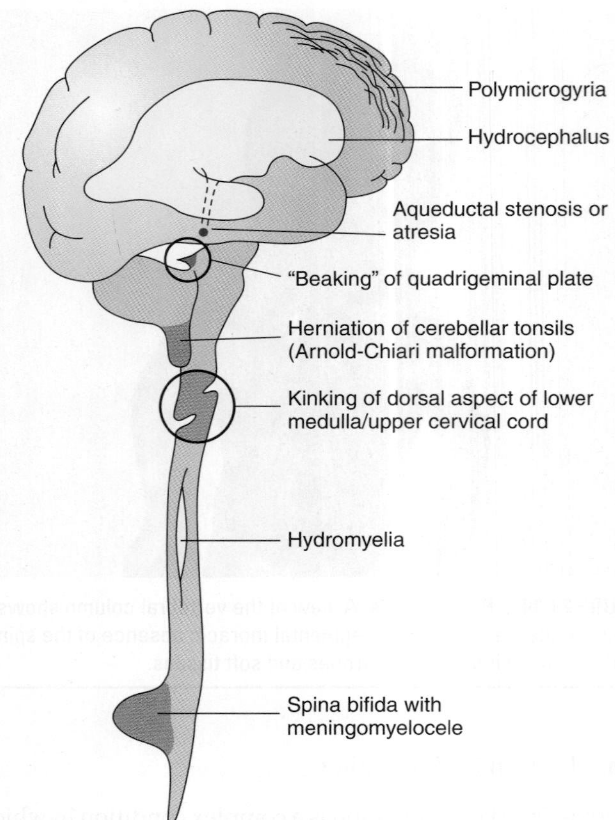

FIGURE 28-105. Arnold-Chiari malformation and associated lesions.

protrusion. The foramina of Magendie and Luschka are compressed by the bony ridge of the foramen magnum, causing hydrocephalus. The cerebellum is flattened to a discoid contour, and the quadrigeminal plate is often deformed by a "beak-shaped" dorsal protrusion of the inferior colliculi.

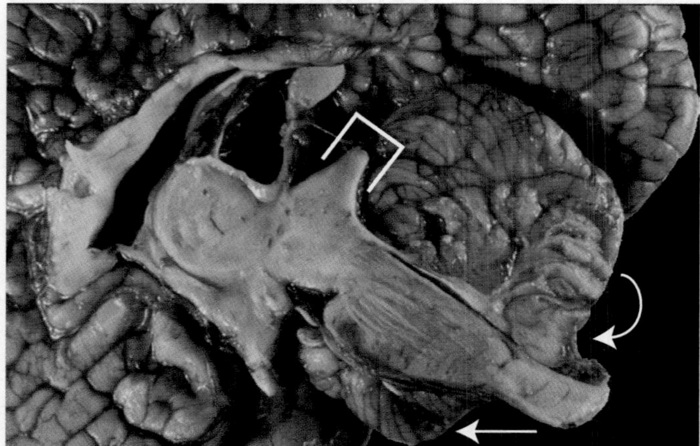

FIGURE 28-106. Arnold-Chiari malformation. The cerebellar vermis is herniated below the level of the foramen magnum (*arrow*). The downward displacement of the dorsal portion of the cord causes the obex of the fourth ventricle to occupy a position below the foramen magnum (*curved arrow*). The midbrain shows extreme "beaking" of the tectum with the four colliculi being replaced by a single pyramidal-shaped structure (*bracket*).

Defects of Segmentation and Cleavage Lead to Loss of Key Central Nervous System Structures

Holoprosencephaly

This term refers to a brain in which the interhemispheric fissure is absent or partly formed as a result of a failure of the telencephalon to divide into the two hemispheres. The holoprosencephaly series of defects are a continuum: complete failure results in **alobar holoprosencephaly,** partial cleavage failure leads to **lobar holoprosencephaly** and, the least severe, and rather subtle, form is failure of olfactory nerves to form, causing **arrhinencephaly.** In alobar holoprosencephaly there is a bulbous horseshoe-shaped cortical dome consisting of fused frontal poles, across which the gyri show an irregular horizontal orientation (Fig. 28-107). A common ventricular chamber is created by lateral displacement of the posterior portions of the telencephalon. Bilobed caudate nuclei and thalami are prominent. In lobar holoprosencephaly, there is partial cleavage in the posterior portion of the telencephalon, but there remains a single gaping ventricular chamber. Holoprosencephaly is rarely compatible with life beyond a few weeks or months, and survival is associated with severe mental retardation and seizures.

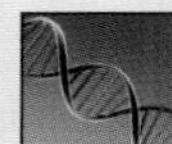

MOLECULAR PATHOGENESIS: About 25% to 50% of patients with holoprosencephaly have numerical or structural chromosomal abnormalities. Monogenic holoprosencephaly is sometimes associated with mutations in *sonic hedgehog*, an important signaling molecule.

Arrhinencephaly

The absence of the olfactory tracts and bulbs (rhinencephalon) is the least severe of the holoprosencephaly defects (Fig. 28-108). It is clinically manifested by lack of a sense of smell **(anosmia)** and may be associated with mental retardation.

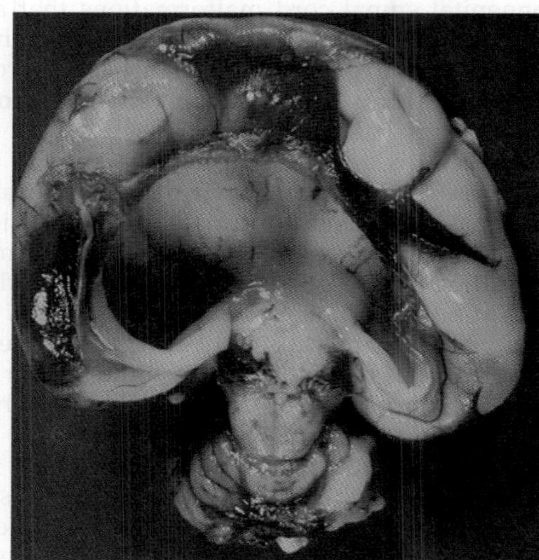

FIGURE 28-107. Holoprosencephaly. The brain exhibits a lack of separation of the hemispheres and a single large ventricle when viewed from an anterior perspective. No interhemispheric fissure is present; therefore, this is alobar holoprosencephaly.

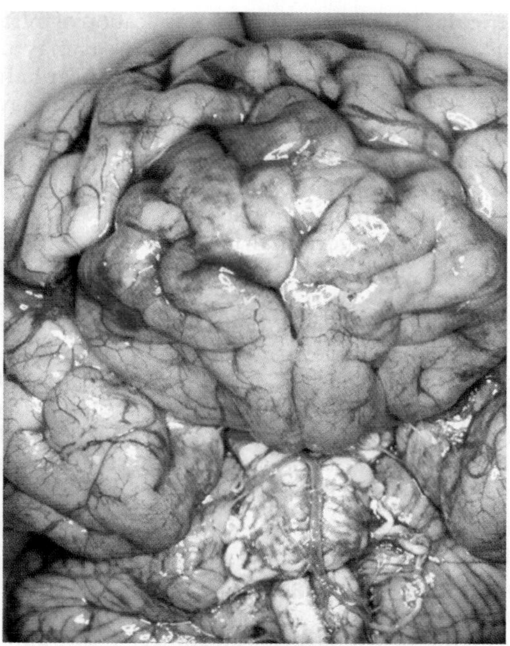

FIGURE 28-108. Arrhinencephaly is the least severe form of holoprosencephaly and consists grossly solely of absence of the olfactory bulbs and nerves, hence the name ("a," *without*, and "rhinencephaly," *nose brain*). There are usually more subtle microscopic abnormalities and most of these individuals have some degree of mental retardation. (Courtesy of Dr. F. Stephen Vogel, Duke University.)

Agenesis of the Corpus Callosum

This anomaly is a regular feature of holoprosencephaly but can also be a solitary lesion. Lack of the corpus callosum may occur without significant impairment of interhemispheric functional coordination, but it is associated with seizures. The corpus callosum physically tethers and functionally interconnects the hemispheres, so its absence permits the lateral ventricles to drift outward and upward, a radiographically diagnostic finding of "bat-wing" ventricles (Fig. 28-109).

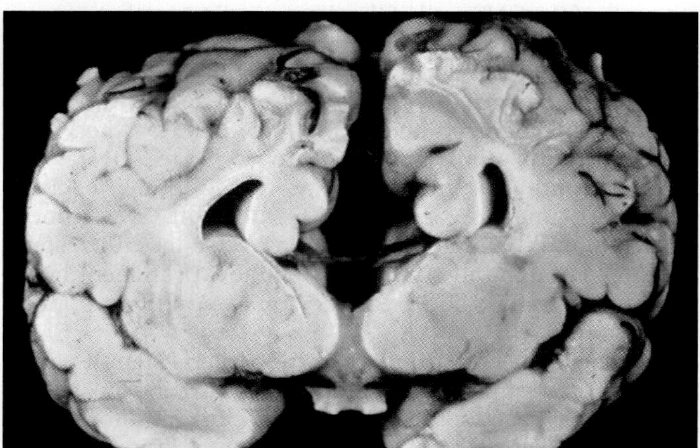

FIGURE 28-109. Congenital absence of the corpus callosum. A coronal section of the brain at the level of the thalamus reveals absence of the corpus callosum and "bat-wing" shape of the lateral ventricles. (Courtesy of Dr. F. Stephen Vogel, Duke University.)

Congenital Atresia of the Aqueduct of Sylvius

This is the most common cause of congenital obstructive hydrocephalus. It may result from deranged mesencephalic (midbrain) development and occurs in 1 in 1000 live births. The brain is enlarged as a result of grotesque enlargement of the ventricles, with thinning of the cerebral cortex and stretching of white matter tracts. The midbrain may show multiple atretic channels or an aqueduct narrowed by gliosis, which may result from developmental failure during segmentation or later in gestation as a result of transplacental transmission of infections that induce ependymitis.

Cortical Malformations Arise From Defects of Neuroglial Proliferation and Migration

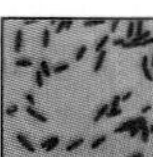

ETIOLOGIC FACTORS: Neuroglial proliferation and migration is a highly patterned process that starts in the first trimester of embryonic development and continues throughout prenatal life. Primitive neurons and glia move centrifugally from the periventricular germinal matrix to populate the cortex. The number of neurons and their positions in the cortex determine the cortical infolding that creates sulci and gyri. These disorders of cortical development are therefore described by the nature and severity of disruption of gyral patterning, as seen by gross inspection. The cortical defect may be global or focal. Portions of the germinal matrix induce formation of specific overlying portions of the cerebral cortex; that is, there is a spatial destiny of the neuroglial cells in a given region of germinal matrix. If a focal region of germinal matrix is destroyed or damaged, the cortical destination of the cells spawned in that region will reflect this damage. Such a failure of focal cortical development caused by damage to the germinal matrix is **schizencephaly,** in which a patch of cortex is "missing." Cortex built from undamaged germinal matrix will be structurally normal. More global, often genetically determined defects of neuroglial proliferation and migration result in a more widespread and severe cortical defect, called lissencephaly, meaning "smooth brain."

- **Lissencephaly** is the most severe congenital disorder of cortical development in which the cortical surface of the cerebral hemispheres is smooth or has imperfectly formed gyri. Some 60% of patients with lissencephaly show deletions in the region of the *LIS1* gene on chromosome 17p13.3, which encodes a protein involved in cytoskeletal dynamics that affects cell proliferation and motility. The white matter contains clusters of neurons that could not successfully migrate to the cortex.
- **Heterotopias** are focal disturbances in neuronal migration that lead to nodules of ectopic neurons and glia, usually in white matter. They are often associated with mental retardation and seizures and may be caused by maternal alcoholism.
- **Polymicrogyria** refers to the presence of small and excessive gyri (Fig. 28-110). The surface of the brain appears to be textured with numerous small bumps on its surface.
- **Pachygyria** is a condition in which the gyri are reduced in number and unusually broad (Fig. 28-111).

Late-Term and Perinatal Insults May Lead to Severe Brain Damage

Sometimes the nervous system develops successfully, only to suffer catastrophic damage late in pregnancy or in the

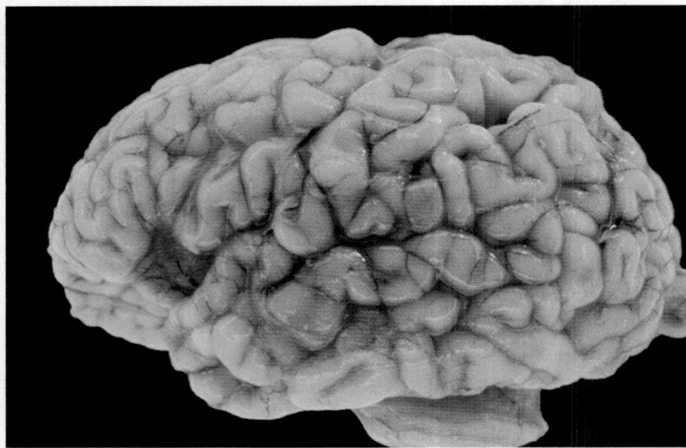

FIGURE 28-110. Polymicrogyria. The surface of the brain exhibits an excessive number of small, irregularly sized, randomly distributed gyral folds.

perinatal period. If the brain is deprived of blood or oxygen, the cerebral hemispheres may liquify, leaving a fluid-filled cranial cavity, a state called **hydranencephaly.** The head circumference reflects the largest size that the brain attained before the insult, and the head can be transilluminated as no tissue remains to block the passage of light through the cranial vault. The cranial sutures may override as the nascent brain degenerates.

Less severe, but still devastating, hypoxia/ischemia may lead to late-term and perinatal cerebral infarcts. The developing brain differs bioenergetically from the adult's, in which gray matter has approximately thrice the blood flow and oxygen consumption as the white matter. In a developing brain, the periventricular germinal matrix and streams of migrating neuroglia equalize bioenergetic demand so that deep structures and cerebral cortex have similar prodigious energy and substrate requirements. The deep periventricular white matter is a watershed perfusion zone and is at highest risk for infarction. This leads to chalky white, sometimes calcific

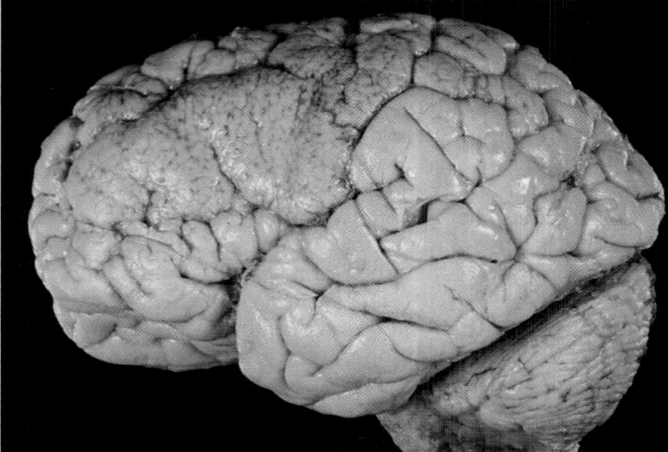

FIGURE 28-111. Pachygyria. Broad textured gyri are seen here in the superior frontal region, indicating a defect in cortical formation. (Courtesy of Dr. F. Stephen Vogel, Duke University.)

periventricular leukomalacia as a complication of intrauterine or perinatal hypoxia ischemia. Infarcted areas may undergo resorption, leading to **multicystic leukoencephalopathy,** which consists of numerous interconnected cystic cavities in the deep white matter near the ventricles.

The germinal matrix is active during the latter phases of gestation but gradually involutes as term approaches. If birth is premature, the premature baby enters the world with a metabolically active germinal matrix perfused by delicate capillaries floating in a frenzied sea of stem cells and newly spawned neuroglia. Such an infant is ill equipped for cerebrovascular regulation. These delicate vessels may be exposed to dramatic swings in perfusion pressure, leading to **germinal matrix hemorrhage.** Hemorrhage may remain confined to a small region of the germinal matrix or it may spread catastrophically as intraventricular hemorrhage. Germinal matrix hemorrhage is among the major challenges in clinical management of premature newborns.

Congenital Defects May Be Associated With Chromosomal Abnormalities

Derangements of the larger autosomes, 1 through 12, are incompatible with sustained intrauterine life: affected fetuses are spontaneously aborted. Structural and functional abnormalities may be attributed to gross chromosomal derangements of the smaller autosomes (e.g., trisomies of chromosomes 13 to 15 and 21 [Down syndrome]). Trisomy 13 or trisomy 15 occurs in 1 per 5000 births, with a modest female predominance. The congenital deformities involve the brain, facial features and extremities: holoprosencephaly, arrhinencephaly, microphthalmia, cyclopia, low-set ears, harelip and cleft palate. The extremities exhibit polydactyly and "rocker bottom" feet.

Central Nervous System Neoplasia

Primary CNS cancers account for about 1.5% of all primary malignant tumors. Metastatic tumors to the CNS are far more common than are primary tumors and are a major problem in clinical management. The broad spectrum of cellular constituents of the CNS—all of the diverse cell types that are represented in the CNS—is mirrored by the wide range of tumor types that arise within the brain and spinal cord and their overlying meninges. Over 130 different types of CNS neoplasms are recognized and formally codified by the World Health Organization, but most are very rare. By far the most common are meningiomas and gliomas, each of which accounts for about one third of all CNS tumors (Table 28-5). While most brain tumors arise in adults, some are more common in childhood, the most prominent being medulloblastoma, pilocytic astrocytoma and diffuse pontine astrocytoma.

Diagnosing a brain tumor involves several steps: (1) generating a preoperative differential diagnosis of the most likely possibilities based on the patient's clinical information (Table 28-6), then (2) biopsy or resection of the lesion to obtain a definitive tissue-based diagnosis upon which further clinical management depends. This approach reflects key characteristics of different types of brain and spinal cord tumors, as well as other types of disease: patient age, location of the lesion within the CNS, specific neuroimaging features, the

Table 28-5

Major Types of Primary Central Nervous System (CNS) Tumors

Major Types of Primary Central Nervous System (CNS) Tumors
Meningioma
Gliomas (including diffuse and circumscribed astrocytomas, oligodendroglioma, ependymoma, choroid plexus tumors, several rare glioma subtypes)
Medulloblastoma and other primitive neuroectodermal tumors
Craniopharyngioma
Germ cell tumors
Hemangioblastoma
Neuronal and mixed glioneuronal tumors
Pineal tumors
Primary CNS lymphoma

nature and time course of preceding clinical signs and symptoms and major elements of the clinical history, such as the presence of a systemic primary tumor or of a tumor predisposition syndrome.

PATIENT AGE: Different types of brain tumors tend to arise at particular ages. Thus, the two most common brain tumors of childhood are medulloblastoma and pilocytic astrocytoma. Several other, rarer tumor types also tend to occur in children, such as diffuse pontine glioma, atypical teratoid/rhabdoid tumor and choroid plexus carcinoma. Similarly, metastatic carcinomas from the lung, breast and colon mainly affect older adults. Still others have a peak incidence in young adulthood, such as ganglioglioma and central neurocytoma. Some tumors may be most common in adults but spare no age group, such as glioblastoma, which is the most common and most malignant type of glioma and may occur at any time in life.

PATIENT GENDER: Most primary brain tumors are more common in males, with two notable exceptions being pituitary adenoma and meningioma, which are more common in young adult and middle-aged to older adult women, respectively. Brain metastases of primary tumors elsewhere follow the gender patterns of incidence of those tumor types (e.g., breast, prostate).

ANATOMIC LOCATION AND COMPARTMENT OF THE LESION: The anatomic location of a lesion includes two components: the general region of the CNS involved, such as the cerebrum, cerebellum or spinal cord, and the anatomic compartment(s), such as intraparenchymal (within the substance of the brain), intraventricular or intradural–extra-axial (inside the spinal dura but outside the spinal cord parenchyma, i.e., located within the spinal subarachnoid space). Such information greatly facilitates formulation of a differential diagnosis. For example, high on the differential diagnosis list for intradural, extra-axial spinal cord masses would be meningioma and peripheral nerve sheath tumors; a mass located within a cerebral lateral ventricle would more likely be one of those entities that frequent this site, such as choroid plexus papilloma, ependymoma, subependymoma, subependymal giant cell astrocytoma, intraventricular (choroid plexus) meningioma and central neurocytoma.

NEUROIMAGING FEATURES: Preoperative evaluation of a CNS lesion provides critical data that bear directly on the differential diagnosis (Table 28-7; Fig 28-112). The most obvious are the number and distribution of the lesion(s), including anatomic location(s) and compartment(s) involved. The nature of the interface between the lesion and the surrounding brain is also important. For example, the border of highly infiltrative tumors, such as fibrillary astrocytomas and lymphomas, is subtle and diffuse, but the interface with the surrounding brain is much more discrete and well circumscribed on preoperative imaging for a metastasis or a minimally infiltrative primary tumor, such as pilocytic astrocytoma or ganglioglioma. The extent of lesion enhancement when a vascular contrast agent is given (e.g., gadolinium for MRI) is also helpful, since some tumor types, such as glioblastoma, meningioma, medulloblastoma and metastatic carcinomas, are more vascular, whereas others usually are not, such as low-grade diffuse fibrillary astrocytoma. Patterns of enhancement can be informative; some tumor types tend to show relatively solid, even enhancement, such as meningiomas and primary CNS lymphoma, but for other types, ring enhancement around a central area of necrosis is typical, such as glioblastoma. Nontumor diseases, many of which mimic tumor radiologically, also often have characteristic enhancement patterns; for example, demyelinating pseudotumor frequently presents as a mass lesion with "open ring" or "C-shaped" enhancement, whereas cerebral abscesses typically show a very smooth-walled enhancing ring (Fig. 28-112).

NATURE AND TIME COURSE OF CLINICAL SIGNS AND SYMPTOMS: In general, a long history, such as several years of poorly controlled seizures, favors more indolent or low-grade disease, whereas a relatively brief history, such as a 2-week history of headache, nausea and emesis and localizing

Table 28-6

Essential Clinical Information

Essential Clinical Information
Patient age and gender
Anatomic location and compartment of the lesion
Neuroimaging (computed tomography, magnetic resonance imaging) features
Nature and time course of presenting signs and symptoms
Relevant clinical history

Table 28-7

Major Neuroimaging (Computed Tomography, Magnetic Resonance Imaging) Features

Major Neuroimaging (Computed Tomography, Magnetic Resonance Imaging) Features
Anatomic location and compartment of the lesion(s)
Nature of the interface between the lesion and the surrounding parenchyma (e.g., sharply circumscribed vs. diffuse)
Presence or absence of enhancement following contrast agent administration
If contrast enhancing, the pattern of enhancement (e.g., solid uniform enhancement, ring enhancement around a central area of necrosis, C-shaped open ring enhancement, enhancing nodule within the wall of a cyst)

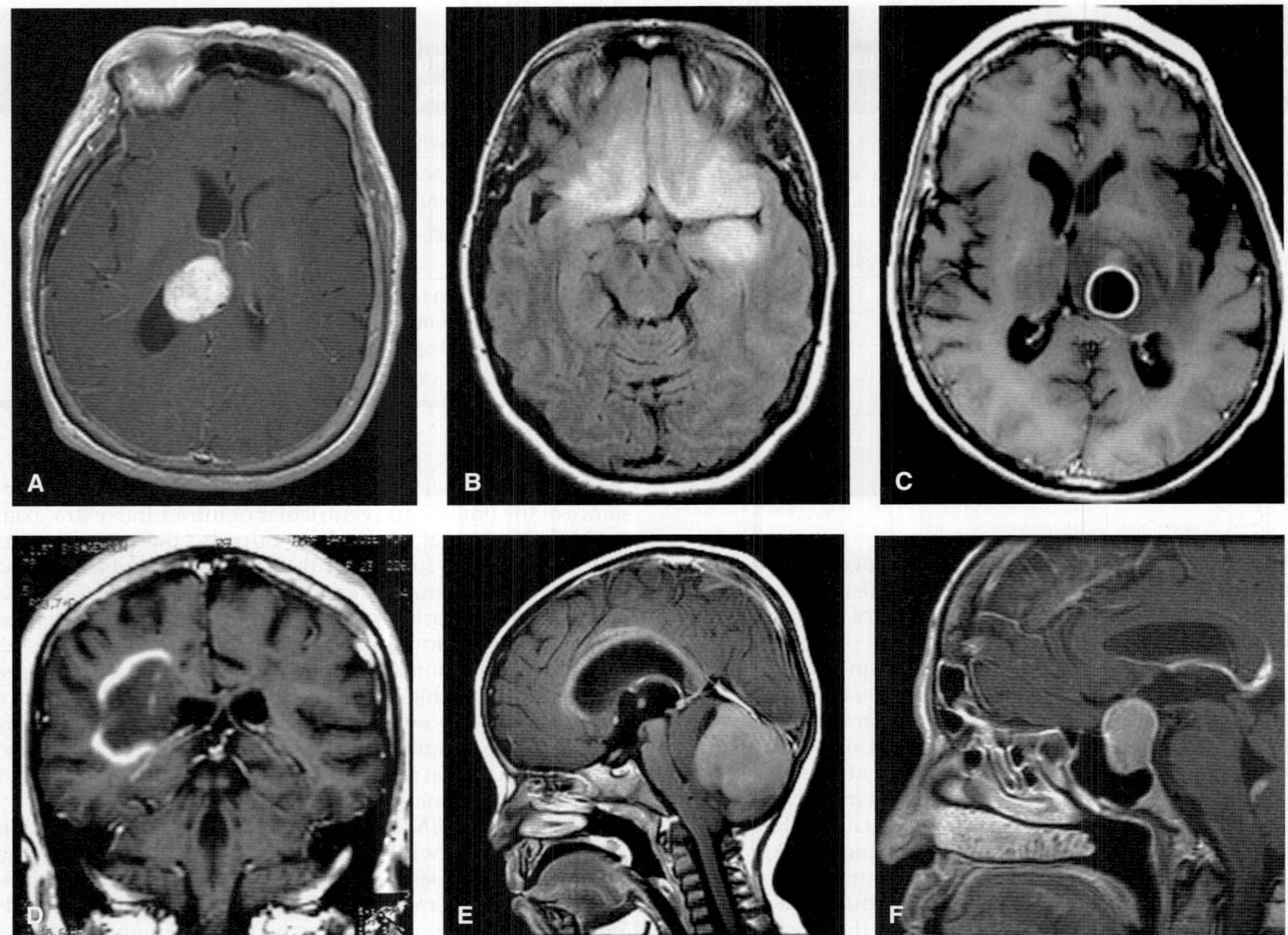

FIGURE 28-112. Neuroimaging—the modern pathologist's gross pathology. Contemporary neuroimaging techniques provide the first look at the "gross pathology" of a central nervous system lesion and constitute a rich source of information that can be utilized by the pathologist to formulate a refined differential diagnosis prior to surgical biopsy and tissue examination. Shown here are representative examples of magnetic resonance images that illustrate the highly informative features of six different brain lesions. **A.** A contrast-enhancing, circumscribed mass located within the lateral ventricle (choroid plexus meningioma). **B.** Diffuse hyperintensity involving both frontal lobes and the left temporal lobe (infiltrating glioma). **C.** Smooth-walled ring-enhancing mass in the left thalamus (pyogenic abscess). **D.** C-shaped open ring-enhancing lesion in the white matter of the right parietal lobe (demyelinating pseudotumor). **E.** Hyperintense midline mass of the cerebellar vermis and fourth ventricle (medulloblastoma). **F.** Contrast-enhancing midline mass of the sellar and suprasellar region (pituitary adenoma).

signs, favors a higher grade and more aggressively expanding lesion.

RELEVANT CLINICAL HISTORY: A clinical history of, for example, a preexisting systemic tumor, prior surgery or chemotherapy or a tumor predisposition syndrome is also useful (Table 28-8).

GRADING OF CENTRAL NERVOUS SYSTEM TUMORS: Tumors in brain and spinal cord are commonly graded according to criteria established by a panel of neuropathologists and neuroscientists convened by the World Health Organization (WHO Classification of Tumours of the Central Nervous System). Tumor grades according to WHO criteria range from I through IV, with I being the lowest grade and IV being the most malignant. The subjective and ill-defined term "benign" should be used with extreme caution, if at all, with respect to CNS tumors, even WHO grade I tumors, because anatomic location, growth pattern and other factors can result in a clinical course for a grade I CNS tumor that entails considerable morbidity and even mortality. For example, most meningiomas are grade I, but those that grow en plaque (flat and plaquelike) along the skull base and surround cranial nerves and blood vessels as they enter and exit the cranial cavity are very difficult to treat by surgery and often do not respond well to radiation or chemotherapy. As well, low-grade diffuse gliomas (WHO grade II), while being the lowest grade for this subtype of glioma, are definitely not "benign" and the vast majority are ultimately lethal.

Table 28-8

Major Nervous System Tumor Predisposition Syndromes

Syndrome	Chromosome Locus	Gene (protein)	Associated Nervous System Tumors
Neurofibromatosis type 1 (NF1)	17q11.2	*NF1* (neurofibromin)	Neurofibromas (dermal and plexiform) Malignant peripheral nerve sheath tumor (MPNST) Pilocytic astrocytoma ("optic glioma") Diffuse astrocytoma Glioblastoma
Neurofibromatosis type 2 (NF2)	22q12	*NF2* (merlin/ schwanomin)	Vestibular schwannomas (bilateral) Other schwannomas Meningiomas (multiple) meningioangiomatosis Ependymoma of spinal cord Diffuse astrocytoma
Schwannomatosis (sometimes referred to as "NF3")	Unknown	Unknown	Schwannomas (multiple, spinal roots, cranial nerves, skin, not vestibular)
von Hippel-Lindau (vHL)	3p25–26	*VHL* (pVHL)	Hemangioblastomas (multiple) of cerebellum, spinal cord, brainstem, retina, spinal peripheral nerve roots Endolymphatic sac tumor
Tuberous sclerosis complex	9q34 16p13.3	*TSC1* (hamartin) *TSC2* (tuberin)	Subependymal giant cell astrocytoma
Li-Fraumeni syndrome	17p13	*TP53* (TP53 protein)	Diffuse astrocytomas, including glioblastoma Medulloblastoma Choroid plexus papilloma Ependymoma Oligodendroglioma Meningioma
Cowden disease	10q23	*PTEN/MMAC1* (PTEN protein)	Dysplastic gangliocytoma of the cerebellum (Lhermitte-Duclos disease)
Turcot type 1 syndrome (mismatch repair [MMR]/ hereditary nonpolyposis colon cancer [HNPCC]–associated Turcot)	3p21.3 2p16 5q11–q13 2q32 7p22	*MLH1* *MSH2* and *MSH6 MSH3* *PMS1* *PMS2* *APC* (APC protein)	Glioblastoma
Turcot type 2 syndrome (familial adenomatous polyposis [FAP]–associated Turcot)	5q21		Medulloblastoma
Nevoid basal cell carcinoma (Gorlin) syndrome	9q22.3	*PTCH* (Ptch protein)	Medulloblastoma
Rhabdoid tumor predisposition syndrome	22q11.2	*INI1* (INI1 protein)	Atypical teratoid/rhabdoid tumor

Meningiomas Are the Most Common Central Nervous System Tumors

Meningiomas are derived from the middle layer of arachnoid (meningothelial) cells that form the outer boundary of the subarachnoid space. Thus, the anatomic locations in which meningiomas arise parallel the distribution of the arachnoid membrane, and these tumors can arise at any CNS site where arachnoid cells are present—including at the dural venous sinuses (such as the superior sagittal sinus), at the cerebral convexity, at the skull base, around the optic nerve, around the spinal cord and even within the choroid plexus in the cerebral ventricles as mentioned earlier.

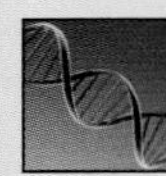

MOLECULAR PATHOGENESIS: Meningiomas typically arise in one of three settings:

- **Sporadic**—most common
- **Iatrogenic**—usually associated with prior cranial irradiation
- **Tumor predisposition syndrome**—most commonly neurofibromatosis type 2 (NF2)

The vast majority of meningiomas arise sporadically. Many such tumors exhibit loss, partial deletion or mutation of the *NF2* locus (22q12), suggesting that perturbations of this tumor suppressor gene are involved not only in NF2-associated tumors but also in the origin of many sporadic meningiomas (and schwannomas).

Induction of meningiomas by radiation therapy generally involves a latent period of a decade or more and is directly related to radiation dosage. Low-dose scalp irradiation for tinea capitis was widely used until around 1960. The average interval between treatment and detection of a meningioma for such patients was 35 years. With higher radiation doses, as are used for head and neck cancers, the interval may be as short as 5 years.

Meningiomas also occur in conjunction with several genetic syndromes, most importantly NF2. Additional rare multiple meningioma syndromes have also been documented.

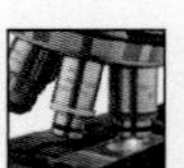

PATHOLOGY: On MRI and gross examination, most meningiomas are well-circumscribed dura-based masses of variable size that compress, but do not invade, underlying brain (Fig. 28-113A, B). The cut surface is fleshy and tan. The classic histologic hallmark of meningiomas is a whorled pattern, often in association with psammoma bodies (laminated, spherical calcospherites) (Fig. 28-113C, D). However, meningiomas can show diverse morphologic patterns, and 13 subtypes are recognized by the WHO (Table 28-9). Most of these are WHO grade I, but two variants, clear cell and chordoid, behave more aggressively (WHO grade II), and two other variants, papillary and rhabdoid, are frankly anaplastic (WHO grade III). Meningiomas typically exhibit focal positivity for epithelial membrane antigen (EMA) (Fig. 28-113C), and their derivation from the cohesive arachnoid barrier cell layer is further reflected by profuse numbers of intercellular junctions seen by electron microscopy (Fig. 28-113E).

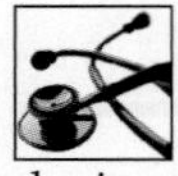

CLINICAL FEATURES: The indolent growth of most meningiomas enables these tumors to enlarge very slowly for years before becoming symptomatic, during which time they displace the brain but do not infiltrate it (Fig. 28-114A, B). Patients frequently have seizures, particularly with tumors at parasagittal sites over the convexity of the hemispheres. In other locations, meningiomas compress a variety of functional structures. Thus, tumors of the olfactory groove produce anosmia; those in the suprasellar region lead to visual deficits by compressing the optic chiasm; meningiomas in the cerebellopontine angle cause cranial nerve dysfunction; and those along the spinal cord compromise spinal nerve root and spinal cord function. Invasion of cranial bone, often accompanied by hyperostosis detected by CT imaging, is relatively common, and growth through the calvarium may create a tumor mass beneath the scalp. In contrast, invasion of the underlying brain by meningiomas is rare, and such aggressive behavior warrants upgrading to WHO grade II (atypical). Tumors that are not completely excised tend to recur, and some may undergo anaplastic progression over time. Anaplastic (malignant) meningiomas (WHO grade III) may also rarely arise de novo.

Table 28-9

Meningioma Subtypes

Meningioma Subtypes
World Health Organization (WHO) Grade I: Benign Meningioma
Meningothelial
Fibrous
Transitional
Psammomatous
Angiomatous
Microcystic
Secretory
Lymphoplasmacyte rich
Metaplastic
WHO Grade II: Atypical Meningioma
Chordoid
Clear cell
WHO Grade III: Anaplastic (Malignant) Meningioma
Rhabdoid
Papillary

Astrocytomas Exhibit a Wide Range of Clinicopathologic Behaviors

Tumors of astrocytic derivation (astrocytomas) are the most common primary brain tumors. They can be divided into two major categories based on how diffusely they infiltrate the brain parenchyma. ***Diffuse astrocytomas*** infiltrate the brain widely and include low-grade fibrillary astrocytoma, anaplastic astrocytoma and the most malignant astrocytic tumor, glioblastoma. Members of the other major category of astrocytomas typically do not infiltrate the CNS but rather are slowly enlarging, compact masses that cause symptoms by compressing adjacent structures. These include pilocytic astrocytoma, pleomorphic xanthoastrocytoma and subependymal giant cell astrocytomas.

Diffuse Astrocytoma

The most salient biological characteristic of diffuse astrocytoma, as the name implies, is the ability of individual tumor cells to infiltrate widely through brain and spinal cord parenchyma (Fig. 28-115). This property reaches its extreme in **gliomatosis cerebri (WHO grade III),** in which

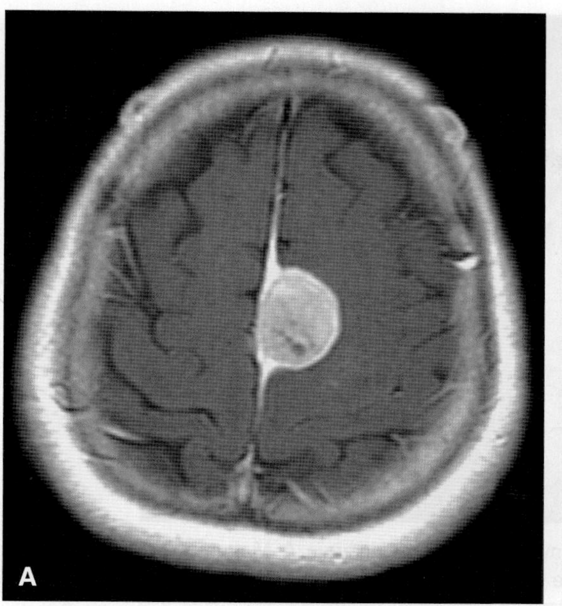

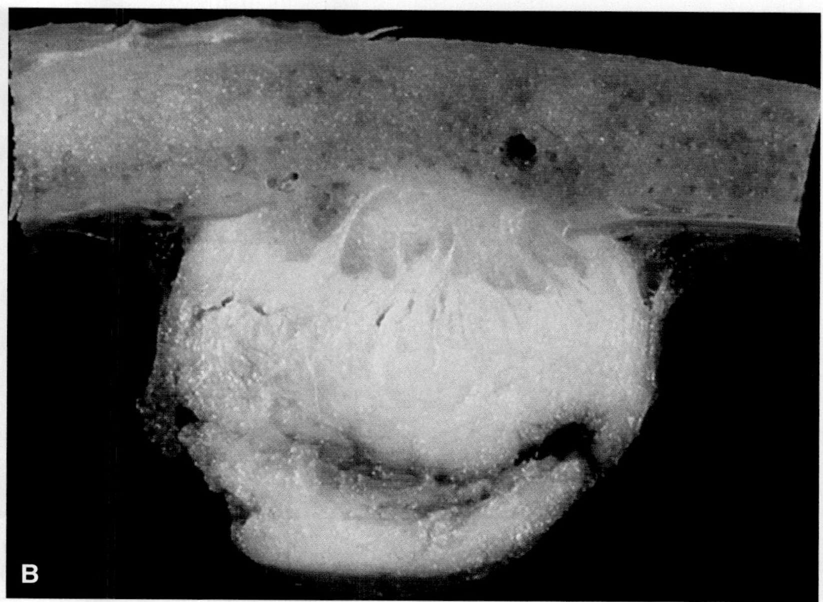

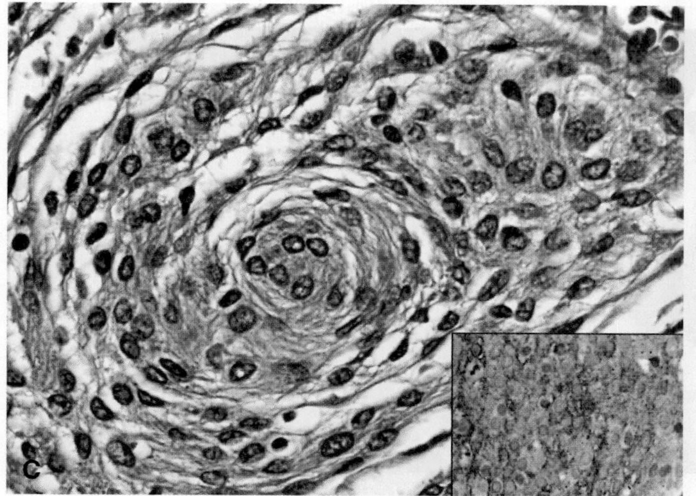

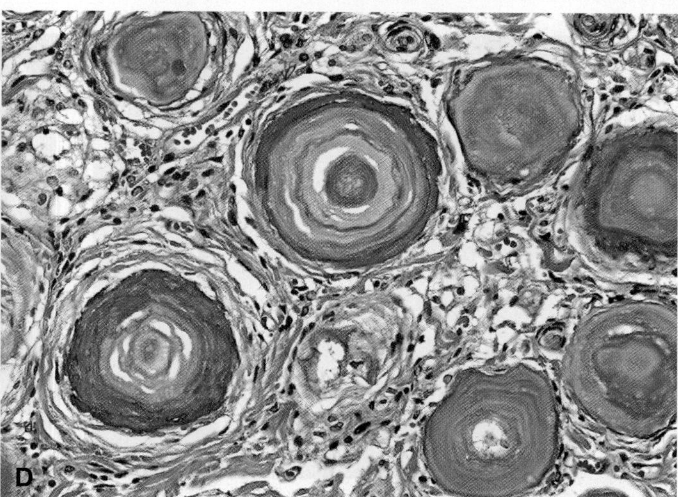

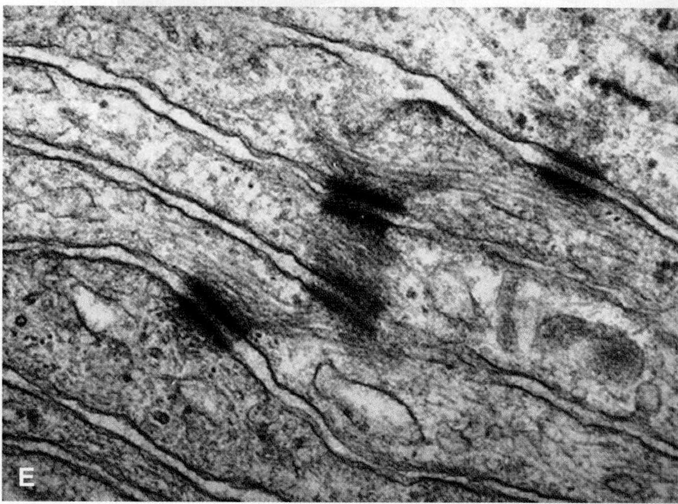

FIGURE 28-113. Meningioma. A. Magnetic resonance imaging showing a superficial dura-based circumscribed mass, with tapering enhancement of the dura adjacent to the site of tumor attachment ("dural tail"); the chief entity in the differential diagnosis for this magnetic resonance appearance is meningioma. **B.** Gross surgical specimen consisting of excised meningioma together with cranial bone and dura. (Courtesy of Dr. F. Stephen Vogel, Duke University.) **C. Histology of meningioma.** Note the whorled, bland, plump spindle cells. Meningiomas are immunopositive for epithelial membrane antigen, which is used as a diagnostic adjunct in difficult cases (*inset*). **D.** Prominent psammoma body formation, typical of the "psammomatous" subtype of meningioma. **E.** The ultrastructural hallmark of meningiomas is numerous intercellular junctions (desmosomes), which tightly bind adjacent meningioma cell processes together.

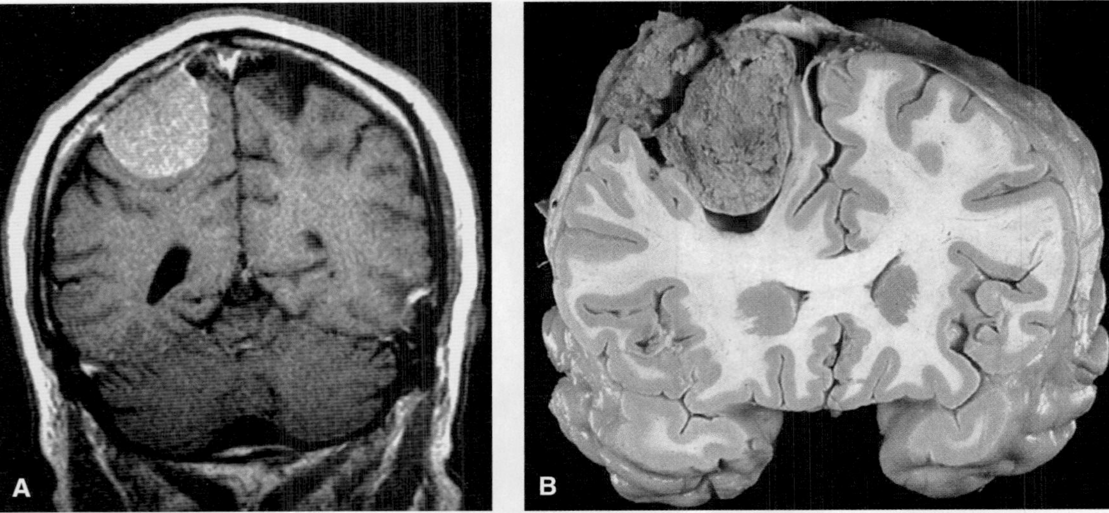

FIGURE 28-114. Meningioma. Meningiomas compress, but do not usually invade, the underlying brain. **A.** Magnetic resonance image. **B.** Gross specimen. (Courtesy of Dr. F. Stephen Vogel, Duke University.)

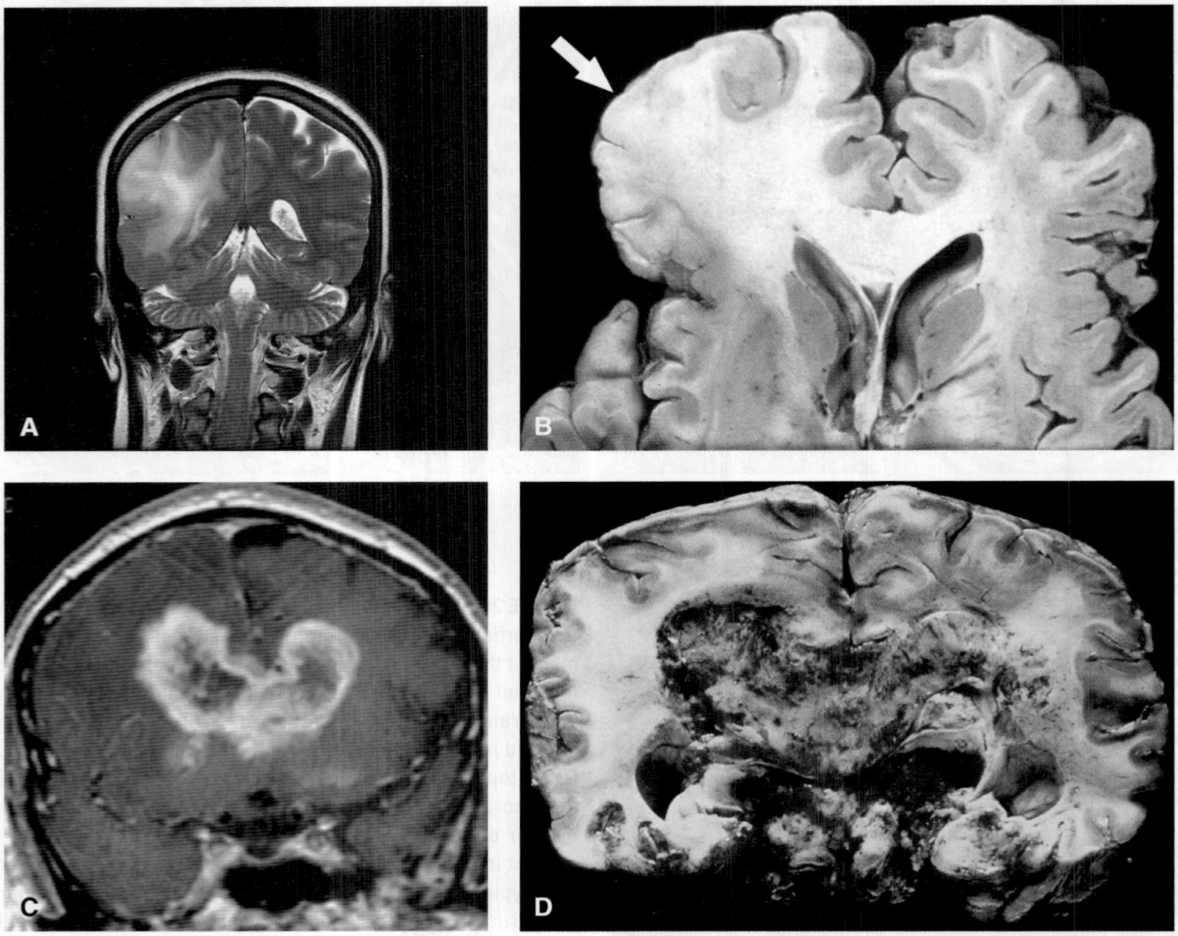

FIGURE 28-115. Gliomas. A. Infiltrating astrocytomas exhibit a diffuse, fuzzy interface with the adjacent brain tissue that is being invaded on magnetic resonance imaging. **B.** One manifestation of diffuse infiltration is "blurring" of the normally sharp interface between the gray matter and white matter as astrocytoma cells overrun the cortex, as seen (*arrow*) in this gross specimen. (Courtesy of Dr. F. Stephen Vogel, Duke University.) **C.** In contrast to low-grade diffuse astrocytomas, **glioblastomas** show prominent irregular ring contrast enhancement and often infiltrate across the corpus callosum to involve the contralateral hemisphere ("butterfly" glioblastoma), as seen in this preoperative magnetic resonance image. **D.** Autopsy gross specimen. (Courtesy of Dr. F. **Stephen Vogel, Duke University.**)

infiltrating glioma cells (usually astrocytes but occasionally oligodendroglia) involve at least three cerebral lobes, and often more, with infiltration into both hemispheres, the brainstem, the cerebellum and even the spinal cord. Diffuse tumor infiltration of brain and spinal cord is a major reason effective treatment is lacking for this class of brain tumors. Glioblastoma typically presents as a large, ring-enhancing mass with an irregular central area of necrosis and prominent edema of surrounding white matter. The infiltrating component of glioblastoma often crosses to the contralateral hemisphere via the corpus callosum; such cases are referred to as "butterfly" glioblastomas based on their appearance on coronal MRI (Fig. 28-115).

PATHOLOGY: Low-grade fibrillary astrocytomas (WHO grade II) have well-differentiated astrocytic tumor cells with very little nuclear atypia and very low cell proliferation. Gemistocytic astrocytoma is a distinctive subtype of low-grade astrocytoma in which the main population of cells exhibits prominent globular cytoplasm laden with glial intermediate filaments (Fig. 28-116). Despite a deceptively bland morphologic appearance, diffuse astrocytomas often undergo anaplastic progression over time, usually several years, into high-grade astrocytoma (anaplastic astrocytoma, WHO grade III) and, ultimately, into glioblastoma (WHO grade IV). This tendency for anaplastic progression is even more pronounced with the gemistocytic variant. **Anaplastic astrocytoma (WHO grade III)** is more cellular than low-grade fibrillary astrocytoma, and individual tumor cells tend to be more pleomorphic (variable in size and shape) (Fig. 28-116). Cell proliferation is elevated and mitotic figures are easily identified. Anaplastic astrocytomas typically progress to glioblastoma within a few years.

Glioblastoma multiforme (GBM; WHO grade IV) is the single most common primary malignant brain tumor, accounting for about 20% of all CNS tumors. GBMs are cytologically highly pleomorphic, with constituent cells varying greatly in size and shape, including large bizarre nuclei and multinucleated cells. They may arise through anaplastic progression from a lower-grade diffuse astrocytoma (secondary glioblastoma; 5% of GBMs) or, much more commonly, de novo (primary glioblastoma; 95% of GBMs). Although usually solitary, they may rarely present as two separate epicenters of enhancement within the brain. Such cases may closely mimic metastases radiologically, with biopsy providing a definitive diagnosis. Mitotic activity in glioblastomas is greatly elevated; additional characteristic features include vascular proliferation and foci of tumor necrosis surrounded by a densely cellular cuff of tumor cells ("pseudopalisading necrosis") (Fig. 28-116C).

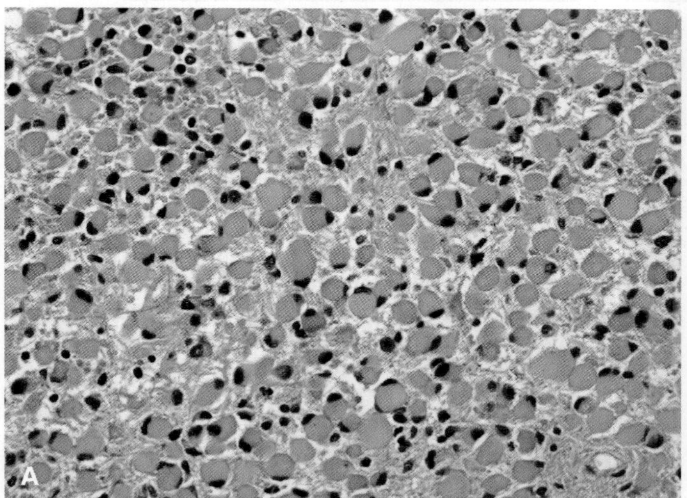

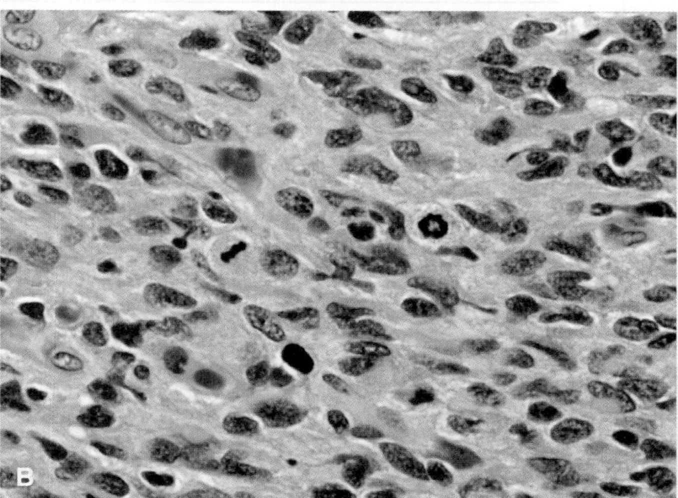

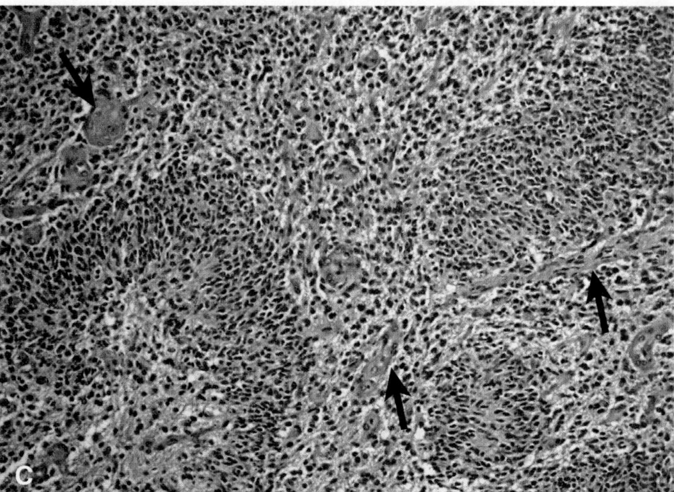

FIGURE 28-116. Diffuse astrocytoma histology. A. Gemistocytic astrocytomas are low-grade (World Health Organization [WHO] grade II) diffuse astrocytomas characterized by prominent globular cytoplasm. **B. Anaplastic astrocytoma (WHO grade III)**, in contrast, is more cellular and more pleomorphic, in addition to having a higher proliferation rate. **C. Glioblastoma (WHO grade IV)** displays foci of tumor necrosis surrounded by hypercellular cuffs of tumor cells ("pseudopalisading necrosis") as well as vascular proliferation (*arrows*).

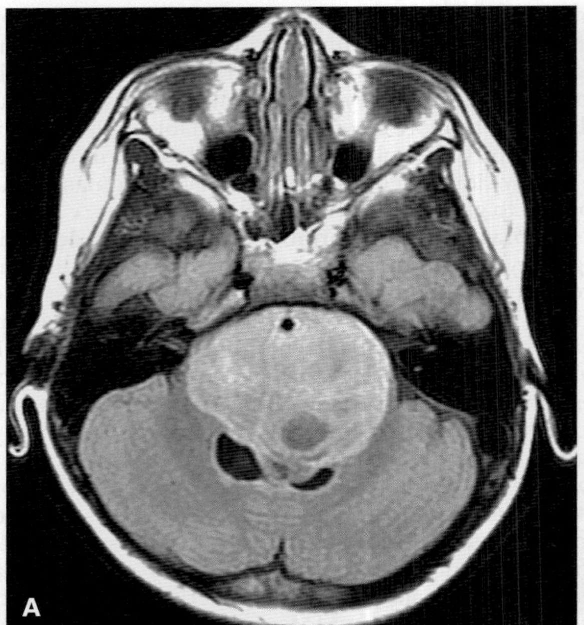

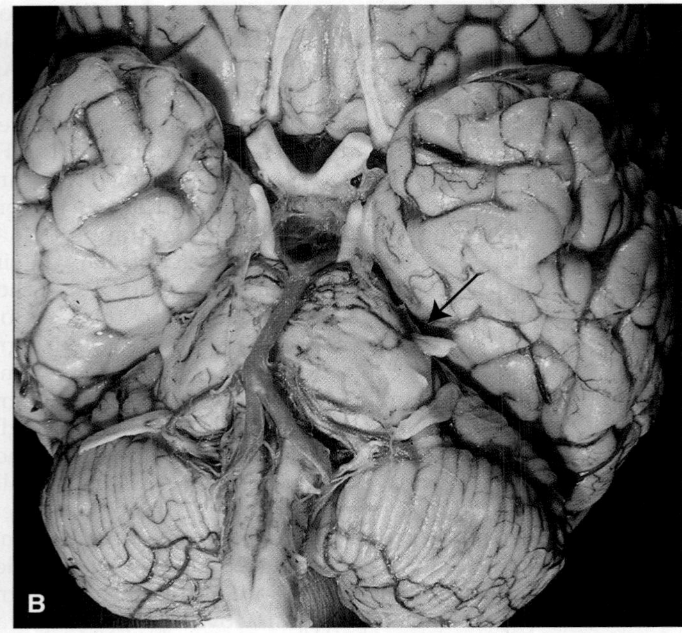

FIGURE 28-117. Diffuse pontine astrocytoma ("pontine glioma"). A diffuse astrocytoma of childhood, diffuse pontine astrocytomas infiltrate and expand the brainstem pons, often to the point of encircling the basilar artery. **A.** Magnetic resonance imaging. **B.** Autopsy gross specimen.

Diffuse pontine astrocytoma (diffuse intrinsic pontine glioma; WHO grade II through IV) is a diffusely infiltrating astrocytoma that arises in, and expands, the pons of the brainstem of young children (Fig. 28-117). The MRI features combined with the clinical features are so characteristic that treatment is usually initiated without biopsy confirmation of the diagnosis. The grade varies from II to IV, but despite aggressive treatment all cases ultimately exhibit lethal growth, infiltration and compromise of vital brainstem structures.

MOLECULAR PATHOGENESIS: *The vast majority of GBMs are sporadic*, but a minority arise in the setting of a genetic tumor predisposition syndrome (Table 28-8). Sporadic GBMs are further stratified into primary (de novo) and secondary (anaplastic progression from lower-grade astrocytoma) subtypes, and molecular characterization reveals differences in the mutations seen in these two major classes. For example, primary GBM is characterized by a higher incidence of amplification of the epidermal growth factor receptor (*EGFR*) gene and mutation of the *PTEN* gene, whereas secondary GBM has a higher incidence of *p53* mutation. More recent molecular and genomic profiling studies have identified mutation of the isocitrate-dehydrogenase genes 1 or 2 (*IDH1, IDH2*), and especially *IDH1*, as a very common signature of low-grade (grade II) and anaplastic (grade III) diffuse gliomas and also of a majority of secondary GBMs that arise from these lower-grade tumors, but not of primary GBMs. Other mutations in specific molecular subsets of GBM include deletion or mutation of the *NF1* gene and amplification of the *ERBB2* gene. Similarly, molecular insight into the basis for resistance to treatment is also beginning to be understood. Recent studies have shown that GBMs can be stratified into two groups based on whether the promotor for the DNA repair gene *MGMT* is methylated, and hence inactivated, or unmethylated, and thus capable of repairing damage caused by chemotherapeutic alkylating agents used for treatment. Patients with *MGMT* promotor methylation (inactivation) respond significantly better to treatment. Contemporary genomic approaches are rapidly enlarging our knowledge of the molecular correlates of diffuse gliomas and other CNS tumors and providing insight into these tumors' genesis and progression, as well as treatment response and resistance.

Pilocytic Astrocytoma (World Health Organization Grade I)

Pilocytic astrocytomas (PAs) are circumscribed gliomas that typically arise in children and young adults and very slowly expand in size. In contrast to diffuse astrocytomas, PAs do not infiltrate brain or spinal cord parenchyma diffusely and are not prone to undergo anaplastic progression to higher-grade tumors. Common anatomic locations include the cerebellum, brainstem, optic nerves and third ventricular region. PAs are contrast enhancing, may be associated with a cystic component and are well circumscribed on preoperative imaging studies (Fig. 28-118).

PATHOLOGY: PAs exhibit a biphasic architectural pattern consisting of compact areas of tumor cells with elongated bipolar cytoplasmic processes (pilocytes) separated by prominent microcysts. The compact areas frequently display prominent **Rosenthal fibers,** a histologic hallmark of pilocytic astrocytoma. Vascular proliferation is typical and correlates with the contrast enhancement seen on

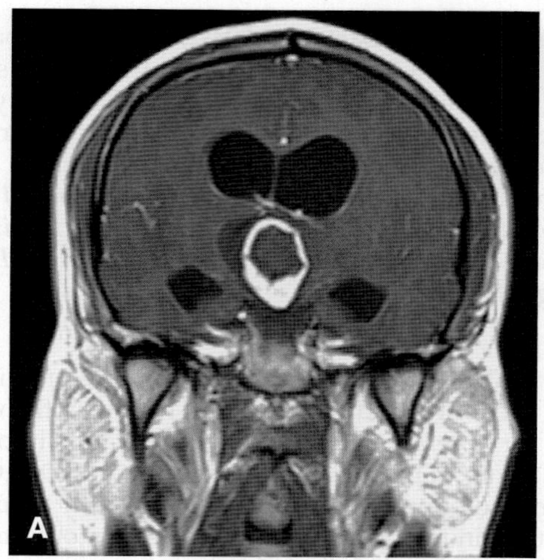

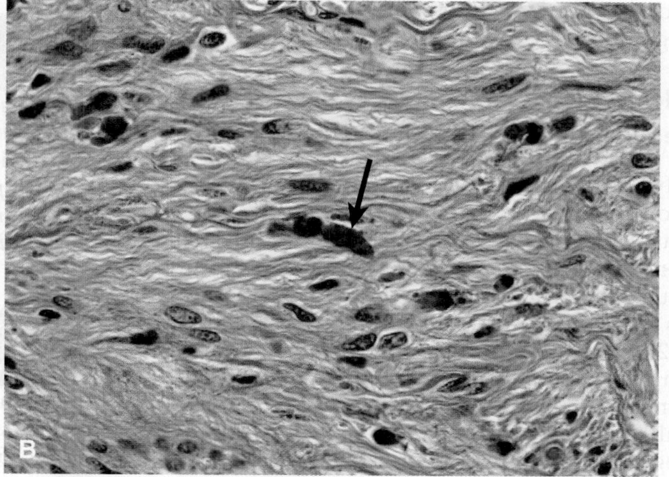

FIGURE 28-118. Pilocytic astrocytoma (World Health Organization grade I). A. Pilocytic astrocytomas are very low-grade circumscribed contrast-enhancing gliomas. **B.** Histologically, the neoplastic pilocytes ("hair cells") exhibit greatly elongated bipolar cytoplasmic processes that are prone to Rosenthal fiber formation (*arrow*).

preoperative MRI studies. Mitotic activity, vascular proliferation and foci of necrosis in pilocytic areas do not have the negative prognostic significance as in diffuse astrocytomas. In favorable anatomic locations, such as the cerebellum, surgical resection may be curative. **Pilomyxoid astrocytoma** (WHO grade II) is a recently recognized variant of PA, primarily arising in the hypothalamic region, that exhibits a more aggressive clinical behavior.

Pleomorphic Xanthoastrocytoma (World Health Organization Grade II)

Pleomorphic xanthoastrocytoma (PXA) is another circumscribed astrocytoma variant of children and young adults (Fig. 28-119A). There is usually a several-year history of poorly controlled seizure activity; the temporal lobe is the most common location. In favorable anatomic locations, PXAs, like PAs, are amenable to surgical resection, although incompletely resected tumors frequently recur, and about 15% of these undergo anaplastic progression to high-grade diffuse astrocytoma.

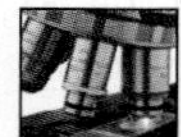

PATHOLOGY: PXA mimics giant cell glioblastoma in its display of strikingly pleomorphic tumor cells (Fig. 28-119B). Unlike glioblastoma, however, mitotic activity is very low, and vascular proliferation and necrosis are usually absent. The characteristic eosinophilic granular bodies, which are also seen in other low-grade circumscribed

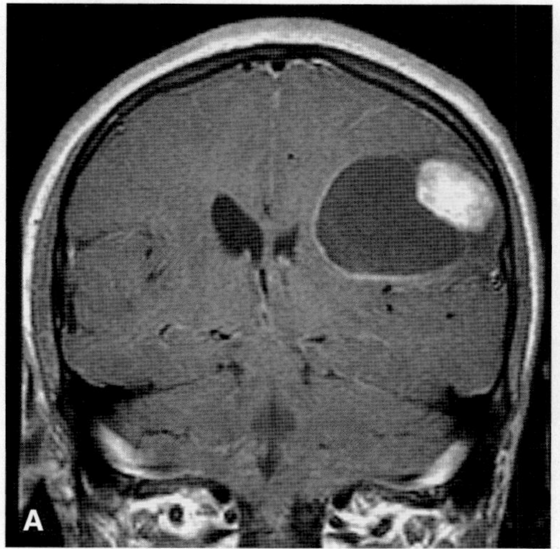

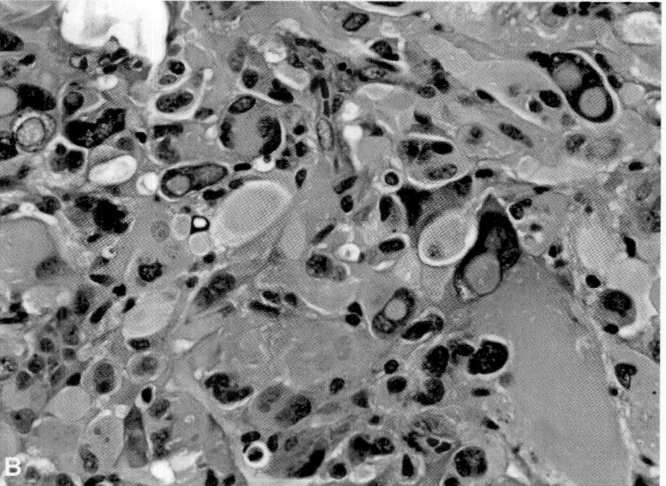

FIGURE 28-119. Pleomorphic xanthoastrocytoma (PXA). A. PXAs are low-grade (World Health Organization grade II) circumscribed astrocytomas that typically display a "cyst with enhancing mural nodule" pattern, similar to other low-grade tumors such as pilocytic astrocytoma and ganglioglioma, on imaging studies. **B.** Microscopically, PXAs superficially resemble giant cell glioblastoma, with strikingly bizarre giant cells (B), but pursue a much more indolent clinical course.

tumors such as pilocytic astrocytoma and ganglioglioma, are a strong signature of PXA.

Subependymal Giant Cell Astrocytoma (World Health Organization Grade I)

Subependymal giant cell astrocytoma (SEGA) is a very indolent low-grade glioma that arises from the wall of the lateral ventricle. It grows slowly within the ventricular cavity until encroachment on the interventricular foramen of Monro causes obstructive hydrocephalus with the attendant signs and symptoms of increased intracranial pressure (Fig. 28-120A). SEGAs are densely compact mixtures of very plump epithelioid cells, often with an elongated spindle cell component (Fig. 28-120B). Based only on histology, SEGA could be misdiagnosed as gemistocytic astrocytoma or ganglioglioma, but the intraventricular location, as readily identified by preoperative imaging and the young patient age, makes misdiagnosis by an informed pathologist highly unlikely. SEGAs are associated with **tuberous sclerosis** and may be the presenting feature in a child with otherwise inconspicuous stigmata of that disease. In keeping with its WHO grade I assignment and favorable location within the lateral ventricle, surgical resection of SEGA is curative.

Oligodendrogliomas (World Health Organization Grade II) Are Often More Indolent Than Diffuse Astrocytomas

Like diffuse astrocytomas, oligodendrogliomas (ODGs) are highly infiltrative. However, their response to treatment and attendant overall survival are much more favorable than for diffuse astrocytomas of comparable grade, so it is critical to distinguish these two types of diffuse glioma.

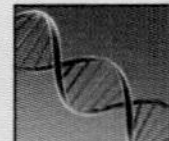

MOLECULAR PATHOGENESIS: The pathogenesis of ODG is unknown, but a translocation between chromosomes 1 and 19 is a very characteristic molecular signature. This translocation results in complete loss of the short arm of chromosome 1 (1p) and the long arm of chromosome 19 (19q). ***Combined deletion of 1p and 19q is a favorable genetic signature in diffuse gliomas and correlates closely with classic ODG morphologic features.***

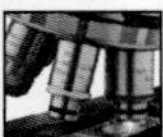

PATHOLOGY: The majority of ODGs arise in adults in the fourth and fifth decades, largely in the white matter of cerebral hemispheres. Infiltration into overlying cerebral cortex is particularly common with ODG. ODGs display a monotonous population of cells with regular round nuclei surrounded by a small rim of clear cytoplasm (referred to as a "perinuclear halo" or "fried egg" appearance) like normal oligodendroglia (Fig. 28-121A). The perinuclear halo is a diagnostically useful artifact of specimen processing by formalin fixation and paraffin embedding. Other characteristic histologic features of ODG include a network of delicate, branching blood vessels ("chicken wire" pattern) and scattered microcalcifications. In areas of cortical infiltration, ODG cells tend to cluster around neuron cell bodies (perineuronal satellitosis) and blood vessels (perivascular satellitosis), and also to form an infiltrating layer just beneath the pia (subpial growth). These features, described by Scherer in 1938, are still referred to as "secondary structures of Scherer." Mitotic activity is inconspicuous in low-grade (WHO grade II) OGD, but these tumors recur and ultimately undergo anaplastic progression.

Anaplastic Oligodendroglioma (World Health Organization Grade III)

Anaplastic oligodendroglioma is distinguished from WHO grade II ODG by increased mitotic activity and the presence

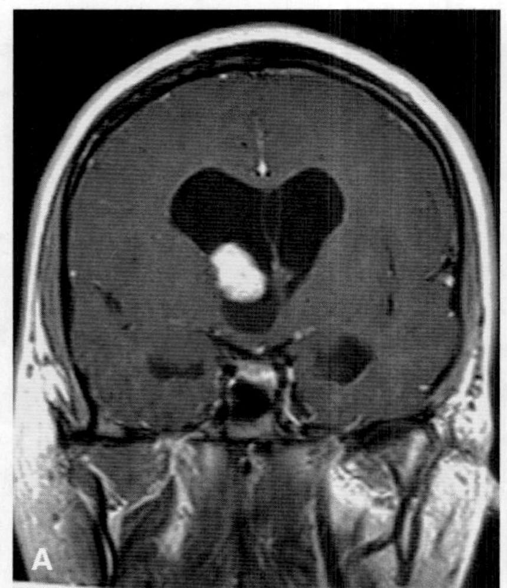

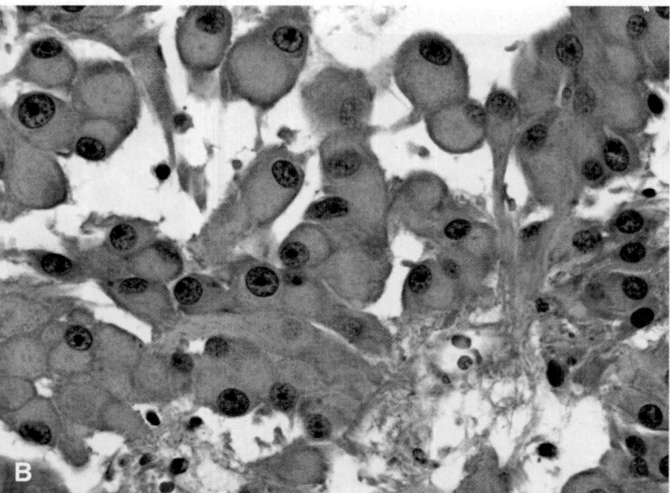

FIGURE 28-120. Subependymal giant cell astrocytoma (SEGA). A. This World Health Organization grade I astrocytoma arises within the lateral ventricle, often obstructing the interventricular foramen of Monro, resulting in obstructive hydrocephalus. **B.** Microscopically, SEGAs have globular eosinophilic cytoplasm and the nuclei often display single prominent nucleoli, thus mimicking gemistocytic astrocytoma or ganglion cell tumor. However, the anatomic location within the cerebral ventricle should preclude misdiagnosis.

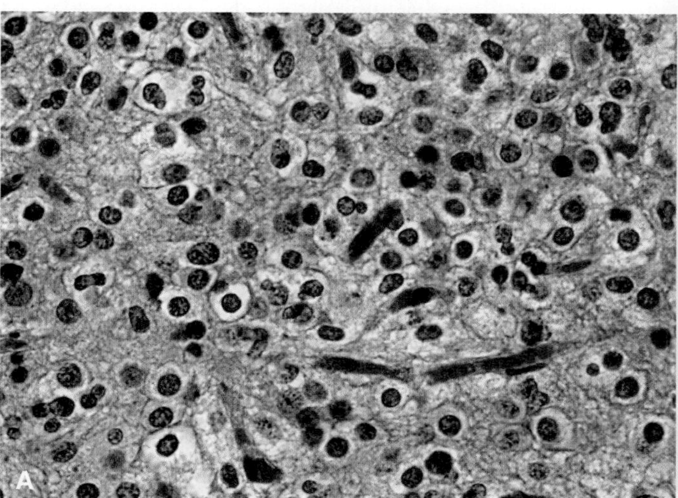

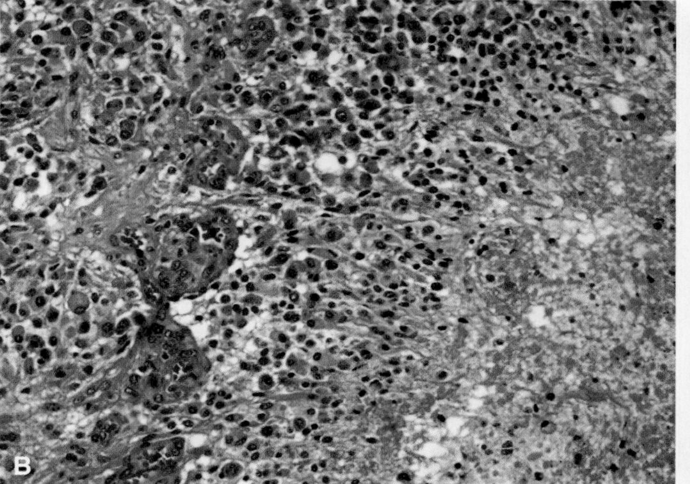

FIGURE 28-121. Oligodendroglioma. A. The cells of **low-grade oligodendroglioma** (World Health Organization grade II) closely resemble normal oligodendrocytes, with regular round nuclei surrounded by perinuclear halos. **B. Anaplastic oligodendroglioma** (AO) displays increased cellularity and brisk mitotic activity, with some tumors also developing foci of necrosis with tumor cell pseudopalisading.

of microvascular proliferation, sometimes accompanied by foci of tumor necrosis (Fig. 28-121B).

Ependymomas (World Health Organization Grade II) Are Derived From Ependymal Lining Cells

These are typically slow-growing neoplasms of children and young adults that originate from the ependymal lining of the cerebral ventricles or central canal of the spinal cord. In children, the posterior fossa fourth ventricle is the preferred location, while in adults most are in the supratentorial compartment and may arise in either the ventricle or in the cerebral hemisphere white matter. Ependymomas of the fourth ventricle tend to fill the ventricle and grow into the lateral recesses, occasionally even flowing through the lateral foramina of Luschka into the subarachnoid space (Fig. 28-122A, B). In the spinal cord, ependymomas are the most common intra-axial tumors, followed by diffuse astrocytoma.

PATHOLOGY: Ependymomas grow as relatively circumscribed masses, and so are amenable to surgical resection. Their primary histologic hallmark is the perivascular pseudorosette, a perivascular cuff of radiating tumor cell cytoplasmic processes (Fig. 28-122C). True ependymal rosettes, in which tumor cells surround a central lumen, can also be seen but are rarer. Ependymomas express epithelial membrane antigen (Fig. 28-122C, *inset*) (EMA) and GFAP (Fig. 28-122D, *inset*). GFAP reactivity is often strongest in the perivascular pseudorosettes, and, unlike the membranous pattern of EMA expression in meningiomas, ependymoma EMA positivity is characteristically in a cytoplasmic dotlike and ringlike distribution. This pattern correlates with the presence of intercellular lumina filled with microvilli and cilia, sealed by intercellular junctional complexes at the ultrastructural level. **Anaplastic ependymoma (WHO grade III)** shows increased mitotic activity and microvascular proliferation.

Myxopapillary Ependymoma (World Health Organization Grade I)

Myxopapillary ependymoma (MPE) is a unique low-grade variant of ependymoma that arises almost exclusively in the spinal cord of adults from ependymal remnants in the conus medullaris or filum terminale (Fig. 28-123A). This tumor slowly enlarges as a discrete, well-circumscribed, elongated mass in the lumbar CSF cistern, covered by an outer layer of investing leptomeninges. Nests and ribbons of epithelioid and spindled ependymal tumor cells are interspersed between myxoid microcysts, and perivascular cuffs of myxoid material also prominent (Fig. 28-123B). The immunophenotype is similar to other ependymomas, with positivity for both glial markers (S-100 protein, GFAP) and epithelial markers (EMA). Because of their circumscription and favorable anatomic location in the lumbar cistern, complete surgical resection is the treatment of choice. In some tumors, microscopic breach of the pial "capsule" may have occurred prior to surgery, resulting in locally disseminated tumor growing around the nerve roots of the cauda equina. Such cases are difficult to treat with conventional irradiation or chemotherapy, as their slow rate of growth makes them relatively resistant to cell cycle inhibitors.

Subependymoma (World Health Organization Grade I)

Subependymoma is another indolent intraventricular glioma of adults (rare cases may arise in the spinal cord). These tumors are often small and asymptomatic and are often incidental findings on imaging studies or at autopsy. Occasionally, however, they enlarge to block the interventricular foramen of Monro or the outlet foramina of the fourth ventricle, resulting in obstructive hydrocephalus (Fig. 28-124A). Subependymomas show scattered clusters of small uniform glial cell nuclei separated by large zones of fibrillary matrix formed by tumor cell cytoplasmic processes (Fig. 28-124B). Surgical resection is curative.

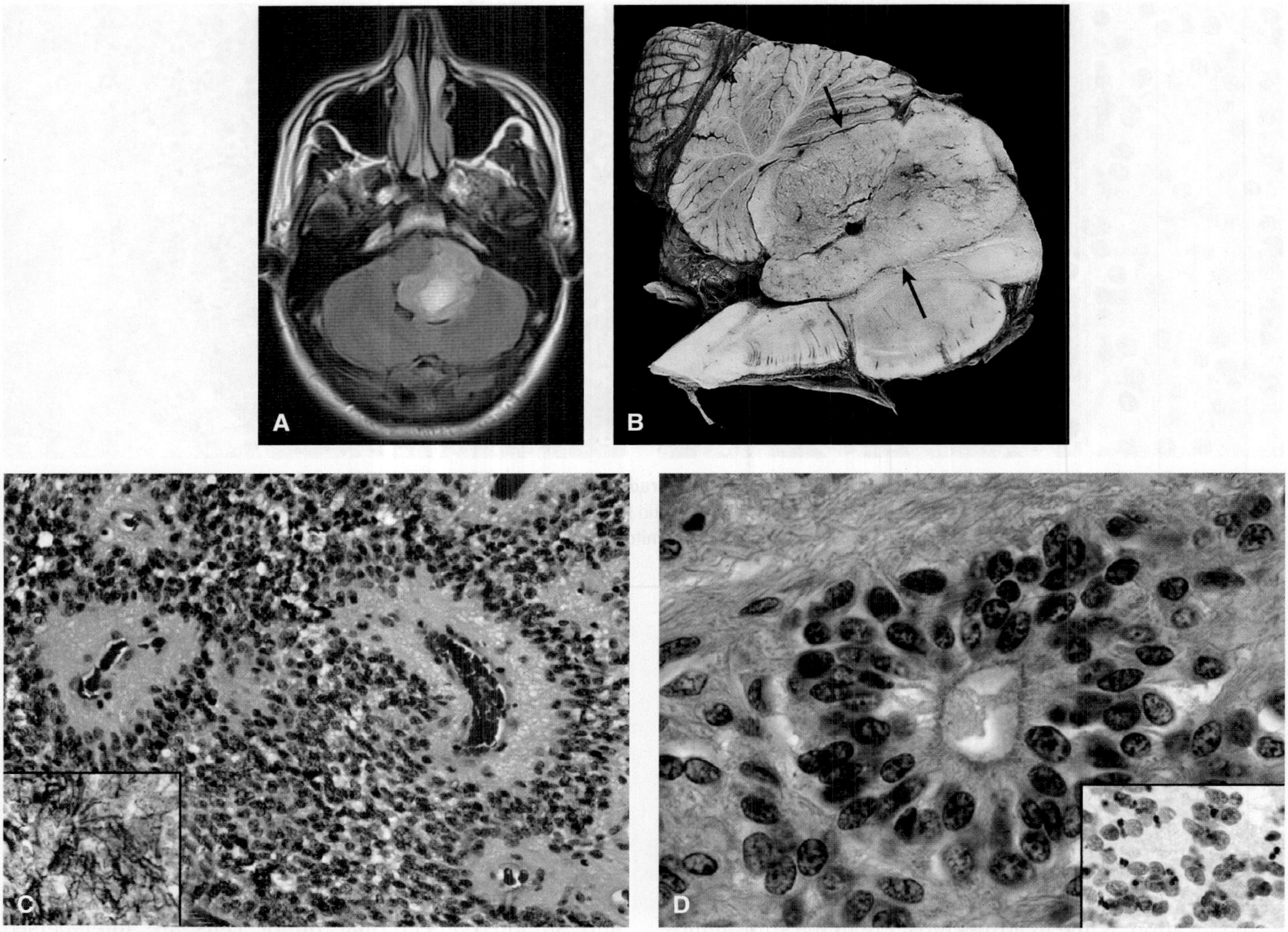

FIGURE 28-122. Ependymoma. A. Ependymomas can arise in the ventricles, the cerebral hemisphere or the spinal cord. Those located within the posterior fossa tend to grow through the ventricular outlet foramina (median foramen of Magendie and lateral foramina of Luschka) into the subarachnoid space, as seen in this magnetic resonance image. **B.** Autopsy gross specimen. Tumor is identified between the arrows. (Courtesy of Dr. F. Stephen Vogel, Duke University.) **C.** Microscopically, the hallmark of ependymomas is the perivascular pseudorosette. The immunophenotype of ependymoma includes dotlike and ringlike positivity for epithelial membrane antigen (*inset*). **D.** Well-formed true ependymal rosette with immunoreactivity of the glial marker glial fibrillary acidic protein (*inset*).

Choroid Plexus Tumors Originate From the Epithelium of the Choroid Plexus

In contrast to other common brain tumors of childhood, which are preferentially located in the posterior fossa (cerebellum, fourth ventricle and brainstem), **choroid plexus papillomas (CPPs; WHO grade I)** in children most commonly arise in the lateral ventricles (Fig. 28-125A). In adults, the fourth ventricle is favored. CPPs are benign and, given their location within the ventricles, are potentially curable by surgery; however, CSF dissemination can occur, significantly worsening the prognosis in such cases.

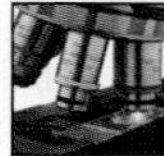

PATHOLOGY: CPP closely recapitulates the papillary architecture of normal choroid plexus, but the tumor cells tend to be more crowded together and commonly assume a columnar rather than cuboidal architecture (Fig. 28-125B). The immunophenotype of CPP includes reactivity for glial markers (S-100 protein, GFAP) and transthyretin (prealbumin). Two higher-grade choroid plexus tumors are recognized: **atypical CPP (WHO grade II),** which displays increased mitotic activity compared to grade I tumors, and **choroid plexus carcinoma (WHO grade III),** in which, in addition to increased mitotic activity, the tumor exhibits loss of papillary architecture with a solid growth pattern and often marked nuclear atypia and cellular pleomorphism (Fig. 28-125C). The latter tumor can invade adjacent brain parenchyma and also has potential for dissemination via the CSF pathways. The choroid plexus may also be the host of several other types of neoplastic and nonneoplastic mass lesions, including "intraventricular" meningioma, metastatic carcinoma (especially renal cell carcinoma) and xanthogranuloma (a reactive mass lesion likely related to microhemorrhage that exhibits prominent cholesterol clefts and an associated multinucleated giant cell reaction).

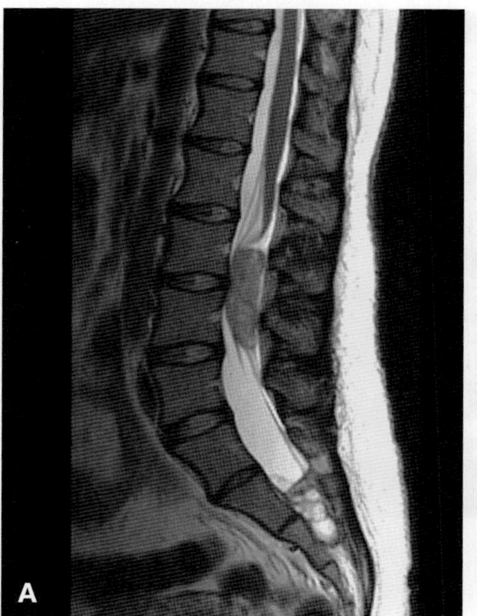

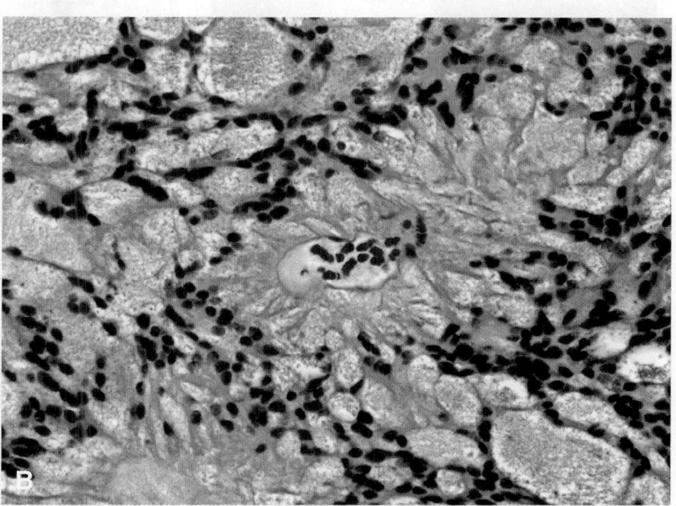

FIGURE 28-123. Myxopapillary ependymoma (MPE). A. MPEs are very low-grade (World Health Organization grade I) ependymal tumors that arise from remnants of the central canal in the spinal cord conus medullaris and filum terminale within the lumbar cistern. **B.** Histologically, prominent myxoid microcysts and perivascular myxoid cuffs separate nests and cords of ependymal cells.

Medulloblastoma and Other Primitive Neuroectodermal Tumors (World Health Organization Grade IV) Are Largely Tumors of Children

A number of different types of primitive neuroectodermal tumor (PNET) are recognized in the WHO classification, but medulloblastoma (MB) is by far the most common and by definition arises in the cerebellum. Its peak incidence is at 7 years, but it can also affect adults in the 20- to 45-year-old age group. Childhood MBs commonly arise in the midline vermis, often expanding to fill the fourth ventricle (Fig. 28-126A). In contrast, adult tumors prefer the cerebellar hemispheres, although there are many exceptions in both children and adults. About one third of patients have

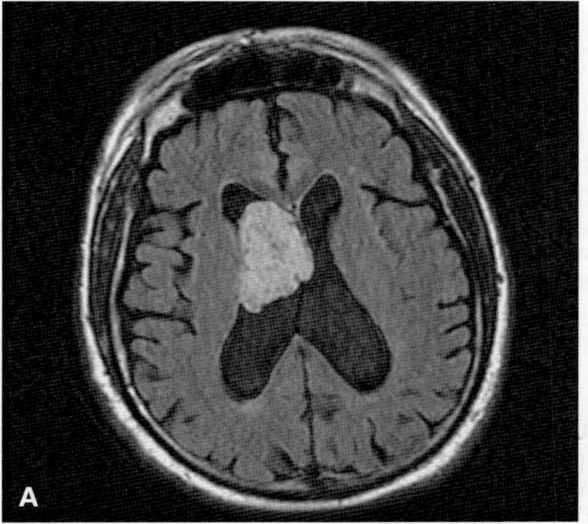

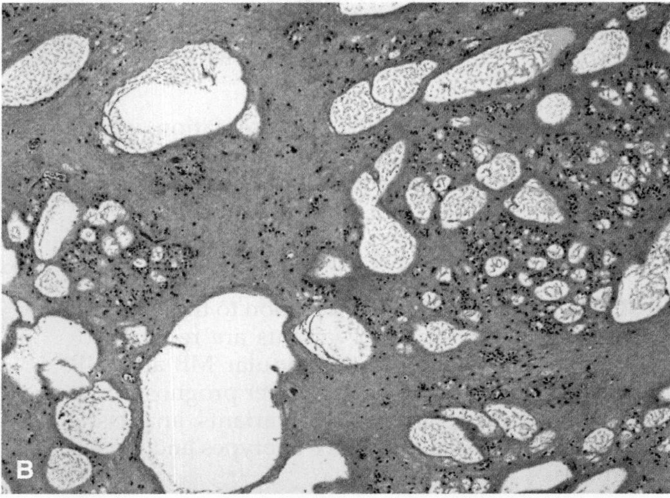

FIGURE 28-124. Subependymoma (SE). A. SE is another very low-grade (World Health Organization grade I) ependymal tumor that arises within the cerebral ventricle (shown in this magnetic resonance imaging scan) or very rarely within the spinal cord (not shown). **B.** Microscopically, SE consists of clusters of small, bland glial nuclei embedded within an abundant finely fibrillar matrix composed of tumor cell processes. Those examples located in the lateral ventricles tend to undergo microcystic degeneration as they enlarge.

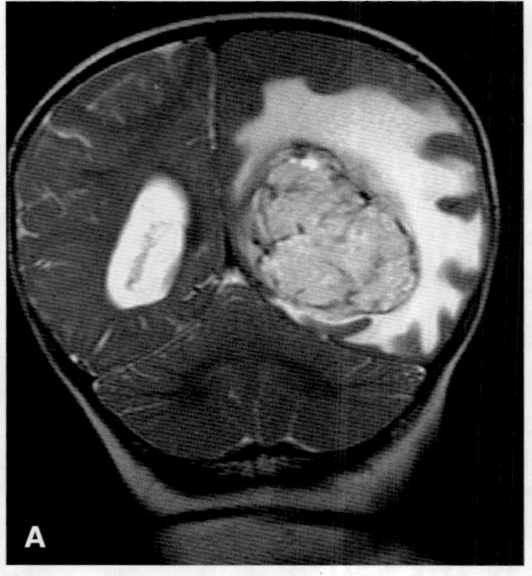

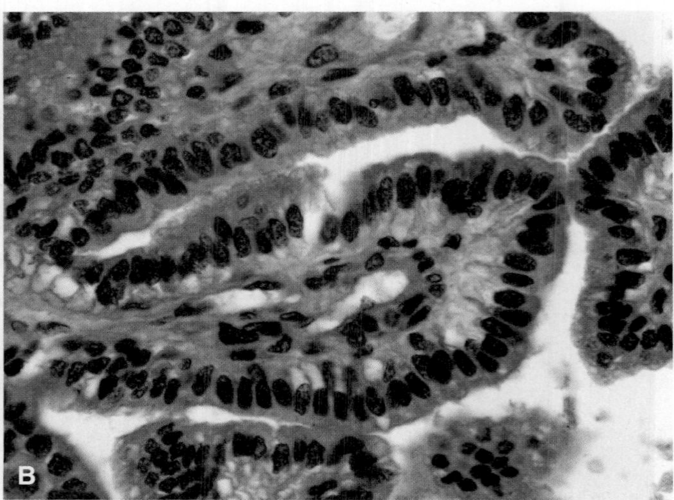

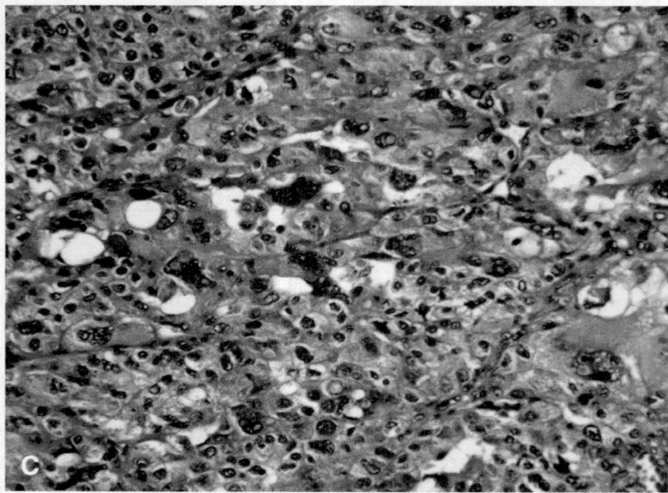

FIGURE 28-125. Choroid plexus papilloma (CPP) and carcinoma (CPC). A. CPP is a low-grade intraventricular tumor that arises from the fourth ventricular choroid plexus in adults and the lateral ventricular choroid plexus in children. **B.** Histologically, **CPP** retains the papillary architecture of choroid plexus, but the cells are more crowded and columnar rather than cuboidal. **C. CPC** is a high-grade tumor that differs from CPP in showing loss of papillary architecture, marked cellular pleomorphism, an increased proliferation rate and a more aggressive clinical course.

leptomeningeal spread at the time of presentation, which is a negative prognostic factor. Poor clinical outcome is associated with only partial surgical resection, large cell or anaplastic morphology and amplification of *MYCN* oncogene.

CLINICAL FEATURES: In addition to the common classic subtype, four MB variants are recognized; two of these, desmoplastic/nodular MB and MB with extensive nodularity, and have a better prognosis than the classic subtype; the remaining two variants, anaplastic and large cell, are the most aggressive subtypes and have a worse prognosis.

PATHOLOGY: MBs are composed of sheets of densely packed malignant small cells with a high nucleus:cytoplasm ratio (Fig. 28-126B). Neuroblastic (Homer Wright type) rosettes are present in about 40% of cases. Cellular proliferation is high. Desmoplastic/nodular MB exhibits a morphologic pattern superficially reminiscent of lymph node tissue, with reticulin-free neurocytic islands ("pale islands") resembling germinal centers (Fig. 28-126C, D). This variant arises predominantly in the cerebellar hemispheres of adults. The closely related MB with extensive nodularity is a tumor of infancy and has a distinctive multinodular appearance on imaging, as well as histologically. **Anaplastic MB and large cell MB** are aggressive variants with overlapping morphologic features (Fig. 28-126E). Anaplastic MB is characterized by marked nuclear pleomorphism, nuclear molding and cell–cell wrapping. In contrast, the large cell variant displays a monomorphous population of large cells whose nuclei exhibit prominent nucleoli. Both variants are characterized by high proliferative activity and abundant apoptosis. The majority of MBs exhibit neuronal differentiation in the form of immunoreactivity for synaptophysin; some also display focal glial differentiation (GFAP immunopositivity). Very rare examples show myogenic differentiation or melanotic differentiation.

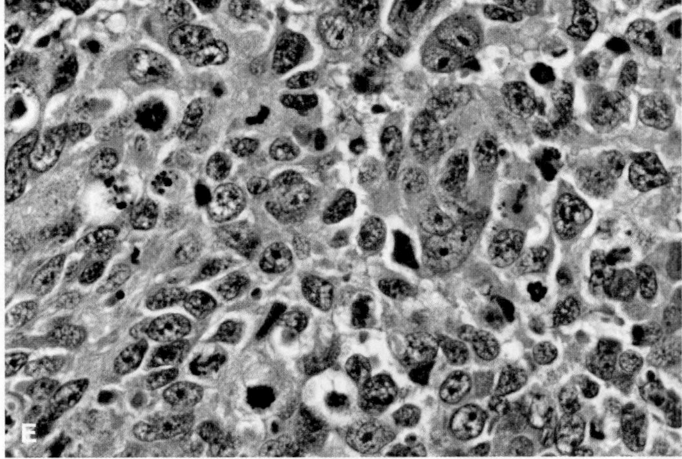

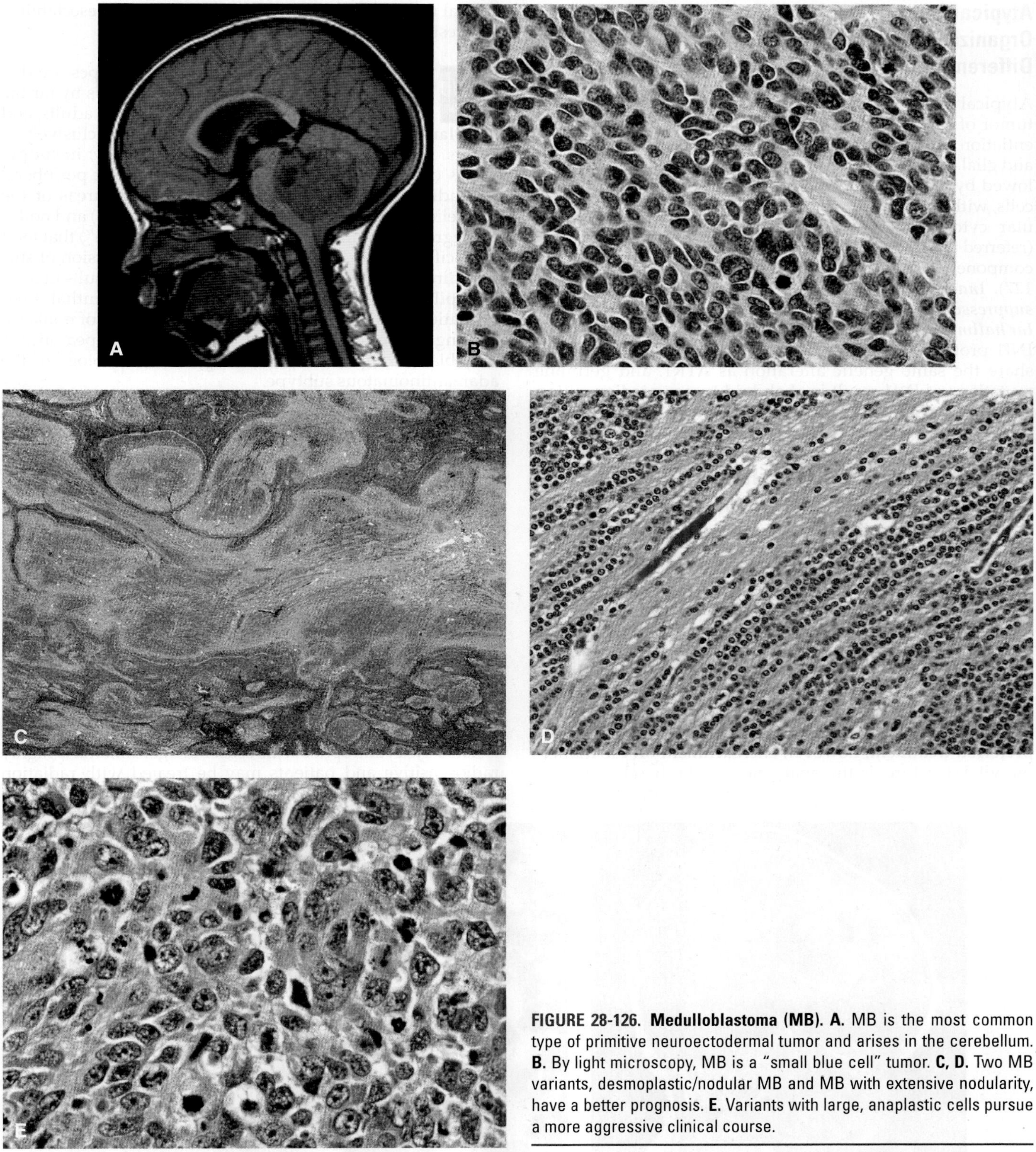

FIGURE 28-126. Medulloblastoma (MB). A. MB is the most common type of primitive neuroectodermal tumor and arises in the cerebellum. **B.** By light microscopy, MB is a "small blue cell" tumor. **C, D.** Two MB variants, desmoplastic/nodular MB and MB with extensive nodularity, have a better prognosis. **E.** Variants with large, anaplastic cells pursue a more aggressive clinical course.

MOLECULAR PATHOGENESIS: MB is thought to arise from stem cells of the fetal external granular layer and/or the periventricular germinal matrix. Molecular studies have implicated two major pathways, *Wnt and sonic hedgehog (SHH)*, in tumor genesis. Differential activation of these pathways likely underlies the different phenotypic subclasses, with the SHH pathway underlying the desmoplastic/nodular MB and MB with extensive nodularity variants, and the Wnt pathway underlying the much more common classic and anaplastic/large cell variants.

Atypical Teratoid/Rhabdoid Tumor (World Health Organization Grade IV) Exhibits Multilineage Differentiation

Atypical teratoid/rhabdoid tumor (ATRT) is a malignant tumor of early childhood characterized by divergent differentiation along rhabdoid, epithelial, mesenchymal, neuronal and glial lines. The posterior fossa is most affected (75%), followed by the supratentorial compartment (25%). Rhabdoid cells, with eccentrically located nuclei and eosinophilic globular cytoplasm, rarely may comprise the entire tumor (referred to as "CNS rhabdoid tumor"), but most often are one component of a heterogeneous malignant neoplasm (Fig. 28-127). ***Inactivation of the INI-1 (hSNF5/SMARCB1) tumor suppressor gene through mutation or deletion is the molecular hallmark of ATRT,*** detected as loss of immunostaining for INI1 protein (Fig. 28-127). Rhabdoid tumors of the kidney share the same genetic alteration as ATRT, and germline mutations of *INI1* result in **rhabdoid tumor predisposition syndrome,** with a propensity for CNS and systemic rhabdoid tumors in infancy.

Craniopharyngiomas (World Health Organization Grade I) Arise in the Sella Turcica and Suprasellar Region

Craniopharyngioma (CP) is a circumscribed epithelial tumor, presumptively derived from Rathke cleft remnants. It arises predominantly in children but also occurs in adults. CP typically exhibits a complex heterogeneous solid and cystic appearance upon preoperative imaging (Fig. 28-128A). Given the origin and expansile growth in the sellar/suprasellar region, CP typically presents with a mixture of endocrine and visual disturbances, referable to compression of the pituitary below and optic chiasm above. Surgical resection is the preferred treatment; however, encroachment on the numerous vital structures in this anatomic neighborhood, including cranial nerves and blood vessels, often hinders resectability, and residual tumor will recur inexorably.

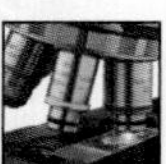

PATHOLOGY: Two morphologic subtypes are distinguished: **adamantinomatous,** which is by far the more common and arises in children and adults, and **papillary,** which is far rarer and arises almost exclusively in adults. The former has distinctive morphology, including sheets of squamous epithelium with prominent peripheral palisading, hydropic degeneration of central areas of the epithelium (referred to as the "stellate reticulum") and nodular aggregates plump keratinocytes ("wet keratin") that tend to calcify (Fig. 28-128B). Long-standing compression of surrounding brain parenchyma characteristically results in reactive piloid astrocytosis with prominent Rosenthal fiber formation. Papillary CP is composed exclusively of nonkeratinizing squamous epithelium. Its histologic appearance is very bland compared to the variegated morphology of the adamantinomatous subtype.

Germinoma (World Health Organization Grade III) and Other Germ Cell Tumors of the Central Nervous System Often Involve the Pineal Gland

Germ cell tumors (GCTs) of the CNS most commonly arise in midline structures, especially the pineal gland and third ventricular region (Fig. 28-129A). **Germinomas** characteristically exhibit a biphasic cell population, with large malignant cells interspersed with swarms of small reactive lymphocytes (Fig. 28-129B). In some cases a granulomatous response may predominate and obscure the neoplastic germ cell component. The tumors are characterized by strong immunoreactivity for OCT3/4 and c-kit, with focal positivity for placental alkaline phosphatase (PLAP) (Fig. 28-129C). In some cases, β-human chorionic gonadotropin (β-HCG) immunostaining identifies isolated syncytiotrophoblastic cells. Pure germinoma is highly radiosensitive and patients may be treated with radiation

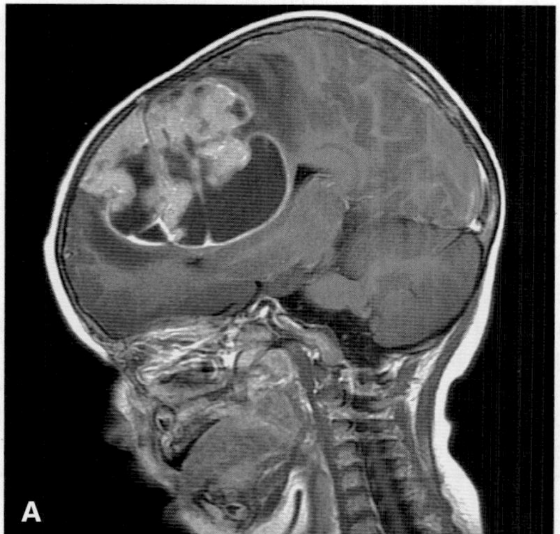

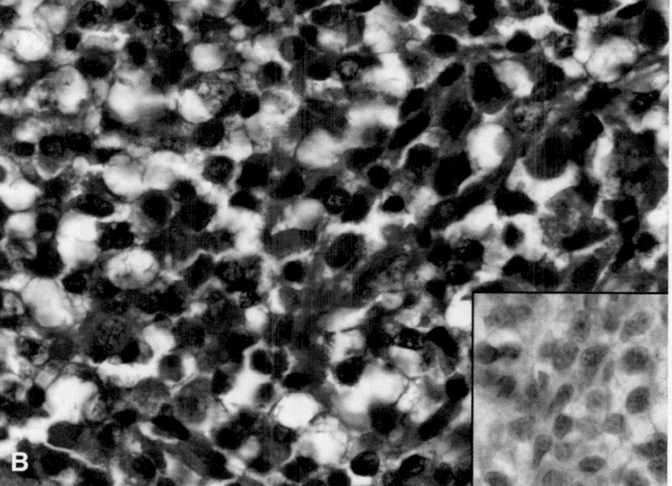

FIGURE 28-127. Atypical teratoid/rhabdoid tumor (ATRT). A. ATRT is a highly malignant neoplasm (World Health Organization grade IV) of early childhood that can arise in the cerebellum or, as illustrated here, in the cerebrum. **B.** The histologic features vary but usually include a rhabdoid cell component featuring plump hypereosinophilic cytoplasm. The molecular signature of ATRT is mutation or deletion of the *INI-1* gene, which can be detected as loss of immunostaining in tumor cell nuclei (*inset*); normal host cells, such as vascular endothelium, serve as positive internal control in this immunostain.

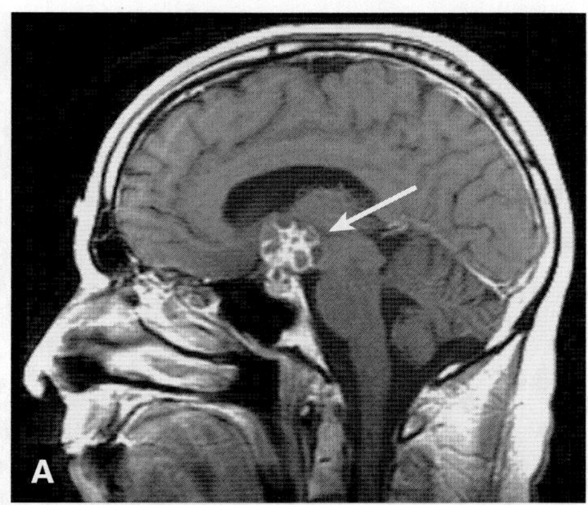

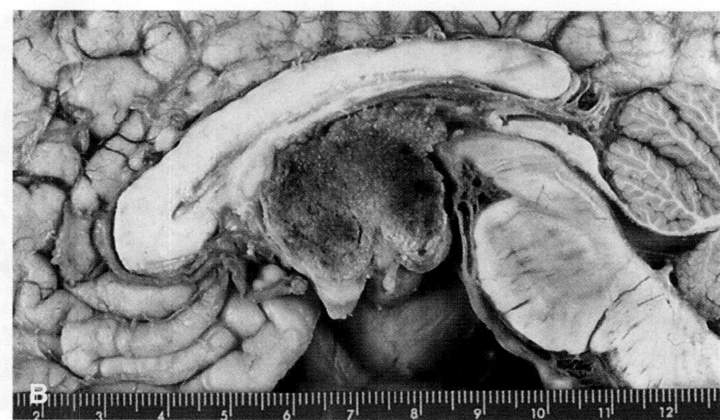

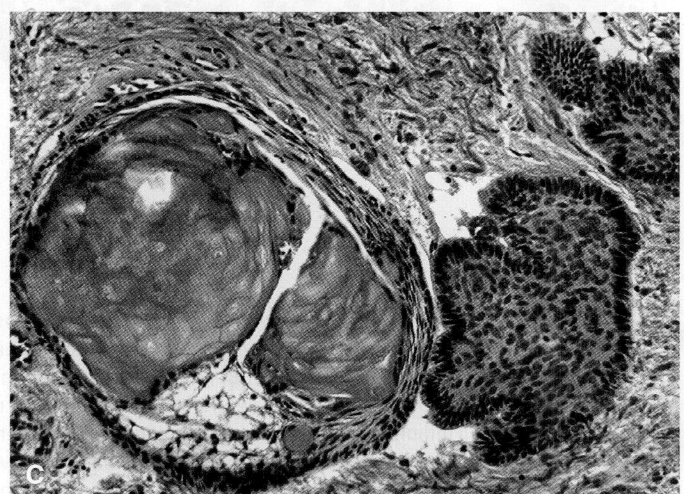

FIGURE 28-128. Craniopharyngioma. A. Craniopharyngiomas arise in the sellar/suprasellar region (*arrow*). **B.** Craniopharyngioma, gross photograph. (Courtesy of Dr. F. Stephen Vogel, Duke University.) **C.** Histologically, craniopharyngiomas are composed of squamous epithelium that displays a number of distinctive morphologic features, including peripheral palisaded nuclei and nodules of plump keratinocytes ("wet keratin") that are prone to calcify.

therapy, chemotherapy or a combination of both. Other germ cell tumors from the pineal region and at other CNS sites include **teratoma** (mature and immature), **yolk sac tumor, embryonal carcinoma** and **choriocarcinoma.** After germinoma, teratoma is the most common of this group to occur as a pure (nonmixed) tumor. The remaining germ cell tumors are mostly encountered in **mixed germ cell tumors.** The prognosis for nongerminomatous GCTs is less favorable than for pure germinoma and is largely dependent on the extent of surgical resection.

Hemangioblastoma (World Health Organization Grade I) Most Often Occurs in the Cerebellum

Hemangioblastomas (HBs) are highly vascular tumors that originate mainly in the cerebellum but also may arise in the spinal cord and brainstem, especially in von Hippel-Lindau disease. HB is one of a number of low-grade circumscribed CNS tumors that present on preoperative imaging studies as a cyst with an enhancing mural nodule (Fig. 28-130A). They typically become apparent clinically as expanding masses in patients 20 to 40 years old. In 20% of cases, HB cells secrete erythropoietin and induce secondary polycythemia. HB can often be cured by surgical resection alone.

PATHOLOGY: HB features vacuolated stromal cells amid a dense capillary vasculature (Fig. 28-130B). The stromal cells are the neoplastic element and are immunoreactive for inhibin-α.

Neuronal Tumors Show Only Neuronal Differentiation and Are Rare

All such tumors are low grade (WHO grade I or II). **Gangliocytoma (WHO grade I)** is a very well-differentiated, circumscribed tumor composed entirely of dysmorphic mature ganglion cells. The temporal lobe is a favored location. **Dysplastic gangliocytoma of the cerebellum (Lhermitte-Duclos disease; WHO grade I)** is a distinctive clinicopathologic entity of the cerebellum characterized by gross enlargement of the folia as easily seen on MRI and disorganized cerebellar cortical histology in which large ganglion cells (derived from granular cell neurons) predominate. A layer of myelinated axons in the outermost part of the molecular layer just beneath the pia is another distinctive feature. An association with **Cowden syndrome** is observed in 50% of patients. Complete surgical resection is curative.

Central neurocytoma (CN; WHO grade II) and **extraventricular neurocytoma (WHO grade II)** are low-grade tumors of young adults that arise from the septum pellucidum, grow into the lateral ventricles and often extend into the third ventricle (Fig. 28-131A). CNs are composed of monomorphous round cells that closely resemble oligodendrocytes (Fig. 28-131B) but, like neurons, strongly express synaptophysin. Extraventricular neurocytomas show similar pathology and behavior but are located in the brain parenchyma rather than the ventricle. Surgery can be curative for small tumors, but partially resected tumors may recur, and central neurocytomas also have the potential for CSF dissemination.

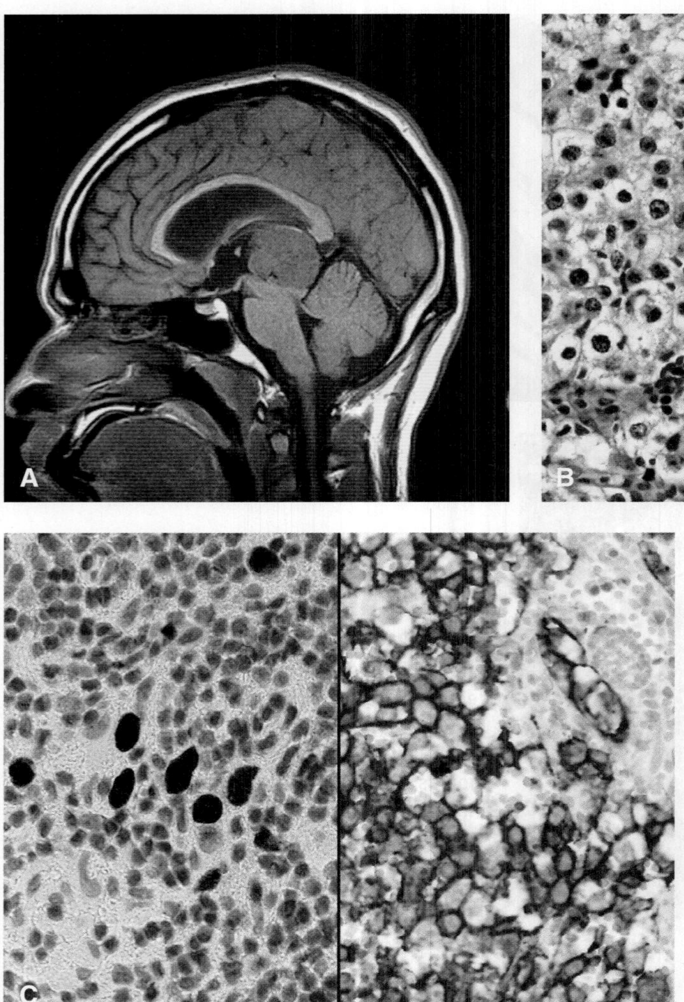

FIGURE 28-129. Germinoma. A. Germ cell tumors most commonly arise in the midline, such as in the pineal gland, as illustrated here. **B.** Microscopically, germinoma, the most common central nervous system germ cell tumor, exhibits a biphasic population of cells: very large germinoma tumor cells and small reactive lymphocytes. **C.** The germinoma immunophenotype includes diagnostically useful nuclear positivity for OCT3/4 (*left panel*) and cytoplasmic positivity for placental alkaline phosphatase (PLAP) (*right panel*).

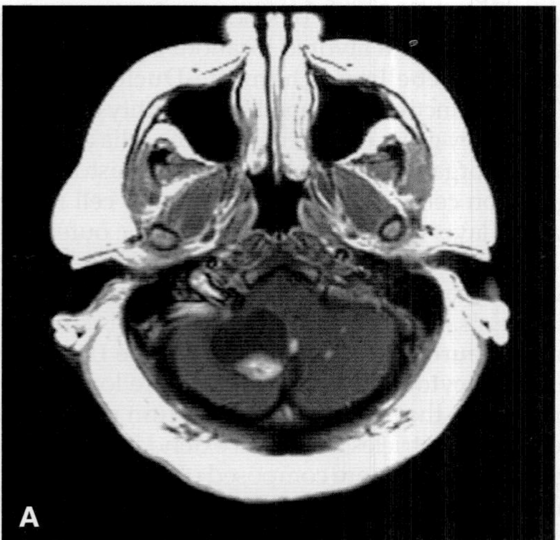

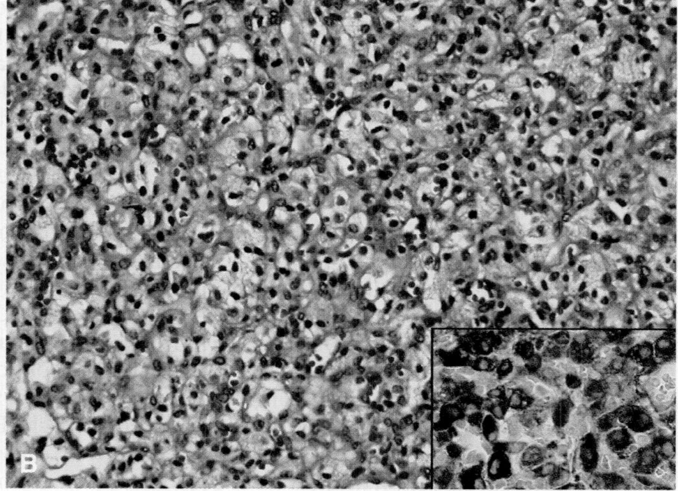

FIGURE 28-130. Hemangioblastoma (HB). A. HB most commonly arises in the cerebellum either sporadically or as part of von Hippel-Lindau disease. A common imaging presentation is as a cyst with a mural nodule. **B.** Microscopically, HB is a highly vascular neoplasm, with the neoplastic stromal cells enmeshed in a dense capillary network. The tumor cells of HB display strong cytoplasmic positivity for inhibin-α (*inset*).

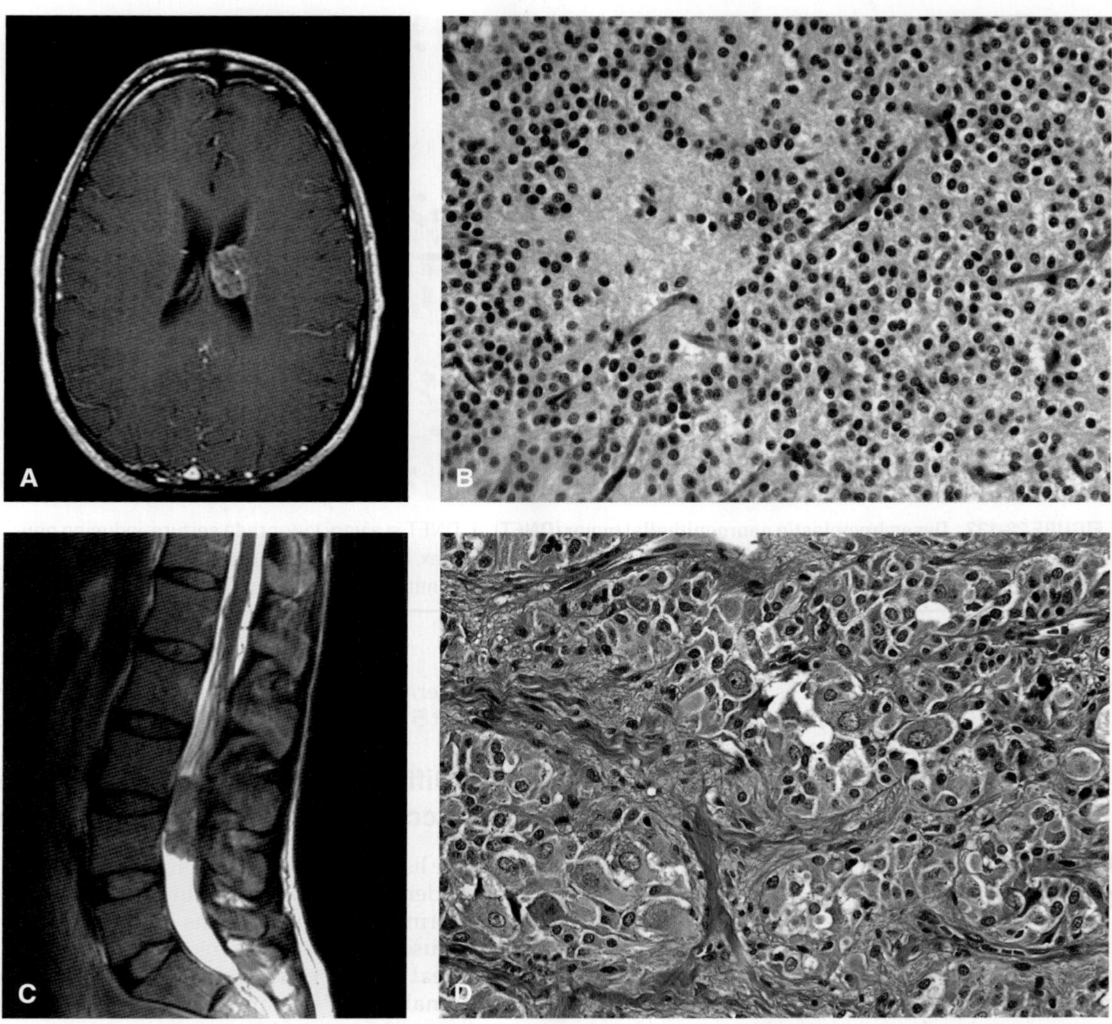

FIGURE 28-131. Neuronal and neuroendocrine tumors. A. Central nervous system neoplasms that exhibit purely neuronal/neuroendocrine differentiation are rare, and the vast majority are low grade. **Central neurocytoma** (CN) is a low-grade neuronal tumor of young adulthood that arises within the lateral ventricle. **B.** CN cells closely mimic oligodendroglioma (compare to Fig. 28-121A) but exhibit a neuronal immunophenotype, including immunoreactivity for synaptophysin. **C. Paraganglioma of the filum terminale** arises, as the name implies, from the distal spinal cord terminus within the lumbar cistern. **D.** Paraganglioma tumor cells exhibit a neuroendocrine phenotype, with strong reactivity for synaptophysin and chromogranin, and frank ganglion cell differentiation is seen in about 25% of cases.

Paraganglioma of the filum terminale (PFT; WHO grade I) is an uncommon neuroendocrine tumor that, similar to myxopapillary ependymoma, arises in the lumbar cistern from the conus medullaris or filum terminale of the spinal cord (Fig. 28-131C). Like paragangliomas arising at other sites in the body, PFTs exhibit a compact acinar ("zellballen") architecture (Fig. 28-131D) with strong immunopositivity for such neuronal markers as synaptophysin and chromogranin, and often show ganglion cell differentiation. Most tumors are "encapsulated" by an investing layer of leptomeninges and are cured by surgical excision.

Mixed Glioneuronal Tumors

Ganglioglioma (GG; WHO grades I and III) is a well-differentiated, circumscribed tumor of neoplastic ganglion cells, with a glioma component. The temporal lobe is its favored location. GG is the most common tumor associated with chronic temporal lobe epilepsy (40% of tumor-associated temporal lobe epilepsy cases). Atypical ganglion cells are intermixed with the glioma element, usually astrocytoma. Although low grade (WHO grade I), GG can progress to **anaplastic ganglioglioma (WHO grade III).** For either grade, the prognosis depends on the extent of surgical resection.

Dysembryoplastic neuroepithelial tumor (DNET; WHO grade I) is a low-grade glioneuronal tumor arising superficially within the cerebral cortex of children (Fig. 28-132A). Its intracortical location correlates with the typical clinical history of long-standing seizures. An additional site of occurrence is in the anterior part of the frontal horn of the lateral ventricle in association with the caudate nucleus and septum pellucidum. It has a multinodular architecture and features prominent nodular aggregates of small rounded oligodendroglial-like cells with interspersed neurons that

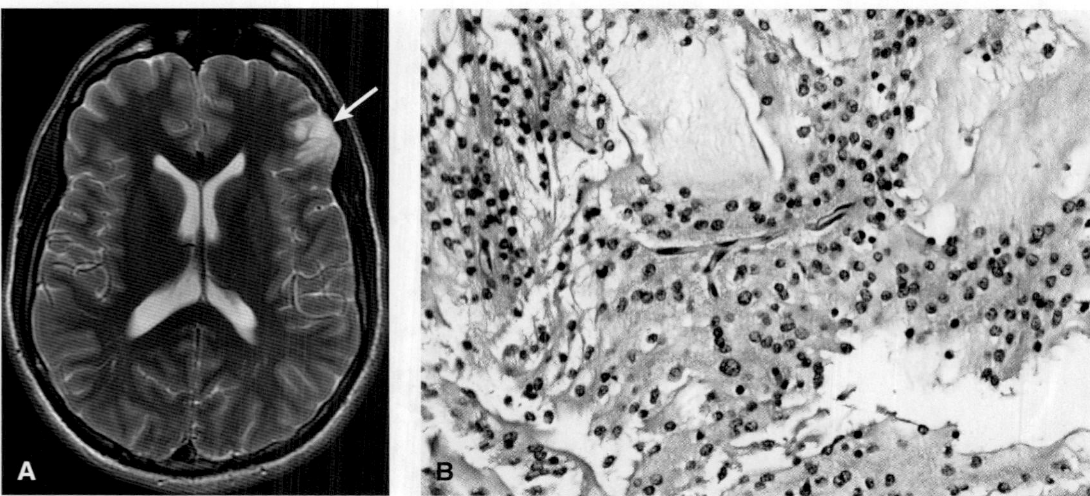

FIGURE 28-132. Dysembryoplastic neuroepithelial tumor (DNET). A. DNET is a very low-grade seizure-inducing neuronal tumor of childhood that arises superficially within the cerebral cortex. **B.** DNET is composed of monotonous round cells that resemble oligodendroglia (B) but is not infiltrative and is potentially curable through surgical resection.

appear to "float" within cystic spaces in the cortical parenchyma (Fig. 28-132B). DNET resembles low-grade oligodendroglioma but lacks the latter's characteristic translocation. Foci of cortical dysplasia may be identified in adjacent peritumoral cortex. Resection is curative.

Pineal Parenchymal Tumors Encompass a Spectrum of Clinical Behavior

Pineal parenchymal tumors (PPTs) range from the very low-grade **pineocytoma (WHO grade I)** to **pineoblastoma,** which is a highly malignant PNET **(WHO grade IV).** In between these two extremes are **pineal parenchymal tumors of intermediate differentiation (PPTIDs; WHO grade II or III).** These are discussed in Chapter 21.

Primary Central Nervous System Lymphomas Are Usually B-Cell Neoplasms

Systemic lymphomas often spread to the CNS, but lymphomas can also originate in the CNS. Primary central nervous system lymphomas (PCNSLs) are tumors of adults and have increased in incidence over the last several decades in both immunocompromised and elderly immunocompetent patients. PCNSLs may present with a wide variety of MRI patterns, including in superficial cortical, deep periventricular or cerebellar location, and as either solitary or multiple lesions (Fig. 28-133A). Definitive pathologic diagnosis is usually made by stereotactic biopsy; surgical resection does not aid survival or response to treatment. PCNSLs are composed of highly infiltrative neoplastic lymphocytes that show prominent invasion and expansion of blood vessel walls (Fig. 28-133B). The vast majority are large cell B-cell tumors and express CD20 and other B-cell markers (Fig. 28-133B). They are highly sensitive to steroids, often decreasing dramatically in size after steroid treatment, but this response is temporary. In addition, steroid therapy can make histologic diagnosis of PCNSL extremely difficult because posttreatment biopsies may show only gliosis and reactive changes. Radiation and/or chemotherapy give a median survival of 70% at 2 years and up to 45% at 5 years in immunocompetent patients.

Many Different Types of Benign (Nonneoplastic) Cysts Occur in the Central Nervous System

These are listed in Table 28-10. Some are degenerative in nature, usually identified as incidental findings on neuroimaging studies performed for other reasons or at autopsy, and only very rarely cause clinical symptoms, such as **choroid plexus cysts** and **pineal gland cysts.** Others, such as **arachnoid cysts** and **ependymal cysts,** are largely asymptomatic but may occasionally require surgical fenestration of the cyst wall to release pressure and relieve mass effect on surrounding structures. The remaining group, also primarily of developmental origin, are

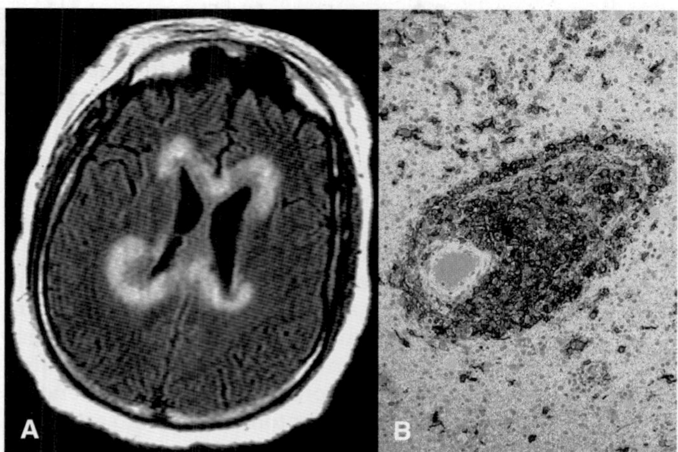

FIGURE 28-133. Primary central nervous system lymphoma (PCNSL). A. One common clinical presentation of PCNSL is as a diffuse periventricular tumor lining the lateral ventricles. **B.** The vast majority of PCNSLs are of diffuse large B-cell phenotype and thus strongly express B-cell markers such as CD20. (Courtesy of Dr. F. Stephen Vogel, Duke University.)

Table 28-10

Central Nervous System Cysts
Choroid plexus cyst
Pineal cyst
Epidermoid cyst
Dermoid cyst
Arachnoid cyst
Ependymal cyst
Neurenteric (enterogenous) cyst
Rathke cyst
Colloid cyst

relatively common causes of mass effect and frequently require simple surgery as definitive treatment. Diagnosis of specific cyst type is based on a combination of anatomic location and histology of the cyst wall lining. For example, three CNS cysts, **Rathke cyst, colloid cyst** and **neurenteric cyst,** share a virtually identical epithelial lining (i.e., ciliated pseudostratified columnar epithelium with goblet cells) but are easily and confidently diagnosed based on anatomic location: Rathke cysts arise in the sellar/suprasellar region, colloid cysts in the roof of the third ventricle near the foramen of Monro and neurenteric cysts in the subarachnoid space anterior to the brainstem medulla or cervical spinal cord (Fig. 28-134). **Epithelial inclusion cysts** (epidermoid and dermoid cysts) are distinguished by their lining and cyst contents, with epidermoids showing only keratinizing stratified squamous epithelium and sheets of anucleate flattened squames for contents, and dermoids displaying a wall that includes dermal appendages, such as sebaceous glands and hair follicles, and contents that include not only anucleate squames but also matted hair (Fig. 28-134).

Metastases to the Central Nervous System Are the Most Common Central Nervous System Tumors

Metastatic tumors far surpass primary CNS tumors in numbers, and CNS metastatic disease is a major clinical problem. Autopsy series show that up to 25% of patients with systemic cancers harbor CNS metastases. The most common site for brain metastasis is at the gray–white junction of the cerebral cortex, but any CNS region may be affected, including the choroid plexus, pineal gland and pituitary gland. The most common primary tumors to involve the CNS are lung (most frequent for both men and women), breast, melanoma, kidney and gastrointestinal tract. Over half of all metastatic disease cases involve multiple metastases (Fig. 28-135A), and metastatic patterns may reflect tumor type. For example, CNS metastases from the gastrointestinal, breast, prostate and uterine cancers are frequently solitary, whereas those from lung carcinoma and melanoma are commonly multiple. A rare extreme form of multiple metastasis, called military metastasis ("carcinomatous encephalitis"), in which innumerable minute metastases shower the brain, is most commonly seen with adenocarcinoma of the lung. Metastases to cranial bones and vertebrae usually originate in the prostate, breast, kidney, thyroid, lung or lymphoma/leukemia (acronym: "Pb KTL"—"lead kettle") (Fig. 28-135B). Breast cancer is frequently the origin of isolated dural metastasis. Isolated metastasis to the leptomeninges and subarachnoid space mostly occurs with lung, breast and gastric adenocarcinomas; hematopoietic neoplasms; and melanoma. Prostate carcinoma frequently metastasizes to the skull and spine, but only rarely involves brain parenchyma. For some very common cancers, such as carcinoma of the uterine cervix, CNS metastasis is extremely rare.

The harmful mass effect on surrounding CNS parenchyma caused by metastatic disease has several underlying etiologic components: (1) tumor growth itself; (2) attendant elicited vasogenic edema in surrounding brain tissue; (3) intratumoral hemorrhage, which can be substantial (primaries especially prone to bleed include melanoma, renal cell carcinoma and choriocarcinoma); and (4) depending on the exact anatomic site of metastasis, obstructive hydrocephalus can be an early contributor to mass effect, as when metastases to the midbrain cause occlusion of the cerebral aqueduct.

Hereditary Intracranial Neoplasms Are Often Associated With Extracranial Tumors

Several hereditary disorders associated with CNS tumors and the genetic bases of the major syndromes are listed in Table 28-8. In some, neoplasms of systemic organs are most prominent, but nervous system tumors also occur. Thus, malignant gliomas occur in Li-Fraumeni syndrome, and medulloblastomas are associated with the gastrointestinal tumors of Turcot syndrome.

Tuberous Sclerosis (Bourneville Disease)

Tuberous sclerosis is an autosomal dominant disease characterized by hamartomas (tubers) of the brain, retina and viscera, as well as various neoplasms. It reflects disordered migration and arrested maturation of neuroectoderm, leading to formation of "tubers" in the cerebral cortex and of subependymal giant cell astrocytomas (Fig. 28-120). The tubers are discrete cortical areas with bizarre cells with neuronal and glial features. The subependymal giant cell astrocytomas resemble "candle drippings." In addition to the intracranial lesions, the syndrome includes (1) facial angiofibromas (adenoma sebaceum), (2) cardiac rhabdomyomas and (3) mesenchymal tumors of the kidney (angiomyolipomas). Most patients have seizures and are mentally retarded. Mutations in two genes are responsible: *TSC1* (9q34) codes for a protein termed hamartin, and *TSC2* (16p13) encodes tuberin, a protein with homology to a guanosine triphosphatase (GTPase)-activating protein. Both genes are tumor suppressors (see Chapter 5).

Sturge-Weber Syndrome (Encephalofacial Angiomatosis)

Sturge-Weber syndrome is a rare, nonfamilial congenital disorder characterized by angiomas of the brain and face. The facial lesion is usually unilateral and is termed a **port wine stain (nevus flammeus).** The leptomeninges exhibit large angiomas, which in severe cases may occupy an entire hemisphere. Cerebral calcification and atrophy often underlie the intracranial angiomas (Fig. 28-136). The link between angiomas of the face and the brain has been attributed to the continuity of the embryologic vascular supply of the telencephalon, the

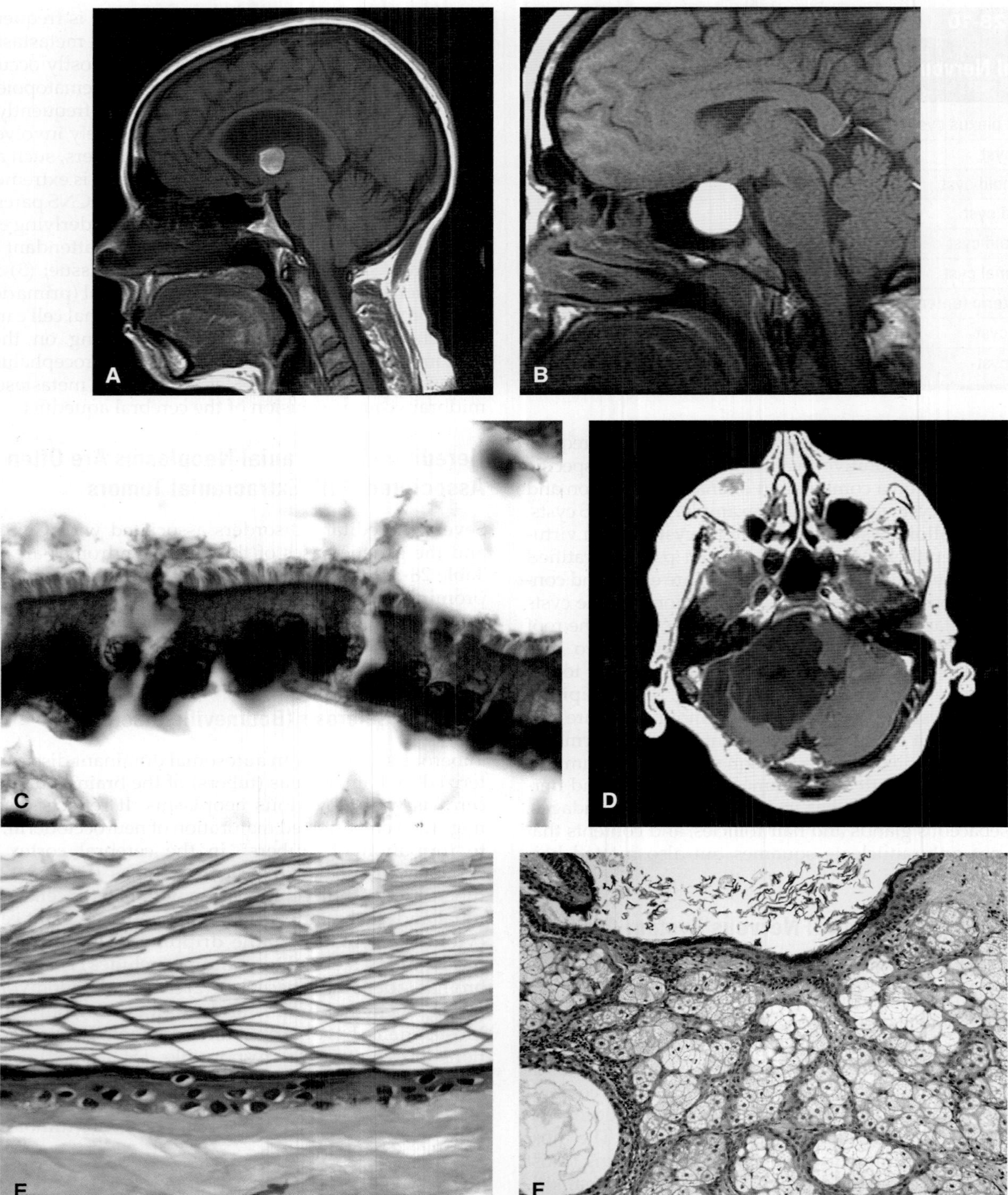

FIGURE 28-134. Cysts of the central nervous system. A. Colloid cysts arise in the rostral roof of the third ventricle. **B. Rathke cysts** are located in the sellar/suprasellar region. **C.** Both of these cysts exhibit a very similar epithelial lining, consisting of ciliated pseudostratified columnar epithelium with goblet cells. **D.** A favored anatomic site for **epidermoid cysts** is the cerebellopontine angle. **E.** Epidermoid cysts differ from dermoid cysts in that the lining of epidermoids is composed of only keratinizing squamous epithelium. **F.** Dermoids also include skin adnexal appendage structures, such as sebaceous glands and hair follicles.

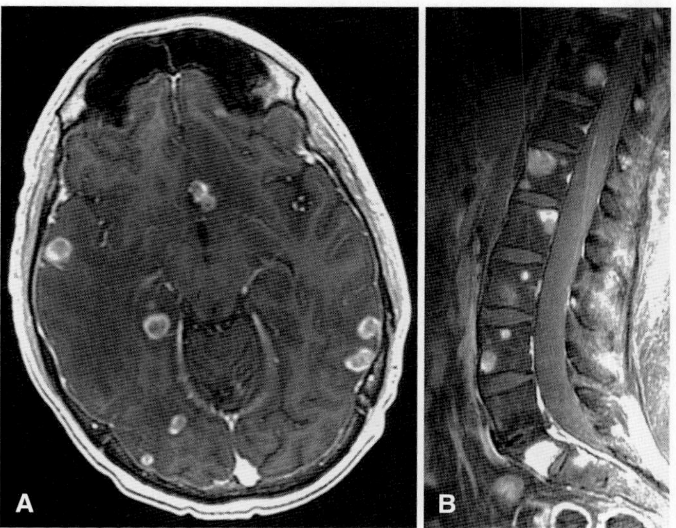

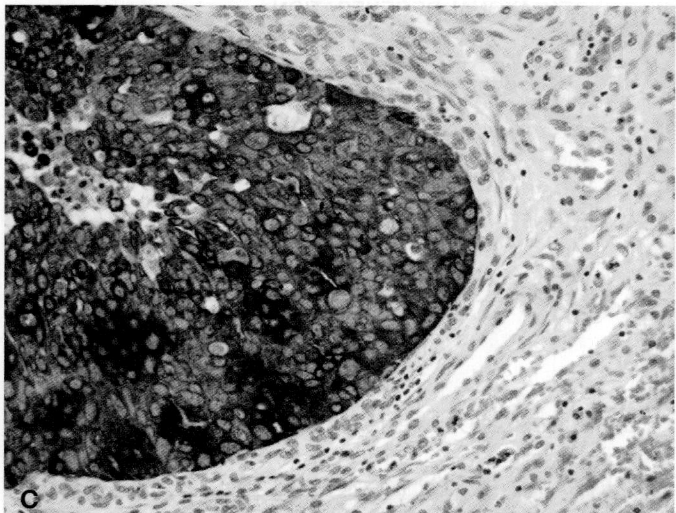

FIGURE 28-135. Metastatic disease. Metastases to the central nervous system commonly produce multiple lesions in both the brain (**A**) and spine (**B**). **C.** Metastatic tumor masses typically show very sharp "pushing" borders with the adjacent brain tissue, as illustrated here with metastatic carcinoma immunostained for keratin.

eye and the overlying skin. In most instances, Sturge-Weber syndrome is associated with mental deficiency.

THE PERIPHERAL NERVOUS SYSTEM

Anatomy

The peripheral nervous system (PNS) is external to the brain and spinal cord and includes (1) cranial nerves, (2) dorsal and ventral spinal roots, (3) spinal nerves and their continuations and (4) ganglia. Peripheral nerves carry somatic motor, somatic sensory, visceral sensory and autonomic fibers.

Somatic motor and preganglionic autonomic fibers arise from neuronal cell bodies within the CNS. The sensory and postganglionic autonomic fibers originate from neuronal cell bodies within ganglia located on cranial nerves, dorsal roots and autonomic nerves. The neurons and satellite cells of the

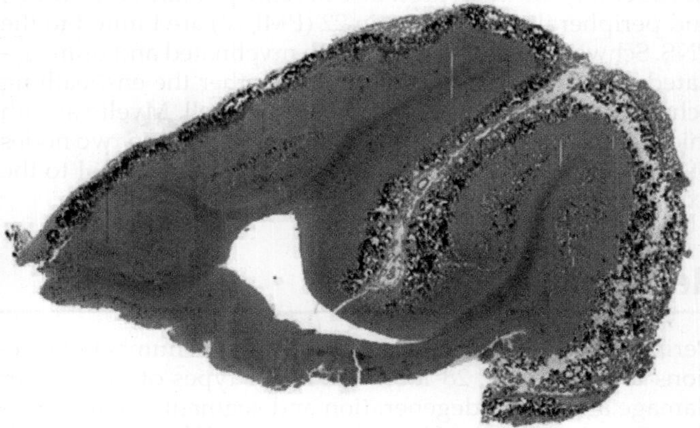

FIGURE 28-136. Sturge-Weber syndrome. Portion of cerebral cortex with overlying capillary angioma involving the leptomeninges and underlying cortical calcification (*purple*).

ganglia and all of the Schwann cells are derived from the neural crest.

Peripheral nerves, but not their ganglia, have a blood-nerve barrier analogous to the blood-brain barrier. Endoneurial connective tissue surrounds the individual nerve fibers, which are bundled into fascicles by the **perineurial sheath.** Epineurial connective tissue binds the fascicles together and contains the nutrient arteries.

Peripheral nerve fibers are either myelinated or unmyelinated (Fig. 28-137). Myelinated fibers are from 1 to 20 μm in diameter, but unmyelinated ones, at 0.4 to 2.4 μm, are much smaller. Myelin is an elaboration of Schwann cell plasmalemma and is necessary for saltatory nerve conduction. Schwann cell–derived PNS myelin and oligodendrocyte-derived CNS myelin have similar lipid composition but differ

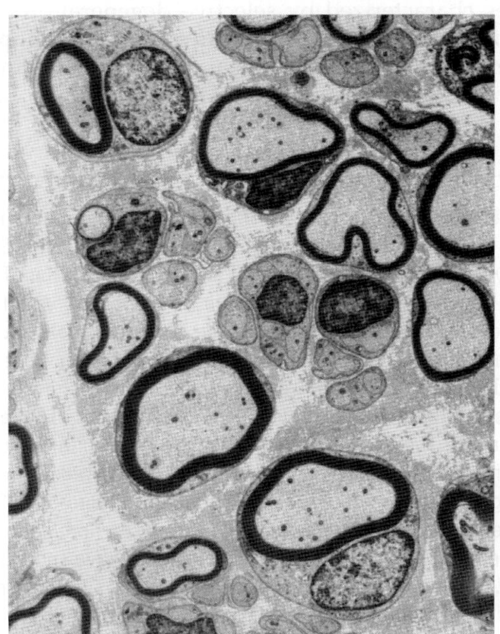

FIGURE 28-137. Structure of peripheral nerve. Electron micrograph of a peripheral nerve shows myelinated fibers interspersed with groups of unmyelinated fibers. Note that unlike myelinated axons, several unmyelinated axons may share a Schwann cell.

considerably in their proteins. Myelin protein zero (MPZ) and peripheral myelin protein 22 (PMP22) are limited to the PNS. Schwann cells ensheathe both myelinated and unmyelinated fibers. The axon determines whether the ensheathing Schwann cell becomes a myelin-forming cell. Myelin sheath thickness, internodal length (i.e., distance between two nodes of Ranvier) and conduction velocity are proportional to the axonal diameter.

Reactions to Injury

Peripheral nerve fibers display only a limited number of reactions to injury (Fig. 28-138). The major types of nerve fiber damage are axonal degeneration and segmental demyelination. Peripheral nerve fibers differ from CNS nerve fibers in having the capacity for functionally significant axonal regeneration and remyelination.

Axonal Degeneration Reflects Direct Injury to the Axon or Neuronal Cell Body

Degeneration (necrosis) of the axon occurs in many neuropathies and may be restricted to the distal axon or involve both the axon and neuronal cell body (Fig. 28-139). Axonal degeneration is quickly followed by breakdown of the myelin sheath and Schwann cell proliferation. Myelin degradation is initiated by Schwann cells and completed by macrophages, which infiltrate the nerve within 3 days after axonal degeneration. If degeneration is restricted to the distal axon, regenerating axons may sprout within 1 week from the intact, proximal axonal stump. There are several types of axonal degeneration.

DISTAL AXONAL DEGENERATION: In many neuropathies, axonal degeneration is limited at first to the distal ends of larger, longer fibers (Fig. 28-138B). Peripheral neuropathies characterized by selective degeneration of distal axons are **dying-back neuropathies (distal axonopathies)** and are typically seen as distal ("length-dependent" or "glove-and-stocking") neuropathies.

In distal axonal degeneration, neuronal cell bodies and proximal axons remain intact. Thus, axon regeneration and return of nerve function may be possible if the cause of the distal axonal degeneration is identified and removed. This must occur before the dying-back degeneration sufficiently extends centripetally to involve the proximal axon and cause death of the neuronal cell body. Recovery is also limited in some dying-back neuropathies because the distal axonal degeneration involves not only the peripherally directed axon

A. INTACT MYELINATED FIBER

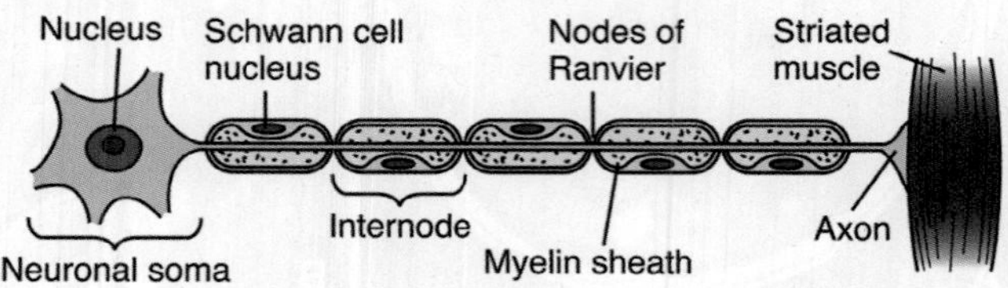

B. DISTAL AXONAL DEGENERATION

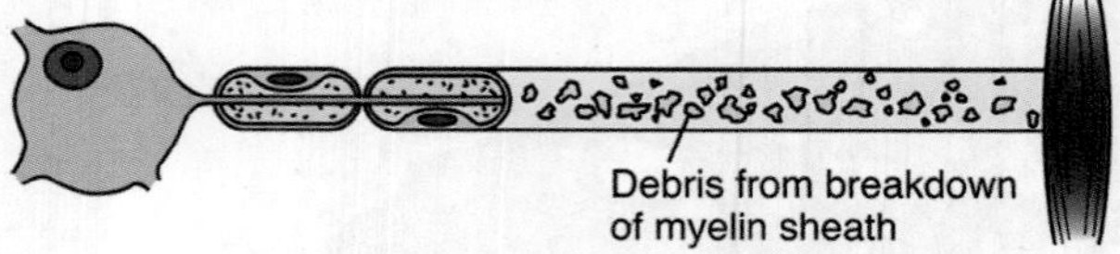

C. DEGENERATION OF CELL BODY AND AXON

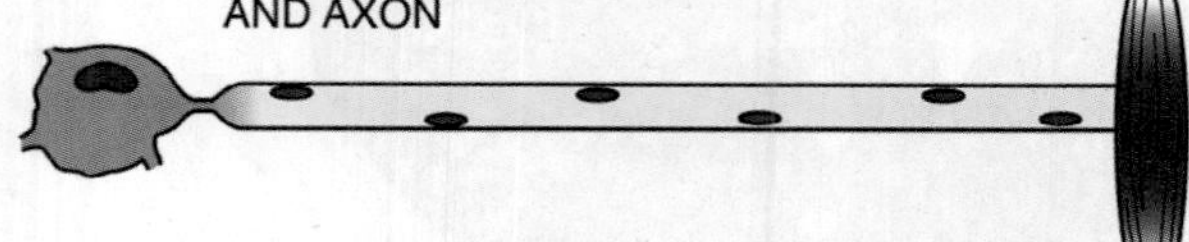

D. SEGMENTAL DEMYELINATION

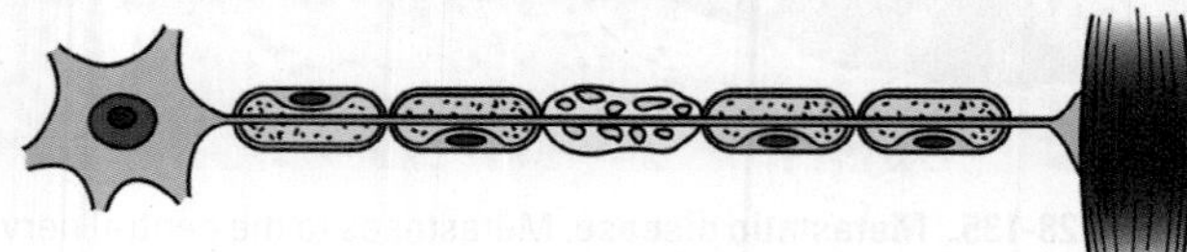

E. REMYELINATION

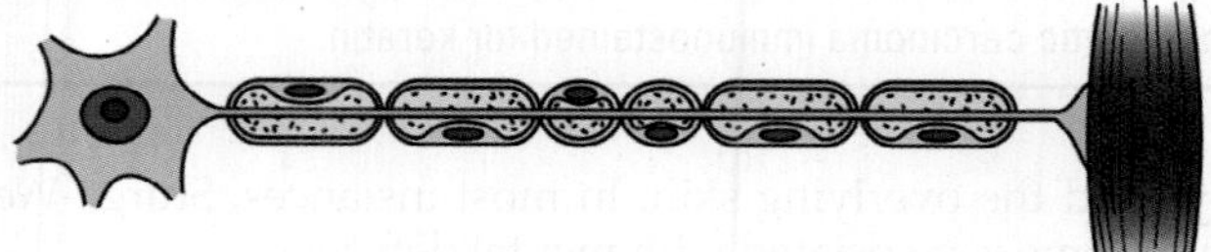

F. REGENERATING AXON

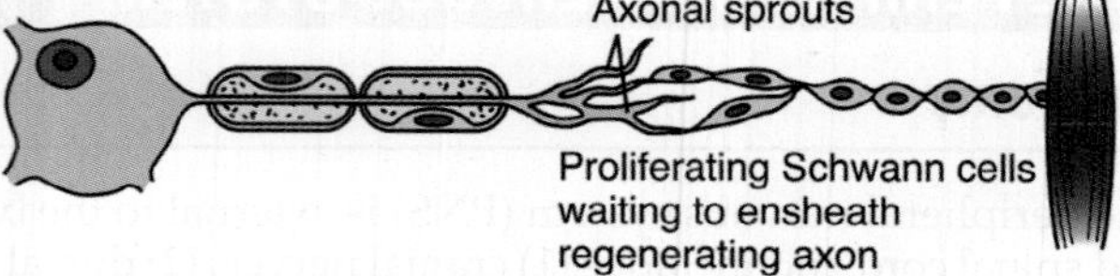

G. REGENERATED NERVE FIBER

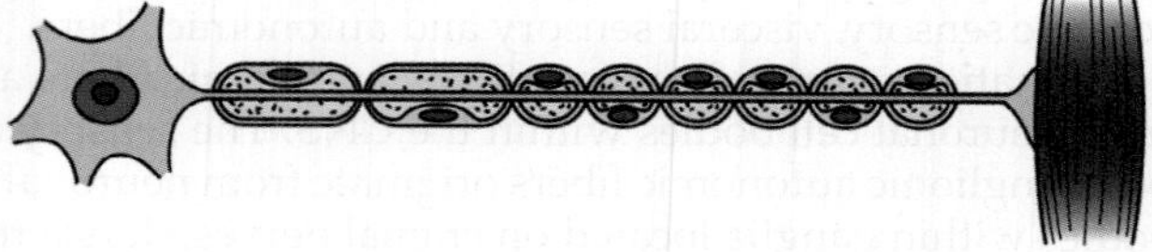

FIGURE 28-138. Basic responses of peripheral nerve fibers to injury. A. Intact myelinated fiber. The axon is insulated by the Schwann cell–derived myelin sheaths. **B. Distal axonal degeneration.** The distal axon has degenerated, and myelin sheaths associated with the distal axon have secondarily degenerated. The striated muscle shows denervation atrophy. **C. Degeneration of cell body and axon.** Degeneration involves the neuronal cell body and its entire axon. The myelin sheaths associated with the axon have also degenerated. **D. Segmental demyelination.** The myelin sheath associated with one Schwann cell has degenerated, leaving a segment of axon uncovered by myelin. The underlying axon remains intact. **E. Remyelination.** Proliferating Schwann cells cover the demyelinated segment of the axon and elaborate new myelin sheaths. The remyelinating Schwann cells have short internodal lengths. **F. Regenerating axon.** Regenerating axons sprout from the distal end of the disrupted axon. Ideally, the regenerating axons reinnervate the distal nerve stump, where they will be ensheathed and myelinated by Schwann cells of the distal stump. **G. Regenerated nerve fiber.** The regenerated portion of the axon is myelinated by Schwann cells with short internodal lengths. The striated muscle is reinnervated.

of the dorsal root–ganglion neuron, but also its centrally directed axon traveling in the dorsal columns of the spinal cord. These centrally directed axons, like other axons within the CNS, have little capacity for regeneration.

NEURONOPATHY: Axonal degeneration may result from death of the neuronal cell body, as in an autoimmune dorsal root ganglionitis (Fig. 28-138C). Neuropathies with selective damage to neuron cell bodies are **neuronopathies** and are much less common than distal axonopathies. There is little potential for recovery of function in neuronopathy because death of the neuronal cell body precludes axonal regeneration.

WALLERIAN DEGENERATION: This term refers to the axonal degeneration that occurs in a nerve distal to a transection or crush of the nerve. If the transection is not too proximal, the nerve may regenerate.

Segmental Demyelination Reflects Direct Schwann Cell Injury or Underlying Axonal Abnormalities

Loss of myelin from one or more internodes (segments) along a myelinated fiber reflects Schwann cell dysfunction (Fig. 28-138D). This condition may be caused by direct injury to the Schwann cell or myelin sheath **(primary demyelination),** or it may result from underlying axonal abnormalities **(secondary demyelination).**

Loss of the myelin sheath is not accompanied by degeneration of the underlying axon. Macrophages infiltrate the nerve and clear the myelin debris. Degeneration of the internodal myelin sheath is followed sequentially by (1) Schwann cell proliferation, (2) remyelination of the demyelinated segments and (3) recovery of function. The remyelinated internodes have shortened internodal lengths (Fig. 28-138E). Repeated episodes of segmental demyelination and remyelination of peripheral nerves, as occurs in chronic demyelinating neuropathies, lead to the accumulation of supernumerary Schwann cells around axons **(onion bulbs)** and clinically apparent nerve enlargement **(hypertrophic neuropathy).**

Peripheral Neuropathies

Peripheral neuropathy is a process that affects the function of one or more peripheral nerves. The disease may be restricted to the PNS, involve both peripheral and central nervous systems or affect multiple organ systems. Peripheral neuropathies are encountered in all age groups and may be hereditary or acquired.

The causes of peripheral neuropathy are many (Table 28-11). ***Diabetes mellitus is the most common cause of generalized peripheral neuropathy in the United States.*** Other common causes include hereditary disorders, alcoholism, chronic renal failure, neurotoxic drugs, autoimmune diseases, paraproteinemia, nutritional deficiencies, infections, cancer and trauma.

Table 28-11

Etiologic Classification of Neuropathies

Immune-mediated neuropathies
Acute inflammatory demyelinating polyradiculoneuropathy (Guillain-Barré syndrome)
Acute motor (and sensory) axonal neuropathy (axonal form of Guillain-Barré syndrome)
Fisher syndrome
Chronic inflammatory demyelinating polyradiculoneuropathy (CIDP)
Multifocal motor neuropathy
Dorsal root ganglionitis (sensory neuronopathy)
Immunoglobulin M (IgM) paraproteinemia-associated demyelinating neuropathy
Vasculitic neuropathy (systemic vasculitis, connective tissue disease, cryoglobulinemia)
Metabolic neuropathies
Diabetic polyneuropathy and mononeuropathies
Uremic neuropathy
Critical illness polyneuropathy
Hypothyroid neuropathy
Acromegalic neuropathy
Nutritional neuropathies
Neuropathy associated with deficiency of vitamin B_1, B_6, B_{12} or E
Copper deficiency myeloneuropathy
Postgastrectomy neuropathy
Alcoholic neuropathy
Toxic and drug-induced neuropathies (see Table 28-12)
Amyloid neuropathy (AL amyloidosis and familial amyloid polyneuropathy)
Hereditary neuropathies (see Table 28-13 and Table 28-14)
Neuropathies associated with infections
Leprosy
Human immunodeficiency virus
Cytomegalovirus
Hepatitis B and C (vasculitic neuropathy or CIDP)
Herpes zoster
Lyme disease
Diphtheria (toxic neuropathy)
Paraneoplastic neuropathy
Sarcoid neuropathy
Radiation neuropathy
Traumatic neuropathy
Chronic idiopathic axonal polyneuropathy

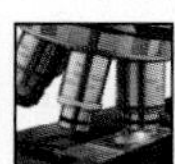

PATHOLOGY: Pathologic findings in most neuropathies are limited to axonal degeneration, segmental demyelination or both. When axonal degeneration predominates, a neuropathy is classified as an **axonal neuropathy;** when segmental demyelination predominates, a neuropathy is a **demyelinating neuropathy.** ***Most (80% to 90%) neuropathies are axonal and of the dying-back type (distal axonal neuropathy).*** Electrophysiologic studies often help to differentiate between axonal and demyelinating neuropathies. Nerve conduction velocity is typically near normal in axonal neuropathies but conspicuously decreased in demyelinating neuropathies. Axonal neuropathies have many causes, but demyelinating neuropathies have a limited number of causes. The distinction between axonal and demyelinating neuropathies is useful clinically. The latter are most likely to be hereditary, immune mediated and inflammatory or IgM paraproteinemia associated.

Many neuropathies do not show additional disease-specific histologies beyond axonal loss or demyelination, so that clinicopathologic correlation is necessary to establish causation. For a small number, a specific origin can be established, such as necrotizing arteritis (vasculitic neuropathy), granulomatous inflammation (leprosy, sarcoid), amyloid deposits (amyloid neuropathy), abnormalities of the myelin sheath (IgM paraproteinemic neuropathy, hereditary neuropathy with liability to pressure palsies) or abnormal accumulations within Schwann cells (leukodystrophy) or axons (giant axonal neuropathy).

CLINICAL FEATURES: The major clinical manifestations of peripheral neuropathy are muscle weakness, muscle atrophy, sensory loss, paresthesia, pain and autonomic dysfunction. Motor, sensory and autonomic functions may be equally or preferentially affected. Sensory abnormalities may reflect predominant involvement of large-diameter fibers (position and vibration sense) or small-diameter fibers (pain and temperature). The neuropathy may be acute (days to weeks), subacute (weeks to months) or chronic (months to years). Disease may be localized to dorsal root ganglia **(sensory neuronopathy),** nerve roots **(radiculopathy),** one nerve **(mononeuropathy)** or several nerves **(mononeuropathy multiplex).** It may also be diffuse and symmetric and involve peripheral nerves **(polyneuropathy)** or nerve roots and peripheral nerves **(polyradiculoneuropathy).**

Diabetic Neuropathy Has Several Clinical Presentations

Peripheral neuropathy is a common complication of type 1 and type 2 diabetes mellitus. The neuropathy may manifest as a distal sensorimotor polyneuropathy, autonomic neuropathy, mononeuropathy or mononeuropathy multiplex. The mononeuropathies may involve cranial nerves (cranial neuropathy), nerve roots or proximal peripheral nerves. ***Distal, predominantly sensory, polyneuropathy is the most common form of diabetic neuropathy.***

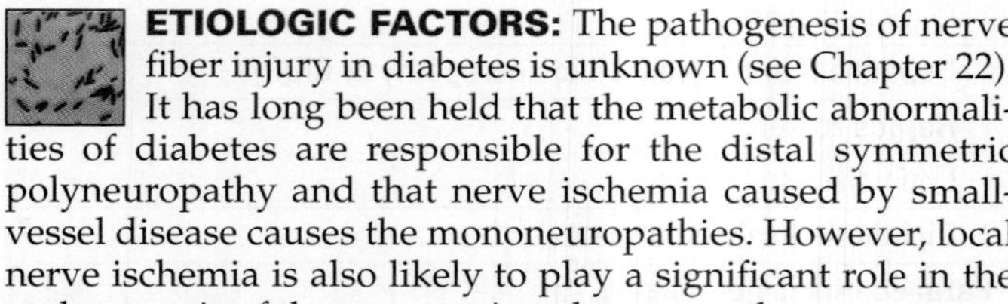

ETIOLOGIC FACTORS: The pathogenesis of nerve fiber injury in diabetes is unknown (see Chapter 22). It has long been held that the metabolic abnormalities of diabetes are responsible for the distal symmetric polyneuropathy and that nerve ischemia caused by small-vessel disease causes the mononeuropathies. However, local nerve ischemia is also likely to play a significant role in the pathogenesis of the symmetric polyneuropathy.

PATHOLOGY: In the distal symmetric polyneuropathy of diabetes, one sees a mixture of axonal degeneration and segmental demyelination, with the former predominating. Axonal loss involves fibers of all sizes but may preferentially affect the large myelinated fibers **(large-fiber neuropathy)** or the small myelinated fibers and unmyelinated fibers **(small-fiber neuropathy).** Occasional neuron loss in the dorsal root ganglia and anterior horns appears to be a consequence of centripetal progression of dying-back axonal degeneration, rather than a neuronopathy.

Uremic Neuropathy Often Complicates Chronic Renal Failure

Uremic neuropathy is a distal sensorimotor axonal polyneuropathy. The pathogenesis of the nerve fiber damage is not known, but the disease usually stabilizes or improves with long-term dialysis. Both distal axonal degeneration and segmental demyelination are seen, with axonal degeneration predominating and preferentially involving large-diameter fibers. The neuropathy resolves after renal transplantation.

Critical Illness Polyneuropathy Is Associated With Sepsis and Multiorgan Failure

Critical illness polyneuropathy is an axonal neuropathy that develops in severely ill patients. The pathogenesis is obscure. The acute, predominantly motor, neuropathy may first be apparent when a patient cannot be weaned from ventilatory support. A **critical illness myopathy** may also occur in these patients.

Alcoholic Neuropathy Is a Frequent Complication of Alcoholism

Alcoholic neuropathy is a distal sensorimotor axonal polyneuropathy that may be attributable to nutritional deficiencies and/or a direct toxic effect of ethanol on the PNS. Peripheral nerves show loss of nerve fibers from axonal degeneration of the dying-back type.

Nutritional Neuropathy Has Multiple Causes

An axonal polyneuropathy may be associated with vitamin deficiencies (B_1, B_6, B_{12} or E), copper deficiency or the post-gastrectomy state. Copper deficiency may be a result of malnutrition, gastric bypass surgery, total parenteral nutrition or excessive ingestion of zinc. Nutritional neuropathy may also complicate bariatric surgery.

Acute Inflammatory Demyelinating Polyradiculoneuropathy (Guillain-Barré Syndrome) Is Immune Mediated

Acute inflammatory demyelinating polyradiculoneuropathy (AIDP) is an acquired, immune-mediated neuropathy that often follows bacterial, viral or mycoplasmal infections. It may also follow immunization or surgery. In most cases, there is an antecedent infection, usually upper respiratory or gastrointestinal. Commonly associated infectious agents include *Campylobacter jejuni*, cytomegalovirus, Epstein-Barr virus and *Mycoplasma pneumoniae*. AIDP is the most common cause in children and adults of the **Guillain-Barré syndrome,** which is an acute symmetric neuromuscular paralysis that often begins distally and ascends proximally. Sensory and autonomic disturbances may also occur. Some 5% of cases present with ophthalmoplegia, ataxia and areflexia **(Fisher syndrome).** Muscular paralysis may cause respiratory embarrassment, and the autonomic involvement may result in cardiac arrhythmias, hypotension or hypertension. Resolution of the neuropathy begins 2 to 4 weeks after onset, and most patients make a good recovery. Characteristically CSF protein is increased, without pleocytosis. The increased protein level is attributable to inflammation of the spinal roots. The pathogenesis of the immunologically mediated demyelination is not known. Both humoral and cellular immune mechanisms have been postulated.

AIDP may affect all levels of the PNS, including spinal roots (polyradiculoneuropathy), ganglia, craniospinal nerves and autonomic nerves. The distribution of lesions varies from case to case. Involved regions show endoneurial infiltrates of lymphocytes and macrophages, segmental demyelination and relative axonal sparing. Lymphoid infiltrates are often perivascular, but there is no true vasculitis. Macrophages are frequently found adjacent to degenerating myelin sheaths and have been observed to strip off and phagocytose the superficial myelin lamellae. Such macrophage-mediated demyelination is rarely observed in other neuropathies.

Guillain-Barré syndrome may also be caused by an immune-mediated axonal neuropathy **(acute motor axonal neuropathy** or **acute motor and sensory axonal neuropathy).** The axonal form of Guillain-Barré syndrome is much less common than the demyelinating form in North America and Europe but is more prevalent in Asia. Patients with the axonal form often have an antecedent *C. jejuni* infection and antiganglioside antibodies (anti-GM1 and others) in their serum. It has been suggested that molecular mimicry between an antigenic component of the infectious agent and an antigenic component of peripheral nerve leads to a cross-reactive immune response that causes axonal injury. Antiganglioside antibodies (anti-GQ1b and others) are also common in the Fisher syndrome.

Chronic inflammatory demyelinating polyradiculoneuropathy (CIDP) is similar to AIDP but has a protracted course with multiple relapses or slow continuous progression. An antecedent upper respiratory or gastrointestinal infection is usually not reported in CIDP. The neuropathy may occur sporadically (idiopathic CIDP) or be associated with paraproteinemia, HIV infection, chronic active hepatitis, connective tissue disease, inflammatory bowel disease or Hodgkin lymphoma. The demyelinating neuropathy is symmetric, sensorimotor and proximal and distal. Rare cases present as a multiple mononeuropathy **(multifocal acquired demyelinating sensory and motor neuropathy).** The nerves and nerve roots in CIDP may show many onion bulbs as a result of recurring episodes of demyelination, Schwann cell proliferation and remyelination. The pathogenesis of this immune-mediated neuropathy is unknown.

Multifocal motor neuropathy is a rare, slowly progressive, demyelinating mononeuropathy multiplex that may be mistaken clinically for motor neuron disease. There is often an associated increased titer of anti-GM_1 antibodies. The demyelinating neuropathy is immune mediated but is considered distinct from CIDP.

Dorsal Root Ganglionitis Is an Immune-Mediated Sensory Neuronopathy

This inflammatory ganglionopathy typically manifests as a subacute or chronic sensory polyneuropathy with sensory ataxia. The pathogenesis of the immune-mediated sensory neuron degeneration is unknown. The disorder may occur sporadically **(idiopathic sensory neuronopathy),** in association with Sjögren syndrome or as a paraneoplastic sensory neuronopathy. The latter is often associated with anti-Hu antibodies (antineuronal autoantibodies) and may be accompanied by a paraneoplastic encephalomyelitis. Dorsal root ganglia show infiltration by lymphocytes and loss of sensory neurons.

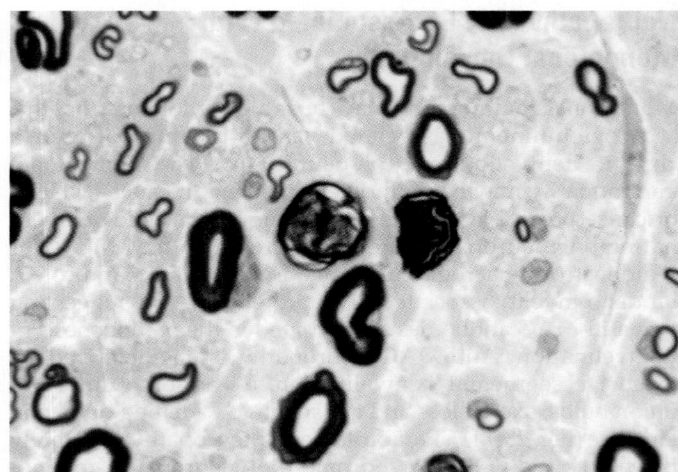

FIGURE 28-139. Axonal degeneration in peripheral nerve. Photomicrograph of a plastic-embedded cross-section of sural nerve shows two degenerating myelinated fibers in the center of the field. The degenerating fibers' axons are gone, and their myelin sheaths are reduced to rounded masses of myelin debris.

Vasculitic Neuropathy Causes Mononeuropathy Multiplex

Necrotizing arteritis may involve the epineurial arteries of nerves as one manifestation of systemic vasculitis (polyarteritis nodosa, Churg-Strauss syndrome, Wegener granulomatosis, microscopic polyangiitis), connective tissue disease (rheumatoid arthritis, systemic lupus erythematosus, Sjögren syndrome), cryoglobulinemia, HIV infection or cancer. In about a third of cases of vasculitic neuropathy, the necrotizing arteritis appears limited to the PNS **(nonsystemic vasculitic neuropathy).** The ischemic neuropathy is characterized pathologically by axonal degeneration (Fig. 28-140).

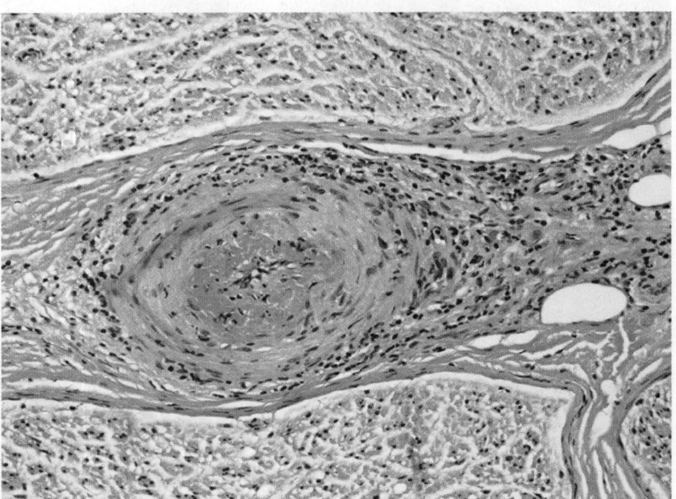

FIGURE 28-140. Vasculitic neuropathy in a patient with polyarteritis nodosa. Photomicrograph of a cross-section of a sural nerve reveals an inflamed epineurial artery with fibrinoid necrosis of its wall.

Neuropathy May Be Associated With Monoclonal Gammopathy

Monoclonal gammopathy may cause an amyloid neuropathy, a cryoglobulinemia-associated vasculitic neuropathy or a chronic demyelinating polyneuropathy. The monoclonal gammopathy may be of undetermined significance (MGUS) or caused by a plasma cell neoplasm. The chronic demyelinating polyneuropathy often occurs with an IgM MGUS or Waldenström macroglobulinemia, in which the paraprotein binds to myelin-associated glycoprotein (MAG), suggesting that anti-MAG antibodies are involved in the pathogenesis of demyelination. Anti-MAG neuropathy is characterized by extensive segmental demyelination, a variable number of onion bulbs, axonal loss and a distinctive widening of myelin lamellae (Fig. 28-141). Paraproteinemic neuropathy may rarely present as the POEMS syndrome (polyneuropathy, organomegaly, endocrinopathy, monoclonal gammopathy and skin changes), in patients with elevated serum levels of vascular endothelial growth factor (VEGF) and a plasma cell disorder.

Amyloid Neuropathy Complicates Light-Chain Amyloidosis and Familial Amyloidosis

In addition to its effects on sensory and motor nerves, amyloid infiltration of the PNS often leads to prominent autonomic dysfunction. Although the disorder may be hereditary, it more often complicates light-chain amyloidosis (AL) in primary systemic amyloidosis or multiple myeloma. A point mutation in the transthyretin gene is responsible for most cases of dominantly inherited, familial amyloid polyneuropathy (see Chapter 23). Mutations of the apolipoprotein A1 gene or gelsolin gene are also associated with familial amyloid polyneuropathy.

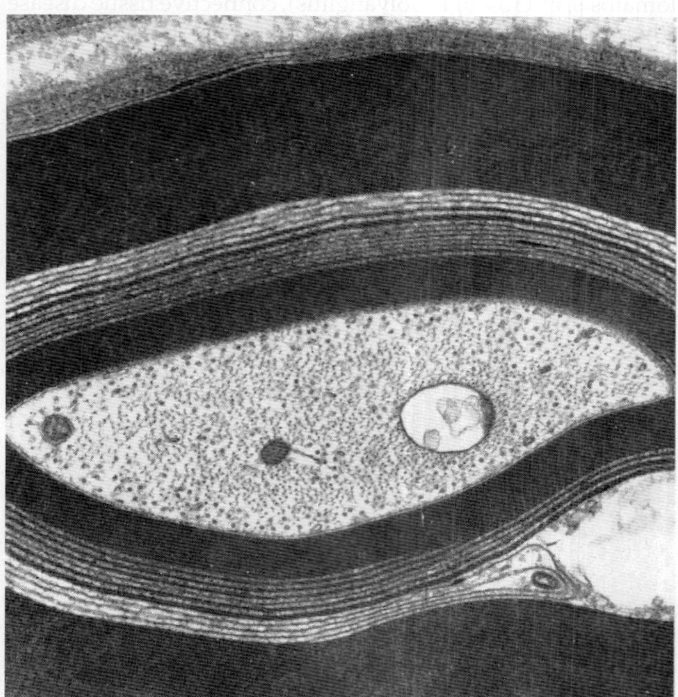

FIGURE 28-141. Paraproteinemic neuropathy. An electron micrograph shows a myelinated fiber with multiple, abnormally widely spaced, myelin lamellae from a patient with an immunoglobulin M monoclonal gammopathy of unknown significance and a chronic demyelinating neuropathy.

Amyloid neuropathy is characterized by deposition of amyloid in peripheral nerves, dorsal root ganglia and autonomic ganglia. The interstitial amyloid deposits are both endoneurial and epineurial and frequently involve blood vessel walls. Amyloid deposition is accompanied by loss of myelinated and unmyelinated fibers. Postulated mechanisms for nerve-fiber damage include direct mechanical injury of nerve fibers and ganglion cells by amyloid deposits and nerve ischemia caused by amyloid infiltration of vasa nervorum.

Carpal tunnel syndrome is a chronic entrapment neuropathy of the median nerve at the wrist. It represents another complication of systemic amyloidosis. Nerve entrapment results from amyloid infiltration of the flexor retinaculum. Many other conditions, including occupational injuries, hypothyroidism, chronic renal failure, pregnancy and rheumatoid arthritis, are also associated with carpal tunnel syndrome.

Paraneoplastic Neuropathy Often Precedes Recognition of Underlying Cancer

Paraneoplastic nervous system diseases include polyneuropathy, chronic encephalomyelitis, necrotizing myelopathy, cerebellar degeneration and the Eaton-Lambert syndrome. Several different clinicopathologic types of paraneoplastic neuropathy have been defined.

- **Paraneoplastic sensorimotor polyneuropathy:** This distal polyneuropathy is the most common form of paraneoplastic neuropathy and is characterized by axonal degeneration and demyelination, mainly the former. The cause of the nerve-fiber degeneration is unknown.
- **Paraneoplastic sensory neuronopathy:** Less commonly, paraneoplastic neuropathy may manifest as a subacute sensory neuronopathy caused by a dorsal root ganglionitis. Similar chronic inflammatory changes may also occur in the CNS **(paraneoplastic encephalomyelitis).** Anti-Hu antibodies are often present in these patients, and small cell carcinoma of the lung is the usual cause. The sensory neuronopathy and encephalitis are thought to be immune mediated.
- **Inflammatory demyelinating polyradiculoneuropathy:** Immune-mediated acute or chronic inflammatory demyelinating polyradiculoneuropathy may be associated with cancer.
- **Paraneoplastic vasculitic neuropathy:** Vasculitic neuropathy may rarely complicate cancer.

Not all paraneoplastic neuropathies result from remote effects of a neoplasm on the nervous system. Tumors may cause neuropathy by direct compression or infiltration of nerves or nerve roots. Cancer patients may also develop chemotherapy-induced toxic neuropathy or radiation-induced neuropathy (brachial or lumbosacral plexopathy).

Toxic Neuropathy Is Often Iatrogenic

A variety of environmental agents and industrial compounds cause peripheral neuropathy (Table 28-12), but most cases of toxic neuropathy are caused by drugs. Almost all toxic

Table 28-12

Agents Associated With Toxic Neuropathy

Drugs	Environmental and Industrial Agents
Amiodarone	Acrylamide
Chloroquine	Allyl chloride
Colchicine	Arsenic
Dapsone	Buckthorn toxin
Disulfiram	Carbon disulfide
Gold salts	Chlordecone
Isoniazid	Dimethylaminopropionitrile
Metronidazole	Diphtheria toxin
Misonidazole	Ethylene oxide
Nitrofurantoin	n-Hexane (glue sniffing)
Nucleoside analogs (antiretrovirals)	Methyl n-butyl ketone
Paclitaxel (taxanes)	Lead
Phenytoin	Mercury
Platinum compounds	Methyl bromide
Podophyllin	Organophosphates
Pyridoxine (vitamin B_6)	Polychlorinated biphenyls
Suramin	Thallium
Thalidomide	Trichloroethylene
Vincristine	Vacor

neuropathies are characterized by axonal degeneration, usually of the dying-back type. Notable exceptions are platinum compounds and pyridoxine, which produce a sensory neuronopathy, and buckthorn toxin and diphtheria toxin, which produce a demyelinating neuropathy. People with hereditary neuropathy may be especially vulnerable to drug-induced peripheral neuropathy.

Table 28-13

Inherited Diseases Associated With Neuropathy

Ataxia-telangiectasia
Abetalipoproteinemia
Acute intermittent porphyria, hereditary coproporphyria, and variegate porphyria
Cerebrotendinous xanthomatosis
Fabry disease (α-galactosidase A deficiency)
Familial amyloid polyneuropathy (transthyretin, apolipoprotein A1, and gelsolin amyloidosis)
Friedreich ataxia
Giant axonal neuropathy
Hereditary motor and sensory neuropathies (Charcot-Marie-Tooth disease)
Hereditary motor neuropathies
Hereditary neuropathy with liability to pressure palsies
Hereditary sensory and autonomic neuropathies
Infantile neuroaxonal dystrophy
Leukodystrophies (metachromatic, globoid cell, and adrenoleukodystrophy)
Refsum disease (phytanic acid storage disease)
Tangier disease

Hereditary Neuropathies Are the Most Common Chronic Neuropathies in Children

Peripheral neuropathy is a manifestation of a variety of inherited diseases (Tables 28-13 and 28-14). The neuropathy may be the sole manifestation of the hereditary disease or just one manifestation of a hereditary multisystem disease.

Table 28-14

Charcot-Marie-Tooth Disease (CMT) and Related Hereditary Motor and Sensory Neuropathies (HMSNs)

Disease	Inheritance	Gene	Pathology
CMT1 (HMSN 1)	Autosomal dominant	Peripheral myelin protein 22 (*PMP22*), myelin protein zero (*MPZ*) and others	Demyelinating neuropathy with onion bulbs; axonal loss also present
CMT2 (HMSN 2)	Autosomal dominant	Mitofusin 2 and others	Axonal neuropathy
CMTX (HMSN X)	X linked	Gap junction protein β1 (connexin 32)	Axonal loss, demyelination, and regenerating axons
Dejerine-Sottas syndrome (congenital hypomyelinating neuropathy)	Autosomal dominant or recessive	*PMP22*, *MPZ*, early growth response 2 (*EGR2*) and others	Demyelinating neuropathy with onion bulbs; axonal loss also present
Hereditary neuropathy with liability to pressure palsies (HNPP)	Autosomal dominant	*PMP22*	Demyelinating neuropathy with tomacula; axonal loss also present

CHARCOT-MARIE-TOOTH DISEASE:

MOLECULAR PATHOGENESIS: Charcot-Marie-Tooth disease (CMT) is a genetically and pathologically heterogeneous group of slowly progressive distal sensorimotor polyneuropathies that manifest in childhood or early adult life. It is the most common inherited neuropathy and among the most common inherited neurologic disorders, with a prevalence of 1 in 2500. CMT may be broadly divided electrophysiologically and pathologically into **demyelinating** and **axonal** subtypes. **CMT1,** the most common subtype, has autosomal dominant inheritance and a chronic demyelinating polyneuropathy with onion bulbs and axonal loss. The less common **CMT2** subtype shows autosomal dominant inheritance and distal axonal degeneration. X-linked **(CMTX)** and autosomal recessive **(CMT4)** subtypes have also been described. Mutations in at least 28 different genes have been associated with the CMT phenotype. Classification is complex, because mutations in different genes may produce the same phenotype, and various mutations in the same gene may produce different phenotypes (Table 28-14). The most common subtype, CMT1, is usually caused by a heterozygous duplication of the peripheral myelin protein 22 gene on chromosome 17. The axonal subtype, CMT2, is frequently caused by a mutation of the gene encoding the mitochondrial fusion protein, mitofusin 2. CMTX is associated with a mutation in the gap junction protein $\beta1$ (connexin 32) gene on the X chromosome.

Dejerine-Sottas syndrome (DSS, CMT3) resembles CMT1 but is much more severe, with onset in early infancy. Peripheral nerves show a severe demyelinating neuropathy with onion bulbs and axonal loss. Several genes are associated with this phenotype (Table 28-14).

Hereditary neuropathy with liability to pressure palsies (HNPP) typically manifests with recurrent mononeuropathies. Nerves show demyelination, distinctive sausage-shaped thickenings (tomacula) of myelin sheaths and axonal loss (tomaculous neuropathy). HNPP is associated with a heterozygous deletion of the peripheral myelin protein 22 gene on chromosome 17.

Neuropathy Is a Complication of HIV Infection

Peripheral neuropathy is a common complaint in persons infected with HIV. The neuropathy may manifest clinically as a distal symmetric polyneuropathy, autonomic neuropathy, lumbosacral polyradiculopathy, mononeuropathy or mononeuropathy multiplex.

- **Distal symmetric polyneuropathy** is the most common type of neuropathy associated with HIV infection. It is characterized by distal axonal degeneration and usually occurs during the later stages of AIDS. The pathogenesis of the axonal degeneration is obscure, and there is no effective therapy.
- **Inflammatory demyelinating polyradiculoneuropathy** associated with AIDS may be acute (AIDP) or chronic (CIDP). The disorder is immunologically mediated. It typically occurs early in the course of HIV infection, before the onset of AIDS. The neuropathy often responds to plasmapheresis, intravenous γ-globulin or corticosteroids.
- **Cytomegalovirus infection** of the PNS is responsible for some of the mononeuropathies and lumbosacral polyradiculopathies associated with AIDS.
- **Vasculitic neuropathy** may cause mononeuropathy and mononeuropathy multiplex in some patients with AIDS.
- **Toxic neuropathy** is caused by several drugs used in the therapy of AIDS (Table 28-12). These antiretroviral-induced axonal neuropathies are clinically similar to AIDS-associated distal symmetric polyneuropathy.
- **Diffuse infiltrative lymphocytosis syndrome** may be complicated by an acute or subacute axonal polyneuropathy. Peripheral nerve shows $CD8^+$ lymphocytic infiltrates.

Chronic Idiopathic Axonal Polyneuropathies Typically Occur in Older Patients

In 10% to 20% of patients with peripheral neuropathy, no cause is apparent despite careful and extensive investigation. These cryptogenic neuropathies are typically chronic, distal, sensory or sensorimotor axonal polyneuropathies and have an indolent course.

Nerve Trauma

Traumatic Neuroma Is a Mass of Regenerating Axons and Scar Tissue

Traumatic neuromas form at the end of the proximal stump of a nerve that has been disrupted physically. After transection of a peripheral nerve, regenerating axonal sprouts arise within 1 week from the distal ends of the intact axons in the proximal nerve stump. If the severed ends of the proximal and distal nerve stumps are closely approximated, regenerating axonal sprouts may find and reinnervate the distal stump. Regenerating axons advance in the distal stump at a rate of about 1 mm/day. However, in many instances, the severed nerve ends are not closely apposed, or there is considerable scar tissue between the two stumps, preventing regenerating sprouts from successfully reinnervating the distal stump. In this situation, the regenerating axons grow haphazardly into the scar tissue at the end of the proximal stump to form a painful swelling known as a **traumatic** or **amputation neuroma.**

Morton Neuroma (Plantar Interdigital Neuroma) Is a Painful Lesion of the Foot

Morton neuroma is a painful, sausage-shaped swelling of the plantar interdigital nerve between the second and third or third and fourth metatarsal bones. It is probably caused by repeated nerve compression. The swelling is not a true neuroma, since it results from endoneurial, perineurial and epineurial fibrosis, rather than a mass of regenerating axons. The fibrotic nerve also shows nerve fiber loss and areas of myxoid degeneration. Morton neuroma is particularly common in women who wear high heels.

Tumors

Primary PNS tumors are of neuronal or nerve sheath origin. The former (e.g., neuroblastoma and ganglioneuroma) usually arise from the adrenal medulla or sympathetic ganglia.

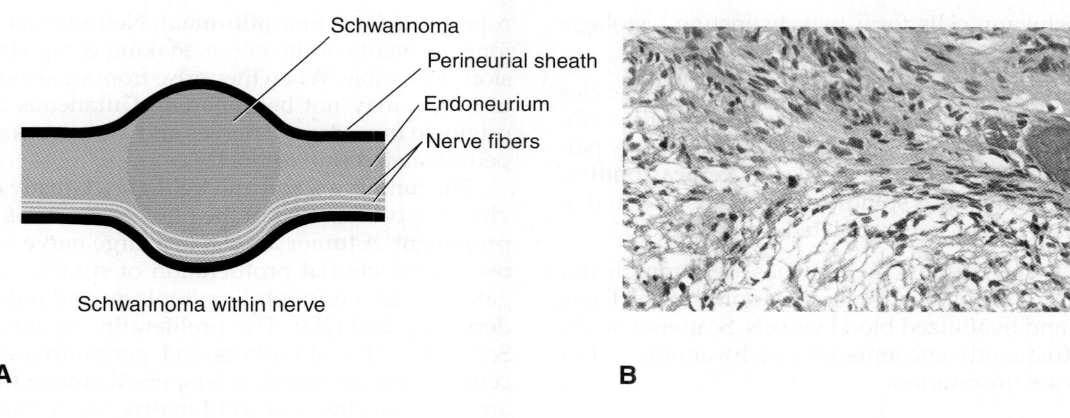

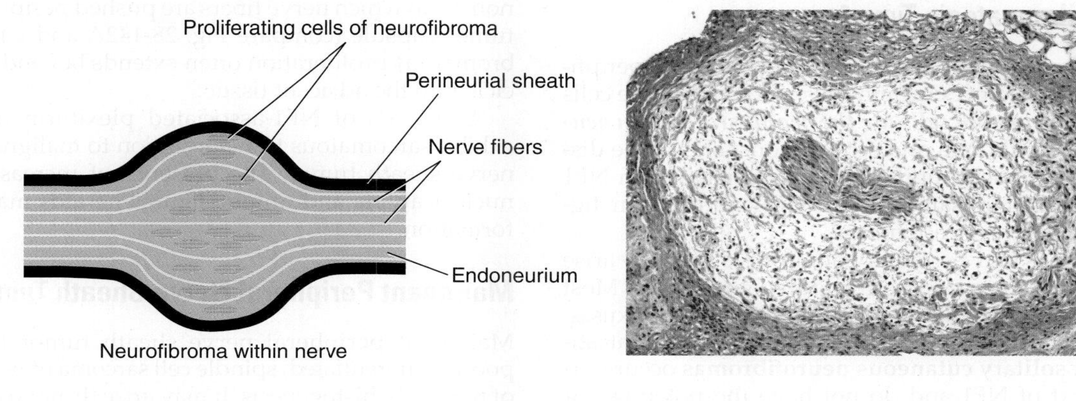

FIGURE 28-142. Growth patterns of schwannoma and neurofibroma within peripheral nerve. A. The cellular proliferation of the schwannoma is well circumscribed and pushes surviving nerve fibers to the periphery of the tumor. **B.** A photomicrograph of a schwannoma shows the characteristically abrupt transition between the compact Antoni type A histologic pattern (*top*) and the spongy Antoni type B histologic pattern (*bottom*). **C.** The cellular proliferation of the neurofibroma is interspersed among the surviving nerve fibers. **D.** Photomicrograph of neurofibroma shows that the proliferating spindle-shaped Schwann cells form small strands that course haphazardly through a myxoid matrix. A small cluster of surviving nerve fibers is in the center of the neurofibroma.

The common nerve sheath tumors are schwannoma and neurofibroma.

Schwannomas May Arise in Any Nerve

Schwannomas are benign, slowly growing, typically encapsulated neoplasms of Schwann cells that originate in cranial nerves, spinal roots or peripheral nerves (Fig. 28-142A). These tumors usually are seen in adults and only very rarely undergo malignant degeneration.

VESTIBULAR SCHWANNOMA (ACOUSTIC SCHWANNOMA): Intracranial schwannomas account for 8% of all primary intracranial tumors. Most arise from the vestibular branch of the eighth cranial nerve within the internal auditory canal or at the meatus and cause unilateral, sensorineural hearing loss, tinnitus and vestibular dysfunction. The slowly growing tumor enlarges the meatus, extends medially into the subarachnoid space of the cerebellopontine angle **(cerebellopontine angle tumor)** and compresses the fifth and seventh cranial nerves, brainstem and cerebellum. The posterior fossa mass may also lead to increased intracranial pressure, hydrocephalus and tonsillar herniation. Most vestibular schwannomas are unilateral and are not associated with NF (see Chapter 6). Bilateral vestibular schwannomas are a defining feature of NF2. The *NF2* gene is also implicated in the development of sporadic schwannomas.

SPINAL AND PERIPHERAL SCHWANNOMAS: Spinal schwannomas are intradural, extramedullary tumors that arise most often from the dorsal (sensory) spinal roots. They produce radicular (root) pain and spinal cord compression. More peripherally located schwannomas usually arise on nerves of the head, neck and extremities.

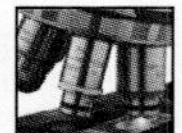

PATHOLOGY: Schwannomas tend to be oval and well demarcated and vary in diameter from a few millimeters to several centimeters. The nerve of origin, if large enough, may be identifiable. The cut surface is firm and tan to gray, and often shows focal hemorrhage, necrosis, xanthomatous change and cystic degeneration. The proliferating Schwann cells form two distinctive histologic patterns (Fig. 28-142B).

- **Antoni A pattern** is characterized by interwoven fascicles of spindle cells with elongated nuclei, eosinophilic cytoplasm and indistinct cytoplasmic borders. Nuclei may palisade in areas to form structures known as **Verocay bodies.**
- **Antoni B pattern** features spindle or oval cells with indistinct cytoplasm in a loose, vacuolated background.

Degenerative changes in schwannomas are common and include collections of foam cells, recent or old hemorrhage, foci of fibrosis and hyalinized blood vessels. Scattered atypical nuclei are frequently encountered in schwannomas, but mitotic figures are uncommon.

Neurofibromas May Be Sporadic or Associated With Neurofibromatosis Type 1

Neurofibromas are benign, slowly growing tumors of peripheral nerve, composed of Schwann cells, perineurial-like cells and fibroblasts. ***Schwann cells are the neoplastic cells in neurofibromas.*** Neurofibroma and schwannoma should be distinguished because neurofibromas are associated with NF1 and have a potential for sarcomatous degeneration to malignant peripheral nerve sheath tumor.

Neurofibromas may be solitary or multiple and may arise on any nerve. They occur in both children and adults. Most commonly, they involve skin, subcutis, major nerve plexuses, large deep nerve trunks, retroperitoneum and gastrointestinal tract. Most **solitary cutaneous neurofibromas** occur outside the context of NF1 and do not have the potential for sarcomatous degeneration. The presence of multiple neurofibromas or one large plexiform neurofibroma is strongly suggestive of NF1 and should prompt a careful search for other stigmata of the disease.

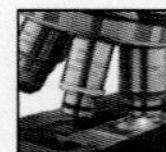

PATHOLOGY: On gross examination, a neurofibroma arising in a large nerve is a poorly circumscribed, fusiform enlargement. The diffuse, intrafascicular growth of tumor within multiple nerve fascicles may so enlarge the fascicles that the nerve looks like a multistranded rope **(plexiform neurofibroma).** Neurofibroma may involve long segments of the nerve, making complete surgical excision impossible. When they arise from small nerves, the nerve of origin may not be apparent. Cutaneous neurofibromas originate from dermal nerves and are seen as soft nodular or pedunculated skin tumors.

The tumors are soft and light gray. Greatly enlarged, individual nerve fascicles of the plexiform neurofibroma may be prominent. A tumor arising in a large nerve is characterized by an endoneurial proliferation of spindle cells with elongated nuclei, eosinophilic cytoplasm and indistinct cell borders (Fig. 28-142D). The proliferating spindle cells include Schwann cells, fibroblasts and perineurial-like cells. Mast cells are also increased. Interspersed among the spindle cells are an extracellular myxoid matrix, wavy bands of collagen and residual nerve fibers. The coursing of nerve fibers through a neurofibroma contrasts with the pattern in schwannomas, in which nerve fibers are pushed peripherally into the tumor capsule (compare Fig. 28-142A and C). The neurofibromatous proliferation often extends beyond the nerve fascicle into the adjacent tissue.

Some 5% of NF1-associated plexiform neurofibromas exhibit sarcomatous transformation to malignant peripheral nerve sheath tumor. The presence of increased cellularity, nuclear atypia and mitotic figures heralds malignant transformation.

Malignant Peripheral Nerve Sheath Tumor

Malignant peripheral nerve sheath tumor (MPNST) is a poorly differentiated, spindle cell sarcoma of peripheral nerve of uncertain histogenesis. It may arise de novo or from malignant transformation of a neurofibroma. MPNST is most common in adults and typically arises in larger nerves of the trunk or proximal limbs. About half of these sarcomas occur in patients with neurofibromatosis. There is an increased incidence of MPNST at sites of previous irradiation.

MPNST appears as an unencapsulated, fusiform enlargement of a nerve. The neoplasm resembles fibrosarcoma, with closely packed spindle cells, nuclear atypia, mitotic figures and often foci of necrosis. It is prone to local recurrence and bloodborne metastases.

29 The Eye

Gordon K. Klintworth

Physical and Chemical Injuries

Physical trauma to the eye commonly causes ecchymosis of the highly vascular eyelids (black eye); when this occurs, other parts of the eye also may be injured. Superficial disruptions of the corneal epithelium follow traumatic abrasions, prolonged wearing of a contact lens, foreign bodies on the eye and exposure to ultraviolet light. The eye is commonly injured by a variety of household and industrial caustic chemicals. The damage created depends on the nature of the chemical.

Blunt trauma increases intraorbital pressure momentarily and may cause the bones in the floor of the orbit to fracture into the maxillary sinus (**blowout fracture**). The inferior rectus muscle may become entrapped in such a fracture, thereby causing the eye to sink into the orbit (**enophthalmos**).

An array of foreign materials can injure the eye. Whereas small particles often lodge in superficial ocular tissues, some penetrate into or through the eye. A foreign particle may damage the eye during entry or because of secondary infection after the introduction of microorganisms. Some foreign bodies provoke a prominent acute inflammatory or granulomatous reaction. Others, such as those containing iron, cause retinal degeneration and even discoloration of ocular tissues (**siderosis bulbi**), effects that may not be evident for several years. Other complications of ocular injuries include cataracts, retinal detachment and glaucoma.

The Eyelids

The important conditions affecting the eyelids include:

Blepharitis is inflammation of the eyelids. It is common and sometimes produces an acute, red, tender, inflammatory mass.

Hordeolum (or sty) refers to an acute, inflammatory, focal lesion of the eyelid. Acute inflammation involving the meibomian glands is termed an **internal hordeolum,** whereas acute folliculitis of the glands of Zeis is an **external hordeolum**.

Chalazion is a granulomatous inflammation centered around the meibomian glands or the glands of Zeis. It is thought to represent a reaction to extruded lipid secretions and usually produces a painless swelling in the eyelid.

Xanthelasma is a yellow plaque of lipid-containing macrophages, usually involving the nasal aspect of the eyelids. It is often seen in older persons and patients with disorders of lipid metabolism (e.g., familial hypercholesterolemia, primary biliary cirrhosis).

The Orbit

Exophthalmos or Proptosis Is Abnormal Forward Protrusion of the Eyeball

The term **exophthalmos** is used mainly when the condition is bilateral; **proptosis** refers to a unilateral protrusion of the eye. Numerous conditions cause forward protrusion of the eye. The most common cause is thyroid disease, followed by orbital dermoid cysts and hemangiomas. Other orbital conditions can cause proptosis: various inflammatory lesions, lymphomas, developmental anomalies, vascular problems and neoplasms. Proptosis also results from lesions of the paranasal sinuses and intracranial cavity.

Exophthalmos of Hyperthyroidism Continues Despite Treatment

Exophthalmos caused by Graves disease may precede or follow other manifestations of thyroid dysfunction. Exophthalmos resulting from thyroid disease usually occurs in early adult life, especially in women (female-to-male ratio, 4:1). It may be severe and progressive, particularly in middle life, when exophthalmos no longer correlates well with the state of thyroid function. Dysthyroid exophthalmos may be associated with edema of the eyelids, chemosis (conjunctival edema) and limitation of ocular motion. Theories of the pathogenesis of hyperthyroidism-related exophthalmos are discussed in Chapter 21.

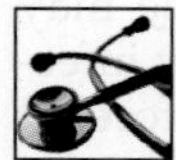

CLINICAL FEATURES: Although exophthalmos of hyperthyroidism is usually bilateral, one eye may be involved earlier or more extensively than the other. Other ocular manifestations of hyperthyroidism include upper eyelid retraction (due to increased sympathetic tone) and a characteristic stare or apparent proptosis resulting from exposure of the conjunctiva above the corneoscleral limbus.

Complications of severe exophthalmos include several potentially blinding complications: corneal exposure with subsequent ulceration, and optic nerve compression. Paradoxically, thyroidectomy may increase the incidence and severity of exophthalmos associated with hyperthyroidism.

Inflammatory Pseudotumor Is a Chronic Idiopathic Inflammatory Condition

Inflammatory pseudotumor is associated with a variable degree of fibrosis. It is a common cause of proptosis and partial immobility of the eyeball.

The Conjunctiva

Conjunctival Hemorrhage May Follow Blunt Trauma, Anoxia or Severe Coughing

Conjunctival hemorrhages also occur spontaneously, often first noted on arising after sleep. They do not extend into the cornea because of the barrier imposed by the close apposition of corneal epithelium to the underlying substantia propria.

Conjunctivitis May Be Infectious or Allergic

Microorganisms lodging on the surface of the eye frequently cause conjunctivitis, keratitis (corneal inflammation) or a corneal ulcer. The conjunctiva, as well as other parts of the eye, may also become infected by hematogenous spread from a focus of infection elsewhere. Iatrogenic eye infections (e.g., with adenovirus) may follow ophthalmic manipulations, such as corneal grafts, intraocular implantation of lens prostheses or use of infected eyedrops or diagnostic instruments.

At some stage in life, virtually everyone has viral or bacterial conjunctivitis. This extremely common eye disease is characterized by hyperemic conjunctival blood vessels (pink eye). The inflammatory exudate that accumulates in the conjunctival sac commonly crusts, causing the eyelids to stick together in the morning. The conjunctival discharge may be purulent, fibrinous, serous or hemorrhagic. Participating inflammatory cells vary with the etiologic agent. As many allergens are seasonal, the allergic conjunctivitis they elicit tends to occur only at particular times of the year.

Trachoma

Trachoma is a chronic, contagious conjunctivitis caused by *Chlamydia trachomatis*. Various serotypes of *C. trachomatis* cause ocular, genital and systemic infections (trachoma, inclusion conjunctivitis and lymphogranuloma venereum; see Chapter 9).

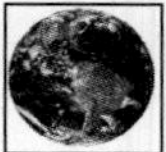

EPIDEMIOLOGY: About 500 million people are afflicted by trachoma, an acute, infectious, fibrosing keratoconjunctivitis caused by *C. trachomatis* (serotypes A, B and C). ***This infection is the most common cause of blindness in the world and is especially prevalent in Asia, the Middle East and parts of Africa.*** The disease has been eradicated in the United States and other developed countries. Trachoma is not very contagious, but overcrowding and poor hygienic conditions favor its transmission by fingers, fomites and flies. Spontaneous healing is common in children, but in adults, the disease progresses more rapidly and rarely heals without treatment.

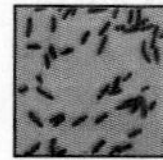

ETIOLOGIC FACTORS: An inflammatory reaction is generated by the immune system in response to *C. trachomatis*. Serial persistent or repetitive inflammatory reactions to different strains of the pathogen are believed to cause the serious cicatricial complications.

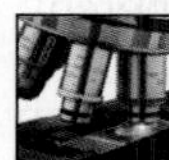

PATHOLOGY: Trachoma is virtually always bilateral and involves the upper half of the conjunctiva more than the lower (Fig. 29-1). The cellular infiltrate is predominantly lymphocytic, and conjunctival lymph follicles with necrotic germinal centers are characteristic. Eventually

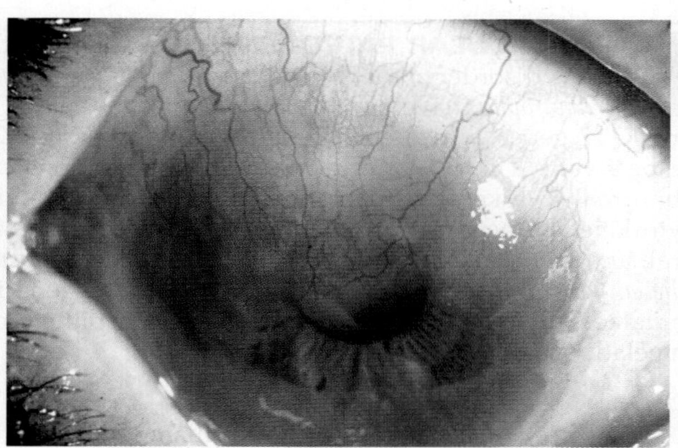

FIGURE 29-1. Trachoma. The cornea of a patient with severe trachoma shows extensive fibrovascular opacity (**pannus**) in the superior cornea.

lymphocytes and blood vessels invade the superior portion of the cornea between the epithelium and Bowman zone (**trachomatous pannus**). Scarring of the conjunctiva and eyelids distorts the eyelids. On microscopic examination, the desquamated conjunctival epithelium exhibits glycogen-rich intracytoplasmic inclusion bodies and large macrophages containing nuclear fragments (Leber cells). Secondary bacterial infections occur commonly.

Other Chlamydial Infections

Chlamydia is responsible for a purulent conjunctivitis (**inclusion blennorrhea**) that develops in newborns, who become infected during passage through the birth canal. The infection is also acquired by swimming in nonchlorinated pools (swimming pool conjunctivitis) or from contact with discharges of infected urethra or cervix.

In adults and older children, *Chlamydia* causes a chronic follicular conjunctivitis with focal lymphoid hyperplasia (**inclusion conjunctivitis**). In contrast to trachoma, the lower tarsal conjunctiva is involved. Scarring and necrosis do not develop, and keratitis is rare and mild.

Ophthalmia Neonatorum

Ophthalmia neonatorum is a severe, acute conjunctivitis with a copious purulent discharge, especially in the newborn, caused by Neisseria gonorrhoeae. The infection, which is a common cause of blindness in some parts of the world, is complicated by corneal ulceration, perforation and scarring and panophthalmitis. Infants usually become infected while passing through the birth canal of an infected mother. Other causative organisms for ophthalmia neonatorum include other pyogenic bacteria and *C. trachomatis.* Today, newborns are usually routinely treated with 5% Betadine eye drops.

Pinguecula and Pterygium

Pinguecula is a yellowish conjunctival lump usually located nasal to the corneoscleral limbus. It is the most common conjunctival lump. It consists of sun-damaged connective tissue identical to that in similarly injured skin (actinic elastosis; see Chapter 24).

Pterygium is a fold of vascularized conjunctiva that grows horizontally onto the cornea in the shape of an insect wing (hence the name). It is often associated with a pinguecula and frequently recurs after excision.

The Cornea

Herpes Simplex Virus Causes Corneal Ulcerations

Herpes simplex virus (HSV) has a predilection for corneal epithelium, where it causes keratitis, but it can invade corneal stroma and occasionally other ocular tissues.

PRIMARY INFECTION BY HERPES SIMPLEX VIRUS TYPE 1: Subclinical or undiagnosed localized ocular lesions are caused by HSV type 1 in childhood. These infections are accompanied by regional lymphadenopathy, systemic infection and fever. Except in newborns infected during passage through an infected mother's birth canal, HSV type 2 rarely causes ocular infection. When it does, it may produce widespread lesions of the cornea and retina. Most corneal lesions due to HSV are asymptomatic plaques of diseased epithelial cells that contain replicating virus. These usually heal without ulceration, but an acute unilateral follicular conjunctivitis may occur. Corneal ulcers appear after serum antibody levels increase.

REACTIVATION OF HERPES SIMPLEX VIRUS INFECTION: Latent in the trigeminal ganglion, HSV may pass down the nerves and reactivate the infection. Unlike primary HSV infection, reactivation disease is characterized by corneal ulceration and a more severe inflammatory reaction. Recurrence of corneal ulcers due to HSV may be precipitated by ultraviolet light, trauma, menstruation, emotional and physical stress, exposure to light or sunlight, vaccination and other factors.

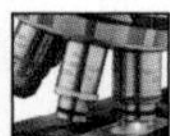

PATHOLOGY: HSV causes multiple, minute, discrete, intraepithelial corneal ulcers (superficial punctate keratopathy). Although some of these lesions heal, others enlarge and eventually coalesce to form linear or branching fissures (dendritic ulcers, from the Greek *dendron,* "tree"). The epithelium between the fissures desquamates, leading to sharply demarcated, irregular geographical ulcers. The corneal ulcers are readily visualized after the cornea is stained with fluorescein. Affected epithelial cells, which may become multinucleated, contain eosinophilic, intranuclear inclusion bodies (Lipschütz bodies).

The lesions of the corneal stroma vary in reactivated HSV infection. Typically, a central disc-shaped corneal opacity develops beneath the epithelium, owing to edema and minimal inflammation (**disciform keratitis**). The corneal stroma may become markedly thinned, and the Descemet membrane may bulge into it (descemetocele). Corneal perforation can also occur.

Onchocerciasis Leads to Blindness in Tropical Regions

The nematode *Onchocerca volvulus,* which is transmitted by bites of infected blackflies, is by far the most important helminthic infection of the eye (see Chapter 9). ***This parasite accounts for blindness in at least half a million people in regions of Africa and Latin America in which it is endemic.*** Microfilaria released from fertilized adult female worms migrate into the superficial cornea, bulbar conjunctiva, aqueous humor and other ocular tissues. The intracorneal microfilaria die and elicit an inflammatory response that leads to corneal opacification and visual impairment (**river blindness**). Less frequently, endophthalmitis, retinal lesions and optic atrophy occur. Treatment with ivermectin is highly effective.

Arcus Lipoides Is a White Arc Due to Lipid Deposition in the Peripheral Cornea

Formerly called **arcus senilis** because of its frequency in the elderly, arcus lipoides may also form an entire ring, in which case the term **annulus lipoides** is more appropriate. Although not necessarily associated with increased serum lipid levels, arcus lipoides accompanies certain disorders of lipid metabolism, and its presence alerts the perceptive clinician to the systemic disorder.

Band Keratopathy Is an Opaque Horizontal Band Across the Cornea

The opacification in band keratopathy may contain calcium phosphate (**calcific band keratopathy**) or noncalcified protein (**chronic actinic keratopathy**).

In **calcific band keratopathy,** calcium phosphate deposits in a horizontal band across the superficial central cornea in conditions associated with hypercalcemia. However, the disorder most often occurs in the absence of hypercalcemia, as in chronic uveitis.

Chronic actinic keratopathy occurs worldwide but is most severe in regions in which people spend a considerable amount of time outdoors. Their unprotected eyes are exposed to excessive ultraviolet light, such as that reflected from desert, water or snow.

Noninflammatory Genetic Corneal Disorders Are Diverse

Most corneal dystrophies have an autosomal dominant or recessive mode of inheritance, but rare cases are X linked recessive. Some of these diseases affect other parts of the body (e.g., Fabry disease, cystinosis, certain types of mucopolysaccharidosis and ichthyosis). Other conditions that primarily affect the cornea were traditionally called corneal dystrophies before the era of molecular genetics and were classified according to the primary corneal layer that is involved: (1) the outer layer composed of epithelium, basement membrane and Bowman layer; (2) the stroma; and (3) the endothelium and Descemet membrane, the basement membrane of the corneal endothelium. However, this classification is now considered somewhat artificial because many corneal dystrophies involve more than one layer.

EPITHELIAL DYSTROPHIES: The different epithelial dystrophies are characterized by a variety of distinct abnormalities, which include microcysts or accumulations of anomalous material within the cytoplasm of the corneal epithelium, defects in the epithelial basement membrane and deposition of a finely fibrillar substance in the Bowman layer. In some epithelial dystrophies, faulty desmosomes may permit adjacent epithelial cells to separate, leading to accumulation of fluid-filled microcysts. Loss of hemidesmosomes between the epithelium and Bowman layer leads to painful, recurrent erosions that begin in early childhood. Although there may be a slow decrease in visual acuity, epithelial dystrophies do not ordinarily cause blindness.

MOLECULAR PATHOGENESIS: Patients with one disorder of the corneal epithelium (*Meesmann dystrophy*) have dominant mutations in the *KRT3* or *KRT12* genes, which encode keratin 3 and keratin 12, respectively. The mutations result in aggregations of abnormal cytokeratin filaments and severely impair cytoskeletal function in the affected cells. In the rare bilateral, autosomal recessive corneal disorder *familial subepithelial corneal dystrophy,* wherein the *TACSTD2* gene is mutated, amyloid is found beneath the corneal epithelium in gelatinous drop-like deposits.

STROMAL DYSTROPHIES: The stromal corneal dystrophies are clear-cut entities in which different substances (amyloid, glycosaminoglycans, proteins or a variety of lipids) accumulate within corneal stroma because of inherited metabolic disorders. Each stromal dystrophy causes a characteristic form of corneal opacification. The age of onset and rate of progression vary with the particular disorder. Although clinical manifestations may be limited to the cornea, other tissues are involved in some of these disorders.

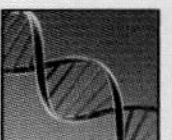

MOLECULAR PATHOGENESIS: Several clinically and histopathologically different inherited corneal disorders, including the granular corneal dystrophies and most lattice corneal dystrophies, result from distinctly different mutations in the same gene, namely, the *TFGBI* gene. Another predominantly stromal corneal dystrophy (macular corneal dystrophy) results from a defect in the *CHST6* gene, which encodes a sulfotransferase that catalyzes sulfation of *N*-acetyl glucosamine and galactose in keratan sulfate. Other corneal stromal diseases are caused by mutations in genes *PIP5K3* (fleck corneal dystrophy), *DCN* (congenital stromal corneal dystrophy) and *UBIAD1* (Schnyder corneal dystrophy).

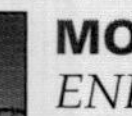

MOLECULAR PATHOGENESIS: *ENDOTHELIAL DYSTROPHIES:* Several different endothelial dystrophies are recognized, usually accompanied by abnormalities in the Descemet membrane. In *Fuchs endothelial corneal dystrophy*, wart-like excrescences form on the Descemet membrane (guttae), and progressive visual loss follows corneal edema and endothelial cell degeneration. Missense mutations in *COL8A2*, the gene encoding the α_2-chain of type VIII collagen, have been identified in some patients with early-onset Fuchs dystrophy and in ***posterior polymorphous corneal dystrophy***, both of which affect the corneal endothelium and Descemet membrane.

The Lens

Cataracts Are Opacifications in the Crystalline Lens

Cataracts are a major cause of visual impairment and blindness throughout the world and are the outcome of numerous conditions.

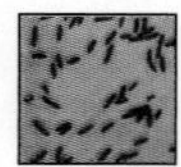

ETIOLOGIC FACTORS: The most common cause of cataracts in the United States is advancing age (age-related cataract). Other cataracts are caused by diabetes, nutritional deficiencies (e.g., deficiencies in riboflavin or tryptophan), toxins (e.g., dinitrophenol, naphthalene, ergot), drugs (e.g., corticosteroids, topical phospholine iodide, phenothiazines) or physical agents (e.g., heat, ultraviolet light, trauma, intraocular surgery and ultrasound).

Cataracts may develop in ocular diseases such as uveitis, intraocular neoplasms, glaucoma, retinitis pigmentosa and retinal detachment. Cataracts also are associated with congenital rubella virus infection, some skin diseases (e.g., atopic dermatitis, scleroderma) and various systemic diseases.

MOLECULAR PATHOGENESIS: A wide variety of cataracts result from genetic disorders, and some of them are associated with other ocular or systemic abnormalities. Cataracts can result from mutations in the heat shock transcription factor-4 *(HSF4)* gene, genes that encode specific lens proteins such as connexins (*GJA3, GJA8*), crystallins (a family of *CRY* genes), a beaded filament structural protein-2 (*BFSP2*), a putative cell-junction protein (*LIM2*) and aquaporin 0 (*MIP*). They also result from genetic mutations and chromosomal anomalies that cause numerous systemic diseases and syndromes.

PATHOLOGY: In the development of cataracts, clefts appear between the lens fibers, and degenerated lens material accumulates in these spaces (morgagnian corpuscles, incipient cataract). Degenerated lens material exerts osmotic pressure, causing the damaged lens to imbibe water and swell. The swollen lens may obstruct the pupil and cause glaucoma (phacomorphic glaucoma).

In a *mature cataract* (Fig. 29-2), the entire lens degenerates, and the lenticular debris escapes into the aqueous humor through the lens capsule, diminishing the volume of the lens (hypermature cataract). After becoming engulfed by macrophages, the extruded lenticular material may obstruct aqueous outflow and produce glaucoma (phacolytic glaucoma). The compressed lens fibers in the center of the lens normally harden with aging (simple nuclear sclerotic cataract) and may become brown or black. If the peripheral part of the lens (lens cortex) becomes liquefied (morgagnian cataract), the sclerotic nucleus may sink within the lens by gravity.

Fortunately, cataractous lenses can be surgically removed, and optical devices can be provided to permit focusing of light on the retina (spectacles, contact lenses, implantation of prosthetic lenses).

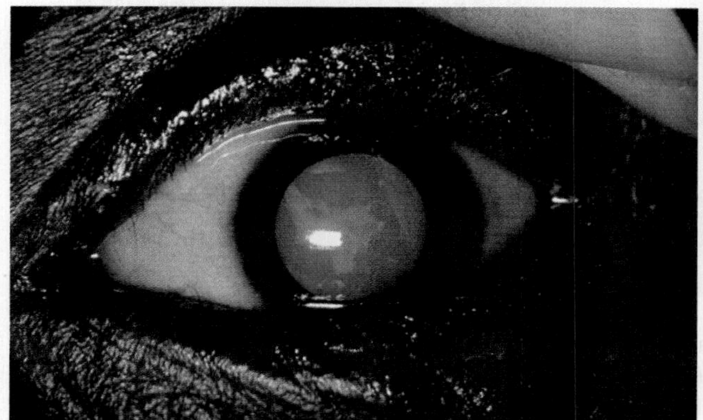

FIGURE 29-2. Cataract. The white appearance of the pupil in this eye is due to complete opacification of the lens ("mature cataract").

Presbyopia Is a Failure of Accommodation as a Result of Aging

With this impairment of vision, the near point of distinct vision becomes located farther from the eye. At the equator of the crystalline lens, the cuboidal subcapsular cells normally differentiate into elongated lens fibers throughout life. Once formed, these lens fibers persist indefinitely. Older fibers become displaced into the center of the lens, causing it to enlarge with age. After this process occurs over many years, the lens loses its elasticity. This effect interferes with the normal tendency of the lens to become spherical, and so diminishes the power of accommodation. As a result, most persons after age 40 years begin to have difficulty reading and require spectacles for near vision.

Phacoanaphylactic Endophthalmitis Is an Autoimmune Granulomatous Reaction to Lens Proteins

In this disorder, an inflammatory lesion occurs around or within the lens (or its remains) in an eye with a traumatized or cataractous lens and sometimes after surgical removal of a cataractous lens. A similar reaction may occur spontaneously in the contralateral eye months or years later. This autoimmune reaction to unique lens proteins, which are normally sequestered from the immune system, can be provoked experimentally by immunization with autologous lens material.

The Uvea

A Variety of Inflammatory Conditions Affect the Uveal Tract

Inflammation of the uvea (**uveitis**) also encompasses inflammation of the iris (**iritis**), the ciliary body (**cyclitis**) and the iris plus the ciliary body (**iridocyclitis**). Inflammation of the iris and ciliary body typically causes a red eye, photophobia, moderate ocular pain, blurred vision, a pericorneal halo, ciliary flush and slight miosis. A flare is common in the anterior chamber on slit-lamp biomicroscopy, and keratic precipitates or a **hypopyon** (leukocytic exudate in the anterior chamber) also develops.

Peripheral anterior synechiae are adhesions between the peripheral iris and the anterior chamber angle. **Posterior synechiae** are adhesions that develop between the iris and the lens. Both types of synechiae are complications of iritis, and both can cause glaucoma.

Sympathetic Ophthalmitis Is an Autoimmune Uveitis

In sympathetic ophthalmitis, the entire uvea develops granulomatous inflammation after a latent period, in response to an injury in the other eye. Perforating ocular injury and prolapse of uveal tissue often lead to a progressive, bilateral, diffuse, granulomatous inflammation of the uvea. This uveitis develops in the originally injured eye (exciting eye) after a latent period of 4 to 8 weeks. The latent period may, however, be as short as 10 days or as long as many years. The uninjured eye (sympathizing eye) becomes affected at the same time as the injured eye, or shortly thereafter. Vitiligo and graying of the eyelashes sometimes accompanies the uveitis. Nodules containing reactive retinal pigment epithelium, macrophages and epithelioid cells commonly appear between the Bruch membrane (**lamina vitrea**) and retinal pigment epithelium (**Dalen-Fuchs nodules**). Experimental studies suggest that the antigen responsible for sympathetic ophthalmitis resides in the photoreceptors of the retina (**arrestin**).

Sarcoidosis Commonly Affects the Eye

Ocular involvement occurs in one fourth to one third of patients with sarcoidosis and is often the initial clinical manifestation. Both eyes are usually affected, most often with a granulomatous uveitis. Although any ocular and orbital tissues may be involved, this granulomatous disease has a predilection for the anterior segment of the eye. Other ocular manifestations of sarcoidosis include calcific band keratopathy, cataracts, retinal vascularization, vitreous hemorrhage and bilateral enlargement of the lacrimal and salivary glands (**Mikulicz syndrome**).

The Retina

Retinal Hemorrhage May Occur in Both Local and Systemic Diseases

The important causes of retinal hemorrhages are hypertension, diabetes mellitus, central retinal vein occlusion, bleeding

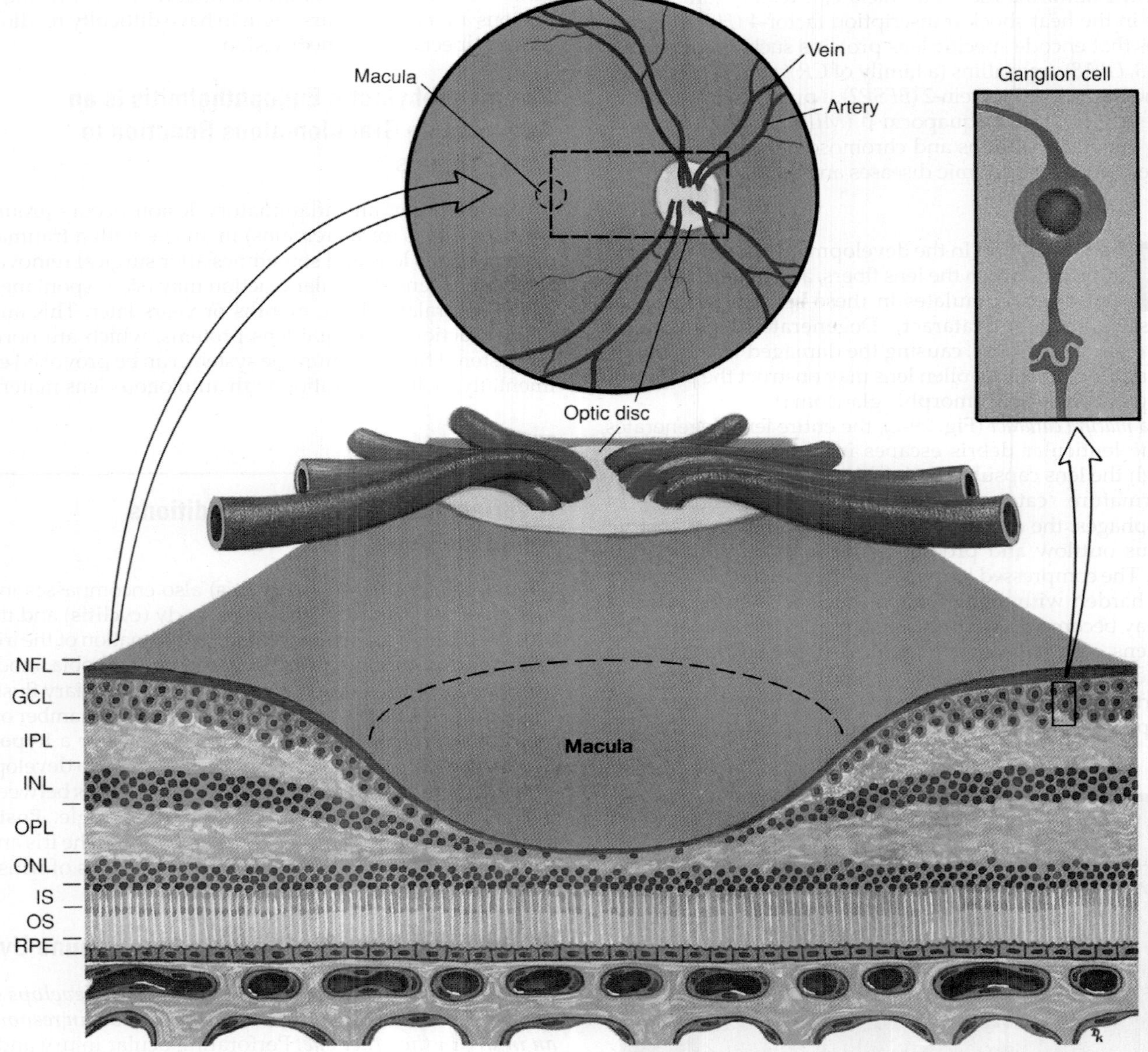

FIGURE 29-3. The normal retina. Constituents of the normal retina are arranged in distinct layers. These include the nerve fiber layer (*NFL*), ganglion cell layer (*GCL*), inner plexiform layer (*IPL*), inner nuclear layer (*INL*), outer plexiform layer (*OPL*), outer nuclear layer (*ONL*), inner segments (*IS*) and outer segments (*OS*) of the photoreceptors and the retinal pigment epithelium (*RPE*). The axons from the ganglion cells enter the nerve fiber layer and converge toward the optic nerve head. The inner retina contains arteries and veins. The retina is thinnest at the center of the macula, where bare photoreceptors rest on the retinal pigment epithelium. Only one cell thick in most of the retina, the ganglion cell layer is multilayered at the macula.

diatheses and trauma, including the "shaken baby syndrome." Appearance varies with cause and location. Hemorrhages in the nerve fiber layer spread between axons and causes a flame-shaped appearance on funduscopy, whereas deep retinal hemorrhages tend to be round. When located between the retinal pigment epithelium and Bruch membrane, blood appears as a dark mass, which may resemble a melanoma.

After accidental or surgical perforation of the globe, choroidal hemorrhages may detach the choroid and displace the retina, vitreous body and lens through the wound.

Retinal Occlusive Vascular Disease Is an Important Cause of Blindness

Vascular occlusion results from thrombosis, embolism, stenosis (as in atherosclerosis), vascular compression, intravascular sludging or coagulation and vasoconstriction (e.g., in hypertensive retinopathy or migraine). Thrombosis of ocular vessels may accompany primary disease of these vessels, as in giant cell arteritis.

Certain disorders of the heart and major vessels, such as the carotid arteries, predispose to emboli that may lodge in the retina and are evident on funduscopic examination at points of vascular bifurcation. Within the optic nerve, emboli in the central retinal artery frequently lodge in the vessel where it passes though the scleral perforations (**lamina cribrosa**).

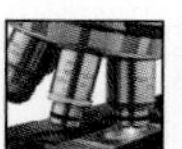

PATHOLOGY: The effect of vascular occlusion depends on the size of the vessel involved, the degree of resultant ischemia and the nature of the embolus. Small emboli often do not interfere with retinal function, whereas septic emboli may cause foci of ocular infection. Retinal ischemia due to any cause frequently leads to white fluffy patches that resemble cotton on ophthalmoscopic examination (**cotton-wool spots**). These round spots, which are seldom wider than the optic nerve head, consist of aggregates of swollen axons in the nerve fiber layer of the retina. Affected axons contain numerous degenerated mitochondria and dense bodies related to the lysosomal system, which accumulate because of impaired axoplasmic flow. Histologically, in cross-section, individual swollen axons resemble cells (cytoid bodies). Cotton-wool spots are reversible if circulation is restored in time.

Central Retinal Artery Occlusion

Like neurons in the rest of the nervous system, those in the retina (Fig. 29-3) are extremely susceptible to hypoxia. Central retinal artery occlusion (Figs. 29-4 and 29-5) may follow thrombosis of the retinal artery, as in atherosclerosis or giant cell arteritis, or embolization to that blood vessel. Intracellular edema, manifested by retinal pallor, is prominent, especially in the macula, where ganglion cells are most numerous. The foveola, the center of the macula, stands out in sharp contrast as a prominent **cherry-red spot,** because of the underlying vascularized choroid. The lack of retinal circulation reduces retinal arterioles to delicate threads (Fig. 29-5).

Permanent blindness follows central retinal artery obstruction, unless the ischemia is of short duration. Unilateral blurred vision, lasting a few minutes **(amaurosis fugax),** occurs with small retinal emboli.

Central Retinal Vein Occlusion

Central retinal vein occlusion results in flame-shaped hemorrhages in the nerve fiber layer of the retina, especially around the optic nerve head. The hemorrhages reflect the high intravascular pressure that dilates and ruptures the veins and collateral vessels (Fig. 29-6). Edema of the optic nerve head and retina occurs because absorption of interstitial fluid is impaired.

Vision is disturbed but may recover surprisingly well, considering the severity of the funduscopic changes. An intractable, closed-angle glaucoma, with severe pain and repeated hemorrhages, commonly ensues 2 to 3 months after central retinal vein occlusion (so-called 100-day glaucoma, thrombotic glaucoma or neovascular glaucoma). This distressing complication is caused by neovascularization of the iris and adhesions between the iris and the anterior chamber angle **(peripheral anterior synechiae).**

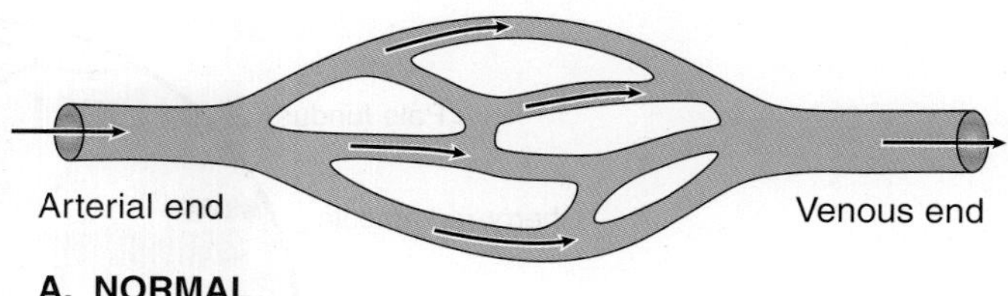

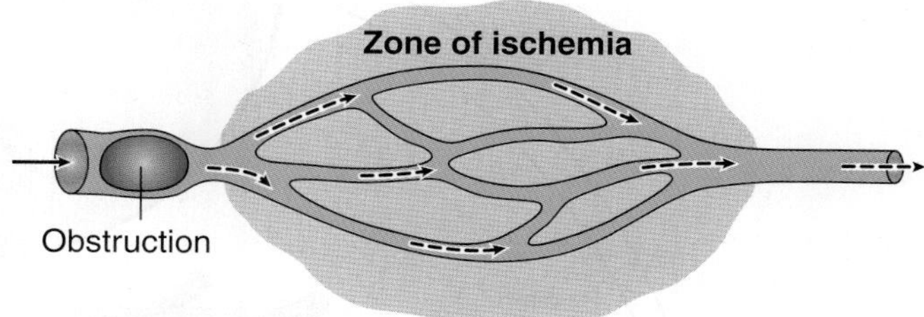

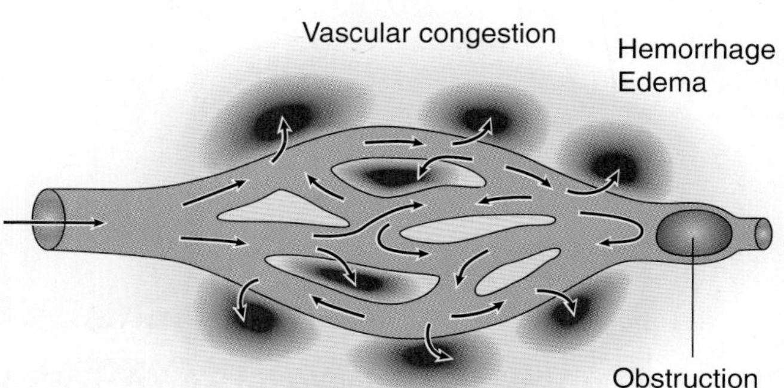

FIGURE 29-4. Occlusion of the retinal artery and vein. A. In the retina, as in other parts of the body, blood normally flows through a capillary network. **B.** When the retinal arteries become occluded (e.g., with an embolus), a zone of retinal ischemia ensues. This is accompanied by impaired neuronal function and visual loss, and the ischemic retina becomes pale. Because the intravascular pressure within the ischemic tissue is low, hemorrhage is inconspicuous. **C.** With retinal vein occlusion, vascular congestion, hemorrhage and edema are prominent, whereas ischemia is mild and neuronal function remains intact.

FIGURE 29-5. Central retinal artery occlusion. When the central retinal artery becomes occluded (e.g., with an embolus), the entire retina becomes edematous and pale. Decreased blood flow makes the retinal vessels less visible on funduscopic examination. The macula becomes cherry-red, owing to the prominent, but normal, underlying vasculature of the choroid.

Hypertensive Retinopathy Correlates With the Severity of Hypertension

Increased blood pressure commonly affects the retina, causing changes that can readily be seen with the ophthalmoscope (Figs. 29-7 and 29-8).

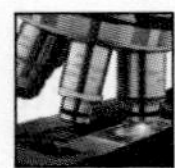

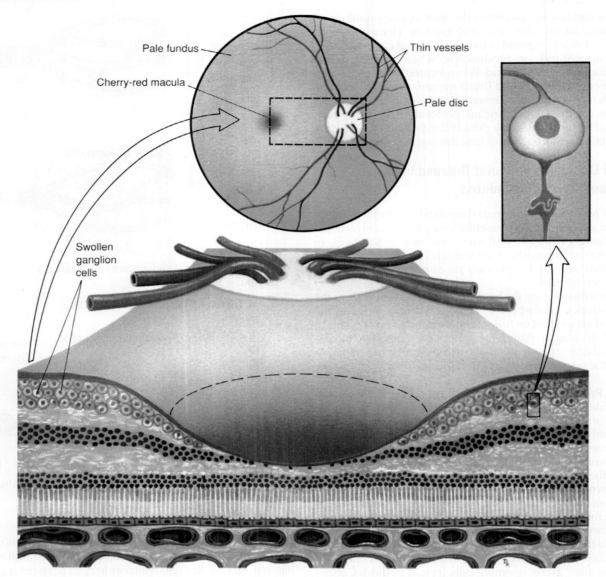

PATHOLOGY: Features of hypertensive retinopathy include:

- **Arteriolar narrowing**
- **Hemorrhages** in the retinal nerve fiber layer (flame-shaped hemorrhages)
- **Exudates,** including some that radiate from the center of the macula (macular star)
- Fluffy white bodies in the superficial retina **(cotton-wool spots)**
- **Microaneurysms**

In the eye, arteriolosclerosis accompanies long-standing hypertension and commonly affects the retinal and choroidal vessels. Lumina of the thickened retinal arterioles become narrowed, increasingly tortuous and of irregular caliber. At sites where arterioles cross veins, the latter appear kinked (**arteriovenous nicking**). However, the venous diameter before the site of compression is not wider than that after it. The kinked appearance of the vein reflects sclerosis within the venous walls, because retinal arteries and veins share a common adventitia at sites of arteriovenous crossings, rather than compression by a taut sclerotic artery.

By funduscopy, abnormal retinal arterioles appear as parallel white lines at sites of vascular crossings (**arterial sheathing**). Initially, the narrowed lumen of the retinal vessels decreases the visibility of the blood column and makes it appear orange on ophthalmoscopic examination (**copper wiring**). However, as the blood column eventually becomes

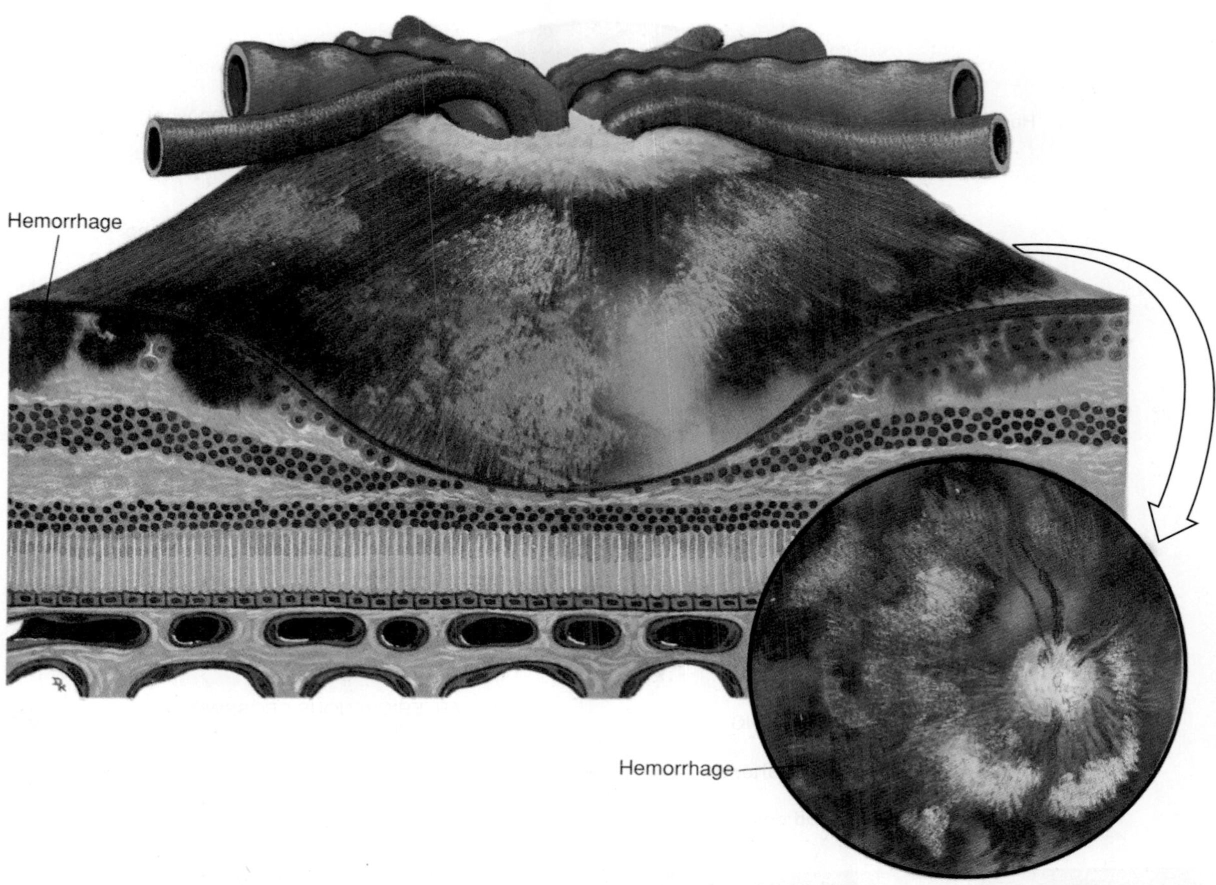

FIGURE 29-6. Central retinal vein occlusion. In contrast to central retinal artery occlusion, central retinal vein occlusion produces considerable vascular engorgement and retinal hemorrhage as a consequence of increased intravascular pressure.

completely obscured, light reflected from the sclerotic vessels appears as threads of silver wire (**silver wiring**).

Small superficial or deep retinal hemorrhages often accompany retinal arteriolosclerosis. **Malignant hypertension** is characterized by necrotizing arteriolitis, with fibrinoid necrosis and thrombosis of precapillary retinal arterioles.

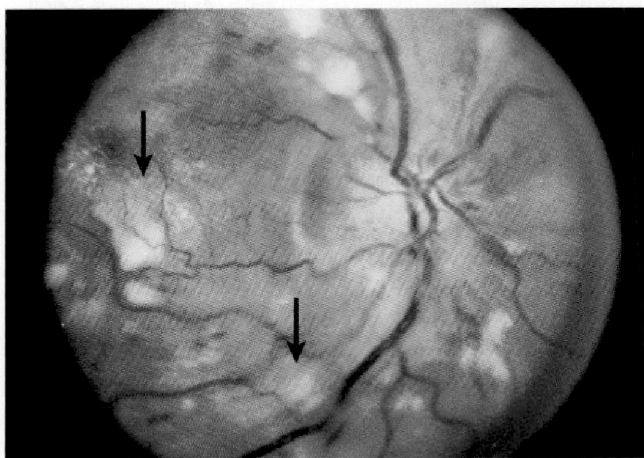

FIGURE 29-7. Hypertensive retinopathy. A photograph of the ocular fundus in a patient with extensive retinopathy. The optic nerve head is edematous; the retina contains numerous "cotton-wool spots" (*arrows*).

Diabetic Retinopathy Is Primarily a Vascular Disease

The eye is frequently involved in diabetes mellitus. Ocular symptoms occur in 20% to 40% of diabetics and may even be evident at the time diabetes is diagnosed. Virtually all patients with type 1 (insulin-dependent) diabetes and many of those with type 2 (non–insulin-dependent) diabetes develop some background retinopathy (see below) within 5 to 15 years of the onset of diabetes (Figs. 29-9 to 29-11). The more dangerous **proliferative retinopathy** does not appear until at least 10 years of diabetes, after which its incidence increases rapidly and remains high for many years. ***In type 1 diabetes, the frequency of proliferative retinopathy correlates with the degree of glycemic control; patients whose diabetes is better controlled develop retinopathy less frequently.*** The relationship between retinal microvascular disease and blood glucose levels in type 2 diabetes is less clear, and other parameters (e.g., blood cholesterol levels, blood pressure) may play more of a role than blood glucose levels.

Retinal ischemia can account for most features of diabetic retinopathy, including the cotton-wool spots, capillary closure, microaneurysms and retinal neovascularization. Ischemia results from narrowing or occlusion of retinal arterioles (as from arteriolosclerosis or platelet and lipid thrombi) or from atherosclerosis of the central retinal or ophthalmic arteries.

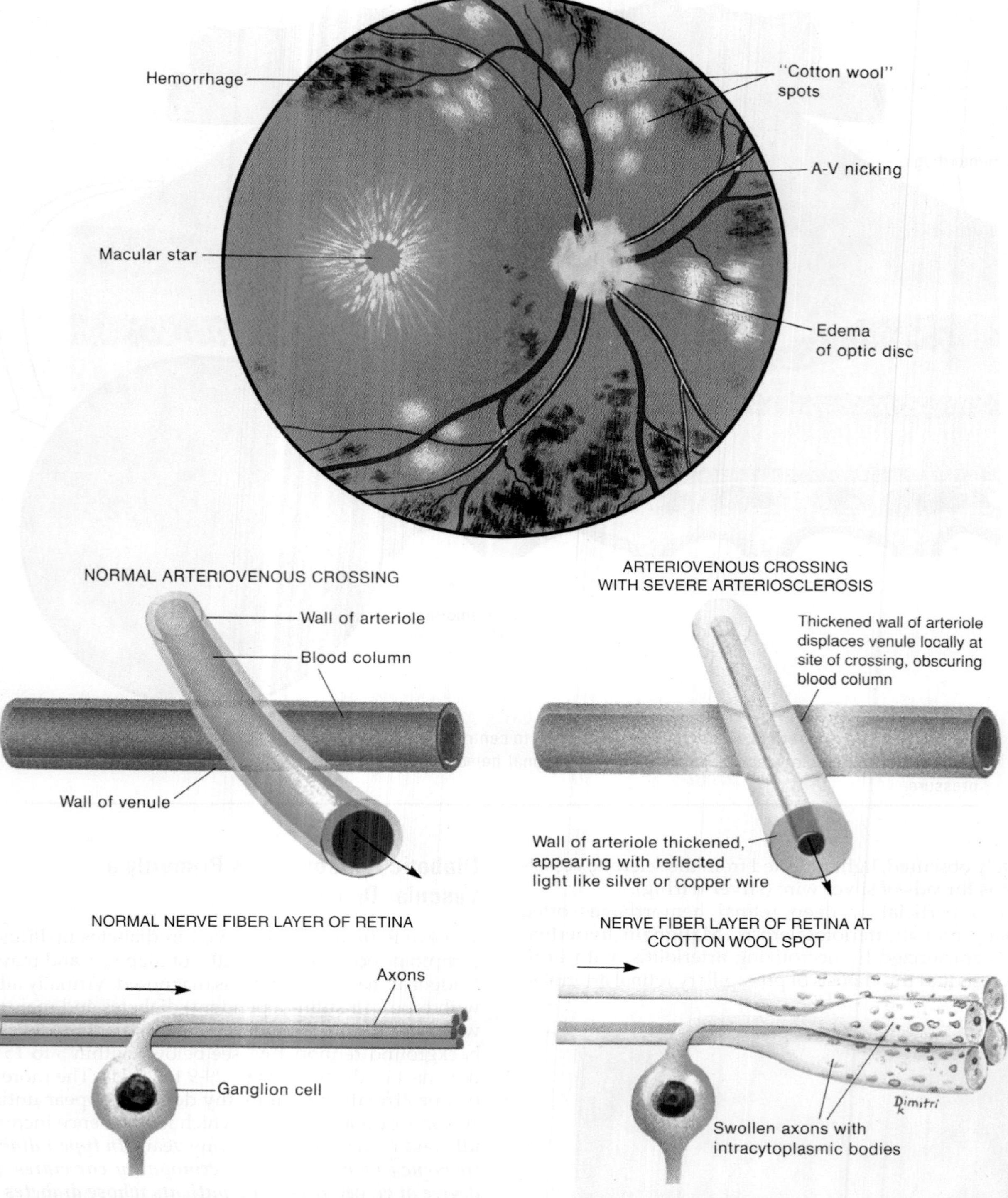

FIGURE 29-8. Hypertensive retinopathy. Various abnormalities develop within the retina in hypertension. The commonly associated arteriolosclerosis affects the appearance of the retinal microvasculature. Light reflected from the thickened arteriolar walls mimics silver or copper wire. Blood flow through the retinal venules is not well visualized at the sites of arteriolar–venular crossings. This effect is due to a thickening of the venular wall rather than to an impediment to blood flow caused by compression; the column of blood proximal to the compression is not wider than the part distal to the crossing. Impaired axoplasmic flow within the nerve fiber layer, caused by ischemia, results in swollen axons with cytoplasmic bodies. Such structures resemble cotton on funduscopy ("cotton-wool spots"). Hemorrhages are common in the retina, and exudates frequently form a star around the macula.

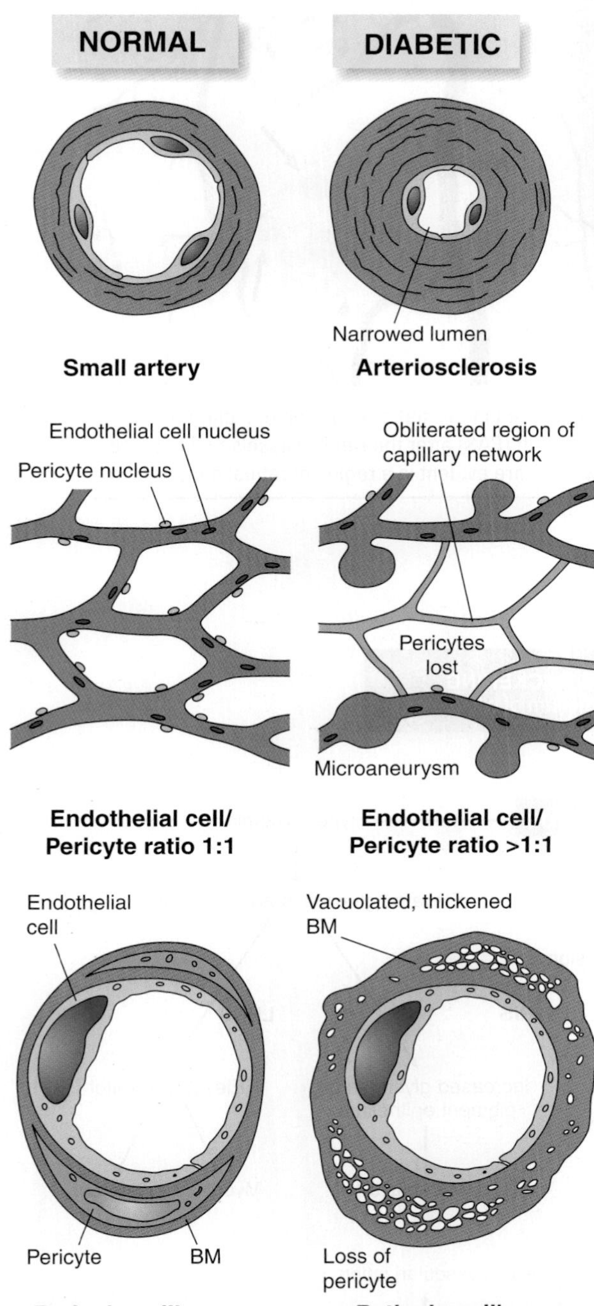

FIGURE 29-9. Diabetic retinopathy. In diabetic retinopathy, the microvasculature is abnormal. Arteriosclerosis narrows the lumen of the small arteries. Pericytes are lost, and the endothelial cell-to-pericyte ratio is greater than 1. Capillary microaneurysms are prominent, and portions of the capillary network become acellular and show no blood flow. The basement membrane (BM) of the retinal capillaries is thickened and vacuolated.

PATHOLOGY: The retinopathy of diabetes is characterized by background and proliferative stages.

BACKGROUND (NONPROLIFERATIVE) DIABETIC RETINOPATHY: This stage exhibits venous engorgement, small hemorrhages (dot and blot hemorrhages), capillary microaneurysms and exudates. These lesions usually do not impair vision unless associated with macular edema. The retinopathy begins at the posterior pole but eventually may involve the entire retina.

On funduscopy, the first discernible clinical abnormality in background diabetic retinopathy is engorged retinal veins, with localized sausage-shaped distentions, coils and loops. This is followed by small hemorrhages in the same areas, mostly in the inner nuclear and outer plexiform layers. With time, "waxy" exudates accumulate, chiefly in the vicinity of the microaneurysms. The retinopathy of elderly diabetic persons frequently displays numerous exudates (**exudative diabetic retinopathy**), which are not seen with type 1 diabetes. Because of the hyperlipoproteinemia of diabetics, the exudates are rich in lipid and thus appear yellowish (**waxy exudates**).

PROLIFERATIVE RETINOPATHY: After many years, diabetic retinopathy becomes proliferative. Delicate new blood vessels grow along with fibrous and glial tissue toward the vitreous body. Retinal neovascularization is a prominent feature of diabetic retinopathy and of other conditions caused by retinal ischemia. Tortuous new vessels first appear on the surface of the retina and optic nerve head and then grow into the vitreous cavity. The newly formed friable vessels bleed easily, and resultant vitreal hemorrhages obscure vision.

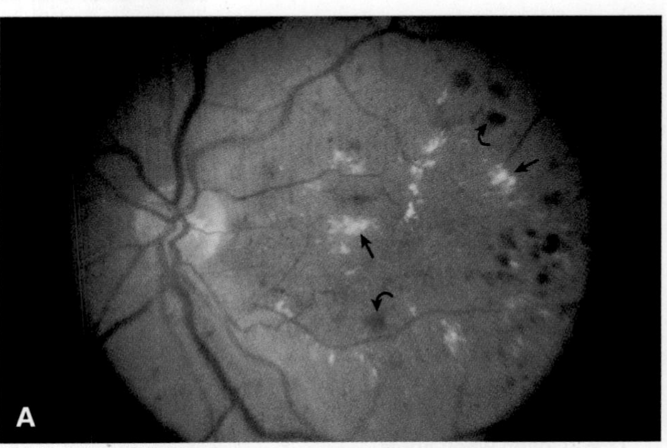

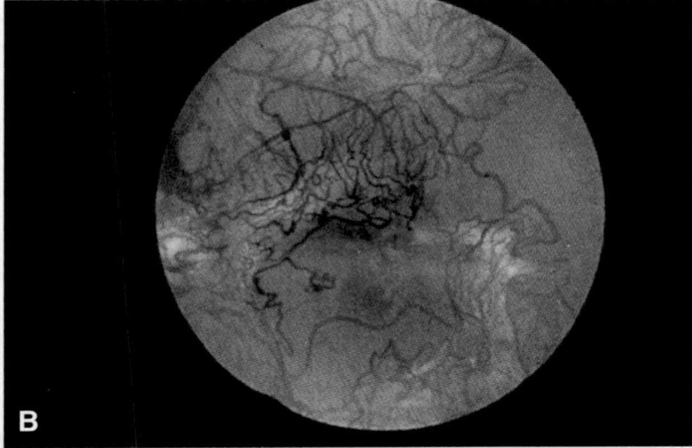

FIGURE 29-10. Diabetic retinopathy. A. The ocular fundus in a patient with background diabetic retinopathy. Several yellowish "hard" exudates (*straight arrows*), which are rich in lipids, are evident, together with several relatively small retinal hemorrhages (*curved arrows*). **B.** A vascular frond (*top half*) has extended anteriorly to the retina in the eye with proliferative diabetic retinopathy.

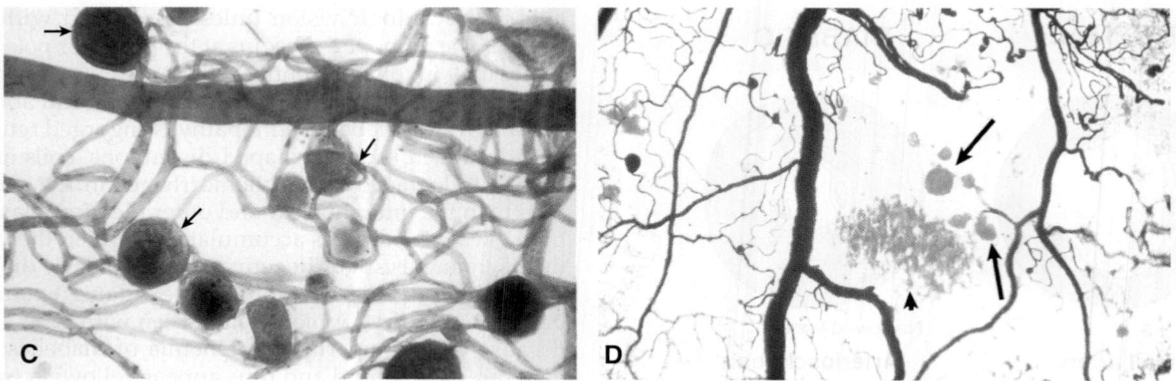

FIGURE 29-10. *(Continued)* **C.** Numerous microaneurysms (*arrows*) are present in this flat preparation of a diabetic retina. **D.** This flat preparation from a diabetic was stained with periodic acid–Schiff (PAS) after the retinal vessels had been perfused with India ink. Microaneurysms (*arrows*) and an exudate (*arrowhead*) are evident in a region of retinal nonperfusion.

BASEMENT MEMBRANE THICKENING
(Retinal capillaries, pigment epithelium of ciliary body)

DIABETES MELLITUS

Hyperlipoproteinemia
Atherosclerosis of central retinal artery/ophthalmic artery
Thrombosis
Arteriolar narrowing
Arteriolosclerosis
Arteriolar occlusion
Hyperglycemia
Elevated glucose in aqueous humor

RETINA
Lipemia retinalis
Retinal ischemia
"Cotton wool" spots
Loss of capillary pericytes
Microaneurysms
Capillary closure
Area of nonperfusion
"Angiogenic factor"
Neovascularization
Preretinal membranes
Retinal detachment

CORNEA
Diabetic keratopathy (?)
Blood staining
Edema

Peripheral neuropathy
Hyphema
Vitreous hemorrhage

IRIS
Increased glycogen in pigment epithelium
"Lacy vacuolization"
Neovascularization
Peripheral anterior synechiae
Glaucoma

LENS
Elevated sorbitol
Myopia
Cataract

BLINDNESS

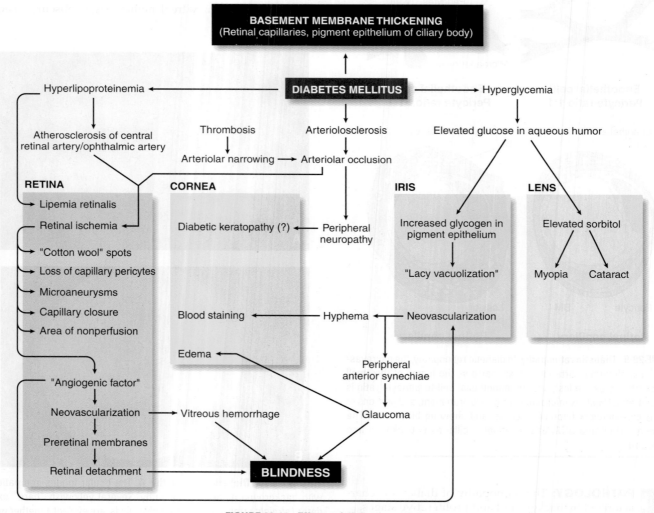

FIGURE 29-11. Effects of diabetes on the eye.

Neovascularization is associated with proliferation and immigration of astrocytes, which grow around the new vessels to form delicate white veils (gliosis). The proliferating fibrovascular and glial tissue contracts, often causing retinal detachment and blindness. Frequently, features of hypertensive and arteriolosclerotic retinopathy are associated with diabetic retinopathy.

Diabetic retinopathy, glaucoma and age-related maculopathy are the leading causes of irreversible blindness in the United States. Blindness in diabetic retinopathy results when the macula is involved, but it also follows vitreous hemorrhage, retinal detachment and glaucoma. Once blindness ensues, it heralds an ominous future for the patient, because death from ischemic heart disease or renal failure often follows. In fact, the mean life expectancy in such cases is less than 6 years, and only one fifth of blind diabetics survive 10 years. Laser phototherapy and strict glycemic control early in the course of proliferative retinopathy have proved effective in controlling this complication.

Diabetic Iridopathy

In diabetics with severe retinopathy, a fibrovascular layer frequently grows along the anterior surface of the iris and in the anterior chamber angle. Because such iris neovascularization (**rubeosis iridis**) occurs in several conditions associated with retinal ischemia, it is believed to be due to an angiogenic factor produced by the ischemic retina.

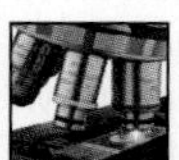

PATHOLOGY: A fibrovascular membrane leads to adhesions between the iris and the cornea **(peripheral anterior synechiae)** and between the iris and lens **(posterior synechiae),** while traction by the fibrovascular membrane pulls the iris pigment epithelium around the pupillary margin **(ectropion uveae).** The friable new vessels on the iris bleed easily and cause **hyphema** (hemorrhage within the anterior chamber of the eye). Neovascularization of the iris is clinically important because it frequently culminates in a blind, painful eye, owing to secondary glaucoma **(neovascular glaucoma).**

Hyperglycemia leads to glycogen storage in the pigmented epithelium of the iris, a phenomenon analogous to that produced in the renal tubules by glycosuria. When tissue sections of diabetic eyes are processed in the usual manner, the pigment epithelium of the iris sometimes contains numerous vacuoles, which imparts a lacy appearance. The vacuoles result from loss of glycogen during preparation of tissue sections. Glycogen storage within the iris pigment epithelium is thought to account for the scattering of iris pigment observed clinically in diabetic patients.

Diabetic Cataracts

Patients with type 1 diabetes often develop bilateral "snowflake" cataracts, a blanket of white needle-shaped opacities in the lens immediately beneath the anterior and posterior lens capsule. The opacities coalesce within a few weeks in adolescents, and within days in children, until the whole lens becomes opaque. Snowflake cataracts can be produced experimentally in young animals and result from an osmotic effect caused by an accumulation of sorbitol, the alcohol derived from glucose (see Chapter 22). The increased sorbitol content of the lens causes imbibition of water and enlargement of the lens.

Age-related cataracts occur in diabetics at an earlier age than in the general population and progress more rapidly to maturity. A sudden temporary myopia, caused by an increase in the refractive power in the lens, may be the presenting manifestation of diabetes.

Other Ophthalmic Manifestations of Diabetes

People with diabetes are at increased risk for inflammation of the anterior segment of the eye, phycomycosis (mucormycosis) of the orbit and primary open-angle glaucoma. They are also prone to the **Argyll Robertson pupil** (unequal and irregularly shaped pupils that react to accommodation but not to light). Cranial nerve palsies occur, especially of the oculomotor nerve. Some patients with long-standing diabetes develop recurrent corneal erosions, which are thought to be due to impaired innervation of the cornea.

The effects of diabetes mellitus on the eye are reviewed in Fig. 29-11.

Retinal Detachment Separates the Sensory Retina From the Pigment Epithelium

During fetal development, the space between the sensory retina and the retinal pigment epithelium is obliterated when these two layers become apposed. However, the sensory retina readily separates from the retinal pigment epithelium when fluid (liquid vitreous, hemorrhage or exudate) accumulates within the potential space between these structures. Such a separation is a common cause of visual impairment and blindness. Laser therapy and surgical approaches have greatly improved the prognosis for patients with detached retina.

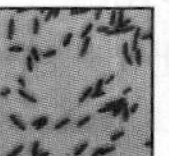

ETIOLOGIC FACTORS: Retinal detachment follows intraocular hemorrhage (e.g., after trauma) and is a potential complication of cataract extractions and several other ocular operations. Factors predisposing to retinal detachment include retinal defects (due to trauma or certain retinal degenerations), vitreous traction, diminished pressure on the retina (e.g., after vitreous loss) and weakening of the fixation of the retina. Full-thickness holes in the retina are not complicated by retinal detachment unless liquid vitreous gains access to the potential space between the retina and the retinal pigment epithelium. Even then, some vitreoretinal traction seems to be necessary for retinal detachment to occur.

The photoreceptors and retinal pigment epithelium normally function as a unit. After they separate in a retinal detachment, oxygen and nutrients that normally reach the outer retina from the choroid must diffuse across a greater distance. This situation causes the photoreceptors to degenerate, after which cyst-like extracellular spaces appear within the retina.

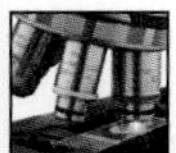

PATHOLOGY: Three varieties of retinal detachment are recognized: rhegmatogenous, tractional and exudative.

RHEGMATOGENOUS RETINAL DETACHMENT: This type of retinal detachment is associated with a retinal tear and also often with degenerative changes in the vitreous body or peripheral retina.

TRACTIONAL RETINAL DETACHMENT: In some cases of retinal detachment the retina is pulled toward the center of the eye by adherent vitreoretinal adhesions, as occurs in

29 | The Eye

proliferative diabetic retinopathy, in retinopathy of prematurity and after intraocular infection.

EXUDATIVE RETINAL DETACHMENT: Accumulation of fluid in the potential space between the sensory retina and the retinal pigment epithelium causes a detached retina in disorders such as choroiditis, choroidal hemangioma and choroidal melanoma.

Retinitis Pigmentosa Is a Heritable Cause of Blindness

Retinitis pigmentosa (pigmentary retinopathy) is a generic term that refers to a variety of bilateral, progressive, degenerative retinopathies characterized clinically by night blindness and constriction of peripheral visual fields and pathologically by loss of retinal photoreceptors (rods and cones) and pigment accumulation within the retina.

The term "retinitis" is a misnomer since inflammation of the retina is not a feature of this disease.

MOLECULAR PATHOGENESIS: A large number of retinal diseases, including retinitis pigmentosa, are caused by mutations in different genes (currently over 200; http://www.sph.uth.tmc.edu/retnet). Some are isolated ocular disorders, with autosomal dominant, autosomal recessive or X-linked recessive inheritance. Some pigmentary retinopathies are associated with neurologic and systemic disorders.

Mutations in at least 48 different genes and loci are associated with nonsyndromic retinitis pigmentosa. Some of the responsible mutated genes encode members of the rod phototransduction cascade, such as rhodopsin (*RHO*) and rod photoreceptor cyclic guanosine 3′,5′-monophosphate (cGMP), phosphodiesterase α and β subunits (*PDE6A, PDE6B*) and photoreceptor structures such as peripherin. How defective proteins in the rod photoreceptors lead to retinitis pigmentosa and the eventual loss of cones remains incompletely understood, but presumably all responsible mutations ultimately cause the death of photoreceptors because of a convergence at a final common point in key metabolic pathways.

PATHOLOGY: In retinitis pigmentosa, destruction of rods, and subsequently cones, is followed by migration of retinal pigment epithelial cells into the sensory retina (Fig. 29-12). Melanin appears within slender processes of spidery cells and accumulates mainly around small branching retinal blood vessels (especially in the equatorial portion of the retina), like spicules of bone. The retinal blood vessels then gradually attenuate, and the optic nerve head acquires a characteristic waxy pallor.

CLINICAL FEATURES: The clinical manifestations of retinitis pigmentosa, including the appearance and distribution of the retinal pigmentation, vary with the causes of the retinopathy. Half of these patients have a family history of the disease. Those with autosomal recessive and X-linked disease are more severely affected and develop night blindness and peripheral field defects in childhood. Autosomal dominant forms of retinitis pigmentosa tend to be less severe, with symptoms beginning later in life. As the condition progresses, contraction of visual fields eventually leads to tunnel vision. Central vision is usually preserved until late in the course of the disease. In some cases, blindness follows macular involvement.

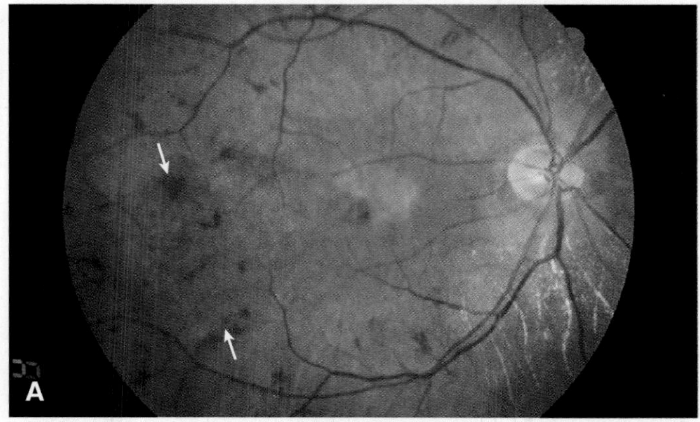

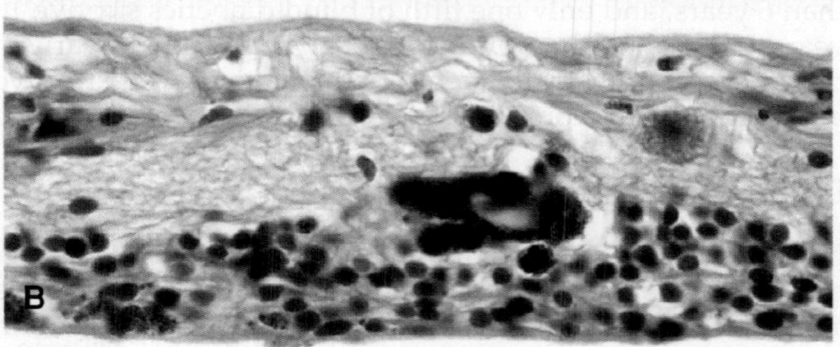

FIGURE 29-12. Retinitis pigmentosa. A. Fundus photograph of the retina of a patient with pigmentary retinopathy (retinitis pigmentosa) shows attenuated retinal vessels and foci of retinal pigmentation (*arrows*). **B.** Microscopic appearance of a severely degenerated retina in pigmentary retinopathy. Note the focal accumulations of pigmented, brown cells (derived from retinal pigmented epithelium) within the retina.

Macular Degeneration Is a Common Cause of Blindness in the Elderly

The center of the macula, the foveola, is the point of greatest visual acuity. In this area, a high concentration of cones rests on the retinal pigment epithelium. Surrounding the macula, the retina has a multilayered concentration of ganglion cells. With aging, in certain drug toxicities (e.g., chloroquine) and in several inherited disorders, the macula degenerates, causing central vision to be impaired.

Age-related macular degeneration currently affects about 15 million people in the United States, and is the most common cause of blindness among individuals of European descent older than age 65. Dry and wet forms of age-related macular degeneration are recognized. The wet variety of this disease accounts for 20% of cases and is associated with subretinal fibrovascular tissue and sometimes bleeding into the subretinal space. Laser photocoagulation and other intraocular antiangiogenic therapies are beneficial in this type of the disorder.

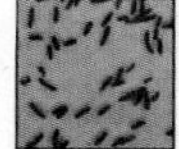

ETIOLOGIC FACTORS: There is general agreement that age-related maculopathy is a multifactorial disease to which environmental and genetic factors contribute. Risk factors include advancing age, smoking, carotid/cardiovascular disease and elevated serum cholesterol levels.

MOLECULAR PATHOGENESIS: A common missense variant of the *CFH* gene that encodes for complement factor H is a risk factor for about 50% of cases of age-related macular degeneration. A susceptibility to age-related macular degeneration has also been associated with mutations or single-nucleotide polymorphisms in *ABCA4* (formerly called *ABCR*), *FBLN5, FBLN6, C3, CST3, LOC387715, TLR4, ERCC6, RAXL1, HTRA1, CX3CR1* and *ESR1* genes and in a mitochondrial gene (*MTTL1*). *ABCA4* encodes a rod cell protein (rim protein) thought to be a transporter involved in molecular recycling. Mutations in this gene may allow degraded material (**drusen**) to accumulate and interfere with retinal function.

Lysosomal Storage Diseases Feature a Cherry-Red Spot at the Macula

In lysosomal storage diseases, including the gangliosidoses, myriad intracytoplasmic lysosomal inclusions within the multilayered ganglion cell layer of the macula impart a striking pallor to the affected retina. As a result, the central foveola appears bright red because of the underlying choroidal vasculature (Fig. 29-13). As mentioned above, a cherry-red spot also occurs at the macula after central retinal artery occlusion because the pale, edematous retina highlights the subfoveolar vascular choroid.

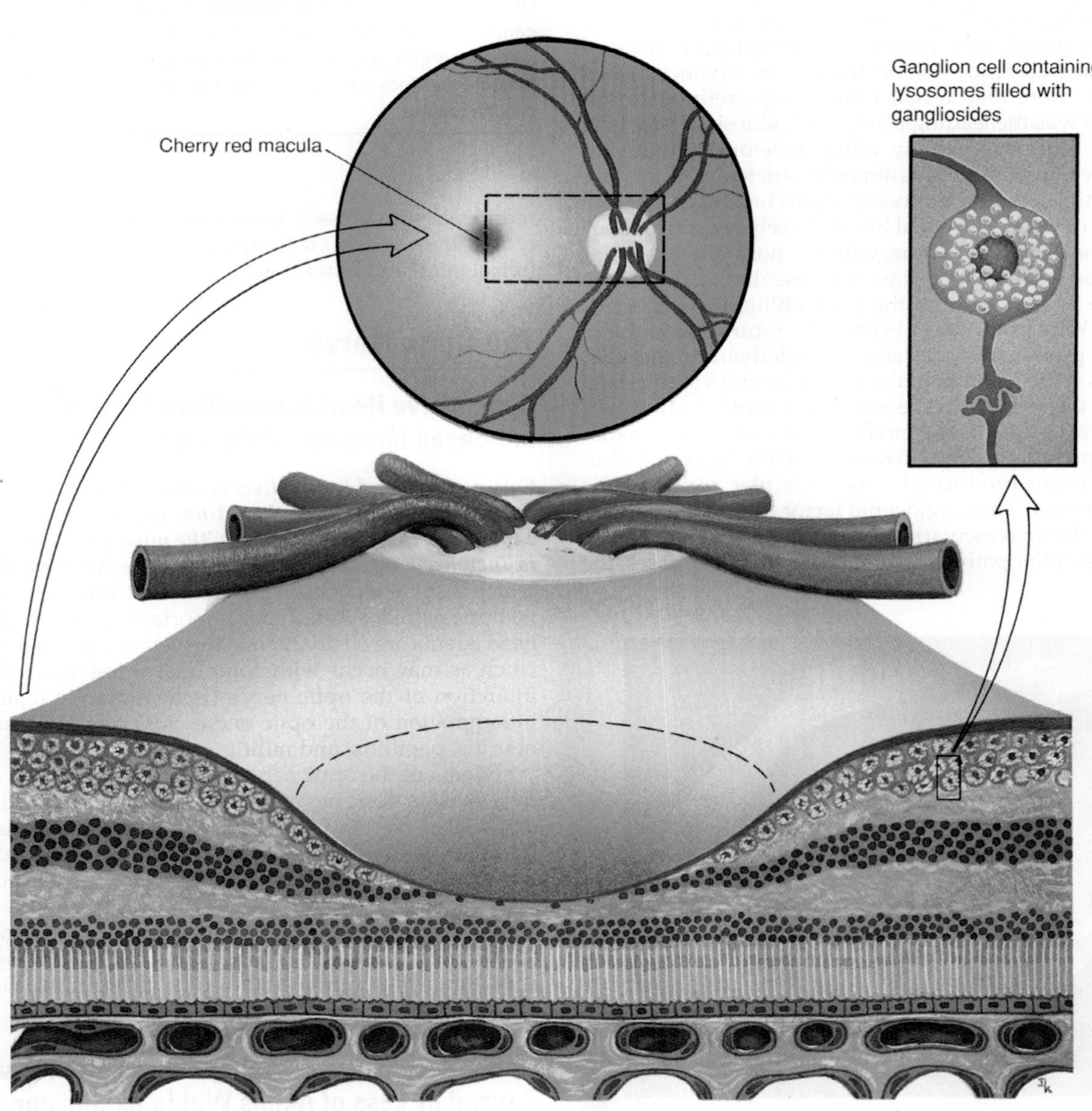

FIGURE 29-13. Cherry-red macula. A cherry-red spot appears at the macula in several lysosomal storage diseases that are characterized by intracytoplasmic accumulations within the retinal ganglion cells, such as Tay-Sachs disease, in which a particular ganglioside is stored (GM_2-ganglioside). The macula develops this appearance because the pallor created by the deposits within the multilayered ganglion cells enhances the visibility of the underlying normal choroidal vasculature.

Angioid Streaks Are Vessel-Like Fractures in the Bruch Membrane

Angioid streaks are seen when the posterior segment of the eye is examined clinically. This occurs when the Bruch membrane fractures, causing characteristic irregular lines that radiate beneath the retina from the optic nerve head (**angioid streaks**). This happens spontaneously in a variety of systemic disorders, most commonly pseudoxanthoma elasticum, sickle cell disease and Paget disease of bone.

Retinopathy of Prematurity Results From Oxygen Toxicity

Retinopathy of prematurity is a bilateral, iatrogenic, retinal disorder that occurs predominantly in premature infants treated with high levels of inspired oxygen after birth. The entity was originally called **retrolental fibroplasia** because of a mass of scarred tissue behind the lens in advanced cases (Fig. 29-14). More than a half century ago, retinopathy of prematurity was the leading cause of blindness in infants in the United States and many other developed countries. Retinopathy of prematurity is almost restricted to premature infants administered high concentrations of oxygen. In such infants, the developing retinal blood vessels become obliterated, and the peripheral retina, which is normally avascular until the end of fetal life, does not vascularize. The more mature the retina, the less the vaso-obliterative effect of hyperoxia. When the infant eventually returns to ambient air, intense proliferation of vascular endothelium and glial cells begins at the junction of the avascular and vascularized portions of the retina. This becomes apparent 5 to 10 weeks after removal of the infant from the incubator and, as in diabetic retinopathy, is thought to result from the liberation of an angiogenic factor produced by the avascular and ischemic peripheral retina. This angiogenic factor is also believed to account for the neovascularization of the iris that sometimes accompanies retinopathy of prematurity. In 25% of cases, the retinopathy progresses to a scarring phase, characterized by retinal detachment, a fibrovascular mass behind the lens (retrolental) and blindness.

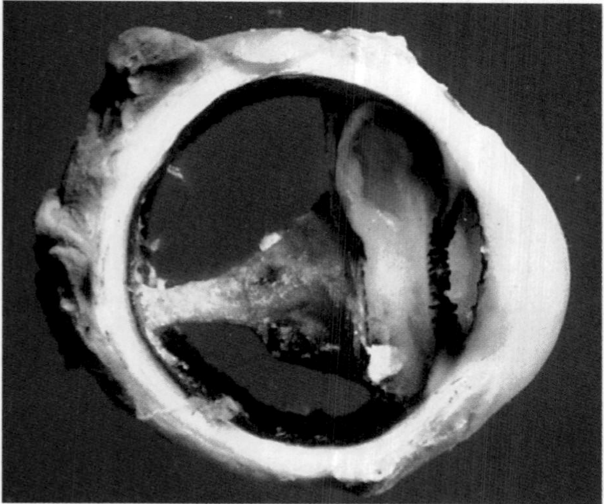

FIGURE 29-14. Retinopathy of prematurity. Horizontal section through an eye with advanced retinopathy of prematurity (retrolental fibroplasia) shows a totally detached retina adherent to a fibrovascular mass behind the lens.

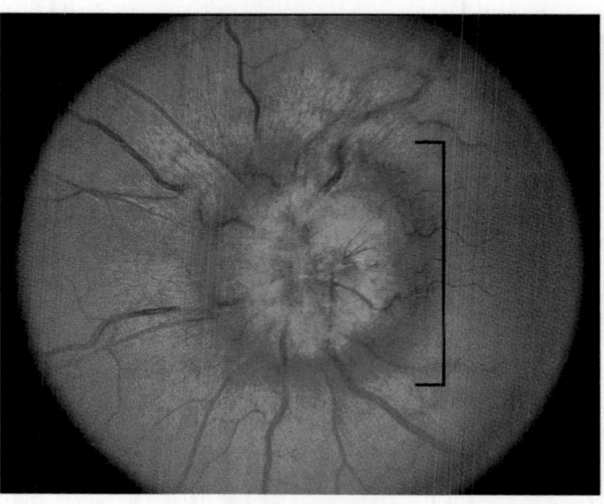

FIGURE 29-15. Chronic papilledema. The optic nerve head (*bracket*) is congested and protrudes anteriorly toward the interior of the eye. It has blurred margins, and the vessels within it are poorly seen. In contrast to acute papilledema, the veins are not so congested, and hemorrhage is not a feature.

The Optic Nerve

Optic Nerve Head Edema Often Reflects Increased Intracranial Pressure

Optic nerve head (optic disc) edema refers to swelling of the optic nerve head where the retinal axons leave the globe. It can result from various causes, the most important of which is increased intracranial pressure. The term **papilledema,** which is still widely used in that context, is imprecise because no optic papilla exists. Other important causes of optic nerve head edema are obstruction to the venous drainage of the eye (such as may occur with compressive lesions of the orbit), infarction of the optic nerve (ischemic optic neuropathy), inflammation of the optic nerve close to the eyeball (optic neuritis, papillitis) and multiple sclerosis.

Edema of the optic nerve head is characterized clinically by a swollen optic nerve head that displays blurred margins and dilated vessels (Fig. 29-15). Frequently, hemorrhages (Fig. 29-16), exudates and cotton-wool spots are seen, and concentric folds of the choroid and retina may surround the nerve head. Acutely, optic nerve head edema results in few, if any, visual symptoms. As the condition becomes established, swelling of the optic nerve head enlarges the normal blind spot. After many months, atrophic changes lead to loss of visual acuity.

Optic Atrophy Is a Thinning of the Optic Nerve Caused by Loss of Axons Within Its Substance

The nerve axons within the optic nerve are lost in many conditions, including long-standing edema of the optic nerve head, optic neuritis, optic nerve compression, glaucoma and retinal degeneration.

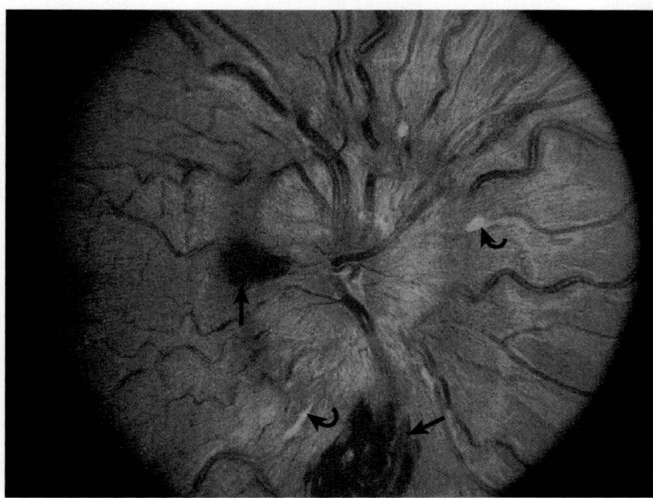

FIGURE 29-16. Hemorrhage in papilledema. The optic nerve head is markedly congested, with dilated veins and a blurred margin. A small hemorrhage is evident within the optic nerve head at its junction with the retina (*straight arrows*). Several small "cotton-wool spots" are present within the adjacent retina (*curved arrows*).

ETIOLOGIC FACTORS: Optic atrophy can also be caused by some drugs, such as ethambutol and isoniazid. The optic nerve head is usually flat and pale in optic atrophy (Fig. 29-17), but when this disorder follows glaucoma, the optic nerve head is excavated **(glaucomatous cupping).**

MOLECULAR PATHOGENESIS: Optic atrophy can follow mutations in *OPA1, OPA3* and *WFS1* genes. Multiple point mutations in the mitochondrial genome are associated with **Leber hereditary optic neuropathy** and three of them account for more than 90% of cases (*MTND1-3460, MTND4-11778* and *MTND6-14484*).

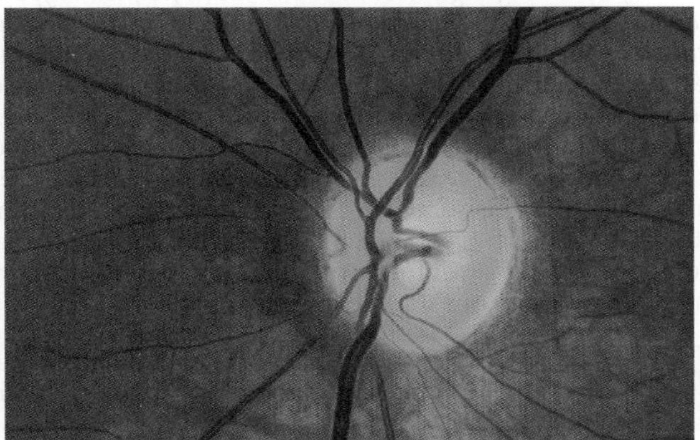

FIGURE 29-17. Optic atrophy. The margin of the optic nerve head is sharply demarcated from the adjacent retina. Because the myelinated axons in the optic nerve are markedly diminished, the optic nerve head appears much whiter than normal.

Glaucoma

Glaucoma refers to a collection of disorders that feature an optic neuropathy accompanied by a characteristic progressive loss of visual field sensitivity and eventual excavation of the optic nerve head. In most cases, glaucoma is produced by increased intraocular pressure (**ocular hypertension**); however, increased intraocular pressure does not necessarily cause glaucoma, and not all patients with glaucoma have elevated intraocular pressure.

After being produced by the ciliary body, the aqueous humor enters the posterior chamber (the space between the iris and the zonules) before passing through the pupil to the anterior chamber (between the iris and the cornea). From that site, it drains into veins by way of the trabecular meshwork and the canal of Schlemm (Fig. 29-18). A delicate balance between production and drainage of the aqueous humor maintains intraocular pressure within its physiologic range (10 to 20 mm Hg). In certain pathologic states, the drainage of aqueous humor from the eye becomes impaired, and intraocular pressure increases. Temporary or permanent impairment of vision results from pressure-induced degenerative changes in the retina and optic nerve head (Fig. 29-19) and from edema and opacification of the cornea.

Glaucoma Is Caused By Obstruction to the Drainage of Aqueous Humor

Glaucoma, one of the most common causes of preventable blindness in the United States, almost always follows a congenital or acquired lesion of the anterior segment of the eye that mechanically obstructs the aqueous drainage. The obstruction may be located between the iris and lens, in the angle of the anterior chamber, in the trabecular meshwork, in the canal of Schlemm or in the venous drainage of the eye.

There Are Several Types of Glaucoma

Congenital Glaucoma (Infantile Glaucoma, Buphthalmos)

Congenital glaucoma is caused by obstruction to aqueous drainage by developmental anomalies. This type of glaucoma develops even though intraocular pressure may not increase until early infancy or childhood. Most cases of congenital glaucoma occur in boys (65%), and an X-linked recessive mode of inheritance is common. The developmental anomaly usually involves both eyes and, although often limited to the angle of the anterior chamber, it may be accompanied by a variety of other ocular malformations. Congenital glaucoma is associated with a deep anterior chamber, corneal cloudiness, sensitivity to bright lights (**photophobia**), excessive tearing and buphthalmos. The term **buphthalmos** (from the Greek *bous*, "ox"; *ophthalmos*, "eye") describes the enlarged eyes of patients with congenital glaucoma that result from expansion caused by increased intraocular pressure beneath a pliable sclera.

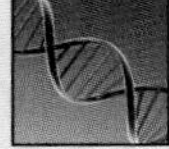

MOLECULAR PATHOGENESIS: Several genes for primary congenital glaucoma have been identified. Homozygous mutations in the cytochrome P4501B1 gene (*CYP1B1*) account for some cases of autosomal

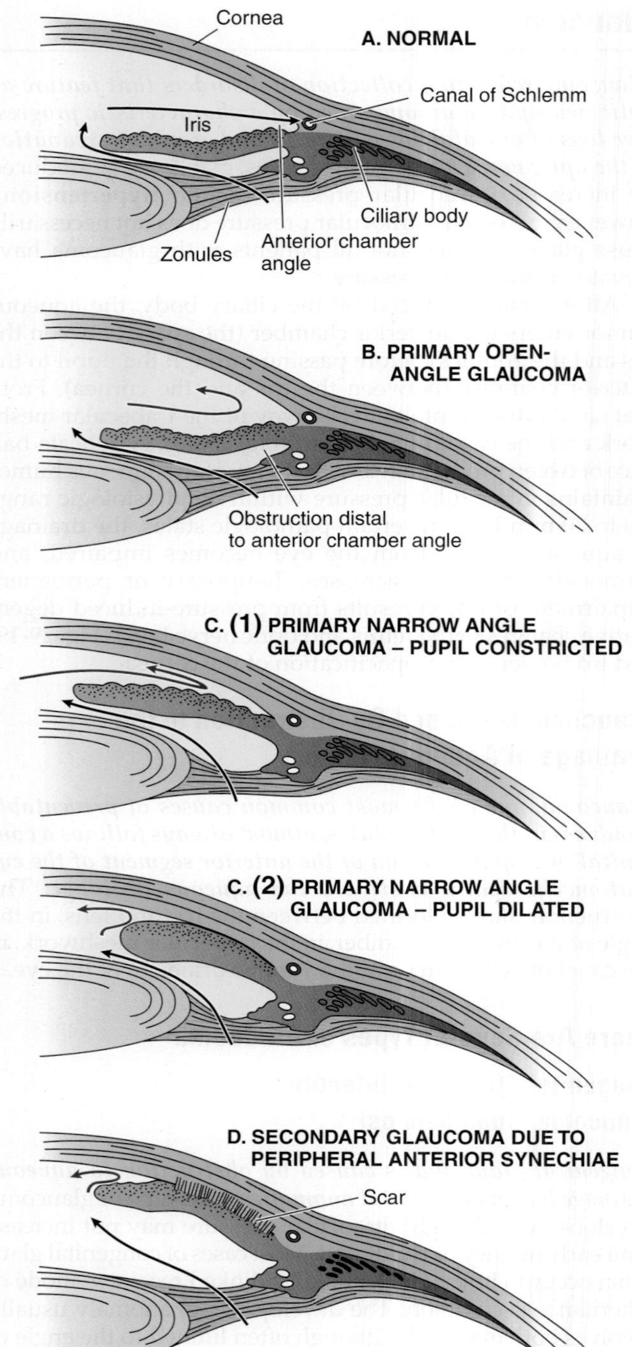

FIGURE 29-18. Pathogenesis of glaucoma. The anterior segment of the eye is affected differently in various forms of glaucoma. **A.** Structure of the normal eye. **B.** In primary open-angle glaucoma, the obstruction to the aqueous outflow is distal to the anterior chamber angle, and the anterior segment resembles that of the normal eye. **C.** In primary narrow-angle glaucoma, the anterior chamber angle is open, but narrower than normal when the pupil is constricted (**C1**). When the pupil becomes dilated in such an eye, the thickened iris obstructs the anterior chamber angle (**C2**), causing increased intraocular pressure. **D.** The anterior chamber angle can become obstructed by a variety of pathologic processes, including an adhesion between the iris and the posterior surface of the cornea (**peripheral anterior synechiae**).

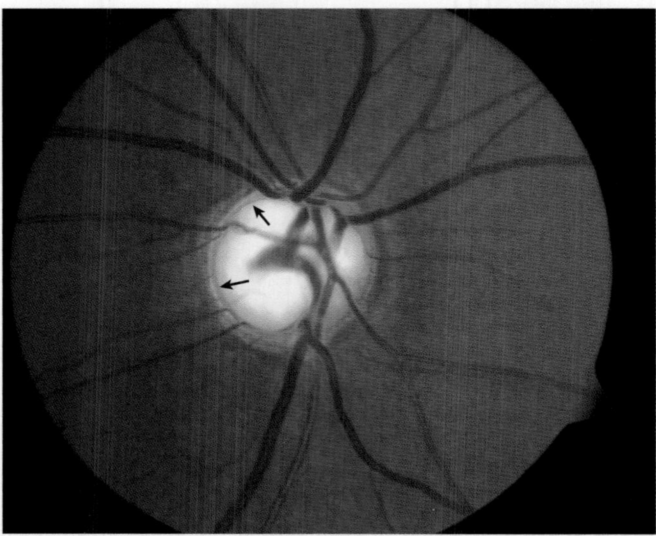

FIGURE 29-19. Optic nerve head in glaucoma. The anterior part of the optic nerve is depressed ("optic cupping"; *arrows*), and the blood vessels crossing the margin of the optic nerve head are displaced to the nasal side. The fundus appears dark because this eye of an African-American patient contains numerous pigmented melanocytes in the choroid.

recessive primary infantile glaucoma. Congenital glaucoma associated with developmental anomalies of the eye (secondary congenital glaucoma) results from mutations in the fork-head transcription factor gene (*FOXC1*), pituitary homeobox 2 gene (*PITX2*) or paired box 6 gene (*PAX6*).

Adult-Onset Primary Glaucoma

Adult-onset primary glaucoma develops in a person with no apparent underlying eye disease. It is subdivided into **primary open-angle glaucoma** (in which the anterior chamber angle is open and appears normal) and **primary closed-angle glaucoma** (in which the anterior chamber is shallower than normal, and the angle is abnormally narrow) (Fig. 29-18).

Primary Open-Angle Glaucoma

Primary open-angle glaucoma is the most frequent type of glaucoma and a major cause of blindness in the United States. It affects 1% to 3% of the population older than 40 years and occurs principally in the sixth decade. The angle of the anterior chamber is open and appears normal, but there is increased resistance to the outflow of the aqueous humor in the vicinity of the canal of Schlemm. The intraocular pressure increases insidiously and asymptomatically, and although almost always bilateral, one eye may be affected more severely than the other. With time, damage to the retina and optic nerve causes irreversible loss of vision.

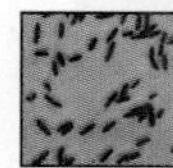

ETIOLOGIC FACTORS: Persons with diabetes mellitus and myopia have increased risk of primary open-angle glaucoma.

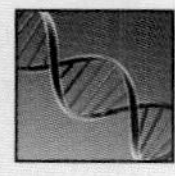

MOLECULAR PATHOGENESIS: Primary open-angle glaucoma has been mapped to at least 13 loci on chromosomes 1, 2, 3, 5, 6, 7, 8, 9, 10 and 20, and three genes have been identified. Some cases of primary open-angle glaucoma are due to numerous different mutations in the *MYOC* (*TGRR*) gene on chromosome 1 (1q21-q31). Primary open-angle glaucoma can occur as a manifestation of the nail–patella syndrome, in association with mutations in the Lim homeobox transcription factor-1 (*LMX1B*) gene. Juvenile-onset primary open-angle glaucoma may result from mutations in the *CRYP1B1, FKHL7, MYOC* and *OPTN* genes.

Primary Closed-Angle Glaucoma

Primary closed-angle glaucoma, differentiated from open-angle glaucoma above, occurs after age 40 years. ***It is the predominant form of primary glaucoma in adults living in Asia.***

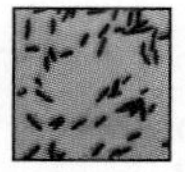

ETIOLOGIC FACTORS: The disorder afflicts persons whose peripheral iris is displaced anteriorly toward the trabecular meshwork, thereby creating an abnormally narrow anterior chamber angle. When the pupil is constricted (miotic), the iris remains stretched so that the chamber angle is not occluded. However, when the pupil dilates (mydriasis), the iris obstructs the drainage of aqueous humor from the eye, resulting in sudden episodes of intraocular hypertension. This is accompanied by ocular pain, and halos or rings are seen around lights. In such persons, intraocular pressure may also increase if the pupil becomes blocked (e.g., by a swollen lens) and aqueous humor accumulates in the posterior chamber.

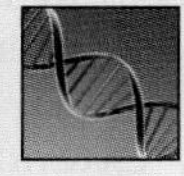

MOLECULAR PATHOGENESIS: Primary closed-angle glaucoma has a familial predisposition, but in contrast to primary open-angle glaucoma, genetic loci have not yet been identified.

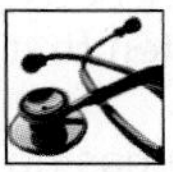

CLINICAL FEATURES: ***Acute closed-angle glaucoma is an ocular emergency, and it is essential to start ocular hypotensive treatment within the first 24 to 48 hours if vision is to be maintained.*** Primary closed-angle glaucoma affects both eyes, but it may become apparent in one eye 2 to 5 years before it is noted in the other. The intraocular pressure is normal between attacks, but after many episodes, adhesions form between the iris and the trabecular meshwork and cornea (**peripheral anterior synechiae**) and accentuate the block to the outflow of aqueous humor.

Low-Tension Glaucoma

In low-tension glaucoma the characteristic visual field defect and all of the ophthalmoscopic features of chronic open-angle glaucoma occur, but without increased intraocular pressure. The characteristic visual field defect and all of the ophthalmoscopic features of chronic simple (open-angle) glaucoma often occur in elderly people who do not show increased intraocular pressure.

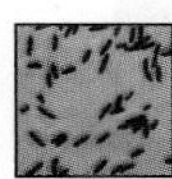

ETIOLOGIC FACTORS: Although some eyes may be hypersensitive to normal intraocular pressure, many cases of low-tension glaucoma probably represent an infarction of the optic nerve head. Susceptibility to normal tension glaucoma is associated with an intronic polymorphism of the *OPA1* gene, as well as with a mutation in the *OPTN* gene.

Secondary Glaucoma

In secondary glaucoma, anterior chamber angles may be open or closed. Because the underlying disorder is usually limited to one eye, secondary glaucoma tends to be unilateral. There are numerous causes of secondary glaucoma including inflammation, hemorrhage, neovascularization of the iris and adhesions.

Effects of Increased Intraocular Pressure

Prolonged ocular hypertension has several effects on the eye:

- In adults, increased intraocular pressure leads to a characteristic cupped excavation of the optic nerve head (glaucomatous cupping), accompanied by a nasal displacement of the retinal blood vessels. In infants, cupping of the optic nerve head tends to be less prominent (Fig. 29-19).
- The cornea or sclera bulges at weak points, such as sites of scars in the outer coat of the eye.
- Optic atrophy, with loss of axons, gliosis and thickening of the pial septa, follows the retinal degeneration and damage to the nerve fibers at the optic nerve head.
- The ganglion cell and nerve fiber layers of the retina degenerate, thereby impairing vision. The outer retina, which derives its nutrition from the underlying choroid, remains intact.
- When intraocular pressure is increased in a child younger than 3 years of age, the pliable eye sometimes enlarges extensively (buphthalmos). After the first few years of life, a rigid sclera prevents glaucomatous eyes from enlarging under the increased pressure.

Myopia

Myopia (also called "nearsightedness") is a refractive ocular abnormality in which light from the visualized object focuses at a point in front of the retina because of a longer than usual anteroposterior diameter of the eye. Myopia affects more than 70 million persons in the United States and is the most common clinically significant disorder of the eye. In Asia it affects an even greater percentage of the population. Treatment requires refractive correction. In addition to glasses and contact lenses, refractive surgery using an excimer laser such as laser-assisted in situ keratomileusis (LASIK) and laser epithelial keratomileusis (LASEK) are popular. Myopia usually begins in young persons and varies in severity. A mild form (stationary or simple myopia) is generally nonprogressive after cessation of body growth, whereas a genetically determined "progressive myopia" is more severe.

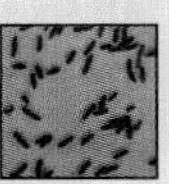 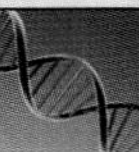

ETIOLOGIC FACTORS AND MOLECULAR PATHOGENESIS: There is strong evidence to implicate excessive accommodation from reading and other near work in childhood in the pathogenesis of myopia. In childhood the vast majority of human eyes with myopia adjust their axial length to the refraction by the anterior segment of the eye (**emmetropization**), and studies in animal models indicate that emmetropization mechanisms elongate the eye. Some nonsyndromic inherited types have been mapped to 14 different loci on various chromosomes. Myopia is also a feature of several systemic diseases, including some disorders of fibrillin (Marfan syndrome), collagen (Stickler syndrome, Knobloch syndrome) and perlecan (Schwartz-Jampel syndrome type I).

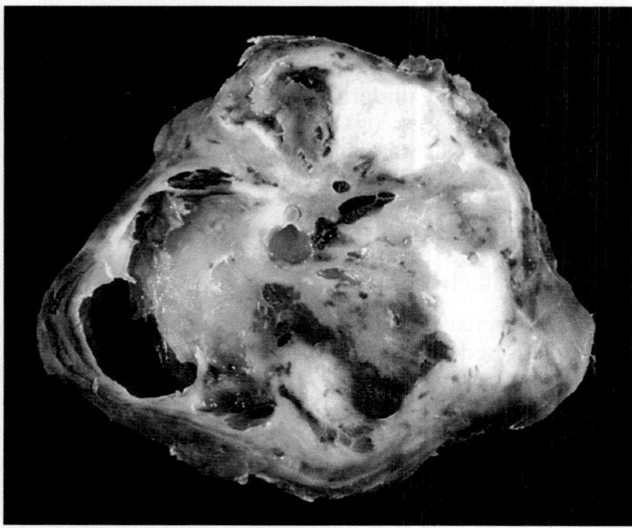

FIGURE 29-20. Phthisis bulbi. Section through an eye with phthisis bulbi, exemplifying the markedly disorganized nature of the intraocular contents of such atrophic disordered globes.

Phthisis Bulbi

Phthisis bulbi refers to a nonspecific, end-stage eye that is disorganized and atrophic. This condition (Fig. 29-20) is most common after trauma to, or inflammation of, the eye. Eyes afflicted with phthisis bulbi are often enucleated. The eye is small and often extremely hard due to intraocular ossification. The choroid and ciliary body are separated from the sclera, which is thickened, wrinkled and indented due to loss of intraocular pressure. The cornea is flattened, shrunken and opaque. Intraocular contents are disorganized by diffuse scarring and detachment of the sensory retina is invariably encountered. If present, the lens is displaced and often calcified. A typical finding in phthisis bulbi is intraocular bone formation, which may be derived from the hyperplastic pigment epithelium.

Ocular Neoplasms

The eye and adjacent structures contain a large number of cell types, and as one might expect, benign and malignant neoplasms arise from them. ***Intraocular neoplasms arise mostly from immature retinal neurons (retinoblastoma) and uveal melanocytes (melanoma).*** Although the retinal pigment epithelium often undergoes reactive proliferation, it seldom becomes neoplastic.

Malignant Melanoma Arises From Melanocytes in the Uvea

Malignant melanoma is the most common primary intraocular malignancy. It may arise from melanocytes in any part of the eye, the choroid being the most common site.

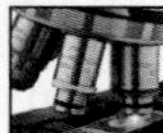

PATHOLOGY: Choroidal melanomas are mostly circumscribed and commonly invade the Bruch membrane, causing a mushroom-shaped mass (Fig. 29-21). By contrast, some tumors are flat (diffuse melanoma) and cause a gradual deterioration of vision over many years. Some do not become apparent until extraocular dissemination has occurred. Orange lipofuscin pigment is sometimes evident over the surface of some choroidal melanomas.

Microscopically, uveal melanomas may be composed mainly of variable numbers of spindle-shaped cells without nucleoli (spindle A cells), spindle-shaped cells with prominent nucleoli (spindle B cells), polygonal cells with distinct cell borders and prominent nucleoli (epithelioid cells) or a fourth cell type that is similar to epithelioid cells but smaller with indistinct cell borders.

Melanomas of the ciliary body and iris may extend circumferentially around the globe (ring melanoma). Melanomas in the iris are usually diagnosed clinically one to two decades earlier than those in the choroid and ciliary body, perhaps because they are more easily seen and are often first observed by the patient.

Lymphatic spread does not occur because the eye has no lymphatic vessels. Aside from hematogenous spread, uveal

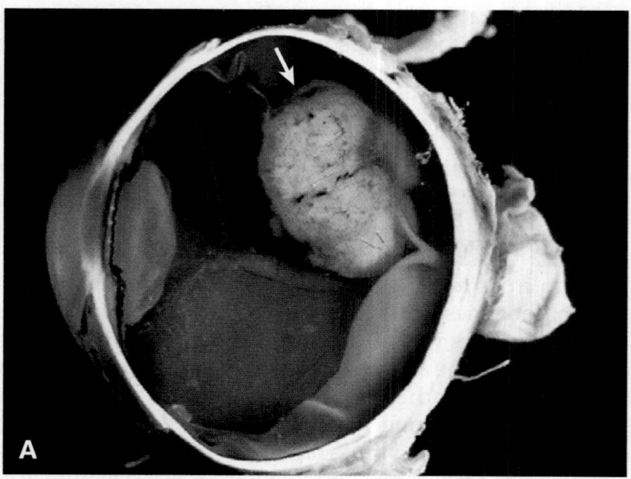

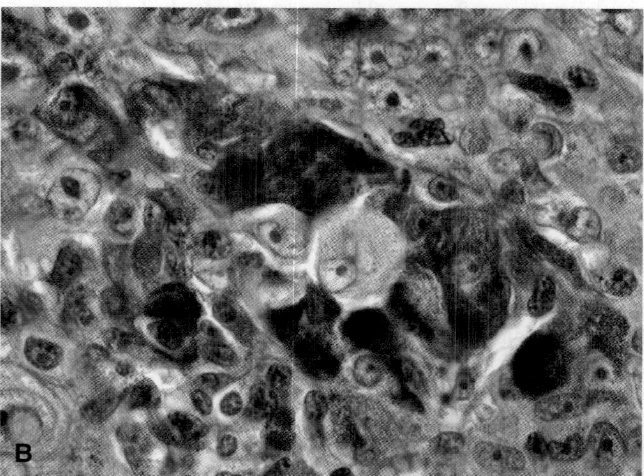

FIGURE 29-21. Malignant melanoma. A. A mushroom-shaped melanoma of the choroid is present in this eye (*arrow*). Choroidal melanomas commonly invade through the Bruch membrane and result in this appearance. **B.** Photomicrograph of a heavily pigmented melanoma of the choroid depicting epithelioid tumor cells with prominent nucleoli.

melanomas disseminate by traversing the sclera to enter the orbital tissues, usually at sites where blood vessels and nerves pass through the sclera. The liver is a common site of metastases, and anecdotally, the diagnosis of metastatic ocular melanoma can be made intuitively by astute clinicians who discover an enlarged liver in a patient with a "glass eye."

CLINICAL FEATURES: Intraocular melanomas may cause cataract, glaucoma, retinal detachment, inflammation and hemorrhage. The options for treating uveal melanomas include enucleation of the eye, radiotherapy and local excision. More than half of patients with uveal melanomas survive for 15 years after enucleation. Prognostic factors include tumor size, tumor location and cell type. Unfavorable indicators are tumor hyperploidy, high mitotic activity, high microvascular density, high tumor-infiltrating lymphocyte counts, chromosome 3 monosomy and high serum melanoma inhibitory activity protein. Deaths have been reported within 5 years from spindle A melanomas, but tumors composed purely of epithelioid cells have the worst prognosis.

Retinoblastomas Originate From Immature Neurons

Retinoblastoma is the most common intraocular malignant neoplasm of childhood, affecting 1:20,000 to 1:34,000 children. It occurs most frequently within the first 2 years of life and may even be found at birth. Most retinoblastomas occur sporadically and are unilateral. Some 6% to 8% of retinoblastomas are inherited. Up to 25% of sporadic retinoblastomas and most inherited retinoblastomas are bilateral.

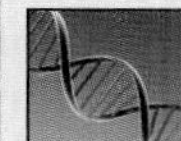

MOLECULAR PATHOGENESIS: Retinoblastomas are related to inherited or acquired deletions of, or mutations in, the retinoblastoma (*Rb*) tumor suppressor gene, located on the long arm of chromosome 13 (13q14) (see Chapter 5). Some patients with retinoblastoma have homologous genomic mutations in the *Rb* gene. Others have a single genomic mutation but the tumors possess an additional one.

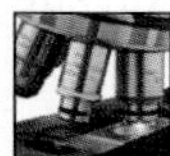

PATHOLOGY: Some retinoblastomas grow toward the vitreous body and can be seen with an ophthalmoscope (**endophytic retinoblastoma**). Others extend between the sensory retina and the retinal pigment epithelium, thereby detaching the retina (**exophytic retinoblastoma**). A few retinoblastomas are both endophytic and exophytic. Rarely, a retinoblastoma spreads diffusely within the retina without forming an obvious mass (**diffuse retinoblastoma**). The retina often contains several distinct foci of tumor in the same eye, some of which represent a multifocal origin, whereas others are tumor implants from dissemination through the vitreous body.

Retinoblastoma is a cream-colored tumor that contains scattered, chalky white, calcified flecks within yellow necrotic zones (Fig. 29-22), which may be detected radiologically. The tumors are intensely cellular and display several morphologic patterns. In some instances, densely packed, round neoplastic cells with hyperchromatic nuclei, scant cytoplasm and abundant mitoses are randomly distributed. In other retinoblastomas, the cells are arranged radially around a central cavity

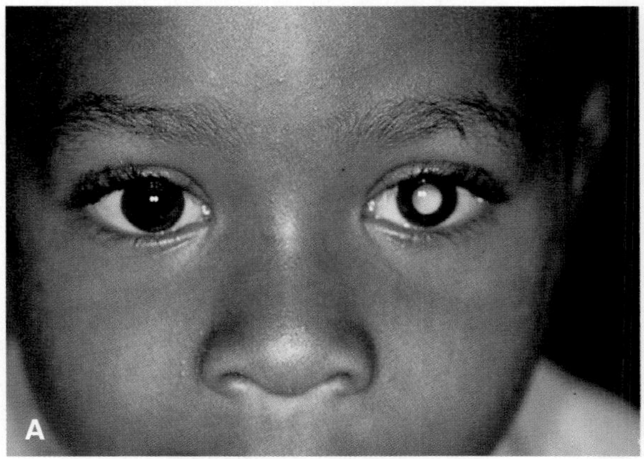

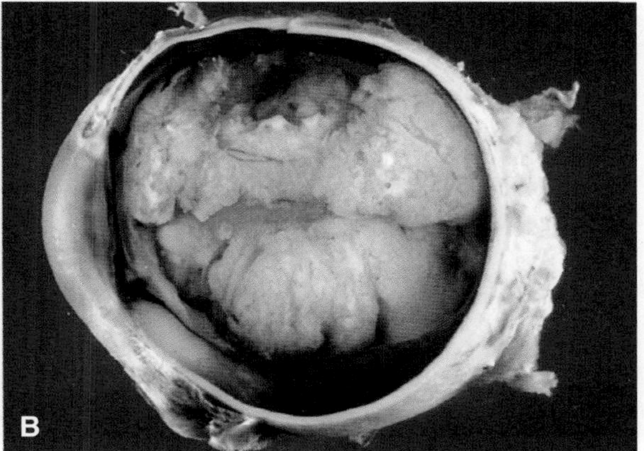

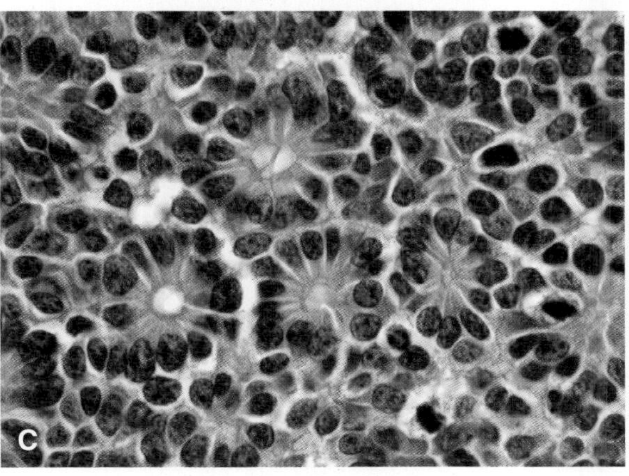

FIGURE 29-22. Retinoblastoma. A. The white pupil (leukocoria) in the left eye is the result of an intraocular retinoblastoma. **B.** This surgically excised eye is almost filled by a cream-colored intraocular retinoblastoma with calcified flecks. **C.** Light microscopic view of a retinoblastoma showing Flexner-Wintersteiner rosettes characterized by cells that are arranged around a central cavity.

(**Flexner-Wintersteiner rosettes**), as they differentiate toward photoreceptors. In some cases, the cellular arrangement resembles a fleur-de-lis (**fleurette**). Viable tumor cells align themselves around blood vessels, and necrotic areas with calcification are seen a short distance from the vascularized regions.

Retinoblastomas disseminate by several routes. They commonly extend into the optic nerve, from where they spread intracranially. They also invade blood vessels, especially in the highly vascular choroid, before metastasizing hematogenously throughout the body. Bone marrow is a common site of blood-borne metastases, but surprisingly, the lung is rarely involved.

CLINICAL FEATURES: Presenting signs include a white pupil (leukocoria), squint (strabismus), poor vision, spontaneous hyphema or a red, painful eye. Secondary glaucoma is a frequent complication. Light entering the eye commonly reflects a yellowish color similar to that from the tapetum of a cat (cat's eye reflex).

Retinoblastomas are almost always fatal if left untreated. However, with early diagnosis and modern therapy, survival is high (about 90%). Rarely, spontaneous regression occurs for reasons that remain unknown. Patients with inherited retinoblastomas, presumably as a consequence of the loss of *Rb* gene function, show increased susceptibility to other malignant tumors, including osteogenic sarcoma, Ewing sarcoma and pinealoblastoma.

Metastatic Tumors to the Eye Are More Common Than Primary Ocular Neoplasms

Sometimes an ocular metastasis may be the initial clinical manifestation of a cancer, but most cases are diagnosed only after death. Leukemias and cancers of the breast and lung usually metastasize to the posterior choroid and account for most cases of intraocular metastases. Neuroblastoma frequently metastasizes to the orbit in infancy and childhood. The orbit may be invaded by malignant neoplasms of the eyelid, conjunctiva, paranasal sinuses, nose, nasopharynx and intracranial cavity.

FIGURE ACKNOWLEDGMENTS

Specific acknowledgment is made for permission to use the following material:

Chapter 1, Figure 1. From Okazaki H, Scheithauer BW. Atlas of Neuropathology. New York: Gower Medical Publishing, 1988. By permission of the author.

Chapter 3, Figure 16. From Okazaki H, Scheithauer BW. Atlas of Neuropathology. New York: Gower Medical Publishing, 1988. By permission of the author.

Chapter 5, Figure 5. From Bullough PG, Vigorita VJ. Atlas of Orthopaedic Pathology. New York: Gower Medical Publishing, 1984.

Chapter 5, Figure 17. From Bullough PG, Boachie-Adjei O. Atlas of Spinal Diseases. New York: Gower Medical Publishing, 1988. Copyright Lippincott Williams & Wilkins.

Chapter 5, Figure 43. From US Mortality Public Use Data Tapes 1960–2002, US Mortality Volumes 1930–1959, National Center for Health Statistics, Centers for Disease Control and Prevention, 2005.

Chapter 6, Figure 30. From Bullough PG, Vigorita VJ. Atlas of Orthopaedic Pathology. New York: Gower Medical Publishing, 1984.

Chapter 7, Figures 3 and 29. Courtesy of UBC Pulmonary Registry, St. Paul's Hospital.

Chapter 7, Figure 5. Courtesy of Dr. Charles Lee, University of British Columbia, Department of Pathology and Laboratory Medicine.

Chapter 7, Figures 6 and 12. Courtesy of Dr. Greg J. Davis, Dept. of Pathology, University of Kentucky College of Medicine.

Chapter 7, Figure 16. Courtesy of Dr. Sean Kelly, Office of Chief Medical Examiner of the City of New York.

Chapter 7, Figure 22. Courtesy of Dr. Ken Berry, Dept. of Pathology, St. Paul's Hospital.

Chapter 7, Figure 34. Courtesy of Dr. Alex Magil, Dept. of Pathology, St. Paul's Hospital.

Chapter 8, Figure 11. From Okazaki H, Scheithauer BW. Atlas of Neuropathology. New York: Gower Medical Publishing, 1988. By permission of the author.

Chapter 8, Figure 13. From McKee PH. Pathology of the Skin. New York: Gower Medical Publishing, 1989. Copyright Lippincott Williams & Wilkins.

Chapter 8, Figure 25. From Shils ME, Shike M, Ross AC, et al., eds. Modern Nutrition in Health and Disease. 10th ed. Philadelphia: Lippincott Williams & Wilkins, 2006: Fig. 38.1C.

Chapter 8, Figure 29. From Shils ME, Shike M, Ross AC, et al., eds. Modern Nutrition in Health and Disease. 10th ed. Philadelphia: Lippincott Williams & Wilkins, 2006: Fig. 38.2C.

Chapter 9, Figures 18A, 18B, 25, 52A, 69, 80, 86, 87, 95A, and 95B. From Farrar WE, Wood MJ, Innes JA, Tubbs H: Infectious Diseases Text and Color Atlas, 2nd ed. New York: Gower Medical Publishing, 1992.

Chapter 12, Figure 40. From Travis WB, Colby TV, Koss MN, et al. Non-neoplastic Disorders of the Lower Respiratory Tract. Washington, DC: American Registry of Pathology, 2002.

Chapter 12, Figure 55. Courtesy of the Armed Forces Institute of Pathology.

Chapter 12, Figure 70. The authors would like to gratefully acknowledge Dr. Anthony Gal for the contribution of Figure 12-70.

Chapter 13, Figure 14. Courtesy of Dr. Cecilia M. Fenoglio-Preiser.

Chapter 13, Figures 15B, 32, 44, 68, and 69. From Mitros FA. Atlas of Gastrointestinal Pathology. New York: Gower Medical Publishing, 1988. Copyright Lippincott Williams & Wilkins.

Chapter 14, Figure 1. From Ross MH, Pawlina W. Histology: A Text and Atlas. 6th Edition. Philadelphia: Lippincott Williams & Wilkins, 2011: 636.

Chapter 14, Figure 58. From Thung SN, Gerber MA. Histopathology of liver transplantation. In Fabry TL, Klion FM, eds. Guide to Liver Transplantation. New York: Igaku-Shoin Medical Publishers, 1992.

Chapter 17, Figures 4 and 10. From Weiss MA, Mills SE. Atlas of Genitourinary Tract Diseases. New York, Gower Medical Publishers, 1988.

Chapter 18, Figures 4, 5, 16, 29, 31, 38A, 50, 76, 77, and 95. Reprinted with permission from Stanley J. Robboy, MD, and Gynecologic Pathology Associates, Durham and Chapel Hill, North Carolina.

Chapter 18, Figures 13, 18, 27, and 30A. From Robboy SJ, Anderson MC, Russell P, eds. Pathology of the Female Reproductive Tract. London: Churchill-Livingstone, 2002: 111–112, 147, 167, 140, 203, 248, 322, 354.

Chapter 21, Figure 13. Sandoz Pharmaceutical Corporation.

Chapter 22, Figure 6. Adapted from Kendall DM, Bergenstal RM. © 2005 International Diabetes Center at Park Nicollet, Minneapolis, MN. All rights reserved. Used with permission.

Chapter 22, Figure 7. Redrawn from Pfeifer MA, Halter JB, Porte D. Insulin secretion in diabetes mellitus. The American Journal of Medicine 1981;70:579–588.

Chapter 22, Figure 14. Courtesy of the American Diabetes Association.

Chapter 24, Figures 9A, 22A, 25A (Courtesy W. Witmer), 26, 32A, 34A, 36A, 38A, 42, 43A, 44, 45, 46, 69A, 70, 71, 72, 79A, and 88A. From Elder AD, Elenitsas R, Johnson BL, et al. Synopsis and Atlas of Lever's Histopathology of the Skin. Philadelphia: Lippincott Williams & Wilkins, 1999:2, clin. fig. IA1; p 163, clin. fig. IVE3; p 167, clin. fig. IVE4.b; p 124, clin. fig. IIIH1.a; p 105, clin. fig. IIIF1.a; p 115, clin. fig. IIIG1.a; p 85, clin. fig. IIIB1a.a; p 219, clin. fig. VE3.a; clin. fig. IVA2.b; p 7, clin. fig. IC1; p 212, fig. VD1.d; p 51, clin. fig. IIE1.f and IIE1.1; p 226, clin. fig. VE5.f; p 283, clin. fig. VIB3.g; p 280, clin. fig. VIB3.q and VIB3.s; p 10, clin. fig. ID1.b; p 31, clin. fig. IIC1.a; clin. fig. IIF2.a; p 96, clin. fig. IIID1.d.

Chapter 26, Figures 20A, 20B, 40A, 52B, 57, and 72A. From Bullough PG: Atlas of Orthopaedic Pathology, 2nd ed. New York, Gower Medical Publishing, 1992. Copyright Lippincott Williams & Wilkins.

Chapter 27, Figure 1. From Ross MH, Pawlina W. Histology: A Text and Atlas. 5th Ed. Philadelphia: Lippincott Williams & Wilkins, 2006.

Chapter 27, Figure 6. Redrawn from Karpati G. Structural and Molecular Basis of Skeletal Muscle Diseases. ISN Neuropath Press, Basel 2002:8, Fig. 2.

Chapter 28, Figures 12, 17, 19A, 19B, 21C, 22B, 24, 25, 26B, 27, 30, 31, 32, 33, 35, 36, 48, 49, 50, 51, 56, 65, 69, 72, 78A, 78B, 79, 80, 82, 86A, 86B, 87, 94, 103, 108, 109, 111, 113B, 114B, 115B, 115D, 122B, 128B, and 133B. Courtesy of Dr. F. Stephen Vogel, Duke University.

INDEX

Note: Page numbers followed by f and t indicates figure and table respectively.

CCS0211